How to use Volume III

This book has important information about the therapeutic equivalence of prescription drugs. It also includes selected state and federal legal requirements that affect the prescribing and dispensing of drugs.

This unique combination makes *USP DI Volume III, Approved Drug Products and Legal Requirements*, a reliable and time saving reference for health care professionals.

On this page, you'll find general information about how to use the two main parts of this book. An illustration showing how the product list for prescription drugs is organized appears on the back of this sheet. For more detailed information about USP and this book, see *Preface* (page v).

About part 1

In this section, you'll find a copy of the FDA's complete listing of approved drug products and their therapeutic equivalence—commonly known as the "Orange Book." It lists the following:

- *Prescription Drug Products*
- *OTC Drug Products*
- *Drug Products with Approval Under Section 505 of the Act Administered by the Center for Biologics Evaluation and Research*
- *Discontinued Drug Products*
- *Orphan Drug Product Designations and Approvals*
- *Drug Products Which Must Demonstrate* in vivo *Bioavailability only if Product Fails to Achieve Adequate Dissolution*
- *Biopharmaceutic Guidance Availability*
- *ANDA Suitability Petitions*

Part 1 also has the following appendixes, addendum, and lists:

- ***Appendix A*** *Product Name Index*
- ***Appendix B*** *Product Name Index Listed by Applicant*
- ***Appendix C*** *Uniform Terms*
- ***Patent and Exclusivity Information Addendum***
- ***Listing of B-rated Drugs***
- ***Listing of "Pre-1938" Products***

About part 2

The second half of this book includes chemistry information, *USP* and *NF* drug standards, and dispensing requirements, as well as relevant state and federal legal requirements.

Part 2 also has information about the USP–Practitioners' Reporting Network and a Medicine Chart, showing actual-size photographs of more than 1,400 widely used capsules and tablets. You'll find a separate index for the part 2 information at the back of the book.

See "Orange Book" illustration on the back of this sheet.

Sample list

Single-ingredient product

Active ingredient

Dosage form; route of administration

Trade or generic names

Applicant   Available strengths

Application number, product number, and approval date

Multiple-ingredient product

Active ingredients, listed alphabetically

To find information about multiple-ingredient products, look under the ingredient that is first alphabetically. For example, if you looked for this drug combination under either Butalbital or Caffeine, you would find a cross reference that says "see Acetaminophen; Butalbital; Caffeine."

Product information—see *Single-ingredient product* listing

PRESCRIPTION DRUG PRODUCTS

I/20   **Approved Drug Products with Therapeutic Equivalence Evaluations**   *USP DI*

ACEBUTOLOL HYDROCHLORIDE

CAPSULE; ORAL

TE	Name / Applicant	Strength	Appl. No. / Date
	SECTRAL		
	WYETH AYERST	EQ 200 MG BASE	N18917 001 DEC 28, 1984
		EQ 400 MG BASE	N18917 003 DEC 28, 1984

ACETAMINOPHEN; ASPIRIN; CODEINE PHOSPHATE

CAPSULE; ORAL

TE	Name / Applicant	Strength	Appl. No. / Date
	ACETAMINOPHEN, ASPIRIN, AND CODEINE PHOSPHATE		
	MIKART	150 MG;180 MG;15 MG	N81095 001 OCT 26, 1990
		150 MG;180 MG;30 MG	N81096 001 OCT 26, 1990
		150 MG;180 MG;60 MG	N81097 001 OCT 26, 1990

ACETAMINOPHEN; BUTALBITAL

CAPSULE; ORAL

TE	Name / Applicant	Strength	Appl. No. / Date
	BANCAP		
AB	FOREST	325 MG;50 MG	N88889 001 JAN 16, 1986
	BUTALBITAL AND ACETAMINOPHEN		
AB	GRAHAM LABS	650 MG;50 MG	N88991 001 JUN 28, 1985
	CONTEN		
AB	GRAHAM LABS	650 MG;50 MG	N89405 001 MAY 15, 1990
	PHRENILIN FORTE		
AB	CARNRICK	650 MG;50 MG	N88831 001 JUN 19, 1985
	TRIAPRIN		
AB	DUNHALL	325 MG;50 MG	N89268 001 JUL 02, 1987

TABLET; ORAL

TE	Name / Applicant	Strength	Appl. No. / Date
	BUTALBITAL AND ACETAMINOPHEN		
AB	DANBURY	325 MG;50 MG	N87550 001 OCT 19, 1984
AB	HALSEY	325 MG;50 MG	N89568 001 OCT 05, 1988
	PHRENILIN		
AB	CARNRICK	325 MG;50 MG	N87811 001 JUN 19, 1985
	SEDAPAP		
	MAYRAND	650 MG;50 MG	N88944 001 OCT 17, 1985

ACETAMINOPHEN; BUTALBITAL; CAFFEINE

CAPSULE; ORAL

TE	Name / Applicant	Strength	Appl. No. / Date
	ACETAMINOPHEN, BUTALBITAL AND CAFFEINE		
AB	GILBERT	325 MG;50 MG;40 MG	N88825 001 DEC 05, 1984
	ACETAMINOPHEN, BUTALBITAL, AND CAFFEINE		
AB	MIKART	325 MG;50 MG;40 MG	N89007 001 MAR 17, 1986
	ANOQUAN		
AB	MALLARD	325 MG;50 MG;40 MG	N87628 001 OCT 01, 1986
	BUTALBITAL, ACETAMINOPHEN, CAFFEINE		
AB	GRAHAM LABS	325 MG;50 MG;40 MG	N88743 001 JUL 18, 1985
AB		325 MG;50 MG;40 MG	N88758 001 MAR 27, 1985
AB		325 MG;50 MG;40 MG	N88765 001 MAR 27, 1985
AB		325 MG;50 MG;40 MG	N89023 001 JUN 19, 1985
AB		325 MG;50 MG;40 MG	N89067 001 APR 19, 1985
AB		325 MG;50 MG;40 MG	N89102 001 JUN 19, 1985
	MEDIGESIC PLUS		
AB	US CHEM MKTG	325 MG;50 MG;40 MG	N89115 001 JAN 14, 1986

TABLET; ORAL

TE	Name / Applicant	Strength	Appl. No. / Date
	ACETAMINOPHEN, BUTALBITAL AND CAFFEINE		
AB	GILBERT	325 MG;50 MG;40 MG	N87629 001 NOV 13, 1984
	BUTALBITAL, ACETAMINOPHEN AND CAFFEINE		
AB	MIKART	325 MG;50 MG;40 MG	N89175 001 JAN 21, 1987
		500 MG;50 MG;40 MG	N89451 001 MAY 23, 1988
	BUTALBITAL, APAP, AND CAFFEINE		
AB	HALSEY	325 MG;50 MG;40 MG	N89536 001 FEB 16, 1988
	ESGIC		
AB	FOREST	325 MG;50 MG;40 MG	N89660 001 DEC 23, 1988
	FIORICET		
AB	SANDOZ	325 MG;50 MG;40 MG	N88616 001 NOV 09, 1984
	REPAN		
AB	GRAHAM LABS	325 MG;50 MG;40 MG	N87804 001 JAN 24, 1985

Therapeutic equivalence codes (TE)

Therapeutically equivalent drug products have TE codes beginning with an "**A**," such as ***AB***. Drug products that are *not* therapeutically equivalent have codes that begin with a "**B**," such as ***BP***.

Drug products offered by a single source do not have TE codes.

VOLUME III

Approved Drug Products and Legal Requirements

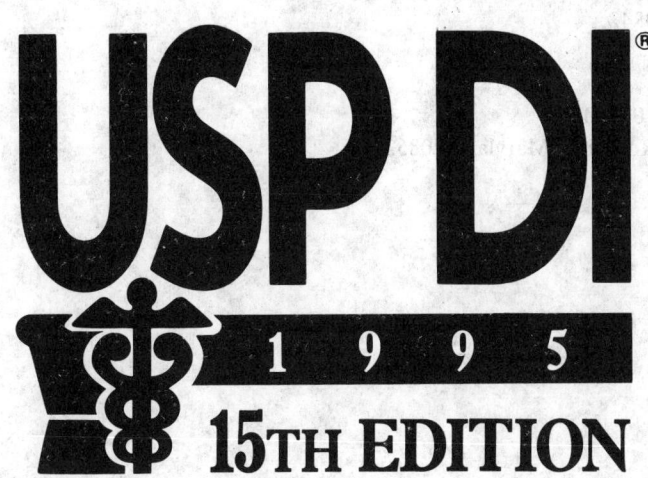

USP DI®

1995

15TH EDITION

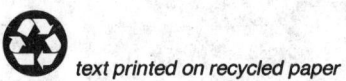

text printed on recycled paper

Turn to the last page for the "Fast-finder" subject guide.

By authority of the United States Pharmacopeial Convention, Inc.

NOTICE AND WARNING

Library of Congress Catalog Card Number 81-640842
ISBN 0-913595-85-3
ISSN 1045-8298

Printed by Rand McNally, Taunton, Massachusetts 02780.
Distributed by USPC, 12601 Twinbrook Parkway, Rockville, Maryland 20852.

Contents

Turn to the last page for the "Fast-finder" subject guide.

USP DI—Volume III
Approved Drug Products and Legal Requirements

Preface

In contrast to "the national consensus" found in Volumes I and II is Volume III of *USP DI.*

Volume III is not a product of the USP Committee of Revision, although some of the Committee's determinations in *USP-NF* are reproduced in it. Rather, Volume III is intended as a service to those who need a convenient source of the legal requirements that affect prescribing/dispensing activities—more convenient, and considerably less expensive than tracking them all down and purchasing them separately.

Volume III contains federal and state requirements relevant to the dispensing situation, including:

- the FDA's "Orange Book," *Approved Drug Products with Therapeutic Equivalence Evaluations.*
- a separate listing of B-rated drugs.
- a list of pre-1938 ("grandfathered") products.
- abstracted *USP-NF* monograph requirements relating to strength, quality, purity, packaging, labeling, and storage.
- selected *USP-NF* General Chapters and General Notices particularly applicable to the practice situation.
- selected portions of the federal Controlled Substance Act Regulations.
- the federal Food, Drug and Cosmetic Act requirements as they relate to human drugs, including the recent drug diversion and sampling amendments.
- the FDA's Current Good Manufacturing Practice Regulations for Finished Pharmaceuticals.

Selected portions of each state's pharmacy practice act and regulations for dispensing, including product selection regulations, are included individually in a special Supplement to the subscribers in that state.

The entire Orange Book and those supplements issued up to our printing deadline are directly reproduced in this 1995 Volume III. Subsequent 1994 supplements will be published in the *USP DI Updates* for 1995.

The Poison Prevention and Packaging Act and the Drug Enforcement Administration regulations are also included in Volume III, where it is believed they will be useful in the prescribing/dispensing interface.

Inclusion of these selected federal statutes and regulations should assist in voluntary compliance. Inclusion of drug standards information from the *United States Pharmacopeia* and the *National Formulary* should assist practitioners in obtaining a better understanding of drug product quality requirements overall.

Acknowledgments—USP wishes to acknowledge the cooperation of the individual State Boards of Pharmacy and the National Association of Boards of Pharmacy, especially its Executive Director, Carmen A. Catizone, in preparation of the state-related materials.

The Food and Drug Administration, in particular the following individuals, was especially helpful in encouraging and facilitating the publication of this volume: Janet Anderson, Susan Daugherty, Donald B. Hare, Gladys Holley, James E. Knoben, Richard Lipov, Miriam McKee, Theodore E. Rushin, George R. Scott, and Robert Tonelli.

FDA's ORANGE BOOK

The Orange Book—The FDA list, *Approved Drug Products with Therapeutic Equivalence Evaluations,* serves two basic purposes:

(1) it identifies the prescription and nonprescription drug products formally approved by the FDA on the basis of safety and effectiveness; and

(2) it provides the FDA's therapeutic equivalence evaluations for those approved multi-source prescription drug products.

In 1984, the Food, Drug and Cosmetic Act was amended by the Drug Price Competition and Patent Term Restoration Act. This law requires the FDA to publish a list of all currently approved drug products and to update it on a monthly basis. The Orange Book and its supplements satisfy this statutory requirement. An addendum providing patent information and identifying those drugs which qualify under this Act for periods of exclusivity is also included.

The Orange Book is referenced in numerous state laws and regulations governing drug substitution in prescribing/dispensing. These are included in the above-mentioned special state *USP DI Updates.*

The following questions and answers were abstracted and compiled from a survey of questions asked by State Boards of Pharmacy and responded to by FDA representatives at the annual meeting of the National Association of Boards of Pharmacy in 1988.

Question: Does the FDA ever plan to cover all legend drugs authorized for manufacturing in the U.S.A.? If not, why not?

Answer: There are two classes of unapproved prescription* drug products that are currently permitted by the FDA to remain on the market:

(1) copies of drugs first marketed before 1938; and (2) certain DESI ineffective products awaiting completion of the FDA's adminstrative procedures. FDA is planning to initiate a program to declare all versions of pre-1938 drugs to be new drugs and require an approved application for a drug product to either stay or come on the market. Products deemed ineffective after the administrative and legal procedures of the DESI process are completed will come off the market. There are currently only a few drugs remaining in this category.

Question: How does the FDA revise its evaluation of a product based on adverse reports?

Answer: Adverse events, including therapeutic failures, may be reported for any drug. (Note: The USP reporting form in the Practitioners' Reporting Network section may be used.) Therapeutic failures occur even when the drug product is not changed, as is evident from the reports we receive. Blood pressures can rise on previously effective therapy; heart failure can worsen on a stable digoxin/diuretic regimen; seizures can break through, etc. We would not consider changing our therapeutic equivalence evaluations unless evidence exists that the adverse reports (e.g., therapeutic failures) were due to the specific drug product rather than to a patient or drug substance problem. If such data were presented to us, we would change the code to therapeutically inequivalent or remove the product from the market.

Question: How long does it take for a drug to appear in the Orange Book?

Answer: The Orange Book is updated monthly. Each cumulative supplement indicates the time period covered by it.

Question: Is the Orange Book an official national compendium and authoritative source which can be used to provide protection in civil suits? Does it have force of law?

Answer: The Orange Book is not an official national compendium. The Orange Book displays the FDA's therapeutic equivalence recommendations on approved multiple source drug products. The FDA's evaluation of therapeutic equivalence is a scientific judgment based upon data submitted to the FDA. Generic substitution is a social and economic policy administered at the state level intended to minimize the cost of drugs to consumers. The programs are administered by the states, because the practices of pharmacy and medicine are state functions.

The question of liability is not one in the FDA's area of expertise. We suggest that counsel in your state be consulted. The Orange Book does not have force of law. The preface of the Orange Book addresses this issue.

Question: Provide tips on how to explain to physicians that drugs that are bioequivalent are indeed therapeutically equivalent. Many believe that drugs are not necessarily therapeutically equivalent, just because they are bioequivalent.

Answer: 1. The FDA is not aware of one clinical study that compared two drug products evaluated by the FDA as bioequivalent/therapeutic equivalent that demonstrates therapeutic inequivalence.

2. In the majority of cases the marketed innovator's product is not the formulation that was tested in clinical trials. The marketed innovator's drug product was shown to be therapeutically equivalent to the formulation that was used in the clinical trials by a bioavailability/bioequivalence study. Therefore, a generic drug product and the innovator's drug product stand in the same relationship to the formulation that was originally tested for safety and effectiveness.

Question: How does the Orange Book relate to and/or impact on state formularies?

Answer: It became apparent to the FDA soon after the repeal of the anti-substitution laws by the states that it could not serve the needs of each state on an individual basis in the preparation of their formularies. In 1978 the Commissioner of Food and Drugs notified appropriate officials of all states of the FDA's intention to provide a list of all prescription drug products that had been approved by the FDA for safety and effectiveness, with therapeutic equivalence recommendations being made on all multiple source drug products in the list. This list could be used by each state in implementing its own law and would relieve the FDA of expending an enormous amount of resources to provide individualized service to all states. Three copies of the Orange Book continue to be sent to state officials for their use in implementing their respective state laws. The states are under no mandate to accept the therapeutic equivalence recommendations in the Orange Book.

Question: What is the applicability of the Orange Book in a community pharmacy setting?

Answer: It was never the FDA's intention to have the Orange Book used in community pharmacies. However, a state could implement its law with this as a requirement.

Question: What is the legal status of pharmaceutical substitution of a different dosage form of a given drug entity? Can the FDA provide any assistance in identifying potential therapeutic problems (or therapeutic comparisons) between available dosage forms?

Answer: The Orange Book does not mandate which drug products may or may not be substituted. The therapeutic equivalence evaluations in the Orange Book are recommendations only. However, the FDA does not recommend substitution between different dosage forms. The Agency has very few bioequivalence studies in its files comparing different dosage forms of a given drug entity.

Question: Does the FDA have any way of identifying which distributors are marketing a given manufacturer's product and providing that information in the Orange Book?

Answer: No. Since an approved supplement is not required for an applicant with an approved drug product to license a distributor, FDA has no good mechanism to monitor distributors and to know when they change manufacturers.

USP-NF requirements—The United States Pharmacopeial Convention is the publisher of the *United States Pharmacopeia* and the *National Formulary*. These texts are recognized as official compendia by the pharmacy and medical professions. They contain standards, specifications, and other requirements relating to drugs and other articles used in medical and pharmacy practice that may be enforceable under various statutes. These requirements are applicable not only when drugs are in the possession of the manufacturer, but at the practice level as well.

Although the standards continue to be applicable when drugs are dispensed or sold, it must also be recognized that most prescriptions today are filled with manufactured products and for the most part physicians and pharmacists rarely compound or analyze drug products. On the other hand, dispensers need to be aware of the quality attributes of products, their packaging and storage requirements, and the other applicable standards to which legal consequences may attach.

In recognition of this need, Volume III presents abstracts of the applicable *USP-NF* standards. Similarly, selected portions of the *USP-NF* General Notices and Chapters that are deemed to be especially relevant are reprinted in Volume III.

The incorporation of these official *USP-NF* materials into *USP DI* is for informational purposes only. Because of varying publication schedules, there may occasionally be a time difference between publication of revisions in the *USP-NF* and the appearance of these changes in *USP DI*. Readers are advised that only the standards as written in the *USP-NF* are regarded as official.

The *USP-NF* material included in *USP DI* is not intended to represent nor shall it be interpreted to be the equivalent of or a substitute for the official *United States Pharmacopeia* and/or *National Formulary*. In the event of any difference or discrepancy between the current official *USP* or *NF* standards and the information contained herein, the context and effect of the official compendia shall prevail.

---

*Editor's note: Relatively few nonprescription medications enter the market through the New Drug Application procedures.

USP People 1990–1995

OFFICERS

Mark Novitch, M.D., *President*, Washington, DC
Donald R. Bennett, M.D., Ph.D., *Vice-President*, Chicago, IL
John T. Fay, Jr., Ph.D., *Treasurer*, San Clemente, CA
Arthur Hull Hayes, Jr., M.D., *Past President*, New Rochelle, NY
Jerome A. Halperin, *Secretary*, Rockville, MD

BOARD OF TRUSTEES

James T. Doluisio, Ph.D.[1], *Chair*, Austin, TX
Donald R. Bennett, M.D., Ph.D., *ex officio*, Chicago, IL
John V. Bergen, Ph.D.[2], *Vice Chair*, Villanova, PA
Edwin D. Bransome, Jr., M.D.[3], Augusta, GA
Jordan L. Cohen, Ph.D.[1], Lexington, KY
J. Richard Crout, M.D.[3], Rockville, MD
John T. Fay, Jr., Ph.D., *ex officio*, San Clemente, CA
Arthur Hull Hayes, Jr., M.D., *ex officio*, New Rochelle, NY
Joseph A. Mollica, Ph.D.[2], Wilmington, DE
Grace Powers Monaco, J.D.[4], Washington, DC
Mark Novitch, M.D., *ex officio*, Washington, DC

GENERAL COMMITTEE OF REVISION

Jerome A. Halperin[5], *Executive Director, USPC, Chairman*
Lee T. Grady, Ph.D.[5], *Director, Drug Standards Division*
Keith W. Johnson[5], *Director, Drug Information Division*
Loyd V. Allen, Jr., Ph.D., Oklahoma City, OK
Jerry R. Allison, Ph.D., New Brunswick, NJ
Thomas J. Ambrosio, Ph.D., Somerville, NJ
Gregory E. Amidon, Ph.D., Kalamazoo, MI
Norman W. Atwater, Ph.D., Hopewell, NJ
Henry L. Avallone, B.Sc., North Brunswick, NJ
Leonard C. Bailey, Ph.D., Piscataway, NJ
John A. Belis, M.D., Hershey, PA
Leslie Z. Benet, Ph.D., San Francisco, CA
Judy P. Boehlert, Ph.D., Nutley, NJ
James C. Boylan, Ph.D., Abbott Park, IL
Lynn R. Brady, Ph.D.[6], (1990–1992), Seattle, WA
R. Edward Branson, Ph.D., Beltsville, MD
William H. Briner, Capt., B.S., Durham, NC
Stephen R. Byrn, Ph.D., West Lafayette, IN
Peter R. Byron, Ph.D., Richmond, VA
Herbert S. Carlin, D.Sc., Florham Park, NJ
Dennis L. Casey, Ph.D., Raritan, NJ
Lester Chafetz, Ph.D., Kansas City, MO
Virginia C. Chamberlain, Ph.D., Rockville, MD
Wei-Wei, Chang, Ph.D., (1992–), Morris Plains, NJ
Mary Beth Chenault, B.S., Harrisonburg, VA
Zak T. Chowhan, Ph.D., Palo Alto, CA
Sebastian G. Ciancio, D.D.S., Buffalo, NY
Murray S. Cooper, Ph.D., Islamorada, FL
Lloyd E. Davis, Ph.D., D.V.M., Urbana, IL
Leon Ellenbogen, Ph.D., Clifton, NJ
R. Michael Enzinger, Ph.D., (1990–1992), Kalamazoo, MI
Clyde R. Erskine, B.S., M.B.A., Newtown Square, PA
Edward A. Fitzgerald, Ph.D., Bethesda, MD
Everett Flanigan, Ph.D., Kankakee, IL
Klaus G. Florey, Ph.D., Princeton, NJ
Thomas S. Foster, Pharm.D., Lexington, KY
Joseph F. Gallelli, Ph.D., Bethesda, MD
Robert L. Garnick, Ph.D., So. San Francisco, CA
Douglas D. Glover, M.D., R.Ph., Morgantown, WV
Alan M. Goldberg, Ph.D., Baltimore, MD
Burton J. Goldstein, M.D., Williams Island, FL
Dennis K. J. Gorecki, Ph.D., Saskatoon, Saskatchewan, Canada
Michael J. Groves, Ph.D., Lake Forest, IL
Robert M. Guthrie, M.D., Columbus, OH
Samir A. Hanna, Ph.D., Lawrenceville, NJ
Stanley L. Hem, Ph.D., West Lafayette, IN
Joy Hochstadt, Ph.D., New York, NY
David W. Hughes, Ph.D., (1990–1993), Nepean, Ontario, Canada
Norman C. Jamieson, Ph.D., St. Louis, MO
Richard D. Johnson, Pharm.D., Ph.D., Kansas City, MO
Judith K. Jones, M.D., Ph.D., Arlington, VA
Stanley A. Kaplan, Ph.D., Baltimore, MD
Herbert E. Kaufman, M.D., New Orleans, LA
Donald Kaye, M.D., Philadelphia, PA
Paul E. Kennedy, Ph.D., West Conshohocken, PA
Jay S. Keystone, M.D., Toronto, Ontario, Canada
Rosalyn C. King, Pharm.D., M.P.H., Silver Spring, MD
Gordon L. Klein, M.D. Galveston, TX
Joseph E. Knapp, Ph.D., Pittsburgh, PA
John B. Landis, Ph.D., (1990–1992), Kalamazoo, MI
Thomas P. Layloff, Ph.D., St. Louis, MO
Lewis J. Leeson, Ph.D., Summit, NJ
John W. Levchuk, Ph.D., Rockville, MD
Robert D. Lindeman, M.D., Albuquerque, NM
Charles H. Lochmüller, Ph.D., Durham, NC
Edward G. Lovering, Ph.D., Nepean, Ontario, Canada
Catherine M. MacLeod, M.D., Chicago, IL
Carol S. Marcus, Ph.D., M.D., Torrance, CA
Tibor I. Matula, Ph.D., (1993–), Ottawa, Ontario, Canada
Thomas Medwick, Ph.D., Piscataway, NJ
Robert F. Morrissey, Ph.D., New Brunswick, NJ
Terry E. Munson, B.S., Fairfax, VA
Harold S. Nelson, M.D., Denver, CO
Wendel L. Nelson, Ph.D., Seattle, WA
Maria I. New, M.D., New York, NY
Sharon C. Northup, Ph.D., Round Lake, IL
Jeffery L. Otto, Ph.D., (1992–), Broomfield, CO
Garnet E. Peck, Ph.D., West Lafayette, IN
Robert V. Petersen, Ph.D., Salt Lake City, UT

[1]Representing pharmacy.
[2]At large.
[3]Representing medicine.
[4]Public member.
[5]12601 Twinbrook Parkway, Rockville, MD 20852.
[6]Deceased.

Rosemary C. Polomano, R.N., M.S.N., Philadelphia, PA
Thomas P. Reinders, Pharm.D., Richmond, VA
Christopher T. Rhodes, Ph.D., West Kingston, RI
Joseph R. Robinson, Ph.D., Madison, WI
Lary A. Robinson, M.D., Tampa, FL
David B. Roll, Ph.D., Salt Lake City, UT
Theodore J. Roseman, Ph.D., Round Lake, IL
Sanford H. Roth, M.D., Phoenix, AZ
Leonard P. Rybak, M.D., Springfield, IL
Ronald J. Sawchuk, Ph.D., Minneapolis, MN
Gordon D. Schiff, M.D., Chicago, IL
Andrew J. Schmitz, Jr., M.S.[6], (1990–1992), Huntington, NY
Ralph F. Shangraw, Ph.D., Baltimore, MD
Albert L. Sheffer, M.D., Boston, MA
Eli Shefter, Ph.D., San Diego, CA
Eric B. Sheinin, Ph.D., Rockville, MD
Robert L. Siegle, M.D., San Antonio, TX
Edward B. Silberstein, M.D., Cincinnati, OH
Joseph E. Sinsheimer, Ph.D., Ann Arbor, MI
Marilyn Dix Smith, Ph.D., Dayton, NJ
Burton E. Sobel, M.D., St. Louis, MO
E. John Staba, Ph.D., Minneapolis, MN
Robert S. Stern, M.D., Boston, MA
James T. Stewart, Ph.D., Athens, GA
Henry S. I. Tan, Ph.D., Cincinnati, OH
Theodore G. Tong, Pharm.D., Tucson, AZ
Salvatore J. Turco, Pharm.D., Philadelphia, PA
Clarence T. Ueda, Pharm.D., Ph.D., Omaha, NE
Elizabeth B. Vadas, Ph.D., Pointe Claire-Dorval, Quebec, Canada
Huib J. M. van de Donk, Ph.D., Bilthoven, The Netherlands
Stanley van den Noort, M.D., Irvine, CA
Vincent S. Venturella, Ph.D., Murray Hill, NJ
Robert E. Vestal, M.D., Boise, ID
James A. Visconti, Ph.D., Columbus, OH
Edward W. Voss, Jr., Ph.D., Urbana, IL
Philip D. Walson, M.D., Columbus, OH
Paul F. White, Ph.D., M.D., Dallas, TX
Robert G. Wolfangel, Ph.D., St. Louis, MO
Manfred E. Wolff, Ph.D., San Diego, CA
Wesley E. Workman, Ph.D., (1992–), St. Louis, MO
Linda R. Wuhl, Ph.D., (1993–), Thousand Oaks, CA
John W. Yarbro, M.D., Ph.D., Springfield, IL
George Zografi, Ph.D., Madison, WI

EXECUTIVE COMMITTEE OF REVISION (1993–1994)

Jerome A. Halperin, *Chair*
Norman W. Atwater, Ph.D.
Clyde R. Erskine, B.S., M.B.A.
Burton J. Goldstein, M.D.
Robert V. Petersen, Ph.D.
Robert S. Stern, M.D.
Paul F. White, Ph.D., M.D.

DRUG INFORMATION DIVISION EXECUTIVE COMMITTEE (1993–1994)

Herbert S. Carlin, D.Sc., *Chair*
James C. Boylan, Ph.D.
Sebastian G. Ciancio, D.D.S.
Lloyd E. Davis, D.V.M., Ph.D.
Jay S. Keystone, M.D.
Robert D. Lindeman, M.D.
Maria I. New, M.D.
Rosemary C. Polomano, R.N., M.S.N.
Thomas P. Reinders, Pharm.D.
Gordon D. Schiff, M.D.
Albert L. Sheffer, M.D.
Theodore G. Tong, Pharm.D.
Robert E. Vestal, M.D.
John W. Yarbro, M.D., Ph.D.

DRUG STANDARDS DIVISION EXECUTIVE COMMITTEE (1993–1994)

James T. Stewart, Ph.D. *Chair*
Jerry R. Allison, Ph.D.
Judy P. Boehlert, Ph.D.
Capt. William H. Briner, B.S.
Herbert S. Carlin, D.Sc.
Lester Chafetz, Ph.D.
Zak T. Chowhan, Ph.D.
Murray S. Cooper, Ph.D.
Klaus G. Florey, Ph.D.
Joseph F. Gallelli, Ph.D.
Robert L. Garnick, Ph.D.
Thomas P. Layloff, Ph.D.
Lewis J. Leeson, Ph.D.
Thomas Medwick, Ph.D.
Robert F. Morrissey, Ph.D.
Sharon C. Northup, Ph.D.
Ralph F. Shangraw, Ph.D.

DRUG NOMENCLATURE COMMITTEE (1993–1994)

Herbert S. Carlin, D.Sc., *Chair*
William M. Heller, Ph.D., *Consultant/Advisor*
Lester Chafetz, Ph.D.
Lloyd E. Davis, D.V.M., Ph.D.
Everett Flanigan, Ph.D.
Douglas D. Glover, M.D.
Richard D. Johnson, Pharm.D., Ph.D.
Edward G. Lovering, Ph.D.
Rosemary C. Polomano, R.N., M.S.N.
Thomas P. Reinders, Pharm.D.
Eric B. Sheinin, Ph.D.
Philip D. Walson, M.D.

DRUG INFORMATION DIVISION ADVISORY PANELS

Members who serve as Chairs are listed first.

The information presented in this text represents an ongoing review of the drugs contained herein and represents a consensus of various viewpoints expressed. The individuals listed below have served on the USP Advisory Panels for the 1993–1994 revision period and have contributed to the development of the 1995 USP DI database. Such listing does not imply that these individuals have reviewed all of the material in this text or that they individually agree with all statements contained herein.

Anesthesiology

Paul F. White, Ph.D., M.D., *Chair*, Dallas, TX; David R. Bevan, M.B., FFARCS, MRCP, Vancouver, British Columbia; Eugene Y. Cheng, M.D., Milwaukee, WI; Charles J. Coté, M.D., Chicago, IL; Robert Feinstein, M.D., St. Louis, MO; Peter S.A. Glass, M.D., Durham, NC; Michael B. Howie, M.D., Columbus, OH; Beverly A. Krause, C.R.N.A., M.S., St. Louis, MO; Carl Lynch, III, M.D., Ph.D., Charlottesville, VA; Carl Rosow, M.D., Ph.D., Boston, MA; Peter S. Sebel, M.B., Ph.D., Atlanta, GA; Walter L. Way, M.D., Greenbrae, CA; Matthew B. Weinger, M.D., San Diego, CA; Richard Weiskopf, M.D., San Francisco, CA; David H. Wong, Pharm.D., M.D., Long Beach, CA

Cardiovascular and Renal Drugs

Burton E. Sobel, M.D., *Chair*, St. Louis, MO; William P. Baker, M.D., Ph.D., Bethesda, MD; Nils U. Bang, M.D., Indianapolis, IN; Emmanuel L. Bravo, M.D., Cleveland, OH; Mary Jo Burgess, M.D., Salt Lake City, UT; James H. Chesebro, M.D., Boston, MA; Peter Corr, Ph.D., St. Louis, MO; Dwain L. Eckberg, M.D., Richmond, VA; Ruth Eshleman, Ph.D., W. Kingston, RI; William H. Frishman, M.D., Bronx, NY; Edward D. Frohlich, M.D., New Orleans, LA; Martha Hill, Ph.D., R.N., Baltimore, MD; Norman M. Kaplan, M.D., Dallas, TX; Michael Lesch, M.D., Detroit, MI; Manuel Martinez-Maldonado, M.D., Decatur, GA; Patrick A. McKee, M.D., Oklahoma City, OK; Dan M. Roden, M.D., Nashville, TN; Michael R. Rosen, M.D., New York, NY; Jane Schultz, R.N., B.S.N., Rochester, MN; Robert L. Talbert, Pharm.D., San Antonio, TX; Raymond L. Woosley, M.D., Ph.D., Washington, DC

Clinical Immunology/Allergy/Rheumatology

Albert L. Sheffer, M.D., *Chair*, Boston, MA; John A. Anderson, M.D., Detroit, MI; Emil Bardana, Jr., M.D., Portland, OR; John Baum, M.D., Rochester, NY; Debra Danoff, M.D., Montreal, Quebec; Daniel G. de Jesus, M.D., Ph.D., Vanier, Ontario; Elliott F. Ellis, M.D., Jacksonville, FL; Patricia A. Fraser, M.D., Boston, MA; Frederick E. Hargreave, M.D., Hamilton, Ontario; Evelyn V. Hess, M.D., Cincinnati, OH; Jean M. Jackson, M.D., Boston, MA; Stephen R. Kaplan, M.D., Buffalo, NY; Sandra M. Koehler, Milwaukee, WI; Richard A. Moscicki, M.D., Newton, MA; Shirley Murphy, M.D., Albuquerque, NM; Gary S. Rachelefsky, M.D., Los Angeles, CA; Robert E. Reisman, M.D., Buffalo, NY; Robert L. Rubin, Ph.D., La Jolla, CA; Daniel J. Stechschulte, M.D., Kansas City, KS; Virginia S. Taggert, Bethesda, MD; Joseph A. Tami, Pharm.D., San Antonio, TX; John H. Toogood, M.D., London, Ontario; Martin D. Valentine, M.D., Baltimore, MD; Michael Weinblatt, M.D., Boston, MA; Dennis Michael Williams, Pharm.D., Chapel Hill, NC; Stewart Wong, Ph.D., Annandale, VA

Clinical Toxicology/Substance Abuse

Theodore G. Tong, Pharm.D., *Chair*, Tucson, AZ; John Ambre, M.D., Ph.D., Chicago, IL; Usoa E. Busto, Pharm.D., Toronto, Ontario; Darryl Inaba, Pharm.D., San Francisco, CA; Edward P. Krenzelok, Pharm.D., Pittsburgh, PA; Michael Montagne, Ph.D., Boston, MA; Sven A. Normann, Pharm.D., Tampa, FL; Gary M. Oderda, Pharm.D., Salt Lake City, UT; Paul Pentel, M.D., Minneapolis, MN; Rose Ann Soloway, R.N., Washington, DC; Daniel A. Spyker, M.D., Ph.D., Rockville, MD; Anthony R. Temple, M.D., Ft. Washington, PA; Anthony Tommasello, Pharm.D., Baltimore, MD; Joseph C. Veltri, Pharm.D., Salt Lake City, UT; William A. Watson, Pharm.D., Kansas City, MO

Consumer Interest/Health Education

Gordon D. Schiff, M.D., *Chair*, Chicago, IL; Michael J. Ackerman, Ph.D., Bethesda, MD; Barbara Aranda-Naranjo, R.N., San Antonio, TX; Frank J. Ascione, Pharm.D., Ph.D., Ann Arbor, MI; Judith I. Brown, Silver Spring, MD; Jose Camacho, Austin, TX; Margaret A. Charters, Ph.D., Syracuse, NY; Jennifer Cross, San Francisco, CA; William G. Harless, Ph.D., Bethesda, MD; Louis H. Kompare, Lake Buena Vista, FL; Margo Kroshus, R.N., B.S.N., Rochester, MN; Marilyn Lister, Wakefield, Quebec; Margaret Lueders, Seattle, WA; Frederick S. Mayer, R.Ph., M.P.H., Sausalito, CA; Nancy Milio, Ph.D., Chapel Hill, NC; Irving Rubin, Port Washington, NY; T. Donald Rucker, Ph.D., River Forest, IL; Stephen B. Soumerai, Sc.D., Boston, MA; Carol A. Vetter, Rockville, MD

Critical Care Medicine

Catherine M. MacLeod, M.D., *Chair*, Chicago, IL; William Banner, Jr., M.D., Salt Lake City, UT; Philip S. Barie, M.D., New York, NY; Thomas P. Bleck, M.D., Charlottesville, VA; Roger C. Bone, M.D., Toledo, OH; Susan S. Fish, Pharm.D., Boston, MA; Edgar R. Gonzalez, Pharm.D., Richmond, VA; Robert Gottesman, Rockville, MD; John W. Hoyt, M.D., Pittsburgh, PA; Sheldon A. Magder, M.D., Montreal, Quebec; Joseph E. Parrillo, M.D., Chicago, IL; Sharon Peters, M.D., St. John's, Newfoundland; Domenic A. Sica, M.D., Richmond, VA; Martin G. Tweeddale, M.B., Ph.D., Vancouver, British Columbia

Dentistry

Sebastian G. Ciancio, D.D.S., *Chair*, Buffalo, NY; Donald F. Adams, D.D.S., Portland, OR; Karen A. Baker, M.S. Pharm., Iowa City, IA; Stephen A. Cooper, D.M.D., Ph.D., Philadelphia, PA; Frederick A. Curro, D.M.D., Ph.D., Jersey City, NJ; Paul J. Desjardins, D.M.D., Ph.D., Newark, NJ; Tommy W. Gage, D.D.S., Ph.D., Dallas, TX; Stephen F. Goodman, D.D.S., New York, NY; Daniel A. Haas, D.D.S., Ph.D., Toronto, Ontario; Richard E. Hall, D.D.S., Ph.D., Buffalo, NY; Lireka P. Joseph, Dr.P.H., Rockville, MD; Janice Lieberman, Fort Lee, NJ; Laurie Lisowski, Lewiston, NY; Clarence L. Trummel, D.D.S., Ph.D., Farmington, CT; Joel M.

Weaver, II, D.D.S., Ph.D., Columbus, OH; Clifford W. Whall, Jr., Ph.D., Chicago, IL; Raymond P. White, Jr., D.D.S., Ph.D., Chapel Hill, NC; Ray C. Williams, D.M.D., Boston, MA

Dermatology
Robert S. Stern, M.D., *Chair*, Boston, MA; Beatrice B. Abrams, Ph.D., Somerville, NJ; Richard D. Baughman, M.D., Hanover, NH; Michael Bigby, M.D., Boston, MA; Janice T. Chussil, R.N., M.S.N., Portland, OR; Stuart Maddin, M.D., Vancouver, British Columbia; Milton Orkin, M.D., Robbinsdale, MN; Neil H. Shear, M.D., Toronto, Ontario; Edgar Benton Smith, M.D., Galveston, TX; Dennis P. West, M.S. Pharm., Lincolnshire, IL; Gail M. Zimmerman, Portland, OR

Diagnostic Agents—Nonradioactive
Robert L. Siegle, M.D., *Chair*, San Antonio, TX; Kaizer Aziz, Ph.D., Rockville, MD; Robert C. Brasch, M.D., San Francisco, CA; Nicholas Harry Malakis, M.D., Bethesda, MD; Robert F. Mattrey, M.D., San Diego, CA; James A. Nelson, M.D., Seattle, WA; Jovitas Skucas, M.D., Rochester, NY; Gerald L. Wolf, Ph.D., M.D., Charlestown, MA

Drug Information Science
James A. Visconti, Ph.D., *Chair*, Columbus, OH; Marie A. Abate, Pharm.D., Morgantown, WV; Ann B. Amerson, Pharm.D., Lexington, KY; Philip O. Anderson, Pharm.D., San Diego, CA; Danial E. Baker, Pharm.D., Spokane, WA; C. David Butler, Pharm.D., M.B.A., Naperville, IL; Linda L. Hart, Pharm.D., Saddle River, NJ; Edward J. Huth, M.D., Philadelphia, PA; John M. Kessler, Pharm.D., Chapel Hill, NC; R. David Lauper, Pharm.D., Emeryville, CA; Domingo R. Martinez, Pharm.D., Birmingham, AL; William F. McGhan, Pharm.D., Ph.D., Philadelphia, PA; John K. Murdoch, B.Sc.Phm., Toronto, Ontario; Kurt A. Proctor, Ph.D., Alexandria, VA; Arnauld F. Scafidi, M.D., M.P.H., Rockville, MD; John A. Scarlett, M.D., Austin, TX; Gary H. Smith, Pharm.D., Tucson, AZ; Dennis F. Thompson, Pharm.D., Oklahoma City, OK; William G. Troutman, Pharm.D., Albuquerque, NM; Lee A. Wanke, M.S., Houston, TX

Drug Utilization Review
Judith K. Jones, M.D., Ph.D., *Chair*, Arlington, VA; John F. Beary, III., M.D., Washington, DC; James L. Blackburn, Pharm.D., Saskatoon, Saskatchewan; Richard S. Blum, M.D., East Hills, NY; Amy Cooper-Outlaw, Pharm.D., Stone Mountain, GA; Joseph W. Cranston, Jr., Ph.D., Chicago, IL; W. Gary Erwin, Pharm.D., Philadelphia, PA; Jere E. Goyan, Ph.D., Saddle River, NJ; Duane M. Kirking, Ph.D., Ann Arbor, MI; Karen E. Koch, Pharm.D., Tupelo, MS; Aida A. LeRoy, Pharm.D., Arlington, VA; Jerome Levine, M.D., Baltimore, MD; Richard W. Lindsay, M.D., Charlottesville, VA; M. Laurie Mashford, M.D., Melbourne, Victoria, Australia; Deborah M. Nadzam, R.N., Ph.D., Oakbrook Terrace, IL; William Z. Potter, M.D., Ph.D., Bethesda, MD; Louise R. Rodriquez, M.S., Washington, DC; Stephen P. Spielberg, M.D., Ph.D., West Point, PA; Suzan M. Streichenwein, M.D., Houston, TX; Brian L. Strom, M.D., Philadelphia, PA; Michael Weintraub, M.D., Rockville, MD; Antonio Carlos Zanini, M.D., Ph.D., Sao Paulo, Brazil

Endocrinology
Maria I. New, M.D., *Chair*, New York, NY; Ronald D. Brown, M.D., Oklahoma City, OK; R. Keith Campbell, Pharm.D., Pullman, WA; David S. Cooper, M.D., Baltimore, MD; Betty J. Dong, Pharm.D., San Francisco, CA; Andrea Dunaif, M.D., New York, NY; Anke A. Ehrhardt, Ph.D., New York, NY; Nadir R. Farid, M.D., Durham, N.C.; John G. Haddad, Jr., M.D., Philadelphia, PA; Michael M. Kaplan, M.D., Southfield, MI; Harold E. Lebovitz, M.D., Brooklyn, NY; Marvin E. Levin, M.D., Chesterfield, MO; Marvin M. Lipman, M.D., Scarsdale, NY; Barbara J. Maschak-Carey, R.N., M.S.N., Philadelphia, PA; James C. Melby, M.D., Boston, MA; Walter J. Meyer, III., M.D., Galveston, TX; Rita Nemchik, R.N., M.S., C.D.E., Florence, NJ; Daniel A. Notterman, M.D., New York, NY; Ron Gershon Rosenfeld, M.D., Stanford, CA; Paul Saenger, M.D., Bronx, NY; Leonard Wartofsky, M.D., Washington, DC

Family Practice
Robert M. Guthrie, M.D., *Chair*, Columbus, OH; Jack A. Brose, D.O., Athens, OH; Jannet M. Carmichael, Pharm.D., Reno, NV; Jacqueline A. Chadwick, M.D., Scottsdale, AZ; Mark E. Clasen, M.D., Ph.D., Dayton, OH; Lloyd P. Haskell, M.D., West Borough, MA; Luis A. Izquierdo-Mora, M.D., Rio Piedras, PR; Edward L. Langston, M.D., Houston, TX; Stephen T. O'Brien, M.D., Enfield, CT; Charles D. Ponte, Pharm.D., Morgantown, WV; Jack M. Rosenberg, Pharm.D., Ph.D., Brooklyn, NY; John F. Sangster, M.D., London, Ontario; Theodore L. Yarboro, Sr., M.D., M.P.H., Sharon, PA

Gastroenterology
Gordon L. Klein, M.D., *Chair*, Galveston, TX; Karl E. Anderson, M.D., Galveston, TX; William Balistreri, M.D., Cincinnati, OH; Paul Bass, Ph.D., Madison, WI; Rosemary R. Berardi, Pharm.D., Ann Arbor, MI; Raymond F. Burk, M.D., Nashville, TN; Thomas Q. Garvey, III, M.D., Potomac, MD; Donald J. Glotzer, M.D., Boston, MA; Flavio Habal, M.D., Toronto, Ontario; Paul E. Hyman, M.D., Torrance, CA; Bernard Mehl, D.P.S., New York, NY; William J. Snape, Jr., M.D., Torrance, CA; Ronald D. Soltis, M.D., Minneapolis, MN; C. Noel Williams, M.D., Halifax, Nova Scotia; Hyman J. Zimmerman, M.D., Bethesda, MD

Geriatrics
Robert E. Vestal, M.D., *Chair*, Boise, ID; Darrell R. Abernethy, M.D., Washington, DC; William B. Abrams, M.D., West Point, PA; Jerry Avorn, M.D., Boston, MA; Robert A. Blouin, Pharm.D., Lexington, KY; S. George Carruthers, M.D., Halifax, Nova Scotia; Lynn E. Chaitovitz, Rockville, MD; Terry Fulmer, R.N., Ph.D., New York, NY; Philip P. Gerbino, Pharm.D., Philadelphia, PA; Pearl S. German, Sc.D., Baltimore, MD; David J. Greenblatt, M.D., Boston, MA; Martin D. Higbee, Pharm.D., Tucson, AZ; Brian B. Hoffman, M.D., Palo Alto, CA; J. Edward Jackson, M.D., San Diego, CA; Joseph V. Levy, Ph.D., San Francisco, CA; Paul A. Mitenko, M.D., FRCPC, Nanaimo, British Columbia; John E. Morley, M.B., B.Ch., St. Louis, MO; Jay Roberts, Ph.D., Philadelphia, PA; Louis J. Rubenstein, R.Ph., Alexandria, VA; Janice B. Schwartz, M.D., San Francisco, CA; Alexander M.M. Shepherd, M.D., San Antonio, TX; William Simonson, Pharm.D., Portland, OR; Daniel S. Sitar, Ph.D., Winnipeg, Manitoba; Mary K. Walker, R.N., Ph.D., Lexington, KY; Alastair J. J. Wood, M.D., Nashville, TN

Hematologic and Neoplastic Disease
John W. Yarbro, M.D., Ph.D., *Chair*, Springfield, IL; Joseph S. Bailes, M.D., McAllen, TX; Laurence H. Baker, D.O., Ann Arbor, MI; Barbara D. Blumberg-Carnes, Albuquerque, NM; Helene G. Brown, B.S., Los Angeles, CA; Nora L. Burnham, Pharm.D., Princeton, NJ; William J. Dana, Pharm.D., Houston, TX; Connie Henke-Yarbro, R.N., B.S.N., Springfield, IL; William H. Hryniuk, M.D., San Diego, CA;

B. J. Kennedy, M.D., Minneapolis, MN; Barnett Kramer, M.D., Rockville, MD; Michael J. Mastrangelo, M.D., Philadelphia, PA; David S. Rosenthal, M.D., Cambridge, MA; Richard L. Schilsky, M.D., Chicago, IL; Rowena N. Schwartz, Pharm.D., Pittsburgh, PA; Roy L. Silverstein, M.D., New York, NY; Samuel G. Taylor, IV, M.D., Chicago, IL; Raymond B. Weiss, M.D., Washington, DC

Infectious Disease Therapy
Donald Kaye, M.D., *Chair*, Philadelphia, PA; Robert Austrian, M.D., Philadelphia, PA; C. Glenn Cobbs, M.D., Birmingham, AL; Joseph W. Cranston, Jr., Ph.D., Chicago, IL; John J. Dennehy, M.D., Danville, PA; Courtney V. Fletcher, Pharm. D., Minneapolis, MN; Earl H. Freimer, M.D., Toledo, OH; Marc LeBel, Pharm.D., Quebec, Quebec; John D. Nelson, M.D., Dallas, TX; Lindsay E. Nicolle, M.D., Winnipeg, Manitoba; Alvin Novick, M.D., New Haven, CT; Charles G. Prober, M.D., Stanford, CA; Douglas D. Richman, M.D., San Diego, CA; Spotswood L. Spruance, M.D., Salt Lake City, UT; Roy T. Steigbigel, M.D., Stony Brook, NY; Paul F. Wehrle, M.D., San Clemente, CA

International Health
Rosalyn C. King, Pharm.D., M.P.H., *Chair*, Silver Spring, MD; Walter M. Batts, Rockville, MD; Eugenie Brown, Pharm.D., Kingston, Jamaica; Alan Cheung, Pharm.D., M.P.H., Washington, DC; Mary Couper, M.D., Geneva, Switzerland; Gabriel Daniel, Washington, DC; S. Albert Edwards, Pharm.D., Lincolnshire, IL; Enrique Fefer, Ph.D., Washington, DC; Peter H. M. Fontilus, Curacao, Netherlands Antilles; Gan Ee Kiang, Penang, Malaysia; Marcellus Grace, Ph.D., New Orleans, LA; George B. Griffenhagen, Washington, DC; Margareta Helling-Borda, Geneva, Switzerland; Thomas Langston, Silver Spring, MD; Thomas Lapnet-Moustapha, Yaounde, Cameroon; David Lee, B.A., M.D., Arlington, VA; Aissatov Lo, Ka-Olack, Senegal; Stuart M. MacLeod, M.D., Hamilton, Ontario; Russell E. Morgan, Jr., Dr.P.H., Chevy Chase, MD; David Ofori-Adjei, M.D., Accra, Ghana; S. Ofosu-Amaah, M.D., New York, NY; James Rankin, Arlington, VA; Olikoye Ransome-Kuti, M.D., Lagos, Nigeria; Budiono Santoso, M.D., Ph.D., Yogyakarta, Indonesia; Carmen Selva, Ph.D., Madrid, Spain; Valentin Vinogradov, Moscow, Russia; Fela Viso-Gurovich, Mexico City, Mexico; William B. Walsh, M.D., Chevy Chase, MD; Lawrence C. Weaver, Ph.D., Minneapolis, MN; Albert I. Wertheimer, Ph.D., Glen Allen, VA

Neurology
Stanley van den Noort, M.D., *Chair*, Irvine, CA; William T. Beaver, M.D., Washington, DC; Elizabeth U. Blalock, M.D., Anaheim, CA; James C. Cloyd, Pharm.D., Minneapolis, MN; David M. Dawson, M.D., West Roxbury, MA; Kevin Farrell, M.D., Vancouver, British Columbia; Kathleen M. Foley, M.D., New York, NY; Anthony E. Lang, M.D., Toronto, Ontario; Ira T. Lott, M.D., Orange, CA; James R. Nelson, M.D., La Jolla, CA; J. Kiffin Penry, M.D., Winston-Salem, NC; Neil H. Raskin, M.D., San Francisco, CA; Alfred J. Spiro, M.D., Bronx, NY; M. DiAnn Turek, R.N., Holt, MI

Nursing Practice
Rosemary C. Polomano, R.N., M.S.N., *Chair*, Philadelpia, PA; Mecca S. Cranley, R.N., Ph.D., Buffalo, NY; Jan M. Ellerhorst-Ryan, R.N., M.S.N., Cincinnati, OH; Linda Felver, Ph.D., R.N., Portland, OR; Hector Hugo Gonzalez, R.N., Ph.D., San Antonio, TX; Mary Harper, R.N., Ph.D., Rockville, MD; Ada K. Jacox, R.N., Ph.D., Baltimore, MD; Patricia Kummeth, R.N., M.S., Rochester, MN; Ida M. Martinson, R.N., Ph.D., San Francisco, CA; Carol P. Patton, R.N., Ph.D., J.D., Detroit, MI; Ginette A. Pepper, R.N., Ph.D., Englewood, CO; Geraldine A. Peterson, R.N., M.A., Potomac, MD; Linda C. Pugh, R.N., Ph.D., York, PA; Sharon S. Rising, R.N., C.N.M., Cheshire, CT; Marjorie Ann Spiro, R.N., B.S., C.S.N., Scarsdale, NY

Nutrition and Electrolytes
Robert D. Lindeman, M.D., *Chair*, Albuquerque, NM; Hans Fisher, Ph.D., New Brunswick, NJ; Walter H. Glinsmann, M.D., Washington, DC; Helen Andrews Guthrie, M.S., Ph.D., State College, PA; Steven B. Heymsfield, M.D., New York, NY; K. N. Jeejeebhoy, M.D., Toronto, Ontario; Leslie M. Klevay, M.D., Grand Forks, ND; Linda S. Knox, M.S.N., Philadelphia, PA; Bonnie Liebman, M.S., Washington, DC; Sudesh K. Mahajan, M.D., Grosse Point Woods, MI; Craig J. McClain, M.D., Lexington, KY; Jay M. Mirtallo, M.S., Columbus, OH; Sohrab Mobarhan, M.D., Maywood, IL; Robert M. Russell, M.D., Boston, MA; Harold H. Sandstead, M.D., Galveston, TX; William J. Stone, M.D., Nashville, TN; Carlos A. Vaamonde, M.D., Miami, FL; Stanley Wallach, M.D., New York, NY

Obstetrics and Gynecology
Douglas D. Glover, M.D., *Chair*, Morgantown, WV; Rudi Ansbacher, M.D., Ann Arbor, MI; Florence Comite, M.D., New Haven, CT; James W. Daly, M.D., Columbia, MO; Marilynn C. Frederiksen, M.D., Chicago, IL; Charles B. Hammond, M.D., Durham, NC; Barbara A. Hayes, M.A., New Rochelle, NY; Art Jacknowitz, Pharm.D., Morgantown, WV; William J. Ledger, M.D., New York, NY; Andre-Marie Leroux, M.D., Ottawa, Ontario; William A. Nahhas, M.D., Dayton, OH; Warren N. Otterson, M.D., Shreveport, LA; Samuel A. Pasquale, M.D., New Brunswick, NJ; Johanna Perlmutter, M.D., Boston, MA; Robert W. Rebar, M.D., Cincinnati, OH; Richard H. Reindollar, M.D., Boston, MA; G. Millard Simmons, M.D., Morgantown, WV; J. Benjamin Younger, M.D., Birmingham, AL

Ophthalmology
Herbert E. Kaufman, M.D., *Chair*, New Orleans, LA; Steven R. Abel, Pharm.D., Indianapolis, IN; Jules Baum, M.D., Boston, MA; Lee R. Duffner, M.D., Miami, FL; David L. Epstein, M.D., Durham, NC; Allan J. Flach, Pharm.D., M.D., Corte Madera, CA; Vincent H. L. Lee, Ph.D., Los Angeles, CA; Steven M. Podos, M.D., New York, NY; Kirk R. Wilhelmus, M.D., Houston, TX; Thom J. Zimmerman, M.D., Ph.D., Louisville, KY

Otorhinolaryngology
Leonard P. Rybak, M.D., Ph.D., *Chair*, Springfield, IL; Robert E. Brummett, Ph.D., Portland, OR; Robert A. Dobie, M.D., San Antonio, TX; Linda J. Gardiner, M.D., Fort Myers, FL; David Hilding, M.D., Price, UT; David B. Hom, M.D., Minneapolis, MN; Helen F. Krause, M.D., Pittsburgh, PA; Richard L. Mabry, M.D., Dallas, TX; Lawrence J. Marentette, M.D., Ann Arbor, MI; Robert A. Mickel, M.D., Ph.D., San Francisco, CA; Randal A. Otto, M.D., San Antonio, TX; Richard W. Waguespack, M.D., Birmingham, AL; William R. Wilson, M.D., Washington, DC

Parasitic Disease
Jay S. Keystone, M.D., *Chair*, Toronto, Ontario; Michele Barry, M.D., New Haven, CT; Frank J. Bia, M.D., M.P.H., Guilford, CT; David Botero, M.D., Medellin, Colombia; David

O. Freedman, M.D., Birmingham, AL; Elaine C. Jong, M.D., Seattle, WA; Dennis D. Juranek, M.D., Atlanta, GA; Donald J. Krogstad, M.D., New Orleans, LA; Douglas W. MacPherson, M.D., Hamilton, Ontario; Edward K. Markell, M.D., Berkeley, CA; Theodore Nash, M.D., Bethesda, MD; Murray Wittner, M.D., Bronx, NY

Patient Counseling (Ad Hoc)
Frank J. Ascione, Pharm.D., Ph.D., *Chair*, Ann Arbor, MI; John E. Arradondo, M.D., Houston, TX; Candace Barnett, Atlanta, GA; Karin Bolte, Washington, DC; Allan H. Bruckheim, M.D., Harrison, NY; Mark Clasen, M.D., Ph.D., Dayton, OH; Amy Cooper-Outlaw, Pharm.D., Stone Mountain, GA; Frederick A. Curro, D.M.D., Ph.D., Jersey City, NJ; Robin DiMatteo, Ph.D., Riverside, CA; Diane B. Ginsburg, Austin, TX; Denise Grimes, R.N., Jackson, MI; Richard Herrier, Tucson, AZ; Barry Kass, R.Ph., Boston, MA; Thomas Kellenberger, Pharm.D., Montvale, NJ; Alice Kimball, Darnestown, MD; Pat Kramer, Bismarck, ND; Patti Kummeth, R.N., Rochester, MN; Ken Leibowitz, Philadelphia, PA; Colleen Lum Lung, R.N., Denver, CO; Louise Matte, Quebec, Canada; Scotti Milley, Richmond, VA; Constance Pavlides, R.N., D.N.Sc., Rockville, MD; Lisa Tedesco, Ph.D., Ann Arbor, MI

Pediatric Anesthesiology (Ad Hoc)
Charles J. Coté, M.D., *Chair*, Chicago, IL, J. Michael Badgwell, M.D., Lubbock, TX; Barbara Brandon, M.D., Pittsburgh, PA; Ryan Cook, M.D., Pittsburgh, PA; John J. Downes, M.D., Philadelphia, PA; Dennis Fisher, M.D., San Francisco, CA; John E. Forestner, M.D., Fort Worth, TX; Helen W. Karl, M.D., Seattle, WA; Harry G. G. Kingston, M.B., Portland, OR; Anne Marie Lynn, M.D., Seattle, WA; Mark Shriner, M.D. Philadelphia, PA; Victoria Simpson, M.D., Ph.D., Denver, CO; Meb Watcha, M.D., St. Louis, MO

Pediatrics
Philip D. Walson, M.D., *Chair*, Columbus, OH; Susan Alpert, Ph.D., M.D., Rockville, MD; Jacob V. Aranda, M.D., Ph.D., Montreal, Quebec; Cheston M. Berlin, Jr., M.D., Hershey, PA; Nancy Jo Braden, M.D., Phoenix, AZ; Patricia J. Bush, Ph.D., Washington, DC; Marion J. Finkel, M.D., Morris Township, NJ; George S. Goldstein, M.D., Briarcliff Manor, NY; Ralph E. Kauffman, M.D., Detroit, MI; Gideon Koren, M.D., Toronto, Ontario; Joan M. Korth-Bradley, Pharm.D., Ph.D., Philadelphia, PA; Richard Leff, Pharm.D., Kansas City, KS; Carolyn Lund, R.N., M.S., San Francisco, CA; Wayne Snodgrass, M.D., Galveston, TX; Celia A. Viets, M.D., Ottawa, Canada; John T. Wilson, M.D., Shreveport, LA; Sumner J. Yaffe, M.D., Bethesda, MD; Karin E. Zenk, Pharm.D., Irvine, CA

Pharmacy Practice
Thomas P. Reinders, Pharm.D., *Chair*, Richmond, VA; Olya Duzey, M.S., Big Rapids, MI; Yves Gariepy, B.Sc.Pharm., Quebec, Quebec; Ned Heltzer, M.S., New Castle, DE; Lester S. Hosto, B.S., Little Rock, AR; Martin J. Jinks, Pharm.D., Pullman, WA; Frederick Klein, B.S., Montvale, NJ; Calvin H. Knowlton, Ph.D., Lumberton, NJ; Patricia A. Kramer, B.S., Bismarck, ND; Dennis McCallum, Pharm.D., Minneapolis, MN; Shirley P. McKee, B.S., Houston, TX; William A. McLean, Pharm.D., Ottawa, Ontario; Gladys Montañez, B.S., Santurce, PR; Donald L. Moore, B.S., Kokomo, IN; John E. Ogden, M.S., Washington, DC; Henry A. Palmer, Ph.D., Storrs, CT; Lorie G. Rice, B.A., M.P.H., San Francisco, CA; Mike R. Sather, M.S., Albuquerque, NM; Albert Sebok, B.S., Hudson, OH; William E. Smith, Pharm.D., Ph.D., Boston, MA; Susan East Torrico, B.S., Orlando, FL; J. Richard Wuest, Pharm.D., Cincinnati, OH; Glenn Y. Yokoyama, Pharm.D., Pasadena, CA

Psychiatric Disease
Burton J. Goldstein, M.D., *Chair*, Williams Island, FL; Magda Campbell, M.D., New York, NY; Alex A. Cardoni, M.S. Pharm., Hartford, CT; James L. Claghorn, M.D., Houston, TX; N. Michael Davis, M.S., Miami, FL; Larry Ereshefsky, Pharm.D., San Antonio, TX; W. Edwin Fann, M.D., Houston, TX; Alan J. Gelenberg, M.D., Tucson, AZ; Tracy R. Gordy, M.D., Austin, TX; Paul Grof, M.D., Ottawa, Ontario; Russell T. Joffe, M.D., Toronto, Ontario; Harriet P. Lefley, Ph.D., Miami, FL; Nathan Rawls, Pharm.D., Memphis, TN; Ruth Robinson, Saskatoon, Saskatchewan; Matthew V. Rudorfer, M.D., Rockville, MD; Karen A. Theesen, Pharm.D., Omaha, NE

Pulmonary Disease
Harold S. Nelson, M.D., *Chair*, Denver, CO; Richard C. Ahrens, M.D., Iowa City, IA; Eugene R. Bleecker, M.D., Baltimore, MD; William W. Busse, M.D., Madison, WI; Christopher Fanta, M.D., Boston, MA; Mary K. Garcia, R.N., Sugarland, TX; Nicholas Gross, M.D., Hines, IL; Leslie Hendeles, Pharm.D., Gainesville, FL; Elliot Israel, M.D., Boston, MA; Susan Janson-Bjerklie, R.N., Ph.D., San Francisco, CA; John W. Jenne, M.D., Hines, IL; H. William Kelly, Pharm.D., Albuquerque, NM; James P. Kemp, M.D., San Diego, CA; Henry Levison, M.D., Toronto, Ontario; Gail Shapiro, M.D., Seattle, WA; Stanley J. Szefler, M.D., Denver, CO

Radiopharmaceuticals
Carol S. Marcus, Ph.D., M.D., *Chair*, Torrance, CA; Capt. William H. Briner, B.S., Durham, NC; Ronald J. Callahan, Ph.D., Boston, MA; Janet F. Eary, M.D., Seattle, WA; Joanna S. Fowler, Ph.D., Upton, NY; David L. Gilday, M.D., Toronto, Ontario; David A. Goodwin, M.D., Palo Alto, CA; David L. Laven, N.Ph., C.R.Ph., FASCP, Bay Pines, FL; Andrea H. McGuire, M.D., Des Moines, IA; Peter Paras, Ph.D., Rockville, MD; Barry A. Siegel, M.D., St. Louis, MO; Edward B. Silberstein, M.D., Cincinnati, OH; Dennis P. Swanson, M.S., Pittsburgh, PA; Mathew L. Thakur, Ph.D., Philadelphia, PA; Henry N. Wellman, M.D., Indianapolis, IN

Surgical Drugs and Devices
Lary A. Robinson, M.D., *Chair*, Tampa, FL; Gregory Alexander, M.D., Rockville, MD; Norman D. Anderson, M.D., Baltimore, MD; Alan R. Dimick, M.D., Birmingham, AL; Jack Hirsh, M.D., Hamilton, Ontario; Manucher J. Javid, M.D., Madison, WI; Henry J. Mann, Pharm.D., Bloomington, MN; Kurt M. W. Niemann, M.D., Birmingham, AL; Robert P. Rapp, Pharm.D., Lexington, KY; Ronald Rubin, M.D., West Newton, MA

Urology
John A. Belis, M.D., *Chair*, Hershey, PA; Culley C. Carson, M.D., Chapel Hill, NC; Richard A. Cohen, M.D., Red Bank, NJ; B. J. Reid Czarapata, R.N., North Potomac, MD; Jean B. de Kernion, M.D., Los Angeles, CA; Warren Heston, Ph.D., New York, NY; Mark V. Jarowenko, M.D., Hershey, PA; Mary Lee, Pharm.D., Chicago, IL; Marguerite C. Lippert, M.D., Charlottesville, VA; Penelope A. Longhurst, Ph.D., Philadelphia, PA; Tom F. Lue, M.D., San Francisco,

CA; Michael G. Mawhinney, Ph.D., Morgantown, WV; Martin G. McLoughlin, M.D., Vancouver, British Columbia; Randall G. Rowland, M.D., Ph.D., Indianapolis, IN; J. Patrick Spirnak, M.D., Cleveland, OH; William F. Tarry, M.D., Morgantown, WV; Keith N. Van Arsdalen, M.D., Philadelphia, PA

Veterinary Medicine

Lloyd E. Davis, D.V.M., Ph.D., *Chair*, Urbana, IL; Arthur L. Aronson, D.V.M., Ph.D., Raleigh, NC; Gordon W. Brumbaugh, D.V.M., Ph.D., College Station, TX; Peter Conlon, D.V.M., Ph.D., Guelph, Ontario; Gordon L. Coppoc, D.V.M., Ph.D., West Lafayette, IN; Sidney A. Ewing, D.V.M., Ph.D., Stillwater, OK; Stuart D. Forney, M.S., Fort Collins, CO; William G. Huber, D.V.M., Ph.D., Sun City West, AZ; Vernon Corey Langston, D.V.M., Ph.D., Mississippi State, MS; Mark G. Papich, D.V.M., Raleigh, NC; John W. Paul, D.V.M., Somerville, NJ; Thomas E. Powers, D.V.M., Ph.D., Columbus, OH; Charles R. Short, D.V.M., Ph.D., Baton Rouge, LA; Richard H. Teske, D.V.M., Ph.D., Rockville, MD; Jeffrey R. Wilcke, D.V.M., M.S., Blacksburg, VA

DRUG INFORMATION DIVISION ADDITIONAL CONTRIBUTORS

The information presented in this text represents an ongoing review of the drugs contained herein and represents a consensus of various viewpoints expressed. In addition to the individuals listed below, many schools, associations, pharmaceutical companies, and governmental agencies have provided comment or otherwise contributed to the development of the 1995 USP DI data base. Such listing does not imply that these individuals have reviewed all of the material in this text or that they individually agree with all statements contained herein.

Donald I. Abrams, M.D., San Francisco, CA
Jonathan Abrams, M.D., Albuquerque, NM
Bruce H. Ackerman, Pharm.D., Philadelphia, PA
N. Franklin Adkinson, M.D., Baltimore, MD
Allen C. Alfrey, M.D., Denver, CO
Joanne Allard, M.D., Toronto, Ontario, Canada
Carmen Allegra, M.D., Bethesda, MD
Mike Apley, D.V.M., Greeley, CO
Martin Bacon, M.D., Bethesda, MD
José M. Ballester, M.D., La Habana, Cuba
Rick Barbarash, Pharm.D., St. Louis, MO
Patsy Barnett, Pharm.D., Birmingham, AL
LuAnne Barron, Birmingham, AL
Robert W. Beightol, Pharm.D., Roanoke, VA
William Bell, M.D., Baltimore, MD
Gladys Bendahan Barchilón, Barcelona, Spain
Patricia Bennett, B.S.Pharm., Cincinnati, OH
David L. Benowitz, M.D., San Francisco, CA
Byron S. Berlin, M.D., Lansing, MI
Frederick A. Berry, M.D., Charlottesville, VA
Ernest Beutler, M.D., La Jolla, CA
Christine A. Bezouska, M.D., Morgantown, WV
S. Bruce Binder, M.D., Ph.D., Dayton, OH
Martin Black, M.D., Philadelphia, PA
Laura Boehnke, Pharm.D., Houston, TX
Halcy Bohen, Ph.D., Washington, DC
Wayne E. Bradley, Duluth, GA
Michael Brady, M.D., Columbus, OH
Edward L. Braud, M.D., Springfield, IL
Robert E. Braun, D.D.S., Buffalo, NY
Kenneth Bridges, M.D., Boston, MA
Paul J. Brown, M.D., Bedford, NH
Louis Buttino, Jr., M.D., Dayton, OH
Wesley G. Byerly, Pharm.D., Winston-Salem, NC
Karim A. Calis, Pharm.D., Bethesda, MD
Mary E. Carman, Ottawa, Ontario
Charles C.J. Carpenter, M.D., Providence, RI
Peggy Carver, M.D., Ann Arbor, MI
Marcel Casavant, M.D., Columbus, OH
Bruce A. Chabner, M.D., Bethesda, MD
Erin S. Champagne, D.V.M., Blacksburg, VA
Chih Wen Chang, Pharm.D., Maywood, IL
Te-Wen Chang, M.D., Boston, MA
Kenneth R. Chapman, M.D., Toronto, Ontario
Bruce D. Cheson, M.D., Bethesda, MD
Henry Chilton, Pharm.D., Winston-Salem, NC
Frank Chytil, Ph.D., Nashville, TN
Scott B. Citino, D.V.M., Yulee, FL
Cyril R. Clarke, Ph.D., Stillwater, OK
Jackson Como, M.D., Birmingham, AL
Betsy Jane Cooper, M.D., Washington, DC
James W. Cooper, Ph.D., Athens, GA
Deborah Cotton, M.D., Boston, MA
Fred F. Cowan, Ph.D., Portland, OR
Donald W. Cox, M.D., Morgantown, WV
Mark V. Crisman, D.V.M., Blacksburg, VA
Craig Darby, R.Ph., Twinsburg, OH
Michael Davidson, D.V.M., Raleigh, NC
Ann J. Davis, M.D., Boston, MA
Janet Davis, M.D., Miami, FL
Ken Davis, M.D., New York, NY
Thomas D. DeCillis, North Port, FL
Carel P. de Haseth, Ph.D., Netherland Antilles
Daniel Deykin, M.D., Boston, MA
Nick Diamant, M.D., Toronto, Ontario Canada
Annette Dickinson, Ph.D., Washington, DC
Barry D. Dickinson, Ph.D., Chicago, IL
Christine Z. Dickinson, M.D., Royal Oak, MI
John B. DiMarco, M.D., Ph.D., Charlottesville, VA
James E. Doherty, M.D., Little Rock, AR
Donald C. Doll, M.D., Columbia, MO
Jerry Dolovich, M.D., Hamilton, Ontario
R. Gordon Douglas, M.D., Rahway, NJ
Ed Drea, Pharm.D., Phoenix, AZ
Bonnie Driggers, R.N., Portland, OR
Marion Dugdale, M.D., Memphis, TN
Carol Duncan, R.N., Portland, OR
Suzanne Eastman, M.S., R.Ph., Columbus, OH
John E. Edwards, Jr., M.D., Torrance, CA
Robert Edwards, Pharm.D., Columbus, OH

Lawrence H. Einhorn, M.D., Indianapolis, IN
Augustin Escalante, M.D., Downey, CA
Gary Euler, Dr.P.H., Atlanta, GA
William Fant, Pharm.D., Cincinnati, OH
Martin N. Farlow, M.D., Indianapolis, IN
R. Edward Faught, M.D., Birmingham, AL
David S. Fedson, M.D., Charlottesville, VA
John P. Feighner, La Mesa, CA
James M. Ferguson, M.D., Salt Lake City, UT
Paul Ferrell, M.D., Bethesda, MD
Anne Gilbert Feuer, R.Ph., Cincinnati, OH
Suzanne Fields, Pharm.D., San Antonio, TX
J.R. Fontilus, M.D., Netherland Antilles
Tammy Fox, R.Ph., Fairfield, OH
Charles W. Francis, M.D., Rochester, NY
Ruth Francis-Floyd, D.V.M., Gainesville, FL
Rudolph M. Franklin, M.D., New Orleans, LA
H. H. Frey, Berlin, Germany
Dorothy Friedberg, M.D., New York, NY
Alan Friedman, M.D., New York, NY
José P.B. Gallardo, R.Ph., Iowa City, IA
Gloria Garber, R.Ph., Cincinnati, OH
Arthur Garson, M.D., Durham, NC
S. Gauthier, M.D., Montreal, PQ, Canada
Edward Genton, M.D., New Orleans, LA
Anne A. Gershon, M.D., New York, NY
Larry N. Gever, Pharm.D., Cranbury, NJ
Michael J. Glade, Ph.D., Chicago, IL
Charles J. Glueck, M.D., Cincinnati, OH
Maryanne Godlewski-Vagnini, R.Ph., Brooklyn, NY
Lewis Goldfrank, M.D., New York, NY
J. Max Goodson, D.D.S., Ph.D., Boston, MA
Fred Gordin, M.D., Washington, DC
John D. Grabenstein, M.S., Fort Sam Houston, TX
Roni Grad, M.D., Albuquerque, NM
Nina M. Graves, Pharm.D., Minneapolis, MN
Terri Graves Davidson, Pharm.D., Atlanta, GA
David Green, M.D., Chicago, IL
Harry Green, M.D., Evansville, IN
Martin D. Green, M.D., Rockville, MD
Philip C. Greig, M.D., Durham, NC
Vincent Habiyambere, M.D., Geneva, Switzerland
Angela M. Hadbavny, Pharm.D., Pittsburgh, PA
Benjamin F. Hammond, D.D.S., Ph.D., Philadelphia, PA
Kenneth R. Hande, M.D., Nashville, TN
Edward A. Hartshorn, Ph.D., League City, TX
Robert C. Hastings, M.D., Carville, LA
William E. Hathaway, Denver, CO
Frederick G. Hayden, M.D., Charlottesville, VA
Cleopatra L. Hazel, Pharm.D., Netherland Antilles
Murk-Hein Heinemann, M.D., New York, NY
Peter Hellyer, D.V.M., Raleigh, NC
Bryan N. Henderson, II, D.D.S., Dallas, TX
William Herbert, M.D., Durham, NC
Barbara Herwaldt, M.D., Atlanta, GA
Monto Ho, M.D., Pittsburgh, PA
Vincent C. Ho, M.D., British Columbia, Canada
M.E. Hoar, Springfield, MA
Robert Hodgeman, M.S., R.Ph., Cincinnati, OH
Gary N. Holland, M.D., Los Angeles, CA
Richard A. Holmes, M.D., Columbia, MO
William Hopkins, Pharm.D., Atlanta, GA
Richard B. Hornick, M.D., Orlando, FL
Raymond W. Houde, M.D., New York, NY
Colin W. Howden, M.D., Columbia, SC
Walter T. Hughes, M.D., Memphis, TN
B. Thomas Hutchinson, M.D., Boston, MA
John Iazzetta, Pharm.D., Toronto, Ontario, Canada
Rodney D. Ice, Ph.D., Atlanta, GA
Frederick Jacobsen, M.D., Washington, DC
Mark Jacobson, M.D., San Francisco, CA
Robert Jacobson, M.D., Carville, LA
Ann L. Janer, M.S., Auburn, AL
Janet P. Jaramilla, Pharm.D., Chicago, IL
James W. Jefferson, M.D., Madison, WI
Alan Jenkins, M.D., Charlottesville, VA
Leslye Johnson, Ph.D., Bethesda, MD
Joseph L. Jorizzo, M.D., Winston-Salem, NC
Gunnar Juliusson, M.D., Ph.D., Huddinge, Sweden
Hugh F. Kabat, Ph.D., Albuquerque, NM
James Kahn, M.D., San Franscisco, CA
Alan Kanada, Pharm.D., Denver, CO
John J. Kavanagh, M.D., Houston, TX
Michael J. Keating, M.D., Houston, TX
Michael Kelley, M.D., Columbus, OH
David C. Kem, M.D., Oklahoma City, OK
N. David Kennedy, R.Ph., Washington, DC
Joseph M. Khoury, M.D., Bethesda, MD
Agnes V. Klein, M.D., Vanier, Ontario
Anne Klibanski, M.D., Boston, MA
Sandra Knowles, B.Pharm., Toronto, Ontario, Canada
John Koepke, Pharm.D., Columbus, OH
Joseph A. Kovacs, M.D., Bethesda, MD
Paul A. Krusinski, M.D., Burlington, VT
Paul B. Kuehn, Ph.D., Woodinville, WA
R.W. Kuncl, M.D., Baltimore, MD
Thomas L. Kurt, M.D., Dallas, TX
Lyle Laird, Pharm.D., San Antonio, TX
John S. Lambert, M.D., Rochester, NY
John R. LaMontagne, Bethesda, MD
Michael Lange, M.D., New York, NY
Victor J. Lanzotti, M.D., Springfield, IL
P. Reed Larsen, M.D., Boston, MA
Eugene Laska, M.D., Orangeburg, NY
Oscar L. Laskin, M.D., East Hanover, NJ
John Laszlo, M.D., Atlanta, GA
Belle Lee, Pharm.D., San Francisco, CA
Ilo E. Leppik, M.D., Minneapolis, MN
Raymond Levy, London, England
Richard A. Lewis, M.D., Houston, TX
William Lieber, M.D., Waterbury, CT
Charles Liebow, II, D.D.S., Ph.D., Buffalo, NY
Christopher D. Lind, M.D., Nashville, TN
Charles H. Livengood, III, M.D., Durham, NC
Don M. Long, M.D., Ph.D., Baltimore, MD
Julio R. Lopez, M.D., Martinez, CA
Colleen Lum Lung, R.N., Denver, CO
Howard I. Maibach, M.D., San Francisco, CA
Marilyn Manco-Johnson, Denver, CO
Victor J. Marder, M.D., Rochester, NY
Joseph E. Margarone, II, D.D.S., Buffalo, NY
Maurie Markman, M.D., Cleveland, OH
Jon Markovitz, M.D., Phoenix, AZ
William C. Matthews, M.D., San Diego, CA
Harry R. Maxon, III, M.D., Cincinnati, OH
Alice Lorraine McAfee, Pharm.D., San Pedro, CA
Lisa Y. McDonald, Pharm.D., Emeryville, CA
Norman L. McElroy, San Jose, CA
Charles McGrath, D.V.M., Blacksburg, VA
Ross E. McKinney, M.D., Durham, NC
Anne McNulty, M.D., Waterbury, CT
Wallace B. Mendelson, M.D. Cleveland, OH
Dean D. Metcalfe, M.D., Bethesda, MD
Donald Miller, Pharm.D., Fargo, ND

John Mills, M.D., Fairfield, Victoria, Australia
Joel S. Mindel, M.D., Ph.D., New York, NY
Bernard L. Mirkin, M.D., Chicago, IL
Janet L. Mitchell, M.D., New York, NY
John R. Modlin, M.D., Hanover, NH
C. Craig Moldenhauer, M.D., San Diego, CA
Garreth A. Moore, Blacksburg, VA
Mary E. Mortensen, M.D., Columbus, OH
Robyn Mueller, R.Ph., Cincinnati, OH
R.I. Ogilvie, M.D., Toronto, Ontario
Linda K. Ohri, Pharm.D., Omaha, NE
James M. Oleske, M.D., Newark, NJ
Robert O'Mara, M.D., Rochester, NY
Michael J. O'Neill, R.Ph., Twinsburg, OH
Walter A. Orenstein, M.D., Atlanta, GA
James R. Oster, M.D., Miami, FL
Judith M. Ozbun, R.Ph., M.S., Fargo, ND
David C. Pang, Ph.D., Chicago, IL
Michael F. Para, M.D., Columbus, OH
Satyapal R. Pareddy, B.Pharm., Brooklyn, NY
Robert C. Park, M.D., Washington, DC
William W. Parmly, M.D., San Francisco, CA
Albert Patterson, Hines, IL
James A. Pederson, M.D., Oklahoma City, OK
Ronald Peterson, M.D., Ph.D., Rochester, MN
Melenie Petropoulos, R.Ph., Twinsburg, OH
Lawrence D. Piro, M.D., La Jolla, CA
Philip A. Pizzo, M.D., Bethesda, MD
Christopher V. Plowe, M.D., Bethesda, MD
Therese Poirier, Pharm.D., Pittsburgh, PA
Michael A. Polis, M.D., Bethesda, MD
James A. Ponto, R.Ph., Iowa City, IA
Carol M. Proudfit, Ph.D., Chicago, IL
Nixa Ramos, Arecibo, Puerto Rico
Norbert P. Rapoza, Ph.D., Chicago, IL
Gary Raskob, M.Sc., Oklahoma City, OK
Terry D. Rees, D.D.S., Dallas, TX
Alfred J. Remillard, Pharm.D., Saskatoon, Saskatchewan, Canada
David Robertson, M.D., Nashville, TN
Robert Roberts, M.D., Houston, TX
Daniel C. Robinson, Pharm.D., Los Angeles, CA
John E. Roney, R.Ph., Cincinnati, OH
Jeff Rosner, R.Ph., Twinsburg, OH
Douglas S. Ross, M.D., Boston, MA
Phillip J. Rubin, M.D., Phoenix, AZ
Michael S. Saag, M.D., Birmingham, AL
Henry S. Sacks, Ph.D., M.D., New York, NY
Sharon Safrin, M.D., San Francisco, CA
Evelyn Salerno, Pharm.D., Hialeah, FL
Hugh A. Sampson, Jr., M.D., Baltimore, MD
Subbiah Sangiah, D.V.M., Ph.D., Stillwater, OK
Victor M. Santana, Memphis, TN
Belinda Sartor, M.D., Shreveport, LA
Donald C. Sawyer, East Lansing, MI
Elliot Schecter, M.D., Oklahoma City, OK
Udo P. Schmiedl, M.D., Ph.D., Seattle, WA
Gabriel Schmunis, M.D., Washington, DC
Steven M. Schnittman, M.D., Rockville, MD
George Schuster, M.D., Augusta, GA
Stephen Schuster, M.D., Philadelphia, PA
Dorothy Schwartz-Porsche, Berlin, Germany
Douglas A. Sears, Tenafly, NJ
Jerome Seidenfeld, Ph.D., Chicago, IL
Charles F. Seifert, Pharm.D., Oklahoma City, OK
Allen Shaughnessy, Pharm.D., Harrisburg, PA
Donald J. Sherrard, M.D., Seattle, WA
Yvonne M. Shevchuk, Pharm.D., Saskatoon, Saskatchewan, Canada
Harold M. Silverman, Pharm.D., Silver Spring, MD
Irv Siven, M.D., New York, NY
Barry H. Smith, M.D., Ph.D., New York, NY
Dance Smith, Pharm.D., Ft. Steilacoom, WA
Geralynn B. Smith, M.S., Detroit, MI
John R. Smith, M.S., Ph.D., Portland, OR
Steven J. Smith, Ph.D., Chicago, IL
Elliott M. Sogol, Ph.D., Research Triangle Park, NC
Nicholas Soter, M.D., New York, NY
William Speliacy, M.D., Tampa, FL
Joan Stachnik, Chicago, IL
William Steers, M.D., Charlottesville, VA
John J. Stern, M.D., Philadelphia, PA
Irwin Strathman, M.D., Lutz, FL
Kris Strohbehn, M.D., Boston, MA
David Stuhr, Denver, CO
Alan Sugar, M.D., Boston, MA
Linda Gore Sutherland, Pharm.D., Laramie, WY
Sandra Tailor, Pharm.D., Toronto, Ontario, Canada
David A. Taylor, M.D., Morgantown, WV
Mary E. Teresi, Iowa City, IA
Cheryl Nunn Thompson, Chicago, IL
John C. Thurman, D.V.M., Urbana, IL
Roger C. Toffle, M.D., Morgantown, WV
Douglas M. Tollefsen, M.D., St. Louis, MO
Eric J. Topol, M.D., Ann Arbor, MI
Jayme Trott, Pharm.D., San Antonio, TX
Donald G. Vidt, M.D., Cleveland, OH
Richard Vogel, D.D.S., Newark, NJ
Georgia Vogelsang, M.D., Baltimore, MD
Paul A. Volberding, M.D., San Francisco, CA
Andrea Wall, R.Ph., Cincinnati, OH
William Warner, Ph.D., New York, NY
Michael Weber, M.D., Irvine, CA
Krisantha Weerasuriya, M.D., Geneva, Switzerland
G. John Weir, M.D., Marshfield, WI
Timothy E. Welty, Pharm.D., Cincinnati, OH
Stanford Wessler, M.D., Rye, NY
Carolyn Westhoff, New York, NY
John White, Pharm.D., Spokane, WA
Richard J. Whitley, M.D., Birmingham, AL
Catherine Wilfert, M.D., Durham, NC
Robert G. Wolfangel, Ph.D., St. Louis, MO
M. Michael Wolfe, M.D., Boston, MA
William Wonderlin, Ph.D., Morgantown, WV
Richard J. Wood, M.D., Boston, MA
Curtis Wright, M.D., Rockville, MD
Catharine Wuest, R.Ph., Cincinnati, OH
Robert Yarchoan, M.D., Bethesda, MD
Stephanie Zarus, Pharm.D., Philadelphia, PA
John M. Zajecka, M.D., Chicago, IL
Frederic J. Zucchero, M.A., R.Ph., Chesterfield, MO
Jane R. Zucker, Atlanta, GA

HEADQUARTERS STAFF

DRUG INFORMATION DIVISION

Director: Keith W. Johnson

Assistant Director: Georgie M. Cathey

Administrative Staff: Jaime A. Ramirez *(Administrative Assistant)*, Albert Crucillo, Mayra L. Rios

Senior Drug Information Specialists: Sandra Lee Boyer, Nancy Lee Dashiell, Debra A. Edwards, Esther H. Klein *(Supervisor)*, Angela Méndez Mayo *(Spanish Publications Coordinator)*

Drug Information Specialists: Katherine M. Bennett, Joyce Carpenter, Ann Corken, Jymeann King, Doris Lee *(Supervisor)*, Robin Schermerhorn, Denise Seldon, Daniel W. Seyoum

Veterinary Drug Information Specialist: Amy Neal

Coordinator, Patient Counseling and Education Programs: Stacy M. Hartranft

Computer Applications: Richard Allen *(Programmer)*, Bernard G. Silverstein *(Computer Applications Specialist)*

Publications Development Staff: Diana M. Blais *(Manager)*, Anne M. Lawrence *(Associate)*, Dorothy Raymond *(Assistant)*, Darcy Schwartz *(Assistant)*

Library Services: Florence A. Hogan *(Manager)*, Terri Rikhy *(Assistant)*, Madeleine Welsch

Research Associate, International Programs: David D. Housley

Research Assistant: Annamarie J. Sibik

Consultants: Janet Elgert, Lourdes de Gonzalez, David W. Hughes, S. Ramakrishnan Iyer, Wanda Janicki, Kate Phelan, Marcelo Vernengo

Scholar in Residence: Patricia J. Bush, Georgetown University

Student Interns/Externs: Robyn Dubinsky, University of Missouri at Kansas City; Rachel Ellis, Nottingham University, England; Kevin Garey, Dalhousie University, Nova Scotia; Bereket Melaku, Howard University; Kavita Nair, University of Toledo; Ken Rogers, University of Arizona; Yván Sánchez-Huamaní, National University of Trujillo, Peru

Visiting Scholars: Giulia Cingolani, Rome, Italy; Elena Oshkalova, Moscow, Russian Federation; Svetlana Udotova, Moscow, Russian Federation

USP ADMINISTRATIVE STAFF

Executive Director: Jerome A. Halperin
Associate Executive Director: Joseph G. Valentino
Assistant Executive Director for Professional and Public Affairs: Jacqueline L. Eng
Director, Finance: Abe Brauner
Director, Operations: J. Robert Strang
Director, Personnel: Arlene Bloom
Director, Fulfillment/Facilities: Drew J. Lutz
Legal: Kim Keller (Staff Attorney), John Lindow (Associate Legal Counsel for Business Affairs), Colleen Ottoson (Staff Attorney)

DRUG STANDARDS DIVISION

Director: Lee T. Grady

Assistant Directors: Charles H. Barnstein *(Revision)*, Barbara B. Hubert, *(Scientific Administration)*, Robert H. King *(Technical Services)*

Senior Scientists: Roger Dabbah, V. Srinivasan, William W. Wright

Scientists: Frank P. Barletta, Vivian A. Gray, W. Larry Paul

Senior Scientific Associate: Todd L. Cecil

Technical Editors: Ann K. Ferguson, Melissa M. Smith

Supervisor of Administration: Anju K. Malhotra

Support Staff: Patricia Barnhill, Glenna Etherton, Theresa H. Lee, Cecilia Luna, Maureen Rawson, Ernestene Williams

Drug Research and Testing Laboratory: Richard F. Lindauer *(Director)*

Hazard Communications: Linda Shear

Consultants: J. Joseph Belson, Zorach R. Glaser, Martin Golden, Aubrey S. Outschoorn

MARKETING

Director: Joan Blitman

Senior Product Manager: Mark A. Sohasky *(Electronic Information)*

Product Manager: Kathleen Bagas *(Publications)*

Marketing Associates: Jennifer C. Glenn, Dana L. McCullah, Steven Saars

Marketing Representative: Susan M. Williams *(Electronic Applications)*

Marketing Communications Manager: Derek Rice

Marketing Research Analyst: Deborah King

PUBLICATION SERVICES

Acting Director: Gail M. Oring

Managing Editors: A. V. Precup *(USP DI)*, Sandra Boynton *(USP-NF)*

Editorial Associates: *USP DI*—Ellen R. Loeb *(Senior Editorial Associate)*, Carol M. Griffin, Carol N. Hankin, Marie Kotomori, Harriet S. Nathanson, Ellen D. Smith, Barbara A. Visco; *USP-NF*—Jesusa D. Cordova *(Senior Editorial Associate)*, Ellen Elovitz, John Pahle, Margaret Kay Walshaw

USAN Staff: Carolyn A. Fleeger *(Editor)*, Gerilynne Seigneur

Typesetting Systems Coordinator: Jean E. Dale

Typesetting Staff: Susan L. Entwistle *(Supervisor)*, Donna Alie, Deborah R. Connelly, Lauren Taylor Davis, Deborah James, M. T. Samahon, Micheline Tranquille

Graphics: Cristy Gonzalez, Todd Hodges, Tia C. Morfessis, Greg Varhola

Word Processing: Barbara A. Bowman *(Supervisor)*, Frances Rampp, Susan Schartman, Jane Shulman

Also Contributing: Barbara Arnold, Proofreading; Brian Dillon and Paul Widem of Editech Services, Inc., Proofreading; Terri A. DeIuliis, Graphics; Michelle Thomas, Clerical Assistance.

PRACTITIONER REPORTING PROGRAMS

Assistant Executive Director for Practitioner Reporting Programs: Diane D. Cousins

Staff: Robin A. Baldwin, Shawn C. Becker, Jean Canada, Alice C. Curtis, Ilze Mohseni, Joanne Pease, Susmita Samanta, Anne Paula Thompson, Mary Susan Zmuda

MEMBERS OF THE USPC AND THE INSTITUTIONS AND ORGANIZATIONS REPRESENTED as of March 15, 1994

Officers and Board of Trustees

President: Mark Novitch, M.D.
Vice President: Donald R. Bennett, M.D., Ph.D.
Treasurer: John T. Fay, Jr., Ph.D.
Trustees Representing Medical Sciences: Edwin D. Bransome, Jr., M.D.; J. Richard Crout, M.D.
Trustees Representing Pharmaceutical Sciences: Jordan L. Cohen, Ph.D.; James T. Doluisio, Ph.D.
Trustee Representing the Public: Grace Powers Monaco, J.D.
Trustees at Large: John V. Bergen, Ph.D.; Joseph A. Mollica, Ph.D.
Past President: Arthur Hull Hayes, Jr., M.D.

United States Government Services

Department of the Army: Col. William O. Hiner, Jr.
Food and Drug Administration: Carl C. Peck, M.D.
Health Care Financing Administration: Robert E. Wren
National Institute of Standards and Technology: Stanley D. Rasberry
Navy Surgeon General's Office/Bureau of Medicine and Surgery: Captain R. Whiten
Office of the Surgeon General, U.S. Air Force: Capt. Edward Zastawny, Pharm.D.
U.S. Office of Consumer Affairs: Howard Seltzer
United States Public Health Service: Richard M. Church
Department of Veterans Affairs: John Ogden

National Organizations

American Association of Pharmaceutical Scientists: Ralph F. Shangraw, Ph.D.
American Chemical Society: Norman C. Jamieson, Ph.D.
American Dental Association: Clifford W. Whall, Ph.D.
American Hospital Association: William R. Reid
American Medical Association: Joseph W. Cranston, Jr., Ph.D.
American Nurses Association: Linda Cronenwett, Ph.D., R.N., F.A.A.N.
American Pharmaceutical Association: Arthur H. Kibbe, Ph.D.
American Society for Clinical Pharmacology & Therapeutics: William J. Mroczek, M.D.
American Society of Consultant Pharmacists: Milton S. Moskowitz
American Society of Hospital Pharmacists: Charles E. Myers
American Society for Pharmacology and Experimental Therapeutics: Kenneth L. Dretchen
American Society for Quality Control: Anthony M. Carfagno
American Veterinary Medical Association: Lloyd Davis, D.V.M., Ph.D.
Animal Health Institute: Martin Terry, D.V.M., Ph.D.
Association of Food and Drug Officials: David R. Work, J.D.
Association of Official Analytical Chemists: Thomas Layloff, Jr.
Chemical Manufacturers Association: Andrew J. Schmitz, Jr. *(deceased)*
Cosmetic, Toiletry & Fragrance Association, Inc.: G.N. McEwen, Jr., Ph.D., J.D.
Council for Responsible Nutrition: Annette Dickinson, Ph.D.
Drug Information Association: Elizabeth B. D'Angelo, Ph.D.
Generic Pharmaceutical Industry Association: William F. Haddad
Health Industry Manufacturers Association: Dee Simons
National Association of Boards of Pharmacy: Carmen Catizone
National Association of Chain Drug Stores, Inc.: Saul Schneider
National Pharmaceutical Alliance: Christina F. Sizemore
National Wholesale Druggists' Association: Bruce R. Siecker, R. Ph., Ph.D.
Nonprescription Drug Manufacturers Association: R. William Soller, Ph.D.
Parenteral Drug Association, Inc.: Peter E. Manni, Ph.D.
Pharmaceutical Manufacturers Association: Maurice Q. Bectel

Other Organizations and Institutions

Alabama

Auburn University, School of Pharmacy: Kenneth N. Barker, Ph.D.
Samford University School of Pharmacy: H. Anthony McBride, Ph.D.
University of Alabama School of Medicine: Robert B. Diasio, M.D.
University of South Alabama, College of Medicine: Samuel J. Strada, Ph.D.
Medical Association of the State of Alabama: Paul A. Palmisano, M.D.
Alabama Pharmaceutical Association: Mitchel C. Rothholz

Alaska

Alaska Pharmaceutical Association: Jackie Warren, R.Ph.

Arizona

University of Arizona, College of Medicine: John D. Palmer, Ph.D., M.D.
University of Arizona, College of Pharmacy: Michael Mayersohn, Ph.D.
Arizona Pharmacy Association: Edward Armstrong

Arkansas

University of Arkansas for Medical Sciences, College of Pharmacy: Kenneth G. Nelson, Ph.D.
Arkansas Pharmacists Association: Norman Canterbury, P.D.

California

Loma Linda University Medical Center: Ralph Cutler, M.D.
Stanford University School of Medicine: Brian B. Hoffman, M.D.
University of California, Davis, School of Medicine: Larry Stark, Ph.D.
University of California, San Diego, School of Medicine: Harold J. Simon, M.D., Ph.D.
University of California, San Francisco, School of Medicine: Walter L. Way, M.D.

University of Southern California, School of Medicine: Wayne R. Bidlack, Ph.D.
University of California, San Francisco, School of Pharmacy: Richard H. Guy, Ph.D.
University of Southern California, School of Pharmacy: Robert T. Koda, Pharm.D., Ph.D.
University of the Pacific, School of Pharmacy: Alice Jean Matuszak, Ph.D.
California Pharmacists Association: Robert P. Marshall, Pharm.D.

Colorado
University of Colorado School of Pharmacy: Merrick Lee Shively, Ph.D.
Colorado Pharmacists Association: Thomas G. Arthur, R.Ph.

Connecticut
University of Connecticut, School of Medicine: Paul F. Davern
University of Connecticut, School of Pharmacy: Karl A. Nieforth, Ph.D.
Connecticut Pharmaceutical Association: Henry A. Palmer, Ph.D.

Delaware
Delaware Pharmaceutical Society: Charles J. O'Connor
Medical Society of Delaware: John M. Levinson, M.D.

District of Columbia
George Washington University: Janet Elgert-Madison, Pharm.D.
Georgetown University, School of Medicine: Arthur Raines, Ph.D.
Howard University, College of Medicine: Sonya K. Sobrian, Ph.D.
Howard University, College of Pharmacy & Pharmacal Sciences: Wendell T. Hill, Jr., Pharm.D.

Florida
Southeastern College of Pharmacy: William D. Hardigan, Ph.D.
University of Florida, College of Medicine: Thomas F. Muther, Ph.D.
University of Florida, College of Pharmacy: Michael A. Schwartz, Ph.D.
University of South Florida, College of Medicine: Joseph J. Krzanowski, Jr., Ph.D.
Florida Pharmacy Association: "Red" Camp

Georgia
Medical College of Georgia, School of Medicine: David W. Hawkins, Pharm.D.
Mercer University School of Medicine: W. Douglas Skelton, M.D.
Mercer University, Southern School of Pharmacy: Hewitt W. Matthews, Ph.D.
Morehouse School of Medicine: Ralph W. Trottier, Jr., Ph.D., J.D.
University of Georgia, College of Pharmacy: Stuart Feldman, Ph.D.
Medical Association of Georgia: E. D. Bransome, Jr., M.D.
Georgia Pharmaceutical Association, Inc.: Larry R. Braden

Idaho
Idaho State University, College of Pharmacy: Eugene I. Isaacson, Ph.D.
Idaho State Pharmaceutical Association: Doris Denney

Illinois
Chicago Medical School/University of Health Sciences: Velayudhan Nair, Ph.D., D.Sc.
Loyola University of Chicago, Stritch School of Medicine: Erwin Coyne, Ph.D.
Northwestern University Medical School: Marilynn C. Frederiksen, M.D.
Rush Medical College of Rush University: Paul G. Pierpaoli, M.S.
Southern Illinois University, School of Medicine: Leonard Rybak, M.D., Ph.D.
University of Chicago, Pritzker School of Medicine: Patrick T. Horn, M.D., Ph.D.
University of Illinois, College of Medicine: Marten M. Kernis, Ph.D.
University of Illinois, College of Pharmacy: Henri R. Manasse, Jr., Ph.D.
Chicago College of Pharmacy: David J. Slatkin, Ph.D.
Illinois Pharmacists Association: Ronald W. Gottrich
Illinois State Medical Society: Vincent A. Costanzo, Jr., M.D.

Indiana
Butler University, College of Pharmacy: Wagar H. Bhatti, Ph.D.
Purdue University, School of Pharmacy and Pharmacal Sciences: Garnet E. Peck, Ph.D.
Indiana State Medical Association: Edward Langston, R.Ph., M.D.

Iowa
Drake University, College of Pharmacy: Sidney L. Finn, Ph.D.
University of Iowa, College of Medicine: John E. Kasik, M.D., Ph.D.
University of Iowa, College of Pharmacy: Robert A. Wiley, Ph.D.
Iowa Pharmacists Association: Steve C. Firman, R.Ph.

Kansas
University of Kansas, School of Pharmacy: Prof. Christopher Riley
Kansas Pharmacists Association: Robert R. Williams

Kentucky
University of Kentucky, College of Medicine: John M. Carney, Ph.D.
University of Kentucky, College of Pharmacy: Patrick P. DeLuca, Ph.D.
University of Louisville, School of Medicine: Peter P. Rowell, Ph.D.
Kentucky Medical Association: Ellsworth C. Seeley, M.D.
Kentucky Pharmacists Association: Chester L. Parker, Pharm.D.

Louisiana
Louisiana State University School of Medicine in New Orleans: Paul L. Kirkendol, Ph.D.
Northeast Louisiana University, School of Pharmacy: William M. Bourn, Ph.D.
Tulane University, School of Medicine: Floyd R. Domer, Ph.D.
Xavier University of Louisiana: Barry A. Bleidt, Ph.D., R.Ph.
Louisiana State Medical Society: Henry W. Jolly, Jr., M.D.
Louisiana Pharmacists Association: Mona J. Davis

Maryland
Johns Hopkins University, School of Medicine: E. Robert Feroli, Jr., Pharm.D.
University of Maryland, School of Medicine: Edson X. Albuquerque, M.D., Ph.D.
Uniformed Services University of the Health Sciences, F. Edward Hebert School of Medicine: Louis R. Cantilena, Jr., M.D., Ph.D.
University of Maryland, Baltimore, School of Pharmacy: Larry L. Augsburger, Ph.D.
Medical and Chirurgical Faculty of the State of Maryland: Frederick Wilhelm, M.D.
Maryland Pharmacists Association: Nicholas C. Lykos, P.D.

Massachusetts
Boston Univeristy, School or Medicine: J. Worth Estes, M.D.
Harvard Medical School: Peter Goldman, M.D.
Massachusetts College of Pharmacy and Allied Health Sciences: David A. Williams, Ph.D.
Northeastern University, College of Pharmacy and Allied Health Professions: John L. Neumeyer, Ph.D.
Tufts University, School of Medicine: John Mazzullo, M.D.
University of Massachusetts Medical School: Brian Johnson, M.D.
Massachusetts Medical Society: Errol Green, M.D.

Michigan
Ferris State University, School of Pharmacy: Gerald W.A. Slywka, Ph.D.
Michigan State University, College of Human Medicine: John Penner, M.D.
University of Michigan, College of Pharmacy: Ara G. Paul, Ph.D.
University of Michigan Medical Center: Jeoffrey K. Stross, M.D.
Wayne State University, School of Medicine: Ralph E. Kauffman, M.D.
Wayne State University, College of Pharmacy and Allied Health Professions: Janardan B. Nagwekar, Ph.D.
Michigan Pharmacists Association: Patrick L. McKercher, Ph.D.

Minnesota
Mayo Medical School: James J. Lipsky, M.D.
University of Minnesota, College of Pharmacy: E. John Staba, Ph.D.
University of Minnesota Medical School, Minneapolis: Jack W. Miller, Ph.D.
Minnesota Medical Association: Harold Seim, M.D.
Minnesota Pharmacists Association: Arnold D. Delger

Mississippi
University of Mississippi, School of Medicine: James L. Achord, M.D.
University of Mississippi, School of Pharmacy: Robert W. Cleary, Ph.D.
Mississippi State Medical Association: Charles L. Mathews
Mississippi Pharmacists Association: Mike Kelly

Missouri

St. Louis College of Pharmacy: John W. Zuzack, Ph.D.
St. Louis University, School of Medicine: Alvin H. Gold, Ph.D.
University of Missouri, Columbia, School of Medicine: John W. Yarbro, M.D.
University of Missouri-Kansas City, School of Medicine: Paul Cuddy, Pharm.D.
University of Missouri, Kansas City, School of Pharmacy: Lester Chafetz, Ph.D.
Washington University, School of Medicine: H. Mitchell Perry, Jr., M.D.
Missouri Pharmaceutical Association: George L. Oestreich

Montana

The University of Montana, School of Pharmacy & Allied Health Sciences: David S. Forbes, Ph.D.

Nebraska

Creighton University, School of Medicine: Michael C. Makoid, Ph.D.
Creighton University School of Pharmacy and Allied Health Professions: Kenneth R. Keefner, Ph.D.
University of Nebraska, College of Medicine: Manuchair Ebadi, Ph.D.
University of Nebraska, College of Pharmacy: Clarence T. Ueda, Pharm.D., Ph.D.
Nebraska Pharmacists Association: Rex C. Higley, R.P.

Nevada

Nevada Pharmacists Association: Steven P. Bradford

New Hampshire

Dartmouth Medical School: James J. Kresel, Ph.D.
New Hampshire Pharmaceutical Association: William J. Lancaster, P.D.

New Jersey

University of Medicine and Dentistry of New Jersey, New Jersey Medical School: Sheldon B. Gertner, Ph.D.
Rutgers, The State University of New Jersey, College of Pharmacy: John L. Colaizzi, Ph.D.
Medical Society of New Jersey: Joseph N. Micale, M.D.
New Jersey Pharmaceutical Association: Stephen J. Csubak, Ph.D.

New Mexico

University of New Mexico, College of Pharmacy: William M. Hadley, Ph.D.
New Mexico Pharmaceutical Association: Hugh Kabat, Ph.D.

New York

Albert Einstein College of Medicine of Yeshiva University: Walter G. Levine, Ph.D.
City University of New York, Mt. Sinai School of Medicine: Joel S. Mindel, M.D., Ph.D.
Columbia University College of Physicians and Surgeons: Michael R. Rosen, M.D.
Cornell University Medical College: Lorraine J. Gudas, Ph.D.
Long Island University, Arnold and Marie Schwartz College of Pharmacy and Health Sciences: Jack M. Rosenberg, Ph.D.
New York Medical College: Mario A. Inchiosa, Jr., Ph.D.
New York University School of Medicine: Norman Altzuler, Ph.D.
State University of New York, Buffalo, School of Medicine: Robert J. McIsaac, Ph.D.
State University of New York, Buffalo, School of Pharmacy: Robert M. Cooper
State University of New York, Health Science Center, Syracuse: Oliver M. Brown, Ph.D.
St. John's University, College of Pharmacy and Allied Health Professions: Albert A. Belmonte, Ph.D.
Union University, Albany College of Pharmacy: David W. Newton, Ph.D.
University of Rochester, School of Medicine and Dentistry: Michael Weintraub, M.D., Ph.D.
Medical Society of the State of New York: Richard S. Blum, M.D.
Pharmaceutical Society of the State of New York: Bruce Moden

North Carolina

Bowman Gray School of Medicine, Wake Forest University: Jack W. Strandhoy, Ph.D.
Campbell University, School of Pharmacy: Antoine Al-Achi, Ph.D.
Duke University Medical Center: William J. Murray, M.D., Ph.D.
East Carolina University, School of Medicine: A-R.A. Abdel-Rahman, Ph.D.
University of North Carolina, Chapel Hill, School of Medicine: George Hatfield, Ph.D.
University of North Carolina, Chapel Hill, School of Pharmacy: Richard J. Kowalsky, Pharm.D.
North Carolina Pharmaceutical Association: George H. Cocolas, Ph.D.
North Carolina Medical Society: T. Reginald Harris, M.D.

North Dakota

University of North Dakota, School of Medicine: David W. Hein, Ph.D.
North Dakota State University, College of Pharmacy: William M. Henderson, Ph.D.
North Dakota Medical Association: Vernon E. Wagner
North Dakota Pharmaceutical Association: William H. Shelver, Ph.D.

Ohio

Case Western Reserve University, School of Medicine: Kenneth A. Scott, Ph.D.
Medical College of Ohio at Toledo: R. Douglas Wilkerson, Ph.D.
Northeastern Ohio University, College of Medicine: Ralph E. Berggren, M.D.
Ohio Northern University, College of Pharmacy: Joseph Theodore, Ph.D.
Ohio State University, College of Medicine: Robert Guthrie, M.D.
Ohio State University, College of Pharmacy: Michael C. Gerald, Ph.D.
University of Cincinnati, College of Medicine: Leonard T. Sigell, Ph.D.
University of Cincinnati, College of Pharmacy: Henry S.I. Tan, Ph.D.
University of Toledo, College of Pharmacy: Norman F. Billups, Ph.D.
Wright State University, School of Medicine: John O. Lindower, M.D., Ph.D.
Ohio State Medical Association: Janet K. Bixel, M.D.
Ohio State Pharmaceutical Association: J. Richard Wuest, Pharm.D.

Oklahoma

University of Oklahoma College of Medicine: Ronald D. Brown, M.D.
Southwestern Oklahoma State University, School of Pharmacy: W. Steven Pray, Ph.D.
University of Oklahoma, College of Pharmacy: Loyd V. Allen, Jr., Ph.D.
Oklahoma State Medical Association: Clinton Nicholas Corder, M.D., Ph.D.
Oklahoma Pharmaceutical Association: Carl D. Lyons

Oregon

Oregon Health Sciences University, School of Medicine: Hall Downes, M.D., Ph.D.
Oregon State University, College of Pharmacy: Randall L. Vanderveen, Ph.D.

Pennsylvania

Duquesne University, School of Pharmacy: Lawrence H. Block, Ph.D.
Hahnemann University, School of Medicine: Vincent J. Zarro, M.D., Ph.D.
Medical College of Pennsylvania: Athole G. McNeil Jacobi, M.D.
Pennsylvania State University, College of Medicine: John D. Connor, Ph.D.
Philadelphia College of Pharmacy and Science: Alfonso R. Gennaro, Ph.D.
Temple University, School of Medicine: Ronald J. Tallarida, Ph.D.
Temple University, School of Pharmacy: Murray Tuckerman, Ph.D.
University of Pennsylvania, School of Medicine: Marilyn E. Hess, Ph.D.
University of Pittsburgh, School of Pharmacy: Terrence L. Schwinghammer, Pharm.D.
Pennsylvania Medical Society: Benjamin Calesnick, M.D.
Pennsylvania Pharmaceutical Association: Joseph A. Mosso, R.Ph.

Puerto Rico
Universidad Central del Caribe, School of Medicine: Jesús Santos-Martínez, Ph.D.
University of Puerto Rico, College of Pharmacy: Benjamin P. de Gracia, Ph.D.
University of Puerto Rico, School of Medicine: Walmor C. De Mello, M.D., Ph.D.

Rhode Island
Brown University Program in Medicine: Darrell R. Abernethy, M.D., Ph.D.
University of Rhode Island, College of Pharmacy: Thomas E. Needham, Ph.D.

South Carolina
Medical University of South Carolina, College of Medicine: Herman B. Daniell, Ph.D.
Medical University of South Carolina, College of Pharmacy: Paul J. Niebergall, Ph.D.
University of South Carolina, College of Pharmacy: Robert L. Beamer, Ph.D.

South Dakota
South Dakota State University, College of Pharmacy: Gary S. Chappell, Ph.D.
South Dakota State Medical Association: Robert D. Johnson
South Dakota Pharmaceutical Association: James Powers

Tennessee
East Tennessee State University, Quillen College of Medicine: Ernest A. Daigneault, Ph.D.
Meharry Medical College, School of Medicine: Dolores C. Shockley, Ph.D.
University of Tennessee, College of Medicine: Murray Heimberg, M.D., Ph.D.
University of Tennessee, College of Pharmacy: Dick R. Gourley, Pharm.D.
Vanderbilt University, School of Medicine: David H. Robertson, M.D.
Tennessee Pharmacists Association: Roger L. Davis, Pharm.D.

Texas
Texas A & M University, College of Medicine: Marsha A. Raebel, Pharm.D.
Texas Southern University, College of Pharmacy and Health Sciences: Eugene Hickman, Ph.D.
University of Houston, College of Pharmacy: Mustafa Lokhandwala, Ph.D.
University of Texas, Austin, College of Pharmacy: James T. Doluisio, Ph.D.
University of Texas, Medical Branch at Galveston: George T. Bryan, M.D.
University of Texas Medical School, Houston: Jacques E. Chelly, M.D., Ph.D.
University of Texas Medical School, San Antonio: Alexander M.M. Shepherd, M.D., Ph.D.
Texas Medical Association: Robert H. Barr, M.D.
Texas Pharmaceutical Association: Shirley McKee, R.Ph.

Utah
University of Utah, College of Pharmacy: David B. Roll, Ph.D.
Utah Pharmaceutical Association: Robert V. Peterson, Ph.D.
Utah Medical Association: David A. Hilding, M.D.

Vermont
University of Vermont, College of Medicine: John J. McCormack, Ph.D.
Vermont Pharmacists Association: Frederick Dobson

Virginia
Medical College of Hampton Roads: William J. Cooke, Ph.D.
Medical College of Virginia/Virginia Commonwealth University, School of Pharmacy: William H. Barr, Pharm.D., Ph.D.
Medical Society of Virginia: Richard W. Lindsay, M.D.
University of Virginia, School of Medicine: Peyton E. Weary, M.D.
Virginia Pharmaceutical Association: Daniel A. Herbert

Washington
Unversity of Washington, School of Pharmacy: Wendel L. Nelson, Ph.D.
Washington State University, College of Pharmacy: Martin J. Jinks, Pharm.D.
Washington State Pharmacists Association: Danial E. Baker

West Virginia
Marshall University, School of Medicine: John L. Szarek, Ph.D.
West Virginia University, School of Medicine: Douglas D. Glover, M.D.
West Virginia University Medical Center, School of Pharmacy: Arthur I. Jacknowitz, Pharm.D.

Wisconsin
Medical College of Wisconsin: Garrett J. Gross, Ph.D.
University of Wisconsin, Madison, School of Pharmacy: Chester A. Bond, Pharm.D.
University of Wisconsin Medical School, Madison: Joseph M. Benforado, M.D.
State Medical Society of Wisconsin: Thomas L. Adams, CAE
Wisconsin Pharmacists Association: Dennis Dziczkowski, R.Ph.

Wyoming
University of Wyoming, School of Pharmacy: Kenneth F. Nelson, Ph.D.
Wyoming Medical Society: R. W. Johnson, Jr.
Wyoming Pharmaceutical Association: Linda G. Sutherland

Members-at-Large

Norman W. Atwater, Ph.D., Hopewell, NJ
Cheston M. Berlin, Jr., M.D., The Milton S. Hershey Medical Center
Fred S. Brinkley, Jr., Texas State Board of Pharmacy
Herbert S. Carlin, D.Sc., Califon, NJ
Jordan Cohen, Ph.D., College of Pharmacy, University of Kentucky
John L. Cova, Ph.D., Health Insurance Association of America
Enrique Fefer, Ph.D., Pan American Health Organization
Leroy Fevang, Canadian Pharmaceutical Association
Klaus G. Florey, Ph.D., Princeton, NJ
Lester Hosto, Ph.D., Arkansas State Board of Pharmacy
Jay S. Keystone, M.D., Toronto General Hospital
Calvin M. Kunin, M.D., Ohio State University
Marvin Lipman, M.D., Scarsdale, NY
Joseph A. Mollica, Ph.D., Montcharin, DE
Stuart L. Nightingale, M.D., Food and Drug Administration
Daniel A. Nona, Ph.D., The American Council on Pharmaceutical Education
Mark Novitch, M.D., Kalamazoo, MI
Charles A. Pergola, SmithKline Beecham Consumer Brands
Donald O. Schiffman, Ph.D., Genealogy Unlimited
Carl E. Trinca, Ph.D., American Association of Colleges of Pharmacy

Members-at-Large (representing other countries that provide legal status to *USP* or *NF*)

Prof. T. D. Arias, Estafeta Universitaria, Panama, Republica De Panama
Keith Bailey, Ph.D., Canadian Bureau of Drug Research
Quintin L. Kintanar, M.D., Ph.D., Department of Health, Metro Manila, Philippines
Marcelo Jorge Vernego, Ph.D., Buenos Aires, Argentina

Members-at-Large (Public)

Clement Bezold, Ph.D., Alternative Futures Association
Alexander Grant, Food and Drug Administration
Grace Powers Monaco, J.D., Washington, DC
Paul G. Rogers, National Council on Patient Information and Education
Frances M. West, J.D., Wilmington, DE

I

Ex-Officio Members

Joseph M. Benforado, M.D., Madison, WI
Joseph P. Buckley, Ph.D., Houston, TX
Estelle G. Cohen, M.A., Baltimore, MD
Leo E. Hollister, M.D., Houston, TX
Paul F. Parker, D.Sc., Lexington, KY

Committee Chairmen

Credentials Committee: Peyton E. Weary, M.D.
Nominating Committee for the General Committee of Revision: Walter L. Way, M.D.
Nominating Committee for Officers and Trustees: Joseph M. Benforado, M.D.
Resolutions Committee: J. Richard Crout, M.D.
General Committee of Revision: Jerome A. Halperin
Constitution and Bylaws Committee: John V. Bergen, Ph.D.

Honorary Members

George F. Archambault, Pharm.D., J.D., Bethesda, MD
William J. Kinnard, Jr., Ph.D., Baltimore, MD
Lloyd C. Miller, Ph.D., Escondido, CA
John H. Moyer, M.D., D.Sc., Palmyra, PA
John A. Owen, Jr., M.D., Charlottesville, VA
Harry C. Shirkey, M.D., Cincinnati, OH
Linwood F. Tice, D.Sc., Philadelphia, PA

Section I

USP DI Volume III Reproduction of

FDA'S APPROVED DRUG PRODUCTS WITH THERAPEUTIC EQUIVALENCE EVALUATIONS

14th EDITION,
incorporating supplements issued
through August 31, 1994

The products in this list have been approved under sections 505 and 507 of the Federal Food, Drug, and Cosmetic Act. This information is current through August 31, 1994. Later Supplements to the FDA's "Orange Book" are provided in the monthly *USP DI Update.*

FOOD AND DRUG ADMINISTRATION
CENTER FOR DRUG EVALUATION AND RESEARCH
APPROVED DRUG PRODUCTS
with
Therapeutic Equivalence Evaluations

CONTENTS

FOOD AND DRUG ADMINISTRATION
CENTER FOR DRUG EVALUATION AND RESEARCH
APPROVED DRUG PRODUCTS
with
Therapeutic Equivalence Evaluations

PREFACE TO FOURTEENTH EDITION

The publication, *Approved Drug Products with Therapeutic Equivalence Evaluations* (the List) identifies drug products approved on the basis of safety and effectiveness by the Food and Drug Administration (FDA) under the Federal Food, Drug, and Cosmetic Act (the Act). Drugs on the market approved only on the basis of safety (covered by the ongoing Drug Efficacy Study Implementation [DESI] review [e.g., Donnatal® Tablets and Librax® Capsules] or products not subject to enforcement action as unapproved drugs or pre-1938 drugs [e.g., Synthroid® Tablets]) are not included in this publication. The main criterion for the inclusion of any product is that the product is the subject of an application with an effective approval that has not been withdrawn for safety or efficacy reasons. Inclusion of products on the List is independent of any current regulatory action through administrative or judicial means against a drug product. In addition, the List contains therapeutic equivalence evaluations for approved multisource prescription drug products. These evaluations have been prepared to serve as public information and advice to state health agencies, prescribers, and pharmacists to promote public education in the area of drug product selection and to foster containment of health costs. Therapeutic equivalence evaluations in this publication are not official FDA actions affecting the legal status of products under the Act.

Background of the Publication. To contain drug costs, virtually every state has adopted laws and/or regulations that encourage the substitution of drug products. These state laws generally require either that substitution be limited to drugs on a specific list (the positive formulary approach) or that it be permitted for all drugs except those prohibited by a particular list (the negative formulary approach). Because of the number of requests in the late 1970s for FDA assistance in preparing both positive and negative formularies, it became apparent that FDA could not serve the needs of each state on an individual basis. The Agency also recognized that providing a single list based on common criteria would be preferable to evaluating drug products on the basis of differing definitions and criteria in various state laws. As a result, on May 31, 1978, the Commissioner of Food and Drugs sent a letter to officials of each state stating FDA's intent to provide a list of all prescription drug products that are approved by FDA for safety and effectiveness, along with therapeutic equivalence determinations for multisource prescription products.

The List was distributed as a proposal in January 1979. It included only currently marketed prescription drug products approved by FDA through new drug applications (NDAs), abbreviated new drug applications (ANDAs), or abbreviated antibiotic applications (AADAs) under the provisions of Section 505 or 507 of the Act.

The therapeutic equivalence evaluations in the List reflect FDA's application of specific criteria to the approved multisource prescription drug products on the List. These evaluations are presented in the form of code letters that indicate the basis for the evaluation made. An explanation of the code appears in the *Introduction.*

A complete discussion of the background and basis of FDA's therapeutic equivalence evaluation policy was published in the *Federal Register* on January 12, 1979 (44 FR 2932). The final rule, which includes FDA's responses to the public comments on the proposal, was published in the *Federal Register* on October 31, 1980 (45 FR 72582). The first publication, October 1980, of the final version of the List incorporated appropriate corrections and additions. Each subsequent edition has included the new approvals and made appropriate changes in data.

On September 24, 1984, the President signed into law the Drug Price Competition and Patent Term Restoration Act (1984 Amendments). The 1984 Amendments require that FDA, among other things, make publicly available a list of approved drug products with monthly supplements. The *Approved Drug Products with Therapeutic Equivalence Evaluations* publication and its monthly Cumulative Supplements satisfy this requirement. The Addendum to this publication identifies drugs that qualify under the 1984 Amendments for periods of exclusivity (during which ANDAs or applications described in Section 505(b)(2) of the Act for those drugs may not be submitted for a specified period of time and if allowed to be submitted would be tentatively approved with a delayed effective date) and provides patent information concerning the listed drugs which also may delay the approval of ANDAs or Section 505(b)(2) applications. The Addendum also provides additional information that may be helpful to those submitting a new drug application to the Agency.

The Agency intends to use this publication to further its objective of obtaining input and comment on the publication itself and related Agency procedures. Therefore, if you have comments on how the publication can be improved, please send them to the Director, Division of Drug Information Resources, Office of Management, Center for Drug Evaluation and Research, HFD-80, 5600 Fishers Lane, Rockville, MD 20857. Comments received are publicly available to the extent allowable under the Freedom of Information regulations.

1. INTRODUCTION

1.1 Content and Exclusion

The List is composed of four parts: (1) approved prescription drug products with therapeutic equivalence evaluations; (2) approved over-the-counter (OTC) drug products for those drugs that may not be marketed without NDAs and ANDAs because they are not covered under the existing OTC monographs; (3) drug products with approval under Section 505 of the Act administered by the Center for Biologics Evaluation and Research; and (4) cumulative list of products that have never been marketed, have been discontinued from marketing or that have had their approvals withdrawn for other than safety or efficacy reasons. This publication also includes indices of prescription and OTC drug products by trade or established name (if no trade name exists) and by applicant name (holder of the approved application). All established names for active ingredients conform to official compendial names or *United States Adopted Names* (USAN) as prescribed in 21 CFR 299.4 (e). The latter list includes applicants' names as abbreviated in this publication; in addition, a list of uniform terms is provided. An Addendum contains drug patent and exclusivity information for the Prescription and OTC Drug Product Lists, and for the Drug Products with Approval under Section 505 of the Act Administered by the Center for Biologics Evaluation and Research.

Prior to the 6th Edition, the publication had excluded OTC drug products and drug products with approval under Section 505 of the Act administered by the Center for Biologics Evaluation and Research, because the main purpose of the publication was to provide information to states regarding FDA's recommendation as to which generic prescription drug products were acceptable candidates for drug product selection. The 1984 Amendments require the Agency to publish an up-to-date list of all marketed drug products, OTC as well as prescription, that have been approved for safety and efficacy and for which new drug applications are required. In general, OTC drug products may be marketed without approved applications if they meet existing OTC drug monographs. The products included in the OTC Drug Product List are limited to those for which approved applications are currently required as a condition of marketing.

Under the 1984 Amendments, some drug products are given tentative approvals with delayed effective dates. Prior to the effective date, the Agency will not represent the drug products with tentative approval in the List; however, they are published in the *FDA Drug and Device Product Approvals* monthly publication. To obtain this publication, see Section 1.12, *Availability of the Publication and Other FDA Reports and Updating Procedures*. When the tentative approval becomes a full approval through a subsequent letter to the applicant holder, the Agency will list the drug product and the final, effective approval date in the appropriate approved drug product list.

Distributors or repackagers of the products on the List are not identified. Because distributors or repackagers are not required to notify FDA when they shift their sources of supply from one approved manufacturer to another, it is not possible to maintain complete information linking the product approval with the distributor or repackager handling the products.

1.2 Therapeutic Equivalence-Related Terms

Pharmaceutical Equivalents. Drug products are considered pharmaceutical equivalents if they contain the same active ingredient(s), are of the same dosage form and are identical in strength or concentration, and route of administration (e.g., chlordiazepoxide hydrochloride, 5mg capsules). Pharmaceutically equivalent drug products are formulated to contain the same amount of active ingredient in the same dosage form and to meet the same or compendial or other applicable standards (i.e., strength, quality, purity, and identity), but they may differ in characteristics such as shape, scoring configuration, packaging, excipients (including colors, flavors, preservatives), expiration time, and, within certain limits, labeling.

Pharmaceutical Alternatives. Drug products are considered pharmaceutical alternatives if they contain the same therapeutic moiety, but are different salts, esters, or complexes of that moiety, or are different dosage forms or strengths (e.g., tetracycline hydrochloride, 250 mg capsules vs. tetracycline phosphate complex, 250 mg capsules; quinidine sulfate, 200 mg tablets vs. quinidine sulfate, 200 mg capsules). Data are generally not available for FDA to make the determination of tablet to capsule bioequivalence. Different dosage forms and strengths within a product line by a single manufacturer are thus pharmaceutical alternatives, as are extended-release products when compared with immediate- or standard-release formulations of the same active ingredient.

Therapeutic Equivalents. Drug products are considered to be therapeutic equivalents only if they are pharmaceutical equivalents and if they can be expected to have the same clinical effect and safety profile when administered to patients under the conditions specified in the labeling.

FDA classifies as therapeutically equivalent those products that meet the following general criteria: (1) they are approved as safe and effective; (2) they are pharmaceutical equivalents in that they (a) contain identical amounts of the same active drug ingredient in the same dosage form and route of administration, and (b) meet compendial or other applicable standards of strength, quality, purity, and identity; (3) they are bioequivalent in that (a) they do not present a known or potential bioequivalence problem, and they meet an acceptable *in vitro* standard, or (b) if they do present such a known or potential problem, they are shown to meet an appropriate bioequivalence standard; (4) they are adequately labeled; and (5) they are manufactured in compliance with Current Good Manufacturing Practice regulations. *The concept of therapeutic equivalence, as used to develop the List, applies only to drug products containing the same active ingredient(s) and does not encompass a comparison of different therapeutic agents used for the same condition (e.g., propoxyphene hydrochloride vs. pentazocine hydrochloride for the treatment of pain).* A single source drug product in the List repackaged and/or distributed by other than the applicant holder is considered to be therapeutically equivalent to the single source drug product. Also, distributors or repackagers of an application holder's drug product are considered to have the same code as the application holder.

FDA considers drug products to be therapeutically equivalent if they meet the criteria outlined above, even though they may differ in certain other characteristics such as shape, scoring configuration, packaging, excipients (including colors, flavors, preservatives), expiration time and minor aspects of labeling (e.g., the presence of specific pharmacokinetic information). When such differences are important in the care of a particular patient, it may be appropriate for the prescribing physician to require that a particular brand be dispensed as a medical necessity. With this limitation, however, FDA believes that products classified as therapeutically equivalent can be substituted with the full expectation that the substituted product will produce the same clinical effect and safety profile as the prescribed product.

Bioavailability. This term means the rate and extent to which the active ingredient or active moiety is absorbed from a drug product and becomes available at the site of action. For drug products that are not intended to be absorbed into the bloodstream, bioavailability may be assessed by measurements intended to reflect the rate and extent to which the active ingredient or active moiety becomes available at the site of action.

Bioequivalent Drug Products. This term describes pharmaceutically equivalent products that display comparable bioavailability when studied under similar experimental conditions. Section 505 (j)(7)(B) of the Act describes one set of conditions under which a test and reference listed drug, see Section 1.4, shall be considered bioequivalent:

> the rate and extent of absorption of the test drug do not show a significant difference from the rate and extent of absorption of the reference drug when administered at the same molar dose of the therapeutic ingredient under similar experimental conditions in either a single dose or multiple doses; or
>
> the extent of absorption of the test drug does not show a significant difference from the extent of absorption of the reference drug when administered at the same molar dose of the therapeutic ingredient under similar experimental conditions in either a single dose or multiple doses and the difference from the reference drug in the rate of absorption of the drug is intentional, is reflected in its proposed labeling, is not essential to the attainment of effective body drug concentrations on chronic use, and is considered medically insignificant for the drug.

Where these above methods are not applicable (e.g., for topically applied products intended for local rather than systemic effect), other *in vivo* tests of bioequivalence may be appropriate.

Bioequivalence may sometimes be demonstrated using an *in vitro* bioequivalence standard, especially when such an *in vitro* test has been correlated with human *in vivo* bioavailability data or in other situations through comparative clinical trials or pharmacodynamic studies.

1.3 Statistical Criteria for Bioequivalence

Under the Drug Price Competition and Patent Term Restoration Act of 1984, manufacturers seeking approval to market a generic drug must submit data demonstrating that the drug product is bioequivalent to the pioneer (innovator) drug product. A major premise underlying the 1984 law is that bioequivalent products are therapeutically equivalent and, therefore, interchangeable.

The standard bioequivalence study is conducted in a crossover fashion in a small number of volunteers, usually with 12 to 24 healthy normal male adults. Single doses of the test and reference drugs are administered and blood or plasma levels of the drug are measured over time. Characteristics of these concentration-time curves, such as the area under the curve (AUC) and the peak blood or plasma concentration (C_{max}), are examined by statistical procedures.

Bioequivalence of different formulations of the same drug substance involves equivalence with respect to the rate and extent of drug absorption. Two formulations whose rate and extent of absorption differ by −20%/+25% or less are generally considered bioequivalent. The use of the −20%/+25% rule is based on a medical decision that, for most drugs, a −20%/+25% difference in the concentration of the active ingredient in blood will not be clinically significant.

In order to verify, for a particular pharmacokinetic parameter, that the −20%/+25% rule is satisfied, two one-sided statistical tests are carried out using the log transformed data from the bioequivalence study. One test is used to verify that the average response for the generic product is no more than 20% below that for the innovator product; the other test is used to verify that the average response for the generic product is no more than 25%

above that for the innovator product. The current practice is to carry out the two one-sided tests at the 0.05 level of significance.

Computationally the two one-sided tests are carried out by computing a 90% confidence interval. For approval of ANDAs, in most cases, the generic manufacturer must show that a 90% confidence interval for the ratio of the mean response (usually AUC and C_{max}) of its product to that of the innovator is within the limits of 0.8 and 1.25, using the log transformed data. If the true average response of the generic product in the population is near 20% below or 25% above the innovator average, one or both of the confidence limits is likely to fall outside the acceptable range and the product will fail the bioequivalence test. Thus, an approved product is likely to differ from that of the innovator by far less than this quantity.

The current practice of carrying out two one-sided tests at the 0.05 level of significance ensures that if the two products truly differ by as much or more than is allowed by the equivalence criteria (usually −20%/+25% of the innovator product average for the bioequivalence parameter, such as AUC or C_{max}) there is no more than a 5% chance that they will be approved as equivalent. This reflects the fact that the primary concern from the regulatory point of view is the protection of the patient against acceptance of bioequivalence if it does not hold true. The results of a bioequivalence study must usually be acceptable for more than one pharmacokinetic parameter. As such, a generic product that truly differs by −20%/+25% or more from the innovator product with respect to one or more pharmacokinetic parameters, would actually have less than a 5% chance of being approved.

1.4 Reference Listed Drug

A reference listed drug means the listed drug identified by FDA as the drug product upon which an applicant relies in seeking approval of its ANDA.

FDA has identified in the Prescription Drug Product List those reference listed drugs to which the *in vivo* bioequivalence, and in some instances the *in vitro* bioequivalence, of the applicant's product is compared. By designating a single reference listed drug against which all generic versions must be shown to be bioequivalent, FDA hopes to avoid possible significant variations among generic drugs and their brand name counterpart. Such variations could result if generic drugs were compared to different reference listed drugs. The reference listed drug is identified by the symbol "+" in the Prescription Drug Product List. These identified reference listed drugs represent the best judgment of the Division of Bioequivalence at this time. The Prescription Drug Product List identifies reference drugs for primarily solid oral dosage forms, injectables, ophthalmics, otics, and topical products. It is recommended that a firm planning to conduct an *in vivo* bioequivalence study, or planning to manufacture a batch of drug product for which *in vivo* waiver of bioequivalence will be requested, contact the Division of Bioequivalence to confirm the appropriate referenced drug.

1.5 General Policies and Legal Status

The List contains public information and advice. It does not mandate the drug products which may be purchased, prescribed, dispensed, or substituted for one another nor does it, conversely, mandate the products that should be avoided. To the extent that the List sets forth FDA's evaluations of the therapeutic equivalence of drug products that have been approved, it contains FDA's advice to the public, to practitioners, and to the states regarding drug product selection. These evaluations do not constitute determinations that any product is in violation of the Act or that any product is preferable to any other. Therapeutic equivalence evaluations are a scientific judgment based upon evidence, while generic substitution may involve social and economic policy administered by the states, intended to reduce the cost of drugs to consumers. To the extent that the List identifies drug products approved under Section 505 or 507 of the Act, it sets forth information that the Agency is required to publish and that the public is entitled to under the Freedom of Information Act. Exclusion of a drug product from the List does not necessarily mean that the drug product is either in violation of Section 505 or 507 of the Act, or that such a product is not safe or effective, or that such a product is not therapeutically equivalent to other drug products. Rather, the exclusion is based on the fact that FDA has not evaluated the safety, effectiveness, and quality of the drug product.

1.6 Practitioner/User Responsibilities

Professional care and judgment should be exercised in using the List. Evaluations of therapeutic equivalence for prescription drugs are based on scientific and medical evaluations by FDA. Products evaluated as therapeutically equivalent can be expected, in the judgment of the FDA, to have equivalent clinical effect and no difference in their potential for adverse effects when used under the conditions of their labeling. However, these products may differ in other characteristics such as shape, scoring configuration, packaging, excipients (including colors, flavors, preservatives), expiration time, and, in some instances, labeling. If products with such differences are substituted for each other, there is a potential for patient confusion due to differences in color or shape of tablets, inability to provide a given dose using a partial tablet if the proper scoring configuration is not available, or decreased patient acceptance of certain products because of flavor. There may also be better stability of one product over another under adverse storage conditions, or allergic reactions in rare cases due to a coloring or a preservative ingredient, as well as differences in cost to the patient.

FDA evaluation of therapeutic equivalence in no way relieves practitioners of their professional responsibilities in prescribing and dispensing such products with due care and with appropriate information to individual patients. In those circumstances where the characteristics of a specific product, other than its active ingredient, are important in the therapy of a particular patient, the physician's specification of that product is appropriate. Pharmacists must also be familiar with the expiration dates and labeling directions for storage of the different products, particularly for reconstituted products, to assure that patients are properly advised when one product is substituted for another.

Multisource and single-source drug products. FDA has evaluated for therapeutic equivalence only multisource prescription drug products, which in virtually all instances means those pharmaceutical equivalents available from more than one manufacturer. For such products, a therapeutic equivalence code is included and, in addition, product information is highlighted in bold face and underlined. Those products with approved applications that are single source (i.e., there is only one approved product available for that active ingredient, dosage form, and route of administration) are also included on the List, but no therapeutic equivalence code is included with such products. However, a single source drug product repackaged and/or distributed by other than the application holder is considered therapeutically equivalent to the single source drug product. Also, distributors or repackagers of an application holder's drug product are considered to have the same code as the application holder. The details of these codes and the policies underlying them are discussed in Section 1.7, *Therapeutic Equivalence Evaluations Codes.*

Products on the List are identified by the names of the holders of approved applications (applicants) who may not necessarily be the manufacturer of the product. The applicant may have had its product manufactured by a contract manufacturer and may simply be distributing the product for which it has obtained approval. In most instances, however, the manufacturer of the product is also the applicant. The name of the manufacturer is permitted by regulation to appear on the label, even when the manufacturer is not the marketer.

Although the products on the List are identified by the names of the applicants, circumstances, such as changing corporate ownership, have sometimes made identification of the applicant difficult. The Agency believes, based on continuing document review and communication with firms, that the applicant designations on the List are, in most cases, correct.

To relate firm name information on a product label to that on the List, the following should be noted: the applicant's name always appears on the List. This applies whether the applicant (firm name on the Form FDA 356h in the application) is the marketer (firm name in largest letters on the label) or not. However, the applicant's name may not always appear on the label of the product.

If the applicant is the marketer, its name appears on the List and on the label; if the applicant is not the marketer, and the Agency is aware of a corporate relationship (e.g., parent and subsidiary) between the applicant and the marketer, the name of the applicant appears on the List and both firm names may appear on the label. Firms with known corporate relationships are displayed in Appendix B. If there is no known corporate relationship between the applicant and the marketer, the applicant's name appears on the List; however, unless the applicant is the manufacturer, packager, or distributor, the applicant's name may not appear on the label. In this case, the practitioner, from labeling alone, will not be able to relate the marketed product to an applicant cited in the List, and hence to a specific approved drug product. In such cases, other references should be used to assure that the product in question is the subject of an approved application.

To relate trade name (proprietary name) information on a product label to that on the List, the following should be noted: if the applicant is the marketer, its name appears on the List and on the label; if the Agency is aware of a corporate relationship between the applicant and the marketer, the trade name (proprietary name) of the drug product (established drug name if no trade name exists) appears on the List. If a corporate relationship exists between an application holder and a marketer and both firms are distributing the drug product, the FDA reserves the right to select the trade name of either the marketer or the application holder to appear on the List. If there is no known corporate relationship between the applicant and the marketer, the established drug name appears on the List.

Every product on the List is subject at all times to regulatory action. From time to time, approved products may be found in violation of one or more provisions of the Act. In such circumstances, the Agency will commence appropriate enforcement action to correct the violation, if necessary, by securing removal of the product from the market by voluntary recall, seizure, or other enforcement actions. Such regulatory actions are, however, independent of the inclusion of a product on the List. The main criterion for inclusion of a product is that it has an application with an effective approval that has not been withdrawn for safety or efficacy reasons. FDA believes that retention of a violative product on the List will not have any significant adverse health consequences, because other legal mechanisms are available to the Agency to prevent the product's actual marketing. FDA may, however, change a product's therapeutic equivalence rating if the circumstances giving rise to the violation change or otherwise call into question the data upon which the Agency's assessment of whether a product meets the criteria for therapeutic equivalence was made.

1.7 Therapeutic Equivalence Evaluations Codes

The two-letter coding system for therapeutic equivalence evaluations is constructed to allow users to determine quickly whether the Agency has evaluated a particular approved product as therapeutically equivalent to other pharmaceutically equivalent products (first letter) and to provide additional information on the basis of FDA's evaluations (second letter). With few exceptions, the therapeutic equivalence evaluation date is the same as the approval date.

The two basic categories into which multisource drugs have been placed are indicated by the first letter as follows:

A—Drug products that FDA considers to be therapeutically equivalent to other pharmaceutically equivalent products, i.e., drug products for which:

(1) there are no known or suspected bioequivalence problems. These are designated **AA, AN, AO, AP,** or **AT,** depending on the dosage form; or

(2) actual or potential bioequivalence problems have been resolved with adequate *in vivo* and/or *in vitro* evidence supporting bioequivalence. These are designated **AB.**

B—Drug products that FDA at this time considers not to be therapeutically equivalent to other pharmaceutically equivalent products, i.e.,

drug products for which actual or potential bioequivalence problems have not been resolved by adequate evidence of bioequivalence. Often the problem is with specific dosage forms rather than with the active ingredients. These are designated **BC, BD, BE, BN, BP, BR, BS, BT, BX,** or **B*.**

Individual drug products have been evaluated as therapeutically equivalent to the reference product in accordance with the definitions and policies outlined below:

"A" CODES

Drug products that are considered to be therapeutically equivalent to other pharmaceutically equivalent products.

"A" products are those for which actual or potential bioequivalence problems have been resolved with adequate *in vivo* and/or *in vitro* evidence supporting bioequivalence. Drug products designated with an **"A"** code fall under one of two main policies:

(1) for those active ingredients or dosage forms for which no *in vivo* bioequivalence issue is known or suspected, the information necessary to show bioequivalence between pharmaceutically equivalent products is presumed and considered self-evident based on other data in the application for some dosage forms (e.g., solutions) or satisfied for solid oral dosage forms by a showing that an acceptable *in vitro* standard is met. A therapeutically equivalent rating is assigned such products so long as they are manufactured in accordance with Current Good Manufacturing Practice regulations and meet the other requirements of their approved applications (these are designated **AA, AN, AO, AP,** or **AT,** depending on the dosage form, as described below); or

(2) for those DESI drug products containing active ingredients on dosage forms that have been identified by FDA as having actual or potential bioequivalence problems and for post-1962 drug products in a dosage form presenting a potential bioequivalence problem, an evaluation of therapeutic equivalence is assigned to pharmaceutical equivalents only if the approved application contains adequate scientific evidence establishing through *in vivo* and/or *in vitro* studies the bioequivalence of the product to a selected reference product (these products are designated as AB).

There are some general principles that may affect the substitution of pharmaceutically equivalent products in specific cases. Prescribers and dispensers of drugs should be alert to these principles so as to deal appropriately with situations that require professional judgment and discretion.

There may be labeling differences among pharmaceutically equivalent products that require attention on the part of the health professional. For example, pharmaceutically equivalent powders to be reconstituted for administration as oral or injectable liquids may vary with respect to their expiration time or storage conditions after reconstitution. An FDA evaluation that such products are therapeutically equivalent is applicable only when each product is reconstituted, stored, and used under the conditions specified in the labeling of that product.

The Agency will use notes in this publication to point out special situations, such as potential differences between two drug products that have been evaluated as bioequivalent and otherwise therapeutically equivalent, when they should be brought to the attention of health professionals. These notes are contained in Section 1.8, *Description of Special Situations.*

For example, though rare, there may be variations among therapeutically equivalent products in their use or in conditions of administration. Such differences may be due to patent or exclusivity rights associated with such use. When such variations may, in the Agency's opinion, affect prescribing or substitution decisions by health professionals, a note will be added to Section 1.8.

Also, there may occasionally arise a situation in which changes in a listed drug product after its approval (for example, a change in dosing interval) may have an impact on the substitutability of already approved generic versions of that product that were rated by the Agency as therapeutically equivalent to the listed product. When such changes in the listed drug product are considered by the Agency to have a significant impact on therapeutic equivalence, the Agency will change the therapeutic equivalence ratings for other versions of the drug product unless the manufacturers of those other versions of the product provide additional information to assure equivalence under the changed conditions. Pending receipt of the additional data, the Agency may add a note to Section 1.8, or, in rare cases, may even change the therapeutic equivalence rating.

In some cases (e.g., Isolyte® S w/ Dextrose 5% in Plastic Container and Plasma-Lyte® 148 and Dextrose 5% in Plastic Container), closely related products are listed as containing the same active ingredients, but in somewhat different amounts. In determining which of these products are pharmaceutically equivalent, the Agency has considered products to be pharmaceutically equivalent with labeled strengths of an ingredient that do not vary by more than 1%.

Different salts and esters of the same therapeutic moiety are regarded as pharmaceutical alternatives. For the purpose of this publication, such products are not considered to be therapeutically equivalent. There are no instances in this List where pharmaceutical alternatives are evaluated or coded with regard to therapeutic equivalence. Anhydrous and hydrated entities are considered pharmaceutical equivalents and must meet the same standards and, where necessary, as in the case of ampicillin/ampicillin trihydrate, their equivalence is supported by appropriate bioavailability/bioequivalence studies.

The codes in this book are not intended to preclude health care professionals from converting pharmaceutically different concentrations into pharmaceutical equivalents using accepted professional practice.

Where package size variations have therapeutic implications, products so packaged have not been considered pharmaceutically equivalent. For example, some oral contraceptives are supplied in 21-tablet and 28-tablet packets; the 28-tablet packets contain 7 placebo or iron tablets. These two packaging configurations are not regarded as pharmaceutically equivalent; thus, they are not designated as therapeutically equivalent.

Preservatives may differ among some therapeutically equivalent drug products. Differences in preservatives and other inactive ingredients do not affect FDA's evaluation of therapeutic equivalence except in cases where these components may influence bioequivalence or routes of administration.

The specific sub-codes for those drugs evaluated as therapeutically equivalent and the policies underlying these sub-codes follow:

AA

Products in conventional dosage forms not presenting bioequivalence problems

Products coded as **AA** contain active ingredients and dosage forms that are not regarded as presenting either actual or potential bioequivalence problems or drug quality or standards issues. However, all solid oral dosage forms must, nonetheless, meet an appropriate *in vitro* test(s) for approval.

AB

Products meeting necessary bioequivalence requirements

Products generally will be coded **AB** if a study is submitted demonstrating bioequivalence. Even though drug products of distributors and/or repackagers are not included in the List, they are considered therapeutically equivalent to the application holder's drug product if the application holder's drug product is rated **AB** or is single source in the List. The only instance in which a multisource product will be rated **AB** on the basis of bioavailability rather than bioequivalence is where the innovator product is the only one listed under that drug ingredient heading and has completed an acceptable bioavailability study. However, it does not signify that this product is therapeutically equivalent to the other drugs under the same heading. Drugs coded **AB** under an ingredient heading are considered therapeutically equivalent only to other drugs coded **AB** under that heading.

AN

Solutions and powders for aerosolization

Uncertainty regarding the therapeutic equivalence of aerosolized products arises primarily because of differences in the drug delivery system. Solutions and powders intended for aerosolization that are marketed for use in any of several delivery systems are considered to be pharmaceutically and therapeutically equivalent and are coded **AN.** Those products that are compatible only with a specific delivery system or those products that are packaged in and with a specific delivery system are coded **BN,** unless they have met an appropriate bioequivalence standard because drug products in their respective delivery systems are not necessarily pharmaceutically equivalent to each other and, therefore, are not therapeutically equivalent.

AO

Injectable oil solutions

The absorption of drugs in injectable (parenteral) oil solutions may vary substantially with the type of oil employed as a vehicle and the concentration of the active ingredient. Injectable oil solutions are therefore considered to be pharmaceutically and therapeutically equivalent only when the active ingredient, its concentration, and the type of oil used as a vehicle are all identical.

AP

Injectable aqueous solutions

It should be noted that even though injectable (parenteral) products under a specific listing may be evaluated as therapeutically equivalent, there may be important differences among the products in the general category, *Injectable; Injection.* For example, some injectable products that are rated therapeutically equivalent are labeled for different routes of administration. In addition, some products evaluated as therapeutically equivalent may have different preservatives or no preservatives at all. Injectable products available as dry powders for reconstitution, concentrated sterile solutions for dilution, or sterile solutions ready for injection are all considered to be pharmaceutically and therapeutically equivalent provided they are designed to produce the same concentration prior to injection and are similarly labeled. Consistent with accepted professional practice, it is the responsibility of the prescriber, dispenser, or individual administering the product to be familiar with a product's labeling to assure that it is given only by the route(s) of administration stated in the labeling.

Certain commonly used large volume intravenous products in glass containers are not included on the List (e.g., dextrose injection 5%, dextrose injection 10%, sodium chloride injection 0.9%) since these products are on the market without FDA approval and the FDA has not published conditions for marketing such parenteral products under approved NDAs. When packaged in plastic containers, however, FDA regulations require approved applications prior to marketing. Approval then depends on, among other things, the extent of the available safety data involving the specific plastic component of the product. All large volume parenteral products are manufactured under similar standards, regardless of whether they are packaged in glass or plastic. Thus, FDA has no reason to believe that the packaging container of large volume parenteral drug products that are pharmaceutically equivalent would have any effect on their therapeutic equivalence.

AT

Topical products

There are a variety of topical dosage forms available for dermatologic, ophthalmic, otic, rectal, and vaginal administration, including solutions, creams, ointments, gels, lotions, pastes, sprays, and suppositories. Even though different topical dosage forms may contain the same active ingredient and potency, these dosage forms are not considered pharmaceutically equivalent. Therefore, they are not considered therapeutically equivalent. All solutions and DESI drug products containing the same active ingredient in the same topical dosage form for which a waiver of *in vivo* bioequivalence has been granted and for which chemistry and manufacturing processes are adequate are considered therapeutically equivalent and coded **AT.** Pharmaceutically equivalent topical products that raise questions of bioequivalence, including all post-1962 topical drug products, are coded **AB** when supported by adequate bioequivalence data, and **BT** in the absence of such data.

"B" CODES

Drug products that FDA at this time considers <u>not to be therapeutically equivalent</u> to other pharmaceutically equivalent products.

"B" products, for which actual or potential bioequivalence problems have not been resolved by adequate evidence of bioequivalence, often have a problem with specific dosage forms rather than with the active ingredients. Drug products designated with a **"B"** code fall under one of three main policies:

(1) the drug products contain active ingredients or are manufactured in dosage forms that have been identified by the Agency as having documented bioequivalence problems or a significant potential for such problems and for which no adequate studies demonstrating bioequivalence have been submitted to FDA; or

(2) the quality standards are inadequate or FDA has an insufficient basis to determine therapeutic equivalence; or

(3) the drug products are under regulatory review.

The specific coding definitions and policies for the **"B"** sub-codes are as follows:

B*

Drug products requiring further FDA investigation and review to determine therapeutic equivalence

The code **B*** is assigned to products that were previously assigned an **A** or **B** code if FDA receives new information that raises a significant question regarding therapeutic equivalence that can be resolved only through further Agency investigation and/or review of data and information submitted by the applicant. The **B*** code signifies that the Agency will take no position regarding the therapeutic equivalence of the product until the Agency completes its investigation and review.

BC

Extended-release dosage forms (capsules, injectables, and tablets)

An extended-release dosage form is defined by the official compendia as one that allows at least a twofold reduction in dosing frequency as compared to that drug presented as a conventional dosage form (e.g., as a solution or a prompt drug-releasing, conventional solid dosage form).

Although bioavailability studies have been conducted on these dosage forms, they are subject to bioavailability differences, primarily because firms developing extended-release products for the same active ingredient rarely employ the same formulation approach. FDA, therefore, does not consider different extended-release dosage forms containing the same active ingredient in equal strength to be therapeutically equivalent unless equivalence between individual products in both rate and extent has been specifically demonstrated through appropriate bioequivalence studies. Extended-release products for which such bioequivalence data have not been submitted are coded **BC,** while those for which such data are available have been coded **AB.**

BD

Active ingredients and dosage forms with documented bioequivalence problems

The **BD** code denotes products containing active ingredients with known bioequivalence problems and for which adequate studies have not been submitted to FDA demonstrating bioequivalence. Where studies showing bioequivalence have been submitted, the product has been coded **AB.**

BE

Delayed-release oral dosage forms

A delayed-release dosage form is defined by the official compendia as one that releases a drug (or drugs) at a time other than promptly after administration. Enteric-coated articles are delayed-release dosage forms.

Drug products in delayed-release dosage forms containing the same active ingredients are subject to significant differences in absorption. Unless otherwise specifically noted, the Agency considers different delayed-release products containing the same active ingredients as presenting a potential bioequivalence problem and codes these products **BE** in the absence of *in vivo* studies showing bioequivalence. If adequate *in vivo* studies have demonstrated the bioequivalence of specific delayed-release products, such products are coded **AB.**

BN

Products in aerosol-nebulizer drug delivery systems

This code applies to drug solutions or powders that are marketed only as a component of, or as compatible with, a specific drug delivery system. There may, for example, be significant differences in the dose of drug and particle size delivered by different products of this type. Therefore, the Agency does not consider different metered aerosol dosage forms containing the same active ingredient(s) in equal strengths to be therapeutically equivalent unless the drug products meet an appropriate bioequivalence standard.

BP

Active ingredients and dosage forms with potential bioequivalence problems

FDA's bioequivalence regulations (21 CFR 320.33) contain criteria and procedures for determining whether a specific active ingredient in a specific dosage form has a potential for causing a bioequivalence problem. It is FDA's policy to consider an ingredient meeting these criteria as having a potential bioequivalence problem even in the absence of positive data demonstrating inequivalence. Pharmaceutically equivalent products containing these ingredients in oral dosage forms are coded **BP** until adequate *in vivo* bioequivalence data are submitted.

Injectable suspensions containing an active ingredient suspended in an aqueous or oleaginous vehicle have also been coded **BP.** Injectable suspensions are subject to bioequivalence problems because differences in particle size, polymorphic structure of the suspended active ingredient, or the suspension formulation can significantly affect the rate of release and absorption. FDA does not consider pharmaceutical equivalents of these products bioequivalent without adequate evidence of bioequivalence.

BR

Suppositories or enemas that deliver drugs for systemic absorption

The absorption of active ingredients from suppositories or enemas that are intended to have a systemic effect (as distinct from suppositories administered for local effect) can vary significantly from product to product. Therefore, FDA considers pharmaceutically equivalent systemic suppositories or enemas bioequivalent only if *in vivo* evidence of bioequivalence is available. In those cases where *in vivo* evidence is available, the product is coded **AB.** If such evidence is not available, the products are coded **BR.**

BS

Products having drug standard deficiencies

If the drug standards for an active ingredient in a particular dosage form are found by FDA to be deficient so as to prevent an FDA evaluation of either pharmaceutical or therapeutic equivalence, all drug products containing that active ingredient in that dosage form are coded **BS.** For example, if the standards permit a wide variation in pharmacologically active components of the active ingredient such that pharmaceutical equivalence is in question, all products containing that active ingredient in that dosage form are coded **BS.**

BT

Topical products with bioequivalence issues

This code applies mainly to post-1962 dermatologic, ophthalmic, otic, rectal, and vaginal products for topical administration, including creams, ointments, gels, lotions, pastes, and sprays, as well as suppositories not intended for systemic drug absorption. Topical products evaluated as having acceptable clinical performance, but that are not bioequivalent to other pharmaceutically equivalent products or that lack sufficient evidence of bioequivalence will be coded **BT.**

BX

Drug products for which the data are insufficient to determine therapeutic equivalence

The code **BX** is assigned to specific drug products for which the data that have been reviewed by the Agency are insufficient to determine therapeutic equivalence under the policies stated in this document. In these situations, the drug products are presumed to be therapeutically inequivalent until the Agency has determined that there is adequate information to make a full evaluation of therapeutic equivalence.

1.8 Description of Special Situations

Certain drugs present special situations that deserve a more complete explanation than can be provided by the two-letter codes used in the List. These drugs have particular problems with standards of identity, analytical methodology, or bioequivalence that are in the process of resolution. The following drugs are in this category:

Amino Acid and Protein Hydrolysate Injections. These products differ in the amount and kinds of amino acids they contain and, therefore, are not considered pharmaceutical equivalents. For this reason, these products are not considered therapeutically equivalent. At the same time, the Agency believes that it is appropriate to point out that where nitrogen balance is the sole therapeutic objective and individual amino acid content is not a consideration, pharmaceutical alternatives with the same total amount of nitrogen content may be considered therapeutically equivalent.

Gaviscon®. Gaviscon® is an OTC product which has been marketed since September 1970. The active ingredients in this product, aluminum hydroxide and magnesium trisilicate, were reviewed by the Agency's OTC Antacid Panel and were considered to be safe and effective ingredients (Category I) by that Panel. However, the tablet failed to pass the antacid test which is required of all antacid products. The Agency, therefore, placed the tablet in Category III for lack of effectiveness. A full NDA with clinical studies was submitted by Marion Laboratories, Inc., and approved by FDA on December 9, 1983. Gaviscon®'s activity in treating reflux acidity is made possible by the physical-chemical properties of the inactive ingredients, sodium bicarbonate and alginic acid. Therefore, *all ANDAs which cite Gaviscon® tablets as the listed drug must contain the inactive ingredients, sodium bicarbonate and alginic acid.* A full NDA will be required to support the effectiveness of the drug product if different inactive ingredients are to be substituted for sodium bicarbonate or alginic acid or if different proportions of these ingredients are to be used.

Theophylline. Studies have suggested that food may significantly alter the absorption of theophylline from some extended-release theophylline drug products. Current research is defining more precisely the relationship between the timing of meals (including type and amount of food) and the rate and extent of absorption of theophylline from the extended-release dosage form. Specific product labeling should be consulted to determine the information available on this subject.

Trazodone Hydrochloride. Generic Trazodone HCl 150 mg tablet entries, marked with a "†", are rated as therapeutically equivalent (**AB**) to Bristol Meyer's Desyrel® (Trazodone HCl) Dividose 150 mg tablets. The therapeutic equivalence determination was made on the basis, among other things, of an acceptable bioequivalence study and acceptable *in vitro* dissolution testing. A patent that exists on the Desyrel® 150 mg tablet scoring design, which enables the patient to break Desyrel® into three 50-mg segments, currently prevents a generic firm from copying this feature. Therefore, a patient will not be able to obtain three 50-mg segments from the generic tablet. Prescribers and dispensers should be aware of this difference and take it into account when writing a prescription or practicing drug product selection.

1.9 Therapeutic Equivalence Code Change for a Drug Entity

The Agency will use the following procedures when, in response to a petition or on its own initiative, it is considering a change in the therapeutic equivalence code for approved multisource drug products. Such changes will generally occur when the Agency becomes aware of new scientific information affecting the therapeutic equivalence of an entire category of drug products in the List (e.g., information concerning the active ingredient or the dosage form), rather than information concerning a single drug product within the category. These procedures will be used when a change in therapeutic equivalence code is under consideration for all drug products found in the Prescription Drug Product List under a specific drug entity and dosage form. The change may be from the code signifying that the drug does not present a bioequivalence problem (e.g., **AA**) to a code signifying a bioequivalence problem (e.g., **BP**), or vice versa. This procedure does not apply to a change of a particular product code (e.g., a change from **BP** to **AB** or from **AB** to **BX**).

Before making a change in a code for an entire category of drugs, the Agency will announce in the *Introduction* to the Cumulative Supplement that it is considering the change, and will invite comment. Comments, along with scientific data, may be sent to the Director, Division of Bioequivalence, Office of Generic Drugs, Center for Drug Evaluation and Research, (MPN-2) HFD-650, 7500 Standish Place, Rockville, MD 20855. The comment period will generally be 60 days in length, and the closing date for comments will be listed in the description of the proposed change for each drug entity.

The most useful type of scientific data submission is an *in vivo* bioavailability/bioequivalence study conducted on batches of the subject drug products. These submissions should present a full description of the analytical procedures and equipment used, a validation of the analytical methodology, including the standard curve, a description of the method of calculating results, and a description of the pharmacokinetic and statistical models used in analyzing the data. Anecdotal or testimonial information is the least useful to the Agency, and such submissions are discouraged. Copies of supporting reports published in the scientific literature or unpublished material, however, are welcome.

1.10 Change of the Therapeutic Equivalence Evaluation for a Single Product

The aforementioned procedure does not apply to a change in a single drug single product code. For example, a change in a single drug product's code from **BP** to **AB** as a result of the submission of a bioequivalence study will not ordinarily be the subject of notice and comment. Likewise, a change in a single drug product's code from **AB** to **BX** (e.g., as a result of new information raising a significant question as to bioequivalence) does not require notice and comment. The Agency's responsibility to provide the public with the Agency's most current information related to therapeutic equivalence may require a change in a drug product's code prior to any formal notice and opportunity for the applicant to be heard. The publication in the *Federal Register* of a Proposal to withdraw approval of a drug product will ordinarily result in a change in a product's code from **AB** to **BX** if this action has not already been taken.

1.11 Availability of Internal Policy and Procedure Guides

The Office of Generic Drugs maintains internal policy and procedure guides. Although these guides are designed for Office personnel and are subject to change without public notice, they are available to members of the public who may wish to know more about the Office's policies and procedures. Copies of these guides may be obtained from the Executive Secretariat Staff, (MNP-1) HFD-8, FDA, Center for Drug Evaluation and Research, 5600 Fishers Lane, Rockville, MD 20857. The Agency welcomes public comment on the policies, procedures, and practices employed in the approval of generic drugs. Such comments may be sent to the Director, Office of Generic Drugs, (MPN-2) HFD-600, 7500 Standish Place, Rockville, MD 20855.

1.12 Availability of the Publication and Other FDA Reports and Updating Procedures

REPORTS AVAILABLE FROM
SUPERINTENDENT OF DOCUMENTS
U.S. GOVERNMENT PRINTING OFFICE
WASHINGTON, DC 20402
(202) 783-3238

- ***Approved Drug Products with Therapeutic Equivalence Evaluations, 14th Edition (1994).*** This publication and its monthly Cumulative Supplements are provided in the subscription price. The Cumulative Supplements provide new drug approval information and, if necessary, revised therapeutic equivalence evaluations and updated patent and exclusivity information. The publication must be used, therefore, in conjunction with the most current Cumulative Supplement.

An updated magnetic tape containing ONLY the Prescription Drug Product List is available quarterly by subscription. Order from the National Technical Information Service. (See the following page).

- ***Recalls - FDA Enforcement Report.*** The FDA Enforcement Report is published weekly and contains information on actions taken in connection with Agency regulatory activities, including recalls and medical device safety alerts voluntarily conducted by firms.

REPORTS AVAILABLE FROM
FREEDOM OF INFORMATION STAFF
5600 FISHERS LANE, HFI-35
ROCKVILLE, MD 20857
(301) 443-6310

• *DESI Drug Products and Known-Related Drug Products that Lack Substantial Evidence of Effectiveness and are Subject to a Notice of Opportunity for Hearing and Those that Already have had Approval Withdrawn.*

• *Inactive Ingredient Guide, 1993.* This guide contains all inactive ingredients present in approved drug products or conditionally approved drug products currently marketed for human use.

• *Phase IV Postapproval Research List.* This report provides monitoring data on the status of postapproval research requested of holders of approved new drug applications.

• *Drug Products that may be Subject to the FDA's Prescription Drug Wrap-Up.*

• *Quality Assurance by Manufacturer.* Under Section 510(h) of the Federal Food, Drug, and Cosmetic Act, every drug establishment registered with the FDA must be inspected at least once every two years to determine if the drugs they market are produced in conformance with current Good Manufacturing Practices. Copies of the inspection reports generated by the FDA District conducting the inspection or any other inspections conducted are available from the local Districts pursuant to the Freedom of Information regulations.

REPORTS AVAILABLE FROM
NATIONAL TECHNICAL
INFORMATION SERVICE
5285 PORT ROYAL ROAD
SPRINGFIELD, VA 22161
(703) 487-4630 (Subscription Department)
(703) 487-4650 (Order Department)

• *Drug/Biologic Quality Reporting System, Annual DQRS Report.*

• *FDA Drug and Device Product Approvals.* Official Agency listing of monthly approval data from the Center for Drug Evaluation and Research, Center for Biologics Evaluation and Research, Center for Veterinary Medicine, and Center for Devices and Radiological Health.

REPORTS AVAILABLE FROM
EXECUTIVE SECRETARIAT STAFF
CENTER FOR DRUG EVALUATION AND
RESEARCH, FDA
5600 FISHERS LANE (HFD-8)
ROCKVILLE, MD 20857
(301) 594-1012

• *Biopharmaceutic Guidelines.* Individual biopharmaceutic guidelines are available at no charge.

• *Clinical Evaluation Guidelines.* Individual clinical guidelines are available at no charge.

Information about other CDER/FDA publications can be obtained from the CDER Executive Secretariat Staff.

2. HOW TO USE THE DRUG PRODUCT LISTS

2.1 Key Sections for Using the Drug Product Lists

This publication contains the illustrations, along with the Drug Product Lists, indices, and lists of abbreviations and terms which facilitate their use.

Illustrations. The annotated Drug Product Illustration and the Therapeutic Equivalence Evaluations Illustration are offered to provide further clarification. These depict the format found in the Prescription Drug Product List (the only List in which therapeutic equivalence evaluation codes are displayed).

Drug Product Lists. The Drug Product Lists, arranged alphabetically by active ingredient, contain product identification information (active ingredients, dosage forms, routes of administration, product names, application holders, strengths) for single and multiple ingredient drug products. Also shown are the application number and drug product number (FDA internal computer data use only) and approval dates for those drug products approved on or after January 1, 1982.

If a prescription drug product is available from more than one source (multisource), a therapeutic equivalence code will appear in front of the applicant's name. If a product is therapeutically equivalent to one or more products or to an appropriate reference, it will be designated with a code beginning with **"A"** and the entry will be underlined for emphasis.

Active ingredient headings for multiple ingredient (combination) drug products are arranged alphabetically. For purposes of this publication, this alphabetical sort takes precedence over United State Pharmacopeia official monograph order (i.e., Reserpine, Hydralazine Hydrochloride, Hydrochlorothiazide). For example, product information labeled as Reserpine, Hydrochlorothiazide and Hydralazine Hydrochloride appears under the active ingredient heading *Hydralazine Hydrochloride; Hydrochlorothiazide; Reserpine.* A cross-reference to the product information (for prescription and OTC products) appears for each additional active ingredient in the product. For combination drug products, the ingredient strengths are separated by semicolons and appear in the same relative sequence as the ingredients in the heading. Available strengths of the dosage form from an applicant appear on separate lines.

To use the Drug Product Lists, determine by alphabetical order the ingredient under which the product information is listed, using the Product Name Index, if appropriate. Then, find the ingredient in the applicable Drug Product List. Proceed to the dosage form and route of administration and compare products within that ingredient heading only. Therapeutic equivalence or inequivalence for prescription products is determined on the basis of the therapeutic equivalence codes provided within that specific dosage form heading. The OTC Drug Product List, Discontinued Drug Product List, and Drug Products with Approval under Section 505 of the Act Administered by the Center for Biologics Evaluation and Research List have their data arranged similarly. The Discontinued Drug Product List contains products that have never been marketed, products discontinued from marketing or products that have had their approval withdrawn for other than safety or effectiveness reasons. All products having a "∂" in the 12th Cumulative Supplement of the 13th Edition List have been added to the Discontinued Drug Product List appearing in the 14th Edition.

USP Monograph Title Additions or Changes. The U.S. Pharmacopeia periodically makes additions to or changes in monograph titles. Some of these additions or changes may affect dosage form terms listed in this publication. Please refer to Section 3.5 for monograph title additions or changes affecting this edition.

Product Name Index (Prescription and OTC Drug Product Lists). This is an index of drug products by established or trade name. The second term of each entry indicates the active ingredient name under which product information can be found in the appropriate Drug Product List. For those drug products with multiple active ingredients, only the first active ingredient (in alphabetical order) will appear. OTC products are so designated.

Product Name Index Listed by Applicant (Prescription and OTC Drug Product Lists). This is an index that cross-references applicants to drug products. The bolded and underlined entry represents the applicant name abbreviation used in this publication. Each complete applicant name that is represented by the abbreviated name is marked with an asterisk (*). Listed under each complete applicant name is the first alphabetically arranged ingredient under which product information can be found in the appropriate Drug Product List. OTC products are so designated. To use the Drug Product Lists, determine by alphabetical order the ingredient under which the product information is listed, using the Product Name Index, if appropriate.

ANDA Suitability Petitions. Under Section 505(j)(2)(C) of the Act, an ANDA applicant may petition FDA for permission to file an ANDA for a drug product that has one different active ingredient in a combination product, or whose route of administration, dosage form, or strength differs from that of the listed drug. These are the only types of changes permitted in an ANDA. This section is comprised of two lists of petitions where the Agency has determined that the referenced product: (1) is suitable for submission as an ANDA (Petitions Approved) or (2) is not suitable for submission as an ANDA (Petitions Denied). The determination that an ANDA will be approved is not made until the ANDA itself is submitted and reviewed by the Agency.

Uniform Terms. To improve readability, uniform terms are used to designate dosage forms, routes of administration, and abbreviations used to express strengths. These terms are listed in Appendix C. In some cases, the terms used may differ from those used in product labels and other labeling.

2.2 DRUG PRODUCT ILLUSTRATION

Single Ingredient

- Active Ingredient → MEPERIDINE HYDROCHLORIDE
- Dosage Form; Route of Administration → INJECTABLE; INJECTION
- Trade or Generic Names → HEXANON; MEPERIDINE HCL
- Therapeutic Equivalence (TE) Code for Multisource Product → AP
- Final Approval Date → AUG 27, 1987
- Single Source Product (No TE Code) → HOLLEY MED
- Reference Drug Symbol → + SFD PHARM
- Applicant
- Available Strength(s) of a Product
- Application Number and Product Number

Product Number Is for FDA Internal Computer Data Use Only

MEPERIDINE HYDROCHLORIDE

INJECTABLE; INJECTION

	HEXANON		
AP	METRO-PHYS	25 MG/ML	N43111 001
AP		50 MG/ML	N43111 002
AP		75 MG/ML	N43111 003 AUG 22, 1983
AP		100 MG/ML	N43111 004 JAN 04, 1985
	MEPERIDINE HCL		
AP	ANDERSON PHARM	25 MG/ML	N42242 001
AP		50 MG/ML	N42296 001
AP		75 MG/ML	N42301 002
AP		100 MG/ML	N42301 003 AUG 27, 1987
	HOLLEY MED	10 MG/ML	N40000 001
AP	PARKLAND	25 MG/ML	N47222 001
	+ SFD PHARM	100 MG/ML	N47100 001
			N47005 001

Multiple Ingredients

With Product Information

- Alphabetically Sorted by Active Ingredient → HYDRALAZINE HYDROCHLORIDE; HYDROCHLOROTHIAZIDE; RESERPINE
- Product Information

HYDRALAZINE HYDROCHLORIDE; HYDROCHLOROTHIAZIDE; RESERPINE

TABLET; ORAL

HYDROCHLOROTHIAZIDE, RESERPINE AND HYDRALAZINE HCL

MADISON	25 MG; 15 MG; 0.1 MG	N41296 001 JAN 18, 1982

With Cross-Reference

- Alphabetically Second Active Ingredient → HYDROCHLOROTHIAZIDE: *MULTIPLE*
- Cross-Reference to Product Information → SEE HYDRALAZINE HYDROCHLORIDE; HYDROCHLOROTHIAZIDE; RESERPINE

HYDROCHLOROTHIAZIDE: *MULTIPLE*

SEE HYDRALAZINE HYDROCHLORIDE; HYDROCHLOROTHIAZIDE; RESERPINE

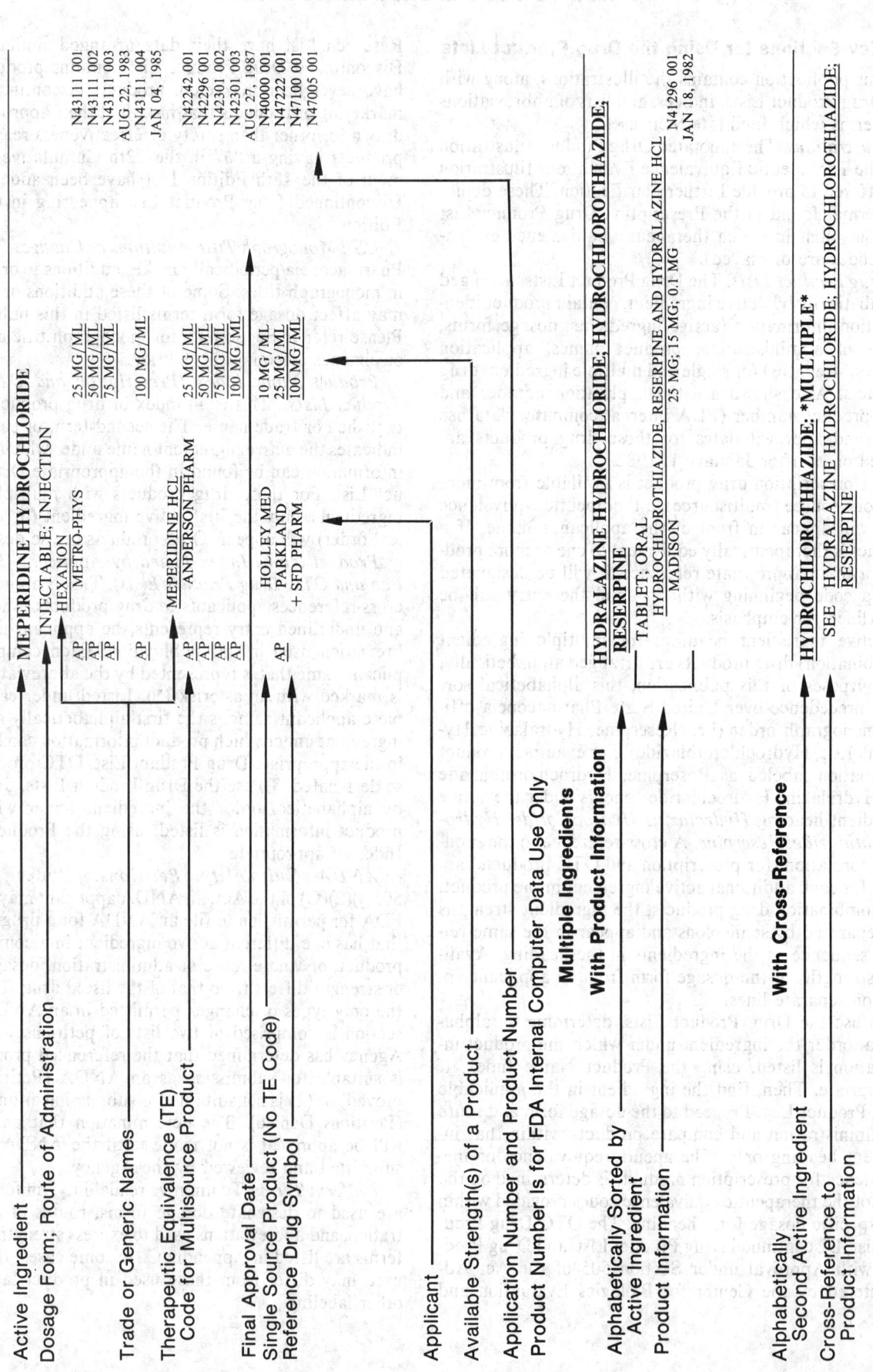

This example is for purposes of illustration only. It does not represent actual products from the Prescription Drug Product list.

2.3 THERAPEUTIC EQUIVALENCE EVALUATIONS ILLUSTRATION

Drug products coded **AB** (or any code beginning with an "**A**") under an ingredient and dosage form heading are considered therapeutically equivalent only to other products coded **AB** (or any code beginning with an "**A**") and **NOT** to those coded **BP** (or any code beginning with a "**B**") and any products not listed. Drug products coded **BP** (or any code beginning with a "**B**") are **NOT** considered therapeutically equivalent to any other product. For a complete explanation of the TE codes refer to Section 1.7 of the *Introduction*.

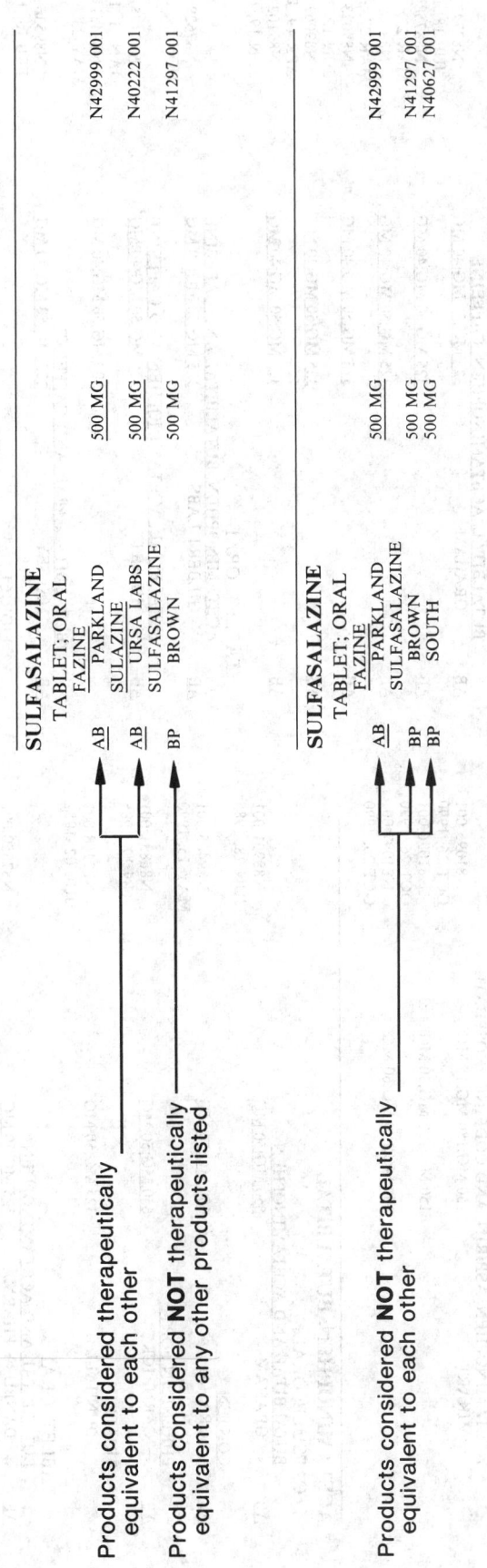

		SULFASALAZINE		
		TABLET; ORAL		
		FAZINE		
Products considered therapeutically equivalent to each other →	AB	PARKLAND	500 MG	N42999 001
		SULAZINE		
	AB	URSA LABS	500 MG	N40222 001
		SULFASALAZINE		
Products considered **NOT** therapeutically equivalent to any other products listed →	BP	BROWN	500 MG	N41297 001

		SULFASALAZINE		
		TABLET; ORAL		
		FAZINE		
Products considered **NOT** therapeutically equivalent to each other →	AB	PARKLAND	500 MG	N42999 001
		SULFASALAZINE		
	BP	BROWN	500 MG	N41297 001
	BP	SOUTH	500 MG	N40627 001

NOTE: Underlining denotes multisource products which are considered therapeutically equivalent.

This example is for purposes of illustration only. It does not represent actual products from the Prescription Drug Product list.

PRESCRIPTION DRUG PRODUCTS

ACEBUTOLOL HYDROCHLORIDE

CAPSULE; ORAL

SECTRAL

TE	Applicant	Strength	Appl No / Date
	WYETH AYERST	EQ 200 MG BASE	N18917 001 DEC 28, 1984
	+	EQ 400 MG BASE	N18917 003 DEC 28, 1984

ACETAMINOPHEN; ASPIRIN; CODEINE PHOSPHATE

CAPSULE; ORAL

ACETAMINOPHEN, ASPIRIN, AND CODEINE PHOSPHATE

TE	Applicant	Strength	Appl No / Date
	MIKART	150 MG;180 MG;15 MG	N81095 001 OCT 26, 1990
		150 MG;180 MG;30 MG	N81096 001 OCT 26, 1990
		150 MG;180 MG;60 MG	N81097 001 OCT 26, 1990

ACETAMINOPHEN; BUTALBITAL

CAPSULE; ORAL

TE	Applicant	Strength	Appl No / Date
	BUTALBITAL AND ACETAMINOPHEN		
AB	GRAHAM	650 MG;50 MG	N88991 001 JUN 28, 1985
	CONTEN		
AB	GRAHAM	650 MG;50 MG	N89405 001 MAY 15, 1990
	PHRENILIN FORTE		
AB	+ CARNRICK	650 MG;50 MG	N88831 001 JUN 19, 1985
	TRIAPRIN		
	DUNHALL	325 MG;50 MG	N89268 001 JUL 02, 1987

TABLET; ORAL

TE	Applicant	Strength	Appl No / Date
	BUTALBITAL AND ACETAMINOPHEN		
AB	DANBURY PHARMA	325 MG;50 MG	N87550 001 OCT 19, 1984
AB	HALSEY	325 MG;50 MG	N89568 001 OCT 05, 1988
	BUTAPAP		
AB	MIKART	325 MG;50 MG	N89987 001 OCT 26, 1992
AB		650 MG;50 MG	N89988 001 OCT 26, 1992
	PHRENILIN		
AB	+ CARNRICK	325 MG;50 MG	N87811 001 JUN 19, 1985
	SEDAPAP		
AB	+ MAYRAND	650 MG;50 MG	N88944 001 OCT 17, 1985

ACETAMINOPHEN; BUTALBITAL; CAFFEINE

CAPSULE; ORAL

TE	Applicant	Strength	Appl No / Date
	ACETAMINOPHEN, BUTALBITAL AND CAFFEINE		
AB	+ GILBERT LABS	325 MG;50 MG;40 MG	N88825 001 DEC 05, 1984
	ACETAMINOPHEN, BUTALBITAL, AND CAFFEINE		
AB	MIKART	325 MG;50 MG;40 MG	N89007 001 MAR 17, 1986
	ANOQUAN		
AB	ROBERTS AND HAUCK	325 MG;50 MG;40 MG	N87628 001 OCT 01, 1986
	BUTALBITAL, ACETAMINOPHEN, CAFFEINE		
AB	GRAHAM	325 MG;50 MG;40 MG	N88743 001 JUL 18, 1985
AB		325 MG;50 MG;40 MG	N88758 001 MAR 27, 1985
AB		325 MG;50 MG;40 MG	N88765 001 MAR 27, 1985
AB		325 MG;50 MG;40 MG	N89023 001 JUN 19, 1985
AB		325 MG;50 MG;40 MG	N89067 001 APR 19, 1985
AB		325 MG;50 MG;40 MG	N89102 001 JUN 19, 1985

TABLET; ORAL

TE	Applicant	Strength	Appl No / Date
	ACETAMINOPHEN, BUTALBITAL AND CAFFEINE		
AB	GILBERT LABS	325 MG;50 MG;40 MG	N87629 001 NOV 13, 1984
	BUTALBITAL, ACETAMINOPHEN AND CAFFEINE		
AB	MIKART	325 MG;50 MG;40 MG	N89175 001 JAN 21, 1987
		500 MG;50 MG;40 MG	N89451 001 MAY 23, 1988
	BUTALBITAL, APAP, AND CAFFEINE		
AB	HALSEY	325 MG;50 MG;40 MG	N89536 001 FEB 16, 1988
	FIORICET		
AB	+ SANDOZ	325 MG;50 MG;40 MG	N88616 001 NOV 09, 1984
	REPAN		
AB	GRAHAM	325 MG;50 MG;40 MG	N87804 001 JAN 24, 1985

ACETAMINOPHEN; BUTALBITAL; CAFFEINE; CODEINE PHOSPHATE

CAPSULE; ORAL

FIORICET W/ CODEINE

TE	Applicant	Strength	Appl No / Date
	+ SANDOZ	325 MG;50 MG;40 MG;30 MG	N20232 001 JUL 30, 1992

Prescription Drug Products *(continued)*

ACETAMINOPHEN; CAFFEINE; DIHYDROCODEINE BITARTRATE

TE	Product / Applicant	Strength	Appl No / Date
	CAPSULE; ORAL		
	COMPAL		
AA	PURDUE FREDERICK	356.4 MG;30 MG;16 MG	N88584 001 MAR 04, 1986
	SYNALGOS-DC-A		
AA	WYETH AYERST	356.4 MG;30 MG;16 MG	N89166 001 MAY 14, 1986

ACETAMINOPHEN; CODEINE PHOSPHATE

TE	Product / Applicant	Strength	Appl No / Date
	CAPSULE; ORAL		
	PHENAPHEN W/ CODEINE NO. 2		
	ROBINS AH	325 MG;15 MG	N84444 001
	PHENAPHEN W/ CODEINE NO. 3		
	ROBINS AH	325 MG;30 MG	N84445 001
	PHENAPHEN W/ CODEINE NO. 4		
	ROBINS AH	325 MG;60 MG	N84446 001
	SOLUTION; ORAL		
	ACETAMINOPHEN AND CODEINE PHOSPHATE		
AA	MIKART	120 MG/5 ML;12 MG/5 ML	N89450 001 OCT 27, 1992
AA	PENNEX	120 MG/5 ML;12 MG/5 ML	N87006 001
AA	PHARM ASSOC	120 MG/5 ML;12 MG/5 ML	N87508 001
	ACETAMINOPHEN W/ CODEINE		
AA	ROXANE	120 MG/5 ML;12 MG/5 ML	N86366 001
	APAP W/ CODEINE		
AA	BARRE	120 MG/5 ML;12 MG/5 ML	N85861 001
	TYLENOL W/ CODEINE		
AA	JOHNSON RW	120 MG/5 ML;12 MG/5 ML	N85057 001
	SUSPENSION; ORAL		
	ACETAMINOPHEN W/ CODEINE PHOSPHATE		
AA	BARRE	120 MG/5 ML;12 MG/5 ML	N85883 001
	CAPITAL AND CODEINE		
AA	CARNRICK	120 MG/5 ML;12 MG/5 ML	N86024 001
	TABLET; ORAL		
	ACETAMINOPHEN AND CODEINE PHOSPHATE		
AA	BARR	300 MG;15 MG	N85795 001
AA		300 MG;30 MG	N85794 001
AA	GENEVA PHARMS	300 MG;30 MG	N81250 001 JUL 16, 1992
AA		300 MG;30 MG	N85291 002
AA		300 MG;60 MG	N81249 001 JUL 16, 1992
AA		300 MG;60 MG	N85964 001
AA	HALSEY	300 MG;60 MG	N86549 001
AA	KV PHARM	300 MG;30 MG	N85288 001
AA		300 MG;60 MG	N85365 001
		325 MG;15 MG	N85364 001
		325 MG;45 MG	N85363 001

ACETAMINOPHEN; CODEINE PHOSPHATE *(continued)*

TE	Product / Applicant	Strength	Appl No / Date
	TABLET; ORAL		
	ACETAMINOPHEN AND CODEINE PHOSPHATE		
AA	MIKART	650 MG;30 MG	N89231 001 MAR 03, 1986
		650 MG;60 MG	N89363 001 SEP 25, 1991
AA	MUTUAL PHARM	300 MG;15 MG	N89671 001 FEB 10, 1988
AA		300 MG;30 MG	N89672 001 FEB 10, 1988
AA		300 MG;60 MG	N89673 001 FEB 10, 1988
AA	PHARMERAL	300 MG;30 MG	N87762 001 DEC 10, 1982
AA	PUREPAC PHARM	300 MG;30 MG	N86681 001
AA		300 MG;60 MG	N86683 001
	ROXANE	500 MG;15 MG	N89511 001 APR 25, 1989
		500 MG;30 MG	N89512 001 APR 25, 1989
		500 MG;60 MG	N89513 001 APR 25, 1989
AA	VINTAGE PHARMS	300 MG;15 MG	N89990 001 SEP 30, 1988
AA		300 MG;30 MG	N89805 001 SEP 30, 1988
AA		300 MG;60 MG	N89828 001 SEP 30, 1988
AA	ZENITH LABS	300 MG;60 MG	N87083 001
	ACETAMINOPHEN AND CODEINE PHOSPHATE #2		
AA	SUPERPHARM	300 MG;15 MG	N89183 001 OCT 18, 1985
	ACETAMINOPHEN AND CODEINE PHOSPHATE #3		
AA	MIKART	300 MG;30 MG	N89238 001 FEB 25, 1986
AA	PUREPAC PHARM	300 MG;30 MG	N89080 001 JUL 17, 1986
AA	SUPERPHARM	300 MG;30 MG	N89184 001 OCT 18, 1985
	ACETAMINOPHEN AND CODEINE PHOSPHATE #4		
AA	MIKART	300 MG;60 MG	N89244 001 FEB 25, 1986
AA	SUPERPHARM	300 MG;60 MG	N89185 001 OCT 18, 1985
	ACETAMINOPHEN AND CODEINE PHOSPHATE NO. 4		
AA	ROXANE	300 MG;60 MG	N84667 001
	ACETAMINOPHEN W/ CODEINE		
AA	BARR	300 MG;60 MG	N87653 001 APR 13, 1982
	ACETAMINOPHEN W/ CODEINE #2		
AA	LEMMON	300 MG;15 MG	N88627 001 MAR 06, 1985

Prescription Drug Products *(continued)*

ACETAMINOPHEN; CODEINE PHOSPHATE *(continued)*

TABLET; ORAL

	ACETAMINOPHEN W/ CODEINE #3		
AA	LEMMON	300 MG;30 MG	N88628 001 MAR 06, 1985
	ACETAMINOPHEN W/ CODEINE #4		
AA	LEMMON	300 MG;60 MG	N88629 001 MAR 06, 1985
	ACETAMINOPHEN W/ CODEINE NO. 2		
AA	ROXANE	300 MG;15 MG	N84659 001
	ACETAMINOPHEN W/ CODEINE NO. 3		
AA	ROXANE	300 MG;30 MG	N84656 001
	ACETAMINOPHEN W/ CODEINE PHOSPHATE		
AA	HALSEY	300 MG;15 MG	N83871 001
AA		300 MG;30 MG	N83872 001
	ACETAMINOPHEN W/ CODEINE PHOSPHATE #3		
AA	ZENITH LABS	300 MG;30 MG	N85868 001
	CAPITAL WITH CODEINE		
	CARNRICK	325 MG;30 MG	N83643 001
	PHENAPHEN-650 W/ CODEINE		
AA	ROBINS AH	650 MG;30 MG	N85856 001
	TYLENOL W/ CODEINE NO. 1		
	+ JOHNSON RW	300 MG;7.5 MG	N85055 001
	TYLENOL W/ CODEINE NO. 2		
AA	JOHNSON RW	300 MG;15 MG	N85055 002
	TYLENOL W/ CODEINE NO. 3		
AA	JOHNSON RW	300 MG;30 MG	N85055 003
	TYLENOL W/ CODEINE NO. 4		
AA	JOHNSON RW	300 MG;60 MG	N85055 004

ACETAMINOPHEN; HYDROCODONE BITARTRATE

CAPSULE; ORAL

	ACETAMINOPHEN AND HYDROCODONE BITARTRATE		
AA	CENT PHARMS	500 MG;5 MG	N88898 001 MAR 27, 1985
AA	GRAHAM	500 MG;5 MG	N87336 001 JUL 08, 1982
AA		500 MG;5 MG	N88956 001 JUL 19, 1985
	ALLAY		
AA	NORTON HN	500 MG;5 MG	N89907 001 JAN 13, 1989
	CO-GESIC		
AA	CENT PHARMS	500 MG;5 MG	N89360 001 MAR 02, 1988
	HYDROCET		
AA	GRAHAM	500 MG;5 MG	N89006 001 AUG 09, 1985

ACETAMINOPHEN; HYDROCODONE BITARTRATE *(continued)*

CAPSULE; ORAL

	HYDROCODONE BITARTRATE AND ACETAMINOPHEN		
AA	MIKART	500 MG;5 MG	N81067 001 NOV 30, 1989
AA		500 MG;5 MG	N81068 001 NOV 30, 1989
AA		500 MG;5 MG	N81069 001 NOV 30, 1989
AA		500 MG;5 MG	N81070 001 NOV 30, 1989
AA		500 MG;5 MG	N89008 001 FEB 21, 1986

ELIXIR; ORAL

	HYDROCODONE BITARTRATE AND ACETAMINOPHEN		
	MIKART	500 MG/15 ML;5 MG/15 ML	N81226 001 OCT 27, 1992
		500 MG/15 ML;5 MG/15 ML	N89557 001 APR 29, 1992
		500 MG/15 ML;7.5 MG/15 ML	N81051 001 AUG 28, 1992

TABLET; ORAL

	ACETAMINOPHEN AND HYDROCODONE BITARTRATE		
AA	GRAHAM	500 MG;5 MG	N87722 001 JUL 09, 1982
	ANEXSIA		
AA	BOEHRINGER MANNHEIM	500 MG;5 MG	N89160 001 APR 23, 1987
	ANEXSIA 7.5/650		
AA	BOEHRINGER MANNHEIM	650 MG;7.5 MG	N89725 001 SEP 30, 1987
	CO-GESIC		
AA	CENT PHARMS	500 MG;5 MG	N87757 001 MAY 03, 1982
	HY-PHEN		
AA	ASCHER	500 MG;5 MG	N87677 001 MAY 03, 1982
	HYDROCODONE BITARTRATE AND ACETAMINOPHEN		
AA	HALSEY	500 MG;5 MG	N89554 001 JUN 12, 1987

Prescription Drug Products *(continued)*

ACETAMINOPHEN; HYDROCODONE BITARTRATE *(continued)*

TABLET; ORAL

	HYDROCODONE BITARTRATE AND ACETAMINOPHEN		
AA	MIKART	500 MG;2.5 MG	N89698 001 AUG 25, 1989
AA		500 MG;5 MG	N89271 001 JUL 16, 1986
AA		500 MG;5 MG	N89697 001 JAN 28, 1992
AA		500 MG;7.5 MG	N89699 001 AUG 25, 1989
AA		650 MG;7.5 MG	N89689 001 JUN 29, 1988
		650 MG;10 MG	N81223 001 MAY 29, 1992
AA	NORTON HN	500 MG;5 MG	N89696 001 APR 21, 1988
AA	VINTAGE PHARMS	500 MG;5 MG	N89831 001 SEP 07, 1988
AA		500 MG;5 MG	N89971 001 DEC 02, 1988
AA	WATSON LABS	500 MG;2.5 MG	N81079 001 AUG 30, 1991
AA		500 MG;5 MG	N89883 001 DEC 01, 1988
AA		500 MG;7.5 MG	N81080 001 AUG 30, 1991
AA		750 MG;7.5 MG	N81083 001 AUG 30, 1991
	HYDROCODONE BITARTRATE W/ ACETAMINOPHEN		
AA	BARR	500 MG;5 MG	N88577 001 DEC 21, 1984
	VICODIN		
AA	KNOLL PHARM	500 MG;5 MG	N88058 001 JAN 07, 1983
	VICODIN ES		
AA	KNOLL PHARM	750 MG;7.5 MG	N89736 001 DEC 09, 1988

ACETAMINOPHEN; OXYCODONE HYDROCHLORIDE

CAPSULE; ORAL

	OXYCODONE AND ACETAMINOPHEN		
AA	HALSEY	500 MG;5 MG	N89994 001 MAY 04, 1989
	TYLOX		
AA	JOHNSON RW	500 MG;5 MG	N88790 001 DEC 12, 1984

SOLUTION; ORAL

	ROXICET		
	ROXANE	325 MG/5 ML;5 MG/5 ML	N89351 001 DEC 03, 1986

ACETAMINOPHEN; OXYCODONE HYDROCHLORIDE *(continued)*

TABLET; ORAL

	OXYCET		
AA	HALSEY	325 MG;5 MG	N87463 001 DEC 07, 1983
	OXYCODONE HCL AND ACETAMINOPHEN		
AA	BARR	325 MG;5 MG	N87406 001
	PERCOCET		
AA	DUPONT MERCK	325 MG;5 MG	N85106 002
	ROXICET		
AA	ROXANE	325 MG;5 MG	N87003 001
	ROXICET 5/500		
	ROXANE	500 MG;5 MG	N89775 001 JAN 12, 1989

ACETAMINOPHEN; PENTAZOCINE HYDROCHLORIDE

TABLET; ORAL

	TALACEN		
	+ STERLING WINTHROP	650 MG;EQ 25 MG BASE	N18458 001 SEP 23, 1982

ACETAMINOPHEN; PROPOXYPHENE HYDROCHLORIDE

TABLET; ORAL

	PROPOXYPHENE HCL AND ACETAMINOPHEN		
AA	GENEVA PHARMS	650 MG;65 MG	N89959 001 JUL 18, 1989
AA	MYLAN	650 MG;65 MG	N83978 001
	WYGESIC		
AA	WYETH AYERST	650 MG;65 MG	N84999 001

ACETAMINOPHEN; PROPOXYPHENE NAPSYLATE

TABLET; ORAL

	DARVOCET-N 100		
AB	+ LILLY	650 MG;100 MG	N17122 002
	DARVOCET-N 50		
AB	LILLY	325 MG;50 MG	N17122 001
	PROPACET 100		
AB	LEMMON	650 MG;100 MG	N70107 001 JUN 12, 1985

Prescription Drug Products *(continued)*

ACETAMINOPHEN; PROPOXYPHENE NAPSYLATE *(continued)*

TABLET; ORAL

PROPOXYPHENE NAPSYLATE AND ACETAMINOPHEN

AB	BARR	325 MG;50 MG	N70115 001 JUN 12, 1985
AB		650 MG;100 MG	N70116 001 JUN 12, 1985
AB		650 MG;100 MG	N70615 001 MAR 21, 1986
AB		650 MG;100 MG	N70771 001 MAR 21, 1986
AB		650 MG;100 MG	N70775 001 MAR 21, 1986
AB	GENEVA PHARMS	650 MG;100 MG	N70443 001 JAN 23, 1986
AB	LEMMON	650 MG;100 MG	N70732 001 JAN 03, 1986
AB	MYLAN	650 MG;100 MG	N70145 001 JUN 12, 1985
AB		650 MG;100 MG	N72195 001 FEB 16, 1988
AB	PUREPAC PHARM	650 MG;100 MG	N70910 001 JAN 02, 1987
AB	SUPERPHARM	650 MG;100 MG	N71319 001 JAN 06, 1987
AB	ZENITH LABS	650 MG;100 MG	N70146 001 AUG 02, 1985

ACETAZOLAMIDE

CAPSULE, EXTENDED RELEASE; ORAL

DIAMOX

	+ LEDERLE	500 MG	N12945 001

TABLET; ORAL

ACETAZOLAMIDE

AB	DANBURY PHARMA	250 MG	N88882 001 OCT 22, 1985
AB	LANNETT	250 MG	N84840 001
AB	MUTUAL PHARM	125 MG	N89752 001 JUN 22, 1988
AB		250 MG	N89753 001 JUN 22, 1988

DIAMOX

AB	LEDERLE	125 MG	N08943 001
AB	+	250 MG	N08943 002

ACETAZOLAMIDE SODIUM

INJECTABLE; INJECTION

DIAMOX

	+ LEDERLE	EQ 500 MG BASE/VIAL	N09388 001 DEC 05, 1990

ACETIC ACID, GLACIAL

SOLUTION; IRRIGATION, URETHRAL

ACETIC ACID 0.25% IN PLASTIC CONTAINER

AT	ABBOTT	250 MG/100 ML	N17656 001
AT	BAXTER	250 MG/100 ML	N18523 001 FEB 19, 1982
AT	MCGAW	250 MG/100 ML	N18161 001

SOLUTION/DROPS; OTIC

ACETASOL

AT	BARRE	2%	N87146 001

ACETIC ACID

AT	THAMES	2%	N88638 001 SEP 06, 1984

VOSOL

AT	+ WALLACE	2%	N12179 001

ACETIC ACID, GLACIAL; ALUMINUM ACETATE

SOLUTION/DROPS; OTIC

ACETIC ACID 2% IN AQUEOUS ALUMINUM ACETATE

AT	BAUSCH AND LOMB	2%;0.79%	N40063 001 FEB 25, 1994

DOMEBORO

AT	+ MILES	2%;0.79%	N84476 001

ACETIC ACID, GLACIAL; DESONIDE

SOLUTION/DROPS; OTIC

TRIDESILON

	+ MILES	2%;0.05%	N17914 001

ACETIC ACID, GLACIAL; HYDROCORTISONE

SOLUTION/DROPS; OTIC

ACETASOL HC

AT	BARRE	2%;1%	N87143 001 JAN 13, 1982

HYDROCORTISONE AND ACETIC ACID

AT	THAMES	2%;1%	N88759 001 MAR 04, 1985

VOSOL HC

AT	+ WALLACE	2%;1%	N12770 001

ACETIC ACID, GLACIAL; HYDROCORTISONE; NEOMYCIN SULFATE

SUSPENSION; OTIC

NEO-CORT-DOME

	+ MILES	2%;1%;EQ 0.35% BASE	N50238 001

Prescription Drug Products *(continued)*

ACETOHEXAMIDE

TABLET; ORAL

	ACETOHEXAMIDE		
AB	BARR	250 MG	N70869 001 FEB 09, 1987
AB		500 MG	N70870 001 FEB 09, 1987
AB	DANBURY PHARMA	250 MG	N71893 001 NOV 25, 1987
AB		500 MG	N71894 001 NOV 25, 1987
	DYMELOR		
AB	LILLY	250 MG	N13378 002
AB	+	500 MG	N13378 001

ACETOHYDROXAMIC ACID

TABLET; ORAL

	LITHOSTAT		
	+ MISSION PHARMA	250 MG	N18749 001 MAY 31, 1983

ACETYLCHOLINE CHLORIDE

POWDER FOR RECONSTITUTION; OPHTHALMIC

	MIOCHOL		
	+ IOLAB	20 MG/VIAL	N16211 001
	MIOCHOL-E		
	+ IOLAB	20 MG/VIAL	N20213 001 SEP 22, 1993

ACETYLCYSTEINE

SOLUTION; INHALATION, ORAL

	ACETYLCYSTEINE		
AN	ABBOTT	10%	N73664 001 AUG 30, 1994
AN		20%	N74037 001 AUG 30, 1994
AN	CETUS BEN VENUE	10%	N72323 001 APR 30, 1992
AN		20%	N72324 001 APR 30, 1992
AN	DUPONT MERCK	10%	N71364 001 MAY 01, 1989
AN		20%	N71365 001 MAY 01, 1989
AN	ROXANE	10%	N72621 001 SEP 30, 1992
AN		20%	N72622 001 SEP 30, 1992

ACETYLCYSTEINE *(continued)*

SOLUTION; INHALATION, ORAL

	MUCOMYST		
AN	+ APOTHECON	10%	N13601 002
AN	+	20%	N13601 001
	MUCOSIL-10		
AN	DEY	10%	N70575 001 OCT 14, 1986
	MUCOSIL-20		
AN	DEY	20%	N70576 001 OCT 14, 1986

ACRIVASTINE; PSEUDOEPHEDRINE HYDROCHLORIDE

CAPSULE; ORAL

	SEMPREX-D		
	+ BURROUGHS WELLCOME	8 MG;60 MG	N19806 001 MAR 25, 1994

ACYCLOVIR

CAPSULE; ORAL

	ZOVIRAX		
	+ BURROUGHS WELLCOME	200 MG	N18828 001 JAN 25, 1985

OINTMENT; TOPICAL

	ZOVIRAX		
	+ BURROUGHS WELLCOME	5%	N18604 001 MAR 29, 1982

SUSPENSION; ORAL

	ZOVIRAX		
	+ BURROUGHS WELLCOME	200 MG/5 ML	N19909 001 DEC 22, 1989

TABLET; ORAL

	ZOVIRAX		
	BURROUGHS WELLCOME	400 MG	N20089 001 APR 30, 1991
	+	800 MG	N20089 002 APR 30, 1991

Prescription Drug Products *(continued)*

ACYCLOVIR SODIUM

INJECTABLE; INJECTION

TE	Product / Applicant	Strength	Appl No / Date
	ZOVIRAX		
	+ BURROUGHS WELLCOME	EQ 500 MG BASE/VIAL	N18603 001 OCT 22, 1982
	+	EQ 1 GM BASE/VIAL	N18603 002 JUN 29, 1989

ADENOSINE

INJECTABLE; INJECTION

TE	Product / Applicant	Strength	Appl No / Date
	ADENOCARD		
	+ MEDCO RES	3 MG/ML	N19937 002 OCT 30, 1989

ALBUMIN CHROMATED CR-51 SERUM

INJECTABLE; INJECTION

TE	Product / Applicant	Strength	Appl No / Date
	CHROMALBIN		
	ISO TEX	100uCi/VIAL	N17835 001

ALBUMIN IODINATED I-125 SERUM

INJECTABLE; INJECTION

TE	Product / Applicant	Strength	Appl No / Date
	RADIOIODINATED SERUM ALBUMIN (HUMAN) IHSA I 125		
	MALLINCKRODT	10uCi/ML	N17844 001
		100uCi/ML	N17844 002
		6.67uCi/ML	N17844 003

ALBUMIN IODINATED I-131 SERUM

INJECTABLE; INJECTION

TE	Product / Applicant	Strength	Appl No / Date
	MEGATOPE		
	ISO TEX	0.5mCi/VIAL	N17837 001
		1mCi/VIAL	N17837 002

ALBUTEROL

AEROSOL, METERED; INHALATION

TE	Product / Applicant	Strength	Appl No / Date
	PROVENTIL		
BN	SCHERING	0.09 MG/INH	N17559 001
	VENTOLIN		
BN	+ GLAXO	0.09 MG/INH	N18473 001

ALBUTEROL SULFATE

CAPSULE; INHALATION

TE	Product / Applicant	Strength	Appl No / Date
	VENTOLIN ROTACAPS		
	+ GLAXO	EQ 0.2 MG BASE	N19489 001 MAY 04, 1988

SOLUTION; INHALATION

TE	Product / Applicant	Strength	Appl No / Date
	ALBUTEROL SULFATE		
AN	COPLEY PHARM	EQ 0.083% BASE	N73495 001 MAY 28, 1993
AN		EQ 0.5% BASE	N73307 001 NOV 27, 1991
AN	DEY	EQ 0.083% BASE	N72652 001 FEB 21, 1992
	PROVENTIL		
AN	+ SCHERING	EQ 0.083% BASE	N19243 002 JAN 14, 1987
AN	+	EQ 0.5% BASE	N19243 001 JAN 14, 1987
	VENTOLIN		
AN	GLAXO	EQ 0.083% BASE	N19773 001 APR 23, 1992
AN		EQ 0.5% BASE	N19269 002 JAN 16, 1987

SYRUP; ORAL

TE	Product / Applicant	Strength	Appl No / Date
	ALBUTEROL SULFATE		
AA	LEMMON	EQ 2 MG BASE/5 ML	N73419 001 MAR 30, 1992
AA	WATSON LABS	EQ 2 MG BASE/5 ML	N73165 001 APR 29, 1993
	PROVENTIL		
AA	SCHERING	EQ 2 MG BASE/5 ML	N18062 001 JAN 19, 1983
	VENTOLIN		
AA	GLAXO	EQ 2 MG BASE/5 ML	N19621 001 JUN 10, 1987

TABLET; ORAL

TE	Product / Applicant	Strength	Appl No / Date
	ALBUTEROL SULFATE		
AB	BIOCRAFT	EQ 2 MG BASE	N72619 001 DEC 05, 1989
AB		EQ 4 MG BASE	N72620 001 DEC 05, 1989
AB	COPLEY PHARM	EQ 2 MG BASE	N72966 001 NOV 22, 1991
AB		EQ 4 MG BASE	N72967 001 NOV 22, 1991
AB	DANBURY PHARMA	EQ 2 MG BASE	N72629 001 JAN 31, 1991
AB		EQ 4 MG BASE	N72630 001 JAN 31, 1991

Prescription Drug Products *(continued)*

ALBUTEROL SULFATE *(continued)*

TABLET; ORAL

	ALBUTEROL SULFATE		
AB	GENEVA PHARMS	EQ 2 MG BASE	N72151 001 DEC 05, 1989
AB		EQ 4 MG BASE	N72152 001 DEC 05, 1989
AB	LEDERLE	EQ 2 MG BASE	N72859 001 DEC 20, 1989
AB		EQ 4 MG BASE	N72860 001 DEC 20, 1989
AB	LEMMON	EQ 2 MG BASE	N72938 001 MAR 30, 1990
AB		EQ 4 MG BASE	N72939 001 MAR 30, 1990
AB	MD PHARM	EQ 2 MG BASE	N73120 001 SEP 29, 1992
AB		EQ 4 MG BASE	N73121 001 SEP 29, 1992
AB	MUTUAL PHARM	EQ 2 MG BASE	N72636 001 DEC 05, 1989
AB		EQ 4 MG BASE	N72637 001 DEC 05, 1989
AB	MYLAN	EQ 2 MG BASE	N72893 001 JAN 17, 1991
AB		EQ 4 MG BASE	N72894 001 JAN 17, 1991
AB	NOVOPHARM	EQ 2 MG BASE	N72779 001 JUN 25, 1993
AB		EQ 4 MG BASE	N72780 001 JUN 25, 1993
AB	SIDMAK LABS NJ	EQ 2 MG BASE	N72316 001 DEC 05, 1989
AB		EQ 4 MG BASE	N72317 001 DEC 05, 1989
AB	WATSON LABS	EQ 2 MG BASE	N72764 001 AUG 28, 1991
AB		EQ 4 MG BASE	N72765 001 AUG 28, 1991
	PROVENTIL		
AB	SCHERING	EQ 2 MG BASE	N17853 001 MAY 07, 1982
AB	+	EQ 4 MG BASE	N17853 002 MAY 07, 1982
	VENTOLIN		
AB	GLAXO	EQ 2 MG BASE	N19112 001 JUL 10, 1986
AB		EQ 4 MG BASE	N19112 002 JUL 10, 1986

ALBUTEROL SULFATE *(continued)*

TABLET, EXTENDED RELEASE; ORAL

	PROVENTIL		
BC	SCHERING	EQ 4 MG BASE	N19383 001 JUL 13, 1987
	VOLMAX		
BC	+ MURO	EQ 4 MG BASE	N19604 002 DEC 23, 1992
	+	EQ 8 MG BASE	N19604 001 DEC 23, 1992

ALCLOMETASONE DIPROPIONATE

CREAM; TOPICAL

	ACLOVATE		
	+ GLAXO	0.05%	N18707 001 DEC 14, 1982

OINTMENT; TOPICAL

	ACLOVATE		
	+ GLAXO	0.05%	N18702 001 DEC 14, 1982

ALCOHOL

INJECTABLE; INJECTION

	ALCOHOL 10% AND DEXTROSE 5%		
	MCGAW	10 ML/100 ML	N04589 006
	ALCOHOL 5% AND DEXTROSE 5%		
AP	MCGAW	5 ML/100 ML	N04589 004
	ALCOHOL 5% IN DEXTROSE 5% IN WATER		
AP	BAXTER	5 ML/100 ML	N83256 001
	ALCOHOL 5% IN D5-W		
AP	ABBOTT	5 ML/100 ML	N83263 001

ALFENTANIL HYDROCHLORIDE

INJECTABLE; INJECTION

	ALFENTA		
	+ JANSSEN	EQ 0.5 MG BASE/ML	N19353 001 DEC 29, 1986

ALGLUCERASE

INJECTABLE; INJECTION

	CEREDASE		
	GENZYME	10 UNITS/ML	N20057 004 MAY 08, 1992
	+	80 UNITS/ML	N20057 003 APR 05, 1991

Prescription Drug Products *(continued)*

ALLOPURINOL

TABLET; ORAL

	ALLOPURINOL		
AB	BARR	100 MG	N70466 001 DEC 24, 1985
AB		300 MG	N70467 001 DEC 24, 1985
AB	DANBURY PHARMA	100 MG	N18832 002 SEP 28, 1984
AB		300 MG	N18877 001 SEP 28, 1984
AB	GENEVA PHARMS	100 MG	N70268 001 DEC 31, 1985
AB		300 MG	N70269 001 DEC 31, 1985
AB	MUTUAL PHARM	100 MG	N71449 001 JAN 09, 1987
AB		300 MG	N71450 001 JAN 09, 1987
AB	MYLAN	100 MG	N18659 001 OCT 24, 1986
AB		300 MG	N18659 002 OCT 24, 1986
AB	PAR PHARM	100 MG	N70150 001 DEC 10, 1985
AB		300 MG	N70147 001 DEC 10, 1985
AB	SUPERPHARM	300 MG	N70951 001 NOV 30, 1988
	LOPURIN		
AB	BOOTS	100 MG	N71586 001 APR 02, 1987
AB		300 MG	N71587 001 APR 02, 1987
	ZYLOPRIM		
AB	BURROUGHS WELLCOME	100 MG	N16084 001
AB +		300 MG	N16084 002

ALPRAZOLAM

CONCENTRATE; ORAL

	ALPRAZOLAM		
	ROXANE	1 MG/ML	N74312 001 OCT 31, 1993

SOLUTION; ORAL

	ALPRAZOLAM		
	ROXANE	0.5 MG/5 ML	N74314 001 OCT 31, 1993

ALPRAZOLAM *(continued)*

TABLET; ORAL

	ALPRAZOLAM		
AB	ALPHAPHARM	0.25 MG	N74046 001 OCT 19, 1993
AB		0.5 MG	N74046 002 OCT 19, 1993
AB		1 MG	N74046 003 OCT 19, 1993
AB	LEDERLE	0.25 MG	N74174 001 OCT 19, 1993
AB		0.5 MG	N74174 002 OCT 19, 1993
AB		1 MG	N74174 003 OCT 19, 1993
AB		2 MG	N74174 004 OCT 19, 1993
AB	MYLAN	0.25 MG	N74215 001 JAN 27, 1994
AB		0.5 MG	N74215 002 JAN 27, 1994
AB		1 MG	N74215 003 JAN 27, 1994
AB		2 MG	N74215 004 JAN 27, 1994
AB	NOVOPHARM	0.25 MG	N74085 001 FEB 16, 1994
AB		0.5 MG	N74085 002 FEB 16, 1994
AB		1 MG	N74085 003 FEB 16, 1994
AB	PUREPAC PHARM	0.25 MG	N74342 001 OCT 31, 1993
AB		0.5 MG	N74342 002 OCT 31, 1993
AB		1 MG	N74342 003 OCT 31, 1993
AB		2 MG	N74342 004 OCT 31, 1993
AB	ROXANE	0.25 MG	N74199 001 OCT 19, 1993
AB		0.5 MG	N74199 002 OCT 19, 1993
AB		1 MG	N74199 003 OCT 19, 1993
AB	ZENITH LABS	0.25 MG	N74294 001 JUL 29, 1994
AB		0.5 MG	N74294 002 JUL 29, 1994
AB		1 MG	N74294 003 JUL 29, 1994
AB		2 MG	N74294 004 JUL 29, 1994

Prescription Drug Products *(continued)*

ALPRAZOLAM *(continued)*

TABLET; ORAL
XANAX

AB	UPJOHN	0.25 MG	N18276 001
AB		0.5 MG	N18276 002
AB	+	1 MG	N18276 003
AB		2 MG	N18276 004 NOV 27, 1985

ALPROSTADIL

INJECTABLE; INJECTION
PROSTIN VR PEDIATRIC

	+ UPJOHN	0.5 MG/ML	N18484 001

ALSEROXYLON

TABLET; ORAL
RAUWILOID

	+ 3M	2 MG	N08867 001

ALTRETAMINE

CAPSULE; ORAL
HEXALEN

	+ US BIOSCIENCE	50 MG	N19926 001 DEC 26, 1990

ALUMINUM ACETATE; *MULTIPLE*

SEE ACETIC ACID, GLACIAL; ALUMINUM ACETATE

AMANTADINE HYDROCHLORIDE

CAPSULE; ORAL
AMANTADINE HCL

AB	INVAMED	100 MG	N71293 001 FEB 18, 1987
AB	ROSEMONT PHARM	100 MG	N70589 001 AUG 05, 1986

SYMADINE

AB	SOLVAY	100 MG	N71000 001 SEP 04, 1986

SYMMETREL

AB	+ DUPONT MERCK	100 MG	N16020 001
AB		100 MG	N17117 001

AMANTADINE HYDROCHLORIDE *(continued)*

SYRUP; ORAL
AMANTADINE HCL

AA	BARRE	50 MG/5 ML	N72655 001 OCT 30, 1990
AA	COPLEY PHARM	50 MG/5 ML	N73115 001 AUG 23, 1991
AA	MIKART	50 MG/5 ML	N74028 001 JUN 28, 1993

SYMMETREL

AA	DUPONT MERCK	50 MG/5 ML	N16023 002
AA		50 MG/5 ML	N17118 001

AMBENONIUM CHLORIDE

TABLET; ORAL
MYTELASE

	STERLING WINTHROP	10 MG	N10155 002

AMCINONIDE

CREAM; TOPICAL
CYCLOCORT

	LEDERLE	0.025%	N18116 001
	+	0.1%	N18116 002

LOTION; TOPICAL
CYCLOCORT

	+ LEDERLE	0.1%	N19729 001 JUN 13, 1988

OINTMENT; TOPICAL
CYCLOCORT

	+ LEDERLE	0.1%	N18498 001

AMIKACIN SULFATE

INJECTABLE; INJECTION
AMIKACIN

AP	BEDFORD	EQ 50 MG BASE/ML	N63313 001 APR 11, 1994
AP		EQ 250 MG BASE/ML	N63315 001 APR 11, 1994
AP	DUPONT MERCK	EQ 50 MG BASE/ML	N63350 001 JUL 30, 1993
AP		EQ 250 MG BASE/ML	N63350 002 JUL 30, 1993
AP	+ ELKINS SINN	EQ 50 MG BASE/ML	N63274 001 MAY 18, 1992
AP	+	EQ 250 MG BASE/ML	N63275 001 MAY 18, 1992
AP	GENSIA	EQ 50 MG BASE/ML	N64045 001 SEP 28, 1993
AP		EQ 250 MG BASE/ML	N64045 002 SEP 28, 1993

Prescription Drug Products *(continued)*

AMILORIDE HYDROCHLORIDE

TABLET; ORAL

AMILORIDE HCL
AB PAR PHARM 5 MG N70346 001 JAN 22, 1986

MIDAMOR
AB + MERCK SHARP DOHME 5 MG N18200 001

AMILORIDE HYDROCHLORIDE; HYDROCHLOROTHIAZIDE

TABLET; ORAL

AMILORIDE HCL AND HYDROCHLOROTHIAZIDE
AB BARR EQ 5 MG ANHYDROUS;50 MG N71111 001 MAY 10, 1988
AB BIOCRAFT EQ 5 MG ANHYDROUS;50 MG N70795 001 APR 17, 1988
AB GENEVA PHARMS EQ 5 MG ANHYDROUS;50 MG N73357 001 NOV 27, 1991
AB MYLAN EQ 5 MG ANHYDROUS;50 MG N73209 001 OCT 31, 1991
AB ROYCE LABS EQ 5 MG ANHYDROUS;50 MG N73334 001 JUL 19, 1991

HYDRO-RIDE
AB PAR PHARM EQ 5 MG ANHYDROUS;50 MG N70347 001 DEC 25, 1990

MODURETIC 5-50
AB + MERCK SHARP DOHME EQ 5 MG ANHYDROUS;50 MG N18201 001

AMINO ACIDS

INJECTABLE; INJECTION

AMINESS 5.2% ESSENTIAL AMINO ACIDS W/ HISTADINE
PHARMACIA 5.2% N18901 001 APR 06, 1984

AMINOSYN II 10%
ABBOTT 10% N19438 005 APR 03, 1986

AMINOSYN II 10% IN PLASTIC CONTAINER
ABBOTT 10% N20015 001 DEC 19, 1991

AMINOSYN II 15% IN PLASTIC CONTAINER
ABBOTT 15% N20041 001 DEC 19, 1991

AMINOSYN II 3.5%
ABBOTT 3.5% N19438 001 APR 03, 1986

AMINO ACIDS *(continued)*

INJECTABLE; INJECTION

AMINOSYN II 5%
ABBOTT 5% N19438 002 APR 03, 1986

AMINOSYN II 7%
ABBOTT 7% N19438 003 APR 03, 1986

AMINOSYN II 8.5%
ABBOTT 8.5% N19438 004 APR 03, 1986

AMINOSYN 10%
ABBOTT 10% N17673 003

AMINOSYN 10% (PH6)
ABBOTT 10% N17673 008 NOV 18, 1985

AMINOSYN 3.5%
ABBOTT 3.5% N17789 004

AMINOSYN 5%
ABBOTT 5% N17673 001

AMINOSYN 7%
ABBOTT 7% N17673 002

AMINOSYN 7% (PH6)
ABBOTT 7% N17673 006 NOV 18, 1985

AMINOSYN 8.5%
ABBOTT 8.5% N17673 004

AMINOSYN 8.5% (PH6)
ABBOTT 8.5% N17673 007 NOV 18, 1985

AMINOSYN-HBC 7%
ABBOTT 7% N19374 001 JUL 12, 1985

AMINOSYN-PF 10%
ABBOTT 10% N19492 002 OCT 17, 1986

AMINOSYN-PF 7%
ABBOTT 7% N19398 001 SEP 06, 1985

AMINOSYN-RF 5.2%
ABBOTT 5.2% N18429 001

BRANCHAMIN 4%
BAXTER 4% N18678 001 SEP 28, 1984

BRANCHAMIN 4% IN PLASTIC CONTAINER
BAXTER 4% N18684 001 SEP 28, 1984

FREAMINE HBC 6.9%
MCGAW 6.9% N16822 006 MAY 17, 1983

FREAMINE III 10%
MCGAW 10% N16822 005

Prescription Drug Products *(continued)*

AMINO ACIDS *(continued)*
INJECTABLE; INJECTION
FREAMINE III 8.5%
MCGAW 8.5% N16822 004
HEPATAMINE 8%
MCGAW 8% N18676 001 AUG 03, 1982
NEPHRAMINE 5.4%
MCGAW 5.4% N17766 001
NOVAMINE 11.4%
PHARMACIA 11.4% N17957 003 AUG 09, 1982
NOVAMINE 15%
PHARMACIA 15% N17957 004 NOV 28, 1986
NOVAMINE 15% SULFITE FREE IN PLASTIC CONTAINER
BAXTER 15% N20107 001 FEB 05, 1993
RENAMIN W/O ELECTROLYTES
BAXTER 6.5% N17493 007 OCT 15, 1982
TRAVASOL 10% IN PLASTIC CONTAINER
BAXTER 10% N18931 003 AUG 23, 1984
TRAVASOL 10% W/O ELECTROLYTES
BAXTER 10% N17493 006
TRAVASOL 5.5% IN PLASTIC CONTAINER
BAXTER 5.5% N18931 001 AUG 23, 1984
TRAVASOL 5.5% W/O ELECTROLYTES
BAXTER 5.5% N17493 004
TRAVASOL 8.5% IN PLASTIC CONTAINER
BAXTER 8.5% N18931 002 AUG 23, 1984
TRAVASOL 8.5% W/O ELECTROLYTES
BAXTER 8.5% N17493 005
TROPHAMINE
MCGAW 6% N19018 001 JUL 20, 1984
TROPHAMINE 10%
MCGAW 10% N19018 003 SEP 07, 1988

AMINO ACIDS; CALCIUM ACETATE; GLYCERIN; MAGNESIUM ACETATE; PHOSPHORIC ACID; POTASSIUM CHLORIDE; SODIUM ACETATE; SODIUM CHLORIDE
INJECTABLE; INJECTION
PROCALAMINE
MCGAW 3%;26 MG/100 ML;3 GM/100 ML;54 MG/100 ML;41 MG/100 ML;150 MG/100 ML;200 MG/100 ML;120 MG/100 ML N18582 001 MAY 08, 1982

AMINO ACIDS; CALCIUM CHLORIDE; DEXTROSE; MAGNESIUM CHLORIDE; POTASSIUM CHLORIDE; POTASSIUM PHOSPHATE, DIBASIC; SODIUM CHLORIDE
INJECTABLE; INJECTION
AMINOSYN II 3.5% W/ ELECTROLYTES IN DEXTROSE 25% W/ CALCIUM IN PLASTIC CONTAINER
ABBOTT 3.5%;36.8 MG/100 ML;25 GM/100 ML;51 MG/100 ML;22.4 MG/100 ML;261 MG/100 ML;205 MG/100 ML N19683 001 NOV 07, 1988
3.5%;36.8 MG/100 ML;25 GM/100 ML;51 MG/100 ML;22.4 MG/100 ML;261 MG/100 ML;205 MG/100 ML N19714 001 SEP 12, 1988
AMINOSYN II 4.25% W/ ELECTROLYTES IN DEXTROSE 20% W/ CALCIUM IN PLASTIC CONTAINER
ABBOTT 4.25%;36.8 MG/100 ML;20 GM/100 ML;51 MG/100 ML;22.4 MG/100 ML;261 MG/100 ML;205 MG/100 ML N19683 002 NOV 07, 1988
4.25%;36.8 MG/100 ML;20 GM/100 ML;51 MG/100 ML;22.4 MG/100 ML;261 MG/100 ML;205 MG/100 ML N19714 002 SEP 12, 1988

Prescription Drug Products *(continued)*

AMINO ACIDS; CALCIUM CHLORIDE; DEXTROSE; MAGNESIUM CHLORIDE; POTASSIUM CHLORIDE; POTASSIUM PHOSPHATE, DIBASIC; SODIUM CHLORIDE *(continued)*

INJECTABLE; INJECTION

AMINOSYN II 4.25% W/ ELECTROLYTES IN DEXTROSE 25% W/ CALCIUM IN PLASTIC CONTAINER

ABBOTT	4.25%;36.8 MG/100 ML;25 GM/100 ML;51 MG/100 ML;22.4 MG/100 ML;261 MG/100 ML;205 MG/100 ML	N19683 003 NOV 07, 1988
	4.25%;36.8 MG/100 ML;25 GM/100 ML;51 MG/100 ML;22.4 MG/100 ML;261 MG/100 ML;205 MG/100 ML	N19714 004 SEP 12, 1988

AMINOSYN II 5% W/ ELECTROLYTES IN DEXTROSE 25% W/ CALCIUM IN PLASTIC CONTAINER

ABBOTT	5%;36.8 MG/100 ML;25 GM/100 ML;51 MG/100 ML;22.4 MG/100 ML;261 MG/100 ML;205 MG/100 ML	N19683 004 NOV 07, 1988
	5%;36.8 MG/100 ML;25 GM/100 ML;51 MG/100 ML;22.4 MG/100 ML;261 MG/100 ML;205 MG/100 ML	N19714 003 SEP 12, 1988

AMINO ACIDS; DEXTROSE

INJECTABLE; INJECTION

AMINOSYN II 3.5% IN DEXTROSE 25% IN PLASTIC CONTAINER

ABBOTT	3.5%;25 GM/100 ML	N19505 002 NOV 07, 1986
	3.5%;25 GM/100 ML	N19681 001 NOV 01, 1988
	3.5%;25 GM/100 ML	N19713 006 SEP 09, 1988

AMINOSYN II 3.5% IN DEXTROSE 5% IN PLASTIC CONTAINER

ABBOTT	3.5%;5 GM/100 ML	N19506 001 NOV 07, 1986
	3.5%;5 GM/100 ML	N19681 002 NOV 01, 1988
	3.5%;5 GM/100 ML	N19713 002 SEP 09, 1988

AMINO ACIDS; DEXTROSE *(continued)*

INJECTABLE; INJECTION

AMINOSYN II 4.25% IN DEXTROSE 10% IN PLASTIC CONTAINER

ABBOTT	4.25%;10 GM/100 ML	N19681 004 NOV 01, 1988
	4.25%;10 GM/100 ML	N19713 001 SEP 09, 1988

AMINOSYN II 4.25% IN DEXTROSE 20% IN PLASTIC CONTAINER

ABBOTT	4.25%;20 GM/100 ML	N19681 005 NOV 01, 1988
	4.25%;20 GM/100 ML	N19713 004 SEP 09, 1988

AMINOSYN II 4.25% IN DEXTROSE 25% IN PLASTIC CONTAINER

ABBOTT	4.25%;25 GM/100 ML	N19504 002 NOV 07, 1986
	4.25%;25 GM/100 ML	N19681 003 NOV 01, 1988
	4.25%;25 GM/100 ML	N19713 005 SEP 09, 1988

AMINOSYN II 5% IN DEXTROSE 25% IN PLASTIC CONTAINER

ABBOTT	5%;25 GM/100 ML	N19681 006 NOV 01, 1988
	5%;25 GM/100 ML	N19713 003 SEP 09, 1988

TRAVASOL 2.75% IN DEXTROSE 10% IN PLASTIC CONTAINER

BAXTER	2.75%;10 GM/100 ML	N19520 002 SEP 23, 1988

TRAVASOL 2.75% IN DEXTROSE 15% IN PLASTIC CONTAINER

BAXTER	2.75%;15 GM/100 ML	N19520 003 SEP 23, 1988

TRAVASOL 2.75% IN DEXTROSE 20% IN PLASTIC CONTAINER

BAXTER	2.75%;20 GM/100 ML	N19520 004 SEP 23, 1988

TRAVASOL 2.75% IN DEXTROSE 25% IN PLASTIC CONTAINER

BAXTER	2.75%;25 GM/100 ML	N19520 005 SEP 23, 1988

TRAVASOL 2.75% IN DEXTROSE 5% IN PLASTIC CONTAINER

BAXTER	2.75%;5 GM/100 ML	N19520 001 SEP 23, 1988

TRAVASOL 4.25% IN DEXTROSE 10% IN PLASTIC CONTAINER

BAXTER	4.25%;10 GM/100 ML	N19520 007 SEP 23, 1988

TRAVASOL 4.25% IN DEXTROSE 15% IN PLASTIC CONTAINER

BAXTER	4.25%;15 GM/100 ML	N19520 008 SEP 23, 1988

TRAVASOL 4.25% IN DEXTROSE 20% IN PLASTIC CONTAINER

BAXTER	4.25%;20 GM/100 ML	N19520 009 SEP 23, 1988

TRAVASOL 4.25% IN DEXTROSE 25% IN PLASTIC CONTAINER

BAXTER	4.25%;25 GM/100 ML	N19520 010 SEP 23, 1988

TRAVASOL 4.25% IN DEXTROSE 5% IN PLASTIC CONTAINER

BAXTER	4.25%;5 GM/100 ML	N19520 006 SEP 23, 1988

Prescription Drug Products *(continued)*

AMINO ACIDS; DEXTROSE; MAGNESIUM CHLORIDE; POTASSIUM ACETATE; POTASSIUM CHLORIDE; POTASSIUM PHOSPHATE, DIBASIC; SODIUM CHLORIDE

INJECTABLE; INJECTION
AMINOSYN II 4.25% W/ ELECT AND ADJUSTED PHOSPHATE IN DEXTROSE 10% IN PLASTIC CONTAINER
ABBOTT 4.25%;10 GM/100 ML;51 MG/100 ML;176.5 MG/100 ML;22.4 MG/100 ML;104.5 MG/100 ML;205 MG/100 ML N19682 003 NOV 01, 1988
4.25%;10 GM/100 ML;51 MG/100 ML;176.5 MG/100 ML;22.4 MG/100 ML;104.5 MG/100 ML;205 MG/100 ML N19712 002 SEP 08, 1988

AMINO ACIDS; DEXTROSE; MAGNESIUM CHLORIDE; POTASSIUM CHLORIDE; SODIUM CHLORIDE; SODIUM PHOSPHATE, DIBASIC

INJECTABLE; INJECTION
AMINOSYN II M 3.5% IN DEXTROSE 5% IN PLASTIC CONTAINER
ABBOTT 3.5%;5 GM/100 ML;30 MG/100 ML;97 MG/100 ML;120 MG/100 ML;49.3 MG/100 ML N19682 001 NOV 01, 1988
AMINOSYN II 3.5% M IN DEXTROSE 5% IN PLASTIC CONTAINER
ABBOTT 3.5%;5 GM/100 ML;30 MG/100 ML;97 MG/100 ML;120 MG/100 ML;49.3 MG/100 ML N19712 001 SEP 08, 1988
AMINOSYN II 4.25% M IN DEXTROSE 10% IN PLASTIC CONTAINER
ABBOTT 4.25%;5 GM/100 ML;30 MG/100 ML;97 MG/100 ML;120 MG/100 ML;49.3 MG/100 ML N19682 002 NOV 01, 1988

AMINO ACIDS; MAGNESIUM ACETATE; PHOSPHORIC ACID; POTASSIUM ACETATE; POTASSIUM CHLORIDE; SODIUM ACETATE

INJECTABLE; INJECTION
FREAMINE III 8.5% W/ ELECTROLYTES
MCGAW 8.5%;110 MG/100 ML;230 MG/100 ML;10 MG/100 ML;440 MG/100 ML;690 MG/100 ML N16822 007 JUL 01, 1988

AMINO ACIDS; MAGNESIUM ACETATE; PHOSPHORIC ACID; POTASSIUM ACETATE; SODIUM CHLORIDE

INJECTABLE; INJECTION
AMINOSYN 3.5% M
ABBOTT 3.5%;21 MG/100 ML;40 MG/100 ML;128 MG/100 ML;234 MG/100 ML N17789 003

AMINO ACIDS; MAGNESIUM ACETATE; PHOSPHORIC ACID; POTASSIUM CHLORIDE; SODIUM ACETATE; SODIUM CHLORIDE

INJECTABLE; INJECTION
FREAMINE III 3% W/ ELECTROLYTES
MCGAW 3%;54 MG/100 ML;40 MG/100 ML;150 MG/100 ML;200 MG/100 ML;120 MG/100 ML N16822 003

AMINO ACIDS; MAGNESIUM CHLORIDE; POTASSIUM CHLORIDE; POTASSIUM PHOSPHATE, DIBASIC; SODIUM CHLORIDE

INJECTABLE; INJECTION
AMINOSYN II 10% W/ ELECTROLYTES
ABBOTT 10%;102 MG/100 ML;45 MG/100 ML;522 MG/100 ML;410 MG/100 ML N19437 004 APR 03, 1986
AMINOSYN II 8.5% W/ ELECTROLYTES
ABBOTT 8.5%;102 MG/100 ML;45 MG/100 ML;522 MG/100 ML;410 MG/100 ML N19437 005 APR 03, 1986

Prescription Drug Products *(continued)*

AMINO ACIDS; MAGNESIUM CHLORIDE; POTASSIUM PHOSPHATE, DIBASIC; SODIUM ACETATE; SODIUM CHLORIDE

INJECTABLE; INJECTION
TRAVASOL 3.5% W/ ELECTROLYTES
BAXTER 3.5%;51 MG/100 ML;131 MG/100 ML;218 MG/100 ML;35 MG/100 ML N17493 003
TRAVASOL 5.5% W/ ELECTROLYTES
BAXTER 5.5%;102 MG/100 ML;522 MG/100 ML;431 MG/100 ML;224 MG/100 ML N17493 001
TRAVASOL 8.5% W/ ELECTROLYTES
BAXTER 8.5%;102 MG/100 ML;522 MG/100 ML;594 MG/100 ML;154 MG/100 ML N17493 002

AMINO ACIDS; MAGNESIUM CHLORIDE; POTASSIUM PHOSPHATE, DIBASIC; SODIUM CHLORIDE

INJECTABLE; INJECTION
AMINOSYN 7% W/ ELECTROLYTES
ABBOTT 7%;102 MG/100 ML;522 MG/100 ML;410 MG/100 ML N17789 002
AMINOSYN 8.5% W/ ELECTROLYTES
ABBOTT 8.5%;102 MG/100 ML;522 MG/100 ML;410 MG/100 ML N17673 005

AMINOCAPROIC ACID

INJECTABLE; INJECTION
AMICAR
AP + IMMUNEX 250 MG/ML N15229 002
AMINOCAPROIC ACID
AP ABBOTT 250 MG/ML N70888 001 JUN 16, 1988
AP ELKINS SINN 250 MG/ML N18590 001 OCT 29, 1982
AP LUITPOLD 250 MG/ML N71192 001 DEC 01, 1987
AMINOCAPROIC ACID IN PLASTIC CONTAINER
AP ABBOTT 250 MG/ML N70010 001 MAR 09, 1987

SYRUP; ORAL
AMICAR
IMMUNEX 1.25 GM/5 ML N15230 002
TABLET; ORAL
AMICAR
+ IMMUNEX 500 MG N15197 001

AMINOGLUTETHIMIDE

TABLET; ORAL
CYTADREN
+ CIBA 250 MG N18202 001

AMINOHIPPURATE SODIUM

INJECTABLE; INJECTION
AMINOHIPPURATE SODIUM
+ MERCK SHARP DOHME 20% N05619 001

AMINOPHYLLINE

INJECTABLE; INJECTION
AMINOPHYLLIN
AP + SEARLE 25 MG/ML N87243 001 MAY 24, 1982
AMINOPHYLLINE
AP ABBOTT 25 MG/ML N87242 001 OCT 26, 1983
AP 25 MG/ML N87601 001 JUL 23, 1982
AP ELKINS SINN 25 MG/ML N87239 001
AP FUJISAWA 25 MG/ML N87200 001
AP 25 MG/ML N88407 001 JAN 25, 1984
AP GENSIA 25 MG/ML N81142 001 SEP 25, 1991
AP INTL MEDICATION 25 MG/ML N87209 001 FEB 01, 1982
AP KING PHARMS 25 MG/ML N86606 001
AP LUITPOLD 25 MG/ML N87240 001
AP 25 MG/ML N87600 001
AP PHARMA SERVE NY 25 MG/ML N87387 001 JUN 03, 1983
AP 25 MG/ML N87392 001 DEC 15, 1983
AP SMITH AND NEPHEW 25 MG/ML N88749 001 MAY 30, 1985
AMINOPHYLLINE IN SODIUM CHLORIDE 0.45%
ABBOTT 100 MG/100 ML N88147 002 MAY 03, 1983
200 MG/100 ML N88147 003 MAY 03, 1982

SOLUTION; ORAL
AMINOPHYLLINE
AA ROXANE 105 MG/5 ML N88126 001 AUG 19, 1983
AMINOPHYLLINE DYE FREE
AA BARRE 105 MG/5 ML N87727 001 APR 16, 1982

Prescription Drug Products *(continued)*

AMINOPHYLLINE *(continued)*

TE	Dosage form / Product / Firm	Strength	Appl. No. / Date
	SUPPOSITORY; RECTAL		
	TRUPHYLLINE		
	G AND W LABS	250 MG	N85498 001 MAR 23, 1983
		500 MG	N85498 002 JAN 03, 1983
	TABLET; ORAL		
	AMINOPHYLLINE		
AB	GENEVA PHARMS	100 MG	N85262 002
AB		200 MG	N85261 002
AB	GLOBAL PHARMS	100 MG	N84574 001
AB		200 MG	N84576 001
BD	HALSEY	100 MG	N84674 001
BD	PHOENIX LABS NY	100 MG	N85409 001
BD		200 MG	N85410 001
AB	+ ROXANE	100 MG	N87500 001 FEB 09, 1982
AB	+	200 MG	N87501 001 FEB 09, 1982
AB	WEST WARD PHARM	100 MG	N84540 001
AB		200 MG	N85003 001
	TABLET, EXTENDED RELEASE; ORAL		
	PHYLLOCONTIN		
	+ PURDUE FREDERICK	225 MG	N86760 001

AMINOSALICYLATE SODIUM

TE	Dosage form / Product / Firm	Strength	Appl. No. / Date
	POWDER; ORAL		
	P.A.S. SODIUM		
AA	CENTURY PHARMS	4 GM/PACKET	N80947 001
	SODIUM AMINOSALICYLATE		
AA	HEXCEL	100%	N80097 001
	TABLET; ORAL		
	SODIUM P.A.S.		
	+ LANNETT	500 MG	N80138 002

AMINOSALICYLATE SODIUM; AMINOSALICYLIC ACID

TE	Dosage form / Product / Firm	Strength	Appl. No. / Date
	TABLET; ORAL		
	NEOPASALATE		
	+ WALLACE	846 MG;112 MG	N80059 002

AMINOSALICYLIC ACID

TE	Dosage form / Product / Firm	Strength	Appl. No. / Date
	GRANULE, DELAYED RELEASE; ORAL		
	PASER		
	+ JACOBUS	4 GM/PACKET	N74346 001 JUN 30, 1994

AMINOSALICYLIC ACID; *MULTIPLE*

SEE AMINOSALICYLATE SODIUM; AMINOSALICYLIC ACID

AMIODARONE HYDROCHLORIDE

TE	Dosage form / Product / Firm	Strength	Appl. No. / Date
	TABLET; ORAL		
	CORDARONE		
	+ WYETH AYERST	200 MG	N18972 001 DEC 24, 1985

AMITRIPTYLINE HYDROCHLORIDE

TE	Dosage form / Product / Firm	Strength	Appl. No. / Date
	CONCENTRATE; ORAL		
	ENDEP		
	ROCHE	40 MG/ML	N85749 001
	INJECTABLE; INJECTION		
	AMITRIPTYLINE HCL		
AP	STERIS	10 MG/ML	N85594 001
	ELAVIL		
AP	+ ZENECA	10 MG/ML	N12704 001
	TABLET; ORAL		
	AMITRIPTYLINE HCL		
AB	BIOCRAFT	10 MG	N84910 003
AB		25 MG	N85031 001
AB		50 MG	N85032 001
AB		75 MG	N85030 001
AB		100 MG	N85836 001
BP	COPLEY PHARM	10 MG	N88421 001 APR 30, 1984
BP		25 MG	N88422 001 APR 30, 1984
BP		50 MG	N88423 001 APR 30, 1984
BP		75 MG	N88424 001 APR 30, 1984
BP		100 MG	N88425 001 APR 30, 1984
BP		150 MG	N88426 001 APR 30, 1984
AB	DANBURY PHARMA	10 MG	N88620 001 MAR 02, 1984
AB		25 MG	N88621 001 MAR 02, 1984
AB		50 MG	N88622 001 MAR 02, 1984
AB		75 MG	N88633 001 MAR 02, 1984
AB		100 MG	N88634 001 MAR 02, 1984
AB		150 MG	N88635 001 MAR 02, 1984

Prescription Drug Products *(continued)*

AMITRIPTYLINE HYDROCHLORIDE *(continued)*

TABLET; ORAL

AMITRIPTYLINE HCL

AB	GENEVA PHARMS	10 MG	N85969 001	
AB		25 MG	N85966 001	
AB		50 MG	N85968 001	
AB		75 MG	N85971 001	
AB		100 MG	N85967 001	
AB		150 MG	N85970 001	
BP	HALSEY	10 MG	N85923 001	
BP		25 MG	N85922 001	
BP		50 MG	N85925 001	
BP		75 MG	N85926 001	MAY 20, 1983
BP		100 MG	N85927 001	MAY 20, 1983
AB	MD PHARM	10 MG	N85864 001	
AB		25 MG	N85935 001	
AB		50 MG	N85936 001	
AB		75 MG	N86337 001	
AB		100 MG	N86336 001	
AB		150 MG	N86335 001	
AB	MUTUAL PHARM	10 MG	N89398 001	JUL 14, 1987
AB		25 MG	N89399 001	JUL 14, 1987
AB		50 MG	N89400 001	JUL 14, 1987
AB		75 MG	N89401 001	JUL 14, 1987
AB		100 MG	N89402 001	JUL 14, 1987
AB		150 MG	N89403 001	JUL 14, 1987
AB	MYLAN	10 MG	N86157 001	
AB		25 MG	N86010 001	
AB		50 MG	N86009 001	
AB		75 MG	N86011 001	
AB		100 MG	N86158 001	
AB		150 MG	N86153 001	
AB	PUREPAC PHARM	10 MG	N88075 001	SEP 16, 1983
AB		25 MG	N88076 001	MAY 20, 1983
AB		50 MG	N88077 001	SEP 16, 1983
AB		75 MG	N88078 001	SEP 16, 1983
AB		100 MG	N88079 001	SEP 16, 1983

AMITRIPTYLINE HYDROCHLORIDE *(continued)*

TABLET; ORAL

AMITRIPTYLINE HCL

AB	ROXANE	10 MG	N86002 001	
AB		25 MG	N85944 001	
AB		50 MG	N85945 001	
AB		75 MG	N86004 001	
AB		100 MG	N86003 001	
AB		150 MG	N86090 001	
AB	SIDMAK LABS NJ	10 MG	N88883 001	SEP 26, 1984
AB		25 MG	N88884 001	SEP 26, 1984
AB		50 MG	N88885 001	SEP 26, 1984
AB		75 MG	N88886 001	SEP 26, 1984
AB		100 MG	N88887 001	SEP 26, 1984
AB		150 MG	N88888 001	SEP 26, 1984
AB	SUPERPHARM	10 MG	N88853 001	NOV 13, 1984
AB		25 MG	N88854 001	NOV 13, 1984
AB		50 MG	N88855 001	NOV 13, 1984
AB		75 MG	N88856 001	NOV 13, 1984
AB		100 MG	N88857 001	NOV 13, 1984

ELAVIL

AB	ZENECA	10 MG	N12703 001	
AB	+	25 MG	N12703 003	
AB		50 MG	N12703 004	
AB		75 MG	N12703 005	
AB		100 MG	N12703 006	
AB		150 MG	N12703 007	

ENDEP

AB	ROCHE	10 MG	N83639 001	
AB		25 MG	N83639 002	
AB		50 MG	N83639 003	
AB		75 MG	N83639 004	
AB		100 MG	N83639 005	
AB		150 MG	N85303 001	

Prescription Drug Products *(continued)*

AMITRIPTYLINE HYDROCHLORIDE; CHLORDIAZEPOXIDE

TABLET; ORAL

CHLORDIAZEPOXIDE AND AMITRIPTYLINE HCL

AB	BARR	EQ 12.5 MG BASE;5 MG	N70765 001 DEC 10, 1986
AB		EQ 25 MG BASE;10 MG	N70766 001 DEC 10, 1986
AB	DANBURY PHARMA	EQ 12.5 MG BASE;5 MG	N72052 001 DEC 16, 1988
AB		EQ 25 MG BASE;10 MG	N72053 001 DEC 16, 1988
AB	MYLAN	EQ 12.5 MG BASE;5 MG	N71296 001 DEC 10, 1986
AB		EQ 25 MG BASE;10 MG	N71297 001 DEC 10, 1986
AB	PAR PHARM	EQ 12.5 MG BASE;5 MG	N72277 001 MAY 09, 1988
AB		EQ 25 MG BASE;10 MG	N72278 001 MAY 09, 1988
	LIMBITROL		
AB	ROCHE	EQ 12.5 MG BASE;5 MG	N16949 001
AB +		EQ 25 MG BASE;10 MG	N16949 002

AMITRIPTYLINE HYDROCHLORIDE; PERPHENAZINE

TABLET; ORAL

	ETRAFON 2-10		
BP	SCHERING	10 MG;2 MG	N14713 007
	ETRAFON 2-25		
BP	SCHERING	25 MG;2 MG	N14713 004
	ETRAFON-A		
BP	SCHERING	10 MG;4 MG	N14713 002
	ETRAFON-FORTE		
BP	SCHERING	25 MG;4 MG	N14713 006
	PERPHENAZINE AND AMITRIPTYLINE HCL		
AB	BARR	10 MG;2 MG	N71077 001 NOV 12, 1986
AB		10 MG;4 MG	N71078 001 NOV 12, 1986
AB		25 MG;2 MG	N70297 001 NOV 12, 1986
AB		25 MG;4 MG	N71079 001 NOV 12, 1986

AMITRIPTYLINE HYDROCHLORIDE; PERPHENAZINE *(continued)*

TABLET; ORAL

PERPHENAZINE AND AMITRIPTYLINE HCL

AB	DANBURY PHARMA	10 MG;2 MG	N72539 001 FEB 15, 1989
AB		10 MG;4 MG	N72540 001 FEB 15, 1989
AB		25 MG;2 MG	N72541 001 FEB 15, 1989
AB		25 MG;4 MG	N72134 001 FEB 15, 1989
AB		50 MG;4 MG	N72135 001 FEB 15, 1989
AB	GENEVA PHARMS	10 MG;2 MG	N71062 001 NOV 27, 1987
AB		10 MG;4 MG	N71862 001 DEC 21, 1987
AB		25 MG;2 MG	N71063 001 NOV 27, 1987
AB		25 MG;4 MG	N71064 001 NOV 27, 1987
AB		50 MG;4 MG	N71863 001 DEC 21, 1987
AB	MYLAN	10 MG;2 MG	N70336 001 NOV 10, 1988
AB		10 MG;4 MG	N71442 001 NOV 10, 1988
AB		25 MG;2 MG	N70337 001 NOV 10, 1988
AB		25 MG;4 MG	N70338 001 NOV 10, 1988
AB		50 MG;4 MG	N71443 001 NOV 10, 1988
AB	ROYCE LABS	10 MG;2 MG	N73007 001 OCT 17, 1991
AB		10 MG;4 MG	N73009 001 OCT 17, 1991
AB		25 MG;2 MG	N73008 001 OCT 17, 1991
AB		25 MG;4 MG	N73010 001 OCT 17, 1991
AB	ZENITH LABS	10 MG;2 MG	N70935 001 SEP 11, 1986
AB		10 MG;4 MG	N70937 001 SEP 11, 1986
AB		25 MG;2 MG	N70936 001 SEP 11, 1986
AB		25 MG;4 MG	N70938 001 SEP 11, 1986
AB		50 MG;4 MG	N70939 001 SEP 12, 1986
	TRIAVIL 2-10		
AB	MERCK SHARP DOHME	10 MG;2 MG	N14715 004

Prescription Drug Products *(continued)*

AMITRIPTYLINE HYDROCHLORIDE; PERPHENAZINE *(continued)*

TABLET; ORAL

	TRIAVIL 2-25		
AB	MERCK SHARP DOHME	25 MG;2 MG	N14715 002
	TRIAVIL 4-10		
AB	MERCK SHARP DOHME	10 MG;4 MG	N14715 003
	TRIAVIL 4-25		
AB	+ MERCK SHARP DOHME	25 MG;4 MG	N14715 005
	TRIAVIL 4-50		
AB	+ MERCK SHARP DOHME	50 MG;4 MG	N14715 006

AMLODIPINE BESYLATE

TABLET; ORAL

	NORVASC		
	PFIZER	EQ 2.5 MG BASE	N19787 001 JUL 31, 1992
		EQ 5 MG BASE	N19787 002 JUL 31, 1992
	+	EQ 10 MG BASE	N19787 003 JUL 31, 1992

AMMONIUM CHLORIDE

INJECTABLE; INJECTION

	AMMONIUM CHLORIDE IN PLASTIC CONTAINER		
	+ ABBOTT	5 MEQ/ML	N88366 001 JUN 13, 1984

AMMONIUM LACTATE

LOTION; TOPICAL

	LAC-HYDRIN		
	+ WESTWOOD SQUIBB	EQ 12% ACID	N19155 001 APR 24, 1985

AMOXAPINE

TABLET; ORAL

	AMOXAPINE		
AB	DANBURY PHARMA	25 MG	N72688 001 AUG 28, 1992
AB		50 MG	N72689 001 AUG 28, 1992
AB		100 MG	N72690 001 AUG 28, 1992
AB		150 MG	N72691 001 AUG 28, 1992

AMOXAPINE *(continued)*

TABLET; ORAL

	AMOXAPINE		
AB	GENEVA PHARMS	25 MG	N72943 001 JUN 28, 1991
AB		50 MG	N72944 001 JUN 28, 1991
AB		100 MG	N72878 001 JUN 28, 1991
AB		150 MG	N72879 001 JUN 28, 1991
AB	WATSON LABS	25 MG	N72418 001 MAY 11, 1989
AB		50 MG	N72419 001 MAY 11, 1989
AB		100 MG	N72420 001 MAY 11, 1989
AB		150 MG	N72421 001 MAY 11, 1989
	ASENDIN		
AB	LEDERLE	25 MG	N18021 001
AB		50 MG	N18021 002
AB		100 MG	N18021 003
AB	+	150 MG	N18021 004

AMOXICILLIN

CAPSULE; ORAL

	AMOXICILLIN		
AB	BIOCRAFT	250 MG	N61926 001
AB		500 MG	N61926 003
AB	CLONMEL	250 MG	N62884 001 FEB 25, 1988
AB		500 MG	N62881 001 FEB 25, 1988
AB	LABS ATRAL	250 MG	N62528 001 AUG 07, 1985
AB		500 MG	N62528 002 AUG 07, 1985
AB	LEMMON	250 MG	N63030 001 FEB 28, 1989
AB		500 MG	N63031 001 FEB 28, 1989
AB	MYLAN	250 MG	N62067 001
AB		500 MG	N62067 002
AB	NOVOPHARM	250 MG	N62853 001 DEC 22, 1987
AB		500 MG	N62854 001 DEC 22, 1987

Prescription Drug Products *(continued)*

AMOXICILLIN *(continued)*

CAPSULE; ORAL

	AMOXIL		
AB	+ SMITHKLINE BEECHAM	250 MG	N50459 001
AB		250 MG	N62216 001
AB	+	500 MG	N50459 002
	COMOX		
AB	COPANOS	250 MG	N62058 001
AB		500 MG	N62058 002
	LAROTID		
AB	SMITHKLINE BEECHAM	250 MG	N62216 003
AB		500 MG	N62216 004
	POLYMOX		
AB	APOTHECON	250 MG	N63099 001 MAR 20, 1992
AB		500 MG	N63099 002 MAR 20, 1992
	TRIMOX		
AB	APOTHECON	250 MG	N61885 001
AB		500 MG	N61885 002
	WYMOX		
AB	WYETH AYERST	250 MG	N62120 001
AB		500 MG	N62120 002

POWDER FOR RECONSTITUTION; ORAL

	AMOXICILLIN		
AB	BIOCRAFT	125 MG/5 ML	N61931 001
AB		250 MG/5 ML	N61931 002
AB	CLONMEL	125 MG/5 ML	N62927 001 NOV 25, 1988
AB		250 MG/5 ML	N62927 002 NOV 25, 1988
AB	MYLAN	125 MG/5 ML	N62090 001
AB		250 MG/5 ML	N62090 002
AB	NOVOPHARM	125 MG/5 ML	N62946 001 NOV 01, 1988
AB		250 MG/5 ML	N63001 001 JAN 06, 1989
	AMOXICILLIN PEDIATRIC		
AB	BIOCRAFT	50 MG/ML	N61931 003 DEC 01, 1982
	AMOXICILLIN TRIHYDRATE		
AB	COPANOS	125 MG/5 ML	N62059 001
AB		250 MG/5 ML	N62059 002

AMOXICILLIN *(continued)*

POWDER FOR RECONSTITUTION; ORAL

	AMOXIL		
AB	+ SMITHKLINE BEECHAM	125 MG/5 ML	N50460 001
AB		125 MG/5 ML	N62226 001
AB	+	250 MG/5 ML	N50460 002
AB	+	50 MG/ML	N50460 005
AB		250 MG/5 ML	N62226 002
AB		50 MG/ML	N62226 005
	LAROTID		
AB	SMITHKLINE BEECHAM	125 MG/5 ML	N62226 003
AB		50 MG/ML	N50460 006
AB		250 MG/5 ML	N62226 004
	TRIMOX		
AB	APOTHECON	125 MG/5 ML	N61886 002
AB		125 MG/5 ML	N62885 001 MAR 08, 1988
AB		50 MG/ML	N61886 001
AB		250 MG/5 ML	N61886 003
AB		250 MG/5 ML	N62885 002 MAR 08, 1988
	WYMOX		
AB	WYETH AYERST	125 MG/5 ML	N62131 001
AB		250 MG/5 ML	N62131 002

TABLET, CHEWABLE; ORAL

	AMOXICILLIN		
AB	BIOCRAFT	250 MG	N64013 001 DEC 22, 1992
	AMOXIL		
AB	+ SMITHKLINE BEECHAM	250 MG	N50542 001
	+	125 MG	N50542 002

AMOXICILLIN; CLAVULANATE POTASSIUM

POWDER FOR RECONSTITUTION; ORAL

	AUGMENTIN '125'		
	+ SMITHKLINE BEECHAM	125 MG/5 ML;EQ 31.25 MG ACID/5 ML	N50575 001 AUG 06, 1984
	AUGMENTIN '250'		
	+ SMITHKLINE BEECHAM	250 MG/5 ML;EQ 62.5 MG ACID/5 ML	N50575 002 AUG 06, 1984

Prescription Drug Products *(continued)*

AMOXICILLIN; CLAVULANATE POTASSIUM *(continued)*

TABLET; ORAL

	AUGMENTIN '250' + SMITHKLINE BEECHAM	250 MG;EQ 125 MG ACID	N50564 001 AUG 06, 1984
	AUGMENTIN '500' + SMITHKLINE BEECHAM	500 MG;EQ 125 MG ACID	N50564 002 AUG 06, 1984

TABLET, CHEWABLE; ORAL

	AUGMENTIN 125 + SMITHKLINE BEECHAM	125 MG;EQ 31.25 MG ACID	N50597 001 JUL 22, 1985
	AUGMENTIN 250 + SMITHKLINE BEECHAM	250 MG;EQ 62.5 MG ACID	N50597 002 JUL 22, 1985

AMPHOTERICIN B

CREAM; TOPICAL

	FUNGIZONE + APOTHECON	3%	N50314 001

INJECTABLE; INJECTION

	AMPHOTERICIN B		
AP	PHARMA TEK	50 MG/VIAL	N63206 001 APR 29, 1992
	FUNGIZONE		
AP	+ APOTHECON	50 MG/VIAL	N60517 001

LOTION; TOPICAL

	FUNGIZONE + APOTHECON	3%	N60570 001

OINTMENT; TOPICAL

	FUNGIZONE + APOTHECON	3%	N50313 001

AMPICILLIN SODIUM

INJECTABLE; INJECTION

	AMPICILLIN SODIUM		
AP	ELKINS SINN	EQ 125 MG BASE/VIAL	N62692 001 JUN 24, 1986
AP		EQ 250 MG BASE/VIAL	N62692 002 JUN 24, 1986
AP		EQ 500 MG BASE/VIAL	N62692 003 JUN 24, 1986
AP		EQ 1 GM BASE/VIAL	N62692 004 JUN 24, 1986
AP		EQ 2 GM BASE/VIAL	N62692 005 JUN 24, 1986
AP		EQ 10 GM BASE/VIAL	N62692 006 JUN 24, 1986

AMPICILLIN SODIUM *(continued)*

INJECTABLE; INJECTION

	AMPICILLIN SODIUM		
AP	HANFORD	EQ 125 MG BASE/VIAL	N63143 001 APR 15, 1993
AP		EQ 250 MG BASE/VIAL	N63145 001 APR 15, 1993
AP		EQ 500 MG BASE/VIAL	N63146 001 APR 15, 1993
AP		EQ 500 MG BASE/VIAL	N63147 001 APR 15, 1993
AP		EQ 1 GM BASE/VIAL	N62772 001 APR 15, 1993
AP		EQ 1 GM BASE/VIAL	N63139 001 APR 15, 1993
AP		EQ 2 GM BASE/VIAL	N63140 001 APR 15, 1993
AP		EQ 2 GM BASE/VIAL	N63141 001 APR 15, 1993
AP		EQ 10 GM BASE/VIAL	N63142 001 APR 15, 1993
AP	IBI SUD	EQ 125 MG BASE/VIAL	N62797 001 JUL 12, 1993
AP		EQ 2 GM BASE/VIAL	N62797 002 JUL 12, 1993
AP	ISTITUTO BIOCHIMICO	EQ 250 MG BASE/VIAL	N62719 001 MAY 12, 1987
AP		EQ 500 MG BASE/VIAL	N62719 003 MAY 12, 1987
AP		EQ 1 GM BASE/VIAL	N62719 002 MAY 12, 1987
AP	MARSAM	EQ 125 MG BASE/VIAL	N62816 001 OCT 24, 1988
AP		EQ 250 MG BASE/VIAL	N62816 002 OCT 24, 1988
AP		EQ 500 MG BASE/VIAL	N62816 003 OCT 24, 1988
AP		EQ 1 GM BASE/VIAL	N62816 004 OCT 24, 1988
AP		EQ 2 GM BASE/VIAL	N62816 005 OCT 24, 1988
AP		EQ 10 GM BASE/VIAL	N62994 001 SEP 15, 1988

Prescription Drug Products *(continued)*

AMPICILLIN SODIUM *(continued)*

INJECTABLE; INJECTION

	OMNIPEN-N		
AP	WYETH AYERST	EQ 125 MG BASE/VIAL	N60626 001
AP		EQ 125 MG BASE/VIAL	N62718 001 DEC 16, 1986
AP		EQ 250 MG BASE/VIAL	N60626 002
AP		EQ 250 MG BASE/VIAL	N62718 002 DEC 16, 1986
AP		EQ 500 MG BASE/VIAL	N60626 003
AP		EQ 500 MG BASE/VIAL	N62718 003 DEC 16, 1986
AP		EQ 1 GM BASE/VIAL	N60626 004
AP		EQ 1 GM BASE/VIAL	N62718 004 DEC 16, 1986
AP		EQ 2 GM BASE/VIAL	N60626 005
AP		EQ 2 GM BASE/VIAL	N62718 005 DEC 16, 1986
	PENBRITIN-S		
AP	WYETH AYERST	EQ 125 MG BASE/VIAL	N50072 001
AP		EQ 250 MG BASE/VIAL	N50072 002
AP		EQ 500 MG BASE/VIAL	N50072 003
AP		EQ 1 GM BASE/VIAL	N50072 004
AP	+	EQ 2 GM BASE/VIAL	N50072 005
	PRINCIPEN		
AP	APOTHECON	EQ 125 MG BASE/VIAL	N61395 001
AP		EQ 125 MG BASE/VIAL	N62860 001 FEB 05, 1988
AP		EQ 250 MG BASE/VIAL	N61395 002
AP		EQ 250 MG BASE/VIAL	N62860 002 FEB 05, 1988
AP		EQ 500 MG BASE/VIAL	N61395 003
AP		EQ 500 MG BASE/VIAL	N62860 003 FEB 05, 1988
AP		EQ 1 GM BASE/VIAL	N61395 004
AP		EQ 1 GM BASE/VIAL	N62738 001 FEB 19, 1987
AP		EQ 1 GM BASE/VIAL	N62860 004 FEB 05, 1988
AP		EQ 2 GM BASE/VIAL	N61395 005
AP		EQ 2 GM BASE/VIAL	N62738 002 FEB 19, 1987
AP		EQ 2 GM BASE/VIAL	N62860 005 FEB 05, 1988
AP	+	EQ 10 GM BASE/VIAL	N61395 006

AMPICILLIN SODIUM *(continued)*

INJECTABLE; INJECTION

	TOTACILLIN-N		
AP	SMITHKLINE BEECHAM	EQ 125 MG BASE/VIAL	N60677 001
AP		EQ 250 MG BASE/VIAL	N60677 002
AP		EQ 500 MG BASE/VIAL	N60677 003
AP		EQ 1 GM BASE/VIAL	N60677 004
AP		EQ 1 GM BASE/VIAL	N62727 001 DEC 19, 1986
AP		EQ 2 GM BASE/VIAL	N60677 005
AP		EQ 2 GM BASE/VIAL	N62727 002 DEC 19, 1986
AP		EQ 10 GM BASE/VIAL	N60677 006

AMPICILLIN SODIUM; SULBACTAM SODIUM

INJECTABLE; INJECTION

	UNASYN		
	+ PFIZER	EQ 1 GM BASE/VIAL;EQ 500 MG BASE/VIAL	N50608 002 DEC 31, 1986
		EQ 1 GM BASE/VIAL;EQ 500 MG BASE/VIAL	N62901 001 NOV 23, 1988
	+	EQ 2 GM BASE/VIAL;EQ 1 GM BASE/VIAL	N50608 001 DEC 31, 1986

AMPICILLIN/AMPICILLIN TRIHYDRATE

CAPSULE; ORAL

	AMPICILLIN		
AB	BIOCRAFT	EQ 250 MG BASE	N61502 001
AB		EQ 500 MG BASE	N61502 002
AB	CLONMEL	EQ 250 MG BASE	N62883 001 FEB 25, 1988
AB		EQ 500 MG BASE	N62882 001 FEB 25, 1988
AB	ZENITH LABS	EQ 250 MG BASE	N60765 001
AB		EQ 500 MG BASE	N60765 002
	AMPICILLIN TRIHYDRATE		
AB	COPANOS	EQ 250 MG BASE	N61602 001
AB		EQ 500 MG BASE	N61602 002
AB	MYLAN	EQ 250 MG BASE	N61755 001
AB		EQ 500 MG BASE	N61755 002
AB	PUREPAC PHARM	EQ 500 MG BASE	N61853 002
	OMNIPEN (AMPICILLIN)		
AB	WYETH AYERST	250 MG	N60624 001
AB		500 MG	N60624 002
	PFIZERPEN-A		
AB	PFIZER	EQ 250 MG BASE	N62050 001
AB		EQ 500 MG BASE	N62050 002

Prescription Drug Products *(continued)*

AMPICILLIN/AMPICILLIN TRIHYDRATE *(continued)*

CAPSULE; ORAL

	PRINCIPEN		
AB	+ APOTHECON	EQ 250 MG BASE	N61392 001
AB		EQ 250 MG BASE	N62888 001 MAR 04, 1988
AB		EQ 500 MG BASE	N61392 002
AB	+	EQ 500 MG BASE	N62888 002 MAR 04, 1988
	TOTACILLIN		
AB	SMITHKLINE BEECHAM	EQ 250 MG BASE	N62212 001
AB		EQ 500 MG BASE	N62212 002

POWDER FOR RECONSTITUTION; ORAL

	AMPICILLIN		
AB	BIOCRAFT	EQ 125 MG BASE/5 ML	N61370 001
AB		EQ 250 MG BASE/5 ML	N61370 002
AB	CLONMEL	EQ 125 MG BASE/5 ML	N62982 001 FEB 10, 1989
AB		EQ 250 MG BASE/5 ML	N62982 002 FEB 10, 1989
	AMPICILLIN TRIHYDRATE		
AB	COPANOS	EQ 125 MG BASE/5 ML	N61601 001
AB		EQ 250 MG BASE/5 ML	N61601 002
AB	MYLAN	EQ 125 MG BASE/5 ML	N61829 002
AB		EQ 250 MG BASE/5 ML	N61829 001
AB	PUREPAC PHARM	EQ 250 MG BASE/5 ML	N61980 002
	OMNIPEN (AMPICILLIN)		
AB	WYETH AYERST	125 MG/5 ML	N60625 002
AB		250 MG/5 ML	N60625 003
AB		100 MG/ML	N60625 001
	PFIZERPEN-A		
AB	PFIZER	EQ 125 MG BASE/5 ML	N62049 001
AB		EQ 250 MG BASE/5 ML	N62049 002
	POLYCILLIN		
AB	+ BRISTOL	EQ 125 MG BASE/5 ML	N50308 001
AB	+	EQ 250 MG BASE/5 ML	N50308 002
AB	+	EQ 500 MG BASE/5 ML	N50308 003
	PRINCIPEN		
AB	APOTHECON	EQ 125 MG BASE/5 ML	N61394 002
AB		EQ 250 MG BASE/5 ML	N61394 003
AB		EQ 100 MG BASE/ML	N61394 001
	TOTACILLIN		
AB	SMITHKLINE BEECHAM	EQ 125 MG BASE/5 ML	N60666 001
AB		EQ 125 MG BASE/5 ML	N62223 001
AB		EQ 250 MG BASE/5 ML	N60666 002
AB		EQ 250 MG BASE/5 ML	N62223 002

AMPICILLIN/AMPICILLIN TRIHYDRATE; PROBENECID

POWDER FOR RECONSTITUTION; ORAL

	POLYCILLIN-PRB		
AB	+ APOTHECON	EQ 3.5 GM BASE/BOT;1 GM/BOT	N61898 001
	PROBAMPACIN		
AB	BIOCRAFT	EQ 3.5 GM BASE/BOT;1 GM/BOT	N61741 001

AMRINONE LACTATE

INJECTABLE; INJECTION

	INOCOR		
	STERLING WINTHROP	EQ 5 MG BASE/ML	N18700 001 JUL 31, 1984

ANISINDIONE

TABLET; ORAL

	MIRADON		
	SCHERING	50 MG	N10909 003

ANTAZOLINE PHOSPHATE; NAPHAZOLINE HYDROCHLORIDE

SOLUTION/DROPS; OPHTHALMIC

	VASOCON-A		
	+ IOLAB	0.5%;0.05%	N18746 001 APR 30, 1990

APRACLONIDINE HYDROCHLORIDE

SOLUTION/DROPS; OPHTHALMIC

	IOPIDINE		
	+ ALCON	EQ 0.5% BASE	N20258 001 JUL 30, 1993
	+	EQ 1% BASE	N19779 001 DEC 31, 1987

APROTININ BOVINE

INJECTABLE; INJECTION

	TRASYLOL		
	+ MILES	10,000KIU/ML	N20304 001 DEC 29, 1993

ARGININE HYDROCHLORIDE

INJECTABLE; INJECTION

	R-GENE 10		
	+ PHARMACIA	10 GM/100 ML	N16931 001

Prescription Drug Products *(continued)*

ASCORBIC ACID; BIOTIN; CYANOCOBALAMIN; DEXPANTHENOL; ERGOCALCIFEROL; FOLIC ACID; NIACINAMIDE; PYRIDOXINE HYDROCHLORIDE; RIBOFLAVIN PHOSPHATE SODIUM; THIAMINE HYDROCHLORIDE; VITAMIN A; VITAMIN E

INJECTABLE; INJECTION

	M.V.I.-12		
AP	+ ASTRA	10 MG/ML;0.006 MG/ML;0.5 MCG/ML;1.5 MG/ML;20IU/ML;0.04 MG/ML;4 MG/ML;0.4 MG/ML;0.36 MG/ML;0.3 MG/ML;330 UNITS/ML;1IU/ML	N08809 004 AUG 08, 1985
	MVC PLUS		
AP	STERIS	10 MG/ML;0.006 MG/ML;0.5 MCG/ML;1.5 MG/ML;20IU/ML;0.04 MG/ML;4 MG/ML;0.4 MG/ML;0.36 MG/ML;0.3 MG/ML;330 UNITS/ML;1IU/ML	N18439 002 AUG 08, 1985

ASCORBIC ACID; BIOTIN; CYANOCOBALAMIN; ERGOCALCIFEROL; FOLIC ACID; NIACINAMIDE; PANTOTHENIC ACID; PHYTONADIONE; PYRIDOXINE; RIBOFLAVIN; THIAMINE; VITAMIN A PALMITATE; VITAMIN E

INJECTABLE; INJECTION

	KABIVITE PED F + W KIT		
	PHARMACIA	80 MG/VIAL;0.02 MG/VIAL;0.001 MG/VIAL;400IU/10 ML;0.14 MG/VIAL;17 MG/VIAL;5 MG/VIAL;0.2 MG/10 ML;1 MG/VIAL;1.4 MG/VIAL;1.2 MG/VIAL;EQ 2300 UNITS BASE/10 ML;7IU/10 ML	N20176 003 DEC 29, 1993

ASPIRIN; *MULTIPLE*

SEE ACETAMINOPHEN; ASPIRIN; CODEINE PHOSPHATE

ASPIRIN; BUTALBITAL

TABLET; ORAL

	AXOTAL		
	+ SAVAGE LABS	650 MG;50 MG	N88305 001 OCT 13, 1983

ASPIRIN; BUTALBITAL; CAFFEINE

CAPSULE; ORAL

	FIORINAL		
AB	+ SANDOZ	325 MG;50 MG;40 MG	N17534 005 APR 16, 1986
	LANORINAL		
AB	LANNETT	325 MG;50 MG;40 MG	N86996 002 OCT 11, 1985

TABLET; ORAL

	ASPIRIN AND CAFFEINE W/ BUTALBITAL		
AB	PUREPAC PHARM	325 MG;50 MG;40 MG	N86710 002 AUG 23, 1983
	BUTAL COMPOUND		
AB	GENEVA PHARMS	325 MG;50 MG;40 MG	N86398 002 APR 06, 1984
	BUTALBITAL COMPOUND		
AB	ZENITH LABS	325 MG;50 MG;40 MG	N85441 002 OCT 31, 1984
	BUTALBITAL W/ ASPIRIN & CAFFEINE		
AB	PHARMERAL	325 MG;50 MG;40 MG	N87048 002 DEC 09, 1983
	BUTALBITAL, ASPIRIN & CAFFEINE		
AB	HALSEY	325 MG;50 MG;40 MG	N89448 001 DEC 01, 1986
	BUTALBITAL, ASPIRIN AND CAFFEINE		
AB	WEST WARD PHARM	325 MG;50 MG;40 MG	N86162 002 FEB 16, 1984
	FIORINAL		
AB	+ SANDOZ	325 MG;50 MG;40 MG	N17534 003 APR 16, 1986
	LANORINAL		
AB	LANNETT	325 MG;50 MG;40 MG	N86986 002 OCT 18, 1985

ASPIRIN; BUTALBITAL; CAFFEINE; CODEINE PHOSPHATE

CAPSULE; ORAL

	FIORINAL W/CODEINE NO 3		
	+ SANDOZ	325 MG;50 MG;40 MG;30 MG	N19429 003 OCT 26, 1990

ASPIRIN; CAFFEINE; DIHYDROCODEINE BITARTRATE

CAPSULE; ORAL

	SYNALGOS-DC		
	WYETH AYERST	356.4 MG;30 MG;16 MG	N11483 004 SEP 06, 1983

Prescription Drug Products *(continued)*

ASPIRIN; CAFFEINE; ORPHENADRINE CITRATE

TABLET; ORAL

	NORGESIC		
	3M	385 MG;30 MG;25 MG	N13416 003 OCT 27, 1982
	NORGESIC FORTE		
	+ 3M	770 MG;60 MG;50 MG	N13416 004 OCT 27, 1982

ASPIRIN; CAFFEINE; PROPOXYPHENE HYDROCHLORIDE

CAPSULE; ORAL

	DARVON COMPOUND		
	LILLY	389 MG;32.4 MG;32 MG	N10996 006 MAR 08, 1983
	DARVON COMPOUND-65		
AA	LILLY	389 MG;32.4 MG;65 MG	N10996 007 MAR 08, 1983
	PROPOXYPHENE COMPOUND 65		
AA	EON LABS	389 MG;32.4 MG;65 MG	N80044 002 SEP 16, 1983
AA	LEMMON	389 MG;32.4 MG;65 MG	N89025 001 MAR 29, 1985
AA	ZENITH LABS	389 MG;32.4 MG;65 MG	N83077 002 DEC 07, 1984
	PROPOXYPHENE COMPOUND-65		
AA	GENEVA PHARMS	389 MG;32.4 MG;65 MG	N83101 002 JUN 24, 1985

ASPIRIN; CARISOPRODOL

TABLET; ORAL

	CARISOPRODOL AND ASPIRIN		
AB	PAR PHARM	325 MG;200 MG	N89594 001 MAR 31, 1989
	SOMA COMPOUND		
AB	+ WALLACE PHARMS	325 MG;200 MG	N12365 005 JUL 11, 1983

ASPIRIN; CARISOPRODOL; CODEINE PHOSPHATE

TABLET; ORAL

	SOMA COMPOUND W/ CODEINE		
	WALLACE PHARMS	325 MG;200 MG;16 MG	N12366 002 JUL 11, 1983

ASPIRIN; HYDROCODONE BITARTRATE

TABLET; ORAL

	AZDONE		
	CENT PHARMS	500 MG;5 MG	N89420 001 JAN 25, 1988

ASPIRIN; MEPROBAMATE

TABLET; ORAL

	EQUAGESIC		
AB	+ WYETH AYERST	325 MG;200 MG	N11702 003 DEC 29, 1983
	MICRAININ		
AB	WALLACE PHARMS	325 MG;200 MG	N84978 001

ASPIRIN; METHOCARBAMOL

TABLET; ORAL

	METHOCARBAMOL AND ASPIRIN		
AB	MCNEIL	325 MG;400 MG	N89193 001 FEB 12, 1986
AB	PAR PHARM	325 MG;400 MG	N89657 001 NOV 04, 1988
AB	ZENITH LABS	325 MG;400 MG	N87211 001 DEC 22, 1982
	ROBAXISAL		
AB	+ ROBINS AH	325 MG;400 MG	N12281 001

ASPIRIN; OXYCODONE HYDROCHLORIDE; OXYCODONE TEREPHTHALATE

TABLET; ORAL

	CODOXY		
AA	HALSEY	325 MG;4.5 MG;0.38 MG	N87464 001 JUL 01, 1982
	OXYCODONE AND ASPIRIN		
AA	BARR	325 MG;4.5 MG;0.38 MG	N87794 001 MAY 26, 1982
	OXYCODONE AND ASPIRIN (HALF-STRENGTH)		
AA	ROXANE	325 MG;2.25 MG;0.19 MG	N87742 001 JUN 04, 1982
	PERCODAN		
AA	DUPONT MERCK	325 MG;4.5 MG;0.38 MG	N07337 006
	PERCODAN-DEMI		
AA	DUPONT MERCK	325 MG;2.25 MG;0.19 MG	N07337 005
	ROXIPRIN		
AA	ROXANE	325 MG;4.5 MG;0.38 MG	N87743 001 JUN 04, 1982

ASPIRIN; PENTAZOCINE HYDROCHLORIDE

TABLET; ORAL

	TALWIN COMPOUND		
	+ STERLING WINTHROP	325 MG;EQ 12.5 MG BASE	N16891 001

ASPIRIN; PROPOXYPHENE HYDROCHLORIDE

CAPSULE; ORAL

	DARVON W/ ASA		
	LILLY	325 MG;65 MG	N10996 005

Prescription Drug Products *(continued)*

ASTEMIZOLE

TABLET; ORAL

HISMANAL

	+ JANSSEN	10 MG	N19402 001 DEC 29, 1988

ATENOLOL

INJECTABLE; INJECTION

TENORMIN

	+ ZENECA	0.5 MG/ML	N19058 001 SEP 13, 1989

TABLET; ORAL

ATENOLOL

AB	APOTHECON	50 MG	N73317 001 MAR 20, 1992
AB		100 MG	N73318 001 MAR 20, 1992
AB	DANBURY PHARMA	50 MG	N73352 001 DEC 27, 1991
AB		100 MG	N73353 001 DEC 27, 1991
AB	GENEVA PHARMS	25 MG	N74052 001 MAY 01, 1992
AB		50 MG	N73025 001 SEP 17, 1991
AB		100 MG	N73026 001 SEP 17, 1991
AB	GENPHARM	50 MG	N74126 001 MAR 23, 1994
AB		100 MG	N74126 002 MAR 23, 1994
AB	INVAMED	25 MG	N74265 001 FEB 28, 1994
AB		50 MG	N74265 002 FEB 28, 1994
AB		100 MG	N74265 003 FEB 28, 1994
AB	IPR	25 MG	N73646 001 JUL 31, 1992
AB		50 MG	N72303 001 JUL 15, 1988
AB		100 MG	N72304 001 JUL 15, 1988
AB	LEDERLE	25 MG	N74099 001 APR 28, 1992
AB		50 MG	N73542 001 DEC 19, 1991
AB		100 MG	N73543 001 DEC 19, 1991

ATENOLOL *(continued)*

TABLET; ORAL

ATENOLOL

AB	MUTUAL PHARM	50 MG	N73475 001 MAR 30, 1993
AB		100 MG	N73476 001 MAR 30, 1993
AB	MYLAN	50 MG	N73456 001 JAN 24, 1992
AB		100 MG	N73457 001 JAN 24, 1992
AB	NOVOPHARM	50 MG	N73315 001 MAY 28, 1993
AB		100 MG	N73316 001 MAY 28, 1993
AB	SCS	50 MG	N73676 001 OCT 30, 1992
AB		100 MG	N73676 002 OCT 30, 1992

TENORMIN

AB	ZENECA	25 MG	N18240 004 APR 09, 1990
AB		50 MG	N18240 001
AB	+	100 MG	N18240 002

ATENOLOL; CHLORTHALIDONE

TABLET; ORAL

ATENOLOL AND CHLORTHALIDONE

AB	DANBURY PHARMA	50 MG;25 MG	N73665 001 JUL 02, 1992
AB		100 MG;25 MG	N73665 002 JUL 02, 1992
AB	IPR	50 MG;25 MG	N72301 001 MAY 31, 1990
AB		100 MG;25 MG	N72302 001 MAY 31, 1990
AB	MUTUAL PHARM	50 MG;25 MG	N73581 001 APR 29, 1993
AB		100 MG;25 MG	N73582 001 APR 29, 1993
AB	MYLAN	50 MG;25 MG	N74203 001 OCT 31, 1993
AB		100 MG;25 MG	N74203 002 OCT 31, 1993

TENORETIC 100

AB	+ ZENECA	100 MG;25 MG	N18760 001 JUN 08, 1984

TENORETIC 50

AB	ZENECA	50 MG;25 MG	N18760 002 JUN 08, 1984

Prescription Drug Products *(continued)*

ATOVAQUONE

TABLET; ORAL
MEPRON
+ BURROUGHS WELLCOME — 250 MG — N20259 001 NOV 25, 1992

ATRACURIUM BESYLATE

INJECTABLE; INJECTION
TRACRIUM
+ BURROUGHS WELLCOME — 10 MG/ML — N18831 001 NOV 23, 1983

ATROPINE

INJECTABLE; INJECTION
ATROPEN

AP	+ SURVIVAL TECH	EQ 2 MG SULFATE/0.7 ML	N17106 001
	ATROPINE		
AP	KALI DUPHAR	EQ 2 MG SULFATE/0.7 ML	N71295 001 JAN 30, 1987

ATROPINE SULFATE; DIFENOXIN HYDROCHLORIDE

TABLET; ORAL
MOTOFEN
+ CARNRICK — 0.025 MG;1 MG — N17744 002

ATROPINE SULFATE; DIPHENOXYLATE HYDROCHLORIDE

CAPSULE; ORAL

	DIPHENOXYLATE HCL W/ ATROPINE SULFATE		
	SCHERER	0.025 MG;2.5 MG	N86440 001
	SOLUTION; ORAL		
	DIPHENOXYLATE HCL AND ATROPINE SULFATE		
AA	ROXANE	0.025 MG/5 ML;2.5 MG/5 ML	N87708 001 MAY 03, 1982
	LOMOTIL		
AA	SEARLE	0.025 MG/5 ML;2.5 MG/5 ML	N12699 001
	TABLET; ORAL		
	DI-ATRO		
AA	MD PHARM	0.025 MG;2.5 MG	N85266 001
	DIPHENOXYLATE HCL AND ATROPINE SULFATE		
AA	BARR	0.025 MG;2.5 MG	N85506 001
AA	INWOOD LABS	0.025 MG;2.5 MG	N85509 001
AA	MYLAN	0.025 MG;2.5 MG	N85762 001
AA	PHARMERAL	0.025 MG;2.5 MG	N85035 001
AA	ROXANE	0.025 MG;2.5 MG	N86057 001
AA	WEST WARD PHARM	0.025 MG;2.5 MG	N87765 001 MAR 15, 1982

ATROPINE SULFATE; DIPHENOXYLATE HYDROCHLORIDE *(continued)*

TABLET; ORAL

	DIPHENOXYLATE HCL W/ ATROPINE SULFATE		
AA	ICN	0.025 MG;2.5 MG	N87195 001 FEB 16, 1982
AA	KV PHARM	0.025 MG;2.5 MG	N85659 001
AA	PRIVATE FORM	0.025 MG;2.5 MG	N85766 001
AA	ZENITH LABS	0.025 MG;2.5 MG	N86727 001
	LOGEN		
AA	SUPERPHARM	0.025 MG;2.5 MG	N88962 001 MAY 10, 1985
	LOMOTIL		
AA	SEARLE	0.025 MG;2.5 MG	N12462 001
	LONOX		
AA	GENEVA PHARMS	0.025 MG;2.5 MG	N85311 002
	LOW-QUEL		
AA	HALSEY	0.025 MG;2.5 MG	N85211 001

ATROPINE SULFATE; EDROPHONIUM CHLORIDE

INJECTABLE; INJECTION
ENLON-PLUS

+ OHMEDA	0.14 MG/ML;10 MG/ML	N19677 001 NOV 06, 1991
+	0.14 MG/ML;10 MG/ML	N19678 001 NOV 06, 1991

ATROPINE SULFATE; MEPERIDINE HYDROCHLORIDE

INJECTABLE; INJECTION
ATROPINE AND DEMEROL

+ STERLING WINTHROP	0.4 MG/ML;50 MG/ML	N87853 001 NOV 26, 1982
+	0.4 MG/ML;75 MG/ML	N87847 001 NOV 26, 1982
+	0.4 MG/ML;100 MG/ML	N87848 001 NOV 26, 1982

AURANOFIN

CAPSULE; ORAL
RIDAURA
+ SMITHKLINE BEECHAM — 3 MG — N18689 001 MAY 24, 1985

AZATADINE MALEATE

TABLET; ORAL
OPTIMINE
+ SCHERING — 1 MG — N17601 001

Prescription Drug Products *(continued)*

AZATADINE MALEATE; PSEUDOEPHEDRINE SULFATE

TABLET, EXTENDED RELEASE; ORAL

	TRINALIN		
	+ SCHERING	1 MG;120 MG	N18506 001 MAR 23, 1982

AZATHIOPRINE

TABLET; ORAL

	IMURAN		
	+ BURROUGHS WELLCOME	50 MG	N16324 001

AZATHIOPRINE SODIUM

INJECTABLE; INJECTION

	IMURAN		
	+ BURROUGHS WELLCOME	EQ 100 MG BASE/VIAL	N17391 001

AZITHROMYCIN DIHYDRATE

CAPSULE; ORAL

	ZITHROMAX		
	+ PFIZER	EQ 250 MG BASE	N50670 001 NOV 01, 1991

AZLOCILLIN SODIUM

INJECTABLE; INJECTION

	AZLIN		
	+ MILES	EQ 2 GM BASE/VIAL	N50562 001 SEP 03, 1982
	+	EQ 3 GM BASE/VIAL	N50562 002 SEP 03, 1982
	+	EQ 4 GM BASE/VIAL	N50562 003 SEP 03, 1982

AZTREONAM

INJECTABLE; INJECTION

	AZACTAM		
	+ SQUIBB	500 MG/VIAL	N50580 001 DEC 31, 1986
	+	1 GM/VIAL	N50580 002 DEC 31, 1986
	+	2 GM/VIAL	N50580 003 DEC 31, 1986
	AZACTAM IN PLASTIC CONTAINER		
	+ SQUIBB	20 MG/ML	N50632 002 MAY 24, 1989
	+	40 MG/ML	N50632 001 MAY 24, 1989

BACAMPICILLIN HYDROCHLORIDE

POWDER FOR RECONSTITUTION; ORAL

	SPECTROBID		
	+ PFIZER	125 MG/5 ML	N50556 001 MAR 23, 1982

TABLET; ORAL

	SPECTROBID		
	+ PFIZER	400 MG	N50520 001

BACITRACIN

INJECTABLE; INJECTION

	BACITRACIN		
AP	+ PFIZER	50,000 UNITS/VIAL	N60282 001
AP	UPJOHN	50,000 UNITS/VIAL	N60733 002
		10,000 UNITS/VIAL	N60733 001

OINTMENT; OPHTHALMIC

	BACITRACIN		
AT	ALTANA	500 UNITS/GM	N61212 001
AT	+ LILLY	500 UNITS/GM	N60687 001

POWDER; FOR RX COMPOUNDING

	BACI-RX		
AA	PHARMA TEK	5,000,000 UNITS/BOT	N61580 001
	BACITRACIN		
AA	BRAE	5,000,000 UNITS/BOT	N61699 001
AA	PADDOCK	5,000,000 UNITS/BOT	N62456 001 JUL 27, 1983

BACITRACIN; HYDROCORTISONE ACETATE; NEOMYCIN SULFATE; POLYMYXIN B SULFATE

OINTMENT; OPHTHALMIC

	BACITRACIN-NEOMYCIN-POLYMYXIN W/ HYDROCORTISONE ACETATE		
AT	+ ALTANA	400 UNITS/GM;1%;EQ 3.5 MG BASE/GM;10,000 UNITS/GM	N60731 002
AT	PHARMADERM	400 UNITS/GM;1%;EQ 3.5 MG BASE/GM;10,000 UNITS/GM	N62166 002

BACITRACIN ZINC

POWDER; FOR RX COMPOUNDING

	ZIBA-RX		
	PHARMA TEK	500,000 UNITS/BOT	N61737 001

Prescription Drug Products *(continued)*

BACITRACIN ZINC; HYDROCORTISONE; NEOMYCIN SULFATE; POLYMYXIN B SULFATE

	OINTMENT; OPHTHALMIC		
	CORTISPORIN		
	+ BURROUGHS WELLCOME	400 UNITS/GM;1%;EQ 3.5 MG BASE/GM;10,000 UNITS/GM	N50416 002
	OINTMENT; TOPICAL		
	CORTISPORIN		
	+ BURROUGHS WELLCOME	400 UNITS/GM;1%;EQ 3.5 MG BASE/GM;5,000 UNITS/GM	N50168 002 MAY 04, 1984

BACITRACIN ZINC; NEOMYCIN SULFATE; POLYMYXIN B SULFATE

	OINTMENT; OPHTHALMIC		
	BACITRACIN-NEOMYCIN-POLYMYXIN		
AT	ALTANA	400 UNITS/GM;EQ 3.5 MG BASE/GM;10,000 UNITS/GM	N60764 002
	NEO-POLYCIN		
	DOW PHARMS	500 UNITS/GM;EQ 3.5 MG BASE/GM;10,000 UNITS/GM	N60647 001
	NEOSPORIN		
AT	+ BURROUGHS WELLCOME	400 UNITS/GM;EQ 3.5 MG BASE/GM;10,000 UNITS/GM	N50417 001

BACITRACIN ZINC; POLYMYXIN B SULFATE

	OINTMENT; OPHTHALMIC		
	OCUMYCIN		
AT	PHARMAFAIR	500 UNITS/GM;10,000 UNITS/GM	N62430 001 APR 08, 1983
	POLYSPORIN		
AT	+ BURROUGHS WELLCOME	500 UNITS/GM;10,000 UNITS/GM	N61229 001

BACLOFEN

	INJECTABLE; INTRATHECAL		
	LIORESAL		
	MEDTRONIC	0.5 MG/ML	N20075 001 JUN 17, 1992
		2 MG/ML	N20075 002 JUN 17, 1992

BACLOFEN *(continued)*

	TABLET; ORAL		
	BACLOFEN		
AB	BIOCRAFT	10 MG	N73043 001 FEB 27, 1992
AB		20 MG	N73044 001 FEB 27, 1992
AB	DANBURY PHARMA	10 MG	N72824 001 SEP 18, 1991
AB		20 MG	N72825 001 SEP 18, 1991
AB	ROYCE LABS	10 MG	N73092 001 JAN 28, 1994
AB		20 MG	N73093 001 JAN 28, 1994
AB	ZENITH LABS	10 MG	N72234 001 JUL 21, 1988
AB		20 MG	N72235 001 JUL 21, 1988
	LIORESAL		
AB	GEIGY	10 MG	N17851 001
AB	+	20 MG	N17851 003 JAN 20, 1982

BECLOMETHASONE DIPROPIONATE

	AEROSOL, METERED; INHALATION		
	BECLOVENT		
BN	GLAXO	0.042 MG/INH	N18153 001
	VANCERIL		
BN	+ SCHERING	0.042 MG/INH	N17573 001
	AEROSOL, METERED; NASAL		
	BECONASE		
BN	+ GLAXO	0.042 MG/INH	N18584 001
	VANCENASE		
BN	SCHERING	0.042 MG/INH	N18521 001

BECLOMETHASONE DIPROPIONATE MONOHYDRATE

	SPRAY, METERED; NASAL		
	BECONASE AQ		
BN	+ GLAXO	EQ 0.042 MG DIPROP/INH	N19389 001 JUL 27, 1987
	VANCENASE AQ		
BN	SCHERING	EQ 0.042 MG DIPROP/INH	N19589 001 DEC 23, 1987

Prescription Drug Products *(continued)*

BENAZEPRIL HYDROCHLORIDE

TABLET; ORAL

	LOTENSIN		
	CIBA	EQ 5 MG BASE	N19851 001 JUN 25, 1991
		EQ 10 MG BASE	N19851 002 JUN 25, 1991
		EQ 20 MG BASE	N19851 003 JUN 25, 1991
	+	EQ 40 MG BASE	N19851 004 JUN 25, 1991

BENAZEPRIL HYDROCHLORIDE; HYDROCHLOROTHIAZIDE

TABLET; ORAL

	LOTENSIN HCT		
	CIBA	5 MG;6.25 MG	N20033 001 MAY 19, 1992
		10 MG;12.5 MG	N20033 002 MAY 19, 1992
		20 MG;12.5 MG	N20033 004 MAY 19, 1992
	+	20 MG;25 MG	N20033 003 MAY 19, 1992

BENDROFLUMETHIAZIDE

TABLET; ORAL

	NATURETIN-10		
	+ SQUIBB	10 MG	N12164 003
	NATURETIN-5		
	SQUIBB	5 MG	N12164 002

BENDROFLUMETHIAZIDE; NADOLOL

TABLET; ORAL

	CORZIDE		
	SQUIBB	5 MG;40 MG	N18647 001 MAY 25, 1983
	+	5 MG;80 MG	N18647 002 MAY 25, 1983

BENTIROMIDE

SOLUTION; ORAL

	CHYMEX		
	SAVAGE LABS	500 MG/7.5 ML	N18366 001 DEC 29, 1983

BENZONATATE

CAPSULE; ORAL

	BENZONATATE		
AA	BANNER PHARMACAPS	100 MG	N81297 001 JAN 29, 1993
	TESSALON		
AA	FOREST LABS	100 MG	N11210 001

BENZOYL PEROXIDE; ERYTHROMYCIN

GEL; TOPICAL

	BENZAMYCIN		
	+ DERMIK	5%;3%	N50557 001 OCT 26, 1984

BENZPHETAMINE HYDROCHLORIDE

TABLET; ORAL

	DIDREX		
	+ UPJOHN	50 MG	N12427 002

BENZQUINAMIDE HYDROCHLORIDE

INJECTABLE; INJECTION

	EMETE-CON		
	+ ROERIG	EQ 50 MG BASE/VIAL	N16820 001

SUPPOSITORY; RECTAL

	EMETE-CON		
	+ ROERIG	EQ 100 MG BASE	N16818 006

BENZTHIAZIDE

TABLET; ORAL

	EXNA		
	+ ROBINS AH	50 MG	N12489 001

BENZTROPINE MESYLATE

INJECTABLE; INJECTION

	COGENTIN		
	+ MERCK SHARP DOHME	1 MG/ML	N12015 001

TABLET; ORAL

	BENZTROPINE MESYLATE		
AA	INVAMED	0.5 MG	N72264 001 FEB 27, 1989
AA		1 MG	N72265 001 FEB 27, 1989
AA		2 MG	N72266 001 FEB 27, 1989

Prescription Drug Products *(continued)*

BENZTROPINE MESYLATE *(continued)*

TABLET; ORAL

BENZTROPINE MESYLATE

AA	MUTUAL PHARM	1 MG	N81264 001 JAN 23, 1992
AA		2 MG	N81265 001 JAN 23, 1992
AA	PAR PHARM	0.5 MG	N88877 001 APR 11, 1985
AA		1 MG	N88894 001 APR 11, 1985
AA		2 MG	N88895 001 APR 11, 1985
AA	SIDMAK LABS NJ	0.5 MG	N89058 001 AUG 10, 1988
AA		1 MG	N89059 001 AUG 10, 1988
AA		2 MG	N89060 001 AUG 10, 1988

COGENTIN

AA	MERCK SHARP DOHME	0.5 MG	N09193 004
AA		1 MG	N09193 003
AA		2 MG	N09193 002

BENZYL PENICILLOYL-POLYLYSINE

INJECTABLE; INJECTION

PRE-PEN

+ SCHWARZ PHARMA	60UMOLAR	N50114 001

BEPRIDIL HYDROCHLORIDE

TABLET; ORAL

VASCOR

JOHNSON RW	200 MG	N19002 001 DEC 28, 1990
	300 MG	N19002 002 DEC 28, 1990
+	400 MG	N19002 003 DEC 28, 1990

BERACTANT

SUSPENSION; INTRATRACHEAL

SURVANTA

+ ROSS LABS	25 MG/ML	N20032 001 JUL 01, 1991

BETA-CAROTENE

CAPSULE; ORAL

SOLATENE

+ ROCHE	30 MG	N17589 001

BETAMETHASONE

SYRUP; ORAL

CELESTONE

SCHERING	0.6 MG/5 ML	N14215 002

TABLET; ORAL

CELESTONE

+ SCHERING	0.6 MG	N12657 003

BETAMETHASONE ACETATE; BETAMETHASONE SODIUM PHOSPHATE

INJECTABLE; INJECTION

CELESTONE SOLUSPAN

+ SCHERING	3 MG/ML;EQ 3 MG BASE/ML	N14602 001

BETAMETHASONE BENZOATE

CREAM; TOPICAL

UTICORT

+ PARKE DAVIS	0.025%	N16998 002

GEL; TOPICAL

UTICORT

+ PARKE DAVIS	0.025%	N17244 001

LOTION; TOPICAL

UTICORT

+ PARKE DAVIS	0.025%	N17528 001

BETAMETHASONE DIPROPIONATE

AEROSOL; TOPICAL

DIPROSONE

+ SCHERING	EQ 0.1% BASE	N17829 001

CREAM; TOPICAL

ALPHATREX

AB	SAVAGE LABS	EQ 0.05% BASE	N19138 001 JUN 26, 1984

BETAMETHASONE DIPROPIONATE

AB	FOUGERA	EQ 0.05% BASE	N19137 001 JUN 26, 1984
AB	LEMMON	EQ 0.05% BASE	N71476 001 AUG 10, 1987
AB	NMC	EQ 0.05% BASE	N70885 001 FEB 03, 1987
AB	TARO	EQ 0.05% BASE	N73552 001 APR 30, 1992
AB	THAMES	EQ 0.05% BASE	N71143 001 JUN 17, 1987

DIPROSONE

AB	+ SCHERING	EQ 0.05% BASE	N17536 001

Prescription Drug Products *(continued)*

BETAMETHASONE DIPROPIONATE *(continued)*

CREAM, AUGMENTED; TOPICAL
DIPROLENE AF
+ SCHERING — EQ 0.05% BASE — N19555 001 APR 27, 1987

GEL; TOPICAL
DIPROLENE
+ SCHERING — EQ 0.05% BASE — N19408 002 NOV 22, 1991

LOTION; TOPICAL
ALPHATREX
AB SAVAGE LABS — EQ 0.05% BASE — N70273 001 AUG 12, 1985

BETAMETHASONE DIPROPIONATE
AB BARRE — EQ 0.05% BASE — N70281 001 JUL 31, 1985
AB CLAY PARK — EQ 0.05% BASE — N72538 001 JAN 31, 1990
AB COPLEY PHARM — EQ 0.05% BASE — N71882 001 JUN 06, 1988
AB FOUGERA — EQ 0.05% BASE — N70275 001 AUG 12, 1985
AB LEMMON — EQ 0.05% BASE — N71467 001 AUG 10, 1987
AB NMC — EQ 0.05% BASE — N71085 001 FEB 03, 1987
AB THAMES — EQ 0.05% BASE — N72276 001 AUG 24, 1988

DIPROSONE
AB + SCHERING — EQ 0.05% BASE — N17781 001

LOTION, AUGMENTED; TOPICAL
DIPROLENE
+ SCHERING — EQ 0.05% BASE — N19716 001 AUG 01, 1988

OINTMENT; TOPICAL
ALPHATREX
AB SAVAGE LABS — EQ 0.05% BASE — N19143 001 SEP 04, 1984

BETAMETHASONE DIPROPIONATE
AB FOUGERA — EQ 0.05% BASE — N19141 001 SEP 04, 1984
AB LEMMON — EQ 0.05% BASE — N71477 001 AUG 10, 1987
AB NMC — EQ 0.05% BASE — N71012 001 FEB 03, 1987

DIPROSONE
AB + SCHERING — EQ 0.05% BASE — N17691 001

OINTMENT, AUGMENTED; TOPICAL
DIPROLENE
+ SCHERING — EQ 0.05% BASE — N18741 001 JUL 27, 1983

BETAMETHASONE DIPROPIONATE; CLOTRIMAZOLE

CREAM; TOPICAL
LOTRISONE
+ SCHERING — EQ 0.05% BASE;1% — N18827 001 JUL 10, 1984

BETAMETHASONE SODIUM PHOSPHATE

INJECTABLE; INJECTION
BETAMETHASONE SODIUM PHOSPHATE
AP STERIS — EQ 3 MG BASE/ML — N85738 001

CELESTONE
AP + SCHERING — EQ 3 MG BASE/ML — N17561 001

BETAMETHASONE SODIUM PHOSPHATE; *MULTIPLE*

SEE BETAMETHASONE ACETATE; BETAMETHASONE SODIUM PHOSPHATE

BETAMETHASONE VALERATE

CREAM; TOPICAL
BETA-VAL
AB LEMMON — EQ 0.1% BASE — N18642 001 MAR 24, 1983

BETADERM
AB ROACO DC — EQ 0.1% BASE — N18839 001 JUN 30, 1983

BETAMETHASONE VALERATE
AB CLAY PARK — EQ 0.1% BASE — N70053 001 JUN 10, 1986
AB FOUGERA — EQ 0.1% BASE — N18861 001 AUG 31, 1983
AB THAMES — EQ 0.1% BASE — N70062 001 MAY 14, 1985

BETATREX
AB SAVAGE LABS — EQ 0.1% BASE — N18862 001 AUG 31, 1983

DERMABET
AB TARO — EQ 0.1% BASE — N72041 001 JAN 06, 1988

VALISONE
AB + SCHERING — EQ 0.1% BASE — N16322 001
EQ 0.01% BASE — N16322 002

VALNAC
AB NMC — EQ 0.1% BASE — N70050 001 OCT 10, 1984

Prescription Drug Products *(continued)*

BETAMETHASONE VALERATE *(continued)*

LOTION; TOPICAL

	BETA-VAL		
AB	LEMMON	EQ 0.1% BASE	N70072 001 JUN 27, 1985
	BETAMETHASONE VALERATE		
AB	BARRE	EQ 0.1% BASE	N70052 001 JUL 31, 1985
AB	COPLEY PHARM	EQ 0.1% BASE	N71883 001 APR 22, 1988
AB	FOUGERA	EQ 0.1% BASE	N18866 001 AUG 31, 1983
AB	PHARMAFAIR	EQ 0.1% BASE	N70484 001 MAY 29, 1987
	BETATREX		
AB	SAVAGE LABS	EQ 0.1% BASE	N18867 001 AUG 31, 1983
	VALISONE		
AB	+ SCHERING	EQ 0.1% BASE	N16932 001

OINTMENT; TOPICAL

	BETA-VAL		
AB	LEMMON	EQ 0.1% BASE	N70069 001 DEC 19, 1985
	BETAMETHASONE VALERATE		
AB	FOUGERA	EQ 0.1% BASE	N18865 001 AUG 31, 1983
AB	NMC	EQ 0.1% BASE	N70051 001 OCT 10, 1984
	BETATREX		
AB	SAVAGE LABS	EQ 0.1% BASE	N18863 001 AUG 31, 1983
	VALISONE		
AB	+ SCHERING	EQ 0.1% BASE	N16740 001

BETAXOLOL HYDROCHLORIDE

SOLUTION/DROPS; OPHTHALMIC

	BETOPTIC		
	+ ALCON	EQ 0.5% BASE	N19270 001 AUG 30, 1985

SUSPENSION/DROPS; OPHTHALMIC

	BETOPTIC S		
	+ ALCON	EQ 0.25% BASE	N19845 001 DEC 29, 1989

TABLET; ORAL

	KERLONE		
	LOREX	10 MG	N19507 001 OCT 27, 1989
	+	20 MG	N19507 002 OCT 27, 1989

BETAXOLOL HYDROCHLORIDE; CHLORTHALIDONE

TABLET; ORAL

	KERLEDEX		
	LOREX	5 MG;12.5 MG	N19807 001 OCT 30, 1992
	+	10 MG;12.5 MG	N19807 002 OCT 30, 1992

BETHANECHOL CHLORIDE

INJECTABLE; INJECTION

	URECHOLINE		
	+ MERCK SHARP DOHME	5 MG/ML	N06536 001

TABLET; ORAL

	BETHANECHOL CHLORIDE		
AA	DANBURY PHARMA	5 MG	N84402 001
AA		10 MG	N84408 001
AA		25 MG	N84441 001
AA		50 MG	N87444 001
AA	SIDMAK LABS NJ	5 MG	N89095 001 DEC 19, 1985
AA		10 MG	N88440 001 MAY 29, 1984
AA		25 MG	N88441 001 MAY 29, 1984
AA		50 MG	N89096 001 DEC 19, 1985
AA	ZENITH LABS	25 MG	N84689 001
	DUVOID		
AA	ROBERTS LABS	10 MG	N86262 001
AA		25 MG	N86263 001
AA		50 MG	N85882 003
	MYOTONACHOL		
AA	GLENWOOD	5 MG	N84188 001
AA		10 MG	N84188 003
AA		25 MG	N84188 004
	URECHOLINE		
AA	MERCK SHARP DOHME	5 MG	N06536 003
AA		10 MG	N06536 002
AA		25 MG	N06536 004
AA		50 MG	N06536 005

Prescription Drug Products *(continued)*

BIOTIN; *MULTIPLE*

SEE ASCORBIC ACID; BIOTIN; CYANOCOBALAMIN; DEXPANTHENOL; ERGOCALCIFEROL; FOLIC ACID; NIACINAMIDE; PYRIDOXINE HYDROCHLORIDE; RIBOFLAVIN PHOSPHATE SODIUM; THIAMINE HYDROCHLORIDE; VITAMIN A; VITAMIN E

SEE ASCORBIC ACID; BIOTIN; CYANOCOBALAMIN; ERGOCALCIFEROL; FOLIC ACID; NIACINAMIDE; PANTOTHENIC ACID; PHYTONADIONE; PYRIDOXINE; RIBOFLAVIN; THIAMINE; VITAMIN A PALMITATE; VITAMIN E

BIPERIDEN HYDROCHLORIDE

TABLET; ORAL
AKINETON

	+ KNOLL PHARM	2 MG	N12003 001

BIPERIDEN LACTATE

INJECTABLE; INJECTION
AKINETON

	+ KNOLL PHARM	5 MG/ML	N12418 002

BISOPROLOL FUMARATE

TABLET; ORAL
ZEBETA

	LEDERLE	5 MG	N19982 002 JUL 31, 1992
	+	10 MG	N19982 001 JUL 31, 1992

BISOPROLOL FUMARATE; HYDROCHLOROTHIAZIDE

TABLET; ORAL
ZIAC

	LEDERLE	2.5 MG;6.25 MG	N20186 003 MAR 26, 1993
		5 MG;6.25 MG	N20186 001 MAR 26, 1993
	+	10 MG;6.25 MG	N20186 002 MAR 26, 1993

BITOLTEROL MESYLATE

AEROSOL, METERED; INHALATION
TORNALATE

	+ STERLING WINTHROP	0.37 MG/INH	N18770 001 DEC 28, 1984

SOLUTION; INHALATION
TORNALATE

	STERLING WINTHROP	0.2%	N19548 001 FEB 19, 1992

BLEOMYCIN SULFATE

INJECTABLE; INJECTION
BLENOXANE

	+ BRISTOL	EQ 15 UNITS BASE/VIAL	N50443 001

BRETYLIUM TOSYLATE

INJECTABLE; INJECTION
BRETYLIUM TOSYLATE

AP	+ ABBOTT	50 MG/ML	N19033 001 APR 29, 1986
AP	ASTRA	50 MG/ML	N71151 001 AUG 10, 1987
AP		50 MG/ML	N71153 001 AUG 10, 1987
AP	ELKINS SINN	50 MG/ML	N70545 001 MAY 14, 1986
AP		50 MG/ML	N70546 001 MAY 14, 1986
AP	INTL MEDICATION	50 MG/ML	N70119 001 APR 29, 1986
AP	LUITPOLD	50 MG/ML	N70891 001 JUL 26, 1988

BRETYLIUM TOSYLATE IN DEXTROSE 5% IN PLASTIC CONTAINER

AP	+ ABBOTT	200 MG/100 ML	N19008 002 APR 29, 1986
AP	+	400 MG/100 ML	N19008 003 APR 29, 1986
AP	BAXTER	200 MG/100 ML	N19837 002 APR 12, 1989
AP		400 MG/100 ML	N19837 001 APR 12, 1989
AP	MCGAW	200 MG/100 ML	N19121 002 APR 29, 1986
AP		400 MG/100 ML	N19121 003 APR 29, 1986
		100 MG/100 ML	N19121 001 APR 29, 1986

BRETYLIUM TOSYLATE IN PLASTIC CONTAINER

AP	+ ABBOTT	50 MG/ML	N19030 001 APR 29, 1986

Prescription Drug Products *(continued)*

BRETYLIUM TOSYLATE *(continued)*

INJECTABLE; INJECTION
BRETYLOL
AP DUPONT MERCK — 50 MG/ML — N17954 001

BROMOCRIPTINE MESYLATE

CAPSULE; ORAL
PARLODEL
+ SANDOZ — EQ 5 MG BASE — N17962 002 MAR 01, 1982

TABLET; ORAL
PARLODEL
+ SANDOZ — EQ 2.5 MG BASE — N17962 001

BROMODIPHENHYDRAMINE HYDROCHLORIDE; CODEINE PHOSPHATE

SYRUP; ORAL
AMBENYL
AA FOREST LABS — 12.5 MG/5 ML;10 MG/5 ML — N09319 006 JAN 10, 1984
BROMANYL
AA BARRE — 12.5 MG/5 ML;10 MG/5 ML — N88343 001 AUG 15, 1984
MYBANIL
AA PENNEX — 12.5 MG/5 ML;10 MG/5 ML — N88626 001 OCT 12, 1984

BROMPHENIRAMINE MALEATE

ELIXIR; ORAL
BROMPHENIRAMINE MALEATE
KV PHARM — 2 MG/5 ML — N85466 001

INJECTABLE; INJECTION
BROMPHENIRAMINE MALEATE
+ STERIS — 10 MG/ML — N83821 001

TABLET; ORAL
BROMPHENIRAMINE MALEATE
AA DANBURY PHARMA — 4 MG — N83123 001
AA NYLOS — 4 MG — N85592 001
AA PHOENIX LABS NY — 4 MG — N85521 001
AA PRIVATE FORM — 4 MG — N85888 001
DIMETANE
AA ROBINS AH — 4 MG — N10799 003
VELTANE
AA LANNETT — 4 MG — N84088 001

BROMPHENIRAMINE MALEATE; CODEINE PHOSPHATE; PHENYLPROPANOLAMINE HYDROCHLORIDE

SYRUP; ORAL
BROMANATE DC
AA BARRE — 2 MG/5 ML;10 MG/5 ML;12.5 MG/5 ML — N88723 001 FEB 25, 1985
DIMETANE-DC
AA ROBINS AH — 2 MG/5 ML;10 MG/5 ML;12.5 MG/5 ML — N11694 006 MAR 29, 1984
MYPHETANE DC
AA PENNEX — 2 MG/5 ML;10 MG/5 ML;12.5 MG/5 ML — N88904 001 FEB 21, 1985

BROMPHENIRAMINE MALEATE; DEXTROMETHORPHAN HYDROBROMIDE; PSEUDOEPHEDRINE HYDROCHLORIDE

SYRUP; ORAL
BROMANATE DM
AA BARRE — 2 MG/5 ML;10 MG/5 ML;30 MG/5 ML — N88722 001 MAR 07, 1985
BROMFED-DM
AA MURO — 2 MG/5 ML;10 MG/5 ML;30 MG/5 ML — N89681 001 DEC 22, 1988
DIMETANE-DX
AA ROBINS AH — 2 MG/5 ML;10 MG/5 ML;30 MG/5 ML — N19279 001 AUG 24, 1984
MYPHETANE DX
AA PENNEX — 2 MG/5 ML;10 MG/5 ML;30 MG/5 ML — N88811 001 JUN 07, 1985

BUCLIZINE HYDROCHLORIDE

TABLET; ORAL
BUCLADIN-S
STUART — 50 MG — N10911 006

BUDESONIDE

AEROSOL, METERED; NASAL
RHINOCORT
+ ASTRA — 0.05 MG/INH — N20233 001 FEB 14, 1994

Prescription Drug Products *(continued)*

BUMETANIDE

INJECTABLE; INJECTION

	BUMEX			
	+ ROCHE	0.25 MG/ML	N18226 001	FEB 28, 1983

TABLET; ORAL

	BUMEX			
	ROCHE	0.5 MG	N18225 002	FEB 28, 1983
		1 MG	N18225 001	FEB 28, 1983
	+	2 MG	N18225 003	JUN 14, 1985

BUPIVACAINE HYDROCHLORIDE

INJECTABLE; INJECTION

	<u>BUPIVACAINE HCL</u>			
<u>AP</u>	ABBOTT	<u>0.25%</u>	N18053 002	
<u>AP</u>		<u>0.25%</u>	N70583 001	FEB 17, 1987
<u>AP</u>		<u>0.25%</u>	N70586 001	MAR 03, 1987
<u>AP</u>		<u>0.25%</u>	N70590 001	FEB 17, 1987
<u>AP</u>		<u>0.5%</u>	N18053 001	
<u>AP</u>		<u>0.5%</u>	N70584 001	FEB 17, 1986
<u>AP</u>		<u>0.5%</u>	N70597 001	MAR 03, 1987
<u>AP</u>		<u>0.5%</u>	N70609 001	MAR 03, 1987
<u>AP</u>		<u>0.75%</u>	N18053 003	
<u>AP</u>		<u>0.75%</u>	N70585 001	MAR 03, 1987
<u>AP</u>		<u>0.75%</u>	N70587 001	MAR 03, 1987
	BUPIVACAINE HCL KIT			
	ABBOTT	0.075%	N19978 001	SEP 03, 1992
		0.114%	N19978 002	SEP 03, 1992
		0.23%	N19978 003	SEP 03, 1992
	<u>MARCAINE HCL</u>			
<u>AP</u>	+ STERLING WINTHROP	<u>0.25%</u>	N16964 001	
<u>AP</u>	+	<u>0.5%</u>	N16964 006	
<u>AP</u>	+	<u>0.75%</u>	N16964 009	

BUPIVACAINE HYDROCHLORIDE *(continued)*

INJECTABLE; INJECTION

	<u>SENSORCAINE</u>			
<u>AP</u>	ASTRA	<u>0.25%</u>	N18304 001	
<u>AP</u>		<u>0.25%</u>	N70552 001	MAY 21, 1986
<u>AP</u>		<u>0.5%</u>	N18304 002	
<u>AP</u>		<u>0.5%</u>	N70553 001	MAY 21, 1986
<u>AP</u>		<u>0.75%</u>	N18304 003	
<u>AP</u>		<u>0.75%</u>	N70554 001	MAY 21, 1986

INJECTABLE; SPINAL

	<u>BUPIVACAINE</u>			
<u>AP</u>	ABBOTT	<u>0.75%</u>	N71810 001	DEC 11, 1987
	<u>MARCAINE</u>			
<u>AP</u>	+ STERLING WINTHROP	<u>0.75%</u>	N18692 001	MAY 04, 1984
	<u>SENSORCAINE</u>			
<u>AP</u>	ASTRA	<u>0.75%</u>	N71202 001	APR 15, 1987

BUPIVACAINE HYDROCHLORIDE; EPINEPHRINE

INJECTABLE; INJECTION

	BUPIVACAINE HCL AND EPINEPHRINE			
	+ ABBOTT	0.25%;0.005 MG/ML	N71165 001	JUN 16, 1988
		0.25%;0.005 MG/ML	N71166 001	JUN 16, 1988
		0.25%;0.005 MG/ML	N71167 001	JUN 16, 1988
	+	0.5%;0.005 MG/ML	N71168 001	JUN 16, 1988
		0.5%;0.005 MG/ML	N71169 001	JUN 16, 1988
		0.5%;0.005 MG/ML	N71170 001	JUN 16, 1988
	+	0.75%;0.005 MG/ML	N71171 001	JUN 16, 1988

BUPIVACAINE HYDROCHLORIDE; EPINEPHRINE BITARTRATE

INJECTABLE; INJECTION

	<u>MARCAINE HCL W/ EPINEPHRINE</u>			
<u>AP</u>	+ STERLING WINTHROP	<u>0.25%;0.0091 MG/ML</u>	N16964 004	
<u>AP</u>	+	<u>0.5%;0.0091 MG/ML</u>	N16964 008	
<u>AP</u>	+	<u>0.75%;0.0091 MG/ML</u>	N16964 010	

Prescription Drug Products *(continued)*

BUPIVACAINE HYDROCHLORIDE; EPINEPHRINE BITARTRATE *(continued)*

INJECTABLE; INJECTION
SENSORCAINE

AP	ASTRA	0.25%;0.0091 MG/ML	N70966 001 OCT 13, 1987
AP		0.25%;0.0091 MG/ML	N70967 001 OCT 13, 1987
AP		0.5%;0.0091 MG/ML	N18304 004 SEP 02, 1983
AP		0.5%;0.0091 MG/ML	N70968 001 OCT 13, 1987
AP		0.75%;0.0091 MG/ML	N18304 005 SEP 02, 1983

BUPRENORPHINE HYDROCHLORIDE

INJECTABLE; INJECTION
BUPRENEX

	+ RECKITT AND COLMAN	EQ 0.3 MG BASE/ML	N18401 001

BUPROPION HYDROCHLORIDE

TABLET; ORAL
WELLBUTRIN

	BURROUGHS WELLCOME	75 MG	N18644 002 DEC 30, 1985
	+	100 MG	N18644 003 DEC 30, 1985

BUSPIRONE HYDROCHLORIDE

TABLET; ORAL
BUSPAR

	BRISTOL MYERS SQUIBB	5 MG	N18731 001 SEP 29, 1986
	+	10 MG	N18731 002 SEP 29, 1986

BUSULFAN

TABLET; ORAL
MYLERAN

	+ BURROUGHS WELLCOME	2 MG	N09386 001

BUTABARBITAL SODIUM

ELIXIR; ORAL

	BUTABARB		
AA	BARRE	30 MG/5 ML	N85873 001
	BUTISOL SODIUM		
AA	WALLACE	30 MG/5 ML	N85380 001
	SARISOL		
AA	HALSEY	30 MG/5 ML	N84723 001

TABLET; ORAL

	BUTABARBITAL		
AA	BUNDY	30 MG	N85550 001
	BUTISOL SODIUM		
AA	WALLACE	15 MG	N00793 002
AA		30 MG	N00793 004
		50 MG	N00793 003
		100 MG	N00793 005
	SARISOL NO. 1		
AA	HALSEY	15 MG	N84719 001
	SARISOL NO. 2		
AA	HALSEY	30 MG	N84719 002
	SODIUM BUTABARBITAL		
AA	LANNETT	15 MG	N85849 001
AA		30 MG	N85866 001
	MARSHALL PHARMA	16.2 MG	N83524 001
		32.4 MG	N83858 001

BUTALBITAL; *MULTIPLE*

SEE ACETAMINOPHEN; BUTALBITAL
SEE ACETAMINOPHEN; BUTALBITAL; CAFFEINE
SEE ACETAMINOPHEN; BUTALBITAL; CAFFEINE; CODEINE PHOSPHATE
SEE ASPIRIN; BUTALBITAL
SEE ASPIRIN; BUTALBITAL; CAFFEINE
SEE ASPIRIN; BUTALBITAL; CAFFEINE; CODEINE PHOSPHATE

BUTOCONAZOLE NITRATE

CREAM; VAGINAL
FEMSTAT

	+ SYNTEX	2%	N19215 001 NOV 25, 1985

Prescription Drug Products *(continued)*

BUTORPHANOL TARTRATE

	INJECTABLE; INJECTION		
	STADOL		
	+ APOTHECON	1 MG/ML	N17857 001
	+	2 MG/ML	N17857 002
	SPRAY, METERED; NASAL		
	STADOL		
	+ BRISTOL MYERS SQUIBB	1 MG/INH	N19890 001 DEC 12, 1991

CAFFEINE; *MULTIPLE*

SEE ACETAMINOPHEN; BUTALBITAL; CAFFEINE
SEE ACETAMINOPHEN; BUTALBITAL; CAFFEINE; CODEINE PHOSPHATE
SEE ACETAMINOPHEN; CAFFEINE; DIHYDROCODEINE BITARTRATE
SEE ASPIRIN; BUTALBITAL; CAFFEINE
SEE ASPIRIN; BUTALBITAL; CAFFEINE; CODEINE PHOSPHATE
SEE ASPIRIN; CAFFEINE; DIHYDROCODEINE BITARTRATE
SEE ASPIRIN; CAFFEINE; ORPHENADRINE CITRATE
SEE ASPIRIN; CAFFEINE; PROPOXYPHENE HYDROCHLORIDE

CAFFEINE; ERGOTAMINE TARTRATE

	SUPPOSITORY; RECTAL		
	CAFERGOT		
BR	+ SANDOZ	100 MG;2 MG	N09000 002
	MIGERGOT		
BR	G AND W LABS	100 MG;2 MG	N86557 001 OCT 04, 1983
	TABLET; ORAL		
	CAFERGOT		
AA	SANDOZ	100 MG;1 MG	N06620 001
	ERCATAB		
AA	GENEVA PHARMS	100 MG;1 MG	N84294 001
	WIGRAINE		
AA	ORGANON	100 MG;1 MG	N86562 001

CALCIFEDIOL

	CAPSULE; ORAL		
	CALDEROL		
	ORGANON	0.02 MG	N18312 001
	+	0.05 MG	N18312 002

CALCIPOTRIENE

	OINTMENT; TOPICAL		
	DOVONEX		
	+ BRISTOL MYERS SQUIBB	0.005%	N20273 001 DEC 29, 1993

CALCITONIN, HUMAN

	INJECTABLE; INJECTION		
	CIBACALCIN		
	+ CIBA	0.5 MG/VIAL	N18470 001 OCT 31, 1986

CALCITONIN, SALMON

	INJECTABLE; INJECTION		
	CALCIMAR		
AP	+ RHONE POULENC RORER	200IU/ML	N17769 001
	MIACALCIN		
AP	SANDOZ	200IU/ML	N17808 002 MAR 29, 1991

CALCITRIOL

	CAPSULE; ORAL		
	ROCALTROL		
	ROCHE	0.25 MCG	N18044 001
	+	0.5 MCG	N18044 002
	INJECTABLE; INJECTION		
	CALCIJEX		
	+ ABBOTT	0.001 MG/ML	N18874 001 SEP 25, 1986
	+	0.002 MG/ML	N18874 002 SEP 25, 1986

CALCIUM ACETATE

	TABLET; ORAL		
	PHOSLO		
	+ BRAINTREE	EQ 169 MG CALCIUM	N19976 001 DEC 10, 1990

CALCIUM ACETATE; *MULTIPLE*

SEE AMINO ACIDS; CALCIUM ACETATE; GLYCERIN; MAGNESIUM ACETATE; PHOSPHORIC ACID; POTASSIUM CHLORIDE; SODIUM ACETATE; SODIUM CHLORIDE

Prescription Drug Products *(continued)*

CALCIUM CHLORIDE; *MULTIPLE*

SEE AMINO ACIDS; CALCIUM CHLORIDE; DEXTROSE; MAGNESIUM CHLORIDE; POTASSIUM CHLORIDE; POTASSIUM PHOSPHATE, DIBASIC; SODIUM CHLORIDE

CALCIUM CHLORIDE; DEXTROSE; GLUTATHIONE DISULFIDE; MAGNESIUM CHLORIDE; POTASSIUM CHLORIDE; SODIUM BICARBONATE; SODIUM CHLORIDE; SODIUM PHOSPHATE

SOLUTION; IRRIGATION

BSS PLUS
AT ALCON — 0.154 MG/ML;0.92 MG/ML;0.184 MG/ML;0.2 MG/ML;0.38 MG/ML;2.1 MG/ML;7.14 MG/ML;0.42 MG/ML — N18469 001

ENDOSOL EXTRA
AT ALLERGAN — 0.154 MG/ML;0.92 MG/ML;0.184 MG/ML;0.2 MG/ML;0.38 MG/ML;2.1 MG/ML;7.14 MG/ML;0.42 MG/ML — N20079 001 NOV 27, 1991

CALCIUM CHLORIDE; DEXTROSE; MAGNESIUM CHLORIDE; POTASSIUM CHLORIDE; SODIUM ACETATE; SODIUM CHLORIDE

INJECTABLE; INJECTION

ISOLYTE R IN DEXTROSE 5% IN PLASTIC CONTAINER
MCGAW — 37 MG/100 ML;5 GM/100 ML;31 MG/100 ML;120 MG/100 ML;330 MG/100 ML;88 MG/100 ML — N19864 001 JUN 10, 1993

ISOLYTE R W/ DEXTROSE 5% IN PLASTIC CONTAINER
MCGAW — 37 MG/100 ML;5 GM/100 ML;31 MG/100 ML;120 MG/100 ML;330 MG/100 ML;88 MG/100 ML — N18271 001

CALCIUM CHLORIDE; DEXTROSE; MAGNESIUM CHLORIDE; POTASSIUM CHLORIDE; SODIUM ACETATE; SODIUM CHLORIDE; SODIUM CITRATE

INJECTABLE; INJECTION

ISOLYTE E IN DEXTROSE 5% IN PLASTIC CONTAINER
MCGAW — 35 MG/100 ML;5 GM/100 ML;30 MG/100 ML;74 MG/100 ML;640 MG/100 ML;500 MG/100 ML;74 MG/100 ML — N19867 001 DEC 20, 1993

ISOLYTE E W/ DEXTROSE 5% IN PLASTIC CONTAINER
MCGAW — 35 MG/100 ML;5 GM/100 ML;30 MG/100 ML;74 MG/100 ML;640 MG/100 ML;500 MG/100 ML;74 MG/100 ML — N18269 002 JAN 17, 1983

CALCIUM CHLORIDE; DEXTROSE; MAGNESIUM CHLORIDE; POTASSIUM CHLORIDE; SODIUM ACETATE; SODIUM CHLORIDE; SODIUM LACTATE

INJECTABLE; INJECTION

PLASMA-LYTE M AND DEXTROSE 5% IN PLASTIC CONTAINER
BAXTER — 37 MG/100 ML;5 GM/100 ML;30 MG/100 ML;119 MG/100 ML;161 MG/100 ML;94 MG/100 ML;138 MG/100 ML — N17390 001

CALCIUM CHLORIDE; DEXTROSE; MAGNESIUM CHLORIDE; SODIUM ACETATE; SODIUM CHLORIDE

SOLUTION; INTRAPERITONEAL

DIALYTE CONCENTRATE W/ DEXTROSE 30% IN PLASTIC CONTAINER
MCGAW — 510 MG/100 ML;30 GM/100 ML;200 MG/100 ML;9.2 GM/100 ML;9.6 GM/100 ML — N18807 001 AUG 26, 1983

510 MG/100 ML;30 GM/100 ML;200 MG/100 ML;9.4 GM/100 ML;11 GM/100 ML — N18807 003 AUG 26, 1983

Prescription Drug Products *(continued)*

CALCIUM CHLORIDE; DEXTROSE; MAGNESIUM CHLORIDE; SODIUM ACETATE; SODIUM CHLORIDE *(continued)*

SOLUTION; INTRAPERITONEAL
DIALYTE CONCENTRATE W/ DEXTROSE 50% IN PLASTIC CONTAINER
MCGAW 510 MG/100 ML;50 GM/100 ML;200 MG/100 ML;9.2 GM/100 ML;9.6 GM/100 ML N18807 002 AUG 26, 1983
510 MG/100 ML;50 GM/100 ML;200 MG/100 ML;9.4 GM/100 ML;11 GM/100 ML N18807 004 AUG 26, 1983

CALCIUM CHLORIDE; DEXTROSE; MAGNESIUM CHLORIDE; SODIUM CHLORIDE; SODIUM LACTATE

SOLUTION; INTRAPERITONEAL
DELFLEX W/ DEXTROSE 1.5% IN PLASTIC CONTAINER
AT FRESENIUS 25.7 MG/100 ML;1.5 GM/100 ML;15.2 MG/100 ML;567 MG/100 ML;392 MG/100 ML N18883 001 NOV 30, 1984
DELFLEX W/ DEXTROSE 1.5% LOW MAGNESIUM IN PLASTIC CONTAINER
AT FRESENIUS 25.7 MG/100 ML;1.5 GM/100 ML;5.08 MG/100 ML;538 MG/100 ML;448 MG/100 ML N18883 004 NOV 30, 1984
DELFLEX W/ DEXTROSE 1.5% LOW MAGNESIUM LOW CALCIUM IN PLASTIC CONTAINER
AT FRESENIUS 18.4 MG/100 ML;1.5 GM/100 ML;5.08 MG/100 ML;538 MG/100 ML;448 MG/100 ML N20171 001 AUG 19, 1992
DELFLEX W/ DEXTROSE 2.5% IN PLASTIC CONTAINER
AT FRESENIUS 25.7 MG/100 ML;2.5 GM/100 ML;15.2 MG/100 ML;567 MG/100 ML;392 MG/100 ML N18883 002 NOV 30, 1984
DELFLEX W/ DEXTROSE 2.5% LOW MAGNESIUM IN PLASTIC CONTAINER
AT FRESENIUS 25.7 MG/100 ML;2.5 GM/100 ML;5.08 MG/100 ML;538 MG/100 ML;448 MG/100 ML N18883 005 NOV 30, 1984

CALCIUM CHLORIDE; DEXTROSE; MAGNESIUM CHLORIDE; SODIUM CHLORIDE; SODIUM LACTATE *(continued)*

SOLUTION; INTRAPERITONEAL
DELFLEX W/ DEXTROSE 2.5% LOW MAGNESIUM LOW CALCIUM IN PLASTIC CONTAINER
FRESENIUS 18.4 MG/100 ML;2.5 GM/100 ML;5.08 MG/100 ML;538 MG/100 ML;448 MG/100 ML N20171 002 AUG 19, 1992
DELFLEX W/ DEXTROSE 4.25% IN PLASTIC CONTAINER
AT FRESENIUS 25.7 MG/100 ML;4.25 GM/100 ML;15.2 MG/100 ML;567 MG/100 ML;392 MG/100 ML N18883 003 NOV 30, 1984
DELFLEX W/ DEXTROSE 4.25% LOW MAGNESIUM IN PLASTIC CONTAINER
AT FRESENIUS 25.7 MG/100 ML;4.25 GM/100 ML;5.08 MG/100 ML;538 MG/100 ML;448 MG/100 ML N18883 006 NOV 30, 1984
DELFLEX W/ DEXTROSE 4.25% LOW MAGNESIUM LOW CALCIUM IN PLASTIC CONTAINER
AT FRESENIUS 18.4 MG/100 ML;4.25 GM/100 ML;5.08 MG/100 ML;538 MG/100 ML;448 MG/100 ML N20171 003 AUG 19, 1992
DIALYTE LM/ DEXTROSE 1.5% IN PLASTIC CONTAINER
MCGAW 26 MG/100 ML;1.5 GM/100 ML;5 MG/100 ML;530 MG/100 ML;450 MG/100 ML N18460 007 JAN 29, 1986
DIALYTE LM/ DEXTROSE 2.5% IN PLASTIC CONTAINER
MCGAW 26 MG/100 ML;2.5 GM/100 ML;5 MG/100 ML;530 MG/100 ML;450 MG/100 ML N18460 005 NOV 02, 1983
DIALYTE LM/ DEXTROSE 4.25% IN PLASTIC CONTAINER
MCGAW 26 MG/100 ML;4.25 GM/100 ML;5 MG/100 ML;530 MG/100 ML;450 MG/100 ML N18460 009 JAN 29, 1986
DIANEAL LOW CALCIUM W/ DEXTROSE 1.5% IN PLASTIC CONTAINER
AT BAXTER 18.3 MG/100 ML;1.5 GM/100 ML;5.08 MG/100 ML;538 MG/100 ML;448 MG/100 ML N20183 001 DEC 04, 1992

Prescription Drug Products *(continued)*

CALCIUM CHLORIDE; DEXTROSE; MAGNESIUM CHLORIDE; SODIUM CHLORIDE; SODIUM LACTATE *(continued)*

SOLUTION; INTRAPERITONEAL

DIANEAL LOW CALCIUM W/ DEXTROSE 2.5% IN PLASTIC CONTAINER

AT BAXTER 18.3 MG/100 ML;2.5 GM/100 ML;5.08 MG/100 ML;538 MG/100 ML;448 MG/100 ML N20183 002 DEC 04, 1992

DIANEAL LOW CALCIUM W/ DEXTROSE 3.5% IN PLASTIC CONTAINER

AT BAXTER 18.3 MG/100 ML;3.5 GM/100 ML;5.08 MG/100 ML;538 MG/100 ML;448 MG/100 ML N20183 003 DEC 04, 1992

DIANEAL LOW CALCIUM W/ DEXTROSE 4.25% IN PLASTIC CONTAINER

AT BAXTER 18.3 MG/100 ML;4.25 GM/100 ML;5.08 MG/100 ML;538 MG/100 ML;448 MG/100 ML N20183 004 DEC 04, 1992

DIANEAL PD-1 W/ DEXTROSE 1.5% IN PLASTIC CONTAINER

AT BAXTER 25.7 MG/100 ML;1.5 GM/100 ML;15.2 MG/100 ML;567 MG/100 ML;392 MG/100 ML N17512 007 JUL 09, 1984

DIANEAL PD-1 W/ DEXTROSE 2.5% IN PLASTIC CONTAINER

AT BAXTER 25.7 MG/100 ML;2.5 GM/100 ML;15.2 MG/100 ML;567 MG/100 ML;392 MG/100 ML N17512 008 JUL 09, 1984

DIANEAL PD-1 W/ DEXTROSE 3.5% IN PLASTIC CONTAINER

AT BAXTER 25.7 MG/100 ML;3.5 GM/100 ML;15.2 MG/100 ML;567 MG/100 ML;392 MG/100 ML N17512 010 NOV 18, 1985

DIANEAL PD-1 W/ DEXTROSE 4.25% IN PLASTIC CONTAINER

AT BAXTER 25.7 MG/100 ML;4.25 GM/100 ML;15.2 MG/100 ML;567 MG/100 ML;392 MG/100 ML N17512 009 JUL 09, 1984

CALCIUM CHLORIDE; DEXTROSE; MAGNESIUM CHLORIDE; SODIUM CHLORIDE; SODIUM LACTATE *(continued)*

SOLUTION; INTRAPERITONEAL

DIANEAL PD-2 W/ DEXTROSE 1.5% IN PLASTIC CONTAINER

AT BAXTER 18.3 MG/100 ML;1.5 GM/100 ML;5.08 MG/100 ML;538 MG/100 ML;448 MG/100 ML N17512 004

AT 25.7 MG/100 ML;1.5 GM/100 ML;5.08 MG/100 ML;538 MG/100 ML;448 MG/100 ML N20163 001 DEC 04, 1992

DIANEAL PD-2 W/ DEXTROSE 2.5% IN PLASTIC CONTAINER

AT BAXTER 25.7 MG/100 ML;2.5 GM/100 ML;5.08 MG/100 ML;538 MG/100 ML;448 MG/100 ML N17512 005

AT 25.7 MG/100 ML;2.5 GM/100 ML;5.08 MG/100 ML;538 MG/100 ML;448 MG/100 ML N20163 002 DEC 04, 1992

DIANEAL PD-2 W/ DEXTROSE 3.5% IN PLASTIC CONTAINER

AT BAXTER 25.7 MG/100 ML;3.5 GM/100 ML;5.08 MG/100 ML;538 MG/100 ML;448 MG/100 ML N17512 011 NOV 18, 1985

DIANEAL PD-2 W/ DEXTROSE 4.25% IN PLASTIC CONTAINER

AT BAXTER 25.7 MG/100 ML;4.25 GM/100 ML;5.08 MG/100 ML;538 MG/100 ML;448 MG/100 ML N17512 006

AT 25.7 MG/100 ML;4.25 GM/100 ML;5.08 MG/100 ML;538 MG/100 ML;448 MG/100 ML N20163 003 DEC 04, 1992

DIANEAL 137 W/ DEXTROSE 1.5% IN PLASTIC CONTAINER

AT BAXTER 25.7 MG/100 ML;1.5 GM/100 ML;15.2 MG/100 ML;567 MG/100 ML;392 MG/100 ML N17512 001

DIANEAL 137 W/ DEXTROSE 2.5% IN PLASTIC CONTAINER

AT BAXTER 25.7 MG/100 ML;2.5 GM/100 ML;15.2 MG/100 ML;567 MG/100 ML;392 MG/100 ML N17512 003

Prescription Drug Products *(continued)*

CALCIUM CHLORIDE; DEXTROSE; MAGNESIUM CHLORIDE; SODIUM CHLORIDE; SODIUM LACTATE *(continued)*

SOLUTION; INTRAPERITONEAL

DIANEAL 137 W/ DEXTROSE 4.25% IN PLASTIC CONTAINER
AT BAXTER 25.7 MG/100 ML;4.25 GM/100 ML;15.2 MG/100 ML;567 MG/100 ML;392 MG/100 ML N17512 002

INPERSOL W/ DEXTROSE 1.5% IN PLASTIC CONTAINER
AT ABBOTT 25.7 MG/100 ML;1.5 GM/100 ML;15.2 MG/100 ML;567 MG/100 ML;392 MG/100 ML N18379 002

INPERSOL W/ DEXTROSE 2.5% IN PLASTIC CONTAINER
AT ABBOTT 25.7 MG/100 ML;2.5 GM/100 ML;15.2 MG/100 ML;567 MG/100 ML;392 MG/100 ML N18379 003

INPERSOL W/ DEXTROSE 3.5% IN PLASTIC CONTAINER
AT ABBOTT 25.7 MG/100 ML;3.5 GM/100 ML;15.2 MG/100 ML;567 MG/100 ML;392 MG/100 ML N18379 007 JUN 24, 1988

INPERSOL W/ DEXTROSE 4.25% IN PLASTIC CONTAINER
AT ABBOTT 25.7 MG/100 ML;4.25 GM/100 ML;15.2 MG/100 ML;567 MG/100 ML;392 MG/100 ML N18379 001

INPERSOL-LC/LM W/ DEXTROSE 1.5% IN PLASTIC CONTAINER
AT ABBOTT 18.4 MG/100 ML;1.5 GM/100 ML;5.08 MG/100 ML;538 MG/100 ML;448 MG/100 ML N20374 001 JUN 13, 1994

INPERSOL-LC/LM W/ DEXTROSE 2.5% IN PLASTIC CONTAINER
AT ABBOTT 18.3 MG/100 ML;2.5 GM/100 ML;5.08 MG/100 ML;538 MG/100 ML;448 MG/100 ML N20374 002 JUN 13, 1994

INPERSOL-LC/LM W/ DEXTROSE 3.5% IN PLASTIC CONTAINER
AT ABBOTT 18.3 MG/100 ML;3.5 GM/100 ML;5.08 MG/100 ML;538 MG/100 ML;448 MG/100 ML N20374 003 JUN 13, 1994

INPERSOL-LC/LM W/ DEXTROSE 4.25% IN PLASTIC CONTAINER
AT ABBOTT 18.4 MG/100 ML;4.25 GM/100 ML;5.08 MG/100 ML;538 MG/100 ML;448 MG/100 ML N20374 004 JUN 13, 1994

CALCIUM CHLORIDE; DEXTROSE; MAGNESIUM CHLORIDE; SODIUM CHLORIDE; SODIUM LACTATE *(continued)*

SOLUTION; INTRAPERITONEAL

INPERSOL-LM W/ DEXTROSE 1.5% IN PLASTIC CONTAINER
AT ABBOTT 25.7 MG/100 ML;1.5 GM/100 ML;5.08 MG/100 ML;538 MG/100 ML;448 MG/100 ML N18379 004 JUL 07, 1982

INPERSOL-LM W/ DEXTROSE 2.5% IN PLASTIC CONTAINER
AT ABBOTT 25.7 MG/100 ML;2.5 GM/100 ML;5.08 MG/100 ML;538 MG/100 ML;448 MG/100 ML N18379 005 JUL 07, 1982

INPERSOL-LM W/ DEXTROSE 3.5% IN PLASTIC CONTAINER
AT ABBOTT 25.7 MG/100 ML;3.5 GM/100 ML;5.08 MG/100 ML;538 MG/100 ML;448 MG/100 ML N18379 008 JUN 24, 1988

INPERSOL-LM W/ DEXTROSE 4.25% IN PLASTIC CONTAINER
AT ABBOTT 25.7 MG/100 ML;4.25 GM/100 ML;5.08 MG/100 ML;538 MG/100 ML;448 MG/100 ML N18379 006 JUL 07, 1982

CALCIUM CHLORIDE; DEXTROSE; POTASSIUM CHLORIDE; SODIUM ACETATE; SODIUM CHLORIDE

INJECTABLE; INJECTION

DEXTROSE 5% IN ACETATED RINGER'S IN PLASTIC CONTAINER
MCGAW 20 MG/100 ML;5 GM/100 ML;30 MG/100 ML;380 MG/100 ML;600 MG/100 ML N18258 001

Prescription Drug Products *(continued)*

CALCIUM CHLORIDE; DEXTROSE; POTASSIUM CHLORIDE; SODIUM CHLORIDE

INJECTABLE; INJECTION

DEXTROSE 5% AND RINGER'S IN PLASTIC CONTAINER

AP ABBOTT 33 MG/100 ML;5 GM/100 ML;30 MG/100 ML;860 MG/100 ML N18254 001

DEXTROSE 5% IN RINGER'S IN PLASTIC CONTAINER

AP BAXTER 33 MG/100 ML;5 GM/100 ML;30 MG/100 ML;860 MG/100 ML N16695 001

AP MCGAW 33 MG/100 ML;5 GM/100 ML;30 MG/100 ML;860 MG/100 ML N18256 001

AP 33 MG/100 ML;5 GM/100 ML;30 MG/100 ML;860 MG/100 ML N20000 001 APR 17, 1992

CALCIUM CHLORIDE; DEXTROSE; POTASSIUM CHLORIDE; SODIUM CHLORIDE; SODIUM LACTATE

INJECTABLE; INJECTION

DEXTROSE 2.5% IN HALF-STRENGTH LACTATED RINGER'S IN PLASTIC CONTAINER

MCGAW 10 MG/100 ML;2.5 GM/100 ML;15 MG/100 ML;300 MG/100 ML;160 MG/100 ML N19634 001 FEB 24, 1988

DEXTROSE 4% IN MODIFIED LACTATED RINGER'S IN PLASTIC CONTAINER

MCGAW 4 MG/100 ML;4 GM/100 ML;6 MG/100 ML;120 MG/100 ML;62 MG/100 ML N19634 002 FEB 24, 1988

DEXTROSE 5% AND LACTATED RINGER'S IN PLASTIC CONTAINER

AP ABBOTT 20 MG/100 ML;5 GM/100 ML;30 MG/100 ML;600 MG/100 ML;310 MG/100 ML N17608 001

DEXTROSE 5% IN LACTATED RINGER'S IN PLASTIC CONTAINER

AP MCGAW 20 MG/100 ML;5 GM/100 ML;30 MG/100 ML;600 MG/100 ML;310 MG/100 ML N17510 001

AP 20 MG/100 ML;5 GM/100 ML;30 MG/100 ML;600 MG/100 ML;310 MG/100 ML N19634 003 FEB 24, 1988

CALCIUM CHLORIDE; DEXTROSE; POTASSIUM CHLORIDE; SODIUM CHLORIDE; SODIUM LACTATE *(continued)*

INJECTABLE; INJECTION

LACTATED RINGER'S AND DEXTROSE 5% IN PLASTIC CONTAINER

AP BAXTER 20 MG/100 ML;5 GM/100 ML;30 MG/100 ML;600 MG/100 ML;310 MG/100 ML N16679 001

POTASSIUM CHLORIDE 10 MEQ IN DEXTROSE 5% AND LACTATED RINGER'S IN PLASTIC CONTAINER

BAXTER 20 MG/100 ML;5 GM/100 ML;105 MG/100 ML;600 MG/100 ML;310 MG/100 ML N19367 002 APR 05, 1985

20 MG/100 ML;5 GM/100 ML;179 MG/100 ML;600 MG/100 ML;310 MG/100 ML N19367 003 APR 05, 1985

POTASSIUM CHLORIDE 15 MEQ IN DEXTROSE 5% AND LACTATED RINGER'S IN PLASTIC CONTAINER

AP BAXTER 20 MG/100 ML;5 GM/100 ML;254 MG/100 ML;600 MG/100 ML;310 MG/100 ML N19367 006 APR 05, 1985

POTASSIUM CHLORIDE 20 MEQ IN DEXTROSE 5% AND LACTATED RINGER'S IN PLASTIC CONTAINER

AP ABBOTT 20 MG/100 ML;5 GM/100 ML;179 MG/100 ML;600 MG/100 ML;310 MG/100 ML N19685 002 OCT 17, 1988

AP 20 MG/100 ML;5 GM/100 ML;328 MG/100 ML;600 MG/100 ML;310 MG/100 ML N19685 008 OCT 17, 1988

AP BAXTER 20 MG/100 ML;5 GM/100 ML;179 MG/100 ML;600 MG/100 ML;310 MG/100 ML N19367 004 APR 05, 1985

AP 20 MG/100 ML;5 GM/100 ML;328 MG/100 ML;600 MG/100 ML;310 MG/100 ML N19367 005 APR 05, 1985

Prescription Drug Products *(continued)*

CALCIUM CHLORIDE; DEXTROSE; POTASSIUM CHLORIDE; SODIUM CHLORIDE; SODIUM LACTATE *(continued)*

INJECTABLE; INJECTION

POTASSIUM CHLORIDE 30 MEQ IN DEXTROSE 5% AND LACTATED RINGER'S IN PLASTIC CONTAINER

AP	BAXTER	20 MG/100 ML;5 GM/100 ML;254 MG/100 ML;600 MG/100 ML;310 MG/100 ML	N19367 007 APR 05, 1985

POTASSIUM CHLORIDE 40 MEQ IN DEXTROSE 5% AND LACTATED RINGER'S IN PLASTIC CONTAINER

AP	ABBOTT	20 MG/100 ML;5 GM/100 ML;328 MG/100 ML;600 MG/100 ML;310 MG/100 ML	N19685 004 OCT 17, 1988
AP	BAXTER	20 MG/100 ML;5 GM/100 ML;328 MG/100 ML;600 MG/100 ML;310 MG/100 ML	N19367 008

POTASSIUM CHLORIDE 5 MEQ IN DEXTROSE 5% AND LACTATED RINGER'S IN PLASTIC CONTAINER

	BAXTER	20 MG/100 ML;5 GM/100 ML;105 MG/100 ML;600 MG/100 ML;310 MG/100 ML	N19367 001 APR 05, 1985

CALCIUM CHLORIDE; MAGNESIUM CHLORIDE; POTASSIUM CHLORIDE; SODIUM ACETATE; SODIUM CHLORIDE

INJECTABLE; INJECTION

TPN ELECTROLYTES IN PLASTIC CONTAINER

	ABBOTT	16.5 MG/ML;25.4 MG/ML;74.6 MG/ML;121 MG/ML;16.1 MG/ML	N18895 001 JUL 20, 1984

CALCIUM CHLORIDE; MAGNESIUM CHLORIDE; POTASSIUM CHLORIDE; SODIUM ACETATE; SODIUM CHLORIDE; SODIUM CITRATE

INJECTABLE; INJECTION

ISOLYTE E IN PLASTIC CONTAINER

	MCGAW	35 MG/100 ML;30 MG/100 ML;74 MG/100 ML;640 MG/100 ML;500 MG/100 ML;74 MG/100 ML	N18899 001 OCT 31, 1983
		35 MG/100 ML;30 MG/100 ML;74 MG/100 ML;640 MG/100 ML;500 MG/100 ML;74 MG/100 ML	N19718 001 SEP 29, 1989

CALCIUM CHLORIDE; MAGNESIUM CHLORIDE; POTASSIUM CHLORIDE; SODIUM ACETATE; SODIUM CHLORIDE; SODIUM LACTATE

INJECTABLE; INJECTION

PLASMA-LYTE R IN PLASTIC CONTAINER

	BAXTER	36.8 MG/100 ML;30.5 MG/100 ML;74.6 MG/100 ML;640 MG/100 ML;496 MG/100 ML;89.6 MG/100 ML	N17438 001

CALCIUM CHLORIDE; MAGNESIUM CHLORIDE; POTASSIUM CHLORIDE; SODIUM CHLORIDE

SOLUTION; PERFUSION, CARDIAC

PLEGISOL IN PLASTIC CONTAINER

	ABBOTT	17.6 MG/100 ML;325.3 MG/100 ML;119.3 MG/100 ML;643 MG/100 ML	N18608 001 FEB 26, 1982

CALCIUM CHLORIDE; POTASSIUM CHLORIDE; SODIUM CHLORIDE

INJECTABLE; INJECTION

RINGER'S IN PLASTIC CONTAINER

AP	ABBOTT	33 MG/100 ML;30 MG/100 ML;860 MG/100 ML	N18251 001
AP	BAXTER	33 MG/100 ML;30 MG/100 ML;860 MG/100 ML	N16693 001

Discontinued Drug Products *(continued)*

CALCIUM CHLORIDE; POTASSIUM CHLORIDE; SODIUM CHLORIDE *(continued)*

INJECTABLE; INJECTION

RINGER'S IN PLASTIC CONTAINER

AP MCGAW 33 MG/100 ML;30 MG/100 ML;860 MG/100 ML N18721 001 NOV 09, 1982

AP 33 MG/100 ML;30 MG/100 ML;860 MG/100 ML N20002 001 APR 17, 1992

SOLUTION; IRRIGATION

RINGER'S IN PLASTIC CONTAINER

AT ABBOTT 33 MG/100 ML;30 MG/100 ML;860 MG/100 ML N17635 001

AT BAXTER 33 MG/100 ML;30 MG/100 ML;860 MG/100 ML N18495 001 FEB 19, 1982

AT MCGAW 33 MG/100 ML;30 MG/100 ML;860 MG/100 ML N18156 001

CALCIUM CHLORIDE; POTASSIUM CHLORIDE; SODIUM CHLORIDE; SODIUM LACTATE

INJECTABLE; INJECTION

LACTATED RINGER'S IN PLASTIC CONTAINER

AP ABBOTT 20 MG/100 ML;30 MG/100 ML;600 MG/100 ML;310 MG/100 ML N17641 001

AP BAXTER 20 MG/100 ML;30 MG/100 ML;600 MG/100 ML;310 MG/100 ML N16682 001

AP MCGAW 20 MG/100 ML;30 MG/100 ML;600 MG/100 ML;310 MG/100 ML N18023 001

AP 20 MG/100 ML;30 MG/100 ML;600 MG/100 ML;310 MG/100 ML N19632 001 FEB 29, 1988

SOLUTION; IRRIGATION

LACTATED RINGER'S IN PLASTIC CONTAINER

AT ABBOTT 20 MG/100 ML;30 MG/100 ML;600 MG/100 ML;310 MG/100 ML N19416 001 JAN 17, 1986

CALCIUM CHLORIDE; POTASSIUM CHLORIDE; SODIUM CHLORIDE; SODIUM LACTATE *(continued)*

SOLUTION; IRRIGATION

LACTATED RINGER'S IN PLASTIC CONTAINER

AT BAXTER 20 MG/100 ML;30 MG/100 ML;600 MG/100 ML;310 MG/100 ML N18494 001 FEB 19, 1982

AT 20 MG/100 ML;30 MG/100 ML;600 MG/100 ML;310 MG/100 ML N18921 001 APR 03, 1984

AT 20 MG/100 ML;30 MG/100 ML;600 MG/100 ML;310 MG/100 ML N19933 001 AUG 29, 1989

AT MCGAW 20 MG/100 ML;30 MG/100 ML;600 MG/100 ML;310 MG/100 ML N18681 001 DEC 27, 1982

CALCIUM GLUCEPTATE

INJECTABLE; INJECTION

CALCIUM GLUCEPTATE

+ ABBOTT EQ 90 MG CALCIUM/5 ML N80001 001

CANDICIDIN

OINTMENT; VAGINAL

VANOBID

+ MERRELL DOW 0.6 MG/GM N61596 001

TABLET; VAGINAL

VANOBID

+ MERRELL DOW 3 MG N61613 001

CAPREOMYCIN SULFATE

INJECTABLE; INJECTION

CAPASTAT SULFATE

+ LILLY EQ 1 GM BASE/VIAL N50095 001

CAPTOPRIL

TABLET; ORAL

CAPOTEN

BRISTOL MYERS SQUIBB 12.5 MG N18343 005 JAN 17, 1985

25 MG N18343 002

50 MG N18343 001

\+ 100 MG N18343 003

Prescription Drug Products *(continued)*

CAPTOPRIL; HYDROCHLOROTHIAZIDE

TABLET; ORAL

	CAPOZIDE 25/15		
	SQUIBB	25 MG;15 MG	N18709 001 OCT 12, 1984
	CAPOZIDE 25/25		
	SQUIBB	25 MG;25 MG	N18709 002 OCT 12, 1984
	CAPOZIDE 50/15		
	SQUIBB	50 MG;15 MG	N18709 004 OCT 12, 1984
	CAPOZIDE 50/25		
	+ SQUIBB	50 MG;25 MG	N18709 003 OCT 12, 1984

CARBACHOL

SOLUTION; INTRAOCULAR

	MIOSTAT		
	+ ALCON	0.01%	N16968 001

CARBAMAZEPINE

SUSPENSION; ORAL

	TEGRETOL		
	+ BASEL PHARMS	100 MG/5 ML	N18927 001 DEC 18, 1987

TABLET; ORAL

	CARBAMAZEPINE		
AB	INWOOD LABS	200 MG	N70231 001 AUG 14, 1986
AB	PUREPAC PHARM	200 MG	N71696 001 NOV 09, 1987
AB	SIDMAK LABS NJ	200 MG	N71479 001 JUL 24, 1987
	EPITOL		
AB	LEMMON	200 MG	N70541 001 SEP 17, 1986
	TEGRETOL		
AB	+ BASEL PHARMS	200 MG	N16608 001

TABLET, CHEWABLE; ORAL

	CARBAMAZEPINE		
AB	WARNER CHILCOTT	100 MG	N71940 001 FEB 01, 1988
	EPITOL		
AB	LEMMON	100 MG	N73524 001 JUL 29, 1992
	TEGRETOL		
AB	+ BASEL PHARMS	100 MG	N18281 001

CARBENICILLIN DISODIUM

INJECTABLE; INJECTION

	GEOPEN		
	+ ROERIG	EQ 1 GM BASE/VIAL	N50306 001
	+	EQ 2 GM BASE/VIAL	N50306 004
	+	EQ 5 GM BASE/VIAL	N50306 002
	+	EQ 10 GM BASE/VIAL	N50306 006
	+	EQ 30 GM BASE/VIAL	N50306 007

CARBENICILLIN INDANYL SODIUM

TABLET; ORAL

	GEOCILLIN		
	+ PFIZER	EQ 382 MG BASE	N50435 001

CARBIDOPA

TABLET; ORAL

	LODOSYN		
	+ MERCK SHARP DOHME	25 MG	N17830 001

CARBIDOPA; LEVODOPA

TABLET; ORAL

	CARBIDOPA AND LEVODOPA		
AB	LEMMON	10 MG;100 MG	N73618 001 AUG 28, 1992
AB		25 MG;100 MG	N73589 001 AUG 28, 1992
AB		25 MG;250 MG	N73607 001 AUG 28, 1992
AB	PUREPAC PHARM	10 MG;100 MG	N74260 001 SEP 03, 1993
AB		25 MG;100 MG	N74260 002 SEP 03, 1993
AB		25 MG;250 MG	N74260 003 SEP 03, 1993
AB	SCS	10 MG;100 MG	N74080 001 MAR 25, 1994
AB		25 MG;100 MG	N74080 002 MAR 25, 1994
AB		25 MG;250 MG	N74080 003 MAR 25, 1994
AB	WATSON LABS	10 MG;100 MG	N73381 001 SEP 28, 1993
AB		25 MG;100 MG	N73382 001 SEP 28, 1993
AB		25 MG;250 MG	N73383 001 SEP 28, 1993

Prescription Drug Products *(continued)*

CARBIDOPA; LEVODOPA *(continued)*
TABLET; ORAL
SINEMET
AB MERCK SHARP DOHME 10 MG;100 MG N17555 001
AB 25 MG;100 MG N17555 003
AB + 25 MG;250 MG N17555 002
TABLET, EXTENDED RELEASE; ORAL
SINEMET CR
MERCK SHARP DOHME 25 MG;100 MG N19856 002 DEC 24, 1992
\+ 50 MG;200 MG N19856 001 MAY 30, 1991

CARBOPLATIN
INJECTABLE; INJECTION
PARAPLATIN
\+ BRISTOL MYERS SQUIBB 50 MG/VIAL N19880 001 MAR 03, 1989
\+ 150 MG/VIAL N19880 002 MAR 03, 1989
\+ 450 MG/VIAL N19880 003 MAR 03, 1989

CARBOPROST TROMETHAMINE
INJECTABLE; INJECTION
HEBAMATE
\+ UPJOHN EQ 0.25 MG BASE/ML N17989 001

CARISOPRODOL
TABLET; ORAL
CARISOPRODOL
AA CHELSEA LABS 350 MG N86179 001
AA DANBURY PHARMA 350 MG N87499 001 APR 20, 1982
AA GENEVA PHARMS 350 MG N81025 001 APR 13, 1989
AA MUTUAL PHARM 350 MG N89346 001 OCT 17, 1991
SOMA
AA WALLACE 350 MG N11792 001

CARISOPRODOL; *MULTIPLE*
SEE ASPIRIN; CARISOPRODOL
SEE ASPIRIN; CARISOPRODOL; CODEINE PHOSPHATE

CARMUSTINE
INJECTABLE; INJECTION
BICNU
\+ BRISTOL 100 MG/VIAL N17422 001

CARTEOLOL HYDROCHLORIDE
SOLUTION/DROPS; OPHTHALMIC
OPTIPRESS
\+ OTSUKA 1% N19972 001 MAY 23, 1990
TABLET; ORAL
CARTROL
ABBOTT 2.5 MG N19204 001 DEC 28, 1988
\+ 5 MG N19204 002 DEC 28, 1988

CEFACLOR
CAPSULE; ORAL
CECLOR
\+ LILLY EQ 250 MG BASE N50521 001
EQ 250 MG BASE N62205 001
\+ EQ 500 MG BASE N50521 002
EQ 500 MG BASE N62205 002
POWDER FOR RECONSTITUTION; ORAL
CECLOR
\+ LILLY EQ 125 MG BASE/5 ML N50522 001
EQ 125 MG BASE/5 ML N62206 001
\+ EQ 187 MG BASE/5 ML N62206 003 APR 20, 1988
\+ EQ 250 MG BASE/5 ML N50522 002
EQ 250 MG BASE/5 ML N62206 002
\+ EQ 375 MG BASE/5 ML N62206 004 APR 20, 1988

CEFADROXIL/CEFADROXIL HEMIHYDRATE
CAPSULE; ORAL
CEFADROXIL
AB APOTHECON EQ 500 MG BASE N62291 001
AB ZENITH LABS EQ 500 MG BASE N62766 001 MAR 03, 1987
DURICEF
AB + BRISTOL MYERS SQUIBB EQ 500 MG BASE N50512 001

Prescription Drug Products *(continued)*

CEFADROXIL/CEFADROXIL HEMIHYDRATE *(continued)*

POWDER FOR RECONSTITUTION; ORAL

	CEFADROXIL		
AB	APOTHECON	EQ 125 MG BASE/5 ML	N62334 001
AB		EQ 250 MG BASE/5 ML	N62334 002
AB		EQ 500 MG BASE/5 ML	N62334 003
	DURICEF		
AB	+ BRISTOL MYERS SQUIBB	EQ 125 MG BASE/5 ML	N50527 002
AB	+	EQ 250 MG BASE/5 ML	N50527 003
AB	+	EQ 500 MG BASE/5 ML	N50527 001

TABLET; ORAL

	CEFADROXIL		
AB	ZENITH LABS	EQ 1 GM BASE	N62774 001 APR 08, 1987
	DURICEF		
AB	+ BRISTOL MYERS SQUIBB	EQ 1 GM BASE	N50528 001
	ULTRACEF		
AB	APOTHECON	EQ 1 GM BASE	N62390 001 JUN 10, 1982

CEFAMANDOLE NAFATE

INJECTABLE; INJECTION

	MANDOL		
	+ LILLY	EQ 500 MG BASE/VIAL	N50504 001
	+	EQ 1 GM BASE/VIAL	N50504 002
		EQ 1 GM BASE/VIAL	N62560 001 SEP 10, 1985
	+	EQ 2 GM BASE/VIAL	N50504 003
		EQ 2 GM BASE/VIAL	N62560 002 SEP 10, 1985
	+	EQ 10 GM BASE/VIAL	N50504 004

CEFAZOLIN SODIUM

INJECTABLE; INJECTION

	ANCEF		
AP	+ SMITHKLINE BEECHAM	EQ 250 MG BASE/VIAL	N50461 001
AP	+	EQ 500 MG BASE/VIAL	N50461 002
AP	+	EQ 1 GM BASE/VIAL	N50461 003
AP	+	EQ 5 GM BASE/VIAL	N50461 004
AP	+	EQ 10 GM BASE/VIAL	N50461 005
	ANCEF IN DEXTROSE 5% IN PLASTIC CONTAINER		
	+ BAXTER	EQ 10 MG BASE/ML	N50566 003 JUN 08, 1983
	+	EQ 20 MG BASE/ML	N50566 004 JUN 08, 1983

CEFAZOLIN SODIUM *(continued)*

INJECTABLE; INJECTION

	ANCEF IN PLASTIC CONTAINER		
	+ BAXTER	EQ 10 MG BASE/ML	N63002 001 MAR 28, 1991
	+	EQ 20 MG BASE/ML	N63002 002 MAR 28, 1991
	CEFAZOLIN SODIUM		
AP	ELKINS SINN	EQ 250 MG BASE/VIAL	N62807 001 JAN 12, 1988
AP		EQ 500 MG BASE/VIAL	N62807 002 JAN 12, 1988
AP		EQ 1 GM BASE/VIAL	N62807 003 JAN 12, 1988
AP		EQ 5 GM BASE/VIAL	N62807 004 JAN 12, 1988
AP		EQ 10 GM BASE/VIAL	N62807 005 JAN 12, 1988
AP		EQ 20 GM BASE/VIAL	N62807 006 JAN 12, 1988
AP	HANFORD	EQ 500 MG BASE/VIAL	N63214 001 DEC 27, 1991
AP		EQ 500 MG BASE/VIAL	N63216 001 DEC 27, 1991
AP		EQ 1 GM BASE/VIAL	N63207 001 DEC 27, 1991
AP		EQ 1 GM BASE/VIAL	N63208 001 DEC 27, 1991
AP		EQ 10 GM BASE/VIAL	N63209 001 DEC 27, 1991
AP	LEMMON	EQ 250 MG BASE/VIAL	N63016 001 MAR 14, 1989
AP		EQ 500 MG BASE/VIAL	N63016 002 MAR 14, 1989
AP		EQ 1 GM BASE/VIAL	N63016 003 MAR 14, 1989
AP		EQ 5 GM BASE/VIAL	N63018 001 MAR 05, 1990
AP		EQ 10 GM BASE/VIAL	N63018 002 MAR 05, 1990
AP	MARSAM	EQ 250 MG BASE/VIAL	N62988 001 DEC 29, 1989
AP		EQ 500 MG BASE/VIAL	N62988 002 DEC 29, 1989
AP		EQ 1 GM BASE/VIAL	N62988 003 DEC 29, 1989
AP		EQ 5 GM BASE/VIAL	N62989 001 DEC 29, 1989
AP		EQ 10 GM BASE/VIAL	N62989 002 DEC 29, 1989
AP		EQ 20 GM BASE/VIAL	N62989 003 DEC 29, 1989

Prescription Drug Products *(continued)*

CEFAZOLIN SODIUM *(continued)*

INJECTABLE; INJECTION

	CEFAZOLIN SODIUM		
AP	SMITHKLINE BEECHAM	EQ 1 GM BASE/VIAL	N64033 001 OCT 31, 1993
	KEFZOL		
AP	LILLY	EQ 250 MG BASE/VIAL	N61773 001
AP		EQ 500 MG BASE/VIAL	N61773 002
AP		EQ 500 MG BASE/VIAL	N62557 001 SEP 10, 1985
AP		EQ 1 GM BASE/VIAL	N61773 003
AP		EQ 1 GM BASE/VIAL	N62557 002 SEP 10, 1985
AP		EQ 10 GM BASE/VIAL	N61773 004
AP		EQ 20 GM BASE/VIAL	N61773 005 SEP 08, 1987
	ZOLICEF		
AP	APOTHECON	EQ 500 MG BASE/VIAL	N62831 001 DEC 09, 1988
AP		EQ 1 GM BASE/VIAL	N62831 002 DEC 09, 1988
AP		EQ 10 GM BASE/VIAL	N62831 003 SEP 25, 1992

CEFIXIME

POWDER FOR RECONSTITUTION; ORAL

SUPRAX		
+ LEDERLE	100 MG/5 ML	N50622 001 APR 28, 1989

TABLET; ORAL

SUPRAX		
+ LEDERLE	200 MG	N50621 001 APR 28, 1989
+	400 MG	N50621 002 APR 28, 1989

CEFMETAZOLE SODIUM

INJECTABLE; INJECTION

ZEFAZONE		
+ UPJOHN	EQ 1 GM BASE/VIAL	N50637 001 DEC 11, 1989
+	EQ 2 GM BASE/VIAL	N50637 002 DEC 11, 1989
ZEFAZONE IN PLASTIC CONTAINER		
UPJOHN	EQ 20 MG BASE/ML	N50683 001 DEC 29, 1992
	EQ 40 MG BASE/ML	N50683 002 DEC 29, 1992

CEFONICID SODIUM

INJECTABLE; INJECTION

MONOCID		
+ SMITHKLINE BEECHAM	EQ 1 GM BASE/VIAL	N50579 002 MAY 23, 1984
	EQ 1 GM BASE/VIAL	N63295 001 JUL 26, 1993
+	EQ 500 MG BASE/VIAL	N50579 001 MAY 23, 1984
+	EQ 10 GM BASE/VIAL	N50579 004 MAY 23, 1984

CEFOPERAZONE SODIUM

INJECTABLE; INJECTION

CEFOBID		
+ PFIZER	EQ 1 GM BASE/VIAL	N50551 001 NOV 18, 1982
+	EQ 2 GM BASE/VIAL	N50551 002 NOV 18, 1982
+	EQ 10 GM BASE/VIAL	N50551 003 MAR 05, 1990
CEFOBID IN PLASTIC CONTAINER		
+ PFIZER	EQ 20 MG BASE/ML	N50613 002 JUL 31, 1987
+	EQ 40 MG BASE/ML	N50613 001 JUL 23, 1986

CEFORANIDE

INJECTABLE; INJECTION

PRECEF		
+ BRISTOL	500 MG/VIAL	N50554 001 MAY 24, 1984
	500 MG/VIAL	N62579 001 NOV 26, 1984
+	1 GM/VIAL	N50554 002 MAY 24, 1984
	1 GM/VIAL	N62579 002 NOV 26, 1984
+	2 GM/VIAL	N50554 003 MAY 24, 1984
	2 GM/VIAL	N62579 003 NOV 26, 1984
+	10 GM/VIAL	N50554 004 MAY 24, 1984
	10 GM/VIAL	N62579 004 NOV 26, 1984
+	20 GM/VIAL	N50554 005 MAY 24, 1984
	20 GM/VIAL	N62579 005 NOV 26, 1984

Prescription Drug Products *(continued)*

CEFOTAXIME SODIUM

INJECTABLE; INJECTION

CLAFORAN		
+ HOECHST ROUSSEL	EQ 500 MG BASE/VIAL	N50547 001
+	EQ 1 GM BASE/VIAL	N50547 002
	EQ 1 GM BASE/VIAL	N62659 001 JAN 13, 1987
+	EQ 2 GM BASE/VIAL	N50547 003
	EQ 2 GM BASE/VIAL	N62659 002 JAN 13, 1987
+	EQ 10 GM BASE/VIAL	N50547 004 DEC 29, 1983
CLAFORAN IN DEXTROSE 5% IN PLASTIC CONTAINER		
+ HOECHST ROUSSEL	EQ 20 MG BASE/ML	N50596 002 MAY 20, 1985
+	EQ 40 MG BASE/ML	N50596 004 MAY 20, 1985
CLAFORAN IN SODIUM CHLORIDE 0.9% IN PLASTIC CONTAINER		
+ HOECHST ROUSSEL	EQ 20 MG BASE/ML	N50596 001 MAY 20, 1985
+	EQ 40 MG BASE/ML	N50596 003 MAY 20, 1985

CEFOTETAN DISODIUM

INJECTABLE; INJECTION

CEFOTAN		
+ ZENECA	EQ 1 GM BASE/VIAL	N50588 001 DEC 27, 1985
	EQ 1 GM BASE/VIAL	N63293 001 APR 29, 1993
+	EQ 2 GM BASE/VIAL	N50588 002 DEC 27, 1985
	EQ 2 GM BASE/VIAL	N63293 002 APR 29, 1993
+	EQ 10 GM BASE/VIAL	N50588 003 APR 25, 1988
CEFOTAN IN PLASTIC CONTAINER		
+ ZENECA	EQ 20 MG BASE/ML	N50694 002 JUL 30, 1993
+	EQ 40 MG BASE/ML	N50694 001 JUL 30, 1993

CEFOXITIN SODIUM

INJECTABLE; INJECTION

MEFOXIN		
+ MERCK SHARP DOHME	EQ 1 GM BASE/VIAL	N50517 001
	EQ 1 GM BASE/VIAL	N62757 001 JAN 08, 1987
+	EQ 2 GM BASE/VIAL	N50517 002
	EQ 2 GM BASE/VIAL	N62757 002 JAN 08, 1987
+	EQ 10 GM BASE/VIAL	N50517 003

CEFOXITIN SODIUM *(continued)*

INJECTABLE; INJECTION

MEFOXIN IN DEXTROSE 5% IN PLASTIC CONTAINER		
+ MERCK SHARP DOHME	EQ 20 MG BASE/ML	N50581 003 SEP 20, 1984
+	EQ 40 MG BASE/ML	N50581 004 SEP 20, 1984
MEFOXIN IN PLASTIC CONTAINER		
MERCK	EQ 20 MG BASE/ML	N63182 001 JAN 25, 1993
	EQ 40 MG BASE/ML	N63182 002 JAN 25, 1993
MEFOXIN IN SODIUM CHLORIDE 0.9% IN PLASTIC CONTAINER		
+ MERCK SHARP DOHME	EQ 20 MG BASE/ML	N50581 002 SEP 20, 1984
+	EQ 40 MG BASE/ML	N50581 001 SEP 20, 1984

CEFPODOXIME PROXETIL

GRANULE, FOR RECONSTITUTION; ORAL

VANTIN		
UPJOHN	EQ 50 MG BASE/5 ML	N50675 001 AUG 07, 1992
+	EQ 100 MG BASE/5 ML	N50675 002 AUG 07, 1992

TABLET; ORAL

VANTIN		
UPJOHN	EQ 100 MG BASE	N50674 001 AUG 07, 1992
+	EQ 200 MG BASE	N50674 002 AUG 07, 1992

CEFPROZIL

POWDER FOR RECONSTITUTION; ORAL

CEFZIL		
BRISTOL MYERS SQUIBB	125 MG/5 ML	N50665 001 DEC 23, 1991
+	250 MG/5 ML	N50665 002 DEC 23, 1991

TABLET; ORAL

CEFZIL		
BRISTOL MYERS SQUIBB	250 MG	N50664 001 DEC 23, 1991
+	500 MG	N50664 002 DEC 23, 1991

Prescription Drug Products *(continued)*

CEFTAZIDIME

INJECTABLE; INJECTION

	FORTAZ		
AP	+ GLAXO	500 MG/VIAL	N50578 001 JUL 19, 1985
AP	+	1 GM/VIAL	N50578 002 JUL 19, 1985
AP	+	2 GM/VIAL	N50578 003 JUL 19, 1985
AP	+	6 GM/VIAL	N50578 004 JUL 19, 1985
	TAZICEF		
AP	SMITHKLINE BEECHAM	500 MG/VIAL	N62662 001 MAR 06, 1986
AP		1 GM/VIAL	N62662 002 MAR 06, 1986
AP		1 GM/VIAL	N64032 001 OCT 31, 1993
AP		2 GM/VIAL	N62662 003 MAR 06, 1986
AP		2 GM/VIAL	N64032 002 OCT 31, 1993
AP		6 GM/VIAL	N62662 004 MAR 06, 1986
	TAZIDIME		
AP	LILLY	500 MG/VIAL	N62640 001 NOV 20, 1985
AP		1 GM/VIAL	N62640 002 NOV 20, 1985
AP		1 GM/VIAL	N62655 001 NOV 20, 1985
AP		2 GM/VIAL	N62640 003 NOV 20, 1985
AP		2 GM/VIAL	N62655 002 NOV 20, 1985
	TAZIDIME IN PLASTIC CONTAINER		
AP	LILLY	1 GM/VIAL	N62739 001 JUL 10, 1986
AP		2 GM/VIAL	N62739 002 JUL 10, 1986

CEFTAZIDIME (ARGININE FORMULATION)

INJECTABLE; INJECTION

	CEPTAZ		
AP	+ GLAXO	1 GM/VIAL	N50646 002 SEP 27, 1990
AP	+	2 GM/VIAL	N50646 003 SEP 27, 1990
AP	+	10 GM/VIAL	N50646 004 SEP 27, 1990
	+	500 MG/VIAL	N50646 001 SEP 27, 1990

CEFTAZIDIME (ARGININE FORMULATION) *(continued)*

INJECTABLE; INJECTION

	PENTACEF		
AP	SMITHKLINE BEECHAM	1 GM/VIAL	N64006 001 MAR 31, 1992
AP		2 GM/VIAL	N64006 002 MAR 31, 1992
AP		10 GM/VIAL	N64008 002 MAR 31, 1992
		6 GM/VIAL	N64008 001 MAR 31, 1992

CEFTAZIDIME SODIUM

INJECTABLE; INJECTION

	CEFTAZIDIME SODIUM IN PLASTIC CONTAINER		
AP	BAXTER	EQ 10 MG BASE/ML	N63221 001 APR 29, 1993
AP		EQ 20 MG BASE/ML	N63221 002 APR 29, 1993
AP		EQ 40 MG BASE/ML	N63221 003 APR 29, 1993
	FORTAZ IN PLASTIC CONTAINER		
AP	+ GLAXO	EQ 10 MG BASE/ML	N50634 001 APR 28, 1989
AP	+	EQ 20 MG BASE/ML	N50634 002 APR 28, 1989
AP	+	EQ 40 MG BASE/ML	N50634 003 APR 28, 1989

CEFTIZOXIME SODIUM

INJECTABLE; INJECTION

	CEFIZOX		
	+ FUJISAWA	EQ 1 GM BASE/VIAL	N50560 002 SEP 15, 1983
		EQ 1 GM BASE/VIAL	N63294 002 MAR 31, 1994
	+	EQ 2 GM BASE/VIAL	N50560 003 SEP 15, 1983
		EQ 2 GM BASE/VIAL	N63294 003 MAR 31, 1994
	+	EQ 500 MG BASE/VIAL	N50560 001 SEP 15, 1983
		EQ 10 GM BASE/VIAL	N50560 005 MAR 19, 1993
	CEFIZOX IN DEXTROSE 5% IN PLASTIC CONTAINER		
	+ FUJISAWA	EQ 20 MG BASE/ML	N50589 001 OCT 03, 1984
	+	EQ 40 MG BASE/ML	N50589 002 OCT 03, 1984

Prescription Drug Products *(continued)*

CEFTRIAXONE SODIUM

INJECTABLE; INJECTION

ROCEPHIN

TE	RLD	Applicant	Strength	Appl No / Approval Date
		ROCHE	EQ 250 MG BASE/VIAL	N63239 001 AUG 13, 1993
			EQ 500 MG BASE/VIAL	N62654 001 APR 30, 1987
			EQ 500 MG BASE/VIAL	N63239 002 AUG 13, 1993
			EQ 1 GM BASE/VIAL	N62654 002 APR 30, 1987
			EQ 1 GM BASE/VIAL	N63239 003 AUG 13, 1993
AP	+		EQ 250 MG BASE/VIAL	N50585 001 DEC 21, 1984
AP	+		EQ 500 MG BASE/VIAL	N50585 002 DEC 21, 1984
AP	+		EQ 1 GM BASE/VIAL	N50585 003 DEC 21, 1984
	+		EQ 2 GM BASE/VIAL	N50585 004 DEC 21, 1984
			EQ 2 GM BASE/VIAL	N62654 003 APR 30, 1987
	+		EQ 10 GM BASE/VIAL	N50585 005 DEC 21, 1984

ROCEPHIN W/ DEXTROSE IN PLASTIC CONTAINER

TE	RLD	Applicant	Strength	Appl No / Approval Date
	+	ROCHE	EQ 20 MG BASE/ML	N50624 002 FEB 11, 1987
	+		EQ 40 MG BASE/ML	N50624 003 FEB 11, 1987

CEFUROXIME AXETIL

POWDER FOR RECONSTITUTION; ORAL

CEFTIN

TE	RLD	Applicant	Strength	Appl No / Approval Date
	+	GLAXO	EQ 125 MG BASE/5 ML	N50672 001 JUN 30, 1994

TABLET; ORAL

CEFTIN

TE	RLD	Applicant	Strength	Appl No / Approval Date
		GLAXO	EQ 125 MG BASE	N50605 001 DEC 28, 1987
			EQ 250 MG BASE	N50605 002 DEC 28, 1987
	+		EQ 500 MG BASE	N50605 003 DEC 28, 1987

CEFUROXIME SODIUM

INJECTABLE; INJECTION

CEFUROXIME

TE	RLD	Applicant	Strength	Appl No / Approval Date
AP		MARSAM	EQ 750 MG BASE/VIAL	N64035 001 FEB 26, 1993
AP			EQ 1.5 GM BASE/VIAL	N64035 002 FEB 26, 1993
AP			EQ 7.5 GM BASE/VIAL	N64036 001 FEB 26, 1993

KEFUROX

TE	RLD	Applicant	Strength	Appl No / Approval Date
AP		LILLY	EQ 750 MG BASE/VIAL	N62591 001 JAN 10, 1986
AP			EQ 750 MG BASE/VIAL	N62592 001 JAN 10, 1986
AP			EQ 1.5 GM BASE/VIAL	N62591 002 JAN 10, 1986
AP			EQ 1.5 GM BASE/VIAL	N62592 002 JAN 10, 1986
AP	+		EQ 7.5 GM BASE/VIAL	N62591 003 DEC 17, 1987

KEFUROX IN PLASTIC CONTAINER

TE	RLD	Applicant	Strength	Appl No / Approval Date
AP		LILLY	EQ 750 MG BASE/VIAL	N62590 001 JAN 10, 1986
AP			EQ 1.5 GM BASE/VIAL	N62590 002 JAN 10, 1986

ZINACEF

TE	RLD	Applicant	Strength	Appl No / Approval Date
AP	+	GLAXO	EQ 750 MG BASE/VIAL	N50558 002 OCT 19, 1983
AP	+		EQ 1.5 GM BASE/VIAL	N50558 003 OCT 19, 1983
AP			EQ 7.5 GM BASE/VIAL	N50558 004 OCT 23, 1986

ZINACEF IN PLASTIC CONTAINER

TE	RLD	Applicant	Strength	Appl No / Approval Date
	+	GLAXO	EQ 15 MG BASE/ML	N50643 001 APR 28, 1989
	+		EQ 30 MG BASE/ML	N50643 002 APR 28, 1989

CELLULOSE SODIUM PHOSPHATE

POWDER; ORAL

CALCIBIND

TE	RLD	Applicant	Strength	Appl No / Approval Date
	+	MISSION PHARMA	300 GM/BOT	N18757 003 OCT 16, 1984

Prescription Drug Products *(continued)*

CEPHALEXIN

CAPSULE; ORAL

CEFANEX

AB	APOTHECON	EQ 250 MG BASE	N63063 001 SEP 29, 1989
AB		EQ 500 MG BASE	N63063 002 SEP 29, 1989

CEPHALEXIN

AB	APOTHECON	EQ 250 MG BASE	N62973 001 NOV 08, 1988
AB		EQ 500 MG BASE	N62974 001 NOV 23, 1988
AB	BARR	EQ 250 MG BASE	N62773 001 JUN 26, 1987
AB		EQ 500 MG BASE	N62775 001 APR 22, 1987
AB	BIOCRAFT	EQ 250 MG BASE	N62702 001 FEB 13, 1987
AB		EQ 500 MG BASE	N62702 002 FEB 13, 1987
AB	LABS ATRAL	EQ 250 MG BASE	N62713 001 JUL 15, 1988
AB		EQ 500 MG BASE	N62713 002 JUL 15, 1988
AB	LEMMON	EQ 250 MG BASE	N62821 001 FEB 05, 1988
AB		EQ 500 MG BASE	N62823 001 FEB 05, 1988
AB	MJ PHARMS	EQ 250 MG BASE	N62791 001 JUN 11, 1987
AB		EQ 500 MG BASE	N62791 002 JUN 11, 1987
AB	NOVOPHARM	EQ 250 MG BASE	N62760 001 APR 24, 1987
AB		EQ 500 MG BASE	N62761 001 APR 24, 1987
AB	PUREPAC PHARM	EQ 250 MG BASE	N62809 001 APR 22, 1987
AB		EQ 500 MG BASE	N62809 002 APR 22, 1987
AB	STEVENS J	EQ 250 MG BASE	N62870 001 MAR 17, 1988
AB		EQ 500 MG BASE	N62869 001 MAR 17, 1988
AB	YOSHITOMI	EQ 250 MG BASE	N62872 001 JUN 20, 1988
AB		EQ 500 MG BASE	N62871 001 JUL 05, 1988
AB	ZENITH LABS	EQ 250 MG BASE	N61969 001
AB		EQ 500 MG BASE	N61969 002

CEPHALEXIN *(continued)*

CAPSULE; ORAL

KEFLEX

AB	+ LILLY	EQ 250 MG BASE	N50405 002
AB		EQ 250 MG BASE	N62118 001
AB	+	EQ 500 MG BASE	N50405 003
AB		EQ 500 MG BASE	N62118 002

POWDER FOR RECONSTITUTION; ORAL

CEPHALEXIN

AB	BARR	EQ 125 MG BASE/5 ML	N62778 001 AUG 06, 1987
AB		EQ 250 MG BASE/5 ML	N62777 001 AUG 06, 1987
AB	BIOCRAFT	EQ 125 MG BASE/5 ML	N62703 001 FEB 13, 1987
AB		EQ 250 MG BASE/5 ML	N62703 002 FEB 13, 1987
AB	LEMMON	EQ 125 MG BASE/5 ML	N62873 001 MAY 23, 1988
AB		EQ 250 MG BASE/5 ML	N62867 001 APR 15, 1988
AB	NOVOPHARM	EQ 125 MG BASE/5 ML	N62767 001 JUN 16, 1987
AB		EQ 250 MG BASE/5 ML	N62768 001 JUN 16, 1987
AB	SQUIBB MARK	EQ 125 MG BASE/5 ML	N62986 001 APR 18, 1991
AB		EQ 250 MG BASE/5 ML	N62987 001 JUL 25, 1989

KEFLEX

AB	+ LILLY	EQ 125 MG BASE/5 ML	N50406 001
AB		EQ 125 MG BASE/5 ML	N62117 002
AB	+	EQ 250 MG BASE/5 ML	N50406 002
AB		EQ 250 MG BASE/5 ML	N62117 003
	+	EQ 100 MG BASE/ML	N50406 003
		EQ 100 MG BASE/ML	N62117 001

TABLET; ORAL

CEPHALEXIN

AB	BARR	EQ 250 MG BASE	N62826 001 AUG 17, 1987
AB		EQ 500 MG BASE	N62827 001 AUG 17, 1987
AB	BIOCRAFT	EQ 250 MG BASE	N63023 001 JAN 12, 1989
AB		EQ 500 MG BASE	N63024 001 JAN 12, 1989

Prescription Drug Products *(continued)*

CEPHALEXIN (*continued*)

TABLET; ORAL

	KEFLET		
AB	+ LILLY	EQ 250 MG BASE	N50440 003 FEB 26, 1987
AB		EQ 250 MG BASE	N62745 001 DEC 01, 1986
AB	+	EQ 500 MG BASE	N50440 001
AB		EQ 500 MG BASE	N62745 002 DEC 01, 1986
	+	EQ 1 GM BASE	N50440 002

CEPHALEXIN HYDROCHLORIDE

TABLET; ORAL

	KEFTAB		
	+ LILLY	EQ 250 MG BASE	N50614 001 OCT 29, 1987
	+	EQ 333 MG BASE	N50614 003 MAY 16, 1988
	+	EQ 500 MG BASE	N50614 002 OCT 29, 1987

CEPHALOGLYCIN

CAPSULE; ORAL

	KAFOCIN		
	+ LILLY	250 MG	N50219 001

CEPHALOTHIN SODIUM

INJECTABLE; INJECTION

	CEPHALOTHIN SODIUM		
AP	ABBOTT	EQ 1 GM BASE/VIAL	N62547 001 SEP 11, 1985
AP		EQ 2 GM BASE/VIAL	N62547 002 SEP 11, 1985
AP	BRISTOL	EQ 1 GM BASE/VIAL	N62464 001 MAY 07, 1984
AP		EQ 2 GM BASE/VIAL	N62464 002 MAY 07, 1984
AP		EQ 4 GM BASE/VIAL	N62464 003 MAY 07, 1984
AP	FUJISAWA	EQ 1 GM BASE/VIAL	N62666 002 JUN 10, 1987
AP		EQ 2 GM BASE/VIAL	N62666 001 JUN 10, 1987

CEPHALOTHIN SODIUM (*continued*)

INJECTABLE; INJECTION

	CEPHALOTHIN SODIUM W/ DEXTROSE IN PLASTIC CONTAINER		
	+ BAXTER	EQ 20 MG BASE/ML	N62422 003 JAN 31, 1984
		EQ 20 MG BASE/ML	N62422 005 JUL 16, 1991
		EQ 20 MG BASE/ML	N62730 001 MAR 05, 1987
	+	EQ 40 MG BASE/ML	N62422 004 JAN 31, 1984
		EQ 40 MG BASE/ML	N62422 006 JUL 16, 1991
		EQ 40 MG BASE/ML	N62730 002 MAR 05, 1987
	CEPHALOTHIN SODIUM W/ SODIUM CHLORIDE IN PLASTIC CONTAINER		
	+ BAXTER	EQ 20 MG BASE/ML	N62422 001 JAN 31, 1984
	+	EQ 40 MG BASE/ML	N62422 002 JAN 31, 1984
	KEFLIN		
AP	+ LILLY	EQ 1 GM BASE/VIAL	N50482 001
AP	+	EQ 2 GM BASE/VIAL	N50482 002
AP	+	EQ 4 GM BASE/VIAL	N50482 003
	+	EQ 20 GM BASE/VIAL	N50482 007
	KEFLIN IN PLASTIC CONTAINER		
AP	+ LILLY	EQ 1 GM BASE/VIAL	N62549 001 SEP 10, 1985
AP	+	EQ 2 GM BASE/VIAL	N62549 002 SEP 10, 1985

CEPHAPIRIN SODIUM

INJECTABLE; INJECTION

	CEFADYL		
	APOTHECON	EQ 500 MG BASE/VIAL	N62961 001 SEP 20, 1988
		EQ 1 GM BASE/VIAL	N61769 001
		EQ 1 GM BASE/VIAL	N62724 001 DEC 23, 1986
		EQ 1 GM BASE/VIAL	N62961 002 SEP 20, 1988
		EQ 2 GM BASE/VIAL	N61769 002
		EQ 2 GM BASE/VIAL	N62724 002 DEC 23, 1986
		EQ 2 GM BASE/VIAL	N62961 003 SEP 20, 1988
		EQ 4 GM BASE/VIAL	N61769 003
		EQ 4 GM BASE/VIAL	N62961 004 SEP 20, 1988

Prescription Drug Products *(continued)*

CEPHRADINE

	CAPSULE; ORAL		
	<u>ANSPOR</u>		
AB	SMITHKLINE BEECHAM	250 MG	N61859 001
AB		500 MG	N61859 002
	<u>CEPHRADINE</u>		
AB	BARR	250 MG	N62850 001 APR 22, 1988
AB		500 MG	N62851 001 APR 22, 1988
AB	BIOCRAFT	250 MG	N62683 001 JAN 09, 1987
AB		500 MG	N62683 002 JAN 09, 1987
AB	ZENITH LABS	250 MG	N62762 001 MAR 06, 1987
AB		500 MG	N62762 002 MAR 06, 1987
	<u>VELOSEF</u>		
AB	+ ERSANA	250 MG	N61764 001
AB	+	500 MG	N61764 002
	INJECTABLE; INJECTION		
	VELOSEF		
	+ SQUIBB	250 MG/VIAL	N61976 001
	+	500 MG/VIAL	N61976 002
	+	1 GM/VIAL	N61976 004
	+	2 GM/VIAL	N61976 003
	+	4 GM/VIAL	N61976 005
	POWDER FOR RECONSTITUTION; ORAL		
	<u>ANSPOR</u>		
AB	SMITHKLINE BEECHAM	125 MG/5 ML	N61866 001
AB		250 MG/5 ML	N61866 002
	<u>CEPHRADINE</u>		
AB	BARR	125 MG/5 ML	N62858 001 MAY 19, 1988
AB		250 MG/5 ML	N62859 001 MAY 19, 1988
AB	BIOCRAFT	125 MG/5 ML	N62693 001 JAN 09, 1987
AB		250 MG/5 ML	N62693 002 JAN 09, 1987
	<u>VELOSEF '125'</u>		
AB	+ ERSANA	125 MG/5 ML	N61763 001
	<u>VELOSEF '250'</u>		
AB	+ ERSANA	250 MG/5 ML	N61763 002

CETYL ALCOHOL; COLFOSCERIL PALMITATE; TYLOXAPOL

	POWDER FOR RECONSTITUTION; INTRATRACHEAL		
	EXOSURF NEONATAL		
	BURROUGHS WELLCOME	12 MG/VIAL;108 MG/ VIAL;8 MG/VIAL	N20044 001 AUG 02, 1990

CHENODIOL

	TABLET; ORAL		
	CHENIX		
	+ SOLVAY	250 MG	N18513 002 JUL 28, 1983

CHLORAMBUCIL

	TABLET; ORAL		
	LEUKERAN		
	+ BURROUGHS WELLCOME	2 MG	N10669 002

CHLORAMPHENICOL

	CAPSULE; ORAL		
	<u>AMPHICOL</u>		
AB	MK LABS	100 MG	N60058 001
AB		250 MG	N60058 002
	<u>CHLORAMPHENICOL</u>		
AB	ZENITH LABS	250 MG	N62247 001
	<u>CHLOROMYCETIN</u>		
AB	+ PARKE DAVIS	100 MG	N60591 003
AB	+	250 MG	N60591 002
		50 MG	N60591 001
	<u>MYCHEL</u>		
AB	RACHELLE	250 MG	N60851 001
	CREAM; TOPICAL		
	CHLOROMYCETIN		
	PARKE DAVIS	1%	N50183 001
	OINTMENT; OPHTHALMIC		
	<u>CHLORAMPHENICOL</u>		
AT	ALTANA	1%	N60133 001
	<u>CHLOROMYCETIN</u>		
AT	PARKE DAVIS	1%	N50156 001
	<u>CHLOROPTIC S.O.P.</u>		
AT	ALLERGAN	1%	N61187 001
	POWDER FOR RECONSTITUTION; OPHTHALMIC		
	CHLOROMYCETIN		
	+ PARKE DAVIS	25 MG/VIAL	N50143 001

CHLORAMPHENICOL *(continued)*

SOLUTION/DROPS; OPHTHALMIC

	CHLORAMPHENICOL		
AT	AKORN	0.5%	N62042 001
AT	STERIS	0.5%	N62628 001 SEP 25, 1985
	CHLOROPTIC		
AT	+ ALLERGAN	0.5%	N50091 001
	OPHTHOCHLOR		
AT	PARKE DAVIS	0.5%	N61220 001
	OPTOMYCIN		
AT	OPTOPICS	0.5%	N62171 001 MAR 31, 1982

SOLUTION/DROPS; OTIC

	CHLOROMYCETIN		
	+ PARKE DAVIS	0.5%	N50205 001

CHLORAMPHENICOL; DESOXYRIBONUCLEASE; FIBRINOLYSIN

OINTMENT; TOPICAL

	ELASE-CHLOROMYCETIN		
	+ PARKE DAVIS	10 MG/GM;666 UNITS/GM;1 UNITS/GM	N50294 001

CHLORAMPHENICOL; HYDROCORTISONE ACETATE

POWDER FOR RECONSTITUTION; OPHTHALMIC

	CHLOROMYCETIN HYDROCORTISONE		
	+ PARKE DAVIS	12.5 MG/VIAL;25 MG/VIAL	N50202 001

CHLORAMPHENICOL; HYDROCORTISONE ACETATE; POLYMYXIN B SULFATE

OINTMENT; OPHTHALMIC

	OPHTHOCORT		
	+ PARKE DAVIS	10 MG/GM;5 MG/GM;10,000 UNITS/GM	N50201 002

CHLORAMPHENICOL PALMITATE

SUSPENSION; ORAL

	CHLOROMYCETIN PALMITATE		
	+ PARKE DAVIS	EQ 150 MG BASE/5 ML	N50152 001
		EQ 150 MG BASE/5 ML	N62301 001

CHLORAMPHENICOL SODIUM SUCCINATE

INJECTABLE; INJECTION

	CHLORAMPHENICOL		
AP	ELKINS SINN	EQ 1 GM BASE/VIAL	N62406 001 NOV 09, 1982
	CHLORAMPHENICOL SODIUM SUCCINATE		
AP	FUJISAWA	EQ 1 GM BASE/VIAL	N62365 001 AUG 25, 1982
AP	GRUPPO LEPETIT	EQ 1 GM BASE/VIAL	N62278 001
	CHLOROMYCETIN		
AP	+ PARKE DAVIS	EQ 1 GM BASE/VIAL	N50155 001

CHLORDIAZEPOXIDE

TABLET; ORAL

	LIBRITABS		
	ROCHE	5 MG	N85482 001
		10 MG	N85481 001
	+	25 MG	N85488 001

CHLORDIAZEPOXIDE; *MULTIPLE*

SEE AMITRIPTYLINE HYDROCHLORIDE; CHLORDIAZEPOXIDE

CHLORDIAZEPOXIDE; ESTROGENS, ESTERIFIED

TABLET; ORAL

	MENRIUM 10-4		
	ROCHE	10 MG;0.4 MG	N14740 006
	MENRIUM 5-2		
	ROCHE	5 MG;0.2 MG	N14740 002
	MENRIUM 5-4		
	+ ROCHE	5 MG;0.4 MG	N14740 004

CHLORDIAZEPOXIDE HYDROCHLORIDE

CAPSULE; ORAL

	CHLORDIAZACHEL		
AB	RACHELLE	5 MG	N85086 001
AB		10 MG	N84639 001
AB		25 MG	N85087 001
	CHLORDIAZEPOXIDE HCL		
AB	BARR	5 MG	N84768 001
AB		10 MG	N83116 001
AB		25 MG	N84769 001
AB	CHELSEA LABS	5 MG	N86383 001
AB		10 MG	N86294 001
AB		25 MG	N86382 001
AB	FERRANTE	5 MG	N85118 001
AB		10 MG	N85119 001
AB		25 MG	N85120 001

Prescription Drug Products *(continued)*

CHLORDIAZEPOXIDE HYDROCHLORIDE *(continued)*

CAPSULE; ORAL

	CHLORDIAZEPOXIDE HCL		
AB	GENEVA PHARMS	5 MG	N84678 001
AB		10 MG	N84041 001
AB		25 MG	N84679 002
AB	GLOBAL PHARMS	5 MG	N86213 001
AB		10 MG	N85113 001
AB		25 MG	N86212 001
AB	HALSEY	5 MG	N85340 001
AB		10 MG	N85339 001
AB		25 MG	N84685 001
AB	MM MAST	10 MG	N86217 001
AB	ROSEMONT PHARM	5 MG	N84644 001
AB		10 MG	N84623 001
AB		25 MG	N84645 001
AB	ZENITH LABS	5 MG	N83741 001
AB		10 MG	N83742 001
AB		25 MG	N83570 001
	LIBRIUM		
AB	ROCHE	5 MG	N85461 001
AB		10 MG	N85472 001
AB	+	25 MG	N85475 001

INJECTABLE; INJECTION

	LIBRIUM		
	+ ROCHE	100 MG/AMP	N12301 001

CHLORHEXIDINE GLUCONATE

SOLUTION; DENTAL

	PERIDEX		
AT	+ PROCTER AND GAMBLE	0.12%	N19028 001 AUG 13, 1986
	PERIOGARD		
AT	COLGATE PALMOLIVE	0.12%	N73695 001 JAN 14, 1994

CHLORMEZANONE

TABLET; ORAL

	TRANCOPAL		
	STERLING WINTHROP	100 MG	N11467 003
		200 MG	N11467 005

CHLOROPROCAINE HYDROCHLORIDE

INJECTABLE; INJECTION

	CHLOROPROCAINE HCL		
AP	ABBOTT	2%	N87447 001 APR 16, 1982
AP		3%	N87446 001 APR 16, 1982
	NESACAINE		
	ASTRA	1%	N09435 001
		2%	N09435 002
	NESACAINE-MPF		
AP	ASTRA	2%	N09435 003
AP		3%	N09435 004

CHLOROQUINE HYDROCHLORIDE

INJECTABLE; INJECTION

	ARALEN HCL		
	+ STERLING WINTHROP	EQ 40 MG BASE/ML	N06002 002

CHLOROQUINE PHOSPHATE

TABLET; ORAL

	ARALEN		
AA	STERLING WINTHROP	EQ 300 MG BASE	N06002 001
	CHLOROQUINE PHOSPHATE		
AA	BIOCRAFT	EQ 150 MG BASE	N87504 001 JAN 13, 1982
AA	DANBURY PHARMA	EQ 150 MG BASE	N87979 001 DEC 21, 1982
AA		EQ 300 MG BASE	N88030 001 DEC 21, 1982
AA	GLOBAL PHARMS	EQ 150 MG BASE	N80880 001
AA	MD PHARM	EQ 150 MG BASE	N87228 001

CHLOROTHIAZIDE

SUSPENSION; ORAL

	DIURIL		
	+ MERCK SHARP DOHME	250 MG/5 ML	N11870 001

TABLET; ORAL

	CHLOROTHIAZIDE		
AB	CAMALL	250 MG	N85569 001
AB	CHELSEA LABS	250 MG	N86795 001 AUG 15, 1983
AB	DANBURY PHARMA	250 MG	N85173 001
AB	MYLAN	250 MG	N84388 001
AB		500 MG	N84217 001
AB	WEST WARD PHARM	250 MG	N86028 001 JUL 14, 1982
AB		500 MG	N87736 001 JUL 14, 1982

Prescription Drug Products *(continued)*

CHLOROTHIAZIDE (*continued*)

	TABLET; ORAL		
	DIURIL		
AB	MERCK SHARP DOHME	250 MG	N11145 004
AB	+	500 MG	N11145 002

CHLOROTHIAZIDE; METHYLDOPA

	TABLET; ORAL		
	ALDOCLOR-150		
	MERCK SHARP DOHME	150 MG;250 MG	N16016 001
	ALDOCLOR-250		
	+ MERCK SHARP DOHME	250 MG;250 MG	N16016 002

CHLOROTHIAZIDE; RESERPINE

	TABLET; ORAL		
	CHLOROTHIAZIDE AND RESERPINE		
BP	WEST WARD PHARM	250 MG;0.125 MG	N88557 001 DEC 22, 1983
BP		500 MG;0.125 MG	N88365 001 DEC 22, 1983
	CHLOROTHIAZIDE-RESERPINE		
BP	MYLAN	250 MG;0.125 MG	N87744 001 MAY 06, 1982
BP		500 MG;0.125 MG	N87745 001 MAY 06, 1982
	DIUPRES-250		
BP	MERCK SHARP DOHME	250 MG;0.125 MG	N11635 003 AUG 26, 1987
	DIUPRES-500		
BP	+ MERCK SHARP DOHME	500 MG;0.125 MG	N11635 006 AUG 26, 1987

CHLOROTHIAZIDE SODIUM

	INJECTABLE; INJECTION		
	DIURIL		
	+ MERCK SHARP DOHME	EQ 500 MG BASE/VIAL	N11145 005

CHLOROTRIANISENE

	CAPSULE; ORAL		
	CHLOROTRIANISENE		
AA	BANNER PHARMACAPS	12 MG	N84652 001
	TACE		
AA	MERRELL DOW	12 MG	N08102 004
		25 MG	N11444 001

CHLOROXINE

	SHAMPOO; TOPICAL		
	CAPITROL		
	+ WESTWOOD SQUIBB	2%	N17594 001

CHLORPHENESIN CARBAMATE

	TABLET; ORAL		
	MAOLATE		
	+ UPJOHN	400 MG	N14217 002

CHLORPHENIRAMINE MALEATE

	INJECTABLE; INJECTION		
	CHLOR-TRIMETON		
AP	+ SCHERING PLOUGH	10 MG/ML	N08826 001
	CHLORPHENIRAMINE MALEATE		
AP	STERIS	10 MG/ML	N83593 001
AP		10 MG/ML	N86096 001
		100 MG/ML	N86095 001
	TABLET; ORAL		
	CHLORPHENIRAMINE MALEATE		
AA	DANBURY PHARMA	4 MG	N80696 001
AA	GENEVA PHARMS	4 MG	N80961 001
AA	GLOBAL PHARMS	4 MG	N80809 001
AA	ICN	4 MG	N80598 001
AA	KV PHARM	4 MG	N87164 001
AA	MARSHALL PHARMA	4 MG	N83286 001
AA	PHARMAVITE	4 MG	N85104 001
AA	PHOENIX LABS NY	4 MG	N85522 001
AA	SUPERPHARM	4 MG	N87747 001 APR 20, 1982
AA	TABLICAPS	4 MG	N83394 001
AA	WEST WARD PHARM	4 MG	N83787 001
	KLOROMIN		
AA	HALSEY	4 MG	N83629 001

CHLORPHENIRAMINE MALEATE; PHENYLPROPANOLAMINE HYDROCHLORIDE

	CAPSULE, EXTENDED RELEASE; ORAL		
	CHLORPHENIRAMINE MALEATE AND PHENYLPROPANOLAMINE HCL		
AB	GENEVA PHARMS	12 MG;75 MG	N88940 001 JAN 26, 1989
	DRIZE		
BC	ASCHER	12 MG;75 MG	N88359 001 FEB 13, 1986
	ORNADE		
AB	+ SMITHKLINE BEECHAM	12 MG;75 MG	N12152 004

CHLORPHENIRAMINE POLISTIREX; HYDROCODONE POLISTIREX

	SUSPENSION, EXTENDED RELEASE; ORAL		
	TUSSIONEX		
	+ FISONS	EQ 8 MG MALEATE/ 5 ML;EQ 10 MG BITARTRATE/5 ML	N19111 001 DEC 31, 1987

Prescription Drug Products *(continued)*

CHLORPROMAZINE

	SUPPOSITORY; RECTAL		
	THORAZINE		
	+ SMITHKLINE BEECHAM	25 MG	N09149 024
	+	100 MG	N09149 033

CHLORPROMAZINE HYDROCHLORIDE

	CAPSULE, EXTENDED RELEASE; ORAL		
	THORAZINE		
	+ SMITHKLINE BEECHAM	30 MG	N11120 016
	+	75 MG	N11120 017
	+	150 MG	N11120 018
	+	200 MG	N11120 019
	+	300 MG	N11120 020
	CONCENTRATE; ORAL		
	CHLORPROMAZINE HCL		
AA	BARRE	100 MG/ML	N86863 001
	CHLORPROMAZINE HCL INTENSOL		
AA	ROXANE	30 MG/ML	N88157 001 APR 27, 1983
AA		100 MG/ML	N88158 001 APR 27, 1983
	SONAZINE		
AA	GENEVA PHARMS	30 MG/ML	N80983 004
AA		100 MG/ML	N80983 005
	THORAZINE		
AA	SMITHKLINE BEECHAM	30 MG/ML	N09149 032
AA		100 MG/ML	N09149 043
	INJECTABLE; INJECTION		
	CHLORPROMAZINE HCL		
AP	ELKINS SINN	25 MG/ML	N83329 001
AP	MARSAM	25 MG/ML	N89563 001 APR 15, 1988
AP	STERIS	25 MG/ML	N80365 001
AP		25 MG/ML	N85591 001
	THORAZINE		
AP	+ SMITHKLINE BEECHAM	25 MG/ML	N09149 011
	SYRUP; ORAL		
	SONAZINE		
AA	GENEVA PHARMS	10 MG/5 ML	N83040 001
	THORAZINE		
AA	SMITHKLINE BEECHAM	10 MG/5 ML	N09149 022

CHLORPROMAZINE HYDROCHLORIDE *(continued)*

	TABLET; ORAL		
	CHLORPROMAZINE HCL		
BP	GENEVA PHARMS	10 MG	N80439 001
BP		25 MG	N80439 002
BP		50 MG	N80439 003
BP		100 MG	N80439 004
BP		200 MG	N80439 005
BP	KV PHARM	10 MG	N85750 002 JAN 04, 1982
BP		25 MG	N85751 001
BP		50 MG	N85484 001
BP		100 MG	N85752 001
BP		200 MG	N85748 002 JAN 04, 1982
BP	LEDERLE	10 MG	N84803 001
BP	ROSEMONT PHARM	10 MG	N83386 001
BP		25 MG	N84112 001
BP		50 MG	N84113 001
BP		100 MG	N84114 001
BP		200 MG	N84115 001
BP	ZENITH LABS	10 MG	N83549 001
BP		25 MG	N83549 002
BP		50 MG	N83549 003
BP		100 MG	N83574 001
BP		200 MG	N83575 001
	THORAZINE		
BP	+ SMITHKLINE BEECHAM	10 MG	N09149 002
BP		25 MG	N09149 007
BP		50 MG	N09149 013
BP	+	100 MG	N09149 018
BP		200 MG	N09149 020

CHLORPROPAMIDE

	TABLET; ORAL		
	CHLORPROPAMIDE		
AB	BARR	100 MG	N88812 001 OCT 19, 1984
AB		100 MG	N89446 001 NOV 17, 1986
AB		250 MG	N88813 001 OCT 19, 1984
AB		250 MG	N89447 001 NOV 17, 1986
AB	DANBURY PHARMA	100 MG	N88852 001 SEP 26, 1984
AB		250 MG	N88826 001 SEP 26, 1984

Prescription Drug Products *(continued)*

CHLORPROPAMIDE *(continued)*

TABLET; ORAL

TE	Product / Applicant	Strength	Appl No	Approval Date
	CHLORPROPAMIDE			
AB	GENEVA PHARMS	100 MG	N88725 001	AUG 31, 1984
AB		250 MG	N88726 001	AUG 31, 1984
AB	HALSEY	100 MG	N89321 001	JAN 16, 1986
AB		250 MG	N88662 001	JAN 09, 1986
AB	LEDERLE	100 MG	N89561 001	SEP 04, 1987
AB		250 MG	N89562 001	SEP 04, 1987
AB	LEMMON	100 MG	N88768 001	OCT 11, 1984
AB	MYLAN	100 MG	N88548 001	JUN 01, 1984
AB		250 MG	N88549 001	JUN 01, 1984
AB	PAR PHARM	100 MG	N88175 001	FEB 27, 1984
AB		250 MG	N88176 001	FEB 27, 1984
AB	SIDMAK LABS NJ	100 MG	N88921 001	APR 12, 1985
AB		250 MG	N88922 001	APR 12, 1985
AB	SUPERPHARM	100 MG	N88694 001	SEP 17, 1984
AB		250 MG	N88695 001	SEP 17, 1984
AB	ZENITH LABS	100 MG	N88840 001	OCT 25, 1984
AB		250 MG	N87353 001	
	DIABINESE			
AB	PFIZER	100 MG	N11641 003	
AB	+	250 MG	N11641 006	
	GLUCAMIDE			
AB	LEMMON	250 MG	N88641 001	OCT 11, 1984

CHLORPROTHIXENE

CONCENTRATE; ORAL

TE	Product / Applicant	Strength	Appl No	Approval Date
	TARACTAN			
	ROCHE	100 MG/5 ML	N16149 002	

INJECTABLE; INJECTION

TE	Product / Applicant	Strength	Appl No	Approval Date
	TARACTAN			
	+ ROCHE	12.5 MG/ML	N12487 001	

CHLORPROTHIXENE *(continued)*

TABLET; ORAL

TE	Product / Applicant	Strength	Appl No	Approval Date
	TARACTAN			
	ROCHE	10 MG	N12486 005	
		25 MG	N12486 004	
		50 MG	N12486 003	
	+	100 MG	N12486 001	

CHLORTETRACYCLINE HYDROCHLORIDE

OINTMENT; OPHTHALMIC

TE	Product / Applicant	Strength	Appl No	Approval Date
	AUREOMYCIN			
	+ LEDERLE	1%	N50404 001	

CHLORTHALIDONE

TABLET; ORAL

TE	Product / Applicant	Strength	Appl No	Approval Date
	CHLORTHALIDONE			
AB	ABBOTT	25 MG	N87364 001	
AB	BARR	25 MG	N87292 001	
AB		50 MG	N87293 001	
AB	CHELSEA LABS	25 MG	N87100 001	
AB	DANBURY PHARMA	25 MG	N87296 001	
AB		25 MG	N87706 001	
AB		50 MG	N87521 001	
AB		50 MG	N87689 001	
AB	EON LABS	50 MG	N87118 001	
AB	GENEVA PHARMS	25 MG	N87380 001	
AB		50 MG	N87381 001	
AB	KV PHARM	25 MG	N87311 001	
AB		50 MG	N87312 001	
AB	LEDERLE	25 MG	N87451 001	
AB		50 MG	N87450 001	
AB	MUTUAL PHARM	25 MG	N89285 001	JUL 21, 1986
AB		25 MG	N89738 001	SEP 19, 1988
AB		50 MG	N89286 001	JUL 21, 1986
AB		50 MG	N89739 001	SEP 19, 1988
AB	MYLAN	25 MG	N87180 001	
AB		50 MG	N86831 001	
AB	PUREPAC PHARM	25 MG	N88139 001	JUL 16, 1986
AB		50 MG	N88140 001	AUG 11, 1983
AB	ROSEMONT PHARM	25 MG	N89051 001	JUN 01, 1987

Prescription Drug Products *(continued)*

CHLORTHALIDONE *(continued)*

TABLET; ORAL

	CHLORTHALIDONE		
AB	SIDMAK LABS NJ	25 MG	N88902 001 SEP 19, 1985
AB		50 MG	N88903 001 SEP 19, 1985
AB	SUPERPHARM	50 MG	N87247 001 FEB 09, 1983
AB	ZENITH LABS	25 MG	N88164 001 JAN 09, 1984
AB		50 MG	N87176 001
AB		50 MG	N87947 001 FEB 27, 1984
	HYGROTON		
AB	RHONE POULENC RORER	25 MG	N12283 004
AB	+	50 MG	N12283 003
	THALITONE		
BX	HORUS THERAP	25 MG	N88051 001 NOV 12, 1982
	+	15 MG	N19574 001 DEC 20, 1988

CHLORTHALIDONE; *MULTIPLE*

SEE ATENOLOL; CHLORTHALIDONE

SEE BETAXOLOL HYDROCHLORIDE; CHLORTHALIDONE

CHLORTHALIDONE; CLONIDINE HYDROCHLORIDE

TABLET; ORAL

	CLONIDINE HCL AND CHLORTHALIDONE		
AB	MYLAN	15 MG;0.1 MG	N71323 001 FEB 09, 1987
AB		15 MG;0.2 MG	N71324 001 FEB 09, 1987
AB		15 MG;0.3 MG	N71325 001 FEB 09, 1987
AB	PAR PHARM	15 MG;0.1 MG	N71179 001 DEC 16, 1987
AB		15 MG;0.2 MG	N71178 001 DEC 16, 1987
AB		15 MG;0.3 MG	N71142 001 DEC 16, 1987
	COMBIPRES		
AB	BOEHRINGER INGELHEIM	15 MG;0.1 MG	N17503 001
AB		15 MG;0.2 MG	N17503 002
AB	+	15 MG;0.3 MG	N17503 003 APR 10, 1984

CHLORTHALIDONE; RESERPINE

TABLET; ORAL

	DEMI-REGROTON		
	RHONE POULENC RORER	25 MG;0.125 MG	N15103 002
	REGROTON		
	+ RHONE POULENC RORER	50 MG;0.25 MG	N15103 001

CHLORZOXAZONE

TABLET; ORAL

	CHLORZOXAZONE		
AA	AMIDE PHARM	250 MG	N88928 001 MAY 08, 1987
AA	BARR	500 MG	N89895 001 MAY 04, 1988
AA	DANBURY PHARMA	250 MG	N86901 001
AA		500 MG	N81019 001 JUL 29, 1991
AA	GENEVA PHARMS	250 MG	N89852 001 MAY 04, 1988
AA		500 MG	N89853 001 MAY 04, 1988
AA	LEMMON	500 MG	N89859 001 MAY 04, 1988
AA	MUTUAL PHARM	500 MG	N89970 001 SEP 27, 1990
AA	OHM	250 MG	N81298 001 DEC 29, 1993
AA		500 MG	N81299 001 DEC 29, 1993
AA	PAR PHARM	250 MG	N87981 001 SEP 20, 1983
AA	ROYCE LABS	500 MG	N81040 001 AUG 22, 1989
	PARAFLEX		
AA	JOHNSON RW	250 MG	N11300 003
	PARAFON FORTE DSC		
AA	JOHNSON RW	500 MG	N11529 002 JUN 15, 1987
	STRIFON FORTE DSC		
AA	FERNDALE LABS	500 MG	N81008 001 DEC 23, 1988

Prescription Drug Products *(continued)*

CHOLESTYRAMINE

BAR, CHEWABLE; ORAL

	CHOLYBAR		
	+ PARKE DAVIS	EQ 4 GM RESIN/BAR	N71621 001 MAY 26, 1988
		EQ 4 GM RESIN/BAR	N71739 001 MAY 26, 1988

POWDER; ORAL

	QUESTRAN		
	+ BRISTOL MYERS	EQ 4 GM RESIN/PACKET	N16640 001
		EQ 4 GM RESIN/SCOOPFUL	N16640 003
	QUESTRAN LIGHT		
	BRISTOL MYERS	EQ 4 GM RESIN/PACKET	N19669 001 DEC 05, 1988
		EQ 4 GM RESIN/SCOOPFUL	N19669 003 DEC 05, 1988

TABLET; ORAL

	QUESTRAN		
	+ BRISTOL MYERS SQUIBB	EQ 1 GM RESIN	N73403 001 APR 28, 1994

CHROMIC CHLORIDE

INJECTABLE; INJECTION

	CHROMIC CHLORIDE		
AP	FUJISAWA	EQ 0.004 MG CHROMIUM/ML	N19271 001 MAY 05, 1987
	CHROMIC CHLORIDE IN PLASTIC CONTAINER		
AP	+ ABBOTT	EQ 0.004 MG CHROMIUM/ML	N18961 001 JUN 26, 1986

CHROMIC PHOSPHATE, P-32

INJECTABLE; INJECTION

	PHOSPHOCOL P32		
	MALLINCKRODT	5mCi/ML	N17084 001

CHYMOPAPAIN

INJECTABLE; INJECTION

	CHYMODIACTIN		
	+ BOOTS	4,000 UNITS/VIAL	N18663 002 AUG 21, 1984

CHYMOTRYPSIN

POWDER FOR RECONSTITUTION; OPHTHALMIC

	CATARASE		
	+ IOLAB	300 UNITS/VIAL	N16938 001
	ZOLYSE		
	ALCON	750 UNITS/VIAL	N11903 001

CICLOPIROX OLAMINE

CREAM; TOPICAL

	LOPROX		
	+ HOECHST ROUSSEL	1%	N18748 001 DEC 30, 1982

LOTION; TOPICAL

	LOPROX		
	+ HOECHST ROUSSEL	1%	N19824 001 DEC 30, 1988

CILASTATIN SODIUM; IMIPENEM

INJECTABLE; INJECTION

	PRIMAXIN		
	+ MERCK SHARP DOHME	EQ 250 MG BASE/VIAL;250 MG/VIAL	N50587 001 NOV 26, 1985
		EQ 250 MG BASE/VIAL;250 MG/VIAL	N62756 001 JAN 08, 1987
	+	EQ 500 MG BASE/VIAL;500 MG/VIAL	N50587 002 NOV 26, 1985
		EQ 500 MG BASE/VIAL;500 MG/VIAL	N50630 001 DEC 14, 1990
		EQ 500 MG BASE/VIAL;500 MG/VIAL	N62756 002 JAN 08, 1987
	+	EQ 750 MG BASE/VIAL;750 MG/VIAL	N50630 002 DEC 14, 1990

CIMETIDINE

TABLET; ORAL

	CIMETIDINE		
AB	ENDO LABS	200 MG	N74281 001 MAY 17, 1994
AB		300 MG	N74281 002 MAY 17, 1994
AB		400 MG	N74281 003 MAY 17, 1994
AB		800 MG	N74329 001 MAY 17, 1994

Prescription Drug Products *(continued)*

CIMETIDINE *(continued)*

TABLET; ORAL

CIMETIDINE

AB MYLAN 200 MG N74246 001 MAY 17, 1994
AB 300 MG N74246 002 MAY 17, 1994
AB 400 MG N74246 003 MAY 17, 1994
AB 800 MG N74246 004 MAY 17, 1994
AB NOVOPHARM 200 MG N74151 001 MAY 17, 1994
AB 300 MG N74151 002 MAY 17, 1994
AB 400 MG N74151 003 MAY 17, 1994
AB 800 MG N74463 001 MAY 17, 1994

TAGAMET

AB SMITHKLINE BEECHAM 200 MG N17920 002
AB 300 MG N17920 003
AB 400 MG N17920 004 DEC 14, 1983
AB + 800 MG N17920 005 APR 30, 1986

CIMETIDINE HYDROCHLORIDE

INJECTABLE; INJECTION

CIMETIDINE HCL

AP ENDO LABS EQ 300 MG BASE/2 ML N74005 001 AUG 31, 1994

TAGAMET

AP + SMITHKLINE BEECHAM EQ 300 MG BASE/2 ML N17939 002

TAGAMET HCL IN SODIUM CHLORIDE 0.9% IN PLASTIC CONTAINER

+ SMITHKLINE BEECHAM EQ 6 MG BASE/ML N19434 001 OCT 31, 1985

SOLUTION; ORAL

CIMETIDINE HCL

AA BARRE EQ 300 MG BASE/5 ML N74176 001 JUN 01, 1994

TAGAMET

AA SMITHKLINE BEECHAM EQ 300 MG BASE/5 ML N17924 001

CINOXACIN

CAPSULE; ORAL

CINOBAC

AB LILLY 250 MG N18067 001
AB + 500 MG N18067 002

CINOXACIN

AB BIOCRAFT 250 MG N73005 001 FEB 28, 1992
AB 500 MG N73006 001 FEB 28, 1992

CIPROFLOXACIN

INJECTABLE; INJECTION

CIPRO

+ MILES 10 MG/ML N19847 001 DEC 26, 1990

CIPRO IN DEXTROSE 5% IN PLASTIC CONTAINER

+ MILES 200 MG/100 ML N19857 001 DEC 26, 1990

CIPRO IN SODIUM CHLORIDE 0.9% IN PLASTIC CONTAINER

+ MILES 200 MG/100 ML N19858 001 DEC 26, 1990

CIPROFLOXACIN HYDROCHLORIDE

SOLUTION/DROPS; OPHTHALMIC

CILOXAN

+ ALCON EQ 0.3% BASE N19992 001 DEC 31, 1990

TABLET; ORAL

CIPRO

MILES EQ 250 MG BASE N19537 002 OCT 22, 1987
EQ 500 MG BASE N19537 003 OCT 22, 1987
+ EQ 750 MG BASE N19537 004 OCT 22, 1987

CISAPRIDE MONOHYDRATE

TABLET; ORAL

PROPULSID

JANSSEN EQ 10 MG BASE N20210 001 JUL 29, 1993
+ EQ 20 MG BASE N20210 002 DEC 23, 1993

Prescription Drug Products *(continued)*

CISPLATIN

INJECTABLE; INJECTION

	Product / Applicant	Strength	Appl No / Date
	PLATINOL		
	+ BRISTOL MYERS	10 MG/VIAL	N18057 001
	+	50 MG/VIAL	N18057 002
	PLATINOL-AQ		
	+ BRISTOL MYERS	1 MG/ML	N18057 004 NOV 08, 1988

CITRIC ACID; GLUCONOLACTONE; MAGNESIUM CARBONATE

SOLUTION; IRRIGATION

	Product / Applicant	Strength	Appl No / Date
	RENACIDIN		
	GUARDIAN LABS	6.602 GM/100 ML;198 MG/100 ML;3.177 GM/100 ML	N19481 001 OCT 02, 1990

CITRIC ACID; MAGNESIUM OXIDE; SODIUM CARBONATE

SOLUTION; IRRIGATION

	Product / Applicant	Strength	Appl No / Date
	<u>IRRIGATING SOLUTION G IN PLASTIC CONTAINER</u>		
<u>AT</u>	BAXTER	<u>3.24 GM/100 ML;380 MG/100 ML;430 MG/100 ML</u>	N18519 001 JUN 22, 1982
	<u>UROLOGIC G IN PLASTIC CONTAINER</u>		
<u>AT</u>	ABBOTT	<u>3.24 GM/100 ML;380 MG/100 ML;430 MG/100 ML</u>	N18904 001 MAY 27, 1983

CLADRIBINE

INJECTABLE; INJECTION

	Product / Applicant	Strength	Appl No / Date
	LEUSTATIN		
	+ JOHNSON RW	1 MG/ML	N20229 001 FEB 26, 1993

CLARITHROMYCIN

GRANULE, FOR RECONSTITUTION; ORAL

	Product / Applicant	Strength	Appl No / Date
	BIAXIN		
	ABBOTT	125 MG/5 ML	N50698 001 DEC 23, 1993
	+	250 MG/5 ML	N50698 002 DEC 23, 1993

CLARITHROMYCIN *(continued)*

TABLET; ORAL

	Product / Applicant	Strength	Appl No / Date
	BIAXIN		
	ABBOTT	250 MG	N50662 001 OCT 31, 1991
		250 MG	N50697 001 DEC 23, 1993
		500 MG	N50662 002 OCT 31, 1991
		500 MG	N50697 002 DEC 23, 1993

CLAVULANATE POTASSIUM; *MULTIPLE*

SEE <u>AMOXICILLIN; CLAVULANATE POTASSIUM</u>

CLAVULANATE POTASSIUM; TICARCILLIN DISODIUM

INJECTABLE; INJECTION

	Product / Applicant	Strength	Appl No / Date
	TIMENTIN		
	+ SMITHKLINE BEECHAM	EQ 1 GM ACID/VIAL;EQ 30 GM BASE/VIAL	N50590 003 AUG 18, 1987
	+	EQ 100 MG ACID/VIAL;EQ 3 GM BASE/VIAL	N50590 001 APR 01, 1985
		EQ 100 MG ACID/VIAL;EQ 3 GM BASE/VIAL	N62691 001 DEC 19, 1986
	+	EQ 200 MG ACID/VIAL;EQ 3 GM BASE/VIAL	N50590 002 APR 01, 1985
	TIMENTIN IN PLASTIC CONTAINER		
	+ SMITHKLINE BEECHAM	EQ 100 MG ACID/100 ML;EQ 3 GM BASE/100 ML	N50658 001 DEC 15, 1989

CLEMASTINE FUMARATE

SYRUP; ORAL

	Product / Applicant	Strength	Appl No / Date
	<u>CLEMASTINE FUMARATE</u>		
<u>AA</u>	BARRE	<u>EQ 0.5 MG BASE/5 ML</u>	N74075 001 OCT 31, 1993
<u>AA</u>	COPLEY PHARM	<u>EQ 0.5 MG BASE/5 ML</u>	N73095 001 APR 21, 1992
<u>AA</u>	LEMMON	<u>EQ 0.5 MG BASE/5 ML</u>	N73399 001 JUN 30, 1994
	<u>TAVIST</u>		
<u>AA</u>	SANDOZ	<u>EQ 0.5 MG BASE/5 ML</u>	N18675 001 JUN 28, 1985

Prescription Drug Products *(continued)*

CLEMASTINE FUMARATE *(continued)*

TABLET; ORAL

	CLEMASTINE FUMARATE		
AB	GENEVA PHARMS	2.68 MG	N73459 001 OCT 31, 1993
AB	LEMMON	2.68 MG	N73283 001 JAN 31, 1992
	TAVIST		
AB	+ SANDOZ	2.68 MG	N17661 001

CLIDINIUM BROMIDE

CAPSULE; ORAL

	QUARZAN		
	ROCHE	2.5 MG	N10355 001
		5 MG	N10355 002

CLINDAMYCIN HYDROCHLORIDE

CAPSULE; ORAL

	CLEOCIN		
AB	+ UPJOHN	EQ 75 MG BASE	N50162 001
AB	+	EQ 150 MG BASE	N50162 002
	CLEOCIN HCL		
	UPJOHN	EQ 300 MG BASE	N50162 003 APR 14, 1988
	CLINDAMYCIN HCL		
AB	BIOCRAFT	EQ 75 MG BASE	N63027 001 SEP 20, 1989
AB		EQ 150 MG BASE	N63029 001 SEP 20, 1989
AB	DANBURY PHARMA	EQ 75 MG BASE	N63082 001 JUL 31, 1991
AB		EQ 150 MG BASE	N63083 001 JUL 31, 1991

CLINDAMYCIN PALMITATE HYDROCHLORIDE

POWDER FOR RECONSTITUTION; ORAL

	CLEOCIN		
	UPJOHN	EQ 75 MG BASE/5 ML	N62644 001 APR 07, 1986

CLINDAMYCIN PHOSPHATE

CREAM; VAGINAL

	CLEOCIN		
	+ UPJOHN	EQ 2% BASE	N50680 001 AUG 11, 1992

GEL; TOPICAL

	CLEOCIN T		
	+ UPJOHN	EQ 1% BASE	N50615 001 JAN 07, 1987

INJECTABLE; INJECTION

	CLEOCIN PHOSPHATE		
AP	+ UPJOHN	EQ 150 MG BASE/ML	N50441 001
AP		EQ 150 MG BASE/ML	N62803 001 OCT 16, 1987
	CLEOCIN PHOSPHATE IN DEXTROSE 5% IN PLASTIC CONTAINER		
AP	+ UPJOHN	EQ 6 MG BASE/ML	N50639 001 AUG 30, 1989
AP	+	EQ 12 MG BASE/ML	N50639 002 AUG 30, 1989
	+	EQ 18 MG BASE/ML	N50639 003 APR 10, 1991
	CLINDAMYCIN PHOSPHATE		
AP	ABBOTT	EQ 150 MG BASE/ML	N62800 001 JUL 24, 1987
AP		EQ 150 MG BASE/ML	N62801 001 JUL 24, 1987
AP		EQ 150 MG BASE/ML	N62943 001 SEP 29, 1988
AP	ASTRA	EQ 150 MG BASE/ML	N62928 001 FEB 13, 1989
AP	BEDFORD	EQ 150 MG BASE/ML	N63163 001 JUN 30, 1994
AP	ELKINS SINN	EQ 150 MG BASE/ML	N62806 001 OCT 15, 1987
AP		EQ 150 MG BASE/ML	N62953 001 APR 21, 1988
AP	GENSIA	EQ 150 MG BASE/ML	N63041 001 DEC 29, 1989
AP		EQ 150 MG BASE/ML	N63282 001 MAY 29, 1992
AP	LEDERLE	EQ 150 MG BASE/ML	N62889 001 APR 25, 1988
AP		EQ 150 MG BASE/ML	N63068 001 AUG 28, 1989
AP	LOCH	EQ 150 MG BASE/ML	N62905 001 MAY 09, 1988
AP	MARSAM	EQ 150 MG BASE/ML	N62913 001 OCT 20, 1988
AP	QUAD PHARMS	EQ 150 MG BASE/ML	N62795 001 DEC 21, 1987

Prescription Drug Products *(continued)*

CLINDAMYCIN PHOSPHATE *(continued)*

	INJECTABLE; INJECTION		
	CLINDAMYCIN PHOSPHATE		
AP	SOLOPAK	EQ 150 MG BASE/ML	N62819 001 MAR 15, 1988
AP		EQ 150 MG BASE/ML	N62852 001 MAR 17, 1988
AP	STERIS	EQ 150 MG BASE/ML	N62900 001 JUN 08, 1988
AP		EQ 150 MG BASE/ML	N63079 001 MAR 05, 1990
	CLINDAMYCIN PHOSPHATE IN DEXTROSE 5%		
AP	FUJISAWA	EQ 900 MG BASE/100 ML	N50635 001 DEC 22, 1989
	CLINDAMYCIN PHOSPHATE IN DEXTROSE 5% IN PLASTIC CONTAINER		
AP	BAXTER	EQ 6 MG BASE/ML	N50648 001 DEC 29, 1989
AP		EQ 900 MG BASE/100 ML	N50648 003 DEC 29, 1989
AP		EQ 12 MG BASE/ML	N50648 002 DEC 29, 1989
	LOTION; TOPICAL		
	CLEOCIN T		
	+ UPJOHN	EQ 1% BASE	N50600 001 MAY 31, 1989
	SOLUTION; TOPICAL		
	CLEOCIN T		
AT	+ UPJOHN	EQ 1% BASE	N50537 001
AT		EQ 1% BASE	N62363 001 FEB 08, 1982
	CLINDA-DERM		
AT	PADDOCK	EQ 1% BASE	N63329 001 SEP 30, 1992
	CLINDAMYCIN PHOSPHATE		
AT	BARRE	EQ 1% BASE	N62811 001 SEP 01, 1988
AT	COPLEY PHARM	EQ 1% BASE	N62944 001 JAN 11, 1989
AT	LEMMON	EQ 1% BASE	N62930 001 JUN 28, 1989
	SWAB; TOPICAL		
	CLEOCIN		
	UPJOHN	EQ 1% BASE	N50537 002 FEB 22, 1994

CLOBETASOL PROPIONATE

	CREAM; TOPICAL		
	CLOBETASOL PROPIONATE		
AB	COPLEY PHARM	0.05%	N74087 001 FEB 16, 1994
AB	NMC	0.05%	N74139 001 AUG 03, 1994
	TEMOVATE		
AB	+ GLAXO	0.05%	N19322 001 DEC 27, 1985
AB	+	0.05%	N20340 001 JUN 17, 1994
	GEL; TOPICAL		
	TEMOVATE		
	+ GLAXO	0.05%	N20337 001 APR 29, 1994
	OINTMENT; TOPICAL		
	CLOBETASOL PROPIONATE		
AB	COPLEY PHARM	0.05%	N74089 001 FEB 16, 1994
AB	NMC	0.05%	N74128 001 AUG 03, 1994
	TEMOVATE		
AB	+ GLAXO	0.05%	N19323 001 DEC 27, 1985
	SOLUTION; TOPICAL		
	TEMOVATE		
	+ GLAXO	0.05%	N19966 001 FEB 22, 1990

CLOCORTOLONE PIVALATE

	CREAM; TOPICAL		
	CLODERM		
	+ HERMAL PHARM	0.1%	N17765 001

CLOFAZIMINE

	CAPSULE; ORAL		
	LAMPRENE		
	GEIGY	50 MG	N19500 002 DEC 15, 1986
	+	100 MG	N19500 001 DEC 15, 1986

Prescription Drug Products *(continued)*

CLOFIBRATE

CAPSULE; ORAL

	ATROMID-S		
AB	+ WYETH AYERST	500 MG	N16099 002
	CLOFIBRATE		
AB	BANNER PHARMACAPS	500 MG	N73396 001 MAR 20, 1992
AB	GENEVA PHARMS	500 MG	N72191 001 MAY 02, 1988
AB	NOVOPHARM	500 MG	N72600 001 JUL 25, 1991
AB	ROSEMONT PHARM	500 MG	N70531 001 JUN 16, 1986

CLOMIPHENE CITRATE

TABLET; ORAL

	CLOMID		
AB	+ MERRELL DOW	50 MG	N16131 002
	MILOPHENE		
AB	MILEX	50 MG	N72196 001 DEC 20, 1988
	SEROPHENE		
AB	SERONO	50 MG	N18361 001 MAR 22, 1982

CLOMIPRAMINE HYDROCHLORIDE

CAPSULE; ORAL

	ANAFRANIL		
	BASEL PHARMS	25 MG	N19906 001 DEC 29, 1989
		50 MG	N19906 002 DEC 29, 1989
	+	75 MG	N19906 003 DEC 29, 1989

CLONAZEPAM

TABLET; ORAL

	KLONOPIN		
	ROCHE	0.5 MG	N17533 001
		1 MG	N17533 002
	+	2 MG	N17533 003

CLONIDINE

FILM, EXTENDED RELEASE; TRANSDERMAL

	CATAPRES-TTS-1		
	+ BOEHRINGER INGELHEIM	0.1 MG/24 HR	N18891 001 OCT 10, 1984
	CATAPRES-TTS-2		
	+ BOEHRINGER INGELHEIM	0.2 MG/24 HR	N18891 002 OCT 10, 1984
	CATAPRES-TTS-3		
	+ BOEHRINGER INGELHEIM	0.3 MG/24 HR	N18891 003 OCT 10, 1984

CLONIDINE HYDROCHLORIDE

TABLET; ORAL

	CATAPRES		
AB	BOEHRINGER INGELHEIM	0.1 MG	N17407 001
AB		0.2 MG	N17407 002
AB	+	0.3 MG	N17407 003
	CLONIDINE HCL		
AB	BARR	0.1 MG	N70925 001 SEP 04, 1987
AB		0.2 MG	N70924 001 SEP 04, 1987
AB		0.3 MG	N70923 001 SEP 04, 1987
AB	DANBURY PHARMA	0.1 MG	N70965 001 JUL 08, 1986
AB		0.2 MG	N70964 001 JUL 08, 1986
AB		0.3 MG	N70963 001 JUL 08, 1986
AB	GENEVA PHARMS	0.1 MG	N70887 001 AUG 31, 1988
AB		0.2 MG	N70886 001 AUG 31, 1988
AB		0.3 MG	N71294 001 AUG 31, 1988
AB	LEDERLE	0.1 MG	N71783 001 APR 05, 1988
AB		0.2 MG	N71784 001 APR 05, 1988
AB		0.3 MG	N71785 001 APR 05, 1988

Prescription Drug Products *(continued)*

CLONIDINE HYDROCHLORIDE *(continued)*

TABLET; ORAL
CLONIDINE HCL

AB	MYLAN	0.1 MG	N70315 001 JUN 09, 1987
AB		0.2 MG	N70316 001 JUN 09, 1987
AB		0.3 MG	N70317 001 JUN 09, 1987
AB	PUREPAC PHARM	0.1 MG	N70974 001 DEC 16, 1986
AB		0.2 MG	N70975 001 DEC 16, 1986
AB		0.3 MG	N70976 001 DEC 16, 1986
AB	WARNER CHILCOTT	0.1 MG	N72138 001 JUN 13, 1988
AB		0.2 MG	N72139 001 JUN 13, 1988
AB		0.3 MG	N72140 001 JUN 13, 1988

CLONIDINE HYDROCHLORIDE; *MULTIPLE*

SEE CHLORTHALIDONE; CLONIDINE HYDROCHLORIDE

CLORAZEPATE DIPOTASSIUM

CAPSULE; ORAL
CLORAZEPATE DIPOTASSIUM

AB	ABLE	3.75 MG	N71777 001 JUL 14, 1987
AB		7.5 MG	N71778 001 JUL 14, 1987
AB		15 MG	N71779 001 JUL 14, 1987
AB	GENEVA PHARMS	3.75 MG	N72219 001 AUG 26, 1988
AB		7.5 MG	N72220 001 AUG 26, 1988
AB		15 MG	N72112 001 AUG 26, 1988
AB	LEDERLE	3.75 MG	N71742 001 DEC 14, 1987
AB		7.5 MG	N71743 001 DEC 14, 1987
AB		15 MG	N71744 001 DEC 14, 1987

CLORAZEPATE DIPOTASSIUM *(continued)*

CAPSULE; ORAL
CLORAZEPATE DIPOTASSIUM

AB	MYLAN	3.75 MG	N71509 001 OCT 19, 1987
AB		7.5 MG	N71510 001 OCT 19, 1987
AB	+	15 MG	N71511 001 OCT 19, 1987
AB	PUREPAC PHARM	7.5 MG	N71925 001 APR 25, 1988
AB		15 MG	N71926 001 APR 25, 1988

TABLET; ORAL
CLORAZEPATE DIPOTASSIUM

AB	ABLE	3.75 MG	N71780 001 JUN 26, 1987
AB		7.5 MG	N71781 001 JUN 26, 1987
AB		15 MG	N71782 001 JUN 26, 1987
AB	GENEVA PHARMS	3.75 MG	N72512 001 MAY 11, 1990
AB		7.5 MG	N72513 001 MAY 11, 1990
AB		15 MG	N72514 001 MAY 11, 1990
AB	MYLAN	3.75 MG	N71856 001 JUL 17, 1987
AB		7.5 MG	N71857 001 JUL 17, 1987
AB		15 MG	N71858 001 JUL 17, 1987
AB	PUREPAC PHARM	3.75 MG	N72330 001 AUG 08, 1988
AB		7.5 MG	N72331 001 AUG 08, 1988
AB		15 MG	N72332 001 AUG 08, 1988
AB	WATSON LABS	3.75 MG	N71852 001 FEB 09, 1988
AB		7.5 MG	N71853 001 FEB 09, 1988
AB		15 MG	N71854 001 FEB 09, 1988

GEN-XENE

AB	ALRA	3.75 MG	N71787 001 APR 26, 1988
AB		7.5 MG	N71788 001 APR 26, 1988
AB		15 MG	N71789 001 APR 26, 1988

Prescription Drug Products *(continued)*

CLORAZEPATE DIPOTASSIUM *(continued)*

TABLET; ORAL

	TRANXENE		
AB	ABBOTT	3.75 MG	N17105 006
AB		7.5 MG	N17105 007
AB	+	15 MG	N17105 008
	TRANXENE SD		
	ABBOTT	11.25 MG	N17105 005
	+	22.5 MG	N17105 004

CLOTRIMAZOLE

CREAM; TOPICAL

	CLOTRIMAZOLE		
AB	TARO	1%	N72640 001 AUG 31, 1993
	LOTRIMIN		
AB	+ SCHERING PLOUGH	1%	N17619 001
	MYCELEX		
BT	MILES	1%	N18183 001

LOTION; TOPICAL

	LOTRIMIN		
	+ SCHERING	1%	N18813 001 FEB 17, 1984

SOLUTION; TOPICAL

	LOTRIMIN		
AT	SCHERING PLOUGH	1%	N17613 001
	MYCELEX		
AT	MILES	1%	N18181 001

TABLET; VAGINAL

	MYCELEX-G		
	MILES	500 MG	N19069 001 APR 19, 1985

TROCHE/LOZENGE; ORAL

	MYCELEX		
	+ MILES	10 MG	N18713 001 JUN 17, 1983

CLOTRIMAZOLE; *MULTIPLE*

SEE BETAMETHASONE DIPROPIONATE; CLOTRIMAZOLE

CLOXACILLIN SODIUM

CAPSULE; ORAL

	CLOXACILLIN SODIUM		
AB	BIOCRAFT	EQ 250 MG BASE	N62240 001
AB		EQ 500 MG BASE	N62240 002

CLOXACILLIN SODIUM *(continued)*

CAPSULE; ORAL

	CLOXAPEN		
AB	SMITHKLINE BEECHAM	EQ 250 MG BASE	N61806 001
AB		EQ 250 MG BASE	N62233 001
AB		EQ 500 MG BASE	N61806 002
AB		EQ 500 MG BASE	N62233 002
	TEGOPEN		
AB	+ APOTHECON	EQ 250 MG BASE	N61452 001
AB	+	EQ 500 MG BASE	N61452 002

POWDER FOR RECONSTITUTION; ORAL

	CLOXACILLIN SODIUM		
AA	BIOCRAFT	EQ 125 MG BASE/5 ML	N62268 001
	TEGOPEN		
AA	APOTHECON	EQ 125 MG BASE/5 ML	N61453 001
AA	BRISTOL	EQ 125 MG BASE/5 ML	N50192 001

CLOZAPINE

TABLET; ORAL

	CLOZARIL		
	SANDOZ	25 MG	N19758 001 SEP 26, 1989
	+	100 MG	N19758 002 SEP 26, 1989

COBALT CHLORIDE, CO-57; CYANOCOBALAMIN; CYANOCOBALAMIN, CO-57; INTRINSIC FACTOR

N/A; N/A

	RUBRATOPE-57 KIT		
	BRACCO	N/A;N/A;N/A;N/A	N16089 001

CODEINE PHOSPHATE; *MULTIPLE*

SEE ACETAMINOPHEN; ASPIRIN; CODEINE PHOSPHATE
SEE ACETAMINOPHEN; BUTALBITAL; CAFFEINE; CODEINE PHOSPHATE
SEE ACETAMINOPHEN; CODEINE PHOSPHATE
SEE ASPIRIN; BUTALBITAL; CAFFEINE; CODEINE PHOSPHATE
SEE ASPIRIN; CARISOPRODOL; CODEINE PHOSPHATE
SEE BROMODIPHENHYDRAMINE HYDROCHLORIDE; CODEINE PHOSPHATE
SEE BROMPHENIRAMINE MALEATE; CODEINE PHOSPHATE; PHENYLPROPANOLAMINE HYDROCHLORIDE

Prescription Drug Products *(continued)*

CODEINE PHOSPHATE; PHENYLEPHRINE HYDROCHLORIDE; PROMETHAZINE HYDROCHLORIDE

SYRUP; ORAL

	PHENERGAN VC W/ CODEINE		
AA	WYETH AYERST	10 MG/5 ML;5 MG/5 ML;6.25 MG/5 ML	N08306 005 APR 02, 1984
	PHERAZINE VC W/ CODEINE		
AA	HALSEY	10 MG/5 ML;5 MG/5 ML;6.25 MG/5 ML	N88870 001 MAR 02, 1987
	PROMETH VC W/ CODEINE		
AA	BARRE	10 MG/5 ML;5 MG/5 ML;6.25 MG/5 ML	N88764 001 OCT 31, 1984
	PROMETHAZINE VC W/ CODEINE		
AA	CENCI	10 MG/5 ML;5 MG/5 ML;6.25 MG/5 ML	N88816 001 NOV 22, 1985
AA	PENNEX	10 MG/5 ML;5 MG/5 ML;6.25 MG/5 ML	N88896 001 JAN 04, 1985

CODEINE PHOSPHATE; PROMETHAZINE HYDROCHLORIDE

SYRUP; ORAL

	PHENERGAN W/ CODEINE		
AA	WYETH AYERST	10 MG/5 ML;6.25 MG/5 ML	N08306 004 APR 02, 1984
	PHERAZINE W/ CODEINE		
AA	HALSEY	10 MG/5 ML;6.25 MG/5 ML	N88739 001 DEC 23, 1988
	PROMETH W/ CODEINE		
AA	BARRE	10 MG/5 ML;6.25 MG/5 ML	N88763 001 OCT 31, 1984
	PROMETHAZINE HCL AND CODEINE PHOSPHATE		
AA	PHARM ASSOC	10 MG/5 ML;6.25 MG/5 ML	N89647 001 DEC 22, 1988
	PROMETHAZINE W/ CODEINE		
AA	CENCI	10 MG/5 ML;6.25 MG/5 ML	N88814 001 NOV 22, 1985
AA	PENNEX	10 MG/5 ML;6.25 MG/5 ML	N88875 001 DEC 17, 1984

CODEINE PHOSPHATE; PSEUDOEPHEDRINE HYDROCHLORIDE; TRIPROLIDINE HYDROCHLORIDE

SYRUP; ORAL

	ACTIFED W/ CODEINE		
AA	BURROUGHS WELLCOME	10 MG/5 ML;30 MG/5 ML;1.25 MG/5 ML	N12575 003 APR 04, 1984
	TRIACIN-C		
AA	BARRE	10 MG/5 ML;30 MG/5 ML;1.25 MG/5 ML	N88704 001 MAR 22, 1985
	TRIPROLIDINE AND PSEUDOEPHEDRINE HYDROCHLORIDES W/ CODEINE		
AA	CENCI	10 MG/5 ML;30 MG/5 ML;1.25 MG/5 ML	N89018 001 JUL 23, 1986
	TRIPROLIDINE HCL, PSEUDOEPHEDRINE HCL AND CODEINE PHOSPHATE		
AA	PENNEX	10 MG/5 ML;30 MG/5 ML;1.25 MG/5 ML	N88833 001 NOV 16, 1984

COLCHICINE; PROBENECID

TABLET; ORAL

	COL-PROBENECID		
BP	DANBURY PHARMA	0.5 MG;500 MG	N84279 001
	COLBENEMID		
BP	+ MERCK SHARP DOHME	0.5 MG;500 MG	N12383 001
	PROBENECID AND COLCHICINE		
BP	GLOBAL PHARMS	0.5 MG;500 MG	N83720 002
BP	ZENITH LABS	0.5 MG;500 MG	N83734 001

COLESTIPOL HYDROCHLORIDE

GRANULE; ORAL

	FLAVORED COLESTID		
	UPJOHN	5 GM/SCOOPFUL	N17563 002
	+	5 GM/PACKET	N17563 001

TABLET; ORAL

	COLESTID		
	UPJOHN	1 GM	N20222 001 JUL 19, 1994

COLFOSCERIL PALMITATE; *MULTIPLE*

SEE CETYL ALCOHOL; COLFOSCERIL PALMITATE; TYLOXAPOL

COLISTIMETHATE SODIUM

INJECTABLE; INJECTION

	COLY-MYCIN M		
	+ PARKE DAVIS	EQ 150 MG BASE/VIAL	N50108 002

Prescription Drug Products *(continued)*

COLISTIN SULFATE

	SUSPENSION; ORAL		
	COLY-MYCIN S		
	PARKE DAVIS	EQ 25 MG BASE/5 ML	N50355 001

COLISTIN SULFATE; HYDROCORTISONE ACETATE; NEOMYCIN SULFATE; THONZONIUM BROMIDE

	SUSPENSION; OTIC		
	COLY-MYCIN S		
	+ PARKE DAVIS	EQ 3 MG BASE/ML;10 MG/ML;EQ 3.3 MG BASE/ML;0.5 MG/ML	N50356 001

COPPER

	INTRAUTERINE DEVICE; INTRAUTERINE		
	COPPER T MODEL TCU 380A		
	+ POPULATION COUNCIL	APPROX 309 MG COPPER	N18680 001 NOV 15, 1984

CORTICOTROPIN

	INJECTABLE; INJECTION		
	<u>ACTH</u>		
<u>AP</u>	PARKE DAVIS	<u>40 UNITS/VIAL</u>	N08317 004
	<u>ACTHAR</u>		
<u>AP</u>	RHONE POULENC RORER	<u>40 UNITS/VIAL</u>	N07504 003
		25 UNITS/VIAL	N07504 002
	CORTICOTROPIN		
BC	ORGANICS IL	40 UNITS/ML	N10831 001
BC	+	80 UNITS/ML	N10831 002
<u>AP</u>	STERIS	<u>40 UNITS/VIAL</u>	N88772 001 NOV 21, 1984
	H.P. ACTHAR GEL		
BC	RHONE POULENC RORER	40 UNITS/ML	N08372 006
BC	+	80 UNITS/ML	N08372 008

CORTISONE ACETATE

	INJECTABLE; INJECTION		
	CORTONE		
	MERCK SHARP DOHME	25 MG/ML	N07110 002
	+	50 MG/ML	N07110 003

CORTISONE ACETATE *(continued)*

	TABLET; ORAL		
	CORTISONE ACETATE		
BP	CHELSEA LABS	25 MG	N85884 001
BP	GLOBAL PHARMS	25 MG	N09458 001
BP	PUREPAC PHARM	25 MG	N80493 001
BP	UPJOHN	25 MG	N08126 001
		5 MG	N08126 003
		10 MG	N08126 004
BP	WEST WARD PHARM	25 MG	N80776 002
	CORTONE		
BP	+ MERCK SHARP DOHME	25 MG	N07750 003

COSYNTROPIN

	INJECTABLE; INJECTION		
	CORTROSYN		
	ORGANON	0.25 MG/VIAL	N16750 001

CROMOLYN SODIUM

	AEROSOL, METERED; INHALATION		
	INTAL		
	+ FISONS	0.8 MG/INH	N18887 001 DEC 05, 1985
	CAPSULE; INHALATION		
	INTAL		
	+ FISONS	20 MG	N16990 001
	CAPSULE; ORAL		
	GASTROCROM		
	+ FISONS	100 MG	N19188 001 DEC 22, 1989
	SOLUTION; INHALATION		
	<u>CROMOLYN SODIUM</u>		
<u>AN</u>	DEY	<u>10 MG/ML</u>	N74209 001 APR 26, 1994
	<u>INTAL</u>		
<u>AN</u>	+ FISONS	<u>10 MG/ML</u>	N18596 001 MAY 28, 1982
	SOLUTION/DROPS; OPHTHALMIC		
	OPTICROM		
	+ FISONS	4%	N18155 001 OCT 03, 1984
	SPRAY, METERED; NASAL		
	NASALCROM		
	+ FISONS	5.2 MG/INH	N18306 001 MAR 18, 1983

Prescription Drug Products *(continued)*

CROTAMITON
CREAM; TOPICAL
EURAX
+ WESTWOOD SQUIBB 10% N06927 001
LOTION; TOPICAL
CROTAN
AT GALDERMA 10% N87204 001
EURAX
AT + WESTWOOD SQUIBB 10% N09112 003

CUPRIC CHLORIDE
INJECTABLE; INJECTION
CUPRIC CHLORIDE IN PLASTIC CONTAINER
+ ABBOTT EQ 0.4 MG COPPER/ML N18960 001 JUN 26, 1986

CUPRIC SULFATE
INJECTABLE; INJECTION
CUPRIC SULFATE
+ FUJISAWA EQ 0.4 MG COPPER/ML N19350 001 MAY 05, 1987

CYANOCOBALAMIN
INJECTABLE; INJECTION
BERUBIGEN
AP UPJOHN 1 MG/ML N06798 001
BETALIN 12
AP LILLY 0.1 MG/ML N80855 001
AP 1 MG/ML N80855 002
COBAVITE
AP STERIS 0.1 MG/ML N83013 001
AP 1 MG/ML N83064 001
CYANOCOBALAMIN
AP AKORN 1 MG/ML N87969 001 NOV 10, 1983
AP DELL LABS 0.1 MG/ML N80689 002
AP 1 MG/ML N80689 003
0.03 MG/ML N80689 001
AP ELKINS SINN 1 MG/ML N80515 002
AP FUJISAWA 0.1 MG/ML N80557 002
AP LUITPOLD 1 MG/ML N80737 001
AP MERRELL DOW 1 MG/ML N80564 001
AP SOLOPAK 1 MG/ML N87551 001 FEB 29, 1984
AP STERIS 0.1 MG/ML N80573 002
AP 0.1 MG/ML N83120 001
AP 1 MG/ML N80573 001
AP 1 MG/ML N83120 002

CYANOCOBALAMIN *(continued)*
INJECTABLE; INJECTION
CYANOCOBALAMIN
AP WYETH AYERST 0.1 MG/ML N80554 001
AP 1 MG/ML N80554 002
RUBRAMIN PC
AP + SQUIBB 0.1 MG/ML N06799 002
AP + 1 MG/ML N06799 004
RUVITE
AP SAVAGE LABS 1 MG/ML N80570 002
SYTOBEX
AP PARKE DAVIS 1 MG/ML N07085 002
VIBISONE
AP FUJISAWA 1 MG/ML N80557 003
TABLET; ORAL
CYANOCOBALAMIN
+ WEST WARD PHARM 1 MG N84264 001

CYANOCOBALAMIN; *MULTIPLE*
SEE ASCORBIC ACID; BIOTIN; CYANOCOBALAMIN; DEXPANTHENOL; ERGOCALCIFEROL; FOLIC ACID; NIACINAMIDE; PYRIDOXINE HYDROCHLORIDE; RIBOFLAVIN PHOSPHATE SODIUM; THIAMINE HYDROCHLORIDE; VITAMIN A; VITAMIN E
SEE ASCORBIC ACID; BIOTIN; CYANOCOBALAMIN; ERGOCALCIFEROL; FOLIC ACID; NIACINAMIDE; PANTOTHENIC ACID; PHYTONADIONE; PYRIDOXINE; RIBOFLAVIN; THIAMINE; VITAMIN A PALMITATE; VITAMIN E
SEE COBALT CHLORIDE, CO-57; CYANOCOBALAMIN; CYANOCOBALAMIN, CO-57; INTRINSIC FACTOR

CYANOCOBALAMIN; CYANOCOBALAMIN, CO-57; CYANOCOBALAMIN, CO-58
N/A; N/A
DICOPAC KIT
AMERSHAM N/A;N/A;N/A N17406 001

CYANOCOBALAMIN; CYANOCOBALAMIN, CO-57; INTRINSIC FACTOR
N/A; N/A
CYANOCOBALAMIN CO 57 SCHILLING TEST KIT
MALLINCKRODT 0.1 MG;0.5uCi;60 MG N16635 001

CYANOCOBALAMIN, CO-57
CAPSULE; ORAL
RUBRATOPE-57
BRACCO 0.5-1uCi N16089 002

Prescription Drug Products *(continued)*

CYANOCOBALAMIN, CO-57; *MULTIPLE*

SEE COBALT CHLORIDE, CO-57; CYANOCOBALAMIN; CYANOCOBALAMIN, CO-57; INTRINSIC FACTOR
SEE CYANOCOBALAMIN; CYANOCOBALAMIN, CO-57; CYANOCOBALAMIN, CO-58
SEE CYANOCOBALAMIN; CYANOCOBALAMIN, CO-57; INTRINSIC FACTOR

CYANOCOBALAMIN, CO-58; *MULTIPLE*

SEE CYANOCOBALAMIN; CYANOCOBALAMIN, CO-57; CYANOCOBALAMIN, CO-58

CYCLACILLIN

TABLET; ORAL

	CYCLACILLIN		
AB	BIOCRAFT	250 MG	N62895 001 AUG 04, 1988
AB		500 MG	N62895 002 AUG 04, 1988
	CYCLAPEN-W		
AB	+ WYETH AYERST	250 MG	N50509 001
AB	+	500 MG	N50509 002

CYCLOBENZAPRINE HYDROCHLORIDE

TABLET; ORAL

	CYCLOBENZAPRINE HCL		
AB	DANBURY PHARMA	10 MG	N71611 001 MAY 03, 1989
AB	GENEVA PHARMS	10 MG	N72854 001 NOV 19, 1991
AB	INVAMED	10 MG	N73683 001 FEB 26, 1993
AB	MYLAN	10 MG	N73144 001 MAY 31, 1991
AB	WATSON LABS	10 MG	N73143 001 NOV 27, 1991
	FLEXERIL		
AB	+ MERCK SHARP DOHME	10 MG	N17821 002

CYCLOPENTOLATE HYDROCHLORIDE

SOLUTION/DROPS; OPHTHALMIC

	AK-PENTOLATE		
AT	AKORN	1%	N85555 001
	CYCLOGYL		
AT	+ ALCON	1%	N84110 001
	+	0.5%	N84109 001
		2%	N84108 001

CYCLOPENTOLATE HYDROCHLORIDE *(continued)*

SOLUTION/DROPS; OPHTHALMIC

	CYCLOPENTOLATE HCL		
AT	STERIS	1%	N89162 001 JAN 24, 1991
	PENTOLAIR		
AT	BAUSCH AND LOMB	1%	N40075 001 APR 29, 1994

CYCLOPENTOLATE HYDROCHLORIDE; PHENYLEPHRINE HYDROCHLORIDE

SOLUTION/DROPS; OPHTHALMIC

	CYCLOMYDRIL		
	+ ALCON	0.2%;1%	N84300 001

CYCLOPHOSPHAMIDE

INJECTABLE; INJECTION

	CYCLOPHOSPHAMIDE		
AP	ELKINS SINN	100 MG/VIAL	N88371 001 JUL 03, 1986
AP		200 MG/VIAL	N88372 001 JUL 03, 1986
AP		500 MG/VIAL	N88373 001 JUL 03, 1986
AP		1 GM/VIAL	N88374 001 SEP 24, 1986
	CYTOXAN		
AP	+ BRISTOL	100 MG/VIAL	N12142 001
AP	+	200 MG/VIAL	N12142 002
AP	+	500 MG/VIAL	N12142 003
AP	+	1 GM/VIAL	N12142 004 AUG 30, 1982
AP	+	2 GM/VIAL	N12142 005 AUG 30, 1982
	LYOPHILIZED CYTOXAN		
AP	+ BRISTOL	100 MG/VIAL	N12142 006 DEC 05, 1985
AP	+	200 MG/VIAL	N12142 007 DEC 10, 1985
AP	+	500 MG/VIAL	N12142 008 JAN 04, 1984
AP	+	1 GM/VIAL	N12142 010 SEP 24, 1985
AP	+	2 GM/VIAL	N12142 009 DEC 10, 1984

Prescription Drug Products *(continued)*

CYCLOPHOSPHAMIDE *(continued)*

INJECTABLE; INJECTION

	NEOSAR		
AP	PHARMACIA	100 MG/VIAL	N40015 001 APR 29, 1993
AP		100 MG/VIAL	N87442 001 FEB 16, 1982
AP		200 MG/VIAL	N40015 002 APR 29, 1993
AP		200 MG/VIAL	N87442 002 FEB 16, 1982
AP		500 MG/VIAL	N40015 003 APR 29, 1993
AP		500 MG/VIAL	N87442 003 FEB 16, 1982
AP		1 GM/VIAL	N40015 004 APR 29, 1993
AP		1 GM/VIAL	N87442 004 JUL 08, 1983
AP		2 GM/VIAL	N40015 005 APR 29, 1993
AP		2 GM/VIAL	N87442 005 MAR 30, 1989

TABLET; ORAL

	CYTOXAN		
	BRISTOL	25 MG	N12141 002
		50 MG	N12141 001

CYCLOSERINE

CAPSULE; ORAL

	SEROMYCIN		
	+ LILLY	250 MG	N60593 001

CYCLOSPORINE

CAPSULE; ORAL

	SANDIMMUNE		
	SANDOZ	25 MG	N50625 001 MAR 02, 1990
	+	100 MG	N50625 002 MAR 02, 1990

INJECTABLE; INJECTION

	SANDIMMUNE		
	+ SANDOZ	50 MG/ML	N50573 001 NOV 14, 1983

SOLUTION; ORAL

	SANDIMMUNE		
	SANDOZ	100 MG/ML	N50574 001 NOV 14, 1983

CYCLOTHIAZIDE

TABLET; ORAL

	ANHYDRON		
	+ LILLY	2 MG	N13157 002

CYPROHEPTADINE HYDROCHLORIDE

SYRUP; ORAL

	CYPROHEPTADINE HCL		
AA	BARRE	2 MG/5 ML	N86833 001
AA	HALSEY	2 MG/5 ML	N89199 001 JUL 03, 1986
	PERIACTIN		
AA	MERCK SHARP DOHME	2 MG/5 ML	N13220 002

TABLET; ORAL

	CYPROHEPTADINE HCL		
AA	ASCOT	4 MG	N87685 001 OCT 25, 1982
AA	CAMALL	4 MG	N88212 001 MAY 26, 1983
AA	DANBURY PHARMA	4 MG	N86580 001
AA	GENEVA PHARMS	4 MG	N86808 001
AA	HALSEY	4 MG	N89057 001 JUL 03, 1986
AA	MD PHARM	4 MG	N87566 001 NOV 10, 1982
AA	PAR PHARM	4 MG	N87129 001
AA	SIDMAK LABS NJ	4 MG	N88205 001 JUL 26, 1983
AA	ZENITH LABS	4 MG	N87056 001
	PERIACTIN		
AA	MERCK SHARP DOHME	4 MG	N12649 001

CYSTEAMINE BITARTRATE

CAPSULE; ORAL

	CYSTAGON		
	MYLAN	EQ 50 MG BASE	N20392 001 AUG 15, 1994
	+	EQ 150 MG BASE	N20392 002 AUG 15, 1994

CYTARABINE

INJECTABLE; INJECTION

	CYTARABINE		
	+ BULL D	20 MG/ML	N71868 001 JUN 04, 1990
	+	20 MG/ML	N72168 001 AUG 31, 1990
	+	20 MG/ML	N72945 001 FEB 28, 1994

Prescription Drug Products *(continued)*

CYTARABINE *(continued)*

INJECTABLE; INJECTION

	CYTARABINE		
AP	CETUS BEN VENUE	100 MG/VIAL	N71471 001 AUG 02, 1989
AP		500 MG/VIAL	N71472 001 AUG 02, 1989
AP		1 GM/VIAL	N74245 001 AUG 31, 1994
AP		2 GM/VIAL	N74245 002 AUG 31, 1994
	CYTOSAR-U		
AP	+ UPJOHN	100 MG/VIAL	N16793 001
AP	+	500 MG/VIAL	N16793 002
AP	+	1 GM/VIAL	N16793 003 DEC 21, 1987
AP	+	2 GM/VIAL	N16793 004 DEC 21, 1987

DACARBAZINE

INJECTABLE; INJECTION

	DTIC-DOME		
	+ MILES	100 MG/VIAL	N17575 001
	+	200 MG/VIAL	N17575 002

DACTINOMYCIN

INJECTABLE; INJECTION

	COSMEGEN		
	+ MERCK SHARP DOHME	0.5 MG/VIAL	N50682 001

DANAZOL

CAPSULE; ORAL

	DANOCRINE		
	STERLING WINTHROP	50 MG	N17557 003
		100 MG	N17557 004
	+	200 MG	N17557 002

DANTROLENE SODIUM

CAPSULE; ORAL

	DANTRIUM		
	PROCTER AND GAMBLE	25 MG	N17443 001
		50 MG	N17443 003
	+	100 MG	N17443 002

INJECTABLE; INJECTION

	DANTRIUM		
	+ PROCTER AND GAMBLE	20 MG/VIAL	N18264 001

DAPIPRAZOLE HYDROCHLORIDE

SOLUTION/DROPS; OPHTHALMIC

	REV-EYES		
	+ ANGELINI	0.5%	N19849 001 DEC 31, 1990

DAPSONE

TABLET; ORAL

	DAPSONE		
	JACOBUS	25 MG	N86841 001
	+	100 MG	N86842 001

DAUNORUBICIN HYDROCHLORIDE

INJECTABLE; INJECTION

	CERUBIDINE		
AP	RHONE POULENC RORER	EQ 20 MG BASE/VIAL	N61876 001
AP	+ WYETH AYERST	EQ 20 MG BASE/VIAL	N50484 001

DEFEROXAMINE MESYLATE

INJECTABLE; INJECTION

	DESFERAL		
	+ CIBA	500 MG/VIAL	N16267 001

DEMECARIUM BROMIDE

SOLUTION/DROPS; OPHTHALMIC

	HUMORSOL		
	+ MERCK SHARP DOHME	0.125%	N11860 002
	+	0.25%	N11860 001

DEMECLOCYCLINE HYDROCHLORIDE

CAPSULE; ORAL

	DECLOMYCIN		
	+ LEDERLE	150 MG	N50262 001

TABLET; ORAL

	DECLOMYCIN		
	LEDERLE	75 MG	N50261 001
		150 MG	N50261 002
	+	300 MG	N50261 003

DESERPIDINE

TABLET; ORAL

	HARMONYL		
	+ ABBOTT	0.25 MG	N10796 002

Prescription Drug Products *(continued)*

DESERPIDINE; HYDROCHLOROTHIAZIDE

	TABLET; ORAL		
	ORETICYL FORTE		
	ABBOTT	0.25 MG;25 MG	N12148 002
	ORETICYL 25		
	ABBOTT	0.125 MG;25 MG	N12148 001
	ORETICYL 50		
	+ ABBOTT	0.125 MG;50 MG	N12148 003

DESERPIDINE; METHYCLOTHIAZIDE

	TABLET; ORAL		
	ENDURONYL		
	ABBOTT	0.25 MG;5 MG	N12775 001
	ENDURONYL FORTE		
	+ ABBOTT	0.5 MG;5 MG	N12775 002

DESFLURANE

	LIQUID; INHALATION		
	SUPRANE		
	OHMEDA	99.9%	N20118 001 SEP 18, 1992

DESIPRAMINE HYDROCHLORIDE

	TABLET; ORAL		
	DESIPRAMINE HCL		
AB	EON LABS	25 MG	N71601 001 JUN 05, 1987
AB		50 MG	N71588 001 JUN 05, 1987
AB		75 MG	N71602 001 OCT 05, 1987
AB		100 MG	N71766 001 OCT 05, 1987
AB	GENEVA PHARMS	10 MG	N72099 001 MAY 24, 1988
AB		25 MG	N72100 001 MAY 24, 1988
AB		50 MG	N72101 001 MAY 24, 1988
AB		75 MG	N72102 001 JUN 20, 1988
AB		100 MG	N72103 001 JUN 20, 1988
AB		150 MG	N72104 001 JUN 20, 1988

DESIPRAMINE HYDROCHLORIDE *(continued)*

	TABLET; ORAL		
	DESIPRAMINE HCL		
AB	SIDMAK LABS NJ	25 MG	N71800 001 DEC 08, 1987
AB		50 MG	N71801 001 DEC 08, 1987
AB		75 MG	N71802 001 DEC 08, 1987
	NORPRAMIN		
AB	MERRELL DOW	10 MG	N14399 007 FEB 11, 1982
AB		25 MG	N14399 001
AB	+	50 MG	N14399 003
AB		75 MG	N14399 004
AB	+	100 MG	N14399 005
AB		150 MG	N14399 006

DESMOPRESSIN ACETATE

	INJECTABLE; INJECTION		
	DDAVP		
	+ RHONE POULENC RORER	0.004 MG/ML	N18938 001 MAR 30, 1984
	SOLUTION; NASAL		
	CONCENTRAID		
BX	FERRING LABS	0.01%	N19776 001 DEC 26, 1990
	DDAVP		
BX	+ RHONE POULENC RORER	0.01%	N17922 001
	SPRAY, METERED; NASAL		
	DDAVP		
	RHONE POULENC RORER	0.01 MG/INH	N17922 002 FEB 06, 1989
	DESMOPRESSIN ACETATE		
	+ RHONE POULENC RORER	0.15 MG/INH	N20355 001 MAR 07, 1994

DESOGESTREL; ETHINYL ESTRADIOL

	TABLET; ORAL-21		
	DESOGEN		
AB	+ ORGANON	0.15 MG;0.03 MG	N20071 001 DEC 10, 1992
	ORTHO-CEPT		
AB	JOHNSON RW	0.15 MG;0.03 MG	N20301 001 DEC 14, 1992

Prescription Drug Products *(continued)*

DESOGESTREL; ETHINYL ESTRADIOL *(continued)*

TABLET; ORAL-28

TE	Product / Applicant	Strength	Appl. No. / Date
	DESOGEN		
AB	ORGANON	0.15 MG;0.03 MG	N20071 002 DEC 10, 1992
	ORTHO-CEPT		
AB	JOHNSON RW	0.15 MG;0.03 MG	N20301 002 DEC 14, 1992

DESONIDE

CREAM; TOPICAL

TE	Product / Applicant	Strength	Appl. No. / Date
	DESONIDE		
AB	COPLEY PHARM	0.05%	N74027 001 SEP 28, 1992
AB	TARO	0.05%	N73548 001 JUN 30, 1992
	DESOWEN		
AB	GALDERMA	0.05%	N19048 001 DEC 14, 1984
	TRIDESILON		
AB	+ MILES	0.05%	N17010 001

LOTION; TOPICAL

TE	Product / Applicant	Strength	Appl. No. / Date
	DESOWEN		
	GALDERMA	0.05%	N72354 001 JAN 24, 1992

OINTMENT; TOPICAL

TE	Product / Applicant	Strength	Appl. No. / Date
	DESONIDE		
AB	TARO	0.05%	N74254 001 AUG 03, 1994
	DESOWEN		
AB	GALDERMA	0.05%	N71425 001 JUN 15, 1988
	TRIDESILON		
AB	+ MILES	0.05%	N17426 001

DESONIDE; *MULTIPLE*

SEE ACETIC ACID, GLACIAL; DESONIDE

DESOXIMETASONE

CREAM; TOPICAL

TE	Product / Applicant	Strength	Appl. No. / Date
	DESOXIMETASONE		
AB	TARO	0.05%	N73210 001 NOV 30, 1990
AB		0.25%	N73193 001 NOV 30, 1990
	TOPICORT		
AB	HOECHST ROUSSEL	0.25%	N17856 001
	TOPICORT LP		
AB	+ HOECHST ROUSSEL	0.05%	N18309 001

DESOXIMETASONE *(continued)*

GEL; TOPICAL

TE	Product / Applicant	Strength	Appl. No. / Date
	TOPICORT		
	HOECHST ROUSSEL	0.05%	N18586 001 MAR 29, 1982

OINTMENT; TOPICAL

TE	Product / Applicant	Strength	Appl. No. / Date
	TOPICORT		
	HOECHST ROUSSEL	0.25%	N18763 001 SEP 30, 1983

DESOXYRIBONUCLEASE; *MULTIPLE*

SEE CHLORAMPHENICOL; DESOXYRIBONUCLEASE; FIBRINOLYSIN

DEXAMETHASONE

AEROSOL; TOPICAL

TE	Product / Applicant	Strength	Appl. No. / Date
	AEROSEB-DEX		
	+ ALLERGAN HERBERT	0.01%	N83296 002
	DECASPRAY		
	+ MERCK SHARP DOHME	0.4%	N12731 002

ELIXIR; ORAL

TE	Product / Applicant	Strength	Appl. No. / Date
	DECADRON		
AA	MERCK SHARP DOHME	0.5 MG/5 ML	N12376 002
	DEXAMETHASONE		
AA	BARRE	0.5 MG/5 ML	N84754 001
AA		0.5 MG/5 ML	N88997 001 OCT 10, 1986
	HEXADROL		
AA	ORGANON	0.5 MG/5 ML	N12674 001
	MYMETHASONE		
AA	PENNEX	0.5 MG/5 ML	N88254 001 JUL 27, 1983

GEL; TOPICAL

TE	Product / Applicant	Strength	Appl. No. / Date
	DECADERM		
	+ MERCK SHARP DOHME	0.1%	N13538 001

SOLUTION; ORAL

TE	Product / Applicant	Strength	Appl. No. / Date
	DEXAMETHASONE		
	ROXANE	0.5 MG/5 ML	N88248 001 SEP 01, 1983
	DEXAMETHASONE INTENSOL		
	ROXANE	0.5 MG/0.5 ML	N88252 001 SEP 01, 1983

SUSPENSION/DROPS; OPHTHALMIC

TE	Product / Applicant	Strength	Appl. No. / Date
	DEXAMETHASONE		
AT	STERIS	0.1%	N89170 001 MAY 09, 1989
	MAXIDEX		
AT	+ ALCON	0.1%	N13422 001

Prescription Drug Products *(continued)*

DEXAMETHASONE *(continued)*

TABLET; ORAL

	DECADRON		
AB	MERCK SHARP DOHME	0.5 MG	N11664 001
AB	+	0.75 MG	N11664 002
AB		1.5 MG	N11664 003
AB		4 MG	N11664 005
BP		0.25 MG	N11664 004
BP	+	6 MG	N11664 006 JUL 30, 1982
	DEXAMETHASONE		
BP	DANBURY PHARMA	0.25 MG	N85455 001
BP		0.5 MG	N85458 001
BP		0.75 MG	N80968 001
BP		1.5 MG	N85456 001
BP	GLOBAL PHARMS	0.75 MG	N85376 001
BP	PAR PHARM	0.25 MG	N88149 001 APR 28, 1983
BP		0.5 MG	N88148 001 APR 28, 1983
BP		0.75 MG	N88160 001 APR 28, 1983
BP		1.5 MG	N88237 001 APR 28, 1983
BP		4 MG	N88238 001 APR 28, 1983
BP		6 MG	N88481 001 NOV 28, 1983
AB	ROXANE	0.5 MG	N84611 001
AB		0.75 MG	N84613 001
AB		1.5 MG	N84610 001
AB		4 MG	N84612 001
BP		6 MG	N88316 001 SEP 15, 1983
		1 MG	N88306 001 SEP 15, 1983
		2 MG	N87916 001 AUG 26, 1982
	DEXONE 0.5		
BP	SOLVAY	0.5 MG	N84991 001
	DEXONE 0.75		
BP	SOLVAY	0.75 MG	N84993 001
	DEXONE 1.5		
BP	SOLVAY	1.5 MG	N84990 001
	DEXONE 4		
BP	SOLVAY	4 MG	N84992 001
	HEXADROL		
BP	ORGANON	0.5 MG	N12675 004
BP		0.75 MG	N12675 007
BP		1.5 MG	N12675 009
BP		4 MG	N12675 010

DEXAMETHASONE; NEOMYCIN SULFATE; POLYMYXIN B SULFATE

OINTMENT; OPHTHALMIC

	DEXACIDIN		
AT	IOLAB	0.1%;EQ 3.5 MG BASE/ GM;10,000 UNITS/GM	N62566 001 FEB 22, 1985
	DEXASPORIN		
AT	BAUSCH AND LOMB	0.1%;EQ 3.5 MG BASE/ GM;10,000 UNITS/GM	N64063 001 JUL 25, 1994
	MAXITROL		
AT	+ ALCON	0.1%;EQ 3.5 MG BASE/ GM;10,000 UNITS/GM	N50065 002
	NEOMYCIN AND POLYMYXIN B SULFATES AND DEXAMETHASONE		
AT	FOUGERA	0.1%;EQ 3.5 MG BASE/ GM;10,000 UNITS/GM	N62938 001 JUL 31, 1989

SUSPENSION/DROPS; OPHTHALMIC

	DEXACIDIN		
AT	IOLAB	0.1%;EQ 3.5 MG BASE/ ML;10,000 UNITS/ML	N62544 001 OCT 29, 1984
	MAXITROL		
AT	+ ALCON	0.1%;EQ 3.5 MG BASE/ ML;10,000 UNITS/ML	N50023 002
AT		0.1%;EQ 3.5 MG BASE/ ML;10,000 UNITS/ML	N62341 001 MAY 22, 1984
	NEOMYCIN AND POLYMYXIN B SULFATES AND DEXAMETHASONE		
AT	STERIS	0.1%;EQ 3.5 MG BASE/ ML;10,000 UNITS/ML	N62721 001 NOV 17, 1986

DEXAMETHASONE; TOBRAMYCIN

OINTMENT; OPHTHALMIC

	TOBRADEX		
	+ ALCON	0.1%;0.3%	N50616 001 SEP 28, 1988

SUSPENSION/DROPS; OPHTHALMIC

	TOBRADEX		
	+ ALCON	0.1%;0.3%	N50592 001 AUG 18, 1988

Prescription Drug Products *(continued)*

DEXAMETHASONE ACETATE

INJECTABLE; INJECTION

	DECADRON-LA		
BP	+ MERCK	EQ 8 MG BASE/ML	N16675 001
	DEXAMETHASONE ACETATE		
BP	STERIS	EQ 8 MG BASE/ML	N84315 001
	+	EQ 16 MG BASE/ML	N87711 001 MAY 24, 1982

DEXAMETHASONE SODIUM PHOSPHATE

AEROSOL; NASAL

	DEXACORT		
	+ MEDEVA	EQ 0.1 MG PHOSPHATE/INH	N14242 001

AEROSOL, METERED; INHALATION

	DEXACORT		
	+ MEDEVA	EQ 0.1 MG PHOSPHATE/INH	N13413 001

CREAM; TOPICAL

	DECADRON		
	+ MERCK SHARP DOHME	EQ 0.1% PHOSPHATE	N11983 002

INJECTABLE; INJECTION

	DECADRON		
AP	MERCK SHARP DOHME	EQ 4 MG PHOSPHATE/ML	N12071 002
AP	+	EQ 24 MG PHOSPHATE/ML	N12071 004
	DEXAMETHASONE		
AP	ELKINS SINN	EQ 4 MG PHOSPHATE/ML	N84282 001
AP		EQ 10 MG PHOSPHATE/ML	N87702 001 SEP 07, 1982
AP	FUJISAWA	EQ 4 MG PHOSPHATE/ML	N88448 001 JAN 25, 1984
AP		EQ 10 MG PHOSPHATE/ML	N88469 001 JAN 25, 1984
	DEXAMETHASONE SODIUM PHOSPHATE		
AP	AKORN	EQ 4 MG PHOSPHATE/ML	N84493 001
AP	DELL LABS	EQ 4 MG PHOSPHATE/ML	N83161 001
AP	FUJISAWA	EQ 4 MG PHOSPHATE/ML	N84916 001
AP	GENSIA	EQ 4 MG PHOSPHATE/ML	N81125 001 AUG 31, 1990
AP		EQ 10 MG PHOSPHATE/ML	N81126 001 AUG 31, 1990
AP	LUITPOLD	EQ 4 MG PHOSPHATE/ML	N87440 001 JUL 21, 1982
AP	STERIS	EQ 4 MG PHOSPHATE/ML	N83702 001
AP		EQ 4 MG PHOSPHATE/ML	N84355 001
AP		EQ 4 MG PHOSPHATE/ML	N89169 001 APR 09, 1986
AP		EQ 10 MG PHOSPHATE/ML	N87668 001 JUL 01, 1982
AP		EQ 24 MG PHOSPHATE/ML	N85606 001

DEXAMETHASONE SODIUM PHOSPHATE *(continued)*

INJECTABLE; INJECTION

	HEXADROL		
AP	+ ORGANON	EQ 4 MG PHOSPHATE/ML	N14694 002
AP	+	EQ 10 MG PHOSPHATE/ML	N14694 003

OINTMENT; OPHTHALMIC

	DECADRON		
AT	+ MERCK SHARP DOHME	EQ 0.05% PHOSPHATE	N11977 001
	DEXAIR		
AT	PHARMAFAIR	EQ 0.05% PHOSPHATE	N88071 001 DEC 28, 1982
	MAXIDEX		
AT	ALCON	EQ 0.05% PHOSPHATE	N83342 001

SOLUTION/DROPS; OPHTHALMIC

	DEXAIR		
	PHARMAFAIR	EQ 0.1% PHOSPHATE	N88433 001 DEC 15, 1983

SOLUTION/DROPS; OPHTHALMIC, OTIC

	DECADRON		
AT	+ MERCK SHARP DOHME	EQ 0.1% PHOSPHATE	N11984 001
	DEXAMETHASONE SODIUM PHOSPHATE		
AT	AKORN	EQ 0.1% PHOSPHATE	N84855 001
AT	STERIS	EQ 0.1% PHOSPHATE	N88771 001 JAN 16, 1985

DEXAMETHASONE SODIUM PHOSPHATE; LIDOCAINE HYDROCHLORIDE

INJECTABLE; INJECTION

	DECADRON W/ XYLOCAINE		
	+ MERCK SHARP DOHME	EQ 4 MG PHOSPHATE/ML;10 MG/ML	N13334 002

DEXAMETHASONE SODIUM PHOSPHATE; NEOMYCIN SULFATE

OINTMENT; OPHTHALMIC

	NEODECADRON		
	+ MERCK SHARP DOHME	EQ 0.05% PHOSPHATE;EQ 3.5 MG BASE/GM	N50324 001

SOLUTION/DROPS; OPHTHALMIC

	NEODECADRON		
AT	+ MERCK SHARP DOHME	EQ 0.1% PHOSPHATE;EQ 3.5 MG BASE/ML	N50322 001
	NEOMYCIN SULFATE-DEXAMETHASONE SODIUM PHOSPHATE		
AT	PHARMAFAIR	EQ 0.1% PHOSPHATE;EQ 3.5 MG BASE/ML	N62539 001 JAN 10, 1985
AT	STERIS	EQ 0.1% PHOSPHATE;EQ 3.5 MG BASE/ML	N62714 001 JUL 21, 1986

Prescription Drug Products *(continued)*

DEXCHLORPHENIRAMINE MALEATE
SYRUP; ORAL
MYLARAMINE
AA PENNEX 2 MG/5 ML N88251 001 MAR 23, 1984
POLARAMINE
AA SCHERING 2 MG/5 ML N86837 001 JUL 19, 1982
TABLET; ORAL
DEXCHLORPHENIRAMINE MALEATE
AA SIDMAK LABS NJ 2 MG N88682 001 JAN 17, 1986
POLARAMINE
AA SCHERING 2 MG N86835 001

DEXPANTHENOL; *MULTIPLE*
SEE ASCORBIC ACID; BIOTIN; CYANOCOBALAMIN; DEXPANTHENOL; ERGOCALCIFEROL; FOLIC ACID; NIACINAMIDE; PYRIDOXINE HYDROCHLORIDE; RIBOFLAVIN PHOSPHATE SODIUM; THIAMINE HYDROCHLORIDE; VITAMIN A; VITAMIN E

DEXTROAMPHETAMINE SULFATE
CAPSULE, EXTENDED RELEASE; ORAL
DEXEDRINE
+ SMITHKLINE BEECHAM 5 MG N17078 001
+ 10 MG N17078 002
+ 15 MG N17078 003
TABLET; ORAL
DEXEDRINE
AA SMITHKLINE BEECHAM 5 MG N84935 001
DEXTROAMPHETAMINE SULFATE
AA HALSEY 10 MG N83930 001
AA MM MAST 5 MG N86521 001
AA REXAR 5 MG N84051 001
AA 10 MG N84051 002

DEXTROMETHORPHAN HYDROBROMIDE; *MULTIPLE*
SEE BROMPHENIRAMINE MALEATE; DEXTROMETHORPHAN HYDROBROMIDE; PSEUDOEPHEDRINE HYDROCHLORIDE

DEXTROMETHORPHAN HYDROBROMIDE; PROMETHAZINE HYDROCHLORIDE
SYRUP; ORAL
PHENERGAN W/ DEXTROMETHORPHAN
AA WYETH AYERST 15 MG/5 ML;6.25 MG/5 ML N11265 002 APR 02, 1984
PHERAZINE DM
AA HALSEY 15 MG/5 ML;6.25 MG/5 ML N88913 001 MAR 02, 1987
PROMETH W/ DEXTROMETHORPHAN
AA BARRE 15 MG/5 ML;6.25 MG/5 ML N88762 001 OCT 31, 1984
PROMETHAZINE W/ DEXTROMETHORPHAN
AA PENNEX 15 MG/5 ML;6.25 MG/5 ML N88864 001 JAN 04, 1985

DEXTROSE
INJECTABLE; INJECTION
DEXTROSE 10% IN PLASTIC CONTAINER
AP ABBOTT 10 GM/100 ML N18080 001
AP BAXTER 10 GM/100 ML N16694 001
AP MCGAW 10 GM/100 ML N18046 001
AP 10 GM/100 ML N19626 004 FEB 02, 1988
DEXTROSE 2.5% IN PLASTIC CONTAINER
MCGAW 2.5 GM/100 ML N18358 001
2.5 GM/100 ML N19626 001 FEB 02, 1988
DEXTROSE 20% IN PLASTIC CONTAINER
AP ABBOTT 20 GM/100 ML N18564 001 MAR 23, 1982
AP BAXTER 20 GM/100 ML N17521 004
DEXTROSE 30% IN PLASTIC CONTAINER
AP ABBOTT 30 GM/100 ML N19345 001 JAN 26, 1985
AP BAXTER 30 GM/100 ML N17521 003
DEXTROSE 40% IN PLASTIC CONTAINER
AP ABBOTT 40 GM/100 ML N18562 001 MAR 23, 1982
AP BAXTER 40 GM/100 ML N17521 002
DEXTROSE 5% IN PLASTIC CONTAINER
AP ABBOTT 50 MG/ML N16367 002
AP 50 MG/ML N19222 001 JUL 13, 1984
AP 5 GM/100 ML N19466 001 JUL 15, 1985
AP 5 GM/100 ML N19479 001 SEP 17, 1985

Prescription Drug Products *(continued)*

DEXTROSE *(continued)*

INJECTABLE; INJECTION

DEXTROSE 5% IN PLASTIC CONTAINER

AP	BAXTER	5 GM/100 ML	N16673 001
AP		50 MG/ML	N16673 003 OCT 30, 1985
AP		5 GM/100 ML	N20179 001 DEC 07, 1992
AP		50 MG/ML	N20179 002 DEC 07, 1992
AP	MCGAW	5 GM/100 ML	N16730 001
AP		50 MG/ML	N16730 002
AP		5 GM/100 ML	N19626 002 FEB 02, 1988

DEXTROSE 50% IN PLASTIC CONTAINER

AP	ABBOTT	50 GM/100 ML	N18563 001 MAR 23, 1982
AP		50 GM/100 ML	N19894 001 DEC 26, 1989
AP	BAXTER	50 GM/100 ML	N17521 001
AP		50 GM/100 ML	N20047 001 JUL 02, 1991

DEXTROSE 60% IN PLASTIC CONTAINER

AP	ABBOTT	60 GM/100 ML	N19346 001 JAN 25, 1985
AP	BAXTER	60 GM/100 ML	N17521 005 MAR 26, 1982
AP		60 GM/100 ML	N20047 002 JUL 02, 1991

DEXTROSE 7.7% IN PLASTIC CONTAINER

	MCGAW	7.7 GM/100 ML	N19626 003 FEB 02, 1988

DEXTROSE 70% IN PLASTIC CONTAINER

AP	ABBOTT	70 GM/100 ML	N18561 001 MAR 23, 1982
AP		70 GM/100 ML	N19893 001 DEC 26, 1989
AP	BAXTER	70 GM/100 ML	N17521 006 MAR 26, 1982
AP		70 GM/100 ML	N20047 003 JUL 02, 1991

DEXTROSE; *MULTIPLE*

SEE AMINO ACIDS; CALCIUM CHLORIDE; DEXTROSE; MAGNESIUM CHLORIDE; POTASSIUM CHLORIDE; POTASSIUM PHOSPHATE, DIBASIC; SODIUM CHLORIDE
SEE AMINO ACIDS; DEXTROSE
SEE AMINO ACIDS; DEXTROSE; MAGNESIUM CHLORIDE; POTASSIUM CHLORIDE; SODIUM CHLORIDE; SODIUM PHOSPHATE, DIBASIC
SEE AMINO ACIDS; DEXTROSE; MAGNESIUM CHLORIDE; POTASSIUM ACETATE; POTASSIUM CHLORIDE; POTASSIUM PHOSPHATE, DIBASIC; SODIUM CHLORIDE
SEE AMINO ACIDS; DEXTROSE; MAGNESIUM CHLORIDE; POTASSIUM CHLORIDE; SODIUM CHLORIDE; SODIUM PHOSPHATE, DIBASIC
SEE CALCIUM CHLORIDE; DEXTROSE; GLUTATHIONE DISULFIDE; MAGNESIUM CHLORIDE; POTASSIUM CHLORIDE; SODIUM BICARBONATE; SODIUM CHLORIDE; SODIUM PHOSPHATE
SEE CALCIUM CHLORIDE; DEXTROSE; MAGNESIUM CHLORIDE; POTASSIUM CHLORIDE; SODIUM ACETATE; SODIUM CHLORIDE
SEE CALCIUM CHLORIDE; DEXTROSE; MAGNESIUM CHLORIDE; POTASSIUM CHLORIDE; SODIUM ACETATE; SODIUM CHLORIDE; SODIUM CITRATE
SEE CALCIUM CHLORIDE; DEXTROSE; MAGNESIUM CHLORIDE; SODIUM CHLORIDE; SODIUM LACTATE
SEE CALCIUM CHLORIDE; DEXTROSE; MAGNESIUM CHLORIDE; SODIUM ACETATE; SODIUM CHLORIDE
SEE CALCIUM CHLORIDE; DEXTROSE; MAGNESIUM CHLORIDE; POTASSIUM CHLORIDE; SODIUM ACETATE; SODIUM CHLORIDE; SODIUM LACTATE
SEE CALCIUM CHLORIDE; DEXTROSE; MAGNESIUM CHLORIDE; SODIUM CHLORIDE; SODIUM LACTATE
SEE CALCIUM CHLORIDE; DEXTROSE; POTASSIUM CHLORIDE; SODIUM CHLORIDE
SEE CALCIUM CHLORIDE; DEXTROSE; POTASSIUM CHLORIDE; SODIUM CHLORIDE; SODIUM LACTATE
SEE CALCIUM CHLORIDE; DEXTROSE; POTASSIUM CHLORIDE; SODIUM ACETATE; SODIUM CHLORIDE
SEE CALCIUM CHLORIDE; DEXTROSE; POTASSIUM CHLORIDE; SODIUM CHLORIDE; SODIUM LACTATE

Prescription Drug Products *(continued)*

DEXTROSE; MAGNESIUM ACETATE; POTASSIUM ACETATE; SODIUM CHLORIDE

INJECTABLE; INJECTION
NORMOSOL-M AND DEXTROSE 5% IN PLASTIC CONTAINER
ABBOTT 5 GM/100 ML;21 MG/
100 ML;128 MG/
100 ML;234 MG/100 ML N17610 001

DEXTROSE; MAGNESIUM ACETATE TETRAHYDRATE; POTASSIUM ACETATE; SODIUM CHLORIDE

INJECTABLE; INJECTION
PLASMA-LYTE 56 AND DEXTROSE 5% IN PLASTIC CONTAINER
BAXTER 5 GM/100 ML;32 MG/
100 ML;128 MG/
100 ML;234 MG/100 ML N17385 001

DEXTROSE; MAGNESIUM CHLORIDE; POTASSIUM CHLORIDE; POTASSIUM PHOSPHATE, DIBASIC; SODIUM ACETATE

INJECTABLE; INJECTION
ISOLYTE P IN DEXTROSE 5% IN PLASTIC CONTAINER
MCGAW 5 GM/100 ML;31 MG/
100 ML;130 MG/
100 ML;26 MG/
100 ML;320 MG/100 ML N19873 001
JUN 10, 1993

ISOLYTE P W/ DEXTROSE 5% IN PLASTIC CONTAINER
MCGAW 5 GM/100 ML;31 MG/
100 ML;130 MG/
100 ML;26 MG/
100 ML;320 MG/100 ML N19025 001
DEC 27, 1984

DEXTROSE; MAGNESIUM CHLORIDE; POTASSIUM CHLORIDE; POTASSIUM PHOSPHATE, DIBASIC; SODIUM CHLORIDE; SODIUM LACTATE; SODIUM PHOSPHATE, MONOBASIC

INJECTABLE; INJECTION
IONOSOL B AND DEXTROSE 5% IN PLASTIC CONTAINER
ABBOTT 5 GM/100 ML;53 MG/
100 ML;100 MG/
100 ML;100 MG/
100 ML;180 MG/
100 ML;280 MG/
100 ML;16 MG/100 ML N19515 001
MAY 08, 1986

DEXTROSE; MAGNESIUM CHLORIDE; POTASSIUM CHLORIDE; POTASSIUM PHOSPHATE, MONOBASIC; SODIUM CHLORIDE; SODIUM LACTATE

INJECTABLE; INJECTION
DEXTROSE 5% AND ELECTROLYTE NO.48 IN PLASTIC CONTAINER
BAXTER 5 GM/100 ML;31 MG/
100 ML;141 MG/
100 ML;20 MG/
100 ML;12 MG/
100 ML;260 MG/100 ML N17484 001

DEXTROSE; MAGNESIUM CHLORIDE; POTASSIUM CHLORIDE; POTASSIUM PHOSPHATE, MONOBASIC; SODIUM LACTATE; SODIUM PHOSPHATE, MONOBASIC

INJECTABLE; INJECTION
IONOSOL MB AND DEXTROSE 5% IN PLASTIC CONTAINER
ABBOTT 5 GM/100 ML;30 MG/
100 ML;141 MG/
100 ML;15 MG/
100 ML;260 MG/
100 ML;25 MG/100 ML N19513 001
MAY 08, 1986

DEXTROSE; MAGNESIUM CHLORIDE; POTASSIUM CHLORIDE; SODIUM ACETATE; SODIUM CHLORIDE

INJECTABLE; INJECTION
ISOLYTE H IN DEXTROSE 5% IN PLASTIC CONTAINER
MCGAW 5 GM/100 ML;30 MG/
100 ML;97 MG/
100 ML;220 MG/
100 ML;140 MG/100 ML N19844 001
JUN 10, 1993

ISOLYTE H W/ DEXTROSE 5% IN PLASTIC CONTAINER
MCGAW 5 GM/100 ML;30 MG/
100 ML;97 MG/
100 ML;220 MG/
100 ML;140 MG/100 ML N18273 001

Prescription Drug Products *(continued)*

DEXTROSE; MAGNESIUM CHLORIDE; POTASSIUM CHLORIDE; SODIUM ACETATE; SODIUM CHLORIDE; SODIUM GLUCONATE

INJECTABLE; INJECTION

ISOLYTE S IN DEXTROSE 5% IN PLASTIC CONTAINER
AP MCGAW 5 GM/100 ML;30 MG/100 ML;37 MG/100 ML;370 MG/100 ML;530 MG/100 ML;500 MG/100 ML N19843 001 AUG 09, 1993

ISOLYTE S W/ DEXTROSE 5% IN PLASTIC CONTAINER
AP MCGAW 5 GM/100 ML;30 MG/100 ML;37 MG/100 ML;370 MG/100 ML;530 MG/100 ML;500 MG/100 ML N18274 001

NORMOSOL-R AND DEXTROSE 5% IN PLASTIC CONTAINER
ABBOTT 5 GM/100 ML;30 MG/100 ML;37 MG/100 ML;222 MG/100 ML;526 MG/100 ML;502 MG/100 ML N17609 001

PLASMA-LYTE 148 AND DEXTROSE 5% IN PLASTIC CONTAINER
AP BAXTER 5 GM/100 ML;30 MG/100 ML;37 MG/100 ML;368 MG/100 ML;526 MG/100 ML;502 MG/100 ML N17451 001

DEXTROSE; POTASSIUM CHLORIDE

INJECTABLE; INJECTION

DEXTROSE 5% AND POTASSIUM CHLORIDE 0.075% IN PLASTIC CONTAINER
AP BAXTER 5 GM/100 ML;75 MG/100 ML N17634 004

DEXTROSE 5% AND POTASSIUM CHLORIDE 0.15% IN PLASTIC CONTAINER
AP BAXTER 5 GM/100 ML;150 MG/100 ML N17634 001

DEXTROSE 5% AND POTASSIUM CHLORIDE 0.224% IN PLASTIC CONTAINER
AP BAXTER 5 GM/100 ML;224 MG/100 ML N17634 003

DEXTROSE 5% AND POTASSIUM CHLORIDE 0.3% IN PLASTIC CONTAINER
AP BAXTER 5 GM/100 ML;300 MG/100 ML N17634 002

POTASSIUM CHLORIDE 0.037% IN DEXTROSE 5% IN PLASTIC CONTAINER
MCGAW 5 GM/100 ML;37 MG/100 ML N19699 001 SEP 29, 1989

POTASSIUM CHLORIDE 0.075% IN DEXTROSE 5% IN PLASTIC CONTAINER
AP MCGAW 5 GM/100 ML;75 MG/100 ML N18744 001 NOV 09, 1982
AP 5 GM/100 ML;75 MG/100 ML N19699 002 SEP 29, 1989

DEXTROSE; POTASSIUM CHLORIDE *(continued)*

INJECTABLE; INJECTION

POTASSIUM CHLORIDE 0.11% IN DEXTROSE 5% IN PLASTIC CONTAINER
MCGAW 5 GM/100 ML;110 MG/100 ML N19699 003 SEP 29, 1989

POTASSIUM CHLORIDE 0.15% IN DEXTROSE 5% IN PLASTIC CONTAINER
AP MCGAW 5 GM/100 ML;150 MG/100 ML N18744 002 NOV 09, 1982
AP 5 GM/100 ML;150 MG/100 ML N19699 004 SEP 29, 1989

POTASSIUM CHLORIDE 0.22% IN DEXTROSE 5% IN PLASTIC CONTAINER
MCGAW 5 GM/100 ML;220 MG/100 ML N18744 003 NOV 09, 1982
5 GM/100 ML;220 MG/100 ML N19699 005 SEP 29, 1989

POTASSIUM CHLORIDE 0.3% IN DEXTROSE 5% IN PLASTIC CONTAINER
AP MCGAW 5 GM/100 ML;300 MG/100 ML N18744 004 NOV 09, 1982
AP 5 GM/100 ML;300 MG/100 ML N19699 006 SEP 29, 1989

POTASSIUM CHLORIDE 20 MEQ IN DEXTROSE 5% IN PLASTIC CONTAINER
ABBOTT 5 GM/100 ML;149 MG/100 ML N18371 001

POTASSIUM CHLORIDE 30 MEQ IN DEXTROSE 5% IN PLASTIC CONTAINER
AP ABBOTT 5 GM/100 ML;224 MG/100 ML N18371 003

POTASSIUM CHLORIDE 40 MEQ IN DEXTROSE 5% IN PLASTIC CONTAINER
ABBOTT 5 GM/100 ML;298 MG/100 ML N18371 002

DEXTROSE; POTASSIUM CHLORIDE; POTASSIUM LACTATE; SODIUM CHLORIDE; SODIUM PHOSPHATE, MONOBASIC

INJECTABLE; INJECTION

IONOSOL T AND DEXTROSE 5% IN PLASTIC CONTAINER
ABBOTT 5 GM/100 ML;111 MG/100 ML;256 MG/100 ML;146 MG/100 ML;207 MG/100 ML N19514 001 MAY 08, 1986

Prescription Drug Products *(continued)*

DEXTROSE; POTASSIUM CHLORIDE; POTASSIUM PHOSPHATE, DIBASIC; SODIUM ACETATE; SODIUM CHLORIDE

INJECTABLE; INJECTION
ISOLYTE M IN DEXTROSE 5% IN PLASTIC CONTAINER
MCGAW — 5 GM/100 ML;150 MG/100 ML;130 MG/100 ML;280 MG/100 ML;91 MG/100 ML — N19870 001 JUN 10, 1993

ISOLYTE M W/ DEXTROSE 5% IN PLASTIC CONTAINER
MCGAW — 5 GM/100 ML;150 MG/100 ML;130 MG/100 ML;280 MG/100 ML;91 MG/100 ML — N18270 001

DEXTROSE; POTASSIUM CHLORIDE; POTASSIUM PHOSPHATE, MONOBASIC; SODIUM CHLORIDE; SODIUM LACTATE

INJECTABLE; INJECTION
DEXTROSE 5% AND ELECTROLYTE NO 75 IN PLASTIC CONTAINER
BAXTER — 5 GM/100 ML;205 MG/100 ML;100 MG/100 ML;120 MG/100 ML;220 MG/100 ML — N18840 001 JUN 29, 1983

DEXTROSE; POTASSIUM CHLORIDE; SODIUM CHLORIDE

INJECTABLE; INJECTION
DEXTROSE 5%, SODIUM CHLORIDE 0.2% AND POTASSIUM CHLORIDE 10 MEQ
AP BAXTER — 5 GM/100 ML;75 MG/100 ML;200 MG/100 ML — N18037 006 APR 13, 1982
AP — 5 GM/100 ML;150 MG/100 ML;200 MG/100 ML — N18037 007 APR 13, 1982

DEXTROSE 5%, SODIUM CHLORIDE 0.2% AND POTASSIUM CHLORIDE 15 MEQ (K)
AP BAXTER — 5 GM/100 ML;224 MG/100 ML;200 MG/100 ML — N18037 004

DEXTROSE 5%, SODIUM CHLORIDE 0.2% AND POTASSIUM CHLORIDE 20 MEQ
AP BAXTER — 5 GM/100 ML;150 MG/100 ML;200 MG/100 ML — N18037 008 APR 13, 1982

DEXTROSE 5%, SODIUM CHLORIDE 0.2% AND POTASSIUM CHLORIDE 20 MEQ (K)
AP BAXTER — 5 GM/100 ML;300 MG/100 ML;200 MG/100 ML — N18037 001

DEXTROSE; POTASSIUM CHLORIDE; SODIUM CHLORIDE *(continued)*

INJECTABLE; INJECTION
DEXTROSE 5%, SODIUM CHLORIDE 0.2% AND POTASSIUM CHLORIDE 30 MEQ
AP BAXTER — 5 GM/100 ML;224 MG/100 ML;200 MG/100 ML — N18037 005 APR 13, 1982

DEXTROSE 5%, SODIUM CHLORIDE 0.2% AND POTASSIUM CHLORIDE 40 MEQ
AP BAXTER — 5 GM/100 ML;300 MG/100 ML;200 MG/100 ML — N18037 009 APR 13, 1982

DEXTROSE 5%, SODIUM CHLORIDE 0.2% AND POTASSIUM CHLORIDE 5 MEQ
AP BAXTER — 5 GM/100 ML;75 MG/100 ML;200 MG/100 ML — N18037 002

DEXTROSE 5%, SODIUM CHLORIDE 0.2% AND POTASSIUM CHLORIDE 5 MEQ (K)
AP BAXTER — 5 GM/100 ML;150 MG/100 ML;200 MG/100 ML — N18037 003

DEXTROSE 5%, SODIUM CHLORIDE 0.2% AND POTASSIUM CHLORIDE 0.075%
AP MCGAW — 5 GM/100 ML;75 MG/100 ML;200 MG/100 ML — N18268 009

DEXTROSE 5%, SODIUM CHLORIDE 0.2% AND POTASSIUM CHLORIDE 0.15% IN PLASTIC CONTAINER
AP MCGAW — 5 GM/100 ML;150 MG/100 ML;200 MG/100 ML — N18268 004

DEXTROSE 5%, SODIUM CHLORIDE 0.2% AND POTASSIUM CHLORIDE 0.224% IN PLASTIC CONTAINER
AP MCGAW — 5 GM/100 ML;220 MG/100 ML;200 MG/100 ML — N18268 005

DEXTROSE 5%, SODIUM CHLORIDE 0.2% AND POTASSIUM CHLORIDE 0.3% IN PLASTIC CONTAINER
AP MCGAW — 5 GM/100 ML;300 MG/100 ML;200 MG/100 ML — N18268 006

DEXTROSE 5%, SODIUM CHLORIDE 0.33% AND POTASSIUM CHLORIDE 10 MEQ IN PLASTIC CONTAINER
AP BAXTER — 5 GM/100 ML;75 MG/100 ML;330 MG/100 ML — N18629 005 MAR 23, 1982
AP — 5 GM/100 ML;150 MG/100 ML;330 MG/100 ML — N18629 002 MAR 23, 1982

DEXTROSE 5%, SODIUM CHLORIDE 0.33% AND POTASSIUM CHLORIDE 15 MEQ IN PLASTIC CONTAINER
AP BAXTER — 5 GM/100 ML;224 MG/100 ML;330 MG/100 ML — N18629 003 MAR 23, 1982

Prescription Drug Products *(continued)*

DEXTROSE; POTASSIUM CHLORIDE; SODIUM CHLORIDE
(continued)

INJECTABLE; INJECTION

<u>DEXTROSE 5%, SODIUM CHLORIDE 0.33% AND POTASSIUM CHLORIDE 20 MEQ IN PLASTIC CONTAINER</u>

<u>AP</u> BAXTER <u>5 GM/100 ML;150 MG/100 ML;330 MG/100 ML</u> N18629 004 MAR 23, 1982

<u>AP</u> <u>5 GM/100 ML;300 MG/100 ML;330 MG/100 ML</u> N18629 006 MAR 23, 1982

<u>DEXTROSE 5%, SODIUM CHLORIDE 0.33% AND POTASSIUM CHLORIDE 30 MEQ IN PLASTIC CONTAINER</u>

<u>AP</u> BAXTER <u>5 GM/100 ML;224 MG/100 ML;330 MG/100 ML</u> N18629 007 MAR 23, 1982

<u>DEXTROSE 5%, SODIUM CHLORIDE 0.33% AND POTASSIUM CHLORIDE 40 MEQ IN PLASTIC CONTAINER</u>

<u>AP</u> BAXTER <u>5 GM/100 ML;300 MG/100 ML;330 MG/100 ML</u> N18629 008 MAR 23, 1982

<u>DEXTROSE 5%, SODIUM CHLORIDE 0.33% AND POTASSIUM CHLORIDE 5 MEQ IN PLASTIC CONTAINER</u>

<u>AP</u> BAXTER <u>5 GM/100 ML;75 MG/100 ML;330 MG/100 ML</u> N18629 001 MAR 23, 1982

<u>DEXTROSE 5%, SODIUM CHLORIDE 0.33% AND POTASSIUM CHLORIDE 0.075% IN PLASTIC CONTAINER</u>

<u>AP</u> MCGAW <u>5 GM/100 ML;75 MG/100 ML;330 MG/100 ML</u> N18268 011 JAN 18, 1986

<u>DEXTROSE 5%, SODIUM CHLORIDE 0.33% AND POTASSIUM CHLORIDE 0.15% IN PLASTIC CONTAINER</u>

<u>AP</u> MCGAW <u>5 GM/100 ML;150 MG/100 ML;330 MG/100 ML</u> N18268 012 JAN 18, 1986

<u>DEXTROSE 5%, SODIUM CHLORIDE 0.33% AND POTASSIUM CHLORIDE 0.22% IN PLASTIC CONTAINER</u>

<u>AP</u> MCGAW <u>5 GM/100 ML;220 MG/100 ML;330 MG/100 ML</u> N18268 013 JAN 18, 1986

<u>DEXTROSE 5%, SODIUM CHLORIDE 0.33% AND POTASSIUM CHLORIDE 0.30% IN PLASTIC CONTAINER</u>

<u>AP</u> MCGAW <u>5 GM/100 ML;300 MG/100 ML;330 MG/100 ML</u> N18268 014 JAN 18, 1986

<u>DEXTROSE 5%, SODIUM CHLORIDE 0.45% AND POTASSIUM CHLORIDE 20 MEQ (K) IN PLASTIC CONTAINER</u>

<u>AP</u> BAXTER <u>5 GM/100 ML;300 MG/100 ML;450 MG/100 ML</u> N18008 010

DEXTROSE; POTASSIUM CHLORIDE; SODIUM CHLORIDE
(continued)

INJECTABLE; INJECTION

<u>DEXTROSE 5%, SODIUM CHLORIDE 0.45% AND POTASSIUM CHLORIDE 0.075%</u>

<u>AP</u> MCGAW <u>5 GM/100 ML;75 MG/100 ML;450 MG/100 ML</u> N18268 010

<u>DEXTROSE 5%, SODIUM CHLORIDE 0.45% AND POTASSIUM CHLORIDE 0.15% IN PLASTIC CONTAINER</u>

<u>AP</u> MCGAW <u>5 GM/100 ML;150 MG/100 ML;450 MG/100 ML</u> N18268 001

DEXTROSE 5%, SODIUM CHLORIDE 0.45% AND POTASSIUM CHLORIDE 0.22% IN PLASTIC CONTAINER

MCGAW 5 GM/100 ML;220 MG/100 ML;450 MG/100 ML N18268 002

<u>DEXTROSE 5%, SODIUM CHLORIDE 0.45% AND POTASSIUM CHLORIDE 0.3% IN PLASTIC CONTAINER</u>

<u>AP</u> MCGAW <u>5 GM/100 ML;300 MG/100 ML;450 MG/100 ML</u> N18268 003

POTASSIUM CHLORIDE 0.037% IN DEXTROSE 10% AND SODIUM CHLORIDE 0.2% IN PLASTIC CONTAINER

MCGAW 10 GM/100 ML;37 MG/100 ML;200 MG/100 ML N19630 031 FEB 17, 1988

POTASSIUM CHLORIDE 0.037% IN DEXTROSE 10% AND SODIUM CHLORIDE 0.45% IN PLASTIC CONTAINER

MCGAW 10 GM/100 ML;37 MG/100 ML;450 MG/100 ML N19630 037 FEB 17, 1988

POTASSIUM CHLORIDE 0.037% IN DEXTROSE 10% AND SODIUM CHLORIDE 0.9% IN PLASTIC CONTAINER

MCGAW 10 GM/100 ML;37 MG/100 ML;900 MG/100 ML N19630 043 FEB 17, 1988

POTASSIUM CHLORIDE 0.037% IN DEXTROSE 5% AND SODIUM CHLORIDE 0.11% IN PLASTIC CONTAINER

MCGAW 5 GM/100 ML;37 MG/100 ML;110 MG/100 ML N19630 001 FEB 17, 1988

POTASSIUM CHLORIDE 0.037% IN DEXTROSE 5% AND SODIUM CHLORIDE 0.2% IN PLASTIC CONTAINER

MCGAW 5 GM/100 ML;37 MG/100 ML;200 MG/100 ML N19630 007 FEB 17, 1988

POTASSIUM CHLORIDE 0.037% IN DEXTROSE 5% AND SODIUM CHLORIDE 0.33% IN PLASTIC CONTAINER

MCGAW 5 GM/100 ML;37 MG/100 ML;330 MG/100 ML N19630 013 FEB 17, 1988

Prescription Drug Products *(continued)*

DEXTROSE; POTASSIUM CHLORIDE; SODIUM CHLORIDE
(continued)

INJECTABLE; INJECTION

POTASSIUM CHLORIDE 0.037% IN DEXTROSE 5% AND SODIUM CHLORIDE 0.45% IN PLASTIC CONTAINER
MCGAW — 5 GM/100 ML;37 MG/100 ML;450 MG/100 ML — N19630 019 — FEB 17, 1988

POTASSIUM CHLORIDE 0.037% IN DEXTROSE 5% AND SODIUM CHLORIDE 0.9% IN PLASTIC CONTAINER
MCGAW — 5 GM/100 ML;37 MG/100 ML;900 MG/100 ML — N19630 025 — FEB 17, 1988

POTASSIUM CHLORIDE 0.075% IN DEXTROSE 10% AND SODIUM CHLORIDE 0.2% IN PLASTIC CONTAINER
MCGAW — 10 GM/100 ML;75 MG/100 ML;200 MG/100 ML — N19630 032 — FEB 17, 1988

POTASSIUM CHLORIDE 0.075% IN DEXTROSE 10% AND SODIUM CHLORIDE 0.45% IN PLASTIC CONTAINER
MCGAW — 10 GM/100 ML;75 MG/100 ML;450 MG/100 ML — N19630 038 — FEB 17, 1988

POTASSIUM CHLORIDE 0.075% IN DEXTROSE 10% AND SODIUM CHLORIDE 0.9% IN PLASTIC CONTAINER
MCGAW — 10 GM/100 ML;75 MG/100 ML;900 MG/100 ML — N19630 044 — FEB 17, 1988

POTASSIUM CHLORIDE 0.075% IN DEXTROSE 3.3% AND SODIUM CHLORIDE 0.3% IN PLASTIC CONTAINER
MCGAW — 3.3 GM/100 ML;75 MG/100 ML;300 MG/100 ML — N19630 049 — MAY 07, 1992

POTASSIUM CHLORIDE 0.075% IN DEXTROSE 5% AND SODIUM CHLORIDE 0.2% IN PLASTIC CONTAINER
AP — MCGAW — 5 GM/100 ML;75 MG/100 ML;200 MG/100 ML — N19630 008 — FEB 17, 1988

POTASSIUM CHLORIDE 0.075% IN DEXTROSE 5% AND SODIUM CHLORIDE 0.33% IN PLASTIC CONTAINER
AP — MCGAW — 5 GM/100 ML;75 MG/100 ML;330 MG/100 ML — N19630 014 — FEB 17, 1988

POTASSIUM CHLORIDE 0.075% IN DEXTROSE 5% AND SODIUM CHLORIDE 0.45% IN PLASTIC CONTAINER
AP — MCGAW — 5 GM/100 ML;75 MG/100 ML;450 MG/100 ML — N19630 020 — FEB 17, 1988

POTASSIUM CHLORIDE 0.075% IN DEXTROSE 5% AND SODIUM CHLORIDE 0.9% IN PLASTIC CONTAINER
AP — MCGAW — 5 GM/100 ML;75 MG/100 ML;900 MG/100 ML — N19630 026 — FEB 17, 1988

DEXTROSE; POTASSIUM CHLORIDE; SODIUM CHLORIDE
(continued)

INJECTABLE; INJECTION

POTASSIUM CHLORIDE 0.075% IN DEXTROSE 5% AND SODIUM CHLORIDE 0.11% IN PLASTIC CONTAINER
MCGAW — 5 GM/100 ML;75 MG/100 ML;110 MG/100 ML — N19630 002 — FEB 17, 1988

POTASSIUM CHLORIDE 0.11% IN DEXTROSE 10% AND SODIUM CHLORIDE 0.2% IN PLASTIC CONTAINER
MCGAW — 10 GM/100 ML;110 MG/100 ML;200 MG/100 ML — N19630 033 — FEB 17, 1988

POTASSIUM CHLORIDE 0.11% IN DEXTROSE 10% AND SODIUM CHLORIDE 0.45% IN PLASTIC CONTAINER
MCGAW — 10 GM/100 ML;110 MG/100 ML;450 MG/100 ML — N19630 039 — FEB 17, 1988

POTASSIUM CHLORIDE 0.11% IN DEXTROSE 10% AND SODIUM CHLORIDE 0.9% IN PLASTIC CONTAINER
MCGAW — 10 GM/100 ML;110 MG/100 ML;900 MG/100 ML — N19630 045 — FEB 17, 1988

POTASSIUM CHLORIDE 0.11% IN DEXTROSE 3.3% AND SODIUM CHLORIDE 0.3% IN PLASTIC CONTAINER
MCGAW — 3.3 GM/100 ML;110 MG/100 ML;300 MG/100 ML — N19630 050 — MAY 07, 1992

POTASSIUM CHLORIDE 0.11% IN DEXTROSE 5% AND SODIUM CHLORIDE 0.11% IN PLASTIC CONTAINER
MCGAW — 5 GM/100 ML;110 MG/100 ML;110 MG/100 ML — N19630 003 — FEB 17, 1988

POTASSIUM CHLORIDE 0.11% IN DEXTROSE 5% AND SODIUM CHLORIDE 0.2% IN PLASTIC CONTAINER
MCGAW — 5 GM/100 ML;110 MG/100 ML;200 MG/100 ML — N19630 009 — FEB 17, 1988

POTASSIUM CHLORIDE 0.11% IN DEXTROSE 5% AND SODIUM CHLORIDE 0.33% IN PLASTIC CONTAINER
MCGAW — 5 GM/100 ML;110 MG/100 ML;330 MG/100 ML — N19630 015 — FEB 17, 1988

POTASSIUM CHLORIDE 0.11% IN DEXTROSE 5% AND SODIUM CHLORIDE 0.45% IN PLASTIC CONTAINER
MCGAW — 5 GM/100 ML;110 MG/100 ML;450 MG/100 ML — N19630 021 — FEB 17, 1988

POTASSIUM CHLORIDE 0.11% IN DEXTROSE 5% AND SODIUM CHLORIDE 0.9% IN PLASTIC CONTAINER
MCGAW — 5 GM/100 ML;110 MG/100 ML;900 MG/100 ML — N19630 027 — FEB 17, 1988

Prescription Drug Products *(continued)*

DEXTROSE; POTASSIUM CHLORIDE; SODIUM CHLORIDE
(continued)
INJECTABLE; INJECTION
POTASSIUM CHLORIDE 0.15% IN DEXTROSE 10% AND SODIUM CHLORIDE 0.2% IN PLASTIC CONTAINER
MCGAW 10 GM/100 ML;150 MG/100 ML;200 MG/100 ML N19630 034 FEB 17, 1988

POTASSIUM CHLORIDE 0.15% IN DEXTROSE 10% AND SODIUM CHLORIDE 0.45% IN PLASTIC CONTAINER
MCGAW 10 GM/100 ML;150 MG/100 ML;450 MG/100 ML N19630 040 FEB 17, 1988

POTASSIUM CHLORIDE 0.15% IN DEXTROSE 10% AND SODIUM CHLORIDE 0.9% IN PLASTIC CONTAINER
MCGAW 10 GM/100 ML;150 MG/100 ML;900 MG/100 ML N19630 046 FEB 17, 1988

POTASSIUM CHLORIDE 0.15% IN DEXTROSE 3.3% AND SODIUM CHLORIDE 0.3% IN PLASTIC CONTAINER
MCGAW 3.3 GM/100 ML;150 MG/100 ML;300 MG/100 ML N19630 051 MAY 07, 1992

POTASSIUM CHLORIDE 0.15% IN DEXTROSE 5% AND SODIUM CHLORIDE 0.2% IN PLASTIC CONTAINER
AP MCGAW 5 GM/100 ML;150 MG/100 ML;200 MG/100 ML N19630 010 FEB 17, 1988

POTASSIUM CHLORIDE 0.15% IN DEXTROSE 5% AND SODIUM CHLORIDE 0.33% IN PLASTIC CONTAINER
AP MCGAW 5 GM/100 ML;150 MG/100 ML;330 MG/100 ML N19630 016 FEB 17, 1988

POTASSIUM CHLORIDE 0.15% IN DEXTROSE 5% AND SODIUM CHLORIDE 0.45% IN PLASTIC CONTAINER
AP MCGAW 5 GM/100 ML;150 MG/100 ML;450 MG/100 ML N19630 022 FEB 17, 1988

POTASSIUM CHLORIDE 0.15% IN DEXTROSE 5% AND SODIUM CHLORIDE 0.9% IN PLASTIC CONTAINER
AP MCGAW 5 GM/100 ML;150 MG/100 ML;900 MG/100 ML N19630 028 FEB 17, 1988

POTASSIUM CHLORIDE 0.15% IN DEXTROSE 5% AND SODIUM CHLORIDE 0.11% IN PLASTIC CONTAINER
MCGAW 5 GM/100 ML;150 MG/100 ML;110 MG/100 ML N19630 004 FEB 17, 1988

DEXTROSE; POTASSIUM CHLORIDE; SODIUM CHLORIDE
(continued)
INJECTABLE; INJECTION
POTASSIUM CHLORIDE 0.22% IN DEXTROSE 10% AND SODIUM CHLORIDE 0.2% IN PLASTIC CONTAINER
MCGAW 10 GM/100 ML;220 MG/100 ML;200 MG/100 ML N19630 035 FEB 17, 1988

POTASSIUM CHLORIDE 0.22% IN DEXTROSE 10% AND SODIUM CHLORIDE 0.45% IN PLASTIC CONTAINER
MCGAW 10 GM/100 ML;220 MG/100 ML;450 MG/100 ML N19630 041 FEB 17, 1988

POTASSIUM CHLORIDE 0.22% IN DEXTROSE 10% AND SODIUM CHLORIDE 0.9% IN PLASTIC CONTAINER
MCGAW 10 GM/100 ML;220 MG/100 ML;900 MG/100 ML N19630 047 FEB 17, 1988

POTASSIUM CHLORIDE 0.22% IN DEXTROSE 3.3% AND SODIUM CHLORIDE 0.3% IN PLASTIC CONTAINER
MCGAW 3.3 GM/100 ML;220 MG/100 ML;300 MG/100 ML N19630 052 MAY 07, 1992

POTASSIUM CHLORIDE 0.22% IN DEXTROSE 5% AND SODIUM CHLORIDE 0.2% IN PLASTIC CONTAINER
MCGAW 5 GM/100 ML;220 MG/100 ML;200 MG/100 ML N19630 011 FEB 17, 1988

POTASSIUM CHLORIDE 0.22% IN DEXTROSE 5% AND SODIUM CHLORIDE 0.33% IN PLASTIC CONTAINER
MCGAW 5 GM/100 ML;220 MG/100 ML;330 MG/100 ML N19630 017 FEB 17, 1988

POTASSIUM CHLORIDE 0.22% IN DEXTROSE 5% AND SODIUM CHLORIDE 0.45% IN PLASTIC CONTAINER
MCGAW 5 GM/100 ML;220 MG/100 ML;450 MG/100 ML N19630 023 FEB 17, 1988

POTASSIUM CHLORIDE 0.22% IN DEXTROSE 5% AND SODIUM CHLORIDE 0.11% IN PLASTIC CONTAINER
MCGAW 5 GM/100 ML;220 MG/100 ML;110 MG/100 ML N19630 005 FEB 17, 1988

POTASSIUM CHLORIDE 0.22% IN DEXTROSE 5% AND SODIUM CHLORIDE 0.9% IN PLASTIC CONTAINER
MCGAW 5 GM/100 ML;220 MG/100 ML;900 MG/100 ML N19630 029 FEB 17, 1988

POTASSIUM CHLORIDE 0.3% IN DEXTROSE 10% AND SODIUM CHLORIDE 0.2% IN PLASTIC CONTAINER
MCGAW 10 GM/100 ML;300 MG/100 ML;200 MG/100 ML N19630 036 FEB 17, 1988

Prescription Drug Products *(continued)*

DEXTROSE; POTASSIUM CHLORIDE; SODIUM CHLORIDE
(continued)

INJECTABLE; INJECTION

POTASSIUM CHLORIDE 0.3% IN DEXTROSE 10% AND SODIUM CHLORIDE 0.45% IN PLASTIC CONTAINER

	MCGAW	10 GM/100 ML;300 MG/ 100 ML;450 MG/100 ML	N19630 042 FEB 17, 1988

POTASSIUM CHLORIDE 0.3% IN DEXTROSE 10% AND SODIUM CHLORIDE 0.9% IN PLASTIC CONTAINER

	MCGAW	10 GM/100 ML;300 MG/ 100 ML;900 MG/100 ML	N19630 048 FEB 17, 1988

POTASSIUM CHLORIDE 0.3% IN DEXTROSE 3.3% AND SODIUM CHLORIDE 0.3% IN PLASTIC CONTAINER

	MCGAW	3.3 GM/100 ML;300 MG/ 100 ML;300 MG/100 ML	N19630 053 MAY 07, 1992

POTASSIUM CHLORIDE 0.3% IN DEXTROSE 5% AND SODIUM CHLORIDE 0.2% IN PLASTIC CONTAINER

AP	MCGAW	5 GM/100 ML;300 MG/ 100 ML;200 MG/100 ML	N19630 012 FEB 17, 1988

POTASSIUM CHLORIDE 0.3% IN DEXTROSE 5% AND SODIUM CHLORIDE 0.33% IN PLASTIC CONTAINER

AP	MCGAW	5 GM/100 ML;300 MG/ 100 ML;330 MG/100 ML	N19630 018 FEB 17, 1988

POTASSIUM CHLORIDE 0.3% IN DEXTROSE 5% AND SODIUM CHLORIDE 0.45% IN PLASTIC CONTAINER

AP	MCGAW	5 GM/100 ML;300 MG/ 100 ML;450 MG/100 ML	N19630 024 FEB 17, 1988

POTASSIUM CHLORIDE 0.3% IN DEXTROSE 5% AND SODIUM CHLORIDE 0.9% IN PLASTIC CONTAINER

AP	MCGAW	5 GM/100 ML;300 MG/ 100 ML;900 MG/100 ML	N19630 030 FEB 17, 1988

POTASSIUM CHLORIDE 0.3% IN DEXTROSE 5% AND SODIUM CHLORIDE 0.11% IN PLASTIC CONTAINER

	MCGAW	5 GM/100 ML;300 MG/ 100 ML;110 MG/100 ML	N19630 006 FEB 17, 1988

POTASSIUM CHLORIDE 10 MEQ IN DEXTROSE 5% AND SODIUM CHLORIDE 0.225% IN PLASTIC CONTAINER

	ABBOTT	5 GM/100 ML;74.5 MG/ 100 ML;225 MG/100 ML	N18365 002 JUL 05, 1983
		5 GM/100 ML;149 MG/ 100 ML;225 MG/100 ML	N18365 006 MAR 28, 1988

DEXTROSE; POTASSIUM CHLORIDE; SODIUM CHLORIDE
(continued)

INJECTABLE; INJECTION

POTASSIUM CHLORIDE 10 MEQ IN DEXTROSE 5% AND SODIUM CHLORIDE 0.3% IN PLASTIC CONTAINER

	ABBOTT	5 GM/100 ML;74.5 MG/ 100 ML;300 MG/100 ML	N18876 001 JAN 17, 1986
		5 GM/100 ML;149 MG/ 100 ML;300 MG/100 ML	N18876 006 MAR 28, 1988

POTASSIUM CHLORIDE 10 MEQ IN DEXTROSE 5% AND SODIUM CHLORIDE 0.45% IN PLASTIC CONTAINER

AP	ABBOTT	5 GM/100 ML;74.5 MG/ 100 ML;450 MG/100 ML	N18362 005 MAR 28, 1988
AP		5 GM/100 ML;74.5 MG/ 100 ML;450 MG/100 ML	N18362 009 JUL 05, 1983

POTASSIUM CHLORIDE 10 MEQ IN DEXTROSE 5% AND SODIUM CHLORIDE 0.9% IN PLASTIC CONTAINER

AP	ABBOTT	5 GM/100 ML;74.5 MG/ 100 ML;900 MG/100 ML	N19691 002 MAR 24, 1988
AP		5 GM/100 ML;149 MG/ 100 ML;900 MG/100 ML	N19691 004 MAR 24, 1988

POTASSIUM CHLORIDE 10 MEQ IN DEXTROSE 5% AND SODIUM CHLORIDE 0.45% IN PLASTIC CONTAINER

AP	BAXTER	5 GM/100 ML;75 MG/ 100 ML;450 MG/100 ML	N18008 005 APR 28, 1982
AP		5 GM/100 ML;150 MG/ 100 ML;450 MG/100 ML	N18008 006 APR 28, 1982

POTASSIUM CHLORIDE 10 MEQ IN DEXTROSE 5% AND SODIUM CHLORIDE 0.9% IN PLASTIC CONTAINER

AP	BAXTER	5 GM/100 ML;75 MG/ 100 ML;900 MG/100 ML	N19308 004 APR 05, 1985
AP		5 GM/100 ML;150 MG/ 100 ML;900 MG/100 ML	N19308 002 APR 05, 1985

POTASSIUM CHLORIDE 15 MEQ IN DEXTROSE 5% AND SODIUM CHLORIDE 0.255% IN PLASTIC CONTAINER

	ABBOTT	5 GM/100 ML;224 MG/ 100 ML;225 MG/100 ML	N18365 008 MAR 28, 1988

POTASSIUM CHLORIDE 15 MEQ IN DEXTROSE 5% AND SODIUM CHLORIDE 0.3% IN PLASTIC CONTAINER

	ABBOTT	5 GM/100 ML;224 MG/ 100 ML;300 MG/100 ML	N18876 007 MAR 28, 1988

Prescription Drug Products *(continued)*

DEXTROSE; POTASSIUM CHLORIDE; SODIUM CHLORIDE
(continued)

INJECTABLE; INJECTION

POTASSIUM CHLORIDE 15 MEQ IN DEXTROSE 5% AND SODIUM CHLORIDE 0.45% IN PLASTIC CONTAINER

AP ABBOTT 5 GM/100 ML;224 MG/100 ML;450 MG/100 ML N18362 006 MAR 28, 1988

POTASSIUM CHLORIDE 15 MEQ IN DEXTROSE 5% AND SODIUM CHLORIDE 0.9% IN PLASTIC CONTAINER

AP ABBOTT 5 GM/100 ML;224 MG/100 ML;900 MG/100 ML N19691 006 MAR 24, 1988

POTASSIUM CHLORIDE 20 MEQ IN DEXTROSE 5% AND SODIUM CHLORIDE 0.225% IN PLASTIC CONTAINER

ABBOTT 5 GM/100 ML;149 MG/100 ML;225 MG/100 ML N18365 001

5 GM/100 ML;298 MG/100 ML;225 MG/100 ML N18365 009 MAR 28, 1988

POTASSIUM CHLORIDE 20 MEQ IN DEXTROSE 5% AND SODIUM CHLORIDE 0.3% IN PLASTIC CONTAINER

ABBOTT 5 GM/100 ML;298 MG/100 ML;300 MG/100 ML N18876 008 MAR 28, 1988

POTASSIUM CHLORIDE 20 MEQ IN DEXTROSE 5% AND SODIUM CHLORIDE 0.45% IN PLASTIC CONTAINER

AP ABBOTT 5 GM/100 ML;149 MG/100 ML;450 MG/100 ML N18362 010 JUL 05, 1983

AP 5 GM/100 ML;298 MG/100 ML;450 MG/100 ML N18362 007 MAR 28, 1988

POTASSIUM CHLORIDE 20 MEQ IN DEXTROSE 5% AND SODIUM CHLORIDE 0.9% IN PLASTIC CONTAINER

AP ABBOTT 5 GM/100 ML;149 MG/100 ML;900 MG/100 ML N19691 005 MAR 24, 1988

AP 5 GM/100 ML;298 MG/100 ML;900 MG/100 ML N19691 008 MAR 24, 1988

POTASSIUM CHLORIDE 20 MEQ IN DEXTROSE 5% AND SODIUM CHLORIDE 0.45% IN PLASTIC CONTAINER

AP BAXTER 5 GM/100 ML;150 MG/100 ML;450 MG/100 ML N18008 007 APR 28, 1982

DEXTROSE; POTASSIUM CHLORIDE; SODIUM CHLORIDE
(continued)

INJECTABLE; INJECTION

POTASSIUM CHLORIDE 20 MEQ IN DEXTROSE 5% AND SODIUM CHLORIDE 0.9% IN PLASTIC CONTAINER

AP BAXTER 5 GM/100 ML;150 MG/100 ML;900 MG/100 ML N19308 005 APR 05, 1985

AP 5 GM/100 ML;300 MG/100 ML;900 MG/100 ML N19308 003 APR 05, 1985

POTASSIUM CHLORIDE 20 MEQ IN DEXTROSE 5% IN SODIUM CHLORIDE 0.3% IN PLASTIC CONTAINER

ABBOTT 5 GM/100 ML;149 MG/100 ML;300 MG/100 ML N18876 002 JAN 17, 1986

POTASSIUM CHLORIDE 30 MEQ IN DEXTROSE 5% AND SODIUM CHLORIDE 0.225% IN PLASTIC CONTAINER

ABBOTT 5 GM/100 ML;224 MG/100 ML;225 MG/100 ML N18365 003 JUL 05, 1983

POTASSIUM CHLORIDE 30 MEQ IN DEXTROSE 5% AND SODIUM CHLORIDE 0.3% IN PLASTIC CONTAINER

ABBOTT INER5 GM/100 ML;224 MG/100 ML;300 MG/100 ML N18876 003 JAN 17, 1986

POTASSIUM CHLORIDE 30 MEQ IN DEXTROSE 5% AND SODIUM CHLORIDE 0.45% IN PLASTIC CONTAINER

AP ABBOTT 5 GM/100 ML;224 MG/100 ML;450 MG/100 ML N18362 002

POTASSIUM CHLORIDE 30 MEQ IN DEXTROSE 5% AND SODIUM CHLORIDE 0.9% IN PLASTIC CONTAINER

AP ABBOTT 5 GM/100 ML;224 MG/100 ML;900 MG/100 ML N19691 007 MAR 24, 1988

POTASSIUM CHLORIDE 30 MEQ IN DEXTROSE 5% AND SODIUM CHLORIDE 0.45% IN PLASTIC CONTAINER

AP BAXTER 5 GM/100 ML;224 MG/100 ML;450 MG/100 ML N18008 008 APR 28, 1982

POTASSIUM CHLORIDE 30 MEQ IN DEXTROSE 5% AND SODIUM CHLORIDE 0.9% IN PLASTIC CONTAINER

AP BAXTER 5 GM/100 ML;224 MG/100 ML;900 MG/100 ML N19308 006 APR 05, 1985

POTASSIUM CHLORIDE 40 MEQ IN DEXTROSE 5% AND SODIUM CHLORIDE 0.225% IN PLASTIC CONTAINER

ABBOTT 5 GM/100 ML;298 MG/100 ML;225 MG/100 ML N18365 004 JUL 05, 1983

Prescription Drug Products *(continued)*

DEXTROSE; POTASSIUM CHLORIDE; SODIUM CHLORIDE
(continued)

INJECTABLE; INJECTION

POTASSIUM CHLORIDE 40 MEQ IN DEXTROSE 5% AND SODIUM CHLORIDE 0.3% IN PLASTIC CONTAINER
- ABBOTT 5 GM/100 ML;298 MG/100 ML;300 MG/100 ML N18876 004 MAR 28, 1988

POTASSIUM CHLORIDE 40 MEQ IN DEXTROSE 5% AND SODIUM CHLORIDE 0.45% IN PLASTIC CONTAINER
- AP ABBOTT 5 GM/100 ML;298 MG/100 ML;450 MG/100 ML N18362 003

POTASSIUM CHLORIDE 40 MEQ IN DEXTROSE 5% AND SODIUM CHLORIDE 0.9% IN PLASTIC CONTAINER
- AP ABBOTT 5 GM/100 ML;298 MG/100 ML;900 MG/100 ML N19691 009 MAR 24, 1988

POTASSIUM CHLORIDE 40 MEQ IN DEXTROSE 5% AND SODIUM CHLORIDE 0.45% IN PLASTIC CONTAINER
- AP BAXTER 5 GM/100 ML;300 MG/100 ML;450 MG/100 ML N18008 009 APR 28, 1982

POTASSIUM CHLORIDE 40 MEQ IN DEXTROSE 5% AND SODIUM CHLORIDE 0.9% IN PLASTIC CONTAINER
- AP BAXTER 5 GM/100 ML;300 MG/100 ML;900 MG/100 ML N19308 007 APR 05, 1985

POTASSIUM CHLORIDE 5 MEQ IN DEXTROSE 5% AND SODIUM CHLORIDE 0.225% IN PLASTIC CONTAINER
- ABBOTT 5 GM/100 ML;74.5 MG/100 ML;225 MG/100 ML N18365 005 MAR 28, 1988
- 5 GM/100 ML;149 MG/100 ML;225 MG/100 ML N18365 007 MAR 28, 1988

POTASSIUM CHLORIDE 5 MEQ IN DEXTROSE 5% AND SODIUM CHLORIDE 0.3% IN PLASTIC CONTAINER
- ABBOTT 5 GM/100 ML;74.5 MG/100 ML;300 MG/100 ML N18876 005 MAR 28, 1988
- 5 GM/100 ML;149 MG/100 ML;300 MG/100 ML N18876 009 MAR 28, 1988

POTASSIUM CHLORIDE 5 MEQ IN DEXTROSE 5% AND SODIUM CHLORIDE 0.45% IN PLASTIC CONTAINER
- AP ABBOTT 5 GM/100 ML;74.5 MG/100 ML;450 MG/100 ML N18362 008 MAR 28, 1988
- AP 5 GM/100 ML;149 MG/100 ML;450 MG/100 ML N18362 004 MAR 28, 1988

DEXTROSE; POTASSIUM CHLORIDE; SODIUM CHLORIDE
(continued)

INJECTABLE; INJECTION

POTASSIUM CHLORIDE 5 MEQ IN DEXTROSE 5% AND SODIUM CHLORIDE 0.9% IN PLASTIC CONTAINER
- AP ABBOTT 5 GM/100 ML;74.5 MG/100 ML;900 MG/100 ML N19691 001 MAR 24, 1988
- AP 5 GM/100 ML;149 MG/100 ML;900 MG/100 ML N19691 003 MAR 24, 1988

POTASSIUM CHLORIDE 5 MEQ IN DEXTROSE 5% AND SODIUM CHLORIDE 0.45% IN PLASTIC CONTAINER
- AP BAXTER 5 GM/100 ML;150 MG/100 ML;450 MG/100 ML N18008 004

POTASSIUM CHLORIDE 5 MEQ IN DEXTROSE 5% AND SODIUM CHLORIDE 0.9% IN PLASTIC CONTAINER
- AP BAXTER 5 GM/100 ML;150 MG/100 ML;900 MG/100 ML N19308 001 APR 05, 1985

DEXTROSE; SODIUM CHLORIDE

INJECTABLE; INJECTION

DEXTROSE 10% AND SODIUM CHLORIDE 0.11% IN PLASTIC CONTAINER
- MCGAW 10 GM/100 ML;110 MG/100 ML N19631 011 FEB 24, 1988

DEXTROSE 10% AND SODIUM CHLORIDE 0.2% IN PLASTIC CONTAINER
- MCGAW 10 GM/100 ML;200 MG/100 ML N18386 001
- 10 GM/100 ML;200 MG/100 ML N19631 012 FEB 24, 1988

DEXTROSE 10% AND SODIUM CHLORIDE 0.33% IN PLASTIC CONTAINER
- MCGAW 10 GM/100 ML;330 MG/100 ML N19631 013 FEB 24, 1988

DEXTROSE 10% AND SODIUM CHLORIDE 0.45% IN PLASTIC CONTAINER
- MCGAW 10 GM/100 ML;450 MG/100 ML N18229 001
- 10 GM/100 ML;450 MG/100 ML N19631 014 FEB 24, 1988

DEXTROSE 10% AND SODIUM CHLORIDE 0.9% IN PLASTIC CONTAINER
- AP BAXTER 10 GM/100 ML;900 MG/100 ML N16696 001
- AP MCGAW 10 GM/100 ML;900 MG/100 ML N18047 001
- AP 10 GM/100 ML;900 MG/100 ML N19631 015 FEB 24, 1988

Prescription Drug Products *(continued)*

DEXTROSE; SODIUM CHLORIDE *(continued)*

INJECTABLE; INJECTION

DEXTROSE 2.5% AND SODIUM CHLORIDE 0.11% IN PLASTIC CONTAINER

	MCGAW	2.5 GM/100 ML;110 MG/ 100 ML	N19631 001 FEB 24, 1988

DEXTROSE 2.5% AND SODIUM CHLORIDE 0.2% IN PLASTIC CONTAINER

	MCGAW	2.5 GM/100 ML;200 MG/ 100 ML	N19631 002 FEB 24, 1988

DEXTROSE 2.5% AND SODIUM CHLORIDE 0.33% IN PLASTIC CONTAINER

	MCGAW	2.5 GM/100 ML;330 MG/ 100 ML	N19631 003 FEB 24, 1988

<u>DEXTROSE 2.5% AND SODIUM CHLORIDE 0.45% IN PLASTIC CONTAINER</u>

AP	ABBOTT	2.5 GM/100 ML;450 MG/ 100 ML	N18096 001
AP	BAXTER	2.5 GM/100 ML;450 MG/ 100 ML	N16697 001
AP	MCGAW	2.5 GM/100 ML;450 MG/ 100 ML	N18030 001
AP		2.5 GM/100 ML;450 MG/ 100 ML	N19631 004 FEB 24, 1988

DEXTROSE 2.5% AND SODIUM CHLORIDE 0.9% IN PLASTIC CONTAINER

	MCGAW	2.5 GM/100 ML;900 MG/ 100 ML	N18376 001
		2.5 GM/100 ML;900 MG/ 100 ML	N19631 005 FEB 24, 1988

DEXTROSE 3.3% AND SODIUM CHLORIDE 0.3% IN PLASTIC CONTAINER

	MCGAW	3.3 GM/100 ML;300 MG/ 100 ML	N19631 016 JAN 19, 1990

DEXTROSE 5% AND SODIUM CHLORIDE 0.11% IN PLASTIC CONTAINER

	MCGAW	5 GM/100 ML;110 MG/ 100 ML	N18030 005
		5 GM/100 ML;110 MG/ 100 ML	N19631 006 FEB 24, 1988

<u>DEXTROSE 5% AND SODIUM CHLORIDE 0.2% IN PLASTIC CONTAINER</u>

AP	MCGAW	5 GM/100 ML;200 MG/ 100 ML	N18030 004
AP		5 GM/100 ML;200 MG/ 100 ML	N19631 007 FEB 24, 1988

DEXTROSE 5% AND SODIUM CHLORIDE 0.225% IN PLASTIC CONTAINER

	ABBOTT	5 GM/100 ML;225 MG/ 100 ML	N17606 001

DEXTROSE 5% AND SODIUM CHLORIDE 0.3% IN PLASTIC CONTAINER

	ABBOTT	5 GM/100 ML;300 MG/ 100 ML	N17799 001

DEXTROSE; SODIUM CHLORIDE *(continued)*

INJECTABLE; INJECTION

<u>DEXTROSE 5% AND SODIUM CHLORIDE 0.33% IN PLASTIC CONTAINER</u>

AP	MCGAW	5 GM/100 ML;330 MG/ 100 ML	N18030 003
AP		5 GM/100 ML;330 MG/ 100 ML	N19631 008 FEB 24, 1988

<u>DEXTROSE 5% AND SODIUM CHLORIDE 0.45% IN PLASTIC CONTAINER</u>

AP	ABBOTT	5 GM/100 ML;450 MG/ 100 ML	N17607 001
AP	MCGAW	5 GM/100 ML;450 MG/ 100 ML	N18030 002
AP		5 GM/100 ML;450 MG/ 100 ML	N19631 009 FEB 24, 1988

<u>DEXTROSE 5% AND SODIUM CHLORIDE 0.9% IN PLASTIC CONTAINER</u>

AP	ABBOTT	5 GM/100 ML;900 MG/ 100 ML	N17585 001
AP	MCGAW	5 GM/100 ML;900 MG/ 100 ML	N18026 001
AP		5 GM/100 ML;900 MG/ 100 ML	N19631 010 FEB 24, 1988

<u>DEXTROSE 5% IN SODIUM CHLORIDE 0.2% IN PLASTIC CONTAINER</u>

AP	BAXTER	5 GM/100 ML;200 MG/ 100 ML	N16689 001

<u>DEXTROSE 5% IN SODIUM CHLORIDE 0.33% IN PLASTIC CONTAINER</u>

AP	BAXTER	5 GM/100 ML;330 MG/ 100 ML	N16687 001

<u>DEXTROSE 5% IN SODIUM CHLORIDE 0.45% IN PLASTIC CONTAINER</u>

AP	BAXTER	5 GM/100 ML;450 MG/ 100 ML	N16683 001

<u>DEXTROSE 5% IN SODIUM CHLORIDE 0.9% IN PLASTIC CONTAINER</u>

AP	BAXTER	5 GM/100 ML;900 MG/ 100 ML	N16678 001

DEXTROTHYROXINE SODIUM

TABLET; ORAL

CHOLOXIN

	BOOTS	1 MG	N12302 005
		2 MG	N12302 002
+		4 MG	N12302 004

Prescription Drug Products *(continued)*

	DEZOCINE		
	INJECTABLE; INJECTION		
	DALGAN		
	+ ASTRA	5 MG/ML	N19082 001 DEC 29, 1989
	+	10 MG/ML	N19082 002 DEC 29, 1989
	+	15 MG/ML	N19082 003 DEC 29, 1989
	DIATRIZOATE MEGLUMINE		
	INJECTABLE; INJECTION		
	ANGIOVIST 282		
AP	BERLEX	60%	N87726 001 SEP 23, 1982
	DIATRIZOATE MEGLUMINE		
	BRACCO	76%	N10040 017
	HYPAQUE		
AP	STERLING WINTHROP	30%	N16403 002
AP		60%	N16403 001
	RENO-M-DIP		
AP	BRACCO	30%	N10040 012
	RENO-M-60		
AP	BRACCO	60%	N10040 016
	UROVIST MEGLUMINE DIU/CT		
AP	BERLEX	30%	N87739 001 SEP 23, 1982
	SOLUTION; URETERAL		
	RENO-M-30		
AT	BRACCO	30%	N10040 021
	UROVIST CYSTO		
AT	BERLEX	30%	N87729 001 SEP 23, 1982
	UROVIST CYSTO PEDIATRIC		
AT	BERLEX	30%	N87731 001 SEP 23, 1982
	SOLUTION; URETHRAL		
	CYSTOGRAFIN		
AT	BRACCO	30%	N10040 018
	CYSTOGRAFIN DILUTE		
	BRACCO	18%	N10040 022 NOV 09, 1982
	HYPAQUE-CYSTO		
AT	STERLING WINTHROP	30%	N16403 003

	DIATRIZOATE MEGLUMINE; DIATRIZOATE SODIUM		
	INJECTABLE; INJECTION		
	ANGIOVIST 292		
AP	BERLEX	52%;8%	N87724 001 SEP 23, 1982
	ANGIOVIST 370		
AP	BERLEX	66%;10%	N87723 001 SEP 23, 1982
	HYPAQUE-76		
AP	STERLING WINTHROP	66%;10%	N86505 001
	MD-60		
AP	MALLINCKRODT	52%;8%	N87074 001
	MD-76		
AP	MALLINCKRODT	66%;10%	N19292 001 SEP 29, 1989
AP		66%;10%	N87073 001
	RENOCAL-76		
AP	BRACCO	66%;10%	N89347 001 JUN 01, 1988
	RENOGRAFIN-60		
AP	BRACCO	52%;8%	N10040 006
	RENOGRAFIN-76		
AP	BRACCO	66%;10%	N10040 001
	RENOVIST		
	BRACCO	34.3%;35%	N10040 020
	RENOVIST II		
	BRACCO	28.5%;29.1%	N10040 019
	SOLUTION; ORAL, RECTAL		
	GASTROGRAFIN		
AA	BRACCO	66%;10%	N11245 003
	GASTROVIST		
AA	BERLEX	66%;10%	N87728 001 SEP 23, 1982
	MD-GASTROVIEW		
AA	MALLINCKRODT	66%;10%	N87388 001
	DIATRIZOATE MEGLUMINE; IODIPAMIDE MEGLUMINE		
	SOLUTION; INTRAUTERINE		
	SINOGRAFIN		
	BRACCO	52.7%;26.8%	N11324 002
	DIATRIZOATE SODIUM		
	INJECTABLE; INJECTION		
	HYPAQUE		
AP	STERLING WINTHROP	50%	N09561 001
		25%	N09561 003
	UROVIST SODIUM 300		
AP	BERLEX	50%	N87725 001 SEP 23, 1982

Prescription Drug Products *(continued)*

DIATRIZOATE SODIUM *(continued)*

POWDER FOR RECONSTITUTION; ORAL, RECTAL

HYPAQUE

TE Code	Applicant	Strength	Appl. No. / Date
	STERLING WINTHROP	100%	N11386 001

SOLUTION; ORAL, RECTAL

HYPAQUE

TE Code	Applicant	Strength	Appl. No. / Date
	STERLING WINTHROP	40%	N11386 003

DIATRIZOATE SODIUM; *MULTIPLE*

SEE DIATRIZOATE MEGLUMINE; DIATRIZOATE SODIUM

DIAZEPAM

CAPSULE, EXTENDED RELEASE; ORAL

VALRELEASE

TE Code	Applicant	Strength	Appl. No. / Date
	+ ROCHE	15 MG	N18179 001

CONCENTRATE; ORAL

DIAZEPAM INTENSOL

TE Code	Applicant	Strength	Appl. No. / Date
	ROXANE	5 MG/ML	N71415 001 APR 03, 1987

INJECTABLE; INJECTION

DIAZEPAM

TE Code	Applicant	Strength	Appl. No. / Date
AP	ABBOTT	5 MG/ML	N71583 001 OCT 13, 1987
AP		5 MG/ML	N71584 001 OCT 13, 1987
AP	ELKINS SINN	5 MG/ML	N70311 001 DEC 16, 1985
AP		5 MG/ML	N70312 001 DEC 16, 1985
AP		5 MG/ML	N70313 001 DEC 16, 1985
AP	FUJISAWA	5 MG/ML	N70662 001 JUN 25, 1986
AP	LEDERLE	5 MG/ML	N71309 001 JUL 17, 1987
AP		5 MG/ML	N71310 001 JUL 17, 1987
AP	MARSAM	5 MG/ML	N72370 001 JAN 29, 1993
AP		5 MG/ML	N72371 001 JAN 29, 1993
AP		5 MG/ML	N72397 001 JAN 29, 1993

DIAZEPAM *(continued)*

INJECTABLE; INJECTION

DIAZEPAM

TE Code	Applicant	Strength	Appl. No. / Date
AP	STERIS	5 MG/ML	N70296 001 FEB 12, 1986
AP		5 MG/ML	N70911 001 AUG 28, 1986
AP		5 MG/ML	N70912 001 AUG 28, 1986
AP		5 MG/ML	N70930 001 DEC 01, 1986
AP	STERLING WINTHROP	5 MG/ML	N72079 001 DEC 20, 1988

VALIUM

TE Code	Applicant	Strength	Appl. No. / Date
AP	+ ROCHE	5 MG/ML	N16087 001

INJECTABLE; INTRAVENOUS

DIZAC

TE Code	Applicant	Strength	Appl. No. / Date
	+ PHARMACIA	5 MG/ML	N19287 001 JUN 18, 1993

SOLUTION; ORAL

DIAZEPAM

TE Code	Applicant	Strength	Appl. No. / Date
	ROXANE	5 MG/5 ML	N70928 001 APR 03, 1987

TABLET; ORAL

DIAZEPAM

TE Code	Applicant	Strength	Appl. No. / Date
AB	BARR	2 MG	N70152 001 NOV 01, 1985
AB		5 MG	N70153 001 NOV 01, 1985
AB		10 MG	N70154 001 NOV 01, 1985
AB	DANBURY PHARMA	2 MG	N71134 001 FEB 03, 1987
AB		5 MG	N71135 001 FEB 03, 1987
AB		10 MG	N71136 001 FEB 03, 1987
AB	GENEVA PHARMS	2 MG	N70302 001 DEC 20, 1985
AB		5 MG	N70303 001 DEC 20, 1985
AB		10 MG	N70304 001 DEC 20, 1985
AB	HALSEY	2 MG	N70987 001 AUG 15, 1986
AB		5 MG	N70996 001 AUG 15, 1986
AB		10 MG	N70956 001 AUG 15, 1986

Prescription Drug Products *(continued)*

DIAZEPAM *(continued)*

TABLET; ORAL

DIAZEPAM

AB	LEDERLE	2 MG	N70226 001 SEP 26, 1985
AB		5 MG	N70227 001 SEP 26, 1985
AB		10 MG	N70228 001 SEP 26, 1985
AB	MYLAN	2 MG	N70323 001 SEP 04, 1985
AB		5 MG	N70324 001 SEP 04, 1985
AB		10 MG	N70325 001 SEP 04, 1985
AB	PAR PHARM	2 MG	N70462 001 FEB 25, 1986
AB		5 MG	N70463 001 FEB 25, 1986
AB		10 MG	N70464 001 FEB 25, 1986
AB	PUREPAC PHARM	2 MG	N70781 001 MAR 19, 1986
AB		5 MG	N70706 001 MAR 19, 1986
AB		10 MG	N70707 001 MAR 19, 1986
AB	ROXANE	2 MG	N70356 001 JUN 17, 1986
AB		5 MG	N70357 001 JUN 17, 1986
AB		10 MG	N70358 001 JUN 17, 1986
AB	ZENITH LABS	2 MG	N71307 001 DEC 10, 1986
AB		5 MG	N71321 001 DEC 10, 1986
AB		10 MG	N70362 001 SEP 04, 1985
AB		10 MG	N71322 001 DEC 10, 1986

VALIUM

AB	ROCHE	2 MG	N13263 002
AB		5 MG	N13263 004
AB	+	10 MG	N13263 006

DIAZOXIDE

CAPSULE; ORAL

PROGLYCEM

	+ BAKER NORTON	50 MG	N17425 001

INJECTABLE; INJECTION

HYPERSTAT

	+ SCHERING	15 MG/ML	N16996 001

SUSPENSION; ORAL

PROGLYCEM

	+ BAKER NORTON	50 MG/ML	N17453 001

DICHLORPHENAMIDE

TABLET; ORAL

DARANIDE

	+ MERCK SHARP DOHME	50 MG	N11366 001

DICLOFENAC POTASSIUM

TABLET; ORAL

CATAFLAM

	GEIGY	25 MG	N20142 001 NOV 24, 1993
	+	50 MG	N20142 002 NOV 24, 1993

DICLOFENAC SODIUM

SOLUTION/DROPS; OPHTHALMIC

VOLTAREN

	CIBA VISION	0.1%	N20037 001 MAR 28, 1991

TABLET, DELAYED RELEASE; ORAL

VOLTAREN

	+ GEIGY	25 MG	N19201 001 JUL 28, 1988
	+	50 MG	N19201 002 JUL 28, 1988
	+	75 MG	N19201 003 JUL 28, 1988

DICLOXACILLIN SODIUM

CAPSULE; ORAL

DICLOXACILLIN SODIUM

AB	BIOCRAFT	EQ 250 MG BASE	N62286 001 JUN 03, 1982
AB		EQ 500 MG BASE	N62286 002 JUN 03, 1982

Prescription Drug Products *(continued)*

DICLOXACILLIN SODIUM *(continued)*

CAPSULE; ORAL

	DYCILL		
AB	SMITHKLINE BEECHAM	EQ 250 MG BASE	N62238 001
AB		EQ 500 MG BASE	N62238 002
	DYNAPEN		
AB	APOTHECON	EQ 250 MG BASE	N61454 001
AB		EQ 500 MG BASE	N61454 003
		EQ 125 MG BASE	N61454 002
	PATHOCIL		
AB	+ WYETH AYERST	EQ 250 MG BASE	N50011 002
AB	+	EQ 500 MG BASE	N50011 003 MAR 28, 1983

POWDER FOR RECONSTITUTION; ORAL

	DYNAPEN		
AB	APOTHECON	EQ 62.5 MG BASE/5 ML	N61455 001
	PATHOCIL		
AB	+ WYETH AYERST	EQ 62.5 MG BASE/5 ML	N50092 001

DICUMAROL

TABLET; ORAL

	DICUMAROL		
	+ ABBOTT	25 MG	N05545 003

DICYCLOMINE HYDROCHLORIDE

CAPSULE; ORAL

	BENTYL		
AB	+ MERRELL DOW	10 MG	N07409 003 OCT 15, 1984
	DICYCLOMINE HCL		
AB	BARR	10 MG	N84505 001 OCT 21, 1986
AB	CHELSEA LABS	10 MG	N85082 001 JUN 19, 1986

INJECTABLE; INJECTION

	BENTYL		
AP	+ MERRELL DOW	10 MG/ML	N08370 001 OCT 15, 1984
	DICYCLOMINE HCL		
AP	STERIS	10 MG/ML	N80614 001 FEB 11, 1986

SYRUP; ORAL

	BENTYL		
AA	MERRELL DOW	10 MG/5 ML	N07961 002 OCT 15, 1984
	DICYCLOMINE HCL		
AA	BARRE	10 MG/5 ML	N84479 001

DICYCLOMINE HYDROCHLORIDE *(continued)*

TABLET; ORAL

	BENTYL		
AB	+ MERRELL DOW	20 MG	N07409 001 OCT 15, 1984
	DICYCLOMINE HCL		
AB	BARR	20 MG	N84600 001 JUL 29, 1985
AB	CHELSEA LABS	20 MG	N85223 001 JUL 30, 1986

DIDANOSINE

POWDER FOR RECONSTITUTION; ORAL

	VIDEX		
	BRISTOL MYERS SQUIBB	10 MG/ML	N20156 001 OCT 09, 1991
		100 MG/PACKET	N20155 003 OCT 09, 1991
		167 MG/PACKET	N20155 004 OCT 09, 1991
		250 MG/PACKET	N20155 005 OCT 09, 1991
	+	375 MG/PACKET	N20155 006 OCT 09, 1991

TABLET, CHEWABLE; ORAL

	VIDEX		
	BRISTOL MYERS SQUIBB	25 MG	N20154 002 OCT 09, 1991
		50 MG	N20154 003 OCT 09, 1991
		100 MG	N20154 004 OCT 09, 1991
	+	150 MG	N20154 005 OCT 09, 1991

DIENESTROL

CREAM; VAGINAL

	DIENESTROL		
AT	JOHNSON RW	0.01%	N06110 005
	DV		
AT	MERRELL DOW	0.01%	N83518 001

SUPPOSITORY; VAGINAL

	DV		
	MERRELL DOW	0.7 MG	N83517 001

Prescription Drug Products *(continued)*

DIETHYLCARBAMAZINE CITRATE
TABLET; ORAL
HETRAZAN
LEDERLE 50 MG N06459 001

DIETHYLPROPION HYDROCHLORIDE
TABLET; ORAL
DIETHYLPROPION HCL
AA CAMALL 25 MG N88267 001 AUG 25, 1983
AA 25 MG N88268 001 AUG 25, 1983
AA MD PHARM 25 MG N85544 001
TENUATE
AA MERRELL DOW 25 MG N11722 002
TEPANIL
AA 3M 25 MG N11673 001
TABLET, EXTENDED RELEASE; ORAL
TENUATE DOSPAN
BC + MERRELL DOW 75 MG N12546 001
TEPANIL TEN-TAB
BC 3M 75 MG N17956 001

DIETHYLSTILBESTROL
TABLET; ORAL
DIETHYLSTILBESTROL
LILLY 1 MG N04041 004
+ 5 MG N04041 005
STILBESTROL
TABLICAPS 0.5 MG N83004 001
TABLET, DELAYED RELEASE; ORAL
DIETHYLSTILBESTROL
+ LILLY 1 MG N04039 004
+ 5 MG N04039 006

DIETHYLSTILBESTROL; METHYLTESTOSTERONE
TABLET; ORAL
TYLOSTERONE
+ LILLY 0.25 MG;5 MG N07661 001

DIETHYLSTILBESTROL DIPHOSPHATE
INJECTABLE; INJECTION
STILPHOSTROL
+ MILES 250 MG/5 ML N10010 001
TABLET; ORAL
STILPHOSTROL
+ MILES 50 MG N10010 002

DIFENOXIN HYDROCHLORIDE; *MULTIPLE*
SEE ATROPINE SULFATE; DIFENOXIN HYDROCHLORIDE

DIFLORASONE DIACETATE
CREAM; TOPICAL
FLORONE
BX + UPJOHN 0.05% N17741 001
PSORCON
BX DERMIK 0.05% N20205 001 NOV 20, 1992
OINTMENT; TOPICAL
FLORONE
+ UPJOHN 0.05% N17994 001
PSORCON
+ UPJOHN 0.05% N19260 001 AUG 28, 1985

DIFLUNISAL
TABLET; ORAL
DIFLUNISAL
AB LEMMON 250 MG N73679 001 JUL 31, 1992
AB 500 MG N73673 001 JUL 31, 1992
AB ROXANE 250 MG N73562 001 NOV 27, 1992
AB 500 MG N73563 001 NOV 27, 1992
DOLOBID
AB MERCK SHARP DOHME 250 MG N18445 001 APR 19, 1982
AB + 500 MG N18445 002 APR 19, 1982

DIGOXIN
CAPSULE; ORAL
LANOXICAPS
BURROUGHS
WELLCOME 0.05 MG N18118 002 JUL 26, 1982
0.1 MG N18118 003 JUL 26, 1982
+ 0.2 MG N18118 001 JUL 26, 1982

Prescription Drug Products *(continued)*

DIGOXIN *(continued)*
INJECTABLE; INJECTION

	DIGOXIN		
AP	ELKINS SINN	0.25 MG/ML	N83391 001
AP	WYETH AYERST	0.25 MG/ML	N84386 001
	LANOXIN		
AP	+ BURROUGHS WELLCOME	0.25 MG/ML	N09330 002
	+	0.1 MG/ML	N09330 004

DIHYDROCODEINE BITARTRATE; *MULTIPLE*
SEE ACETAMINOPHEN; CAFFEINE; DIHYDROCODEINE BITARTRATE
SEE ASPIRIN; CAFFEINE; DIHYDROCODEINE BITARTRATE

DIHYDROERGOTAMINE MESYLATE
INJECTABLE; INJECTION

	D.H.E. 45		
	+ SANDOZ	1 MG/ML	N05929 001

DILTIAZEM HYDROCHLORIDE
CAPSULE, EXTENDED RELEASE; ORAL

	CARDIZEM CD		
BC	+ CARDERM	120 MG	N20062 001 AUG 10, 1992
BC	+	180 MG	N20062 002 DEC 27, 1991
BC	+	240 MG	N20062 003 DEC 27, 1991
	+	300 MG	N20062 004 DEC 27, 1991
	CARDIZEM SR		
AB	+ MARION MERRELL DOW	60 MG	N19471 001 JAN 23, 1989
AB	+	90 MG	N19471 002 JAN 23, 1989
AB	+	120 MG	N19471 003 JAN 23, 1989
	DILACOR XR		
BC	RHONE POULENC RORER	120 MG	N20092 001 MAY 29, 1992
BC		180 MG	N20092 002 MAY 29, 1992
BC		240 MG	N20092 003 MAY 29, 1992

DILTIAZEM HYDROCHLORIDE *(continued)*
CAPSULE, EXTENDED RELEASE; ORAL

	DILTIAZEM HCL		
AB	PROGRAPHARM	60 MG	N74079 001 NOV 30, 1993
AB		90 MG	N74079 002 NOV 30, 1993
AB		120 MG	N74079 003 NOV 30, 1993

INJECTABLE; INJECTION

	CARDIZEM		
	+ MARION MERRELL DOW	5 MG/ML	N20027 001 OCT 24, 1991

TABLET; ORAL

	CARDIZEM		
AB	MARION MERRELL DOW	30 MG	N18602 001 NOV 05, 1982
AB		60 MG	N18602 002 NOV 05, 1982
AB		90 MG	N18602 003 DEC 08, 1986
AB	+	120 MG	N18602 004 DEC 08, 1986
	DILTIAZEM HCL		
AB	APOTHECON	30 MG	N74051 001 MAR 31, 1993
AB		60 MG	N74051 002 MAR 31, 1993
AB		90 MG	N74051 003 MAR 31, 1993
AB		120 MG	N74051 004 MAR 31, 1993
AB	COPLEY PHARM	30 MG	N74067 001 NOV 05, 1992
AB		60 MG	N74067 002 NOV 05, 1992
AB		90 MG	N74067 003 NOV 05, 1992
AB		120 MG	N74067 004 NOV 05, 1992
AB	LEDERLE	30 MG	N74093 001 NOV 05, 1992
AB		60 MG	N74093 002 NOV 05, 1992
AB		90 MG	N74093 003 NOV 05, 1992
AB		120 MG	N74093 004 NOV 05, 1992

Prescription Drug Products *(continued)*

DILTIAZEM HYDROCHLORIDE *(continued)*

TABLET; ORAL
DILTIAZEM HCL

AB	MYLAN	30 MG	N73185 001 NOV 05, 1992
AB		60 MG	N73186 001 NOV 05, 1992
AB		90 MG	N72837 001 MAR 30, 1992
AB		120 MG	N72838 001 MAR 30, 1992
AB	NOVOPHARM	30 MG	N74084 001 FEB 25, 1994
AB		60 MG	N74084 002 FEB 25, 1994

DIMENHYDRINATE

INJECTABLE; INJECTION
DIMENHYDRINATE

AP	ELKINS SINN	50 MG/ML	N84767 001
AP	STERIS	50 MG/ML	N80615 001
AP		50 MG/ML	N83531 001
AP	WYETH AYERST	50 MG/ML	N84316 001

DIMERCAPROL

INJECTABLE; INJECTION
BAL

	+ BECTON DICKINSON	10%	N05939 001

DIMETHYL SULFOXIDE

SOLUTION; INTRAVESICAL
RIMSO-50

	RES INDS	50%	N17788 001

DINOPROSTONE

GEL; ENDOCERVICAL
PREPIDIL

	+ UPJOHN	0.5 MG/3 GM	N19617 001 DEC 09, 1992

SUPPOSITORY; VAGINAL
PROSTIN E2

	+ UPJOHN	20 MG	N17810 001

DIPHENHYDRAMINE HYDROCHLORIDE

CAPSULE; ORAL
BENADRYL

AA	PARKE DAVIS	25 MG	N05845 007
AA		50 MG	N05845 001

DIPHENHYDRAMINE HCL

AA	BARR	25 MG	N84506 001
AA		50 MG	N80738 001
AA	CHELSEA LABS	50 MG	N85083 001
AA	DANBURY PHARMA	25 MG	N80728 001
AA		50 MG	N80727 001
AA	EON LABS	25 MG	N80845 002
AA		50 MG	N80845 001
AA	GENEVA PHARMS	25 MG	N80832 001
AA		50 MG	N80832 002
AA	GLOBAL PHARMS	25 MG	N80807 001
AA		50 MG	N80807 002
AA	HALSEY	50 MG	N87914 001 JUN 04, 1984
AA	ICN	25 MG	N80596 001
AA		50 MG	N80592 001
AA	LNK	25 MG	N87977 001 JAN 27, 1983
AA		50 MG	N87978 001 JAN 27, 1983
AA	MK LABS	25 MG	N83087 001
AA		50 MG	N83087 002
AA	MUTUAL PHARM	25 MG	N89488 001 JAN 02, 1987
AA		50 MG	N89489 001 JAN 02, 1987
AA	NEWTRON PHARMS	25 MG	N86543 001
AA		50 MG	N86544 001
AA	PRIVATE FORM	25 MG	N83027 001
AA		50 MG	N83027 002
AA	PUREPAC PHARM	25 MG	N85156 001
AA		50 MG	N85150 001
AA	SUPERPHARM	25 MG	N89040 001 MAY 15, 1985
AA	WEST WARD PHARM	50 MG	N83567 001
AA	ZENITH LABS	25 MG	N80762 001
AA		50 MG	N80762 002

ELIXIR; ORAL
BELIX

AA	HALSEY	12.5 MG/5 ML	N86586 001 OCT 03, 1983

BENADRYL

AA	PARKE DAVIS	12.5 MG/5 ML	N05845 004

DIBENIL

AA	CENCI	12.5 MG/5 ML	N88304 001 DEC 16, 1983

Prescription Drug Products *(continued)*

DIPHENHYDRAMINE HYDROCHLORIDE *(continued)*

ELIXIR; ORAL

	DIPHENHYDRAMINE HCL		
AA	BUNDY	12.5 MG/5 ML	N83674 001
AA	CENCI	12.5 MG/5 ML	N87941 001 DEC 17, 1982
AA	LANNETT	12.5 MG/5 ML	N80939 002
AA	MK LABS	12.5 MG/5 ML	N83088 002
AA	PHARM ASSOC	12.5 MG/5 ML	N87513 001 FEB 10, 1982
AA	PUREPAC PHARM	12.5 MG/5 ML	N83237 001 JAN 25, 1982
AA	ROXANE	12.5 MG/5 ML	N80643 001
	HYDRAMINE		
AA	BARRE	12.5 MG/5 ML	N80763 002

INJECTABLE; INJECTION

	BENADRYL		
AP	+ PARKE DAVIS	10 MG/ML	N06146 001
AP	+	50 MG/ML	N06146 002
AP	+	50 MG/ML	N09486 001
	DIPHENHYDRAMINE HCL		
AP	ELKINS SINN	50 MG/ML	N80817 002
AP	FUJISAWA	50 MG/ML	N80586 002
AP	INTL MEDICATION	50 MG/ML	N84094 001
AP	STERIS	10 MG/ML	N80873 001
AP		10 MG/ML	N83533 001
AP		50 MG/ML	N80873 002
AP	WYETH AYERST	50 MG/ML	N80577 001

DIPHENIDOL HYDROCHLORIDE

TABLET; ORAL

	VONTROL		
	+ SMITHKLINE BEECHAM	EQ 25 MG BASE	N16033 001

DIPHENOXYLATE HYDROCHLORIDE; *MULTIPLE*

SEE ATROPINE SULFATE; DIPHENOXYLATE HYDROCHLORIDE

DIPIVEFRIN HYDROCHLORIDE

SOLUTION/DROPS; OPHTHALMIC

	DIPIVEFRIN HCL		
AT	ALCON	0.1%	N73636 001 JUN 30, 1994
	PROPINE		
AT	+ ALLERGAN	0.1%	N18239 001

DIPYRIDAMOLE

INJECTABLE; INJECTION

	IV PERSANTINE		
	+ BOEHRINGER INGELHEIM	5 MG/ML	N19817 001 DEC 13, 1990

TABLET; ORAL

	DIPYRIDAMOLE		
AB	BARR	25 MG	N87184 001 OCT 03, 1990
AB		50 MG	N87716 001 OCT 03, 1990
AB		75 MG	N87717 001 OCT 03, 1990
AB	GENEVA PHARMS	25 MG	N86944 002 APR 16, 1991
AB		50 MG	N87562 001 FEB 25, 1992
AB		75 MG	N87561 001 FEB 25, 1992
AB	LEDERLE	25 MG	N88999 001 FEB 05, 1991
AB		50 MG	N89000 001 FEB 05, 1991
AB		75 MG	N89001 001 FEB 05, 1991
AB	PUREPAC PHARM	25 MG	N89425 001 JUL 12, 1990
AB		50 MG	N89426 001 JUL 12, 1990
AB		75 MG	N89427 001 JUL 12, 1990
	PERSANTINE		
AB	BOEHRINGER INGELHEIM	25 MG	N12836 003 DEC 22, 1986
AB	+	50 MG	N12836 004 FEB 06, 1987
AB		75 MG	N12836 005 FEB 06, 1987

DISOPYRAMIDE PHOSPHATE

CAPSULE; ORAL

	DISOPYRAMIDE PHOSPHATE		
AB	BARR	EQ 100 MG BASE	N70351 001 DEC 17, 1985
AB		EQ 150 MG BASE	N70352 001 DEC 17, 1985

Prescription Drug Products *(continued)*

DISOPYRAMIDE PHOSPHATE *(continued)*

CAPSULE; ORAL

	DISOPYRAMIDE PHOSPHATE		
AB	BIOCRAFT	EQ 100 MG BASE	N70101 001 FEB 22, 1985
AB		EQ 150 MG BASE	N70102 001 FEB 22, 1985
AB	DANBURY PHARMA	EQ 100 MG BASE	N70173 001 MAY 31, 1985
AB		EQ 150 MG BASE	N70174 001 MAY 31, 1985
AB	GENEVA PHARMS	EQ 100 MG BASE	N70470 001 DEC 10, 1985
AB		EQ 150 MG BASE	N70471 001 DEC 10, 1985
AB	SUPERPHARM	EQ 100 MG BASE	N70940 001 FEB 09, 1987
AB	ZENITH LABS	EQ 100 MG BASE	N70186 001 NOV 18, 1985
AB		EQ 150 MG BASE	N70187 001 NOV 18, 1985
	NORPACE		
AB	SEARLE	EQ 100 MG BASE	N17447 001
AB	+	EQ 150 MG BASE	N17447 002

CAPSULE, EXTENDED RELEASE; ORAL

	DISOPYRAMIDE PHOSPHATE		
AB	KV PHARM	EQ 150 MG BASE	N71200 001 DEC 15, 1987
B*		EQ 100 MG BASE	N71929 001 AUG 19, 1988
	NORPACE CR		
AB	SEARLE	EQ 100 MG BASE	N18655 001 JUL 20, 1982
AB	+	EQ 150 MG BASE	N18655 002 JUL 20, 1982

DISULFIRAM

TABLET; ORAL

	ANTABUSE		
BX	WYETH AYERST	250 MG	N07883 003
BX	+	500 MG	N07883 002
	DISULFIRAM		
BX	DANBURY PHARMA	250 MG	N86889 001
BX		500 MG	N86890 001
BX	PAR PHARM	250 MG	N88792 001 AUG 14, 1984
BX		500 MG	N88793 001 AUG 14, 1984
BX	SIDMAK LABS NJ	250 MG	N88482 001 DEC 08, 1983
BX		500 MG	N88483 001 DEC 08, 1983

DIVALPROEX SODIUM

CAPSULE, DELAYED REL PELLETS; ORAL

	DEPAKOTE		
	+ ABBOTT	EQ 125 MG BASE	N19680 001 SEP 12, 1989

TABLET, DELAYED RELEASE; ORAL

	DEPAKOTE		
	ABBOTT	EQ 125 MG BASE	N18723 003 OCT 26, 1984
		EQ 250 MG BASE	N18723 001 MAR 10, 1983
	+	EQ 500 MG BASE	N18723 002 MAR 10, 1983

DOBUTAMINE HYDROCHLORIDE

INJECTABLE; INJECTION

	DOBUTAMINE HCL		
AP	ABBOTT	EQ 12.5 MG BASE/ML	N74086 001 NOV 29, 1993
AP	GENSIA	EQ 12.5 MG BASE/ML	N74206 001 OCT 19, 1993
AP	STERIS	EQ 12.5 MG BASE/ML	N74114 001 NOV 30, 1993
	DOBUTAMINE HCL IN DEXTROSE 5%		
AP	+ ABBOTT	EQ 50 MG BASE/100 ML	N20269 001 OCT 19, 1993
AP	+	EQ 100 MG BASE/100 ML	N20269 002 OCT 19, 1993
AP	+	EQ 200 MG BASE/100 ML	N20269 003 OCT 19, 1993
	DOBUTAMINE HCL IN DEXTROSE 5% IN PLASTIC CONTAINER		
AP	ABBOTT	EQ 50 MG BASE/100 ML	N20201 003 OCT 19, 1993
AP		EQ 100 MG BASE/100 ML	N20201 002 OCT 19, 1993
AP		EQ 200 MG BASE/100 ML	N20201 001 OCT 19, 1993
AP		EQ 400 MG BASE/100 ML	N20201 006 JUL 07, 1994
AP	+ BAXTER	EQ 50 MG BASE/100 ML	N20255 001 OCT 19, 1993
AP	+	EQ 100 MG BASE/100 ML	N20255 003 OCT 19, 1993
AP	+	EQ 200 MG BASE/100 ML	N20255 004 OCT 19, 1993
AP	+	EQ 400 MG BASE/100 ML	N20255 005 OCT 19, 1993
	DOBUTREX		
AP	+ LILLY	EQ 12.5 MG BASE/ML	N17820 002

Prescription Drug Products *(continued)*

DOPAMINE HYDROCHLORIDE

INJECTABLE; INJECTION

	DOPAMINE		
AP	ELKINS SINN	40 MG/ML	N18398 001
AP		80 MG/ML	N18398 002 MAR 22, 1982
	DOPAMINE HCL		
AP	ABBOTT	80 MG/100 ML	N18132 002 FEB 04, 1982
AP		160 MG/100 ML	N18132 003 FEB 04, 1982
AP		40 MG/ML	N18132 001
AP		40 MG/ML	N70656 001 JAN 24, 1989
AP		80 MG/ML	N18132 004 JUL 09, 1982
AP		80 MG/ML	N70657 001 JAN 24, 1989
AP	ASTRA	40 MG/ML	N18656 001 JUN 28, 1983
AP		80 MG/ML	N70091 001 OCT 23, 1985
AP		160 MG/ML	N70092 001 OCT 23, 1985
AP	FUJISAWA	80 MG/ML	N70013 001 JUN 12, 1985
AP	GENSIA	40 MG/ML	N72999 001 OCT 23, 1991
AP		80 MG/ML	N73000 001 OCT 23, 1991
AP	INTL MEDICATION	40 MG/ML	N18014 001
AP	LUITPOLD	40 MG/ML	N70799 001 FEB 11, 1987
AP		80 MG/ML	N70820 001 FEB 11, 1987
AP		160 MG/ML	N70826 001 FEB 11, 1987
AP	SMITH AND NEPHEW	40 MG/ML	N70046 001 AUG 29, 1985
AP		80 MG/ML	N70047 001 AUG 29, 1985
	DOPAMINE HCL AND DEXTROSE 5%		
AP	MCGAW	80 MG/100 ML	N19099 002 OCT 15, 1986
AP		320 MG/100 ML	N19099 004 OCT 15, 1986
	DOPAMINE HCL AND DEXTROSE 5% IN PLASTIC CONTAINER		
AP	MCGAW	160 MG/100 ML	N19099 003 OCT 15, 1986
	+	40 MG/100 ML	N19099 001 OCT 15, 1986

DOPAMINE HYDROCHLORIDE *(continued)*

INJECTABLE; INJECTION

	DOPAMINE HCL IN DEXTROSE 5% IN PLASTIC CONTAINER		
AP	+ ABBOTT	80 MG/100 ML	N18826 001 SEP 30, 1983
AP	+	160 MG/100 ML	N18826 002 SEP 30, 1983
AP	+	320 MG/100 ML	N18826 003 SEP 30, 1983
AP	BAXTER	80 MG/100 ML	N19615 001 MAR 27, 1987
AP		160 MG/100 ML	N19615 002 MAR 27, 1987
AP		320 MG/100 ML	N19615 003 MAR 27, 1987
		640 MG/100 ML	N19615 004 MAR 27, 1987
	INTROPIN		
AP	+ DUPONT MERCK	40 MG/ML	N17395 001
AP	+	80 MG/ML	N17395 002
AP	+	160 MG/ML	N17395 003

DOXACURIUM CHLORIDE

INJECTABLE; INJECTION

	NUROMAX		
	+ BURROUGHS WELLCOME	EQ 1 MG BASE/ML	N19946 001 MAR 07, 1991

DOXAPRAM HYDROCHLORIDE

INJECTABLE; INJECTION

	DOPRAM		
AP	+ ROBINS AH	20 MG/ML	N14879 001
	DOXAPRAM HCL		
AP	STERIS	20 MG/ML	N73529 001 JAN 30, 1992

DOXAZOSIN MESYLATE

TABLET; ORAL

	CARDURA		
	PFIZER	EQ 1 MG BASE	N19668 001 NOV 02, 1990
		EQ 2 MG BASE	N19668 002 NOV 02, 1990
		EQ 4 MG BASE	N19668 003 NOV 02, 1990
		EQ 8 MG BASE	N19668 004 NOV 02, 1990

Prescription Drug Products *(continued)*

DOXEPIN HYDROCHLORIDE

CAPSULE; ORAL

DOXEPIN HCL

AB	DANBURY PHARMA	EQ 10 MG BASE	N71485 001 APR 30, 1987
AB		EQ 25 MG BASE	N71486 001 APR 30, 1987
AB		EQ 50 MG BASE	N71238 001 APR 30, 1987
AB		EQ 75 MG BASE	N71326 001 APR 30, 1987
AB		EQ 100 MG BASE	N71239 001 APR 30, 1987
AB	GENEVA PHARMS	EQ 10 MG BASE	N71487 001 MAR 02, 1987
AB		EQ 25 MG BASE	N70827 001 MAY 15, 1986
AB		EQ 50 MG BASE	N70828 001 MAY 15, 1986
AB		EQ 75 MG BASE	N70825 001 MAY 15, 1986
AB		EQ 100 MG BASE	N71562 001 MAR 02, 1987
AB	LEDERLE	EQ 10 MG BASE	N71685 001 JAN 05, 1988
AB		EQ 25 MG BASE	N71686 001 JAN 05, 1988
AB		EQ 50 MG BASE	N71673 001 JAN 05, 1988
AB		EQ 75 MG BASE	N71674 001 JAN 05, 1988
AB		EQ 100 MG BASE	N71675 001 JAN 05, 1988
AB		EQ 150 MG BASE	N71676 001 JAN 05, 1988
AB	MYLAN	EQ 10 MG BASE	N70789 001 MAY 13, 1986
AB		EQ 25 MG BASE	N70790 001 MAY 13, 1986
AB		EQ 50 MG BASE	N70791 001 MAY 13, 1986
AB		EQ 75 MG BASE	N70792 001 MAY 13, 1986
AB		EQ 100 MG BASE	N70793 001 MAY 13, 1986

DOXEPIN HYDROCHLORIDE *(continued)*

CAPSULE; ORAL

DOXEPIN HCL

AB	PAR PHARM	EQ 10 MG BASE	N71697 001 NOV 09, 1987
AB		EQ 25 MG BASE	N71437 001 NOV 09, 1987
AB		EQ 50 MG BASE	N71595 001 NOV 09, 1987
AB		EQ 75 MG BASE	N71608 001 NOV 09, 1987
AB		EQ 100 MG BASE	N71422 001 NOV 09, 1987
AB		EQ 150 MG BASE	N71669 001 NOV 09, 1987
AB	PUREPAC PHARM	EQ 10 MG BASE	N73054 001 DEC 28, 1990
AB		EQ 25 MG BASE	N72109 001 DEC 28, 1990
AB		EQ 50 MG BASE	N73055 001 DEC 28, 1990
AB		EQ 100 MG BASE	N72110 001 SEP 08, 1988
AB	ROYCE LABS	EQ 10 MG BASE	N72985 001 MAR 29, 1991
AB		EQ 25 MG BASE	N72986 001 MAR 29, 1991
AB		EQ 50 MG BASE	N72987 001 MAR 29, 1991
	SINEQUAN		
AB	PFIZER	EQ 10 MG BASE	N16798 003
AB	+	EQ 25 MG BASE	N16798 001
AB		EQ 50 MG BASE	N16798 002
AB		EQ 75 MG BASE	N16798 006
AB	+	EQ 100 MG BASE	N16798 005
AB		EQ 150 MG BASE	N16798 007

CONCENTRATE; ORAL

DOXEPIN HCL

AA	COPLEY PHARM	EQ 10 MG BASE/ML	N71609 001 NOV 09, 1987
AA	PENNEX	EQ 10 MG BASE/ML	N71918 001 JUL 20, 1988
	SINEQUAN		
AA	PFIZER	EQ 10 MG BASE/ML	N17516 001

CREAM; TOPICAL

ZONALON

	+ GENDERM	5%	N20126 001 APR 01, 1994

Prescription Drug Products *(continued)*

DOXORUBICIN HYDROCHLORIDE

INJECTABLE; INJECTION

	ADRIAMYCIN PFS		
	+ PHARMACIA	200 MG/100 ML	N50629 002 MAY 03, 1988
		200 MG/100 ML	N63165 002 JAN 30, 1991
AP	+	2 MG/ML	N50629 001 DEC 23, 1987
AP		2 MG/ML	N63165 001 JAN 30, 1991
	ADRIAMYCIN RDF		
AP	+ PHARMACIA	10 MG/VIAL	N50467 001
AP	+	20 MG/VIAL	N50467 003 MAY 20, 1985
AP	+	50 MG/VIAL	N50467 002
	+	150 MG/VIAL	N50467 004 JUL 22, 1987
	DOXORUBICIN HCL		
AP	CETUS BEN VENUE	2 MG/ML	N62975 001 MAR 17, 1989
AP		10 MG/VIAL	N62921 001 MAR 17, 1989
AP		20 MG/VIAL	N62921 002 MAR 17, 1989
AP		50 MG/VIAL	N62921 003 MAR 17, 1989
AP	PHARMACHEMIE (NL)	10 MG/VIAL	N63097 001 MAY 21, 1990
AP		20 MG/VIAL	N63097 002 MAY 21, 1990
AP		50 MG/VIAL	N63097 003 MAY 21, 1990
	RUBEX		
AP	BRISTOL MYERS	10 MG/VIAL	N62926 001 APR 13, 1989
AP		50 MG/VIAL	N62926 002 APR 13, 1989
		100 MG/VIAL	N62926 003 APR 13, 1989

DOXYCYCLINE

CAPSULE; ORAL

	DOXYCYCLINE MONOHYDRATE		
	+ VINTAGE PHARMS	EQ 100 MG BASE	N50641 001 DEC 29, 1989

POWDER FOR RECONSTITUTION; ORAL

	DOXYCHEL		
AB	RACHELLE	EQ 25 MG BASE/5 ML	N61720 001
	VIBRAMYCIN		
AB	+ PFIZER	EQ 25 MG BASE/5 ML	N50006 001

DOXYCYCLINE CALCIUM

SUSPENSION; ORAL

	VIBRAMYCIN		
	+ PFIZER	EQ 50 MG BASE/5 ML	N50480 001

DOXYCYCLINE HYCLATE

CAPSULE; ORAL

	DOXY-LEMMON		
AB	LEMMON	EQ 50 MG BASE	N62497 001 AUG 23, 1984
AB		EQ 100 MG BASE	N62497 002 JUN 15, 1984
	DOXYCHEL HYCLATE		
AB	RACHELLE	EQ 50 MG BASE	N61717 001
AB		EQ 100 MG BASE	N61717 002
	DOXYCYCLINE HYCLATE		
AB	BARR	EQ 50 MG BASE	N62418 001 JAN 28, 1983
AB		EQ 100 MG BASE	N62418 002 JAN 28, 1983
AB	CHELSEA LABS	EQ 50 MG BASE	N62142 001
AB		EQ 100 MG BASE	N62142 002
AB	DANBURY PHARMA	EQ 50 MG BASE	N62031 002 OCT 13, 1982
AB		EQ 100 MG BASE	N62031 001
AB	HALSEY	EQ 50 MG BASE	N62119 002 MAY 24, 1985
AB		EQ 100 MG BASE	N62119 001 MAY 24, 1985
AB	MUTUAL PHARM	EQ 50 MG BASE	N62675 001 JUL 10, 1986
AB		EQ 100 MG BASE	N62676 001 JUL 10, 1986
AB	MYLAN	EQ 50 MG BASE	N62337 001 MAR 29, 1982
AB		EQ 100 MG BASE	N62337 002 MAR 29, 1982
AB	PRIVATE FORM	EQ 50 MG BASE	N62631 001 JUL 24, 1986
AB		EQ 100 MG BASE	N62631 002 JUL 24, 1986
AB	PUREPAC PHARM	EQ 50 MG BASE	N62479 001 DEC 23, 1983
AB		EQ 100 MG BASE	N62479 002 DEC 23, 1983
AB	WEST WARD PHARM	EQ 50 MG BASE	N62396 002 NOV 07, 1984
AB		EQ 100 MG BASE	N62396 001 MAY 07, 1984

Prescription Drug Products *(continued)*

DOXYCYCLINE HYCLATE *(continued)*

CAPSULE; ORAL

DOXYCYCLINE HYCLATE
- AB ZENITH LABS — EQ 50 MG BASE — N62500 001 SEP 11, 1984
- AB — EQ 100 MG BASE — N62500 002 SEP 11, 1984

VIBRAMYCIN
- AB PFIZER — EQ 50 MG BASE — N50007 001
- AB + — EQ 100 MG BASE — N50007 002

CAPSULE, COATED PELLETS; ORAL

DORYX
- AB + FAULDING — EQ 100 MG BASE — N50582 001 JUL 22, 1985
- AB PARKE DAVIS — EQ 100 MG BASE — N62653 001 OCT 30, 1985

DOXYCYCLINE HYCLATE
- AB SIDMAK LABS NJ — EQ 100 MG BASE — N63187 001 JUN 30, 1992

INJECTABLE; INJECTION

DOXY 100
- AP FUJISAWA — EQ 100 MG BASE/VIAL — N62475 001 DEC 09, 1983

DOXY 200
- AP FUJISAWA — EQ 200 MG BASE/VIAL — N62475 002 DEC 09, 1983

DOXYCHEL HYCLATE
- AP RACHELLE — EQ 100 MG BASE/VIAL — N61953 001

DOXYCYCLINE
- AP BEN VENUE — EQ 100 MG BASE/VIAL — N62569 001 MAR 09, 1988
- AP — EQ 200 MG BASE/VIAL — N62569 002 MAR 09, 1988
- AP ELKINS SINN — EQ 100 MG BASE/VIAL — N62450 001 OCT 27, 1983
- AP — EQ 200 MG BASE/VIAL — N62450 002 OCT 27, 1983

DOXYCYCLINE HYCLATE
- AP LEDERLE — EQ 100 MG BASE/VIAL — N62992 001 FEB 16, 1989
- AP — EQ 200 MG BASE/VIAL — N62992 002 FEB 16, 1989

VIBRAMYCIN
- AP + PFIZER — EQ 100 MG BASE/VIAL — N50442 002
- AP + — EQ 200 MG BASE/VIAL — N50442 001

DOXYCYCLINE HYCLATE *(continued)*

TABLET; ORAL

DOXY-LEMMON
- AB LEMMON — EQ 100 MG BASE — N62581 001 MAR 15, 1985

DOXY-TABS
- AB RACHELLE — EQ 100 MG BASE — N62269 001
- AB — EQ 100 MG BASE — N62269 002 NOV 08, 1982

DOXYCYCLINE HYCLATE
- AB BARR — EQ 100 MG BASE — N62391 001 SEP 30, 1982
- AB DANBURY PHARMA — EQ 100 MG BASE — N62421 001 FEB 02, 1983
- AB MUTUAL PHARM — EQ 100 MG BASE — N62677 001 JUL 10, 1986
- AB MYLAN — EQ 100 MG BASE — N62432 001 FEB 15, 1983
- AB SUPERPHARM — EQ 100 MG BASE — N62494 001 FEB 20, 1985
- AB VINTAGE PHARMS — EQ 100 MG BASE — N62538 001 APR 07, 1986
- AB ZENITH LABS — EQ 100 MG BASE — N62505 001 SEP 11, 1984

VIBRA-TABS
- AB + PFIZER — EQ 100 MG BASE — N50533 001

DRONABINOL

CAPSULE; ORAL

MARINOL
- UNIMED INC — 2.5 MG — N18651 001 MAY 31, 1985
- 5 MG — N18651 002 MAY 31, 1985
- \+ — 10 MG — N18651 003 MAY 31, 1985

DROPERIDOL

INJECTABLE; INJECTION

DROPERIDOL
- AP ABBOTT — 2.5 MG/ML — N71981 001 FEB 29, 1988
- AP ASTRA — 2.5 MG/ML — N72018 001 OCT 20, 1988
- AP — 2.5 MG/ML — N72019 001 OCT 19, 1988
- AP — 2.5 MG/ML — N72021 001 OCT 19, 1988
- AP DUPONT MERCK — 2.5 MG/ML — N71645 001 APR 07, 1988

Prescription Drug Products *(continued)*

DROPERIDOL *(continued)*
INJECTABLE; INJECTION
DROPERIDOL
AP LUITPOLD 2.5 MG/ML N72123 001 OCT 24, 1988
AP 2.5 MG/ML N72335 001 OCT 24, 1988
AP SOLOPAK 2.5 MG/ML N71754 001 SEP 06, 1988
AP 2.5 MG/ML N71755 001 SEP 06, 1988
AP STERIS 2.5 MG/ML N73520 001 NOV 27, 1991
AP 2.5 MG/ML N73521 001 NOV 27, 1991
AP 2.5 MG/ML N73523 001 NOV 27, 1991
INAPSINE
AP + JANSSEN 2.5 MG/ML N16796 001

DROPERIDOL; FENTANYL CITRATE
INJECTABLE; INJECTION
FENTANYL CITRATE AND DROPERIDOL
AP ABBOTT 2.5 MG/ML;EQ 0.05 MG BASE/ML N71982 001 MAY 04, 1988
AP ASTRA 2.5 MG/ML;EQ 0.05 MG BASE/ML N72026 001 APR 13, 1989
AP 2.5 MG/ML;EQ 0.05 MG BASE/ML N72027 001 APR 13, 1989
INNOVAR
AP + JANSSEN 2.5 MG/ML;EQ 0.05 MG BASE/ML N16049 001

DYCLONINE HYDROCHLORIDE
SOLUTION; TOPICAL
DYCLONE
ASTRA 0.5% N09925 002
1% N09925 001

DYPHYLLINE
INJECTABLE; INJECTION
NEOTHYLLINE
+ LEMMON 250 MG/ML N09088 001
TABLET; ORAL
DILOR
BP SAVAGE LABS 200 MG N84514 001
DILOR-400
BP SAVAGE LABS 400 MG N84751 001
LUFYLLIN
BP WALLACE 200 MG N84566 001
BP 400 MG N84566 002
NEOTHYLLINE
BP LEMMON 200 MG N07794 001
BP + 400 MG N07794 002

ECHOTHIOPHATE IODIDE
POWDER FOR RECONSTITUTION; OPHTHALMIC
PHOSPHOLINE IODIDE
WYETH AYERST 0.03% N11963 002
0.06% N11963 004
0.125% N11963 001
0.25% N11963 003

ECONAZOLE NITRATE
CREAM; TOPICAL
SPECTAZOLE
+ JOHNSON RW 1% N18751 001 DEC 23, 1982

EDETATE CALCIUM DISODIUM
INJECTABLE; INJECTION
CALCIUM DISODIUM VERSENATE
+ 3M 200 MG/ML N08922 001

EDETATE DISODIUM
INJECTABLE; INJECTION
EDETATE DISODIUM
AP STERIS 150 MG/ML N80391 001
ENDRATE
AP + ABBOTT 150 MG/ML N11355 001
SODIUM VERSENATE
+ 3M 200 MG/ML N10573 001

Prescription Drug Products *(continued)*

EDROPHONIUM CHLORIDE
INJECTABLE; INJECTION
ENLON
AP OHMEDA 10 MG/ML N88873 001 AUG 06, 1985
REVERSOL
AP ORGANON 10 MG/ML N89624 001 MAY 13, 1988
TENSILON
AP + ROCHE 10 MG/ML N07959 001

EDROPHONIUM CHLORIDE; *MULTIPLE*
SEE ATROPINE SULFATE; EDROPHONIUM CHLORIDE

ENALAPRIL MALEATE
TABLET; ORAL
VASOTEC
MERCK 2.5 MG N18998 005 JUL 26, 1988
5 MG N18998 001 DEC 24, 1985
10 MG N18998 002 DEC 24, 1985
+ 20 MG N18998 003 DEC 24, 1985

ENALAPRIL MALEATE; HYDROCHLOROTHIAZIDE
TABLET; ORAL
VASERETIC
+ MERCK 10 MG;25 MG N19221 001 OCT 31, 1986

ENALAPRILAT
INJECTABLE; INJECTION
VASOTEC
+ MERCK 1.25 MG/ML N19309 001 FEB 09, 1988

ENFLURANE
LIQUID; INHALATION
ENFLURANE
AN ABBOTT 99.9% N70803 001 SEP 08, 1987
AN INHALON 99.9% N74396 001 JUL 29, 1994
ETHRANE
AN OHMEDA 99.9% N17087 001

ENOXACIN
TABLET; ORAL
PENETREX
RHONE POULENC RORER 200 MG N19616 004 DEC 31, 1991
+ 400 MG N19616 005 DEC 31, 1991

ENOXAPARIN SODIUM
INJECTABLE; INJECTION
LOVENOX
RHONE POULENC RORER 30 MG/0.3 ML N20164 001 MAR 29, 1993

EPINEPHRINE
INJECTABLE; INJECTION
EPIPEN
+ SURVIVAL TECH 1 MG/ML N19430 001 DEC 22, 1987
EPIPEN JR.
+ SURVIVAL TECH 0.5 MG/ML N19430 002 DEC 22, 1987
SUS-PHRINE
+ FOREST LABS 5 MG/ML N07942 001

EPINEPHRINE; *MULTIPLE*
SEE BUPIVACAINE HYDROCHLORIDE; EPINEPHRINE

EPINEPHRINE; LIDOCAINE HYDROCHLORIDE
INJECTABLE; INJECTION
ALPHACAINE HCL W/ EPINEPHRINE
AP CARLISLE 0.01 MG/ML;2% N84720 001
AP 0.02 MG/ML;2% N84732 001
LIDOCAINE HCL AND EPINEPHRINE
AP ABBOTT 0.005 MG/ML;0.5% N89635 001 JUN 21, 1988
AP 0.005 MG/ML;1% N89649 001 JUN 21, 1988
AP 0.005 MG/ML;1.5% N88571 001 SEP 13, 1985
AP 0.005 MG/ML;1.5% N89645 001 JUN 21, 1988
AP 0.005 MG/ML;1.5% N89650 001 JUN 21, 1988
AP 0.005 MG/ML;2% N89651 001 JUN 21, 1988
AP 0.01 MG/ML;1% N89644 001 JUN 21, 1988
AP 0.01 MG/ML;2% N89646 001 JUN 21, 1988

Prescription Drug Products *(continued)*

EPINEPHRINE; LIDOCAINE HYDROCHLORIDE *(continued)*

INJECTABLE; INJECTION

TE	Product / Applicant	Strength	Appl No / Date
	LIDOCAINE HCL AND EPINEPHRINE		
AP	ELKINS SINN	0.01 MG/ML;1%	N80406 001
AP		0.01 MG/ML;2%	N80406 002
AP	GRAHAM CHEM	0.01 MG/ML;2%	N80504 004 OCT 19, 1983
AP		0.02 MG/ML;2%	N80504 005 OCT 19, 1983
	STERLING WINTHROP	0.02 MG/ML;2%	N40057 001 FEB 26, 1993
AP		0.01 MG/ML;2%	N40057 002 FEB 26, 1993
	LIDOCAINE HCL W/ EPINEPHRINE		
AP	ABBOTT	0.01 MG/ML;1%	N83154 001
AP	DELL LABS	0.01 MG/ML;1%	N83389 001
AP		0.01 MG/ML;2%	N83390 001
AP	INTL MEDICATION	0.01 MG/ML;1%	N86402 001
AP	STERIS	0.01 MG/ML;1%	N80377 003
AP		0.01 MG/ML;2%	N80377 004
	LIDOCATON		
AP	PHARMATON	0.01 MG/ML;2%	N84729 001 AUG 17, 1983
AP		0.02 MG/ML;2%	N84728 001 AUG 17, 1983
	OCTOCAINE		
AP	NOVOCOL	0.01 MG/ML;2%	N84048 001
AP	+	0.02 MG/ML;2%	N84048 002
	XYLOCAINE W/ EPINEPHRINE		
AP	+ ASTRA	0.005 MG/ML;0.5%	N06488 012
AP	+	0.005 MG/ML;1%	N06488 018 NOV 13, 1986
AP	+	0.005 MG/ML;1.5%	N06488 017
AP	+	0.005 MG/ML;2%	N06488 019 NOV 13, 1986
AP	+	0.01 MG/ML;1%	N06488 004
AP	+	0.01 MG/ML;2%	N06488 003

EPINEPHRINE BITARTRATE; *MULTIPLE*

SEE BUPIVACAINE HYDROCHLORIDE; EPINEPHRINE BITARTRATE

EPINEPHRINE BITARTRATE; ETIDOCAINE HYDROCHLORIDE

INJECTABLE; INJECTION

TE	Product / Applicant	Strength	Appl No / Date
	DURANEST		
	+ ASTRA	0.005 MG/ML;1%	N17751 006
	+	0.005 MG/ML;1.5%	N17751 007

EPINEPHRINE BITARTRATE; LIDOCAINE HYDROCHLORIDE

INJECTABLE; INJECTION

TE	Product / Applicant	Strength	Appl No / Date
	LIGNOSPAN FORTE		
	+ DEPROCO	EQ 0.02 MG BASE/ML;2%	N88389 001 JAN 22, 1985
	LIGNOSPAN STANDARD		
	+ DEPROCO	EQ 0.01 MG BASE/ML;2%	N88390 001 JAN 22, 1985

EPINEPHRINE BITARTRATE; PRILOCAINE HYDROCHLORIDE

INJECTABLE; INJECTION

TE	Product / Applicant	Strength	Appl No / Date
	CITANEST FORTE		
	+ ASTRA	0.005 MG/ML;4%	N14763 008

ERGOCALCIFEROL

CAPSULE; ORAL

TE	Product / Applicant	Strength	Appl No / Date
	DRISDOL		
AA	STERLING WINTHROP	50,000IU	N03444 001
	VITAMIN D		
AA	BANNER PHARMACAPS	50,000IU	N80704 001
AA	GLOBAL PHARMS	50,000IU	N80951 001

ERGOCALCIFEROL; *MULTIPLE*

SEE ASCORBIC ACID; BIOTIN; CYANOCOBALAMIN; DEXPANTHENOL; ERGOCALCIFEROL; FOLIC ACID; NIACINAMIDE; PYRIDOXINE HYDROCHLORIDE; RIBOFLAVIN PHOSPHATE SODIUM; THIAMINE HYDROCHLORIDE; VITAMIN A; VITAMIN E

SEE ASCORBIC ACID; BIOTIN; CYANOCOBALAMIN; ERGOCALCIFEROL; FOLIC ACID; NIACINAMIDE; PANTOTHENIC ACID; PHYTONADIONE; PYRIDOXINE; RIBOFLAVIN; THIAMINE; VITAMIN A PALMITATE; VITAMIN E

ERGOLOID MESYLATES

CAPSULE; ORAL

TE	Product / Applicant	Strength	Appl No / Date
	HYDERGINE LC		
	+ SANDOZ	1 MG	N18706 001 JAN 18, 1983

SOLUTION; ORAL

TE	Product / Applicant	Strength	Appl No / Date
	HYDERGINE		
	SANDOZ	1 MG/ML	N18418 001

Prescription Drug Products *(continued)*

ERGOLOID MESYLATES *(continued)*

TABLET; ORAL

ERGOLOID MESYLATES

AB	BARR	1 MG	N88891 001 NOV 01, 1985
AB	DANBURY PHARMA	1 MG	N87244 001 AUG 16, 1982
AB	MUTUAL PHARM	1 MG	N81113 001 OCT 31, 1991

HYDERGINE

AB	+ SANDOZ	1 MG	N17993 001

TABLET; SUBLINGUAL

ERGOLOID MESYLATES

AA	BARR	0.5 MG	N87407 001
AA		1 MG	N87552 001
AA	DANBURY PHARMA	0.5 MG	N87233 001
AA		1 MG	N87183 001
AA	KV PHARM	0.5 MG	N85899 001
AA		1 MG	N85900 001

GERIMAL

AA	CHELSEA LABS	0.5 MG	N86189 001
AA		1 MG	N86188 001

HYDERGINE

AA	SANDOZ	0.5 MG	N09087 002
AA		1 MG	N09087 001

HYDROGENATED ERGOT ALKALOIDS

AA	ZENITH LABS	1 MG	N87185 001

ERGOTAMINE TARTRATE

AEROSOL, METERED; INHALATION

MEDIHALER ERGOTAMINE

	+ 3M	0.36 MG/INH	N12102 001

TABLET; SUBLINGUAL

ERGOMAR

AA	LOTUS BIOCHEM	2 MG	N87693 001 FEB 24, 1983

ERGOSTAT

AA	PARKE DAVIS	2 MG	N88337 001 JUN 08, 1984

WIGRETTES

AA	ORGANON	2 MG	N86750 001 JUL 29, 1982

ERGOTAMINE TARTRATE; *MULTIPLE*

SEE CAFFEINE; ERGOTAMINE TARTRATE

ERYTHROMYCIN

CAPSULE, DELAYED REL PELLETS; ORAL

ERYC

AB	FAULDING	250 MG	N50536 001
AB	+ PARKE DAVIS	250 MG	N62338 001
AB		250 MG	N62618 001 SEP 25, 1985

ERYTHROMYCIN

AB	ABBOTT	250 MG	N62746 001 DEC 22, 1986
AB	BARR	250 MG	N63098 001 MAY 04, 1989

GEL; TOPICAL

EMGEL

AT	GLAXO	2%	N63107 001 AUG 23, 1991

ERYGEL

AT	+ ALLERGAN HERBERT	2%	N50617 001 OCT 21, 1987

ERYTHROMYCIN

AT	STIEFEL	2%	N63211 001 JAN 29, 1993

LOTION; TOPICAL

E-SOLVE 2

	+ SYOSSET	2%	N62467 001 JUL 03, 1985

OINTMENT; OPHTHALMIC

ERYTHROMYCIN

AT	BAUSCH AND LOMB	0.5%	N64067 001 JUL 29, 1994
AT	FOUGERA	0.5%	N62447 001 SEP 26, 1983

ILOTYCIN

AT	+ DISTA	0.5%	N50368 001

OINTMENT; TOPICAL

AKNE-MYCIN

	+ HERMAL PHARM	2%	N50584 001 JAN 10, 1985

SOLUTION; TOPICAL

A/T/S

AT	HOECHST ROUSSEL	2%	N62405 001 NOV 18, 1982

C-SOLVE-2

AT	SYOSSET	2%	N62468 001 JUL 03, 1985

ERYDERM

AT	ABBOTT	2%	N62290 001

ERYMAX

AT	ALLERGAN HERBERT	2%	N62508 002 JUL 11, 1985

Prescription Drug Products *(continued)*

ERYTHROMYCIN *(continued)*

SOLUTION; TOPICAL

	ERYTHRA-DERM			
AT	PADDOCK	2%	N62687 001	FEB 05, 1988
	ERYTHROMYCIN			
AT	BARRE	1.5%	N62328 001	APR 19, 1982
AT		2%	N62326 001	APR 19, 1982
AT	BAUSCH AND LOMB	2%	N64039 001	JAN 27, 1994
AT	CLAY PARK	2%	N63038 001	JAN 11, 1991
AT	PENNEX	2%	N62825 001	OCT 23, 1987
	SANSAC			
AT	GALDERMA	2%	N62522 001	JAN 24, 1985
	STATICIN			
AT	+ WESTWOOD SQUIBB	1.5%	N50526 001	
	T-STAT			
AT	+ WESTWOOD SQUIBB	2%	N62436 001	MAR 09, 1983

SWAB; TOPICAL

	C-SOLVE-2			
AT	SYOSSET	2%	N62751 001	JUL 30, 1993
	ERYCETTE			
AT	+ JOHNSON RW	2%	N50594 001	FEB 15, 1985
	T-STAT			
AT	WESTWOOD SQUIBB	2%	N62748 001	JUL 23, 1987

TABLET; ORAL

	ERYTHROMYCIN			
	ABBOTT	250 MG	N61621 001	
	+	500 MG	N61621 002	

TABLET, COATED PARTICLES; ORAL

	PCE			
	+ ABBOTT	333 MG	N50611 001	SEP 09, 1986
	+	500 MG	N50611 002	AUG 22, 1990

ERYTHROMYCIN *(continued)*

TABLET, DELAYED RELEASE; ORAL

	E-BASE			
AB	BARR	333 MG	N63028 001	MAY 15, 1990
AB		333 MG	N63086 001	MAY 15, 1990
AB		500 MG	N62999 001	NOV 25, 1988
	E-MYCIN			
AB	BOOTS	250 MG	N60272 001	
AB	+	333 MG	N60272 002	
	ERY-TAB			
AB	ABBOTT	250 MG	N62298 001	
AB		333 MG	N62298 003	MAR 29, 1982
AB		500 MG	N62298 002	
	ILOTYCIN			
AB	DISTA	250 MG	N61910 001	
	ROBIMYCIN			
AB	ROBINS AH	250 MG	N61633 001	

ERYTHROMYCIN; *MULTIPLE*

SEE BENZOYL PEROXIDE; ERYTHROMYCIN

ERYTHROMYCIN ESTOLATE

CAPSULE; ORAL

	ERYTHROMYCIN ESTOLATE		
AB	BARR	EQ 125 MG BASE	N62162 001
AB		EQ 250 MG BASE	N62162 002
AB	DANBURY PHARMA	EQ 250 MG BASE	N62087 001
AB	ZENITH LABS	EQ 250 MG BASE	N62237 001
	ILOSONE		
AB	DISTA	EQ 125 MG BASE	N61897 001
AB	+	EQ 250 MG BASE	N61897 002

DROPS; ORAL

	ILOSONE		
	+ DISTA	EQ 100 MG BASE/ML	N61894 003

POWDER FOR RECONSTITUTION; ORAL

	ILOSONE		
	+ DISTA	EQ 125 MG BASE/5 ML	N61893 001

Prescription Drug Products *(continued)*

ERYTHROMYCIN ESTOLATE *(continued)*

	SUSPENSION; ORAL		
	ERYTHROMYCIN ESTOLATE		
AB	BARR	EQ 125 MG BASE/5 ML	N62169 001 OCT 17, 1990
AB		EQ 250 MG BASE/5 ML	N62169 002 OCT 17, 1990
AB	BARRE	EQ 125 MG BASE/5 ML	N62353 001 NOV 18, 1982
AB		EQ 250 MG BASE/5 ML	N62409 001 DEC 16, 1982
	ILOSONE		
AB	DISTA	EQ 125 MG BASE/5 ML	N61894 001
AB	+	EQ 250 MG BASE/5 ML	N61894 002
	TABLET; ORAL		
	ILOSONE		
	+ DISTA	EQ 500 MG BASE	N61896 001
	TABLET, CHEWABLE; ORAL		
	ILOSONE		
	DISTA	EQ 125 MG BASE	N61895 001
	+	EQ 250 MG BASE	N61895 002

ERYTHROMYCIN ETHYLSUCCINATE

	DROPS; ORAL		
	PEDIAMYCIN		
	+ ROSS LABS	EQ 100 MG BASE/2.5 ML	N62305 002
	GRANULE; ORAL		
	E.E.S.		
AB	+ ABBOTT	EQ 200 MG BASE/5 ML	N50207 001
	ERYPED		
	ABBOTT	EQ 400 MG BASE/5 ML	N50207 002
	ERYTHROMYCIN ETHYLSUCCINATE		
AB	BARR	EQ 200 MG BASE/5 ML	N62055 001
	PEDIAMYCIN		
AB	ROSS LABS	EQ 200 MG BASE/5 ML	N62305 001
	SUSPENSION; ORAL		
	E.E.S. 200		
AB	ABBOTT	EQ 200 MG BASE/5 ML	N61639 001
	E.E.S. 400		
AB	+ ABBOTT	EQ 400 MG BASE/5 ML	N61639 002
	ERYTHROMYCIN ETHYLSUCCINATE		
AB	BARRE	EQ 200 MG BASE/5 ML	N62200 001
AB		EQ 400 MG BASE/5 ML	N62200 002
	PEDIAMYCIN		
AB	ROSS LABS	EQ 200 MG BASE/5 ML	N62304 001
	PEDIAMYCIN 400		
AB	ROSS LABS	EQ 400 MG BASE/5 ML	N62304 002
	WYAMYCIN E		
AB	WYETH AYERST	EQ 200 MG BASE/5 ML	N62123 002
AB		EQ 400 MG BASE/5 ML	N62123 001

ERYTHROMYCIN ETHYLSUCCINATE *(continued)*

	TABLET; ORAL		
	E.E.S. 400		
AB	+ ABBOTT	EQ 400 MG BASE	N61905 002 AUG 12, 1982
	ERYTHROMYCIN ETHYLSUCCINATE		
AB	BARR	EQ 400 MG BASE	N62256 001
AB	MYLAN	EQ 400 MG BASE	N62847 001 SEP 14, 1988
	TABLET, CHEWABLE; ORAL		
	E.E.S.		
AB	+ ABBOTT	EQ 200 MG BASE	N50297 002
	ERYPED		
AB	ABBOTT	EQ 200 MG BASE	N50297 003 JUL 05, 1988
	PEDIAMYCIN		
AB	ROSS LABS	EQ 200 MG BASE	N62306 001

ERYTHROMYCIN ETHYLSUCCINATE; SULFISOXAZOLE ACETYL

	GRANULE; ORAL		
	ERYTHROMYCIN ETHYLSUCCINATE AND SULFISOXAZOLE ACETYL		
AB	BARR	EQ 200 MG BASE/5 ML;EQ 600 MG BASE/5 ML	N62759 001 MAY 20, 1988
	ERYZOLE		
AB	ALRA	EQ 200 MG BASE/5 ML;EQ 600 MG BASE/5 ML	N62758 001 JUN 15, 1988
	PEDIAZOLE		
AB	+ ROSS LABS	EQ 200 MG BASE/5 ML;EQ 600 MG BASE/5 ML	N50529 001

ERYTHROMYCIN GLUCEPTATE

	INJECTABLE; INJECTION		
	ILOTYCIN GLUCEPTATE		
	+ DISTA	EQ 250 MG BASE/VIAL	N50370 001
	+	EQ 500 MG BASE/VIAL	N50370 002
	+	EQ 1 GM BASE/VIAL	N50370 003

ERYTHROMYCIN LACTOBIONATE

	INJECTABLE; INJECTION		
	ERYTHROCIN		
AP	+ ABBOTT	EQ 500 MG BASE/VIAL	N50182 002
AP		EQ 500 MG BASE/VIAL	N50609 001 SEP 24, 1986
AP		EQ 500 MG BASE/VIAL	N62586 001 JAN 04, 1988
AP		EQ 500 MG BASE/VIAL	N62638 001 OCT 31, 1986

Prescription Drug Products *(continued)*

ERYTHROMYCIN LACTOBIONATE *(continued)*

	INJECTABLE; INJECTION		
	ERYTHROCIN		
AP	+ ABBOTT	EQ 1 GM BASE/VIAL	N50182 003
AP		EQ 1 GM BASE/VIAL	N50609 002 SEP 24, 1986
AP		EQ 1 GM BASE/VIAL	N62586 002 JAN 04, 1988
AP		EQ 1 GM BASE/VIAL	N62638 002 OCT 31, 1986
	ERYTHROMYCIN		
AP	ELKINS SINN	EQ 500 MG BASE/VIAL	N62563 001 MAR 28, 1985
AP		EQ 1 GM BASE/VIAL	N62563 002 MAR 28, 1985
	ERYTHROMYCIN LACTOBIONATE		
AP	GENSIA	EQ 500 MG BASE/VIAL	N63253 001 JUL 30, 1993
AP		EQ 1 GM BASE/VIAL	N63253 002 JUL 30, 1993
AP	LEDERLE	EQ 500 MG BASE/VIAL	N62993 001 MAY 09, 1989
AP		EQ 1 GM BASE/VIAL	N62993 002 MAY 09, 1989

ERYTHROMYCIN STEARATE

	TABLET; ORAL		
	ERYTHROCIN STEARATE		
AB	ABBOTT	EQ 250 MG BASE	N60359 001
AB	+	EQ 500 MG BASE	N60359 003
	ERYTHROMYCIN STEARATE		
AB	BARR	EQ 250 MG BASE	N61591 001
AB		EQ 500 MG BASE	N63179 001 MAY 15, 1990
AB	CHELSEA LABS	EQ 250 MG BASE	N62121 002
AB		EQ 500 MG BASE	N62121 001
AB	MYLAN	EQ 250 MG BASE	N61505 001
AB		EQ 500 MG BASE	N61505 002
AB	ZENITH LABS	EQ 250 MG BASE	N61461 001
AB		EQ 500 MG BASE	N61461 002
	ETHRIL 250		
AB	SQUIBB	EQ 250 MG BASE	N61605 001
	ETHRIL 500		
AB	SQUIBB	EQ 500 MG BASE	N61605 002
	WYAMYCIN S		
AB	WYETH AYERST	EQ 250 MG BASE	N61675 001
AB		EQ 500 MG BASE	N61675 002

ESMOLOL HYDROCHLORIDE

	INJECTABLE; INJECTION		
	BREVIBLOC		
	+ OHMEDA	10 MG/ML	N19386 001 AUG 15, 1988
	+	250 MG/ML	N19386 002 DEC 31, 1986

ESTAZOLAM

	TABLET; ORAL		
	PROSOM		
	ABBOTT	1 MG	N19080 001 DEC 26, 1990
		2 MG	N19080 002 DEC 26, 1990

ESTRADIOL

	CREAM; VAGINAL		
	ESTRACE		
	+ BRISTOL MYERS SQUIBB	0.01%	N86069 001 JAN 31, 1984
	FILM, EXTENDED RELEASE; TRANSDERMAL		
	ESTRADERM		
	+ CIBA	0.05 MG/24 HR	N19081 002 SEP 10, 1986
	+	0.1 MG/24 HR	N19081 003 SEP 10, 1986
	TABLET; ORAL		
	ESTRACE		
	BRISTOL MYERS SQUIBB	0.5 MG	N81295 001 JUN 30, 1993
		1 MG	N84499 001
	+	2 MG	N84500 001

ESTRADIOL CYPIONATE

	INJECTABLE; INJECTION		
	DEPO-ESTRADIOL		
AO	+ UPJOHN	5 MG/ML	N85470 003
	+	1 MG/ML	N85470 001
	+	3 MG/ML	N85470 002
	ESTRADIOL CYPIONATE		
AO	STERIS	5 MG/ML	N85620 001

Prescription Drug Products *(continued)*

ESTRADIOL CYPIONATE; TESTOSTERONE CYPIONATE

	INJECTABLE; INJECTION		
	DEPO-TESTADIOL		
AO	+ UPJOHN	2 MG/ML;50 MG/ML	N17968 001
	TESTOSTERONE CYPIONATE-ESTRADIOL CYPIONATE		
AO	STERIS	2 MG/ML;50 MG/ML	N85603 001 MAR 13, 1986

ESTRADIOL VALERATE

	INJECTABLE; INJECTION		
	DELESTROGEN		
AO	+ SQUIBB	10 MG/ML	N09402 002
AO	+	20 MG/ML	N09402 004
AO	+	40 MG/ML	N09402 003
	ESTRADIOL VALERATE		
AO	STERIS	10 MG/ML	N83546 001
AO		20 MG/ML	N83547 001
AO		40 MG/ML	N83714 001

ESTRADIOL VALERATE; TESTOSTERONE ENANTHATE

	INJECTABLE; INJECTION		
	DITATE-DS		
	+ SAVAGE LABS	8 MG/ML;180 MG/ML	N86423 001
	TESTOSTERONE ENANTHATE AND ESTRADIOL VALERATE		
	+ STERIS	4 MG/ML;90 MG/ML	N85865 001

ESTRAMUSTINE PHOSPHATE SODIUM

	CAPSULE; ORAL		
	EMCYT		
	+ PHARMACIA	EQ 140 MG PHOSPHATE	N18045 001

ESTROGENS, CONJUGATED

	CREAM; TOPICAL, VAGINAL		
	PREMARIN		
	+ AYERST	0.625 MG/GM	N20216 001
	INJECTABLE; INJECTION		
	PREMARIN		
	+ WYETH AYERST	25 MG/VIAL	N10402 001
	TABLET; ORAL		
	PREMARIN		
	WYETH AYERST	0.3 MG	N04782 003
	+	0.625 MG	N04782 004
		0.9 MG	N04782 005 JAN 26, 1984
	+	1.25 MG	N04782 001
		2.5 MG	N04782 002

ESTROGENS, CONJUGATED; MEPROBAMATE

	TABLET; ORAL		
	PMB 200		
	+ WYETH AYERST	0.45 MG;200 MG	N10971 005
	PMB 400		
	+ WYETH AYERST	0.45 MG;400 MG	N10971 003

ESTROGENS, ESTERIFIED

	TABLET; ORAL		
	ESTRATAB		
BS	SOLVAY	0.3 MG	N86715 001
BS	+	0.625 MG	N83209 001
BS		1.25 MG	N83856 001
BS	+	2.5 MG	N83857 001
	MENEST		
BS	SMITHKLINE BEECHAM	0.3 MG	N84951 001
BS		0.625 MG	N84948 001
BS		1.25 MG	N84950 001
BS		2.5 MG	N84949 001

ESTROGENS, ESTERIFIED; *MULTIPLE*

SEE CHLORDIAZEPOXIDE; ESTROGENS, ESTERIFIED

ESTRONE

	INJECTABLE; INJECTION		
	ESTROGENIC SUBSTANCE		
BP	WYETH AYERST	2 MG/ML	N83488 001
	ESTRONE		
	+ STERIS	5 MG/ML	N85239 001
	NATURAL ESTROGENIC SUBSTANCE-ESTRONE		
BP	STERIS	2 MG/ML	N85237 001 NOV 23, 1982
	THEELIN		
BP	+ PARKE DAVIS	2 MG/ML	N03977 002

Prescription Drug Products *(continued)*

ESTROPIPATE

	CREAM; VAGINAL		
	OGEN		
	+ ABBOTT	1.5 MG/GM	N84710 001
	TABLET; ORAL		
	ESTROPIPATE		
AB	WATSON LABS	0.75 MG	N81213 001 SEP 23, 1993
AB		1.5 MG	N81214 001 SEP 23, 1993
AB		3 MG	N81215 001 SEP 23, 1993
AB		6 MG	N81216 001 SEP 23, 1993
	OGEN .625		
AB	ABBOTT	0.75 MG	N83220 001
	OGEN 1.25		
AB	ABBOTT	1.5 MG	N83220 002
	OGEN 2.5		
AB	+ ABBOTT	3 MG	N83220 003
	OGEN 5		
AB	ABBOTT	6 MG	N83220 004
	ORTHO-EST		
AB	JOHNSON RW	0.75 MG	N89567 001 FEB 27, 1991
AB		1.5 MG	N89582 001 JUL 17, 1991

ETHACRYNATE SODIUM

	INJECTABLE; INJECTION		
	EDECRIN		
	+ MERCK SHARP DOHME	EQ 50 MG ACID/VIAL	N16093 001

ETHACRYNIC ACID

	TABLET; ORAL		
	EDECRIN		
	MERCK SHARP DOHME	25 MG	N16092 001
	+	50 MG	N16092 002

ETHAMBUTOL HYDROCHLORIDE

	TABLET; ORAL		
	MYAMBUTOL		
	LEDERLE	100 MG	N16320 001
	+	400 MG	N16320 003

ETHANOLAMINE OLEATE

	INJECTABLE; INJECTION		
	ETHAMOLIN		
	+ REED AND CARNRICK	50 MG/ML	N19357 001 DEC 22, 1988

ETHCHLORVYNOL

	CAPSULE; ORAL		
	ETHCHLORVYNOL		
AA	BANNER PHARMACAPS	200 MG	N84463 002
AA		500 MG	N84463 003
AA		750 MG	N84463 004
		100 MG	N84463 001
	PLACIDYL		
AA	ABBOTT	200 MG	N10021 007
AA		500 MG	N10021 002
AA		750 MG	N10021 010

ETHINYL ESTRADIOL

	TABLET; ORAL		
	ESTINYL		
	SCHERING	0.02 MG	N05292 001
		0.05 MG	N05292 002
	+	0.5 MG	N05292 003

ETHINYL ESTRADIOL; *MULTIPLE*

SEE DESOGESTREL; ETHINYL ESTRADIOL

ETHINYL ESTRADIOL; ETHYNODIOL DIACETATE

	TABLET; ORAL-21		
	DEMULEN 1/35-21		
AB	+ SEARLE	0.035 MG;1 MG	N18168 001
	DEMULEN 1/50-21		
AB	+ SEARLE	0.05 MG;1 MG	N16927 001
	ETHYNODIOL DIACETATE AND ETHINYL ESTRADIOL 1/35-21		
AB	WATSON LABS	0.035 MG;1 MG	N72720 001 DEC 30, 1991
	ETHYNODIOL DIACETATE AND ETHINYL ESTRADIOL 1/50-21		
AB	WATSON LABS	0.05 MG;1 MG	N72722 001 DEC 30, 1991

Prescription Drug Products *(continued)*

ETHINYL ESTRADIOL; ETHYNODIOL DIACETATE *(continued)*

TABLET; ORAL-28

	DEMULEN 1/35-28		
AB	SEARLE	0.035 MG;1 MG	N18160 001
	DEMULEN 1/50-28		
AB	SEARLE	0.05 MG;1 MG	N16936 001
	ETHYNODIOL DIACETATE AND ETHINYL ESTRADIOL 1/35-28		
AB	WATSON LABS	0.035 MG;1 MG	N72721 001 DEC 30, 1991
	ETHYNODIOL DIACETATE AND ETHINYL ESTRADIOL 1/50-28		
AB	WATSON LABS	0.05 MG;1 MG	N72723 001 DEC 30, 1991

ETHINYL ESTRADIOL; FERROUS FUMARATE; NORETHINDRONE ACETATE

TABLET; ORAL-28

	LOESTRIN FE 1.5/30		
	+ PARKE DAVIS	0.03 MG;75 MG;1.5 MG	N17355 001
	LOESTRIN FE 1/20		
	+ PARKE DAVIS	0.02 MG;75 MG;1 MG	N17354 001

ETHINYL ESTRADIOL; LEVONORGESTREL

TABLET; ORAL-21

	LEVORA 0.15/30-21		
AB	SYNTEX	0.03 MG;0.15 MG	N73592 001 DEC 13, 1993
	NORDETTE-21		
AB	+ WYETH AYERST	0.03 MG;0.15 MG	N18668 001 MAY 10, 1982
	TRIPHASIL-21		
	+ WYETH AYERST	0.03 MG,0.04 MG,0.03 MG;0.05 MG,0.075 MG,0.125 MG	N19192 001 NOV 01, 1984

TABLET; ORAL-28

	LEVORA 0.15/30-28		
AB	SYNTEX	0.03 MG;0.15 MG	N73594 001 DEC 13, 1993
	NORDETTE-28		
AB	WYETH AYERST	0.03 MG;0.15 MG	N18782 001 JUL 21, 1982
	TRIPHASIL-28		
	WYETH AYERST	0.03 MG,0.04 MG,0.03 MG;0.05 MG,0.075 MG,0.125 MG	N19190 001 NOV 01, 1984

ETHINYL ESTRADIOL; NORETHINDRONE

TABLET; ORAL-21

	BREVICON 21-DAY		
AB	SYNTEX	0.035 MG;0.5 MG	N17566 001
	GENCEPT 0.5/35-21		
AB	GENCON	0.035 MG;0.5 MG	N72692 001 FEB 28, 1992
	GENCEPT 1/35-21		
AB	GENCON	0.035 MG;1 MG	N72693 001 FEB 28, 1992
	GENCEPT 10/11-21		
AB	GENCON	0.035 MG;0.5 MG AND 1 MG	N72694 001 FEB 28, 1992
	MODICON 21		
AB	JOHNSON RW	0.035 MG;0.5 MG	N17488 001
	NORCEPT-E 1/35 21		
AB	GYNOPHARMA	0.035 MG;1 MG	N71545 001 FEB 09, 1989
	NORETHIN 1/35E-21		
AB	ROBERTS LABS	0.035 MG;1 MG	N71480 001 APR 12, 1988
	NORETHINDRONE AND ETHINYL ESTRADIOL		
AB	WATSON LABS	0.035 MG;1 MG	N70685 001 JAN 29, 1987
AB		0.035 MG;0.5 MG	N70684 001 JAN 29, 1987
	NORETHINDRONE AND ETHINYL ESTRADIOL (10/11)		
AB	WATSON LABS	0.035 MG;0.5 MG AND 1 MG	N71043 001 APR 01, 1988
	NORETHINDRONE AND ETHINYL ESTRADIOL (7/14)		
AB	WATSON LABS	0.035 MG;0.5 MG AND 1 MG	N71041 001 SEP 24, 1991
	NORINYL 1+35 21-DAY		
AB	SYNTEX	0.035 MG;1 MG	N17565 001
	ORTHO-NOVUM 1/35-21		
AB	+ JOHNSON RW	0.035 MG;1 MG	N17489 002
	ORTHO-NOVUM 10/11-21		
AB	+ JOHNSON RW	0.035 MG;0.5 MG AND 1 MG	N18354 001 JAN 11, 1982
	ORTHO-NOVUM 7/14-21		
AB	+ JOHNSON RW	0.035 MG;0.5 MG AND 1 MG	N19004 001 APR 04, 1984
	ORTHO-NOVUM 7/7/7-21		
	+ JOHNSON RW	0.035 MG;0.5 MG, 0.75 MG AND 1 MG	N18985 001 APR 04, 1984
	OVCON-35		
	+ MEAD JOHNSON	0.035 MG;0.4 MG	N18127 001
	OVCON-50		
	+ MEAD JOHNSON	0.05 MG;1 MG	N18128 001
	TRI-NORINYL 21-DAY		
	+ SYNTEX	0.035 MG;0.5 MG AND 1 MG	N18977 001 APR 13, 1984

Prescription Drug Products *(continued)*

ETHINYL ESTRADIOL; NORETHINDRONE *(continued)*

TABLET; ORAL-28

	BREVICON 28-DAY		
AB	SYNTEX	0.035 MG;0.5 MG	N17743 001
	GENCEPT 0.5/35-28		
AB	GENCON	0.035 MG;0.5 MG	N72695 001 FEB 28, 1992
	GENCEPT 1/35-28		
AB	GENCON	0.035 MG;1 MG	N72696 001 FEB 28, 1992
	GENCEPT 10/11-28		
AB	GENCON	0.035 MG;0.5 MG AND 1 MG	N72697 001 FEB 28, 1992
	MODICON 28		
AB	JOHNSON RW	0.035 MG;0.5 MG	N17735 001
	NORCEPT-E 1/35 28		
AB	GYNOPHARMA	0.035 MG;1 MG	N71546 001 FEB 09, 1989
	NORETHIN 1/35E-28		
AB	ROBERTS LABS	0.035 MG;1 MG	N71481 001 APR 12, 1988
	NORETHINDRONE AND ETHINYL ESTRADIOL		
AB	WATSON LABS	0.035 MG;1 MG	N70687 001 JAN 29, 1987
AB		0.035 MG;0.5 MG	N70686 001 JAN 29, 1987
	NORETHINDRONE AND ETHINYL ESTRADIOL (10/11)		
AB	WATSON LABS	0.035 MG;0.5 MG AND 1 MG	N71044 001 APR 01, 1988
	NORETHINDRONE AND ETHINYL ESTRADIOL (7/14)		
AB	WATSON LABS	0.035 MG;0.5 MG AND 1 MG	N71042 001 SEP 24, 1991
	NORINYL 1+35 28-DAY		
AB	SYNTEX	0.035 MG;1 MG	N17565 002
	ORTHO-NOVUM 1/35-28		
AB	JOHNSON RW	0.035 MG;1 MG	N17919 002
	ORTHO-NOVUM 10/11-28 IN PLASTIC CONTAINER		
AB	JOHNSON RW	0.035 MG;0.5 MG AND 1 MG	N18354 002 JAN 11, 1982
	ORTHO-NOVUM 7/14-28		
AB	+ JOHNSON RW	0.035 MG;0.5 MG AND 1 MG	N19004 002 APR 04, 1984
	ORTHO-NOVUM 7/7/7-28		
	JOHNSON RW	0.035 MG;0.5 MG, 0.75 MG AND 1 MG	N18985 002 APR 04, 1984
	OVCON-35		
	MEAD JOHNSON	0.035 MG;0.4 MG	N17716 001
	OVCON-50		
	MEAD JOHNSON	0.05 MG;1 MG	N17576 001
	TRI-NORINYL 28-DAY		
	SYNTEX	0.035 MG;0.5 MG AND 1 MG	N18977 002 APR 13, 1984

ETHINYL ESTRADIOL; NORETHINDRONE ACETATE

TABLET; ORAL-21

	LOESTRIN 21 1.5/30		
	+ PARKE DAVIS	0.03 MG;1.5 MG	N17875 001
	LOESTRIN 21 1/20		
	+ PARKE DAVIS	0.02 MG;1 MG	N17876 001

ETHINYL ESTRADIOL; NORGESTIMATE

TABLET; ORAL-21

	ORTHO CYCLEN-21		
	+ JOHNSON RW	0.035 MG;0.25 MG	N19653 001 DEC 29, 1989
	ORTHO TRI-CYCLEN		
	+ JOHNSON RW	0.035 MG;0.18 MG,0.215 MG,0.25 MG	N19697 002 JUL 03, 1992

TABLET; ORAL-28

	ORTHO CYCLEN-28		
	JOHNSON RW	0.035 MG;0.25 MG	N19653 002 DEC 29, 1989
	ORTHO TRI-CYCLEN		
	JOHNSON RW	0.035 MG;0.18 MG,0.215 MG,0.25 MG	N19697 001 JUL 03, 1992

ETHINYL ESTRADIOL; NORGESTREL

TABLET; ORAL-21

	LO/OVRAL		
	+ WYETH AYERST	0.03 MG;0.3 MG	N17612 001
	OVRAL		
	+ WYETH AYERST	0.05 MG;0.5 MG	N16672 001

TABLET; ORAL-28

	LO/OVRAL-28		
	WYETH AYERST	0.03 MG;0.3 MG	N17802 001
	OVRAL-28		
	WYETH AYERST	0.05 MG;0.5 MG	N16806 001

ETHIODIZED OIL

OIL; INTRALYMPHATIC, INTRAUTERINE

	ETHIODOL		
	SAVAGE LABS	99%	N09190 001

Prescription Drug Products *(continued)*

ETHIONAMIDE
TABLET; ORAL
TRECATOR-SC
WYETH AYERST 250 MG N13026 002

ETHOPROPAZINE HYDROCHLORIDE
TABLET; ORAL
PARSIDOL
PARKE DAVIS 10 MG N09078 003
50 MG N09078 006
100 MG N09078 008

ETHOSUXIMIDE
CAPSULE; ORAL
ZARONTIN
+ PARKE DAVIS 250 MG N12380 001
SYRUP; ORAL
ETHOSUXIMIDE
AA COPLEY PHARM 250 MG/5 ML N81306 001 JUL 30, 1993
ZARONTIN
AA PARKE DAVIS 250 MG/5 ML N80258 001

ETHOTOIN
TABLET; ORAL
PEGANONE
ABBOTT 250 MG N10841 001
+ 500 MG N10841 003

ETHYNODIOL DIACETATE; *MULTIPLE*
SEE ETHINYL ESTRADIOL; ETHYNODIOL DIACETATE

ETIDOCAINE HYDROCHLORIDE
INJECTABLE; INJECTION
DURANEST
+ ASTRA 1% N17751 005

ETIDOCAINE HYDROCHLORIDE; *MULTIPLE*
SEE EPINEPHRINE BITARTRATE; ETIDOCAINE HYDROCHLORIDE

ETIDRONATE DISODIUM
INJECTABLE; INJECTION
DIDRONEL
+ MGI 50 MG/ML N19545 001 APR 20, 1987
TABLET; ORAL
DIDRONEL
PROCTER AND GAMBLE 200 MG N17831 001
+ 400 MG N17831 002

ETODOLAC
CAPSULE; ORAL
LODINE
WYETH AYERST 200 MG N18922 002 JAN 31, 1991
+ 300 MG N18922 003 JAN 31, 1991
TABLET; ORAL
LODINE
+ WYETH AYERST 400 MG N18922 004 JUL 29, 1993

ETOMIDATE
INJECTABLE; INJECTION
AMIDATE
+ ABBOTT 2 MG/ML N18227 001 SEP 07, 1982

ETOPOSIDE
CAPSULE; ORAL
VEPESID
+ BRISTOL 50 MG N19557 001 DEC 30, 1986
INJECTABLE; INJECTION
ETOPOSIDE
AP GENSIA 20 MG/ML N74284 001 FEB 10, 1994
VEPESID
AP + BRISTOL 20 MG/ML N18768 001 NOV 10, 1983

ETRETINATE
CAPSULE; ORAL
TEGISON
ROCHE 10 MG N19369 001 SEP 30, 1986
+ 25 MG N19369 002 SEP 30, 1986

Prescription Drug Products *(continued)*

FAMCICLOVIR

	TABLET; ORAL		
	FAMVIR		
	+ SMITHKLINE BEECHAM	500 MG	N20363 002 JUN 29, 1994

FAMOTIDINE

	INJECTABLE; INJECTION		
	PEPCID		
	+ MERCK	10 MG/ML	N19510 001 NOV 04, 1986
	PEPCID IN PLASTIC CONTAINER		
	+ MERCK	0.4 MG/ML	N20249 001 FEB 18, 1994
	POWDER FOR RECONSTITUTION; ORAL		
	PEPCID		
	+ MERCK	40 MG/5 ML	N19527 001 FEB 02, 1987
	TABLET; ORAL		
	PEPCID		
	MERCK	20 MG	N19462 001 OCT 15, 1986
	+	40 MG	N19462 002 OCT 15, 1986

FELBAMATE

	SUSPENSION; ORAL		
	FELBATOL		
	+ WALLACE	600 MG/5 ML	N20189 003 JUL 29, 1993
	TABLET; ORAL		
	FELBATOL		
	WALLACE	400 MG	N20189 001 JUL 29, 1993
	+	600 MG	N20189 002 JUL 29, 1993

FELODIPINE

	TABLET, EXTENDED RELEASE; ORAL		
	PLENDIL		
	MERCK	5 MG	N19834 001 JUL 25, 1991
		10 MG	N19834 002 JUL 25, 1991

FENFLURAMINE HYDROCHLORIDE

	TABLET; ORAL		
	PONDIMIN		
	+ ROBINS AH	20 MG	N16618 001

FENOFIBRATE

	CAPSULE; ORAL		
	LIPIDIL		
	+ LABS FOURNIER	100 MG	N19304 001 DEC 31, 1993

FENOPROFEN CALCIUM

	CAPSULE; ORAL		
	FENOPROFEN CALCIUM		
AB	DANBURY PHARMA	EQ 200 MG BASE	N72981 001 AUG 19, 1991
AB		EQ 300 MG BASE	N72982 001 AUG 19, 1991
AB	GENEVA PHARMS	EQ 200 MG BASE	N72394 001 OCT 17, 1988
AB		EQ 300 MG BASE	N72395 001 OCT 17, 1988
AB	PAR PHARM	EQ 200 MG BASE	N72437 001 AUG 22, 1988
AB		EQ 300 MG BASE	N72438 001 AUG 22, 1988
AB	WATSON LABS	EQ 200 MG BASE	N72294 001 AUG 17, 1988
AB		EQ 300 MG BASE	N72293 001 AUG 17, 1988
	NALFON		
AB	+ DISTA	EQ 300 MG BASE	N17604 002
	NALFON 200		
AB	DISTA	EQ 200 MG BASE	N17604 003
	TABLET; ORAL		
	FENOPROFEN CALCIUM		
AB	CHELSEA LABS	EQ 600 MG BASE	N72407 001 AUG 17, 1988
AB	DANBURY PHARMA	EQ 600 MG BASE	N72602 001 OCT 11, 1988
AB	GENEVA PHARMS	EQ 600 MG BASE	N72396 001 OCT 17, 1988
AB	LEDERLE	EQ 600 MG BASE	N72326 001 AUG 17, 1988
AB	MUTUAL PHARM	EQ 600 MG BASE	N72902 001 DEC 21, 1990
AB	MYLAN	EQ 600 MG BASE	N72267 001 AUG 17, 1988

Prescription Drug Products *(continued)*

FENOPROFEN CALCIUM *(continued)*

TABLET; ORAL

FENOPROFEN CALCIUM

AB	PAR PHARM	EQ 600 MG BASE	N72429 001 AUG 17, 1988
AB	PUREPAC PHARM	EQ 600 MG BASE	N72274 001 MAY 02, 1988
AB	WATSON LABS	EQ 600 MG BASE	N72165 001 AUG 17, 1988
AB	ZENITH LABS	EQ 600 MG BASE	N72557 001 AUG 29, 1988

NALFON

AB	+ DISTA	EQ 600 MG BASE	N17710 001

FENTANYL

FILM, EXTENDED RELEASE; TRANSDERMAL

DURAGESIC

+ ALZA	0.6 MG/24 HR	N19813 004 AUG 07, 1990
+	1.2 MG/24 HR	N19813 003 AUG 07, 1990
+	1.8 MG/24 HR	N19813 002 AUG 07, 1990
+	2.4 MG/24 HR	N19813 001 AUG 07, 1990

FENTANYL CITRATE

INJECTABLE; INJECTION

FENTANYL CITRATE

AP	ABBOTT	EQ 0.05 MG BASE/ML	N19115 001 JAN 12, 1985
AP		EQ 0.05 MG BASE/ML	N70636 001 APR 30, 1990
AP		EQ 0.05 MG BASE/ML	N70637 001 APR 30, 1990
AP	ELKINS SINN	EQ 0.05 MG BASE/ML	N19101 001 JUL 11, 1984
AP	STERIS	EQ 0.05 MG BASE/ML	N73488 001 JUN 30, 1992
AP	STERLING WINTHROP	EQ 0.05 MG BASE/ML	N72786 001 SEP 24, 1991

SUBLIMAZE

AP	+ JANSSEN	EQ 0.05 MG BASE/ML	N16619 001

TROCHE/LOZENGE; ORAL

FENTANYL

ANESTA	EQ 0.2 MG BASE	N20195 001 OCT 04, 1993
	EQ 0.3 MG BASE	N20195 002 OCT 04, 1993
+	EQ 0.4 MG BASE	N20195 003 OCT 04, 1993

FENTANYL CITRATE; *MULTIPLE*

SEE DROPERIDOL; FENTANYL CITRATE

FERROUS FUMARATE; *MULTIPLE*

SEE ETHINYL ESTRADIOL; FERROUS FUMARATE; NORETHINDRONE ACETATE

FIBRINOLYSIN; *MULTIPLE*

SEE CHLORAMPHENICOL; DESOXYRIBONUCLEASE; FIBRINOLYSIN

FINASTERIDE

TABLET; ORAL

PROSCAR

+ MERCK SHARP DOHME	5 MG	N20180 001 JUN 19, 1992

FLAVOXATE HYDROCHLORIDE

TABLET; ORAL

URISPAS

+ SMITHKLINE BEECHAM	100 MG	N16769 001

FLECAINIDE ACETATE

TABLET; ORAL

TAMBOCOR

3M	50 MG	N18830 004 AUG 23, 1988
	100 MG	N18830 001 OCT 31, 1985
+	150 MG	N18830 003 JUN 03, 1988

FLOSEQUINAN

TABLET; ORAL

MANOPLAX

BOOTS	50 MG	N19960 001 DEC 30, 1992
	75 MG	N19960 002 DEC 30, 1992
+	100 MG	N19960 003 DEC 30, 1992

FLOXURIDINE

INJECTABLE; INJECTION

FUDR

+ ROCHE	500 MG/VIAL	N16929 001

Prescription Drug Products *(continued)*

FLUCONAZOLE
INJECTABLE; INJECTION
DIFLUCAN
+ PFIZER 2 MG/ML N19950 001 JAN 29, 1990

POWDER FOR RECONSTITUTION; ORAL
DIFLUCAN
PFIZER 50 MG/5 ML N20090 001 DEC 23, 1993
\+ 200 MG/5 ML N20090 002 DEC 23, 1993

TABLET; ORAL
DIFLUCAN
PFIZER 50 MG N19949 001 JAN 29, 1990
100 MG N19949 002 JAN 29, 1990
150 MG N20322 001 JUN 30, 1994
\+ 200 MG N19949 003 JAN 29, 1990

FLUCYTOSINE
CAPSULE; ORAL
ANCOBON
ROCHE 250 MG N17001 001
\+ 500 MG N17001 002

FLUDARABINE PHOSPHATE
INJECTABLE; INJECTION
FLUDARA
+ BERLEX 50 MG/VIAL N20038 001 APR 18, 1991

FLUDEOXYGLUCOSE, F-18
INJECTABLE; INJECTION
FLUDEOXYGLUCOSE F 18
+ DOWNSTATE CLINCL 6.8-35.7mCi/ML N20306 001 AUG 19, 1994

FLUDROCORTISONE ACETATE
TABLET; ORAL
FLORINEF
+ SQUIBB 0.1 MG N10060 001

FLUMAZENIL
INJECTABLE; INJECTION
ROMAZICON
+ ROCHE 0.1 MG/ML N20073 001 DEC 20, 1991

FLUNISOLIDE
AEROSOL, METERED; INHALATION
AEROBID
+ SYNTEX 0.25 MG/INH N18340 001 AUG 17, 1984

SPRAY, METERED; NASAL
NASALIDE
+ SYNTEX 0.025 MG/INH N18148 001

FLUOCINOLONE ACETONIDE
CREAM; TOPICAL
FLUOCET
AT NMC 0.025% N88360 001 JAN 16, 1984

FLUOCINOLONE ACETONIDE
AT CLAY PARK 0.01% N86810 001 MAR 04, 1982
AT 0.025% N86811 001 MAR 04, 1982
AT FOUGERA 0.01% N88170 001 DEC 16, 1982
AT 0.025% N88169 001 DEC 16, 1982
AT G AND W LABS 0.01% N89526 001 JUL 26, 1988
AT 0.025% N89525 001 JUL 26, 1988
AT NMC 0.01% N88361 001 JAN 16, 1984
AT THAMES 0.01% N87102 001 APR 27, 1982
AT 0.025% N87104 001 APR 27, 1982

FLUONID
AT ALLERGAN HERBERT 0.025% N87156 002 SEP 06, 1984

SYNALAR
AT + SYNTEX 0.01% N12787 004
AT + 0.025% N12787 002

SYNALAR-HP
+ SYNTEX 0.2% N16161 002

SYNEMOL
AT + SYNTEX 0.025% N12787 005

FLUOCINOLONE ACETONIDE *(continued)*

OIL; TOPICAL

	Product / Applicant	Strength	Appl No / Approval Date
	DERMA-SMOOTHE/FS		
	+ HILL DERMAC	0.01%	N19452 001 FEB 03, 1988

OINTMENT; TOPICAL

	Product / Applicant	Strength	Appl No / Approval Date
	FLUOCINOLONE ACETONIDE		
AT	FOUGERA	0.025%	N88168 001 DEC 16, 1982
AT	G AND W LABS	0.025%	N89524 001 JUL 26, 1988
	FLUONID		
AT	ALLERGAN HERBERT	0.025%	N87157 001 SEP 06, 1984
	SYNALAR		
AT	+ SYNTEX	0.025%	N13960 001

SHAMPOO; TOPICAL

	Product / Applicant	Strength	Appl No / Approval Date
	FS SHAMPOO		
	+ HILL DERMAC	0.01%	N20001 001 AUG 27, 1990

SOLUTION; TOPICAL

	Product / Applicant	Strength	Appl No / Approval Date
	FLUOCINOLONE ACETONIDE		
AT	BARRE	0.01%	N87159 001 JUN 16, 1982
AT	BAUSCH AND LOMB	0.01%	N40059 001 DEC 20, 1993
AT	FOUGERA	0.01%	N88167 001 DEC 16, 1982
AT	PHARMADERM	0.01%	N88048 001 DEC 16, 1982
AT	THAMES	0.01%	N89124 001 SEP 11, 1985
	FLUONID		
AT	ALLERGAN HERBERT	0.01%	N87158 001 MAR 17, 1983
	SYNALAR		
AT	+ SYNTEX	0.01%	N15296 001

FLUOCINOLONE ACETONIDE; NEOMYCIN SULFATE

CREAM; TOPICAL

	Product / Applicant	Strength	Appl No / Approval Date
	NEO-SYNALAR		
	+ HAMILTON PHARMA CA	0.025%;EQ 3.5 MG BASE/GM	N60700 001

FLUOCINONIDE

CREAM; TOPICAL

	Product / Applicant	Strength	Appl No / Approval Date
	FLUOCINONIDE		
AB	LEMMON	0.05%	N72488 001 FEB 06, 1989
AB		0.05%	N72490 001 FEB 07, 1989
AB	NMC	0.05%	N73085 001 FEB 14, 1992
AB	TARO	0.05%	N19117 001 JUN 26, 1984
AB	THAMES	0.05%	N71500 001 JUN 10, 1987
AB	TICAN	0.05%	N72494 001 JAN 19, 1989
	LIDEX		
AB	+ SYNTEX	0.05%	N16908 002
	LIDEX-E		
AB	SYNTEX	0.05%	N16908 003

GEL; TOPICAL

	Product / Applicant	Strength	Appl No / Approval Date
	FLUOCINONIDE		
AB	LEMMON	0.05%	N72537 001 FEB 07, 1989
	LIDEX		
AB	+ SYNTEX	0.05%	N17373 001

OINTMENT; TOPICAL

	Product / Applicant	Strength	Appl No / Approval Date
	FLUOCINONIDE		
AB	LEMMON	0.05%	N73481 001 DEC 27, 1991
	LIDEX		
AB	+ SYNTEX	0.05%	N16909 002

SOLUTION; TOPICAL

	Product / Applicant	Strength	Appl No / Approval Date
	FLUOCINONIDE		
AT	BARRE	0.05%	N71535 001 DEC 02, 1988
AT	COPLEY PHARM	0.05%	N72522 001 SEP 28, 1990
AT	LEMMON	0.05%	N72511 001 FEB 07, 1989
AT	THAMES	0.05%	N72857 001 AUG 02, 1989
	LIDEX		
AT	+ SYNTEX	0.05%	N18849 001 APR 06, 1984

FLUORESCEIN SODIUM

INJECTABLE; INJECTION

	Product / Applicant	Strength	Appl No / Approval Date
	FUNDUSCEIN-25		
	+ IOLAB	25%	N17869 001

Prescription Drug Products *(continued)*

FLUOROMETHOLONE

OINTMENT; OPHTHALMIC

	FML		
	+ ALLERGAN	0.1%	N17760 001 SEP 04, 1985

SUSPENSION/DROPS; OPHTHALMIC

	FLUOR-OP		
AB	IOLAB	0.1%	N70185 001 FEB 27, 1986
	FML		
AB	+ ALLERGAN	0.1%	N16851 002 JUL 28, 1982
	FML FORTE		
	ALLERGAN	0.25%	N19216 001 APR 23, 1986

FLUOROMETHOLONE; SULFACETAMIDE SODIUM

SUSPENSION/DROPS; OPHTHALMIC

	FML-S		
	+ ALLERGAN	0.1%;10%	N19525 001 SEP 29, 1989

FLUOROMETHOLONE ACETATE

SUSPENSION/DROPS; OPHTHALMIC

	FLAREX		
	+ ALCON	0.1%	N19079 001 FEB 11, 1986

FLUOROMETHOLONE ACETATE; TOBRAMYCIN

SUSPENSION/DROPS; OPHTHALMIC

	TOBRASONE		
	+ ALCON	0.1%;0.3%	N50628 001 JUL 21, 1989

FLUOROURACIL

CREAM; TOPICAL

	EFUDEX		
	+ ROCHE	5%	N16831 003
	FLUOROPLEX		
	+ ALLERGAN HERBERT	1%	N16988 001

FLUOROURACIL *(continued)*

INJECTABLE; INJECTION

	ADRUCIL		
AP	+ PHARMACIA	50 MG/ML	N40023 001 OCT 18, 1991
AP		50 MG/ML	N81222 001 JUN 28, 1991
AP		50 MG/ML	N81225 001 AUG 28, 1991
	FLUOROURACIL		
AP	BEN VENUE	50 MG/ML	N89508 001 JAN 26, 1988
AP	ROCHE	50 MG/ML	N12209 001
AP	SMITH AND NEPHEW	50 MG/ML	N88767 001 DEC 28, 1984
AP		50 MG/ML	N89434 001 MAR 26, 1987
AP	STERIS	50 MG/ML	N87792 001 OCT 13, 1982

SOLUTION; TOPICAL

	EFUDEX		
	+ ROCHE	2%	N16831 001
	+	5%	N16831 002
	FLUOROPLEX		
	+ ALLERGAN HERBERT	1%	N16765 001

FLUOXETINE HYDROCHLORIDE

CAPSULE; ORAL

	PROZAC		
	LILLY	EQ 10 MG BASE	N18936 006 DEC 23, 1992
	+	EQ 20 MG BASE	N18936 001 DEC 29, 1987

SOLUTION; ORAL

	PROZAC		
	LILLY	EQ 20 MG BASE/5 ML	N20101 001 APR 24, 1991

FLUOXYMESTERONE

TABLET; ORAL

	FLUOXYMESTERONE		
BP	ROSEMONT PHARM	10 MG	N88342 001 OCT 21, 1983
	HALOTESTIN		
BP	+ UPJOHN	10 MG	N10611 010
		2 MG	N10611 002
		5 MG	N10611 006

Prescription Drug Products *(continued)*

FLUPHENAZINE DECANOATE

	INJECTABLE; INJECTION		
	FLUPHENAZINE DECANOATE		
A0	FUJISAWA	25 MG/ML	N71413 001 JUL 14, 1987
	PROLIXIN DECANOATE		
AO	+ APOTHECON	25 MG/ML	N16727 001

FLUPHENAZINE ENANTHATE

	INJECTABLE; INJECTION		
	PROLIXIN ENANTHATE		
	+ APOTHECON	25 MG/ML	N16110 001

FLUPHENAZINE HYDROCHLORIDE

	CONCENTRATE; ORAL		
	FLUPHENAZINE HCL		
AA	COPLEY PHARM	5 MG/ML	N73058 001 AUG 30, 1991
	PERMITIL		
AA	SCHERING	5 MG/ML	N16008 001
	PROLIXIN		
AA	APOTHECON	5 MG/ML	N70533 001 NOV 07, 1985
	ELIXIR; ORAL		
	FLUPHENAZINE HCL		
AA	COPLEY PHARM	2.5 MG/5 ML	N81310 001 APR 29, 1993
	PROLIXIN		
AA	APOTHECON	2.5 MG/5 ML	N12145 003
	INJECTABLE; INJECTION		
	FLUPHENAZINE HCL		
AP	FUJISAWA	2.5 MG/ML	N89556 001 APR 16, 1987
	PROLIXIN		
AP	+ APOTHECON	2.5 MG/ML	N11751 005
	TABLET; ORAL		
	FLUPHENAZINE HCL		
AB	GENEVA PHARMS	1 MG	N89583 001 OCT 16, 1987
AB		2.5 MG	N89584 001 OCT 16, 1987
AB		5 MG	N89585 001 OCT 16, 1987
AB		10 MG	N89586 001 OCT 16, 1987

FLUPHENAZINE HYDROCHLORIDE *(continued)*

	TABLET; ORAL		
	FLUPHENAZINE HCL		
AB	MYLAN	1 MG	N89801 001 AUG 12, 1988
AB		2.5 MG	N89802 001 AUG 12, 1988
AB		5 MG	N89803 001 AUG 12, 1988
AB		10 MG	N89804 001 AUG 12, 1988
AB	PAR PHARM	1 MG	N89740 001 AUG 25, 1988
AB		2.5 MG	N89741 001 AUG 25, 1988
AB		5 MG	N89742 001 AUG 25, 1988
AB		10 MG	N89743 001 AUG 25, 1988
	PERMITIL		
BP	SCHERING	2.5 MG	N12034 004
BP		5 MG	N12034 005
BP		10 MG	N12034 006
	PROLIXIN		
AB	APOTHECON	1 MG	N11751 004
AB		2.5 MG	N11751 001
AB		5 MG	N11751 003
AB	+	10 MG	N11751 002

FLURANDRENOLIDE

	CREAM; TOPICAL		
	CORDRAN SP		
	+ LILLY	0.025%	N12806 003
	+	0.05%	N12806 002
	LOTION; TOPICAL		
	CORDRAN		
AT	+ LILLY	0.05%	N13790 001
	FLURANDRENOLIDE		
AT	BARRE	0.05%	N87203 001 APR 29, 1982
	OINTMENT; TOPICAL		
	CORDRAN		
	+ LILLY	0.025%	N12806 004
	+	0.05%	N12806 001
	TAPE; TOPICAL		
	CORDRAN		
	+ LILLY	0.004 MG/SQ CM	N16455 001

Prescription Drug Products *(continued)*

FLURANDRENOLIDE; NEOMYCIN SULFATE

CREAM; TOPICAL

	CORDRAN-N		
	+ LILLY	0.05%;EQ 3.5 MG BASE/GM	N50346 001

OINTMENT; TOPICAL

	CORDRAN-N		
	+ LILLY	0.05%;EQ 3.5 MG BASE/GM	N50345 001

FLURAZEPAM HYDROCHLORIDE

CAPSULE; ORAL

	DALMANE		
AB	ROCHE	15 MG	N16721 001
AB	+	30 MG	N16721 002
	FLURAZEPAM HCL		
AB	BARR	15 MG	N70454 001 AUG 04, 1986
AB		30 MG	N70455 001 AUG 04, 1986
AB	CHELSEA LABS	15 MG	N72368 001 MAR 30, 1989
AB		30 MG	N72369 001 MAR 30, 1989
AB	DANBURY PHARMA	15 MG	N71205 001 NOV 25, 1986
AB		30 MG	N71068 001 NOV 25, 1986
AB	GENEVA PHARMS	15 MG	N71716 001 JUL 31, 1991
AB		30 MG	N71717 001 JUL 31, 1991
AB	HALSEY	15 MG	N71808 001 JAN 07, 1988
AB		30 MG	N71809 001 JAN 07, 1988
AB	MYLAN	15 MG	N70344 001 NOV 27, 1985
AB		30 MG	N70345 001 NOV 27, 1985
AB	PAR PHARM	15 MG	N70444 001 MAR 20, 1986
AB		30 MG	N70445 001 MAR 20, 1986
AB	PUREPAC PHARM	15 MG	N71927 001 SEP 09, 1987
AB		30 MG	N71551 001 SEP 09, 1987
AB	SUPERPHARM	15 MG	N71659 001 AUG 04, 1988
AB		30 MG	N71660 001 AUG 04, 1988

FLURAZEPAM HYDROCHLORIDE *(continued)*

CAPSULE; ORAL

	FLURAZEPAM HCL		
AB	WARNER CHILCOTT	15 MG	N71767 001 DEC 04, 1987
AB		30 MG	N71768 001 DEC 04, 1987
AB	WEST WARD PHARM	15 MG	N71107 001 DEC 08, 1986
AB		30 MG	N71108 001 DEC 08, 1986

FLURBIPROFEN

TABLET; ORAL

	ANSAID		
AB	UPJOHN	50 MG	N18766 002 OCT 31, 1988
AB	+	100 MG	N18766 003 OCT 31, 1988
	FLURBIPROFEN		
AB	MYLAN	50 MG	N74358 001 JUN 20, 1994
AB		100 MG	N74358 002 JUN 20, 1994

FLURBIPROFEN SODIUM

SOLUTION/DROPS; OPHTHALMIC

	OCUFEN		
	+ ALLERGAN	0.03%	N19404 001 DEC 31, 1986

FLUTAMIDE

CAPSULE; ORAL

	EULEXIN		
	+ SCHERING	125 MG	N18554 001 JAN 27, 1989

FLUTICASONE PROPIONATE

CREAM; TOPICAL

	CUTIVATE		
	+ GLAXO	0.05%	N19958 001 DEC 18, 1990

OINTMENT; TOPICAL

	CUTIVATE		
	+ GLAXO	0.005%	N19957 001 DEC 14, 1990

Prescription Drug Products *(continued)*

FLUVASTATIN SODIUM

	CAPSULE; ORAL		
	LESCOL		
	SANDOZ	EQ 20 MG BASE	N20261 001 DEC 31, 1993
	+	EQ 40 MG BASE	N20261 002 DEC 31, 1993

FOLIC ACID

	INJECTABLE; INJECTION		
	FOLIC ACID		
AP	FUJISAWA	5 MG/ML	N89202 001 FEB 18, 1986
AP	LOCH	5 MG/ML	N81066 001 DEC 29, 1993
	FOLVITE		
AP	+ LEDERLE	5 MG/ML	N05897 008
	TABLET; ORAL		
	FOLIC ACID		
AA	DANBURY PHARMA	1 MG	N80680 001
AA	GLOBAL PHARMS	1 MG	N80686 001
AA	HALSEY	1 MG	N83598 001
AA	ICN	1 MG	N80903 001
AA	MK LABS	1 MG	N83526 001
AA	PRIVATE FORM	1 MG	N85061 001
AA	TABLICAPS	1 MG	N83133 002
AA	VINTAGE PHARMS	1 MG	N86296 001
AA	WEST WARD PHARM	1 MG	N80600 001
AA	ZENITH LABS	1 MG	N83000 001
	FOLICET		
AA	MISSION PHARMA	1 MG	N87438 001
	FOLVITE		
AA	LEDERLE	1 MG	N05897 004

FOLIC ACID; *MULTIPLE*

SEE ASCORBIC ACID; BIOTIN; CYANOCOBALAMIN; DEXPANTHENOL; ERGOCALCIFEROL; FOLIC ACID; NIACINAMIDE; PYRIDOXINE HYDROCHLORIDE; RIBOFLAVIN PHOSPHATE SODIUM; THIAMINE HYDROCHLORIDE; VITAMIN A; VITAMIN E

SEE ASCORBIC ACID; BIOTIN; CYANOCOBALAMIN; ERGOCALCIFEROL; FOLIC ACID; NIACINAMIDE; PANTOTHENIC ACID; PHYTONADIONE; PYRIDOXINE; RIBOFLAVIN; THIAMINE; VITAMIN A PALMITATE; VITAMIN E

FOSCARNET SODIUM

	INJECTABLE; INJECTION		
	FOSCAVIR		
	+ ASTRA	24 MG/ML	N20068 001 SEP 27, 1991

FOSINOPRIL SODIUM

	TABLET; ORAL		
	MONOPRIL		
	BRISTOL MYERS SQUIBB	10 MG	N19915 002 MAY 16, 1991
	+	20 MG	N19915 003 MAY 16, 1991

FURAZOLIDONE

	SUSPENSION; ORAL		
	FUROXONE		
	+ ROBERTS LABS	50 MG/15 ML	N11323 002
	TABLET; ORAL		
	FUROXONE		
	+ ROBERTS LABS	100 MG	N11270 002

FUROSEMIDE

	INJECTABLE; INJECTION		
	FUROSEMIDE		
AP	ABBOTT	10 MG/ML	N18667 001 MAY 28, 1982
AP	ASTRA	10 MG/ML	N70095 001 SEP 09, 1985
AP		10 MG/ML	N70096 001 SEP 09, 1985
AP	ELKINS SINN	10 MG/ML	N18267 001
AP	FUJISAWA	10 MG/ML	N18902 001 MAY 22, 1984
AP	INTL MEDICATION	10 MG/ML	N18025 001
AP	LEDERLE	10 MG/ML	N71439 001 SEP 14, 1990
AP	LUITPOLD	10 MG/ML	N18579 001 NOV 30, 1983
AP	MARSAM	10 MG/ML	N74017 001 JUN 30, 1994
AP	SMITH AND NEPHEW	10 MG/ML	N70078 001 FEB 05, 1986
AP	STERIS	10 MG/ML	N70019 001 SEP 22, 1986
AP		10 MG/ML	N70604 001 JAN 02, 1987

Prescription Drug Products *(continued)*

FUROSEMIDE *(continued)*

INJECTABLE; INJECTION

	FUROSEMIDE		
AP	STERLING WINTHROP	10 MG/ML	N70578 001 JUL 08, 1987
AP		10 MG/ML	N72080 001 AUG 13, 1991
	LASIX		
AP	+ HOECHST ROUSSEL	10 MG/ML	N16363 001

SOLUTION; ORAL

	FUROSEMIDE		
AA	PENNEX	10 MG/ML	N70655 001 OCT 02, 1987
AA	ROXANE	10 MG/ML	N70434 001 APR 22, 1987
		40 MG/5 ML	N70433 001 APR 22, 1987
	LASIX		
AA	HOECHST ROUSSEL	10 MG/ML	N17688 001

TABLET; ORAL

	FUROSEMIDE		
AB	BARR	20 MG	N70043 001 SEP 26, 1985
AB		40 MG	N18790 001 NOV 29, 1983
AB		80 MG	N70100 001 JAN 26, 1988
AB	DANBURY PHARMA	20 MG	N70412 001 FEB 26, 1986
AB		40 MG	N70413 001 FEB 26, 1986
AB		80 MG	N71594 001 FEB 09, 1988
AB	GENEVA PHARMS	20 MG	N18569 002
AB		40 MG	N18569 001
AB		80 MG	N18569 005 AUG 14, 1984
AB	INTL MEDICATION	20 MG	N18753 001 FEB 28, 1984
AB		40 MG	N18753 002 FEB 28, 1984
AB	KALAPHARM	20 MG	N18868 001 JUN 28, 1983
AB		40 MG	N18868 002 JUN 28, 1983
AB	LEDERLE	20 MG	N18415 001 JUL 27, 1982
AB		40 MG	N18415 002 JUL 27, 1982
AB		80 MG	N18415 003 NOV 26, 1984

FUROSEMIDE *(continued)*

TABLET; ORAL

	FUROSEMIDE		
AB	MYLAN	20 MG	N18487 001
AB		40 MG	N18487 002
AB		80 MG	N70082 001 OCT 29, 1986
AB	ROXANE	20 MG	N18823 001 NOV 10, 1983
AB		40 MG	N18823 002 NOV 10, 1983
AB		80 MG	N70086 001 JAN 24, 1986
AB	SUPERPHARM	20 MG	N18370 002 JUN 26, 1984
AB		40 MG	N18370 001 FEB 10, 1983
AB	WATSON LABS	20 MG	N70449 001 NOV 22, 1985
AB		20 MG	N71379 001 JAN 02, 1987
AB		40 MG	N70450 001 NOV 22, 1985
AB		80 MG	N70528 001 JAN 07, 1986
AB	ZENITH LABS	20 MG	N18413 001 NOV 30, 1983
AB		40 MG	N18413 002 NOV 30, 1983
	LASIX		
AB	HOECHST ROUSSEL	20 MG	N16273 002
AB		40 MG	N16273 001
AB	+	80 MG	N16273 003

GABAPENTIN

CAPSULE; ORAL

	NEURONTIN		
	PARKE DAVIS	100 MG	N20235 001 DEC 30, 1993
		300 MG	N20235 002 DEC 30, 1993
	+	400 MG	N20235 003 DEC 30, 1993

GADODIAMIDE

INJECTABLE; INJECTION

	OMNISCAN		
	STERLING WINTHROP	287 MG/ML	N20123 001 JAN 08, 1993

Prescription Drug Products *(continued)*

GADOPENTETATE DIMEGLUMINE

	INJECTABLE; INJECTION		
	MAGNEVIST		
	+ BERLEX	469.01 MG/ML	N19596 001 JUN 02, 1988

GADOTERIDOL

	INJECTABLE; INJECTION		
	PROHANCE		
	BRACCO	279.3 MG/ML	N20131 001 NOV 16, 1992

GALLAMINE TRIETHIODIDE

	INJECTABLE; INJECTION		
	FLAXEDIL		
	+ DAVIS AND GECK	20 MG/ML	N07842 001
	+	100 MG/ML	N07842 002

GALLIUM CITRATE, GA-67

	INJECTABLE; INJECTION		
	GALLIUM CITRATE GA 67		
BS	DUPONT	2mCi/ML	N17478 001
BS	MALLINCKRODT	2mCi/ML	N18058 001
	NEOSCAN		
BS	MEDI PHYSICS	2mCi/ML	N17655 001

GALLIUM NITRATE

	INJECTABLE; INJECTION		
	GANITE		
	+ FUJISAWA	25 MG/ML	N19961 002 JAN 17, 1991

GANCICLOVIR SODIUM

	INJECTABLE; INJECTION		
	CYTOVENE		
	+ SYNTEX	EQ 500 MG BASE/VIAL	N19661 001 JUN 23, 1989

GEMFIBROZIL

	CAPSULE; ORAL		
	GEMFIBROZIL		
AB	MYLAN	300 MG	N73466 001 JAN 25, 1993
AB	PUREPAC PHARM	300 MG	N72929 001 JAN 29, 1993

GEMFIBROZIL *(continued)*

	CAPSULE; ORAL		
	LOPID		
AB	+ PARKE DAVIS	300 MG	N18422 002
	TABLET; ORAL		
	GEMFIBROZIL		
AB	LEDERLE	600 MG	N74270 001 SEP 27, 1993
AB	LEMMON	600 MG	N74256 001 OCT 31, 1993
AB	PUREPAC PHARM	600 MG	N74360 001 AUG 31, 1994
	LOPID		
AB	+ PARKE DAVIS	600 MG	N18422 003 NOV 20, 1986

GENTAMICIN SULFATE

	CREAM; TOPICAL		
	GARAMYCIN		
AT	+ SCHERING	EQ 0.1% BASE	N60462 001
	GENTAMICIN		
AT	CLAY PARK	EQ 0.1% BASE	N62307 001
	GENTAMICIN SULFATE		
AT	BAUSCH AND LOMB	EQ 0.1% BASE	N64056 001 APR 29, 1994
AT	FOUGERA	EQ 0.1% BASE	N62531 001 JUL 05, 1984
AT	NMC	EQ 0.1% BASE	N62471 001 SEP 27, 1983
AT	THAMES	EQ 0.1% BASE	N62427 001 MAY 26, 1983
	INJECTABLE; INJECTION		
	APOGEN		
AP	KING PHARMS	EQ 10 MG BASE/ML	N62289 001
AP		EQ 40 MG BASE/ML	N62289 002
	BRISTAGEN		
AP	BRISTOL	EQ 40 MG BASE/ML	N62288 001
	GARAMYCIN		
AP	+ SCHERING	EQ 1 MG BASE/ML	N61716 002
AP	+	EQ 10 MG BASE/ML	N61739 001
AP	+	EQ 40 MG BASE/ML	N61716 001
	GENTAFAIR		
AP	PHARMAFAIR	EQ 40 MG BASE/ML	N62493 001 AUG 28, 1985
	GENTAMICIN		
AP	INTL MEDICATION	EQ 1 MG BASE/ML	N62325 003 JUN 23, 1982
AP		EQ 100 MG BASE/100 ML	N62325 004 JUN 23, 1982
AP		EQ 40 MG BASE/ML	N62325 001

Prescription Drug Products *(continued)*

GENTAMICIN SULFATE *(continued)*

INJECTABLE; INJECTION

GENTAMICIN SULFATE

AP	ABBOTT	EQ 60 MG BASE/100 ML	N62413 006 AUG 11, 1983
AP		EQ 70 MG BASE/100 ML	N62413 007 AUG 11, 1983
AP		EQ 80 MG BASE/100 ML	N62413 008 AUG 11, 1983
AP		EQ 90 MG BASE/100 ML	N62413 009 AUG 11, 1983
AP		EQ 100 MG BASE/100 ML	N62413 010 AUG 11, 1983
AP		EQ 1.2 MG BASE/ML	N62413 001 AUG 11, 1983
AP		EQ 1.4 MG BASE/ML	N62413 002 AUG 11, 1983
AP		EQ 1.6 MG BASE/ML	N62413 003 AUG 11, 1983
AP		EQ 1.8 MG BASE/ML	N62413 004 AUG 11, 1983
AP		EQ 2 MG BASE/ML	N62413 005 AUG 11, 1983
AP		EQ 10 MG BASE/ML	N62420 001 AUG 15, 1983
AP		EQ 10 MG BASE/ML	N62612 004 FEB 20, 1986
AP		EQ 40 MG BASE/ML	N62420 002 AUG 15, 1983
AP	ELKINS SINN	EQ 10 MG BASE/ML	N62251 002
AP		EQ 40 MG BASE/ML	N62251 001
AP	FUJISAWA	EQ 10 MG BASE/ML	N62356 001 MAR 04, 1982
AP		EQ 40 MG BASE/ML	N62356 002 MAR 04, 1982
AP		EQ 40 MG BASE/ML	N62366 001 AUG 04, 1983
AP	GENSIA	EQ 10 MG BASE/ML	N63149 001 NOV 21, 1991
AP		EQ 40 MG BASE/ML	N63106 002 NOV 21, 1991
AP	KALAPHARM	EQ 40 MG BASE/ML	N62354 001 APR 05, 1982
AP	PHARM SPECLTS ASSOC	EQ 40 MG BASE/ML	N62340 001 MAR 28, 1983
AP	SOLOPAK	EQ 10 MG BASE/ML	N62507 001 JUN 06, 1985
AP		EQ 40 MG BASE/ML	N62507 002 JUN 06, 1985
AP	STERIS	EQ 10 MG BASE/ML	N62318 002
AP		EQ 40 MG BASE/ML	N62318 001

GENTAMICIN SULFATE *(continued)*

INJECTABLE; INJECTION

GENTAMICIN SULFATE IN SODIUM CHLORIDE 0.9% IN PLASTIC CONTAINER

AP	ABBOTT	EQ 60 MG BASE/100 ML	N62414 006 AUG 15, 1983
AP		EQ 70 MG BASE/100 ML	N62414 007 AUG 15, 1983
AP		EQ 80 MG BASE/100 ML	N62414 008 AUG 15, 1983
AP		EQ 90 MG BASE/100 ML	N62414 009 AUG 15, 1983
AP		EQ 100 MG BASE/100 ML	N62414 010 AUG 15, 1983
AP		EQ 1.2 MG BASE/ML	N62414 001 AUG 15, 1983
AP		EQ 1.4 MG BASE/ML	N62414 002 AUG 15, 1983
AP		EQ 1.6 MG BASE/ML	N62414 003 AUG 15, 1983
AP		EQ 1.8 MG BASE/ML	N62414 004 AUG 15, 1983
AP		EQ 2 MG BASE/ML	N62414 005 AUG 15, 1983
AP	MCGAW	EQ 40 MG BASE/100 ML	N62814 008 AUG 28, 1987
AP		EQ 60 MG BASE/100 ML	N62814 009 AUG 28, 1987
AP		EQ 70 MG BASE/100 ML	N62814 010 AUG 28, 1987
AP		EQ 0.8 MG BASE/ML	N62814 001 AUG 28, 1987
AP		EQ 80 MG BASE/100 ML	N62814 011 AUG 28, 1987
AP		EQ 90 MG BASE/100 ML	N62814 012 AUG 28, 1987
AP		EQ 100 MG BASE/100 ML	N62814 013 AUG 28, 1987
AP		EQ 1.2 MG BASE/ML	N62814 002 AUG 28, 1987
AP		EQ 120 MG BASE/100 ML	N62814 014 AUG 28, 1987
AP		EQ 1.4 MG BASE/ML	N62814 003 AUG 28, 1987
AP		EQ 1.6 MG BASE/ML	N62814 004 AUG 28, 1987
AP		EQ 1.8 MG BASE/ML	N62814 005 AUG 28, 1987
AP		EQ 2 MG BASE/ML	N62814 006 AUG 28, 1987
AP		EQ 2.4 MG BASE/ML	N62814 007 AUG 28, 1987

Prescription Drug Products *(continued)*

GENTAMICIN SULFATE *(continued)*

	INJECTABLE; INJECTION		
	ISOTONIC GENTAMICIN SULFATE IN PLASTIC CONTAINER		
AP	BAXTER	EQ 40 MG BASE/100 ML	N62373 003 SEP 07, 1982
AP		EQ 60 MG BASE/100 ML	N62373 004 SEP 07, 1982
AP		EQ 0.8 MG BASE/ML	N62373 001 SEP 07, 1982
AP		EQ 80 MG BASE/100 ML	N62373 002 SEP 07, 1982
AP		EQ 100 MG BASE/100 ML	N62373 005 SEP 07, 1982
AP		EQ 120 MG BASE/100 ML	N62373 006 SEP 07, 1982
AP		EQ 1.2 MG BASE/ML	N62373 007 SEP 07, 1982
AP		EQ 1.6 MG BASE/ML	N62373 008 SEP 07, 1982
AP		EQ 2 MG BASE/ML	N62373 009 SEP 07, 1982
AP		EQ 2.4 MG BASE/ML	N62373 010 SEP 07, 1982
	U-GENCIN		
AP	UPJOHN	EQ 10 MG BASE/ML	N62248 001
AP		EQ 40 MG BASE/ML	N62248 002
	INJECTABLE; INTRATHECAL		
	GARAMYCIN		
	+ SCHERING	EQ 2 MG BASE/ML	N50505 001
	OINTMENT; OPHTHALMIC		
	GARAMYCIN		
AT	+ SCHERING	EQ 0.3% BASE	N50425 001
	GENTACIDIN		
AT	IOLAB	EQ 0.3% BASE	N62501 001 JUL 26, 1984
	OINTMENT; TOPICAL		
	GARAMYCIN		
AT	+ SCHERING	EQ 0.1% BASE	N60463 001
	GENTAMICIN		
AT	CLAY PARK	EQ 0.1% BASE	N62351 001 FEB 18, 1982
	GENTAMICIN SULFATE		
AT	BAUSCH AND LOMB	EQ 0.1% BASE	N64054 001 APR 29, 1994
AT	FOUGERA	EQ 0.1% BASE	N62533 001 OCT 05, 1984
AT	NMC	EQ 0.1% BASE	N62496 001 MAR 14, 1984
AT	PHARMADERM	EQ 0.1% BASE	N62534 001 OCT 10, 1984

GENTAMICIN SULFATE *(continued)*

	OINTMENT; TOPICAL		
	GENTAMICIN SULFATE		
AT	THAMES	EQ 0.1% BASE	N62477 001 DEC 23, 1983
	SOLUTION/DROPS; OPHTHALMIC		
	GARAMYCIN		
AT	+ SCHERING	EQ 0.3% BASE	N50039 002
	GENOPTIC		
AT	ALLERGAN	EQ 0.3% BASE	N62452 001 OCT 10, 1984
	GENTACIDIN		
AT	IOLAB	EQ 0.3% BASE	N62480 001 MAR 30, 1984
	GENTAMICIN SULFATE		
AT	AKORN	EQ 0.3% BASE	N62635 001 JAN 08, 1987
AT	BAUSCH AND LOMB	EQ 0.3% BASE	N64048 001 MAY 11, 1994
AT	STERIS	EQ 0.3% BASE	N62523 001 NOV 25, 1985

GENTAMICIN SULFATE; PREDNISOLONE ACETATE

	OINTMENT; OPHTHALMIC		
	PRED-G		
	+ ALLERGAN	EQ 0.3% BASE;0.6%	N50612 001 DEC 01, 1989
	SUSPENSION/DROPS; OPHTHALMIC		
	PRED-G		
	+ ALLERGAN	EQ 0.3% BASE;1%	N50586 001 JUN 10, 1988

GENTIAN VIOLET

	SUPPOSITORY; VAGINAL		
	GVS		
	+ SAVAGE LABS	0.4%	N83513 001

GLIPIZIDE

	TABLET; ORAL		
	GLIPIZIDE		
AB	MYLAN	5 MG	N74226 001 MAY 10, 1994
AB		10 MG	N74226 002 MAY 10, 1994

Prescription Drug Products *(continued)*

GLIPIZIDE *(continued)*

TABLET; ORAL
GLUCOTROL

AB	PFIZER	5 MG	N17783 001 MAY 08, 1984
AB	+	10 MG	N17783 002 MAY 08, 1984
		2.5 MG	N17783 003 MAY 11, 1993

TABLET, EXTENDED RELEASE; ORAL
GLUCOTROL XL

	+ PFIZER	5 MG	N20329 001 APR 26, 1994
	+	10 MG	N20329 002 APR 26, 1994

GLUCAGON HYDROCHLORIDE

INJECTABLE; INJECTION
GLUCAGON

	+ LILLY	EQ 1 MG BASE/VIAL	N12122 001
		EQ 10 MG BASE/VIAL	N12122 002

GLUCONOLACTONE; *MULTIPLE*

SEE CITRIC ACID; GLUCONOLACTONE; MAGNESIUM CARBONATE

GLUTATHIONE DISULFIDE; *MULTIPLE*

SEE CALCIUM CHLORIDE; DEXTROSE; GLUTATHIONE DISULFIDE; MAGNESIUM CHLORIDE; POTASSIUM CHLORIDE; SODIUM BICARBONATE; SODIUM CHLORIDE; SODIUM PHOSPHATE

GLUTETHIMIDE

TABLET; ORAL
GLUTETHIMIDE

AA	DANBURY PHARMA	500 MG	N84362 001
AA	GENEVA PHARMS	500 MG	N83234 002
AA	HALSEY	500 MG	N89459 001 OCT 10, 1986
		250 MG	N89458 001 OCT 10, 1986
AA	MD PHARM	500 MG	N85171 001

GLYBURIDE

TABLET; ORAL
DIABETA

BX	HOECHST ROUSSEL	1.25 MG	N17532 001 MAY 01, 1984
BX		2.5 MG	N17532 002 MAY 01, 1984
BX		5 MG	N17532 003 MAY 01, 1984

GLYNASE

	UPJOHN	1.5 MG	N20051 001 MAR 04, 1992
		3 MG	N20051 002 MAR 04, 1992
		4.5 MG	N20051 003 SEP 24, 1993
	+	6 MG	N20051 004 SEP 24, 1993

MICRONASE

BX	UPJOHN	1.25 MG	N17498 001 MAY 01, 1984
BX		2.5 MG	N17498 002 MAY 01, 1984
BX	+	5 MG	N17498 003 MAY 01, 1984

GLYCERIN; *MULTIPLE*

SEE AMINO ACIDS; CALCIUM ACETATE; GLYCERIN; MAGNESIUM ACETATE; PHOSPHORIC ACID; POTASSIUM CHLORIDE; SODIUM ACETATE; SODIUM CHLORIDE

GLYCINE

SOLUTION; IRRIGATION
AMINOACETIC ACID 1.5% IN PLASTIC CONTAINER

AT	BAXTER	1.5 GM/100 ML	N17865 001

GLYCINE 1.5% IN PLASTIC CONTAINER

AT	ABBOTT	1.5 GM/100 ML	N17633 001
AT		1.5 GM/100 ML	N18315 001
AT	BAXTER	1.5 GM/100 ML	N18522 001 FEB 19, 1982
AT	MCGAW	1.5 GM/100 ML	N16784 001

Prescription Drug Products *(continued)*

GLYCOPYRROLATE

	INJECTABLE; INJECTION		
	GLYCOPYRROLATE		
AP	ABBOTT	0.2 MG/ML	N89393 001 JUN 15, 1988
AP	GENSIA	0.2 MG/ML	N81169 001 SEP 10, 1991
AP	LUITPOLD	0.2 MG/ML	N89335 001 JUL 23, 1986
AP	STERIS	0.2 MG/ML	N86947 001 JUN 24, 1983
	ROBINUL		
AP	+ ROBINS AH	0.2 MG/ML	N17558 001
	TABLET; ORAL		
	GLYCOPYRROLATE		
AA	DANBURY PHARMA	1 MG	N86902 001
AA		2 MG	N86900 001
	ROBINUL		
AA	ROBINS AH	1 MG	N12827 001
	ROBINUL FORTE		
AA	ROBINS AH	2 MG	N12827 002

GONADORELIN ACETATE

	INJECTABLE; INJECTION		
	LUTREPULSE KIT		
	+ FERRING LABS	0.8 MG/VIAL	N19687 001 OCT 10, 1989
	+	3.2 MG/VIAL	N19687 002 OCT 10, 1989

GONADORELIN HYDROCHLORIDE

	INJECTABLE; INJECTION		
	FACTREL		
	WYETH AYERST	EQ 0.1 MG BASE/VIAL	N18123 001 SEP 30, 1982
		EQ 0.5 MG BASE/VIAL	N18123 003 SEP 30, 1982

GONADOTROPIN, CHORIONIC

	INJECTABLE; INJECTION		
	A.P.L.		
AP	+ WYETH AYERST	5,000 UNITS/VIAL	N17055 001
AP	+	10,000 UNITS/VIAL	N17055 002
AP	+	20,000 UNITS/VIAL	N17055 003
	CHORIONIC GONADOTROPIN		
AP	FUJISAWA	10,000 UNITS/VIAL	N17067 002
AP	STERIS	5,000 UNITS/VIAL	N17016 006
AP		10,000 UNITS/VIAL	N17016 007
AP		20,000 UNITS/VIAL	N17016 004
	+	2,000 UNITS/VIAL	N17016 011 FEB 16, 1990
	+	15,000 UNITS/VIAL	N17016 010 FEB 15, 1985
	PREGNYL		
AP	ORGANON	10,000 UNITS/VIAL	N17692 001

GOSERELIN ACETATE

	IMPLANT; IMPLANTATION		
	ZOLADEX		
	+ ZENECA	EQ 3.6 MG BASE	N19726 001 DEC 29, 1989

GRAMICIDIN; NEOMYCIN SULFATE; POLYMYXIN B SULFATE

	SOLUTION/DROPS; OPHTHALMIC		
	NEOMYCIN AND POLYMYXIN B SULFATES AND GRAMICIDIN		
AT	IPHARM	0.025 MG/ML;EQ 1.75 MG BASE/ML;10,000 UNITS/ML	N62818 001 OCT 11, 1988
AT	STERIS	0.025 MG/ML;EQ 1.75 MG BASE/ML;10,000 UNITS/ML	N62788 001 JUN 11, 1987
	NEOSPORIN		
AT	+ BURROUGHS WELLCOME	0.025 MG/ML;EQ 1.75 MG BASE/ML;10,000 UNITS/ML	N60582 001

GRANISETRON HYDROCHLORIDE

	INJECTABLE; INJECTION		
	KYTRIL		
	+ SMITHKLINE BEECHAM	EQ 1 MG BASE/ML	N20239 002 MAR 11, 1994

Prescription Drug Products *(continued)*

GRISEOFULVIN, MICROCRYSTALLINE

	CAPSULE; ORAL		
	GRISACTIN		
	+ WYETH AYERST	250 MG	N50051 001
	SUSPENSION; ORAL		
	GRIFULVIN V		
	+ JOHNSON RW	125 MG/5 ML	N50448 001
		125 MG/5 ML	N62483 001 JAN 26, 1984
	TABLET; ORAL		
	FULVICIN-U/F		
AB	SCHERING	250 MG	N60569 002
AB	+	500 MG	N60569 001
	GRIFULVIN V		
AB	JOHNSON RW	250 MG	N60618 002
AB		250 MG	N62279 002
AB		500 MG	N60618 003
AB		500 MG	N62279 003
		125 MG	N60618 001
		125 MG	N62279 001
	GRISACTIN		
AB	WYETH AYERST	500 MG	N60212 001

GRISEOFULVIN, ULTRAMICROCRYSTALLINE

	TABLET; ORAL		
	FULVICIN P/G		
AB	+ SCHERING	125 MG	N61996 001
AB	+	250 MG	N61996 002
	FULVICIN P/G 165		
AB	+ SCHERING	165 MG	N61996 003 APR 06, 1982
	FULVICIN P/G 330		
AB	+ SCHERING	330 MG	N61996 004 APR 06, 1982
	GRIS-PEG		
AB	ALLERGAN HERBERT	125 MG	N50475 001
AB		250 MG	N50475 002
	GRISACTIN ULTRA		
AB	WYETH AYERST	125 MG	N62178 001
AB		165 MG	N62438 001 NOV 17, 1983
AB		250 MG	N62178 002
AB		330 MG	N62438 002 NOV 17, 1983
	ULTRAGRIS-165		
AB	SIDMAK LABS NJ	165 MG	N62645 001 JUN 30, 1992
	ULTRAGRIS-330		
AB	SIDMAK LABS NJ	330 MG	N62646 001 JUN 30, 1992

GUANABENZ ACETATE

	TABLET; ORAL		
	GUANABENZ ACETATE		
AB	COPLEY PHARM	EQ 4 MG BASE	N74267 001 JUN 01, 1994
AB		EQ 8 MG BASE	N74267 002 JUN 01, 1994
AB	WATSON LABS	EQ 4 MG BASE	N74025 001 FEB 28, 1994
AB		EQ 8 MG BASE	N74025 002 FEB 28, 1994
	WYTENSIN		
AB	WYETH AYERST	EQ 4 MG BASE	N18587 001 SEP 07, 1982
AB	+	EQ 8 MG BASE	N18587 002 SEP 07, 1982

GUANADREL SULFATE

	TABLET; ORAL		
	HYLOREL		
	UPJOHN	10 MG	N18104 001 DEC 29, 1982
	+	25 MG	N18104 002 DEC 29, 1982

GUANETHIDINE MONOSULFATE

	TABLET; ORAL		
	ISMELIN		
	CIBA	EQ 10 MG SULFATE	N12329 001
	+	EQ 25 MG SULFATE	N12329 002

GUANETHIDINE MONOSULFATE; HYDROCHLOROTHIAZIDE

	TABLET; ORAL		
	ESIMIL		
	CIBA	10 MG;25 MG	N13553 001

GUANFACINE HYDROCHLORIDE

	TABLET; ORAL		
	TENEX		
	ROBINS AH	1 MG	N19032 001 OCT 27, 1986
		2 MG	N19032 002 NOV 07, 1988

GUANIDINE HYDROCHLORIDE

	TABLET; ORAL		
	GUANIDINE HCL		
	SCHERING	125 MG	N01546 001

Prescription Drug Products *(continued)*

HALAZEPAM

TABLET; ORAL

	PAXIPAM		
	SCHERING	20 MG	N17736 003
	+	40 MG	N17736 004

HALCINONIDE

CREAM; TOPICAL

	HALOG		
AT	+ WESTWOOD SQUIBB	0.1%	N17556 001
		0.025%	N17818 001
	HALOG-E		
AT	WESTWOOD SQUIBB	0.1%	N18234 001

OINTMENT; TOPICAL

	HALOG		
	+ WESTWOOD SQUIBB	0.1%	N17824 001

SOLUTION; TOPICAL

	HALOG		
	WESTWOOD SQUIBB	0.1%	N17823 001

HALOBETASOL PROPIONATE

CREAM; TOPICAL

	ULTRAVATE		
	+ WESTWOOD SQUIBB	0.05%	N19967 001 DEC 27, 1990

OINTMENT; TOPICAL

	ULTRAVATE		
	+ WESTWOOD SQUIBB	0.05%	N19968 001 DEC 17, 1990

HALOPERIDOL

TABLET; ORAL

	HALDOL		
AB	JOHNSON RW	0.5 MG	N15921 001
AB		1 MG	N15921 002
AB		2 MG	N15921 003
AB	+	5 MG	N15921 004
AB		10 MG	N15921 005
AB	+	20 MG	N15921 006 FEB 02, 1982

HALOPERIDOL *(continued)*

TABLET; ORAL

	HALOPERIDOL		
AB	BARR	0.5 MG	N71156 001 JAN 02, 1987
AB		1 MG	N71157 001 JAN 02, 1987
AB		2 MG	N71172 001 JAN 02, 1987
AB		5 MG	N71212 001 JAN 07, 1988
AB		10 MG	N71173 001 JAN 07, 1988
AB		20 MG	N71177 001 JAN 07, 1988
AB	DANBURY PHARMA	0.5 MG	N70981 001 MAR 06, 1987
AB		1 MG	N70982 001 MAR 06, 1987
AB		2 MG	N70983 001 MAR 06, 1987
AB		5 MG	N70984 001 MAR 06, 1987
AB		10 MG	N72113 001 AUG 27, 1991
AB		20 MG	N72353 001 AUG 27, 1991
AB	GENEVA PHARMS	0.5 MG	N71206 001 NOV 17, 1986
AB		1 MG	N71207 001 NOV 17, 1986
AB		2 MG	N71208 001 NOV 17, 1986
AB		5 MG	N71209 001 NOV 17, 1986
AB		10 MG	N71210 001 MAR 11, 1988
AB		20 MG	N71211 001 MAR 11, 1988
AB	MYLAN	0.5 MG	N70276 001 JUN 10, 1986
AB		1 MG	N70277 001 JUN 10, 1986
AB		2 MG	N70278 001 JUN 10, 1986
AB		5 MG	N70279 001 JUN 10, 1986

Prescription Drug Products *(continued)*

HALOPERIDOL *(continued)*

TABLET; ORAL

HALOPERIDOL

AB	PAR PHARM	0.5 MG	N71233 001 NOV 03, 1986
AB		1 MG	N71234 001 NOV 03, 1986
AB		2 MG	N71235 001 NOV 03, 1986
AB		5 MG	N71236 001 NOV 03, 1986
AB		10 MG	N71237 001 JUL 20, 1987
AB	PUREPAC PHARM	0.5 MG	N71071 001 NOV 03, 1986
AB		1 MG	N71072 001 NOV 03, 1986
AB		2 MG	N71073 001 NOV 03, 1986
AB		5 MG	N71074 001 NOV 03, 1986
AB		10 MG	N71075 001 AUG 04, 1987
AB		20 MG	N71076 001 AUG 04, 1987
AB	ROXANE	0.5 MG	N71128 001 FEB 17, 1987
AB		1 MG	N71129 001 FEB 17, 1987
AB		2 MG	N71130 001 FEB 17, 1987
AB		5 MG	N71131 001 FEB 17, 1987
AB		10 MG	N71132 001 MAY 12, 1987
AB		20 MG	N71133 001 MAY 12, 1987
AB	SCS	0.5 MG	N70720 001 JUN 10, 1986
AB		1 MG	N70721 001 JUN 10, 1986
AB		2 MG	N70722 001 JUN 10, 1986
AB		5 MG	N70723 001 JUN 10, 1986
AB		10 MG	N70724 001 JUN 10, 1986
AB		20 MG	N70725 001 SEP 24, 1986

HALOPERIDOL DECANOATE

INJECTABLE; INJECTION

HALDOL DECANOATE 50

	+ JOHNSON RW	EQ 50 MG BASE/ML	N18701 001 JAN 14, 1986

HALOPERIDOL LACTATE

CONCENTRATE; ORAL

	HALDOL		
AA	JOHNSON RW	EQ 2 MG BASE/ML	N15922 001
	HALOPERIDOL		
AA	BARRE	EQ 2 MG BASE/ML	N70318 001 APR 11, 1986
AA	COPLEY PHARM	EQ 2 MG BASE/ML	N71617 001 DEC 01, 1988
AA	LEMMON	EQ 2 MG BASE/ML	N71015 001 AUG 25, 1987
AA	PHARM ASSOC	EQ 2 MG BASE/ML	N73037 001 FEB 26, 1993
AA	SCS	EQ 2 MG BASE/ML	N70726 001 JUN 10, 1986
AA	SILARX	EQ 2 MG BASE/ML	N73364 001 SEP 28, 1993
	HALOPERIDOL INTENSOL		
AA	ROXANE	EQ 2 MG BASE/ML	N72045 001 APR 12, 1988

INJECTABLE; INJECTION

	HALDOL		
AP	+ JOHNSON RW	EQ 5 MG BASE/ML	N15923 001
	HALOPERIDOL		
AP	MARSAM	EQ 5 MG BASE/ML	N72516 001 FEB 25, 1993
AP		EQ 5 MG BASE/ML	N72517 001 FEB 25, 1993
AP	SOLOPAK	EQ 5 MG BASE/ML	N70800 001 DEC 14, 1987
AP		EQ 5 MG BASE/ML	N70801 001 DEC 14, 1987
AP		EQ 5 MG BASE/ML	N70864 001 DEC 14, 1987
AP	STERIS	EQ 5 MG BASE/ML	N70713 001 MAY 17, 1988
AP		EQ 5 MG BASE/ML	N70714 001 MAY 17, 1988
AP		EQ 5 MG BASE/ML	N70744 001 MAY 17, 1988

Prescription Drug Products *(continued)*

HALOPROGIN

	CREAM; TOPICAL		
	HALOTEX		
	+ WESTWOOD SQUIBB	1%	N16942 001
	SOLUTION; TOPICAL		
	HALOTEX		
	+ WESTWOOD SQUIBB	1%	N16943 001

HALOTHANE

	LIQUID; INHALATION		
	FLUOTHANE		
AN	WYETH AYERST	99.99%	N11338 001
	HALOTHANE		
AN	ABBOTT	99.99%	N83254 001
AN	BH	99.99%	N84977 001
AN	HALOCARBON	99.99%	N80810 001

HEPARIN CALCIUM

	INJECTABLE; INJECTION		
	CALCIPARINE		
	+ CHOAY	25,000 UNITS/ML	N18237 001

HEPARIN SODIUM

	INJECTABLE; INJECTION		
	HEP FLUSH KIT IN PLASTIC CONTAINER		
AP	FUJISAWA	10 UNITS/ML	N17029 017 DEC 05, 1985
AP		100 UNITS/ML	N17029 018 DEC 05, 1985
	HEP-LOCK		
AP	ELKINS SINN	10 UNITS/ML	N17037 007
AP		100 UNITS/ML	N17037 006
	HEP-LOCK U/P		
AP	ELKINS SINN	10 UNITS/ML	N17037 010 JUN 10, 1983
AP		100 UNITS/ML	N17037 011 JUN 10, 1983
	HEPARIN LOCK FLUSH		
AP	ABBOTT	10 UNITS/ML	N05264 001
AP	FUJISAWA	10 UNITS/ML	N17029 007 MAY 06, 1982
AP		100 UNITS/ML	N17029 006

HEPARIN SODIUM *(continued)*

	INJECTABLE; INJECTION		
	HEPARIN LOCK FLUSH		
AP	SMITH AND NEPHEW	10 UNITS/ML	N87904 001 APR 20, 1983
AP		10 UNITS/ML	N88458 001 JUL 26, 1984
AP		10 UNITS/ML	N88580 001 OCT 25, 1984
AP		100 UNITS/ML	N87906 001 APR 20, 1983
AP		100 UNITS/ML	N88460 001 JUL 26, 1984
AP		100 UNITS/ML	N88581 001 OCT 25, 1984
AP	SOLOPAK	10 UNITS/ML	N87903 001 APR 20, 1983
AP		10 UNITS/ML	N88457 001 OCT 25, 1984
AP		100 UNITS/ML	N87905 001 APR 20, 1983
AP		100 UNITS/ML	N88459 001 JUL 26, 1984
AP	STERLING WINTHROP	10 UNITS/ML	N88097 001 APR 28, 1983
AP		10 UNITS/ML	N88346 001 MAY 18, 1983
AP		100 UNITS/ML	N88098 001 APR 28, 1983
AP		100 UNITS/ML	N88347 001 MAY 18, 1983
AP	+ WYETH AYERST	10 UNITS/ML	N17007 008
AP	+	100 UNITS/ML	N17007 009
	HEPARIN LOCK FLUSH IN PLASTIC CONTAINER		
AP	ABBOTT	10 UNITS/ML	N05264 015 MAY 21, 1985
AP		100 UNITS/ML	N05264 016 MAY 21, 1985
	HEPARIN SODIUM		
AP	+ ABBOTT	2,500 UNITS/ML	N05264 014 APR 07, 1986
	+	2,000 UNITS/ML	N05264 013 APR 07, 1986
AP	AKORN	1,000 UNITS/ML	N17486 001
AP		5,000 UNITS/ML	N17486 002
AP		10,000 UNITS/ML	N17486 003
AP		20,000 UNITS/ML	N17486 004
AP		40,000 UNITS/ML	N17486 005
AP	DELL LABS	1,000 UNITS/ML	N17540 001
AP		5,000 UNITS/ML	N17540 002
AP		10,000 UNITS/ML	N17540 003
AP		20,000 UNITS/ML	N17540 004
AP		40,000 UNITS/ML	N17540 005

Prescription Drug Products *(continued)*

HEPARIN SODIUM *(continued)*

INJECTABLE; INJECTION

HEPARIN SODIUM

AP	ELKINS SINN	1,000 UNITS/ML	N17037 001
AP		5,000 UNITS/ML	N17037 002
AP		10,000 UNITS/ML	N17037 003
AP		10,000 UNITS/ML	N17037 013 APR 07, 1986
AP	FUJISAWA	1,000 UNITS/ML	N17029 001
AP		1,000 UNITS/ML	N17979 001
AP		5,000 UNITS/ML	N17651 006
AP		10,000 UNITS/ML	N17029 003
AP		10,000 UNITS/ML	N17979 002
AP	LILLY	1,000 UNITS/ML	N05521 001
AP		10,000 UNITS/ML	N05521 002
AP		20,000 UNITS/ML	N05521 004
AP	ORGANON	1,000 UNITS/ML	N00552 008
AP		5,000 UNITS/ML	N00552 009
AP		10,000 UNITS/ML	N00552 010
AP	PHARM SPECLTS ASSOC	1,000 UNITS/ML	N17780 001
AP		5,000 UNITS/ML	N17780 002
AP		10,000 UNITS/ML	N17780 003
AP		20,000 UNITS/ML	N17780 004
AP	PHARMA SERVE NY	1,000 UNITS/ML	N86129 001
AP	SMITH AND NEPHEW	1,000 UNITS/ML	N88239 001 JUL 26, 1984
AP	SOLOPAK	1,000 UNITS/ML	N87043 001
AP		5,000 UNITS/ML	N87077 001
AP		10,000 UNITS/ML	N87107 001
AP		5,000 UNITS/0.5 ML	N87395 001
AP		10,000 UNITS/0.5 ML	N87363 001
AP	STERIS	1,000 UNITS/ML	N17064 002
AP		5,000 UNITS/ML	N17064 003
AP		10,000 UNITS/ML	N17064 004
AP		20,000 UNITS/ML	N17064 005
AP		40,000 UNITS/ML	N17064 006
AP	STERLING WINTHROP	2,500 UNITS/ML	N88099 001 APR 28, 1983
AP		5,000 UNITS/ML	N88100 001 APR 28, 1983
AP	+ UPJOHN	1,000 UNITS/ML	N04570 001
AP	+	5,000 UNITS/ML	N04570 002
AP	+	10,000 UNITS/ML	N04570 003
AP	WYETH AYERST	1,000 UNITS/ML	N17007 001
AP		2,500 UNITS/ML	N17007 007
AP		5,000 UNITS/ML	N17007 002
AP		10,000 UNITS/ML	N17007 004
AP	+	20,000 UNITS/ML	N17007 006
	+	7,500 UNITS/ML	N17007 003

HEPARIN SODIUM *(continued)*

INJECTABLE; INJECTION

	HEPARIN SODIUM IN PLASTIC CONTAINER		
AP	FUJISAWA	1,000 UNITS/ML	N17029 013 DEC 05, 1985
AP		5,000 UNITS/ML	N17029 014 DEC 05, 1985
AP		10,000 UNITS/ML	N17029 015 DEC 05, 1985
AP		20,000 UNITS/ML	N17029 016 DEC 05, 1985
	HEPARIN SODIUM PRESERVATIVE FREE		
AP	FUJISAWA	1,000 UNITS/ML	N17029 010 APR 28, 1986
AP	MARSAM	1,000 UNITS/ML	N89464 001 JUN 03, 1986
AP	STERLING WINTHROP	10,000 UNITS/ML	N89522 001 MAY 04, 1987
	HEPARIN SODIUM 10,000 UNITS IN DEXTROSE 5%		
AP	ABBOTT	10,000 UNITS/100 ML	N18911 006 JAN 30, 1985
	HEPARIN SODIUM 1000 UNITS AND DEXTROSE 5% IN PLASTIC CONTAINER		
AP	MCGAW	200 UNITS/100 ML	N19130 001 DEC 31, 1984
	HEPARIN SODIUM 1000 UNITS AND SODIUM CHLORIDE 0.9% IN PLASTIC CONTAINER		
AP	BAXTER	200 UNITS/100 ML	N18609 001 APR 28, 1982
	HEPARIN SODIUM 1000 UNITS IN SODIUM CHLORIDE 0.9% IN PLASTIC CONTAINER		
AP	ABBOTT	200 UNITS/100 ML	N18916 010 JUN 23, 1989
AP	MCGAW	200 UNITS/100 ML	N19042 001 MAR 29, 1985
AP		200 UNITS/100 ML	N19953 001
	HEPARIN SODIUM 12,500 UNITS IN DEXTROSE 5%		
AP	ABBOTT	5,000 UNITS/100 ML	N18911 007 JAN 30, 1985
	HEPARIN SODIUM 12,500 UNITS IN SODIUM CHLORIDE 0.45% IN PLASTIC CONTAINER		
AP	ABBOTT	5,000 UNITS/100 ML	N18916 006 JAN 31, 1984
	HEPARIN SODIUM 12500 UNITS IN SODIUM CHLORIDE 0.45% IN PLASTIC CONTAINER		
AP	MCGAW	5,000 UNITS/100 ML	N19802 001 JUL 20, 1992
	HEPARIN SODIUM 20,000 UNITS AND DEXTROSE 5% IN PLASTIC CONTAINER		
AP	BAXTER	4,000 UNITS/100 ML	N18814 001 OCT 31, 1983

Prescription Drug Products *(continued)*

HEPARIN SODIUM *(continued)*

INJECTABLE; INJECTION

HEPARIN SODIUM 20,000 UNITS IN DEXTROSE 5% IN PLASTIC CONTAINER

AP ABBOTT 4,000 UNITS/100 ML N19805 001 JAN 25, 1989

HEPARIN SODIUM 2000 UNITS AND SODIUM CHLORIDE 0.9% IN PLASTIC CONTAINER

AP BAXTER 200 UNITS/100 ML N18609 002 APR 28, 1982

HEPARIN SODIUM 2000 UNITS IN DEXTROSE 5% IN PLASTIC CONTAINER

AP MCGAW 200 UNITS/100 ML N19130 003 DEC 31, 1984

HEPARIN SODIUM 2000 UNITS IN SODIUM CHLORIDE 0.9% IN PLASTIC CONTAINER

AP ABBOTT 200 UNITS/100 ML N18916 011 JUN 23, 1989

AP MCGAW 200 UNITS/100 ML N19042 002 MAR 29, 1985

HEPARIN SODIUM 20000 UNITS IN DEXTROSE 5% IN PLASTIC CONTAINER

AP MCGAW 4,000 UNITS/100 ML N19952 001 JUL 20, 1992

HEPARIN SODIUM 25,000 UNITS AND DEXTROSE 5% IN PLASTIC CONTAINER

AP BAXTER 5,000 UNITS/100 ML N18814 003 JUL 09, 1985

AP 10,000 UNITS/100 ML N18814 004 JUL 02, 1987

HEPARIN SODIUM 25,000 UNITS IN DEXTROSE 5%

AP ABBOTT 5,000 UNITS/100 ML N18911 009 JAN 30, 1985

AP 10,000 UNITS/100 ML N18911 008 JAN 30, 1985

HEPARIN SODIUM 25,000 UNITS IN DEXTROSE 5% IN PLASTIC CONTAINER

AP ABBOTT 5,000 UNITS/100 ML N19805 002 JAN 25, 1989

HEPARIN SODIUM 25,000 UNITS IN SODIUM CHLORIDE 0.45% IN PLASTIC CONTAINER

AP ABBOTT 5,000 UNITS/100 ML N18916 007 JAN 31, 1984

AP 10,000 UNITS/100 ML N18916 008 JAN 31, 1984

HEPARIN SODIUM 25000 UNITS IN DEXTROSE 5% IN PLASTIC CONTAINER

AP MCGAW 5,000 UNITS/100 ML N19134 001 MAR 29, 1985

AP 5,000 UNITS/100 ML N19952 004 JUL 20, 1992

AP 10,000 UNITS/100 ML N19952 005 JUL 20, 1992

HEPARIN SODIUM *(continued)*

INJECTABLE; INJECTION

HEPARIN SODIUM 25000 UNITS IN SODIUM CHLORIDE 0.45% IN PLASTIC CONTAINER

AP MCGAW 5,000 UNITS/100 ML N19802 005 JUL 20, 1992

AP 10,000 UNITS/100 ML N19802 002 JUL 20, 1992

HEPARIN SODIUM 25000 UNITS IN SODIUM CHLORIDE 0.9% IN PLASTIC CONTAINER

MCGAW 5,000 UNITS/100 ML N19802 003 JUL 20, 1992

HEPARIN SODIUM 5000 UNITS IN DEXTROSE 5% IN PLASTIC CONTAINER

AP MCGAW 1,000 UNITS/100 ML N19130 002 DEC 31, 1984

HEPFLUSH-10

AP FUJISAWA 10 UNITS/ML N17651 009 JUN 26, 1984

LIQUAEMIN LOCK FLUSH

AP ORGANON 100 UNITS/ML N00552 007

LIQUAEMIN SODIUM

AP ORGANON 1,000 UNITS/ML N00552 004

AP 5,000 UNITS/ML N00552 003

AP 10,000 UNITS/ML N00552 005

SODIUM HEPARIN

AP BAXTER 1,000 UNITS/ML N17036 001

HEXACHLOROPHENE

AEROSOL; TOPICAL

SEPTISOL

+ VESTAL LABS 0.23% N17424 001

EMULSION; TOPICAL

PHISOHEX

+ STERLING WINTHROP 3% N06882 001

SOAP; TOPICAL

GAMOPHEN

+ ARBROOK 2% N06270 003

SPONGE; TOPICAL

E-Z SCRUB

+ DESERET 450 MG N17452 001

PRE-OP

AT + DAVIS AND GECK 480 MG N17433 001

PRE-OP II

AT DAVIS AND GECK 480 MG N17433 002

Prescription Drug Products *(continued)*

HISTRELIN ACETATE

	INJECTABLE; INJECTION		
	SUPPRELIN		
	+ ROBERTS LABS	EQ 0.2 MG BASE/ML	N19836 001 DEC 24, 1991
	+	EQ 0.5 MG BASE/ML	N19836 002 DEC 24, 1991
	+	EQ 1 MG BASE/ML	N19836 003 DEC 24, 1991

HOMATROPINE METHYLBROMIDE

	TABLET; ORAL		
	HOMAPIN-10		
	MISSION PHARMA	10 MG	N86308 001
	HOMAPIN-5		
	MISSION PHARMA	5 MG	N86309 001

HOMATROPINE METHYLBROMIDE; HYDROCODONE BITARTRATE

	SYRUP; ORAL		
	HYCODAN		
AA	DUPONT MERCK	1.5 MG/5 ML;5 MG/5 ML	N05213 002 JUL 26, 1988
	HYDROCODONE COMPOUND		
AA	BARRE	1.5 MG/5 ML;5 MG/5 ML	N88017 001 JUL 05, 1983
	HYDROPANE		
AA	HALSEY	1.5 MG/5 ML;5 MG/5 ML	N88066 001 JUN 28, 1985
	MYCODONE		
AA	PENNEX	1.5 MG/5 ML;5 MG/5 ML	N88008 001 MAR 03, 1983
	TABLET; ORAL		
	HYCODAN		
AA	DUPONT MERCK	1.5 MG;5 MG	N05213 001 JUL 26, 1988
	TUSSIGON		
AA	DANIELS PHARMS	1.5 MG;5 MG	N88508 001 JUL 30, 1985

HYALURONIDASE

	INJECTABLE; INJECTION		
	WYDASE		
	+ WYETH AYERST	150 UNITS/ML	N06343 002
	+	150 UNITS/VIAL	N06343 006
	+	1,500 UNITS/VIAL	N06343 005

HYDRALAZINE HYDROCHLORIDE

	INJECTABLE; INJECTION		
	APRESOLINE		
AP	+ CIBA	20 MG/ML	N08303 003
	HYDRALAZINE HCL		
AP	SOLOPAK	20 MG/ML	N88517 001 AUG 22, 1985
	TABLET; ORAL		
	APRESOLINE		
AA	CIBA	10 MG	N08303 004
AA		25 MG	N08303 001
AA		50 MG	N08303 002
AA		100 MG	N08303 005
	DRALZINE		
AA	LEMMON	25 MG	N84301 001
	HYDRALAZINE HCL		
AA	AMIDE PHARM	25 MG	N88560 001 OCT 04, 1984
AA		50 MG	N88649 001 OCT 18, 1984
AA	BARR	10 MG	N88728 001 APR 11, 1985
AA		25 MG	N84106 002
AA		50 MG	N84107 002
AA		100 MG	N88729 001 APR 11, 1985
AA	CAMALL	10 MG	N88846 001 FEB 26, 1985
AA		25 MG	N88847 001 FEB 26, 1985
AA		50 MG	N88848 001 FEB 26, 1985
AA		100 MG	N88849 001 FEB 26, 1985
AA	DANBURY PHARMA	25 MG	N84504 001
AA		50 MG	N84503 001
AA	GENEVA PHARMS	10 MG	N83241 001
AA		25 MG	N83560 001
AA		50 MG	N83561 001
AA	GLOBAL PHARMS	25 MG	N84922 001
AA		50 MG	N84923 001
AA	HALSEY	10 MG	N89218 001 JAN 22, 1986
AA		25 MG	N89130 001 JAN 15, 1986
AA		50 MG	N89222 001 JAN 22, 1986
AA		100 MG	N89178 001 JAN 15, 1986
AA	LEDERLE	25 MG	N86243 001
AA		50 MG	N86242 002

Prescription Drug Products *(continued)*

HYDRALAZINE HYDROCHLORIDE *(continued)*

TABLET; ORAL

	HYDRALAZINE HCL		
AA	MUTUAL PHARM	10 MG	N89359 001 JUL 25, 1986
AA		25 MG	N89258 001 MAY 05, 1986
AA		50 MG	N89259 001 MAY 05, 1986
AA	PAR PHARM	10 MG	N87836 001 OCT 05, 1982
AA		25 MG	N86961 002
AA		50 MG	N86962 001
AA		100 MG	N88391 001 SEP 27, 1983
AA	PUREPAC PHARM	25 MG	N88177 001 JUL 29, 1983
AA	SIDMAK LABS NJ	10 MG	N89097 001 DEC 18, 1985
AA		25 MG	N88467 001 MAY 01, 1984
AA		50 MG	N88468 001 MAY 01, 1984
AA		100 MG	N89098 001 DEC 18, 1985
AA	ZENITH LABS	10 MG	N84443 001
AA		25 MG	N84437 001
AA		50 MG	N84469 002
AA		100 MG	N84581 001

HYDRALAZINE HYDROCHLORIDE; HYDROCHLOROTHIAZIDE

CAPSULE; ORAL

	APRESAZIDE		
AB	CIBA	25 MG;25 MG	N84735 001
AB		50 MG;50 MG	N84810 001
AB	+	100 MG;50 MG	N84811 001
	HYDRA-ZIDE		
AB	PAR PHARM	25 MG;25 MG	N88957 001 OCT 21, 1985
AB		50 MG;50 MG	N88946 001 OCT 21, 1985
AB		100 MG;50 MG	N88961 001 OCT 21, 1985
	HYDRALAZINE HCL AND HYDROCHLOROTHIAZIDE		
AB	SOLVAY	25 MG;25 MG	N87608 001 FEB 08, 1982
AB		50 MG;50 MG	N87213 001 FEB 08, 1982
AB	SUPERPHARM	50 MG;50 MG	N89201 001 FEB 09, 1987

HYDRALAZINE HYDROCHLORIDE; HYDROCHLOROTHIAZIDE *(continued)*

CAPSULE; ORAL

	HYDRALAZINE HCL W/ HYDROCHLOROTHIAZIDE 25/25		
AB	ZENITH LABS	25 MG;25 MG	N88356 001 APR 10, 1984
	HYDRALAZINE HCL W/ HYDROCHLOROTHIAZIDE 50/50		
AB	ZENITH LABS	50 MG;50 MG	N88357 001 APR 10, 1984

TABLET; ORAL

	APRESOLINE-ESIDRIX		
	+ CIBA	25 MG;15 MG	N12026 002

HYDRALAZINE HYDROCHLORIDE; HYDROCHLOROTHIAZIDE; RESERPINE

TABLET; ORAL

	CAM-AP-ES		
BP	CAMALL	25 MG;15 MG;0.1 MG	N84897 001
	HYDRALAZINE HCL, HYDROCHLOROTHIAZIDE AND RESERPINE		
BP	ZENITH LABS	25 MG;15 MG;0.1 MG	N84291 001
	HYDROSERPINE PLUS (R-H-H)		
BP	ZENITH LABS	25 MG;15 MG;0.1 MG	N83877 001
	RESERPINE, HYDRALAZINE HCL AND HYDROCHLOROTHIAZIDE		
BP	BARR	25 MG;15 MG;0.1 MG	N88570 001 APR 10, 1984
BP	DANBURY PHARMA	25 MG;15 MG;0.1 MG	N85549 001
BP	SOLVAY	25 MG;15 MG;0.1 MG	N88376 001 OCT 28, 1983
	SER-AP-ES		
BP	+ CIBA	25 MG;15 MG;0.1 MG	N12193 005
	UNIPRES		
BP	SOLVAY	25 MG;15 MG;0.1 MG	N86298 001

HYDROCHLOROTHIAZIDE

SOLUTION; ORAL

	HYDROCHLOROTHIAZIDE		
	ROXANE	50 MG/5 ML	N88587 001 JUL 02, 1984

TABLET; ORAL

	ESIDRIX		
AB	CIBA	25 MG	N11793 005
AB		50 MG	N11793 008
AB		100 MG	N11793 009
	HYDRO-D		
AB	HALSEY	25 MG	N86504 001
AB		50 MG	N83891 002

Prescription Drug Products *(continued)*

HYDROCHLOROTHIAZIDE *(continued)*

TABLET; ORAL

HYDROCHLOROTHIAZIDE

AB		ASCOT	50 MG	N87540 001 FEB 03, 1982
AB		BARR	25 MG	N83972 001
AB			50 MG	N83972 002
AB			50 MG	N84771 001
AB			100 MG	N83972 003
AB		CAMALL	25 MG	N85683 001
AB			50 MG	N83965 001
AB			50 MG	N85672 001
AB		DANBURY PHARMA	25 MG	N81189 001 JAN 24, 1992
AB			50 MG	N83232 001
AB			100 MG	N81190 001 JAN 24, 1992
AB		EON LABS	50 MG	N85219 001
AB		GENEVA PHARMS	25 MG	N87565 001 MAR 09, 1982
AB			50 MG	N84912 001
AB		GLOBAL PHARMS	25 MG	N84029 001
AB			50 MG	N83607 002
AB			100 MG	N85098 001
AB		INWOOD LABS	25 MG	N85067 001
AB		LEDERLE	25 MG	N87059 001
AB			50 MG	N87068 001
AB			100 MG	N87060 001
AB		MM MAST	25 MG	N86192 001
AB			50 MG	N86192 002
AB		PHARMERAL	25 MG	N84325 001
AB			50 MG	N84324 001
AB		PRIVATE FORM	25 MG	N85181 001
AB			50 MG	N85182 001
AB			50 MG	N86597 001
AB		PUREPAC PHARM	25 MG	N85054 002
AB			50 MG	N85208 001
AB		ROXANE	50 MG	N84536 002
AB		SUPERPHARM	25 MG	N88827 001 DEC 28, 1984
AB			50 MG	N88828 001 DEC 28, 1984
AB			100 MG	N88829 001 DEC 28, 1984
AB		WEST WARD PHARM	25 MG	N84899 001
AB			50 MG	N84878 001
AB		ZENITH LABS	25 MG	N83177 001
AB			50 MG	N83177 002
AB			100 MG	N85022 001

HYDRODIURIL

AB		MERCK SHARP DOHME	25 MG	N11835 003
AB	+		50 MG	N11835 006
AB			100 MG	N11835 007

HYDROCHLOROTHIAZIDE *(continued)*

TABLET; ORAL

ORETIC

AB	ABBOTT	25 MG	N11971 001
AB		50 MG	N11971 002

HYDROCHLOROTHIAZIDE; *MULTIPLE*

SEE AMILORIDE HYDROCHLORIDE; HYDROCHLOROTHIAZIDE
SEE BENAZEPRIL HYDROCHLORIDE; HYDROCHLOROTHIAZIDE
SEE BISOPROLOL FUMARATE; HYDROCHLOROTHIAZIDE
SEE CAPTOPRIL; HYDROCHLOROTHIAZIDE
SEE DESERPIDINE; HYDROCHLOROTHIAZIDE
SEE ENALAPRIL MALEATE; HYDROCHLOROTHIAZIDE
SEE GUANETHIDINE MONOSULFATE; HYDROCHLOROTHIAZIDE
SEE HYDRALAZINE HYDROCHLORIDE; HYDROCHLOROTHIAZIDE
SEE HYDRALAZINE HYDROCHLORIDE; HYDROCHLOROTHIAZIDE; RESERPINE
SEE HYDRALAZINE HYDROCHLORIDE; HYDROCHLOROTHIAZIDE

HYDROCHLOROTHIAZIDE; LISINOPRIL

TABLET; ORAL

		PRINZIDE 10-12.5		
AB		MERCK	12.5 MG;10 MG	N19778 003 NOV 18, 1993
		PRINZIDE 20-12.5		
AB		MERCK	12.5 MG;20 MG	N19778 001 FEB 16, 1989
		PRINZIDE 20-25		
AB	+	MERCK	25 MG;20 MG	N19778 002 FEB 16, 1989
		ZESTORETIC 10-12.5		
AB		ZENECA	12.5 MG;10 MG	N19888 003 NOV 18, 1993
		ZESTORETIC 20-12.5		
AB		ZENECA	12.5 MG;20 MG	N19888 001 SEP 20, 1990
		ZESTORETIC 20-25		
AB		ZENECA	25 MG;20 MG	N19888 002 JUL 20, 1989

Prescription Drug Products *(continued)*

HYDROCHLOROTHIAZIDE; METHYLDOPA

TABLET; ORAL

	ALDORIL D30		
AB	MERCK SHARP DOHME	30 MG;500 MG	N13402 003
	ALDORIL D50		
AB	+ MERCK SHARP DOHME	50 MG;500 MG	N13402 004
	ALDORIL 15		
AB	MERCK SHARP DOHME	15 MG;250 MG	N13402 001
	ALDORIL 25		
AB	MERCK SHARP DOHME	25 MG;250 MG	N13402 002
	METHYLDOPA AND HYDROCHLOROTHIAZIDE		
AB	DANBURY PHARMA	15 MG;250 MG	N70958 001 FEB 06, 1989
AB		25 MG;250 MG	N70959 001 JAN 19, 1989
AB		30 MG;500 MG	N71069 001 JAN 19, 1989
AB		50 MG;500 MG	N70960 001 FEB 06, 1989
AB	GENEVA PHARMS	15 MG;250 MG	N70182 001 JAN 15, 1986
AB		25 MG;250 MG	N70183 001 JAN 15, 1986
AB		30 MG;500 MG	N70543 001 JAN 15, 1986
AB		50 MG;500 MG	N70544 001 JAN 15, 1986
AB	INVAMED	15 MG;250 MG	N70829 001 MAR 09, 1987
AB		25 MG;250 MG	N70830 001 MAR 09, 1987
AB	LEDERLE	15 MG;250 MG	N72507 001 JUN 02, 1989
AB		25 MG;250 MG	N72508 001 JUN 02, 1989
AB		30 MG;500 MG	N72509 001 JUN 02, 1989
AB		50 MG;500 MG	N72510 001 JUN 02, 1989
AB	MYLAN	15 MG;250 MG	N70264 001 JAN 23, 1986
AB		25 MG;250 MG	N70265 001 JAN 23, 1986
AB	NOVOPHARM	15 MG;250 MG	N71819 001 APR 08, 1988
AB		25 MG;250 MG	N71820 001 APR 08, 1988
AB		30 MG;500 MG	N71821 001 APR 08, 1988
AB		50 MG;500 MG	N71822 001 APR 08, 1988

HYDROCHLOROTHIAZIDE; METHYLDOPA *(continued)*

TABLET; ORAL

	METHYLDOPA AND HYDROCHLOROTHIAZIDE		
AB	PAR PHARM	15 MG;250 MG	N70616 001 FEB 02, 1987
AB		25 MG;250 MG	N70612 001 FEB 02, 1987
AB		30 MG;500 MG	N70613 001 FEB 02, 1987
AB		50 MG;500 MG	N70614 001 FEB 02, 1987
AB	PARKE DAVIS	15 MG;250 MG	N71897 001 NOV 23, 1987
AB		25 MG;250 MG	N71898 001 NOV 23, 1987
AB		30 MG;500 MG	N71899 001 NOV 23, 1987
AB		50 MG;500 MG	N71900 001 NOV 23, 1987
AB	PUREPAC PHARM	15 MG;250 MG	N70853 001 OCT 08, 1986
AB		25 MG;250 MG	N70688 001 APR 24, 1986
AB		30 MG;500 MG	N70854 001 OCT 08, 1986
AB	WATSON LABS	15 MG;250 MG	N71920 001 AUG 29, 1988
AB		25 MG;250 MG	N71921 001 AUG 29, 1988
AB		30 MG;500 MG	N71922 001 AUG 29, 1988
AB		50 MG;500 MG	N71923 001 AUG 29, 1988
AB	ZENITH LABS	15 MG;250 MG	N71458 001 MAR 08, 1988
AB		25 MG;250 MG	N71459 001 MAR 08, 1988
AB		30 MG;500 MG	N71460 001 MAR 08, 1988
AB		50 MG;500 MG	N71461 001 MAR 08, 1988

HYDROCHLOROTHIAZIDE; METOPROLOL TARTRATE

TABLET; ORAL

	LOPRESSOR HCT 100/25		
	CIBA	25 MG;100 MG	N18303 002 DEC 31, 1984
	LOPRESSOR HCT 100/50		
	+ CIBA	50 MG;100 MG	N18303 003 DEC 31, 1984
	LOPRESSOR HCT 50/25		
	CIBA	25 MG;50 MG	N18303 001 DEC 31, 1984

Prescription Drug Products *(continued)*

HYDROCHLOROTHIAZIDE; PROPRANOLOL HYDROCHLORIDE

	CAPSULE, EXTENDED RELEASE; ORAL		
	INDERIDE LA 120/50		
	+ WYETH AYERST	50 MG;120 MG	N19059 002 JUL 03, 1985
	INDERIDE LA 160/50		
	+ WYETH AYERST	50 MG;160 MG	N19059 003 JUL 03, 1985
	INDERIDE LA 80/50		
	+ WYETH AYERST	50 MG;80 MG	N19059 001 JUL 03, 1985
	TABLET; ORAL		
	INDERIDE-40/25		
AB	WYETH AYERST	25 MG;40 MG	N18031 001
	INDERIDE-80/25		
AB	+ WYETH AYERST	25 MG;80 MG	N18031 002
	PROPRANOLOL HCL AND HYDROCHLOROTHIAZIDE		
AB	BARR	25 MG;40 MG	N70704 001 OCT 01, 1986
AB		25 MG;80 MG	N70705 001 OCT 01, 1986
AB	CHELSEA LABS	25 MG;40 MG	N70301 001 APR 18, 1986
AB		25 MG;80 MG	N70305 001 APR 18, 1986
AB	DANBURY PHARMA	25 MG;40 MG	N71498 001 DEC 18, 1991
AB		25 MG;80 MG	N71501 001 DEC 18, 1991
AB	GENEVA PHARMS	25 MG;40 MG	N71060 001 AUG 26, 1987
AB		25 MG;80 MG	N71061 001 AUG 26, 1987
AB	MYLAN	25 MG;40 MG	N70946 001 MAR 04, 1987
AB		25 MG;80 MG	N70947 001 APR 01, 1987
AB	PUREPAC PHARM	25 MG;40 MG	N70851 001 MAY 15, 1986
AB		25 MG;80 MG	N70852 001 MAY 15, 1986
AB	SIDMAK LABS NJ	25 MG;40 MG	N72042 001 MAR 14, 1988
AB		25 MG;80 MG	N72043 001 MAR 14, 1988
AB	WARNER CHILCOTT	25 MG;40 MG	N71771 001 JAN 26, 1988
AB		25 MG;80 MG	N71772 001 JAN 26, 1988
AB	ZENITH LABS	25 MG;40 MG	N71552 001 DEC 01, 1988
AB		25 MG;80 MG	N71553 001 DEC 01, 1988

HYDROCHLOROTHIAZIDE; RESERPINE

	TABLET; ORAL		
	HYDRO-RESERP		
BP	CAMALL	50 MG;0.125 MG	N84714 002 JUN 29, 1982
	HYDROCHLOROTHIAZIDE W/ RESERPINE		
BP	DANBURY PHARMA	25 MG;0.125 MG	N84466 001
BP		50 MG;0.125 MG	N84467 001
BP	ZENITH LABS	25 MG;0.125 MG	N83571 001
BP		50 MG;0.125 MG	N83573 001
		25 MG;0.1 MG	N83572 001
		50 MG;0.1 MG	N83568 001
	HYDROPRES 25		
BP	MERCK SHARP DOHME	25 MG;0.125 MG	N11958 002
	HYDROPRES 50		
BP	MERCK SHARP DOHME	50 MG;0.125 MG	N11958 003
	RESERPINE AND HYDROCHLOROTHIAZIDE-50		
BP	WEST WARD PHARM	50 MG;0.125 MG	N88189 001 MAY 10, 1984

HYDROCHLOROTHIAZIDE; SPIRONOLACTONE

	TABLET; ORAL		
	ALDACTAZIDE		
AB	SEARLE	25 MG;25 MG	N12616 004 DEC 30, 1982
	+	50 MG;50 MG	N12616 005 DEC 30, 1982
	SPIRONOLACTONE AND HYDROCHLOROTHIAZIDE		
AB	BARR	25 MG;25 MG	N87267 001
AB	MUTUAL PHARM	25 MG;25 MG	N89534 001 JUL 02, 1987
AB	MYLAN	25 MG;25 MG	N86513 001
AB	PUREPAC PHARM	25 MG;25 MG	N87999 001 NOV 06, 1985
	SPIRONOLACTONE W/ HYDROCHLOROTHIAZIDE		
AB	GENEVA PHARMS	25 MG;25 MG	N86881 001
AB	PARKE DAVIS	25 MG;25 MG	N87948 001 FEB 22, 1983
AB	ZENITH LABS	25 MG;25 MG	N87004 002 MAY 24, 1982
	SPIRONOLACTONE/HYDROCHLOROTHIAZIDE		
AB	DANBURY PHARMA	25 MG;25 MG	N87398 001

HYDROCHLOROTHIAZIDE; TIMOLOL MALEATE

	TABLET; ORAL		
	TIMOLIDE 10-25		
	+ MERCK SHARP DOHME	25 MG;10 MG	N18061 001

Prescription Drug Products *(continued)*

HYDROCHLOROTHIAZIDE; TRIAMTERENE

CAPSULE; ORAL

	DYAZIDE		
	SMITHKLINE BEECHAM	25 MG;37.5 MG	N16042 003 MAR 03, 1994
	TRIAMTERENE AND HYDROCHLOROTHIAZIDE		
	+ GENEVA PHARMS	25 MG;50 MG	N73191 001 JUL 31, 1991

TABLET; ORAL

	MAXZIDE		
AB	+ MYLAN	50 MG;75 MG	N19129 001 OCT 22, 1984
	MAXZIDE-25		
AB	MYLAN	25 MG;37.5 MG	N19129 003 MAY 13, 1988
	TRIAMTERENE AND HYDROCHLOROTHIAZIDE		
AB	BARR	50 MG;75 MG	N71251 001 APR 17, 1988
AB	DANBURY PHARMA	50 MG;75 MG	N71969 001 APR 17, 1988
AB	GENEVA PHARMS	25 MG;37.5 MG	N73281 001 APR 30, 1992
AB		50 MG;75 MG	N72011 001 JUN 17, 1988
B*	PAR PHARM	50 MG;75 MG	N72337 001 MAY 11, 1988
AB	WATSON LABS	25 MG;37.5 MG	N73449 001 SEP 23, 1993
AB		50 MG;75 MG	N71851 001 NOV 30, 1988

HYDROCODONE BITARTRATE; *MULTIPLE*

SEE ACETAMINOPHEN; HYDROCODONE BITARTRATE
SEE ASPIRIN; HYDROCODONE BITARTRATE
SEE HOMATROPINE METHYLBROMIDE; HYDROCODONE BITARTRATE

HYDROCODONE BITARTRATE; PHENYLPROPANOLAMINE HYDROCHLORIDE

SYRUP; ORAL

	HYCOMINE		
	DUPONT MERCK	5 MG/5 ML;25 MG/5 ML	N19410 001 AUG 17, 1990
	HYCOMINE PEDIATRIC		
	DUPONT MERCK	2.5 MG/5 ML;12.5 MG/5 ML	N19411 001 AUG 17, 1990

HYDROCODONE POLISTIREX; *MULTIPLE*

SEE CHLORPHENIRAMINE POLISTIREX; HYDROCODONE POLISTIREX

HYDROCORTISONE

AEROSOL; TOPICAL

	AEROSEB-HC		
	+ ALLERGAN HERBERT	0.5%	N85805 001

CREAM; TOPICAL

	ALA-CORT		
AT	DEL RAY LABS	1%	N80706 006
	ANUSOL HC		
AT	PARKE DAVIS	2.5%	N88250 001 JUN 06, 1984
	CORT-DOME		
AT	MILES	0.5%	N09585 003
AT		1%	N09585 001
	DERMACORT		
AT	SOLVAY	1%	N83011 002
	FLEXICORT		
AT	WESTWOOD SQUIBB	0.5%	N87136 003 APR 08, 1982
AT		1%	N87136 002 APR 08, 1982
AT		2.5%	N87136 001 APR 08, 1982
	HC (HYDROCORTISONE)		
AT	C AND M PHARMA	0.5%	N80482 003
AT		1%	N80482 004
	HI-COR		
AT	C AND M PHARMA	2.5%	N80483 001
	HYDROCORTISONE		
AT	ALTANA	0.5%	N80848 002
AT		1%	N80848 003
AT	AMBIX	1%	N86080 001
AT		2.5%	N86271 001
AT	BARRE	2.5%	N89682 001 MAR 10, 1988
AT	CLAY PARK	0.5%	N84970 002
AT		1%	N85026 001
AT		2.5%	N85025 001
AT	EVERYLIFE	1%	N80452 002
AT	FOUGERA	1%	N80693 003
AT		2.5%	N89414 001 DEC 16, 1986
AT	G AND W LABS	1%	N84059 001
AT	INGRAM PHARM	0.5%	N80456 002
AT		1%	N80456 003

Prescription Drug Products *(continued)*

HYDROCORTISONE *(continued)*

	CREAM; TOPICAL		
	HYDROCORTISONE		
AT	NMC	1%	N87795 001
			MAY 03, 1983
AT		2.5%	N89754 001
			FEB 01, 1989
AT	PHARMADERM	2.5%	N89413 001
			DEC 16, 1986
AT	SYOSSET	0.5%	N85527 001
AT		1%	N85733 001
AT	THAMES	1%	N86155 001
AT		2.5%	N88799 001
			NOV 09, 1984
AT	TOPIDERM	1%	N89273 001
			FEB 17, 1989
	HYTONE		
AT	+ DERMIK	1%	N80472 003
AT	+	2.5%	N80472 004
	NOGENIC HC		
AT	SYOSSET	1%	N87427 001
			APR 04, 1988
	NUTRACORT		
AT	GALDERMA	0.5%	N80442 002
AT		1%	N80442 003
	PENECORT		
AT	ALLERGAN HERBERT	1%	N88216 001
			JUN 06, 1984
	PROCTOCORT		
AT	SOLVAY	1%	N83011 001
	SYNACORT		
AT	SYNTEX	1%	N87458 001
AT		2.5%	N87457 001
	ENEMA; RECTAL		
	CORTENEMA		
	+ SOLVAY	100 MG/60 ML	N16199 001
	HYDROCORTISONE		
AT	COPLEY PHARM	100 MG/60 ML	N74171 001
			MAY 27, 1994
	GEL; TOPICAL		
	PENECORT		
	+ ALLERGAN HERBERT	1%	N88215 001
			JUN 06, 1984

HYDROCORTISONE *(continued)*

	LOTION; TOPICAL		
	ACTICORT		
AT	BAKER NORTON	1%	N86535 001
	ALA-CORT		
AT	DEL RAY LABS	1%	N83201 001
	ALA-SCALP		
	DEL RAY LABS	2%	N83231 001
	BETA-HC		
AT	BETA DERMAC	1%	N89495 001
			JAN 25, 1988
	CETACORT		
AT	GALDERMA	0.5%	N80426 002
AT		1%	N80426 001
	DERMACORT		
AT	SOLVAY	0.5%	N84573 002
AT		1%	N86462 001
	EPICORT		
AT	BLULINE	0.5%	N83219 002
	GLYCORT		
AT	HERAN	1%	N87489 001
			OCT 03, 1983
	HYDROCORTISONE		
AT	CLAY PARK	0.5%	N85662 001
AT	MERICON	0.5%	N85282 001
AT		1%	N85282 002
			FEB 26, 1987
	HYTONE		
AT	+ DERMIK	1%	N80473 003
AT	+	2.5%	N80473 004
			NOV 30, 1982
	NUTRACORT		
AT	GALDERMA	0.5%	N80443 002
AT		1%	N80443 003
AT		2.5%	N87644 001
			AUG 24, 1982
	STIE-CORT		
AT	STIEFEL	1%	N89066 001
			NOV 25, 1985
AT		2.5%	N89074 001
			NOV 26, 1985
	OINTMENT; TOPICAL		
	CORTRIL		
AT	PFIPHARMECS	1%	N09176 001
AT		2.5%	N09176 002
	HC (HYDROCORTISONE)		
AT	C AND M PHARMA	1%	N80481 002

Prescription Drug Products *(continued)*

HYDROCORTISONE *(continued)*

OINTMENT; TOPICAL

	<u>HYDROCORTISONE</u>		
AT	ALTANA	1%	N80489 003
AT		1%	N80692 001
AT	AMBIX	1%	N86079 001
AT		2.5%	N86272 001
AT	CLAY PARK	2.5%	N85027 001
		0.5%	N84969 003
AT	FOUGERA	2.5%	N81203 001 MAY 28, 1993
AT	NMC	1%	N87796 001 OCT 13, 1982
AT	THAMES	1%	N86257 001
	<u>HYDROCORTISONE IN ABSORBASE</u>		
AT	CAROLINA MEDCL	1%	N88138 001 SEP 06, 1985
	<u>HYTONE</u>		
AT	+ DERMIK	1%	N80474 003
AT	+	2.5%	N80474 004
	<u>PENECORT</u>		
AT	ALLERGAN HERBERT	2.5%	N88217 001 JUN 06, 1984

POWDER; FOR RX COMPOUNDING

	<u>H-CORT</u>		
AA	TORCH LABS	100%	N87834 001 MAR 29, 1982
	<u>HYDROCORTISONE</u>		
AA	PADDOCK	100%	N88082 001 APR 08, 1983
AA	PHARMA TEK	100%	N85982 001

SOLUTION; TOPICAL

	<u>PENECORT</u>		
AT	ALLERGAN HERBERT	1%	N88214 001 JUN 06, 1984
	<u>TEXACORT</u>		
AT	GENDERM	1%	N80425 001
		2.5%	N81271 001 APR 17, 1992

TABLET; ORAL

	CORTEF		
BP	UPJOHN	10 MG	N08697 001
BP		20 MG	N08697 002
		5 MG	N08697 003
	HYDROCORTISONE		
BP	GLOBAL PHARMS	20 MG	N80781 001
BP	LANNETT	20 MG	N85070 001
BP	PUREPAC PHARM	10 MG	N84247 003 AUG 31, 1982
BP		20 MG	N84247 002
BP	WEST WARD PHARM	20 MG	N83365 001

HYDROCORTISONE *(continued)*

TABLET; ORAL

	HYDROCORTONE		
BP	MERCK SHARP DOHME	10 MG	N08506 007
BP	+	20 MG	N08506 011

HYDROCORTISONE; *MULTIPLE*

SEE <u>ACETIC ACID, GLACIAL; HYDROCORTISONE</u>

SEE <u>ACETIC ACID, GLACIAL; HYDROCORTISONE; NEOMYCIN SULFATE</u>

SEE <u>BACITRACIN ZINC; HYDROCORTISONE; NEOMYCIN SULFATE; POLYMYXIN B SULFATE</u>

HYDROCORTISONE; NEOMYCIN SULFATE

CREAM; TOPICAL

	NEO-CORT-DOME		
	+ MILES	0.5%;EQ 3.5 MG BASE/GM	N50237 006 JUN 05, 1984
	+	1%;EQ 3.5 MG BASE/GM	N50237 005 JUN 05, 1984

HYDROCORTISONE; NEOMYCIN SULFATE; POLYMYXIN B SULFATE

SOLUTION/DROPS; OTIC

	<u>CORTISPORIN</u>		
AT	+ BURROUGHS WELLCOME	<u>1%;EQ 3.5 MG BASE/ ML;10,000 UNITS/ML</u>	N50479 001
	<u>NEO-OTOSOL-HC</u>		
AT	STERIS	<u>1%;EQ 3.5 MG BASE/ ML;10,000 UNITS/ML</u>	N62423 001 AUG 25, 1983
	<u>OTOCORT</u>		
AT	STERIS	<u>1%;EQ 3.5 MG BASE/ ML;10,000 UNITS/ML</u>	N60730 002

SUSPENSION; OTIC

	<u>CORTISPORIN</u>		
AT	+ BURROUGHS WELLCOME	<u>1%;EQ 3.5 MG BASE/ ML;10,000 UNITS/ML</u>	N60613 001
	<u>NEOMYCIN AND POLYMYXIN B SULFATES AND HYDROCORTISONE</u>		
AT	STERIS	<u>1%;EQ 3.5 MG BASE/ ML;10,000 UNITS/ML</u>	N62488 001 NOV 06, 1985
	<u>OTOCORT</u>		
AT	STERIS	<u>1%;EQ 3.5 MG BASE/ ML;10,000 UNITS/ML</u>	N62521 001 JUL 11, 1985

Prescription Drug Products *(continued)*

HYDROCORTISONE; NEOMYCIN SULFATE; POLYMYXIN B SULFATE *(continued)*

SUSPENSION; OTIC

	PEDIOTIC		
AT	BURROUGHS WELLCOME	1%;EQ 3.5 MG BASE/ML;10,000 UNITS/ML	N62822 001 SEP 29, 1987

SUSPENSION/DROPS; OPHTHALMIC

	CORTISPORIN		
AT	+ BURROUGHS WELLCOME	1%;EQ 3.5 MG BASE/ML;10,000 UNITS/ML	N50169 001
	NEOMYCIN AND POLYMYXIN B SULFATES AND HYDROCORTISONE		
AT	STERIS	1%;EQ 3.5 MG BASE/ML;10,000 UNITS/ML	N62874 001 MAY 11, 1988

HYDROCORTISONE; POLYMYXIN B SULFATE

SOLUTION/DROPS; OTIC

	OTOBIOTIC		
AT	+ SCHERING	5 MG/ML;EQ 10,000 UNITS BASE/ML	N62302 001
	PYOCIDIN		
AT	FOREST LABS	5 MG/ML;EQ 10,000 UNITS BASE/ML	N61606 001

HYDROCORTISONE; TETRACYCLINE HYDROCHLORIDE

OINTMENT; OPHTHALMIC

	ACHROMYCIN		
	+ LEDERLE	1.5%;1%	N50272 001

HYDROCORTISONE; UREA

CREAM; TOPICAL

	ALPHADERM		
AT	VIVAN	1%;10%	N86008 001
	CALMURID HC		
AT	+ PHARMACIA	1%;10%	N83947 001

HYDROCORTISONE ACETATE

AEROSOL; RECTAL

	CORTIFOAM		
	+ REED AND CARNRICK	10%	N17351 001 FEB 10, 1982

CREAM; TOPICAL

	HEMSOL-HC		
AT	ABLE	1%	N81274 001 JUN 19, 1992
	HYDROCORTISONE ACETATE		
AT	+ CENCI	1%	N80419 001 JAN 25, 1982
AT	PUREPAC PHARM	1%	N86052 001
		0.5%	N86050 001

INJECTABLE; INJECTION

	HYDROCORTISONE ACETATE		
BP	AKORN	25 MG/ML	N09637 001
BP		50 MG/ML	N09637 002
BP	STERIS	25 MG/ML	N83128 001
BP		25 MG/ML	N83759 001
BP		50 MG/ML	N83759 002
	HYDROCORTONE		
BP	MERCK SHARP DOHME	25 MG/ML	N08228 001
BP	+	50 MG/ML	N08228 004

LOTION; TOPICAL

	DRICORT		
	+ INGRAM PHARM	0.5%	N86207 001

OINTMENT; OPHTHALMIC

	HYDROCORTISONE ACETATE		
	+ ALTANA	0.5%	N80828 001

PASTE; TOPICAL

	ORABASE HCA		
	HOYT LABS	0.5%	N83205 001

POWDER; FOR RX COMPOUNDING

	HYDROCORTISONE ACETATE		
	PHARMA TEK	100%	N85981 001

HYDROCORTISONE ACETATE; *MULTIPLE*

SEE BACITRACIN; HYDROCORTISONE ACETATE; NEOMYCIN SULFATE; POLYMYXIN B SULFATE
SEE CHLORAMPHENICOL; HYDROCORTISONE ACETATE
SEE CHLORAMPHENICOL; HYDROCORTISONE ACETATE; POLYMYXIN B SULFATE
SEE COLISTIN SULFATE; HYDROCORTISONE ACETATE; NEOMYCIN SULFATE; THONZONIUM BROMIDE

Prescription Drug Products *(continued)*

HYDROCORTISONE ACETATE; NEOMYCIN SULFATE
OINTMENT; TOPICAL
NEO-CORTEF
+ UPJOHN 1%;EQ 3.5 MG BASE/GM N60751 002
SUSPENSION/DROPS; OPHTHALMIC
COR-OTICIN
+ AKORN 1.5%;EQ 3.5 MG BASE/ML N60188 001

HYDROCORTISONE ACETATE; NEOMYCIN SULFATE; POLYMYXIN B SULFATE
CREAM; TOPICAL
CORTISPORIN
BURROUGHS WELLCOME 0.5%;EQ 3.5 MG BASE/GM;10,000 UNITS/GM N50218 001 AUG 09, 1985

HYDROCORTISONE ACETATE; OXYTETRACYCLINE HYDROCHLORIDE
SUSPENSION/DROPS; OPHTHALMIC
TERRA-CORTRIL
+ PFIZER 1.5%;EQ 5 MG BASE/ML N61016 001

HYDROCORTISONE ACETATE; PRAMOXINE HYDROCHLORIDE
AEROSOL; TOPICAL
EPIFOAM
BX REED AND CARNRICK 1%;1% N86457 001
HYDROCORTISONE ACETATE 1% AND PRAMOXINE HCL 1%
BX COPLEY PHARM 1%;1% N89440 001 MAY 17, 1988
PROCTOFOAM HC
BX REED AND CARNRICK 1%;1% N86195 001
CREAM; TOPICAL
PRAMOSONE
FERNDALE LABS 0.5%;1% N83778 001
1%;1% N85368 001
LOTION; TOPICAL
PRAMOSONE
FERNDALE LABS 1%;1% N85980 001
2.5%;1% N85979 001

HYDROCORTISONE ACETATE; UREA
CREAM; TOPICAL
CARMOL HC
AT + SYNTEX 1%;10% N80505 001
U-CORT
AT THAMES 1%;10% N89472 001 JUN 13, 1988

HYDROCORTISONE BUTYRATE
CREAM; TOPICAL
LOCOID
+ YAMANOUCHI 0.1% N18514 001 MAR 31, 1982
SOLUTION; TOPICAL
LOCOID
+ YAMANOUCHI 0.1% N19116 001 FEB 25, 1987

HYDROCORTISONE CYPIONATE
SUSPENSION; ORAL
CORTEF
+ UPJOHN EQ 10 MG BASE/5 ML N09900 001

HYDROCORTISONE SODIUM PHOSPHATE
INJECTABLE; INJECTION
HYDROCORTONE
+ MERCK SHARP DOHME EQ 50 MG BASE/ML N12052 001

HYDROCORTISONE SODIUM SUCCINATE
INJECTABLE; INJECTION
A-HYDROCORT
AP ABBOTT EQ 100 MG BASE/VIAL N85928 001
AP EQ 100 MG BASE/VIAL N85929 001
AP EQ 100 MG BASE/VIAL N89577 001 APR 11, 1989
AP EQ 250 MG BASE/VIAL N85930 001
AP EQ 500 MG BASE/VIAL N85931 001
AP EQ 1 GM BASE/VIAL N85932 001
HYDROCORTISONE SODIUM SUCCINATE
AP ELKINS SINN EQ 1 GM BASE/VIAL N87569 001
AP INTL MEDICATION EQ 100 MG BASE/VIAL N87532 001 MAR 19, 1982
AP STERIS EQ 100 MG BASE/VIAL N84737 002
AP EQ 100 MG BASE/VIAL N84738 001
AP EQ 250 MG BASE/VIAL N84737 001
AP EQ 500 MG BASE/VIAL N84747 001
AP EQ 1 GM BASE/VIAL N84748 001
SOLU-CORTEF
AP + UPJOHN EQ 100 MG BASE/VIAL N09866 001
AP + EQ 250 MG BASE/VIAL N09866 002
AP + EQ 500 MG BASE/VIAL N09866 003
AP + EQ 1 GM BASE/VIAL N09866 004

Prescription Drug Products *(continued)*

HYDROCORTISONE VALERATE

CREAM; TOPICAL
WESTCORT
+ WESTWOOD SQUIBB 0.2% N17950 001
OINTMENT; TOPICAL
WESTCORT
+ WESTWOOD SQUIBB 0.2% N18726 001 AUG 08, 1983

HYDROFLUMETHIAZIDE

TABLET; ORAL
DIUCARDIN
AB WYETH AYERST 50 MG N83383 001
HYDROFLUMETHIAZIDE
AB PAR PHARM 50 MG N88850 001 MAY 31, 1985
SALURON
AB + ROBERTS LABS 50 MG N11949 001

HYDROFLUMETHIAZIDE; RESERPINE

TABLET; ORAL
RESERPINE AND HYDROFLUMETHIAZIDE
BP PAR PHARM 50 MG;0.125 MG N88907 001 SEP 20, 1985
BP ZENITH LABS 50 MG;0.125 MG N88932 001 JAN 11, 1985
SALUTENSIN
BP + ROBERTS LABS 50 MG;0.125 MG N12359 003
SALUTENSIN-DEMI
ROBERTS LABS 25 MG;0.125 MG N12359 004

HYDROMORPHONE HYDROCHLORIDE

INJECTABLE; INJECTION
DILAUDID-HP
+ KNOLL PHARM 10 MG/ML N19034 001 JAN 11, 1984
+ 250 MG/VIAL N19034 002 AUG 04, 1994
SOLUTION; ORAL
DILAUDID
KNOLL PHARM 5 MG/5 ML N19891 001 DEC 07, 1992
TABLET; ORAL
DILAUDID
+ KNOLL PHARM 8 MG N19892 001 DEC 07, 1992

HYDROXOCOBALAMIN

INJECTABLE; INJECTION
ALPHAREDISOL
AP + MERCK SHARP DOHME 1 MG/ML N80778 001
HYDROXOCOBALAMIN
AP STERIS 1 MG/ML N85528 001
AP 1 MG/ML N85998 001

HYDROXYAMPHETAMINE HYDROBROMIDE

SOLUTION/DROPS; OPHTHALMIC
PAREDRINE
+ PHARMICS 1% N00004 004

HYDROXYAMPHETAMINE HYDROBROMIDE; TROPICAMIDE

SOLUTION/DROPS; OPHTHALMIC
PAREMYD
ALLERGAN 1%;0.25% N19261 001 JAN 30, 1992

HYDROXYCHLOROQUINE SULFATE

TABLET; ORAL
PLAQUENIL
+ STERLING WINTHROP 200 MG N09768 001

HYDROXYPROGESTERONE CAPROATE

INJECTABLE; INJECTION
HYDROXYPROGESTERONE CAPROATE
AO AKORN 125 MG/ML N18004 001
AO + STERIS 125 MG/ML N17439 001
+ 250 MG/ML N17439 002

HYDROXYPROPYL CELLULOSE

INSERT; OPHTHALMIC
LACRISERT
MERCK 5 MG N18771 001

HYDROXYUREA

CAPSULE; ORAL
HYDREA
SQUIBB 500 MG N16295 001

Prescription Drug Products *(continued)*

HYDROXYZINE HYDROCHLORIDE

INJECTABLE; INJECTION

TE	Product / Applicant	Strength	Appl No / Date
	HYDROXYZINE		
AP	ELKINS SINN	50 MG/ML	N85551 002
	HYDROXYZINE HCL		
AP	ABBOTT	50 MG/ML	N86821 001
AP	ELKINS SINN	25 MG/ML	N85551 001
AP	FUJISAWA	25 MG/ML	N87329 001
AP		25 MG/ML	N88184 001 MAR 31, 1983
AP		50 MG/ML	N87329 002
AP		50 MG/ML	N88185 001 MAR 31, 1983
AP	LUITPOLD	25 MG/ML	N87408 001
AP		50 MG/ML	N87408 002
AP	PHARMAFAIR	50 MG/ML	N88881 001 FEB 14, 1986
AP	SOLOPAK	25 MG/ML	N86822 001
AP		25 MG/ML	N87591 001
AP		50 MG/ML	N87310 001
AP		50 MG/ML	N87593 001
AP		50 MG/ML	N87595 001
AP		50 MG/ML	N87596 001
AP	STERIS	25 MG/ML	N85778 001
AP		25 MG/ML	N87274 001
AP		50 MG/ML	N85779 001
AP		50 MG/ML	N87274 002
AP	STERLING WINTHROP	25 MG/ML	N87416 001
AP		50 MG/ML	N87546 001
	VISTARIL		
AP	+ PFIZER	25 MG/ML	N11111 001
AP	+	50 MG/ML	N11111 002

SYRUP; ORAL

TE	Product / Applicant	Strength	Appl No / Date
	ATARAX		
AA	ROERIG	10 MG/5 ML	N10485 001
	HYDROXYZINE HCL		
AA	BARRE	10 MG/5 ML	N86880 001
AA		10 MG/5 ML	N88785 001 FEB 03, 1988
AA	KV PHARM	10 MG/5 ML	N87730 001 JUL 01, 1982
AA	PENNEX	10 MG/5 ML	N87294 001 APR 12, 1982

HYDROXYZINE HYDROCHLORIDE *(continued)*

TABLET; ORAL

TE	Product / Applicant	Strength	Appl No / Date
	ATARAX		
AB	+ ROERIG	10 MG	N10392 001
AB	+	25 MG	N10392 004
AB	+	50 MG	N10392 006
AB	+	100 MG	N10392 005
	HYDROXYZINE HCL		
AB	AMIDE PHARM	10 MG	N89071 001 JUL 22, 1986
AB		25 MG	N89072 001 JUL 22, 1986
AB		50 MG	N89073 001 JUL 22, 1986
AB	DANBURY PHARMA	10 MG	N88348 001 SEP 15, 1983
AB		25 MG	N88349 001 SEP 15, 1983
AB		50 MG	N88350 001 SEP 15, 1983
AB	GENEVA PHARMS	10 MG	N87869 001 DEC 20, 1982
AB		25 MG	N87870 001 DEC 20, 1982
AB		50 MG	N87871 001 DEC 20, 1982
AB	HALSEY	10 MG	N89366 001 MAY 02, 1988
AB		25 MG	N89117 001 MAY 02, 1988
AB		50 MG	N89396 001 MAY 02, 1988
AB	KV PHARM	10 MG	N87819 001 JUN 23, 1982
AB		25 MG	N87820 001 JUN 23, 1982
AB		50 MG	N87821 001 JUN 23, 1982
AB		100 MG	N87822 001 JUN 23, 1982
AB	MUTUAL PHARM	10 MG	N89381 001 MAY 19, 1986
AB		25 MG	N89382 001 MAY 19, 1986
AB		50 MG	N89383 001 MAY 19, 1986
AB	PAR PHARM	10 MG	N87602 001 JAN 22, 1982
AB		25 MG	N87603 001 JAN 22, 1982
AB		50 MG	N87604 001 JAN 22, 1982

Prescription Drug Products *(continued)*

HYDROXYZINE HYDROCHLORIDE *(continued)*

	TABLET; ORAL		
	HYDROXYZINE HCL		
AB	PUREPAC PHARM	10 MG	N88120 001 SEP 25, 1984
AB		25 MG	N88121 001 SEP 25, 1984
AB		50 MG	N88122 001 SEP 25, 1984
AB	ROYCE LABS	10 MG	N81149 001 MAR 18, 1994
AB		25 MG	N81150 001 MAR 18, 1994
AB		50 MG	N81151 001 MAR 18, 1994
AB	SIDMAK LABS NJ	10 MG	N88617 001 JAN 10, 1986
AB		25 MG	N88618 001 JAN 10, 1986
AB		50 MG	N88619 001 JAN 10, 1986
AB	SUPERPHARM	10 MG	N88794 001 DEC 05, 1984
AB		25 MG	N88795 001 DEC 05, 1984
AB		50 MG	N88796 001 DEC 05, 1984
AB	ZENITH LABS	10 MG	N87216 001
AB		25 MG	N87410 001
AB		50 MG	N87411 001

HYDROXYZINE PAMOATE

	CAPSULE; ORAL		
	HY-PAM		
AB	EON LABS	EQ 25 MG HCL	N87479 001
	HYDROXYZINE PAMOATE		
AB	BARR	EQ 25 MG HCL	N88496 001 JUN 15, 1984
AB		EQ 50 MG HCL	N88487 001 JUN 15, 1984
AB		EQ 100 MG HCL	N88488 001 JUN 15, 1984
AB	DANBURY PHARMA	EQ 25 MG HCL	N81165 001 JUL 31, 1991
AB		EQ 50 MG HCL	N87767 001 AUG 16, 1982
AB		EQ 100 MG HCL	N87790 001 AUG 16, 1982
AB	EON LABS	EQ 50 MG HCL	N86183 001

HYDROXYZINE PAMOATE *(continued)*

	CAPSULE; ORAL		
	HYDROXYZINE PAMOATE		
AB	GENEVA PHARMS	EQ 25 MG HCL	N81127 001 JUN 28, 1991
AB		EQ 50 MG HCL	N81128 001 JUN 28, 1991
AB		EQ 100 MG HCL	N81129 001 JUN 28, 1991
AB	VANGARD	EQ 50 MG HCL	N88393 001 SEP 19, 1983
AB	ZENITH LABS	EQ 25 MG HCL	N87761 001 MAR 05, 1982
AB		EQ 50 MG HCL	N87760 001 MAR 05, 1982
	VISTARIL		
AB	PFIZER	EQ 25 MG HCL	N11459 002
AB	+	EQ 50 MG HCL	N11459 004
AB		EQ 100 MG HCL	N11459 006
	SUSPENSION; ORAL		
	VISTARIL		
	PFIZER	EQ 25 MG HCL/5 ML	N11795 001

IBUPROFEN

	SUSPENSION; ORAL		
	CHILDREN'S ADVIL		
BX	WHITEHALL LABS	100 MG/5 ML	N19833 002 SEP 19, 1989
	PEDIA PROFEN		
BX	+ MCNEIL	100 MG/5 ML	N19842 001 SEP 19, 1989
	RUFEN		
BX	BOOTS	100 MG/5 ML	N19784 001 DEC 18, 1989
	TABLET; ORAL		
	IBU-TAB		
AB	ALRA	400 MG	N71058 001 AUG 11, 1988
AB		600 MG	N71059 001 AUG 11, 1988
AB		800 MG	N71965 001 AUG 11, 1988

Prescription Drug Products *(continued)*

IBUPROFEN *(continued)*

TABLET; ORAL

IBUPROFEN

AB	BARR	400 MG	N70079 001	JUL 24, 1985
AB		600 MG	N70080 001	JUL 24, 1985
AB		800 MG	N71448 001	FEB 18, 1987
AB	BOOTS	400 MG	N70083 001	FEB 22, 1985
AB	DANBURY PHARMA	400 MG	N70436 001	AUG 21, 1985
AB		600 MG	N70437 001	AUG 21, 1985
AB		800 MG	N71547 001	JUL 02, 1987
AB	GENEVA PHARMS	300 MG	N70734 001	JUN 12, 1986
AB		400 MG	N70735 001	JUN 12, 1986
AB		600 MG	N70736 001	JUN 12, 1986
AB		800 MG	N72169 001	DEC 11, 1987
AB	HALSEY	300 MG	N71028 001	MAR 23, 1987
AB		400 MG	N71029 001	MAR 23, 1987
AB		600 MG	N71030 001	MAR 23, 1987
AB		800 MG	N72137 001	FEB 05, 1988
AB	INTERPHARM	400 MG	N71334 001	NOV 25, 1986
AB		600 MG	N71335 001	NOV 25, 1986
AB		800 MG	N71935 001	OCT 13, 1987
AB	INVAMED	400 MG	N72064 001	JAN 14, 1988
AB		600 MG	N72065 001	JAN 14, 1988
AB		800 MG	N71938 001	JAN 14, 1988
AB	LEDERLE	400 MG	N70629 001	SEP 19, 1986
AB		600 MG	N70630 001	SEP 19, 1986

IBUPROFEN *(continued)*

TABLET; ORAL

IBUPROFEN

AB	LEMMON	400 MG	N73343 001	JUN 30, 1992
AB		600 MG	N73344 001	JUN 30, 1992
AB		800 MG	N73345 001	JUN 30, 1992
AB	MUTUAL PHARM	300 MG	N71230 001	OCT 22, 1986
AB		400 MG	N71231 001	OCT 22, 1986
AB		600 MG	N71232 001	OCT 22, 1986
AB		800 MG	N72004 001	NOV 18, 1987
AB	MYLAN	400 MG	N70045 001	SEP 24, 1985
AB		600 MG	N70057 001	SEP 24, 1985
AB		800 MG	N71999 001	DEC 03, 1987
AB	NORTON HN	400 MG	N71145 001	SEP 23, 1986
AB		600 MG	N71146 001	SEP 23, 1986
AB		800 MG	N71769 001	MAY 08, 1987
AB	OHM	400 MG	N70818 001	DEC 26, 1985
AB	PAR PHARM	400 MG	N70329 001	AUG 06, 1985
AB		600 MG	N70330 001	AUG 06, 1985
AB		800 MG	N70986 001	JUL 25, 1986
AB	PRIVATE FORM	300 MG	N71266 001	OCT 15, 1986
AB		400 MG	N71267 001	OCT 15, 1986
AB		600 MG	N71268 001	OCT 15, 1986
AB		800 MG	N72300 001	JUL 01, 1988

Prescription Drug Products *(continued)*

IBUPROFEN *(continued)*

TABLET; ORAL

	IBUPROFEN		
AB	PUREPAC PHARM	300 MG	N71123 001 SEP 19, 1986
AB		400 MG	N71124 001 SEP 19, 1986
AB		600 MG	N71125 001 SEP 19, 1986
AB		800 MG	N71964 001 FEB 01, 1988
AB	SIDMAK LABS NJ	400 MG	N71666 001 JUN 18, 1987
AB		600 MG	N71667 001 JUN 18, 1987
AB		800 MG	N71668 001 JUN 18, 1987
AB	VINTAGE PHARMS	400 MG	N71644 001 FEB 01, 1988
	IBUPROHM		
AB	OHM	400 MG	N70469 001 AUG 29, 1985
	MOTRIN		
AB	UPJOHN	300 MG	N17463 003
AB		400 MG	N17463 002
AB		600 MG	N17463 004
AB	+	800 MG	N17463 005 MAY 22, 1985
	RUFEN		
AB	BOOTS	400 MG	N18197 001
AB		600 MG	N70088 001 FEB 08, 1985
AB		600 MG	N70099 001 MAR 29, 1985
AB		800 MG	N70745 001 JUL 23, 1986

IDARUBICIN HYDROCHLORIDE

INJECTABLE; INJECTION

	IDAMYCIN		
	+ PHARMACIA	5 MG/VIAL	N50661 002 SEP 27, 1990
	+	10 MG/VIAL	N50661 001 SEP 27, 1990

IDOXURIDINE

SOLUTION/DROPS; OPHTHALMIC

	DENDRID		
AT	ALCON	0.1%	N14169 001
	HERPLEX		
AT	+ ALLERGAN	0.1%	N13935 002

IFOSFAMIDE

INJECTABLE; INJECTION

	IFEX		
	+ BRISTOL MYERS SQUIBB	1 GM/VIAL	N19763 001 DEC 30, 1988
	+	3 GM/VIAL	N19763 002 DEC 30, 1988

IMIGLUCERASE

INJECTABLE; INJECTION

	CEREZYME		
	+ GENZYME	200 UNITS/VIAL	N20367 001 MAY 23, 1994

IMIPENEM; *MULTIPLE*

SEE CILASTATIN SODIUM; IMIPENEM

IMIPRAMINE HYDROCHLORIDE

CONCENTRATE; ORAL

	IMIPRAMINE HCL		
	CIBA	25 MG/ML	N86765 001

INJECTABLE; INJECTION

	TOFRANIL		
	+ GEIGY	12.5 MG/ML	N11838 002

TABLET; ORAL

	IMIPRAMINE HCL		
AB	BIOCRAFT	10 MG	N83729 001
AB		25 MG	N83729 004
AB		50 MG	N83729 003
AB	EON LABS	10 MG	N85200 001
AB		25 MG	N84869 002
AB		50 MG	N85133 001
AB	GENEVA PHARMS	10 MG	N84936 002
AB		25 MG	N83745 001
AB		50 MG	N84937 001
AB	MUTUAL PHARM	10 MG	N81048 001 JUN 05, 1990
AB		25 MG	N81049 001 JUN 05, 1990
AB		50 MG	N81050 001 JUN 05, 1990

Prescription Drug Products *(continued)*

IMIPRAMINE HYDROCHLORIDE *(continued)*

	TABLET; ORAL		
	IMIPRAMINE HCL		
AB	PAR PHARM	10 MG	N88292 001 OCT 21, 1983
AB		10 MG	N89422 001 JUL 14, 1987
AB		25 MG	N88262 001 OCT 21, 1983
AB		25 MG	N89497 001 JUL 14, 1987
AB		50 MG	N88276 001 OCT 21, 1983
AB	ROXANE	10 MG	N83799 001
AB		25 MG	N83799 002
AB		50 MG	N83799 003
	JANIMINE		
AB	ABBOTT	10 MG	N17895 001
AB		25 MG	N17895 002
AB		50 MG	N17895 003
	TOFRANIL		
AB	GEIGY	10 MG	N87844 001 MAY 22, 1984
AB		25 MG	N87845 001 MAY 22, 1984
AB	+	50 MG	N87846 001 MAY 22, 1984

IMIPRAMINE PAMOATE

	CAPSULE; ORAL		
	TOFRANIL-PM		
	GEIGY	EQ 75 MG HCL	N17090 001
		EQ 100 MG HCL	N17090 004
		EQ 125 MG HCL	N17090 003
	+	EQ 150 MG HCL	N17090 002

INDAPAMIDE

	TABLET; ORAL		
	LOZOL		
	RHONE POULENC RORER	1.25 MG	N18538 002 APR 29, 1993
	+	2.5 MG	N18538 001 JUL 06, 1983

INDECAINIDE HYDROCHLORIDE

	TABLET, EXTENDED RELEASE; ORAL		
	DECABID		
	LILLY	EQ 50 MG BASE	N19693 001 DEC 29, 1989
		EQ 75 MG BASE	N19693 002 DEC 29, 1989
	+	EQ 100 MG BASE	N19693 003 DEC 29, 1989

INDIUM IN-111 OXYQUINOLINE

	INJECTABLE; INJECTION		
	INDIUM IN-111 OXYQUINOLINE		
	AMERSHAM	1mCi/ML	N19044 001 DEC 23, 1985

INDIUM IN-111 PENTETATE DISODIUM

	INJECTABLE; INTRATHECAL		
	MPI INDIUM DTPA IN 111		
	MEDI PHYSICS	1mCi/ML	N17707 001 FEB 18, 1982

INDIUM IN-111 PENTETREOTIDE KIT

	INJECTABLE; INJECTION		
	OCTREOSCAN		
	MALLINCKRODT	3mCi/ML	N20314 001 JUN 02, 1994

INDOCYANINE GREEN

	INJECTABLE; INJECTION		
	CARDIO-GREEN		
	+ BECTON DICKINSON	25 MG/VIAL	N11525 001
	+	50 MG/VIAL	N11525 002

INDOMETHACIN

	CAPSULE; ORAL		
	INDO-LEMMON		
AB	LEMMON	25 MG	N70266 001 NOV 07, 1985
AB		50 MG	N70267 001 NOV 07, 1985
	INDOCIN		
AB	MERCK	25 MG	N16059 001
AB	+	50 MG	N16059 002

Prescription Drug Products *(continued)*

INDOMETHACIN *(continued)*

CAPSULE; ORAL

INDOMETHACIN

AB	BARR	25 MG	N70067 001 OCT 03, 1986
AB		50 MG	N70068 001 OCT 03, 1986
AB	DANBURY PHARMA	25 MG	N72996 001 JUL 31, 1991
AB		50 MG	N72997 001 JUL 31, 1991
AB	GENEVA PHARMS	25 MG	N70673 001 APR 29, 1987
AB		50 MG	N70674 001 APR 29, 1987
AB	HALSEY	25 MG	N70782 001 JUN 03, 1987
AB		50 MG	N70635 001 JUN 03, 1987
AB	LEDERLE	25 MG	N18851 001 MAY 18, 1984
AB		50 MG	N18851 002 MAY 18, 1984
AB	MUTUAL PHARM	25 MG	N70899 001 FEB 09, 1987
AB		50 MG	N70900 001 FEB 09, 1987
AB	MYLAN	25 MG	N18858 001 APR 20, 1984
AB		50 MG	N18858 002 APR 20, 1984
AB		50 MG	N70624 001 SEP 04, 1985
AB	NOVOPHARM	25 MG	N71342 001 APR 18, 1988
AB		50 MG	N71343 001 APR 18, 1988
AB	PAR PHARM	25 MG	N18829 002 AUG 06, 1984
AB		50 MG	N18829 001 AUG 06, 1984
AB		50 MG	N70651 001 MAR 05, 1986
AB	PARKE DAVIS	25 MG	N18806 001 NOV 23, 1984
AB		50 MG	N18806 002 NOV 23, 1984
AB	SIDMAK LABS NJ	25 MG	N71148 001 MAR 18, 1987
AB		50 MG	N71149 001 MAR 18, 1987
AB	WATSON LABS	25 MG	N70529 001 OCT 18, 1985
AB		50 MG	N70530 001 OCT 18, 1985
AB	ZENITH LABS	25 MG	N70719 001 FEB 12, 1986
AB		50 MG	N70756 001 FEB 12, 1986

CAPSULE, EXTENDED RELEASE; ORAL

	INDOCIN SR		
AB	+ MERCK	75 MG	N18185 001 FEB 23, 1982
	INDOMETHACIN		
AB	INWOOD LABS	75 MG	N72410 001 MAR 15, 1989

SUPPOSITORY; RECTAL

	INDOCIN		
AB	+ MERCK	50 MG	N17814 001 AUG 13, 1984
	INDOMETHEGAN		
AB	G AND W LABS	50 MG	N73314 001 AUG 31, 1992

SUSPENSION; ORAL

	INDOCIN		
AB	+ MERCK	25 MG/5 ML	N18332 001 OCT 10, 1985
	INDOMETHACIN		
AB	ROXANE	25 MG/5 ML	N71412 001 MAR 18, 1987

INDOMETHACIN SODIUM

INJECTABLE; INJECTION

	INDOCIN I.V.		
	+ MERCK	EQ 1 MG BASE/VIAL	N18878 001 JAN 30, 1985

INSULIN BIOSYNTHETIC HUMAN

INJECTABLE; INJECTION

	HUMULIN R		
	+ LILLY	500 UNITS/ML	N18780 004 MAR 31, 1994

INSULIN PORK

INJECTABLE; INJECTION

	ILETIN I		
	+ LILLY	500 UNITS/ML	N17931 001

Prescription Drug Products *(continued)*

INSULIN PURIFIED PORK
INJECTABLE; INJECTION
ILETIN II
+ LILLY 500 UNITS/ML N18344 002

INTRINSIC FACTOR; *MULTIPLE*
SEE COBALT CHLORIDE, CO-57; CYANOCOBALAMIN; CYANOCOBALAMIN, CO-57; INTRINSIC FACTOR
SEE CYANOCOBALAMIN; CYANOCOBALAMIN, CO-57; INTRINSIC FACTOR

INULIN
INJECTABLE; INJECTION
INULIN AND SODIUM CHLORIDE
+ ISO TEX 100 MG/ML N02282 001

IOBENGUANE SULFATE I 131
INJECTABLE; INJECTION
IOBENGUANE SULFATE I 131
CIS 2.3mCi/ML N20084 001 MAR 25, 1994

IOCETAMIC ACID
TABLET; ORAL
CHOLEBRINE
+ MALLINCKRODT 750 MG N17129 001

IODAMIDE MEGLUMINE
INJECTABLE; INJECTION
RENOVUE-DIP
+ BRACCO 24% N17903 001
RENOVUE-65
+ BRACCO 65% N17902 001

IODIPAMIDE MEGLUMINE
INJECTABLE; INJECTION
CHOLOGRAFIN MEGLUMINE
+ BRACCO 10.3% N09321 007
+ 52% N09321 003

IODIPAMIDE MEGLUMINE; *MULTIPLE*
SEE DIATRIZOATE MEGLUMINE; IODIPAMIDE MEGLUMINE

IODOHIPPURATE SODIUM, I-131
INJECTABLE; INJECTION
HIPPURAN I 131
MALLINCKRODT 0.25mCi/ML N16666 001
HIPPUTOPE
BRACCO 1-2mCi/VIAL N15419 002
IODOHIPPURATE SODIUM I 131
SORIN BIOMEDICA (US) 0.2mCi/ML N17313 001

IOFETAMINE HYDROCHLORIDE I-123
INJECTABLE; INJECTION
SPECTAMINE
IMP 1mCi/ML N19432 001 DEC 24, 1987

IOHEXOL
INJECTABLE; INJECTION
OMNIPAQUE 140
+ STERLING WINTHROP 30.2% N18956 005 NOV 30, 1988
OMNIPAQUE 210
+ STERLING WINTHROP 45.3% N18956 006 JUN 30, 1989
SOLUTION; INJECTION, ORAL
OMNIPAQUE 350
+ STERLING WINTHROP 75.5% N18956 004 DEC 26, 1985
SOLUTION; INJECTION, ORAL, RECTAL
OMNIPAQUE 180
+ STERLING WINTHROP 38.8% N18956 001 DEC 26, 1985
OMNIPAQUE 240
+ STERLING WINTHROP 51.8% N18956 002 DEC 26, 1985
OMNIPAQUE 300
+ STERLING WINTHROP 64.7% N18956 003 DEC 26, 1985
SOLUTION; URETHRAL
OMNIPAQUE 70
+ STERLING WINTHROP 15.1% N18956 007 JUN 01, 1994

Prescription Drug Products *(continued)*

IOPAMIDOL

INJECTABLE; INJECTION

ISOVUE-M 200		
+ BRACCO	41%	N18735 001 DEC 31, 1985
ISOVUE-M 300		
+ BRACCO	61%	N18735 004 DEC 31, 1985
ISOVUE-128		
+ BRACCO	26%	N18735 005 OCT 21, 1986
ISOVUE-200		
+ BRACCO	41%	N18735 006 JUL 07, 1987
ISOVUE-250		
+ BRACCO	51%	N18735 007 JUL 06, 1992
ISOVUE-300		
+ BRACCO	61%	N18735 002 DEC 31, 1985
ISOVUE-370		
+ BRACCO	76%	N18735 003 DEC 31, 1985

IOPANOIC ACID

TABLET; ORAL

TELEPAQUE		
STERLING WINTHROP	500 MG	N08032 001

IOTHALAMATE MEGLUMINE

INJECTABLE; INJECTION

CONRAY		
+ MALLINCKRODT	60%	N13295 001
CONRAY 30		
+ MALLINCKRODT	30%	N16983 001
CONRAY 43		
+ MALLINCKRODT	43%	N13295 002

SOLUTION; INTRAVESICAL

CYSTO-CONRAY II		
MALLINCKRODT	17.2%	N17057 002

SOLUTION; INTRAVESICAL, URETERAL

CYSTO-CONRAY		
MALLINCKRODT	43%	N17057 001

IOTHALAMATE MEGLUMINE; IOTHALAMATE SODIUM

INJECTABLE; INJECTION

VASCORAY		
+ MALLINCKRODT	52%;26%	N16783 001

IOTHALAMATE SODIUM

INJECTABLE; INJECTION

ANGIO-CONRAY		
+ MALLINCKRODT	80%	N13319 001
CONRAY 325		
+ MALLINCKRODT	54.3%	N17685 001
CONRAY 400		
+ MALLINCKRODT	66.8%	N14295 001

IOTHALAMATE SODIUM; *MULTIPLE*

SEE <u>IOTHALAMATE MEGLUMINE; IOTHALAMATE SODIUM</u>

IOTHALAMATE SODIUM, I-125

INJECTABLE; INJECTION

GLOFIL-125		
ISO TEX	250-300uCi/ML	N17279 001

IOVERSOL

INJECTABLE; INJECTION

OPTIRAY 160		
+ MALLINCKRODT	34%	N19710 003 DEC 30, 1988
OPTIRAY 240		
+ MALLINCKRODT	51%	N19710 002 DEC 30, 1988
OPTIRAY 300		
+ MALLINCKRODT	64%	N19710 004 JAN 22, 1992
OPTIRAY 320		
+ MALLINCKRODT	68%	N19710 001 DEC 30, 1988
OPTIRAY 350		
+ MALLINCKRODT	74%	N19710 005 JAN 22, 1992

IOXAGLATE MEGLUMINE; IOXAGLATE SODIUM

INJECTABLE; INJECTION

HEXABRIX		
+ MALLINCKRODT	39.3%;19.6%	N18905 002 JUL 26, 1985

IOXAGLATE SODIUM; *MULTIPLE*

SEE <u>IOXAGLATE MEGLUMINE; IOXAGLATE SODIUM</u>

IPODATE CALCIUM

GRANULE; ORAL

ORAGRAFIN CALCIUM		
BRACCO	3 GM/PACKET	N12968 001

Prescription Drug Products *(continued)*

IPODATE SODIUM

CAPSULE; ORAL

	BILIVIST		
AA	BERLEX	500 MG	N87768 001 AUG 11, 1982
	ORAGRAFIN SODIUM		
AA	BRACCO	500 MG	N12967 001

IPRATROPIUM BROMIDE

AEROSOL, METERED; INHALATION

	ATROVENT		
	BOEHRINGER INGELHEIM	0.018 MG/INH	N19085 001 DEC 29, 1986

SOLUTION; INHALATION

	ATROVENT		
	+ BOEHRINGER INGELHEIM	0.02%	N20228 001 SEP 29, 1993

IRON DEXTRAN

INJECTABLE; INJECTION

	INFED		
BP	+ SCHEIN	EQ 50 MG IRON/ML	N17441 001
	PROFERDEX		
BP	LOTUS BIOCHEM	EQ 50 MG IRON/ML	N17807 001

ISOETHARINE HYDROCHLORIDE

SOLUTION; INHALATION

	BETA-2		
AN	NEPHRON	1%	N86711 001
	BRONKOSOL		
AN	+ STERLING WINTHROP	1%	N12339 008
	ISOETHARINE HCL		
AN	+ ASTRA	0.125%	N89615 001 JUN 13, 1991
AN	+	0.167%	N89616 001 JUN 13, 1991
AN	+	0.2%	N89617 001 JUN 13, 1991
AN	+	0.25%	N89618 001 JUN 13, 1991
	+	0.062%	N89614 001 JUN 13, 1991
AN	BARRE	1%	N87101 001

ISOETHARINE HYDROCHLORIDE *(continued)*

SOLUTION; INHALATION

	ISOETHARINE HCL		
AN	INTL MEDICATION	0.08%	N86651 002
AN		0.1%	N86651 003
AN		0.167%	N86651 005
AN		0.2%	N86651 006
AN		0.25%	N86651 007
AN		1%	N86651 008
	+	0.077%	N86651 001
	+	0.143%	N86651 004
AN	ROXANE	0.1%	N87396 001
AN		0.125%	N87025 001
AN		0.167%	N88226 001 SEP 16, 1983
AN		0.2%	N87324 001
AN		0.25%	N88275 001 JUN 03, 1983
AN		1%	N86899 001
	ISOETHARINE HCL S/F		
AN	+ DEY	0.08%	N89817 001 NOV 22, 1988
AN	+	0.1%	N89818 001 NOV 22, 1988
AN	+	0.25%	N89820 001 NOV 22, 1988
AN	+	1%	N89252 001 SEP 15, 1986
AN	+	0.17%	N89819 001 NOV 22, 1988

ISOETHARINE MESYLATE

AEROSOL, METERED; INHALATION

	BRONKOMETER		
	+ STERLING WINTHROP	0.34 MG/INH	N12339 007

ISOFLURANE

LIQUID; INHALATION

	FORANE		
AN	+ OHMEDA	99.9%	N17624 001
	ISOFLURANE		
AN	ABBOTT	99.9%	N74097 001 JAN 25, 1993

ISOFLUROPHATE

OINTMENT; OPHTHALMIC

	FLOROPRYL		
	+ MERCK SHARP DOHME	0.025%	N10656 001

Prescription Drug Products *(continued)*

ISONIAZID

INJECTABLE; INJECTION
NYDRAZID
+ APOTHECON 100 MG/ML N08662 001

SYRUP; ORAL
ISONIAZID
AA CAROLINA MEDCL 50 MG/5 ML N88235 001 NOV 10, 1983
LANIAZID
AA LANNETT 50 MG/5 ML N89243 001 FEB 03, 1986

TABLET; ORAL
ISONIAZID

AA	BARR	100 MG	N80936 001
AA		300 MG	N80937 002
AA	DANBURY PHARMA	50 MG	N80522 001
AA		100 MG	N80523 001
AA		300 MG	N80521 001
AA	DURAMED	100 MG	N88231 001 MAR 17, 1983
AA		300 MG	N88119 001 MAR 17, 1983
AA	+ EON LABS	100 MG	N08678 002
AA	+	300 MG	N08678 003
AA	GLOBAL PHARMS	100 MG	N80153 001
AA	HALSEY	50 MG	N83632 001
AA		100 MG	N80136 001
AA		300 MG	N83633 001
AA	PHOENIX LABS NY	50 MG	N80368 001
AA		100 MG	N80368 002
AA	WEST WARD PHARM	100 MG	N80212 001
AA		300 MG	N87425 001
AA	ZENITH LABS	100 MG	N80270 001
AA		300 MG	N83610 001

LANIAZID

AA	LANNETT	50 MG	N80140 001
AA		100 MG	N80140 002
AA		300 MG	N89776 001 JUN 13, 1988

ISONIAZID; PYRAZINAMIDE; RIFAMPIN

TABLET; ORAL
RIFATER
+ MARION MERRELL DOW 50 MG;300 MG;120 MG N50705 001 MAY 31, 1994

ISONIAZID; RIFAMPIN

CAPSULE; ORAL
RIFAMATE
+ DOW PHARMS 150 MG;300 MG N61884 001

ISOPROTERENOL HYDROCHLORIDE

AEROSOL, METERED; INHALATION
ISOPROTERENOL HCL

BN	BARRE	0.12 MG/INH	N85904 001
BN	+ 3M	0.12 MG/INH	N10375 004

ISUPREL
+ STERLING WINTHROP 0.131 MG/INH N11178 001

INJECTABLE; INJECTION
ISOPROTERENOL HCL

AP	ABBOTT	0.2 MG/ML	N83346 001
		0.02 MG/ML	N83283 001
AP	ELKINS SINN	0.2 MG/ML	N83486 001
AP	INTL MEDICATION	0.2 MG/ML	N83724 001

ISUPREL
AP + STERLING WINTHROP 0.2 MG/ML N10515 001

SOLUTION; INHALATION
AEROLONE
+ LILLY 0.25% N07245 001

TABLET; RECTAL, SUBLINGUAL
ISUPREL

; INHALATION STERLING WINTHROP	10 MG	N06328 001
+ STERLING WINTHROP	0.5%	N06327 002
+	1%	N06327 003

ISOPROTERENOL HYDROCHLORIDE; PHENYLEPHRINE BITARTRATE

AEROSOL, METERED; INHALATION
DUO-MEDIHALER
+ 3M 0.16 MG/INH;0.24 MG/INH N13296 001

ISOPROTERENOL SULFATE

AEROSOL, METERED; INHALATION
MEDIHALER-ISO
+ 3M 0.08 MG/INH N10375 003

ISOSORBIDE

SOLUTION; ORAL
ISMOTIC
ALCON 100 GM/220 ML N17063 001

ISOSORBIDE DINITRATE

CAPSULE, EXTENDED RELEASE; ORAL

TE	Product / Applicant	Strength	Appl No	Approval Date
	DILATRATE-SR			
BC	REED AND CARNRICK	40 MG	N19790 001	SEP 02, 1988
	ISORDIL			
BC	+ WYETH AYERST	40 MG	N12882 002	JUL 29, 1988

TABLET; ORAL

TE	Product / Applicant	Strength	Appl No	Approval Date
	ISORDIL			
AB	WYETH AYERST	5 MG	N12093 007	JUL 29, 1988
AB		10 MG	N12093 002	JUL 29, 1988
AB		20 MG	N12093 006	JUL 29, 1988
AB	+	30 MG	N12093 005	JUL 29, 1988
AB		40 MG	N12093 001	JUL 29, 1988
	ISOSORBIDE DINITRATE			
AB	BARR	5 MG	N86166 002	SEP 19, 1986
AB		10 MG	N86169 001	SEP 19, 1986
AB		20 MG	N86167 001	SEP 19, 1986
AB		30 MG	N87564 001	SEP 18, 1986
AB	DANBURY PHARMA	5 MG	N86034 001	JAN 06, 1988
AB		10 MG	N86032 001	JAN 07, 1988
AB	GENEVA PHARMS	5 MG	N86221 001	JAN 07, 1988
AB		10 MG	N86223 001	JAN 07, 1988
AB		20 MG	N89367 001	APR 07, 1988
AB	PAR PHARM	5 MG	N86923 001	MAR 12, 1987
AB		10 MG	N86925 001	MAR 12, 1987
AB		20 MG	N87537 001	OCT 02, 1987
AB		30 MG	N87946 001	JAN 12, 1988

ISOSORBIDE DINITRATE *(continued)*

TABLET; ORAL

TE	Product / Applicant	Strength	Appl No	Approval Date
	ISOSORBIDE DINITRATE			
AB	WEST WARD PHARM	5 MG	N86067 001	OCT 29, 1987
AB		10 MG	N86066 001	OCT 29, 1987
AB		20 MG	N88088 001	NOV 02, 1987
	SORBITRATE			
AB	ZENECA	20 MG	N86405 002	AUG 21, 1990
AB		30 MG	N88124 001	AUG 21, 1990
AB		40 MG	N88125 001	AUG 21, 1990

TABLET; SUBLINGUAL

TE	Product / Applicant	Strength	Appl No	Approval Date
	ISORDIL			
AB	WYETH AYERST	2.5 MG	N12940 004	JUL 29, 1988
AB		5 MG	N12940 003	JUL 29, 1988
AB	+	10 MG	N12940 005	JUL 29, 1988
	ISOSORBIDE DINITRATE			
AB	BARR	2.5 MG	N84204 001	SEP 18, 1986
AB		5 MG	N86168 001	SEP 18, 1986
AB		10 MG	N87545 001	SEP 18, 1986
AB	DANBURY PHARMA	2.5 MG	N86033 001	FEB 26, 1988
AB		5 MG	N86031 001	SEP 29, 1987
AB	GENEVA PHARMS	2.5 MG	N86225 001	FEB 19, 1988
AB		5 MG	N86222 001	FEB 19, 1988
AB	WEST WARD PHARM	2.5 MG	N86054 001	OCT 29, 1987
AB		5 MG	N86055 001	NOV 02, 1987

TABLET, EXTENDED RELEASE; ORAL

TE	Product / Applicant	Strength	Appl No	Approval Date
	ISORDIL			
	+ WYETH AYERST	40 MG	N12882 001	JUL 29, 1988

Prescription Drug Products *(continued)*

ISOSORBIDE MONONITRATE

TABLET; ORAL

ISMO

AB + WYETH 20 MG N19091 001 DEC 30, 1991

MONOKET

AB SCHWARZ PHARMA 20 MG N20215 001 JUN 30, 1993

10 MG N20215 002 JUN 30, 1993

TABLET, EXTENDED RELEASE; ORAL

IMDUR

SCHERING PLOUGH 60 MG N20225 002 AUG 12, 1993

ISOSULFAN BLUE

INJECTABLE; INJECTION

LYMPHAZURIN

\+ HIRSCH INDS 1% N18310 001

ISOTRETINOIN

CAPSULE; ORAL

ACCUTANE

ROCHE 10 MG N18662 002 MAY 07, 1982

20 MG N18662 004 MAR 28, 1983

\+ 40 MG N18662 003 MAY 07, 1982

ISRADIPINE

CAPSULE; ORAL

DYNACIRC

SANDOZ 2.5 MG N19546 001 DEC 20, 1990

\+ 5 MG N19546 002 DEC 20, 1990

TABLET, EXTENDED RELEASE; ORAL

DYNACIRC CR

\+ SANDOZ 5 MG N20336 001 JUN 01, 1994

\+ 10 MG N20336 002 JUN 01, 1994

ITRACONAZOLE

CAPSULE; ORAL

SPORANOX

\+ JANSSEN 100 MG N20083 001 SEP 11, 1992

KANAMYCIN SULFATE

CAPSULE; ORAL

KANTREX

\+ APOTHECON EQ 500 MG BASE N62726 001 MAR 06, 1987

INJECTABLE; INJECTION

KANAMYCIN

AP ELKINS SINN EQ 75 MG BASE/2 ML N62324 001

AP EQ 500 MG BASE/2 ML N62324 002

AP EQ 1 GM BASE/3 ML N62324 003

KANAMYCIN SULFATE

AP LOCH EQ 75 MG BASE/2 ML N63021 001 JUL 31, 1992

AP EQ 500 MG BASE/2 ML N63022 001 JUL 31, 1992

AP EQ 1 GM BASE/3 ML N63025 001 JUL 31, 1992

AP PHARMAFAIR EQ 75 MG BASE/2 ML N62668 001 MAY 07, 1987

AP EQ 500 MG BASE/2 ML N62672 001 MAY 07, 1987

AP EQ 1 GM BASE/3 ML N62669 001 MAY 07, 1987

AP SOLOPAK EQ 75 MG BASE/2 ML N62605 003 FEB 26, 1986

AP EQ 500 MG BASE/2 ML N62605 001 FEB 26, 1986

AP EQ 1 GM BASE/3 ML N62605 002 FEB 26, 1986

AP STERIS EQ 1 GM BASE/3 ML N62520 003 MAY 09, 1985

KANTREX

AP + APOTHECON EQ 75 MG BASE/2 ML N61901 003

AP + EQ 500 MG BASE/2 ML N61901 001

AP + EQ 1 GM BASE/3 ML N61901 002

KETAMINE HYDROCHLORIDE

INJECTABLE; INJECTION

KETALAR

\+ PARKE DAVIS EQ 10 MG BASE/ML N16812 001

\+ EQ 50 MG BASE/ML N16812 002

\+ EQ 100 MG BASE/ML N16812 003

Prescription Drug Products *(continued)*

KETOCONAZOLE

CREAM; TOPICAL
NIZORAL

TE	Applicant	Strength	Appl No / Date
	+ JANSSEN	2%	N19084 001 DEC 31, 1985
		2%	N19576 001 OCT 22, 1987
		2%	N19648 001 SEP 25, 1987

SHAMPOO; TOPICAL
NIZORAL

TE	Applicant	Strength	Appl No / Date
	+ JANSSEN	2%	N19927 001 AUG 31, 1990

TABLET; ORAL
NIZORAL

TE	Applicant	Strength	Appl No / Date
	+ JANSSEN	200 MG	N18533 001

KETOPROFEN

CAPSULE; ORAL
KETOPROFEN

TE	Applicant	Strength	Appl No / Date
AB	BIOCRAFT	25 MG	N73515 001 DEC 22, 1992
AB		50 MG	N73516 001 DEC 22, 1992
AB		75 MG	N73517 001 DEC 22, 1992
AB	LEDERLE	25 MG	N74014 001 JAN 29, 1993
AB		50 MG	N74014 002 JAN 29, 1993
AB		75 MG	N74014 003 JAN 29, 1993

ORUDIS

TE	Applicant	Strength	Appl No / Date
AB	WYETH AYERST	25 MG	N18754 001 JUL 31, 1987
AB		50 MG	N18754 002 JAN 09, 1986
AB	+	75 MG	N18754 003 JAN 09, 1986

CAPSULE, EXTENDED RELEASE; ORAL
ORUVAIL

TE	Applicant	Strength	Appl No / Date
	+ WYETH AYERST	200 MG	N19816 001 SEP 24, 1993

KETOROLAC TROMETHAMINE

INJECTABLE; INJECTION
TORADOL

TE	Applicant	Strength	Appl No / Date
	+ SYNTEX	15 MG/ML	N19698 001 NOV 30, 1989
	+	30 MG/ML	N19698 002 NOV 30, 1989

SOLUTION/DROPS; OPHTHALMIC
ACULAR

TE	Applicant	Strength	Appl No / Date
	SYNTEX	0.5%	N19700 001 NOV 09, 1992

TABLET; ORAL
TORADOL

TE	Applicant	Strength	Appl No / Date
	+ SYNTEX	10 MG	N19645 001 DEC 20, 1991

KRYPTON, KR-81M

GAS; INHALATION
MPI KRYPTON 81M GAS GENERATOR

TE	Applicant	Strength	Appl No / Date
	MEDI PHYSICS	N/A	N18088 001

LABETALOL HYDROCHLORIDE

INJECTABLE; INJECTION
NORMODYNE

TE	Applicant	Strength	Appl No / Date
AP	+ SCHERING	5 MG/ML	N18686 001 AUG 01, 1984

TRANDATE

TE	Applicant	Strength	Appl No / Date
AP	GLAXO	5 MG/ML	N19425 001 DEC 31, 1985

TABLET; ORAL
NORMODYNE

TE	Applicant	Strength	Appl No / Date
AB	SCHERING	100 MG	N18687 001 AUG 31, 1987
AB		200 MG	N18687 002 AUG 01, 1984
AB	+	300 MG	N18687 003 AUG 01, 1984

TRANDATE

TE	Applicant	Strength	Appl No / Date
AB	GLAXO	100 MG	N18716 001 MAY 24, 1985
AB		200 MG	N18716 002 AUG 01, 1984
AB		300 MG	N18716 003 AUG 01, 1984

Prescription Drug Products *(continued)*

LACTULOSE

SOLUTION; ORAL

	CHRONULAC		
AA	MERRELL DOW	10 GM/15 ML	N17884 001
	CONSTILAC		
AA	ALRA	10 GM/15 ML	N71054 001 JUL 26, 1988
	CONSTULOSE		
AA	BARRE	10 GM/15 ML	N70288 001 AUG 15, 1988
	DUPHALAC		
AA	SOLVAY	10 GM/15 ML	N72372 001 MAR 22, 1989
	EVALOSE		
AA	COPLEY PHARM	10 GM/15 ML	N73497 001 MAY 28, 1993
	LACTULOSE		
AA	PACO	10 GM/15 ML	N73160 001 AUG 25, 1992
AA	ROXANE	10 GM/15 ML	N73591 001 MAY 29, 1992
AA	UDL	10 GM/15 ML	N74138 001 SEP 30, 1992
	LAXILOSE		
AA	TECHNILAB	10 GM/15 ML	N73686 001 MAY 28, 1993

SOLUTION; ORAL, RECTAL

	ACILAC		
AA	TECHNILAB	10 GM/15 ML	N73685 001 MAY 28, 1993
	CEPHULAC		
AA	MERRELL DOW	10 GM/15 ML	N17657 001
	CHOLAC		
AA	ALRA	10 GM/15 ML	N71331 001 JUL 26, 1988
	ENULOSE		
AA	BARRE	10 GM/15 ML	N71548 001 AUG 15, 1988
	HEPTALAC		
AA	COPLEY PHARM	10 GM/15 ML	N73504 001 MAY 28, 1993
	LACTULOSE		
AA	PACO	10 GM/15 ML	N72029 001 AUG 25, 1992
AA	ROXANE	10 GM/15 ML	N73590 001 MAY 29, 1992

LEUCOVORIN CALCIUM

INJECTABLE; INJECTION

	LEUCOVORIN CALCIUM		
AP	BEN VENUE	EQ 50 MG BASE/VIAL	N89384 001 SEP 14, 1987
AP		EQ 100 MG BASE/VIAL	N89717 001 MAR 28, 1988
AP	ELKINS SINN	EQ 50 MG BASE/VIAL	N70480 001 JAN 02, 1987
AP		EQ 100 MG BASE/VIAL	N81224 001 JUN 03, 1994
AP	GENSIA	EQ 50 MG BASE/VIAL	N81278 001 SEP 28, 1993
AP		EQ 100 MG BASE/VIAL	N81277 001 SEP 28, 1993
AP	+ IMMUNEX	EQ 50 MG BASE/VIAL	N08107 002
AP	+	EQ 100 MG BASE/VIAL	N08107 004 MAY 23, 1988
	+	EQ 350 MG BASE/VIAL	N08107 005 APR 05, 1989
	WELLCOVORIN		
AP	BURROUGHS WELLCOME	EQ 50 MG BASE/VIAL	N89465 001 JAN 23, 1989
AP		EQ 100 MG BASE/VIAL	N89834 001 JAN 23, 1989
	+	EQ 5 MG BASE/ML	N87439 001 OCT 19, 1982
	+	EQ 25 MG BASE/VIAL	N89833 001 JAN 23, 1989

POWDER FOR RECONSTITUTION; ORAL

	LEUCOVORIN CALCIUM		
	IMMUNEX	EQ 60 MG BASE/VIAL	N08107 003 JAN 30, 1987

TABLET; ORAL

	LEUCOVORIN CALCIUM		
AB	BARR	EQ 5 MG BASE	N71198 001 SEP 24, 1987
AB		EQ 25 MG BASE	N71199 001 SEP 24, 1987
AB	IMMUNEX	EQ 10 MG BASE	N71962 001 NOV 19, 1987
AB	+	EQ 15 MG BASE	N71104 001 MAR 04, 1987
BX		EQ 5 MG BASE	N18459 001 JAN 30, 1986

Prescription Drug Products *(continued)*

LEUCOVORIN CALCIUM *(continued)*

TABLET; ORAL

TE	Product / Applicant	Strength	Appl No / Date
	LEUCOVORIN CALCIUM		
AB	ROXANE	EQ 5 MG BASE	N72733 001 FEB 22, 1993
AB		EQ 10 MG BASE	N72734 001 FEB 22, 1993
AB		EQ 15 MG BASE	N72735 001 FEB 22, 1993
AB		EQ 25 MG BASE	N72736 001 FEB 22, 1993
	WELLCOVORIN		
AB	BURROUGHS WELLCOME	EQ 5 MG BASE	N18342 001 JUL 08, 1983
AB	+	EQ 25 MG BASE	N18342 002 JUL 08, 1983

LEUPROLIDE ACETATE

INJECTABLE; INJECTION

TE	Product / Applicant	Strength	Appl No / Date
	LUPRON		
	+ TAP PHARMS	5 MG/ML	N19010 001 APR 09, 1985
		5 MG/ML	N20263 001 APR 16, 1993
	LUPRON DEPOT		
	+ TAP PHARMS	7.5 MG/VIAL	N19732 001 JAN 26, 1989
	+	3.75 MG/VIAL	N20011 001 OCT 22, 1990
	LUPRON DEPOT-PED		
	+ TAP PHARMS	7.5 MG/VIAL	N20263 002 APR 16, 1993
	+	3.75 MG/VIAL&7.5 MG/VIAL	N20263 003 APR 16, 1993
	+	7.5 MG/VIAL&7.5 MG/VIAL	N20263 004 APR 16, 1993

LEVAMISOLE HYDROCHLORIDE

TABLET; ORAL

TE	Product / Applicant	Strength	Appl No / Date
	ERGAMISOL		
	JANSSEN	EQ 50 MG BASE	N20035 001 JUN 18, 1990

LEVOBUNOLOL HYDROCHLORIDE

SOLUTION/DROPS; OPHTHALMIC

TE	Product / Applicant	Strength	Appl No / Date
	BETAGAN		
AT	+ ALLERGAN	0.25%	N19814 001 JUN 28, 1989
AT	+	0.5%	N19219 002 DEC 19, 1985
	LEVOBUNOLOL HCL		
AT	BAUSCH AND LOMB	0.25%	N74307 001 MAR 04, 1994
AT		0.5%	N74326 001 MAR 04, 1994

LEVOCABASTINE HYDROCHLORIDE

SUSPENSION/DROPS; OPHTHALMIC

TE	Product / Applicant	Strength	Appl No / Date
	LIVOSTIN		
	+ IOLAB	EQ 0.05% BASE	N20219 001 NOV 10, 1993

LEVOCARNITINE

INJECTABLE; INJECTION

TE	Product / Applicant	Strength	Appl No / Date
	CARNITOR		
	SIGMA TAU	200 MG/ML	N20182 001 DEC 16, 1992

SOLUTION; ORAL

TE	Product / Applicant	Strength	Appl No / Date
	CARNITOR		
	SIGMA TAU	1 GM/10 ML	N18948 002 APR 27, 1988
		1 GM/10 ML	N19257 001 APR 10, 1986

TABLET; ORAL

TE	Product / Applicant	Strength	Appl No / Date
	CARNITOR		
	SIGMA TAU	330 MG	N18948 001 DEC 27, 1985

LEVODOPA

CAPSULE; ORAL

TE	Product / Applicant	Strength	Appl No / Date
	DOPAR		
	ROBERTS LABS	100 MG	N16913 003
		250 MG	N16913 001
	+	500 MG	N16913 002

TABLET; ORAL

TE	Product / Applicant	Strength	Appl No / Date
	DOPAR		
BD	ROBERTS LABS	250 MG	N16913 004
BD		500 MG	N16913 005
	LARODOPA		
BD	ROCHE	250 MG	N16912 003
BD		500 MG	N16912 004
		100 MG	N16912 005

Prescription Drug Products *(continued)*

LEVODOPA; *MULTIPLE*

SEE CARBIDOPA; LEVODOPA

LEVOMETHADYL ACETATE HYDROCHLORIDE

CONCENTRATE; ORAL

	ORLAAM		
	BIODEVELOPMENT	10 MG/ML	N20315 001 JUL 09, 1993

LEVONORDEFRIN; MEPIVACAINE HYDROCHLORIDE

INJECTABLE; INJECTION

	CARBOCAINE W/ NEO-COBEFRIN		
AP	+ COOK WAITE	0.05 MG/ML;2%	N12125 002
	ISOCAINE HCL W/ LEVONORDEFRIN		
AP	NOVOCOL	0.05 MG/ML;2%	N84697 001
	MEPIVACAINE HCL W/ LEVONORDEFRIN		
AP	GRAHAM CHEM	0.05 MG/ML;2%	N84850 002 OCT 21, 1983
	POLOCAINE W/ LEVONORDEFRIN		
AP	ASTRA	0.05 MG/ML;2%	N89517 001 APR 14, 1988
	SCANDONEST L		
AP	DEPROCO	0.05 MG/ML;2%	N88388 001 OCT 10, 1984

LEVONORGESTREL

IMPLANT; IMPLANTATION

	NORPLANT SYSTEM		
	WYETH AYERST	36 MG/IMPLANT	N20088 001 DEC 10, 1990

LEVONORGESTREL; *MULTIPLE*

SEE ETHINYL ESTRADIOL; LEVONORGESTREL

LEVORPHANOL TARTRATE

INJECTABLE; INJECTION

	LEVO-DROMORAN		
	+ ROCHE	2 MG/ML	N08719 001 DEC 19, 1991

TABLET; ORAL

	LEVO-DROMORAN		
	+ ROCHE	2 MG	N08720 001 DEC 19, 1991

LIDOCAINE

AEROSOL; ORAL

	XYLOCAINE		
	ASTRA	10%	N14394 001

OINTMENT; TOPICAL

	ALPHACAINE		
AT	CARLISLE	5%	N84944 001
AT		5%	N84946 001
AT		5%	N84947 001
	LIDOCAINE		
AT	FOUGERA	5%	N80198 001
AT	GRAHAM CHEM	5%	N80210 001
AT	THAMES	5%	N86724 001
	XYLOCAINE		
AT	+ ASTRA	5%	N08048 001

SOLUTION; TOPICAL

	XYLOCAINE		
	+ ASTRA	5%	N14127 001

LIDOCAINE; PRILOCAINE

CREAM; TOPICAL

	EMLA		
	+ ASTRA	2.5%;2.5%	N19941 001 DEC 30, 1992

LIDOCAINE HYDROCHLORIDE

INJECTABLE; INJECTION

	ALPHACAINE HCL		
AP	CARLISLE	2%	N84721 001
	LIDOCAINE HCL		
AP	ABBOTT	0.5%	N88328 001 MAY 17, 1984
AP		1%	N80408 001
AP		1%	N83158 001
AP		1%	N88329 001 MAY 17, 1984
AP		1.5%	N80408 002
AP		2%	N83158 002
AP		2%	N88294 001 MAY 17, 1984
AP		2%	N88331 001 MAY 17, 1984
AP		4%	N88295 001 MAY 17, 1984
AP		20%	N83158 003
AP		20%	N89362 001 MAY 25, 1988
AP	AKORN	1%	N85037 001
AP		2%	N85037 002

LIDOCAINE HYDROCHLORIDE (*continued*)

INJECTABLE; INJECTION

	LIDOCAINE HCL		
AP	DELL LABS	1%	N83387 001
AP		2%	N83388 001
AP	ELKINS SINN	1%	N80407 001
AP		1%	N84625 001
AP		2%	N80407 002
AP		2%	N84625 002
AP	FUJISAWA	1%	N80404 002
AP		2%	N17508 001
AP		2%	N17584 001
AP		2%	N80404 003
AP		2%	N80420 004
AP		4%	N17508 002
AP		4%	N17584 002
AP		20%	N17508 004
AP	GRAHAM CHEM	2%	N80504 001
AP	INTL MEDICATION	1%	N17701 002
AP		1%	N83173 001
AP		2%	N17701 001
AP		2%	N83173 002
AP		20%	N17702 001
AP	LUITPOLD	1%	N80850 001
AP		2%	N83198 001
AP	STERIS	1%	N80377 001
AP		2%	N80377 002
AP	WYETH AYERST	1%	N83083 001
AP		2%	N83083 002
	LIDOCAINE HCL IN PLASTIC CONTAINER		
AP	ABBOTT	0.5%	N88325 001 JUL 31, 1984
AP		1%	N88299 001 JUL 31, 1984
AP		1.5%	N88326 001 JUL 31, 1984
AP		2%	N88327 001 JUL 31, 1984
AP		10%	N88367 001 JUL 31, 1984
AP		20%	N88368 001 JUL 31, 1984
AP	FUJISAWA	1%	N88586 001 JUL 24, 1985
	LIDOCAINE HCL 0.2% AND DEXTROSE 5% IN PLASTIC CONTAINER		
AP	BAXTER	200 MG/100 ML	N18461 002
AP	MCGAW	200 MG/100 ML	N18967 001 MAR 30, 1984
AP		200 MG/100 ML	N19830 002 APR 08, 1992
	LIDOCAINE HCL 0.2% IN DEXTROSE 5%		
AP	ABBOTT	200 MG/100 ML	N83158 005

LIDOCAINE HYDROCHLORIDE (*continued*)

INJECTABLE; INJECTION

	LIDOCAINE HCL 0.2% IN DEXTROSE 5% IN PLASTIC CONTAINER		
AP	ABBOTT	200 MG/100 ML	N18388 001
	LIDOCAINE HCL 0.4% AND DEXTROSE 5% IN PLASTIC CONTAINER		
AP	BAXTER	400 MG/100 ML	N18461 003
AP	MCGAW	400 MG/100 ML	N18967 002 MAR 30, 1984
AP		400 MG/100 ML	N19830 003 APR 08, 1992
	LIDOCAINE HCL 0.4% IN DEXTROSE 5%		
AP	ABBOTT	400 MG/100 ML	N83158 006
	LIDOCAINE HCL 0.4% IN DEXTROSE 5% IN PLASTIC CONTAINER		
AP	ABBOTT	400 MG/100 ML	N18388 002
	LIDOCAINE HCL 0.8% AND DEXTROSE 5% IN PLASTIC CONTAINER		
AP	BAXTER	800 MG/100 ML	N18461 004 FEB 22, 1982
AP	MCGAW	800 MG/100 ML	N18967 003 MAR 30, 1984
AP		800 MG/100 ML	N19830 004 APR 08, 1992
	LIDOCAINE HCL 0.8% IN DEXTROSE 5% IN PLASTIC CONTAINER		
AP	ABBOTT	800 MG/100 ML	N18388 003 NOV 05, 1982
	LIDOCATON		
AP	PHARMATON	2%	N84727 001 AUG 17, 1983
	LIDOPEN		
AP	SURVIVAL TECH	10%	N17549 001
	XYLOCAINE		
AP	+ ASTRA	0.5%	N06488 008
AP	+	1%	N06488 007
AP		1%	N16801 005 JAN 19, 1988
AP	+	1.5%	N06488 010
AP	+	2%	N06488 002
AP		2%	N16801 001
AP		4%	N16801 002
AP	+	10%	N16801 003
AP	+	20%	N16801 004
	XYLOCAINE 4%		
AP	+ ASTRA	4%	N10417 001

INJECTABLE; SPINAL

	LIDOCAINE HCL AND DEXTROSE 7.5%		
AP	ABBOTT	5%	N83914 001
	XYLOCAINE W/ DEXTROSE 7.5%		
	+ ASTRA	1.5%	N16297 001
	XYLOCAINE 5% W/ GLUCOSE 7.5%		
AP	+ ASTRA	5%	N10496 002 JUL 07, 1982

Prescription Drug Products *(continued)*

LIDOCAINE HYDROCHLORIDE *(continued)*

	JELLY; TOPICAL		
	LIDOCAINE HCL		
AT	COPLEY PHARM	2%	N81318 001 APR 29, 1993
AT	INTL MEDICATION	2%	N86283 001
	XYLOCAINE		
AT	+ ASTRA	2%	N08816 001
	SOLUTION; ORAL		
	LIDOCAINE HCL VISCOUS		
AT	BARRE	2%	N86578 001
AT	INTL MEDICATION	2%	N86389 001 FEB 02, 1982
	LIDOCAINE VISCOUS		
AT	ROXANE	2%	N88802 001 APR 26, 1985
	MYLOCAINE		
AT	PENNEX	2%	N87872 001 NOV 18, 1982
	XYLOCAINE VISCOUS		
AT	+ ASTRA	2%	N09470 001
	SOLUTION; TOPICAL		
	ANESTACON		
AT	+ ALCON	2%	N80429 001
	LARYNG-O-JET KIT		
AT	INTL MEDICATION	4%	N86364 001
	LIDOCAINE HCL		
AT	ROXANE	4%	N88803 001 APR 03, 1985
	LTA II KIT		
AT	ABBOTT	4%	N80409 001
AT		4%	N88542 001 JUL 31, 1984
	MYLOCAINE		
AT	PENNEX	4%	N87881 001 NOV 18, 1982
	PEDIATRIC LTA KIT		
AT	ABBOTT	2%	N85995 001
	XYLOCAINE 4%		
AT	+ ASTRA	4%	N10417 002

LIDOCAINE HYDROCHLORIDE; *MULTIPLE*

SEE DEXAMETHASONE SODIUM PHOSPHATE; LIDOCAINE HYDROCHLORIDE

SEE EPINEPHRINE; LIDOCAINE HYDROCHLORIDE

SEE EPINEPHRINE BITARTRATE; LIDOCAINE HYDROCHLORIDE

LIDOCAINE HYDROCHLORIDE; OXYTETRACYCLINE

	INJECTABLE; INJECTION		
	TERRAMYCIN		
	PFIZER	2%;50 MG/ML	N60567 001
		2%;125 MG/ML	N60567 002

LINCOMYCIN HYDROCHLORIDE

	CAPSULE; ORAL		
	LINCOCIN		
	UPJOHN	EQ 250 MG BASE	N50316 001
	+	EQ 500 MG BASE	N50316 002
	INJECTABLE; INJECTION		
	LINCOCIN		
AP	+ UPJOHN	EQ 300 MG BASE/ML	N50317 001
	LINCOMYCIN HCL		
AP	STERIS	EQ 300 MG BASE/ML	N63180 001 APR 16, 1991

LINDANE

	CREAM; TOPICAL		
	KWELL		
	+ REED AND CARNRICK	1%	N06309 001
		1%	N84218 001
	LOTION; TOPICAL		
	KWELL		
AT	+ REED AND CARNRICK	1%	N06309 003
AT		1%	N84218 002
	LINDANE		
AT	BARRE	1%	N87313 001
AT	PENNEX	1%	N88190 001 AUG 16, 1984
	SCABENE		
AT	STIEFEL	1%	N86769 001
	SHAMPOO; TOPICAL		
	KWELL		
AT	+ REED AND CARNRICK	1%	N10718 001
AT		1%	N84219 001
	LINDANE		
AT	BARRE	1%	N87266 001
AT	PENNEX	1%	N88191 001 SEP 18, 1984
	SCABENE		
AT	STIEFEL	1%	N87940 001 APR 08, 1983

Prescription Drug Products *(continued)*

LIOTHYRONINE SODIUM

	INJECTABLE; INJECTION		
	TRIOSTAT		
	+ SMITHKLINE BEECHAM	EQ 0.01 MG BASE/ML	N20105 001 DEC 31, 1991
	TABLET; ORAL		
	CYTOMEL		
	SMITHKLINE BEECHAM	EQ 0.005 MG BASE	N10379 001
		EQ 0.025 MG BASE	N10379 002
	+	EQ 0.05 MG BASE	N10379 003

LIOTRIX (T4;T3)

	TABLET; ORAL		
	THYROLAR-0.25		
	FOREST LABS	0.0125 MG;0.0031 MG	N16807 001
	THYROLAR-0.5		
	FOREST LABS	0.025 MG;0.00625 MG	N16807 005
	THYROLAR-1		
	FOREST LABS	0.05 MG;0.0125 MG	N16807 004
	THYROLAR-2		
	FOREST LABS	0.1 MG;0.025 MG	N16807 002
	THYROLAR-3		
	+ FOREST LABS	0.15 MG;0.0375 MG	N16807 003

LISINOPRIL

	TABLET; ORAL		
	PRINIVIL		
AB	MERCK	2.5 MG	N19558 006 JAN 28, 1994
AB		5 MG	N19558 001 DEC 29, 1987
AB		10 MG	N19558 002 DEC 29, 1987
AB		20 MG	N19558 003 DEC 29, 1987
AB		40 MG	N19558 004 OCT 25, 1988
	ZESTRIL		
AB	ZENECA	2.5 MG	N19777 005 APR 29, 1993
AB		5 MG	N19777 001 MAY 19, 1988
AB		10 MG	N19777 002 MAY 19, 1988
AB		20 MG	N19777 003 MAY 19, 1988
AB	+	40 MG	N19777 004 MAY 19, 1988

LISINOPRIL; *MULTIPLE*

SEE <u>HYDROCHLOROTHIAZIDE; LISINOPRIL</u>

LITHIUM CARBONATE

	CAPSULE; ORAL		
	ESKALITH		
AB	+ SMITHKLINE BEECHAM	300 MG	N16860 001
	LITHIUM CARBONATE		
AB	ROXANE	300 MG	N17812 001
		150 MG	N17812 002 JAN 28, 1987
		600 MG	N17812 003 JAN 28, 1987
	LITHONATE		
AB	SOLVAY	300 MG	N16782 001
	TABLET; ORAL		
	LITHIUM CARBONATE		
AB	PFIZER	300 MG	N16834 001
AB	ROXANE	300 MG	N18558 001 JAN 29, 1982
	LITHOTABS		
AB	SOLVAY	300 MG	N16980 001
	TABLET, EXTENDED RELEASE; ORAL		
	ESKALITH CR		
	+ SMITHKLINE BEECHAM	450 MG	N18152 001 MAR 29, 1982

LITHIUM CITRATE

	SYRUP; ORAL		
	CIBALITH-S		
AA	CIBA	EQ 300 MG CARBONATE/5 ML	N17672 001
	LITHIUM CITRATE		
AA	PENNEX	EQ 300 MG CARBONATE/5 ML	N70755 001 MAY 21, 1986
AA	ROXANE	EQ 300 MG CARBONATE/5 ML	N18421 001

LODOXAMIDE TROMETHAMINE

	SOLUTION/DROPS; OPHTHALMIC		
	ALOMIDE		
	+ ALCON	EQ 0.1% BASE	N20191 001 SEP 23, 1993

Prescription Drug Products *(continued)*

LOMEFLOXACIN HYDROCHLORIDE

	TABLET; ORAL		
	MAXAQUIN		
	+ SEARLE	EQ 400 MG BASE	N20013 001 FEB 21, 1992

LOMUSTINE

	CAPSULE; ORAL		
	CEENU		
	BRISTOL	10 MG	N17588 001
		40 MG	N17588 002
	+	100 MG	N17588 003

LOPERAMIDE HYDROCHLORIDE

	CAPSULE; ORAL		
	IMODIUM		
AB	+ JANSSEN	2 MG	N17694 001
	LOPERAMIDE HCL		
AB	GENEVA PHARMS	2 MG	N72993 001 AUG 28, 1992
AB	LEMMON	2 MG	N73192 001 APR 30, 1992
AB	MYLAN	2 MG	N72741 001 SEP 18, 1991
AB	NOVOPHARM	2 MG	N73122 001 AUG 30, 1991
AB	ROXANE	2 MG	N73080 001 NOV 27, 1991

LORACARBEF

	CAPSULE; ORAL		
	LORABID		
	+ LILLY	200 MG	N50668 001 DEC 31, 1991
	POWDER FOR RECONSTITUTION; ORAL		
	LORABID		
	LILLY	100 MG/5 ML	N50667 001 DEC 31, 1991
	+	200 MG/5 ML	N50667 002 DEC 31, 1991

LORATADINE

	TABLET; ORAL		
	CLARITIN		
	+ SCHERING	10 MG	N19658 001 APR 12, 1993

LORAZEPAM

	CONCENTRATE; ORAL		
	LORAZEPAM INTENSOL		
	ROXANE	2 MG/ML	N72755 001 JUN 28, 1991
	INJECTABLE; INJECTION		
	ATIVAN		
AP	+ WYETH AYERST	2 MG/ML	N18140 001
AP	+	4 MG/ML	N18140 002
	LORAZEPAM		
AP	ABBOTT	2 MG/ML	N74280 001 MAY 27, 1994
AP		2 MG/ML	N74282 001 MAY 27, 1994
AP		4 MG/ML	N74280 002 MAY 27, 1994
AP		4 MG/ML	N74282 002 MAY 27, 1994
AP	STERIS	2 MG/ML	N74276 001 APR 15, 1994
AP		4 MG/ML	N74276 002 APR 15, 1994
AP	STERLING WINTHROP	2 MG/ML	N74243 001 APR 12, 1994
AP		2 MG/ML	N74300 001 APR 12, 1994
AP		4 MG/ML	N74243 002 APR 12, 1994
	TABLET; ORAL		
	ATIVAN		
AB	WYETH AYERST	0.5 MG	N17794 001
AB		1 MG	N17794 002
AB	+	2 MG	N17794 003
	LORAZEPAM		
AB	BARR	0.5 MG	N70472 001 DEC 10, 1985
AB		1 MG	N70473 001 DEC 10, 1985
AB		2 MG	N70474 001 DEC 10, 1985
AB	DANBURY PHARMA	0.5 MG	N71117 001 JUL 24, 1986
AB		1 MG	N71118 001 JUL 24, 1986
AB		2 MG	N71110 001 JUL 24, 1986

LORAZEPAM (*continued*)
TABLET; ORAL
LORAZEPAM

AB	GENEVA PHARMS	0.5 MG	N71193 001 APR 15, 1988
AB		1 MG	N71194 001 APR 15, 1988
AB		2 MG	N71195 001 APR 15, 1988
AB	HALSEY	0.5 MG	N71434 001 SEP 01, 1987
AB		1 MG	N71435 001 SEP 01, 1987
AB		2 MG	N71436 001 SEP 01, 1987
AB	MUTUAL PHARM	0.5 MG	N72553 001 MAR 29, 1991
AB		1 MG	N72554 001 MAR 29, 1991
AB		2 MG	N72555 001 MAR 29, 1991
AB	MYLAN	0.5 MG	N71589 001 OCT 13, 1987
AB		1 MG	N71590 001 OCT 13, 1987
AB		2 MG	N71591 001 OCT 13, 1987
AB	PUREPAC PHARM	0.5 MG	N71403 001 APR 21, 1987
AB		1 MG	N71404 001 APR 21, 1987
AB		2 MG	N71141 001 APR 21, 1987
AB	ROYCE LABS	0.5 MG	N72926 001 OCT 31, 1991
AB		1 MG	N72927 001 OCT 31, 1991
AB		2 MG	N72928 001 OCT 31, 1991
AB	SUPERPHARM	0.5 MG	N71245 001 FEB 09, 1987
AB		1 MG	N71246 001 FEB 09, 1987
AB		2 MG	N71247 001 FEB 09, 1987
AB	WATSON LABS	0.5 MG	N71086 001 MAR 23, 1987
AB		1 MG	N71087 001 MAR 23, 1987
AB		2 MG	N71088 001 MAR 23, 1987

LOVASTATIN
TABLET; ORAL
MEVACOR

	MERCK	10 MG	N19643 002 MAR 28, 1991
		20 MG	N19643 003 AUG 31, 1987
	+	40 MG	N19643 004 DEC 14, 1988

LOXAPINE HYDROCHLORIDE
CONCENTRATE; ORAL
LOXITANE C

	LEDERLE	EQ 25 MG BASE/ML	N17658 001

INJECTABLE; INJECTION
LOXITANE IM

	+ LEDERLE	EQ 50 MG BASE/ML	N18039 001

LOXAPINE SUCCINATE
CAPSULE; ORAL
LOXAPINE SUCCINATE

AB	WATSON LABS	EQ 5 MG BASE	N72204 001 JUN 15, 1988
AB		EQ 10 MG BASE	N72205 001 JUN 15, 1988
AB		EQ 25 MG BASE	N72206 001 JUN 15, 1988
AB		EQ 50 MG BASE	N72062 001 JUN 15, 1988

LOXITANE

AB	LEDERLE	EQ 5 MG BASE	N17525 001
AB		EQ 10 MG BASE	N17525 002
AB	+	EQ 25 MG BASE	N17525 003
AB		EQ 50 MG BASE	N17525 004

LYPRESSIN
SOLUTION; NASAL
DIAPID

	+ SANDOZ	0.185 MG/ML	N16755 001

MAFENIDE ACETATE
CREAM; TOPICAL
SULFAMYLON

	+ HICKAM	EQ 85 MG BASE/GM	N16763 001

Prescription Drug Products *(continued)*

MAGNESIUM ACETATE; *MULTIPLE*

SEE AMINO ACIDS; CALCIUM ACETATE; GLYCERIN; MAGNESIUM ACETATE; PHOSPHORIC ACID; POTASSIUM CHLORIDE; SODIUM ACETATE; SODIUM CHLORIDE

SEE AMINO ACIDS; MAGNESIUM ACETATE; PHOSPHORIC ACID; POTASSIUM ACETATE; POTASSIUM CHLORIDE; SODIUM ACETATE

SEE AMINO ACIDS; MAGNESIUM ACETATE; PHOSPHORIC ACID; POTASSIUM ACETATE; SODIUM CHLORIDE

SEE AMINO ACIDS; MAGNESIUM ACETATE; PHOSPHORIC ACID; POTASSIUM CHLORIDE; SODIUM ACETATE; SODIUM CHLORIDE

SEE DEXTROSE; MAGNESIUM ACETATE; POTASSIUM ACETATE; SODIUM CHLORIDE

MAGNESIUM ACETATE TETRAHYDRATE; *MULTIPLE*

SEE DEXTROSE; MAGNESIUM ACETATE TETRAHYDRATE; POTASSIUM ACETATE; SODIUM CHLORIDE

MAGNESIUM ACETATE TETRAHYDRATE; POTASSIUM ACETATE; SODIUM CHLORIDE

INJECTABLE; INJECTION

PLASMA-LYTE 56 IN PLASTIC CONTAINER

BAXTER	32 MG/100 ML;128 MG/100 ML;234 MG/100 ML	N19047 001 JUN 15, 1984

MAGNESIUM CARBONATE; *MULTIPLE*

SEE CITRIC ACID; GLUCONOLACTONE; MAGNESIUM CARBONATE

MAGNESIUM CHLORIDE; *MULTIPLE*

SEE AMINO ACIDS; CALCIUM CHLORIDE; DEXTROSE; MAGNESIUM CHLORIDE; POTASSIUM CHLORIDE; POTASSIUM PHOSPHATE, DIBASIC; SODIUM CHLORIDE

SEE AMINO ACIDS; DEXTROSE; MAGNESIUM CHLORIDE; POTASSIUM CHLORIDE; SODIUM CHLORIDE; SODIUM PHOSPHATE, DIBASIC

SEE AMINO ACIDS; DEXTROSE; MAGNESIUM CHLORIDE; POTASSIUM ACETATE; POTASSIUM CHLORIDE; POTASSIUM PHOSPHATE, DIBASIC; SODIUM CHLORIDE

SEE AMINO ACIDS; DEXTROSE; MAGNESIUM CHLORIDE; POTASSIUM CHLORIDE; SODIUM CHLORIDE; SODIUM PHOSPHATE, DIBASIC

SEE AMINO ACIDS; MAGNESIUM CHLORIDE; POTASSIUM CHLORIDE; POTASSIUM PHOSPHATE, DIBASIC; SODIUM CHLORIDE

SEE AMINO ACIDS; MAGNESIUM CHLORIDE; POTASSIUM PHOSPHATE, DIBASIC; SODIUM ACETATE; SODIUM CHLORIDE

SEE AMINO ACIDS; MAGNESIUM CHLORIDE; POTASSIUM PHOSPHATE, DIBASIC; SODIUM CHLORIDE

SEE CALCIUM CHLORIDE; DEXTROSE; GLUTATHIONE DISULFIDE; MAGNESIUM CHLORIDE; POTASSIUM CHLORIDE; SODIUM BICARBONATE; SODIUM CHLORIDE; SODIUM PHOSPHATE

SEE CALCIUM CHLORIDE; DEXTROSE; MAGNESIUM CHLORIDE; POTASSIUM CHLORIDE; SODIUM ACETATE; SODIUM CHLORIDE

SEE CALCIUM CHLORIDE; DEXTROSE; MAGNESIUM CHLORIDE; POTASSIUM CHLORIDE; SODIUM ACETATE; SODIUM CHLORIDE; SODIUM CITRATE

SEE CALCIUM CHLORIDE; DEXTROSE; MAGNESIUM CHLORIDE; SODIUM CHLORIDE; SODIUM LACTATE

SEE CALCIUM CHLORIDE; DEXTROSE; MAGNESIUM CHLORIDE; SODIUM ACETATE; SODIUM CHLORIDE

SEE CALCIUM CHLORIDE; DEXTROSE; MAGNESIUM CHLORIDE; POTASSIUM CHLORIDE; SODIUM ACETATE; SODIUM CHLORIDE; SODIUM LACTATE

SEE CALCIUM CHLORIDE; DEXTROSE; MAGNESIUM CHLORIDE; SODIUM CHLORIDE; SODIUM LACTATE

SEE CALCIUM CHLORIDE; MAGNESIUM CHLORIDE; POTASSIUM CHLORIDE; SODIUM ACETATE; SODIUM CHLORIDE; SODIUM CITRATE

Prescription Drug Products *(continued)*

MAGNESIUM CHLORIDE; *MULTIPLE* *(continued)*

SEE CALCIUM CHLORIDE; MAGNESIUM CHLORIDE; POTASSIUM CHLORIDE; SODIUM ACETATE; SODIUM CHLORIDE
SEE CALCIUM CHLORIDE; MAGNESIUM CHLORIDE; POTASSIUM CHLORIDE; SODIUM ACETATE; SODIUM CHLORIDE; SODIUM LACTATE
SEE CALCIUM CHLORIDE; MAGNESIUM CHLORIDE; POTASSIUM CHLORIDE; SODIUM CHLORIDE
SEE DEXTROSE; MAGNESIUM CHLORIDE; POTASSIUM CHLORIDE; SODIUM ACETATE; SODIUM CHLORIDE
SEE DEXTROSE; MAGNESIUM CHLORIDE; POTASSIUM CHLORIDE; SODIUM ACETATE; SODIUM CHLORIDE; SODIUM GLUCONATE
SEE DEXTROSE; MAGNESIUM CHLORIDE; POTASSIUM CHLORIDE; POTASSIUM PHOSPHATE, DIBASIC; SODIUM ACETATE
SEE DEXTROSE; MAGNESIUM CHLORIDE; POTASSIUM CHLORIDE; SODIUM ACETATE; SODIUM CHLORIDE; SODIUM GLUCONATE
SEE DEXTROSE; MAGNESIUM CHLORIDE; POTASSIUM CHLORIDE; POTASSIUM PHOSPHATE, DIBASIC; SODIUM CHLORIDE; SODIUM LACTATE; SODIUM PHOSPHATE, MONOBASIC
SEE DEXTROSE; MAGNESIUM CHLORIDE; POTASSIUM CHLORIDE; POTASSIUM PHOSPHATE, MONOBASIC; SODIUM LACTATE; SODIUM PHOSPHATE, MONOBASIC
SEE DEXTROSE; MAGNESIUM CHLORIDE; POTASSIUM CHLORIDE; POTASSIUM PHOSPHATE, MONOBASIC; SODIUM CHLORIDE; SODIUM LACTATE

MAGNESIUM CHLORIDE; POTASSIUM CHLORIDE; POTASSIUM PHOSPHATE, MONOBASIC; SODIUM ACETATE; SODIUM CHLORIDE; SODIUM GLUCONATE; SODIUM PHOSPHATE, DIBASIC

INJECTABLE; INJECTION

ISOLYTE S PH 7.4 IN PLASTIC CONTAINER

	MCGAW	30 MG/100 ML;37 MG/ 100 ML;0.82 MG/ 100 ML;370 MG/ 100 ML;530 MG/ 100 ML;500 MG/ 100 ML;12 MG/100 ML	N19006 001 APR 04, 1984
		30 MG/100 ML;37 MG/ 100 ML;0.82 MG/ 100 ML;370 MG/ 100 ML;530 MG/ 100 ML;500 MG/ 100 ML;12 MG/100 ML	N19696 001 SEP 29, 1989

MAGNESIUM CHLORIDE; POTASSIUM CHLORIDE; SODIUM ACETATE; SODIUM CHLORIDE; SODIUM GLUCONATE

INJECTABLE; INJECTION

ISOLYTE S IN PLASTIC CONTAINER

AP	MCGAW	30 MG/100 ML;37 MG/ 100 ML;370 MG/ 100 ML;530 MG/ 100 ML;500 MG/100 ML	N18252 001
AP		30 MG/100 ML;37 MG/ 100 ML;370 MG/ 100 ML;530 MG/ 100 ML;500 MG/100 ML	N19711 001 SEP 29, 1989

NORMOSOL-R IN PLASTIC CONTAINER

	ABBOTT	30 MG/100 ML;37 MG/ 100 ML;222 MG/ 100 ML;526 MG/ 100 ML;502 MG/100 ML	N17586 001

PLASMA-LYTE A IN PLASTIC CONTAINER

AP	BAXTER	30 MG/100 ML;37 MG/ 100 ML;368 MG/ 100 ML;526 MG/ 100 ML;502 MG/100 ML	N17378 002 NOV 22, 1982

PLASMA-LYTE 148 IN WATER IN PLASTIC CONTAINER

AP	BAXTER	30 MG/100 ML;37 MG/ 100 ML;368 MG/ 100 ML;526 MG/ 100 ML;502 MG/100 ML	N17378 001

SOLUTION; IRRIGATION

PHYSIOLYTE IN PLASTIC CONTAINER

AT	MCGAW	30 MG/100 ML;37 MG/ 100 ML;370 MG/ 100 ML;530 MG/ 100 ML;500 MG/100 ML	N19024 001 JUN 08, 1984

PHYSIOSOL IN PLASTIC CONTAINER

AT	ABBOTT	30 MG/100 ML;37 MG/ 100 ML;222 MG/ 100 ML;526 MG/ 100 ML;502 MG/100 ML	N17637 002 JUL 08, 1982

PHYSIOSOL PH 7.4 IN PLASTIC CONTAINER

	ABBOTT	30 MG/100 ML;37 MG/ 100 ML;222 MG/ 100 ML;526 MG/ 100 ML;502 MG/100 ML	N18406 002 JUL 08, 1982

Prescription Drug Products *(continued)*

MAGNESIUM CHLORIDE; POTASSIUM CHLORIDE; SODIUM ACETATE; SODIUM CHLORIDE; SODIUM GLUCONATE *(continued)*

SOLUTION; IRRIGATION

SYNOVALYTE IN PLASTIC CONTAINER

AT	BAXTER	30 MG/100 ML;37 MG/100 ML;368 MG/100 ML;526 MG/100 ML;502 MG/100 ML	N19326 001 JAN 25, 1985

MAGNESIUM OXIDE; *MULTIPLE*

SEE CITRIC ACID; MAGNESIUM OXIDE; SODIUM CARBONATE

MAGNESIUM SULFATE

INJECTABLE; INJECTION

MAGNESIUM SULFATE

	FUJISAWA	500 MG/ML	N19316 001 SEP 08, 1986

MAGNESIUM SULFATE IN PLASTIC CONTAINER

	ABBOTT	4 GM/100 ML	N20309 001 JUN 24, 1994
		80 MG/ML	N20309 002 JUN 24, 1994

MAGNESIUM SULFATE; POTASSIUM CHLORIDE; POTASSIUM PHOSPHATE, MONOBASIC; SODIUM CHLORIDE; SODIUM PHOSPHATE

SOLUTION; IRRIGATION

TIS-U-SOL

AT	BAXTER	20 MG/100 ML;40 MG/100 ML;6.25 MG/100 ML;800 MG/100 ML;8.75 MG/100 ML	N18508 001 FEB 19, 1982

TIS-U-SOL IN PLASTIC CONTAINER

AT	BAXTER	20 MG/100 ML;40 MG/100 ML;6.25 MG/100 ML;800 MG/100 ML;8.75 MG/100 ML	N18336 001

MALATHION

LOTION; TOPICAL

OVIDE

	+ GENDERM	0.5%	N18613 001 AUG 02, 1982

MANGANESE CHLORIDE

INJECTABLE; INJECTION

MANGANESE CHLORIDE IN PLASTIC CONTAINER

	ABBOTT	EQ 0.1 MG MANGANESE/ML	N18962 001 JUN 26, 1986

MANGANESE SULFATE

INJECTABLE; INJECTION

MANGANESE SULFATE

	FUJISAWA	EQ 0.1 MG MANGANESE/ML	N19228 001 MAY 05, 1987

MANNITOL

INJECTABLE; INJECTION

MANNITOL 10%

AP	ABBOTT	10 GM/100 ML	N16269 002
AP	MCGAW	10 GM/100 ML	N16080 002

MANNITOL 10% IN PLASTIC CONTAINER

AP	ABBOTT	10 GM/100 ML	N19603 002 JAN 08, 1987
AP	MCGAW	10 GM/100 ML	N20006 002 JUL 26, 1993

MANNITOL 10% W/ DEXTROSE 5% IN DISTILLED WATER

AP	MCGAW	10 GM/100 ML	N16080 006

MANNITOL 15%

AP	ABBOTT	15 GM/100 ML	N16269 003
AP	MCGAW	15 GM/100 ML	N16080 003

MANNITOL 15% IN PLASTIC CONTAINER

AP	ABBOTT	15 GM/100 ML	N19603 003 JAN 08, 1990
AP	MCGAW	15 GM/100 ML	N20006 003 JUL 26, 1993

MANNITOL 15% W/ DEXTROSE 5% IN SODIUM CHLORIDE 0.45%

AP	MCGAW	15 GM/100 ML	N16080 005

MANNITOL 20%

AP	ABBOTT	20 GM/100 ML	N16269 004
AP	MCGAW	20 GM/100 ML	N14738 001
AP		20 GM/100 ML	N16080 004

MANNITOL 20% IN PLASTIC CONTAINER

AP	ABBOTT	20 GM/100 ML	N19603 004 JAN 08, 1990
AP	MCGAW	20 GM/100 ML	N20006 004 JUL 26, 1993

Prescription Drug Products *(continued)*

MANNITOL *(continued)*

INJECTABLE; INJECTION

MANNITOL 25%

AP	ABBOTT	12.5 GM/50 ML	N16269 005
AP	ASTRA	12.5 GM/50 ML	N89239 001 MAY 06, 1987
AP		12.5 GM/50 ML	N89240 001 MAY 06, 1987
AP	FUJISAWA	12.5 GM/50 ML	N80677 001
AP	INTL MEDICATION	12.5 GM/50 ML	N83051 001
AP	LUITPOLD	12.5 GM/50 ML	N87409 001 JAN 21, 1982
AP	STERIS	12.5 GM/50 ML	N87460 001 JUN 27, 1983

MANNITOL 5%

AP	ABBOTT	5 GM/100 ML	N16269 001
AP	MCGAW	5 GM/100 ML	N16080 001

MANNITOL 5% IN PLASTIC CONTAINER

AP	ABBOTT	5 GM/100 ML	N19603 001 JAN 08, 1987
AP	MCGAW	5 GM/100 ML	N20006 001 JUL 26, 1993

MANNITOL 5% W/ DEXTROSE 5% IN SODIUM CHLORIDE 0.12%

AP	MCGAW	5 GM/100 ML	N16080 007

OSMITROL 10% IN WATER

AP	BAXTER	10 GM/100 ML	N13684 002

OSMITROL 10% IN WATER IN PLASTIC CONTAINER

AP	BAXTER	10 GM/100 ML	N13684 006

OSMITROL 15% IN WATER

AP	BAXTER	15 GM/100 ML	N13684 004

OSMITROL 15% IN WATER IN PLASTIC CONTAINER

AP	BAXTER	15 GM/100 ML	N13684 008

OSMITROL 20% IN WATER

AP	BAXTER	20 GM/100 ML	N13684 003

OSMITROL 20% IN WATER IN PLASTIC CONTAINER

AP	BAXTER	20 GM/100 ML	N13684 007

OSMITROL 5% IN WATER

AP	BAXTER	5 GM/100 ML	N13684 001

OSMITROL 5% IN WATER IN PLASTIC CONTAINER

AP	BAXTER	5 GM/100 ML	N13684 005

SOLUTION; IRRIGATION

RESECTISOL IN PLASTIC CONTAINER

	MCGAW	5 GM/100 ML	N16772 002

MANNITOL; SORBITOL

SOLUTION; IRRIGATION

SORBITOL-MANNITOL IN PLASTIC CONTAINER

AT	ABBOTT	540 MG/100 ML;2.7 GM/100 ML	N17636 001
AT		540 MG/100 ML;2.7 GM/100 ML	N18316 001

MAPROTILINE HYDROCHLORIDE

TABLET; ORAL

LUDIOMIL

AB	CIBA	25 MG	N17543 001
AB	+	50 MG	N17543 002
AB		75 MG	N17543 003 SEP 30, 1982

MAPROTILINE HCL

AB	MYLAN	25 MG	N72284 001 OCT 03, 1988
AB		50 MG	N72285 001 OCT 03, 1988
AB		75 MG	N72286 001 OCT 03, 1988
AB	WATSON LABS	25 MG	N72162 001 JUN 01, 1988
AB		50 MG	N72163 001 JUN 01, 1988
AB		75 MG	N72164 001 JUN 01, 1988

MASOPROCOL

CREAM; TOPICAL

ACTINEX

	+ BLOCK DRUG	10%	N19940 001 SEP 04, 1992

MAZINDOL

TABLET; ORAL

MAZANOR

BP	WYETH AYERST	1 MG	N17980 002

SANOREX

BP	SANDOZ	1 MG	N17247 001
	+	2 MG	N17247 002

MEBENDAZOLE

TABLET, CHEWABLE; ORAL

VERMOX

	+ JANSSEN	100 MG	N17481 001

MECAMYLAMINE HYDROCHLORIDE

TABLET; ORAL

INVERSINE

	+ MERCK SHARP DOHME	2.5 MG	N10251 001

Prescription Drug Products *(continued)*

MECHLORETHAMINE HYDROCHLORIDE

	INJECTABLE; INJECTION		
	MUSTARGEN		
	+ MERCK SHARP DOHME	10 MG/VIAL	N06695 001

MECLIZINE HYDROCHLORIDE

	TABLET; ORAL		
	ANTIVERT		
AA	ROERIG	12.5 MG	N10721 006
AA		25 MG	N10721 004
AA		50 MG	N10721 001 JAN 20, 1982
	MECLIZINE HCL		
AA	BUNDY	12.5 MG	N84382 001
AA		25 MG	N84872 001
AA	CAMALL	12.5 MG	N85253 001
AA		25 MG	N85252 001
AA	CHELSEA LABS	12.5 MG	N85269 001
AA		25 MG	N85740 001
AA	GENEVA PHARMS	12.5 MG	N84843 002 MAY 22, 1989
AA		25 MG	N84092 003 MAY 22, 1989
AA	KV PHARM	12.5 MG	N85524 001
AA		25 MG	N85523 001
AA	PAR PHARM	12.5 MG	N87127 001
AA		25 MG	N87128 001
AA		50 MG	N89674 001 MAR 31, 1988
AA	SIDMAK LABS NJ	12.5 MG	N88732 001 DEC 11, 1985
AA		25 MG	N88734 001 DEC 11, 1985
AA	ZENITH LABS	12.5 MG	N83784 001
AA		12.5 MG	N84975 001
AA		25 MG	N84657 001
	TABLET, CHEWABLE; ORAL		
	ANTIVERT		
AA	ROERIG	25 MG	N10721 005
	MECLIZINE HCL		
AA	SIDMAK LABS NJ	25 MG	N88733 001 DEC 11, 1985
AA	ZENITH LABS	25 MG	N84976 001

MECLOCYCLINE SULFOSALICYLATE

	CREAM; TOPICAL		
	MECLAN		
	+ JOHNSON RW	1%	N50518 001

MECLOFENAMATE SODIUM

	CAPSULE; ORAL		
	MECLOFENAMATE SODIUM		
AB	BARR	EQ 50 MG BASE	N72848 001 MAR 20, 1989
AB		EQ 100 MG BASE	N72809 001 MAR 20, 1989
AB	DANBURY PHARMA	EQ 50 MG BASE	N71468 001 APR 15, 1987
AB		EQ 100 MG BASE	N71469 001 APR 15, 1987
AB	GENEVA PHARMS	EQ 50 MG BASE	N72262 001 NOV 29, 1988
AB		EQ 100 MG BASE	N72263 001 NOV 29, 1988
AB	MYLAN	EQ 50 MG BASE	N71080 001 SEP 03, 1986
AB		EQ 100 MG BASE	N71081 001 SEP 03, 1986
	MECLOMEN		
AB	PARKE DAVIS	EQ 50 MG BASE	N18006 001
AB	+	EQ 100 MG BASE	N18006 002

MEDROXYPROGESTERONE ACETATE

	INJECTABLE; INJECTION		
	DEPO-PROVERA		
	+ UPJOHN	100 MG/ML	N12541 002
	+	150 MG/ML	N20246 001 OCT 29, 1992
	+	400 MG/ML	N12541 003
	TABLET; ORAL		
	AMEN		
BP	CARNRICK	10 MG	N83242 001
	CURRETAB		
BP	SOLVAY	10 MG	N85686 001
	CYCRIN		
AB	WYETH AYERST	2.5 MG	N81239 001 OCT 30, 1992
AB		5 MG	N81240 001 OCT 30, 1992
AB		10 MG	N89386 001 SEP 09, 1987
	MEDROXYPROGESTERONE ACETATE		
BP	ROSEMONT PHARM	10 MG	N88484 001 JUL 26, 1984

Prescription Drug Products *(continued)*

MEDROXYPROGESTERONE ACETATE *(continued)*

TABLET; ORAL

	PROVERA		
AB	UPJOHN	2.5 MG	N11839 001
AB		5 MG	N11839 003
AB	+	10 MG	N11839 004

MEDRYSONE

SUSPENSION/DROPS; OPHTHALMIC

	HMS		
	+ ALLERGAN	1%	N16624 003

MEFENAMIC ACID

CAPSULE; ORAL

	PONSTEL		
	+ PARKE DAVIS	250 MG	N15034 003

MEFLOQUINE HYDROCHLORIDE

TABLET; ORAL

	LARIAM		
	+ ROCHE	250 MG	N19591 001 MAY 02, 1989

MEGESTROL ACETATE

SUSPENSION; ORAL

	MEGACE		
	+ BRISTOL MYERS SQUIBB	40 MG/ML	N20264 001 SEP 10, 1993

TABLET; ORAL

	MEGACE		
AB	MEAD JOHNSON	20 MG	N16979 001
AB	+	40 MG	N16979 002
	MEGESTROL ACETATE		
AB	PAR PHARM	20 MG	N72422 001 AUG 08, 1988
AB		40 MG	N72423 001 AUG 08, 1988

MELPHALAN

TABLET; ORAL

	ALKERAN		
	+ BURROUGHS WELLCOME	2 MG	N14691 002

MELPHALAN HYDROCHLORIDE

INJECTABLE; INJECTION

	ALKERAN		
	BURROUGHS WELLCOME	EQ 50 MG BASE/VIAL	N20207 001 NOV 18, 1992

MENOTROPINS (FSH;LH)

INJECTABLE; INJECTION

	PERGONAL		
	+ SERONO	75IU/AMP;75IU/AMP	N17646 001
	+	150IU/AMP;150IU/AMP	N17646 002 MAY 20, 1985

MEPENZOLATE BROMIDE

TABLET; ORAL

	CANTIL		
	MERRELL DOW	25 MG	N10679 003

MEPERIDINE HYDROCHLORIDE

INJECTABLE; INJECTION

	DEMEROL		
AP	+ STERLING WINTHROP	25 MG/ML	N05010 007
AP	+	50 MG/ML	N05010 002
AP	+	75 MG/ML	N05010 009
AP	+	100 MG/ML	N05010 003
	MEPERIDINE HCL		
AP	+ ABBOTT	10 MG/ML	N88432 001 AUG 16, 1984
AP	ASTRA	10 MG/ML	N81002 001 JUL 30, 1993
AP		50 MG/ML	N89784 001 MAR 31, 1989
AP		100 MG/ML	N89788 001 MAR 31, 1989
AP	ELKINS SINN	25 MG/ML	N80445 001
AP		50 MG/ML	N80445 002
AP		75 MG/ML	N80445 003
AP		100 MG/ML	N80445 004
AP	INTL MEDICATION	10 MG/ML	N81309 001 AUG 30, 1993
AP	STERIS	10 MG/ML	N73443 001 MAR 17, 1992
AP		50 MG/ML	N73444 001 MAR 17, 1992
AP		100 MG/ML	N73445 001 MAR 17, 1992

Prescription Drug Products *(continued)*

MEPERIDINE HYDROCHLORIDE *(continued)*

	INJECTABLE; INJECTION		
	MEPERIDINE HCL		
AP	WYETH AYERST	25 MG/ML	N80455 007
AP		50 MG/ML	N80455 008
AP		75 MG/ML	N80455 009
AP		100 MG/ML	N80455 010
	SYRUP; ORAL		
	DEMEROL		
AA	STERLING WINTHROP	50 MG/5 ML	N05010 005
	MEPERIDINE HCL		
AA	ROXANE	50 MG/5 ML	N88744 001 JAN 30, 1985
	TABLET; ORAL		
	DEMEROL		
AA	STERLING WINTHROP	50 MG	N05010 001
AA		100 MG	N05010 004
	MEPERIDINE HCL		
AA	BARR	50 MG	N88639 001 JUL 02, 1984
AA		100 MG	N88640 001 SEP 19, 1984
AA	HALSEY	50 MG	N80448 001
AA		100 MG	N80448 002
AA	WYETH AYERST	50 MG	N80454 001

MEPERIDINE HYDROCHLORIDE; *MULTIPLE*

SEE ATROPINE SULFATE; MEPERIDINE HYDROCHLORIDE

MEPERIDINE HYDROCHLORIDE; PROMETHAZINE HYDROCHLORIDE

	INJECTABLE; INJECTION		
	MEPERGAN		
	+ WYETH AYERST	25 MG/ML;25 MG/ML	N11730 001

MEPHENTERMINE SULFATE

	INJECTABLE; INJECTION		
	WYAMINE SULFATE		
	+ WYETH AYERST	EQ 15 MG BASE/ML	N08248 002
	+	EQ 30 MG BASE/ML	N08248 001

MEPHENYTOIN

	TABLET; ORAL		
	MESANTOIN		
	SANDOZ	100 MG	N06008 001

MEPIVACAINE HYDROCHLORIDE

	INJECTABLE; INJECTION		
	CARBOCAINE		
AP	+ COOK WAITE	3%	N12125 003
AP	+ STERLING WINTHROP	1%	N12250 001
AP	+	1.5%	N12250 005
AP	+	2%	N12250 002
	ISOCAINE HCL		
AP	NOVOCOL	3%	N80925 001
	MEPIVACAINE HCL		
AP	GRAHAM CHEM	3%	N83559 001
AP	INTL MEDICATION	1%	N87509 001 OCT 05, 1982
AP	STERIS	1%	N88769 001 NOV 20, 1984
AP		2%	N88770 001 NOV 20, 1984
	POLOCAINE		
AP	ASTRA	1%	N89407 001 DEC 01, 1986
AP		2%	N89410 001 DEC 01, 1986
AP		3%	N88653 001 AUG 21, 1984
	POLOCAINE-MPF		
AP	ASTRA	1%	N89406 001 DEC 01, 1986
AP		1.5%	N89408 001 DEC 01, 1986
AP		2%	N89409 001 DEC 01, 1986
	SCANDONEST PLAIN		
AP	DEPROCO	3%	N88387 001 OCT 10, 1984

MEPIVACAINE HYDROCHLORIDE; *MULTIPLE*

SEE LEVONORDEFRIN; MEPIVACAINE HYDROCHLORIDE

MEPROBAMATE

	CAPSULE, EXTENDED RELEASE; ORAL		
	MEPROSPAN		
	WALLACE PHARMS	200 MG	N11284 001
	+	400 MG	N11284 002

Prescription Drug Products *(continued)*

MEPROBAMATE *(continued)*

TABLET; ORAL

	AMOSENE		
AA	FERNDALE LABS	400 MG	N84030 001
	EQUANIL		
AA	WYETH AYERST	200 MG	N10028 005
AA		400 MG	N10028 004
	MEPROBAMATE		
AA	BARR	200 MG	N80699 001
AA		400 MG	N80699 002
AA		600 MG	N84230 001
AA	CHELSEA LABS	200 MG	N85720 001
AA		400 MG	N85721 001
AA	DANBURY PHARMA	200 MG	N83304 001
AA		400 MG	N83308 001
AA		600 MG	N84274 001
AA	EON LABS	200 MG	N14547 002
AA		400 MG	N14547 001
AA	GENEVA PHARMS	400 MG	N80655 001
AA	GLOBAL PHARMS	200 MG	N14322 002
AA		400 MG	N14322 001
AA	LANNETT	200 MG	N14882 002
AA		400 MG	N14882 001
AA	MK LABS	200 MG	N14368 004
AA		400 MG	N14368 002
AA	MYLAN	400 MG	N83618 001
AA	PHARMAVITE	400 MG	N84438 001
AA	PUREPAC PHARM	200 MG	N84804 001
AA		400 MG	N84804 002
AA	ROXANE	600 MG	N84332 001
AA	TABLICAPS	400 MG	N83494 001
AA	WEST WARD PHARM	200 MG	N15417 003
AA		400 MG	N15417 002
AA	ZENITH LABS	600 MG	N84181 001
AA	1ST TX	400 MG	N83343 001
	MILTOWN		
AA	WALLACE PHARMS	200 MG	N09698 004
AA		400 MG	N09698 002
AA		600 MG	N83919 001
	NEURAMATE		
AA	HALSEY	200 MG	N14359 002
AA		400 MG	N14359 001
	TRANMEP		
AA	SOLVAY	400 MG	N16249 001

MEPROBAMATE; *MULTIPLE*

SEE ASPIRIN; MEPROBAMATE
SEE ESTROGENS, CONJUGATED; MEPROBAMATE

MERCAPTOPURINE

TABLET; ORAL

PURINETHOL		
+ BURROUGHS WELLCOME	50 MG	N09053 002

MERSALYL SODIUM; THEOPHYLLINE

INJECTABLE; INJECTION

MERSALYL-THEOPHYLLINE		
+ STERIS	100 MG/ML;50 MG/ML	N84875 001

MESALAMINE

CAPSULE, EXTENDED RELEASE; ORAL

PENTASA		
+ MARION MERRELL DOW	250 MG	N20049 001 MAY 10, 1993

ENEMA; RECTAL

ROWASA		
+ SOLVAY	4 GM/60 ML	N19618 001 DEC 24, 1987

SUPPOSITORY; RECTAL

ROWASA		
+ SOLVAY	500 MG	N19919 001 DEC 18, 1990

TABLET, DELAYED RELEASE; ORAL

ASACOL		
+ PROCTER AND GAMBLE	400 MG	N19651 001 JAN 31, 1992

MESNA

INJECTABLE; INJECTION

MESNEX		
+ ASTA	100 MG/ML	N19884 001 DEC 30, 1988

MESORIDAZINE BESYLATE

CONCENTRATE; ORAL

SERENTIL		
SANDOZ	EQ 25 MG BASE/ML	N16997 001

INJECTABLE; INJECTION

SERENTIL		
+ SANDOZ	EQ 25 MG BASE/ML	N16775 001

Prescription Drug Products *(continued)*

MESORIDAZINE BESYLATE *(continued)*

TABLET; ORAL
SERENTIL

	SANDOZ	EQ 10 MG BASE	N16774 001
		EQ 25 MG BASE	N16774 002
		EQ 50 MG BASE	N16774 003
	+	EQ 100 MG BASE	N16774 004

MESTRANOL; NORETHINDRONE

TABLET; ORAL-21

	NORETHIN 1/50M-21		
AB	ROBERTS LABS	0.05 MG;1 MG	N71539 001 APR 12, 1988
	NORETHINDRONE AND MESTRANOL		
AB	WATSON LABS	0.05 MG;1 MG	N70758 001 JUL 01, 1988
	NORINYL 1+50 21-DAY		
AB	SYNTEX	0.05 MG;1 MG	N13625 002
	ORTHO-NOVUM 1/50 21		
AB	+ JOHNSON RW	0.05 MG;1 MG	N12728 004

TABLET; ORAL-28

	NORETHIN 1/50M-28		
AB	ROBERTS LABS	0.05 MG;1 MG	N71540 001 APR 12, 1988
	NORETHINDRONE AND MESTRANOL		
AB	WATSON LABS	0.05 MG;1 MG	N70759 001 JUL 01, 1988
	NORINYL 1+50 28-DAY		
AB	SYNTEX	0.05 MG;1 MG	N16659 001
	ORTHO-NOVUM 1/50 28		
AB	JOHNSON RW	0.05 MG;1 MG	N16709 001

METAPROTERENOL SULFATE

AEROSOL, METERED; INHALATION
ALUPENT

	+ BOEHRINGER INGELHEIM	0.65 MG/INH	N16402 001

SOLUTION; INHALATION
ALUPENT

AN	+ BOEHRINGER INGELHEIM	0.4%	N18761 002 OCT 10, 1986
AN	+	0.6%	N18761 001 JUN 30, 1983
AN	+	5%	N17659 001

METAPROTERENOL SULFATE *(continued)*

SOLUTION; INHALATION

	METAPROTERENOL SULFATE		
AN	ASTRA	0.4%	N71275 001 JUL 27, 1988
AN		0.6%	N71018 001 JUL 27, 1988
AN	DEY	0.4%	N71786 001 AUG 05, 1988
AN		0.6%	N70804 001 AUG 17, 1987
AN		5%	N70805 001 AUG 17, 1987
AN	PACO	0.4%	N71855 001 JUL 14, 1988
AN		0.6%	N71726 001 JUL 14, 1988
	PROMETA		
AN	MURO	5%	N73340 001 MAR 30, 1992

SYRUP; ORAL

	ALUPENT		
AA	BOEHRINGER INGELHEIM	10 MG/5 ML	N17571 001
	METAPROTERENOL SULFATE		
AA	BIOCRAFT	10 MG/5 ML	N72761 001 FEB 27, 1992
AA	COPLEY PHARM	10 MG/5 ML	N73034 001 AUG 30, 1991
AA	PENNEX	10 MG/5 ML	N71656 001 OCT 13, 1987
AA	SILARX	10 MG/5 ML	N73632 001 JUL 22, 1992
	PROMETA		
AA	MURO	10 MG/5 ML	N72023 001 SEP 15, 1988

TABLET; ORAL

	ALUPENT		
AB	BOEHRINGER INGELHEIM	10 MG	N15874 002
AB	+	20 MG	N15874 001
	METAPROTERENOL SULFATE		
AB	BIOCRAFT	10 MG	N72519 001 MAR 30, 1990
AB		20 MG	N72520 001 MAR 30, 1990
AB	DANBURY PHARMA	10 MG	N73013 001 JAN 31, 1991
AB		20 MG	N72795 001 JAN 31, 1991

Prescription Drug Products *(continued)*

METAPROTERENOL SULFATE *(continued)*

TABLET; ORAL

	METAPROTERENOL SULFATE		
AB	PAR PHARM	10 MG	N72024 001 JUN 28, 1988
AB		20 MG	N72025 001 JUN 28, 1988

METARAMINOL BITARTRATE

INJECTABLE; INJECTION

	ARAMINE		
AP	+ MERCK SHARP DOHME	EQ 10 MG BASE/ML	N09509 002 DEC 22, 1987
	METARAMINOL BITARTRATE		
AP	FUJISAWA	EQ 10 MG BASE/ML	N80722 001

METAXALONE

TABLET; ORAL

	SKELAXIN		
	CARNRICK	400 MG	N13217 001

METHACHOLINE CHLORIDE

POWDER FOR RECONSTITUTION; INHALATION

	PROVOCHOLINE		
	ROCHE	100 MG/VIAL	N19193 001 OCT 31, 1986

METHADONE HYDROCHLORIDE

CONCENTRATE; ORAL

	METHADONE HCL INTENSOL		
AA	ROXANE	10 MG/ML	N89897 001 SEP 06, 1988
	METHADOSE		
AA	MALLINCKRODT	10 MG/ML	N17116 002

INJECTABLE; INJECTION

	DOLOPHINE HCL		
	+ LILLY	10 MG/ML	N06134 006

SOLUTION; ORAL

	METHADONE HCL		
	ROXANE	5 MG/5 ML	N87393 001
		10 MG/5 ML	N87997 001 AUG 30, 1982

SYRUP; ORAL

	DOLOPHINE HCL		
	LILLY	10 MG/30 ML	N06134 004

METHADONE HYDROCHLORIDE *(continued)*

TABLET; ORAL

	DOLOPHINE HCL		
AA	LILLY	5 MG	N06134 002
AA		10 MG	N06134 010
	METHADONE HCL		
AA	ROXANE	5 MG	N88108 001 MAR 08, 1983
AA		10 MG	N88109 001 MAR 08, 1983
	METHADOSE		
AA	MALLINCKRODT	5 MG	N40050 001 APR 15, 1993
AA		10 MG	N40050 002 APR 15, 1993

TABLET, DISPERSIBLE; ORAL

	METHADONE HCL		
AA	LILLY	40 MG	N17058 001
	METHADOSE		
AA	MALLINCKRODT	40 MG	N74184 001 APR 29, 1993

METHAMPHETAMINE HYDROCHLORIDE

TABLET; ORAL

	DESOXYN		
AA	ABBOTT	5 MG	N05378 002
	METHAMPHETAMINE HCL		
AA	REXAR	5 MG	N84931 001
		10 MG	N84931 002

TABLET, EXTENDED RELEASE; ORAL

	DESOXYN		
	ABBOTT	5 MG	N05378 004
		10 MG	N05378 003
		15 MG	N05378 005

METHANTHELINE BROMIDE

TABLET; ORAL

	BANTHINE		
	ROBERTS LABS	50 MG	N07390 001

METHAZOLAMIDE

TABLET; ORAL

	METHAZOLAMIDE		
AB	COPLEY PHARM	25 MG	N40001 001 JUN 30, 1993
AB		50 MG	N40001 002 JUN 30, 1993

Prescription Drug Products *(continued)*

METHAZOLAMIDE *(continued)*

TABLET; ORAL

	METHAZOLAMIDE		
AB	GENEVA PHARMS	25 MG	N40036 001 JUN 30, 1993
AB		50 MG	N40036 002 JUN 30, 1993
AB	MIKART	25 MG	N40062 001 JAN 27, 1994
AB		50 MG	N40062 002 JAN 27, 1994
	NEPTAZANE		
AB	LEDERLE	25 MG	N11721 002 NOV 25, 1991
AB	+	50 MG	N11721 001

METHENAMINE HIPPURATE

TABLET; ORAL

	HIPREX		
AB	+ MERRELL DOW	1 GM	N17681 001
	UREX		
AB	3M	1 GM	N16151 001

METHICILLIN SODIUM

INJECTABLE; INJECTION

	STAPHCILLIN		
	+ APOTHECON	EQ 900 MG BASE/VIAL	N61449 001
	+	EQ 3.6 GM BASE/VIAL	N61449 002
	+	EQ 5.4 GM BASE/VIAL	N61449 003

METHIMAZOLE

TABLET; ORAL

	TAPAZOLE		
	LILLY	5 MG	N07517 002
		10 MG	N07517 004

METHOCARBAMOL

INJECTABLE; INJECTION

	METHOCARBAMOL		
AP	MARSAM	100 MG/ML	N89849 001 DEC 27, 1991
AP	STERIS	100 MG/ML	N86459 001
	ROBAXIN		
AP	+ ROBINS AH	100 MG/ML	N11790 001

METHOCARBAMOL *(continued)*

TABLET; ORAL

	FORBAXIN		
AA	FOREST LABS	750 MG	N85136 001
	METHOCARBAMOL		
AA	BARR	750 MG	N84486 001
AA	CHELSEA LABS	500 MG	N85180 001
AA		750 MG	N85192 001
AA	DANBURY PHARMA	500 MG	N84277 001
AA		750 MG	N84276 002
AA	EON LABS	500 MG	N87283 001
AA		750 MG	N87282 001
AA	GENEVA PHARMS	500 MG	N84616 001
AA		750 MG	N84615 001
AA	GLOBAL PHARMS	500 MG	N84927 001
AA		750 MG	N84928 001
AA	INWOOD LABS	500 MG	N85137 001
AA	KV PHARM	500 MG	N85660 001
AA		750 MG	N85658 001
AA	LANNETT	750 MG	N84756 001
AA	LEDERLE	500 MG	N85961 001
AA		750 MG	N85963 001
AA	NYLOS	750 MG	N85033 001
AA	PAR PHARM	500 MG	N86989 001
AA		750 MG	N86988 001
AA	PUREPAC PHARM	500 MG	N85718 001
AA		750 MG	N85718 002
AA	SUPERPHARM	500 MG	N87589 001 JAN 22, 1982
AA		750 MG	N87590 001 JAN 22, 1982
AA	TABLICAPS	500 MG	N84846 001
AA	WEST WARD PHARM	500 MG	N85159 001
AA		750 MG	N85123 001
AA	ZENITH LABS	500 MG	N84648 001
AA		750 MG	N84649 001
	ROBAXIN		
AA	ROBINS AH	500 MG	N11011 004
	ROBAXIN-750		
AA	ROBINS AH	750 MG	N11011 006

METHOCARBAMOL; *MULTIPLE*

SEE ASPIRIN; METHOCARBAMOL

METHOHEXITAL SODIUM

INJECTABLE; INJECTION

	BREVITAL SODIUM		
	LILLY	500 MG/VIAL	N11559 001
		2.5 GM/VIAL	N11559 002
		5 GM/VIAL	N11559 003

Prescription Drug Products *(continued)*

METHOTREXATE SODIUM

INJECTABLE; INJECTION

	FOLEX		
AP	PHARMACIA	EQ 50 MG BASE/VIAL	N87695 002 APR 08, 1983
AP		EQ 100 MG BASE/VIAL	N87695 003 APR 08, 1983
		EQ 25 MG BASE/VIAL	N87695 001 APR 08, 1983
		EQ 250 MG BASE/VIAL	N88954 001 OCT 24, 1985
	FOLEX PFS		
AP	PHARMACIA	EQ 25 MG BASE/ML	N81242 001 AUG 23, 1991
	METHOTREXATE LPF		
AP	+ LEDERLE	EQ 25 MG BASE/ML	N11719 007 MAR 31, 1982
	METHOTREXATE SODIUM		
AP	BEN VENUE	EQ 25 MG BASE/ML	N89340 001 SEP 16, 1986
AP		EQ 25 MG BASE/ML	N89341 001 SEP 16, 1986
AP		EQ 25 MG BASE/ML	N89342 001 SEP 16, 1986
AP		EQ 25 MG BASE/ML	N89343 001 SEP 16, 1986
AP	+ LEDERLE	EQ 25 MG BASE/ML	N11719 005
AP	+	EQ 50 MG BASE/VIAL	N11719 003
AP	+	EQ 100 MG BASE/VIAL	N11719 006
	+	EQ 2.5 MG BASE/ML	N11719 004
	+	EQ 20 MG BASE/VIAL	N11719 001
	+	EQ 1 GM BASE/VIAL	N11719 009 APR 07, 1988
AP	NORBROOK	EQ 25 MG BASE/ML	N88648 001 MAY 09, 1986
AP	PHARMACHEMIE (US)	EQ 25 MG BASE/ML	N89158 001 JUL 08, 1988
	MEXATE-AQ		
AP	BRISTOL MYERS	EQ 25 MG BASE/ML	N88760 001 FEB 14, 1985
	MEXATE-AQ PRESERVED		
AP	BRISTOL MYERS	EQ 25 MG BASE/ML	N89887 001 APR 14, 1989

TABLET; ORAL

	METHOTREXATE SODIUM		
AB	BARR	EQ 2.5 MG BASE	N81099 001 OCT 15, 1990
AB	+ LEDERLE	EQ 2.5 MG BASE	N08085 002
AB	MYLAN	EQ 2.5 MG BASE	N81235 001 MAY 15, 1992
AB	ROXANE	EQ 2.5 MG BASE	N40054 001 AUG 01, 1994

METHOTRIMEPRAZINE

INJECTABLE; INJECTION

	LEVOPROME		
	+ LEDERLE	20 MG/ML	N15865 001

METHOXAMINE HYDROCHLORIDE

INJECTABLE; INJECTION

	VASOXYL		
	+ BURROUGHS WELLCOME	20 MG/ML	N06772 001

METHOXSALEN

CAPSULE; ORAL

	8-MOP		
	+ ICN	10 MG	N09048 001

CAPSULE, LIQUID FILLED; ORAL

	OXSORALEN-ULTRA		
	+ ICN	10 MG	N19600 001 OCT 30, 1986

LOTION; TOPICAL

	OXSORALEN		
	+ ICN	1%	N09048 002

METHOXYFLURANE

LIQUID; INHALATION

	PENTHRANE		
	ABBOTT	99.9%	N13056 001

METHSCOPOLAMINE BROMIDE

TABLET; ORAL

	METHSCOPOLAMINE BROMIDE		
AA	PRIVATE FORM	2.5 MG	N80970 001
	PAMINE		
AA	BRADLEY	2.5 MG	N08848 001

METHSUXIMIDE

CAPSULE; ORAL

	CELONTIN		
	PARKE DAVIS	150 MG	N10596 007
	+	300 MG	N10596 008

Prescription Drug Products *(continued)*

METHYCLOTHIAZIDE

TABLET; ORAL

	AQUATENSEN			
AB	WALLACE	5 MG	N17364 001	
	ENDURON			
AB	ABBOTT	2.5 MG	N12524 001	
AB	+	5 MG	N12524 004	
	METHYCLOTHIAZIDE			
AB	CHELSEA LABS	5 MG	N88724 001	SEP 06, 1984
AB	GENEVA PHARMS	2.5 MG	N89835 001	AUG 18, 1988
AB		5 MG	N89837 001	AUG 18, 1988
AB	MYLAN	5 MG	N87672 001	AUG 17, 1982
AB	PAR PHARM	2.5 MG	N89135 001	FEB 12, 1986
AB		5 MG	N89136 001	FEB 12, 1986
AB	ZENITH LABS	2.5 MG	N87913 001	JUN 03, 1982
AB		5 MG	N87786 001	MAY 18, 1982

METHYCLOTHIAZIDE; *MULTIPLE*

SEE DESERPIDINE; METHYCLOTHIAZIDE

METHYCLOTHIAZIDE; RESERPINE

TABLET; ORAL

	DIUTENSEN-R		
	+ WALLACE	2.5 MG;0.1 MG	N12708 005

METHYLDOPA

SUSPENSION; ORAL

	ALDOMET		
	+ MERCK SHARP DOHME	250 MG/5 ML	N18389 001

TABLET; ORAL

	ALDOMET		
AB	MERCK SHARP DOHME	125 MG	N13400 003
AB		250 MG	N13400 001
AB	+	500 MG	N13400 002

METHYLDOPA *(continued)*

TABLET; ORAL

	METHYLDOPA			
AB	BARR	125 MG	N70073 001	OCT 09, 1986
AB		250 MG	N70060 001	OCT 09, 1986
AB		500 MG	N70074 001	OCT 09, 1986
AB	DANBURY PHARMA	250 MG	N70703 001	JUN 06, 1986
AB		500 MG	N70625 001	JUN 06, 1986
AB	GENEVA PHARMS	125 MG	N71700 001	MAR 02, 1988
AB		250 MG	N18934 001	JUN 29, 1984
AB		500 MG	N18934 002	JUN 29, 1984
AB	HALSEY	125 MG	N71751 001	MAR 28, 1988
AB		250 MG	N71752 001	MAR 28, 1988
AB		500 MG	N71753 001	MAR 28, 1988
AB	LEDERLE	125 MG	N70070 003	OCT 15, 1985
AB		250 MG	N70084 001	OCT 15, 1985
AB		500 MG	N70085 001	OCT 15, 1985
AB	MYLAN	250 MG	N70075 001	APR 18, 1985
AB		500 MG	N70076 001	APR 18, 1985
AB	NOVOPHARM	125 MG	N71105 001	DEC 05, 1986
AB		250 MG	N71106 001	DEC 05, 1986
AB		500 MG	N71067 001	DEC 05, 1986
AB	PAR PHARM	125 MG	N70535 001	JAN 02, 1987
AB		250 MG	N70536 001	JAN 02, 1987
AB		500 MG	N70537 001	JAN 02, 1987

Prescription Drug Products *(continued)*

METHYLDOPA *(continued)*

TABLET; ORAL

METHYLDOPA

AB	PUREPAC PHARM	125 MG	N70749 001 FEB 07, 1986
AB		250 MG	N70750 001 FEB 07, 1986
AB		500 MG	N70452 001 FEB 07, 1986
AB	SIDMAK LABS NJ	125 MG	N72126 001 JUL 07, 1988
AB		250 MG	N72127 001 JUL 07, 1988
AB		500 MG	N72128 001 JUL 07, 1988
AB	SUPERPHARM	250 MG	N70669 001 JUN 23, 1989
AB		500 MG	N70670 001 JUN 23, 1989
AB	ZENITH LABS	250 MG	N70098 001 FEB 20, 1986
AB		500 MG	N70343 001 FEB 20, 1986

METHYLDOPA; *MULTIPLE*

SEE CHLOROTHIAZIDE; METHYLDOPA

SEE HYDROCHLOROTHIAZIDE; METHYLDOPA

METHYLDOPATE HYDROCHLORIDE

INJECTABLE; INJECTION

	ALDOMET		
AP	+ MERCK SHARP DOHME	50 MG/ML	N13401 001
	METHYLDOPATE HCL		
AP	ABBOTT	50 MG/ML	N70698 001 JUN 15, 1987
AP		50 MG/ML	N70699 001 JUN 15, 1987
AP	DUPONT MERCK	50 MG/ML	N70691 001 JUN 19, 1987
AP		50 MG/ML	N70849 001 JUN 19, 1987
AP	ELKINS SINN	50 MG/ML	N70291 001 JUL 01, 1986
AP	GENSIA	50 MG/ML	N72974 001 NOV 22, 1991
AP	LUITPOLD	50 MG/ML	N71279 001 OCT 02, 1987
AP	MARSAM	50 MG/ML	N71812 001 DEC 22, 1987
AP	SMITH AND NEPHEW	50 MG/ML	N70841 001 JAN 02, 1987

METHYLERGONOVINE MALEATE

INJECTABLE; INJECTION

	METHERGINE		
	+ SANDOZ	0.2 MG/ML	N06035 004

TABLET; ORAL

	METHERGINE		
	SANDOZ	0.2 MG	N06035 003

METHYLPHENIDATE HYDROCHLORIDE

TABLET; ORAL

	METHYLPHENIDATE HCL		
AB	MD PHARM	5 MG	N86429 001
AB		10 MG	N85799 001
AB		20 MG	N86428 001
	RITALIN		
AB	CIBA	5 MG	N10187 003
AB		10 MG	N10187 006
AB	+	20 MG	N10187 010

TABLET, EXTENDED RELEASE; ORAL

	METHYLPHENIDATE HCL		
AB	MD PHARM	20 MG	N89601 001 JUN 01, 1988
	RITALIN-SR		
AB	+ CIBA	20 MG	N18029 001 MAR 30, 1982

METHYLPREDNISOLONE

TABLET; ORAL

	MEDROL		
AB	UPJOHN	4 MG	N11153 001
AB		16 MG	N11153 003
AB		24 MG	N11153 005
AB	+	32 MG	N11153 006
		2 MG	N11153 002
		8 MG	N11153 004
	METHYLPREDNISOLONE		
AB	DURAMED	4 MG	N88497 001 FEB 21, 1984
AB	PAR PHARM	16 MG	N89207 001 APR 25, 1988
AB		24 MG	N89208 001 APR 25, 1988
AB		32 MG	N89209 001 APR 25, 1988

Prescription Drug Products *(continued)*

METHYLPREDNISOLONE ACETATE

INJECTABLE; INJECTION

	DEPO-MEDROL		
BP	UPJOHN	20 MG/ML	N11757 002
BP		40 MG/ML	N11757 001
BP	+	80 MG/ML	N11757 004
	METHYLPREDNISOLONE ACETATE		
BP	AKORN	40 MG/ML	N86903 001 OCT 20, 1982
BP		80 MG/ML	N86903 002 OCT 20, 1982
BP	STERIS	20 MG/ML	N85597 001
BP		40 MG/ML	N85600 001
BP		80 MG/ML	N85595 001

OINTMENT; TOPICAL

	MEDROL ACETATE		
	+ UPJOHN	0.25%	N12421 001

METHYLPREDNISOLONE ACETATE; NEOMYCIN SULFATE

CREAM; TOPICAL

	NEO-MEDROL ACETATE		
	+ UPJOHN	0.25%;EQ 3.5 MG BASE/GM	N60611 002
		1%;EQ 3.5 MG BASE/GM	N60611 001

METHYLPREDNISOLONE SODIUM SUCCINATE

INJECTABLE; INJECTION

	A-METHAPRED		
AP	ABBOTT	EQ 40 MG BASE/VIAL	N85853 001
AP		EQ 125 MG BASE/VIAL	N85855 001
AP		EQ 500 MG BASE/VIAL	N85854 001
AP		EQ 500 MG BASE/VIAL	N89173 001 AUG 18, 1987
AP		EQ 1 GM BASE/VIAL	N85852 001
AP		EQ 1 GM BASE/VIAL	N89174 001 AUG 18, 1987
	METHYLPREDNISOLONE SODIUM SUCCINATE		
AP	GENSIA	EQ 125 MG BASE/VIAL	N81266 001 NOV 30, 1992
AP		EQ 500 MG BASE/VIAL	N81267 001 NOV 30, 1992
AP		EQ 1 GM BASE/VIAL	N81268 001 NOV 30, 1992
AP	STERIS	EQ 40 MG BASE/VIAL	N86953 001 JUL 22, 1982
AP		EQ 125 MG BASE/VIAL	N87030 001 JUL 22, 1982
AP		EQ 500 MG BASE/VIAL	N88523 001 JUL 24, 1984
AP		EQ 1 GM BASE/VIAL	N88524 001 JUL 24, 1984

METHYLPREDNISOLONE SODIUM SUCCINATE *(continued)*

INJECTABLE; INJECTION

	SOLU-MEDROL		
AP	UPJOHN	EQ 40 MG BASE/VIAL	N11856 003
AP		EQ 125 MG BASE/VIAL	N11856 004
AP		EQ 500 MG BASE/VIAL	N11856 005
AP		EQ 1 GM BASE/VIAL	N11856 006
		EQ 2 GM BASE/VIAL	N11856 007 FEB 27, 1985

METHYLTESTOSTERONE

CAPSULE; ORAL

	TESTRED		
BP	+ ICN	10 MG	N83976 001
	VIRILON		
BP	STAR PHARMS FL	10 MG	N87750 001 NOV 24, 1982

TABLET; BUCCAL

	ORETON		
	+ SCHERING	10 MG	N80281 001

TABLET; BUCCAL/SUBLINGUAL

	METHYLTESTOSTERONE		
BP	GLOBAL PHARMS	10 MG	N84287 001
BP	+ LILLY	10 MG	N80256 001

TABLET; ORAL

	ANDROID 10		
AB	ICN	10 MG	N86450 001
	ANDROID 25		
AB	ICN	25 MG	N87147 001
	METHYLTESTOSTERONE		
BP	GLOBAL PHARMS	10 MG	N80767 002
BP		25 MG	N84310 001
BP	LANNETT	10 MG	N87092 001 NOV 05, 1982
BP		25 MG	N87111 001 JAN 27, 1983
BP	LILLY	25 MG	N80256 002
	ORETON METHYL		
BP	SCHERING	10 MG	N03158 001
BP	+	25 MG	N03158 002

METHYLTESTOSTERONE; *MULTIPLE*

SEE DIETHYLSTILBESTROL; METHYLTESTOSTERONE

METHYSERGIDE MALEATE

TABLET; ORAL

	SANSERT		
	SANDOZ	2 MG	N12516 001

Prescription Drug Products *(continued)*

METIPRANOLOL HYDROCHLORIDE

SOLUTION/DROPS; OPHTHALMIC

	OPTIPRANOLOL		
	+ BAUSCH AND LOMB	0.3%	N19907 001 DEC 29, 1989

METOCLOPRAMIDE HYDROCHLORIDE

CONCENTRATE; ORAL

	METOCLOPRAMIDE INTENSOL		
	ROXANE	EQ 10 MG BASE/ML	N72995 001 JAN 30, 1992

INJECTABLE; INJECTION

	METOCLOPRAMIDE HCL		
AP	ABBOTT	EQ 10 MG BASE/2 ML	N70505 001 JUN 23, 1989
AP		EQ 10 MG BASE/2 ML	N70506 001 JUN 22, 1989
AP		EQ 10 MG BASE/2 ML	N73117 001 JAN 17, 1991
AP		EQ 10 MG BASE/2 ML	N73118 001 JAN 17, 1991
AP	BULL D	EQ 10 MG BASE/2 ML	N71990 001 JAN 18, 1989
AP	CETUS BEN VENUE	EQ 10 MG BASE/2 ML	N72155 001 MAR 30, 1992
AP		EQ 10 MG BASE/2 ML	N72244 001 MAR 30, 1992
AP		EQ 10 MG BASE/2 ML	N72247 001 MAY 18, 1992
AP	DUPONT MERCK	EQ 10 MG BASE/2 ML	N70847 001 NOV 07, 1988
AP		EQ 10 MG BASE/2 ML	N71291 001 MAR 03, 1989
AP	GENSIA	EQ 10 MG BASE/2 ML	N73135 001 NOV 27, 1991
AP	SMITH AND NEPHEW	EQ 10 MG BASE/2 ML	N70623 001 MAR 02, 1987
	REGLAN		
AP	+ ROBINS AH	EQ 10 MG BASE/2 ML	N17862 001

SOLUTION; ORAL

	METOCLOPRAMIDE HCL		
AA	BARRE	EQ 5 MG BASE/5 ML	N71340 001 AUG 18, 1988
AA	BIOCRAFT	EQ 5 MG BASE/5 ML	N70819 001 JUL 10, 1987
AA	LEMMON	EQ 5 MG BASE/5 ML	N71315 001 JUN 30, 1993
AA	LIQUIPHARM	EQ 5 MG BASE/5 ML	N71402 001 JUN 25, 1993

METOCLOPRAMIDE HYDROCHLORIDE *(continued)*

SOLUTION; ORAL

	METOCLOPRAMIDE HCL		
AA	PENNEX	EQ 5 MG BASE/5 ML	N70949 001 MAR 06, 1987
AA	PHARM ASSOC	EQ 5 MG BASE/5 ML	N72744 001 MAY 28, 1991
AA	ROXANE	EQ 5 MG BASE/5 ML	N72038 001 DEC 05, 1988
AA	SILARX	EQ 5 MG BASE/5 ML	N73680 001 OCT 27, 1992
	REGLAN		
AA	+ ROBINS AH	EQ 5 MG BASE/5 ML	N18821 001 MAR 25, 1983

TABLET; ORAL

	MAXOLON		
AB	KING PHARMS	EQ 10 MG BASE	N70106 001 MAR 04, 1986
	METOCLOPRAMIDE HCL		
AB	BIOCRAFT	EQ 5 MG BASE	N72801 001 JUN 15, 1993
AB		EQ 10 MG BASE	N70184 001 JUL 29, 1985
AB	DANBURY PHARMA	EQ 10 MG BASE	N70511 001 JAN 22, 1986
AB	GENEVA PHARMS	EQ 10 MG BASE	N72215 001 JAN 30, 1990
AB	HALSEY	EQ 10 MG BASE	N70906 001 OCT 28, 1986
AB	INVAMED	EQ 5 MG BASE	N72436 001 JUN 22, 1989
AB		EQ 10 MG BASE	N70850 001 FEB 03, 1987
AB	LEDERLE	EQ 10 MG BASE	N72639 001 MAY 09, 1991
AB	MUTUAL PHARM	EQ 10 MG BASE	N71536 001 APR 28, 1993
AB	PUREPAC PHARM	EQ 10 MG BASE	N70581 001 OCT 17, 1985
AB	SCHERING	EQ 10 MG BASE	N70598 001 FEB 02, 1987
AB	SIDMAK LABS NJ	EQ 10 MG BASE	N71250 001 FEB 03, 1988
AB	SUPERPHARM	EQ 10 MG BASE	N70926 001 JUN 26, 1987
AB	WATSON LABS	EQ 10 MG BASE	N70645 001 MAY 11, 1987
	REGLAN		
AB	ROBINS AH	EQ 5 MG BASE	N17854 002 MAY 05, 1987
AB	+	EQ 10 MG BASE	N17854 001

Prescription Drug Products *(continued)*

METOCURINE IODIDE

INJECTABLE; INJECTION

	METUBINE IODIDE		
	+ LILLY	2 MG/ML	N06632 003

METOLAZONE

TABLET; ORAL

	MYKROX		
	FISONS	0.5 MG	N19532 001 OCT 30, 1987
	ZAROXOLYN		
	FISONS	2.5 MG	N17386 001
		5 MG	N17386 002
	+	10 MG	N17386 003

METOPROLOL FUMARATE

TABLET, EXTENDED RELEASE; ORAL

	LOPRESSOR		
	GEIGY	EQ 100 MG TARTRATE	N19786 001 DEC 27, 1989
		EQ 200 MG TARTRATE	N19786 002 DEC 27, 1989
		EQ 300 MG TARTRATE	N19786 003 DEC 27, 1989
	+	EQ 400 MG TARTRATE	N19786 004 DEC 27, 1989

METOPROLOL SUCCINATE

TABLET, EXTENDED RELEASE; ORAL

	TOPROL XL		
	+ HASSLE AB	EQ 50 MG TARTRATE	N19962 001 JAN 10, 1992
	+	EQ 100 MG TARTRATE	N19962 002 JAN 10, 1992
	+	EQ 200 MG TARTRATE	N19962 003 JAN 10, 1992

METOPROLOL TARTRATE

INJECTABLE; INJECTION

	LOPRESSOR		
AP	+ GEIGY	1 MG/ML	N18704 001 MAR 30, 1984
	METOPROLOL TARTRATE		
AP	STERIS	1 MG/ML	N74032 001 DEC 21, 1993
AP	STERLING WINTHROP	1 MG/ML	N74133 001 DEC 21, 1993

METOPROLOL TARTRATE *(continued)*

TABLET; ORAL

	LOPRESSOR		
AB	+ GEIGY	50 MG	N17963 001
AB	+	100 MG	N17963 002
	METOPROLOL TARTRATE		
AB	APOTHECON	50 MG	N74258 001 JAN 27, 1994
AB		100 MG	N74258 002 JAN 27, 1994
AB	COPLEY PHARM	50 MG	N74333 001 JAN 27, 1994
AB		100 MG	N74333 002 JAN 27, 1994
AB	GENEVA PHARMS	50 MG	N73288 001 MAR 25, 1994
AB		100 MG	N73289 001 MAR 25, 1994
AB	MUTUAL PHARM	50 MG	N73653 001 DEC 21, 1993
AB		100 MG	N73654 001 DEC 21, 1993
AB	MYLAN	50 MG	N73666 001 DEC 21, 1993
AB		100 MG	N73666 002 DEC 21, 1993
AB	PUREPAC PHARM	50 MG	N74380 001 JUL 29, 1994
AB		100 MG	N74380 002 JUL 29, 1994
AB	WATSON LABS	50 MG	N74217 001 MAY 27, 1994
AB		100 MG	N74217 002 MAY 27, 1994

METOPROLOL TARTRATE; *MULTIPLE*

SEE HYDROCHLOROTHIAZIDE; METOPROLOL TARTRATE

METRIZAMIDE

INJECTABLE; INJECTION

	AMIPAQUE		
	+ STERLING WINTHROP	3.75 GM/VIAL	N17982 001
	+	6.75 GM/VIAL	N17982 002

Prescription Drug Products *(continued)*

METRONIDAZOLE

GEL; TOPICAL

METROGEL

	+ GALDERMA	0.75%	N19737 001 NOV 22, 1988

GEL; VAGINAL

METROGEL

	+ CURATEK	0.75%	N20208 001 AUG 17, 1992

INJECTABLE; INJECTION

FLAGYL I.V. RTU IN PLASTIC CONTAINER

AP	+ SCS	500 MG/100 ML	N18353 002
AP		500 MG/100 ML	N18657 001

METRO I.V.

AP	MCGAW	500 MG/100 ML	N18674 001 AUG 31, 1982

METRO I.V. IN PLASTIC CONTAINER

AP	+ MCGAW	500 MG/100 ML	N18900 001 SEP 29, 1983

METRONIDAZOLE

AP	ABBOTT	500 MG/100 ML	N18889 001 NOV 18, 1983
AP	ELKINS SINN	500 MG/100 ML	N18907 001 MAR 30, 1984
AP	STERIS	500 MG/100 ML	N70042 001 DEC 20, 1984
AP		500 MG/100 ML	N70170 001 APR 01, 1986

METRONIDAZOLE IN PLASTIC CONTAINER

AP	ABBOTT	500 MG/100 ML	N18890 002 NOV 18, 1983

TABLET; ORAL

FLAGYL

AB	SEARLE	250 MG	N12623 001
AB	+	500 MG	N12623 003

METRONIDAZOLE

AB	BARR	250 MG	N18818 001 FEB 16, 1983
AB		500 MG	N18818 002 FEB 16, 1983
AB	DANBURY PHARMA	250 MG	N18764 001 SEP 17, 1982
AB		500 MG	N18764 002 DEC 20, 1982
AB	EON LABS	250 MG	N18620 001 MAR 04, 1982
AB		500 MG	N18620 002 JUN 02, 1983

METRONIDAZOLE *(continued)*

TABLET; ORAL

METRONIDAZOLE

AB	GENEVA PHARMS	250 MG	N18740 001 OCT 22, 1982
AB		500 MG	N18740 002 OCT 22, 1982
AB	HALSEY	250 MG	N70021 001 APR 02, 1985
AB		500 MG	N70593 001 FEB 27, 1986
AB	LNK	250 MG	N19029 001 APR 10, 1984
AB	MUTUAL PHARM	250 MG	N70772 001 JUL 16, 1986
AB		500 MG	N70773 001 JUL 16, 1986
AB	PAR PHARM	250 MG	N18845 001 AUG 18, 1983
AB		250 MG	N70040 001 JAN 29, 1985
AB		500 MG	N18930 001 AUG 18, 1983
AB		500 MG	N70039 001 JAN 29, 1985
AB	SIDMAK LABS NJ	250 MG	N70027 001 NOV 06, 1984
AB		500 MG	N70033 001 DEC 06, 1984
AB	ZENITH LABS	250 MG	N18517 001
AB		500 MG	N18517 002 MAY 05, 1982

METRYL

AB	LEMMON	250 MG	N70035 001 DEC 20, 1984

METRYL 500

AB	LEMMON	500 MG	N70044 001 FEB 08, 1985

PROTOSTAT

AB	JOHNSON RW	250 MG	N18871 001 MAR 02, 1983
AB		500 MG	N18871 002 MAR 02, 1983

METRONIDAZOLE HYDROCHLORIDE

INJECTABLE; INJECTION

FLAGYL I.V.

	+ SCS	EQ 500 MG BASE/VIAL	N18353 001

Prescription Drug Products *(continued)*

METYRAPONE

	TABLET; ORAL		
	METOPIRONE		
	CIBA	250 MG	N12911 001

METYROSINE

	CAPSULE; ORAL		
	DEMSER		
	+ MERCK SHARP DOHME	250 MG	N17871 001

MEXILETINE HYDROCHLORIDE

	CAPSULE; ORAL		
	MEXITIL		
	BOEHRINGER INGELHEIM	150 MG	N18873 002 DEC 30, 1985
		200 MG	N18873 003 DEC 30, 1985
	+	250 MG	N18873 004 DEC 30, 1985

MEZLOCILLIN SODIUM MONOHYDRATE

	INJECTABLE; INJECTION		
	MEZLIN		
	+ MILES	EQ 1 GM BASE/VIAL	N50549 001
		EQ 1 GM BASE/VIAL	N62372 005 JAN 13, 1983
	+	EQ 2 GM BASE/VIAL	N50549 002
		EQ 2 GM BASE/VIAL	N62372 001 MAY 13, 1982
	+	EQ 3 GM BASE/VIAL	N50549 003
		EQ 3 GM BASE/VIAL	N62372 002 MAY 13, 1982
		EQ 3 GM BASE/VIAL	N62697 001 JAN 22, 1987
	+	EQ 4 GM BASE/VIAL	N50549 004
		EQ 4 GM BASE/VIAL	N62372 003 MAY 13, 1982
		EQ 4 GM BASE/VIAL	N62697 002 JAN 22, 1987
	+	EQ 20 GM BASE/VIAL	N50549 005 MAR 02, 1988
		EQ 20 GM BASE/VIAL	N62372 004 MAR 02, 1988

MICONAZOLE

	INJECTABLE; INJECTION		
	MONISTAT		
	+ JANSSEN	10 MG/ML	N18040 001

MICONAZOLE NITRATE

	CREAM; TOPICAL		
	MONISTAT-DERM		
	+ JOHNSON RW	2%	N17494 001
	CREAM, SUPPOSITORY; TOPICAL, VAGINAL		
	MONISTAT DUAL-PAK		
	+ JOHNSON RW	2%;200 MG	N18888 002 OCT 17, 1988
	SUPPOSITORY; VAGINAL		
	MICONAZOLE NITRATE		
AB	ABLE	200 MG	N73508 001 NOV 19, 1993
	MONISTAT 3		
AB	+ JOHNSON RW	200 MG	N18888 001 AUG 15, 1984
	TAMPON; VAGINAL		
	MONISTAT 5		
	+ JOHNSON RW	100 MG	N18592 001 OCT 27, 1989

MIDAZOLAM HYDROCHLORIDE

	INJECTABLE; INJECTION		
	VERSED		
	+ ROCHE	EQ 1 MG BASE/ML	N18654 002 MAY 26, 1987
	+	EQ 5 MG BASE/ML	N18654 001 DEC 20, 1985

MILRINONE LACTATE

	INJECTABLE; INJECTION		
	PRIMACOR		
	+ STERLING WINTHROP	EQ 1 MG BASE/ML	N19436 001 DEC 31, 1987
	PRIMACOR IN DEXTROSE 5% IN PLASTIC CONTAINER		
	+ STERLING WINTHROP	EQ 20 MG BASE/100 ML	N20343 003 AUG 09, 1994

MINOCYCLINE HYDROCHLORIDE

	CAPSULE; ORAL		
	MINOCIN		
AB	LEDERLE	EQ 50 MG BASE	N50649 001 MAY 31, 1990
AB	+	EQ 100 MG BASE	N50649 002 MAY 31, 1990

Prescription Drug Products *(continued)*

MINOCYCLINE HYDROCHLORIDE *(continued)*

	CAPSULE; ORAL		
	MINOCYCLINE HCL		
AB	BIOCRAFT	EQ 50 MG BASE	N63011 001 MAR 02, 1992
AB		EQ 100 MG BASE	N63009 001 MAR 02, 1992
AB	DANBURY PHARMA	EQ 50 MG BASE	N63181 001 DEC 30, 1991
AB		EQ 100 MG BASE	N63065 001 DEC 30, 1991
AB	WARNER CHILCOTT	EQ 50 MG BASE	N63066 001 AUG 14, 1990
AB		EQ 100 MG BASE	N63067 001 JUL 31, 1990
	INJECTABLE; INJECTION		
	MINOCIN		
	+ LEDERLE	EQ 100 MG BASE/VIAL	N50444 001
	SUSPENSION; ORAL		
	MINOCIN		
	+ LEDERLE	EQ 50 MG BASE/5 ML	N50445 001
	TABLET; ORAL		
	MINOCYCLINE HCL		
	LEDERLE	EQ 50 MG BASE	N50451 003 AUG 10, 1982
		EQ 100 MG BASE	N50451 002 AUG 10, 1982

MINOXIDIL

	SOLUTION; TOPICAL		
	ROGAINE		
	+ UPJOHN	2%	N19501 001 AUG 17, 1988
	TABLET; ORAL		
	LONITEN		
AB	UPJOHN	2.5 MG	N18154 001
AB	+	10 MG	N18154 003
	MINOXIDIL		
AB	DANBURY PHARMA	2.5 MG	N71344 001 MAR 03, 1987
AB		10 MG	N71345 001 MAR 03, 1987
AB	PAR PHARM	2.5 MG	N71826 001 NOV 14, 1988
AB		10 MG	N71839 001 NOV 14, 1988

MISOPROSTOL

	TABLET; ORAL		
	CYTOTEC		
	SEARLE	0.1 MG	N19268 003 SEP 21, 1990
	+	0.2 MG	N19268 001 DEC 27, 1988

MITOMYCIN

	INJECTABLE; INJECTION		
	MUTAMYCIN		
AP	+ BRISTOL	5 MG/VIAL	N50450 001
AP	+	20 MG/VIAL	N50450 002
AP	BRISTOL MYERS	5 MG/VIAL	N62336 001
AP		20 MG/VIAL	N62336 002
		40 MG/VIAL	N62336 003 MAR 10, 1988

MITOTANE

	TABLET; ORAL		
	LYSODREN		
	+ BRISTOL	500 MG	N16885 001

MITOXANTRONE HYDROCHLORIDE

	INJECTABLE; INJECTION		
	NOVANTRONE		
	+ IMMUNEX	EQ 2 MG BASE/ML	N19297 001 DEC 23, 1987

MIVACURIUM CHLORIDE

	INJECTABLE; INJECTION		
	MIVACRON		
	BURROUGHS WELLCOME	EQ 2 MG BASE/ML	N20098 001 JAN 22, 1992
	MIVACRON IN DEXTROSE 5% IN PLASTIC CONTAINER		
	BURROUGHS WELLCOME	EQ 0.5 MG BASE/ML	N20098 002 JAN 22, 1992
		EQ 50 MG BASE/100 ML	N20098 003 JAN 22, 1992

Prescription Drug Products *(continued)*

MOLINDONE HYDROCHLORIDE

CONCENTRATE; ORAL
MOBAN
DUPONT MERCK 20 MG/ML N17938 001

TABLET; ORAL
MOBAN
DUPONT MERCK 5 MG N17111 004
10 MG N17111 005
+ 25 MG N17111 006
50 MG N17111 007
+ 100 MG N17111 008

MOMETASONE FUROATE

CREAM; TOPICAL
ELOCON
+ SCHERING 0.1% N19625 001 MAY 06, 1987

LOTION; TOPICAL
ELOCON
+ SCHERING 0.1% N19796 001 MAR 30, 1989

OINTMENT; TOPICAL
ELOCON
+ SCHERING 0.1% N19543 001 APR 30, 1987

MONOBENZONE

CREAM; TOPICAL
BENOQUIN
+ ICN 20% N08173 003

MONOCTANOIN

LIQUID; PERFUSION, BILIARY
MOCTANIN
ETHITEK 100% N19368 001 OCT 29, 1985

MORICIZINE HYDROCHLORIDE

TABLET; ORAL
ETHMOZINE
ROBERTS LABS 200 MG N19753 001 JUN 19, 1990
250 MG N19753 002 JUN 19, 1990
300 MG N19753 003 JUN 19, 1990

MORPHINE SULFATE

INJECTABLE; INJECTION
ASTRAMORPH PF
AP ASTRA 0.5 MG/ML N71050 001 OCT 07, 1986
AP 0.5 MG/ML N71051 001 OCT 07, 1986
AP 1 MG/ML N71052 001 OCT 07, 1986
AP 1 MG/ML N71053 001 OCT 07, 1986
DURAMORPH PF
AP + ELKINS SINN 0.5 MG/ML N18565 001 SEP 18, 1984
AP + 1 MG/ML N18565 002 SEP 18, 1984
INFUMORPH
+ ELKINS SINN 10 MG/ML N18565 003 JUL 19, 1991
+ 25 MG/ML N18565 004 JUL 19, 1991
MORPHINE SULFATE
AP ABBOTT 0.5 MG/ML N19917 001 OCT 30, 1992
AP 0.5 MG/ML N71849 001 MAY 11, 1988
AP 0.5 MG/ML N73509 001 SEP 30, 1992
AP 1 MG/ML N19916 001 OCT 30, 1992
AP 1 MG/ML N71850 001 MAY 11, 1988
AP 1 MG/ML N73510 001 SEP 30, 1992
AP STERIS 0.5 MG/ML N73373 001 SEP 30, 1991
AP 0.5 MG/ML N73375 001 SEP 30, 1991
AP 1 MG/ML N73374 001 SEP 30, 1991
AP 1 MG/ML N73376 001 SEP 30, 1991
SURVIVAL TECH 15 MG/ML N19999 001 JUL 12, 1990

Prescription Drug Products *(continued)*

MORPHINE SULFATE (*continued*)

TABLET, EXTENDED RELEASE; ORAL

	MS CONTIN		
BC	+ PURDUE FREDERICK	30 MG	N19516 001 MAY 29, 1987
BC	+	60 MG	N19516 002 APR 08, 1988
BC	+	100 MG	N19516 004 JAN 16, 1990
	+	15 MG	N19516 003 SEP 12, 1989
	+	200 MG	N19516 005 NOV 08, 1993
	ORAMORPH SR		
BC	ROXANE	30 MG	N19977 001 AUG 15, 1991
BC		60 MG	N19977 002 AUG 15, 1991
BC		100 MG	N19977 003 AUG 15, 1991

MOXALACTAM DISODIUM

INJECTABLE; INJECTION

MOXAM		
+ LILLY	EQ 250 MG BASE/VIAL	N50550 001
+	EQ 500 MG BASE/VIAL	N50550 002
+	EQ 1 GM BASE/VIAL	N50550 003
+	EQ 2 GM BASE/VIAL	N50550 004
+	EQ 10 GM BASE/VIAL	N50550 008

MUPIROCIN

OINTMENT; TOPICAL

BACTROBAN		
+ SMITHKLINE BEECHAM	2%	N50591 001 DEC 31, 1987

NABUMETONE

TABLET; ORAL

RELAFEN		
SMITHKLINE BEECHAM	500 MG	N19583 001 DEC 24, 1991
+	750 MG	N19583 002 DEC 24, 1991

NADOLOL

TABLET; ORAL

	CORGARD		
AB	SQUIBB	20 MG	N18063 005 OCT 28, 1986
AB		40 MG	N18063 001
AB		40 MG	N18064 001
AB		80 MG	N18063 002
AB		80 MG	N18064 002
AB		120 MG	N18063 003
AB		120 MG	N18064 003
AB	+	160 MG	N18063 004
AB		160 MG	N18064 004
	NADOLOL		
AB	COPLEY PHARM	80 MG	N74368 001 AUG 31, 1994
AB		120 MG	N74368 002 AUG 31, 1994
AB		160 MG	N74368 003 AUG 31, 1994
AB	MYLAN	20 MG	N74172 001 OCT 31, 1993
AB		40 MG	N74172 002 OCT 31, 1993
AB		80 MG	N74172 003 OCT 31, 1993

NADOLOL; *MULTIPLE*

SEE BENDROFLUMETHIAZIDE; NADOLOL

NAFARELIN ACETATE

SPRAY, METERED; NASAL

SYNAREL		
+ SYNTEX	EQ 0.2 MG BASE/INH	N19886 001 FEB 13, 1990
	EQ 0.2 MG BASE/INH	N20109 001 FEB 26, 1992

Prescription Drug Products *(continued)*

NAFCILLIN SODIUM

CAPSULE; ORAL

	UNIPEN		
	+ WYETH AYERST	EQ 250 MG BASE	N50111 001

INJECTABLE; INJECTION

	NAFCIL		
AP	APOTHECON	EQ 500 MG BASE/VIAL	N61984 001
AP		EQ 500 MG BASE/VIAL	N62527 001 AUG 02, 1984
AP		EQ 1 GM BASE/VIAL	N61984 002
AP		EQ 1 GM BASE/VIAL	N62527 002 AUG 02, 1984
AP		EQ 1 GM BASE/VIAL	N62732 001 DEC 23, 1986
AP		EQ 2 GM BASE/VIAL	N61984 003
AP		EQ 2 GM BASE/VIAL	N62527 003 AUG 02, 1984
AP		EQ 2 GM BASE/VIAL	N62732 002 DEC 23, 1986
AP		EQ 4 GM BASE/VIAL	N61984 005
AP		EQ 10 GM BASE/VIAL	N62527 004 AUG 02, 1984
	NAFCILLIN SODIUM		
AP	MARSAM	EQ 500 MG BASE/VIAL	N62844 001 OCT 26, 1988
AP		EQ 1 GM BASE/VIAL	N62844 002 OCT 26, 1988
AP		EQ 2 GM BASE/VIAL	N62844 004 OCT 26, 1988
AP		EQ 4 GM BASE/VIAL	N62844 005 OCT 26, 1988
AP		EQ 10 GM BASE/VIAL	N63008 001 SEP 29, 1988
	+	EQ 1.5 GM BASE/VIAL	N62844 003 OCT 26, 1988
	NALLPEN		
AP	SMITHKLINE BEECHAM	EQ 500 MG BASE/VIAL	N61999 001
AP		EQ 1 GM BASE/VIAL	N61999 002
AP		EQ 1 GM BASE/VIAL	N62755 001 DEC 19, 1986
AP		EQ 2 GM BASE/VIAL	N61999 003
AP		EQ 2 GM BASE/VIAL	N62755 002 DEC 19, 1986
AP		EQ 10 GM BASE/VIAL	N61999 004
	NALLPEN IN PLASTIC CONTAINER		
	+ BAXTER	EQ 20 MG BASE/ML	N50655 001 OCT 31, 1989
	+	EQ 40 MG BASE/ML	N50655 002 OCT 31, 1989

NAFCILLIN SODIUM *(continued)*

INJECTABLE; INJECTION

	UNIPEN		
AP	+ WYETH AYERST	EQ 500 MG BASE/VIAL	N50320 001
AP		EQ 500 MG BASE/VIAL	N62717 001 DEC 16, 1986
AP	+	EQ 1 GM BASE/VIAL	N62717 002 DEC 16, 1986
AP	+	EQ 2 GM BASE/VIAL	N50320 003
AP		EQ 2 GM BASE/VIAL	N62717 004 DEC 16, 1986
AP	+	EQ 4 GM BASE/VIAL	N50320 004
AP		EQ 10 GM BASE/VIAL	N50320 005
	UNIPEN IN PLASTIC CONTAINER		
AP	WYETH AYERST	EQ 1 GM BASE/VIAL	N50320 002

TABLET; ORAL

	UNIPEN		
	+ WYETH AYERST	EQ 500 MG BASE	N50462 001

NAFTIFINE HYDROCHLORIDE

CREAM; TOPICAL

	NAFTIN		
	+ ALLERGAN HERBERT	1%	N19599 001 FEB 29, 1988

GEL; TOPICAL

	NAFTIN		
	+ ALLERGAN HERBERT	1%	N19356 001 JUN 18, 1990

NALBUPHINE HYDROCHLORIDE

INJECTABLE; INJECTION

	NALBUPHINE HCL		
AP	ABBOTT	10 MG/ML	N70914 001 FEB 03, 1989
AP		10 MG/ML	N70915 001 FEB 03, 1989
AP		20 MG/ML	N70916 001 FEB 03, 1989
AP		20 MG/ML	N70917 001 FEB 03, 1989
AP		20 MG/ML	N70918 001 FEB 03, 1989
AP	ASTRA	10 MG/ML	N72070 001 APR 10, 1989
AP		20 MG/ML	N72073 001 APR 10, 1989
	NALBUPHINE HYDROCHLORIDE		
	ABBOTT	1.5 MG/ML	N20200 001 MAR 12, 1993

Prescription Drug Products *(continued)*

NALBUPHINE HYDROCHLORIDE *(continued)*

INJECTABLE; INJECTION

NUBAIN

AP	+ DUPONT MERCK	10 MG/ML	N18024 001
AP	+	20 MG/ML	N18024 002 MAY 27, 1982

NALIDIXIC ACID

SUSPENSION; ORAL

NEGGRAM

	+ STERLING WINTHROP	250 MG/5 ML	N17430 001

TABLET; ORAL

NALIDIXIC ACID

AB	BARR	250 MG	N70270 001 JUN 29, 1988
AB		500 MG	N70271 001 JUN 29, 1988
AB		1 GM	N70272 001 JUN 29, 1988
AB	DANBURY PHARMA	250 MG	N71936 001 JUN 29, 1988
AB		500 MG	N72061 001 JUN 29, 1988
AB		1 GM	N71919 001 JUN 29, 1988

NEGGRAM

AB	STERLING WINTHROP	250 MG	N14214 002
AB		500 MG	N14214 004
AB	+	1 GM	N14214 005

NALOXONE HYDROCHLORIDE

INJECTABLE; INJECTION

NALOXONE

AP	ELKINS SINN	0.4 MG/ML	N70298 001 SEP 24, 1986
AP		0.4 MG/ML	N70299 001 SEP 24, 1986
AP	WYETH AYERST	0.02 MG/ML	N70188 001 SEP 24, 1986
AP		0.02 MG/ML	N70189 001 SEP 24, 1986
AP		0.4 MG/ML	N70190 001 SEP 24, 1986
AP		0.4 MG/ML	N70191 001 SEP 24, 1986

NALOXONE HYDROCHLORIDE *(continued)*

INJECTABLE; INJECTION

NALOXONE HCL

AP	ABBOTT	0.02 MG/ML	N70252 001 JAN 16, 1987
AP		0.02 MG/ML	N70253 001 JAN 16, 1987
AP		0.4 MG/ML	N70254 001 JAN 07, 1987
AP		0.4 MG/ML	N70255 001 JAN 07, 1987
AP		0.4 MG/ML	N70256 001 JAN 07, 1987
AP		0.4 MG/ML	N70257 001 JAN 07, 1987
AP	ASTRA	0.02 MG/ML	N72081 001 APR 11, 1989
AP		0.4 MG/ML	N72086 001 APR 11, 1989
AP		1 MG/ML	N72091 001 APR 11, 1989
AP	ELKINS SINN	0.02 MG/ML	N71272 001 MAY 24, 1988
AP		1 MG/ML	N71273 001 MAY 24, 1988
AP		1 MG/ML	N71274 001 MAY 24, 1988
AP		1 MG/ML	N71287 001 MAY 24, 1988
AP	FUJISAWA	0.02 MG/ML	N70648 001 NOV 17, 1986
AP		0.4 MG/ML	N70649 001 NOV 17, 1986
AP	INTL MEDICATION	0.4 MG/ML	N70639 001 SEP 24, 1986
AP		1 MG/ML	N72076 001 MAR 24, 1988
AP	MARSAM	0.4 MG/ML	N71811 001 JUL 19, 1988
AP	SMITH AND NEPHEW	0.02 MG/ML	N71671 001 NOV 17, 1987
AP		0.4 MG/ML	N71681 001 NOV 17, 1987
AP		0.4 MG/ML	N71682 001 NOV 17, 1987
AP	SOLOPAK	0.02 MG/ML	N71672 001 NOV 17, 1987
AP		0.4 MG/ML	N71683 001 NOV 17, 1987
AP	STERIS	0.4 MG/ML	N71339 001 NOV 18, 1987

Prescription Drug Products *(continued)*

NALOXONE HYDROCHLORIDE *(continued)*

INJECTABLE; INJECTION

	NALOXONE HCL		
AP	STERLING WINTHROP	0.02 MG/ML	N70171 001 SEP 24, 1986
AP		0.4 MG/ML	N70172 001 SEP 24, 1986
	NARCAN		
AP	+ DUPONT MERCK	0.02 MG/ML	N16636 002
AP	+	0.4 MG/ML	N16636 001
AP	+	1 MG/ML	N16636 003 JUN 14, 1982

NALOXONE HYDROCHLORIDE; PENTAZOCINE HYDROCHLORIDE

TABLET; ORAL

	TALWIN NX		
	+ STERLING WINTHROP	EQ 0.5 MG BASE;EQ 50 MG BASE	N18733 001 DEC 16, 1982

NALTREXONE HYDROCHLORIDE

TABLET; ORAL

	TREXAN		
	+ DUPONT MERCK	50 MG	N18932 001 NOV 20, 1984

NANDROLONE DECANOATE

INJECTABLE; INJECTION

	DECA-DURABOLIN		
AO	+ ORGANON	50 MG/ML	N13132 001 JUN 12, 1986
AO	+	100 MG/ML	N13132 002 JUN 12, 1986
AO	+	200 MG/ML	N13132 003 JUN 12, 1986
	NANDROLONE DECANOATE		
AO	AKORN	100 MG/ML	N87519 001 SEP 28, 1983
AO	STERIS	50 MG/ML	N86385 001 JAN 13, 1984
AO		50 MG/ML	N87598 001 OCT 06, 1983
AO		50 MG/ML	N88554 001 FEB 10, 1986
AO		100 MG/ML	N86598 001 JAN 13, 1984
AO		100 MG/ML	N87599 001 OCT 06, 1983
AO		200 MG/ML	N88128 001 DEC 05, 1983

NANDROLONE PHENPROPIONATE

INJECTABLE; INJECTION

	DURABOLIN		
AO	+ ORGANON	25 MG/ML	N11891 001
	DURABOLIN-50		
AO	+ ORGANON	50 MG/ML	N11891 002
	NANDROLONE PHENPROPIONATE		
AO	STERIS	25 MG/ML	N86386 001 JUN 17, 1983
AO		50 MG/ML	N87488 001 JUN 17, 1983

NAPHAZOLINE HYDROCHLORIDE

SOLUTION/DROPS; OPHTHALMIC

	ALBALON		
AT	ALLERGAN	0.1%	N80248 001
	NAFAZAIR		
AT	BAUSCH AND LOMB	0.1%	N40073 001 MAY 25, 1994
	NAPHAZOLINE HCL		
AT	AKORN	0.1%	N83590 001
	NAPHCON FORTE		
AT	+ ALCON	0.1%	N80229 001
	OPCON		
AT	BAUSCH AND LOMB	0.1%	N87506 001
	VASOCON		
AT	IOLAB	0.1%	N80235 002 MAR 24, 1983

NAPHAZOLINE HYDROCHLORIDE; *MULTIPLE*

SEE ANTAZOLINE PHOSPHATE; NAPHAZOLINE HYDROCHLORIDE

NAPROXEN

SUSPENSION; ORAL

	NAPROSYN		
AB	+ SYNTEX	25 MG/ML	N18965 001 MAR 23, 1987
	NAPROXEN		
AB	ROXANE	25 MG/ML	N74190 001 MAR 30, 1994

TABLET; ORAL

	NAPROSYN		
AB	SYNTEX	250 MG	N17581 002
AB		375 MG	N17581 003
AB	+	500 MG	N17581 004 APR 15, 1982

Prescription Drug Products *(continued)*

NAPROXEN *(continued)*

TABLET; ORAL

NAPROXEN

AB	COPLEY PHARM	250 MG	N74207 001 DEC 21, 1993
AB		375 MG	N74207 002 DEC 21, 1993
AB		500 MG	N74207 003 DEC 21, 1993
AB	GENEVA PHARMS	250 MG	N74140 001 DEC 21, 1993
AB		375 MG	N74140 002 DEC 21, 1993
AB		500 MG	N74140 003 DEC 21, 1993
AB	HAMILTON PHARMS	250 MG	N74110 001 OCT 30, 1992
AB		375 MG	N74110 002 OCT 30, 1992
AB		500 MG	N74110 003 OCT 30, 1992
AB	LEDERLE	250 MG	N74105 001 DEC 21, 1993
AB		375 MG	N74105 002 DEC 21, 1993
AB		500 MG	N74105 003 DEC 21, 1993
AB	LEMMON	250 MG	N74201 001 DEC 21, 1993
AB		375 MG	N74201 002 DEC 21, 1993
AB		500 MG	N74201 003 DEC 21, 1993
AB	MYLAN	250 MG	N74121 001 DEC 21, 1993
AB		375 MG	N74121 002 DEC 21, 1993
AB		500 MG	N74121 003 DEC 21, 1993
AB	NOVOPHARM	250 MG	N74129 001 DEC 21, 1993
AB		375 MG	N74129 002 DEC 21, 1993
AB		500 MG	N74129 003 DEC 21, 1993
AB	PUREPAC PHARM	250 MG	N74263 001 DEC 21, 1993
AB		375 MG	N74263 002 DEC 21, 1993
AB		500 MG	N74263 003 DEC 21, 1993

NAPROXEN *(continued)*

TABLET; ORAL

NAPROXEN

AB	ROXANE	250 MG	N74211 001 FEB 28, 1994
AB		375 MG	N74211 002 FEB 28, 1994
AB		500 MG	N74211 003 FEB 28, 1994

NAPROXEN SODIUM

TABLET; ORAL

	ANAPROX		
AB	SYNTEX	EQ 250 MG BASE	N18164 001
	ANAPROX DS		
AB	+ SYNTEX	EQ 500 MG BASE	N18164 003 SEP 30, 1987
	NAPROXEN SODIUM		
AB	COPLEY PHARM	EQ 250 MG BASE	N74289 001 JAN 27, 1994
AB		EQ 500 MG BASE	N74289 002 JAN 27, 1994
AB	DANBURY PHARMA	EQ 250 MG BASE	N74195 001 DEC 21, 1993
AB		EQ 500 MG BASE	N74195 002 DEC 21, 1993
AB	GENEVA PHARMS	EQ 250 MG BASE	N74162 001 DEC 21, 1993
AB		EQ 500 MG BASE	N74162 002 DEC 21, 1993
AB	HAMILTON PHARMS	EQ 250 MG BASE	N74106 001 AUG 31, 1993
AB		EQ 500 MG BASE	N74106 002 AUG 31, 1993
AB	LEMMON	EQ 250 MG BASE	N74198 001 DEC 21, 1993
AB		EQ 500 MG BASE	N74198 002 DEC 21, 1993
AB	MYLAN	EQ 250 MG BASE	N74367 001 AUG 31, 1994
AB		EQ 500 MG BASE	N74367 002 AUG 31, 1994
AB	NOVOPHARM	EQ 250 MG BASE	N74142 001 DEC 21, 1993
AB		EQ 500 MG BASE	N74142 002 DEC 21, 1993

Prescription Drug Products *(continued)*

NAPROXEN SODIUM *(continued)*

TABLET; ORAL

	NAPROXEN SODIUM		
AB	ROXANE	EQ 250 MG BASE	N74257 001 DEC 21, 1993
AB		EQ 500 MG BASE	N74257 002 DEC 21, 1993

NATAMYCIN

SUSPENSION/DROPS; OPHTHALMIC

	NATACYN		
	+ ALCON	5%	N50514 001

NEDOCROMIL SODIUM

AEROSOL, METERED; INHALATION

	TILADE		
	+ FISONS	1.75 MG/INH	N19660 001 DEC 30, 1992

NEOMYCIN SULFATE

INJECTABLE; INJECTION

	MYCIFRADIN		
AP	+ UPJOHN	EQ 350 MG BASE/VIAL	N60477 001
	NEOMYCIN SULFATE		
AP	PFIZER	EQ 350 MG BASE/VIAL	N61084 001
AP	SQUIBB	EQ 350 MG BASE/VIAL	N60366 001

POWDER; FOR RX COMPOUNDING

	NEO-RX		
AA	PHARMA TEK	100%	N61579 001
	NEOMYCIN SULFATE		
AA	PADDOCK	100%	N62385 001 JUN 01, 1982

SOLUTION; ORAL

	MYCIFRADIN		
	UPJOHN	EQ 87.5 MG BASE/5 ML	N50285 001

TABLET; ORAL

	NEOMYCIN SULFATE		
AA	BIOCRAFT	EQ 350 MG BASE	N60304 001
AA	LILLY	EQ 350 MG BASE	N60385 001

NEOMYCIN SULFATE; *MULTIPLE*

SEE ACETIC ACID, GLACIAL; HYDROCORTISONE; NEOMYCIN SULFATE
SEE BACITRACIN; HYDROCORTISONE ACETATE; NEOMYCIN SULFATE; POLYMYXIN B SULFATE
SEE BACITRACIN ZINC; HYDROCORTISONE; NEOMYCIN SULFATE; POLYMYXIN B SULFATE
SEE BACITRACIN ZINC; NEOMYCIN SULFATE; POLYMYXIN B SULFATE
SEE COLISTIN SULFATE; HYDROCORTISONE ACETATE; NEOMYCIN SULFATE; THONZONIUM BROMIDE
SEE DEXAMETHASONE; NEOMYCIN SULFATE; POLYMYXIN B SULFATE
SEE DEXAMETHASONE SODIUM PHOSPHATE; NEOMYCIN SULFATE
SEE FLUOCINOLONE ACETONIDE; NEOMYCIN SULFATE
SEE FLURANDRENOLIDE; NEOMYCIN SULFATE
SEE GRAMICIDIN; NEOMYCIN SULFATE; POLYMYXIN B SULFATE
SEE HYDROCORTISONE; NEOMYCIN SULFATE
SEE HYDROCORTISONE; NEOMYCIN SULFATE; POLYMYXIN B SULFATE
SEE HYDROCORTISONE ACETATE; NEOMYCIN SULFATE
SEE HYDROCORTISONE ACETATE; NEOMYCIN SULFATE; POLYMYXIN B SULFATE
SEE METHYLPREDNISOLONE ACETATE; NEOMYCIN SULFATE

NEOMYCIN SULFATE; POLYMYXIN B SULFATE

OINTMENT; OPHTHALMIC

	STATROL		
	+ ALCON	EQ 3.5 MG BASE/GM;10,000 UNITS/GM	N50344 002

SOLUTION; IRRIGATION

	NEOMYCIN AND POLYMYXIN B SULFATES		
AT	STERIS	EQ 40 MG BASE/ML;200,000 UNITS/ML	N62664 001 APR 08, 1986
	NEOSPORIN G.U. IRRIGANT		
AT	BURROUGHS WELLCOME	EQ 40 MG BASE/ML;200,000 UNITS/ML	N60707 001

SOLUTION/DROPS; OPHTHALMIC

	STATROL		
	ALCON	EQ 3.5 MG BASE/ML;16,250 UNITS/ML	N50456 001
		EQ 3.5 MG BASE/ML;16,250 UNITS/ML	N62339 001 NOV 30, 1984

Prescription Drug Products *(continued)*

NEOMYCIN SULFATE; POLYMYXIN B SULFATE; PREDNISOLONE ACETATE

SUSPENSION/DROPS; OPHTHALMIC
POLY-PRED
+ ALLERGAN — EQ 0.35% BASE;10,000 UNITS/ML;0.5% — N50081 002

NETILMICIN SULFATE

INJECTABLE; INJECTION
NETROMYCIN
+ SCHERING — EQ 100 MG BASE/ML — N50544 003 FEB 28, 1983

NIACIN

TABLET; ORAL
NIACIN

AA	DANBURY PHARMA	500 MG	N83305 001
AA	GLOBAL PHARMS	500 MG	N83115 001
AA	HALSEY	500 MG	N83453 001
AA	MK LABS	500 MG	N83525 001
AA	PUREPAC PHARM	500 MG	N83271 001
AA	TABLICAPS	500 MG	N84237 001
AA	WOCKHARDT	500 MG	N81134 001 APR 28, 1992

NICOLAR

AA	RHONE POULENC RORER	500 MG	N83823 001

NIACINAMIDE; *MULTIPLE*

SEE ASCORBIC ACID; BIOTIN; CYANOCOBALAMIN; DEXPANTHENOL; ERGOCALCIFEROL; FOLIC ACID; NIACINAMIDE; PYRIDOXINE HYDROCHLORIDE; RIBOFLAVIN PHOSPHATE SODIUM; THIAMINE HYDROCHLORIDE; VITAMIN A; VITAMIN E

SEE ASCORBIC ACID; BIOTIN; CYANOCOBALAMIN; ERGOCALCIFEROL; FOLIC ACID; NIACINAMIDE; PANTOTHENIC ACID; PHYTONADIONE; PYRIDOXINE; RIBOFLAVIN; THIAMINE; VITAMIN A PALMITATE; VITAMIN E

NICARDIPINE HYDROCHLORIDE

CAPSULE; ORAL
CARDENE

	SYNTEX	20 MG	N19488 001 DEC 21, 1988
	+	30 MG	N19488 002 DEC 21, 1988

NICARDIPINE HYDROCHLORIDE *(continued)*

CAPSULE, EXTENDED RELEASE; ORAL
CARDENE SR

	+ SYNTEX	30 MG	N20005 001 FEB 21, 1992
	+	45 MG	N20005 002 FEB 21, 1992
	+	60 MG	N20005 003 FEB 21, 1992

INJECTABLE; INJECTION
CARDENE
SYNTEX — 2.5 MG/ML — N19734 001 JAN 30, 1992

NICLOSAMIDE

TABLET, CHEWABLE; ORAL
NICLOCIDE
+ MILES — 500 MG — N18669 001 MAY 14, 1982

NICOTINE

FILM, EXTENDED RELEASE; TRANSDERMAL
HABITROL

BC	+ BASEL PHARMS	7 MG/24 HR	N20076 001 NOV 27, 1991
BC	+	14 MG/24 HR	N20076 002 NOV 27, 1991
BC	+	21 MG/24 HR	N20076 003 NOV 27, 1991

NICODERM

BC	+ MARION MERRELL DOW	7 MG/24 HR	N20165 001 NOV 07, 1991
BC	+	14 MG/24 HR	N20165 002 NOV 07, 1991
BC	+	21 MG/24 HR	N20165 003 NOV 07, 1991

NICOTROL

	+ PHARMACIA	5 MG/16 HR	N20150 001 APR 22, 1992
	+	10 MG/16 HR	N20150 002 APR 22, 1992
	+	15 MG/16 HR	N20150 003 APR 22, 1992

PROSTEP

	+ ELAN PHARM	11 MG/24 HR	N19983 001 JAN 28, 1992
	+	22 MG/24 HR	N19983 002 JAN 28, 1992

Prescription Drug Products *(continued)*

NICOTINE POLACRILEX

GUM, CHEWING; BUCCAL

	NICORETTE		
	+ MERRELL DOW	EQ 2 MG BASE	N18612 001 JAN 13, 1984
	NICORETTE DS		
	+ MERRELL DOW	EQ 4 MG BASE	N20066 001 JUN 08, 1992

NIFEDIPINE

CAPSULE; ORAL

	ADALAT		
AB	MILES	10 MG	N19478 001 NOV 27, 1985
AB		20 MG	N19478 002 SEP 17, 1986
	NIFEDIPINE		
AB	CHASE LABS NJ	10 MG	N72409 001 JUL 04, 1990
AB		20 MG	N73421 001 JUN 19, 1991
AB	FLEMINGTON PHARM	10 MG	N72781 001 JUL 30, 1993
AB	NOVOPHARM	10 MG	N72651 001 FEB 19, 1992
AB	PUREPAC PHARM	10 MG	N72579 001 JAN 08, 1991
AB		20 MG	N72556 001 SEP 20, 1990
AB	SCHERER	10 MG	N73250 001 OCT 08, 1991
AB		20 MG	N74045 001 APR 30, 1992
	PROCARDIA		
AB	PFIZER	10 MG	N18482 001
AB	+	20 MG	N18482 002 JUL 24, 1986

TABLET, EXTENDED RELEASE; ORAL

	ADALAT CC		
BC	MILES	30 MG	N20198 001 APR 21, 1993
BC		60 MG	N20198 002 APR 21, 1993
BC		90 MG	N20198 003 APR 21, 1993
	PROCARDIA XL		
BC	+ PFIZER	30 MG	N19684 001 SEP 06, 1989
BC	+	60 MG	N19684 002 SEP 06, 1989
BC	+	90 MG	N19684 003 SEP 06, 1989

NIMODIPINE

CAPSULE; ORAL

	NIMOTOP		
	+ MILES	30 MG	N18869 001 DEC 28, 1988

NITROFURANTOIN

SUSPENSION; ORAL

	FURADANTIN		
	+ PROCTER AND GAMBLE	25 MG/5 ML	N09175 001

TABLET; ORAL

	FURADANTIN		
AB	PROCTER AND GAMBLE	50 MG	N08693 001
AB	+	100 MG	N08693 002
	NITROFURANTOIN		
AB	CIRCA	50 MG	N80447 001
AB	WHITEWORTH TOWNE	100 MG	N84085 002

NITROFURANTOIN; NITROFURANTOIN, MACROCRYSTALLINE

CAPSULE; ORAL

	MACROBID		
	+ PROCTER AND GAMBLE	75 MG;25 MG	N20064 001 DEC 24, 1991

NITROFURANTOIN, MACROCRYSTALLINE

CAPSULE; ORAL

	MACRODANTIN		
AB	PROCTER AND GAMBLE	25 MG	N16620 003
AB		50 MG	N16620 001
AB	+	100 MG	N16620 002
	NITROFURANTOIN		
AB	DANBURY PHARMA	25 MG	N73696 001 DEC 31, 1992
AB		50 MG	N73696 002 DEC 31, 1992
AB		100 MG	N73696 003 DEC 31, 1992
AB	ZENITH LABS	50 MG	N73671 001 JAN 28, 1993
AB		100 MG	N73652 001 JAN 28, 1993

NITROFURANTOIN, MACROCRYSTALLINE; *MULTIPLE*

SEE NITROFURANTOIN; NITROFURANTOIN, MACROCRYSTALLINE

Prescription Drug Products *(continued)*

NITROFURAZONE

	CREAM; TOPICAL		
	FURACIN		
	+ ROBERTS LABS	0.2%	N83789 001
	OINTMENT; TOPICAL		
	FURACIN		
AT	+ ROBERTS LABS	0.2%	N05795 001
	NITROFURAZONE		
AT	AMBIX	0.2%	N86077 001
AT	+ CLAY PARK	0.2%	N84968 001
AT	THAMES	0.2%	N86156 001
AT	WENDT	0.2%	N86766 001
	POWDER; TOPICAL		
	FURACIN		
	ROBERTS LABS	0.2%	N83791 001
	SOLUTION; TOPICAL		
	NITROFURAZONE		
AT	+ CLAY PARK	0.2%	N85130 001
AT	WENDT	0.2%	N87081 001

NITROGLYCERIN

	AEROSOL; ORAL		
	NITROLINGUAL		
	+ G POHL BOSKAMP	0.4 MG/SPRAY	N18705 001 OCT 31, 1985
	INJECTABLE; INJECTION		
	NITRO IV		
AP	G POHL BOSKAMP	5 MG/ML	N18672 002 AUG 30, 1983
	NITRO-BID		
AP	MARION MERRELL DOW	5 MG/ML	N18621 001 JAN 05, 1982
	NITROGLYCERIN		
AP	+ ABBOTT	5 MG/ML	N18531 001
AP	FUJISAWA	5 MG/ML	N70077 001 DEC 13, 1985
AP	LUITPOLD	5 MG/ML	N72034 001 MAY 24, 1988
AP	SMITH AND NEPHEW	5 MG/ML	N70633 001 JUN 19, 1986

NITROGLYCERIN *(continued)*

	INJECTABLE; INJECTION		
	NITROGLYCERIN IN DEXTROSE 5%		
AP	ABBOTT	10 MG/100 ML	N71846 001 AUG 31, 1990
AP		20 MG/100 ML	N71847 001 AUG 31, 1990
AP		40 MG/100 ML	N71848 001 AUG 31, 1990
AP	+ BAXTER	10 MG/100 ML	N19970 001 DEC 29, 1989
AP	+	20 MG/100 ML	N19970 002 DEC 29, 1989
AP	+	40 MG/100 ML	N19970 003 DEC 29, 1989
	NITROSTAT		
AP	PARKE DAVIS	5 MG/ML	N18588 002 DEC 23, 1983
	+	0.8 MG/ML	N18588 001
	TRIDIL		
AP	DUPONT MERCK	5 MG/ML	N18537 001
	+	0.5 MG/ML	N18537 002 JUN 16, 1983
	OINTMENT; TRANSDERMAL		
	NITROGLYCERIN		
	ALTANA	2%	N87355 001 JUL 08, 1988

NIZATIDINE

	CAPSULE; ORAL		
	AXID		
	LILLY	150 MG	N19508 001 APR 12, 1988
	+	300 MG	N19508 002 APR 12, 1988

NOREPINEPHRINE BITARTRATE

	INJECTABLE; INJECTION		
	LEVOPHED		
	+ STERLING WINTHROP	EQ 1 MG BASE/ML	N07513 001

NOREPINEPHRINE BITARTRATE; PROCAINE HYDROCHLORIDE; PROPOXYCAINE HYDROCHLORIDE

	INJECTABLE; INJECTION		
	RAVOCAINE AND NOVOCAIN W/ LEVOPHED		
	STERLING WINTHROP	EQ 0.033 MG BASE/ML;2%;0.4%	N08592 003

Prescription Drug Products *(continued)*

NORETHINDRONE

	TABLET; ORAL		
	NOR-Q.D.		
	SYNTEX	0.35 MG	N17060 001
	TABLET; ORAL-28		
	MICRONOR		
	+ JOHNSON RW	0.35 MG	N16954 001

NORETHINDRONE; *MULTIPLE*

SEE ETHINYL ESTRADIOL; NORETHINDRONE

SEE MESTRANOL; NORETHINDRONE

NORETHINDRONE ACETATE

	TABLET; ORAL		
	AYGESTIN		
AB	WYETH AYERST	5 MG	N18405 001 APR 21, 1982
	NORLUTATE		
AB	+ PARKE DAVIS	5 MG	N12184 002

NORETHINDRONE ACETATE; *MULTIPLE*

SEE ETHINYL ESTRADIOL; FERROUS FUMARATE; NORETHINDRONE ACETATE

SEE ETHINYL ESTRADIOL; NORETHINDRONE ACETATE

NORFLOXACIN

	SOLUTION/DROPS; OPHTHALMIC		
	CHIBROXIN		
	+ MERCK	0.3%	N19757 001 JUN 17, 1991
	TABLET; ORAL		
	NOROXIN		
	+ MERCK	400 MG	N19384 002 OCT 31, 1986

NORGESTIMATE; *MULTIPLE*

SEE ETHINYL ESTRADIOL; NORGESTIMATE

NORGESTREL

	TABLET; ORAL		
	OVRETTE		
	+ WYETH AYERST	0.075 MG	N17031 001

NORGESTREL; *MULTIPLE*

SEE ETHINYL ESTRADIOL; NORGESTREL

NORTRIPTYLINE HYDROCHLORIDE

	CAPSULE; ORAL		
	AVENTYL HCL		
BD	LILLY	EQ 10 MG BASE	N14684 001
BD		EQ 25 MG BASE	N14684 002
	NORTRIPTYLINE HCL		
AB	DANBURY PHARMA	EQ 10 MG BASE	N73553 001 MAR 30, 1992
AB		EQ 25 MG BASE	N73554 001 MAR 30, 1992
AB		EQ 50 MG BASE	N73555 001 MAR 30, 1992
AB		EQ 75 MG BASE	N73556 001 MAR 30, 1992
AB	GENEVA PHARMS	EQ 10 MG BASE	N74054 001 DEC 31, 1992
AB		EQ 25 MG BASE	N74054 002 DEC 31, 1992
AB		EQ 50 MG BASE	N74054 003 DEC 31, 1992
AB		EQ 75 MG BASE	N74054 004 DEC 31, 1992
AB	MYLAN	EQ 10 MG BASE	N74234 001 JUL 26, 1993
AB		EQ 25 MG BASE	N74234 002 JUL 26, 1993
AB		EQ 50 MG BASE	N74234 003 JUL 26, 1993
AB		EQ 75 MG BASE	N74234 004 JUL 26, 1993
	PAMELOR		
AB	SANDOZ	EQ 10 MG BASE	N18013 001
AB		EQ 25 MG BASE	N18013 002
AB		EQ 50 MG BASE	N18013 004
AB	+	EQ 75 MG BASE	N18013 003
	SOLUTION; ORAL		
	AVENTYL HCL		
AA	LILLY	EQ 10 MG BASE/5 ML	N14685 001
	PAMELOR		
AA	SANDOZ	EQ 10 MG BASE/5 ML	N18012 001

NOVOBIOCIN SODIUM

	CAPSULE; ORAL		
	ALBAMYCIN		
	+ UPJOHN	EQ 250 MG BASE	N50339 001

Prescription Drug Products *(continued)*

NYSTATIN

	CREAM; TOPICAL		
	MYCOSTATIN		
AT	+ SQUIBB	100,000 UNITS/GM	N60575 001
	MYKINAC		
AT	NMC	100,000 UNITS/GM	N62387 001 JUL 29, 1982
	NILSTAT		
AT	LEDERLE	100,000 UNITS/GM	N61445 001
	NYSTATIN		
AT	ALTANA	100,000 UNITS/GM	N62129 001
AT	BARRE	100,000 UNITS/GM	N62949 001 JUN 13, 1988
AT	CLAY PARK	100,000 UNITS/GM	N62225 001
AT	LEMMON	100,000 UNITS/GM	N61966 001
AT	TARO	100,000 UNITS/GM	N64022 001 JAN 29, 1993
AT	THAMES	100,000 UNITS/GM	N62457 001 JUL 28, 1983
	OINTMENT; TOPICAL		
	MYCOSTATIN		
AT	+ SQUIBB	100,000 UNITS/GM	N60571 001
	MYKINAC		
AT	NMC	100,000 UNITS/GM	N62731 001 SEP 22, 1986
	NILSTAT		
AT	LEDERLE	100,000 UNITS/GM	N61444 001
	NYSTATIN		
AT	ALTANA	100,000 UNITS/GM	N62124 002 SEP 23, 1982
AT	BARRE	100,000 UNITS/GM	N62840 001 NOV 13, 1987
AT	CLAY PARK	100,000 UNITS/GM	N62472 001 FEB 13, 1984
	PASTILLE; ORAL		
	MYCOSTATIN		
	+ SQUIBB	200,000 UNITS	N50619 001 APR 09, 1987
	POWDER; ORAL		
	NILSTAT		
AA	LEDERLE	100%	N50576 001 DEC 22, 1983
	NYSTATIN		
AA	PADDOCK	100%	N62613 001 NOV 26, 1985
	POWDER; TOPICAL		
	MYCOSTATIN		
	WESTWOOD SQUIBB	100,000 UNITS/GM	N60578 001

NYSTATIN *(continued)*

	SUSPENSION; ORAL		
	MYCOSTATIN		
AA	APOTHECON	100,000 UNITS/ML	N61533 001
	NILSTAT		
AA	LEDERLE	100,000 UNITS/ML	N50299 001
	NYSTATIN		
AA	BARRE	100,000 UNITS/ML	N62349 001 JUL 14, 1982
AA		100,000 UNITS/ML	N62571 001 OCT 29, 1985
AA	BAUSCH AND LOMB	100,000 UNITS/ML	N64042 001 FEB 28, 1994
AA	BIOCRAFT	100,000 UNITS/ML	N62670 001 JUN 18, 1987
AA	FOUGERA	100,000 UNITS/ML	N62517 001 JUN 07, 1984
AA	LEMMON	100,000 UNITS/ML	N62776 001 DEC 17, 1987
AA	PENNEX	100,000 UNITS/ML	N62512 001 OCT 29, 1984
AA	ROXANE	100,000 UNITS/ML	N62832 001 DEC 27, 1991
AA	THAMES	100,000 UNITS/ML	N62876 001 FEB 29, 1988
	NYSTEX		
AA	SAVAGE LABS	100,000 UNITS/ML	N62519 001 JUL 06, 1984
	TABLET; ORAL		
	MYCOSTATIN		
AA	SQUIBB	500,000 UNITS	N60574 001
	NILSTAT		
AA	LEDERLE	500,000 UNITS	N61151 001
	NYSTATIN		
AA	EON LABS	500,000 UNITS	N62065 001
AA	LEMMON	500,000 UNITS	N62506 001 JAN 16, 1984
AA	MUTUAL PHARM	500,000 UNITS	N62838 001 DEC 22, 1988
AA	PAR PHARM	500,000 UNITS	N62474 001 DEC 22, 1983
AA	ROSEMONT PHARM	500,000 UNITS	N62524 001 NOV 26, 1985

Prescription Drug Products *(continued)*

NYSTATIN *(continued)*

TABLET; VAGINAL

	KOROSTATIN		
AT	HOLLAND RANTOS	100,000 UNITS	N61718 001
	MYCOSTATIN		
AT	SQUIBB	100,000 UNITS	N60577 001
	NILSTAT		
AT	LEDERLE	100,000 UNITS	N61325 001
	NYSTATIN		
AT	FOUGERA	100,000 UNITS	N62459 001 NOV 09, 1983
AT	LEMMON	100,000 UNITS	N62502 001 DEC 23, 1983
AT	PHARMADERM	100,000 UNITS	N62460 001 NOV 09, 1983
AT	SIDMAK LABS NJ	100,000 UNITS	N62615 001 OCT 17, 1985

NYSTATIN; TRIAMCINOLONE ACETONIDE

CREAM; TOPICAL

	MYCO-TRIACET II		
AT	LEMMON	100,000 UNITS/GM;0.1%	N61954 002 SEP 20, 1985
	MYCOLOG-II		
AT	+ APOTHECON	100,000 UNITS/GM;0.1%	N60576 002 MAY 01, 1985
AT		100,000 UNITS/GM;0.1%	N62606 001 MAY 15, 1985
	MYKACET		
AT	NMC	100,000 UNITS/GM;0.1%	N62367 001 MAY 28, 1985
	MYTREX F		
AT	SAVAGE LABS	100,000 UNITS/GM;0.1%	N62597 001 OCT 08, 1985
	NYSTATIN AND TRIAMCINOLONE ACETONIDE		
AT	TARO	100,000 UNITS/GM;0.1%	N62364 001 DEC 22, 1987
AT	THAMES	100,000 UNITS/GM;0.1%	N62347 001 MAR 30, 1987
	NYSTATIN-TRIAMCINOLONE ACETONIDE		
AT	FOUGERA	100,000 UNITS/GM;0.1%	N62599 001 OCT 08, 1985

OINTMENT; TOPICAL

	MYCO-TRIACET II		
AT	LEMMON	100,000 UNITS/GM;0.1%	N62045 002 NOV 26, 1985
	MYCOLOG-II		
AT	+ WESTWOOD SQUIBB	100,000 UNITS/GM;0.1%	N60572 001 JUN 28, 1985

NYSTATIN; TRIAMCINOLONE ACETONIDE *(continued)*

OINTMENT; TOPICAL

	MYKACET		
AT	NMC	100,000 UNITS/GM;0.1%	N62733 001 MAR 09, 1987
	MYTREX F		
AT	SAVAGE LABS	100,000 UNITS/GM;0.1%	N62601 001 OCT 09, 1985
	NYSTATIN AND TRIAMCINOLONE ACETONIDE		
AT	CLAY PARK	100,000 UNITS/GM;0.1%	N62280 002 OCT 10, 1985
AT	PHARMAFAIR	100,000 UNITS/GM;0.1%	N62656 001 JUL 30, 1986
AT	TARO	100,000 UNITS/GM;0.1%	N63305 001 MAR 29, 1993
	NYSTATIN-TRIAMCINOLONE ACETONIDE		
AT	FOUGERA	100,000 UNITS/GM;0.1%	N62602 001 OCT 09, 1985

OCTREOTIDE ACETATE

INJECTABLE; INJECTION

	SANDOSTATIN		
	+ SANDOZ	EQ 0.05 MG BASE/ML	N19667 001 OCT 21, 1988
	+	EQ 0.1 MG BASE/ML	N19667 002 OCT 21, 1988
		EQ 0.2 MG BASE/ML	N19667 004 JUN 12, 1991
	+	EQ 0.5 MG BASE/ML	N19667 003 OCT 21, 1988
		EQ 1 MG BASE/ML	N19667 005 JUN 12, 1991

OFLOXACIN

INJECTABLE; INJECTION

	FLOXIN		
	JOHNSON RW	20 MG/ML	N20087 002 MAR 31, 1992
		40 MG/ML	N20087 003 MAR 31, 1992
	FLOXIN IN DEXTROSE 5%		
	JOHNSON RW	400 MG/100 ML	N20087 001 MAR 31, 1992
	FLOXIN IN DEXTROSE 5% IN PLASTIC CONTAINER		
	JOHNSON RW	4 MG/ML	N20087 004 MAR 31, 1992
		400 MG/100 ML	N20087 005 MAR 31, 1992

Prescription Drug Products *(continued)*

OFLOXACIN *(continued)*
SOLUTION/DROPS; OPHTHALMIC
OCUFLOX
+ ALLERGAN 0.3% N19921 001 JUL 30, 1993

TABLET; ORAL
FLOXIN
JOHNSON RW 200 MG N19735 001 DEC 28, 1990
300 MG N19735 002 DEC 28, 1990
+ 400 MG N19735 003 DEC 28, 1990

OLSALAZINE SODIUM
CAPSULE; ORAL
DIPENTUM
+ PHARMACIA 250 MG N19715 001 JUL 31, 1990

OMEPRAZOLE
CAPSULE, DELAYED REL PELLETS; ORAL
PRILOSEC
+ ASTRA MERCK 20 MG N19810 001 SEP 14, 1989

ONDANSETRON HYDROCHLORIDE
INJECTABLE; INJECTION
ZOFRAN
+ GLAXO EQ 2 MG BASE/ML N20007 001 JAN 04, 1991

TABLET; ORAL
ZOFRAN
GLAXO EQ 4 MG BASE N20103 001 DEC 31, 1992
+ EQ 8 MG BASE N20103 002 DEC 31, 1992

ORPHENADRINE CITRATE
INJECTABLE; INJECTION
NORFLEX
AP + 3M 30 MG/ML N13055 001
ORPHENADRINE CITRATE
AP STERIS 30 MG/ML N84779 001 MAR 15, 1982
AP 30 MG/ML N87062 001
TABLET, EXTENDED RELEASE; ORAL
NORFLEX
+ 3M 100 MG N12157 001

ORPHENADRINE CITRATE; *MULTIPLE*
SEE ASPIRIN; CAFFEINE; ORPHENADRINE CITRATE

OXACILLIN SODIUM
CAPSULE; ORAL
BACTOCILL
AB SMITHKLINE BEECHAM EQ 250 MG BASE N61336 001
AB EQ 250 MG BASE N62241 001
AB EQ 500 MG BASE N61336 002
AB EQ 500 MG BASE N62241 002
OXACILLIN SODIUM
AB BIOCRAFT EQ 250 MG BASE N62222 001
AB EQ 500 MG BASE N62222 002
PROSTAPHLIN
AB APOTHECON EQ 250 MG BASE N61450 002
AB + EQ 500 MG BASE N61450 001
INJECTABLE; INJECTION
BACTOCILL
AP + SMITHKLINE BEECHAM EQ 500 MG BASE/VIAL N61334 009 MAR 26, 1982
AP + EQ 1 GM BASE/VIAL N61334 006 MAR 26, 1982
AP + EQ 1 GM BASE/VIAL N62736 001 DEC 19, 1986
AP + EQ 2 GM BASE/VIAL N61334 007 MAR 26, 1982
AP + EQ 2 GM BASE/VIAL N62736 002 DEC 19, 1986
AP + EQ 4 GM BASE/VIAL N61334 008 MAR 26, 1982
AP + EQ 10 GM BASE/VIAL N61334 010
BACTOCILL IN PLASTIC CONTAINER
+ BAXTER EQ 20 MG BASE/ML N50640 001 OCT 26, 1989
+ EQ 40 MG BASE/ML N50640 002 OCT 26, 1989
OXACILLIN SODIUM
AP APOTHECON EQ 250 MG BASE/VIAL N61490 001
AP EQ 500 MG BASE/VIAL N61490 002
AP EQ 1 GM BASE/VIAL N61490 003
AP EQ 1 GM BASE/VIAL N62737 001 DEC 23, 1986
AP EQ 2 GM BASE/VIAL N62737 002 DEC 23, 1986
AP EQ 10 GM BASE/VIAL N61490 006 MAY 09, 1991

Prescription Drug Products *(continued)*

OXACILLIN SODIUM *(continued)*

INJECTABLE; INJECTION

	OXACILLIN SODIUM		
AP	MARSAM	EQ 250 MG BASE/VIAL	N62856 001 OCT 26, 1988
AP		EQ 500 MG BASE/VIAL	N62856 002 OCT 26, 1988
AP		EQ 1 GM BASE/VIAL	N62856 003 OCT 26, 1988
AP		EQ 2 GM BASE/VIAL	N62856 004 OCT 26, 1988
AP		EQ 4 GM BASE/VIAL	N62856 005 OCT 26, 1988
AP		EQ 10 GM BASE/VIAL	N62984 001 SEP 29, 1988

POWDER FOR RECONSTITUTION; ORAL

	BACTOCILL		
AA	SMITHKLINE BEECHAM	EQ 250 MG BASE/5 ML	N62321 001
	OXACILLIN SODIUM		
AA	BIOCRAFT	EQ 250 MG BASE/5 ML	N62252 001
	PROSTAPHLIN		
AA	APOTHECON	EQ 250 MG BASE/5 ML	N61457 001

OXAMNIQUINE

CAPSULE; ORAL

	VANSIL		
	+ PFIZER	250 MG	N18069 001

OXANDROLONE

TABLET; ORAL

	OXANDRIN		
	+ BIO TECH GEN	2.5 MG	N13718 001

OXAPROZIN

TABLET; ORAL

	DAYPRO		
	+ SEARLE	600 MG	N18841 004 OCT 29, 1992

OXAZEPAM

CAPSULE; ORAL

	OXAZEPAM		
AB	BARR	10 MG	N70957 001 AUG 10, 1987
AB		15 MG	N71025 001 AUG 10, 1987
AB		30 MG	N71026 001 AUG 10, 1987

OXAZEPAM *(continued)*

CAPSULE; ORAL

	OXAZEPAM		
AB	DANBURY PHARMA	10 MG	N72952 001 SEP 28, 1990
AB		15 MG	N72953 001 SEP 28, 1990
AB		30 MG	N72954 001 SEP 28, 1990
AB	GENEVA PHARMS	10 MG	N71813 001 APR 19, 1988
AB		15 MG	N71756 001 APR 19, 1988
AB		30 MG	N71814 001 APR 19, 1988
AB	PUREPAC PHARM	10 MG	N72251 001 APR 14, 1988
AB		15 MG	N72252 001 APR 14, 1988
AB		30 MG	N72253 001 APR 14, 1988
AB	ZENITH LABS	10 MG	N70943 001 AUG 03, 1987
AB		15 MG	N70944 001 AUG 03, 1987
AB		30 MG	N70945 001 AUG 03, 1987
	SERAX		
AB	WYETH AYERST	10 MG	N15539 002
AB		15 MG	N15539 004
AB	+	30 MG	N15539 006

TABLET; ORAL

	OXAZEPAM		
AB	BARR	15 MG	N70683 001 JAN 16, 1987
AB	DANBURY PHARMA	15 MG	N71494 001 APR 21, 1987
AB	PARKE DAVIS	15 MG	N71508 001 FEB 02, 1987
	SERAX		
AB	+ WYETH AYERST	15 MG	N15539 008

OXICONAZOLE NITRATE

CREAM; TOPICAL

	OXISTAT		
	+ GLAXO	EQ 1% BASE	N19828 001 DEC 30, 1988

LOTION; TOPICAL

	OXISTAT		
	+ GLAXO	EQ 1% BASE	N20209 001 SEP 30, 1992

Prescription Drug Products *(continued)*

OXTRIPHYLLINE

SOLUTION; ORAL
CHOLEDYL
PARKE DAVIS — 100 MG/5 ML — N09268 012 — NOV 27, 1984

SYRUP; ORAL
CHOLEDYL
PARKE DAVIS — 50 MG/5 ML — N09268 011

TABLET, DELAYED RELEASE; ORAL
CHOLEDYL
+ PARKE DAVIS — 100 MG — N09268 003
+ — 200 MG — N09268 007

TABLET, EXTENDED RELEASE; ORAL
CHOLEDYL SA
+ PARKE DAVIS — 400 MG — N87863 001 — MAY 24, 1983
+ — 600 MG — N86742 001

OXYBUTYNIN CHLORIDE

SYRUP; ORAL
DITROPAN
MARION MERRELL DOW — 5 MG/5 ML — N18211 001

TABLET; ORAL
DITROPAN
AB + MARION MERRELL DOW — 5 MG — N17577 001
OXYBUTYNIN CHLORIDE
AB SIDMAK LABS NJ — 5 MG — N71655 001 — NOV 14, 1988

OXYCODONE HYDROCHLORIDE; *MULTIPLE*

SEE ACETAMINOPHEN; OXYCODONE HYDROCHLORIDE
SEE ASPIRIN; OXYCODONE HYDROCHLORIDE; OXYCODONE TEREPHTHALATE

OXYCODONE TEREPHTHALATE; *MULTIPLE*

SEE ASPIRIN; OXYCODONE HYDROCHLORIDE; OXYCODONE TEREPHTHALATE

OXYMETHOLONE

TABLET; ORAL
ANADROL-50
+ SYNTEX — 50 MG — N16848 001

OXYMORPHONE HYDROCHLORIDE

INJECTABLE; INJECTION
NUMORPHAN
+ DUPONT MERCK — 1 MG/ML — N11707 002
+ — 1.5 MG/ML — N11707 001

SUPPOSITORY; RECTAL
NUMORPHAN
+ DUPONT MERCK — 5 MG — N11738 004

OXYPHENCYCLIMINE HYDROCHLORIDE

TABLET; ORAL
DARICON
PFIZER — 10 MG — N11612 001

OXYTETRACYCLINE

TABLET; ORAL
TERRAMYCIN
+ PFIZER — 250 MG — N50287 001

OXYTETRACYCLINE; *MULTIPLE*

SEE LIDOCAINE HYDROCHLORIDE; OXYTETRACYCLINE

OXYTETRACYCLINE CALCIUM

SYRUP; ORAL
TERRAMYCIN
+ PFIZER — EQ 125 MG BASE/5 ML — N60595 001

OXYTETRACYCLINE HYDROCHLORIDE

CAPSULE; ORAL
OXY-KESSO-TETRA
AB MK LABS — EQ 250 MG BASE — N60179 001
OXYTETRACYCLINE HCL
AB GLOBAL PHARMS — EQ 250 MG BASE — N60760 001
AB PROTER — EQ 250 MG BASE — N60869 001
AB WEST WARD PHARM — EQ 250 MG BASE — N60770 001
TERRAMYCIN
AB + PFIZER — EQ 250 MG BASE — N50286 002

INJECTABLE; INJECTION
TERRAMYCIN
+ PFIZER — EQ 250 MG BASE/VIAL — N60586 001
+ — EQ 500 MG BASE/VIAL — N60586 002

OXYTETRACYCLINE HYDROCHLORIDE; *MULTIPLE*

SEE HYDROCORTISONE ACETATE; OXYTETRACYCLINE HYDROCHLORIDE

Prescription Drug Products *(continued)*

OXYTETRACYCLINE HYDROCHLORIDE; POLYMYXIN B SULFATE

OINTMENT; OPHTHALMIC
TERRAMYCIN W/ POLYMYXIN B SULFATE

	+ PFIZER	EQ 5 MG BASE/GM;10,000 UNITS/GM	N61015 001

OINTMENT; OTIC
TERRAMYCIN W/ POLYMYXIN

	+ PFIZER	EQ 5 MG BASE/GM;10,000 UNITS/GM	N61841 001

TABLET; VAGINAL
TERRAMYCIN-POLYMYXIN

	PFIZER	EQ 100 MG BASE;100,000 UNITS	N61009 001

OXYTOCIN

INJECTABLE; INJECTION

	OXYTOCIN		
AP	FUJISAWA	10USP UNITS/ML	N18248 001
AP	WYETH AYERST	10USP UNITS/ML	N18243 001
	PITOCIN		
AP	+ PARKE DAVIS	10USP UNITS/ML	N18261 001
	SYNTOCINON		
AP	SANDOZ	10USP UNITS/ML	N18245 001

SOLUTION; NASAL
SYNTOCINON

	+ SANDOZ	40USP UNITS/ML	N12285 001

PACLITAXEL

INJECTABLE; INJECTION
TAXOL

	BRISTOL MYERS SQUIBB	6 MG/ML	N20262 001 DEC 29, 1992

PAMIDRONATE DISODIUM

INJECTABLE; INJECTION
AREDIA

	+ CIBA GEIGY	30 MG/VIAL	N20036 001 OCT 31, 1991
	+	60 MG/VIAL	N20036 003 MAY 06, 1993
	+	90 MG/VIAL	N20036 004 MAY 06, 1993

PANCURONIUM BROMIDE

INJECTABLE; INJECTION

	PANCURONIUM		
AP	ELKINS SINN	1 MG/ML	N72058 001 MAR 23, 1988
AP		2 MG/ML	N72059 001 MAR 23, 1988
AP		2 MG/ML	N72060 001 MAR 23, 1988
	PANCURONIUM BROMIDE		
AP	ABBOTT	1 MG/ML	N72320 001 JAN 19, 1989
AP		2 MG/ML	N72321 001 JAN 19, 1989
AP	ASTRA	1 MG/ML	N72210 001 MAR 31, 1988
AP		2 MG/ML	N72211 001 MAR 31, 1988
AP		2 MG/ML	N72213 001 MAR 31, 1988
AP	GENSIA	1 MG/ML	N72759 001 JUL 31, 1990
AP		2 MG/ML	N72760 001 JUL 31, 1990
	PAVULON		
AP	+ ORGANON	1 MG/ML	N17015 002
AP	+	2 MG/ML	N17015 001

PANTOTHENIC ACID; *MULTIPLE*

SEE ASCORBIC ACID; BIOTIN; CYANOCOBALAMIN; ERGOCALCIFEROL; FOLIC ACID; NIACINAMIDE; PANTOTHENIC ACID; PHYTONADIONE; PYRIDOXINE; RIBOFLAVIN; THIAMINE; VITAMIN A PALMITATE; VITAMIN E

PARAMETHADIONE

CAPSULE; ORAL
PARADIONE

	ABBOTT	150 MG	N06800 003
		300 MG	N06800 001

PAROMOMYCIN SULFATE

CAPSULE; ORAL
HUMATIN

	+ PARKE DAVIS	EQ 250 MG BASE	N60521 001
		EQ 250 MG BASE	N62310 001

Prescription Drug Products *(continued)*

PAROXETINE HYDROCHLORIDE

	TABLET; ORAL		
	PAXIL		
	SMITHKLINE BEECHAM	EQ 20 MG BASE	N20031 002 DEC 29, 1992
	+	EQ 30 MG BASE	N20031 003 DEC 29, 1992

PEGADEMASE BOVINE

	INJECTABLE; INJECTION		
	ADAGEN		
	+ ENZON	250 UNITS/ML	N19818 001 MAR 21, 1990

PEMOLINE

	TABLET; ORAL		
	CYLERT		
	ABBOTT	18.75 MG	N16832 001
		37.5 MG	N16832 002
	+	75 MG	N16832 003
	TABLET, CHEWABLE; ORAL		
	CYLERT		
	+ ABBOTT	37.5 MG	N17703 001

PENBUTOLOL SULFATE

	TABLET; ORAL		
	LEVATOL		
	+ REED AND CARNRICK	20 MG	N18976 004 JAN 05, 1989

PENICILLAMINE

	CAPSULE; ORAL		
	CUPRIMINE		
	MERCK SHARP DOHME	125 MG	N19853 002
	+	250 MG	N19853 001
	TABLET; ORAL		
	DEPEN 250		
	+ WALLACE	250 MG	N19854 001

PENICILLIN G BENZATHINE

	INJECTABLE; INJECTION		
	BICILLIN L-A		
BC	+ WYETH AYERST	600,000 UNITS/ML	N50141 001
	+	300,000 UNITS/ML	N50141 003
	PERMAPEN		
BC	PFIZER	600,000 UNITS/ML	N60014 001

PENICILLIN G BENZATHINE; PENICILLIN G PROCAINE

	INJECTABLE; INJECTION		
	BICILLIN C-R		
	+ WYETH AYERST	150,000 UNITS/ML;150,000 UNITS/ML	N50138 002
	+	300,000 UNITS/ML;300,000 UNITS/ML	N50138 001
	BICILLIN C-R 900/300		
	+ WYETH AYERST	900,000 UNITS/2 ML;300,000 UNITS/2 ML	N50138 003

PENICILLIN G POTASSIUM

	INJECTABLE; INJECTION		
	PENICILLIN G POTASSIUM		
AP	+ LILLY	1,000,000 UNITS/VIAL	N60384 002
AP	+	5,000,000 UNITS/VIAL	N60384 001
AP	+	20,000,000 UNITS/VIAL	N60384 005
AP		20,000,000 UNITS/VIAL	N60601 001
	+	200,000 UNITS/VIAL	N60384 004
	+	500,000 UNITS/VIAL	N60384 003
AP	MARSAM	1,000,000 UNITS/VIAL	N62991 001 SEP 13, 1988
AP		5,000,000 UNITS/VIAL	N62991 002 SEP 13, 1988
AP		20,000,000 UNITS/VIAL	N62991 004 SEP 13, 1988
		10,000,000 UNITS/VIAL	N62991 003 SEP 13, 1988
AP	PFIZER	20,000,000 UNITS/VIAL	N60074 003
	PENICILLIN G POTASSIUM IN PLASTIC CONTAINER		
	+ BAXTER	20,000 UNITS/ML	N50638 001 JUN 25, 1990
	+	40,000 UNITS/ML	N50638 002 JUN 25, 1990
	+	60,000 UNITS/ML	N50638 003 JUN 25, 1990
	PFIZERPEN		
AP	PFIZER	1,000,000 UNITS/VIAL	N60657 001
AP		5,000,000 UNITS/VIAL	N60657 002
AP		20,000,000 UNITS/VIAL	N60657 003
	POWDER FOR RECONSTITUTION; ORAL		
	PENICILLIN		
AA	BIOCRAFT	400,000 UNITS/5 ML	N60307 004
		200,000 UNITS/5 ML	N60307 002
	PENICILLIN-2		
	BIOCRAFT	250,000 UNITS/5 ML	N60307 003
	PFIZERPEN G		
AA	PFIZER	400,000 UNITS/5 ML	N60587 001

Prescription Drug Products *(continued)*

PENICILLIN G POTASSIUM *(continued)*

TABLET; ORAL

	PENICILLIN G POTASSIUM		
AB	BIOCRAFT	200,000 UNITS	N60306 001
AB		250,000 UNITS	N60306 002
AB		400,000 UNITS	N60306 003
AB		500,000 UNITS	N60306 004
AB	DISTA	250,000 UNITS	N60403 001
AB	MYLAN	200,000 UNITS	N60781 001
AB		250,000 UNITS	N60781 002
AB		400,000 UNITS	N60781 003
AB		500,000 UNITS	N60781 005
AB		800,000 UNITS	N60781 004
AB	WYETH AYERST	200,000 UNITS	N60413 001
AB		250,000 UNITS	N60413 002
AB		400,000 UNITS	N60413 003
AB	ZENITH LABS	400,000 UNITS	N60073 004
	PFIZERPEN G		
AB	PFIZER	200,000 UNITS	N60075 003
AB		250,000 UNITS	N60075 004
AB		400,000 UNITS	N60075 005
AB	+	800,000 UNITS	N60075 006
		50,000 UNITS	N60075 001
		100,000 UNITS	N60075 002

PENICILLIN G PROCAINE

INJECTABLE; INJECTION

	PENICILLIN G PROCAINE		
	PFIZER	300,000 UNITS/VIAL	N60099 001
	+	1,500,000 UNITS/VIAL	N60099 002
	PFIZERPEN-AS		
AP	+ PFIZER	300,000 UNITS/ML	N60286 001
AP	+	600,000 UNITS/ML	N60286 002
	WYCILLIN		
AP	WYETH AYERST	300,000 UNITS/ML	N60101 002
AP		600,000 UNITS/ML	N60101 001

PENICILLIN G PROCAINE; *MULTIPLE*

SEE PENICILLIN G BENZATHINE; PENICILLIN G PROCAINE

PENICILLIN G SODIUM

INJECTABLE; INJECTION

	PENICILLIN G SODIUM		
	+ MARSAM	5,000,000 UNITS/VIAL	N63014 001 SEP 13, 1988
	+ UPJOHN	1,000,000 UNITS/VIAL	N61046 001

PENICILLIN V POTASSIUM

POWDER FOR RECONSTITUTION; ORAL

	BEEPEN-VK		
AA	SMITHKLINE BEECHAM	EQ 125 MG BASE/5 ML	N62270 001
AA		EQ 250 MG BASE/5 ML	N62270 002
	LEDERCILLIN VK		
AA	LEDERLE	EQ 125 MG BASE/5 ML	N60136 001
AA		EQ 250 MG BASE/5 ML	N60136 002
	PEN-VEE K		
AA	WYETH AYERST	EQ 125 MG BASE/5 ML	N60007 001
AA		EQ 250 MG BASE/5 ML	N60007 002
	PENICILLIN V POTASSIUM		
AA	CLONMEL	EQ 125 MG BASE/5 ML	N62981 001 FEB 10, 1989
AA		EQ 250 MG BASE/5 ML	N62981 002 FEB 10, 1989
AA	COPANOS	EQ 125 MG BASE/5 ML	N61529 001
AA		EQ 250 MG BASE/5 ML	N61529 002
AA	MYLAN	EQ 125 MG BASE/5 ML	N61624 002
AA		EQ 250 MG BASE/5 ML	N61624 001
	PENICILLIN-VK		
AA	BIOCRAFT	EQ 125 MG BASE/5 ML	N60456 001
AA		EQ 250 MG BASE/5 ML	N60456 002
	PFIZERPEN VK		
AA	PFIZER	EQ 125 MG BASE/5 ML	N61815 001
AA		EQ 250 MG BASE/5 ML	N61815 002
	V-CILLIN K		
AA	LILLY	EQ 125 MG BASE/5 ML	N60004 001
AA		EQ 250 MG BASE/5 ML	N60004 002

TABLET; ORAL

	BEEPEN-VK		
AB	SMITHKLINE BEECHAM	EQ 250 MG BASE	N62273 001
AB		EQ 500 MG BASE	N62273 002
	BETAPEN-VK		
AB	APOTHECON	EQ 250 MG BASE	N61411 001
AB		EQ 500 MG BASE	N61411 002
AB	BRISTOL	EQ 250 MG BASE	N61150 001
AB		EQ 500 MG BASE	N61150 002
	LEDERCILLIN VK		
AB	LEDERLE	EQ 250 MG BASE	N60134 001
AB		EQ 500 MG BASE	N60134 002
	PEN-VEE K		
AB	WYETH AYERST	EQ 250 MG BASE	N60006 002
AB		EQ 500 MG BASE	N60006 003

Prescription Drug Products *(continued)*

PENICILLIN V POTASSIUM *(continued)*

	TABLET; ORAL		
	PENICILLIN V POTASSIUM		
AB	CLONMEL	EQ 250 MG BASE	N62936 001 NOV 25, 1988
AB		EQ 500 MG BASE	N62935 001 NOV 23, 1988
AB	COPANOS	EQ 250 MG BASE	N61528 001
AB		EQ 500 MG BASE	N61528 002
AB	MYLAN	EQ 250 MG BASE	N61530 001
AB		EQ 500 MG BASE	N61530 002
AB	ZENITH LABS	EQ 125 MG BASE	N60518 001
AB		EQ 250 MG BASE	N60518 002
AB		EQ 500 MG BASE	N60518 003
	PENICILLIN-VK		
AB	BIOCRAFT	EQ 250 MG BASE	N60711 002
AB		EQ 500 MG BASE	N60711 003
	PFIZERPEN VK		
AB	PFIZER	EQ 250 MG BASE	N61836 001
AB		EQ 500 MG BASE	N61836 002
	UTICILLIN VK		
AB	UPJOHN	EQ 250 MG BASE	N61651 001
	V-CILLIN K		
AB	+ LILLY	EQ 125 MG BASE	N60003 001
AB	+	EQ 250 MG BASE	N60003 002
AB	+	EQ 500 MG BASE	N60003 003

PENTAGASTRIN

	INJECTABLE; INJECTION		
	PEPTAVLON		
	+ WYETH AYERST	0.25 MG/ML	N17048 001

PENTAMIDINE ISETHIONATE

	INJECTABLE; IM-IV		
	PENTAM 300		
	+ FUJISAWA	300 MG/VIAL	N19264 001 OCT 16, 1984
	INJECTABLE; INJECTION		
	PENTACARINAT		
AP	RHONE POULENC RORER	300 MG/VIAL	N73447 001 APR 28, 1994
	PENTAMIDINE ISETHIONATE		
AP	ABBOTT	300 MG/VIAL	N73479 001 JUN 30, 1992
	POWDER FOR RECONSTITUTION; INHALATION		
	NEBUPENT		
	FUJISAWA	300 MG/VIAL	N19887 001 JUN 15, 1989

PENTAZOCINE HYDROCHLORIDE; *MULTIPLE*

SEE ACETAMINOPHEN; PENTAZOCINE HYDROCHLORIDE
SEE ASPIRIN; PENTAZOCINE HYDROCHLORIDE
SEE NALOXONE HYDROCHLORIDE; PENTAZOCINE HYDROCHLORIDE

PENTAZOCINE LACTATE

	INJECTABLE; INJECTION		
	TALWIN		
	+ STERLING WINTHROP	EQ 30 MG BASE/ML	N16194 001

PENTOBARBITAL

	ELIXIR; ORAL		
	NEMBUTAL		
	ABBOTT	18.2 MG/5 ML	N83244 001

PENTOBARBITAL SODIUM

	CAPSULE; ORAL		
	NEMBUTAL SODIUM		
AA	ABBOTT	50 MG	N84093 001
AA		100 MG	N83245 001
		30 MG	N84095 001
	SODIUM PENTOBARBITAL		
AA	HALSEY	100 MG	N84677 001
AA	ICN	100 MG	N83264 001
AA	ZENITH LABS	50 MG	N83461 001
AA		100 MG	N83461 002
	INJECTABLE; INJECTION		
	NEMBUTAL SODIUM		
AP	+ ABBOTT	50 MG/ML	N83246 001
	SODIUM PENTOBARBITAL		
AP	WYETH AYERST	50 MG/ML	N83261 001
	SUPPOSITORY; RECTAL		
	NEMBUTAL		
	+ ABBOTT	30 MG	N83247 001 JAN 25, 1982
	+	60 MG	N83247 002 JAN 25, 1982
	+	120 MG	N83247 003 JAN 25, 1982
	+	200 MG	N83247 004 JAN 25, 1982

PENTOSTATIN

	INJECTABLE; INJECTION		
	NIPENT		
	+ PARKE DAVIS	10 MG/VIAL	N20122 001 OCT 11, 1991

Prescription Drug Products *(continued)*

PENTOXIFYLLINE

TABLET, EXTENDED RELEASE; ORAL
TRENTAL
+ HOECHST ROUSSEL 400 MG N18631 001 AUG 30, 1984

PERFLUBRON

LIQUID; ORAL
IMAGENT
+ ALLIANCE PHARM 100% N20091 001 AUG 13, 1993

PERGOLIDE MESYLATE

TABLET; ORAL
PERMAX
LILLY EQ 0.05 MG BASE N19385 001 DEC 30, 1988
EQ 0.25 MG BASE N19385 002 DEC 30, 1988
+ EQ 1 MG BASE N19385 003 DEC 30, 1988

PERINDOPRIL ERBUMINE

TABLET; ORAL
ACEON
JOHNSON RW 2 MG N20184 001 DEC 30, 1993
4 MG N20184 002 DEC 30, 1993
+ 8 MG N20184 003 DEC 30, 1993

PERMETHRIN

CREAM; TOPICAL
ELIMITE
+ BURROUGHS WELLCOME 5% N19855 001 AUG 25, 1989

PERPHENAZINE

CONCENTRATE; ORAL
TRILAFON
SCHERING 16 MG/5 ML N11557 001

INJECTABLE; INJECTION
TRILAFON
+ SCHERING 5 MG/ML N11213 002

PERPHENAZINE *(continued)*

TABLET; ORAL
PERPHENAZINE
AB GENEVA PHARMS 2 MG N89683 001 DEC 08, 1988
AB 4 MG N89684 001 DEC 08, 1988
AB 8 MG N89685 001 DEC 08, 1988
AB 16 MG N89686 001 DEC 08, 1988
AB ZENITH LABS 2 MG N89707 001 SEP 10, 1987
AB 4 MG N89708 001 SEP 10, 1987
AB 8 MG N89456 001 SEP 10, 1987
AB 16 MG N89457 001 SEP 10, 1987
TRILAFON
AB SCHERING 2 MG N10775 001
AB 4 MG N10775 002
AB 8 MG N10775 003
AB + 16 MG N10775 004

PERPHENAZINE; *MULTIPLE*

SEE AMITRIPTYLINE HYDROCHLORIDE; PERPHENAZINE

PHENACEMIDE

TABLET; ORAL
PHENURONE
+ ABBOTT 500 MG N07707 001

PHENAZOPYRIDINE HYDROCHLORIDE; SULFAMETHOXAZOLE

TABLET; ORAL
AZO GANTANOL
+ ROCHE 100 MG;500 MG N13294 001 SEP 10, 1987

PHENAZOPYRIDINE HYDROCHLORIDE; SULFISOXAZOLE

TABLET; ORAL
AZO GANTRISIN
+ ROCHE 50 MG;500 MG N19358 001 AUG 31, 1990

PHENDIMETRAZINE TARTRATE

CAPSULE; ORAL

	PHENAZINE		
AA	MM MAST	35 MG	N86523 001
AA		35 MG	N86524 001
AA		35 MG	N86525 001
	PHENDIMETRAZINE TARTRATE		
AA	EON LABS	35 MG	N85633 001
AA		35 MG	N85694 001
AA		35 MG	N85695 001
AA		35 MG	N85702 001
	X-TROZINE		
AA	REXAR	35 MG	N87394 001 SEP 22, 1982

CAPSULE, EXTENDED RELEASE; ORAL

	PHENDIMETRAZINE TARTRATE		
BC	EON LABS	105 MG	N18074 001
BC	+ GENEVA PHARMS	105 MG	N87378 001
BC	GRAHAM	105 MG	N87214 001 MAY 26, 1982
BC		105 MG	N88020 001 AUG 16, 1982
BC		105 MG	N88021 001 SEP 21, 1982
BC		105 MG	N88028 001 AUG 16, 1982
BC		105 MG	N88062 001 SEP 13, 1982
BC		105 MG	N88063 001 SEP 10, 1982
BC		105 MG	N88111 001 OCT 18, 1982
	X-TROZINE L.A.		
BC	REXAR	105 MG	N87371 001 AUG 24, 1982

TABLET; ORAL

	BONTRIL PDM		
AA	CARNRICK	35 MG	N85272 001
	CAM-METRAZINE		
AA	CAMALL	35 MG	N83922 001
AA		35 MG	N85318 001
AA		35 MG	N85320 001
AA		35 MG	N85321 001
AA		35 MG	N85511 001
AA		35 MG	N85756 001
	PHENAZINE		
AA	MM MAST	35 MG	N87305 001
	PHENAZINE-35		
AA	CAMALL	35 MG	N85512 001

PHENDIMETRAZINE TARTRATE *(continued)*

TABLET; ORAL

	PHENDIMETRAZINE TARTRATE		
AA	CAMALL	35 MG	N85761 001
AA		35 MG	N85941 001 JUN 27, 1983
AA	EON LABS	35 MG	N85402 001
AA		35 MG	N85497 001
AA		35 MG	N85588 001
AA		35 MG	N85830 001
AA	INWOOD LABS	35 MG	N84740 001
AA		35 MG	N84741 001
AA		35 MG	N84742 001
AA		35 MG	N84743 001
AA	KV PHARM	35 MG	N84138 001
AA		35 MG	N84141 001
AA		35 MG	N85525 001
AA	MFG CHEMISTS	35 MG	N85914 001
AA	MIKART	35 MG	N89452 001 OCT 30, 1991
AA	PRIVATE FORM	35 MG	N85697 001
AA	ROSEMONT PHARM	35 MG	N84399 001
	PLEGINE		
AA	WYETH AYERST	35 MG	N12248 001
	STATOBEX		
AA	LEMMON	35 MG	N86013 001
	X-TROZINE		
AA	REXAR	35 MG	N86550 001
AA		35 MG	N86551 001
AA		35 MG	N86552 001
AA		35 MG	N86553 001
AA		35 MG	N86554 001

PHENELZINE SULFATE

TABLET; ORAL

	NARDIL		
	+ PARKE DAVIS	EQ 15 MG BASE	N11909 002

PHENOXYBENZAMINE HYDROCHLORIDE

CAPSULE; ORAL

	DIBENZYLINE		
	+ SMITHKLINE BEECHAM	10 MG	N08708 001

PHENSUXIMIDE

CAPSULE; ORAL

	MILONTIN		
	+ PARKE DAVIS	500 MG	N08855 004

Prescription Drug Products *(continued)*

PHENTERMINE HYDROCHLORIDE

CAPSULE; ORAL

	ADIPEX-P		
AA	LEMMON	37.5 MG	N88023 001 AUG 02, 1983
	DAPEX-37.5		
AA	FERNDALE LABS	37.5 MG	N88414 001 OCT 19, 1983
	FASTIN		
AA	SMITHKLINE BEECHAM	30 MG	N17352 001
	OBY-TRIM		
AA	REXAR	30 MG	N87764 001 MAR 18, 1982
	ONA-MAST		
AA	MM MAST	30 MG	N86511 001
AA		30 MG	N86516 001
	PHENTERMINE HCL		
AA	CAMALL	15 MG	N86735 001
AA		30 MG	N85411 001
AA		30 MG	N85417 001
AA		30 MG	N86732 002
AA		30 MG	N87215 001
AA		30 MG	N87226 001
AA		37.5 MG	N87915 001 DEC 22, 1983
AA		37.5 MG	N87918 001 DEC 22, 1983
AA		37.5 MG	N87930 001 OCT 14, 1983
AA		37.5 MG	N88610 001 JUN 04, 1984
AA		37.5 MG	N88611 001 JUN 04, 1984
AA		37.5 MG	N88625 001 AUG 23, 1984
		18.75 MG	N88576 001 MAY 23, 1984
AA	EON LABS	15 MG	N87301 001
AA		30 MG	N86945 001 JUL 20, 1983
AA		30 MG	N87190 001
AA		30 MG	N87208 001
AA		30 MG	N87223 001
AA	LEMMON	30 MG	N87777 001 NOV 01, 1985
AA		30 MG	N88612 001 APR 04, 1984
AA		30 MG	N88613 001 APR 09, 1984
AA		30 MG	N88614 001 APR 09, 1984

PHENTERMINE HYDROCHLORIDE *(continued)*

CAPSULE; ORAL

	PHENTERMINE HCL		
AA	ROSEMONT PHARM	30 MG	N84487 001 APR 09, 1982
AA		30 MG	N88797 001 DEC 10, 1984

TABLET; ORAL

	ADIPEX-P		
AA	LEMMON	37.5 MG	N85128 001
	ONA MAST		
AA	MM MAST	8 MG	N86260 001
	PHENTERMINE HCL		
AA	CAMALL	8 MG	N83923 001
AA		8 MG	N85319 001
AA		37.5 MG	N87805 001 DEC 06, 1982
AA		37.5 MG	N88596 001 APR 04, 1984
AA	ROSEMONT PHARM	8 MG	N83804 001
AA		37.5 MG	N88910 001 JUL 17, 1985
AA		37.5 MG	N88917 001 JUL 17, 1985
	UMI-PEX 30		
	FERNDALE LABS	30 MG	N88605 001 SEP 28, 1987

PHENTERMINE RESIN COMPLEX

CAPSULE, EXTENDED RELEASE; ORAL

	IONAMIN-15		
	FISONS	EQ 15 MG BASE	N11613 004
	IONAMIN-30		
	+ FISONS	EQ 30 MG BASE	N11613 002

PHENTOLAMINE MESYLATE

INJECTABLE; INJECTION

	REGITINE		
	+ CIBA	5 MG/VIAL	N08278 003

PHENYLBUTAZONE

CAPSULE; ORAL

	PHENYLBUTAZONE		
	+ BARR	100 MG	N88994 001 DEC 04, 1985

TABLET; ORAL

	PHENYLBUTAZONE		
	+ BARR	100 MG	N88863 001 DEC 04, 1985

Prescription Drug Products *(continued)*

PHENYLEPHRINE BITARTRATE; *MULTIPLE*
SEE ISOPROTERENOL HYDROCHLORIDE; PHENYLEPHRINE BITARTRATE

PHENYLEPHRINE HYDROCHLORIDE; *MULTIPLE*
SEE CODEINE PHOSPHATE; PHENYLEPHRINE HYDROCHLORIDE; PROMETHAZINE HYDROCHLORIDE
SEE CYCLOPENTOLATE HYDROCHLORIDE; PHENYLEPHRINE HYDROCHLORIDE

PHENYLEPHRINE HYDROCHLORIDE; PROMETHAZINE HYDROCHLORIDE
SYRUP; ORAL
PHENERGAN VC
AA WYETH AYERST 5 MG/5 ML;6.25 MG/5 ML N08604 003 APR 02, 1984
PHERAZINE VC
AA HALSEY 5 MG/5 ML;6.25 MG/5 ML N88868 001 MAR 02, 1987
PROMETH VC PLAIN
AA BARRE 5 MG/5 ML;6.25 MG/5 ML N88761 001 NOV 08, 1984
PROMETHAZINE VC PLAIN
AA CENCI 5 MG/5 ML;6.25 MG/5 ML N88815 001 NOV 22, 1985
AA PENNEX 5 MG/5 ML;6.25 MG/5 ML N88897 001 JAN 04, 1985

PHENYLEPHRINE HYDROCHLORIDE; PYRILAMINE MALEATE
SOLUTION/DROPS; OPHTHALMIC
PREFRIN-A
ALLERGAN 0.12%;0.1% N07953 001

PHENYLPROPANOLAMINE HYDROCHLORIDE; *MULTIPLE*
SEE BROMPHENIRAMINE MALEATE; CODEINE PHOSPHATE; PHENYLPROPANOLAMINE HYDROCHLORIDE
SEE CHLORPHENIRAMINE MALEATE; PHENYLPROPANOLAMINE HYDROCHLORIDE
SEE HYDROCODONE BITARTRATE; PHENYLPROPANOLAMINE HYDROCHLORIDE

PHENYTOIN
SUSPENSION; ORAL
DILANTIN-125
AB + PARKE DAVIS 125 MG/5 ML N08762 001
PHENYTOIN
AB BARRE 125 MG/5 ML N89892 001 SEP 25, 1992

TABLET, CHEWABLE; ORAL
DILANTIN
+ PARKE DAVIS 50 MG N84427 001

PHENYTOIN SODIUM
INJECTABLE; INJECTION
DILANTIN
AP + PARKE DAVIS 50 MG/ML N10151 001
PHENYTOIN
AP ELKINS SINN 50 MG/ML N84307 001
PHENYTOIN SODIUM
AP ABBOTT 50 MG/ML N89521 001 MAR 17, 1987
AP FUJISAWA 50 MG/ML N89003 001 MAY 31, 1985
AP MARSAM 50 MG/ML N89501 001 OCT 13, 1987
AP 50 MG/ML N89779 001 NOV 27, 1992
AP SMITH AND NEPHEW 50 MG/ML N88519 001 DEC 19, 1984
AP SOLOPAK 50 MG/ML N88520 001 DEC 17, 1984
AP STERIS 50 MG/ML N85434 001
AP WINTHROP 50 MG/ML N89744 001 DEC 18, 1987

PHENYTOIN SODIUM, EXTENDED
CAPSULE; ORAL
DILANTIN
PARKE DAVIS 30 MG N84349 001
+ 100 MG N84349 002

PHENYTOIN SODIUM, PROMPT
CAPSULE; ORAL
PROMPT PHENYTOIN SODIUM
BX + DANBURY PHARMA 100 MG N80905 001
BX ZENITH LABS 100 MG N80259 001

Prescription Drug Products *(continued)*

PHOSPHORIC ACID; *MULTIPLE*

SEE AMINO ACIDS; CALCIUM ACETATE; GLYCERIN; MAGNESIUM ACETATE; PHOSPHORIC ACID; POTASSIUM CHLORIDE; SODIUM ACETATE; SODIUM CHLORIDE

SEE AMINO ACIDS; MAGNESIUM ACETATE; PHOSPHORIC ACID; POTASSIUM ACETATE; POTASSIUM CHLORIDE; SODIUM ACETATE

SEE AMINO ACIDS; MAGNESIUM ACETATE; PHOSPHORIC ACID; POTASSIUM ACETATE; SODIUM CHLORIDE

SEE AMINO ACIDS; MAGNESIUM ACETATE; PHOSPHORIC ACID; POTASSIUM CHLORIDE; SODIUM ACETATE; SODIUM CHLORIDE

PHYTONADIONE

INJECTABLE; INJECTION

	AQUAMEPHYTON		
BP	+ MERCK SHARP DOHME	1 MG/0.5 ML	N12223 002
BP	+	10 MG/ML	N12223 001
	KONAKION		
BP	ROCHE	1 MG/0.5 ML	N11745 001
BP		10 MG/ML	N11745 003
	PHYTONADIONE		
BP	INTL MEDICATION	1 MG/0.5 ML	N83722 001
	VITAMIN K1		
BP	ABBOTT	1 MG/0.5 ML	N87954 001 JUL 25, 1983
BP		10 MG/ML	N87955 001 JUL 25, 1983

TABLET; ORAL

	MEPHYTON		
	+ MERCK SHARP DOHME	5 MG	N10104 003

PHYTONADIONE; *MULTIPLE*

SEE ASCORBIC ACID; BIOTIN; CYANOCOBALAMIN; ERGOCALCIFEROL; FOLIC ACID; NIACINAMIDE; PANTOTHENIC ACID; PHYTONADIONE; PYRIDOXINE; RIBOFLAVIN; THIAMINE; VITAMIN A PALMITATE; VITAMIN E

PILOCARPINE

INSERT, EXTENDED RELEASE; OPHTHALMIC

OCUSERT PILO-20		
+ ALZA	5 MG	N17431 001
OCUSERT PILO-40		
+ ALZA	11 MG	N17548 001

PILOCARPINE HYDROCHLORIDE

GEL; OPHTHALMIC

PILOPINE HS		
+ ALCON	4%	N18796 001 OCT 01, 1984

TABLET; ORAL

SALAGEN		
+ MGI	5 MG	N20237 001 MAR 22, 1994

PIMOZIDE

TABLET; ORAL

ORAP		
+ LEMMON	2 MG	N17473 001 JUL 31, 1984

PINACIDIL

CAPSULE, EXTENDED RELEASE; ORAL

PINDAC		
+ LEO PHARM	12.5 MG	N19456 001 DEC 28, 1989
+	25 MG	N19456 002 DEC 28, 1989

PINDOLOL

TABLET; ORAL

	PINDOLOL		
AB	GENEVA PHARMS	5 MG	N73608 001 MAR 29, 1993
AB		10 MG	N73609 001 MAR 29, 1993
AB	GENPHARM	5 MG	N74013 001 SEP 24, 1992
AB		10 MG	N74018 001 SEP 24, 1992
AB	MUTUAL PHARM	5 MG	N74063 001 JAN 27, 1994
AB		10 MG	N74063 002 JAN 27, 1994
AB	MYLAN	5 MG	N74019 001 SEP 03, 1992
AB		10 MG	N74019 002 SEP 03, 1992
AB	NOVOPHARM	5 MG	N73661 001 OCT 31, 1993
AB		10 MG	N73661 002 OCT 31, 1993

Prescription Drug Products *(continued)*

PINDOLOL *(continued)*

	TABLET; ORAL		
	PINDOLOL		
AB	PUREPAC PHARM	5 MG	N74125 001 APR 28, 1993
AB		10 MG	N74125 002 APR 28, 1993
AB	ZENITH LABS	5 MG	N73687 001 FEB 26, 1993
AB		10 MG	N73687 002 FEB 26, 1993
	VISKEN		
AB	SANDOZ	5 MG	N18285 001 SEP 03, 1982
AB	+	10 MG	N18285 002 SEP 03, 1982

PIPECURONIUM BROMIDE

	INJECTABLE; INJECTION		
	ARDUAN		
	+ ORGANON	10 MG/VIAL	N19638 001 JUN 26, 1990

PIPERACILLIN SODIUM

	INJECTABLE; INJECTION		
	PIPRACIL		
	+ LEDERLE	EQ 2 GM BASE/VIAL	N50545 002
		EQ 2 GM BASE/VIAL	N62750 001 OCT 13, 1987
	+	EQ 3 GM BASE/VIAL	N50545 003
		EQ 3 GM BASE/VIAL	N62750 002 OCT 13, 1987
	+	EQ 4 GM BASE/VIAL	N50545 004
		EQ 4 GM BASE/VIAL	N62750 003 OCT 13, 1987

PIPERACILLIN SODIUM; TAZOBACTAM SODIUM

	INJECTABLE; INJECTION		
	ZOSYN		
	+ LEDERLE	EQ 2 GM BASE/VIAL;EQ 250 MG BASE/VIAL	N50684 001 OCT 22, 1993
	+	EQ 3 GM BASE/VIAL;EQ 375 MG BASE/VIAL	N50684 002 OCT 22, 1993
	+	EQ 4 GM BASE/VIAL;EQ 500 MG BASE/VIAL	N50684 003 OCT 22, 1993
	+	EQ 36 GM BASE/VIAL;EQ 4.5 GM BASE/VIAL	N50684 004 OCT 22, 1993

PIPERAZINE CITRATE

	SYRUP; ORAL		
	MULTIFUGE		
AA	BLULINE	EQ 500 MG BASE/5 ML	N09452 001
	PIPERAZINE CITRATE		
AA	LANNETT	EQ 500 MG BASE/5 ML	N80963 001
AA	LUITPOLD	EQ 500 MG BASE/5 ML	N80671 001
	TABLET; ORAL		
	PIPERAZINE CITRATE		
	GLOBAL PHARMS	EQ 250 MG BASE	N80874 001

PIPOBROMAN

	TABLET; ORAL		
	VERCYTE		
	+ ABBOTT	25 MG	N16245 002

PIRBUTEROL ACETATE

	AEROSOL, METERED; INHALATION		
	MAXAIR		
	+ 3M	EQ 0.2 MG BASE/INH	N19009 001 DEC 30, 1986
	+	EQ 0.2 MG BASE/INH	N20014 001 NOV 30, 1992

PIROXICAM

	CAPSULE; ORAL		
	FELDENE		
AB	PFIZER	10 MG	N18147 002 APR 06, 1982
AB	+	20 MG	N18147 003 APR 06, 1982
	PIROXICAM		
AB	COPLEY PHARM	10 MG	N74103 001 AUG 28, 1992
AB		20 MG	N74103 002 AUG 28, 1992
AB	GENPHARM	10 MG	N74043 001 SEP 22, 1992
AB		20 MG	N74043 002 SEP 22, 1992
AB	LEMMON	10 MG	N74131 001 DEC 11, 1992
AB		20 MG	N74131 002 DEC 11, 1992
AB	MEPHA	10 MG	N74116 001 JUN 15, 1993
AB		20 MG	N74118 001 JUN 15, 1993

Prescription Drug Products *(continued)*

PIROXICAM *(continued)*

CAPSULE; ORAL

PIROXICAM

TE	Applicant	Strength	Appl. No. / Date
AB	MUTUAL PHARM	10 MG	N73535 001 MAR 12, 1993
AB		20 MG	N73536 001 MAR 12, 1993
AB	MYLAN	10 MG	N74102 001 JUL 31, 1992
AB		20 MG	N74102 002 JUL 31, 1992
AB	NOVOPHARM	10 MG	N73637 001 JAN 28, 1994
AB		20 MG	N73638 001 JAN 28, 1994
AB	ROXANE	10 MG	N73651 001 FEB 26, 1993
AB		20 MG	N73651 002 FEB 26, 1993
AB	SCS	10 MG	N74036 001 MAY 29, 1992
AB		20 MG	N74036 002 MAY 29, 1992

PLICAMYCIN

INJECTABLE; INJECTION

MITHRACIN

TE	Applicant	Strength	Appl. No. / Date
	+ MILES	2.5 MG/VIAL	N50109 001

PODOFILOX

SOLUTION; TOPICAL

CONDYLOX

TE	Applicant	Strength	Appl. No. / Date
	+ OCLASSEN	0.5%	N19795 001 DEC 13, 1990

POLYESTRADIOL PHOSPHATE

INJECTABLE; INJECTION

ESTRADURIN

TE	Applicant	Strength	Appl. No. / Date
	+ WYETH AYERST	40 MG/AMP	N10753 001

POLYETHYLENE GLYCOL 3350; POTASSIUM CHLORIDE; SODIUM BICARBONATE; SODIUM CHLORIDE

POWDER FOR RECONSTITUTION; ORAL

NULYTELY

TE	Applicant	Strength	Appl. No. / Date
	BRAINTREE	420 GM/BOT;1.48 GM/ BOT;5.72 GM/ BOT;11.2 GM/BOT	N19797 001 APR 22, 1991

POLYETHYLENE GLYCOL 3350; POTASSIUM CHLORIDE; SODIUM BICARBONATE; SODIUM CHLORIDE; SODIUM SULFATE

SOLUTION; ORAL

OCL

TE	Applicant	Strength	Appl. No. / Date
	ABBOTT	6 GM/100 ML;75 MG/ 100 ML;168 MG/ 100 ML;146 MG/ 100 ML;1.29 GM/100 ML	N19284 001 APR 30, 1986

POLYETHYLENE GLYCOL 3350; POTASSIUM CHLORIDE; SODIUM BICARBONATE; SODIUM CHLORIDE; SODIUM SULFATE, ANHYDROUS

POWDER FOR RECONSTITUTION; ORAL

TE	Applicant	Strength	Appl. No. / Date
	CO-LAV		
AA	COPLEY PHARM	240 GM/BOT;2.98 GM/ BOT;6.72 GM/ BOT;5.84 GM/ BOT;22.72 GM/BOT	N73428 001 JAN 28, 1992
	COLOVAGE		
AA	DYNAPHARM	227.1 GM/PACKET;2.82 GM/ PACKET;6.36 GM/ PACKET;5.53 GM/ PACKET;21.5 GM/PACKET	N71320 001 APR 20, 1988
	COLYTE		
AA	REED AND CARNRICK	227.1 GM/BOT;2.82 GM/ BOT;6.36 GM/ BOT;5.53 GM/ BOT;21.5 GM/BOT	N18983 010 JAN 31, 1989
AA		240 GM/BOT;2.98 GM/ BOT;6.72 GM/ BOT;5.84 GM/ BOT;22.72 GM/BOT	N18983 007 JUN 12, 1987
	COLYTE-FLAVORED		
AA	REED AND CARNRICK	227.1 GM/BOT;2.82 GM/ BOT;6.36 GM/ BOT;5.53 GM/ BOT;21.5 GM/BOT	N18983 008 NOV 14, 1991
AA		240 GM/BOT;2.98 GM/ BOT;6.72 GM/ BOT;5.84 GM/ BOT;22.72 GM/BOT	N18983 009 NOV 14, 1991

Prescription Drug Products *(continued)*

POLYETHYLENE GLYCOL 3350; POTASSIUM CHLORIDE; SODIUM BICARBONATE; SODIUM CHLORIDE; SODIUM SULFATE, ANHYDROUS *(continued)*

POWDER FOR RECONSTITUTION; ORAL

	E-Z-EM PREP LYTE		
AA	E Z EM	236 GM/BOT;2.97 GM/BOT;6.74 GM/BOT;5.86 GM/BOT;22.74 GM/BOT	N71278 001 NOV 21, 1988
	GLYCOPREP		
AA	GOLDLINE	236 GM/BOT;2.97 GM/BOT;6.74 GM/BOT;5.86 GM/BOT;22.74 GM/BOT	N72319 001 DEC 23, 1988
	GO-EVAC		
AA	COPLEY PHARM	236 GM/BOT;2.97 GM/BOT;6.74 GM/BOT;5.86 GM/BOT;22.74 GM/BOT	N73433 001 APR 28, 1992
	GOLYTELY		
AA	BRAINTREE	236 GM/BOT;2.97 GM/BOT;6.74 GM/BOT;5.86 GM/BOT;22.74 GM/BOT	N19011 001 JUL 13, 1984
	PEG-LYTE		
AA	INVAMED	236 GM/BOT;2.97 GM/BOT;6.74 GM/BOT;5.86 GM/BOT;22.74 GM/BOT	N73098 001 AUG 31, 1993

POLYMYXIN B SULFATE

INJECTABLE; INJECTION

	AEROSPORIN		
AP	+ BURROUGHS WELLCOME	500,000 UNITS/VIAL	N62036 001
	POLYMIXIN B SULFATE		
AP	PFIZER	500,000 UNITS/VIAL	N60716 001

POWDER; FOR RX COMPOUNDING

	POLY-RX		
AA	PHARMA TEK	100,000,000 UNITS/BOT	N61578 001
	POLYMIXIN B SULFATE		
AA	PADDOCK	100,000,000 UNITS/BOT	N62455 001 JUL 27, 1983

POLYMYXIN B SULFATE; *MULTIPLE*

SEE BACITRACIN; HYDROCORTISONE ACETATE; NEOMYCIN SULFATE; POLYMYXIN B SULFATE
SEE BACITRACIN ZINC; HYDROCORTISONE; NEOMYCIN SULFATE; POLYMYXIN B SULFATE
SEE BACITRACIN ZINC; NEOMYCIN SULFATE; POLYMYXIN B SULFATE
SEE BACITRACIN ZINC; POLYMYXIN B SULFATE
SEE CHLORAMPHENICOL; HYDROCORTISONE ACETATE; POLYMYXIN B SULFATE
SEE DEXAMETHASONE; NEOMYCIN SULFATE; POLYMYXIN B SULFATE
SEE GRAMICIDIN; NEOMYCIN SULFATE; POLYMYXIN B SULFATE
SEE HYDROCORTISONE; NEOMYCIN SULFATE; POLYMYXIN B SULFATE
SEE HYDROCORTISONE; POLYMYXIN B SULFATE
SEE HYDROCORTISONE ACETATE; NEOMYCIN SULFATE; POLYMYXIN B SULFATE
SEE NEOMYCIN SULFATE; POLYMYXIN B SULFATE
SEE NEOMYCIN SULFATE; POLYMYXIN B SULFATE; PREDNISOLONE ACETATE
SEE OXYTETRACYCLINE HYDROCHLORIDE; POLYMYXIN B SULFATE

POLYMYXIN B SULFATE; TRIMETHOPRIM SULFATE

SOLUTION/DROPS; OPHTHALMIC

	POLYTRIM		
	ALLERGAN	10,000 UNITS/ML;EQ 1 MG BASE/ML	N50567 001 OCT 20, 1988

POLYTHIAZIDE

TABLET; ORAL

	RENESE		
	PFIZER	1 MG	N12845 001
		2 MG	N12845 002
	+	4 MG	N12845 003

POLYTHIAZIDE; PRAZOSIN HYDROCHLORIDE

CAPSULE; ORAL

	MINIZIDE		
	PFIZER	0.5 MG;1 MG	N17986 001
		0.5 MG;2 MG	N17986 002
	+	0.5 MG;5 MG	N17986 003

Prescription Drug Products *(continued)*

POLYTHIAZIDE; RESERPINE

TABLET; ORAL
RENESE-R

	+ PFIZER	2 MG;0.25 MG	N13636 001

POTASSIUM ACETATE

INJECTABLE; INJECTION
POTASSIUM ACETATE IN PLASTIC CONTAINER

	+ ABBOTT	2 MEQ/ML	N18896 001 JUL 20, 1984

POTASSIUM ACETATE; *MULTIPLE*

SEE AMINO ACIDS; DEXTROSE; MAGNESIUM CHLORIDE; POTASSIUM ACETATE; POTASSIUM CHLORIDE; POTASSIUM PHOSPHATE, DIBASIC; SODIUM CHLORIDE
SEE AMINO ACIDS; MAGNESIUM ACETATE; PHOSPHORIC ACID; POTASSIUM ACETATE; POTASSIUM CHLORIDE; SODIUM ACETATE
SEE AMINO ACIDS; MAGNESIUM ACETATE; PHOSPHORIC ACID; POTASSIUM ACETATE; SODIUM CHLORIDE
SEE DEXTROSE; MAGNESIUM ACETATE; POTASSIUM ACETATE; SODIUM CHLORIDE
SEE DEXTROSE; MAGNESIUM ACETATE TETRAHYDRATE; POTASSIUM ACETATE; SODIUM CHLORIDE
SEE MAGNESIUM ACETATE TETRAHYDRATE; POTASSIUM ACETATE; SODIUM CHLORIDE

POTASSIUM AMINOSALICYLATE

CAPSULE; ORAL
PASKALIUM

	GLENWOOD	500 MG	N09395 004

TABLET; ORAL
PASKALIUM

	GLENWOOD	1 GM	N09395 003

POTASSIUM CHLORIDE

CAPSULE, EXTENDED RELEASE; ORAL
K-LEASE

AB	SAVAGE LABS	8 MEQ	N73398 001 JAN 28, 1992
AB		10 MEQ	N72427 001 MAR 28, 1990

MICRO-K

AB	ROBINS AH	8 MEQ	N18238 001

POTASSIUM CHLORIDE *(continued)*

CAPSULE, EXTENDED RELEASE; ORAL
MICRO-K 10

AB	+ ROBINS AH	10 MEQ	N18238 002 MAY 14, 1984

POTASSIUM CHLORIDE

AB	KV PHARM	10 MEQ	N70980 001 FEB 17, 1987

GRANULE, FOR RECONSTITUTION ER; ORAL
MICRO-K LS

	+ ROBINS AH	20 MEQ/PACKET	N19561 003 AUG 26, 1988

INJECTABLE; INJECTION
POTASSIUM CHLORIDE

AP	+ ABBOTT	2 MEQ/ML	N80205 001
AP		2 MEQ/ML	N83345 002
	+	1.5 MEQ/ML	N83345 001
AP	AKORN	2 MEQ/ML	N88286 001 SEP 05, 1985
AP	BAXTER	2 MEQ/ML	N85499 001
AP	FUJISAWA	2 MEQ/ML	N80225 001
AP		2 MEQ/ML	N84290 001
AP		2 MEQ/ML	N87787 001 APR 20, 1982
AP		2 MEQ/ML	N87817 001 OCT 20, 1982
AP		3 MEQ/ML	N80225 003
AP	INTL MEDICATION	2 MEQ/ML	N83163 001
AP	LUITPOLD	2 MEQ/ML	N87584 001
AP		2 MEQ/ML	N87585 001
AP	MCGAW	2 MEQ/ML	N85870 001
	+ MILES	4 MEQ/ML	N80195 004
AP	PHARMA SERVE NY	2 MEQ/ML	N86297 001
AP		2 MEQ/ML	N87362 001 MAR 08, 1983
AP	STERIS	2 MEQ/ML	N86208 001
AP		2 MEQ/ML	N89163 001 MAR 10, 1988
AP		2 MEQ/ML	N89421 001 JAN 02, 1987
AP	+	3 MEQ/ML	N86210 001

POTASSIUM CHLORIDE IN PLASTIC CONTAINER

AP	FUJISAWA	2 MEQ/ML	N88901 001 JAN 25, 1985
AP		2 MEQ/ML	N88908 001 JAN 25, 1985

Prescription Drug Products *(continued)*

POTASSIUM CHLORIDE *(continued)*

INJECTABLE; INJECTION

	POTASSIUM CHLORIDE 10 MEQ IN PLASTIC CONTAINER		
AP	ABBOTT	745 MG/100 ML	N20161 001 NOV 30, 1992
AP		14.9 MG/ML	N20161 005 NOV 30, 1992
AP	BAXTER	746 MG/100 ML	N19904 005 DEC 17, 1990
AP		14.9 MG/ML	N19904 001 DEC 26, 1989
	POTASSIUM CHLORIDE 20 MEQ IN PLASTIC CONTAINER		
AP	ABBOTT	1.49 GM/100 ML	N20161 002 NOV 30, 1992
	BAXTER	29.8 MG/ML	N19904 002 DEC 26, 1989
AP		1.49 GM/100 ML	N19904 006 DEC 17, 1990
	POTASSIUM CHLORIDE 30 MEQ IN PLASTIC CONTAINER		
	BAXTER	2.24 GM/100 ML	N19904 003 DEC 26, 1989
	POTASSIUM CHLORIDE 40 MEQ IN PLASTIC CONTAINER		
	BAXTER	2.98 GM/100 ML	N19904 004 DEC 26, 1989

TABLET, EXTENDED RELEASE; ORAL

	K+10		
BC	ALRA	10 MEQ	N70999 001 OCT 22, 1987
	K+8		
AB	ALRA	8 MEQ	N70998 001 JAN 25, 1993
	K-DUR 10		
BC	SCHERING	10 MEQ	N19439 002 JUN 13, 1986
	K-DUR 20		
	SCHERING	20 MEQ	N19439 001 JUN 13, 1986
	K-TAB		
BC	+ ABBOTT	10 MEQ	N18279 001
	KAON CL		
	SAVAGE LABS	6.7 MEQ	N17046 001
	KAON CL-10		
BC	SAVAGE LABS	10 MEQ	N17046 002
	KLOR-CON		
AB	UPSHER SMITH	8 MEQ	N19123 001 APR 17, 1986
BC		10 MEQ	N19123 002 APR 17, 1986
	KLOTRIX		
BC	APOTHECON	10 MEQ	N17850 001

POTASSIUM CHLORIDE *(continued)*

TABLET, EXTENDED RELEASE; ORAL

	POTASSIUM CHLORIDE		
BC	ABBOTT	8 MEQ	N18279 002 AUG 01, 1988
AB	COPLEY PHARM	8 MEQ	N70618 001 SEP 09, 1987
	SLOW-K		
AB	+ CIBA	8 MEQ	N17476 002
	TEN-K		
BC	CIBA	10 MEQ	N19381 001 APR 16, 1986

POTASSIUM CHLORIDE; *MULTIPLE*

SEE AMINO ACIDS; CALCIUM ACETATE; GLYCERIN; MAGNESIUM ACETATE; PHOSPHORIC ACID; POTASSIUM CHLORIDE; SODIUM ACETATE; SODIUM CHLORIDE

SEE AMINO ACIDS; CALCIUM CHLORIDE; DEXTROSE; MAGNESIUM CHLORIDE; POTASSIUM CHLORIDE; POTASSIUM PHOSPHATE, DIBASIC; SODIUM CHLORIDE

SEE AMINO ACIDS; DEXTROSE; MAGNESIUM CHLORIDE; POTASSIUM CHLORIDE; SODIUM CHLORIDE; SODIUM PHOSPHATE, DIBASIC

SEE AMINO ACIDS; DEXTROSE; MAGNESIUM CHLORIDE; POTASSIUM ACETATE; POTASSIUM CHLORIDE; POTASSIUM PHOSPHATE, DIBASIC; SODIUM CHLORIDE

SEE AMINO ACIDS; DEXTROSE; MAGNESIUM CHLORIDE; POTASSIUM CHLORIDE; SODIUM CHLORIDE; SODIUM PHOSPHATE, DIBASIC

SEE AMINO ACIDS; MAGNESIUM ACETATE; PHOSPHORIC ACID; POTASSIUM ACETATE; POTASSIUM CHLORIDE; SODIUM ACETATE

SEE AMINO ACIDS; MAGNESIUM ACETATE; PHOSPHORIC ACID; POTASSIUM CHLORIDE; SODIUM ACETATE; SODIUM CHLORIDE

SEE AMINO ACIDS; MAGNESIUM CHLORIDE; POTASSIUM CHLORIDE; POTASSIUM PHOSPHATE, DIBASIC; SODIUM CHLORIDE

SEE CALCIUM CHLORIDE; DEXTROSE; GLUTATHIONE DISULFIDE; MAGNESIUM CHLORIDE; POTASSIUM CHLORIDE; SODIUM BICARBONATE; SODIUM CHLORIDE; SODIUM PHOSPHATE

Prescription Drug Products *(continued)*

POTASSIUM CHLORIDE; *MULTIPLE* *(continued)*

SEE CALCIUM CHLORIDE; DEXTROSE; MAGNESIUM CHLORIDE; POTASSIUM CHLORIDE; SODIUM ACETATE; SODIUM CHLORIDE
SEE CALCIUM CHLORIDE; DEXTROSE; MAGNESIUM CHLORIDE; POTASSIUM CHLORIDE; SODIUM ACETATE; SODIUM CHLORIDE; SODIUM CITRATE
SEE CALCIUM CHLORIDE; DEXTROSE; MAGNESIUM CHLORIDE; POTASSIUM CHLORIDE; SODIUM ACETATE; SODIUM CHLORIDE; SODIUM LACTATE
SEE CALCIUM CHLORIDE; DEXTROSE; POTASSIUM CHLORIDE; SODIUM CHLORIDE
SEE CALCIUM CHLORIDE; DEXTROSE; POTASSIUM CHLORIDE; SODIUM CHLORIDE; SODIUM LACTATE
SEE CALCIUM CHLORIDE; DEXTROSE; POTASSIUM CHLORIDE; SODIUM ACETATE; SODIUM CHLORIDE
SEE CALCIUM CHLORIDE; DEXTROSE; POTASSIUM CHLORIDE; SODIUM CHLORIDE; SODIUM LACTATE
SEE CALCIUM CHLORIDE; MAGNESIUM CHLORIDE; POTASSIUM CHLORIDE; SODIUM ACETATE; SODIUM CHLORIDE; SODIUM CITRATE
SEE CALCIUM CHLORIDE; MAGNESIUM CHLORIDE; POTASSIUM CHLORIDE; SODIUM ACETATE; SODIUM CHLORIDE
SEE CALCIUM CHLORIDE; MAGNESIUM CHLORIDE; POTASSIUM CHLORIDE; SODIUM ACETATE; SODIUM CHLORIDE; SODIUM LACTATE
SEE CALCIUM CHLORIDE; MAGNESIUM CHLORIDE; POTASSIUM CHLORIDE; SODIUM CHLORIDE
SEE CALCIUM CHLORIDE; POTASSIUM CHLORIDE; SODIUM CHLORIDE
SEE CALCIUM CHLORIDE; POTASSIUM CHLORIDE; SODIUM CHLORIDE; SODIUM LACTATE
SEE DEXTROSE; MAGNESIUM CHLORIDE; POTASSIUM CHLORIDE; SODIUM ACETATE; SODIUM CHLORIDE
SEE DEXTROSE; MAGNESIUM CHLORIDE; POTASSIUM CHLORIDE; SODIUM ACETATE; SODIUM CHLORIDE; SODIUM GLUCONATE
SEE DEXTROSE; MAGNESIUM CHLORIDE; POTASSIUM CHLORIDE; POTASSIUM PHOSPHATE, DIBASIC; SODIUM ACETATE
SEE DEXTROSE; MAGNESIUM CHLORIDE; POTASSIUM CHLORIDE; SODIUM ACETATE; SODIUM CHLORIDE; SODIUM GLUCONATE

POTASSIUM CHLORIDE; *MULTIPLE* *(continued)*

SEE DEXTROSE; MAGNESIUM CHLORIDE; POTASSIUM CHLORIDE; POTASSIUM PHOSPHATE, DIBASIC; SODIUM CHLORIDE; SODIUM LACTATE; SODIUM PHOSPHATE, MONOBASIC
SEE DEXTROSE; MAGNESIUM CHLORIDE; POTASSIUM CHLORIDE; POTASSIUM PHOSPHATE, MONOBASIC; SODIUM LACTATE; SODIUM PHOSPHATE, MONOBASIC
SEE DEXTROSE; MAGNESIUM CHLORIDE; POTASSIUM CHLORIDE; POTASSIUM PHOSPHATE, MONOBASIC; SODIUM CHLORIDE; SODIUM LACTATE
SEE DEXTROSE; POTASSIUM CHLORIDE
SEE DEXTROSE; POTASSIUM CHLORIDE; POTASSIUM LACTATE; SODIUM CHLORIDE; SODIUM PHOSPHATE, MONOBASIC
SEE DEXTROSE; POTASSIUM CHLORIDE; POTASSIUM PHOSPHATE, DIBASIC; SODIUM ACETATE; SODIUM CHLORIDE
SEE DEXTROSE; POTASSIUM CHLORIDE; POTASSIUM PHOSPHATE, MONOBASIC; SODIUM CHLORIDE; SODIUM LACTATE
SEE DEXTROSE; POTASSIUM CHLORIDE; SODIUM CHLORIDE
SEE MAGNESIUM CHLORIDE; POTASSIUM CHLORIDE; POTASSIUM PHOSPHATE, MONOBASIC; SODIUM ACETATE; SODIUM CHLORIDE; SODIUM GLUCONATE; SODIUM PHOSPHATE, DIBASIC
SEE MAGNESIUM CHLORIDE; POTASSIUM CHLORIDE; SODIUM ACETATE; SODIUM CHLORIDE; SODIUM GLUCONATE
SEE MAGNESIUM SULFATE; POTASSIUM CHLORIDE; POTASSIUM PHOSPHATE, MONOBASIC; SODIUM CHLORIDE; SODIUM PHOSPHATE
SEE POLYETHYLENE GLYCOL 3350; POTASSIUM CHLORIDE; SODIUM BICARBONATE; SODIUM CHLORIDE; SODIUM SULFATE, ANHYDROUS
SEE POLYETHYLENE GLYCOL 3350; POTASSIUM CHLORIDE; SODIUM BICARBONATE; SODIUM CHLORIDE
SEE POLYETHYLENE GLYCOL 3350; POTASSIUM CHLORIDE; SODIUM BICARBONATE; SODIUM CHLORIDE; SODIUM SULFATE
SEE POLYETHYLENE GLYCOL 3350; POTASSIUM CHLORIDE; SODIUM BICARBONATE; SODIUM CHLORIDE; SODIUM SULFATE, ANHYDROUS

Prescription Drug Products *(continued)*

POTASSIUM CHLORIDE; SODIUM CHLORIDE

INJECTABLE; INJECTION

POTASSIUM CHLORIDE 0.037% IN SODIUM CHLORIDE 0.9% IN PLASTIC CONTAINER

	MCGAW	37 MG/100 ML;900 MG/100 ML	N19708 001 SEP 29, 1989

POTASSIUM CHLORIDE 0.075% IN SODIUM CHLORIDE 0.9% IN PLASTIC CONTAINER

	MCGAW	75 MG/100 ML;900 MG/100 ML	N19708 002 SEP 29, 1989

POTASSIUM CHLORIDE 0.11% IN SODIUM CHLORIDE 0.9% IN PLASTIC CONTAINER

	MCGAW	110 MG/100 ML;900 MG/100 ML	N19708 003 SEP 29, 1989

POTASSIUM CHLORIDE 0.15% IN SODIUM CHLORIDE 0.9% IN PLASTIC CONTAINER

AP	MCGAW	150 MG/100 ML;900 MG/100 ML	N19708 004 SEP 29, 1989

POTASSIUM CHLORIDE 0.22% IN SODIUM CHLORIDE 0.9% IN PLASTIC CONTAINER

	MCGAW	220 MG/100 ML;900 MG/100 ML	N19708 005 SEP 29, 1989

POTASSIUM CHLORIDE 0.3% IN SODIUM CHLORIDE 0.9% IN PLASTIC CONTAINER

AP	MCGAW	300 MG/100 ML;900 MG/100 ML	N19708 006 SEP 29, 1989

POTASSIUM CHLORIDE 20 MEQ IN SODIUM CHLORIDE 0.9% IN PLASTIC CONTAINER

AP	ABBOTT	149 MG/100 ML;900 MG/100 ML	N19686 001 OCT 17, 1988

POTASSIUM CHLORIDE 40 MEQ IN SODIUM CHLORIDE 0.9% IN PLASTIC CONTAINER

AP	ABBOTT	298 MG/100 ML;900 MG/100 ML	N19686 002 OCT 17, 1988

SODIUM CHLORIDE 0.9% AND POTASSIUM CHLORIDE 0.15% IN PLASTIC CONTAINER

AP	BAXTER	150 MG/100 ML;900 MG/100 ML	N17648 001

SODIUM CHLORIDE 0.9% AND POTASSIUM CHLORIDE 0.224%

	BAXTER	224 MG/100 ML;900 MG/100 ML	N17648 003

SODIUM CHLORIDE 0.9% AND POTASSIUM CHLORIDE 0.3% IN PLASTIC CONTAINER

AP	BAXTER	300 MG/100 ML;900 MG/100 ML	N17648 002

POTASSIUM CHLORIDE; SODIUM CHLORIDE; TROMETHAMINE

INJECTABLE; INJECTION

THAM-E

+ ABBOTT	370 MG/VIAL;1.75 GM/VIAL;36 GM/VIAL	N13025 001

POTASSIUM CITRATE

TABLET, EXTENDED RELEASE; ORAL

POTASSIUM CITRATE

	UNIV TX	5 MEQ	N19071 001 AUG 30, 1985
+		10 MEQ	N19071 002 AUG 31, 1992

POTASSIUM LACTATE; *MULTIPLE*

SEE DEXTROSE; POTASSIUM CHLORIDE; POTASSIUM LACTATE; SODIUM CHLORIDE; SODIUM PHOSPHATE, MONOBASIC

POTASSIUM PERCHLORATE

CAPSULE; ORAL

PERCHLORACAP

MALLINCKRODT	200 MG	N17551 001

POTASSIUM PHOSPHATE, DIBASIC; *MULTIPLE*

SEE AMINO ACIDS; CALCIUM CHLORIDE; DEXTROSE; MAGNESIUM CHLORIDE; POTASSIUM CHLORIDE; POTASSIUM PHOSPHATE, DIBASIC; SODIUM CHLORIDE

SEE AMINO ACIDS; DEXTROSE; MAGNESIUM CHLORIDE; POTASSIUM ACETATE; POTASSIUM CHLORIDE; POTASSIUM PHOSPHATE, DIBASIC; SODIUM CHLORIDE

SEE AMINO ACIDS; MAGNESIUM CHLORIDE; POTASSIUM CHLORIDE; POTASSIUM PHOSPHATE, DIBASIC; SODIUM CHLORIDE

SEE AMINO ACIDS; MAGNESIUM CHLORIDE; POTASSIUM PHOSPHATE, DIBASIC; SODIUM ACETATE; SODIUM CHLORIDE

SEE AMINO ACIDS; MAGNESIUM CHLORIDE; POTASSIUM PHOSPHATE, DIBASIC; SODIUM CHLORIDE

SEE DEXTROSE; MAGNESIUM CHLORIDE; POTASSIUM CHLORIDE; POTASSIUM PHOSPHATE, DIBASIC; SODIUM ACETATE

SEE DEXTROSE; MAGNESIUM CHLORIDE; POTASSIUM CHLORIDE; POTASSIUM PHOSPHATE, DIBASIC; SODIUM CHLORIDE; SODIUM LACTATE; SODIUM PHOSPHATE, MONOBASIC

SEE DEXTROSE; POTASSIUM CHLORIDE; POTASSIUM PHOSPHATE, DIBASIC; SODIUM ACETATE; SODIUM CHLORIDE

Prescription Drug Products *(continued)*

POTASSIUM PHOSPHATE, MONOBASIC; *MULTIPLE*

SEE DEXTROSE; MAGNESIUM CHLORIDE; POTASSIUM CHLORIDE; POTASSIUM PHOSPHATE, MONOBASIC; SODIUM LACTATE; SODIUM PHOSPHATE, MONOBASIC

SEE DEXTROSE; MAGNESIUM CHLORIDE; POTASSIUM CHLORIDE; POTASSIUM PHOSPHATE, MONOBASIC; SODIUM CHLORIDE; SODIUM LACTATE

SEE DEXTROSE; POTASSIUM CHLORIDE; POTASSIUM PHOSPHATE, MONOBASIC; SODIUM CHLORIDE; SODIUM LACTATE

SEE MAGNESIUM CHLORIDE; POTASSIUM CHLORIDE; POTASSIUM PHOSPHATE, MONOBASIC; SODIUM ACETATE; SODIUM CHLORIDE; SODIUM GLUCONATE; SODIUM PHOSPHATE, DIBASIC

SEE MAGNESIUM SULFATE; POTASSIUM CHLORIDE; POTASSIUM PHOSPHATE, MONOBASIC; SODIUM CHLORIDE; SODIUM PHOSPHATE

POVIDONE-IODINE

SOLUTION/DROPS; OPHTHALMIC
BETADINE
+ PURDUE FREDERICK 5% N18634 001 DEC 17, 1986

PRALIDOXIME CHLORIDE

INJECTABLE; INJECTION
PRALIDOXIME CHLORIDE
+ SURVIVAL TECH 300 MG/ML N18986 001 APR 26, 1983
PROTOPAM CHLORIDE
+ WYETH AYERST 1 GM/VIAL N14134 001

PRAMOXINE HYDROCHLORIDE; *MULTIPLE*

SEE HYDROCORTISONE ACETATE; PRAMOXINE HYDROCHLORIDE

PRAVASTATIN SODIUM

TABLET; ORAL
PRAVACHOL
BRISTOL MYERS SQUIBB 10 MG N19898 002 OCT 31, 1991
20 MG N19898 003 OCT 31, 1991
+ 40 MG N19898 004 MAR 22, 1993

PRAZIQUANTEL

TABLET; ORAL
BILTRICIDE
+ MILES 600 MG N18714 001 DEC 29, 1982

PRAZOSIN HYDROCHLORIDE

CAPSULE; ORAL
MINIPRESS
AB PFIZER EQ 1 MG BASE N17442 002
AB + EQ 2 MG BASE N17442 003
AB EQ 5 MG BASE N17442 001
PRAZOSIN HCL
AB DANBURY PHARMA EQ 1 MG BASE N72352 001 MAY 16, 1989
AB EQ 2 MG BASE N72333 001 MAY 16, 1989
AB EQ 5 MG BASE N72609 001 MAY 16, 1989
AB GENEVA PHARMS EQ 1 MG BASE N72576 001 MAY 16, 1989
AB EQ 2 MG BASE N72577 001 MAY 16, 1989
AB EQ 5 MG BASE N72578 001 MAY 16, 1989
AB LEDERLE EQ 1 MG BASE N72705 001 MAY 16, 1989
AB EQ 2 MG BASE N72706 001 MAY 16, 1989
AB EQ 5 MG BASE N72707 001 MAY 16, 1989
AB MYLAN EQ 1 MG BASE N72573 001 MAY 16, 1989
AB EQ 2 MG BASE N72574 001 MAY 16, 1989
AB EQ 5 MG BASE N72575 001 MAY 16, 1989
AB PUREPAC PHARM EQ 1 MG BASE N72991 001 MAY 16, 1989
AB EQ 2 MG BASE N72921 001 MAY 16, 1989
AB EQ 5 MG BASE N72992 001 MAY 16, 1989
AB ZENITH LABS EQ 1 MG BASE N71994 001 SEP 12, 1988
AB EQ 2 MG BASE N71995 001 MAY 16, 1989
AB EQ 5 MG BASE N71745 001 MAY 16, 1989

Prescription Drug Products *(continued)*

PRAZOSIN HYDROCHLORIDE *(continued)*

TABLET, EXTENDED RELEASE; ORAL

	MINIPRESS XL		
	+ PFIZER	2.5 MG	N19775 001 JAN 29, 1992
	+	5 MG	N19775 002 JAN 29, 1992

PRAZOSIN HYDROCHLORIDE; *MULTIPLE*

SEE POLYTHIAZIDE; PRAZOSIN HYDROCHLORIDE

PREDNICARBATE

CREAM; TOPICAL

	DERMATOP		
	HOECHST ROUSSEL	0.1%	N20279 001 OCT 29, 1993

PREDNISOLONE

SYRUP; ORAL

	PRELONE		
	MURO	5 MG/5 ML	N89654 001 JAN 17, 1989
		15 MG/5 ML	N89081 001 FEB 04, 1986

TABLET; ORAL

	CORTALONE		
BX	HALSEY	1 MG	N80304 003
BX		2.5 MG	N80304 002
BX		5 MG	N80304 001
	PREDNISOLONE		
BX	CHELSEA LABS	5 MG	N85085 002
BX	DANBURY PHARMA	5 MG	N80354 001
BX	EVERYLIFE	2.5 MG	N84439 002
BX		5 MG	N84439 003
BX	GENEVA PHARMS	5 MG	N80339 001
BX	GLOBAL PHARMS	5 MG	N80780 001
BX	LANNETT	5 MG	N80531 002
BX	MARSHALL PHARMA	2.5 MG	N80562 001
BX		5 MG	N80307 001
BX		5 MG	N80562 002
BX	PHOENIX LABS NY	5 MG	N80322 001
BX	PUREPAC PHARM	5 MG	N80325 001
BX	ROXANE	5 MG	N80327 002
BX	SPERTI	1 MG	N80358 001
BX		2.5 MG	N80358 002
BX		5 MG	N80358 003
BX	ZENITH LABS	5 MG	N80378 001

PREDNISOLONE ACETATE

INJECTABLE; INJECTION

	PREDNISOLONE ACETATE		
	+ STERIS	25 MG/ML	N83398 001
		25 MG/ML	N83654 001
	+	40 MG/ML	N83767 001
		50 MG/ML	N83764 001
	+	50 MG/ML	N85781 001

SUSPENSION/DROPS; OPHTHALMIC

	ECONOPRED		
	+ ALCON	0.125%	N17468 001
	ECONOPRED PLUS		
AT	ALCON	1%	N17469 001
	PRED FORTE		
AT	+ ALLERGAN	1%	N17011 001
	PRED MILD		
	+ ALLERGAN	0.12%	N17100 001

PREDNISOLONE ACETATE; *MULTIPLE*

SEE GENTAMICIN SULFATE; PREDNISOLONE ACETATE

SEE NEOMYCIN SULFATE; POLYMYXIN B SULFATE; PREDNISOLONE ACETATE

PREDNISOLONE ACETATE; SULFACETAMIDE SODIUM

OINTMENT; OPHTHALMIC

	BLEPHAMIDE S.O.P.		
	+ ALLERGAN	0.2%;10%	N87748 001 DEC 03, 1986
	CETAPRED		
	ALCON	0.25%;10%	N87771 001 AUG 06, 1993
	METIMYD		
AT	+ SCHERING	0.5%;10%	N10210 002
	VASOCIDIN		
AT	IOLAB	0.5%;10%	N88791 001 OCT 05, 1984

SUSPENSION/DROPS; OPHTHALMIC

	BLEPHAMIDE		
	ALLERGAN	0.2%;10%	N12813 002
	ISOPTO CETAPRED		
	+ ALCON	0.25%;10%	N87547 001
	METIMYD		
AT	+ SCHERING	0.5%;10%	N10210 001
	PREDAMIDE		
AT	AKORN	0.5%;10%	N88059 001 JUL 29, 1983
	SULPHRIN		
AT	BAUSCH AND LOMB	0.5%;10%	N88089 001 DEC 28, 1982

Prescription Drug Products *(continued)*

PREDNISOLONE SODIUM PHOSPHATE

	INJECTABLE; INJECTION		
	HYDELTRASOL		
AP	+ MERCK SHARP DOHME	EQ 20 MG PHOSPHATE/ML	N11583 002
	PREDNISOLONE SODIUM PHOSPHATE		
AP	STERIS	EQ 20 MG PHOSPHATE/ML	N80517 001
	SOLUTION; ORAL		
	PEDIAPRED		
	FISONS	EQ 5 MG BASE/5 ML	N19157 001 MAY 28, 1986
	SOLUTION/DROPS; OPHTHALMIC		
	INFLAMASE FORTE		
AT	+ IOLAB	EQ 0.9% PHOSPHATE	N80751 002
	INFLAMASE MILD		
AT	+ IOLAB	EQ 0.11% PHOSPHATE	N80751 001
	PREDNISOLONE SODIUM PHOSPHATE		
AT	AKORN	EQ 0.11% PHOSPHATE	N83358 001
AT		EQ 0.9% PHOSPHATE	N83358 002
AT	BAUSCH AND LOMB	EQ 0.11% PHOSPHATE	N40065 001 JUL 29, 1994
AT		EQ 0.9% PHOSPHATE	N40070 001 JUL 29, 1994
AT	STERIS	EQ 0.11% PHOSPHATE	N81043 001 OCT 24, 1991
AT		EQ 0.9% PHOSPHATE	N81044 001 OCT 24, 1991

PREDNISOLONE SODIUM PHOSPHATE; SULFACETAMIDE SODIUM

	SOLUTION/DROPS; OPHTHALMIC		
	SULFACETAMIDE SODIUM AND PREDNISOLONE SODIUM PHOSPHATE		
AT	STERIS	EQ 0.23% PHOSPHATE;10%	N73630 001 MAY 27, 1993
	VASOCIDIN		
AT	+ IOLAB	EQ 0.23% PHOSPHATE;10%	N18988 001 AUG 26, 1988

PREDNISOLONE TEBUTATE

	INJECTABLE; INJECTION		
	HYDELTRA-TBA		
BP	+ MERCK SHARP DOHME	20 MG/ML	N10562 001
	PREDNISOLONE TEBUTATE		
BP	STERIS	20 MG/ML	N83362 001 FEB 17, 1984

PREDNISONE

	SOLUTION; ORAL		
	PREDNISONE		
	ROXANE	5 MG/5 ML	N88703 001 NOV 08, 1984
	PREDNISONE INTENSOL		
	ROXANE	5 MG/ML	N88810 001 FEB 20, 1985
	SYRUP; ORAL		
	LIQUID PRED		
	MURO	5 MG/5 ML	N87611 002 SEP 07, 1982
	TABLET; ORAL		
	CORTAN		
BX	HALSEY	20 MG	N87480 001
	DELTASONE		
AB	+ UPJOHN	2.5 MG	N09986 005
AB	+	5 MG	N09986 002
AB	+	10 MG	N09986 006
AB	+	20 MG	N09986 007
AB	+	50 MG	N09986 008
	METICORTEN		
AB	+ SCHERING	1 MG	N09766 002
	ORASONE		
AB	SOLVAY	1 MG	N83009 001
AB		5 MG	N83009 002
AB		10 MG	N83009 003
AB		20 MG	N83009 004
AB		50 MG	N85999 001
	PREDNICEN-M		
AB	CENT PHARMS	5 MG	N84655 001
	PREDNISONE		
AB	BARR	5 MG	N80701 001
AB		10 MG	N86595 001
AB		20 MG	N84634 001
AB	CHELSEA LABS	5 MG	N85084 002
AB		10 MG	N87773 001 JUL 13, 1982
AB		20 MG	N86813 001
AB		50 MG	N87772 001 JUL 13, 1982
AB	DANBURY PHARMA	5 MG	N80356 001
AB		10 MG	N85162 001
AB		20 MG	N85161 001
BX	EVERYLIFE	1 MG	N84440 001
BX		2.5 MG	N84440 002
BX		5 MG	N84440 003

PREDNISONE *(continued)*

TABLET; ORAL
PREDNISONE

AB	GENEVA PHARMS	5 MG	N80336 002
AB		10 MG	N89983 001 JAN 12, 1989
AB		20 MG	N85813 001
AB		50 MG	N89984 001 JAN 12, 1989
AB	GLOBAL PHARMS	5 MG	N80782 001
AB	HALSEY	5 MG	N80300 001
AB	INTERPHARM	5 MG	N89597 001 OCT 05, 1987
AB		10 MG	N89598 001 OCT 05, 1987
AB		20 MG	N89599 001 OCT 05, 1987
BX	LANNETT	5 MG	N80514 001
BX		20 MG	N84275 001
BX	MARSHALL PHARMA	5 MG	N80301 001
AB	MUTUAL PHARM	5 MG	N89245 001 DEC 04, 1985
AB		10 MG	N89246 001 DEC 04, 1985
AB		20 MG	N89247 001 DEC 04, 1985
BX	PHARMAVITE	5 MG	N84662 002
BX	PHOENIX LABS NY	5 MG	N80321 001
BX		20 MG	N83807 001
AB	PRIVATE FORM	5 MG	N80209 001
AB	PUREPAC PHARM	5 MG	N80353 001
AB		10 MG	N86062 001
AB		20 MG	N86061 001
AB	ROXANE	1 MG	N87800 001 APR 22, 1982
AB		2.5 MG	N87801 001 APR 22, 1982
AB		5 MG	N80352 001
AB		10 MG	N84122 001
AB		20 MG	N87342 001
AB		50 MG	N84283 001
AB	SUPERPHARM	5 MG	N88865 001 OCT 25, 1984
AB		10 MG	N88866 001 OCT 25, 1984
AB		20 MG	N88867 001 OCT 25, 1984
AB	WEST WARD PHARM	5 MG	N80292 001
AB		10 MG	N88832 001 DEC 04, 1985
AB		20 MG	N83677 001
AB		50 MG	N88465 001 JUN 01, 1984

PREDNISONE *(continued)*

TABLET; ORAL
PREDNISONE

BX	ZENITH LABS	5 MG	N80283 001
BX		10 MG	N84133 001

PRILOCAINE; *MULTIPLE*

SEE LIDOCAINE; PRILOCAINE

PRILOCAINE HYDROCHLORIDE

INJECTABLE; INJECTION
CITANEST PLAIN

	+ ASTRA	4%	N14763 007

PRILOCAINE HYDROCHLORIDE; *MULTIPLE*

SEE EPINEPHRINE BITARTRATE; PRILOCAINE HYDROCHLORIDE

PRIMAQUINE PHOSPHATE

TABLET; ORAL
PRIMAQUINE

	STERLING WINTHROP	EQ 15 MG BASE	N08316 001

PRIMIDONE

SUSPENSION; ORAL
MYSOLINE

	WYETH AYERST	250 MG/5 ML	N10401 001

TABLET; ORAL
MYSOLINE

AB	+ WYETH AYERST	250 MG	N09170 002
	+	50 MG	N09170 003

PRIMIDONE

AB	DANBURY PHARMA	250 MG	N83551 001
AB	LANNETT	250 MG	N84903 001

PROBENECID

TABLET; ORAL
BENEMID

AB	+ MERCK SHARP DOHME	500 MG	N07898 004

PROBALAN

AB	LANNETT	500 MG	N80966 001

PROBENECID

AB	DANBURY PHARMA	500 MG	N84442 004 MAR 29, 1983
AB	MYLAN	500 MG	N84211 002 JUN 02, 1982
AB	ZENITH LABS	500 MG	N83740 001 MAY 09, 1984

Prescription Drug Products *(continued)*

PROBENECID; *MULTIPLE*

SEE AMPICILLIN/AMPICILLIN TRIHYDRATE; PROBENECID
SEE COLCHICINE; PROBENECID

PROBUCOL

TABLET; ORAL

LORELCO

	MERRELL DOW	250 MG	N17535 001
	+	500 MG	N17535 002 JUL 06, 1988

PROCAINAMIDE HYDROCHLORIDE

CAPSULE; ORAL

PROCAINAMIDE HCL

AB	DANBURY PHARMA	250 MG	N83287 001
AB		375 MG	N84403 001
AB		500 MG	N84280 001
AB	GENEVA PHARMS	250 MG	N89219 001 JUL 01, 1986
AB		375 MG	N89220 001 JUL 01, 1986
AB		500 MG	N89221 001 JUL 01, 1986
AB	LANNETT	250 MG	N83693 001
AB		500 MG	N84696 001
AB	ZENITH LABS	250 MG	N84604 001
AB		375 MG	N84595 001
AB		500 MG	N84606 001

PRONESTYL

AB	APOTHECON	250 MG	N07335 001
AB		375 MG	N07335 004
AB	+	500 MG	N07335 003

INJECTABLE; INJECTION

PROCAINAMIDE HCL

AP	ABBOTT	100 MG/ML	N89069 001 FEB 12, 1986
AP		500 MG/ML	N89070 001 FEB 12, 1986
AP	ELKINS SINN	100 MG/ML	N89029 001 APR 17, 1986
AP		500 MG/ML	N89030 001 APR 17, 1986
AP	INTL MEDICATION	100 MG/ML	N88636 001 JUL 31, 1984
AP		500 MG/ML	N88637 001 JUL 31, 1984

PROCAINAMIDE HYDROCHLORIDE *(continued)*

INJECTABLE; INJECTION

PROCAINAMIDE HCL

AP	SMITH AND NEPHEW	100 MG/ML	N88530 001 MAR 04, 1985
AP		500 MG/ML	N88531 001 MAR 04, 1985
AP	SOLOPAK	500 MG/ML	N88532 001 MAR 04, 1985
AP	STERIS	100 MG/ML	N87079 001
AP		500 MG/ML	N87080 001
AP	WINTHROP	500 MG/ML	N89537 001 AUG 25, 1987

PRONESTYL

AP	+ APOTHECON	100 MG/ML	N07335 002
AP	+	500 MG/ML	N07335 005

TABLET; ORAL

PRONESTYL

	SQUIBB	250 MG	N17371 001
		375 MG	N17371 002
	+	500 MG	N17371 003

TABLET, EXTENDED RELEASE; ORAL

PROCAINAMIDE HCL

AB	COPLEY PHARM	500 MG	N88974 001 JUL 22, 1985
AB		750 MG	N89438 001 MAR 23, 1987
AB	DANBURY PHARMA	250 MG	N89026 001 OCT 22, 1985
AB		500 MG	N89027 001 OCT 22, 1985
AB		750 MG	N89042 001 OCT 22, 1985
AB	GENEVA PHARMS	250 MG	N89369 001 AUG 14, 1987
AB		500 MG	N89370 001 JAN 09, 1987
AB		750 MG	N89371 001 AUG 14, 1987
AB	INVAMED	500 MG	N89284 001 JUN 23, 1986
AB	INWOOD LABS	500 MG	N89840 001 MAR 06, 1989
AB	SIDMAK LABS NJ	250 MG	N88958 001 DEC 02, 1985
AB		500 MG	N88959 001 DEC 02, 1985

Prescription Drug Products *(continued)*

PROCAINAMIDE HYDROCHLORIDE *(continued)*

TABLET, EXTENDED RELEASE; ORAL

	PROCAN SR		
AB	PARKE DAVIS	250 MG	N86468 001
AB		500 MG	N86065 001
AB		750 MG	N87510 001 APR 01, 1982
	+	1 GM	N88489 001 JAN 16, 1985
	PRONESTYL-SR		
BC	BRISTOL MYERS SQUIBB	500 MG	N87361 001

PROCAINE HYDROCHLORIDE

INJECTABLE; INJECTION

	NOVOCAIN		
AP	+ STERLING WINTHROP	1%	N85362 003
AP	+	2%	N85362 004
	+	10%	N86797 001
	PROCAINE HCL		
AP	ABBOTT	1%	N80416 001
AP		2%	N80416 002
AP	ELKINS SINN	1%	N83315 001
AP		2%	N83315 002
AP	FUJISAWA	1%	N80384 002
AP		1%	N80421 001
AP		2%	N80384 003
AP		2%	N80421 002
AP	STERIS	1%	N80658 001
AP		1%	N83535 001
AP		2%	N80658 002
AP		2%	N83535 002

PROCAINE HYDROCHLORIDE; *MULTIPLE*

SEE NOREPINEPHRINE BITARTRATE; PROCAINE HYDROCHLORIDE; PROPOXYCAINE HYDROCHLORIDE

PROCAINE HYDROCHLORIDE; TETRACYCLINE HYDROCHLORIDE

INJECTABLE; INJECTION

	TETRACYN		
	PFIZER	40 MG/VIAL;250 MG/VIAL	N60285 003

PROCARBAZINE HYDROCHLORIDE

CAPSULE; ORAL

	MATULANE		
	+ ROCHE	EQ 50 MG BASE	N16785 001

PROCHLORPERAZINE

SUPPOSITORY; RECTAL

	COMPAZINE		
AB	+ SMITHKLINE BEECHAM	25 MG	N11127 002
		2.5 MG	N11127 003
		5 MG	N11127 001
	PROCHLORPERAZINE		
AB	G AND W LABS	25 MG	N40058 001 NOV 24, 1993

PROCHLORPERAZINE EDISYLATE

INJECTABLE; INJECTION

	COMPAZINE		
AP	+ SMITHKLINE BEECHAM	EQ 5 MG BASE/ML	N10742 002
	PROCHLORPERAZINE		
AP	ELKINS SINN	EQ 5 MG BASE/ML	N87759 001 OCT 01, 1982
	PROCHLORPERAZINE EDISYLATE		
AP	ELKINS SINN	EQ 5 MG BASE/ML	N89903 001 AUG 29, 1989
AP	MARSAM	EQ 5 MG BASE/ML	N89675 001 DEC 05, 1988
AP	SMITH AND NEPHEW	EQ 5 MG BASE/ML	N89251 001 DEC 04, 1986
AP	STERIS	EQ 5 MG BASE/ML	N89530 001 JUL 08, 1987
AP		EQ 5 MG BASE/ML	N89605 001 JUL 08, 1987
AP		EQ 5 MG BASE/ML	N89606 001 JUL 08, 1987
AP	STERLING WINTHROP	EQ 5 MG BASE/ML	N89703 001 APR 07, 1988
AP	WYETH AYERST	EQ 5 MG BASE/ML	N86348 001

SYRUP; ORAL

	COMPAZINE		
	SMITHKLINE BEECHAM	EQ 5 MG BASE/5 ML	N11188 001

PROCHLORPERAZINE MALEATE

CAPSULE, EXTENDED RELEASE; ORAL

	COMPAZINE		
	SMITHKLINE BEECHAM	EQ 10 MG BASE	N11000 001
		EQ 15 MG BASE	N11000 002
		EQ 30 MG BASE	N11000 003

Prescription Drug Products *(continued)*

PROCHLORPERAZINE MALEATE *(continued)*

TABLET; ORAL
COMPAZINE
SMITHKLINE

	BEECHAM	EQ 5 MG BASE	N10571 001
		EQ 10 MG BASE	N10571 002
	+	EQ 25 MG BASE	N10571 003

PROCYCLIDINE HYDROCHLORIDE

TABLET; ORAL
KEMADRIN
BURROUGHS

	WELLCOME	5 MG	N09818 003

PROGESTERONE

INJECTABLE; INJECTION
PROGESTERONE

AO	+ LILLY	50 MG/ML	N09238 001
AO	STERIS	50 MG/ML	N17362 002

INSERT, EXTENDED RELEASE; INTRAUTERINE
PROGESTASERT

	ALZA	38 MG	N17553 001

PROMAZINE HYDROCHLORIDE

INJECTABLE; INJECTION

	PROMAZINE HCL		
AP	STERIS	50 MG/ML	N84517 001
		25 MG/ML	N84510 001
	SPARINE		
AP	+ WYETH AYERST	50 MG/ML	N10349 006

TABLET; ORAL
SPARINE

	WYETH AYERST	25 MG	N10348 001
		50 MG	N10348 002
		100 MG	N10348 003

PROMETHAZINE HYDROCHLORIDE

INJECTABLE; INJECTION
PHENERGAN

AP	+ WYETH AYERST	25 MG/ML	N08857 002
AP	+	50 MG/ML	N08857 003

PROMETHAZINE HYDROCHLORIDE *(continued)*

INJECTABLE; INJECTION

	PROMETHAZINE HCL		
AP	AKORN	25 MG/ML	N83955 002
AP		50 MG/ML	N83955 001
AP	ELKINS SINN	25 MG/ML	N83312 001
AP		50 MG/ML	N83312 002
AP	MARSAM	25 MG/ML	N89463 001 MAY 02, 1988
AP		50 MG/ML	N89477 001 MAY 02, 1988
AP	STERIS	25 MG/ML	N83532 001
AP		25 MG/ML	N84591 001
AP		50 MG/ML	N80629 002
AP		50 MG/ML	N83532 002
AP	STERLING WINTHROP	50 MG/ML	N83838 002

SUPPOSITORY; RECTAL

	PHENERGAN		
BR	WYETH AYERST	25 MG	N10926 001
BR	+	50 MG	N11689 001
		12.5 MG	N10926 002
	PROMETHACON		
BR	POLYMEDICA	25 MG	N84901 001
BR		50 MG	N84902 001
	PROMETHEGAN		
BR	G AND W LABS	50 MG	N87165 001 AUG 14, 1987

SYRUP; ORAL

	PHENERGAN FORTIS		
AA	WYETH AYERST	25 MG/5 ML	N08381 003
	PHENERGAN PLAIN		
AA	WYETH AYERST	6.25 MG/5 ML	N08381 004 APR 18, 1984
	PROMETH		
AA	BARRE	6.25 MG/5 ML	N85953 001
AA		25 MG/5 ML	N84772 001
	PROMETHAZINE		
AA	CENCI	6.25 MG/5 ML	N89013 001 SEP 20, 1985
	PROMETHAZINE HCL		
AA	WHITEWORTH TOWNE	6.25 MG/5 ML	N86395 001
	PROMETHAZINE PLAIN		
AA	PENNEX	6.25 MG/5 ML	N87953 001 NOV 15, 1982

Prescription Drug Products *(continued)*

PROMETHAZINE HYDROCHLORIDE *(continued)*

TABLET; ORAL

	PHENERGAN		
BP	WYETH AYERST	12.5 MG	N07935 002
BP		25 MG	N07935 003
BP	+	50 MG	N07935 004
	PROMETHAZINE HCL		
BP	DANBURY PHARMA	12.5 MG	N83712 001
BP		25 MG	N83426 001
BP		50 MG	N83711 001
BP	GENEVA PHARMS	25 MG	N84234 001
BP		50 MG	N84176 001
BP	GLOBAL PHARMS	25 MG	N84214 002 JUL 07, 1982
BP	LANNETT	12.5 MG	N80949 001
BP		25 MG	N80949 002
BP		50 MG	N80949 003
BP	PRIVATE FORM	25 MG	N83658 001
BP	ZENITH LABS	12.5 MG	N83604 001
BP		25 MG	N83603 001

PROMETHAZINE HYDROCHLORIDE; *MULTIPLE*

SEE CODEINE PHOSPHATE; PHENYLEPHRINE HYDROCHLORIDE; PROMETHAZINE HYDROCHLORIDE

SEE CODEINE PHOSPHATE; PROMETHAZINE HYDROCHLORIDE

SEE DEXTROMETHORPHAN HYDROBROMIDE; PROMETHAZINE HYDROCHLORIDE

SEE MEPERIDINE HYDROCHLORIDE; PROMETHAZINE HYDROCHLORIDE

SEE PHENYLEPHRINE HYDROCHLORIDE; PROMETHAZINE HYDROCHLORIDE

PROPAFENONE HYDROCHLORIDE

TABLET; ORAL

	RYTHMOL		
	KNOLL PHARM	150 MG	N19151 001 NOV 27, 1989
		225 MG	N19151 003 NOV 20, 1992
	+	300 MG	N19151 002 NOV 27, 1989

PROPANTHELINE BROMIDE

TABLET; ORAL

	PRO-BANTHINE		
AA	ROBERTS LABS	7.5 MG	N08732 003
AA		15 MG	N08732 002
	PROPANTHELINE BROMIDE		
AA	DANBURY PHARMA	15 MG	N83029 002
AA	GLOBAL PHARMS	15 MG	N84541 002
AA	PAR PHARM	15 MG	N88377 001 DEC 08, 1983
AA	ROXANE	7.5 MG	N80927 001
AA		15 MG	N80927 002
AA	TABLICAPS	15 MG	N84428 001

PROPARACAINE HYDROCHLORIDE

SOLUTION/DROPS; OPHTHALMIC

	ALCAINE		
AT	ALCON	0.5%	N80027 001
	OPHTHAINE		
AT	+ SQUIBB	0.5%	N08883 001
	OPHTHETIC		
AT	ALLERGAN	0.5%	N12583 001
	PARACAINE		
AT	OPTOPICS	0.5%	N87681 001 AUG 05, 1982

PROPIOLACTONE

SOLUTION; IRRIGATION

	BETAPRONE		
	FOREST LABS	N/A	N11657 001

PROPIOMAZINE HYDROCHLORIDE

INJECTABLE; INJECTION

	LARGON		
	+ WYETH AYERST	20 MG/ML	N12382 002

PROPOFOL

INJECTABLE; INJECTION

	DIPRIVAN		
	+ ZENECA	10 MG/ML	N19627 001 OCT 02, 1989

PROPOXYCAINE HYDROCHLORIDE; *MULTIPLE*

SEE NOREPINEPHRINE BITARTRATE; PROCAINE HYDROCHLORIDE; PROPOXYCAINE HYDROCHLORIDE

Prescription Drug Products *(continued)*

PROPOXYPHENE HYDROCHLORIDE
CAPSULE; ORAL
DARVON
AA LILLY 32 MG N10997 001
AA 65 MG N10997 003
DOLENE
AA LEDERLE 65 MG N80530 001
KESSO-GESIC
AA MK LABS 65 MG N83544 001
PROPHENE 65
AA HALSEY 65 MG N83538 002
PROPOXYPHENE HCL
AA DANBURY PHARMA 65 MG N80908 002
AA GENEVA PHARMS 65 MG N83125 002
AA GLOBAL PHARMS 65 MG N83317 001
AA ICN 65 MG N80783 001
AA LEMMON 65 MG N88615 001 OCT 22, 1984
AA MYLAN 32 MG N83528 001
AA PUREPAC PHARM 65 MG N83278 001
AA ROXANE 32 MG N83089 001
AA 65 MG N83089 002
AA WEST WARD PHARM 65 MG N83501 001
AA WHITEWORTH TOWNE 65 MG N84551 001
AA ZENITH LABS 32 MG N83597 001
AA 65 MG N80269 001

PROPOXYPHENE HYDROCHLORIDE; *MULTIPLE*
SEE ACETAMINOPHEN; PROPOXYPHENE HYDROCHLORIDE
SEE ASPIRIN; CAFFEINE; PROPOXYPHENE HYDROCHLORIDE
SEE ASPIRIN; PROPOXYPHENE HYDROCHLORIDE

PROPOXYPHENE NAPSYLATE
SUSPENSION; ORAL
DARVON-N
+ LILLY 50 MG/5 ML N16861 001
TABLET; ORAL
DARVON-N
+ LILLY 100 MG N16862 002

PROPOXYPHENE NAPSYLATE; *MULTIPLE*
SEE ACETAMINOPHEN; PROPOXYPHENE NAPSYLATE

PROPRANOLOL HYDROCHLORIDE
CAPSULE, EXTENDED RELEASE; ORAL
INDERAL LA
AB + WYETH AYERST 60 MG N18553 004 MAR 18, 1987
AB + 80 MG N18553 002 APR 19, 1983
AB + 120 MG N18553 003 APR 19, 1983
AB + 160 MG N18553 001 APR 19, 1983
PROPRANOLOL HCL
AB INWOOD LABS 60 MG N72499 001 APR 11, 1989
AB 80 MG N72500 001 APR 11, 1989
AB 120 MG N72501 001 APR 11, 1989
AB 160 MG N72502 001 APR 11, 1989
CONCENTRATE; ORAL
PROPRANOLOL HCL INTENSOL
ROXANE 80 MG/ML N71388 001 MAY 15, 1987
INJECTABLE; INJECTION
INDERAL
AP + WYETH AYERST 1 MG/ML N16419 001
PROPRANOLOL HCL
AP SMITH AND NEPHEW 1 MG/ML N70137 001 APR 15, 1986
AP SOLOPAK 1 MG/ML N70136 001 APR 15, 1986
SOLUTION; ORAL
PROPRANOLOL HCL
ROXANE 20 MG/5 ML N70979 001 MAY 15, 1987
40 MG/5 ML N70690 001 MAY 15, 1987
TABLET; ORAL
INDERAL
AB + WYETH AYERST 10 MG N16418 001
AB 20 MG N16418 003
AB 40 MG N16418 002
AB 60 MG N16418 009 OCT 18, 1982
AB + 80 MG N16418 004

Prescription Drug Products *(continued)*

PROPRANOLOL HYDROCHLORIDE *(continued)*

TABLET; ORAL

PROPRANOLOL HCL

AB	BARR	10 MG	N70319 001 OCT 22, 1985
AB		20 MG	N70320 001 OCT 22, 1985
AB		40 MG	N70103 001 OCT 22, 1985
AB		60 MG	N70321 001 SEP 24, 1986
AB		80 MG	N70322 001 AUG 04, 1986
AB	DANBURY PHARMA	10 MG	N70175 001 MAY 13, 1986
AB		20 MG	N70176 001 MAY 13, 1986
AB		40 MG	N70177 001 MAY 13, 1986
AB		60 MG	N71098 001 OCT 06, 1986
AB		80 MG	N70178 001 MAY 13, 1986
AB	GENEVA PHARMS	10 MG	N70663 001 JUN 13, 1986
AB		20 MG	N70664 001 JUN 13, 1986
AB		40 MG	N70665 001 JUN 13, 1986
AB		60 MG	N70666 001 OCT 10, 1986
AB		80 MG	N70667 001 JUN 13, 1986
AB	INTERPHARM	10 MG	N71368 001 MAY 05, 1987
AB		20 MG	N71369 001 MAY 05, 1987
AB		40 MG	N71370 001 MAY 05, 1987
AB		80 MG	N71371 001 MAY 05, 1987
AB	INVAMED	10 MG	N71658 001 JUL 05, 1988
AB		20 MG	N71687 001 JUL 05, 1988
AB		40 MG	N71688 001 JUL 05, 1988
AB		60 MG	N72197 001 JUL 05, 1988
AB		80 MG	N71689 001 JUL 05, 1988
AB		90 MG	N72198 001 JUL 05, 1988

PROPRANOLOL HYDROCHLORIDE *(continued)*

TABLET; ORAL

PROPRANOLOL HCL

AB	LEDERLE	10 MG	N70125 001 JUL 30, 1985
AB		20 MG	N70126 001 JUL 30, 1985
AB		40 MG	N70127 001 JUL 30, 1985
AB		60 MG	N71495 001 DEC 31, 1987
AB		80 MG	N70128 001 JUL 30, 1985
AB		90 MG	N71496 001 DEC 31, 1987
AB	LEMMON	40 MG	N70234 001 JUN 23, 1986
AB	MYLAN	10 MG	N70211 001 NOV 19, 1985
AB		20 MG	N70212 001 NOV 19, 1985
AB		40 MG	N70213 001 NOV 19, 1985
AB		80 MG	N70214 001 NOV 19, 1985
AB	PAR PHARM	10 MG	N70217 001 AUG 01, 1986
AB		20 MG	N70218 001 AUG 01, 1986
AB		40 MG	N70219 001 AUG 01, 1986
AB		60 MG	N70220 001 SEP 24, 1986
AB		80 MG	N70221 001 APR 14, 1986
AB		90 MG	N71288 001 OCT 22, 1986
AB	PARKE DAVIS	20 MG	N70439 001 SEP 15, 1986
AB		40 MG	N70440 001 SEP 15, 1986
AB		60 MG	N70441 001 SEP 24, 1986
AB		80 MG	N70442 001 SEP 15, 1986

Prescription Drug Products *(continued)*

PROPRANOLOL HYDROCHLORIDE *(continued)*

TABLET; ORAL
PROPRANOLOL HCL

AB	PUREPAC PHARM	10 MG	N70814 001 NOV 03, 1986
AB		20 MG	N70815 001 NOV 03, 1986
AB		40 MG	N70816 001 NOV 03, 1986
AB		60 MG	N70817 001 NOV 03, 1986
AB		80 MG	N70757 001 NOV 03, 1986
AB	ROXANE	10 MG	N70516 001 JUL 07, 1986
AB		20 MG	N70517 001 JUL 07, 1986
AB		40 MG	N70518 001 JUL 07, 1986
AB		60 MG	N70519 001 SEP 24, 1986
AB		80 MG	N70520 001 JUL 07, 1986
AB		90 MG	N70521 001 SEP 24, 1986
AB	SIDMAK LABS NJ	10 MG	N71972 001 APR 06, 1988
AB		20 MG	N71973 001 APR 06, 1988
AB		40 MG	N71974 001 APR 06, 1988
AB		60 MG	N71975 001 APR 06, 1988
AB		80 MG	N71976 001 APR 06, 1988
AB		90 MG	N71977 001 APR 06, 1988
AB	WARNER CHILCOTT	10 MG	N70438 001 SEP 15, 1986
AB	WATSON LABS	10 MG	N70548 001 JUL 10, 1986
AB		20 MG	N70549 001 APR 11, 1986
AB		40 MG	N70550 001 APR 11, 1986
AB		60 MG	N71791 001 JUL 15, 1987
AB		80 MG	N70551 001 JUL 10, 1986
AB		90 MG	N71792 001 JUL 15, 1987

PROPRANOLOL HYDROCHLORIDE *(continued)*

TABLET; ORAL
PROPRANOLOL HCL

AB	ZENITH LABS	10 MG	N72063 001 JUL 29, 1988
AB		20 MG	N72066 001 JUL 29, 1988
AB		40 MG	N72067 001 JUL 29, 1988
AB		80 MG	N72069 001 JUL 29, 1988

PROPRANOLOL HYDROCHLORIDE; *MULTIPLE*

SEE HYDROCHLOROTHIAZIDE; PROPRANOLOL HYDROCHLORIDE

PROPYLTHIOURACIL

TABLET; ORAL
PROPYLTHIOURACIL

BD	BARR	50 MG	N83982 001
BD	GLOBAL PHARMS	50 MG	N80159 001
BD	HALSEY	50 MG	N80015 001
BD	+ LEDERLE	50 MG	N06188 001
BD	LILLY	50 MG	N06213 001
BD	PUREPAC PHARM	50 MG	N80172 001
BD	WEST WARD PHARM	50 MG	N80154 001

PROTAMINE SULFATE

INJECTABLE; INJECTION
PROTAMINE SULFATE

AP	ELKINS SINN	10 MG/ML	N89474 001 NOV 05, 1986
AP		10 MG/ML	N89475 001 NOV 05, 1986
AP	FUJISAWA	10 MG/ML	N89454 001 APR 07, 1987
AP	+ LILLY	10 MG/ML	N06460 002

PROTIRELIN

INJECTABLE; INJECTION

	THYPINONE		
AP	+ ABBOTT	0.5 MG/ML	N17638 001
	THYREL TRH		
AP	FERRING LABS	0.5 MG/ML	N18087 001

PROTOKYLOL HYDROCHLORIDE

TABLET; ORAL
VENTAIRE

	MARION MERRELL DOW	2 MG	N83459 001

Prescription Drug Products *(continued)*

PROTRIPTYLINE HYDROCHLORIDE

TABLET; ORAL

	VIVACTIL		
	MERCK SHARP DOHME	5 MG	N16012 001
	+	10 MG	N16012 002

PSEUDOEPHEDRINE HYDROCHLORIDE

CAPSULE, EXTENDED RELEASE; ORAL

	NOVAFED		
	DOW PHARMS	120 MG	N17603 001

PSEUDOEPHEDRINE HYDROCHLORIDE; *MULTIPLE*

SEE ACRIVASTINE; PSEUDOEPHEDRINE HYDROCHLORIDE

SEE BROMPHENIRAMINE MALEATE; DEXTROMETHORPHAN HYDROBROMIDE; PSEUDOEPHEDRINE HYDROCHLORIDE

SEE CODEINE PHOSPHATE; PSEUDOEPHEDRINE HYDROCHLORIDE; TRIPROLIDINE HYDROCHLORIDE

PSEUDOEPHEDRINE HYDROCHLORIDE; TERFENADINE

TABLET, EXTENDED RELEASE; ORAL

	SELDANE-D		
	MERRELL DOW	120 MG;60 MG	N19664 001 AUG 19, 1991

PSEUDOEPHEDRINE HYDROCHLORIDE; TRIPROLIDINE HYDROCHLORIDE

SYRUP; ORAL

	ACTAHIST		
AA	CENCI	30 MG/5 ML;1.25 MG/5 ML	N88344 001 FEB 09, 1984
	TRILITRON		
AA	NEWTRON PHARMS	30 MG/5 ML;1.25 MG/5 ML	N88474 001 FEB 12, 1985

TABLET; ORAL

	CORPHED		
AA	GENEVA PHARMS	60 MG;2.5 MG	N88602 001 APR 11, 1985
	PSEUDOEPHEDRINE HCL AND TRIPROLIDINE HCL		
AA	EON LABS	60 MG;2.5 MG	N88193 001 MAY 17, 1983
	TRILITRON		
AA	NEWTRON PHARMS	60 MG;2.5 MG	N88515 001 JAN 09, 1985
	TRIPHED		
AA	LEMMON	60 MG;2.5 MG	N88630 001 MAY 17, 1984

PSEUDOEPHEDRINE HYDROCHLORIDE; TRIPROLIDINE HYDROCHLORIDE *(continued)*

TABLET; ORAL

	TRIPROLIDINE HCL AND PSEUDOEPHEDRINE HCL		
AA	SUPERPHARM	60 MG;2.5 MG	N88578 001 FEB 21, 1985
AA	ZENITH LABS	60 MG;2.5 MG	N85273 001 DEC 12, 1984

PSEUDOEPHEDRINE SULFATE; *MULTIPLE*

SEE AZATADINE MALEATE; PSEUDOEPHEDRINE SULFATE

PYRAZINAMIDE

TABLET; ORAL

	PYRAZINAMIDE		
AB	+ LEDERLE	500 MG	N80157 001
AB	MIKART	500 MG	N81319 001 JUN 30, 1992

PYRAZINAMIDE; *MULTIPLE*

SEE ISONIAZID; PYRAZINAMIDE; RIFAMPIN

PYRIDOSTIGMINE BROMIDE

INJECTABLE; INJECTION

	MESTINON		
AP	+ ROCHE	5 MG/ML	N09830 001
	REGONOL		
AP	ORGANON	5 MG/ML	N17398 001

SYRUP; ORAL

	MESTINON		
	ROCHE	60 MG/5 ML	N15193 001

TABLET; ORAL

	MESTINON		
	+ ROCHE	60 MG	N09829 002

TABLET, EXTENDED RELEASE; ORAL

	MESTINON		
	+ ROCHE	180 MG	N11665 001

PYRIDOXINE; *MULTIPLE*

SEE ASCORBIC ACID; BIOTIN; CYANOCOBALAMIN; ERGOCALCIFEROL; FOLIC ACID; NIACINAMIDE; PANTOTHENIC ACID; PHYTONADIONE; PYRIDOXINE; RIBOFLAVIN; THIAMINE; VITAMIN A PALMITATE; VITAMIN E

Prescription Drug Products *(continued)*

PYRIDOXINE HYDROCHLORIDE

INJECTABLE; INJECTION

	PYRIDOXINE HCL		
AP	AKORN	100 MG/ML	N87967 001 OCT 01, 1982
AP	DELL LABS	100 MG/ML	N83772 001
		50 MG/ML	N83771 001
AP	FUJISAWA	100 MG/ML	N80618 001
AP	+ STERIS	100 MG/ML	N80572 001
AP		100 MG/ML	N83760 001

PYRIDOXINE HYDROCHLORIDE; *MULTIPLE*

SEE ASCORBIC ACID; BIOTIN; CYANOCOBALAMIN; DEXPANTHENOL; ERGOCALCIFEROL; FOLIC ACID; NIACINAMIDE; PYRIDOXINE HYDROCHLORIDE; RIBOFLAVIN PHOSPHATE SODIUM; THIAMINE HYDROCHLORIDE; VITAMIN A; VITAMIN E

PYRILAMINE MALEATE

TABLET; ORAL

	PYRILAMINE MALEATE		
	GLOBAL PHARMS	25 MG	N80808 001

PYRILAMINE MALEATE; *MULTIPLE*

SEE PHENYLEPHRINE HYDROCHLORIDE; PYRILAMINE MALEATE

PYRIMETHAMINE

TABLET; ORAL

	DARAPRIM		
	BURROUGHS WELLCOME	25 MG	N08578 001

PYRIMETHAMINE; SULFADOXINE

TABLET; ORAL

	FANSIDAR		
	+ ROCHE	25 MG;500 MG	N18557 001

QUAZEPAM

TABLET; ORAL

	DORAL		
	WALLACE	7.5 MG	N18708 003 FEB 26, 1987
	+	15 MG	N18708 001 DEC 27, 1985

QUINAPRIL HYDROCHLORIDE

TABLET; ORAL

	ACCUPRIL		
	PARKE DAVIS	EQ 5 MG BASE	N19885 001 NOV 19, 1991
		EQ 10 MG BASE	N19885 002 NOV 19, 1991
		EQ 20 MG BASE	N19885 003 NOV 19, 1991
		EQ 40 MG BASE	N19885 004 NOV 19, 1991

QUINESTROL

TABLET; ORAL

	ESTROVIS		
	PARKE DAVIS	0.1 MG	N16768 002

QUINETHAZONE

TABLET; ORAL

	HYDROMOX		
	LEDERLE	50 MG	N13264 001

QUINIDINE GLUCONATE

INJECTABLE; INJECTION

	QUINIDINE GLUCONATE		
	+ LILLY	80 MG/ML	N07529 002 FEB 10, 1989

TABLET, EXTENDED RELEASE; ORAL

	QUINAGLUTE		
AB	+ BERLEX	324 MG	N16647 001
	QUINALAN		
BC	LANNETT	324 MG	N88081 001 FEB 10, 1986
	QUINIDINE GLUCONATE		
AB	DANBURY PHARMA	324 MG	N87810 001 SEP 29, 1982
AB	GENEVA PHARMS	324 MG	N89894 001 DEC 15, 1988
AB	HALSEY	324 MG	N89476 001 APR 10, 1987
AB	MUTUAL PHARM	324 MG	N89338 001 FEB 11, 1987

QUINIDINE POLYGALACTURONATE

TABLET; ORAL

	CARDIOQUIN		
	PURDUE FREDERICK	275 MG	N11642 002

Prescription Drug Products *(continued)*

QUINIDINE SULFATE

	CAPSULE; ORAL		
	CIN-QUIN		
AB	SOLVAY	200 MG	N85296 001
		300 MG	N85297 001
	QUINIDINE SULFATE		
AB	+ LILLY	200 MG	N85103 001
	TABLET; ORAL		
	QUINIDINE SULFATE		
AB	BARR	200 MG	N84177 001
AB	CHELSEA LABS	200 MG	N85140 002
AB	DANBURY PHARMA	100 MG	N85584 001
AB		200 MG	N83288 001
AB		300 MG	N85583 001
AB	EON LABS	200 MG	N84631 001
AB		300 MG	N88072 001 SEP 26, 1983
AB	GENEVA PHARMS	200 MG	N84914 001
AB		300 MG	N89839 001 SEP 29, 1988
AB	GLOBAL PHARMS	200 MG	N83347 001
AB	HALSEY	200 MG	N83583 001
AB	ICN	200 MG	N83393 001
AB	KV PHARM	200 MG	N85276 001
AB	LANNETT	200 MG	N83743 001
AB	LEDERLE	200 MG	N87011 001
AB	+ LILLY	200 MG	N85038 001
AB	MUTUAL PHARM	100 MG	N81029 001 APR 14, 1989
AB		200 MG	N81030 001 APR 14, 1989
AB		300 MG	N81031 001 APR 14, 1989
AB	PHARMAVITE	200 MG	N84627 001
AB	PHOENIX LABS NY	200 MG	N83963 001
AB	PRIVATE FORM	200 MG	N83808 001
AB	PUREPAC PHARM	200 MG	N84003 001
AB	ROXANE	200 MG	N83640 001
AB		300 MG	N85632 001
AB	SMITHKLINE BEECHAM	200 MG	N85175 001
AB	SUPERPHARM	200 MG	N88973 001 APR 10, 1985
AB	WEST WARD PHARM	200 MG	N83862 001
AB	ZENITH LABS	200 MG	N84549 001
AB	1ST TX	200 MG	N85068 001
	QUINORA		
AB	+ KEY PHARMS	300 MG	N85222 001

QUINIDINE SULFATE *(continued)*

	TABLET, EXTENDED RELEASE; ORAL		
	QUINIDEX		
AB	+ ROBINS AH	300 MG	N12796 002
	QUINIDINE SULFATE		
AB	COPLEY PHARM	300 MG	N40045 001 JUN 30, 1994

RAMIPRIL

	CAPSULE; ORAL		
	ALTACE		
	HOECHST ROUSSEL	1.25 MG	N19901 001 JAN 28, 1991
		2.5 MG	N19901 002 JAN 28, 1991
		5 MG	N19901 003 JAN 28, 1991
	+	10 MG	N19901 004 JAN 28, 1991

RANITIDINE HYDROCHLORIDE

	CAPSULE; ORAL		
	ZANTAC 150		
	GLAXO	EQ 150 MG BASE	N20095 001 MAR 08, 1994
	ZANTAC 300		
	+ GLAXO	EQ 300 MG BASE	N20095 002 MAR 08, 1994
	GRANULE, EFFERVESCENT; ORAL		
	ZANTAC 150		
	+ GLAXO	EQ 150 MG BASE/PACKET	N20251 002 MAR 31, 1994
	INJECTABLE; INJECTION		
	ZANTAC		
	+ GLAXO	EQ 25 MG BASE/ML	N19090 001 OCT 19, 1984
	ZANTAC IN PLASTIC CONTAINER		
	+ GLAXO	EQ 1 MG BASE/ML	N19593 002 SEP 27, 1991
	SYRUP; ORAL		
	ZANTAC		
	GLAXO	EQ 15 MG BASE/ML	N19675 001 DEC 30, 1988

Prescription Drug Products *(continued)*

RANITIDINE HYDROCHLORIDE *(continued)*

TABLET; ORAL
ZANTAC 150
GLAXO EQ 150 MG BASE N18703 001 JUN 09, 1983
ZANTAC 300
+ GLAXO EQ 300 MG BASE N18703 002 DEC 09, 1985
TABLET, EFFERVESCENT; ORAL
ZANTAC 150
+ GLAXO EQ 150 MG BASE N20251 001 MAR 31, 1994

RAUWOLFIA SERPENTINA

TABLET; ORAL
HIWOLFIA
BP BOWMAN PHARMS 50 MG N09276 005
RAUDIXIN
BP APOTHECON 50 MG N08842 001
BP + 100 MG N08842 002
RAUVAL
BP VALE 50 MG N09108 002
BP 100 MG N09108 004
RAUWOLFIA SERPENTINA
BP DANBURY PHARMA 50 MG N80907 001
BP GLOBAL PHARMS 50 MG N09273 001
BP 100 MG N09273 002
BP HALSEY 50 MG N80498 001
BP 100 MG N80498 002

RESCINNAMINE

TABLET; ORAL
MODERIL
PFIZER 0.25 MG N10686 003
0.5 MG N10686 006

RESERPINE

ELIXIR; ORAL
SERPASIL
CIBA 0.2 MG/4 ML N09115 005
TABLET; ORAL
RESERPINE
BP EON LABS 0.1 MG N09838 001
BP 0.25 MG N09838 002
BP GLOBAL PHARMS 0.1 MG N09627 001
BP 0.25 MG N09627 002
BP PUREPAC PHARM 0.1 MG N80753 002
BP 0.25 MG N80753 001
SERPALAN
BP LANNETT 0.1 MG N10124 001
BP 0.25 MG N10124 002
SERPASIL
BP CIBA 0.1 MG N09115 001
BP + 0.25 MG N09115 003
SERPIVITE
BP VITARINE 0.25 MG N09645 002

RESERPINE; *MULTIPLE*

SEE CHLOROTHIAZIDE; RESERPINE
SEE CHLORTHALIDONE; RESERPINE
SEE HYDRALAZINE HYDROCHLORIDE; HYDROCHLOROTHIAZIDE; RESERPINE
SEE HYDROCHLOROTHIAZIDE; RESERPINE
SEE HYDROFLUMETHIAZIDE; RESERPINE
SEE METHYCLOTHIAZIDE; RESERPINE
SEE POLYTHIAZIDE; RESERPINE

RESERPINE; TRICHLORMETHIAZIDE

TABLET; ORAL
METATENSIN #2
MERRELL DOW 0.1 MG;2 MG N12972 001
METATENSIN #4
MERRELL DOW 0.1 MG;4 MG N12972 002

RIBAVIRIN

POWDER FOR RECONSTITUTION; INHALATION
VIRAZOLE
+ VIRATEK 6 GM/VIAL N18859 001 DEC 31, 1985

Prescription Drug Products *(continued)*

RIBOFLAVIN; *MULTIPLE*
SEE ASCORBIC ACID; BIOTIN; CYANOCOBALAMIN; ERGOCALCIFEROL; FOLIC ACID; NIACINAMIDE; PANTOTHENIC ACID; PHYTONADIONE; PYRIDOXINE; RIBOFLAVIN; THIAMINE; VITAMIN A PALMITATE; VITAMIN E

RIBOFLAVIN PHOSPHATE SODIUM; *MULTIPLE*
SEE ASCORBIC ACID; BIOTIN; CYANOCOBALAMIN; DEXPANTHENOL; ERGOCALCIFEROL; FOLIC ACID; NIACINAMIDE; PYRIDOXINE HYDROCHLORIDE; RIBOFLAVIN PHOSPHATE SODIUM; THIAMINE HYDROCHLORIDE; VITAMIN A; VITAMIN E

RIFABUTIN

	CAPSULE; ORAL		
	MYCOBUTIN		
	+ PHARMACIA	150 MG	N50689 001 DEC 23, 1992

RIFAMPIN

	CAPSULE; ORAL		
	RIFADIN		
AB	+ MERRELL DOW	300 MG	N50420 001
		150 MG	N62303 001
	RIMACTANE		
AB	CIBA	300 MG	N50429 001
	INJECTABLE; INJECTION		
	RIFADIN		
	+ MERRELL DOW	600 MG/VIAL	N50627 001 MAY 25, 1989

RIFAMPIN; *MULTIPLE*
SEE ISONIAZID; PYRAZINAMIDE; RIFAMPIN
SEE ISONIAZID; RIFAMPIN

RIMANTADINE HYDROCHLORIDE

	SYRUP; ORAL		
	FLUMADINE		
	+ FOREST LABS	50 MG/5 ML	N19650 001 SEP 17, 1993
	TABLET; ORAL		
	FLUMADINE		
	+ FOREST LABS	100 MG	N19649 001 SEP 17, 1993

RISPERIDONE

	TABLET; ORAL		
	RISPERDAL		
	JANSSEN	1 MG	N20272 001 DEC 29, 1993
		2 MG	N20272 002 DEC 29, 1993
		3 MG	N20272 003 DEC 29, 1993
	+	4 MG	N20272 004 DEC 29, 1993

RITODRINE HYDROCHLORIDE

	INJECTABLE; INJECTION		
	RITODRINE HCL		
AP	ABBOTT	10 MG/ML	N71618 001 FEB 28, 1991
AP		15 MG/ML	N71619 001 FEB 28, 1991
	RITODRINE HCL IN DEXTROSE 5% IN PLASTIC CONTAINER		
	+ ABBOTT	30 MG/100 ML	N71438 001 JAN 22, 1991
	YUTOPAR		
AP	+ ASTRA	10 MG/ML	N18580 001
AP	+	15 MG/ML	N18580 002
	TABLET; ORAL		
	YUTOPAR		
	ASTRA	10 MG	N18555 001

ROCURONIUM BROMIDE

	INJECTABLE; INJECTION		
	ZEMURON		
	+ ORGANON	10 MG/ML	N20214 002 MAR 17, 1994
	ZEMURON (P/F)		
	+ ORGANON	10 MG/ML	N20214 001 MAR 17, 1994

RUBIDIUM CHLORIDE RB-82

	INJECTABLE; INJECTION		
	CARDIOGEN-82		
	BRACCO	N/A	N19414 001 DEC 29, 1989

Prescription Drug Products *(continued)*

SAFFLOWER OIL; SOYBEAN OIL
INJECTABLE; INJECTION

	LIPOSYN II 10%		
	+ ABBOTT	5%;5%	N18997 001 AUG 27, 1984
	LIPOSYN II 20%		
	+ ABBOTT	10%;10%	N18991 001 AUG 27, 1984

SALMETEROL XINAFOATE
AEROSOL, METERED; INHALATION

	SEREVENT		
	+ GLAXO	EQ 0.021 MG BASE/INH	N20236 001 FEB 04, 1994

SCOPOLAMINE
FILM, EXTENDED RELEASE; TRANSDERMAL

	TRANSDERM-SCOP		
	+ CIBA	0.5 MG/24 HR	N17874 001

SECOBARBITAL SODIUM
CAPSULE; ORAL

	SECOBARBITAL SODIUM		
AA	EVERYLIFE	100 MG	N85895 001
AA	ICN	100 MG	N85477 001
AA	ZENITH LABS	100 MG	N85869 001
	SECONAL SODIUM		
AA	LILLY	100 MG	N86101 002 OCT 03, 1983
		50 MG	N86101 001 OCT 03, 1983
	SODIUM SECOBARBITAL		
AA	HALSEY	100 MG	N84676 001
AA	WEST WARD PHARM	100 MG	N84926 001

INJECTABLE; INJECTION

	SECOBARBITAL SODIUM		
	+ ELKINS SINN	100 MG/VIAL	N83281 001
	SODIUM SECOBARBITAL		
	+ WYETH AYERST	50 MG/ML	N83262 001

SECRETIN
INJECTABLE; INJECTION

	SECRETIN-FERRING		
	+ FERRING LABS	75CU/VIAL	N18290 001

SELEGILINE HYDROCHLORIDE
TABLET; ORAL

	ELDEPRYL		
	+ SOMERSET	5 MG	N19334 001 JUN 05, 1989

SELENIUM SULFIDE
LOTION/SHAMPOO; TOPICAL

	EXSEL		
AT	ALLERGAN HERBERT	2.5%	N83892 001
	SELENIUM SULFIDE		
AT	BARRE	2.5%	N84394 001
AT	CLAY PARK	2.5%	N89996 001 JAN 10, 1991
AT	SYOSSET	2.5%	N85777 001
	SELSUN		
AT	+ ABBOTT	2.5%	N07936 001

SELENOMETHIONINE, SE-75
INJECTABLE; INJECTION

	SELENOMETHIONINE SE 75		
	CIS	500uCi/ML	N17322 001

SERMORELIN ACETATE
INJECTABLE; INJECTION

	GEREF		
	+ SERONO	EQ 0.05 MG BASE/AMP	N19863 001 DEC 28, 1990

SERTRALINE HYDROCHLORIDE
TABLET; ORAL

	ZOLOFT		
	PFIZER	EQ 50 MG BASE	N19839 001 DEC 30, 1991
		EQ 100 MG BASE	N19839 002 DEC 30, 1991

SILVER SULFADIAZINE

CREAM; TOPICAL

	SILVADENE		
AB	+ MARION MERRELL DOW	1%	N17381 001
	SSD		
AB	BOOTS	1%	N18578 001 FEB 25, 1982
	THERMAZENE		
AB	SHERWOOD MEDCL	1%	N18810 001 DEC 23, 1985

SIMVASTATIN

TABLET; ORAL

ZOCOR		
MERCK	5 MG	N19766 001 DEC 23, 1991
	10 MG	N19766 002 DEC 23, 1991
	20 MG	N19766 003 DEC 23, 1991
	40 MG	N19766 004 DEC 23, 1991

SINCALIDE

INJECTABLE; INJECTION

KINEVAC		
+ BRACCO	0.005 MG/VIAL	N17697 001

SODIUM ACETATE; *MULTIPLE*

SEE AMINO ACIDS; CALCIUM ACETATE; GLYCERIN; MAGNESIUM ACETATE; PHOSPHORIC ACID; POTASSIUM CHLORIDE; SODIUM ACETATE; SODIUM CHLORIDE

SEE AMINO ACIDS; MAGNESIUM ACETATE; PHOSPHORIC ACID; POTASSIUM ACETATE; POTASSIUM CHLORIDE; SODIUM ACETATE

SEE AMINO ACIDS; MAGNESIUM ACETATE; PHOSPHORIC ACID; POTASSIUM CHLORIDE; SODIUM ACETATE; SODIUM CHLORIDE

SEE AMINO ACIDS; MAGNESIUM CHLORIDE; POTASSIUM PHOSPHATE, DIBASIC; SODIUM ACETATE; SODIUM CHLORIDE

SEE CALCIUM CHLORIDE; DEXTROSE; MAGNESIUM CHLORIDE; POTASSIUM CHLORIDE; SODIUM ACETATE; SODIUM CHLORIDE

SODIUM ACETATE; *MULTIPLE* *(continued)*

SEE CALCIUM CHLORIDE; DEXTROSE; MAGNESIUM CHLORIDE; POTASSIUM CHLORIDE; SODIUM ACETATE; SODIUM CHLORIDE; SODIUM CITRATE

SEE CALCIUM CHLORIDE; DEXTROSE; MAGNESIUM CHLORIDE; SODIUM ACETATE; SODIUM CHLORIDE

SEE CALCIUM CHLORIDE; DEXTROSE; MAGNESIUM CHLORIDE; POTASSIUM CHLORIDE; SODIUM ACETATE; SODIUM CHLORIDE; SODIUM LACTATE

SEE CALCIUM CHLORIDE; DEXTROSE; POTASSIUM CHLORIDE; SODIUM ACETATE; SODIUM CHLORIDE

SEE CALCIUM CHLORIDE; MAGNESIUM CHLORIDE; POTASSIUM CHLORIDE; SODIUM ACETATE; SODIUM CHLORIDE; SODIUM CITRATE

SEE CALCIUM CHLORIDE; MAGNESIUM CHLORIDE; POTASSIUM CHLORIDE; SODIUM ACETATE; SODIUM CHLORIDE

SEE CALCIUM CHLORIDE; MAGNESIUM CHLORIDE; POTASSIUM CHLORIDE; SODIUM ACETATE; SODIUM CHLORIDE; SODIUM LACTATE

SEE DEXTROSE; MAGNESIUM CHLORIDE; POTASSIUM CHLORIDE; SODIUM ACETATE; SODIUM CHLORIDE

SEE DEXTROSE; MAGNESIUM CHLORIDE; POTASSIUM CHLORIDE; SODIUM ACETATE; SODIUM CHLORIDE; SODIUM GLUCONATE

SEE DEXTROSE; MAGNESIUM CHLORIDE; POTASSIUM CHLORIDE; POTASSIUM PHOSPHATE, DIBASIC; SODIUM ACETATE

SEE DEXTROSE; MAGNESIUM CHLORIDE; POTASSIUM CHLORIDE; SODIUM ACETATE; SODIUM CHLORIDE; SODIUM GLUCONATE

SEE DEXTROSE; POTASSIUM CHLORIDE; POTASSIUM PHOSPHATE, DIBASIC; SODIUM ACETATE; SODIUM CHLORIDE

SEE MAGNESIUM CHLORIDE; POTASSIUM CHLORIDE; POTASSIUM PHOSPHATE, MONOBASIC; SODIUM ACETATE; SODIUM CHLORIDE; SODIUM GLUCONATE; SODIUM PHOSPHATE, DIBASIC

SEE MAGNESIUM CHLORIDE; POTASSIUM CHLORIDE; SODIUM ACETATE; SODIUM CHLORIDE; SODIUM GLUCONATE

SODIUM ACETATE, ANHYDROUS

INJECTABLE; INJECTION

SODIUM ACETATE IN PLASTIC CONTAINER		
+ ABBOTT	2 MEQ/ML	N18893 001 MAY 04, 1983

Prescription Drug Products *(continued)*

SODIUM BENZOATE; SODIUM PHENYLACETATE

SOLUTION; ORAL

	UCEPHAN		
	+ MCGAW	100 MG/ML;100 MG/ML	N19530 001 DEC 23, 1987

SODIUM BICARBONATE; *MULTIPLE*

SEE CALCIUM CHLORIDE; DEXTROSE; GLUTATHIONE DISULFIDE; MAGNESIUM CHLORIDE; POTASSIUM CHLORIDE; SODIUM BICARBONATE; SODIUM CHLORIDE; SODIUM PHOSPHATE

SEE POLYETHYLENE GLYCOL 3350; POTASSIUM CHLORIDE; SODIUM BICARBONATE; SODIUM CHLORIDE; SODIUM SULFATE, ANHYDROUS

SEE POLYETHYLENE GLYCOL 3350; POTASSIUM CHLORIDE; SODIUM BICARBONATE; SODIUM CHLORIDE

SEE POLYETHYLENE GLYCOL 3350; POTASSIUM CHLORIDE; SODIUM BICARBONATE; SODIUM CHLORIDE; SODIUM SULFATE

SEE POLYETHYLENE GLYCOL 3350; POTASSIUM CHLORIDE; SODIUM BICARBONATE; SODIUM CHLORIDE; SODIUM SULFATE, ANHYDROUS

SODIUM BICARBONATE; TARTARIC ACID

GRANULE, EFFERVESCENT; ORAL

	BAROS		
	LAFAYETTE PHARMS	460 MG/GM;420 MG/GM	N18509 001 AUG 07, 1985

SODIUM CARBONATE; *MULTIPLE*

SEE CITRIC ACID; MAGNESIUM OXIDE; SODIUM CARBONATE

SODIUM CHLORIDE

INJECTABLE; INJECTION

	BACTERIOSTATIC SODIUM CHLORIDE 0.9% IN PLASTIC CONTAINER		
AP	ABBOTT	9 MG/ML	N18800 001 OCT 29, 1982
AP	FUJISAWA	9 MG/ML	N88911 001 FEB 07, 1985
	SODIUM CHLORIDE		
	MCGAW	20 GM/100 ML	N17038 001
	SODIUM CHLORIDE IN PLASTIC CONTAINER		
	ABBOTT	2.5 MEQ/ML	N18897 001 JUL 20, 1984

SODIUM CHLORIDE *(continued)*

INJECTABLE; INJECTION

	SODIUM CHLORIDE 0.45% IN PLASTIC CONTAINER		
AP	ABBOTT	450 MG/100 ML	N18090 001
AP		450 MG/100 ML	N19759 001 JUN 08, 1988
AP	BAXTER	450 MG/100 ML	N18016 001
AP	MCGAW	450 MG/100 ML	N18184 001
AP		450 MG/100 ML	N19635 001 MAR 09, 1988
	SODIUM CHLORIDE 0.9% IN PLASTIC CONTAINER		
AP	ABBOTT	900 MG/100 ML	N16366 001
AP		9 MG/ML	N18803 001 OCT 29, 1982
AP		9 MG/ML	N19217 001 JUL 13, 1984
AP		900 MG/100 ML	N19465 001 JUL 15, 1985
AP		900 MG/100 ML	N19480 001 SEP 17, 1985
AP	BAXTER	900 MG/100 ML	N16677 001
AP		9 MG/ML	N16677 004 OCT 30, 1985
AP		900 MG/100 ML	N20178 001 DEC 07, 1992
AP		9 MG/ML	N20178 002 DEC 07, 1992
AP	FUJISAWA	9 MG/ML	N88912 001 JAN 10, 1985
AP	MCGAW	900 MG/100 ML	N17464 001
AP		900 MG/100 ML	N19635 002 MAR 09, 1988
	SODIUM CHLORIDE 3% IN PLASTIC CONTAINER		
	BAXTER	3 GM/100 ML	N19022 001 NOV 01, 1983
	SODIUM CHLORIDE 5% IN PLASTIC CONTAINER		
	BAXTER	5 GM/100 ML	N19022 002 NOV 01, 1983

SOLUTION FOR SLUSH; IRRIGATION

	SODIUM CHLORIDE 0.9% IN STERILE PLASTIC CONTAINER		
	BAXTER	900 MG/100 ML	N19319 002 MAY 17, 1985

SOLUTION; IRRIGATION

	SODIUM CHLORIDE 0.45% IN PLASTIC CONTAINER		
AT	ABBOTT	450 MG/100 ML	N17670 001
AT	BAXTER	450 MG/100 ML	N17864 001
AT		450 MG/100 ML	N18497 001 FEB 19, 1982

Prescription Drug Products *(continued)*

SODIUM CHLORIDE *(continued)*

SOLUTION; IRRIGATION
SODIUM CHLORIDE 0.9% IN PLASTIC CONTAINER

AT	ABBOTT	900 MG/100 ML	N17514 001
AT		900 MG/100 ML	N18314 001
AT	BAXTER	900 MG/100 ML	N17427 001
AT		900 MG/100 ML	N17867 001
AT	MCGAW	900 MG/100 ML	N16733 001

SODIUM CHLORIDE; *MULTIPLE*

SEE AMINO ACIDS; CALCIUM ACETATE; GLYCERIN; MAGNESIUM ACETATE; PHOSPHORIC ACID; POTASSIUM CHLORIDE; SODIUM ACETATE; SODIUM CHLORIDE
SEE AMINO ACIDS; CALCIUM CHLORIDE; DEXTROSE; MAGNESIUM CHLORIDE; POTASSIUM CHLORIDE; POTASSIUM PHOSPHATE, DIBASIC; SODIUM CHLORIDE
SEE AMINO ACIDS; DEXTROSE; MAGNESIUM CHLORIDE; POTASSIUM CHLORIDE; SODIUM CHLORIDE; SODIUM PHOSPHATE, DIBASIC
SEE AMINO ACIDS; DEXTROSE; MAGNESIUM CHLORIDE; POTASSIUM ACETATE; POTASSIUM CHLORIDE; POTASSIUM PHOSPHATE, DIBASIC; SODIUM CHLORIDE
SEE AMINO ACIDS; DEXTROSE; MAGNESIUM CHLORIDE; POTASSIUM CHLORIDE; SODIUM CHLORIDE; SODIUM PHOSPHATE, DIBASIC
SEE AMINO ACIDS; MAGNESIUM ACETATE; PHOSPHORIC ACID; POTASSIUM ACETATE; SODIUM CHLORIDE
SEE AMINO ACIDS; MAGNESIUM ACETATE; PHOSPHORIC ACID; POTASSIUM CHLORIDE; SODIUM ACETATE; SODIUM CHLORIDE
SEE AMINO ACIDS; MAGNESIUM CHLORIDE; POTASSIUM CHLORIDE; POTASSIUM PHOSPHATE, DIBASIC; SODIUM CHLORIDE
SEE AMINO ACIDS; MAGNESIUM CHLORIDE; POTASSIUM PHOSPHATE, DIBASIC; SODIUM ACETATE; SODIUM CHLORIDE
SEE AMINO ACIDS; MAGNESIUM CHLORIDE; POTASSIUM PHOSPHATE, DIBASIC; SODIUM CHLORIDE
SEE CALCIUM CHLORIDE; DEXTROSE; GLUTATHIONE DISULFIDE; MAGNESIUM CHLORIDE; POTASSIUM CHLORIDE; SODIUM BICARBONATE; SODIUM CHLORIDE; SODIUM PHOSPHATE

SODIUM CHLORIDE; *MULTIPLE* *(continued)*

SEE CALCIUM CHLORIDE; DEXTROSE; MAGNESIUM CHLORIDE; POTASSIUM CHLORIDE; SODIUM ACETATE; SODIUM CHLORIDE
SEE CALCIUM CHLORIDE; DEXTROSE; MAGNESIUM CHLORIDE; POTASSIUM CHLORIDE; SODIUM ACETATE; SODIUM CHLORIDE; SODIUM CITRATE
SEE CALCIUM CHLORIDE; DEXTROSE; MAGNESIUM CHLORIDE; SODIUM CHLORIDE; SODIUM LACTATE
SEE CALCIUM CHLORIDE; DEXTROSE; MAGNESIUM CHLORIDE; SODIUM ACETATE; SODIUM CHLORIDE
SEE CALCIUM CHLORIDE; DEXTROSE; MAGNESIUM CHLORIDE; POTASSIUM CHLORIDE; SODIUM ACETATE; SODIUM CHLORIDE; SODIUM LACTATE
SEE CALCIUM CHLORIDE; DEXTROSE; MAGNESIUM CHLORIDE; SODIUM CHLORIDE; SODIUM LACTATE
SEE CALCIUM CHLORIDE; DEXTROSE; POTASSIUM CHLORIDE; SODIUM CHLORIDE
SEE CALCIUM CHLORIDE; DEXTROSE; POTASSIUM CHLORIDE; SODIUM CHLORIDE; SODIUM LACTATE
SEE CALCIUM CHLORIDE; DEXTROSE; POTASSIUM CHLORIDE; SODIUM ACETATE; SODIUM CHLORIDE
SEE CALCIUM CHLORIDE; DEXTROSE; POTASSIUM CHLORIDE; SODIUM CHLORIDE; SODIUM LACTATE
SEE CALCIUM CHLORIDE; MAGNESIUM CHLORIDE; POTASSIUM CHLORIDE; SODIUM ACETATE; SODIUM CHLORIDE; SODIUM CITRATE
SEE CALCIUM CHLORIDE; MAGNESIUM CHLORIDE; POTASSIUM CHLORIDE; SODIUM ACETATE; SODIUM CHLORIDE
SEE CALCIUM CHLORIDE; MAGNESIUM CHLORIDE; POTASSIUM CHLORIDE; SODIUM ACETATE; SODIUM CHLORIDE; SODIUM LACTATE
SEE CALCIUM CHLORIDE; MAGNESIUM CHLORIDE; POTASSIUM CHLORIDE; SODIUM CHLORIDE
SEE CALCIUM CHLORIDE; POTASSIUM CHLORIDE; SODIUM CHLORIDE
SEE CALCIUM CHLORIDE; POTASSIUM CHLORIDE; SODIUM CHLORIDE; SODIUM LACTATE
SEE DEXTROSE; MAGNESIUM ACETATE; POTASSIUM ACETATE; SODIUM CHLORIDE
SEE DEXTROSE; MAGNESIUM ACETATE TETRAHYDRATE; POTASSIUM ACETATE; SODIUM CHLORIDE

Prescription Drug Products *(continued)*

SODIUM CHLORIDE; *MULTIPLE* *(continued)*

SEE DEXTROSE; MAGNESIUM CHLORIDE; POTASSIUM CHLORIDE; SODIUM ACETATE; SODIUM CHLORIDE

SEE DEXTROSE; MAGNESIUM CHLORIDE; POTASSIUM CHLORIDE; SODIUM ACETATE; SODIUM CHLORIDE; SODIUM GLUCONATE

SEE DEXTROSE; MAGNESIUM CHLORIDE; POTASSIUM CHLORIDE; POTASSIUM PHOSPHATE, DIBASIC; SODIUM CHLORIDE; SODIUM LACTATE; SODIUM PHOSPHATE, MONOBASIC

SEE DEXTROSE; MAGNESIUM CHLORIDE; POTASSIUM CHLORIDE; POTASSIUM PHOSPHATE, MONOBASIC; SODIUM CHLORIDE; SODIUM LACTATE

SEE DEXTROSE; POTASSIUM CHLORIDE; POTASSIUM LACTATE; SODIUM CHLORIDE; SODIUM PHOSPHATE, MONOBASIC

SEE DEXTROSE; POTASSIUM CHLORIDE; POTASSIUM PHOSPHATE, DIBASIC; SODIUM ACETATE; SODIUM CHLORIDE

SEE DEXTROSE; POTASSIUM CHLORIDE; POTASSIUM PHOSPHATE, MONOBASIC; SODIUM CHLORIDE; SODIUM LACTATE

SEE DEXTROSE; POTASSIUM CHLORIDE; SODIUM CHLORIDE

SEE DEXTROSE; SODIUM CHLORIDE

SEE MAGNESIUM ACETATE TETRAHYDRATE; POTASSIUM ACETATE; SODIUM CHLORIDE

SEE MAGNESIUM CHLORIDE; POTASSIUM CHLORIDE; POTASSIUM PHOSPHATE, MONOBASIC; SODIUM ACETATE; SODIUM CHLORIDE; SODIUM GLUCONATE; SODIUM PHOSPHATE, DIBASIC

SEE MAGNESIUM CHLORIDE; POTASSIUM CHLORIDE; SODIUM ACETATE; SODIUM CHLORIDE; SODIUM GLUCONATE

SEE MAGNESIUM SULFATE; POTASSIUM CHLORIDE; POTASSIUM PHOSPHATE, MONOBASIC; SODIUM CHLORIDE; SODIUM PHOSPHATE

SEE POLYETHYLENE GLYCOL 3350; POTASSIUM CHLORIDE; SODIUM BICARBONATE; SODIUM CHLORIDE; SODIUM SULFATE, ANHYDROUS

SEE POLYETHYLENE GLYCOL 3350; POTASSIUM CHLORIDE; SODIUM BICARBONATE; SODIUM CHLORIDE

SEE POLYETHYLENE GLYCOL 3350; POTASSIUM CHLORIDE; SODIUM BICARBONATE; SODIUM CHLORIDE; SODIUM SULFATE

SEE POLYETHYLENE GLYCOL 3350; POTASSIUM CHLORIDE; SODIUM BICARBONATE; SODIUM CHLORIDE; SODIUM SULFATE, ANHYDROUS

SEE POTASSIUM CHLORIDE; SODIUM CHLORIDE

SEE POTASSIUM CHLORIDE; SODIUM CHLORIDE; TROMETHAMINE

SODIUM CHROMATE, CR-51

INJECTABLE; INJECTION

	CHROMITOPE SODIUM		
	BRACCO	250uCi/VIAL	N13993 001
		1mCi/VIAL	N13993 003
	SODIUM CHROMATE CR 51		
	MALLINCKRODT	100uCi/ML	N16708 001

SODIUM CITRATE; *MULTIPLE*

SEE CALCIUM CHLORIDE; DEXTROSE; MAGNESIUM CHLORIDE; POTASSIUM CHLORIDE; SODIUM ACETATE; SODIUM CHLORIDE; SODIUM CITRATE

SEE CALCIUM CHLORIDE; MAGNESIUM CHLORIDE; POTASSIUM CHLORIDE; SODIUM ACETATE; SODIUM CHLORIDE; SODIUM CITRATE

SODIUM GLUCONATE; *MULTIPLE*

SEE DEXTROSE; MAGNESIUM CHLORIDE; POTASSIUM CHLORIDE; SODIUM ACETATE; SODIUM CHLORIDE; SODIUM GLUCONATE

SEE MAGNESIUM CHLORIDE; POTASSIUM CHLORIDE; POTASSIUM PHOSPHATE, MONOBASIC; SODIUM ACETATE; SODIUM CHLORIDE; SODIUM GLUCONATE; SODIUM PHOSPHATE, DIBASIC

SEE MAGNESIUM CHLORIDE; POTASSIUM CHLORIDE; SODIUM ACETATE; SODIUM CHLORIDE; SODIUM GLUCONATE

SODIUM IODIDE, I-123

CAPSULE; ORAL

	SODIUM IODIDE I 123		
AA	GOLDEN PHARMS	100uCi	N18671 001 MAY 27, 1982
AA		200uCi	N18671 002 MAY 27, 1982
AA	MALLINCKRODT	100uCi	N71909 001 FEB 28, 1989
AA		200uCi	N71910 001 FEB 28, 1989
AA	MEDI PHYSICS	100uCi	N17630 001

SOLUTION; ORAL

	SODIUM IODIDE I 123		
	MEDI PHYSICS	2mCi/ML	N17630 002

Prescription Drug Products *(continued)*

SODIUM IODIDE, I-131

CAPSULE; ORAL

	IODOTOPE		
	BRACCO	8-100uCi	N10929 001
		1-50mCi	N10929 003
	SODIUM IODIDE I 131		
	CIS	100uCi	N17316 002
	MALLINCKRODT	0.8-100mCi	N16517 001
		15-100uCi	N16517 002

SOLUTION; ORAL

	IODOTOPE		
	BRACCO	7-106mCi/BOT	N10929 002
	SODIUM IODIDE I 131		
	CIS	50mCi/ML	N17315 001
	MALLINCKRODT	3.5-150mCi/VIAL	N16515 001

SODIUM LACTATE

INJECTABLE; INJECTION

	SODIUM LACTATE IN PLASTIC CONTAINER		
	ABBOTT	5 MEQ/ML	N18947 001 SEP 05, 1984
	SODIUM LACTATE 0.167 MOLAR IN PLASTIC CONTAINER		
AP	ABBOTT	1.87 GM/100 ML	N18249 001
AP	BAXTER	1.87 GM/100 ML	N16692 001
AP	MCGAW	1.87 GM/100 ML	N18186 001
	SODIUM LACTATE 1/6 MOLAR IN PLASTIC CONTAINER		
AP	MCGAW	1.87 GM/100 ML	N20004 001 APR 21, 1992

SODIUM LACTATE; *MULTIPLE*

SEE CALCIUM CHLORIDE; DEXTROSE; MAGNESIUM CHLORIDE; SODIUM CHLORIDE; SODIUM LACTATE

SEE CALCIUM CHLORIDE; DEXTROSE; MAGNESIUM CHLORIDE; POTASSIUM CHLORIDE; SODIUM ACETATE; SODIUM CHLORIDE; SODIUM LACTATE

SEE CALCIUM CHLORIDE; DEXTROSE; MAGNESIUM CHLORIDE; SODIUM CHLORIDE; SODIUM LACTATE

SEE CALCIUM CHLORIDE; DEXTROSE; POTASSIUM CHLORIDE; SODIUM CHLORIDE; SODIUM LACTATE

SEE CALCIUM CHLORIDE; MAGNESIUM CHLORIDE; POTASSIUM CHLORIDE; SODIUM ACETATE; SODIUM CHLORIDE; SODIUM LACTATE

SEE CALCIUM CHLORIDE; POTASSIUM CHLORIDE; SODIUM CHLORIDE; SODIUM LACTATE

SODIUM LACTATE; *MULTIPLE* *(continued)*

SEE DEXTROSE; MAGNESIUM CHLORIDE; POTASSIUM CHLORIDE; POTASSIUM PHOSPHATE, DIBASIC; SODIUM CHLORIDE; SODIUM LACTATE; SODIUM PHOSPHATE, MONOBASIC

SEE DEXTROSE; MAGNESIUM CHLORIDE; POTASSIUM CHLORIDE; POTASSIUM PHOSPHATE, MONOBASIC; SODIUM LACTATE; SODIUM PHOSPHATE, MONOBASIC

SEE DEXTROSE; MAGNESIUM CHLORIDE; POTASSIUM CHLORIDE; POTASSIUM PHOSPHATE, MONOBASIC; SODIUM CHLORIDE; SODIUM LACTATE

SEE DEXTROSE; POTASSIUM CHLORIDE; POTASSIUM PHOSPHATE, MONOBASIC; SODIUM CHLORIDE; SODIUM LACTATE

SODIUM NITROPRUSSIDE

INJECTABLE; INJECTION

	NIPRIDE		
AP	+ ROCHE	50 MG/VIAL	N17546 001
	NITROPRESS		
AP	+ ABBOTT	25 MG/ML	N71961 001 AUG 01, 1988
AP		50 MG/VIAL	N70566 001 JUN 09, 1986
AP		50 MG/VIAL	N71555 001 NOV 16, 1987
	SODIUM NITROPRUSSIDE		
AP	ELKINS SINN	50 MG/VIAL	N18581 001 JUL 28, 1982
AP	GENSIA	25 MG/ML	N73465 001 MAR 30, 1992

SODIUM PHENYLACETATE; *MULTIPLE*

SEE SODIUM BENZOATE; SODIUM PHENYLACETATE

SODIUM PHOSPHATE; *MULTIPLE*

SEE CALCIUM CHLORIDE; DEXTROSE; GLUTATHIONE DISULFIDE; MAGNESIUM CHLORIDE; POTASSIUM CHLORIDE; SODIUM BICARBONATE; SODIUM CHLORIDE; SODIUM PHOSPHATE

SEE MAGNESIUM SULFATE; POTASSIUM CHLORIDE; POTASSIUM PHOSPHATE, MONOBASIC; SODIUM CHLORIDE; SODIUM PHOSPHATE

Prescription Drug Products *(continued)*

SODIUM PHOSPHATE, DIBASIC; *MULTIPLE*

SEE AMINO ACIDS; DEXTROSE; MAGNESIUM CHLORIDE; POTASSIUM CHLORIDE; SODIUM CHLORIDE; SODIUM PHOSPHATE, DIBASIC

SEE MAGNESIUM CHLORIDE; POTASSIUM CHLORIDE; POTASSIUM PHOSPHATE, MONOBASIC; SODIUM ACETATE; SODIUM CHLORIDE; SODIUM GLUCONATE; SODIUM PHOSPHATE, DIBASIC

SODIUM PHOSPHATE, DIBASIC; SODIUM PHOSPHATE, MONOBASIC

INJECTABLE; INJECTION
SODIUM PHOSPHATES IN PLASTIC CONTAINER

	ABBOTT	142 MG/ML;276 MG/ML	N18892 001 MAY 10, 1983

SODIUM PHOSPHATE, MONOBASIC; *MULTIPLE*

SEE DEXTROSE; MAGNESIUM CHLORIDE; POTASSIUM CHLORIDE; POTASSIUM PHOSPHATE, DIBASIC; SODIUM CHLORIDE; SODIUM LACTATE; SODIUM PHOSPHATE, MONOBASIC

SEE DEXTROSE; MAGNESIUM CHLORIDE; POTASSIUM CHLORIDE; POTASSIUM PHOSPHATE, MONOBASIC; SODIUM LACTATE; SODIUM PHOSPHATE, MONOBASIC

SEE DEXTROSE; POTASSIUM CHLORIDE; POTASSIUM LACTATE; SODIUM CHLORIDE; SODIUM PHOSPHATE, MONOBASIC

SEE SODIUM PHOSPHATE, DIBASIC; SODIUM PHOSPHATE, MONOBASIC

SODIUM PHOSPHATE, P-32

SOLUTION; INJECTION
SODIUM PHOSPHATE P 32

	MALLINCKRODT	0.67mCi/ML	N11777 001

SODIUM POLYSTYRENE SULFONATE

POWDER; ORAL, RECTAL

	KAYEXALATE		
AA	STERLING WINTHROP	453.6 GM/BOT	N11287 001
	SODIUM POLYSTYRENE SULFONATE		
AA	CAROLINA MEDCL	454 GM/BOT	N89910 001 JAN 19, 1989

SODIUM POLYSTYRENE SULFONATE *(continued)*

SUSPENSION; ORAL, RECTAL

	SODIUM POLYSTYRENE SULFONATE		
AA	ROXANE	15 GM/60 ML	N89049 001 NOV 17, 1986
	SPS		
AA	CAROLINA MEDCL	15 GM/60 ML	N87859 001 DEC 08, 1982

SODIUM SULFATE; *MULTIPLE*

SEE POLYETHYLENE GLYCOL 3350; POTASSIUM CHLORIDE; SODIUM BICARBONATE; SODIUM CHLORIDE; SODIUM SULFATE

SODIUM SULFATE, ANHYDROUS; *MULTIPLE*

SEE POLYETHYLENE GLYCOL 3350; POTASSIUM CHLORIDE; SODIUM BICARBONATE; SODIUM CHLORIDE; SODIUM SULFATE, ANHYDROUS

SODIUM TETRADECYL SULFATE

INJECTABLE; INJECTION
SOTRADECOL

+	ELKINS SINN	1%	N05970 004
+		3%	N05970 005

SODIUM THIOSULFATE

INJECTABLE; INJECTION
SODIUM THIOSULFATE

	US ARMY	250 MG/ML	N20166 001 FEB 14, 1992

SOMATREM

INJECTABLE; INJECTION
PROTROPIN

+	GENENTECH	5 MG/VIAL	N19107 001 OCT 17, 1985
+		10 MG/VIAL	N19107 002 OCT 24, 1989

Prescription Drug Products *(continued)*

SOMATROPIN, BIOSYNTHETIC
INJECTABLE; INJECTION
HUMATROPE
BX + LILLY 5 MG/VIAL N19640 004 MAR 08, 1987
NUTROPIN
BX GENENTECH 5 MG/VIAL N20168 001 NOV 17, 1993
+ 10 MG/VIAL N20168 002 NOV 17, 1993

SORBITOL
SOLUTION; IRRIGATION
SORBITOL 3.3% IN PLASTIC CONTAINER
MCGAW 3.3 GM/100 ML N16741 001
SORBITOL 3% IN PLASTIC CONTAINER
BAXTER 3 GM/100 ML N17863 001

SORBITOL; *MULTIPLE*
SEE <u>MANNITOL; SORBITOL</u>

SOTALOL HYDROCHLORIDE
TABLET; ORAL
BETAPACE
BERLEX 80 MG N19865 001 OCT 30, 1992
120 MG N19865 005 APR 20, 1994
160 MG N19865 002 OCT 30, 1992
+ 240 MG N19865 003 OCT 30, 1992

SOYBEAN OIL
INJECTABLE; INJECTION
<u>INTRALIPID 10%</u>
<u>AP</u> PHARMACIA <u>10%</u> N17643 001
<u>INTRALIPID 20%</u>
<u>AP</u> PHARMACIA <u>20%</u> N18449 001
INTRALIPID 30%
PHARMACIA 30% N19942 001 DEC 30, 1993
<u>LIPOSYN III 10%</u>
<u>AP</u> ABBOTT <u>10%</u> N18969 001 SEP 24, 1984
<u>LIPOSYN III 20%</u>
<u>AP</u> ABBOTT <u>20%</u> N18970 001 SEP 25, 1984

SOYBEAN OIL *(continued)*
INJECTABLE; INJECTION
<u>NUTRILIPID 10%</u>
<u>AP</u> MCGAW <u>10%</u> N19531 001 MAY 28, 1993
<u>NUTRILIPID 20%</u>
<u>AP</u> MCGAW <u>20%</u> N19531 002 MAY 28, 1993
<u>SOYACAL 10%</u>
<u>AP</u> ALPHA THERAPEUTIC <u>10%</u> N18465 001 JUN 29, 1983
<u>SOYACAL 20%</u>
<u>AP</u> ALPHA THERAPEUTIC <u>20%</u> N18786 001 JUN 29, 1983
<u>TRAVAMULSION 10%</u>
<u>AP</u> BAXTER <u>10%</u> N18660 001 FEB 26, 1982

SOYBEAN OIL; *MULTIPLE*
SEE <u>SAFFLOWER OIL; SOYBEAN OIL</u>

SPECTINOMYCIN HYDROCHLORIDE
INJECTABLE; INJECTION
TROBICIN
+ UPJOHN EQ 2 GM BASE/VIAL N50347 001
+ EQ 4 GM BASE/VIAL N50347 002

SPIRONOLACTONE
TABLET; ORAL
<u>ALDACTONE</u>
<u>AB</u> + SEARLE <u>25 MG</u> N12151 009 DEC 30, 1983
50 MG N12151 008 DEC 30, 1982
100 MG N12151 010 DEC 30, 1983
<u>SPIRONOLACTONE</u>
<u>AB</u> BARR <u>25 MG</u> N87265 001
<u>AB</u> GENEVA PHARMS <u>25 MG</u> N86809 001
<u>AB</u> MUTUAL PHARM <u>25 MG</u> N89424 001 JUL 23, 1986
<u>AB</u> MYLAN <u>25 MG</u> N87086 001
<u>AB</u> PUREPAC PHARM <u>25 MG</u> N87998 001 OCT 14, 1983
<u>AB</u> SUPERPHARM <u>25 MG</u> N89364 001 NOV 07, 1986
<u>AB</u> ZENITH LABS <u>25 MG</u> N87108 001

SPIRONOLACTONE; *MULTIPLE*
SEE <u>HYDROCHLOROTHIAZIDE; SPIRONOLACTONE</u>

Prescription Drug Products *(continued)*

STANOZOLOL
TABLET; ORAL
WINSTROL
+ STERLING WINTHROP 2 MG N12885 001 MAY 14, 1984

STAVUDINE
CAPSULE; ORAL
ZERIT
BRISTOL MYERS SQUIBB 15 MG N20412 002 JUN 24, 1994
20 MG N20412 003 JUN 24, 1994
30 MG N20412 004 JUN 24, 1994
\+ 40 MG N20412 005 JUN 24, 1994

STREPTOMYCIN SULFATE
INJECTABLE; INJECTION
STREPTOMYCIN SULFATE
AP LILLY EQ 1 GM BASE/VIAL N60107 001
AP EQ 5 GM BASE/VIAL N60107 002
EQ 1 GM BASE/2 ML N60404 001
AP + PFIZER EQ 1 GM BASE/VIAL N60076 001
AP + EQ 5 GM BASE/VIAL N60076 002
EQ 1 GM BASE/2.5 ML N60111 001

STREPTOZOCIN
INJECTABLE; INJECTION
ZANOSAR
+ UPJOHN 1 GM/VIAL N50577 001 MAY 07, 1982

STRONTIUM CHLORIDE, SR-89
INJECTABLE; INJECTION
METASTRON
MEDI PHYSICS 1mCi/ML N20134 001 JUN 18, 1993

SUCCIMER
CAPSULE; ORAL
CHEMET
+ MCNEIL 100 MG N19998 002 JAN 30, 1991

SUCCINYLCHOLINE CHLORIDE
INJECTABLE; INJECTION
ANECTINE
AP BURROUGHS WELLCOME 20 MG/ML N08453 002
\+ 500 MG/VIAL N08453 001
\+ 1 GM/VIAL N08453 004
QUELICIN
AP + ABBOTT 20 MG/ML N08845 001
AP + 100 MG/ML N08845 004
\+ 50 MG/ML N08845 002
SUCCINYLCHOLINE CHLORIDE
AP ORGANON 20 MG/ML N80997 001
SUCOSTRIN
AP SQUIBB 20 MG/ML N08847 001
AP 100 MG/ML N08847 003

SUCRALFATE
SUSPENSION; ORAL
CARAFATE
+ MARION MERRELL DOW 1 GM/10 ML N19183 001 DEC 16, 1993
TABLET; ORAL
CARAFATE
+ BLUE RIDGE 1 GM N18333 001

SUFENTANIL CITRATE
INJECTABLE; INJECTION
SUFENTA
+ JANSSEN EQ 0.05 MG BASE/ML N19050 001 MAY 04, 1984

SULBACTAM SODIUM; *MULTIPLE*
SEE AMPICILLIN SODIUM; SULBACTAM SODIUM

SULCONAZOLE NITRATE
CREAM; TOPICAL
EXELDERM
+ WESTWOOD SQUIBB 1% N18737 001 FEB 28, 1989

Prescription Drug Products *(continued)*

SULFACETAMIDE SODIUM

OINTMENT; OPHTHALMIC

	BLEPH-10		
AT	ALLERGAN	10%	N84015 001
	CETAMIDE		
AT	ALCON	10%	N80021 001
	SODIUM SULAMYD		
AT	+ SCHERING	10%	N05963 002
	SULFACETAMIDE SODIUM		
AT	ALTANA	10%	N80029 001

SOLUTION/DROPS; OPHTHALMIC

	BLEPH-10		
AT	ALLERGAN	10%	N80028 001
	BLEPH-30		
AT	ALLERGAN	30%	N80028 002
	ISOPTO CETAMIDE		
AT	+ ALCON	15%	N80020 002
	OCUSULF-10		
AT	OPTOPICS	10%	N80660 001
	OCUSULF-30		
AT	OPTOPICS	30%	N80660 002
	SODIUM SULAMYD		
AT	+ SCHERING	10%	N05963 001
AT	+	30%	N05963 003
	SODIUM SULFACETAMIDE		
AT	AKORN	10%	N83021 001
AT		15%	N83021 002
AT		30%	N83021 003
	SULF-10		
AT	IOLAB	10%	N80025 001
	SULFACEL-15		
AT	OPTOPICS	15%	N80024 001
	SULFACETAMIDE SODIUM		
AT	PHARMAFAIR	10%	N88947 001 MAY 17, 1985
AT	STERIS	10%	N89560 001 OCT 18, 1988
AT		30%	N89068 001 MAY 05, 1987
	SULFAIR 10		
AT	PHARMAFAIR	10%	N87949 001 DEC 13, 1982
	SULTEN-10		
AT	BAUSCH AND LOMB	10%	N87818 001 FEB 03, 1983

SULFACETAMIDE SODIUM; *MULTIPLE*

SEE FLUOROMETHOLONE; SULFACETAMIDE SODIUM
SEE PREDNISOLONE ACETATE; SULFACETAMIDE SODIUM
SEE PREDNISOLONE SODIUM PHOSPHATE; SULFACETAMIDE SODIUM

SULFACYTINE

TABLET; ORAL

	RENOQUID		
	+ GLENWOOD	250 MG	N17569 001

SULFADIAZINE

TABLET; ORAL

	SULFADIAZINE		
AB	+ EON LABS	500 MG	N40091 001 JUL 29, 1994
AA	GLOBAL PHARMS	500 MG	N80081 001
AB	LANNETT	500 MG	N80084 001

SULFADIAZINE; SULFAMERAZINE

SUSPENSION; ORAL

	SULFONAMIDES DUPLEX		
	LILLY	250 MG/5 ML;250 MG/5 ML	N06317 007

SULFADOXINE; *MULTIPLE*

SEE PYRIMETHAMINE; SULFADOXINE

SULFAMERAZINE; *MULTIPLE*

SEE SULFADIAZINE; SULFAMERAZINE

SULFAMETHIZOLE

TABLET; ORAL

	THIOSULFIL		
	+ WYETH AYERST	500 MG	N08565 004

SULFAMETHOXAZOLE

SUSPENSION; ORAL

	GANTANOL		
	ROCHE	500 MG/5 ML	N13664 002

TABLET; ORAL

	GANTANOL		
AB	+ ROCHE	500 MG	N12715 002
	SULFAMETHOXAZOLE		
AB	GENEVA PHARMS	500 MG	N85844 001

SULFAMETHOXAZOLE; *MULTIPLE*

SEE PHENAZOPYRIDINE HYDROCHLORIDE; SULFAMETHOXAZOLE

Prescription Drug Products *(continued)*

SULFAMETHOXAZOLE; TRIMETHOPRIM

INJECTABLE; INJECTION

	BACTRIM		
AP	ROCHE	80 MG/ML;16 MG/ML	N18374 001
	SEPTRA		
AP	BURROUGHS WELLCOME	80 MG/ML;16 MG/ML	N18452 001
	SULFAMETHOXAZOLE AND TRIMETHOPRIM		
AP	CETUS BEN VENUE	80 MG/ML;16 MG/ML	N72383 001 APR 29, 1992
AP	ELKINS SINN	80 MG/ML;16 MG/ML	N70627 001 DEC 29, 1987
AP		80 MG/ML;16 MG/ML	N70628 001 DEC 29, 1987
AP	GENSIA	80 MG/ML;16 MG/ML	N73303 001 OCT 31, 1991
AP	STERIS	80 MG/ML;16 MG/ML	N71556 001 DEC 29, 1987
AP	STERLING WINTHROP	80 MG/ML;16 MG/ML	N73199 001 SEP 11, 1992

SUSPENSION; ORAL

	BACTRIM PEDIATRIC		
AB	+ ROCHE	200 MG/5 ML;40 MG/5 ML	N17560 002
	COTRIM PEDIATRIC		
AB	LEMMON	200 MG/5 ML;40 MG/5 ML	N70028 001 JUN 02, 1987
	SEPTRA		
AB	BURROUGHS WELLCOME	200 MG/5 ML;40 MG/5 ML	N17598 001
	SEPTRA GRAPE		
AB	BURROUGHS WELLCOME	200 MG/5 ML;40 MG/5 ML	N17598 002 FEB 12, 1986
	SMZ-TMP		
AB	BIOCRAFT	200 MG/5 ML;40 MG/5 ML	N18812 001 JAN 28, 1983
	SMZ-TMP PEDIATRIC		
AB	BIOCRAFT	200 MG/5 ML;40 MG/5 ML	N18812 002 JUN 10, 1983
	SULFATRIM		
AB	BARRE	200 MG/5 ML;40 MG/5 ML	N18615 002 JAN 07, 1983
	SULFATRIM PEDIATRIC		
AB	BARRE	200 MG/5 ML;40 MG/5 ML	N18615 001 JAN 07, 1983
	TRIMETH/SULFA		
AB	BARRE	200 MG/5 ML;40 MG/5 ML	N72289 001 MAY 23, 1988
AB	NASKA	200 MG/5 ML;40 MG/5 ML	N72399 001 MAY 23, 1988

SULFAMETHOXAZOLE; TRIMETHOPRIM *(continued)*

TABLET; ORAL

	BACTRIM		
AB	ROCHE	400 MG;80 MG	N17377 001
	BACTRIM DS		
AB	+ ROCHE	800 MG;160 MG	N17377 002
	COTRIM		
AB	LEMMON	400 MG;80 MG	N70034 001 MAY 16, 1985
	COTRIM D.S.		
AB	LEMMON	800 MG;160 MG	N70048 001 MAR 18, 1985
	SEPTRA		
AB	BURROUGHS WELLCOME	400 MG;80 MG	N17376 001
	SEPTRA DS		
AB	BURROUGHS WELLCOME	800 MG;160 MG	N17376 002
	SMZ-TMP		
AB	BIOCRAFT	400 MG;80 MG	N18242 001
AB		800 MG;160 MG	N18242 002
	SULFAMETHOPRIM		
AB	PAR PHARM	400 MG;80 MG	N70022 001 FEB 15, 1985
	SULFAMETHOPRIM-DS		
AB	PAR PHARM	800 MG;160 MG	N70032 001 FEB 15, 1985
	SULFAMETHOXAZOLE AND TRIMETHOPRIM		
AB	BARR	400 MG;80 MG	N70006 001 NOV 14, 1984
AB	DANBURY PHARMA	400 MG;80 MG	N18852 001 MAY 09, 1983
AB	GENEVA PHARMS	400 MG;80 MG	N70889 001 NOV 13, 1986
AB		800 MG;160 MG	N70890 001 NOV 13, 1986
AB	MUTUAL PHARM	400 MG;80 MG	N71016 001 AUG 25, 1986
AB		800 MG;160 MG	N71017 001 AUG 25, 1986
AB	ROXANE	400 MG;80 MG	N72768 001 AUG 30, 1991
AB	SIDMAK LABS NJ	400 MG;80 MG	N70215 001 SEP 10, 1985
AB		800 MG;160 MG	N70216 001 SEP 10, 1985

Prescription Drug Products *(continued)*

SULFAMETHOXAZOLE; TRIMETHOPRIM *(continued)*

TABLET; ORAL

SULFAMETHOXAZOLE AND TRIMETHOPRIM DOUBLE STRENGTH

AB	BARR	800 MG;160 MG	N70007 001 NOV 14, 1984
AB	DANBURY PHARMA	800 MG;160 MG	N18854 001 MAY 09, 1983
AB	EON LABS	800 MG;160 MG	N18598 004 MAY 19, 1982
AB	PLANTEX	800 MG;160 MG	N70037 001 JUN 02, 1987
AB	ROXANE	800 MG;160 MG	N72769 001 AUG 30, 1991

SULFAMETHOXAZOLE AND TRIMETHOPRIM SINGLE STRENGTH

AB	PLANTEX	400 MG;80 MG	N70030 001 JUN 02, 1987

SULFATRIM-DS

AB	SUPERPHARM	800 MG;160 MG	N70066 001 JUN 24, 1985

SULFATRIM-SS

AB	SUPERPHARM	400 MG;80 MG	N70065 002 JUN 24, 1985

SULFANILAMIDE

CREAM; VAGINAL

AVC

AT	+ MERRELL DOW	15%	N06530 003 JAN 27, 1987

SULFANILAMIDE

AT	LEMMON	15%	N88718 001 SEP 19, 1985

SUPPOSITORY; VAGINAL

AVC

	MERRELL DOW	1.05 GM	N06530 004 JAN 27, 1987

SULFAPYRIDINE

TABLET; ORAL

SULFAPYRIDINE

	LILLY	500 MG	N00159 001

SULFASALAZINE

SUSPENSION; ORAL

AZULFIDINE

	+ PHARMACIA	250 MG/5 ML	N86983 001

TABLET; ORAL

AZULFIDINE

AB	+ PHARMACIA	500 MG	N07073 001

SULFASALAZINE

AB	CHELSEA LABS	500 MG	N85828 001
AB	DANBURY PHARMA	500 MG	N87197 001
AB	LEDERLE	500 MG	N80197 001
AB	MUTUAL PHARM	500 MG	N89590 001 OCT 19, 1987
AB	SUPERPHARM	500 MG	N89339 001 OCT 26, 1987

TABLET, DELAYED RELEASE; ORAL

AZULFIDINE EN-TABS

	+ PHARMACIA	500 MG	N07073 002 APR 06, 1983

SULFINPYRAZONE

CAPSULE; ORAL

ANTURANE

AB	+ CIBA	200 MG	N11556 004

SULFINPYRAZONE

AB	BARR	200 MG	N87666 001 SEP 17, 1982
AB	PAR PHARM	200 MG	N88934 001 SEP 06, 1985
AB	ZENITH LABS	200 MG	N87770 001 NOV 19, 1982

TABLET; ORAL

ANTURANE

AB	+ CIBA	100 MG	N11556 003

SULFINPYRAZONE

AB	BARR	100 MG	N87665 001 SEP 17, 1982
AB	DANBURY PHARMA	100 MG	N87667 001 MAY 26, 1982
AB	PAR PHARM	100 MG	N88933 001 SEP 06, 1985
AB	ZENITH LABS	100 MG	N87769 001 JUN 01, 1982

Prescription Drug Products *(continued)*

SULFISOXAZOLE

TABLET; ORAL

	GANTRISIN		
AB	+ ROCHE	500 MG	N06525 001
	SOSOL		
AB	MK LABS	500 MG	N80036 001
	SULFISOXAZOLE		
AB	GENEVA PHARMS	500 MG	N85628 001
AB	GLOBAL PHARMS	500 MG	N80109 001
AB	ICN	500 MG	N80268 002
AB	PUREPAC PHARM	500 MG	N80087 001
AB	ROXANE	500 MG	N80082 001
AB	ZENITH LABS	500 MG	N80142 001

SULFISOXAZOLE; *MULTIPLE*

SEE PHENAZOPYRIDINE HYDROCHLORIDE; SULFISOXAZOLE

SULFISOXAZOLE ACETYL

SUSPENSION; ORAL

	GANTRISIN PEDIATRIC		
	+ ROCHE	EQ 500 MG BASE/5 ML	N09182 004

SYRUP; ORAL

	GANTRISIN		
	+ ROCHE	EQ 500 MG BASE/5 ML	N09182 002

SULFISOXAZOLE ACETYL; *MULTIPLE*

SEE ERYTHROMYCIN ETHYLSUCCINATE; SULFISOXAZOLE ACETYL

SULFISOXAZOLE DIOLAMINE

SOLUTION/DROPS; OPHTHALMIC

	GANTRISIN		
	+ ROCHE	EQ 4% BASE	N07757 002

SULINDAC

TABLET; ORAL

	CLINORIL		
AB	MERCK	150 MG	N17911 001
AB	+	200 MG	N17911 002

SULINDAC *(continued)*

TABLET; ORAL

	SULINDAC		
AB	DANBURY PHARMA	150 MG	N71891 001 APR 03, 1990
AB		200 MG	N71795 001 APR 03, 1990
AB	GENEVA PHARMS	150 MG	N72712 001 AUG 30, 1991
AB		200 MG	N72713 001 AUG 30, 1991
AB	LEDERLE	150 MG	N73261 001 SEP 06, 1991
AB		200 MG	N73262 001 SEP 06, 1991
AB	LEMMON	150 MG	N72972 001 FEB 28, 1992
AB		200 MG	N72973 001 FEB 28, 1992
AB	MUTUAL PHARM	150 MG	N72050 001 APR 17, 1991
AB		200 MG	N72051 001 APR 17, 1991
AB	MYLAN	150 MG	N73038 001 JUN 22, 1993
AB		200 MG	N73039 001 JUN 22, 1993
AB	WARNER CHILCOTT	150 MG	N72710 001 MAR 25, 1991
AB		200 MG	N72711 001 MAR 25, 1991

SUMATRIPTAN SUCCINATE

INJECTABLE; INJECTION

	IMITREX		
	GLAXO	EQ 6 MG BASE/0.5 ML	N20080 001 DEC 28, 1992

SUPROFEN

SOLUTION/DROPS; OPHTHALMIC

	PROFENAL		
	ALCON	1%	N19387 001 DEC 23, 1988

SUTILAINS

OINTMENT; TOPICAL

	TRAVASE		
	BOOTS	82,000 UNITS/GM	N12828 001

Prescription Drug Products *(continued)*

TACRINE HYDROCHLORIDE

	CAPSULE; ORAL		
	COGNEX		
	PARKE DAVIS	EQ 10 MG BASE	N20070 001 SEP 09, 1993
		EQ 20 MG BASE	N20070 002 SEP 09, 1993
		EQ 30 MG BASE	N20070 003 SEP 09, 1993
	+	EQ 40 MG BASE	N20070 004 SEP 09, 1993

TACROLIMUS

	CAPSULE; ORAL		
	PROGRAF		
	+ FUJISAWA	EQ 1 MG BASE	N50708 001 APR 08, 1994
	+	EQ 5 MG BASE	N50708 002 APR 08, 1994
	INJECTABLE; INJECTION		
	PROGRAF		
	+ FUJISAWA	EQ 5 MG BASE/ML	N50709 001 APR 08, 1994

TAMOXIFEN CITRATE

	TABLET; ORAL		
	NOLVADEX		
	+ ZENECA	EQ 10 MG BASE	N17970 001
	+	EQ 20 MG BASE	N17970 002 MAR 21, 1994

TARTARIC ACID; *MULTIPLE*

SEE <u>SODIUM BICARBONATE; TARTARIC ACID</u>

TAZOBACTAM SODIUM; *MULTIPLE*

SEE <u>PIPERACILLIN SODIUM; TAZOBACTAM SODIUM</u>

TECHNETIUM TC-99M ALBUMIN AGGREGATED KIT

	INJECTABLE; INJECTION		
	AN-MAA		
BS	SORIN BIOMEDICA (US)	N/A	N17792 001
	MACROTEC		
BS	BRACCO	N/A	N17833 001
	PULMOLITE		
BS	DUPONT	N/A	N17776 001
	TECHNESCAN MAA		
BS	MALLINCKRODT	N/A	N17842 001

TECHNETIUM TC-99M ALBUMIN AGGREGATED KIT *(continued)*

	INJECTABLE; INJECTION		
	TECHNETIUM TC 99M ALBUMIN AGGREGATED KIT		
BS	MERCK SHARP DOHME	N/A	N17881 001 DEC 30, 1987

TECHNETIUM TC-99M ALBUMIN COLLOID KIT

	INJECTABLE; INJECTION		
	MICROLITE		
	DUPONT	N/A	N18263 001 MAR 25, 1983

TECHNETIUM TC-99M ALBUMIN KIT

	INJECTABLE; INJECTION		
	TECHNETIUM TC 99M HSA		
	MEDI PHYSICS	N/A	N17775 001

TECHNETIUM TC-99M DISOFENIN KIT

	INJECTABLE; INJECTION		
	HEPATOLITE		
	DUPONT	N/A	N18467 001 MAR 16, 1982

TECHNETIUM TC-99M EXAMETAZIME KIT

	INJECTABLE; INJECTION		
	CERETEC		
	AMERSHAM	N/A	N19829 001 DEC 30, 1988

TECHNETIUM TC-99M GLUCEPTATE KIT

	INJECTABLE; INJECTION		
	<u>GLUCOSCAN</u>		
<u>AP</u>	DUPONT	<u>N/A</u>	N17907 001
	<u>TECHNESCAN GLUCEPTATE</u>		
<u>AP</u>	MERCK SHARP DOHME	<u>N/A</u>	N18272 001 JAN 27, 1982

TECHNETIUM TC-99M LIDOFENIN KIT

	INJECTABLE; INJECTION		
	TECHNESCAN HIDA		
	MERCK	N/A	N18489 001 OCT 31, 1986

Prescription Drug Products *(continued)*

TECHNETIUM TC-99M MEBROFENIN KIT

INJECTABLE; INJECTION

	CHOLETEC		
	BRACCO	N/A	N18963 001 JAN 21, 1987

TECHNETIUM TC-99M MEDRONATE KIT

INJECTABLE; INJECTION

	AN-MDP		
AP	CIS	N/A	N18124 001
	MDP-SQUIBB		
AP	BRACCO	N/A	N18107 001
	OSTEOLITE		
AP	DUPONT	N/A	N17972 001
	TECHNESCAN MDP KIT		
AP	MERCK SHARP DOHME	N/A	N18035 001
	TECHNETIUM TC 99M MPI MDP		
AP	MEDI PHYSICS	N/A	N18141 001

TECHNETIUM TC-99M MERTIATIDE KIT

INJECTABLE; INJECTION

	TECHNESCAN MAG3		
	MALLINCKRODT	N/A	N19882 001 JUN 15, 1990

TECHNETIUM TC-99M OXIDRONATE KIT

INJECTABLE; INJECTION

	TECHNESCAN HDP		
	MALLINCKRODT	N/A	N18321 001

TECHNETIUM TC-99M PENTETATE KIT

INJECTABLE; INJECTION

	AN-DTPA		
AP	CIS	N/A	N17714 001
	MPI DTPA KIT - CHELATE		
AP	MEDI PHYSICS	N/A	N17255 001
	TECHNESCAN DTPA KIT		
AP	MERCK	N/A	N18511 001 DEC 29, 1989
	TECHNETIUM TC-99M PENTETATE KIT		
AP	MEDI PHYSICS	N/A	N17264 002

TECHNETIUM TC-99M PYRO/TRIMETA PHOSPHATES KIT

INJECTABLE; INJECTION

	PYROLITE		
	DUPONT	N/A	N17684 001

TECHNETIUM TC-99M PYROPHOSPHATE KIT

INJECTABLE; INJECTION

	PHOSPHOTEC		
AP	BRACCO	N/A	N17680 001
	TECHNESCAN PYP KIT		
AP	MALLINCKRODT	N/A	N17538 001

TECHNETIUM TC-99M RED BLOOD CELL KIT

INJECTABLE; INJECTION

	RBC-SCAN		
	CADEMA	N/A	N20063 001 JUN 11, 1992
	ULTRATAG		
	MALLINCKRODT	N/A	N19981 001 JUN 10, 1991

TECHNETIUM TC-99M SESTAMIBI KIT

INJECTABLE; INJECTION

	CARDIOLITE		
	DUPONT	N/A	N19785 001 DEC 21, 1990

TECHNETIUM TC-99M SODIUM PERTECHNETATE

SOLUTION; INJECTION, ORAL

	SODIUM PERTECHNETATE TC 99M		
	MALLINCKRODT	10-60mCi/ML	N17725 001

TECHNETIUM TC-99M SODIUM PERTECHNETATE GENERATOR

SOLUTION; INJECTION, ORAL

	TECHNETIUM TC 99M GENERATOR		
	DUPONT	0.0083-2.7 CI/GENERATOR	N17771 001
	MEDI PHYSICS	830-16,600mCi/GENERATOR	N17693 001
	ULTRA-TECHNEKOW FM		
	MALLINCKRODT	0.25-3 CI/GENERATOR	N17243 002

TECHNETIUM TC-99M SUCCIMER KIT

INJECTABLE; INJECTION

	MPI DMSA KIDNEY REAGENT		
	MEDI PHYSICS	N/A	N17944 001 MAY 18, 1982

TECHNETIUM TC-99M SULFUR COLLOID

SOLUTION; ORAL

	TECHNETIUM TC 99M SULFUR COLLOID		
	MALLINCKRODT	3mCi/ML	N17724 001

Prescription Drug Products *(continued)*

TECHNETIUM TC-99M SULFUR COLLOID KIT

SOLUTION; INJECTION, ORAL

	AN-SULFUR COLLOID		
AP	CIS	N/A	N17858 001
	TECHNECOLL		
AP	MALLINCKRODT	N/A	N17059 001
	TECHNETIUM TC 99M TSC		
AP	MEDI PHYSICS	N/A	N17784 001
	TESULOID		
AP	BRACCO	N/A	N16923 001

TECHNETIUM TC-99M TEBOROXIME KIT

INJECTABLE; INJECTION

	CARDIOTEC		
	BRACCO	N/A	N19928 001 DEC 19, 1990

TEMAZEPAM

CAPSULE; ORAL

	RESTORIL		
AB	SANDOZ	15 MG	N18163 001
AB	+	30 MG	N18163 002
		7.5 MG	N18163 003 OCT 25, 1991
	TEMAZEPAM		
AB	BARR	15 MG	N71174 001 JUL 10, 1986
AB		30 MG	N71175 001 JUL 10, 1986
AB	DANBURY PHARMA	15 MG	N71446 001 MAY 21, 1993
AB		30 MG	N71447 001 MAY 21, 1993
AB	GENEVA PHARMS	15 MG	N71427 001 JAN 12, 1988
AB		30 MG	N71428 001 JAN 12, 1988
AB	MYLAN	15 MG	N70919 001 JUL 07, 1986
AB		30 MG	N70920 001 JUL 07, 1986
AB	PAR PHARM	15 MG	N71456 001 APR 21, 1987
AB		30 MG	N71457 001 APR 21, 1987
AB	PUREPAC PHARM	15 MG	N71638 001 AUG 07, 1987
AB		30 MG	N71620 001 AUG 07, 1987

TENIPOSIDE

INJECTABLE; INJECTION

	VUMON		
	BRISTOL MYERS SQUIBB	10 MG/ML	N20119 001 JUL 14, 1992

TERAZOSIN HYDROCHLORIDE

TABLET; ORAL

	HYTRIN		
	ABBOTT	EQ 1 MG BASE	N19057 001 AUG 07, 1987
		EQ 1 MG BASE	N20223 001 SEP 29, 1993
	+	EQ 2 MG BASE	N19057 002 AUG 07, 1987
		EQ 2 MG BASE	N20223 002 SEP 29, 1993
		EQ 5 MG BASE	N19057 003 AUG 07, 1987
		EQ 5 MG BASE	N20223 003 SEP 29, 1993
		EQ 10 MG BASE	N19057 004 AUG 07, 1987
		EQ 10 MG BASE	N20223 004 SEP 29, 1993

TERBINAFINE HYDROCHLORIDE

CREAM; TOPICAL

	LAMISIL		
	+ SANDOZ	1%	N20192 001 DEC 30, 1992

TERBUTALINE SULFATE

AEROSOL, METERED; INHALATION

	BRETHAIRE		
	GEIGY	0.2 MG/INH	N18762 001 AUG 17, 1984

INJECTABLE; INJECTION

	BRETHINE		
AP	+ GEIGY	1 MG/ML	N18571 001
	BRICANYL		
AP	MERRELL DOW	1 MG/ML	N17466 001

TABLET; ORAL

	BRETHINE		
BP	GEIGY	2.5 MG	N17849 001
BP	+	5 MG	N17849 002
	BRICANYL		
BP	MERRELL DOW	2.5 MG	N17618 001
BP		5 MG	N17618 002

Prescription Drug Products *(continued)*

TERCONAZOLE
CREAM; VAGINAL
TERAZOL 3
+ JOHNSON RW 0.8% N19964 001 FEB 21, 1991
TERAZOL 7
+ JOHNSON RW 0.4% N19579 001 DEC 31, 1987
SUPPOSITORY; VAGINAL
TERAZOL 3
+ JOHNSON RW 80 MG N19641 001 MAY 24, 1988

TERFENADINE
TABLET; ORAL
SELDANE
+ MERRELL DOW 60 MG N18949 001 MAY 08, 1985

TERFENADINE; *MULTIPLE*
SEE PSEUDOEPHEDRINE HYDROCHLORIDE; TERFENADINE

TERIPARATIDE ACETATE
INJECTABLE; INJECTION
PARATHAR
+ RHONE POULENC RORER 200 UNITS/VIAL N19498 001 DEC 23, 1987

TESTOLACTONE
TABLET; ORAL
TESLAC
+ SQUIBB 50 MG N16118 001

TESTOSTERONE
FILM, EXTENDED RELEASE; TRANSDERMAL
TESTODERM
+ ALZA 4 MG/24 HR N19762 001 OCT 12, 1993
+ 6 MG/24 HR N19762 002 OCT 12, 1993
INJECTABLE; INJECTION
TESTOSTERONE
+ STERIS 100 MG/ML N86417 001 JUL 07, 1983
PELLET; IMPLANTATION
TESTOSTERONE
BARTOR 75 MG N80911 001

TESTOSTERONE CYPIONATE
INJECTABLE; INJECTION
DEPO-TESTOSTERONE
AO + UPJOHN 100 MG/ML N85635 002
AO + 200 MG/ML N85635 003
TESTOSTERONE CYPIONATE
AO STERIS 100 MG/ML N86029 001
AO 200 MG/ML N86030 001

TESTOSTERONE CYPIONATE; *MULTIPLE*
SEE ESTRADIOL CYPIONATE; TESTOSTERONE CYPIONATE

TESTOSTERONE ENANTHATE
INJECTABLE; INJECTION
DELATESTRYL
AO + BTG PHARMS 200 MG/ML N09165 003
TESTOSTERONE ENANTHATE
AO STERIS 200 MG/ML N85598 001
100 MG/ML N85599 001

TESTOSTERONE ENANTHATE; *MULTIPLE*
SEE ESTRADIOL VALERATE; TESTOSTERONE ENANTHATE

TESTOSTERONE PROPIONATE
INJECTABLE; INJECTION
TESTOSTERONE PROPIONATE
+ STERIS 25 MG/ML N80188 001
50 MG/ML N80188 002
+ 100 MG/ML N80188 003

TETRACYCLINE HYDROCHLORIDE
CAPSULE; ORAL
ACHROMYCIN V
AB LEDERLE 250 MG N50278 003
AB + 500 MG N50278 001
BRISTACYCLINE
AB BRISTOL 250 MG N61658 001
AB 250 MG N61888 001
AB 500 MG N61658 002
AB 500 MG N61888 002
PANMYCIN
AB UPJOHN 250 MG N60347 001
ROBITET
AB WYETH AYERST 250 MG N61734 001
AB 500 MG N61734 002
SUMYCIN
AB APOTHECON 250 MG N60429 001
AB 500 MG N60429 003

Prescription Drug Products *(continued)*

TETRACYCLINE HYDROCHLORIDE *(continued)*

	CAPSULE; ORAL		
	TETRACYCLINE HCL		
AB	BARR	250 MG	N61837 001
AB		500 MG	N61837 002
AB	DANBURY PHARMA	250 MG	N62343 001
AB		500 MG	N62343 002
AB	EON LABS	250 MG	N61471 001
AB	GLOBAL PHARMS	250 MG	N60469 001
AB		500 MG	N60469 003
		100 MG	N60469 002
AB	HALSEY	250 MG	N60736 001
AB		500 MG	N60736 002
AB	LABS ATRAL	250 MG	N62752 001 AUG 12, 1988
AB		500 MG	N62752 002 AUG 12, 1988
AB	MK LABS	250 MG	N60173 002
		125 MG	N60173 001
AB	MM MAST	250 MG	N62085 001
AB	MYLAN	250 MG	N60783 001
AB		500 MG	N60783 002
AB	PRIVATE FORM	250 MG	N62686 001 JUL 24, 1986
AB		500 MG	N62686 002 JUL 24, 1986
AB	PUREPAC PHARM	250 MG	N60290 001
AB		500 MG	N60290 002
AB	ROXANE	500 MG	N61214 002
AB	SUPERPHARM	250 MG	N62540 001 MAR 21, 1985
AB		500 MG	N62540 002 MAR 21, 1985
AB	WARNER CHILCOTT	250 MG	N62300 001
AB		500 MG	N62300 002
AB	WEST WARD PHARM	250 MG	N60768 001
AB		500 MG	N60768 002
AB	WYETH AYERST	250 MG	N61685 001
AB		500 MG	N61685 002
AB	ZENITH LABS	250 MG	N60704 001
AB		500 MG	N60704 002
	TETRACYN		
AB	PFIPHARMECS	250 MG	N60082 003
AB		500 MG	N60082 004
	FIBER, EXTENDED RELEASE; PERIODONTAL		
	ACTISITE		
	+ ON SITE	12.7 MG/FIBER	N50653 001 MAR 25, 1994

TETRACYCLINE HYDROCHLORIDE *(continued)*

	INJECTABLE; INJECTION		
	ACHROMYCIN		
AP	+ LEDERLE	250 MG/VIAL	N50273 002
AP		500 MG/VIAL	N50273 003
	TETRACYN		
AP	PFIZER	250 MG/VIAL	N60096 001
AP		500 MG/VIAL	N60096 002
	OINTMENT; OPHTHALMIC, OTIC		
	ACHROMYCIN		
	+ LEDERLE	10 MG/GM	N50266 001
	POWDER FOR RECONSTITUTION; TOPICAL		
	TOPICYCLINE		
	ROBERTS LABS	2.2 MG/ML	N50493 001
	SUSPENSION/DROPS; OPHTHALMIC		
	ACHROMYCIN		
	+ LEDERLE	1%	N50268 001
	SYRUP; ORAL		
	ACHROMYCIN V		
AB	+ LEDERLE	125 MG/5 ML	N50263 002
	SUMYCIN		
AB	SQUIBB	125 MG/5 ML	N60400 001
	TETRACYCLINE HCL		
AB	BARRE	125 MG/5 ML	N60633 001
AB	MK LABS	125 MG/5 ML	N60174 001
AB	PUREPAC PHARM	125 MG/5 ML	N60291 001
	TETRACYN		
AB	PFIPHARMECS	125 MG/5 ML	N60095 001
	TETRAMED		
AB	ZENITH LABS	125 MG/5 ML	N61468 001
	TABLET; ORAL		
	SUMYCIN		
	APOTHECON	50 MG	N61147 003
		100 MG	N61147 002
		250 MG	N61147 001
	+	500 MG	N61147 004

TETRACYCLINE HYDROCHLORIDE; *MULTIPLE*

SEE HYDROCORTISONE; TETRACYCLINE HYDROCHLORIDE

SEE PROCAINE HYDROCHLORIDE; TETRACYCLINE HYDROCHLORIDE

Prescription Drug Products *(continued)*

TETRACYCLINE PHOSPHATE COMPLEX

	CAPSULE; ORAL		
	TETREX		
	BRISTOL	EQ 100 MG HCL	N61653 001
		EQ 250 MG HCL	N61653 002
	+	EQ 250 MG HCL	N61889 002
		EQ 500 MG HCL	N61653 003
		EQ 500 MG HCL	N61889 001

TETRAHYDROZOLINE HYDROCHLORIDE

	SOLUTION; NASAL		
	TYZINE		
	+ KEY PHARMS	0.05%	N86576 002
		0.1%	N86576 001
	SPRAY; NASAL		
	TYZINE		
	+ KEY PHARMS	0.1%	N86576 003

THALLOUS CHLORIDE, TL-201

	INJECTABLE; INJECTION		
	THALLOUS CHLORIDE TL 201		
AP	DUPONT	1mCi/ML	N17806 001
AP	MALLINCKRODT	1mCi/ML	N18150 001
	MEDI PHYSICS	2mCi/ML	N18110 001 FEB 01, 1982

THEOPHYLLINE

	CAPSULE; ORAL		
	BRONKODYL		
BP	STERLING WINTHROP	100 MG	N85264 001
BP		200 MG	N85264 002
	ELIXOPHYLLIN		
BX	FOREST LABS	100 MG	N85545 001 JUL 31, 1984
BX	+	200 MG	N83921 001 JUL 31, 1984
	THEOPHYLLINE		
BP	KV PHARM	100 MG	N85263 001
BP		200 MG	N85263 002
	CAPSULE, EXTENDED RELEASE; ORAL		
	AEROLATE III		
	+ FLEMING PHARMS	65 MG	N85075 003 NOV 24, 1986
	AEROLATE JR		
BC	FLEMING PHARMS	130 MG	N85075 002 NOV 24, 1986
	AEROLATE SR		
BC	FLEMING PHARMS	260 MG	N85075 001 NOV 24, 1986

THEOPHYLLINE *(continued)*

	CAPSULE, EXTENDED RELEASE; ORAL		
	ELIXOPHYLLIN SR		
BC	FOREST LABS	125 MG	N86826 001 JAN 29, 1985
BC		250 MG	N86826 002 JAN 29, 1985
	SLO-BID		
AB	RHONE POULENC RORER	100 MG	N87892 001 JAN 31, 1985
AB		125 MG	N89540 001 MAY 10, 1989
AB		200 MG	N87893 001 JAN 31, 1985
AB	+	300 MG	N87894 001 JAN 31, 1985
BC	+	50 MG	N88269 001 JAN 31, 1985
BC		75 MG	N89539 001 MAY 10, 1989
	SLO-PHYLLIN		
BC	RHONE POULENC RORER	125 MG	N85203 001 MAY 24, 1982
BC		250 MG	N85205 001 MAY 24, 1982
		60 MG	N85206 001 MAY 24, 1982
	SOMOPHYLLIN-CRT		
BC	GRAHAM	50 MG	N87763 001 FEB 27, 1985
BC		100 MG	N87194 001
BC		200 MG	N88382 001 FEB 27, 1985
BC		250 MG	N87193 001
BC		300 MG	N88383 001 FEB 27, 1985
	THEO-DUR		
BC	KEY PHARMS	50 MG	N88022 001 SEP 10, 1985
BC		75 MG	N88015 001 SEP 10, 1985
BC		125 MG	N88016 001 SEP 10, 1985
BC		200 MG	N87995 001 SEP 10, 1985

THEOPHYLLINE *(continued)*

CAPSULE, EXTENDED RELEASE; ORAL

	THEO-24		
BC	WHITBY	100 MG	N87942 001 AUG 22, 1983
BC		200 MG	N87943 001 AUG 22, 1983
BC		300 MG	N87944 001 AUG 22, 1983
		400 MG	N81034 001 FEB 28, 1992
	THEOCLEAR L.A.-130		
BC	+ CENT PHARMS	130 MG	N86569 001 MAY 27, 1982
	THEOCLEAR L.A.-260		
BC	+ CENT PHARMS	260 MG	N86569 002 MAY 27, 1982
	THEOPHYLLINE		
AB	INWOOD LABS	100 MG	N40052 001 FEB 14, 1994
AB		125 MG	N40052 002 FEB 14, 1994
AB		200 MG	N40052 003 FEB 14, 1994
AB		300 MG	N40052 004 FEB 14, 1994
	THEOVENT		
BC	SCHERING	125 MG	N87010 001 JAN 31, 1985
BC		250 MG	N87910 001 JAN 31, 1985

ELIXIR; ORAL

	ELIXOMIN		
AA	CENCI	80 MG/15 ML	N88303 001 JAN 25, 1984
	ELIXOPHYLLIN		
AA	FOREST LABS	80 MG/15 ML	N85186 001
	THEOPHYLLINE		
AA	BARRE	80 MG/15 ML	N85863 001
AA	HALSEY	80 MG/15 ML	N85169 001
AA	PENNEX	80 MG/15 ML	N86748 001
AA	PHARM ASSOC	80 MG/15 ML	N86720 001
AA	THAMES	80 MG/15 ML	N89626 001 OCT 28, 1988

THEOPHYLLINE *(continued)*

INJECTABLE; INJECTION

	THEOPHYLLINE AND DEXTROSE 5% IN PLASTIC CONTAINER		
AP	+ BAXTER	40 MG/100 ML	N18649 001 JUL 26, 1982
AP	+	80 MG/100 ML	N18649 002 JUL 26, 1982
AP	+	160 MG/100 ML	N18649 003 JUL 26, 1982
AP	+	200 MG/100 ML	N18649 004 JUL 26, 1982
AP	+	320 MG/100 ML	N18649 006 NOV 13, 1985
AP	+	400 MG/100 ML	N18649 005 JUL 26, 1982
AP		4 MG/ML	N18649 007 JUL 26, 1982
	THEOPHYLLINE IN DEXTROSE 5% IN PLASTIC CONTAINER		
AP	ABBOTT	40 MG/100 ML	N19211 001 DEC 14, 1984
AP		80 MG/100 ML	N19211 002 DEC 14, 1984
AP		160 MG/100 ML	N19211 003 DEC 14, 1984
AP		200 MG/100 ML	N19211 004 DEC 14, 1984
AP		320 MG/100 ML	N19211 006 JAN 20, 1988
AP		400 MG/100 ML	N19211 005 DEC 14, 1984
AP		4 MG/ML	N19211 007 DEC 14, 1984
	THEOPHYLLINE 0.04% AND DEXTROSE 5% IN PLASTIC CONTAINER		
AP	MCGAW	40 MG/100 ML	N19083 001 NOV 07, 1984
AP		40 MG/100 ML	N19826 001 AUG 14, 1992
	THEOPHYLLINE 0.08% AND DEXTROSE 5% IN PLASTIC CONTAINER		
AP	MCGAW	80 MG/100 ML	N19083 002 NOV 07 1984
AP		80 MG/100 ML	N19826 002 AUG 14, 1992
	THEOPHYLLINE 0.16% AND DEXTROSE 5% IN PLASTIC CONTAINER		
AP	MCGAW	160 MG/100 ML	N19083 003 NOV 07, 1984
AP		160 MG/100 ML	N19826 003 AUG 14, 1992
	THEOPHYLLINE 0.2% AND DEXTROSE 5% IN PLASTIC CONTAINER		
AP	MCGAW	200 MG/100 ML	N19212 001 NOV 07, 1984
AP		200 MG/100 ML	N19826 004 AUG 14, 1992

Prescription Drug Products *(continued)*

THEOPHYLLINE *(continued)*

INJECTABLE; INJECTION

	THEOPHYLLINE 0.32% AND DEXTROSE 5% IN PLASTIC CONTAINER		
AP	MCGAW	320 MG/100 ML	N19826 006 AUG 14, 1992
	THEOPHYLLINE 0.4% AND DEXTROSE 5% IN PLASTIC CONTAINER		
AP	MCGAW	400 MG/100 ML	N19212 002 NOV 07, 1984
AP		4 MG/ML	N19212 003 NOV 07, 1984
AP		400 MG/100 ML	N19826 005 AUG 14, 1992

SOLUTION; ORAL

	AEROLATE		
	FLEMING PHARMS	150 MG/15 ML	N89141 001 DEC 03, 1986
	THEOLAIR		
AA	3M	80 MG/15 ML	N86107 001
	THEOPHYLLINE		
AA	ROXANE	80 MG/15 ML	N87449 001 SEP 15, 1983

SUSPENSION; ORAL

	ELIXICON		
	FOREST LABS	100 MG/5 ML	N85502 001

SYRUP; ORAL

	AQUAPHYLLIN		
AA	FERNDALE LABS	80 MG/15 ML	N87917 001 JAN 18, 1983
	SLO-PHYLLIN		
AA	RHONE POULENC RORER	80 MG/15 ML	N85187 001
	THEOCLEAR-80		
AA	CENT PHARMS	80 MG/15 ML	N87095 001 MAR 01, 1982

TABLET; ORAL

	QUIBRON-T		
	+ ROBERTS LABS	300 MG	N88656 001 AUG 22, 1985
	SLO-PHYLLIN		
	+ RHONE POULENC RORER	100 MG	N85202 001
	+	200 MG	N85204 001
	THEOLAIR		
	+ 3M	125 MG	N86399 001
	+	250 MG	N86399 002

THEOPHYLLINE *(continued)*

TABLET, EXTENDED RELEASE; ORAL

	LABID		
BC	+ PROCTER AND GAMBLE	250 MG	N87225 001
	QUIBRON-T/SR		
BC	ROBERTS LABS	300 MG	N87563 001 JUN 21, 1983
	SUSTAIRE		
BC	ROERIG	100 MG	N85665 001
BC		300 MG	N85665 002
	T-PHYL		
BC	PURDUE FREDERICK	200 MG	N88253 001 AUG 17, 1983
	THEO-DUR		
AB	+ KEY PHARMS	100 MG	N85328 001
AB	+	200 MG	N86998 001
AB	+	300 MG	N85328 002
AB	+	450 MG	N89131 001 JUN 25, 1986
	THEOCHRON		
AB	INWOOD LABS	100 MG	N88320 001 FEB 21, 1985
AB		200 MG	N88321 001 FEB 21, 1985
AB		300 MG	N87400 002 JAN 11, 1983
	THEOLAIR-SR		
BC	3M	200 MG	N88369 001 JUL 16, 1987
BC		250 MG	N86363 002 JUL 16, 1987
BC		300 MG	N88364 001 JUL 16, 1987
	+	500 MG	N89132 001 JUL 16, 1987
	THEOPHYLLINE		
AB	SIDMAK LABS NJ	100 MG	N89807 001 APR 30, 1990
AB		200 MG	N89808 001 APR 30, 1990
AB		300 MG	N89763 001 APR 30, 1990
AB		450 MG	N81236 001 NOV 09, 1992
	UNIPHYL		
	+ PURDUE FREDERICK	400 MG	N87571 001 SEP 01, 1982

THEOPHYLLINE; *MULTIPLE*

SEE MERSALYL SODIUM; THEOPHYLLINE

Prescription Drug Products *(continued)*

THEOPHYLLINE SODIUM GLYCINATE
TABLET; ORAL
ASBRON
+ DORSEY — EQ 150 MG BASE — N85148 001

THIABENDAZOLE
SUSPENSION; ORAL
MINTEZOL
+ MERCK SHARP DOHME — 500 MG/5 ML — N16097 001
TABLET, CHEWABLE; ORAL
MINTEZOL
MERCK SHARP DOHME — 500 MG — N16096 001

THIAMINE; *MULTIPLE*
SEE ASCORBIC ACID; BIOTIN; CYANOCOBALAMIN; ERGOCALCIFEROL; FOLIC ACID; NIACINAMIDE; PANTOTHENIC ACID; PHYTONADIONE; PYRIDOXINE; RIBOFLAVIN; THIAMINE; VITAMIN A PALMITATE; VITAMIN E

THIAMINE HYDROCHLORIDE
INJECTABLE; INJECTION
BETALIN S
AP + LILLY — 100 MG/ML — N80853 001
THIAMINE HCL
AP AKORN — 100 MG/ML — N87968 001 OCT 01, 1982
AP DELL LABS — 100 MG/ML — N83775 001
AP ELKINS SINN — 100 MG/ML — N80575 001
AP FUJISAWA — 100 MG/ML — N80556 001
AP STERIS — 100 MG/ML — N80571 001
AP — 100 MG/ML — N83534 001
+ — 200 MG/ML — N80571 002
200 MG/ML — N83534 002
AP WYETH AYERST — 100 MG/ML — N80553 001

THIAMINE HYDROCHLORIDE; *MULTIPLE*
SEE ASCORBIC ACID; BIOTIN; CYANOCOBALAMIN; DEXPANTHENOL; ERGOCALCIFEROL; FOLIC ACID; NIACINAMIDE; PYRIDOXINE HYDROCHLORIDE; RIBOFLAVIN PHOSPHATE SODIUM; THIAMINE HYDROCHLORIDE; VITAMIN A; VITAMIN E

THIAMYLAL SODIUM
INJECTABLE; INJECTION
SURITAL
+ PARKE DAVIS — 1 GM/VIAL — N07600 003
+ — 5 GM/VIAL — N07600 005
+ — 10 GM/VIAL — N07600 009

THIETHYLPERAZINE MALATE
INJECTABLE; INJECTION
TORECAN
+ SANDOZ — 5 MG/ML — N12754 002

THIETHYLPERAZINE MALEATE
SUPPOSITORY; RECTAL
TORECAN
SANDOZ — 10 MG — N13247 001
TABLET; ORAL
TORECAN
SANDOZ — 10 MG — N12753 001

THIOGUANINE
TABLET; ORAL
THIOGUANINE
BURROUGHS WELLCOME — 40 MG — N12429 001

THIOPENTAL SODIUM
SUSPENSION; RECTAL
PENTOTHAL
ABBOTT — 400 MG/GM — N11679 001

THIORIDAZINE
SUSPENSION; ORAL
MELLARIL-S
SANDOZ — EQ 25 MG HCL/5 ML — N17923 001
+ — EQ 100 MG HCL/5 ML — N17923 002

THIORIDAZINE HYDROCHLORIDE
CONCENTRATE; ORAL
MELLARIL
AA SANDOZ — 30 MG/ML — N11808 012
AA — 100 MG/ML — N11808 018
THIORIDAZINE HCL
AA BARRE — 100 MG/ML — N88229 001 AUG 23, 1983
AA COPLEY PHARM — 30 MG/ML — N89602 001 NOV 09, 1987
AA — 100 MG/ML — N89603 001 NOV 09, 1987
THIORIDAZINE HCL INTENSOL
AA ROXANE — 30 MG/ML — N88941 001 DEC 16, 1985
AA — 100 MG/ML — N88942 001 DEC 16, 1985

Prescription Drug Products *(continued)*

THIORIDAZINE HYDROCHLORIDE *(continued)*

TABLET; ORAL

	MELLARIL			
AB	SANDOZ	10 MG	N11808 003	
AB		15 MG	N11808 016	
AB	+	25 MG	N11808 006	
AB		50 MG	N11808 011	
AB	+	100 MG	N11808 009	
AB		150 MG	N11808 017	
AB	+	200 MG	N11808 015	
	THIORIDAZINE HCL			
AB	BARR	10 MG	N88375 001	NOV 18, 1983
AB		15 MG	N88461 001	NOV 18, 1983
AB		25 MG	N87264 001	NOV 18, 1983
AB		50 MG	N88370 001	NOV 18, 1983
AB		100 MG	N88379 001	NOV 16, 1983
AB		150 MG	N88737 001	SEP 26, 1984
AB		200 MG	N88738 001	OCT 16, 1984
AB	BIOCRAFT	10 MG	N88493 001	MAY 17, 1985
AB		100 MG	N88456 001	MAY 17, 1985
AB	CHELSEA LABS	10 MG	N88561 001	MAY 11, 1984
AB		25 MG	N88567 001	MAY 11, 1984
AB		50 MG	N88563 001	MAY 11, 1984
AB		100 MG	N88564 001	MAY 11, 1984
AB	DANBURY PHARMA	10 MG	N88476 001	NOV 08, 1983
AB		15 MG	N88477 001	NOV 08, 1983
AB		25 MG	N88478 001	NOV 08, 1983
AB		25 MG	N88755 001	JUL 24, 1984
AB		50 MG	N88479 001	NOV 08, 1983
AB		100 MG	N88736 001	JUL 24, 1984

THIORIDAZINE HYDROCHLORIDE *(continued)*

TABLET; ORAL

	THIORIDAZINE HCL			
AB		150 MG	N88869 001	JUN 28, 1985
AB		200 MG	N88872 001	APR 26, 1985
AB	GENEVA PHARMS	10 MG	N88131 001	AUG 30, 1983
AB		15 MG	N88132 001	AUG 30, 1983
AB		25 MG	N88133 001	AUG 30, 1983
AB		50 MG	N88134 001	AUG 30, 1983
AB		100 MG	N88135 001	NOV 20, 1984
AB		150 MG	N88136 001	SEP 17, 1986
AB		200 MG	N88137 001	SEP 17, 1986
AB	MUTUAL PHARM	10 MG	N89431 001	AUG 01, 1986
AB		25 MG	N89432 001	AUG 01, 1986
AB		50 MG	N89433 001	AUG 01, 1986
AB		100 MG	N89953 001	OCT 07, 1988
AB	MYLAN	10 MG	N88001 001	MAR 15, 1983
AB		25 MG	N88002 001	MAR 15, 1983
AB		50 MG	N88003 001	MAR 15, 1983
AB		100 MG	N88004 001	NOV 18, 1983
AB	SUPERPHARM	10 MG	N89103 001	JUL 02, 1985
AB		25 MG	N89104 001	JUL 02, 1985
AB		50 MG	N89105 001	JUL 02, 1985
AB	ZENITH LABS	10 MG	N88270 001	APR 14, 1983
AB		15 MG	N88271 001	APR 14, 1983
AB		25 MG	N88272 001	APR 14, 1983
AB		50 MG	N88194 001	APR 14, 1983

Prescription Drug Products *(continued)*

THIOTEPA

INJECTABLE; INJECTION
THIOTEPA

	+ IMMUNEX	15 MG/VIAL	N11683 001

THIOTHIXENE

CAPSULE; ORAL

	NAVANE		
AB	ROERIG	1 MG	N16584 001
AB		2 MG	N16584 002
AB	+	5 MG	N16584 003
AB		10 MG	N16584 004
		20 MG	N16584 005
	THIOTHIXENE		
AB	DANBURY PHARMA	1 MG	N70600 001 JUN 05, 1987
AB		2 MG	N70601 001 JUN 05, 1987
AB		5 MG	N70602 001 JUN 05, 1987
AB		10 MG	N70603 001 JUN 05, 1987
AB	GENEVA PHARMS	1 MG	N71610 001 JUN 24, 1987
AB		2 MG	N71570 001 JUN 24, 1987
AB		5 MG	N71529 001 JUN 24, 1987
AB		10 MG	N71530 001 JUN 24, 1987
AB	MYLAN	1 MG	N71090 001 JUN 23, 1987
AB		2 MG	N71091 001 JUN 23, 1987
AB		5 MG	N71092 001 JUN 23, 1987
AB		10 MG	N71093 001 JUN 23, 1987

THIOTHIXENE HYDROCHLORIDE

CONCENTRATE; ORAL

	NAVANE		
AA	ROERIG	EQ 5 MG BASE/ML	N16758 001
	THIOTHIXENE HCL		
AA	BARRE	EQ 5 MG BASE/ML	N70969 001 OCT 16, 1987
AA	COPLEY PHARM	EQ 5 MG BASE/ML	N71554 001 OCT 16, 1987
AA	LEMMON	EQ 5 MG BASE/ML	N71184 001 JUN 22, 1987

THIOTHIXENE HYDROCHLORIDE *(continued)*

CONCENTRATE; ORAL

	THIOTHIXENE HCL INTENSOL		
AA	ROXANE	EQ 5 MG BASE/ML	N73494 001 JUN 30, 1992

INJECTABLE; INJECTION

	NAVANE		
	+ ROERIG	EQ 2 MG BASE/ML	N16904 001
	+	EQ 10 MG BASE/VIAL	N16904 002

THONZONIUM BROMIDE; *MULTIPLE*

SEE COLISTIN SULFATE; HYDROCORTISONE ACETATE; NEOMYCIN SULFATE; THONZONIUM BROMIDE

THYROGLOBULIN

TABLET; ORAL
THYROGLOBULIN

	+ GLOBAL PHARMS	64.8 MG	N80151 001

THYROTROPIN

INJECTABLE; INJECTION
THYTROPAR

	+ ARMOUR	10IU/VIAL	N08682 001

TICARCILLIN DISODIUM

INJECTABLE; INJECTION
TICAR

	+ SMITHKLINE BEECHAM	EQ 1 GM BASE/VIAL	N50497 001
	+	EQ 3 GM BASE/VIAL	N50497 002
		EQ 3 GM BASE/VIAL	N62690 001 DEC 19, 1986
	+	EQ 6 GM BASE/VIAL	N50497 003
	+	EQ 20 GM BASE/VIAL	N50497 004
	+	EQ 30 GM BASE/VIAL	N50497 005 APR 04, 1984

TICARCILLIN DISODIUM; *MULTIPLE*

SEE CLAVULANATE POTASSIUM; TICARCILLIN DISODIUM

TICLOPIDINE HYDROCHLORIDE

TABLET; ORAL
TICLID

	+ SYNTEX	250 MG	N19979 002 OCT 31, 1991

Prescription Drug Products *(continued)*

TIMOLOL MALEATE

	SOLUTION/DROPS; OPHTHALMIC		
	TIMOPTIC		
	+ MERCK	EQ 0.25% BASE	N18086 001
	+	EQ 0.5% BASE	N18086 002
	TIMOPTIC IN OCUDOSE		
	+ MERCK	EQ 0.25% BASE	N19463 001 NOV 05, 1986
	+	EQ 0.5% BASE	N19463 002 NOV 05, 1986
	TIMOPTIC-XE		
	+ MERCK	EQ 0.25% BASE	N20330 001 NOV 04, 1993
	+	EQ 0.5% BASE	N20330 002 NOV 04, 1993
	TABLET; ORAL		
	BLOCADREN		
AB	MERCK SHARP DOHME	5 MG	N18017 001
AB		10 MG	N18017 002
AB	+	20 MG	N18017 004
	TIMOLOL MALEATE		
AB	DANBURY PHARMA	5 MG	N72917 001 JUL 31, 1991
AB		10 MG	N72918 001 JUL 31, 1991
AB		20 MG	N72919 001 JUL 31, 1991
AB	GENEVA PHARMS	5 MG	N72550 001 APR 13, 1989
AB		10 MG	N72551 001 APR 13, 1989
AB		20 MG	N72552 001 APR 13, 1989
AB	MYLAN	5 MG	N72666 001 JUN 08, 1990
AB		10 MG	N72667 001 JUN 08, 1990
AB		20 MG	N72668 001 JUN 08, 1990
AB	NOVOPHARM	5 MG	N72648 001 JUN 16, 1993
AB		10 MG	N72649 001 JUN 16, 1993
AB		20 MG	N72650 001 JUN 16, 1993

TIMOLOL MALEATE; *MULTIPLE*

SEE HYDROCHLOROTHIAZIDE; TIMOLOL MALEATE

TIOCONAZOLE

	OINTMENT; VAGINAL		
	VAGISTAT-1		
	+ BRISTOL MYERS SQUIBB	6.5%	N19355 001 DEC 30, 1986

TIOPRONIN

	TABLET; ORAL		
	TIOPRONIN		
	+ UNIV TX	100 MG	N19569 001 AUG 11, 1988

TOBRAMYCIN

	OINTMENT; OPHTHALMIC		
	TOBREX		
	+ ALCON	0.3%	N50555 001
	SOLUTION/DROPS; OPHTHALMIC		
	TOBRAMYCIN		
AT	BAUSCH AND LOMB	0.3%	N64052 001 NOV 29, 1993
AT	STERIS	0.3%	N63176 001 MAY 25, 1994
	TOBREX		
AT	+ ALCON	0.3%	N50541 001
AT		0.3%	N62535 001 DEC 13, 1984

TOBRAMYCIN; *MULTIPLE*

SEE DEXAMETHASONE; TOBRAMYCIN

SEE FLUOROMETHOLONE ACETATE; TOBRAMYCIN

TOBRAMYCIN SULFATE

	INJECTABLE; INJECTION		
	NEBCIN		
AP	+ LILLY	EQ 10 MG BASE/ML	N50477 005
AP		EQ 10 MG BASE/ML	N62008 004
AP		EQ 10 MG BASE/ML	N62707 001 APR 29, 1987
AP	+	EQ 40 MG BASE/ML	N62008 001
	+	EQ 1.2 GM BASE/VIAL	N50519 001

Prescription Drug Products *(continued)*

TOBRAMYCIN SULFATE *(continued)*

INJECTABLE; INJECTION

TOBRAMYCIN SULFATE

AP	ABBOTT	EQ 10 MG BASE/ML	N63080 001 APR 30, 1991
AP		EQ 10 MG BASE/ML	N63112 001 APR 30, 1991
AP		EQ 40 MG BASE/ML	N63111 001 APR 30, 1991
AP		EQ 40 MG BASE/ML	N63116 001 MAY 18, 1992
AP		EQ 40 MG BASE/ML	N63161 001 MAY 29, 1991
AP	APOTHECON	EQ 10 MG BASE/ML	N64021 001 MAY 31, 1994
AP		EQ 40 MG BASE/ML	N64021 002 MAY 31, 1994
AP		EQ 40 MG BASE/ML	N64026 001 MAY 31, 1994
AP	ELKINS SINN	EQ 10 MG BASE/ML	N63128 001 NOV 27, 1991
AP		EQ 40 MG BASE/ML	N63127 001 NOV 27, 1991
AP	GENSIA	EQ 40 MG BASE/ML	N63100 001 JAN 30, 1992
AP	LEDERLE	EQ 10 MG BASE/ML	N63113 001 APR 26, 1991
AP		EQ 40 MG BASE/ML	N63117 001 APR 26, 1991
AP		EQ 40 MG BASE/ML	N63118 001 JUL 29, 1991
AP	MARSAM	EQ 10 MG BASE/ML	N62945 001 AUG 09, 1989
AP		EQ 40 MG BASE/ML	N62945 002 AUG 09, 1989

TOBRAMYCIN SULFATE IN SODIUM CHLORIDE 0.9% IN PLASTIC CONTAINER

	+ ABBOTT	EQ 80 MG BASE/100 ML	N63081 001 JUL 31, 1990
	+	EQ 1.2 MG BASE/ML	N63081 003 JUL 31, 1990
	+	EQ 1.6 MG BASE/ML	N63081 006 JUN 02, 1993

TOCAINIDE HYDROCHLORIDE

TABLET; ORAL

TONOCARD

	MERCK SHARP DOHME	400 MG	N18257 001 NOV 09, 1984
	+	600 MG	N18257 002 NOV 09, 1984

TOLAZAMIDE

TABLET; ORAL

TOLAZAMIDE

AB	BARR	100 MG	N70162 001 JAN 14, 1986
AB		250 MG	N70163 001 JAN 14, 1986
AB		500 MG	N70164 001 JAN 14, 1986
AB	DANBURY PHARMA	100 MG	N70513 001 JAN 09, 1986
AB		250 MG	N70514 001 JAN 09, 1986
AB		500 MG	N70515 001 JAN 09, 1986
AB	GENEVA PHARMS	100 MG	N71633 001 DEC 09, 1987
AB		250 MG	N70289 001 MAR 13, 1986
AB		500 MG	N70290 001 MAR 13, 1986
AB	MUTUAL PHARM	100 MG	N71357 001 JUL 16, 1987
AB		250 MG	N71358 001 JUL 16, 1987
AB		500 MG	N71359 001 JUL 16, 1987
AB	MYLAN	250 MG	N70259 001 JAN 02, 1986
AB		500 MG	N70913 001 MAR 17, 1986
AB	PAR PHARM	100 MG	N70159 001 JAN 06, 1986
AB		250 MG	N70160 001 JAN 06, 1986
AB		500 MG	N70161 001 JAN 06, 1986
AB	ZENITH LABS	100 MG	N18894 001 NOV 02, 1984
AB		250 MG	N18894 002 NOV 02, 1984
AB		500 MG	N18894 003 NOV 02, 1984

TOLINASE

AB	UPJOHN	100 MG	N15500 002
AB		250 MG	N15500 004
AB	+	500 MG	N15500 005

TOLAZOLINE HYDROCHLORIDE

INJECTABLE; INJECTION

PRISCOLINE

	+ CIBA	25 MG/ML	N06403 005 FEB 22, 1985

Prescription Drug Products *(continued)*

TOLBUTAMIDE

TABLET; ORAL

	ORINASE		
AB	+ UPJOHN	500 MG	N10670 001
		250 MG	N10670 002
	TOLBUTAMIDE		
AB	BARR	500 MG	N87121 001
AB	CHELSEA LABS	500 MG	N86109 001
AB	DANBURY PHARMA	500 MG	N87318 001
AB	EON LABS	500 MG	N12678 001
AB	GENEVA PHARMS	500 MG	N86574 001
AB	LEDERLE	500 MG	N86926 001
AB	MYLAN	500 MG	N86445 001
AB	PUREPAC PHARM	500 MG	N88950 001 JUN 17, 1985
AB	SUPERPHARM	500 MG	N88893 001 NOV 19, 1984
AB	ZENITH LABS	500 MG	N87093 001

TOLBUTAMIDE SODIUM

INJECTABLE; INJECTION

	ORINASE DIAGNOSTIC		
	+ UPJOHN	EQ 1 GM BASE/VIAL	N12095 001

TOLMETIN SODIUM

CAPSULE; ORAL

	TOLECTIN DS		
AB	+ JOHNSON RW	EQ 400 MG BASE	N18084 001
	TOLMETIN SODIUM		
AB	BAKER NORTON	EQ 400 MG BASE	N73392 001 JAN 24, 1992
AB	GENEVA PHARMS	EQ 400 MG BASE	N73462 001 APR 30, 1992
AB	LEMMON	EQ 400 MG BASE	N73519 001 MAY 29, 1992
AB	MUTUAL PHARM	EQ 400 MG BASE	N73311 001 NOV 27, 1991
AB	MYLAN	EQ 400 MG BASE	N73393 001 MAY 27, 1993
AB	NOVOPHARM	EQ 400 MG BASE	N73290 001 NOV 27, 1991
AB	PUREPAC PHARM	EQ 400 MG BASE	N73308 001 JAN 24, 1992

TOLMETIN SODIUM *(continued)*

TABLET; ORAL

	TOLECTIN		
AB	JOHNSON RW	EQ 200 MG BASE	N17628 001
	TOLECTIN 600		
AB	+ JOHNSON RW	EQ 600 MG BASE	N17628 002 MAR 08, 1989
	TOLMETIN SODIUM		
AB	GENEVA PHARMS	EQ 200 MG BASE	N73588 001 JUL 31, 1992
AB		EQ 600 MG BASE	N74002 001 SEP 27, 1993
AB	MUTUAL PHARM	EQ 200 MG BASE	N73310 001 NOV 27, 1991
AB	MYLAN	EQ 600 MG BASE	N74473 001 AUG 30, 1994
AB	PUREPAC PHARM	EQ 600 MG BASE	N73527 001 JUN 30, 1992

TORSEMIDE

INJECTABLE; INJECTION

	DEMADEX		
	+ BOEHRINGER MANNHEIM	10 MG/ML	N20137 002 AUG 23, 1993

TABLET; ORAL

	DEMADEX		
	BOEHRINGER MANNHEIM	5 MG	N20136 001 AUG 23, 1993
		10 MG	N20136 002 AUG 23, 1993
		20 MG	N20136 003 AUG 23, 1993
	+	100 MG	N20136 004 AUG 23, 1993

TRANEXAMIC ACID

INJECTABLE; INJECTION

	CYKLOKAPRON		
	+ PHARMACIA	100 MG/ML	N19281 001 DEC 30, 1986

TABLET; ORAL

	CYKLOKAPRON		
	+ PHARMACIA	500 MG	N19280 001 DEC 30, 1986

Prescription Drug Products *(continued)*

TRANYLCYPROMINE SULFATE

TABLET; ORAL

PARNATE

	+ SMITH KLINE FRENCH	EQ 10 MG BASE	N12342 003 AUG 16, 1985

TRAZODONE HYDROCHLORIDE

TABLET; ORAL

DESYREL

AB	APOTHECON	50 MG	N18207 001
AB	+	100 MG	N18207 002
AB		150 MG	N18207 003 MAR 25, 1985
		300 MG	N18207 004 NOV 07, 1988

TRAZODONE HCL

AB	BARR	50 MG	N71258 001 MAR 25, 1987
AB		100 MG	N71196 001 MAR 25, 1987
AB	DANBURY PHARMA	50 MG	N70857 001 OCT 10, 1986
AB		100 MG	N70858 001 OCT 10, 1986
AB	GENEVA PHARMS	50 MG	N72484 001 APR 30, 1990
AB		100 MG	N72483 001 APR 30, 1990
AB	LEMMON	50 MG	N72192 001 FEB 02, 1989
AB		100 MG	N72193 001 FEB 02, 1989
AB	MUTUAL PHARM	50 MG	N73136 001 MAR 24, 1993
AB		100 MG	N73137 001 MAR 24, 1993
AB	MYLAN	50 MG	N71405 001 FEB 27, 1991
AB		100 MG	N71406 001 FEB 27, 1991
AB	PUREPAC PHARM	50 MG	N71636 001 APR 18, 1988
AB		100 MG	N71514 001 APR 18, 1988
AB	SIDMAK LABS NJ	50 MG	N71523 001 DEC 11, 1987
AB		100 MG	N71524 001 DEC 11, 1987

TRAZON-150

AB	SIDMAK LABS NJ	150 MG†	N71525 001 MAR 09, 1988

†SEE SECTION 1.8 OF INTRODUCTION

TRETINOIN

CREAM; TOPICAL

RETIN-A

	+ JOHNSON RW	0.025%	N19049 001 SEP 16, 1988
	+	0.05%	N17522 001
	+	0.1%	N17340 001

GEL; TOPICAL

RETIN-A

	+ JOHNSON RW	0.01%	N17955 001
	+	0.025%	N17579 002

SOLUTION; TOPICAL

RETIN-A

	+ JOHNSON RW	0.05%	N16921 001

TRIAMCINOLONE

TABLET; ORAL

ARISTOCORT

BP	LEDERLE	2 MG	N11161 004
BP		4 MG	N11161 007
BP	+	8 MG	N11161 011
		1 MG	N11161 009

KENACORT

BP	SQUIBB	4 MG	N11283 006
BP		8 MG	N11283 010

TRIAMCINOLONE

BP	DANBURY PHARMA	4 MG	N84270 001
BP	GLOBAL PHARMS	4 MG	N84340 001
BP	LEMMON	4 MG	N84775 001
BP	PUREPAC PHARM	2 MG	N84020 002
BP		4 MG	N84020 003
BP	ROXANE	2 MG	N84708 001
BP		4 MG	N84709 001
BP		8 MG	N84707 001
BP	ZENITH LABS	4 MG	N83750 001

TRIAMCINOLONE ACETONIDE

AEROSOL; TOPICAL

KENALOG

	+ APOTHECON	0.147 MG/GM	N12104 001

AEROSOL, METERED; INHALATION

AZMACORT

	+ RHONE POULENC RORER	0.1 MG/INH	N18117 001 APR 23, 1982

Prescription Drug Products *(continued)*

TRIAMCINOLONE ACETONIDE *(continued)*

	AEROSOL, METERED; NASAL			
	NASACORT			
	+ RHONE POULENC RORER	0.055 MG/INH	N19798 001	JUL 11, 1991
	CREAM; TOPICAL			
	ARISTOCORT			
AT	LEDERLE	0.025%	N83017 003	
AT		0.1%	N83016 004	
AT		0.5%	N83015 002	
	ARISTOCORT A			
AT	LEDERLE	0.025%	N83017 004	
AT		0.025%	N88818 001	OCT 16, 1984
AT		0.1%	N83016 005	
AT		0.1%	N88819 001	OCT 16, 1984
AT		0.5%	N83015 003	
AT		0.5%	N88820 001	OCT 16, 1984
	FLUTEX			
AT	SYOSSET	0.025%	N85539 001	
AT		0.1%	N85539 002	
AT		0.5%	N85539 003	
	KENALOG			
AT	+ APOTHECON	0.025%	N11601 003	
AT	+	0.1%	N11601 006	
AT	+	0.5%	N83943 001	
	KENALOG-H			
AT	WESTWOOD SQUIBB	0.1%	N86240 001	
	TRIACET			
AT	LEMMON	0.025%	N84908 001	
AT		0.1%	N84908 002	
AT		0.5%	N84908 003	
	TRIAMCINOLONE ACETONIDE			
AT	ALTANA	0.025%	N85692 001	
AT		0.1%	N85692 003	
AT		0.5%	N85692 002	
AT	AMBIX	0.025%	N87932 001	MAY 09, 1983
AT	CLAY PARK	0.025%	N86415 001	
AT		0.1%	N86414 001	
AT		0.5%	N86413 001	
AT	G AND W LABS	0.025%	N89797 001	MAY 31, 1991
AT		0.1%	N89798 001	MAY 31, 1991
AT	NMC	0.025%	N87797 001	JUN 07, 1982
AT		0.1%	N87798 001	JUN 04, 1982

TRIAMCINOLONE ACETONIDE *(continued)*

	CREAM; TOPICAL			
	TRIAMCINOLONE ACETONIDE			
AT	THAMES	0.025%	N86277 001	
AT		0.1%	N86276 001	
AT		0.5%	N86275 001	
AT	TOPIDERM	0.025%	N89274 001	FEB 21, 1989
AT		0.1%	N89275 001	FEB 21, 1989
AT		0.5%	N89276 001	FEB 21, 1989
	TRIATEX			
AT	SYOSSET	0.025%	N87430 001	NOV 01, 1988
AT		0.1%	N87429 001	NOV 01, 1988
AT		0.5%	N87428 001	NOV 01, 1988
	TRIDERM			
AT	DEL RAY LABS	0.1%	N88042 001	MAR 19, 1984
	TRYMEX			
AT	SAVAGE LABS	0.025%	N88196 001	MAR 25, 1983
AT		0.1%	N88197 001	MAR 25, 1983
	INJECTABLE; INJECTION			
	KENALOG-10			
	+ WESTWOOD SQUIBB	10 MG/ML	N12041 001	
	KENALOG-40			
BP	WESTWOOD SQUIBB	40 MG/ML	N14901 001	
	TRIAMCINOLONE ACETONIDE			
	PARNELL	3 MG/ML	N19503 001	OCT 16, 1987
BP	STERIS	40 MG/ML	N85825 001	
	LOTION; TOPICAL			
	KENALOG			
AT	WESTWOOD SQUIBB	0.025%	N84343 001	
AT	+	0.1%	N84343 002	
	TRIAMCINOLONE ACETONIDE			
AT	BARRE	0.025%	N87191 001	SEP 08, 1982
AT		0.1%	N87192 001	SEP 08, 1982
AT	PENNEX	0.025%	N88450 001	APR 01, 1985
AT		0.1%	N88451 001	APR 03, 1985
AT	THAMES	0.1%	N89129 001	AUG 14, 1986

Prescription Drug Products *(continued)*

TRIAMCINOLONE ACETONIDE *(continued)*

OINTMENT; TOPICAL

	ARISTOCORT		
AT	LEDERLE	0.1%	N80750 004
AT		0.5%	N80745 002
	ARISTOCORT A		
AT	LEDERLE	0.1%	N80750 003
AT		0.1%	N88780 001 OCT 01, 1984
AT		0.5%	N80745 003
	FLUTEX		
AT	SYOSSET	0.025%	N87375 001 NOV 01, 1988
AT		0.1%	N87377 001 NOV 01, 1988
AT		0.5%	N87376 001 NOV 01, 1988
	KENALOG		
AT	+ APOTHECON	0.025%	N11600 003
AT	+	0.1%	N11600 001
AT	+	0.5%	N83944 001
	TRIAMCINOLONE ACETONIDE		
AT	ALTANA	0.025%	N85691 001
AT		0.1%	N85691 003
AT		0.5%	N85691 002
AT	BARRE	0.5%	N89913 001 DEC 23, 1988
AT	CLAY PARK	0.025%	N87356 001
AT		0.1%	N87357 001
AT		0.5%	N87385 001
AT	G AND W LABS	0.025%	N89795 001 DEC 23, 1988
AT		0.1%	N89796 001 DEC 23, 1988
AT	NMC	0.1%	N87799 001 JUN 07, 1982
AT	THAMES	0.1%	N87902 001 DEC 27, 1982
	TRYMEX		
AT	SAVAGE LABS	0.025%	N88693 001 AUG 02, 1984
AT		0.1%	N88691 001 AUG 02, 1984

PASTE; DENTAL

	KENALOG IN ORABASE		
AT	+ SQUIBB	0.1%	N12097 001
	ORACORT		
AT	TARO	0.1%	N70730 001 OCT 01, 1986
	ORALONE		
AT	THAMES	0.1%	N71383 001 JUL 06, 1987

TRIAMCINOLONE ACETONIDE; *MULTIPLE*

SEE NYSTATIN; TRIAMCINOLONE ACETONIDE

TRIAMCINOLONE DIACETATE

INJECTABLE; INJECTION

	ARISTOCORT		
BP	+ LEDERLE	25 MG/ML	N11685 003
BP	+	40 MG/ML	N12802 001
	TRIAMCINOLONE DIACETATE		
BP	AKORN	25 MG/ML	N85122 001
BP		40 MG/ML	N86394 001
BP	STERIS	40 MG/ML	N84072 001
BP		40 MG/ML	N85529 001

SYRUP; ORAL

	ARISTOCORT		
	LEDERLE	2 MG/5 ML	N11960 004
	KENACORT		
	SQUIBB	EQ 4 MG BASE/5 ML	N12515 001

TRIAMCINOLONE HEXACETONIDE

INJECTABLE; INJECTION

	ARISTOSPAN		
	+ LEDERLE	5 MG/ML	N16466 001
	+	20 MG/ML	N16466 002

TRIAMTERENE

CAPSULE; ORAL

	DYRENIUM		
	SMITHKLINE BEECHAM	50 MG	N13174 001
		100 MG	N13174 002

TRIAMTERENE; *MULTIPLE*

SEE HYDROCHLOROTHIAZIDE; TRIAMTERENE

TRIAZOLAM

TABLET; ORAL

	HALCION		
AB	UPJOHN	0.125 MG	N17892 003 APR 26, 1985
AB		0.25 MG	N17892 001 NOV 15, 1982

Prescription Drug Products *(continued)*

TRIAZOLAM *(continued)*

TABLET; ORAL

TE	Product / Applicant	Strength	Appl. No.
	TRIAZOLAM		
AB	ALPHAPHARM	0.125 MG	N74031 001 MAR 25, 1994
AB		0.25 MG	N74031 002 MAR 25, 1994
AB	ROXANE	0.125 MG	N74224 001 JUN 01, 1994
AB		0.25 MG	N74224 002 JUN 01, 1994

TRICHLORMETHIAZIDE

TABLET; ORAL

TE	Product / Applicant	Strength	Appl. No.
	METAHYDRIN		
BP	MERRELL DOW	2 MG	N12594 001 JUN 16, 1988
BP		4 MG	N12594 002 JUN 16, 1988
	NAQUA		
BP	SCHERING	2 MG	N12265 001
BP	+	4 MG	N12265 002
	TRICHLOREX		
BP	LANNETT	4 MG	N83436 001
BP		4 MG	N85630 001
	TRICHLORMAS		
BP	MM MAST	4 MG	N86259 001
	TRICHLORMETHIAZIDE		
BP	CAMALL	4 MG	N85568 001
BP	DANBURY PHARMA	2 MG	N83847 001
BP		4 MG	N83855 001
BP	GLOBAL PHARMS	4 MG	N83967 001
BP	PAR PHARM	2 MG	N87007 001
BP		4 MG	N87005 001

TRICHLORMETHIAZIDE; *MULTIPLE*

SEE RESERPINE; TRICHLORMETHIAZIDE

TRIENTINE HYDROCHLORIDE

CAPSULE; ORAL

TE	Product / Applicant	Strength	Appl. No.
	SYPRINE		
	+ MERCK SHARP DOHME	250 MG	N19194 001 NOV 08, 1985

TRIETHANOLAMINE POLYPEPTIDE OLEATE CONDENSATE

SOLUTION/DROPS; OTIC

TE	Product / Applicant	Strength	Appl. No.
	CERUMENEX		
	+ PURDUE FREDERICK	10%	N11340 002

TRIFLUOPERAZINE HYDROCHLORIDE

CONCENTRATE; ORAL

TE	Product / Applicant	Strength	Appl. No.
	STELAZINE		
AA	SMITHKLINE BEECHAM	EQ 10 MG BASE/ML	N11552 006
	TRIFLUOPERAZINE HCL		
AA	GENEVA PHARMS	EQ 10 MG BASE/ML	N85787 001 APR 15, 1982

INJECTABLE; INJECTION

TE	Product / Applicant	Strength	Appl. No.
	STELAZINE		
	+ SMITHKLINE BEECHAM	EQ 2 MG BASE/ML	N11552 005

TABLET; ORAL

TE	Product / Applicant	Strength	Appl. No.
	STELAZINE		
AB	SMITHKLINE BEECHAM	EQ 1 MG BASE	N11552 001
AB		EQ 2 MG BASE	N11552 002
AB		EQ 5 MG BASE	N11552 003
AB	+	EQ 10 MG BASE	N11552 004
	TRIFLUOPERAZINE HCL		
AB	GENEVA PHARMS	EQ 1 MG BASE	N85785 001
AB		EQ 2 MG BASE	N85786 001
AB		EQ 5 MG BASE	N85789 001
AB		EQ 10 MG BASE	N85788 001
AB	ZENITH LABS	EQ 1 MG BASE	N87612 001 NOV 19, 1982
AB		EQ 2 MG BASE	N87613 001 NOV 19, 1982
AB		EQ 5 MG BASE	N87328 001 NOV 19, 1982
AB		EQ 10 MG BASE	N87614 001 NOV 19, 1982

TRIFLUPROMAZINE HYDROCHLORIDE

INJECTABLE; INJECTION

TE	Product / Applicant	Strength	Appl. No.
	VESPRIN		
	+ APOTHECON	10 MG/ML	N11325 004
	+	20 MG/ML	N11325 001

TRIFLURIDINE

SOLUTION/DROPS; OPHTHALMIC

TE	Product / Applicant	Strength	Appl. No.
	VIROPTIC		
	BURROUGHS WELLCOME	1%	N18299 001

Prescription Drug Products *(continued)*

TRIHEXYPHENIDYL HYDROCHLORIDE

	CAPSULE, EXTENDED RELEASE; ORAL		
	ARTANE		
	+ LEDERLE	5 MG	N12947 001
	ELIXIR; ORAL		
	ARTANE		
AA	LEDERLE	2 MG/5 ML	N06773 009
	TRIHEXYPHENIDYL HCL		
AA	LIQUIPHARM	2 MG/5 ML	N89514 001 APR 07, 1989
	TABLET; ORAL		
	ARTANE		
AA	LEDERLE	2 MG	N06773 005
AA		5 MG	N06773 003
	TRIHEXYPHENIDYL HCL		
AA	DANBURY PHARMA	2 MG	N84363 001
AA		5 MG	N84364 001
AA	NYLOS	5 MG	N85622 001

TRILOSTANE

	CAPSULE; ORAL		
	MODRASTANE		
	STERLING WINTHROP	30 MG	N18719 002 DEC 31, 1984
	+	60 MG	N18719 001 DEC 31, 1984

TRIMEPRAZINE TARTRATE

	CAPSULE, EXTENDED RELEASE; ORAL		
	TEMARIL		
	+ ALLERGAN HERBERT	EQ 5 MG BASE	N11316 004
	SYRUP; ORAL		
	TEMARIL		
	ALLERGAN HERBERT	EQ 2.5 MG BASE/5 ML	N11316 003
	TABLET; ORAL		
	TEMARIL		
	ALLERGAN HERBERT	EQ 2.5 MG BASE	N11316 001

TRIMETHADIONE

	CAPSULE; ORAL		
	TRIDIONE		
	+ ABBOTT	300 MG	N05856 005
	SOLUTION; ORAL		
	TRIDIONE		
	ABBOTT	200 MG/5 ML	N05856 002
	TABLET; ORAL		
	TRIDIONE		
	+ ABBOTT	150 MG	N05856 009

TRIMETHAPHAN CAMSYLATE

	INJECTABLE; INJECTION		
	ARFONAD		
	+ ROCHE	50 MG/ML	N08983 001

TRIMETHOBENZAMIDE HYDROCHLORIDE

	INJECTABLE; INJECTION		
	TIGAN		
AP	+ SMITHKLINE BEECHAM	100 MG/ML	N17530 001
	TRIMETHOBENZAMIDE HCL		
AP	SMITH AND NEPHEW	100 MG/ML	N88960 001 APR 04, 1986
AP	SOLOPAK	100 MG/ML	N89094 001 APR 04, 1986
AP	STERIS	100 MG/ML	N86577 001 OCT 19, 1982
AP		100 MG/ML	N87939 001 DEC 28, 1982
AP	STERLING WINTHROP	100 MG/ML	N88804 001 APR 03, 1987

TRIMETHOPRIM

	TABLET; ORAL		
	PROLOPRIM		
AB	BURROUGHS WELLCOME	100 MG	N17943 001
AB		200 MG	N17943 003 JUL 14, 1982
	TRIMETHOPRIM		
AB	BARR	100 MG	N70494 001 JAN 22, 1986
AB	BIOCRAFT	100 MG	N18679 001 JUL 30, 1982
AB		200 MG	N71259 001 JUN 18, 1987
AB	DANBURY PHARMA	100 MG	N70049 001 JUN 06, 1985
	TRIMPEX		
AB	ROCHE	100 MG	N17952 001
	TRIMPEX 200		
AB	+ ROCHE	200 MG	N17952 002 NOV 09, 1982

TRIMETHOPRIM; *MULTIPLE*

SEE SULFAMETHOXAZOLE; TRIMETHOPRIM

TRIMETHOPRIM SULFATE; *MULTIPLE*

SEE POLYMYXIN B SULFATE; TRIMETHOPRIM SULFATE

Prescription Drug Products *(continued)*

TRIMETREXATE GLUCURONATE

INJECTABLE; INJECTION

	NEUTREXIN		
	+ US BIOSCIENCE	EQ 25 MG BASE/VIAL	N20326 001 DEC 17, 1993

TRIMIPRAMINE MALEATE

CAPSULE; ORAL

	SURMONTIL		
	WYETH AYERST	EQ 25 MG BASE	N16792 001
		EQ 50 MG BASE	N16792 002
	+	EQ 100 MG BASE	N16792 003 SEP 15, 1982

TRIOXSALEN

TABLET; ORAL

	TRISORALEN		
	ICN	5 MG	N12697 001

TRIPELENNAMINE CITRATE

ELIXIR; ORAL

	PBZ		
	GEIGY	EQ 25 MG HCL/5 ML	N05914 004

TRIPELENNAMINE HYDROCHLORIDE

TABLET; ORAL

	PBZ		
AA	GEIGY	50 MG	N05914 002
		25 MG	N83149 001
	TRIPELENNAMINE HCL		
AA	DANBURY PHARMA	50 MG	N80713 001
AA	GLOBAL PHARMS	50 MG	N80785 001
AA	LANNETT	50 MG	N83557 001
AA	NYLOS	50 MG	N85412 001

TABLET, EXTENDED RELEASE; ORAL

	PBZ-SR		
	GEIGY	100 MG	N10533 001

TRIPLE SULFA (SULFABENZAMIDE;SULFACETAMIDE;SULFATHIAZOLE)

CREAM; VAGINAL

	GYNE-SULF		
AT	G AND W LABS	3.7%;2.86%;3.42%	N88607 001 JUN 09, 1986
	SULTRIN		
AT	+ JOHNSON RW	3.7%;2.86%;3.42%	N05794 001

TRIPLE SULFA (SULFABENZAMIDE;SULFACETAMIDE;SULFATHIAZOLE) *(continued)*

CREAM; VAGINAL

	TRIPLE SULFA		
AT	CLAY PARK	3.7%;2.86%;3.42%	N87285 001 NOV 15, 1982
AT	FOUGERA	3.7%;2.86%;3.42%	N86424 001
AT	NMC	3.7%;2.86%;3.42%	N87864 001 SEP 01, 1982
	TRYSUL		
AT	SAVAGE LABS	3.7%;2.86%;3.42%	N87887 001 JUL 23, 1982

TABLET; VAGINAL

	SULTRIN		
	+ JOHNSON RW	184 MG;143.75 MG;172.5 MG	N05794 002

TRIPROLIDINE HYDROCHLORIDE

SYRUP; ORAL

	TRIPROLIDINE HCL		
	HALSEY	1.25 MG/5 ML	N88735 001 JAN 17, 1985

TABLET; ORAL

	TRIPROLIDINE HCL		
	DANBURY PHARMA	2.5 MG	N85094 001

TRIPROLIDINE HYDROCHLORIDE; *MULTIPLE*

SEE CODEINE PHOSPHATE; PSEUDOEPHEDRINE HYDROCHLORIDE; TRIPROLIDINE HYDROCHLORIDE

SEE PSEUDOEPHEDRINE HYDROCHLORIDE; TRIPROLIDINE HYDROCHLORIDE

TRISULFAPYRIMIDINES (SULFADIAZINE; SULFAMERAZINE; SULFAMETHAZINE)

SUSPENSION; ORAL

	NEOTRIZINE		
AB	+ LILLY	167 MG/5 ML;167 MG/5 ML;167 MG/5 ML	N06317 012
	TERFONYL		
AB	SQUIBB	167 MG/5 ML;167 MG/5 ML;167 MG/5 ML	N06904 002

TABLET; ORAL

	NEOTRIZINE		
AB	+ LILLY	167 MG;167 MG;167 MG	N06317 011
	SULFA-TRIPLE #2		
AB	GLOBAL PHARMS	167 MG;167 MG;167 MG	N80079 001
	TERFONYL		
AB	SQUIBB	167 MG;167 MG;167 MG	N06904 001
	TRIPLE SULFOID		
AB	VALE	167 MG;167 MG;167 MG	N80094 001

Prescription Drug Products *(continued)*

TROLEANDOMYCIN
CAPSULE; ORAL
TAO
+ ROERIG — EQ 250 MG BASE — N50336 002

TROMETHAMINE
INJECTABLE; INJECTION
THAM
+ ABBOTT — 3.6 GM/100 ML — N13025 002

TROMETHAMINE; *MULTIPLE*
SEE POTASSIUM CHLORIDE; SODIUM CHLORIDE; TROMETHAMINE

TROPICAMIDE
SOLUTION/DROPS; OPHTHALMIC

	MYDRIACYL		
AT	+ ALCON	0.5%	N84305 001
AT	+	1%	N84306 001
	TROPICAMIDE		
AT	AKORN	1%	N88447 001 AUG 28, 1985
AT	BAUSCH AND LOMB	0.5%	N40067 001 JUL 27, 1994
AT		1%	N40064 001 JUL 27, 1994
AT	OPTOPICS	0.5%	N87636 001 JUL 30, 1982
AT		1%	N87637 001 AUG 09, 1982
AT	STERIS	0.5%	N89171 001 DEC 28, 1990
AT		1%	N89172 001 DEC 28, 1990

TROPICAMIDE; *MULTIPLE*
SEE HYDROXYAMPHETAMINE HYDROBROMIDE; TROPICAMIDE

TUBOCURARINE CHLORIDE
INJECTABLE; INJECTION

	TUBOCURARINE CHLORIDE		
AP	ABBOTT	3 MG/ML	N06095 001
AP	LILLY	3 MG/ML	N06325 001
AP	+ SQUIBB	3 MG/ML	N05657 001

TYLOXAPOL; *MULTIPLE*
SEE CETYL ALCOHOL; COLFOSCERIL PALMITATE; TYLOXAPOL

TYROPANOATE SODIUM
CAPSULE; ORAL
BILOPAQUE
STERLING WINTHROP — 750 MG — N13731 001

URACIL MUSTARD
CAPSULE; ORAL
URACIL MUSTARD
ROBERTS LABS — 1 MG — N12892 001

UREA
INJECTABLE; INJECTION
UREAPHIL
+ ABBOTT — 40 GM/VIAL — N12154 001

UREA; *MULTIPLE*
SEE HYDROCORTISONE; UREA
SEE HYDROCORTISONE ACETATE; UREA

UROFOLLITROPIN
INJECTABLE; INJECTION
METRODIN
+ SERONO — 75IU/AMP — N19415 002 SEP 18, 1986

URSODIOL
CAPSULE; ORAL
ACTIGALL
+ CIBA — 300 MG — N19594 002 DEC 31, 1987

VALPROIC ACID
CAPSULE; ORAL

	DEPAKENE		
AB	+ ABBOTT	250 MG	N18081 001
	VALPROIC ACID		
AB	BANNER PHARMACAPS	250 MG	N73484 001 JUN 29, 1993
AB	PAR PHARM	250 MG	N70431 001 FEB 28, 1986
AB	ROSEMONT PHARM	250 MG	N70631 001 JUN 11, 1987
AB	SCHERER	250 MG	N70195 001 JUL 02, 1987
AB		250 MG	N73229 001 OCT 29, 1991

Prescription Drug Products *(continued)*

VALPROIC ACID *(continued)*

SYRUP; ORAL

	DEPAKENE		
AA	ABBOTT	250 MG/5 ML	N18082 001
	MYPROIC ACID		
AA	PENNEX	250 MG/5 ML	N70868 001 JUL 01, 1986
	VALPROIC ACID		
AA	COPLEY PHARM	250 MG/5 ML	N73178 001 AUG 25, 1992

VANCOMYCIN HYDROCHLORIDE

CAPSULE; ORAL

	VANCOCIN HCL		
	LILLY	EQ 125 MG BASE	N50606 001 APR 15, 1986
	+	EQ 250 MG BASE	N50606 002 APR 15, 1986

INJECTABLE; INJECTION

	LYPHOCIN		
AP	FUJISAWA	EQ 500 MG BASE/VIAL	N62663 001 MAR 17, 1987
AP		EQ 1 GM BASE/VIAL	N62663 002 JUL 31, 1987
AP		EQ 5 GM BASE/VIAL	N62663 003 JUN 03, 1988
	VANCOCIN HCL		
AP	+ LILLY	EQ 500 MG BASE/VIAL	N60180 001
AP		EQ 500 MG BASE/VIAL	N62476 001 MAR 15, 1984
AP		EQ 500 MG BASE/VIAL	N62716 001 MAR 13, 1987
AP		EQ 500 MG BASE/VIAL	N62812 001 NOV 17, 1987
AP	+	EQ 1 GM BASE/VIAL	N60180 002 MAR 21, 1986
AP		EQ 1 GM BASE/VIAL	N62476 002 MAR 21, 1986
AP		EQ 1 GM BASE/VIAL	N62716 002 MAR 13, 1987
AP		EQ 1 GM BASE/VIAL	N62812 002 NOV 17, 1987
AP	+	EQ 10 GM BASE/VIAL	N62812 003 NOV 17, 1987
	VANCOCIN HCL IN PLASTIC CONTAINER		
	+ LILLY	EQ 500 MG BASE/100 ML	N50671 001 APR 29, 1993

VANCOMYCIN HYDROCHLORIDE *(continued)*

INJECTABLE; INJECTION

	VANCOLED		
AP	LEDERLE	EQ 500 MG BASE/VIAL	N62682 001 JUL 22, 1986
AP		EQ 1 GM BASE/VIAL	N62682 002 MAR 30, 1988
AP	+	EQ 5 GM BASE/VIAL	N62682 004 MAY 11, 1988
AP		EQ 10 GM BASE/VIAL	N62682 005 MAY 11, 1988
	+	EQ 2 GM BASE/VIAL	N62682 003 MAY 11, 1988
	VANCOMYCIN HCL		
AP	ABBOTT	EQ 500 MG BASE/VIAL	N62911 001 AUG 04, 1988
AP		EQ 500 MG BASE/VIAL	N62931 001 OCT 29, 1992
AP		EQ 1 GM BASE/VIAL	N62912 001 AUG 04, 1988
AP		EQ 1 GM BASE/VIAL	N62933 001 OCT 29, 1992
AP		EQ 5 GM BASE/VIAL	N63076 001 DEC 21, 1990
AP	ELKINS SINN	EQ 500 MG BASE/VIAL	N62879 001 AUG 02, 1988
AP		EQ 1 GM BASE/VIAL	N62879 002 AUG 02, 1988

POWDER FOR RECONSTITUTION; ORAL

	VANCOCIN HCL		
AB	LILLY	EQ 250 MG BASE/5 ML	N61667 002 JUL 13, 1983
AB		EQ 500 MG BASE/6 ML	N61667 001
	VANCOLED		
AB	LEDERLE	EQ 250 MG BASE/5 ML	N63321 002 OCT 15, 1993
AB		EQ 500 MG BASE/6 ML	N63321 003 OCT 15, 1993

VECURONIUM BROMIDE

INJECTABLE; INJECTION

	NORCURON		
	ORGANON	10 MG/VIAL	N18776 002 APR 30, 1984
		20 MG/VIAL	N18776 003 JAN 03, 1992

Prescription Drug Products *(continued)*

VENLAFAXINE HYDROCHLORIDE

TABLET; ORAL

TE	Product / Applicant	Strength	Appl No / Approval Date
	EFFEXOR		
	+ WYETH AYERST	EQ 25 MG BASE	N20151 002 DEC 28, 1993
		EQ 37.5 MG BASE	N20151 006 DEC 28, 1993
		EQ 50 MG BASE	N20151 003 DEC 28, 1993
		EQ 75 MG BASE	N20151 004 DEC 28, 1993
	+	EQ 100 MG BASE	N20151 005 DEC 28, 1993

VERAPAMIL HYDROCHLORIDE

CAPSULE, EXTENDED RELEASE; ORAL

TE	Product / Applicant	Strength	Appl No / Approval Date
	VERELAN		
	+ ELAN PHARM	120 MG	N19614 001 MAY 29, 1990
	+	180 MG	N19614 003 JAN 09, 1992
	+	240 MG	N19614 002 MAY 29, 1990

INJECTABLE; INJECTION

TE	Product / Applicant	Strength	Appl No / Approval Date
	ISOPTIN		
AP	+ KNOLL PHARM	2.5 MG/ML	N18485 001
	VERAPAMIL HCL		
AP	ABBOTT	2.5 MG/ML	N70737 001 MAY 06, 1987
AP		2.5 MG/ML	N70738 001 MAY 06, 1987
AP		2.5 MG/ML	N70739 001 MAY 06, 1987
AP		2.5 MG/ML	N70740 001 MAY 06, 1987
AP	INTL MEDICATION	2.5 MG/ML	N70451 001 DEC 16, 1985
AP	LUITPOLD	2.5 MG/ML	N70225 001 NOV 12, 1985
AP		2.5 MG/ML	N70617 001 NOV 12, 1985
AP	MARSAM	2.5 MG/ML	N72233 001 FEB 26, 1993
AP		2.5 MG/ML	N73485 001 SEP 27, 1993
AP	SMITH AND NEPHEW	2.5 MG/ML	N70696 001 JUL 31, 1987
AP	SOLOPAK	2.5 MG/ML	N70695 001 JUL 31, 1987
AP	STERLING WINTHROP	2.5 MG/ML	N70577 001 FEB 02, 1987

VERAPAMIL HYDROCHLORIDE (*continued*)

TABLET; ORAL

TE	Product / Applicant	Strength	Appl No / Approval Date
	CALAN		
AB	SEARLE	40 MG	N18817 003 FEB 23, 1988
AB		80 MG	N18817 001 SEP 10, 1984
AB		120 MG	N18817 002 SEP 10, 1984
	ISOPTIN		
AB	KNOLL PHARM	40 MG	N18593 003 NOV 23, 1987
AB		80 MG	N18593 001 MAR 08, 1982
AB	+	120 MG	N18593 002 MAR 08, 1982
	VERAPAMIL HCL		
AB	BARR	80 MG	N70482 001 SEP 24, 1986
AB		120 MG	N70483 001 SEP 24, 1986
AB	DANBURY PHARMA	80 MG	N70855 001 SEP 24, 1986
AB		120 MG	N70856 001 SEP 24, 1986
AB	GENEVA PHARMS	40 MG	N73168 001 JUL 31, 1992
AB		80 MG	N71423 001 MAY 24, 1988
AB		120 MG	N71424 001 MAY 25, 1988
AB	LEDERLE	80 MG	N71880 001 APR 05, 1988
AB		120 MG	N71881 001 APR 05, 1988
AB	MUTUAL PHARM	80 MG	N71488 001 JAN 13, 1988
AB		120 MG	N71489 001 JAN 13, 1988
AB	MYLAN	80 MG	N71482 001 FEB 15, 1989
AB		120 MG	N71483 001 FEB 15, 1989
AB	PUREPAC PHARM	80 MG	N71019 001 SEP 24, 1986
AB		120 MG	N70468 001 SEP 24, 1986
AB	SIDMAK LABS NJ	80 MG	N72124 001 JAN 26, 1989
AB		120 MG	N72125 001 JAN 26, 1989

Prescription Drug Products *(continued)*

VERAPAMIL HYDROCHLORIDE *(continued)*

TABLET; ORAL

VERAPAMIL HCL

AB	WATSON LABS	40 MG	N72923 001 JUN 29, 1993
AB		40 MG	N72924 001 JUN 29, 1993
AB		80 MG	N70995 001 OCT 01, 1986
AB		80 MG	N71366 001 OCT 01, 1986
AB		120 MG	N70994 001 OCT 01, 1986
AB		120 MG	N71367 001 OCT 01, 1986

TABLET, EXTENDED RELEASE; ORAL

ISOPTIN SR

AB	+ KNOLL PHARM	180 MG	N19152 002 DEC 15, 1989
AB	+	240 MG	N19152 001 DEC 16, 1986
	+	120 MG	N19152 003 MAR 06, 1991

VERAPAMIL HCL

AB	BAKER NORTON	180 MG	N74330 001 JAN 31, 1994
AB		240 MG	N73568 001 JUL 31, 1992

VIDARABINE

INJECTABLE; INJECTION

VIRA-A

	+ PARKE DAVIS	EQ 187.4 MG BASE/ML	N50523 001

OINTMENT; OPHTHALMIC

VIRA-A

	+ PARKE DAVIS	3%	N50486 001

VINBLASTINE SULFATE

INJECTABLE; INJECTION

VELBAN

AP	+ LILLY	10 MG/VIAL	N12665 001

VINBLASTINE SULFATE

AP	BEN VENUE	10 MG/VIAL	N89395 001 APR 09, 1987
AP	FAULDING	10 MG/VIAL	N89565 001 AUG 18, 1987
	+ FUJISAWA	1 MG/ML	N89515 001 APR 29, 1987

VINCRISTINE SULFATE

INJECTABLE; INJECTION

ONCOVIN

AP	+ LILLY	1 MG/ML	N14103 003 MAR 07, 1984

VINCASAR PFS

AP	PHARMACIA	1 MG/ML	N71426 001 JUL 17, 1987

VINCREX

AP	+ BRISTOL	5 MG/VIAL	N70867 001 JUL 12, 1988

VINCRISTINE SULFATE

AP	BULL D	5 MG/VIAL	N71561 001 APR 11, 1988
	+	1 MG/VIAL	N71559 001 APR 11, 1988
	+	2 MG/VIAL	N71560 001 APR 11, 1988

VINCRISTINE SULFATE PFS

AP	FAULDING	1 MG/ML	N71484 001 APR 19, 1988

VITAMIN A

CAPSULE; ORAL

AQUASOL A

AA	ASTRA	50,000USP UNITS	N83080 001
		25,000USP UNITS	N83080 002

VITAMIN A

AA	BANNER PHARMACAPS	50,000USP UNITS	N83973 001
AA	GLOBAL PHARMS	50,000USP UNITS	N80952 001
AA	WEST WARD PHARM	50,000USP UNITS	N80985 001

VITAMIN A; *MULTIPLE*

SEE ASCORBIC ACID; BIOTIN; CYANOCOBALAMIN; DEXPANTHENOL; ERGOCALCIFEROL; FOLIC ACID; NIACINAMIDE; PYRIDOXINE HYDROCHLORIDE; RIBOFLAVIN PHOSPHATE SODIUM; THIAMINE HYDROCHLORIDE; VITAMIN A; VITAMIN E

Prescription Drug Products *(continued)*

VITAMIN A PALMITATE

CAPSULE; ORAL

	DEL-VI-A		
AA	DEL RAY LABS	EQ 50,000 UNITS BASE	N80830 001
	VITAMIN A		
AA	BANNER PHARMACAPS	EQ 50,000 UNITS BASE	N80702 001
AA	GLOBAL PHARMS	EQ 50,000 UNITS BASE	N80953 001
AA		EQ 50,000 UNITS BASE	N80955 001
AA	MK LABS	EQ 50,000 UNITS BASE	N83457 001
		EQ 25,000 UNITS BASE	N83457 002
AA	WEST WARD PHARM	EQ 50,000 UNITS BASE	N80967 001
	VITAMIN A PALMITATE		
AA	ARCUM	EQ 50,000 UNITS BASE	N83311 001
AA		EQ 50,000 UNITS BASE	N83321 001
AA	BANNER PHARMACAPS	EQ 50,000 UNITS BASE	N83948 001

INJECTABLE; INJECTION

	AQUASOL A		
	ASTRA	EQ 50,000 UNITS BASE/ML	N06823 001

VITAMIN A PALMITATE; *MULTIPLE*

SEE ASCORBIC ACID; BIOTIN; CYANOCOBALAMIN; ERGOCALCIFEROL; FOLIC ACID; NIACINAMIDE; PANTOTHENIC ACID; PHYTONADIONE; PYRIDOXINE; RIBOFLAVIN; THIAMINE; VITAMIN A PALMITATE; VITAMIN E

VITAMIN E; *MULTIPLE*

SEE ASCORBIC ACID; BIOTIN; CYANOCOBALAMIN; DEXPANTHENOL; ERGOCALCIFEROL; FOLIC ACID; NIACINAMIDE; PYRIDOXINE HYDROCHLORIDE; RIBOFLAVIN PHOSPHATE SODIUM; THIAMINE HYDROCHLORIDE; VITAMIN A; VITAMIN E

SEE ASCORBIC ACID; BIOTIN; CYANOCOBALAMIN; ERGOCALCIFEROL; FOLIC ACID; NIACINAMIDE; PANTOTHENIC ACID; PHYTONADIONE; PYRIDOXINE; RIBOFLAVIN; THIAMINE; VITAMIN A PALMITATE; VITAMIN E

WARFARIN SODIUM

TABLET; ORAL

	COUMADIN		
	DUPONT MERCK	1 MG	N09218 022 MAR 01, 1990
+		2 MG	N09218 013
		2.5 MG	N09218 018
		4 MG	N09218 023 AUG 24, 1993
		5 MG	N09218 007
		7.5 MG	N09218 016
+		10 MG	N09218 005

WATER FOR INJECTION, STERILE

LIQUID; N/A

	BACTERIOSTATIC WATER FOR INJECTION IN PLASTIC CONTAINER		
AP	ABBOTT	100%	N18802 001 OCT 27, 1982
AP	FUJISAWA	100%	N89099 001 DEC 29, 1987
AP		100%	N89100 001 DEC 29, 1987
	STERILE WATER FOR INJECTION IN PLASTIC CONTAINER		
AP	ABBOTT	100%	N18233 001
AP		100%	N18801 001 OCT 27, 1982
AP		100%	N19869 001 DEC 26, 1989
AP	BAXTER	100%	N18632 001 JUN 30, 1982
AP		100%	N18632 002 APR 19, 1988
AP	FUJISAWA	100%	N88400 001 JAN 16, 1984
AP	MCGAW	100%	N19077 001 MAR 02, 1984
AP		100%	N19633 001 FEB 29, 1988

WATER FOR IRRIGATION, STERILE

LIQUID; IRRIGATION

	STERILE WATER		
AT	BAXTER	100%	N17428 001
	STERILE WATER IN PLASTIC CONTAINER		
AT	ABBOTT	100%	N17513 001
AT		100%	N18313 001
AT	BAXTER	100%	N17866 001
AT	MCGAW	100%	N16734 001

XENON, XE-127

GAS; INHALATION

	XENON XE 127		
	MALLINCKRODT	10mCi/VIAL	N18536 002 OCT 01, 1982
		5mCi/VIAL	N18536 001 OCT 01, 1982

Prescription Drug Products *(continued)*

XENON, XE-133

	GAS; INHALATION		
	XENON XE 133		
AA	DUPONT	10mCi/VIAL	N17284 001
AA		20mCi/VIAL	N17284 002
	GENERAL ELECTRIC	1-2.5 CI/AMP	N17550 003
		5 CI/CYLINDER	N17550 001
AA	MALLINCKRODT	10mCi/VIAL	N18327 001 MAR 09, 1982
AA		20mCi/VIAL	N18327 002 MAR 09, 1982
AA	MEDI PHYSICS	10mCi/VIAL	N17687 002
AA		20mCi/VIAL	N17687 003
		1 CI/AMP	N17256 002

XYLOSE

	POWDER; ORAL		
	XYLO-PFAN		
AA	SAVAGE LABS	25 GM/BOT	N17605 001
	XYLOSE		
AA	LYNE	25 GM/BOT	N18856 001 MAR 26, 1987

ZALCITABINE

	TABLET; ORAL		
	HIVID		
	ROCHE	0.375 MG	N20199 001 JUN 19, 1992
	+	0.75 MG	N20199 002 JUN 19, 1992

ZIDOVUDINE

	CAPSULE; ORAL		
	RETROVIR		
	+ BURROUGHS WELLCOME	100 MG	N19655 001 MAR 19, 1987
	INJECTABLE; INJECTION		
	RETROVIR		
	+ BURROUGHS WELLCOME	10 MG/ML	N19951 001 FEB 02, 1990
	SYRUP; ORAL		
	RETROVIR		
	BURROUGHS WELLCOME	50 MG/5 ML	N19910 001 SEP 28, 1989

ZINC CHLORIDE

	INJECTABLE; INJECTION		
	ZINC CHLORIDE IN PLASTIC CONTAINER		
	+ ABBOTT	EQ 1 MG ZINC/ML	N18959 001 JUN 26, 1986

ZOLPIDEM TARTRATE

	TABLET; ORAL		
	AMBIEN		
	LOREX	5 MG	N19908 001 DEC 16, 1992
	+	10 MG	N19908 002 DEC 16, 1992

OTC DRUG PRODUCTS

ACETAMINOPHEN

SUPPOSITORY; RECTAL
ACEPHEN
+ G AND W LABS 120 MG N18060 001
120 MG N72218 001 MAR 27, 1992
+ 325 MG N18060 003 DEC 18, 1986
325 MG N72344 001 MAR 27, 1992
+ 650 MG N18060 002
650 MG N72237 001 MAR 27, 1992
ACETAMINOPHEN
ROXANE 120 MG N71010 001 MAY 12, 1987
650 MG N71011 001 MAY 12, 1987
SUPPOSITORIA 120 MG N70607 001 APR 06, 1987
650 MG N70608 001 DEC 01, 1986
UPSHER SMITH 120 MG N18337 003 SEP 12, 1983
325 MG N18337 002
650 MG N18337 001
INFANTS' FEVERALL
UPSHER SMITH 80 MG N18337 004 AUG 26, 1992
NEOPAP
POLYMEDICA 120 MG N16401 001
TABLET, EXTENDED RELEASE; ORAL
TYLENOL
+ MCNEIL 650 MG N19872 001 JUN 08, 1994

ACETAMINOPHEN; DEXBROMPHENIRAMINE MALEATE; PSEUDOEPHEDRINE SULFATE

TABLET, EXTENDED RELEASE; ORAL
DRIXORAL PLUS
+ SCHERING PLOUGH 500 MG;3 MG;60 MG N19453 001 MAY 22, 1987

ALUMINUM HYDROXIDE; MAGNESIUM TRISILICATE

TABLET, CHEWABLE; ORAL
FOAMCOAT
GUARDIAN DRUG 80 MG;20 MG N71793 001 SEP 04, 1987
FOAMICON
INVAMED 80 MG;20 MG N72687 001 JUN 28, 1989
GAVISCON
+ MARION MERRELL
DOW 80 MG;20 MG N18685 001 DEC 09, 1983
GAVISCON-2
+ MARION MERRELL
DOW 160 MG;40 MG N18685 002 DEC 09, 1983

ASPIRIN

TABLET, EXTENDED RELEASE; ORAL
MEASURIN
+ STERLING WINTHROP 650 MG N16030 002
8-HOUR BAYER
+ STERLING WINTHROP 650 MG N16030 001

AVOBENZONE; OCTYL METHOXYCINNAMATE; OXYBENZONE

LOTION; TOPICAL
SHADE UVAGUARD
PLOUGH 3%;7.5%;3% N20045 001 DEC 07, 1992

AVOBENZONE; PADIMATE O

LOTION; TOPICAL
PHOTOPLEX
+ ALLERGAN HERBERT 3%;7% N19459 001 SEP 30, 1988

BACITRACIN

OINTMENT; TOPICAL
BACITRACIN
+ NASKA 500 UNITS/GM N62857 001 NOV 13, 1987

BACITRACIN ZINC; NEOMYCIN SULFATE; POLYMYXIN B SULFATE

OINTMENT; TOPICAL
BACITRACIN ZINC-NEOMYCIN SULFATE-POLYMYXIN B SULFATE
+ NASKA 400 UNITS/GM;EQ 3.5 MG BASE/GM;5,000 UNITS/GM N62833 001 NOV 09, 1987

OTC Drug Products *(continued)*

BACITRACIN ZINC; POLYMYXIN B SULFATE

OINTMENT; TOPICAL

BACITRACIN ZINC-POLYMYXIN B SULFATE		
+ NASKA	500 UNITS/GM;10,000 UNITS/GM	N62849 001 NOV 13, 1987

BROMPHENIRAMINE MALEATE

TABLET, EXTENDED RELEASE; ORAL

DIMETANE		
+ ROBINS AH	8 MG	N10799 010 JUN 10, 1983
+	12 MG	N10799 011 JUN 10, 1983

BROMPHENIRAMINE MALEATE; PHENYLPROPANOLAMINE HYDROCHLORIDE

ELIXIR; ORAL

DIMETAPP		
+ ROBINS AH	2 MG/5 ML;12.5 MG/5 ML	N13087 003 MAR 29, 1984

TABLET, EXTENDED RELEASE; ORAL

BROMATAPP		
COPLEY PHARM	12 MG;75 MG	N71099 001 JUL 02, 1987
DIMETAPP		
+ ROBINS AH	12 MG;75 MG	N12436 003 MAY 14, 1985

CHLORHEXIDINE GLUCONATE

AEROSOL; TOPICAL

EXIDINE		
+ XTTRIUM	4%	N19127 001 DEC 24, 1984

SOLUTION; TOPICAL

BRIAN CARE		
BRIAN	4%	N71419 001 DEC 17, 1987
CHG SCRUB		
HUNTINGTON LABS	4%	N19258 002 JUL 22, 1986
CIDA-STAT		
HUNTINGTON LABS	2%	N19258 001 JUL 22, 1986
EXIDINE		
+ XTTRIUM	2%	N19422 001 DEC 17, 1985
	4%	N19125 001 DEC 24, 1984

CHLORHEXIDINE GLUCONATE *(continued)*

SOLUTION; TOPICAL

HIBICLENS		
+ ZENECA	4%	N17768 001
HIBISTAT		
+ ZENECA	0.5%	N18300 001
MICROCOL		
JOHNSON AND JOHNSON	0.5%	N72292 001 JAN 28, 1992
MICRODERM		
JOHNSON AND JOHNSON	4%	N72255 001 APR 15, 1991
STERI-STAT		
MATRIX MEDCL	4%	N70104 001 JUL 24, 1986

SPONGE; TOPICAL

BIOSCRUB		
GRIFFEN	4%	N19822 001 MAR 31, 1989
CHLORHEXIDINE GLUCONATE		
DESERET	4%	N72525 001 OCT 24, 1989
KENDALL	4%	N19490 001 MAR 27, 1987
HIBICLENS		
+ ZENECA	4%	N18423 001
MICRODERM		
JOHNSON AND JOHNSON	4%	N72295 001 FEB 28, 1991
PHARMASEAL SCRUB CARE		
BAXTER	4%	N19793 001 DEC 02, 1988

CHLORPHENIRAMINE MALEATE

CAPSULE, EXTENDED RELEASE; ORAL

CHLORPHENIRAMINE MALEATE		
GENEVA PHARMS	12 MG	N70797 001 AUG 12, 1988
TELDRIN		
+ SMITHKLINE	12 MG	N17369 002

TABLET, EXTENDED RELEASE; ORAL

CHLOR-TRIMETON		
+ SCHERING PLOUGH	8 MG	N07638 001
+	12 MG	N07638 002

OTC Drug Products *(continued)*

CHLORPHENIRAMINE MALEATE; PHENYLPROPANOLAMINE HYDROCHLORIDE

CAPSULE, EXTENDED RELEASE; ORAL
COLD CAPSULE IV
+ GRAHAM 12 MG;75 MG N18793 001 APR 25, 1985
COLD CAPSULE V
GRAHAM 8 MG;75 MG N18794 001 APR 23, 1985
CONTAC
+ SMITHKLINE 8 MG;75 MG N18099 001
PHENYLPROPANOLAMINE HCL W/ CHLORPHENIRAMINE MALEATE
CENT PHARMS 8 MG;75 MG N18809 001 MAY 07, 1984

TABLET, EXTENDED RELEASE; ORAL
DEMAZIN
+ SCHERING PLOUGH 4 MG;25 MG N18556 001 MAY 14, 1984
PHENYLPROPANOLAMINE HCL/CHLORPHENIRAMINE
DORSEY 12 MG;75 MG N19613 001
TRIAMINIC-12
+ SANDOZ 12 MG;75 MG N18115 001

CHLORPHENIRAMINE MALEATE; PSEUDOEPHEDRINE HYDROCHLORIDE

CAPSULE, EXTENDED RELEASE; ORAL
CODIMAL-L.A. 12
CENT PHARMS 12 MG;120 MG N18935 001 APR 15, 1985
PSEUDOEPHEDRINE HCL AND CHLORPHENIRAMINE MALEATE
KV PHARM 12 MG;120 MG N71455 001 MAR 01, 1989
PSEUDOEPHEDRINE HCL/CHLORPHENIRAMINE MALEATE
+ GRAHAM 8 MG;120 MG N18844 001 MAR 20, 1985
+ 12 MG;120 MG N18843 001 MAR 18, 1985
PSEUDOEPHEDRINE HYDROCHLORIDE AND CHLORPHENIRAMINE MALEATE
CENT PHARMS 8 MG;120 MG N19428 001 AUG 02, 1988

CHLORPHENIRAMINE MALEATE; PSEUDOEPHEDRINE SULFATE

TABLET, EXTENDED RELEASE; ORAL
CHLOR-TRIMETON
+ SCHERING PLOUGH 8 MG;120 MG N18397 001

CLEMASTINE FUMARATE

TABLET; ORAL
CLEMASTINE FUMARATE
GENEVA PHARMS 1.34 MG N73458 001 OCT 31, 1993
LEMMON 1.34 MG N73282 002 DEC 03, 1992
TAVIST-1
SANDOZ 1.34 MG N17661 003 AUG 21, 1992

CLEMASTINE FUMARATE; PHENYLPROPANOLAMINE HYDROCHLORIDE

TABLET, EXTENDED RELEASE; ORAL
TAVIST-D
SANDOZ 1.34 MG;75 MG N18298 002 AUG 21, 1992

CLOTRIMAZOLE

CREAM; TOPICAL
CLOTRIMAZOLE
TARO 1% N72640 002 AUG 31, 1993
LOTRIMIN AF
+ SCHERING PLOUGH 1% N17619 002 OCT 27, 1989
MYCELEX
MILES 1% N18183 002 APR 01, 1991

CREAM; VAGINAL
CLOTRIMAZOLE
NMC 1% N74165 001 JUL 16, 1993
GYNE-LOTRIMIN
+ SCHERING PLOUGH 1% N18052 002 NOV 30, 1990
MYCELEX-7
MILES 1% N18230 002 DEC 26, 1991

CREAM, SUPPOSITORY; TOPICAL, VAGINAL
GYNE-LOTRIMIN COMBINATION PACK
+ SCHERING PLOUGH 1%;100 MG N20289 002 APR 26, 1993
MYCELEX-7 COMBINATION PACK
MILES 1%;100 MG N20389 002 JUN 23, 1994

OTC Drug Products *(continued)*

CLOTRIMAZOLE *(continued)*

LOTION; TOPICAL
- LOTRIMIN AF
  - + SCHERING — 1% — N18813 002 — OCT 27, 1989

SOLUTION; TOPICAL
- LOTRIMIN AF
  - + SCHERING PLOUGH — 1% — N17613 002 — OCT 27, 1989
- MYCELEX
  - MILES — 1% — N18181 002 — APR 01, 1991

TABLET; VAGINAL
- GYNE-LOTRIMIN
  - + SCHERING PLOUGH — 100 MG — N17717 002 — NOV 30, 1990
- MYCELEX-7
  - MILES — 100 MG — N18182 002 — DEC 26, 1991

DEXBROMPHENIRAMINE MALEATE; *MULTIPLE*

SEE ACETAMINOPHEN; DEXBROMPHENIRAMINE MALEATE; PSEUDOEPHEDRINE SULFATE

DEXBROMPHENIRAMINE MALEATE; PSEUDOEPHEDRINE SULFATE

TABLET, EXTENDED RELEASE; ORAL
- BROMPHERIL
  - COPLEY PHARM — 6 MG;120 MG — N89116 001 — JAN 22, 1987
- DISOBROM
  - GENEVA PHARMS — 6 MG;120 MG — N70770 001 — SEP 30, 1991
- DISOPHROL
  - SCHERING PLOUGH — 6 MG;120 MG — N13483 004 — SEP 13, 1982
- DRIXORAL
  - + SCHERING PLOUGH — 6 MG;120 MG — N13483 003 — SEP 13, 1982

DEXTROMETHORPHAN POLISTIREX

SUSPENSION, EXTENDED RELEASE; ORAL
- DELSYM
  - + FISONS — EQ 30 MG HBR/5 ML — N18658 001

DIPHENHYDRAMINE HYDROCHLORIDE

SYRUP; ORAL
- ANTITUSSIVE
  - PERRIGO — 12.5 MG/5 ML — N71292 001 — APR 10, 1987
- BELDIN
  - HALSEY — 12.5 MG/5 ML — N89179 001 — JUN 05, 1986
- BENYLIN
  - + PARKE DAVIS — 12.5 MG/5 ML — N06514 004
- DIPHEN
  - PENNEX — 12.5 MG/5 ML — N70118 001 — OCT 01, 1985
- DIPHENHYDRAMINE HCL
  - CUMBERLAND SWAN — 12.5 MG/5 ML — N73611 001 — AUG 20, 1992
  - HI TECH PHARMA — 12.5 MG/5 ML — N72416 001 — SEP 28, 1990
- HYDRAMINE
  - BARRE — 12.5 MG/5 ML — N70205 001 — JAN 28, 1986
- SILPHEN
  - SILARX — 12.5 MG/5 ML — N72646 001 — FEB 27, 1992
- VICKS FORMULA 44
  - VICKS — 12.5 MG/5 ML — N70524 001 — JAN 14, 1987

DIPHENHYDRAMINE HYDROCHLORIDE; PSEUDOEPHEDRINE HYDROCHLORIDE

SOLUTION; ORAL
- BENYLIN
  - + PARKE DAVIS — 12.5 MG/5 ML;30 MG/5 ML — N19014 001 — JUN 11, 1985

DOXYLAMINE SUCCINATE

TABLET; ORAL
- DOXYLAMINE SUCCINATE
  - COPLEY PHARM — 25 MG — N88900 002 — FEB 12, 1988
- UNISOM
  - + PFIZER — 25 MG — N18066 001

OTC Drug Products *(continued)*

EPINEPHRINE

AEROSOL, METERED; INHALATION

BRONKAID MIST
+ STERLING WINTHROP 0.25 MG/INH N16803 001

EPINEPHRINE
BARRE 0.2 MG/INH N87907 001 MAY 23, 1984

PRIMATENE MIST
+ WHITEHALL LABS 0.2 MG/INH N16126 001

EPINEPHRINE BITARTRATE

AEROSOL, METERED; INHALATION

BRONITIN MIST
WHITEHALL LABS 0.3 MG/INH N16126 002

MEDIHALER-EPI
+ 3M 0.3 MG/INH N10374 003

IBUPROFEN

CAPSULE; ORAL

MIDOL
+ WINTHROP 200 MG N70626 001 SEP 02, 1987
200 MG N71002 001 SEP 02, 1987

TABLET; ORAL

ACHES-N-PAIN
LEDERLE 200 MG N71065 001 MAY 28, 1987

ADVIL
WHITEHALL LABS 200 MG N18989 001 MAY 18, 1984

CAP-PROFEN
PERRIGO 200 MG N72097 001 DEC 08, 1987

IBU-TAB 200
ALRA 200 MG N71057 001 AUG 11, 1988

IBUPRIN
SIDMAK LABS NJ 200 MG N71773 001 JUL 16, 1987

IBUPROFEN
BARR 200 MG N70493 001 DEC 24, 1985
200 MG N70908 001 SEP 26, 1986
200 MG N71462 001 OCT 02, 1986

IBUPROFEN *(continued)*

TABLET; ORAL

IBUPROFEN
DANBURY PHARMA 200 MG N70435 001 MAR 05, 1986
200 MG N71905 001 MAR 08, 1988
GENEVA PHARMS 200 MG N70733 001 SEP 19, 1986
HALSEY 200 MG N71027 001 SEP 29, 1987
INTERPHARM 200 MG N71333 001 FEB 17, 1987
200 MG N72199 001 MAY 23, 1988
INVAMED 200 MG N71807 001 FEB 25, 1988
MCNEIL 200 MG N73019 001 MAR 30, 1994
MUTUAL PHARM 200 MG N71229 001 APR 01, 1987
200 MG N72249 001 JAN 10, 1989
MYLAN 200 MG N71870 001 MAY 05, 1988
NORTON HN 200 MG N71144 001 JAN 20, 1987
200 MG N72901 001 DEC 19, 1991
200 MG N72903 001 DEC 19, 1991
OHM 200 MG N71163 001 JUL 15, 1986
PAR PHARM 200 MG N70481 001 SEP 24, 1986
200 MG N70985 001 OCT 02, 1987
200 MG N71575 001 MAY 08, 1987
PERRIGO 200 MG N72096 001 DEC 08, 1987
200 MG N72098 001 DEC 08, 1987
PRIVATE FORM 200 MG N71732 001 SEP 10, 1987
200 MG N71735 001 SEP 10, 1987
200 MG N72299 001 JUL 01, 1988
200 MG N73691 001 FEB 25, 1994

OTC Drug Products *(continued)*

IBUPROFEN *(continued)*

TABLET; ORAL

IBUPROFEN		
PUREPAC PHARM	200 MG	N71122 001 OCT 03, 1986
	200 MG	N71664 001 FEB 03, 1987
TAG PHARMS	200 MG	N73141 001 MAY 29, 1992
VINTAGE PHARMS	200 MG	N71639 001 FEB 02, 1988
IBUPROHM		
OHM	200 MG	N71214 001 DEC 01, 1986
MEDIPREN		
MCNEIL	200 MG	N70475 001 FEB 06, 1986
	200 MG	N71215 001 JUN 26, 1986
MIDOL		
WINTHROP	200 MG	N70591 001 SEP 02, 1987
	200 MG	N71001 001 SEP 02, 1987
NUPRIN		
+ BRISTOL MYERS	200 MG	N72035 001 FEB 16, 1988
	200 MG	N72036 001 FEB 16, 1988
PROFEN		
PRIVATE FORM	200 MG	N71265 001 OCT 15, 1986
TAB-PROFEN		
PERRIGO	200 MG	N72095 001 DEC 08, 1987

IBUPROFEN; PSEUDOEPHEDRINE HYDROCHLORIDE

TABLET; ORAL

ADVIL COLD AND SINUS		
+ WHITEHALL LABS	200 MG;30 MG	N19771 001 SEP 19, 1989
SINE-AID IB		
MCNEIL	200 MG;30 MG	N19899 001 DEC 31, 1992

INSULIN BIOSYNTHETIC HUMAN

INJECTABLE; INJECTION

HUMULIN R		
+ LILLY	100 UNITS/ML	N18780 001 OCT 28, 1982
NOVOLIN R		
NOVO NORDISK	100 UNITS/ML	N19938 001 JUN 25, 1991

INSULIN BIOSYNTHETIC HUMAN; INSULIN SUSP ISOPHANE BIOSYNTHETIC HUMAN

INJECTABLE; INJECTION

HUMULIN 50/50		
LILLY	50 UNITS/ML;50 UNITS/ML	N20100 001 APR 29, 1992
HUMULIN 70/30		
+ LILLY	30 UNITS/ML;70 UNITS/ML	N19717 001 APR 25, 1989
NOVOLIN 70/30		
NOVO NORDISK	30 UNITS/ML;70 UNITS/ML	N19991 001 JUN 25, 1991

INSULIN PORK

INJECTABLE; INJECTION

INSULIN		
+ NOVO NORDISK	100 UNITS/ML	N17926 003

INSULIN PURIFIED BEEF

INJECTABLE; INJECTION

REGULAR ILETIN II		
+ LILLY	100 UNITS/ML	N18478 001

INSULIN PURIFIED PORK

INJECTABLE; INJECTION

REGULAR ILETIN II (PORK)		
+ LILLY	100 UNITS/ML	N18344 001
REGULAR PURIFIED PORK INSULIN		
NOVO NORDISK	100 UNITS/ML	N18381 001
VELOSULIN		
NOVO NORDISK	100 UNITS/ML	N18193 001

INSULIN PURIFIED PORK; INSULIN SUSP ISOPHANE PURIFIED PORK

INJECTABLE; INJECTION

INSULIN NORDISK MIXTARD (PORK)		
+ NOVO NORDISK	30 UNITS/ML;70 UNITS/ML	N18195 001

OTC Drug Products *(continued)*

INSULIN SEMISYNTHETIC PURIFIED HUMAN
INJECTABLE; INJECTION
NOVOLIN R
+ NOVO NORDISK — 100 UNITS/ML — N18778 001 AUG 30, 1983
VELOSULIN HUMAN
+ NOVO NORDISK — 100 UNITS/ML — N19450 001 MAY 30, 1986

INSULIN SEMISYNTHETIC PURIFIED HUMAN; INSULIN SUSP ISOPHANE SEMISYNTHETIC PURIFIED HUMAN
INJECTABLE; INJECTION
MIXTARD HUMAN 70/30
+ NOVO NORDISK — 30 UNITS/ML;70 UNITS/ML — N19585 001 MAR 11, 1988
NOVOLIN 70/30
+ NOVO NORDISK — 30 UNITS/ML;70 UNITS/ML — N19441 001 JUL 11, 1986

INSULIN SUSP ISOPHANE BEEF
INJECTABLE; INJECTION
NPH INSULIN
+ NOVO NORDISK — 100 UNITS/ML — N17929 003

INSULIN SUSP ISOPHANE BEEF/PORK
INJECTABLE; INJECTION
NPH ILETIN I (BEEF-PORK)
+ LILLY — 40 UNITS/ML — N17936 001
+ — 100 UNITS/ML — N17936 002

INSULIN SUSP ISOPHANE BIOSYNTHETIC HUMAN
INJECTABLE; INJECTION
HUMULIN N
+ LILLY — 100 UNITS/ML — N18781 001 OCT 28, 1982
NOVOLIN N
NOVO NORDISK — 100 UNITS/ML — N19959 001 JUL 01, 1991

INSULIN SUSP ISOPHANE BIOSYNTHETIC HUMAN; *MULTIPLE*
SEE <u>INSULIN BIOSYNTHETIC HUMAN; INSULIN SUSP ISOPHANE BIOSYNTHETIC HUMAN</u>

INSULIN SUSP ISOPHANE PURIFIED BEEF
INJECTABLE; INJECTION
NPH ILETIN II
+ LILLY — 100 UNITS/ML — N18479 001

INSULIN SUSP ISOPHANE PURIFIED PORK
INJECTABLE; INJECTION
INSULIN INSULATARD NPH NORDISK
+ NOVO NORDISK — 100 UNITS/ML — N18194 001
NPH PURIFIED PORK ISOPHANE INSULIN
+ NOVO NORDISK — 100 UNITS/ML — N18623 001

INSULIN SUSP ISOPHANE PURIFIED PORK; *MULTIPLE*
SEE <u>INSULIN PURIFIED PORK; INSULIN SUSP ISOPHANE PURIFIED PORK</u>

INSULIN SUSP ISOPHANE SEMISYNTHETIC PURIFIED HUMAN
INJECTABLE; INJECTION
INSULATARD NPH HUMAN
+ NOVO NORDISK — 100 UNITS/ML — N19449 001 MAY 30, 1986
NOVOLIN N
+ NOVO NORDISK — 100 UNITS/ML — N19065 001 JAN 23, 1985

INSULIN SUSP ISOPHANE SEMISYNTHETIC PURIFIED HUMAN; *MULTIPLE*
SEE <u>INSULIN SEMISYNTHETIC PURIFIED HUMAN; INSULIN SUSP ISOPHANE SEMISYNTHETIC PURIFIED HUMAN</u>

INSULIN SUSP PROTAMINE ZINC PURIFIED BEEF
INJECTABLE; INJECTION
PROTAMINE ZINC AND ILETIN II
+ LILLY — 100 UNITS/ML — N18476 001
PROTAMINE ZINC INSULIN
SQUIBB — 100 UNITS/ML — N17928 003
+ — 40 UNITS/ML — N17928 001

INSULIN ZINC SUSP BEEF
INJECTABLE; INJECTION
LENTE INSULIN
+ NOVO NORDISK — 100 UNITS/ML — N17998 003

INSULIN ZINC SUSP BIOSYNTHETIC HUMAN
INJECTABLE; INJECTION
HUMULIN L
+ LILLY — 100 UNITS/ML — N19377 002 SEP 30, 1985
NOVOLIN L
NOVO NORDISK — 100 UNITS/ML — N19965 001 JUN 25, 1991

OTC Drug Products *(continued)*

INSULIN ZINC SUSP EXTENDED BEEF

INJECTABLE; INJECTION
ULTRALENTE INSULIN
+ NOVO NORDISK 100 UNITS/ML N17997 003

INSULIN ZINC SUSP EXTENDED BIOSYNTHETIC HUMAN

INJECTABLE; INJECTION
HUMULIN U
+ LILLY 100 UNITS/ML N19571 002 JUN 10, 1987

INSULIN ZINC SUSP EXTENDED PURIFIED BEEF

INJECTABLE; INJECTION
ULTRALENTE
+ NOVO NORDISK 100 UNITS/ML N18385 001

INSULIN ZINC SUSP PROMPT BEEF

INJECTABLE; INJECTION
SEMILENTE INSULIN
+ NOVO NORDISK 100 UNITS/ML N17996 003

INSULIN ZINC SUSP PROMPT PURIFIED PORK

INJECTABLE; INJECTION
SEMILENTE
+ NOVO NORDISK 100 UNITS/ML N18382 001

INSULIN ZINC SUSP PURIFIED BEEF

INJECTABLE; INJECTION
LENTE ILETIN II
+ LILLY 100 UNITS/ML N18477 001

INSULIN ZINC SUSP PURIFIED PORK

INJECTABLE; INJECTION
LENTE
NOVO NORDISK 100 UNITS/ML N18383 001
LENTE ILETIN II (PORK)
+ LILLY 100 UNITS/ML N18347 001

INSULIN ZINC SUSP SEMISYNTHETIC PURIFIED HUMAN

INJECTABLE; INJECTION
NOVOLIN L
NOVO NORDISK 100 UNITS/ML N18777 001 AUG 30, 1983

LOPERAMIDE HYDROCHLORIDE

SOLUTION; ORAL
IMODIUM A-D
+ MCNEIL 1 MG/5 ML N19487 001 MAR 01, 1988

LOPERAMIDE HCL
BARRE 1 MG/5 ML N73187 001 SEP 15, 1992
PERRIGO 1 MG/5 ML N73243 001 JAN 21, 1992
ROXANE 1 MG/5 ML N73079 001 APR 30, 1992
WATSON LABS 1 MG/5 ML N73062 001 MAY 28, 1993

TABLET; ORAL
IMODIUM A-D
+ MCNEIL 2 MG N19860 001 NOV 22, 1989

LOPERAMIDE HCL
ABLE 2 MG N73528 001 NOV 30, 1993
NOVOPHARM 2 MG N73254 001 JUL 30, 1993
OHM 2 MG N74091 001 DEC 10, 1992
PERRIGO 2 MG N74194 001 OCT 30, 1992

MAGNESIUM TRISILICATE; *MULTIPLE*

SEE ALUMINUM HYDROXIDE; MAGNESIUM TRISILICATE

MICONAZOLE NITRATE

CREAM; VAGINAL
MICONAZOLE NITRATE
COPLEY PHARM 2% N74030 001 OCT 30, 1992

MONISTAT 7
+ JOHNSON RW 2% N17450 002 FEB 15, 1991

CREAM, SUPPOSITORY; TOPICAL, VAGINAL
MONISTAT 7 COMBINATION PACK
+ ADV CARE 2%;100 MG N20288 002 APR 26, 1993

SUPPOSITORY; VAGINAL
MICONAZOLE NITRATE
ABLE 100 MG N73507 001 NOV 19, 1993

MONISTAT 7
+ JOHNSON RW 100 MG N18520 002 FEB 15, 1991

OTC Drug Products *(continued)*

NAPHAZOLINE HYDROCHLORIDE; PHENIRAMINE MALEATE
SOLUTION/DROPS; OPHTHALMIC
NAPHCON-A
+ ALCON 0.025%;0.3% N20226 001 JUN 08, 1994
OPCON-A
+ BAUSCH AND LOMB 0.027%;0.315% N20065 001 JUN 08, 1994

NAPROXEN SODIUM
TABLET; ORAL
ALEVE
HAMILTON PHARMS EQ 200 MG BASE N20204 002 JAN 11, 1994

NEOMYCIN SULFATE; *MULTIPLE*
SEE BACITRACIN ZINC; NEOMYCIN SULFATE; POLYMYXIN B SULFATE

NONOXYNOL-9
SPONGE; VAGINAL
TODAY
+ WHITEHALL LABS 1 GM N18683 001 APR 01, 1983

OCTYL METHOXYCINNAMATE; *MULTIPLE*
SEE AVOBENZONE; OCTYL METHOXYCINNAMATE; OXYBENZONE

OXYBENZONE; *MULTIPLE*
SEE AVOBENZONE; OCTYL METHOXYCINNAMATE; OXYBENZONE

OXYMETAZOLINE HYDROCHLORIDE
SOLUTION/DROPS; OPHTHALMIC
OCUCLEAR
SCHERING PLOUGH 0.025% N18471 001 MAY 30, 1986
VISINE L.R.
+ PFIZER 0.025% N19407 001 MAR 31, 1989

PADIMATE O; *MULTIPLE*
SEE AVOBENZONE; PADIMATE O

PERMETHRIN
LOTION; TOPICAL
NIX
+ WARNER WELLCOME 1% N19918 001 MAY 02, 1990

PHENIRAMINE MALEATE; *MULTIPLE*
SEE NAPHAZOLINE HYDROCHLORIDE; PHENIRAMINE MALEATE

PHENYLPROPANOLAMINE HYDROCHLORIDE; *MULTIPLE*
SEE BROMPHENIRAMINE MALEATE; PHENYLPROPANOLAMINE HYDROCHLORIDE
SEE CHLORPHENIRAMINE MALEATE; PHENYLPROPANOLAMINE HYDROCHLORIDE
SEE CLEMASTINE FUMARATE; PHENYLPROPANOLAMINE HYDROCHLORIDE

POLYMYXIN B SULFATE; *MULTIPLE*
SEE BACITRACIN ZINC; NEOMYCIN SULFATE; POLYMYXIN B SULFATE
SEE BACITRACIN ZINC; POLYMYXIN B SULFATE

POTASSIUM IODIDE
SOLUTION; ORAL
POTASSIUM IODIDE
+ ROXANE 1 GM/ML N18551 001 FEB 19, 1982

TABLET; ORAL
IOSAT
ANBEX 130 MG N18664 001 OCT 14, 1982
THYRO-BLOCK
+ WALLACE 130 MG N18307 001

POVIDONE-IODINE
SOLUTION; TOPICAL
E-Z PREP
+ BECTON DICKINSON 10% N19382 001 JUL 25, 1989
POVIDONE IODINE
+ BAXTER 1% N19522 001 MAR 31, 1989

POVIDONE-IODINE *(continued)*
SPONGE; TOPICAL
E-Z PREP
\+ BECTON DICKINSON 5% N19382 002 JUL 25, 1989
E-Z PREP 220
\+ BECTON DICKINSON 5% N19382 003 JUL 25, 1989
E-Z SCRUB 201
\+ BECTON DICKINSON 20% N19240 001 NOV 29, 1985
E-Z SCRUB 241
\+ BECTON DICKINSON 10% N19476 001 JAN 07, 1987

PSEUDOEPHEDRINE HYDROCHLORIDE
TABLET, EXTENDED RELEASE; ORAL
EFIDAC/24
\+ CIBA 240 MG N20021 002 DEC 15, 1992
SUDAFED 12 HOUR
\+ WARNER WELLCOME 120 MG N73585 001 OCT 31, 1991

PSEUDOEPHEDRINE HYDROCHLORIDE; *MULTIPLE*
SEE CHLORPHENIRAMINE MALEATE; PSEUDOEPHEDRINE HYDROCHLORIDE
SEE DIPHENHYDRAMINE HYDROCHLORIDE; PSEUDOEPHEDRINE HYDROCHLORIDE
SEE IBUPROFEN; PSEUDOEPHEDRINE HYDROCHLORIDE

PSEUDOEPHEDRINE HYDROCHLORIDE; TRIPROLIDINE HYDROCHLORIDE
CAPSULE, EXTENDED RELEASE; ORAL
TRIPROLIDINE AND PSEUDOEPHRINE HCL
KV PHARM 120 MG;5 MG N71798 001 MAR 16, 1989
TABLET, EXTENDED RELEASE; ORAL
TRIPROLIDINE AND PSEUDOEPHEDRINE HYDROCHLORIDES
\+ KV PHARM 120 MG;5 MG N72758 001 NOV 25, 1991

PSEUDOEPHEDRINE SULFATE
TABLET, EXTENDED RELEASE; ORAL
AFRINOL
\+ SCHERING PLOUGH 120 MG N18191 001

PSEUDOEPHEDRINE SULFATE; *MULTIPLE*
SEE ACETAMINOPHEN; DEXBROMPHENIRAMINE MALEATE; PSEUDOEPHEDRINE SULFATE
SEE CHLORPHENIRAMINE MALEATE; PSEUDOEPHEDRINE SULFATE
SEE DEXBROMPHENIRAMINE MALEATE; PSEUDOEPHEDRINE SULFATE

PYRITHIONE ZINC
LOTION; TOPICAL
HEAD & SHOULDERS CONDITIONER
\+ PROCTER AND GAMBLE 0.3% N19412 002 MAR 10, 1986

SODIUM CHLORIDE
AEROSOL, METERED; INHALATION
BRONCHO SALINE
BLAIREX 0.9% N19912 001 SEP 03, 1992

SODIUM MONOFLUOROPHOSPHATE
GEL; DENTAL
EXTRA-STRENGTH AIM
\+ CHESEBROUGH PONDS 1.2% N19518 002 AUG 06, 1986
PASTE; DENTAL
EXTRA-STRENGTH AIM
CHESEBROUGH PONDS 1.2% N19518 001 JUN 03, 1987

TRIPROLIDINE HYDROCHLORIDE; *MULTIPLE*
SEE PSEUDOEPHEDRINE HYDROCHLORIDE; TRIPROLIDINE HYDROCHLORIDE

DRUG PRODUCTS WITH APPROVAL UNDER SECTION 505 OF THE ACT ADMINISTERED BY THE CENTER FOR BIOLOGICS EVALUATION AND RESEARCH

ANTICOAGULANT CITRATE DEXTROSE SOLUTION USP
INJECTABLE; INJECTION
NONE
CUTTER BIO — N 71497

ANTICOAGULANT CITRATE DEXTROSE SOLUTION USP
INJECTABLE; INJECTION
NONE
CUTTER BIO — N 10102

ANTICOAGULANT CITRATE DEXTROSE SOLUTION USP
INJECTABLE; INJECTION
NONE
DELMED — N 11912

ANTICOAGULANT CITRATE DEXTROSE SOLUTION USP
INJECTABLE; INJECTION
NONE
TRAVENOL LABS — N 10855

ANTICOAGULANT CITRATE DEXTROSE SOLUTION USP
INJECTABLE; INJECTION
NONE
TRAVENOL LABS — N 16918

ANTICOAGULANT CITRATE PHOSPHATE DEXTROSE ADENINE SOLUTION
INJECTABLE; INJECTION
NONE
DELMED — N 78519

ANTICOAGULANT CITRATE PHOSPHATE DEXTROSE ADENINE SOLUTION
INJECTABLE; INJECTION
NONE
TERUMO — N 82528, NOV 03, 1982

ANTICOAGULANT CITRATE PHOSPHATE DEXTROSE ADENINE SOLUTION
INJECTABLE; INJECTION
NONE
TRAVENOL LABS — N 77420

ANTICOAGULANT CITRATE PHOSPHATE DEXTROSE ADENINE SOLUTION USP
INJECTABLE; INJECTION
BLOOD PACK UNIT CPDA-1 IN PLASTIC CONTAINER
BAXTER HLTHCARE — N 940404, JUL 28, 1994

ANTICOAGULANT CITRATE PHOSPHATE DEXTROSE ADENINE-1 SOLUTION
INJECTABLE; INJECTION
NONE
CUTTER BIO — N 08077

ANTICOAGULANT CITRATE PHOSPHATE DEXTROSE SOLUTION USP
INJECTABLE; INJECTION
NONE
CUTTER BIO — N 16527

ANTICOAGULANT CITRATE PHOSPHATE DEXTROSE SOLUTION USP
INJECTABLE; INJECTION
NONE
CUTTER BIO — N 80222, AUG 23, 1982

ANTICOAGULANT CITRATE PHOSPHATE DEXTROSE SOLUTION USP
INJECTABLE; INJECTION
NONE
DELMED — N 16907

ANTICOAGULANT CITRATE PHOSPHATE DEXTROSE SOLUTION USP
INJECTABLE; INJECTION
NONE
TERUMO — N 781211

ANTICOAGULANT CITRATE PHOSPHATE DEXTROSE SOLUTION USP
INJECTABLE; INJECTION
NONE
TRAVENOL LABS — N 17401

ANTICOAGULANT CITRATE PHOSPHATE DEXTROSE SOLUTION USP
INJECTABLE; INJECTION
NONE
TRAVENOL LABS — N 811012, JUN 28, 1983

ANTICOAGULANT CITRATE PHOSPHATE DEXTROSE SOLUTION USP WITH: AS-1: DEXTROSE USP; SODIUM CHLORIDE USP; MANNITOL USP; ADENINE
INJECTABLE; INJECTION
ADSOL RED BLOOD CELL PRESERVATIVE SOLUTION
TRAVENOL LABS — 2.2 GM/100 ML;0.9 GM/100 ML;0.75 GM/100 ML;0.027 GM/100 ML — N 811104, MAY 16, 1983

ANTICOAGULANT CITRATE PHOSPHATE DEXTROSE SOLUTION USP WITH: AS-5: DEXTROSE USP; SODIUM CHLORIDE USP; MANNITOL USP; ADENINE
INJECTABLE; INJECTION
OPTISOL RED BLOOD CELL PRESERVATIVE SOLUTION
TERUMO — 0.9 GM/100 ML;0.877 GM/100 ML;0.525 GM/100 ML;0.03 GM/100 ML — N 880217, OCT 07, 1988

Drug Products with Approval Under Section 505 of the Act Administered by the Center for Biologics Evaluation and Research *(continued)*

ANTICOAGULANT CITRATE PHOSPHATE DOUBLE DEXTROSE SOLUTION WITH: AS-2: CITRIC ACID USP; DIBASIC SODIUM PHOSPHATE USP; SODIUM CHLORIDE USP; ADENINE; DEXTROSE USP; SODIUM CITRATE USP

INJECTABLE; INJECTION
AS-2 NUTRICEL ADDITIVE SYSTEM
CUTTER BIO — 0.042 GM/100 ML;0.285 GM/100 ML;0.718 GM/100 ML;0.017 GM/100 ML;0.396 GM/100 ML;0.588 GM/100 ML — N 82915 SEP 22, 1983

ANTICOAGULANT CITRATE PHOSPHATE DOUBLE DEXTROSE SOLUTION WITH: AS-3: CITRIC ACID USP; MONOBASIC SODIUM PHOSPHATE USP; SODIUM CHLORIDE USP; ADENINE; DEXTROSE USP; SODIUM CITRATE USP

INJECTABLE; INJECTION
AS-3 NUTRICEL ADDITIVE SYSTEM
CUTTER BIO — 0.042 GM/100 ML;0.276 GM/100 ML;0.410 GM/100 ML;0.30 GM/100 ML;1.10 GM/100 ML;0.588 GM/100 ML — N 82915 OCT 19, 1984

ANTICOAGULANT HEPARIN SOLUTION USP

INJECTABLE; INJECTION
NONE
DELMED — N 77822

ANTICOAGULANT HEPARIN SOLUTION USP

INJECTABLE; INJECTION
NONE
TRAVENOL LABS — N 811217 MAY 16, 1983

ANTICOAGULANT SODIUM CITRATE SOLUTION USP

INJECTABLE; INJECTION
NONE
ALPHA THERPTC — N 81416 OCT 12, 1983

ANTICOAGULANT SODIUM CITRATE SOLUTION USP

INJECTABLE; INJECTION
NONE
CUTTER BIO — N 76305

ANTICOAGULANT SODIUM CITRATE SOLUTION USP

INJECTABLE; INJECTION
NONE
DELMED — N 16702

ANTICOAGULANT SODIUM CITRATE SOLUTION USP

INJECTABLE; INJECTION
NONE
TERUMO — N 781214

ANTICOAGULANT SODIUM CITRATE SOLUTION USP

INJECTABLE; INJECTION
NONE
TRAVENOL LABS — N 77923

CDP BLOOD BAG UNIT

INJECTABLE; INJECTION
CDP BLOOD BAG UNIT IN PLASTIC CONTAINER
BAXTER HLTHCARE — N900224 DEC 27, 1991

DEXTRAN 1 IN SODIUM CHLORIDE 0.6%

INJECTABLE; INJECTION
PROMIT
PHARMACIA LABS — 150 MG/ML;6 MG/ML — N 83715 OCT 30, 1984

DEXTRAN 40, 10% IN DEXTROSE 5%

INJECTABLE; INJECTION
GENTRAN 40
TRAVENOL LABS — 10 GM/100 ML;5 GM/100 ML — N 16628

DEXTRAN 40, 10% IN DEXTROSE 5%

INJECTABLE; INJECTION
GENTRAN 40
TRAVENOL LABS — 10 GM/100 ML;5 GM/100 ML — N 84619 FEB 22, 1985

DEXTRAN 40, 10% IN DEXTROSE 5%

INJECTABLE; INJECTION
LMD IN PLASTIC CONTAINER
ABBOTT LABS — 10 GM/100 ML;5 GM/100 ML — N 72563 OCT 30, 1992

DEXTRAN 40, 10% IN DEXTROSE 5%

INJECTABLE; INJECTION
RHEDMACRODEX
PHARMACIA LABS — 10 GM/100 ML;5 GM/100 ML — N 14716

DEXTRAN 40, 10% IN DEXTROSE 5%

INJECTABLE; INJECTION
NONE
ABBOTT LABS — 10 GM/100 ML;5 GM/100 ML — N 16375

Drug Products with Approval Under Section 505 of the Act Administered by the Center for Biologics Evaluation and Research *(continued)*

DEXTRAN 40, 10% IN DEXTROSE 5%
INJECTABLE; INJECTION
NONE
AMERICAN MCGAW — 10 GM/100 ML;5 GM/100 ML — N 16767

DEXTRAN 40, 10% IN DEXTROSE 5%
INJECTABLE; INJECTION
NONE
CUTTER BIO — 10 GM/100 ML;5 GM/100 ML — N 16653

DEXTRAN 40, 10% IN DEXTROSE 5%
INJECTABLE; INJECTION
NONE
PHARMACHEM — 10 GM/100 ML;0.9 GM/100 ML — N 16836

DEXTRAN 40, 10% IN SODIUM CHLORIDE 0.9%
INJECTABLE; INJECTION
GENTRAN 40
TRAVENOL — 10 GM/100 ML;0.9 GM/100 ML — N 16628

DEXTRAN 40, 10% IN SODIUM CHLORIDE 0.9%
INJECTABLE; INJECTION
GENTRAN 40
TRAVENOL LABS — 10 GM/100 ML;0.9 GM/100 ML — N 84620 FEB 22, 1985

DEXTRAN 40, 10% IN SODIUM CHLORIDE 0.9%
INJECTABLE; INJECTION
LMD IN PLASTIC CONTAINER
ABBOTT LABS — 10 GM/100 ML;0.9 GM/100 ML — N 72562 OCT 30, 1992

DEXTRAN 40, 10% IN SODIUM CHLORIDE 0.9%
INJECTABLE; INJECTION
RHEOMACRODEX
PHARMACIA LABS — 10 GM/100 ML;0.9 GM/100 ML — N 14716

DEXTRAN 40, 10% IN SODIUM CHLORIDE 0.9%
INJECTABLE; INJECTION
NONE
ABBOTT LABS — 10 GM/100 ML;0.9 GM/100 ML — N 16375

DEXTRAN 40, 10% IN SODIUM CHLORIDE 0.9%
INJECTABLE; INJECTION
NONE
AMERICAN MCGAW — 10 GM/100 ML;0.9 GM/100 ML — N 16767

DEXTRAN 40, 10% IN SODIUM CHLORIDE 0.9%
INJECTABLE; INJECTION
NONE
CUTTER LABS — 10 GM/100 ML;0.9 GM/100 ML — N 16653 OCT 30, 1992

DEXTRAN 40, 10% IN SODIUM CHLORIDE 0.9%
INJECTABLE; INJECTION
NONE
PHARMACHEM — 10 GM/100 ML;0.9 GM/100 ML — N 16836

DEXTRAN 70, 6% IN DEXTROSE 5%
INJECTABLE; INJECTION
MACRODEX
PHARMACIA INC — 6 GM/100 ML;5 GM/100 ML — N 06826

DEXTRAN 70, 6% IN SODIUM CHLORIDE 0.9%
INJECTABLE; INJECTION
MACRODEX
PHARMACIA INC — 6 GM/100 ML;0.9 GM/100 ML — N 06826

DEXTRAN 70, 6% IN SODIUM CHLORIDE 0.9%
INJECTABLE; INJECTION
NONE
AMERICAN MCGAW — 6 GM/100 ML;0.9 GM/100 ML — N 09024

DEXTRAN 70, 6% IN SODIUM CHLORIDE 0.9%
INJECTABLE; INJECTION
NONE
CUTTER BIO — 6 GM/100 ML;0.9 GM/100 ML — N 08716

DEXTRAN 75, 6% IN DEXTROSE 5%
INJECTABLE; INJECTION
NONE
ABBOTT LABS — 6 GM/100 ML;5 GM/100 ML — N 08819

Drug Products with Approval Under Section 505 of the Act Administered by the Center for Biologics Evaluation and Research *(continued)*

DEXTRAN 75, 6% IN SODIUM CHLORIDE 0.9%
INJECTABLE; INJECTION
GENTRAN 75
TRAVENOL LABS 6 GM/100 ML;0.9 GM/100 ML N 16607

DEXTRAN 75, 6% IN SODIUM CHLORIDE 0.9%
INJECTABLE; INJECTION
NONE
ABBOTT LABS 6 GM/100 ML;0.9 GM/100 ML N 08819

DEXTRAN 75, 6% IN SODIUM CHLORIDE 0.9%
INJECTABLE; INJECTION
NONE
ABBOTT LABS 6 GM/100 ML;0.9 GM/100 ML N 18253
FEB 04, 1983

DEXTRAN 75, 6% IN SODIUM CHLORIDE 0.9%
INJECTABLE; INJECTION
NONE
PHARMACHEM 6 GM/100 ML;0.9 GM/100 ML N 08564

DEXTRAN 75, 6% IN SODIUM CHLORIDE 0.9%
INJECTABLE; INJECTION
NONE
PHARMACHEM 6 GM/100 ML;0.9 GM/100 ML N 16759

DEXTRAN 75, 6% INVERTED SUGAR 10% IN SODIUM CHLORIDE 0.9%
INJECTABLE; INJECTION
6% GENTRAN 75 AND 10% TRAVERT
TRAVENOL LABS 6 GM/100 ML;10 GM/100 ML;0.9 GM/100 ML N 08788

HETASTARCH 6% IN SODIUM CHLORIDE 0.9%
INJECTABLE; INJECTION
HESPAN
AM CRITICAL CARE 6 GM/100 ML;0.9 GM/100 ML N 16889

HETASTARCH 6% IN SODIUM CHLORIDE 0.9%
INJECTABLE; INJECTION
HESPAN IN PLASTIC CONTAINER
DUPONT MERCK PHARM 6 GM/ 100 ML;0.9 GM/100 ML N 890105
APR 04, 1991

INDIUM IN^{111} CHLORIDE
SOLUTION; INJECTION
INDICLOR
AMERSHAM N/A N 19862
DEC 29,1992

PENTASTARCH 10% IN SODIUM CHLORIDE 0.9%
INJECTABLE; INJECTION
PENTASPAN
DUPONT CRI CARE 10 GM/100 ML;0.9 GM/100 ML N 841207
MAY 19, 1987

PENTASTARCH 10% IN SODIUM CHLORIDE 0.9%
INJECTABLE; INJECTION
PENTASPAN IN PLASTIC CONTAINER
DUPONT MERCK PHARM 10 GM/100 ML;0.9 GM/100 ML N 890104
APR 04, 1991

PERFLUORODECALIN; PERFLUOROTRI-N-PROPYLAMINE
INJECTABLE; INJECTION
FLUOSOL
ALPHA THERPTC 17.5 GM/100 ML;7.5 GM/100 ML N 860909
DEC 26, 1989

RED CELL PRESERVATION SOLUTION SYSTEM
INJECTABLE; INJECTION
ADSOL IN PLASTIC CONTAINER
BAXTER HLTH CARE N900223
DEC 27, 1991

UROKINASE
INJECTABLE; INJECTION
ABBOKINASE OPEN-CATHETER
ABBOTT LABS 5000 IU/VIAL N 761021
DEC 15, 1983

UROKINASE
INJECTABLE; INJECTION
ABBOKINASE
ABBOTT LABS 250,000 IU/VIAL N 761021

UROKINASE
INJECTABLE; INJECTION
BREOKINASE
STERLING DRUG 250,000 IU/VIAL N 17873

DISCONTINUED DRUG PRODUCTS

ACETAMINOPHEN

INJECTABLE; INJECTION
  INJECTAPAP
    JOHNSON RW   100 MG/ML   N17785 001 MAR 07, 1986
SUPPOSITORY; RECTAL
  TYLENOL
    MCNEIL   120 MG   N17756 002
              650 MG   N17756 001

ACETAMINOPHEN; ASPIRIN; CODEINE PHOSPHATE

CAPSULE; ORAL
  CODEINE, ASPIRIN, APAP FORMULA NO. 2
    1ST TX   150 MG;180 MG;15 MG   N85640 001
  CODEINE, ASPIRIN, APAP FORMULA NO. 3
    1ST TX   150 MG;180 MG;30 MG   N85639 001
  CODEINE, ASPIRIN, APAP FORMULA NO. 4
    1ST TX   150 MG;180 MG;60 MG   N85638 001

ACETAMINOPHEN; BUTALBITAL

CAPSULE; ORAL
  BANCAP
    FOREST PHARMS   325 MG;50 MG   N88889 001 JAN 16, 1986

ACETAMINOPHEN; BUTALBITAL; CAFFEINE

CAPSULE; ORAL
  MEDIGESIC PLUS
    US CHEM   325 MG;50 MG;40 MG   N89115 001 JAN 14, 1986
TABLET; ORAL
  ESGIC
    FOREST PHARMS   325 MG;50 MG;40 MG   N89660 001 DEC 23, 1988

ACETAMINOPHEN; CODEINE PHOSPHATE

CAPSULE; ORAL
  ACETAMINOPHEN AND CODEINE PHOSPHATE
    LEMMON   300 MG;30 MG   N88324 001 DEC 29, 1983
  ACETAMINOPHEN W/ CODEINE #2
    LEMMON   300 MG;15 MG   N88537 001 JUN 04, 1984
  ACETAMINOPHEN W/ CODEINE #4
    LEMMON   300 MG;60 MG   N88599 001 JUN 01, 1984
  PROVAL #3
    SOLVAY   325 MG;30 MG   N85685 001

ACETAMINOPHEN; CODEINE PHOSPHATE (*continued*)

CAPSULE; ORAL
  TYLENOL W/ CODEINE NO. 3
    JOHNSON RW   300 MG;30 MG   N87422 001
  TYLENOL W/ CODEINE NO. 4
    JOHNSON RW   300 MG;60 MG   N87421 001
TABLET; ORAL
  ACETAMINOPHEN AND CODEINE PHOSPHATE
    DURAMED   300 MG;15 MG   N88353 001 FEB 06, 1984
               300 MG;30 MG   N88354 001 FEB 06, 1984
               300 MG;60 MG   N88355 001 FEB 06, 1984
    EON LABS   300 MG;15 MG   N87433 001
                300 MG;30 MG   N85917 001
                300 MG;60 MG   N87423 001
    WARNER CHILCOTT   300 MG;15 MG   N85992 001
                       300 MG;30 MG   N85218 002
  ACETAMINOPHEN AND CODEINE PHOSPHATE #3
    SUPERPHARM   300 MG;30 MG   N89253 001 MAY 19, 1986
  ACETAMINOPHEN AND CODEINE PHOSPHATE #4
    SUPERPHARM   300 MG;60 MG   N89254 001 MAY 19, 1986
  ACETAMINOPHEN AND CODEINE PHOSPHATE NO. 2
    AM THERAP   300 MG;15 MG   N89478 001 MAR 03, 1987
                 300 MG;15 MG   N89481 001 MAR 03, 1987
  ACETAMINOPHEN AND CODEINE PHOSPHATE NO. 3
    AM THERAP   300 MG;30 MG   N89479 001 MAR 03, 1987
                 300 MG;30 MG   N89482 001 MAR 03, 1987
  ACETAMINOPHEN AND CODEINE PHOSPHATE NO. 4
    AM THERAP   300 MG;60 MG   N89480 001 MAR 03, 1987
                 300 MG;60 MG   N89483 001 MAR 03, 1987
  ACETAMINOPHEN W/ CODEINE
    LEDERLE   300 MG;30 MG   N87141 001
  ACETAMINOPHEN W/ CODEINE PHOSPHATE
    CHELSEA LABS   300 MG;15 MG   N87277 001 MAY 26, 1982
                    300 MG;30 MG   N87276 001 MAY 26, 1982
                    300 MG;60 MG   N87275 001 MAY 26, 1982

Discontinued Drug Products *(continued)*

ACETAMINOPHEN; CODEINE PHOSPHATE *(continued)*

TABLET; ORAL

ACETAMINOPHEN W/ CODEINE PHOSPHATE		
ROSEMONT PHARM	300 MG;30 MG	N87919 001 JUN 22, 1982
	300 MG;60 MG	N87920 001 JUN 22, 1982
VITARINE	300 MG;30 MG	N85676 001
WARNER CHILCOTT	300 MG;60 MG	N87306 001
WHITEWORTH TOWNE	300 MG;30 MG	N84360 001
	300 MG;60 MG	N85607 001
APAP W/ CODEINE PHOSPHATE		
EVERYLIFE	325 MG;30 MG	N85217 001
CODEINE PHOSPHATE AND ACETAMINOPHEN		
ICN	300 MG;30 MG	N85896 001
EMPRACET W/ CODEINE PHOSPHATE #3		
BURROUGHS WELLCOME	300 MG;30 MG	N83951 001
EMPRACET W/ CODEINE PHOSPHATE #4		
BURROUGHS WELLCOME	300 MG;60 MG	N83951 002
PAPA-DEINE #3		
VANGARD	300 MG;30 MG	N88037 001 MAR 20, 1984
PAPA-DEINE #4		
VANGARD	300 MG;60 MG	N88715 001 MAR 20, 1984
TYLENOL W/ CODEINE		
JOHNSON RW	325 MG;30 MG	N85056 003
	325 MG;7.5 MG	N85056 001
	325 MG;15 MG	N85056 002
	325 MG;60 MG	N85056 004

ACETAMINOPHEN; HYDROCODONE BITARTRATE

CAPSULE; ORAL

BANCAP HC		
FOREST PHARMS	500 MG;5 MG	N87961 001 MAR 17, 1983

TABLET; ORAL

DURADYNE DHC		
FOREST PHARMS	500 MG;5 MG	N87809 001 MAR 17, 1983
HYDROCODONE BITARTRATE AND ACETAMINOPHEN		
ROSEMONT PHARM	500 MG;5 MG	N89290 001 MAY 29, 1987
	500 MG;5 MG	N89291 001 MAY 29, 1987
NORCET		
ABANA	500 MG;5 MG	N88871 001 MAY 15, 1986

ACETAMINOPHEN; HYDROCODONE BITARTRATE *(continued)*

TABLET; ORAL

TYCOLET		
JOHNSON RW	500 MG;5 MG	N89385 001 AUG 27, 1986
VICODIN		
KNOLL PHARM	500 MG;5 MG	N85667 001

ACETAMINOPHEN; OXYCODONE HYDROCHLORIDE

CAPSULE; ORAL

TYLOX-325		
JOHNSON RW	325 MG;5 MG	N88246 001 NOV 08, 1984

TABLET; ORAL

OXYCODONE 2.5/APAP 500		
DUPONT MERCK	500 MG;2.5 MG	N85910 001
OXYCODONE 5/APAP 500		
DUPONT MERCK	500 MG;5 MG	N85911 001

ACETAMINOPHEN; OXYCODONE HYDROCHLORIDE; OXYCODONE TEREPHTHALATE

CAPSULE; ORAL

TYLOX		
JOHNSON RW	500 MG;4.5 MG;0.38 MG	N85375 001

ACETAMINOPHEN; PROPOXYPHENE HYDROCHLORIDE

TABLET; ORAL

DARVOCET		
LILLY	325 MG;32.5 MG	N16844 001
DOLENE AP-65		
LEDERLE	650 MG;65 MG	N85100 001
PROPOXYPHENE HCL AND ACETAMINOPHEN		
MYLAN	325 MG;32 MG	N83689 001

ACETAMINOPHEN; PROPOXYPHENE NAPSYLATE

TABLET; ORAL

PROPOXYPHENE NAPSYLATE AND ACETAMINOPHEN		
CIRCA	325 MG;50 MG	N70398 001 DEC 18, 1986
	650 MG;100 MG	N70399 001 DEC 18, 1986
HALSEY	325 MG;50 MG	N72105 001 MAY 13, 1988
	650 MG;100 MG	N72106 001 MAY 13, 1988

Discontinued Drug Products *(continued)*

ACETAZOLAMIDE
TABLET; ORAL
ACETAZOLAMIDE
ALRA 250 MG N83320 001
ASCOT 250 MG N87686 001 OCT 20, 1982
CIRCA 250 MG N84498 002
VANGARD 250 MG N87654 001 FEB 05, 1982

ACETAZOLAMIDE SODIUM
INJECTABLE; INJECTION
ACETAZOLAMIDE SODIUM
QUAD PHARMS EQ 500 MG BASE/VIAL N89619 001 JAN 13, 1988

ACETIC ACID, GLACIAL
SOLUTION/DROPS; OTIC
ACETIC ACID
KV PHARM 2% N85493 001
ORLEX
PROCTER AND GAMBLE 2% N86845 001

ACETIC ACID, GLACIAL; ALUMINUM ACETATE
SOLUTION/DROPS; OTIC
BOROFAIR
PHARMAFAIR 2%;0.79% N88606 001 AUG 21, 1985

ACETIC ACID, GLACIAL; HYDROCORTISONE
SOLUTION/DROPS; OTIC
ACETIC ACID W/ HYDROCORTISONE
KV PHARM 2%;1% N85492 001
ORLEX HC
PROCTER AND GAMBLE 2%;1% N86844 001

ACETOHEXAMIDE
TABLET; ORAL
ACETOHEXAMIDE
ROSEMONT PHARM 250 MG N70753 001 NOV 03, 1986
500 MG N70754 001 NOV 03, 1986

ACETOPHENAZINE MALEATE
TABLET; ORAL
TINDAL
SCHERING 20 MG N12254 002

ACETRIZOATE SODIUM
SOLUTION; INTRAUTERINE
SALPIX
JOHNSON RW 53% N09008 001

ACETYLCYSTEINE
SOLUTION; INHALATION, ORAL
ACETYLCYSTEINE
QUAD PHARMS 10% N71740 001 AUG 11, 1987
20% N71741 001 AUG 11, 1987

ACETYLCYSTEINE; ISOPROTERENOL HYDROCHLORIDE
SOLUTION; INHALATION
MUCOMYST W/ ISOPROTERENOL
MEAD JOHNSON 10%;0.05% N17366 001

ACETYLDIGITOXIN
TABLET; ORAL
ACYLANID
SANDOZ 0.1 MG N09436 001

ACRISORCIN
CREAM; TOPICAL
AKRINOL
SCHERING 2 MG/GM N12470 001

ACYCLOVIR SODIUM
INJECTABLE; INJECTION
ZOVIRAX
BURROUGHS WELLCOME EQ 250 MG BASE/VIAL N18603 003 AUG 30, 1983

ALBUMIN CHROMATED CR-51 SERUM
INJECTABLE; INJECTION
CHROMALBIN
ISO TEX 250uCi/VIAL N17835 002
500uCi/VIAL N17835 003

Discontinued Drug Products *(continued)*

ALBUMIN IODINATED I-125 SERUM

INJECTABLE; INJECTION
ALBUMOTOPE 125 I
ISO TEX 5-50uCi/AMP N17836 001
RADIO-IODINATED (I 125) SERUM ALBUMIN (HUMAN)
MILES 2.5uCi/AMP N17846 001

ALBUMIN IODINATED I-131 SERUM

INJECTABLE; INJECTION
MEGATOPE
ISO TEX 20uCi/AMP N17837 005
5uCi/AMP N17837 004
2mCi/VIAL N17837 003

ALBUTEROL SULFATE

TABLET; ORAL
ALBUTEROL SULFATE
AM THERAP EQ 2 MG BASE N72449 001 DEC 05, 1989
EQ 4 MG BASE N72450 001 DEC 05, 1989
WARNER CHILCOTT EQ 2 MG BASE N72817 001 JAN 09, 1990
EQ 4 MG BASE N72818 001 JAN 09, 1990

ALCOHOL

INJECTABLE; INJECTION
ALCOHOL 5% IN DEXTROSE 5%
MILES 5 ML/100 ML N83483 001

ALKAVERVIR

TABLET; ORAL
VERILOID
3M 2 MG N07336 002
3 MG N07336 003

ALLOPURINOL

TABLET; ORAL
ALLOPURINOL
CHELSEA LABS 100 MG N18785 001 SEP 28, 1984
300 MG N18785 002 SEP 28, 1984

ALLOPURINOL *(continued)*

TABLET; ORAL
ALLOPURINOL
CIRCA 100 MG N18241 001 NOV 16, 1984
300 MG N18241 002 NOV 16, 1984
PUREPAC PHARM 100 MG N70579 001 APR 14, 1986
300 MG N70580 001 APR 14, 1986
SUPERPHARM 100 MG N70950 001 NOV 30, 1988
LOPURIN
BOOTS 100 MG N18297 001
300 MG N18297 002

ALSEROXYLON

TABLET; ORAL
RAUTENSIN
DORSEY 2 MG N09215 001

ALUMINUM ACETATE; *MULTIPLE*

SEE <u>ACETIC ACID, GLACIAL; ALUMINUM ACETATE</u>

ALUMINUM HYDROXIDE; MAGNESIUM TRISILICATE

TABLET, CHEWABLE; ORAL
ALUMINUM HYDROXIDE AND MAGNESIUM TRISILICATE
PENNEX 80 MG;20 MG N89449 001 NOV 27, 1987

AMANTADINE HYDROCHLORIDE

CAPSULE; ORAL
AMANTADINE HCL
CIRCA 100 MG N71382 001 JAN 21, 1987

TABLET; ORAL
SYMMETREL
DUPONT MERCK 100 MG N18101 001

Discontinued Drug Products *(continued)*

AMDINOCILLIN
INJECTABLE; INJECTION
COACTIN
ROCHE — 250 MG/VIAL — N50565 001 DEC 21, 1984
500 MG/VIAL — N50565 002 DEC 21, 1984
1 GM/VIAL — N50565 003 DEC 21, 1984

AMIKACIN SULFATE
INJECTABLE; INJECTION
AMIKIN
APOTHECON — EQ 50 MG BASE/ML — N50495 001
EQ 250 MG BASE/ML — N50495 002
BRISTOL — EQ 50 MG BASE/ML — N62562 001 SEP 20, 1984
EQ 250 MG BASE/ML — N62562 002 SEP 20, 1984
AMIKIN IN SODIUM CHLORIDE 0.9% IN PLASTIC CONTAINER
BRISTOL — EQ 5 MG BASE/ML — N50618 002 NOV 30, 1987
EQ 10 MG BASE/ML — N50618 001 NOV 30, 1987

AMINO ACIDS
INJECTABLE; INJECTION
AMINOSYN II 3.5% IN PLASTIC CONTAINER
ABBOTT — 3.5% — N19491 001 OCT 10, 1986
AMINOSYN 3.5% IN PLASTIC CONTAINER
ABBOTT — 3.5% — N18804 001 MAY 15, 1984
3.5% — N18875 001 AUG 08, 1984
AMINOSYN-HBC 7% IN PLASTIC CONTAINER
ABBOTT — 7% — N19400 001 JUL 23, 1986
FREAMINE II 8.5%
MCGAW — 8.5% — N16822 002
FREAMINE 8.5%
MCGAW — 8.5% — N16822 001
NEOPHAM 6.4%
PHARMACIA — 6.4% — N18792 001 JAN 17, 1984
NOVAMINE 8.5%
PHARMACIA — 8.5% — N17957 002 AUG 09, 1982

AMINO ACIDS; DEXTROSE
INJECTABLE; INJECTION
AMINOSYN II 5% IN DEXTROSE 25% IN PLASTIC CONTAINER
ABBOTT — 5%;25 GM/100 ML — N19565 001 DEC 17, 1986
AMINOSYN 3.5% W/ DEXTROSE 25% IN PLASTIC CONTAINER
ABBOTT — 3.5%;25 GM/100 ML — N19118 001 OCT 11, 1984
AMINOSYN 3.5% W/ DEXTROSE 5% IN PLASTIC CONTAINER
ABBOTT — 3.5%;5 GM/100 ML — N19120 001 OCT 11, 1984
AMINOSYN 4.25% W/ DEXTROSE 25% IN PLASTIC CONTAINER
ABBOTT — 4.25%;25 GM/100 ML — N19119 001 OCT 11, 1984

AMINO ACIDS; DEXTROSE; MAGNESIUM CHLORIDE; POTASSIUM CHLORIDE; POTASSIUM PHOSPHATE, DIBASIC; SODIUM CHLORIDE
INJECTABLE; INJECTION
AMINOSYN II 3.5% W/ ELECTROLYTES IN DEXTROSE 25% IN PLASTIC CONTAINER
ABBOTT — 3.5%;25 GM/100 ML;51 MG/100 ML;22.4 MG/100 ML;261 MG/100 ML;205 MG/100 ML — N19564 002 DEC 16, 1986
AMINOSYN II 4.25% W/ ELECTROLYTES IN DEXTROSE 25% IN PLASTIC CONTAINER
ABBOTT — 4.25%;25 GM/100 ML;51 MG/100 ML;22.4 MG/100 ML;261 MG/100 ML;205 MG/100 ML — N19564 004 DEC 16, 1986

AMINO ACIDS; DEXTROSE; MAGNESIUM CHLORIDE; POTASSIUM CHLORIDE; SODIUM CHLORIDE; SODIUM PHOSPHATE, DIBASIC
INJECTABLE; INJECTION
AMINOSYN II 3.5% M IN DEXTROSE 5% IN PLASTIC CONTAINER
ABBOTT — 3.5%;5 GM/100 ML;30 MG/100 ML;97 MG/100 ML;120 MG/100 ML;49.3 MG/100 ML — N19564 001 DEC 16, 1986
AMINOSYN II 4.25% M IN DEXTROSE 10% IN PLASTIC CONTAINER
ABBOTT — 4.25%;10 GM/100 ML;30 MG/100 ML;97 MG/100 ML;120 MG/100 ML;49.3 MG/100 ML — N19564 003 DEC 16, 1986

Discontinued Drug Products *(continued)*

AMINO ACIDS; MAGNESIUM ACETATE; PHOSPHORIC ACID; POTASSIUM ACETATE; SODIUM CHLORIDE

INJECTABLE; INJECTION
AMINOSYN 3.5% M IN PLASTIC CONTAINER
ABBOTT 3.5%;21 MG/100 ML;40 MG/100 ML;128 MG/100 ML;234 MG/100 ML N18804 002 MAY 15, 1984
3.5%;21 MG/100 ML;40 MG/100 ML;128 MG/100 ML;234 MG/100 ML N18875 002 AUG 08, 1984

AMINO ACIDS; MAGNESIUM ACETATE; POTASSIUM ACETATE; SODIUM CHLORIDE

INJECTABLE; INJECTION
AMINOSYN 3.5% M
ABBOTT 3.5%;21 MG/100 ML;128 MG/100 ML;234 MG/100 ML N17789 005

AMINO ACIDS; MAGNESIUM ACETATE; POTASSIUM ACETATE; SODIUM CHLORIDE; SODIUM PHOSPHATE, DIBASIC

INJECTABLE; INJECTION
AMINOSYN II 3.5% M IN PLASTIC CONTAINER
ABBOTT 3.5%;32 MG/100 ML;128 MG/100 ML;222 MG/100 ML;49 MG/100 ML N19493 001 OCT 16, 1986

AMINO ACIDS; MAGNESIUM CHLORIDE; POTASSIUM ACETATE; POTASSIUM CHLORIDE; SODIUM ACETATE

INJECTABLE; INJECTION
VEINAMINE 8%
PHARMACIA 8%;61 MG/100 ML;211 MG/100 ML;56 MG/100 ML;388 MG/100 ML N17957 001

AMINO ACIDS; MAGNESIUM CHLORIDE; POTASSIUM CHLORIDE; POTASSIUM PHOSPHATE, DIBASIC; SODIUM CHLORIDE

INJECTABLE; INJECTION
AMINOSYN II 7% W/ ELECTROLYTES
ABBOTT 7%;102 MG/100 ML;45 MG/100 ML;522 MG/100 ML;410 MG/100 ML N19437 006 APR 03, 1986

AMINO ACIDS; MAGNESIUM CHLORIDE; POTASSIUM CHLORIDE; SODIUM CHLORIDE; SODIUM PHOSPHATE, DIBASIC

INJECTABLE; INJECTION
AMINOSYN II 3.5% M
ABBOTT 3.5%;30 MG/100 ML;97 MG/100 ML;120 MG/100 ML;49 MG/100 ML N19437 007 APR 03, 1986

AMINOCAPROIC ACID

INJECTABLE; INJECTION
AMINOCAPROIC ACID
FUJISAWA 250 MG/ML N70522 001 JUN 17, 1986
QUAD PHARMS 250 MG/ML N70694 001 MAR 04, 1986

AMINOHIPPURATE SODIUM

INJECTABLE; INJECTION
AMINOHIPPURATE SODIUM
QUAD PHARMS 20% N89821 001 JUL 14, 1988

AMINOPHYLLINE

ENEMA; RECTAL
SOMOPHYLLIN
FISONS 300 MG/5 ML N18232 001 APR 02, 1982

INJECTABLE; INJECTION
AMINOPHYLLIN
SEARLE 25 MG/ML N87621 001 MAY 24, 1982
AMINOPHYLLINE
FUJISAWA 25 MG/ML N84568 001
25 MG/ML N87250 001 JAN 06, 1982
25 MG/ML N87431 001
25 MG/ML N87886 001 AUG 30, 1983
INTL MEDICATION 25 MG/ML N87867 001 NOV 10, 1983
25 MG/ML N87868 001 NOV 10, 1983
SMITH AND NEPHEW 25 MG/ML N88429 001 MAY 30, 1985

Discontinued Drug Products *(continued)*

AMINOPHYLLINE *(continued)*

INJECTABLE; INJECTION
AMINOPHYLLINE IN SODIUM CHLORIDE 0.45% IN PLASTIC CONTAINER
ABBOTT 100 MG/100 ML N18924 001 DEC 12, 1984
200 MG/100 ML N18924 002 DEC 12, 1984
400 MG/100 ML N18924 003 DEC 12, 1984
500 MG/100 ML N18924 004 DEC 12, 1984

SOLUTION; ORAL
AMINOPHYLLINE
PENNEX 105 MG/5 ML N88156 001 DEC 05, 1983
SOMOPHYLLIN
FISONS 105 MG/5 ML N86466 001
SOMOPHYLLIN-DF
FISONS 105 MG/5 ML N87045 001

TABLET; ORAL
AMINOPHYLLIN
SEARLE 100 MG N02386 002
200 MG N02386 003
AMINOPHYLLINE
ASCOT 100 MG N87522 001 FEB 12, 1982
200 MG N87523 001 FEB 12, 1982
BARR 100 MG N88297 001 AUG 19, 1983
200 MG N88298 001 AUG 19, 1983
CHELSEA LABS 100 MG N85567 001
200 MG N85564 001
DURAMED 100 MG N88182 001 MAR 31, 1983
200 MG N88183 001 MAR 31, 1983
GENEVA PHARMS 100 MG N85261 003
ICN 200 MG N84563 001
KV PHARM 100 MG N85284 001
200 MG N85289 001
LANNETT 100 MG N84588 001
200 MG N84588 002
PAL PAK 100 MG N84533 001
PANRAY 100 MG N84552 001
200 MG N84552 002
PUREPAC PHARM 100 MG N84699 001
200 MG N85333 001

AMINOPHYLLINE *(continued)*

TABLET; ORAL
AMINOPHYLLINE
VANGARD 100 MG N88314 001 OCT 03, 1983
200 MG N88319 001 OCT 03, 1983

TABLET, DELAYED RELEASE; ORAL
AMINOPHYLLINE
GLOBAL PHARMS 100 MG N84577 001
200 MG N84575 001
TABLICAPS 100 MG N84632 002
VALE 100 MG N84531 001
200 MG N84530 001

AMINOSALICYLATE SODIUM

TABLET; ORAL
PARASAL SODIUM
PANRAY 500 MG N06811 006
1 GM N06811 011
TEEBACIN
CONSOLIDATED
MIDLAND 500 MG N07320 002

AMINOSALICYLIC ACID

TABLET; ORAL
PARASAL
PANRAY 500 MG N06811 001
1 GM N06811 002

AMINOSALICYLIC ACID RESIN COMPLEX

POWDER; ORAL
REZIPAS
SQUIBB EQ 500 MG BASE/GM N09052 001

AMITRIPTYLINE HYDROCHLORIDE

TABLET; ORAL
AMITID
SQUIBB 10 MG N86454 001
25 MG N86454 002
50 MG N86454 003
75 MG N86454 004
100 MG N86454 005

Discontinued Drug Products *(continued)*

AMITRIPTYLINE HYDROCHLORIDE *(continued)*

TABLET; ORAL

AMITRIL

WARNER CHILCOTT	10 MG	N83939 001
	25 MG	N83937 001
	50 MG	N83938 002
	75 MG	N84957 001
	100 MG	N85093 001
	150 MG	N86295 001

AMITRIPTYLINE HCL

AM THERAP	25 MG	N88672 001 NOV 20, 1984
	50 MG	N88673 001 NOV 20, 1984
	75 MG	N88674 001 NOV 20, 1984
	100 MG	N88675 001 NOV 20, 1984
BARR	10 MG	N85744 001
	25 MG	N85627 001
	50 MG	N85745 001
	75 MG	N85743 001
	100 MG	N85742 002 MAY 11, 1982
	150 MG	N89423 001 FEB 17, 1987
CHELSEA LABS	10 MG	N85816 001
	25 MG	N85817 001
	50 MG	N85815 001
	75 MG	N85819 001
	100 MG	N85820 001
	150 MG	N85821 001
LEDERLE	10 MG	N86744 001
	10 MG	N87366 001 JAN 04, 1982
	25 MG	N86746 001
	25 MG	N87367 001 MAY 03, 1982
	50 MG	N86743 001
	50 MG	N87181 001 JAN 04, 1982
	75 MG	N86745 001
	75 MG	N87369 001 JAN 04, 1982
	100 MG	N86747 001
	100 MG	N87368 001 MAY 03, 1982
	150 MG	N87370 001 JAN 04, 1982

AMITRIPTYLINE HYDROCHLORIDE *(continued)*

TABLET; ORAL

AMITRIPTYLINE HCL

LEMMON	10 MG	N86610 001
	25 MG	N86859 001
	50 MG	N86857 001
	75 MG	N86860 001
	100 MG	N86854 001
	150 MG	N86853 001
PAR PHARM	10 MG	N88697 001 SEP 25, 1984
	25 MG	N88698 001 SEP 25, 1984
	50 MG	N88699 001 SEP 25, 1984
	75 MG	N88700 001 SEP 25, 1984
	100 MG	N88701 001 SEP 25, 1984
	150 MG	N88702 001 SEP 25, 1984
PUREPAC PHARM	10 MG	N88084 001 JUL 18, 1983
	25 MG	N88085 001 JUL 18, 1983
	50 MG	N88105 001 JUL 18, 1983
	75 MG	N88106 001 JUL 18, 1983
	100 MG	N88107 001 JUL 18, 1983
ROSEMONT PHARM	25 MG	N87775 001 FEB 10, 1982
ROXANE	10 MG	N86144 001
	25 MG	N86145 001
	50 MG	N86143 001
	75 MG	N86147 001
	100 MG	N86146 001
	150 MG	N86148 001
VANGARD	10 MG	N87632 001 FEB 01, 1982
	50 MG	N87616 001 FEB 08, 1982
	75 MG	N87617 001 FEB 05, 1982
	100 MG	N87639 001 FEB 08, 1982
WEST WARD PHARM	10 MG	N87647 001 MAR 05, 1982
	25 MG	N87278 001
	50 MG	N87557 001 MAR 05, 1982

Discontinued Drug Products *(continued)*

AMITRIPTYLINE HYDROCHLORIDE; CHLORDIAZEPOXIDE

TABLET; ORAL
CHLORDIAZEPOXIDE AND AMITRIPTYLINE HCL

ROSEMONT PHARM	EQ 12.5 MG BASE;5 MG	N70477 001 JAN 12, 1988
	EQ 25 MG BASE;10 MG	N70478 001 JAN 12, 1988

AMITRIPTYLINE HYDROCHLORIDE; PERPHENAZINE

TABLET; ORAL
PERPHENAZINE AND AMITRIPTYLINE HCL

CHELSEA LABS	50 MG;4 MG	N71558 001 MAR 02, 1987
CIRCA	10 MG;2 MG	N70373 001 AUG 25, 1986
	10 MG;4 MG	N70375 001 AUG 25, 1986
	25 MG;2 MG	N70374 001 AUG 25, 1986
	25 MG;4 MG	N70376 001 AUG 25, 1986
	50 MG;4 MG	N70377 001 NOV 04, 1986
PAR PHARM	10 MG;2 MG	N70565 001 SEP 11, 1986
	10 MG;4 MG	N70620 001 SEP 11, 1986
	25 MG;2 MG	N70621 001 SEP 11, 1986
	25 MG;4 MG	N70595 001 SEP 11, 1986
	50 MG;4 MG	N70574 001 SEP 11, 1986

AMMONIUM CHLORIDE

INJECTABLE; INJECTION

AMMONIUM CHLORIDE		
ABBOTT	5 MEQ/ML	N83130 001
SEARLE	3 MEQ/ML	N86205 001
AMMONIUM CHLORIDE 0.9% IN NORMAL SALINE		
MCGAW	900 MG/100 ML	N06580 001
AMMONIUM CHLORIDE 2.14%		
MCGAW	40 MEQ/100 ML	N85734 001

AMODIAQUINE HYDROCHLORIDE

TABLET; ORAL
CAMOQUIN HCL

PARKE DAVIS	EQ 200 MG BASE	N06441 001

AMOXICILLIN

CAPSULE; ORAL

TRIMOX		
APOTHECON	250 MG	N62098 001
	250 MG	N62152 001
	500 MG	N62098 002
	500 MG	N62152 002
UTIMOX		
PARKE DAVIS	250 MG	N62107 001
	500 MG	N62107 002

POWDER FOR RECONSTITUTION; ORAL

POLYMOX		
APOTHECON	125 MG/5 ML	N61851 001
	125 MG/5 ML	N62323 001
	250 MG/5 ML	N61851 002
	250 MG/5 ML	N62323 002
TRIMOX		
APOTHECON	125 MG/5 ML	N62099 001
	125 MG/5 ML	N62154 001
	250 MG/5 ML	N62099 002
	250 MG/5 ML	N62154 002
UTIMOX		
PARKE DAVIS	125 MG/5 ML	N62127 001
	250 MG/5 ML	N62127 002

AMPHETAMINE ADIPATE; AMPHETAMINE SULFATE; DEXTROAMPHETAMINE ADIPATE; DEXTROAMPHETAMINE SULFATE

CAPSULE; ORAL
DELCOBESE

LEMMON	1.25 MG;1.25 MG;1.25 MG;1.25 MG	N83564 001
	2.5 MG;2.5 MG;2.5 MG;2.5 MG	N83564 002
	3.75 MG;3.75 MG;3.75 MG;3.75 MG	N83564 003
	5 MG;5 MG;5 MG;5 MG	N83564 004

TABLET; ORAL
DELCOBESE

LEMMON	1.25 MG;1.25 MG;1.25 MG;1.25 MG	N83563 004
	2.5 MG;2.5 MG;2.5 MG;2.5 MG	N83563 003
	3.75 MG;3.75 MG;3.75 MG;3.75 MG	N83563 002
	5 MG;5 MG;5 MG;5 MG	N83563 001

AMPHETAMINE RESIN COMPLEX; DEXTROAMPHETAMINE RESIN COMPLEX

CAPSULE, EXTENDED RELEASE; ORAL

BIPHETAMINE 12.5		
FISONS	EQ 6.25 MG BASE;EQ 6.25 MG BASE	N10093 007
BIPHETAMINE 20		
FISONS	EQ 10 MG BASE;EQ 10 MG BASE	N10093 003
BIPHETAMINE 7.5		
FISONS	EQ 3.75 MG BASE;EQ 3.75 MG BASE	N10093 009

AMPHETAMINE SULFATE

TABLET; ORAL

AMPHETAMINE SULFATE		
LANNETT	5 MG	N83901 001 AUG 31, 1984
	10 MG	N83901 002 AUG 31, 1984

AMPHETAMINE SULFATE; *MULTIPLE*

SEE AMPHETAMINE ADIPATE; AMPHETAMINE SULFATE; DEXTROAMPHETAMINE ADIPATE; DEXTROAMPHETAMINE SULFATE

AMPHOTERICIN B

INJECTABLE; INJECTION

AMPHOTERICIN B		
FUJISAWA	50 MG/VIAL	N62728 001 APR 13, 1987

AMPICILLIN SODIUM

INJECTABLE; INJECTION

AMPICILLIN SODIUM		
COPANOS	EQ 125 MG BASE/VIAL	N61936 005
	EQ 250 MG BASE/VIAL	N61936 001
	EQ 500 MG BASE/VIAL	N61936 002
	EQ 1 GM BASE/VIAL	N61936 003
	EQ 2 GM BASE/VIAL	N61936 004
INTL MEDICATION	EQ 1 GM BASE/VIAL	N62634 002 JAN 09, 1987
	EQ 2 GM BASE/VIAL	N62634 003 JAN 09, 1987

AMPICILLIN SODIUM *(continued)*

INJECTABLE; INJECTION

AMPICILLIN SODIUM		
LILLY	EQ 500 MG BASE/VIAL	N62565 001 APR 04, 1985
	EQ 1 GM BASE/VIAL	N62565 002 APR 04, 1985
	EQ 2 GM BASE/VIAL	N62565 003 JUN 24, 1986
PENBRITIN-S		
WYETH AYERST	EQ 4 GM BASE/VIAL	N50072 006
POLYCILLIN-N		
BRISTOL	EQ 125 MG BASE/VIAL	N50309 001
	EQ 250 MG BASE/VIAL	N50309 002
	EQ 500 MG BASE/VIAL	N50309 003
	EQ 1 GM BASE/VIAL	N50309 004
	EQ 2 GM BASE/VIAL	N50309 005

AMPICILLIN SODIUM; SULBACTAM SODIUM

INJECTABLE; INJECTION

UNASYN		
PFIZER	EQ 500 MG BASE/VIAL;EQ 250 MG BASE/VIAL	N50608 003 DEC 31, 1986

AMPICILLIN/AMPICILLIN TRIHYDRATE

CAPSULE; ORAL

AMCILL		
PARKE DAVIS	EQ 250 MG BASE	N62041 001
	EQ 500 MG BASE	N62041 002
AMPICILLIN		
LEDERLE	EQ 250 MG BASE	N62208 001
	EQ 500 MG BASE	N62208 002
VITARINE	EQ 250 MG BASE	N61387 001
	EQ 500 MG BASE	N61387 003
AMPICILLIN TRIHYDRATE		
PUREPAC PHARM	EQ 250 MG BASE	N61853 001
PENBRITIN		
WYETH AYERST	EQ 250 MG BASE	N60908 001
	EQ 500 MG BASE	N60908 002
POLYCILLIN		
BRISTOL	EQ 250 MG BASE	N50310 001
	EQ 500 MG BASE	N50310 002
PRINCIPEN '250'		
APOTHECON	EQ 250 MG BASE	N50056 001
	EQ 250 MG BASE	N62157 002
PRINCIPEN '500'		
APOTHECON	EQ 500 MG BASE	N50056 002
	EQ 500 MG BASE	N62157 001

Discontinued Drug Products *(continued)*

AMPICILLIN/AMPICILLIN TRIHYDRATE *(continued)*

CAPSULE; ORAL		
TOTACILLIN		
SMITHKLINE BEECHAM	EQ 250 MG BASE	N60060 001
	EQ 500 MG BASE	N60060 002
POWDER FOR RECONSTITUTION; ORAL		
AMCILL		
PARKE DAVIS	EQ 125 MG BASE/5 ML	N62030 001
	EQ 250 MG BASE/5 ML	N62030 002
AMPICILLIN TRIHYDRATE		
PUREPAC PHARM	EQ 125 MG BASE/5 ML	N61980 001
OMNIPEN (AMPICILLIN)		
WYETH AYERST	500 MG/5 ML	N60625 004
PENBRITIN		
WYETH AYERST	EQ 125 MG BASE/5 ML	N50019 002
	EQ 250 MG BASE/5 ML	N50019 003
	EQ 100 MG BASE/ML	N50019 001
POLYCILLIN		
APOTHECON	EQ 125 MG BASE/5 ML	N62297 001
	EQ 250 MG BASE/5 ML	N62297 002
BRISTOL	EQ 100 MG BASE/ML	N50308 004
PRINCIPEN '125'		
APOTHECON	EQ 125 MG BASE/5 ML	N60127 002
	EQ 125 MG BASE/5 ML	N62151 001
PRINCIPEN '250'		
APOTHECON	EQ 250 MG BASE/5 ML	N60127 001
	EQ 250 MG BASE/5 ML	N62151 002
TABLET, CHEWABLE; ORAL		
POLYCILLIN		
BRISTOL	EQ 125 MG BASE	N50093 001

AMPICILLIN/AMPICILLIN TRIHYDRATE; PROBENECID

CAPSULE; ORAL		
PRINCIPEN W/ PROBENECID		
APOTHECON	EQ 389 MG BASE;111 MG	N50488 001
	EQ 389 MG BASE;111 MG	N62150 001
POWDER FOR RECONSTITUTION; ORAL		
POLYCILLIN-PRB		
BRISTOL	EQ 3.5 GM BASE/BOT;1 GM/BOT	N50457 001

ANILERIDINE HYDROCHLORIDE

TABLET; ORAL		
LERITINE		
MERCK SHARP DOHME	EQ 25 MG BASE	N10585 002

ANILERIDINE PHOSPHATE

INJECTABLE; INJECTION		
LERITINE		
MERCK SHARP DOHME	EQ 25 MG BASE/ML	N10520 003

ANISOTROPINE METHYLBROMIDE

TABLET; ORAL		
ANISOTROPINE METHYLBROMIDE		
CIRCA	50 MG	N86046 001
VALPIN 50		
DUPONT MERCK	50 MG	N13428 001

ASCORBIC ACID; BIOTIN; CYANOCOBALAMIN; DEXPANTHENOL; ERGOCALCIFEROL; FOLIC ACID; NIACINAMIDE; PYRIDOXINE; RIBOFLAVIN PHOSPHATE SODIUM; THIAMINE; VITAMIN A; VITAMIN E

INJECTABLE; INJECTION		
M.V.I.-12 LYOPHILIZED		
ASTRA	100 MG/VIAL;0.06 MG/VIAL;0.005 MG/VIAL;15 MG/VIAL;5 UGM/VIAL;0.4 MG/VIAL;40 MG/VIAL;4 MG/VIAL;3.6 MG/VIAL;3 MG/VIAL;1 MG/VIAL;10 MG/VIAL	N18933 002 AUG 08, 1985

ASCORBIC ACID; BIOTIN; CYANOCOBALAMIN; DEXPANTHENOL; ERGOCALCIFEROL; FOLIC ACID; NIACINAMIDE; PYRIDOXINE HYDROCHLORIDE; RIBOFLAVIN PHOSPHATE SODIUM; THIAMINE HYDROCHLORIDE; VITAMIN A PALMITATE; VITAMIN E

INJECTABLE; INJECTION		
BEROCCA PN		
ROCHE	50 MG/ML;0.03 MG/ML;0.0025 MG/ML;7.5 MG/ML;100IU/ML;0.2 MG/ML;20 MG/ML;2 MG/ML;1.8 MG/ML;1.5 MG/ML;1,650IU/ML;5IU/ML	N06071 003 OCT 10, 1985

Discontinued Drug Products *(continued)*

ASCORBIC ACID; BIOTIN; CYANOCOBALAMIN; DEXPANTHENOL; ERGOCALCIFEROL; FOLIC ACID; NIACINAMIDE; PYRIDOXINE HYDROCHLORIDE; RIBOFLAVIN PHOSPHATE SODIUM; THIAMINE HYDROCHLORIDE; VITAMIN A; VITAMIN E

INJECTABLE; INJECTION
M.V.C. 9+3
FUJISAWA — 10 MG/ML;0.006 MG/ML;0.5 MCG/ML;1.5 MG/ML;20IU/ML;0.04 MG/ML;4 MG/ML;0.4 MG/ML;0.36 MG/ML;0.3 MG/ML;330 UNITS/ML;1IU/ML — N18440 002 AUG 08, 1985

ASPIRIN; *MULTIPLE*
SEE ACETAMINOPHEN; ASPIRIN; CODEINE PHOSPHATE

ASPIRIN; BUTALBITAL; CAFFEINE

CAPSULE; ORAL
BUTALBITAL, ASPIRIN AND CAFFEINE
CHELSEA LABS — 325 MG;50 MG;40 MG — N86231 002 FEB 12, 1985

TABLET; ORAL
BUTALBITAL ASPIRIN AND CAFFEINE
QUANTUM PHARMICS — 325 MG;50 MG;40 MG — N88972 001 JUN 18, 1985
BUTALBITAL, ASPIRIN AND CAFFEINE
CHELSEA LABS — 325 MG;50 MG;40 MG — N86237 002 MAR 23, 1984

ASPIRIN; CAFFEINE; ORPHENADRINE CITRATE

TABLET; ORAL
ORPHENGESIC
PAR PHARM — 385 MG;30 MG;25 MG — N71642 001 JUN 23, 1987
ORPHENGESIC FORTE
PAR PHARM — 770 MG;60 MG;50 MG — N71643 001 JUN 23, 1987

ASPIRIN; CAFFEINE; PROPOXYPHENE HYDROCHLORIDE

CAPSULE; ORAL
COMPOUND 65
ALRA — 389 MG;32.4 MG;65 MG — N84553 002 AUG 17, 1983
PROPOXYPHENE HCL W/ ASPIRIN AND CAFFEINE
CHELSEA LABS — 389 MG;32.4 MG;65 MG — N85732 002 SEP 03, 1984

ASPIRIN; CARISOPRODOL

TABLET; ORAL
CARISOPRODOL COMPOUND
CIRCA — 325 MG;200 MG — N88809 001 OCT 03, 1985

ASPIRIN; HYDROCODONE BITARTRATE

TABLET; ORAL
VICOPRIN
KNOLL PHARM — 500 MG;5 MG — N86333 001 SEP 14, 1983

ASPIRIN; MEPROBAMATE

TABLET; ORAL
MEPRO-ASPIRIN
EON LABS — 325 MG;200 MG — N89127 001 MAR 02, 1987
MEPROBAMATE AND ASPIRIN
PAR PHARM — 325 MG;200 MG — N89126 001 AUG 19, 1986
Q-GESIC
QUANTUM PHARMICS — 325 MG;200 MG — N88740 001 JUN 01, 1984

ASPIRIN; PROPOXYPHENE NAPSYLATE

CAPSULE; ORAL
DARVON-N W/ ASA
LILLY — 325 MG;100 MG — N16829 001

TABLET; ORAL
DARVON-N W/ ASA
LILLY — 325 MG;100 MG — N16863 001

ATROPINE SULFATE

AEROSOL, METERED; INHALATION
ATROPINE SULFATE
US ARMY — EQ 0.36 MG BASE/INH — N20056 001 SEP 19, 1990

ATROPINE SULFATE; DIFENOXIN HYDROCHLORIDE

TABLET; ORAL
MOTOFEN HALF-STRENGTH
CARNRICK — 0.025 MG;0.5 MG — N17744 001

Discontinued Drug Products *(continued)*

ATROPINE SULFATE; DIPHENOXYLATE HYDROCHLORIDE

SOLUTION; ORAL
COLONAID
WALLACE — 0.025 MG/5 ML;2.5 MG/5 ML — N85735 001
LOMANATE
BARRE — 0.025 MG/5 ML;2.5 MG/5 ML — N85746 001

TABLET; ORAL
COLONAID
WALLACE — 0.025 MG;2.5 MG — N85737 001
DIPHENOXYLATE HCL AND ATROPINE SULFATE
ASCOT — 0.025 MG;2.5 MG — N87934 001 JUL 19, 1983
CHELSEA LABS — 0.025 MG;2.5 MG — N85876 001
HEATHER — 0.025 MG;2.5 MG — N86798 001
LEDERLE — 0.025 MG;2.5 MG — N86950 001
PARKE DAVIS — 0.025 MG;2.5 MG — N87131 001
DIPHENOXYLATE HCL W/ ATROPINE SULFATE
EON LABS — 0.025 MG;2.5 MG — N86173 001
ROSEMONT PHARM — 0.025 MG;2.5 MG — N87842 001 MAR 29, 1982
LO-TROL
VANGARD — 0.025 MG;2.5 MG — N88009 001 MAR 25, 1983
LOFENE
LANNETT — 0.025 MG;2.5 MG — N85372 001

ATROPINE SULFATE; MEPERIDINE HYDROCHLORIDE

INJECTABLE; INJECTION
MEPERIDINE AND ATROPINE SULFATE
WYETH AYERST — 0.4 MG/ML;50 MG/ML — N85121 001
0.4 MG/ML;75 MG/ML — N85121 002
0.4 MG/ML;100 MG/ML — N85121 003

AZATHIOPRINE

TABLET; ORAL
IMURAN
BURROUGHS WELLCOME — 25 MG — N16324 002

AZATHIOPRINE SODIUM

INJECTABLE; INJECTION
AZATHIOPRINE
QUAD PHARMS — EQ 100 MG BASE/VIAL — N71056 001 JUN 08, 1988

AZLOCILLIN SODIUM

INJECTABLE; INJECTION
AZLIN
MILES — EQ 2 GM BASE/VIAL — N62388 001 SEP 08, 1982
EQ 2 GM BASE/VIAL — N62417 001 OCT 12, 1982
EQ 3 GM BASE/VIAL — N62388 002 SEP 08, 1982
EQ 3 GM BASE/VIAL — N62417 002 OCT 12, 1982
EQ 4 GM BASE/VIAL — N62388 003 SEP 08, 1982
EQ 4 GM BASE/VIAL — N62417 003 OCT 12, 1982

AZTREONAM

INJECTABLE; INJECTION
AZACTAM IN PLASTIC CONTAINER
SQUIBB — 10 MG/ML — N50632 003 MAY 24, 1989

BACAMPICILLIN HYDROCHLORIDE

TABLET; ORAL
SPECTROBID
PFIZER — 800 MG — N50520 002 SEP 12, 1983

BACITRACIN

INJECTABLE; INJECTION
BACITRACIN
QUAD PHARMS — 10,000 UNITS/VIAL — N62696 001 APR 17, 1987
50,000 UNITS/VIAL — N62696 002 APR 17, 1987

OINTMENT; OPHTHALMIC
BACIGUENT
UPJOHN — 500 UNITS/GM — N60734 001
BACITRACIN
PHARMADERM — 500 UNITS/GM — N62158 001
PHARMAFAIR — 500 UNITS/GM — N62453 001 MAR 28, 1984

OINTMENT; TOPICAL
BACITRACIN
COMBE — 500 UNITS/GM — N62799 001 MAY 14, 1987

Discontinued Drug Products *(continued)*

BACITRACIN; NEOMYCIN SULFATE; POLYMYXIN B SULFATE
OINTMENT; OPHTHALMIC
MYCITRACIN
UPJOHN 500 UNITS/GM;EQ 3.5 MG BASE/GM;10,000 UNITS/GM N61048 001

BACITRACIN; POLYMYXIN B SULFATE
AEROSOL; TOPICAL
LANABIOTIC
COMBE 500 UNITS/GM;5,000 UNITS/GM N50598 001 SEP 22, 1986

BACITRACIN ZINC; HYDROCORTISONE; NEOMYCIN SULFATE; POLYMYXIN B SULFATE
OINTMENT; OPHTHALMIC
ZINC BACITRACIN,NEOMYCIN SULFATE,POLYMYXIN B SULFATE & HYDROCORTISONE
PHARMAFAIR 400 UNITS/GM;1%;EQ 3.5 MG BASE/GM;10,000 UNITS/GM N62389 001 JUL 02, 1982
OINTMENT; TOPICAL
NEOMYCIN & POLYMYXIN B SULFATES & BACITRACIN ZINC & HYDROCORTISONE
PHARMAFAIR 400 UNITS/GM;1%;EQ 3.5 MG BASE/GM;5,000 UNITS/GM N62381 001 SEP 06, 1985

BACITRACIN ZINC; LIDOCAINE; NEOMYCIN SULFATE; POLYMYXIN B SULFATE
OINTMENT; TOPICAL
LANABIOTIC
COMBE 400 UNITS/GM;40 MG/GM;EQ 5 MG BASE/GM;5,000 UNITS/GM N62499 001 JUN 03, 1985

BACITRACIN ZINC; NEOMYCIN SULFATE; POLYMYXIN B SULFATE
OINTMENT; OPHTHALMIC
BACITRACIN ZINC-NEOMYCIN SULFATE-POLYMYXIN B SULFATE
PHARMAFAIR 400 UNITS/GM;EQ 3.5 MG BASE/GM;10,000 UNITS/GM N62386 001 SEP 09, 1982
BACITRACIN-NEOMYCIN-POLYMYXIN
PHARMADERM 400 UNITS/GM;EQ 3.5 MG BASE/GM;5,000 UNITS/GM N62167 001

BACLOFEN
TABLET; ORAL
BACLOFEN
ROSEMONT PHARM 10 MG N71260 001 MAY 06, 1988
20 MG N71261 001 MAY 06, 1988

BENDROFLUMETHIAZIDE
TABLET; ORAL
NATURETIN-2.5
SQUIBB 2.5 MG N12164 001

BENOXINATE HYDROCHLORIDE
SOLUTION/DROPS; OPHTHALMIC
BENOXINATE HCL
SOLA BARNES HIND 0.4% N84149 001

BENTONITE; SULFUR
POWDER; TOPICAL
BENSULFOID
POYTHRESS 66.64%;33.32% N02918 001

BENZPHETAMINE HYDROCHLORIDE
TABLET; ORAL
DIDREX
UPJOHN 25 MG N12427 003

Discontinued Drug Products *(continued)*

BENZTHIAZIDE
TABLET; ORAL
AQUATAG
SOLVAY 25 MG N16001 001
50 MG N16001 002
BENZTHIAZIDE
PRIVATE FORM 50 MG N83206 001
FOVANE
PFIZER 50 MG N12128 002
URESE
PFIZER 25 MG N12128 003

BENZTROPINE MESYLATE
TABLET; ORAL
BENZTROPINE MESYLATE
QUANTUM PHARMICS 0.5 MG N88514 001 JAN 31, 1984
1 MG N88510 001 JAN 31, 1984
2 MG N88511 001 JAN 31, 1984
ROSEMONT PHARM 0.5 MG N89211 001 JUN 14, 1988
1 MG N89212 001 JUN 14, 1988
2 MG N89213 001 JUN 14, 1988

BENZYL BENZOATE
EMULSION; TOPICAL
BENZYL BENZOATE
LANNETT 50% N84535 001

BEPRIDIL HYDROCHLORIDE
TABLET; ORAL
BEPADIN
WALLACE 200 MG N19001 001 DEC 28, 1990
300 MG N19001 002 DEC 28, 1990
400 MG N19001 003 DEC 28, 1990

BETAMETHASONE
CREAM; TOPICAL
CELESTONE
SCHERING 0.2% N14762 001

BETAMETHASONE BENZOATE
OINTMENT; TOPICAL
UTICORT
PARKE DAVIS 0.025% N18089 001

BETAMETHASONE DIPROPIONATE
CREAM; TOPICAL
BETAMETHASONE DIPROPIONATE
CLAY PARK EQ 0.05% BASE N72536 001 JAN 31, 1990
PHARMADERM EQ 0.05% BASE N19136 001 JUN 26, 1984
CREAM, AUGMENTED; TOPICAL
DIPROLENE
SCHERING EQ 0.05% BASE N19408 001 JAN 31, 1986
LOTION; TOPICAL
BETAMETHASONE DIPROPIONATE
PHARMADERM EQ 0.05% BASE N70274 001 AUG 12, 1985
OINTMENT; TOPICAL
BETAMETHASONE DIPROPIONATE
CLAY PARK EQ 0.05% BASE N72526 001 JAN 31, 1990
PHARMADERM EQ 0.05% BASE N19140 001 SEP 04, 1984

BETAMETHASONE VALERATE
CREAM; TOPICAL
BETAMETHASONE VALERATE
PHARMADERM EQ 0.1% BASE N18860 002 AUG 31, 1983
PHARMAFAIR EQ 0.1% BASE N70485 001 MAY 29, 1987
LOTION; TOPICAL
BETAMETHASONE VALERATE
PHARMADERM EQ 0.1% BASE N18870 001 AUG 31, 1983
OINTMENT; TOPICAL
BETAMETHASONE VALERATE
CLAY PARK EQ 0.1% BASE N71478 001 DEC 23, 1987
PHARMADERM EQ 0.1% BASE N18864 001 AUG 31, 1983
PHARMAFAIR EQ 0.1% BASE N70486 001 MAY 29, 1987

Discontinued Drug Products *(continued)*

BETAZOLE HYDROCHLORIDE

INJECTABLE; INJECTION
HISTALOG
LILLY 50 MG/ML N09344 001

BETHANECHOL CHLORIDE

INJECTABLE; INJECTION
BETHANECHOL CHLORIDE
QUAD PHARMS 5 MG/ML N89815 001 APR 12, 1988

TABLET; ORAL
BETHANECHOL CHLORIDE

ASCOT	10 MG	N88288 001 JUN 08, 1983
	25 MG	N88289 001 JUN 08, 1983
CHELSEA LABS	5 MG	N85841 001
	10 MG	N85842 001
	25 MG	N85839 001
CIRCA	5 MG	N85230 002
	10 MG	N85228 001
	25 MG	N85229 001
	50 MG	N87397 001
EON LABS	5 MG	N84353 001
	10 MG	N84378 001
	10 MG	N84379 001
	25 MG	N84383 001
	25 MG	N84384 001
LANNETT	5 MG	N84702 001
	10 MG	N84712 001
	25 MG	N84074 001

BETHANIDINE SULFATE

TABLET; ORAL
TENATHAN

ROBINS AH	10 MG	N17675 001
	25 MG	N17675 002

BIOTIN; *MULTIPLE*

SEE ASCORBIC ACID; BIOTIN; CYANOCOBALAMIN; DEXPANTHENOL; ERGOCALCIFEROL; FOLIC ACID; NIACINAMIDE; PYRIDOXINE HYDROCHLORIDE; RIBOFLAVIN PHOSPHATE SODIUM; THIAMINE HYDROCHLORIDE; VITAMIN A; VITAMIN E

SEE ASCORBIC ACID; BIOTIN; CYANOCOBALAMIN; DEXPANTHENOL; ERGOCALCIFEROL; FOLIC ACID; NIACINAMIDE; PYRIDOXINE HYDROCHLORIDE; RIBOFLAVIN PHOSPHATE SODIUM; THIAMINE HYDROCHLORIDE; VITAMIN A PALMITATE; VITAMIN E

SEE ASCORBIC ACID; BIOTIN; CYANOCOBALAMIN; DEXPANTHENOL; ERGOCALCIFEROL; FOLIC ACID; NIACINAMIDE; PYRIDOXINE; RIBOFLAVIN PHOSPHATE SODIUM; THIAMINE; VITAMIN A; VITAMIN E

BRETYLIUM TOSYLATE

INJECTABLE; INJECTION
BRETYLIUM TOSYLATE

ASTRA	50 MG/ML	N71152 001 AUG 10, 1987
FUJISAWA	50 MG/ML	N70134 001 APR 29, 1986
	100 MG/ML	N71298 001 FEB 13, 1987
QUAD PHARMS	50 MG/ML	N71181 001 FEB 16, 1988

BRETYLIUM TOSYLATE IN DEXTROSE 5%

ABBOTT	800 MG/100 ML	N19005 001 APR 29, 1986
	200 MG/100 ML	N19005 002 APR 29, 1986
	400 MG/100 ML	N19005 003 APR 29, 1986

BRETYLIUM TOSYLATE IN DEXTROSE 5% IN PLASTIC CONTAINER
ABBOTT 800 MG/100 ML N19008 001 APR 29, 1986

BROMODIPHENHYDRAMINE HYDROCHLORIDE

CAPSULE; ORAL
AMBODRYL
PARKE DAVIS 25 MG N07984 001

Discontinued Drug Products *(continued)*

BROMPHENIRAMINE MALEATE
ELIXIR; ORAL
BROMPHENIRAMINE MALEATE
BARRE 2 MG/5 ML N86936 001
PHARM ASSOC 2 MG/5 ML N87517 001
ROSEMONT PHARM 2 MG/5 ML N87964 001 JAN 25, 1983
INJECTABLE; INJECTION
BROMPHENIRAMINE MALEATE
STERIS 100 MG/ML N83820 001
DIMETANE-TEN
WYETH AYERST 10 MG/ML N11418 002
TABLET; ORAL
BROMPHENIRAMINE MALEATE
ANABOLIC 4 MG N86187 001
BARR 4 MG N84468 001
CHELSEA LABS 4 MG N85769 001
GENEVA PHARMS 4 MG N83215 001
NEWTRON PHARMS 4 MG N86987 001
PAR PHARM 4 MG N87009 001
PIONEER PHARMS 4 MG N88604 001 JUL 13, 1984
VITARINE 4 MG N85850 001
ZENITH LABS 4 MG N84351 001

BROMPHENIRAMINE MALEATE; PHENYLPROPANOLAMINE HYDROCHLORIDE
ELIXIR; ORAL
BIPHETAP
PENNEX 4 MG/5 ML;25 MG/5 ML N88687 001 SEP 26, 1984
BROMANATE
BARRE 4 MG/5 ML;25 MG/5 ML N88688 001 FEB 06, 1985

BUPROPION HYDROCHLORIDE
TABLET; ORAL
WELLBUTRIN
BURROUGHS WELLCOME 50 MG N18644 001 DEC 30, 1985

BUTABARBITAL SODIUM
CAPSULE; ORAL
BUTICAPS
WALLACE 15 MG N85381 001
30 MG N85381 002
50 MG N85381 003
100 MG N85381 004
ELIXIR; ORAL
BUTABARBITAL SODIUM
PENNEX 30 MG/5 ML N85383 001
BUTALAN
LANNETT 33.3 MG/5 ML N85880 001
TABLET; ORAL
BUTABARBITAL SODIUM
CHELSEA LABS 15 MG N85764 001
30 MG N85772 001
EON LABS 15 MG N85938 001
30 MG N85934 001
GENEVA PHARMS 15 MG N84292 003 FEB 09, 1982
30 MG N84272 002
LEMMON 15 MG N88632 001 MAY 18, 1985
30 MG N88631 001 MAY 01, 1985
SOLVAY 16.2 MG N83606 001
32.4 MG N83898 001
48.6 MG N83897 001
97.2 MG N83896 001
WHITEWORTH TOWNE 15 MG N83325 002
30 MG N83337 001
SODIUM BUTABARBITAL
LANNETT 100 MG N85881 001
WEST WARD PHARM 15 MG N85418 001
30 MG N85432 001
ZENITH LABS 15 MG N83484 001
30 MG N84040 001

BUTALBITAL; *MULTIPLE*
SEE ACETAMINOPHEN; BUTALBITAL
SEE ACETAMINOPHEN; BUTALBITAL; CAFFEINE
SEE ASPIRIN; BUTALBITAL; CAFFEINE

BUTOCONAZOLE NITRATE
SUPPOSITORY; VAGINAL
FEMSTAT
SYNTEX 100 MG N19359 001 NOV 25, 1985

Discontinued Drug Products *(continued)*

CAFFEINE; *MULTIPLE*
SEE ACETAMINOPHEN; BUTALBITAL; CAFFEINE
SEE ASPIRIN; BUTALBITAL; CAFFEINE
SEE ASPIRIN; CAFFEINE; ORPHENADRINE CITRATE
SEE ASPIRIN; CAFFEINE; PROPOXYPHENE HYDROCHLORIDE

CALCITONIN, SALMON
INJECTABLE; INJECTION
CALCIMAR
RHONE POULENC RORER — 400IU/VIAL — N17497 001
MIACALCIN
SANDOZ — 100IU/ML — N17808 001 JUL 03, 1986

CALCIUM; MEGLUMINE; METRIZOIC ACID
INJECTABLE; INJECTION
ISOPAQUE 280
STERLING WINTHROP — 0.35 MG/ML;140.1 MG/ML;461.8 MG/ML — N17506 001

CALCIUM CHLORIDE; DEXTROSE; MAGNESIUM CHLORIDE; SODIUM ACETATE; SODIUM CHLORIDE
SOLUTION; INTRAPERITONEAL
DIALYTE LM/ DEXTROSE 2.5% IN PLASTIC CONTAINER
MCGAW — 29 MG/100 ML;2.5 GM/100 ML;15 MG/100 ML;610 MG/100 ML;560 MG/100 ML — N18460 006 JAN 29, 1986
DIALYTE W/ DEXTROSE 1.5% IN PLASTIC CONTAINER
MCGAW — 29 MG/100 ML;1.5 GM/100 ML;15 MG/100 ML;610 MG/100 ML;560 MG/100 ML — N18460 001
DIALYTE W/ DEXTROSE 4.25% IN PLASTIC CONTAINER
MCGAW — 29 MG/100 ML;4.25 GM/100 ML;15 MG/100 ML;610 MG/100 ML;560 MG/100 ML — N18460 003

CALCIUM CHLORIDE; DEXTROSE; MAGNESIUM CHLORIDE; SODIUM CHLORIDE; SODIUM LACTATE
SOLUTION; INTRAPERITONEAL
DIALYTE LM/ DEXTROSE 1.5% IN PLASTIC CONTAINER
MCGAW — 26 MG/100 ML;1.5 GM/100 ML;15 MG/100 ML;560 MG/100 ML;390 MG/100 ML — N18460 002
DIALYTE LM/ DEXTROSE 2.5% IN PLASTIC CONTAINER
MCGAW — 26 MG/100 ML;5 GM/100 ML;5 MG/100 ML;530 MG/100 ML;450 MG/100 ML — N18460 008 JAN 29, 1986
DIALYTE LM/ DEXTROSE 4.25% IN PLASTIC CONTAINER
MCGAW — 26 MG/100 ML;4.25 GM/100 ML;15 MG/100 ML;560 MG/100 ML;390 MG/100 ML — N18460 004

CALCIUM CHLORIDE; DEXTROSE; POTASSIUM CHLORIDE; SODIUM CHLORIDE; SODIUM LACTATE
INJECTABLE; INJECTION
DEXTROSE 5% IN LACTATED RINGER'S IN PLASTIC CONTAINER
MILES — 20 MG/100 ML;5 GM/100 ML;30 MG/100 ML;600 MG/100 ML;310 MG/100 ML — N18499 001
POTASSIUM CHLORIDE 10 MEQ IN DEXTROSE 5% AND LACTATED RINGER'S IN PLASTIC CONTAINER
ABBOTT — 20 MG/100 ML;5 GM/100 ML;104 MG/100 ML;600 MG/100 ML;310 MG/100 ML — N19685 005 OCT 17, 1988
20 MG/100 ML;5 GM/100 ML;179 MG/100 ML;600 MG/100 ML;310 MG/100 ML — N19685 006 OCT 17, 1988
POTASSIUM CHLORIDE 15 MEQ IN DEXTROSE 5% AND LACTATED RINGER'S IN PLASTIC CONTAINER
ABBOTT — 20 MG/100 ML;5 GM/100 ML;254 MG/100 ML;600 MG/100 ML;310 MG/100 ML — N19685 007 OCT 17, 1988

Discontinued Drug Products *(continued)*

CALCIUM CHLORIDE; DEXTROSE; POTASSIUM CHLORIDE; SODIUM CHLORIDE; SODIUM LACTATE *(continued)*

INJECTABLE; INJECTION
POTASSIUM CHLORIDE 30 MEQ IN DEXTROSE 5% AND LACTATED RINGER'S IN PLASTIC CONTAINER
ABBOTT — 20 MG/100 ML;5 GM/100 ML;254 MG/100 ML;600 MG/100 ML;310 MG/100 ML — N19685 003 — OCT 17, 1988
POTASSIUM CHLORIDE 5 MEQ IN DEXTROSE 5% AND LACTATED RINGER'S IN PLASTIC CONTAINER
ABBOTT — 20 MG/100 ML;5 GM/100 ML;104 MG/100 ML;600 MG/100 ML;310 MG/100 ML — N19685 001 — OCT 17, 1988

CALCIUM CHLORIDE; DEXTROSE; SODIUM CHLORIDE; SODIUM LACTATE

SOLUTION; INTRAPERITONEAL
INPERSOL-ZM W/ DEXTROSE 1.5% IN PLASTIC CONTAINER
ABBOTT — 25.7 MG/100 ML;1.5 GM/100 ML;538 MG/100 ML;448 MG/100 ML — N19395 001 — MAR 26, 1986
INPERSOL-ZM W/ DEXTROSE 2.5% IN PLASTIC CONTAINER
ABBOTT — 25.7 MG/100 ML;2.5 GM/100 ML;538 MG/100 ML;448 MG/100 ML — N19395 002 — MAR 26, 1986
INPERSOL-ZM W/ DEXTROSE 4.25% IN PLASTIC CONTAINER
ABBOTT — 25.7 MG/100 ML;4.25 GM/100 ML;538 MG/100 ML;448 MG/100 ML — N19395 003 — MAR 26, 1986

CALCIUM CHLORIDE; MAGNESIUM CHLORIDE; POTASSIUM CHLORIDE; SODIUM ACETATE; SODIUM CHLORIDE

INJECTABLE; INJECTION
TPN ELECTROLYTES IN PLASTIC CONTAINER
ABBOTT — 16.5 MG/ML;25.4 MG/ML;74.6 MG/ML;121 MG/ML;16.1 MG/ML — N19399 001 — JUN 16, 1986

CALCIUM CHLORIDE; POTASSIUM CHLORIDE; SODIUM ACETATE; SODIUM CHLORIDE

INJECTABLE; INJECTION
ACETATED RINGER'S IN PLASTIC CONTAINER
MCGAW — 20 MG/100 ML;30 MG/100 ML;380 MG/100 ML;600 MG/100 ML — N18725 001 — NOV 29, 1982

CALCIUM CHLORIDE; POTASSIUM CHLORIDE; SODIUM CHLORIDE

SOLUTION; IRRIGATION
RINGER'S IN PLASTIC CONTAINER
ABBOTT — 33 MG/100 ML;30 MG/100 ML;860 MG/100 ML — N18462 001

CALCIUM CHLORIDE; POTASSIUM CHLORIDE; SODIUM CHLORIDE; SODIUM LACTATE

INJECTABLE; INJECTION
LACTATED RINGER'S IN PLASTIC CONTAINER
ABBOTT — 20 MG/100 ML;30 MG/100 ML;600 MG/100 ML;310 MG/100 ML — N19485 001 — OCT 24, 1985
MILES — 20 MG/100 ML;30 MG/100 ML;600 MG/100 ML;310 MG/100 ML — N18417 001

CALCIUM GLUCEPTATE

INJECTABLE; INJECTION
CALCIUM GLUCEPTATE
ABBOTT — EQ 90 MG CALCIUM/5 ML — N83159 001
FUJISAWA — EQ 90 MG CALCIUM/5 ML — N89373 001 — APR 30, 1987
LILLY — EQ 90 MG CALCIUM/5 ML — N06470 001

CALCIUM METRIZOATE; MEGLUMINE METRIZOATE; METRIZOATE MAGNESIUM; METRIZOATE SODIUM

INJECTABLE; INJECTION
ISOPAQUE 440
STERLING WINTHROP — 0.78 MG/ML;75.9 MG/ML;0.15 MG/ML;16.6 MG/ML — N16847 001

Discontinued Drug Products *(continued)*

CAPTOPRIL
TABLET; ORAL
CAPOTEN
BRISTOL MYERS SQUIBB — 37.5 MG — N18343 006 SEP 17, 1986

CARBACHOL
SOLUTION; INTRAOCULAR
CARBACHOL
PHARMAFAIR — 0.01% — N70292 001 MAY 21, 1986

CARBAMAZEPINE
TABLET; ORAL
CARBAMAZEPINE
ROSEMONT PHARM — 200 MG — N70300 001 MAY 15, 1986
WARNER CHILCOTT — 200 MG — N70429 001 JAN 02, 1987

CARBENICILLIN DISODIUM
INJECTABLE; INJECTION
PYOPEN
SMITHKLINE BEECHAM — EQ 1 GM BASE/VIAL — N50298 001
EQ 2 GM BASE/VIAL — N50298 002
EQ 5 GM BASE/VIAL — N50298 003
EQ 10 GM BASE/VIAL — N50298 006
EQ 20 GM BASE/VIAL — N50298 007

CARBINOXAMINE MALEATE
TABLET; ORAL
CLISTIN
JOHNSON RW — 4 MG — N08915 001

CARISOPRODOL
CAPSULE; ORAL
SOMA
WALLACE — 250 MG — N11792 003
TABLET; ORAL
CARISOPRODOL
CIRCA — 350 MG — N85433 001
EON LABS — 350 MG — N89566 001 AUG 30, 1988
PIONEER PHARMS — 350 MG — N89390 001 OCT 13, 1988
RELA
SCHERING — 350 MG — N12155 001

CARISOPRODOL; *MULTIPLE*
SEE ASPIRIN; CARISOPRODOL

CARPHENAZINE MALEATE
CONCENTRATE; ORAL
PROKETAZINE
WYETH AYERST — 50 MG/ML — N14173 001
TABLET; ORAL
PROKETAZINE
WYETH AYERST — 12.5 MG — N12768 001
25 MG — N12768 002
50 MG — N12768 004

CARPROFEN
TABLET; ORAL
RIMADYL
ROCHE — 100 MG — N18550 002 DEC 31, 1987
150 MG — N18550 003 DEC 31, 1987

CARTEOLOL HYDROCHLORIDE
TABLET; ORAL
CARTROL
ABBOTT — 10 MG — N19204 003 DEC 28, 1988

Discontinued Drug Products *(continued)*

CEFADROXIL/CEFADROXIL HEMIHYDRATE

CAPSULE; ORAL

CEFADROXIL			
BIOCRAFT	EQ 500 MG BASE	N62695 001	FEB 10, 1989
PUREPAC PHARM	EQ 500 MG BASE	N63017 001	JAN 05, 1989
DURICEF			
BRISTOL MYERS SQUIBB	EQ 250 MG BASE	N50512 002	
ULTRACEF			
BRISTOL	EQ 500 MG BASE	N62378 001	MAR 16, 1982

POWDER FOR RECONSTITUTION; ORAL

CEFADROXIL			
BIOCRAFT	EQ 125 MG BASE/5 ML	N62698 001	MAR 01, 1989
	EQ 250 MG BASE/5 ML	N62698 002	MAR 01, 1989
	EQ 500 MG BASE/5 ML	N62698 003	MAR 01, 1989
ULTRACEF			
BRISTOL	EQ 125 MG BASE/5 ML	N62376 001	MAR 16, 1982
	EQ 250 MG BASE/5 ML	N62376 002	MAR 16, 1982
	EQ 500 MG BASE/5 ML	N62376 003	MAR 16, 1982

TABLET; ORAL

ULTRACEF			
BRISTOL	EQ 1 GM BASE	N62408 001	AUG 31, 1982

CEFAZOLIN SODIUM

INJECTABLE; INJECTION

ANCEF IN SODIUM CHLORIDE 0.9% IN PLASTIC CONTAINER			
BAXTER	EQ 10 MG BASE/ML	N50566 001	JUN 08, 1983
	EQ 20 MG BASE/ML	N50566 002	JUN 08, 1983

CEFAZOLIN SODIUM *(continued)*

INJECTABLE; INJECTION

CEFAZOLIN SODIUM			
BEN VENUE	EQ 500 MG BASE/VIAL	N62894 002	JUL 21, 1988
	EQ 1 GM BASE/VIAL	N62894 003	JUL 21, 1988
	EQ 10 GM BASE/VIAL	N62894 005	JUL 21, 1988
	EQ 250 MG BASE/VIAL	N62894 001	JUL 21, 1988
	EQ 5 GM BASE/VIAL	N62894 004	JUL 21, 1988
FUJISAWA	EQ 500 MG BASE/VIAL	N62688 002	NOV 17, 1986
	EQ 1 GM BASE/VIAL	N62688 003	NOV 17, 1986
	EQ 10 GM BASE/VIAL	N62688 004	NOV 17, 1986
	EQ 20 GM BASE/VIAL	N62688 005	AUG 03, 1987

CEFMENOXIME HYDROCHLORIDE

INJECTABLE; INJECTION

CEFMAX			
TAP PHARMS	EQ 500 MG BASE/VIAL	N50571 001	DEC 30, 1987
	EQ 1 GM BASE/VIAL	N50571 002	DEC 30, 1987
	EQ 2 GM BASE/VIAL	N50571 003	DEC 30, 1987

CEFONICID SODIUM

INJECTABLE; INJECTION

MONOCID			
SMITHKLINE BEECHAM	EQ 2 GM BASE/VIAL	N50579 003	MAY 23, 1984

CEFOTIAM HYDROCHLORIDE

INJECTABLE; INJECTION

CERADON			
TAKEDA	EQ 1 GM BASE/VIAL	N50601 001	DEC 30, 1988

Discontinued Drug Products *(continued)*

CEFPIRAMIDE SODIUM

INJECTABLE; INJECTION
CEFPIRAMIDE SODIUM

WYETH AYERST	EQ 1 GM BASE/VIAL	N50633 002 JAN 31, 1989
	EQ 2 GM BASE/VIAL	N50633 003 JAN 31, 1989
	EQ 10 GM BASE/VIAL	N50633 005 JAN 31, 1989

CEFPODOXIME PROXETIL

GRANULE, FOR RECONSTITUTION; ORAL
BANAN

SANKYO	EQ 50 MG BASE/5 ML	N50688 002 AUG 07, 1992
	EQ 100 MG BASE/5 ML	N50688 001 AUG 07, 1992

TABLET; ORAL
BANAN

SANKYO	EQ 100 MG BASE	N50687 001 AUG 07, 1992
	EQ 200 MG BASE	N50687 002 AUG 07, 1992

CEFTRIAXONE SODIUM

INJECTABLE; INJECTION
ROCEPHIN

ROCHE	EQ 250 MG BASE/VIAL	N62510 001 MAR 12, 1985
	EQ 500 MG BASE/VIAL	N62510 002 MAR 12, 1985
	EQ 1 GM BASE/VIAL	N62510 003 MAR 12, 1985

ROCEPHIN W/ DEXTROSE IN PLASTIC CONTAINER

ROCHE	EQ 10 MG BASE/ML	N50624 001 FEB 11, 1987

CELLULOSE SODIUM PHOSPHATE

POWDER; ORAL
CALCIBIND

MISSION PHARMA	2.5 GM/PACKET	N18757 002 DEC 28, 1982

CEPHALEXIN

POWDER FOR RECONSTITUTION; ORAL
CEPHALEXIN

VITARINE	EQ 125 MG BASE/5 ML	N62779 001 DEC 22, 1987
	EQ 250 MG BASE/5 ML	N62781 001 DEC 22, 1987

TABLET; ORAL
CEPHALEXIN

VITARINE	EQ 250 MG BASE	N62863 001 AUG 11, 1988
	EQ 500 MG BASE	N62863 002 AUG 11, 1988
	EQ 1 GM BASE	N62863 003 AUG 11, 1988

CEPHALOTHIN SODIUM

INJECTABLE; INJECTION
CEPHALOTHIN

INTL MEDICATION	EQ 1 GM BASE/VIAL	N62426 002 MAY 03, 1985
	EQ 2 GM BASE/VIAL	N62426 003 MAY 03, 1985
	EQ 500 MG BASE/VIAL	N62426 001 MAY 03, 1985
	EQ 4 GM BASE/VIAL	N62426 004 MAY 03, 1985

CEPHALOTHIN SODIUM

ABBOTT	EQ 1 GM BASE/VIAL	N62548 001 SEP 11, 1985
	EQ 2 GM BASE/VIAL	N62548 002 SEP 11, 1985

SEFFIN

GLAXO	EQ 1 GM BASE/VIAL	N62435 001 NOV 15, 1983
	EQ 2 GM BASE/VIAL	N62435 002 NOV 15, 1983
	EQ 10 GM BASE/VIAL	N62435 003 NOV 15, 1983

CEPHAPIRIN SODIUM

INJECTABLE; INJECTION
CEFADYL

APOTHECON	EQ 500 MG BASE/VIAL	N50446 005
	EQ 1 GM BASE/VIAL	N50446 001
	EQ 2 GM BASE/VIAL	N50446 002
	EQ 4 GM BASE/VIAL	N50446 003
	EQ 20 GM BASE/VIAL	N50446 004

Discontinued Drug Products *(continued)*

CEPHAPIRIN SODIUM *(continued)*
INJECTABLE; INJECTION
CEPHAPIRIN SODIUM
ELKINS SINN — EQ 500 MG BASE/VIAL — N62720 001 JUL 02, 1987
EQ 1 GM BASE/VIAL — N62720 002 JUL 02, 1987
EQ 2 GM BASE/VIAL — N62720 003 JUL 02, 1987
EQ 20 GM BASE/VIAL — N62720 004 JUL 02, 1987
FUJISAWA — EQ 500 MG BASE/VIAL — N62723 001 NOV 17, 1986
EQ 1 GM BASE/VIAL — N62723 002 NOV 17, 1986
EQ 2 GM BASE/VIAL — N62723 003 NOV 17, 1986
EQ 4 GM BASE/VIAL — N62723 004 NOV 17, 1986
EQ 20 GM BASE/VIAL — N62723 005 NOV 17, 1986

CEPHRADINE
CAPSULE; ORAL
CEPHRADINE
VITARINE — 250 MG — N62813 001 FEB 25, 1988
500 MG — N62813 002 FEB 25, 1988
VELOSEF '250'
ERSANA — 250 MG — N50548 001
VELOSEF '500'
ERSANA — 500 MG — N50548 002
TABLET; ORAL
VELOSEF
SQUIBB — 1 GM — N50530 001

CERULETIDE DIETHYLAMINE
INJECTABLE; INJECTION
TYMTRAN
PHARMACIA — 0.02 MG/ML — N18296 001

CHLOPHEDIANOL HYDROCHLORIDE
SYRUP; ORAL
ULO
3M — 25 MG/5 ML — N12126 001

CHLORAMPHENICOL
INJECTABLE; INJECTION
CHLOROMYCETIN
PARKE DAVIS — 250 MG/ML — N50153 001
OINTMENT; OPHTHALMIC
CHLOROFAIR
PHARMAFAIR — 1% — N62439 001 APR 21, 1983
ECONOCHLOR
ALCON — 1% — N61648 001
SOLUTION/DROPS; OPHTHALMIC
CHLOROFAIR
PHARMAFAIR — 0.5% — N62437 001 APR 14, 1983
ECONOCHLOR
ALCON — 0.5% — N61645 001

CHLORAMPHENICOL; POLYMYXIN B SULFATE
OINTMENT; OPHTHALMIC
CHLOROMYXIN
PARKE DAVIS — 1%;10,000 UNITS/GM — N50203 002

CHLORAMPHENICOL; PREDNISOLONE
OINTMENT; OPHTHALMIC
CHLOROPTIC-P S.O.P.
ALLERGAN — 1%;0.5% — N61188 001

CHLORAMPHENICOL SODIUM SUCCINATE
INJECTABLE; INJECTION
MYCHEL-S
ANGUS — EQ 1 GM BASE/VIAL — N60132 001

CHLORDIAZEPOXIDE
CAPSULE, EXTENDED RELEASE; ORAL
LIBRELEASE
ROCHE — 30 MG — N17813 001 SEP 12, 1983

CHLORDIAZEPOXIDE; *MULTIPLE*
SEE AMITRIPTYLINE HYDROCHLORIDE; CHLORDIAZEPOXIDE

Discontinued Drug Products *(continued)*

CHLORDIAZEPOXIDE HYDROCHLORIDE

CAPSULE; ORAL

A-POXIDE		
ABBOTT	5 MG	N85447 001
	5 MG	N85517 001
	10 MG	N85447 002
	10 MG	N85518 001
	25 MG	N85447 003
	25 MG	N85513 001
CHLORDIAZEPOXIDE HCL		
ASCOT	5 MG	N87525 001 JAN 07, 1982
	10 MG	N87524 001 JAN 07, 1982
	25 MG	N87512 001 JAN 07, 1982
EON LABS	5 MG	N84919 001
	10 MG	N84920 001
	25 MG	N84823 001
LEDERLE	5 MG	N86892 001
	5 MG	N87234 001
	10 MG	N86876 001
	10 MG	N87037 001
	25 MG	N86893 001
	25 MG	N87231 001
LEMMON	5 MG	N88705 001 JAN 18, 1985
	10 MG	N88706 001 JAN 18, 1985
	25 MG	N86494 001
	25 MG	N88707 001 JAN 18, 1985
MYLAN	5 MG	N84886 001
	10 MG	N84601 001
	25 MG	N84887 001
PARKE DAVIS	5 MG	N85163 001
	10 MG	N84598 001
	25 MG	N85164 001
PIONEER PHARMS	10 MG	N89533 001 JUL 15, 1988
	25 MG	N89558 001 JUL 15, 1988
PUREPAC PHARM	5 MG	N85155 001
	10 MG	N84939 002
	25 MG	N85144 001
ROXANE	5 MG	N84706 001
	10 MG	N84700 001
	25 MG	N84705 001

CHLORDIAZEPOXIDE HYDROCHLORIDE *(continued)*

CAPSULE; ORAL

CHLORDIAZEPOXIDE HCL		
SUPERPHARM	5 MG	N88987 001 APR 25, 1985
	10 MG	N88986 001 APR 25, 1985
	25 MG	N88988 001 APR 25, 1985
VANGARD	5 MG	N88129 001 MAR 28, 1983
	10 MG	N88010 001 MAR 28, 1983
	25 MG	N88130 001 MAR 28, 1983
WEST WARD PHARM	5 MG	N85014 001
	10 MG	N85000 001
	25 MG	N85294 001
LIBRIUM		
ROCHE	5 MG	N12249 002
	10 MG	N12249 001
	25 MG	N12249 003
LYGEN		
ALRA	5 MG	N85107 001
	10 MG	N85009 001
	25 MG	N85108 001

CHLORHEXIDINE GLUCONATE

SOLUTION; TOPICAL

EXIDINE		
XTTRIUM	2.5%	N19421 001 DEC 17, 1985

TINCTURE; TOPICAL

HIBITANE		
ZENECA	0.5%	N18049 001

CHLORMERODRIN, HG-197

INJECTABLE; INJECTION

CHLORMERODRIN HG 197		
BRACCO	0.6-1.4mCi/ML	N17269 001

CHLOROQUINE PHOSPHATE

TABLET; ORAL

CHLOROQUINE PHOSPHATE		
PUREPAC PHARM	EQ 150 MG BASE	N80886 001
WEST WARD PHARM	EQ 150 MG BASE	N83082 001

Discontinued Drug Products *(continued)*

CHLOROQUINE PHOSPHATE; PRIMAQUINE PHOSPHATE

TABLET; ORAL
ARALEN PHOSPHATE W/ PRIMAQUINE PHOSPHATE

STERLING WINTHROP	EQ 300 MG BASE;EQ 45 MG BASE	N14860 002

CHLOROTHIAZIDE

TABLET; ORAL
CHLOROTHIAZIDE

CHELSEA LABS	500 MG	N86796 001 AUG 15, 1983
CIRCA	250 MG	N85165 001
	500 MG	N84026 001 SEP 01, 1982
EON LABS	250 MG	N85485 001
LEDERLE	250 MG	N86940 001
	500 MG	N86938 001

CHLOROTHIAZIDE; METHYLDOPA

TABLET; ORAL
METHYLDOPA AND CHLOROTHIAZIDE

PAR PHARM	150 MG;250 MG	N70783 001 NOV 06, 1987
	250 MG;250 MG	N70654 001 NOV 06, 1987

CHLOROTHIAZIDE; RESERPINE

TABLET; ORAL
CHLOROTHIAZIDE W/ RESERPINE

CIRCA	250 MG;0.125 MG	N84853 001
	500 MG;0.125 MG	N88151 001 JUN 09, 1983

CHLOROTRIANISENE

CAPSULE; ORAL
TACE

MERRELL DOW	72 MG	N16235 001

CHLORPHENIRAMINE MALEATE

CAPSULE, EXTENDED RELEASE; ORAL
TELDRIN

SMITHKLINE	8 MG	N17369 001

INJECTABLE; INJECTION
CHLOR-TRIMETON

SCHERING PLOUGH	100 MG/ML	N08794 001

CHLORPHENIRAMINE MALEATE

BEL MAR	10 MG/ML	N80821 001
ELKINS SINN	10 MG/ML	N80797 001

PYRIDAMAL 100

BEL MAR	100 MG/ML	N83733 001

SYRUP; ORAL
CHLOR-TRIMETON

SCHERING	2 MG/5 ML	N06921 006

CHLORPHENIRAMINE MALEATE

PHARM ASSOC	2 MG/5 ML	N87520 001 FEB 10, 1982

TABLET; ORAL
ANTAGONATE

MILES	4 MG	N83381 001

CHLOR-TRIMETON

SCHERING	4 MG	N06921 002

CHLORPHENIRAMINE MALEATE

ANABOLIC	4 MG	N83078 001
BARR	4 MG	N80700 001
BELL PHARMA	4 MG	N83062 001
CHELSEA LABS	4 MG	N85139 001
CIRCA	4 MG	N80791 001
ELKINS SINN	4 MG	N80938 001
LEDERLE	4 MG	N86941 001
NEWTRON PHARMS	4 MG	N86519 001
PANRAY	4 MG	N83243 001
PHARMERAL	4 MG	N83753 001
PIONEER PHARMS	4 MG	N88556 001 JUL 13, 1984
PRIVATE FORM	4 MG	N80786 001
PUREPAC PHARM	4 MG	N86306 001
ROXANE	4 MG	N80626 001
VITARINE	4 MG	N85837 001
ZENITH LABS	4 MG	N80779 001

PHENETRON

LANNETT	4 MG	N80846 001

CHLORPHENIRAMINE MALEATE; PHENYLPROPANOLAMINE HYDROCHLORIDE

CAPSULE, EXTENDED RELEASE; ORAL
CHLOROHENIRAMINE MALEATE AND PHENYLPROPANOLAMINE HCL

CHELSEA LABS	12 MG;75 MG	N88681 001 SEP 29, 1987

Discontinued Drug Products *(continued)*

CHLORPHENIRAMINE MALEATE; PSEUDOEPHEDRINE HYDROCHLORIDE

CAPSULE, EXTENDED RELEASE; ORAL		
ISOCLOR		
FISONS	8 MG;120 MG	N18747 001 MAR 06, 1986

CHLORPHENIRAMINE POLISTIREX; CODEINE POLISTIREX

SUSPENSION, EXTENDED RELEASE; ORAL		
PENNTUSS		
FISONS	EQ 4 MG MALEATE/ 5 ML;EQ 10 MG BASE/ 5 ML	N18928 001 AUG 14, 1985

CHLORPHENIRAMINE POLISTIREX; PHENYLPROPANOLAMINE POLISTIREX

SUSPENSION, EXTENDED RELEASE; ORAL		
CORSYM		
FISONS	EQ 4 MG MALEATE/ 5 ML;EQ 37.5 MG HCL/ 5 ML	N18050 001 JAN 04, 1984

CHLORPHENTERMINE HYDROCHLORIDE

TABLET; ORAL		
PRE-SATE		
PARKE DAVIS	EQ 65 MG BASE	N14696 001

CHLORPROMAZINE HYDROCHLORIDE

CONCENTRATE; ORAL		
CHLORPROMAZINE HCL		
PENNEX	30 MG/ML	N87032 001 JUL 08, 1982
	100 MG/ML	N87053 001
INJECTABLE; INJECTION		
CHLORPROMAZINE HCL		
FUJISAWA	25 MG/ML	N84911 001
WYETH AYERST	25 MG/ML	N80370 001
SYRUP; ORAL		
CHLORPROMAZINE HCL		
BARRE	10 MG/5 ML	N86712 001

CHLORPROMAZINE HYDROCHLORIDE *(continued)*

TABLET; ORAL		
CHLORPROMAZINE HCL		
BOOTS	10 MG	N84414 001
	25 MG	N84415 001
	50 MG	N84411 001
	100 MG	N84412 001
	200 MG	N84413 001
CHELSEA LABS	10 MG	N85959 001
	25 MG	N85956 001
	50 MG	N85960 001
	100 MG	N85957 001
	200 MG	N85958 001
LEDERLE	25 MG	N84801 001
	50 MG	N84800 001
	100 MG	N84789 001
	200 MG	N84802 001
PRIVATE FORM	25 MG	N80340 001
	50 MG	N80340 002
	200 MG	N80340 003
PUREPAC PHARM	10 MG	N80403 004
	25 MG	N80403 001
	50 MG	N80403 002
	100 MG	N80403 003
	200 MG	N80403 005
ROXANE	10 MG	N85331 001
	25 MG	N85331 002
	50 MG	N85331 003
	100 MG	N85331 004
	200 MG	N85331 005
VANGARD	10 MG	N88038 001 AUG 16, 1982
	25 MG	N87645 001
	50 MG	N87646 001
WEST WARD PHARM	10 MG	N87783 001 SEP 16, 1982
	25 MG	N87865 001 SEP 16, 1982
	50 MG	N87878 001 SEP 15, 1982
	100 MG	N87884 001 SEP 15, 1982
	200 MG	N87880 001 SEP 16, 1982
PROMAPAR		
PARKE DAVIS	10 MG	N86886 001
	25 MG	N84423 001
	50 MG	N86887 001
	100 MG	N86888 001
	200 MG	N86885 001

Discontinued Drug Products *(continued)*

CHLORPROPAMIDE

TABLET; ORAL
CHLORPROPAMIDE

CHELSEA LABS	100 MG	N86865 001 SEP 24, 1984
	250 MG	N86866 001
CIRCA	100 MG	N88608 001 APR 12, 1984
	250 MG	N88568 001 APR 12, 1984
DURAMED	100 MG	N88918 001 OCT 16, 1984
	250 MG	N88919 001 OCT 16, 1984
EON LABS	250 MG	N84669 001
ROSEMONT PHARM	100 MG	N88708 001 AUG 30, 1984
	250 MG	N88709 001 AUG 30, 1984

CHLORTHALIDONE

TABLET; ORAL
CHLORTHALIDONE

ABBOTT	50 MG	N87384 001
ASCOT	25 MG	N87698 001 OCT 20, 1982
	50 MG	N87699 001 OCT 20, 1982
CHELSEA LABS	50 MG	N87082 001
CIRCA	25 MG	N87050 001
	50 MG	N87029 001
LEMMON	50 MG	N88651 001 MAY 30, 1985
PIONEER PHARMS	50 MG	N89591 001 JUL 21, 1988
ROSEMONT PHARM	50 MG	N89052 001 JUN 01, 1987
SUPERPHARM	25 MG	N87473 001 FEB 09, 1983
VANGARD	25 MG	N88012 001 JUL 14, 1982
	50 MG	N88073 001 MAR 25, 1983
WARNER CHILCOTT	25 MG	N87515 001 JAN 24, 1983
	50 MG	N87516 001 FEB 09, 1983
ZENITH LABS	25 MG	N87555 001

CHLORTHALIDONE; METOPROLOL TARTRATE

CAPSULE; ORAL
LOPRESSIDONE

CIBA	25 MG;100 MG	N19451 001 DEC 31, 1987
	25 MG;200 MG	N19451 002 DEC 31, 1987

CHLORZOXAZONE

TABLET; ORAL
CHLORZOXAZONE

CHELSEA LABS	250 MG	N86948 001 AUG 09, 1982
PIONEER PHARMS	250 MG	N89592 001 JAN 06, 1989
	500 MG	N89948 001 JAN 06, 1989

CHYMOPAPAIN

INJECTABLE; INJECTION

CHYMODIACTIN		
BOOTS	10,000 UNITS/VIAL	N18663 001 NOV 10, 1982
DISCASE		
BOOTS	12,500 UNITS/VIAL	N18625 001 JAN 18, 1984

CHYMOTRYPSIN

POWDER FOR RECONSTITUTION; OPHTHALMIC

ALPHA CHYMAR		
SOLA BARNES HIND	750 UNITS/VIAL	N11837 001
CATARASE		
IOLAB	150 UNITS/VIAL	N18121 001

CISPLATIN

INJECTABLE; INJECTION
PLATINOL-AQ

BRISTOL MYERS	0.5 MG/ML	N18057 003 JUL 18, 1984

CLEMASTINE FUMARATE

TABLET; ORAL

CLEMASTINE FUMARATE		
LEMMON	1.34 MG	N73282 001 JAN 31, 1992
TAVIST-1		
SANDOZ	1.34 MG	N17661 002

Discontinued Drug Products *(continued)*

CLEMASTINE FUMARATE; PHENYLPROPANOLAMINE HYDROCHLORIDE

TABLET, EXTENDED RELEASE; ORAL

TAVIST D

SANDOZ	EQ 1 MG BASE;75 MG	N18298 001 DEC 15, 1982

CLINDAMYCIN HYDROCHLORIDE

CAPSULE; ORAL

CLEOCIN

UPJOHN	EQ 75 MG BASE	N61809 001
	EQ 150 MG BASE	N61809 002

CLINDAMYCIN PALMITATE HYDROCHLORIDE

POWDER FOR RECONSTITUTION; ORAL

CLEOCIN

UPJOHN	EQ 75 MG BASE/5 ML	N61827 001

CLINDAMYCIN PHOSPHATE

INJECTABLE; INJECTION

CLEOCIN PHOSPHATE		
UPJOHN	EQ 150 MG BASE/ML	N61839 001
CLINDAMYCIN PHOSPHATE		
DUPONT MERCK	EQ 150 MG BASE/ML	N62908 001 FEB 01, 1989
FUJISAWA	EQ 150 MG BASE/ML	N62747 001 JUN 03, 1988
QUAD PHARMS	EQ 150 MG BASE/ML	N62877 001 MAR 15, 1988
CLINDAMYCIN PHOSPHATE IN DEXTROSE 5%		
FUJISAWA	EQ 12 MG BASE/ML	N50636 001 DEC 22, 1989

CLIOQUINOL; NYSTATIN

OINTMENT; TOPICAL

NYSTAFORM

MILES	10 MG/GM;100,000 UNITS/GM	N50235 001

CLOFIBRATE

CAPSULE; ORAL

CLOFIBRATE

CHELSEA LABS	500 MG	N71603 001 SEP 18, 1987

CLONIDINE HYDROCHLORIDE

TABLET; ORAL

CLONIDINE HCL

AM THERAP	0.1 MG	N70881 001 JUL 08, 1986
	0.2 MG	N70882 001 JUL 08, 1986
	0.3 MG	N70883 001 JUL 08, 1986
BIOCRAFT	0.1 MG	N70747 001 JUL 08, 1986
	0.2 MG	N70702 001 JUL 08, 1986
	0.3 MG	N70659 001 JUL 08, 1986
CIRCA	0.1 MG	N70395 001 MAR 23, 1987
	0.2 MG	N70396 001 MAR 23, 1987
	0.3 MG	N70397 001 MAR 23, 1987
DURAMED	0.1 MG	N71103 001 AUG 14, 1986
	0.2 MG	N71102 001 AUG 14, 1986
	0.3 MG	N71101 001 AUG 14, 1986
INTERPHARM	0.1 MG	N71252 001 OCT 01, 1986
	0.2 MG	N71253 001 OCT 01, 1986
	0.3 MG	N71254 001 OCT 01, 1986
PAR PHARM	0.1 MG	N70461 001 JUL 08, 1986
	0.2 MG	N70460 001 JUL 08, 1986
	0.3 MG	N70459 001 JUL 08, 1986

CLORAZEPATE DIPOTASSIUM

CAPSULE; ORAL

CLORAZEPATE DIPOTASSIUM

AM THERAP	3.75 MG	N71429 001 JUN 23, 1987
	7.5 MG	N71430 001 JUN 23, 1987
	15 MG	N71431 001 JUN 23, 1987

Discontinued Drug Products *(continued)*

CLORAZEPATE DIPOTASSIUM (*continued*)

CAPSULE; ORAL
CLORAZEPATE DIPOTASSIUM

CHELSEA LABS	3.75 MG	N71878 001 MAR 15, 1988
	7.5 MG	N71879 001 MAR 15, 1988
	15 MG	N71860 001 MAR 15, 1988
PUREPAC PHARM	3.75 MG	N71924 001 APR 25, 1988
QUANTUM PHARMICS	3.75 MG	N71549 001 SEP 12, 1988
	7.5 MG	N71550 001 SEP 12, 1988
	15 MG	N71522 001 SEP 12, 1988
ROSEMONT PHARM	3.75 MG	N71242 001 JUN 23, 1987
	7.5 MG	N71243 001 JUN 23, 1987
	15 MG	N71244 001 JUN 23, 1987
SEARLE	3.75 MG	N71727 001 DEC 18, 1987
	7.5 MG	N71728 001 DEC 18, 1987
	15 MG	N71729 001 DEC 18, 1987
WARNER CHILCOTT	3.75 MG	N71774 001 MAR 01, 1988
	7.5 MG	N71775 001 MAR 01, 1988
	15 MG	N71776 001 MAR 01, 1988

TRANXENE

ABBOTT	3.75 MG	N17105 001
	7.5 MG	N17105 002
	15 MG	N17105 003

TABLET; ORAL
CLORAZEPATE DIPOTASSIUM

AM THERAP	3.75 MG	N71747 001 JUN 23, 1987
	7.5 MG	N71748 001 JUN 23, 1987
	15 MG	N71749 001 JUN 23, 1987

CLORAZEPATE DIPOTASSIUM (*continued*)

TABLET; ORAL
CLORAZEPATE DIPOTASSIUM

LEDERLE	3.75 MG	N72013 001 DEC 15, 1987
	7.5 MG	N72014 001 DEC 15, 1987
	15 MG	N72015 001 DEC 15, 1987
QUANTUM PHARMICS	3.75 MG	N71730 001 OCT 26, 1987
	7.5 MG	N71731 001 OCT 26, 1987
	15 MG	N71702 001 OCT 26, 1987
WARNER CHILCOTT	3.75 MG	N71828 001 MAR 03, 1988
	7.5 MG	N71829 001 MAR 03, 1988
	15 MG	N71830 001 MAR 03, 1988

CLOXACILLIN SODIUM

POWDER FOR RECONSTITUTION; ORAL
CLOXACILLIN SODIUM

NOVOPHARM	EQ 125 MG BASE/5 ML	N62978 001 APR 06, 1989

COBALT CHLORIDE, CO-60; CYANOCOBALAMIN; CYANOCOBALAMIN, CO-60; INTRINSIC FACTOR

N/A; N/A
RUBRATOPE-60 KIT

BRACCO	N/A;N/A;N/A;N/A	N16090 001

CODEINE PHOSPHATE; *MULTIPLE*

SEE ACETAMINOPHEN; ASPIRIN; CODEINE PHOSPHATE
SEE ACETAMINOPHEN; CODEINE PHOSPHATE

CODEINE POLISTIREX; *MULTIPLE*

SEE CHLORPHENIRAMINE POLISTIREX; CODEINE POLISTIREX

Discontinued Drug Products *(continued)*

COLCHICINE; PROBENECID

TABLET; ORAL

PROBEN-C		
CHELSEA LABS	0.5 MG;500 MG	N85552 001
PROBENECID AND COLCHICINE		
BEECHAM	0.5 MG;500 MG	N84321 001
EON LABS	0.5 MG;500 MG	N86130 001
PROBENECID W/ COLCHICINE		
CIRCA	0.5 MG;500 MG	N83221 001
LEDERLE	0.5 MG;500 MG	N86954 001

COPPER

INTRAUTERINE DEVICE; INTRAUTERINE

CU-7		
SEARLE	89 MG	N17408 001
TATUM-T		
SEARLE	120 MG	N18205 001

CORTICOTROPIN

INJECTABLE; INJECTION

ACTH		
PARKE DAVIS	25 UNITS/VIAL	N08317 002
PURIFIED CORTROPHIN GEL		
ORGANON	40 UNITS/ML	N08975 001
	80 UNITS/ML	N08975 002

CORTICOTROPIN-ZINC HYDROXIDE

INJECTABLE; INJECTION

CORTROPHIN-ZINC		
ORGANON	40 UNITS/ML	N09854 001

CORTISONE ACETATE

INJECTABLE; INJECTION

CORTISONE ACETATE		
STERIS	25 MG/ML	N83147 003
	25 MG/ML	N85677 001
	50 MG/ML	N83147 004
	50 MG/ML	N85677 002
UPJOHN	25 MG/ML	N08126 002

CORTISONE ACETATE *(continued)*

TABLET; ORAL

CORTISONE ACETATE		
BARR	25 MG	N83471 001
ELKINS SINN	25 MG	N80836 001
EVERYLIFE	25 MG	N84246 001
HEATHER	25 MG	N85736 001
INWOOD LABS	25 MG	N80731 001
LANNETT	25 MG	N80694 001
PANRAY	25 MG	N08284 001
	5 MG	N08284 002
VITARINE	25 MG	N80333 001
WHITEWORTH TOWNE	25 MG	N80341 001
ZENITH LABS	25 MG	N80630 001
	25 MG	N83536 001

CRYPTENAMINE ACETATES

INJECTABLE; INJECTION

UNITENSEN		
WALLACE	260CSR UNIT/ML	N08814 001

CRYPTENAMINE TANNATES

TABLET; ORAL

UNITENSEN		
WALLACE	260CSR UNIT	N09217 001

CYANOCOBALAMIN

INJECTABLE; INJECTION

CYANOCOBALAMIN		
FUJISAWA	0.03 MG/ML	N80510 003
	0.1 MG/ML	N80510 001
	1 MG/ML	N80510 002
	1 MG/ML	N83075 001
LUITPOLD	0.03 MG/ML	N80668 001
REDISOL		
MERCK SHARP DOHME	1 MG/ML	N06668 010
RUBIVITE		
BEL MAR	0.03 MG/ML	N10791 004
	0.1 MG/ML	N10791 002
	1 MG/ML	N10791 003
	0.05 MG/ML	N10791 001
	0.12 MG/ML	N10791 005
VI-TWEL		
BERLEX	1 MG/ML	N07012 002

Discontinued Drug Products *(continued)*

CYANOCOBALAMIN; *MULTIPLE*

SEE ASCORBIC ACID; BIOTIN; CYANOCOBALAMIN; DEXPANTHENOL; ERGOCALCIFEROL; FOLIC ACID; NIACINAMIDE; PYRIDOXINE HYDROCHLORIDE; RIBOFLAVIN PHOSPHATE SODIUM; THIAMINE HYDROCHLORIDE; VITAMIN A; VITAMIN E

SEE ASCORBIC ACID; BIOTIN; CYANOCOBALAMIN; DEXPANTHENOL; ERGOCALCIFEROL; FOLIC ACID; NIACINAMIDE; PYRIDOXINE HYDROCHLORIDE; RIBOFLAVIN PHOSPHATE SODIUM; THIAMINE HYDROCHLORIDE; VITAMIN A PALMITATE; VITAMIN E

SEE ASCORBIC ACID; BIOTIN; CYANOCOBALAMIN; DEXPANTHENOL; ERGOCALCIFEROL; FOLIC ACID; NIACINAMIDE; PYRIDOXINE; RIBOFLAVIN PHOSPHATE SODIUM; THIAMINE; VITAMIN A; VITAMIN E

SEE COBALT CHLORIDE, CO-60; CYANOCOBALAMIN; CYANOCOBALAMIN, CO-60; INTRINSIC FACTOR

CYANOCOBALAMIN; TANNIC ACID; ZINC ACETATE

INJECTABLE; INJECTION
DEPINAR

ARMOUR	0.5 MG/ML;2.3 MG/ML;1 MG/ML	N11208 001

CYANOCOBALAMIN, CO-60

CAPSULE; ORAL
RUBRATOPE-60

BRACCO	0.5-1uCi	N16090 002

CYANOCOBALAMIN, CO-60; *MULTIPLE*

SEE COBALT CHLORIDE, CO-60; CYANOCOBALAMIN; CYANOCOBALAMIN, CO-60; INTRINSIC FACTOR

CYCLACILLIN

POWDER FOR RECONSTITUTION; ORAL
CYCLAPEN-W

WYETH AYERST	125 MG/5 ML	N50508 001
	250 MG/5 ML	N50508 002
	500 MG/5 ML	N50508 003

CYCLIZINE LACTATE

INJECTABLE; INJECTION
MAREZINE

BURROUGHS WELLCOME	50 MG/ML	N09495 001

CYCLOBENZAPRINE HYDROCHLORIDE

TABLET; ORAL
FLEXERIL

MERCK SHARP DOHME	5 MG	N17821 001

CYCLOPENTOLATE HYDROCHLORIDE

SOLUTION/DROPS; OPHTHALMIC
CYCLOPENTOLATE HCL

SOLA BARNES HIND	1%	N84150 001
	1%	N84863 001

PENTOLAIR

PHARMAFAIR	1%	N88150 001 FEB 25, 1983
	0.5%	N88643 001 FEB 09, 1987

CYCLOTHIAZIDE

TABLET; ORAL
FLUIDIL

PHARMACIA	2 MG	N18173 001

CYCRIMINE HYDROCHLORIDE

TABLET; ORAL
PAGITANE

LILLY	1.25 MG	N08951 001
	2.5 MG	N08951 002

CYPROHEPTADINE HYDROCHLORIDE

SYRUP; ORAL
CYPROHEPTADINE HCL

NASKA	2 MG/5 ML	N89021 001 DEC 21, 1987
PENNEX	2 MG/5 ML	N87001 001 NOV 04, 1982

TABLET; ORAL
CYPROHEPTADINE HCL

AM THERAP	4 MG	N88798 001 FEB 15, 1985
CHELSEA LABS	4 MG	N86165 001
CIRCA	4 MG	N85245 001
DURAMED	4 MG	N88232 001 OCT 25, 1983
KV PHARM	4 MG	N86737 001
MYLAN	4 MG	N86678 001
PIONEER PHARMS	4 MG	N87839 001 FEB 08, 1984
SUPERPHARM	4 MG	N87405 001
VITARINE	4 MG	N87284 001

Discontinued Drug Products *(continued)*

CYSTEINE HYDROCHLORIDE
INJECTABLE; INJECTION
CYSTEINE HCL
PHARMACIA 7.25% N19523 001 OCT 22, 1986

CYTARABINE
INJECTABLE; INJECTION
CYTARABINE
QUAD PHARMS 100 MG/VIAL N71248 001 DEC 30, 1987
500 MG/VIAL N71249 001 DEC 30, 1987

DACARBAZINE
INJECTABLE; INJECTION
DACARBAZINE
FUJISAWA 100 MG/VIAL N70962 001 AUG 28, 1986
200 MG/VIAL N70990 001 AUG 28, 1986
QUAD PHARMS 100 MG/VIAL N70821 001 OCT 09, 1986
200 MG/VIAL N70822 001 OCT 09, 1986
500 MG/VIAL N71563 001 MAY 06, 1988

DANAZOL
CAPSULE; ORAL
DANAZOL
AM THERAP 200 MG N71569 001 DEC 30, 1987

DECAMETHONIUM BROMIDE
INJECTABLE; INJECTION
SYNCURINE
BURROUGHS WELLCOME 1 MG/ML N06931 002

DEMECLOCYCLINE HYDROCHLORIDE
SYRUP; ORAL
DECLOMYCIN
LEDERLE 75 MG/5 ML N50257 001

DESERPIDINE
TABLET; ORAL
HARMONYL
ABBOTT 0.1 MG N10796 001

DESERPIDINE; METHYCLOTHIAZIDE
TABLET; ORAL
METHYCLOTHIAZIDE AND DESERPIDINE
CIRCA 0.25 MG;5 MG N88486 001 AUG 10, 1984
0.5 MG;5 MG N88452 001 AUG 10, 1984

DESIPRAMINE HYDROCHLORIDE
CAPSULE; ORAL
PERTOFRANE
RHONE POULENC RORER 25 MG N13621 001
50 MG N13621 002
TABLET; ORAL
DESIPRAMINE HCL
ROSEMONT PHARM 25 MG N71864 001 SEP 09, 1987
50 MG N71865 001 SEP 09, 1987
75 MG N71866 001 SEP 09, 1987
100 MG N71867 001 SEP 09, 1987

DESLANOSIDE
INJECTABLE; INJECTION
CEDILANID-D
SANDOZ 0.2 MG/ML N09282 002

DESOXIMETASONE
OINTMENT; TOPICAL
TOPICORT
HOECHST ROUSSEL 0.05% N18594 001 JAN 17, 1985

DESOXYCORTICOSTERONE ACETATE
INJECTABLE; INJECTION
DOCA
ORGANON 5 MG/ML N01104 001
PELLET; IMPLANTATION
PERCORTEN
CIBA 125 MG N05151 001

Discontinued Drug Products *(continued)*

DESOXYCORTICOSTERONE PIVALATE

INJECTABLE; INJECTION		
PERCORTEN		
CIBA	25 MG/ML	N08822 001

DEXAMETHASONE

TABLET; ORAL		
DEXAMETHASONE		
BARR	0.25 MG	N84013 001
	0.25 MG	N84764 001
	0.5 MG	N84084 001
	0.5 MG	N84766 001
	0.75 MG	N84081 001
	0.75 MG	N84765 001
	1.5 MG	N84086 001
	1.5 MG	N84763 001
CHELSEA LABS	0.75 MG	N85818 001
	1.5 MG	N85840 001
CIRCA	0.75 MG	N84457 001
GENEVA PHARMS	0.75 MG	N80399 001
PHOENIX LABS NY	0.75 MG	N83806 001
PRIVATE FORM	0.75 MG	N83420 001
ROXANE	0.25 MG	N84614 001
UPSHER SMITH	0.75 MG	N87534 001
	1.5 MG	N87533 001
WHITEWORTH TOWNE	0.75 MG	N84327 001

DEXAMETHASONE; NEOMYCIN SULFATE; POLYMYXIN B SULFATE

OINTMENT; OPHTHALMIC		
DEXASPORIN		
PHARMAFAIR	0.1%;EQ 3.5 MG BASE/ GM;10,000 UNITS/GM	N62411 001 MAY 16, 1983
SUSPENSION/DROPS; OPHTHALMIC		
DEXASPORIN		
PHARMAFAIR	0.1%;EQ 3.5 MG BASE/ ML;10,000 UNITS/ML	N62428 001 MAY 18, 1983

DEXAMETHASONE SODIUM PHOSPHATE

INJECTABLE; INJECTION		
DEXACEN-4		
CENT PHARMS	EQ 4 MG PHOSPHATE/ML	N84342 001
DEXAMETHASONE SODIUM PHOSPHATE		
BEL MAR	EQ 4 MG PHOSPHATE/ML	N84752 001
FUJISAWA	EQ 4 MG PHOSPHATE/ML	N87065 001
INTL MEDICATION	EQ 20 MG PHOSPHATE/ML	N88522 001 FEB 17, 1984
QUAD PHARMS	EQ 4 MG PHOSPHATE/ML	N89280 001 MAR 18, 1987
	EQ 20 MG PHOSPHATE/ML	N89282 001 MAR 18, 1987
	EQ 10 MG PHOSPHATE/ML	N89281 001 MAR 18, 1987
	EQ 24 MG PHOSPHATE/ML	N89372 001 MAR 18, 1987
WYETH AYERST	EQ 4 MG PHOSPHATE/ML	N85641 001
HEXADROL		
ORGANON	EQ 20 MG PHOSPHATE/ML	N14694 004
SOLUTION/DROPS; OPHTHALMIC		
DEXAMETHASONE SODIUM PHOSPHATE		
SOLA BARNES HIND	EQ 0.1% PHOSPHATE	N84170 001
	EQ 0.1% PHOSPHATE	N84173 001

DEXBROMPHENIRAMINE MALEATE

SYRUP; ORAL		
DISOMER		
SCHERING	2 MG/5 ML	N11814 002
TABLET; ORAL		
DISOMER		
SCHERING	2 MG	N11814 001

DEXBROMPHENIRAMINE MALEATE; PSEUDOEPHEDRINE SULFATE

TABLET; ORAL		
DISOPHROL		
SCHERING	2 MG;60 MG	N12394 002
TABLET, EXTENDED RELEASE; ORAL		
RESPORAL		
PIONEER PHARMS	6 MG;120 MG	N89139 001 JUN 16, 1988

Discontinued Drug Products *(continued)*

DEXPANTHENOL; *MULTIPLE*

SEE ASCORBIC ACID; BIOTIN; CYANOCOBALAMIN; DEXPANTHENOL; ERGOCALCIFEROL; FOLIC ACID; NIACINAMIDE; PYRIDOXINE HYDROCHLORIDE; RIBOFLAVIN PHOSPHATE SODIUM; THIAMINE HYDROCHLORIDE; VITAMIN A; VITAMIN E

SEE ASCORBIC ACID; BIOTIN; CYANOCOBALAMIN; DEXPANTHENOL; ERGOCALCIFEROL; FOLIC ACID; NIACINAMIDE; PYRIDOXINE HYDROCHLORIDE; RIBOFLAVIN PHOSPHATE SODIUM; THIAMINE HYDROCHLORIDE; VITAMIN A PALMITATE; VITAMIN E

SEE ASCORBIC ACID; BIOTIN; CYANOCOBALAMIN; DEXPANTHENOL; ERGOCALCIFEROL; FOLIC ACID; NIACINAMIDE; PYRIDOXINE; RIBOFLAVIN PHOSPHATE SODIUM; THIAMINE; VITAMIN A; VITAMIN E

DEXTROAMPHETAMINE ADIPATE; *MULTIPLE*

SEE AMPHETAMINE ADIPATE; AMPHETAMINE SULFATE; DEXTROAMPHETAMINE ADIPATE; DEXTROAMPHETAMINE SULFATE

DEXTROAMPHETAMINE RESIN COMPLEX; *MULTIPLE*

SEE AMPHETAMINE RESIN COMPLEX; DEXTROAMPHETAMINE RESIN COMPLEX

DEXTROAMPHETAMINE SULFATE

CAPSULE; ORAL		
DEXAMPEX		
LEMMON	15 MG	N85355 001
ELIXIR; ORAL		
DEXEDRINE		
SMITHKLINE BEECHAM	5 MG/5 ML	N83902 001
TABLET; ORAL		
DEXAMPEX		
LEMMON	5 MG	N83735 001
	10 MG	N83735 002
DEXTROAMPHETAMINE SULFATE		
GENEVA PHARMS	5 MG	N85370 001
	10 MG	N85371 001
LANNETT	5 MG	N83903 001
	10 MG	N83903 003
	15 MG	N85652 001
PUREPAC PHARM	5 MG	N84125 001
VITARINE	5 MG	N84986 001
	10 MG	N85892 001
FERNDEX		
FERNDALE LABS	5 MG	N84001 001

DEXTROAMPHETAMINE SULFATE; *MULTIPLE*

SEE AMPHETAMINE ADIPATE; AMPHETAMINE SULFATE; DEXTROAMPHETAMINE ADIPATE; DEXTROAMPHETAMINE SULFATE

DEXTROSE

INJECTABLE; INJECTION		
DEXTROSE 10% IN PLASTIC CONTAINER		
MILES	10 GM/100 ML	N18504 001
DEXTROSE 38.5% IN PLASTIC CONTAINER		
ABBOTT	38.5 GM/100 ML	N18923 001 SEP 19, 1984
DEXTROSE 50% IN PLASTIC CONTAINER		
ABBOTT	500 MG/ML	N19445 001 JUN 03, 1986
DEXTROSE 60%		
MCGAW	60 GM/100 ML	N17995 002 SEP 22, 1982
DEXTROSE 60% IN PLASTIC CONTAINER		
MCGAW	60 GM/100 ML	N17995 001

DEXTROSE; *MULTIPLE*

SEE AMINO ACIDS; DEXTROSE

SEE AMINO ACIDS; DEXTROSE; MAGNESIUM CHLORIDE; POTASSIUM CHLORIDE; SODIUM CHLORIDE; SODIUM PHOSPHATE, DIBASIC

SEE AMINO ACIDS; DEXTROSE; MAGNESIUM CHLORIDE; POTASSIUM CHLORIDE; POTASSIUM PHOSPHATE, DIBASIC; SODIUM CHLORIDE

SEE CALCIUM CHLORIDE; DEXTROSE; MAGNESIUM CHLORIDE; SODIUM ACETATE; SODIUM CHLORIDE

SEE CALCIUM CHLORIDE; DEXTROSE; MAGNESIUM CHLORIDE; SODIUM CHLORIDE; SODIUM LACTATE

SEE CALCIUM CHLORIDE; DEXTROSE; POTASSIUM CHLORIDE; SODIUM CHLORIDE; SODIUM LACTATE

SEE CALCIUM CHLORIDE; DEXTROSE; SODIUM CHLORIDE; SODIUM LACTATE

Discontinued Drug Products *(continued)*

DEXTROSE; POTASSIUM CHLORIDE; SODIUM CHLORIDE

INJECTABLE; INJECTION

DEXTROSE 5%, SODIUM CHLORIDE 0.45% AND POTASSIUM CHLORIDE 15 MEQ IN PLASTIC CONTAINER

BAXTER 5 GM/100 ML;224 MG/100 ML;450 MG/100 ML N18008 003

DEXTROSE 5%, SODIUM CHLORIDE 0.45% AND POTASSIUM CHLORIDE 20 MEQ (K) IN PLASTIC CONTAINER

BAXTER 5 GM/100 ML;300 MG/100 ML;450 MG/100 ML N18008 001

DEXTROSE 5%, SODIUM CHLORIDE 0.45% AND POTASSIUM CHLORIDE 5 MEQ IN PLASTIC CONTAINER

BAXTER 5 GM/100 ML;75 MG/100 ML;450 MG/100 ML N18008 002

DEXTROSE; SODIUM CHLORIDE

INJECTABLE; INJECTION

DEXTROSE 3.3% AND SODIUM CHLORIDE 0.3% IN PLASTIC CONTAINER

ABBOTT 3.3 GM/100 ML;300 MG/100 ML N18055 001

DEXTROSE 5% AND SODIUM CHLORIDE 0.2% IN PLASTIC CONTAINER

MILES 5 GM/100 ML;200 MG/100 ML N18399 001

DEXTROSE 5% AND SODIUM CHLORIDE 0.225% IN PLASTIC CONTAINER

ABBOTT 5 GM/100 ML;225 MG/100 ML N19482 001 OCT 04, 1985

DEXTROSE 5% AND SODIUM CHLORIDE 0.3% IN PLASTIC CONTAINER

ABBOTT 5 GM/100 ML;300 MG/100 ML N19486 001 OCT 04, 1985

MILES 5 GM/100 ML;300 MG/100 ML N18501 001

DEXTROSE 5% AND SODIUM CHLORIDE 0.45% IN PLASTIC CONTAINER

ABBOTT 5 GM/100 ML;450 MG/100 ML N19484 001 OCT 04, 1985

MILES 5 GM/100 ML;450 MG/100 ML N18400 001

DEXTROSE 5% AND SODIUM CHLORIDE 0.9% IN PLASTIC CONTAINER

ABBOTT 5 GM/100 ML;900 MG/100 ML N19483 001 OCT 04, 1985

MILES 5 GM/100 ML;900 MG/100 ML N18500 001

DEXTROTHYROXINE SODIUM

TABLET; ORAL

CHOLOXIN

BOOTS 6 MG N12302 006

DIATRIZOATE MEGLUMINE

INJECTABLE; INJECTION

CARDIOGRAFIN

BRACCO 85% N11620 002

DIATRIZOATE MEGLUMINE; DIATRIZOATE SODIUM

INJECTABLE; INJECTION

DIATRIZOATE-60

INTL MEDICATION 52%;8% N88166 001 JUN 17, 1983

HYPAQUE-M,75%

STERLING WINTHROP 50%;25% N10220 003

HYPAQUE-M,90%

STERLING WINTHROP 60%;30% N10220 002

DIATRIZOATE SODIUM

INJECTABLE; INJECTION

MD-50

MALLINCKRODT 50% N87075 001

SOLUTION; URETERAL

HYPAQUE SODIUM 20%

STERLING WINTHROP 20% N09561 002

DIATRIZOATE SODIUM; *MULTIPLE*

SEE DIATRIZOATE MEGLUMINE; DIATRIZOATE SODIUM

DIAZEPAM

INJECTABLE; INJECTION

DIAZEPAM

LEDERLE 5 MG/ML N71308 001 JUL 17, 1987

US ARMY 5 MG/ML N20124 001 DEC 05, 1990

WARNER CHILCOTT 5 MG/ML N71613 001 OCT 22, 1987

5 MG/ML N71614 001 OCT 22, 1987

TABLET; ORAL

DIAZEPAM

CHELSEA LABS 2 MG N70456 001 NOV 01, 1985

5 MG N70457 001 NOV 01, 1985

10 MG N70458 001 NOV 01, 1985

Discontinued Drug Products *(continued)*

DIAZEPAM *(continued)*

TABLET; ORAL

DIAZEPAM

DURAMED	2 MG	N70894 001 AUG 27, 1986
	5 MG	N70895 001 AUG 27, 1986
	10 MG	N70896 001 AUG 27, 1986
FERNDALE LABS	2 MG	N70903 001 APR 01, 1987
	5 MG	N70904 001 APR 01, 1987
	10 MG	N70905 001 APR 01, 1987
MARTEC	10 MG	N72402 001 APR 25, 1989
PIONEER PHARMS	2 MG	N70787 001 AUG 02, 1988
	5 MG	N70788 001 AUG 02, 1988
	10 MG	N70776 001 AUG 02, 1988
WARNER CHILCOTT	2 MG	N70209 001 SEP 04, 1985
	5 MG	N70210 001 SEP 04, 1985
	10 MG	N70222 001 SEP 04, 1985
ZENITH LABS	2 MG	N70360 001 SEP 04, 1985
	5 MG	N70361 001 SEP 04, 1985

Q-PAM

QUANTUM PHARMICS	2 MG	N70423 001 DEC 12, 1985
	2 MG	N72431 001 APR 29, 1988
	5 MG	N70424 001 DEC 12, 1985
	5 MG	N72432 001 APR 29, 1988
	10 MG	N70425 001 DEC 12, 1985
	10 MG	N72433 001 APR 29, 1988

DIAZOXIDE

CAPSULE; ORAL

PROGLYCEM

BAKER NORTON	100 MG	N17425 002

INJECTABLE; INJECTION

DIAZOXIDE

FUJISAWA	15 MG/ML	N71519 001 AUG 26, 1987
QUAD PHARMS	15 MG/ML	N71908 001 JAN 26, 1988

DIBUCAINE HYDROCHLORIDE

INJECTABLE; INJECTION

HEAVY SOLUTION NUPERCAINE

CIBA	2.5 MG/ML	N06203 001

DICLOXACILLIN SODIUM

CAPSULE; ORAL

DYCILL

SMITHKLINE BEECHAM	EQ 250 MG BASE	N60254 002
	EQ 500 MG BASE	N60254 003

POWDER FOR RECONSTITUTION; ORAL

DYNAPEN

BRISTOL	EQ 62.5 MG BASE/5 ML	N50337 002

DICUMAROL

CAPSULE; ORAL

DICUMAROL

LILLY	25 MG	N05509 003
	50 MG	N05509 001

TABLET; ORAL

DICUMAROL

ABBOTT	50 MG	N05545 004
	100 MG	N05545 005

DICYCLOMINE HYDROCHLORIDE

CAPSULE; ORAL

DICYCLOMINE HCL

CIRCA	10 MG	N83179 001 FEB 12, 1986
PIONEER PHARMS	10 MG	N89361 001 JAN 10, 1989

Discontinued Drug Products *(continued)*

DICYCLOMINE HYDROCHLORIDE *(continued)*
TABLET; ORAL
DICYCLOMINE HCL

CIRCA	20 MG	N84361 001 FEB 06, 1986
PIONEER PHARMS	20 MG	N88585 001 AUG 20, 1986

DIENESTROL
CREAM; VAGINAL
ESTRAGUARD

SOLVAY	0.01%	N84436 001

DIETHYLPROPION HYDROCHLORIDE
TABLET; ORAL
DIETHYLPROPION HCL

CHELSEA LABS	25 MG	N85741 001
EON LABS	25 MG	N85916 001
LEMMON	25 MG	N88642 001 SEP 20, 1984

TENUATE

MERRELL DOW	25 MG	N17668 001

TABLET, EXTENDED RELEASE; ORAL
TENUATE

MERRELL DOW	75 MG	N17669 001

DIETHYLSTILBESTROL
INJECTABLE; INJECTION
STILBESTROL

SQUIBB	0.2 MG/ML	N04056 003
	0.5 MG/ML	N04056 004
	1 MG/ML	N04056 005
	5 MG/ML	N04056 006

SUPPOSITORY; VAGINAL
DIETHYLSTILBESTROL

LILLY	0.1 MG	N04040 001
	0.5 MG	N04040 002

STILBESTROL

SQUIBB	0.1 MG	N04056 001
	0.5 MG	N04056 002

DIETHYLSTILBESTROL *(continued)*
TABLET; ORAL
DIETHYLSTILBESTROL

LILLY	0.1 MG	N04041 002
	0.5 MG	N04041 003

STILBESTROL

TABLICAPS	1 MG	N83002 001
	5 MG	N83006 001

STILBETIN

SQUIBB	0.1 MG	N04056 007
	0.5 MG	N04056 008
	1 MG	N04056 009
	5 MG	N04056 010
	0.25 MG	N04056 017

TABLET, DELAYED RELEASE; ORAL
DIETHYLSTILBESTROL

LILLY	0.1 MG	N04039 002
	0.5 MG	N04039 003
	0.25 MG	N04039 005

STILBESTROL

TABLICAPS	0.5 MG	N83003 001
	1 MG	N83005 001
	5 MG	N83007 001

STILBETIN

SQUIBB	0.1 MG	N04056 011
	0.5 MG	N04056 012
	1 MG	N04056 013
	5 MG	N04056 014

DIFENOXIN HYDROCHLORIDE; *MULTIPLE*
SEE ATROPINE SULFATE; DIFENOXIN HYDROCHLORIDE

DIFLORASONE DIACETATE
CREAM; TOPICAL
DIFLORASONE DIACETATE

UPJOHN	0.05%	N19259 001 AUG 28, 1985

DIGITOXIN
INJECTABLE; INJECTION
CRYSTODIGIN

LILLY	0.2 MG/ML	N84100 005

Discontinued Drug Products *(continued)*

DIGOXIN

CAPSULE; ORAL		
LANOXICAPS		
BURROUGHS WELLCOME	0.15 MG	N18118 004 SEP 24, 1984
INJECTABLE; INJECTION		
DIGOXIN		
FUJISAWA	0.25 MG/ML	N83217 001

DIHYDROERGOTAMINE MESYLATE; HEPARIN SODIUM; LIDOCAINE HYDROCHLORIDE

INJECTABLE; INJECTION		
EMBOLEX		
SANDOZ	0.5 MG/0.7 ML;5,000 UNITS/ 0.7 ML;7.46 MG/0.7 ML	N18885 002 NOV 30, 1984
	0.5 MG/0.5 ML;2,500 UNITS/ 0.5 ML;5.33 MG/0.5 ML	N18885 001 NOV 30, 1984

DILTIAZEM HYDROCHLORIDE

CAPSULE, EXTENDED RELEASE; ORAL		
CARDIZEM SR		
MARION MERRELL DOW	180 MG	N19471 004 JAN 23, 1989

DIMENHYDRINATE

LIQUID; ORAL		
DIMENHYDRINATE		
ALRA	12.5 MG/4 ML	N80715 001
TABLET; ORAL		
DIMENHYDRINATE		
ANABOLIC	50 MG	N85985 001
CHELSEA LABS	50 MG	N85166 001
HEATHER	50 MG	N80841 001

DINOPROST TROMETHAMINE

INJECTABLE; INJECTION		
PROSTIN F2 ALPHA		
UPJOHN	EQ 5 MG BASE/ML	N17434 001

DIPHEMANIL METHYLSULFATE

TABLET; ORAL		
PRANTAL		
SCHERING	100 MG	N08114 004

DIPHENHYDRAMINE HYDROCHLORIDE

CAPSULE; ORAL		
DIPHENHYDRAMINE HCL		
ALRA	25 MG	N80519 004
	50 MG	N80519 003
ANABOLIC	25 MG	N83634 001
	50 MG	N83275 001
CHELSEA LABS	25 MG	N85138 001
CIRCA	25 MG	N83797 001
	50 MG	N83797 002
ELKINS SINN	25 MG	N85701 001
	50 MG	N85701 002
HEATHER	25 MG	N84524 001
	50 MG	N83953 001
LANNETT	25 MG	N80868 001
	50 MG	N80868 002
LEDERLE	25 MG	N86874 001
	50 MG	N86875 001
LEMMON	25 MG	N85874 001
	50 MG	N85874 002
PERRIGO	25 MG	N83061 001
	50 MG	N83061 002
PIONEER PHARMS	25 MG	N89101 001 DEC 20, 1985
	50 MG	N88880 001 DEC 20, 1985
ROXANE	50 MG	N80635 001
SUPERPHARM	50 MG	N89041 001 MAY 15, 1985
VANGARD	25 MG	N88034 001 OCT 27, 1982
	50 MG	N87630 001
WHITEWORTH TOWNE	25 MG	N83441 001
	50 MG	N80800 001
ELIXIR; ORAL		
DIPHEN		
ROSEMONT PHARM	12.5 MG/5 ML	N84640 001
DIPHENHYDRAMINE HCL		
KV PHARM	12.5 MG/5 ML	N85621 001
LEDERLE	12.5 MG/5 ML	N86937 001
NASKA	12.5 MG/5 ML	N88680 001 MAY 31, 1985
PERRIGO	12.5 MG/5 ML	N83063 001
PRIVATE FORM	12.5 MG/5 ML	N85287 001
INJECTABLE; INJECTION		
DIPHENHYDRAMINE HCL		
BEL MAR	10 MG/ML	N80822 001
ELKINS SINN	50 MG/ML	N83183 001
FUJISAWA	10 MG/ML	N87066 001
SYRUP; ORAL		
DIPHENHYDRAMINE HCL		
BARRE	12.5 MG/5 ML	N70497 001 APR 25, 1989

DIPHENOXYLATE HYDROCHLORIDE; *MULTIPLE*

SEE ATROPINE SULFATE; DIPHENOXYLATE HYDROCHLORIDE

DIPHENYLPYRALINE HYDROCHLORIDE

CAPSULE, EXTENDED RELEASE; ORAL

HISPRIL		
SMITHKLINE BEECHAM	5 MG	N11945 001

DISOPYRAMIDE PHOSPHATE

CAPSULE; ORAL

DISOPYRAMIDE PHOSPHATE		
CIRCA	EQ 100 MG BASE	N70240 001 FEB 02, 1986
	EQ 150 MG BASE	N70241 001 FEB 02, 1986
INTERPHARM	EQ 100 MG BASE	N71190 001 JAN 15, 1987
	EQ 150 MG BASE	N71191 001 JAN 15, 1987
MYLAN	EQ 100 MG BASE	N70138 001 JUN 14, 1985
	EQ 150 MG BASE	N70139 001 JUN 14, 1985
SUPERPHARM	EQ 150 MG BASE	N70941 001 FEB 09, 1987

DISULFIRAM

TABLET; ORAL

DISULFIRAM		
CHELSEA LABS	250 MG	N87973 001 AUG 05, 1983
	500 MG	N87974 001 AUG 05, 1983

DIVALPROEX SODIUM

TABLET, DELAYED RELEASE; ORAL

DEPAKOTE CP		
ABBOTT	EQ 250 MG BASE	N19794 001 JUL 11, 1990
	EQ 500 MG BASE	N19794 002 JUL 11, 1990

DOPAMINE HYDROCHLORIDE

INJECTABLE; INJECTION

DOPAMINE HCL		
ASTRA	40 MG/ML	N70087 001 OCT 23, 1985
	80 MG/ML	N70089 001 OCT 23, 1985
	80 MG/ML	N70090 001 OCT 23, 1985
	160 MG/ML	N70093 001 OCT 23, 1985
	160 MG/ML	N70094 001 OCT 23, 1985
FUJISAWA	40 MG/ML	N18549 001 MAR 11, 1983
	40 MG/ML	N70012 001 JUN 12, 1985
	40 MG/ML	N70058 001 MAR 20, 1985
	80 MG/ML	N70059 001 MAR 20, 1985
	160 MG/ML	N70364 001 DEC 04, 1985
SMITH AND NEPHEW	40 MG/ML	N70011 001 AUG 29, 1985
WARNER CHILCOTT	40 MG/ML	N18138 001
	40 MG/ML	N70558 001 SEP 20, 1985
	80 MG/ML	N70559 001 SEP 20, 1985

DOXEPIN HYDROCHLORIDE

CAPSULE; ORAL

DOXEPIN HCL		
BARR	EQ 25 MG BASE	N71502 001 FEB 18, 1988
	EQ 50 MG BASE	N71653 001 FEB 18, 1988
	EQ 75 MG BASE	N71654 001 FEB 18, 1988
	EQ 100 MG BASE	N71521 001 FEB 18, 1988

Discontinued Drug Products *(continued)*

DOXEPIN HYDROCHLORIDE *(continued)*

CAPSULE; ORAL		
DOXEPIN HCL		
CHELSEA LABS	EQ 10 MG BASE	N70952 001 MAR 04, 1987
	EQ 25 MG BASE	N70953 001 MAY 15, 1986
	EQ 50 MG BASE	N70954 001 MAY 15, 1986
	EQ 75 MG BASE	N71763 001 FEB 09, 1988
	EQ 100 MG BASE	N70955 001 MAY 15, 1986
	EQ 150 MG BASE	N71764 001 FEB 09, 1988
FISONS	EQ 10 MG BASE	N16987 001
	EQ 25 MG BASE	N16987 002
	EQ 50 MG BASE	N16987 003
	EQ 75 MG BASE	N16987 006
	EQ 100 MG BASE	N16987 004
	EQ 150 MG BASE	N16987 007 APR 13, 1987
PUREPAC PHARM	EQ 75 MG BASE	N72386 001 SEP 08, 1988
	EQ 150 MG BASE	N72387 001 SEP 08, 1988
QUANTUM PHARMICS	EQ 10 MG BASE	N70972 001 SEP 29, 1987
	EQ 25 MG BASE	N70973 001 SEP 29, 1987
	EQ 50 MG BASE	N70931 001 SEP 29, 1987
	EQ 75 MG BASE	N70932 001 SEP 29, 1987
	EQ 100 MG BASE	N72375 001 MAR 15, 1989
	EQ 150 MG BASE	N72376 001 MAR 15, 1989

DOXYCYCLINE HYCLATE

CAPSULE; ORAL		
DOXYCYCLINE HYCLATE		
HEATHER	EQ 50 MG BASE	N62463 001 DEC 07, 1983
	EQ 100 MG BASE	N62463 002 DEC 07, 1983
INTERPHARM	EQ 50 MG BASE	N62763 001 SEP 02, 1988
	EQ 100 MG BASE	N62763 002 SEP 02, 1988

DOXYCYCLINE HYCLATE *(continued)*

CAPSULE; ORAL		
DOXYCYCLINE HYCLATE		
PAR PHARM	EQ 50 MG BASE	N62434 001 OCT 19, 1984
	EQ 100 MG BASE	N62442 001 DEC 22, 1983
SUPERPHARM	EQ 50 MG BASE	N62469 001 OCT 31, 1984
	EQ 100 MG BASE	N62469 002 OCT 31, 1984
WARNER CHILCOTT	EQ 50 MG BASE	N62594 001 DEC 05, 1985
	EQ 100 MG BASE	N62594 002 DEC 05, 1985
INJECTABLE; INJECTION		
DOXYCYCLINE HYCLATE		
QUAD PHARMS	EQ 100 MG BASE/VIAL	N62643 001 FEB 13, 1986
	EQ 200 MG BASE/VIAL	N62643 002 FEB 13, 1986
TABLET; ORAL		
DOXY-TABS		
RACHELLE	EQ 50 MG BASE	N62269 003
DOXYCYCLINE HYCLATE		
CHELSEA LABS	EQ 50 MG BASE	N62392 001 MAR 31, 1983
	EQ 100 MG BASE	N62392 002 MAR 31, 1983
HEATHER	EQ 100 MG BASE	N62462 001 MAY 11, 1983
INTERPHARM	EQ 100 MG BASE	N62764 001 SEP 02, 1988
WARNER CHILCOTT	EQ 100 MG BASE	N62593 001 AUG 28, 1985

DOXYLAMINE SUCCINATE

CAPSULE; ORAL		
UNISOM		
PFIZER	25 MG	N19440 001 FEB 05, 1986
TABLET; ORAL		
DECAPRYN		
MERRELL DOW	25 MG	N06412 014
	12.5 MG	N06412 015
DOXY-SLEEP-AID		
PAR PHARM	25 MG	N70156 001 JUL 02, 1987
DOXYLAMINE SUCCINATE		
QUANTUM PHARMICS	25 MG	N88603 001 AUG 07, 1984

Discontinued Drug Products *(continued)*

DROMOSTANOLONE PROPIONATE
INJECTABLE; INJECTION
DROLBAN
LILLY 50 MG/ML N12936 001

DROPERIDOL
INJECTABLE; INJECTION
DROPERIDOL
ASTRA 2.5 MG/ML N72020 001 OCT 19, 1988
FUJISAWA 2.5 MG/ML N70992 001 NOV 17, 1986
2.5 MG/ML N70993 001 NOV 17, 1986
QUAD PHARMS 2.5 MG/ML N71941 001 AUG 17, 1988
2.5 MG/ML N71942 001 AUG 17, 1988
SMITH AND NEPHEW 2.5 MG/ML N71750 001 SEP 06, 1988

DROPERIDOL; FENTANYL CITRATE
INJECTABLE; INJECTION
FENTANYL CITRATE AND DROPERIDOL
ASTRA 2.5 MG/ML;EQ 0.05 MG BASE/ML N72028 001 APR 13, 1989

DYDROGESTERONE
TABLET; ORAL
GYNOREST
SOLVAY 5 MG N17388 001
10 MG N17388 002

DYPHYLLINE
ELIXIR; ORAL
NEOTHYLLINE
LEMMON 160 MG/15 ML N07794 003

EDETATE CALCIUM DISODIUM
TABLET; ORAL
CALCIUM DISODIUM VERSENATE
3M 500 MG N08922 002

EDETATE DISODIUM
INJECTABLE; INJECTION
DISODIUM EDETATE
STERIS 150 MG/ML N84356 001

EFLORNITHINE HYDROCHLORIDE
INJECTABLE; INJECTION
ORNIDYL
MERRELL DOW 200 MG/ML N19879 002 NOV 28, 1990

ENCAINIDE HYDROCHLORIDE
CAPSULE; ORAL
ENKAID
BRISTOL 25 MG N18981 002 DEC 24, 1986
35 MG N18981 003 DEC 24, 1986
50 MG N18981 004 DEC 24, 1986

EPINEPHRINE; ETIDOCAINE HYDROCHLORIDE
INJECTABLE; INJECTION
DURANEST
ASTRA 0.005 MG/ML;0.5% N17751 004

EPINEPHRINE; LIDOCAINE HYDROCHLORIDE
INJECTABLE; INJECTION
LIDOCAINE HCL W/ EPINEPHRINE
BEL MAR 0.01 MG/ML;1% N80820 001
0.01 MG/ML;2% N80757 001
STERIS 0.01 MG/ML;1% N85463 001
XYLOCAINE W/ EPINEPHRINE
ASTRA 0.005 MG/ML;1% N10418 006
0.005 MG/ML;1.5% N10418 010
0.005 MG/ML;2% N10418 008
0.02 MG/ML;2% N06488 005

EPINEPHRINE; PROCAINE HYDROCHLORIDE
INJECTABLE; INJECTION
PROCAINE HCL W/ EPINEPHRINE
BEL MAR 0.02 MG/ML;1% N80758 001
0.02 MG/ML;2% N80759 001

ERGOCALCIFEROL
CAPSULE; ORAL
DELTALIN
LILLY 50,000IU N80884 001
VITAMIN D
CHASE CHEM 50,000IU N80747 001
EVERYLIFE 50,000IU N80956 001
LANNETT 50,000IU N80825 001
VITARINE 50,000IU N84053 001
WEST WARD PHARM 50,000IU N83102 001

ERGOCALCIFEROL; *MULTIPLE*

SEE ASCORBIC ACID; BIOTIN; CYANOCOBALAMIN; DEXPANTHENOL; ERGOCALCIFEROL; FOLIC ACID; NIACINAMIDE; PYRIDOXINE HYDROCHLORIDE; RIBOFLAVIN PHOSPHATE SODIUM; THIAMINE HYDROCHLORIDE; VITAMIN A; VITAMIN E

SEE ASCORBIC ACID; BIOTIN; CYANOCOBALAMIN; DEXPANTHENOL; ERGOCALCIFEROL; FOLIC ACID; NIACINAMIDE; PYRIDOXINE HYDROCHLORIDE; RIBOFLAVIN PHOSPHATE SODIUM; THIAMINE HYDROCHLORIDE; VITAMIN A PALMITATE; VITAMIN E

SEE ASCORBIC ACID; BIOTIN; CYANOCOBALAMIN; DEXPANTHENOL; ERGOCALCIFEROL; FOLIC ACID; NIACINAMIDE; PYRIDOXINE; RIBOFLAVIN PHOSPHATE SODIUM; THIAMINE; VITAMIN A; VITAMIN E

ERGOLOID MESYLATES

TABLET; ORAL		
ERGOLOID MESYLATES		
CIRCA	1 MG	N86433 001 MAY 27, 1982
GERIMAL		
CHELSEA LABS	1 MG	N88207 001 MAR 22, 1984
HYDERGINE		
SANDOZ	0.5 MG	N17993 003
TABLET; SUBLINGUAL		
ALKERGOT		
EON LABS	0.5 MG	N85153 001
	1 MG	N87417 001
CIRCANOL		
3M	0.5 MG	N84868 001
	1 MG	N85809 001
DEAPRIL-ST		
BRISTOL MYERS SQUIBB	1 MG	N85020 002
ERGOLOID MESYLATES		
CIRCA	0.5 MG	N84930 001
	1 MG	N85177 001
KV PHARM	0.5 MG	N86265 001
	1 MG	N86264 001
LEDERLE	0.5 MG	N86984 001
	1 MG	N86985 001
SUPERPHARM	0.5 MG	N89233 001 SEP 23, 1986
	1 MG	N89234 001 SEP 23, 1986

ERGOLOID MESYLATES *(continued)*

TABLET; SUBLINGUAL		
ERGOLOID MESYLATES		
VANGARD	0.5 MG	N88013 001 SEP 20, 1982
	1 MG	N88014 001 SEP 20, 1982
HYDROGENATED ERGOT ALKALOIDS		
ZENITH LABS	0.5 MG	N87186 001

ERYTHROMYCIN

CAPSULE, DELAYED REL PELLETS; ORAL		
ERYC		
PARKE DAVIS	250 MG	N62546 001 JUL 25, 1985
ERYC SPRINKLES		
FAULDING	125 MG	N50593 001 JUL 22, 1985
ERYC 125		
PARKE DAVIS	125 MG	N62648 001 OCT 24, 1985
OINTMENT; OPHTHALMIC		
ERYTHROMYCIN		
PHARMADERM	5 MG/GM	N62446 001 SEP 26, 1983
PHARMAFAIR	5 MG/GM	N62481 001 APR 05, 1984
POWDER; FOR RX COMPOUNDING		
ERYTHROMYCIN		
PADDOCK	100%	N50610 001 NOV 07, 1986
SOLUTION; TOPICAL		
ERYTHROMYCIN		
BARRE	2%	N62327 001 APR 19, 1982
	2%	N62342 001 FEB 25, 1982
	2%	N62957 001 JUL 21, 1988
LILLY	2%	N50532 001
PHARMAFAIR	2%	N62616 001 JUL 25, 1985
	1.5%	N62485 001 JUL 11, 1984
TABLET, DELAYED RELEASE; ORAL		
R-P MYCIN		
SOLVAY	250 MG	N61659 001

Discontinued Drug Products *(continued)*

ERYTHROMYCIN ESTOLATE

SUSPENSION; ORAL		
ERYTHROMYCIN ESTOLATE		
LIFE LABS	EQ 250 MG BASE/5 ML	N62362 001 DEC 17, 1982

ERYTHROMYCIN ESTOLATE; SULFISOXAZOLE ACETYL

SUSPENSION; ORAL		
ILOSONE SULFA		
LILLY	EQ 125 MG BASE/5 ML;EQ 600 MG BASE/5 ML	N50599 001 SEP 29, 1989

ERYTHROMYCIN ETHYLSUCCINATE

SUSPENSION; ORAL		
E-MYCIN E		
UPJOHN	EQ 200 MG BASE/5 ML	N62198 001
	EQ 400 MG BASE/5 ML	N62198 002
ERYTHROMYCIN ETHYLSUCCINATE		
DISTA	EQ 200 MG BASE/5 ML	N62177 001
	EQ 400 MG BASE/5 ML	N62177 002
KV PHARM	EQ 200 MG BASE/5 ML	N62047 001
	EQ 400 MG BASE/5 ML	N62047 002
NASKA	EQ 400 MG BASE/5 ML	N62674 001 MAR 10, 1987
PARKE DAVIS	EQ 200 MG BASE/5 ML	N62231 001
	EQ 400 MG BASE/5 ML	N62231 002
PHARMAFAIR	EQ 200 MG BASE/5 ML	N62559 001 MAR 15, 1985
	EQ 400 MG BASE/5 ML	N62558 001 MAR 15, 1985
TABLET; ORAL		
E.E.S. 400		
ABBOTT	EQ 400 MG BASE	N61905 001

ERYTHROMYCIN LACTOBIONATE

INJECTABLE; INJECTION		
ERYTHROMYCIN LACTOBIONATE		
FUJISAWA	EQ 500 MG BASE/VIAL	N62604 001 NOV 24, 1986
	EQ 1 GM BASE/VIAL	N62604 002 NOV 24, 1986
QUAD PHARMS	EQ 500 MG BASE/VIAL	N62660 001 NOV 24, 1986
	EQ 1 GM BASE/VIAL	N62660 003 NOV 24, 1986

ERYTHROMYCIN STEARATE

TABLET; ORAL		
BRISTAMYCIN		
BRISTOL	EQ 250 MG BASE	N61304 001
	EQ 250 MG BASE	N61887 001
ERYPAR		
PARKE DAVIS	EQ 250 MG BASE	N62032 001
	EQ 500 MG BASE	N62032 002
WARNER CHILCOTT	EQ 250 MG BASE	N62322 001
ERYTHROCIN STEARATE		
ABBOTT	EQ 125 MG BASE	N60359 002
ERYTHROMYCIN STEARATE		
LEDERLE	EQ 250 MG BASE	N62089 001
	EQ 500 MG BASE	N62089 002
PUREPAC PHARM	EQ 250 MG BASE	N61743 001
PFIZER-E		
PFIZER	EQ 250 MG BASE	N61791 001
	EQ 500 MG BASE	N61791 002

ESMOLOL HYDROCHLORIDE

INJECTABLE; INJECTION		
BREVIBLOC		
OHMEDA	100 MG/ML	N19386 003 DEC 31, 1986

ESTRADIOL CYPIONATE

INJECTABLE; INJECTION		
ESTRADIOL CYPIONATE		
QUAD PHARMS	5 MG/ML	N89310 001 FEB 09, 1987

ESTRADIOL VALERATE; TESTOSTERONE ENANTHATE

INJECTABLE; INJECTION		
DELADUMONE		
SQUIBB	4 MG/ML;90 MG/ML	N09545 001
DELADUMONE OB		
SQUIBB	8 MG/ML;180 MG/ML	N09545 002
TESTOSTERONE ENANTHATE AND ESTRADIOL VALERATE		
STERIS	8 MG/ML;180 MG/ML	N85860 001

ESTROGENS, CONJUGATED; MEPROBAMATE

TABLET; ORAL		
MILPREM-200		
WALLACE PHARMS	0.45 MG;200 MG	N11045 002
MILPREM-400		
WALLACE PHARMS	0.45 MG;400 MG	N11045 001

Discontinued Drug Products *(continued)*

ESTROGENS, ESTERIFIED

TABLET; ORAL
AMNESTROGEN
SQUIBB 0.625 MG N83266 002
1.25 MG N83266 003
2.5 MG N83266 004
0.3 MG N83266 001
ESTERIFIED ESTROGENS
GENEVA PHARMS 1.25 MG N85302 001
PRIVATE FORM 0.625 MG N83414 001
1.25 MG N83765 001
2.5 MG N85907 001
EVEX
SYNTEX 0.625 MG N84215 001
1.25 MG N83376 002
FEMOGEN
PRIVATE FORM 0.625 MG N85076 001
1.25 MG N85008 001
2.5 MG N85007 001

ESTRONE

INJECTABLE; INJECTION
ESTRONE
STERIS 2 MG/ML N83397 001
THEELIN
PARKE DAVIS 1 MG/ML N03977 001
5 MG/ML N03977 003

ETHAMBUTOL HYDROCHLORIDE

TABLET; ORAL
MYAMBUTOL
LEDERLE 200 MG N16320 002
500 MG N16320 004

ETHCHLORVYNOL

CAPSULE; ORAL
PLACIDYL
ABBOTT 100 MG N10021 004

ETHINAMATE

CAPSULE; ORAL
VALMID
DISTA 500 MG N09750 001

ETHINYL ESTRADIOL

TABLET; ORAL
FEMINONE
UPJOHN 0.05 MG N16649 001
LYNORAL
ORGANON 0.05 MG N05490 002
0.01 MG N05490 003

ETHINYL ESTRADIOL; FERROUS FUMARATE; NORETHINDRONE

TABLET; ORAL-28
NORQUEST FE
SYNTEX 0.035 MG;75 MG;1 MG N18926 001
JUL 18, 1986

ETHINYL ESTRADIOL; FERROUS FUMARATE; NORETHINDRONE ACETATE

TABLET; ORAL-28
NORLESTRIN FE 1/50
PARKE DAVIS 0.05 MG;75 MG;1 MG N16766 001
NORLESTRIN FE 2.5/50
PARKE DAVIS 0.05 MG;75 MG;2.5 MG N16854 001

ETHINYL ESTRADIOL; FLUOXYMESTERONE

TABLET; ORAL
HALODRIN
UPJOHN 0.02 MG;1 MG N11267 001

ETHINYL ESTRADIOL; NORETHINDRONE

TABLET; ORAL-21
N.E.E. 1/35 21
LPI 0.035 MG;1 MG N71541 001
DEC 14, 1987

TABLET; ORAL-28
N.E.E. 1/35 28
LPI 0.035 MG;1 MG N71542 001
DEC 14, 1987

ETHINYL ESTRADIOL; NORETHINDRONE ACETATE

TABLET; ORAL-21
NORLESTRIN 21 1/50
PARKE DAVIS 0.05 MG;1 MG N16749 001
NORLESTRIN 21 2.5/50
PARKE DAVIS 0.05 MG;2.5 MG N16852 001
TABLET; ORAL-28
NORLESTRIN 28 1/50
PARKE DAVIS 0.05 MG;1 MG N16723 001

Discontinued Drug Products *(continued)*

ETHOXZOLAMIDE
TABLET; ORAL
CARDASE
UPJOHN — 62.5 MG — N11047 002
CARDRASE
UPJOHN — 125 MG — N11047 001
ETHAMIDE
ALLERGAN — 125 MG — N16144 001

ETHYLESTRENOL
ELIXIR; ORAL
MAXIBOLIN
ORGANON — 2 MG/5 ML — N14006 002
TABLET; ORAL
MAXIBOLIN
ORGANON — 2 MG — N14005 002

ETHYNODIOL DIACETATE; MESTRANOL
TABLET; ORAL-20
OVULEN
SEARLE — 1 MG;0.1 MG — N16029 002
TABLET; ORAL-21
OVULEN-21
SEARLE — 1 MG;0.1 MG — N16029 003
TABLET; ORAL-28
OVULEN-28
SEARLE — 1 MG;0.1 MG — N16705 001

ETIDOCAINE HYDROCHLORIDE
INJECTABLE; INJECTION
DURANEST
ASTRA — 0.5% — N17751 003

ETIDOCAINE HYDROCHLORIDE; *MULTIPLE*
SEE <u>EPINEPHRINE; ETIDOCAINE HYDROCHLORIDE</u>

ETOPOSIDE
CAPSULE; ORAL
VEPESID
BRISTOL — 100 MG — N19557 002 DEC 30, 1986

FENFLURAMINE HYDROCHLORIDE
TABLET, EXTENDED RELEASE; ORAL
PONDIMIN
ROBINS AH — 60 MG — N16618 003 JUL 27, 1982

FENOPROFEN CALCIUM
CAPSULE; ORAL
FENOPROFEN CALCIUM
AM THERAP — EQ 200 MG BASE — N72307 001 AUG 22, 1988
EQ 300 MG BASE — N72308 001 AUG 22, 1988
HALSEY — EQ 200 MG BASE — N72355 001 AUG 17, 1988
EQ 300 MG BASE — N72356 001 AUG 17, 1988
QUANTUM PHARMICS — EQ 200 MG BASE — N72214 001 AUG 17, 1988
EQ 300 MG BASE — N71738 001 AUG 17, 1988
WARNER CHILCOTT — EQ 200 MG BASE — N72946 001 APR 30, 1991
EQ 300 MG BASE — N72472 001 APR 30, 1991
TABLET; ORAL
FENOPROFEN CALCIUM
AM THERAP — EQ 600 MG BASE — N72309 001 AUG 17, 1988
HALSEY — EQ 600 MG BASE — N72357 001 AUG 17, 1988
QUANTUM PHARMICS — EQ 600 MG BASE — N72194 001 AUG 17, 1988
ROSEMONT PHARM — EQ 600 MG BASE — N72362 001 AUG 17, 1988

Discontinued Drug Products *(continued)*

FENTANYL CITRATE; *MULTIPLE*
SEE DROPERIDOL; FENTANYL CITRATE

FERROUS CITRATE, FE-59
INJECTABLE; INJECTION
FERROUS CITRATE FE 59
MALLINCKRODT 25uCi/ML N16729 001

FERROUS FUMARATE; *MULTIPLE*
SEE ETHINYL ESTRADIOL; FERROUS FUMARATE; NORETHINDRONE ACETATE
SEE ETHINYL ESTRADIOL; FERROUS FUMARATE; NORETHINDRONE

FERROUS SULFATE; FOLIC ACID
CAPSULE; ORAL
FOLVRON
LEDERLE 182 MG;0.33 MG N06012 003

FIBRINOGEN, I-125
INJECTABLE; INJECTION
IBRIN
AMERSHAM 154uCi/VIAL N17879 001
RADIONUCLIDE-LABELED (125 I) FIBRINOGEN (HUMAN) SENSOR
ABBOTT 140uCi/ML N17787 001

FLOSEQUINAN
TABLET; ORAL
MANOPLAX
BOOTS 125 MG N19960 004
DEC 30, 1992

FLOXURIDINE
INJECTABLE; INJECTION
FLOXURIDINE
QUAD PHARMS 500 MG/VIAL N71055 001
AUG 24, 1987

FLUMETHASONE PIVALATE
CREAM; TOPICAL
LOCORTEN
CIBA 0.03% N16379 001

FLUOCINOLONE ACETONIDE
CREAM; TOPICAL
FLUOCINOLONE ACETONIDE
PHARMADERM 0.01% N88047 001
DEC 16, 1982
0.025% N88045 001
DEC 16, 1982
PHARMAFAIR 0.01% N88499 001
AUG 02, 1984
0.025% N88506 001
AUG 02, 1984
ROSEMONT PHARM 0.01% N88757 001
FEB 11, 1985
0.025% N88756 001
MAR 28, 1985

FLUOCINOLONE ACETONIDE *(continued)*

CREAM; TOPICAL
  FLUOTREX
    SAVAGE LABS 0.01% N88174 001 MAY 06, 1983
    0.025% N88173 001 MAR 09, 1983

GEL; TOPICAL
  FLUONID
    ALLERGAN HERBERT 0.025% N87300 001 MAY 27, 1982

OINTMENT; TOPICAL
  FLUOCINOLONE ACETONIDE
    PHARMADERM 0.025% N88046 001 DEC 16, 1982
    PHARMAFAIR 0.025% N88507 001 FEB 27, 1984
    ROSEMONT PHARM 0.025% N88742 001 FEB 08, 1985
  FLUOTREX
    SAVAGE LABS 0.025% N88172 001 MAR 09, 1983

SOLUTION; TOPICAL
  FLUOCINOLONE ACETONIDE
    PENNEX 0.01% N88312 001 JAN 27, 1984
    PHARMAFAIR 0.01% N88449 001 FEB 08, 1984
  FLUOTREX
    SAVAGE LABS 0.01% N88171 001 MAR 09, 1983

FLUOCINONIDE

CREAM; TOPICAL
  FLUOCINONIDE
    CLAY PARK 0.05% N71790 001 JUL 13, 1988

FLUOROMETHOLONE

CREAM; TOPICAL
  OXYLONE
    UPJOHN 0.025% N11748 001

FLUOROURACIL

INJECTABLE; INJECTION
  ADRUCIL
    PHARMACIA 50 MG/ML N17959 001
  FLUOROURACIL
    ABIC 50 MG/ML N88929 001 MAR 04, 1986
    FUJISAWA 50 MG/ML N89152 001 MAR 21, 1986
    50 MG/ML N89428 001 JAN 12, 1987
    50 MG/ML N89519 001 MAR 12, 1987
    MARCHAR 50 MG/ML N87791 001 JAN 18, 1983
    QUAD PHARMS 50 MG/ML N89368 001 FEB 03, 1987
    50 MG/ML N89455 001 FEB 03, 1987
    SMITH AND NEPHEW 50 MG/ML N88766 001 DEC 28, 1984

FLUOXYMESTERONE

TABLET; ORAL
  ANDROID-F
    ICN 10 MG N87196 001
  FLUOXYMESTERONE
    CIRCA 2 MG N88260 001 DEC 06, 1983
    5 MG N88265 001 DEC 06, 1983
    10 MG N88309 001 DEC 06, 1983
    ICN 10 MG N88221 001 MAY 05, 1983
  ORA-TESTRYL
    SQUIBB 2 MG N11359 001
    5 MG N11359 002

Discontinued Drug Products *(continued)*

FLUOXYMESTERONE; *MULTIPLE*

SEE ETHINYL ESTRADIOL; FLUOXYMESTERONE

FLUPHENAZINE DECANOATE

INJECTABLE; INJECTION			
FLUPHENAZINE			
QUAD PHARMS	25 MG/ML	N70762 001	FEB 20, 1986

FLUPHENAZINE HYDROCHLORIDE

INJECTABLE; INJECTION			
FLUPHENAZINE HCL			
QUAD PHARMS	2.5 MG/ML	N89800 001	JUN 08, 1988
TABLET; ORAL			
FLUPHENAZINE HCL			
CIRCA	1 MG	N88555 001	DEC 18, 1987
	2.5 MG	N88544 001	DEC 18, 1987
	5 MG	N88527 001	DEC 18, 1987
	10 MG	N88550 001	DEC 18, 1987
PERMITIL			
SCHERING	0.25 MG	N12034 001	
TABLET, EXTENDED RELEASE; ORAL			
PERMITIL			
SCHERING	1 MG	N12419 004	

FLUPREDNISOLONE

TABLET; ORAL			
ALPHADROL			
UPJOHN	1.5 MG	N12259 002	

FLURAZEPAM HYDROCHLORIDE

CAPSULE; ORAL			
FLURAZEPAM HCL			
ROSEMONT PHARM	15 MG	N70562 001	JUL 09, 1987
	30 MG	N70563 001	JUL 09, 1987

FOLIC ACID

TABLET; ORAL			
FOLIC ACID			
ANABOLIC	1 MG	N84915 001	
BARR	1 MG	N89177 001	JAN 08, 1986
CHELSEA LABS	1 MG	N85141 002	
CIRCA	1 MG	N83141 001	
EON LABS	1 MG	N84472 001	
EVERYLIFE	1 MG	N80755 001	
LANNETT	1 MG	N80816 001	
LILLY	1 MG	N06135 003	
PHARMERAL	1 MG	N84158 001	
PIONEER PHARMS	1 MG	N88949 001	SEP 13, 1985
PUREPAC PHARM	1 MG	N80784 001	
ROSEMONT PHARM	1 MG	N87828 001	MAY 13, 1982
UDL	1 MG	N88199 001	MAR 29, 1983
VANGARD	1 MG	N88730 001	MAR 23, 1984
WHITEWORTH TOWNE	1 MG	N80691 002	

Discontinued Drug Products *(continued)*

FOLIC ACID; *MULTIPLE*

SEE ASCORBIC ACID; BIOTIN; CYANOCOBALAMIN; DEXPANTHENOL; ERGOCALCIFEROL; FOLIC ACID; NIACINAMIDE; PYRIDOXINE HYDROCHLORIDE; RIBOFLAVIN PHOSPHATE SODIUM; THIAMINE HYDROCHLORIDE; VITAMIN A; VITAMIN E

SEE ASCORBIC ACID; BIOTIN; CYANOCOBALAMIN; DEXPANTHENOL; ERGOCALCIFEROL; FOLIC ACID; NIACINAMIDE; PYRIDOXINE HYDROCHLORIDE; RIBOFLAVIN PHOSPHATE SODIUM; THIAMINE HYDROCHLORIDE; VITAMIN A PALMITATE; VITAMIN E

SEE ASCORBIC ACID; BIOTIN; CYANOCOBALAMIN; DEXPANTHENOL; ERGOCALCIFEROL; FOLIC ACID; NIACINAMIDE; PYRIDOXINE; RIBOFLAVIN PHOSPHATE SODIUM; THIAMINE; VITAMIN A; VITAMIN E

SEE FERROUS SULFATE; FOLIC ACID

FUROSEMIDE

INJECTABLE; INJECTION
FUROSEMIDE

ASTRA	10 MG/ML	N70014 001 SEP 09, 1985
FUJISAWA	10 MG/ML	N18507 001 JUL 30, 1982
	10 MG/ML	N19036 001 AUG 13, 1984
ORGANON	10 MG/ML	N70017 001 DEC 15, 1986
SMITH AND NEPHEW	10 MG/ML	N70023 001 FEB 05, 1986
WARNER CHILCOTT	10 MG/ML	N18420 001 FEB 26, 1982
WYETH AYERST	10 MG/ML	N18670 001 JUL 20, 1982

FUROSEMIDE *(continued)*

TABLET; ORAL
FUROSEMIDE

CHELSEA LABS	20 MG	N18369 001 MAY 14, 1982
	40 MG	N18369 002 MAY 14, 1982
EON LABS	40 MG	N18750 002 JUL 30, 1984
WARNER CHILCOTT	20 MG	N18419 001 JAN 31, 1983
	40 MG	N18419 002 JAN 31, 1983
	80 MG	N18419 003 NOV 13, 1984

GALLIUM CITRATE, GA-67

INJECTABLE; INJECTION
GALLIUM CITRATE GA 67

MEDI PHYSICS	1mCi/ML	N17700 001

GEMFIBROZIL

CAPSULE; ORAL
LOPID

PARKE DAVIS	200 MG	N18422 001

GENTAMICIN SULFATE

CREAM; TOPICAL
GENTAFAIR

PHARMAFAIR	EQ 0.1% BASE	N62458 001 SEP 01, 1983

GENTAMICIN SULFATE

PHARMADERM	EQ 1 MG BASE/GM	N62530 001 JUL 05, 1984

INJECTABLE; INJECTION
GENTAMICIN SULFATE

WYETH AYERST	EQ 10 MG BASE/ML	N62264 001
	EQ 40 MG BASE/ML	N62264 002

Discontinued Drug Products *(continued)*

GENTAMICIN SULFATE *(continued)*

INJECTABLE; INJECTION

GENTAMICIN SULFATE IN SODIUM CHLORIDE 0.9% IN PLASTIC CONTAINER

ABBOTT	EQ 60 MG BASE/100 ML	N62588 006 JAN 06, 1986
	EQ 70 MG BASE/100 ML	N62588 007 JAN 06, 1986
	EQ 80 MG BASE/100 ML	N62588 008 JAN 06, 1986
	EQ 90 MG BASE/100 ML	N62588 009 JAN 06, 1986
	EQ 100 MG BASE/100 ML	N62588 010 JAN 06, 1986
	EQ 1.2 MG BASE/ML	N62588 001 JAN 06, 1986
	EQ 1.4 MG BASE/ML	N62588 002 JAN 06, 1986
	EQ 1.6 MG BASE/ML	N62588 003 JAN 06, 1986
	EQ 1.8 MG BASE/ML	N62588 004 JAN 06, 1986
	EQ 2 MG BASE/ML	N62588 005 JAN 06, 1986

OINTMENT; OPHTHALMIC

GENTAFAIR

PHARMAFAIR	EQ 3 MG BASE/GM	N62443 001 MAY 26, 1983

OINTMENT; TOPICAL

GENTAFAIR

PHARMAFAIR	EQ 0.1% BASE	N62444 001 MAY 26, 1983

SOLUTION/DROPS; OPHTHALMIC

GENTAFAIR

PHARMAFAIR	EQ 0.3% BASE	N62440 001 MAY 03, 1983

GENTAMICIN SULFATE

PACO	EQ 3 MG BASE/ML	N62932 001 NOV 07, 1988

GENTIAN VIOLET

TAMPON; VAGINAL

GENAPAX

KEY PHARMS	5 MG	N85017 001

GLUCAGON HYDROCHLORIDE

INJECTABLE; INJECTION

GLUCAGON

QUAD PHARMS	EQ 1 MG BASE/VIAL	N71022 001 MAR 04, 1987
	EQ 10 MG BASE/VIAL	N71023 001 MAR 04, 1987

GLUTETHIMIDE

CAPSULE; ORAL

DORIDEN

RHONE POULENC RORER	500 MG	N09519 008

TABLET; ORAL

DORIDEN

RHONE POULENC RORER	250 MG	N09519 002
	500 MG	N09519 005

GLUTETHIMIDE

CHELSEA LABS	500 MG	N85763 001
LANNETT	250 MG	N83475 001
	500 MG	N85571 001
VITARINE	500 MG	N87297 001

GLYBURIDE

TABLET; ORAL

GLUBATE

HOECHST ROUSSEL	1.5 MG	N20055 001 APR 17, 1992
	3 MG	N20055 002 APR 17, 1992

GLYCOPYRROLATE

INJECTABLE; INJECTION

GLYCOPYRROLATE

FUJISAWA	0.2 MG/ML	N88475 001 JUN 12, 1984
QUAD PHARMS	0.2 MG/ML	N89397 001 DEC 09, 1986

ROBINUL

ROBINS AH	0.2 MG/ML	N14764 001

TABLET; ORAL

GLYCOPYRROLATE

CHELSEA LABS	2 MG	N86178 001
CIRCA	2 MG	N85563 001
	1 MG	N85562 001

GONADORELIN HYDROCHLORIDE
INJECTABLE; INJECTION
FACTREL
WYETH AYERST — EQ 0.2 MG BASE/VIAL — N18123 002 SEP 30, 1982

GONADOTROPIN, CHORIONIC
INJECTABLE; INJECTION
CHORIONIC GONADOTROPIN

BEL MAR	5,000 UNITS/VIAL	N17054 001
	10,000 UNITS/VIAL	N17054 002
FUJISAWA	5,000 UNITS/VIAL	N17067 001
	20,000 UNITS/VIAL	N17067 003
	15,000 UNITS/VIAL	N17067 004
QUAD PHARMS	5,000 UNITS/VIAL	N89312 001 DEC 04, 1986
	5,000 UNITS/VIAL	N89313 001 DEC 04, 1986
	10,000 UNITS/VIAL	N89314 001 DEC 04, 1986
	10,000 UNITS/VIAL	N89315 001 DEC 04, 1986
	20,000 UNITS/VIAL	N89316 001 DEC 04, 1986
STERIS	2,000 UNITS/VIAL	N17016 009 DEC 27, 1984

FOLLUTEIN
SQUIBB — 10,000 UNITS/VIAL — N17056 001

GRAMICIDIN; NEOMYCIN SULFATE; POLYMYXIN B SULFATE
SOLUTION/DROPS; OPHTHALMIC
NEO-POLYCIN
DOW PHARMS — 0.025 MG/ML;EQ 1.75 MG BASE/ML;10,000 UNITS/ML — N60427 001
NEOMYCIN SULFATE AND POLYMYXIN B SULFATE GRAMICIDIN
PHARMAFAIR — 0.025 MG/ML;EQ 1.75 MG BASE/ML;10,000 UNITS/ML — N62383 001 AUG 31, 1982

GRANISETRON HYDROCHLORIDE
INJECTABLE; INJECTION
KYTRIL
SMITHKLINE BEECHAM — EQ 3 MG BASE/ML — N20239 001 DEC 29, 1993

GRISEOFULVIN, MICROCRYSTALLINE
CAPSULE; ORAL
GRISACTIN
WYETH AYERST — 125 MG — N50051 002

GUANABENZ ACETATE
TABLET; ORAL
WYTENSIN
WYETH AYERST — EQ 16 MG BASE — N18587 003 SEP 07, 1982

GUANETHIDINE MONOSULFATE
TABLET; ORAL
GUANETHIDINE MONOSULFATE

CIRCA	EQ 10 MG SULFATE	N86113 001 MAR 26, 1985
	EQ 25 MG SULFATE	N86114 001 MAR 26, 1985

GUANFACINE HYDROCHLORIDE
TABLET; ORAL
TENEX
ROBINS AH — 3 MG — N19032 003 NOV 07, 1988

HALCINONIDE
OINTMENT; TOPICAL
HALOG
BRISTOL MYERS SQUIBB — 0.025% — N18125 001

HALOFANTRINE HYDROCHLORIDE
TABLET; ORAL
HALFAN
SMITHKLINE BEECHAM — 250 MG — N20250 001 JUL 24, 1992

Discontinued Drug Products *(continued)*

HALOPERIDOL

TABLET; ORAL

HALDOL SOLUTAB		
JOHNSON RW	1 MG	N17079 001
HALOPERIDOL		
CIRCA	0.5 MG	N71571 001 JUN 03, 1988
	1 MG	N71572 001 JUN 03, 1988
	2 MG	N71573 001 JUN 03, 1988
	5 MG	N71374 001 JUN 03, 1988
	10 MG	N71375 001 JUN 03, 1988
	20 MG	N71376 001 JUN 03, 1988
DURAMED	0.5 MG	N71216 001 DEC 04, 1986
	1 MG	N71217 001 DEC 04, 1986
	2 MG	N71218 001 DEC 04, 1986
	5 MG	N71219 001 DEC 04, 1986
	10 MG	N71220 001 JUL 07, 1987
	20 MG	N71221 001 JUL 07, 1987
LEDERLE	0.5 MG	N72727 001 SEP 19, 1989
	1 MG	N72728 001 SEP 19, 1989
	2 MG	N72729 001 SEP 19, 1989
	5 MG	N72730 001 SEP 19, 1989
	10 MG	N72731 001 SEP 19, 1989
	20 MG	N72732 001 SEP 19, 1989
PAR PHARM	20 MG	N71328 001 JUL 20, 1987
QUANTUM PHARMICS	0.5 MG	N71255 001 FEB 17, 1987
	1 MG	N71269 001 FEB 17, 1987
	2 MG	N71256 001 FEB 17, 1987
	5 MG	N71257 001 FEB 17, 1987

HALOPERIDOL *(continued)*

TABLET; ORAL

HALOPERIDOL		
ROYCE LABS	0.5 MG	N71722 001 DEC 24, 1987
	1 MG	N71723 001 DEC 24, 1987
	2 MG	N71724 001 DEC 24, 1987
	5 MG	N71725 001 DEC 24, 1987
	10 MG	N72121 001 DEC 24, 1987
	20 MG	N72122 001 DEC 24, 1987

HALOPERIDOL LACTATE

CONCENTRATE; ORAL

HALOPERIDOL		
PENNEX	EQ 2 MG BASE/ML	N70710 001 MAR 07, 1986

INJECTABLE; INJECTION

HALOPERIDOL		
FUJISAWA	EQ 5 MG BASE/ML	N71187 001 JAN 20, 1987
QUAD PHARMS	EQ 5 MG BASE/ML	N71082 001 JAN 02, 1987
SMITH AND NEPHEW	EQ 5 MG BASE/ML	N70802 001 DEC 14, 1987

HEPARIN SODIUM

INJECTABLE; INJECTION

HEPARIN LOCK FLUSH		
ABBOTT	100 UNITS/ML	N05264 010
FUJISAWA	100 UNITS/ML	N17651 010
INTL MEDICATION	10 UNITS/ML	N86357 001
	500 UNITS/ML	N86357 002
LUITPOLD	10 UNITS/ML	N89063 001 OCT 09, 1985
	100 UNITS/ML	N89064 001 OCT 09, 1985
PARKE DAVIS	10 UNITS/ML	N17346 006
SMITH AND NEPHEW	10 UNITS/ML	N87958 001 APR 20, 1983
	100 UNITS/ML	N87959 001 APR 20, 1983
STERIS	100 UNITS/ML	N17064 001

Discontinued Drug Products *(continued)*

HEPARIN SODIUM *(continued)*

INJECTABLE; INJECTION

HEPARIN LOCK FLUSH PRESERVATIVE FREE

FUJISAWA	10 UNITS/ML	N17029 011 SEP 22, 1987
	100 UNITS/ML	N17029 012 SEP 22, 1987

HEPARIN LOCK FLUSH PRESERVATIVE FREE IN PLASTIC CONTAINER

FUJISAWA	10 UNITS/ML	N17029 008 SEP 22, 1987
	100 UNITS/ML	N17029 009 SEP 22, 1987

HEPARIN SODIUM

CHAMBERLIN PARENTERL	1,000 UNITS/ML	N17130 001
	5,000 UNITS/ML	N17130 002
	10,000 UNITS/ML	N17130 003
	20,000 UNITS/ML	N17130 004
FUJISAWA	1,000 UNITS/ML	N17033 001
	1,000 UNITS/ML	N17651 005
	5,000 UNITS/ML	N17029 002
	5,000 UNITS/ML	N17979 003
	10,000 UNITS/ML	N17651 003
	20,000 UNITS/ML	N17651 008
LUITPOLD	1,000 UNITS/ML	N87452 001 OCT 31, 1983
PARKE DAVIS	1,000 UNITS/ML	N17346 001
	5,000 UNITS/ML	N17346 002
	7,500 UNITS/ML	N17346 003
	10,000 UNITS/ML	N17346 004
	20,000 UNITS/ML	N17346 005
PHARM SPECLTS ASSOC	40,000 UNITS/ML	N17780 005
STERIS	7,500 UNITS/ML	N17064 019
	2,500 UNITS/ML	N17064 015
	3,000 UNITS/ML	N17064 016
	4,000 UNITS/ML	N17064 017
	6,000 UNITS/ML	N17064 018
WYETH AYERST	15,000 UNITS/ML	N17007 005

HEPARIN SODIUM 10,000 UNITS IN DEXTROSE 5% IN PLASTIC CONTAINER

ABBOTT	10,000 UNITS/100 ML	N19339 003 MAR 27, 1985
BAXTER	2,000 UNITS/100 ML	N18814 002 JUL 09, 1985

HEPARIN SODIUM 10,000 UNITS IN SODIUM CHLORIDE 0.45%

ABBOTT	10,000 UNITS/100 ML	N18911 001 JAN 30, 1985
	10,000 UNITS/100 ML	N18916 005 JAN 31, 1984

HEPARIN SODIUM *(continued)*

INJECTABLE; INJECTION

HEPARIN SODIUM 10,000 UNITS IN SODIUM CHLORIDE 0.9%

ABBOTT	10,000 UNITS/100 ML	N18911 003 JAN 30, 1985
	10,000 UNITS/100 ML	N18916 002 JAN 31, 1984

HEPARIN SODIUM 12,500 UNITS IN DEXTROSE 5% IN PLASTIC CONTAINER

ABBOTT	5,000 UNITS/100 ML	N19339 001 MAR 27, 1985

HEPARIN SODIUM 12,500 UNITS IN SODIUM CHLORIDE 0.9%

ABBOTT	5,000 UNITS/100 ML	N18911 005 JAN 30, 1985
	5,000 UNITS/100 ML	N18916 003 JAN 31, 1984

HEPARIN SODIUM 25,000 UNITS IN DEXTROSE 5% IN PLASTIC CONTAINER

ABBOTT	5,000 UNITS/100 ML	N19339 004 MAR 27, 1985
	10,000 UNITS/100 ML	N19339 002 MAR 27, 1985

HEPARIN SODIUM 25,000 UNITS IN SODIUM CHLORIDE 0.9%

ABBOTT	5,000 UNITS/100 ML	N18911 004 JAN 30, 1985

HEPARIN SODIUM 25,000 UNITS IN SODIUM CHLORIDE 0.9% IN PLASTIC CONTAINER

ABBOTT	5,000 UNITS/100 ML	N18916 009 JAN 31, 1984

HEPARIN SODIUM 25000 UNITS IN SODIUM CHLORIDE 0.9% IN PLASTIC CONTAINER

MCGAW	5,000 UNITS/100 ML	N19135 001 MAR 29, 1985

HEPARIN SODIUM 5,000 UNITS IN SODIUM CHLORIDE 0.45%

ABBOTT	100 UNITS/ML	N18916 004 JAN 31, 1984

HEPARIN SODIUM 5000 UNITS AND SODIUM CHLORIDE 0.9% IN PLASTIC CONTAINER

BAXTER	500 UNITS/100 ML	N18609 003 APR 28, 1982

HEPARIN SODIUM 5000 UNITS IN SODIUM CHLORIDE 0.45%

ABBOTT	100 UNITS/ML	N18911 002 JAN 30, 1985

HEPARIN SODIUM 5000 UNITS IN SODIUM CHLORIDE 0.9%

ABBOTT	1,000 UNITS/100 ML	N18916 001 JAN 31, 1984

HEPARIN SODIUM 5000 UNITS IN SODIUM CHLORIDE 0.9% IN PLASTIC CONTAINER

MCGAW	1,000 UNITS/100 ML	N19042 004 MAR 29, 1985

Discontinued Drug Products *(continued)*

HEPARIN SODIUM *(continued)*

INJECTABLE; INJECTION		
LIPO-HEPIN		
3M	1,000 UNITS/ML	N17027 006
	5,000 UNITS/ML	N17027 008
	5,000 UNITS/0.5 ML	N17027 002
	10,000 UNITS/ML	N17027 009
	7,500 UNITS/0.5 ML	N17027 010
	10,000 UNITS/0.5 ML	N17027 003
	20,000 UNITS/ML	N17027 007
	20,000 UNITS/0.5 ML	N17027 004
	40,000 UNITS/ML	N17027 005
	1,000 UNITS/0.5 ML	N17027 001
	15,000 UNITS/0.5 ML	N17027 011
LIQUAEMIN SODIUM		
ORGANON	20,000 UNITS/ML	N00552 001
	40,000 UNITS/ML	N00552 002
LIQUAEMIN SODIUM PRESERVATIVE FREE		
ORGANON	1,000 UNITS/ML	N00552 011 APR 11, 1986
	5,000 UNITS/ML	N00552 012 APR 11, 1986
	10,000 UNITS/ML	N00552 013 APR 11, 1986
PANHEPRIN		
ABBOTT	1,000 UNITS/ML	N05264 004
	5,000 UNITS/ML	N05264 006
	10,000 UNITS/ML	N05264 007
	20,000 UNITS/ML	N05264 008
	40,000 UNITS/ML	N05264 009
SODIUM HEPARIN		
FUJISAWA	5,000 UNITS/ML	N17033 002
	10,000 UNITS/ML	N17033 003
	20,000 UNITS/ML	N17033 004

HEPARIN SODIUM; *MULTIPLE*

SEE <u>DIHYDROERGOTAMINE MESYLATE; HEPARIN SODIUM; LIDOCAINE HYDROCHLORIDE</u>

HETACILLIN

POWDER FOR RECONSTITUTION; ORAL		
VERSAPEN		
BRISTOL	EQ 112.5 MG AMPICIL/ML	N50060 003
	EQ 112.5 MG AMPICIL/ML	N61398 001
	EQ 112.5 MG AMPICIL/5 ML	N50060 001
	EQ 225 MG AMPICIL/5 ML	N61398 002

HETACILLIN POTASSIUM

CAPSULE; ORAL		
VERSAPEN-K		
BRISTOL	EQ 450 MG AMPICIL	N61396 002
	EQ 225 MG AMPICIL	N61396 001

HEXACHLOROPHENE

AEROSOL; TOPICAL		
TURGEX		
XTTRIUM	3%	N18375 001
EMULSION; TOPICAL		
HEXA-GERM		
HUNTINGTON LABS	3%	N17411 001
PHISOHEX		
STERLING WINTHROP	3%	N08402 001
SOY-DOME		
MILES	3%	N17405 001
TURGEX		
XTTRIUM	3%	N19055 001 NOV 30, 1984
SOLUTION; TOPICAL		
DIAL		
DIAL	0.25%	N17421 002
GERMA-MEDICA		
HUNTINGTON LABS	1%	N17412 001
GERMA-MEDICA "MG"		
HUNTINGTON LABS	0.25%	N17412 002
SEPTI-SOFT		
CALGON	0.25%	N17460 001
SEPTISOL		
VESTAL LABS	0.25%	N17423 001
SPONGE; TOPICAL		
HEXASCRUB		
PROF DISPOSABLES	3%	N18363 001
PHISO-SCRUB		
STERLING WINTHROP	3%	N17446 001
SCRUBTEAM SURGICAL SPONGEBRUSH		
3M	330 MG	N17413 001

HEXAFLUORENIUM BROMIDE

INJECTABLE; INJECTION		
MYLAXEN		
WALLACE	20 MG/ML	N09789 003

HEXOCYCLIUM METHYLSULFATE

TABLET; ORAL		
TRAL		
ABBOTT	25 MG	N10599 001

Discontinued Drug Products *(continued)*

HEXYLCAINE HYDROCHLORIDE
SOLUTION; TOPICAL
CYCLAINE
MERCK SHARP DOHME 5% N08472 001

HISTAMINE PHOSPHATE
INJECTABLE; INJECTION
HISTAMINE PHOSPHATE
LILLY EQ 0.1 MG BASE/ML N00734 003
EQ 0.2 MG BASE/ML N00734 002
EQ 1 MG BASE/ML N00734 001

HOMATROPINE METHYLBROMIDE
TABLET, CHEWABLE; ORAL
EQUIPIN
MISSION PHARMA 3 MG N86310 001

HYDRALAZINE HYDROCHLORIDE
INJECTABLE; INJECTION
HYDRALAZINE HCL
FUJISAWA 20 MG/ML N89532 001 AUG 11, 1987
SMITH AND NEPHEW 20 MG/ML N88518 001 APR 20, 1984

TABLET; ORAL
HYDRALAZINE HCL
ASCOT 25 MG N88310 001 DEC 19, 1984
50 MG N88311 001 DEC 19, 1984
CHELSEA LABS 25 MG N85532 002 MAY 24, 1982
50 MG N85533 002 MAY 25, 1982
EON LABS 50 MG N85088 001
PUREPAC PHARM 50 MG N88178 001 AUG 15, 1983
QUANTUM PHARMICS 10 MG N88671 001 MAY 01, 1984
25 MG N88657 001 JUN 15, 1984
50 MG N88652 001 MAY 08, 1984
100 MG N88686 001 MAY 01, 1984

HYDRALAZINE HYDROCHLORIDE *(continued)*
TABLET; ORAL
HYDRALAZINE HCL
ROSEMONT PHARM 25 MG N87780 001 MAR 29, 1982
50 MG N87751 001 MAR 29, 1982
SUPERPHARM 10 MG N88787 001 AUG 28, 1984
25 MG N88788 001 AUG 28, 1984
50 MG N88789 001 AUG 28, 1984
VANGARD 25 MG N87712 001
50 MG N87908 001 MAY 07, 1982
VITARINE 25 MG N86088 001
WEST WARD PHARM 25 MG N88240 001 MAY 27, 1983
50 MG N88241 001 MAY 27, 1983

HYDRALAZINE HYDROCHLORIDE; HYDROCHLOROTHIAZIDE
CAPSULE; ORAL
HYDRALAZINE HCL AND HYDROCHLOROTHIAZIDE
CIRCA 25 MG;25 MG N85457 001 MAR 04, 1982
100 MG;50 MG N85440 001 MAR 04, 1982
50 MG;50 MG N85446 001 MAR 04, 1982
SOLVAY 100 MG;50 MG N87609 001 FEB 08, 1982
SUPERPHARM 25 MG;25 MG N89200 001 FEB 09, 1987
HYDRALAZINE HCL W/ HYDROCHLOROTHIAZIDE 100/50
ZENITH LABS 100 MG;50 MG N88358 001 APR 10, 1984

TABLET; ORAL
HYDRALAZINE AND HYDROCHLORTHIAZIDE
CHELSEA LABS 25 MG;15 MG N85827 001
HYDROCHLOROTHIAZIDE W/ HYDRALAZINE
CIRCA 25 MG;15 MG N85373 001

Discontinued Drug Products *(continued)*

HYDRALAZINE HYDROCHLORIDE; HYDROCHLOROTHIAZIDE; RESERPINE

TABLET; ORAL

HYDRALAZINE HCL-HYDROCHLOROTHIAZIDE-RESERPINE		
MYLAN	25 MG;15 MG;0.1 MG	N87085 001
HYDRALAZINE, HYDROCHLOROTHIAZIDE W/ RESERPINE		
CHELSEA LABS	25 MG;15 MG;0.1 MG	N85771 001
HYDRAP-ES		
EON LABS	25 MG;15 MG;0.1 MG	N84876 001
HYDROCHLOROTHIAZIDE W/ RESERPINE AND HYDRALAZINE		
CIRCA	25 MG;15 MG;0.1 MG	N83770 001
RESERPINE, HYDRALAZINE HCL AND HYDROCHLOROTHIAZIDE		
DANBURY PHARMA	25 MG;15 MG;0.1 MG	N87556 001
RESERPINE, HYDROCHLOROTHIAZIDE, AND HYDRALAZINE HCL		
LEDERLE	25 MG;15 MG;0.1 MG	N87709 001 MAY 13, 1982
SER-A-GEN		
SOLVAY	25 MG;15 MG;0.1 MG	N87210 001
UNIPRES		
SOLVAY	25 MG;15 MG;0.1 MG	N85893 001

HYDRALAZINE HYDROCHLORIDE; RESERPINE

TABLET; ORAL

DRALSERP		
EON LABS	25 MG;0.1 MG	N84617 001
SERPASIL-APRESOLINE		
CIBA	25 MG;0.1 MG	N09296 004
	50 MG;0.2 MG	N09296 002

HYDROCHLOROTHIAZIDE

SOLUTION; ORAL

HYDROCHLOROTHIAZIDE		
PENNEX	50 MG/5 ML	N89661 001 JUN 20, 1988
HYDROCHLOROTHIAZIDE INTENSOL		
ROXANE	100 MG/ML	N88588 001 JUL 02, 1984

TABLET; ORAL

HYDROCHLOROTHIAZIDE		
ALRA	25 MG	N86369 001
	50 MG	N83554 001
ASCOT	25 MG	N87539 001 FEB 03, 1982
CHELSEA LABS	25 MG	N85232 002
	50 MG	N85233 001
	50 MG	N86087 001
	50 MG	N86594 001
	100 MG	N87002 001

HYDROCHLOROTHIAZIDE (*continued*)

TABLET; ORAL

HYDROCHLOROTHIAZIDE		
CIRCA	25 MG	N83458 001
	50 MG	N83456 001
	100 MG	N85099 001
ELKINS SINN	50 MG	N85152 002
EON LABS	25 MG	N83899 001
HEATHER	50 MG	N84135 001
INWOOD LABS	25 MG	N84776 001
	50 MG	N84776 002
LEMMON	25 MG	N88924 001 FEB 07, 1985
	50 MG	N88923 001 FEB 07, 1985
MYLAN	25 MG	N84880 001
	50 MG	N85112 001
ROSEMONT PHARM	25 MG	N87827 001 APR 19, 1982
	50 MG	N87752 001 APR 19, 1982
ROXANE	25 MG	N85004 001
	50 MG	N85005 001
SOLVAY	25 MG	N85323 001
VANGARD	25 MG	N87638 001
	50 MG	N87610 001
WARNER CHILCOTT	25 MG	N87586 001 MAY 03, 1982
	50 MG	N87587 001 MAY 03, 1982
WHITEWORTH TOWNE	25 MG	N83809 002
	50 MG	N83809 001
	100 MG	N85347 001
ZENITH LABS	50 MG	N84658 001
ZIDE		
SOLVAY	50 MG	N83925 001

HYDROCHLOROTHIAZIDE; *MULTIPLE*

SEE HYDRALAZINE HYDROCHLORIDE; HYDROCHLOROTHIAZIDE

SEE HYDRALAZINE HYDROCHLORIDE; HYDROCHLOROTHIAZIDE; RESERPINE

SEE HYDRALAZINE HYDROCHLORIDE; HYDROCHLOROTHIAZIDE

Discontinued Drug Products *(continued)*

HYDROCHLOROTHIAZIDE; LABETALOL HYDROCHLORIDE

TABLET; ORAL
NORMOZIDE
SCHERING — 25 MG;100 MG — N19046 001 — APR 06, 1987
25 MG;200 MG — N19046 002 — APR 06, 1987
25 MG;300 MG — N19046 003 — APR 06, 1987
25 MG;400 MG — N19046 004 — APR 06, 1987
TRANDATE HCT
GLAXO — 25 MG;100 MG — N19174 001 — APR 10, 1987
25 MG;200 MG — N19174 002 — APR 10, 1987
25 MG;300 MG — N19174 003 — APR 10, 1987
25 MG;400 MG — N19174 004 — APR 10, 1987

HYDROCHLOROTHIAZIDE; METHYLDOPA

TABLET; ORAL
METHYLDOPA AND HYDROCHLOROTHIAZIDE
CIRCA — 50 MG;500 MG — N70368 001 — APR 16, 1986
15 MG;250 MG — N70365 001 — MAR 19, 1986
25 MG;250 MG — N70366 001 — APR 16, 1986
30 MG;500 MG — N70367 001 — MAR 19, 1986
PUREPAC PHARM — 50 MG;500 MG — N70689 001 — APR 24, 1986

HYDROCHLOROTHIAZIDE; PINDOLOL

TABLET; ORAL
VISKAZIDE
SANDOZ — 25 MG;5 MG — N18872 001 — JUL 22, 1987
25 MG;10 MG — N18872 002 — JUL 22, 1987

HYDROCHLOROTHIAZIDE; PROPRANOLOL HYDROCHLORIDE

TABLET; ORAL
PROPRANOLOL HCL & HYDROCHLOROTHIAZIDE
DURAMED — 25 MG;40 MG — N71126 001 — MAR 02, 1987
25 MG;80 MG — N71127 001 — MAR 02, 1987

HYDROCHLOROTHIAZIDE; RESERPINE

TABLET; ORAL
H.R.-50
WHITEWORTH TOWNE — 50 MG;0.125 MG — N85338 001
HYDRO-SERP "25"
EON LABS — 25 MG;0.125 MG — N84827 001
HYDRO-SERP "50"
EON LABS — 50 MG;0.125 MG — N85213 001
HYDROCHLOROTHIAZIDE W/ RESERPINE
CHELSEA LABS — 25 MG;0.125 MG — N86330 002
50 MG;0.125 MG — N86331 001
CIRCA — 25 MG;0.125 MG — N85317 001
50 MG;0.125 MG — N83666 001
PHARMERAL — 25 MG;0.125 MG — N85421 001
50 MG;0.125 MG — N85420 001
ROXANE — 50 MG;0.125 MG — N84603 001
RESERPINE AND HYDROCHLOROTHIAZIDE
BARR — 25 MG;0.125 MG — N84580 001
50 MG;0.125 MG — N84579 001
GENEVA PHARMS — 50 MG;0.125 MG — N88200 001 — JAN 31, 1984
SERPASIL-ESIDRIX #1
CIBA — 25 MG;0.1 MG — N11878 003
SERPASIL-ESIDRIX #2
CIBA — 50 MG;0.1 MG — N11878 005

HYDROCHLOROTHIAZIDE; SPIRONOLACTONE

TABLET; ORAL
SPIRONOLACTONE + HYDROCHLOROTHIAZIDE
ASCOT — 25 MG;25 MG — N88025 001 — NOV 23, 1984
SPIRONOLACTONE AND HYDROCHLOROTHIAZIDE
SUPERPHARM — 25 MG;25 MG — N89137 001 — AUG 26, 1985
SPIRONOLACTONE W/ HYDROCHLOROTHIAZIDE
CHELSEA LABS — 25 MG;25 MG — N86026 001
CIRCA — 25 MG;25 MG — N85974 001
LEDERLE — 25 MG;25 MG — N87511 001
PUREPAC PHARM — 25 MG;25 MG — N88054 001 — AUG 18, 1983
ROSEMONT PHARM — 25 MG;25 MG — N87651 001
UPSHER SMITH — 25 MG;25 MG — N87553 001
VANGARD — 25 MG;25 MG — N87655 001

Discontinued Drug Products *(continued)*

HYDROCHLOROTHIAZIDE; TRIAMTERENE

CAPSULE; ORAL
  DYAZIDE
    SMITHKLINE
      BEECHAM — 25 MG;50 MG — N16042 002
  TRIAMTERENE AND HYDROCHLOROTHIAZIDE
    VITARINE — 25 MG;50 MG — N71737 001 FEB 12, 1988

TABLET; ORAL
  TRIAMTERENE AND HYDROCHLOROTHIAZIDE
    AM THERAP — 50 MG;75 MG — N72022 001 APR 17, 1988
    QUANTUM PHARMICS — 50 MG;75 MG — N71980 001 APR 17, 1988

HYDROCODONE BITARTRATE; *MULTIPLE*

SEE ACETAMINOPHEN; HYDROCODONE BITARTRATE
SEE ASPIRIN; HYDROCODONE BITARTRATE

HYDROCORTAMATE HYDROCHLORIDE

OINTMENT; TOPICAL
  MAGNACORT
    PFIZER — 0.5% — N10554 001

HYDROCORTISONE

CREAM; TOPICAL
  ELDECORT
    ELDER — 1% — N80459 001
    2.5% — N84055 001
  H-CORT
    PHARM ASSOC — 0.5% — N86823 001
  HC #1
    MILES — 0.5% — N80438 001
  HC #4
    MILES — 1% — N80438 002
  HYDROCORTISONE
    BIOCRAFT — 0.5% — N80400 002
    1% — N80400 003
    2.5% — N80400 004
    EVERYLIFE — 0.5% — N80452 001
    LEMMON — 1% — N85191 001
    NASKA — 1% — N89706 001 MAR 10, 1988
    PHARMADERM — 1% — N88845 001 FEB 27, 1986
    PHARMAFAIR — 1% — N87838 001 JUL 28, 1982

HYDROCORTISONE *(continued)*

CREAM; TOPICAL
  HYDROCORTISONE
    ROSEMONT PHARM — 1% — N88027 001 SEP 27, 1983
    2.5% — N88029 001 SEP 27, 1983
    STIEFEL — 1% — N86170 001
    THAMES — 0.5% — N86154 001
    WHITEWORTH TOWNE — 1% — N80496 002
  SYNACORT
    SYNTEX — 0.5% — N87459 001

GEL; TOPICAL
  NUTRACORT
    GALDERMA — 1% — N84698 001

INJECTABLE; INJECTION
  CORTEF
    UPJOHN — 50 MG/ML — N09864 001

LOTION; TOPICAL
  BALNEOL-HC
    SOLVAY — 1% — N88041 001 DEC 03, 1982
  CORT-DOME
    MILES — 0.5% — N09895 003
    1% — N09895 001
  H-CORT
    PHARM ASSOC — 0.5% — N86824 001
  HYDROCORTISONE
    BARRE — 0.5% — N87317 001 JUN 07, 1982
    1% — N87315 001 JUN 07, 1982
    CLAY PARK — 1% — N85663 001
    NASKA — 1% — N89705 001 APR 25, 1988
    THAMES — 1% — N89024 001 FEB 12, 1986

OINTMENT; TOPICAL
  HC (HYDROCORTISONE)
    C AND M PHARMA — 0.5% — N80481 001
  HYDROCORTISONE
    ALTANA — 0.5% — N80489 002
    CLAY PARK — 1% — N85028 001
    NASKA — 1% — N89704 001 MAR 10, 1988
    PHARMADERM — 1% — N88842 001 FEB 09, 1987
    ROSEMONT PHARM — 1% — N88061 001 SEP 27, 1983
    2.5% — N88039 001 SEP 27, 1983

Discontinued Drug Products *(continued)*

HYDROCORTISONE *(continued)*

OINTMENT; TOPICAL
HYDROCORTISONE
THAMES 0.5% N86256 001

TABLET; ORAL
CORTRIL
PFIZER 10 MG N09127 005
20 MG N09127 003
HYDROCORTISONE
ANABOLIC 20 MG N83140 001
BARR 20 MG N83999 001
DANBURY PHARMA 20 MG N80355 001
ELKINS SINN 20 MG N80624 001
EON LABS 20 MG N80642 002
FERRANTE 10 MG N80568 001
20 MG N80568 002
INWOOD LABS 20 MG N80732 001
PANRAY 10 MG N09659 001
20 MG N09659 002
PARKE DAVIS 20 MG N84243 001
PUREPAC PHARM 20 MG N80395 001
ROXANE 10 MG N88539 001
MAR 21, 1984
WHITEWORTH TOWNE 10 MG N80344 001
20 MG N80344 002

TABLET; VAGINAL
CORTRIL
PFIPHARMECS 10 MG N09796 001

HYDROCORTISONE; *MULTIPLE*

SEE ACETIC ACID, GLACIAL; HYDROCORTISONE
SEE BACITRACIN ZINC; HYDROCORTISONE; NEOMYCIN SULFATE; POLYMYXIN B SULFATE

HYDROCORTISONE; NEOMYCIN SULFATE; POLYMYXIN B SULFATE

SOLUTION/DROPS; OTIC
NEOMYCIN SULFATE-POLYMYXIN B SULFATE-HYDROCORTISONE
PHARMAFAIR 1%;EQ 3.5 MG BASE/ML;10,000 UNITS/ML N62394 001
SEP 29, 1982

SUSPENSION; OTIC
NEOMYCIN SULFATE, POLYMYXIN B SULFATE & HYDROCORTISONE
PHARMAFAIR 1%;EQ 3.5 MG BASE/ML;10,000 UNITS/ML N62617 001
SEP 18, 1985
OTICAIR
PHARMAFAIR 1%;EQ 3.5 MG BASE/ML;10,000 UNITS/ML N62399 001
NOV 18, 1982
OTOBIONE
SCHERING 1%;EQ 3.5 MG BASE/ML;10,000 UNITS/ML N61816 001

SUSPENSION/DROPS; OPHTHALMIC
NEOMYCIN SULFATE-POLYMYXIN B SULFATE-HYDROCORTISONE
PHARMAFAIR 1%;EQ 3.5 MG BASE/ML;10,000 UNITS/ML N62623 001
SEP 24, 1985

HYDROCORTISONE ACETATE

CREAM; TOPICAL
HYDROCORTISONE ACETATE
PARKE DAVIS 1% N89914 001
JAN 03, 1989

INJECTABLE; INJECTION
CORTEF ACETATE
UPJOHN 50 MG/ML N09378 002
CORTRIL
PFIZER 25 MG/ML N09164 001
HYDROCORTISONE ACETATE
BEL MAR 25 MG/ML N83739 001
50 MG/ML N83739 002
STERIS 50 MG/ML N85214 001

OINTMENT; OPHTHALMIC, OTIC
HYDROCORTONE
MERCK SHARP DOHME 1.5% N09018 003

OINTMENT; TOPICAL
CORTEF ACETATE
UPJOHN EQ 1% BASE N08917 002
2.5% N08917 001

Discontinued Drug Products *(continued)*

HYDROCORTISONE ACETATE; NEOMYCIN SULFATE

CREAM; TOPICAL
NEO-CORTEF
UPJOHN 1%;EQ 3.5 MG BASE/GM N61049 001
2.5%;EQ 3.5 MG BASE/GM N61049 002

OINTMENT; OPHTHALMIC
NEO-CORTEF
UPJOHN 0.5%;EQ 3.5 MG BASE/GM N60610 001
1.5%;EQ 3.5 MG BASE/GM N60610 002

OINTMENT; TOPICAL
NEO-CORTEF
UPJOHN 0.5%;EQ 3.5 MG BASE/GM N60751 001
2.5%;EQ 3.5 MG BASE/GM N60751 003

SUSPENSION/DROPS; OPHTHALMIC
NEO-CORTEF
UPJOHN 0.5%;EQ 3.5 MG BASE/ML N60612 002
1.5%;EQ 3.5 MG BASE/ML N60612 001

HYDROCORTISONE ACETATE; PRAMOXINE HYDROCHLORIDE

LOTION; TOPICAL
PRAMOSONE
FERNDALE LABS 0.5%;1% N83213 002

HYDROCORTISONE BUTYRATE

CREAM; TOPICAL
LOCOID
GALDERMA 0.1% N18795 001 JAN 07, 1983

OINTMENT; TOPICAL
LOCOID
GALDERMA 0.1% N19106 001 JUL 03, 1984
YAMANOUCHI 0.1% N18652 001 OCT 29, 1982

SOLUTION; TOPICAL
LOCOID
GALDERMA 0.1% N19819 001 SEP 15, 1988

HYDROCORTISONE SODIUM PHOSPHATE

INJECTABLE; INJECTION
HYDROCORTISONE SODIUM PHOSPHATE
QUAD PHARMS EQ 50 MG BASE/ML N89581 001 MAY 28, 1987

HYDROCORTISONE SODIUM SUCCINATE

INJECTABLE; INJECTION
A-HYDROCORT
ABBOTT EQ 250 MG BASE/VIAL N89578 001 APR 11, 1989
EQ 500 MG BASE/VIAL N89579 001 APR 11, 1989
EQ 1 GM BASE/VIAL N89580 001 APR 11, 1989
HYDROCORTISONE SODIUM SUCCINATE
ELKINS SINN EQ 100 MG BASE/VIAL N86619 001
EQ 250 MG BASE/VIAL N87567 001
EQ 500 MG BASE/VIAL N87568 001
FUJISAWA EQ 100 MG BASE/VIAL N88667 001 JUN 08, 1984
EQ 100 MG BASE/VIAL N88712 001 JUN 08, 1984
EQ 250 MG BASE/VIAL N88668 001 JUN 08, 1984
EQ 500 MG BASE/VIAL N88669 001 JUN 08, 1984
EQ 1 GM BASE/VIAL N88670 001 JUN 08, 1984

HYDROFLUMETHIAZIDE

TABLET; ORAL
HYDROFLUMETHIAZIDE
CHELSEA LABS 50 MG N88528 001 AUG 15, 1984
CIRCA 50 MG N88031 001 APR 06, 1983

HYDROFLUMETHIAZIDE; RESERPINE

TABLET; ORAL
HYDROFLUMETHIAZIDE AND RESERPINE
CIRCA 50 MG;0.125 MG N88110 001 MAR 22, 1983
25 MG;0.125 MG N88127 001 MAR 22, 1983
ROSEMONT PHARM 50 MG;0.125 MG N88195 001 OCT 26, 1983

HYDROXOCOBALAMIN

INJECTABLE; INJECTION
HYDROXOCOBALAMIN
FUJISAWA 1 MG/ML N84921 001
HYDROXOMIN
BEL MAR 1 MG/ML N84629 001

Discontinued Drug Products *(continued)*

HYDROXYPROGESTERONE CAPROATE

INJECTABLE; INJECTION

DELALUTIN		
SQUIBB	125 MG/ML	N10347 004
	125 MG/ML	N16911 001
	250 MG/ML	N10347 002
	250 MG/ML	N16911 002
HYDROXYPROGESTERONE CAPROATE		
QUAD PHARMS	125 MG/ML	N89330 001 JAN 02, 1987
	250 MG/ML	N89331 001 JAN 02, 1987

HYDROXYSTILBAMIDINE ISETHIONATE

INJECTABLE; INJECTION

HYDROXYSTILBAMIDINE ISETHIONATE		
MERRELL DOW	225 MG/AMP	N09166 001

HYDROXYZINE HYDROCHLORIDE

INJECTABLE; INJECTION

HYDROXYZINE HCL		
ALTANA	25 MG/ML	N87273 001 APR 20, 1982
	50 MG/ML	N87273 002 APR 20, 1982
PHARMAFAIR	25 MG/ML	N88862 001 FEB 14, 1986
	25 MG/ML	N89106 001 FEB 14, 1986
	50 MG/ML	N89107 001 FEB 14, 1986
SMITH AND NEPHEW	25 MG/ML	N87592 001
WYETH AYERST	25 MG/ML	N86258 001
	50 MG/ML	N86258 002
ORGATRAX		
ORGANON	25 MG/ML	N87014 001
	50 MG/ML	N87014 002

TABLET; ORAL

HYDROXYZINE HCL		
BARR	10 MG	N88409 001 NOV 15, 1983
	25 MG	N87857 001 APR 18, 1983
	50 MG	N87860 001 APR 18, 1983
	100 MG	N87862 001 APR 18, 1983
CHELSEA LABS	10 MG	N86827 001
	25 MG	N86829 001
	50 MG	N86836 001

HYDROXYZINE HYDROCHLORIDE *(continued)*

TABLET; ORAL

HYDROXYZINE HCL		
EON LABS	10 MG	N87246 002
	25 MG	N85247 001
	50 MG	N87245 001
QUANTUM PHARMICS	10 MG	N88540 001 OCT 22, 1985
	25 MG	N88551 001 OCT 22, 1985
	50 MG	N88529 001 OCT 22, 1985
ROSEMONT PHARM	10 MG	N89121 001 MAR 20, 1986
	25 MG	N89122 001 MAR 20, 1986
	50 MG	N89123 001 MAR 20, 1986

HYDROXYZINE PAMOATE

CAPSULE; ORAL

HY-PAM "25"		
LEMMON	EQ 25 MG HCL	N88713 001 MAR 04, 1985
HYDROXYZINE PAMOATE		
CHELSEA LABS	EQ 25 MG HCL	N86840 001 JUL 01, 1982
	EQ 50 MG HCL	N86705 001 JUL 01, 1982
	EQ 100 MG HCL	N86728 001 OCT 05, 1982
CIRCA	EQ 25 MG HCL	N86698 001
	EQ 50 MG HCL	N86695 001
	EQ 100 MG HCL	N86697 001
DURAMED	EQ 25 MG HCL	N88593 001 FEB 29, 1984
	EQ 50 MG HCL	N88594 001 FEB 29, 1984
	EQ 100 MG HCL	N88595 001 FEB 29, 1984
PAR PHARM	EQ 25 MG HCL	N87656 001 JUN 11, 1982
	EQ 25 MG HCL	N89145 001 MAR 17, 1986
	EQ 50 MG HCL	N87657 001 JUN 11, 1982
	EQ 50 MG HCL	N89146 001 MAR 17, 1986
	EQ 100 MG HCL	N87658 001 JUN 11, 1982

Discontinued Drug Products *(continued)*

HYDROXYZINE PAMOATE *(continued)*

CAPSULE; ORAL
HYDROXYZINE PAMOATE

SUPERPHARM	EQ 25 MG HCL	N89031 001 JAN 02, 1987
	EQ 50 MG HCL	N89032 001 JAN 02, 1987
	EQ 100 MG HCL	N89033 001 JAN 02, 1987
VANGARD	EQ 25 MG HCL	N88392 001 SEP 19, 1983

IBUPROFEN

TABLET; ORAL
IBUPROFEN

BOOTS	600 MG	N70556 001 JUN 14, 1985
	800 MG	N71264 001 JUL 25, 1986
CHELSEA LABS	200 MG	N71765 001 SEP 04, 1987
	300 MG	N71338 001 DEC 01, 1986
	400 MG	N70038 001 SEP 06, 1985
	600 MG	N70041 001 SEP 06, 1985
	800 MG	N71911 001 OCT 13, 1987
MCNEIL	400 MG	N70081 001 JUN 16, 1986
	600 MG	N70476 001 JUN 16, 1986
PAR PHARM	300 MG	N70328 001 AUG 06, 1985
SUPERPHARM	600 MG	N70709 001 APR 25, 1986
ZENITH LABS	200 MG	N71154 001 OCT 27, 1987
	200 MG	N72040 001 APR 29, 1988

NUPRIN

UPJOHN	200 MG	N19012 001 MAY 18, 1984
	200 MG	N19012 003 JUL 29, 1987

RUFEN

BOOTS	600 MG	N18197 002 MAR 05, 1984

IDOXURIDINE

OINTMENT; OPHTHALMIC
STOXIL

SMITHKLINE BEECHAM	0.5%	N15868 001

SOLUTION/DROPS; OPHTHALMIC
STOXIL

SMITHKLINE BEECHAM	0.1%	N13934 001

IMIPRAMINE HYDROCHLORIDE

TABLET; ORAL
IMIPRAMINE HCL

CHELSEA LABS	10 MG	N85875 001
	25 MG	N85878 001
	50 MG	N85877 001
CIRCA	10 MG	N85220 001
	25 MG	N84252 002
	50 MG	N85221 001
LEDERLE	10 MG	N86269 001
	25 MG	N86267 001
	50 MG	N86268 001
ROSEMONT PHARM	25 MG	N87776 001 FEB 10, 1982
VANGARD	10 MG	N88036 001 NOV 03, 1982
	25 MG	N87619 001 FEB 09, 1982
	50 MG	N87631 001 JAN 04, 1982
WEST WARD PHARM	25 MG	N88222 001 MAY 26, 1983
	50 MG	N88223 001 MAY 26, 1983

PRAMINE

ALRA	10 MG	N83827 001
	25 MG	N83827 002
	50 MG	N83827 003

PRESAMINE

RHONE POULENC RORER	10 MG	N11836 006
	25 MG	N11836 003
	50 MG	N11836 007

INDOCYANINE GREEN

INJECTABLE; INJECTION
CARDIO-GREEN

BECTON DICKINSON	10 MG/VIAL	N11525 003
	40 MG/VIAL	N11525 004

Discontinued Drug Products *(continued)*

INDOMETHACIN
CAPSULE; ORAL
INDOMETHACIN

CHELSEA LABS	25 MG	N18690 001 JUL 31, 1984
	50 MG	N18690 002 JUL 31, 1984
	50 MG	N71635 001 MAY 18, 1987
CIRCA	25 MG	N70784 001 AUG 20, 1986
	50 MG	N70785 001 AUG 20, 1986
DURAMED	25 MG	N70326 001 OCT 18, 1985
	50 MG	N70327 001 OCT 18, 1985
PIONEER PHARMS	25 MG	N70813 001 AUG 11, 1986
	50 MG	N70592 001 AUG 11, 1986
ROXANE	25 MG	N70353 001 JUN 18, 1985
	50 MG	N70354 001 JUN 18, 1985
SUPERPHARM	25 MG	N70487 001 OCT 10, 1986
	50 MG	N70488 001 OCT 10, 1986
ZENITH LABS	25 MG	N18730 001 MAY 04, 1984
	50 MG	N18730 002 MAY 04, 1984

INSULIN BIOSYNTHETIC HUMAN
INJECTABLE; INJECTION
HUMULIN BR
LILLY 100 UNITS/ML N19529 001 APR 28, 1986

INSULIN PORK
INJECTABLE; INJECTION
INSULIN
NOVO NORDISK 40 UNITS/ML N17926 001

INSULIN SUSP ISOPHANE BEEF
INJECTABLE; INJECTION
NPH INSULIN
NOVO NORDISK 40 UNITS/ML N17929 001

INSULIN SUSP ISOPHANE PURIFIED PORK
INJECTABLE; INJECTION
NPH ILETIN II (PORK)
LILLY 100 UNITS/ML N18345 001

INSULIN SUSP PROTAMINE ZINC BEEF/PORK
INJECTABLE; INJECTION
PROTAMINE, ZINC & ILETIN I (BEEF-PORK)
LILLY 40 UNITS/ML N17932 001
100 UNITS/ML N17932 002

INSULIN SUSP PROTAMINE ZINC PURIFIED PORK
INJECTABLE; INJECTION
PROTAMINE ZINC AND ILETIN II (PORK)
LILLY 100 UNITS/ML N18346 001

INSULIN ZINC SUSP BEEF
INJECTABLE; INJECTION
LENTE INSULIN
NOVO NORDISK 40 UNITS/ML N17998 001

INSULIN ZINC SUSP EXTENDED BIOSYNTHETIC HUMAN
INJECTABLE; INJECTION
HUMULIN U
LILLY 40 UNITS/ML N19571 001 JUN 10, 1987

INSULIN ZINC SUSP PURIFIED BEEF/PORK
INJECTABLE; INJECTION
LENTARD
NOVO NORDISK 100 UNITS/ML N18384 001

INTRINSIC FACTOR; *MULTIPLE*
SEE COBALT CHLORIDE, CO-60; CYANOCOBALAMIN; CYANOCOBALAMIN, CO-60; INTRINSIC FACTOR

INVERT SUGAR
INJECTABLE; INJECTION
TRAVERT 10% IN PLASTIC CONTAINER
BAXTER 10 GM/100 ML N16717 001

IODIPAMIDE SODIUM
INJECTABLE; INJECTION
CHOLOGRAFIN SODIUM
BRACCO 20% N09321 001

Discontinued Drug Products *(continued)*

IODOHIPPURATE SODIUM, I-123
INJECTABLE; INJECTION
NEPHROFLOW
MEDI PHYSICS 1mCi/ML N18289 001 DEC 28, 1984

IODOXAMATE MEGLUMINE
INJECTABLE; INJECTION
CHOLOVUE
BRACCO 9.9% N18077 001
40.3% N18076 001

IOPHENDYLATE
INJECTABLE; INJECTION
PANTOPAQUE
ALCON 100% N05319 001

IOTROLAN
INJECTABLE; INTRATHECAL
OSMOVIST
BERLEX EQ 190 MG IODINE/ML N19580 001 DEC 07, 1989
EQ 240 MG IODINE/ML N19580 002 DEC 07, 1989

IRON DEXTRAN
INJECTABLE; INJECTION
IRON DEXTRAN
FISONS EQ 50 MG IRON/ML N10787 002

ISOETHARINE HYDROCHLORIDE
SOLUTION; INHALATION
BRONKOSOL
STERLING WINTHROP 0.25% N12339 009
ISOETHARINE HCL
ASTRA 0.25% N88472 001 MAR 14, 1984
0.062% N87937 001 NOV 15, 1982
0.125% N87938 001 NOV 15, 1982
0.167% N88470 001 MAR 14, 1984
0.2% N88471 001 MAR 14, 1984

ISOETHARINE HYDROCHLORIDE *(continued)*
SOLUTION; INHALATION
ISOETHARINE HCL
BAXTER 0.08% N88144 001 JUL 29, 1983
0.25% N88146 001 AUG 01, 1983
0.14% N88145 001 MAR 26, 1984
DEY 0.08% N88187 001 DEC 03, 1982
0.25% N88188 001 DEC 03, 1982
1% N86763 001
0.1% N87389 001
0.17% N87390 001
PARKE DAVIS 1% N85889 001
0.5% N85997 001

ISOETHARINE MESYLATE
AEROSOL, METERED; INHALATION
ISOETHARINE MESYLATE
BARRE 0.34 MG/INH N87858 001 AUG 21, 1984

ISONIAZID
INJECTABLE; INJECTION
ISONIAZID
QUAD PHARMS 100 MG/ML N89816 001 OCT 28, 1988
RIMIFON
ROCHE 100 MG/ML N08420 003
25 MG/ML N08420 002
SYRUP; ORAL
RIMIFON
ROCHE 50 MG/5 ML N08420 001
TABLET; ORAL
DOW-ISONIAZID
DOW PHARMS 300 MG N80330 002
HYZYD
WALLACE 100 MG N80134 003
300 MG N80134 004
INH
CIBA 300 MG N80935 001

ISONIAZID (*continued*)

TABLET; ORAL
ISONIAZID

ANABOLIC	100 MG	N84050 001
CHELSEA LABS	100 MG	N85790 001
	300 MG	N85784 001
CIRCA	100 MG	N80401 001
	300 MG	N83178 001
LILLY	100 MG	N08499 002
	300 MG	N08499 003
MK LABS	100 MG	N80941 001
PANRAY	50 MG	N08428 001
	100 MG	N08428 002
	300 MG	N08428 003
PERRIGO	100 MG	N83060 001
PHARMAVITE	100 MG	N85091 001
PUREPAC PHARM	50 MG	N80132 003 JUL 14, 1982
	100 MG	N80132 004 JUL 14, 1982
WHITEWORTH TOWNE	100 MG	N80120 002
NYDRAZID		
SQUIBB	100 MG	N08392 003
STANOZIDE		
EVERYLIFE	100 MG	N80126 001
	300 MG	N80126 002

ISOPROPAMIDE IODIDE

TABLET; ORAL
DARBID

SMITHKLINE BEECHAM	EQ 5 MG BASE	N10744 001

ISOPROTERENOL HYDROCHLORIDE

AEROSOL; INHALATION		
NORISODRINE AEROTROL		
ABBOTT	0.25%	N16814 001
INJECTABLE; INJECTION		
ISOPROTERENOL HCL		
FUJISAWA	0.2 MG/ML	N83431 001
SOLUTION; INHALATION		
ISOPROTERENOL HCL		
ARMOUR	0.031%	N87935 001 NOV 18, 1982
	0.062%	N87936 001 NOV 18, 1982
DEY	0.5%	N86764 001 JAN 04, 1982
PARKE DAVIS	0.5%	N85540 001
	0.25%	N85994 001

ISOPROTERENOL HYDROCHLORIDE (*continued*)

SOLUTION; INHALATION		
VAPO-ISO		
FISONS	0.5%	N16813 001
TABLET; RECTAL, SUBLINGUAL		
ISUPREL		
STERLING WINTHROP	15 MG	N06328 002

ISOPROTERENOL HYDROCHLORIDE; *MULTIPLE*

SEE <u>ACETYLCYSTEINE; ISOPROTERENOL HYDROCHLORIDE</u>

ISOPROTERENOL SULFATE

POWDER; INHALATION
NORISODRINE

ABBOTT	10%	N06905 003
	25%	N06905 002

ISOSORBIDE DINITRATE

TABLET; ORAL
ISOSORBIDE DINITRATE

SUPERPHARM	5 MG	N89190 001 FEB 17, 1987
	10 MG	N89191 001 FEB 17, 1987
	20 MG	N89192 001 FEB 17, 1987

ISOSORBIDE MONONITRATE

TABLET, EXTENDED RELEASE; ORAL
IMDUR

SCHERING PLOUGH	30 MG	N20225 001 AUG 12, 1993

KANAMYCIN SULFATE

CAPSULE; ORAL
KANTREX

APOTHECON	EQ 500 MG BASE	N60516 001
	EQ 500 MG BASE	N61911 001

Discontinued Drug Products *(continued)*

KANAMYCIN SULFATE *(continued)*

INJECTABLE; INJECTION

KANAMYCIN SULFATE		
FUJISAWA	EQ 75 MG BASE/2 ML	N62504 001 APR 05, 1984
	EQ 500 MG BASE/2 ML	N62504 002 APR 05, 1984
	EQ 1 GM BASE/3 ML	N62504 003 APR 05, 1984
INTL MEDICATION	EQ 500 MG BASE/2 ML	N62466 001 SEP 30, 1983
	EQ 1 GM BASE/3 ML	N62466 002 SEP 30, 1983
QUAD PHARMS	EQ 75 MG BASE/2 ML	N62642 001 FEB 03, 1986
	EQ 500 MG BASE/2 ML	N62642 002 FEB 03, 1986
	EQ 1 GM BASE/3 ML	N62642 003 FEB 03, 1986
WARNER CHILCOTT	EQ 1 GM BASE/3 ML	N63092 001 OCT 11, 1989
KANTREX		
APOTHECON	EQ 75 MG BASE/2 ML	N61655 003
	EQ 75 MG BASE/2 ML	N62564 001 SEP 21, 1984
	EQ 500 MG BASE/2 ML	N61655 001
	EQ 500 MG BASE/2 ML	N62564 002 SEP 21, 1984
	EQ 1 GM BASE/3 ML	N61655 002
	EQ 1 GM BASE/3 ML	N62564 003 SEP 21, 1984
KLEBCIL		
KING PHARMS	EQ 75 MG BASE/2 ML	N62170 001
	EQ 500 MG BASE/2 ML	N62170 002
	EQ 1 GM BASE/3 ML	N62170 003

KETAMINE HYDROCHLORIDE

INJECTABLE; INJECTION

KETAMINE HCL		
QUAD PHARMS	EQ 10 MG BASE/ML	N71949 001 APR 11, 1988
	EQ 50 MG BASE/ML	N71950 001 APR 11, 1988
	EQ 100 MG BASE/ML	N71951 001 APR 11, 1988

KETOCONAZOLE

SUSPENSION; ORAL

NIZORAL		
JANSSEN	100 MG/5 ML	N70767 001 NOV 07, 1986

LABETALOL HYDROCHLORIDE

TABLET; ORAL

NORMODYNE		
SCHERING	400 MG	N18687 004 AUG 01, 1984
TRANDATE		
GLAXO	400 MG	N18716 004 AUG 01, 1984

LABETALOL HYDROCHLORIDE; *MULTIPLE*

SEE HYDROCHLOROTHIAZIDE; LABETALOL HYDROCHLORIDE

LACTULOSE

SOLUTION; ORAL

LACTULOSE		
PENNEX	10 GM/15 ML	N71841 001 SEP 22, 1988

SOLUTION; ORAL, RECTAL

GENERLAC		
PENNEX	10 GM/15 ML	N71842 001 SEP 27, 1988
LACTULOSE		
SOLVAY	10 GM/15 ML	N17906 001
PORTALAC		
SOLVAY	10 GM/15 ML	N72374 001 MAR 22, 1989

LEUCOVORIN CALCIUM

INJECTABLE; INJECTION

LEUCOVORIN CALCIUM		
ABIC	EQ 3 MG BASE/ML	N89352 001 JUN 01, 1988
	EQ 50 MG BASE/VIAL	N89353 001 JUN 01, 1988
FUJISAWA	EQ 50 MG BASE/VIAL	N88939 001 DEC 01, 1986
IMMUNEX	EQ 3 MG BASE/ML	N08107 001
QUAD PHARMS	EQ 50 MG BASE/VIAL	N89496 001 MAR 05, 1987
	EQ 5 MG BASE/ML	N89503 001 OCT 05, 1987
	EQ 5 MG BASE/ML	N89504 001 DEC 22, 1987
	EQ 100 MG BASE/VIAL	N89636 001 DEC 24, 1987

Discontinued Drug Products *(continued)*

LEUCOVORIN CALCIUM *(continued)*

TABLET; ORAL
LEUCOVORIN CALCIUM

PAR PHARM	EQ 5 MG BASE	N71600 001 OCT 14, 1987
	EQ 25 MG BASE	N71598 001 OCT 14, 1987

LEVALLORPHAN TARTRATE

INJECTABLE; INJECTION
LORFAN

ROCHE	1 MG/ML	N10423 001

LEVODOPA

CAPSULE; ORAL
BENDOPA

ICN	100 MG	N16948 003
	250 MG	N16948 001
	500 MG	N16948 002

LARODOPA

ROCHE	100 MG	N16912 002
	250 MG	N16912 001
	500 MG	N16912 006

LEVONORDEFRIN; MEPIVACAINE HYDROCHLORIDE

INJECTABLE; INJECTION
ARESTOCAINE HCL W/ LEVONORDEFRIN

SOLVAY	0.05 MG/ML;2%	N85010 001

LEVONORDEFRIN; PROCAINE HYDROCHLORIDE; PROPOXYCAINE HYDROCHLORIDE

INJECTABLE; INJECTION
RAVOCAINE AND NOVOCAIN W/ NEO-COBEFRIN

STERLING WINTHROP	0.05 MG/ML;2%;0.4%	N08592 007

LEVONORGESTREL

IMPLANT; IMPLANTATION
NORPLANT

POPULATION COUNCIL	36 MG/IMPLANT	N19897 001 DEC 10, 1990

LEVOPROPOXYPHENE NAPSYLATE, ANHYDROUS

CAPSULE; ORAL
NOVRAD

LILLY	EQ 50 MG BASE	N12928 006
	EQ 100 MG BASE	N12928 004

SUSPENSION; ORAL
NOVRAD

LILLY	EQ 50 MG BASE/5 ML	N12928 002

LIDOCAINE

SUPPOSITORY; RECTAL
XYLOCAINE

ASTRA	100 MG	N13077 001

LIDOCAINE; *MULTIPLE*

SEE <u>BACITRACIN ZINC; LIDOCAINE; NEOMYCIN SULFATE; POLYMYXIN BSULFATE</u>

LIDOCAINE HYDROCHLORIDE

INJECTABLE; INJECTION
LIDOCAINE HCL

ABBOTT	1.5%	N88330 001 MAY 17, 1984
	10%	N87980 001 FEB 02, 1983
BEL MAR	1%	N80710 001
	2%	N80760 001
ELKINS SINN	4%	N84626 001
	0.5%	N85131 001
FUJISAWA	1%	N80390 001
	1%	N80420 001
	1%	N86761 001
	1.5%	N80420 005
	2%	N80390 002
	2%	N80420 002
	2%	N86761 002
INTL MEDICATION	4%	N17702 002
	1 GM/VIAL	N18543 001
	2 GM/VIAL	N18543 002
MILES	1%	N80414 001
	2%	N80414 002
SEARLE	1%	N83135 001
	2%	N83135 002
STERIS	1%	N83627 001
	2%	N83627 002

LIDOCAINE HCL 0.1% AND DEXTROSE 5% IN PLASTIC CONTAINER

BAXTER	100 MG/100 ML	N18461 001

Discontinued Drug Products *(continued)*

LIDOCAINE HYDROCHLORIDE *(continued)*

INJECTABLE; INJECTION
LIDOCAINE HCL 0.2% IN DEXTROSE 5% IN PLASTIC CONTAINER
ABBOTT 200 MG/100 ML N18954 001 JUL 09, 1985
XYLOCAINE
ASTRA 1% N10418 005
1.5% N10418 009
2% N10418 007
SOLUTION; TOPICAL
LARYNGOTRACHEAL ANESTHESIA KIT
KENDALL 4% N87931 001 JUN 10, 1983
LIDOCAINE HCL
PACO 4% N89688 001 JUN 30, 1989
PEDIATRIC LTA KIT
ABBOTT 2% N88572 001 JUL 31, 1984

LIDOCAINE HYDROCHLORIDE; *MULTIPLE*

SEE DIHYDROERGOTAMINE MESYLATE; HEPARIN SODIUM; LIDOCAINE HYDROCHLORIDE
SEE EPINEPHRINE; LIDOCAINE HYDROCHLORIDE

LINCOMYCIN HYDROCHLORIDE

INJECTABLE; INJECTION
LINCOMYCIN HCL
QUAD PHARMS EQ 300 MG BASE/ML N62784 001 MAR 14, 1988

LINDANE

LOTION; TOPICAL
GAMENE
SOLA BARNES HIND 1% N84989 001
SHAMPOO; TOPICAL
GAMENE
SOLA BARNES HIND 1% N84988 001

LIOTHYRONINE SODIUM

TABLET; ORAL
LIOTHYRONINE SODIUM
CIRCA EQ 0.025 MG BASE N85755 001 JAN 25, 1982
EQ 0.05 MG BASE N85753 001 FEB 03, 1982

LIOTRIX (T4;T3)

TABLET; ORAL
EUTHROID-0.5
PARKE DAVIS 0.03 MG;0.0075 MG N16680 001
EUTHROID-1
PARKE DAVIS 0.06 MG;0.015 MG N16680 002
EUTHROID-2
PARKE DAVIS 0.12 MG;0.03 MG N16680 003
EUTHROID-3
PARKE DAVIS 0.18 MG;0.045 MG N16680 004
THYROLAR-5
FOREST LABS 0.25 MG;0.0625 MG N16807 006

LITHIUM CARBONATE

CAPSULE; ORAL
LITHIUM CARBONATE
CIRCA 300 MG N70407 001 MAR 19, 1987
ROSEMONT PHARM 300 MG N72542 001 FEB 01, 1989
TABLET; ORAL
ESKALITH
SMITHKLINE BEECHAM 300 MG N17971 001
LITHANE
MILES 300 MG N18833 001 JUL 18, 1985
TABLET, EXTENDED RELEASE; ORAL
LITHOBID
CIBA 300 MG N18027 001

LOPERAMIDE HYDROCHLORIDE

CAPSULE; ORAL
IMODIUM
JANSSEN 2 MG N17690 001
SOLUTION; ORAL
IMODIUM
JANSSEN 1 MG/5 ML N19037 001 JUL 31, 1984

LORAZEPAM

TABLET; ORAL
LORAZ
QUANTUM PHARMICS 0.5 MG N70200 001 AUG 09, 1985
1 MG N70201 001 AUG 09, 1985
2 MG N70202 001 AUG 09, 1985

Discontinued Drug Products *(continued)*

LORAZEPAM *(continued)*

TABLET; ORAL

LORAZEPAM

AM THERAP	0.5 MG	N70727 001 MAR 07, 1986
	1 MG	N70728 001 MAR 07, 1986
	2 MG	N70729 001 MAR 07, 1986
PAR PHARM	0.5 MG	N70675 001 DEC 01, 1986
	1 MG	N70676 001 DEC 01, 1986
	2 MG	N70677 001 DEC 01, 1986
ROSEMONT PHARM	1 MG	N70539 001 DEC 22, 1986
	2 MG	N70540 001 DEC 22, 1986
WARNER CHILCOTT	1 MG	N71038 001 JAN 12, 1988
	2 MG	N71039 001 JAN 12, 1988

LOXAPINE SUCCINATE

TABLET; ORAL

LOXITANE

LEDERLE	EQ 10 MG BASE	N17525 006
	EQ 25 MG BASE	N17525 007
	EQ 50 MG BASE	N17525 008

MAGNESIUM ACETATE; *MULTIPLE*

SEE AMINO ACIDS; MAGNESIUM ACETATE; PHOSPHORIC ACID; POTASSIUM ACETATE; SODIUM CHLORIDE

SEE AMINO ACIDS; MAGNESIUM ACETATE; POTASSIUM ACETATE; SODIUM CHLORIDE

SEE AMINO ACIDS; MAGNESIUM ACETATE; POTASSIUM ACETATE; SODIUM CHLORIDE; SODIUM PHOSPHATE, DIBASIC

MAGNESIUM CHLORIDE; *MULTIPLE*

SEE AMINO ACIDS; DEXTROSE; MAGNESIUM CHLORIDE; POTASSIUM CHLORIDE; SODIUM CHLORIDE; SODIUM PHOSPHATE, DIBASIC

SEE AMINO ACIDS; DEXTROSE; MAGNESIUM CHLORIDE; POTASSIUM CHLORIDE; POTASSIUM PHOSPHATE, DIBASIC; SODIUM CHLORIDE

SEE AMINO ACIDS; MAGNESIUM CHLORIDE; POTASSIUM ACETATE; POTASSIUM CHLORIDE; SODIUM ACETATE

SEE AMINO ACIDS; MAGNESIUM CHLORIDE; POTASSIUM CHLORIDE; SODIUM CHLORIDE; SODIUM PHOSPHATE, DIBASIC

SEE AMINO ACIDS; MAGNESIUM CHLORIDE; POTASSIUM CHLORIDE; POTASSIUM PHOSPHATE, DIBASIC; SODIUM CHLORIDE

SEE CALCIUM CHLORIDE; DEXTROSE; MAGNESIUM CHLORIDE; SODIUM ACETATE; SODIUM CHLORIDE

SEE CALCIUM CHLORIDE; DEXTROSE; MAGNESIUM CHLORIDE; SODIUM CHLORIDE; SODIUM LACTATE

SEE CALCIUM CHLORIDE; MAGNESIUM CHLORIDE; POTASSIUM CHLORIDE; SODIUM ACETATE; SODIUM CHLORIDE

MAGNESIUM CHLORIDE; POTASSIUM CHLORIDE; SODIUM ACETATE; SODIUM CHLORIDE; SODIUM GLUCONATE

SOLUTION; IRRIGATION

PHYSIOSOL IN PLASTIC CONTAINER

ABBOTT	14 MG/100 ML;37 MG/100 ML;222 MG/100 ML;526 MG/100 ML;502 MG/100 ML	N18406 001

MAGNESIUM TRISILICATE; *MULTIPLE*

SEE ALUMINUM HYDROXIDE; MAGNESIUM TRISILICATE

MANNITOL

INJECTABLE; INJECTION

MANNITOL 10%		
MILES	10 GM/100 ML	N16472 002
MANNITOL 15%		
MILES	15 GM/100 ML	N16472 005
MANNITOL 20%		
MILES	20 GM/100 ML	N16472 004
MANNITOL 25%		
FUJISAWA	12.5 GM/50 ML	N86754 001
MERCK SHARP DOHME	12.5 GM/50 ML	N05620 001

Discontinued Drug Products *(continued)*

MANNITOL *(continued)*

SOLUTION; IRRIGATION

RESECTISOL

MCGAW	5 GM/100 ML	N16704 002

MANNITOL; SORBITOL

SOLUTION; IRRIGATION

SORBITOL-MANNITOL

ABBOTT	540 MG/100 ML;2.7 GM/100 ML	N80224 001

MAPROTILINE HYDROCHLORIDE

TABLET; ORAL

MAPROTILINE HCL

AM THERAP	25 MG	N72129 001 JAN 14, 1988
	50 MG	N72130 001 JAN 14, 1988
	75 MG	N72131 001 JAN 14, 1988
CIRCA	25 MG	N71943 001 DEC 30, 1987
	50 MG	N71944 001 DEC 30, 1987
	75 MG	N71945 001 DEC 30, 1987

MAZINDOL

TABLET; ORAL

MAZANOR

WYETH AYERST	2 MG	N17980 001

MEBUTAMATE

TABLET; ORAL

DORMATE

WALLACE PHARMS	600 MG	N17374 001

MECLIZINE HYDROCHLORIDE

TABLET; ORAL

MECLIZINE HCL

ANABOLIC	25 MG	N85891 001
CIRCA	12.5 MG	N85195 001
SUPERPHARM	12.5 MG	N89113 001 AUG 20, 1985
	25 MG	N89114 001 AUG 20, 1985

MECLIZINE HYDROCHLORIDE *(continued)*

TABLET; ORAL

MECLIZINE HCL

UDL	12.5 MG	N88256 001 JUN 13, 1983
	25 MG	N88257 001 JUN 13, 1983
VANGARD	12.5 MG	N87877 001 APR 20, 1982
	25 MG	N87620 001 JAN 04, 1982

TABLET, CHEWABLE; ORAL

MECLIZINE HCL

ANABOLIC	25 MG	N86392 001

MECLOFENAMATE SODIUM

CAPSULE; ORAL

MECLODIUM

QUANTUM PHARMICS	EQ 50 MG BASE	N71380 001 JUL 14, 1987
	EQ 100 MG BASE	N71381 001 JUL 14, 1987

MECLOFENAMATE SODIUM

AM THERAP	EQ 50 MG BASE	N71362 001 FEB 10, 1987
	EQ 100 MG BASE	N71363 001 FEB 10, 1987
CHELSEA LABS	EQ 50 MG BASE	N71640 001 AUG 11, 1987
	EQ 100 MG BASE	N71641 001 AUG 11, 1987
CIRCA	EQ 50 MG BASE	N70400 001 NOV 25, 1986
	EQ 100 MG BASE	N70401 001 NOV 25, 1986
PAR PHARM	EQ 50 MG BASE	N72077 001 MAR 10, 1988
	EQ 100 MG BASE	N72078 001 MAR 10, 1988
ROSEMONT PHARM	EQ 50 MG BASE	N71007 001 MAR 25, 1988
	EQ 100 MG BASE	N71008 001 MAR 25, 1988
VITARINE	EQ 50 MG BASE	N71710 001 JUN 15, 1988
	EQ 100 MG BASE	N71684 001 JUN 15, 1988

Discontinued Drug Products *(continued)*

MEFLOQUINE HYDROCHLORIDE

TABLET; ORAL
MEFLOQUINE HCL

US ARMY	250 MG	N19578 001 MAY 02, 1989

MEGESTROL ACETATE

TABLET; ORAL
MEGESTROL ACETATE

ROSEMONT PHARM	20 MG	N70646 001 OCT 02, 1987
	40 MG	N70647 001 OCT 02, 1987

MEGLUMINE; *MULTIPLE*

SEE CALCIUM; MEGLUMINE; METRIZOIC ACID

MEGLUMINE METRIZOATE; *MULTIPLE*

SEE CALCIUM METRIZOATE; MEGLUMINE METRIZOATE; METRIZOATE MAGNESIUM; METRIZOATE SODIUM

MENADIOL SODIUM DIPHOSPHATE

INJECTABLE; INJECTION
KAPPADIONE

LILLY	10 MG/ML	N05725 001

SYNKAYVITE

ROCHE	10 MG/ML	N03718 006
	5 MG/ML	N03718 004
	37.5 MG/ML	N03718 008

TABLET; ORAL
SYNKAYVITE

ROCHE	5 MG	N03718 010

MENADIONE

TABLET; ORAL
MENADIONE

LILLY	5 MG	N02139 003

MEPENZOLATE BROMIDE

SOLUTION; ORAL
CANTIL

MERRELL DOW	25 MG/5 ML	N10679 004

MEPERIDINE HYDROCHLORIDE

INJECTABLE; INJECTION
MEPERIDINE HCL

ASTRA	25 MG/ML	N89781 001 MAR 31, 1989
	50 MG/ML	N89782 001 MAR 31, 1989
	50 MG/ML	N89783 001 MAR 31, 1989
	75 MG/ML	N89785 001 MAR 31, 1989
	100 MG/ML	N89786 001 MAR 31, 1989
	100 MG/ML	N89787 001 MAR 31, 1989
ELKINS SINN	25 MG/ML	N88279 001 JUN 15, 1984
	50 MG/ML	N88280 001 JUN 15, 1984
	75 MG/ML	N88281 001 JUN 15, 1984
	100 MG/ML	N88282 001 JUN 15, 1984
INTL MEDICATION	10 MG/ML	N86332 001
KNOLL PHARM	25 MG/ML	N80388 001
	50 MG/ML	N80385 001
	50 MG/ML	N80387 001
	75 MG/ML	N80389 001
	100 MG/ML	N80386 001
PARKE DAVIS	50 MG/ML	N80364 002
	75 MG/ML	N80364 003
	100 MG/ML	N80364 001

MEPERIDINE HYDROCHLORIDE; *MULTIPLE*

SEE ATROPINE SULFATE; MEPERIDINE HYDROCHLORIDE

MEPIVACAINE HYDROCHLORIDE

INJECTABLE; INJECTION
ARESTOCAINE HCL

SOLVAY	3%	N84777 002 APR 18, 1982

MEPIVACAINE HYDROCHLORIDE; *MULTIPLE*

SEE LEVONORDEFRIN; MEPIVACAINE HYDROCHLORIDE

MEPREDNISONE

TABLET; ORAL
BETAPAR

SCHERING	4 MG	N16053 002

Discontinued Drug Products *(continued)*

MEPROBAMATE

CAPSULE; ORAL		
EQUANIL		
WYETH AYERST	400 MG	N12455 002
TABLET; ORAL		
BAMATE		
ALRA	200 MG	N80380 001
	400 MG	N80380 002
MEPRIAM		
LEMMON	400 MG	N16069 001
MEPROBAMATE		
ANABOLIC	200 MG	N84220 001
	400 MG	N84589 001
CHELSEA LABS	600 MG	N85719 001
ELKINS SINN	200 MG	N15426 002
	400 MG	N15426 001
HEATHER	400 MG	N16928 003
	600 MG	N84329 001
ICN	200 MG	N15139 006
	400 MG	N15139 005
KM LEE	400 MG	N89538 001 NOV 25, 1987
LEDERLE	400 MG	N86299 001
MALLARD	400 MG	N15072 002
PARKE DAVIS	200 MG	N84744 001
	400 MG	N84744 002
PERRIGO	200 MG	N84546 001
	400 MG	N84547 001
PHARMERAL	400 MG	N84153 001
PRIVATE FORM	400 MG	N14601 001
ROSEMONT PHARM	200 MG	N87825 001 MAR 18, 1982
	400 MG	N87826 001 MAR 18, 1982
SOLVAY	200 MG	N84435 001
STANLABS	200 MG	N14474 002
	400 MG	N14474 004
VANGARD	400 MG	N88011 001 JUL 14, 1982
WHITEWORTH TOWNE	200 MG	N83830 001
	400 MG	N83442 001
ZENITH LABS	200 MG	N15438 001
	400 MG	N15438 002
TRANMEP		
SOLVAY	400 MG	N84369 001

MEPROBAMATE; *MULTIPLE*

SEE <u>ASPIRIN; MEPROBAMATE</u>

SEE <u>ESTROGENS, CONJUGATED; MEPROBAMATE</u>

MESTRANOL; *MULTIPLE*

SEE <u>ETHYNODIOL DIACETATE; MESTRANOL</u>

MESTRANOL; NORETHINDRONE

TABLET; ORAL-20		
NORINYL		
SYNTEX	0.1 MG;2 MG	N13625 004
TABLET; ORAL-21		
NORINYL 1+80 21-DAY		
SYNTEX	0.08 MG;1 MG	N16724 001
ORTHO-NOVUM 1/80 21		
JOHNSON RW	0.08 MG;1 MG	N16715 001
ORTHO-NOVUM 10-21		
JOHNSON RW	0.06 MG;10 MG	N12728 001
ORTHO-NOVUM 2-21		
JOHNSON RW	0.1 MG;2 MG	N12728 005
TABLET; ORAL-28		
NORINYL 1+80 28-DAY		
SYNTEX	0.08 MG;1 MG	N16725 001
ORTHO-N0VUM 1/80 28		
JOHNSON RW	0.08 MG;1 MG	N16715 002

MESTRANOL; NORETHYNODREL

TABLET; ORAL		
ENOVID		
SEARLE	0.075 MG;5 MG	N10976 008
	0.15 MG;9.85 MG	N10976 005
TABLET; ORAL-20		
ENOVID		
SEARLE	0.075 MG;5 MG	N10976 004
ENOVID-E		
SEARLE	0.1 MG;2.5 MG	N10976 006
TABLET; ORAL-21		
ENOVID-E 21		
SEARLE	0.1 MG;2.5 MG	N10976 007

METAPROTERENOL SULFATE

SOLUTION; INHALATION		
METAPROTERENOL SULFATE		
DEY	0.33%	N71806 001 AUG 05, 1988
	0.5%	N71805 001 AUG 05, 1988
PENNEX	5%	N72190 001 JUN 07, 1988

Discontinued Drug Products *(continued)*

METAPROTERENOL SULFATE *(continued)*

TABLET; ORAL

METAPROTERENOL SULFATE		
AM THERAP	10 MG	N72054 001 JUN 23, 1988
	20 MG	N72055 001 JUN 23, 1988
ROSEMONT PHARM	10 MG	N71013 001 JAN 25, 1988
	20 MG	N71014 001 JAN 25, 1988

METARAMINOL BITARTRATE

INJECTABLE; INJECTION

METARAMINOL BITARTRATE		
ELKINS SINN	EQ 10 MG BASE/ML	N83363 001
FUJISAWA	EQ 10 MG BASE/ML	N80431 001
SEARLE	EQ 10 MG BASE/ML	N86418 001
	EQ 20 MG BASE/ML	N86418 002

METHACYCLINE HYDROCHLORIDE

CAPSULE; ORAL

RONDOMYCIN		
WALLACE	EQ 140 MG BASE	N60641 001
	EQ 280 MG BASE	N60641 002

SYRUP; ORAL

RONDOMYCIN		
WALLACE	EQ 70 MG BASE/5 ML	N60641 003

METHADONE HYDROCHLORIDE

TABLET, DISPERSIBLE; ORAL

WESTADONE		
EON LABS	2.5 MG	N17108 001
	5 MG	N17108 002
	10 MG	N17108 003
	40 MG	N17108 004

METHAMPHETAMINE HYDROCHLORIDE

TABLET; ORAL

METHAMPEX		
LEMMON	10 MG	N83889 001
METHAMPHETAMINE HCL		
LEMMON	5 MG	N86359 001

METHARBITAL

TABLET; ORAL

GEMONIL		
ABBOTT	100 MG	N08322 001

METHDILAZINE

TABLET, CHEWABLE; ORAL

TACARYL		
WESTWOOD SQUIBB	3.6 MG	N11950 009

METHDILAZINE HYDROCHLORIDE

SYRUP; ORAL

METHDILAZINE HCL		
BARRE	4 MG/5 ML	N87122 001
TACARYL		
WESTWOOD SQUIBB	4 MG/5 ML	N11950 007

TABLET; ORAL

TACARYL		
WESTWOOD SQUIBB	8 MG	N11950 006

METHICILLIN SODIUM

INJECTABLE; INJECTION

STAPHCILLIN		
BRISTOL	EQ 900 MG BASE/VIAL	N50117 001
	EQ 3.6 GM BASE/VIAL	N50117 002
	EQ 5.4 GM BASE/VIAL	N50117 003

METHIXENE HYDROCHLORIDE

TABLET; ORAL

TREST		
SANDOZ	1 MG	N13420 001

METHOCARBAMOL

TABLET; ORAL

DELAXIN		
FERNDALE LABS	500 MG	N85454 001
METHOCARBAMOL		
AM THERAP	500 MG	N89417 001 FEB 11, 1987
	750 MG	N89418 001 FEB 11, 1987
ASCOT	500 MG	N87660 001 OCT 27, 1982
	750 MG	N87661 001 OCT 27, 1982
BARR	500 MG	N84488 001
CIRCA	500 MG	N83605 001
	750 MG	N83605 002
HEATHER	500 MG	N84675 001
	750 MG	N84924 001
MYLAN	500 MG	N84259 001
	750 MG	N84323 001

Discontinued Drug Products *(continued)*

METHOCARBAMOL *(continued)*

TABLET; ORAL
METHOCARBAMOL

PHARMERAL	500 MG	N84231 002
	750 MG	N84471 001
PIONEER PHARMS	500 MG	N88731 001 DEC 13, 1985
	750 MG	N89082 001 DEC 13, 1985
ROXANE	500 MG	N88646 001 FEB 29, 1984
	750 MG	N88647 001 FEB 29, 1984
SOLVAY	500 MG	N84448 001
	750 MG	N84449 001
UPSHER SMITH	500 MG	N87453 001
	750 MG	N87454 001

METHOTREXATE SODIUM

INJECTABLE; INJECTION
ABITREXATE

ABIC	EQ 25 MG BASE/ML	N89161 001 MAR 10, 1987
	EQ 50 MG BASE/VIAL	N89354 001 JUL 17, 1987
	EQ 100 MG BASE/VIAL	N89355 001 JUL 17, 1987
	EQ 250 MG BASE/VIAL	N89356 001 JUL 17, 1987

FOLEX PFS

PHARMACIA	EQ 25 MG BASE/ML	N89180 001 JAN 03, 1986

METHOTREXATE SODIUM

FUJISAWA	EQ 25 MG BASE/ML	N89263 001 JUN 13, 1986
	EQ 25 MG BASE/ML	N89322 001 JUN 13, 1986
	EQ 20 MG BASE/VIAL	N88935 001 OCT 11, 1985
	EQ 50 MG BASE/VIAL	N88936 001 OCT 11, 1985
	EQ 100 MG BASE/VIAL	N88937 001 OCT 11, 1985
	EQ 2.5 MG BASE/ML	N89323 001 JUN 13, 1986

METHOTREXATE SODIUM *(continued)*

INJECTABLE; INJECTION
METHOTREXATE SODIUM

QUAD PHARMS	EQ 25 MG BASE/ML	N89308 001 JUL 10, 1986
	EQ 25 MG BASE/ML	N89309 001 JUL 10, 1986
	EQ 20 MG BASE/VIAL	N89293 001 JUL 10, 1986
	EQ 50 MG BASE/VIAL	N89294 001 JUL 10, 1986
	EQ 100 MG BASE/VIAL	N89295 001 JUL 10, 1986
	EQ 250 MG BASE/VIAL	N89296 001 JUL 10, 1986

MEXATE

BRISTOL	EQ 20 MG BASE/VIAL	N86358 001
	EQ 50 MG BASE/VIAL	N86358 002
	EQ 100 MG BASE/VIAL	N86358 003
	EQ 250 MG BASE/VIAL	N86358 004

METHOXAMINE HYDROCHLORIDE

INJECTABLE; INJECTION
VASOXYL

BURROUGHS WELLCOME	10 MG/ML	N06772 002

METHOXSALEN

CAPSULE; ORAL
METHOXSALEN

GENEVA PHARMS	10 MG	N87781 001 JUN 08, 1982

METHYCLOTHIAZIDE

TABLET; ORAL
METHYCLOTHIAZIDE

CHELSEA LABS	2.5 MG	N88750 001 SEP 06, 1984
CIRCA	2.5 MG	N85487 001 MAR 11, 1982
	5 MG	N85476 001 MAR 11, 1982
MYLAN	2.5 MG	N87671 001 AUG 17, 1982
ROSEMONT PHARM	5 MG	N88745 001 MAR 21, 1985

METHYCLOTHIAZIDE; *MULTIPLE*

SEE DESERPIDINE; METHYCLOTHIAZIDE

Discontinued Drug Products *(continued)*

METHYCLOTHIAZIDE; PARGYLINE HYDROCHLORIDE

TABLET; ORAL
EUTRON
ABBOTT 5 MG;25 MG N16047 001

METHYLDOPA

TABLET; ORAL
METHYLDOPA
CHELSEA LABS 125 MG N70260 001 JUN 24, 1985
250 MG N70261 001 JUN 24, 1985
500 MG N70262 001 JUN 24, 1985
CIRCA 125 MG N70245 001 FEB 25, 1986
250 MG N70246 001 FEB 25, 1986
500 MG N70247 001 FEB 25, 1986
DURAMED 250 MG N71006 001 DEC 16, 1986
500 MG N71009 001 DEC 16, 1986
PARKE DAVIS 125 MG N70331 001 APR 15, 1986
250 MG N70332 001 APR 15, 1986
500 MG N70333 001 APR 15, 1986
ROXANE 125 MG N70192 001 APR 25, 1986
250 MG N70193 001 APR 25, 1986
500 MG N70194 001 APR 25, 1986

METHYLDOPA; *MULTIPLE*

SEE CHLOROTHIAZIDE; METHYLDOPA
SEE HYDROCHLOROTHIAZIDE; METHYLDOPA

METHYLDOPATE HYDROCHLORIDE

INJECTABLE; INJECTION
METHYLDOPATE HCL
FUJISAWA 50 MG/ML N70652 001 JUN 03, 1986
QUAD PHARMS 50 MG/ML N71024 001 SEP 18, 1986

METHYLPREDNISOLONE

TABLET; ORAL
METHYLPREDNISOLONE
CHELSEA LABS 4 MG N86161 001 FEB 09, 1982
16 MG N86159 001 FEB 09, 1982
EON LABS 4 MG N87341 001
HEATHER 4 MG N85650 001

METHYLPREDNISOLONE; NEOMYCIN SULFATE

OINTMENT; OPHTHALMIC
NEO-MEDROL
UPJOHN 0.1%;EQ 3.5 MG BASE/GM N60645 001

METHYLPREDNISOLONE ACETATE

ENEMA; RECTAL
MEDROL
UPJOHN 40 MG/BOT N18102 001

INJECTABLE; INJECTION
M-PREDROL
BEL MAR 40 MG/ML N86666 001
80 MG/ML N87135 001
METHYLPREDNISOLONE ACETATE
STERIS 40 MG/ML N85374 001
80 MG/ML N86507 001
20 MG/ML N87248 001

OINTMENT; TOPICAL
MEDROL ACETATE
UPJOHN 1% N12421 002

METHYLPREDNISOLONE SODIUM SUCCINATE

INJECTABLE; INJECTION
A-METHAPRED
ABBOTT EQ 40 MG BASE/VIAL N89573 001 FEB 22, 1991
EQ 125 MG BASE/VIAL N89574 001 FEB 22, 1991
EQ 500 MG BASE/VIAL N89575 001 FEB 22, 1991
EQ 1 GM BASE/VIAL N89576 001 FEB 22, 1991

Discontinued Drug Products *(continued)*

METHYLPREDNISOLONE SODIUM SUCCINATE *(continued)*

INJECTABLE; INJECTION
METHYLPREDNISOLONE

ELKINS SINN	EQ 125 MG BASE/VIAL	N86906 002
	EQ 500 MG BASE/VIAL	N86906 003
	EQ 1 GM BASE/VIAL	N86906 004
ORGANON	EQ 500 MG BASE/VIAL	N87535 001 JUN 25, 1982
	EQ 1 GM BASE/VIAL	N87535 002 JUN 25, 1982

METHYLPREDNISOLONE SODIUM SUCCINATE

ELKINS SINN	EQ 40 MG BASE/VIAL	N86906 001
FUJISAWA	EQ 40 MG BASE/VIAL	N88676 001 JUN 08, 1984
	EQ 40 MG BASE/VIAL	N89143 001 MAR 28, 1986
	EQ 125 MG BASE/VIAL	N88677 001 JUN 08, 1984
	EQ 125 MG BASE/VIAL	N89144 001 MAR 28, 1986
	EQ 500 MG BASE/VIAL	N88678 001 JUN 08, 1984
	EQ 500 MG BASE/VIAL	N89186 001 MAR 28, 1986
	EQ 500 MG BASE/VIAL	N89187 001 MAR 28, 1986
	EQ 1 GM BASE/VIAL	N88679 001 JUN 08, 1984
	EQ 1 GM BASE/VIAL	N89188 001 MAR 28, 1986
	EQ 1 GM BASE/VIAL	N89189 001 MAR 28, 1986
INTL MEDICATION	EQ 40 MG BASE/VIAL	N87812 001 FEB 09, 1983
	EQ 125 MG BASE/VIAL	N87813 001 FEB 09, 1983
	EQ 500 MG BASE/VIAL	N87851 001 FEB 09, 1983
	EQ 1 GM BASE/VIAL	N87852 001 FEB 09, 1983
QUAD PHARMS	EQ 40 MG BASE/VIAL	N89264 001 JAN 22, 1986
	EQ 125 MG BASE/VIAL	N89265 001 JAN 22, 1986
	EQ 500 MG BASE/VIAL	N89266 001 JAN 22, 1986
	EQ 1 GM BASE/VIAL	N89267 001 JAN 22, 1986

METHYLTESTOSTERONE

CAPSULE; ORAL
METHYLTESTOSTERONE

HEATHER	10 MG	N84967 001

TABLET; BUCCAL
ANDROID 5

ICN	5 MG	N87222 001

TABLET; BUCCAL/SUBLINGUAL
METANDREN

CIBA	5 MG	N03240 004
	10 MG	N03240 005

METHYLTESTOSTERONE

PRIVATE FORM	5 MG	N83836 001
PUREPAC PHARM	10 MG	N80308 001
	10 MG	N80475 001
ROSEMONT PHARM	10 MG	N80271 001
TABLICAPS	10 MG	N85125 001

TABLET; ORAL
METANDREN

CIBA	10 MG	N03240 001
	25 MG	N03240 003

METHYLTESTOSTERONE

DANBURY PHARMA	10 MG	N80933 001
	25 MG	N80931 001
INWOOD LABS	10 MG	N80839 001
	25 MG	N80973 001
KV PHARM	10 MG	N84312 001
PARKE DAVIS	10 MG	N84244 001
	25 MG	N84241 001
PRIVATE FORM	10 MG	N80214 002
	25 MG	N80214 003
	5 MG	N80214 001
PUREPAC PHARM	10 MG	N80309 001
	10 MG	N80475 002
	25 MG	N80310 001
	25 MG	N80475 003
TABLICAPS	10 MG	N80313 001
	25 MG	N85270 001
WEST WARD PHARM	10 MG	N84331 001
	25 MG	N84331 002
	25 MG	N84642 001

METHYPRYLON

CAPSULE; ORAL
NOLUDAR

ROCHE	300 MG	N09660 008

ELIXIR; ORAL
NOLUDAR

ROCHE	50 MG/5 ML	N09660 007

Discontinued Drug Products *(continued)*

METHYPRYLON *(continued)*

TABLET; ORAL
NOLUDAR

ROCHE	50 MG	N09660 002
	200 MG	N09660 004

METOCLOPRAMIDE HYDROCHLORIDE

INJECTABLE; INJECTION
METOCLOPRAMIDE HCL

FUJISAWA	EQ 10 MG BASE/2 ML	N70293 001 JAN 24, 1986
NORBROOK	EQ 10 MG BASE/2 ML	N70892 001 AUG 26, 1988
QUAD PHARMS	EQ 10 MG BASE/2 ML	N70671 001 MAY 27, 1986
SMITH AND NEPHEW	EQ 10 MG BASE/2 ML	N70622 001 MAR 02, 1987

REGLAN

ROBINS AH	EQ 10 MG BASE/ML	N17862 004 MAY 28, 1987

SOLUTION; ORAL
METOCLOPRAMIDE HCL

PACO	EQ 5 MG BASE/5 ML	N71665 001 DEC 05, 1988

TABLET; ORAL
CLOPRA

QUANTUM PHARMICS	EQ 10 MG BASE	N70294 001 JUL 29, 1985
	EQ 5 MG BASE	N72384 001 JUN 02, 1988

CLOPRA-"YELLOW"

QUANTUM PHARMICS	EQ 10 MG BASE	N70632 001 OCT 28, 1985

METOCLOPRAMIDE HCL

BARR	EQ 10 MG BASE	N70660 001 FEB 10, 1987
CHELSEA LABS	EQ 10 MG BASE	N70453 001 JUN 06, 1986
CIRCA	EQ 10 MG BASE	N70363 001 MAR 02, 1987
INTERPHARM	EQ 10 MG BASE	N71213 001 SEP 24, 1986
PAR PHARM	EQ 10 MG BASE	N70342 001 MAR 25, 1986
ROSEMONT PHARM	EQ 10 MG BASE	N70339 001 JUL 29, 1985

METOCURINE IODIDE

INJECTABLE; INJECTION
METOCURINE IODIDE

QUAD PHARMS	2 MG/ML	N89443 001 JUN 01, 1988

METOLAZONE

TABLET; ORAL
DIULO

SCS	2.5 MG	N18535 001
	5 MG	N18535 002
	10 MG	N18535 003

METOPROLOL TARTRATE; *MULTIPLE*

SEE CHLORTHALIDONE; METOPROLOL TARTRATE

METRIZAMIDE

INJECTABLE; INJECTION
AMIPAQUE

STERLING WINTHROP	2.5 GM/VIAL	N17982 003 SEP 12, 1983
	13.5 GM/VIAL	N17982 004 SEP 12, 1983

METRIZOATE MAGNESIUM; *MULTIPLE*

SEE CALCIUM METRIZOATE; MEGLUMINE METRIZOATE; METRIZOATE MAGNESIUM; METRIZOATE SODIUM

METRIZOATE SODIUM; *MULTIPLE*

SEE CALCIUM METRIZOATE; MEGLUMINE METRIZOATE; METRIZOATE MAGNESIUM; METRIZOATE SODIUM

METRIZOIC ACID; *MULTIPLE*

SEE CALCIUM; MEGLUMINE; METRIZOIC ACID

METRONIDAZOLE

INJECTABLE; INJECTION
METRONIDAZOLE

FUJISAWA	500 MG/100 ML	N70071 001 DEC 03, 1984
INTL MEDICATION	500 MG/100 ML	N70004 001 MAY 08, 1985

Discontinued Drug Products *(continued)*

METRONIDAZOLE (*continued*)
TABLET; ORAL
METRONIDAZOLE
CHELSEA LABS 250 MG N18599 001 SEP 17, 1982
500 MG N18599 002 FEB 13, 1984
SUPERPHARM 250 MG N70008 001 DEC 11, 1984
500 MG N70009 001 DEC 11, 1984
SATRIC
SAVAGE LABS 250 MG N70029 001 MAR 19, 1985
500 MG N70731 001 JUN 08, 1987

METRONIDAZOLE HYDROCHLORIDE
INJECTABLE; INJECTION
METRONIDAZOLE HCL
FUJISAWA EQ 500 MG BASE/VIAL N70295 001 OCT 15, 1985

MEZLOCILLIN SODIUM MONOHYDRATE
INJECTABLE; INJECTION
MEZLIN
MILES EQ 1 GM BASE/VIAL N62333 001
EQ 2 GM BASE/VIAL N62333 002
EQ 3 GM BASE/VIAL N62333 003
EQ 4 GM BASE/VIAL N62333 004

MICONAZOLE NITRATE
LOTION; TOPICAL
MONISTAT-DERM
JOHNSON RW 2% N17739 001

MILRINONE LACTATE
INJECTABLE; INJECTION
PRIMACOR IN DEXTROSE 5% IN PLASTIC CONTAINER
STERLING WINTHROP EQ 10 MG BASE/100 ML N20343 001 AUG 09, 1994
EQ 15 MG BASE/100 ML N20343 002 AUG 09, 1994

MINOCYCLINE HYDROCHLORIDE
CAPSULE; ORAL
MINOCIN
LEDERLE EQ 50 MG BASE N50315 002
EQ 100 MG BASE N50315 001
INJECTABLE; INJECTION
MINOCIN
LEDERLE EQ 100 MG BASE/VIAL N62139 001

MINOXIDIL
TABLET; ORAL
MINODYL
QUANTUM PHARMICS 2.5 MG N72153 001 JUL 13, 1988
10 MG N71534 001 MAR 19, 1987
MINOXIDIL
ROSEMONT PHARM 2.5 MG N71537 001 DEC 16, 1988
ROYCE LABS 2.5 MG N71799 001 NOV 10, 1987
10 MG N71796 001 NOV 10, 1987

MOLINDONE HYDROCHLORIDE
CAPSULE; ORAL
MOBAN
DUPONT MERCK 5 MG N17111 001
10 MG N17111 002
25 MG N17111 003

NABILONE
CAPSULE; ORAL
CESAMET
LILLY 1 MG N18677 001 DEC 26, 1985

NAFCILLIN SODIUM
INJECTABLE; INJECTION
UNIPEN
WYETH AYERST EQ 20 GM BASE/VIAL N50320 006
POWDER FOR RECONSTITUTION; ORAL
UNIPEN
WYETH AYERST EQ 250 MG BASE/5 ML N50199 001

Discontinued Drug Products *(continued)*

NALBUPHINE HYDROCHLORIDE

INJECTABLE; INJECTION

NALBUPHINE		
FUJISAWA	10 MG/ML	N70751 001 JUL 02, 1986
	20 MG/ML	N70752 001 SEP 24, 1986
QUAD PHARMS	10 MG/ML	N70692 001 MAR 25, 1986
	20 MG/ML	N70693 001 SEP 24, 1986
NALBUPHINE HCL		
ASTRA	10 MG/ML	N72071 001 APR 10, 1989
	10 MG/ML	N72072 001 APR 10, 1989
	20 MG/ML	N72074 001 APR 10, 1989
	20 MG/ML	N72075 001 APR 10, 1989

NALOXONE HYDROCHLORIDE

INJECTABLE; INJECTION

NALOXONE		
ELKINS SINN	0.4 MG/ML	N70496 001 SEP 24, 1986
NALOXONE HCL		
ASTRA	0.02 MG/ML	N72082 001 APR 11, 1989
	0.02 MG/ML	N72083 001 APR 11, 1989
	0.02 MG/ML	N72084 001 APR 11, 1989
	0.02 MG/ML	N72085 001 APR 11, 1989
	0.4 MG/ML	N72087 001 APR 11, 1989
	0.4 MG/ML	N72088 001 APR 11, 1989
	0.4 MG/ML	N72089 001 APR 11, 1989
	0.4 MG/ML	N72090 001 APR 11, 1989
	1 MG/ML	N72092 001 APR 11, 1989
	1 MG/ML	N72093 001 APR 11, 1989
FUJISAWA	0.02 MG/ML	N70661 001 NOV 17, 1986
	1 MG/ML	N71604 001 DEC 16, 1988

NALOXONE HYDROCHLORIDE (*continued*)

INJECTABLE; INJECTION

NALOXONE HCL		
INTL MEDICATION	0.4 MG/ML	N70417 001 SEP 24, 1986
	1 MG/ML	N72115 001 APR 27, 1988
QUAD PHARMS	0.02 MG/ML	N70678 001 DEC 18, 1986
	0.4 MG/ML	N70679 001 DEC 18, 1986
	1 MG/ML	N70680 001 DEC 18, 1986
NARCAN		
DUPONT MERCK	0.4 MG/ML	N71083 001 JUL 28, 1988
	1 MG/ML	N71084 001 JUL 28, 1988
	1 MG/ML	N71311 001 JUL 28, 1988

NANDROLONE DECANOATE

INJECTABLE; INJECTION

NANDDROLONE DECANOATE		
QUAD PHARMS	50 MG/ML	N89248 001 JUN 25, 1986
NANDROLONE DECANOATE		
FUJISAWA	100 MG/ML	N88290 001 OCT 03, 1983
	200 MG/ML	N88317 001 OCT 14, 1983
QUAD PHARMS	100 MG/ML	N89249 001 JUN 25, 1986
	200 MG/ML	N89250 001 JUN 25, 1986

NANDROLONE PHENPROPIONATE

INJECTABLE; INJECTION

NANDROLONE PHENPROPIONATE		
QUAD PHARMS	25 MG/ML	N89297 001 OCT 01, 1986
	50 MG/ML	N89298 001 OCT 01, 1986

NAPHAZOLINE HYDROCHLORIDE

SOLUTION/DROPS; OPHTHALMIC

NAFAZAIR		
PHARMAFAIR	0.1%	N88101 001 APR 15, 1983

Discontinued Drug Products *(continued)*

NEOMYCIN SULFATE

POWDER; FOR RX COMPOUNDING		
NEOMYCIN SULFATE		
ELKINS SINN	100%	N61698 001
TABLET; ORAL		
MYCIFRADIN		
UPJOHN	EQ 350 MG BASE	N60520 001
NEOBIOTIC		
PFIZER	EQ 350 MG BASE	N60475 001
NEOMYCIN SULFATE		
EON LABS	EQ 350 MG BASE	N61586 001
LANNETT	EQ 350 MG BASE	N60607 001
ROXANE	EQ 350 MG BASE	N62173 001
SQUIBB	EQ 350 MG BASE	N60365 001

NEOMYCIN SULFATE; *MULTIPLE*

SEE BACITRACIN; NEOMYCIN SULFATE; POLYMYXIN B SULFATE
SEE BACITRACIN ZINC; HYDROCORTISONE; NEOMYCIN SULFATE; POLYMYXIN B SULFATE
SEE BACITRACIN ZINC; LIDOCAINE; NEOMYCIN SULFATE; POLYMYXIN BSULFATE
SEE BACITRACIN ZINC; NEOMYCIN SULFATE; POLYMYXIN B SULFATE
SEE DEXAMETHASONE; NEOMYCIN SULFATE; POLYMYXIN B SULFATE
SEE GRAMICIDIN; NEOMYCIN SULFATE; POLYMYXIN B SULFATE
SEE HYDROCORTISONE; NEOMYCIN SULFATE; POLYMYXIN B SULFATE
SEE HYDROCORTISONE ACETATE; NEOMYCIN SULFATE
SEE METHYLPREDNISOLONE; NEOMYCIN SULFATE

NEOMYCIN SULFATE; PREDNISOLONE ACETATE

OINTMENT; OPHTHALMIC		
NEO-DELTA-CORTEF		
UPJOHN	EQ 3.5 MG BASE/GM;0.25%	N61039 002
	EQ 3.5 MG BASE/GM;0.5%	N61039 001
SUSPENSION/DROPS; OPHTHALMIC		
NEO-DELTA-CORTEF		
UPJOHN	EQ 3.5 MG BASE/ML;0.25%	N61037 001

NEOMYCIN SULFATE; PREDNISOLONE SODIUM PHOSPHATE

OINTMENT; OPHTHALMIC		
NEO-HYDELTRASOL		
MERCK SHARP DOHME	EQ 3.5 MG BASE/GM;EQ 0.25% PHOSPHATE	N50378 001

NEOMYCIN SULFATE; TRIAMCINOLONE ACETONIDE

CREAM; TOPICAL		
MYTREX A		
SAVAGE LABS	EQ 3.5 MG BASE/GM;0.1%	N62598 001 JUL 21, 1986
NEOMYCIN SULFATE-TRIAMCINOLONE ACETONIDE		
FOUGERA	EQ 3.5 MG BASE/GM;0.1%	N62600 001 JUL 21, 1986
PHARMADERM	EQ 3.5 MG BASE/GM;0.1%	N62595 001 JUL 21, 1986
OINTMENT; TOPICAL		
MYTREX A		
SAVAGE LABS	EQ 3.5 MG BASE/GM;0.1%	N62609 001 MAY 23, 1986
NEOMYCIN SULFATE-TRIAMCINOLONE ACETONIDE		
FOUGERA	EQ 3.5 MG BASE/GM;0.1%	N62608 001 MAY 23, 1986
PHARMADERM	EQ 3.5 MG BASE/GM;0.1%	N62607 001 MAY 23, 1986

NETILMICIN SULFATE

INJECTABLE; INJECTION		
NETROMYCIN		
SCHERING	EQ 10 MG BASE/ML	N50544 001 FEB 28, 1983
	EQ 25 MG BASE/ML	N50544 002 FEB 28, 1983

NIACIN

CAPSULE; ORAL		
WAMPOCAP		
WALLACE	500 MG	N11073 003
TABLET; ORAL		
NIACIN		
CHELSEA LABS	500 MG	N85172 001
CIRCA	500 MG	N83136 001
EVERYLIFE	500 MG	N83203 001
GENEVA PHARMS	500 MG	N83306 001
WEST WARD PHARM	500 MG	N83718 001
ZENITH LABS	500 MG	N83180 001

Discontinued Drug Products *(continued)*

NIACINAMIDE; *MULTIPLE*

SEE ASCORBIC ACID; BIOTIN; CYANOCOBALAMIN; DEXPANTHENOL; ERGOCALCIFEROL; FOLIC ACID; NIACINAMIDE; PYRIDOXINE HYDROCHLORIDE; RIBOFLAVIN PHOSPHATE SODIUM; THIAMINE HYDROCHLORIDE; VITAMIN A; VITAMIN E

SEE ASCORBIC ACID; BIOTIN; CYANOCOBALAMIN; DEXPANTHENOL; ERGOCALCIFEROL; FOLIC ACID; NIACINAMIDE; PYRIDOXINE HYDROCHLORIDE; RIBOFLAVIN PHOSPHATE SODIUM; THIAMINE HYDROCHLORIDE; VITAMIN A PALMITATE; VITAMIN E

SEE ASCORBIC ACID; BIOTIN; CYANOCOBALAMIN; DEXPANTHENOL; ERGOCALCIFEROL; FOLIC ACID; NIACINAMIDE; PYRIDOXINE; RIBOFLAVIN PHOSPHATE SODIUM; THIAMINE; VITAMIN A; VITAMIN E

NITROFURANTOIN

CAPSULE; ORAL		
NITROFURANTOIN		
CIRCA	50 MG	N84326 001
	100 MG	N84326 002
TABLET; ORAL		
FURALAN		
LANNETT	50 MG	N80017 001
	100 MG	N80017 002
NITROFURANTOIN		
CHELSEA LABS	50 MG	N85797 001
	100 MG	N85796 001
CIRCA	100 MG	N80447 002
ELKINS SINN	50 MG	N80003 001
	100 MG	N80003 002
EON LABS	50 MG	N80043 001
	100 MG	N80043 002
ZENITH LABS	50 MG	N80078 002
	100 MG	N80078 001

NITROFURANTOIN SODIUM

INJECTABLE; INJECTION		
IVADANTIN		
PROCTER AND GAMBLE	EQ 180 MG BASE/VIAL	N12402 001

NITROFURANTOIN, MACROCRYSTALLINE

CAPSULE; ORAL		
NITROFURANTOIN MACROCRYSTALLINE		
CIRCA	50 MG	N70248 001 JUN 24, 1988
	100 MG	N70249 001 JUN 24, 1988

NITROFURAZONE

DRESSING; TOPICAL		
ACTIN-N		
SHERWOOD MEDCL	0.2%	N17343 001
OINTMENT; TOPICAL		
NITROFURAZONE		
LANNETT	0.2%	N84393 001

NITROGLYCERIN

INJECTABLE; INJECTION		
NITRO-BID		
MARION MERRELL DOW	10 MG/ML	N71159 001 FEB 28, 1990
NITROGLYCERIN		
FUJISAWA	5 MG/ML	N71203 001 MAY 08, 1987
INTL MEDICATION	5 MG/ML	N70026 001 SEP 10, 1985
LUITPOLD	5 MG/ML	N71492 001 MAY 24, 1988
QUAD PHARMS	5 MG/ML	N71094 001 JUL 31, 1987
	10 MG/ML	N71095 001 JUL 31, 1987
SMITH AND NEPHEW	5 MG/ML	N70634 001 JUN 19, 1986
NITROL		
RORER	0.8 MG/ML	N18774 001 JAN 19, 1983
NITRONAL		
G POHL BOSKAMP	1 MG/ML	N18672 001 AUG 30, 1983
NITROSTAT		
PARKE DAVIS	5 MG/ML	N70863 001 JAN 08, 1987
	10 MG/ML	N70871 001 JAN 08, 1987
	10 MG/ML	N70872 001 JAN 08, 1987

Discontinued Drug Products *(continued)*

NORETHINDRONE
TABLET; ORAL
NORLUTIN
PARKE DAVIS 5 MG N10895 002

NORETHINDRONE; *MULTIPLE*
SEE ETHINYL ESTRADIOL; FERROUS FUMARATE; NORETHINDRONE
SEE ETHINYL ESTRADIOL; NORETHINDRONE
SEE MESTRANOL; NORETHINDRONE

NORETHINDRONE ACETATE; *MULTIPLE*
SEE ETHINYL ESTRADIOL; FERROUS FUMARATE; NORETHINDRONE ACETATE
SEE ETHINYL ESTRADIOL; NORETHINDRONE ACETATE

NORETHYNODREL; *MULTIPLE*
SEE MESTRANOL; NORETHYNODREL

NYSTATIN
CREAM; TOPICAL
CANDEX
MILES 100,000 UNITS/GM N61810 001
LOTION; TOPICAL
CANDEX
MILES 100,000 UNITS/ML N50233 001
POWDER; ORAL
BARSTATIN 100
BARLAN 100% N62489 001 APR 27, 1988
SUPPOSITORY; VAGINAL
NYSERT
PROCTER AND GAMBLE 100,000 UNITS N50478 001
SUSPENSION; ORAL
NYSTATIN
PENNEX 100,000 UNITS/ML N62835 001 NOV 19, 1987
PHARMADERM 100,000 UNITS/ML N62518 001 JUL 06, 1984
PHARMAFAIR 100,000 UNITS/ML N62541 001 JAN 16, 1985

NYSTATIN *(continued)*
TABLET; ORAL
NYSTATIN
CHELSEA LABS 500,000 UNITS N62402 001 DEC 16, 1982
QUANTUM PHARMICS 500,000 UNITS N62525 001 OCT 29, 1984
TABLET; VAGINAL
NYSTATIN
CHELSEA LABS 100,000 UNITS N62176 001
EON LABS 100,000 UNITS N61965 001
QUANTUM PHARMICS 100,000 UNITS N62509 001 APR 03, 1984

NYSTATIN; *MULTIPLE*
SEE CLIOQUINOL; NYSTATIN

NYSTATIN; TRIAMCINOLONE ACETONIDE
CREAM; TOPICAL
NYSTATIN AND TRIAMCINOLONE ACETONIDE
BARRE 100,000 UNITS/GM;0.1% N63010 001 DEC 20, 1988
CLAY PARK 100,000 UNITS/GM;0.1% N62186 002 JUN 06, 1985
PHARMAFAIR 100,000 UNITS/GM;0.1% N62657 001 JUL 30, 1986
NYSTATIN-TRIAMCINOLONE ACETONIDE
PHARMADERM 100,000 UNITS/GM;0.1% N62596 001 OCT 08, 1985
OINTMENT; TOPICAL
NYSTATIN-TRIAMCINOLONE ACETONIDE
PHARMADERM 100,000 UNITS/GM;0.1% N62603 001 OCT 09, 1985

ORPHENADRINE CITRATE
TABLET, EXTENDED RELEASE; ORAL
ORPHENADRINE CITRATE
ASCOT 100 MG N88067 001 APR 06, 1983
CIRCA 100 MG N84303 001
GENEVA PHARMS 100 MG N85046 001

ORPHENADRINE CITRATE; *MULTIPLE*
SEE ASPIRIN; CAFFEINE; ORPHENADRINE CITRATE

Discontinued Drug Products *(continued)*

ORPHENADRINE HYDROCHLORIDE

TABLET; ORAL
DISIPAL
3M — 50 MG — N10653 001

OXACILLIN SODIUM

CAPSULE; ORAL
PROSTAPHLIN
BRISTOL — EQ 500 MG BASE — N50118 002

INJECTABLE; INJECTION
OXACILLIN SODIUM

APOTHECON	EQ 250 MG BASE/VIAL	N50195 001
	EQ 500 MG BASE/VIAL	N50195 002
	EQ 1 GM BASE/VIAL	N50195 003
	EQ 2 GM BASE/VIAL	N50195 004
	EQ 4 GM BASE/VIAL	N50195 005
ELKINS SINN	EQ 250 MG BASE/VIAL	N62711 001 FEB 03, 1989
	EQ 500 MG BASE/VIAL	N62711 002 FEB 03, 1989
	EQ 1 GM BASE/VIAL	N62711 003 FEB 03, 1989
	EQ 2 GM BASE/VIAL	N62711 004 FEB 03, 1989
	EQ 4 GM BASE/VIAL	N62711 005 FEB 03, 1989
	EQ 10 GM BASE/VIAL	N62711 006 FEB 03, 1989

POWDER FOR RECONSTITUTION; ORAL
PROSTAPHLIN
BRISTOL — EQ 250 MG BASE/5 ML — N50194 001

OXAZEPAM

CAPSULE; ORAL
OXAZEPAM

AM THERAP	10 MG	N71955 001 MAR 03, 1988
	15 MG	N71956 001 MAR 03, 1988
	30 MG	N71957 001 MAR 03, 1988
MYLAN	10 MG	N71713 001 OCT 20, 1987
	15 MG	N71714 001 OCT 20, 1987
	30 MG	N71715 001 OCT 20, 1987

OXAZEPAM *(continued)*

CAPSULE; ORAL
ZAXOPAM

QUANTUM PHARMICS	10 MG	N70650 001 MAR 01, 1988
	15 MG	N70640 001 MAR 01, 1988
	30 MG	N70641 001 MAR 01, 1988

OXPRENOLOL HYDROCHLORIDE

CAPSULE; ORAL
TRASICOR

CIBA	20 MG	N18166 001 DEC 28, 1983
	40 MG	N18166 002 DEC 28, 1983
	80 MG	N18166 003 DEC 28, 1983
	160 MG	N18166 004 DEC 28, 1983

OXTRIPHYLLINE

SOLUTION; ORAL
OXTRIPHYLLINE
PENNEX — 100 MG/5 ML — N88243 001 DEC 05, 1983

SYRUP; ORAL
OXTRIPHYLLINE PEDIATRIC
PENNEX — 50 MG/5 ML — N88242 001 DEC 05, 1983

TABLET, DELAYED RELEASE; ORAL
OXTRIPHYLLINE

CIRCA	100 MG	N87866 001 AUG 25, 1983
	200 MG	N87835 001 AUG 25, 1983

OXYBUTYNIN CHLORIDE

TABLET; ORAL
OXYBUTYNIN CHLORIDE

CIRCA	5 MG	N72485 001 APR 19, 1989
QUANTUM PHARMICS	5 MG	N72296 001 DEC 08, 1988
ROSEMONT PHARM	5 MG	N70746 001 MAR 10, 1988

Discontinued Drug Products *(continued)*

OXYCODONE HYDROCHLORIDE; *MULTIPLE*
SEE ACETAMINOPHEN; OXYCODONE HYDROCHLORIDE
SEE ACETAMINOPHEN; OXYCODONE HYDROCHLORIDE; OXYCODONE TEREPHTHALATE

OXYCODONE TEREPHTHALATE; *MULTIPLE*
SEE ACETAMINOPHEN; OXYCODONE HYDROCHLORIDE; OXYCODONE TEREPHTHALATE

OXYPHENBUTAZONE

TABLET; ORAL		
OXYPHENBUTAZONE		
CIRCA	100 MG	N88399 001 SEP 17, 1984
TANDEARIL		
GEIGY	100 MG	N12542 004 SEP 03, 1982

OXYPHENONIUM BROMIDE

TABLET; ORAL		
ANTRENYL		
CIBA	5 MG	N08492 002

OXYTETRACYCLINE HYDROCHLORIDE

CAPSULE; ORAL		
OXYTETRACYCLINE HCL		
PUREPAC PHARM	EQ 250 MG BASE	N60634 001
TERRAMYCIN		
PFIZER	EQ 125 MG BASE	N50286 001

OXYTOCIN

INJECTABLE; INJECTION		
OXYTOCIN 10 USP UNITS IN DEXTROSE 5%		
ABBOTT	1USP UNITS/100 ML	N19185 004 MAR 29, 1985
	2USP UNITS/100 ML	N19185 003 MAR 29, 1985
OXYTOCIN 20 USP UNITS IN DEXTROSE 5%		
ABBOTT	2USP UNITS/100 ML	N19185 002 MAR 29, 1985
OXYTOCIN 5 USP UNITS IN DEXTROSE 5%		
ABBOTT	1USP UNITS/100 ML	N19185 001 MAR 29, 1985

PANCURONIUM BROMIDE

INJECTABLE; INJECTION		
PANCURONIUM BROMIDE		
ASTRA	2 MG/ML	N72212 001 MAR 31, 1988
QUAD PHARMS	2 MG/ML	N72208 001 JUN 03, 1988
	1 MG/ML	N72209 001 JUN 03, 1988

PARAMETHADIONE

SOLUTION; ORAL		
PARADIONE		
ABBOTT	300 MG/ML	N06800 002

PARAMETHASONE ACETATE

TABLET; ORAL		
HALDRONE		
LILLY	1 MG	N12772 005
	2 MG	N12772 006

PARGYLINE HYDROCHLORIDE

TABLET; ORAL		
EUTONYL		
ABBOTT	10 MG	N13448 002
	25 MG	N13448 003
	50 MG	N13448 004

PARGYLINE HYDROCHLORIDE; *MULTIPLE*
SEE METHYCLOTHIAZIDE; PARGYLINE HYDROCHLORIDE

PAROMOMYCIN SULFATE

SYRUP; ORAL		
HUMATIN		
PARKE DAVIS	EQ 125 MG BASE/5 ML	N60522 001

PAROXETINE HYDROCHLORIDE

TABLET; ORAL		
PAXIL		
SMITHKLINE BEECHAM	EQ 10 MG BASE	N20031 001 DEC 29, 1992
	EQ 40 MG BASE	N20031 005 DEC 29, 1992
	EQ 50 MG BASE	N20031 004 DEC 29, 1992

Discontinued Drug Products *(continued)*

PENBUTOLOL SULFATE

TABLET; ORAL
LEVATOL
REED AND CARNRICK 10 MG N18976 001 DEC 30, 1987

PENICILLIN G BENZATHINE

INJECTABLE; INJECTION
BICILLIN L-A
WYETH AYERST 300,000 UNITS/ML N50131 001

SUSPENSION; ORAL
BICILLIN
WYETH AYERST 300,000 UNITS/5 ML N50126 002

TABLET; ORAL
BICILLIN
WYETH AYERST 200,000 UNITS N50128 001

PENICILLIN G POTASSIUM

INJECTABLE; INJECTION
PENICILLIN G POTASSIUM
APOTHECON 1,000,000 UNITS/VIAL N60362 001
5,000,000 UNITS/VIAL N60362 003
10,000,000 UNITS/VIAL N60362 004
20,000,000 UNITS/VIAL N60362 002
COPANOS 1,000,000 UNITS/VIAL N60806 002
5,000,000 UNITS/VIAL N60806 003
10,000,000 UNITS/VIAL N60806 004
500,000 UNITS/VIAL N60806 001
PARKE DAVIS 1,000,000 UNITS/VIAL N62003 001
5,000,000 UNITS/VIAL N62003 002

POWDER FOR RECONSTITUTION; ORAL
PENICILLIN G POTASSIUM
MYLAN 200,000 UNITS/5 ML N60752 003
250,000 UNITS/5 ML N60752 002
400,000 UNITS/5 ML N60752 001
PUREPAC PHARM 250,000 UNITS/5 ML N61740 001
400,000 UNITS/5 ML N61740 002
PENTIDS '200'
APOTHECON 200,000 UNITS/5 ML N62149 001
PENTIDS '400'
APOTHECON 400,000 UNITS/5 ML N62149 002

PENICILLIN G POTASSIUM *(continued)*

TABLET; ORAL
PENICILLIN G POTASSIUM
APOTHECON 250,000 UNITS N60392 003
PUREPAC PHARM 200,000 UNITS N61588 001
250,000 UNITS N61588 002
400,000 UNITS N61588 003
PENTIDS '200'
APOTHECON 200,000 UNITS N62155 001
PENTIDS '250'
APOTHECON 250,000 UNITS N62155 002
PENTIDS '400'
APOTHECON 400,000 UNITS N60392 004
400,000 UNITS N62155 003
PENTIDS '800'
APOTHECON 800,000 UNITS N60392 005
800,000 UNITS N62155 004

PENICILLIN G PROCAINE

INJECTABLE; INJECTION
DURACILLIN A.S.
LILLY 300,000 UNITS/ML N60093 001
PENICILLIN G PROCAINE
COPANOS 300,000 UNITS/ML N60800 001
600,000 UNITS/1.2 ML N60800 002
PARKE DAVIS 300,000 UNITS/ML N62029 001

PENICILLIN G SODIUM

INJECTABLE; INJECTION
PENICILLIN G SODIUM
COPANOS 5,000,000 UNITS/VIAL N61051 001
SQUIBB 5,000,000 UNITS/VIAL N61935 001

PENICILLIN V

POWDER FOR RECONSTITUTION; ORAL
V-CILLIN
LILLY 125 MG/0.6 ML N60002 001

PENICILLIN V POTASSIUM

POWDER FOR RECONSTITUTION; ORAL
BETAPEN-VK
APOTHECON EQ 125 MG BASE/5 ML N61149 001
EQ 250 MG BASE/5 ML N61149 002
PENAPAR-VK
PARKE DAVIS EQ 125 MG BASE/5 ML N62002 001
EQ 250 MG BASE/5 ML N62002 002
PENICILLIN V POTASSIUM
PUREPAC PHARM EQ 125 MG BASE/5 ML N61758 001
EQ 250 MG BASE/5 ML N61758 002

Discontinued Drug Products *(continued)*

PENICILLIN V POTASSIUM *(continued)*

POWDER FOR RECONSTITUTION; ORAL		
VEETIDS '125'		
APOTHECON	EQ 125 MG BASE/5 ML	N61206 001
	EQ 125 MG BASE/5 ML	N62153 001
VEETIDS '250'		
APOTHECON	EQ 250 MG BASE/5 ML	N61206 002
	EQ 250 MG BASE/5 ML	N62153 002
TABLET; ORAL		
PEN-VEE K		
WYETH AYERST	EQ 125 MG BASE	N60006 001
PENAPAR-VK		
PARKE DAVIS	EQ 250 MG BASE	N62001 001
	EQ 500 MG BASE	N62001 002
PENICILLIN V POTASSIUM		
PUREPAC PHARM	EQ 125 MG BASE	N61571 001
	EQ 250 MG BASE	N61571 002
	EQ 500 MG BASE	N61571 003
UTICILLIN VK		
UPJOHN	EQ 500 MG BASE	N61651 002
VEETIDS '250'		
APOTHECON	EQ 250 MG BASE	N61164 001
	EQ 250 MG BASE	N62156 002
VEETIDS '500'		
APOTHECON	EQ 500 MG BASE	N61164 002
	EQ 500 MG BASE	N62156 001

PENTAZOCINE HYDROCHLORIDE

TABLET; ORAL		
TALWIN 50		
STERLING WINTHROP	EQ 50 MG BASE	N16732 001

PENTETATE CALCIUM TRISODIUM YB-169

INJECTABLE; INJECTION		
YTTERBIUM YB 169 DTPA		
3M	2mCi/ML	N17518 001

PENTOBARBITAL SODIUM

CAPSULE; ORAL		
PENTOBARBITAL SODIUM		
LANNETT	100 MG	N85915 001
	50 MG	N85937 001
VITARINE	100 MG	N83284 001
WHITEWORTH TOWNE	100 MG	N83338 001

PENTOBARBITAL SODIUM *(continued)*

CAPSULE; ORAL		
SODIUM PENTOBARBITAL		
ANABOLIC	100 MG	N84590 001
CHELSEA LABS	100 MG	N85791 001
ELKINS SINN	100 MG	N83368 001
EVERYLIFE	100 MG	N83259 001
PARKE DAVIS	100 MG	N84156 001
PERRIGO	100 MG	N84560 001
PUREPAC PHARM	100 MG	N83301 001
WYETH AYERST	100 MG	N83239 001
INJECTABLE; INJECTION		
PENTOBARBITAL SODIUM		
ELKINS SINN	50 MG/ML	N83270 001
TABLET; ORAL		
PENTOBARBITAL SODIUM		
VITARINE	100 MG	N83285 001
SODIUM PENTOBARBITAL		
ANABOLIC	100 MG	N84238 001

PENTOLINIUM TARTRATE

INJECTABLE; INJECTION		
ANSOLYSEN		
WYETH AYERST	10 MG/ML	N09372 001

PERMETHRIN

LOTION; TOPICAL		
NIX		
BURROUGHS WELLCOME	1%	N19435 001 MAR 31, 1986

PERPHENAZINE

SYRUP; ORAL		
TRILAFON		
SCHERING	2 MG/5 ML	N11294 002
TABLET, EXTENDED RELEASE; ORAL		
TRILAFON		
SCHERING	8 MG	N11361 002

PERPHENAZINE; *MULTIPLE*

SEE AMITRIPTYLINE HYDROCHLORIDE; PERPHENAZINE

Discontinued Drug Products *(continued)*

PHENDIMETRAZINE TARTRATE

CAPSULE; ORAL		
PHENDIMETRAZINE TARTRATE		
VITARINE	35 MG	N85634 001
	35 MG	N85645 001
	35 MG	N85670 001
	35 MG	N86403 001
	35 MG	N86408 001
	35 MG	N86410 001
	35 MG	N87424 001
SPRX-3		
SOLVAY	35 MG	N85897 001
STATOBEX		
LEMMON	35 MG	N85507 001
CAPSULE, EXTENDED RELEASE; ORAL		
MELFIAT-105		
SOLVAY	105 MG	N87487 001 OCT 13, 1982
SPRX-105		
SOLVAY	105 MG	N88024 001 DEC 22, 1982
TABLET; ORAL		
ADPHEN		
FERNDALE LABS	35 MG	N83655 001
ALPHAZINE		
EON LABS	35 MG	N85034 001
DI-METREX		
PRIVATE FORM	35 MG	N85698 001
MELFIAT		
SOLVAY	35 MG	N83790 002
METRA		
FOREST PHARMS	35 MG	N83754 001
PHENDIMETRAZINE TARTRATE		
ANABOLIC	35 MG	N86020 001
BARR	35 MG	N83644 001
	35 MG	N83684 001
	35 MG	N83686 001
	35 MG	N83687 001
	35 MG	N84831 001
	35 MG	N84834 001
	35 MG	N84835 001
CHELSEA LABS	35 MG	N85767 001
	35 MG	N85768 001
	35 MG	N85770 001
	35 MG	N85773 001
FERNDALE LABS	35 MG	N86834 001 SEP 15, 1983
GENEVA PHARMS	35 MG	N86365 001
	35 MG	N86370 001
PRIVATE FORM	35 MG	N85199 001
ROSEMONT PHARM	35 MG	N83805 001
	35 MG	N84398 001

PHENDIMETRAZINE TARTRATE *(continued)*

TABLET; ORAL		
PHENDIMETRAZINE TARTRATE		
SOLVAY	35 MG	N83790 001
	35 MG	N83993 001
VITARINE	35 MG	N85519 001
	35 MG	N86005 001
	35 MG	N86106 001
ZENITH LABS	35 MG	N83682 001
	35 MG	N85611 001
	35 MG	N85612 001
STATOBEX-G		
LEMMON	35 MG	N85095 001

PHENINDIONE

TABLET; ORAL		
HEDULIN		
MERRELL DOW	50 MG	N08767 002

PHENMETRAZINE HYDROCHLORIDE

TABLET; ORAL		
PRELUDIN		
BOEHRINGER INGELHEIM	25 MG	N10460 005
TABLET, EXTENDED RELEASE; ORAL		
PRELUDIN		
BOEHRINGER INGELHEIM	50 MG	N11752 004
	75 MG	N11752 003

PHENPROCOUMON

TABLET; ORAL		
LIQUAMAR		
ORGANON	3 MG	N11228 001

Discontinued Drug Products *(continued)*

PHENTERMINE HYDROCHLORIDE

CAPSULE; ORAL		
OBESTIN-30		
FERNDALE LABS	30 MG	N87144 001
PHENTERMINE HCL		
CHELSEA LABS	30 MG	N86740 001 MAR 21, 1985
DURAMED	30 MG	N88948 001 APR 25, 1986
LANNETT	30 MG	N87022 001 FEB 03, 1983
LEMMON	30 MG	N86911 001
	30 MG	N87126 001
ROSEMONT PHARM	30 MG	N88430 001 MAR 27, 1984
VITARINE	30 MG	N87202 001
	30 MG	N87235 001
ZENITH LABS	30 MG	N86329 001
TABLET; ORAL		
PHENTERMINE HCL		
CHELSEA LABS	8 MG	N85739 001
EON LABS	8 MG	N85671 001
	8 MG	N85689 001
VITARINE	8 MG	N86453 001
	8 MG	N86456 001
ZENITH LABS	8 MG	N85553 001
TORA		
SOLVAY	8 MG	N84035 001

PHENTERMINE RESIN COMPLEX

CAPSULE, EXTENDED RELEASE; ORAL		
PHENTERMINE RESIN 30		
QUANTUM PHARMICS	EQ 30 MG BASE	N89120 001 FEB 04, 1988

PHENYL AMINOSALICYLATE

POWDER; ORAL		
PHENY-PAS-TEBAMIN		
PURDUE FREDERICK	50%	N11695 002
TABLET; ORAL		
PHENY-PAS-TEBAMIN		
PURDUE FREDERICK	500 MG	N11695 003

PHENYLBUTAZONE

CAPSULE; ORAL		
AZOLID		
RHONE POULENC RORER	100 MG	N87260 001
BUTAZOLIDIN		
GEIGY	100 MG	N08319 009
PHENYLBUTAZONE		
CHELSEA LABS	100 MG	N87756 001 DEC 17, 1982
GENEVA PHARMS	100 MG	N87774 001 JUN 16, 1982
ZENITH LABS	100 MG	N88218 001 JUN 24, 1983
TABLET; ORAL		
AZOLID		
RHONE POULENC RORER	100 MG	N87091 001
BUTAZOLIDIN		
GEIGY	100 MG	N08319 008
PHENYLBUTAZONE		
CHELSEA LABS	100 MG	N86151 001
DANBURY PHARMA	100 MG	N87674 001 APR 21, 1982
GENEVA PHARMS	100 MG	N84339 001

PHENYLPROPANOLAMINE HYDROCHLORIDE; *MULTIPLE*

SEE BROMPHENIRAMINE MALEATE; PHENYLPROPANOLAMINE HYDROCHLORIDE

SEE CHLORPHENIRAMINE MALEATE; PHENYLPROPANOLAMINE HYDROCHLORIDE

SEE CLEMASTINE FUMARATE; PHENYLPROPANOLAMINE HYDROCHLORIDE

PHENYLPROPANOLAMINE POLISTIREX; *MULTIPLE*

SEE CHLORPHENIRAMINE POLISTIREX; PHENYLPROPANOLAMINE POLISTIREX

PHENYTOIN

SUSPENSION; ORAL		
DILANTIN-30		
PARKE DAVIS	30 MG/5 ML	N08762 002

Discontinued Drug Products *(continued)*

PHENYTOIN SODIUM

INJECTABLE; INJECTION

PHENYTOIN SODIUM		
SMITH AND NEPHEW	50 MG/ML	N88521 001 DEC 18, 1984
WARNER CHILCOTT	50 MG/ML	N89900 001 MAR 30, 1990

PHENYTOIN SODIUM, EXTENDED

CAPSULE; ORAL

EXTENDED PHENYTOIN SODIUM		
SIDMAK LABS NJ	100 MG	N89441 001 DEC 18, 1986
PHENYTEX		
CIRCA	100 MG	N88711 001 DEC 21, 1984

PHENYTOIN SODIUM, PROMPT

CAPSULE; ORAL

DIPHENYLAN SODIUM		
LANNETT	100 MG	N80857 002
	30 MG	N80857 001
PHENYTOIN SODIUM		
CHELSEA LABS	100 MG	N85894 001
PHARMERAL	100 MG	N85435 001

PHOSPHORIC ACID; *MULTIPLE*

SEE AMINO ACIDS; MAGNESIUM ACETATE; PHOSPHORIC ACID; POTASSIUM ACETATE; SODIUM CHLORIDE

PHYTONADIONE

INJECTABLE; INJECTION

PHYTONADIONE		
SMITHKLINE BEECHAM	10 MG/ML	N84060 002
	1 MG/0.5 ML	N84060 001
VITAMIN K1		
ABBOTT	10 MG/ML	N87956 001 JUL 25, 1983

PINDOLOL; *MULTIPLE*

SEE HYDROCHLOROTHIAZIDE; PINDOLOL

PIPERACETAZINE

TABLET; ORAL

QUIDE		
DOW PHARMS	10 MG	N13615 001
	25 MG	N13615 002

PIPERAZINE CITRATE

SYRUP; ORAL

ANTEPAR		
BURROUGHS WELLCOME	EQ 500 MG BASE/5 ML	N09102 001
BRYREL		
STERLING WINTHROP	EQ 500 MG BASE/5 ML	N17796 001
PIPERAZINE CITRATE		
BARRE	EQ 500 MG BASE/5 ML	N80774 001
VERMIDOL		
SOLVAY	EQ 500 MG BASE/5 ML	N80992 001

TABLET; ORAL

ANTEPAR		
BURROUGHS WELLCOME	EQ 500 MG BASE	N09102 003

PIPOBROMAN

TABLET; ORAL

VERCYTE		
ABBOTT	10 MG	N16245 001

POLYETHYLENE GLYCOL 3350; POTASSIUM CHLORIDE; SODIUM BICARBONATE; SODIUM CHLORIDE; SODIUM SULFATE, ANHYDROUS

POWDER FOR RECONSTITUTION; ORAL

COLYTE		
REED AND CARNRICK	120 GM/PACKET;1.49 GM/PACKET;3.36 GM/PACKET;2.92 GM/PACKET;11.36 GM/PACKET	N18983 005 OCT 26, 1984
	227.1 GM/PACKET;2.82 GM/PACKET;6.36 GM/PACKET;5.53 GM/PACKET;21.5 GM/PACKET	N18983 004 OCT 26, 1984
	360 GM/PACKET;4.47 GM/PACKET;10.08 GM/PACKET;8.76 GM/PACKET;34.08 GM/PACKET	N18983 006 OCT 26, 1984

Discontinued Drug Products *(continued)*

POLYMYXIN B SULFATE; *MULTIPLE*

SEE BACITRACIN; NEOMYCIN SULFATE; POLYMYXIN B SULFATE
SEE BACITRACIN; POLYMYXIN B SULFATE
SEE BACITRACIN ZINC; HYDROCORTISONE; NEOMYCIN SULFATE; POLYMYXIN B SULFATE
SEE BACITRACIN ZINC; LIDOCAINE; NEOMYCIN SULFATE; POLYMYXIN BSULFATE
SEE BACITRACIN ZINC; NEOMYCIN SULFATE; POLYMYXIN B SULFATE
SEE CHLORAMPHENICOL; POLYMYXIN B SULFATE
SEE DEXAMETHASONE; NEOMYCIN SULFATE; POLYMYXIN B SULFATE
SEE GRAMICIDIN; NEOMYCIN SULFATE; POLYMYXIN B SULFATE
SEE HYDROCORTISONE; NEOMYCIN SULFATE; POLYMYXIN B SULFATE

POTASSIUM ACETATE; *MULTIPLE*

SEE AMINO ACIDS; MAGNESIUM ACETATE; PHOSPHORIC ACID; POTASSIUM ACETATE; SODIUM CHLORIDE
SEE AMINO ACIDS; MAGNESIUM ACETATE; POTASSIUM ACETATE; SODIUM CHLORIDE
SEE AMINO ACIDS; MAGNESIUM ACETATE; POTASSIUM ACETATE; SODIUM CHLORIDE; SODIUM PHOSPHATE, DIBASIC
SEE AMINO ACIDS; MAGNESIUM CHLORIDE; POTASSIUM ACETATE; POTASSIUM CHLORIDE; SODIUM ACETATE

POTASSIUM AMINOSALICYLATE

POWDER; ORAL
POTASSIUM AMINOSALICYLATE

HEXCEL	100%	N80098 001

POTASSIUM CHLORIDE

INJECTABLE; INJECTION
POTASSIUM CHLORIDE

ABBOTT	1 MEQ/ML	N80205 003
	1 MEQ/ML	N83345 003
	2.4 MEQ/ML	N80205 004
	3.2 MEQ/ML	N80205 005
ELKINS SINN	2 MEQ/ML	N80203 001
FUJISAWA	2 MEQ/ML	N80204 001
	2 MEQ/ML	N86713 001
	2 MEQ/ML	N86714 001
	2 MEQ/ML	N87885 001
		FEB 03, 1983
LILLY	2 MEQ/ML	N07865 002

POTASSIUM CHLORIDE *(continued)*

INJECTABLE; INJECTION
POTASSIUM CHLORIDE

LUITPOLD	2 MEQ/ML	N80221 001
	2 MEQ/ML	N80736 001
MILES	1 MEQ/ML	N80195 002
	2 MEQ/ML	N80195 001
	3 MEQ/ML	N80195 003
SEARLE	1 MEQ/ML	N86219 001
	2 MEQ/ML	N86219 002
	2 MEQ/ML	N86220 002
	3 MEQ/ML	N86219 003
	3 MEQ/ML	N86220 001
	4 MEQ/ML	N86219 004

POTASSIUM CHLORIDE; *MULTIPLE*

SEE AMINO ACIDS; DEXTROSE; MAGNESIUM CHLORIDE; POTASSIUM CHLORIDE; SODIUM CHLORIDE; SODIUM PHOSPHATE, DIBASIC
SEE AMINO ACIDS; DEXTROSE; MAGNESIUM CHLORIDE; POTASSIUM CHLORIDE; POTASSIUM PHOSPHATE, DIBASIC; SODIUM CHLORIDE
SEE AMINO ACIDS; MAGNESIUM CHLORIDE; POTASSIUM ACETATE; POTASSIUM CHLORIDE; SODIUM ACETATE
SEE AMINO ACIDS; MAGNESIUM CHLORIDE; POTASSIUM CHLORIDE; SODIUM CHLORIDE; SODIUM PHOSPHATE, DIBASIC
SEE AMINO ACIDS; MAGNESIUM CHLORIDE; POTASSIUM CHLORIDE; POTASSIUM PHOSPHATE, DIBASIC; SODIUM CHLORIDE
SEE CALCIUM CHLORIDE; DEXTROSE; POTASSIUM CHLORIDE; SODIUM CHLORIDE; SODIUM LACTATE
SEE CALCIUM CHLORIDE; MAGNESIUM CHLORIDE; POTASSIUM CHLORIDE; SODIUM ACETATE; SODIUM CHLORIDE
SEE CALCIUM CHLORIDE; POTASSIUM CHLORIDE; SODIUM CHLORIDE; SODIUM LACTATE
SEE CALCIUM CHLORIDE; POTASSIUM CHLORIDE; SODIUM ACETATE; SODIUM CHLORIDE
SEE CALCIUM CHLORIDE; POTASSIUM CHLORIDE; SODIUM CHLORIDE
SEE DEXTROSE; POTASSIUM CHLORIDE; SODIUM CHLORIDE
SEE MAGNESIUM CHLORIDE; POTASSIUM CHLORIDE; SODIUM ACETATE; SODIUM CHLORIDE; SODIUM GLUCONATE
SEE POLYETHYLENE GLYCOL 3350; POTASSIUM CHLORIDE; SODIUM BICARBONATE; SODIUM CHLORIDE; SODIUM SULFATE, ANHYDROUS

Discontinued Drug Products *(continued)*

POTASSIUM CHLORIDE; SODIUM CHLORIDE
INJECTABLE; INJECTION
SODIUM CHLORIDE 0.9% AND POTASSIUM CHLORIDE 0.075%
BAXTER — 75 MG/100 ML;900 MG/100 ML — N17648 004
MCGAW — 75 MG/100 ML;900 MG/100 ML — N18722 001 NOV 09, 1982
SODIUM CHLORIDE 0.9% AND POTASSIUM CHLORIDE 0.15%
MCGAW — 150 MG/100 ML;900 MG/100 ML — N18722 002 NOV 09, 1982
SODIUM CHLORIDE 0.9% AND POTASSIUM CHLORIDE 0.22% IN PLASTIC CONTAINER
MCGAW — 220 MG/100 ML;900 MG/100 ML — N18722 003 NOV 09, 1982
SODIUM CHLORIDE 0.9% AND POTASSIUM CHLORIDE 0.3%
MCGAW — 300 MG/100 ML;900 MG/100 ML — N18722 004 NOV 09, 1982

POTASSIUM CITRATE
POWDER FOR RECONSTITUTION; ORAL
POTASSIUM CITRATE
UNIV TX — 10 MEQ/PACKET — N19647 002 OCT 13, 1988
20 MEQ/PACKET — N19647 001 OCT 13, 1988

POTASSIUM PHOSPHATE, DIBASIC; *MULTIPLE*
SEE AMINO ACIDS; DEXTROSE; MAGNESIUM CHLORIDE; POTASSIUM CHLORIDE; POTASSIUM PHOSPHATE, DIBASIC; SODIUM CHLORIDE
SEE AMINO ACIDS; MAGNESIUM CHLORIDE; POTASSIUM CHLORIDE; POTASSIUM PHOSPHATE, DIBASIC; SODIUM CHLORIDE

PRALIDOXIME CHLORIDE
INJECTABLE; INJECTION
PRALIDOXIME CHLORIDE
QUAD PHARMS — 1 GM/VIAL — N72224 001 NOV 23, 1988
WYETH AYERST — 300 MG/ML — N18799 001 DEC 13, 1982
TABLET; ORAL
PROTOPAM CHLORIDE
WYETH AYERST — 500 MG — N14122 002

PRAMOXINE HYDROCHLORIDE; *MULTIPLE*
SEE HYDROCORTISONE ACETATE; PRAMOXINE HYDROCHLORIDE

PRAZEPAM
CAPSULE; ORAL
CENTRAX
PARKE DAVIS — 5 MG — N18144 001
10 MG — N18144 002
20 MG — N18144 003 MAY 10, 1982
PRAZEPAM
ROSEMONT PHARM — 5 MG — N70427 001 NOV 06, 1987
10 MG — N70428 001 NOV 06, 1987
TABLET; ORAL
CENTRAX
PARKE DAVIS — 10 MG — N17415 001

PRAZOSIN HYDROCHLORIDE
CAPSULE; ORAL
PRAZOSIN HCL
AM THERAP — EQ 1 MG BASE — N72782 001 MAY 16, 1989
EQ 2 MG BASE — N72783 001 MAY 16, 1989
EQ 5 MG BASE — N72784 001 MAY 16, 1989

PREDNICARBATE
OINTMENT; TOPICAL
DERMATOP
HOECHST ROUSSEL — 0.1% — N19568 001 SEP 23, 1991

Discontinued Drug Products *(continued)*

PREDNISOLONE

CREAM; TOPICAL		
METI-DERM		
SCHERING	0.5%	N10209 002
TABLET; ORAL		
DELTA-CORTEF		
UPJOHN	5 MG	N09987 004
FERNISOLONE-P		
FERNDALE LABS	5 MG	N83941 001
PREDNISOLONE		
BARR	5 MG	N84426 002
BUNDY	5 MG	N83675 001
CHELSEA LABS	5 MG	N85415 001
	5 MG	N85416 001
ELKINS SINN	5 MG	N80625 001
EON LABS	5 MG	N84773 001
EVERYLIFE	1 MG	N84439 001
HEATHER	5 MG	N80326 001
ICN	5 MG	N80236 001
INWOOD LABS	5 MG	N80748 001
LEMMON	5 MG	N80398 001
PANRAY	1 MG	N80351 001
	5 MG	N80351 002
PERRIGO	5 MG	N84542 001
PRIVATE FORM	5 MG	N80211 001
SUPERPHARM	5 MG	N88892 001 FEB 26, 1985
TABLICAPS	5 MG	N85170 001
UDL	5 MG	N87987 001 JAN 18, 1983
VITARINE	5 MG	N80534 001
WEST WARD PHARM	5 MG	N80324 001
WHITEWORTH TOWNE	5 MG	N80342 001
STERANE		
PFIZER	5 MG	N09996 001

PREDNISOLONE; *MULTIPLE*

SEE CHLORAMPHENICOL; PREDNISOLONE

PREDNISOLONE ACETATE

INJECTABLE; INJECTION		
METICORTELONE		
SCHERING	25 MG/ML	N10255 002
PREDNISOLONE ACETATE		
AKORN	25 MG/ML	N83032 001
	50 MG/ML	N84492 001
BEL MAR	25 MG/ML	N83738 001
	50 MG/ML	N83738 002
CENT PHARMS	25 MG/ML	N84717 001
	50 MG/ML	N84717 002

PREDNISOLONE ACETATE *(continued)*

INJECTABLE; INJECTION		
STERANE		
PFIZER	25 MG/ML	N11446 001

PREDNISOLONE ACETATE; *MULTIPLE*

SEE NEOMYCIN SULFATE; PREDNISOLONE ACETATE

PREDNISOLONE ACETATE; SULFACETAMIDE SODIUM

OINTMENT; OPHTHALMIC		
PREDSULFAIR		
PHARMAFAIR	0.5%;10%	N88032 001 APR 15, 1983
SUSPENSION/DROPS; OPHTHALMIC		
PREDSULFAIR		
PHARMAFAIR	0.5%;10%	N88007 001 APR 19, 1983
PREDSULFAIR II		
PHARMAFAIR	0.2%;10%	N88837 001 DEC 24, 1985

PREDNISOLONE SODIUM PHOSPHATE

OINTMENT; OPHTHALMIC, OTIC		
HYDELTRASOL		
MERCK SHARP DOHME	EQ 0.25% PHOSPHATE	N11028 001
SOLUTION/DROPS; OPHTHALMIC		
METRETON		
SCHERING	EQ 0.5% PHOSPHATE	N83834 001
PREDAIR		
PHARMAFAIR	EQ 0.11% PHOSPHATE	N88415 001 FEB 29, 1984
PREDAIR FORTE		
PHARMAFAIR	EQ 0.9% PHOSPHATE	N88165 001 MAR 28, 1983
PREDNISOLONE SODIUM PHOSPHATE		
SOLA BARNES HIND	EQ 0.11% PHOSPHATE	N84171 001
	EQ 0.9% PHOSPHATE	N84168 001
	EQ 0.9% PHOSPHATE	N84169 001
	EQ 0.9% PHOSPHATE	N84172 001

PREDNISOLONE SODIUM PHOSPHATE; *MULTIPLE*

SEE NEOMYCIN SULFATE; PREDNISOLONE SODIUM PHOSPHATE

Discontinued Drug Products *(continued)*

PREDNISONE

SOLUTION; ORAL		
PREDNISONE		
PENNEX	5 MG/5 ML	N89726 001 AUG 02, 1988
TABLET; ORAL		
DELTA-DOME		
MILES	5 MG	N80293 001
FERNISONE		
FERNDALE LABS	5 MG	N83364 001
METICORTEN		
SCHERING	5 MG	N09766 001
PARACORT		
PARKE DAVIS	5 MG	N10962 002
PREDNISONE		
AM THERAP	5 MG	N89387 001 NOV 06, 1986
	10 MG	N89388 001 NOV 06, 1986
	20 MG	N89389 001 NOV 06, 1986
BARR	50 MG	N86596 001
BUNDY	5 MG	N83676 001
DANBURY PHARMA	50 MG	N86867 001
DURAMED	5 MG	N88394 001 OCT 04, 1983
	10 MG	N88395 001 OCT 04, 1983
	20 MG	N88396 001 OCT 04, 1983
ELKINS SINN	5 MG	N80491 001
	20 MG	N85811 001
EON LABS	5 MG	N84774 001
FERRANTE	2.5 MG	N80563 001
	5 MG	N80563 002
HEATHER	5 MG	N80320 001
	10 MG	N84341 001
	20 MG	N84417 001
	20 MG	N85543 001
	50 MG	N86946 001
ICN	5 MG	N80237 001
INWOOD LABS	1 MG	N80328 001
	2.5 MG	N80306 001
	5 MG	N80279 001
KV PHARM	5 MG	N84236 001
LEDERLE	5 MG	N86968 001
LEMMON	5 MG	N80397 001
NYLOS	5 MG	N85115 001
PANRAY	1 MG	N80350 001
	2.5 MG	N80350 002
	5 MG	N80350 003
PERRIGO	5 MG	N83059 001

PREDNISONE *(continued)*

TABLET; ORAL		
PREDNISONE		
PRIVATE FORM	20 MG	N85151 001
REXALL	5 MG	N80232 001
ROXANE	20 MG	N17109 001
	25 MG	N87833 001 MAY 04, 1982
SPERTI	1 MG	N80359 001
	2.5 MG	N80359 002
	5 MG	N80359 003
UDL	5 MG	N87984 001 JAN 18, 1983
	10 MG	N87985 001 JAN 18, 1983
	20 MG	N87986 001 JAN 18, 1983
UPSHER SMITH	5 MG	N87471 001
	20 MG	N87470 001
VANGARD	5 MG	N87682 001 JAN 15, 1982
	20 MG	N87701 001 JAN 15, 1982
VITARINE	5 MG	N80334 001
	5 MG	N80506 001
WHITEWORTH TOWNE	2.5 MG	N84913 001
	5 MG	N80343 001
	10 MG	N89028 001 JUL 24, 1986
	20 MG	N84913 002
ZENITH LABS	20 MG	N84134 001
1ST TX	5 MG	N80371 001
SERVISONE		
LEDERLE	5 MG	N80223 001

PRILOCAINE HYDROCHLORIDE

INJECTABLE; INJECTION		
CITANEST		
ASTRA	1%	N14763 004
	2%	N14763 005
	3%	N14763 003

PRIMAQUINE PHOSPHATE; *MULTIPLE*

SEE CHLOROQUINE PHOSPHATE; PRIMAQUINE PHOSPHATE

PRIMIDONE

TABLET; ORAL		
PRIMIDONE		
CIRCA	250 MG	N85052 001

Discontinued Drug Products *(continued)*

PROBENECID

TABLET; ORAL
PROBENECID

CHELSEA LABS	500 MG	N86150 002 APR 23, 1982
LEDERLE	500 MG	N86917 001

PROBENECID; *MULTIPLE*

SEE AMPICILLIN/AMPICILLIN TRIHYDRATE; PROBENECID
SEE COLCHICINE; PROBENECID

PROCAINAMIDE HYDROCHLORIDE

CAPSULE; ORAL
PROCAINAMIDE HCL

ASCOT	250 MG	N87542 001 JAN 08, 1982
	375 MG	N87697 001 MAR 01, 1983
	500 MG	N87543 001 JAN 08, 1982
CHELSEA LABS	250 MG	N85167 001
	375 MG	N87020 001
	500 MG	N87021 001
CIRCA	250 MG	N83795 001
	500 MG	N84357 001
LEDERLE	250 MG	N86942 001
	375 MG	N86952 001
	500 MG	N86943 001
ROXANE	250 MG	N88989 001 APR 26, 1985
	500 MG	N88990 001 APR 26, 1985
VANGARD	250 MG	N87643 001 JUN 01, 1982
	500 MG	N87875 001 JUN 01, 1982

PROCAN

PARKE DAVIS	250 MG	N85804 001
	375 MG	N87502 001
	500 MG	N85079 001

PROCAPAN

PANRAY	250 MG	N83553 002

PROCAINAMIDE HYDROCHLORIDE *(continued)*

INJECTABLE; INJECTION
PROCAINAMIDE HCL

FUJISAWA	100 MG/ML	N89415 001 NOV 17, 1986
	500 MG/ML	N89416 001 NOV 17, 1986
PHARMAFAIR	100 MG/ML	N88824 001 NOV 20, 1985
	500 MG/ML	N88830 001 NOV 20, 1985
QUAD PHARMS	100 MG/ML	N89256 001 MAY 30, 1986
	500 MG/ML	N89257 001 MAY 30, 1986
WARNER CHILCOTT	100 MG/ML	N89528 001 MAY 03, 1988
	500 MG/ML	N89529 001 MAY 03, 1988

TABLET, EXTENDED RELEASE; ORAL
PROCAINAMIDE HCL

CIRCA	250 MG	N88533 001 DEC 03, 1984
	500 MG	N88534 001 DEC 03, 1984
	750 MG	N88535 001 NOV 03, 1984
	1 GM	N89520 001 JAN 15, 1987

PROCAINE HYDROCHLORIDE

INJECTABLE; INJECTION
PROCAINE HCL

BEL MAR	1%	N80711 001
	2%	N80756 001
MILES	1%	N80415 001
	2%	N80415 002
SEARLE	1%	N86202 001
	2%	N86202 002

PROCAINE HYDROCHLORIDE; *MULTIPLE*

SEE EPINEPHRINE; PROCAINE HYDROCHLORIDE
SEE LEVONORDEFRIN; PROCAINE HYDROCHLORIDE; PROPOXYCAINE HYDROCHLORIDE

Discontinued Drug Products *(continued)*

PROCAINE HYDROCHLORIDE; TETRACYCLINE HYDROCHLORIDE

INJECTABLE; INJECTION
ACHROMYCIN
LEDERLE — 40 MG/VIAL;100 MG/VIAL — N50276 001
40 MG/VIAL;250 MG/VIAL — N50276 003
TETRACYN
PFIZER — 40 MG/VIAL;100 MG/VIAL — N60285 002

PROCAINE MERETHOXYLLINE; THEOPHYLLINE

INJECTABLE; INJECTION
DICURIN PROCAINE
LILLY — 100 MG/ML;50 MG/ML — N08869 001

PROCHLORPERAZINE EDISYLATE

CONCENTRATE; ORAL
COMPAZINE
SMITH KLINE FRENCH — EQ 10 MG BASE/ML — N11276 001
PROCHLORPERAZINE
BARRE — EQ 10 MG BASE/ML — N87153 001 JUN 08, 1982
PROCHLORPERAZINE EDISYLATE
PENNEX — EQ 10 MG BASE/ML — N88598 001 OCT 25, 1984

INJECTABLE; INJECTION
PROCHLORPERAZINE EDISYLATE
ELKINS SINN — EQ 5 MG BASE/ML — N89523 001 MAY 03, 1988
QUAD PHARMS — EQ 5 MG BASE/ML — N89637 001 FEB 01, 1988
EQ 5 MG BASE/ML — N89638 001 FEB 01, 1988

SYRUP; ORAL
PROCHLORPERAZINE EDISYLATE
BARRE — EQ 5 MG BASE/5 ML — N87154 001 SEP 01, 1982
PENNEX — EQ 5 MG BASE/5 ML — N88597 001 OCT 25, 1984

PROCHLORPERAZINE MALEATE

CAPSULE, EXTENDED RELEASE; ORAL
COMPAZINE
SMITHKLINE BEECHAM — EQ 75 MG BASE — N11000 004

TABLET; ORAL
PROCHLORPERAZINE
CIRCA — EQ 5 MG BASE — N85580 001
EQ 10 MG BASE — N85178 001
EQ 25 MG BASE — N85579 001
PROCHLORPERAZINE MALEATE
DURAMED — EQ 5 MG BASE — N89484 001 JAN 20, 1987
EQ 10 MG BASE — N89485 001 JAN 20, 1987
EQ 25 MG BASE — N89486 001 JAN 20, 1987

PROCYCLIDINE HYDROCHLORIDE

TABLET; ORAL
KEMADRIN
BURROUGHS WELLCOME — 2 MG — N09818 005

PROGESTERONE

INJECTABLE; INJECTION
PROGESTERONE
LILLY — 25 MG/ML — N09238 002

PROMAZINE HYDROCHLORIDE

CONCENTRATE; ORAL
SPARINE
WYETH AYERST — 30 MG/ML — N10942 001
100 MG/ML — N10942 004

INJECTABLE; INJECTION
SPARINE
WYETH AYERST — 25 MG/ML — N10349 008

SYRUP; ORAL
SPARINE
WYETH AYERST — 10 MG/5 ML — N10942 003

TABLET; ORAL
SPARINE
WYETH AYERST — 10 MG — N10348 006
200 MG — N10348 004

PROMETHAZINE HYDROCHLORIDE

INJECTABLE; INJECTION		
PROMETHAZINE HCL		
KNOLL PHARM	25 MG/ML	N84223 001
	50 MG/ML	N84222 001
ZIPAN-25		
ALTANA	25 MG/ML	N83997 001
ZIPAN-50		
ALTANA	50 MG/ML	N83997 002
SYRUP; ORAL		
MYMETHAZINE FORTIS		
ROSEMONT PHARM	25 MG/5 ML	N87996 001 JAN 18, 1983
PROMETHAZINE HCL		
KV PHARM	6.25 MG/5 ML	N85388 001
	25 MG/5 ML	N85385 001
PHARM ASSOC	6.25 MG/5 ML	N87518 001
TABLET; ORAL		
PROMETHAZINE HCL		
BARR	12.5 MG	N84555 001
	25 MG	N84554 001
	50 MG	N84557 001
BOOTS	12.5 MG	N84160 001
	25 MG	N84166 001
	50 MG	N84539 001
CHELSEA LABS	12.5 MG	N85986 001
	25 MG	N85684 001
	50 MG	N85664 001
CIRCA	12.5 MG	N83401 001
	25 MG	N83204 001
	50 MG	N83403 001
EON LABS	25 MG	N85146 001
	50 MG	N85146 002
GENEVA PHARMS	12.5 MG	N84233 001
LEMMON	25 MG	N89109 001 SEP 10, 1985
PRIVATE FORM	12.5 MG	N83214 001
TABLICAPS	12.5 MG	N84080 001
	25 MG	N84027 001
ZENITH LABS	50 MG	N83613 001
REMSED		
DUPONT MERCK	25 MG	N83176 002
	50 MG	N83176 001

PROPANTHELINE BROMIDE

INJECTABLE; INJECTION		
PRO-BANTHINE		
SEARLE	30 MG/VIAL	N08843 001
TABLET; ORAL		
PROPANTHELINE BROMIDE		
ASCOT	15 MG	N87663 001 OCT 25, 1982
CIRCA	15 MG	N83151 001
GENEVA PHARMS	15 MG	N80928 001
HEATHER	15 MG	N85780 001
MYLAN	15 MG	N83706 001
PRIVATE FORM	15 MG	N80977 001

PROPARACAINE HYDROCHLORIDE

SOLUTION/DROPS; OPHTHALMIC		
KAINAIR		
PHARMAFAIR	0.5%	N88087 001 JUN 07, 1983
PROPARACAINE HCL		
SOLA BARNES HIND	0.5%	N84144 001
	0.5%	N84151 001

PROPOXYCAINE HYDROCHLORIDE; *MULTIPLE*

SEE LEVONORDEFRIN; PROCAINE HYDROCHLORIDE; PROPOXYCAINE HYDROCHLORIDE

PROPOXYPHENE HYDROCHLORIDE

CAPSULE; ORAL		
PROPOXYPHENE HCL		
ALRA	65 MG	N83184 001
ANABOLIC	65 MG	N83185 001
BARR	65 MG	N83186 001
CHELSEA LABS	65 MG	N85190 001
EON LABS	32 MG	N84014 001
	65 MG	N83688 001
	65 MG	N83870 002
	65 MG	N86495 001
MYLAN	65 MG	N83299 001
PRIVATE FORM	32 MG	N83464 001
	65 MG	N83113 001
PROPOXYPHENE HCL 65		
WARNER CHILCOTT	65 MG	N83786 001

PROPOXYPHENE HYDROCHLORIDE; *MULTIPLE*

SEE ACETAMINOPHEN; PROPOXYPHENE HYDROCHLORIDE

SEE ASPIRIN; CAFFEINE; PROPOXYPHENE HYDROCHLORIDE

Discontinued Drug Products *(continued)*

PROPOXYPHENE NAPSYLATE; *MULTIPLE*

SEE ACETAMINOPHEN; PROPOXYPHENE NAPSYLATE
SEE ASPIRIN; PROPOXYPHENE NAPSYLATE

PROPRANOLOL HYDROCHLORIDE

INJECTABLE; INJECTION
PROPRANOLOL HCL

SMITH AND NEPHEW	1 MG/ML	N70135 001	APR 15, 1986

SOLUTION; ORAL
PROPRANOLOL HCL

PENNEX	20 MG/5 ML	N71984 001	MAR 03, 1989
	40 MG/5 ML	N71985 001	MAR 03, 1989

SUSPENSION; ORAL
INDERAL

WYETH AYERST	10 MG/ML	N19536 001	DEC 12, 1986

TABLET; ORAL
INDERAL

WYETH AYERST	90 MG	N16418 010	OCT 18, 1982

PROPRANOLOL HCL

CHELSEA LABS	10 MG	N70140 001	JUL 30, 1985
	20 MG	N70141 001	JUL 30, 1985
	40 MG	N70142 001	JUL 30, 1985
	60 MG	N70143 001	JAN 15, 1987
	80 MG	N70144 001	JUL 30, 1985
CIRCA	10 MG	N70378 001	MAR 19, 1987
	20 MG	N70379 001	MAR 19, 1987
	40 MG	N70380 001	MAR 19, 1987
	60 MG	N70381 001	MAR 19, 1987
	80 MG	N70382 001	MAR 19, 1987
DANBURY PHARMA	90 MG	N71183 001	OCT 06, 1986

PROPRANOLOL HYDROCHLORIDE *(continued)*

TABLET; ORAL
PROPRANOLOL HCL

DURAMED	10 MG	N70306 001	SEP 09, 1985
	20 MG	N70307 001	SEP 09, 1985
	40 MG	N70308 001	SEP 09, 1985
	60 MG	N70309 001	OCT 01, 1986
	80 MG	N70310 001	SEP 09, 1985
	90 MG	N71327 001	OCT 01, 1986
LEDERLE	10 MG	N72117 001	JUN 23, 1988
	20 MG	N72118 001	JUN 23, 1988
	40 MG	N72119 001	JUN 23, 1988
	80 MG	N72120 001	JUN 23, 1988
LEMMON	10 MG	N70232 001	OCT 07, 1987
	20 MG	N70233 001	JUN 23, 1986
MYLAN	60 MG	N72275 001	JUN 09, 1989
SCHERING	10 MG	N70120 001	AUG 06, 1985
	20 MG	N70121 001	AUG 06, 1985
	40 MG	N70122 001	AUG 06, 1985
	60 MG	N70123 001	OCT 29, 1986
	80 MG	N70124 001	AUG 06, 1985
SUPERPHARM	10 MG	N71515 001	JUN 08, 1988
	20 MG	N71516 001	JUN 08, 1988
	40 MG	N71517 001	JUN 08, 1988
	80 MG	N71518 001	JUN 08, 1988
ZENITH LABS	60 MG	N72068 001	JUL 29, 1988

PROPRANOLOL HYDROCHLORIDE; *MULTIPLE*

SEE HYDROCHLOROTHIAZIDE; PROPRANOLOL HYDROCHLORIDE

Discontinued Drug Products *(continued)*

PROPYLIODONE

SUSPENSION; INTRATRACHEAL

DIONOSIL AQUEOUS		
GLAXO	50%	N09309 001
DIONOSIL OILY		
GLAXO	60%	N09309 002

PROPYLTHIOURACIL

TABLET; ORAL

PROPYLTHIOURACIL		
ANABOLIC	50 MG	N80285 001
BOOTS	50 MG	N84075 001
CHELSEA LABS	50 MG	N85201 001
DANBURY PHARMA	50 MG	N80932 001
LANNETT	50 MG	N80016 001
PERRIGO	50 MG	N84543 001
TABLICAPS	50 MG	N80840 001
ZENITH LABS	50 MG	N80215 001

PROTAMINE SULFATE

INJECTABLE; INJECTION

PROTAMINE SULFATE		
QUAD PHARMS	50 MG/VIAL	N89307 001 MAY 30, 1986
	10 MG/ML	N89306 001 MAY 30, 1986
UPJOHN	50 MG/VIAL	N07413 001
	250 MG/VIAL	N07413 002 AUG 02, 1984

PROTEIN HYDROLYSATE

INJECTABLE; INJECTION

AMINOSOL 5%		
ABBOTT	5%	N05932 012 JAN 31, 1985
HYPROTIGEN 5%		
MCGAW	5%	N06170 003 JAN 10, 1984

PSEUDOEPHEDRINE HYDROCHLORIDE

CAPSULE, EXTENDED RELEASE; ORAL

SUDAFED 12 HOUR		
BURROUGHS WELLCOME	120 MG	N17941 002

PSEUDOEPHEDRINE HYDROCHLORIDE; *MULTIPLE*

SEE <u>CHLORPHENIRAMINE MALEATE; PSEUDOEPHEDRINE HYDROCHLORIDE</u>

PSEUDOEPHEDRINE HYDROCHLORIDE; TRIPROLIDINE HYDROCHLORIDE

CAPSULE, EXTENDED RELEASE; ORAL

ACTIFED		
BURROUGHS WELLCOME	120 MG;5 MG	N18996 001 JUN 17, 1985

SYRUP; ORAL

HISTAFED		
CENCI	30 MG/5 ML;1.25 MG/5 ML	N88283 001 APR 20, 1984
MYFED		
ROSEMONT PHARM	30 MG/5 ML;1.25 MG/5 ML	N88116 001 MAR 04, 1983

TABLET; ORAL

ALLERFED		
PRIVATE FORM	60 MG;2.5 MG	N88860 001 JAN 31, 1985
TRIPROLIDINE AND PSEUDOEPHEDRINE		
CIRCA	60 MG;2.5 MG	N88318 002 JAN 13, 1984
WEST WARD PHARM	60 MG;2.5 MG	N88117 001 APR 19, 1983

PSEUDOEPHEDRINE POLISTIREX

SUSPENSION, EXTENDED RELEASE; ORAL

PSEUDO-12		
FISONS	EQ 60 MG HCL/5 ML	N19401 001 JUN 19, 1987

PSEUDOEPHEDRINE SULFATE; *MULTIPLE*

SEE <u>DEXBROMPHENIRAMINE MALEATE; PSEUDOEPHEDRINE SULFATE</u>

PYRIDOSTIGMINE BROMIDE

TABLET; ORAL

PYRIDOSTIGMINE BROMIDE		
SOLVAY	30 MG	N89572 001 NOV 27, 1990

PYRIDOXINE; *MULTIPLE*

SEE <u>ASCORBIC ACID; BIOTIN; CYANOCOBALAMIN; DEXPANTHENOL; ERGOCALCIFEROL; FOLIC ACID; NIACINAMIDE; PYRIDOXINE; RIBOFLAVIN PHOSPHATE SODIUM; THIAMINE; VITAMIN A; VITAMIN E</u>

Discontinued Drug Products *(continued)*

PYRIDOXINE HYDROCHLORIDE
INJECTABLE; INJECTION
HEXA-BETALIN
LILLY 100 MG/ML N80854 001
PYRIDOXINE HCL
BEL MAR 100 MG/ML N80761 001
ELKINS SINN 100 MG/ML N80581 001
LUITPOLD 100 MG/ML N80669 001

PYRIDOXINE HYDROCHLORIDE; *MULTIPLE*
SEE ASCORBIC ACID; BIOTIN; CYANOCOBALAMIN; DEXPANTHENOL; ERGOCALCIFEROL; FOLIC ACID; NIACINAMIDE; PYRIDOXINE HYDROCHLORIDE; RIBOFLAVIN PHOSPHATE SODIUM; THIAMINE HYDROCHLORIDE; VITAMIN A; VITAMIN E
SEE ASCORBIC ACID; BIOTIN; CYANOCOBALAMIN; DEXPANTHENOL; ERGOCALCIFEROL; FOLIC ACID; NIACINAMIDE; PYRIDOXINE HYDROCHLORIDE; RIBOFLAVIN PHOSPHATE SODIUM; THIAMINE HYDROCHLORIDE; VITAMIN A PALMITATE; VITAMIN E

PYRILAMINE MALEATE
TABLET; ORAL
PYRILAMINE MALEATE
CHELSEA LABS 25 MG N85231 001

PYRVINIUM PAMOATE
SUSPENSION; ORAL
POVAN
PARKE DAVIS EQ 50 MG BASE/5 ML N11964 001
TABLET; ORAL
POVAN
PARKE DAVIS EQ 50 MG BASE N12485 002

QUINESTROL
TABLET; ORAL
ESTROVIS
PARKE DAVIS 0.2 MG N16768 003

QUINETHAZONE; RESERPINE
TABLET; ORAL
HYDROMOX R
LEDERLE 50 MG;0.125 MG N13927 001

QUINIDINE GLUCONATE
TABLET; ORAL
QUINACT
BERLEX 266 MG N85978 001
400 MG N86099 001
TABLET, EXTENDED RELEASE; ORAL
DURAQUIN
WARNER CHILCOTT 330 MG N17917 001
QUINATIME
CIRCA 324 MG N87448 001
QUINIDINE GLUCONATE
ASCOT 324 MG N88582 001 JUN 17, 1985
CHELSEA LABS 324 MG N87785 001 JAN 24, 1983
ROXANE 324 MG N88431 001 JAN 06, 1984
SUPERPHARM 324 MG N89164 001 NOV 21, 1985

QUINIDINE SULFATE
TABLET; ORAL
CIN-QUIN
SOLVAY 200 MG N84932 001
100 MG N85299 001
300 MG N85298 001
QUINIDINE SULFATE
ELKINS SINN 200 MG N83622 001
EVERYLIFE 200 MG N83439 001
LEDERLE 200 MG N86176 001
PERRIGO 200 MG N85322 001
ROSEMONT PHARM 200 MG N87837 001 APR 14, 1982
VANGARD 200 MG N87909 001 JUL 13, 1982
WARNER CHILCOTT 200 MG N83879 001
WHITEWORTH TOWNE 200 MG N85444 001
QUINORA
KEY PHARMS 200 MG N83576 001

RANITIDINE HYDROCHLORIDE
INJECTABLE; INJECTION
ZANTAC IN PLASTIC CONTAINER
GLAXO EQ 50 MG BASE/100 ML N19593 001 DEC 17, 1986

Discontinued Drug Products *(continued)*

RAUWOLFIA SERPENTINA

TABLET; ORAL

HIWOLFIA		
BOWMAN PHARMS	50 MG	N09276 003
	100 MG	N09276 004
HYSERPIN		
PHYS PRODS VA	50 MG	N10581 001
KOGLUCOID		
PANRAY	50 MG	N09278 001
	100 MG	N09278 002
RAUSERPIN		
FERNDALE LABS	50 MG	N09926 002
	100 MG	N09926 004
RAUWOLFIA SERPENTINA		
BUNDY	50 MG	N09477 001
	100 MG	N09477 002
DANBURY PHARMA	100 MG	N80914 001
ICN	50 MG	N09668 001
	100 MG	N09668 002
PRIVATE FORM	50 MG	N80583 001
	100 MG	N80583 002
PUREPAC PHARM	50 MG	N80842 001
	100 MG	N80842 002
SOLVAY	50 MG	N80500 001
	100 MG	N80500 002
TABLICAPS	50 MG	N83867 001
	100 MG	N83444 001
ZENITH LABS	50 MG	N11521 001
	100 MG	N11521 002
WOLFINA		
FOREST PHARMS	50 MG	N09255 008
	100 MG	N09255 006

RESCINNAMINE

CAPSULE; ORAL

CINNASIL		
PANRAY	0.5 MG	N84736 001

RESERPINE

INJECTABLE; INJECTION

SANDRIL		
LILLY	2.5 MG/ML	N10012 001
SERPASIL		
CIBA	2.5 MG/ML	N09434 002

RESERPINE *(continued)*

TABLET; ORAL

HISERPIA		
BOWMAN PHARMS	0.1 MG	N09631 002
	0.25 MG	N09631 004
RAU-SED		
SQUIBB	0.1 MG	N09357 001
	0.25 MG	N09357 004
	0.5 MG	N09357 006
	1 MG	N09357 008
RESERPINE		
BARR	0.25 MG	N80721 002
BELL PHARMA	0.1 MG	N83058 001
	0.25 MG	N83058 002
BUNDY	0.1 MG	N09663 001
	0.25 MG	N09663 003
CHELSEA LABS	0.25 MG	N85401 001
DANBURY PHARMA	0.1 MG	N80679 001
	0.25 MG	N80393 001
	1 MG	N80749 001
ELKINS SINN	0.1 MG	N83145 001
	0.25 MG	N83145 002
EVERYLIFE	0.1 MG	N10441 001
	0.25 MG	N10441 002
	0.5 MG	N10441 003
	1 MG	N10441 004
HALSEY	0.1 MG	N80457 002
	0.25 MG	N80457 001
	1 MG	N80457 003
ICN	0.1 MG	N09667 001
	0.25 MG	N09667 002
LEMMON	0.1 MG	N89020 001 MAR 07, 1985
	0.25 MG	N89019 001 MAR 07, 1985
MARSHALL PHARMA	0.1 MG	N80492 001
	0.25 MG	N80492 002
MK LABS	0.1 MG	N80525 002
	0.25 MG	N80525 001
MYLAN	1 MG	N84974 001
PHARMAVITE	0.25 MG	N84663 001
PRIVATE FORM	0.1 MG	N86117 001
	0.25 MG	N80582 001
	0.25 MG	N85775 001
	1 MG	N80582 002
REXALL	0.25 MG	N80637 001
ROXANE	0.1 MG	N09859 001
	0.25 MG	N09859 002
SOLVAY	0.25 MG	N80446 001
TABLICAPS	0.25 MG	N85207 001
WEST WARD PHARM	0.1 MG	N80975 001
	0.25 MG	N80975 002
	1 MG	N80975 003

Discontinued Drug Products *(continued)*

RESERPINE *(continued)*

TABLET; ORAL
RESERPINE
WHITEWORTH TOWNE 0.1 MG N80723 001
0.25 MG N80723 002
1 MG N80723 003
ZENITH LABS 0.1 MG N11185 001
0.25 MG N11185 002
SANDRIL
LILLY 0.1 MG N09376 004
0.25 MG N09376 001
SERPANRAY
PANRAY 0.1 MG N09391 001
0.25 MG N09391 002
1 MG N09391 004
SERPASIL
CIBA 1 MG N09115 004
SERPATE
VALE 0.1 MG N09453 001
0.25 MG N09453 002

RESERPINE; *MULTIPLE*

SEE CHLOROTHIAZIDE; RESERPINE
SEE HYDRALAZINE HYDROCHLORIDE; HYDROCHLOROTHIAZIDE; RESERPINE
SEE HYDRALAZINE HYDROCHLORIDE; RESERPINE
SEE HYDROCHLOROTHIAZIDE; RESERPINE
SEE HYDROFLUMETHIAZIDE; RESERPINE
SEE QUINETHAZONE; RESERPINE

RESERPINE; TRICHLORMETHIAZIDE

TABLET; ORAL
NAQUIVAL
SCHERING 0.1 MG;4 MG N12265 003
TRICHLORMETHIAZIDE W/ RESERPINE
CIRCA 0.1 MG;4 MG N85248 001

RIBOFLAVIN PHOSPHATE SODIUM; *MULTIPLE*

SEE ASCORBIC ACID; BIOTIN; CYANOCOBALAMIN; DEXPANTHENOL; ERGOCALCIFEROL; FOLIC ACID; NIACINAMIDE; PYRIDOXINE HYDROCHLORIDE; RIBOFLAVIN PHOSPHATE SODIUM; THIAMINE HYDROCHLORIDE; VITAMIN A; VITAMIN E
SEE ASCORBIC ACID; BIOTIN; CYANOCOBALAMIN; DEXPANTHENOL; ERGOCALCIFEROL; FOLIC ACID; NIACINAMIDE; PYRIDOXINE HYDROCHLORIDE; RIBOFLAVIN PHOSPHATE SODIUM; THIAMINE HYDROCHLORIDE; VITAMIN A PALMITATE; VITAMIN E
SEE ASCORBIC ACID; BIOTIN; CYANOCOBALAMIN; DEXPANTHENOL; ERGOCALCIFEROL; FOLIC ACID; NIACINAMIDE; PYRIDOXINE; RIBOFLAVIN PHOSPHATE SODIUM; THIAMINE; VITAMIN A; VITAMIN E

RISPERIDONE

TABLET; ORAL
RISPERDAL
JANSSEN 5 MG N20272 005
DEC 29, 1993

RITODRINE HYDROCHLORIDE

INJECTABLE; INJECTION
RITODRINE HCL
FUJISAWA 10 MG/ML N71188 001
JUL 23, 1987
15 MG/ML N71189 001
JUL 23, 1987
QUAD PHARMS 10 MG/ML N70700 001
OCT 06, 1986
15 MG/ML N70701 001
OCT 06, 1986

ROSE BENGAL SODIUM, I-131

INJECTABLE; INJECTION
ROBENGATOPE
BRACCO 0.5mCi/VIAL N16224 001
1mCi/VIAL N16224 002
2mCi/VIAL N16224 003
SODIUM ROSE BENGAL I 131
SORIN BIOMEDICA (US) 0.5mCi/ML N17318 001

Discontinued Drug Products *(continued)*

SAFFLOWER OIL
INJECTABLE; INJECTION
LIPOSYN 10%
ABBOTT 10% N18203 001
LIPOSYN 20%
ABBOTT 20% N18614 001

SARALASIN ACETATE
INJECTABLE; INJECTION
SARENIN
PROCTER AND GAMBLE EQ 0.6 MG BASE/ML N18009 001

SECOBARBITAL SODIUM
CAPSULE; ORAL
SECOBARBITAL SODIUM
LANNETT 100 MG N85903 001
50 MG N85909 001
PARKE DAVIS 100 MG N84762 001
PUREPAC PHARM 100 MG N85867 001
VITARINE 100 MG N85898 001
100 MG N86273 001
WHITEWORTH TOWNE 100 MG N85798 001
WYETH AYERST 100 MG N86390 001
SODIUM SECOBARBITAL
ANABOLIC 100 MG N84422 001
BARR 100 MG N84225 001
CHELSEA LABS 100 MG N85792 001
KV PHARM 100 MG N85285 001
PERRIGO 100 MG N84561 001
INJECTABLE; INJECTION
SECONAL SODIUM
LILLY 50 MG/ML N07392 002
SUPPOSITORY; RECTAL
SECONAL SODIUM
LILLY 30 MG N86530 001
60 MG N86530 002
120 MG N86530 003
200 MG N86530 004

SELENIUM SULFIDE
LOTION/SHAMPOO; TOPICAL
SELENIUM SULFIDE
PENNEX 2.5% N88228 001
SEP 01, 1983
THAMES 2.5% N86209 001

SELENOMETHIONINE, SE-75
INJECTABLE; INJECTION
SELENOMETHIONINE SE 75
MALLINCKRODT 100uCi/ML N17098 001
MEDI PHYSICS 250uCi/ML N17257 001
SETHOTOPE
BRACCO 85-550uCi/ML N17047 001

SERACTIDE ACETATE
INJECTABLE; INJECTION
ACTHAR GEL-SYNTHETIC
ARMOUR 40 UNITS/ML N17861 001
80 UNITS/ML N17861 002

SERTRALINE HYDROCHLORIDE
TABLET; ORAL
ZOLOFT
PFIZER EQ 150 MG BASE N19839 003
DEC 30, 1991
EQ 200 MG BASE N19839 004
DEC 30, 1991

SILVER SULFADIAZINE
DRESSING; TOPICAL
SILDIMAC
ENQUAY 1% N19608 001
NOV 30, 1989

SODIUM ACETATE; *MULTIPLE*
SEE AMINO ACIDS; MAGNESIUM CHLORIDE; POTASSIUM ACETATE; POTASSIUM CHLORIDE; SODIUM ACETATE
SEE CALCIUM CHLORIDE; DEXTROSE; MAGNESIUM CHLORIDE; SODIUM ACETATE; SODIUM CHLORIDE
SEE CALCIUM CHLORIDE; MAGNESIUM CHLORIDE; POTASSIUM CHLORIDE; SODIUM ACETATE; SODIUM CHLORIDE
SEE CALCIUM CHLORIDE; POTASSIUM CHLORIDE; SODIUM ACETATE; SODIUM CHLORIDE
SEE MAGNESIUM CHLORIDE; POTASSIUM CHLORIDE; SODIUM ACETATE; SODIUM CHLORIDE; SODIUM GLUCONATE

SODIUM BICARBONATE
INJECTABLE; INJECTION
SODIUM BICARBONATE IN PLASTIC CONTAINER
ABBOTT 0.9 MEQ/ML N19443 001
JUN 03, 1986
1 MEQ/ML N19443 002
JUN 03, 1986

Discontinued Drug Products *(continued)*

SODIUM BICARBONATE; *MULTIPLE*

SEE POLYETHYLENE GLYCOL 3350; POTASSIUM CHLORIDE; SODIUM BICARBONATE; SODIUM CHLORIDE; SODIUM SULFATE, ANHYDROUS

SODIUM CHLORIDE

INJECTABLE; INJECTION

BACTERIOSTATIC SODIUM CHLORIDE 0.9% IN PLASTIC CONTAINER

FUJISAWA	9 MG/ML	N88909 001 FEB 07, 1985

SODIUM CHLORIDE

ABBOTT	20 GM/100 ML	N17013 001

SODIUM CHLORIDE 0.45% IN PLASTIC CONTAINER

MILES	450 MG/100 ML	N18503 001

SODIUM CHLORIDE 0.9% IN PLASTIC CONTAINER

ABBOTT	9 MG/ML	N19218 001 JUL 13, 1984
MILES	900 MG/100 ML	N18502 001

SODIUM CHLORIDE 23.4% IN PLASTIC CONTAINER

FUJISAWA	234 MG/ML	N19329 001 APR 22, 1987

SODIUM CHLORIDE 3% IN PLASTIC CONTAINER

MCGAW	3 GM/100 ML	N19635 003 MAR 09, 1988

SODIUM CHLORIDE 5% IN PLASTIC CONTAINER

MCGAW	5 GM/100 ML	N19635 004 MAR 09, 1988

SOLUTION; IRRIGATION

SODIUM CHLORIDE IN PLASTIC CONTAINER

MILES	900 MG/100 ML	N18247 001

SODIUM CHLORIDE 0.45% IN PLASTIC CONTAINER

ABBOTT	450 MG/100 ML	N18380 001

SODIUM CHLORIDE; *MULTIPLE*

SEE AMINO ACIDS; DEXTROSE; MAGNESIUM CHLORIDE; POTASSIUM CHLORIDE; SODIUM CHLORIDE; SODIUM PHOSPHATE, DIBASIC

SEE AMINO ACIDS; DEXTROSE; MAGNESIUM CHLORIDE; POTASSIUM CHLORIDE; POTASSIUM PHOSPHATE, DIBASIC; SODIUM CHLORIDE

SEE AMINO ACIDS; MAGNESIUM ACETATE; PHOSPHORIC ACID; POTASSIUM ACETATE; SODIUM CHLORIDE

SEE AMINO ACIDS; MAGNESIUM ACETATE; POTASSIUM ACETATE; SODIUM CHLORIDE

SEE AMINO ACIDS; MAGNESIUM ACETATE; POTASSIUM ACETATE; SODIUM CHLORIDE; SODIUM PHOSPHATE, DIBASIC

SODIUM CHLORIDE; *MULTIPLE* *(continued)*

SEE AMINO ACIDS; MAGNESIUM CHLORIDE; POTASSIUM CHLORIDE; SODIUM CHLORIDE; SODIUM PHOSPHATE, DIBASIC

SEE AMINO ACIDS; MAGNESIUM CHLORIDE; POTASSIUM CHLORIDE; POTASSIUM PHOSPHATE, DIBASIC; SODIUM CHLORIDE

SEE CALCIUM CHLORIDE; DEXTROSE; MAGNESIUM CHLORIDE; SODIUM ACETATE; SODIUM CHLORIDE

SEE CALCIUM CHLORIDE; DEXTROSE; MAGNESIUM CHLORIDE; SODIUM CHLORIDE; SODIUM LACTATE

SEE CALCIUM CHLORIDE; DEXTROSE; POTASSIUM CHLORIDE; SODIUM CHLORIDE; SODIUM LACTATE

SEE CALCIUM CHLORIDE; DEXTROSE; SODIUM CHLORIDE; SODIUM LACTATE

SEE CALCIUM CHLORIDE; MAGNESIUM CHLORIDE; POTASSIUM CHLORIDE; SODIUM ACETATE; SODIUM CHLORIDE

SEE CALCIUM CHLORIDE; POTASSIUM CHLORIDE; SODIUM CHLORIDE; SODIUM LACTATE

SEE CALCIUM CHLORIDE; POTASSIUM CHLORIDE; SODIUM ACETATE; SODIUM CHLORIDE

SEE CALCIUM CHLORIDE; POTASSIUM CHLORIDE; SODIUM CHLORIDE

SEE DEXTROSE; POTASSIUM CHLORIDE; SODIUM CHLORIDE

SEE DEXTROSE; SODIUM CHLORIDE

SEE MAGNESIUM CHLORIDE; POTASSIUM CHLORIDE; SODIUM ACETATE; SODIUM CHLORIDE; SODIUM GLUCONATE

SEE POLYETHYLENE GLYCOL 3350; POTASSIUM CHLORIDE; SODIUM BICARBONATE; SODIUM CHLORIDE; SODIUM SULFATE, ANHYDROUS

SEE POTASSIUM CHLORIDE; SODIUM CHLORIDE

SODIUM CHROMATE, CR-51

INJECTABLE; INJECTION

CHROMITOPE SODIUM

BRACCO	2mCi/VIAL	N13993 002

SODIUM GLUCONATE; *MULTIPLE*

SEE MAGNESIUM CHLORIDE; POTASSIUM CHLORIDE; SODIUM ACETATE; SODIUM CHLORIDE; SODIUM GLUCONATE

Discontinued Drug Products *(continued)*

SODIUM IODIDE, I-123
CAPSULE; ORAL
SODIUM IODIDE I 123
GOLDEN PHARMS 400uCi N18671 003 MAY 27, 1982

SODIUM IODIDE, I-131
CAPSULE; ORAL
SODIUM IODIDE I 131
CIS 50uCi N17316 001
MALLINCKRODT 0.8-100mCi N16515 002

SODIUM LACTATE; *MULTIPLE*
SEE CALCIUM CHLORIDE; DEXTROSE; MAGNESIUM CHLORIDE; SODIUM CHLORIDE; SODIUM LACTATE
SEE CALCIUM CHLORIDE; DEXTROSE; POTASSIUM CHLORIDE; SODIUM CHLORIDE; SODIUM LACTATE
SEE CALCIUM CHLORIDE; DEXTROSE; SODIUM CHLORIDE; SODIUM LACTATE
SEE CALCIUM CHLORIDE; POTASSIUM CHLORIDE; SODIUM CHLORIDE; SODIUM LACTATE

SODIUM NITROPRUSSIDE
INJECTABLE; INJECTION
NITROPRESS
ABBOTT 50 MG/VIAL N18450 001
SODIUM NITROPRUSSIDE
FUJISAWA 50 MG/VIAL N70031 001 JAN 17, 1985

SODIUM PHOSPHATE, DIBASIC; *MULTIPLE*
SEE AMINO ACIDS; DEXTROSE; MAGNESIUM CHLORIDE; POTASSIUM CHLORIDE; SODIUM CHLORIDE; SODIUM PHOSPHATE, DIBASIC
SEE AMINO ACIDS; MAGNESIUM ACETATE; POTASSIUM ACETATE; SODIUM CHLORIDE; SODIUM PHOSPHATE, DIBASIC
SEE AMINO ACIDS; MAGNESIUM CHLORIDE; POTASSIUM CHLORIDE; SODIUM CHLORIDE; SODIUM PHOSPHATE, DIBASIC

SODIUM PHOSPHATE, P-32
SOLUTION; INJECTION, ORAL
PHOSPHOTOPE
BRACCO 1-8mCi/VIAL N10927 001
SODIUM PHOSPHATE P 32
MALLINCKRODT 1.5mCi/VIAL N11777 002

SODIUM POLYSTYRENE SULFONATE
POWDER; ORAL, RECTAL
SODIUM POLYSTYRENE SULFONATE
PENNEX 453.6 GM/BOT N88786 001 SEP 11, 1984

SUSPENSION; ORAL, RECTAL
SODIUM POLYSTYRENE SULFONATE
PENNEX 15 GM/60 ML N88717 001 SEP 11, 1984
ROXANE 15 GM/60 ML N88453 001 NOV 17, 1983

SODIUM SUCCINATE
INJECTABLE; INJECTION
SODIUM SUCCINATE
ELKINS SINN 30% N80516 001

SODIUM SULFATE, ANHYDROUS; *MULTIPLE*
SEE POLYETHYLENE GLYCOL 3350; POTASSIUM CHLORIDE; SODIUM BICARBONATE; SODIUM CHLORIDE; SODIUM SULFATE, ANHYDROUS

SOMATROPIN
INJECTABLE; INJECTION
ASELLACRIN 10
SERONO 10IU/VIAL N17726 001
ASELLACRIN 2
SERONO 2IU/VIAL N17726 002 JUL 21, 1983
CRESCORMON
GENENTECH 4IU/VIAL N17992 001

SOMATROPIN, BIOSYNTHETIC
INJECTABLE; INJECTION
HUMATROPE
LILLY 2 MG/VIAL N19640 001 JUN 23, 1987

SORBITOL
SOLUTION; IRRIGATION
SORBITOL 3% IN PLASTIC CONTAINER
BAXTER 3 GM/100 ML N18512 001 MAY 27, 1982

SORBITOL; *MULTIPLE*
SEE MANNITOL; SORBITOL

Discontinued Drug Products *(continued)*

SOTALOL HYDROCHLORIDE
TABLET; ORAL
BETAPACE
BERLEX 320 MG N19865 004 OCT 30, 1992

SOYBEAN OIL
INJECTABLE; INJECTION
TRAVAMULSION 20%
BAXTER 20% N18758 001 FEB 15, 1983

SPIRONOLACTONE
TABLET; ORAL
SPIRONOLACTONE
ASCOT 25 MG N87687 001 OCT 20, 1982
CHELSEA LABS 25 MG N87078 001
CIRCA 25 MG N86898 002 MAR 02, 1982
LEDERLE 25 MG N87634 001
PUREPAC PHARM 25 MG N88053 001 AUG 25, 1983
UPSHER SMITH 25 MG N87554 001
VANGARD 25 MG N87648 001 FEB 01, 1982
WARNER CHILCOTT 25 MG N87952 001 NOV 18, 1982

SPIRONOLACTONE; *MULTIPLE*
SEE HYDROCHLOROTHIAZIDE; SPIRONOLACTONE

STAVUDINE
CAPSULE; ORAL
ZERIT
BRISTOL MYERS SQUIBB 5 MG N20412 001 JUN 24, 1994

STREPTOMYCIN SULFATE
INJECTABLE; INJECTION
STREPTOMYCIN SULFATE
COPANOS EQ 500 MG BASE/ML N60684 001

SUCCINYLCHOLINE CHLORIDE
INJECTABLE; INJECTION
ANECTINE
BURROUGHS WELLCOME 50 MG/ML N08453 003
SUCCINYLCHOLINE CHLORIDE
INTL MEDICATION 100 MG/VIAL N85400 001 FEB 04, 1982

SULBACTAM SODIUM; *MULTIPLE*
SEE AMPICILLIN SODIUM; SULBACTAM SODIUM

SULCONAZOLE NITRATE
SOLUTION; TOPICAL
EXELDERM
WESTWOOD SQUIBB 1% N18738 001 AUG 30, 1985

SULFACETAMIDE SODIUM
OINTMENT; OPHTHALMIC
SULFAIR 10
PHARMAFAIR 10% N88000 001 DEC 22, 1982
SOLUTION/DROPS; OPHTHALMIC
SODIUM SULFACETAMIDE
SOLA BARNES HIND 30% N84146 001
30% N84147 001
10% N84143 001
10% N84145 001
SULFAIR FORTE
PHARMAFAIR 30% N88385 001 OCT 13, 1983
SULFAIR-15
PHARMAFAIR 15% N88186 001 MAY 25, 1983

SULFACETAMIDE SODIUM; *MULTIPLE*
SEE PREDNISOLONE ACETATE; SULFACETAMIDE SODIUM

SULFADIAZINE
TABLET; ORAL
SULFADIAZINE
ABBOTT 300 MG N04125 005
EVERYLIFE 500 MG N80088 001
LEDERLE 500 MG N04054 001
LILLY 500 MG N04122 002

Discontinued Drug Products *(continued)*

SULFADIAZINE SODIUM
INJECTABLE; INJECTION
SULFADIAZINE SODIUM
LEDERLE 250 MG/ML N04054 002

SULFAMETER
TABLET; ORAL
SULLA
BERLEX 500 MG N16000 002

SULFAMETHIZOLE
TABLET; ORAL
MICROSUL
FOREST PHARMS 1 GM N86012 001
PROKLAR
FOREST PHARMS 500 MG N80273 001
THIOSULFIL
WYETH AYERST 250 MG N08565 001

SULFAMETHOXAZOLE
TABLET; ORAL
GANTANOL-DS
ROCHE 1 GM N12715 003
SULFAMETHOXAZOLE
ASCOT 500 MG N87662 001 OCT 20, 1982
BARR 500 MG N87189 001 JUL 25, 1983
CIRCA 500 MG N85053 001
1 GM N86000 001
HEATHER 500 MG N86163 001
UROBAK
SHIONOGI 500 MG N87307 001

SULFAMETHOXAZOLE; TRIMETHOPRIM
INJECTABLE; INJECTION
SULFAMETHOPRIM
QUAD PHARMS 80 MG/ML;16 MG/ML N71341 001 AUG 07, 1987

SULFAMETHOXAZOLE AND TRIMETHOPRIM
FUJISAWA 80 MG/ML;16 MG/ML N70223 001 DEC 29, 1987

SULFAMETHOXAZOLE; TRIMETHOPRIM *(continued)*
SUSPENSION; ORAL
BACTRIM
ROCHE 200 MG/5 ML;40 MG/5 ML N17560 001
SULMEPRIM
ROSEMONT PHARM 200 MG/5 ML;40 MG/5 ML N70063 001 AUG 01, 1986

SULMEPRIM PEDIATRIC
ROSEMONT PHARM 200 MG/5 ML;40 MG/5 ML N70064 001 AUG 01, 1986

TRIMETH/SULFA
BARRE 200 MG/5 ML;40 MG/5 ML N72398 001 MAY 23, 1988

TABLET; ORAL
SULFAMETHOXAZOLE & TRIMETHOPRIM
HEATHER 400 MG;80 MG N18946 001 AUG 10, 1984
800 MG;160 MG N18946 002 AUG 10, 1984

SULFAMETHOXAZOLE AND TRIMETHOPRIM
CHELSEA LABS 400 MG;80 MG N70002 001 NOV 07, 1984
800 MG;160 MG N70000 001 NOV 07, 1984
EON LABS 400 MG;80 MG N18598 003 MAY 19, 1982
INTERPHARM 400 MG;80 MG N71299 001 OCT 27, 1987
800 MG;160 MG N71300 001 OCT 27, 1987
MARTEC 400 MG;80 MG N72408 001 DEC 07, 1988
ROSEMONT PHARM 400 MG;80 MG N70203 001 NOV 08, 1985
800 MG;160 MG N70204 001 NOV 08, 1985

SULFAMETHOXAZOLE AND TRIMETHOPRIM DOUBLE STRENGTH
MARTEC 800 MG;160 MG N72417 001 DEC 07, 1988

UROPLUS DS
SHIONOGI 800 MG;160 MG N71816 001 SEP 28, 1987

UROPLUS SS
SHIONOGI 400 MG;80 MG N71815 001 SEP 28, 1987

Discontinued Drug Products *(continued)*

SULFAPHENAZOLE
SUSPENSION; ORAL
SULFABID
PURDUE FREDERICK 500 MG/5 ML N13093 001
TABLET; ORAL
SULFABID
PURDUE FREDERICK 500 MG N13092 002

SULFASALAZINE
SUSPENSION; ORAL
AZULFIDINE
PHARMACIA 250 MG/5 ML N18605 001
TABLET; ORAL
S.A.S.-500
SOLVAY 500 MG N83450 001
SULFASALAZINE
CIRCA 500 MG N84964 001
EON LABS 500 MG N86184 001
TABLET, DELAYED RELEASE; ORAL
SULFASALAZINE
CIRCA 500 MG N88052 001 MAY 24, 1983

SULFINPYRAZONE
CAPSULE; ORAL
SULFINPYRAZONE
VANGARD 200 MG N88666 001 FEB 17, 1984

SULFISOXAZOLE
TABLET; ORAL
SOXAZOLE
ALRA 500 MG N80366 001
SULFALAR
PARKE DAVIS 500 MG N84955 001
SULFISOXAZOLE
BARR 500 MG N84031 001
CHELSEA LABS 500 MG N85534 001
HEATHER 500 MG N80189 001
LANNETT 500 MG N80085 001
LEDERLE 500 MG N87649 001
PHARMERAL 500 MG N84385 001
VITARINE 500 MG N87332 001
WEST WARD PHARM 500 MG N80379 001
SULSOXIN
SOLVAY 500 MG N80040 001

SULFISOXAZOLE ACETYL
EMULSION; ORAL
LIPO GANTRISIN
ROCHE EQ 1 GM BASE/5 ML N09182 009

SULFISOXAZOLE ACETYL; *MULTIPLE*
SEE ERYTHROMYCIN ESTOLATE; SULFISOXAZOLE ACETYL

SULFISOXAZOLE DIOLAMINE
INJECTABLE; INJECTION
GANTRISIN
ROCHE EQ 400 MG BASE/ML N06917 001
OINTMENT; OPHTHALMIC
GANTRISIN
ROCHE EQ 4% BASE N08414 002
SOLUTION/DROPS; OPHTHALMIC
SULFISOXAZOLE DIOLAMINE
SOLA BARNES HIND EQ 4% BASE N84148 001

SULFOXONE SODIUM
TABLET, DELAYED RELEASE; ORAL
DIASONE SODIUM
ABBOTT 165 MG N06044 003

SULFUR; *MULTIPLE*
SEE BENTONITE; SULFUR

SUPROFEN
CAPSULE; ORAL
SUPROL
JOHNSON RW 200 MG N18217 001 DEC 24, 1985

TALBUTAL
TABLET; ORAL
LOTUSATE
STERLING WINTHROP 120 MG N09410 005

TANNIC ACID; *MULTIPLE*
SEE CYANOCOBALAMIN; TANNIC ACID; ZINC ACETATE

TECHNETIUM TC-99M ALBUMIN AGGREGATED
INJECTABLE; INJECTION
TC 99M-LUNGAGGREGATE
MEDI PHYSICS 5mCi/ML N17848 001

Discontinued Drug Products *(continued)*

TECHNETIUM TC-99M ALBUMIN AGGREGATED KIT

INJECTABLE; INJECTION
A-N STANNOUS AGGREGATED ALBUMIN
GOLDEN PHARMS N/A N17916 001
LUNGAGGREGATE REAGENT
MEDI PHYSICS N/A N17838 001
TECHNETIUM TC 99M MAA
MEDI PHYSICS N/A N17773 001

TECHNETIUM TC-99M ALBUMIN MICROSPHERES KIT

INJECTABLE; INJECTION
INSTANT MICROSPHERES
3M N/A N17832 001

TECHNETIUM TC-99M ETIDRONATE KIT

INJECTABLE; INJECTION
CINTICHEM TECHNETIUM 99M HEDSPA
MEDI PHYSICS N/A N17653 001
MPI STANNOUS DIPHOSPHONATE
MEDI PHYSICS N/A N17667 001
OSTEOSCAN
MALLINCKRODT N/A N17454 001
TECHNETIUM TC 99M DIPHOSPHONATE-TIN KIT
MEDI PHYSICS N/A N17562 001

TECHNETIUM TC-99M FERPENTETATE KIT

INJECTABLE; INJECTION
RENOTEC
BRACCO N/A N17045 001

TECHNETIUM TC-99M MEDRONATE KIT

INJECTABLE; INJECTION
AMERSCAN MDP KIT
AMERSHAM N/A N18335 001
AUG 05, 1982

TECHNETIUM TC-99M POLYPHOSPHATE KIT

INJECTABLE; INJECTION
SODIUM POLYPHOSPHATE-TIN KIT
MEDI PHYSICS N/A N17664 001

TECHNETIUM TC-99M PYROPHOSPHATE KIT

INJECTABLE; INJECTION
AN-PYROTEC
CIS N/A N19039 001
JUN 30, 1987

TECHNETIUM TC-99M SODIUM PERTECHNETATE

SOLUTION; INJECTION, ORAL
SODIUM PERTECHNETATE TC 99M
CIS 12mCi/ML N17321 001
24mCi/ML N17321 002
48mCi/ML N17321 003
MEDI PHYSICS 2-100mCi/ML N17471 001

TECHNETIUM TC-99M SODIUM PERTECHNETATE GENERATOR

SOLUTION; INJECTION, ORAL
MINITEC
BRACCO 0.22-2.22 CI/GENERATOR N17339 001

TECHNETIUM TC-99M SULFUR COLLOID

SOLUTION; INJECTION, ORAL
TECHNETIUM TC 99M SULFUR COLLOID
MEDI PHYSICS 4mCi/ML N17456 001

TEMAFLOXACIN HYDROCHLORIDE

TABLET; ORAL
OMNIFLOX
ABBOTT EQ 400 MG BASE N20043 003
JAN 30, 1992
EQ 600 MG BASE N20043 004
JAN 30, 1992

TEMAZEPAM

CAPSULE; ORAL
TEMAZ
QUANTUM PHARMICS 15 MG N70564 001
OCT 15, 1985
30 MG N70547 001
OCT 15, 1985
TEMAZEPAM
CIRCA 15 MG N70383 001
MAR 23, 1987
30 MG N70384 001
MAR 23, 1987
DURAMED 15 MG N71708 001
SEP 29, 1988
30 MG N71709 001
SEP 29, 1988
ROSEMONT PHARM 15 MG N70489 001
JUL 07, 1986
30 MG N70490 001
JUL 07, 1986

Discontinued Drug Products *(continued)*

TERBUTALINE SULFATE
AEROSOL, METERED; INHALATION
BRICANYL
MERRELL DOW 0.2 MG/INH N18000 001 MAR 19, 1985

TESTOLACTONE
INJECTABLE; INJECTION
TESLAC
SQUIBB 100 MG/ML N16119 001
TABLET; ORAL
TESLAC
SQUIBB 250 MG N16118 002

TESTOSTERONE
INJECTABLE; INJECTION
TESTOSTERONE
STERIS 25 MG/ML N86420 001 MAY 10, 1983
50 MG/ML N86419 001 AUG 23, 1983

TESTOSTERONE CYPIONATE
INJECTABLE; INJECTION
DEPO-TESTOSTERONE
UPJOHN 50 MG/ML N85635 001
TESTOSTERONE CYPIONATE
QUAD PHARMS 100 MG/ML N89326 001 OCT 28, 1988
200 MG/ML N89327 001 OCT 28, 1988
STERIS 100 MG/ML N84401 001
200 MG/ML N84401 002

TESTOSTERONE ENANTHATE
INJECTABLE; INJECTION
DELATESTRYL
BTG PHARMS 200 MG/ML N09165 001
TESTOSTERONE ENANTHATE
QUAD PHARMS 100 MG/ML N89324 001 SEP 16, 1986
200 MG/ML N89325 001 SEP 16, 1986
STERIS 100 MG/ML N83667 001
200 MG/ML N83667 002

TESTOSTERONE ENANTHATE; *MULTIPLE*
SEE ESTRADIOL VALERATE; TESTOSTERONE ENANTHATE

TESTOSTERONE PROPIONATE
INJECTABLE; INJECTION
TESTOSTERONE PROPIONATE
BEL MAR 25 MG/ML N80741 001
50 MG/ML N80742 001
100 MG/ML N80743 001
ELKINS SINN 25 MG/ML N80276 001
LILLY 50 MG/ML N80254 002
QUAD PHARMS 100 MG/ML N89283 001 NOV 03, 1986
STERIS 25 MG/ML N85490 001
50 MG/ML N85490 002
100 MG/ML N83595 003

TETRACYCLINE HYDROCHLORIDE
CAPSULE; ORAL
CYCLOPAR
WARNER CHILCOTT 250 MG N61725 001
250 MG N62175 001
250 MG N62332 001
500 MG N61725 002
500 MG N62332 002
RETET
SOLVAY 250 MG N61443 001
500 MG N61443 002
SUMYCIN
APOTHECON 100 MG N60429 002
125 MG N60429 004
TETRACHEL
ANGUS 250 MG N60343 001
500 MG N60343 003
TETRACYCLINE HCL
BOOTS 250 MG N61802 001
500 MG N61802 002
CHELSEA LABS 250 MG N62103 001
500 MG N62103 002
ELKINS SINN 250 MG N60059 001
HEATHER 250 MG N61148 001
500 MG N61148 002
ICN 250 MG N60471 001
500 MG N60471 002
TABLET; ORAL
PANMYCIN
UPJOHN 250 MG N61705 001
500 MG N61705 002

TETRACYCLINE HYDROCHLORIDE; *MULTIPLE*
SEE PROCAINE HYDROCHLORIDE; TETRACYCLINE HYDROCHLORIDE

Discontinued Drug Products *(continued)*

TETRACYCLINE PHOSPHATE COMPLEX

CAPSULE; ORAL		
TETREX		
BRISTOL	EQ 250 MG HCL	N50212 002
	EQ 500 MG HCL	N50212 003

THALLOUS CHLORIDE, TL-201

INJECTABLE; INJECTION		
THALLOUS CHLORIDE TL 201		
BRACCO	1mCi/ML	N18548 001 DEC 30, 1982

THEOPHYLLINE

CAPSULE; ORAL		
SOMOPHYLLIN-T		
FISONS	100 MG	N87155 001 FEB 25, 1985
	200 MG	N87155 002 FEB 25, 1985
	250 MG	N87155 003 FEB 25, 1985
THEOPHYLLINE		
SCHERER	100 MG	N84731 002 NOV 07, 1986
	200 MG	N84731 001 NOV 07, 1986
	250 MG	N84731 003 NOV 07, 1986
CAPSULE, EXTENDED RELEASE; ORAL		
THEOBID		
WHITBY	260 MG	N85983 001 MAR 20, 1985
THEOBID JR.		
WHITBY	130 MG	N87854 001 MAR 20, 1985
THEOPHYL-SR		
JOHNSON RW	125 MG	N86480 001 FEB 08, 1985
	250 MG	N86471 001 FEB 08, 1985
THEOPHYLLINE		
CENT PHARMS	125 MG	N88654 001 FEB 12, 1985
	250 MG	N88689 001 FEB 12, 1985
EON LABS	260 MG	N87462 001 MAY 11, 1982
THEOPHYLLINE-SR		
SCHERER	300 MG	N88255 001 JUN 12, 1986

THEOPHYLLINE (*continued*)

ELIXIR; ORAL		
LANOPHYLLIN		
LANNETT	80 MG/15 ML	N84578 001
THEOLIXIR		
PANRAY	80 MG/15 ML	N84559 001
THEOPHYL-225		
JOHNSON RW	112.5 MG/15 ML	N86485 001
THEOPHYLLINE		
BARRE	80 MG/15 ML	N89223 001 MAY 27, 1988
CENCI	80 MG/15 ML	N87679 001 APR 15, 1982
PERRIGO	80 MG/15 ML	N85952 001
ROXANE	80 MG/15 ML	N84739 001
SYRUP; ORAL		
ACCURBRON		
MERRELL DOW	150 MG/15 ML	N88746 001 NOV 22, 1985
THEOPHYLLINE		
BARRE	150 MG/15 ML	N86545 001
	80 MG/15 ML	N86001 001
TABLET; ORAL		
THEOCLEAR-100		
CENT PHARMS	100 MG	N85353 002
THEOCLEAR-200		
CENT PHARMS	200 MG	N85353 001
THEOPHYL-225		
JOHNSON RW	225 MG	N84726 001
TABLET, CHEWABLE; ORAL		
THEOPHYL		
JOHNSON RW	100 MG	N86506 001 SEP 12, 1985
TABLET, EXTENDED RELEASE; ORAL		
DURAPHYL		
FOREST LABS	100 MG	N88503 001 APR 03, 1985
	200 MG	N88504 001 APR 03, 1985
	300 MG	N88505 001 APR 03, 1985

THEOPHYLLINE; *MULTIPLE*

SEE <u>PROCAINE MERETHOXYLLINE; THEOPHYLLINE</u>

THEOPHYLLINE SODIUM GLYCINATE

ELIXIR; ORAL		
SYNOPHYLATE		
CENT PHARMS	EQ 165 MG BASE/15 ML	N06333 008

Discontinued Drug Products *(continued)*

THIAMINE; *MULTIPLE*

SEE ASCORBIC ACID; BIOTIN; CYANOCOBALAMIN; DEXPANTHENOL; ERGOCALCIFEROL; FOLIC ACID; NIACINAMIDE; PYRIDOXINE; RIBOFLAVIN PHOSPHATE SODIUM; THIAMINE; VITAMIN A; VITAMIN E

THIAMINE HYDROCHLORIDE

INJECTABLE; INJECTION
THIAMINE HCL

BEL MAR	100 MG/ML	N80718 001
	200 MG/ML	N80712 001
FUJISAWA	100 MG/ML	N80509 001
LUITPOLD	100 MG/ML	N80667 001
PARKE DAVIS	100 MG/ML	N80770 001

THIAMINE HYDROCHLORIDE; *MULTIPLE*

SEE ASCORBIC ACID; BIOTIN; CYANOCOBALAMIN; DEXPANTHENOL; ERGOCALCIFEROL; FOLIC ACID; NIACINAMIDE; PYRIDOXINE HYDROCHLORIDE; RIBOFLAVIN PHOSPHATE SODIUM; THIAMINE HYDROCHLORIDE; VITAMIN A; VITAMIN E

SEE ASCORBIC ACID; BIOTIN; CYANOCOBALAMIN; DEXPANTHENOL; ERGOCALCIFEROL; FOLIC ACID; NIACINAMIDE; PYRIDOXINE HYDROCHLORIDE; RIBOFLAVIN PHOSPHATE SODIUM; THIAMINE HYDROCHLORIDE; VITAMIN A PALMITATE; VITAMIN E

THIORIDAZINE HYDROCHLORIDE

CONCENTRATE; ORAL
THIORIDAZINE HCL

BARRE	30 MG/ML	N87766 001 APR 26, 1983
GENEVA PHARMS	30 MG/ML	N88307 001 NOV 23, 1983
	100 MG/ML	N88308 001 NOV 23, 1983
PENNEX	30 MG/ML	N88258 001 JUL 25, 1983
	100 MG/ML	N88227 001 JUL 05, 1983

THIORIDAZINE HYDROCHLORIDE *(continued)*

TABLET; ORAL
THIORIDAZINE HCL

CHELSEA LABS	15 MG	N88562 001 MAY 11, 1984
CIRCA	10 MG	N88412 001 SEP 12, 1983
	15 MG	N88345 001 JUL 28, 1983
	25 MG	N88296 001 JUL 28, 1983
	50 MG	N88323 001 JUL 28, 1983
	100 MG	N88284 001 AUG 25, 1983
	150 MG	N88410 001 MAR 05, 1984
	200 MG	N88381 001 MAR 14, 1984
MYLAN	10 MG	N88332 001 JUN 27, 1983
	25 MG	N88333 001 JUN 27, 1983
	50 MG	N88334 001 JUN 27, 1983
	100 MG	N88335 001 NOV 18, 1983
PAR PHARM	10 MG	N88351 001 DEC 05, 1983
	15 MG	N88352 001 DEC 05, 1983
	25 MG	N88336 001 DEC 05, 1983
	50 MG	N88322 001 DEC 05, 1983
	100 MG	N88480 001 DEC 29, 1983
	150 MG	N89764 001 FEB 09, 1988
	200 MG	N89765 001 FEB 09, 1988
ROXANE	10 MG	N88663 001 MAR 15, 1984
	25 MG	N88664 001 MAR 15, 1984
	50 MG	N88665 001 MAR 15, 1984
	100 MG	N89048 001 FEB 26, 1985

Discontinued Drug Products *(continued)*

THIORIDAZINE HYDROCHLORIDE *(continued)*

TABLET; ORAL
THIORIDAZINE HCL

WEST WARD PHARM	10 MG	N88658 001 MAR 26, 1984
	15 MG	N88659 001 MAR 26, 1984
	25 MG	N88660 001 MAR 26, 1984
	50 MG	N88661 001 MAR 26, 1984
ZENITH LABS	100 MG	N88273 001 OCT 03, 1983

THIOTHIXENE

CAPSULE; ORAL
THIOTHIXENE

AM THERAP	2 MG	N71885 001 AUG 12, 1987
	5 MG	N71886 001 AUG 12, 1987
	10 MG	N71887 001 AUG 12, 1987
	1 MG	N71884 001 AUG 12, 1987
	20 MG	N72200 001 DEC 17, 1987
CHELSEA LABS	2 MG	N71626 001 JUN 25, 1987
	5 MG	N71627 001 JUN 25, 1987
	10 MG	N71628 001 JUN 25, 1987

THIOTHIXENE HYDROCHLORIDE

CONCENTRATE; ORAL
THIOTHIXENE HCL

PACO	EQ 1 MG BASE/ML	N71917 001 SEP 20, 1989
	EQ 5 MG BASE/ML	N71939 001 DEC 16, 1988

THYROGLOBULIN

TABLET; ORAL
PROLOID

PARKE DAVIS	16 MG	N02245 009
	32 MG	N02245 005
	65 MG	N02245 002
	100 MG	N02245 008
	130 MG	N02245 010
	200 MG	N02245 007
	325 MG	N02245 004

TICLOPIDINE HYDROCHLORIDE

TABLET; ORAL
TICLID

SYNTEX	125 MG	N19979 001 MAR 24, 1993

TIMOLOL MALEATE

TABLET; ORAL
TIMOLOL MALEATE

CIRCA	5 MG	N72269 001 APR 11, 1989
	10 MG	N72270 001 APR 11, 1989
	20 MG	N72271 001 APR 11, 1989
QUANTUM PHARMICS	5 MG	N72466 001 MAY 19, 1989
	10 MG	N72467 001 MAY 19, 1989
	20 MG	N72468 001 MAY 19, 1989
ROSEMONT PHARM	5 MG	N72001 001 APR 11, 1989
	10 MG	N72002 001 APR 11, 1989
	20 MG	N72003 001 APR 11, 1989

TIOCONAZOLE

CREAM; TOPICAL
TZ-3

PFIZER	1%	N18682 001 FEB 18, 1983

TOLAZAMIDE

TABLET; ORAL
TOLAZAMIDE

CIRCA	100 MG	N70242 001 AUG 01, 1986
	250 MG	N70243 001 AUG 01, 1986
	500 MG	N70244 001 AUG 01, 1986

Discontinued Drug Products *(continued)*

TOLAZAMIDE *(continued)*

TABLET; ORAL
TOLAZAMIDE

DURAMED	100 MG	N70165 001 JAN 10, 1986
	250 MG	N70166 001 JAN 10, 1986
	500 MG	N70167 001 JAN 10, 1986
INTERPHARM	250 MG	N71270 001 SEP 23, 1986
	500 MG	N71271 001 SEP 23, 1986
ROSEMONT PHARM	100 MG	N71355 001 JAN 11, 1988
	250 MG	N70168 001 APR 02, 1986
	500 MG	N70169 001 APR 02, 1986
SUPERPHARM	250 MG	N70763 001 JUN 16, 1986
	500 MG	N70764 001 JUN 16, 1986

TOLBUTAMIDE

TABLET; ORAL
TOLBUTAMIDE

ALRA	500 MG	N86141 001
ASCOT	500 MG	N87541 001 MAR 01, 1983
CIRCA	500 MG	N89111 001 MAY 29, 1987
	250 MG	N89110 001 MAY 29, 1987
PARKE DAVIS	500 MG	N86047 001
VANGARD	500 MG	N87876 001 APR 20, 1982

TRAZODONE HYDROCHLORIDE

TABLET; ORAL
TRAZODONE HCL

AM THERAP	50 MG	N71139 001 OCT 29, 1986
	100 MG	N71140 001 OCT 29, 1986
CIRCA	50 MG	N71112 001 NOV 17, 1986
	100 MG	N71113 001 NOV 17, 1986

TRAZODONE HYDROCHLORIDE *(continued)*

TABLET; ORAL
TRAZODONE HCL

QUANTUM PHARMICS	100 MG	N70921 001 DEC 01, 1986
ROSEMONT PHARM	50 MG	N70491 001 APR 29, 1987
	100 MG	N70492 001 APR 29, 1987

TRIALODINE

QUANTUM PHARMICS	50 MG	N70942 001 DEC 01, 1986

TRETINOIN

SWAB; TOPICAL
RETIN-A

JOHNSON RW	0.05%	N16921 002

TRIAMCINOLONE

TABLET; ORAL
ARISTOCORT

LEDERLE	16 MG	N11161 010

KENACORT

SQUIBB	2 MG	N11283 008
	1 MG	N11283 003

TRIAMCINOLONE

BARR	2 MG	N84286 001
	2 MG	N84318 001
	4 MG	N84267 001
	4 MG	N84319 001
	8 MG	N84268 001
	8 MG	N84320 001
CHELSEA LABS	4 MG	N85834 001
GENEVA PHARMS	4 MG	N85601 001
MYLAN	2 MG	N84406 001

Discontinued Drug Products *(continued)*

TRIAMCINOLONE ACETONIDE

CREAM; TOPICAL		
TRIACORT		
SOLVAY	0.1%	N87113 001
TRIAMCINOLONE ACETONIDE		
PENNEX	0.025%	N88094 001 SEP 01, 1983
	0.1%	N88095 001 SEP 01, 1983
	0.5%	N88096 001 SEP 01, 1983
PHARMADERM	0.025%	N87990 001 JUL 07, 1983
	0.1%	N87991 001 JUL 07, 1983
	0.5%	N87992 001 JUL 07, 1983
PHARMAFAIR	0.025%	N87921 001 AUG 10, 1982
	0.1%	N87912 001 AUG 10, 1982
	0.5%	N87922 001 AUG 10, 1982
TRYMEX		
SAVAGE LABS	0.5%	N88198 001 MAR 25, 1983
GEL; TOPICAL		
ARISTOGEL		
LEDERLE	0.1%	N83380 001
LOTION; TOPICAL		
KENALOG		
WESTWOOD SQUIBB	0.025%	N11602 003
	0.1%	N11602 001
OINTMENT; TOPICAL		
ARISTOCORT A		
LEDERLE	0.5%	N88781 001 OCT 05, 1984
TRIAMCINOLONE ACETONIDE		
PENNEX	0.025%	N88090 001 SEP 01, 1983
	0.1%	N88091 001 SEP 01, 1983
	0.5%	N88092 001 SEP 01, 1983
PHARMADERM	0.025%	N88692 001 AUG 02, 1984
	0.1%	N88690 001 AUG 02, 1984

TRIAMCINOLONE ACETONIDE; *MULTIPLE*

SEE NEOMYCIN SULFATE; TRIAMCINOLONE ACETONIDE
SEE NYSTATIN; TRIAMCINOLONE ACETONIDE

TRIAMTERENE; *MULTIPLE*

SEE HYDROCHLOROTHIAZIDE; TRIAMTERENE

TRIAZOLAM

TABLET; ORAL		
HALCION		
UPJOHN	0.5 MG	N17892 002 NOV 15, 1982

TRICHLORMETHIAZIDE

TABLET; ORAL		
TRICHLORMETHIAZIDE		
CHELSEA LABS	4 MG	N85962 001
	2 MG	N86458 001
CIRCA	4 MG	N83462 001
EON LABS	4 MG	N86171 001

TRICHLORMETHIAZIDE; *MULTIPLE*

SEE RESERPINE; TRICHLORMETHIAZIDE

TRICLOFOS SODIUM

SOLUTION; ORAL		
TRICLOS		
MERRELL DOW	1.5 GM/15 ML	N16830 001
TABLET; ORAL		
TRICLOS		
MERRELL DOW	750 MG	N16809 002

TRIDIHEXETHYL CHLORIDE

INJECTABLE; INJECTION		
PATHILON		
LEDERLE	10 MG/ML	N09729 001
TABLET; ORAL		
PATHILON		
LEDERLE	25 MG	N09489 005

Discontinued Drug Products *(continued)*

TRIFLUOPERAZINE HYDROCHLORIDE
CONCENTRATE; ORAL
TRIFLUOPERAZINE HCL
PENNEX EQ 10 MG BASE/ML N88143 001 JUL 26, 1983
INJECTABLE; INJECTION
TRIFLUOPERAZINE HCL
QUAD PHARMS EQ 2 MG BASE/ML N89893 001 OCT 17, 1988
TABLET; ORAL
TRIFLUOPERAZINE HCL
CIRCA EQ 1 MG BASE N85975 001 JUN 23, 1988
EQ 2 MG BASE N85976 001 JUN 23, 1988
EQ 5 MG BASE N85973 001 JUN 23, 1988
EQ 10 MG BASE N88710 001 JUN 23, 1988
DURAMED EQ 1 MG BASE N88967 001 APR 23, 1985
EQ 2 MG BASE N88968 001 APR 23, 1985
EQ 5 MG BASE N88969 001 APR 23, 1985
EQ 10 MG BASE N88970 001 APR 23, 1985

TRIFLUPROMAZINE
SUSPENSION; ORAL
VESPRIN
APOTHECON EQ 50 MG HCL/5 ML N11491 004

TRIFLUPROMAZINE HYDROCHLORIDE
INJECTABLE; INJECTION
VESPRIN
APOTHECON 3 MG/ML N11325 005
TABLET; ORAL
VESPRIN
SQUIBB 10 MG N11123 001
25 MG N11123 002
50 MG N11123 003

TRIHEXYPHENIDYL HYDROCHLORIDE
CAPSULE, EXTENDED RELEASE; ORAL
ARTANE
LEDERLE 5 MG N06773 010
TABLET; ORAL
TREMIN
SCHERING 2 MG N80381 001
5 MG N80381 003
TRIHEXYPHENIDYL HCL
CIRCA 2 MG N85117 001
5 MG N85105 001
VANGARD 2 MG N88035 001 JUL 30, 1982

TRIMEPRAZINE TARTRATE
SYRUP; ORAL
TRIMEPRAZINE TARTRATE
BARRE EQ 2.5 MG BASE/5 ML N85015 001 FEB 18, 1982
PENNEX EQ 2.5 MG BASE/5 ML N88285 001 APR 11, 1985

TRIMETHOBENZAMIDE HYDROCHLORIDE
INJECTABLE; INJECTION
TRIMETHOBENZAMIDE HCL
SMITH AND NEPHEW 100 MG/ML N89043 001 APR 04, 1986

TRIMETHOPRIM
TABLET; ORAL
TRIMETHOPRIM
BARR 200 MG N70495 001 SEP 24, 1986

TRIMETHOPRIM; *MULTIPLE*
SEE SULFAMETHOXAZOLE; TRIMETHOPRIM

TRIMIPRAMINE MALEATE
CAPSULE; ORAL
TRIMIPRAMINE MALEATE
ROSEMONT PHARM EQ 25 MG BASE N71283 001 DEC 08, 1987
EQ 50 MG BASE N71284 001 DEC 08, 1987
EQ 100 MG BASE N71285 001 DEC 08, 1987

Discontinued Drug Products *(continued)*

TRIPELENNAMINE HYDROCHLORIDE

TABLET; ORAL
TRIPELENNAMINE HCL

ANABOLIC	50 MG	N83037 001
BARR	50 MG	N80744 001
CHELSEA LABS	50 MG	N85188 001
CIRCA	50 MG	N80790 001
HEATHER	50 MG	N83989 001
PARKE DAVIS	50 MG	N83626 001
	25 MG	N83625 001

TABLET, EXTENDED RELEASE; ORAL
PBZ-SR

GEIGY	50 MG	N10533 002

TRIPLE SULFA (SULFABENZAMIDE;SULFACETAMIDE;SULFATHIAZOLE)

CREAM; VAGINAL
VAGILIA

LEMMON	3.7%;2.86%;3.42%	N88821 001 NOV 09, 1987

TABLET; VAGINAL
TRIPLE SULFA

FOUGERA	184 MG;143.75 MG;172.5 MG	N88463 001 JAN 03, 1985
PHARMADERM	184 MG;143.75 MG;172.5 MG	N88462 001 JAN 03, 1985

TRIPROLIDINE HYDROCHLORIDE

SYRUP; ORAL
ACTIDIL

BURROUGHS WELLCOME	1.25 MG/5 ML	N11496 002 JUL 01, 1983

MYIDYL

ROSEMONT PHARM	1.25 MG/5 ML	N87963 001 JAN 18, 1983

TRIPROLIDINE HCL

BARRE	1.25 MG/5 ML	N85940 001
PHARM ASSOC	1.25 MG/5 ML	N87514 001 FEB 10, 1982

TABLET; ORAL
ACTIDIL

BURROUGHS WELLCOME	2.5 MG	N11110 002 JUL 01, 1983

TRIPROLIDINE HCL

VITARINE	2.5 MG	N85610 001

TRIPROLIDINE HYDROCHLORIDE; *MULTIPLE*

SEE PSEUDOEPHEDRINE HYDROCHLORIDE; TRIPROLIDINE HYDROCHLORIDE

TRISULFAPYRIMIDINES (SULFADIAZINE;SULFAMERAZINE;SULFAMETHAZI

SUSPENSION; ORAL
LANTRISUL

LANNETT	167 MG/5 ML;167 MG/5 ML;167	N80123 002

SULFALOID

FOREST PHARMS	167 MG/5 ML;167 MG/5 ML;167	N80100 001

SULFOSE

WYETH AYERST	167 MG/5 ML;167 MG/5 ML;167	N80013 002

TRIPLE SULFA

BARRE	167 MG/5 ML;167 MG/5 ML;167	N80280 001

TRIPLE SULFAS

LEDERLE	167 MG/5 ML;167 MG/5 ML;167	N06920 003

TABLET; ORAL
SULFALOID

FOREST PHARMS	167 MG;167 MG;167 MG	N80099 001

SULFOSE

WYETH AYERST	167 MG;167 MG;167 MG	N80013 001

TRIPLE SULFA

PUREPAC PHARM	167 MG;167 MG;167 MG	N80086 001

TRIPLE SULFAS

LEDERLE	167 MG;167 MG;167 MG	N06920 002

TROLEANDOMYCIN

SUSPENSION; ORAL
TAO

PFIZER	EQ 125 MG BASE/5 ML	N50332 001

TROPICAMIDE

SOLUTION/DROPS; OPHTHALMIC
MYDRIACYL

ALCON	0.5%	N12111 002
	1%	N12111 004

MYDRIAFAIR

PHARMAFAIR	0.5%	N88274 001 SEP 16, 1983
	1%	N88230 001 SEP 16, 1983

Discontinued Drug Products *(continued)*

TUBOCURARINE CHLORIDE
INJECTABLE; INJECTION
TUBOCURARINE CHLORIDE

QUAD PHARMS	3 MG/ML	N89442 001 AUG 12, 1988

UNDECOYLIUM CHLORIDE; UNDECOYLIUM CHLORIDE IODINE COMPLEX
SOLUTION; TOPICAL
VIRAC REX

CHESEBROUGH PONDS	0.5%;1.8%	N11914 001

UNDECOYLIUM CHLORIDE IODINE COMPLEX; *MULTIPLE*
SEE UNDECOYLIUM CHLORIDE; UNDECOYLIUM CHLORIDE IODINE COMPLEX

UREA
INJECTABLE; INJECTION
STERILE UREA

ABBOTT	40 GM/VIAL	N17698 001

URSODIOL
CAPSULE; ORAL
ACTIGALL

CIBA	150 MG	N19594 001 DEC 31, 1987

VANCOMYCIN HYDROCHLORIDE
INJECTABLE; INJECTION

VANCOMYCIN HCL		
QUAD PHARMS	EQ 500 MG BASE/VIAL	N62845 001 JUL 15, 1988
	EQ 1 GM BASE/VIAL	N62845 002 JUL 15, 1988
VANCOR		
PHARMACIA	EQ 500 MG BASE/VIAL	N62956 001 AUG 01, 1988
	EQ 1 GM BASE/VIAL	N62956 002 AUG 01, 1988

VASOPRESSIN TANNATE
INJECTABLE; INJECTION
PITRESSIN TANNATE

PARKE DAVIS	5PRESSOR UNITS/ML	N03402 001

VENLAFAXINE HYDROCHLORIDE
TABLET; ORAL
EFFEXOR

WYETH AYERST	EQ 12.5 MG BASE	N20151 001 DEC 28, 1993

VERAPAMIL HYDROCHLORIDE
INJECTABLE; INJECTION

CALAN		
SEARLE	2.5 MG/ML	N18925 001 MAR 30, 1984
	2.5 MG/ML	N19038 001 MAR 30, 1984
VERAPAMIL HCL		
FUJISAWA	2.5 MG/ML	N70348 001 MAY 01, 1986
QUAD PHARMS	2.5 MG/ML	N70672 001 MAR 07, 1986
SMITH AND NEPHEW	2.5 MG/ML	N70697 001 JUL 31, 1987

TABLET; ORAL

CALAN		
SEARLE	160 MG	N18817 004 FEB 23, 1988
VERAPAMIL HCL		
CHELSEA LABS	40 MG	N72799 001 APR 28, 1989
WARNER CHILCOTT	80 MG	N70340 001 SEP 24, 1986
	120 MG	N70341 001 SEP 24, 1986

VERATRUM VIRIDE
TABLET; ORAL
VERTAVIS

WALLACE	130CSR UNIT	N05691 002

VINBLASTINE SULFATE
INJECTABLE; INJECTION
VINBLASTINE SULFATE

FUJISAWA	10 MG/VIAL	N89011 001 NOV 18, 1985
QUAD PHARMS	10 MG/VIAL	N89365 001 AUG 07, 1986
	1 MG/ML	N89311 001 MAR 23, 1987

Discontinued Drug Products *(continued)*

VINCRISTINE SULFATE

INJECTABLE; INJECTION		
ONCOVIN		
LILLY	1 MG/VIAL	N14103 001
	5 MG/VIAL	N14103 002
VINCRISTINE SULFATE		
ABIC	1 MG/ML	N70873 001 FEB 19, 1987
FUJISAWA	1 MG/ML	N70411 001 SEP 10, 1986
QUAD PHARMS	1 MG/ML	N70777 001 APR 29, 1986
	1 MG/ML	N70778 001 MAY 01, 1986
	1 MG/VIAL	N71222 001 MAR 07, 1988
	5 MG/VIAL	N71937 001 MAR 07, 1988
	2 MG/VIAL	N71223 001 MAR 07, 1988

VIOMYCIN SULFATE

INJECTABLE; INJECTION		
VIOCIN SULFATE		
PFIZER	EQ 1 GM BASE/VIAL	N61086 001
	EQ 5 GM BASE/VIAL	N61086 002

VITAMIN A

CAPSULE; ORAL		
VITAMIN A		
CHASE CHEM	50,000IU	N83351 001
EVERYLIFE	50,000IU	N83134 001

VITAMIN A; *MULTIPLE*

SEE ASCORBIC ACID; BIOTIN; CYANOCOBALAMIN; DEXPANTHENOL; ERGOCALCIFEROL; FOLIC ACID; NIACINAMIDE; PYRIDOXINE HYDROCHLORIDE; RIBOFLAVIN PHOSPHATE SODIUM; THIAMINE HYDROCHLORIDE; VITAMIN A; VITAMIN E

SEE ASCORBIC ACID; BIOTIN; CYANOCOBALAMIN; DEXPANTHENOL; ERGOCALCIFEROL; FOLIC ACID; NIACINAMIDE; PYRIDOXINE; RIBOFLAVIN PHOSPHATE SODIUM; THIAMINE; VITAMIN A; VITAMIN E

VITAMIN A PALMITATE

CAPSULE; ORAL		
AFAXIN		
STERLING WINTHROP	EQ 50,000 UNITS BASE	N83187 001
ALPHALIN		
LILLY	EQ 50,000 UNITS BASE	N80883 001
VI-DOM-A		
MILES	EQ 50,000 UNITS BASE	N80972 001
VITAMIN A		
CHASE CHEM	EQ 50,000 UNITS BASE	N80746 001
	EQ 50,000 UNITS BASE	N83207 001
ELKINS SINN	EQ 50,000 UNITS BASE	N85479 001
EVERYLIFE	EQ 50,000 UNITS BASE	N80943 001
	EQ 50,000 UNITS BASE	N83114 001
SQUIBB	EQ 50,000 UNITS BASE	N80860 001
WHARTON LABS	EQ 50,000 UNITS BASE	N83665 001
ZENITH LABS	EQ 50,000 UNITS BASE	N83035 001
	EQ 50,000 UNITS BASE	N83190 001
VITAMIN A PALMITATE		
BANNER PHARMACAPS	EQ 50,000 UNITS BASE	N83981 001
VITAMIN A SOLUBILIZED		
LEMMON	EQ 50,000 UNITS BASE	N80921 001
INJECTABLE; INJECTION		
VITAMIN A PALMITATE		
BEL MAR	EQ 50,000 UNITS BASE/ML	N80819 001

VITAMIN A PALMITATE; *MULTIPLE*

SEE ASCORBIC ACID; BIOTIN; CYANOCOBALAMIN; DEXPANTHENOL; ERGOCALCIFEROL; FOLIC ACID; NIACINAMIDE; PYRIDOXINE HYDROCHLORIDE; RIBOFLAVIN PHOSPHATE SODIUM; THIAMINE HYDROCHLORIDE; VITAMIN A PALMITATE; VITAMIN E

VITAMIN E; *MULTIPLE*

SEE ASCORBIC ACID; BIOTIN; CYANOCOBALAMIN; DEXPANTHENOL; ERGOCALCIFEROL; FOLIC ACID; NIACINAMIDE; PYRIDOXINE HYDROCHLORIDE; RIBOFLAVIN PHOSPHATE SODIUM; THIAMINE HYDROCHLORIDE; VITAMIN A; VITAMIN E

SEE ASCORBIC ACID; BIOTIN; CYANOCOBALAMIN; DEXPANTHENOL; ERGOCALCIFEROL; FOLIC ACID; NIACINAMIDE; PYRIDOXINE HYDROCHLORIDE; RIBOFLAVIN PHOSPHATE SODIUM; THIAMINE HYDROCHLORIDE; VITAMIN A PALMITATE; VITAMIN E

SEE ASCORBIC ACID; BIOTIN; CYANOCOBALAMIN; DEXPANTHENOL; ERGOCALCIFEROL; FOLIC ACID; NIACINAMIDE; PYRIDOXINE; RIBOFLAVIN PHOSPHATE SODIUM; THIAMINE; VITAMIN A; VITAMIN E

Discontinued Drug Products *(continued)*

WARFARIN POTASSIUM
TABLET; ORAL
ATHROMBIN-K

PURDUE FREDERICK	2 MG	N11771 007
	5 MG	N11771 004
	10 MG	N11771 005
	25 MG	N11771 006

WARFARIN SODIUM
INJECTABLE; INJECTION
COUMADIN

DUPONT MERCK	50 MG/VIAL	N09218 020
	75 MG/VIAL	N09218 012

TABLET; ORAL
ATHROMBIN

PURDUE FREDERICK	5 MG	N11771 003
	10 MG	N11771 002
	25 MG	N11771 001

PANWARFIN

ABBOTT	2 MG	N17020 001
	2.5 MG	N17020 002
	5 MG	N17020 003
	7.5 MG	N17020 004
	10 MG	N17020 005

WARFARIN SODIUM

CIRCA	2 MG	N86123 001 AUG 17, 1982
	2.5 MG	N86120 001 AUG 17, 1982
	5 MG	N86119 001 AUG 17, 1982
	7.5 MG	N86118 001 AUG 17, 1982
	10 MG	N86122 001 AUG 17, 1982
ROSEMONT PHARM	2 MG	N88719 001 JUN 27, 1985
	2.5 MG	N88720 001 AUG 06, 1985
	5 MG	N88721 001 JUL 02, 1985

WATER FOR IRRIGATION, STERILE
LIQUID; IRRIGATION
STERILE WATER IN PLASTIC CONTAINER

MILES	100%	N18246 001

XENON, XE-133
GAS; INHALATION
XENON XE 133-V.S.S.

MEDI PHYSICS	10mCi/VIAL	N17687 001

INJECTABLE; INJECTION
XENON XE 133

DUPONT	6.3mCi/ML	N17283 001
MEDI PHYSICS	1.3-1.7 CI/AMP	N17256 001

SOLUTION; INHALATION, INJECTION
XENEISOL

MALLINCKRODT	18-25mCi/AMP	N17262 002

ZINC ACETATE; *MULTIPLE*
SEE CYANOCOBALAMIN; TANNIC ACID; ZINC ACETATE

ZINC SULFATE
INJECTABLE; INJECTION
ZINC SULFATE

FUJISAWA	EQ 1 MG ZINC/ML	N19229 002 MAY 05, 1987

USP MONOGRAPH TITLE ADDITIONS OR CHANGES

The U.S. Pharmacopeia (USP) periodically makes additions to or changes in monograph titles. Some of these additions or changes may affect dosage form terms listed in this publication. The Cumulative Supplement lists, in a section similar to this one, applicable monograph title and dosage form additions or changes as soon as the modified USP Monograph is official. The monograph title additions or changes remain in that section of the Cumulative Supplement and in each succeeding supplement of that edition. Once the next edition of *Approved Drug Products with Therapeutic Equivalence Evaluations* is published, the products affected by the title additions or changes are displayed with the new dosage form in the appropriate drug list. It is possible for these additions or changes to be displayed in that section before all applicant holders have made labeling modifications; therefore, as notification to the reader, all monograph title additions or changes appearing in the 12th Cumulative Supplement of the previous Edition (14th), are listed below.

FORMER USP MONOGRAPH TITLE (FORMER ADP DOSAGE FORM; ROUTE)	NEW USP MONOGRAPH TITLE (NEW ADP DOSAGE FORM; ROUTE)

There were no additions or changes for this Section in 1994.

CUMULATIVE LIST OF ORPHAN PRODUCT DESIGNATIONS AND APPROVALS

[Through August 31, 1994]

NAME *Generic/Chemical* *TN=Trade Name*	INDICATION DESIGNATED	SPONSOR AND ADDRESS *DD=Date Designated* *MA=Marketing Approval*
2-0-DESULFATED HEPARIN TN= AEROPIN	TREATMENT OF CYSTIC FIBROSIS.	KENNEDY & HOIDAL, MDs. 7702 PARHAM ROAD RICHMOND VA 23294 DD 09/17/93
2-CHLORODEOXYADENOSINE	TREATMENT OF ACUTE MYELOID LEUKEMIA.	R.W. JOHNSON RESEARCH INSTITUTE ROUTE 202 SOUTH, P.O. BOX 670 RARITAN NJ 08869-0670 DD 07/20/90
24,25 DIHYDROXYCHOLECAL-CIFEROL	TREATMENT OF UREMIC OSTEODYSTROPHY.	LEMMON COMPANY 650 CATHILL ROAD SELLERSVILLE PA 18960 DD 02/27/87
3,4-DIAMINOPYRIDINE	TREATMENT OF LAMBERT-EATON MYASTHENIC SYNDROME.	JACOBUS PHARMACEUTICAL COMPANY P.O. BOX 5290 PRINCETON NJ 08540 DD 12/18/90
4-AMINOPYRIDINE	RELIEF OF SYMPTOMS OF MULTIPLE SCLEROSIS.	ELAN PHARMACEUTICAL RESEARCH 1300 GOULD DRIVE GAINESVILLE GA 30501 DD 06/02/87
4-AMINOSALICYLIC ACID TN= PAMISYL (P-D), REZI-PAS (SQUIBB)	TREATMENT OF MILD TO MODERATE ULCERATIVE COLITIS IN PATIENTS INTOLERANT TO SULFASALAZINE.	BEEKEN, WARREN, M.D. UNIVERSITY OF VERMONT BURLINGTON VT 05405-0068 DD 12/13/89
4-METHYLPYRAZOLE	TREATMENT OF METHANOL OR ETHYLENE GLYCOL POISON-ING.	ORPHAN MEDICAL 13911 RIDGEDALE DRIVE MINNETONKA MN 55305 DD 12/22/88
5-AZA-2'-DEOXYCYTIDINE	TREATMENT OF ACUTE LEUKEMIA.	PHARMACHEMIE U.S.A., INCORP. P.O. BOX 145 ORADELL NJ 07049 DD 08/03/87
5a8, MONOCLONAL ANTI-BODY TO CD4	FOR USE IN POST-EXPOSURE PROPHYLAXIS FOR OCCUPA-TIONAL EXPOSURE TO HUMAN IMMUNODEFICIENCY VIRUS.	BIOGEN, INC. 14 CAMBRIDGE CENTER CAMBRIDGE MA 02142 DD 12/20/93
6-METHYLENANDROSTA-1,4-DIENE-3,1,7-DIONE	HORMONAL THERAPY OF METASTATIC CARCINOMA OF THE BREAST.	ADRIA LABORATORIES, INC. P.O. BOX 16529 COLUMBUS OH 43216-6529 DD 09/19/91
8-METHOXSALEN TN= UVADEX	FOR USE IN CONJUNCTION WITH THE UVAR PHOTOPHERESIS TO TREAT DIFFUSE SYSTEMIC SCLEROSIS.	THERAKOS, INCORPORATED 201 BRANDYWINE PARKWAY WEST CHESTER PA 19380 DD 06/22/93
8-METHOXSALEN TN= UVADEX	FOR THE PREVENTION OF ACUTE REJECTION OF CARDIAC ALLOGRAFTS.	THERAKOS, INCORPORATED 201 BRANDYWINE PARKWAY WEST CHESTER PA 19380 DD 05/12/94
9-CIS RETINOIC ACID	TREATMENT OF ACUTE PROMYELOCYTIC LEUKEMIA.	LIGAND PHARMACEUTICALS, INC. 9393 TOWNE CENTRE DRIVE SUITE 100 SAN DIEGO CA 92121 DD 04/10/92
9-[3-PYRIDYLMETHYL]-9-DEA-ZAGUANINE	TREATMENT OF CUTANEOUS T-CELL LYMPHOMA.	BIOCRYST PHARMACEUTICALS, INCORPORATED 2190 PARKWAY LAKE DRIVE BIRMINGHAM AL 35244 DD 10/05/93
ACETYLCYSTEINE TN= MUCOMYST/MUCO-MYST 10 IV	INTRAVENOUS TREATMENT OF PATIENTS PRESENTING WITH MODERATE TO SEVERE ACETAMINOPHEN OVERDOSE.	APOTHECON P.O. BOX 4500 PRINCETON NJ 08543-4500 DD 08/13/87

CUMULATIVE LIST OF ORPHAN PRODUCT DESIGNATIONS AND APPROVALS *(continued)*

NAME *Generic/Chemical* *TN= Trade Name*	**INDICATION DESIGNATED**	**SPONSOR AND ADDRESS** *DD=Date Designated* *MA=Marketing Approval*
ACONIAZIDE	TREATMENT OF TUBERCULOSIS.	LINCOLN DIAGNOSTICS P.O. BOX 1128 DECATUR IL 62525 DD 06/20/88
AI-RSA	TREATMENT OF AUTOIMMUNE UVEITIS.	AUTOIMMUNE, INC. 10 VINING STREET BOSTON MA 02115 DD 10/08/92
ALDESLEUKIN TN= PROLEUKIN	TREATMENT OF METASTATIC RENAL CELL CARCINOMA.	CHIRON CORPORATION 4560 HORTON STREET EMERYVILLE CA 94608-2916 DD 09/14/88 MA 05/05/92
ALDESLEUKIN TN= PROLEUKIN	TREATMENT OF PRIMARY IMMUNODEFICIENCY DISEASE ASSOCIATED WITH T-CELL DEFECTS.	CHIRON CORPORATION 4560 HORTON STREET EMERYVILLE CA 94608 DD 03/22/89
ALGLUCERASE INJECTION TN= CEREDASE	REPLACEMENT THERAPY IN PATIENTS WITH GAUCHER'S DISEASE TYPE I.	GENZYME CORPORATION ONE KENDALL SQUARE CAMBRIDGE MA 02139 DD 03/11/85 MA 04/05/91
ALL-TRANS RETINOIC ACID TN= VEASNOID	TREATMENT OF ACUTE PROMYELOCYTIC LEUKEMIA.	HOFFMANN-LA ROCHE, INC. 340 KINGSLAND STREET NUTLEY NJ 07110 DD 10/24/90
ALLOPURINOL SODIUM TN= ZYLOPRIM FOR INJECTION	MANAGEMENT OF PATIENTS WITH LEUKEMIA, LYMPHOMA, AND SOLID TUMOR MALIGNANCIES WHO ARE RECEIVING CANCER THERAPY WHICH CAUSES ELEVATIONS OF SERUM AND URINARY URIC ACID LEVELS AND WHO CANNOT TOLERATE ORAL THERAPY.	BURROUGHS WELLCOME COMPANY 3030 CORNWALLIS ROAD RESEARCH TRIANGLE PK NC 27709 DD 10/16/92
ALPHA-1-ANTITRYPSIN (RECOMBINANT DNA ORIGIN)	SUPPLEMENTATION THERAPY FOR ALPHA-1-ANTITRYPSIN DEFICIENCY IN THE ZZ PHENOTYPE POPULATION.	COOPER DEVELOPMENT COMPANY 455 EAST MIDDLEFIELD ROAD MOUNTAIN VIEW CA 94034 DD 01/01/84
ALPHA-1-PROTEINASE INHIBITOR TN= PROLASTIN	REPLACEMENT THERAPY IN THE ALPHA-1-PROTEINASE INHIBITOR CONGENITAL DEFICIENCY STATE.	MILES, INC. 4TH & PARKER STREETS BERKELEY CA 94710 DD 12/07/84 MA 12/02/87
ALPHA-GALACTOSIDASE A TN= FABRase	TREATMENT OF FABRY'S DISEASE.	DESNICK, ROBERT J., M.D. MOUNT SINAI SCHOOL OF MEDICINE NEW YORK NY 10029-6574 DD 07/20/90
ALPHA-GALACTOSIDASE A TN= CC-GALACTOSIDASE	TREATMENT OF ALPHA-GALACTOSIDASE A DEFICIENCY (FABRY'S DISEASE).	CALHOUN, DAVID H., PH.D. CONVENT AVE. & 138TH STREET NEW YORK NY 10031-9127 DD 06/17/91
ALPROSTADIL TN= VASOPROST	TREATMENT OF SEVERE PERIPHERAL ARTERIAL OCCLUSIVE DISEASE (CRITICAL LIMB ISCHEMIA) IN PATIENTS WHERE OTHER PROCEDURES, GRAFTS OR ANGIOPLASTY, ARE NOT INDICATED.	SCHWARZ PHARMA 5600 WEST COUNTY LINE ROAD MEQUON WI 53092 DD 10/20/93
ALTRETAMINE TN= HEXALEN	TREATMENT OF ADVANCED ADENOCARCINOMA OF THE OVARY.	U.S. BIOSCIENCE, INC. 100 FRONT STREET WEST CONSHOHOCKEN PA 19428 DD 02/09/84 MA 12/26/90
AMILORIDE HCL SOLUTION FOR INHALATION	TREATMENT OF CYSTIC FIBROSIS.	GLAXO, INC. 5 MOORE DRIVE RESEARCH TRIANGLE PK NC 27709 DD 07/18/90
AMINOSALICYLATE SODIUM	TREATMENT OF CROHN'S DISEASE.	SYNCOM PHARMACEUTICALS, INC. 155 PASSAIC AVENUE FAIRFIELD NJ 07004 DD 04/06/93
AMINOSALICYLIC ACID TN= PASER GRANULES	TREATMENT OF TUBERCULOSIS INFECTIONS.	JACOBUS PHARMACEUTICAL COMPANY 37 CLEVELAND LANE PRINCETON NJ 08540 DD 02/19/92 MA 06/30/94

CUMULATIVE LIST OF ORPHAN PRODUCT DESIGNATIONS AND APPROVALS *(continued)*

NAME *Generic/Chemical* *TN=Trade Name*	INDICATION DESIGNATED	SPONSOR AND ADDRESS *DD=Date Designated* *MA=Marketing Approval*
AMINOSIDINE TN= GABBROMICINA	TREATMENT OF TUBERCULOSIS.	KANYOK, THOMAS P., PHARM.D UNIVERSITY OF ILLINOIS AT CHICAGO CHICAGO IL 60612 DD 05/14/93
AMINOSIDINE TN= GABBROMICINA	TREATMENT OF MYCOBACTERIUM AVIUM COMPLEX.	KANYOK, THOMAS P., PHARM.D. UNIVERSITY OF ILLINOIS AT CHICAGO CHICAGO IL 60612 DD 11/15/93
AMIODARONE TN= AMIO-AQUEOUS	TREATMENT OF INCESSANT VENTRICULAR TACHYCARDIA.	ACADEMIC PHARMACEUTICALS, INC. 25720 SAUNDERS ROAD NORTH LAKE FOREST IL 60045 DD 08/17/93
AMIODARONE HCL TN= CORDARONE	FOR THE ACUTE TREATMENT AND PROPHYLAXIS OF LIFE-THREATENING VENTRICULAR TACHYCARDIA OR VENTRICULAR FIBRILLATION.	WYETH-AYERST LABORATORIES P.O. BOX 8299 PHILADELPHIA PA 19101-1245 DD 03/16/94
AMMONIUM TETRATHIOMOLYBDATE	TREATMENT OF WILSON'S DISEASE.	BREWER, GEORGE J., M.D. UNIVERSITY OF MICHIGAN MEDICAL SCHOOL ANN ARBOR MI 48109-0618 DD 01/31/94
AMPHOTERICIN B LIPID COMPLEX TN= ABLC	TREATMENT OF CRYPTOCOCCAL MENINGITIS.	THE LIPOSOME COMPANY ONE RESEARCH WAY PRINCETON NJ 08540-6619 DD 12/05/91
AMSACRINE TN= AMSIDYL	TREATMENT OF ACUTE ADULT LEUKEMIA.	WARNER-LAMBERT COMPANY 2800 PLYMOUTH ROAD, P.O. BOX 1047 ANN ARBOR MI 48106-1047 DD 12/07/84
ANAGRELIDE	TREATMENT OF POLYCYTHEMIA VERA.	ROBERTS PHARMACEUTICAL CORP. 6 INDUSTRIAL WAY WEST EATONTOWN NJ 07724 DD 06/11/85
ANAGRELIDE	TREATMENT OF ESSENTIAL THROMBOCYTHEMIA (ET).	ROBERTS PHARMACEUTICAL CORP. 6 INDUSTRIAL WAY WEST EATONTOWN NJ 07724 DD 01/27/88
ANAGRELIDE	TREATMENT OF THROMBOCYTOSIS IN CHRONIC MYELOGENOUS LEUKEMIA.	ROBERTS PHARMACEUTICAL CORP. 6 INDUSTRIAL WAY WEST EATONTOWN NJ 07724 DD 07/14/86
ANANAIN, COMOSAIN TN= VIANAIN	FOR THE ENZYMATIC DEBRIDEMENT OF SEVERE BURNS.	GENZYME CORPORATION ONE KENDALL SQUARE CAMBRIDGE MA 02139 DD 01/21/92
ANARITIDE ACETATE TN= AURICULIN	IMPROVEMENT OF EARLY RENAL ALLOGRAFT FUNCTION FOLLOWING RENAL TRANSPLANTATION.	SCIOS NOVA, INC. 2450 BAYSHORE PARKWAY MOUNTAIN VIEW CA 94043 DD 04/10/92
ANARITIDE ACETATE TN= AURICULIN	TREATMENT OF PATIENTS WITH ACUTE RENAL FAILURE.	SCIOS NOVA, INC. 2450 BAYSHORE PARKWAY MOUNTAIN VIEW CA 94043 DD 08/27/92
ANCROD TN= ARVIN	FOR USE AS AN ANTITHROMBOTIC IN PATIENTS WITH HEPARIN INDUCED THROMBOCYTOPENIA OR THROMBOSIS WHO REQUIRE IMMEDIATE AND CONTINUED ANTICOAGULATION.	KNOLL PHARMACEUTICALS 30 NORTH JEFFERSON ROAD WHIPPANY NJ 07981 DD 10/20/89
ANTI PAN T LYMPHOCYTE MONOCLONAL ANTIBODY TN= ANTI-T LYMPHOCYTE IMMUNOTOXIN XMMLY-H65-RTA	FOR EX-VIVO TREATMENT TO ELIMINATE MATURE T CELLS FROM POTENTIAL BONE MARROW GRAFTS.	XOMA CORPORATION 2910 SEVENTH STREET BERKELEY CA 94710 DD 01/29/86

CUMULATIVE LIST OF ORPHAN PRODUCT DESIGNATIONS AND APPROVALS *(continued)*

NAME *Generic/Chemical* *TN=Trade Name*	**INDICATION DESIGNATED**	**SPONSOR AND ADDRESS** *DD=Date Designated* *MA=Marketing Approval*
ANTI PAN T LYMPHOCYTE MONOCLONAL ANTIBODY TN= ANTI-T LYMPHOCYTE IMMUNOTOXIN XMMLY-H65-RTA	FOR IN-VIVO TREATMENT OF BONE MARROW RECIPIENTS TO PREVENT GRAFT REJECTION AND GRAFT VS. HOST DISEASE (GVHD).	XOMA CORPORATION 2910 SEVENTH STREET BERKELEY CA 94710 DD 01/29/86
ANTI-CD45 MONOCLONAL ANTIBODIES	PREVENTION OF ACUTE GRAFT REJECTION OF HUMAN ORGAN TRANSPLANTS.	BAXTER HEALTHCARE CORPORATION 1620 WAUKEGAN ROAD MCGAW PARK IL 60085 DD 09/10/90
ANTI-TAP-72 IMMUNOTOXIN TN= XOMAZYME-791	TREATMENT OF METASTATIC COLORECTAL ADENOCARCINOMA.	XOMA CORPORATION 2910 SEVENTH STREET BERKELEY CA 94710 DD 03/06/87
ANTI-THYMOCYTE SERUM TN= NASHVILLE RABBIT ANTI-THYMOCYTE SERUM	TREATMENT OF ALLOGRAFT REJECTION, INCLUDING SOLID ORGAN (KIDNEY, LIVER, HEART, LUNG, AND PANCREAS) AND BONE MARROW TRANSPLANTATION.	APPLIED MEDICAL RESEARCH 1600 HAYES STREET NASHVILLE TN 37203 DD 06/02/93
ANTIEPILEPSIRINE	TREATMENT OF DRUG RESISTANT GENERALIZED TONIC-CLONIC (GTC) EPILEPSY IN CHILDREN AND ADULTS.	CHILDREN'S HOSPITAL 700 CHILDREN'S DRIVE COLUMBUS OH 43205 DD 03/23/89
ANTIHEMOPHILIC FACTOR (RECOMBINANT) TN= KOGENATE	PROPHYLAXIS AND TREATMENT OF BLEEDING IN INDIVIDUALS WITH HEMOPHILIA A OR FOR PROPHYLAXIS WHEN SURGERY IS REQUIRED IN INDIVIDUALS WITH HEMOPHILIA A.	MILES, INC. 4TH & PARKER STREETS BERKELEY CA 94701 DD 09/25/89 MA 02/25/93
ANTIHEMOPHILIC FACTOR, HUMAN TN= HUMATE P	TREATMENT OF PATIENTS WITH VON WILLEBRAND'S DISEASE.	BEHRINGWERKE AKTIENGESELLSCHAFT (AG) 500 ARCOLA ROAD, P.O. BOX 1200 COLLEGEVILLE PA 19426-0107 DD 10/16/92
ANTIMELANOMA ANTIBODY XMMME-001-DTPA 111 INDIUM TN= ANTIMELANOMA ANTIBODY XMMME-001-DTPA 111 INDIUM	DIAGNOSTIC USE IN IMAGING SYSTEMIC AND NODAL MELANOMA METASTASIS.	XOMA CORPORATION 2910 SEVENTH STREET BERKELEY CA 94710 DD 11/14/84
ANTIMELANOMA ANTIBODY XMMME-001-RTA TN= ANTIMELANOMA ANTIBODY XMMME-001-RTA	TREATMENT OF STAGE III MELANOMA NOT AMENABLE TO SURGICAL RESECTION.	XOMA CORPORATION 2910 SEVENTH SREET BERKELEY CA 94710 DD 11/14/84
ANTITHROMBIN III (HUMAN) TN= THROMBATE III	REPLACEMENT THERAPY IN CONGENITAL DEFICIENCY OF AT-III FOR PREVENTION AND TREATMENT OF THROMBOSIS AND PULMONARY EMBOLI.	MILES, INC. P.O. BOX 1986 BERKELEY CA 94701 DD 11/26/84 MA 12/30/91
ANTITHROMBIN III CONCENTRATE IV TN= KYBERNIN	PROPHYLAXIS AND TREATMENT OF THROMBOEMBOLIC EPISODES IN PATIENTS WITH GENETIC AT-III DEFICIENCY.	HOECHST-ROUSSEL PHARMACEUTICAL ROUTE 202-206 NORTH SOMERVILLE NJ 08876 DD 07/02/85
ANTITHROMBIN III HUMAN TN= ATnativ	FOR THE TREATMENT OF PATIENTS WITH HEREDITARY ANTITHROMBIN III DEFICIENCY IN CONNECTION WITH SURGICAL OR OBSTETRICAL PROCEDURES OR WHEN THEY SUFFER FROM THROMBOEMBOLISM.	KABIVITRUM, INC. P.O. BOX 430 DANVILLE CA 94526 DD 02/08/85 MA 12/13/89
ANTITHROMBIN III HUMAN TN= ANTITHROMBIN III HUMAN	PREVENTING OR ARRESTING EPISODES OF THROMBOSIS IN PATIENTS WITH CONGENITAL AT-III DEFICIENCY AND/OR TO PREVENT THE OCCURRENCE OF THROMBOSIS IN PATIENTS WITH AT-III DEFICIENCY WHO HAVE UNDERGONE TRAUMA OR WHO ARE ABOUT TO UNDERGO SURGERY OR PARTURITION.	AMERICAN NATIONAL RED CROSS 9312 OLD GEORGETOWN ROAD BETHESDA MD 20814 DD 01/02/86
ANTIVENIN, POLYVALENT CROTALID (OVINE) FAB TN= CROTAB	TREATMENT OF ENVENOMATIONS INFLICTED BY NORTH AMERICAN CROTALID SNAKES.	THERAPEUTIC ANTIBODIES INC. 1500 21ST AVENUE SOUTH SOUTE 310 NASHVILLE TN 37212 DD 01/12/94
ANTIVENOM (CROTALIDAE) PURIFIED (AVIAN)	TREATMENT OF ENVENOMATION BY POISONOUS SNAKES BELONGING TO THE CROTALIDAE FAMILY.	OPHIDIAN PHARMACEUTICALS, INC. 5445 EAST CHERYL PARKWAY MADISON WI 53711 DD 02/12/91

CUMULATIVE LIST OF ORPHAN PRODUCT DESIGNATIONS AND APPROVALS *(continued)*

NAME *Generic/Chemical* *TN=Trade Name*	INDICATION DESIGNATED	SPONSOR AND ADDRESS *DD=Date Designated* *MA=Marketing Approval*
APOMORPHINE HCL	TREATMENT OF THE ON-OFF FLUCTUATIONS ASSOCIATED WITH LATE-STAGE PARKINSON'S DISEASE.	FORUM PRODUCTS, INC. 33 FLYING POINT ROAD SOUTHAMPTON NY 11968 DD 04/22/93
APROTININ TN= TRASYLOL	FOR PROPHYLACTIC USE TO REDUCE PERIOPERATIVE BLOOD LOSS AND THE HOMOLOGOUS BLOOD TRANSFUSION REQUIREMENT IN PATIENTS UNDERGOING CARDIOPULMONARY BYPASS SURGERY IN THE COURSE OF REPEAT CORONARY ARTERY BYPASS GRAFT SURGERY, AND IN SELECTED CASES OF PRIMARY CORONARY ARTERY BYPASS GRAFT SURGERY WHERE THE RISK OF BLEEDING IS ESPECIALLY HIGH (IMPAIRED HEMOSTASIS, E.G., PRESENCE OF ASPIRIN OR OTHER COAGULOPATHY) OR WHERE TRANSFUSION IS UNAVAILABLE OR UNACCEPTABLE.	MILES, INC. 400 MORGAN LANE WEST HAVEN CT 06516 DD 11/17/94 MA 12/29/93
ARGININE BUTYRATE	TREATMENT OF BETA-HEMOGLOBINOPATHIES AND BETA-THALASSEMIA.	PERRINE, SUSAN P., M.D. BOSTON UNIVERSITY, CANCER RES. CTR. BOSTON MA 02118 DD 04/07/92
ARGININE BUTYRATE	TREATMENT OF SICKLE CELL DISEASE AND BETA THALASSEMIA.	VERTEX PHARMACEUTICALS INC. 40 ALLSTON STREET CAMBRIDGE MA 02139-4211 DD 05/25/94
ATOVAQUONE TN= MEPRON	TREATMENT OF AIDS ASSOCIATED PNEUMOCYSTIS CARINII PNEUMONIA (PCP).	BURROUGHS WELLCOME COMPANY 3030 CORNWALLIS ROAD RESEARCH TRIANGLE PK NC 27709 DD 09/10/90 MA 11/25/92
ATOVAQUONE TN= MEPRON	PREVENTION OF PNEUMOCYSTIS CARINII PNEUMONIA (PCP) IN HIGH-RISK, HIV-INFECTED PATIENTS DEFINED BY A HISTORY OF ONE OR MORE EPISODES OF PCP AND/OR A PERIPHERAL CD4+ (T4 HELPHER/INDUCER) LYMPHOCYTE COUNT LESS THAN OR EQUAL TO 200/MM3.	BURROUGHS WELLCOME COMPANY 3030 CORNWALLIS ROAD RESEARCH TRIANGLE PK NC 27709 DD 08/14/91
ATOVAQUONE TN= MEPRON	TREATMENT AND SUPPRESSION OF TOXOPLASMA GONDII ENCEPHALITIS.	BURROUGHS WELLCOME COMPANY 3030 CORNWALLIS ROAD RESEARCH TRIANGLE PK NC 27709 DD 03/16/93
ATOVAQUONE TN= MEPRON	PRIMARY PROPHYLAXIS OF HIV-INFECTED PERSONS AT HIGH RISK FOR DEVELOPING TOXOPLASMA GONDII ENCEPHALITIS.	BURROUGHS WELLCOME COMPANY 3030 CORNWALLIS ROAD RESEARCH TRIANGLE PK NC 27709 DD 03/16/93
AUTOLYMPHOCYTE THERAPY	TREATMENT OF RENAL CELL CARCINOMA.	CELLCOR INCORPORATED 200 WELLS AVENUE NEWTON MA 02159 DD 07/12/94
BACITRACIN TN= ALTRACIN	ANTIBIOTIC-ASSOCIATED PSEUDOMEMBRANOUS ENTEROCOLITIS CAUSED BY TOXINS A AND B ELABORATED BY CLOSTRIDIUM DIFFICILE.	A.L. LABORATORIES, INC. ONE EXECUTIVE DR., P.O. BOX 1399 FORT LEE NJ 07024 DD 03/13/84
BACLOFEN TN= LIORESAL INTRATHECAL	TREATMENT OF INTRACTABLE SPASTICITY CAUSED BY SPINAL CORD INJURY, MULTIPLE SCLEROSIS, AND OTHER SPINAL DISEASES (INCLUDING SPINAL ISCHEMIA, SPINAL TUMOR, TRANSVERSE MYELITIS, CERVICAL SPONDYLOSIS, AND DEGENERATIVE MYELOPATHY).	MEDTRONIC, INC. 7000 CENTRAL AVE N.E. MINNEAPOLIS MN 55432 DD 11/10/87 MA 06/25/92
BACLOFEN	TREATMENT OF INTRACTABLE SPASTICITY DUE TO MULTIPLE SCLEROSIS OR SPINAL CORD INJURY.	INFUSAID, INC. 1400 PROVIDENCE HIGHWAY NORWOOD MA 02062 DD 12/16/91
BENZOATE AND PHENYLACETATE TN= UCEPHAN	ADJUNCTIVE THERAPY IN THE PREVENTION AND TREATMENT OF HYPERAMMONEMIA IN PATIENTS WITH UREA CYCLE ENZYMOPATHY (UCE) DUE TO CARBAMYLPHOSPHATE SYNTHETASE, ORNITHINE, TRANSCARBAMYLASE, OR ARGINOSUCCINATE SYNTHETASE DEFICIENCY.	KENDALL McGAW LABORATORIES 2525 McGAW AVENUE, P.O. BOX 19791 IRVINE CA 92713-9791 DD 01/21/86 MA 12/23/87
BENZYLPENICILLIN, BENZYLPENICILLOIC, BENZYLPENILLOIC ACID TN= PRE-PEN/MDM	ASSESSING THE RISK OF ADMINISTRATING PENICILLIN WHEN IT IS THE PREFERRED DRUG OF CHOICE IN ADULT PATIENTS WHO HAVE PREVIOUSLY RECEIVED PENICILLIN AND HAVE A HISTORY OF CLINICAL SENSITIVITY.	KREMERS-URBAN COMPANY P.O. BOX 2038 MILWAUKEE WI 53201 DD 09/29/87

CUMULATIVE LIST OF ORPHAN PRODUCT DESIGNATIONS AND APPROVALS *(continued)*

NAME *Generic/Chemical* *TN=Trade Name*	INDICATION DESIGNATED	SPONSOR AND ADDRESS *DD=Date Designated* *MA=Marketing Approval*
BERACTANT TN= SURVANTA INTRATRA-CHEAL SUSPENSION	TREATMENT OF NEONATAL RESPIRATORY DISTRESS SYNDROME (RDS).	ROSS LABORATORIES 625 CLEVELAND AVENUE COLUMBUS OH 43215 DD 02/05/86 MA 07/01/91
BERACTANT TN= SURVANTA INTRATRA-CHEAL SUSPENSION	PREVENTION OF NEONATAL RESPIRATORY DISTRESS SYNDROME (RDS).	ROSS LABORATORIES 625 CLEVELAND AVENUE COLUMBUS OH 43215 DD 02/05/86 MA 07/01/91
BERACTANT TN= SURVANTA INTRATRA-CHEAL SUSPENSION	TREATMENT OF FULL-TERM NEWBORN INFANTS WITH RESPIRATORY FAILURE CAUSED BY MECONIUM ASPIRATION SYNDROME, PERSISTENT PULMONARY HYPERTENSION OF THE NEWBORN, OR PNEUMONIA AND SEPSIS.	ROSS LABORATORIES 625 CLEVELAND AVENUE COLUMBUS OH 43215 DD 12/20/93
BETAINE	TREATMENT OF HOMOCYSTINURIA.	ORPHAN MEDICAL 13911 RIDGEDALE DRIVE MINNETONKA MN 55305 DD 05/16/94
BIODEL IMPLANT/CARMUS-TINE (BCNU) TN= GLIADEL.	FOR THE LOCALIZED PLACEMENT IN THE BRAIN FOR THE TREATMENT OF RECURRENT MALIGNANT GLIOMA	GUILFORD PHARMACEUTICALS, INC. 6611 TRIBUTARY STREET BALTIMORE MD 21224 DD 12/13/89
BISPECIFIC ANTIBODY 520C9x22	IN VIVO SEROTHERAPY OF PATIENTS WITH OVARIAN CANCER.	MEDAREX 12 COMMERCE AVENUE WEST LEBANON NH 03784 DD 10/05/93
BLEOMYCIN SULFATE TN= BLENOXANE	TREATMENT OF MALIGNANT PLEURAL EFFUSION.	BRISTOL-MYERS SQUIBB P.O. BOX 4000 PRINCETON NJ 08543-4000 DD 09/17/93
BOTULINUM TOXIN TYPE A TN= BOTOX	TREATMENT OF BLEPHAROSPASM ASSOCIATED WITH DYSTONIA IN ADULTS (PATIENTS 12 YEARS OF AGE AND ABOVE).	ALLERGAN, INC. 2525 DUPONT DRIVE, P.O. BOX 19534 IRVINE CA 92713-9534 DD 03/22/84 MA 12/29/89
BOTULINUM TOXIN TYPE A TN= BOTOX	TREATMENT OF STRABISMUS ASSOCIATED WITH DYSTONIA IN ADULTS (PATIENTS 12 YEARS OF AGE AND ABOVE).	ALLERGAN, INC. 2525 DUPONT DRIVE, P.O. BOX 19534 IRVINE CA 92713-9534 DD 03/22/84 MA 12/29/89
BOTULINUM TOXIN TYPE A TN= BOXTOX	TREATMENT OF CERVICAL DYSTONIA.	ALLERGAN, INC. 2525 DUPONT DRIVE, P.O. BOX 19534 IRVINE CA 92713-9534 DD 08/20/86
BOTULINUM TOXIN TYPE A TN= DYSPORT	TREATMENT OF ESSENTIAL BLEPHAROSPASM.	PORTON INTERNATIONAL, INC. 816 CONNECTICUT AVENUE NW WASHINGTON DC 20006 DD 03/23/89
BOTULINUM TOXIN TYPE A TN= BOTOX	TREATMENT OF DYNAMIC MUSCLE CONTRACTURE IN PEDIATRIC CEREBRAL PALSY PATIENTS.	ALLERGAN, INC. 2525 DUPONT DR., P.O. BOX 19534 IRVINE CA 92713-9534 DD 12/06/91
BOTULINUM TOXIN TYPE A	TREATMENT OF SYNKINETIC CLOSURE OF THE EYELID ASSOCIATED WITH VII CRANIAL NERVE ABERRANT REGENERATION.	ASSOCIATED SYNAPSE BIOLOGICS 68 HARRISON AVENUE BOSTON MA 02111 DD 09/15/92
BOTULINUM TOXIN TYPE B	TREATMENT OF CERVICAL DYSTONIA.	ATHENA NEUROSCIENCES, INC. 800F GATEWAY BOULEVARD SOUTH SAN FRANCISCO CA 94080 DD 01/16/92
BOTULINUM TOXIN TYPE F	TREATMENT OF ESSENTIAL BLEPHAROSPASM.	PORTON INTERNATIONAL, INC. 816 CONNECTICUT AVENUE N.W. WASHINGTON DC 20006 DD 12/05/91
BOTULINUM TOXIN TYPE F	TREATMENT OF SPASMODIC TORTICOLLIS (CERVICAL DYSTONIA).	PORTON INTERNATIONAL, INC. 816 CONNECTICUT AVENUE N.W. WASHINGTON DC 20006 DD 10/24/91

CUMULATIVE LIST OF ORPHAN PRODUCT DESIGNATIONS AND APPROVALS *(continued)*

NAME *Generic/Chemical* *TN=Trade Name*	INDICATION DESIGNATED	SPONSOR AND ADDRESS *DD=Date Designated* *MA=Marketing Approval*
BOTULISM IMMUNE GLOBULIN	TREATMENT OF INFANT BOTULISM.	CALIFORNIA DEPT HEALTH SERVICE 2151 BERKELEY WAY BERKELEY CA 94704 DD 01/31/89
BOVINE COLOSTRUM	TREATMENT OF AIDS-RELATED DIARRHEA.	HASTINGS, DONALD, DVM 1030 NORTH PARKVIEW DRIVE BISMARCK ND 58501 DD 11/19/90
BOVINE IMMUNOGLOBULIN CONCENTRATE, CRYPTOSPORIDIUM PARVUM TN= SPORIDIN-G	TREATMENT AND SYMPTOMATIC RELIEF OF CRYPTOSPORIDIUM PARVUM INFECTION OF THE GASTROINTESTINAL TRACT IN IMMUNOCOMPROMISED PATIENTS.	GALAGEN, INCORPORATED 4001 LEXINGTON AVENUE NORTH ARDEN HILLS MN 55126-2998 DD 03/01/94
BOVINE WHEY PROTEIN CONCENTRATE TN= IMMUNO-C	TREATMENT OF CRYPTOSPORIDIOSIS CAUSED BY THE PRESENCE OF CRYPTOSPORIDIUM PARVUM IN THE GASTROINTESTINAL TRACT OF PATIENTS WHO ARE IMMUNODEFICIENT/IMMUNOCOMPROMISED OR IMMUNOCOMPETENT.	BIOMUNE SYSTEMS, INCORPORATED 40 EAST SOUTH TEMPLE, SUITE 310 SALT LAKE CITY UT 84111 DD 09/30/93
BRANCHED CHAIN AMINO ACIDS	TREATMENT OF AMYOTROPHIC LATERAL SCLEROSIS.	MOUNT SINAI MEDICAL CENTER ONE GUSTAVE L. LEVY PLACE NEW YORK NY 10029-6574 DD 12/23/88
BROMHEXINE	TREATMENT OF MILD TO MODERATE KERATOCONJUNCTIVITIS SICCA IN PATIENTS WITH SJOGREN'S SYNDROME.	BOEHRINGER INGELHEIM 900 RIDGEBURY ROAD, BOX 368 RIDGEFIELD CT 06877 DD 05/15/89
BUPRENORPHINE HYDROCHLORIDE	TREATMENT OF OPIATE ADDICTION IN OPIATE USERS.	RECKITT & COLMAN PHARMACEUTICALS, INC. 1901 HUGUENOT ROAD RICHMOND VA 23235 DD 06/15/94
BUSULFAN	FOR USE AS PREPARATIVE THERAPY FOR MALIGNANCIES TREATED WITH BONE MARROW TRANSPLANTATION.	SPARTA PHARMACEUTICALS, INC. P.O. BOX 13288 RESEARCH TRIANGLE PK NC 27709 DD 04/21/94
BUSULFAN	AS PREPARATIVE THERAPY IN THE TREATMENT OF MALIGNANCIES WITH BONE MARROW TRANSPLANTATION.	ORPHAN MEDICAL 13911 RIDGEDALE DRIVE MINNETONKA MN 55305 DD 07/28/94
BUTYRYLCHOLINESTERASE	FOR THE REDUCTION AND CLEARANCE OF TOXIC BLOOD LEVELS OF COCAINE ENCOUNTERED DURING A DRUG OVERDOSE.	PHARMAVENE, INC. 35 WEST WATKINS MILL ROAD GAITHERSBURG MD 20878 DD 03/25/92
BUTYRYLCHOLINESTERASE	TREATMENT OF POST-SURGICAL APNEA.	PHARMAVENE, INC. 35 WEST WATKINS MILL ROAD GAITHERSBURG MD 20878 DD 09/30/92
C1-ESTERASE-INHIBITOR, HUMAN, PASTEURIZED	PREVENTION AND/OR TREATMENT OF ACUTE ATTACKS OF HEREDITARY ANGIOEDEMA.	BEHRINGWERKE AKTIENGESELLSCHAFT (AG) P.O. BOX 575 OCEANSIDE NY 11572 DD 10/16/92
C1-INHIBITOR TN= C1-INHIBITOR (HUMAN) VAPOR HEATED, IMMUNO	PREVENTION OF ACUTE ATTACKS OF ANGIOEDEMA, INCLUDING SHORT-TERM PROPHYLAXIS FOR PATIENTS REQUIRING DENTAL OR OTHER SURGICAL PROCEDURES.	IMMUNO CLINICAL RESEARCH CORP. 750 LEXINGTON AVENUE, 19TH FLOOR NEW YORK NY 10022 DD 08/30/90
C1-INHIBITOR TN= C1-INHIBITOR (HUMAN) VAPOR HEATED, IMMUNO	TREATMENT OF ACUTE ATTACKS OF ANGIOEDEMA.	OSTERREICHISCHES INSTITUTE FUR HAEMODER. 750 LEXINGTON AVENUE, 19TH FLOOR NEW YORK NY 10022 DD 08/30/90
CAFFEINE TN= NEOCAF	TREATMENT OF APNEA OF PREMATURITY.	O.P.R. DEVELOPMENT, L.P. 1501 WAKARUSA DRIVE LAWRENCE KS 66047 DD 09/20/88

CUMULATIVE LIST OF ORPHAN PRODUCT DESIGNATIONS AND APPROVALS *(continued)*

NAME *Generic/Chemical* *TN=Trade Name*	INDICATION DESIGNATED	SPONSOR AND ADDRESS *DD=Date Designated* *MA=Marketing Approval*
CALCITONIN SALMON NASAL SPRAY TN= MIACALCIN NASAL SPRAY	TREATMENT OF SYMPTOMATIC PAGET'S DISEASE (OSTEITIS DEFORMANS).	SANDOZ PHARMACEUTICALS CORP. 59 ROUTE 10 EAST HANOVER NJ 07936-1080 DD 10/29/90
CALCITONIN-HUMAN FOR INJECTION TN= CIBACALCIN	TREATMENT OF SYMPTOMATIC PAGET'S DISEASE (OSTEITIS DEFORMANS).	CIBA-GEIGY CORPORATION 556 MORRIS AVE SUMMIT NJ 07901 DD 01/20/87 MA 10/31/86
CALCIUM ACETATE TN= PHOS-LO	TREATMENT OF HYPERPHOSPHATEMIA IN END STAGE RENAL FAILURE.	BRAINTREE LABORATORIES 60 COLUMBIAN STREET P.O. BOX 361 BRAINTREE MA 02184 DD 12/22/88 MA 12/10/90
CALCIUM ACETATE	TREATMENT OF HYPERPHOSPHATEMIA IN END STAGE RENAL DISEASE (ESRD).	PHARMEDIC COMPANY 417 HARVESTER COURT DEERFIELD IL 60015 DD 06/27/89
CALCIUM CARBONATE TN= R & D CALCIUM CARBONATE/600	TREATMENT OF HYPERPHOSPHATEMIA IN PATIENTS WITH END STAGE RENAL DISEASE.	R & D LABORATORIES, INC. 4204 GLENCOE AVENUE MARINA DEL REY CA 90292 DD 06/06/90
CALCIUM GLUCONATE GEL TN= H-F GEL	FOR USE IN THE EMERGENCY TOPICAL TREATMENT OF HYDROGEN FLUORIDE (HYDROFLUORIC ACID) BURNS.	LTR PHARMACEUTICALS, INC. 145 SAKONNET BLVD. NARRAGANSETT RI 02882 DD 05/21/91
CALCIUM GLUCONATE GEL 2.5%	EMERGENCY TOPICAL TREATMENT OF HYDROGEN FLUORIDE (HYDROFLUORIC ACID) BURNS.	PADDOCK LABORATORIES, INC. 3101 LOUISIANA AVE. N. MINNEAPOLIS MN 55427 DD 09/10/90
CARBOVIR	TREATMENT OF PERSONS WITH AIDS AND IN PATIENTS WITH SYMPTOMATIC HIV INFECTION AND A CD4 COUNT LESS THAN 200/MM3.	GLAXO, INC. 5 MOORE DRIVE, P.O. BOX 13358 RESEARCH TRIANGLE PK NC 27709 DD 12/13/89
CASCARA SAGRADA FLUID EXTRACT	TREATMENT OF ORAL DRUG OVERDOSAGE TO SPEED LOWER BOWEL EVACUATION.	INTRAMED CORPORATION 102 TREMONT WAY AUGUSTA GA 30907 DD 03/21/89
CCD 1042	TREATMENT OF INFANTILE SPASMS.	COCENSYS, INC. 213 TECHNOLOGY DRIVE IRVINE CA 92718 DD 05/25/94
CD5-T LYMPHOCYTE IMMUNOTOXIN TN= XOMAZYME-H65	TREATMENT OF GRAFT VERSUS HOST DISEASE (GVHD) AND/OR REJECTION IN PATIENTS WHO HAVE RECEIVED BONE MARROW TRANSPLANTS.	XOMA CORPORATION 2910 SEVENTH STREET BERKELEY CA 94710 DD 08/27/87
CERAMIDE TRIHEXOSIDASE/ALPHA-GALACTOSIDASE A	TREATMENT OF FABRY'S DISEASE.	GENZYME CORPORATION ONE KENDALL SQUARE CAMBRIDGE MA 02139-1562 DD 01/19/88
CHENODIOL TN= CHENIX	FOR PATIENTS WITH RADIOLUCENT STONES IN WELL OPACIFYING GALLBLADDERS, IN WHOM ELECTIVE SURGERY WOULD BE UNDERTAKEN EXCEPT FOR THE PRESENCE OF INCREASED SURGICAL RISK DUE TO SYSTEMIC DISEASE OR AGE.	SOLVAY 901 SAWYER ROAD MARIETTA GA 30062-2224 DD 09/21/84 MA 07/28/83
CHIMERIC (MURINE VARIABLE, HUMAN CONSTANT) MAB TO CD20	TREATMENT OF NON-HODGKIN'S B-CELL LYMPHOMA.	IDEC PHARMACEUTICALS CORPORATION 11011 TORREYANA ROAD SAN DIEGO CA 92121 DD 06/13/94
CHIMERIC M-T412 (HUMAN-MURINE) IgG MONOCLONAL ANTI-CD4	TREATMENT OF MULTIPLE SCLEROSIS.	CENTOCOR, INC. 244 GREAT VALLEY PARKWAY MALVERN PA 19355 DD 06/05/91
CHLORHEXIDINE GLUCONATE MOUTHRINSE TN= PERIDEX	FOR USE IN THE AMELIORATION OF ORAL MUCOSITIS ASSOCIATED WITH CYTOREDUCTIVE THERAPY USED IN CONDITIONING PATIENTS FOR BONE MARROW TRANSPLANTATION THERAPY.	PROCTER & GAMBLE COMPANY 11370 REED HARTMAN HIGHWAY CINCINNATI OH 45241-2422 DD 08/18/86

CUMULATIVE LIST OF ORPHAN PRODUCT DESIGNATIONS AND APPROVALS *(continued)*

NAME *Generic/Chemical* *TN=Trade Name*	INDICATION DESIGNATED	SPONSOR AND ADDRESS *DD=Date Designated* *MA=Marketing Approval*
CHOLINE CHLORIDE	TREATMENT OF CHOLINE DEFICIENCY, SPECIFICALLY THE CHOLINE DEFICIENCY, HEPATIC STEATOSIS, AND CHOLESTASIS, ASSOCIATED WITH LONG-TERM PARENTERAL NUTRITION.	BUCHMAN, ALAN, M.D. 6550 FANNIN, SUITE 1122 HOUSTON TX 77030 DD 02/10/94
CILIARY NEUROTROPHIC FACTOR	TREATMENT OF AMYOTROPHIC LATERAL SCLEROSIS.	REGENERON PHARMACEUTICALS, INC 777 OLD SAW MILL RIVER ROAD TARRYTOWN NY 10591-6707 DD 01/30/92
CILIARY NEUROTROPHIC FACTOR, RECOMBINANT HUMAN	TREATMENT OF SPINAL MUSCULAR ATROPHIES.	SYNTEX-SYNERGEN NEUROSCIENCE 1885 33RD STREET BOULDER CO 80301 DD 04/02/92
CILIARY NEUROTROPHIC FACTOR, RECOMBINANT HUMAN	TREATMENT OF MOTOR NEURON DISEASE (INCLUDING AMYOTROPHIC LATERAL SCLEROSIS, PROGRESSIVE MUSCULAR ATROPHY, PROGRESSIVE BULBAR PALSY, AND PRIMARY LATERAL SCLEROSIS).	SYNTEX-SYNERGEN NEUROSCIENCE 1885 33RD STREET BOULDER CO 80301 DD 05/08/92
CITRIC ACID, GLUCONO-DELTA-LACTONE AND MAGNESIUM CARBONATE TN= RENACIDIN IRRIGATION	TREATMENT OF RENAL AND BLADDER CALCULI OF THE APATITE OR STRUVITE VARIETY.	UNITED-GUARDIAN, INC. P.O. BOX 2500 SMITHTOWN NY 11787 DD 08/28/89 MA 10/02/90
CLADRIBINE TN= LEUSTATIN INJECTION	TREATMENT OF HAIRY CELL LEUKEMIA.	R.W. JOHNSON RESEARCH INSTITUTE ROUTE 202, P.O. BOX 300 RARITAN NJ 08869-0602 DD 11/15/90 MA 02/26/93
CLADRIBINE TN= LEUSTATIN INJECTION	TREATMENT OF CHRONIC LYMPHOCYTIC LEUKEMIA.	R.W. JOHNSON RESEARCH INSTITUTE ROUTE 202, P.O. BOX 300 RARITAN NJ 08869-0602 DD 12/31/90
CLADRIBINE TN= LEUSTATIN INJECTION	TREATMENT OF NON-HODGKIN'S LYMPHOMA.	R.W. JOHNSON RESEARCH INSTITUTE ROUTE 202 SOUTH, P.O. BOX 300 RARITAN NJ 08869-0602 DD 04/19/93
CLADRIBINE TN= LEUSTATIN	TREATMENT OF THE CHRONIC PROGRESSIVE FORM OF MULTIPLE SCLEROSIS.	R.W. JOHNSON RESEARCH INSTITUTE 700 ROUTE 200 SOUTH P.O. BOX 670 RARITAN NJ 08869-0670 DD 04/19/94
CLINDAMYCIN TN= CLEOCIN	TREATMENT OF PNEUMOCYSTIS CARINII PNEUMONIA ASSOCIATED WITH AIDS PATIENTS.	UPJOHN COMPANY 7000 PORTAGE ROAD KALAMAZOO MI 49001 DD 10/28/88
CLINDAMYCIN TN= CLEOCIN	PREVENTION OF PNEUMOCYSTIS CARINII PNEUMONIA IN AIDS PATIENTS.	UPJOHN COMPANY 7000 PORTAGE ROAD KALAMAZOO MI 49001 DD 10/28/88
CLOFAZIMINE TN= LAMPRENE	TREATMENT OF LEPROMATOUS LEPROSY, INCLUDING DAPSONE-RESISTANT LEPROMATOUS LEPROSY AND LEPROMATOUS LEPROSY COMPLICATED BY ERYTHEMA NODOSUM LEPROSUM.	CIBA-GEIGY CORPORATION 556 MORRIS AVE SUMMIT NJ 07901 DD 06/11/84 MA 12/15/86
CLONAZEPAM TN= KLONOPIN	TREATMENT OF HYPEREKPLEXIA (STARTLE DISEASE).	HOFFMAN-LA ROCHE, INCORPORATED 340 KINGSLAND STREET NUTLEY NJ 07110-1199 DD 08/04/94
CLONIDINE HYDROCHLORIDE (EPIDURAL INJECTION)	EPIDURAL ADMINISTRATION FOR THE TREATMENT OF PAIN IN CANCER PATIENTS TOLERANT TO OR UNRESPONSIVE TO INTRASPINAL OPIATES.	FUJISAWA PHARMACEUTICAL CO. 3 PARKWAY NORTH DEERFIELD IL 60015-2548 DD 01/24/89
COAGULATION FACTOR IX TN= MONONINE	REPLACEMENT TREATMENT AND PROPHYLAXIS OF THE HEMORRHAGIC COMPLICATIONS OF HEMOPHILIA B.	ARMOUR PHARMACEUTICAL COMPANY 500 ARCOLA ROAD, P.O. BOX 1200 COLLEGEVILLE PA 19426-0107 DD 06/27/89 MA 08/20/92

CUMULATIVE LIST OF ORPHAN PRODUCT DESIGNATIONS AND APPROVALS *(continued)*

NAME *Generic/Chemical* *TN=Trade Name*	INDICATION DESIGNATED	SPONSOR AND ADDRESS *DD=Date Designated* *MA=Marketing Approval*
COAGULATION FACTOR IX (HUMAN) TN= ALPHANINE	FOR USE AS REPLACEMENT THERAPY IN PATIENTS WITH HEMOPHILIA B FOR THE PREVENTION AND CONTROL OF BLEEDING EPISODES, AND DURING SURGERY TO CORRECT DEFECTIVE HEMOSTASIS.	ALPHA THERAPEUTIC CORPORATION 555 VALLEY BLVD LOS ANGELES CA 90032 DD 07/05/90 MA 12/31/90
COLCHICINE	ARRESTING THE PROGRESSION OF NEUROLOGIC DISABILITY CAUSED BY CHRONIC PROGRESSIVE MULTIPLE SCLEROSIS.	PHARMACONTROL CORPORATION 661 PALISADE AVE., P.O. BOX 931 ENGLEWOOD CLIFFS NJ 07632 DD 12/09/85
COLFOSCERIL PALMITATE, CETYL ALCOHOL, TYLOXAPOL TN= EXOSURF NEONATAL FOR INTRATRACHEAL SUSPENSION	PREVENTION OF HYALINE MEMBRANE DISEASE (HMD), ALSO KNOWN AS RESPIRATORY DISTRESS SYNDROME (RDS), IN INFANTS BORN AT 32 WEEKS GESTATION OR LESS.	BURROUGHS WELLCOME COMPANY 3030 CORNWALLIS ROAD RESEARCH TRIANGLE PK NC 27709 DD 10/20/89 MA 08/02/90
COLFOSCERIL PALMITATE, CETYL ALCOHOL, TYLOXAPOL TN= EXOSURF NEONATAL FOR INTRATRACHEAL SUSPENSION	TREATMENT OF ESTABLISHED HYALINE MEMBRANE DISEASE (HMD) AT ALL GESTATIONAL AGES.	BURROUGHS WELLCOME COMPANY 3030 CORNWALLIS ROAD RESEARCH TRIANGLE PK NC 27709 DD 10/20/89 MA 08/02/90
COLFOSCERIL PALMITATE, CETYL ALCOHOL, TYLOXAPOL TN= EXOSURF	TREATMENT OF ADULT RESPIRATORY DISTRESS SYNDROME.	BURROUGHS WELLCOME COMPANY 3030 CORNWALLIS ROAD RESEARCH TRIANGLE PK NC 27709 DD 01/11/93
COPOLYMER 1 (COP 1)	TREATMENT OF MULTIPLE SCLEROSIS.	LEMMON COMPANY 650 CATHILL ROAD SELLERSVILLE PA 18960 DD 11/12/87
CORTICORELIN OVINE TRIFLUTATE TN= ACTHREL	FOR USE IN DIFFERENTIATING PITUITARY AND ECTOPIC PRODUCTION OF ACTH IN PATIENTS WITH ACTH-DEPENDENT CUSHINGS SYNDROME.	FERRING LABORATORIES, INC. 400 RELLA BOULEVARD, SUITE 201 SUFFERN NY 10901 DD 11/24/89
CROMOLYN SODIUM TN= GASTROCROM	TREATMENT OF MASTOCYTOSIS.	FISONS CORPORATION 755 JEFFERSON RD., P.O. BOX 1710 ROCHESTER NY 14603 DD 03/08/84 MA 12/22/89
CROMOLYN SODIUM 4% OPHTHALMIC SOLUTION TN= OPTICROM 4% OPHTHALMIC SOLUTION	TREATMENT OF VERNAL KERATOCONJUNCTIVITIS (VKC).	FISONS CORPORATION 755 JEFFERSON RD., P.O. BOX 1710 ROCHESTER NY 14603 DD 07/24/85 MA 10/03/84
CRYPTOSPORIDIUM HYPERIMMUNE BOVINE COLOSTRUM IgG CONCENTRATE	TREATMENT OF DIARRHEA IN AIDS PATIENTS CAUSED BY INFECTION WITH CRYPTOSPORIDIUM PARVUM.	IMMUCELL CORPORATION 56 EVERGREEN DRIVE PORTLAND ME 04103-1066 DD 12/30/91
CY-1503	TREATMENT OF POST-ISCHEMIC PULMONARY REPERFUSION EDEMA FOLLOWING SURGICAL TREATMENT FOR CHRONIC THROMBOEMBOLIC PULMONARY HYPERTENSION.	CYTEL CORPORATION 3525 JOHN HOPKINS COURT SAN DIEGO CA 92121 DD 12/22/93
CY-1899	TREATMENT OF CHRONIC ACTIVE HEPATITIS B INFECTION IN HLA-A2 POSITIVE PATIENTS.	CYTEL CORPORATION 3525 JOHN HOPKINS COURT SAN DIEGO CA 92121 DD 03/16/94
CYCLOSPORINE 2% OPHTHALMIC OINTMENT TN= SANDIMMUNE	TREATMENT OF PATIENTS AT HIGH RISK OF GRAFT REJECTION FOLLOWING PENETRATING KERATOPLASTY.	SANDOZ PHARMACEUTICALS CORP. 59 ROUTE 10 EAST HANOVER NJ 07936 DD 08/01/91
CYCLOSPORINE 2% OPHTHALMIC OINTMENT TN= SANDIMMUNE	FOR USE IN CORNEAL MELTING SYNDROMES OF KNOWN OR PRESUMED IMMUNOLOGIC ETIOPATHOGENESIS, INCLUDING MOOREN'S ULCER.	SANDOZ PHARMACEUTICALS CORP. 59 ROUTE 10 EAST HANOVER NJ 07936 DD 08/01/91
CYCLOSPORINE OPHTHALMIC TN= OPTIMMUNE	TREATMENT OF SEVERE KERATOCONJUNCTIVITIS SICCA ASSOCIATED WITH SJOGREN'S SYNDROME.	UNIVERSITY OF GEORGIA COLLEGE OF VETERINARY MEDICINE ATHENS GA 30602-7390 DD 11/09/88

CUMULATIVE LIST OF ORPHAN PRODUCT DESIGNATIONS AND APPROVALS *(continued)*

NAME *Generic/Chemical* *TN=Trade Name*	INDICATION DESIGNATED	SPONSOR AND ADDRESS *DD=Date Designated* *MA=Marketing Approval*
CYSTEAMINE	TREATMENT OF NEPHROPATHIC CYSTINOSIS.	THOENE, JESS, M.D. UNIVERSITY OF MICHIGAN ANN ARBOR MI 48109-2029 DD 05/01/86
CYSTEAMINE	TREATMENT OF NEPHROPATHIC CYSTINOSIS.	MYLAN LABORATORIES, INC 781 CHESTNUT RIDGE ROAD P.O. BOX 4310 MORGANTOWN WV 26504-4310 DD 01/25/91
CYSTIC FIBROSIS GENE THERAPY	TREATMENT OF CYSTIC FIBROSIS.	GENZYME CORPORATION ONE KENDALL SQUARE CAMBRIDGE MA 02139-1562 DD 06/30/92
CYSTIC FIBROSIS TRANS-MEMBRANE CONDUCT-ANCE REGULATOR	FOR CYSTIC FIBROSIS TRANSMEMBRANE CONDUCTANCE REGULATOR PROTEIN REPLACEMENT THERAPY IN CYSTIC FIBROSIS PATIENTS.	GENZYME CORPORATION ONE KENDALL SQUARE CAMBRIDGE MA 02139 DD 01/14/92
CYSTIC FIBROSIS TRANS-MEMBRANE CONDUCT-ANCE REGULATOR GENE	TREATMENT OF CYSTIC FIBROSIS.	GENETIC THERAPY, INC. 19 FIRSTFIELD ROAD GAITHERSBURG MD 20878 DD 01/08/93
CYTOMEGALOVIRUS IM-MUNE GLOBULIN (HU-MAN)	PREVENTION OR ATTENUATION OF PRIMARY CYTOMEGALOVIRUS DISEASE IN IMMUNOSUPPRESSED RECIPIENTS OF ORGAN TRANSPLANTS.	MASS PUB HEALTH BIO LABS 305 SOUTH STREET BOSTON MA 02130 DD 08/03/87 MA 04/17/90
CYTOMEGALOVIRUS IM-MUNE GLOBULIN INTRA-VENOUS (HUMAN)	FOR USE IN CONJUNCTION WITH GANCICLOVIR SODIUM FOR THE TREATMENT OF CYTOMEGALOVIRUS PNEUMONIA IN BONE MARROW TRANSPLANT PATIENTS.	MILES, INC. 4TH & PARKER STREETS BERKELEY CA 94701 DD 01/28/91
DAPSONE USP TN= DAPSONE	PROPHYLAXIS FOR PNEUMOCYSTIS CARINII PNEUMONIA.	JACOBUS PHARMACEUTICAL COMPANY P.O. BOX 5290 PRINCETON NJ 08540 DD 12/24/91
DAPSONE USP TN= DAPSONE	FOR THE COMBINATION TREATMENT OF PNEUMOCYSTIS CARINII PNEUMONIA IN CONJUNCTION WITH TRIMETHOPRIM.	JACOBUS PHARMACEUTICAL COMPANY P.O. BOX 5290 PRINCETON NJ 08540 DD 01/08/92
DEFIBROTIDE	TREATMENT OF THROMBOTIC THROMBOCYTOPENIC PURPURA.	CRINOS INTERNATIONAL VIA BELVEDERE 1 VILLA GUARDIA, ITALY 22079 DD 07/05/85
DEHYDREX	TREATMENT OF RECURRENT CORNEAL EROSION UNRESPONSIVE TO CONVENTIONAL THERAPY.	HOLLES LABORATORIES, INC. 30 FOREST NOTCH COHASSET MA 02025 DD 03/05/90
DEHYDROEPIANDROS-TERONE	TREATMENT OF SYSTEMIC LUPUS ERYTHEMATOSUS (SLE) AND THE REDUCTION THE USE OF STEROIDS IN STEROID-DEPENDENT SLE PATIENTS.	GENELABS TECHNOLOGIES, INC. 505 PENOBSCOT DRIVE REDWOOD CITY CA 94063 DD 07/13/94
DEPOFOAM ENCAPSULATED CYTARABINE	TREATMENT OF NEOPLASTIC MENINGITIS.	DEPOTECH CORPORATION 11025 NORTH TORREY PINES ROAD, SUITE 100 LA JOLLA CA 92037 DD 06/02/93
DESLORELIN TN= SOMAGARD	TREATMENT OF CENTRAL PRECOCIOUS PUBERTY.	ROBERTS PHARMACEUTICAL CORP. 6 INDUSTRIAL WAY WEST EATONTOWN NJ 07724 DD 11/05/87
DESMOPRESSIN ACETATE TN= DDAVP HIGH CONCEN-TRATION (1.5 MG/ML) NA-SAL SPRAY	TREATMENT OF MILD HEMOPHILIA A AND VON WILLEBRAND'S DISEASE.	RHONE-POULENC RORER PHARM. 500 ARCOLA ROAD COLLEGEVILLE PA 19426 DD 01/22/91
DEXRAZOXANE FOR INJEC-TION TN= ZINECARD	FOR THE PREVENTION OF CARDIOMYOPATHY ASSOCIATED WITH DOXORUBICIN ADMINISTRATION.	ADRIA LABORATORIES, INC. P.O. BOX 16529 COLUMBUS OH 43216-6529 DD 12/17/91

CUMULATIVE LIST OF ORPHAN PRODUCT DESIGNATIONS AND APPROVALS *(continued)*

NAME *Generic/Chemical* *TN=Trade Name*	INDICATION DESIGNATED	SPONSOR AND ADDRESS *DD=Date Designated* *MA=Marketing Approval*
DEXTRAN AND DEFEROXAMINE TN= BIO-RESCUE	TREATMENT OF ACUTE IRON POISONING.	BIOMEDICAL FRONTIERS, INC. 1095 10TH AVENUE S.E. MINNEAPOLIS MN 55414 DD 03/08/91
DEXTRAN SULFATE (INHALED, AEROSOLIZED) TN= UENDEX	AS AN ADJUNCT TO THE TREATMENT OF CYSTIC FIBROSIS.	KENNEDY & HOIDAL, MDs. 7702 PARHAM ROAD RICHMOND VA 23294 DD 10/05/90
DEXTRAN SULFATE SODIUM	TREATMENT OF ACQUIRED IMMUNODEFICIENCY SYNDROME (AIDS).	UENO FINE CHEMICALS 2-31 KORAIBASHI, HIGASHI-KU OSAKA 541, JAPAN DD 11/19/87
DIANEAL PD-2 PERITONEAL DIALYSIS SOLN WITH 1.1% AMINO ACIDS TN= NUTRINEAL PD-2 PERITONEAL DIALYSIS SOLN WITH 1.1% AMINO ACID	FOR USE AS A NUTRITIONAL SUPPLEMENT FOR THE TREATMENT OF MALNOURISHMENT IN PATIENTS UNDERGOING CONTINUOUS AMBULATORY PERITONEAL DIALYSIS.	BAXTER HEALTHCARE CORPORATION ROUTE 120 AND WILSON ROAD ROUND LAKE IL 60073-0490 DD 06/11/92
DIAZEPAM VISCOUS SOLUTION FOR RECTAL ADMINISTRATION TN= DIASTAT	TREATMENT OF ACUTE REPETITIVE SEIZURES.	ATHENA NEUROSCIENCES, INC. 800F GATEWAY BOULEVARD SOUTH SAN FRANCISCO CA 94080 DD 02/25/92
DIBROMODULCITOL TN= MITOLACTOL	TREATMENT OF RECURRENT INVASIVE OR METASTATIC SQUAMOUS CARCINOMA OF THE CERVIX.	BIOPHARMACEUTICS, INC. 990 STATION ROAD BELLPORT NY 11713 DD 01/23/89
DIETHYLDITHIOCARBAMATE TN= IMUTHIOL	TREATMENT OF ACQUIRED IMMUNODEFICIENCY SYNDROME (AIDS).	CONNAUGHT LABORATORIES ROUTE 611, P.O. BOX 187 SWIFTWATER PA 18370-0187 DD 04/03/86
DIGOXIN IMMUNE FAB (OVINE) TN= DIGIDOTE	TREATMENT OF LIFE-THREATENING ACUTE CARDIAC GLYCOSIDE INTOXICATION MANIFESTED BY CONDUCTION DISORDERS, ECTOPIC VENTRICULAR ACTIVITY AND (IN SOME CASES) HYPERKALEMIA.	BOEHRINGER MANNHEIM CORP. 1301 PICCARD DRIVE ROCKVILLE MD 20850 DD 03/11/85
DIGOXIN IMMUNE FAB (OVINE) TN= DIGIBIND	TREATMENT OF POTENTIALLY LIFE THREATENING DIGITALIS INTOXICATION IN PATIENTS WHO ARE REFRACTORY TO MANAGEMENT BY CONVENTIONAL THERAPY.	BURROUGHS WELLCOME COMPANY 3030 CORNWALLIS ROAD RESEARCH TRIANGLE PK NC 27709 DD 11/01/84 MA 03/21/86
DIPALMITOYLPHOSPHATIDYLCHOLINE/PHOSPHATIDYLGLYCEROL TN= ALEC	PREVENTION AND TREATMENT OF NEONATAL RESPIRATORY DISTRESS SYNDROME (RDS).	FORUM PRODUCTS, INC. 33 FLYING POINT ROAD SOUTHAMPTON NY 11968 DD 07/28/88
DISACCHARIDE TRIPEPTIDE GLYCEROL DIPALMITOYL TN= ImmTher	TREATMENT OF PULMONARY AND HEPATIC METASTASES IN PATIENTS WITH COLORECTAL ADENOCARCINOMA.	IMMUNO THERAPEUTICS, INC. 3505 RIVERVIEW CIRCLE MOORHEAD MN 56560-5560 DD 03/01/90
DISODIUM CLODRONATE	TREATMENT OF HYPERCALCEMIA OF MALIGNANCY.	DISCOVERY EXPERIMENTAL & DEVELOPMENT, INC 29949 S.R. 54 WEST WESLEY CHAPEL FL 33543 DD 06/16/93
DISODIUM CLODRONATE TETRAHYDRATE TN= BONEFOS	TREATMENT OF INCREASED BONE RESORPTION DUE TO MALIGNANCY.	LEIRAS, INCORPORATED 1805 CENTENNIAL PARK DRIVE, SUITE 450 RESTON VA 22091 DD 03/05/90
DISODIUM SILIBININ DIHEMISUCCINATE TN= LEGALON	TREATMENT OF HEPATIC INTOXICATION BY AMANITA PHALLOIDES (MUSHROOM POISONING).	PHARMAQUEST CORPORATION 4470 REDWOOD HIGHWAY SAN RAFAEL CA 94903 DD 07/10/86
DORNASE ALFA TN= PULMOZYME	TO REDUCE MUCOUS VISCOSITY AND ENABLE THE CLEARANCE OF AIRWAY SECRETIONS IN PATIENTS WITH CYSTIC FIBROSIS.	GENETECH, INC. 460 POINT SAN BRUNO BOULEVARD SOUTH SAN FRANCISCO CA 94080 DD 01/16/91 MA 12/30/93
DRONABINOL TN= MARINOL	FOR THE STIMULATION OF APPETITE AND PREVENTION OF WEIGHT LOSS IN PATIENTS WITH A CONFIRMED DIAGNOSIS OF ACQUIRED IMMUNODEFICIENCY SYNDROME (AIDS).	UNIMED, INC. 2150 EAST LAKE COOK ROAD BUFFALO GROVE IL 60089 DD 01/15/91 MA 12/22/92

CUMULATIVE LIST OF ORPHAN PRODUCT DESIGNATIONS AND APPROVALS *(continued)*

NAME *Generic/Chemical* *TN=Trade Name*	INDICATION DESIGNATED	SPONSOR AND ADDRESS *DD=Date Designated* *MA=Marketing Approval*
DYNAMINE	TREATMENT OF LAMBERT EATON MYASTHENIC SYNDROME.	MAYO FOUNDATION 200 S.W. 1ST AVENUE ROCHESTER MN 55905 DD 02/05/90
DYNAMINE	TREATMENT OF HEREDITARY MOTOR AND SENSORY NEUROPATHY TYPE I (CHARCOT-MARIE-TOOTH DISEASE).	MAYO FOUNDATION 200 S.W. 1ST AVENUE ROCHESTER MN 55905 DD 10/16/91
EFLORNITHINE HCL TN= ORNIDYL	TREATMENT OF TRYPANOSOMA BRUCEI GAMBIENSE INFECTION (SLEEPING SICKNESS).	MARION MERRELL DOW, INC. P.O. BOX 9707, MARION PARK DRIVE KANSAS CITY MO 64134-0707 DD 04/23/86 MA 11/28/90
ELLIOTT'S B SOLUTION	TREATMENT OF ACUTE LYMPHOCYTIC LEUKEMIAS AND ACUTE LYMPHOBLASTIC LYMPHOMAS.	ORPHAN MEDICAL 13911 RIDGEDALE DRIVE MINNETONKA MN 55305 DD 08/24/94
EPIDERMAL GROWTH FACTOR (HUMAN)	ACCELERATION OF CORNEAL EPITHELIAL REGENERATION AND THE HEALING OF STROMAL TISSUE IN THE CONDITION OF NON-HEALING CORNEAL DEFECTS.	CHIRON OPHTHALMICS 9342 JERONIMO ROAD IRVINE CA 92718-1903 DD 10/05/87
EPOETIN ALFA TN= EPOGEN	TREATMENT OF ANEMIA ASSOCIATED WITH END STAGE RENAL DISEASE (ESRD).	AMGEN, INC. 1840 DEHAVILLAND DRIVE THOUSAND OAKS CA 91320-1789 DD 04/10/86 MA 06/01/89
EPOETIN ALFA TN= EPOGEN	TREATMENT OF ANEMIA ASSOCIATED WITH HIV INFECTION OR HIV TREATMENT.	AMGEN, INC. 1840 DEHAVILLAND DRIVE THOUSAND OAKS CA 91320-1789 DD 07/01/91 MA 12/31/90
EPOETIN ALFA	TREATMENT OF MYELODYSPLASTIC SYNDROME.	R.W. JOHNSON RESEARCH INSTITUTE ROUTE 202, P.O. BOX 300 RARITAN NJ 08869-0602 DD 12/20/93
EPOETIN ALFA TN= PROCRIT	TREATMENT OF ANEMIA ASSOCIATED WITH END STAGE RENAL DISEASE.	R.W. JOHNSON RESEARCH INSTITUTE ROUTE 202, P.O. BOX 300 RARITAN NJ 08869-0602 DD 08/27/87
EPOETIN ALFA TN= PROCRIT	TREATMENT OF ANEMIA OF PREMATURITY IN PRETERM INFANTS.	R.W. JOHNSON RESEARCH INSTITUTE ROUTE 202, P.O. BOX 300 RARITAN NJ 08869-0602 DD 07/21/88
EPOETIN ALFA TN= PROCRIT	TREATMENT OF HIV ASSOCIATED ANEMIA RELATED TO HIV INFECTION OR HIV TREATMENT.	R.W. JOHNSON RESEARCH INSTITUTE ROUTE 202, P.O. BOX 300 RARITAN NJ 08869-0602 DD 03/07/89
EPOETIN BETA TN= MAROGEN	TREATMENT OF ANEMIA ASSOCIATED WITH END STAGE RENAL DISEASE (ESRD).	CHUGAI-USA, INC. 3780 HAWTHORN COURT WAUKEGAN IL 60087 DD 10/22/87
EPOPROSTENOL TN= FLOLAN	TREATMENT OF PRIMARY PULMONARY HYPERTENSION (PPH).	BURROUGHS WELLCOME COMPANY 3030 CORNWALLIS ROAD RESEARCH TRIANGLE PK NC 27709 DD 09/25/85
EPOPROSTENOL TN= FLOLAN	REPLACEMENT OF HEPARIN IN PATIENTS REQUIRING HEMODIALYSIS AND WHO ARE AT INCREASED RISK OF HEMORRHAGE.	BURROUGHS WELLCOME COMPANY 3030 CORNWALLIS ROAD RESEARCH TRIANGLE PK NC 27709 DD 03/29/84
ERWINIA L-ASPARAGINASE TN= ERWINASE	TREATMENT OF ACUTE LYMPHOCYTIC LEUKEMIA.	PORTON INTERNATIONAL, INC. 816 CONNECTICUT AVENUE NW WASHINGTON DC 20006 DD 07/30/86
ERYTHROPOIETIN (RECOMBINANT HUMAN)	TREATMENT OF ANEMIA ASSOCIATED WITH END STAGE RENAL DISEASE.	MCDONNELL DOUGLAS CORP P.O. BOX 516 ST. LOUIS MO 63166 DD 08/19/87

CUMULATIVE LIST OF ORPHAN PRODUCT DESIGNATIONS AND APPROVALS *(continued)*

NAME *Generic/Chemical* *TN= Trade Name*	INDICATION DESIGNATED	SPONSOR AND ADDRESS *DD= Date Designated* *MA= Marketing Approval*
ETHANOLAMINE OLEATE TN= ETHAMOLIN	TREATMENT OF PATIENTS WITH ESOPHAGEAL VARICES THAT HAVE RECENTLY BLED, TO PREVENT REBLEEDING.	BLOCK DRUG COMPANY, INC. 257 CORNELISON AVENUE JERSEY CITY NJ 07302 DD 03/22/84 MA 12/12/88
ETHINYL ESTRADIOL, USP	TREATMENT OF TURNER'S SYNDROME.	BIO-TECHNOLOGY GENERAL CORP. 70 WOOD AVENUE, SOUTH ISELIN NJ 08830 DD 06/22/88
ETHIOFOS TN= ETHYOL	FOR USE AS A CHEMOPROTECTIVE AGENT FOR CISPLATIN IN THE TREATMENT OF ADVANCED OVARIAN CARCINOMA.	U.S. BIOSCIENCE, INC. 100 FRONT STREET WEST CONSHOHOCKEN PA 19428 DD 05/30/90
ETHIOFOS TN= ETHYOL	FOR USE AS A CHEMOPROTECTIVE AGENT FOR CYCLOPHOSPHAMIDE IN THE TREATMENT OF ADVANCED OVARIAN CARCINOMA.	U.S. BIOSCIENCE, INC. 100 FRONT STREET WEST CONSHOHOCKEN PA 19428 DD 05/30/90
ETHIOFOS TN= ETHYOL	FOR USE AS A CHEMOPROTECTIVE AGENT FOR CISPLATIN IN THE TREATMENT OF METASTATIC MELANOMA.	U.S. BIOSCIENCE, INC. 100 FRONT STREET WEST CONSHOHOCKEN PA 19428 DD 05/30/90
ETIDRONATE DISODIUM TN= DIDRONEL	TREATMENT OF HYPERCALCEMIA OF A MALIGNANCY INADEQUATELY MANAGED BY DIETARY MODIFICATION AND/OR ORAL HYDRATION.	MGI PHARMA, INC. 9900 BREN ROAD EAST, SUITE 300E MINNEAPOLIS MN 55343-9667 DD 03/21/86 MA 04/21/87
FACTOR VIIa (RECOMBINANT, DNA ORIGIN)	TREATMENT OF PATIENTS WITH HEMOPHILIA A AND B WITH AND WITHOUT ANTIBODIES AGAINST FACTORS VIII/IX, AND PATIENTS WITH VON WILLEBRAND'S DISEASE.	NOVO NORDISK PHARMACEUTICALS 100 OVERLOOK CENTER, SUITE 200 PRINCETON NJ 08540-7810 DD 06/06/88
FACTOR XIII (PLACENTA-DERIVED) TN= FIBROGAMMIN P	TREATMENT OF CONGENITAL FACTOR XIII DEFICIENCY.	HOECHST-ROUSSEL PHARMACEUTICAL ROUTE 202-206, P.O. BOX 2500 SOMERVILLE NJ 08876-1258 DD 01/16/85
FELBAMATE TN= FELBATOL	TREATMENT OF LENNOX-GASTAUT SYNDROME.	WALLACE LABORATORIES 301B COLLEGE ROAD EAST PRINCETON NJ 08540 DD 01/24/89 MA 07/29/93
FGN-1	FOR THE SUPPRESSION AND CONTROL OF COLONIC ADENOMATOUS POLYPS IN THE INHERITED DISEASE ADENOMATOUS POLYPOSIS COLI.	CELL PATHWAYS, INC. 1700 BROADWAY, SUITE 2000 DENVER CO 80290 DD 02/14/94
FIAU	ADJUNCTIVE TREATMENT OF CHRONIC ACTIVE HEPATITIS B.	OCLASSEN PHARMACEUTICALS, INC. 100 PELICAN WAY SAN RAFAEL CA 94901 DD 07/24/92
FIBRONECTIN (HUMAN PLASMA)	TREATMENT OF NON-HEALING CORNEAL ULCERS OR EPITHELIAL DEFECTS WHICH HAVE BEEN UNRESPONSIVE TO CONVENTIONAL THERAPY AND THE UNDERLYING CAUSE HAS BEEN ELIMINATED.	NEW YORK BLOOD CENTER 310 E. 67TH STREET NEW YORK NY 10021 DD 09/05/88
FIBRONECTIN (PLASMA DERIVED)	TREATMENT OF NON-HEALING CORNEAL ULCERS OR EPITHELIAL DEFECTS WHICH ARE UNRESPONSIVE TO CONVENTIONAL THERAPY AND FOR WHICH ANY INFECTIOUS CAUSE OF THE DEFECT HAS BEEN ELIMINATED.	CHIRON OPHTHALMICS 9342 JERONIMO ROAD IRVINE CA 92718-1903 DD 12/05/88
FILGRASTIM TN= NEUPOGEN	TREATMENT OF MYELODYSPLASTIC SYNDROME.	AMGEN, INC. 1840 DEHAVILLAND DRIVE THOUSAND OAKS CA 91320-1789 DD 08/30/90
FILGRASTIM TN= NEUPOGEN	TREATMENT OF PATIENTS WITH SEVERE CHRONIC NEUTROPENIA (ABSOLUTE NEUTROPHIL COUNT LESS THAN 500/MM3).	AMGEN, INC. 1840 DEHAVILLAND DRIVE THOUSAND OAKS CA 91320-1789 DD 11/07/90
FILGRASTIM TN= NEUPOGEN	TREATMENT OF NEUTROPENIA ASSOCIATED WITH BONE MARROW TRANSPLANTS.	AMGEN, INC. 1840 DEHAVILLAND DRIVE THOUSAND OAKS CA 91320-1789 DD 10/01/90

CUMULATIVE LIST OF ORPHAN PRODUCT DESIGNATIONS AND APPROVALS *(continued)*

NAME *Generic/Chemical* *TN=Trade Name*	INDICATION DESIGNATED	SPONSOR AND ADDRESS *DD=Date Designated* *MA=Marketing Approval*
FILGRASTIM TN= NEUPOGEN	TREATMENT OF PATIENTS WITH ACQUIRED IMMUNODEFICIENCY SYNDROME (AIDS) WHO, IN ADDITION, ARE AFFLICTED WITH CYTOMEGALOVIRUS RETINITIS (CMV RETINITIS) AND ARE BEING TREATED WITH GANCICLOVIR.	AMGEN, INC. 1840 DEHAVILLAND DRIVE THOUSAND OAKS CA 91320-1789 DD 09/03/91
FLUDARABINE PHOSPHATE TN= FLUDARA	TREATMENT OF CHRONIC LYMPHOCYTIC LEUKEMIA (CLL), INCLUDING REFRACTORY CLL.	BERLEX LABORATORIES, INC. 15049 SAN PABLO AVENUE P.O. BOX 4099 RICHMOND CA 94804-0099 DD 04/18/89 MA 04/18/91
FLUDARABINE PHOSPHATE TN= FLUDARA	TREATMENT AND MANAGEMENT OF PATIENTS WITH NON-HODGKINS LYMPHOMA.	BERLEX LABORATORIES, INC. 15049 SAN PABLO AVENUE P.O. BOX 4099 RICHMOND CA 94804-0099 DD 04/18/89
FLUMECINOL TN= ZIXORYN	TREATMENT OF HYPERBILIRUBINEMIA IN NEWBORN INFANTS UNRESPONSIVE TO PHOTOTHERAPY.	FARMACON, INC. 90 GROVE STREET, SUITE 109 RIDGEFIELD CT 06877-4118 DD 01/15/85
FLUNARIZINE TN= SIBELIUM	TREATMENT OF ALTERNATING HEMIPLEGIA.	JANSSEN RESEARCH FOUNDATION 1125 TRENTON-HARBOURTON ROAD P.O. BOX 200 TITUSVILLE NJ 08560-0200 DD 01/06/86
FLUOROURACIL TN= ADRUCIL	FOR USE IN COMBINATION WITH LEUCOVORIN FOR THERAPY OF METASTATIC ADENOCARCINOMA OF THE COLON AND RECTUM.	LEDERLE LABORATORIES DIVISION AMERICAN CYANAMIDE COMPANY PEARL RIVER NY 10965 DD 02/06/89
FLUOROURACIL	FOR USE IN COMBINATION WITH INTERFERON ALPHA-2A, RECOMBINANT, FOR THE TREATMENT OF ESOPHAGEAL CARCINOMA.	HOFFMANN-LA ROCHE, INC. 340 KINGSLAND STREET NUTLEY NJ 07110-1199 DD 10/27/89
FLUOROURACIL	FOR USE IN COMBINATION WITH INTERFERON ALPHA-2A, RECOMBINANT, FOR THE TREATMENT OF ADVANCED COLORECTAL CARCINOMA.	HOFFMANN-LA ROCHE, INC. 340 KINGSLAND STREET NUTLEY NJ 07110-1199 DD 04/18/90
FOSPHENYTOIN	ACUTE TREATMENT OF PATIENTS WITH STATUS EPILEPTICUS OF THE GRAND MAL TYPE.	WARNER-LAMBERT COMPANY 2800 PLYMOUTH ROAD ANN ARBOR MI 48105-2430 DD 06/04/91
GALLIUM NITRATE INJECTION TN= GANITE	TREATMENT OF HYPERCALCEMIA OF MALIGNANCY.	FUJISAWA PHARMACEUTICAL CO. 3 PARKWAY NORTH DEERFIELD IL 60015-2548 DD 12/05/88 MA 01/17/91
GAMMALINOLENIC ACID	TREATMENT OF JUVENILE RHEUMATOID ARTHRITIS.	ZURIER, ROBERT B., M.D. 55 LAKE AVE. UNIV. OF MASS. MED. CTR. WORCESTER MA 01655 DD 07/27/94
GENTAMICIN IMPREGNATED PMMA BEADS ON SURGICAL WIRE TN= SEPTOPAL	TREATMENT OF CHRONIC OSTEOMYELITIS OF POST-TRAUMATIC, POSTOPERATIVE, OR HEMATOGENOUS ORIGIN.	EM INDUSTRIES, INC. 5 SKYLINE DRIVE HAWTHORNE NY 10532 DD 01/31/91
GENTAMICIN LIPOSOME INJECTION TN= MAITEC	TREATMENT OF DISSEMINATED MYCOBACTERIUM AVIUM-INTRACELLULARE INFECTION.	THE LIPOSOME COMPANY, INC. ONE RESEARCH WAY PRINCETON NJ 08540 DD 07/10/90
GONADORELIN ACETATE TN= LUTREPULSE	INDUCTION OF OVULATION IN WOMEN WITH HYPOTHALAMIC AMENORRHEA DUE TO A DEFICIENCY OR ABSENCE IN THE QUANTITY OR PULSE PATTERN OF ENDOGENOUS GNRH SECRETION.	FERRING LABORATORIES, INC. 400 RELLA BOULEVARD, SUITE 201 SUFFERN NY 10901-4249 DD 04/22/87 MA 10/10/89
GOSSYPOL	TREATMENT OF CANCER OF THE ADRENAL CORTEX.	REIDENBERG, MARCUS M., M.D. 525 EAST 68TH STREET, BOX 70 NEW YORK NY 10021 DD 10/22/90
GROUP B STREPTOCOCCUS IMMUNE GLOBULIN	TREATMENT OF NEONATES FOR DISSEMINATED GROUP B STREPTOCOCCAL INFECTION.	UNIVAX BIOLOGICS, INC. 12280 WILKINS AVENUE ROCKVILLE MD 20852 DD 05/08/90

CUMULATIVE LIST OF ORPHAN PRODUCT DESIGNATIONS AND APPROVALS *(continued)*

NAME *Generic/Chemical* *TN=Trade Name*	INDICATION DESIGNATED	SPONSOR AND ADDRESS *DD=Date Designated* *MA=Marketing Approval*
GROWTH HORMONE RELEASING FACTOR	FOR THE LONG-TERM TREATMENT OF CHILDREN WHO HAVE GROWTH FAILURE DUE TO A LACK OF ADEQUATE ENDOGENOUS GROWTH HORMONE SECRETION.	FUJISAWA PHARMACEUTICAL CO. 3 PARKWAY NORTH DEERFIELD IL 60015-2548 DD 08/07/89
GUANETHIDINE MONOSULFATE TN= ISMELIN	TREATMENT OF MODERATE TO SEVERE REFLEX SYMPATHETIC DYSTROPHY AND CAUSALGIA.	CIBA-GEIGY CORPORATION 556 MORRIS AVENUE SUMMIT NJ 07901 DD 01/06/86
HALOFANTRINE TN= HALFAN	TREATMENT OF MILD TO MODERATE ACUTE MALARIA CAUSED BY SUSCEPTIBLE STRAINS OF P. FALCIPARUM AND P. VIVAX.	SMITHKLINE BEECHAM P.O. BOX 1510 KING OF PRUSSIA PA 19406 DD 11/04/91 MA 07/24/92
HEME ARGINATE TN= NORMOSANG	TREATMENT OF SYMPTOMATIC STAGE OF ACUTE PORPHYRIA.	LEIRAS, INCORPORATED 1850 CENTENNIAL PARK DRIVE, SUITE 450 RESTON VA 22091 DD 03/01/94
HEME ARGINATE TN= NORMOSANG	TREATMENT OF MYELODYSPLASTIC SYNDROMES.	LEIRAS, INCORPORATED 1850 CENTENNIAL PARK DRIVE SUITE 450 RESTON VA 22091 DD 03/01/94
HEMIN TN= PANHEMATIN	AMELIORIATION OF RECURRENT ATTACKS OF ACUTE INTERMITTENT PORPHYRIA (AIP) TEMPORARILY RELATED TO THE MENSTRUAL CYCLE IN SUSCEPTIBLE WOMEN AND SIMILAR SYMPTOMS WHICH OCCUR IN OTHER PATIENTS WITH AIP, PORPHYRIA VARIEGATA AND HEREDITA COPROPORPHYRIA.	ABBOTT LABORATORIES DIAGNOSTICS DIVISION ABBOTT PARK IL 60064 DD 03/16/84 MA 07/20/83
HEMIN AND ZINC MESOPORPHYRIN TN= HEMEX	TREATMENT OF ACUTE PORPHYRIC SYNDROMES.	BONKOVSKY, HERBERT L., M.D. UNIV. OF MASS. MED. CTR. WORCESTER MA 01655 DD 12/20/93
HERPES SIMPLEX VIRUS GENE	TREATMENT OF PRIMARY AND METASTATIC BRAIN TUMORS.	GENETIC THERAPY, INC. 19 FIRSTFIELD ROAD GAITHERSBURG MD 20878 DD 10/16/92
HISTRELIN	TREATMENT OF ACUTE INTERMITTENT PORPHYRIA, HEREDITARY COPROPORPHYRIA, AND VARIEGATE PORPHYRIA.	ANDERSON, KARL E., M.D. U. OF TEXAS MEDICAL BRANCH GALVESTON TX 77550 DD 05/03/91
HISTRELIN ACETATE TN= SUPPRELIN INJECTION	TREATMENT OF CENTRAL PRECOCIOUS PUBERTY.	ROBERTS PHARMACEUTICAL CORP. 6 INDUSTRIAL WAY WEST EATONTOWN NJ 07724 DD 08/10/88 MA 12/24/91
HIV NEUTRALIZING ANTIBODIES TN= IMMUPATH	TREATMENT OF ACQUIRED IMMUNODEFICIENCY SYNDROME (AIDS).	HEMACARE CORPORATION 4954 VAN NUYS BOULEVARD SHERMAN OAKS CA 91403 DD 03/24/92
HUMAN IMMUNODEFICIENCY VIRUS IMMUNE GLOBULIN	TREATMENT OF AIDS.	NORTH AMERICAN BIOLOGICALS, INC. 16500 N.W. 15TH AVENUE MIAMI FL 33169 DD 11/21/89
HUMAN IMMUNODEFICIENCY VIRUS IMMUNE GLOBULIN	TREATMENT OF HIV-INFECTED PREGNANT WOMEN AND INFANTS OF HIV-INFECTED MOTHERS.	NORTH AMERICAN BIOLOGICALS, INC. 16500 N.W. 15TH AVENUE MIAMI FL 33169 DD 03/25/92
HUMAN T-LYMPHOTROPIC VIRUS TYPE III gp160 ANTIGENS TN= VAXSYN HIV-1	TREATMENT OF ACQUIRED IMMUNODEFICIENCY SYNDROME (AIDS).	MICROGENESYS, INC. 1000 RESEARCH PARKWAY MERIDEN CT 06450 DD 11/20/89
HUMAN THYROID STIMULATING HORMONE (TSH) TN= THYROGEN	AS AN ADJUNCT IN THE DIAGNOSIS OF THYROID CANCER.	GENZYME CORPORATION ONE KENDALL SQUARE CAMBRIDGE MA 02139 DD 02/24/92

CUMULATIVE LIST OF ORPHAN PRODUCT DESIGNATIONS AND APPROVALS *(continued)*

NAME *Generic/Chemical* *TN=Trade Name*	INDICATION DESIGNATED	SPONSOR AND ADDRESS *DD=Date Designated* *MA=Marketing Approval*
HUMANIZED ANTI-TAC	PREVENTION OF ACUTE RENAL ALLOGRAFT REJECTION.	HOFFMANN-LA ROCHE, INC. 340 KINGSLAND STREET NUTLEY NJ 07110 DD 03/05/93
HUMANIZED ANTI-TAC	PREVENTION OF ACUTE GRAFT-VS-HOST DISEASE FOLLOWING BONE MARROW TRANSPLANTATION.	HOFFMANN-LA ROCHE, INC. 340 KINGSLAND STREET NUTLEY NJ 07110 DD 03/05/93
HYDROXYCOBALAMIN/SODIUM THIOSULFATE	TREATMENT OF SEVERE ACUTE CYANIDE POISONING.	YAMIN, MICHAEL A., PH.D. C/O INNAPHARMA, INC. 75 MONTEBELLO ROAD SUFFERN NY 10901 DD 10/04/85
HYDROXYUREA TN= HYDREA	TREATMENT OF PATIENTS WITH SICKLE CELL ANEMIA AS SHOWN BY THE PRESENCE OF HEMOGLOBIN S.	BRISTOL-MYERS SQUIBB 2400 WEST LLOYD EXPRESSWAY EVANSVILLE IN 47721-0001 DD 10/01/90
I-131 RADIOLABELED B1 MONOCLONAL ANTIBODY	TREATMENT OF NON-HODGKIN'S B-CELL LYMPHOMA.	COULTER CORPORATION 11800 S.W. 147 AVENUE P.O. BOX 169015 MIAMI FL 33116-9015 DD 05/16/94
IDARUBICIN TN= IDAMYCIN	TREATMENT OF MYELODYSPLASTIC SYNDROMES.	ADRIA LABORATORIES, INC. P.O. BOX 16529 COLUMBUS OH 43216-6529 DD 12/01/92
IDARUBICIN TN= IDAMYCIN	TREATMENT OF CHRONIC MYELOGENOUS LEUKEMIA.	ADRIA LABORATORIES, INC. P.O. BOX 16529 COLUMBUS OH 42316-6529 DD 12/02/92
IDARUBICIN HCL FOR INJECTION TN= IDAMYCIN	TREATMENT OF ACUTE MYELOGENOUS LEUKEMIA (AML), ALSO REFERRED TO AS ACUTE NONLYMPHOCYTIC LEUKEMIA (ANLL).	ADRIA LABORATORIES, INC. P.O. BOX 16529 COLUMBUS OH 43216-6529 DD 07/25/88 MA 09/27/90
IDARUBICIN HCL FOR INJECTION TN= IDAMYCIN	TREATMENT OF ACUTE LYMPHOBLASTIC LEUKEMIA IN PEDIATRIC PATIENTS.	ADRIA LABORATORIES, INC. P.O. BOX 16529 COLUMBUS OH 43216-6529 DD 02/12/91
IFOSFAMIDE TN= IFEX	IN COMBINATION WITH CERTAIN OTHER APPROVED ANTINEOPLASTIC AGENTS, FOR THIRD LINE CHEMOTHERAPY IN THE TREATMENT OF GERM CELL TESTICULAR CANCER.	BRISTOL-MYERS SQUIBB 5 RESEARCH PARKWAY, P.O. BOX 5100 WALLINGFORD CT 06492-7660 DD 01/20/87 MA 12/30/88
IFOSFAMIDE TN= IFEX	TREATMENT OF BONE SARCOMAS.	BRISTOL-MYERS SQUIBB 5 RESEARCH PARKWAY, P.O. BOX 5100 WALLINGFORD CT 06492-7660 DD 08/07/85
IFOSFAMIDE TN= IFEX	TREATMENT OF SOFT TISSUE SARCOMAS.	BRISTOL-MYERS SQUIBB 5 RESEARCH PARKWAY, P.O. BOX 5100 WALLINGFORD CT 06492 DD 08/07/85
IMCIROMAB PENTETATE TN= MYOSCINT	DETECTING EARLY NECROSIS AS AN INDICATION OF REJECTION OF ORTHOTOPIC CARDIAC TRANSPLANTS.	CENTOCOR, INC. 244 GREAT VALLEY PARKWAY MALVERN PA 19355-1307 DD 01/25/89
IMIGLUCERASE TN= CEREZYME	FOR REPLACEMENT THERAPY IN PATIENTS WITH TYPES I, II, AND III GAUCHER'S DISEASE.	GENZYME CORPORATION ONE KENDALL SQUARE CAMBRIDGE MA 02139 DD 11/05/91 MA 05/23/94
IMMUNE GLOBULIN INTRAVENOUS (HUMAN) TN= IVEEGAM, IMMUNO	TREATMENT OF JUVENILE RHEUMATOID ARTHRITIS.	IMMUNO CLINICAL RESEARCH CORP. 155 EAST 56TH STREET NEW YORK NY 10022 DD 12/16/92

CUMULATIVE LIST OF ORPHAN PRODUCT DESIGNATIONS AND APPROVALS *(continued)*

NAME *Generic/Chemical* *TN=Trade Name*	INDICATION DESIGNATED	SPONSOR AND ADDRESS *DD=Date Designated* *MA=Marketing Approval*
IMMUNE GLOBULIN INTRAVENOUS (HUMAN) TN= IVEEGAM, IMMUNO	TREATMENT OF POLYMYOSITIS/DERMATOMYOSITIS.	IMMUNO CLINICAL RESEARCH CORP. 155 EAST 56TH STREET NEW YORK NY 10022 DD 10/13/92
IMMUNE GLOBULIN INTRAVENOUS (HUMAN) TN= IMMUNE GLOBULIN INTRAVENOUS (HUMAN) IMMUNO, IVEEGAM	TREATMENT OF PATIENTS WITH ACUTE MYOCARDITIS.	IMMUNO CLINICAL RESEARCH CORP. 750 LEXINGTON AVENUE NEW YORK NY 10022 DD 11/22/93
IMMUNE GLOBULIN INTRAVENOUS HUMAN TN= GAMIMUNE N	INFECTION PROPHYLAXIS IN PEDIATRIC PATIENTS AFFECTED WITH THE HUMAN IMMUNODEFICIENCY VIRUS.	MILES, INC. 4TH & PARKER STREETS BERKELEY CA 94710 DD 02/18/93
IMPORTED FIRE ANT VENOM, ALLERGENIC EXTRACT	FOR SKIN TESTING OF VICTIMS OF FIRE ANT STINGS TO CONFIRM FIRE ANT SENSITIVITY AND IF POSITIVE, FOR USE AS IMMUNOTHERAPY FOR THE PREVENTION OF IgE-MEDIATED ANAPHYLACTIC REACTIONS.	ALK LABORATORIES, INC. 132 RESEARCH DRIVE MILFORD CT 06460 DD 05/12/92
INDIUM IN 111 MURINE MONOCLONAL ANTIBODY FAB TO MYOSIN TN= MYOSCINT	TO AID IN THE DIAGNOSIS OF MYOCARDITIS.	CENTOCOR, INC. 244 GREAT VALLEY PARKWAY MALVERN PA 19355 DD 08/07/89
INDIUM In-111 ALTUMOMAB PENTETATE TN= HYBRI-CEAker	DETECTION OF SUSPECTED AND PREVIOUSLY UNIDENTIFIED TUMOR FOCI OF RECURRENT COLORECTAL CARCINOMA.	HYBRITECH, INC. 11095 TORREYANNA ROAD SAN DIEGO CA 92196-9006 DD 02/06/90
INOSINE PRANOBEX TN= ISOPRINOSINE	TREATMENT OF SUBACUTE SCLEROSING PANENCEPHALITIS (SSPE).	NEWPORT PHARMACEUTICALS 897 WEST SIXTEENTH STREET NEWPORT BEACH CA 92663 DD 09/20/88
INSULIN-LIKE GROWTH FACTOR-1 TN= MYOTROPHIN	TREATMENT OF AMYOTROPHIC LATERAL SCLEROSIS (ALS).	CEPHALON, INC. 145 BRANDYWINE PARKWAY WEST CHESTER PA 19380-4245 DD 08/05/91
INTERFERON ALFA-2A (RECOMBINANT) TN= ROFERON-A	TREATMENT OF AIDS RELATED KAPOSI'S SARCOMA.	HOFFMANN-LA ROCHE, INC. 340 KINGSLAND STREET NUTLEY NJ 07110 DD 12/14/87 MA 11/21/88
INTERFERON ALFA-2A (RECOMBINANT) TN= ROFERON-A	TREATMENT OF RENAL CELL CARCINOMA.	HOFFMANN-LA ROCHE, INC. 340 KINGSLAND STREET NUTLEY NJ 07110-1199 DD 04/18/88
INTERFERON ALFA-2A (RECOMBINANT) TN= ROFERON A	TREATMENT OF CHRONIC MYELOGENOUS LEUKEMIA.	HOFFMANN-LA ROCHE, INC. 340 KINGSLAND STREET NUTLEY NJ 07110-1199 DD 06/06/89
INTERFERON ALFA-2A (RECOMBINANT) TN= ROFERON-A	FOR USE IN COMBINATION WITH FLUOROURACIL FOR THE TREATMENT OF ESOPHAGEAL CARCINOMA.	HOFFMANN-LA ROCHE, INC. 340 KINGSLAND STREET NUTLEY NJ 07110-1199 DD 10/27/89
INTERFERON ALFA-2A (RECOMBINANT) TN= ROFERON-A	FOR THE CONCOMITANT ADMINISTRATION WITH TECELEUKIN FOR THE TREATMENT OF METASTATIC RENAL CELL CARCINOMA.	HOFFMANN-LA ROCHE, INC. 340 KINGSLAND STREET NUTLEY NJ 07119-1199 DD 05/02/90
INTERFERON ALFA-2A (RECOMBINANT) TN= ROFERON-A	FOR THE TREATMENT OF METASTATIC MALIGNANT MELANOMA IN COMBINATION WITH TECELEUKIN.	HOFFMANN-LA ROCHE, INC. 340 KINGSLAND STREET NUTLEY NJ 07110-1199 DD 05/11/90
INTERFERON ALFA-2B (RECOMBINANT) TN= INTRON A	TREATMENT OF CHRONIC MYELOGENOUS LEUKEMIA (CML).	SCHERING CORPORATION 2000 GALLOPING HILL ROAD KENILWORTH NJ 07033 DD 06/22/87
INTERFERON ALFA-2B (RECOMBINANT) TN= INTRON A	TREATMENT OF AIDS-RELATED KAPOSI'S SARCOMA.	SCHERING CORPORATION 2000 GALLOPING HILL ROAD KENILWORTH NJ 07033 DD 06/24/87 MA 11/21/88

CUMULATIVE LIST OF ORPHAN PRODUCT DESIGNATIONS AND APPROVALS *(continued)*

NAME *Generic/Chemical* *TN=Trade Name*	INDICATION DESIGNATED	SPONSOR AND ADDRESS *DD=Date Designated* *MA=Marketing Approval*
INTERFERON ALFA-2B (RECOMBINANT) TN= INTRON A	TREATMENT OF ACUTE HEPATITIS B.	SCHERING CORPORATION 2000 GALLOPING HILL ROAD KENILWORTH NJ 07033 DD 11/17/88
INTERFERON ALFA-NL TN= WELLFERON	TREATMENT OF AIDS RELATED KAPOSI'S SARCOMA.	BURROUGHS WELLCOME COMPANY 3030 CORNWALLIS ROAD RESEARCH TRIANGLE PK NC 27709 DD 08/25/86
INTERFERON ALFA-NL TN= WELLFERON	TREATMENT OF HUMAN PAPILLOMAVIRUS (HPV) IN PATIENTS WITH SEVERE RESISTANT/RECURRENT RESPIRATORY (LARYNGEAL) PAPILLOMATOSIS.	BURROUGHS WELLCOME COMPANY 3030 CORNWALLIS ROAD RESEARCH TRIANGLE PK NC 27709 DD 10/16/87
INTERFERON BETA (RECOMBINANT HUMAN)	TREATMENT OF MULTIPLE SCLEROSIS.	BIOGEN, INC. 14 CAMBRIDGE CENTER CAMBRIDGE MA 02142 DD 12/16/91
INTERFERON BETA (RECOMBINANT HUMAN)	TREATMENT OF ACUTE NON-A, NON-B HEPATITIS.	BIOGEN, INC. 14 CAMBRIDGE CENTER CAMBRIDGE MA 02142 DD 07/24/92
INTERFERON BETA (RECOMBINANT HUMAN)	TREATMENT OF PRIMARY BRAIN TUMORS.	BIOGEN, INC. 14 CAMBRIDGE CENTER CAMBRIDGE MA 02142 DD 01/13/93
INTERFERON BETA (RECOMBINANT) TN= r-IFN-beta	SYSTEMIC TREATMENT OF CUTANEOUS T-CELL LYMPHOMA.	BIOGEN, INC. 14 CAMBRIDGE CENTER CAMBRIDGE MA 02142 DD 04/18/91
INTERFERON BETA (RECOMBINANT) TN= r-IFN-beta	SYSTEMIC TREATMENT OF CUTANEOUS MALIGNANT MELANOMA.	BIOGEN, INC. 14 CAMBRIDGE CENTER CAMBRIDGE MA 02142 DD 04/03/91
INTERFERON BETA (RECOMBINANT) TN= r-IFN-beta	FOR THE INTRALESIONAL AND/OR SYSTEMIC TREATMENT OF AIDS-RELATED KAPOSI'S SARCOMA.	BIOGEN, INC. 14 CAMBRIDGE CENTER CAMBRIDGE MA 02142 DD 05/09/91
INTERFERON BETA (RECOMBINANT) TN= r-IFN-beta	SYSTEMIC TREATMENT OF METASTATIC RENAL CELL CARCINOMA.	BIOGEN, INC. 14 CAMBRIDGE CENTER CAMBRIDGE MA 02142 DD 02/12/91
INTERFERON BETA (RECOMBINANT) TN= R-FRONE	TREATMENT OF SYMPTOMATIC PATIENTS WITH ACQUIRED IMMUNODEFICIENCY SYNDROME INCLUDING ALL PATIENTS WITH CD4 T-CELL COUNTS LESS THAN 200 CELLS PER MM3.	SERONO LABORATORIES, INC. 100 LONGWATER CIRCLE NORWELL MA 02061 DD 12/02/92
INTERFERON BETA, RECOMBINANT HUMAN TN= BETASERON	TREATMENT OF MULTIPLE SCLEROSIS.	CHIRON CORPORATION 4560 HORTON STREET EMERYVILLE CA 94608 DD 11/17/88 MA 07/23/93
INTERFERON GAMMA 1-B TN= ACTIMMUNE	TREATMENT OF CHRONIC GRANULOMATOUS DISEASE.	GENENTECH, INC. 460 POINT SAN BRUNO BOULEVARD SOUTH SAN FRANCISCO CA 94080 DD 09/30/88 MA 12/20/90
INTERLEUKIN-1 RECEPTOR ANTAGONIST, HUMAN RECOMBINANT TN= ANTRIL	TREATMENT OF JUVENILE RHEUMATOID ARTHRITIS.	SYNERGEN, INC. 1885 33RD STREET BOULDER CO 80301 DD 09/23/91
INTERLEUKIN-1 RECEPTOR ANTAGONIST, HUMAN RECOMBINANT TN= ANTRIL	PREVENTION AND TREATMENT OF GRAFT VERSUS HOST DISEASE IN TRANSPLANT RECIPIENTS.	SYNERGEN, INC. 1885 33RD STREET BOULDER CO 80301 DD 10/16/92
INTERLEUKIN-2 TN= TECELEUKIN	TREATMENT OF METASTATIC RENAL CELL CARCINOMA.	HOFFMANN-LA ROCHE, INC. 340 KINGSLAND STREET NUTLEY NJ 07110-1199 DD 02/05/90
INTERLEUKIN-2 TN= TELELEUKIN	TREATMENT OF METASTATIC MALIGNANT MELANOMA.	HOFFMANN-LA ROCHE, INC. 340 KINGSLAND STREET NUTLEY NJ 07110-1199 DD 02/06/90

CUMULATIVE LIST OF ORPHAN PRODUCT DESIGNATIONS AND APPROVALS *(continued)*

NAME *Generic/Chemical* *TN=Trade Name*	INDICATION DESIGNATED	SPONSOR AND ADDRESS *DD=Date Designated* *MA=Marketing Approval*
INTERLEUKIN-2 TN= TECELEUKIN	IN COMBINATION WITH INTERFERON ALFA-2A FOR THE TREATMENT OF METASTATIC RENAL CELL CARCINOMA.	HOFFMANN-LA ROCHE, INC. 340 KINGSLAND STREET NUTLEY NJ 07110-1199 DD 05/03/90
INTERLEUKIN-2 TN= TECELEUKIN	IN COMBINATION WITH INTERFERON ALFA-2A FOR THE TREATMENT OF METASTATIC MALIGNANT MELANOMA.	HOFFMANN-LA ROCHE, INC. 340 KINGSLAND STREET NUTLEY NJ 07110-1199 DD 05/11/90
INTERLEUKIN-3 HUMAN, RECOMBINANT	FOR SEQUENTIAL ADMINISTRATION WITH SARGRAMOSTIM TO ACCELERATE NEUTROPHIL AND PLATELET RECOVERY IN PATIENTS UNDERGOING AUTOLOGOUS BONE MARROW TRANSPLANTATION FOR THE TREATMENT OF HODGKIN'S DISEASE OR NON-HODGKIN'S LYMPHOMA.	SANDOZ PHARMACEUTICALS CORP. 59 ROUTE 10 EAST HANOVER NJ 07936-1080 DD 09/30/93
IODINE 131 6B-IODOMETHYL-19-NORCHOLESTEROL	ADRENAL CORTICAL IMAGING.	BEIERWALTES, WILLIAM, M.D. 1405 E. ANN STREET ANN ARBOR MI 48109 DD 08/01/84
IODINE 131 METAIODOBENZYLGUANIDINE SULFATE	DIAGNOSTIC ADJUNCT IN PATIENTS WITH PHEOCHROMOCYTOMA.	BEIERWALTES, WILLIAM, M.D. 1405 E. ANN STREET ANN ARBOR MI 48109 DD 11/14/84
IODINE I 123 MURINE MONOCLONAL ANTIBODY TO ALPHA-FETOPROTEIN	DETECTION OF HEPATOCELLULAR CARCINOMA AND HEPATOBLASTOMA.	IMMUNOMEDICS, INC. 300 AMERICAN ROAD MORRIS PLAINS NJ 07950 DD 09/30/88
IODINE I 123 MURINE MONOCLONAL ANTIBODY TO ALPHA-FETOPROTEIN	DETECTION OF ALPHA-FETOPROTEIN PRODUCING GERM CELL TUMORS.	IMMUNOMEDICS, INC. 300 AMERICAN ROAD MORRIS PLAINS NJ 07950 DD 09/30/88
IODINE I 123 MURINE MONOCLONAL ANTIBODY TO HCG	DETECTION OF HCG PRODUCING TUMORS SUCH AS GERM CELL AND TROPHOBLASTIC CELL TUMORS.	IMMUNOMEDICS, INC. 300 AMERICAN ROAD MORRIS PLAINS NJ 07950 DD 11/07/88
IODINE I 131 MURINE MONOCLONAL ANTIBODY IgG2a TO B CELL TN= IMMURAIT, LL-2-I-131	TREATMENT OF B-CELL LEUKEMIA AND B-CELL LYMPHOMA.	IMMUNOMEDICS, INC. 300 AMERICAN ROAD MORRIS PLAINS NJ 07950 DD 09/18/89
IODINE I 131 MURINE MONOCLONAL ANTIBODY TO ALPHA-FETOPROTEIN	TREATMENT OF HEPATOCELLULAR CARCINOMA AND HEPATOBLASTOMA.	IMMUNOMEDICS, INC. 300 AMERICAN ROAD MORRIS PLAINS NJ 07950 DD 09/30/88
IODINE I 131 MURINE MONOCLONAL ANTIBODY TO ALPHA-FETOPROTEIN	TREATMENT OF ALPHA-FETOPROTEIN PRODUCING GERM CELL TUMORS.	IMMUNOMEDICS, INC. 300 AMERICAN ROAD MORRIS PLAINS NJ 07950 DD 09/30/88
IODINE I 131 MURINE MONOCLONAL ANTIBODY TO HCG	TREATMENT OF HCG PRODUCING TUMORS SUCH AS GERM CELL AND TROPHOBLASTIC CELL TUMORS.	IMMUNOMEDICS, INC. 300 AMERICAN ROAD MORRIS PLAINS NJ 07950 DD 11/07/88
ISOBUTYRAMIDE TN= ISOBUTYRAMIDE ORAL SOLUTION	TREATMENT OF BETA-HEMOGLOBINOPATHIES AND BETA-THALASSEMIA SYNDROMES.	PERRINE, SUSAN P., M.D. BOSTON UNIVERSITY, CANCER RES. CTR. BOSTON MA 02118 DD 12/18/92
ISOBUTYRAMIDE	TREATMENT OF SICKLE CELL DISEASE AND BETA THALASSEMIA.	VERTEX PHARMACEUTICALS INC. 40 ALLSTON STREET CAMBRIDGE MA 02139-4211 DD 05/25/94
L-2 OXOTHIAZOLIDINE-4-CARBOXYLIC ACID TN= PROCYSTEINE	TREATMENT OF ADULT RESPIRATORY DISTRESS SYNDROME.	FREE RADICAL SCIENCES, INC. 245 FIRST STREET CAMBRIDGE MA 02142 DD 06/14/94
L-5 HYDROXYTRYPTOPHAN	TREATMENT OF POSTANOXIC INTENTION MYOCLONUS.	CIRCA PHARMACEUTICALS, INC. 33 RALPH AVENUE P.O. BOX 30 COPIAQUE NY 11726 DD 11/01/84

CUMULATIVE LIST OF ORPHAN PRODUCT DESIGNATIONS AND APPROVALS *(continued)*

NAME *Generic/Chemical* *TN=Trade Name*	**INDICATION DESIGNATED**	**SPONSOR AND ADDRESS** *DD=Date Designated* *MA=Marketing Approval*
L-BACLOFEN	TREATMENT OF TRIGEMINAL NEURALGIA.	FROMM, GERHARD, M.D. UNIVERSITY OF PITTSBURGH PITTSBURGH PA 15261 DD 07/13/90
L-BACLOFEN TN= NEURALGON	TREATMENT OF INTRACTABLE SPASTICITY ASSOCIATED WITH SPINAL CORD INJURY OR MULTIPLE SCLEROSIS.	WTD, INCORPORATED 8819 NORTH PIONEER ROAD PEORIA IL 61615 DD 12/17/91
L-BACLOFEN TN= NEURALGON	TREATMENT OF INTRACTABLE SPASTICITY IN CHILDREN WITH CEREBRAL PALSY.	WTD, INCORPORATED 8819 NORTH PIONEER ROAD PEORIA IL 61615 DD 01/30/92
L-CYCLOSERINE	TREATMENT OF GAUCHER'S DISEASE.	ORPHAN MEDICAL 13911 RIDGEDALE DRIVE MINNETONKA MN 55305 DD 08/01/89
L-CYSTEINE	FOR THE PREVENTION AND LESSENING OF PHOTOSENSITIVITY IN ERYTHROPOIETIC PROTOPORPHYRIA.	TYSON AND ASSOCIATES 12832 SOUTH CHADRON AVENUE HAWTHORNE CA 90250 DD 05/16/94
L-LEUCOVORIN TN= ISOVORIN	FOR USE IN CONJUNCTION WITH HIGH-DOSE METHOTREXATE IN THE TREATMENT OF OSTEOSARCOMA.	LEDERLE LABORATORIES DIVISION AMERICAN CYANAMID CORPORATION PEARL RIVER NY 10965 DD 08/01/91
L-LEUCOVORIN TN= ISOVORIN	FOR USE IN COMBINATION CHEMOTHERAPY WITH THE APPROVED AGENT 5-FLUOROURACIL IN THE PALLIATIVE TREATMENT OF METASTATIC ADENOCARCINOMA OF THE COLON AND RECTUM.	LEDERLE LABORATORIES DIVISION AMERICAN CYANAMIDE COMPANY PEARL RIVER NY 10965 DD 12/18/90
L-THREONINE TN= THREOSTAT	TREATMENT OF AMYOTROPHIC LATERAL SCLEROSIS.	TYSON AND ASSOCIATES 12832 CHADRON AVENUE HAWTHORNE CA 90250 DD 02/06/89
L-THREONINE	TREATMENT SPASTICITY ASSOCIATED WITH FAMILIAL SPASTIC PARAPARESIS.	INTERNEURON PHARMACEUTICALS 99 HAYDEN AVENUE, SUITE 340 LEXINGTON MA 02173 DD 07/24/92
LACTOBIN TN= LACTOBIN	TREAMENT OF AIDS-ASSOCIATED DIARRHEA UNRESPONSIVE TO INITIAL ANTIDIARRHEAL THERAPY.	ROXANE LABORATORIES, INC. 1809 WILSON ROAD, P.O. BOX 16532 COLUMBUS OH 43216-6532 DD 09/12/90
LEUCOVORIN TN= LEUCOVORIN CALCIUM	FOR USE IN COMBINATION WITH 5-FLUOROURACIL FOR THE TREATMENT OF METASTATIC COLORECTAL CANCER.	LEDERLE LABORATORIES DIVISION N. MIDDLETOWN ROAD PEARL RIVER NY 10965 DD 12/08/86 MA 12/12/91
LEUCOVORIN TN= LEUCOVORIN CALCIUM	FOR RESCUE USE AFTER HIGH DOSE METHOTREXATE THERAPY IN THE TREATMENT OF OSTEOSARCOMA.	LEDERLE LABORATORIES DIVISION AMERICAN CYANAMID COMPANY PEARL RIVER NY 10965 DD 08/17/88 MA 08/31/88
LEUCOVORIN CALCIUM TN= WELLCOVORIN	FOR USE IN COMBINATION WITH 5-FLUOROURACIL FOR THE TREATMENT OF METASTATIC COLORECTAL CANCER.	BURROUGHS WELLCOME COMPANY 3030 CORNWALLIS ROAD RESEARCH TRIANGLE PK NC 27709 DD 06/23/88
LEUPEPTIN	AS AN ADJUNCT TO MICROSURGICAL PERIPHERAL NERVE REPAIR.	RESEARCH TRIANGLE PHARMACEUTICALS 4364 SOUTH ALSTON AVENUE DURHAM NC 27713 DD 09/18/90
LEUPROLIDE ACETATE TN= LUPRON INJECTION	TREATMENT OF CENTRAL PRECOCIOUS PUBERTY.	TAP PHARMACEUTICALS, INC. 2355 WAUKEGAN ROAD DEERFIELD IL 60015 DD 07/25/88 MA 04/16/93
LEVOCARNITINE TN= VITA CARN	TREATMENT OF GENETIC CARNITINE DEFICIENCY.	SIGMA-TAU PHARMACEUTICALS, INC. 200 ORCHARD RIDGE DRIVE SUITE 300 GAITHERSBURG MD 20878-1978 DD 02/28/84 MA 04/10/86

CUMULATIVE LIST OF ORPHAN PRODUCT DESIGNATIONS AND APPROVALS *(continued)*

NAME *Generic/Chemical* *TN=Trade Name*	INDICATION DESIGNATED	SPONSOR AND ADDRESS *DD=Date Designated* *MA=Marketing Approval*
LEVOCARNITINE TN= CARNITOR	TREATMENT OF PRIMARY AND SECONDARY CARNITINE DEFICIENCY OF GENETIC ORIGIN.	SIGMA-TAU PHARMACEUTICALS, INC. 200 ORCHARD RIDGE DRIVE SUITE 300 GAITHERSBURG MD 20878-1978 DD 07/26/84 MA 12/16/92
LEVOCARNITINE TN= CARNITOR	TREATMENT OF MANIFESTATIONS OF CARNITINE DEFICIENCY IN PATIENTS WITH END STAGE RENAL DISEASE (ESRD) WHO REQUIRE DIALYSIS	SIGMA-TAU PHARMACEUTICALS, INC. 200 ORCHARD RIDGE DRIVE SUITE 300 GAITHERSBURG MD 20878-1978 DD 09/06/88
LEVOCARNITINE TN= VITACARN	FOR THE PREVENTION OF SECONDARY CARNITINE DEFICIENCY IN VALPROIC ACID TOXICITY.	SIGMA-TAU PHARMACEUTICALS, INC. 200 ORCHARD RIDGE DRIVE SUITE 300 GAITHERSBURG MD 20878-1978 DD 11/15/89
LEVOCARNITINE TN= VITACARN	FOR THE TREATMENT OF SECONDARY CARNITINE DEFICIENCY IN VALPROIC ACID TOXICITY	SIGMA-TAU PHARMACEUTICALS, INC. 200 ORCHARD RIDGE DRIVE SUITE 300 GAITHERSBURG MD 20878-1978 DD 11/15/89
LEVOCARNITINE TN= CARNITOR	TREATMENT OF PEDIATRIC CARDIOMYOPATHY.	SIGMA-TAU PHARMACEUTICALS, INC. 200 ORCHARD RIDGE DRIVE SUITE 300 GAITHERSBURG MD 20878 DD 11/22/93
LEVOMETHADYL ACETATE HYDROCHLORIDE TN= ORLAAM	TREATMENT OF HEROIN ADDICTS SUITABLE FOR MAINTENANCE ON OPIATE AGONISTS.	BIODEVELOPMENT CORPORATION 1300 NORTH 17TH STREET, SUITE 300 ARLINGTON VA 22209-2306 DD 01/24/84 MA 07/09/93
LIOTHYRONINE SODIUM INJECTION TN= TRIOSTAT	TREATMENT OF MYXEDEMA COMA/PRECOMA.	SMITHKLINE BEECHAM P.O. BOX 1510 KING OF PRUSSIA PA 19406 DD 07/30/90 MA 12/31/91
LIPOSOMAL DAUNORUBICIN TN= DAUNOXOME	TREATMENT OF PATIENTS WITH ADVANCED HIV-ASSOCIATED KAPOSI'S SARCOMA.	VESTAR, INC. 650 CLIFFSIDE DRIVE SAN DIMAS CA 91773 DD 05/14/93
LIPOSOME ENCAPSULATED RECOMBINANT INTERLEUKIN-2	TREATMENT OF BRAIN AND CNS TUMORS.	ONCOTHERAPEUTICS, INC. 1002 EASTPARK BOULEVARD CRANBURY NJ 08512 DD 11/25/91
LIPOSOME ENCAPSULATED RECOMBINANT INTERLEUKIN-2	TREATMENT OF CANCERS OF THE KIDNEY AND RENAL PELVIS.	ONCOTHERAPEUTICS, INC. 1002 EASTPARK BOULEVARD CRANBURY NJ 08512 DD 06/20/94
LODOXAMIDE TROMETHAMINE TN= ALOMIDE OPHTHALMIC SOLUTION	TREATMENT OF VERNAL KERATOCONJUNCTIVITIS.	ALCON LABORATORIES, INC. 6201 SOUTH FREEWAY FORT WORTH TX 76134 DD 10/16/91
MAFENIDE ACETATE SOLUTION TN= SULFAMYLON SOLUTION	FOR USE IN THE PREVENTION OF GRAFT LOSS OF MESHED AUTOGRAFTS ON EXCISED BURN WOUNDS.	DOW B. HICKAM, INC. 10410 CORPORATE DRIVE SUGAR LAND TX 77478 DD 07/18/90
MATRIX METALLOPROTEINASE INHIBITOR TN= GALARDIN	TREATMENT OF CORNEAL ULCERS.	GLYCOMED, INC 860 ATLANTIC AVENUE ALAMEDA CA 94501 DD 12/05/91
MAZINDOL TN= SANOREX	TREATMENT OF DUCHENNE MUSCULAR DYSTROPHY (DMD).	COLLIPP, PLATON J., M.D. 176 MEMORIAL DRIVE JESUP GA 31545 DD 12/08/86
MEFLOQUINE HCL TN= MEPHAQUIN	TREATMENT OF CHLOROQUINE-RESISTANT FALCIPARUMMALARIA.	MEPHA AG 4143 DORNACH, POSTFASH 137 AESCH BASEL, SWITZED DD 07/22/87

CUMULATIVE LIST OF ORPHAN PRODUCT DESIGNATIONS AND APPROVALS *(continued)*

NAME *Generic/Chemical* *TN=Trade Name*	INDICATION DESIGNATED	SPONSOR AND ADDRESS *DD=Date Designated* *MA=Marketing Approval*
MEFLOQUINE HCL TN= LARIAM	TREATMENT OF ACUTE MALARIA DUE TO PLASMODIUM FALCIPARUM AND PLASMODIUM VIVAX.	HOFFMANN-LA ROCHE, INC. 340 KINGSLAND STREET NUTLEY NJ 07110 DD 04/13/88 MA 05/02/89
MEFLOQUINE HCL TN= LARIAM	PROPHYLAXIS OF PLASMODIUM FALCIPARUM MALARIA WHICH IS RESISTANT TO OTHER AVAILABLE DRUGS.	HOFFMANN-LA ROCHE, INC. 340 KINGSLAND STREET NUTLEY NJ 07110 DD 04/13/88 MA 05/02/89
MEFLOQUINE HCL TN= MEPHAQUIN	PREVENTION OF CHLOROQUINE-RESISTANT FALCIPARUM MALARIA.	MEPHA AG 4143 DORNACH, POSTFASH 137 AESCH BASEL, SWITZED DD 07/22/87
MEGESTROL ACETATE TN= MEGACE	TREATMENT OF PATIENTS WITH ANOREXIA, CACHEXIA, OR SIGNIFICANT WEIGHT LOSS (=/10% OF BASELINE BODY WEIGHT) AND CONFIRMED DIAGNOSIS OF ACQUIRED IMMUNODEFICIENCY SYNDROME (AIDS).	BRISTOL-MYERS SQUIBB 2400 WEST LLOYD EXPRESSWAY EVANSVILLE IN 47721-0001 DD 04/13/88
MELANOMA VACCINE TN= MELACINE	TREATMENT OF STAGE III - IV MELANOMA.	RIBI IMMUNOCHEM RESEARCH, INC. P.O. BOX 1409 HAMILTON MT 59840 DD 12/20/89
MELATONIN	TREATMENT OF CIRCADIAN RHYTHM SLEEP DISORDERS IN BLIND PEOPLE WITH NO LIGHT PERCEPTION.	SACK, ROBERT, M.D. 3181 S.W. SAM JACKSON PARK ROAD PORTLAND OR 97201-3098 DD 11/15/93
MELPHALAN TN= ALKERAN FOR INJECTION	TREATMENT OF PATIENTS WITH MULTIPLE MYELOMA FOR WHOM ORAL THERAPY IS INAPPROPRIATE.	BURROUGHS WELLCOME COMPANY 3030 CORNWALLIS ROAD RESEARCH TRIANGLE PK NC 27709 DD 02/24/92 MA 11/18/92
MELPHALAN TN= ALKERAN FOR INJECTION	FOR USE IN HYPERTHERMIC REGIONAL LIMB PERFUSION TO TREAT METASTATIC MELANOMA OF THE EXTREMITY.	BURROUGHS WELLCOME COMPANY 3030 CORNWALLIS ROAD RESEARCH TRIANGLE PK IL 27709 DD 03/03/92
MESNA TN= MESNEX	FOR USE AS A PROPHYLACTIC AGENT IN REDUCING THE INCIDENCE OF IFOSFAMIDE-INDUCED HEMORRHAGIC CYSTITIS.	DEGUSSA CORPORATION 65 CHALLENGER ROAD RIDGEFIELD NJ 07660 DD 12/16/87
MESNA	INHIBITION OF THE UROTOXIC EFFECTS INDUCED BY OXAZAPHOSPHORINE COMPOUNDS SUCH AS CYCLOPHOSPHAMIDE.	ASTA MEDICAL 401 HACKENSACK AVENUE HACKENSACK NJ 07601 DD 12/16/87
METHOTREXATE TN= RHEUMATREX	TREATMENT OF JUVENILE RHEUMATOID ARTHRITIS.	LEDERLE LABORATORIES 401 N. MIDDLETOWN ROAD PEARL RIVER NY 10965-1299 DD 08/23/93
METHOTREXATE SODIUM TN= METHOTREXATE	TREATMENT OF OSTEOGENIC SARCOMA.	LEDERLE LABORATORIES DIVISION AMERICAN CYANAMIDE COMPANY PEARL RIVER NY 10965 DD 10/21/85 MA 04/07/88
METHOTREXATE USP WITH LAUROCAPRAM TN= METHOTREXATE/AZONE	TOPICAL TREATMENT OF MYCOSIS FUNGOIDES.	DISCOVERY THERAPEUTICS, INC. 911 EAST LEIGH STREET RICHMOND VA 23219 DD 10/15/90
METRONIDAZOLE TN= METROGEL.	TREATMENT OF PERIORAL DERMATITIS.	CURATEK PHARMACEUTICALS 1965 PRATT BLOULEVARD ELK GROVE VILLAGE IL 60007 DD 10/24/91
METRONIDAZOLE (TOPICAL) TN= METROGEL	TREATMENT OF ACNE ROSACEA	GALDERMA LABORATORIES, INC. P.O. BOX 331329 FORT WORTH TX 76163 DD 10/22/87 MA 11/22/88
METRONIDAZOLE (TOPICAL) TN= FLAGYL	TREATMENT OF GRADE III AND IV, ANAEROBICALLY INFECTED, DECUBITUS ULCERS.	G.D. SEARLE & COMPANY 4901 SEARLE PARKWAY SKOKIE IL 60077 DD 11/24/87
MICROBUBBLE CONTRAST AGENT TN= FILMIX NEUROSONOGRAPHIC CONTRAST AGENT	INTRAOPERATIVE AID IN THE IDENTIFICATION AND LOCALIZATION OF INTRACRANIAL TUMORS.	CAV-CON, INC. 55 KNOLLWOOD ROAD FARMINGTON CT 06032 DD 11/16/90

CUMULATIVE LIST OF ORPHAN PRODUCT DESIGNATIONS AND APPROVALS *(continued)*

NAME *Generic/Chemical* *TN= Trade Name*	**INDICATION DESIGNATED**	**SPONSOR AND ADDRESS** *DD=Date Designated* *MA=Marketing Approval*
MIDODRINE HCL TN= AMATINE	TREATMENT OF IDIOPATHIC ORTHOSTATIC HYPOTENSION.	ROBERTS PHARMACEUTICAL CORP. 6 INDUSTRIAL WAY WEST EATONTOWN NJ 07724 DD 06/21/85
MINOCYCLINE HCL TN= MINOCIN INTRAVENOUS	TREATMENT OF CHRONIC MALIGNANT PLEURAL EFFUSION.	LEDERLE LABORATORIES DIVISION AMERICAN CYANAMID COMPANY PEARL RIVER NY 10965 DD 06/19/92
MITOGUAZONE	TREATMENT OF DIFFUSE NON-HODGKIN'S LYMPHOMA, INCLUDING AIDS-RELATED DIFFUSE NON-HODGKIN'S LYMPHOMA.	CTRC RESEARCH FOUNDATION 11812 BECKET STREET POTOMAC MD 20854 DD 03/18/94
MITOXANTRONE HCL TN= NOVANTRONE	TREATMENT OF ACUTE MYELOGENOUS LEUKEMIA (AML), ALSO REFERRED TO AS ACUTE NONLYMPHOCYTIC LEUKEMIA (ANLL).	LEDERLE LABORATORIES DIVISION AMERICAN CYANAMIDE COMPANY PEARL RIVER NY 10965 DD 07/13/87 MA 12/23/87
MODAFINIL	TREATMENT OF EXCESSIVE DAYTIME SLEEPINESS IN NARCOLEPSY.	CEPHALON, INC. 145 BRANDYWINE PARKWAY WEST CHESTER PA 19380-4245 DD 03/15/93
MONOCLONAL ANTIBODIES (MURINE OR HUMAN) B-CELL LYMPHOMA	TREATMENT OF B-CELL LYMPHOMA.	IDEC PHARMACEUTICAL CORP. 11011 TORREYANA ROAD SAN DIEGO CA 92121 DD 05/06/86
MONOCLONAL ANTIBODIES PM-81 AND AML-2-23	FOR THE EXOGENOUS DEPLETION OF CD14 AND CD15 POSITIVE ACUTE MYELOID LEUKEMIC BONE MARROW CELLS FROM PATIENTS UNDERGOING BONE MARROW TRANSPLANTATION.	MEDAREX, INC. 12 COMMERCE AVENUE WEST LEBANON NH 03784 DD 03/12/90
MONOCLONAL ANTIBODY 17-1A TN= PANOREX	TREATMENT OF PANCREATIC CANCER.	CENTOCOR, INC. 244 GREAT VALLEY PARKWAY MALVERN PA 19355 DD 04/04/88
MONOCLONAL ANTIBODY FOR IMMUNIZATION AGAINST LUPUS NEPHRITIS	TREATMENT OF LUPUS NEPHRITIS.	MEDCLONE, INC. 2435 MILITARY AVENUE LOS ANGELES CA 90064 DD 01/07/93
MONOCLONAL ANTIBODY PM-81	ADJUNCTIVE TREATMENT OF ACUTE MYELOGENOUS LEUKEMIA.	MEDAREX, INC. 12 COMMERCE AVENUE WEST LEBANON NH 03784 DD 06/27/91
MONOCLONAL ANTIBODY TO CYTOMEGALOVIRUS (HUMAN)	PROPHYLAXIS OF CYTOMEGALOVIRUS DISEASE IN PATIENTS UNDERGOING SOLID ORGAN TRANSPLANTATION.	PROTEIN DESIGN LABS, INC. 2375 GARCIA AVENUE MOUNTAIN VIEW CA 94043 DD 09/13/91
MONOCLONAL ANTIBODY TO CYTOMEGALOVIRUS (HUMAN)	TREATMENT OF CYTOMEGALOVIRUS RETINITIS IN PATIENTS WITH ACQUIRED IMMUNODEFICIENCY SYNDROME.	PROTEIN DESIGN LABS, INC. 2375 GARCIA AVENUE MOUNTAIN VIEW CA 94043 DD 11/15/91
MONOCLONAL ANTIBODY TO HEPATITIS B VIRUS (HUMAN)	PROPHYLAXIS OF HEPATITIS B REINFECTION IN PATIENTS UNDERGOING LIVER TRANSPLANTATION SECONDARY TO END-STAGE CHRONIC HEPATITIS B INFECTION.	PROTEIN DESIGN LABS, INC. 2375 GARCIA AVENUE MOUNTAIN VIEW CA 94043 DD 06/17/91
MONOLAURIN TN= GLYLORIN	TREATMENT OF CONGENITAL PRIMARY ICHTHYOSIS.	CELLEGY PHARMACEUTICALS, INC. 371 BEL MARIN KEYS, SUITE 210 NOVATO CA 94949 DD 04/29/93
MONOOCTANOIN TN= MOCTANIN	DISSOLUTION OF CHOLESTEROL GALLSTONES RETAINED IN THE COMMON BILE DUCT.	ETHITEK PHARMACEUTICALS, INC. 7855 GROSS POINT ROAD, UNIT L SKOKIE IL 60077 DD 05/30/84 MA 10/31/85
MORPHINE SULFATE CONCENTRATE (PRESERVATIVE FREE) TN= INFUMORPH	FOR USE IN MICROINFUSION DEVICES FOR INTRASPINAL ADMINISTRATION IN THE TREATMENT OF INTRACTABLE CHRONIC PAIN.	ELKINS-SINN, INC. 2 ESTERBROOK LANE CHERRY HILL NJ 08003-4099 DD 07/12/90 MA 07/19/91
MUCOID EXOPOLYSACCHARIDE PSEUDOMONAS HYPERIMMUNE GLOBULIN TN= MEPIG	TREATMENT OF PULMONARY INFECTIONS DUE TO PSEUDOMONAS AERUGINOSA IN PATIENTS WITH CYSTIC FIBROSIS.	UNIVAX BIOLOGICS, INC. 12280 WILKINS AVENUE ROCKVILLE MD 20852 DD 01/09/91

CUMULATIVE LIST OF ORPHAN PRODUCT DESIGNATIONS AND APPROVALS *(continued)*

NAME *Generic/Chemical* *TN=Trade Name*	INDICATION DESIGNATED	SPONSOR AND ADDRESS *DD=Date Designated* *MA=Marketing Approval*
MUCOID EXOPOLYSACCHARIDE PSEUDOMONAS HYPERIMMUNE GLOBULIN TN= MEPIG	PREVENTION OF PULMONARY INFECTIONS DUE TO PSEUDOMONAS AERUGINOSA IN PATIENTS WITH CYSTIC FIBROSIS.	UNIVAX BIOLOGICS, INC. 12280 WILKINS AVENUE ROCKVILLE MD 20852 DD 11/07/90
MULTI-VITAMIN INFUSION (NEONATAL FORMULA)	FOR ESTABLISHMENT AND MAINTENANCE OF TOTAL PARENTERAL NUTRITION IN VERY LOW BIRTH WEIGHT INFANTS.	ASTRA PHARMACEUTICAL PRODUCTS, INC. 50 OTIS STREET WESTBOROUGH MA 01581-4500 DD 12/12/89
MYELIN	TREATMENT OF MULTIPLE SCLEROSIS.	AUTOIMMUNE, INC. 128 SPRING STREET LEXINGTON MA 02173 DD 06/27/91
MYTOMYCIN-C	TREATMENT OF REFRACTORY GLAUCOMA AS AN ADJUNCT TO AB EXTERNO GLAUCOMA SURGERY.	IOP INCORPORATED 3100 AIRWAY AVENUE COSTA MESA CA 92626 DD 08/20/93
N-TRIFLUOROACETYLADRIAMYCIN-14-VALERATE	TREATMENT OF CARCINOMA IN SITU OF THE URINARY BLADDER.	ANTHRA PHARMACEUTICALS, INC. 19 CARSON ROAD PRINCETON NJ 08540 DD 05/23/94
NAFARELIN ACETATE TN= SYNAREL NASAL SOLUTION	TREATMENT OF CENTRAL PRECOCIOUS PUBERTY.	SYNTEX (USA), INC. 3401 HILLVIEW AVENUE PALO ALTO CA 94303 DD 07/20/88 MA 02/26/92
NALTREXONE HCL TN= TREXAN	BLOCKADE OF THE PHARMACOLOGICAL EFFECTS OF EXOGENOUSLY ADMINISTERED OPIOIDS AS AN ADJUNCT TO THE MAINTENANCE OF THE OPIOID-FREE STATE IN DETOXIFIED FORMERLY OPIOID-DEPENDENT INDIVIDUALS.	DU PONT PHARMACEUTICALS E.I. du PONT de NEMOURS & CO. WILMINGTON DE 19880-0026 DD 03/11/85 MA 11/30/84
NEBACUMAB TN= CENTOXIN	TREATMENT OF PATIENTS WITH GRAM-NEGATIVE BACTEREMIA WHICH HAS PROGRESSED TO ENDOTOXIN SHOCK.	CENTOCOR, INC. 2OO GREAT VALLEY PARKWAY MALVERN PA 19355-1307 DD 10/01/86
NG-29 TN= SOMATREL	DIAGNOSTIC MEASURE OF THE CAPACITY OF THE PITUITARY GLAND TO RELEASE GROWTH HORMONE.	FERRING LABORATORIES, INC. 400 RELLA BOULEVARD, SUITE 201 SUFFERN NY 10901 DD 08/08/89
NIFEDIPINE	TREATMENT OF INTERSTITIAL CYSTITIS.	FLEISCHMANN, JONATHAN, M.D. 3395 SCRANTON ROAD CLEVELAND OH 44109 DD 06/13/91
NITRIC OXIDE	TREATMENT OF PERSISTENT PULMONARY HYPERTENSION IN THE NEWBORN.	OHMEDA PHARMACEUTICAL PRODUCTS DIVISION 110 ALLEN ROAD, P.O. BOX 804 LIBERTY CORNER NJ 07938-0804 DD 06/22/93
OFLOXACIN SOLUTION	TREATMENT OF BACTERIAL CORNEAL ULCERS.	ALLERGAN, INC. 2525 DUPONT DRIVE IRVINE CA 92715 DD 04/18/91
OM 401 TN= DREPANOL	PROPHYLACTIC TREATMENT OF SICKLE CELL DISEASE.	OMEX INTERNATIONAL, INC. 6001 SAVOY, SUITE 110 HOUSTON TX 77036 DD 10/24/91
OXALIPLATIN	TREATMENT OF OVARIAN CANCER.	AXION PHARMACEUTICALS 395 OYSTER POINT BOULEVARD SUITE 405 SOUTH SAN FRANCISCO CA 94080 DD 10/06/92
OXANDROLONE TN= OXANDRIN	TREATMENT OF SHORT STATURE ASSOCIATED WITH TURNER'S SYNDROME.	BIO-TECHNOLOGY GENERAL CORP. 70 WOOD AVENUE, SOUTH ISELIN NJ 08830 DD 07/05/90
OXANDROLONE	TREATMENT OF CONSTITUTIONAL DELAY OF GROWTH AND PUBERTY.	BIO-TECHNOLOGY GENERAL CORP. 70 WOOD AVENUE, SOUTH ISELIN NJ 08830 DD 10/05/90

CUMULATIVE LIST OF ORPHAN PRODUCT DESIGNATIONS AND APPROVALS *(continued)*

NAME *Generic/Chemical* *TN=Trade Name*	INDICATION DESIGNATED	SPONSOR AND ADDRESS *DD=Date Designated* *MA=Marketing Approval*
OXANDROLONE TN= OXANDRIN	ADJUNCTIVE THERAPY FOR AIDS PATIENTS SUFFERING FROM HIV-WASTING SYNDROME.	BIO-TECHNOLOGY GENERAL CORP. 70 WOOD AVENUE, SOUTH ISELIN NJ 08830 DD 09/06/91
OXANDROLONE TN= HEPANDRIN	TREATMENT OF MODERATE/SEVERE ACUTE ALCOHOLIC HEPATITIS IN THE PRESENCE OF MODERATE PROTEIN CALORIE MALNUTRITION.	BIO-TECHNOLOGY GENERAL CORP. 700 WOOD AVENUE SOUTH ISELIN NJ 08830 DD 03/18/94
OXYMORPHONE HCL TN= NUMORPHAN H.P.	RELIEF OF SEVERE INTRACTABLE PAIN IN NARCOTIC-TOLERANT PATIENTS.	DU PONT MERCK PHARMACEUTICALS P.O. BOX 80027 WILMINGTON DE 19880-0027 DD 03/19/85
OncoRad OV103	TREATMENT OF OVARIAN CANCER.	CYTOGEN CORPORATION 600 COLLEGE ROAD EAST PRINCETON NJ 08540-5308 DD 04/24/90
PEG-GLUCOCEREBROSIDASE	FOR USE AS CHRONIC ENZYME REPLACEMENT THERAPY IN PATIENTS WITH GAUCHER'S DISEASE WHO ARE DEFICIENT IN GLUCOCEREBROSIDASE.	ENZON, INC. 40 KINGSBRIDGE ROAD PISCATAWAY NJ 08854-3998 DD 12/09/92
PEG-INTERLEUKIN-2	TREATMENT OF PRIMARY IMMUNODEFICIENCIES ASSOCIATED WITH T-CELL DEFECTS.	CHIRON CORPORATION 4560 HORTON STREET EMERYVILLE CA 94608 DD 02/01/90
PEGADEMASE BOVINE TN= ADAGEN	ENZYME REPLACEMENT THERAPY FOR ADA DEFICIENCY IN PATIENTS WITH SEVERE COMBINED IMMUNODEFICIENCY (SCID).	ENZON, INC. 40 KINGSBRIDGE ROAD PISCATAWAY NJ 08854-3998 DD 05/29/94 MA 03/21/90
PEG-L-ASPARAGINASE	TREATMENT OF ACUTE LYMPHOCYTIC LEUKEMIA (ALL).	ENZON, INC. 40 KINGSBRIDGE ROAD PISCATAWAY NJ 08854-3998 DD 10/20/89
PENTAMIDINE ISETHIONATE TN= PENTAM 300	TREATMENT OF PNEUMOCYSTIS CARINII PNEUMONIA.	FUJISAWA PHARMACEUTICAL CO. 3 PARKWAY NORTH DEERFIELD IL 60015-2548 DD 02/28/84 MA 10/16/84
PENTAMIDINE ISETHIONATE	TREATMENT OF PNEUMOCYSTIS CARINII PNEUMONIA.	RHONE-POULENC RORER PHARM. 500 ARCOLA ROAD COLLEGEVILLE PA 19426 DD 10/29/84
PENTAMIDINE ISETHIONATE TN= NEBUPENT	PREVENTION OF PNEUMOCYSTIS CARINII PNEUMONIA IN PATIENTS AT HIGH RISK OF DEVELOPING THIS DISEASE.	FUJISAWA PHARMACEUTICAL CO. 3 PARKWAY NORTH DEERFIELD IL 60015-2548 DD 01/12/88 MA 06/15/89
PENTAMIDINE ISETHIONATE (INHALATION) TN= PNEUMOPENT	PREVENTION OF PNEUMOCYSTIS CARINII PNEUMONIA IN PATIENTS AT HIGH RISK OF DEVELOPING THIS DISEASE.	FISONS CORPORATION 755 JEFFERSON RD., P.O. BOX 1710 ROCHESTER NY 14603 DD 10/05/87
PENTASTARCH TN= PENTASPAN	ADJUNCT IN LEUKAPHERESIS TO IMPROVE THE HARVESTING AND INCREASE THE YIELD OF LEUKOCYTES BY CENTRIFUGAL MEANS.	DU PONT PHARMACEUTICALS E.I. du PONT de NEMOURS & CO. WILMINGTON DE 19898 DD 08/28/85 MA 05/19/87
PENTOSAN POLYSULPHATE TN= ELMIRON	TREATMENT OF INTERSTITIAL CYSTITIS.	BAKER NORTON PHARMACEUTICALS 8800 NORTHWEST 36TH STREET MIAMI FL 33178 DD 08/07/85
PENTOSTATIN	TREATMENT OF PATIENTS WITH CHRONIC LYMPHOCYTIC LEUKEMIA.	WARNER-LAMBERT COMPANY 2800 PLYMOUTH ROAD ANN ARBOR MI 48106-1047 DD 01/29/91
PENTOSTATIN FOR INJECTION TN= NIPENT	TREATMENT OF HAIRY CELL LEUKEMIA.	WARNER-LAMBERT COMPANY 2800 PLYMOUTH RD., P.O. BOX 1047 ANN ARBOR MI 48106 DD 09/10/87 MA 10/11/91

CUMULATIVE LIST OF ORPHAN PRODUCT DESIGNATIONS AND APPROVALS *(continued)*

NAME *Generic/Chemical* *TN=Trade Name*	INDICATION DESIGNATED	SPONSOR AND ADDRESS *DD=Date Designated* *MA=Marketing Approval*
PERFOSFAMIDE TN= PERGAMID	FOR USE IN THE EX-VIVO TREATMENT OF AUTOLOGOUS BONE MARROW AND SUBSEQUENT REINFUSION IN PATIENTS WITH ACUTE MYELOGENOUS LEUKEMIA (AML), ALSO REFERRED TO AS ACUTE NONLYMPHOCYTIC LEUKEMIA (ANLL).	SCIOS NOVA, INC. 2450 BAYSHORE PARKWAY MOUNTAIN VIEW CA 94043 DD 12/04/89
PHOSPHOCYSTEAMINE	TREATMENT OF CYSTINOSIS	MEDEA RESEARCH LABORATORIES 200 WILSON STREET, BLDG D-6 PORT JEFFERSON NY 11776 DD 09/12/88
PHYSOSTIGMINE SALICYLATE TN= ANTILIRIUM	FRIEDREICH'S AND OTHER INHERITED ATAXIAS.	FOREST PHARMACEUTICALS, INC. 150 EAST 58TH STREET NEW YORK NY 10155 DD 01/16/85
PILOCARPINE HCl	TREATMENT OF XEROSTOMIA INDUCED BY RADIATION THERAPY FOR HEAD AND NECK CANCER.	MGI PHARMA, INC. SUITE 300 E, 9900 BREN ROAD EAST MINNEAPOLIS MN 55343-9667 DD 09/24/90
PILOCARPINE HCL	TREATMENT OF XEROSTOMIA AND KERATOCONJUNCTIVITIS SICCA IN SJOGREN'S SYNDROME PATIENTS.	MGI PHARMA, INC. 9900 BREN ROAD EAST, SUITE 900E MINNEAPOLIS MN 55343-9667 DD 02/28/92
PIRACETAM TN= NOOTROPIL	TREATMENT OF MYOCLONUS.	UCB PHARMACEUTICALS, INC. P.O. BOX 4410 HAMPTON VA 23664 DD 10/02/87
PIRITREXIM ISETHIONATE	TREATMENT OF INFECTIONS CAUSED BY PNEUMOCYSTIS CARINII, TOXOPLASMA GONDII, AND MYCOBACTERIUM AVIUM-INTRACELLULARE.	BURROUGHS WELLCOME COMPANY 3030 CORNWALLIS ROAD RESEARCH TRIANGLE PK NC 27709 DD 06/13/88
POLOXAMER 188 TN= RHEOTHRX COPOLYMER	TREATMENT OF SICKLE CELL CRISIS.	BURROUGHS WELLCOME COMPANY 3030 CORNWALLIS ROAD RESEARCH TRIANGLE PK NC 27709 DD 06/27/89
POLOXAMER 188 TN= RHEOTHRX COPOLYMER	TREATMENT OF SEVERE BURNS REQUIRING HOSPITALIZATION.	BURROUGHS WELLCOME COMPANY 3030 CORNWALLIS ROAD RESEARCH TRIANGLE PK NC 27709 DD 02/22/90
POLOXAMER 331 TN= PROTOX	INITIAL THERAPY OF TOXOPLASMOSIS IN PATIENTS WITH ACQUIRED IMMUNODEFICIENCY SYNDROME (AIDS).	CYTRX CORPORATION 150 TECHNOLOGY PARKWAY NORCROSS GA 30092 DD 03/21/91
POLY I: POLY C12U TN= AMPLIGEN	TREATMENT OF ACQUIRED IMMUNODEFICIENCY SYNDROME (AIDS).	HEM PHARMACEUTICALS CORP. 1617 JFK BOULEVARD, SUITE 600 PHILADELPHIA PA 19103 DD 07/19/88
POLY I: POLY C12U TN= AMPLIGEN	TREATMENT OF RENAL CELL CARCINOMA.	HEM PHARMACEUTICALS CORP. 1617 JFK BOULEVARD, SUITE 600 PHILADELPHIA PA 19103 DD 05/20/91
POLY I: POLY C12U TN= AMPLIGEN	TREATMENT OF CHRONIC FATIGUE SYNDROME.	HEM PHARMACEUTICALS CORP. ONE PENN CENTER, SUITE 660 PHILADELPHIA PA 19103 DD 12/09/93
POLYMERIC OXYGEN	TREATMENT OF SICKLE CELL ANEMIA.	CAPMED USA P.O. BOX 14 BRYN MAWR PA 19010 DD 03/25/92
PORFIMER SODIUM TN= PHOTOFRIN	FOR THE PHOTODYNAMIC THERAPY OF PATIENTS WITH PRIMARY OR RECURRENT OBSTRUCTING (EITHER PARTIALLY OR COMPLETELY) ESOPHAGEAL CARCINOMA.	QLT PHOTOTHERAPEUTICS, INC. 401 NORTH MIDDLETOWN ROAD PEARL RIVER NY 10965 DD 06/06/89
PORFIMER SODIUM TN= PHOTOFRIN	FOR THE PHOTODYNAMIC THERAPY OF PATIENTS WITH TRANSITIONAL CELL CARCINOMA IN SITU OF URINARY BLADDER.	QLT PHOTOTHERAPEUTICS, INC. 401 NORTH MIDDLETOWN ROAD PEARL RIVER NY 10965 DD 116/15/89

CUMULATIVE LIST OF ORPHAN PRODUCT DESIGNATIONS AND APPROVALS *(continued)*

NAME *Generic/Chemical* *TN=Trade Name*	INDICATION DESIGNATED	SPONSOR AND ADDRESS *DD=Date Designated* *MA=Marketing Approval*
POTASSIUM CITRATE TN= UROCIT-K	PREVENTION OF URIC ACID NEPHROLITHIASIS.	UNIV. OF TEXAS HEALTH SCIENCES 5323 HARRY HINES BLVD DALLAS TX 75235 DD 11/01/84 MA 08/30/85
POTASSIUM CITRATE TN= UROCIT-K	PREVENTION OF CALCIUM RENAL STONES IN PATIENTS WITH HYPOCITRATURIA.	UNIV. OF TEXAS HEALTH SCIENCES 5323 HARRY HINES BLVD DALLAS TX 75235 DD 09/16/85 MA 08/30/85
POTASSIUM CITRATE TN= UROCIT K	AVOIDANCE OF THE COMPLICATION OF CALCIUM STONE FORMATION IN PATIENTS WITH URIC LITHIASIS.	UNIV. OF TEXAS HEALTH SCIENCES 5323 HARRY HINES BLVD. DALLAS TX 75235 DD 05/29/84 MA 08/30/85
PPI-002	TREATMENT OF MALIGNANT MESOTHELIOMA.	CANCER THERAPY AND RESEARCH CENTER 14960 OMICRON SAN ANTONIO TX 78245-3217 DD 05/11/92
PR-122 (REDOX-PHENYTOIN)	FOR THE EMERGENCY RESCUE TREATMENT OF STATUS EPILEPTICUS, GRAND MAL TYPE.	PHARMOS 2 INNOVATION DRIVE ALACHUA FL 32615 DD 07/05/90
PR-225 (REDOX-ACYCLOVIR)	TREATMENT OF HERPES SIMPLEX ENCEPHALITIS IN INDIVIDUALS AFFLICTED WITH AIDS.	PHARMOS 2 INNOVATION DRIVE ALACHUA FL 32615 DD 05/29/90
PR-239 (REDOX PENICILLIN G)	TREATMENT OF AIDS ASSOCIATED NEUROSYPHILIS.	PHARMOS 2 INNOVATION DRIVE ALACHUA FL 32615 DD 05/23/90
PR-320 (MOLECUSOL-CARBAMAZEPINE)	FOR THE EMERGENCY RESCUE TREATMENT OF STATUS EPILEPTICUS, GRAND MAL TYPE.	PHARMOS 2 INNOVATION DRIVE ALACHUA FL 32615 DD 07/20/90
PREDNIMUSTINE TN= STERECYT	TREATMENT OF MALIGNANT NON-HODGKIN'S LYMPHOMAS.	KABI PHARMACIA 800 CENTENNIAL AVENUE PISCATAWAY NJ 08855-1327 DD 06/17/85
PRIMAQUINE PHOSPHATE	FOR USE IN COMBINATION WITH CLINDAMYCIN HYDROCHLORIDE IN THE TREATMENT OF PNEUMOCYSTIS CARINII PNEUMONIA ASSOCIATED WITH ACQUIRED IMMUNODEFICIENCY SYNDROME.	STERLING WINTHROP INC. 90 PARK AVENUE NEW YORK NY 10016 DD 07/23/93
PROPAMIDINE ISETHIONATE 0.1% OPHTHALMIC SOLUTION TN= BROLENE	TREATMENT OF ACANTHAMOEBA KERATITIS.	BAUSH & LOMB PHARMACEUTICALS 1400 NORTH GOODMAN STREET ROCHESTER NY 14692 DD 03/10/88
PROTEIN C CONCENTRATE TN= PROTEIN C CONCENTRATE (HUMAN) VAPOR HEATED, IMMUNO	FOR REPLACEMENT THERAPY IN PATIENTS WITH CONGENITAL OR ACQUIRED PROTEIN C DEFICIENCY FOR THE PREVENTION AND TREATMENT OF WARFARIN-INDUCED SKIN NECROSIS DURING ORAL ANTICOAGULATION.	IMMUNO CLINICAL RESEARCH CORP. 750 LEXINGTON AVENUE, 19TH FLOOR NEW YORK NY 10022 DD 06/19/92
PROTEIN C CONCENTRATE TN= PROTEIN C CONCENTRATE (HUMAN) VAPOR HEATED, IMMUNO	FOR USE IN THE PREVENTION AND TREATMENT OF PURPURA FULMINANS IN MENINGOCOCCEMIA.	IMMUNO CLINICAL RESEARCH CORP. 750 LEXINGTON AVENUE, 19TH FLOOR NEW YORK NY 10022 DD 04/22/93
PROTEIN C CONCENTRATE TN= PROTEIN C CONCENTRATE (HUMAN) VAPOR HEATED, IMMUNO	FOR REPLACEMENT THERAPY IN CONGENITAL PROTEIN C DEFICIENCY FOR THE PREVENTION AND TREATMENT OF THROMBOSIS, PULMONARY EMBOLI, AND PURPURA FULMINANS.	IMMUNO CLINICAL RESEARCH CORP. 750 LEXINGTON AVENUE, 19TH FLOOR NEW YORK NY 10022 DD 06/23/92
PROTIRELIN	PREVENTION OF INFANT RESPIRATORY DISTRESS SYNDROME ASSOCIATED WITH PREMATURITY.	UCB PHARMACEUTICALS, INC. 5505-A ROBIN HOOD ROAD NORFOLK VA 23513 DD 08/24/93

CUMULATIVE LIST OF ORPHAN PRODUCT DESIGNATIONS AND APPROVALS *(continued)*

NAME *Generic/Chemical* *TN=Trade Name*	INDICATION DESIGNATED	SPONSOR AND ADDRESS *DD=Date Designated* *MA=Marketing Approval*
PULMONARY SURFACTANT REPLACEMENT	PREVENTION AND TREATMENT OF INFANT RESPIRATORY DISTRESS SYNDROME (RDS).	SCIOS NOVA, INC. 2450 BAYSHORE PARKWAY MOUNTAIN VIEW CA 94043 DD 12/05/88
PULMONARY SUFACTANT REPLACMENT, PORCINE TN= CUROSURF	FOR THE TREATMENT AND PREVENTION OF RESPIRATORY DISTRESS SYNDROME IN PREMATURE INFANTS.	CHIESI PHARMACEUTICALS, INC. 150 DANBURY ROAD RIDGEFIELD CT 06877 DD 08/02/93
RECOMBINANT HUMAN CD4 IMMUNOGLOBULIN G	TREATMENT OF ACQUIRED IMMUNODEFICIENCY SYNDROME (AIDS) RESULTING FROM INFECTION WITH THE HUMAN IMMUNODEFICIENCY VIRUS (HIV-1).	GENENTECH, INC. 460 POINT SAN BRUNO BOULEVARD SO. SAN FRANCISCO CA 94080 DD 08/30/90
RECOMBINANT HUMAN GEL-SOLIN	TREATMENT OF THE RESPIRATORY SYMTOMS OF CYSTIC FI-BROSIS.	BIOGEN, INC. 14 CAMBRIDGE CENTER CAMBRIDGE MA 02124 DD 01/12/94
RECOMBINANT RETROVIRAL VECTOR—GLUCOCERE-BROSIDASE	FOR USE AS ENZYME REPLACEMENT THERAPY FOR PA-TIENTS WITH TYPES I, II, OR III GAUCHER DISEASE.	GENETIC THERAPY, INC. 938 CLOPPER ROAD GAITHERSBURG MD 20878 DD 11/15/93
RECOMBINANT SECRETORY LEUCOCYTE PROTEASE INHIBITOR	TREATMENT OF CONGENITAL ALPHA-1 ANTITRYPSIN DEFI-CIENCY.	SYNERGEN, INC. 1885 33RD STREET BOULDER CO 80301 DD 03/29/91
RECOMBINANT SECRETORY LEUCOCYTE PROTEASE INHIBITOR	TREATMENT OF CYSTIC FIBROSIS.	SYNERGEN, INC. 1885 33RD STREET BOULDER CO 80301 DD 03/29/91
RECOMBINANT SOLUBLE HUMAN CD 4 (rCD4)	TREATMENT OF AIDS IN PATIENTS INFECTED WITH HIV VI-RUS.	GENENTECH, INC. 460 POINT SAN BRUNO BOULEVARD SOUTH SAN FRANCISCO CA 94080 DD 03/23/89
RECOMBINANT SOLUBLE HUMAN CD4 TN= RECEPTIN	TREATMENT OF ACQUIRED IMMUNODEFICIENCY SYNDROME (AIDS).	BIOGEN, INC. 14 CAMBRIDGE CENTER CAMBRIDGE MA 02142 DD 11/20/89
RECOMBINANT VACCINIA (HUMAN PAPILLOMAVI-RUS) TN= TA-HPV	TREATMENT OF CERVICAL CANCER.	CANTAB PHARMACEUTICALS RESEARCH, LTD. 184 CAMBRIDGE SCIENCE PARK CAMBRIDGE CB4 4GN UK DD 08/24/94
REDUCED L-GLUTATHIONE TN= CACHEXON	TREATMENT OF AIDS-ASSOCIATED CACHEXIA.	TELLURIDE PHARMACEUTICAL CORPORATION 146 FLANDERS DRIVE HILLSBOROUGH NJ 08876-4656 DD 02/14/94
RESPIRATORY SYNCYTIAL VIRUS IMMUNE GLOBU-LIN (HUMAN) TN= HYPERMUNE RSV	PROPHYLAXIS OF RESPIRATORY SYNCYTIAL VIRUS (RSV) LOWER RESPIRATORY TRACT INFECTIONS IN INFANTS AND YOUNG CHILDREN AT HIGH RISK OF RSV DISEASE.	MEDIMMUNE, INC. 35 WEST WATKINS MILL ROAD GAITHERSBURG MD 20878 DD 09/27/90
RESPIRATORY SYNCYTIAL VIRUS IMMUNE GLOBU-LIN (HUMAN) TN= HYPERMUNE RSV	TREATMENT OF RESPIRATORY SYNCYTIAL VIRUS (RSV) LOWER RESPIRATORY TRACT INFECTIONS IN HOSPITAL-IZED INFANTS AND YOUNG CHILDREN.	MEDIMMUNE, INC. 35 WEST WATKINS MILL ROAD GAITHERSBURG MD 20878 DD 09/27/90
RIBAVIRIN TN= VIRAZOLE	TREATMENT OF HEMORRHAGIC FEVER WITH RENAL SYN-DROME.	ICN PHARMACEUTICALS, INC. 3300 HYLAND AVENUE COSTA MESA CA 92626 DD 04/12/91
RICIN (BLOCKED) CONJU-GATED MURINE MCA (ANTI-B4)	TREATMENT OF B-CELL LEUKEMIA AND B-CELL LYMPHOMA.	IMMUNOGEN, INC. 148 SIDNEY STREET CAMBRIDGE MA 02139 DD 11/17/88
RICIN (BLOCKED) CONJU-GATED MURINE MCA (ANTI-B4)	FOR THE EX-VIVO PURGING OF LEUKEMIC CELLS FROM THE BONE MARROW OF NON-T CELL ACUTE LYMPHOCYTIC LEUKEMIA PATIENTS WHO ARE IN COMPLETE REMIS-SION.	IMMUNOGEN, INC. 148 SIDNEY STREET CAMBRIDGE MA 02139 DD 01/24/91

CUMULATIVE LIST OF ORPHAN PRODUCT DESIGNATIONS AND APPROVALS *(continued)*

NAME *Generic/Chemical* *TN=Trade Name*	INDICATION DESIGNATED	SPONSOR AND ADDRESS *DD=Date Designated* *MA=Marketing Approval*
RICIN (BLOCKED) CONJUGATED MURINE MCA (ANTI-MY9)	TREATMENT OF MYELOID LEUKEMIA, INCLUDING AML, AND BLAST CRISIS OF CML.	IMMUNOGEN, INC. 148 SIDNEY STREET CAMBRIDGE MA 02139 DD 08/03/89
RICIN (BLOCKED) CONJUGATED MURINE MCA (ANTI-MY9)	FOR USE IN THE EX-VIVO TREATMENT OF AUTOLOGOUS BONE MARROW AND SUBSEQUENT REINFUSION IN PATIENTS WITH ACUTE MYELOGENOUS LEUKEMIA (AML).	IMMUNOGEN, INC. 148 SIDNEY STREET CAMBRIDGE MA 02139 DD 02/01/90
RICIN (BLOCKED) CONJUGATED MURINE MCA (N901)	TREATMENT OF SMALL CELL LUNG CANCER.	IMMUNOGEN, INC. 148 SIDNEY STREET CAMBRIDGE MA 02139 DD 01/25/91
RIFABUTIN	TREATMENT OF DISSEMINATED MYCOBACTERIUM AVIUM COMPLEX (MAC) DISEASE	ADRIA LABORATORIES, INC. P.O. BOX 16529 COLUMBUS OH 43216-6529 DD 12/18/89
RIFABUTIN TN= MYCOBUTIN	PREVENTION OF DISSEMINATED MYCOBACTERIUM AVIUM COMPLEX (MAC) DISEASE IN PATIENTS WITH ADVANCED HIV INFECTION.	ADRIA LABORATORIES, INC. P.O. BOX 16529 COLUMBUS OH 43216-6529 DD 12/18/89 MA 12/23/92
RIFAMPIN TN= RIFADIN I.V.	ANTITUBERCULOSIS TREATMENT WHERE USE OF THE ORAL FORM OF THE DRUG IS NOT FEASIBLE.	MARION MERRELL DOW, INC. P.O. BOX 9707, MARION PARK DRIVE KANSAS CITY MO 64134-0707 DD 12/09/85 MA 05/25/89
RIFAMPIN, ISONIAZID, PYRAZINAMIDE TN= RIFATER II	SHORT COURSE TREATMENT OF TUBERCULOSIS.	MARION MERRELL DOW, INC. P.O. BOX 9627 KANSAS CITY MO 64134-0627 DD 09/12/85
RII RETINAMIDE	TREATMENT OF MYELODYSPLASTIC SYNDROMES.	SPARTA PHARMACEUTICALS, INCORPORATED P.O. BOX 13288 RESEARCH TRIANGLE PK NC 27709 DD 05/06/93
RILUZOLE	TREATMENT OF AMYOTROPHIC LATERAL SCLEROSIS.	RHONE-POULENC RORER PHARM. 500 ARCOLA ROAD, P.O. BOX 1200 COLLEGEVILLE PA 19426-0107 DD 03/16/93
ROQUINIMEX TN= LINOMIDE	TO PROLONG TIME TO RELAPSE IN LEUKEMIA PATIENTS WHO HAVE UNDERGONE AUTOLOGOUS BONE MARROW TRANSPLANTATION.	KABI PHARMACIA, INC. 800 CENTENNIAL AVENUE PISCATAWAY NJ 08855-1327 DD 07/01/93
Rho IMMUNE GLOBULIN (HUMAN) TN= WINRho SD	TREATMENT OF IMMUNE THROMBOCYTOPENIC PURPURA.	RH PHARMACEUTICALS, INC. 104 CHANCELLOR MATHESON ROAD WINNIPEG, MANITOBA DD 11/09/93
SARGRAMOSTIM TN= LEUKINE	TREATMENT OF NEUTROPENIA ASSOCIATED WITH BONE MARROW TRANSPLANT, FOR THE TREATMENT OF GRAFT FAILURE AND DELAY OF ENGRAFTMENT, AND FOR THE PROMOTION OF EARLY ENGRAFTMENT.	IMMUNEX CORPORATION 51 UNIVERSITY STREET SEATTLE WA 98101 DD 05/03/90 MA 03/05/91
SATUMOMAB PENDETIDE TN= ONCOSCINT CR/OV	DETECTION OF OVARIAN CARCINOMA.	CYTOGEN CORPORATION 201 COLLEGE ROAD EAST PRINCETON NJ 08540-5308 DD 09/25/89 MA 12/29/92
SECALCIFEROL TN= OSTEO-D	TREATMENT OF FAMILIAL HYPOPHOSPHATEMIC RICKETS.	LEMMON COMPANY 650 CATHILL ROAD SELLERSVILLE PA 18960 DD 07/26/93
SECRETORY LEUKOCYTE PROTEASE INHIBITOR	TREATMENT OF BRONCHOPULMONARY DYSPLASIA.	SYNERGEN, INC. 1885 33RD STREET BOULDER CO 80301-2546 DD 06/30/92
SELEGILINE HCL TN= ELDEPRYL	ADJUVANT TO LEVODOPA AND CARBIDOPA TREATMENT OF IDIOPATHIC PARKINSON'S DISEASE (PARALYSIS AGITANS), POSTENCEPHALITIC PARKINSONISM, AND SYMPTOMATIC PARKINSONISM.	SOMERSET PHARMACEUTICALS, INC. 777 SOUTH HARBOR ISLAND BOULEVARD TAMPA FL 33602 DD 11/07/84 MA 06/05/89

CUMULATIVE LIST OF ORPHAN PRODUCT DESIGNATIONS AND APPROVALS *(continued)*

NAME *Generic/Chemical* *TN=Trade Name*	INDICATION DESIGNATED	SPONSOR AND ADDRESS *DD=Date Designated* *MA=Marketing Approval*
SERMORELIN ACETATE TN= GEREF	TREATMENT OF IDIOPATHIC OR ORGANIC GROWTH HORMONE DEFICIENCY (GHD) IN CHILDREN WITH GROWTH FAILURE.	SERONO LABORATORIES, INC. 100 LONGWATER CIRCLE NORWELL MA 02061 DD 09/14/88
SERMORELIN ACETATE TN= GEREF	ADJUNCT TO GONADOTROPIN THERAPY IN THE INDUCTION OF OVULATION IN WOMEN WITH ANOVULATORY OR OLIGO-OVULATORY INFERTILITY WHO FAIL TO OVULATE IN RESPONSE TO ADEQUATE TREATMENT WITH CLOMIPHENE CITRATE ALONE AND GONADOTROPIN THERAPY ALONE.	SERONO LABORATORIES, INC. 100 LONGWATER CIRCLE NORWELL MA 02061 DD 02/13/90
SERMORELIN ACETATE TN= GEREF	TREATMENT OF AIDS-ASSOCIATED CATABOLISM/WEIGHT LOSS.	SERONO LABORATORIES, INC. 100 LONGWATER CIRCLE NORWELL MA 02061 DD 12/05/91
SERRATIA MARCESCENS EXTRACT (POLYRIBOSOMES) TN= IMUVERT	TREATMENT OF PRIMARY BRAIN MALIGNANCIES.	CELL TECHNOLOGY, INC. 1668 VALTEC LANE BOULDER CO 80306 DD 09/07/88
SHORT CHAIN FATTY ACID SOLUTION	TREATMENT OF THE ACTIVE PHASE OF ULCERATIVE COLITIS WITH INVOLVEMENT RESTRICTED TO THE LEFT SIDE OF THE COLON.	ORPHAN MEDICAL 13911 RIDGEDALE DRIVE MINNETONKA MN 55305 DD 05/29/90
SK&F 110679	FOR THE LONG TERM TREATMENT OF CHILDREN WHO HAVE GROWTH FAILURE DUE TO A LACK OF ADEQUATE ENDOGENOUS GROWTH HORMONE SECRETION.	SMITHKLINE BEECHAM P.O. BOX 1510 KING OF PRUSSIA PA 19406 DD 05/23/90
SODIUM BENZOATE/SODIUM PHENYLACETATE	TREATMENT OF UREA CYCLE DISORDERS: CARBAMYLPHOSPHATE SYNTHETASE DEFICIENCY, ORNITHINE TRANSCARBAMYLASE DEFICIENCY, AND ARGININOSUCCINIC ACID SYNTHETASE DEFICIENCY.	BRUSILOW, SAUL W., M.D. JOHNS HOPKINS MEDICAL INSTITUTIONS BALTIMORE MD 21205 DD 11/22/93
SODIUM DICHLOROACETATE	TREATMENT OF CONGENITAL LACTIC ACIDOSIS.	STACPOOLE, PETER, M.D. U. OF FLORIDA, P.O. BOX 100226 GAINESVILLE FL 32610-0226 DD 06/11/90
SODIUM DICHLOROACETATE	TREATMENT OF HOMOZYGOUS FAMILIAL HYPERCHOLESTEROLEMIA.	STACPOOLE, PETER, M.D. U. OF FLORIDA, P.O. BOX 100226 GAINESVILLE FL 32610-0226 DD 06/11/90
SODIUM MONOMERCAPTOUNDECAHYDRO-CLOSO-DO DECABORATE TN= BOROCELL	FOR USE IN BORON NEUTRON CAPTURE THERAPY (BNCT) IN THE TREATMENT OF GLIOBLASTOMA MULTIFORME.	NEUTRON TECH. CORP.& NEUTRON R&D PARTNER 877 MAIN STREET BOISE ID 83702 DD 04/15/92
SODIUM PHENYLBUTYRATE	TREATMENT FOR SICKLING DISORDERS, WHICH INCLUDE S-S HEMOGLOBINOPATHY, S-C HEMOGLOBINOPATHY, AND S-THALASSEMIA HEMOGLOBINOPATHY.	BRUSILOW, SAUL W., M.D. JOHNS HOPKINS MEDICAL INSTITUTIONS BALTIMORE MD 21205 DD 07/02/92
SODIUM PHENYLBUTYRATE	TREATMENT OF UREA CYCLE DISORDERS: CARBAMYLPHOSPHATE SYNTHETASE DEFICIENCY, ORNITHINE TRANSCARBAMYLASE DEFICIENCY, AND ARGINIOSUCCINIC ACID SYNTHETASE DEFICIENCY.	BRUSILOW, SAUL W., M.D. JOHNS HOPKINS MEDICAL INSTITUTIONS BALTIMORE MD 21205 DD 11/22/93
SODIUM TETRADECYL SULFATE TN= SOTRADECOL	TREATMENT OF BLEEDING ESOPHAGEAL VARICES.	ELKINS-SINN, INC. 2 ESTERBROOK LANE CHERRY HILL NJ 08003-4099 DD 06/10/86
SODIUM/GAMMA HYDROXYBUTYRATE	TREATMENT OF NARCOLEPSY AND THE AUXILIARY SYMPTOMS OF CATAPLEXY, SLEEP PARALYSIS, HYPNAGOGIC HALLUCINATIONS AND AUTOMATIC BEHAVIOR.	BIOCRAFT LABORATORIES, INC. 18-01 RIVER ROAD FAIR LAWN NJ 07410 DD 12/22/87
SOMATOSTATIN TN= ZECNIL	ADJUNCT TO THE NON-OPERATIVE MANAGEMENT OF SECRETING CUTANEOUS FISTULAS OF THE STOMACH, DUODENUM, SMALL INTESTINE (JEJUNUM AND ILEUM), OR PANCREAS	FERRING LABORATORIES, INC. 400 RELLA BOULEVARD, SUITE 201 SUFFERN NY 10901 DD 06/20/88

CUMULATIVE LIST OF ORPHAN PRODUCT DESIGNATIONS AND APPROVALS *(continued)*

NAME *Generic/Chemical* *TN=Trade Name*	INDICATION DESIGNATED	SPONSOR AND ADDRESS *DD=Date Designated* *MA=Marketing Approval*
SOMATREM FOR INJECTION TN= PROTROPIN	FOR LONG-TERM TREATMENT OF CHILDREN WHO HAVE GROWTH FAILURE DUE TO A LACK OF ADEQUATE ENDOGENOUS GROWTH HORMONE SECRETION.	GENENTECH, INC. 460 POINT SAN BRUNO BOULEVARD SOUTH SAN FRANCISCO CA 94080 DD 12/09/85 MA 10/17/85
SOMATREM FOR INJECTION TN= PROTROPIN	TREATMENT OF SHORT STATURE ASSOCIATED WITH TURNER'S SYNDROME.	GENENTECH, INC. 460 POINT SAN BRUNO BOULEVARD SOUTH SAN FRANCISCO CA 94080 DD 12/09/85
SOMATROPIN TN= SAIZEN	TREATMENT OF IDIOPATHIC OR ORGANIC GROWTH HORMONE DEFICIENCY IN CHILDREN WITH GROWTH FAILURE.	SERONO LABORATORIES, INC. 100 LONGWATER CIRCLE NORWELL MA 02061 DD 03/06/87
SOMATROPIN TN= PROTROPIN II	FOR USE IN THE LONG-TERM TREATMENT OF CHILDREN WHO HAVE GROWTH FAILURE DUE TO A LACK OF ADEQUATE ENDOGENOUS GROWTH HORMONE SECRETION.	GENENTECH, INC. 460 POINT SAN BRUNO BOULEVARD SOUTH SAN FRANCISCO CA 94080 DD 03/06/87
SOMATROPIN TN= NORDITROPIN	TREATMENT OF GROWTH FAILURE IN CHILDREN DUE TO INADEQUATE GROWTH HORMONE SECRETION.	NOVO NORDISK PHARMACEUTICALS 100 OVERLOOK CENTER, SUITE 200 PRINCETON NJ 08540-7810 DD 07/10/87
SOMATROPIN TN= NORDITROPIN	TREATMENT OF SHORT STATURE ASSOCIATED WITH TURNER'S SYNDROME.	NOVO NORDISK PHARMACEUTICALS 100 OVERLOOK CENTER, SUITE 200 PRINCETON NJ 08540-7810 DD 11/05/87
SOMATROPIN TN= NORDITROPIN	ADJUNCT FOR THE INDUCTION OF OVULATION IN WOMEN WITH INFERTILITY DUE TO HYPOGONADOTROPIC HYPOGONADISM OR BILATERAL TUBAL OCCLUSION OR UNEXPLAINED INFERTILITY, WHO ARE UNDERGOING IN VIVO OR IN VITRO FERTILIZATION PROCEDURES	NOVO NORDISK PHARMACEUTICALS 100 OVERLOOK CENTER, SUITE 200 PRINCETON NJ 08540-7810 DD 09/01/87
SOMATROPIN TN= SAIZEN	FOR THE ENHANCEMENT OF NITROGEN RETENTION IN HOSPITALIZED PATIENTS SUFFERING FROM SEVERE BURNS.	SERONO LABORATORIES, INC. 100 LONGWATER CIRCLE NORWELL MA 02061 DD 05/03/89
SOMATROPIN TN= HUMATROPE	TREATMENT OF SHORT STATURE ASSOCIATED WITH TURNER'S SYNDROME.	ELI LILLY AND COMPANY LILLY CORPORATE CENTER INDIANAPOLIS IN 46285 DD 05/08/90
SOMATROPIN TN= BIOTROPIN	TREATMENT OF CACHEXIA ASSOCIATED WITH AIDS.	BIO-TECHNOLOGY GENERAL CORPORATION 1250 BROADWAY, 20TH FLOOR NEW YORK NY 10001 DD 02/12/93
SOMATROPIN FOR INJECTION TN= HUMATROPE	LONG-TERM TREATMENT OF CHILDREN WHO HAVE GROWTH FAILURE DUE TO INADEQUATE SECRETION OF NORMAL ENDOGENOUS GROWTH HORMONE.	ELI LILLY AND COMPANY LILLY CORPORATE CENTER INDIANAPOLIS IN 46285 DD 06/12/86 MA 03/08/87
SOMATROPIN FOR INJECTION TN= NUTROPIN	TREATMENT OF GROWTH RETARDATION ASSOCIATED WITH CHRONIC RENAL FAILURE.	GENENTECH, INC. 460 POINT SAN BRUNO BOULEVARD SOUTH SAN FRANCISCO CA 94080 DD 08/04/89
SOMATROPIN FOR INJECTION TN= NUTROPIN	TREATMENT OF SHORT STATURE ASSOCIATED WITH TURNER'S SYNDROME.	GENENTECH, INC. 460 POINT SAN BRUNO BOULEVARD SOUTH SAN FRANCISCO CA 94080 DD 03/23/89
SOMATROPIN FOR INJECTION TN= SAIZEN	TREATMENT OF AIDS-ASSOCIATED CATABOLISM/WEIGHT LOSS.	SERONO LABORATORIES, INC. 100 LONGWATER CIRCLE NORWELL MA 02061 DD 11/15/91
SOTALOL HCL TN= BETAPACE	TREATMENT OF LIFE-THREATENING VENTRICULAR TACHYARRHYTHMIAS.	BERLEX LABORATORIES 300 FAIRFIELD ROAD WAYNE NJ 07470-4100 DD 09/23/88 MA 10/30/92
SOTALOL HCL TN= BETAPACE	PREVENTION OF LIFE THREATENING VENTRICULAR TACHYARRHYTHMIAS.	BERLEX LABORATORIES 300 FAIRFIELD ROAD WAYNE NJ 07470-4100 DD 09/23/88

CUMULATIVE LIST OF ORPHAN PRODUCT DESIGNATIONS AND APPROVALS *(continued)*

NAME *Generic/Chemical* *TN=Trade Name*	**INDICATION DESIGNATED**	**SPONSOR AND ADDRESS** *DD=Date Designated* *MA=Marketing Approval*
ST1-RTA IMMUNOTOXIN (SR 44163)	TREATMENT OF PATIENTS WITH B-CHRONIC LYMPHOCYTIC LEUKEMIA (CLL).	SANOFI PHARMACEUTICALS, INC. 101 PARK AVENUE NEW YORK NY 10178 DD 08/12/87
ST1-RTA IMMUNOTOXIN (SR-44163)	PREVENTION OF ACUTE GRAFT VERSUS HOST DISEASE (GVHD) IN ALLOGENIC BONE MARROW TRANSPLANTATION.	SANOFI PHARMACEUTICALS, INC. 101 PARK AVENUE NEW YORK NY 10178 DD 08/12/87
SUCCIMER TN= CHEMET CAPSULES	TREATMENT OF LEAD POISONING IN CHILDREN.	MCNEIL CONSUMER PRODUCTS CO. CAMP HILL ROAD FORT WASHINGTON PA 19034 DD 05/09/84 MA 01/30/91
SUCCIMER TN= CHEMET	PREVENTION OF CYSTINE KIDNEY STONE FORMATION IN PATIENTS WITH HOMOZYGOUS CYSTINURIA WHO ARE PRONE TO STONE DEVELOPMENT.	MCNEIL CONSUMER PRODUCTS CO. CAMP HILL ROAD FORT WASHINGTON PA 19034 DD 11/05/90
SUCCIMER TN= CHEMET	TREATMENT OF MERCURY INTOXICATION.	MCNEIL CONSUMER PRODUCTS CO. CAMP HILL ROAD FORT WASHINGTON PA 19034 DD 03/22/91
SUCRALFATE	TREATMENT OF ORAL MUCOSITIS AND STOMATITIS FOLLOWING RADIATION THERAPY FOR HEAD AND NECK CANCER.	FUISZ TECHNOLOGIES, LTD. 3810 CONCORDE PARKWAY SUITE 100 CHANTILLY VA 22021 DD 07/15/93
SUCRALFATE SUSPENSION	TREATMENT OF ORAL COMPLICATIONS OF CHEMOTHERAPY IN BONE MARROW TRANSPLANT PATIENTS.	DARBY PHARMACEUTICALS, INC. 100 BANKS AVENUE ROCKVILLE CENTRE NY 11570 DD 03/12/90
SUCRALFATE SUSPENSION	TREATMENT OF ORAL ULCERATIONS AND DYSPHAGIA IN PATIENTS WITH EPIDERMOLYSIS BULLOSA.	DARBY PHARMACEUTICALS, INC. 100 BANKS AVENUE ROCKVILLE CENTRE NY 11570 DD 03/04/91
SUCRASE (YEAST-DERIVED) TN= SACARASA	TREATMENT OF CONGENITAL SUCRASE-ISOMALTASE DEFICIENCY.	TREEM, WILLIAM R., M.D. HARTFORD HOSPITAL HARTFORD CT 06115 DD 12/10/93
SULFADIAZINE	FOR USE IN COMBINATION WITH PYRIMETHAMINE FOR THE TREATMENT OF TOXOPLASMA GONDII ENCEPHALITIS IN PATIENTS WITH AND WITHOUT ACQUIRED IMMUNODEFICIENCY SYNDROME.	EON LABS MANUFACTURING, INC. 227-15 NORTH CONDUIT AVENUE LAURELTON NY 11413 DD 03/14/94 MA 07/29/94
SULFAPYRIDINE	TREATMENT OF DERMATITIS HERPETIFORMIS.	JACOBUS PHARMACEUTICAL COMPANY P.O. BOX 5290 PRINCETON NJ 08540 DD 09/10/90
SUPEROXIDE DISMUTASE (HUMAN)	PROTECTION OF DONOR ORGAN TISSUE FROM DAMAGE OR INJURY MEDIATED BY OXYGEN-DERIVED FREE RADICALS THAT ARE GENERATED DURING THE NECESSARY PERIODS OF ISCHEMIA (HYPOXIA, ANOXIA), AND ESPECIALLY REPERFUSION, ASSOCIATED WITH THE OPERATIVE PROCEDURE.	PHARMACIA-CHIRON PARTNERSHIP 4560 HORTON STREET EMERYVILLE CA 94608 DD 03/06/85
SUPEROXIDE DISMUTASE (RECOMBINANT HUMAN)	PREVENTION OF REPERFUSION INJURY TO DONOR ORGAN TISSUE.	BIO-TECHNOLOGY GENERAL CORP. 70 WOOD AVENUE, SOUTH ISELIN NJ 08830 DD 05/17/88
SUPEROXIDE DISMUTASE (RECOMBINANT HUMAN)	FOR THE PREVENTION OF BRONCHOPULMONARY DYSPLASIA IN PREMATURE NEONATES WEIGHING LESS THAN 1500 GRAMS.	BIO-TECHNOLOGY GENERAL CORP. 70 WOOD AVENUE, SOUTH ISELIN NJ 08830 DD 04/18/91
SURFACE ACTIVE EXTRACT OF SALINE LAVAGE OF BOVINE LUNGS TN= INFASURF	TREATMENT AND PREVENTION OF RESPIRATORY FAILURE DUE TO PULMONARY SURFACTANT DEFICIENCY IN PRETERM INFANTS.	ONY, INC. 1576 SWEET HOME ROAD AMHERST NY 14228 DD 06/07/85
T4 ENDONUCLEASE V, LIPOSOME ENCAPSULATED	TO PREVENT CUTANEOUS NEOPLASMS AND OTHER SKIN ABNORMALITIES IN XERODERMA PIGMENTOSUM.	APPLIED GENETICS, INC. 205 BUFFALO AVENUE FREEPORT NY 11520 DD 06/27/89

CUMULATIVE LIST OF ORPHAN PRODUCT DESIGNATIONS AND APPROVALS *(continued)*

NAME *Generic/Chemical* *TN=Trade Name*	INDICATION DESIGNATED	SPONSOR AND ADDRESS *DD=Date Designated* *MA=Marketing Approval*
TECHNETIUM TC 99M ANTI-MELANOMA MURINE MONOCLONAL ANTIBODY TN= ONCOTRAC MELANOMA IMAGING KIT	FOR USE IN DETECTING, BY IMAGING, METASTASES OF MALIGNANT MELANOMA.	NEORX CORPORATION 410 WEST HARRISON SEATTLE WA 98119 DD 06/02/87
TECHNETIUM Tc-99m MURINE MONOCLONAL ANTIBODY (IgG2a) TO B CE TN= IMMURAID-LL-2[99mTc]	DIAGNOSTIC IMAGING IN THE EVALUATION OF THE EXTENT OF DISEASE IN PATIENTS WITH HISTOLOGICALLY CONFIRMED DIAGNOSIS OF NON-HODGKIN'S B-CELL LYMPHOMA, ACUTE B-CELL LYMPHOBLASTIC LEUKEMIA (IN CHILDREN AND ADULTS), AND CHRONIC B-CELL LYMPHOCYTIC LEUKEMIA.	IMMUNOMEDICS, INC. 300 AMERICAN ROAD MORRIS PLAINS NJ 07950 DD 04/07/92
TECHNETIUM Tc-99m MURINE MONOCLONAL ANTIBODY TO HUMAN AFP TN= ImmuRAID, AFP-Tc99m	DETECTION OF HEPATOCELLULAR CARCINOMA AND HEPATOBLASTOMA.	IMMUNOMEDICS, INC. 300 AMERICAN ROAD MORRIS PLAINS NJ 07950 DD 08/01/89
TECHNETIUM Tc-99m MURINE MONOCLONAL ANTIBODY TO HUMAN AFP TN= ImmuRAID, AFP-Tc99m	DETECTION OF ALPHA-FETOPROTEIN PRODUCING GERM CELL TUMORS.	IMMUNOMEDICS, INC. 300 AMERICAN ROAD MORRIS PLAINS NJ 07950 DD 08/01/89
TECHNETIUM Tc-99m MURINE MONOCLONAL ANTIBODY TO hCG TN= ImmuRAID, hCG-Tc-99m	DETECTION OF HCG PRODUCING TUMORS SUCH AS GERM CELL AND TROPHOBLASTIC CELL TUMORS.	IMMUNOMEDICS, INC. 300 AMERICAN ROAD MORRIS PLAINS NJ 07950 DD 08/07/89
TENIPOSIDE TN= VUMON FOR INJECTION	TREATMENT OF REFRACTORY CHILDHOOD ACUTE LYMPHOCYTIC LEUKEMIA (ALL).	BRISTOL-MYERS SQUIBB 5 RESEARCH PARKWAY, P.O. BOX 5100 WALLINGFORD CT 06492-7660 DD 11/01/84 MA 07/14/92
TERIPARATIDE TN= PARATHAR	DIAGNOSTIC AGENT TO ASSIST IN ESTABLISHING THE DIAGNOSIS IN PATIENTS PRESENTING WITH CLINICAL AND LABORATORY EVIDENCE OF HYPOCALCEMIA DUE TO EITHER HYPOPARATHYROIDISM OR PSEUDOHYPOPARATHYROIDISM.	RHONE-POULENC RORER PHARM. 500 ARCOLA ROAD COLLEGEVILLE PA 19426 DD 01/09/87 MA 12/23/87
TERLIPRESSIN TN= GLYPRESSIN	TREATMENT OF BLEEDING ESOPHAGEAL VARICES.	FERRING LABORATORIES, INC. 400 RELLA BOULEVARD, SUITE 201 SUFFERN NY 10901 DD 03/06/86
TESTOSTERONE PROPIONATE OINTMENT 2%	TREATMENT OF VULVAR DYSTROPHIES.	STAR PHARMACEUTICALS, INC. 1990 N.W. 44TH STREET POMPANO BEACH FL 33064 DD 07/31/91
TESTOSTERONE SUBLINGUAL	TREATMENT OF CONSTITUTIONAL DELAY OF GROWTH AND PUBERTY IN BOYS.	BIO-TECHNOLOGY GENERAL CORP. 70 WOOD AVENUE, SOUTH ISELIN NJ 08830 DD 01/16/91
THALIDOMIDE	TREATMENT OF GRAFT VERSUS HOST DISEASE (GVHD) IN PATIENTS RECEIVING BONE MARROW TRANSPLANTATION (BMT).	PEDIATRIC PHARMACEUTICALS, INC. 718 BRADFORD AVENUE WESTFIELD NJ 07090 DD 09/19/88
THALIDOMIDE	PREVENTION OF GRAFT VERSUS HOST DISEASE (GVHD) IN PATIENTS RECEIVING BONE MARROW TRANSPLANTATION.	PEDIATRIC PHARMACEUTICALS, INC. 718 BRADFORD AVENUE WESTFIELD NJ 07090 DD 09/19/88
THALIDOMIDE	TREATMENT AND MAINTENANCE OF REACTIONAL LEPROMATOUS LEPROSY.	PEDIATRIC PHARMACEUTICALS, INC. 718 BRADFORD AVENUE WESTFIELD NJ 07090 DD 11/15/88
THALIDOMIDE	TREATMENT OF GRAFT VERSUS HOST DISEASE.	ANDRULIS PHARMACEUTICALS CORPORATION 11800 BALTIMORE AVENUE BELTSVILLE MD 20705 DD 03/05/90
THALIDOMIDE	PREVENTION OF GRAFT VERSUS HOST DISEASE.	ANDRULIS PHARMACEUTICALS CORPORATION 11800 BALTIMORE AVENUE BELTSVILLE MD 20705 DD 03/05/90

CUMULATIVE LIST OF ORPHAN PRODUCT DESIGNATIONS AND APPROVALS *(continued)*

NAME *Generic/Chemical* *TN=Trade Name*	INDICATION DESIGNATED	SPONSOR AND ADDRESS *DD=Date Designated* *MA=Marketing Approval*
THALIDOMIDE	TREATMENT OF THE CLINICAL MANIFESTATIONS OF MYCOBACTERIAL INFECTION CAUSED BY MYCOBACTERIUM TUBERCULOSIS AND NON-TUBERCULOUS MYCOBACTERIA.	CELGENE CORPORATION 7 POWDER HORN DRIVE WARREN NJ 07059 DD 01/12/93
THYMOSIN ALPHA-1	TREATMENT OF CHRONIC ACTIVE HEPATITIS B.	ALPHA 1 BIOMEDICALS, INC. 6903 ROCKLEDGE DRIVE, SUITE 1200 BETHESDA MD 20817-1818 DD 05/03/91
TIOPRONIN TN= THIOLA	PREVENTION OF CYSTINE NEPHROLITHIASIS IN PATIENTS WITH HOMOZYGOUS CYSTINURIA.	PAK, CHARLES Y.C., M.D. 5323 HARRY HINES BOULEVARD DALLAS TX 75235 DD 01/17/86 MA 08/11/88
TIRATRICOL TN= TRIACANA	FOR USE IN COMBINATION WITH LEVO-THYROXINE TO SUPPRESS THYROID STIMULATING HORMONE (TSH) IN PATIENTS WITH WELL-DIFFERENTIATED THYROID CANCER WHO ARE INTOLERANT TO ADEQUATE DOSES OF LEVOTHYROXINE ALONE.	MARCOFINA LABORATORIES 48 BIS RUE DES BELLES FEUILLES 75116 PARIS, FRANCE DD 08/13/91
TIZANIDINE HCL TN= ZANAFLEX	TREATMENT OF SPASTICITY ASSOCIATED WITH MULTIPLE SCLEROSIS AND SPINAL CORD INJURY.	ATHENA NEUROSCIENCES, INC. 800F GATEWAY BOULEVARD SOUTH SAN FRANCISCO CA 94080 DD 01/31/94
TOPIRAMATE TN= TOPIMAX	TREATMENT OF LENNOX-GASTAUT SYNDROME.	R.W. JOHNSON RESEARCH INSTITUTE WELSH AND MCKEAN ROADS SPRING HOUSE PA 19477-0776 DD 11/25/92
TOREMIFENE	HORMONAL THERAPY OF METASTATIC CARCINOMA OF THE BREAST.	ADRIA LABORATORIES, INC. P.O. BOX 16529 COLUMBUS OH 43216-6529 DD 09/19/91
TOREMIFENE TN= ESTRINEX	TREATMENT OF DESMOID TUMORS.	ADRIA LABORATORIES P.O. BOX 16529 COLUMBUS OH 43216-6529 DD 08/17/93
TRANEXAMIC ACID TN= CYKLOKAPRON	TREATMENT OF HEREDITARY ANGIONEUROTIC EDEMA.	KABIVITRUM, INC. P.O. BOX 430 DANVILLE CA 94526 DD 09/09/85
TRANEXAMIC ACID TN= CYKLOKAPRON	TREATMENT OF PATIENTS UNDERGOING PROSTATECTOMY WHERE THERE IS HEMORRHAGE OR RISK OF HEMORRHAGE AS A RESULT OF INCREASED FIBRINOLYSIS OR FIBRINOGENOLYSIS.	R & R REGISTRATIONS P.O. BOX 262069 SAN DIEGO CA 92196-2069 DD 07/23/87
TRANEXAMIC ACID TN= CYKLOKAPRON	TREATMENT OF PATIENTS WITH CONGENITAL COAGULOPATHIES WHO ARE UNDERGOING SURGICAL PROCEDURES E.G. DENTAL EXTRACTIONS.	KABIVITRUM, INC. P.O. BOX 262069 SAN DIEGO CA 92196 DD 10/29/85 MA 12/30/86
TRANSFORMING GROWTH FACTOR-BETA 2	TREATMENT OF FULL THICKNESS MACULAR HOLES.	CELTRIX PHARMACEUTICALS, INC. 3055 PATRICK HENRY DRIVE SANTA CLARA CA 95054 DD 12/18/92
TREOSULFAN TN= OVASTAT	TREATMENT OF OVARIAN CANCER.	MEDAC GmbH C/O PRINCETON REG. ASSOC. 65 SOUTH MAIN STREET PENNINGTON NJ 08534 DD 05/16/94
TRETINOIN	TREATMENT OF SQUAMOUS METAPLASIA OF THE OCULAR SURFACE EPITHELIA (CONJUNCTIVA AND/OR CORNEA) WITH MUCOUS DEFICIENCY AND KERATINIZATION.	HANNAN OPHTHALMIC MARKETING SERVICES, INC 163 MEETINGHOUSE ROAD DUXBURY MA 02332 DD 04/15/85
TRETINOIN TN= TRETINOIN LF, IV	TREATMENT OF ACUTE AND CHRONIC LEUKEMIA.	ARGUS PHARMACEUTICALS, INC. 3400 RESEARCH FOREST DRIVE THE WOODLANDS TX 77381 DD 01/14/93
TRIENTINE HCL TN= CUPRID	TREATMENT OF PATIENTS WITH WILSON'S DISEASE WHO ARE INTOLERANT, OR INADEQUATELY RESPONSIVE TO PENICILLAMINE.	MERCK SHARP & DOHME RESEARCH DIVISION OF MERCK AND COMPANY WEST POINT PA 19486 DD 12/24/84 MA 11/08/85

CUMULATIVE LIST OF ORPHAN PRODUCT DESIGNATIONS AND APPROVALS *(continued)*

NAME *Generic/Chemical* *TN=Trade Name*	**INDICATION DESIGNATED**	**SPONSOR AND ADDRESS** *DD=Date Designated* *MA=Marketing Approval*
TRIMETREXATE GLUCURONATE	TREATMENT OF PNEUMOCYSTIS CARINII PNEUMONIA (PCP) IN AIDS PATIENTS.	U.S. BIOSCIENCE, INC. ONE TOWER BRIDGE 100 FRONT STREET WEST CONSHOHOCKEN PA 19428 DD 05/15/86
TRIMETREXATE GLUCURONATE	TREATMENT OF METASTATIC CARCINOMA OF THE HEAD AND NECK (I.E.,BUCCAL CAVITY PHARYNX, AND LARYNX).	U.S. BIOSCIENCE, INC. ONE TOWER BRIDGE 100 FRONT STREET WEST CONSHOHOCKEN PA 19428 DD 07/25/85
TRIMETREXATE GLUCURONATE	TREATMENT OF METASTATIC COLORECTAL ADENOCARCINOMA.	U.S. BIOSCIENCE, INC. ONE TOWER BRIDGE 100 FRONT STREET WEST CONSHOHOCKEN PA 19428 DD 07/25/85
TRIMETREXATE GLUCURONATE	TREATMENT OF PANCREATIC ADENOCARCINOMA.	U.S. BIOSCIENCE, INC. ONE TOWER BRIDGE 100 FRONT STREET WEST CONSHOHOCKEN PA 19428 DD 07/25/85
TRIMETREXATE GLUCURONATE	TREATMENT OF PATIENTS WITH ADVANCED NON-SMALL CELL CARCINOMA OF THE LUNG.	U.S. BIOSCIENCE, INC. ONE TOWER BRIDGE 100 FRONT STREET WEST CONSHOHOCKEN PA 19428 DD 01/13/88
TRIPTORELIN PAMOATE TN= DECAPEPTYL INJECTION	FOR USE IN THE PALLIATIVE TREATMENT OF ADVANCED OVARIAN CARCINOMA OF EPITHELIAL ORIGIN.	ORGANON, INC. 375 MT. PLEASANT AVENUE WEST ORANGE NJ 07052 DD 08/10/90
TRISACCHARIDES A AND B TN= BIOSYNJECT	TREATMENT OF MODERATE TO SEVERE CLINICAL FORMS OF HEMOLYTICDISEASE OF THE NEWBORN ARISING FROM PLACENTAL TRANSFER OF ANTIBODIES AGAINST BLOOD GROUP SUBSTANCES A AND B.	CHEMBIOMED, LTD. P.O. BOX 8050, EDMONTON, ALBERTA CANADA T6H4NP DD 04/12/87
TRISACCHARIDES A AND B TN= BIOSYNJECT	FOR USE IN ABO-INCOMPATIBLE SOLID ORGAN TRANSPLANTATION, INCLUDING KIDNEY, HEART, LIVER AND PANCREAS.	CHEMBIOMED, LTD. P.O. BOX 8050, EDMONTON, ALBERTA CANADA T6H4N9 DD 04/20/87
TRISACCHARIDES A AND B TN= BIOSYNJECT	PREVENTION OF ABO MEDICAL HEMOLYTIC REACTIONS ARISING FROM ABO-INCOMPATIBLE BONE MARROW TRANSPLANTATION.	CHEMBIOMED, LTD. P.O. BOX 8050, EDMONTON, ALBERTA CANADA DD 04/15/88
TROLEANDOMYCIN	TREATMENT OF SEVERE STEROID-REQUIRING ASTHMA.	SZEFLER, STANLEY M., M.D. 1400 JACKSON STREET DENVER CO 80206 DD 09/21/89
TUMOR NECROSIS FACTOR-BINDING PROTEIN 1	TREATMENT OF SYMPTOMATIC PATIENTS WITH ACQUIRED IMMUNODEFICIENCY SYNDROME INCLUDING ALL PATIENTS WITH CD4 COUNTS LESS THAN 200 CELLS PER MM3.	SERONO LABORATORIES, INC. 100 LONGWATER CIRCLE NORWELL MA 02061 DD 01/06/93
TUMOR NECROSIS FACTOR-BINDING PROTEIN II	TREATMENT OF SYMPTOMATIC PATIENTS WITH THE ACQUIRED IMMUNODEFICIENCY SYNDROME INCLUDING ALL PATIENTS WITH CD4 T-CELL COUNTS LESS THAN 200 CELLS PER MM3.	SERONO LABORATORIES, INC. 100 LONGWATER CIRCLE NORWELL MA 02061 DD 01/06/93
UROFOLLITROPIN TN= METRODIN	INDUCTION OF OVULATION IN PATIENTS WITH POLYCYSTIC OVARIAN DISEASE WHO HAVE AN ELEVATED LH/FSH RATIO AND WHO HAVE FAILED TO RESPOND TO ADEQUATE CLOMIPHENE CITRATE THERAPY.	SERONO LABORATORIES, INC. 100 LONGWATER CIRCLE NORWELL MA 02061 DD 11/25/87 MA 09/18/86
UROGASTRONE	ACCELERATION OF CORNEAL EPITHELIAL REGENERATION AND HEALING OF STROMAL INCISIONS FROM CORNEAL TRANSPLANT SURGERY.	CHIRON OPHTHALMICS 9342 JERONIMO ROAD IRVINE CA 92718-1903 DD 11/01/84
URSODEOXYCHOLIC ACID TN= URSOFALK	TREATMENT OF PATIENTS WITH PRIMARY BILIARY CIRRHOSIS.	INTERFALK U.S., INC. 25 MARGARET STREET PLATTSBURGH NY 12901-1206 DD 06/20/91
URSODIOL TN= ACTIGALL	MANAGEMENT OF THE CLINICAL SIGNS AND SYMPTOMS ASSOCIATED WITH PRIMARY BILIARY CIRRHOSIS.	CIBA-GEIGY CORPORATION 556 MORRIS AVENUE SUMMIT NJ 07901 DD 02/19/91

CUMULATIVE LIST OF ORPHAN PRODUCT DESIGNATIONS AND APPROVALS *(continued)*

NAME *Generic/Chemical* *TN=Trade Name*	**INDICATION DESIGNATED**	**SPONSOR AND ADDRESS** *DD=Date Designated* *MA=Marketing Approval*
VASOACTIVE INTESTINAL POLYPEPTIDE	TREATMENT OF ACUTE ESOPHAGEAL FOOD IMPACTION.	RESEARCH TRIANGLE PHARMACEUTICALS 200 WESTPARK CORPORATE CENTER DURHAM NC 27713 DD 06/23/93
ZALCITABINE	TREATMENT OF ACQUIRED IMMUNODEFICIENCY SYNDROME (AIDS).	NATIONAL CANCER INSTITUTE, DCT NIH, EXEC. PLAZA N., ROOM 7-18 BETHESDA MD 20892 DD 12/09/86
ZALCITABINE TN= HIVID	TREATMENT OF ACQUIRED IMMUNODEFICIENCY SYNDROME (AIDS).	HOFFMANN-LA ROCHE, INC. 340 KINGSLAND STREET NUTLEY NJ 07110-1199 DD 06/28/88 MA 06/19/92
ZIDOVUDINE TN= RETROVIR	TREATMENT OF ACQUIRED IMMUNODEFICIENCY SYNDROME (AIDS).	BURROUGHS WELLCOME COMPANY 3030 CORNWALLIS ROAD RESEARCH TRIANGLE PK NC 27709 DD 07/17/85 MA 03/19/87
ZIDOVUDINE TN= RETROVIR	TREATMENT OF AIDS RELATED COMPLEX (ARC).	BURROUGHS WELLCOME COMPANY 3030 CORNWALLIS ROAD RESEARCH TRIANGLE PK NC 27709 DD 05/12/87 MA 03/19/87
ZINC ACETATE	TREATMENT OF WILSON'S DISEASE.	LEMMON COMPANY 650 CATHILL ROAD SELLERSVILLE PA 18960 DD 11/06/85

DRUG PRODUCTS WHICH MUST DEMONSTRATE *IN VIVO* BIOAVAILABILITY ONLY IF PRODUCT FAILS TO ACHIEVE ADEQUATE DISSOLUTION

Acetaminophen; Aspirin; Butalbital
Capsule or Tablet; Oral
160-165 mg; 160-165 mg; 50 mg

Acetaminophen; Aspirin; Butalbital
Capsule or Tablet; Oral
325 mg; 325 mg; 50 mg

Acetaminophen; Aspirin; Butalbital; Caffeine
Capsule or Tablet; Oral
160-165 mg; 160-165 mg; 50 mg; 40 mg

Acetaminophen; Aspirin; Butalbital; Caffeine
Capsule or Tablet; Oral
325 mg; 325 mg; 50 mg; 40 mg

Acetaminophen; Butalbital
Capsule or Tablet; Oral
325 mg; 50 mg
650 mg; 50 mg

Acetaminophen; Butalbital; Caffeine
Capsule or Tablet; Oral
325 mg; 50 mg; 40 mg
650 mg; 50 mg; 40 mg

Aminophylline
Tablet; Oral
100 mg
200 mg

Aspirin; Butalbital;
Capsule or Tablet; Oral
325 mg; 50 mg
650 mg; 50 mg

Aspirin; Butalbital; Caffeine
Capsule or Tablet; Oral
325 mg; 50 mg; 40 mg
650 mg; 50 mg; 40 mg

Aspirin; Caffeine; Carisoprodol
Tablet; Oral
160 mg; 32 mg; 200 mg

Aspirin; Caffeine; Carisoprodol; Codeine Phosphate
Tablet; Oral
160 mg; 32 mg; 200 mg; 16 mg

Aspirin; Carisoprodol
Tablet; Oral
325 mg; 200 mg

Aspirin; Carisoprodol; Codeine Phosphate
Tablet; Oral
325 mg; 200 mg; 16 mg

Aspirin; Meprobamate
Tablet; Oral
325 mg; 200 mg

Aspirin; Methocarbamol
Tablet; Oral
325 mg; 400 mg

Chlorothiazide
Tablet; Oral
250 mg

Hydroxyzine Hydrochloride
Tablet; Oral
10 mg; 25 mg;
50 mg; 100 mg

Prednisone
Tablet; Oral
1 mg; 2.5 mg; 5 mg; 10 mg;
20 mg; 25 mg; 50 mg

BIOPHARMACEUTIC GUIDANCE AVAILABILITY

THE FOLLOWING IS A LIST OF GUIDANCES AVAILABLE FOR *IN VIVO* BIOEQUIVALENCE STUDIES AND *IN VITRO* DISSOLUTION TESTING. COMMENTS AND SUGGESTIONS CONCERNING THESE GUIDANCES ARE ENCOURAGED AND SHOULD BE SENT TO THE DIVISION OF BIOEQUIVALENCE (HFD-650, MPN-2 ROOM 279) 5600 FISHERS LANE, ROCKVILLE, MD 20857.

DRUG NAME (DOSAGE FORM)	DATE	REVISED DATE
ACETAMINOPHEN WITH PROPOXYPHENE NAPSYLATE (TABLET)	MAR 26, 1980	
ACETOHEXAMIDE (TABLET)	NOV 15, 1985	AUG 01, 1988
ALBUTEROL (METERED DOSE INHALER - *IN VIVO*)	JAN 27, 1994	
ALBUTEROL AND METAPROTERENOL SULFATE (METERED DOSE INHALER - *IN VITRO*)	JUN 27, 1989	
ALBUTEROL SULFATE (TABLET)	MAY 29, 1987	
ALLOPURINOL (TABLET)	JUL 15, 1985	
ALPRAZOLAM (TABLET)	NOV 27, 1992	
AMILORIDE HYDROCHLORIDE (TABLET)	MAR 29, 1985	
AMINOPHYLLINE (SUPPOSITORY)	JUL 05, 1983	
AMITRIPTYLINE HYDROCHLORIDE (TABLET)	JUL 05, 1983	
AMITRIPTYLINE AND PERPHENAZINE (TABLET)	AUG 27,1987	
AMOXAPINE (TABLET)	SEP 10, 1987	AUG 05, 1988
AMOXICILLIN (CAPSULE, SUSPENSION AND TABLET)	AUG 18, 1987	JUN 10, 1988
ANTIFUNGAL (DRAFT GUIDANCE) (TOPICAL)	FEB 24, 1990	
ANTIFUNGAL (DRAFT GUIDANCE) (VAGINAL)	FEB 24, 1990	
ATENOLOL (TABLET)	OCT 06, 1988	
BACLOFEN (TABLET)	MAY 05, 1986	
BUMETANIDE (TABLET)	APR 23, 1993	
BUSIPRONE HYDROCHLORIDE (TABLET)	AUG 13, 1993	
CAPTOPRIL (TABLET)	MAY 13, 1993	
CARBAMAZEPINE (TABLET)	SEP 30, 1987	JAN 20, 1988
CARBIDOPA AND LEVODOPA (TABLET)	JUN 19, 1992	
CEFACLOR (CAPSULE AND SUSPENSION)	APR 23, 1993	
CEFADROXIL (CAPSULE, SUSPENSION, AND TABLET)	OCT 07, 1986	
CEPHALEXIN (CAPSULE AND TABLET)	AUG 13, 1986	MAR 19, 1987
CEPHRADINE (CAPSULE AND SUSPENSION)	SEP 10, 1986	
CHLORDIAZEPOXIDE (TABLET)	JUL 05, 1983	
CHLORDIAZEPOXIDE HYDROCHLORIDE (CAPSULE)	JUL 05, 1983	
CHLORPROPAMIDE (TABLET)	JUL 05, 1983	
CHLORTHALIDONE (TABLET)	JUL 05, 1983	
CHOLESTRYRAMINE (POWDER)	JUL 15, 1993	
CIMETIDINE (TABLET)	JUN 12, 1992	
CLINDAMYCIN HYDROCHLORIDE (CAPSULE)	MAY 31, 1988	
CLOFIBRATE (CAPSULE)	APR 07, 1986	
CLONIDINE HYDROCHLORIDE (TABLET)	DEC 05, 1986	
CLORAZEPATE DIPOTASSIUM (CAPSULE AND TABLET)	MAR 10, 1986	FEB 17, 1987
CORTICOSTEROID *IN VITRO* AND *IN VIVO* INTERIM (TOPICAL)	JUL 01, 1992	
CYCLOBENZAPRINE HYDROCHLORIDE (TABLET)	DEC 18, 1987	JAN 25, 1988
DESIPRAMINE HYDROCHLORIDE (TABLET)	APR 28, 1987	SEP 22, 1987
DIAZEPAM (TABLET)	JUL 08, 1985	
DICLOFENAC SODIUM (TABLET)	DEC 24, 1992	
DICYCLOMINE HYDROCHLORIDE (CAPSULE AND TABLET)	AUG 10, 1984	
DIFLUNISAL (TABLET)	MAY 16, 1992	
DILTIAZEM HYDROCHLORIDE (TABLET)	MAY 16, 1992	
DIPYRIDAMOLE (TABLET)	JUL 05, 1983	SEP 25, 1987
DISOPYRAMIDE PHOSPHATE (CAPSULE)	JUL 09, 1985	
DISSOLUTION TESTING (GENERAL)	APR 01, 1978	
DOXEPIN HYDROCHLORIDE (CAPSULE)	APR 02, 1985	OCT 09, 1986
DOXYCYCLINE HYCLATE (CAPSULE AND TABLET)	APR 11, 1988	
ERYTHROMYCIN (CAPSULE, DELAYED RELEASE PELLETS)	SEP 21, 1988	
ESTROGENS, CONJUGATED (TABLET)	AUG 21, 1991	
ESTROPIPATE (TABLET)	AUG 26, 1992	
ETHINYL ESTRADIOL AND NORETHINDRONE (TABLET)	MAR 18, 1988	
FENOPROFEN (CAPSULE AND TABLET)	AUG 27, 1987	FEB 03, 1988
FLURAZEPAM HYDROCHLORIDE (CAPSULE)	OCT 15, 1985	
FLURBIPROFEN (TABLET)	DEC 24, 1992	
GEMFIBROZIL (CAPSULE AND TABLET)	JUN 23, 1989	JUN 15, 1992
GLIPIZIDE (TABLET)	APR 23, 1993	
GLYBURIDE (TABLET)	APR 23, 1993	

GUANABENZ ACETATE (TABLET)	APR 23, 1993	
HALOPERIDOL (TABLET)	APR 30, 1987	
HYDROCHLOROTHIAZIDE (TABLET)	JUL 25, 1983	SEP 28, 1987
HYDROXYZINE HYDROCHLORIDE (TABLET, DISSOLUTION ONLY)	JAN 27, 1981	
HYDROXYZINE PAMOATE (CAPSULE)	JUL 26, 1983	SEP 28, 1987
INDAPAMIDE (TABLET)	APR 23, 1993	
INDOMETHACIN (CAPSULE)	APR 06, 1985	JAN 27, 1988
ISOPROPAMIDE IODIDE (TABLET)	MAY 12, 1982	
ISOSORBIDE DINITRATE (CAPSULE, EXTENDED RELEASE AND TABLET, EXTENDED RELEASE)	NOV 06, 1985	
ISOSORBIDE DINITRATE (CHEWABLE TABLET, ORAL TABLET, AND SUBLINGUAL TABLET)	JUN 04, 1985	SEP 22, 1987
KETOPROFEN (CAPSULE)	APR 23, 1993	
LEUCOVORIN CALCIUM (TABLET)	APR 28, 1987	AUG 04, 1988
LORAZEPAM (TABLET)	DEC 03, 1984	SEP 16, 1987
LOXAPINE SUCCINATE (CAPSULE)	SEP 10, 1987	
MAPROTILINE HYDROCHLORIDE (TABLET)	AUG 27, 1987	
MECLOFENAMATE SODIUM (CAPSULE)	NOV 12, 1986	
MEDROXYPROGESTERONE ACETATE (TABLET)	DEC 24, 1986	SEP 17, 1987
MEGESTROL ACETATE (TABLET)	AUG 17, 1987	
MESTRANOL AND NORETHINDRONE (TABLET)	MAY 13, 1988	
METAPROTERENOL SULFATE (TABLET)	MAR 18, 1988	
METHYLPREDNISOLONE (TABLET)	JUN 12, 1986	
METOCLOPRAMIDE HYDROCHLORIDE (TABLET)	DEC 27, 1984	
METOPROLOL TARTRATE (TABLET)	JUN 12, 1992	
MINOXIDIL (TABLET)	APR 02, 1986	
NADOLOL (TABLET)	MAY 16, 1992	
NAFCILLIN SODIUM (CAPSULE AND TABLET)	SEP 10, 1987	
NALIDIXIC ACID (TABLET)	AUG 19, 1987	
NAPROXEN (TABLET)	JUN 12, 1992	
NITROFURANTOIN (CAPSULE, MACROCRYSTALLINE)	OCT 29, 1985	
NITROGLYCERIN (OINTMENT)	DEC 17, 1986	
NORTRIPTYLINE HYDROCHLORIDE (CAPSULE)	JUN 12, 1992	
ORAL EXTENDED (CONTROLLED RELEASE)	SEP 09, 1993	
ORPHENADRINE CITRATE (TABLET)	JUL 22, 1983	
PERPHENAZINE (TABLET)	AUG 27, 1987	
PHENYLBUTAZONE (CAPSULE AND TABLET)	JUL 15, 1983	SEP 28, 1987
PHENYTOIN (SUSPENSION AND CHEWABLE TABLET)	MAR 04, 1994	
PHENYTOIN SODIUM (CAPSULE, EXTENDED AND PROMPT)	MAR 04, 1994	
PINDOLOL (TABLET)	APR 23, 1993	
PIROXICAM (CAPSULE)	JUN 15, 1992	
POTASSIUM CHLORIDE (CAPSULE, SLOW RELEASE AND TABLET, SLOW RELEASE)	JAN 17, 1987	
PRAZEPAM (CAPSULE AND TABLET)	JUL 26, 1988	
PREDNISONE (TABLET--DISSOLUTION ONLY)	JUL 10, 1985	
PROBENECID (TABLET)	JUL 26, 1983	
PROCAINAMIDE HYDROCHLORIDE (TABLET)	JUL 25, 1983	SEP 28, 1987
PROPRANOLOL HYDROCHLORIDE (TABLET)	MAY 19, 1984	
PROPYLTHIOURACIL (TABLET)	AUG 13, 1986	
QUINIDINE GLUCONATE (TABLET, EXTENDED RELEASE)	JUN 15, 1987	SEP 22, 1987
RANITIDINE HYDROCHLORIDE (TABLET)	APR 23, 1993	
RIFAMPIN (CAPSULE)	SEP 08, 1988	
RITODRINE HYDROCHLORIDE (TABLET)	AUG 27, 1987	
SILVER SULFADIAZINE (CREAM)	MAY 07, 1987	
SPIRONOLACTONE (TABLET)	JUL 25, 1983	
STATISTICAL PROCEDURE FOR BIOEQUIVALENCE STUDIES USING A STANDARD TWO-TREATMENT CROSSOVER DESIGN	JUL 01, 1992	
SULFASALAZINE (TABLET)	OCT 08, 1987	
SULFINPYRAZONE (CAPSULE AND TABLET)	JUL 15, 1983	SEP 25, 1987
SULFONES (TABLET)	NOV 07, 1986	
SULINDAC (TABLET)	SEP 28, 1987	JUL 18, 1988
TEMAZEPAM (CAPSULE)	AUG 08, 1985	
TERFENADINE (TABLET)	JUN 12, 1992	
THEOPHYLLINE (TABLET)	NOV 01, 1984	
TIMOLOL MALEATE (TABLET)	AUG 09, 1988	
TOLAZAMIDE (TABLET)	AUG 22, 1984	
TOLBUTAMIDE (TABLET)	DEC 01, 1983	
TOLMETIN SODIUM (CAPSULE AND TABLET)	APR 20, 1989	
TRAZODONE HYDROCHLORIDE (TABLET)	NOV 15, 1985	APR 30, 1986

TRIAZOLAM (TABLET)	DEC 24, 1992	
TRIMIPRAMINE MALEATE (CAPSULE)	NOV 03, 1986	AUG 18, 1987
VERAPAMIL (TABLET)	JUL 18, 1985	
WAIVER POLICY (DRAFT GUIDANCE)	JUN 23, 1989	

ANDA SUITABILITY PETITIONS

THE FOLLOWING ARE TWO LISTS OF PETITIONS FILED UNDER SECTION 505(j)(2)(C) OF THE ACT WHERE THE AGENCY HAS DETERMINED THAT THE REFERENCED PRODUCT: (1) IS SUITABLE FOR SUBMISSION AS AN ANDA (PETITIONS APPROVED) OR (2) IS NOT SUITABLE FOR SUBMISSION AS AN ANDA (PETITIONS DENIED). THE DETERMINATION THAT AN ANDA WILL BE APPROVED IS NOT MADE UNTIL THE ANDA ITSELF IS SUBMITTED AND REVIEWED BY THE AGENCY. A COPY OF EACH PETITION IS LISTED BY DOCKET NUMBER ON PUBLIC DISPLAY IN FDA'S DOCKETS MANAGEMENT BRANCH, HFA-305, ROOM 4-62, 5600 FISHERS LANE, ROCKVILLE, MD 20857.

PETITIONS APPROVED

DRUG NAME DOSAGE FORM; ROUTE	STRENGTH (CONTAINER SIZE)	DOCKET NUMBER	PETITIONER	REASON FOR PETITION	STATUS
ACETAMINOPHEN SUPPOSITORY; RECTAL	80 MG	85 P-0403/CP	UPSHER SMITH	NEW STRENGTH	APPROVED OCT 16, 1985
ACETAMINOPHEN; ASPIRIN; CODEINE PHOSPHATE TABLET; ORAL	325 MG 325 MG 30 MG	86 P-0361/CP	BOCK PHARMA	NEW DOSAGE FORM NEW STRENGTH	APPROVED DEC 16, 1987
ACETAMINOPHEN; ASPIRIN; HYDROCODONE BITARTRATE CAPSULE; ORAL	150 MG 180 MG 2.5 MG	92 P-0282/CP3	MIKART	NEW COMBINATION	APPROVED NOV 10, 1993
ACETAMINOPHEN; ASPIRIN; HYDROCODONE BITARTRATE CAPSULE; ORAL	150 MG 180 MG 5 MG	92 P-0282/CP1	MIKART	NEW COMBINATION	APPROVED NOV 10, 1993
ACETAMINOPHEN; ASPIRIN; HYDROCODONE BITARTRATE CAPSULE; ORAL	150 MG 180 MG 7.5 MG	92 P-0282/CP2	MIKART	NEW COMBINATION NEW STRENGTH	APPROVED NOV 10, 1993
ACETAMINOPHEN; ASPIRIN; HYDROCODONE BITARTRATE CAPSULE; ORAL	150 MG 180 MG 10 MG	92 P-0282/CP4	MIKART	NEW COMBINATION	APPROVED NOV 10, 1993
ACETAMINOPHEN; ASPIRIN; HYDROCODONE BITARTRATE TABLET; ORAL	150 MG 180 MG 2.5 MG	92 P-0282/CP3	MIKART	NEW COMBINATION NEW DOSAGE FORM	APPROVED NOV 10, 1993
ACETAMINOPHEN; ASPIRIN; HYDROCODONE BITARTRATE TABLET; ORAL	150 MG 180 MG 5 MG	92 P-0282/CP1	MIKART	NEW COMBINATION NEW DOSAGE FORM	APPROVED NOV 10, 1993
ACETAMINOPHEN; ASPIRIN; HYDROCODONE BITARTRATE TABLET; ORAL	150 MG 180 MG 7.5 MG	92 P-0282/CP2	MIKART	NEW COMBINATION NEW DOSAGE FORM NEW STRENGTH	APPROVED NOV 10, 1993
ACETAMINOPHEN; ASPIRIN; HYDROCODONE BITARTRATE TABLET; ORAL	150 MG 180 MG 10 MG	92 P-0282/CP4	MIKART	NEW COMBINATION NEW DOSAGE FORM	APPROVED NOV 10, 1993
ACETAMINOPHEN; BUTALBITAL; CAFFEINE CAPSULE; ORAL	500 MG 50 MG 40 MG	89 P-0345/CP	MALLARD	NEW DOSAGE FORM	APPROVED OCT 27, 1989
ACETAMINOPHEN; BUTALBITAL; CAFFEINE CODEINE PHOSPHATE CAPSULE; ORAL	325 MG 50 MG 40 MG 30 MG	91 P-069/CP2	KING & SPAULDING	NEW COMBINATION	APPROVED DEC 10, 1991
ACETAMINOPHEN; CODEINE PHOSPHATE CAPSULE; ORAL	500 MG 30 MG	84 P-0228/CP	RW JOHNSON	NEW DOSAGE FORM NEW STRENGTH	APPROVED JUN 02, 1986

ANDA SUITABILITY PETITIONS

PETITIONS APPROVED *(continued)*

DRUG NAME DOSAGE FORM; ROUTE	STRENGTH (CONTAINER SIZE)	DOCKET NUMBER	PETITIONER	REASON FOR PETITION	STATUS
ACETAMINOPHEN; CODEINE PHOSPHATE CAPSULE; ORAL	500 MG 60 MG	84 P-0228/CP	RW JOHNSON	NEW DOSAGE FORM NEW STRENGTH	APPROVED JUN 02, 1986
ACETAMINOPHEN; CODEINE PHOSPHATE CAPSULE; ORAL	500 MG 45 MG	93 P-0314/CP1	MIKART	NEW DOSAGE FORM NEW STRENGTH	APPROVED NOV 10, 1993
ACETAMINOPHEN; CODEINE PHOSPHATE CAPSULE; ORAL	650 MG 15 MG	86 P-0200/CP	MIKART	NEW DOSAGE FORM NEW STRENGTH	APPROVED OCT 03, 1986
ACETAMINOPHEN; CODEINE PHOSPHATE SOFT GELATIN CAPSULE; ORAL	300 MG 30 MG	85 P-0543/CP	SOFTAN	NEW DOSAGE FORM	APPROVED MAR 18, 1986
ACETAMINOPHEN; CODEINE PHOSPHATE SOFT GELATIN CAPSULE; ORAL	500 MG 7.5 MG	85 P-0543/ CP0002	SOFTAN	NEW DOSAGE FORM NEW STRENGTH	APPROVED MAR 19, 1986
ACETAMINOPHEN; CODEINE PHOSPHATE SOFT GELATIN CAPSULE; ORAL	500 MG 15 MG	85 P-0543/ CP0002	SOFTAN	NEW DOSAGE FORM NEW STRENGTH	APPROVED MAR 19, 1986
ACETAMINOPHEN; CODEINE PHOSPHATE SOLUTION; ORAL	160 MG/5 ML 6 MG/5 ML	86 P-0133/CP	KLEINFELD, KAPLAN AND BECKER	NEW STRENGTH	APPROVED MAY 21, 1986
ACETAMINOPHEN; CODEINE PHOSPHATE SYRUP; ORAL	160 MG/5 ML 6 MG/5 ML	87 P-0323/CP	KLEINFELD, KAPLAN AND BECKER	NEW DOSAGE FORM NEW STRENGTH	APPROVED NOV 04, 1987
ACETAMINOPHEN; CODEINE PHOSPHATE TABLET; ORAL	500 MG 7.5 MG	91 P-0514/CP1	SOFTAN	NEW STRENGTH	APPROVED JUN 03, 1992
ACETAMINOPHEN; CODEINE PHOSPHATE TABLET; ORAL	500 MG 45 MG	93 P-0314/CP1	MIKART	NEW STRENGTH	APPROVED NOV 10, 1993
ACETAMINOPHEN; CODEINE PHOSPHATE TABLET; ORAL	650 MG 15 MG	86 P-0200/CP	MIKART	NEW STRENGTH	APPROVED OCT 03, 1986
ACETAMINOPHEN; HYDROCODONE BITARTRATE CAPSULE; ORAL	650 MG 7.5 MG	85 P-0390/CP	UAD LABS	NEW DOSAGE FORM NEW STRENGTH	APPROVED MAR 17, 1987
ACETAMINOPHEN; HYDROCODONE BITARTRATE ELIXIR; ORAL	500 MG/15 ML 7.5 MG/15 ML	85 P-0439/ CP0003	RUSS PHARMS	NEW DOSAGE FORM NEW STRENGTH	APPROVED APR 01, 1987
ACETAMINOPHEN; HYDROCODONE BITARTRATE SOLUTION; ORAL	325 MG/15 ML 2.5 MG/15 ML	87 P-0129/ CP0002	MIKART	NEW STRENGTH	APPROVED JUN 08, 1987
ACETAMINOPHEN; HYDROCODONE BITARTRATE SOLUTION; ORAL	325 MG/15 ML 5 MG/15 ML	87 P-0129/ CP0002	MIKART	NEW STRENGTH	APPROVED JUN 08, 1987
ACETAMINOPHEN; HYDROCODONE BITARTRATE SOLUTION; ORAL	325 MG/15 ML 7.5 MG/15 ML	87 P-0129/ CP0002	MIKART	NEW STRENGTH	APPROVED JUN 08, 1987
ACETAMINOPHEN; HYDROCODONE BITARTRATE SOLUTION; ORAL	325 MG/15 ML 10 MG/15 ML	87 P-0129/ CP0002	MIKART	NEW STRENGTH	APPROVED JUN 08, 1987

ANDA SUITABILITY PETITIONS

PETITIONS APPROVED *(continued)*

DRUG NAME DOSAGE FORM; ROUTE	STRENGTH (CONTAINER SIZE)	DOCKET NUMBER	PETITIONER	REASON FOR PETITION	STATUS
ACETAMINOPHEN; HYDROCODONE BITARTRATE SOLUTION; ORAL	500 MG/15 ML 5 MG/15 ML	84 P-0391/CP	UAD LABS	NEW DOSAGE FORM	APPROVED JUL 02, 1985
ACETAMINOPHEN; HYDROCODONE BITARTRATE TABLET; ORAL	325 MG 2.5 MG	87 P-0129/CP	MIKART	NEW STRENGTH	APPROVED JUN 08, 1987
ACETAMINOPHEN; HYDROCODONE BITARTRATE TABLET; ORAL	325 MG 5 MG	87 P-0129/CP	MIKART	NEW STRENGTH	APPROVED JUN 08, 1987
ACETAMINOPHEN; HYDROCODONE BITARTRATE TABLET; ORAL	325 MG 7.5 MG	87 P-0129/CP	MIKART	NEW STRENGTH	APPROVED JUN 08, 1987
ACETAMINOPHEN; HYDROCODONE BITARTRATE TABLET; ORAL	325 MG 10 MG	87 P-0129/CP	MIKART	NEW STRENGTH	APPROVED JUN 08, 1987
ACETAMINOPHEN; HYDROCODONE BITARTRATE TABLET; ORAL	500 MG 10 MG	87 P-0170/CP	LUCHEM	NEW STRENGTH	APPROVED JUL 07, 1987
ACETAMINOPHEN; HYDROCODONE BITARTRATE TABLET; ORAL	650 MG 10 MG	88 P-0416/CP	MORAVEC	NEW STRENGTH	APPROVED MAR 01, 1989
ACETAMINOPHEN; HYDROCODONE BITARTRATE TABLET; ORAL	660 MG 10 MG	91 P-0004/ CP1	KNOLL	NEW STRENGTH	APPROVED OCT 27, 1992
ACETAMINOPHEN; OXYCODONE HYDROCHLO- RIDE SOFT GELATIN CAPSULE; ORAL	500 MG 5 MG	85 P-0543/ CP0003	SOFTAN	NEW DOSAGE FORM	APPROVED MAR 18, 1986
ACETAMINOPHEN; PROPOXYPHENE HYDROCHLO- RIDE SOFT GELATIN CAPSULE; ORAL	500 MG 32 MG	85 P-0581/CP	SOFTAN	NEW DOSAGE FORM NEW STRENGTH	APPROVED MAR 18, 1986
ACETYLCYSTEINE SOLUTION; INHALATION	20%	88 P-0237/CP	DEY	NEW STRENGTH	APPROVED NOV 29, 1988
ACYCLOVIR TABLET; ORAL	200 MG	93 P-0339/CP1	NOVOPHARM	NEW DOSAGE FORM	APPROVED FEB 08, 1994
ACYCLOVIR SODIUM INJECTABLE; INJECTION	25 MG/ML (20 ML/VIAL) (40 ML/VIAL)	93 P-0469/CP1	FAULDING	NEW DOSAGE FORM	APPROVED JUN 09, 1994
ACYCLOVIR SODIUM INJECTABLE; INJECTION	EQ 50 MG BASE/ML (10 ML/VIAL) (20 ML/VIAL)	92 P-0468/CP1	BULL	NEW DOSAGE FORM	APPROVED SEP 01, 1993
ALBUTEROL SULFATE CAPSULE, EXTENDED RELEASE; ORAL	EQ 4 MG BASE	91 P-0348/CP1	HAMER	NEW DOSAGE FORM	APPROVED MAR 17, 1992
ALBUTEROL SULFATE SOLUTION; ORAL	2 MG/5 ML	89 P-0447/CP	BIOCRAFT	NEW DOSAGE FORM	APPROVED MAR 15, 1990
ALPRAZOLAM CONCENTRATE; ORAL	1 MG/ML	92 P-0050/ CP1	ROXANE	NEW DOSAGE FORM	APPROVED DEC 15, 1992
ALPRAZOLAM SOLUTION; ORAL	0.5 MG/5 ML	92 P-0050/ CP2	ROXANE	NEW DOSAGE FORM	APPROVED DEC 15, 1992
AMINOCAPROIC ACID INJECTABLE; INJECTION	500 MG/ML (10 ML/VIAL)	85 P-0308/CP	ABBOTT	NEW STRENGTH	APPROVED FEB 12, 1986
AMINOPHYLLINE INJECTABLE; INJECTION	10 MG/ML (10 ML/VIAL)	85 P-0459/CP	ABBOTT	NEW STRENGTH	APPROVED FEB 12, 1986
AMINOPHYLLINE INJECTABLE; INJECTION	10 MG/ML (10 ML/VIAL)	87 P-0103/CP	LYPHOMED	NEW STRENGTH	APPROVED JUL 07, 1987

ANDA SUITABILITY PETITIONS

PETITIONS APPROVED *(continued)*

DRUG NAME DOSAGE FORM; ROUTE	STRENGTH (CONTAINER SIZE)	DOCKET NUMBER	PETITIONER	REASON FOR PETITION	STATUS
AMINOPHYLLINE INJECTABLE; INJECTION	50 MG/ML (20 ML/VIAL)	85 P-0459/CP	ABBOTT	NEW STRENGTH	APPROVED FEB 12, 1986
AMINOSALICYLIC ACID GRANULES, ENTERIC-COATED; ORAL	4 GM/PACKET	92 P-0356/ CP1	JACOBUS	NEW DOSAGE FORM NEW STRENGTH	APPROVED MAR 03, 1993
ASPIRIN; CAFFEINE; DIHYDROCODEINE BITARTRATE TABLET; ORAL	356.4 MG 30 MG 16 MG	86 P-0359/CP	CENTRAL PHARMS	NEW DOSAGE FORM	APPROVED SEP 29, 1986
ASPIRIN; HYDROCODONE BITARTRATE TABLET; ORAL	325 MG 5 MG	87 P-0376/ CP0002	ANABOLIC	NEW STRENGTH	APPROVED FEB 12, 1988
ASPIRIN; HYDROCODONE BITARTRATE TABLET; ORAL	500 MG 7.5 MG	87 P-0100/CP	KING AND SPAULDING	NEW STRENGTH	APPROVED APR 24, 1987
ASPIRIN; HYDROCODONE BITARTRATE TABLET; ORAL	650 MG 5 MG	87 P-0376/CP	ANABOLIC	NEW STRENGTH	APPROVED FEB 12, 1988
ASPIRIN; HYDROCODONE BITARTRATE TABLET; ORAL	650 MG 7.5 MG	90 P-0050/CP	MASON PHARMS	NEW STRENGTH	APPROVED JUN 01, 1990
AZATADINE MALEATE; PHENYLPROPANOLAMINE HYDROCHLORIDE CAPSULE, EXTENDED RELEASE; ORAL	1 MG 75 MG	85 P-0492/CP	SKF	NEW COMBINATION NEW DOSAGE FORM	APPROVED JAN 28, 1986
BENZTROPINE MESYLATE SYRUP; ORAL	0.5 MG/5 ML	85 P-0423/CP	RIM CONSULTING	NEW DOSAGE FORM	APPROVED OCT 16, 1985
BRETYLIUM TOSYLATE INJECTABLE; INJECTION	200 MG/ML (5 ML/CONTAINER)	87 P-0228/CP	ASTRA	NEW STRENGTH	APPROVED OCT 06, 1987
BRETYLIUM TOSYLATE INJECTABLE; INJECTION	200 MG/ML (10 ML/CONTAINER)	85 P-0546/CP	INTL MEDICATION	NEW STRENGTH	APPROVED JAN 20, 1987
BRETYLIUM TOSYLATE IN DEXTROSE 5% INJECTABLE; INJECTION	10 MG/ML (50 ML/CONTAINER)	87 P-0065/CP	LYPHOMED	NEW STRENGTH	APPROVED APR 27, 1987
BRETYLIUM TOSYLATE IN DEXTROSE 5% INJECTABLE; INJECTION	10 MG/ML (100 ML/CONTAINER)	87 P-0128/CP	LYPHOMED	NEW STRENGTH	APPROVED JUL 22, 1987
BROMPHENIRAMINE MALEATE; PSEUDOEPHEDRINE HYDROCHLORIDE CAPSULE, EXTENDED RELEASE; ORAL	12 MG 120 MG	85 P-0095/CP	UAD LABS	NEW COMBINATION NEW DOSAGE FORM	APPROVED DEC 13, 1985
CARBAMAZINE SUSPENSION; ORAL	200 MG/5 ML	89 P-0399/CP	GUIDELINES	NEW DOSAGE FORM	APPROVED MAY 16, 1991
CARBOPLATIN INJECTABLE; INJECTION	10 MG/ML (5 ML/VIAL) (15 ML/VIAL) (45 ML/VIAL)	92 P-0467/ CP1	BULL	NEW DOSAGE FORM	APPROVED MAY 20, 1993
CARMUSTINE, STERILE INJECTABLE; INJECTION	200 MG/VIAL	88 P-0410/CP	QUAD	NEW STRENGTH	APPROVED FEB 13, 1989
CHLORHEXIDINE GLUCONATE SOLUTION; TOPICAL	1.5%	84 P-0417/CP	PARKE DAVIS	NEW STRENGTH	APPROVED SEP 18, 1985
CHLORHEXIDINE GLUCONATE SPRAY; TOPICAL	0.5%	88 P-0036/CP	ARENT, FOX, KINTNER, PLOTKIN & KAHN	NEW DOSAGE FORM	APPROVED AUG 19, 1988

ANDA SUITABILITY PETITIONS

PETITIONS APPROVED *(continued)*

DRUG NAME DOSAGE FORM; ROUTE	STRENGTH (CONTAINER SIZE)	DOCKET NUMBER	PETITIONER	REASON FOR PETITION	STATUS
CHLORHEXIDINE GLUCONATE TOWELETTE; TOPICAL	4%	88 P-0295/CP	BRIAN	NEW STRENGTH	APPROVED NOV 03, 1988
CHLORPHENIRAMINE MALEATE; PHENYLPROPANOLAMINE HYDROCHLORIDE CAPSULE, EXTENDED RELEASE; ORAL	10 MG 75 MG	85 P-0149/CP	DURA PHARMS	NEW STRENGTH	APPROVED DEC 13, 1985
CHLORPHENIRAMINE MALEATE; PSEUDOEPHEDRINE HYDROCHLORIDE TABLET, EXTENDED RELEASE; ORAL	12 MG 120 MG	87 P-0165/CP	SANDOZ	NEW DOSAGE FORM	APPROVED MAY 19, 1987
CHLORPROMAZINE HYDROCHLORIDE SOLUTION; ORAL	25 MG/5 ML	92 P-0284/CP1	UDL	NEW STRENGTH	APPROVED JAN 07, 1993
CHLORZOXAZONE CAPSULE; ORAL	250 MG	90 P-0084/CP0001	MIKART	NEW DOSAGE FORM	APPROVED MAY 24, 1990
CHLORZOXAZONE CAPSULE; ORAL	500 MG	82 N-0032/CP0006	MIKART	NEW DOSAGE FORM	APPROVED JAN 13, 1988
CHLORZOXAZONE TABLET; ORAL	750 MG	91 P-0153/CP1	MIKART	NEW STRENGTH	APPROVED JUN 03, 1992
CHOLESTYRAMINE CAPSULE; ORAL	EQ 500 MG RESIN	86 P-0474/CP	BRISTOL MYERS	NEW DOSAGE FORM NEW STRENGTH	APPROVED JAN 30, 1987
CHOLESTYRAMINE GEL; ORAL	EQ 4 GM RESIN/CONTAINER	87 P-0301/CP	CIBA	NEW DOSAGE FORM	APPROVED NOV 04, 1987
CHOLESTYRAMINE TABLET; ORAL	EQ 800 MG RESIN	86 P-0475/CP	BRISTOL MYERS	NEW DOSAGE FORM NEW STRENGTH	APPROVED JAN 30, 1987
CHOLESTYRAMINE TABLET; ORAL	EQ 1 GM RESIN	87 P-0324/CP	BRISTOL MYERS	NEW DOSAGE FORM NEW STRENGTH	APPROVED DEC 08, 1987
CIMETIDINE TABLET, EFFERVESCENT; ORAL	200 MG 300 MG 400 MG 800 MG	93 P-0048/CP1	FLEMINGTON PHARM	NEW DOSAGE FORM	APPROVED SEP 18, 1993
CIMETIDINE HYDROCHLORIDE IN SODIUM CHLORIDE 0.9% IN PLASTIC CONTAINER INJECTABLE; INJECTION	90 MG/100 ML* 120 MG/100 ML* 180 MG/100 ML* 240 MG/100 ML* 360 MG/100 ML* 480 MG/100 ML* (*EQ xxMG BASE/100 ML)	92 P-0337/CP1	ABBOTT	NEW STRENGTH	APPROVED OCT 26, 1992
CISPLATIN INJECTABLE; INJECTION	1 MG/ML (10 ML/VIAL) (50 ML/VIAL) (100 ML/VIAL)	87 P-0421/CP	BULL	NEW DOSAGE FORM NEW STRENGTH	APPROVED FEB 29, 1988
CISPLATIN INJECTABLE; INJECTION	1 MG/ML (20 ML/VIAL)	88 P-0010/CP	LYPHOMED	NEW DOSAGE FORM NEW STRENGTH	APPROVED APR 01, 1988
CISPLATIN INJECTABLE; INJECTION	1 MG/ML (100 ML/VIAL) (500 ML/VIAL)	87 P-0130/CP	BAXTER	NEW DOSAGE FORM NEW STRENGTH	APPROVED OCT 06, 1987

ANDA SUITABILITY PETITIONS

PETITIONS APPROVED *(continued)*

DRUG NAME DOSAGE FORM; ROUTE	STRENGTH (CONTAINER SIZE)	DOCKET NUMBER	PETITIONER	REASON FOR PETITION	STATUS
CISPLATIN INJECTABLE; INJECTION	1 MG/ML (200 ML/VIAL)	93 P-0084/CP1	FUJISAWA	NEW STRENGTH	APPROVED NOV 10, 1993
CISPLATIN INJECTABLE; INJECTION	20 MG/VIAL	87 P-0291/CP	LYPHOMED	NEW STRENGTH	APPROVED NOV 03, 1987
CISPLATIN INJECTABLE; INJECTION	100 MG/VIAL	86 P-0395/CP	BEN VENUE	NEW STRENGTH	APPROVED DEC 08, 1986
CLEMASTINE FUMARATE; PHENYLPROPANOLAMINE HYDROCHLORIDE CAPSULE, EXTENDED RELEASE; ORAL	1.34 MG 75 MG	88 P-0350/CP	SCI CONSULTING	NEW DOSAGE FORM	APPROVED DEC 13, 1988
CLEMASTINE FUMARATE; PSEUDOEPHEDRINE HYDROCHLORIDE TABLET, EXTENDED RELEASE; ORAL	EQ 1 MG BASE 120 MG	87 P-0314/CP	DORSEY	NEW COMBINATION	APPROVED NOV 03, 1987
CLOBETASOL PROPIONATE LOTION; TOPICAL	0.05%	90 P-0198/CP1	KROSS	NEW DOSAGE FORM	APPROVED MAR 14, 1991
CODEINE PHOSPHATE; DEXBROMPHENIRAMINE MALEATE; PHENYLPROPANOLAMINE HYDROCHLORIDE SYRUP; ORAL	10 MG/5 ML 1 MG/5 ML 12.5 MG/5 ML	85 P-0269/CP	BOCK PHARMA	NEW COMBINATION	APPROVED DEC 06, 1985
CYCLOPHOSPHAMIDE INJECTABLE; INJECTION	20 MG/ML (250 ML/CONTAINER)	88 P-0379/CP	BAXTER	NEW DOSAGE FORM NEW STRENGTH	APPROVED MAR 01, 1989
CYCLOPHOSPHAMIDE INJECTABLE; INJECTION	20 MG/ML (500 ML/CONTAINER)	88 P-0011/CP	BAXTER	NEW DOSAGE FORM	APPROVED JUN 10, 1988
CYCLOPHOSPHAMIDE INJECTABLE; INJECTION	100 MG/VIAL	90 P-0250/CP1	PHARMA-CHEMIE	NEW DOSAGE FORM	APPROVED MAY 07, 1991
CYCLOPHOSPHAMIDE INJECTABLE; INJECTION	200 MG/VIAL	90 P-0250/CP2	PHARMA-CHEMIE	NEW DOSAGE FORM	APPROVED MAY 07, 1991
CYCLOPHOSPHAMIDE INJECTABLE; INJECTION	500 MG/VIAL	90 P-0250/CP3	PHARMA-CHEMIE	NEW DOSAGE FORM	APPROVED MAY 07, 1991
CYCLOPHOSPHAMIDE INJECTABLE; INJECTION	1 GM/VIAL	90 P-0250/CP4	PHARMA-CHEMIE	NEW DOSAGE FORM	APPROVED MAY 07, 1991
CYTARABINE INJECTABLE; INJECTION	20 MG/ML (5 ML/VIAL)	86 P-0130/CP	QUAD	NEW DOSAGE FORM	APPROVED AUG 21, 1986
CYTARABINE INJECTABLE; INJECTION	20 MG/ML (12.5 ML/VIAL)	92 P-0381/CP1	BRISTOL MYERS SQUIBB	NEW DOSAGE FORM NEW STRENGTH	APPROVED MAR 18, 1993
CYTARABINE INJECTABLE; INJECTION	20 MG/ML (25 ML/VIAL)	86 P-0130/CP	QUAD	NEW DOSAGE FORM	APPROVED AUG 21, 1986
CYTARABINE INJECTABLE; INJECTION	20 MG/ML (50 ML/CONTAINER)	86 P-0428/CP0002	ADRIA	NEW DOSAGE FORM NEW STRENGTH	APPROVED MAY 07, 1987
CYTARABINE INJECTABLE; INJECTION	20 MG/ML (100 ML/CONTAINER)	86 P-0428/CP0005	ADRIA	NEW DOSAGE FORM	APPROVED OCT 28, 1991
CYTARABINE INJECTABLE; INJECTION	1 GM/VIAL	86 P-0313/CP	QUAD	NEW STRENGTH	APPROVED MAY 07, 1987
DESONIDE LOTION; TOPICAL	0.05%	87 P-0105/CP	OWEN	NEW DOSAGE FORM	APPROVED SEP 10, 1987

ANDA SUITABILITY PETITIONS

PETITIONS APPROVED *(continued)*

DRUG NAME DOSAGE FORM; ROUTE	STRENGTH (CONTAINER SIZE)	DOCKET NUMBER	PETITIONER	REASON FOR PETITION	STATUS
DEXBROMPHENIRAMINE MALEATE; PHENYLPROPANOLAMINE HYDROCHLORIDE CAPSULE, EXTENDED RELEASE; ORAL	6 MG 75 MG	85 P-0238/ CP0002	BOCK PHARMA	NEW COMBINATION	APPROVED DEC 13, 1985
DEXBROMPHENIRAMINE MALEATE; PHENYLPROPANOLAMINE HYDROCHLORIDE CAPSULE, EXTENDED RELEASE; ORAL	6 MG 75 MG	87 P-0265/CP	BOCK PHARMA	NEW COMBINATION NEW DOSAGE FORM	APPROVED NOV 04, 1987
DEXBROMPHENIRAMINE MALEATE; PSEUDOEPHEDRINE HYDROCHLORIDE CAPSULE, EXTENDED RELEASE; ORAL	6 MG 120 MG	85 P-0140/CP	CENTRAL PHARMS	NEW COMBINATION NEW DOSAGE FORM	APPROVED DEC 13, 1985
DEXBROMPHENIRAMINE MALEATE; PSEUDOEPHEDRINE SULFATE CAPSULE, EXTENDED RELEASE; ORAL	6 MG 120 MG	85 P-0140/ CP0002	CENTRAL PHARMS	NEW DOSAGE FORM	APPROVED JAN 22, 1986
DEXTROMETHORPHAN POLISTIREX SUSPENSION, EXTENDED RELEASE; ORAL	EQ 15 MG HBR/5 ML	87 P-0088/CP	KING AND SPAULDING	NEW STRENGTH	APPROVED APR 27, 1987
DIAZEPAM INTENSOL SOLUTION (CONCENTRATE); ORAL	5 MG/ML	85 P-0566/CP	ROXANE	NEW DOSAGE FORM	APPROVED MAR 18, 1986
DIAZEPAM SYRUP; ORAL	2 MG/5 ML	85 P-0499/CP	CAROLINA MEDCL	NEW DOSAGE FORM	APPROVED FEB 28, 1986
DIPHENHYDRAMINE HYDROCHLORIDE CONCENTRATE; ORAL	50 MG/ML	84 P-0174/CP	ROXANE	NEW STRENGTH	APPROVED SEP 11, 1985
DISOPYRAMIDE PHOSPHATE TABLET, EXTENDED RELEASE; ORAL	200 MG 300 MG	84 N-0116/CP	BIOCRAFT	NEW DOSAGE FORM NEW STRENGTH	APPROVED JUN 03, 1986
DISULFIRAM SUSPENSION; ORAL	500 MG/30 ML	85 P-0215/CP	PADDOCK	NEW DOSAGE FORM	APPROVED OCT 08, 1985
DOBUTAMINE HYDOCHLORIDE INJECTABLE; INJECTION	EQ 12.5 MG BASE/ML (40 ML/VIAL)	92 P-0365/ CP1	LYPHOMED	NEW STRENGTH	APPROVED FEB 11, 1993
DOBUTAMINE HYDROCHLORIDE INJECTABLE; INJECTION	EQ 12.5 MG BASE/ML (100 ML/CONTAINER)	93 P-0045/CP1	MARSAM	NEW STRENGTH	APPROVED SEP 10, 1993
DOPAMINE HYDROCHLORIDE INJECTABLE; INJECTION	5 MG/ML	90 P-0137/ CP1	ABBOTT	NEW STRENGTH	APPROVED APR 10, 1991
ESTRADIOL FILM, EXTENDED RELEASE; TRANSDERMAL	0.067 MG/24 HR	90 P-0125/ CP1	NOVEN PHARMS	NEW STRENGTH	APPROVED MAR 14, 1991
ESTRADIOL FILM, EXTENDED RELEASE; TRANSDERMAL	0.084 MG/24 HR	90 P-0125/ CP2	NOVEN PHARMS	NEW STRENGTH	APPROVED MAR 14, 1991
ESTRADIOL TABLET; ORAL	0.5 MG	84 P-0308/CP	KEY PHARMS	NEW STRENGTH	APPROVED MAR 24, 1986
ESTRADIOL TABLET; ORAL	1.5 MG	93 P-0344/CP1	BRISTOL MYERS SQUIBB	NEW STRENGTH	APPROVED JUN 08, 1994
ETOPOSIDE INJECTABLE; INJECTION	20 MG/ML (12.5 MG/VIAL)	92 P-0355/ CP1	LEDERLE	NEW STRENGTH	APPROVED JAN 07, 1993

ANDA SUITABILITY PETITIONS

PETITIONS APPROVED (continued)

DRUG NAME DOSAGE FORM; ROUTE	STRENGTH (CONTAINER SIZE)	DOCKET NUMBER	PETITIONER	REASON FOR PETITION	STATUS
ETOPOSIDE INJECTABLE; INJECTION	20 MG/ML (25 ML/VIAL)	91 P-0041/ CP1	ADRIA	NEW STRENGTH	APPROVED MAY 22, 1991
ETOPOSIDE INJECTABLE; INJECTION	20 MG/ML (50 ML/CONTAINER)	91 P-0460/ CP1	ABBOTT	NEW STRENGTH	APPROVED FEB 11, 1993
FENOPROFEN CALCIUM TABLET; ORAL	EQ 200 MG BASE EQ 300 MG BASE	87 P-0133/CP	BARR	NEW STRENGTH	APPROVED AUG 04, 1987
FLOXURIDINE INJECTABLE; INJECTION	100 MG/ML	86 P-0242/CP	QUAD	NEW DOSAGE FORM	APPROVED AUG 15, 1986
FLUOCINONIDE LOTION; TOPICAL	0.05%	87 P-0004/CP	HAMER	NEW DOSAGE FORM	APPROVED SEP 10, 1987
FLUOROURACIL INJECTABLE; INJECTION	25 MG/ML	85 P-0208/CP	INTL PHARM	NEW STRENGTH	APPROVED OCT 08, 1985
FLUOROURACIL INJECTABLE; INJECTION	50 MG/ML (5 ML/VIAL)	88 P-0052/CP	BEN VENUE	NEW STRENGTH	APPROVED MAR 21, 1988
FLUOROURACIL INJECTABLE; INJECTION	50 MG/ML (20 ML/VIAL)	86 P-0080/CP	BEN VENUE	NEW STRENGTH	APPROVED APR 02, 1986
FLUOROURACIL INJECTABLE; INJECTION	50 MG/ML (50 ML/VIAL)	86 P-0490/CP	ADRIA	NEW STRENGTH	APPROVED JAN 09, 1987
FLUOROURACIL INJECTABLE; INJECTION	50 MG/ML (100 ML/VIAL)	85 P-0221/CP	LYPHOMED	NEW STRENGTH	APPROVED FEB 18, 1986
FLUOROURACIL INJECTABLE; INJECTION	50 MG/ML (250 ML/VIAL)	88 P-0146/CP	BAXTER	NEW STRENGTH	APPROVED JUN 10, 1988
FLURAZEPAM HYDROCHLO-RIDE CONCENTRATE; ORAL	30 MG/ML	85 P-0081/CP	ROXANE	NEW DOSAGE FORM	APPROVED JUL 10, 1985
FLURAZEPAM HYDROCHLO-RIDE SOLUTION; ORAL	15 MG/5 ML	85 P-0091/CP	ROXANE	NEW DOSAGE FORM	APPROVED OCT 25, 1985
FUROSEMIDE CONCENTRATE; ORAL	80 MG/ML	85 P-0106/CP	ROXANE	NEW STRENGTH	APPROVED SEP 19, 1985
FUROSEMIDE SOLUTION; ORAL	40 MG/5 ML	85 P-0106/ CP0002	ROXANE	NEW STRENGTH	APPROVED SEP 19, 1985
GLUCAGON HYDROCHLORIDE INJECTABLE; INJECTION	EQ 2 MG BASE/VIAL	86 P-0411/CP	KING AND SPAULDING	NEW STRENGTH	APPROVED OCT 30, 1986
HALOPERIDOL CONCENTRATE; ORAL	EQ 0.5 MG/5 ML	89 P-0088/CP	UDL	NEW STRENGTH	APPROVED MAY 11, 1989
HALOPERIDOL DECANOATE INJECTABLE; INJECTION	EQ 50 MG BASE/ML (2 ML/CONTAINER)	88 P-0411/CP	QUAD	NEW STRENGTH	APPROVED FEB 13, 1989
HALOPERIDOL LACTATE SOLUTION; ORAL	EQ 2 MG BASE/5 ML	85 P-0076/ CP0002	ROXANE	NEW STRENGTH	APPROVED MAR 28, 1986
HALOPERIDOL LACTATE SOLUTION; ORAL	EQ 5 MG BASE/5 ML	85 P-0080/CP	ROXANE	NEW DOSAGE FORM	APPROVED SEP 19, 1985
HALOPERIDOL LACTATE IN-TENSOL CONCENTRATE; ORAL	EQ 5 MG BASE/ML	85 P-0076/CP	ROXANE	NEW STRENGTH	APPROVED DEC 08, 1986
HOMATROPINE METHYLBROM-IDE; HYDROCODONE BITARTRATE SOFT GELATIN CAPSULE; ORAL	1.5 MG 5 MG	88 P-0061/CP	KLEINFELD, KAPLAN AND BECKER	NEW DOSAGE FORM	APPROVED MAY 12, 1988
HYDRALAZINE HYDROCHLO-RIDE SOLUTION; ORAL	25 MG/5 ML	85 P-0074/CP	ROXANE	NEW DOSAGE FORM	APPROVED JUL 03, 1985
HYDROCHLOROTHIAZIDE; PROPRANOLOL HYDROCHLO-RIDE SOLUTION; ORAL	25 MG/5 ML 40 MG/5 ML	87 P-0399/CP	BURDITT, BOWLES, RADZIUS AND RUBERRY	NEW DOSAGE FORM	APPROVED FEB 16, 1988

ANDA SUITABILITY PETITIONS

PETITIONS APPROVED *(continued)*

DRUG NAME DOSAGE FORM; ROUTE	STRENGTH (CONTAINER SIZE)	DOCKET NUMBER	PETITIONER	REASON FOR PETITION	STATUS
HYDROCHLOROTHIAZIDE; PROPRANOLOL HYDROCHLORIDE SOLUTION; ORAL	25 MG/5 ML 80 MG/5 ML	87 P-0399/CP	BURDITT, BOWLES, RADZIUS AND RUBERRY	NEW DOSAGE FORM	APPROVED FEB 16, 1988
HYDROCHLOROTHIAZIDE; TRIAMTERENE CAPSULE; ORAL	50 MG 75 MG	86 P-0427/CP	PAR	NEW DOSAGE FORM	APPROVED DEC 11, 1986
HYDROCHLOROTHIAZIDE; TRIAMTERENE TABLET; ORAL	25 MG 50 MG	87 P-0335/CP	PAR	NEW DOSAGE FORM	APPROVED FEB 26, 1988
HYDROCORTISONE SOLUTION; TOPICAL	2.5%	89 P-0175/CP	GENDERM	NEW STRENGTH	APPROVED JAN 11, 1990
HYDROCORTISONE ACETATE AEROSOL; TOPICAL	2.5%	92 P-0101/CP1	HOGAN & HARTSON	NEW DOSAGE FORM	APPROVED JUL 08, 1992
HYDROCORTISONE ACETATE CREAM; TOPICAL	2.5%	90 P-0049/CP	FERNDALE	NEW STRENGTH	APPROVED JUN 22, 1990
HYDROCORTISONE ACETATE LOTION; TOPICAL	1%	90 P-0049/CP	FERNDALE	NEW DOSAGE FORM	APPROVED JUN 22, 1990
HYDROCORTISONE ACETATE LOTION; TOPICAL	2.5%	90 P-0049/CP	FERNDALE	NEW DOSAGE FORM	APPROVED JUN 22, 1990
HYDROCORTISONE ACETATE OINTMENT; TOPICAL	1%	90 P-0154/CP1	FERNDALE	NEW DOSAGE FORM	APPROVED DEC 07, 1990
HYDROCORTISONE VALERATE LOTION; TOPICAL	0.2%	89 P-0028/CP	MCKENNA, CONNER & CUNEO	NEW DOSAGE FORM	APPROVED MAY 10, 1989
HYDROCORTISONE VALERATE SOLUTION; TOPICAL	0.2%	89 P-0029/CP	MCKENNA, CONNER & CUNEO	NEW DOSAGE FORM	APPROVED MAY 10, 1989
IBUPROFEN CAPSULE; ORAL	200 MG	84 P-0383/CP	STERLING	NEW DOSAGE FORM	APPROVED JUN 25, 1985
IBUPROFEN SOFT GELATIN CAPSULE; ORAL	200 MG	87 P-0232/CP	SIDMAK	NEW DOSAGE FORM	APPROVED OCT 06, 1987
IBUPROFEN SOFT GELATIN CAPSULE; ORAL	300 MG 400 MG 600 MG	85 P-0563/CP	SOFTAN	NEW DOSAGE FORM	APPROVED MAR 19, 1986
IBUPROFEN SOFT GELATIN CAPSULE; ORAL	800 MG	87 P-0242/CP	SIDMAK	NEW DOSAGE FORM	APPROVED OCT 06, 1987
ISONIAZID CONCENTRATE; ORAL	50 MG/ML	85 P-0468/CP	CAROLINA MEDCL	NEW STRENGTH	APPROVED DEC 13, 1985
ISOSORBIDE DINITRATE TABLET, EXTENDED RELEASE; ORAL	60 MG	89 P-0485/CP	ADRIA	NEW STRENGTH	APPROVED JUN 01, 1990
LACTULOSE CRYSTAL; ORAL	10 GM/PACKET	92 P-0370/CP1	BENNETT AND COMPANY	NEW DOSAGE FORM	APPROVED JAN 07, 1993
LEUCOVORIN CALCIUM INJECTABLE; INJECTION	EQ 1 MG BASE/ML	86 P-0149/CP	ROXANE	NEW DOSAGE FORM	APPROVED JUL 25, 1988
LEUCOVORIN CALCIUM INJECTABLE; INJECTION	EQ 5 MG BASE/ML (10 ML/VIAL)	86 P-0241/CP	QUAD	NEW STRENGTH	APPROVED JUL 28, 1987
LEUCOVORIN CALCIUM INJECTABLE; INJECTION	EQ 5 MG BASE/ML (20 ML/VIAL)	86 P-0241/CP	QUAD	NEW STRENGTH	APPROVED JUL 28, 1987
LEUCOVORIN CALCIUM INJECTABLE; INJECTION	EQ 200 MG BASE/VIAL	91 P-0235/CP1	CETUS	NEW STRENGTH	APPROVED DEC 10, 1991
LOPERAMIDE HYDROCHLORIDE TABLET; EFFERVESCENT; ORAL	1 MG	93 P-0332/CP1	ELLIS PHARM CONSULTING	NEW DOSAGE FORM	APPROVED FEB 08, 1994

ANDA SUITABILITY PETITIONS

PETITIONS APPROVED *(continued)*

DRUG NAME DOSAGE FORM; ROUTE	STRENGTH (CONTAINER SIZE)	DOCKET NUMBER	PETITIONER	REASON FOR PETITION	STATUS
LOPERAMIDE HYDROCHLO- RIDE TABLET; ORAL	2 MG	87 P-0268/CP	KROSS	NEW DOSAGE FORM	APPROVED OCT 06, 1987
LORAZEPAM SOFT GELATIN CAPSULE; ORAL	0.5 MG 1 MG 2 MG	87 P-0037/CP	APPLIED LABS	NEW DOSAGE FORM	APPROVED MAR 10, 1987
LORAZEPAM SOLUTION; ORAL	1 MG/5 ML	86 P-0292/CP	ROXANE	NEW DOSAGE FORM	APPROVED OCT 15, 1986
LORAZEPAM SOLUTION (CONCENTRATE); ORAL	2 MG/ML	86 P-0291/CP	ROXANE	NEW DOSAGE FORM	APPROVED OCT 15, 1986
LORAZEPAM TABLET; ORAL	0.5 MG 1 MG 2 MG	85 P-0515/CP	WYETH AYERST	NEW DOSAGE FORM	APPROVED FEB 25, 1986
MEPERIDINE HYDROCHLO- RIDE CONCENTRATE; ORAL	100 MG/ML	84 P-0175/CP	ROXANE	NEW STRENGTH	APPROVED JUN 07, 1985
MEPERIDINE HYDROCHLO- RIDE INJECTABLE; INJECTION	10 MG/ML (50 ML/CONTAINER)	88 P-0008/CP	LYPHOMED	NEW STRENGTH	APPROVED APR 01, 1988
METHYLDOPATE HYDROCHLO- RIDE IN DEXTROSE 5% INJECTABLE; INJECTION	2.5 MG/ML (100 ML/CONTAINER)	86 P-0410/ CP0002	KING AND SPAULDING	NEW STRENGTH	APPROVED MAR 10, 1987
METHYLDOPATE HYDROCHLO- RIDE IN DEXTROSE 5% INJECTABLE; INJECTION	5 MG/ML (100 ML/CONTAINER)	86 P-0410/ CP0003	KING AND SPAULDING	NEW STRENGTH	APPROVED MAR 10, 1987
METHYLPHENIDATE HYDRO- CHLORIDE TABLET, EXTENDED RELEASE; ORAL	10 MG	92 P-0400/ CP1	MD PHARM	NEW STRENGTH	APPROVED MAR 22, 1993
METHYLTESTOSTERONE CAPSULE; ORAL	25 MG	85 P-0067/CP	STAR PHARMS	NEW DOSAGE FORM	APPROVED AUG 23, 1985
METHYLTESTOSTERONE CAPSULE; ORAL	25 MG	93 P-0459/CP1	ICN	NEW DOSAGE FORM	APPROVED JUN 08, 1994
METOCLOPRAMIDE HYDRO- CHLORIDE INJECTABLE; INJECTION	5 MG/ML (20 ML/VIAL)	86 P-0036/CP	DUPONT	NEW STRENGTH	APPROVED MAR 18, 1986
METOCLOPRAMIDE HYDRO- CHLORIDE INJECTABLE; INJECTION	5 MG/ML (50 ML/VIAL)	85 P-0545/CP	LYPHOMED	NEW STRENGTH	APPROVED FEB 28, 1986
METOCLOPRAMIDE HYDRO- CHLORIDE INJECTABLE; INJECTION	5 MG/ML (50 ML/VIAL) (100 ML/VIAL)	85 P-0540/CP	QUAD	NEW STRENGTH	APPROVED FEB 28, 1986
METOCLOPRAMIDE HYDRO- CHLORIDE INTENSOL CONCENTRATE; ORAL	10 MG/ML	88 P-0164/CP	ROXANE	NEW STRENGTH	APPROVED JUN 28, 1988
MICONAZOLE NITRATE CREAM; VAGINAL	4%	84 P-0398/CP	RW JOHNSON	NEW STRENGTH	APPROVED MAR 31, 1986
MORPHINE SULFATE CAPSULE, EXTENDED RE- LEASE; ORAL	15 MG 60 MG 100 MG	93 P-0446/CP1	PHARMA CONSULT	NEW DOSAGE FORM	APPROVED JUN 08, 1994
MORPHINE SULFATE CAPSULE, EXTENDED RE- LEASE; ORAL	30 MG	89 P-0071/CP	OXFORD RES INTL	NEW DOSAGE FORM	APPROVED MAY 10, 1989
NALBUPHINE HYDROCHLO- RIDE INJECTABLE; INJECTION	10 MG/ML (2 ML/CONTAINER)	92 P-0224/CP	STERLING	NEW STRENGTH	APPROVED SEP 11, 1992
NIFEDIPINE CAPSULE, EXTENDED RELEASE; ORAL	30 MG 60 MG 90 MG	90 P-0436/CP1	KV	NEW DOSAGE FORM	APPROVED OCT 23, 1991

ANDA SUITABILITY PETITIONS

PETITIONS APPROVED *(continued)*

DRUG NAME DOSAGE FORM; ROUTE	STRENGTH (CONTAINER SIZE)	DOCKET NUMBER	PETITIONER	REASON FOR PETITION	STATUS
NIFEDIPINE TABLET; ORAL	10 MG 20 MG	87 P-0340/CP	PAR	NEW DOSAGE FORM	APPROVED DEC 11, 1987
NITROGLYCERIN IN DEXTROSE 5% INJECTABLE; INJECTION	0.5 MG/ML (100 ML/CONTAINER)	86 P-0099/ CP0004	ABBOTT	NEW STRENGTH	APPROVED FEB 02, 1987
NITROGLYCERIN IN DEXTROSE 5% INJECTABLE; INJECTION	100 MCG/ML (50 ML/CONTAINER)	91 P-0387/CP1	ABBOTT	NEW STRENGTH	APPROVED FEB 18, 1992
NITROGLYCERIN IN DEXTROSE 5% INJECTABLE; INJECTION	100 MCG/ML (100 ML/CONTAINER)	91 P-0387/CP1	ABBOTT	NEW STRENGTH	APPROVED FEB 18, 1992
NITROGLYCERIN IN DEXTROSE 5% INJECTABLE; INJECTION	10 MG/100 ML (500 ML/CONTAINER)	86 P-0099/CP	ABBOTT	NEW STRENGTH	APPROVED APR 01, 1986
NITROGLYCERIN IN DEXTROSE 5% INJECTABLE; INJECTION	40 MG/100 ML (500 ML/CONTAINER)	86 P-0099/ CP0003	ABBOTT	NEW STRENGTH	APPROVED APR 01, 1986
NITROGLYCERIN IN DEXTROSE 5% INJECTABLE; INJECTION	0.05 MG/ML (500 ML/CONTAINER)	89 P-0422/CP	LYPHOMED	NEW STRENGTH	APPROVED APR 20, 1990
NITROGLYCERIN IN DEXTROSE 5% INJECTABLE; INJECTION	0.2 MG/ML (500 ML/CONTAINER)	89 P-0422/CP	LYPHOMED	NEW STRENGTH	APPROVED APR 20, 1990
NITROGLYCERIN OINTMENT; TOPICAL	4%	87 P-0184/CP	FOREST	NEW STRENGTH	APPROVED SEP 15, 1987
OXAZEPAM TABLET; ORAL	15 MG 30 MG	85 P-0516/CP	WYETH AYERST	NEW DOSAGE FORM	APPROVED FEB 25, 1986
PANCURONIUM BROMIDE INJECTABLE; INJECTION	0.1 MG/ML	91 P-0006/ CP1	LYPHOMED	NEW STRENGTH	APPROVED OCT 28, 1991
PENTAMIDINE ISETHIONATE INJECTABLE; INJECTION	100 MG/ML (3 ML/VIAL)	89 P-0435/CP	ASTRA	NEW DOSAGE FORM	APPROVED JAN 18, 1990
PENTETATE PENTASODIUM; STANNOUS CHLORIDE (TECHNETIUM TC-99M PENTETATE KIT) INJECTABLE; INJECTION	10 MG 0.55 MG	89 P-0113/CP	CADEMA MED PRODS	NEW STRENGTH	APPROVED JUL 14, 1989
PHENYTOIN SODIUM INJECTABLE; INJECTION	100 MG/VIAL 250 MG/VIAL	87 P-0367/CP	LYPHOMED	NEW DOSAGE FORM	APPROVED FEB 16, 1988
POLYETHYLENE GLYCOL 3350; POTASSIUM CHLORIDE; SODIUM BICARBONATE; SODIUM CHLORIDE; SODIUM SULFATE IN PLASTIC CONTAINER POWDER FOR RECONSTITUTION; ORAL	59 GM/PACKET 0.7425 GM/PACKET 1.685 GM/PACKET 1.465 GM/PACKET 5.685 GM/PACKET	88 P-0419/CP	GUIDELINES	NEW STRENGTH	APPROVED MAR 01, 1989
PREDNISOLONE SYRUP; ORAL	10 MG/5 ML	92 P-0439/ CP1	WE PHARMS	NEW STRENGTH	APPROVED MAY 20, 1993
PREDNISOLONE SODIUM PHOSPHATE SOLUTION; ORAL	EQ 5 MG BASE/ML	88 P-0235/CP	PAN AM PHARMS	NEW STRENGTH	APPROVED AUG 24, 1988
PREDNISOLONE SODIUM PHOSPHATE SOLUTION; ORAL	EQ 15 MG BASE/5 ML	87 P-0235/CP	FISONS	NEW STRENGTH	APPROVED NOV 04, 1987
PREDNISONE CAPSULE; ORAL	1 MG 2.5 MG 5 MG 10 MG 20 MG 25 MG 50 MG	88 P-0391/CP	ASCHER	NEW DOSAGE FORM	APPROVED MAR 01, 1989

ANDA SUITABILITY PETITIONS

PETITIONS APPROVED *(continued)*

DRUG NAME DOSAGE FORM; ROUTE	STRENGTH (CONTAINER SIZE)	DOCKET NUMBER	PETITIONER	REASON FOR PETITION	STATUS
PREDNISONE TABLET, CHEWABLE; ORAL	1 MG 2.5 MG 20 MG 50 MG	93 P-0333/CP1	DURA	NEW DOSAGE FORM	APPROVED JUN 08, 1994
PREDNISONE TABLET, CHEWABLE; ORAL	1 MG 5 MG 10 MG	92 P-0336/CP1	WE PHARMS	NEW DOSAGE FORM	APPROVED NOV 10, 1993
PROBUCOL TABLET; ORAL	500 MG	85 P-0337/CP	MERRELL DOW	NEW STRENGTH	APPROVED OCT 25, 1985
PROCAINAMIDE HYDROCHLORIDE TABLET, EXTENDED RELEASE; ORAL	375 MG	85 P-0125/CP	KEY PHARMS	NEW STRENGTH	APPROVED SEP 19, 1985
PROMETHAZINE HYDROCHLORIDE INJECTABLE; INJECTION	25 MG/ML (2 ML/VIAL)	87 P-0087/CP	LYPHOMED	NEW STRENGTH	APPROVED MAY 01, 1987
PROMETHAZINE HYDROCHLORIDE INJECTABLE; INJECTION	50 MG/ML (2 ML/VIAL)	87 P-0087/ CP0002	LYPHOMED	NEW STRENGTH	APPROVED MAY 01, 1987
PROPRANOLOL HYDROCHLORIDE CAPSULE; ORAL	10 MG 20 MG 40 MG 60 MG 80 MG 90 MG	86 P-0045/CP	NUTRIPHARM LABS	NEW DOSAGE FORM	APPROVED MAR 19, 1986
PROPRANOLOL HYDROCHLORIDE TABLET, EFFERVESCENT; ORAL	10 MG 20 MG 60 MG 80 MG 90 MG	93 P-0049/CP1	FLEMINGTON PHARM	NEW DOSAGE FORM NEW STRENGTH	APPROVED SEP 01, 1993
PROPRANOLOL HYDROCHLORIDE TABLET, EFFERVESCENT; ORAL	40 MG	92 P-0332/ CP1	FLEMINGTON PHARM	NEW DOSAGE FORM	APPROVED NOV 25, 1992
PROPRANOLOL HYDROCHLORIDE TABLET, EXTENDED RELEASE; ORAL	80 MG 120 MG 160 MG	85 P-0197/CP	FOREST	NEW DOSAGE FORM	APPROVED SEP 27, 1985
PROPRANOLOL HYDROCHLORIDE TABLET, EXTENDED RELEASE; ORAL	160 MG	85 P-0129/CP	VEREX LABS	NEW DOSAGE FORM	APPROVED SEP 25, 1985
PROTIRELIN INJECTABLE; INJECTION	0.2 MG/ML	90 P-0214/ CP1	FERRING	NEW STRENGTH	APPROVED DEC 21, 1990
PSEUDOEPHEDRINE HYDROCHLORIDE TABLET, EXTENDED RELEASE; ORAL	120 MG	87 P-0297/CP	HLTH PLCY NTWK	NEW DOSAGE FORM	APPROVED NOV 03, 1987
PSEUDOEPHEDRINE HYDROCHLORIDE; TERFENADINE CAPSULE, EXTENDED RELEASE; ORAL	120 MG 60 MG	93 P-0367/CP1	EURAND AMERICA	NEW DOSAGE FORM	APPROVED FEB 08, 1994
PSEUDOEPHEDRINE HYDROCHLORIDE; TRIPROLIDINE HYDROCHLORIDE TABLET, EXTENDED RELEASE; ORAL	120 MG 5 MG	87 P-0296/CP	HLTH PLCY NTWK	NEW DOSAGE FORM	APPROVED NOV 03, 1987
QUINIDINE GLUCONATE TABLET, EXTENDED RELEASE; ORAL	648 MG	87 P-0276/CP	FOREST	NEW STRENGTH	APPROVED NOV 22, 1988

ANDA SUITABILITY PETITIONS

PETITIONS APPROVED *(continued)*

DRUG NAME DOSAGE FORM; ROUTE	STRENGTH (CONTAINER SIZE)	DOCKET NUMBER	PETITIONER	REASON FOR PETITION	STATUS
QUINIDINE SULFATE CAPSULE, EXTENDED RE- LEASE; ORAL	300 MG	88 P-0277/CP	ROBINS	NEW DOSAGE FORM	APPROVED DEC 13, 1988
RITODRINE HYDROCHLORIDE IN DEXTROSE 5% INJECTABLE; INJECTION	30 MG/100 ML (500 ML/CONTAINER)	86 P-0100/CP	ABBOTT	NEW STRENGTH	APPROVED MAY 07, 1986
SCOPOLAMINE TRANSDERMAL SYSTEM/24 HOUR FILM, EXTENDED RELEASE; PERCUTANEOUS	1 MG	85 P-0168/CP	CIBA	NEW STRENGTH (DOSING INTERVAL)	APPROVED SEP 27, 1985
SODIUM CHLORIDE 0.9% IN PLASTIC CONTAINER INJECTABLE; INJECTION	900 MG/100 ML (100 ML/VIAL)	87 P-0391/CP	LYPHOMED	NEW STRENGTH	APPROVED AUG 11, 1988
SODIUM NITROPRUSSIDE INJECTABLE; INJECTION	0.5 MG/ML	90 P-0179/ CP1	ABBOTT	NEW STRENGTH	APPROVED DEC 21, 1990
SPIRONOLACTONE SUSPENSION; ORAL	25 MG/5 ML	86 P-0055/CP	CAROLINA MEDCL	NEW DOSAGE FORM	APPROVED MAR 28, 1986
SPIRONOLACTONE SYRUP; ORAL	25 MG/5 ML	85 P-0510/CP	CAROLINA MEDCL	NEW DOSAGE FORM	APPROVED JAN 22, 1986
STERILE WATER IN PLASTIC CONTAINER INJECTABLE; INJECTION	100% (100 ML/CONTAINER)	87 P-0392/CP	LYPHOMED	NEW STRENGTH	APPROVED AUG 11, 1988
TAMOXIFEN CITRATE TABLET; ORAL	EQ 20 MG BASE	92 P-0269/ CP1	KROSS	NEW STRENGTH	APPROVED OCT 26, 1992
TECHNETIUM TC99 MEDRONATE KIT INJECTABLE: INJECTION	N/A	91 P-0040/CP1	ABARIS	NEW STRENGTH	APPROVED OCT 28, 1991
TERBUTALINE SULFATE INJECTABLE; INJECTION	1 MG (0.25 ML/CONTAINER)	92 P-0430/CP1	STERLING WINTHROP	NEW STRENGTH	APPROVED MAR 18, 1993
TERFENADINE CAPSULE: ORAL	60 MG	91 P-0087/CP1	ARTHUR A. CHECCHI	NEW DOSAGE FORM	APPROVED OCT 28, 1991
THEOPHYLLINE CAPSULE; ORAL	150 MG 300 MG	85 P-0175/CP	MEAD JOHNSON	NEW STRENGTH	APPROVED OCT 08, 1985
THEOPHYLLINE CAPSULE, EXTENDED RE- LEASE; ORAL	400 MG	86 P-0471/ CP0002	SEARLE	NEW STRENGTH	APPROVED MAR 10, 1987
THEOPHYLLINE CAPSULE, EXTENDED RE- LEASE; ORAL	450 MG	88 P-0119/CP	RIKER LABS	NEW STRENGTH	APPROVED MAY 11, 1988
THEOPHYLLINE CAPSULE, EXTENDED RE- LEASE; ORAL	500 MG	88 P-0226/CP	SAVAGE	NEW STRENGTH	APPROVED AUG 25, 1988
THEOPHYLLINE SOLUTION; ORAL	160 MG/15 ML	88 P-0301/CP	FLEMING	NEW STRENGTH	APPROVED NOV 04, 1988
THEOPHYLLINE TABLET; ORAL	150 MG	89 P-0499/CP	SCI CONSULTING	NEW STRENGTH	APPROVED MAY 03, 1990
THEOPHYLLINE TABLET, EXTENDED RELEASE; ORAL	600 MG	85 P-0580/CP	PURDUE FREDERICK	NEW STRENGTH	APPROVED OCT 24, 1986
THEOPHYLLINE TABLET, EXTENDED RELEASE; ORAL	800 MG	91 P-0209/CP1	PURDUE FREDERICK	NEW STRENGTH	APPROVED DEC 10, 1991
THIOTEPA, STERILE INJECTABLE; INJECTION	30 MG/VIAL 60 MG/VIAL	88 P-0412/CP	QUAD	NEW STRENGTH	APPROVED MAR 01, 1989
THIOTEPA, STERILE (WITH DILUENT) INJECTABLE; INJECTION	15 MG/VIAL	87 P-0382/CP	LYPHOMED	NEW DOSAGE FORM	APPROVED MAY 12, 1988

ANDA SUITABILITY PETITIONS

PETITIONS APPROVED *(continued)*

DRUG NAME DOSAGE FORM; ROUTE	STRENGTH (CONTAINER SIZE)	DOCKET NUMBER	PETITIONER	REASON FOR PETITION	STATUS
THIOTHIXENE HYDROCHLORIDE SOLUTION; ORAL	5 MG/5 ML	86 P-0178/CP	ELLIS PHARM	NEW STRENGTH	APPROVED JUN 04, 1986
TOLMETIN SODIUM TABLET; ORAL	EQ 400 MG BASE	90 P-0011/CP	QUANTUM PHARMICS	NEW STRENGTH	APPROVED MAY 03, 1990
TRIAMCINOLONE ACETONIDE CREAM; TOPICAL	0.05%	86 P-0360/CP	CAROLINA MEDCL	NEW STRENGTH	APPROVED OCT 15, 1986
TRIAMCINOLONE ACETONIDE LOTION; TOPICAL	0.5%	87 P-0019/CP	HAMER	NEW STRENGTH	APPROVED SEP 11, 1987
TRIAMCINOLONE ACETONIDE OINTMENT; TOPICAL	0.05%	86 P-0360/CP	CAROLINA MEDCL	NEW STRENGTH	APPROVED OCT 15, 1986
TRIAZOLAM SOLUTION; ORAL	0.125 MG/5 ML	92 P-0048/ CP2	ROXANE	NEW DOSAGE FORM	APPROVED SEP 11, 1992
TRIMETHOPRIM SOLUTION; ORAL	25 MG/5 ML	92 P-0500/ CP1	ASCENT PHARMS	NEW DOSAGE FORM	APPROVED MAY 20, 1993
VERAPAMIL HYDROCHLORIDE CAPSULE, EXTENDED RELEASE; ORAL	120 MG 240 MG	87 P-0233/CP	SEARLE	NEW DOSAGE FORM NEW STRENGTH	APPROVED FEB 26, 1988
VERAPAMIL HYDROCHLORIDE SOLUTION; ORAL	40 MG/5 ML 80 MG/5 ML	87 P-0101/CP	PHARM BASICS	NEW DOSAGE FORM	APPROVED SEP 10, 1987
VERAPAMIL HYDROCHLORIDE TABLET, EXTENDED RELEASE; ORAL	120 MG	89 P-0220/CP	LEDERLE	NEW STRENGTH	APPROVED JAN 11, 1990
VINBLASTINE SULFATE INJECTABLE; INJECTION	1 MG/ML (10 ML/VIAL)	86 P-0056/CP	QUAD	NEW DOSAGE FORM	APPROVED MAR 28, 1986
VINBLASTINE SULFATE INJECTABLE; INJECTION	1 MG/ML (25 ML/VIAL)	87 P-0112/CP	QUAD	NEW DOSAGE FORM NEW STRENGTH	APPROVED JUN 08, 1987
VINBLASTINE SULFATE INJECTABLE; INJECTION	1 MG/ML (30 ML/VIAL)	87 P-0211/CP	LYPHOMED	NEW STRENGTH	APPROVED JUL 28, 1987
VINCRISTINE SULFATE INJECTABLE; INJECTION	1 MG/ML (1.5 ML/CONTAINER)	87 P-0210/CP	LYPHOMED	NEW STRENGTH	APPROVED JUL 28, 1987
XENON XE 133 GAS; INHALATION	150 MCI/VIAL 250 MCI/VIAL	86 P-0041/CP	MEDI NUCLR	NEW STRENGTH	APPROVED OCT 15, 1986
XENON XE 133 INJECTABLE; INJECTION	60 MCI/VIAL 150 MCI/VIAL	86 P-0342/CP	MEDI NUCLR	NEW STRENGTH	APPROVED SEP 11, 1987

ANDA SUITABILITY PETITIONS

PETITIONS DENIED

DRUG NAME DOSAGE FORM; ROUTE	STRENGTH (CONTAINER SIZE)	DOCKET NUMBER	PETITIONER	REASON FOR PETITION	STATUS
ACETAMINOPHEN; DIHYDROCODEINE BITARTRATE CAPSULE; ORAL	356.4 MG 20 MG	86 P-0040/CP	DUNHALL	NEW COMBINATION NEW STRENGTH	DENIED FEB 12, 1987
ACETAMINOPHEN; HYDROCODONE BITARTRATE TABLET; ORAL	650 MG 10 MG	85 P-0015/CP	APPLIED LABS	NEW STRENGTH	DENIED NOV 07, 1985
ACETAMINOPHEN; METHOCARBAMOL TABLET; ORAL	325 MG 400 MG	85 P-0102/CP	RW JOHNSON	NEW COMBINATION	DENIED JUN 24, 1986
ALBUTEROL SULFATE CAPSULE, EXTENDED RELEASE; ORAL	EQ 4 MG BASE	89 P-0207/CP	PARTICLE DYNAMICS	NEW DOSAGE FORM	DENIED DEC 13, 1991

ANDA SUITABILITY PETITIONS

PETITIONS DENIED *(continued)*

DRUG NAME DOSAGE FORM; ROUTE	STRENGTH (CONTAINER SIZE)	DOCKET NUMBER	PETITIONER	REASON FOR PETITION	STATUS
ALLOPURINOL SODIUM INJECTABLE; INJECTION	500 MG (30 ML/VIAL)	89 P-0103/CP	BURROUGHS WELLCOME	NEW DOSAGE FORM NEW INGREDIENT (NEW SALT) NEW ROUTE OF ADMINISTRA- TION	DENIED JUL 14, 1989
AMINOCAPROIC ACID INJECTABLE; INJECTION	500 MG/ML	85 P-0064/CP	JAMES E. MURRAY	NEW STRENGTH	DENIED MAY 29, 1985
AMINOPHYLLINE INJECTABLE; INJECTION	10 MG/ML 50 MG/ML	85 P-0066/CP	JAMES E. MURRAY	NEW STRENGTH	DENIED MAY 03, 1985
5-AMINOSALICYLIC ACID SUPPOSITORY; RECTAL	500 MG	84 P-0425/CP	REID ROWELL	NEW INGREDIENT	DENIED JUN 05, 1986
ASPIRIN; BUTALBITAL; CAFFEINE; CODEINE PHOSPHATE CAPSULE; ORAL	325 MG 50 MG 40 MG 7.5 MG	85 P-0101/CP	SANDOZ	NEW COMBINATION	DENIED SEP 11, 1985
ASPIRIN; BUTALBITAL; CAFFEINE; CODEINE PHOSPHATE CAPSULE; ORAL	325 MG 50 MG 40 MG 15 MG	85 P-0101/CP	SANDOZ	NEW COMBINATION	DENIED SEP 11, 1985
ASPIRIN; BUTALBITAL; CAFFEINE; CODEINE PHOSPHATE CAPSULE; ORAL	325 MG 50 MG 40 MG 30 MG	85 P-0101/CP	SANDOZ	NEW COMBINATION	DENIED SEP 11, 1985
ASPIRIN; BUTALBITAL; CAFFEINE; CODEINE PHOSPHATE CAPSULE; ORAL	325 MG 50 MG 40 MG 60 MG	85 P-0101/ CP0002	SANDOZ	NEW COMBINATION	DENIED SEP 11, 1985
ASPIRIN; CAFFEINE; HYDROCODONE BITARTRATE TABLET; ORAL	224 MG 32 MG 5 MG	86 P-0243/CP	MASON PHARMS	NEW COMBINATION NEW DOSAGE FORM NEW STRENGTH	DENIED JUN 12, 1987
ASPIRIN; CAFFEINE; HYDROCODONE BITARTRATE TABLET; ORAL	325 MG 30 MG 5 MG	85 P-0455/CP	CENTRAL PHARMS	NEW COMBINATION NEW DOSAGE FORM NEW STRENGTH	DENIED JUN 08, 1987
ASPIRIN; CAFFEINE; HYDROCODONE BITARTRATE TABLET; ORAL	356.4 MG 30 MG 5 MG	86 P-0243/ CP0002	MASON PHARMS	NEW COMBINATION NEW DOSAGE FORM	DENIED JUN 16, 1987
ASPIRIN; CHLORZOXAZONE TABLET; ORAL	325 MG 250 MG	85 P-0071/CP	RW JOHNSON	NEW COMBINATION	DENIED SEP 03, 1985
BENZOYL METRONIDAZOLE SUSPENSION; ORAL	200 MG/5 ML	85 P-0258/CP	APKON LABS	NEW INGREDIENT (NEW ESTER)	DENIED MAR 19, 1986
BETAMETHASONE DIPROPIONATE; MICONAZOLE NITRATE CREAM; TOPICAL	0.05% 2%	85 P-0271/CP	RW JOHNSON	NEW COMBINATION	DENIED APR 18, 1986
BRETYLIUM TOSYLATE INJECTABLE; INJECTION	2 MG/ML	85 P-0063/CP	MARK W. LOTZ	NEW STRENGTH	DENIED MAY 29, 1985

ANDA SUITABILITY PETITIONS

PETITIONS DENIED *(continued)*

DRUG NAME DOSAGE FORM; ROUTE	STRENGTH (CONTAINER SIZE)	DOCKET NUMBER	PETITIONER	REASON FOR PETITION	STATUS
BRETYLIUM TOSYLATE INJECTABLE; INJECTION	4 MG/ML	85 P-0063/ CP0002	MARK W. LOTZ	NEW STRENGTH	DENIED MAY 29, 1985
BRETYLIUM TOSYLATE INJECTABLE; INJECTION	8 MG/ML	85 P-0063/ CP0003	MARK W. LOTZ	NEW STRENGTH	DENIED MAY 29, 1985
BRETYLIUM TOSYLATE INJECTABLE; INJECTION	10 MG/ML	85 P-0063/ CP0004	MARK W. LOTZ	NEW STRENGTH	DENIED MAY 29, 1985
BROMDIPHENHYDRAMINE HYDROCHLORIDE; HYDROCODONE BITARTRATE SOLUTION; ORAL	12.5 MG/5 ML 2.5 MG/5 ML	85 P-0255/CP	MIKART	NEW COMBINATION	DENIED MAY 11, 1988
BROMDIPHENHYDRAMINE HYDROCHLORIDE; HYDROCODONE BITARTRATE SYRUP; ORAL	12.5 MG/5 ML 2.5 MG/5 ML	85 P-0255/CP	MIKART	NEW COMBINATION	DENIED MAY 11, 1988
BROMPHENIRAMINE MALEATE; HYDROCODONE BITARTRATE; PHENYLPROPANOLAMINE HYDROCHLORIDE SYRUP; ORAL	2 MG/5 ML 2.5 MG/5 ML 12.5 MG/5 ML	85 P-0237/CP	MIKART	NEW COMBINATION	DENIED MAY 11, 1988
CAFFEINE; ERGOTAMINE TARTRATE; PENTOBARBITAL SODIUM SUPPOSITORY; RECTAL	200 MG 2 MG 60 MG	85 P-0433/ CP0002	SANDOZ	NEW COMBINATION	DENIED NOV 08, 1985
CAFFEINE; ERGOTAMINE TARTRATE; PENTOBARBITAL SODIUM TABLET; ORAL	100 MG 1 MG 30 MG	85 P-0433/CP	SANDOZ	NEW COMBINATION	DENIED NOV 08, 1985
CHOLECALCIFEROL CAPSULE; ORAL	1.25 MG	84 P-0161/CP	PHARMACAPS	NEW INGREDIENT	DENIED FEB 13, 1986
CHOLINE MAGNESIUM TRISALICYLATE; CODEINE PHOSPHATE TABLET; ORAL	500 MG 30 MG	85 P-0142/CP	PURDUE FREDERICK	NEW COMBINATION	DENIED JUL 21, 1986
CHOLINE MAGNESIUM TRISALICYLATE; CODEINE PHOSPHATE TABLET; ORAL	500 MG 60 MG	85 P-0142/CP	PURDUE FREDERICK	NEW COMBINATION	DENIED JUL 21, 1986
CLONIDINE HYDROCHLORIDE CAPSULE, EXTENDED RELEASE; ORAL	0.2 MG	88 P-0365/CP	BOEHRINGER INGELHEIM	NEW DOSAGE FORM	DENIED JAN 11, 1990
CODEINE PHOSPHATE; IBUPROFEN CAPSULE; ORAL	30 MG 200 MG	84 P-0388/CP	RW JOHNSON	NEW COMBINATION	DENIED SEP 16, 1985
CODEINE PHOSPHATE; IBUPROFEN CAPSULE; ORAL	60 MG 200 MG	84 P-0388/CP	RW JOHNSON	NEW COMBINATION	DENIED SEP 16, 1985
CODEINE PHOSPHATE; IBUPROFEN TABLET; ORAL	30 MG 200 MG	84 P-0388/CP	RW JOHNSON	NEW COMBINATION	DENIED SEP 16, 1985
CODEINE PHOSPHATE; IBUPROFEN TABLET; ORAL	60 MG 200 MG	84 P-0388/CP	RW JOHNSON	NEW COMBINATION	DENIED SEP 16, 1985
CROTAMITON GEL; TOPICAL	10 MG	92 P-0249/CP1	HAMER	NEW DOSAGE FORM	DENIED NOV 10, 1993
CYCLOBENZAPRINE HYDROCHLORIDE TABLET; ORAL	15 MG	86 P-0386/CP	CENTRAL PHARMS	NEW STRENGTH	DENIED AUG 15, 1988

ANDA SUITABILITY PETITIONS

PETITIONS DENIED *(continued)*

DRUG NAME DOSAGE FORM; ROUTE	STRENGTH (CONTAINER SIZE)	DOCKET NUMBER	PETITIONER	REASON FOR PETITION	STATUS
CYCLOPHOSPHAMIDE INJECTABLE; INJECTION	100 MG/ML (1 ML/VIAL) (2 ML/VIAL)	87 P-0283/CP	LYPHOMED	NEW DOSAGE FORM NEW STRENGTH	DENIED JAN 21, 1988
CYCLOPHOSPHAMIDE INJECTABLE; INJECTION	500 MG/ML (1 ML/VIAL) (2 ML/VIAL) (4 ML/VIAL)	87 P-0283/CP	LYPHOMED	NEW DOSAGE FORM NEW STRENGTH	DENIED JAN 21, 1988
DEXTROMETHORPHAN HYDROBROMIDE TABLET, EXTENDED RELEASE; ORAL	60 MG	85 P-0135/CP	CIBA	NEW DOSAGE FORM NEW INGREDIENT	DENIED JUL 17, 1986
DIATRIZOATE MEGLUMINE; LIDOCAINE HYDROCHLORIDE INJECTABLE; INJECTION	60% 1.5 MG/ML	84 P-0325/CP	COOK	NEW COMBINATION	DENIED SEP 03, 1985
DIAZEPAM INTENSOL CONCENTRATE; ORAL	10 MG/ML	85 P-0075/CP	ROXANE	NEW DOSAGE FORM	DENIED SEP 24, 1985
DIPHENHYDRAMINE HYDROCHLORIDE CAPSULE, EXTENDED RELEASE; ORAL	75 MG	87 P-0355/CP	PARKE DAVIS	NEW DOSAGE FORM NEW STRENGTH	DENIED MAY 11, 1988
TRI-PHASIC CONTRACEPTIVE TABLET; ORAL (21 AND 28 DAYS) ETHINYL ESTRADIOL; NORETHINDRONE ETHINYL ESTRADIOL; NORETHINDRONE ETHINYL ESTRADIOL; NORETHINDRONE	 0.05 MG 0.5 MG 0.05 MG 0.75 MG 0.05 MG 1 MG	84 P-0443/CP	RW JOHNSON	NEW STRENGTH (DOSE SCHEDULE)	DENIED SEP 03, 1985
ETOPOSIDE INJECTABLE; INJECTION	20 MG/ML (50 ML/VIAL)	91 P-0076/CP1	ADRIA	NEW STRENGTH	DENIED FEB 19, 1992
FLUPHENAZINE HYDROCHLORIDE INJECTABLE; INJECTION	5 MG/ML	85 P-0019/CP	SQUIBB	NEW STRENGTH	DENIED OCT 25, 1985
FUROSEMIDE INJECTABLE; INJECTION	1 MG/ML	90 P-0313/CP1	LYPHOMED	NEW STRENGTH	DENIED OCT 28, 1991
HEPARIN SODIUM INJECTABLE; INJECTION	2,000 UNITS/ML 4,000 UNITS/ML	85 P-0065/CP	ABBOTT	NEW STRENGTH	DENIED MAY 29, 1985
HYDROCHLOROTHIAZIDE; PROPRANOLOL HYDROCHLORIDE; TRIAMTERENE CAPSULE, EXTENDED RELEASE; ORAL	50 MG 80 MG 75 MG	85 P-0571/CP	WYETH AYERST	NEW COMBINATION	DENIED MAY 16, 1986
HYDROCHLOROTHIAZIDE; PROPRANOLOL HYDROCHLORIDE; TRIAMTERENE CAPSULE, EXTENDED RELEASE; ORAL	50 MG 120 MG 75 MG	85 P-0571/CP	WYETH AYERST	NEW COMBINATION	DENIED MAY 16, 1986
HYDROCHLOROTHIAZIDE; PROPRANOLOL HYDROCHLORIDE; TRIAMTERENE CAPSULE, EXTENDED RELEASE; ORAL	50 MG 160 MG 75 MG	85 P-0571/CP	WYETH AYERST	NEW COMBINATION	DENIED MAY 16, 1986
HYDROCODONE BITARTRATE; PHENYLEPHRINE HYDROCHLORIDE; PROMETHAZINE HYDROCHLORIDE SYRUP; ORAL	1.66 MG/5 ML 5 MG/5 ML 6.25 MG/5 ML	85 P-0389/CP	UAD LABS	NEW COMBINATION	DENIED MAY 11, 1988

ANDA SUITABILITY PETITIONS

PETITIONS DENIED *(continued)*

DRUG NAME DOSAGE FORM; ROUTE	STRENGTH (CONTAINER SIZE)	DOCKET NUMBER	PETITIONER	REASON FOR PETITION	STATUS
HYDROCODONE BITARTRATE; PROMETHAZINE HYDROCHLORIDE SOLUTION; ORAL	2.5 MG/5 ML 6.25 MG/5 ML	85 P-0256/CP	MIKART	NEW COMBINATION	DENIED MAY 11, 1988
HYDROCORTISONE; SALICYLIC ACID; SULFUR CREAM; TOPICAL	0.25% 2.35% 4%	86 P-0439/CP	C&M PHARMA	NEW COMBINATION	DENIED MAY 06, 1987
HYDROCORTISONE ACETATE SUPPOSITORY; RECTAL	1%	85 P-0088/CP	PARKE DAVIS	NEW DOSAGE FORM NEW ROUTE OF ADMINISTRATION	DENIED SEP 16, 1986
IBUPROFEN LIQUID; ORAL	200 MG/5 ML	88 P-0291/ CP0001	BIOCRAFT	NEW DOSAGE FORM	DENIED DEC 15, 1988
IBUPROFEN LIQUID; ORAL	400 MG/10 ML	88 P-0291/ CP0002	BIOCRAFT	NEW DOSAGE FORM	DENIED DEC 15, 1988
IBUPROFEN; OXYCODONE HYDROCHLORIDE CAPSULE; ORAL	200 MG 5 MG	85 P-0141/CP	DUPONT	NEW COMBINATION	DENIED SEP 27, 1985
IBUPROFEN; OXYCODONE HYDROCHLORIDE TABLET; ORAL	200 MG 5 MG	85 P-0141/CP	DUPONT	NEW COMBINATION	DENIED SEP 27, 1985
INDOMETHACIN TABLET; ORAL	25 MG 50 MG	85 P-0025/CP	VEREX LABS	NEW DOSAGE FORM	DENIED MAR 31, 1986
INDOMETHACIN TABLET, EXTENDED RELEASE; ORAL	75 MG	85 P-0026/CP	VEREX LABS	NEW DOSAGE FORM	DENIED SEP 16, 1985
INDOMETHACIN TABLET, EXTENDED RELEASE; ORAL	75 MG	85 P-0180/CP	FOREST	NEW DOSAGE FORM	DENIED APR 07, 1986
INDOMETHACIN INTENSOL SOLUTION (CONCENTRATE); ORAL	50 MG/ML	85 P-0077/CP	ROXANE	NEW DOSAGE FORM	DENIED APR 07, 1986
MAGNESIUM ASCORBATE INJECTABLE; INJECTION	10% 20%	88 P-0200/CP	RIM CONSULTING	NEW INGREDIENT	DENIED JUN 10, 1988
METOCLOPRAMIDE HYDROCHLORIDE INJECTABLE; INJECTION	1 MG/ML (50 ML/VIAL) (75 ML/VIAL) (100 ML/VIAL)	86 P-0015/CP	INTL MEDICATION	NEW STRENGTH	DENIED APR 25, 1986
METOCLOPRAMIDE HYDROCHLORIDE INJECTABLE; INJECTION	1 MG/ML (50 ML/VIAL) (75 ML/VIAL) (100 ML/VIAL)	87 P-0090/CP	INTL MEDICATION	NEW STRENGTH	DENIED FEB 08, 1988
METOCLOPRAMIDE HYDROCHLORIDE INJECTABLE; INJECTION	10 MG/ML	85 P-0062/CP	MARK W. LOTZ	NEW STRENGTH	DENIED MAY 29, 1985
METOCLOPRAMIDE HYDROCHLORIDE INJECTABLE; INJECTION	10 MG/ML	85 P-0457/CP	ABBOTT	NEW STRENGTH	DENIED APR 18, 1986
METOCLOPRAMIDE HYDROCHLORIDE INJECTABLE; INJECTION	20 MG/ML	85 P-0062/ CP0002	MARK W. LOTZ	NEW STRENGTH	DENIED MAY 29, 1985
METOCLOPRAMIDE HYDROCHLORIDE INJECTABLE; INJECTION	20 MG/ML	85 P-0457/ CP0002	ABBOTT	NEW STRENGTH	DENIED APR 18, 1986
METRONIDAZOLE SPONGE; VAGINAL	50-125 MG/SPONGE	85 P-0117/CP	VLI	NEW DOSAGE FORM	DENIED OCT 08, 1985

ANDA SUITABILITY PETITIONS

PETITIONS DENIED *(continued)*

DRUG NAME DOSAGE FORM; ROUTE	STRENGTH (CONTAINER SIZE)	DOCKET NUMBER	PETITIONER	REASON FOR PETITION	STATUS
NITROGLYCERIN FILM, EXTENDED RELEASE; PERCUTANEOUS	NONE GIVEN	84 P-0302/CP	KEY PHARMS	NEW DOSAGE FORM (NEW MATRIX)	DENIED JUL 29, 1985
PHENYLEPHRINE HYDROCHLORIDE; SULFATHIAZOLE NASAL SUSPENSION; TOPICAL	0.5% 5%	85 P-0205/CP	TANYA W. ROSS	NEW COMBINATION NEW DOSAGE FORM	DENIED NOV 14, 1985
PHENYLPROPANOLAMINE HYDROCHLORIDE FILM, EXTENDED RELEASE; PERCUTANEOUS	150 MG	88 P-0265/CP	BIO AMERICAN	NEW DOSAGE FORM NEW STRENGTH	DENIED OCT 07, 1988
PROCAINAMIDE HYDROCHLORIDE TABLET, EXTENDED RELEASE; ORAL	500 MG 750 MG 1,000 MG	85 P-0181/CP	FOREST	NEW DOSAGE FORM	DENIED APR 21, 1987
PROCAINAMIDE HYDROCHLORIDE TABLET, EXTENDED RELEASE; ORAL	500 MG 750 MG 1,000 MG	86 P-0328/CP	KV	NEW DOSAGE FORM	DENIED APR 21, 1987
PSEUDOEPHEDRINE POLISTIREX CAPSULE, EXTENDED RELEASE; ORAL	60 MG	85 P-0334/CP	PENNWALT	NEW INGREDIENT NEW SALT	DENIED MAR 19, 1986
TEMAZEPAM SOFT GELATIN CAPSULE; ORAL	10 MG 20 MG	85 P-0016/CP	WYETH AYERST	NEW DOSAGE FORM NEW STRENGTH	DENIED SEP 29, 1986
TRIAMCINOLONE ACETONIDE SUSPENSION; INJECTION	2.5 MG/ML	85 P-0001/CP	GENDERM	NEW STRENGTH	DENIED MAR 04, 1985
TRIAMCINOLONE ACETONIDE SUSPENSION; INJECTION	3 MG/ML	84 P-0240/CP	PHARM BASICS	NEW STRENGTH	DENIED MAR 04, 1985

APPENDIX A
PRODUCT NAME INDEX

A

A.P.L., GONADOTROPIN, CHORIONIC
A-HYDROCORT, HYDROCORTISONE SODIUM SUCCINATE
A-METHAPRED, METHYLPREDNISOLONE SODIUM SUCCINATE
A-N STANNOUS AGGREGATED ALBUMIN, TECHNETIUM TC-99M ALBUMIN AGGREGATED KIT
A-POXIDE, CHLORDIAZEPOXIDE HYDROCHLORIDE
A/T/S, ERYTHROMYCIN
ABITREXATE, METHOTREXATE SODIUM
ACCUPRIL, QUINAPRIL HYDROCHLORIDE
ACCURBRON, THEOPHYLLINE
ACCUTANE, ISOTRETINOIN
ACEON, PERINDOPRIL ERBUMINE
ACEPHEN, ACETAMINOPHEN (OTC)
ACETAMINOPHEN, ACETAMINOPHEN (OTC)
ACETAMINOPHEN AND CODEINE PHOSPHATE, ACETAMINOPHEN
ACETAMINOPHEN AND CODEINE PHOSPHATE #2, ACETAMINOPHEN
ACETAMINOPHEN AND CODEINE PHOSPHATE #3, ACETAMINOPHEN
ACETAMINOPHEN AND CODEINE PHOSPHATE #4, ACETAMINOPHEN
ACETAMINOPHEN AND CODEINE PHOSPHATE NO. 2, ACETAMINOPHEN
ACETAMINOPHEN AND CODEINE PHOSPHATE NO. 3, ACETAMINOPHEN
ACETAMINOPHEN AND CODEINE PHOSPHATE NO. 4, ACETAMINOPHEN
ACETAMINOPHEN AND HYDROCODONE BITARTRATE, ACETAMINOPHEN
ACETAMINOPHEN W/ CODEINE, ACETAMINOPHEN
ACETAMINOPHEN W/ CODEINE #2, ACETAMINOPHEN
ACETAMINOPHEN W/ CODEINE #3, ACETAMINOPHEN
ACETAMINOPHEN W/ CODEINE #4, ACETAMINOPHEN
ACETAMINOPHEN W/ CODEINE NO. 2, ACETAMINOPHEN
ACETAMINOPHEN W/ CODEINE NO. 3, ACETAMINOPHEN
ACETAMINOPHEN W/ CODEINE PHOSPHATE, ACETAMINOPHEN
ACETAMINOPHEN W/ CODEINE PHOSPHATE #3, ACETAMINOPHEN
ACETAMINOPHEN, ASPIRIN, AND CODEINE PHOSPHATE, ACETAMINOPHEN
ACETAMINOPHEN, BUTALBITAL AND CAFFEINE, ACETAMINOPHEN
ACETAMINOPHEN, BUTALBITAL, AND CAFFEINE, ACETAMINOPHEN
ACETASOL, ACETIC ACID, GLACIAL
ACETASOL HC, ACETIC ACID, GLACIAL
ACETATED RINGER'S IN PLASTIC CONTAINER, CALCIUM CHLORIDE
ACETAZOLAMIDE, ACETAZOLAMIDE
ACETAZOLAMIDE SODIUM, ACETAZOLAMIDE SODIUM
ACETIC ACID, ACETIC ACID, GLACIAL
ACETIC ACID W/ HYDROCORTISONE, ACETIC ACID, GLACIAL
ACETIC ACID 0.25% IN PLASTIC CONTAINER, ACETIC ACID, GLACIAL
ACETIC ACID 2% IN AQUEOUS ALUMINUM ACETATE, ACETIC ACID, GLACIAL
ACETOHEXAMIDE, ACETOHEXAMIDE
ACETYLCYSTEINE, ACETYLCYSTEINE
ACHES-N-PAIN, IBUPROFEN (OTC)
ACHROMYCIN, HYDROCORTISONE
ACHROMYCIN, PROCAINE HYDROCHLORIDE
ACHROMYCIN, TETRACYCLINE HYDROCHLORIDE
ACHROMYCIN V, TETRACYCLINE HYDROCHLORIDE
ACILAC, LACTULOSE
ACLOVATE, ALCLOMETASONE DIPROPIONATE
ACTAHIST, PSEUDOEPHEDRINE HYDROCHLORIDE
ACTH, CORTICOTROPIN
ACTHAR, CORTICOTROPIN
ACTHAR GEL-SYNTHETIC, SERACTIDE ACETATE
ACTICORT, HYDROCORTISONE
ACTIDIL, TRIPROLIDINE HYDROCHLORIDE (OTC)
ACTIFED, PSEUDOEPHEDRINE HYDROCHLORIDE (OTC)
ACTIFED W/ CODEINE, CODEINE PHOSPHATE
ACTIGALL, URSODIOL
ACTIN-N, NITROFURAZONE
ACTINEX, MASOPROCOL
ACTISITE, TETRACYCLINE HYDROCHLORIDE
ACULAR, KETOROLAC TROMETHAMINE
ACYLANID, ACETYLDIGITOXIN
ADAGEN, PEGADEMASE BOVINE
ADALAT, NIFEDIPINE
ADALAT CC, NIFEDIPINE
ADENOCARD, ADENOSINE
ADIPEX-P, PHENTERMINE HYDROCHLORIDE
ADPHEN, PHENDIMETRAZINE TARTRATE
ADRIAMYCIN PFS, DOXORUBICIN HYDROCHLORIDE
ADRIAMYCIN RDF, DOXORUBICIN HYDROCHLORIDE
ADRUCIL, FLUOROURACIL
ADVIL, IBUPROFEN (OTC)
ADVIL COLD AND SINUS, IBUPROFEN (OTC)
AEROBID, FLUNISOLIDE
AEROLATE, THEOPHYLLINE
AEROLATE III, THEOPHYLLINE
AEROLATE JR, THEOPHYLLINE
AEROLATE SR, THEOPHYLLINE
AEROLONE, ISOPROTERENOL HYDROCHLORIDE
AEROSEB-DEX, DEXAMETHASONE
AEROSEB-HC, HYDROCORTISONE
AEROSPORIN, POLYMYXIN B SULFATE
AFAXIN, VITAMIN A PALMITATE
AFRINOL, PSEUDOEPHEDRINE SULFATE (OTC)
AK-PENTOLATE, CYCLOPENTOLATE HYDROCHLORIDE
AKINETON, BIPERIDEN HYDROCHLORIDE
AKINETON, BIPERIDEN LACTATE
AKNE-MYCIN, ERYTHROMYCIN
AKRINOL, ACRISORCIN
ALA-CORT, HYDROCORTISONE
ALA-SCALP, HYDROCORTISONE
ALBALON, NAPHAZOLINE HYDROCHLORIDE
ALBAMYCIN, NOVOBIOCIN SODIUM
ALBUMOTOPE 125 I, ALBUMIN IODINATED I-125 SERUM
ALBUTEROL SULFATE, ALBUTEROL SULFATE
ALCAINE, PROPARACAINE HYDROCHLORIDE
ALCOHOL 10% AND DEXTROSE 5%, ALCOHOL
ALCOHOL 5% AND DEXTROSE 5%, ALCOHOL
ALCOHOL 5% IN DEXTROSE 5%, ALCOHOL
ALCOHOL 5% IN DEXTROSE 5% IN WATER, ALCOHOL
ALCOHOL 5% IN D5-W, ALCOHOL
ALDACTAZIDE, HYDROCHLOROTHIAZIDE
ALDACTONE, SPIRONOLACTONE
ALDOCLOR-150, CHLOROTHIAZIDE
ALDOCLOR-250, CHLOROTHIAZIDE
ALDOMET, METHYLDOPA
ALDOMET, METHYLDOPATE HYDROCHLORIDE

APPENDIX A
PRODUCT NAME INDEX *(continued)*

ALDORIL D30, HYDROCHLOROTHIAZIDE
ALDORIL D50, HYDROCHLOROTHIAZIDE
ALDORIL 15, HYDROCHLOROTHIAZIDE
ALDORIL 25, HYDROCHLOROTHIAZIDE
ALEVE, NAPROXEN SODIUM
ALFENTA, ALFENTANIL HYDROCHLORIDE
ALKERAN, MELPHALAN
ALKERAN, MELPHALAN HYDROCHLORIDE
ALKERGOT, ERGOLOID MESYLATES
ALLAY, ACETAMINOPHEN
ALLERFED, PSEUDOEPHEDRINE HYDROCHLORIDE
ALLOPURINOL, ALLOPURINOL
ALOMIDE, LODOXAMIDE TROMETHAMINE
ALPHA CHYMAR, CHYMOTRYPSIN
ALPHACAINE, LIDOCAINE
ALPHACAINE HCL, LIDOCAINE HYDROCHLORIDE
ALPHACAINE HCL W/ EPINEPHRINE, EPINEPHRINE
ALPHADERM, HYDROCORTISONE
ALPHADROL, FLUPREDNISOLONE
ALPHALIN, VITAMIN A PALMITATE
ALPHAREDISOL, HYDROXOCOBALAMIN
ALPHATREX, BETAMETHASONE DIPROPIONATE
ALPHAZINE, PHENDIMETRAZINE TARTRATE
ALPRAZOLAM, ALPRAZOLAM
ALTACE, RAMIPRIL
ALUMINUM HYDROXIDE AND MAGNESIUM TRISILICATE, ALUMINUM HYDROXIDE (OTC)
ALUPENT, METAPROTERENOL SULFATE
AMANTADINE HCL, AMANTADINE HYDROCHLORIDE
AMBENYL, BROMODIPHENHYDRAMINE HYDROCHLORIDE
AMBIEN, ZOLPIDEM TARTRATE
AMBODRYL, BROMODIPHENHYDRAMINE HYDROCHLORIDE
AMCILL, AMPICILLIN/AMPICILLIN TRIHYDRATE
AMEN, MEDROXYPROGESTERONE ACETATE
AMERSCAN MDP KIT, TECHNETIUM TC-99M MEDRONATE KIT
AMICAR, AMINOCAPROIC ACID
AMIDATE, ETOMIDATE
AMIKACIN, AMIKACIN SULFATE
AMIKIN, AMIKACIN SULFATE
AMIKIN IN SODIUM CHLORIDE 0.9%, AMIKACIN SULFATE
AMILORIDE HCL, AMILORIDE HYDROCHLORIDE
AMILORIDE HCL AND HYDROCHLOROTHIAZIDE, AMILORIDE HYDROCHLORIDE
AMINESS 5.2% ESSENTIAL AMINO ACIDS W/ HISTADINE, AMINO ACIDS
AMINOACETIC ACID 1.5% IN PLASTIC CONTAINER, GLYCINE
AMINOCAPROIC ACID, AMINOCAPROIC ACID
AMINOHIPPURATE SODIUM, AMINOHIPPURATE SODIUM
AMINOPHYLLIN, AMINOPHYLLINE
AMINOPHYLLINE, AMINOPHYLLINE
AMINOPHYLLINE DYE FREE, AMINOPHYLLINE
AMINOPHYLLINE IN SODIUM CHLORIDE 0.45%, AMINOPHYLLINE
AMINOPHYLLINE IN SODIUM CHLORIDE 0.45% IN PLASTIC CONTAINER, AMINOPHYLLINE
AMINOSOL 5%, PROTEIN HYDROLYSATE
AMINOSYN II M 3.5% IN DEXTROSE 5%, AMINO ACIDS
AMINOSYN II 10%, AMINO ACIDS
AMINOSYN II 10% W/ ELECTROLYTES, AMINO ACIDS
AMINOSYN II 15%, AMINO ACIDS
AMINOSYN II 3.5%, AMINO ACIDS
AMINOSYN II 3.5% IN DEXTROSE 25%, AMINO ACIDS
AMINOSYN II 3.5% IN DEXTROSE 5%, AMINO ACIDS
AMINOSYN II 3.5% M, AMINO ACIDS
AMINOSYN II 3.5% M IN DEXTROSE 5%, AMINO ACIDS
AMINOSYN II 3.5% W/ ELECTROLYTES IN DEXTROSE 25%, AMINO ACIDS
AMINOSYN II 3.5% W/ ELECTROLYTES IN DEXTROSE 25% W/ CALCIUM, AMINO ACIDS
AMINOSYN II 4.25% IN DEXTROSE 10%, AMINO ACIDS
AMINOSYN II 4.25% IN DEXTROSE 20%, AMINO ACIDS
AMINOSYN II 4.25% IN DEXTROSE 25%, AMINO ACIDS
AMINOSYN II 4.25% M IN DEXTROSE 10%, AMINO ACIDS
AMINOSYN II 4.25% W/ ELECT AND ADJUSTED PHOSPHATE IN DEXTROSE 10%, AMINO ACIDS
AMINOSYN II 4.25% W/ ELECTROLYTES IN DEXTROSE 20% W/ CALCIUM, AMINO ACIDS
AMINOSYN II 4.25% W/ ELECTROLYTES IN DEXTROSE 25%, AMINO ACIDS
AMINOSYN II 4.25% W/ ELECTROLYTES IN DEXTROSE 25% W/ CALCIUM, AMINO ACIDS
AMINOSYN II 5%, AMINO ACIDS
AMINOSYN II 5% IN DEXTROSE 25%, AMINO ACIDS
AMINOSYN II 5% W/ ELECTROLYTES IN DEXTROSE 25% W/ CALCIUM, AMINO ACIDS
AMINOSYN II 7%, AMINO ACIDS
AMINOSYN II 7% W/ ELECTROLYTES, AMINO ACIDS
AMINOSYN II 8.5%, AMINO ACIDS
AMINOSYN II 8.5% W/ ELECTROLYTES, AMINO ACIDS
AMINOSYN 10%, AMINO ACIDS
AMINOSYN 10% (PH6), AMINO ACIDS
AMINOSYN 3.5%, AMINO ACIDS
AMINOSYN 3.5% IN PLASTIC CONTAINER, AMINO ACIDS
AMINOSYN 3.5% M, AMINO ACIDS
AMINOSYN 3.5% M IN PLASTIC CONTAINER, AMINO ACIDS
AMINOSYN 3.5% W/ DEXTROSE 25% IN PLASTIC CONTAINER, AMINO ACIDS
AMINOSYN 3.5% W/ DEXTROSE 5% IN PLASTIC CONTAINER, AMINO ACIDS
AMINOSYN 4.25% W/ DEXTROSE 25% IN PLASTIC CONTAINER, AMINO ACIDS
AMINOSYN 5%, AMINO ACIDS
AMINOSYN 7%, AMINO ACIDS
AMINOSYN 7% (PH6), AMINO ACIDS
AMINOSYN 7% W/ ELECTROLYTES, AMINO ACIDS
AMINOSYN 8.5%, AMINO ACIDS
AMINOSYN 8.5% (PH6), AMINO ACIDS
AMINOSYN 8.5% W/ ELECTROLYTES, AMINO ACIDS
AMINOSYN-HBC 7%, AMINO ACIDS
AMINOSYN-HBC 7% IN PLASTIC CONTAINER, AMINO ACIDS
AMINOSYN-PF 10%, AMINO ACIDS
AMINOSYN-PF 7%, AMINO ACIDS
AMINOSYN-RF 5.2%, AMINO ACIDS
AMIPAQUE, METRIZAMIDE
AMITID, AMITRIPTYLINE HYDROCHLORIDE
AMITRIL, AMITRIPTYLINE HYDROCHLORIDE
AMITRIPTYLINE HCL, AMITRIPTYLINE HYDROCHLORIDE
AMMONIUM CHLORIDE, AMMONIUM CHLORIDE
AMMONIUM CHLORIDE IN PLASTIC CONTAINER, AMMONIUM CHLORIDE
AMMONIUM CHLORIDE 0.9% IN NORMAL SALINE, AMMONIUM CHLORIDE
AMMONIUM CHLORIDE 2.14%, AMMONIUM CHLORIDE
AMNESTROGEN, ESTROGENS, ESTERIFIED
AMOSENE, MEPROBAMATE
AMOXAPINE, AMOXAPINE
AMOXICILLIN, AMOXICILLIN
AMOXICILLIN PEDIATRIC, AMOXICILLIN
AMOXICILLIN TRIHYDRATE, AMOXICILLIN
AMOXIL, AMOXICILLIN
AMPHETAMINE SULFATE, AMPHETAMINE SULFATE
AMPHICOL, CHLORAMPHENICOL
AMPHOTERICIN B, AMPHOTERICIN B
AMPICILLIN, AMPICILLIN/AMPICILLIN TRIHYDRATE
AMPICILLIN SODIUM, AMPICILLIN SODIUM
AMPICILLIN TRIHYDRATE, AMPICILLIN/AMPICILLIN TRIHYDRATE

APPENDIX A
PRODUCT NAME INDEX *(continued)*

AN-DTPA, TECHNETIUM TC-99M PENTETATE KIT
AN-MAA, TECHNETIUM TC-99M ALBUMIN AGGREGATED KIT
AN-MDP, TECHNETIUM TC-99M MEDRONATE KIT
AN-PYROTEC, TECHNETIUM TC-99M PYROPHOSPHATE KIT
AN-SULFUR COLLOID, TECHNETIUM TC-99M SULFUR COLLOID KIT
ANADROL-50, OXYMETHOLONE
ANAFRANIL, CLOMIPRAMINE HYDROCHLORIDE
ANAPROX, NAPROXEN SODIUM
ANAPROX DS, NAPROXEN SODIUM
ANCEF, CEFAZOLIN SODIUM
ANCEF IN DEXTROSE 5% IN PLASTIC CONTAINER, CEFAZOLIN SODIUM
ANCEF IN SODIUM CHLORIDE 0.9% IN PLASTIC CONTAINER, CEFAZOLIN SODIUM
ANCOBON, FLUCYTOSINE
ANDROID 10, METHYLTESTOSTERONE
ANDROID 25, METHYLTESTOSTERONE
ANDROID 5, METHYLTESTOSTERONE
ANDROID-F, FLUOXYMESTERONE
ANECTINE, SUCCINYLCHOLINE CHLORIDE
ANESTACON, LIDOCAINE HYDROCHLORIDE
ANEXSIA, ACETAMINOPHEN
ANEXSIA 7.5/650, ACETAMINOPHEN
ANGIO-CONRAY, IOTHALAMATE SODIUM
ANGIOVIST 282, DIATRIZOATE MEGLUMINE
ANGIOVIST 292, DIATRIZOATE MEGLUMINE
ANGIOVIST 370, DIATRIZOATE MEGLUMINE
ANHYDRON, CYCLOTHIAZIDE
ANISOTROPINE METHYLBROMIDE, ANISOTROPINE METHYLBROMIDE
ANOQUAN, ACETAMINOPHEN
ANSAID, FLURBIPROFEN
ANSOLYSEN, PENTOLINIUM TARTRATE
ANSPOR, CEPHRADINE
ANTABUSE, DISULFIRAM
ANTAGONATE, CHLORPHENIRAMINE MALEATE
ANTEPAR, PIPERAZINE CITRATE
ANTITUSSIVE, DIPHENHYDRAMINE HYDROCHLORIDE (OTC)
ANTIVERT, MECLIZINE HYDROCHLORIDE
ANTRENYL, OXYPHENONIUM BROMIDE
ANTURANE, SULFINPYRAZONE
ANUSOL HC, HYDROCORTISONE
APAP W/ CODEINE, ACETAMINOPHEN
APAP W/ CODEINE PHOSPHATE, ACETAMINOPHEN
APOGEN, GENTAMICIN SULFATE
APRESAZIDE, HYDRALAZINE HYDROCHLORIDE
APRESOLINE, HYDRALAZINE HYDROCHLORIDE
APRESOLINE-ESIDRIX, HYDRALAZINE HYDROCHLORIDE
AQUAMEPHYTON, PHYTONADIONE
AQUAPHYLLIN, THEOPHYLLINE
AQUASOL A, VITAMIN A
AQUASOL A, VITAMIN A PALMITATE
AQUATAG, BENZTHIAZIDE
AQUATENSEN, METHYCLOTHIAZIDE
ARALEN, CHLOROQUINE PHOSPHATE
ARALEN HCL, CHLOROQUINE HYDROCHLORIDE
ARALEN PHOSPHATE W/ PRIMAQUINE PHOSPHATE, CHLOROQUINE PHOSPHATE
ARAMINE, METARAMINOL BITARTRATE
ARDUAN, PIPECURONIUM BROMIDE
AREDIA, PAMIDRONATE DISODIUM
ARESTOCAINE HCL, MEPIVACAINE HYDROCHLORIDE
ARESTOCAINE HCL W/ LEVONORDEFRIN, LEVONORDEFRIN
ARFONAD, TRIMETHAPHAN CAMSYLATE
ARISTOCORT, TRIAMCINOLONE
ARISTOCORT, TRIAMCINOLONE ACETONIDE
ARISTOCORT, TRIAMCINOLONE DIACETATE
ARISTOCORT A, TRIAMCINOLONE ACETONIDE
ARISTOGEL, TRIAMCINOLONE ACETONIDE
ARISTOSPAN, TRIAMCINOLONE HEXACETONIDE
ARTANE, TRIHEXYPHENIDYL HYDROCHLORIDE
ASACOL, MESALAMINE
ASBRON, THEOPHYLLINE SODIUM GLYCINATE
ASELLACRIN 10, SOMATROPIN
ASELLACRIN 2, SOMATROPIN
ASENDIN, AMOXAPINE
ASPIRIN AND CAFFEINE W/ BUTALBITAL, ASPIRIN
ASTRAMORPH PF, MORPHINE SULFATE
ATARAX, HYDROXYZINE HYDROCHLORIDE
ATENOLOL, ATENOLOL
ATENOLOL AND CHLORTHALIDONE, ATENOLOL
ATHROMBIN, WARFARIN SODIUM
ATHROMBIN-K, WARFARIN POTASSIUM
ATIVAN, LORAZEPAM
ATROMID-S, CLOFIBRATE
ATROPEN, ATROPINE
ATROPINE, ATROPINE
ATROPINE AND DEMEROL, ATROPINE SULFATE
ATROPINE SULFATE, ATROPINE SULFATE
ATROVENT, IPRATROPIUM BROMIDE
AUGMENTIN 125, AMOXICILLIN
AUGMENTIN 250, AMOXICILLIN
AUGMENTIN '125', AMOXICILLIN
AUGMENTIN '250', AMOXICILLIN
AUGMENTIN '500', AMOXICILLIN
AUREOMYCIN, CHLORTETRACYCLINE HYDROCHLORIDE
AVC, SULFANILAMIDE
AVENTYL HCL, NORTRIPTYLINE HYDROCHLORIDE
AXID, NIZATIDINE
AXOTAL, ASPIRIN
AYGESTIN, NORETHINDRONE ACETATE
AZACTAM, AZTREONAM
AZATHIOPRINE, AZATHIOPRINE SODIUM
AZDONE, ASPIRIN
AZLIN, AZLOCILLIN SODIUM
AZMACORT, TRIAMCINOLONE ACETONIDE
AZO GANTANOL, PHENAZOPYRIDINE HYDROCHLORIDE
AZO GANTRISIN, PHENAZOPYRIDINE HYDROCHLORIDE
AZOLID, PHENYLBUTAZONE
AZULFIDINE, SULFASALAZINE
AZULFIDINE EN-TABS, SULFASALAZINE

B

BACI-RX, BACITRACIN
BACIGUENT, BACITRACIN
BACITRACIN, BACITRACIN
BACITRACIN, BACITRACIN (OTC)
BACITRACIN ZINC-NEOMYCIN SULFATE-POLYMYXIN B SULFATE, BACITRACIN ZINC
BACITRACIN ZINC-NEOMYCIN SULFATE-POLYMYXIN B SULFATE, BACITRACIN ZINC (OTC)
BACITRACIN ZINC-POLYMYXIN B SULFATE, BACITRACIN ZINC (OTC)
BACITRACIN-NEOMYCIN-POLYMYXIN, BACITRACIN ZINC
BACITRACIN-NEOMYCIN-POLYMYXIN W/ HYDROCORTISONE ACETATE, BACITRACIN
BACLOFEN, BACLOFEN
BACTERIOSTATIC SODIUM CHLORIDE 0.9%, SODIUM CHLORIDE
BACTERIOSTATIC SODIUM CHLORIDE 0.9% IN PLASTIC CONTAINER, SODIUM CHLORIDE
BACTERIOSTATIC WATER FOR INJECTION, WATER FOR INJECTION, STERILE
BACTOCILL, OXACILLIN SODIUM
BACTRIM, SULFAMETHOXAZOLE

APPENDIX A
PRODUCT NAME INDEX *(continued)*

BACTRIM DS, SULFAMETHOXAZOLE
BACTRIM PEDIATRIC, SULFAMETHOXAZOLE
BACTROBAN, MUPIROCIN
BAL, DIMERCAPROL
BALNEOL-HC, HYDROCORTISONE
BAMATE, MEPROBAMATE
BANAN, CEFPODOXIME PROXETIL
BANCAP, ACETAMINOPHEN
BANCAP HC, ACETAMINOPHEN
BANTHINE, METHANTHELINE BROMIDE
BAROS, SODIUM BICARBONATE
BARSTATIN 100, NYSTATIN
BECLOVENT, BECLOMETHASONE DIPROPIONATE
BECONASE, BECLOMETHASONE DIPROPIONATE
BECONASE AQ, BECLOMETHASONE DIPROPIONATE MONOHYDRATE
BEEPEN-VK, PENICILLIN V POTASSIUM
BELDIN, DIPHENHYDRAMINE HYDROCHLORIDE (OTC)
BELIX, DIPHENHYDRAMINE HYDROCHLORIDE
BENADRYL, DIPHENHYDRAMINE HYDROCHLORIDE
BENDOPA, LEVODOPA
BENEMID, PROBENECID
BENOQUIN, MONOBENZONE
BENOXINATE HCL, BENOXINATE HYDROCHLORIDE
BENSULFOID, BENTONITE
BENTYL, DICYCLOMINE HYDROCHLORIDE
BENYLIN, DIPHENHYDRAMINE HYDROCHLORIDE (OTC)
BENZAMYCIN, BENZOYL PEROXIDE
BENZONATATE, BENZONATATE
BENZTHIAZIDE, BENZTHIAZIDE
BENZTROPINE MESYLATE, BENZTROPINE MESYLATE
BENZYL BENZOATE, BENZYL BENZOATE
BEPADIN, BEPRIDIL HYDROCHLORIDE
BEROCCA PN, ASCORBIC ACID
BERUBIGEN, CYANOCOBALAMIN
BETA-HC, HYDROCORTISONE
BETA-VAL, BETAMETHASONE VALERATE
BETA-2, ISOETHARINE HYDROCHLORIDE
BETADERM, BETAMETHASONE VALERATE
BETADINE, POVIDONE-IODINE
BETAGAN, LEVOBUNOLOL HYDROCHLORIDE
BETALIN S, THIAMINE HYDROCHLORIDE
BETALIN 12, CYANOCOBALAMIN
BETAMETHASONE DIPROPIONATE, BETAMETHASONE DIPROPIONATE
BETAMETHASONE SODIUM PHOSPHATE, BETAMETHASONE SODIUM PHOSPHATE
BETAMETHASONE VALERATE, BETAMETHASONE VALERATE
BETAPACE, SOTALOL HYDROCHLORIDE
BETAPAR, MEPREDNISONE
BETAPEN-VK, PENICILLIN V POTASSIUM
BETAPRONE, PROPIOLACTONE
BETATREX, BETAMETHASONE VALERATE
BETHANECHOL CHLORIDE, BETHANECHOL CHLORIDE
BETOPTIC, BETAXOLOL HYDROCHLORIDE
BETOPTIC S, BETAXOLOL HYDROCHLORIDE
BIAXIN, CLARITHROMYCIN
BICILLIN, PENICILLIN G BENZATHINE
BICILLIN C-R, PENICILLIN G BENZATHINE
BICILLIN C-R 900/300, PENICILLIN G BENZATHINE
BICILLIN L-A, PENICILLIN G BENZATHINE
BICNU, CARMUSTINE
BILIVIST, IPODATE SODIUM
BILOPAQUE, TYROPANOATE SODIUM
BILTRICIDE, PRAZIQUANTEL
BIOSCRUB, CHLORHEXIDINE GLUCONATE (OTC)
BIPHETAMINE 12.5, AMPHETAMINE RESIN COMPLEX
BIPHETAMINE 20, AMPHETAMINE RESIN COMPLEX
BIPHETAMINE 7.5, AMPHETAMINE RESIN COMPLEX
BIPHETAP, BROMPHENIRAMINE MALEATE
BLENOXANE, BLEOMYCIN SULFATE
BLEPH-10, SULFACETAMIDE SODIUM
BLEPH-30, SULFACETAMIDE SODIUM
BLEPHAMIDE, PREDNISOLONE ACETATE
BLEPHAMIDE S.O.P., PREDNISOLONE ACETATE
BLOCADREN, TIMOLOL MALEATE
BONTRIL PDM, PHENDIMETRAZINE TARTRATE
BOROFAIR, ACETIC ACID, GLACIAL
BRANCHAMIN 4%, AMINO ACIDS
BRETHAIRE, TERBUTALINE SULFATE
BRETHINE, TERBUTALINE SULFATE
BRETYLIUM TOSYLATE, BRETYLIUM TOSYLATE
BRETYLIUM TOSYLATE IN DEXTROSE 5%, BRETYLIUM TOSYLATE
BRETYLIUM TOSYLATE IN DEXTROSE 5% IN PLASTIC CONTAINER, BRETYLIUM TOSYLATE
BRETYLOL, BRETYLIUM TOSYLATE
BREVIBLOC, ESMOLOL HYDROCHLORIDE
BREVICON 21-DAY, ETHINYL ESTRADIOL
BREVICON 28-DAY, ETHINYL ESTRADIOL
BREVITAL SODIUM, METHOHEXITAL SODIUM
BRIAN CARE, CHLORHEXIDINE GLUCONATE (OTC)
BRICANYL, TERBUTALINE SULFATE
BRISTACYCLINE, TETRACYCLINE HYDROCHLORIDE
BRISTAGEN, GENTAMICIN SULFATE
BRISTAMYCIN, ERYTHROMYCIN STEARATE
BROMANATE, BROMPHENIRAMINE MALEATE
BROMANATE DC, BROMPHENIRAMINE MALEATE
BROMANATE DM, BROMPHENIRAMINE MALEATE
BROMANYL, BROMODIPHENHYDRAMINE HYDROCHLORIDE
BROMATAPP, BROMPHENIRAMINE MALEATE (OTC)
BROMFED-DM, BROMPHENIRAMINE MALEATE
BROMPHENIRAMINE MALEATE, BROMPHENIRAMINE MALEATE
BROMPHERIL, DEXBROMPHENIRAMINE MALEATE (OTC)
BRONCHO SALINE, SODIUM CHLORIDE (OTC)
BRONITIN MIST, EPINEPHRINE BITARTRATE (OTC)
BRONKAID MIST, EPINEPHRINE (OTC)
BRONKODYL, THEOPHYLLINE
BRONKOMETER, ISOETHARINE MESYLATE
BRONKOSOL, ISOETHARINE HYDROCHLORIDE
BRYREL, PIPERAZINE CITRATE
BSS PLUS, CALCIUM CHLORIDE
BUCLADIN-S, BUCLIZINE HYDROCHLORIDE
BUMEX, BUMETANIDE
BUPIVACAINE, BUPIVACAINE HYDROCHLORIDE
BUPIVACAINE HCL, BUPIVACAINE HYDROCHLORIDE
BUPIVACAINE HCL AND EPINEPHRINE, BUPIVACAINE HYDROCHLORIDE
BUPIVACAINE HCL KIT, BUPIVACAINE HYDROCHLORIDE
BUPRENEX, BUPRENORPHINE HYDROCHLORIDE
BUSPAR, BUSPIRONE HYDROCHLORIDE
BUTABARB, BUTABARBITAL SODIUM
BUTABARBITAL, BUTABARBITAL SODIUM
BUTABARBITAL SODIUM, BUTABARBITAL SODIUM
BUTAL COMPOUND, ASPIRIN
BUTALAN, BUTABARBITAL SODIUM
BUTALBITAL AND ACETAMINOPHEN, ACETAMINOPHEN
BUTALBITAL ASPIRIN AND CAFFEINE, ASPIRIN
BUTALBITAL COMPOUND, ASPIRIN
BUTALBITAL W/ ASPIRIN & CAFFEINE, ASPIRIN
BUTALBITAL, ACETAMINOPHEN AND CAFFEINE, ACETAMINOPHEN
BUTALBITAL, ACETAMINOPHEN, CAFFEINE, ACETAMINOPHEN
BUTALBITAL, APAP, AND CAFFEINE, ACETAMINOPHEN
BUTALBITAL, ASPIRIN & CAFFEINE, ASPIRIN
BUTALBITAL, ASPIRIN AND CAFFEINE, ASPIRIN
BUTAPAP, ACETAMINOPHEN
BUTAZOLIDIN, PHENYLBUTAZONE
BUTICAPS, BUTABARBITAL SODIUM
BUTISOL SODIUM, BUTABARBITAL SODIUM

APPENDIX A
PRODUCT NAME INDEX *(continued)*

C

C-SOLVE-2, ERYTHROMYCIN
CAFERGOT, CAFFEINE
CALAN, VERAPAMIL HYDROCHLORIDE
CALCIBIND, CELLULOSE SODIUM PHOSPHATE
CALCIJEX, CALCITRIOL
CALCIMAR, CALCITONIN, SALMON
CALCIPARINE, HEPARIN CALCIUM
CALCIUM DISODIUM VERSENATE, EDETATE CALCIUM DISODIUM
CALCIUM GLUCEPTATE, CALCIUM GLUCEPTATE
CALDEROL, CALCIFEDIOL
CALMURID HC, HYDROCORTISONE
CAM-AP-ES, HYDRALAZINE HYDROCHLORIDE
CAM-METRAZINE, PHENDIMETRAZINE TARTRATE
CAMOQUIN HCL, AMODIAQUINE HYDROCHLORIDE
CANDEX, NYSTATIN
CANTIL, MEPENZOLATE BROMIDE
CAP-PROFEN, IBUPROFEN (OTC)
CAPASTAT SULFATE, CAPREOMYCIN SULFATE
CAPITAL AND CODEINE, ACETAMINOPHEN
CAPITAL WITH CODEINE, ACETAMINOPHEN
CAPITROL, CHLOROXINE
CAPOTEN, CAPTOPRIL
CAPOZIDE 25/15, CAPTOPRIL
CAPOZIDE 25/25, CAPTOPRIL
CAPOZIDE 50/15, CAPTOPRIL
CAPOZIDE 50/25, CAPTOPRIL
CARAFATE, SUCRALFATE
CARBACHOL, CARBACHOL
CARBAMAZEPINE, CARBAMAZEPINE
CARBIDOPA AND LEVODOPA, CARBIDOPA
CARBOCAINE, MEPIVACAINE HYDROCHLORIDE
CARBOCAINE W/ NEO-COBEFRIN, LEVONORDEFRIN
CARDASE, ETHOXZOLAMIDE
CARDENE, NICARDIPINE HYDROCHLORIDE
CARDENE SR, NICARDIPINE HYDROCHLORIDE
CARDIO-GREEN, INDOCYANINE GREEN
CARDIOGEN-82, RUBIDIUM CHLORIDE RB-82
CARDIOGRAFIN, DIATRIZOATE MEGLUMINE
CARDIOLITE, TECHNETIUM TC-99M SESTAMIBI KIT
CARDIOQUIN, QUINIDINE POLYGALACTURONATE
CARDIOTEC, TECHNETIUM TC-99M TEBOROXIME KIT
CARDIZEM, DILTIAZEM HYDROCHLORIDE
CARDIZEM CD, DILTIAZEM HYDROCHLORIDE
CARDIZEM SR, DILTIAZEM HYDROCHLORIDE
CARDRASE, ETHOXZOLAMIDE
CARDURA, DOXAZOSIN MESYLATE
CARISOPRODOL, CARISOPRODOL
CARISOPRODOL AND ASPIRIN, ASPIRIN
CARISOPRODOL COMPOUND, ASPIRIN
CARMOL HC, HYDROCORTISONE ACETATE
CARNITOR, LEVOCARNITINE
CARTROL, CARTEOLOL HYDROCHLORIDE
CATAFLAM, DICLOFENAC POTASSIUM
CATAPRES, CLONIDINE HYDROCHLORIDE
CATAPRES-TTS-1, CLONIDINE
CATAPRES-TTS-2, CLONIDINE
CATAPRES-TTS-3, CLONIDINE
CATARASE, CHYMOTRYPSIN
CECLOR, CEFACLOR
CEDILANID-D, DESLANOSIDE
CEENU, LOMUSTINE
CEFADROXIL, CEFADROXIL/CEFADROXIL HEMIHYDRATE
CEFADYL, CEPHAPIRIN SODIUM
CEFANEX, CEPHALEXIN
CEFAZOLIN SODIUM, CEFAZOLIN SODIUM
CEFIZOX, CEFTIZOXIME SODIUM
CEFIZOX IN DEXTROSE 5% IN PLASTIC CONTAINER, CEFTIZOXIME SODIUM
CEFMAX, CEFMENOXIME HYDROCHLORIDE
CEFOBID, CEFOPERAZONE SODIUM
CEFOTAN, CEFOTETAN DISODIUM
CEFPIRAMIDE SODIUM, CEFPIRAMIDE SODIUM
CEFTAZIDIME SODIUM, CEFTAZIDIME SODIUM
CEFTIN, CEFUROXIME AXETIL
CEFUROXIME, CEFUROXIME SODIUM
CEFZIL, CEFPROZIL
CELESTONE, BETAMETHASONE
CELESTONE, BETAMETHASONE SODIUM PHOSPHATE
CELESTONE SOLUSPAN, BETAMETHASONE ACETATE
CELONTIN, METHSUXIMIDE
CENTRAX, PRAZEPAM
CEPHALEXIN, CEPHALEXIN
CEPHALOTHIN, CEPHALOTHIN SODIUM
CEPHALOTHIN SODIUM, CEPHALOTHIN SODIUM
CEPHALOTHIN SODIUM W/ DEXTROSE, CEPHALOTHIN SODIUM
CEPHALOTHIN SODIUM W/ SODIUM CHLORIDE, CEPHALOTHIN SODIUM
CEPHAPIRIN SODIUM, CEPHAPIRIN SODIUM
CEPHRADINE, CEPHRADINE
CEPHULAC, LACTULOSE
CEPTAZ, CEFTAZIDIME (ARGININE FORMULATION)
CERADON, CEFOTIAM HYDROCHLORIDE
CEREDASE, ALGLUCERASE
CERETEC, TECHNETIUM TC-99M EXAMETAZIME KIT
CEREZYME, IMIGLUCERASE
CERUBIDINE, DAUNORUBICIN HYDROCHLORIDE
CERUMENEX, TRIETHANOLAMINE POLYPEPTIDE OLEATE CONDENSATE
CESAMET, NABILONE
CETACORT, HYDROCORTISONE
CETAMIDE, SULFACETAMIDE SODIUM
CETAPRED, PREDNISOLONE ACETATE
CHEMET, SUCCIMER
CHENIX, CHENODIOL
CHG SCRUB, CHLORHEXIDINE GLUCONATE (OTC)
CHIBROXIN, NORFLOXACIN
CHILDREN'S ADVIL, IBUPROFEN
CHLOR-TRIMETON, CHLORPHENIRAMINE MALEATE
CHLOR-TRIMETON, CHLORPHENIRAMINE MALEATE (OTC)
CHLORAMPHENICOL, CHLORAMPHENICOL
CHLORAMPHENICOL, CHLORAMPHENICOL SODIUM SUCCINATE
CHLORAMPHENICOL SODIUM SUCCINATE, CHLORAMPHENICOL SODIUM SUCCINATE
CHLORDIAZACHEL, CHLORDIAZEPOXIDE HYDROCHLORIDE
CHLORDIAZEPOXIDE AND AMITRIPTYLINE HCL, AMITRIPTYLINE HYDROCHLORIDE
CHLORDIAZEPOXIDE HCL, CHLORDIAZEPOXIDE HYDROCHLORIDE
CHLORHEXIDINE GLUCONATE, CHLORHEXIDINE GLUCONATE (OTC)
CHLORMERODRIN HG 197, CHLORMERODRIN, HG-197
CHLOROFAIR, CHLORAMPHENICOL
CHLOROHENIRAMINE MALEATE AND PHENYLPROPANOLAMINE HCL, CHLORPHENIRAMINE MALEATE
CHLOROMYCETIN, CHLORAMPHENICOL
CHLOROMYCETIN, CHLORAMPHENICOL SODIUM SUCCINATE
CHLOROMYCETIN HYDROCORTISONE, CHLORAMPHENICOL
CHLOROMYCETIN PALMITATE, CHLORAMPHENICOL PALMITATE
CHLOROMYXIN, CHLORAMPHENICOL
CHLOROPROCAINE HCL, CHLOROPROCAINE HYDROCHLORIDE
CHLOROPTIC, CHLORAMPHENICOL

APPENDIX A
PRODUCT NAME INDEX *(continued)*

CHLOROPTIC S.O.P., CHLORAMPHENICOL
CHLOROPTIC-P S.O.P., CHLORAMPHENICOL
CHLOROQUINE PHOSPHATE, CHLOROQUINE PHOSPHATE
CHLOROTHIAZIDE, CHLOROTHIAZIDE
CHLOROTHIAZIDE AND RESERPINE, CHLOROTHIAZIDE
CHLOROTHIAZIDE W/ RESERPINE, CHLOROTHIAZIDE
CHLOROTHIAZIDE-RESERPINE, CHLOROTHIAZIDE
CHLOROTRIANISENE, CHLOROTRIANISENE
CHLORPHENIRAMINE MALEATE, CHLORPHENIRAMINE MALEATE
CHLORPHENIRAMINE MALEATE, CHLORPHENIRAMINE MALEATE (OTC)
CHLORPHENIRAMINE MALEATE AND PHENYLPROPANOLAMINE HCL, CHLORPHENIRAMINE MALEATE
CHLORPROMAZINE HCL, CHLORPROMAZINE HYDROCHLORIDE
CHLORPROMAZINE HCL INTENSOL, CHLORPROMAZINE HYDROCHLORIDE
CHLORPROPAMIDE, CHLORPROPAMIDE
CHLORTHALIDONE, CHLORTHALIDONE
CHLORZOXAZONE, CHLORZOXAZONE
CHOLAC, LACTULOSE
CHOLEBRINE, IOCETAMIC ACID
CHOLEDYL, OXTRIPHYLLINE
CHOLEDYL SA, OXTRIPHYLLINE
CHOLETEC, TECHNETIUM TC-99M MEBROFENIN KIT
CHOLOGRAFIN MEGLUMINE, IODIPAMIDE MEGLUMINE
CHOLOGRAFIN SODIUM, IODIPAMIDE SODIUM
CHOLOVUE, IODOXAMATE MEGLUMINE
CHOLOXIN, DEXTROTHYROXINE SODIUM
CHOLYBAR, CHOLESTYRAMINE
CHORIONIC GONADOTROPIN, GONADOTROPIN, CHORIONIC
CHROMALBIN, ALBUMIN CHROMATED CR-51 SERUM
CHROMIC CHLORIDE, CHROMIC CHLORIDE
CHROMITOPE SODIUM, SODIUM CHROMATE, CR-51
CHRONULAC, LACTULOSE
CHYMEX, BENTIROMIDE
CHYMODIACTIN, CHYMOPAPAIN
CIBACALCIN, CALCITONIN, HUMAN
CIBALITH-S, LITHIUM CITRATE
CIDA-STAT, CHLORHEXIDINE GLUCONATE (OTC)
CILOXAN, CIPROFLOXACIN HYDROCHLORIDE
CIMETIDINE, CIMETIDINE
CIMETIDINE HCL, CIMETIDINE HYDROCHLORIDE
CIN-QUIN, QUINIDINE SULFATE
CINNASIL, RESCINNAMINE
CINOBAC, CINOXACIN
CINOXACIN, CINOXACIN
CINTICHEM TECHNETIUM 99M HEDSPA, TECHNETIUM TC-99M ETIDRONATE KIT
CIPRO, CIPROFLOXACIN
CIPRO, CIPROFLOXACIN HYDROCHLORIDE
CIPRO IN DEXTROSE 5%, CIPROFLOXACIN
CIPRO IN SODIUM CHLORIDE 0.9%, CIPROFLOXACIN
CIRCANOL, ERGOLOID MESYLATES
CITANEST, PRILOCAINE HYDROCHLORIDE
CITANEST FORTE, EPINEPHRINE BITARTRATE
CITANEST PLAIN, PRILOCAINE HYDROCHLORIDE
CLAFORAN, CEFOTAXIME SODIUM
CLAFORAN IN DEXTROSE 5%, CEFOTAXIME SODIUM
CLAFORAN IN SODIUM CHLORIDE 0.9%, CEFOTAXIME SODIUM
CLARITIN, LORATADINE
CLEMASTINE FUMARATE, CLEMASTINE FUMARATE
CLEMASTINE FUMARATE, CLEMASTINE FUMARATE (OTC)
CLEOCIN, CLINDAMYCIN HYDROCHLORIDE
CLEOCIN, CLINDAMYCIN PALMITATE HYDROCHLORIDE
CLEOCIN, CLINDAMYCIN PHOSPHATE
CLEOCIN HCL, CLINDAMYCIN HYDROCHLORIDE
CLEOCIN PHOSPHATE, CLINDAMYCIN PHOSPHATE
CLEOCIN PHOSPHATE IN DEXTROSE 5%, CLINDAMYCIN PHOSPHATE
CLEOCIN T, CLINDAMYCIN PHOSPHATE
CLINDA-DERM, CLINDAMYCIN PHOSPHATE
CLINDAMYCIN HCL, CLINDAMYCIN HYDROCHLORIDE
CLINDAMYCIN PHOSPHATE, CLINDAMYCIN PHOSPHATE
CLINDAMYCIN PHOSPHATE IN DEXTROSE 5%, CLINDAMYCIN PHOSPHATE
CLINORIL, SULINDAC
CLISTIN, CARBINOXAMINE MALEATE
CLOBETASOL PROPIONATE, CLOBETASOL PROPIONATE
CLODERM, CLOCORTOLONE PIVALATE
CLOFIBRATE, CLOFIBRATE
CLOMID, CLOMIPHENE CITRATE
CLONIDINE HCL, CLONIDINE HYDROCHLORIDE
CLONIDINE HCL AND CHLORTHALIDONE, CHLORTHALIDONE
CLOPRA, METOCLOPRAMIDE HYDROCHLORIDE
CLOPRA"-YELLOW", METOCLOPRAMIDE HYDROCHLORIDE
CLORAZEPATE DIPOTASSIUM, CLORAZEPATE DIPOTASSIUM
CLOTRIMAZOLE, CLOTRIMAZOLE
CLOXACILLIN SODIUM, CLOXACILLIN SODIUM
CLOXAPEN, CLOXACILLIN SODIUM
CLOZARIL, CLOZAPINE
CO-GESIC, ACETAMINOPHEN
CO-LAV, POLYETHYLENE GLYCOL 3350
COACTIN, AMDINOCILLIN
COBAVITE, CYANOCOBALAMIN
CODEINE PHOSPHATE AND ACETAMINOPHEN, ACETAMINOPHEN
CODEINE, ASPIRIN, APAP FORMULA NO. 2, ACETAMINOPHEN
CODEINE, ASPIRIN, APAP FORMULA NO. 3, ACETAMINOPHEN
CODEINE, ASPIRIN, APAP FORMULA NO. 4, ACETAMINOPHEN
CODIMAL-L.A. 12, CHLORPHENIRAMINE MALEATE (OTC)
CODOXY, ASPIRIN
COGENTIN, BENZTROPINE MESYLATE
COGNEX, TACRINE HYDROCHLORIDE
COL-PROBENECID, COLCHICINE
COLBENEMID, COLCHICINE
COLD CAPSULE IV, CHLORPHENIRAMINE MALEATE (OTC)
COLD CAPSULE V, CHLORPHENIRAMINE MALEATE (OTC)
COLESTID, COLESTIPOL HYDROCHLORIDE
COLONAID, ATROPINE SULFATE
COLOVAGE, POLYETHYLENE GLYCOL 3350
COLY-MYCIN M, COLISTIMETHATE SODIUM
COLY-MYCIN S, COLISTIN SULFATE
COLYTE, POLYETHYLENE GLYCOL 3350
COLYTE-FLAVORED, POLYETHYLENE GLYCOL 3350
COMBIPRES, CHLORTHALIDONE
COMOX, AMOXICILLIN
COMPAL, ACETAMINOPHEN
COMPAZINE, PROCHLORPERAZINE
COMPAZINE, PROCHLORPERAZINE EDISYLATE
COMPAZINE, PROCHLORPERAZINE MALEATE
COMPOUND 65, ASPIRIN
CONCENTRAID, DESMOPRESSIN ACETATE
CONDYLOX, PODOFILOX
CONRAY, IOTHALAMATE MEGLUMINE
CONRAY 30, IOTHALAMATE MEGLUMINE
CONRAY 325, IOTHALAMATE SODIUM
CONRAY 400, IOTHALAMATE SODIUM
CONRAY 43, IOTHALAMATE MEGLUMINE
CONSTILAC, LACTULOSE
CONSTULOSE, LACTULOSE

APPENDIX A
PRODUCT NAME INDEX *(continued)*

CONTAC, CHLORPHENIRAMINE MALEATE (OTC)
CONTEN, ACETAMINOPHEN
COPPER T MODEL TCU 380A, COPPER
COR-OTICIN, HYDROCORTISONE ACETATE
CORDARONE, AMIODARONE HYDROCHLORIDE
CORDRAN, FLURANDRENOLIDE
CORDRAN SP, FLURANDRENOLIDE
CORDRAN-N, FLURANDRENOLIDE
CORGARD, NADOLOL
CORPHED, PSEUDOEPHEDRINE HYDROCHLORIDE
CORSYM, CHLORPHENIRAMINE POLISTIREX (OTC)
CORT-DOME, HYDROCORTISONE
CORTALONE, PREDNISOLONE
CORTAN, PREDNISONE
CORTEF, HYDROCORTISONE
CORTEF, HYDROCORTISONE CYPIONATE
CORTEF ACETATE, HYDROCORTISONE ACETATE
CORTENEMA, HYDROCORTISONE
CORTICOTROPIN, CORTICOTROPIN
CORTIFOAM, HYDROCORTISONE ACETATE
CORTISONE ACETATE, CORTISONE ACETATE
CORTISPORIN, BACITRACIN ZINC
CORTISPORIN, HYDROCORTISONE
CORTISPORIN, HYDROCORTISONE ACETATE
CORTONE, CORTISONE ACETATE
CORTRIL, HYDROCORTISONE
CORTRIL, HYDROCORTISONE ACETATE
CORTROPHIN-ZINC, CORTICOTROPIN-ZINC HYDROXIDE
CORTROSYN, COSYNTROPIN
CORZIDE, BENDROFLUMETHIAZIDE
COSMEGEN, DACTINOMYCIN
COTRIM, SULFAMETHOXAZOLE
COTRIM D.S., SULFAMETHOXAZOLE
COTRIM PEDIATRIC, SULFAMETHOXAZOLE
COUMADIN, WARFARIN SODIUM
CRESCORMON, SOMATROPIN
CROMOLYN SODIUM, CROMOLYN SODIUM
CROTAN, CROTAMITON
CRYSTODIGIN, DIGITOXIN
CU-7, COPPER
CUPRIC CHLORIDE, CUPRIC CHLORIDE
CUPRIC SULFATE, CUPRIC SULFATE
CUPRIMINE, PENICILLAMINE
CURRETAB, MEDROXYPROGESTERONE ACETATE
CUTIVATE, FLUTICASONE PROPIONATE
CYANOCOBALAMIN, CYANOCOBALAMIN
CYANOCOBALAMIN CO 57 SCHILLING TEST KIT, CYANOCOBALAMIN
CYCLACILLIN, CYCLACILLIN
CYCLAINE, HEXYLCAINE HYDROCHLORIDE
CYCLAPEN-W, CYCLACILLIN
CYCLOBENZAPRINE HCL, CYCLOBENZAPRINE HYDROCHLORIDE
CYCLOCORT, AMCINONIDE
CYCLOGYL, CYCLOPENTOLATE HYDROCHLORIDE
CYCLOMYDRIL, CYCLOPENTOLATE HYDROCHLORIDE
CYCLOPAR, TETRACYCLINE HYDROCHLORIDE
CYCLOPENTOLATE HCL, CYCLOPENTOLATE HYDROCHLORIDE
CYCLOPHOSPHAMIDE, CYCLOPHOSPHAMIDE
CYCRIN, MEDROXYPROGESTERONE ACETATE
CYKLOKAPRON, TRANEXAMIC ACID
CYLERT, PEMOLINE
CYPROHEPTADINE HCL, CYPROHEPTADINE HYDROCHLORIDE
CYSTAGON, CYSTEAMINE BITARTRATE
CYSTEINE HCL, CYSTEINE HYDROCHLORIDE
CYSTO-CONRAY, IOTHALAMATE MEGLUMINE
CYSTO-CONRAY II, IOTHALAMATE MEGLUMINE
CYSTOGRAFIN, DIATRIZOATE MEGLUMINE
CYSTOGRAFIN DILUTE, DIATRIZOATE MEGLUMINE
CYTADREN, AMINOGLUTETHIMIDE
CYTARABINE, CYTARABINE
CYTOMEL, LIOTHYRONINE SODIUM
CYTOSAR-U, CYTARABINE
CYTOTEC, MISOPROSTOL
CYTOVENE, GANCICLOVIR SODIUM
CYTOXAN, CYCLOPHOSPHAMIDE

D

D.H.E. 45, DIHYDROERGOTAMINE MESYLATE
DACARBAZINE, DACARBAZINE
DALGAN, DEZOCINE
DALMANE, FLURAZEPAM HYDROCHLORIDE
DANAZOL, DANAZOL
DANOCRINE, DANAZOL
DANTRIUM, DANTROLENE SODIUM
DAPEX-37.5, PHENTERMINE HYDROCHLORIDE
DAPSONE, DAPSONE
DARANIDE, DICHLORPHENAMIDE
DARAPRIM, PYRIMETHAMINE
DARBID, ISOPROPAMIDE IODIDE
DARICON, OXYPHENCYCLIMINE HYDROCHLORIDE
DARVOCET, ACETAMINOPHEN
DARVOCET-N 100, ACETAMINOPHEN
DARVOCET-N 50, ACETAMINOPHEN
DARVON, PROPOXYPHENE HYDROCHLORIDE
DARVON COMPOUND, ASPIRIN
DARVON COMPOUND-65, ASPIRIN
DARVON W/ ASA, ASPIRIN
DARVON-N, PROPOXYPHENE NAPSYLATE
DARVON-N W/ ASA, ASPIRIN
DAYPRO, OXAPROZIN
DDAVP, DESMOPRESSIN ACETATE
DEAPRIL-ST, ERGOLOID MESYLATES
DECA-DURABOLIN, NANDROLONE DECANOATE
DECABID, INDECAINIDE HYDROCHLORIDE
DECADERM, DEXAMETHASONE
DECADRON, DEXAMETHASONE
DECADRON, DEXAMETHASONE SODIUM PHOSPHATE
DECADRON W/ XYLOCAINE, DEXAMETHASONE SODIUM PHOSPHATE
DECADRON-LA, DEXAMETHASONE ACETATE
DECAPRYN, DOXYLAMINE SUCCINATE
DECASPRAY, DEXAMETHASONE
DECLOMYCIN, DEMECLOCYCLINE HYDROCHLORIDE
DEL-VI-A, VITAMIN A PALMITATE
DELADUMONE, ESTRADIOL VALERATE
DELADUMONE OB, ESTRADIOL VALERATE
DELALUTIN, HYDROXYPROGESTERONE CAPROATE
DELATESTRYL, TESTOSTERONE ENANTHATE
DELAXIN, METHOCARBAMOL
DELCOBESE, AMPHETAMINE ADIPATE
DELESTROGEN, ESTRADIOL VALERATE
DELFLEX W/ DEXTROSE 1.5% IN PLASTIC CONTAINER, CALCIUM CHLORIDE
DELFLEX W/ DEXTROSE 1.5% LOW MAGNESIUM IN PLASTIC CONTAINER, CALCIUM CHLORIDE
DELFLEX W/ DEXTROSE 1.5% LOW MAGNESIUM LOW CALCIUM, CALCIUM CHLORIDE
DELFLEX W/ DEXTROSE 2.5% IN PLASTIC CONTAINER, CALCIUM CHLORIDE
DELFLEX W/ DEXTROSE 2.5% LOW MAGNESIUM IN PLASTIC CONTAINER, CALCIUM CHLORIDE
DELFLEX W/ DEXTROSE 2.5% LOW MAGNESIUM LOW CALCIUM, CALCIUM CHLORIDE
DELFLEX W/ DEXTROSE 4.25% IN PLASTIC CONTAINER, CALCIUM CHLORIDE
DELFLEX W/ DEXTROSE 4.25% LOW MAGNESIUM IN PLASTIC CONTAINER, CALCIUM CHLORIDE
DELFLEX W/ DEXTROSE 4.25% LOW MAGNESIUM LOW CALCIUM, CALCIUM CHLORIDE

APPENDIX A
PRODUCT NAME INDEX *(continued)*

DELSYM, DEXTROMETHORPHAN POLISTIREX (OTC)
DELTA-CORTEF, PREDNISOLONE
DELTA-DOME, PREDNISONE
DELTALIN, ERGOCALCIFEROL
DELTASONE, PREDNISONE
DEMADEX, TORSEMIDE
DEMAZIN, CHLORPHENIRAMINE MALEATE (OTC)
DEMEROL, MEPERIDINE HYDROCHLORIDE
DEMI-REGROTON, CHLORTHALIDONE
DEMSER, METYROSINE
DEMULEN 1/35-21, ETHINYL ESTRADIOL
DEMULEN 1/35-28, ETHINYL ESTRADIOL
DEMULEN 1/50-21, ETHINYL ESTRADIOL
DEMULEN 1/50-28, ETHINYL ESTRADIOL
DENDRID, IDOXURIDINE
DEPAKENE, VALPROIC ACID
DEPAKOTE, DIVALPROEX SODIUM
DEPAKOTE CP, DIVALPROEX SODIUM
DEPEN 250, PENICILLAMINE
DEPINAR, CYANOCOBALAMIN
DEPO-ESTRADIOL, ESTRADIOL CYPIONATE
DEPO-MEDROL, METHYLPREDNISOLONE ACETATE
DEPO-PROVERA, MEDROXYPROGESTERONE ACETATE
DEPO-TESTADIOL, ESTRADIOL CYPIONATE
DEPO-TESTOSTERONE, TESTOSTERONE CYPIONATE
DERMA-SMOOTHE/FS, FLUOCINOLONE ACETONIDE
DERMABET, BETAMETHASONE VALERATE
DERMACORT, HYDROCORTISONE
DERMATOP, PREDNICARBATE
DESFERAL, DEFEROXAMINE MESYLATE
DESIPRAMINE HCL, DESIPRAMINE HYDROCHLORIDE
DESMOPRESSIN ACETATE, DESMOPRESSIN ACETATE
DESOGEN, DESOGESTREL
DESONIDE, DESONIDE
DESOWEN, DESONIDE
DESOXIMETASONE, DESOXIMETASONE
DESOXYN, METHAMPHETAMINE HYDROCHLORIDE
DESYREL, TRAZODONE HYDROCHLORIDE
DEXACEN-4, DEXAMETHASONE SODIUM PHOSPHATE
DEXACIDIN, DEXAMETHASONE
DEXACORT, DEXAMETHASONE SODIUM PHOSPHATE
DEXAIR, DEXAMETHASONE SODIUM PHOSPHATE
DEXAMETHASONE, DEXAMETHASONE
DEXAMETHASONE, DEXAMETHASONE SODIUM PHOSPHATE
DEXAMETHASONE ACETATE, DEXAMETHASONE ACETATE
DEXAMETHASONE INTENSOL, DEXAMETHASONE
DEXAMETHASONE SODIUM PHOSPHATE, DEXAMETHASONE SODIUM PHOSPHATE
DEXAMPEX, DEXTROAMPHETAMINE SULFATE
DEXASPORIN, DEXAMETHASONE
DEXCHLORPHENIRAMINE MALEATE, DEXCHLORPHENIRAMINE MALEATE
DEXEDRINE, DEXTROAMPHETAMINE SULFATE
DEXONE 0.5, DEXAMETHASONE
DEXONE 0.75, DEXAMETHASONE
DEXONE 1.5, DEXAMETHASONE
DEXONE 4, DEXAMETHASONE
DEXTROAMPHETAMINE SULFATE, DEXTROAMPHETAMINE SULFATE
DEXTROSE 10%, DEXTROSE
DEXTROSE 10% AND SODIUM CHLORIDE 0.11%, DEXTROSE
DEXTROSE 10% AND SODIUM CHLORIDE 0.2%, DEXTROSE
DEXTROSE 10% AND SODIUM CHLORIDE 0.33%, DEXTROSE
DEXTROSE 10% AND SODIUM CHLORIDE 0.45%, DEXTROSE
DEXTROSE 10% AND SODIUM CHLORIDE 0.9%, DEXTROSE
DEXTROSE 10% AND SODIUM CHLORIDE 0.9% IN PLASTIC CONTAINER, DEXTROSE
DEXTROSE 10% IN PLASTIC CONTAINER, DEXTROSE
DEXTROSE 2.5%, DEXTROSE
DEXTROSE 2.5% AND SODIUM CHLORIDE 0.11%, DEXTROSE
DEXTROSE 2.5% AND SODIUM CHLORIDE 0.2%, DEXTROSE
DEXTROSE 2.5% AND SODIUM CHLORIDE 0.33%, DEXTROSE
DEXTROSE 2.5% AND SODIUM CHLORIDE 0.45%, DEXTROSE
DEXTROSE 2.5% AND SODIUM CHLORIDE 0.45% IN PLASTIC CONTAINER, DEXTROSE
DEXTROSE 2.5% AND SODIUM CHLORIDE 0.9%, DEXTROSE
DEXTROSE 2.5% IN HALF-STRENGTH LACTATED RINGER'S, CALCIUM CHLORIDE
DEXTROSE 20% IN PLASTIC CONTAINER, DEXTROSE
DEXTROSE 3.3% AND SODIUM CHLORIDE 0.3%, DEXTROSE
DEXTROSE 3.3% AND SODIUM CHLORIDE 0.3% IN PLASTIC CONTAINER, DEXTROSE
DEXTROSE 30% IN PLASTIC CONTAINER, DEXTROSE
DEXTROSE 38.5% IN PLASTIC CONTAINER, DEXTROSE
DEXTROSE 4% IN MODIFIED LACTATED RINGER'S, CALCIUM CHLORIDE
DEXTROSE 40% IN PLASTIC CONTAINER, DEXTROSE
DEXTROSE 5%, DEXTROSE
DEXTROSE 5% AND ELECTROLYTE NO 75, DEXTROSE
DEXTROSE 5% AND ELECTROLYTE NO.48 IN PLASTIC CONTAINER, DEXTROSE
DEXTROSE 5% AND LACTATED RINGER'S IN PLASTIC CONTAINER, CALCIUM CHLORIDE
DEXTROSE 5% AND POTASSIUM CHLORIDE 0.075% IN PLASTIC CONTAINER, DEXTROSE
DEXTROSE 5% AND POTASSIUM CHLORIDE 0.15% IN PLASTIC CONTAINER, DEXTROSE
DEXTROSE 5% AND POTASSIUM CHLORIDE 0.224% IN PLASTIC CONTAINER, DEXTROSE
DEXTROSE 5% AND POTASSIUM CHLORIDE 0.3% IN PLASTIC CONTAINER, DEXTROSE
DEXTROSE 5% AND RINGER'S IN PLASTIC CONTAINER, CALCIUM CHLORIDE
DEXTROSE 5% AND SODIUM CHLORIDE 0.11%, DEXTROSE
DEXTROSE 5% AND SODIUM CHLORIDE 0.11% IN PLASTIC CONTAINER, DEXTROSE
DEXTROSE 5% AND SODIUM CHLORIDE 0.2%, DEXTROSE
DEXTROSE 5% AND SODIUM CHLORIDE 0.2% IN PLASTIC CONTAINER, DEXTROSE
DEXTROSE 5% AND SODIUM CHLORIDE 0.225%, DEXTROSE
DEXTROSE 5% AND SODIUM CHLORIDE 0.225% IN PLASTIC CONTAINER, DEXTROSE
DEXTROSE 5% AND SODIUM CHLORIDE 0.3%, DEXTROSE
DEXTROSE 5% AND SODIUM CHLORIDE 0.3% IN PLASTIC CONTAINER, DEXTROSE
DEXTROSE 5% AND SODIUM CHLORIDE 0.33%, DEXTROSE
DEXTROSE 5% AND SODIUM CHLORIDE 0.33% IN PLASTIC CONTAINER, DEXTROSE
DEXTROSE 5% AND SODIUM CHLORIDE 0.45%, DEXTROSE
DEXTROSE 5% AND SODIUM CHLORIDE 0.45% IN PLASTIC CONTAINER, DEXTROSE
DEXTROSE 5% AND SODIUM CHLORIDE 0.9%, DEXTROSE
DEXTROSE 5% AND SODIUM CHLORIDE 0.9% IN PLASTIC CONTAINER, DEXTROSE
DEXTROSE 5% IN ACETATED RINGER'S IN PLASTIC CONTAINER, CALCIUM CHLORIDE
DEXTROSE 5% IN LACTATED RINGER'S, CALCIUM CHLORIDE
DEXTROSE 5% IN LACTATED RINGER'S IN PLASTIC CONTAINER, CALCIUM CHLORIDE
DEXTROSE 5% IN PLASTIC CONTAINER, DEXTROSE
DEXTROSE 5% IN RINGER'S, CALCIUM CHLORIDE

APPENDIX A
PRODUCT NAME INDEX *(continued)*

DEXTROSE 5% IN RINGER'S IN PLASTIC CONTAINER, CALCIUM CHLORIDE
DEXTROSE 5% IN SODIUM CHLORIDE 0.2% IN PLASTIC CONTAINER, DEXTROSE
DEXTROSE 5% IN SODIUM CHLORIDE 0.33% IN PLASTIC CONTAINER, DEXTROSE
DEXTROSE 5% IN SODIUM CHLORIDE 0.45% IN PLASTIC CONTAINER, DEXTROSE
DEXTROSE 5% IN SODIUM CHLORIDE 0.9% IN PLASTIC CONTAINER, DEXTROSE
DEXTROSE 5%, SODIUM CHLORIDE 0.2% AND POTASSIUM CHLORIDE 0.075%, DEXTROSE
DEXTROSE 5%, SODIUM CHLORIDE 0.2% AND POTASSIUM CHLORIDE 0.15%, DEXTROSE
DEXTROSE 5%, SODIUM CHLORIDE 0.2% AND POTASSIUM CHLORIDE 0.224%, DEXTROSE
DEXTROSE 5%, SODIUM CHLORIDE 0.2% AND POTASSIUM CHLORIDE 0.3%, DEXTROSE
DEXTROSE 5%, SODIUM CHLORIDE 0.2% AND POTASSIUM CHLORIDE 10 MEQ, DEXTROSE
DEXTROSE 5%, SODIUM CHLORIDE 0.2% AND POTASSIUM CHLORIDE 15 MEQ (K), DEXTROSE
DEXTROSE 5%, SODIUM CHLORIDE 0.2% AND POTASSIUM CHLORIDE 20 MEQ (K), DEXTROSE
DEXTROSE 5%, SODIUM CHLORIDE 0.2% AND POTASSIUM CHLORIDE 20 MEQ, DEXTROSE
DEXTROSE 5%, SODIUM CHLORIDE 0.2% AND POTASSIUM CHLORIDE 30 MEQ, DEXTROSE
DEXTROSE 5%, SODIUM CHLORIDE 0.2% AND POTASSIUM CHLORIDE 40 MEQ, DEXTROSE
DEXTROSE 5%, SODIUM CHLORIDE 0.2% AND POTASSIUM CHLORIDE 5 MEQ (K), DEXTROSE
DEXTROSE 5%, SODIUM CHLORIDE 0.2% AND POTASSIUM CHLORIDE 5 MEQ, DEXTROSE
DEXTROSE 5%, SODIUM CHLORIDE 0.33% AND POTASSIUM CHLORIDE 0.075%, DEXTROSE
DEXTROSE 5%, SODIUM CHLORIDE 0.33% AND POTASSIUM CHLORIDE 0.15%, DEXTROSE
DEXTROSE 5%, SODIUM CHLORIDE 0.33% AND POTASSIUM CHLORIDE 0.22%, DEXTROSE
DEXTROSE 5%, SODIUM CHLORIDE 0.33% AND POTASSIUM CHLORIDE 0.30%, DEXTROSE
DEXTROSE 5%, SODIUM CHLORIDE 0.33% AND POTASSIUM CHLORIDE 10 MEQ, DEXTROSE
DEXTROSE 5%, SODIUM CHLORIDE 0.33% AND POTASSIUM CHLORIDE 15 MEQ, DEXTROSE
DEXTROSE 5%, SODIUM CHLORIDE 0.33% AND POTASSIUM CHLORIDE 20 MEQ, DEXTROSE
DEXTROSE 5%, SODIUM CHLORIDE 0.33% AND POTASSIUM CHLORIDE 30 MEQ, DEXTROSE
DEXTROSE 5%, SODIUM CHLORIDE 0.33% AND POTASSIUM CHLORIDE 40 MEQ, DEXTROSE
DEXTROSE 5%, SODIUM CHLORIDE 0.33% AND POTASSIUM CHLORIDE 5 MEQ, DEXTROSE
DEXTROSE 5%, SODIUM CHLORIDE 0.45% AND POTASSIUM CHLORIDE 0.075%, DEXTROSE
DEXTROSE 5%, SODIUM CHLORIDE 0.45% AND POTASSIUM CHLORIDE 0.15%, DEXTROSE
DEXTROSE 5%, SODIUM CHLORIDE 0.45% AND POTASSIUM CHLORIDE 0.22%, DEXTROSE
DEXTROSE 5%, SODIUM CHLORIDE 0.45% AND POTASSIUM CHLORIDE 0.3%, DEXTROSE
DEXTROSE 5%, SODIUM CHLORIDE 0.45% AND POTASSIUM CHLORIDE 15 MEQ, DEXTROSE
DEXTROSE 5%, SODIUM CHLORIDE 0.45% AND POTASSIUM CHLORIDE 20 MEQ (K), DEXTROSE
DEXTROSE 5%, SODIUM CHLORIDE 0.45% AND POTASSIUM CHLORIDE 20 MEQ (K), DEXTROSE
DEXTROSE 5%, SODIUM CHLORIDE 0.45% AND POTASSIUM CHLORIDE 5 MEQ, DEXTROSE
DEXTROSE 50%, DEXTROSE
DEXTROSE 50% IN PLASTIC CONTAINER, DEXTROSE
DEXTROSE 60%, DEXTROSE
DEXTROSE 60% IN PLASTIC CONTAINER, DEXTROSE
DEXTROSE 7.7%, DEXTROSE
DEXTROSE 70%, DEXTROSE
DEXTROSE 70% IN PLASTIC CONTAINER, DEXTROSE
DI-ATRO, ATROPINE SULFATE
DI-METREX, PHENDIMETRAZINE TARTRATE
DIABETA, GLYBURIDE
DIABINESE, CHLORPROPAMIDE
DIAL, HEXACHLOROPHENE
DIALYTE CONCENTRATE W/ DEXTROSE 30% IN PLASTIC CONTAINER, CALCIUM CHLORIDE
DIALYTE CONCENTRATE W/ DEXTROSE 50% IN PLASTIC CONTAINER, CALCIUM CHLORIDE
DIALYTE LM/ DEXTROSE 1.5%, CALCIUM CHLORIDE
DIALYTE LM/ DEXTROSE 2.5%, CALCIUM CHLORIDE
DIALYTE LM/ DEXTROSE 4.25%, CALCIUM CHLORIDE
DIALYTE W/ DEXTROSE 1.5% IN PLASTIC CONTAINER, CALCIUM CHLORIDE
DIALYTE W/ DEXTROSE 4.25% IN PLASTIC CONTAINER, CALCIUM CHLORIDE
DIAMOX, ACETAZOLAMIDE
DIAMOX, ACETAZOLAMIDE SODIUM
DIANEAL LOW CALCIUM W/ DEXTROSE 1.5%, CALCIUM CHLORIDE
DIANEAL LOW CALCIUM W/ DEXTROSE 2.5%, CALCIUM CHLORIDE
DIANEAL LOW CALCIUM W/ DEXTROSE 3.5%, CALCIUM CHLORIDE
DIANEAL LOW CALCIUM W/ DEXTROSE 4.25%, CALCIUM CHLORIDE
DIANEAL PD-1 W/ DEXTROSE 1.5% IN PLASTIC CONTAINER, CALCIUM CHLORIDE
DIANEAL PD-1 W/ DEXTROSE 2.5% IN PLASTIC CONTAINER, CALCIUM CHLORIDE
DIANEAL PD-1 W/ DEXTROSE 3.5%, CALCIUM CHLORIDE
DIANEAL PD-1 W/ DEXTROSE 4.25% IN PLASTIC CONTAINER, CALCIUM CHLORIDE
DIANEAL PD-2 W/ DEXTROSE 1.5%, CALCIUM CHLORIDE
DIANEAL PD-2 W/ DEXTROSE 2.5%, CALCIUM CHLORIDE
DIANEAL PD-2 W/ DEXTROSE 2.5% IN PLASTIC CONTAINER, CALCIUM CHLORIDE
DIANEAL PD-2 W/ DEXTROSE 3.5%, CALCIUM CHLORIDE
DIANEAL PD-2 W/ DEXTROSE 4.25%, CALCIUM CHLORIDE
DIANEAL PD-2 W/ DEXTROSE 4.25% IN PLASTIC CONTAINER, CALCIUM CHLORIDE
DIANEAL 137 W/ DEXTROSE 1.5% IN PLASTIC CONTAINER, CALCIUM CHLORIDE
DIANEAL 137 W/ DEXTROSE 2.5% IN PLASTIC CONTAINER, CALCIUM CHLORIDE
DIANEAL 137 W/ DEXTROSE 4.25% IN PLASTIC CONTAINER, CALCIUM CHLORIDE
DIAPID, LYPRESSIN
DIASONE SODIUM, SULFOXONE SODIUM
DIATRIZOATE MEGLUMINE, DIATRIZOATE MEGLUMINE
DIATRIZOATE-60, DIATRIZOATE MEGLUMINE
DIAZEPAM, DIAZEPAM
DIAZEPAM INTENSOL, DIAZEPAM
DIAZOXIDE, DIAZOXIDE
DIBENIL, DIPHENHYDRAMINE HYDROCHLORIDE
DIBENZYLINE, PHENOXYBENZAMINE HYDROCHLORIDE
DICLOXACILLIN SODIUM, DICLOXACILLIN SODIUM
DICOPAC KIT, CYANOCOBALAMIN
DICUMAROL, DICUMAROL
DICURIN PROCAINE, PROCAINE MERETHOXYLLINE
DICYCLOMINE HCL, DICYCLOMINE HYDROCHLORIDE
DIDREX, BENZPHETAMINE HYDROCHLORIDE
DIDRONEL, ETIDRONATE DISODIUM
DIENESTROL, DIENESTROL
DIETHYLPROPION HCL, DIETHYLPROPION HYDROCHLORIDE
DIETHYLSTILBESTROL, DIETHYLSTILBESTROL

APPENDIX A
PRODUCT NAME INDEX *(continued)*

DIFLORASONE DIACETATE, DIFLORASONE DIACETATE
DIFLUCAN, FLUCONAZOLE
DIFLUNISAL, DIFLUNISAL
DIGOXIN, DIGOXIN
DILACOR XR, DILTIAZEM HYDROCHLORIDE
DILANTIN, PHENYTOIN
DILANTIN, PHENYTOIN SODIUM
DILANTIN, PHENYTOIN SODIUM, EXTENDED
DILANTIN-125, PHENYTOIN
DILANTIN-30, PHENYTOIN
DILATRATE-SR, ISOSORBIDE DINITRATE
DILAUDID, HYDROMORPHONE HYDROCHLORIDE
DILAUDID-HP, HYDROMORPHONE HYDROCHLORIDE
DILOR, DYPHYLLINE
DILOR-400, DYPHYLLINE
DILTIAZEM HCL, DILTIAZEM HYDROCHLORIDE
DIMENHYDRINATE, DIMENHYDRINATE
DIMETANE, BROMPHENIRAMINE MALEATE
DIMETANE, BROMPHENIRAMINE MALEATE (OTC)
DIMETANE-DC, BROMPHENIRAMINE MALEATE
DIMETANE-DX, BROMPHENIRAMINE MALEATE
DIMETANE-TEN, BROMPHENIRAMINE MALEATE
DIMETAPP, BROMPHENIRAMINE MALEATE (OTC)
DIONOSIL AQUEOUS, PROPYLIODONE
DIONOSIL OILY, PROPYLIODONE
DIPENTUM, OLSALAZINE SODIUM
DIPHEN, DIPHENHYDRAMINE HYDROCHLORIDE
DIPHEN, DIPHENHYDRAMINE HYDROCHLORIDE (OTC)
DIPHENHYDRAMINE HCL, DIPHENHYDRAMINE HYDROCHLORIDE
DIPHENHYDRAMINE HCL, DIPHENHYDRAMINE HYDROCHLORIDE (OTC)
DIPHENOXYLATE HCL AND ATROPINE SULFATE, ATROPINE SULFATE
DIPHENOXYLATE HCL W/ ATROPINE SULFATE, ATROPINE SULFATE
DIPHENYLAN SODIUM, PHENYTOIN SODIUM, PROMPT
DIPIVEFRIN HCL, DIPIVEFRIN HYDROCHLORIDE
DIPRIVAN, PROPOFOL
DIPROLENE, BETAMETHASONE DIPROPIONATE
DIPROLENE AF, BETAMETHASONE DIPROPIONATE
DIPROSONE, BETAMETHASONE DIPROPIONATE
DIPYRIDAMOLE, DIPYRIDAMOLE
DISCASE, CHYMOPAPAIN
DISIPAL, ORPHENADRINE HYDROCHLORIDE
DISOBROM, DEXBROMPHENIRAMINE MALEATE (OTC)
DISODIUM EDETATE, EDETATE DISODIUM
DISOMER, DEXBROMPHENIRAMINE MALEATE
DISOPHROL, DEXBROMPHENIRAMINE MALEATE (OTC)
DISOPYRAMIDE PHOSPHATE, DISOPYRAMIDE PHOSPHATE
DISULFIRAM, DISULFIRAM
DITATE-DS, ESTRADIOL VALERATE
DITROPAN, OXYBUTYNIN CHLORIDE
DIUCARDIN, HYDROFLUMETHIAZIDE
DIULO, METOLAZONE
DIUPRES-250, CHLOROTHIAZIDE
DIUPRES-500, CHLOROTHIAZIDE
DIURIL, CHLOROTHIAZIDE
DIURIL, CHLOROTHIAZIDE SODIUM
DIUTENSEN-R, METHYCLOTHIAZIDE
DIZAC, DIAZEPAM
DOBUTAMINE HCL, DOBUTAMINE HYDROCHLORIDE
DOBUTAMINE HCL IN DEXTROSE 5%, DOBUTAMINE HYDROCHLORIDE
DOBUTREX, DOBUTAMINE HYDROCHLORIDE
DOCA, DESOXYCORTICOSTERONE ACETATE
DOLENE, PROPOXYPHENE HYDROCHLORIDE
DOLENE AP-65, ACETAMINOPHEN
DOLOBID, DIFLUNISAL
DOLOPHINE HCL, METHADONE HYDROCHLORIDE
DOMEBORO, ACETIC ACID, GLACIAL
DOPAMINE, DOPAMINE HYDROCHLORIDE
DOPAMINE HCL, DOPAMINE HYDROCHLORIDE
DOPAMINE HCL AND DEXTROSE 5%, DOPAMINE HYDROCHLORIDE
DOPAMINE HCL IN DEXTROSE 5%, DOPAMINE HYDROCHLORIDE
DOPAR, LEVODOPA
DOPRAM, DOXAPRAM HYDROCHLORIDE
DORAL, QUAZEPAM
DORIDEN, GLUTETHIMIDE
DORMATE, MEBUTAMATE
DORYX, DOXYCYCLINE HYCLATE
DOVONEX, CALCIPOTRIENE
DOW-ISONIAZID, ISONIAZID
DOXAPRAM HCL, DOXAPRAM HYDROCHLORIDE
DOXEPIN HCL, DOXEPIN HYDROCHLORIDE
DOXORUBICIN HCL, DOXORUBICIN HYDROCHLORIDE
DOXY 100, DOXYCYCLINE HYCLATE
DOXY 200, DOXYCYCLINE HYCLATE
DOXY-LEMMON, DOXYCYCLINE HYCLATE
DOXY-SLEEP-AID, DOXYLAMINE SUCCINATE (OTC)
DOXY-TABS, DOXYCYCLINE HYCLATE
DOXYCHEL, DOXYCYCLINE
DOXYCHEL HYCLATE, DOXYCYCLINE HYCLATE
DOXYCYCLINE, DOXYCYCLINE HYCLATE
DOXYCYCLINE HYCLATE, DOXYCYCLINE HYCLATE
DOXYCYCLINE MONOHYDRATE, DOXYCYCLINE
DOXYLAMINE SUCCINATE, DOXYLAMINE SUCCINATE
DOXYLAMINE SUCCINATE, DOXYLAMINE SUCCINATE (OTC)
DRALSERP, HYDRALAZINE HYDROCHLORIDE
DRALZINE, HYDRALAZINE HYDROCHLORIDE
DRICORT, HYDROCORTISONE ACETATE
DRISDOL, ERGOCALCIFEROL
DRIXORAL, DEXBROMPHENIRAMINE MALEATE (OTC)
DRIXORAL PLUS, ACETAMINOPHEN (OTC)
DRIZE, CHLORPHENIRAMINE MALEATE
DROLBAN, DROMOSTANOLONE PROPIONATE
DROPERIDOL, DROPERIDOL
DTIC-DOME, DACARBAZINE
DUO-MEDIHALER, ISOPROTERENOL HYDROCHLORIDE
DUPHALAC, LACTULOSE
DURABOLIN, NANDROLONE PHENPROPIONATE
DURABOLIN-50, NANDROLONE PHENPROPIONATE
DURACILLIN A.S., PENICILLIN G PROCAINE
DURADYNE DHC, ACETAMINOPHEN
DURAGESIC, FENTANYL
DURAMORPH PF, MORPHINE SULFATE
DURANEST, EPINEPHRINE
DURANEST, EPINEPHRINE BITARTRATE
DURANEST, ETIDOCAINE HYDROCHLORIDE
DURAPHYL, THEOPHYLLINE
DURAQUIN, QUINIDINE GLUCONATE
DURICEF, CEFADROXIL/CEFADROXIL HEMIHYDRATE
DUVOID, BETHANECHOL CHLORIDE
DV, DIENESTROL
DYAZIDE, HYDROCHLOROTHIAZIDE
DYCILL, DICLOXACILLIN SODIUM
DYCLONE, DYCLONINE HYDROCHLORIDE
DYMELOR, ACETOHEXAMIDE
DYNACIRC, ISRADIPINE
DYNACIRC CR, ISRADIPINE
DYNAPEN, DICLOXACILLIN SODIUM
DYRENIUM, TRIAMTERENE

E

E.E.S., ERYTHROMYCIN ETHYLSUCCINATE
E.E.S. 200, ERYTHROMYCIN ETHYLSUCCINATE
E.E.S. 400, ERYTHROMYCIN ETHYLSUCCINATE

APPENDIX A
PRODUCT NAME INDEX *(continued)*

E-BASE, ERYTHROMYCIN
E-MYCIN, ERYTHROMYCIN
E-MYCIN E, ERYTHROMYCIN ETHYLSUCCINATE
E-SOLVE 2, ERYTHROMYCIN
E-Z PREP, POVIDONE-IODINE (OTC)
E-Z PREP 220, POVIDONE-IODINE (OTC)
E-Z SCRUB, HEXACHLOROPHENE
E-Z SCRUB 201, POVIDONE-IODINE (OTC)
E-Z SCRUB 241, POVIDONE-IODINE (OTC)
E-Z-EM PREP LYTE, POLYETHYLENE GLYCOL 3350
ECONOCHLOR, CHLORAMPHENICOL
ECONOPRED, PREDNISOLONE ACETATE
ECONOPRED PLUS, PREDNISOLONE ACETATE
EDECRIN, ETHACRYNATE SODIUM
EDECRIN, ETHACRYNIC ACID
EDETATE DISODIUM, EDETATE DISODIUM
EFFEXOR, VENLAFAXINE HYDROCHLORIDE
EFIDAC/24, PSEUDOEPHEDRINE HYDROCHLORIDE (OTC)
EFUDEX, FLUOROURACIL
ELASE-CHLOROMYCETIN, CHLORAMPHENICOL
ELAVIL, AMITRIPTYLINE HYDROCHLORIDE
ELDECORT, HYDROCORTISONE
ELDEPRYL, SELEGILINE HYDROCHLORIDE
ELIMITE, PERMETHRIN
ELIXICON, THEOPHYLLINE
ELIXOMIN, THEOPHYLLINE
ELIXOPHYLLIN, THEOPHYLLINE
ELIXOPHYLLIN SR, THEOPHYLLINE
ELOCON, MOMETASONE FUROATE
EMBOLEX, DIHYDROERGOTAMINE MESYLATE
EMCYT, ESTRAMUSTINE PHOSPHATE SODIUM
EMETE-CON, BENZQUINAMIDE HYDROCHLORIDE
EMGEL, ERYTHROMYCIN
EMLA, LIDOCAINE
EMPRACET W/ CODEINE PHOSPHATE #3, ACETAMINOPHEN
EMPRACET W/ CODEINE PHOSPHATE #4, ACETAMINOPHEN
ENDEP, AMITRIPTYLINE HYDROCHLORIDE
ENDOSOL EXTRA, CALCIUM CHLORIDE
ENDRATE, EDETATE DISODIUM
ENDURON, METHYCLOTHIAZIDE
ENDURONYL, DESERPIDINE
ENDURONYL FORTE, DESERPIDINE
ENFLURANE, ENFLURANE
ENKAID, ENCAINIDE HYDROCHLORIDE
ENLON, EDROPHONIUM CHLORIDE
ENLON-PLUS, ATROPINE SULFATE
ENOVID, MESTRANOL
ENOVID-E, MESTRANOL
ENOVID-E 21, MESTRANOL
ENULOSE, LACTULOSE
EPICORT, HYDROCORTISONE
EPIFOAM, HYDROCORTISONE ACETATE
EPINEPHRINE, EPINEPHRINE (OTC)
EPIPEN, EPINEPHRINE
EPIPEN JR., EPINEPHRINE
EPITOL, CARBAMAZEPINE
EQUAGESIC, ASPIRIN
EQUANIL, MEPROBAMATE
EQUIPIN, HOMATROPINE METHYLBROMIDE
ERCATAB, CAFFEINE
ERGAMISOL, LEVAMISOLE HYDROCHLORIDE
ERGOLOID MESYLATES, ERGOLOID MESYLATES
ERGOMAR, ERGOTAMINE TARTRATE
ERGOSTAT, ERGOTAMINE TARTRATE
ERY-TAB, ERYTHROMYCIN
ERYC, ERYTHROMYCIN
ERYC SPRINKLES, ERYTHROMYCIN
ERYC 125, ERYTHROMYCIN
ERYCETTE, ERYTHROMYCIN
ERYDERM, ERYTHROMYCIN
ERYGEL, ERYTHROMYCIN
ERYMAX, ERYTHROMYCIN
ERYPAR, ERYTHROMYCIN STEARATE
ERYPED, ERYTHROMYCIN ETHYLSUCCINATE
ERYTHRA-DERM, ERYTHROMYCIN
ERYTHROCIN, ERYTHROMYCIN LACTOBIONATE
ERYTHROCIN STEARATE, ERYTHROMYCIN STEARATE
ERYTHROMYCIN, ERYTHROMYCIN
ERYTHROMYCIN, ERYTHROMYCIN LACTOBIONATE
ERYTHROMYCIN ESTOLATE, ERYTHROMYCIN ESTOLATE
ERYTHROMYCIN ETHYLSUCCINATE, ERYTHROMYCIN ETHYLSUCCINATE
ERYTHROMYCIN ETHYLSUCCINATE AND SULFISOXAZOLE ACETYL, ERYTHROMYCIN ETHYLSUCCINATE
ERYTHROMYCIN LACTOBIONATE, ERYTHROMYCIN LACTOBIONATE
ERYTHROMYCIN STEARATE, ERYTHROMYCIN STEARATE
ERYZOLE, ERYTHROMYCIN ETHYLSUCCINATE
ESGIC, ACETAMINOPHEN
ESIDRIX, HYDROCHLOROTHIAZIDE
ESIMIL, GUANETHIDINE MONOSULFATE
ESKALITH, LITHIUM CARBONATE
ESKALITH CR, LITHIUM CARBONATE
ESTERIFIED ESTROGENS, ESTROGENS, ESTERIFIED
ESTINYL, ETHINYL ESTRADIOL
ESTRACE, ESTRADIOL
ESTRADERM, ESTRADIOL
ESTRADIOL CYPIONATE, ESTRADIOL CYPIONATE
ESTRADIOL VALERATE, ESTRADIOL VALERATE
ESTRADURIN, POLYESTRADIOL PHOSPHATE
ESTRAGUARD, DIENESTROL
ESTRATAB, ESTROGENS, ESTERIFIED
ESTROGENIC SUBSTANCE, ESTRONE
ESTRONE, ESTRONE
ESTROPIPATE, ESTROPIPATE
ESTROVIS, QUINESTROL
ETHAMIDE, ETHOXZOLAMIDE
ETHAMOLIN, ETHANOLAMINE OLEATE
ETHCHLORVYNOL, ETHCHLORVYNOL
ETHIODOL, ETHIODIZED OIL
ETHMOZINE, MORICIZINE HYDROCHLORIDE
ETHOSUXIMIDE, ETHOSUXIMIDE
ETHRANE, ENFLURANE
ETHRIL 250, ERYTHROMYCIN STEARATE
ETHRIL 500, ERYTHROMYCIN STEARATE
ETHYNODIOL DIACETATE AND ETHINYL ESTRADIOL 1/35-21, ETHINYL ESTRADIOL
ETHYNODIOL DIACETATE AND ETHINYL ESTRADIOL 1/35-28, ETHINYL ESTRADIOL
ETHYNODIOL DIACETATE AND ETHINYL ESTRADIOL 1/50-21, ETHINYL ESTRADIOL
ETHYNODIOL DIACETATE AND ETHINYL ESTRADIOL 1/50-28, ETHINYL ESTRADIOL
ETOPOSIDE, ETOPOSIDE
ETRAFON 2-10, AMITRIPTYLINE HYDROCHLORIDE
ETRAFON 2-25, AMITRIPTYLINE HYDROCHLORIDE
ETRAFON-A, AMITRIPTYLINE HYDROCHLORIDE
ETRAFON-FORTE, AMITRIPTYLINE HYDROCHLORIDE
EULEXIN, FLUTAMIDE
EURAX, CROTAMITON
EUTHROID-0.5, LIOTRIX (T4;T3)
EUTHROID-1, LIOTRIX (T4;T3)
EUTHROID-2, LIOTRIX (T4;T3)
EUTHROID-3, LIOTRIX (T4;T3)
EUTONYL, PARGYLINE HYDROCHLORIDE
EUTRON, METHYCLOTHIAZIDE
EVALOSE, LACTULOSE
EVEX, ESTROGENS, ESTERIFIED
EXELDERM, SULCONAZOLE NITRATE
EXIDINE, CHLORHEXIDINE GLUCONATE (OTC)

APPENDIX A
PRODUCT NAME INDEX *(continued)*

EXNA, BENZTHIAZIDE
EXOSURF NEONATAL, CETYL ALCOHOL
EXSEL, SELENIUM SULFIDE
EXTENDED PHENYTOIN SODIUM, PHENYTOIN SODIUM, EXTENDED
EXTRA-STRENGTH AIM, SODIUM MONOFLUOROPHOSPHATE (OTC)

F

FACTREL, GONADORELIN HYDROCHLORIDE
FAMVIR, FAMCICLOVIR
FANSIDAR, PYRIMETHAMINE
FASTIN, PHENTERMINE HYDROCHLORIDE
FELBATOL, FELBAMATE
FELDENE, PIROXICAM
FEMINONE, ETHINYL ESTRADIOL
FEMOGEN, ESTROGENS, ESTERIFIED
FEMSTAT, BUTOCONAZOLE NITRATE
FENOPROFEN CALCIUM, FENOPROFEN CALCIUM
FENTANYL, FENTANYL CITRATE
FENTANYL CITRATE, FENTANYL CITRATE
FENTANYL CITRATE AND DROPERIDOL, DROPERIDOL
FERNDEX, DEXTROAMPHETAMINE SULFATE
FERNISOLONE-P, PREDNISOLONE
FERNISONE, PREDNISONE
FERROUS CITRATE FE 59, FERROUS CITRATE, FE-59
FIORICET, ACETAMINOPHEN
FIORICET W/ CODEINE, ACETAMINOPHEN
FIORINAL, ASPIRIN
FIORINAL W/CODEINE NO 3, ASPIRIN
FLAGYL, METRONIDAZOLE
FLAGYL I.V., METRONIDAZOLE HYDROCHLORIDE
FLAGYL I.V. RTU, METRONIDAZOLE
FLAGYL I.V. RTU IN PLASTIC CONTAINER, METRONIDAZOLE
FLAREX, FLUOROMETHOLONE ACETATE
FLAVORED COLESTID, COLESTIPOL HYDROCHLORIDE
FLAXEDIL, GALLAMINE TRIETHIODIDE
FLEXERIL, CYCLOBENZAPRINE HYDROCHLORIDE
FLEXICORT, HYDROCORTISONE
FLORINEF, FLUDROCORTISONE ACETATE
FLORONE, DIFLORASONE DIACETATE
FLOROPRYL, ISOFLUROPHATE
FLOXIN, OFLOXACIN
FLOXIN IN DEXTROSE 5%, OFLOXACIN
FLOXURIDINE, FLOXURIDINE
FLUDARA, FLUDARABINE PHOSPHATE
FLUDEOXYGLUCOSE F 18, FLUDEOXYGLUCOSE, F-18
FLUIDIL, CYCLOTHIAZIDE
FLUMADINE, RIMANTADINE HYDROCHLORIDE
FLUOCET, FLUOCINOLONE ACETONIDE
FLUOCINOLONE ACETONIDE, FLUOCINOLONE ACETONIDE
FLUOCINONIDE, FLUOCINONIDE
FLUONID, FLUOCINOLONE ACETONIDE
FLUOR-OP, FLUOROMETHOLONE
FLUOROPLEX, FLUOROURACIL
FLUOROURACIL, FLUOROURACIL
FLUOTHANE, HALOTHANE
FLUOTREX, FLUOCINOLONE ACETONIDE
FLUOXYMESTERONE, FLUOXYMESTERONE
FLUPHENAZINE, FLUPHENAZINE DECANOATE
FLUPHENAZINE DECANOATE, FLUPHENAZINE DECANOATE
FLUPHENAZINE HCL, FLUPHENAZINE HYDROCHLORIDE
FLURANDRENOLIDE, FLURANDRENOLIDE
FLURAZEPAM HCL, FLURAZEPAM HYDROCHLORIDE
FLURBIPROFEN, FLURBIPROFEN
FLUTEX, TRIAMCINOLONE ACETONIDE
FML, FLUOROMETHOLONE
FML FORTE, FLUOROMETHOLONE
FML-S, FLUOROMETHOLONE
FOAMCOAT, ALUMINUM HYDROXIDE (OTC)
FOAMICON, ALUMINUM HYDROXIDE (OTC)
FOLEX, METHOTREXATE SODIUM
FOLEX PFS, METHOTREXATE SODIUM
FOLIC ACID, FOLIC ACID
FOLICET, FOLIC ACID
FOLLUTEIN, GONADOTROPIN, CHORIONIC
FOLVITE, FOLIC ACID
FOLVRON, FERROUS SULFATE
FORANE, ISOFLURANE
FORBAXIN, METHOCARBAMOL
FORTAZ, CEFTAZIDIME
FORTAZ, CEFTAZIDIME SODIUM
FOSCAVIR, FOSCARNET SODIUM
FOVANE, BENZTHIAZIDE
FREAMINE HBC 6.9%, AMINO ACIDS
FREAMINE II 8.5%, AMINO ACIDS
FREAMINE III 10%, AMINO ACIDS
FREAMINE III 3% W/ ELECTROLYTES, AMINO ACIDS
FREAMINE III 8.5%, AMINO ACIDS
FREAMINE III 8.5% W/ ELECTROLYTES, AMINO ACIDS
FREAMINE 8.5%, AMINO ACIDS
FS SHAMPOO, FLUOCINOLONE ACETONIDE
FUDR, FLOXURIDINE
FULVICIN P/G, GRISEOFULVIN, ULTRAMICROCRYSTALLINE
FULVICIN P/G 165, GRISEOFULVIN, ULTRAMICROCRYSTALLINE
FULVICIN P/G 330, GRISEOFULVIN, ULTRAMICROCRYSTALLINE
FULVICIN-U/F, GRISEOFULVIN, MICROCRYSTALLINE
FUNDUSCEIN-25, FLUORESCEIN SODIUM
FUNGIZONE, AMPHOTERICIN B
FURACIN, NITROFURAZONE
FURADANTIN, NITROFURANTOIN
FURALAN, NITROFURANTOIN
FUROSEMIDE, FUROSEMIDE
FUROXONE, FURAZOLIDONE

G

GALLIUM CITRATE GA 67, GALLIUM CITRATE, GA-67
GAMENE, LINDANE
GAMOPHEN, HEXACHLOROPHENE
GANITE, GALLIUM NITRATE
GANTANOL, SULFAMETHOXAZOLE
GANTANOL-DS, SULFAMETHOXAZOLE
GANTRISIN, SULFISOXAZOLE
GANTRISIN, SULFISOXAZOLE ACETYL
GANTRISIN, SULFISOXAZOLE DIOLAMINE
GANTRISIN PEDIATRIC, SULFISOXAZOLE ACETYL
GARAMYCIN, GENTAMICIN SULFATE
GASTROCROM, CROMOLYN SODIUM
GASTROGRAFIN, DIATRIZOATE MEGLUMINE
GASTROVIST, DIATRIZOATE MEGLUMINE
GAVISCON, ALUMINUM HYDROXIDE (OTC)
GAVISCON-2, ALUMINUM HYDROXIDE (OTC)
GEMFIBROZIL, GEMFIBROZIL
GEMONIL, METHARBITAL
GEN-XENE, CLORAZEPATE DIPOTASSIUM
GENAPAX, GENTIAN VIOLET
GENCEPT 0.5/35-21, ETHINYL ESTRADIOL
GENCEPT 0.5/35-28, ETHINYL ESTRADIOL
GENCEPT 1/35-21, ETHINYL ESTRADIOL
GENCEPT 1/35-28, ETHINYL ESTRADIOL
GENCEPT 10/11-21, ETHINYL ESTRADIOL
GENCEPT 10/11-28, ETHINYL ESTRADIOL

APPENDIX A
PRODUCT NAME INDEX *(continued)*

GENERLAC, LACTULOSE
GENOPTIC, GENTAMICIN SULFATE
GENTACIDIN, GENTAMICIN SULFATE
GENTAFAIR, GENTAMICIN SULFATE
GENTAMICIN, GENTAMICIN SULFATE
GENTAMICIN SULFATE, GENTAMICIN SULFATE
GENTAMICIN SULFATE IN SODIUM CHLORIDE 0.9%, GENTAMICIN SULFATE
GEOCILLIN, CARBENICILLIN INDANYL SODIUM
GEOPEN, CARBENICILLIN DISODIUM
GEREF, SERMORELIN ACETATE
GERIMAL, ERGOLOID MESYLATES
GERMA-MEDICA, HEXACHLOROPHENE
GERMA-MEDICA "MG", HEXACHLOROPHENE
GLIPIZIDE, GLIPIZIDE
GLOFIL-125, IOTHALAMATE SODIUM, I-125
GLUBATE, GLYBURIDE
GLUCAGON, GLUCAGON HYDROCHLORIDE
GLUCAMIDE, CHLORPROPAMIDE
GLUCOSCAN, TECHNETIUM TC-99M GLUCEPTATE KIT
GLUCOTROL, GLIPIZIDE
GLUCOTROL XL, GLIPIZIDE
GLUTETHIMIDE, GLUTETHIMIDE
GLYCINE 1.5%, GLYCINE
GLYCINE 1.5% IN PLASTIC CONTAINER, GLYCINE
GLYCOPREP, POLYETHYLENE GLYCOL 3350
GLYCOPYRROLATE, GLYCOPYRROLATE
GLYCORT, HYDROCORTISONE
GLYNASE, GLYBURIDE
GO-EVAC, POLYETHYLENE GLYCOL 3350
GOLYTELY, POLYETHYLENE GLYCOL 3350
GRIFULVIN V, GRISEOFULVIN, MICROCRYSTALLINE
GRIS-PEG, GRISEOFULVIN, ULTRAMICROCRYSTALLINE
GRISACTIN, GRISEOFULVIN, MICROCRYSTALLINE
GRISACTIN ULTRA, GRISEOFULVIN, ULTRAMICROCRYSTALLINE
GUANABENZ ACETATE, GUANABENZ ACETATE
GUANETHIDINE MONOSULFATE, GUANETHIDINE MONOSULFATE
GUANIDINE HCL, GUANIDINE HYDROCHLORIDE
GVS, GENTIAN VIOLET
GYNE-LOTRIMIN, CLOTRIMAZOLE (OTC)
GYNE-LOTRIMIN COMBINATION PACK, CLOTRIMAZOLE
GYNE-SULF, TRIPLE SULFA (SULFABENZAMIDE;SULFACETAMIDE;SULFATHIAZOLE)
GYNOREST, DYDROGESTERONE

H

H.P. ACTHAR GEL, CORTICOTROPIN
H.R.-50, HYDROCHLOROTHIAZIDE
H-CORT, HYDROCORTISONE
HABITROL, NICOTINE
HALCION, TRIAZOLAM
HALDOL, HALOPERIDOL
HALDOL, HALOPERIDOL LACTATE
HALDOL DECANOATE 50, HALOPERIDOL DECANOATE
HALDOL SOLUTAB, HALOPERIDOL
HALDRONE, PARAMETHASONE ACETATE
HALFAN, HALOFANTRINE HYDROCHLORIDE
HALODRIN, ETHINYL ESTRADIOL
HALOG, HALCINONIDE
HALOG-E, HALCINONIDE
HALOPERIDOL, HALOPERIDOL
HALOPERIDOL, HALOPERIDOL LACTATE
HALOPERIDOL INTENSOL, HALOPERIDOL LACTATE
HALOTESTIN, FLUOXYMESTERONE
HALOTEX, HALOPROGIN
HALOTHANE, HALOTHANE
HARMONYL, DESERPIDINE
HC (HYDROCORTISONE), HYDROCORTISONE
HC (HYDROCORTISONE), HYDROCORTISONE (OTC)
HC #1, HYDROCORTISONE
HC #4, HYDROCORTISONE
HEAD & SHOULDERS CONDITIONER, PYRITHIONE ZINC
HEAVY SOLUTION NUPERCAINE, DIBUCAINE HYDROCHLORIDE
HEBAMATE, CARBOPROST TROMETHAMINE
HEDULIN, PHENINDIONE
HEMSOL-HC, HYDROCORTISONE ACETATE
HEP FLUSH KIT, HEPARIN SODIUM
HEP-LOCK, HEPARIN SODIUM
HEP-LOCK U/P, HEPARIN SODIUM
HEPARIN LOCK FLUSH, HEPARIN SODIUM
HEPARIN LOCK FLUSH PRESERVATIVE FREE, HEPARIN SODIUM
HEPARIN SODIUM, HEPARIN SODIUM
HEPARIN SODIUM PRESERVATIVE FREE, HEPARIN SODIUM
HEPARIN SODIUM 10,000 UNITS IN DEXTROSE 5%, HEPARIN SODIUM
HEPARIN SODIUM 10,000 UNITS IN DEXTROSE 5% IN PLASTIC CONTAINER, HEPARIN SODIUM
HEPARIN SODIUM 10,000 UNITS IN SODIUM CHLORIDE 0.45%, HEPARIN SODIUM
HEPARIN SODIUM 10,000 UNITS IN SODIUM CHLORIDE 0.9%, HEPARIN SODIUM
HEPARIN SODIUM 1000 UNITS AND DEXTROSE 5% IN PLASTIC CONTAINER, HEPARIN SODIUM
HEPARIN SODIUM 1000 UNITS AND SODIUM CHLORIDE 0.9%, HEPARIN SODIUM
HEPARIN SODIUM 1000 UNITS IN SODIUM CHLORIDE 0.9%, HEPARIN SODIUM
HEPARIN SODIUM 12,500 UNITS IN DEXTROSE 5%, HEPARIN SODIUM
HEPARIN SODIUM 12,500 UNITS IN DEXTROSE 5% IN PLASTIC CONTAINER, HEPARIN SODIUM
HEPARIN SODIUM 12,500 UNITS IN SODIUM CHLORIDE 0.45%, HEPARIN SODIUM
HEPARIN SODIUM 12,500 UNITS IN SODIUM CHLORIDE 0.9%, HEPARIN SODIUM
HEPARIN SODIUM 12500 UNITS IN SODIUM CHLORIDE 0.45%, HEPARIN SODIUM
HEPARIN SODIUM 20,000 UNITS AND DEXTROSE 5% IN PLASTIC CONTAINER, HEPARIN SODIUM
HEPARIN SODIUM 20,000 UNITS IN DEXTROSE 5%, HEPARIN SODIUM
HEPARIN SODIUM 2000 UNITS AND SODIUM CHLORIDE 0.9%, HEPARIN SODIUM
HEPARIN SODIUM 2000 UNITS IN DEXTROSE 5% IN PLASTIC CONTAINER, HEPARIN SODIUM
HEPARIN SODIUM 2000 UNITS IN SODIUM CHLORIDE 0.9%, HEPARIN SODIUM
HEPARIN SODIUM 20000 UNITS IN DEXTROSE 5%, HEPARIN SODIUM
HEPARIN SODIUM 25,000 UNITS AND DEXTROSE 5%, HEPARIN SODIUM
HEPARIN SODIUM 25,000 UNITS IN DEXTROSE 5%, HEPARIN SODIUM
HEPARIN SODIUM 25,000 UNITS IN DEXTROSE 5% IN PLASTIC CONTAINER, HEPARIN SODIUM
HEPARIN SODIUM 25,000 UNITS IN SODIUM CHLORIDE 0.45%, HEPARIN SODIUM
HEPARIN SODIUM 25,000 UNITS IN SODIUM CHLORIDE 0.9%, HEPARIN SODIUM
HEPARIN SODIUM 25000 UNITS IN DEXTROSE 5%, HEPARIN SODIUM
HEPARIN SODIUM 25000 UNITS IN DEXTROSE 5% IN PLASTIC CONTAINER, HEPARIN SODIUM
HEPARIN SODIUM 25000 UNITS IN SODIUM CHLORIDE 0.45%, HEPARIN SODIUM

APPENDIX A
PRODUCT NAME INDEX *(continued)*

HEPARIN SODIUM 25000 UNITS IN SODIUM CHLORIDE 0.9%, HEPARIN SODIUM
HEPARIN SODIUM 5,000 UNITS IN SODIUM CHLORIDE 0.45%, HEPARIN SODIUM
HEPARIN SODIUM 5000 UNITS AND SODIUM CHLORIDE 0.9%, HEPARIN SODIUM
HEPARIN SODIUM 5000 UNITS IN DEXTROSE 5% IN PLASTIC CONTAINER, HEPARIN SODIUM
HEPARIN SODIUM 5000 UNITS IN SODIUM CHLORIDE 0.45%, HEPARIN SODIUM
HEPARIN SODIUM 5000 UNITS IN SODIUM CHLORIDE 0.9%, HEPARIN SODIUM
HEPATAMINE 8%, AMINO ACIDS
HEPATOLITE, TECHNETIUM TC-99M DISOFENIN KIT
HEPFLUSH-10, HEPARIN SODIUM
HEPTALAC, LACTULOSE
HERPLEX, IDOXURIDINE
HETRAZAN, DIETHYLCARBAMAZINE CITRATE
HEXA-BETALIN, PYRIDOXINE HYDROCHLORIDE
HEXA-GERM, HEXACHLOROPHENE
HEXABRIX, IOXAGLATE MEGLUMINE
HEXADROL, DEXAMETHASONE
HEXADROL, DEXAMETHASONE SODIUM PHOSPHATE
HEXALEN, ALTRETAMINE
HEXASCRUB, HEXACHLOROPHENE
HI-COR, HYDROCORTISONE
HIBICLENS, CHLORHEXIDINE GLUCONATE (OTC)
HIBISTAT, CHLORHEXIDINE GLUCONATE (OTC)
HIBITANE, CHLORHEXIDINE GLUCONATE (OTC)
HIPPURAN I 131, IODOHIPPURATE SODIUM, I-131
HIPPUTOPE, IODOHIPPURATE SODIUM, I-131
HIPREX, METHENAMINE HIPPURATE
HISERPIA, RESERPINE
HISMANAL, ASTEMIZOLE
HISPRIL, DIPHENYLPYRALINE HYDROCHLORIDE
HISTAFED, PSEUDOEPHEDRINE HYDROCHLORIDE
HISTALOG, BETAZOLE HYDROCHLORIDE
HISTAMINE PHOSPHATE, HISTAMINE PHOSPHATE
HIVID, ZALCITABINE
HIWOLFIA, RAUWOLFIA SERPENTINA
HMS, MEDRYSONE
HOMAPIN-10, HOMATROPINE METHYLBROMIDE
HOMAPIN-5, HOMATROPINE METHYLBROMIDE
HUMATIN, PAROMOMYCIN SULFATE
HUMATROPE, SOMATROPIN, BIOSYNTHETIC
HUMORSOL, DEMECARIUM BROMIDE
HUMULIN BR, INSULIN BIOSYNTHETIC HUMAN (OTC)
HUMULIN L, INSULIN ZINC SUSP BIOSYNTHETIC HUMAN (OTC)
HUMULIN N, INSULIN SUSP ISOPHANE BIOSYNTHETIC HUMAN (OTC)
HUMULIN R, INSULIN BIOSYNTHETIC HUMAN
HUMULIN R, INSULIN BIOSYNTHETIC HUMAN (OTC)
HUMULIN U, INSULIN ZINC SUSP EXTENDED BIOSYNTHETIC HUMAN (OTC)
HUMULIN 50/50, INSULIN BIOSYNTHETIC HUMAN (OTC)
HUMULIN 70/30, INSULIN BIOSYNTHETIC HUMAN (OTC)
HY-PAM, HYDROXYZINE PAMOATE
HY-PAM "25", HYDROXYZINE PAMOATE
HY-PHEN, ACETAMINOPHEN
HYCODAN, HOMATROPINE METHYLBROMIDE
HYCOMINE, HYDROCODONE BITARTRATE
HYCOMINE PEDIATRIC, HYDROCODONE BITARTRATE
HYDELTRA-TBA, PREDNISOLONE TEBUTATE
HYDELTRASOL, PREDNISOLONE SODIUM PHOSPHATE
HYDERGINE, ERGOLOID MESYLATES
HYDERGINE LC, ERGOLOID MESYLATES
HYDRA-ZIDE, HYDRALAZINE HYDROCHLORIDE
HYDRALAZINE AND HYDROCHLORTHIAZIDE, HYDRALAZINE HYDROCHLORIDE
HYDRALAZINE HCL, HYDRALAZINE HYDROCHLORIDE
HYDRALAZINE HCL AND HYDROCHLOROTHIAZIDE, HYDRALAZINE HYDROCHLORIDE
HYDRALAZINE HCL W/ HYDROCHLOROTHIAZIDE 100/50, HYDRALAZINE HYDROCHLORIDE
HYDRALAZINE HCL W/ HYDROCHLOROTHIAZIDE 25/25, HYDRALAZINE HYDROCHLORIDE
HYDRALAZINE HCL W/ HYDROCHLOROTHIAZIDE 50/50, HYDRALAZINE HYDROCHLORIDE
HYDRALAZINE HCL-HYDROCHLOROTHIAZIDE-RESERPINE, HYDRALAZINE HYDROCHLORIDE
HYDRALAZINE HCL, HYDROCHLOROTHIAZIDE AND RESERPINE, HYDRALAZINE HYDROCHLORIDE
HYDRALAZINE, HYDROCHLOROTHIAZIDE W/ RESERPINE, HYDRALAZINE HYDROCHLORIDE
HYDRAMINE, DIPHENHYDRAMINE HYDROCHLORIDE
HYDRAMINE, DIPHENHYDRAMINE HYDROCHLORIDE (OTC)
HYDRAP-ES, HYDRALAZINE HYDROCHLORIDE
HYDREA, HYDROXYUREA
HYDRO-D, HYDROCHLOROTHIAZIDE
HYDRO-RESERP, HYDROCHLOROTHIAZIDE
HYDRO-RIDE, AMILORIDE HYDROCHLORIDE
HYDRO-SERP "25", HYDROCHLOROTHIAZIDE
HYDRO-SERP "50", HYDROCHLOROTHIAZIDE
HYDROCET, ACETAMINOPHEN
HYDROCHLOROTHIAZIDE, HYDROCHLOROTHIAZIDE
HYDROCHLOROTHIAZIDE INTENSOL, HYDROCHLOROTHIAZIDE
HYDROCHLOROTHIAZIDE W/ HYDRALAZINE, HYDRALAZINE HYDROCHLORIDE
HYDROCHLOROTHIAZIDE W/ RESERPINE, HYDROCHLOROTHIAZIDE
HYDROCHLOROTHIAZIDE W/ RESERPINE AND HYDRALAZINE, HYDRALAZINE HYDROCHLORIDE
HYDROCODONE BITARTRATE AND ACETAMINOPHEN, ACETAMINOPHEN
HYDROCODONE BITARTRATE W/ ACETAMINOPHEN, ACETAMINOPHEN
HYDROCODONE COMPOUND, HOMATROPINE METHYLBROMIDE
HYDROCORTISONE, HYDROCORTISONE
HYDROCORTISONE ACETATE, HYDROCORTISONE ACETATE
HYDROCORTISONE ACETATE 1% AND PRAMOXINE HCL 1%, HYDROCORTISONE ACETATE
HYDROCORTISONE AND ACETIC ACID, ACETIC ACID, GLACIAL
HYDROCORTISONE IN ABSORBASE, HYDROCORTISONE
HYDROCORTISONE SODIUM PHOSPHATE, HYDROCORTISONE SODIUM PHOSPHATE
HYDROCORTISONE SODIUM SUCCINATE, HYDROCORTISONE SODIUM SUCCINATE
HYDROCORTONE, HYDROCORTISONE
HYDROCORTONE, HYDROCORTISONE ACETATE
HYDROCORTONE, HYDROCORTISONE SODIUM PHOSPHATE
HYDRODIURIL, HYDROCHLOROTHIAZIDE
HYDROFLUMETHIAZIDE, HYDROFLUMETHIAZIDE
HYDROFLUMETHIAZIDE AND RESERPINE, HYDROFLUMETHIAZIDE
HYDROGENATED ERGOT ALKALOIDS, ERGOLOID MESYLATES
HYDROMOX, QUINETHAZONE
HYDROMOX R, QUINETHAZONE
HYDROPANE, HOMATROPINE METHYLBROMIDE
HYDROPRES 25, HYDROCHLOROTHIAZIDE
HYDROPRES 50, HYDROCHLOROTHIAZIDE
HYDROSERPINE PLUS (R-H-H), HYDRALAZINE HYDROCHLORIDE
HYDROXOCOBALAMIN, HYDROXOCOBALAMIN
HYDROXOMIN, HYDROXOCOBALAMIN
HYDROXYPROGESTERONE CAPROATE, HYDROXYPROGESTERONE CAPROATE
HYDROXYSTILBAMIDINE ISETHIONATE, HYDROXYSTILBAMIDINE ISETHIONATE

APPENDIX A
PRODUCT NAME INDEX *(continued)*

HYDROXYZINE, HYDROXYZINE HYDROCHLORIDE
HYDROXYZINE HCL, HYDROXYZINE HYDROCHLORIDE
HYDROXYZINE PAMOATE, HYDROXYZINE PAMOATE
HYGROTON, CHLORTHALIDONE
HYLOREL, GUANADREL SULFATE
HYPAQUE, DIATRIZOATE MEGLUMINE
HYPAQUE, DIATRIZOATE SODIUM
HYPAQUE SODIUM 20%, DIATRIZOATE SODIUM
HYPAQUE-CYSTO, DIATRIZOATE MEGLUMINE
HYPAQUE-M,75%, DIATRIZOATE MEGLUMINE
HYPAQUE-M,90%, DIATRIZOATE MEGLUMINE
HYPAQUE-76, DIATRIZOATE MEGLUMINE
HYPERSTAT, DIAZOXIDE
HYPROTIGEN 5%, PROTEIN HYDROLYSATE
HYSERPIN, RAUWOLFIA SERPENTINA
HYTONE, HYDROCORTISONE
HYTRIN, TERAZOSIN HYDROCHLORIDE
HYZYD, ISONIAZID

I

IBRIN, FIBRINOGEN, I-125
IBU-TAB, IBUPROFEN
IBU-TAB 200, IBUPROFEN (OTC)
IBUPRIN, IBUPROFEN (OTC)
IBUPROFEN, IBUPROFEN
IBUPROFEN, IBUPROFEN (OTC)
IBUPROHM, IBUPROFEN
IBUPROHM, IBUPROFEN (OTC)
IDAMYCIN, IDARUBICIN HYDROCHLORIDE
IFEX, IFOSFAMIDE
ILETIN I, INSULIN PORK
ILETIN II, INSULIN PURIFIED PORK
ILOSONE, ERYTHROMYCIN ESTOLATE
ILOSONE SULFA, ERYTHROMYCIN ESTOLATE
ILOTYCIN, ERYTHROMYCIN
ILOTYCIN GLUCEPTATE, ERYTHROMYCIN GLUCEPTATE
IMAGENT, PERFLUBRON
IMDUR, ISOSORBIDE MONONITRATE
IMIPRAMINE HCL, IMIPRAMINE HYDROCHLORIDE
IMITREX, SUMATRIPTAN SUCCINATE
IMODIUM, LOPERAMIDE HYDROCHLORIDE
IMODIUM A-D, LOPERAMIDE HYDROCHLORIDE (OTC)
IMURAN, AZATHIOPRINE
IMURAN, AZATHIOPRINE SODIUM
INAPSINE, DROPERIDOL
INDERAL, PROPRANOLOL HYDROCHLORIDE
INDERAL LA, PROPRANOLOL HYDROCHLORIDE
INDERIDE LA 120/50, HYDROCHLOROTHIAZIDE
INDERIDE LA 160/50, HYDROCHLOROTHIAZIDE
INDERIDE LA 80/50, HYDROCHLOROTHIAZIDE
INDERIDE-40/25, HYDROCHLOROTHIAZIDE
INDERIDE-80/25, HYDROCHLOROTHIAZIDE
INDIUM IN-111 OXYQUINOLINE, INDIUM IN-111 OXYQUINOLINE
INDO-LEMMON, INDOMETHACIN
INDOCIN, INDOMETHACIN
INDOCIN I.V., INDOMETHACIN SODIUM
INDOCIN SR, INDOMETHACIN
INDOMETHACIN, INDOMETHACIN
INDOMETHEGAN, INDOMETHACIN
INFANTS' FEVERALL, ACETAMINOPHEN
INFED, IRON DEXTRAN
INFLAMASE FORTE, PREDNISOLONE SODIUM PHOSPHATE
INFLAMASE MILD, PREDNISOLONE SODIUM PHOSPHATE
INFUMORPH, MORPHINE SULFATE
INH, ISONIAZID
INJECTAPAP, ACETAMINOPHEN
INNOVAR, DROPERIDOL
INOCOR, AMRINONE LACTATE
INPERSOL W/ DEXTROSE 1.5%, CALCIUM CHLORIDE
INPERSOL W/ DEXTROSE 2.5%, CALCIUM CHLORIDE
INPERSOL W/ DEXTROSE 3.5%, CALCIUM CHLORIDE
INPERSOL W/ DEXTROSE 4.25%, CALCIUM CHLORIDE
INPERSOL-LC/LM W/ DEXTROSE 1.5%, CALCIUM CHLORIDE
INPERSOL-LC/LM W/ DEXTROSE 2.5%, CALCIUM CHLORIDE
INPERSOL-LC/LM W/ DEXTROSE 3.5%, CALCIUM CHLORIDE
INPERSOL-LC/LM W/ DEXTROSE 4.25%, CALCIUM CHLORIDE
INPERSOL-LM W/ DEXTROSE 1.5%, CALCIUM CHLORIDE
INPERSOL-LM W/ DEXTROSE 2.5%, CALCIUM CHLORIDE
INPERSOL-LM W/ DEXTROSE 3.5%, CALCIUM CHLORIDE
INPERSOL-LM W/ DEXTROSE 4.25%, CALCIUM CHLORIDE
INPERSOL-ZM W/ DEXTROSE 1.5% IN PLASTIC CONTAINER, CALCIUM CHLORIDE
INPERSOL-ZM W/ DEXTROSE 2.5% IN PLASTIC CONTAINER, CALCIUM CHLORIDE
INPERSOL-ZM W/ DEXTROSE 4.25% IN PLASTIC CONTAINER, CALCIUM CHLORIDE
INSTANT MICROSPHERES, TECHNETIUM TC-99M ALBUMIN MICROSPHERES KIT
INSULATARD NPH HUMAN, INSULIN SUSP ISOPHANE SEMISYNTHETIC PURIFIED HUMAN (OTC)
INSULIN, INSULIN PORK (OTC)
INSULIN INSULATARD NPH NORDISK, INSULIN SUSP ISOPHANE PURIFIED PORK (OTC)
INSULIN NORDISK MIXTARD (PORK), INSULIN PURIFIED PORK (OTC)
INTAL, CROMOLYN SODIUM
INTRALIPID 10%, SOYBEAN OIL
INTRALIPID 20%, SOYBEAN OIL
INTRALIPID 30%, SOYBEAN OIL
INTROPIN, DOPAMINE HYDROCHLORIDE
INULIN AND SODIUM CHLORIDE, INULIN
INVERSINE, MECAMYLAMINE HYDROCHLORIDE
IOBENGUANE SULFATE I 131, IOBENGUANE SULFATE I 131
IODOHIPPURATE SODIUM I 131, IODOHIPPURATE SODIUM, I-131
IODOTOPE, SODIUM IODIDE, I-131
IONAMIN-15, PHENTERMINE RESIN COMPLEX
IONAMIN-30, PHENTERMINE RESIN COMPLEX
IONOSOL B AND DEXTROSE 5%, DEXTROSE
IONOSOL MB AND DEXTROSE 5%, DEXTROSE
IONOSOL T AND DEXTROSE 5%, DEXTROSE
IOPIDINE, APRACLONIDINE HYDROCHLORIDE
IOSAT, POTASSIUM IODIDE (OTC)
IRON DEXTRAN, IRON DEXTRAN
IRRIGATING SOLUTION G IN PLASTIC CONTAINER, CITRIC ACID
ISMELIN, GUANETHIDINE MONOSULFATE
ISMO, ISOSORBIDE MONONITRATE
ISMOTIC, ISOSORBIDE
ISOCAINE HCL, MEPIVACAINE HYDROCHLORIDE
ISOCAINE HCL W/ LEVONORDEFRIN, LEVONORDEFRIN
ISOCLOR, CHLORPHENIRAMINE MALEATE (OTC)
ISOETHARINE HCL, ISOETHARINE HYDROCHLORIDE
ISOETHARINE HCL S/F, ISOETHARINE HYDROCHLORIDE
ISOETHARINE MESYLATE, ISOETHARINE MESYLATE
ISOFLURANE, ISOFLURANE
ISOLYTE E, CALCIUM CHLORIDE
ISOLYTE E IN DEXTROSE 5%, CALCIUM CHLORIDE
ISOLYTE E IN PLASTIC CONTAINER, CALCIUM CHLORIDE
ISOLYTE E W/ DEXTROSE 5% IN PLASTIC CONTAINER, CALCIUM CHLORIDE
ISOLYTE H IN DEXTROSE 5%, DEXTROSE
ISOLYTE H W/ DEXTROSE 5%, DEXTROSE

APPENDIX A
PRODUCT NAME INDEX *(continued)*

ISOLYTE M IN DEXTROSE 5%, DEXTROSE
ISOLYTE M W/ DEXTROSE 5% IN PLASTIC CONTAINER, DEXTROSE
ISOLYTE P IN DEXTROSE 5%, DEXTROSE
ISOLYTE P W/ DEXTROSE 5% IN PLASTIC CONTAINER, DEXTROSE
ISOLYTE R IN DEXTROSE 5%, CALCIUM CHLORIDE
ISOLYTE R W/ DEXTROSE 5%, CALCIUM CHLORIDE
ISOLYTE S, MAGNESIUM CHLORIDE
ISOLYTE S IN DEXTROSE 5%, DEXTROSE
ISOLYTE S IN PLASTIC CONTAINER, MAGNESIUM CHLORIDE
ISOLYTE S PH 7.4, MAGNESIUM CHLORIDE
ISOLYTE S PH 7.4 IN PLASTIC CONTAINER, MAGNESIUM CHLORIDE
ISOLYTE S W/ DEXTROSE 5% IN PLASTIC CONTAINER, DEXTROSE
ISONIAZID, ISONIAZID
ISOPAQUE 280, CALCIUM
ISOPAQUE 440, CALCIUM METRIZOATE
ISOPROTERENOL HCL, ISOPROTERENOL HYDROCHLORIDE
ISOPTIN, VERAPAMIL HYDROCHLORIDE
ISOPTIN SR, VERAPAMIL HYDROCHLORIDE
ISOPTO CETAMIDE, SULFACETAMIDE SODIUM
ISOPTO CETAPRED, PREDNISOLONE ACETATE
ISORDIL, ISOSORBIDE DINITRATE
ISOSORBIDE DINITRATE, ISOSORBIDE DINITRATE
ISOTONIC GENTAMICIN SULFATE IN PLASTIC CONTAINER, GENTAMICIN SULFATE
ISOVUE-M 200, IOPAMIDOL
ISOVUE-M 300, IOPAMIDOL
ISOVUE-128, IOPAMIDOL
ISOVUE-200, IOPAMIDOL
ISOVUE-250, IOPAMIDOL
ISOVUE-300, IOPAMIDOL
ISOVUE-370, IOPAMIDOL
ISUPREL, ISOPROTERENOL HYDROCHLORIDE
IV PERSANTINE, DIPYRIDAMOLE
IVADANTIN, NITROFURANTOIN SODIUM

J

JANIMINE, IMIPRAMINE HYDROCHLORIDE

K

K+10, POTASSIUM CHLORIDE
K+8, POTASSIUM CHLORIDE
K-DUR 10, POTASSIUM CHLORIDE
K-DUR 20, POTASSIUM CHLORIDE
K-LEASE, POTASSIUM CHLORIDE
K-TAB, POTASSIUM CHLORIDE
KABIVITE PED F + W KIT, ASCORBIC ACID
KAFOCIN, CEPHALOGLYCIN
KAINAIR, PROPARACAINE HYDROCHLORIDE
KANAMYCIN, KANAMYCIN SULFATE
KANAMYCIN SULFATE, KANAMYCIN SULFATE
KANTREX, KANAMYCIN SULFATE
KAON CL, POTASSIUM CHLORIDE
KAON CL-10, POTASSIUM CHLORIDE
KAPPADIONE, MENADIOL SODIUM DIPHOSPHATE
KAYEXALATE, SODIUM POLYSTYRENE SULFONATE
KEFLET, CEPHALEXIN
KEFLEX, CEPHALEXIN
KEFLIN, CEPHALOTHIN SODIUM
KEFTAB, CEPHALEXIN HYDROCHLORIDE
KEFUROX, CEFUROXIME SODIUM
KEFUROX IN PLASTIC CONTAINER, CEFUROXIME SODIUM
KEFZOL, CEFAZOLIN SODIUM
KEMADRIN, PROCYCLIDINE HYDROCHLORIDE
KENACORT, TRIAMCINOLONE
KENACORT, TRIAMCINOLONE DIACETATE
KENALOG, TRIAMCINOLONE ACETONIDE
KENALOG IN ORABASE, TRIAMCINOLONE ACETONIDE
KENALOG-H, TRIAMCINOLONE ACETONIDE
KENALOG-10, TRIAMCINOLONE ACETONIDE
KENALOG-40, TRIAMCINOLONE ACETONIDE
KERLEDEX, BETAXOLOL HYDROCHLORIDE
KERLONE, BETAXOLOL HYDROCHLORIDE
KESSO-GESIC, PROPOXYPHENE HYDROCHLORIDE
KETALAR, KETAMINE HYDROCHLORIDE
KETAMINE HCL, KETAMINE HYDROCHLORIDE
KETOPROFEN, KETOPROFEN
KINEVAC, SINCALIDE
KLEBCIL, KANAMYCIN SULFATE
KLONOPIN, CLONAZEPAM
KLOR-CON, POTASSIUM CHLORIDE
KLOROMIN, CHLORPHENIRAMINE MALEATE
KLOTRIX, POTASSIUM CHLORIDE
KOGLUCOID, RAUWOLFIA SERPENTINA
KONAKION, PHYTONADIONE
KOROSTATIN, NYSTATIN
KWELL, LINDANE
KYTRIL, GRANISETRON HYDROCHLORIDE

L

LABID, THEOPHYLLINE
LAC-HYDRIN, AMMONIUM LACTATE
LACRISERT, HYDROXYPROPYL CELLULOSE
LACTATED RINGER'S, CALCIUM CHLORIDE
LACTATED RINGER'S AND DEXTROSE 5% IN PLASTIC CONTAINER, CALCIUM CHLORIDE
LACTATED RINGER'S IN PLASTIC CONTAINER, CALCIUM CHLORIDE
LACTULOSE, LACTULOSE
LAMISIL, TERBINAFINE HYDROCHLORIDE
LAMPRENE, CLOFAZIMINE
LANABIOTIC, BACITRACIN (OTC)
LANABIOTIC, BACITRACIN ZINC (OTC)
LANIAZID, ISONIAZID
LANOPHYLLIN, THEOPHYLLINE
LANORINAL, ASPIRIN
LANOXICAPS, DIGOXIN
LANOXIN, DIGOXIN
LANTRISUL, TRISULFAPYRIMIDINES (SULFADIAZINE;SULFAMERAZINE;SULFAMETHAZINE)
LARGON, PROPIOMAZINE HYDROCHLORIDE
LARIAM, MEFLOQUINE HYDROCHLORIDE
LARODOPA, LEVODOPA
LAROTID, AMOXICILLIN
LARYNG-O-JET KIT, LIDOCAINE HYDROCHLORIDE
LARYNGOTRACHEAL ANESTHESIA KIT, LIDOCAINE HYDROCHLORIDE
LASIX, FUROSEMIDE
LAXILOSE, LACTULOSE
LEDERCILLIN VK, PENICILLIN V POTASSIUM
LENTARD, INSULIN ZINC SUSP PURIFIED BEEF/PORK (OTC)
LENTE, INSULIN ZINC SUSP PURIFIED PORK (OTC)
LENTE ILETIN II, INSULIN ZINC SUSP PURIFIED BEEF (OTC)
LENTE ILETIN II (PORK), INSULIN ZINC SUSP PURIFIED PORK (OTC)
LENTE INSULIN, INSULIN ZINC SUSP BEEF (OTC)
LERITINE, ANILERIDINE HYDROCHLORIDE
LERITINE, ANILERIDINE PHOSPHATE
LESCOL, FLUVASTATIN SODIUM

APPENDIX A
PRODUCT NAME INDEX *(continued)*

LEUCOVORIN CALCIUM, LEUCOVORIN CALCIUM
LEUKERAN, CHLORAMBUCIL
LEUSTATIN, CLADRIBINE
LEVATOL, PENBUTOLOL SULFATE
LEVO-DROMORAN, LEVORPHANOL TARTRATE
LEVOBUNOLOL HCL, LEVOBUNOLOL HYDROCHLORIDE
LEVOPHED, NOREPINEPHRINE BITARTRATE
LEVOPROME, METHOTRIMEPRAZINE
LEVORA 0.15/30-21, ETHINYL ESTRADIOL
LEVORA 0.15/30-28, ETHINYL ESTRADIOL
LIBRELEASE, CHLORDIAZEPOXIDE
LIBRITABS, CHLORDIAZEPOXIDE
LIBRIUM, CHLORDIAZEPOXIDE HYDROCHLORIDE
LIDEX, FLUOCINONIDE
LIDEX-E, FLUOCINONIDE
LIDOCAINE, LIDOCAINE
LIDOCAINE HCL, LIDOCAINE HYDROCHLORIDE
LIDOCAINE HCL AND DEXTROSE 7.5%, LIDOCAINE HYDROCHLORIDE
LIDOCAINE HCL AND EPINEPHRINE, EPINEPHRINE
LIDOCAINE HCL IN PLASTIC CONTAINER, LIDOCAINE HYDROCHLORIDE
LIDOCAINE HCL VISCOUS, LIDOCAINE HYDROCHLORIDE
LIDOCAINE HCL W/ EPINEPHRINE, EPINEPHRINE
LIDOCAINE HCL 0.1% AND DEXTROSE 5% IN PLASTIC CONTAINER, LIDOCAINE HYDROCHLORIDE
LIDOCAINE HCL 0.2% AND DEXTROSE 5%, LIDOCAINE HYDROCHLORIDE
LIDOCAINE HCL 0.2% AND DEXTROSE 5% IN PLASTIC CONTAINER, LIDOCAINE HYDROCHLORIDE
LIDOCAINE HCL 0.2% IN DEXTROSE 5%, LIDOCAINE HYDROCHLORIDE
LIDOCAINE HCL 0.2% IN DEXTROSE 5% IN PLASTIC CONTAINER, LIDOCAINE HYDROCHLORIDE
LIDOCAINE HCL 0.4% AND DEXTROSE 5%, LIDOCAINE HYDROCHLORIDE
LIDOCAINE HCL 0.4% AND DEXTROSE 5% IN PLASTIC CONTAINER, LIDOCAINE HYDROCHLORIDE
LIDOCAINE HCL 0.4% IN DEXTROSE 5%, LIDOCAINE HYDROCHLORIDE
LIDOCAINE HCL 0.4% IN DEXTROSE 5% IN PLASTIC CONTAINER, LIDOCAINE HYDROCHLORIDE
LIDOCAINE HCL 0.8% AND DEXTROSE 5%, LIDOCAINE HYDROCHLORIDE
LIDOCAINE HCL 0.8% AND DEXTROSE 5% IN PLASTIC CONTAINER, LIDOCAINE HYDROCHLORIDE
LIDOCAINE HCL 0.8% IN DEXTROSE 5% IN PLASTIC CONTAINER, LIDOCAINE HYDROCHLORIDE
LIDOCAINE VISCOUS, LIDOCAINE HYDROCHLORIDE
LIDOCATON, EPINEPHRINE
LIDOCATON, LIDOCAINE HYDROCHLORIDE
LIDOPEN, LIDOCAINE HYDROCHLORIDE
LIGNOSPAN FORTE, EPINEPHRINE BITARTRATE
LIGNOSPAN STANDARD, EPINEPHRINE BITARTRATE
LIMBITROL, AMITRIPTYLINE HYDROCHLORIDE
LINCOCIN, LINCOMYCIN HYDROCHLORIDE
LINCOMYCIN HCL, LINCOMYCIN HYDROCHLORIDE
LINDANE, LINDANE
LIORESAL, BACLOFEN
LIOTHYRONINE SODIUM, LIOTHYRONINE SODIUM
LIPIDIL, FENOFIBRATE
LIPO GANTRISIN, SULFISOXAZOLE ACETYL
LIPO-HEPIN, HEPARIN SODIUM
LIPOSYN II 10%, SAFFLOWER OIL
LIPOSYN II 20%, SAFFLOWER OIL
LIPOSYN III 10%, SOYBEAN OIL
LIPOSYN III 20%, SOYBEAN OIL
LIPOSYN 10%, SAFFLOWER OIL
LIPOSYN 20%, SAFFLOWER OIL
LIQUAEMIN LOCK FLUSH, HEPARIN SODIUM
LIQUAEMIN SODIUM, HEPARIN SODIUM
LIQUAEMIN SODIUM PRESERVATIVE FREE, HEPARIN SODIUM
LIQUAMAR, PHENPROCOUMON
LIQUID PRED, PREDNISONE
LITHANE, LITHIUM CARBONATE
LITHIUM CARBONATE, LITHIUM CARBONATE
LITHIUM CITRATE, LITHIUM CITRATE
LITHOBID, LITHIUM CARBONATE
LITHONATE, LITHIUM CARBONATE
LITHOSTAT, ACETOHYDROXAMIC ACID
LITHOTABS, LITHIUM CARBONATE
LIVOSTIN, LEVOCABASTINE HYDROCHLORIDE
LO-TROL, ATROPINE SULFATE
LO/OVRAL, ETHINYL ESTRADIOL
LO/OVRAL-28, ETHINYL ESTRADIOL
LOCOID, HYDROCORTISONE BUTYRATE
LOCORTEN, FLUMETHASONE PIVALATE
LODINE, ETODOLAC
LODOSYN, CARBIDOPA
LOESTRIN FE 1.5/30, ETHINYL ESTRADIOL
LOESTRIN FE 1/20, ETHINYL ESTRADIOL
LOESTRIN 21 1.5/30, ETHINYL ESTRADIOL
LOESTRIN 21 1/20, ETHINYL ESTRADIOL
LOFENE, ATROPINE SULFATE
LOGEN, ATROPINE SULFATE
LOMANATE, ATROPINE SULFATE
LOMOTIL, ATROPINE SULFATE
LONITEN, MINOXIDIL
LONOX, ATROPINE SULFATE
LOPERAMIDE HCL, LOPERAMIDE HYDROCHLORIDE
LOPERAMIDE HCL, LOPERAMIDE HYDROCHLORIDE (OTC)
LOPID, GEMFIBROZIL
LOPRESSIDONE, CHLORTHALIDONE
LOPRESSOR, METOPROLOL FUMARATE
LOPRESSOR, METOPROLOL TARTRATE
LOPRESSOR HCT 100/25, HYDROCHLOROTHIAZIDE
LOPRESSOR HCT 100/50, HYDROCHLOROTHIAZIDE
LOPRESSOR HCT 50/25, HYDROCHLOROTHIAZIDE
LOPROX, CICLOPIROX OLAMINE
LOPURIN, ALLOPURINOL
LORABID, LORACARBEF
LORAZ, LORAZEPAM
LORAZEPAM, LORAZEPAM
LORAZEPAM INTENSOL, LORAZEPAM
LORELCO, PROBUCOL
LORFAN, LEVALLORPHAN TARTRATE
LOTENSIN, BENAZEPRIL HYDROCHLORIDE
LOTENSIN HCT, BENAZEPRIL HYDROCHLORIDE
LOTRIMIN, CLOTRIMAZOLE
LOTRIMIN AF, CLOTRIMAZOLE (OTC)
LOTRISONE, BETAMETHASONE DIPROPIONATE
LOTUSATE, TALBUTAL
LOVENOX, ENOXAPARIN SODIUM
LOW-QUEL, ATROPINE SULFATE
LOXAPINE SUCCINATE, LOXAPINE SUCCINATE
LOXITANE, LOXAPINE SUCCINATE
LOXITANE C, LOXAPINE HYDROCHLORIDE
LOXITANE IM, LOXAPINE HYDROCHLORIDE
LOZOL, INDAPAMIDE
LTA II KIT, LIDOCAINE HYDROCHLORIDE
LUDIOMIL, MAPROTILINE HYDROCHLORIDE
LUFYLLIN, DYPHYLLINE
LUNGAGGREGATE REAGENT, TECHNETIUM TC-99M ALBUMIN AGGREGATED KIT
LUPRON, LEUPROLIDE ACETATE
LUPRON DEPOT, LEUPROLIDE ACETATE
LUPRON DEPOT-PED, LEUPROLIDE ACETATE
LUTREPULSE KIT, GONADORELIN ACETATE
LYGEN, CHLORDIAZEPOXIDE HYDROCHLORIDE
LYMPHAZURIN, ISOSULFAN BLUE
LYNORAL, ETHINYL ESTRADIOL

APPENDIX A
PRODUCT NAME INDEX *(continued)*

LYOPHILIZED CYTOXAN, CYCLOPHOSPHAMIDE
LYPHOCIN, VANCOMYCIN HYDROCHLORIDE
LYSODREN, MITOTANE

M

M.V.C. 9+3, ASCORBIC ACID
M.V.I.-12, ASCORBIC ACID
M.V.I.-12 LYOPHILIZED, ASCORBIC ACID
M-PREDROL, METHYLPREDNISOLONE ACETATE
MACROBID, NITROFURANTOIN
MACRODANTIN, NITROFURANTOIN, MACROCRYSTALLINE
MACROTEC, TECHNETIUM TC-99M ALBUMIN AGGREGATED KIT
MAGNACORT, HYDROCORTAMATE HYDROCHLORIDE
MAGNESIUM SULFATE, MAGNESIUM SULFATE
MAGNEVIST, GADOPENTETATE DIMEGLUMINE
MANDOL, CEFAMANDOLE NAFATE
MANGANESE CHLORIDE, MANGANESE CHLORIDE
MANGANESE SULFATE, MANGANESE SULFATE
MANNITOL 10%, MANNITOL
MANNITOL 10% W/ DEXTROSE 5% IN DISTILLED WATER, MANNITOL
MANNITOL 15%, MANNITOL
MANNITOL 15% W/ DEXTROSE 5% IN SODIUM CHLORIDE 0.45%, MANNITOL
MANNITOL 20%, MANNITOL
MANNITOL 25%, MANNITOL
MANNITOL 5%, MANNITOL
MANNITOL 5% W/ DEXTROSE 5% IN SODIUM CHLORIDE 0.12%, MANNITOL
MANOPLAX, FLOSEQUINAN
MAOLATE, CHLORPHENESIN CARBAMATE
MAPROTILINE HCL, MAPROTILINE HYDROCHLORIDE
MARCAINE, BUPIVACAINE HYDROCHLORIDE
MARCAINE HCL, BUPIVACAINE HYDROCHLORIDE
MARCAINE HCL W/ EPINEPHRINE, BUPIVACAINE HYDROCHLORIDE
MAREZINE, CYCLIZINE LACTATE
MARINOL, DRONABINOL
MATULANE, PROCARBAZINE HYDROCHLORIDE
MAXAIR, PIRBUTEROL ACETATE
MAXAQUIN, LOMEFLOXACIN HYDROCHLORIDE
MAXIBOLIN, ETHYLESTRENOL
MAXIDEX, DEXAMETHASONE
MAXIDEX, DEXAMETHASONE SODIUM PHOSPHATE
MAXITROL, DEXAMETHASONE
MAXOLON, METOCLOPRAMIDE HYDROCHLORIDE
MAXZIDE, HYDROCHLOROTHIAZIDE
MAXZIDE-25, HYDROCHLOROTHIAZIDE
MAZANOR, MAZINDOL
MD-GASTROVIEW, DIATRIZOATE MEGLUMINE
MD-50, DIATRIZOATE SODIUM
MD-60, DIATRIZOATE MEGLUMINE
MD-76, DIATRIZOATE MEGLUMINE
MDP-SQUIBB, TECHNETIUM TC-99M MEDRONATE KIT
MEASURIN, ASPIRIN (OTC)
MECLAN, MECLOCYCLINE SULFOSALICYLATE
MECLIZINE HCL, MECLIZINE HYDROCHLORIDE
MECLODIUM, MECLOFENAMATE SODIUM
MECLOFENAMATE SODIUM, MECLOFENAMATE SODIUM
MECLOMEN, MECLOFENAMATE SODIUM
MEDIGESIC PLUS, ACETAMINOPHEN
MEDIHALER ERGOTAMINE, ERGOTAMINE TARTRATE
MEDIHALER-EPI, EPINEPHRINE BITARTRATE (OTC)
MEDIHALER-ISO, ISOPROTERENOL SULFATE
MEDIPREN, IBUPROFEN (OTC)
MEDROL, METHYLPREDNISOLONE
MEDROL, METHYLPREDNISOLONE ACETATE
MEDROL ACETATE, METHYLPREDNISOLONE ACETATE
MEDROXYPROGESTERONE ACETATE, MEDROXYPROGESTERONE ACETATE
MEFLOQUINE HCL, MEFLOQUINE HYDROCHLORIDE
MEFOXIN, CEFOXITIN SODIUM
MEFOXIN IN DEXTROSE 5% IN PLASTIC CONTAINER, CEFOXITIN SODIUM
MEFOXIN IN SODIUM CHLORIDE 0.9% IN PLASTIC CONTAINER, CEFOXITIN SODIUM
MEGACE, MEGESTROL ACETATE
MEGATOPE, ALBUMIN IODINATED I-131 SERUM
MEGESTROL ACETATE, MEGESTROL ACETATE
MELFIAT, PHENDIMETRAZINE TARTRATE
MELFIAT-105, PHENDIMETRAZINE TARTRATE
MELLARIL, THIORIDAZINE HYDROCHLORIDE
MELLARIL-S, THIORIDAZINE
MENADIONE, MENADIONE
MENEST, ESTROGENS, ESTERIFIED
MENRIUM 10-4, CHLORDIAZEPOXIDE
MENRIUM 5-2, CHLORDIAZEPOXIDE
MENRIUM 5-4, CHLORDIAZEPOXIDE
MEPERGAN, MEPERIDINE HYDROCHLORIDE
MEPERIDINE AND ATROPINE SULFATE, ATROPINE SULFATE
MEPERIDINE HCL, MEPERIDINE HYDROCHLORIDE
MEPHYTON, PHYTONADIONE
MEPIVACAINE HCL, MEPIVACAINE HYDROCHLORIDE
MEPIVACAINE HCL W/ LEVONORDEFRIN, LEVONORDEFRIN
MEPRIAM, MEPROBAMATE
MEPRO-ASPIRIN, ASPIRIN
MEPROBAMATE, MEPROBAMATE
MEPROBAMATE AND ASPIRIN, ASPIRIN
MEPRON, ATOVAQUONE
MEPROSPAN, MEPROBAMATE
MERSALYL-THEOPHYLLINE, MERSALYL SODIUM
MESANTOIN, MEPHENYTOIN
MESNEX, MESNA
MESTINON, PYRIDOSTIGMINE BROMIDE
METAHYDRIN, TRICHLORMETHIAZIDE
METANDREN, METHYLTESTOSTERONE
METAPROTERENOL SULFATE, METAPROTERENOL SULFATE
METARAMINOL BITARTRATE, METARAMINOL BITARTRATE
METASTRON, STRONTIUM CHLORIDE, SR-89
METATENSIN #2, RESERPINE
METATENSIN #4, RESERPINE
METHADONE HCL, METHADONE HYDROCHLORIDE
METHADONE HCL INTENSOL, METHADONE HYDROCHLORIDE
METHADOSE, METHADONE HYDROCHLORIDE
METHAMPEX, METHAMPHETAMINE HYDROCHLORIDE
METHAMPHETAMINE HCL, METHAMPHETAMINE HYDROCHLORIDE
METHAZOLAMIDE, METHAZOLAMIDE
METHDILAZINE HCL, METHDILAZINE HYDROCHLORIDE
METHERGINE, METHYLERGONOVINE MALEATE
METHOCARBAMOL, METHOCARBAMOL
METHOCARBAMOL AND ASPIRIN, ASPIRIN
METHOTREXATE LPF, METHOTREXATE SODIUM
METHOTREXATE SODIUM, METHOTREXATE SODIUM
METHOXSALEN, METHOXSALEN
METHSCOPOLAMINE BROMIDE, METHSCOPOLAMINE BROMIDE
METHYCLOTHIAZIDE, METHYCLOTHIAZIDE
METHYCLOTHIAZIDE AND DESERPIDINE, DESERPIDINE
METHYLDOPA, METHYLDOPA
METHYLDOPA AND CHLOROTHIAZIDE, CHLOROTHIAZIDE
METHYLDOPA AND HYDROCHLOROTHIAZIDE, HYDROCHLOROTHIAZIDE

APPENDIX A
PRODUCT NAME INDEX *(continued)*

METHYLDOPATE HCL, METHYLDOPATE HYDROCHLORIDE
METHYLPHENIDATE HCL, METHYLPHENIDATE HYDROCHLORIDE
METHYLPREDNISOLONE, METHYLPREDNISOLONE
METHYLPREDNISOLONE, METHYLPREDNISOLONE SODIUM SUCCINATE
METHYLPREDNISOLONE ACETATE, METHYLPREDNISOLONE ACETATE
METHYLPREDNISOLONE SODIUM SUCCINATE, METHYLPREDNISOLONE SODIUM SUCCINATE
METHYLTESTOSTERONE, METHYLTESTOSTERONE
METI-DERM, PREDNISOLONE
METICORTELONE, PREDNISOLONE ACETATE
METICORTEN, PREDNISONE
METIMYD, PREDNISOLONE ACETATE
METOCLOPRAMIDE HCL, METOCLOPRAMIDE HYDROCHLORIDE
METOCLOPRAMIDE INTENSOL, METOCLOPRAMIDE HYDROCHLORIDE
METOCURINE IODIDE, METOCURINE IODIDE
METOPIRONE, METYRAPONE
METOPROLOL TARTRATE, METOPROLOL TARTRATE
METRA, PHENDIMETRAZINE TARTRATE
METRETON, PREDNISOLONE SODIUM PHOSPHATE
METRO I.V., METRONIDAZOLE
METRO I.V. IN PLASTIC CONTAINER, METRONIDAZOLE
METRODIN, UROFOLLITROPIN
METROGEL, METRONIDAZOLE
METRONIDAZOLE, METRONIDAZOLE
METRONIDAZOLE HCL, METRONIDAZOLE HYDROCHLORIDE
METRYL, METRONIDAZOLE
METRYL 500, METRONIDAZOLE
METUBINE IODIDE, METOCURINE IODIDE
MEVACOR, LOVASTATIN
MEXATE, METHOTREXATE SODIUM
MEXATE-AQ, METHOTREXATE SODIUM
MEXATE-AQ PRESERVED, METHOTREXATE SODIUM
MEXITIL, MEXILETINE HYDROCHLORIDE
MEZLIN, MEZLOCILLIN SODIUM MONOHYDRATE
MIACALCIN, CALCITONIN, SALMON
MICONAZOLE NITRATE, MICONAZOLE NITRATE
MICONAZOLE NITRATE, MICONAZOLE NITRATE (OTC)
MICRAININ, ASPIRIN
MICRO-K, POTASSIUM CHLORIDE
MICRO-K LS, POTASSIUM CHLORIDE
MICRO-K 10, POTASSIUM CHLORIDE
MICROCOL, CHLORHEXIDINE GLUCONATE (OTC)
MICRODERM, CHLORHEXIDINE GLUCONATE (OTC)
MICROLITE, TECHNETIUM TC-99M ALBUMIN COLLOID KIT
MICRONASE, GLYBURIDE
MICRONOR, NORETHINDRONE
MICROSUL, SULFAMETHIZOLE
MIDAMOR, AMILORIDE HYDROCHLORIDE
MIDOL, IBUPROFEN (OTC)
MIGERGOT, CAFFEINE
MILONTIN, PHENSUXIMIDE
MILOPHENE, CLOMIPHENE CITRATE
MILPREM-200, ESTROGENS, CONJUGATED
MILPREM-400, ESTROGENS, CONJUGATED
MILTOWN, MEPROBAMATE
MINIPRESS, PRAZOSIN HYDROCHLORIDE
MINIPRESS XL, PRAZOSIN HYDROCHLORIDE
MINITEC, TECHNETIUM TC-99M SODIUM PERTECHNETATE GENERATOR
MINIZIDE, POLYTHIAZIDE
MINOCIN, MINOCYCLINE HYDROCHLORIDE
MINOCYCLINE HCL, MINOCYCLINE HYDROCHLORIDE
MINODYL, MINOXIDIL
MINOXIDIL, MINOXIDIL
MINTEZOL, THIABENDAZOLE
MIOCHOL, ACETYLCHOLINE CHLORIDE
MIOCHOL-E, ACETYLCHOLINE CHLORIDE
MIOSTAT, CARBACHOL
MIRADON, ANISINDIONE
MITHRACIN, PLICAMYCIN
MIVACRON, MIVACURIUM CHLORIDE
MIVACRON IN DEXTROSE 5%, MIVACURIUM CHLORIDE
MIXTARD HUMAN 70/30, INSULIN SEMISYNTHETIC PURIFIED HUMAN (OTC)
MOBAN, MOLINDONE HYDROCHLORIDE
MOCTANIN, MONOCTANOIN
MODERIL, RESCINNAMINE
MODICON 21, ETHINYL ESTRADIOL
MODICON 28, ETHINYL ESTRADIOL
MODRASTANE, TRILOSTANE
MODURETIC 5-50, AMILORIDE HYDROCHLORIDE
MONISTAT, MICONAZOLE
MONISTAT DUAL-PAK, MICONAZOLE NITRATE
MONISTAT 3, MICONAZOLE NITRATE
MONISTAT 5, MICONAZOLE NITRATE
MONISTAT 7, MICONAZOLE NITRATE (OTC)
MONISTAT 7 COMBINATION PACK, MICONAZOLE NITRATE
MONISTAT-DERM, MICONAZOLE NITRATE
MONOCID, CEFONICID SODIUM
MONOKET, ISOSORBIDE MONONITRATE
MONOPRIL, FOSINOPRIL SODIUM
MORPHINE SULFATE, MORPHINE SULFATE
MOTOFEN, ATROPINE SULFATE
MOTOFEN HALF-STRENGTH, ATROPINE SULFATE
MOTRIN, IBUPROFEN
MOXAM, MOXALACTAM DISODIUM
MPI DMSA KIDNEY REAGENT, TECHNETIUM TC-99M SUCCIMER KIT
MPI DTPA KIT - CHELATE, TECHNETIUM TC-99M PENTETATE KIT
MPI INDIUM DTPA IN 111, INDIUM IN-111 PENTETATE DISODIUM
MPI KRYPTON 81M GAS GENERATOR, KRYPTON, KR-81M
MPI STANNOUS DIPHOSPHONATE, TECHNETIUM TC-99M ETIDRONATE KIT
MS CONTIN, MORPHINE SULFATE
MUCOMYST, ACETYLCYSTEINE
MUCOMYST W/ ISOPROTERENOL, ACETYLCYSTEINE
MUCOSIL-10, ACETYLCYSTEINE
MUCOSIL-20, ACETYLCYSTEINE
MULTIFUGE, PIPERAZINE CITRATE
MUSTARGEN, MECHLORETHAMINE HYDROCHLORIDE
MUTAMYCIN, MITOMYCIN
MVC PLUS, ASCORBIC ACID
MYAMBUTOL, ETHAMBUTOL HYDROCHLORIDE
MYBANIL, BROMODIPHENHYDRAMINE HYDROCHLORIDE
MYCELEX, CLOTRIMAZOLE
MYCELEX, CLOTRIMAZOLE (OTC)
MYCELEX-G, CLOTRIMAZOLE
MYCELEX-7, CLOTRIMAZOLE (OTC)
MYCELEX-7 COMBINATION PACK, CLOTRIMAZOLE
MYCHEL, CHLORAMPHENICOL
MYCHEL-S, CHLORAMPHENICOL SODIUM SUCCINATE
MYCIFRADIN, NEOMYCIN SULFATE
MYCITRACIN, BACITRACIN
MYCO-TRIACET II, NYSTATIN
MYCOBUTIN, RIFABUTIN
MYCODONE, HOMATROPINE METHYLBROMIDE
MYCOLOG-II, NYSTATIN
MYCOSTATIN, NYSTATIN
MYDRIACYL, TROPICAMIDE
MYDRIAFAIR, TROPICAMIDE
MYFED, PSEUDOEPHEDRINE HYDROCHLORIDE (OTC)
MYIDYL, TRIPROLIDINE HYDROCHLORIDE

APPENDIX A
PRODUCT NAME INDEX *(continued)*

MYKACET, NYSTATIN
MYKINAC, NYSTATIN
MYKROX, METOLAZONE
MYLARAMINE, DEXCHLORPHENIRAMINE MALEATE
MYLAXEN, HEXAFLUORENIUM BROMIDE
MYLERAN, BUSULFAN
MYLOCAINE, LIDOCAINE HYDROCHLORIDE
MYMETHASONE, DEXAMETHASONE
MYMETHAZINE FORTIS, PROMETHAZINE HYDROCHLORIDE
MYOTONACHOL, BETHANECHOL CHLORIDE
MYPHETANE DC, BROMPHENIRAMINE MALEATE
MYPHETANE DX, BROMPHENIRAMINE MALEATE
MYPROIC ACID, VALPROIC ACID
MYSOLINE, PRIMIDONE
MYTELASE, AMBENONIUM CHLORIDE
MYTREX A, NEOMYCIN SULFATE
MYTREX F, NYSTATIN

N

N.E.E. 1/35 21, ETHINYL ESTRADIOL
N.E.E. 1/35 28, ETHINYL ESTRADIOL
NADOLOL, NADOLOL
NAFAZAIR, NAPHAZOLINE HYDROCHLORIDE
NAFCIL, NAFCILLIN SODIUM
NAFCILLIN SODIUM, NAFCILLIN SODIUM
NAFTIN, NAFTIFINE HYDROCHLORIDE
NALBUPHINE, NALBUPHINE HYDROCHLORIDE
NALBUPHINE HCL, NALBUPHINE HYDROCHLORIDE
NALBUPHINE HYDROCHLORIDE, NALBUPHINE HYDROCHLORIDE
NALFON, FENOPROFEN CALCIUM
NALFON 200, FENOPROFEN CALCIUM
NALIDIXIC ACID, NALIDIXIC ACID
NALLPEN, NAFCILLIN SODIUM
NALOXONE, NALOXONE HYDROCHLORIDE
NALOXONE HCL, NALOXONE HYDROCHLORIDE
NANDDROLONE DECANOATE, NANDROLONE DECANOATE
NANDROLONE DECANOATE, NANDROLONE DECANOATE
NANDROLONE PHENPROPIONATE, NANDROLONE PHENPROPIONATE
NAPHAZOLINE HCL, NAPHAZOLINE HYDROCHLORIDE
NAPHCON FORTE, NAPHAZOLINE HYDROCHLORIDE
NAPHCON-A, NAPHAZOLINE HYDROCHLORIDE
NAPROSYN, NAPROXEN
NAPROXEN, NAPROXEN
NAPROXEN SODIUM, NAPROXEN SODIUM
NAQUA, TRICHLORMETHIAZIDE
NAQUIVAL, RESERPINE
NARCAN, NALOXONE HYDROCHLORIDE
NARDIL, PHENELZINE SULFATE
NASACORT, TRIAMCINOLONE ACETONIDE
NASALCROM, CROMOLYN SODIUM
NASALIDE, FLUNISOLIDE
NATACYN, NATAMYCIN
NATURAL ESTROGENIC SUBSTANCE-ESTRONE, ESTRONE
NATURETIN-10, BENDROFLUMETHIAZIDE
NATURETIN-2.5, BENDROFLUMETHIAZIDE
NATURETIN-5, BENDROFLUMETHIAZIDE
NAVANE, THIOTHIXENE
NAVANE, THIOTHIXENE HYDROCHLORIDE
NEBCIN, TOBRAMYCIN SULFATE
NEBUPENT, PENTAMIDINE ISETHIONATE
NEGGRAM, NALIDIXIC ACID
NEMBUTAL, PENTOBARBITAL
NEMBUTAL, PENTOBARBITAL SODIUM
NEMBUTAL SODIUM, PENTOBARBITAL SODIUM
NEO-CORT-DOME, ACETIC ACID, GLACIAL
NEO-CORT-DOME, HYDROCORTISONE
NEO-CORTEF, HYDROCORTISONE ACETATE
NEO-DELTA-CORTEF, NEOMYCIN SULFATE
NEO-HYDELTRASOL, NEOMYCIN SULFATE
NEO-MEDROL, METHYLPREDNISOLONE
NEO-MEDROL ACETATE, METHYLPREDNISOLONE ACETATE
NEO-OTOSOL-HC, HYDROCORTISONE
NEO-POLYCIN, BACITRACIN ZINC
NEO-POLYCIN, GRAMICIDIN
NEO-RX, NEOMYCIN SULFATE
NEO-SYNALAR, FLUOCINOLONE ACETONIDE
NEOBIOTIC, NEOMYCIN SULFATE
NEODECADRON, DEXAMETHASONE SODIUM PHOSPHATE
NEOMYCIN & POLYMYXIN B SULFATES & BACITRACIN ZINC & HYDROCORTISONE, BACITRACIN ZINC
NEOMYCIN AND POLYMYXIN B SULFATES, NEOMYCIN SULFATE
NEOMYCIN AND POLYMYXIN B SULFATES AND DEXAMETHASONE, DEXAMETHASONE
NEOMYCIN AND POLYMYXIN B SULFATES AND GRAMICIDIN, GRAMICIDIN
NEOMYCIN AND POLYMYXIN B SULFATES AND HYDROCORTISONE, HYDROCORTISONE
NEOMYCIN SULFATE, NEOMYCIN SULFATE
NEOMYCIN SULFATE AND POLYMYXIN B SULFATE GRAMICIDIN, GRAMICIDIN
NEOMYCIN SULFATE-DEXAMETHASONE SODIUM PHOSPHATE, DEXAMETHASONE SODIUM PHOSPHATE
NEOMYCIN SULFATE-POLYMYXIN B SULFATE-HYDROCORTISONE, HYDROCORTISONE
NEOMYCIN SULFATE-TRIAMCINOLONE ACETONIDE, NEOMYCIN SULFATE
NEOMYCIN SULFATE, POLYMYXIN B SULFATE & HYDROCORTISONE, HYDROCORTISONE
NEOPAP, ACETAMINOPHEN (OTC)
NEOPASALATE, AMINOSALICYLATE SODIUM
NEOPHAM 6.4%, AMINO ACIDS
NEOSAR, CYCLOPHOSPHAMIDE
NEOSCAN, GALLIUM CITRATE, GA-67
NEOSPORIN, BACITRACIN ZINC
NEOSPORIN, GRAMICIDIN
NEOSPORIN G.U. IRRIGANT, NEOMYCIN SULFATE
NEOTHYLLINE, DYPHYLLINE
NEOTRIZINE, TRISULFAPYRIMIDINES (SULFADIAZINE;SULFAMERAZINE;SULFAMETHAZINE)
NEPHRAMINE 5.4%, AMINO ACIDS
NEPHROFLOW, IODOHIPPURATE SODIUM, I-123
NEPTAZANE, METHAZOLAMIDE
NESACAINE, CHLOROPROCAINE HYDROCHLORIDE
NESACAINE-MPF, CHLOROPROCAINE HYDROCHLORIDE
NETROMYCIN, NETILMICIN SULFATE
NEURAMATE, MEPROBAMATE
NEURONTIN, GABAPENTIN
NEUTREXIN, TRIMETREXATE GLUCURONATE
NIACIN, NIACIN
NICLOCIDE, NICLOSAMIDE
NICODERM, NICOTINE
NICOLAR, NIACIN
NICORETTE, NICOTINE POLACRILEX
NICORETTE DS, NICOTINE POLACRILEX
NICOTROL, NICOTINE
NIFEDIPINE, NIFEDIPINE
NILSTAT, NYSTATIN
NIMOTOP, NIMODIPINE
NIPENT, PENTOSTATIN
NIPRIDE, SODIUM NITROPRUSSIDE
NITRO IV, NITROGLYCERIN
NITRO-BID, NITROGLYCERIN
NITROFURANTOIN, NITROFURANTOIN
NITROFURANTOIN, NITROFURANTOIN, MACROCRYSTALLINE

APPENDIX A
PRODUCT NAME INDEX *(continued)*

NITROFURANTOIN MACROCRYSTALLINE, NITROFURANTOIN, MACROCRYSTALLINE
NITROFURAZONE, NITROFURAZONE
NITROGLYCERIN, NITROGLYCERIN
NITROGLYCERIN IN DEXTROSE 5%, NITROGLYCERIN
NITROL, NITROGLYCERIN
NITROLINGUAL, NITROGLYCERIN
NITRONAL, NITROGLYCERIN
NITROPRESS, SODIUM NITROPRUSSIDE
NITROSTAT, NITROGLYCERIN
NIX, PERMETHRIN
NIX, PERMETHRIN (OTC)
NIZORAL, KETOCONAZOLE
NOGENIC HC, HYDROCORTISONE
NOLUDAR, METHYPRYLON
NOLVADEX, TAMOXIFEN CITRATE
NOR-Q.D., NORETHINDRONE
NORCEPT-E 1/35 21, ETHINYL ESTRADIOL
NORCEPT-E 1/35 28, ETHINYL ESTRADIOL
NORCET, ACETAMINOPHEN
NORCURON, VECURONIUM BROMIDE
NORDETTE-21, ETHINYL ESTRADIOL
NORDETTE-28, ETHINYL ESTRADIOL
NORETHIN 1/35E-21, ETHINYL ESTRADIOL
NORETHIN 1/35E-28, ETHINYL ESTRADIOL
NORETHIN 1/50M-21, MESTRANOL
NORETHIN 1/50M-28, MESTRANOL
NORETHINDRONE AND ETHINYL ESTRADIOL, ETHINYL ESTRADIOL
NORETHINDRONE AND ETHINYL ESTRADIOL (10/11), ETHINYL ESTRADIOL
NORETHINDRONE AND ETHINYL ESTRADIOL (7/14), ETHINYL ESTRADIOL
NORETHINDRONE AND MESTRANOL, MESTRANOL
NORFLEX, ORPHENADRINE CITRATE
NORGESIC, ASPIRIN
NORGESIC FORTE, ASPIRIN
NORINYL, MESTRANOL
NORINYL 1+35 21-DAY, ETHINYL ESTRADIOL
NORINYL 1+35 28-DAY, ETHINYL ESTRADIOL
NORINYL 1+50 21-DAY, MESTRANOL
NORINYL 1+50 28-DAY, MESTRANOL
NORINYL 1+80 21-DAY, MESTRANOL
NORINYL 1+80 28-DAY, MESTRANOL
NORISODRINE, ISOPROTERENOL SULFATE
NORISODRINE AEROTROL, ISOPROTERENOL HYDROCHLORIDE
NORLESTRIN FE 1/50, ETHINYL ESTRADIOL
NORLESTRIN FE 2.5/50, ETHINYL ESTRADIOL
NORLESTRIN 21 1/50, ETHINYL ESTRADIOL
NORLESTRIN 21 2.5/50, ETHINYL ESTRADIOL
NORLESTRIN 28 1/50, ETHINYL ESTRADIOL
NORLUTATE, NORETHINDRONE ACETATE
NORLUTIN, NORETHINDRONE
NORMODYNE, LABETALOL HYDROCHLORIDE
NORMOSOL-M AND DEXTROSE 5%, DEXTROSE
NORMOSOL-R AND DEXTROSE 5% IN PLASTIC CONTAINER, DEXTROSE
NORMOSOL-R IN PLASTIC CONTAINER, MAGNESIUM CHLORIDE
NORMOZIDE, HYDROCHLOROTHIAZIDE
NOROXIN, NORFLOXACIN
NORPACE, DISOPYRAMIDE PHOSPHATE
NORPACE CR, DISOPYRAMIDE PHOSPHATE
NORPLANT, LEVONORGESTREL
NORPLANT SYSTEM, LEVONORGESTREL
NORPRAMIN, DESIPRAMINE HYDROCHLORIDE
NORQUEST FE, ETHINYL ESTRADIOL
NORTRIPTYLINE HCL, NORTRIPTYLINE HYDROCHLORIDE
NORVASC, AMLODIPINE BESYLATE
NOVAFED, PSEUDOEPHEDRINE HYDROCHLORIDE
NOVAMINE 11.4%, AMINO ACIDS
NOVAMINE 15%, AMINO ACIDS
NOVAMINE 15% SULFITE FREE, AMINO ACIDS
NOVAMINE 8.5%, AMINO ACIDS
NOVANTRONE, MITOXANTRONE HYDROCHLORIDE
NOVOCAIN, PROCAINE HYDROCHLORIDE
NOVOLIN L, INSULIN ZINC SUSP BIOSYNTHETIC HUMAN (OTC)
NOVOLIN L, INSULIN ZINC SUSP SEMISYNTHETIC PURIFIED HUMAN (OTC)
NOVOLIN N, INSULIN SUSP ISOPHANE BIOSYNTHETIC HUMAN (OTC)
NOVOLIN N, INSULIN SUSP ISOPHANE SEMISYNTHETIC PURIFIED HUMAN (OTC)
NOVOLIN R, INSULIN BIOSYNTHETIC HUMAN (OTC)
NOVOLIN R, INSULIN SEMISYNTHETIC PURIFIED HUMAN (OTC)
NOVOLIN 70/30, INSULIN BIOSYNTHETIC HUMAN (OTC)
NOVOLIN 70/30, INSULIN SEMISYNTHETIC PURIFIED HUMAN (OTC)
NOVRAD, LEVOPROPOXYPHENE NAPSYLATE, ANHYDROUS
NPH ILETIN I (BEEF-PORK), INSULIN SUSP ISOPHANE BEEF/PORK (OTC)
NPH ILETIN II, INSULIN SUSP ISOPHANE PURIFIED BEEF (OTC)
NPH ILETIN II (PORK), INSULIN SUSP ISOPHANE PURIFIED PORK (OTC)
NPH INSULIN, INSULIN SUSP ISOPHANE BEEF (OTC)
NPH PURIFIED PORK ISOPHANE INSULIN, INSULIN SUSP ISOPHANE PURIFIED PORK (OTC)
NUBAIN, NALBUPHINE HYDROCHLORIDE
NULYTELY, POLYETHYLENE GLYCOL 3350
NUMORPHAN, OXYMORPHONE HYDROCHLORIDE
NUPRIN, IBUPROFEN (OTC)
NUROMAX, DOXACURIUM CHLORIDE
NUTRACORT, HYDROCORTISONE
NUTRILIPID 10%, SOYBEAN OIL
NUTRILIPID 20%, SOYBEAN OIL
NUTROPIN, SOMATROPIN, BIOSYNTHETIC
NYDRAZID, ISONIAZID
NYSERT, NYSTATIN
NYSTAFORM, CLIOQUINOL
NYSTATIN, NYSTATIN
NYSTATIN AND TRIAMCINOLONE ACETONIDE, NYSTATIN
NYSTATIN-TRIAMCINOLONE ACETONIDE, NYSTATIN
NYSTEX, NYSTATIN

O

OBESTIN-30, PHENTERMINE HYDROCHLORIDE
OBY-TRIM, PHENTERMINE HYDROCHLORIDE
OCL, POLYETHYLENE GLYCOL 3350
OCTOCAINE, EPINEPHRINE
OCTREOSCAN, INDIUM IN-111 PENTETREOTIDE KIT
OCUCLEAR, OXYMETAZOLINE HYDROCHLORIDE (OTC)
OCUFEN, FLURBIPROFEN SODIUM
OCUFLOX, OFLOXACIN
OCUMYCIN, BACITRACIN ZINC
OCUSERT PILO-20, PILOCARPINE
OCUSERT PILO-40, PILOCARPINE
OCUSULF-10, SULFACETAMIDE SODIUM
OCUSULF-30, SULFACETAMIDE SODIUM
OGEN, ESTROPIPATE
OGEN .625, ESTROPIPATE
OGEN 1.25, ESTROPIPATE
OGEN 2.5, ESTROPIPATE
OGEN 5, ESTROPIPATE
OMNIFLOX, TEMAFLOXACIN HYDROCHLORIDE

APPENDIX A
PRODUCT NAME INDEX *(continued)*

OMNIPAQUE 140, IOHEXOL
OMNIPAQUE 180, IOHEXOL
OMNIPAQUE 210, IOHEXOL
OMNIPAQUE 240, IOHEXOL
OMNIPAQUE 300, IOHEXOL
OMNIPAQUE 350, IOHEXOL
OMNIPAQUE 70, IOHEXOL
OMNIPEN (AMPICILLIN), AMPICILLIN/AMPICILLIN TRIHYDRATE
OMNIPEN-N, AMPICILLIN SODIUM
OMNISCAN, GADODIAMIDE
ONA MAST, PHENTERMINE HYDROCHLORIDE
ONA-MAST, PHENTERMINE HYDROCHLORIDE
ONCOVIN, VINCRISTINE SULFATE
OPCON, NAPHAZOLINE HYDROCHLORIDE
OPCON-A, NAPHAZOLINE HYDROCHLORIDE
OPHTHAINE, PROPARACAINE HYDROCHLORIDE
OPHTHETIC, PROPARACAINE HYDROCHLORIDE
OPHTHOCHLOR, CHLORAMPHENICOL
OPHTHOCORT, CHLORAMPHENICOL
OPTICROM, CROMOLYN SODIUM
OPTIMINE, AZATADINE MALEATE
OPTIPRANOLOL, METIPRANOLOL HYDROCHLORIDE
OPTIPRESS, CARTEOLOL HYDROCHLORIDE
OPTIRAY 160, IOVERSOL
OPTIRAY 240, IOVERSOL
OPTIRAY 300, IOVERSOL
OPTIRAY 320, IOVERSOL
OPTIRAY 350, IOVERSOL
OPTOMYCIN, CHLORAMPHENICOL
ORA-TESTRYL, FLUOXYMESTERONE
ORABASE HCA, HYDROCORTISONE ACETATE
ORACORT, TRIAMCINOLONE ACETONIDE
ORAGRAFIN CALCIUM, IPODATE CALCIUM
ORAGRAFIN SODIUM, IPODATE SODIUM
ORALONE, TRIAMCINOLONE ACETONIDE
ORAMORPH SR, MORPHINE SULFATE
ORAP, PIMOZIDE
ORASONE, PREDNISONE
ORETIC, HYDROCHLOROTHIAZIDE
ORETICYL FORTE, DESERPIDINE
ORETICYL 25, DESERPIDINE
ORETICYL 50, DESERPIDINE
ORETON, METHYLTESTOSTERONE
ORETON METHYL, METHYLTESTOSTERONE
ORGATRAX, HYDROXYZINE HYDROCHLORIDE
ORINASE, TOLBUTAMIDE
ORINASE DIAGNOSTIC, TOLBUTAMIDE SODIUM
ORLAAM, LEVOMETHADYL ACETATE HYDROCHLORIDE
ORLEX, ACETIC ACID, GLACIAL
ORLEX HC, ACETIC ACID, GLACIAL
ORNADE, CHLORPHENIRAMINE MALEATE
ORNIDYL, EFLORNITHINE HYDROCHLORIDE
ORPHENADRINE CITRATE, ORPHENADRINE CITRATE
ORPHENGESIC, ASPIRIN
ORPHENGESIC FORTE, ASPIRIN
ORTHO CYCLEN-21, ETHINYL ESTRADIOL
ORTHO CYCLEN-28, ETHINYL ESTRADIOL
ORTHO TRI-CYCLEN, ETHINYL ESTRADIOL
ORTHO-CEPT, DESOGESTREL
ORTHO-EST, ESTROPIPATE
ORTHO-NOVUM 1/35-21, ETHINYL ESTRADIOL
ORTHO-NOVUM 1/35-28, ETHINYL ESTRADIOL
ORTHO-NOVUM 1/50 21, MESTRANOL
ORTHO-NOVUM 1/50 28, MESTRANOL
ORTHO-NOVUM 1/80 21, MESTRANOL
ORTHO-NOVUM 10-21, MESTRANOL
ORTHO-NOVUM 10/11-21, ETHINYL ESTRADIOL
ORTHO-NOVUM 10/11-28, ETHINYL ESTRADIOL
ORTHO-NOVUM 2-21, MESTRANOL
ORTHO-NOVUM 7/14-21, ETHINYL ESTRADIOL
ORTHO-NOVUM 7/14-28, ETHINYL ESTRADIOL
ORTHO-NOVUM 7/7/7-21, ETHINYL ESTRADIOL
ORTHO-NOVUM 7/7/7-28, ETHINYL ESTRADIOL
ORTHO-N0VUM 1/80 28, MESTRANOL
ORUDIS, KETOPROFEN
ORUVAIL, KETOPROFEN
OSMITROL 10% IN WATER, MANNITOL
OSMITROL 10% IN WATER IN PLASTIC CONTAINER, MANNITOL
OSMITROL 15% IN WATER, MANNITOL
OSMITROL 15% IN WATER IN PLASTIC CONTAINER, MANNITOL
OSMITROL 20% IN WATER, MANNITOL
OSMITROL 20% IN WATER IN PLASTIC CONTAINER, MANNITOL
OSMITROL 5% IN WATER, MANNITOL
OSMITROL 5% IN WATER IN PLASTIC CONTAINER, MANNITOL
OSMOVIST, IOTROLAN
OSTEOLITE, TECHNETIUM TC-99M MEDRONATE KIT
OSTEOSCAN, TECHNETIUM TC-99M ETIDRONATE KIT
OTICAIR, HYDROCORTISONE
OTOBIONE, HYDROCORTISONE
OTOBIOTIC, HYDROCORTISONE
OTOCORT, HYDROCORTISONE
OVCON-35, ETHINYL ESTRADIOL
OVCON-50, ETHINYL ESTRADIOL
OVIDE, MALATHION
OVRAL, ETHINYL ESTRADIOL
OVRAL-28, ETHINYL ESTRADIOL
OVRETTE, NORGESTREL
OVULEN, ETHYNODIOL DIACETATE
OVULEN-21, ETHYNODIOL DIACETATE
OVULEN-28, ETHYNODIOL DIACETATE
OXACILLIN SODIUM, OXACILLIN SODIUM
OXANDRIN, OXANDROLONE
OXAZEPAM, OXAZEPAM
OXISTAT, OXICONAZOLE NITRATE
OXSORALEN, METHOXSALEN
OXSORALEN-ULTRA, METHOXSALEN
OXTRIPHYLLINE, OXTRIPHYLLINE
OXTRIPHYLLINE PEDIATRIC, OXTRIPHYLLINE
OXY-KESSO-TETRA, OXYTETRACYCLINE HYDROCHLORIDE
OXYBUTYNIN CHLORIDE, OXYBUTYNIN CHLORIDE
OXYCET, ACETAMINOPHEN
OXYCODONE AND ACETAMINOPHEN, ACETAMINOPHEN
OXYCODONE AND ASPIRIN, ASPIRIN
OXYCODONE AND ASPIRIN (HALF-STRENGTH), ASPIRIN
OXYCODONE HCL AND ACETAMINOPHEN, ACETAMINOPHEN
OXYCODONE 2.5/APAP 500, ACETAMINOPHEN
OXYCODONE 5/APAP 500, ACETAMINOPHEN
OXYLONE, FLUOROMETHOLONE
OXYPHENBUTAZONE, OXYPHENBUTAZONE
OXYTETRACYCLINE HCL, OXYTETRACYCLINE HYDROCHLORIDE
OXYTOCIN, OXYTOCIN
OXYTOCIN 10 USP UNITS IN DEXTROSE 5%, OXYTOCIN
OXYTOCIN 20 USP UNITS IN DEXTROSE 5%, OXYTOCIN
OXYTOCIN 5 USP UNITS IN DEXTROSE 5%, OXYTOCIN

P

P.A.S. SODIUM, AMINOSALICYLATE SODIUM
PAGITANE, CYCRIMINE HYDROCHLORIDE
PAMELOR, NORTRIPTYLINE HYDROCHLORIDE
PAMINE, METHSCOPOLAMINE BROMIDE
PANCURONIUM, PANCURONIUM BROMIDE
PANCURONIUM BROMIDE, PANCURONIUM BROMIDE
PANHEPRIN, HEPARIN SODIUM

APPENDIX A
PRODUCT NAME INDEX *(continued)*

PANMYCIN, TETRACYCLINE HYDROCHLORIDE
PANTOPAQUE, IOPHENDYLATE
PANWARFIN, WARFARIN SODIUM
PAPA-DEINE #3, ACETAMINOPHEN
PAPA-DEINE #4, ACETAMINOPHEN
PARACAINE, PROPARACAINE HYDROCHLORIDE
PARACORT, PREDNISONE
PARADIONE, PARAMETHADIONE
PARAFLEX, CHLORZOXAZONE
PARAFON FORTE DSC, CHLORZOXAZONE
PARAPLATIN, CARBOPLATIN
PARASAL, AMINOSALICYLIC ACID
PARASAL SODIUM, AMINOSALICYLATE SODIUM
PARATHAR, TERIPARATIDE ACETATE
PAREDRINE, HYDROXYAMPHETAMINE HYDROBROMIDE
PAREMYD, HYDROXYAMPHETAMINE HYDROBROMIDE
PARLODEL, BROMOCRIPTINE MESYLATE
PARNATE, TRANYLCYPROMINE SULFATE
PARSIDOL, ETHOPROPAZINE HYDROCHLORIDE
PASER, AMINOSALICYLIC ACID
PASKALIUM, POTASSIUM AMINOSALICYLATE
PATHILON, TRIDIHEXETHYL CHLORIDE
PATHOCIL, DICLOXACILLIN SODIUM
PAVULON, PANCURONIUM BROMIDE
PAXIL, PAROXETINE HYDROCHLORIDE
PAXIPAM, HALAZEPAM
PBZ, TRIPELENNAMINE CITRATE
PBZ, TRIPELENNAMINE HYDROCHLORIDE
PBZ-SR, TRIPELENNAMINE HYDROCHLORIDE
PCE, ERYTHROMYCIN
PEDIA PROFEN, IBUPROFEN
PEDIAMYCIN, ERYTHROMYCIN ETHYLSUCCINATE
PEDIAMYCIN 400, ERYTHROMYCIN ETHYLSUCCINATE
PEDIAPRED, PREDNISOLONE SODIUM PHOSPHATE
PEDIATRIC LTA KIT, LIDOCAINE HYDROCHLORIDE
PEDIAZOLE, ERYTHROMYCIN ETHYLSUCCINATE
PEDIOTIC, HYDROCORTISONE
PEG-LYTE, POLYETHYLENE GLYCOL 3350
PEGANONE, ETHOTOIN
PEN-VEE K, PENICILLIN V POTASSIUM
PENAPAR-VK, PENICILLIN V POTASSIUM
PENBRITIN, AMPICILLIN/AMPICILLIN TRIHYDRATE
PENBRITIN-S, AMPICILLIN SODIUM
PENECORT, HYDROCORTISONE
PENETREX, ENOXACIN
PENICILLIN, PENICILLIN G POTASSIUM
PENICILLIN G POTASSIUM, PENICILLIN G POTASSIUM
PENICILLIN G PROCAINE, PENICILLIN G PROCAINE
PENICILLIN G SODIUM, PENICILLIN G SODIUM
PENICILLIN V POTASSIUM, PENICILLIN V POTASSIUM
PENICILLIN-VK, PENICILLIN V POTASSIUM
PENICILLIN-2, PENICILLIN G POTASSIUM
PENNTUSS, CHLORPHENIRAMINE POLISTIREX (OTC)
PENTACARINAT, PENTAMIDINE ISETHIONATE
PENTACEF, CEFTAZIDIME (ARGININE FORMULATION)
PENTAM 300, PENTAMIDINE ISETHIONATE
PENTAMIDINE ISETHIONATE, PENTAMIDINE ISETHIONATE
PENTASA, MESALAMINE
PENTHRANE, METHOXYFLURANE
PENTIDS '200', PENICILLIN G POTASSIUM
PENTIDS '250', PENICILLIN G POTASSIUM
PENTIDS '400', PENICILLIN G POTASSIUM
PENTIDS '800', PENICILLIN G POTASSIUM
PENTOBARBITAL SODIUM, PENTOBARBITAL SODIUM
PENTOLAIR, CYCLOPENTOLATE HYDROCHLORIDE
PENTOTHAL, THIOPENTAL SODIUM
PEPCID, FAMOTIDINE
PEPTAVLON, PENTAGASTRIN
PERCHLORACAP, POTASSIUM PERCHLORATE
PERCOCET, ACETAMINOPHEN
PERCODAN, ASPIRIN
PERCODAN-DEMI, ASPIRIN
PERCORTEN, DESOXYCORTICOSTERONE ACETATE
PERCORTEN, DESOXYCORTICOSTERONE PIVALATE
PERGONAL, MENOTROPINS (FSH;LH)
PERIACTIN, CYPROHEPTADINE HYDROCHLORIDE
PERIDEX, CHLORHEXIDINE GLUCONATE
PERIOGARD, CHLORHEXIDINE GLUCONATE
PERMAPEN, PENICILLIN G BENZATHINE
PERMAX, PERGOLIDE MESYLATE
PERMITIL, FLUPHENAZINE HYDROCHLORIDE
PERPHENAZINE, PERPHENAZINE
PERPHENAZINE AND AMITRIPTYLINE HCL, AMITRIPTYLINE HYDROCHLORIDE
PERSANTINE, DIPYRIDAMOLE
PERTOFRANE, DESIPRAMINE HYDROCHLORIDE
PFIZER-E, ERYTHROMYCIN STEARATE
PFIZERPEN, PENICILLIN G POTASSIUM
PFIZERPEN G, PENICILLIN G POTASSIUM
PFIZERPEN VK, PENICILLIN V POTASSIUM
PFIZERPEN-A, AMPICILLIN/AMPICILLIN TRIHYDRATE
PFIZERPEN-AS, PENICILLIN G PROCAINE
PHARMASEAL SCRUB CARE, CHLORHEXIDINE GLUCONATE (OTC)
PHENAPHEN W/ CODEINE NO. 2, ACETAMINOPHEN
PHENAPHEN W/ CODEINE NO. 3, ACETAMINOPHEN
PHENAPHEN W/ CODEINE NO. 4, ACETAMINOPHEN
PHENAPHEN-650 W/ CODEINE, ACETAMINOPHEN
PHENAZINE, PHENDIMETRAZINE TARTRATE
PHENAZINE-35, PHENDIMETRAZINE TARTRATE
PHENDIMETRAZINE TARTRATE, PHENDIMETRAZINE TARTRATE
PHENERGAN, PROMETHAZINE HYDROCHLORIDE
PHENERGAN FORTIS, PROMETHAZINE HYDROCHLORIDE
PHENERGAN PLAIN, PROMETHAZINE HYDROCHLORIDE
PHENERGAN VC, PHENYLEPHRINE HYDROCHLORIDE
PHENERGAN VC W/ CODEINE, CODEINE PHOSPHATE
PHENERGAN W/ CODEINE, CODEINE PHOSPHATE
PHENERGAN W/ DEXTROMETHORPHAN, DEXTROMETHORPHAN HYDROBROMIDE
PHENETRON, CHLORPHENIRAMINE MALEATE
PHENTERMINE HCL, PHENTERMINE HYDROCHLORIDE
PHENTERMINE RESIN 30, PHENTERMINE RESIN COMPLEX
PHENURONE, PHENACEMIDE
PHENY-PAS-TEBAMIN, PHENYL AMINOSALICYLATE
PHENYLBUTAZONE, PHENYLBUTAZONE
PHENYLPROPANOLAMINE HCL W/ CHLORPHENIRAMINE MALEATE, CHLORPHENIRAMINE MALEATE (OTC)
PHENYLPROPANOLAMINE HCL/CHLORPHENIRAMINE, CHLORPHENIRAMINE MALEATE (OTC)
PHENYTEX, PHENYTOIN SODIUM, EXTENDED
PHENYTOIN, PHENYTOIN
PHENYTOIN, PHENYTOIN SODIUM
PHENYTOIN SODIUM, PHENYTOIN SODIUM
PHENYTOIN SODIUM, PHENYTOIN SODIUM, PROMPT
PHERAZINE DM, DEXTROMETHORPHAN HYDROBROMIDE
PHERAZINE VC, PHENYLEPHRINE HYDROCHLORIDE
PHERAZINE VC W/ CODEINE, CODEINE PHOSPHATE
PHERAZINE W/ CODEINE, CODEINE PHOSPHATE
PHISO-SCRUB, HEXACHLOROPHENE
PHISOHEX, HEXACHLOROPHENE
PHOSLO, CALCIUM ACETATE
PHOSPHOCOL P32, CHROMIC PHOSPHATE, P-32
PHOSPHOLINE IODIDE, ECHOTHIOPHATE IODIDE
PHOSPHOTEC, TECHNETIUM TC-99M PYROPHOSPHATE KIT
PHOSPHOTOPE, SODIUM PHOSPHATE, P-32
PHOTOPLEX, AVOBENZONE (OTC)
PHRENILIN, ACETAMINOPHEN
PHRENILIN FORTE, ACETAMINOPHEN

APPENDIX A
PRODUCT NAME INDEX *(continued)*

PHYLLOCONTIN, AMINOPHYLLINE
PHYSIOLYTE IN PLASTIC CONTAINER, MAGNESIUM CHLORIDE
PHYSIOSOL IN PLASTIC CONTAINER, MAGNESIUM CHLORIDE
PHYSIOSOL PH 7.4, MAGNESIUM CHLORIDE
PHYTONADIONE, PHYTONADIONE
PILOPINE HS, PILOCARPINE HYDROCHLORIDE
PINDAC, PINACIDIL
PINDOLOL, PINDOLOL
PIPERAZINE CITRATE, PIPERAZINE CITRATE
PIPRACIL, PIPERACILLIN SODIUM
PIROXICAM, PIROXICAM
PITOCIN, OXYTOCIN
PITRESSIN TANNATE, VASOPRESSIN TANNATE
PLACIDYL, ETHCHLORVYNOL
PLAQUENIL, HYDROXYCHLOROQUINE SULFATE
PLASMA-LYTE A IN PLASTIC CONTAINER, MAGNESIUM CHLORIDE
PLASMA-LYTE M AND DEXTROSE 5% IN PLASTIC CONTAINER, CALCIUM CHLORIDE
PLASMA-LYTE R IN PLASTIC CONTAINER, CALCIUM CHLORIDE
PLASMA-LYTE 148 AND DEXTROSE 5% IN PLASTIC CONTAINER, DEXTROSE
PLASMA-LYTE 148 IN WATER IN PLASTIC CONTAINER, MAGNESIUM CHLORIDE
PLASMA-LYTE 56 AND DEXTROSE 5% IN PLASTIC CONTAINER, DEXTROSE
PLASMA-LYTE 56 IN PLASTIC CONTAINER, MAGNESIUM ACETATE TETRAHYDRATE
PLATINOL, CISPLATIN
PLATINOL-AQ, CISPLATIN
PLEGINE, PHENDIMETRAZINE TARTRATE
PLEGISOL, CALCIUM CHLORIDE
PLENDIL, FELODIPINE
PMB 200, ESTROGENS, CONJUGATED
PMB 400, ESTROGENS, CONJUGATED
POLARAMINE, DEXCHLORPHENIRAMINE MALEATE
POLOCAINE, MEPIVACAINE HYDROCHLORIDE
POLOCAINE W/ LEVONORDEFRIN, LEVONORDEFRIN
POLOCAINE-MPF, MEPIVACAINE HYDROCHLORIDE
POLY-PRED, NEOMYCIN SULFATE
POLY-RX, POLYMYXIN B SULFATE
POLYCILLIN, AMPICILLIN/AMPICILLIN TRIHYDRATE
POLYCILLIN-N, AMPICILLIN SODIUM
POLYCILLIN-PRB, AMPICILLIN/AMPICILLIN TRIHYDRATE
POLYMIXIN B SULFATE, POLYMYXIN B SULFATE
POLYMOX, AMOXICILLIN
POLYSPORIN, BACITRACIN ZINC
POLYTRIM, POLYMYXIN B SULFATE
PONDIMIN, FENFLURAMINE HYDROCHLORIDE
PONSTEL, MEFENAMIC ACID
PORTALAC, LACTULOSE
POTASSIUM ACETATE IN PLASTIC CONTAINER, POTASSIUM ACETATE
POTASSIUM AMINOSALICYLATE, POTASSIUM AMINOSALICYLATE
POTASSIUM CHLORIDE, POTASSIUM CHLORIDE
POTASSIUM CHLORIDE IN PLASTIC CONTAINER, POTASSIUM CHLORIDE
POTASSIUM CHLORIDE 0.037% IN DEXTROSE 10% AND SODIUM CHLORIDE 0.2%, DEXTROSE
POTASSIUM CHLORIDE 0.037% IN DEXTROSE 10% AND SODIUM CHLORIDE 0.45%, DEXTROSE
POTASSIUM CHLORIDE 0.037% IN DEXTROSE 10% AND SODIUM CHLORIDE 0.9%, DEXTROSE
POTASSIUM CHLORIDE 0.037% IN DEXTROSE 5%, DEXTROSE
POTASSIUM CHLORIDE 0.037% IN DEXTROSE 5% AND SODIUM CHLORIDE 0.11%, DEXTROSE
POTASSIUM CHLORIDE 0.037% IN DEXTROSE 5% AND SODIUM CHLORIDE 0.2%, DEXTROSE
POTASSIUM CHLORIDE 0.037% IN DEXTROSE 5% AND SODIUM CHLORIDE 0.33%, DEXTROSE
POTASSIUM CHLORIDE 0.037% IN DEXTROSE 5% AND SODIUM CHLORIDE 0.45%, DEXTROSE
POTASSIUM CHLORIDE 0.037% IN DEXTROSE 5% AND SODIUM CHLORIDE 0.9%, DEXTROSE
POTASSIUM CHLORIDE 0.037% IN SODIUM CHLORIDE 0.9%, POTASSIUM CHLORIDE
POTASSIUM CHLORIDE 0.075% IN DEXTROSE 10% AND SODIUM CHLORIDE 0.2%, DEXTROSE
POTASSIUM CHLORIDE 0.075% IN DEXTROSE 10% AND SODIUM CHLORIDE 0.45%, DEXTROSE
POTASSIUM CHLORIDE 0.075% IN DEXTROSE 10% AND SODIUM CHLORIDE 0.9%, DEXTROSE
POTASSIUM CHLORIDE 0.075% IN DEXTROSE 3.3% AND SODIUM CHLORIDE 0.3%, DEXTROSE
POTASSIUM CHLORIDE 0.075% IN DEXTROSE 5%, DEXTROSE
POTASSIUM CHLORIDE 0.075% IN DEXTROSE 5% AND SODIUM CHLORIDE 0.11%, DEXTROSE
POTASSIUM CHLORIDE 0.075% IN DEXTROSE 5% AND SODIUM CHLORIDE 0.2%, DEXTROSE
POTASSIUM CHLORIDE 0.075% IN DEXTROSE 5% AND SODIUM CHLORIDE 0.33%, DEXTROSE
POTASSIUM CHLORIDE 0.075% IN DEXTROSE 5% AND SODIUM CHLORIDE 0.45%, DEXTROSE
POTASSIUM CHLORIDE 0.075% IN DEXTROSE 5% AND SODIUM CHLORIDE 0.9%, DEXTROSE
POTASSIUM CHLORIDE 0.075% IN SODIUM CHLORIDE 0.9%, POTASSIUM CHLORIDE
POTASSIUM CHLORIDE 0.11% IN DEXTROSE 10% AND SODIUM CHLORIDE 0.2%, DEXTROSE
POTASSIUM CHLORIDE 0.11% IN DEXTROSE 10% AND SODIUM CHLORIDE 0.45%, DEXTROSE
POTASSIUM CHLORIDE 0.11% IN DEXTROSE 10% AND SODIUM CHLORIDE 0.9%, DEXTROSE
POTASSIUM CHLORIDE 0.11% IN DEXTROSE 3.3% AND SODIUM CHLORIDE 0.3%, DEXTROSE
POTASSIUM CHLORIDE 0.11% IN DEXTROSE 5%, DEXTROSE
POTASSIUM CHLORIDE 0.11% IN DEXTROSE 5% AND SODIUM CHLORIDE 0.11%, DEXTROSE
POTASSIUM CHLORIDE 0.11% IN DEXTROSE 5% AND SODIUM CHLORIDE 0.2%, DEXTROSE
POTASSIUM CHLORIDE 0.11% IN DEXTROSE 5% AND SODIUM CHLORIDE 0.33%, DEXTROSE
POTASSIUM CHLORIDE 0.11% IN DEXTROSE 5% AND SODIUM CHLORIDE 0.45%, DEXTROSE
POTASSIUM CHLORIDE 0.11% IN DEXTROSE 5% AND SODIUM CHLORIDE 0.9%, DEXTROSE
POTASSIUM CHLORIDE 0.11% IN SODIUM CHLORIDE 0.9%, POTASSIUM CHLORIDE
POTASSIUM CHLORIDE 0.15% IN DEXTROSE 10% AND SODIUM CHLORIDE 0.2%, DEXTROSE
POTASSIUM CHLORIDE 0.15% IN DEXTROSE 10% AND SODIUM CHLORIDE 0.45%, DEXTROSE
POTASSIUM CHLORIDE 0.15% IN DEXTROSE 10% AND SODIUM CHLORIDE 0.9%, DEXTROSE
POTASSIUM CHLORIDE 0.15% IN DEXTROSE 3.3% AND SODIUM CHLORIDE 0.3%, DEXTROSE
POTASSIUM CHLORIDE 0.15% IN DEXTROSE 5%, DEXTROSE
POTASSIUM CHLORIDE 0.15% IN DEXTROSE 5% AND SODIUM CHLORIDE 0.11%, DEXTROSE
POTASSIUM CHLORIDE 0.15% IN DEXTROSE 5% AND SODIUM CHLORIDE 0.2%, DEXTROSE
POTASSIUM CHLORIDE 0.15% IN DEXTROSE 5% AND SODIUM CHLORIDE 0.33%, DEXTROSE
POTASSIUM CHLORIDE 0.15% IN DEXTROSE 5% AND SODIUM CHLORIDE 0.45%, DEXTROSE

APPENDIX A
PRODUCT NAME INDEX *(continued)*

POTASSIUM CHLORIDE 0.15% IN DEXTROSE 5% AND SODIUM CHLORIDE 0.9%, DEXTROSE
POTASSIUM CHLORIDE 0.15% IN SODIUM CHLORIDE 0.9%, POTASSIUM CHLORIDE
POTASSIUM CHLORIDE 0.22% IN DEXTROSE 10% AND SODIUM CHLORIDE 0.2%, DEXTROSE
POTASSIUM CHLORIDE 0.22% IN DEXTROSE 10% AND SODIUM CHLORIDE 0.45%, DEXTROSE
POTASSIUM CHLORIDE 0.22% IN DEXTROSE 10% AND SODIUM CHLORIDE 0.9%, DEXTROSE
POTASSIUM CHLORIDE 0.22% IN DEXTROSE 3.3% AND SODIUM CHLORIDE 0.3%, DEXTROSE
POTASSIUM CHLORIDE 0.22% IN DEXTROSE 5%, DEXTROSE
POTASSIUM CHLORIDE 0.22% IN DEXTROSE 5% AND SODIUM CHLORIDE 0.11%, DEXTROSE
POTASSIUM CHLORIDE 0.22% IN DEXTROSE 5% AND SODIUM CHLORIDE 0.2%, DEXTROSE
POTASSIUM CHLORIDE 0.22% IN DEXTROSE 5% AND SODIUM CHLORIDE 0.33%, DEXTROSE
POTASSIUM CHLORIDE 0.22% IN DEXTROSE 5% AND SODIUM CHLORIDE 0.45%, DEXTROSE
POTASSIUM CHLORIDE 0.22% IN DEXTROSE 5% AND SODIUM CHLORIDE 0.9%, DEXTROSE
POTASSIUM CHLORIDE 0.22% IN SODIUM CHLORIDE 0.9%, POTASSIUM CHLORIDE
POTASSIUM CHLORIDE 0.3% IN DEXTROSE 10% AND SODIUM CHLORIDE 0.2%, DEXTROSE
POTASSIUM CHLORIDE 0.3% IN DEXTROSE 10% AND SODIUM CHLORIDE 0.45%, DEXTROSE
POTASSIUM CHLORIDE 0.3% IN DEXTROSE 10% AND SODIUM CHLORIDE 0.9%, DEXTROSE
POTASSIUM CHLORIDE 0.3% IN DEXTROSE 3.3% AND SODIUM CHLORIDE 0.3%, DEXTROSE
POTASSIUM CHLORIDE 0.3% IN DEXTROSE 5%, DEXTROSE
POTASSIUM CHLORIDE 0.3% IN DEXTROSE 5% AND SODIUM CHLORIDE 0.11%, DEXTROSE
POTASSIUM CHLORIDE 0.3% IN DEXTROSE 5% AND SODIUM CHLORIDE 0.2%, DEXTROSE
POTASSIUM CHLORIDE 0.3% IN DEXTROSE 5% AND SODIUM CHLORIDE 0.33%, DEXTROSE
POTASSIUM CHLORIDE 0.3% IN DEXTROSE 5% AND SODIUM CHLORIDE 0.45%, DEXTROSE
POTASSIUM CHLORIDE 0.3% IN DEXTROSE 5% AND SODIUM CHLORIDE 0.9%, DEXTROSE
POTASSIUM CHLORIDE 0.3% IN SODIUM CHLORIDE 0.9%, POTASSIUM CHLORIDE
POTASSIUM CHLORIDE 10 MEQ, POTASSIUM CHLORIDE
POTASSIUM CHLORIDE 10 MEQ IN DEXTROSE 5% AND LACTATED RINGER'S, CALCIUM CHLORIDE
POTASSIUM CHLORIDE 10 MEQ IN DEXTROSE 5% AND SODIUM CHLORIDE 0.225%, DEXTROSE
POTASSIUM CHLORIDE 10 MEQ IN DEXTROSE 5% AND SODIUM CHLORIDE 0.3%, DEXTROSE
POTASSIUM CHLORIDE 10 MEQ IN DEXTROSE 5% AND SODIUM CHLORIDE 0.45%, DEXTROSE
POTASSIUM CHLORIDE 10 MEQ IN DEXTROSE 5% AND SODIUM CHLORIDE 0.9%, DEXTROSE
POTASSIUM CHLORIDE 15 MEQ IN DEXTROSE 5% AND LACTATED RINGER'S, CALCIUM CHLORIDE
POTASSIUM CHLORIDE 15 MEQ IN DEXTROSE 5% AND SODIUM CHLORIDE 0.225%, DEXTROSE
POTASSIUM CHLORIDE 15 MEQ IN DEXTROSE 5% AND SODIUM CHLORIDE 0.3%, DEXTROSE
POTASSIUM CHLORIDE 15 MEQ IN DEXTROSE 5% AND SODIUM CHLORIDE 0.45%, DEXTROSE
POTASSIUM CHLORIDE 15 MEQ IN DEXTROSE 5% AND SODIUM CHLORIDE 0.9%, DEXTROSE
POTASSIUM CHLORIDE 20 MEQ, POTASSIUM CHLORIDE
POTASSIUM CHLORIDE 20 MEQ IN DEXTROSE 5%, DEXTROSE
POTASSIUM CHLORIDE 20 MEQ IN DEXTROSE 5% AND LACTATED RINGER'S, CALCIUM CHLORIDE
POTASSIUM CHLORIDE 20 MEQ IN DEXTROSE 5% AND SODIUM CHLORIDE 0.225%, DEXTROSE
POTASSIUM CHLORIDE 20 MEQ IN DEXTROSE 5% AND SODIUM CHLORIDE 0.3%, DEXTROSE
POTASSIUM CHLORIDE 20 MEQ IN DEXTROSE 5% AND SODIUM CHLORIDE 0.45%, DEXTROSE
POTASSIUM CHLORIDE 20 MEQ IN DEXTROSE 5% AND SODIUM CHLORIDE 0.9%, DEXTROSE
POTASSIUM CHLORIDE 20 MEQ IN DEXTROSE 5% IN SODIUM CHLORIDE 0.3%, DEXTROSE
POTASSIUM CHLORIDE 20 MEQ IN SODIUM CHLORIDE 0.9%, POTASSIUM CHLORIDE
POTASSIUM CHLORIDE 30 MEQ, POTASSIUM CHLORIDE
POTASSIUM CHLORIDE 30 MEQ IN DEXTROSE 5%, DEXTROSE
POTASSIUM CHLORIDE 30 MEQ IN DEXTROSE 5% AND LACTATED RINGER'S, CALCIUM CHLORIDE
POTASSIUM CHLORIDE 30 MEQ IN DEXTROSE 5% AND SODIUM CHLORIDE 0.225%, DEXTROSE
POTASSIUM CHLORIDE 30 MEQ IN DEXTROSE 5% AND SODIUM CHLORIDE 0.3%, DEXTROSE
POTASSIUM CHLORIDE 30 MEQ IN DEXTROSE 5% AND SODIUM CHLORIDE 0.45%, DEXTROSE
POTASSIUM CHLORIDE 30 MEQ IN DEXTROSE 5% AND SODIUM CHLORIDE 0.9%, DEXTROSE
POTASSIUM CHLORIDE 40 MEQ, POTASSIUM CHLORIDE
POTASSIUM CHLORIDE 40 MEQ IN DEXTROSE 5%, DEXTROSE
POTASSIUM CHLORIDE 40 MEQ IN DEXTROSE 5% AND LACTATED RINGER'S, CALCIUM CHLORIDE
POTASSIUM CHLORIDE 40 MEQ IN DEXTROSE 5% AND SODIUM CHLORIDE 0.225%, DEXTROSE
POTASSIUM CHLORIDE 40 MEQ IN DEXTROSE 5% AND SODIUM CHLORIDE 0.3%, DEXTROSE
POTASSIUM CHLORIDE 40 MEQ IN DEXTROSE 5% AND SODIUM CHLORIDE 0.45%, DEXTROSE
POTASSIUM CHLORIDE 40 MEQ IN DEXTROSE 5% AND SODIUM CHLORIDE 0.9%, DEXTROSE
POTASSIUM CHLORIDE 40 MEQ IN SODIUM CHLORIDE 0.9%, POTASSIUM CHLORIDE
POTASSIUM CHLORIDE 5 MEQ IN DEXTROSE 5% AND LACTATED RINGER'S, CALCIUM CHLORIDE
POTASSIUM CHLORIDE 5 MEQ IN DEXTROSE 5% AND SODIUM CHLORIDE 0.225%, DEXTROSE
POTASSIUM CHLORIDE 5 MEQ IN DEXTROSE 5% AND SODIUM CHLORIDE 0.3%, DEXTROSE
POTASSIUM CHLORIDE 5 MEQ IN DEXTROSE 5% AND SODIUM CHLORIDE 0.45%, DEXTROSE
POTASSIUM CHLORIDE 5 MEQ IN DEXTROSE 5% AND SODIUM CHLORIDE 0.9%, DEXTROSE
POTASSIUM CITRATE, POTASSIUM CITRATE
POTASSIUM IODIDE, POTASSIUM IODIDE (OTC)
POVAN, PYRVINIUM PAMOATE
POVIDONE IODINE, POVIDONE-IODINE (OTC)
PRALIDOXIME CHLORIDE, PRALIDOXIME CHLORIDE
PRAMINE, IMIPRAMINE HYDROCHLORIDE
PRAMOSONE, HYDROCORTISONE ACETATE
PRANTAL, DIPHEMANIL METHYLSULFATE
PRAVACHOL, PRAVASTATIN SODIUM
PRAZEPAM, PRAZEPAM
PRAZOSIN HCL, PRAZOSIN HYDROCHLORIDE
PRE-OP, HEXACHLOROPHENE
PRE-OP II, HEXACHLOROPHENE
PRE-PEN, BENZYL PENICILLOYL-POLYLYSINE
PRE-SATE, CHLORPHENTERMINE HYDROCHLORIDE
PRECEF, CEFORANIDE
PRED FORTE, PREDNISOLONE ACETATE
PRED MILD, PREDNISOLONE ACETATE
PRED-G, GENTAMICIN SULFATE
PREDAIR, PREDNISOLONE SODIUM PHOSPHATE

APPENDIX A
PRODUCT NAME INDEX *(continued)*

PREDAIR FORTE, PREDNISOLONE SODIUM PHOSPHATE
PREDAMIDE, PREDNISOLONE ACETATE
PREDNICEN-M, PREDNISONE
PREDNISOLONE, PREDNISOLONE
PREDNISOLONE ACETATE, PREDNISOLONE ACETATE
PREDNISOLONE SODIUM PHOSPHATE, PREDNISOLONE SODIUM PHOSPHATE
PREDNISOLONE TEBUTATE, PREDNISOLONE TEBUTATE
PREDNISONE, PREDNISONE
PREDNISONE INTENSOL, PREDNISONE
PREDSULFAIR, PREDNISOLONE ACETATE
PREDSULFAIR II, PREDNISOLONE ACETATE
PREFRIN-A, PHENYLEPHRINE HYDROCHLORIDE
PREGNYL, GONADOTROPIN, CHORIONIC
PRELONE, PREDNISOLONE
PRELUDIN, PHENMETRAZINE HYDROCHLORIDE
PREMARIN, ESTROGENS, CONJUGATED
PREPIDIL, DINOPROSTONE
PRESAMINE, IMIPRAMINE HYDROCHLORIDE
PRILOSEC, OMEPRAZOLE
PRIMACOR, MILRINONE LACTATE
PRIMACOR IN DEXTROSE 5%, MILRINONE LACTATE
PRIMAQUINE, PRIMAQUINE PHOSPHATE
PRIMATENE MIST, EPINEPHRINE (OTC)
PRIMAXIN, CILASTATIN SODIUM
PRIMIDONE, PRIMIDONE
PRINCIPEN, AMPICILLIN SODIUM
PRINCIPEN, AMPICILLIN/AMPICILLIN TRIHYDRATE
PRINCIPEN '125', AMPICILLIN/AMPICILLIN TRIHYDRATE
PRINCIPEN '250', AMPICILLIN/AMPICILLIN TRIHYDRATE
PRINCIPEN '500', AMPICILLIN/AMPICILLIN TRIHYDRATE
PRINCIPEN W/ PROBENECID, AMPICILLIN/AMPICILLIN TRIHYDRATE
PRINIVIL, LISINOPRIL
PRINZIDE 10-12.5, HYDROCHLOROTHIAZIDE
PRINZIDE 20-12.5, HYDROCHLOROTHIAZIDE
PRINZIDE 20-25, HYDROCHLOROTHIAZIDE
PRISCOLINE, TOLAZOLINE HYDROCHLORIDE
PRO-BANTHINE, PROPANTHELINE BROMIDE
PROBALAN, PROBENECID
PROBAMPACIN, AMPICILLIN/AMPICILLIN TRIHYDRATE
PROBEN-C, COLCHICINE
PROBENECID, PROBENECID
PROBENECID AND COLCHICINE, COLCHICINE
PROBENECID W/ COLCHICINE, COLCHICINE
PROCAINAMIDE HCL, PROCAINAMIDE HYDROCHLORIDE
PROCAINE HCL, PROCAINE HYDROCHLORIDE
PROCAINE HCL W/ EPINEPHRINE, EPINEPHRINE
PROCALAMINE, AMINO ACIDS
PROCAN, PROCAINAMIDE HYDROCHLORIDE
PROCAN SR, PROCAINAMIDE HYDROCHLORIDE
PROCAPAN, PROCAINAMIDE HYDROCHLORIDE
PROCARDIA, NIFEDIPINE
PROCARDIA XL, NIFEDIPINE
PROCHLORPERAZINE, PROCHLORPERAZINE
PROCHLORPERAZINE, PROCHLORPERAZINE EDISYLATE
PROCHLORPERAZINE, PROCHLORPERAZINE MALEATE
PROCHLORPERAZINE EDISYLATE, PROCHLORPERAZINE EDISYLATE
PROCHLORPERAZINE MALEATE, PROCHLORPERAZINE MALEATE
PROCTOCORT, HYDROCORTISONE
PROCTOFOAM HC, HYDROCORTISONE ACETATE
PROFEN, IBUPROFEN (OTC)
PROFENAL, SUPROFEN
PROFERDEX, IRON DEXTRAN
PROGESTASERT, PROGESTERONE
PROGESTERONE, PROGESTERONE
PROGLYCEM, DIAZOXIDE
PROGRAF, TACROLIMUS
PROHANCE, GADOTERIDOL
PROKETAZINE, CARPHENAZINE MALEATE
PROKLAR, SULFAMETHIZOLE
PROLIXIN, FLUPHENAZINE HYDROCHLORIDE
PROLIXIN DECANOATE, FLUPHENAZINE DECANOATE
PROLIXIN ENANTHATE, FLUPHENAZINE ENANTHATE
PROLOID, THYROGLOBULIN
PROLOPRIM, TRIMETHOPRIM
PROMAPAR, CHLORPROMAZINE HYDROCHLORIDE
PROMAZINE HCL, PROMAZINE HYDROCHLORIDE
PROMETA, METAPROTERENOL SULFATE
PROMETH, PROMETHAZINE HYDROCHLORIDE
PROMETH VC PLAIN, PHENYLEPHRINE HYDROCHLORIDE
PROMETH VC W/ CODEINE, CODEINE PHOSPHATE
PROMETH W/ CODEINE, CODEINE PHOSPHATE
PROMETH W/ DEXTROMETHORPHAN, DEXTROMETHORPHAN HYDROBROMIDE
PROMETHACON, PROMETHAZINE HYDROCHLORIDE
PROMETHAZINE, PROMETHAZINE HYDROCHLORIDE
PROMETHAZINE HCL, PROMETHAZINE HYDROCHLORIDE
PROMETHAZINE HCL AND CODEINE PHOSPHATE, CODEINE PHOSPHATE
PROMETHAZINE PLAIN, PROMETHAZINE HYDROCHLORIDE
PROMETHAZINE VC PLAIN, PHENYLEPHRINE HYDROCHLORIDE
PROMETHAZINE VC W/ CODEINE, CODEINE PHOSPHATE
PROMETHAZINE W/ CODEINE, CODEINE PHOSPHATE
PROMETHAZINE W/ DEXTROMETHORPHAN, DEXTROMETHORPHAN HYDROBROMIDE
PROMETHEGAN, PROMETHAZINE HYDROCHLORIDE
PROMPT PHENYTOIN SODIUM, PHENYTOIN SODIUM, PROMPT
PRONESTYL, PROCAINAMIDE HYDROCHLORIDE
PRONESTYL-SR, PROCAINAMIDE HYDROCHLORIDE
PROPACET 100, ACETAMINOPHEN
PROPANTHELINE BROMIDE, PROPANTHELINE BROMIDE
PROPARACAINE HCL, PROPARACAINE HYDROCHLORIDE
PROPHENE 65, PROPOXYPHENE HYDROCHLORIDE
PROPINE, DIPIVEFRIN HYDROCHLORIDE
PROPOXYPHENE COMPOUND 65, ASPIRIN
PROPOXYPHENE COMPOUND-65, ASPIRIN
PROPOXYPHENE HCL, PROPOXYPHENE HYDROCHLORIDE
PROPOXYPHENE HCL AND ACETAMINOPHEN, ACETAMINOPHEN
PROPOXYPHENE HCL W/ ASPIRIN AND CAFFEINE, ASPIRIN
PROPOXYPHENE HCL 65, PROPOXYPHENE HYDROCHLORIDE
PROPOXYPHENE NAPSYLATE AND ACETAMINOPHEN, ACETAMINOPHEN
PROPRANOLOL HCL, PROPRANOLOL HYDROCHLORIDE
PROPRANOLOL HCL & HYDROCHLOROTHIAZIDE, HYDROCHLOROTHIAZIDE
PROPRANOLOL HCL AND HYDROCHLOROTHIAZIDE, HYDROCHLOROTHIAZIDE
PROPRANOLOL HCL INTENSOL, PROPRANOLOL HYDROCHLORIDE
PROPULSID, CISAPRIDE MONOHYDRATE
PROPYLTHIOURACIL, PROPYLTHIOURACIL
PROSCAR, FINASTERIDE
PROSOM, ESTAZOLAM
PROSTAPHLIN, OXACILLIN SODIUM
PROSTEP, NICOTINE
PROSTIN E2, DINOPROSTONE
PROSTIN F2 ALPHA, DINOPROST TROMETHAMINE
PROSTIN VR PEDIATRIC, ALPROSTADIL
PROTAMINE SULFATE, PROTAMINE SULFATE
PROTAMINE ZINC AND ILETIN II, INSULIN SUSP PROTAMINE ZINC PURIFIED BEEF (OTC)
PROTAMINE ZINC AND ILETIN II (PORK), INSULIN SUSP PROTAMINE ZINC PURIFIED PORK (OTC)

APPENDIX A
PRODUCT NAME INDEX *(continued)*

PROTAMINE ZINC INSULIN, INSULIN SUSP PROTAMINE ZINC PURIFIED BEEF (OTC)
PROTAMINE, ZINC & ILETIN I (BEEF-PORK), INSULIN SUSP PROTAMINE ZINC BEEF/PORK (OTC)
PROTOPAM CHLORIDE, PRALIDOXIME CHLORIDE
PROTOSTAT, METRONIDAZOLE
PROTROPIN, SOMATREM
PROVAL #3, ACETAMINOPHEN
PROVENTIL, ALBUTEROL
PROVENTIL, ALBUTEROL SULFATE
PROVERA, MEDROXYPROGESTERONE ACETATE
PROVOCHOLINE, METHACHOLINE CHLORIDE
PROZAC, FLUOXETINE HYDROCHLORIDE
PSEUDO-12, PSEUDOEPHEDRINE POLISTIREX (OTC)
PSEUDOEPHEDRINE HCL AND CHLORPHENIRAMINE MALEATE, CHLORPHENIRAMINE MALEATE (OTC)
PSEUDOEPHEDRINE HCL AND TRIPROLIDINE HCL, PSEUDOEPHEDRINE HYDROCHLORIDE
PSEUDOEPHEDRINE HCL/CHLORPHENIRAMINE MALEATE, CHLORPHENIRAMINE MALEATE (OTC)
PSEUDOEPHEDRINE HYDROCHLORIDE AND CHLORPHENIRAMINE MALEATE, CHLORPHENIRAMINE MALEATE (OTC)
PSORCON, DIFLORASONE DIACETATE
PULMOLITE, TECHNETIUM TC-99M ALBUMIN AGGREGATED KIT
PURIFIED CORTROPHIN GEL, CORTICOTROPIN
PURINETHOL, MERCAPTOPURINE
PYOCIDIN, HYDROCORTISONE
PYOPEN, CARBENICILLIN DISODIUM
PYRAZINAMIDE, PYRAZINAMIDE
PYRIDAMAL 100, CHLORPHENIRAMINE MALEATE
PYRIDOSTIGMINE BROMIDE, PYRIDOSTIGMINE BROMIDE
PYRIDOXINE HCL, PYRIDOXINE HYDROCHLORIDE
PYRILAMINE MALEATE, PYRILAMINE MALEATE
PYROLITE, TECHNETIUM TC-99M PYRO/TRIMETA PHOSPHATES KIT

Q

Q-GESIC, ASPIRIN
Q-PAM, DIAZEPAM
QUARZAN, CLIDINIUM BROMIDE
QUELICIN, SUCCINYLCHOLINE CHLORIDE
QUESTRAN, CHOLESTYRAMINE
QUESTRAN LIGHT, CHOLESTYRAMINE
QUIBRON-T, THEOPHYLLINE
QUIBRON-T/SR, THEOPHYLLINE
QUIDE, PIPERACETAZINE
QUINACT, QUINIDINE GLUCONATE
QUINAGLUTE, QUINIDINE GLUCONATE
QUINALAN, QUINIDINE GLUCONATE
QUINATIME, QUINIDINE GLUCONATE
QUINIDEX, QUINIDINE SULFATE
QUINIDINE GLUCONATE, QUINIDINE GLUCONATE
QUINIDINE SULFATE, QUINIDINE SULFATE
QUINORA, QUINIDINE SULFATE

R

R-GENE 10, ARGININE HYDROCHLORIDE
R-P MYCIN, ERYTHROMYCIN
RADIO-IODINATED (I 125) SERUM ALBUMIN (HUMAN), ALBUMIN IODINATED I-125 SERUM
RADIOIODINATED SERUM ALBUMIN (HUMAN) IHSA I 125, ALBUMIN IODINATED I-125 SERUM
RADIONUCLIDE-LABELED (125 I) FIBRINOGEN (HUMAN) SENSOR, FIBRINOGEN, I-125
RAU-SED, RESERPINE
RAUDIXIN, RAUWOLFIA SERPENTINA
RAUSERPIN, RAUWOLFIA SERPENTINA
RAUTENSIN, ALSEROXYLON
RAUVAL, RAUWOLFIA SERPENTINA
RAUWILOID, ALSEROXYLON
RAUWOLFIA SERPENTINA, RAUWOLFIA SERPENTINA
RAVOCAINE AND NOVOCAIN W/ LEVOPHED, NOREPINEPHRINE BITARTRATE
RAVOCAINE AND NOVOCAIN W/ NEO-COBEFRIN, LEVONORDEFRIN
RBC-SCAN, TECHNETIUM TC-99M RED BLOOD CELL KIT
REDISOL, CYANOCOBALAMIN
REGITINE, PHENTOLAMINE MESYLATE
REGLAN, METOCLOPRAMIDE HYDROCHLORIDE
REGONOL, PYRIDOSTIGMINE BROMIDE
REGROTON, CHLORTHALIDONE
REGULAR ILETIN II, INSULIN PURIFIED BEEF (OTC)
REGULAR ILETIN II (PORK), INSULIN PURIFIED PORK (OTC)
REGULAR PURIFIED PORK INSULIN, INSULIN PURIFIED PORK (OTC)
RELA, CARISOPRODOL
RELAFEN, NABUMETONE
REMSED, PROMETHAZINE HYDROCHLORIDE
RENACIDIN, CITRIC ACID
RENAMIN W/O ELECTROLYTES, AMINO ACIDS
RENESE, POLYTHIAZIDE
RENESE-R, POLYTHIAZIDE
RENO-M-DIP, DIATRIZOATE MEGLUMINE
RENO-M-30, DIATRIZOATE MEGLUMINE
RENO-M-60, DIATRIZOATE MEGLUMINE
RENOCAL-76, DIATRIZOATE MEGLUMINE
RENOGRAFIN-60, DIATRIZOATE MEGLUMINE
RENOGRAFIN-76, DIATRIZOATE MEGLUMINE
RENOQUID, SULFACYTINE
RENOTEC, TECHNETIUM TC-99M FERPENTETATE KIT
RENOVIST, DIATRIZOATE MEGLUMINE
RENOVIST II, DIATRIZOATE MEGLUMINE
RENOVUE-DIP, IODAMIDE MEGLUMINE
RENOVUE-65, IODAMIDE MEGLUMINE
REPAN, ACETAMINOPHEN
RESECTISOL, MANNITOL
RESERPINE, RESERPINE
RESERPINE AND HYDROCHLOROTHIAZIDE, HYDROCHLOROTHIAZIDE
RESERPINE AND HYDROCHLOROTHIAZIDE-50, HYDROCHLOROTHIAZIDE
RESERPINE AND HYDROFLUMETHIAZIDE, HYDROFLUMETHIAZIDE
RESERPINE, HYDRALAZINE HCL AND HYDROCHLOROTHIAZIDE, HYDRALAZINE HYDROCHLORIDE
RESERPINE, HYDROCHLOROTHIAZIDE, AND HYDRALAZINE HCL, HYDRALAZINE HYDROCHLORIDE
RESPORAL, DEXBROMPHENIRAMINE MALEATE (OTC)
RESTORIL, TEMAZEPAM
RETET, TETRACYCLINE HYDROCHLORIDE
RETIN-A, TRETINOIN
RETROVIR, ZIDOVUDINE
REV-EYES, DAPIPRAZOLE HYDROCHLORIDE
REVERSOL, EDROPHONIUM CHLORIDE
REZIPAS, AMINOSALICYLIC ACID RESIN COMPLEX
RHINOCORT, BUDESONIDE
RIDAURA, AURANOFIN
RIFADIN, RIFAMPIN
RIFAMATE, ISONIAZID
RIFATER, ISONIAZID
RIMACTANE, RIFAMPIN

APPENDIX A
PRODUCT NAME INDEX *(continued)*

RIMADYL, CARPROFEN
RIMIFON, ISONIAZID
RIMSO-50, DIMETHYL SULFOXIDE
RINGER'S, CALCIUM CHLORIDE
RINGER'S IN PLASTIC CONTAINER, CALCIUM CHLORIDE
RISPERDAL, RISPERIDONE
RITALIN, METHYLPHENIDATE HYDROCHLORIDE
RITALIN-SR, METHYLPHENIDATE HYDROCHLORIDE
RITODRINE HCL, RITODRINE HYDROCHLORIDE
RITODRINE HCL IN DEXTROSE 5% IN PLASTIC CONTAINER, RITODRINE HYDROCHLORIDE
ROBAXIN, METHOCARBAMOL
ROBAXIN-750, METHOCARBAMOL
ROBAXISAL, ASPIRIN
ROBENGATOPE, ROSE BENGAL SODIUM, I-131
ROBIMYCIN, ERYTHROMYCIN
ROBINUL, GLYCOPYRROLATE
ROBINUL FORTE, GLYCOPYRROLATE
ROBITET, TETRACYCLINE HYDROCHLORIDE
ROCALTROL, CALCITRIOL
ROCEPHIN, CEFTRIAXONE SODIUM
ROCEPHIN W/ DEXTROSE, CEFTRIAXONE SODIUM
ROGAINE, MINOXIDIL
ROMAZICON, FLUMAZENIL
RONDOMYCIN, METHACYCLINE HYDROCHLORIDE
ROWASA, MESALAMINE
ROXICET, ACETAMINOPHEN
ROXICET 5/500, ACETAMINOPHEN
ROXIPRIN, ASPIRIN
RUBEX, DOXORUBICIN HYDROCHLORIDE
RUBIVITE, CYANOCOBALAMIN
RUBRAMIN PC, CYANOCOBALAMIN
RUBRATOPE-57, CYANOCOBALAMIN, CO-57
RUBRATOPE-57 KIT, COBALT CHLORIDE, CO-57
RUBRATOPE-60, CYANOCOBALAMIN, CO-60
RUBRATOPE-60 KIT, COBALT CHLORIDE, CO-60
RUFEN, IBUPROFEN
RUVITE, CYANOCOBALAMIN
RYTHMOL, PROPAFENONE HYDROCHLORIDE

S

S.A.S.-500, SULFASALAZINE
SALAGEN, PILOCARPINE HYDROCHLORIDE
SALPIX, ACETRIZOATE SODIUM
SALURON, HYDROFLUMETHIAZIDE
SALUTENSIN, HYDROFLUMETHIAZIDE
SALUTENSIN-DEMI, HYDROFLUMETHIAZIDE
SANDIMMUNE, CYCLOSPORINE
SANDOSTATIN, OCTREOTIDE ACETATE
SANDRIL, RESERPINE
SANOREX, MAZINDOL
SANSAC, ERYTHROMYCIN
SANSERT, METHYSERGIDE MALEATE
SARENIN, SARALASIN ACETATE
SARISOL, BUTABARBITAL SODIUM
SARISOL NO. 1, BUTABARBITAL SODIUM
SARISOL NO. 2, BUTABARBITAL SODIUM
SATRIC, METRONIDAZOLE
SCABENE, LINDANE
SCANDONEST L, LEVONORDEFRIN
SCANDONEST PLAIN, MEPIVACAINE HYDROCHLORIDE
SCRUBTEAM SURGICAL SPONGEBRUSH, HEXACHLOROPHENE
SECOBARBITAL SODIUM, SECOBARBITAL SODIUM
SECONAL SODIUM, SECOBARBITAL SODIUM
SECRETIN-FERRING, SECRETIN
SECTRAL, ACEBUTOLOL HYDROCHLORIDE
SEDAPAP, ACETAMINOPHEN
SEFFIN, CEPHALOTHIN SODIUM
SELDANE, TERFENADINE
SELDANE-D, PSEUDOEPHEDRINE HYDROCHLORIDE
SELENIUM SULFIDE, SELENIUM SULFIDE
SELENOMETHIONINE SE 75, SELENOMETHIONINE, SE-75
SELSUN, SELENIUM SULFIDE
SEMILENTE, INSULIN ZINC SUSP PROMPT PURIFIED PORK (OTC)
SEMILENTE INSULIN, INSULIN ZINC SUSP PROMPT BEEF (OTC)
SEMPREX-D, ACRIVASTINE
SENSORCAINE, BUPIVACAINE HYDROCHLORIDE
SEPTI-SOFT, HEXACHLOROPHENE
SEPTISOL, HEXACHLOROPHENE
SEPTRA, SULFAMETHOXAZOLE
SEPTRA DS, SULFAMETHOXAZOLE
SEPTRA GRAPE, SULFAMETHOXAZOLE
SER-A-GEN, HYDRALAZINE HYDROCHLORIDE
SER-AP-ES, HYDRALAZINE HYDROCHLORIDE
SERAX, OXAZEPAM
SERENTIL, MESORIDAZINE BESYLATE
SEREVENT, SALMETEROL XINAFOATE
SEROMYCIN, CYCLOSERINE
SEROPHENE, CLOMIPHENE CITRATE
SERPALAN, RESERPINE
SERPANRAY, RESERPINE
SERPASIL, RESERPINE
SERPASIL-APRESOLINE, HYDRALAZINE HYDROCHLORIDE
SERPASIL-ESIDRIX #1, HYDROCHLOROTHIAZIDE
SERPASIL-ESIDRIX #2, HYDROCHLOROTHIAZIDE
SERPATE, RESERPINE
SERPIVITE, RESERPINE
SERVISONE, PREDNISONE
SETHOTOPE, SELENOMETHIONINE, SE-75
SHADE UVAGUARD, AVOBENZONE (OTC)
SILDIMAC, SILVER SULFADIAZINE
SILPHEN, DIPHENHYDRAMINE HYDROCHLORIDE (OTC)
SILVADENE, SILVER SULFADIAZINE
SINE-AID IB, IBUPROFEN (OTC)
SINEMET, CARBIDOPA
SINEMET CR, CARBIDOPA
SINEQUAN, DOXEPIN HYDROCHLORIDE
SINOGRAFIN, DIATRIZOATE MEGLUMINE
SKELAXIN, METAXALONE
SLO-BID, THEOPHYLLINE
SLO-PHYLLIN, THEOPHYLLINE
SLOW-K, POTASSIUM CHLORIDE
SMZ-TMP, SULFAMETHOXAZOLE
SMZ-TMP PEDIATRIC, SULFAMETHOXAZOLE
SODIUM ACETATE IN PLASTIC CONTAINER, SODIUM ACETATE, ANHYDROUS
SODIUM AMINOSALICYLATE, AMINOSALICYLATE SODIUM
SODIUM BICARBONATE IN PLASTIC CONTAINER, SODIUM BICARBONATE
SODIUM BUTABARBITAL, BUTABARBITAL SODIUM
SODIUM CHLORIDE, SODIUM CHLORIDE
SODIUM CHLORIDE IN PLASTIC CONTAINER, SODIUM CHLORIDE
SODIUM CHLORIDE 0.45%, SODIUM CHLORIDE
SODIUM CHLORIDE 0.45% IN PLASTIC CONTAINER, SODIUM CHLORIDE
SODIUM CHLORIDE 0.9%, SODIUM CHLORIDE
SODIUM CHLORIDE 0.9% AND POTASSIUM CHLORIDE 0.075%, POTASSIUM CHLORIDE
SODIUM CHLORIDE 0.9% AND POTASSIUM CHLORIDE 0.15%, POTASSIUM CHLORIDE
SODIUM CHLORIDE 0.9% AND POTASSIUM CHLORIDE 0.22%, POTASSIUM CHLORIDE
SODIUM CHLORIDE 0.9% AND POTASSIUM CHLORIDE 0.224%, POTASSIUM CHLORIDE
SODIUM CHLORIDE 0.9% AND POTASSIUM CHLORIDE 0.3%, POTASSIUM CHLORIDE

APPENDIX A
PRODUCT NAME INDEX (continued)

SODIUM CHLORIDE 0.9% IN PLASTIC CONTAINER, SODIUM CHLORIDE
SODIUM CHLORIDE 0.9% IN STERILE PLASTIC CONTAINER, SODIUM CHLORIDE
SODIUM CHLORIDE 23.4%, SODIUM CHLORIDE
SODIUM CHLORIDE 3%, SODIUM CHLORIDE
SODIUM CHLORIDE 3% IN PLASTIC CONTAINER, SODIUM CHLORIDE
SODIUM CHLORIDE 5%, SODIUM CHLORIDE
SODIUM CHLORIDE 5% IN PLASTIC CONTAINER, SODIUM CHLORIDE
SODIUM CHROMATE CR 51, SODIUM CHROMATE, CR-51
SODIUM HEPARIN, HEPARIN SODIUM
SODIUM IODIDE I 123, SODIUM IODIDE, I-123
SODIUM IODIDE I 131, SODIUM IODIDE, I-131
SODIUM LACTATE IN PLASTIC CONTAINER, SODIUM LACTATE
SODIUM LACTATE 0.167 MOLAR IN PLASTIC CONTAINER, SODIUM LACTATE
SODIUM LACTATE 1/6 MOLAR, SODIUM LACTATE
SODIUM NITROPRUSSIDE, SODIUM NITROPRUSSIDE
SODIUM P.A.S., AMINOSALICYLATE SODIUM
SODIUM PENTOBARBITAL, PENTOBARBITAL SODIUM
SODIUM PERTECHNETATE TC 99M, TECHNETIUM TC-99M SODIUM PERTECHNETATE
SODIUM PHOSPHATE P 32, SODIUM PHOSPHATE, P-32
SODIUM PHOSPHATES IN PLASTIC CONTAINER, SODIUM PHOSPHATE, DIBASIC
SODIUM POLYPHOSPHATE-TIN KIT, TECHNETIUM TC-99M POLYPHOSPHATE KIT
SODIUM POLYSTYRENE SULFONATE, SODIUM POLYSTYRENE SULFONATE
SODIUM ROSE BENGAL I 131, ROSE BENGAL SODIUM, I-131
SODIUM SECOBARBITAL, SECOBARBITAL SODIUM
SODIUM SUCCINATE, SODIUM SUCCINATE
SODIUM SULAMYD, SULFACETAMIDE SODIUM
SODIUM SULFACETAMIDE, SULFACETAMIDE SODIUM
SODIUM THIOSULFATE, SODIUM THIOSULFATE
SODIUM VERSENATE, EDETATE DISODIUM
SOLATENE, BETA-CAROTENE
SOLU-CORTEF, HYDROCORTISONE SODIUM SUCCINATE
SOLU-MEDROL, METHYLPREDNISOLONE SODIUM SUCCINATE
SOMA, CARISOPRODOL
SOMA COMPOUND, ASPIRIN
SOMA COMPOUND W/ CODEINE, ASPIRIN
SOMOPHYLLIN, AMINOPHYLLINE
SOMOPHYLLIN-CRT, THEOPHYLLINE
SOMOPHYLLIN-DF, AMINOPHYLLINE
SOMOPHYLLIN-T, THEOPHYLLINE
SONAZINE, CHLORPROMAZINE HYDROCHLORIDE
SORBITOL 3.3% IN PLASTIC CONTAINER, SORBITOL
SORBITOL 3% IN PLASTIC CONTAINER, SORBITOL
SORBITOL-MANNITOL, MANNITOL
SORBITOL-MANNITOL IN PLASTIC CONTAINER, MANNITOL
SORBITRATE, ISOSORBIDE DINITRATE
SOSOL, SULFISOXAZOLE
SOTRADECOL, SODIUM TETRADECYL SULFATE
SOXAZOLE, SULFISOXAZOLE
SOY-DOME, HEXACHLOROPHENE
SOYACAL 10%, SOYBEAN OIL
SOYACAL 20%, SOYBEAN OIL
SPARINE, PROMAZINE HYDROCHLORIDE
SPECTAMINE, IOFETAMINE HYDROCHLORIDE I-123
SPECTAZOLE, ECONAZOLE NITRATE
SPECTROBID, BACAMPICILLIN HYDROCHLORIDE
SPIRONOLACTONE, SPIRONOLACTONE
SPIRONOLACTONE + HYDROCHLOROTHIAZIDE, HYDROCHLOROTHIAZIDE
SPIRONOLACTONE AND HYDROCHLOROTHIAZIDE, HYDROCHLOROTHIAZIDE
SPIRONOLACTONE W/ HYDROCHLOROTHIAZIDE, HYDROCHLOROTHIAZIDE
SPIRONOLACTONE/HYDROCHLOROTHIAZIDE, HYDROCHLOROTHIAZIDE
SPORANOX, ITRACONAZOLE
SPRX-105, PHENDIMETRAZINE TARTRATE
SPRX-3, PHENDIMETRAZINE TARTRATE
SPS, SODIUM POLYSTYRENE SULFONATE
SSD, SILVER SULFADIAZINE
STADOL, BUTORPHANOL TARTRATE
STANOZIDE, ISONIAZID
STAPHCILLIN, METHICILLIN SODIUM
STATICIN, ERYTHROMYCIN
STATOBEX, PHENDIMETRAZINE TARTRATE
STATOBEX-G, PHENDIMETRAZINE TARTRATE
STATROL, NEOMYCIN SULFATE
STELAZINE, TRIFLUOPERAZINE HYDROCHLORIDE
STERANE, PREDNISOLONE
STERANE, PREDNISOLONE ACETATE
STERI-STAT, CHLORHEXIDINE GLUCONATE (OTC)
STERILE UREA, UREA
STERILE WATER, WATER FOR IRRIGATION, STERILE
STERILE WATER FOR INJECTION, WATER FOR INJECTION, STERILE
STERILE WATER FOR INJECTION IN PLASTIC CONTAINER, WATER FOR INJECTION, STERILE
STERILE WATER IN PLASTIC CONTAINER, WATER FOR IRRIGATION, STERILE
STIE-CORT, HYDROCORTISONE
STILBESTROL, DIETHYLSTILBESTROL
STILBETIN, DIETHYLSTILBESTROL
STILPHOSTROL, DIETHYLSTILBESTROL DIPHOSPHATE
STOXIL, IDOXURIDINE
STREPTOMYCIN SULFATE, STREPTOMYCIN SULFATE
STRIFON FORTE DSC, CHLORZOXAZONE
SUBLIMAZE, FENTANYL CITRATE
SUCCINYLCHOLINE CHLORIDE, SUCCINYLCHOLINE CHLORIDE
SUCOSTRIN, SUCCINYLCHOLINE CHLORIDE
SUDAFED 12 HOUR, PSEUDOEPHEDRINE HYDROCHLORIDE (OTC)
SUFENTA, SUFENTANIL CITRATE
SULF-10, SULFACETAMIDE SODIUM
SULFA-TRIPLE #2, TRISULFAPYRIMIDINES (SULFADIAZINE;SULFAMERAZINE;SULFAMETHAZINE)
SULFABID, SULFAPHENAZOLE
SULFACEL-15, SULFACETAMIDE SODIUM
SULFACETAMIDE SODIUM, SULFACETAMIDE SODIUM
SULFACETAMIDE SODIUM AND PREDNISOLONE SODIUM PHOSPHATE, PREDNISOLONE SODIUM PHOSPHATE
SULFADIAZINE, SULFADIAZINE
SULFADIAZINE SODIUM, SULFADIAZINE SODIUM
SULFAIR FORTE, SULFACETAMIDE SODIUM
SULFAIR 10, SULFACETAMIDE SODIUM
SULFAIR-15, SULFACETAMIDE SODIUM
SULFALAR, SULFISOXAZOLE
SULFALOID, TRISULFAPYRIMIDINES (SULFADIAZINE;SULFAMERAZINE;SULFAMETHAZINE)
SULFAMETHOPRIM, SULFAMETHOXAZOLE
SULFAMETHOPRIM-DS, SULFAMETHOXAZOLE
SULFAMETHOXAZOLE, SULFAMETHOXAZOLE
SULFAMETHOXAZOLE & TRIMETHOPRIM, SULFAMETHOXAZOLE
SULFAMETHOXAZOLE AND TRIMETHOPRIM, SULFAMETHOXAZOLE
SULFAMETHOXAZOLE AND TRIMETHOPRIM DOUBLE STRENGTH, SULFAMETHOXAZOLE
SULFAMETHOXAZOLE AND TRIMETHOPRIM SINGLE STRENGTH, SULFAMETHOXAZOLE
SULFAMYLON, MAFENIDE ACETATE
SULFANILAMIDE, SULFANILAMIDE
SULFAPYRIDINE, SULFAPYRIDINE

APPENDIX A
PRODUCT NAME INDEX *(continued)*

SULFASALAZINE, SULFASALAZINE
SULFATRIM, SULFAMETHOXAZOLE
SULFATRIM PEDIATRIC, SULFAMETHOXAZOLE
SULFATRIM-DS, SULFAMETHOXAZOLE
SULFATRIM-SS, SULFAMETHOXAZOLE
SULFINPYRAZONE, SULFINPYRAZONE
SULFISOXAZOLE, SULFISOXAZOLE
SULFISOXAZOLE DIOLAMINE, SULFISOXAZOLE DIOLAMINE
SULFONAMIDES DUPLEX, SULFADIAZINE
SULFOSE, TRISULFAPYRIMIDINES (SULFADIAZINE;SULFAMERAZINE;SULFAMETHAZINE)
SULINDAC, SULINDAC
SULLA, SULFAMETER
SULMEPRIM, SULFAMETHOXAZOLE
SULMEPRIM PEDIATRIC, SULFAMETHOXAZOLE
SULPHRIN, PREDNISOLONE ACETATE
SULSOXIN, SULFISOXAZOLE
SULTEN-10, SULFACETAMIDE SODIUM
SULTRIN, TRIPLE SULFA (SULFABENZAMIDE;SULFACETAMIDE;SULFATHIAZOLE)
SUMYCIN, TETRACYCLINE HYDROCHLORIDE
SUPPRELIN, HISTRELIN ACETATE
SUPRANE, DESFLURANE
SUPRAX, CEFIXIME
SUPROL, SUPROFEN
SURITAL, THIAMYLAL SODIUM
SURMONTIL, TRIMIPRAMINE MALEATE
SURVANTA, BERACTANT
SUS-PHRINE, EPINEPHRINE
SUSTAIRE, THEOPHYLLINE
SYMADINE, AMANTADINE HYDROCHLORIDE
SYMMETREL, AMANTADINE HYDROCHLORIDE
SYNACORT, HYDROCORTISONE
SYNALAR, FLUOCINOLONE ACETONIDE
SYNALAR-HP, FLUOCINOLONE ACETONIDE
SYNALGOS-DC, ASPIRIN
SYNALGOS-DC-A, ACETAMINOPHEN
SYNAREL, NAFARELIN ACETATE
SYNCURINE, DECAMETHONIUM BROMIDE
SYNEMOL, FLUOCINOLONE ACETONIDE
SYNKAYVITE, MENADIOL SODIUM DIPHOSPHATE
SYNOPHYLATE, THEOPHYLLINE SODIUM GLYCINATE
SYNOVALYTE IN PLASTIC CONTAINER, MAGNESIUM CHLORIDE
SYNTOCINON, OXYTOCIN
SYPRINE, TRIENTINE HYDROCHLORIDE
SYTOBEX, CYANOCOBALAMIN

T

T-PHYL, THEOPHYLLINE
T-STAT, ERYTHROMYCIN
TAB-PROFEN, IBUPROFEN (OTC)
TACARYL, METHDILAZINE
TACARYL, METHDILAZINE HYDROCHLORIDE
TACE, CHLOROTRIANISENE
TAGAMET, CIMETIDINE
TAGAMET, CIMETIDINE HYDROCHLORIDE
TAGAMET HCL IN SODIUM CHLORIDE 0.9%, CIMETIDINE HYDROCHLORIDE
TALACEN, ACETAMINOPHEN
TALWIN, PENTAZOCINE LACTATE
TALWIN COMPOUND, ASPIRIN
TALWIN NX, NALOXONE HYDROCHLORIDE
TALWIN 50, PENTAZOCINE HYDROCHLORIDE
TAMBOCOR, FLECAINIDE ACETATE
TANDEARIL, OXYPHENBUTAZONE
TAO, TROLEANDOMYCIN
TAPAZOLE, METHIMAZOLE
TARACTAN, CHLORPROTHIXENE
TATUM-T, COPPER
TAVIST, CLEMASTINE FUMARATE
TAVIST D, CLEMASTINE FUMARATE
TAVIST-D, CLEMASTINE FUMARATE (OTC)
TAVIST-1, CLEMASTINE FUMARATE
TAVIST-1, CLEMASTINE FUMARATE (OTC)
TAXOL, PACLITAXEL
TAZICEF, CEFTAZIDIME
TAZIDIME, CEFTAZIDIME
TC 99M-LUNGAGGREGATE, TECHNETIUM TC-99M ALBUMIN AGGREGATED
TECHNECOLL, TECHNETIUM TC-99M SULFUR COLLOID KIT
TECHNESCAN DTPA KIT, TECHNETIUM TC-99M PENTETATE KIT
TECHNESCAN GLUCEPTATE, TECHNETIUM TC-99M GLUCEPTATE KIT
TECHNESCAN HDP, TECHNETIUM TC-99M OXIDRONATE KIT
TECHNESCAN HIDA, TECHNETIUM TC-99M LIDOFENIN KIT
TECHNESCAN MAA, TECHNETIUM TC-99M ALBUMIN AGGREGATED KIT
TECHNESCAN MAG3, TECHNETIUM TC-99M MERTIATIDE KIT
TECHNESCAN MDP KIT, TECHNETIUM TC-99M MEDRONATE KIT
TECHNESCAN PYP KIT, TECHNETIUM TC-99M PYROPHOSPHATE KIT
TECHNETIUM TC 99M ALBUMIN AGGREGATED KIT, TECHNETIUM TC-99M ALBUMIN AGGREGATED KIT
TECHNETIUM TC 99M DIPHOSPHONATE-TIN KIT, TECHNETIUM TC-99M ETIDRONATE KIT
TECHNETIUM TC 99M GENERATOR, TECHNETIUM TC-99M SODIUM PERTECHNETATE GENERATOR
TECHNETIUM TC 99M HSA, TECHNETIUM TC-99M ALBUMIN KIT
TECHNETIUM TC 99M MAA, TECHNETIUM TC-99M ALBUMIN AGGREGATED KIT
TECHNETIUM TC 99M MPI MDP, TECHNETIUM TC-99M MEDRONATE KIT
TECHNETIUM TC 99M SULFUR COLLOID, TECHNETIUM TC-99M SULFUR COLLOID
TECHNETIUM TC 99M TSC, TECHNETIUM TC-99M SULFUR COLLOID KIT
TECHNETIUM TC-99M PENTETATE KIT, TECHNETIUM TC-99M PENTETATE KIT
TEEBACIN, AMINOSALICYLATE SODIUM
TEGISON, ETRETINATE
TEGOPEN, CLOXACILLIN SODIUM
TEGRETOL, CARBAMAZEPINE
TELDRIN, CHLORPHENIRAMINE MALEATE (OTC)
TELEPAQUE, IOPANOIC ACID
TEMARIL, TRIMEPRAZINE TARTRATE
TEMAZ, TEMAZEPAM
TEMAZEPAM, TEMAZEPAM
TEMOVATE, CLOBETASOL PROPIONATE
TEN-K, POTASSIUM CHLORIDE
TENATHAN, BETHANIDINE SULFATE
TENEX, GUANFACINE HYDROCHLORIDE
TENORETIC 100, ATENOLOL
TENORETIC 50, ATENOLOL
TENORMIN, ATENOLOL
TENSILON, EDROPHONIUM CHLORIDE
TENUATE, DIETHYLPROPION HYDROCHLORIDE
TENUATE DOSPAN, DIETHYLPROPION HYDROCHLORIDE
TEPANIL, DIETHYLPROPION HYDROCHLORIDE
TEPANIL TEN-TAB, DIETHYLPROPION HYDROCHLORIDE
TERAZOL 3, TERCONAZOLE
TERAZOL 7, TERCONAZOLE
TERFONYL, TRISULFAPYRIMIDINES (SULFADIAZINE;SULFAMERAZINE;SULFAMETHAZINE)

APPENDIX A
PRODUCT NAME INDEX *(continued)*

TERRA-CORTRIL, HYDROCORTISONE ACETATE
TERRAMYCIN, LIDOCAINE HYDROCHLORIDE
TERRAMYCIN, OXYTETRACYCLINE
TERRAMYCIN, OXYTETRACYCLINE CALCIUM
TERRAMYCIN, OXYTETRACYCLINE HYDROCHLORIDE
TERRAMYCIN W/ POLYMYXIN, OXYTETRACYCLINE HYDROCHLORIDE
TERRAMYCIN W/ POLYMYXIN B SULFATE, OXYTETRACYCLINE HYDROCHLORIDE
TERRAMYCIN-POLYMYXIN, OXYTETRACYCLINE HYDROCHLORIDE
TESLAC, TESTOLACTONE
TESSALON, BENZONATATE
TESTODERM, TESTOSTERONE
TESTOSTERONE, TESTOSTERONE
TESTOSTERONE CYPIONATE, TESTOSTERONE CYPIONATE
TESTOSTERONE CYPIONATE-ESTRADIOL CYPIONATE, ESTRADIOL CYPIONATE
TESTOSTERONE ENANTHATE, TESTOSTERONE ENANTHATE
TESTOSTERONE ENANTHATE AND ESTRADIOL VALERATE, ESTRADIOL VALERATE
TESTOSTERONE PROPIONATE, TESTOSTERONE PROPIONATE
TESTRED, METHYLTESTOSTERONE
TESULOID, TECHNETIUM TC-99M SULFUR COLLOID KIT
TETRACHEL, TETRACYCLINE HYDROCHLORIDE
TETRACYCLINE HCL, TETRACYCLINE HYDROCHLORIDE
TETRACYN, PROCAINE HYDROCHLORIDE
TETRACYN, TETRACYCLINE HYDROCHLORIDE
TETRAMED, TETRACYCLINE HYDROCHLORIDE
TETREX, TETRACYCLINE PHOSPHATE COMPLEX
TEXACORT, HYDROCORTISONE
THALITONE, CHLORTHALIDONE
THALLOUS CHLORIDE TL 201, THALLOUS CHLORIDE, TL-201
THAM, TROMETHAMINE
THAM-E, POTASSIUM CHLORIDE
THEELIN, ESTRONE
THEO-DUR, THEOPHYLLINE
THEO-24, THEOPHYLLINE
THEOBID, THEOPHYLLINE
THEOBID JR., THEOPHYLLINE
THEOCHRON, THEOPHYLLINE
THEOCLEAR L.A.-130, THEOPHYLLINE
THEOCLEAR L.A.-260, THEOPHYLLINE
THEOCLEAR-100, THEOPHYLLINE
THEOCLEAR-200, THEOPHYLLINE
THEOCLEAR-80, THEOPHYLLINE
THEOLAIR, THEOPHYLLINE
THEOLAIR-SR, THEOPHYLLINE
THEOLIXIR, THEOPHYLLINE
THEOPHYL, THEOPHYLLINE
THEOPHYL-SR, THEOPHYLLINE
THEOPHYL-225, THEOPHYLLINE
THEOPHYLLINE, THEOPHYLLINE
THEOPHYLLINE AND DEXTROSE 5%, THEOPHYLLINE
THEOPHYLLINE IN DEXTROSE 5%, THEOPHYLLINE
THEOPHYLLINE IN DEXTROSE 5% IN PLASTIC CONTAINER, THEOPHYLLINE
THEOPHYLLINE 0.04% AND DEXTROSE 5%, THEOPHYLLINE
THEOPHYLLINE 0.04% AND DEXTROSE 5% IN PLASTIC CONTAINER, THEOPHYLLINE
THEOPHYLLINE 0.08% AND DEXTROSE 5%, THEOPHYLLINE
THEOPHYLLINE 0.08% AND DEXTROSE 5% IN PLASTIC CONTAINER, THEOPHYLLINE
THEOPHYLLINE 0.16% AND DEXTROSE 5%, THEOPHYLLINE
THEOPHYLLINE 0.16% AND DEXTROSE 5% IN PLASTIC CONTAINER, THEOPHYLLINE
THEOPHYLLINE 0.2% AND DEXTROSE 5%, THEOPHYLLINE
THEOPHYLLINE 0.2% AND DEXTROSE 5% IN PLASTIC CONTAINER, THEOPHYLLINE
THEOPHYLLINE 0.32% AND DEXTROSE 5%, THEOPHYLLINE
THEOPHYLLINE 0.4% AND DEXTROSE 5%, THEOPHYLLINE
THEOPHYLLINE 0.4% AND DEXTROSE 5% IN PLASTIC CONTAINER, THEOPHYLLINE
THEOPHYLLINE-SR, THEOPHYLLINE
THEOVENT, THEOPHYLLINE
THERMAZENE, SILVER SULFADIAZINE
THIAMINE HCL, THIAMINE HYDROCHLORIDE
THIOGUANINE, THIOGUANINE
THIORIDAZINE HCL, THIORIDAZINE HYDROCHLORIDE
THIORIDAZINE HCL INTENSOL, THIORIDAZINE HYDROCHLORIDE
THIOSULFIL, SULFAMETHIZOLE
THIOTEPA, THIOTEPA
THIOTHIXENE, THIOTHIXENE
THIOTHIXENE HCL, THIOTHIXENE HYDROCHLORIDE
THIOTHIXENE HCL INTENSOL, THIOTHIXENE HYDROCHLORIDE
THORAZINE, CHLORPROMAZINE
THORAZINE, CHLORPROMAZINE HYDROCHLORIDE
THYPINONE, PROTIRELIN
THYREL TRH, PROTIRELIN
THYRO-BLOCK, POTASSIUM IODIDE (OTC)
THYROGLOBULIN, THYROGLOBULIN
THYROLAR-0.25, LIOTRIX (T4;T3)
THYROLAR-0.5, LIOTRIX (T4;T3)
THYROLAR-1, LIOTRIX (T4;T3)
THYROLAR-2, LIOTRIX (T4;T3)
THYROLAR-3, LIOTRIX (T4;T3)
THYROLAR-5, LIOTRIX (T4;T3)
THYTROPAR, THYROTROPIN
TICAR, TICARCILLIN DISODIUM
TICLID, TICLOPIDINE HYDROCHLORIDE
TIGAN, TRIMETHOBENZAMIDE HYDROCHLORIDE
TILADE, NEDOCROMIL SODIUM
TIMENTIN, CLAVULANATE POTASSIUM
TIMOLIDE 10-25, HYDROCHLOROTHIAZIDE
TIMOLOL MALEATE, TIMOLOL MALEATE
TIMOPTIC, TIMOLOL MALEATE
TIMOPTIC IN OCUDOSE, TIMOLOL MALEATE
TIMOPTIC-XE, TIMOLOL MALEATE
TINDAL, ACETOPHENAZINE MALEATE
TIOPRONIN, TIOPRONIN
TIS-U-SOL, MAGNESIUM SULFATE
TIS-U-SOL IN PLASTIC CONTAINER, MAGNESIUM SULFATE
TOBRADEX, DEXAMETHASONE
TOBRAMYCIN, TOBRAMYCIN
TOBRAMYCIN SULFATE, TOBRAMYCIN SULFATE
TOBRAMYCIN SULFATE IN SODIUM CHLORIDE 0.9%, TOBRAMYCIN SULFATE
TOBRASONE, FLUOROMETHOLONE ACETATE
TOBREX, TOBRAMYCIN
TODAY, NONOXYNOL-9 (OTC)
TOFRANIL, IMIPRAMINE HYDROCHLORIDE
TOFRANIL-PM, IMIPRAMINE PAMOATE
TOLAZAMIDE, TOLAZAMIDE
TOLBUTAMIDE, TOLBUTAMIDE
TOLECTIN, TOLMETIN SODIUM
TOLECTIN DS, TOLMETIN SODIUM
TOLECTIN 600, TOLMETIN SODIUM
TOLINASE, TOLAZAMIDE
TOLMETIN SODIUM, TOLMETIN SODIUM
TONOCARD, TOCAINIDE HYDROCHLORIDE
TOPICORT, DESOXIMETASONE
TOPICORT LP, DESOXIMETASONE

APPENDIX A
PRODUCT NAME INDEX *(continued)*

TOPICYCLINE, TETRACYCLINE HYDROCHLORIDE
TOPROL XL, METOPROLOL SUCCINATE
TORA, PHENTERMINE HYDROCHLORIDE
TORADOL, KETOROLAC TROMETHAMINE
TORECAN, THIETHYLPERAZINE MALATE
TORECAN, THIETHYLPERAZINE MALEATE
TORNALATE, BITOLTEROL MESYLATE
TOTACILLIN, AMPICILLIN/AMPICILLIN TRIHYDRATE
TOTACILLIN-N, AMPICILLIN SODIUM
TPN ELECTROLYTES IN PLASTIC CONTAINER, CALCIUM CHLORIDE
TRACRIUM, ATRACURIUM BESYLATE
TRAL, HEXOCYCLIUM METHYLSULFATE
TRANCOPAL, CHLORMEZANONE
TRANDATE, LABETALOL HYDROCHLORIDE
TRANDATE HCT, HYDROCHLOROTHIAZIDE
TRANMEP, MEPROBAMATE
TRANSDERM-SCOP, SCOPOLAMINE
TRANXENE, CLORAZEPATE DIPOTASSIUM
TRANXENE SD, CLORAZEPATE DIPOTASSIUM
TRASICOR, OXPRENOLOL HYDROCHLORIDE
TRASYLOL, APROTININ BOVINE
TRAVAMULSION 10%, SOYBEAN OIL
TRAVAMULSION 20%, SOYBEAN OIL
TRAVASE, SUTILAINS
TRAVASOL 10%, AMINO ACIDS
TRAVASOL 10% W/O ELECTROLYTES, AMINO ACIDS
TRAVASOL 2.75% IN DEXTROSE 10%, AMINO ACIDS
TRAVASOL 2.75% IN DEXTROSE 15%, AMINO ACIDS
TRAVASOL 2.75% IN DEXTROSE 20%, AMINO ACIDS
TRAVASOL 2.75% IN DEXTROSE 25%, AMINO ACIDS
TRAVASOL 2.75% IN DEXTROSE 5%, AMINO ACIDS
TRAVASOL 3.5% W/ ELECTROLYTES, AMINO ACIDS
TRAVASOL 4.25% IN DEXTROSE 10%, AMINO ACIDS
TRAVASOL 4.25% IN DEXTROSE 15%, AMINO ACIDS
TRAVASOL 4.25% IN DEXTROSE 20%, AMINO ACIDS
TRAVASOL 4.25% IN DEXTROSE 25%, AMINO ACIDS
TRAVASOL 4.25% IN DEXTROSE 5%, AMINO ACIDS
TRAVASOL 5.5%, AMINO ACIDS
TRAVASOL 5.5% W/ ELECTROLYTES, AMINO ACIDS
TRAVASOL 5.5% W/O ELECTROLYTES, AMINO ACIDS
TRAVASOL 8.5%, AMINO ACIDS
TRAVASOL 8.5% W/ ELECTROLYTES, AMINO ACIDS
TRAVASOL 8.5% W/O ELECTROLYTES, AMINO ACIDS
TRAVERT 10%, INVERT SUGAR
TRAZODONE HCL, TRAZODONE HYDROCHLORIDE
TRAZON-150, TRAZODONE HYDROCHLORIDE
TRECATOR-SC, ETHIONAMIDE
TREMIN, TRIHEXYPHENIDYL HYDROCHLORIDE
TRENTAL, PENTOXIFYLLINE
TREST, METHIXENE HYDROCHLORIDE
TREXAN, NALTREXONE HYDROCHLORIDE
TRI-NORINYL 21-DAY, ETHINYL ESTRADIOL
TRI-NORINYL 28-DAY, ETHINYL ESTRADIOL
TRIACET, TRIAMCINOLONE ACETONIDE
TRIACIN-C, CODEINE PHOSPHATE
TRIACORT, TRIAMCINOLONE ACETONIDE
TRIALODINE, TRAZODONE HYDROCHLORIDE
TRIAMCINOLONE, TRIAMCINOLONE
TRIAMCINOLONE ACETONIDE, TRIAMCINOLONE ACETONIDE
TRIAMCINOLONE DIACETATE, TRIAMCINOLONE DIACETATE
TRIAMINIC-12, CHLORPHENIRAMINE MALEATE (OTC)
TRIAMTERENE AND HYDROCHLOROTHIAZIDE, HYDROCHLOROTHIAZIDE
TRIAPRIN, ACETAMINOPHEN
TRIATEX, TRIAMCINOLONE ACETONIDE
TRIAVIL 2-10, AMITRIPTYLINE HYDROCHLORIDE
TRIAVIL 2-25, AMITRIPTYLINE HYDROCHLORIDE
TRIAVIL 4-10, AMITRIPTYLINE HYDROCHLORIDE
TRIAVIL 4-25, AMITRIPTYLINE HYDROCHLORIDE
TRIAVIL 4-50, AMITRIPTYLINE HYDROCHLORIDE
TRIAZOLAM, TRIAZOLAM
TRICHLOREX, TRICHLORMETHIAZIDE
TRICHLORMAS, TRICHLORMETHIAZIDE
TRICHLORMETHIAZIDE, TRICHLORMETHIAZIDE
TRICHLORMETHIAZIDE W/ RESERPINE, RESERPINE
TRICLOS, TRICLOFOS SODIUM
TRIDERM, TRIAMCINOLONE ACETONIDE
TRIDESILON, ACETIC ACID, GLACIAL
TRIDESILON, DESONIDE
TRIDIL, NITROGLYCERIN
TRIDIONE, TRIMETHADIONE
TRIFLUOPERAZINE HCL, TRIFLUOPERAZINE HYDROCHLORIDE
TRIHEXYPHENIDYL HCL, TRIHEXYPHENIDYL HYDROCHLORIDE
TRILAFON, PERPHENAZINE
TRILITRON, PSEUDOEPHEDRINE HYDROCHLORIDE
TRIMEPRAZINE TARTRATE, TRIMEPRAZINE TARTRATE
TRIMETH/SULFA, SULFAMETHOXAZOLE
TRIMETHOBENZAMIDE HCL, TRIMETHOBENZAMIDE HYDROCHLORIDE
TRIMETHOPRIM, TRIMETHOPRIM
TRIMIPRAMINE MALEATE, TRIMIPRAMINE MALEATE
TRIMOX, AMOXICILLIN
TRIMPEX, TRIMETHOPRIM
TRIMPEX 200, TRIMETHOPRIM
TRINALIN, AZATADINE MALEATE
TRIOSTAT, LIOTHYRONINE SODIUM
TRIPELENNAMINE HCL, TRIPELENNAMINE HYDROCHLORIDE
TRIPHASIL-21, ETHINYL ESTRADIOL
TRIPHASIL-28, ETHINYL ESTRADIOL
TRIPHED, PSEUDOEPHEDRINE HYDROCHLORIDE
TRIPLE SULFA, TRIPLE SULFA (SULFABENZAMIDE;SULFACETAMIDE;SULFATHIAZOLE)
TRIPLE SULFA, TRISULFAPYRIMIDINES (SULFADIAZINE;SULFAMERAZINE;SULFAMETHAZINE)
TRIPLE SULFAS, TRISULFAPYRIMIDINES (SULFADIAZINE;SULFAMERAZINE;SULFAMETHAZINE)
TRIPLE SULFOID, TRISULFAPYRIMIDINES (SULFADIAZINE;SULFAMERAZINE;SULFAMETHAZINE)
TRIPROLIDINE AND PSEUDOEPHEDRINE, PSEUDOEPHEDRINE HYDROCHLORIDE
TRIPROLIDINE AND PSEUDOEPHEDRINE, PSEUDOEPHEDRINE HYDROCHLORIDE (OTC)
TRIPROLIDINE AND PSEUDOEPHEDRINE HYDROCHLORIDES, PSEUDOEPHEDRINE HYDROCHLORIDE (OTC)
TRIPROLIDINE AND PSEUDOEPHEDRINE HYDROCHLORIDES W/ CODEINE, CODEINE PHOSPHATE
TRIPROLIDINE AND PSEUDOEPHRINE HCL, PSEUDOEPHEDRINE HYDROCHLORIDE (OTC)
TRIPROLIDINE HCL, TRIPROLIDINE HYDROCHLORIDE
TRIPROLIDINE HCL AND PSEUDOEPHEDRINE HCL, PSEUDOEPHEDRINE HYDROCHLORIDE
TRIPROLIDINE HCL, PSEUDOEPHEDRINE HCL AND CODEINE PHOSPHATE, CODEINE PHOSPHATE
TRISORALEN, TRIOXSALEN
TROBICIN, SPECTINOMYCIN HYDROCHLORIDE
TROPHAMINE, AMINO ACIDS
TROPHAMINE 10%, AMINO ACIDS
TROPICAMIDE, TROPICAMIDE
TRUPHYLLINE, AMINOPHYLLINE
TRYMEX, TRIAMCINOLONE ACETONIDE
TRYSUL, TRIPLE SULFA (SULFABENZAMIDE;SULFACETAMIDE;SULFATHIAZOLE)
TUBOCURARINE CHLORIDE, TUBOCURARINE CHLORIDE
TURGEX, HEXACHLOROPHENE
TUSSIGON, HOMATROPINE METHYLBROMIDE

APPENDIX A
PRODUCT NAME INDEX *(continued)*

TUSSIONEX, CHLORPHENIRAMINE POLISTIREX
TYCOLET, ACETAMINOPHEN
TYLENOL, ACETAMINOPHEN
TYLENOL, ACETAMINOPHEN (OTC)
TYLENOL W/ CODEINE, ACETAMINOPHEN
TYLENOL W/ CODEINE NO. 1, ACETAMINOPHEN
TYLENOL W/ CODEINE NO. 2, ACETAMINOPHEN
TYLENOL W/ CODEINE NO. 3, ACETAMINOPHEN
TYLENOL W/ CODEINE NO. 4, ACETAMINOPHEN
TYLOSTERONE, DIETHYLSTILBESTROL
TYLOX, ACETAMINOPHEN
TYLOX-325, ACETAMINOPHEN
TYMTRAN, CERULETIDE DIETHYLAMINE
TYZINE, TETRAHYDROZOLINE HYDROCHLORIDE
TZ-3, TIOCONAZOLE (OTC)

U

U-CORT, HYDROCORTISONE ACETATE
U-GENCIN, GENTAMICIN SULFATE
UCEPHAN, SODIUM BENZOATE
ULO, CHLOPHEDIANOL HYDROCHLORIDE
ULTRA-TECHNEKOW FM, TECHNETIUM TC-99M SODIUM PERTECHNETATE GENERATOR
ULTRACEF, CEFADROXIL/CEFADROXIL HEMIHYDRATE
ULTRAGRIS-165, GRISEOFULVIN, ULTRAMICROCRYSTALLINE
ULTRAGRIS-330, GRISEOFULVIN, ULTRAMICROCRYSTALLINE
ULTRALENTE, INSULIN ZINC SUSP EXTENDED PURIFIED BEEF (OTC)
ULTRALENTE INSULIN, INSULIN ZINC SUSP EXTENDED BEEF (OTC)
ULTRATAG, TECHNETIUM TC-99M RED BLOOD CELL KIT
ULTRAVATE, HALOBETASOL PROPIONATE
UMI-PEX 30, PHENTERMINE HYDROCHLORIDE
UNASYN, AMPICILLIN SODIUM
UNIPEN, NAFCILLIN SODIUM
UNIPHYL, THEOPHYLLINE
UNIPRES, HYDRALAZINE HYDROCHLORIDE
UNISOM, DOXYLAMINE SUCCINATE (OTC)
UNITENSEN, CRYPTENAMINE ACETATES
UNITENSEN, CRYPTENAMINE TANNATES
URACIL MUSTARD, URACIL MUSTARD
UREAPHIL, UREA
URECHOLINE, BETHANECHOL CHLORIDE
URESE, BENZTHIAZIDE
UREX, METHENAMINE HIPPURATE
URISPAS, FLAVOXATE HYDROCHLORIDE
UROBAK, SULFAMETHOXAZOLE
UROLOGIC G IN PLASTIC CONTAINER, CITRIC ACID
UROPLUS DS, SULFAMETHOXAZOLE
UROPLUS SS, SULFAMETHOXAZOLE
UROVIST CYSTO, DIATRIZOATE MEGLUMINE
UROVIST CYSTO PEDIATRIC, DIATRIZOATE MEGLUMINE
UROVIST MEGLUMINE DIU/CT, DIATRIZOATE MEGLUMINE
UROVIST SODIUM 300, DIATRIZOATE SODIUM
UTICILLIN VK, PENICILLIN V POTASSIUM
UTICORT, BETAMETHASONE BENZOATE
UTIMOX, AMOXICILLIN

V

V-CILLIN, PENICILLIN V
V-CILLIN K, PENICILLIN V POTASSIUM
VAGILIA, TRIPLE SULFA (SULFABENZAMIDE;SULFACETAMIDE;SULFATHIAZOLE)
VAGISTAT-1, TIOCONAZOLE
VALISONE, BETAMETHASONE VALERATE
VALIUM, DIAZEPAM
VALMID, ETHINAMATE
VALNAC, BETAMETHASONE VALERATE
VALPIN 50, ANISOTROPINE METHYLBROMIDE
VALPROIC ACID, VALPROIC ACID
VALRELEASE, DIAZEPAM
VANCENASE, BECLOMETHASONE DIPROPIONATE
VANCENASE AQ, BECLOMETHASONE DIPROPIONATE MONOHYDRATE
VANCERIL, BECLOMETHASONE DIPROPIONATE
VANCOCIN HCL, VANCOMYCIN HYDROCHLORIDE
VANCOLED, VANCOMYCIN HYDROCHLORIDE
VANCOMYCIN HCL, VANCOMYCIN HYDROCHLORIDE
VANCOR, VANCOMYCIN HYDROCHLORIDE
VANOBID, CANDICIDIN
VANSIL, OXAMNIQUINE
VANTIN, CEFPODOXIME PROXETIL
VAPO-ISO, ISOPROTERENOL HYDROCHLORIDE
VASCOR, BEPRIDIL HYDROCHLORIDE
VASCORAY, IOTHALAMATE MEGLUMINE
VASERETIC, ENALAPRIL MALEATE
VASOCIDIN, PREDNISOLONE ACETATE
VASOCIDIN, PREDNISOLONE SODIUM PHOSPHATE
VASOCON, NAPHAZOLINE HYDROCHLORIDE
VASOCON-A, ANTAZOLINE PHOSPHATE
VASOTEC, ENALAPRIL MALEATE
VASOTEC, ENALAPRILAT
VASOXYL, METHOXAMINE HYDROCHLORIDE
VEETIDS '125', PENICILLIN V POTASSIUM
VEETIDS '250', PENICILLIN V POTASSIUM
VEETIDS '500', PENICILLIN V POTASSIUM
VEINAMINE 8%, AMINO ACIDS
VELBAN, VINBLASTINE SULFATE
VELOSEF, CEPHRADINE
VELOSEF '125', CEPHRADINE
VELOSEF '250', CEPHRADINE
VELOSEF '500', CEPHRADINE
VELOSULIN, INSULIN PURIFIED PORK (OTC)
VELOSULIN HUMAN, INSULIN SEMISYNTHETIC PURIFIED HUMAN (OTC)
VELTANE, BROMPHENIRAMINE MALEATE
VENTAIRE, PROTOKYLOL HYDROCHLORIDE
VENTOLIN, ALBUTEROL
VENTOLIN, ALBUTEROL SULFATE
VENTOLIN ROTACAPS, ALBUTEROL SULFATE
VEPESID, ETOPOSIDE
VERAPAMIL HCL, VERAPAMIL HYDROCHLORIDE
VERCYTE, PIPOBROMAN
VERELAN, VERAPAMIL HYDROCHLORIDE
VERILOID, ALKAVERVIR
VERMIDOL, PIPERAZINE CITRATE
VERMOX, MEBENDAZOLE
VERSAPEN, HETACILLIN
VERSAPEN-K, HETACILLIN POTASSIUM
VERSED, MIDAZOLAM HYDROCHLORIDE
VERTAVIS, VERATRUM VIRIDE
VESPRIN, TRIFLUPROMAZINE
VESPRIN, TRIFLUPROMAZINE HYDROCHLORIDE
VI-DOM-A, VITAMIN A PALMITATE
VI-TWEL, CYANOCOBALAMIN
VIBISONE, CYANOCOBALAMIN
VIBRA-TABS, DOXYCYCLINE HYCLATE
VIBRAMYCIN, DOXYCYCLINE
VIBRAMYCIN, DOXYCYCLINE CALCIUM
VIBRAMYCIN, DOXYCYCLINE HYCLATE
VICKS FORMULA 44, DIPHENHYDRAMINE HYDROCHLORIDE (OTC)
VICODIN, ACETAMINOPHEN
VICODIN ES, ACETAMINOPHEN
VICOPRIN, ASPIRIN
VIDEX, DIDANOSINE

APPENDIX A
PRODUCT NAME INDEX *(continued)*

VINBLASTINE SULFATE, VINBLASTINE SULFATE
VINCASAR PFS, VINCRISTINE SULFATE
VINCREX, VINCRISTINE SULFATE
VINCRISTINE SULFATE, VINCRISTINE SULFATE
VINCRISTINE SULFATE PFS, VINCRISTINE SULFATE
VIOCIN SULFATE, VIOMYCIN SULFATE
VIRA-A, VIDARABINE
VIRAC REX, UNDECOYLIUM CHLORIDE
VIRAZOLE, RIBAVIRIN
VIRILON, METHYLTESTOSTERONE
VIROPTIC, TRIFLURIDINE
VISINE L.R., OXYMETAZOLINE HYDROCHLORIDE (OTC)
VISKAZIDE, HYDROCHLOROTHIAZIDE
VISKEN, PINDOLOL
VISTARIL, HYDROXYZINE HYDROCHLORIDE
VISTARIL, HYDROXYZINE PAMOATE
VITAMIN A, VITAMIN A
VITAMIN A, VITAMIN A PALMITATE
VITAMIN A PALMITATE, VITAMIN A PALMITATE
VITAMIN A SOLUBILIZED, VITAMIN A PALMITATE
VITAMIN D, ERGOCALCIFEROL
VITAMIN K1, PHYTONADIONE
VIVACTIL, PROTRIPTYLINE HYDROCHLORIDE
VOLMAX, ALBUTEROL SULFATE
VOLTAREN, DICLOFENAC SODIUM
VONTROL, DIPHENIDOL HYDROCHLORIDE
VOSOL, ACETIC ACID, GLACIAL
VOSOL HC, ACETIC ACID, GLACIAL
VUMON, TENIPOSIDE

W

WAMPOCAP, NIACIN
WARFARIN SODIUM, WARFARIN SODIUM
WELLBUTRIN, BUPROPION HYDROCHLORIDE
WELLCOVORIN, LEUCOVORIN CALCIUM
WESTADONE, METHADONE HYDROCHLORIDE
WESTCORT, HYDROCORTISONE VALERATE
WIGRAINE, CAFFEINE
WIGRETTES, ERGOTAMINE TARTRATE
WINSTROL, STANOZOLOL
WOLFINA, RAUWOLFIA SERPENTINA
WYAMINE SULFATE, MEPHENTERMINE SULFATE
WYAMYCIN E, ERYTHROMYCIN ETHYLSUCCINATE
WYAMYCIN S, ERYTHROMYCIN STEARATE
WYCILLIN, PENICILLIN G PROCAINE
WYDASE, HYALURONIDASE
WYGESIC, ACETAMINOPHEN
WYMOX, AMOXICILLIN
WYTENSIN, GUANABENZ ACETATE

X

X-TROZINE, PHENDIMETRAZINE TARTRATE
X-TROZINE L.A., PHENDIMETRAZINE TARTRATE
XANAX, ALPRAZOLAM
XENEISOL, XENON, XE-133
XENON XE 127, XENON, XE-127
XENON XE 133, XENON, XE-133
XENON XE 133-V.S.S., XENON, XE-133
XYLO-PFAN, XYLOSE
XYLOCAINE, LIDOCAINE
XYLOCAINE, LIDOCAINE HYDROCHLORIDE
XYLOCAINE VISCOUS, LIDOCAINE HYDROCHLORIDE
XYLOCAINE W/ DEXTROSE 7.5%, LIDOCAINE HYDROCHLORIDE
XYLOCAINE W/ EPINEPHRINE, EPINEPHRINE
XYLOCAINE 4%, LIDOCAINE HYDROCHLORIDE
XYLOCAINE 5% W/ GLUCOSE 7.5%, LIDOCAINE HYDROCHLORIDE
XYLOSE, XYLOSE

Y

YTTERBIUM YB 169 DTPA, PENTETATE CALCIUM TRISODIUM YB-169
YUTOPAR, RITODRINE HYDROCHLORIDE

Z

ZANOSAR, STREPTOZOCIN
ZANTAC, RANITIDINE HYDROCHLORIDE
ZANTAC 150, RANITIDINE HYDROCHLORIDE
ZANTAC 300, RANITIDINE HYDROCHLORIDE
ZARONTIN, ETHOSUXIMIDE
ZAROXOLYN, METOLAZONE
ZAXOPAM, OXAZEPAM
ZEBETA, BISOPROLOL FUMARATE
ZEFAZONE, CEFMETAZOLE SODIUM
ZEMURON, ROCURONIUM BROMIDE
ZEMURON (P/F), ROCURONIUM BROMIDE
ZERIT, STAVUDINE
ZESTORETIC 10-12.5, HYDROCHLOROTHIAZIDE
ZESTORETIC 20-12.5, HYDROCHLOROTHIAZIDE
ZESTORETIC 20-25, HYDROCHLOROTHIAZIDE
ZESTRIL, LISINOPRIL
ZIAC, BISOPROLOL FUMARATE
ZIBA-RX, BACITRACIN ZINC
ZIDE, HYDROCHLOROTHIAZIDE
ZINACEF, CEFUROXIME SODIUM
ZINC BACITRACIN,NEOMYCIN SULFATE,POLYMYXIN B SULFATE & HYDROCORTISONE, BACITRACIN ZINC
ZINC CHLORIDE, ZINC CHLORIDE
ZINC SULFATE, ZINC SULFATE
ZIPAN-25, PROMETHAZINE HYDROCHLORIDE
ZIPAN-50, PROMETHAZINE HYDROCHLORIDE
ZITHROMAX, AZITHROMYCIN DIHYDRATE
ZOCOR, SIMVASTATIN
ZOFRAN, ONDANSETRON HYDROCHLORIDE
ZOLADEX, GOSERELIN ACETATE
ZOLICEF, CEFAZOLIN SODIUM
ZOLOFT, SERTRALINE HYDROCHLORIDE
ZOLYSE, CHYMOTRYPSIN
ZONALON, DOXEPIN HYDROCHLORIDE
ZOSYN, PIPERACILLIN SODIUM
ZOVIRAX, ACYCLOVIR
ZOVIRAX, ACYCLOVIR SODIUM
ZYLOPRIM, ALLOPURINOL

8

8-HOUR BAYER, ASPIRIN (OTC)
8-MOP, METHOXSALEN

APPENDIX B
PRODUCT NAME INDEX
LISTED BY APPLICANT

A

ABANA
* ABANA PHARMACEUTICALS INC
  NORCET, ACETAMINOPHEN

ABBOTT
* ABBOTT LABORATORIES
  A-METHAPRED, METHYLPREDNISOLONE SODIUM SUCCINATE
  ACETYLCYSTEINE, ACETYLCYSTEINE
  BUPIVACAINE HCL KIT, BUPIVACAINE HYDROCHLORIDE
  DOBUTAMINE HCL, DOBUTAMINE HYDROCHLORIDE
  DOBUTAMINE HCL IN DEXTROSE 5%, DOBUTAMINE HYDROCHLORIDE
  HYTRIN, TERAZOSIN HYDROCHLORIDE
  INPERSOL-LC/LM W/ DEXTROSE 1.5%, CALCIUM CHLORIDE
  INPERSOL-LC/LM W/ DEXTROSE 2.5%, CALCIUM CHLORIDE
  INPERSOL-LC/LM W/ DEXTROSE 3.5%, CALCIUM CHLORIDE
  INPERSOL-LC/LM W/ DEXTROSE 4.25%, CALCIUM CHLORIDE
  ISOFLURANE, ISOFLURANE
  LORAZEPAM, LORAZEPAM
  MAGNESIUM SULFATE, MAGNESIUM SULFATE
  NALBUPHINE HYDROCHLORIDE, NALBUPHINE HYDROCHLORIDE
  PENTAMIDINE ISETHIONATE, PENTAMIDINE ISETHIONATE
  POTASSIUM CHLORIDE 10 MEQ, POTASSIUM CHLORIDE
  POTASSIUM CHLORIDE 20 MEQ, POTASSIUM CHLORIDE
* ABBOTT LABORATORIES HOSP PRODUCTS DIV
  A-HYDROCORT, HYDROCORTISONE SODIUM SUCCINATE
  A-METHAPRED, METHYLPREDNISOLONE SODIUM SUCCINATE
  AMIDATE, ETOMIDATE
  AMINOCAPROIC ACID, AMINOCAPROIC ACID
  AMINOSYN II M 3.5% IN DEXTROSE 5%, AMINO ACIDS
  AMINOSYN II 10%, AMINO ACIDS
  AMINOSYN II 15%, AMINO ACIDS
  AMINOSYN II 3.5% IN DEXTROSE 25%, AMINO ACIDS
  AMINOSYN II 3.5% IN DEXTROSE 5%, AMINO ACIDS
  AMINOSYN II 3.5% M IN DEXTROSE 5%, AMINO ACIDS
  AMINOSYN II 3.5% W/ ELECTROLYTES IN DEXTROSE 25% W/ CALCIUM, AMINO ACIDS
  AMINOSYN II 4.25% IN DEXTROSE 10%, AMINO ACIDS
  AMINOSYN II 4.25% IN DEXTROSE 20%, AMINO ACIDS
  AMINOSYN II 4.25% IN DEXTROSE 25%, AMINO ACIDS
  AMINOSYN II 4.25% M IN DEXTROSE 10%, AMINO ACIDS
  AMINOSYN II 4.25% W/ ELECT AND ADJUSTED PHOSPHATE IN DEXTROSE 10%, AMINO ACIDS
  AMINOSYN II 4.25% W/ ELECTROLYTES IN DEXTROSE 20% W/ CALCIUM, AMINO ACIDS
  AMINOSYN II 4.25% W/ ELECTROLYTES IN DEXTROSE 25% W/ CALCIUM, AMINO ACIDS
  AMINOSYN II 5% IN DEXTROSE 25%, AMINO ACIDS
  AMINOSYN II 5% W/ ELECTROLYTES IN DEXTROSE 25% W/ CALCIUM, AMINO ACIDS
  AMINOSYN-HBC 7%, AMINO ACIDS
  BUPIVACAINE HCL AND EPINEPHRINE, BUPIVACAINE HYDROCHLORIDE
  CALCIJEX, CALCITRIOL
  CHROMIC CHLORIDE, CHROMIC CHLORIDE
  CLINDAMYCIN PHOSPHATE, CLINDAMYCIN PHOSPHATE
  CUPRIC CHLORIDE, CUPRIC CHLORIDE
  DEXTROSE 5% IN PLASTIC CONTAINER, DEXTROSE
  DEXTROSE 50%, DEXTROSE
  DEXTROSE 70%, DEXTROSE
  DIAZEPAM, DIAZEPAM
  DOPAMINE HCL, DOPAMINE HYDROCHLORIDE
  ERYTHROCIN, ERYTHROMYCIN LACTOBIONATE
  FENTANYL CITRATE, FENTANYL CITRATE
  FENTANYL CITRATE AND DROPERIDOL, DROPERIDOL
  HEPARIN LOCK FLUSH, HEPARIN SODIUM
  HEPARIN SODIUM, HEPARIN SODIUM
  HEPARIN SODIUM 20,000 UNITS IN DEXTROSE 5%, HEPARIN SODIUM
  HEPARIN SODIUM 25,000 UNITS IN DEXTROSE 5%, HEPARIN SODIUM
  LIDOCAINE HCL, LIDOCAINE HYDROCHLORIDE
  LIDOCAINE HCL AND EPINEPHRINE, EPINEPHRINE
  MANGANESE CHLORIDE, MANGANESE CHLORIDE
  METOCLOPRAMIDE HCL, METOCLOPRAMIDE HYDROCHLORIDE
  MORPHINE SULFATE, MORPHINE SULFATE
  NALBUPHINE HCL, NALBUPHINE HYDROCHLORIDE
  NITROGLYCERIN IN DEXTROSE 5%, NITROGLYCERIN
  NITROPRESS, SODIUM NITROPRUSSIDE
  PANCURONIUM BROMIDE, PANCURONIUM BROMIDE
  PANHEPRIN, HEPARIN SODIUM
  PENTHRANE, METHOXYFLURANE
  PENTOTHAL, THIOPENTAL SODIUM
  POTASSIUM ACETATE IN PLASTIC CONTAINER, POTASSIUM ACETATE
  POTASSIUM CHLORIDE 10 MEQ IN DEXTROSE 5% AND LACTATED RINGER'S, CALCIUM CHLORIDE
  POTASSIUM CHLORIDE 15 MEQ IN DEXTROSE 5% AND LACTATED RINGER'S, CALCIUM CHLORIDE
  POTASSIUM CHLORIDE 20 MEQ IN DEXTROSE 5% AND LACTATED RINGER'S, CALCIUM CHLORIDE
  POTASSIUM CHLORIDE 20 MEQ IN SODIUM CHLORIDE 0.9%, POTASSIUM CHLORIDE
  POTASSIUM CHLORIDE 30 MEQ IN DEXTROSE 5% AND LACTATED RINGER'S, CALCIUM CHLORIDE
  POTASSIUM CHLORIDE 40 MEQ IN DEXTROSE 5% AND LACTATED RINGER'S, CALCIUM CHLORIDE
  POTASSIUM CHLORIDE 40 MEQ IN SODIUM CHLORIDE 0.9%, POTASSIUM CHLORIDE
  POTASSIUM CHLORIDE 5 MEQ IN DEXTROSE 5% AND LACTATED RINGER'S, CALCIUM CHLORIDE
  QUELICIN, SUCCINYLCHOLINE CHLORIDE

APPENDIX B
PRODUCT NAME INDEX
LISTED BY APPLICANT *(continued)*

RITODRINE HCL, RITODRINE HYDROCHLORIDE
RITODRINE HCL IN DEXTROSE 5% IN PLASTIC CONTAINER, RITODRINE HYDROCHLORIDE
SODIUM ACETATE IN PLASTIC CONTAINER, SODIUM ACETATE, ANHYDROUS
SODIUM CHLORIDE IN PLASTIC CONTAINER, SODIUM CHLORIDE
SODIUM CHLORIDE 0.45%, SODIUM CHLORIDE
SODIUM CHLORIDE 0.9% IN PLASTIC CONTAINER, SODIUM CHLORIDE
SODIUM LACTATE IN PLASTIC CONTAINER, SODIUM LACTATE
SODIUM PHOSPHATES IN PLASTIC CONTAINER, SODIUM PHOSPHATE, DIBASIC
STERILE WATER FOR INJECTION, WATER FOR INJECTION, STERILE
THAM, TROMETHAMINE
THAM-E, POTASSIUM CHLORIDE
TOBRAMYCIN SULFATE, TOBRAMYCIN SULFATE
TOBRAMYCIN SULFATE IN SODIUM CHLORIDE 0.9%, TOBRAMYCIN SULFATE
TPN ELECTROLYTES IN PLASTIC CONTAINER, CALCIUM CHLORIDE
TUBOCURARINE CHLORIDE, TUBOCURARINE CHLORIDE
UREAPHIL, UREA
VANCOMYCIN HCL, VANCOMYCIN HYDROCHLORIDE
ZINC CHLORIDE, ZINC CHLORIDE

* ABBOTT LABORATORIES PHARMACEUTICAL PRODUCTS DIV
A-HYDROCORT, HYDROCORTISONE SODIUM SUCCINATE
A-METHAPRED, METHYLPREDNISOLONE SODIUM SUCCINATE
A-POXIDE, CHLORDIAZEPOXIDE HYDROCHLORIDE
ACETIC ACID 0.25% IN PLASTIC CONTAINER, ACETIC ACID, GLACIAL
ALCOHOL 5% IN D5-W, ALCOHOL
AMINOCAPROIC ACID, AMINOCAPROIC ACID
AMINOPHYLLINE, AMINOPHYLLINE
AMINOPHYLLINE IN SODIUM CHLORIDE 0.45%, AMINOPHYLLINE
AMINOPHYLLINE IN SODIUM CHLORIDE 0.45% IN PLASTIC CONTAINER, AMINOPHYLLINE
AMINOSOL 5%, PROTEIN HYDROLYSATE
AMINOSYN II 10%, AMINO ACIDS
AMINOSYN II 10% W/ ELECTROLYTES, AMINO ACIDS
AMINOSYN II 3.5%, AMINO ACIDS
AMINOSYN II 3.5% IN DEXTROSE 25%, AMINO ACIDS
AMINOSYN II 3.5% IN DEXTROSE 5%, AMINO ACIDS
AMINOSYN II 3.5% M, AMINO ACIDS
AMINOSYN II 3.5% M IN DEXTROSE 5%, AMINO ACIDS
AMINOSYN II 3.5% W/ ELECTROLYTES IN DEXTROSE 25%, AMINO ACID
AMINOSYN II 4.25% IN DEXTROSE 25%, AMINO ACIDS
AMINOSYN II 4.25% M IN DEXTROSE 10%, AMINO ACIDS
AMINOSYN II 4.25% W/ ELECTROLYTES IN DEXTROSE 25%, AMINO ACIDS
AMINOSYN II 5%, AMINO ACIDS
AMINOSYN II 5% IN DEXTROSE 25%, AMINO ACIDS
AMINOSYN II 7%, AMINO ACIDS
AMINOSYN II 7% W/ ELECTROLYTES, AMINO ACIDS
AMINOSYN II 8.5%, AMINO ACIDS
AMINOSYN II 8.5% W/ ELECTROLYTES, AMINO ACIDS
AMINOSYN 10%, AMINO ACIDS
AMINOSYN 10% (PH6), AMINO ACIDS
AMINOSYN 3.5%, AMINO ACIDS
AMINOSYN 3.5% IN PLASTIC CONTAINER, AMINO ACIDS
AMINOSYN 3.5% M, AMINO ACIDS
AMINOSYN 3.5% M IN PLASTIC CONTAINER, AMINO ACIDS
AMINOSYN 3.5% W/ DEXTROSE 25% IN PLASTIC CONTAINER, AMINO ACIDS
AMINOSYN 3.5% W/ DEXTROSE 5% IN PLASTIC CONTAINER, AMINO ACIDS
AMINOSYN 4.25% W/ DEXTROSE 25% IN PLASTIC CONTAINER, AMINO ACIDS
AMINOSYN 5%, AMINO ACIDS
AMINOSYN 7%, AMINO ACIDS
AMINOSYN 7% (PH6), AMINO ACIDS
AMINOSYN 7% W/ ELECTROLYTES, AMINO ACIDS
AMINOSYN 8.5%, AMINO ACIDS
AMINOSYN 8.5% (PH6), AMINO ACIDS
AMINOSYN 8.5% W/ ELECTROLYTES, AMINO ACIDS
AMINOSYN-HBC 7% IN PLASTIC CONTAINER, AMINO ACIDS
AMINOSYN-PF 10%, AMINO ACIDS
AMINOSYN-PF 7%, AMINO ACIDS
AMINOSYN-RF 5.2%, AMINO ACIDS
AMMONIUM CHLORIDE, AMMONIUM CHLORIDE
AMMONIUM CHLORIDE IN PLASTIC CONTAINER, AMMONIUM CHLORIDE
BACTERIOSTATIC SODIUM CHLORIDE 0.9%, SODIUM CHLORIDE
BACTERIOSTATIC WATER FOR INJECTION, WATER FOR INJECTION, STERILE
BIAXIN, CLARITHROMYCIN
BRETYLIUM TOSYLATE, BRETYLIUM TOSYLATE
BRETYLIUM TOSYLATE IN DEXTROSE 5%, BRETYLIUM TOSYLATE
BRETYLIUM TOSYLATE IN DEXTROSE 5% IN PLASTIC CONTAINER, BRETYLIUM TOSYLATE
BUPIVACAINE, BUPIVACAINE HYDROCHLORIDE
BUPIVACAINE HCL, BUPIVACAINE HYDROCHLORIDE
CALCIUM GLUCEPTATE, CALCIUM GLUCEPTATE
CARTROL, CARTEOLOL HYDROCHLORIDE
CEPHALOTHIN SODIUM, CEPHALOTHIN SODIUM
CHLOROPROCAINE HCL, CHLOROPROCAINE HYDROCHLORIDE
CHLORTHALIDONE, CHLORTHALIDONE
CLINDAMYCIN PHOSPHATE, CLINDAMYCIN PHOSPHATE
CYLERT, PEMOLINE
DEPAKENE, VALPROIC ACID
DEPAKOTE, DIVALPROEX SODIUM
DEPAKOTE CP, DIVALPROEX SODIUM
DESOXYN, METHAMPHETAMINE HYDROCHLORIDE
DEXTROSE 10% IN PLASTIC CONTAINER, DEXTROSE
DEXTROSE 2.5% AND SODIUM CHLORIDE 0.45% IN PLASTIC CONTAINER, DEXTROSE
DEXTROSE 20% IN PLASTIC CONTAINER, DEXTROSE
DEXTROSE 3.3% AND SODIUM CHLORIDE 0.3% IN PLASTIC CONTAINER, DEXTROSE
DEXTROSE 30% IN PLASTIC CONTAINER, DEXTROSE
DEXTROSE 38.5% IN PLASTIC CONTAINER, DEXTROSE
DEXTROSE 40% IN PLASTIC CONTAINER, DEXTROSE
DEXTROSE 5%, DEXTROSE
DEXTROSE 5% AND LACTATED RINGER'S IN PLASTIC CONTAINER, CALCIUM CHLORIDE
DEXTROSE 5% AND RINGER'S IN PLASTIC CONTAINER, CALCIUM CHLORIDE
DEXTROSE 5% AND SODIUM CHLORIDE 0.225%, DEXTROSE

APPENDIX B
PRODUCT NAME INDEX
LISTED BY APPLICANT *(continued)*

DEXTROSE 5% AND SODIUM CHLORIDE 0.225% IN PLASTIC CONTAINER, DEXTROSE
DEXTROSE 5% AND SODIUM CHLORIDE 0.3%, DEXTROSE
DEXTROSE 5% AND SODIUM CHLORIDE 0.3% IN PLASTIC CONTAINER, DEXTROSE
DEXTROSE 5% AND SODIUM CHLORIDE 0.45%, DEXTROSE
DEXTROSE 5% AND SODIUM CHLORIDE 0.45% IN PLASTIC CONTAINER, DEXTROSE
DEXTROSE 5% AND SODIUM CHLORIDE 0.9%, DEXTROSE
DEXTROSE 5% AND SODIUM CHLORIDE 0.9% IN PLASTIC CONTAINER, DEXTROSE
DEXTROSE 5% IN PLASTIC CONTAINER, DEXTROSE
DEXTROSE 50% IN PLASTIC CONTAINER, DEXTROSE
DEXTROSE 60% IN PLASTIC CONTAINER, DEXTROSE
DEXTROSE 70% IN PLASTIC CONTAINER, DEXTROSE
DIASONE SODIUM, SULFOXONE SODIUM
DICUMAROL, DICUMAROL
DOPAMINE HCL, DOPAMINE HYDROCHLORIDE
DOPAMINE HCL IN DEXTROSE 5%, DOPAMINE HYDROCHLORIDE
DROPERIDOL, DROPERIDOL
E.E.S., ERYTHROMYCIN ETHYLSUCCINATE
E.E.S. 200, ERYTHROMYCIN ETHYLSUCCINATE
E.E.S. 400, ERYTHROMYCIN ETHYLSUCCINATE
ENDRATE, EDETATE DISODIUM
ENDURON, METHYCLOTHIAZIDE
ENDURONYL, DESERPIDINE
ENDURONYL FORTE, DESERPIDINE
ENFLURANE, ENFLURANE
ERY-TAB, ERYTHROMYCIN
ERYDERM, ERYTHROMYCIN
ERYPED, ERYTHROMYCIN ETHYLSUCCINATE
ERYTHROCIN, ERYTHROMYCIN LACTOBIONATE
ERYTHROCIN STEARATE, ERYTHROMYCIN STEARATE
ERYTHROMYCIN, ERYTHROMYCIN
EUTONYL, PARGYLINE HYDROCHLORIDE
EUTRON, METHYCLOTHIAZIDE
FENTANYL CITRATE, FENTANYL CITRATE
FUROSEMIDE, FUROSEMIDE
GEMONIL, METHARBITAL
GENTAMICIN SULFATE, GENTAMICIN SULFATE
GENTAMICIN SULFATE IN SODIUM CHLORIDE 0.9%, GENTAMICIN SULFATE
GLYCINE 1.5%, GLYCINE
GLYCINE 1.5% IN PLASTIC CONTAINER, GLYCINE
GLYCOPYRROLATE, GLYCOPYRROLATE
HALOTHANE, HALOTHANE
HARMONYL, DESERPIDINE
HEPARIN SODIUM 10,000 UNITS IN DEXTROSE 5%, HEPARIN SODIUM
HEPARIN SODIUM 10,000 UNITS IN DEXTROSE 5% IN PLASTIC CONTAINER, HEPARIN SODIUM
HEPARIN SODIUM 10,000 UNITS IN SODIUM CHLORIDE 0.45%, HEPARIN SODIUM
HEPARIN SODIUM 10,000 UNITS IN SODIUM CHLORIDE 0.9%, HEPARIN SODIUM
HEPARIN SODIUM 1000 UNITS IN SODIUM CHLORIDE 0.9%, HEPARIN SODIUM
HEPARIN SODIUM 12,500 UNITS IN DEXTROSE 5%, HEPARIN SODIUM
HEPARIN SODIUM 12,500 UNITS IN DEXTROSE 5% IN PLASTIC CONTAINER, HEPARIN SODIUM
HEPARIN SODIUM 12,500 UNITS IN SODIUM CHLORIDE 0.45%, HEPARIN SODIUM
HEPARIN SODIUM 12,500 UNITS IN SODIUM CHLORIDE 0.9%, HEPARIN SODIUM
HEPARIN SODIUM 2000 UNITS IN SODIUM CHLORIDE 0.9%, HEPARIN SODIUM
HEPARIN SODIUM 25,000 UNITS IN DEXTROSE 5%, HEPARIN SODIUM
HEPARIN SODIUM 25,000 UNITS IN DEXTROSE 5% IN PLASTIC CONTAINER, HEPARIN SODIUM
HEPARIN SODIUM 25,000 UNITS IN SODIUM CHLORIDE 0.45%, HEPARIN SODIUM
HEPARIN SODIUM 25,000 UNITS IN SODIUM CHLORIDE 0.9%, HEPARIN SODIUM
HEPARIN SODIUM 5,000 UNITS IN SODIUM CHLORIDE 0.45%, HEPARIN SODIUM
HEPARIN SODIUM 5000 UNITS IN SODIUM CHLORIDE 0.45%, HEPARIN SODIUM
HEPARIN SODIUM 5000 UNITS IN SODIUM CHLORIDE 0.9%, HEPARIN SODIUM
HYDROXYZINE HCL, HYDROXYZINE HYDROCHLORIDE
HYTRIN, TERAZOSIN HYDROCHLORIDE
INPERSOL W/ DEXTROSE 1.5%, CALCIUM CHLORIDE
INPERSOL W/ DEXTROSE 2.5%, CALCIUM CHLORIDE
INPERSOL W/ DEXTROSE 3.5%, CALCIUM CHLORIDE
INPERSOL W/ DEXTROSE 4.25%, CALCIUM CHLORIDE
INPERSOL-LM W/ DEXTROSE 1.5%, CALCIUM CHLORIDE
INPERSOL-LM W/ DEXTROSE 2.5%, CALCIUM CHLORIDE
INPERSOL-LM W/ DEXTROSE 3.5%, CALCIUM CHLORIDE
INPERSOL-LM W/ DEXTROSE 4.25%, CALCIUM CHLORIDE
INPERSOL-ZM W/ DEXTROSE 1.5% IN PLASTIC CONTAINER, CALCIUM CHLORIDE
INPERSOL-ZM W/ DEXTROSE 2.5% IN PLASTIC CONTAINER, CALCIUM CHLORIDE
INPERSOL-ZM W/ DEXTROSE 4.25% IN PLASTIC CONTAINER, CALCIUM CHLORIDE
IONOSOL B AND DEXTROSE 5%, DEXTROSE
IONOSOL MB AND DEXTROSE 5%, DEXTROSE
IONOSOL T AND DEXTROSE 5%, DEXTROSE
ISOPROTERENOL HCL, ISOPROTERENOL HYDROCHLORIDE
JANIMINE, IMIPRAMINE HYDROCHLORIDE
K-TAB, POTASSIUM CHLORIDE
LACTATED RINGER'S, CALCIUM CHLORIDE
LACTATED RINGER'S IN PLASTIC CONTAINER, CALCIUM CHLORIDE
LIDOCAINE HCL, LIDOCAINE HYDROCHLORIDE
LIDOCAINE HCL AND DEXTROSE 7.5%, LIDOCAINE HYDROCHLORIDE
LIDOCAINE HCL AND EPINEPHRINE, EPINEPHRINE
LIDOCAINE HCL IN PLASTIC CONTAINER, LIDOCAINE HYDROCHLORIDE
LIDOCAINE HCL W/ EPINEPHRINE, EPINEPHRINE
LIDOCAINE HCL 0.2% IN DEXTROSE 5%, LIDOCAINE HYDROCHLORIDE
LIDOCAINE HCL 0.2% IN DEXTROSE 5% IN PLASTIC CONTAINER, LIDOCAINE HYDROCHLORIDE
LIDOCAINE HCL 0.4% IN DEXTROSE 5%, LIDOCAINE HYDROCHLORIDE
LIDOCAINE HCL 0.4% IN DEXTROSE 5% IN PLASTIC CONTAINER, LIDOCAINE HYDROCHLORIDE
LIDOCAINE HCL 0.8% IN DEXTROSE 5% IN PLASTIC CONTAINER, LIDOCAINE HYDROCHLORIDE
LIPOSYN II 10%, SAFFLOWER OIL

APPENDIX B
PRODUCT NAME INDEX
LISTED BY APPLICANT *(continued)*

LIPOSYN II 20%, SAFFLOWER OIL
LIPOSYN III 10%, SOYBEAN OIL
LIPOSYN III 20%, SOYBEAN OIL
LIPOSYN 10%, SAFFLOWER OIL
LIPOSYN 20%, SAFFLOWER OIL
LTA II KIT, LIDOCAINE HYDROCHLORIDE
MANNITOL 10%, MANNITOL
MANNITOL 15%, MANNITOL
MANNITOL 20%, MANNITOL
MANNITOL 25%, MANNITOL
MANNITOL 5%, MANNITOL
MEPERIDINE HCL, MEPERIDINE HYDROCHLORIDE
METHYLDOPATE HCL, METHYLDOPATE HYDROCHLORIDE
METRONIDAZOLE, METRONIDAZOLE
MORPHINE SULFATE, MORPHINE SULFATE
NALOXONE HCL, NALOXONE HYDROCHLORIDE
NEMBUTAL, PENTOBARBITAL
NEMBUTAL, PENTOBARBITAL SODIUM
NEMBUTAL SODIUM, PENTOBARBITAL SODIUM
NITROGLYCERIN, NITROGLYCERIN
NITROPRESS, SODIUM NITROPRUSSIDE
NORISODRINE, ISOPROTERENOL SULFATE
NORISODRINE AEROTROL, ISOPROTERENOL HYDROCHLORIDE
NORMOSOL-M AND DEXTROSE 5%, DEXTROSE
NORMOSOL-R AND DEXTROSE 5% IN PLASTIC CONTAINER, DEXTROSE
NORMOSOL-R IN PLASTIC CONTAINER, MAGNESIUM CHLORIDE
OCL, POLYETHYLENE GLYCOL 3350
OGEN, ESTROPIPATE
OGEN .625, ESTROPIPATE
OGEN 1.25, ESTROPIPATE
OGEN 2.5, ESTROPIPATE
OGEN 5, ESTROPIPATE
OMNIFLOX, TEMAFLOXACIN HYDROCHLORIDE
ORETIC, HYDROCHLOROTHIAZIDE
ORETICYL FORTE, DESERPIDINE
ORETICYL 25, DESERPIDINE
ORETICYL 50, DESERPIDINE
OXYTOCIN 10 USP UNITS IN DEXTROSE 5%, OXYTOCIN
OXYTOCIN 20 USP UNITS IN DEXTROSE 5%, OXYTOCIN
OXYTOCIN 5 USP UNITS IN DEXTROSE 5%, OXYTOCIN
PANWARFIN, WARFARIN SODIUM
PARADIONE, PARAMETHADIONE
PCE, ERYTHROMYCIN
PEDIATRIC LTA KIT, LIDOCAINE HYDROCHLORIDE
PEGANONE, ETHOTOIN
PHENURONE, PHENACEMIDE
PHENYTOIN SODIUM, PHENYTOIN SODIUM
PHYSIOSOL IN PLASTIC CONTAINER, MAGNESIUM CHLORIDE
PHYSIOSOL PH 7.4, MAGNESIUM CHLORIDE
PLACIDYL, ETHCHLORVYNOL
PLEGISOL, CALCIUM CHLORIDE
POTASSIUM CHLORIDE, POTASSIUM CHLORIDE
POTASSIUM CHLORIDE 10 MEQ IN DEXTROSE 5% AND SODIUM CHLORIDE 0.225%, DEXTROSE
POTASSIUM CHLORIDE 10 MEQ IN DEXTROSE 5% AND SODIUM CHLORIDE 0.3%, DEXTROSE
POTASSIUM CHLORIDE 10 MEQ IN DEXTROSE 5% AND SODIUM CHLORIDE 0.45%, DEXTROSE
POTASSIUM CHLORIDE 10 MEQ IN DEXTROSE 5% AND SODIUM CHLORIDE 0.9%, DEXTROSE
POTASSIUM CHLORIDE 15 MEQ IN DEXTROSE 5% AND SODIUM CHLORIDE 0.225%, DEXTROSE
POTASSIUM CHLORIDE 15 MEQ IN DEXTROSE 5% AND SODIUM CHLORIDE 0.3%, DEXTROSE
POTASSIUM CHLORIDE 15 MEQ IN DEXTROSE 5% AND SODIUM CHLORIDE 0.45%, DEXTROSE
POTASSIUM CHLORIDE 15 MEQ IN DEXTROSE 5% AND SODIUM CHLORIDE 0.9%, DEXTROSE
POTASSIUM CHLORIDE 20 MEQ IN DEXTROSE 5%, DEXTROSE
POTASSIUM CHLORIDE 20 MEQ IN DEXTROSE 5% AND SODIUM CHLORIDE 0.225%, DEXTROSE
POTASSIUM CHLORIDE 20 MEQ IN DEXTROSE 5% AND SODIUM CHLORIDE 0.3%, DEXTROSE
POTASSIUM CHLORIDE 20 MEQ IN DEXTROSE 5% AND SODIUM CHLORIDE 0.45%, DEXTROSE
POTASSIUM CHLORIDE 20 MEQ IN DEXTROSE 5% AND SODIUM CHLORIDE 0.9%, DEXTROSE
POTASSIUM CHLORIDE 20 MEQ IN DEXTROSE 5% IN SODIUM CHLORIDE 0.3%, DEXTROSE
POTASSIUM CHLORIDE 30 MEQ IN DEXTROSE 5%, DEXTROSE
POTASSIUM CHLORIDE 30 MEQ IN DEXTROSE 5% AND SODIUM CHLORIDE 0.225%, DEXTROSE
POTASSIUM CHLORIDE 30 MEQ IN DEXTROSE 5% AND SODIUM CHLORIDE 0.3%, DEXTROSE
POTASSIUM CHLORIDE 30 MEQ IN DEXTROSE 5% AND SODIUM CHLORIDE 0.45%, DEXTROSE
POTASSIUM CHLORIDE 30 MEQ IN DEXTROSE 5% AND SODIUM CHLORIDE 0.9%, DEXTROSE
POTASSIUM CHLORIDE 40 MEQ IN DEXTROSE 5%, DEXTROSE
POTASSIUM CHLORIDE 40 MEQ IN DEXTROSE 5% AND SODIUM CHLORIDE 0.225%, DEXTROSE
POTASSIUM CHLORIDE 40 MEQ IN DEXTROSE 5% AND SODIUM CHLORIDE 0.3%, DEXTROSE
POTASSIUM CHLORIDE 40 MEQ IN DEXTROSE 5% AND SODIUM CHLORIDE 0.45%, DEXTROSE
POTASSIUM CHLORIDE 40 MEQ IN DEXTROSE 5% AND SODIUM CHLORIDE 0.9%, DEXTROSE
POTASSIUM CHLORIDE 5 MEQ IN DEXTROSE 5% AND SODIUM CHLORIDE 0.225%, DEXTROSE
POTASSIUM CHLORIDE 5 MEQ IN DEXTROSE 5% AND SODIUM CHLORIDE 0.3%, DEXTROSE
POTASSIUM CHLORIDE 5 MEQ IN DEXTROSE 5% AND SODIUM CHLORIDE 0.45%, DEXTROSE
POTASSIUM CHLORIDE 5 MEQ IN DEXTROSE 5% AND SODIUM CHLORIDE 0.9%, DEXTROSE
PROCAINAMIDE HCL, PROCAINAMIDE HYDROCHLORIDE
PROCAINE HCL, PROCAINE HYDROCHLORIDE
PROSOM, ESTAZOLAM
RADIONUCLIDE-LABELED (125 I) FIBRINOGEN (HUMAN) SENSOR, FIBRINOGEN, I-125
RINGER'S IN PLASTIC CONTAINER, CALCIUM CHLORIDE
SELSUN, SELENIUM SULFIDE
SODIUM BICARBONATE IN PLASTIC CONTAINER, SODIUM BICARBONATE
SODIUM CHLORIDE, SODIUM CHLORIDE
SODIUM CHLORIDE 0.45% IN PLASTIC CONTAINER, SODIUM CHLORIDE
SODIUM CHLORIDE 0.9%, SODIUM CHLORIDE
SODIUM CHLORIDE 0.9% IN PLASTIC CONTAINER, SODIUM CHLORIDE
SODIUM LACTATE 0.167 MOLAR IN PLASTIC CONTAINER, SODIUM LACTATE

APPENDIX B
PRODUCT NAME INDEX
LISTED BY APPLICANT *(continued)*

SORBITOL-MANNITOL, MANNITOL
SORBITOL-MANNITOL IN PLASTIC CONTAINER, MANNITOL
STERILE UREA, UREA
STERILE WATER, WATER FOR IRRIGATION, STERILE
STERILE WATER FOR INJECTION, WATER FOR INJECTION, STERILE
STERILE WATER IN PLASTIC CONTAINER, WATER FOR IRRIGATION, STERILE
SULFADIAZINE, SULFADIAZINE
THEOPHYLLINE IN DEXTROSE 5%, THEOPHYLLINE
THEOPHYLLINE IN DEXTROSE 5% IN PLASTIC CONTAINER, THEOPHYLLINE
THYPINONE, PROTIRELIN
TPN ELECTROLYTES IN PLASTIC CONTAINER, CALCIUM CHLORIDE
TRAL, HEXOCYCLIUM METHYLSULFATE
TRANXENE, CLORAZEPATE DIPOTASSIUM
TRANXENE SD, CLORAZEPATE DIPOTASSIUM
TRIDIONE, TRIMETHADIONE
UROLOGIC G IN PLASTIC CONTAINER, CITRIC ACID
VERAPAMIL HCL, VERAPAMIL HYDROCHLORIDE
VERCYTE, PIPOBROMAN
VITAMIN K1, PHYTONADIONE

ABIC
* ABIC LTD
ABITREXATE, METHOTREXATE SODIUM
FLUOROURACIL, FLUOROURACIL
LEUCOVORIN CALCIUM, LEUCOVORIN CALCIUM
VINCRISTINE SULFATE, VINCRISTINE SULFATE

ABLE
* ABLE LABORATORIES INC
CLORAZEPATE DIPOTASSIUM, CLORAZEPATE DIPOTASSIUM
HEMSOL-HC, HYDROCORTISONE ACETATE
LOPERAMIDE HCL, LOPERAMIDE HYDROCHLORIDE
MICONAZOLE NITRATE, MICONAZOLE NITRATE

ADV CARE
* ADVANCED CARE PRODUCTS DIV ORTHO PHARMACEUTICAL CORP
MONISTAT 7 COMBINATION PACK, MICONAZOLE NITRATE

AKORN
* AKORN INC
AK-PENTOLATE, CYCLOPENTOLATE HYDROCHLORIDE
CHLORAMPHENICOL, CHLORAMPHENICOL
COR-OTICIN, HYDROCORTISONE ACETATE
CYANOCOBALAMIN, CYANOCOBALAMIN
DEXAMETHASONE SODIUM PHOSPHATE, DEXAMETHASONE SODIUM PHOSPHATE
GENTAMICIN SULFATE, GENTAMICIN SULFATE
HEPARIN SODIUM, HEPARIN SODIUM
HYDROCORTISONE ACETATE, HYDROCORTISONE ACETATE
HYDROXYPROGESTERONE CAPROATE, HYDROXYPROGESTERONE CAPROATE
LIDOCAINE HCL, LIDOCAINE HYDROCHLORIDE
METHYLPREDNISOLONE ACETATE, METHYLPREDNISOLONE ACETATE
NANDROLONE DECANOATE, NANDROLONE DECANOATE
NAPHAZOLINE HCL, NAPHAZOLINE HYDROCHLORIDE
POTASSIUM CHLORIDE, POTASSIUM CHLORIDE
PREDAMIDE, PREDNISOLONE ACETATE
PREDNISOLONE ACETATE, PREDNISOLONE ACETATE
PREDNISOLONE SODIUM PHOSPHATE, PREDNISOLONE SODIUM PHOSPHATE
PROMETHAZINE HCL, PROMETHAZINE HYDROCHLORIDE
PYRIDOXINE HCL, PYRIDOXINE HYDROCHLORIDE
SODIUM SULFACETAMIDE, SULFACETAMIDE SODIUM
THIAMINE HCL, THIAMINE HYDROCHLORIDE
TRIAMCINOLONE DIACETATE, TRIAMCINOLONE DIACETATE
TROPICAMIDE, TROPICAMIDE

ALCON
* ALCON LABORATORIES INC
ALCAINE, PROPARACAINE HYDROCHLORIDE
ALOMIDE, LODOXAMIDE TROMETHAMINE
ANESTACON, LIDOCAINE HYDROCHLORIDE
BETOPTIC, BETAXOLOL HYDROCHLORIDE
BETOPTIC S, BETAXOLOL HYDROCHLORIDE
BSS PLUS, CALCIUM CHLORIDE
CETAMIDE, SULFACETAMIDE SODIUM
CETAPRED, PREDNISOLONE ACETATE
CILOXAN, CIPROFLOXACIN HYDROCHLORIDE
CYCLOGYL, CYCLOPENTOLATE HYDROCHLORIDE
CYCLOMYDRIL, CYCLOPENTOLATE HYDROCHLORIDE
DENDRID, IDOXURIDINE
DIPIVEFRIN HCL, DIPIVEFRIN HYDROCHLORIDE
ECONOCHLOR, CHLORAMPHENICOL
ECONOPRED, PREDNISOLONE ACETATE
ECONOPRED PLUS, PREDNISOLONE ACETATE
FLAREX, FLUOROMETHOLONE ACETATE
IOPIDINE, APRACLONIDINE HYDROCHLORIDE
ISMOTIC, ISOSORBIDE
ISOPTO CETAMIDE, SULFACETAMIDE SODIUM
ISOPTO CETAPRED, PREDNISOLONE ACETATE
MAXIDEX, DEXAMETHASONE
MAXIDEX, DEXAMETHASONE SODIUM PHOSPHATE
MAXITROL, DEXAMETHASONE
MIOSTAT, CARBACHOL
MYDRIACYL, TROPICAMIDE
NAPHCON FORTE, NAPHAZOLINE HYDROCHLORIDE
NAPHCON-A, NAPHAZOLINE HYDROCHLORIDE
NATACYN, NATAMYCIN
PANTOPAQUE, IOPHENDYLATE
PILOPINE HS, PILOCARPINE HYDROCHLORIDE
PROFENAL, SUPROFEN
STATROL, NEOMYCIN SULFATE
TOBRADEX, DEXAMETHASONE
TOBRASONE, FLUOROMETHOLONE ACETATE
TOBREX, TOBRAMYCIN
ZOLYSE, CHYMOTRYPSIN

ALLERGAN
* ALLERGAN INC
OCUFLOX, OFLOXACIN
* ALLERGAN MEDICAL OPTICS
ENDOSOL EXTRA, CALCIUM CHLORIDE
* ALLERGAN PHARMACEUTICAL
ALBALON, NAPHAZOLINE HYDROCHLORIDE
BETAGAN, LEVOBUNOLOL HYDROCHLORIDE
BLEPH-10, SULFACETAMIDE SODIUM
BLEPH-30, SULFACETAMIDE SODIUM
BLEPHAMIDE, PREDNISOLONE ACETATE
BLEPHAMIDE S.O.P., PREDNISOLONE ACETATE

APPENDIX B
PRODUCT NAME INDEX
LISTED BY APPLICANT *(continued)*

CHLOROPTIC, CHLORAMPHENICOL
CHLOROPTIC S.O.P., CHLORAMPHENICOL
CHLOROPTIC-P S.O.P., CHLORAMPHENICOL
ETHAMIDE, ETHOXZOLAMIDE
FML, FLUOROMETHOLONE
FML FORTE, FLUOROMETHOLONE
FML-S, FLUOROMETHOLONE
GENOPTIC, GENTAMICIN SULFATE
HERPLEX, IDOXURIDINE
HMS, MEDRYSONE
OCUFEN, FLURBIPROFEN SODIUM
OPHTHETIC, PROPARACAINE HYDROCHLORIDE
PAREMYD, HYDROXYAMPHETAMINE HYDROBROMIDE
POLY-PRED, NEOMYCIN SULFATE
POLYTRIM, POLYMYXIN B SULFATE
PRED FORTE, PREDNISOLONE ACETATE
PRED MILD, PREDNISOLONE ACETATE
PRED-G, GENTAMICIN SULFATE
PREFRIN-A, PHENYLEPHRINE HYDROCHLORIDE
PROPINE, DIPIVEFRIN HYDROCHLORIDE

ALLERGAN HERBERT
* ALLERGAN HERBERT DIV ALLERGAN INC
AEROSEB-DEX, DEXAMETHASONE
AEROSEB-HC, HYDROCORTISONE
ERYGEL, ERYTHROMYCIN
ERYMAX, ERYTHROMYCIN
EXSEL, SELENIUM SULFIDE
FLUONID, FLUOCINOLONE ACETONIDE
FLUOROPLEX, FLUOROURACIL
GRIS-PEG, GRISEOFULVIN, ULTRAMICROCRYSTALLINE
PENECORT, HYDROCORTISONE
PHOTOPLEX, AVOBENZONE (OTC)
* ALLERGAN HERBERT SKIN CARE DIV ALLERGAN INC
FLUOROPLEX, FLUOROURACIL
NAFTIN, NAFTIFINE HYDROCHLORIDE
PENECORT, HYDROCORTISONE
TEMARIL, TRIMEPRAZINE TARTRATE

ALLIANCE PHARM
* ALLIANCE PHARMACEUTICAL CORP
IMAGENT, PERFLUBRON

ALPHA THERAPEUTIC
* ALPHA THERAPEUTIC CORP
SOYACAL 10%, SOYBEAN OIL
SOYACAL 20%, SOYBEAN OIL

ALPHAPHARM
* ALPHAPHARM PARTY LTD
ALPRAZOLAM, ALPRAZOLAM
TRIAZOLAM, TRIAZOLAM

ALRA
* ALRA LABORATORIES INC
ACETAZOLAMIDE, ACETAZOLAMIDE
BAMATE, MEPROBAMATE
CHOLAC, LACTULOSE
COMPOUND 65, ASPIRIN
CONSTILAC, LACTULOSE
DIMENHYDRINATE, DIMENHYDRINATE
DIPHENHYDRAMINE HCL, DIPHENHYDRAMINE HYDROCHLORIDE
ERYZOLE, ERYTHROMYCIN ETHYLSUCCINATE
GEN-XENE, CLORAZEPATE DIPOTASSIUM
HYDROCHLOROTHIAZIDE, HYDROCHLOROTHIAZIDE
IBU-TAB, IBUPROFEN
IBU-TAB 200, IBUPROFEN (OTC)
K+10, POTASSIUM CHLORIDE
K+8, POTASSIUM CHLORIDE
LYGEN, CHLORDIAZEPOXIDE HYDROCHLORIDE
PRAMINE, IMIPRAMINE HYDROCHLORIDE
PROPOXYPHENE HCL, PROPOXYPHENE HYDROCHLORIDE
SOXAZOLE, SULFISOXAZOLE
TOLBUTAMIDE, TOLBUTAMIDE

ALTANA
* ALTANA INC
BACITRACIN, BACITRACIN
BACITRACIN-NEOMYCIN-POLYMYXIN, BACITRACIN ZINC
BACITRACIN-NEOMYCIN-POLYMYXIN W/ HYDROCORTISONE ACETATE, BACITRACIN
CHLORAMPHENICOL, CHLORAMPHENICOL
HYDROCORTISONE, HYDROCORTISONE
HYDROCORTISONE ACETATE, HYDROCORTISONE ACETATE
HYDROXYZINE HCL, HYDROXYZINE HYDROCHLORIDE
NITROGLYCERIN, NITROGLYCERIN
NYSTATIN, NYSTATIN
SULFACETAMIDE SODIUM, SULFACETAMIDE SODIUM
TRIAMCINOLONE ACETONIDE, TRIAMCINOLONE ACETONIDE
ZIPAN-25, PROMETHAZINE HYDROCHLORIDE
ZIPAN-50, PROMETHAZINE HYDROCHLORIDE

ALZA
* ALZA CORP
DURAGESIC, FENTANYL
OCUSERT PILO-20, PILOCARPINE
OCUSERT PILO-40, PILOCARPINE
PROGESTASERT, PROGESTERONE
TESTODERM, TESTOSTERONE

AM THERAP
* AMERICAN THERAPEUTICS INC
ACETAMINOPHEN AND CODEINE PHOSPHATE NO. 2, ACETAMINOPHEN
ACETAMINOPHEN AND CODEINE PHOSPHATE NO. 3, ACETAMINOPHEN
ACETAMINOPHEN AND CODEINE PHOSPHATE NO. 4, ACETAMINOPHEN
ALBUTEROL SULFATE, ALBUTEROL SULFATE
AMITRIPTYLINE HCL, AMITRIPTYLINE HYDROCHLORIDE
CLONIDINE HCL, CLONIDINE HYDROCHLORIDE
CLORAZEPATE DIPOTASSIUM, CLORAZEPATE DIPOTASSIUM
CYPROHEPTADINE HCL, CYPROHEPTADINE HYDROCHLORIDE
DANAZOL, DANAZOL
FENOPROFEN CALCIUM, FENOPROFEN CALCIUM
LORAZEPAM, LORAZEPAM
MAPROTILINE HCL, MAPROTILINE HYDROCHLORIDE
MECLOFENAMATE SODIUM, MECLOFENAMATE SODIUM
METAPROTERENOL SULFATE, METAPROTERENOL SULFATE
METHOCARBAMOL, METHOCARBAMOL
OXAZEPAM, OXAZEPAM
PRAZOSIN HCL, PRAZOSIN HYDROCHLORIDE

APPENDIX B
PRODUCT NAME INDEX
LISTED BY APPLICANT *(continued)*

PREDNISONE, PREDNISONE
THIOTHIXENE, THIOTHIXENE
TRAZODONE HCL, TRAZODONE HYDROCHLORIDE
TRIAMTERENE AND HYDROCHLOROTHIAZIDE, HYDROCHLOROTHIAZIDE

AMBIX
* AMBIX LABORATORIES DIV ORGANICS CORP AMERICA
HYDROCORTISONE, HYDROCORTISONE
NITROFURAZONE, NITROFURAZONE
TRIAMCINOLONE ACETONIDE, TRIAMCINOLONE ACETONIDE

AMERSHAM
* AMERSHAM CORP SUB RADIOCHEMICAL CENTER
AMERSCAN MDP KIT, TECHNETIUM TC-99M MEDRONATE KIT
CERETEC, TECHNETIUM TC-99M EXAMETAZIME KIT
DICOPAC KIT, CYANOCOBALAMIN
IBRIN, FIBRINOGEN, I-125
INDIUM IN-111 OXYQUINOLINE, INDIUM IN-111 OXYQUINOLINE

AMIDE PHARM
* AMIDE PHARMACEUTICAL INC
CHLORZOXAZONE, CHLORZOXAZONE
HYDRALAZINE HCL, HYDRALAZINE HYDROCHLORIDE
HYDROXYZINE HCL, HYDROXYZINE HYDROCHLORIDE

ANABOLIC
* ANABOLIC INC
BROMPHENIRAMINE MALEATE, BROMPHENIRAMINE MALEATE
CHLORPHENIRAMINE MALEATE, CHLORPHENIRAMINE MALEATE
DIMENHYDRINATE, DIMENHYDRINATE
DIPHENHYDRAMINE HCL, DIPHENHYDRAMINE HYDROCHLORIDE
FOLIC ACID, FOLIC ACID
HYDROCORTISONE, HYDROCORTISONE
ISONIAZID, ISONIAZID
MECLIZINE HCL, MECLIZINE HYDROCHLORIDE
MEPROBAMATE, MEPROBAMATE
PHENDIMETRAZINE TARTRATE, PHENDIMETRAZINE TARTRATE
PROPOXYPHENE HCL, PROPOXYPHENE HYDROCHLORIDE
PROPYLTHIOURACIL, PROPYLTHIOURACIL
SODIUM PENTOBARBITAL, PENTOBARBITAL SODIUM
SODIUM SECOBARBITAL, SECOBARBITAL SODIUM
TRIPELENNAMINE HCL, TRIPELENNAMINE HYDROCHLORIDE

ANBEX
* ANBEX INC
IOSAT, POTASSIUM IODIDE (OTC)

ANESTA
* ANESTA CORP
FENTANYL, FENTANYL CITRATE

ANGELINI
* ANGELINI PHARMACEUTICALS INC
REV-EYES, DAPIPRAZOLE HYDROCHLORIDE

ANGUS
* ANGUS CHEMICAL CO
MYCHEL-S, CHLORAMPHENICOL SODIUM SUCCINATE
TETRACHEL, TETRACYCLINE HYDROCHLORIDE

APOTHECON
* APOTHECON INC DIV BRISTOL MYERS SQUIBB
AMIKIN, AMIKACIN SULFATE
BETAPEN-VK, PENICILLIN V POTASSIUM
CEFADROXIL, CEFADROXIL/CEFADROXIL HEMIHYDRATE
CEFADYL, CEPHAPIRIN SODIUM
CEFANEX, CEPHALEXIN
CEPHALEXIN, CEPHALEXIN
DESYREL, TRAZODONE HYDROCHLORIDE
DYNAPEN, DICLOXACILLIN SODIUM
FUNGIZONE, AMPHOTERICIN B
KANTREX, KANAMYCIN SULFATE
KENALOG, TRIAMCINOLONE ACETONIDE
METOPROLOL TARTRATE, METOPROLOL TARTRATE
MUCOMYST, ACETYLCYSTEINE
MYCOLOG-II, NYSTATIN
MYCOSTATIN, NYSTATIN
NAFCIL, NAFCILLIN SODIUM
NYDRAZID, ISONIAZID
PENICILLIN G POTASSIUM, PENICILLIN G POTASSIUM
POLYCILLIN, AMPICILLIN/AMPICILLIN TRIHYDRATE
POLYCILLIN-PRB, AMPICILLIN/AMPICILLIN TRIHYDRATE
POLYMOX, AMOXICILLIN
PRINCIPEN, AMPICILLIN SODIUM
PRINCIPEN, AMPICILLIN/AMPICILLIN TRIHYDRATE
PROLIXIN, FLUPHENAZINE HYDROCHLORIDE
PROLIXIN DECANOATE, FLUPHENAZINE DECANOATE
PROLIXIN ENANTHATE, FLUPHENAZINE ENANTHATE
PRONESTYL, PROCAINAMIDE HYDROCHLORIDE
PROSTAPHLIN, OXACILLIN SODIUM
RAUDIXIN, RAUWOLFIA SERPENTINA
STADOL, BUTORPHANOL TARTRATE
STAPHCILLIN, METHICILLIN SODIUM
TEGOPEN, CLOXACILLIN SODIUM
TOBRAMYCIN SULFATE, TOBRAMYCIN SULFATE
TRIMOX, AMOXICILLIN
ULTRACEF, CEFADROXIL/CEFADROXIL HEMIHYDRATE
VESPRIN, TRIFLUPROMAZINE HYDROCHLORIDE
ZOLICEF, CEFAZOLIN SODIUM
* APOTHECON SUB BRISTOL MYERS SQUIBB CO
ATENOLOL, ATENOLOL
DILTIAZEM HCL, DILTIAZEM HYDROCHLORIDE
KLOTRIX, POTASSIUM CHLORIDE
OXACILLIN SODIUM, OXACILLIN SODIUM
PENICILLIN G POTASSIUM, PENICILLIN G POTASSIUM
PENTIDS '200', PENICILLIN G POTASSIUM
PENTIDS '250', PENICILLIN G POTASSIUM
PENTIDS '400', PENICILLIN G POTASSIUM
PENTIDS '800', PENICILLIN G POTASSIUM
PRINCIPEN '125', AMPICILLIN/AMPICILLIN TRIHYDRATE
PRINCIPEN '250', AMPICILLIN/AMPICILLIN TRIHYDRATE
PRINCIPEN '500', AMPICILLIN/AMPICILLIN TRIHYDRATE
PRINCIPEN W/ PROBENECID, AMPICILLIN/AMPICILLIN TRIHYDRATE
SUMYCIN, TETRACYCLINE HYDROCHLORIDE
TRIMOX, AMOXICILLIN
VEETIDS '125', PENICILLIN V POTASSIUM
VEETIDS '250', PENICILLIN V POTASSIUM

APPENDIX B
PRODUCT NAME INDEX
LISTED BY APPLICANT *(continued)*

VEETIDS '500', PENICILLIN V POTASSIUM
VESPRIN, TRIFLUPROMAZINE

ARBROOK
* ARBROOK INC
GAMOPHEN, HEXACHLOROPHENE

ARCUM
* ARCUM PHARMACEUTICAL CORP
VITAMIN A PALMITATE, VITAMIN A PALMITATE

ARMOUR
* ARMOUR PHARMACEUTICAL CO
ACTHAR GEL-SYNTHETIC, SERACTIDE ACETATE
DEPINAR, CYANOCOBALAMIN
ISOPROTERENOL HCL, ISOPROTERENOL HYDROCHLORIDE
THYTROPAR, THYROTROPIN

ASCHER
* BF ASCHER AND CO INC
DRIZE, CHLORPHENIRAMINE MALEATE
HY-PHEN, ACETAMINOPHEN

ASCOT
* ASCOT HOSP PHARMACEUTICALS INC DIV TRAVENOL LABORATORIES I
ACETAZOLAMIDE, ACETAZOLAMIDE
AMINOPHYLLINE, AMINOPHYLLINE
BETHANECHOL CHLORIDE, BETHANECHOL CHLORIDE
CHLORDIAZEPOXIDE HCL, CHLORDIAZEPOXIDE HYDROCHLORIDE
CHLORTHALIDONE, CHLORTHALIDONE
CYPROHEPTADINE HCL, CYPROHEPTADINE HYDROCHLORIDE
DIPHENOXYLATE HCL AND ATROPINE SULFATE, ATROPINE SULFATE
HYDRALAZINE HCL, HYDRALAZINE HYDROCHLORIDE
HYDROCHLOROTHIAZIDE, HYDROCHLOROTHIAZIDE
METHOCARBAMOL, METHOCARBAMOL
ORPHENADRINE CITRATE, ORPHENADRINE CITRATE
PROCAINAMIDE HCL, PROCAINAMIDE HYDROCHLORIDE
PROPANTHELINE BROMIDE, PROPANTHELINE BROMIDE
QUINIDINE GLUCONATE, QUINIDINE GLUCONATE
SPIRONOLACTONE, SPIRONOLACTONE
SPIRONOLACTONE + HYDROCHLOROTHIAZIDE, HYDROCHLOROTHIAZIDE
SULFAMETHOXAZOLE, SULFAMETHOXAZOLE
TOLBUTAMIDE, TOLBUTAMIDE

ASTA
* ASTA PHARMA AG
MESNEX, MESNA

ASTRA
* ASTRA USA INC
AQUASOL A, VITAMIN A
AQUASOL A, VITAMIN A PALMITATE
ASTRAMORPH PF, MORPHINE SULFATE
BRETYLIUM TOSYLATE, BRETYLIUM TOSYLATE
CITANEST, PRILOCAINE HYDROCHLORIDE
CITANEST FORTE, EPINEPHRINE BITARTRATE
CITANEST PLAIN, PRILOCAINE HYDROCHLORIDE
CLINDAMYCIN PHOSPHATE, CLINDAMYCIN PHOSPHATE
DALGAN, DEZOCINE
DOPAMINE HCL, DOPAMINE HYDROCHLORIDE
DROPERIDOL, DROPERIDOL
DURANEST, EPINEPHRINE
DURANEST, EPINEPHRINE BITARTRATE
DURANEST, ETIDOCAINE HYDROCHLORIDE
DYCLONE, DYCLONINE HYDROCHLORIDE
EMLA, LIDOCAINE
FENTANYL CITRATE AND DROPERIDOL, DROPERIDOL
FOSCAVIR, FOSCARNET SODIUM
FUROSEMIDE, FUROSEMIDE
ISOETHARINE HCL, ISOETHARINE HYDROCHLORIDE
M.V.I.-12, ASCORBIC ACID
M.V.I.-12 LYOPHILIZED, ASCORBIC ACID
MANNITOL 25%, MANNITOL
MEPERIDINE HCL, MEPERIDINE HYDROCHLORIDE
METAPROTERENOL SULFATE, METAPROTERENOL SULFATE
NALBUPHINE HCL, NALBUPHINE HYDROCHLORIDE
NALOXONE HCL, NALOXONE HYDROCHLORIDE
NESACAINE, CHLOROPROCAINE HYDROCHLORIDE
NESACAINE-MPF, CHLOROPROCAINE HYDROCHLORIDE
PANCURONIUM BROMIDE, PANCURONIUM BROMIDE
POLOCAINE, MEPIVACAINE HYDROCHLORIDE
POLOCAINE W/ LEVONORDEFRIN, LEVONORDEFRIN
POLOCAINE-MPF, MEPIVACAINE HYDROCHLORIDE
RHINOCORT, BUDESONIDE
SENSORCAINE, BUPIVACAINE HYDROCHLORIDE
XYLOCAINE, LIDOCAINE
XYLOCAINE, LIDOCAINE HYDROCHLORIDE
XYLOCAINE VISCOUS, LIDOCAINE HYDROCHLORIDE
XYLOCAINE W/ DEXTROSE 7.5%, LIDOCAINE HYDROCHLORIDE
XYLOCAINE W/ EPINEPHRINE, EPINEPHRINE
XYLOCAINE 4%, LIDOCAINE HYDROCHLORIDE
XYLOCAINE 5% W/ GLUCOSE 7.5%, LIDOCAINE HYDROCHLORIDE
YUTOPAR, RITODRINE HYDROCHLORIDE

ASTRA MERCK
* ASTRA MERCK GROUP OF MERCK AND CO INC
PRILOSEC, OMEPRAZOLE

AYERST
* AYERST LABORATORIES INC
PREMARIN, ESTROGENS, CONJUGATED

B

BAKER NORTON
* BAKER NORTON
PROGLYCEM, DIAZOXIDE
* BAKER NORTON PHARMACEUTICALS INC
ACTICORT, HYDROCORTISONE
TOLMETIN SODIUM, TOLMETIN SODIUM
VERAPAMIL HCL, VERAPAMIL HYDROCHLORIDE

BANNER PHARMACAPS
* BANNER PHARMACAPS INC
BENZONATATE, BENZONATATE
CHLOROTRIANISENE, CHLOROTRIANISENE
CLOFIBRATE, CLOFIBRATE
ETHCHLORVYNOL, ETHCHLORVYNOL

APPENDIX B
PRODUCT NAME INDEX
LISTED BY APPLICANT *(continued)*

VALPROIC ACID, VALPROIC ACID
VITAMIN A, VITAMIN A
VITAMIN A, VITAMIN A PALMITATE
VITAMIN A PALMITATE, VITAMIN A PALMITATE
VITAMIN D, ERGOCALCIFEROL

BARLAN
* BARLAN PHARMACAL CO INC
BARSTATIN 100, NYSTATIN

BARR
* BARR LABORATORIES INC
ACETAMINOPHEN AND CODEINE PHOSPHATE, ACETAMINOPHEN
ACETAMINOPHEN W/ CODEINE, ACETAMINOPHEN
ACETOHEXAMIDE, ACETOHEXAMIDE
ALLOPURINOL, ALLOPURINOL
AMILORIDE HCL AND HYDROCHLOROTHIAZIDE, AMILORIDE HYDROCHLORIDE
AMINOPHYLLINE, AMINOPHYLLINE
AMITRIPTYLINE HCL, AMITRIPTYLINE HYDROCHLORIDE
BROMPHENIRAMINE MALEATE, BROMPHENIRAMINE MALEATE
CEPHALEXIN, CEPHALEXIN
CEPHRADINE, CEPHRADINE
CHLORDIAZEPOXIDE AND AMITRIPTYLINE HCL, AMITRIPTYLINE HYDROCHLORIDE
CHLORDIAZEPOXIDE HCL, CHLORDIAZEPOXIDE HYDROCHLORIDE
CHLORPHENIRAMINE MALEATE, CHLORPHENIRAMINE MALEATE
CHLORPROPAMIDE, CHLORPROPAMIDE
CHLORTHALIDONE, CHLORTHALIDONE
CHLORZOXAZONE, CHLORZOXAZONE
CLONIDINE HCL, CLONIDINE HYDROCHLORIDE
CORTISONE ACETATE, CORTISONE ACETATE
DEXAMETHASONE, DEXAMETHASONE
DIAZEPAM, DIAZEPAM
DICYCLOMINE HCL, DICYCLOMINE HYDROCHLORIDE
DIPHENHYDRAMINE HCL, DIPHENHYDRAMINE HYDROCHLORIDE
DIPHENOXYLATE HCL AND ATROPINE SULFATE, ATROPINE SULFATE
DIPYRIDAMOLE, DIPYRIDAMOLE
DISOPYRAMIDE PHOSPHATE, DISOPYRAMIDE PHOSPHATE
DOXEPIN HCL, DOXEPIN HYDROCHLORIDE
DOXYCYCLINE HYCLATE, DOXYCYCLINE HYCLATE
E-BASE, ERYTHROMYCIN
ERGOLOID MESYLATES, ERGOLOID MESYLATES
ERYTHROMYCIN, ERYTHROMYCIN
ERYTHROMYCIN ESTOLATE, ERYTHROMYCIN ESTOLATE
ERYTHROMYCIN ETHYLSUCCINATE, ERYTHROMYCIN ETHYLSUCCINATE
ERYTHROMYCIN ETHYLSUCCINATE AND SULFISOXAZOLE ACETYL, ERYTHROMYCIN ETHYLSUCCINATE
ERYTHROMYCIN STEARATE, ERYTHROMYCIN STEARATE
FLURAZEPAM HCL, FLURAZEPAM HYDROCHLORIDE
FOLIC ACID, FOLIC ACID
FUROSEMIDE, FUROSEMIDE
HALOPERIDOL, HALOPERIDOL
HYDRALAZINE HCL, HYDRALAZINE HYDROCHLORIDE
HYDROCHLOROTHIAZIDE, HYDROCHLOROTHIAZIDE
HYDROCODONE BITARTRATE W/ ACETAMINOPHEN, ACETAMINOPHEN
HYDROCORTISONE, HYDROCORTISONE
HYDROXYZINE HCL, HYDROXYZINE HYDROCHLORIDE
HYDROXYZINE PAMOATE, HYDROXYZINE PAMOATE
IBUPROFEN, IBUPROFEN
IBUPROFEN, IBUPROFEN (OTC)
INDOMETHACIN, INDOMETHACIN
ISONIAZID, ISONIAZID
ISOSORBIDE DINITRATE, ISOSORBIDE DINITRATE
LEUCOVORIN CALCIUM, LEUCOVORIN CALCIUM
LORAZEPAM, LORAZEPAM
MECLOFENAMATE SODIUM, MECLOFENAMATE SODIUM
MEPERIDINE HCL, MEPERIDINE HYDROCHLORIDE
MEPROBAMATE, MEPROBAMATE
METHOCARBAMOL, METHOCARBAMOL
METHOTREXATE SODIUM, METHOTREXATE SODIUM
METHYLDOPA, METHYLDOPA
METOCLOPRAMIDE HCL, METOCLOPRAMIDE HYDROCHLORIDE
METRONIDAZOLE, METRONIDAZOLE
NALIDIXIC ACID, NALIDIXIC ACID
OXAZEPAM, OXAZEPAM
OXYCODONE AND ASPIRIN, ASPIRIN
OXYCODONE HCL AND ACETAMINOPHEN, ACETAMINOPHEN
PERPHENAZINE AND AMITRIPTYLINE HCL, AMITRIPTYLINE HYDROCHLORIDE
PHENDIMETRAZINE TARTRATE, PHENDIMETRAZINE TARTRATE
PHENYLBUTAZONE, PHENYLBUTAZONE
PREDNISOLONE, PREDNISOLONE
PREDNISONE, PREDNISONE
PROMETHAZINE HCL, PROMETHAZINE HYDROCHLORIDE
PROPOXYPHENE HCL, PROPOXYPHENE HYDROCHLORIDE
PROPOXYPHENE NAPSYLATE AND ACETAMINOPHEN, ACETAMINOPHEN
PROPRANOLOL HCL, PROPRANOLOL HYDROCHLORIDE
PROPRANOLOL HCL AND HYDROCHLOROTHIAZIDE, HYDROCHLOROTHIAZIDE
PROPYLTHIOURACIL, PROPYLTHIOURACIL
QUINIDINE SULFATE, QUINIDINE SULFATE
RESERPINE, RESERPINE
RESERPINE AND HYDROCHLOROTHIAZIDE, HYDROCHLOROTHIAZIDE
RESERPINE, HYDRALAZINE HCL AND HYDROCHLOROTHIAZIDE, HYDRALAZINE HYDROCHLORIDE
SODIUM SECOBARBITAL, SECOBARBITAL SODIUM
SPIRONOLACTONE, SPIRONOLACTONE
SPIRONOLACTONE AND HYDROCHLOROTHIAZIDE, HYDROCHLOROTHIAZIDE
SULFAMETHOXAZOLE, SULFAMETHOXAZOLE
SULFAMETHOXAZOLE AND TRIMETHOPRIM, SULFAMETHOXAZOLE
SULFAMETHOXAZOLE AND TRIMETHOPRIM DOUBLE STRENGTH, SULFAMETHOXAZOLE
SULFINPYRAZONE, SULFINPYRAZONE
SULFISOXAZOLE, SULFISOXAZOLE
TEMAZEPAM, TEMAZEPAM
TETRACYCLINE HCL, TETRACYCLINE HYDROCHLORIDE

APPENDIX B
PRODUCT NAME INDEX
LISTED BY APPLICANT *(continued)*

THIORIDAZINE HCL, THIORIDAZINE HYDROCHLORIDE
TOLAZAMIDE, TOLAZAMIDE
TOLBUTAMIDE, TOLBUTAMIDE
TRAZODONE HCL, TRAZODONE HYDROCHLORIDE
TRIAMCINOLONE, TRIAMCINOLONE
TRIAMTERENE AND HYDROCHLOROTHIAZIDE, HYDROCHLOROTHIAZIDE
TRIMETHOPRIM, TRIMETHOPRIM
TRIPELENNAMINE HCL, TRIPELENNAMINE HYDROCHLORIDE
VERAPAMIL HCL, VERAPAMIL HYDROCHLORIDE

BARRE
* BARRE NATIONAL INC
ACETAMINOPHEN W/ CODEINE PHOSPHATE, ACETAMINOPHEN
ACETASOL, ACETIC ACID, GLACIAL
ACETASOL HC, ACETIC ACID, GLACIAL
AMANTADINE HCL, AMANTADINE HYDROCHLORIDE
AMINOPHYLLINE DYE FREE, AMINOPHYLLINE
APAP W/ CODEINE, ACETAMINOPHEN
BETAMETHASONE DIPROPIONATE, BETAMETHASONE DIPROPIONATE
BETAMETHASONE VALERATE, BETAMETHASONE VALERATE
BROMANATE, BROMPHENIRAMINE MALEATE
BROMANATE DC, BROMPHENIRAMINE MALEATE
BROMANATE DM, BROMPHENIRAMINE MALEATE
BROMANYL, BROMODIPHENHYDRAMINE HYDROCHLORIDE
BROMPHENIRAMINE MALEATE, BROMPHENIRAMINE MALEATE
BUTABARB, BUTABARBITAL SODIUM
CHLORPROMAZINE HCL, CHLORPROMAZINE HYDROCHLORIDE
CIMETIDINE HCL, CIMETIDINE HYDROCHLORIDE
CLEMASTINE FUMARATE, CLEMASTINE FUMARATE
CLINDAMYCIN PHOSPHATE, CLINDAMYCIN PHOSPHATE
CONSTULOSE, LACTULOSE
CYPROHEPTADINE HCL, CYPROHEPTADINE HYDROCHLORIDE
DEXAMETHASONE, DEXAMETHASONE
DICYCLOMINE HCL, DICYCLOMINE HYDROCHLORIDE
DIPHENHYDRAMINE HCL, DIPHENHYDRAMINE HYDROCHLORIDE (OTC)
ENULOSE, LACTULOSE
EPINEPHRINE, EPINEPHRINE (OTC)
ERYTHROMYCIN, ERYTHROMYCIN
ERYTHROMYCIN ESTOLATE, ERYTHROMYCIN ESTOLATE
ERYTHROMYCIN ETHYLSUCCINATE, ERYTHROMYCIN ETHYLSUCCINATE
FLUOCINOLONE ACETONIDE, FLUOCINOLONE ACETONIDE
FLUOCINONIDE, FLUOCINONIDE
FLURANDRENOLIDE, FLURANDRENOLIDE
HALOPERIDOL, HALOPERIDOL LACTATE
HYDRAMINE, DIPHENHYDRAMINE HYDROCHLORIDE (OTC)
HYDRAMINE, DIPHENHYDRAMINE HYDROCHLORIDE
HYDROCODONE COMPOUND, HOMATROPINE METHYLBROMIDE
HYDROCORTISONE, HYDROCORTISONE
HYDROXYZINE HCL, HYDROXYZINE HYDROCHLORIDE
ISOETHARINE HCL, ISOETHARINE HYDROCHLORIDE
ISOETHARINE MESYLATE, ISOETHARINE MESYLATE
ISOPROTERENOL HCL, ISOPROTERENOL HYDROCHLORIDE
LIDOCAINE HCL VISCOUS, LIDOCAINE HYDROCHLORIDE
LINDANE, LINDANE
LOMANATE, ATROPINE SULFATE
LOPERAMIDE HCL, LOPERAMIDE HYDROCHLORIDE (OTC)
METHDILAZINE HCL, METHDILAZINE HYDROCHLORIDE
METOCLOPRAMIDE HCL, METOCLOPRAMIDE HYDROCHLORIDE
NYSTATIN, NYSTATIN
NYSTATIN AND TRIAMCINOLONE ACETONIDE, NYSTATIN
PHENYTOIN, PHENYTOIN
PIPERAZINE CITRATE, PIPERAZINE CITRATE
PROCHLORPERAZINE, PROCHLORPERAZINE EDISYLATE
PROCHLORPERAZINE EDISYLATE, PROCHLORPERAZINE EDISYLATE
PROMETH, PROMETHAZINE HYDROCHLORIDE
PROMETH VC PLAIN, PHENYLEPHRINE HYDROCHLORIDE
PROMETH VC W/ CODEINE, CODEINE PHOSPHATE
PROMETH W/ CODEINE, CODEINE PHOSPHATE
PROMETH W/ DEXTROMETHORPHAN, DEXTROMETHORPHAN HYDROBROMIDE
SELENIUM SULFIDE, SELENIUM SULFIDE
SULFATRIM, SULFAMETHOXAZOLE
SULFATRIM PEDIATRIC, SULFAMETHOXAZOLE
TETRACYCLINE HCL, TETRACYCLINE HYDROCHLORIDE
THEOPHYLLINE, THEOPHYLLINE
THIORIDAZINE HCL, THIORIDAZINE HYDROCHLORIDE
THIOTHIXENE HCL, THIOTHIXENE HYDROCHLORIDE
TRIACIN-C, CODEINE PHOSPHATE
TRIAMCINOLONE ACETONIDE, TRIAMCINOLONE ACETONIDE
TRIMEPRAZINE TARTRATE, TRIMEPRAZINE TARTRATE
TRIMETH/SULFA, SULFAMETHOXAZOLE
TRIPLE SULFA, TRISULFAPYRIMIDINES (SULFADIAZINE;SULFAMERAZINE;SULFAMETHAZINE)
TRIPROLIDINE HCL, TRIPROLIDINE HYDROCHLORIDE

BARTOR
* BARTOR PHARMACAL CO
TESTOSTERONE, TESTOSTERONE

BASEL PHARMS
* BASEL PHARMACEUTICALS DIV CIBA GEIGY CORP
ANAFRANIL, CLOMIPRAMINE HYDROCHLORIDE
HABITROL, NICOTINE
TEGRETOL, CARBAMAZEPINE

BAUSCH AND LOMB
* BAUSCH AND LOMB INC
OPCON-A, NAPHAZOLINE HYDROCHLORIDE
SULPHRIN, PREDNISOLONE ACETATE
SULTEN-10, SULFACETAMIDE SODIUM
* BAUSCH AND LOMB PHARMACEUTICALS INC
ACETIC ACID 2% IN AQUEOUS ALUMINUM ACETATE, ACETIC ACID, GLACIAL
DEXASPORIN, DEXAMETHASONE

APPENDIX B
PRODUCT NAME INDEX
LISTED BY APPLICANT *(continued)*

ERYTHROMYCIN, ERYTHROMYCIN
FLUOCINOLONE ACETONIDE, FLUOCINOLONE ACETONIDE
GENTAMICIN SULFATE, GENTAMICIN SULFATE
LEVOBUNOLOL HCL, LEVOBUNOLOL HYDROCHLORIDE
NAFAZAIR, NAPHAZOLINE HYDROCHLORIDE
NYSTATIN, NYSTATIN
OPCON, NAPHAZOLINE HYDROCHLORIDE
OPTIPRANOLOL, METIPRANOLOL HYDROCHLORIDE
PENTOLAIR, CYCLOPENTOLATE HYDROCHLORIDE
PREDNISOLONE SODIUM PHOSPHATE, PREDNISOLONE SODIUM PHOSPHATE
TOBRAMYCIN, TOBRAMYCIN
TROPICAMIDE, TROPICAMIDE

BAXTER

* BAXTER HEALTHCARE CORP
ACETIC ACID 0.25% IN PLASTIC CONTAINER, ACETIC ACID, GLACIAL
ALCOHOL 5% IN DEXTROSE 5% IN WATER, ALCOHOL
AMINOACETIC ACID 1.5% IN PLASTIC CONTAINER, GLYCINE
ANCEF, CEFAZOLIN SODIUM
ANCEF IN DEXTROSE 5% IN PLASTIC CONTAINER, CEFAZOLIN SODIUM
ANCEF IN SODIUM CHLORIDE 0.9% IN PLASTIC CONTAINER, CEFAZOLIN SODIUM
BACTOCILL, OXACILLIN SODIUM
BRANCHAMIN 4%, AMINO ACIDS
BRETYLIUM TOSYLATE IN DEXTROSE 5%, BRETYLIUM TOSYLATE
CEFTAZIDIME SODIUM, CEFTAZIDIME SODIUM
CEPHALOTHIN SODIUM W/ DEXTROSE, CEPHALOTHIN SODIUM
CEPHALOTHIN SODIUM W/ SODIUM CHLORIDE, CEPHALOTHIN SODIUM
CLINDAMYCIN PHOSPHATE IN DEXTROSE 5%, CLINDAMYCIN PHOSPHATE
DEXTROSE 10% AND SODIUM CHLORIDE 0.9% IN PLASTIC CONTAINER, DEXTROSE
DEXTROSE 10% IN PLASTIC CONTAINER, DEXTROSE
DEXTROSE 2.5% AND SODIUM CHLORIDE 0.45% IN PLASTIC CONTAINER, DEXTROSE
DEXTROSE 20% IN PLASTIC CONTAINER, DEXTROSE
DEXTROSE 30% IN PLASTIC CONTAINER, DEXTROSE
DEXTROSE 40% IN PLASTIC CONTAINER, DEXTROSE
DEXTROSE 5%, DEXTROSE
DEXTROSE 5% AND ELECTROLYTE NO 75, DEXTROSE
DEXTROSE 5% AND ELECTROLYTE NO.48 IN PLASTIC CONTAINER, DEXTROSE
DEXTROSE 5% AND POTASSIUM CHLORIDE 0.075% IN PLASTIC CONTAINER, DEXTROSE
DEXTROSE 5% AND POTASSIUM CHLORIDE 0.15% IN PLASTIC CONTAINER, DEXTROSE
DEXTROSE 5% AND POTASSIUM CHLORIDE 0.224% IN PLASTIC CONTAINER, DEXTROSE
DEXTROSE 5% AND POTASSIUM CHLORIDE 0.3% IN PLASTIC CONTAINER, DEXTROSE
DEXTROSE 5% IN RINGER'S IN PLASTIC CONTAINER, CALCIUM CHLORIDE
DEXTROSE 5% IN SODIUM CHLORIDE 0.2% IN PLASTIC CONTAINER, DEXTROSE
DEXTROSE 5% IN SODIUM CHLORIDE 0.33% IN PLASTIC CONTAINER, DEXTROSE
DEXTROSE 5% IN SODIUM CHLORIDE 0.45% IN PLASTIC CONTAINER, DEXTROSE
DEXTROSE 5% IN SODIUM CHLORIDE 0.9% IN PLASTIC CONTAINER, DEXTROSE
DEXTROSE 5%, SODIUM CHLORIDE 0.2% AND POTASSIUM CHLORIDE 10 MEQ, DEXTROSE
DEXTROSE 5%, SODIUM CHLORIDE 0.2% AND POTASSIUM CHLORIDE 15 MEQ (K), DEXTROSE
DEXTROSE 5%, SODIUM CHLORIDE 0.2% AND POTASSIUM CHLORIDE 20 MEQ, DEXTROSE
DEXTROSE 5%, SODIUM CHLORIDE 0.2% AND POTASSIUM CHLORIDE 20 MEQ (K), DEXTROSE
DEXTROSE 5%, SODIUM CHLORIDE 0.2% AND POTASSIUM CHLORIDE 30 MEQ, DEXTROSE
DEXTROSE 5%, SODIUM CHLORIDE 0.2% AND POTASSIUM CHLORIDE 40 MEQ, DEXTROSE
DEXTROSE 5%, SODIUM CHLORIDE 0.2% AND POTASSIUM CHLORIDE 5 MEQ, DEXTROSE
DEXTROSE 5%, SODIUM CHLORIDE 0.2% AND POTASSIUM CHLORIDE 5 MEQ (K), DEXTROSE
DEXTROSE 5%, SODIUM CHLORIDE 0.33% AND POTASSIUM CHLORIDE 10 MEQ, DEXTROSE
DEXTROSE 5%, SODIUM CHLORIDE 0.33% AND POTASSIUM CHLORIDE 15 MEQ, DEXTROSE
DEXTROSE 5%, SODIUM CHLORIDE 0.33% AND POTASSIUM CHLORIDE 20 MEQ, DEXTROSE
DEXTROSE 5%, SODIUM CHLORIDE 0.33% AND POTASSIUM CHLORIDE 30 MEQ, DEXTROSE
DEXTROSE 5%, SODIUM CHLORIDE 0.33% AND POTASSIUM CHLORIDE 40 MEQ, DEXTROSE
DEXTROSE 5%, SODIUM CHLORIDE 0.33% AND POTASSIUM CHLORIDE 5 MEQ, DEXTROSE
DEXTROSE 5%, SODIUM CHLORIDE 0.45% AND POTASSIUM CHLORIDE 15 MEQ, DEXTROSE
DEXTROSE 5%, SODIUM CHLORIDE 0.45% AND POTASSIUM CHLORIDE 20 MEQ (K), DEXTROSE
DEXTROSE 5%, SODIUM CHLORIDE 0.45% AND POTASSIUM CHLORIDE 20 MEQ (K), DEXTROSE
DEXTROSE 5%, SODIUM CHLORIDE 0.45% AND POTASSIUM CHLORIDE 5 MEQ, DEXTROSE
DEXTROSE 50%, DEXTROSE
DEXTROSE 60%, DEXTROSE
DEXTROSE 60% IN PLASTIC CONTAINER, DEXTROSE
DEXTROSE 70%, DEXTROSE
DEXTROSE 70% IN PLASTIC CONTAINER, DEXTROSE
DIANEAL LOW CALCIUM W/ DEXTROSE 1.5%, CALCIUM CHLORIDE
DIANEAL LOW CALCIUM W/ DEXTROSE 2.5%, CALCIUM CHLORIDE
DIANEAL LOW CALCIUM W/ DEXTROSE 3.5%, CALCIUM CHLORIDE
DIANEAL LOW CALCIUM W/ DEXTROSE 4.25%, CALCIUM CHLORIDE
DIANEAL PD-1 W/ DEXTROSE 1.5% IN PLASTIC CONTAINER, CALCIUM CHLORIDE
DIANEAL PD-1 W/ DEXTROSE 2.5% IN PLASTIC CONTAINER, CALCIUM CHLORIDE
DIANEAL PD-1 W/ DEXTROSE 3.5%, CALCIUM CHLORIDE
DIANEAL PD-1 W/ DEXTROSE 4.25% IN PLASTIC CONTAINER, CALCIUM CHLORIDE
DIANEAL PD-2 W/ DEXTROSE 1.5%, CALCIUM CHLORIDE
DIANEAL PD-2 W/ DEXTROSE 2.5%, CALCIUM CHLORIDE
DIANEAL PD-2 W/ DEXTROSE 2.5% IN PLASTIC CONTAINER, CALCIUM CHLORIDE
DIANEAL PD-2 W/ DEXTROSE 3.5%, CALCIUM CHLORIDE

APPENDIX B
PRODUCT NAME INDEX
LISTED BY APPLICANT *(continued)*

DIANEAL PD-2 W/ DEXTROSE 4.25%, CALCIUM CHLORIDE
DIANEAL PD-2 W/ DEXTROSE 4.25% IN PLASTIC CONTAINER, CALCIUM CHLORIDE
DIANEAL 137 W/ DEXTROSE 1.5% IN PLASTIC CONTAINER, CALCIUM CHLORIDE
DIANEAL 137 W/ DEXTROSE 2.5% IN PLASTIC CONTAINER, CALCIUM CHLORIDE
DIANEAL 137 W/ DEXTROSE 4.25% IN PLASTIC CONTAINER, CALCIUM CHLORIDE
DOBUTAMINE HCL IN DEXTROSE 5%, DOBUTAMINE HYDROCHLORIDE
DOPAMINE HCL IN DEXTROSE 5%, DOPAMINE HYDROCHLORIDE
GLYCINE 1.5%, GLYCINE
HEPARIN SODIUM 10,000 UNITS IN DEXTROSE 5%, HEPARIN SODIUM
HEPARIN SODIUM 1000 UNITS AND SODIUM CHLORIDE 0.9%, HEPARIN SODIUM
HEPARIN SODIUM 20,000 UNITS AND DEXTROSE 5% IN PLASTIC CONTAINER, HEPARIN SODIUM
HEPARIN SODIUM 2000 UNITS AND SODIUM CHLORIDE 0.9%, HEPARIN SODIUM
HEPARIN SODIUM 25,000 UNITS AND DEXTROSE 5%, HEPARIN SODIUM
HEPARIN SODIUM 5000 UNITS AND SODIUM CHLORIDE 0.9%, HEPARIN SODIUM
IRRIGATING SOLUTION G IN PLASTIC CONTAINER, CITRIC ACID
ISOETHARINE HCL, ISOETHARINE HYDROCHLORIDE
ISOTONIC GENTAMICIN SULFATE IN PLASTIC CONTAINER, GENTAMICIN SULFATE
LACTATED RINGER'S, CALCIUM CHLORIDE
LACTATED RINGER'S AND DEXTROSE 5% IN PLASTIC CONTAINER, CALCIUM CHLORIDE
LACTATED RINGER'S IN PLASTIC CONTAINER, CALCIUM CHLORIDE
LIDOCAINE HCL 0.1% AND DEXTROSE 5% IN PLASTIC CONTAINER, LIDOCAINE HYDROCHLORIDE
LIDOCAINE HCL 0.2% AND DEXTROSE 5% IN PLASTIC CONTAINER, LIDOCAINE HYDROCHLORIDE
LIDOCAINE HCL 0.4% AND DEXTROSE 5% IN PLASTIC CONTAINER, LIDOCAINE HYDROCHLORIDE
LIDOCAINE HCL 0.8% AND DEXTROSE 5% IN PLASTIC CONTAINER, LIDOCAINE HYDROCHLORIDE
NALLPEN, NAFCILLIN SODIUM
NITROGLYCERIN IN DEXTROSE 5%, NITROGLYCERIN
NOVAMINE 15% SULFITE FREE, AMINO ACIDS
OSMITROL 10% IN WATER, MANNITOL
OSMITROL 10% IN WATER IN PLASTIC CONTAINER, MANNITOL
OSMITROL 15% IN WATER, MANNITOL
OSMITROL 15% IN WATER IN PLASTIC CONTAINER, MANNITOL
OSMITROL 20% IN WATER, MANNITOL
OSMITROL 20% IN WATER IN PLASTIC CONTAINER, MANNITOL
OSMITROL 5% IN WATER, MANNITOL
OSMITROL 5% IN WATER IN PLASTIC CONTAINER, MANNITOL
PENICILLIN G POTASSIUM, PENICILLIN G POTASSIUM
PLASMA-LYTE A IN PLASTIC CONTAINER, MAGNESIUM CHLORIDE
PLASMA-LYTE M AND DEXTROSE 5% IN PLASTIC CONTAINER, CALCIUM CHLORIDE
PLASMA-LYTE R IN PLASTIC CONTAINER, CALCIUM CHLORIDE
PLASMA-LYTE 148 AND DEXTROSE 5% IN PLASTIC CONTAINER, DEXTROSE
PLASMA-LYTE 148 IN WATER IN PLASTIC CONTAINER, MAGNESIUM CHLORIDE
PLASMA-LYTE 56 AND DEXTROSE 5% IN PLASTIC CONTAINER, DEXTROS
PLASMA-LYTE 56 IN PLASTIC CONTAINER, MAGNESIUM ACETATE TETRAHYDRATE
POTASSIUM CHLORIDE, POTASSIUM CHLORIDE
POTASSIUM CHLORIDE 10 MEQ, POTASSIUM CHLORIDE
POTASSIUM CHLORIDE 10 MEQ IN DEXTROSE 5% AND LACTATED RINGER'S, CALCIUM CHLORIDE
POTASSIUM CHLORIDE 10 MEQ IN DEXTROSE 5% AND SODIUM CHLORIDE 0.45%, DEXTROSE
POTASSIUM CHLORIDE 10 MEQ IN DEXTROSE 5% AND SODIUM CHLORIDE 0.9%, DEXTROSE
POTASSIUM CHLORIDE 15 MEQ IN DEXTROSE 5% AND LACTATED RINGER'S, CALCIUM CHLORIDE
POTASSIUM CHLORIDE 20 MEQ, POTASSIUM CHLORIDE
POTASSIUM CHLORIDE 20 MEQ IN DEXTROSE 5% AND LACTATED RINGER'S, CALCIUM CHLORIDE
POTASSIUM CHLORIDE 20 MEQ IN DEXTROSE 5% AND SODIUM CHLORIDE 0.45%, DEXTROSE
POTASSIUM CHLORIDE 20 MEQ IN DEXTROSE 5% AND SODIUM CHLORIDE 0.9%, DEXTROSE
POTASSIUM CHLORIDE 30 MEQ, POTASSIUM CHLORIDE
POTASSIUM CHLORIDE 30 MEQ IN DEXTROSE 5% AND LACTATED RINGER'S, CALCIUM CHLORIDE
POTASSIUM CHLORIDE 30 MEQ IN DEXTROSE 5% AND SODIUM CHLORIDE 0.45%, DEXTROSE
POTASSIUM CHLORIDE 30 MEQ IN DEXTROSE 5% AND SODIUM CHLORIDE 0.9%, DEXTROSE
POTASSIUM CHLORIDE 40 MEQ, POTASSIUM CHLORIDE
POTASSIUM CHLORIDE 40 MEQ IN DEXTROSE 5% AND LACTATED RINGER'S, CALCIUM CHLORIDE
POTASSIUM CHLORIDE 40 MEQ IN DEXTROSE 5% AND SODIUM CHLORIDE 0.45%, DEXTROSE
POTASSIUM CHLORIDE 40 MEQ IN DEXTROSE 5% AND SODIUM CHLORIDE 0.9%, DEXTROSE
POTASSIUM CHLORIDE 5 MEQ IN DEXTROSE 5% AND LACTATED RINGER'S, CALCIUM CHLORIDE
POTASSIUM CHLORIDE 5 MEQ IN DEXTROSE 5% AND SODIUM CHLORIDE 0.45%, DEXTROSE
POTASSIUM CHLORIDE 5 MEQ IN DEXTROSE 5% AND SODIUM CHLORIDE 0.9%, DEXTROSE
RENAMIN W/O ELECTROLYTES, AMINO ACIDS
RINGER'S IN PLASTIC CONTAINER, CALCIUM CHLORIDE
SODIUM CHLORIDE 0.45%, SODIUM CHLORIDE
SODIUM CHLORIDE 0.45% IN PLASTIC CONTAINER, SODIUM CHLORIDE
SODIUM CHLORIDE 0.9%, SODIUM CHLORIDE
SODIUM CHLORIDE 0.9% AND POTASSIUM CHLORIDE 0.075%, POTASSIUM CHLORIDE
SODIUM CHLORIDE 0.9% AND POTASSIUM CHLORIDE 0.15%, POTASSIUM CHLORIDE
SODIUM CHLORIDE 0.9% AND POTASSIUM CHLORIDE 0.224%, POTASSIUM CHLORIDE
SODIUM CHLORIDE 0.9% AND POTASSIUM CHLORIDE 0.3%, POTASSIUM CHLORIDE
SODIUM CHLORIDE 0.9% IN PLASTIC CONTAINER, SODIUM CHLORIDE
SODIUM CHLORIDE 0.9% IN STERILE PLASTIC CONTAINER, SODIUM CHLORIDE

APPENDIX B
PRODUCT NAME INDEX
LISTED BY APPLICANT *(continued)*

SODIUM CHLORIDE 3% IN PLASTIC CONTAINER, SODIUM CHLORIDE
SODIUM CHLORIDE 5% IN PLASTIC CONTAINER, SODIUM CHLORIDE
SODIUM HEPARIN, HEPARIN SODIUM
SODIUM LACTATE 0.167 MOLAR IN PLASTIC CONTAINER, SODIUM LACTATE
SORBITOL 3% IN PLASTIC CONTAINER, SORBITOL
STERILE WATER, WATER FOR IRRIGATION, STERILE
STERILE WATER FOR INJECTION, WATER FOR INJECTION, STERILE
STERILE WATER FOR INJECTION IN PLASTIC CONTAINER, WATER FOR INJECTION, STERILE
STERILE WATER IN PLASTIC CONTAINER, WATER FOR IRRIGATION, STERILE
SYNOVALYTE IN PLASTIC CONTAINER, MAGNESIUM CHLORIDE
THEOPHYLLINE AND DEXTROSE 5%, THEOPHYLLINE
TIS-U-SOL, MAGNESIUM SULFATE
TIS-U-SOL IN PLASTIC CONTAINER, MAGNESIUM SULFATE
TRAVAMULSION 10%, SOYBEAN OIL
TRAVAMULSION 20%, SOYBEAN OIL
TRAVASOL 10%, AMINO ACIDS
TRAVASOL 10% W/O ELECTROLYTES, AMINO ACIDS
TRAVASOL 2.75% IN DEXTROSE 10%, AMINO ACIDS
TRAVASOL 2.75% IN DEXTROSE 15%, AMINO ACIDS
TRAVASOL 2.75% IN DEXTROSE 20%, AMINO ACIDS
TRAVASOL 2.75% IN DEXTROSE 25%, AMINO ACIDS
TRAVASOL 2.75% IN DEXTROSE 5%, AMINO ACIDS
TRAVASOL 3.5% W/ ELECTROLYTES, AMINO ACIDS
TRAVASOL 4.25% IN DEXTROSE 10%, AMINO ACIDS
TRAVASOL 4.25% IN DEXTROSE 15%, AMINO ACIDS
TRAVASOL 4.25% IN DEXTROSE 20%, AMINO ACIDS
TRAVASOL 4.25% IN DEXTROSE 25%, AMINO ACIDS
TRAVASOL 4.25% IN DEXTROSE 5%, AMINO ACIDS
TRAVASOL 5.5%, AMINO ACIDS
TRAVASOL 5.5% W/ ELECTROLYTES, AMINO ACIDS
TRAVASOL 5.5% W/O ELECTROLYTES, AMINO ACIDS
TRAVASOL 8.5%, AMINO ACIDS
TRAVASOL 8.5% W/ ELECTROLYTES, AMINO ACIDS
TRAVASOL 8.5% W/O ELECTROLYTES, AMINO ACIDS
TRAVERT 10%, INVERT SUGAR

* BAXTER HEALTHCARE CORP PHARMASEAL DIV
PHARMASEAL SCRUB CARE, CHLORHEXIDINE GLUCONATE (OTC)
POVIDONE IODINE, POVIDONE-IODINE (OTC)

BECTON DICKINSON

* BECTON DICKINSON AND CO
E-Z PREP, POVIDONE-IODINE (OTC)
E-Z PREP 220, POVIDONE-IODINE (OTC)
E-Z SCRUB 201, POVIDONE-IODINE (OTC)
E-Z SCRUB 241, POVIDONE-IODINE (OTC)

* BECTON DICKINSON MICROBIOLOGY SYSTEMS
BAL, DIMERCAPROL
CARDIO-GREEN, INDOCYANINE GREEN

BEDFORD

* BEDFORD LABORATORIES DIV BEN VENUE LABORATORIES INC
AMIKACIN, AMIKACIN SULFATE
CLINDAMYCIN PHOSPHATE, CLINDAMYCIN PHOSPHATE

BEECHAM

* BEECHAM LABORATORIES DIV BEECHAM INC
PROBENECID AND COLCHICINE, COLCHICINE

BEL MAR

* BEL MAR LABORATORIES INC
CHLORPHENIRAMINE MALEATE, CHLORPHENIRAMINE MALEATE
CHORIONIC GONADOTROPIN, GONADOTROPIN, CHORIONIC
DEXAMETHASONE SODIUM PHOSPHATE, DEXAMETHASONE SODIUM PHOSPHATE
DIPHENHYDRAMINE HCL, DIPHENHYDRAMINE HYDROCHLORIDE
HYDROCORTISONE ACETATE, HYDROCORTISONE ACETATE
HYDROXOMIN, HYDROXOCOBALAMIN
LIDOCAINE HCL, LIDOCAINE HYDROCHLORIDE
LIDOCAINE HCL W/ EPINEPHRINE, EPINEPHRINE
M-PREDROL, METHYLPREDNISOLONE ACETATE
PREDNISOLONE ACETATE, PREDNISOLONE ACETATE
PROCAINE HCL, PROCAINE HYDROCHLORIDE
PROCAINE HCL W/ EPINEPHRINE, EPINEPHRINE
PYRIDAMAL 100, CHLORPHENIRAMINE MALEATE
PYRIDOXINE HCL, PYRIDOXINE HYDROCHLORIDE
RUBIVITE, CYANOCOBALAMIN
TESTOSTERONE PROPIONATE, TESTOSTERONE PROPIONATE
THIAMINE HCL, THIAMINE HYDROCHLORIDE
VITAMIN A PALMITATE, VITAMIN A PALMITATE

BELL PHARMA

* BELL PHARMACAL CORP
CHLORPHENIRAMINE MALEATE, CHLORPHENIRAMINE MALEATE
RESERPINE, RESERPINE

BEN VENUE

* BEN VENUE LABORATORIES INC
CEFAZOLIN SODIUM, CEFAZOLIN SODIUM
DOXYCYCLINE, DOXYCYCLINE HYCLATE
FLUOROURACIL, FLUOROURACIL
LEUCOVORIN CALCIUM, LEUCOVORIN CALCIUM
METHOTREXATE SODIUM, METHOTREXATE SODIUM
VINBLASTINE SULFATE, VINBLASTINE SULFATE

BERLEX

* BERLEX LABORATORIES INC SUB SCHERING AG
ANGIOVIST 282, DIATRIZOATE MEGLUMINE
ANGIOVIST 292, DIATRIZOATE MEGLUMINE
ANGIOVIST 370, DIATRIZOATE MEGLUMINE
BETAPACE, SOTALOL HYDROCHLORIDE
BILIVIST, IPODATE SODIUM
FLUDARA, FLUDARABINE PHOSPHATE
GASTROVIST, DIATRIZOATE MEGLUMINE
MAGNEVIST, GADOPENTETATE DIMEGLUMINE
OSMOVIST, IOTROLAN
QUINACT, QUINIDINE GLUCONATE
QUINAGLUTE, QUINIDINE GLUCONATE
SULLA, SULFAMETER
UROVIST CYSTO, DIATRIZOATE MEGLUMINE
UROVIST CYSTO PEDIATRIC, DIATRIZOATE MEGLUMINE
UROVIST MEGLUMINE DIU/CT, DIATRIZOATE MEGLUMINE
UROVIST SODIUM 300, DIATRIZOATE SODIUM
VI-TWEL, CYANOCOBALAMIN

BETA DERMAC

* BETA DERMACEUTICALS INC
BETA-HC, HYDROCORTISONE

APPENDIX B
PRODUCT NAME INDEX
LISTED BY APPLICANT *(continued)*

BH
* BH CHEMICALS INC
  HALOTHANE, HALOTHANE

BIO TECH GEN
* BIO TECHNOLOGY GENERAL CORP
  OXANDRIN, OXANDROLONE

BIOCRAFT
* BIOCRAFT LABORATORIES INC
  ALBUTEROL SULFATE, ALBUTEROL SULFATE
  AMILORIDE HCL AND HYDROCHLOROTHIAZIDE, AMILORIDE HYDROCHLORIDE
  AMITRIPTYLINE HCL, AMITRIPTYLINE HYDROCHLORIDE
  AMOXICILLIN, AMOXICILLIN
  AMOXICILLIN PEDIATRIC, AMOXICILLIN
  AMPICILLIN, AMPICILLIN/AMPICILLIN TRIHYDRATE
  BACLOFEN, BACLOFEN
  CEFADROXIL, CEFADROXIL/CEFADROXIL HEMIHYDRATE
  CEPHALEXIN, CEPHALEXIN
  CEPHRADINE, CEPHRADINE
  CHLOROQUINE PHOSPHATE, CHLOROQUINE PHOSPHATE
  CINOXACIN, CINOXACIN
  CLINDAMYCIN HCL, CLINDAMYCIN HYDROCHLORIDE
  CLONIDINE HCL, CLONIDINE HYDROCHLORIDE
  CLOXACILLIN SODIUM, CLOXACILLIN SODIUM
  CYCLACILLIN, CYCLACILLIN
  DICLOXACILLIN SODIUM, DICLOXACILLIN SODIUM
  DISOPYRAMIDE PHOSPHATE, DISOPYRAMIDE PHOSPHATE
  HYDROCORTISONE, HYDROCORTISONE
  IMIPRAMINE HCL, IMIPRAMINE HYDROCHLORIDE
  KETOPROFEN, KETOPROFEN
  METAPROTERENOL SULFATE, METAPROTERENOL SULFATE
  METOCLOPRAMIDE HCL, METOCLOPRAMIDE HYDROCHLORIDE
  MINOCYCLINE HCL, MINOCYCLINE HYDROCHLORIDE
  NEOMYCIN SULFATE, NEOMYCIN SULFATE
  NYSTATIN, NYSTATIN
  OXACILLIN SODIUM, OXACILLIN SODIUM
  PENICILLIN, PENICILLIN G POTASSIUM
  PENICILLIN G POTASSIUM, PENICILLIN G POTASSIUM
  PENICILLIN-VK, PENICILLIN V POTASSIUM
  PENICILLIN-2, PENICILLIN G POTASSIUM
  PROBAMPACIN, AMPICILLIN/AMPICILLIN TRIHYDRATE
  SMZ-TMP, SULFAMETHOXAZOLE
  SMZ-TMP PEDIATRIC, SULFAMETHOXAZOLE
  THIORIDAZINE HCL, THIORIDAZINE HYDROCHLORIDE
  TRIMETHOPRIM, TRIMETHOPRIM

BIODEVELOPMENT
* BIODEVELOPMENT CORP
  ORLAAM, LEVOMETHADYL ACETATE HYDROCHLORIDE

BLAIREX
* BLAIREX LABORATORIES INC
  BRONCHO SALINE, SODIUM CHLORIDE (OTC)

BLOCK DRUG
* BLOCK DRUG CO INC
  ACTINEX, MASOPROCOL

BLUE RIDGE
* BLUE RIDGE LABORATORIES INC
  CARAFATE, SUCRALFATE

BLULINE
* BLULINE LABORATORIES INC
  EPICORT, HYDROCORTISONE
  MULTIFUGE, PIPERAZINE CITRATE

BOEHRINGER INGELHEIM
* BOEHRINGER INGELHEIM PHARMACEUTICALS INC
  ALUPENT, METAPROTERENOL SULFATE
  ATROVENT, IPRATROPIUM BROMIDE
  CATAPRES, CLONIDINE HYDROCHLORIDE
  CATAPRES-TTS-1, CLONIDINE
  CATAPRES-TTS-2, CLONIDINE
  CATAPRES-TTS-3, CLONIDINE
  COMBIPRES, CHLORTHALIDONE
  IV PERSANTINE, DIPYRIDAMOLE
  MEXITIL, MEXILETINE HYDROCHLORIDE
  PERSANTINE, DIPYRIDAMOLE
  PRELUDIN, PHENMETRAZINE HYDROCHLORIDE

BOEHRINGER MANNHEIM
* BOEHRINGER MANNHEIM PHARMACEUTICALS CORP
  ANEXSIA, ACETAMINOPHEN
  ANEXSIA 7.5/650, ACETAMINOPHEN
  DEMADEX, TORSEMIDE

BOOTS
* BOOTS PHARMACEUTICALS INC
  CHLORPROMAZINE HCL, CHLORPROMAZINE HYDROCHLORIDE
  CHOLOXIN, DEXTROTHYROXINE SODIUM
  CHYMODIACTIN, CHYMOPAPAIN
  DISCASE, CHYMOPAPAIN
  E-MYCIN, ERYTHROMYCIN
  IBUPROFEN, IBUPROFEN
  LOPURIN, ALLOPURINOL
  MANOPLAX, FLOSEQUINAN
  PROMETHAZINE HCL, PROMETHAZINE HYDROCHLORIDE
  PROPYLTHIOURACIL, PROPYLTHIOURACIL
  RUFEN, IBUPROFEN
  SSD, SILVER SULFADIAZINE
  TETRACYCLINE HCL, TETRACYCLINE HYDROCHLORIDE
  TRAVASE, SUTILAINS

BOWMAN PHARMS
* BOWMAN PHARMACEUTICALS INC
  HISERPIA, RESERPINE
  HIWOLFIA, RAUWOLFIA SERPENTINA

BRACCO
* BRACCO DIAGNOSTICS INC
  CARDIOGEN-82, RUBIDIUM CHLORIDE RB-82
  CARDIOGRAFIN, DIATRIZOATE MEGLUMINE
  CARDIOTEC, TECHNETIUM TC-99M TEBOROXIME KIT
  CHLORMERODRIN HG 197, CHLORMERODRIN, HG-197
  CHOLETEC, TECHNETIUM TC-99M MEBROFENIN KIT
  CHOLOGRAFIN MEGLUMINE, IODIPAMIDE MEGLUMINE

APPENDIX B
PRODUCT NAME INDEX
LISTED BY APPLICANT *(continued)*

CHOLOGRAFIN SODIUM, IODIPAMIDE SODIUM
CHOLOVUE, IODOXAMATE MEGLUMINE
CHROMITOPE SODIUM, SODIUM CHROMATE, CR-51
CYSTOGRAFIN, DIATRIZOATE MEGLUMINE
CYSTOGRAFIN DILUTE, DIATRIZOATE MEGLUMINE
DIATRIZOATE MEGLUMINE, DIATRIZOATE MEGLUMINE
GASTROGRAFIN, DIATRIZOATE MEGLUMINE
HIPPUTOPE, IODOHIPPURATE SODIUM, I-131
IODOTOPE, SODIUM IODIDE, I-131
ISOVUE-M 200, IOPAMIDOL
ISOVUE-M 300, IOPAMIDOL
ISOVUE-128, IOPAMIDOL
ISOVUE-200, IOPAMIDOL
ISOVUE-250, IOPAMIDOL
ISOVUE-300, IOPAMIDOL
ISOVUE-370, IOPAMIDOL
KINEVAC, SINCALIDE
MACROTEC, TECHNETIUM TC-99M ALBUMIN AGGREGATED KIT
MDP-SQUIBB, TECHNETIUM TC-99M MEDRONATE KIT
MINITEC, TECHNETIUM TC-99M SODIUM PERTECHNETATE GENERATOR
ORAGRAFIN CALCIUM, IPODATE CALCIUM
ORAGRAFIN SODIUM, IPODATE SODIUM
PHOSPHOTEC, TECHNETIUM TC-99M PYROPHOSPHATE KIT
PHOSPHOTOPE, SODIUM PHOSPHATE, P-32
PROHANCE, GADOTERIDOL
RENO-M-DIP, DIATRIZOATE MEGLUMINE
RENO-M-30, DIATRIZOATE MEGLUMINE
RENO-M-60, DIATRIZOATE MEGLUMINE
RENOCAL-76, DIATRIZOATE MEGLUMINE
RENOGRAFIN-60, DIATRIZOATE MEGLUMINE
RENOGRAFIN-76, DIATRIZOATE MEGLUMINE
RENOTEC, TECHNETIUM TC-99M FERPENTETATE KIT
RENOVIST, DIATRIZOATE MEGLUMINE
RENOVIST II, DIATRIZOATE MEGLUMINE
RENOVUE-DIP, IODAMIDE MEGLUMINE
RENOVUE-65, IODAMIDE MEGLUMINE
ROBENGATOPE, ROSE BENGAL SODIUM, I-131
RUBRATOPE-57, CYANOCOBALAMIN, CO-57
RUBRATOPE-57 KIT, COBALT CHLORIDE, CO-57
RUBRATOPE-60, CYANOCOBALAMIN, CO-60
RUBRATOPE-60 KIT, COBALT CHLORIDE, CO-60
SETHOTOPE, SELENOMETHIONINE, SE-75
SINOGRAFIN, DIATRIZOATE MEGLUMINE
TESULOID, TECHNETIUM TC-99M SULFUR COLLOID KIT
THALLOUS CHLORIDE TL 201, THALLOUS CHLORIDE, TL-201

BRADLEY
* BRADLEY PHARMACEUTICALS INC
PAMINE, METHSCOPOLAMINE BROMIDE

BRAE
* BRAE LABORATORIES INC
BACITRACIN, BACITRACIN

BRAINTREE
* BRAINTREE LABORATORIES INC
GOLYTELY, POLYETHYLENE GLYCOL 3350
NULYTELY, POLYETHYLENE GLYCOL 3350
PHOSLO, CALCIUM ACETATE

BRIAN
* BRIAN PHARMACEUTICALS INC
BRIAN CARE, CHLORHEXIDINE GLUCONATE (OTC)

BRISTOL
* BRISTOL LABORATORIES INC DIV BRISTOL MYERS CO
AMIKIN, AMIKACIN SULFATE
AMIKIN IN SODIUM CHLORIDE 0.9%, AMIKACIN SULFATE
BETAPEN-VK, PENICILLIN V POTASSIUM
BICNU, CARMUSTINE
BLENOXANE, BLEOMYCIN SULFATE
BRISTACYCLINE, TETRACYCLINE HYDROCHLORIDE
BRISTAGEN, GENTAMICIN SULFATE
BRISTAMYCIN, ERYTHROMYCIN STEARATE
CEENU, LOMUSTINE
CEPHALOTHIN SODIUM, CEPHALOTHIN SODIUM
CYTOXAN, CYCLOPHOSPHAMIDE
DYNAPEN, DICLOXACILLIN SODIUM
ENKAID, ENCAINIDE HYDROCHLORIDE
LYOPHILIZED CYTOXAN, CYCLOPHOSPHAMIDE
LYSODREN, MITOTANE
MEXATE, METHOTREXATE SODIUM
MUTAMYCIN, MITOMYCIN
POLYCILLIN, AMPICILLIN/AMPICILLIN TRIHYDRATE
POLYCILLIN-N, AMPICILLIN SODIUM
POLYCILLIN-PRB, AMPICILLIN/AMPICILLIN TRIHYDRATE
PRECEF, CEFORANIDE
PROSTAPHLIN, OXACILLIN SODIUM
STAPHCILLIN, METHICILLIN SODIUM
TEGOPEN, CLOXACILLIN SODIUM
TETREX, TETRACYCLINE PHOSPHATE COMPLEX
ULTRACEF, CEFADROXIL/CEFADROXIL HEMIHYDRATE
VEPESID, ETOPOSIDE
VERSAPEN, HETACILLIN
VERSAPEN-K, HETACILLIN POTASSIUM
VINCREX, VINCRISTINE SULFATE

BRISTOL MYERS
* BRISTOL MYERS CO
MEXATE-AQ, METHOTREXATE SODIUM
MEXATE-AQ PRESERVED, METHOTREXATE SODIUM
MUTAMYCIN, MITOMYCIN
PLATINOL, CISPLATIN
PLATINOL-AQ, CISPLATIN
QUESTRAN, CHOLESTYRAMINE
QUESTRAN LIGHT, CHOLESTYRAMINE
* BRISTOL MYERS PRODUCTS INC
NUPRIN, IBUPROFEN (OTC)
* BRISTOL MYERS US PHARMACEUTICAL AND NUTRITION GROUP
RUBEX, DOXORUBICIN HYDROCHLORIDE

BRISTOL MYERS SQUIBB
* BRISTOL MYERS SQUIBB
CAPOTEN, CAPTOPRIL
HALOG, HALCINONIDE
MONOPRIL, FOSINOPRIL SODIUM
PRAVACHOL, PRAVASTATIN SODIUM
PRONESTYL-SR, PROCAINAMIDE HYDROCHLORIDE
* BRISTOL MYERS SQUIBB CO
DURICEF, CEFADROXIL/CEFADROXIL HEMIHYDRATE
ESTRACE, ESTRADIOL
QUESTRAN, CHOLESTYRAMINE
* BRISTOL MYERS SQUIBB CO PHARMACEUTICAL RESEARCH INSTITUTE
BUSPAR, BUSPIRONE HYDROCHLORIDE
CEFZIL, CEFPROZIL
DEAPRIL-ST, ERGOLOID MESYLATES

APPENDIX B
PRODUCT NAME INDEX
LISTED BY APPLICANT *(continued)*

DOVONEX, CALCIPOTRIENE
ESTRACE, ESTRADIOL
IFEX, IFOSFAMIDE
MEGACE, MEGESTROL ACETATE
PARAPLATIN, CARBOPLATIN
STADOL, BUTORPHANOL TARTRATE
TAXOL, PACLITAXEL
VAGISTAT-1, TIOCONAZOLE
VIDEX, DIDANOSINE
VUMON, TENIPOSIDE
ZERIT, STAVUDINE

BTG PHARMS
* BTG PHARMACEUTICALS CORP SUB BIOTECHNOLOGY GENERAL CORP
DELATESTRYL, TESTOSTERONE ENANTHATE

BULL D
* DAVID BULL LABORATORIES PARTY LTD
CYTARABINE, CYTARABINE
METOCLOPRAMIDE HCL, METOCLOPRAMIDE HYDROCHLORIDE
VINCRISTINE SULFATE, VINCRISTINE SULFATE

BUNDY
* CM BUNDY CO
BUTABARBITAL, BUTABARBITAL SODIUM
DIPHENHYDRAMINE HCL, DIPHENHYDRAMINE HYDROCHLORIDE
MECLIZINE HCL, MECLIZINE HYDROCHLORIDE
PREDNISOLONE, PREDNISOLONE
PREDNISONE, PREDNISONE
RAUWOLFIA SERPENTINA, RAUWOLFIA SERPENTINA
RESERPINE, RESERPINE

BURROUGHS WELLCOME
* BURROUGHS WELLCOME CO
ACTIDIL, TRIPROLIDINE HYDROCHLORIDE (OTC)
ACTIFED, PSEUDOEPHEDRINE HYDROCHLORIDE (OTC)
ACTIFED W/ CODEINE, CODEINE PHOSPHATE
AEROSPORIN, POLYMYXIN B SULFATE
ALKERAN, MELPHALAN
ALKERAN, MELPHALAN HYDROCHLORIDE
ANECTINE, SUCCINYLCHOLINE CHLORIDE
ANTEPAR, PIPERAZINE CITRATE
CORTISPORIN, BACITRACIN ZINC
CORTISPORIN, HYDROCORTISONE
CORTISPORIN, HYDROCORTISONE ACETATE
DARAPRIM, PYRIMETHAMINE
ELIMITE, PERMETHRIN
EMPRACET W/ CODEINE PHOSPHATE #3, ACETAMINOPHEN
EMPRACET W/ CODEINE PHOSPHATE #4, ACETAMINOPHEN
EXOSURF NEONATAL, CETYL ALCOHOL
IMURAN, AZATHIOPRINE
IMURAN, AZATHIOPRINE SODIUM
KEMADRIN, PROCYCLIDINE HYDROCHLORIDE
LANOXICAPS, DIGOXIN
LANOXIN, DIGOXIN
LEUKERAN, CHLORAMBUCIL
MAREZINE, CYCLIZINE LACTATE
MEPRON, ATOVAQUONE
MIVACRON, MIVACURIUM CHLORIDE
MIVACRON IN DEXTROSE 5%, MIVACURIUM CHLORIDE
MYLERAN, BUSULFAN
NEOSPORIN, BACITRACIN ZINC
NEOSPORIN, GRAMICIDIN
NEOSPORIN G.U. IRRIGANT, NEOMYCIN SULFATE
NIX, PERMETHRIN
NUROMAX, DOXACURIUM CHLORIDE
PEDIOTIC, HYDROCORTISONE
POLYSPORIN, BACITRACIN ZINC
PROLOPRIM, TRIMETHOPRIM
PURINETHOL, MERCAPTOPURINE
RETROVIR, ZIDOVUDINE
SEMPREX-D, ACRIVASTINE
SEPTRA, SULFAMETHOXAZOLE
SEPTRA DS, SULFAMETHOXAZOLE
SEPTRA GRAPE, SULFAMETHOXAZOLE
SUDAFED 12 HOUR, PSEUDOEPHEDRINE HYDROCHLORIDE (OTC)
SYNCURINE, DECAMETHONIUM BROMIDE
THIOGUANINE, THIOGUANINE
TRACRIUM, ATRACURIUM BESYLATE
VASOXYL, METHOXAMINE HYDROCHLORIDE
VIROPTIC, TRIFLURIDINE
WELLBUTRIN, BUPROPION HYDROCHLORIDE
WELLCOVORIN, LEUCOVORIN CALCIUM
ZOVIRAX, ACYCLOVIR
ZOVIRAX, ACYCLOVIR SODIUM
ZYLOPRIM, ALLOPURINOL

C

C AND M PHARMA
* C AND M PHARMACAL INC
HC (HYDROCORTISONE), HYDROCORTISONE
HC (HYDROCORTISONE), HYDROCORTISONE (OTC)
HI-COR, HYDROCORTISONE

CADEMA
* CADEMA MEDICAL PRODUCTS INC
RBC-SCAN, TECHNETIUM TC-99M RED BLOOD CELL KIT

CALGON
* CALGON CORP DIV MERCK AND CO INC
SEPTI-SOFT, HEXACHLOROPHENE

CAMALL
* CAMALL CO INC
CAM-AP-ES, HYDRALAZINE HYDROCHLORIDE
CAM-METRAZINE, PHENDIMETRAZINE TARTRATE
CHLOROTHIAZIDE, CHLOROTHIAZIDE
CYPROHEPTADINE HCL, CYPROHEPTADINE HYDROCHLORIDE
DIETHYLPROPION HCL, DIETHYLPROPION HYDROCHLORIDE
HYDRALAZINE HCL, HYDRALAZINE HYDROCHLORIDE
HYDRO-RESERP, HYDROCHLOROTHIAZIDE
HYDROCHLOROTHIAZIDE, HYDROCHLOROTHIAZIDE
MECLIZINE HCL, MECLIZINE HYDROCHLORIDE
PHENAZINE-35, PHENDIMETRAZINE TARTRATE
PHENDIMETRAZINE TARTRATE, PHENDIMETRAZINE TARTRATE
PHENTERMINE HCL, PHENTERMINE HYDROCHLORIDE
TRICHLORMETHIAZIDE, TRICHLORMETHIAZIDE

APPENDIX B
PRODUCT NAME INDEX
LISTED BY APPLICANT *(continued)*

CARDERM
* CARDERM CAPITAL LP
  CARDIZEM CD, DILTIAZEM HYDROCHLORIDE

CARLISLE
* CARLISLE LABORATORIES INC
  ALPHACAINE, LIDOCAINE
  ALPHACAINE HCL, LIDOCAINE HYDROCHLORIDE
  ALPHACAINE HCL W/ EPINEPHRINE, EPINEPHRINE

CARNRICK
* CARNRICK LABORATORIES INC DIV GW CARNRICK CO
  AMEN, MEDROXYPROGESTERONE ACETATE
  BONTRIL PDM, PHENDIMETRAZINE TARTRATE
  CAPITAL AND CODEINE, ACETAMINOPHEN
  CAPITAL WITH CODEINE, ACETAMINOPHEN
  MOTOFEN, ATROPINE SULFATE
  MOTOFEN HALF-STRENGTH, ATROPINE SULFATE
  PHRENILIN, ACETAMINOPHEN
  PHRENILIN FORTE, ACETAMINOPHEN
  SKELAXIN, METAXALONE

CAROLINA MEDCL
* CAROLINA MEDICAL PRODUCTS CO
  HYDROCORTISONE IN ABSORBASE, HYDROCORTISONE
  ISONIAZID, ISONIAZID
  SODIUM POLYSTYRENE SULFONATE, SODIUM POLYSTYRENE SULFONATE
  SPS, SODIUM POLYSTYRENE SULFONATE

CENCI
* CENCI POWDER PRODUCTS INC
  THEOPHYLLINE, THEOPHYLLINE
* HR CENCI LABORATORIES INC
  ACTAHIST, PSEUDOEPHEDRINE HYDROCHLORIDE
  DIBENIL, DIPHENHYDRAMINE HYDROCHLORIDE
  DIPHENHYDRAMINE HCL, DIPHENHYDRAMINE HYDROCHLORIDE
  ELIXOMIN, THEOPHYLLINE
  HISTAFED, PSEUDOEPHEDRINE HYDROCHLORIDE
  HYDROCORTISONE ACETATE, HYDROCORTISONE ACETATE
  PROMETHAZINE, PROMETHAZINE HYDROCHLORIDE
  PROMETHAZINE VC PLAIN, PHENYLEPHRINE HYDROCHLORIDE
  PROMETHAZINE VC W/ CODEINE, CODEINE PHOSPHATE
  PROMETHAZINE W/ CODEINE, CODEINE PHOSPHATE
  TRIPROLIDINE AND PSEUDOEPHEDRINE HYDROCHLORIDES W/ CODEINE, CODEINE PHOSPHATE

CENT PHARMS
* CENTRAL PHARMACEUTICALS INC
  ACETAMINOPHEN AND HYDROCODONE BITARTRATE, ACETAMINOPHEN
  AZDONE, ASPIRIN
  CO-GESIC, ACETAMINOPHEN
  CODIMAL-L.A. 12, CHLORPHENIRAMINE MALEATE (OTC)
  DEXACEN-4, DEXAMETHASONE SODIUM PHOSPHATE
  PHENYLPROPANOLAMINE HCL W/ CHLORPHENIRAMINE MALEATE, CHLORPHENIRAMINE MALEATE (OTC)
  PREDNICEN-M, PREDNISONE
  PREDNISOLONE ACETATE, PREDNISOLONE ACETATE
  PSEUDOEPHEDRINE HYDROCHLORIDE AND CHLORPHENIRAMINE MALEATE, CHLORPHENIRAMINE MALEATE (OTC)
  SYNOPHYLATE, THEOPHYLLINE SODIUM GLYCINATE
  THEOCLEAR L.A.-130, THEOPHYLLINE
  THEOCLEAR L.A.-260, THEOPHYLLINE
  THEOCLEAR-100, THEOPHYLLINE
  THEOCLEAR-200, THEOPHYLLINE
  THEOCLEAR-80, THEOPHYLLINE
  THEOPHYLLINE, THEOPHYLLINE

CENTURY PHARMS
* CENTURY PHARMACEUTICALS INC
  P.A.S. SODIUM, AMINOSALICYLATE SODIUM

CETUS BEN VENUE
* CETUS BEN VENUE THERAPEUTICS
  ACETYLCYSTEINE, ACETYLCYSTEINE
  CYTARABINE, CYTARABINE
  DOXORUBICIN HCL, DOXORUBICIN HYDROCHLORIDE
  METOCLOPRAMIDE HCL, METOCLOPRAMIDE HYDROCHLORIDE
  SULFAMETHOXAZOLE AND TRIMETHOPRIM, SULFAMETHOXAZOLE

CHAMBERLIN PARENTERL
* CHAMBERLIN PARENTERAL CORP
  HEPARIN SODIUM, HEPARIN SODIUM

CHASE CHEM
* CHASE CHEMICAL CO LP
  VITAMIN A, VITAMIN A
  VITAMIN A, VITAMIN A PALMITATE
  VITAMIN D, ERGOCALCIFEROL

CHASE LABS NJ
* CHASE LABORATORIES INC
  NIFEDIPINE, NIFEDIPINE

CHELSEA LABS
* CHELSEA LABORATORIES INC
  ACETAMINOPHEN W/ CODEINE PHOSPHATE, ACETAMINOPHEN
  ALLOPURINOL, ALLOPURINOL
  AMINOPHYLLINE, AMINOPHYLLINE
  AMITRIPTYLINE HCL, AMITRIPTYLINE HYDROCHLORIDE
  BETHANECHOL CHLORIDE, BETHANECHOL CHLORIDE
  BROMPHENIRAMINE MALEATE, BROMPHENIRAMINE MALEATE
  BUTABARBITAL SODIUM, BUTABARBITAL SODIUM
  BUTALBITAL, ASPIRIN AND CAFFEINE, ASPIRIN
  CARISOPRODOL, CARISOPRODOL
  CHLORDIAZEPOXIDE HCL, CHLORDIAZEPOXIDE HYDROCHLORIDE
  CHLOROHENIRAMINE MALEATE AND PHENYLPROPANOLAMINE HCL, CHLORPHENIRAMINE MALEATE
  CHLOROTHIAZIDE, CHLOROTHIAZIDE
  CHLORPHENIRAMINE MALEATE, CHLORPHENIRAMINE MALEATE
  CHLORPROMAZINE HCL, CHLORPROMAZINE HYDROCHLORIDE
  CHLORPROPAMIDE, CHLORPROPAMIDE
  CHLORTHALIDONE, CHLORTHALIDONE
  CHLORZOXAZONE, CHLORZOXAZONE

APPENDIX B
PRODUCT NAME INDEX
LISTED BY APPLICANT *(continued)*

CLOFIBRATE, CLOFIBRATE
CLORAZEPATE DIPOTASSIUM, CLORAZEPATE DIPOTASSIUM
CORTISONE ACETATE, CORTISONE ACETATE
CYPROHEPTADINE HCL, CYPROHEPTADINE HYDROCHLORIDE
DEXAMETHASONE, DEXAMETHASONE
DIAZEPAM, DIAZEPAM
DICYCLOMINE HCL, DICYCLOMINE HYDROCHLORIDE
DIETHYLPROPION HCL, DIETHYLPROPION HYDROCHLORIDE
DIMENHYDRINATE, DIMENHYDRINATE
DIPHENHYDRAMINE HCL, DIPHENHYDRAMINE HYDROCHLORIDE
DIPHENOXYLATE HCL AND ATROPINE SULFATE, ATROPINE SULFATE
DISULFIRAM, DISULFIRAM
DOXEPIN HCL, DOXEPIN HYDROCHLORIDE
DOXYCYCLINE HYCLATE, DOXYCYCLINE HYCLATE
ERYTHROMYCIN STEARATE, ERYTHROMYCIN STEARATE
FENOPROFEN CALCIUM, FENOPROFEN CALCIUM
FLURAZEPAM HCL, FLURAZEPAM HYDROCHLORIDE
FOLIC ACID, FOLIC ACID
FUROSEMIDE, FUROSEMIDE
GERIMAL, ERGOLOID MESYLATES
GLUTETHIMIDE, GLUTETHIMIDE
GLYCOPYRROLATE, GLYCOPYRROLATE
HYDRALAZINE AND HYDROCHLORTHIAZIDE, HYDRALAZINE HYDROCHLORID
HYDRALAZINE HCL, HYDRALAZINE HYDROCHLORIDE
HYDRALAZINE, HYDROCHLOROTHIAZIDE W/ RESERPINE, HYDRALAZINE HYDROCHLORIDE
HYDROCHLOROTHIAZIDE, HYDROCHLOROTHIAZIDE
HYDROCHLOROTHIAZIDE W/ RESERPINE, HYDROCHLOROTHIAZIDE
HYDROFLUMETHIAZIDE, HYDROFLUMETHIAZIDE
HYDROXYZINE HCL, HYDROXYZINE HYDROCHLORIDE
HYDROXYZINE PAMOATE, HYDROXYZINE PAMOATE
IBUPROFEN, IBUPROFEN
IBUPROFEN, IBUPROFEN (OTC)
IMIPRAMINE HCL, IMIPRAMINE HYDROCHLORIDE
INDOMETHACIN, INDOMETHACIN
ISONIAZID, ISONIAZID
MECLIZINE HCL, MECLIZINE HYDROCHLORIDE
MECLOFENAMATE SODIUM, MECLOFENAMATE SODIUM
MEPROBAMATE, MEPROBAMATE
METHOCARBAMOL, METHOCARBAMOL
METHYCLOTHIAZIDE, METHYCLOTHIAZIDE
METHYLDOPA, METHYLDOPA
METHYLPREDNISOLONE, METHYLPREDNISOLONE
METOCLOPRAMIDE HCL, METOCLOPRAMIDE HYDROCHLORIDE
METRONIDAZOLE, METRONIDAZOLE
NIACIN, NIACIN
NITROFURANTOIN, NITROFURANTOIN
NYSTATIN, NYSTATIN
PERPHENAZINE AND AMITRIPTYLINE HCL, AMITRIPTYLINE HYDROCHLORIDE
PHENDIMETRAZINE TARTRATE, PHENDIMETRAZINE TARTRATE
PHENTERMINE HCL, PHENTERMINE HYDROCHLORIDE
PHENYLBUTAZONE, PHENYLBUTAZONE
PHENYTOIN SODIUM, PHENYTOIN SODIUM, PROMPT
PREDNISOLONE, PREDNISOLONE
PREDNISONE, PREDNISONE
PROBEN-C, COLCHICINE
PROBENECID, PROBENECID
PROCAINAMIDE HCL, PROCAINAMIDE HYDROCHLORIDE
PROMETHAZINE HCL, PROMETHAZINE HYDROCHLORIDE
PROPOXYPHENE HCL, PROPOXYPHENE HYDROCHLORIDE
PROPOXYPHENE HCL W/ ASPIRIN AND CAFFEINE, ASPIRIN
PROPRANOLOL HCL, PROPRANOLOL HYDROCHLORIDE
PROPRANOLOL HCL AND HYDROCHLOROTHIAZIDE, HYDROCHLOROTHIAZIDE
PROPYLTHIOURACIL, PROPYLTHIOURACIL
PYRILAMINE MALEATE, PYRILAMINE MALEATE
QUINIDINE GLUCONATE, QUINIDINE GLUCONATE
QUINIDINE SULFATE, QUINIDINE SULFATE
RESERPINE, RESERPINE
SODIUM PENTOBARBITAL, PENTOBARBITAL SODIUM
SODIUM SECOBARBITAL, SECOBARBITAL SODIUM
SPIRONOLACTONE, SPIRONOLACTONE
SPIRONOLACTONE W/ HYDROCHLOROTHIAZIDE, HYDROCHLOROTHIAZIDE
SULFAMETHOXAZOLE AND TRIMETHOPRIM, SULFAMETHOXAZOLE
SULFASALAZINE, SULFASALAZINE
SULFISOXAZOLE, SULFISOXAZOLE
TETRACYCLINE HCL, TETRACYCLINE HYDROCHLORIDE
THIORIDAZINE HCL, THIORIDAZINE HYDROCHLORIDE
THIOTHIXENE, THIOTHIXENE
TOLBUTAMIDE, TOLBUTAMIDE
TRIAMCINOLONE, TRIAMCINOLONE
TRICHLORMETHIAZIDE, TRICHLORMETHIAZIDE
TRIPELENNAMINE HCL, TRIPELENNAMINE HYDROCHLORIDE
VERAPAMIL HCL, VERAPAMIL HYDROCHLORIDE

CHESEBROUGH PONDS
* CHESEBROUGH PONDS INC
EXTRA-STRENGTH AIM, SODIUM MONOFLUOROPHOSPHATE (OTC)
VIRAC REX, UNDECOYLIUM CHLORIDE

CHOAY
* CHOAY LABORATORIES INC DIV ELF SANOFI INC
CALCIPARINE, HEPARIN CALCIUM

CIBA
* CIBA CONSUMER PHARMACEUTICALS DIV CIBA GEIGY
EFIDAC/24, PSEUDOEPHEDRINE HYDROCHLORIDE (OTC)
TRANSDERM-SCOP, SCOPOLAMINE
* CIBA PHARMACEUTICAL CO DIV CIBA GEIGY CORP
ACTIGALL, URSODIOL
ANTRENYL, OXYPHENONIUM BROMIDE
ANTURANE, SULFINPYRAZONE
APRESAZIDE, HYDRALAZINE HYDROCHLORIDE
APRESOLINE, HYDRALAZINE HYDROCHLORIDE
APRESOLINE-ESIDRIX, HYDRALAZINE HYDROCHLORIDE
CIBACALCIN, CALCITONIN, HUMAN

APPENDIX B
PRODUCT NAME INDEX
LISTED BY APPLICANT *(continued)*

CIBALITH-S, LITHIUM CITRATE
CYTADREN, AMINOGLUTETHIMIDE
DESFERAL, DEFEROXAMINE MESYLATE
ESIDRIX, HYDROCHLOROTHIAZIDE
ESIMIL, GUANETHIDINE MONOSULFATE
ESTRADERM, ESTRADIOL
HEAVY SOLUTION NUPERCAINE, DIBUCAINE HYDROCHLORIDE
IMIPRAMINE HCL, IMIPRAMINE HYDROCHLORIDE
INH, ISONIAZID
ISMELIN, GUANETHIDINE MONOSULFATE
LITHOBID, LITHIUM CARBONATE
LOCORTEN, FLUMETHASONE PIVALATE
LOPRESSIDONE, CHLORTHALIDONE
LOPRESSOR HCT 100/25, HYDROCHLOROTHIAZIDE
LOPRESSOR HCT 100/50, HYDROCHLOROTHIAZIDE
LOPRESSOR HCT 50/25, HYDROCHLOROTHIAZIDE
LOTENSIN, BENAZEPRIL HYDROCHLORIDE
LOTENSIN HCT, BENAZEPRIL HYDROCHLORIDE
LUDIOMIL, MAPROTILINE HYDROCHLORIDE
METANDREN, METHYLTESTOSTERONE
METOPIRONE, METYRAPONE
PERCORTEN, DESOXYCORTICOSTERONE ACETATE
PERCORTEN, DESOXYCORTICOSTERONE PIVALATE
PRISCOLINE, TOLAZOLINE HYDROCHLORIDE
REGITINE, PHENTOLAMINE MESYLATE
RIMACTANE, RIFAMPIN
RITALIN, METHYLPHENIDATE HYDROCHLORIDE
RITALIN-SR, METHYLPHENIDATE HYDROCHLORIDE
SER-AP-ES, HYDRALAZINE HYDROCHLORIDE
SERPASIL, RESERPINE
SERPASIL-APRESOLINE, HYDRALAZINE HYDROCHLORIDE
SERPASIL-ESIDRIX #1, HYDROCHLOROTHIAZIDE
SERPASIL-ESIDRIX #2, HYDROCHLOROTHIAZIDE
SLOW-K, POTASSIUM CHLORIDE
TEN-K, POTASSIUM CHLORIDE
TRASICOR, OXPRENOLOL HYDROCHLORIDE

CIBA GEIGY
* CIBA GEIGY CORP PHARMACEUTICAL DIV
AREDIA, PAMIDRONATE DISODIUM

CIBA VISION
* CIBA VISION OPHTHALMICS DIV CIBA VISION CORP
VOLTAREN, DICLOFENAC SODIUM

CIRCA
* CIRCA PHARMACEUTICALS INC
ACETAZOLAMIDE, ACETAZOLAMIDE
ALLOPURINOL, ALLOPURINOL
AMANTADINE HCL, AMANTADINE HYDROCHLORIDE
ANISOTROPINE METHYLBROMIDE, ANISOTROPINE METHYLBROMIDE
BETHANECHOL CHLORIDE, BETHANECHOL CHLORIDE
CARISOPRODOL, CARISOPRODOL
CARISOPRODOL COMPOUND, ASPIRIN
CHLOROTHIAZIDE, CHLOROTHIAZIDE
CHLOROTHIAZIDE W/ RESERPINE, CHLOROTHIAZIDE
CHLORPHENIRAMINE MALEATE, CHLORPHENIRAMINE MALEATE
CHLORPROPAMIDE, CHLORPROPAMIDE
CHLORTHALIDONE, CHLORTHALIDONE
CLONIDINE HCL, CLONIDINE HYDROCHLORIDE
CYPROHEPTADINE HCL, CYPROHEPTADINE HYDROCHLORIDE
DEXAMETHASONE, DEXAMETHASONE
DICYCLOMINE HCL, DICYCLOMINE HYDROCHLORIDE
DIPHENHYDRAMINE HCL, DIPHENHYDRAMINE HYDROCHLORIDE
DISOPYRAMIDE PHOSPHATE, DISOPYRAMIDE PHOSPHATE
ERGOLOID MESYLATES, ERGOLOID MESYLATES
FLUOXYMESTERONE, FLUOXYMESTERONE
FLUPHENAZINE HCL, FLUPHENAZINE HYDROCHLORIDE
FOLIC ACID, FOLIC ACID
GLYCOPYRROLATE, GLYCOPYRROLATE
GUANETHIDINE MONOSULFATE, GUANETHIDINE MONOSULFATE
HALOPERIDOL, HALOPERIDOL
HYDRALAZINE HCL AND HYDROCHLOROTHIAZIDE, HYDRALAZINE HYDROCHLORIDE
HYDROCHLOROTHIAZIDE, HYDROCHLOROTHIAZIDE
HYDROCHLOROTHIAZIDE W/ HYDRALAZINE, HYDRALAZINE HYDROCHLORID
HYDROCHLOROTHIAZIDE W/ RESERPINE, HYDROCHLOROTHIAZIDE
HYDROCHLOROTHIAZIDE W/ RESERPINE AND HYDRALAZINE, HYDRALAZINE HYDROCHLORIDE
HYDROFLUMETHIAZIDE, HYDROFLUMETHIAZIDE
HYDROFLUMETHIAZIDE AND RESERPINE, HYDROFLUMETHIAZIDE
HYDROXYZINE PAMOATE, HYDROXYZINE PAMOATE
IMIPRAMINE HCL, IMIPRAMINE HYDROCHLORIDE
INDOMETHACIN, INDOMETHACIN
ISONIAZID, ISONIAZID
LIOTHYRONINE SODIUM, LIOTHYRONINE SODIUM
LITHIUM CARBONATE, LITHIUM CARBONATE
MAPROTILINE HCL, MAPROTILINE HYDROCHLORIDE
MECLIZINE HCL, MECLIZINE HYDROCHLORIDE
MECLOFENAMATE SODIUM, MECLOFENAMATE SODIUM
METHOCARBAMOL, METHOCARBAMOL
METHYCLOTHIAZIDE, METHYCLOTHIAZIDE
METHYCLOTHIAZIDE AND DESERPIDINE, DESERPIDINE
METHYLDOPA, METHYLDOPA
METHYLDOPA AND HYDROCHLOROTHIAZIDE, HYDROCHLOROTHIAZIDE
METOCLOPRAMIDE HCL, METOCLOPRAMIDE HYDROCHLORIDE
NIACIN, NIACIN
NITROFURANTOIN, NITROFURANTOIN
NITROFURANTOIN MACROCRYSTALLINE, NITROFURANTOIN, MACROCRYSTALLINE
ORPHENADRINE CITRATE, ORPHENADRINE CITRATE
OXTRIPHYLLINE, OXTRIPHYLLINE
OXYBUTYNIN CHLORIDE, OXYBUTYNIN CHLORIDE
OXYPHENBUTAZONE, OXYPHENBUTAZONE
PERPHENAZINE AND AMITRIPTYLINE HCL, AMITRIPTYLINE HYDROCHLORIDE
PHENYTEX, PHENYTOIN SODIUM, EXTENDED
PRIMIDONE, PRIMIDONE
PROBENECID W/ COLCHICINE, COLCHICINE
PROCAINAMIDE HCL, PROCAINAMIDE HYDROCHLORIDE
PROCHLORPERAZINE, PROCHLORPERAZINE MALEATE
PROMETHAZINE HCL, PROMETHAZINE HYDROCHLORIDE
PROPANTHELINE BROMIDE, PROPANTHELINE BROMIDE

APPENDIX B
PRODUCT NAME INDEX
LISTED BY APPLICANT *(continued)*

PROPOXYPHENE NAPSYLATE AND ACETAMINOPHEN, ACETAMINOPHEN
PROPRANOLOL HCL, PROPRANOLOL HYDROCHLORIDE
QUINATIME, QUINIDINE GLUCONATE
SPIRONOLACTONE, SPIRONOLACTONE
SPIRONOLACTONE W/ HYDROCHLOROTHIAZIDE, HYDROCHLOROTHIAZIDE
SULFAMETHOXAZOLE, SULFAMETHOXAZOLE
SULFASALAZINE, SULFASALAZINE
TEMAZEPAM, TEMAZEPAM
THIORIDAZINE HCL, THIORIDAZINE HYDROCHLORIDE
TIMOLOL MALEATE, TIMOLOL MALEATE
TOLAZAMIDE, TOLAZAMIDE
TOLBUTAMIDE, TOLBUTAMIDE
TRAZODONE HCL, TRAZODONE HYDROCHLORIDE
TRICHLORMETHIAZIDE, TRICHLORMETHIAZIDE
TRICHLORMETHIAZIDE W/ RESERPINE, RESERPINE
TRIFLUOPERAZINE HCL, TRIFLUOPERAZINE HYDROCHLORIDE
TRIHEXYPHENIDYL HCL, TRIHEXYPHENIDYL HYDROCHLORIDE
TRIPELENNAMINE HCL, TRIPELENNAMINE HYDROCHLORIDE
TRIPROLIDINE AND PSEUDOEPHEDRINE, PSEUDOEPHEDRINE HYDROCHLORIDE (OTC)
WARFARIN SODIUM, WARFARIN SODIUM

CIS
* CIS BIOINDUSTRIES COMPAGNIE
SODIUM IODIDE I 131, SODIUM IODIDE, I-131
* CIS US INC
AN-DTPA, TECHNETIUM TC-99M PENTETATE KIT
AN-MDP, TECHNETIUM TC-99M MEDRONATE KIT
AN-PYROTEC, TECHNETIUM TC-99M PYROPHOSPHATE KIT
AN-SULFUR COLLOID, TECHNETIUM TC-99M SULFUR COLLOID KIT
IOBENGUANE SULFATE I 131, IOBENGUANE SULFATE I 131
SELENOMETHIONINE SE 75, SELENOMETHIONINE, SE-75
SODIUM PERTECHNETATE TC 99M, TECHNETIUM TC-99M SODIUM PERTECHNETATE

CLAY PARK
* CLAY PARK LABORATORIES INC
BETAMETHASONE DIPROPIONATE, BETAMETHASONE DIPROPIONATE
BETAMETHASONE VALERATE, BETAMETHASONE VALERATE
ERYTHROMYCIN, ERYTHROMYCIN
FLUOCINOLONE ACETONIDE, FLUOCINOLONE ACETONIDE
FLUOCINONIDE, FLUOCINONIDE
GENTAMICIN, GENTAMICIN SULFATE
HYDROCORTISONE, HYDROCORTISONE
NITROFURAZONE, NITROFURAZONE
NYSTATIN, NYSTATIN
NYSTATIN AND TRIAMCINOLONE ACETONIDE, NYSTATIN
SELENIUM SULFIDE, SELENIUM SULFIDE
TRIAMCINOLONE ACETONIDE, TRIAMCINOLONE ACETONIDE
TRIPLE SULFA, TRIPLE SULFA (SULFABENZAMIDE;SULFACETAMIDE;SULFATHIAZOLE)

CLONMEL
* CLONMEL HEALTH CARE
AMOXICILLIN, AMOXICILLIN
AMPICILLIN, AMPICILLIN/AMPICILLIN TRIHYDRATE
PENICILLIN V POTASSIUM, PENICILLIN V POTASSIUM

COLGATE PALMOLIVE
* COLGATE PALMOLIVE CO
PERIOGARD, CHLORHEXIDINE GLUCONATE

COMBE
* COMBE INC
BACITRACIN, BACITRACIN (OTC)
LANABIOTIC, BACITRACIN (OTC)
LANABIOTIC, BACITRACIN ZINC (OTC)

CONSOLIDATED MIDLAND
* CONSOLIDATED MIDLAND CORP
TEEBACIN, AMINOSALICYLATE SODIUM

COOK WAITE
* COOK WAITE LABORATORIES INC SUB STERLING DRUG INC
CARBOCAINE, MEPIVACAINE HYDROCHLORIDE
CARBOCAINE W/ NEO-COBEFRIN, LEVONORDEFRIN

COPANOS
* JOHN D COPANOS AND CO INC
AMOXICILLIN TRIHYDRATE, AMOXICILLIN
AMPICILLIN SODIUM, AMPICILLIN SODIUM
AMPICILLIN TRIHYDRATE, AMPICILLIN/AMPICILLIN TRIHYDRATE
COMOX, AMOXICILLIN
PENICILLIN G POTASSIUM, PENICILLIN G POTASSIUM
PENICILLIN G PROCAINE, PENICILLIN G PROCAINE
PENICILLIN G SODIUM, PENICILLIN G SODIUM
PENICILLIN V POTASSIUM, PENICILLIN V POTASSIUM
STREPTOMYCIN SULFATE, STREPTOMYCIN SULFATE

COPLEY PHARM
* COPLEY PHARMACEUTICAL INC
ALBUTEROL SULFATE, ALBUTEROL SULFATE
AMANTADINE HCL, AMANTADINE HYDROCHLORIDE
AMITRIPTYLINE HCL, AMITRIPTYLINE HYDROCHLORIDE
BETAMETHASONE DIPROPIONATE, BETAMETHASONE DIPROPIONATE
BETAMETHASONE VALERATE, BETAMETHASONE VALERATE
BROMATAPP, BROMPHENIRAMINE MALEATE (OTC)
BROMPHERIL, DEXBROMPHENIRAMINE MALEATE (OTC)
CLEMASTINE FUMARATE, CLEMASTINE FUMARATE
CLINDAMYCIN PHOSPHATE, CLINDAMYCIN PHOSPHATE
CLOBETASOL PROPIONATE, CLOBETASOL PROPIONATE
CO-LAV, POLYETHYLENE GLYCOL 3350
DESONIDE, DESONIDE
DILTIAZEM HCL, DILTIAZEM HYDROCHLORIDE
DOXEPIN HCL, DOXEPIN HYDROCHLORIDE
DOXYLAMINE SUCCINATE, DOXYLAMINE SUCCINATE (OTC)
ETHOSUXIMIDE, ETHOSUXIMIDE
EVALOSE, LACTULOSE

APPENDIX B
PRODUCT NAME INDEX
LISTED BY APPLICANT *(continued)*

FLUOCINONIDE, FLUOCINONIDE
FLUPHENAZINE HCL, FLUPHENAZINE HYDROCHLORIDE
GO-EVAC, POLYETHYLENE GLYCOL 3350
GUANABENZ ACETATE, GUANABENZ ACETATE
HALOPERIDOL, HALOPERIDOL LACTATE
HEPTALAC, LACTULOSE
HYDROCORTISONE, HYDROCORTISONE
HYDROCORTISONE ACETATE 1% AND PRAMOXINE HCL 1%, HYDROCORTISONE ACETATE
LIDOCAINE HCL, LIDOCAINE HYDROCHLORIDE
METAPROTERENOL SULFATE, METAPROTERENOL SULFATE
METHAZOLAMIDE, METHAZOLAMIDE
METOPROLOL TARTRATE, METOPROLOL TARTRATE
MICONAZOLE NITRATE, MICONAZOLE NITRATE (OTC)
NADOLOL, NADOLOL
NAPROXEN, NAPROXEN
NAPROXEN SODIUM, NAPROXEN SODIUM
PIROXICAM, PIROXICAM
POTASSIUM CHLORIDE, POTASSIUM CHLORIDE
PROCAINAMIDE HCL, PROCAINAMIDE HYDROCHLORIDE
QUINIDINE SULFATE, QUINIDINE SULFATE
THIORIDAZINE HCL, THIORIDAZINE HYDROCHLORIDE
THIOTHIXENE HCL, THIOTHIXENE HYDROCHLORIDE
VALPROIC ACID, VALPROIC ACID

CUMBERLAND SWAN
* CUMBERLAND SWAN INC
DIPHENHYDRAMINE HCL, DIPHENHYDRAMINE HYDROCHLORIDE (OTC)

CURATEK
* CURATEK PHARMACEUTICALS LTD PARTNERSHIP
METROGEL, METRONIDAZOLE

D

DANBURY PHARMA
* DANBURY PHARMACAL INC
ACETAZOLAMIDE, ACETAZOLAMIDE
ACETOHEXAMIDE, ACETOHEXAMIDE
ALBUTEROL SULFATE, ALBUTEROL SULFATE
ALLOPURINOL, ALLOPURINOL
AMITRIPTYLINE HCL, AMITRIPTYLINE HYDROCHLORIDE
AMOXAPINE, AMOXAPINE
ATENOLOL, ATENOLOL
ATENOLOL AND CHLORTHALIDONE, ATENOLOL
BACLOFEN, BACLOFEN
BETHANECHOL CHLORIDE, BETHANECHOL CHLORIDE
BROMPHENIRAMINE MALEATE, BROMPHENIRAMINE MALEATE
BUTALBITAL AND ACETAMINOPHEN, ACETAMINOPHEN
CARISOPRODOL, CARISOPRODOL
CHLORDIAZEPOXIDE AND AMITRIPTYLINE HCL, AMITRIPTYLINE HYDROCHLORIDE
CHLOROQUINE PHOSPHATE, CHLOROQUINE PHOSPHATE
CHLOROTHIAZIDE, CHLOROTHIAZIDE
CHLORPHENIRAMINE MALEATE, CHLORPHENIRAMINE MALEATE
CHLORPROPAMIDE, CHLORPROPAMIDE
CHLORTHALIDONE, CHLORTHALIDONE
CHLORZOXAZONE, CHLORZOXAZONE
CLINDAMYCIN HCL, CLINDAMYCIN HYDROCHLORIDE
CLONIDINE HCL, CLONIDINE HYDROCHLORIDE
COL-PROBENECID, COLCHICINE
CYCLOBENZAPRINE HCL, CYCLOBENZAPRINE HYDROCHLORIDE
CYPROHEPTADINE HCL, CYPROHEPTADINE HYDROCHLORIDE
DEXAMETHASONE, DEXAMETHASONE
DIAZEPAM, DIAZEPAM
DIPHENHYDRAMINE HCL, DIPHENHYDRAMINE HYDROCHLORIDE
DISOPYRAMIDE PHOSPHATE, DISOPYRAMIDE PHOSPHATE
DISULFIRAM, DISULFIRAM
DOXEPIN HCL, DOXEPIN HYDROCHLORIDE
DOXYCYCLINE HYCLATE, DOXYCYCLINE HYCLATE
ERGOLOID MESYLATES, ERGOLOID MESYLATES
ERYTHROMYCIN ESTOLATE, ERYTHROMYCIN ESTOLATE
FENOPROFEN CALCIUM, FENOPROFEN CALCIUM
FLURAZEPAM HCL, FLURAZEPAM HYDROCHLORIDE
FOLIC ACID, FOLIC ACID
FUROSEMIDE, FUROSEMIDE
GLUTETHIMIDE, GLUTETHIMIDE
GLYCOPYRROLATE, GLYCOPYRROLATE
HALOPERIDOL, HALOPERIDOL
HYDRALAZINE HCL, HYDRALAZINE HYDROCHLORIDE
HYDROCHLOROTHIAZIDE, HYDROCHLOROTHIAZIDE
HYDROCHLOROTHIAZIDE W/ RESERPINE, HYDROCHLOROTHIAZIDE
HYDROCORTISONE, HYDROCORTISONE
HYDROXYZINE HCL, HYDROXYZINE HYDROCHLORIDE
HYDROXYZINE PAMOATE, HYDROXYZINE PAMOATE
IBUPROFEN, IBUPROFEN
IBUPROFEN, IBUPROFEN (OTC)
INDOMETHACIN, INDOMETHACIN
ISONIAZID, ISONIAZID
ISOSORBIDE DINITRATE, ISOSORBIDE DINITRATE
LORAZEPAM, LORAZEPAM
MECLOFENAMATE SODIUM, MECLOFENAMATE SODIUM
MEPROBAMATE, MEPROBAMATE
METAPROTERENOL SULFATE, METAPROTERENOL SULFATE
METHOCARBAMOL, METHOCARBAMOL
METHYLDOPA, METHYLDOPA
METHYLDOPA AND HYDROCHLOROTHIAZIDE, HYDROCHLOROTHIAZIDE
METHYLTESTOSTERONE, METHYLTESTOSTERONE
METOCLOPRAMIDE HCL, METOCLOPRAMIDE HYDROCHLORIDE
METRONIDAZOLE, METRONIDAZOLE
MINOCYCLINE HCL, MINOCYCLINE HYDROCHLORIDE
MINOXIDIL, MINOXIDIL
NALIDIXIC ACID, NALIDIXIC ACID
NAPROXEN SODIUM, NAPROXEN SODIUM
NIACIN, NIACIN
NITROFURANTOIN, NITROFURANTOIN, MACROCRYSTALLINE

APPENDIX B
PRODUCT NAME INDEX
LISTED BY APPLICANT *(continued)*

NORTRIPTYLINE HCL, NORTRIPTYLINE HYDROCHLORIDE
OXAZEPAM, OXAZEPAM
PERPHENAZINE AND AMITRIPTYLINE HCL, AMITRIPTYLINE HYDROCHLORIDE
PHENYLBUTAZONE, PHENYLBUTAZONE
PRAZOSIN HCL, PRAZOSIN HYDROCHLORIDE
PREDNISOLONE, PREDNISOLONE
PREDNISONE, PREDNISONE
PRIMIDONE, PRIMIDONE
PROBENECID, PROBENECID
PROCAINAMIDE HCL, PROCAINAMIDE HYDROCHLORIDE
PROMETHAZINE HCL, PROMETHAZINE HYDROCHLORIDE
PROMPT PHENYTOIN SODIUM, PHENYTOIN SODIUM, PROMPT
PROPANTHELINE BROMIDE, PROPANTHELINE BROMIDE
PROPOXYPHENE HCL, PROPOXYPHENE HYDROCHLORIDE
PROPRANOLOL HCL, PROPRANOLOL HYDROCHLORIDE
PROPRANOLOL HCL AND HYDROCHLOROTHIAZIDE, HYDROCHLOROTHIAZIDE
PROPYLTHIOURACIL, PROPYLTHIOURACIL
QUINIDINE GLUCONATE, QUINIDINE GLUCONATE
QUINIDINE SULFATE, QUINIDINE SULFATE
RAUWOLFIA SERPENTINA, RAUWOLFIA SERPENTINA
RESERPINE, RESERPINE
RESERPINE, HYDRALAZINE HCL AND HYDROCHLOROTHIAZIDE, HYDRALAZINE HYDROCHLORIDE
SPIRONOLACTONE/HYDROCHLOROTHIAZIDE, HYDROCHLOROTHIAZIDE
SULFAMETHOXAZOLE AND TRIMETHOPRIM, SULFAMETHOXAZOLE
SULFAMETHOXAZOLE AND TRIMETHOPRIM DOUBLE STRENGTH, SULFAMETHOXAZOLE
SULFASALAZINE, SULFASALAZINE
SULFINPYRAZONE, SULFINPYRAZONE
SULINDAC, SULINDAC
TEMAZEPAM, TEMAZEPAM
TETRACYCLINE HCL, TETRACYCLINE HYDROCHLORIDE
THIORIDAZINE HCL, THIORIDAZINE HYDROCHLORIDE
THIOTHIXENE, THIOTHIXENE
TIMOLOL MALEATE, TIMOLOL MALEATE
TOLAZAMIDE, TOLAZAMIDE
TOLBUTAMIDE, TOLBUTAMIDE
TRAZODONE HCL, TRAZODONE HYDROCHLORIDE
TRIAMCINOLONE, TRIAMCINOLONE
TRIAMTERENE AND HYDROCHLOROTHIAZIDE, HYDROCHLOROTHIAZIDE
TRICHLORMETHIAZIDE, TRICHLORMETHIAZIDE
TRIHEXYPHENIDYL HCL, TRIHEXYPHENIDYL HYDROCHLORIDE
TRIMETHOPRIM, TRIMETHOPRIM
TRIPELENNAMINE HCL, TRIPELENNAMINE HYDROCHLORIDE
TRIPROLIDINE HCL, TRIPROLIDINE HYDROCHLORIDE
VERAPAMIL HCL, VERAPAMIL HYDROCHLORIDE

DANIELS PHARMS
* DANIELS PHARMACEUTICALS INC
TUSSIGON, HOMATROPINE METHYLBROMIDE

DAVIS AND GECK
* DAVIS AND GECK DIV AMERICAN CYANAMID CO
FLAXEDIL, GALLAMINE TRIETHIODIDE
PRE-OP, HEXACHLOROPHENE
PRE-OP II, HEXACHLOROPHENE

DEL RAY LABS
* DEL RAY LABORATORIES INC
ALA-CORT, HYDROCORTISONE
ALA-SCALP, HYDROCORTISONE
DEL-VI-A, VITAMIN A PALMITATE
TRIDERM, TRIAMCINOLONE ACETONIDE

DELL LABS
* DELL LABORATORIES INC
CYANOCOBALAMIN, CYANOCOBALAMIN
DEXAMETHASONE SODIUM PHOSPHATE, DEXAMETHASONE SODIUM PHOSPHATE
HEPARIN SODIUM, HEPARIN SODIUM
LIDOCAINE HCL, LIDOCAINE HYDROCHLORIDE
LIDOCAINE HCL W/ EPINEPHRINE, EPINEPHRINE
PYRIDOXINE HCL, PYRIDOXINE HYDROCHLORIDE
THIAMINE HCL, THIAMINE HYDROCHLORIDE

DEPROCO
* DEPROCO INC
LIGNOSPAN FORTE, EPINEPHRINE BITARTRATE
LIGNOSPAN STANDARD, EPINEPHRINE BITARTRATE
SCANDONEST L, LEVONORDEFRIN
SCANDONEST PLAIN, MEPIVACAINE HYDROCHLORIDE

DERMIK
* DERMIK LABORATORIES INC SUB RORER
BENZAMYCIN, BENZOYL PEROXIDE
HYTONE, HYDROCORTISONE
PSORCON, DIFLORASONE DIACETATE

DESERET
* DESERET MEDICAL INC DIV BECTON DICKINSON AND CO
CHLORHEXIDINE GLUCONATE, CHLORHEXIDINE GLUCONATE (OTC)
E-Z SCRUB, HEXACHLOROPHENE

DEY
* DEY LABORATORIES INC
ALBUTEROL SULFATE, ALBUTEROL SULFATE
CROMOLYN SODIUM, CROMOLYN SODIUM
ISOETHARINE HCL, ISOETHARINE HYDROCHLORIDE
ISOETHARINE HCL S/F, ISOETHARINE HYDROCHLORIDE
ISOPROTERENOL HCL, ISOPROTERENOL HYDROCHLORIDE
METAPROTERENOL SULFATE, METAPROTERENOL SULFATE
MUCOSIL-10, ACETYLCYSTEINE
MUCOSIL-20, ACETYLCYSTEINE

DIAL
* DIAL CORP DIV GREYHOUND CO
DIAL, HEXACHLOROPHENE

DISTA
* DISTA PRODUCTS CO DIV ELI LILLY AND CO
ERYTHROMYCIN ETHYLSUCCINATE, ERYTHROMYCIN ETHYLSUCCINATE
ILOSONE, ERYTHROMYCIN ESTOLATE
ILOTYCIN, ERYTHROMYCIN

APPENDIX B
PRODUCT NAME INDEX
LISTED BY APPLICANT *(continued)*

ILOTYCIN GLUCEPTATE, ERYTHROMYCIN GLUCEPTATE
NALFON, FENOPROFEN CALCIUM
NALFON 200, FENOPROFEN CALCIUM
PENICILLIN G POTASSIUM, PENICILLIN G POTASSIUM
VALMID, ETHINAMATE

DORSEY
* DORSEY LABORATORIES DIV SANDOZ WANDER INC
ASBRON, THEOPHYLLINE SODIUM GLYCINATE
PHENYLPROPANOLAMINE HCL/ CHLORPHENIRAMINE, CHLORPHENIRAMINE MALEATE (OTC)
RAUTENSIN, ALSEROXYLON

DOW PHARMS
* DOW PHARMACEUTICALS CORP SUB DOW CHEMICAL CO
DOW-ISONIAZID, ISONIAZID
NEO-POLYCIN, BACITRACIN ZINC
NEO-POLYCIN, GRAMICIDIN
NOVAFED, PSEUDOEPHEDRINE HYDROCHLORIDE
QUIDE, PIPERACETAZINE
RIFAMATE, ISONIAZID

DOWNSTATE CLINCL
* DOWNSTATE CLINICAL PET CENTER
FLUDEOXYGLUCOSE F 18, FLUDEOXYGLUCOSE, F-18

DUNHALL
* DUNHALL PHARMACEUTICALS INC
TRIAPRIN, ACETAMINOPHEN

DUPONT
* DUPONT RADIOPHARMACEUTICALS DIV
CARDIOLITE, TECHNETIUM TC-99M SESTAMIBI KIT
GALLIUM CITRATE GA 67, GALLIUM CITRATE, GA-67
GLUCOSCAN, TECHNETIUM TC-99M GLUCEPTATE KIT
HEPATOLITE, TECHNETIUM TC-99M DISOFENIN KIT
MICROLITE, TECHNETIUM TC-99M ALBUMIN COLLOID KIT
OSTEOLITE, TECHNETIUM TC-99M MEDRONATE KIT
PULMOLITE, TECHNETIUM TC-99M ALBUMIN AGGREGATED KIT
PYROLITE, TECHNETIUM TC-99M PYRO/TRIMETA PHOSPHATES KIT
TECHNETIUM TC 99M GENERATOR, TECHNETIUM TC-99M SODIUM PERTECHNETATE GENERATOR
THALLOUS CHLORIDE TL 201, THALLOUS CHLORIDE, TL-201
XENON XE 133, XENON, XE-133

DUPONT MERCK
* DUPONT MERCK PHARMACEUTICAL CO
ACETYLCYSTEINE, ACETYLCYSTEINE
AMIKACIN, AMIKACIN SULFATE
BRETYLOL, BRETYLIUM TOSYLATE
CLINDAMYCIN PHOSPHATE, CLINDAMYCIN PHOSPHATE
COUMADIN, WARFARIN SODIUM
DROPERIDOL, DROPERIDOL
HYCODAN, HOMATROPINE METHYLBROMIDE
HYCOMINE, HYDROCODONE BITARTRATE
HYCOMINE PEDIATRIC, HYDROCODONE BITARTRATE
INTROPIN, DOPAMINE HYDROCHLORIDE
METHYLDOPATE HCL, METHYLDOPATE HYDROCHLORIDE
METOCLOPRAMIDE HCL, METOCLOPRAMIDE HYDROCHLORIDE
MOBAN, MOLINDONE HYDROCHLORIDE
NARCAN, NALOXONE HYDROCHLORIDE
NUBAIN, NALBUPHINE HYDROCHLORIDE
NUMORPHAN, OXYMORPHONE HYDROCHLORIDE
OXYCODONE 2.5/APAP 500, ACETAMINOPHEN
OXYCODONE 5/APAP 500, ACETAMINOPHEN
PERCOCET, ACETAMINOPHEN
PERCODAN, ASPIRIN
PERCODAN-DEMI, ASPIRIN
REMSED, PROMETHAZINE HYDROCHLORIDE
SYMMETREL, AMANTADINE HYDROCHLORIDE
TREXAN, NALTREXONE HYDROCHLORIDE
TRIDIL, NITROGLYCERIN
VALPIN 50, ANISOTROPINE METHYLBROMIDE

DURAMED
* DURAMED PHARMACEUTICALS INC
ACETAMINOPHEN AND CODEINE PHOSPHATE, ACETAMINOPHEN
AMINOPHYLLINE, AMINOPHYLLINE
CHLORPROPAMIDE, CHLORPROPAMIDE
CLONIDINE HCL, CLONIDINE HYDROCHLORIDE
CYPROHEPTADINE HCL, CYPROHEPTADINE HYDROCHLORIDE
DIAZEPAM, DIAZEPAM
HALOPERIDOL, HALOPERIDOL
HYDROXYZINE PAMOATE, HYDROXYZINE PAMOATE
INDOMETHACIN, INDOMETHACIN
ISONIAZID, ISONIAZID
METHYLDOPA, METHYLDOPA
METHYLPREDNISOLONE, METHYLPREDNISOLONE
PHENTERMINE HCL, PHENTERMINE HYDROCHLORIDE
PREDNISONE, PREDNISONE
PROCHLORPERAZINE MALEATE, PROCHLORPERAZINE MALEATE
PROPRANOLOL HCL, PROPRANOLOL HYDROCHLORIDE
PROPRANOLOL HCL & HYDROCHLOROTHIAZIDE, HYDROCHLOROTHIAZIDE
TEMAZEPAM, TEMAZEPAM
TOLAZAMIDE, TOLAZAMIDE
TRIFLUOPERAZINE HCL, TRIFLUOPERAZINE HYDROCHLORIDE

DYNAPHARM
* DYNAPHARM INC
COLOVAGE, POLYETHYLENE GLYCOL 3350

E

E Z EM
* E Z EM CO INC
E-Z-EM PREP LYTE, POLYETHYLENE GLYCOL 3350

ELAN PHARM
* ELAN PHARMACEUTICAL RESEARCH CORP
PROSTEP, NICOTINE
VERELAN, VERAPAMIL HYDROCHLORIDE

ELDER
* ELDER PHARMACEUTICALS LTD
ELDECORT, HYDROCORTISONE

APPENDIX B
PRODUCT NAME INDEX
LISTED BY APPLICANT *(continued)*

ELKINS SINN
* ELKINS SINN INC DIV AH ROBINS CO INC
AMIKACIN, AMIKACIN SULFATE
AMINOCAPROIC ACID, AMINOCAPROIC ACID
AMINOPHYLLINE, AMINOPHYLLINE
AMPICILLIN SODIUM, AMPICILLIN SODIUM
BRETYLIUM TOSYLATE, BRETYLIUM TOSYLATE
CEFAZOLIN SODIUM, CEFAZOLIN SODIUM
CEPHAPIRIN SODIUM, CEPHAPIRIN SODIUM
CHLORAMPHENICOL, CHLORAMPHENICOL SODIUM SUCCINATE
CHLORPHENIRAMINE MALEATE, CHLORPHENIRAMINE MALEATE
CHLORPROMAZINE HCL, CHLORPROMAZINE HYDROCHLORIDE
CLINDAMYCIN PHOSPHATE, CLINDAMYCIN PHOSPHATE
CORTISONE ACETATE, CORTISONE ACETATE
CYANOCOBALAMIN, CYANOCOBALAMIN
CYCLOPHOSPHAMIDE, CYCLOPHOSPHAMIDE
DEXAMETHASONE, DEXAMETHASONE SODIUM PHOSPHATE
DIAZEPAM, DIAZEPAM
DIGOXIN, DIGOXIN
DIMENHYDRINATE, DIMENHYDRINATE
DIPHENHYDRAMINE HCL, DIPHENHYDRAMINE HYDROCHLORIDE
DOPAMINE, DOPAMINE HYDROCHLORIDE
DOXYCYCLINE, DOXYCYCLINE HYCLATE
DURAMORPH PF, MORPHINE SULFATE
ERYTHROMYCIN, ERYTHROMYCIN LACTOBIONATE
FENTANYL CITRATE, FENTANYL CITRATE
FUROSEMIDE, FUROSEMIDE
GENTAMICIN SULFATE, GENTAMICIN SULFATE
HEP-LOCK, HEPARIN SODIUM
HEP-LOCK U/P, HEPARIN SODIUM
HEPARIN SODIUM, HEPARIN SODIUM
HYDROCHLOROTHIAZIDE, HYDROCHLOROTHIAZIDE
HYDROCORTISONE, HYDROCORTISONE
HYDROCORTISONE SODIUM SUCCINATE, HYDROCORTISONE SODIUM SUCCINATE
HYDROXYZINE, HYDROXYZINE HYDROCHLORIDE
HYDROXYZINE HCL, HYDROXYZINE HYDROCHLORIDE
INFUMORPH, MORPHINE SULFATE
ISOPROTERENOL HCL, ISOPROTERENOL HYDROCHLORIDE
KANAMYCIN, KANAMYCIN SULFATE
LEUCOVORIN CALCIUM, LEUCOVORIN CALCIUM
LIDOCAINE HCL, LIDOCAINE HYDROCHLORIDE
LIDOCAINE HCL AND EPINEPHRINE, EPINEPHRINE
MEPERIDINE HCL, MEPERIDINE HYDROCHLORIDE
MEPROBAMATE, MEPROBAMATE
METARAMINOL BITARTRATE, METARAMINOL BITARTRATE
METHYLDOPATE HCL, METHYLDOPATE HYDROCHLORIDE
METHYLPREDNISOLONE, METHYLPREDNISOLONE SODIUM SUCCINATE
METHYLPREDNISOLONE SODIUM SUCCINATE, METHYLPREDNISOLONE SODIUM SUCCINATE
METRONIDAZOLE, METRONIDAZOLE
NALOXONE, NALOXONE HYDROCHLORIDE
NALOXONE HCL, NALOXONE HYDROCHLORIDE
NEOMYCIN SULFATE, NEOMYCIN SULFATE
NITROFURANTOIN, NITROFURANTOIN
OXACILLIN SODIUM, OXACILLIN SODIUM
PANCURONIUM, PANCURONIUM BROMIDE
PENTOBARBITAL SODIUM, PENTOBARBITAL SODIUM
PHENYTOIN, PHENYTOIN SODIUM
POTASSIUM CHLORIDE, POTASSIUM CHLORIDE
PREDNISOLONE, PREDNISOLONE
PREDNISONE, PREDNISONE
PROCAINAMIDE HCL, PROCAINAMIDE HYDROCHLORIDE
PROCAINE HCL, PROCAINE HYDROCHLORIDE
PROCHLORPERAZINE, PROCHLORPERAZINE EDISYLATE
PROCHLORPERAZINE EDISYLATE, PROCHLORPERAZINE EDISYLATE
PROMETHAZINE HCL, PROMETHAZINE HYDROCHLORIDE
PROTAMINE SULFATE, PROTAMINE SULFATE
PYRIDOXINE HCL, PYRIDOXINE HYDROCHLORIDE
QUINIDINE SULFATE, QUINIDINE SULFATE
RESERPINE, RESERPINE
SECOBARBITAL SODIUM, SECOBARBITAL SODIUM
SODIUM NITROPRUSSIDE, SODIUM NITROPRUSSIDE
SODIUM PENTOBARBITAL, PENTOBARBITAL SODIUM
SODIUM SUCCINATE, SODIUM SUCCINATE
SOTRADECOL, SODIUM TETRADECYL SULFATE
SULFAMETHOXAZOLE AND TRIMETHOPRIM, SULFAMETHOXAZOLE
TESTOSTERONE PROPIONATE, TESTOSTERONE PROPIONATE
TETRACYCLINE HCL, TETRACYCLINE HYDROCHLORIDE
THIAMINE HCL, THIAMINE HYDROCHLORIDE
TOBRAMYCIN SULFATE, TOBRAMYCIN SULFATE
VANCOMYCIN HCL, VANCOMYCIN HYDROCHLORIDE
VITAMIN A, VITAMIN A PALMITATE

ENDO LABS
* ENDO LABORATORIES LLC
CIMETIDINE, CIMETIDINE
CIMETIDINE HCL, CIMETIDINE HYDROCHLORIDE

ENQUAY
* ENQUAY PHARMACEUTICAL ASSOC
SILDIMAC, SILVER SULFADIAZINE

ENZON
* ENZON INC
ADAGEN, PEGADEMASE BOVINE

EON LABS
* EON LABORATORIES MANUFACTURING INC
ACETAMINOPHEN AND CODEINE PHOSPHATE, ACETAMINOPHEN
ALKERGOT, ERGOLOID MESYLATES
ALPHAZINE, PHENDIMETRAZINE TARTRATE
BETHANECHOL CHLORIDE, BETHANECHOL CHLORIDE
BUTABARBITAL SODIUM, BUTABARBITAL SODIUM
CARISOPRODOL, CARISOPRODOL
CHLORDIAZEPOXIDE HCL, CHLORDIAZEPOXIDE HYDROCHLORIDE
CHLOROTHIAZIDE, CHLOROTHIAZIDE
CHLORPROPAMIDE, CHLORPROPAMIDE
CHLORTHALIDONE, CHLORTHALIDONE
DESIPRAMINE HCL, DESIPRAMINE HYDROCHLORIDE
DIETHYLPROPION HCL, DIETHYLPROPION HYDROCHLORIDE
DIPHENHYDRAMINE HCL, DIPHENHYDRAMINE HYDROCHLORIDE

APPENDIX B
PRODUCT NAME INDEX
LISTED BY APPLICANT *(continued)*

DIPHENOXYLATE HCL W/ ATROPINE SULFATE, ATROPINE SULFATE
DRALSERP, HYDRALAZINE HYDROCHLORIDE
FOLIC ACID, FOLIC ACID
FUROSEMIDE, FUROSEMIDE
HY-PAM, HYDROXYZINE PAMOATE
HYDRALAZINE HCL, HYDRALAZINE HYDROCHLORIDE
HYDRAP-ES, HYDRALAZINE HYDROCHLORIDE
HYDRO-SERP "25", HYDROCHLOROTHIAZIDE
HYDRO-SERP "50", HYDROCHLOROTHIAZIDE
HYDROCHLOROTHIAZIDE, HYDROCHLOROTHIAZIDE
HYDROCORTISONE, HYDROCORTISONE
HYDROXYZINE HCL, HYDROXYZINE HYDROCHLORIDE
HYDROXYZINE PAMOATE, HYDROXYZINE PAMOATE
IMIPRAMINE HCL, IMIPRAMINE HYDROCHLORIDE
ISONIAZID, ISONIAZID
MEPRO-ASPIRIN, ASPIRIN
MEPROBAMATE, MEPROBAMATE
METHOCARBAMOL, METHOCARBAMOL
METHYLPREDNISOLONE, METHYLPREDNISOLONE
METRONIDAZOLE, METRONIDAZOLE
NEOMYCIN SULFATE, NEOMYCIN SULFATE
NITROFURANTOIN, NITROFURANTOIN
NYSTATIN, NYSTATIN
PHENDIMETRAZINE TARTRATE, PHENDIMETRAZINE TARTRATE
PHENTERMINE HCL, PHENTERMINE HYDROCHLORIDE
PREDNISOLONE, PREDNISOLONE
PREDNISONE, PREDNISONE
PROBENECID AND COLCHICINE, COLCHICINE
PROMETHAZINE HCL, PROMETHAZINE HYDROCHLORIDE
PROPOXYPHENE COMPOUND 65, ASPIRIN
PROPOXYPHENE HCL, PROPOXYPHENE HYDROCHLORIDE
PSEUDOEPHEDRINE HCL AND TRIPROLIDINE HCL, PSEUDOEPHEDRINE HYDROCHLORIDE
QUINIDINE SULFATE, QUINIDINE SULFATE
RESERPINE, RESERPINE
SULFADIAZINE, SULFADIAZINE
SULFAMETHOXAZOLE AND TRIMETHOPRIM, SULFAMETHOXAZOLE
SULFAMETHOXAZOLE AND TRIMETHOPRIM DOUBLE STRENGTH, SULFAMETHOXAZOLE
SULFASALAZINE, SULFASALAZINE
TETRACYCLINE HCL, TETRACYCLINE HYDROCHLORIDE
THEOPHYLLINE, THEOPHYLLINE
TOLBUTAMIDE, TOLBUTAMIDE
TRICHLORMETHIAZIDE, TRICHLORMETHIAZIDE
WESTADONE, METHADONE HYDROCHLORIDE

ERSANA
* ERSANA INC SUB ER SQUIBB AND SONS
VELOSEF, CEPHRADINE
VELOSEF '125', CEPHRADINE
VELOSEF '250', CEPHRADINE
VELOSEF '500', CEPHRADINE

ETHITEK
* ETHITEK PHARMACEUTICALS CO
MOCTANIN, MONOCTANOIN

EVERYLIFE
* EVERYLIFE
APAP W/ CODEINE PHOSPHATE, ACETAMINOPHEN
CORTISONE ACETATE, CORTISONE ACETATE
FOLIC ACID, FOLIC ACID
HYDROCORTISONE, HYDROCORTISONE
NIACIN, NIACIN
PREDNISOLONE, PREDNISOLONE
PREDNISONE, PREDNISONE
QUINIDINE SULFATE, QUINIDINE SULFATE
RESERPINE, RESERPINE
SECOBARBITAL SODIUM, SECOBARBITAL SODIUM
SODIUM PENTOBARBITAL, PENTOBARBITAL SODIUM
STANOZIDE, ISONIAZID
SULFADIAZINE, SULFADIAZINE
VITAMIN A, VITAMIN A
VITAMIN A, VITAMIN A PALMITATE
VITAMIN D, ERGOCALCIFEROL

F

FAULDING
* FH FAULDING AND CO LTD
DORYX, DOXYCYCLINE HYCLATE
ERYC, ERYTHROMYCIN
ERYC SPRINKLES, ERYTHROMYCIN
VINBLASTINE SULFATE, VINBLASTINE SULFATE
VINCRISTINE SULFATE PFS, VINCRISTINE SULFATE

FERNDALE LABS
* FERNDALE LABORATORIES INC
ADPHEN, PHENDIMETRAZINE TARTRATE
AMOSENE, MEPROBAMATE
AQUAPHYLLIN, THEOPHYLLINE
DAPEX-37.5, PHENTERMINE HYDROCHLORIDE
DELAXIN, METHOCARBAMOL
DIAZEPAM, DIAZEPAM
FERNDEX, DEXTROAMPHETAMINE SULFATE
FERNISOLONE-P, PREDNISOLONE
FERNISONE, PREDNISONE
OBESTIN-30, PHENTERMINE HYDROCHLORIDE
PHENDIMETRAZINE TARTRATE, PHENDIMETRAZINE TARTRATE
PRAMOSONE, HYDROCORTISONE ACETATE
RAUSERPIN, RAUWOLFIA SERPENTINA
STRIFON FORTE DSC, CHLORZOXAZONE
UMI-PEX 30, PHENTERMINE HYDROCHLORIDE

FERRANTE
* FERRANTE JOHN J
CHLORDIAZEPOXIDE HCL, CHLORDIAZEPOXIDE HYDROCHLORIDE
HYDROCORTISONE, HYDROCORTISONE
PREDNISONE, PREDNISONE

FERRING LABS
* FERRING LABORATORIES INC
CONCENTRAID, DESMOPRESSIN ACETATE
LUTREPULSE KIT, GONADORELIN ACETATE
SECRETIN-FERRING, SECRETIN
THYREL TRH, PROTIRELIN

FISONS
* FISONS CORP
BIPHETAMINE 12.5, AMPHETAMINE RESIN COMPLEX
BIPHETAMINE 20, AMPHETAMINE RESIN COMPLEX
BIPHETAMINE 7.5, AMPHETAMINE RESIN COMPLEX

APPENDIX B
PRODUCT NAME INDEX
LISTED BY APPLICANT *(continued)*

CORSYM, CHLORPHENIRAMINE POLISTIREX (OTC)
DELSYM, DEXTROMETHORPHAN POLISTIREX (OTC)
DOXEPIN HCL, DOXEPIN HYDROCHLORIDE
GASTROCROM, CROMOLYN SODIUM
INTAL, CROMOLYN SODIUM
IONAMIN-15, PHENTERMINE RESIN COMPLEX
IONAMIN-30, PHENTERMINE RESIN COMPLEX
IRON DEXTRAN, IRON DEXTRAN
ISOCLOR, CHLORPHENIRAMINE MALEATE (OTC)
MYKROX, METOLAZONE
NASALCROM, CROMOLYN SODIUM
OPTICROM, CROMOLYN SODIUM
PEDIAPRED, PREDNISOLONE SODIUM PHOSPHATE
PENNTUSS, CHLORPHENIRAMINE POLISTIREX (OTC)
PSEUDO-12, PSEUDOEPHEDRINE POLISTIREX (OTC)
SOMOPHYLLIN, AMINOPHYLLINE
SOMOPHYLLIN-DF, AMINOPHYLLINE
SOMOPHYLLIN-T, THEOPHYLLINE
TILADE, NEDOCROMIL SODIUM
TUSSIONEX, CHLORPHENIRAMINE POLISTIREX
VAPO-ISO, ISOPROTERENOL HYDROCHLORIDE
ZAROXOLYN, METOLAZONE

FLEMING PHARMS
* FLEMING AND CO PHARMACEUTICALS INC
AEROLATE, THEOPHYLLINE
AEROLATE III, THEOPHYLLINE
AEROLATE JR, THEOPHYLLINE
AEROLATE SR, THEOPHYLLINE

FLEMINGTON PHARM
* FLEMINGTON PHARMACEUTICAL CORP
NIFEDIPINE, NIFEDIPINE

FOREST LABS
* FOREST LABORATORIES INC
AMBENYL, BROMODIPHENHYDRAMINE HYDROCHLORIDE
BETAPRONE, PROPIOLACTONE
DURAPHYL, THEOPHYLLINE
ELIXICON, THEOPHYLLINE
ELIXOPHYLLIN, THEOPHYLLINE
ELIXOPHYLLIN SR, THEOPHYLLINE
FLUMADINE, RIMANTADINE HYDROCHLORIDE
FORBAXIN, METHOCARBAMOL
PYOCIDIN, HYDROCORTISONE
SUS-PHRINE, EPINEPHRINE
TESSALON, BENZONATATE
THYROLAR-0.25, LIOTRIX (T4;T3)
THYROLAR-0.5, LIOTRIX (T4;T3)
THYROLAR-1, LIOTRIX (T4;T3)
THYROLAR-2, LIOTRIX (T4;T3)
THYROLAR-3, LIOTRIX (T4;T3)
THYROLAR-5, LIOTRIX (T4;T3)

FOREST PHARMS
* FOREST PHARMACEUTICALS INC
BANCAP, ACETAMINOPHEN
BANCAP HC, ACETAMINOPHEN
DURADYNE DHC, ACETAMINOPHEN
ESGIC, ACETAMINOPHEN
METRA, PHENDIMETRAZINE TARTRATE
MICROSUL, SULFAMETHIZOLE
PROKLAR, SULFAMETHIZOLE
SULFALOID, TRISULFAPYRIMIDINES (SULFADIAZINE;SULFAMERAZINE;SULFAMETHAZINE)
WOLFINA, RAUWOLFIA SERPENTINA

FOUGERA
* E FOUGERA DIV ALTANA INC
BETAMETHASONE DIPROPIONATE, BETAMETHASONE DIPROPIONATE
BETAMETHASONE VALERATE, BETAMETHASONE VALERATE
ERYTHROMYCIN, ERYTHROMYCIN
FLUOCINOLONE ACETONIDE, FLUOCINOLONE ACETONIDE
GENTAMICIN SULFATE, GENTAMICIN SULFATE
HYDROCORTISONE, HYDROCORTISONE
LIDOCAINE, LIDOCAINE
NEOMYCIN AND POLYMYXIN B SULFATES AND DEXAMETHASONE, DEXAMETHASONE
NEOMYCIN SULFATE-TRIAMCINOLONE ACETONIDE, NEOMYCIN SULFATE
NYSTATIN, NYSTATIN
NYSTATIN-TRIAMCINOLONE ACETONIDE, NYSTATIN
TRIPLE SULFA, TRIPLE SULFA (SULFABENZAMIDE;SULFACETAMIDE;SULFATHIAZOLE)

FRESENIUS
* FRESENIUS USA INC
DELFLEX W/ DEXTROSE 1.5% IN PLASTIC CONTAINER, CALCIUM CHLORIDE
DELFLEX W/ DEXTROSE 1.5% LOW MAGNESIUM IN PLASTIC CONTAINER, CALCIUM CHLORIDE
DELFLEX W/ DEXTROSE 1.5% LOW MAGNESIUM LOW CALCIUM, CALCIUM CHLORIDE
DELFLEX W/ DEXTROSE 2.5% IN PLASTIC CONTAINER, CALCIUM CHLORIDE
DELFLEX W/ DEXTROSE 2.5% LOW MAGNESIUM IN PLASTIC CONTAINER, CALCIUM CHLORIDE
DELFLEX W/ DEXTROSE 2.5% LOW MAGNESIUM LOW CALCIUM, CALCIUM CHLORIDE
DELFLEX W/ DEXTROSE 4.25% IN PLASTIC CONTAINER, CALCIUM CHLORIDE
DELFLEX W/ DEXTROSE 4.25% LOW MAGNESIUM IN PLASTIC CONTAINER, CALCIUM CHLORIDE
DELFLEX W/ DEXTROSE 4.25% LOW MAGNESIUM LOW CALCIUM, CALCIUM CHLORIDE

FUJISAWA
* FUJISAWA USA INC
AMINOCAPROIC ACID, AMINOCAPROIC ACID
AMINOPHYLLINE, AMINOPHYLLINE
AMPHOTERICIN B, AMPHOTERICIN B
BACTERIOSTATIC SODIUM CHLORIDE 0.9%, SODIUM CHLORIDE
BACTERIOSTATIC SODIUM CHLORIDE 0.9% IN PLASTIC CONTAINER, SODIUM CHLORIDE
BACTERIOSTATIC WATER FOR INJECTION, WATER FOR INJECTION, STERILE
BRETYLIUM TOSYLATE, BRETYLIUM TOSYLATE
CALCIUM GLUCEPTATE, CALCIUM GLUCEPTATE
CEFAZOLIN SODIUM, CEFAZOLIN SODIUM
CEFIZOX, CEFTIZOXIME SODIUM
CEFIZOX IN DEXTROSE 5% IN PLASTIC CONTAINER, CEFTIZOXIME SODIUM
CEPHALOTHIN SODIUM, CEPHALOTHIN SODIUM
CEPHAPIRIN SODIUM, CEPHAPIRIN SODIUM
CHLORAMPHENICOL SODIUM SUCCINATE, CHLORAMPHENICOL SODIUM SUCCINATE
CHLORPROMAZINE HCL, CHLORPROMAZINE HYDROCHLORIDE
CHORIONIC GONADOTROPIN, GONADOTROPIN, CHORIONIC

APPENDIX B
PRODUCT NAME INDEX
LISTED BY APPLICANT *(continued)*

CHROMIC CHLORIDE, CHROMIC CHLORIDE
CLINDAMYCIN PHOSPHATE, CLINDAMYCIN PHOSPHATE
CLINDAMYCIN PHOSPHATE IN DEXTROSE 5%, CLINDAMYCIN PHOSPHATE
CUPRIC SULFATE, CUPRIC SULFATE
CYANOCOBALAMIN, CYANOCOBALAMIN
DACARBAZINE, DACARBAZINE
DEXAMETHASONE, DEXAMETHASONE SODIUM PHOSPHATE
DEXAMETHASONE SODIUM PHOSPHATE, DEXAMETHASONE SODIUM PHOSPHATE
DIAZEPAM, DIAZEPAM
DIAZOXIDE, DIAZOXIDE
DIGOXIN, DIGOXIN
DIPHENHYDRAMINE HCL, DIPHENHYDRAMINE HYDROCHLORIDE
DOPAMINE HCL, DOPAMINE HYDROCHLORIDE
DOXY 100, DOXYCYCLINE HYCLATE
DOXY 200, DOXYCYCLINE HYCLATE
DROPERIDOL, DROPERIDOL
ERYTHROMYCIN LACTOBIONATE, ERYTHROMYCIN LACTOBIONATE
FLUOROURACIL, FLUOROURACIL
FLUPHENAZINE DECANOATE, FLUPHENAZINE DECANOATE
FLUPHENAZINE HCL, FLUPHENAZINE HYDROCHLORIDE
FOLIC ACID, FOLIC ACID
FUROSEMIDE, FUROSEMIDE
GANITE, GALLIUM NITRATE
GENTAMICIN SULFATE, GENTAMICIN SULFATE
GLYCOPYRROLATE, GLYCOPYRROLATE
HALOPERIDOL, HALOPERIDOL LACTATE
HEP FLUSH KIT, HEPARIN SODIUM
HEPARIN LOCK FLUSH, HEPARIN SODIUM
HEPARIN LOCK FLUSH PRESERVATIVE FREE, HEPARIN SODIUM
HEPARIN SODIUM, HEPARIN SODIUM
HEPARIN SODIUM PRESERVATIVE FREE, HEPARIN SODIUM
HEPFLUSH-10, HEPARIN SODIUM
HYDRALAZINE HCL, HYDRALAZINE HYDROCHLORIDE
HYDROCORTISONE SODIUM SUCCINATE, HYDROCORTISONE SODIUM SUCCINATE
HYDROXOCOBALAMIN, HYDROXOCOBALAMIN
HYDROXYZINE HCL, HYDROXYZINE HYDROCHLORIDE
ISOPROTERENOL HCL, ISOPROTERENOL HYDROCHLORIDE
KANAMYCIN SULFATE, KANAMYCIN SULFATE
LEUCOVORIN CALCIUM, LEUCOVORIN CALCIUM
LIDOCAINE HCL, LIDOCAINE HYDROCHLORIDE
LIDOCAINE HCL IN PLASTIC CONTAINER, LIDOCAINE HYDROCHLORIDE
LYPHOCIN, VANCOMYCIN HYDROCHLORIDE
M.V.C. 9+3, ASCORBIC ACID
MAGNESIUM SULFATE, MAGNESIUM SULFATE
MANGANESE SULFATE, MANGANESE SULFATE
MANNITOL 25%, MANNITOL
METARAMINOL BITARTRATE, METARAMINOL BITARTRATE
METHOTREXATE SODIUM, METHOTREXATE SODIUM
METHYLDOPATE HCL, METHYLDOPATE HYDROCHLORIDE
METHYLPREDNISOLONE SODIUM SUCCINATE, METHYLPREDNISOLONE SODIUM SUCCINATE
METOCLOPRAMIDE HCL, METOCLOPRAMIDE HYDROCHLORIDE
METRONIDAZOLE, METRONIDAZOLE
METRONIDAZOLE HCL, METRONIDAZOLE HYDROCHLORIDE
NALBUPHINE, NALBUPHINE HYDROCHLORIDE
NALOXONE HCL, NALOXONE HYDROCHLORIDE
NANDROLONE DECANOATE, NANDROLONE DECANOATE
NEBUPENT, PENTAMIDINE ISETHIONATE
NITROGLYCERIN, NITROGLYCERIN
OXYTOCIN, OXYTOCIN
PENTAM 300, PENTAMIDINE ISETHIONATE
PHENYTOIN SODIUM, PHENYTOIN SODIUM
POTASSIUM CHLORIDE, POTASSIUM CHLORIDE
POTASSIUM CHLORIDE IN PLASTIC CONTAINER, POTASSIUM CHLORIDE
PROCAINAMIDE HCL, PROCAINAMIDE HYDROCHLORIDE
PROCAINE HCL, PROCAINE HYDROCHLORIDE
PROGRAF, TACROLIMUS
PROTAMINE SULFATE, PROTAMINE SULFATE
PYRIDOXINE HCL, PYRIDOXINE HYDROCHLORIDE
RITODRINE HCL, RITODRINE HYDROCHLORIDE
SODIUM CHLORIDE 0.9% IN PLASTIC CONTAINER, SODIUM CHLORIDE
SODIUM CHLORIDE 23.4%, SODIUM CHLORIDE
SODIUM HEPARIN, HEPARIN SODIUM
SODIUM NITROPRUSSIDE, SODIUM NITROPRUSSIDE
STERILE WATER FOR INJECTION IN PLASTIC CONTAINER, WATER FOR INJECTION, STERILE
SULFAMETHOXAZOLE AND TRIMETHOPRIM, SULFAMETHOXAZOLE
THIAMINE HCL, THIAMINE HYDROCHLORIDE
VERAPAMIL HCL, VERAPAMIL HYDROCHLORIDE
VIBISONE, CYANOCOBALAMIN
VINBLASTINE SULFATE, VINBLASTINE SULFATE
VINCRISTINE SULFATE, VINCRISTINE SULFATE
ZINC SULFATE, ZINC SULFATE

G

G AND W LABS

* G AND W LABORATORIES INC
ACEPHEN, ACETAMINOPHEN (OTC)
FLUOCINOLONE ACETONIDE, FLUOCINOLONE ACETONIDE
GYNE-SULF, TRIPLE SULFA (SULFABENZAMIDE;SULFACETAMIDE;SULFATHIAZOLE)
HYDROCORTISONE, HYDROCORTISONE
INDOMETHEGAN, INDOMETHACIN
MIGERGOT, CAFFEINE
PROCHLORPERAZINE, PROCHLORPERAZINE
PROMETHEGAN, PROMETHAZINE HYDROCHLORIDE
TRIAMCINOLONE ACETONIDE, TRIAMCINOLONE ACETONIDE
TRUPHYLLINE, AMINOPHYLLINE

G POHL BOSKAMP

* G POHL BOSKAMP GMBH AND CO
NITRO IV, NITROGLYCERIN
NITROLINGUAL, NITROGLYCERIN
NITRONAL, NITROGLYCERIN

APPENDIX B
PRODUCT NAME INDEX
LISTED BY APPLICANT *(continued)*

GALDERMA
* GALDERMA LABORATORIES INC
  CETACORT, HYDROCORTISONE
  CROTAN, CROTAMITON
  DESOWEN, DESONIDE
  LOCOID, HYDROCORTISONE BUTYRATE
  METROGEL, METRONIDAZOLE
  NUTRACORT, HYDROCORTISONE
  SANSAC, ERYTHROMYCIN

GEIGY
* GEIGY PHARMACEUTICALS DIV CIBA GEIGY CORP
  BRETHAIRE, TERBUTALINE SULFATE
  BRETHINE, TERBUTALINE SULFATE
  BUTAZOLIDIN, PHENYLBUTAZONE
  CATAFLAM, DICLOFENAC POTASSIUM
  LAMPRENE, CLOFAZIMINE
  LIORESAL, BACLOFEN
  LOPRESSOR, METOPROLOL FUMARATE
  LOPRESSOR, METOPROLOL TARTRATE
  PBZ, TRIPELENNAMINE CITRATE
  PBZ, TRIPELENNAMINE HYDROCHLORIDE
  PBZ-SR, TRIPELENNAMINE HYDROCHLORIDE
  TANDEARIL, OXYPHENBUTAZONE
  TOFRANIL, IMIPRAMINE HYDROCHLORIDE
  TOFRANIL-PM, IMIPRAMINE PAMOATE
  VOLTAREN, DICLOFENAC SODIUM

GENCON
* GENCON PHARMACEUTICALS INC
  GENCEPT 0.5/35-21, ETHINYL ESTRADIOL
  GENCEPT 0.5/35-28, ETHINYL ESTRADIOL
  GENCEPT 1/35-21, ETHINYL ESTRADIOL
  GENCEPT 1/35-28, ETHINYL ESTRADIOL
  GENCEPT 10/11-21, ETHINYL ESTRADIOL
  GENCEPT 10/11-28, ETHINYL ESTRADIOL

GENDERM
* GENDERM CORP
  OVIDE, MALATHION
  TEXACORT, HYDROCORTISONE
  ZONALON, DOXEPIN HYDROCHLORIDE

GENENTECH
* GENENTECH INC
  CRESCORMON, SOMATROPIN
  NUTROPIN, SOMATROPIN, BIOSYNTHETIC
  PROTROPIN, SOMATREM

GENERAL ELECTRIC
* GENERAL ELECTRIC CO
  XENON XE 133, XENON, XE-133

GENEVA PHARMS
* GENEVA PHARMACEUTICALS INC
  ACETAMINOPHEN AND CODEINE PHOSPHATE, ACETAMINOPHEN
  ALBUTEROL SULFATE, ALBUTEROL SULFATE
  ALLOPURINOL, ALLOPURINOL
  AMILORIDE HCL AND HYDROCHLOROTHIAZIDE, AMILORIDE HYDROCHLORIDE
  AMINOPHYLLINE, AMINOPHYLLINE
  AMITRIPTYLINE HCL, AMITRIPTYLINE HYDROCHLORIDE
  AMOXAPINE, AMOXAPINE
  ATENOLOL, ATENOLOL
  BROMPHENIRAMINE MALEATE, BROMPHENIRAMINE MALEATE
  BUTABARBITAL SODIUM, BUTABARBITAL SODIUM
  BUTAL COMPOUND, ASPIRIN
  CARISOPRODOL, CARISOPRODOL
  CHLORDIAZEPOXIDE HCL, CHLORDIAZEPOXIDE HYDROCHLORIDE
  CHLORPHENIRAMINE MALEATE, CHLORPHENIRAMINE MALEATE (OTC)
  CHLORPHENIRAMINE MALEATE, CHLORPHENIRAMINE MALEATE
  CHLORPHENIRAMINE MALEATE AND PHENYLPROPANOLAMINE HCL, CHLORPHENIRAMINE MALEATE
  CHLORPROMAZINE HCL, CHLORPROMAZINE HYDROCHLORIDE
  CHLORPROPAMIDE, CHLORPROPAMIDE
  CHLORTHALIDONE, CHLORTHALIDONE
  CHLORZOXAZONE, CHLORZOXAZONE
  CLEMASTINE FUMARATE, CLEMASTINE FUMARATE
  CLOFIBRATE, CLOFIBRATE
  CLONIDINE HCL, CLONIDINE HYDROCHLORIDE
  CLORAZEPATE DIPOTASSIUM, CLORAZEPATE DIPOTASSIUM
  CORPHED, PSEUDOEPHEDRINE HYDROCHLORIDE
  CYCLOBENZAPRINE HCL, CYCLOBENZAPRINE HYDROCHLORIDE
  CYPROHEPTADINE HCL, CYPROHEPTADINE HYDROCHLORIDE
  DESIPRAMINE HCL, DESIPRAMINE HYDROCHLORIDE
  DEXAMETHASONE, DEXAMETHASONE
  DEXTROAMPHETAMINE SULFATE, DEXTROAMPHETAMINE SULFATE
  DIAZEPAM, DIAZEPAM
  DIPHENHYDRAMINE HCL, DIPHENHYDRAMINE HYDROCHLORIDE
  DIPYRIDAMOLE, DIPYRIDAMOLE
  DISOBROM, DEXBROMPHENIRAMINE MALEATE (OTC)
  DISOPYRAMIDE PHOSPHATE, DISOPYRAMIDE PHOSPHATE
  DOXEPIN HCL, DOXEPIN HYDROCHLORIDE
  ERCATAB, CAFFEINE
  ESTERIFIED ESTROGENS, ESTROGENS, ESTERIFIED
  FENOPROFEN CALCIUM, FENOPROFEN CALCIUM
  FLUPHENAZINE HCL, FLUPHENAZINE HYDROCHLORIDE
  FLURAZEPAM HCL, FLURAZEPAM HYDROCHLORIDE
  FUROSEMIDE, FUROSEMIDE
  GLUTETHIMIDE, GLUTETHIMIDE
  HALOPERIDOL, HALOPERIDOL
  HYDRALAZINE HCL, HYDRALAZINE HYDROCHLORIDE
  HYDROCHLOROTHIAZIDE, HYDROCHLOROTHIAZIDE
  HYDROXYZINE HCL, HYDROXYZINE HYDROCHLORIDE
  HYDROXYZINE PAMOATE, HYDROXYZINE PAMOATE
  IBUPROFEN, IBUPROFEN
  IBUPROFEN, IBUPROFEN (OTC)
  IMIPRAMINE HCL, IMIPRAMINE HYDROCHLORIDE
  INDOMETHACIN, INDOMETHACIN
  ISOSORBIDE DINITRATE, ISOSORBIDE DINITRATE
  LONOX, ATROPINE SULFATE
  LOPERAMIDE HCL, LOPERAMIDE HYDROCHLORIDE
  LORAZEPAM, LORAZEPAM
  MECLIZINE HCL, MECLIZINE HYDROCHLORIDE
  MECLOFENAMATE SODIUM, MECLOFENAMATE SODIUM
  MEPROBAMATE, MEPROBAMATE
  METHAZOLAMIDE, METHAZOLAMIDE

APPENDIX B
PRODUCT NAME INDEX
LISTED BY APPLICANT *(continued)*

METHOCARBAMOL, METHOCARBAMOL
METHOXSALEN, METHOXSALEN
METHYCLOTHIAZIDE, METHYCLOTHIAZIDE
METHYLDOPA, METHYLDOPA
METHYLDOPA AND HYDROCHLOROTHIAZIDE, HYDROCHLOROTHIAZIDE
METOCLOPRAMIDE HCL, METOCLOPRAMIDE HYDROCHLORIDE
METOPROLOL TARTRATE, METOPROLOL TARTRATE
METRONIDAZOLE, METRONIDAZOLE
NAPROXEN, NAPROXEN
NAPROXEN SODIUM, NAPROXEN SODIUM
NIACIN, NIACIN
NORTRIPTYLINE HCL, NORTRIPTYLINE HYDROCHLORIDE
ORPHENADRINE CITRATE, ORPHENADRINE CITRATE
OXAZEPAM, OXAZEPAM
PERPHENAZINE, PERPHENAZINE
PERPHENAZINE AND AMITRIPTYLINE HCL, AMITRIPTYLINE HYDROCHLORIDE
PHENDIMETRAZINE TARTRATE, PHENDIMETRAZINE TARTRATE
PHENYLBUTAZONE, PHENYLBUTAZONE
PINDOLOL, PINDOLOL
PRAZOSIN HCL, PRAZOSIN HYDROCHLORIDE
PREDNISOLONE, PREDNISOLONE
PREDNISONE, PREDNISONE
PROCAINAMIDE HCL, PROCAINAMIDE HYDROCHLORIDE
PROMETHAZINE HCL, PROMETHAZINE HYDROCHLORIDE
PROPANTHELINE BROMIDE, PROPANTHELINE BROMIDE
PROPOXYPHENE COMPOUND-65, ASPIRIN
PROPOXYPHENE HCL, PROPOXYPHENE HYDROCHLORIDE
PROPOXYPHENE HCL AND ACETAMINOPHEN, ACETAMINOPHEN
PROPOXYPHENE NAPSYLATE AND ACETAMINOPHEN, ACETAMINOPHEN
PROPRANOLOL HCL, PROPRANOLOL HYDROCHLORIDE
PROPRANOLOL HCL AND HYDROCHLOROTHIAZIDE, HYDROCHLOROTHIAZIDE
QUINIDINE GLUCONATE, QUINIDINE GLUCONATE
QUINIDINE SULFATE, QUINIDINE SULFATE
RESERPINE AND HYDROCHLOROTHIAZIDE, HYDROCHLOROTHIAZIDE
SONAZINE, CHLORPROMAZINE HYDROCHLORIDE
SPIRONOLACTONE, SPIRONOLACTONE
SPIRONOLACTONE W/ HYDROCHLOROTHIAZIDE, HYDROCHLOROTHIAZIDE
SULFAMETHOXAZOLE, SULFAMETHOXAZOLE
SULFAMETHOXAZOLE AND TRIMETHOPRIM, SULFAMETHOXAZOLE
SULFISOXAZOLE, SULFISOXAZOLE
SULINDAC, SULINDAC
TEMAZEPAM, TEMAZEPAM
THIORIDAZINE HCL, THIORIDAZINE HYDROCHLORIDE
THIOTHIXENE, THIOTHIXENE
TIMOLOL MALEATE, TIMOLOL MALEATE
TOLAZAMIDE, TOLAZAMIDE
TOLBUTAMIDE, TOLBUTAMIDE
TOLMETIN SODIUM, TOLMETIN SODIUM
TRAZODONE HCL, TRAZODONE HYDROCHLORIDE
TRIAMCINOLONE, TRIAMCINOLONE
TRIAMTERENE AND HYDROCHLOROTHIAZIDE, HYDROCHLOROTHIAZIDE
TRIFLUOPERAZINE HCL, TRIFLUOPERAZINE HYDROCHLORIDE
VERAPAMIL HCL, VERAPAMIL HYDROCHLORIDE

GENPHARM
* GENPHARM INC PHARMACEUTICALS
ATENOLOL, ATENOLOL
PINDOLOL, PINDOLOL
PIROXICAM, PIROXICAM

GENSIA
* GENSIA INC
AMIKACIN, AMIKACIN SULFATE
AMINOPHYLLINE, AMINOPHYLLINE
CLINDAMYCIN PHOSPHATE, CLINDAMYCIN PHOSPHATE
DEXAMETHASONE SODIUM PHOSPHATE, DEXAMETHASONE SODIUM PHOSPHATE
DOBUTAMINE HCL, DOBUTAMINE HYDROCHLORIDE
DOPAMINE HCL, DOPAMINE HYDROCHLORIDE
ERYTHROMYCIN LACTOBIONATE, ERYTHROMYCIN LACTOBIONATE
ETOPOSIDE, ETOPOSIDE
GENTAMICIN SULFATE, GENTAMICIN SULFATE
GLYCOPYRROLATE, GLYCOPYRROLATE
LEUCOVORIN CALCIUM, LEUCOVORIN CALCIUM
METHYLDOPATE HCL, METHYLDOPATE HYDROCHLORIDE
METHYLPREDNISOLONE SODIUM SUCCINATE, METHYLPREDNISOLONE SODIUM SUCCINATE
METOCLOPRAMIDE HCL, METOCLOPRAMIDE HYDROCHLORIDE
PANCURONIUM BROMIDE, PANCURONIUM BROMIDE
SODIUM NITROPRUSSIDE, SODIUM NITROPRUSSIDE
SULFAMETHOXAZOLE AND TRIMETHOPRIM, SULFAMETHOXAZOLE
TOBRAMYCIN SULFATE, TOBRAMYCIN SULFATE
* GENSIA LABORATORIES LTD
LEUCOVORIN CALCIUM, LEUCOVORIN CALCIUM

GENZYME
* GENZYME CORP
CEREDASE, ALGLUCERASE
CEREZYME, IMIGLUCERASE

GILBERT LABS
* GILBERT LABORATORIES
ACETAMINOPHEN, BUTALBITAL AND CAFFEINE, ACETAMINOPHEN

GLAXO
* GLAXO INC
ACLOVATE, ALCLOMETASONE DIPROPIONATE
BECLOVENT, BECLOMETHASONE DIPROPIONATE
BECONASE, BECLOMETHASONE DIPROPIONATE
BECONASE AQ, BECLOMETHASONE DIPROPIONATE MONOHYDRATE
CEFTIN, CEFUROXIME AXETIL
CEPTAZ, CEFTAZIDIME (ARGININE FORMULATION)
CUTIVATE, FLUTICASONE PROPIONATE
DIONOSIL AQUEOUS, PROPYLIODONE
DIONOSIL OILY, PROPYLIODONE
EMGEL, ERYTHROMYCIN
FORTAZ, CEFTAZIDIME
FORTAZ, CEFTAZIDIME SODIUM
IMITREX, SUMATRIPTAN SUCCINATE

APPENDIX B
PRODUCT NAME INDEX
LISTED BY APPLICANT *(continued)*

OXISTAT, OXICONAZOLE NITRATE
SEFFIN, CEPHALOTHIN SODIUM
SEREVENT, SALMETEROL XINAFOATE
TEMOVATE, CLOBETASOL PROPIONATE
TRANDATE, LABETALOL HYDROCHLORIDE
TRANDATE HCT, HYDROCHLOROTHIAZIDE
VENTOLIN, ALBUTEROL
VENTOLIN, ALBUTEROL SULFATE
VENTOLIN ROTACAPS, ALBUTEROL SULFATE
ZANTAC, RANITIDINE HYDROCHLORIDE
ZANTAC 150, RANITIDINE HYDROCHLORIDE
ZANTAC 300, RANITIDINE HYDROCHLORIDE
ZINACEF, CEFUROXIME SODIUM
ZOFRAN, ONDANSETRON HYDROCHLORIDE

GLENWOOD
* GLENWOOD INC
MYOTONACHOL, BETHANECHOL CHLORIDE
PASKALIUM, POTASSIUM AMINOSALICYLATE
RENOQUID, SULFACYTINE

GLOBAL PHARMS
* GLOBAL PHARMACEUTICAL CORP
AMINOPHYLLINE, AMINOPHYLLINE
CHLORDIAZEPOXIDE HCL, CHLORDIAZEPOXIDE HYDROCHLORIDE
CHLOROQUINE PHOSPHATE, CHLOROQUINE PHOSPHATE
CHLORPHENIRAMINE MALEATE, CHLORPHENIRAMINE MALEATE
CORTISONE ACETATE, CORTISONE ACETATE
DEXAMETHASONE, DEXAMETHASONE
DIPHENHYDRAMINE HCL, DIPHENHYDRAMINE HYDROCHLORIDE
FOLIC ACID, FOLIC ACID
HYDRALAZINE HCL, HYDRALAZINE HYDROCHLORIDE
HYDROCHLOROTHIAZIDE, HYDROCHLOROTHIAZIDE
HYDROCORTISONE, HYDROCORTISONE
ISONIAZID, ISONIAZID
MEPROBAMATE, MEPROBAMATE
METHOCARBAMOL, METHOCARBAMOL
METHYLTESTOSTERONE, METHYLTESTOSTERONE
NIACIN, NIACIN
OXYTETRACYCLINE HCL, OXYTETRACYCLINE HYDROCHLORIDE
PIPERAZINE CITRATE, PIPERAZINE CITRATE
PREDNISOLONE, PREDNISOLONE
PREDNISONE, PREDNISONE
PROBENECID AND COLCHICINE, COLCHICINE
PROMETHAZINE HCL, PROMETHAZINE HYDROCHLORIDE
PROPANTHELINE BROMIDE, PROPANTHELINE BROMIDE
PROPOXYPHENE HCL, PROPOXYPHENE HYDROCHLORIDE
PROPYLTHIOURACIL, PROPYLTHIOURACIL
PYRILAMINE MALEATE, PYRILAMINE MALEATE
QUINIDINE SULFATE, QUINIDINE SULFATE
RAUWOLFIA SERPENTINA, RAUWOLFIA SERPENTINA
RESERPINE, RESERPINE
SULFA-TRIPLE #2, TRISULFAPYRIMIDINES (SULFADIAZINE;SULFAMERAZINE;SULFAMETHAZINE)
SULFADIAZINE, SULFADIAZINE
SULFISOXAZOLE, SULFISOXAZOLE
TETRACYCLINE HCL, TETRACYCLINE HYDROCHLORIDE
THYROGLOBULIN, THYROGLOBULIN
TRIAMCINOLONE, TRIAMCINOLONE
TRICHLORMETHIAZIDE, TRICHLORMETHIAZIDE
TRIPELENNAMINE HCL, TRIPELENNAMINE HYDROCHLORIDE
VITAMIN A, VITAMIN A
VITAMIN A, VITAMIN A PALMITATE
VITAMIN D, ERGOCALCIFEROL

GOLDEN PHARMS
* GOLDEN PHARMACEUTICALS INC
A-N STANNOUS AGGREGATED ALBUMIN, TECHNETIUM TC-99M ALBUMIN AGGREGATED KIT
SODIUM IODIDE I 123, SODIUM IODIDE, I-123

GOLDLINE
* GOLDLINE LABORATORIES INC
GLYCOPREP, POLYETHYLENE GLYCOL 3350

GRAHAM
* DM GRAHAM LABORATORIES INC
ACETAMINOPHEN AND HYDROCODONE BITARTRATE, ACETAMINOPHEN
BUTALBITAL AND ACETAMINOPHEN, ACETAMINOPHEN
BUTALBITAL, ACETAMINOPHEN, CAFFEINE, ACETAMINOPHEN
COLD CAPSULE IV, CHLORPHENIRAMINE MALEATE (OTC)
COLD CAPSULE V, CHLORPHENIRAMINE MALEATE (OTC)
CONTEN, ACETAMINOPHEN
HYDROCET, ACETAMINOPHEN
PHENDIMETRAZINE TARTRATE, PHENDIMETRAZINE TARTRATE
PSEUDOEPHEDRINE HCL/CHLORPHENIRAMINE MALEATE, CHLORPHENIRAMINE MALEATE (OTC)
REPAN, ACETAMINOPHEN
SOMOPHYLLIN-CRT, THEOPHYLLINE

GRAHAM CHEM
* GRAHAM CHEMICAL CO
LIDOCAINE, LIDOCAINE
LIDOCAINE HCL, LIDOCAINE HYDROCHLORIDE
LIDOCAINE HCL AND EPINEPHRINE, EPINEPHRINE
MEPIVACAINE HCL, MEPIVACAINE HYDROCHLORIDE
MEPIVACAINE HCL W/ LEVONORDEFRIN, LEVONORDEFRIN

GRIFFEN
* KW GRIFFEN CO
BIOSCRUB, CHLORHEXIDINE GLUCONATE (OTC)

GRUPPO LEPETIT
* GRUPPO LEPETIT SPA SUB MERRELL DOW PHARMACEUTICALS INC
CHLORAMPHENICOL SODIUM SUCCINATE, CHLORAMPHENICOL SODIUM SUCCINATE

GUARDIAN DRUG
* GUARDIAN DRUG CO INC
FOAMCOAT, ALUMINUM HYDROXIDE (OTC)

GUARDIAN LABS
* GUARDIAN LABORATORIES DIV UNITED GUARDIAN INC
RENACIDIN, CITRIC ACID

APPENDIX B
PRODUCT NAME INDEX
LISTED BY APPLICANT *(continued)*

GYNOPHARMA
* GYNOPHARMA INC
NORCEPT-E 1/35 21, ETHINYL ESTRADIOL
NORCEPT-E 1/35 28, ETHINYL ESTRADIOL

H

HALOCARBON
* HALOCARBON LABORATORIES DIV HALOCARBON PRODUCTS CORP
HALOTHANE, HALOTHANE

HALSEY
* HALSEY DRUG CO INC
ACETAMINOPHEN AND CODEINE PHOSPHATE, ACETAMINOPHEN
ACETAMINOPHEN W/ CODEINE PHOSPHATE, ACETAMINOPHEN
AMINOPHYLLINE, AMINOPHYLLINE
AMITRIPTYLINE HCL, AMITRIPTYLINE HYDROCHLORIDE
BELDIN, DIPHENHYDRAMINE HYDROCHLORIDE (OTC)
BELIX, DIPHENHYDRAMINE HYDROCHLORIDE
BUTALBITAL AND ACETAMINOPHEN, ACETAMINOPHEN
BUTALBITAL, APAP, AND CAFFEINE, ACETAMINOPHEN
BUTALBITAL, ASPIRIN & CAFFEINE, ASPIRIN
CHLORDIAZEPOXIDE HCL, CHLORDIAZEPOXIDE HYDROCHLORIDE
CHLORPROPAMIDE, CHLORPROPAMIDE
CODOXY, ASPIRIN
CORTALONE, PREDNISOLONE
CORTAN, PREDNISONE
CYPROHEPTADINE HCL, CYPROHEPTADINE HYDROCHLORIDE
DEXTROAMPHETAMINE SULFATE, DEXTROAMPHETAMINE SULFATE
DIAZEPAM, DIAZEPAM
DIPHENHYDRAMINE HCL, DIPHENHYDRAMINE HYDROCHLORIDE
DOXYCYCLINE HYCLATE, DOXYCYCLINE HYCLATE
FENOPROFEN CALCIUM, FENOPROFEN CALCIUM
FLURAZEPAM HCL, FLURAZEPAM HYDROCHLORIDE
FOLIC ACID, FOLIC ACID
GLUTETHIMIDE, GLUTETHIMIDE
HYDRALAZINE HCL, HYDRALAZINE HYDROCHLORIDE
HYDRO-D, HYDROCHLOROTHIAZIDE
HYDROCODONE BITARTRATE AND ACETAMINOPHEN, ACETAMINOPHEN
HYDROPANE, HOMATROPINE METHYLBROMIDE
HYDROXYZINE HCL, HYDROXYZINE HYDROCHLORIDE
IBUPROFEN, IBUPROFEN
IBUPROFEN, IBUPROFEN (OTC)
INDOMETHACIN, INDOMETHACIN
ISONIAZID, ISONIAZID
KLOROMIN, CHLORPHENIRAMINE MALEATE
LORAZEPAM, LORAZEPAM
LOW-QUEL, ATROPINE SULFATE
MEPERIDINE HCL, MEPERIDINE HYDROCHLORIDE
METHYLDOPA, METHYLDOPA
METOCLOPRAMIDE HCL, METOCLOPRAMIDE HYDROCHLORIDE
METRONIDAZOLE, METRONIDAZOLE
NEURAMATE, MEPROBAMATE
NIACIN, NIACIN
OXYCET, ACETAMINOPHEN
OXYCODONE AND ACETAMINOPHEN, ACETAMINOPHEN
PHERAZINE DM, DEXTROMETHORPHAN HYDROBROMIDE
PHERAZINE VC, PHENYLEPHRINE HYDROCHLORIDE
PHERAZINE VC W/ CODEINE, CODEINE PHOSPHATE
PHERAZINE W/ CODEINE, CODEINE PHOSPHATE
PREDNISONE, PREDNISONE
PROPHENE 65, PROPOXYPHENE HYDROCHLORIDE
PROPOXYPHENE NAPSYLATE AND ACETAMINOPHEN, ACETAMINOPHEN
PROPYLTHIOURACIL, PROPYLTHIOURACIL
QUINIDINE GLUCONATE, QUINIDINE GLUCONATE
QUINIDINE SULFATE, QUINIDINE SULFATE
RAUWOLFIA SERPENTINA, RAUWOLFIA SERPENTINA
RESERPINE, RESERPINE
SARISOL, BUTABARBITAL SODIUM
SARISOL NO. 1, BUTABARBITAL SODIUM
SARISOL NO. 2, BUTABARBITAL SODIUM
SODIUM PENTOBARBITAL, PENTOBARBITAL SODIUM
SODIUM SECOBARBITAL, SECOBARBITAL SODIUM
TETRACYCLINE HCL, TETRACYCLINE HYDROCHLORIDE
THEOPHYLLINE, THEOPHYLLINE
TRIPROLIDINE HCL, TRIPROLIDINE HYDROCHLORIDE

HAMILTON PHARMA CA
* HAMILTON PHARMA INC
NEO-SYNALAR, FLUOCINOLONE ACETONIDE

HAMILTON PHARMS
* HAMILTON PHARMACEUTICALS LTD
ALEVE, NAPROXEN SODIUM
NAPROXEN, NAPROXEN
NAPROXEN SODIUM, NAPROXEN SODIUM

HANFORD
* GC HANFORD MANUFACTURING CO
AMPICILLIN SODIUM, AMPICILLIN SODIUM
CEFAZOLIN SODIUM, CEFAZOLIN SODIUM

HASSLE AB
* AB HASSLE
TOPROL XL, METOPROLOL SUCCINATE

HEATHER
* HEATHER DRUG CO INC
CORTISONE ACETATE, CORTISONE ACETATE
DIMENHYDRINATE, DIMENHYDRINATE
DIPHENHYDRAMINE HCL, DIPHENHYDRAMINE HYDROCHLORIDE
DIPHENOXYLATE HCL AND ATROPINE SULFATE, ATROPINE SULFATE
DOXYCYCLINE HYCLATE, DOXYCYCLINE HYCLATE
HYDROCHLOROTHIAZIDE, HYDROCHLOROTHIAZIDE
MEPROBAMATE, MEPROBAMATE
METHOCARBAMOL, METHOCARBAMOL
METHYLPREDNISOLONE, METHYLPREDNISOLONE
METHYLTESTOSTERONE, METHYLTESTOSTERONE
PREDNISOLONE, PREDNISOLONE
PREDNISONE, PREDNISONE
PROPANTHELINE BROMIDE, PROPANTHELINE BROMIDE

APPENDIX B
PRODUCT NAME INDEX
LISTED BY APPLICANT *(continued)*

SULFAMETHOXAZOLE, SULFAMETHOXAZOLE
SULFAMETHOXAZOLE & TRIMETHOPRIM, SULFAMETHOXAZOLE
SULFISOXAZOLE, SULFISOXAZOLE
TETRACYCLINE HCL, TETRACYCLINE HYDROCHLORIDE
TRIPELENNAMINE HCL, TRIPELENNAMINE HYDROCHLORIDE

HERAN
* HERAN PHARMACEUTICAL INC
GLYCORT, HYDROCORTISONE

HERMAL PHARM
* HERMAL PHARMACEUTICAL LABORATORIES INC
AKNE-MYCIN, ERYTHROMYCIN
CLODERM, CLOCORTOLONE PIVALATE

HEXCEL
* HEXCEL CHEMICAL PRODUCTS
POTASSIUM AMINOSALICYLATE, POTASSIUM AMINOSALICYLATE
SODIUM AMINOSALICYLATE, AMINOSALICYLATE SODIUM

HI TECH PHARMA
* HI TECH PHARMACAL CO INC
DIPHENHYDRAMINE HCL, DIPHENHYDRAMINE HYDROCHLORIDE (OTC)

HICKAM
* DOW B HICKAM INC
SULFAMYLON, MAFENIDE ACETATE

HILL DERMAC
* HILL DERMACEUTICALS INC
DERMA-SMOOTHE/FS, FLUOCINOLONE ACETONIDE
FS SHAMPOO, FLUOCINOLONE ACETONIDE

HIRSCH INDS
* HIRSCH INDUSTRIES INC
LYMPHAZURIN, ISOSULFAN BLUE

HOECHST ROUSSEL
* HOECHST ROUSSEL PHARMACEUTICALS INC
A/T/S, ERYTHROMYCIN
ALTACE, RAMIPRIL
CLAFORAN, CEFOTAXIME SODIUM
CLAFORAN IN DEXTROSE 5%, CEFOTAXIME SODIUM
CLAFORAN IN SODIUM CHLORIDE 0.9%, CEFOTAXIME SODIUM
DERMATOP, PREDNICARBATE
DIABETA, GLYBURIDE
GLUBATE, GLYBURIDE
LASIX, FUROSEMIDE
LOPROX, CICLOPIROX OLAMINE
TOPICORT, DESOXIMETASONE
TOPICORT LP, DESOXIMETASONE
TRENTAL, PENTOXIFYLLINE

HOLLAND RANTOS
* HOLLAND RANTOS CO INC
KOROSTATIN, NYSTATIN

HORUS THERAP
* HORUS THERAPEUTICS INC
THALITONE, CHLORTHALIDONE

HOYT LABS
* HOYT LABORATORIES DIV COLGATE PALMOLIVE CO
ORABASE HCA, HYDROCORTISONE ACETATE

HUNTINGTON LABS
* HUNTINGTON LABORATORIES INC
CHG SCRUB, CHLORHEXIDINE GLUCONATE (OTC)
CIDA-STAT, CHLORHEXIDINE GLUCONATE (OTC)
GERMA-MEDICA, HEXACHLOROPHENE
GERMA-MEDICA "MG", HEXACHLOROPHENE
HEXA-GERM, HEXACHLOROPHENE

I

IBI SUD
* IBI SUD SPA
AMPICILLIN SODIUM, AMPICILLIN SODIUM

ICN
* ICN PHARMACEUTICALS INC
AMINOPHYLLINE, AMINOPHYLLINE
ANDROID 10, METHYLTESTOSTERONE
ANDROID 25, METHYLTESTOSTERONE
ANDROID 5, METHYLTESTOSTERONE
ANDROID-F, FLUOXYMESTERONE
BENDOPA, LEVODOPA
BENOQUIN, MONOBENZONE
CHLORPHENIRAMINE MALEATE, CHLORPHENIRAMINE MALEATE
CODEINE PHOSPHATE AND ACETAMINOPHEN, ACETAMINOPHEN
DIPHENHYDRAMINE HCL, DIPHENHYDRAMINE HYDROCHLORIDE
DIPHENOXYLATE HCL W/ ATROPINE SULFATE, ATROPINE SULFATE
FLUOXYMESTERONE, FLUOXYMESTERONE
FOLIC ACID, FOLIC ACID
MEPROBAMATE, MEPROBAMATE
OXSORALEN, METHOXSALEN
OXSORALEN-ULTRA, METHOXSALEN
PREDNISOLONE, PREDNISOLONE
PREDNISONE, PREDNISONE
PROPOXYPHENE HCL, PROPOXYPHENE HYDROCHLORIDE
QUINIDINE SULFATE, QUINIDINE SULFATE
RAUWOLFIA SERPENTINA, RAUWOLFIA SERPENTINA
RESERPINE, RESERPINE
SECOBARBITAL SODIUM, SECOBARBITAL SODIUM
SODIUM PENTOBARBITAL, PENTOBARBITAL SODIUM
SULFISOXAZOLE, SULFISOXAZOLE
TESTRED, METHYLTESTOSTERONE
TETRACYCLINE HCL, TETRACYCLINE HYDROCHLORIDE
TRISORALEN, TRIOXSALEN
8-MOP, METHOXSALEN

IMMUNEX
* IMMUNEX CORP
AMICAR, AMINOCAPROIC ACID
LEUCOVORIN CALCIUM, LEUCOVORIN CALCIUM
NOVANTRONE, MITOXANTRONE HYDROCHLORIDE
THIOTEPA, THIOTEPA

IMP
* IMP INC
SPECTAMINE, IOFETAMINE HYDROCHLORIDE I-123

INGRAM PHARM
* INGRAM PHARMACEUTICAL CO
DRICORT, HYDROCORTISONE ACETATE
HYDROCORTISONE, HYDROCORTISONE

APPENDIX B
PRODUCT NAME INDEX
LISTED BY APPLICANT *(continued)*

INHALON
* INHALON PHARMACEUTICALS INC
  ENFLURANE, ENFLURANE

INTERPHARM
* INTERPHARM INC
  CLONIDINE HCL, CLONIDINE HYDROCHLORIDE
  DISOPYRAMIDE PHOSPHATE, DISOPYRAMIDE PHOSPHATE
  DOXYCYCLINE HYCLATE, DOXYCYCLINE HYCLATE
  IBUPROFEN, IBUPROFEN
  IBUPROFEN, IBUPROFEN (OTC)
  METOCLOPRAMIDE HCL, METOCLOPRAMIDE HYDROCHLORIDE
  PREDNISONE, PREDNISONE
  PROPRANOLOL HCL, PROPRANOLOL HYDROCHLORIDE
  SULFAMETHOXAZOLE AND TRIMETHOPRIM, SULFAMETHOXAZOLE
  TOLAZAMIDE, TOLAZAMIDE

INTL MEDICATION
* INTERNATIONAL MEDICATION SYSTEMS LTD
  AMINOPHYLLINE, AMINOPHYLLINE
  AMPICILLIN SODIUM, AMPICILLIN SODIUM
  BRETYLIUM TOSYLATE, BRETYLIUM TOSYLATE
  CEPHALOTHIN, CEPHALOTHIN SODIUM
  DEXAMETHASONE SODIUM PHOSPHATE, DEXAMETHASONE SODIUM PHOSPHATE
  DIATRIZOATE-60, DIATRIZOATE MEGLUMINE
  DIPHENHYDRAMINE HCL, DIPHENHYDRAMINE HYDROCHLORIDE
  DOPAMINE HCL, DOPAMINE HYDROCHLORIDE
  FUROSEMIDE, FUROSEMIDE
  GENTAMICIN, GENTAMICIN SULFATE
  HEPARIN LOCK FLUSH, HEPARIN SODIUM
  HYDROCORTISONE SODIUM SUCCINATE, HYDROCORTISONE SODIUM SUCCINATE
  ISOETHARINE HCL, ISOETHARINE HYDROCHLORIDE
  ISOPROTERENOL HCL, ISOPROTERENOL HYDROCHLORIDE
  KANAMYCIN SULFATE, KANAMYCIN SULFATE
  LARYNG-O-JET KIT, LIDOCAINE HYDROCHLORIDE
  LIDOCAINE HCL, LIDOCAINE HYDROCHLORIDE
  LIDOCAINE HCL VISCOUS, LIDOCAINE HYDROCHLORIDE
  LIDOCAINE HCL W/ EPINEPHRINE, EPINEPHRINE
  MANNITOL 25%, MANNITOL
  MEPERIDINE HCL, MEPERIDINE HYDROCHLORIDE
  MEPIVACAINE HCL, MEPIVACAINE HYDROCHLORIDE
  METHYLPREDNISOLONE SODIUM SUCCINATE, METHYLPREDNISOLONE SODIUM SUCCINATE
  METRONIDAZOLE, METRONIDAZOLE
  NALOXONE HCL, NALOXONE HYDROCHLORIDE
  NITROGLYCERIN, NITROGLYCERIN
  PHYTONADIONE, PHYTONADIONE
  POTASSIUM CHLORIDE, POTASSIUM CHLORIDE
  PROCAINAMIDE HCL, PROCAINAMIDE HYDROCHLORIDE
  SUCCINYLCHOLINE CHLORIDE, SUCCINYLCHOLINE CHLORIDE
  VERAPAMIL HCL, VERAPAMIL HYDROCHLORIDE

INVAMED
* INVAMED INC
  AMANTADINE HCL, AMANTADINE HYDROCHLORIDE
  ATENOLOL, ATENOLOL
  BENZTROPINE MESYLATE, BENZTROPINE MESYLATE
  CYCLOBENZAPRINE HCL, CYCLOBENZAPRINE HYDROCHLORIDE
  FOAMICON, ALUMINUM HYDROXIDE (OTC)
  IBUPROFEN, IBUPROFEN
  IBUPROFEN, IBUPROFEN (OTC)
  METHYLDOPA AND HYDROCHLOROTHIAZIDE, HYDROCHLOROTHIAZIDE
  METOCLOPRAMIDE HCL, METOCLOPRAMIDE HYDROCHLORIDE
  PEG-LYTE, POLYETHYLENE GLYCOL 3350
  PROCAINAMIDE HCL, PROCAINAMIDE HYDROCHLORIDE
  PROPRANOLOL HCL, PROPRANOLOL HYDROCHLORIDE

INWOOD LABS
* INWOOD LABORATORIES INC SUB FOREST LABORATORIES INC
  CARBAMAZEPINE, CARBAMAZEPINE
  CORTISONE ACETATE, CORTISONE ACETATE
  DIPHENOXYLATE HCL AND ATROPINE SULFATE, ATROPINE SULFATE
  HYDROCHLOROTHIAZIDE, HYDROCHLOROTHIAZIDE
  HYDROCORTISONE, HYDROCORTISONE
  INDOMETHACIN, INDOMETHACIN
  METHOCARBAMOL, METHOCARBAMOL
  METHYLTESTOSTERONE, METHYLTESTOSTERONE
  PHENDIMETRAZINE TARTRATE, PHENDIMETRAZINE TARTRATE
  PREDNISOLONE, PREDNISOLONE
  PREDNISONE, PREDNISONE
  PROCAINAMIDE HCL, PROCAINAMIDE HYDROCHLORIDE
  PROPRANOLOL HCL, PROPRANOLOL HYDROCHLORIDE
  THEOCHRON, THEOPHYLLINE
  THEOPHYLLINE, THEOPHYLLINE

IOLAB
* IOLAB CORP
  LIVOSTIN, LEVOCABASTINE HYDROCHLORIDE
* IOLAB PHARMACEUTICALS SUB JOHNSON AND JOHNSON CO
  CATARASE, CHYMOTRYPSIN
  DEXACIDIN, DEXAMETHASONE
  FLUOR-OP, FLUOROMETHOLONE
  FUNDUSCEIN-25, FLUORESCEIN SODIUM
  GENTACIDIN, GENTAMICIN SULFATE
  INFLAMASE FORTE, PREDNISOLONE SODIUM PHOSPHATE
  INFLAMASE MILD, PREDNISOLONE SODIUM PHOSPHATE
  MIOCHOL, ACETYLCHOLINE CHLORIDE
  MIOCHOL-E, ACETYLCHOLINE CHLORIDE
  SULF-10, SULFACETAMIDE SODIUM
  VASOCIDIN, PREDNISOLONE ACETATE
  VASOCIDIN, PREDNISOLONE SODIUM PHOSPHATE
  VASOCON, NAPHAZOLINE HYDROCHLORIDE
  VASOCON-A, ANTAZOLINE PHOSPHATE

IPHARM
* IPHARM DIV LYPHOMED INC
  NEOMYCIN AND POLYMYXIN B SULFATES AND GRAMICIDIN, GRAMICIDIN

IPR
* IPR PHARMACEUTICALS INC
  ATENOLOL, ATENOLOL
  ATENOLOL AND CHLORTHALIDONE, ATENOLOL

APPENDIX B
PRODUCT NAME INDEX
LISTED BY APPLICANT *(continued)*

ISO TEX
* ISO TEX DIAGNOSTICS INC
ALBUMOTOPE 125 I, ALBUMIN IODINATED I-125 SERUM
CHROMALBIN, ALBUMIN CHROMATED CR-51 SERUM
GLOFIL-125, IOTHALAMATE SODIUM, I-125
INULIN AND SODIUM CHLORIDE, INULIN
MEGATOPE, ALBUMIN IODINATED I-131 SERUM

ISTITUTO BIOCHIMICO
* ISTITUTO BIOCHIMICO ITALIANO GIOVANNI LORENZINI SPA
AMPICILLIN SODIUM, AMPICILLIN SODIUM

J

JACOBUS
* JACOBUS PHARMACEUTICAL CO
DAPSONE, DAPSONE
PASER, AMINOSALICYLIC ACID

JANSSEN
* JANSSEN PHARMACEUTICA INC
ALFENTA, ALFENTANIL HYDROCHLORIDE
HISMANAL, ASTEMIZOLE
IMODIUM, LOPERAMIDE HYDROCHLORIDE
INAPSINE, DROPERIDOL
INNOVAR, DROPERIDOL
MONISTAT, MICONAZOLE
NIZORAL, KETOCONAZOLE
SUBLIMAZE, FENTANYL CITRATE
SUFENTA, SUFENTANIL CITRATE
* JANSSEN RESEARCH FDN DIV JOHNSON AND JOHNSON
ERGAMISOL, LEVAMISOLE HYDROCHLORIDE
PROPULSID, CISAPRIDE MONOHYDRATE
RISPERDAL, RISPERIDONE
SPORANOX, ITRACONAZOLE
VERMOX, MEBENDAZOLE

JOHNSON AND JOHNSON
* JOHNSON AND JOHNSON MEDICAL INC
MICROCOL, CHLORHEXIDINE GLUCONATE (OTC)
MICRODERM, CHLORHEXIDINE GLUCONATE (OTC)

JOHNSON RW
* RW JOHNSON PHARMACEUTICAL RESEARCH INSTITUTE DIV ORTHO PHA
ACEON, PERINDOPRIL ERBUMINE
CLISTIN, CARBINOXAMINE MALEATE
DIENESTROL, DIENESTROL
ERYCETTE, ERYTHROMYCIN
FLOXIN, OFLOXACIN
FLOXIN IN DEXTROSE 5%, OFLOXACIN
GRIFULVIN V, GRISEOFULVIN, MICROCRYSTALLINE
HALDOL, HALOPERIDOL
HALDOL, HALOPERIDOL LACTATE
HALDOL DECANOATE 50, HALOPERIDOL DECANOATE
HALDOL SOLUTAB, HALOPERIDOL
INJECTAPAP, ACETAMINOPHEN
LEUSTATIN, CLADRIBINE
MECLAN, MECLOCYCLINE SULFOSALICYLATE
MICRONOR, NORETHINDRONE
MODICON 21, ETHINYL ESTRADIOL
MODICON 28, ETHINYL ESTRADIOL
MONISTAT DUAL-PAK, MICONAZOLE NITRATE
MONISTAT 3, MICONAZOLE NITRATE
MONISTAT 5, MICONAZOLE NITRATE
MONISTAT 7, MICONAZOLE NITRATE (OTC)
MONISTAT-DERM, MICONAZOLE NITRATE
ORTHO CYCLEN-21, ETHINYL ESTRADIOL
ORTHO CYCLEN-28, ETHINYL ESTRADIOL
ORTHO TRI-CYCLEN, ETHINYL ESTRADIOL
ORTHO-CEPT, DESOGESTREL
ORTHO-EST, ESTROPIPATE
ORTHO-NOVUM 1/35-21, ETHINYL ESTRADIOL
ORTHO-NOVUM 1/35-28, ETHINYL ESTRADIOL
ORTHO-NOVUM 1/50 21, MESTRANOL
ORTHO-NOVUM 1/50 28, MESTRANOL
ORTHO-NOVUM 1/80 21, MESTRANOL
ORTHO-NOVUM 10-21, MESTRANOL
ORTHO-NOVUM 10/11-21, ETHINYL ESTRADIOL
ORTHO-NOVUM 10/11-28, ETHINYL ESTRADIOL
ORTHO-NOVUM 2-21, MESTRANOL
ORTHO-NOVUM 7/14-21, ETHINYL ESTRADIOL
ORTHO-NOVUM 7/14-28, ETHINYL ESTRADIOL
ORTHO-NOVUM 7/7/7-21, ETHINYL ESTRADIOL
ORTHO-NOVUM 7/7/7-28, ETHINYL ESTRADIOL
ORTHO-N0VUM 1/80 28, MESTRANOL
PARAFLEX, CHLORZOXAZONE
PARAFON FORTE DSC, CHLORZOXAZONE
PROTOSTAT, METRONIDAZOLE
RETIN-A, TRETINOIN
SALPIX, ACETRIZOATE SODIUM
SPECTAZOLE, ECONAZOLE NITRATE
SULTRIN, TRIPLE SULFA (SULFABENZAMIDE;SULFACETAMIDE;SULFATHIAZOLE)
SUPROL, SUPROFEN
TERAZOL 3, TERCONAZOLE
TERAZOL 7, TERCONAZOLE
THEOPHYL, THEOPHYLLINE
THEOPHYL-SR, THEOPHYLLINE
THEOPHYL-225, THEOPHYLLINE
TOLECTIN, TOLMETIN SODIUM
TOLECTIN DS, TOLMETIN SODIUM
TOLECTIN 600, TOLMETIN SODIUM
TYCOLET, ACETAMINOPHEN
TYLENOL W/ CODEINE, ACETAMINOPHEN
TYLENOL W/ CODEINE NO. 1, ACETAMINOPHEN
TYLENOL W/ CODEINE NO. 2, ACETAMINOPHEN
TYLENOL W/ CODEINE NO. 3, ACETAMINOPHEN
TYLENOL W/ CODEINE NO. 4, ACETAMINOPHEN
TYLOX, ACETAMINOPHEN
TYLOX-325, ACETAMINOPHEN
VASCOR, BEPRIDIL HYDROCHLORIDE

K

KALAPHARM
* KALAPHARM INC
FUROSEMIDE, FUROSEMIDE
GENTAMICIN SULFATE, GENTAMICIN SULFATE

KALI DUPHAR
* KALI DUPHAR INC
ATROPINE, ATROPINE

KENDALL
* KENDALL CO
CHLORHEXIDINE GLUCONATE, CHLORHEXIDINE GLUCONATE (OTC)
LARYNGOTRACHEAL ANESTHESIA KIT, LIDOCAINE HYDROCHLORIDE

APPENDIX B
PRODUCT NAME INDEX
LISTED BY APPLICANT *(continued)*

KEY PHARMS
* KEY PHARMACEUTICALS INC SUB SCHERING PLOUGH CORP
GENAPAX, GENTIAN VIOLET
QUINORA, QUINIDINE SULFATE
THEO-DUR, THEOPHYLLINE
TYZINE, TETRAHYDROZOLINE HYDROCHLORIDE

KING PHARMS
* KING PHARMACEUTICALS INC
AMINOPHYLLINE, AMINOPHYLLINE
APOGEN, GENTAMICIN SULFATE
KLEBCIL, KANAMYCIN SULFATE
MAXOLON, METOCLOPRAMIDE HYDROCHLORIDE

KM LEE
* KM LEE LABORATORIES INC
MEPROBAMATE, MEPROBAMATE

KNOLL PHARM
* KNOLL PHARMACEUTICAL CO UNIT BASF K AND CORP
AKINETON, BIPERIDEN HYDROCHLORIDE
AKINETON, BIPERIDEN LACTATE
DILAUDID, HYDROMORPHONE HYDROCHLORIDE
DILAUDID-HP, HYDROMORPHONE HYDROCHLORIDE
ISOPTIN, VERAPAMIL HYDROCHLORIDE
ISOPTIN SR, VERAPAMIL HYDROCHLORIDE
MEPERIDINE HCL, MEPERIDINE HYDROCHLORIDE
PROMETHAZINE HCL, PROMETHAZINE HYDROCHLORIDE
RYTHMOL, PROPAFENONE HYDROCHLORIDE
VICODIN, ACETAMINOPHEN
VICODIN ES, ACETAMINOPHEN
VICOPRIN, ASPIRIN

KV PHARM
* KV PHARMACEUTICAL CO
ACETAMINOPHEN AND CODEINE PHOSPHATE, ACETAMINOPHEN
ACETIC ACID, ACETIC ACID, GLACIAL
ACETIC ACID W/ HYDROCORTISONE, ACETIC ACID, GLACIAL
AMINOPHYLLINE, AMINOPHYLLINE
BROMPHENIRAMINE MALEATE, BROMPHENIRAMINE MALEATE
CHLORPHENIRAMINE MALEATE, CHLORPHENIRAMINE MALEATE
CHLORPROMAZINE HCL, CHLORPROMAZINE HYDROCHLORIDE
CHLORTHALIDONE, CHLORTHALIDONE
CYPROHEPTADINE HCL, CYPROHEPTADINE HYDROCHLORIDE
DIPHENHYDRAMINE HCL, DIPHENHYDRAMINE HYDROCHLORIDE
DIPHENOXYLATE HCL W/ ATROPINE SULFATE, ATROPINE SULFATE
DISOPYRAMIDE PHOSPHATE, DISOPYRAMIDE PHOSPHATE
ERGOLOID MESYLATES, ERGOLOID MESYLATES
ERYTHROMYCIN ETHYLSUCCINATE, ERYTHROMYCIN ETHYLSUCCINATE
HYDROXYZINE HCL, HYDROXYZINE HYDROCHLORIDE
MECLIZINE HCL, MECLIZINE HYDROCHLORIDE
METHOCARBAMOL, METHOCARBAMOL
METHYLTESTOSTERONE, METHYLTESTOSTERONE
PHENDIMETRAZINE TARTRATE, PHENDIMETRAZINE TARTRATE
POTASSIUM CHLORIDE, POTASSIUM CHLORIDE
PREDNISONE, PREDNISONE
PROMETHAZINE HCL, PROMETHAZINE HYDROCHLORIDE
PSEUDOEPHEDRINE HCL AND CHLORPHENIRAMINE MALEATE, CHLORPHENIRAMINE MALEATE (OTC)
QUINIDINE SULFATE, QUINIDINE SULFATE
SODIUM SECOBARBITAL, SECOBARBITAL SODIUM
THEOPHYLLINE, THEOPHYLLINE
TRIPROLIDINE AND PSEUDOEPHEDRINE HYDROCHLORIDES, PSEUDOEPHEDRINE HYDROCHLORIDE (OTC)
TRIPROLIDINE AND PSEUDOEPHRINE HCL, PSEUDOEPHEDRINE HYDROCHLORIDE (OTC)

L

LABS ATRAL
* LABORATORIOS ATRAL SARL
AMOXICILLIN, AMOXICILLIN
CEPHALEXIN, CEPHALEXIN
TETRACYCLINE HCL, TETRACYCLINE HYDROCHLORIDE

LABS FOURNIER
* LABORATOIRES FOURNIER SCA
LIPIDIL, FENOFIBRATE

LAFAYETTE PHARMS
* LAFAYETTE PHARMACEUTICALS INC
BAROS, SODIUM BICARBONATE

LANNETT
* LANNETT CO INC
ACETAZOLAMIDE, ACETAZOLAMIDE
AMINOPHYLLINE, AMINOPHYLLINE
AMPHETAMINE SULFATE, AMPHETAMINE SULFATE
BENZYL BENZOATE, BENZYL BENZOATE
BETHANECHOL CHLORIDE, BETHANECHOL CHLORIDE
BUTALAN, BUTABARBITAL SODIUM
CORTISONE ACETATE, CORTISONE ACETATE
DEXTROAMPHETAMINE SULFATE, DEXTROAMPHETAMINE SULFATE
DIPHENHYDRAMINE HCL, DIPHENHYDRAMINE HYDROCHLORIDE
DIPHENYLAN SODIUM, PHENYTOIN SODIUM, PROMPT
FOLIC ACID, FOLIC ACID
FURALAN, NITROFURANTOIN
GLUTETHIMIDE, GLUTETHIMIDE
HYDROCORTISONE, HYDROCORTISONE
LANIAZID, ISONIAZID
LANOPHYLLIN, THEOPHYLLINE
LANORINAL, ASPIRIN
LANTRISUL, TRISULFAPYRIMIDINES (SULFADIAZINE;SULFAMERAZINE;SULFAMETHAZINE)
LOFENE, ATROPINE SULFATE
MEPROBAMATE, MEPROBAMATE
METHOCARBAMOL, METHOCARBAMOL
METHYLTESTOSTERONE, METHYLTESTOSTERONE
NEOMYCIN SULFATE, NEOMYCIN SULFATE
NITROFURAZONE, NITROFURAZONE
PENTOBARBITAL SODIUM, PENTOBARBITAL SODIUM
PHENETRON, CHLORPHENIRAMINE MALEATE

APPENDIX B
PRODUCT NAME INDEX
LISTED BY APPLICANT *(continued)*

PHENTERMINE HCL, PHENTERMINE HYDROCHLORIDE
PIPERAZINE CITRATE, PIPERAZINE CITRATE
PREDNISOLONE, PREDNISOLONE
PREDNISONE, PREDNISONE
PRIMIDONE, PRIMIDONE
PROBALAN, PROBENECID
PROCAINAMIDE HCL, PROCAINAMIDE HYDROCHLORIDE
PROMETHAZINE HCL, PROMETHAZINE HYDROCHLORIDE
PROPYLTHIOURACIL, PROPYLTHIOURACIL
QUINALAN, QUINIDINE GLUCONATE
QUINIDINE SULFATE, QUINIDINE SULFATE
SECOBARBITAL SODIUM, SECOBARBITAL SODIUM
SERPALAN, RESERPINE
SODIUM BUTABARBITAL, BUTABARBITAL SODIUM
SODIUM P.A.S., AMINOSALICYLATE SODIUM
SULFADIAZINE, SULFADIAZINE
SULFISOXAZOLE, SULFISOXAZOLE
TRICHLOREX, TRICHLORMETHIAZIDE
TRIPELENNAMINE HCL, TRIPELENNAMINE HYDROCHLORIDE
VELTANE, BROMPHENIRAMINE MALEATE
VITAMIN D, ERGOCALCIFEROL

LEDERLE
* LEDERLE LABORATORIES DIV AMERICAN CYANAMID CO
ACETAMINOPHEN W/ CODEINE, ACETAMINOPHEN
ACHES-N-PAIN, IBUPROFEN (OTC)
ACHROMYCIN, HYDROCORTISONE
ACHROMYCIN, PROCAINE HYDROCHLORIDE
ACHROMYCIN, TETRACYCLINE HYDROCHLORIDE
ACHROMYCIN V, TETRACYCLINE HYDROCHLORIDE
ALBUTEROL SULFATE, ALBUTEROL SULFATE
ALPRAZOLAM, ALPRAZOLAM
AMITRIPTYLINE HCL, AMITRIPTYLINE HYDROCHLORIDE
AMPICILLIN, AMPICILLIN/AMPICILLIN TRIHYDRATE
ARISTOCORT, TRIAMCINOLONE
ARISTOCORT, TRIAMCINOLONE ACETONIDE
ARISTOCORT, TRIAMCINOLONE DIACETATE
ARISTOCORT A, TRIAMCINOLONE ACETONIDE
ARISTOGEL, TRIAMCINOLONE ACETONIDE
ARISTOSPAN, TRIAMCINOLONE HEXACETONIDE
ARTANE, TRIHEXYPHENIDYL HYDROCHLORIDE
ASENDIN, AMOXAPINE
ATENOLOL, ATENOLOL
AUREOMYCIN, CHLORTETRACYCLINE HYDROCHLORIDE
CHLORDIAZEPOXIDE HCL, CHLORDIAZEPOXIDE HYDROCHLORIDE
CHLOROTHIAZIDE, CHLOROTHIAZIDE
CHLORPHENIRAMINE MALEATE, CHLORPHENIRAMINE MALEATE
CHLORPROMAZINE HCL, CHLORPROMAZINE HYDROCHLORIDE
CHLORPROPAMIDE, CHLORPROPAMIDE
CHLORTHALIDONE, CHLORTHALIDONE
CLONIDINE HCL, CLONIDINE HYDROCHLORIDE
CLORAZEPATE DIPOTASSIUM, CLORAZEPATE DIPOTASSIUM
CYCLOCORT, AMCINONIDE
DECLOMYCIN, DEMECLOCYCLINE HYDROCHLORIDE
DIAMOX, ACETAZOLAMIDE
DIAMOX, ACETAZOLAMIDE SODIUM
DIAZEPAM, DIAZEPAM
DILTIAZEM HCL, DILTIAZEM HYDROCHLORIDE
DIPHENHYDRAMINE HCL, DIPHENHYDRAMINE HYDROCHLORIDE
DIPHENOXYLATE HCL AND ATROPINE SULFATE, ATROPINE SULFATE
DIPYRIDAMOLE, DIPYRIDAMOLE
DOLENE, PROPOXYPHENE HYDROCHLORIDE
DOLENE AP-65, ACETAMINOPHEN
DOXEPIN HCL, DOXEPIN HYDROCHLORIDE
ERGOLOID MESYLATES, ERGOLOID MESYLATES
ERYTHROMYCIN STEARATE, ERYTHROMYCIN STEARATE
FENOPROFEN CALCIUM, FENOPROFEN CALCIUM
FOLVITE, FOLIC ACID
FOLVRON, FERROUS SULFATE
FUROSEMIDE, FUROSEMIDE
GEMFIBROZIL, GEMFIBROZIL
HALOPERIDOL, HALOPERIDOL
HETRAZAN, DIETHYLCARBAMAZINE CITRATE
HYDRALAZINE HCL, HYDRALAZINE HYDROCHLORIDE
HYDROCHLOROTHIAZIDE, HYDROCHLOROTHIAZIDE
HYDROMOX, QUINETHAZONE
HYDROMOX R, QUINETHAZONE
IBUPROFEN, IBUPROFEN
IMIPRAMINE HCL, IMIPRAMINE HYDROCHLORIDE
INDOMETHACIN, INDOMETHACIN
KETOPROFEN, KETOPROFEN
LEDERCILLIN VK, PENICILLIN V POTASSIUM
LEVOPROME, METHOTRIMEPRAZINE
LOXITANE, LOXAPINE SUCCINATE
LOXITANE C, LOXAPINE HYDROCHLORIDE
LOXITANE IM, LOXAPINE HYDROCHLORIDE
MEPROBAMATE, MEPROBAMATE
METHOCARBAMOL, METHOCARBAMOL
METHOTREXATE LPF, METHOTREXATE SODIUM
METHOTREXATE SODIUM, METHOTREXATE SODIUM
METHYLDOPA, METHYLDOPA
METHYLDOPA AND HYDROCHLOROTHIAZIDE, HYDROCHLOROTHIAZIDE
METOCLOPRAMIDE HCL, METOCLOPRAMIDE HYDROCHLORIDE
MINOCIN, MINOCYCLINE HYDROCHLORIDE
MINOCYCLINE HCL, MINOCYCLINE HYDROCHLORIDE
MYAMBUTOL, ETHAMBUTOL HYDROCHLORIDE
NAPROXEN, NAPROXEN
NEPTAZANE, METHAZOLAMIDE
NILSTAT, NYSTATIN
PATHILON, TRIDIHEXETHYL CHLORIDE
PIPRACIL, PIPERACILLIN SODIUM
PRAZOSIN HCL, PRAZOSIN HYDROCHLORIDE
PREDNISONE, PREDNISONE
PROBENECID, PROBENECID
PROBENECID W/ COLCHICINE, COLCHICINE
PROCAINAMIDE HCL, PROCAINAMIDE HYDROCHLORIDE
PROPRANOLOL HCL, PROPRANOLOL HYDROCHLORIDE
PROPYLTHIOURACIL, PROPYLTHIOURACIL
PYRAZINAMIDE, PYRAZINAMIDE
QUINIDINE SULFATE, QUINIDINE SULFATE
RESERPINE, HYDROCHLOROTHIAZIDE, AND HYDRALAZINE HCL, HYDRALAZINE HYDROCHLORIDE
SERVISONE, PREDNISONE

APPENDIX B
PRODUCT NAME INDEX
LISTED BY APPLICANT *(continued)*

SPIRONOLACTONE, SPIRONOLACTONE
SPIRONOLACTONE W/ HYDROCHLOROTHIAZIDE, HYDROCHLOROTHIAZIDE
SULFADIAZINE, SULFADIAZINE
SULFADIAZINE SODIUM, SULFADIAZINE SODIUM
SULFASALAZINE, SULFASALAZINE
SULFISOXAZOLE, SULFISOXAZOLE
SULINDAC, SULINDAC
SUPRAX, CEFIXIME
TOLBUTAMIDE, TOLBUTAMIDE
TRIPLE SULFAS, TRISULFAPYRIMIDINES (SULFADIAZINE;SULFAMERAZINE;SULFAMETHAZINE)
VANCOLED, VANCOMYCIN HYDROCHLORIDE
VERAPAMIL HCL, VERAPAMIL HYDROCHLORIDE
ZEBETA, BISOPROLOL FUMARATE
ZIAC, BISOPROLOL FUMARATE
ZOSYN, PIPERACILLIN SODIUM

* LEDERLE PARENTERALS INC
CLINDAMYCIN PHOSPHATE, CLINDAMYCIN PHOSPHATE
DOXYCYCLINE HYCLATE, DOXYCYCLINE HYCLATE
ERYTHROMYCIN LACTOBIONATE, ERYTHROMYCIN LACTOBIONATE
FUROSEMIDE, FUROSEMIDE
TOBRAMYCIN SULFATE, TOBRAMYCIN SULFATE
VANCOLED, VANCOMYCIN HYDROCHLORIDE

* LEDERLE PIPERACILLIN INC DIV AMERICAN CYANAMID CO
PIPRACIL, PIPERACILLIN SODIUM

LEMMON

* LEMMON CO SUB TEVA PHARMACEUTICALS
ACETAMINOPHEN AND CODEINE PHOSPHATE, ACETAMINOPHEN
ACETAMINOPHEN W/ CODEINE #2, ACETAMINOPHEN
ACETAMINOPHEN W/ CODEINE #3, ACETAMINOPHEN
ACETAMINOPHEN W/ CODEINE #4, ACETAMINOPHEN
ADIPEX-P, PHENTERMINE HYDROCHLORIDE
ALBUTEROL SULFATE, ALBUTEROL SULFATE
AMITRIPTYLINE HCL, AMITRIPTYLINE HYDROCHLORIDE
AMOXICILLIN, AMOXICILLIN
BETA-VAL, BETAMETHASONE VALERATE
BETAMETHASONE DIPROPIONATE, BETAMETHASONE DIPROPIONATE
BUTABARBITAL SODIUM, BUTABARBITAL SODIUM
CARBIDOPA AND LEVODOPA, CARBIDOPA
CEFAZOLIN SODIUM, CEFAZOLIN SODIUM
CEPHALEXIN, CEPHALEXIN
CHLORDIAZEPOXIDE HCL, CHLORDIAZEPOXIDE HYDROCHLORIDE
CHLORPROPAMIDE, CHLORPROPAMIDE
CHLORTHALIDONE, CHLORTHALIDONE
CHLORZOXAZONE, CHLORZOXAZONE
CLEMASTINE FUMARATE, CLEMASTINE FUMARATE
CLEMASTINE FUMARATE, CLEMASTINE FUMARATE (OTC)
CLEMASTINE FUMARATE, CLEMASTINE FUMARATE
CLINDAMYCIN PHOSPHATE, CLINDAMYCIN PHOSPHATE
COTRIM, SULFAMETHOXAZOLE
COTRIM D.S., SULFAMETHOXAZOLE
COTRIM PEDIATRIC, SULFAMETHOXAZOLE
DELCOBESE, AMPHETAMINE ADIPATE
DEXAMPEX, DEXTROAMPHETAMINE SULFATE
DIETHYLPROPION HCL, DIETHYLPROPION HYDROCHLORIDE
DIFLUNISAL, DIFLUNISAL
DIPHENHYDRAMINE HCL, DIPHENHYDRAMINE HYDROCHLORIDE
DOXY-LEMMON, DOXYCYCLINE HYCLATE
DRALZINE, HYDRALAZINE HYDROCHLORIDE
EPITOL, CARBAMAZEPINE
FLUOCINONIDE, FLUOCINONIDE
GEMFIBROZIL, GEMFIBROZIL
GLUCAMIDE, CHLORPROPAMIDE
HALOPERIDOL, HALOPERIDOL LACTATE
HY-PAM "25", HYDROXYZINE PAMOATE
HYDROCHLOROTHIAZIDE, HYDROCHLOROTHIAZIDE
HYDROCORTISONE, HYDROCORTISONE
IBUPROFEN, IBUPROFEN
INDO-LEMMON, INDOMETHACIN
LOPERAMIDE HCL, LOPERAMIDE HYDROCHLORIDE
MEPRIAM, MEPROBAMATE
METHAMPEX, METHAMPHETAMINE HYDROCHLORIDE
METHAMPHETAMINE HCL, METHAMPHETAMINE HYDROCHLORIDE
METOCLOPRAMIDE HCL, METOCLOPRAMIDE HYDROCHLORIDE
METRYL, METRONIDAZOLE
METRYL 500, METRONIDAZOLE
MYCO-TRIACET II, NYSTATIN
NAPROXEN, NAPROXEN
NAPROXEN SODIUM, NAPROXEN SODIUM
NEOTHYLLINE, DYPHYLLINE
NYSTATIN, NYSTATIN
ORAP, PIMOZIDE
PHENTERMINE HCL, PHENTERMINE HYDROCHLORIDE
PIROXICAM, PIROXICAM
PREDNISOLONE, PREDNISOLONE
PREDNISONE, PREDNISONE
PROMETHAZINE HCL, PROMETHAZINE HYDROCHLORIDE
PROPACET 100, ACETAMINOPHEN
PROPOXYPHENE COMPOUND 65, ASPIRIN
PROPOXYPHENE HCL, PROPOXYPHENE HYDROCHLORIDE
PROPOXYPHENE NAPSYLATE AND ACETAMINOPHEN, ACETAMINOPHEN
PROPRANOLOL HCL, PROPRANOLOL HYDROCHLORIDE
RESERPINE, RESERPINE
STATOBEX, PHENDIMETRAZINE TARTRATE
STATOBEX-G, PHENDIMETRAZINE TARTRATE
SULFANILAMIDE, SULFANILAMIDE
SULINDAC, SULINDAC
THIOTHIXENE HCL, THIOTHIXENE HYDROCHLORIDE
TOLMETIN SODIUM, TOLMETIN SODIUM
TRAZODONE HCL, TRAZODONE HYDROCHLORIDE
TRIACET, TRIAMCINOLONE ACETONIDE
TRIAMCINOLONE, TRIAMCINOLONE
TRIPHED, PSEUDOEPHEDRINE HYDROCHLORIDE
VAGILIA, TRIPLE SULFA (SULFABENZAMIDE;SULFACETAMIDE;SULFATHIAZOLE)
VITAMIN A SOLUBILIZED, VITAMIN A PALMITATE

LEO PHARM

* LEO PHARMACEUTICAL PRODUCTS LTD
PINDAC, PINACIDIL

LIFE LABS

* LIFE LABORATORIES INC
ERYTHROMYCIN ESTOLATE, ERYTHROMYCIN ESTOLATE

APPENDIX B
PRODUCT NAME INDEX
LISTED BY APPLICANT *(continued)*

LILLY
* ELI LILLY AND CO
AEROLONE, ISOPROTERENOL HYDROCHLORIDE
ALPHALIN, VITAMIN A PALMITATE
AMPICILLIN SODIUM, AMPICILLIN SODIUM
ANHYDRON, CYCLOTHIAZIDE
AVENTYL HCL, NORTRIPTYLINE HYDROCHLORIDE
AXID, NIZATIDINE
BACITRACIN, BACITRACIN
BETALIN S, THIAMINE HYDROCHLORIDE
BETALIN 12, CYANOCOBALAMIN
BREVITAL SODIUM, METHOHEXITAL SODIUM
CALCIUM GLUCEPTATE, CALCIUM GLUCEPTATE
CAPASTAT SULFATE, CAPREOMYCIN SULFATE
CECLOR, CEFACLOR
CESAMET, NABILONE
CINOBAC, CINOXACIN
CORDRAN, FLURANDRENOLIDE
CORDRAN SP, FLURANDRENOLIDE
CORDRAN-N, FLURANDRENOLIDE
CRYSTODIGIN, DIGITOXIN
DARVOCET, ACETAMINOPHEN
DARVOCET-N 100, ACETAMINOPHEN
DARVOCET-N 50, ACETAMINOPHEN
DARVON-N, PROPOXYPHENE NAPSYLATE
DARVON-N W/ ASA, ASPIRIN
DECABID, INDECAINIDE HYDROCHLORIDE
DELTALIN, ERGOCALCIFEROL
DICUMAROL, DICUMAROL
DICURIN PROCAINE, PROCAINE MERETHOXYLLINE
DIETHYLSTILBESTROL, DIETHYLSTILBESTROL
DOBUTREX, DOBUTAMINE HYDROCHLORIDE
DOLOPHINE HCL, METHADONE HYDROCHLORIDE
DROLBAN, DROMOSTANOLONE PROPIONATE
DURACILLIN A.S., PENICILLIN G PROCAINE
ERYTHROMYCIN, ERYTHROMYCIN
FOLIC ACID, FOLIC ACID
GLUCAGON, GLUCAGON HYDROCHLORIDE
HALDRONE, PARAMETHASONE ACETATE
HEPARIN SODIUM, HEPARIN SODIUM
HEXA-BETALIN, PYRIDOXINE HYDROCHLORIDE
HISTALOG, BETAZOLE HYDROCHLORIDE
HISTAMINE PHOSPHATE, HISTAMINE PHOSPHATE
HUMATROPE, SOMATROPIN, BIOSYNTHETIC
HUMULIN BR, INSULIN BIOSYNTHETIC HUMAN (OTC)
HUMULIN L, INSULIN ZINC SUSP BIOSYNTHETIC HUMAN (OTC)
HUMULIN N, INSULIN SUSP ISOPHANE BIOSYNTHETIC HUMAN (OTC)
HUMULIN R, INSULIN BIOSYNTHETIC HUMAN (OTC)
HUMULIN R, INSULIN BIOSYNTHETIC HUMAN
HUMULIN U, INSULIN ZINC SUSP EXTENDED BIOSYNTHETIC HUMAN (OTC)
HUMULIN 50/50, INSULIN BIOSYNTHETIC HUMAN (OTC)
HUMULIN 70/30, INSULIN BIOSYNTHETIC HUMAN (OTC)
ILETIN I, INSULIN PORK
ILETIN II, INSULIN PURIFIED PORK
ILOSONE SULFA, ERYTHROMYCIN ESTOLATE
ISONIAZID, ISONIAZID
KAFOCIN, CEPHALOGLYCIN
KAPPADIONE, MENADIOL SODIUM DIPHOSPHATE
KEFLET, CEPHALEXIN
KEFLEX, CEPHALEXIN
KEFLIN, CEPHALOTHIN SODIUM
KEFTAB, CEPHALEXIN HYDROCHLORIDE
KEFUROX, CEFUROXIME SODIUM
KEFUROX IN PLASTIC CONTAINER, CEFUROXIME SODIUM
KEFZOL, CEFAZOLIN SODIUM
LENTE ILETIN II, INSULIN ZINC SUSP PURIFIED BEEF (OTC)
LENTE ILETIN II (PORK), INSULIN ZINC SUSP PURIFIED PORK (OTC
LORABID, LORACARBEF
MANDOL, CEFAMANDOLE NAFATE
MENADIONE, MENADIONE
METHADONE HCL, METHADONE HYDROCHLORIDE
METHYLTESTOSTERONE, METHYLTESTOSTERONE
METUBINE IODIDE, METOCURINE IODIDE
MOXAM, MOXALACTAM DISODIUM
NEBCIN, TOBRAMYCIN SULFATE
NEOMYCIN SULFATE, NEOMYCIN SULFATE
NEOTRIZINE, TRISULFAPYRIMIDINES (SULFADIAZINE;SULFAMERAZINE;SULFAMETHAZINE)
NPH ILETIN I (BEEF-PORK), INSULIN SUSP ISOPHANE BEEF/PORK (OTC)
NPH ILETIN II, INSULIN SUSP ISOPHANE PURIFIED BEEF (OTC)
NPH ILETIN II (PORK), INSULIN SUSP ISOPHANE PURIFIED PORK (OTC)
ONCOVIN, VINCRISTINE SULFATE
PAGITANE, CYCRIMINE HYDROCHLORIDE
PENICILLIN G POTASSIUM, PENICILLIN G POTASSIUM
PERMAX, PERGOLIDE MESYLATE
POTASSIUM CHLORIDE, POTASSIUM CHLORIDE
PROGESTERONE, PROGESTERONE
PROPYLTHIOURACIL, PROPYLTHIOURACIL
PROTAMINE SULFATE, PROTAMINE SULFATE
PROTAMINE ZINC AND ILETIN II, INSULIN SUSP PROTAMINE ZINC PURIFIED BEEF (OTC)
PROTAMINE ZINC AND ILETIN II (PORK), INSULIN SUSP PROTAMINE ZINC PURIFIED PORK (OTC)
PROTAMINE, ZINC & ILETIN I (BEEF-PORK), INSULIN SUSP PROTAMINE ZINC BEEF/PORK (OTC)
PROZAC, FLUOXETINE HYDROCHLORIDE
QUINIDINE GLUCONATE, QUINIDINE GLUCONATE
QUINIDINE SULFATE, QUINIDINE SULFATE
REGULAR ILETIN II, INSULIN PURIFIED BEEF (OTC)
REGULAR ILETIN II (PORK), INSULIN PURIFIED PORK (OTC)
SANDRIL, RESERPINE
SECONAL SODIUM, SECOBARBITAL SODIUM
SEROMYCIN, CYCLOSERINE
STREPTOMYCIN SULFATE, STREPTOMYCIN SULFATE
SULFADIAZINE, SULFADIAZINE
SULFAPYRIDINE, SULFAPYRIDINE
SULFONAMIDES DUPLEX, SULFADIAZINE
TAPAZOLE, METHIMAZOLE
TAZIDIME, CEFTAZIDIME
TESTOSTERONE PROPIONATE, TESTOSTERONE PROPIONATE
TUBOCURARINE CHLORIDE, TUBOCURARINE CHLORIDE
TYLOSTERONE, DIETHYLSTILBESTROL
V-CILLIN, PENICILLIN V
V-CILLIN K, PENICILLIN V POTASSIUM
VANCOCIN HCL, VANCOMYCIN HYDROCHLORIDE
VELBAN, VINBLASTINE SULFATE
* ELI LILLY INDUSTRIES INC
DARVON, PROPOXYPHENE HYDROCHLORIDE
DARVON COMPOUND, ASPIRIN
DARVON COMPOUND-65, ASPIRIN

APPENDIX B
PRODUCT NAME INDEX
LISTED BY APPLICANT *(continued)*

DARVON W/ ASA, ASPIRIN
DARVON-N, PROPOXYPHENE NAPSYLATE
DYMELOR, ACETOHEXAMIDE
NOVRAD, LEVOPROPOXYPHENE NAPSYLATE, ANHYDROUS
* LILLY RESEARCH LABORATORIES DIV ELI LILLY CO
PROZAC, FLUOXETINE HYDROCHLORIDE

LIQUIPHARM
* LIQUIPHARM INC
METOCLOPRAMIDE HCL, METOCLOPRAMIDE HYDROCHLORIDE
TRIHEXYPHENIDYL HCL, TRIHEXYPHENIDYL HYDROCHLORIDE

LNK
* LNK INTERNATIONAL INC
DIPHENHYDRAMINE HCL, DIPHENHYDRAMINE HYDROCHLORIDE
METRONIDAZOLE, METRONIDAZOLE

LOCH
* LOCH PHARMACEUTICALS INC
CLINDAMYCIN PHOSPHATE, CLINDAMYCIN PHOSPHATE
FOLIC ACID, FOLIC ACID
KANAMYCIN SULFATE, KANAMYCIN SULFATE

LOREX
* LOREX PHARMACEUTICALS INC
AMBIEN, ZOLPIDEM TARTRATE
KERLEDEX, BETAXOLOL HYDROCHLORIDE
KERLONE, BETAXOLOL HYDROCHLORIDE

LOTUS BIOCHEM
* LOTUS BIOCHEMICAL CORP
ERGOMAR, ERGOTAMINE TARTRATE
PROFERDEX, IRON DEXTRAN

LPI
* LPI HOLDINGS INC
N.E.E. 1/35 21, ETHINYL ESTRADIOL
N.E.E. 1/35 28, ETHINYL ESTRADIOL

LUITPOLD
* LUITPOLD PHARMACEUTICALS INC
AMINOCAPROIC ACID, AMINOCAPROIC ACID
AMINOPHYLLINE, AMINOPHYLLINE
BRETYLIUM TOSYLATE, BRETYLIUM TOSYLATE
CYANOCOBALAMIN, CYANOCOBALAMIN
DEXAMETHASONE SODIUM PHOSPHATE, DEXAMETHASONE SODIUM PHOSPHATE
DOPAMINE HCL, DOPAMINE HYDROCHLORIDE
DROPERIDOL, DROPERIDOL
FUROSEMIDE, FUROSEMIDE
GLYCOPYRROLATE, GLYCOPYRROLATE
HEPARIN LOCK FLUSH, HEPARIN SODIUM
HEPARIN SODIUM, HEPARIN SODIUM
HYDROXYZINE HCL, HYDROXYZINE HYDROCHLORIDE
LIDOCAINE HCL, LIDOCAINE HYDROCHLORIDE
MANNITOL 25%, MANNITOL
METHYLDOPATE HCL, METHYLDOPATE HYDROCHLORIDE
NITROGLYCERIN, NITROGLYCERIN
PIPERAZINE CITRATE, PIPERAZINE CITRATE
POTASSIUM CHLORIDE, POTASSIUM CHLORIDE
PYRIDOXINE HCL, PYRIDOXINE HYDROCHLORIDE
THIAMINE HCL, THIAMINE HYDROCHLORIDE
VERAPAMIL HCL, VERAPAMIL HYDROCHLORIDE

LYNE
* LYNE LABORATORIES INC
XYLOSE, XYLOSE

M

MALLARD
* MALLARD INC
MEPROBAMATE, MEPROBAMATE

MALLINCKRODT
* MALLINCKRODT CHEMICAL INC
METHADOSE, METHADONE HYDROCHLORIDE
* MALLINCKRODT INC
FERROUS CITRATE FE 59, FERROUS CITRATE, FE-59
MD-50, DIATRIZOATE SODIUM
OCTREOSCAN, INDIUM IN-111 PENTETREOTIDE KIT
OSTEOSCAN, TECHNETIUM TC-99M ETIDRONATE KIT
SELENOMETHIONINE SE 75, SELENOMETHIONINE, SE-75
XENEISOL, XENON, XE-133
* MALLINCKRODT MEDICAL INC
ANGIO-CONRAY, IOTHALAMATE SODIUM
CHOLEBRINE, IOCETAMIC ACID
CONRAY, IOTHALAMATE MEGLUMINE
CONRAY 30, IOTHALAMATE MEGLUMINE
CONRAY 325, IOTHALAMATE SODIUM
CONRAY 400, IOTHALAMATE SODIUM
CONRAY 43, IOTHALAMATE MEGLUMINE
CYANOCOBALAMIN CO 57 SCHILLING TEST KIT, CYANOCOBALAMIN
CYSTO-CONRAY, IOTHALAMATE MEGLUMINE
CYSTO-CONRAY II, IOTHALAMATE MEGLUMINE
GALLIUM CITRATE GA 67, GALLIUM CITRATE, GA-67
HEXABRIX, IOXAGLATE MEGLUMINE
HIPPURAN I 131, IODOHIPPURATE SODIUM, I-131
MD-GASTROVIEW, DIATRIZOATE MEGLUMINE
MD-60, DIATRIZOATE MEGLUMINE
MD-76, DIATRIZOATE MEGLUMINE
OPTIRAY 160, IOVERSOL
OPTIRAY 240, IOVERSOL
OPTIRAY 300, IOVERSOL
OPTIRAY 320, IOVERSOL
OPTIRAY 350, IOVERSOL
PERCHLORACAP, POTASSIUM PERCHLORATE
PHOSPHOCOL P32, CHROMIC PHOSPHATE, P-32
RADIOIODINATED SERUM ALBUMIN (HUMAN) IHSA I 125, ALBUMIN IODINATED I-125 SERUM
SODIUM CHROMATE CR 51, SODIUM CHROMATE, CR-51
SODIUM IODIDE I 123, SODIUM IODIDE, I-123
SODIUM IODIDE I 131, SODIUM IODIDE, I-131
SODIUM PERTECHNETATE TC 99M, TECHNETIUM TC-99M SODIUM PERTECHNETATE
SODIUM PHOSPHATE P 32, SODIUM PHOSPHATE, P-32
TECHNECOLL, TECHNETIUM TC-99M SULFUR COLLOID KIT
TECHNESCAN HDP, TECHNETIUM TC-99M OXIDRONATE KIT
TECHNESCAN MAA, TECHNETIUM TC-99M ALBUMIN AGGREGATED KIT
TECHNESCAN MAG3, TECHNETIUM TC-99M MERTIATIDE KIT

APPENDIX B
PRODUCT NAME INDEX
LISTED BY APPLICANT *(continued)*

TECHNESCAN PYP KIT, TECHNETIUM TC-99M PYROPHOSPHATE KIT
TECHNETIUM TC 99M SULFUR COLLOID, TECHNETIUM TC-99M SULFUR COLLOID
THALLOUS CHLORIDE TL 201, THALLOUS CHLORIDE, TL-201
ULTRA-TECHNEKOW FM, TECHNETIUM TC-99M SODIUM PERTECHNETATE GENERATOR
ULTRATAG, TECHNETIUM TC-99M RED BLOOD CELL KIT
VASCORAY, IOTHALAMATE MEGLUMINE
XENON XE 127, XENON, XE-127
XENON XE 133, XENON, XE-133

MARCHAR
* MARCHAR LABORATORIES INC LTD
FLUOROURACIL, FLUOROURACIL

MARION MERRELL DOW
* MARION MERRELL DOW INC
CARAFATE, SUCRALFATE
CARDIZEM, DILTIAZEM HYDROCHLORIDE
CARDIZEM SR, DILTIAZEM HYDROCHLORIDE
DITROPAN, OXYBUTYNIN CHLORIDE
GAVISCON, ALUMINUM HYDROXIDE (OTC)
GAVISCON-2, ALUMINUM HYDROXIDE (OTC)
NICODERM, NICOTINE
NITRO-BID, NITROGLYCERIN
PENTASA, MESALAMINE
RIFATER, ISONIAZID
SILVADENE, SILVER SULFADIAZINE
VENTAIRE, PROTOKYLOL HYDROCHLORIDE

MARSAM
* MARSAM PHARMACEUTICALS INC
AMPICILLIN SODIUM, AMPICILLIN SODIUM
CEFAZOLIN SODIUM, CEFAZOLIN SODIUM
CEFUROXIME, CEFUROXIME SODIUM
CHLORPROMAZINE HCL, CHLORPROMAZINE HYDROCHLORIDE
CLINDAMYCIN PHOSPHATE, CLINDAMYCIN PHOSPHATE
DIAZEPAM, DIAZEPAM
FUROSEMIDE, FUROSEMIDE
HALOPERIDOL, HALOPERIDOL LACTATE
HEPARIN SODIUM PRESERVATIVE FREE, HEPARIN SODIUM
METHOCARBAMOL, METHOCARBAMOL
METHYLDOPATE HCL, METHYLDOPATE HYDROCHLORIDE
NAFCILLIN SODIUM, NAFCILLIN SODIUM
NALOXONE HCL, NALOXONE HYDROCHLORIDE
OXACILLIN SODIUM, OXACILLIN SODIUM
PENICILLIN G POTASSIUM, PENICILLIN G POTASSIUM
PENICILLIN G SODIUM, PENICILLIN G SODIUM
PHENYTOIN SODIUM, PHENYTOIN SODIUM
PROCHLORPERAZINE EDISYLATE, PROCHLORPERAZINE EDISYLATE
PROMETHAZINE HCL, PROMETHAZINE HYDROCHLORIDE
TOBRAMYCIN SULFATE, TOBRAMYCIN SULFATE
VERAPAMIL HCL, VERAPAMIL HYDROCHLORIDE

MARSHALL PHARMA
* MARSHALL PHARMACAL CORP
CHLORPHENIRAMINE MALEATE, CHLORPHENIRAMINE MALEATE
PREDNISOLONE, PREDNISOLONE
PREDNISONE, PREDNISONE
RESERPINE, RESERPINE
SODIUM BUTABARBITAL, BUTABARBITAL SODIUM

MARTEC
* MARTEC PHARMACEUTICALS INC
DIAZEPAM, DIAZEPAM
SULFAMETHOXAZOLE AND TRIMETHOPRIM, SULFAMETHOXAZOLE
SULFAMETHOXAZOLE AND TRIMETHOPRIM DOUBLE STRENGTH, SULFAMETHOXAZOLE

MATRIX MEDCL
* MATRIX MEDICAL CORP
STERI-STAT, CHLORHEXIDINE GLUCONATE (OTC)

MAYRAND
* MAYRAND INC
SEDAPAP, ACETAMINOPHEN

MCGAW
* MCGAW INC
ACETATED RINGER'S IN PLASTIC CONTAINER, CALCIUM CHLORIDE
ACETIC ACID 0.25% IN PLASTIC CONTAINER, ACETIC ACID, GLACIAL
ALCOHOL 10% AND DEXTROSE 5%, ALCOHOL
ALCOHOL 5% AND DEXTROSE 5%, ALCOHOL
AMMONIUM CHLORIDE 0.9% IN NORMAL SALINE, AMMONIUM CHLORIDE
AMMONIUM CHLORIDE 2.14%, AMMONIUM CHLORIDE
BRETYLIUM TOSYLATE IN DEXTROSE 5%, BRETYLIUM TOSYLATE
DEXTROSE 10%, DEXTROSE
DEXTROSE 10% AND SODIUM CHLORIDE 0.11%, DEXTROSE
DEXTROSE 10% AND SODIUM CHLORIDE 0.2%, DEXTROSE
DEXTROSE 10% AND SODIUM CHLORIDE 0.33%, DEXTROSE
DEXTROSE 10% AND SODIUM CHLORIDE 0.45%, DEXTROSE
DEXTROSE 10% AND SODIUM CHLORIDE 0.9%, DEXTROSE
DEXTROSE 10% AND SODIUM CHLORIDE 0.9% IN PLASTIC CONTAINER, DEXTROSE
DEXTROSE 10% IN PLASTIC CONTAINER, DEXTROSE
DEXTROSE 2.5%, DEXTROSE
DEXTROSE 2.5% AND SODIUM CHLORIDE 0.11%, DEXTROSE
DEXTROSE 2.5% AND SODIUM CHLORIDE 0.2%, DEXTROSE
DEXTROSE 2.5% AND SODIUM CHLORIDE 0.33%, DEXTROSE
DEXTROSE 2.5% AND SODIUM CHLORIDE 0.45%, DEXTROSE
DEXTROSE 2.5% AND SODIUM CHLORIDE 0.45% IN PLASTIC CONTAINER, DEXTROSE
DEXTROSE 2.5% AND SODIUM CHLORIDE 0.9%, DEXTROSE
DEXTROSE 2.5% IN HALF-STRENGTH LACTATED RINGER'S, CALCIUM CHLORIDE
DEXTROSE 3.3% AND SODIUM CHLORIDE 0.3%, DEXTROSE
DEXTROSE 4% IN MODIFIED LACTATED RINGER'S, CALCIUM CHLORIDE
DEXTROSE 5%, DEXTROSE

APPENDIX B
PRODUCT NAME INDEX
LISTED BY APPLICANT *(continued)*

DEXTROSE 5% AND SODIUM CHLORIDE 0.11%, DEXTROSE
DEXTROSE 5% AND SODIUM CHLORIDE 0.11% IN PLASTIC CONTAINER, DEXTROSE
DEXTROSE 5% AND SODIUM CHLORIDE 0.2%, DEXTROSE
DEXTROSE 5% AND SODIUM CHLORIDE 0.2% IN PLASTIC CONTAINER, DEXTROSE
DEXTROSE 5% AND SODIUM CHLORIDE 0.33%, DEXTROSE
DEXTROSE 5% AND SODIUM CHLORIDE 0.33% IN PLASTIC CONTAINER, DEXTROSE
DEXTROSE 5% AND SODIUM CHLORIDE 0.45%, DEXTROSE
DEXTROSE 5% AND SODIUM CHLORIDE 0.45% IN PLASTIC CONTAINER, DEXTROSE
DEXTROSE 5% AND SODIUM CHLORIDE 0.9%, DEXTROSE
DEXTROSE 5% IN ACETATED RINGER'S IN PLASTIC CONTAINER, CALCIUM CHLORIDE
DEXTROSE 5% IN LACTATED RINGER'S, CALCIUM CHLORIDE
DEXTROSE 5% IN LACTATED RINGER'S IN PLASTIC CONTAINER, CALCIUM CHLORIDE
DEXTROSE 5% IN PLASTIC CONTAINER, DEXTROSE
DEXTROSE 5% IN RINGER'S, CALCIUM CHLORIDE
DEXTROSE 5% IN RINGER'S IN PLASTIC CONTAINER, CALCIUM CHLORIDE
DEXTROSE 5%, SODIUM CHLORIDE 0.2% AND POTASSIUM CHLORIDE 0.075%, DEXTROSE
DEXTROSE 5%, SODIUM CHLORIDE 0.2% AND POTASSIUM CHLORIDE 0.15%, DEXTROSE
DEXTROSE 5%, SODIUM CHLORIDE 0.2% AND POTASSIUM CHLORIDE 0.224%, DEXTROSE
DEXTROSE 5%, SODIUM CHLORIDE 0.2% AND POTASSIUM CHLORIDE 0.3%, DEXTROSE
DEXTROSE 5%, SODIUM CHLORIDE 0.33% AND POTASSIUM CHLORIDE 0.075%, DEXTROSE
DEXTROSE 5%, SODIUM CHLORIDE 0.33% AND POTASSIUM CHLORIDE 0.15%, DEXTROSE
DEXTROSE 5%, SODIUM CHLORIDE 0.33% AND POTASSIUM CHLORIDE 0.22%, DEXTROSE
DEXTROSE 5%, SODIUM CHLORIDE 0.33% AND POTASSIUM CHLORIDE 0.30%, DEXTROSE
DEXTROSE 5%, SODIUM CHLORIDE 0.45% AND POTASSIUM CHLORIDE 0.075%, DEXTROSE
DEXTROSE 5%, SODIUM CHLORIDE 0.45% AND POTASSIUM CHLORIDE 0.15%, DEXTROSE
DEXTROSE 5%, SODIUM CHLORIDE 0.45% AND POTASSIUM CHLORIDE 0.22%, DEXTROSE
DEXTROSE 5%, SODIUM CHLORIDE 0.45% AND POTASSIUM CHLORIDE 0.3%, DEXTROSE
DEXTROSE 60%, DEXTROSE
DEXTROSE 60% IN PLASTIC CONTAINER, DEXTROSE
DEXTROSE 7.7%, DEXTROSE
DIALYTE CONCENTRATE W/ DEXTROSE 30% IN PLASTIC CONTAINER, CALCIUM CHLORIDE
DIALYTE CONCENTRATE W/ DEXTROSE 50% IN PLASTIC CONTAINER, CALCIUM CHLORIDE
DIALYTE LM/ DEXTROSE 1.5%, CALCIUM CHLORIDE
DIALYTE LM/ DEXTROSE 2.5%, CALCIUM CHLORIDE
DIALYTE LM/ DEXTROSE 4.25%, CALCIUM CHLORIDE
DIALYTE W/ DEXTROSE 1.5% IN PLASTIC CONTAINER, CALCIUM CHLORIDE
DIALYTE W/ DEXTROSE 4.25% IN PLASTIC CONTAINER, CALCIUM CHLORIDE
DOPAMINE HCL AND DEXTROSE 5%, DOPAMINE HYDROCHLORIDE
FREAMINE HBC 6.9%, AMINO ACIDS
FREAMINE II 8.5%, AMINO ACIDS
FREAMINE III 10%, AMINO ACIDS
FREAMINE III 3% W/ ELECTROLYTES, AMINO ACIDS
FREAMINE III 8.5%, AMINO ACIDS
FREAMINE III 8.5% W/ ELECTROLYTES, AMINO ACIDS
FREAMINE 8.5%, AMINO ACIDS
GENTAMICIN SULFATE IN SODIUM CHLORIDE 0.9%, GENTAMICIN SULFATE
GLYCINE 1.5% IN PLASTIC CONTAINER, GLYCINE
HEPARIN SODIUM 1000 UNITS AND DEXTROSE 5% IN PLASTIC CONTAINER, HEPARIN SODIUM
HEPARIN SODIUM 1000 UNITS IN SODIUM CHLORIDE 0.9%, HEPARIN SODIUM
HEPARIN SODIUM 12500 UNITS IN SODIUM CHLORIDE 0.45%, HEPARIN SODIUM
HEPARIN SODIUM 2000 UNITS IN DEXTROSE 5% IN PLASTIC CONTAINER, HEPARIN SODIUM
HEPARIN SODIUM 2000 UNITS IN SODIUM CHLORIDE 0.9%, HEPARIN SODIUM
HEPARIN SODIUM 20000 UNITS IN DEXTROSE 5%, HEPARIN SODIUM
HEPARIN SODIUM 25000 UNITS IN DEXTROSE 5%, HEPARIN SODIUM
HEPARIN SODIUM 25000 UNITS IN DEXTROSE 5% IN PLASTIC CONTAINER, HEPARIN SODIUM
HEPARIN SODIUM 25000 UNITS IN SODIUM CHLORIDE 0.45%, HEPARIN SODIUM
HEPARIN SODIUM 25000 UNITS IN SODIUM CHLORIDE 0.9%, HEPARIN SODIUM
HEPARIN SODIUM 5000 UNITS IN DEXTROSE 5% IN PLASTIC CONTAINER, HEPARIN SODIUM
HEPARIN SODIUM 5000 UNITS IN SODIUM CHLORIDE 0.9%, HEPARIN SODIUM
HEPATAMINE 8%, AMINO ACIDS
HYPROTIGEN 5%, PROTEIN HYDROLYSATE
ISOLYTE E, CALCIUM CHLORIDE
ISOLYTE E IN DEXTROSE 5%, CALCIUM CHLORIDE
ISOLYTE E IN PLASTIC CONTAINER, CALCIUM CHLORIDE
ISOLYTE E W/ DEXTROSE 5% IN PLASTIC CONTAINER, CALCIUM CHLORIDE
ISOLYTE H IN DEXTROSE 5%, DEXTROSE
ISOLYTE H W/ DEXTROSE 5%, DEXTROSE
ISOLYTE M IN DEXTROSE 5%, DEXTROSE
ISOLYTE M W/ DEXTROSE 5% IN PLASTIC CONTAINER, DEXTROSE
ISOLYTE P IN DEXTROSE 5%, DEXTROSE
ISOLYTE P W/ DEXTROSE 5% IN PLASTIC CONTAINER, DEXTROSE
ISOLYTE R IN DEXTROSE 5%, CALCIUM CHLORIDE
ISOLYTE R W/ DEXTROSE 5%, CALCIUM CHLORIDE
ISOLYTE S, MAGNESIUM CHLORIDE
ISOLYTE S IN DEXTROSE 5%, DEXTROSE
ISOLYTE S IN PLASTIC CONTAINER, MAGNESIUM CHLORIDE
ISOLYTE S PH 7.4, MAGNESIUM CHLORIDE
ISOLYTE S PH 7.4 IN PLASTIC CONTAINER, MAGNESIUM CHLORIDE
ISOLYTE S W/ DEXTROSE 5% IN PLASTIC CONTAINER, DEXTROSE
LACTATED RINGER'S, CALCIUM CHLORIDE
LACTATED RINGER'S IN PLASTIC CONTAINER, CALCIUM CHLORIDE
LIDOCAINE HCL 0.2% AND DEXTROSE 5%, LIDOCAINE HYDROCHLORIDE
LIDOCAINE HCL 0.2% AND DEXTROSE 5% IN PLASTIC CONTAINER, LIDOCAINE HYDROCHLORIDE

APPENDIX B
PRODUCT NAME INDEX
LISTED BY APPLICANT *(continued)*

LIDOCAINE HCL 0.4% AND DEXTROSE 5%, LIDOCAINE HYDROCHLORIDE
LIDOCAINE HCL 0.4% AND DEXTROSE 5% IN PLASTIC CONTAINER, LIDOCAINE HYDROCHLORIDE
LIDOCAINE HCL 0.8% AND DEXTROSE 5%, LIDOCAINE HYDROCHLORIDE
LIDOCAINE HCL 0.8% AND DEXTROSE 5% IN PLASTIC CONTAINER, LIDOCAINE HYDROCHLORIDE
MANNITOL 10%, MANNITOL
MANNITOL 10% W/ DEXTROSE 5% IN DISTILLED WATER, MANNITOL
MANNITOL 15%, MANNITOL
MANNITOL 15% W/ DEXTROSE 5% IN SODIUM CHLORIDE 0.45%, MANNITOL
MANNITOL 20%, MANNITOL
MANNITOL 5%, MANNITOL
MANNITOL 5% W/ DEXTROSE 5% IN SODIUM CHLORIDE 0.12%, MANNITO
METRO I.V., METRONIDAZOLE
METRO I.V. IN PLASTIC CONTAINER, METRONIDAZOLE
NEPHRAMINE 5.4%, AMINO ACIDS
NUTRILIPID 10%, SOYBEAN OIL
NUTRILIPID 20%, SOYBEAN OIL
PHYSIOLYTE IN PLASTIC CONTAINER, MAGNESIUM CHLORIDE
POTASSIUM CHLORIDE, POTASSIUM CHLORIDE
POTASSIUM CHLORIDE 0.037% IN DEXTROSE 10% AND SODIUM CHLORIDE 0.2%, DEXTROSE
POTASSIUM CHLORIDE 0.037% IN DEXTROSE 10% AND SODIUM CHLORIDE 0.45%, DEXTROSE
POTASSIUM CHLORIDE 0.037% IN DEXTROSE 10% AND SODIUM CHLORIDE 0.9%, DEXTROSE
POTASSIUM CHLORIDE 0.037% IN DEXTROSE 5%, DEXTROSE
POTASSIUM CHLORIDE 0.037% IN DEXTROSE 5% AND SODIUM CHLORIDE 0.11%, DEXTROSE
POTASSIUM CHLORIDE 0.037% IN DEXTROSE 5% AND SODIUM CHLORIDE 0.2%, DEXTROSE
POTASSIUM CHLORIDE 0.037% IN DEXTROSE 5% AND SODIUM CHLORIDE 0.33%, DEXTROSE
POTASSIUM CHLORIDE 0.037% IN DEXTROSE 5% AND SODIUM CHLORIDE 0.45%, DEXTROSE
POTASSIUM CHLORIDE 0.037% IN DEXTROSE 5% AND SODIUM CHLORIDE 0.9%, DEXTROSE
POTASSIUM CHLORIDE 0.037% IN SODIUM CHLORIDE 0.9%, POTASSIUM CHLORIDE
POTASSIUM CHLORIDE 0.075% IN DEXTROSE 10% AND SODIUM CHLORIDE 0.2%, DEXTROSE
POTASSIUM CHLORIDE 0.075% IN DEXTROSE 10% AND SODIUM CHLORIDE 0.45%, DEXTROSE
POTASSIUM CHLORIDE 0.075% IN DEXTROSE 10% AND SODIUM CHLORIDE 0.9%, DEXTROSE
POTASSIUM CHLORIDE 0.075% IN DEXTROSE 3.3% AND SODIUM CHLORIDE 0.3%, DEXTROSE
POTASSIUM CHLORIDE 0.075% IN DEXTROSE 5%, DEXTROSE
POTASSIUM CHLORIDE 0.075% IN DEXTROSE 5% AND SODIUM CHLORIDE 0.11%, DEXTROSE
POTASSIUM CHLORIDE 0.075% IN DEXTROSE 5% AND SODIUM CHLORIDE 0.2%, DEXTROSE
POTASSIUM CHLORIDE 0.075% IN DEXTROSE 5% AND SODIUM CHLORIDE 0.33%, DEXTROSE
POTASSIUM CHLORIDE 0.075% IN DEXTROSE 5% AND SODIUM CHLORIDE 0.45%, DEXTROSE
POTASSIUM CHLORIDE 0.075% IN DEXTROSE 5% AND SODIUM CHLORIDE 0.9%, DEXTROSE
POTASSIUM CHLORIDE 0.075% IN SODIUM CHLORIDE 0.9%, POTASSIUM CHLORIDE
POTASSIUM CHLORIDE 0.11% IN DEXTROSE 10% AND SODIUM CHLORIDE 0.2%, DEXTROSE
POTASSIUM CHLORIDE 0.11% IN DEXTROSE 10% AND SODIUM CHLORIDE 0.45%, DEXTROSE
POTASSIUM CHLORIDE 0.11% IN DEXTROSE 10% AND SODIUM CHLORIDE 0.9%, DEXTROSE
POTASSIUM CHLORIDE 0.11% IN DEXTROSE 3.3% AND SODIUM CHLORIDE 0.3%, DEXTROSE
POTASSIUM CHLORIDE 0.11% IN DEXTROSE 5%, DEXTROSE
POTASSIUM CHLORIDE 0.11% IN DEXTROSE 5% AND SODIUM CHLORIDE 0.11%, DEXTROSE
POTASSIUM CHLORIDE 0.11% IN DEXTROSE 5% AND SODIUM CHLORIDE 0.2%, DEXTROSE
POTASSIUM CHLORIDE 0.11% IN DEXTROSE 5% AND SODIUM CHLORIDE 0.33%, DEXTROSE
POTASSIUM CHLORIDE 0.11% IN DEXTROSE 5% AND SODIUM CHLORIDE 0.45%, DEXTROSE
POTASSIUM CHLORIDE 0.11% IN DEXTROSE 5% AND SODIUM CHLORIDE 0.9%, DEXTROSE
POTASSIUM CHLORIDE 0.11% IN SODIUM CHLORIDE 0.9%, POTASSIUM CHLORIDE
POTASSIUM CHLORIDE 0.15% IN DEXTROSE 10% AND SODIUM CHLORIDE 0.2%, DEXTROSE
POTASSIUM CHLORIDE 0.15% IN DEXTROSE 10% AND SODIUM CHLORIDE 0.45%, DEXTROSE
POTASSIUM CHLORIDE 0.15% IN DEXTROSE 10% AND SODIUM CHLORIDE 0.9%, DEXTROSE
POTASSIUM CHLORIDE 0.15% IN DEXTROSE 3.3% AND SODIUM CHLORIDE 0.3%, DEXTROSE
POTASSIUM CHLORIDE 0.15% IN DEXTROSE 5%, DEXTROSE
POTASSIUM CHLORIDE 0.15% IN DEXTROSE 5% AND SODIUM CHLORIDE 0.11%, DEXTROSE
POTASSIUM CHLORIDE 0.15% IN DEXTROSE 5% AND SODIUM CHLORIDE 0.2%, DEXTROSE
POTASSIUM CHLORIDE 0.15% IN DEXTROSE 5% AND SODIUM CHLORIDE 0.33%, DEXTROSE
POTASSIUM CHLORIDE 0.15% IN DEXTROSE 5% AND SODIUM CHLORIDE 0.45%, DEXTROSE
POTASSIUM CHLORIDE 0.15% IN DEXTROSE 5% AND SODIUM CHLORIDE 0.9%, DEXTROSE
POTASSIUM CHLORIDE 0.15% IN SODIUM CHLORIDE 0.9%, POTASSIUM CHLORIDE
POTASSIUM CHLORIDE 0.22% IN DEXTROSE 10% AND SODIUM CHLORIDE 0.2%, DEXTROSE
POTASSIUM CHLORIDE 0.22% IN DEXTROSE 10% AND SODIUM CHLORIDE 0.45%, DEXTROSE
POTASSIUM CHLORIDE 0.22% IN DEXTROSE 10% AND SODIUM CHLORIDE 0.9%, DEXTROSE
POTASSIUM CHLORIDE 0.22% IN DEXTROSE 3.3% AND SODIUM CHLORIDE 0.3%, DEXTROSE
POTASSIUM CHLORIDE 0.22% IN DEXTROSE 5%, DEXTROSE
POTASSIUM CHLORIDE 0.22% IN DEXTROSE 5% AND SODIUM CHLORIDE 0.11%, DEXTROSE
POTASSIUM CHLORIDE 0.22% IN DEXTROSE 5% AND SODIUM CHLORIDE 0.2%, DEXTROSE
POTASSIUM CHLORIDE 0.22% IN DEXTROSE 5% AND SODIUM CHLORIDE 0.33%, DEXTROSE
POTASSIUM CHLORIDE 0.22% IN DEXTROSE 5% AND SODIUM CHLORIDE 0.45%, DEXTROSE
POTASSIUM CHLORIDE 0.22% IN DEXTROSE 5% AND SODIUM CHLORIDE 0.9%, DEXTROSE
POTASSIUM CHLORIDE 0.22% IN SODIUM CHLORIDE 0.9%, POTASSIUM CHLORIDE

APPENDIX B
PRODUCT NAME INDEX
LISTED BY APPLICANT *(continued)*

POTASSIUM CHLORIDE 0.3% IN DEXTROSE 10% AND SODIUM CHLORIDE 0.2%, DEXTROSE
POTASSIUM CHLORIDE 0.3% IN DEXTROSE 10% AND SODIUM CHLORIDE 0.45%, DEXTROSE
POTASSIUM CHLORIDE 0.3% IN DEXTROSE 10% AND SODIUM CHLORIDE 0.9%, DEXTROSE
POTASSIUM CHLORIDE 0.3% IN DEXTROSE 3.3% AND SODIUM CHLORIDE 0.3%, DEXTROSE
POTASSIUM CHLORIDE 0.3% IN DEXTROSE 5%, DEXTROSE
POTASSIUM CHLORIDE 0.3% IN DEXTROSE 5% AND SODIUM CHLORIDE 0.11%, DEXTROSE
POTASSIUM CHLORIDE 0.3% IN DEXTROSE 5% AND SODIUM CHLORIDE 0.2%, DEXTROSE
POTASSIUM CHLORIDE 0.3% IN DEXTROSE 5% AND SODIUM CHLORIDE 0.33%, DEXTROSE
POTASSIUM CHLORIDE 0.3% IN DEXTROSE 5% AND SODIUM CHLORIDE 0.45%, DEXTROSE
POTASSIUM CHLORIDE 0.3% IN DEXTROSE 5% AND SODIUM CHLORIDE 0.9%, DEXTROSE
POTASSIUM CHLORIDE 0.3% IN SODIUM CHLORIDE 0.9%, POTASSIUM CHLORIDE
PROCALAMINE, AMINO ACIDS
RESECTISOL, MANNITOL
RINGER'S, CALCIUM CHLORIDE
RINGER'S IN PLASTIC CONTAINER, CALCIUM CHLORIDE
SODIUM CHLORIDE, SODIUM CHLORIDE
SODIUM CHLORIDE 0.45%, SODIUM CHLORIDE
SODIUM CHLORIDE 0.45% IN PLASTIC CONTAINER, SODIUM CHLORIDE
SODIUM CHLORIDE 0.9%, SODIUM CHLORIDE
SODIUM CHLORIDE 0.9% AND POTASSIUM CHLORIDE 0.075%, POTASSIUM CHLORIDE
SODIUM CHLORIDE 0.9% AND POTASSIUM CHLORIDE 0.15%, POTASSIUM CHLORIDE
SODIUM CHLORIDE 0.9% AND POTASSIUM CHLORIDE 0.22%, POTASSIUM CHLORIDE
SODIUM CHLORIDE 0.9% AND POTASSIUM CHLORIDE 0.3%, POTASSIUM CHLORIDE
SODIUM CHLORIDE 0.9% IN PLASTIC CONTAINER, SODIUM CHLORIDE
SODIUM CHLORIDE 3%, SODIUM CHLORIDE
SODIUM CHLORIDE 5%, SODIUM CHLORIDE
SODIUM LACTATE 0.167 MOLAR IN PLASTIC CONTAINER, SODIUM LACTATE
SODIUM LACTATE 1/6 MOLAR, SODIUM LACTATE
SORBITOL 3.3% IN PLASTIC CONTAINER, SORBITOL
STERILE WATER FOR INJECTION, WATER FOR INJECTION, STERILE
STERILE WATER FOR INJECTION IN PLASTIC CONTAINER, WATER FOR INJECTION, STERILE
STERILE WATER IN PLASTIC CONTAINER, WATER FOR IRRIGATION, STERILE
THEOPHYLLINE 0.04% AND DEXTROSE 5%, THEOPHYLLINE
THEOPHYLLINE 0.04% AND DEXTROSE 5% IN PLASTIC CONTAINER, THEOPHYLLINE
THEOPHYLLINE 0.08% AND DEXTROSE 5%, THEOPHYLLINE
THEOPHYLLINE 0.08% AND DEXTROSE 5% IN PLASTIC CONTAINER, THEOPHYLLINE
THEOPHYLLINE 0.16% AND DEXTROSE 5%, THEOPHYLLINE
THEOPHYLLINE 0.16% AND DEXTROSE 5% IN PLASTIC CONTAINER, THEOPHYLLINE
THEOPHYLLINE 0.2% AND DEXTROSE 5%, THEOPHYLLINE
THEOPHYLLINE 0.2% AND DEXTROSE 5% IN PLASTIC CONTAINER, THEOPHYLLINE
THEOPHYLLINE 0.32% AND DEXTROSE 5%, THEOPHYLLINE
THEOPHYLLINE 0.4% AND DEXTROSE 5%, THEOPHYLLINE
THEOPHYLLINE 0.4% AND DEXTROSE 5% IN PLASTIC CONTAINER, THEOPHYLLINE
TROPHAMINE, AMINO ACIDS
TROPHAMINE 10%, AMINO ACIDS
UCEPHAN, SODIUM BENZOATE

MCNEIL
* MCNEIL CONSUMER PRODUCTS CO DIV MCNEILAB INC
CHEMET, SUCCIMER
IBUPROFEN, IBUPROFEN
IMODIUM A-D, LOPERAMIDE HYDROCHLORIDE (OTC)
MEDIPREN, IBUPROFEN (OTC)
METHOCARBAMOL AND ASPIRIN, ASPIRIN
PEDIA PROFEN, IBUPROFEN
SINE-AID IB, IBUPROFEN (OTC)
TYLENOL, ACETAMINOPHEN
TYLENOL, ACETAMINOPHEN (OTC)

MD PHARM
* MD PHARMACEUTICAL INC
ALBUTEROL SULFATE, ALBUTEROL SULFATE
AMITRIPTYLINE HCL, AMITRIPTYLINE HYDROCHLORIDE
CHLOROQUINE PHOSPHATE, CHLOROQUINE PHOSPHATE
CYPROHEPTADINE HCL, CYPROHEPTADINE HYDROCHLORIDE
DI-ATRO, ATROPINE SULFATE
DIETHYLPROPION HCL, DIETHYLPROPION HYDROCHLORIDE
GLUTETHIMIDE, GLUTETHIMIDE
METHYLPHENIDATE HCL, METHYLPHENIDATE HYDROCHLORIDE

MEAD JOHNSON
* MEAD JOHNSON AND CO SUB BRISTOL MYERS CO
MEGACE, MEGESTROL ACETATE
MUCOMYST W/ ISOPROTERENOL, ACETYLCYSTEINE
OVCON-35, ETHINYL ESTRADIOL
OVCON-50, ETHINYL ESTRADIOL

MEDCO RES
* MEDCO RESEARCH INC
ADENOCARD, ADENOSINE

MEDEVA
* MEDEVA INC
DEXACORT, DEXAMETHASONE SODIUM PHOSPHATE

MEDI PHYSICS
* MEDI PHYSICS INC
CINTICHEM TECHNETIUM 99M HEDSPA, TECHNETIUM TC-99M ETIDRONATE KIT
GALLIUM CITRATE GA 67, GALLIUM CITRATE, GA-67
LUNGAGGREGATE REAGENT, TECHNETIUM TC-99M ALBUMIN AGGREGATED KIT
METASTRON, STRONTIUM CHLORIDE, SR-89
MPI DMSA KIDNEY REAGENT, TECHNETIUM TC-99M SUCCIMER KIT
MPI DTPA KIT - CHELATE, TECHNETIUM TC-99M PENTETATE KIT

APPENDIX B
PRODUCT NAME INDEX
LISTED BY APPLICANT *(continued)*

MPI INDIUM DTPA IN 111, INDIUM IN-111 PENTETATE DISODIUM
MPI KRYPTON 81M GAS GENERATOR, KRYPTON, KR-81M
MPI STANNOUS DIPHOSPHONATE, TECHNETIUM TC-99M ETIDRONATE KIT
NEOSCAN, GALLIUM CITRATE, GA-67
NEPHROFLOW, IODOHIPPURATE SODIUM, I-123
SELENOMETHIONINE SE 75, SELENOMETHIONINE, SE-75
SODIUM IODIDE I 123, SODIUM IODIDE, I-123
SODIUM PERTECHNETATE TC 99M, TECHNETIUM TC-99M SODIUM PERTECHNETATE
SODIUM POLYPHOSPHATE-TIN KIT, TECHNETIUM TC-99M POLYPHOSPHATE KIT
TC 99M-LUNGAGGREGATE, TECHNETIUM TC-99M ALBUMIN AGGREGATED
TECHNETIUM TC 99M DIPHOSPHONATE-TIN KIT, TECHNETIUM TC-99M ETIDRONATE KIT
TECHNETIUM TC 99M GENERATOR, TECHNETIUM TC-99M SODIUM PERTECHNETATE GENERATOR
TECHNETIUM TC 99M HSA, TECHNETIUM TC-99M ALBUMIN KIT
TECHNETIUM TC 99M MAA, TECHNETIUM TC-99M ALBUMIN AGGREGATED KIT
TECHNETIUM TC 99M MPI MDP, TECHNETIUM TC-99M MEDRONATE KIT
TECHNETIUM TC 99M SULFUR COLLOID, TECHNETIUM TC-99M SULFUR COLLOID
TECHNETIUM TC 99M TSC, TECHNETIUM TC-99M SULFUR COLLOID KIT
TECHNETIUM TC-99M PENTETATE KIT, TECHNETIUM TC-99M PENTETATE KIT
THALLOUS CHLORIDE TL 201, THALLOUS CHLORIDE, TL-201
XENON XE 133, XENON, XE-133
XENON XE 133-V.S.S., XENON, XE-133

MEDTRONIC
* MEDTRONIC INC
LIORESAL, BACLOFEN

MEPHA
* MEPHA AG
PIROXICAM, PIROXICAM

MERCK
* MERCK RESEARCH LABORATORIES DIV MERCK AND CO INC
CHIBROXIN, NORFLOXACIN
CLINORIL, SULINDAC
DECADRON-LA, DEXAMETHASONE ACETATE
INDOCIN, INDOMETHACIN
INDOCIN I.V., INDOMETHACIN SODIUM
INDOCIN SR, INDOMETHACIN
LACRISERT, HYDROXYPROPYL CELLULOSE
MEFOXIN, CEFOXITIN SODIUM
MEVACOR, LOVASTATIN
NOROXIN, NORFLOXACIN
PEPCID, FAMOTIDINE
PLENDIL, FELODIPINE
PRINIVIL, LISINOPRIL
PRINZIDE 10-12.5, HYDROCHLOROTHIAZIDE
PRINZIDE 20-12.5, HYDROCHLOROTHIAZIDE
PRINZIDE 20-25, HYDROCHLOROTHIAZIDE
TECHNESCAN DTPA KIT, TECHNETIUM TC-99M PENTETATE KIT
TECHNESCAN HIDA, TECHNETIUM TC-99M LIDOFENIN KIT
TIMOPTIC, TIMOLOL MALEATE
TIMOPTIC IN OCUDOSE, TIMOLOL MALEATE
TIMOPTIC-XE, TIMOLOL MALEATE
VASERETIC, ENALAPRIL MALEATE
VASOTEC, ENALAPRIL MALEATE
VASOTEC, ENALAPRILAT
ZOCOR, SIMVASTATIN

MERCK SHARP DOHME
* MERCK SHARP AND DOHME DIV MERCK AND CO INC
ALDOCLOR-150, CHLOROTHIAZIDE
ALDOCLOR-250, CHLOROTHIAZIDE
ALDOMET, METHYLDOPA
ALDOMET, METHYLDOPATE HYDROCHLORIDE
ALDORIL D30, HYDROCHLOROTHIAZIDE
ALDORIL D50, HYDROCHLOROTHIAZIDE
ALDORIL 15, HYDROCHLOROTHIAZIDE
ALDORIL 25, HYDROCHLOROTHIAZIDE
ALPHAREDISOL, HYDROXOCOBALAMIN
AMINOHIPPURATE SODIUM, AMINOHIPPURATE SODIUM
AQUAMEPHYTON, PHYTONADIONE
ARAMINE, METARAMINOL BITARTRATE
BENEMID, PROBENECID
BLOCADREN, TIMOLOL MALEATE
COGENTIN, BENZTROPINE MESYLATE
COLBENEMID, COLCHICINE
CORTONE, CORTISONE ACETATE
COSMEGEN, DACTINOMYCIN
CUPRIMINE, PENICILLAMINE
CYCLAINE, HEXYLCAINE HYDROCHLORIDE
DARANIDE, DICHLORPHENAMIDE
DECADERM, DEXAMETHASONE
DECADRON, DEXAMETHASONE
DECADRON, DEXAMETHASONE SODIUM PHOSPHATE
DECADRON W/ XYLOCAINE, DEXAMETHASONE SODIUM PHOSPHATE
DECASPRAY, DEXAMETHASONE
DEMSER, METYROSINE
DIUPRES-250, CHLOROTHIAZIDE
DIUPRES-500, CHLOROTHIAZIDE
DIURIL, CHLOROTHIAZIDE
DIURIL, CHLOROTHIAZIDE SODIUM
DOLOBID, DIFLUNISAL
EDECRIN, ETHACRYNATE SODIUM
EDECRIN, ETHACRYNIC ACID
FLEXERIL, CYCLOBENZAPRINE HYDROCHLORIDE
FLOROPRYL, ISOFLUROPHATE
HUMORSOL, DEMECARIUM BROMIDE
HYDELTRA-TBA, PREDNISOLONE TEBUTATE
HYDELTRASOL, PREDNISOLONE SODIUM PHOSPHATE
HYDROCORTONE, HYDROCORTISONE
HYDROCORTONE, HYDROCORTISONE ACETATE
HYDROCORTONE, HYDROCORTISONE SODIUM PHOSPHATE
HYDRODIURIL, HYDROCHLOROTHIAZIDE
HYDROPRES 25, HYDROCHLOROTHIAZIDE
HYDROPRES 50, HYDROCHLOROTHIAZIDE
INVERSINE, MECAMYLAMINE HYDROCHLORIDE
LERITINE, ANILERIDINE HYDROCHLORIDE
LERITINE, ANILERIDINE PHOSPHATE
LODOSYN, CARBIDOPA
MANNITOL 25%, MANNITOL
MEFOXIN, CEFOXITIN SODIUM
MEFOXIN IN DEXTROSE 5% IN PLASTIC CONTAINER, CEFOXITIN SODIU

APPENDIX B
PRODUCT NAME INDEX
LISTED BY APPLICANT *(continued)*

MEFOXIN IN SODIUM CHLORIDE 0.9% IN PLASTIC CONTAINER, CEFOXITIN SODIUM
MEPHYTON, PHYTONADIONE
MIDAMOR, AMILORIDE HYDROCHLORIDE
MINTEZOL, THIABENDAZOLE
MODURETIC 5-50, AMILORIDE HYDROCHLORIDE
MUSTARGEN, MECHLORETHAMINE HYDROCHLORIDE
NEO-HYDELTRASOL, NEOMYCIN SULFATE
NEODECADRON, DEXAMETHASONE SODIUM PHOSPHATE
PERIACTIN, CYPROHEPTADINE HYDROCHLORIDE
PRIMAXIN, CILASTATIN SODIUM
PROSCAR, FINASTERIDE
REDISOL, CYANOCOBALAMIN
SINEMET, CARBIDOPA
SINEMET CR, CARBIDOPA
SYPRINE, TRIENTINE HYDROCHLORIDE
TECHNESCAN GLUCEPTATE, TECHNETIUM TC-99M GLUCEPTATE KIT
TECHNESCAN MDP KIT, TECHNETIUM TC-99M MEDRONATE KIT
TECHNETIUM TC 99M ALBUMIN AGGREGATED KIT, TECHNETIUM TC-99M ALBUMIN AGGREGATED KIT
TIMOLIDE 10-25, HYDROCHLOROTHIAZIDE
TONOCARD, TOCAINIDE HYDROCHLORIDE
TRIAVIL 2-10, AMITRIPTYLINE HYDROCHLORIDE
TRIAVIL 2-25, AMITRIPTYLINE HYDROCHLORIDE
TRIAVIL 4-10, AMITRIPTYLINE HYDROCHLORIDE
TRIAVIL 4-25, AMITRIPTYLINE HYDROCHLORIDE
TRIAVIL 4-50, AMITRIPTYLINE HYDROCHLORIDE
URECHOLINE, BETHANECHOL CHLORIDE
VIVACTIL, PROTRIPTYLINE HYDROCHLORIDE

MERICON
* MERICON INDUSTRIES INC
HYDROCORTISONE, HYDROCORTISONE

MERRELL DOW
* MERRELL DOW PHARMACEUTICALS INC SUB DOW CHEMICAL CO
ACCURBRON, THEOPHYLLINE
AVC, SULFANILAMIDE
BENTYL, DICYCLOMINE HYDROCHLORIDE
BRICANYL, TERBUTALINE SULFATE
CANTIL, MEPENZOLATE BROMIDE
CEPHULAC, LACTULOSE
CHRONULAC, LACTULOSE
CLOMID, CLOMIPHENE CITRATE
CYANOCOBALAMIN, CYANOCOBALAMIN
DECAPRYN, DOXYLAMINE SUCCINATE
DV, DIENESTROL
HEDULIN, PHENINDIONE
HIPREX, METHENAMINE HIPPURATE
HYDROXYSTILBAMIDINE ISETHIONATE, HYDROXYSTILBAMIDINE ISETHIONATE
LORELCO, PROBUCOL
METAHYDRIN, TRICHLORMETHIAZIDE
METATENSIN #2, RESERPINE
METATENSIN #4, RESERPINE
NICORETTE, NICOTINE POLACRILEX
NICORETTE DS, NICOTINE POLACRILEX
NORPRAMIN, DESIPRAMINE HYDROCHLORIDE
ORNIDYL, EFLORNITHINE HYDROCHLORIDE
RIFADIN, RIFAMPIN
SELDANE, TERFENADINE
SELDANE-D, PSEUDOEPHEDRINE HYDROCHLORIDE
TACE, CHLOROTRIANISENE
TENUATE, DIETHYLPROPION HYDROCHLORIDE
TENUATE DOSPAN, DIETHYLPROPION HYDROCHLORIDE
TRICLOS, TRICLOFOS SODIUM
VANOBID, CANDICIDIN

MFG CHEMISTS
* MANUFACTURING CHEMISTS INC
PHENDIMETRAZINE TARTRATE, PHENDIMETRAZINE TARTRATE

MGI
* MGI PHARMA INC
DIDRONEL, ETIDRONATE DISODIUM
SALAGEN, PILOCARPINE HYDROCHLORIDE

MIKART
* MIKART INC
ACETAMINOPHEN AND CODEINE PHOSPHATE, ACETAMINOPHEN
ACETAMINOPHEN AND CODEINE PHOSPHATE #3, ACETAMINOPHEN
ACETAMINOPHEN AND CODEINE PHOSPHATE #4, ACETAMINOPHEN
ACETAMINOPHEN, ASPIRIN, AND CODEINE PHOSPHATE, ACETAMINOPHEN
ACETAMINOPHEN, BUTALBITAL, AND CAFFEINE, ACETAMINOPHEN
AMANTADINE HCL, AMANTADINE HYDROCHLORIDE
BUTALBITAL, ACETAMINOPHEN AND CAFFEINE, ACETAMINOPHEN
BUTAPAP, ACETAMINOPHEN
HYDROCODONE BITARTRATE AND ACETAMINOPHEN, ACETAMINOPHEN
METHAZOLAMIDE, METHAZOLAMIDE
PHENDIMETRAZINE TARTRATE, PHENDIMETRAZINE TARTRATE
PYRAZINAMIDE, PYRAZINAMIDE

MILES
* MILES INC
MITHRACIN, PLICAMYCIN
* MILES LABORATORIES INC
ALCOHOL 5% IN DEXTROSE 5%, ALCOHOL
DEXTROSE 10% IN PLASTIC CONTAINER, DEXTROSE
DEXTROSE 5% AND SODIUM CHLORIDE 0.2% IN PLASTIC CONTAINER, DEXTROSE
DEXTROSE 5% AND SODIUM CHLORIDE 0.3% IN PLASTIC CONTAINER, DEXTROSE
DEXTROSE 5% AND SODIUM CHLORIDE 0.45% IN PLASTIC CONTAINER, DEXTROSE
DEXTROSE 5% AND SODIUM CHLORIDE 0.9% IN PLASTIC CONTAINER, DEXTROSE
DEXTROSE 5% IN LACTATED RINGER'S IN PLASTIC CONTAINER, CALCIUM CHLORIDE
LACTATED RINGER'S IN PLASTIC CONTAINER, CALCIUM CHLORIDE
LIDOCAINE HCL, LIDOCAINE HYDROCHLORIDE
MANNITOL 10%, MANNITOL
MANNITOL 15%, MANNITOL
MANNITOL 20%, MANNITOL
POTASSIUM CHLORIDE, POTASSIUM CHLORIDE
PROCAINE HCL, PROCAINE HYDROCHLORIDE
SODIUM CHLORIDE IN PLASTIC CONTAINER, SODIUM CHLORIDE

APPENDIX B
PRODUCT NAME INDEX
LISTED BY APPLICANT *(continued)*

SODIUM CHLORIDE 0.45% IN PLASTIC CONTAINER, SODIUM CHLORIDE
SODIUM CHLORIDE 0.9% IN PLASTIC CONTAINER, SODIUM CHLORIDE
STERILE WATER IN PLASTIC CONTAINER, WATER FOR IRRIGATION, STERILE

* MILES PHARMACEUTICAL DIV MILES INC
ADALAT, NIFEDIPINE
ADALAT CC, NIFEDIPINE
ANTAGONATE, CHLORPHENIRAMINE MALEATE
AZLIN, AZLOCILLIN SODIUM
BILTRICIDE, PRAZIQUANTEL
CANDEX, NYSTATIN
CIPRO, CIPROFLOXACIN
CIPRO, CIPROFLOXACIN HYDROCHLORIDE
CIPRO IN DEXTROSE 5%, CIPROFLOXACIN
CIPRO IN SODIUM CHLORIDE 0.9%, CIPROFLOXACIN
CORT-DOME, HYDROCORTISONE
DELTA-DOME, PREDNISONE
DOMEBORO, ACETIC ACID, GLACIAL
DTIC-DOME, DACARBAZINE
HC #1, HYDROCORTISONE
HC #4, HYDROCORTISONE
LITHANE, LITHIUM CARBONATE
MEZLIN, MEZLOCILLIN SODIUM MONOHYDRATE
MYCELEX, CLOTRIMAZOLE
MYCELEX, CLOTRIMAZOLE (OTC)
MYCELEX-G, CLOTRIMAZOLE
MYCELEX-7, CLOTRIMAZOLE (OTC)
MYCELEX-7 COMBINATION PACK, CLOTRIMAZOLE
NEO-CORT-DOME, ACETIC ACID, GLACIAL
NEO-CORT-DOME, HYDROCORTISONE
NICLOCIDE, NICLOSAMIDE
NIMOTOP, NIMODIPINE
NYSTAFORM, CLIOQUINOL
RADIO-IODINATED (I 125) SERUM ALBUMIN (HUMAN), ALBUMIN IODINATED I-125 SERUM
SOY-DOME, HEXACHLOROPHENE
STILPHOSTROL, DIETHYLSTILBESTROL DIPHOSPHATE
TRASYLOL, APROTININ BOVINE
TRIDESILON, ACETIC ACID, GLACIAL
TRIDESILON, DESONIDE
VI-DOM-A, VITAMIN A PALMITATE

MILEX
* MILEX PRODUCTS INC
MILOPHENE, CLOMIPHENE CITRATE

MISSION PHARMA
* MISSION PHARMACAL CO
CALCIBIND, CELLULOSE SODIUM PHOSPHATE
EQUIPIN, HOMATROPINE METHYLBROMIDE
FOLICET, FOLIC ACID
HOMAPIN-10, HOMATROPINE METHYLBROMIDE
HOMAPIN-5, HOMATROPINE METHYLBROMIDE
LITHOSTAT, ACETOHYDROXAMIC ACID

MJ PHARMS
* MJ PHARMACEUTICALS LTD
CEPHALEXIN, CEPHALEXIN

MK LABS
* MK LABORATORIES INC
AMPHICOL, CHLORAMPHENICOL
DIPHENHYDRAMINE HCL, DIPHENHYDRAMINE HYDROCHLORIDE
FOLIC ACID, FOLIC ACID
ISONIAZID, ISONIAZID
KESSO-GESIC, PROPOXYPHENE HYDROCHLORIDE
MEPROBAMATE, MEPROBAMATE
NIACIN, NIACIN
OXY-KESSO-TETRA, OXYTETRACYCLINE HYDROCHLORIDE
RESERPINE, RESERPINE
SOSOL, SULFISOXAZOLE
TETRACYCLINE HCL, TETRACYCLINE HYDROCHLORIDE
VITAMIN A, VITAMIN A PALMITATE

MM MAST
* MM MAST AND CO
CHLORDIAZEPOXIDE HCL, CHLORDIAZEPOXIDE HYDROCHLORIDE
DEXTROAMPHETAMINE SULFATE, DEXTROAMPHETAMINE SULFATE
HYDROCHLOROTHIAZIDE, HYDROCHLOROTHIAZIDE
ONA MAST, PHENTERMINE HYDROCHLORIDE
ONA-MAST, PHENTERMINE HYDROCHLORIDE
PHENAZINE, PHENDIMETRAZINE TARTRATE
TETRACYCLINE HCL, TETRACYCLINE HYDROCHLORIDE
TRICHLORMAS, TRICHLORMETHIAZIDE

MURO
* MURO PHARMACEUTICAL INC
BROMFED-DM, BROMPHENIRAMINE MALEATE
LIQUID PRED, PREDNISONE
PRELONE, PREDNISOLONE
PROMETA, METAPROTERENOL SULFATE
VOLMAX, ALBUTEROL SULFATE

MUTUAL PHARM
* MUTUAL PHARMACEUTICAL CO INC
ACETAMINOPHEN AND CODEINE PHOSPHATE, ACETAMINOPHEN
ACETAZOLAMIDE, ACETAZOLAMIDE
ALBUTEROL SULFATE, ALBUTEROL SULFATE
ALLOPURINOL, ALLOPURINOL
AMITRIPTYLINE HCL, AMITRIPTYLINE HYDROCHLORIDE
ATENOLOL, ATENOLOL
ATENOLOL AND CHLORTHALIDONE, ATENOLOL
BENZTROPINE MESYLATE, BENZTROPINE MESYLATE
CARISOPRODOL, CARISOPRODOL
CHLORTHALIDONE, CHLORTHALIDONE
CHLORZOXAZONE, CHLORZOXAZONE
DIPHENHYDRAMINE HCL, DIPHENHYDRAMINE HYDROCHLORIDE
DOXYCYCLINE HYCLATE, DOXYCYCLINE HYCLATE
ERGOLOID MESYLATES, ERGOLOID MESYLATES
FENOPROFEN CALCIUM, FENOPROFEN CALCIUM
HYDRALAZINE HCL, HYDRALAZINE HYDROCHLORIDE
HYDROXYZINE HCL, HYDROXYZINE HYDROCHLORIDE
IBUPROFEN, IBUPROFEN
IBUPROFEN, IBUPROFEN (OTC)
IMIPRAMINE HCL, IMIPRAMINE HYDROCHLORIDE
INDOMETHACIN, INDOMETHACIN
LORAZEPAM, LORAZEPAM
METOCLOPRAMIDE HCL, METOCLOPRAMIDE HYDROCHLORIDE
METOPROLOL TARTRATE, METOPROLOL TARTRATE
METRONIDAZOLE, METRONIDAZOLE
NYSTATIN, NYSTATIN

APPENDIX B
PRODUCT NAME INDEX
LISTED BY APPLICANT *(continued)*

PINDOLOL, PINDOLOL
PIROXICAM, PIROXICAM
PREDNISONE, PREDNISONE
QUINIDINE GLUCONATE, QUINIDINE GLUCONATE
QUINIDINE SULFATE, QUINIDINE SULFATE
SPIRONOLACTONE, SPIRONOLACTONE
SPIRONOLACTONE AND HYDROCHLOROTHIAZIDE, HYDROCHLOROTHIAZIDE
SULFAMETHOXAZOLE AND TRIMETHOPRIM, SULFAMETHOXAZOLE
SULFASALAZINE, SULFASALAZINE
SULINDAC, SULINDAC
THIORIDAZINE HCL, THIORIDAZINE HYDROCHLORIDE
TOLAZAMIDE, TOLAZAMIDE
TOLMETIN SODIUM, TOLMETIN SODIUM
TRAZODONE HCL, TRAZODONE HYDROCHLORIDE
VERAPAMIL HCL, VERAPAMIL HYDROCHLORIDE

MYLAN
* MYLAN PHARMACEUTICALS INC
ALBUTEROL SULFATE, ALBUTEROL SULFATE
ALLOPURINOL, ALLOPURINOL
ALPRAZOLAM, ALPRAZOLAM
AMILORIDE HCL AND HYDROCHLOROTHIAZIDE, AMILORIDE HYDROCHLORIDE
AMITRIPTYLINE HCL, AMITRIPTYLINE HYDROCHLORIDE
AMOXICILLIN, AMOXICILLIN
AMPICILLIN TRIHYDRATE, AMPICILLIN/AMPICILLIN TRIHYDRATE
ATENOLOL, ATENOLOL
ATENOLOL AND CHLORTHALIDONE, ATENOLOL
CHLORDIAZEPOXIDE AND AMITRIPTYLINE HCL, AMITRIPTYLINE HYDROCHLORIDE
CHLORDIAZEPOXIDE HCL, CHLORDIAZEPOXIDE HYDROCHLORIDE
CHLOROTHIAZIDE, CHLOROTHIAZIDE
CHLOROTHIAZIDE-RESERPINE, CHLOROTHIAZIDE
CHLORPROPAMIDE, CHLORPROPAMIDE
CHLORTHALIDONE, CHLORTHALIDONE
CIMETIDINE, CIMETIDINE
CLONIDINE HCL, CLONIDINE HYDROCHLORIDE
CLONIDINE HCL AND CHLORTHALIDONE, CHLORTHALIDONE
CLORAZEPATE DIPOTASSIUM, CLORAZEPATE DIPOTASSIUM
CYCLOBENZAPRINE HCL, CYCLOBENZAPRINE HYDROCHLORIDE
CYPROHEPTADINE HCL, CYPROHEPTADINE HYDROCHLORIDE
CYSTAGON, CYSTEAMINE BITARTRATE
DIAZEPAM, DIAZEPAM
DILTIAZEM HCL, DILTIAZEM HYDROCHLORIDE
DIPHENOXYLATE HCL AND ATROPINE SULFATE, ATROPINE SULFATE
DISOPYRAMIDE PHOSPHATE, DISOPYRAMIDE PHOSPHATE
DOXEPIN HCL, DOXEPIN HYDROCHLORIDE
DOXYCYCLINE HYCLATE, DOXYCYCLINE HYCLATE
ERYTHROMYCIN ETHYLSUCCINATE, ERYTHROMYCIN ETHYLSUCCINATE
ERYTHROMYCIN STEARATE, ERYTHROMYCIN STEARATE
FENOPROFEN CALCIUM, FENOPROFEN CALCIUM
FLUPHENAZINE HCL, FLUPHENAZINE HYDROCHLORIDE
FLURAZEPAM HCL, FLURAZEPAM HYDROCHLORIDE
FLURBIPROFEN, FLURBIPROFEN
FUROSEMIDE, FUROSEMIDE
GEMFIBROZIL, GEMFIBROZIL
GLIPIZIDE, GLIPIZIDE
HALOPERIDOL, HALOPERIDOL
HYDRALAZINE HCL-HYDROCHLOROTHIAZIDE-RESERPINE, HYDRALAZINE HYDROCHLORIDE
HYDROCHLOROTHIAZIDE, HYDROCHLOROTHIAZIDE
IBUPROFEN, IBUPROFEN
IBUPROFEN, IBUPROFEN (OTC)
INDOMETHACIN, INDOMETHACIN
LOPERAMIDE HCL, LOPERAMIDE HYDROCHLORIDE
LORAZEPAM, LORAZEPAM
MAPROTILINE HCL, MAPROTILINE HYDROCHLORIDE
MAXZIDE, HYDROCHLOROTHIAZIDE
MAXZIDE-25, HYDROCHLOROTHIAZIDE
MECLOFENAMATE SODIUM, MECLOFENAMATE SODIUM
MEPROBAMATE, MEPROBAMATE
METHOCARBAMOL, METHOCARBAMOL
METHOTREXATE SODIUM, METHOTREXATE SODIUM
METHYCLOTHIAZIDE, METHYCLOTHIAZIDE
METHYLDOPA, METHYLDOPA
METHYLDOPA AND HYDROCHLOROTHIAZIDE, HYDROCHLOROTHIAZIDE
METOPROLOL TARTRATE, METOPROLOL TARTRATE
NADOLOL, NADOLOL
NAPROXEN, NAPROXEN
NAPROXEN SODIUM, NAPROXEN SODIUM
NORTRIPTYLINE HCL, NORTRIPTYLINE HYDROCHLORIDE
OXAZEPAM, OXAZEPAM
PENICILLIN G POTASSIUM, PENICILLIN G POTASSIUM
PENICILLIN V POTASSIUM, PENICILLIN V POTASSIUM
PERPHENAZINE AND AMITRIPTYLINE HCL, AMITRIPTYLINE HYDROCHLORIDE
PINDOLOL, PINDOLOL
PIROXICAM, PIROXICAM
PRAZOSIN HCL, PRAZOSIN HYDROCHLORIDE
PROBENECID, PROBENECID
PROPANTHELINE BROMIDE, PROPANTHELINE BROMIDE
PROPOXYPHENE HCL, PROPOXYPHENE HYDROCHLORIDE
PROPOXYPHENE HCL AND ACETAMINOPHEN, ACETAMINOPHEN
PROPOXYPHENE NAPSYLATE AND ACETAMINOPHEN, ACETAMINOPHEN
PROPRANOLOL HCL, PROPRANOLOL HYDROCHLORIDE
PROPRANOLOL HCL AND HYDROCHLOROTHIAZIDE, HYDROCHLOROTHIAZIDE
RESERPINE, RESERPINE
SPIRONOLACTONE, SPIRONOLACTONE
SPIRONOLACTONE AND HYDROCHLOROTHIAZIDE, HYDROCHLOROTHIAZIDE
SULINDAC, SULINDAC
TEMAZEPAM, TEMAZEPAM
TETRACYCLINE HCL, TETRACYCLINE HYDROCHLORIDE
THIORIDAZINE HCL, THIORIDAZINE HYDROCHLORIDE
THIOTHIXENE, THIOTHIXENE
TIMOLOL MALEATE, TIMOLOL MALEATE

APPENDIX B
PRODUCT NAME INDEX
LISTED BY APPLICANT *(continued)*

TOLAZAMIDE, TOLAZAMIDE
TOLBUTAMIDE, TOLBUTAMIDE
TOLMETIN SODIUM, TOLMETIN SODIUM
TRAZODONE HCL, TRAZODONE HYDROCHLORIDE
TRIAMCINOLONE, TRIAMCINOLONE
VERAPAMIL HCL, VERAPAMIL HYDROCHLORIDE

N

NASKA
* NASKA PHARMACAL CO INC DIV RUGBY DARBY GROUP COSMETICS
BACITRACIN, BACITRACIN (OTC)
BACITRACIN ZINC-NEOMYCIN SULFATE-POLYMYXIN B SULFATE, BACITRACIN ZINC (OTC)
BACITRACIN ZINC-POLYMYXIN B SULFATE, BACITRACIN ZINC (OTC)
CYPROHEPTADINE HCL, CYPROHEPTADINE HYDROCHLORIDE
DIPHENHYDRAMINE HCL, DIPHENHYDRAMINE HYDROCHLORIDE
ERYTHROMYCIN ETHYLSUCCINATE, ERYTHROMYCIN ETHYLSUCCINATE
HYDROCORTISONE, HYDROCORTISONE
TRIMETH/SULFA, SULFAMETHOXAZOLE

NEPHRON
* NEPHRON CORP
BETA-2, ISOETHARINE HYDROCHLORIDE

NEWTRON PHARMS
* NEWTRON PHARMACEUTICALS INC
BROMPHENIRAMINE MALEATE, BROMPHENIRAMINE MALEATE
CHLORPHENIRAMINE MALEATE, CHLORPHENIRAMINE MALEATE
DIPHENHYDRAMINE HCL, DIPHENHYDRAMINE HYDROCHLORIDE
TRILITRON, PSEUDOEPHEDRINE HYDROCHLORIDE

NMC
* NMC LABORATORIES INC
BETAMETHASONE DIPROPIONATE, BETAMETHASONE DIPROPIONATE
BETAMETHASONE VALERATE, BETAMETHASONE VALERATE
CLOBETASOL PROPIONATE, CLOBETASOL PROPIONATE
CLOTRIMAZOLE, CLOTRIMAZOLE
FLUOCET, FLUOCINOLONE ACETONIDE
FLUOCINOLONE ACETONIDE, FLUOCINOLONE ACETONIDE
FLUOCINONIDE, FLUOCINONIDE
GENTAMICIN SULFATE, GENTAMICIN SULFATE
HYDROCORTISONE, HYDROCORTISONE
MYKACET, NYSTATIN
MYKINAC, NYSTATIN
TRIAMCINOLONE ACETONIDE, TRIAMCINOLONE ACETONIDE
TRIPLE SULFA, TRIPLE SULFA (SULFABENZAMIDE;SULFACETAMIDE;SULFATHIAZOLE)
VALNAC, BETAMETHASONE VALERATE

NORBROOK
* NORBROOK LABORATORIES LTD
METHOTREXATE SODIUM, METHOTREXATE SODIUM
METOCLOPRAMIDE HCL, METOCLOPRAMIDE HYDROCHLORIDE

NORTON HN
* HN NORTON AND CO
ALLAY, ACETAMINOPHEN
HYDROCODONE BITARTRATE AND ACETAMINOPHEN, ACETAMINOPHEN
IBUPROFEN, IBUPROFEN
IBUPROFEN, IBUPROFEN (OTC)

NOVO NORDISK
* NOVO NORDISK PHARMACEUTICAL INC
INSULATARD NPH HUMAN, INSULIN SUSP ISOPHANE SEMISYNTHETIC PURIFIED HUMAN (OTC)
INSULIN, INSULIN PORK (OTC)
INSULIN INSULATARD NPH NORDISK, INSULIN SUSP ISOPHANE PURIFIED PORK (OTC)
INSULIN NORDISK MIXTARD (PORK), INSULIN PURIFIED PORK (OTC)
LENTARD, INSULIN ZINC SUSP PURIFIED BEEF/PORK (OTC)
LENTE, INSULIN ZINC SUSP PURIFIED PORK (OTC)
LENTE INSULIN, INSULIN ZINC SUSP BEEF (OTC)
MIXTARD HUMAN 70/30, INSULIN SEMISYNTHETIC PURIFIED HUMAN (OTC)
NOVOLIN L, INSULIN ZINC SUSP BIOSYNTHETIC HUMAN (OTC)
NOVOLIN L, INSULIN ZINC SUSP SEMISYNTHETIC PURIFIED HUMAN (OTC)
NOVOLIN N, INSULIN SUSP ISOPHANE SEMISYNTHETIC PURIFIED HUMAN (OTC)
NOVOLIN N, INSULIN SUSP ISOPHANE BIOSYNTHETIC HUMAN (OTC)
NOVOLIN R, INSULIN BIOSYNTHETIC HUMAN (OTC)
NOVOLIN R, INSULIN SEMISYNTHETIC PURIFIED HUMAN (OTC)
NOVOLIN 70/30, INSULIN BIOSYNTHETIC HUMAN (OTC)
NOVOLIN 70/30, INSULIN SEMISYNTHETIC PURIFIED HUMAN (OTC)
NPH INSULIN, INSULIN SUSP ISOPHANE BEEF (OTC)
NPH PURIFIED PORK ISOPHANE INSULIN, INSULIN SUSP ISOPHANE PURIFIED PORK (OTC)
REGULAR PURIFIED PORK INSULIN, INSULIN PURIFIED PORK (OTC)
SEMILENTE, INSULIN ZINC SUSP PROMPT PURIFIED PORK (OTC)
SEMILENTE INSULIN, INSULIN ZINC SUSP PROMPT BEEF (OTC)
ULTRALENTE, INSULIN ZINC SUSP EXTENDED PURIFIED BEEF (OTC)
ULTRALENTE INSULIN, INSULIN ZINC SUSP EXTENDED BEEF (OTC)
VELOSULIN, INSULIN PURIFIED PORK (OTC)
VELOSULIN HUMAN, INSULIN SEMISYNTHETIC PURIFIED HUMAN (OTC)

NOVOCOL
* NOVOCOL PHARMACEUTICAL INC
ISOCAINE HCL, MEPIVACAINE HYDROCHLORIDE
ISOCAINE HCL W/ LEVONORDEFRIN, LEVONORDEFRIN
OCTOCAINE, EPINEPHRINE

NOVOPHARM
* NOVOPHARM LTD
ALBUTEROL SULFATE, ALBUTEROL SULFATE
ALPRAZOLAM, ALPRAZOLAM
AMOXICILLIN, AMOXICILLIN

APPENDIX B
PRODUCT NAME INDEX
LISTED BY APPLICANT *(continued)*

ATENOLOL, ATENOLOL
CEPHALEXIN, CEPHALEXIN
CIMETIDINE, CIMETIDINE
CLOFIBRATE, CLOFIBRATE
CLOXACILLIN SODIUM, CLOXACILLIN SODIUM
DILTIAZEM HCL, DILTIAZEM HYDROCHLORIDE
INDOMETHACIN, INDOMETHACIN
LOPERAMIDE HCL, LOPERAMIDE HYDROCHLORIDE
METHYLDOPA, METHYLDOPA
METHYLDOPA AND HYDROCHLOROTHIAZIDE, HYDROCHLOROTHIAZIDE
NAPROXEN, NAPROXEN
NAPROXEN SODIUM, NAPROXEN SODIUM
NIFEDIPINE, NIFEDIPINE
PINDOLOL, PINDOLOL
PIROXICAM, PIROXICAM
TIMOLOL MALEATE, TIMOLOL MALEATE
TOLMETIN SODIUM, TOLMETIN SODIUM

NYLOS
* NYLOS TRADING CO INC
BROMPHENIRAMINE MALEATE, BROMPHENIRAMINE MALEATE
METHOCARBAMOL, METHOCARBAMOL
PREDNISONE, PREDNISONE
TRIHEXYPHENIDYL HCL, TRIHEXYPHENIDYL HYDROCHLORIDE
TRIPELENNAMINE HCL, TRIPELENNAMINE HYDROCHLORIDE

O

OCLASSEN
* OCLASSEN PHARMACEUTICALS INC
CONDYLOX, PODOFILOX

OHM
* OHM LABORATORIES INC
CHLORZOXAZONE, CHLORZOXAZONE
IBUPROFEN, IBUPROFEN
IBUPROFEN, IBUPROFEN (OTC)
IBUPROHM, IBUPROFEN
IBUPROHM, IBUPROFEN (OTC)
LOPERAMIDE HCL, LOPERAMIDE HYDROCHLORIDE (OTC)

OHMEDA
* OHMEDA PHARMACEUTICAL PRODUCTS DIV INC
BREVIBLOC, ESMOLOL HYDROCHLORIDE
ENLON, EDROPHONIUM CHLORIDE
ENLON-PLUS, ATROPINE SULFATE
ETHRANE, ENFLURANE
FORANE, ISOFLURANE
SUPRANE, DESFLURANE

ON SITE
* ON SITE THERAPEUTICS INC
ACTISITE, TETRACYCLINE HYDROCHLORIDE

OPTOPICS
* OPTOPICS LABORATORIES CORP
OCUSULF-10, SULFACETAMIDE SODIUM
OCUSULF-30, SULFACETAMIDE SODIUM
OPTOMYCIN, CHLORAMPHENICOL
PARACAINE, PROPARACAINE HYDROCHLORIDE
SULFACEL-15, SULFACETAMIDE SODIUM
TROPICAMIDE, TROPICAMIDE

ORGANICS IL
* ORGANICS LA GRANGE INC
CORTICOTROPIN, CORTICOTROPIN

ORGANON
* ORGANON INC SUB AKZONA INC
ARDUAN, PIPECURONIUM BROMIDE
CALDEROL, CALCIFEDIOL
CORTROPHIN-ZINC, CORTICOTROPIN-ZINC HYDROXIDE
CORTROSYN, COSYNTROPIN
DECA-DURABOLIN, NANDROLONE DECANOATE
DESOGEN, DESOGESTREL
DOCA, DESOXYCORTICOSTERONE ACETATE
DURABOLIN, NANDROLONE PHENPROPIONATE
DURABOLIN-50, NANDROLONE PHENPROPIONATE
FUROSEMIDE, FUROSEMIDE
HEPARIN SODIUM, HEPARIN SODIUM
HEXADROL, DEXAMETHASONE
HEXADROL, DEXAMETHASONE SODIUM PHOSPHATE
LIQUAEMIN LOCK FLUSH, HEPARIN SODIUM
LIQUAEMIN SODIUM, HEPARIN SODIUM
LIQUAEMIN SODIUM PRESERVATIVE FREE, HEPARIN SODIUM
LIQUAMAR, PHENPROCOUMON
LYNORAL, ETHINYL ESTRADIOL
MAXIBOLIN, ETHYLESTRENOL
METHYLPREDNISOLONE, METHYLPREDNISOLONE SODIUM SUCCINATE
NORCURON, VECURONIUM BROMIDE
ORGATRAX, HYDROXYZINE HYDROCHLORIDE
PAVULON, PANCURONIUM BROMIDE
PREGNYL, GONADOTROPIN, CHORIONIC
PURIFIED CORTROPHIN GEL, CORTICOTROPIN
REGONOL, PYRIDOSTIGMINE BROMIDE
REVERSOL, EDROPHONIUM CHLORIDE
SUCCINYLCHOLINE CHLORIDE, SUCCINYLCHOLINE CHLORIDE
WIGRAINE, CAFFEINE
WIGRETTES, ERGOTAMINE TARTRATE
ZEMURON, ROCURONIUM BROMIDE
ZEMURON (P/F), ROCURONIUM BROMIDE

OTSUKA
* OTSUKA AMERICA PHARMACEUTICAL INC
OPTIPRESS, CARTEOLOL HYDROCHLORIDE

P

PACO
* PACO PHARMACEUTICAL SERVICES INC
LACTULOSE, LACTULOSE
* PACO RESEARCH CORP
GENTAMICIN SULFATE, GENTAMICIN SULFATE
LIDOCAINE HCL, LIDOCAINE HYDROCHLORIDE
METAPROTERENOL SULFATE, METAPROTERENOL SULFATE
METOCLOPRAMIDE HCL, METOCLOPRAMIDE HYDROCHLORIDE
THIOTHIXENE HCL, THIOTHIXENE HYDROCHLORIDE

PADDOCK
* PADDOCK LABORATORIES INC
BACITRACIN, BACITRACIN
CLINDA-DERM, CLINDAMYCIN PHOSPHATE
ERYTHRA-DERM, ERYTHROMYCIN

APPENDIX B
PRODUCT NAME INDEX
LISTED BY APPLICANT *(continued)*

ERYTHROMYCIN, ERYTHROMYCIN
HYDROCORTISONE, HYDROCORTISONE
NEOMYCIN SULFATE, NEOMYCIN SULFATE
NYSTATIN, NYSTATIN
POLYMIXIN B SULFATE, POLYMYXIN B SULFATE

PAL PAK
* PAL PAK INC
AMINOPHYLLINE, AMINOPHYLLINE

PANRAY
* PANRAY CORP SUB ORMONT DRUG AND CHEMICAL CO INC
AMINOPHYLLINE, AMINOPHYLLINE
CHLORPHENIRAMINE MALEATE, CHLORPHENIRAMINE MALEATE
CINNASIL, RESCINNAMINE
CORTISONE ACETATE, CORTISONE ACETATE
HYDROCORTISONE, HYDROCORTISONE
ISONIAZID, ISONIAZID
KOGLUCOID, RAUWOLFIA SERPENTINA
PARASAL, AMINOSALICYLIC ACID
PARASAL SODIUM, AMINOSALICYLATE SODIUM
PREDNISOLONE, PREDNISOLONE
PREDNISONE, PREDNISONE
PROCAPAN, PROCAINAMIDE HYDROCHLORIDE
SERPANRAY, RESERPINE
THEOLIXIR, THEOPHYLLINE

PAR PHARM
* PAR PHARMACEUTICAL INC
ALLOPURINOL, ALLOPURINOL
AMILORIDE HCL, AMILORIDE HYDROCHLORIDE
AMITRIPTYLINE HCL, AMITRIPTYLINE HYDROCHLORIDE
BENZTROPINE MESYLATE, BENZTROPINE MESYLATE
BROMPHENIRAMINE MALEATE, BROMPHENIRAMINE MALEATE
CARISOPRODOL AND ASPIRIN, ASPIRIN
CHLORDIAZEPOXIDE AND AMITRIPTYLINE HCL, AMITRIPTYLINE HYDROCHLORIDE
CHLORPROPAMIDE, CHLORPROPAMIDE
CHLORZOXAZONE, CHLORZOXAZONE
CLONIDINE HCL, CLONIDINE HYDROCHLORIDE
CLONIDINE HCL AND CHLORTHALIDONE, CHLORTHALIDONE
CYPROHEPTADINE HCL, CYPROHEPTADINE HYDROCHLORIDE
DEXAMETHASONE, DEXAMETHASONE
DIAZEPAM, DIAZEPAM
DISULFIRAM, DISULFIRAM
DOXEPIN HCL, DOXEPIN HYDROCHLORIDE
DOXY-SLEEP-AID, DOXYLAMINE SUCCINATE (OTC)
DOXYCYCLINE HYCLATE, DOXYCYCLINE HYCLATE
FENOPROFEN CALCIUM, FENOPROFEN CALCIUM
FLUPHENAZINE HCL, FLUPHENAZINE HYDROCHLORIDE
FLURAZEPAM HCL, FLURAZEPAM HYDROCHLORIDE
HALOPERIDOL, HALOPERIDOL
HYDRA-ZIDE, HYDRALAZINE HYDROCHLORIDE
HYDRALAZINE HCL, HYDRALAZINE HYDROCHLORIDE
HYDRO-RIDE, AMILORIDE HYDROCHLORIDE
HYDROFLUMETHIAZIDE, HYDROFLUMETHIAZIDE
HYDROXYZINE HCL, HYDROXYZINE HYDROCHLORIDE
HYDROXYZINE PAMOATE, HYDROXYZINE PAMOATE
IBUPROFEN, IBUPROFEN
IBUPROFEN, IBUPROFEN (OTC)
IMIPRAMINE HCL, IMIPRAMINE HYDROCHLORIDE
INDOMETHACIN, INDOMETHACIN
ISOSORBIDE DINITRATE, ISOSORBIDE DINITRATE
LEUCOVORIN CALCIUM, LEUCOVORIN CALCIUM
LORAZEPAM, LORAZEPAM
MECLIZINE HCL, MECLIZINE HYDROCHLORIDE
MECLOFENAMATE SODIUM, MECLOFENAMATE SODIUM
MEGESTROL ACETATE, MEGESTROL ACETATE
MEPROBAMATE AND ASPIRIN, ASPIRIN
METAPROTERENOL SULFATE, METAPROTERENOL SULFATE
METHOCARBAMOL, METHOCARBAMOL
METHOCARBAMOL AND ASPIRIN, ASPIRIN
METHYCLOTHIAZIDE, METHYCLOTHIAZIDE
METHYLDOPA, METHYLDOPA
METHYLDOPA AND CHLOROTHIAZIDE, CHLOROTHIAZIDE
METHYLDOPA AND HYDROCHLOROTHIAZIDE, HYDROCHLOROTHIAZIDE
METHYLPREDNISOLONE, METHYLPREDNISOLONE
METOCLOPRAMIDE HCL, METOCLOPRAMIDE HYDROCHLORIDE
METRONIDAZOLE, METRONIDAZOLE
MINOXIDIL, MINOXIDIL
NYSTATIN, NYSTATIN
ORPHENGESIC, ASPIRIN
ORPHENGESIC FORTE, ASPIRIN
PERPHENAZINE AND AMITRIPTYLINE HCL, AMITRIPTYLINE HYDROCHLORIDE
PROPANTHELINE BROMIDE, PROPANTHELINE BROMIDE
PROPRANOLOL HCL, PROPRANOLOL HYDROCHLORIDE
RESERPINE AND HYDROFLUMETHIAZIDE, HYDROFLUMETHIAZIDE
SULFAMETHOPRIM, SULFAMETHOXAZOLE
SULFAMETHOPRIM-DS, SULFAMETHOXAZOLE
SULFINPYRAZONE, SULFINPYRAZONE
TEMAZEPAM, TEMAZEPAM
THIORIDAZINE HCL, THIORIDAZINE HYDROCHLORIDE
TOLAZAMIDE, TOLAZAMIDE
TRIAMTERENE AND HYDROCHLOROTHIAZIDE, HYDROCHLOROTHIAZIDE
TRICHLORMETHIAZIDE, TRICHLORMETHIAZIDE
VALPROIC ACID, VALPROIC ACID

PARKE DAVIS
* PARKE DAVIS DIV WARNER LAMBERT CO
ACTH, CORTICOTROPIN
AMBODRYL, BROMODIPHENHYDRAMINE HYDROCHLORIDE
AMCILL, AMPICILLIN/AMPICILLIN TRIHYDRATE
ANUSOL HC, HYDROCORTISONE
BENADRYL, DIPHENHYDRAMINE HYDROCHLORIDE
BENYLIN, DIPHENHYDRAMINE HYDROCHLORIDE (OTC)
CAMOQUIN HCL, AMODIAQUINE HYDROCHLORIDE
CELONTIN, METHSUXIMIDE
CENTRAX, PRAZEPAM
CHLORDIAZEPOXIDE HCL, CHLORDIAZEPOXIDE HYDROCHLORIDE
CHLOROMYCETIN, CHLORAMPHENICOL
CHOLEDYL, OXTRIPHYLLINE
CHOLEDYL SA, OXTRIPHYLLINE

APPENDIX B
PRODUCT NAME INDEX
LISTED BY APPLICANT *(continued)*

CHOLYBAR, CHOLESTYRAMINE
COLY-MYCIN S, COLISTIN SULFATE
DILANTIN, PHENYTOIN
DILANTIN, PHENYTOIN SODIUM
DILANTIN, PHENYTOIN SODIUM, EXTENDED
DILANTIN-125, PHENYTOIN
DILANTIN-30, PHENYTOIN
DIPHENOXYLATE HCL AND ATROPINE SULFATE, ATROPINE SULFATE
DORYX, DOXYCYCLINE HYCLATE
ERGOSTAT, ERGOTAMINE TARTRATE
ERYC, ERYTHROMYCIN
ERYC 125, ERYTHROMYCIN
ERYPAR, ERYTHROMYCIN STEARATE
ERYTHROMYCIN ETHYLSUCCINATE, ERYTHROMYCIN ETHYLSUCCINATE
ESTROVIS, QUINESTROL
EUTHROID-0.5, LIOTRIX (T4;T3)
EUTHROID-1, LIOTRIX (T4;T3)
EUTHROID-2, LIOTRIX (T4;T3)
EUTHROID-3, LIOTRIX (T4;T3)
HEPARIN LOCK FLUSH, HEPARIN SODIUM
HEPARIN SODIUM, HEPARIN SODIUM
HUMATIN, PAROMOMYCIN SULFATE
HYDROCORTISONE, HYDROCORTISONE
HYDROCORTISONE ACETATE, HYDROCORTISONE ACETATE
INDOMETHACIN, INDOMETHACIN
ISOPROTERENOL HCL, ISOPROTERENOL HYDROCHLORIDE
KETALAR, KETAMINE HYDROCHLORIDE
LOESTRIN FE 1.5/30, ETHINYL ESTRADIOL
LOESTRIN FE 1/20, ETHINYL ESTRADIOL
LOESTRIN 21 1/20, ETHINYL ESTRADIOL
LOPID, GEMFIBROZIL
MECLOMEN, MECLOFENAMATE SODIUM
MEPERIDINE HCL, MEPERIDINE HYDROCHLORIDE
MEPROBAMATE, MEPROBAMATE
METHYLDOPA, METHYLDOPA
METHYLDOPA AND HYDROCHLOROTHIAZIDE, HYDROCHLOROTHIAZIDE
METHYLTESTOSTERONE, METHYLTESTOSTERONE
MILONTIN, PHENSUXIMIDE
NARDIL, PHENELZINE SULFATE
NITROSTAT, NITROGLYCERIN
NORLUTATE, NORETHINDRONE ACETATE
NORLUTIN, NORETHINDRONE
OXAZEPAM, OXAZEPAM
PARACORT, PREDNISONE
PARSIDOL, ETHOPROPAZINE HYDROCHLORIDE
PENAPAR-VK, PENICILLIN V POTASSIUM
PENICILLIN G POTASSIUM, PENICILLIN G POTASSIUM
PENICILLIN G PROCAINE, PENICILLIN G PROCAINE
PITOCIN, OXYTOCIN
PITRESSIN TANNATE, VASOPRESSIN TANNATE
PONSTEL, MEFENAMIC ACID
POVAN, PYRVINIUM PAMOATE
PRE-SATE, CHLORPHENTERMINE HYDROCHLORIDE
PROCAN, PROCAINAMIDE HYDROCHLORIDE
PROCAN SR, PROCAINAMIDE HYDROCHLORIDE
PROLOID, THYROGLOBULIN
PROMAPAR, CHLORPROMAZINE HYDROCHLORIDE
PROPRANOLOL HCL, PROPRANOLOL HYDROCHLORIDE
SECOBARBITAL SODIUM, SECOBARBITAL SODIUM
SODIUM PENTOBARBITAL, PENTOBARBITAL SODIUM
SPIRONOLACTONE W/ HYDROCHLOROTHIAZIDE, HYDROCHLOROTHIAZIDE
SULFALAR, SULFISOXAZOLE
SURITAL, THIAMYLAL SODIUM
SYTOBEX, CYANOCOBALAMIN
THEELIN, ESTRONE
THIAMINE HCL, THIAMINE HYDROCHLORIDE
TOLBUTAMIDE, TOLBUTAMIDE
TRIPELENNAMINE HCL, TRIPELENNAMINE HYDROCHLORIDE
UTICORT, BETAMETHASONE BENZOATE
UTIMOX, AMOXICILLIN
VIRA-A, VIDARABINE
ZARONTIN, ETHOSUXIMIDE

* PARKE DAVIS LABORATORIES DIV WARNER LAMBERT CO
NORLESTRIN FE 1/50, ETHINYL ESTRADIOL
NORLESTRIN FE 2.5/50, ETHINYL ESTRADIOL
NORLESTRIN 21 1/50, ETHINYL ESTRADIOL
NORLESTRIN 21 2.5/50, ETHINYL ESTRADIOL
NORLESTRIN 28 1/50, ETHINYL ESTRADIOL

* PARKE DAVIS PHARMACEUTICAL RESEARCH DIV WARNER LAMBERT CO
ACCUPRIL, QUINAPRIL HYDROCHLORIDE
CHLOROMYCETIN, CHLORAMPHENICOL
CHLOROMYCETIN, CHLORAMPHENICOL SODIUM SUCCINATE
CHLOROMYCETIN HYDROCORTISONE, CHLORAMPHENICOL
CHLOROMYCETIN PALMITATE, CHLORAMPHENICOL PALMITATE
CHLOROMYXIN, CHLORAMPHENICOL
COGNEX, TACRINE HYDROCHLORIDE
COLY-MYCIN M, COLISTIMETHATE SODIUM
ELASE-CHLOROMYCETIN, CHLORAMPHENICOL
ISOETHARINE HCL, ISOETHARINE HYDROCHLORIDE
LOESTRIN 21 1.5/30, ETHINYL ESTRADIOL
NEURONTIN, GABAPENTIN
NIPENT, PENTOSTATIN
OPHTHOCHLOR, CHLORAMPHENICOL
OPHTHOCORT, CHLORAMPHENICOL
UTICORT, BETAMETHASONE BENZOATE

PARNELL
* PARNELL PHARMACEUTICALS INC
TRIAMCINOLONE ACETONIDE, TRIAMCINOLONE ACETONIDE

PENNEX
* PENNEX PHARMACEUTICALS INC
ACETAMINOPHEN AND CODEINE PHOSPHATE, ACETAMINOPHEN
AMINOPHYLLINE, AMINOPHYLLINE
BIPHETAP, BROMPHENIRAMINE MALEATE
BUTABARBITAL SODIUM, BUTABARBITAL SODIUM
CHLORPROMAZINE HCL, CHLORPROMAZINE HYDROCHLORIDE
CYPROHEPTADINE HCL, CYPROHEPTADINE HYDROCHLORIDE
DIPHEN, DIPHENHYDRAMINE HYDROCHLORIDE (OTC)
DOXEPIN HCL, DOXEPIN HYDROCHLORIDE
ERYTHROMYCIN, ERYTHROMYCIN
FLUOCINOLONE ACETONIDE, FLUOCINOLONE ACETONIDE
FUROSEMIDE, FUROSEMIDE
GENERLAC, LACTULOSE

APPENDIX B
PRODUCT NAME INDEX
LISTED BY APPLICANT *(continued)*

HALOPERIDOL, HALOPERIDOL LACTATE
HYDROCHLOROTHIAZIDE, HYDROCHLOROTHIAZIDE
HYDROXYZINE HCL, HYDROXYZINE HYDROCHLORIDE
LACTULOSE, LACTULOSE
LINDANE, LINDANE
LITHIUM CITRATE, LITHIUM CITRATE
METAPROTERENOL SULFATE, METAPROTERENOL SULFATE
METOCLOPRAMIDE HCL, METOCLOPRAMIDE HYDROCHLORIDE
MYBANIL, BROMODIPHENHYDRAMINE HYDROCHLORIDE
MYCODONE, HOMATROPINE METHYLBROMIDE
MYLARAMINE, DEXCHLORPHENIRAMINE MALEATE
MYLOCAINE, LIDOCAINE HYDROCHLORIDE
MYMETHASONE, DEXAMETHASONE
MYPHETANE DC, BROMPHENIRAMINE MALEATE
MYPHETANE DX, BROMPHENIRAMINE MALEATE
MYPROIC ACID, VALPROIC ACID
NYSTATIN, NYSTATIN
OXTRIPHYLLINE, OXTRIPHYLLINE
OXTRIPHYLLINE PEDIATRIC, OXTRIPHYLLINE
PREDNISONE, PREDNISONE
PROCHLORPERAZINE EDISYLATE, PROCHLORPERAZINE EDISYLATE
PROMETHAZINE PLAIN, PROMETHAZINE HYDROCHLORIDE
PROMETHAZINE VC PLAIN, PHENYLEPHRINE HYDROCHLORIDE
PROMETHAZINE VC W/ CODEINE, CODEINE PHOSPHATE
PROMETHAZINE W/ CODEINE, CODEINE PHOSPHATE
PROMETHAZINE W/ DEXTROMETHORPHAN, DEXTROMETHORPHAN HYDROBROMIDE
PROPRANOLOL HCL, PROPRANOLOL HYDROCHLORIDE
SELENIUM SULFIDE, SELENIUM SULFIDE
SODIUM POLYSTYRENE SULFONATE, SODIUM POLYSTYRENE SULFONATE
THEOPHYLLINE, THEOPHYLLINE
THIORIDAZINE HCL, THIORIDAZINE HYDROCHLORIDE
TRIAMCINOLONE ACETONIDE, TRIAMCINOLONE ACETONIDE
TRIFLUOPERAZINE HCL, TRIFLUOPERAZINE HYDROCHLORIDE
TRIMEPRAZINE TARTRATE, TRIMEPRAZINE TARTRATE
TRIPROLIDINE HCL, PSEUDOEPHEDRINE HCL AND CODEINE PHOSPHATE, CODEINE PHOSPHATE

* PENNEX PRODUCTS CO INC
ALUMINUM HYDROXIDE AND MAGNESIUM TRISILICATE, ALUMINUM HYDROXIDE (OTC)

PERRIGO

* L PERRIGO CO
ANTITUSSIVE, DIPHENHYDRAMINE HYDROCHLORIDE (OTC)
CAP-PROFEN, IBUPROFEN (OTC)
DIPHENHYDRAMINE HCL, DIPHENHYDRAMINE HYDROCHLORIDE
IBUPROFEN, IBUPROFEN (OTC)
ISONIAZID, ISONIAZID
LOPERAMIDE HCL, LOPERAMIDE HYDROCHLORIDE (OTC)
MEPROBAMATE, MEPROBAMATE
PREDNISOLONE, PREDNISOLONE
PREDNISONE, PREDNISONE
PROPYLTHIOURACIL, PROPYLTHIOURACIL
QUINIDINE SULFATE, QUINIDINE SULFATE
SODIUM PENTOBARBITAL, PENTOBARBITAL SODIUM
SODIUM SECOBARBITAL, SECOBARBITAL SODIUM
TAB-PROFEN, IBUPROFEN (OTC)
THEOPHYLLINE, THEOPHYLLINE

PFIPHARMECS

* PFIPHARMECS DIV PFIZER INC
CORTRIL, HYDROCORTISONE
TETRACYN, TETRACYCLINE HYDROCHLORIDE

PFIZER

* PFIZER CENTRAL RESEARCH
DIFLUCAN, FLUCONAZOLE
ZOLOFT, SERTRALINE HYDROCHLORIDE
* PFIZER CHEMICALS DIV PFIZER INC
DIFLUCAN, FLUCONAZOLE
ZITHROMAX, AZITHROMYCIN DIHYDRATE
* PFIZER INC
DIFLUCAN, FLUCONAZOLE
GLUCOTROL, GLIPIZIDE
GLUCOTROL XL, GLIPIZIDE
LITHIUM CARBONATE, LITHIUM CARBONATE
MINIPRESS XL, PRAZOSIN HYDROCHLORIDE
NORVASC, AMLODIPINE BESYLATE
* PFIZER LABORATORIES DIV PFIZER INC
BACITRACIN, BACITRACIN
CARDURA, DOXAZOSIN MESYLATE
CEFOBID, CEFOPERAZONE SODIUM
CORTRIL, HYDROCORTISONE
CORTRIL, HYDROCORTISONE ACETATE
DARICON, OXYPHENCYCLIMINE HYDROCHLORIDE
DIABINESE, CHLORPROPAMIDE
FELDENE, PIROXICAM
FOVANE, BENZTHIAZIDE
GEOCILLIN, CARBENICILLIN INDANYL SODIUM
MAGNACORT, HYDROCORTAMATE HYDROCHLORIDE
MINIPRESS, PRAZOSIN HYDROCHLORIDE
MINIZIDE, POLYTHIAZIDE
MODERIL, RESCINNAMINE
NEOBIOTIC, NEOMYCIN SULFATE
NEOMYCIN SULFATE, NEOMYCIN SULFATE
PENICILLIN G POTASSIUM, PENICILLIN G POTASSIUM
PENICILLIN G PROCAINE, PENICILLIN G PROCAINE
PERMAPEN, PENICILLIN G BENZATHINE
PFIZER-E, ERYTHROMYCIN STEARATE
PFIZERPEN, PENICILLIN G POTASSIUM
PFIZERPEN G, PENICILLIN G POTASSIUM
PFIZERPEN VK, PENICILLIN V POTASSIUM
PFIZERPEN-A, AMPICILLIN/AMPICILLIN TRIHYDRATE
PFIZERPEN-AS, PENICILLIN G PROCAINE
POLYMIXIN B SULFATE, POLYMYXIN B SULFATE
PROCARDIA, NIFEDIPINE
PROCARDIA XL, NIFEDIPINE
RENESE, POLYTHIAZIDE
RENESE-R, POLYTHIAZIDE
SINEQUAN, DOXEPIN HYDROCHLORIDE
SPECTROBID, BACAMPICILLIN HYDROCHLORIDE
STERANE, PREDNISOLONE
STERANE, PREDNISOLONE ACETATE
STREPTOMYCIN SULFATE, STREPTOMYCIN SULFATE
TAO, TROLEANDOMYCIN

APPENDIX B
PRODUCT NAME INDEX
LISTED BY APPLICANT *(continued)*

TERRA-CORTRIL, HYDROCORTISONE ACETATE
TERRAMYCIN, LIDOCAINE HYDROCHLORIDE
TERRAMYCIN, OXYTETRACYCLINE
TERRAMYCIN, OXYTETRACYCLINE CALCIUM
TERRAMYCIN, OXYTETRACYCLINE HYDROCHLORIDE
TERRAMYCIN W/ POLYMYXIN, OXYTETRACYCLINE HYDROCHLORIDE
TERRAMYCIN W/ POLYMYXIN B SULFATE, OXYTETRACYCLINE HYDROCHLORIDE
TERRAMYCIN-POLYMYXIN, OXYTETRACYCLINE HYDROCHLORIDE
TETRACYN, PROCAINE HYDROCHLORIDE
TETRACYN, TETRACYCLINE HYDROCHLORIDE
TZ-3, TIOCONAZOLE (OTC)
UNASYN, AMPICILLIN SODIUM
UNISOM, DOXYLAMINE SUCCINATE (OTC)
URESE, BENZTHIAZIDE
VANSIL, OXAMNIQUINE
VIBRA-TABS, DOXYCYCLINE HYCLATE
VIBRAMYCIN, DOXYCYCLINE
VIBRAMYCIN, DOXYCYCLINE CALCIUM
VIBRAMYCIN, DOXYCYCLINE HYCLATE
VIOCIN SULFATE, VIOMYCIN SULFATE
VISINE L.R., OXYMETAZOLINE HYDROCHLORIDE (OTC)
VISTARIL, HYDROXYZINE HYDROCHLORIDE
VISTARIL, HYDROXYZINE PAMOATE

PHARM ASSOC
* PHARMACEUTICAL ASSOC INC DIV BEACH PRODUCTS
ACETAMINOPHEN AND CODEINE PHOSPHATE, ACETAMINOPHEN
BROMPHENIRAMINE MALEATE, BROMPHENIRAMINE MALEATE
CHLORPHENIRAMINE MALEATE, CHLORPHENIRAMINE MALEATE
DIPHENHYDRAMINE HCL, DIPHENHYDRAMINE HYDROCHLORIDE
H-CORT, HYDROCORTISONE
HALOPERIDOL, HALOPERIDOL LACTATE
METOCLOPRAMIDE HCL, METOCLOPRAMIDE HYDROCHLORIDE
PROMETHAZINE HCL, PROMETHAZINE HYDROCHLORIDE
PROMETHAZINE HCL AND CODEINE PHOSPHATE, CODEINE PHOSPHATE
THEOPHYLLINE, THEOPHYLLINE
TRIPROLIDINE HCL, TRIPROLIDINE HYDROCHLORIDE

PHARM SPECLTS ASSOC
* PHARMACEUTICAL SPECIALIST ASSOC
GENTAMICIN SULFATE, GENTAMICIN SULFATE
HEPARIN SODIUM, HEPARIN SODIUM

PHARMA SERVE NY
* PHARMA SERVE INC SUB TORIGIAN LABORATORIES
AMINOPHYLLINE, AMINOPHYLLINE
HEPARIN SODIUM, HEPARIN SODIUM
POTASSIUM CHLORIDE, POTASSIUM CHLORIDE

PHARMA TEK
* PHARMA TEK INC
AMPHOTERICIN B, AMPHOTERICIN B
BACI-RX, BACITRACIN
HYDROCORTISONE, HYDROCORTISONE
HYDROCORTISONE ACETATE, HYDROCORTISONE ACETATE
NEO-RX, NEOMYCIN SULFATE
POLY-RX, POLYMYXIN B SULFATE
ZIBA-RX, BACITRACIN ZINC

PHARMACHEMIE (NL)
* PHARMACHEMIE BV
DOXORUBICIN HCL, DOXORUBICIN HYDROCHLORIDE

PHARMACHEMIE (US)
* PHARMACHEMIE USA INC
METHOTREXATE SODIUM, METHOTREXATE SODIUM

PHARMACIA
* PHARMACIA INC
ADRIAMYCIN PFS, DOXORUBICIN HYDROCHLORIDE
ADRIAMYCIN RDF, DOXORUBICIN HYDROCHLORIDE
ADRUCIL, FLUOROURACIL
AMINESS 5.2% ESSENTIAL AMINO ACIDS W/ HISTADINE, AMINO ACIDS
AZULFIDINE, SULFASALAZINE
AZULFIDINE EN-TABS, SULFASALAZINE
CALMURID HC, HYDROCORTISONE
CYKLOKAPRON, TRANEXAMIC ACID
CYSTEINE HCL, CYSTEINE HYDROCHLORIDE
DIPENTUM, OLSALAZINE SODIUM
DIZAC, DIAZEPAM
EMCYT, ESTRAMUSTINE PHOSPHATE SODIUM
FLUIDIL, CYCLOTHIAZIDE
FOLEX, METHOTREXATE SODIUM
FOLEX PFS, METHOTREXATE SODIUM
IDAMYCIN, IDARUBICIN HYDROCHLORIDE
INTRALIPID 10%, SOYBEAN OIL
INTRALIPID 20%, SOYBEAN OIL
INTRALIPID 30%, SOYBEAN OIL
KABIVITE PED F + W KIT, ASCORBIC ACID
MYCOBUTIN, RIFABUTIN
NEOPHAM 6.4%, AMINO ACIDS
NEOSAR, CYCLOPHOSPHAMIDE
NICOTROL, NICOTINE
NOVAMINE 11.4%, AMINO ACIDS
NOVAMINE 15%, AMINO ACIDS
NOVAMINE 8.5%, AMINO ACIDS
R-GENE 10, ARGININE HYDROCHLORIDE
TYMTRAN, CERULETIDE DIETHYLAMINE
VANCOR, VANCOMYCIN HYDROCHLORIDE
VEINAMINE 8%, AMINO ACIDS
VINCASAR PFS, VINCRISTINE SULFATE

PHARMADERM
* PHARMADERM DIV ALTANA INC
BACITRACIN, BACITRACIN
BACITRACIN-NEOMYCIN-POLYMYXIN, BACITRACIN ZINC
BACITRACIN-NEOMYCIN-POLYMYXIN W/ HYDROCORTISONE ACETATE, BACITRACIN
BETAMETHASONE DIPROPIONATE, BETAMETHASONE DIPROPIONATE
BETAMETHASONE VALERATE, BETAMETHASONE VALERATE
ERYTHROMYCIN, ERYTHROMYCIN
FLUOCINOLONE ACETONIDE, FLUOCINOLONE ACETONIDE
GENTAMICIN SULFATE, GENTAMICIN SULFATE
HYDROCORTISONE, HYDROCORTISONE
NEOMYCIN SULFATE-TRIAMCINOLONE ACETONIDE, NEOMYCIN SULFATE
NYSTATIN, NYSTATIN

APPENDIX B
PRODUCT NAME INDEX
LISTED BY APPLICANT *(continued)*

NYSTATIN-TRIAMCINOLONE ACETONIDE, NYSTATIN
TRIAMCINOLONE ACETONIDE, TRIAMCINOLONE ACETONIDE
TRIPLE SULFA, TRIPLE SULFA (SULFABENZAMIDE;SULFACETAMIDE;SULFATHIAZOLE)

PHARMAFAIR
* PHARMAFAIR INC
BACITRACIN, BACITRACIN
BACITRACIN ZINC-NEOMYCIN SULFATE-POLYMYXIN B SULFATE, BACITRACIN ZINC
BETAMETHASONE VALERATE, BETAMETHASONE VALERATE
BOROFAIR, ACETIC ACID, GLACIAL
CARBACHOL, CARBACHOL
CHLOROFAIR, CHLORAMPHENICOL
DEXAIR, DEXAMETHASONE SODIUM PHOSPHATE
DEXASPORIN, DEXAMETHASONE
ERYTHROMYCIN, ERYTHROMYCIN
ERYTHROMYCIN ETHYLSUCCINATE, ERYTHROMYCIN ETHYLSUCCINATE
FLUOCINOLONE ACETONIDE, FLUOCINOLONE ACETONIDE
GENTAFAIR, GENTAMICIN SULFATE
HYDROCORTISONE, HYDROCORTISONE
HYDROXYZINE HCL, HYDROXYZINE HYDROCHLORIDE
KAINAIR, PROPARACAINE HYDROCHLORIDE
KANAMYCIN SULFATE, KANAMYCIN SULFATE
MYDRIAFAIR, TROPICAMIDE
NAFAZAIR, NAPHAZOLINE HYDROCHLORIDE
NEOMYCIN & POLYMYXIN B SULFATES & BACITRACIN ZINC & HYDROCORTISONE, BACITRACIN ZINC
NEOMYCIN SULFATE AND POLYMYXIN B SULFATE GRAMICIDIN, GRAMICIDIN
NEOMYCIN SULFATE-DEXAMETHASONE SODIUM PHOSPHATE, DEXAMETHASONE SODIUM PHOSPHATE
NEOMYCIN SULFATE-POLYMYXIN B SULFATE-HYDROCORTISONE, HYDROCORTISONE
NEOMYCIN SULFATE, POLYMYXIN B SULFATE & HYDROCORTISONE, HYDROCORTISONE
NYSTATIN, NYSTATIN
NYSTATIN AND TRIAMCINOLONE ACETONIDE, NYSTATIN
OCUMYCIN, BACITRACIN ZINC
OTICAIR, HYDROCORTISONE
PENTOLAIR, CYCLOPENTOLATE HYDROCHLORIDE
PREDAIR, PREDNISOLONE SODIUM PHOSPHATE
PREDAIR FORTE, PREDNISOLONE SODIUM PHOSPHATE
PREDSULFAIR, PREDNISOLONE ACETATE
PREDSULFAIR II, PREDNISOLONE ACETATE
PROCAINAMIDE HCL, PROCAINAMIDE HYDROCHLORIDE
SULFACETAMIDE SODIUM, SULFACETAMIDE SODIUM
SULFAIR FORTE, SULFACETAMIDE SODIUM
SULFAIR 10, SULFACETAMIDE SODIUM
SULFAIR-15, SULFACETAMIDE SODIUM
TRIAMCINOLONE ACETONIDE, TRIAMCINOLONE ACETONIDE
ZINC BACITRACIN,NEOMYCIN SULFATE,POLYMYXIN B SULFATE & HYDROCORTISONE, BACITRACIN ZINC

PHARMATON
* PHARMATON LTD
LIDOCATON, EPINEPHRINE
LIDOCATON, LIDOCAINE HYDROCHLORIDE

PHARMAVITE
* PHARMAVITE PHARMACEUTICALS
CHLORPHENIRAMINE MALEATE, CHLORPHENIRAMINE MALEATE
ISONIAZID, ISONIAZID
MEPROBAMATE, MEPROBAMATE
PREDNISONE, PREDNISONE
QUINIDINE SULFATE, QUINIDINE SULFATE
RESERPINE, RESERPINE

PHARMERAL
* PHARMERAL INC
ACETAMINOPHEN AND CODEINE PHOSPHATE, ACETAMINOPHEN
BUTALBITAL W/ ASPIRIN & CAFFEINE, ASPIRIN
CHLORPHENIRAMINE MALEATE, CHLORPHENIRAMINE MALEATE
DIPHENOXYLATE HCL AND ATROPINE SULFATE, ATROPINE SULFATE
FOLIC ACID, FOLIC ACID
HYDROCHLOROTHIAZIDE, HYDROCHLOROTHIAZIDE
HYDROCHLOROTHIAZIDE W/ RESERPINE, HYDROCHLOROTHIAZIDE
MEPROBAMATE, MEPROBAMATE
METHOCARBAMOL, METHOCARBAMOL
PHENYTOIN SODIUM, PHENYTOIN SODIUM, PROMPT
SULFISOXAZOLE, SULFISOXAZOLE

PHARMICS
* PHARMICS INC
PAREDRINE, HYDROXYAMPHETAMINE HYDROBROMIDE

PHOENIX LABS NY
* PHOENIX LABORATORIES INC
AMINOPHYLLINE, AMINOPHYLLINE
BROMPHENIRAMINE MALEATE, BROMPHENIRAMINE MALEATE
CHLORPHENIRAMINE MALEATE, CHLORPHENIRAMINE MALEATE
DEXAMETHASONE, DEXAMETHASONE
ISONIAZID, ISONIAZID
PREDNISOLONE, PREDNISOLONE
PREDNISONE, PREDNISONE
QUINIDINE SULFATE, QUINIDINE SULFATE

PHYS PRODS VA
* PHYSICIANS PRODUCTS CO INC DIV INTERNATIONAL LATEX CORP
HYSERPIN, RAUWOLFIA SERPENTINA

PIONEER PHARMS
* PIONEER PHARMACEUTICALS INC
BROMPHENIRAMINE MALEATE, BROMPHENIRAMINE MALEATE
CARISOPRODOL, CARISOPRODOL
CHLORDIAZEPOXIDE HCL, CHLORDIAZEPOXIDE HYDROCHLORIDE
CHLORPHENIRAMINE MALEATE, CHLORPHENIRAMINE MALEATE
CHLORTHALIDONE, CHLORTHALIDONE
CHLORZOXAZONE, CHLORZOXAZONE
CYPROHEPTADINE HCL, CYPROHEPTADINE HYDROCHLORIDE

APPENDIX B
PRODUCT NAME INDEX
LISTED BY APPLICANT *(continued)*

DIAZEPAM, DIAZEPAM
DICYCLOMINE HCL, DICYCLOMINE HYDROCHLORIDE
DIPHENHYDRAMINE HCL, DIPHENHYDRAMINE HYDROCHLORIDE
FOLIC ACID, FOLIC ACID
INDOMETHACIN, INDOMETHACIN
METHOCARBAMOL, METHOCARBAMOL
RESPORAL, DEXBROMPHENIRAMINE MALEATE (OTC)

PLANTEX
* PLANTEX USA INC DIV IKAPHARM INC
SULFAMETHOXAZOLE AND TRIMETHOPRIM DOUBLE STRENGTH, SULFAMETHOXAZOLE
SULFAMETHOXAZOLE AND TRIMETHOPRIM SINGLE STRENGTH, SULFAMETHOXAZOLE

PLOUGH
* PLOUGH INC DIV SCHERING PLOUGH INC
SHADE UVAGUARD, AVOBENZONE (OTC)

POLYMEDICA
* POLYMEDICA INDUSTRIES INC
NEOPAP, ACETAMINOPHEN (OTC)
PROMETHACON, PROMETHAZINE HYDROCHLORIDE

POPULATION COUNCIL
* POPULATION COUNCIL
NORPLANT, LEVONORGESTREL
* POPULATION COUNCIL CENTER FOR BIOMEDICAL RESEARCH
COPPER T MODEL TCU 380A, COPPER

POYTHRESS
* WILLIAM P POYTHRESS AND CO INC
BENSULFOID, BENTONITE

PRIVATE FORM
* PRIVATE FORMULATIONS INC
ALLERFED, PSEUDOEPHEDRINE HYDROCHLORIDE
BENZTHIAZIDE, BENZTHIAZIDE
BROMPHENIRAMINE MALEATE, BROMPHENIRAMINE MALEATE
CHLORPHENIRAMINE MALEATE, CHLORPHENIRAMINE MALEATE
CHLORPROMAZINE HCL, CHLORPROMAZINE HYDROCHLORIDE
DEXAMETHASONE, DEXAMETHASONE
DI-METREX, PHENDIMETRAZINE TARTRATE
DIPHENHYDRAMINE HCL, DIPHENHYDRAMINE HYDROCHLORIDE
DIPHENOXYLATE HCL W/ ATROPINE SULFATE, ATROPINE SULFATE
DOXYCYCLINE HYCLATE, DOXYCYCLINE HYCLATE
ESTERIFIED ESTROGENS, ESTROGENS, ESTERIFIED
FEMOGEN, ESTROGENS, ESTERIFIED
FOLIC ACID, FOLIC ACID
HYDROCHLOROTHIAZIDE, HYDROCHLOROTHIAZIDE
IBUPROFEN, IBUPROFEN
IBUPROFEN, IBUPROFEN (OTC)
MEPROBAMATE, MEPROBAMATE
METHSCOPOLAMINE BROMIDE, METHSCOPOLAMINE BROMIDE
METHYLTESTOSTERONE, METHYLTESTOSTERONE
PHENDIMETRAZINE TARTRATE, PHENDIMETRAZINE TARTRATE
PREDNISOLONE, PREDNISOLONE
PREDNISONE, PREDNISONE
PROFEN, IBUPROFEN (OTC)
PROMETHAZINE HCL, PROMETHAZINE HYDROCHLORIDE
PROPANTHELINE BROMIDE, PROPANTHELINE BROMIDE
PROPOXYPHENE HCL, PROPOXYPHENE HYDROCHLORIDE
QUINIDINE SULFATE, QUINIDINE SULFATE
RAUWOLFIA SERPENTINA, RAUWOLFIA SERPENTINA
RESERPINE, RESERPINE
TETRACYCLINE HCL, TETRACYCLINE HYDROCHLORIDE

PROCTER AND GAMBLE
* PROCTER AND GAMBLE CO
HEAD & SHOULDERS CONDITIONER, PYRITHIONE ZINC
PERIDEX, CHLORHEXIDINE GLUCONATE
* PROCTER AND GAMBLE PHARMACEUTICALS INC SUB PROCTER AND GAM
ASACOL, MESALAMINE
DANTRIUM, DANTROLENE SODIUM
DIDRONEL, ETIDRONATE DISODIUM
FURADANTIN, NITROFURANTOIN
IVADANTIN, NITROFURANTOIN SODIUM
LABID, THEOPHYLLINE
MACROBID, NITROFURANTOIN
MACRODANTIN, NITROFURANTOIN, MACROCRYSTALLINE
NYSERT, NYSTATIN
ORLEX, ACETIC ACID, GLACIAL
ORLEX HC, ACETIC ACID, GLACIAL
SARENIN, SARALASIN ACETATE

PROF DISPOSABLES
* PROFESSIONAL DISPOSABLES INC
HEXASCRUB, HEXACHLOROPHENE

PROGRAPHARM
* PROGRAPHARM USA LTD
DILTIAZEM HCL, DILTIAZEM HYDROCHLORIDE

PROTER
* PROTER LABORATORY SPA
OXYTETRACYCLINE HCL, OXYTETRACYCLINE HYDROCHLORIDE

PURDUE FREDERICK
* PURDUE FREDERICK CO
ATHROMBIN, WARFARIN SODIUM
ATHROMBIN-K, WARFARIN POTASSIUM
BETADINE, POVIDONE-IODINE
CARDIOQUIN, QUINIDINE POLYGALACTURONATE
CERUMENEX, TRIETHANOLAMINE POLYPEPTIDE OLEATE CONDENSATE
COMPAL, ACETAMINOPHEN
MS CONTIN, MORPHINE SULFATE
PHENY-PAS-TEBAMIN, PHENYL AMINOSALICYLATE
PHYLLOCONTIN, AMINOPHYLLINE
SULFABID, SULFAPHENAZOLE
T-PHYL, THEOPHYLLINE
UNIPHYL, THEOPHYLLINE

PUREPAC PHARM
* PUREPAC PHARMACEUTICAL CO DIV PUREPAC INC
ACETAMINOPHEN AND CODEINE PHOSPHATE, ACETAMINOPHEN
ACETAMINOPHEN AND CODEINE PHOSPHATE #3, ACETAMINOPHEN

APPENDIX B
PRODUCT NAME INDEX
LISTED BY APPLICANT *(continued)*

ALLOPURINOL, ALLOPURINOL
ALPRAZOLAM, ALPRAZOLAM
AMINOPHYLLINE, AMINOPHYLLINE
AMITRIPTYLINE HCL, AMITRIPTYLINE HYDROCHLORIDE
AMPICILLIN TRIHYDRATE, AMPICILLIN/AMPICILLIN TRIHYDRATE
ASPIRIN AND CAFFEINE W/ BUTALBITAL, ASPIRIN
CARBAMAZEPINE, CARBAMAZEPINE
CARBIDOPA AND LEVODOPA, CARBIDOPA
CEFADROXIL, CEFADROXIL/CEFADROXIL HEMIHYDRATE
CEPHALEXIN, CEPHALEXIN
CHLORDIAZEPOXIDE HCL, CHLORDIAZEPOXIDE HYDROCHLORIDE
CHLOROQUINE PHOSPHATE, CHLOROQUINE PHOSPHATE
CHLORPHENIRAMINE MALEATE, CHLORPHENIRAMINE MALEATE
CHLORPROMAZINE HCL, CHLORPROMAZINE HYDROCHLORIDE
CHLORTHALIDONE, CHLORTHALIDONE
CLONIDINE HCL, CLONIDINE HYDROCHLORIDE
CLORAZEPATE DIPOTASSIUM, CLORAZEPATE DIPOTASSIUM
CORTISONE ACETATE, CORTISONE ACETATE
DEXTROAMPHETAMINE SULFATE, DEXTROAMPHETAMINE SULFATE
DIAZEPAM, DIAZEPAM
DIPHENHYDRAMINE HCL, DIPHENHYDRAMINE HYDROCHLORIDE
DIPYRIDAMOLE, DIPYRIDAMOLE
DOXEPIN HCL, DOXEPIN HYDROCHLORIDE
DOXYCYCLINE HYCLATE, DOXYCYCLINE HYCLATE
ERYTHROMYCIN STEARATE, ERYTHROMYCIN STEARATE
FENOPROFEN CALCIUM, FENOPROFEN CALCIUM
FLURAZEPAM HCL, FLURAZEPAM HYDROCHLORIDE
FOLIC ACID, FOLIC ACID
GEMFIBROZIL, GEMFIBROZIL
HALOPERIDOL, HALOPERIDOL
HYDRALAZINE HCL, HYDRALAZINE HYDROCHLORIDE
HYDROCHLOROTHIAZIDE, HYDROCHLOROTHIAZIDE
HYDROCORTISONE, HYDROCORTISONE
HYDROCORTISONE ACETATE, HYDROCORTISONE ACETATE
HYDROXYZINE HCL, HYDROXYZINE HYDROCHLORIDE
IBUPROFEN, IBUPROFEN
IBUPROFEN, IBUPROFEN (OTC)
ISONIAZID, ISONIAZID
LORAZEPAM, LORAZEPAM
MEPROBAMATE, MEPROBAMATE
METHOCARBAMOL, METHOCARBAMOL
METHYLDOPA, METHYLDOPA
METHYLDOPA AND HYDROCHLOROTHIAZIDE, HYDROCHLOROTHIAZIDE
METHYLTESTOSTERONE, METHYLTESTOSTERONE
METOCLOPRAMIDE HCL, METOCLOPRAMIDE HYDROCHLORIDE
METOPROLOL TARTRATE, METOPROLOL TARTRATE
NAPROXEN, NAPROXEN
NIACIN, NIACIN
NIFEDIPINE, NIFEDIPINE
OXAZEPAM, OXAZEPAM
OXYTETRACYCLINE HCL, OXYTETRACYCLINE HYDROCHLORIDE
PENICILLIN G POTASSIUM, PENICILLIN G POTASSIUM
PENICILLIN V POTASSIUM, PENICILLIN V POTASSIUM
PINDOLOL, PINDOLOL
PRAZOSIN HCL, PRAZOSIN HYDROCHLORIDE
PREDNISOLONE, PREDNISOLONE
PREDNISONE, PREDNISONE
PROPOXYPHENE HCL, PROPOXYPHENE HYDROCHLORIDE
PROPOXYPHENE NAPSYLATE AND ACETAMINOPHEN, ACETAMINOPHEN
PROPRANOLOL HCL, PROPRANOLOL HYDROCHLORIDE
PROPRANOLOL HCL AND HYDROCHLOROTHIAZIDE, HYDROCHLOROTHIAZIDE
PROPYLTHIOURACIL, PROPYLTHIOURACIL
QUINIDINE SULFATE, QUINIDINE SULFATE
RAUWOLFIA SERPENTINA, RAUWOLFIA SERPENTINA
RESERPINE, RESERPINE
SECOBARBITAL SODIUM, SECOBARBITAL SODIUM
SODIUM PENTOBARBITAL, PENTOBARBITAL SODIUM
SPIRONOLACTONE, SPIRONOLACTONE
SPIRONOLACTONE AND HYDROCHLOROTHIAZIDE, HYDROCHLOROTHIAZIDE
SPIRONOLACTONE W/ HYDROCHLOROTHIAZIDE, HYDROCHLOROTHIAZIDE
SULFISOXAZOLE, SULFISOXAZOLE
TEMAZEPAM, TEMAZEPAM
TETRACYCLINE HCL, TETRACYCLINE HYDROCHLORIDE
TOLBUTAMIDE, TOLBUTAMIDE
TOLMETIN SODIUM, TOLMETIN SODIUM
TRAZODONE HCL, TRAZODONE HYDROCHLORIDE
TRIAMCINOLONE, TRIAMCINOLONE
TRIPLE SULFA, TRISULFAPYRIMIDINES (SULFADIAZINE;SULFAMERAZINE;SULFAMETHAZINE)
VERAPAMIL HCL, VERAPAMIL HYDROCHLORIDE

Q

QUAD PHARMS

* QUAD PHARMACEUTICALS INC
ACETAZOLAMIDE SODIUM, ACETAZOLAMIDE SODIUM
ACETYLCYSTEINE, ACETYLCYSTEINE
AMINOCAPROIC ACID, AMINOCAPROIC ACID
AMINOHIPPURATE SODIUM, AMINOHIPPURATE SODIUM
AZATHIOPRINE, AZATHIOPRINE SODIUM
BACITRACIN, BACITRACIN
BETHANECHOL CHLORIDE, BETHANECHOL CHLORIDE
BRETYLIUM TOSYLATE, BRETYLIUM TOSYLATE
CHORIONIC GONADOTROPIN, GONADOTROPIN, CHORIONIC
CLINDAMYCIN PHOSPHATE, CLINDAMYCIN PHOSPHATE
CYTARABINE, CYTARABINE
DACARBAZINE, DACARBAZINE
DEXAMETHASONE SODIUM PHOSPHATE, DEXAMETHASONE SODIUM PHOSPHATE
DIAZOXIDE, DIAZOXIDE
DOXYCYCLINE HYCLATE, DOXYCYCLINE HYCLATE
DROPERIDOL, DROPERIDOL

APPENDIX B
PRODUCT NAME INDEX
LISTED BY APPLICANT *(continued)*

ERYTHROMYCIN LACTOBIONATE, ERYTHROMYCIN LACTOBIONATE
ESTRADIOL CYPIONATE, ESTRADIOL CYPIONATE
FLOXURIDINE, FLOXURIDINE
FLUOROURACIL, FLUOROURACIL
FLUPHENAZINE, FLUPHENAZINE DECANOATE
FLUPHENAZINE HCL, FLUPHENAZINE HYDROCHLORIDE
GLUCAGON, GLUCAGON HYDROCHLORIDE
GLYCOPYRROLATE, GLYCOPYRROLATE
HALOPERIDOL, HALOPERIDOL LACTATE
HYDROCORTISONE SODIUM PHOSPHATE, HYDROCORTISONE SODIUM PHOSPHATE
HYDROXYPROGESTERONE CAPROATE, HYDROXYPROGESTERONE CAPROATE
ISONIAZID, ISONIAZID
KANAMYCIN SULFATE, KANAMYCIN SULFATE
KETAMINE HCL, KETAMINE HYDROCHLORIDE
LEUCOVORIN CALCIUM, LEUCOVORIN CALCIUM
LINCOMYCIN HCL, LINCOMYCIN HYDROCHLORIDE
METHOTREXATE SODIUM, METHOTREXATE SODIUM
METHYLDOPATE HCL, METHYLDOPATE HYDROCHLORIDE
METHYLPREDNISOLONE SODIUM SUCCINATE, METHYLPREDNISOLONE SODIUM SUCCINATE
METOCLOPRAMIDE HCL, METOCLOPRAMIDE HYDROCHLORIDE
METOCURINE IODIDE, METOCURINE IODIDE
NALBUPHINE, NALBUPHINE HYDROCHLORIDE
NALOXONE HCL, NALOXONE HYDROCHLORIDE
NANDDROLONE DECANOATE, NANDROLONE DECANOATE
NANDROLONE DECANOATE, NANDROLONE DECANOATE
NANDROLONE PHENPROPIONATE, NANDROLONE PHENPROPIONATE
NITROGLYCERIN, NITROGLYCERIN
PANCURONIUM BROMIDE, PANCURONIUM BROMIDE
PRALIDOXIME CHLORIDE, PRALIDOXIME CHLORIDE
PROCAINAMIDE HCL, PROCAINAMIDE HYDROCHLORIDE
PROCHLORPERAZINE EDISYLATE, PROCHLORPERAZINE EDISYLATE
PROTAMINE SULFATE, PROTAMINE SULFATE
RITODRINE HCL, RITODRINE HYDROCHLORIDE
SULFAMETHOPRIM, SULFAMETHOXAZOLE
TESTOSTERONE CYPIONATE, TESTOSTERONE CYPIONATE
TESTOSTERONE ENANTHATE, TESTOSTERONE ENANTHATE
TESTOSTERONE PROPIONATE, TESTOSTERONE PROPIONATE
TRIFLUOPERAZINE HCL, TRIFLUOPERAZINE HYDROCHLORIDE
TUBOCURARINE CHLORIDE, TUBOCURARINE CHLORIDE
VANCOMYCIN HCL, VANCOMYCIN HYDROCHLORIDE
VERAPAMIL HCL, VERAPAMIL HYDROCHLORIDE
VINBLASTINE SULFATE, VINBLASTINE SULFATE
VINCRISTINE SULFATE, VINCRISTINE SULFATE

QUANTUM PHARMICS
* QUANTUM PHARMICS LTD
BENZTROPINE MESYLATE, BENZTROPINE MESYLATE

BUTALBITAL ASPIRIN AND CAFFEINE, ASPIRIN
CLOPRA, METOCLOPRAMIDE HYDROCHLORIDE
CLOPRA-"YELLOW", METOCLOPRAMIDE HYDROCHLORIDE
CLORAZEPATE DIPOTASSIUM, CLORAZEPATE DIPOTASSIUM
DOXEPIN HCL, DOXEPIN HYDROCHLORIDE
DOXYLAMINE SUCCINATE, DOXYLAMINE SUCCINATE
FENOPROFEN CALCIUM, FENOPROFEN CALCIUM
HALOPERIDOL, HALOPERIDOL
HYDRALAZINE HCL, HYDRALAZINE HYDROCHLORIDE
HYDROXYZINE HCL, HYDROXYZINE HYDROCHLORIDE
LORAZ, LORAZEPAM
MECLODIUM, MECLOFENAMATE SODIUM
MINODYL, MINOXIDIL
NYSTATIN, NYSTATIN
OXYBUTYNIN CHLORIDE, OXYBUTYNIN CHLORIDE
PHENTERMINE RESIN 30, PHENTERMINE RESIN COMPLEX
Q-GESIC, ASPIRIN
Q-PAM, DIAZEPAM
TEMAZ, TEMAZEPAM
TIMOLOL MALEATE, TIMOLOL MALEATE
TRAZODONE HCL, TRAZODONE HYDROCHLORIDE
TRIALODINE, TRAZODONE HYDROCHLORIDE
TRIAMTERENE AND HYDROCHLOROTHIAZIDE, HYDROCHLOROTHIAZIDE
ZAXOPAM, OXAZEPAM

R

RACHELLE
* RACHELLE LABORATORIES INC
CHLORDIAZACHEL, CHLORDIAZEPOXIDE HYDROCHLORIDE
DOXY-TABS, DOXYCYCLINE HYCLATE
DOXYCHEL, DOXYCYCLINE
DOXYCHEL HYCLATE, DOXYCYCLINE HYCLATE
MYCHEL, CHLORAMPHENICOL

RECKITT AND COLMAN
* RECKITT AND COLMAN PHARMACEUTICALS INC
BUPRENEX, BUPRENORPHINE HYDROCHLORIDE

REED AND CARNRICK
* REED AND CARNRICK DIV BLOCK DRUG CO INC
CORTIFOAM, HYDROCORTISONE ACETATE
LEVATOL, PENBUTOLOL SULFATE
* REED AND CARNRICK PHARMACEUTICALS DIV BLOCK DRUG CO INC
COLYTE, POLYETHYLENE GLYCOL 3350
COLYTE-FLAVORED, POLYETHYLENE GLYCOL 3350
DILATRATE-SR, ISOSORBIDE DINITRATE
EPIFOAM, HYDROCORTISONE ACETATE
ETHAMOLIN, ETHANOLAMINE OLEATE
KWELL, LINDANE
PROCTOFOAM HC, HYDROCORTISONE ACETATE

RES INDS
* RESEARCH INDUSTRIES CORP
RIMSO-50, DIMETHYL SULFOXIDE

REXALL
* REXALL DRUG CO
PREDNISONE, PREDNISONE
RESERPINE, RESERPINE

APPENDIX B
PRODUCT NAME INDEX
LISTED BY APPLICANT *(continued)*

REXAR
* REXAR PHARMACAL CORP
 DEXTROAMPHETAMINE SULFATE, DEXTROAMPHETAMINE SULFATE
 METHAMPHETAMINE HCL, METHAMPHETAMINE HYDROCHLORIDE
 OBY-TRIM, PHENTERMINE HYDROCHLORIDE
 X-TROZINE, PHENDIMETRAZINE TARTRATE
 X-TROZINE L.A., PHENDIMETRAZINE TARTRATE

RHONE POULENC RORER
* RHONE POULENC RORER PHARMACEUTICALS INC
 ACTHAR, CORTICOTROPIN
 AZMACORT, TRIAMCINOLONE ACETONIDE
 AZOLID, PHENYLBUTAZONE
 CALCIMAR, CALCITONIN, SALMON
 CERUBIDINE, DAUNORUBICIN HYDROCHLORIDE
 DDAVP, DESMOPRESSIN ACETATE
 DEMI-REGROTON, CHLORTHALIDONE
 DESMOPRESSIN ACETATE, DESMOPRESSIN ACETATE
 DILACOR XR, DILTIAZEM HYDROCHLORIDE
 DORIDEN, GLUTETHIMIDE
 H.P. ACTHAR GEL, CORTICOTROPIN
 HYGROTON, CHLORTHALIDONE
 LOVENOX, ENOXAPARIN SODIUM
 LOZOL, INDAPAMIDE
 NASACORT, TRIAMCINOLONE ACETONIDE
 NICOLAR, NIACIN
 PARATHAR, TERIPARATIDE ACETATE
 PENETREX, ENOXACIN
 PENTACARINAT, PENTAMIDINE ISETHIONATE
 PERTOFRANE, DESIPRAMINE HYDROCHLORIDE
 PRESAMINE, IMIPRAMINE HYDROCHLORIDE
 REGROTON, CHLORTHALIDONE
 SLO-BID, THEOPHYLLINE
 SLO-PHYLLIN, THEOPHYLLINE

ROACO DC
* TJ ROACO LTD
 BETADERM, BETAMETHASONE VALERATE

ROBERTS AND HAUCK
* ROBERTS AND HAUCK PHARMACEUTICALS INC
 ANOQUAN, ACETAMINOPHEN

ROBERTS LABS
* ROBERTS LABORATORIES INC
 BANTHINE, METHANTHELINE BROMIDE
 DOPAR, LEVODOPA
 DUVOID, BETHANECHOL CHLORIDE
 ETHMOZINE, MORICIZINE HYDROCHLORIDE
 FURACIN, NITROFURAZONE
 FUROXONE, FURAZOLIDONE
 NORETHIN 1/35E-21, ETHINYL ESTRADIOL
 NORETHIN 1/35E-28, ETHINYL ESTRADIOL
 NORETHIN 1/50M-21, MESTRANOL
 NORETHIN 1/50M-28, MESTRANOL
 PRO-BANTHINE, PROPANTHELINE BROMIDE
 QUIBRON-T, THEOPHYLLINE
 QUIBRON-T/SR, THEOPHYLLINE
 SALURON, HYDROFLUMETHIAZIDE
 SALUTENSIN, HYDROFLUMETHIAZIDE
 SALUTENSIN-DEMI, HYDROFLUMETHIAZIDE
 SUPPRELIN, HISTRELIN ACETATE
 TOPICYCLINE, TETRACYCLINE HYDROCHLORIDE
 URACIL MUSTARD, URACIL MUSTARD

ROBINS AH
* AH ROBINS CO
 DIMETANE, BROMPHENIRAMINE MALEATE
 DIMETANE, BROMPHENIRAMINE MALEATE (OTC)
 DIMETANE-DC, BROMPHENIRAMINE MALEATE
 DIMETANE-DX, BROMPHENIRAMINE MALEATE
 DIMETAPP, BROMPHENIRAMINE MALEATE (OTC)
 DOPRAM, DOXAPRAM HYDROCHLORIDE
 EXNA, BENZTHIAZIDE
 MICRO-K, POTASSIUM CHLORIDE
 MICRO-K LS, POTASSIUM CHLORIDE
 MICRO-K 10, POTASSIUM CHLORIDE
 PHENAPHEN W/ CODEINE NO. 2, ACETAMINOPHEN
 PHENAPHEN W/ CODEINE NO. 3, ACETAMINOPHEN
 PHENAPHEN W/ CODEINE NO. 4, ACETAMINOPHEN
 PHENAPHEN-650 W/ CODEINE, ACETAMINOPHEN
 PONDIMIN, FENFLURAMINE HYDROCHLORIDE
 QUINIDEX, QUINIDINE SULFATE
 REGLAN, METOCLOPRAMIDE HYDROCHLORIDE
 ROBAXIN, METHOCARBAMOL
 ROBAXIN-750, METHOCARBAMOL
 ROBAXISAL, ASPIRIN
 ROBIMYCIN, ERYTHROMYCIN
 ROBINUL, GLYCOPYRROLATE
 ROBINUL FORTE, GLYCOPYRROLATE
 TENATHAN, BETHANIDINE SULFATE
 TENEX, GUANFACINE HYDROCHLORIDE

ROCHE
* HOFFMANN LAROCHE INC
 ACCUTANE, ISOTRETINOIN
 ANCOBON, FLUCYTOSINE
 ARFONAD, TRIMETHAPHAN CAMSYLATE
 AZO GANTANOL, PHENAZOPYRIDINE HYDROCHLORIDE
 AZO GANTRISIN, PHENAZOPYRIDINE HYDROCHLORIDE
 BACTRIM, SULFAMETHOXAZOLE
 BACTRIM DS, SULFAMETHOXAZOLE
 BACTRIM PEDIATRIC, SULFAMETHOXAZOLE
 BEROCCA PN, ASCORBIC ACID
 BUMEX, BUMETANIDE
 COACTIN, AMDINOCILLIN
 EFUDEX, FLUOROURACIL
 ENDEP, AMITRIPTYLINE HYDROCHLORIDE
 FANSIDAR, PYRIMETHAMINE
 FLUOROURACIL, FLUOROURACIL
 FUDR, FLOXURIDINE
 GANTANOL, SULFAMETHOXAZOLE
 GANTANOL-DS, SULFAMETHOXAZOLE
 GANTRISIN, SULFISOXAZOLE
 GANTRISIN, SULFISOXAZOLE ACETYL
 GANTRISIN, SULFISOXAZOLE DIOLAMINE
 GANTRISIN PEDIATRIC, SULFISOXAZOLE ACETYL
 HIVID, ZALCITABINE
 KLONOPIN, CLONAZEPAM
 KONAKION, PHYTONADIONE
 LARIAM, MEFLOQUINE HYDROCHLORIDE
 LARODOPA, LEVODOPA
 LEVO-DROMORAN, LEVORPHANOL TARTRATE
 LIBRELEASE, CHLORDIAZEPOXIDE
 LIBRIUM, CHLORDIAZEPOXIDE HYDROCHLORIDE
 LIMBITROL, AMITRIPTYLINE HYDROCHLORIDE
 LIPO GANTRISIN, SULFISOXAZOLE ACETYL
 LORFAN, LEVALLORPHAN TARTRATE
 MATULANE, PROCARBAZINE HYDROCHLORIDE
 MENRIUM 10-4, CHLORDIAZEPOXIDE

APPENDIX B
PRODUCT NAME INDEX
LISTED BY APPLICANT *(continued)*

MENRIUM 5-2, CHLORDIAZEPOXIDE
MENRIUM 5-4, CHLORDIAZEPOXIDE
MESTINON, PYRIDOSTIGMINE BROMIDE
NIPRIDE, SODIUM NITROPRUSSIDE
NOLUDAR, METHYPRYLON
PROVOCHOLINE, METHACHOLINE CHLORIDE
QUARZAN, CLIDINIUM BROMIDE
RIMADYL, CARPROFEN
RIMIFON, ISONIAZID
ROCALTROL, CALCITRIOL
ROCEPHIN, CEFTRIAXONE SODIUM
ROCEPHIN W/ DEXTROSE, CEFTRIAXONE SODIUM
ROMAZICON, FLUMAZENIL
SOLATENE, BETA-CAROTENE
SYNKAYVITE, MENADIOL SODIUM DIPHOSPHATE
TARACTAN, CHLORPROTHIXENE
TEGISON, ETRETINATE
TENSILON, EDROPHONIUM CHLORIDE
TRIMPEX, TRIMETHOPRIM
TRIMPEX 200, TRIMETHOPRIM
VALIUM, DIAZEPAM
VALRELEASE, DIAZEPAM
VERSED, MIDAZOLAM HYDROCHLORIDE
* ROCHE LABORATORIES DIV HOFFMANN LAROCHE INC
ROCEPHIN, CEFTRIAXONE SODIUM
* ROCHE PRODUCTS INC
DALMANE, FLURAZEPAM HYDROCHLORIDE
LIBRITABS, CHLORDIAZEPOXIDE
LIBRIUM, CHLORDIAZEPOXIDE HYDROCHLORIDE

ROERIG
* ROERIG DIV PFIZER INC
ANTIVERT, MECLIZINE HYDROCHLORIDE
ATARAX, HYDROXYZINE HYDROCHLORIDE
EMETE-CON, BENZQUINAMIDE HYDROCHLORIDE
GEOPEN, CARBENICILLIN DISODIUM
NAVANE, THIOTHIXENE
NAVANE, THIOTHIXENE HYDROCHLORIDE
SUSTAIRE, THEOPHYLLINE
TAO, TROLEANDOMYCIN

RORER
* RORER PHARMACEUTICAL CORP SUB RORER GROUP
NITROL, NITROGLYCERIN

ROSEMONT PHARM
* ROSEMONT PHARMACEUTICAL CORP
ACETAMINOPHEN W/ CODEINE PHOSPHATE, ACETAMINOPHEN
ACETOHEXAMIDE, ACETOHEXAMIDE
AMANTADINE HCL, AMANTADINE HYDROCHLORIDE
AMITRIPTYLINE HCL, AMITRIPTYLINE HYDROCHLORIDE
BACLOFEN, BACLOFEN
BENZTROPINE MESYLATE, BENZTROPINE MESYLATE
BROMPHENIRAMINE MALEATE, BROMPHENIRAMINE MALEATE
CARBAMAZEPINE, CARBAMAZEPINE
CHLORDIAZEPOXIDE AND AMITRIPTYLINE HCL, AMITRIPTYLINE HYDROCHLORIDE
CHLORDIAZEPOXIDE HCL, CHLORDIAZEPOXIDE HYDROCHLORIDE
CHLORPROMAZINE HCL, CHLORPROMAZINE HYDROCHLORIDE
CHLORPROPAMIDE, CHLORPROPAMIDE
CHLORTHALIDONE, CHLORTHALIDONE
CLOFIBRATE, CLOFIBRATE
CLORAZEPATE DIPOTASSIUM, CLORAZEPATE DIPOTASSIUM
DESIPRAMINE HCL, DESIPRAMINE HYDROCHLORIDE
DIPHEN, DIPHENHYDRAMINE HYDROCHLORIDE
DIPHENOXYLATE HCL W/ ATROPINE SULFATE, ATROPINE SULFATE
FENOPROFEN CALCIUM, FENOPROFEN CALCIUM
FLUOCINOLONE ACETONIDE, FLUOCINOLONE ACETONIDE
FLUOXYMESTERONE, FLUOXYMESTERONE
FLURAZEPAM HCL, FLURAZEPAM HYDROCHLORIDE
FOLIC ACID, FOLIC ACID
HYDRALAZINE HCL, HYDRALAZINE HYDROCHLORIDE
HYDROCHLOROTHIAZIDE, HYDROCHLOROTHIAZIDE
HYDROCODONE BITARTRATE AND ACETAMINOPHEN, ACETAMINOPHEN
HYDROCORTISONE, HYDROCORTISONE
HYDROFLUMETHIAZIDE AND RESERPINE, HYDROFLUMETHIAZIDE
HYDROXYZINE HCL, HYDROXYZINE HYDROCHLORIDE
IMIPRAMINE HCL, IMIPRAMINE HYDROCHLORIDE
LITHIUM CARBONATE, LITHIUM CARBONATE
LORAZEPAM, LORAZEPAM
MECLOFENAMATE SODIUM, MECLOFENAMATE SODIUM
MEDROXYPROGESTERONE ACETATE, MEDROXYPROGESTERONE ACETATE
MEGESTROL ACETATE, MEGESTROL ACETATE
MEPROBAMATE, MEPROBAMATE
METAPROTERENOL SULFATE, METAPROTERENOL SULFATE
METHYCLOTHIAZIDE, METHYCLOTHIAZIDE
METHYLTESTOSTERONE, METHYLTESTOSTERONE
METOCLOPRAMIDE HCL, METOCLOPRAMIDE HYDROCHLORIDE
MINOXIDIL, MINOXIDIL
MYFED, PSEUDOEPHEDRINE HYDROCHLORIDE (OTC)
MYIDYL, TRIPROLIDINE HYDROCHLORIDE
MYMETHAZINE FORTIS, PROMETHAZINE HYDROCHLORIDE
NYSTATIN, NYSTATIN
OXYBUTYNIN CHLORIDE, OXYBUTYNIN CHLORIDE
PHENDIMETRAZINE TARTRATE, PHENDIMETRAZINE TARTRATE
PHENTERMINE HCL, PHENTERMINE HYDROCHLORIDE
PRAZEPAM, PRAZEPAM
QUINIDINE SULFATE, QUINIDINE SULFATE
SPIRONOLACTONE W/ HYDROCHLOROTHIAZIDE, HYDROCHLOROTHIAZIDE
SULFAMETHOXAZOLE AND TRIMETHOPRIM, SULFAMETHOXAZOLE
SULMEPRIM, SULFAMETHOXAZOLE
SULMEPRIM PEDIATRIC, SULFAMETHOXAZOLE
TEMAZEPAM, TEMAZEPAM
TIMOLOL MALEATE, TIMOLOL MALEATE
TOLAZAMIDE, TOLAZAMIDE
TRAZODONE HCL, TRAZODONE HYDROCHLORIDE
TRIMIPRAMINE MALEATE, TRIMIPRAMINE MALEATE
VALPROIC ACID, VALPROIC ACID
WARFARIN SODIUM, WARFARIN SODIUM

ROSS LABS
* ROSS LABORATORIES DIV ABBOTT LABORATORIES INC
PEDIAMYCIN, ERYTHROMYCIN ETHYLSUCCINATE
PEDIAMYCIN 400, ERYTHROMYCIN ETHYLSUCCINATE

APPENDIX B
PRODUCT NAME INDEX
LISTED BY APPLICANT *(continued)*

PEDIAZOLE, ERYTHROMYCIN ETHYLSUCCINATE
SURVANTA, BERACTANT

ROXANE
* ROXANE LABORATORIES INC
ACETAMINOPHEN, ACETAMINOPHEN (OTC)
ACETAMINOPHEN AND CODEINE PHOSPHATE, ACETAMINOPHEN
ACETAMINOPHEN AND CODEINE PHOSPHATE NO. 4, ACETAMINOPHEN
ACETAMINOPHEN W/ CODEINE, ACETAMINOPHEN
ACETAMINOPHEN W/ CODEINE NO. 2, ACETAMINOPHEN
ACETAMINOPHEN W/ CODEINE NO. 3, ACETAMINOPHEN
ACETYLCYSTEINE, ACETYLCYSTEINE
ALPRAZOLAM, ALPRAZOLAM
AMINOPHYLLINE, AMINOPHYLLINE
AMITRIPTYLINE HCL, AMITRIPTYLINE HYDROCHLORIDE
CHLORDIAZEPOXIDE HCL, CHLORDIAZEPOXIDE HYDROCHLORIDE
CHLORPHENIRAMINE MALEATE, CHLORPHENIRAMINE MALEATE
CHLORPROMAZINE HCL, CHLORPROMAZINE HYDROCHLORIDE
CHLORPROMAZINE HCL INTENSOL, CHLORPROMAZINE HYDROCHLORIDE
DEXAMETHASONE, DEXAMETHASONE
DEXAMETHASONE INTENSOL, DEXAMETHASONE
DIAZEPAM, DIAZEPAM
DIAZEPAM INTENSOL, DIAZEPAM
DIFLUNISAL, DIFLUNISAL
DIPHENHYDRAMINE HCL, DIPHENHYDRAMINE HYDROCHLORIDE
DIPHENOXYLATE HCL AND ATROPINE SULFATE, ATROPINE SULFATE
FUROSEMIDE, FUROSEMIDE
HALOPERIDOL, HALOPERIDOL
HALOPERIDOL INTENSOL, HALOPERIDOL LACTATE
HYDROCHLOROTHIAZIDE, HYDROCHLOROTHIAZIDE
HYDROCHLOROTHIAZIDE INTENSOL, HYDROCHLOROTHIAZIDE
HYDROCHLOROTHIAZIDE W/ RESERPINE, HYDROCHLOROTHIAZIDE
HYDROCORTISONE, HYDROCORTISONE
IMIPRAMINE HCL, IMIPRAMINE HYDROCHLORIDE
INDOMETHACIN, INDOMETHACIN
ISOETHARINE HCL, ISOETHARINE HYDROCHLORIDE
LACTULOSE, LACTULOSE
LEUCOVORIN CALCIUM, LEUCOVORIN CALCIUM
LIDOCAINE HCL, LIDOCAINE HYDROCHLORIDE
LIDOCAINE VISCOUS, LIDOCAINE HYDROCHLORIDE
LITHIUM CARBONATE, LITHIUM CARBONATE
LITHIUM CITRATE, LITHIUM CITRATE
LOPERAMIDE HCL, LOPERAMIDE HYDROCHLORIDE (OTC)
LOPERAMIDE HCL, LOPERAMIDE HYDROCHLORIDE
LORAZEPAM INTENSOL, LORAZEPAM
MEPERIDINE HCL, MEPERIDINE HYDROCHLORIDE
MEPROBAMATE, MEPROBAMATE
METHADONE HCL, METHADONE HYDROCHLORIDE
METHADONE HCL INTENSOL, METHADONE HYDROCHLORIDE
METHOCARBAMOL, METHOCARBAMOL
METHOTREXATE SODIUM, METHOTREXATE SODIUM
METHYLDOPA, METHYLDOPA
METOCLOPRAMIDE HCL, METOCLOPRAMIDE HYDROCHLORIDE
METOCLOPRAMIDE INTENSOL, METOCLOPRAMIDE HYDROCHLORIDE
NAPROXEN, NAPROXEN
NAPROXEN SODIUM, NAPROXEN SODIUM
NEOMYCIN SULFATE, NEOMYCIN SULFATE
NYSTATIN, NYSTATIN
ORAMORPH SR, MORPHINE SULFATE
OXYCODONE AND ASPIRIN (HALF-STRENGTH), ASPIRIN
PIROXICAM, PIROXICAM
POTASSIUM IODIDE, POTASSIUM IODIDE (OTC)
PREDNISOLONE, PREDNISOLONE
PREDNISONE, PREDNISONE
PREDNISONE INTENSOL, PREDNISONE
PROCAINAMIDE HCL, PROCAINAMIDE HYDROCHLORIDE
PROPANTHELINE BROMIDE, PROPANTHELINE BROMIDE
PROPOXYPHENE HCL, PROPOXYPHENE HYDROCHLORIDE
PROPRANOLOL HCL, PROPRANOLOL HYDROCHLORIDE
PROPRANOLOL HCL INTENSOL, PROPRANOLOL HYDROCHLORIDE
QUINIDINE GLUCONATE, QUINIDINE GLUCONATE
QUINIDINE SULFATE, QUINIDINE SULFATE
RESERPINE, RESERPINE
ROXICET, ACETAMINOPHEN
ROXICET 5/500, ACETAMINOPHEN
ROXIPRIN, ASPIRIN
SODIUM POLYSTYRENE SULFONATE, SODIUM POLYSTYRENE SULFONATE
SULFAMETHOXAZOLE AND TRIMETHOPRIM, SULFAMETHOXAZOLE
SULFAMETHOXAZOLE AND TRIMETHOPRIM DOUBLE STRENGTH, SULFAMETHOXAZOLE
SULFISOXAZOLE, SULFISOXAZOLE
TETRACYCLINE HCL, TETRACYCLINE HYDROCHLORIDE
THEOPHYLLINE, THEOPHYLLINE
THIORIDAZINE HCL, THIORIDAZINE HYDROCHLORIDE
THIORIDAZINE HCL INTENSOL, THIORIDAZINE HYDROCHLORIDE
THIOTHIXENE HCL INTENSOL, THIOTHIXENE HYDROCHLORIDE
TRIAMCINOLONE, TRIAMCINOLONE
TRIAZOLAM, TRIAZOLAM

ROYCE LABS
* ROYCE LABORATORIES INC
AMILORIDE HCL AND HYDROCHLOROTHIAZIDE, AMILORIDE HYDROCHLORIDE
BACLOFEN, BACLOFEN
CHLORZOXAZONE, CHLORZOXAZONE
DOXEPIN HCL, DOXEPIN HYDROCHLORIDE
HALOPERIDOL, HALOPERIDOL
HYDROXYZINE HCL, HYDROXYZINE HYDROCHLORIDE
LORAZEPAM, LORAZEPAM
MINOXIDIL, MINOXIDIL
PERPHENAZINE AND AMITRIPTYLINE HCL, AMITRIPTYLINE HYDROCHLORIDE

APPENDIX B
PRODUCT NAME INDEX
LISTED BY APPLICANT *(continued)*

S

SANDOZ
* SANDOZ PHARMACEUTICALS CORP DIV SANDOZ INC
ACYLANID, ACETYLDIGITOXIN
CAFERGOT, CAFFEINE
CEDILANID-D, DESLANOSIDE
CLOZARIL, CLOZAPINE
D.H.E. 45, DIHYDROERGOTAMINE MESYLATE
DIAPID, LYPRESSIN
DYNACIRC, ISRADIPINE
DYNACIRC CR, ISRADIPINE
EMBOLEX, DIHYDROERGOTAMINE MESYLATE
FIORICET, ACETAMINOPHEN
FIORICET W/ CODEINE, ACETAMINOPHEN
FIORINAL, ASPIRIN
FIORINAL W/CODEINE NO 3, ASPIRIN
HYDERGINE, ERGOLOID MESYLATES
HYDERGINE LC, ERGOLOID MESYLATES
LAMISIL, TERBINAFINE HYDROCHLORIDE
LESCOL, FLUVASTATIN SODIUM
MELLARIL, THIORIDAZINE HYDROCHLORIDE
MELLARIL-S, THIORIDAZINE
MESANTOIN, MEPHENYTOIN
METHERGINE, METHYLERGONOVINE MALEATE
MIACALCIN, CALCITONIN, SALMON
PAMELOR, NORTRIPTYLINE HYDROCHLORIDE
PARLODEL, BROMOCRIPTINE MESYLATE
RESTORIL, TEMAZEPAM
SANDIMMUNE, CYCLOSPORINE
SANDOSTATIN, OCTREOTIDE ACETATE
SANOREX, MAZINDOL
SANSERT, METHYSERGIDE MALEATE
SERENTIL, MESORIDAZINE BESYLATE
SYNTOCINON, OXYTOCIN
TAVIST, CLEMASTINE FUMARATE
TAVIST D, CLEMASTINE FUMARATE
TAVIST-D, CLEMASTINE FUMARATE (OTC)
TAVIST-1, CLEMASTINE FUMARATE
TAVIST-1, CLEMASTINE FUMARATE (OTC)
TORECAN, THIETHYLPERAZINE MALEATE
TORECAN, THIETHYLPERAZINE MALATE
TORECAN, THIETHYLPERAZINE MALEATE
TREST, METHIXENE HYDROCHLORIDE
TRIAMINIC-12, CHLORPHENIRAMINE MALEATE (OTC)
VISKAZIDE, HYDROCHLOROTHIAZIDE
VISKEN, PINDOLOL

SANKYO
* SANKYO USA CORP
BANAN, CEFPODOXIME PROXETIL

SAVAGE LABS
* SAVAGE LABORATORIES INC DIV ALTANA INC
ALPHATREX, BETAMETHASONE DIPROPIONATE
AXOTAL, ASPIRIN
BETATREX, BETAMETHASONE VALERATE
CHYMEX, BENTIROMIDE
DILOR, DYPHYLLINE
DILOR-400, DYPHYLLINE
DITATE-DS, ESTRADIOL VALERATE
ETHIODOL, ETHIODIZED OIL
FLUOTREX, FLUOCINOLONE ACETONIDE
GVS, GENTIAN VIOLET
K-LEASE, POTASSIUM CHLORIDE
KAON CL, POTASSIUM CHLORIDE
KAON CL-10, POTASSIUM CHLORIDE
MYTREX A, NEOMYCIN SULFATE
MYTREX F, NYSTATIN
NYSTEX, NYSTATIN
RUVITE, CYANOCOBALAMIN
SATRIC, METRONIDAZOLE
TRYMEX, TRIAMCINOLONE ACETONIDE
TRYSUL, TRIPLE SULFA (SULFABENZAMIDE;SULFACETAMIDE;SULFATHIAZOLE)
XYLO-PFAN, XYLOSE

SCHEIN
* SCHEIN PHARMACEUTICAL INC
INFED, IRON DEXTRAN

SCHERER
* RP SCHERER CORP
NIFEDIPINE, NIFEDIPINE
* RP SCHERER NORTH AMERICA
NIFEDIPINE, NIFEDIPINE
VALPROIC ACID, VALPROIC ACID
* RP SCHERER NORTH AMERICA DIV RP SCHERER CORP
DIPHENOXYLATE HCL W/ ATROPINE SULFATE, ATROPINE SULFATE
THEOPHYLLINE, THEOPHYLLINE
THEOPHYLLINE-SR, THEOPHYLLINE
VALPROIC ACID, VALPROIC ACID

SCHERING
* SCHERING CORP
GUANIDINE HCL, GUANIDINE HYDROCHLORIDE
LOTRISONE, BETAMETHASONE DIPROPIONATE
VALISONE, BETAMETHASONE VALERATE
* SCHERING CORP SUB SCHERING PLOUGH CORP
AKRINOL, ACRISORCIN
BETAPAR, MEPREDNISONE
CELESTONE, BETAMETHASONE
CELESTONE, BETAMETHASONE SODIUM PHOSPHATE
CELESTONE SOLUSPAN, BETAMETHASONE ACETATE
CHLOR-TRIMETON, CHLORPHENIRAMINE MALEATE
CLARITIN, LORATADINE
DIPROLENE, BETAMETHASONE DIPROPIONATE
DIPROLENE AF, BETAMETHASONE DIPROPIONATE
DIPROSONE, BETAMETHASONE DIPROPIONATE
DISOMER, DEXBROMPHENIRAMINE MALEATE
DISOPHROL, DEXBROMPHENIRAMINE MALEATE (OTC)
ELOCON, MOMETASONE FUROATE
ESTINYL, ETHINYL ESTRADIOL
ETRAFON 2-10, AMITRIPTYLINE HYDROCHLORIDE
ETRAFON 2-25, AMITRIPTYLINE HYDROCHLORIDE
ETRAFON-A, AMITRIPTYLINE HYDROCHLORIDE
ETRAFON-FORTE, AMITRIPTYLINE HYDROCHLORIDE
EULEXIN, FLUTAMIDE
FULVICIN P/G, GRISEOFULVIN, ULTRAMICROCRYSTALLINE
FULVICIN P/G 165, GRISEOFULVIN, ULTRAMICROCRYSTALLINE
FULVICIN P/G 330, GRISEOFULVIN, ULTRAMICROCRYSTALLINE
FULVICIN-U/F, GRISEOFULVIN, MICROCRYSTALLINE
GARAMYCIN, GENTAMICIN SULFATE
HYPERSTAT, DIAZOXIDE
K-DUR 10, POTASSIUM CHLORIDE
K-DUR 20, POTASSIUM CHLORIDE
LOTRIMIN, CLOTRIMAZOLE
LOTRIMIN AF, CLOTRIMAZOLE (OTC)
METI-DERM, PREDNISOLONE

APPENDIX B
PRODUCT NAME INDEX
LISTED BY APPLICANT *(continued)*

METICORTELONE, PREDNISOLONE ACETATE
METICORTEN, PREDNISONE
METIMYD, PREDNISOLONE ACETATE
METOCLOPRAMIDE HCL, METOCLOPRAMIDE HYDROCHLORIDE
METRETON, PREDNISOLONE SODIUM PHOSPHATE
MIRADON, ANISINDIONE
NAQUA, TRICHLORMETHIAZIDE
NAQUIVAL, RESERPINE
NETROMYCIN, NETILMICIN SULFATE
NORMODYNE, LABETALOL HYDROCHLORIDE
NORMOZIDE, HYDROCHLOROTHIAZIDE
OPTIMINE, AZATADINE MALEATE
ORETON, METHYLTESTOSTERONE
ORETON METHYL, METHYLTESTOSTERONE
OTOBIONE, HYDROCORTISONE
OTOBIOTIC, HYDROCORTISONE
PAXIPAM, HALAZEPAM
PERMITIL, FLUPHENAZINE HYDROCHLORIDE
POLARAMINE, DEXCHLORPHENIRAMINE MALEATE
PRANTAL, DIPHEMANIL METHYLSULFATE
PROPRANOLOL HCL, PROPRANOLOL HYDROCHLORIDE
PROVENTIL, ALBUTEROL
PROVENTIL, ALBUTEROL SULFATE
RELA, CARISOPRODOL
SODIUM SULAMYD, SULFACETAMIDE SODIUM
THEOVENT, THEOPHYLLINE
TINDAL, ACETOPHENAZINE MALEATE
TREMIN, TRIHEXYPHENIDYL HYDROCHLORIDE
TRILAFON, PERPHENAZINE
TRINALIN, AZATADINE MALEATE
VALISONE, BETAMETHASONE VALERATE
VANCENASE, BECLOMETHASONE DIPROPIONATE
VANCENASE AQ, BECLOMETHASONE DIPROPIONATE MONOHYDRATE
VANCERIL, BECLOMETHASONE DIPROPIONATE

SCHERING PLOUGH
* SCHERING PLOUGH CORP
IMDUR, ISOSORBIDE MONONITRATE
* SCHERING PLOUGH HEALTHCARE PRODUCTS INC
AFRINOL, PSEUDOEPHEDRINE SULFATE (OTC)
CHLOR-TRIMETON, CHLORPHENIRAMINE MALEATE (OTC)
CHLOR-TRIMETON, CHLORPHENIRAMINE MALEATE
CHLOR-TRIMETON, CHLORPHENIRAMINE MALEATE (OTC)
DEMAZIN, CHLORPHENIRAMINE MALEATE (OTC)
DISOPHROL, DEXBROMPHENIRAMINE MALEATE (OTC)
DRIXORAL, DEXBROMPHENIRAMINE MALEATE (OTC)
DRIXORAL PLUS, ACETAMINOPHEN (OTC)
GYNE-LOTRIMIN, CLOTRIMAZOLE (OTC)
GYNE-LOTRIMIN COMBINATION PACK, CLOTRIMAZOLE
LOTRIMIN, CLOTRIMAZOLE
LOTRIMIN AF, CLOTRIMAZOLE (OTC)
OCUCLEAR, OXYMETAZOLINE HYDROCHLORIDE (OTC)

SCHWARZ PHARMA
* SCHWARZ PHARMA DIV KREMERS URBAN CO
MONOKET, ISOSORBIDE MONONITRATE
PRE-PEN, BENZYL PENICILLOYL-POLYLYSINE

SCS
* SCS PHARMACEUTICALS
ATENOLOL, ATENOLOL
CARBIDOPA AND LEVODOPA, CARBIDOPA
DIULO, METOLAZONE
FLAGYL I.V., METRONIDAZOLE HYDROCHLORIDE
FLAGYL I.V. RTU, METRONIDAZOLE
FLAGYL I.V. RTU IN PLASTIC CONTAINER, METRONIDAZOLE
HALOPERIDOL, HALOPERIDOL
HALOPERIDOL, HALOPERIDOL LACTATE
PIROXICAM, PIROXICAM

SEARLE
* GD SEARLE AND CO
ALDACTONE, SPIRONOLACTONE
AMINOPHYLLIN, AMINOPHYLLINE
AMMONIUM CHLORIDE, AMMONIUM CHLORIDE
CALAN, VERAPAMIL HYDROCHLORIDE
CLORAZEPATE DIPOTASSIUM, CLORAZEPATE DIPOTASSIUM
CU-7, COPPER
CYTOTEC, MISOPROSTOL
DAYPRO, OXAPROZIN
DEMULEN 1/35-21, ETHINYL ESTRADIOL
DEMULEN 1/35-28, ETHINYL ESTRADIOL
DEMULEN 1/50-21, ETHINYL ESTRADIOL
DEMULEN 1/50-28, ETHINYL ESTRADIOL
ENOVID, MESTRANOL
ENOVID-E, MESTRANOL
ENOVID-E 21, MESTRANOL
FLAGYL, METRONIDAZOLE
LIDOCAINE HCL, LIDOCAINE HYDROCHLORIDE
LOMOTIL, ATROPINE SULFATE
MAXAQUIN, LOMEFLOXACIN HYDROCHLORIDE
METARAMINOL BITARTRATE, METARAMINOL BITARTRATE
NORPACE, DISOPYRAMIDE PHOSPHATE
NORPACE CR, DISOPYRAMIDE PHOSPHATE
OVULEN, ETHYNODIOL DIACETATE
OVULEN-21, ETHYNODIOL DIACETATE
OVULEN-28, ETHYNODIOL DIACETATE
POTASSIUM CHLORIDE, POTASSIUM CHLORIDE
PRO-BANTHINE, PROPANTHELINE BROMIDE
PROCAINE HCL, PROCAINE HYDROCHLORIDE
TATUM-T, COPPER
* GD SEARLE PHARMACEUTICALS INC
ALDACTAZIDE, HYDROCHLOROTHIAZIDE

SERONO
* SERONO LABORATORIES INC
ASELLACRIN 10, SOMATROPIN
ASELLACRIN 2, SOMATROPIN
GEREF, SERMORELIN ACETATE
METRODIN, UROFOLLITROPIN
PERGONAL, MENOTROPINS (FSH;LH)
SEROPHENE, CLOMIPHENE CITRATE

SHERWOOD MEDCL
* SHERWOOD MEDICAL CO
ACTIN-N, NITROFURAZONE
THERMAZENE, SILVER SULFADIAZINE

SHIONOGI
* SHIONOGI USA INC
UROBAK, SULFAMETHOXAZOLE
UROPLUS DS, SULFAMETHOXAZOLE
UROPLUS SS, SULFAMETHOXAZOLE

APPENDIX B
PRODUCT NAME INDEX
LISTED BY APPLICANT *(continued)*

SIDMAK LABS NJ
* SIDMAK LABORATORIES INC
ALBUTEROL SULFATE, ALBUTEROL SULFATE
AMITRIPTYLINE HCL, AMITRIPTYLINE HYDROCHLORIDE
BENZTROPINE MESYLATE, BENZTROPINE MESYLATE
BETHANECHOL CHLORIDE, BETHANECHOL CHLORIDE
CARBAMAZEPINE, CARBAMAZEPINE
CHLORPROPAMIDE, CHLORPROPAMIDE
CHLORTHALIDONE, CHLORTHALIDONE
CYPROHEPTADINE HCL, CYPROHEPTADINE HYDROCHLORIDE
DESIPRAMINE HCL, DESIPRAMINE HYDROCHLORIDE
DEXCHLORPHENIRAMINE MALEATE, DEXCHLORPHENIRAMINE MALEATE
DISULFIRAM, DISULFIRAM
DOXYCYCLINE HYCLATE, DOXYCYCLINE HYCLATE
EXTENDED PHENYTOIN SODIUM, PHENYTOIN SODIUM, EXTENDED
HYDRALAZINE HCL, HYDRALAZINE HYDROCHLORIDE
HYDROXYZINE HCL, HYDROXYZINE HYDROCHLORIDE
IBUPRIN, IBUPROFEN (OTC)
IBUPROFEN, IBUPROFEN
INDOMETHACIN, INDOMETHACIN
MECLIZINE HCL, MECLIZINE HYDROCHLORIDE
METHYLDOPA, METHYLDOPA
METOCLOPRAMIDE HCL, METOCLOPRAMIDE HYDROCHLORIDE
METRONIDAZOLE, METRONIDAZOLE
NYSTATIN, NYSTATIN
OXYBUTYNIN CHLORIDE, OXYBUTYNIN CHLORIDE
PROCAINAMIDE HCL, PROCAINAMIDE HYDROCHLORIDE
PROPRANOLOL HCL, PROPRANOLOL HYDROCHLORIDE
PROPRANOLOL HCL AND HYDROCHLOROTHIAZIDE, HYDROCHLOROTHIAZIDE
SULFAMETHOXAZOLE AND TRIMETHOPRIM, SULFAMETHOXAZOLE
THEOPHYLLINE, THEOPHYLLINE
TRAZODONE HCL, TRAZODONE HYDROCHLORIDE
TRAZON-150, TRAZODONE HYDROCHLORIDE
ULTRAGRIS-165, GRISEOFULVIN, ULTRAMICROCRYSTALLINE
ULTRAGRIS-330, GRISEOFULVIN, ULTRAMICROCRYSTALLINE
VERAPAMIL HCL, VERAPAMIL HYDROCHLORIDE

SIGMA TAU
* SIGMA TAU PHARMACEUTICALS INC
CARNITOR, LEVOCARNITINE

SILARX
* SILARX PHARMACEUTICALS INC
HALOPERIDOL, HALOPERIDOL LACTATE
METAPROTERENOL SULFATE, METAPROTERENOL SULFATE
METOCLOPRAMIDE HCL, METOCLOPRAMIDE HYDROCHLORIDE
SILPHEN, DIPHENHYDRAMINE HYDROCHLORIDE (OTC)

SMITH AND NEPHEW
* SMITH AND NEPHEW SOLOPAK DIV SMITH AND NEPHEW
AMINOPHYLLINE, AMINOPHYLLINE
DOPAMINE HCL, DOPAMINE HYDROCHLORIDE
DROPERIDOL, DROPERIDOL
FLUOROURACIL, FLUOROURACIL
FUROSEMIDE, FUROSEMIDE
HALOPERIDOL, HALOPERIDOL LACTATE
HEPARIN LOCK FLUSH, HEPARIN SODIUM
HEPARIN SODIUM, HEPARIN SODIUM
HYDRALAZINE HCL, HYDRALAZINE HYDROCHLORIDE
HYDROXYZINE HCL, HYDROXYZINE HYDROCHLORIDE
METHYLDOPATE HCL, METHYLDOPATE HYDROCHLORIDE
METOCLOPRAMIDE HCL, METOCLOPRAMIDE HYDROCHLORIDE
NALOXONE HCL, NALOXONE HYDROCHLORIDE
NITROGLYCERIN, NITROGLYCERIN
PHENYTOIN SODIUM, PHENYTOIN SODIUM
PROCAINAMIDE HCL, PROCAINAMIDE HYDROCHLORIDE
PROCHLORPERAZINE EDISYLATE, PROCHLORPERAZINE EDISYLATE
PROPRANOLOL HCL, PROPRANOLOL HYDROCHLORIDE
TRIMETHOBENZAMIDE HCL, TRIMETHOBENZAMIDE HYDROCHLORIDE
VERAPAMIL HCL, VERAPAMIL HYDROCHLORIDE

SMITH KLINE FRENCH
* SMITH KLINE AND FRENCH LABORATORY CO SUB SMITHKLINE BECKMA
COMPAZINE, PROCHLORPERAZINE EDISYLATE
PARNATE, TRANYLCYPROMINE SULFATE

SMITHKLINE
* SMITHKLINE CONSUMER PRODUCTS DIV SMITHKLINE AND FRENCH LAB
CONTAC, CHLORPHENIRAMINE MALEATE (OTC)
TELDRIN, CHLORPHENIRAMINE MALEATE (OTC)

SMITHKLINE BEECHAM
* SMITHKLINE BEECHAM INC
AUGMENTIN 125, AMOXICILLIN
AUGMENTIN 250, AMOXICILLIN
* SMITHKLINE BEECHAM PHARMACEUTICALS
AMOXIL, AMOXICILLIN
ANCEF, CEFAZOLIN SODIUM
ANSPOR, CEPHRADINE
AUGMENTIN '125', AMOXICILLIN
AUGMENTIN '250', AMOXICILLIN
AUGMENTIN '500', AMOXICILLIN
BACTOCILL, OXACILLIN SODIUM
BACTROBAN, MUPIROCIN
BEEPEN-VK, PENICILLIN V POTASSIUM
CEFAZOLIN SODIUM, CEFAZOLIN SODIUM
CLOXAPEN, CLOXACILLIN SODIUM
COMPAZINE, PROCHLORPERAZINE
COMPAZINE, PROCHLORPERAZINE EDISYLATE
COMPAZINE, PROCHLORPERAZINE MALEATE
CYTOMEL, LIOTHYRONINE SODIUM
DARBID, ISOPROPAMIDE IODIDE
DEXEDRINE, DEXTROAMPHETAMINE SULFATE
DIBENZYLINE, PHENOXYBENZAMINE HYDROCHLORIDE
DYAZIDE, HYDROCHLOROTHIAZIDE
DYCILL, DICLOXACILLIN SODIUM
DYRENIUM, TRIAMTERENE
ESKALITH, LITHIUM CARBONATE
ESKALITH CR, LITHIUM CARBONATE
FASTIN, PHENTERMINE HYDROCHLORIDE

APPENDIX B
PRODUCT NAME INDEX
LISTED BY APPLICANT *(continued)*

HALFAN, HALOFANTRINE HYDROCHLORIDE
HISPRIL, DIPHENYLPYRALINE HYDROCHLORIDE
KYTRIL, GRANISETRON HYDROCHLORIDE
LAROTID, AMOXICILLIN
MENEST, ESTROGENS, ESTERIFIED
MONOCID, CEFONICID SODIUM
NALLPEN, NAFCILLIN SODIUM
ORNADE, CHLORPHENIRAMINE MALEATE
PAXIL, PAROXETINE HYDROCHLORIDE
PENTACEF, CEFTAZIDIME (ARGININE FORMULATION)
PHYTONADIONE, PHYTONADIONE
PYOPEN, CARBENICILLIN DISODIUM
QUINIDINE SULFATE, QUINIDINE SULFATE
RELAFEN, NABUMETONE
RIDAURA, AURANOFIN
STELAZINE, TRIFLUOPERAZINE HYDROCHLORIDE
STOXIL, IDOXURIDINE
TAGAMET, CIMETIDINE
TAGAMET, CIMETIDINE HYDROCHLORIDE
TAGAMET HCL IN SODIUM CHLORIDE 0.9%, CIMETIDINE HYDROCHLORID
TAZICEF, CEFTAZIDIME
THORAZINE, CHLORPROMAZINE
THORAZINE, CHLORPROMAZINE HYDROCHLORIDE
TICAR, TICARCILLIN DISODIUM
TIGAN, TRIMETHOBENZAMIDE HYDROCHLORIDE
TIMENTIN, CLAVULANATE POTASSIUM
TOTACILLIN, AMPICILLIN/AMPICILLIN TRIHYDRATE
TOTACILLIN-N, AMPICILLIN SODIUM
TRIOSTAT, LIOTHYRONINE SODIUM
URISPAS, FLAVOXATE HYDROCHLORIDE
VONTROL, DIPHENIDOL HYDROCHLORIDE

* SMITHKLINE BEECHAM PHARMACEUTICALS CO
FAMVIR, FAMCICLOVIR
MONOCID, CEFONICID SODIUM
TAZICEF, CEFTAZIDIME

SOLA BARNES HIND

* SOLA BARNES HIND
ALPHA CHYMAR, CHYMOTRYPSIN
BENOXINATE HCL, BENOXINATE HYDROCHLORIDE
CYCLOPENTOLATE HCL, CYCLOPENTOLATE HYDROCHLORIDE
DEXAMETHASONE SODIUM PHOSPHATE, DEXAMETHASONE SODIUM PHOSPHATE
GAMENE, LINDANE
PREDNISOLONE SODIUM PHOSPHATE, PREDNISOLONE SODIUM PHOSPHATE
PROPARACAINE HCL, PROPARACAINE HYDROCHLORIDE
SODIUM SULFACETAMIDE, SULFACETAMIDE SODIUM
SULFISOXAZOLE DIOLAMINE, SULFISOXAZOLE DIOLAMINE

SOLOPAK

* SOLOPAK LABORATORIES INC
CLINDAMYCIN PHOSPHATE, CLINDAMYCIN PHOSPHATE
DROPERIDOL, DROPERIDOL
GENTAMICIN SULFATE, GENTAMICIN SULFATE
HALOPERIDOL, HALOPERIDOL LACTATE
HYDRALAZINE HCL, HYDRALAZINE HYDROCHLORIDE
HYDROXYZINE HCL, HYDROXYZINE HYDROCHLORIDE
KANAMYCIN SULFATE, KANAMYCIN SULFATE

* SOLOPAK MEDICAL PRODUCTS INC
CYANOCOBALAMIN, CYANOCOBALAMIN
HALOPERIDOL, HALOPERIDOL LACTATE
HEPARIN LOCK FLUSH, HEPARIN SODIUM
HEPARIN SODIUM, HEPARIN SODIUM
HYDROXYZINE HCL, HYDROXYZINE HYDROCHLORIDE
NALOXONE HCL, NALOXONE HYDROCHLORIDE
PHENYTOIN SODIUM, PHENYTOIN SODIUM
PROCAINAMIDE HCL, PROCAINAMIDE HYDROCHLORIDE
PROPRANOLOL HCL, PROPRANOLOL HYDROCHLORIDE
TRIMETHOBENZAMIDE HCL, TRIMETHOBENZAMIDE HYDROCHLORIDE
VERAPAMIL HCL, VERAPAMIL HYDROCHLORIDE

SOLVAY

* SOLVAY PHARMACEUTICALS
AQUATAG, BENZTHIAZIDE
ARESTOCAINE HCL, MEPIVACAINE HYDROCHLORIDE
ARESTOCAINE HCL W/ LEVONORDEFRIN, LEVONORDEFRIN
BALNEOL-HC, HYDROCORTISONE
BUTABARBITAL SODIUM, BUTABARBITAL SODIUM
CHENIX, CHENODIOL
CIN-QUIN, QUINIDINE SULFATE
CORTENEMA, HYDROCORTISONE
CURRETAB, MEDROXYPROGESTERONE ACETATE
DERMACORT, HYDROCORTISONE
DEXONE 0.5, DEXAMETHASONE
DEXONE 0.75, DEXAMETHASONE
DEXONE 1.5, DEXAMETHASONE
DEXONE 4, DEXAMETHASONE
DUPHALAC, LACTULOSE
ESTRAGUARD, DIENESTROL
ESTRATAB, ESTROGENS, ESTERIFIED
GYNOREST, DYDROGESTERONE
HYDRALAZINE HCL AND HYDROCHLOROTHIAZIDE, HYDRALAZINE HYDROCHLORIDE
HYDROCHLOROTHIAZIDE, HYDROCHLOROTHIAZIDE
LACTULOSE, LACTULOSE
LITHONATE, LITHIUM CARBONATE
LITHOTABS, LITHIUM CARBONATE
MELFIAT, PHENDIMETRAZINE TARTRATE
MELFIAT-105, PHENDIMETRAZINE TARTRATE
MEPROBAMATE, MEPROBAMATE
METHOCARBAMOL, METHOCARBAMOL
ORASONE, PREDNISONE
PHENDIMETRAZINE TARTRATE, PHENDIMETRAZINE TARTRATE
PORTALAC, LACTULOSE
PROCTOCORT, HYDROCORTISONE
PROVAL #3, ACETAMINOPHEN
PYRIDOSTIGMINE BROMIDE, PYRIDOSTIGMINE BROMIDE
R-P MYCIN, ERYTHROMYCIN
RAUWOLFIA SERPENTINA, RAUWOLFIA SERPENTINA
RESERPINE, RESERPINE
RESERPINE, HYDRALAZINE HCL AND HYDROCHLOROTHIAZIDE, HYDRALAZINE HYDROCHLORIDE
RETET, TETRACYCLINE HYDROCHLORIDE
ROWASA, MESALAMINE
S.A.S.-500, SULFASALAZINE
SER-A-GEN, HYDRALAZINE HYDROCHLORIDE
SPRX-105, PHENDIMETRAZINE TARTRATE

APPENDIX B
PRODUCT NAME INDEX
LISTED BY APPLICANT *(continued)*

SPRX-3, PHENDIMETRAZINE TARTRATE
SULSOXIN, SULFISOXAZOLE
SYMADINE, AMANTADINE HYDROCHLORIDE
TORA, PHENTERMINE HYDROCHLORIDE
TRANMEP, MEPROBAMATE
TRIACORT, TRIAMCINOLONE ACETONIDE
UNIPRES, HYDRALAZINE HYDROCHLORIDE
VERMIDOL, PIPERAZINE CITRATE
ZIDE, HYDROCHLOROTHIAZIDE

SOMERSET
* SOMERSET PHARMACEUTICALS INC
ELDEPRYL, SELEGILINE HYDROCHLORIDE

SORIN BIOMEDICA (US)
* SORIN BIOMEDICA SPA
AN-MAA, TECHNETIUM TC-99M ALBUMIN AGGREGATED KIT
IODOHIPPURATE SODIUM I 131, IODOHIPPURATE SODIUM, I-131
SODIUM ROSE BENGAL I 131, ROSE BENGAL SODIUM, I-131

SPERTI
* SPERTI DRUG PRODUCTS INC
PREDNISOLONE, PREDNISOLONE
PREDNISONE, PREDNISONE

SQUIBB
* ER SQUIBB AND SONS INC
AMITID, AMITRIPTYLINE HYDROCHLORIDE
AMNESTROGEN, ESTROGENS, ESTERIFIED
AZACTAM, AZTREONAM
CAPOZIDE 25/15, CAPTOPRIL
CAPOZIDE 25/25, CAPTOPRIL
CAPOZIDE 50/15, CAPTOPRIL
CAPOZIDE 50/25, CAPTOPRIL
CORGARD, NADOLOL
CORZIDE, BENDROFLUMETHIAZIDE
DELADUMONE, ESTRADIOL VALERATE
DELADUMONE OB, ESTRADIOL VALERATE
DELALUTIN, HYDROXYPROGESTERONE CAPROATE
DELESTROGEN, ESTRADIOL VALERATE
ETHRIL 250, ERYTHROMYCIN STEARATE
ETHRIL 500, ERYTHROMYCIN STEARATE
FLORINEF, FLUDROCORTISONE ACETATE
FOLLUTEIN, GONADOTROPIN, CHORIONIC
HYDREA, HYDROXYUREA
KENACORT, TRIAMCINOLONE
KENACORT, TRIAMCINOLONE DIACETATE
KENALOG IN ORABASE, TRIAMCINOLONE ACETONIDE
MYCOSTATIN, NYSTATIN
NATURETIN-10, BENDROFLUMETHIAZIDE
NATURETIN-2.5, BENDROFLUMETHIAZIDE
NATURETIN-5, BENDROFLUMETHIAZIDE
NEOMYCIN SULFATE, NEOMYCIN SULFATE
NYDRAZID, ISONIAZID
OPHTHAINE, PROPARACAINE HYDROCHLORIDE
ORA-TESTRYL, FLUOXYMESTERONE
PRONESTYL, PROCAINAMIDE HYDROCHLORIDE
PROTAMINE ZINC INSULIN, INSULIN SUSP PROTAMINE ZINC PURIFIED BEEF (OTC)
RAU-SED, RESERPINE
REZIPAS, AMINOSALICYLIC ACID RESIN COMPLEX
RUBRAMIN PC, CYANOCOBALAMIN
STILBESTROL, DIETHYLSTILBESTROL
STILBETIN, DIETHYLSTILBESTROL
SUCOSTRIN, SUCCINYLCHOLINE CHLORIDE
SUMYCIN, TETRACYCLINE HYDROCHLORIDE
TERFONYL, TRISULFAPYRIMIDINES (SULFADIAZINE;SULFAMERAZINE;SULFAMETHAZINE)
TESLAC, TESTOLACTONE
TUBOCURARINE CHLORIDE, TUBOCURARINE CHLORIDE
VELOSEF, CEPHRADINE
VESPRIN, TRIFLUPROMAZINE HYDROCHLORIDE
VITAMIN A, VITAMIN A PALMITATE
* SQUIBB SPA
PENICILLIN G SODIUM, PENICILLIN G SODIUM

SQUIBB MARK
* SQUIBB MARK DIV ER SQUIBB AND SONS INC
CEPHALEXIN, CEPHALEXIN

STANLABS
* STANLABS PHARMACEUTICAL CO SUB SIMPAK CORP
MEPROBAMATE, MEPROBAMATE

STAR PHARMS FL
* STAR PHARMACEUTICALS INC
VIRILON, METHYLTESTOSTERONE

STERIS
* STERIS LABORATORIES INC
AMITRIPTYLINE HCL, AMITRIPTYLINE HYDROCHLORIDE
BETAMETHASONE SODIUM PHOSPHATE, BETAMETHASONE SODIUM PHOSPHATE
BROMPHENIRAMINE MALEATE, BROMPHENIRAMINE MALEATE
CHLORAMPHENICOL, CHLORAMPHENICOL
CHLORPHENIRAMINE MALEATE, CHLORPHENIRAMINE MALEATE
CHLORPROMAZINE HCL, CHLORPROMAZINE HYDROCHLORIDE
CHORIONIC GONADOTROPIN, GONADOTROPIN, CHORIONIC
CLINDAMYCIN PHOSPHATE, CLINDAMYCIN PHOSPHATE
COBAVITE, CYANOCOBALAMIN
CORTICOTROPIN, CORTICOTROPIN
CORTISONE ACETATE, CORTISONE ACETATE
CYANOCOBALAMIN, CYANOCOBALAMIN
CYCLOPENTOLATE HCL, CYCLOPENTOLATE HYDROCHLORIDE
DEXAMETHASONE, DEXAMETHASONE
DEXAMETHASONE ACETATE, DEXAMETHASONE ACETATE
DEXAMETHASONE SODIUM PHOSPHATE, DEXAMETHASONE SODIUM PHOSPHATE
DIAZEPAM, DIAZEPAM
DICYCLOMINE HCL, DICYCLOMINE HYDROCHLORIDE
DIMENHYDRINATE, DIMENHYDRINATE
DIPHENHYDRAMINE HCL, DIPHENHYDRAMINE HYDROCHLORIDE
DISODIUM EDETATE, EDETATE DISODIUM
DOBUTAMINE HCL, DOBUTAMINE HYDROCHLORIDE
DOXAPRAM HCL, DOXAPRAM HYDROCHLORIDE
DROPERIDOL, DROPERIDOL
EDETATE DISODIUM, EDETATE DISODIUM
ESTRADIOL CYPIONATE, ESTRADIOL CYPIONATE
ESTRADIOL VALERATE, ESTRADIOL VALERATE
ESTRONE, ESTRONE
FENTANYL CITRATE, FENTANYL CITRATE

APPENDIX B
PRODUCT NAME INDEX
LISTED BY APPLICANT *(continued)*

FLUOROURACIL, FLUOROURACIL
FUROSEMIDE, FUROSEMIDE
GENTAMICIN SULFATE, GENTAMICIN SULFATE
GLYCOPYRROLATE, GLYCOPYRROLATE
HALOPERIDOL, HALOPERIDOL LACTATE
HEPARIN LOCK FLUSH, HEPARIN SODIUM
HEPARIN SODIUM, HEPARIN SODIUM
HYDROCORTISONE ACETATE, HYDROCORTISONE ACETATE
HYDROCORTISONE SODIUM SUCCINATE, HYDROCORTISONE SODIUM SUCCINATE
HYDROXOCOBALAMIN, HYDROXOCOBALAMIN
HYDROXYPROGESTERONE CAPROATE, HYDROXYPROGESTERONE CAPROATE
HYDROXYZINE HCL, HYDROXYZINE HYDROCHLORIDE
KANAMYCIN SULFATE, KANAMYCIN SULFATE
LIDOCAINE HCL, LIDOCAINE HYDROCHLORIDE
LIDOCAINE HCL W/ EPINEPHRINE, EPINEPHRINE
LINCOMYCIN HCL, LINCOMYCIN HYDROCHLORIDE
LORAZEPAM, LORAZEPAM
MANNITOL 25%, MANNITOL
MEPERIDINE HCL, MEPERIDINE HYDROCHLORIDE
MEPIVACAINE HCL, MEPIVACAINE HYDROCHLORIDE
MERSALYL-THEOPHYLLINE, MERSALYL SODIUM
METHOCARBAMOL, METHOCARBAMOL
METHYLPREDNISOLONE ACETATE, METHYLPREDNISOLONE ACETATE
METHYLPREDNISOLONE SODIUM SUCCINATE, METHYLPREDNISOLONE SODIUM SUCCINATE
METOPROLOL TARTRATE, METOPROLOL TARTRATE
METRONIDAZOLE, METRONIDAZOLE
MORPHINE SULFATE, MORPHINE SULFATE
MVC PLUS, ASCORBIC ACID
NALOXONE HCL, NALOXONE HYDROCHLORIDE
NANDROLONE DECANOATE, NANDROLONE DECANOATE
NANDROLONE PHENPROPIONATE, NANDROLONE PHENPROPIONATE
NATURAL ESTROGENIC SUBSTANCE-ESTRONE, ESTRONE
NEO-OTOSOL-HC, HYDROCORTISONE
NEOMYCIN AND POLYMYXIN B SULFATES, NEOMYCIN SULFATE
NEOMYCIN AND POLYMYXIN B SULFATES AND DEXAMETHASONE, DEXAMETHASONE
NEOMYCIN AND POLYMYXIN B SULFATES AND GRAMICIDIN, GRAMICIDIN
NEOMYCIN AND POLYMYXIN B SULFATES AND HYDROCORTISONE, HYDROCORTISONE
NEOMYCIN SULFATE-DEXAMETHASONE SODIUM PHOSPHATE, DEXAMETHASONE SODIUM PHOSPHATE
ORPHENADRINE CITRATE, ORPHENADRINE CITRATE
OTOCORT, HYDROCORTISONE
PHENYTOIN SODIUM, PHENYTOIN SODIUM
POTASSIUM CHLORIDE, POTASSIUM CHLORIDE
PREDNISOLONE ACETATE, PREDNISOLONE ACETATE
PREDNISOLONE SODIUM PHOSPHATE, PREDNISOLONE SODIUM PHOSPHATE
PREDNISOLONE TEBUTATE, PREDNISOLONE TEBUTATE
PROCAINAMIDE HCL, PROCAINAMIDE HYDROCHLORIDE
PROCAINE HCL, PROCAINE HYDROCHLORIDE
PROCHLORPERAZINE EDISYLATE, PROCHLORPERAZINE EDISYLATE
PROGESTERONE, PROGESTERONE
PROMAZINE HCL, PROMAZINE HYDROCHLORIDE
PROMETHAZINE HCL, PROMETHAZINE HYDROCHLORIDE
PYRIDOXINE HCL, PYRIDOXINE HYDROCHLORIDE
SULFACETAMIDE SODIUM, SULFACETAMIDE SODIUM
SULFACETAMIDE SODIUM AND PREDNISOLONE SODIUM PHOSPHATE, PREDNISOLONE SODIUM PHOSPHATE
SULFAMETHOXAZOLE AND TRIMETHOPRIM, SULFAMETHOXAZOLE
TESTOSTERONE, TESTOSTERONE
TESTOSTERONE CYPIONATE, TESTOSTERONE CYPIONATE
TESTOSTERONE CYPIONATE-ESTRADIOL CYPIONATE, ESTRADIOL CYPIONATE
TESTOSTERONE ENANTHATE, TESTOSTERONE ENANTHATE
TESTOSTERONE ENANTHATE AND ESTRADIOL VALERATE, ESTRADIOL VALERATE
TESTOSTERONE PROPIONATE, TESTOSTERONE PROPIONATE
THIAMINE HCL, THIAMINE HYDROCHLORIDE
TOBRAMYCIN, TOBRAMYCIN
TRIAMCINOLONE ACETONIDE, TRIAMCINOLONE ACETONIDE
TRIAMCINOLONE DIACETATE, TRIAMCINOLONE DIACETATE
TRIMETHOBENZAMIDE HCL, TRIMETHOBENZAMIDE HYDROCHLORIDE
TROPICAMIDE, TROPICAMIDE

STERLING WINTHROP
* STERLING WINTHROP INC
AFAXIN, VITAMIN A PALMITATE
AMIPAQUE, METRIZAMIDE
ARALEN, CHLOROQUINE PHOSPHATE
ARALEN HCL, CHLOROQUINE HYDROCHLORIDE
ARALEN PHOSPHATE W/ PRIMAQUINE PHOSPHATE, CHLOROQUINE PHOSPHATE
ATROPINE AND DEMEROL, ATROPINE SULFATE
BILOPAQUE, TYROPANOATE SODIUM
BRONKAID MIST, EPINEPHRINE (OTC)
BRONKODYL, THEOPHYLLINE
BRONKOMETER, ISOETHARINE MESYLATE
BRONKOSOL, ISOETHARINE HYDROCHLORIDE
BRYREL, PIPERAZINE CITRATE
CARBOCAINE, MEPIVACAINE HYDROCHLORIDE
DANOCRINE, DANAZOL
DEMEROL, MEPERIDINE HYDROCHLORIDE
DIAZEPAM, DIAZEPAM
DRISDOL, ERGOCALCIFEROL
FENTANYL CITRATE, FENTANYL CITRATE
FUROSEMIDE, FUROSEMIDE
HEPARIN LOCK FLUSH, HEPARIN SODIUM
HEPARIN SODIUM, HEPARIN SODIUM
HEPARIN SODIUM PRESERVATIVE FREE, HEPARIN SODIUM
HYDROXYZINE HCL, HYDROXYZINE HYDROCHLORIDE
HYPAQUE, DIATRIZOATE MEGLUMINE
HYPAQUE, DIATRIZOATE SODIUM
HYPAQUE SODIUM 20%, DIATRIZOATE SODIUM
HYPAQUE-CYSTO, DIATRIZOATE MEGLUMINE
HYPAQUE-M,75%, DIATRIZOATE MEGLUMINE
HYPAQUE-M,90%, DIATRIZOATE MEGLUMINE
HYPAQUE-76, DIATRIZOATE MEGLUMINE

APPENDIX B
PRODUCT NAME INDEX
LISTED BY APPLICANT *(continued)*

INOCOR, AMRINONE LACTATE
ISOPAQUE 280, CALCIUM
ISOPAQUE 440, CALCIUM METRIZOATE
ISUPREL, ISOPROTERENOL HYDROCHLORIDE
KAYEXALATE, SODIUM POLYSTYRENE SULFONATE
LEVOPHED, NOREPINEPHRINE BITARTRATE
LIDOCAINE HCL AND EPINEPHRINE, EPINEPHRINE
LORAZEPAM, LORAZEPAM
LOTUSATE, TALBUTAL
MARCAINE, BUPIVACAINE HYDROCHLORIDE
MARCAINE HCL, BUPIVACAINE HYDROCHLORIDE
MARCAINE HCL W/ EPINEPHRINE, BUPIVACAINE HYDROCHLORIDE
MEASURIN, ASPIRIN (OTC)
METOPROLOL TARTRATE, METOPROLOL TARTRATE
MODRASTANE, TRILOSTANE
MYTELASE, AMBENONIUM CHLORIDE
NALOXONE HCL, NALOXONE HYDROCHLORIDE
NEGGRAM, NALIDIXIC ACID
NOVOCAIN, PROCAINE HYDROCHLORIDE
OMNIPAQUE 140, IOHEXOL
OMNIPAQUE 180, IOHEXOL
OMNIPAQUE 210, IOHEXOL
OMNIPAQUE 240, IOHEXOL
OMNIPAQUE 300, IOHEXOL
OMNIPAQUE 350, IOHEXOL
OMNIPAQUE 70, IOHEXOL
PHISO-SCRUB, HEXACHLOROPHENE
PHISOHEX, HEXACHLOROPHENE
PLAQUENIL, HYDROXYCHLOROQUINE SULFATE
PRIMACOR, MILRINONE LACTATE
PRIMAQUINE, PRIMAQUINE PHOSPHATE
PROCHLORPERAZINE EDISYLATE, PROCHLORPERAZINE EDISYLATE
PROMETHAZINE HCL, PROMETHAZINE HYDROCHLORIDE
RAVOCAINE AND NOVOCAIN W/ LEVOPHED, NOREPINEPHRINE BITARTRAT
RAVOCAINE AND NOVOCAIN W/ NEO-COBEFRIN, LEVONORDEFRIN
SULFAMETHOXAZOLE AND TRIMETHOPRIM, SULFAMETHOXAZOLE
TALACEN, ACETAMINOPHEN
TALWIN, PENTAZOCINE LACTATE
TALWIN COMPOUND, ASPIRIN
TALWIN NX, NALOXONE HYDROCHLORIDE
TALWIN 50, PENTAZOCINE HYDROCHLORIDE
TELEPAQUE, IOPANOIC ACID
TORNALATE, BITOLTEROL MESYLATE
TRANCOPAL, CHLORMEZANONE
TRIMETHOBENZAMIDE HCL, TRIMETHOBENZAMIDE HYDROCHLORIDE
VERAPAMIL HCL, VERAPAMIL HYDROCHLORIDE
WINSTROL, STANOZOLOL
8-HOUR BAYER, ASPIRIN (OTC)

* STERLING WINTHROP INC PHARMACEUTICALS RESEARCH DIV
OMNISCAN, GADODIAMIDE
PRIMACOR IN DEXTROSE 5%, MILRINONE LACTATE
TORNALATE, BITOLTEROL MESYLATE

STEVENS J

* JEROME STEVENS PHARMACEUTICALS INC
CEPHALEXIN, CEPHALEXIN

STIEFEL

* STIEFEL LABORATORIES INC
ERYTHROMYCIN, ERYTHROMYCIN
HYDROCORTISONE, HYDROCORTISONE
SCABENE, LINDANE
STIE-CORT, HYDROCORTISONE

STUART

* STUART PHARMACEUTICALS DIV ICI AMERICAS
BUCLADIN-S, BUCLIZINE HYDROCHLORIDE

SUPERPHARM

* SUPERPHARM CORP
ACETAMINOPHEN AND CODEINE PHOSPHATE #2, ACETAMINOPHEN
ACETAMINOPHEN AND CODEINE PHOSPHATE #3, ACETAMINOPHEN
ACETAMINOPHEN AND CODEINE PHOSPHATE #4, ACETAMINOPHEN
ALLOPURINOL, ALLOPURINOL
AMITRIPTYLINE HCL, AMITRIPTYLINE HYDROCHLORIDE
CHLORDIAZEPOXIDE HCL, CHLORDIAZEPOXIDE HYDROCHLORIDE
CHLORPHENIRAMINE MALEATE, CHLORPHENIRAMINE MALEATE
CHLORPROPAMIDE, CHLORPROPAMIDE
CHLORTHALIDONE, CHLORTHALIDONE
CYPROHEPTADINE HCL, CYPROHEPTADINE HYDROCHLORIDE
DIPHENHYDRAMINE HCL, DIPHENHYDRAMINE HYDROCHLORIDE
DISOPYRAMIDE PHOSPHATE, DISOPYRAMIDE PHOSPHATE
DOXYCYCLINE HYCLATE, DOXYCYCLINE HYCLATE
ERGOLOID MESYLATES, ERGOLOID MESYLATES
FLURAZEPAM HCL, FLURAZEPAM HYDROCHLORIDE
FUROSEMIDE, FUROSEMIDE
HYDRALAZINE HCL, HYDRALAZINE HYDROCHLORIDE
HYDRALAZINE HCL AND HYDROCHLOROTHIAZIDE, HYDRALAZINE HYDROCHLORIDE
HYDROCHLOROTHIAZIDE, HYDROCHLOROTHIAZIDE
HYDROXYZINE HCL, HYDROXYZINE HYDROCHLORIDE
HYDROXYZINE PAMOATE, HYDROXYZINE PAMOATE
IBUPROFEN, IBUPROFEN
INDOMETHACIN, INDOMETHACIN
ISOSORBIDE DINITRATE, ISOSORBIDE DINITRATE
LOGEN, ATROPINE SULFATE
LORAZEPAM, LORAZEPAM
MECLIZINE HCL, MECLIZINE HYDROCHLORIDE
METHOCARBAMOL, METHOCARBAMOL
METHYLDOPA, METHYLDOPA
METOCLOPRAMIDE HCL, METOCLOPRAMIDE HYDROCHLORIDE
METRONIDAZOLE, METRONIDAZOLE
PREDNISOLONE, PREDNISOLONE
PREDNISONE, PREDNISONE
PROPOXYPHENE NAPSYLATE AND ACETAMINOPHEN, ACETAMINOPHEN
PROPRANOLOL HCL, PROPRANOLOL HYDROCHLORIDE
QUINIDINE GLUCONATE, QUINIDINE GLUCONATE
QUINIDINE SULFATE, QUINIDINE SULFATE
SPIRONOLACTONE, SPIRONOLACTONE
SPIRONOLACTONE AND HYDROCHLOROTHIAZIDE, HYDROCHLOROTHIAZIDE
SULFASALAZINE, SULFASALAZINE
SULFATRIM-DS, SULFAMETHOXAZOLE
SULFATRIM-SS, SULFAMETHOXAZOLE
TETRACYCLINE HCL, TETRACYCLINE HYDROCHLORIDE

APPENDIX B
PRODUCT NAME INDEX
LISTED BY APPLICANT *(continued)*

THIORIDAZINE HCL, THIORIDAZINE HYDROCHLORIDE
TOLAZAMIDE, TOLAZAMIDE
TOLBUTAMIDE, TOLBUTAMIDE
TRIPROLIDINE HCL AND PSEUDOEPHEDRINE HCL, PSEUDOEPHEDRINE HYDROCHLORIDE

SUPPOSITORIA
* SUPPOSITORIA LABORATORIES INC
ACETAMINOPHEN, ACETAMINOPHEN (OTC)

SURVIVAL TECH
* SURVIVAL TECHNOLOGY INC
ATROPEN, ATROPINE
EPIPEN, EPINEPHRINE
EPIPEN JR., EPINEPHRINE
LIDOPEN, LIDOCAINE HYDROCHLORIDE
MORPHINE SULFATE, MORPHINE SULFATE
PRALIDOXIME CHLORIDE, PRALIDOXIME CHLORIDE

SYNTEX
* SYNTEX (FP) INC
ANAPROX, NAPROXEN SODIUM
ANAPROX DS, NAPROXEN SODIUM
BREVICON 21-DAY, ETHINYL ESTRADIOL
BREVICON 28-DAY, ETHINYL ESTRADIOL
LEVORA 0.15/30-21, ETHINYL ESTRADIOL
LEVORA 0.15/30-28, ETHINYL ESTRADIOL
NAPROSYN, NAPROXEN
NOR-Q.D., NORETHINDRONE
NORINYL 1+35 21-DAY, ETHINYL ESTRADIOL
NORINYL 1+35 28-DAY, ETHINYL ESTRADIOL
NORINYL 1+50 28-DAY, MESTRANOL
NORINYL 1+80 21-DAY, MESTRANOL
NORINYL 1+80 28-DAY, MESTRANOL
NORQUEST FE, ETHINYL ESTRADIOL
TRI-NORINYL 21-DAY, ETHINYL ESTRADIOL
TRI-NORINYL 28-DAY, ETHINYL ESTRADIOL
* SYNTEX LABORATORIES INC SUB SYNTEX CORP
ACULAR, KETOROLAC TROMETHAMINE
AEROBID, FLUNISOLIDE
ANADROL-50, OXYMETHOLONE
CARDENE, NICARDIPINE HYDROCHLORIDE
CARDENE SR, NICARDIPINE HYDROCHLORIDE
CARMOL HC, HYDROCORTISONE ACETATE
CYTOVENE, GANCICLOVIR SODIUM
EVEX, ESTROGENS, ESTERIFIED
FEMSTAT, BUTOCONAZOLE NITRATE
LIDEX, FLUOCINONIDE
LIDEX-E, FLUOCINONIDE
NAPROSYN, NAPROXEN
NASALIDE, FLUNISOLIDE
NORINYL, MESTRANOL
NORINYL 1+50 21-DAY, MESTRANOL
SYNACORT, HYDROCORTISONE
SYNALAR, FLUOCINOLONE ACETONIDE
SYNALAR-HP, FLUOCINOLONE ACETONIDE
SYNAREL, NAFARELIN ACETATE
SYNEMOL, FLUOCINOLONE ACETONIDE
TICLID, TICLOPIDINE HYDROCHLORIDE
TORADOL, KETOROLAC TROMETHAMINE

SYOSSET
* SYOSSET LABORATORIES INC
C-SOLVE-2, ERYTHROMYCIN
E-SOLVE 2, ERYTHROMYCIN
FLUTEX, TRIAMCINOLONE ACETONIDE
HYDROCORTISONE, HYDROCORTISONE
NOGENIC HC, HYDROCORTISONE
SELENIUM SULFIDE, SELENIUM SULFIDE
TRIATEX, TRIAMCINOLONE ACETONIDE

T

TABLICAPS
* TABLICAPS INC
AMINOPHYLLINE, AMINOPHYLLINE
CHLORPHENIRAMINE MALEATE, CHLORPHENIRAMINE MALEATE
FOLIC ACID, FOLIC ACID
MEPROBAMATE, MEPROBAMATE
METHOCARBAMOL, METHOCARBAMOL
METHYLTESTOSTERONE, METHYLTESTOSTERONE
NIACIN, NIACIN
PREDNISOLONE, PREDNISOLONE
PROMETHAZINE HCL, PROMETHAZINE HYDROCHLORIDE
PROPANTHELINE BROMIDE, PROPANTHELINE BROMIDE
PROPYLTHIOURACIL, PROPYLTHIOURACIL
RAUWOLFIA SERPENTINA, RAUWOLFIA SERPENTINA
RESERPINE, RESERPINE
STILBESTROL, DIETHYLSTILBESTROL

TAG PHARMS
* TAG PHARMACEUTICALS INC
IBUPROFEN, IBUPROFEN (OTC)

TAKEDA
* TAKEDA CHEMICAL INDUSTRIES LTD
CERADON, CEFOTIAM HYDROCHLORIDE

TAP PHARMS
* TAP PHARMACEUTICALS INC
CEFMAX, CEFMENOXIME HYDROCHLORIDE
LUPRON, LEUPROLIDE ACETATE
LUPRON DEPOT, LEUPROLIDE ACETATE
LUPRON DEPOT-PED, LEUPROLIDE ACETATE

TARO
* TARO PHARMACEUTICALS USA INC
BETAMETHASONE DIPROPIONATE, BETAMETHASONE DIPROPIONATE
CLOTRIMAZOLE, CLOTRIMAZOLE
DERMABET, BETAMETHASONE VALERATE
DESONIDE, DESONIDE
DESOXIMETASONE, DESOXIMETASONE
FLUOCINONIDE, FLUOCINONIDE
NYSTATIN, NYSTATIN
NYSTATIN AND TRIAMCINOLONE ACETONIDE, NYSTATIN
ORACORT, TRIAMCINOLONE ACETONIDE

TECHNILAB
* TECHNILAB INC
ACILAC, LACTULOSE
LAXILOSE, LACTULOSE

THAMES
* THAMES PHARMACAL CO INC
ACETIC ACID, ACETIC ACID, GLACIAL
BETAMETHASONE DIPROPIONATE, BETAMETHASONE DIPROPIONATE
BETAMETHASONE VALERATE, BETAMETHASONE VALERATE

APPENDIX B
PRODUCT NAME INDEX
LISTED BY APPLICANT *(continued)*

FLUOCINOLONE ACETONIDE, FLUOCINOLONE ACETONIDE
FLUOCINONIDE, FLUOCINONIDE
GENTAMICIN SULFATE, GENTAMICIN SULFATE
HYDROCORTISONE, HYDROCORTISONE
HYDROCORTISONE AND ACETIC ACID, ACETIC ACID, GLACIAL
LIDOCAINE, LIDOCAINE
NITROFURAZONE, NITROFURAZONE
NYSTATIN, NYSTATIN
NYSTATIN AND TRIAMCINOLONE ACETONIDE, NYSTATIN
ORALONE, TRIAMCINOLONE ACETONIDE
SELENIUM SULFIDE, SELENIUM SULFIDE
THEOPHYLLINE, THEOPHYLLINE
TRIAMCINOLONE ACETONIDE, TRIAMCINOLONE ACETONIDE
U-CORT, HYDROCORTISONE ACETATE

TICAN
* TICAN PHARMACEUTICALS LTD
FLUOCINONIDE, FLUOCINONIDE

TOPIDERM
* TOPIDERM INC
HYDROCORTISONE, HYDROCORTISONE
TRIAMCINOLONE ACETONIDE, TRIAMCINOLONE ACETONIDE

TORCH LABS
* TORCH LABORATORIES INC
H-CORT, HYDROCORTISONE

U

UDL
* UDL LABORATORIES INC
FOLIC ACID, FOLIC ACID
LACTULOSE, LACTULOSE
MECLIZINE HCL, MECLIZINE HYDROCHLORIDE
PREDNISOLONE, PREDNISOLONE
PREDNISONE, PREDNISONE

UNIMED INC
* UNIMED INC
MARINOL, DRONABINOL

UNIV TX
* UNIV TEXAS HEALTH SCIENCE CENTER
POTASSIUM CITRATE, POTASSIUM CITRATE
TIOPRONIN, TIOPRONIN

UPJOHN
* UPJOHN CO
ALBAMYCIN, NOVOBIOCIN SODIUM
ALPHADROL, FLUPREDNISOLONE
ANSAID, FLURBIPROFEN
BACIGUENT, BACITRACIN
BACITRACIN, BACITRACIN
BERUBIGEN, CYANOCOBALAMIN
CARDASE, ETHOXZOLAMIDE
CARDRASE, ETHOXZOLAMIDE
CLEOCIN, CLINDAMYCIN HYDROCHLORIDE
CLEOCIN, CLINDAMYCIN PALMITATE HYDROCHLORIDE
CLEOCIN, CLINDAMYCIN PHOSPHATE
CLEOCIN HCL, CLINDAMYCIN HYDROCHLORIDE
CLEOCIN PHOSPHATE, CLINDAMYCIN PHOSPHATE
CLEOCIN PHOSPHATE IN DEXTROSE 5%, CLINDAMYCIN PHOSPHATE
CLEOCIN T, CLINDAMYCIN PHOSPHATE
COLESTID, COLESTIPOL HYDROCHLORIDE
CORTEF, HYDROCORTISONE
CORTEF, HYDROCORTISONE CYPIONATE
CORTEF ACETATE, HYDROCORTISONE ACETATE
CORTISONE ACETATE, CORTISONE ACETATE
CYTOSAR-U, CYTARABINE
DELTA-CORTEF, PREDNISOLONE
DELTASONE, PREDNISONE
DEPO-ESTRADIOL, ESTRADIOL CYPIONATE
DEPO-MEDROL, METHYLPREDNISOLONE ACETATE
DEPO-PROVERA, MEDROXYPROGESTERONE ACETATE
DEPO-TESTADIOL, ESTRADIOL CYPIONATE
DEPO-TESTOSTERONE, TESTOSTERONE CYPIONATE
DIDREX, BENZPHETAMINE HYDROCHLORIDE
DIFLORASONE DIACETATE, DIFLORASONE DIACETATE
E-MYCIN E, ERYTHROMYCIN ETHYLSUCCINATE
FEMINONE, ETHINYL ESTRADIOL
FLAVORED COLESTID, COLESTIPOL HYDROCHLORIDE
FLORONE, DIFLORASONE DIACETATE
GLYNASE, GLYBURIDE
HALCION, TRIAZOLAM
HALODRIN, ETHINYL ESTRADIOL
HALOTESTIN, FLUOXYMESTERONE
HEBAMATE, CARBOPROST TROMETHAMINE
HEPARIN SODIUM, HEPARIN SODIUM
HYLOREL, GUANADREL SULFATE
LINCOCIN, LINCOMYCIN HYDROCHLORIDE
LONITEN, MINOXIDIL
MAOLATE, CHLORPHENESIN CARBAMATE
MEDROL, METHYLPREDNISOLONE
MEDROL, METHYLPREDNISOLONE ACETATE
MEDROL ACETATE, METHYLPREDNISOLONE ACETATE
MICRONASE, GLYBURIDE
MOTRIN, IBUPROFEN
MYCIFRADIN, NEOMYCIN SULFATE
MYCITRACIN, BACITRACIN
NEO-CORTEF, HYDROCORTISONE ACETATE
NEO-DELTA-CORTEF, NEOMYCIN SULFATE
NEO-MEDROL, METHYLPREDNISOLONE
NEO-MEDROL ACETATE, METHYLPREDNISOLONE ACETATE
NUPRIN, IBUPROFEN (OTC)
ORINASE, TOLBUTAMIDE
ORINASE DIAGNOSTIC, TOLBUTAMIDE SODIUM
OXYLONE, FLUOROMETHOLONE
PANMYCIN, TETRACYCLINE HYDROCHLORIDE
PENICILLIN G SODIUM, PENICILLIN G SODIUM
PREPIDIL, DINOPROSTONE
PROSTIN E2, DINOPROSTONE
PROSTIN F2 ALPHA, DINOPROST TROMETHAMINE
PROSTIN VR PEDIATRIC, ALPROSTADIL
PROTAMINE SULFATE, PROTAMINE SULFATE
PROVERA, MEDROXYPROGESTERONE ACETATE
PSORCON, DIFLORASONE DIACETATE
ROGAINE, MINOXIDIL
SOLU-CORTEF, HYDROCORTISONE SODIUM SUCCINATE
SOLU-MEDROL, METHYLPREDNISOLONE SODIUM SUCCINATE

APPENDIX B
PRODUCT NAME INDEX
LISTED BY APPLICANT *(continued)*

TOLINASE, TOLAZAMIDE
TROBICIN, SPECTINOMYCIN HYDROCHLORIDE
U-GENCIN, GENTAMICIN SULFATE
UTICILLIN VK, PENICILLIN V POTASSIUM
XANAX, ALPRAZOLAM
ZANOSAR, STREPTOZOCIN
ZEFAZONE, CEFMETAZOLE SODIUM
* UPJOHN MANUFACTURING CO
CLEOCIN, CLINDAMYCIN HYDROCHLORIDE
CLEOCIN, CLINDAMYCIN PALMITATE HYDROCHLORIDE
CLEOCIN PHOSPHATE, CLINDAMYCIN PHOSPHATE
* UPJOHN TRADING CORP
VANTIN, CEFPODOXIME PROXETIL

UPSHER SMITH
* UPSHER SMITH LABORATORIES INC
ACETAMINOPHEN, ACETAMINOPHEN (OTC)
DEXAMETHASONE, DEXAMETHASONE
INFANTS' FEVERALL, ACETAMINOPHEN
KLOR-CON, POTASSIUM CHLORIDE
METHOCARBAMOL, METHOCARBAMOL
PREDNISONE, PREDNISONE
SPIRONOLACTONE, SPIRONOLACTONE
SPIRONOLACTONE W/ HYDROCHLOROTHIAZIDE, HYDROCHLOROTHIAZIDE

US ARMY
* UNITED STATES ARMY OFFICE SURGEON GENERAL
ATROPINE SULFATE, ATROPINE SULFATE
DIAZEPAM, DIAZEPAM
SODIUM THIOSULFATE, SODIUM THIOSULFATE
* UNITED STATES ARMY WALTER REED ARMY INSTITUTE RESEARCH
MEFLOQUINE HCL, MEFLOQUINE HYDROCHLORIDE

US BIOSCIENCE
* US BIOSCIENCE INC
HEXALEN, ALTRETAMINE
NEUTREXIN, TRIMETREXATE GLUCURONATE

US CHEM
* US CHEMICAL MARKETING GROUP INC
MEDIGESIC PLUS, ACETAMINOPHEN

V

VALE
* VALE CHEMICAL CO INC
AMINOPHYLLINE, AMINOPHYLLINE
RAUVAL, RAUWOLFIA SERPENTINA
SERPATE, RESERPINE
TRIPLE SULFOID, TRISULFAPYRIMIDINES (SULFADIAZINE;SULFAMERAZINE;SULFAMETHAZINE)

VANGARD
* VANGARD LABORATORIES INC DIV MIDWAY MEDICAL CO
ACETAZOLAMIDE, ACETAZOLAMIDE
AMINOPHYLLINE, AMINOPHYLLINE
AMITRIPTYLINE HCL, AMITRIPTYLINE HYDROCHLORIDE
CHLORDIAZEPOXIDE HCL, CHLORDIAZEPOXIDE HYDROCHLORIDE
CHLORPROMAZINE HCL, CHLORPROMAZINE HYDROCHLORIDE
CHLORTHALIDONE, CHLORTHALIDONE
DIPHENHYDRAMINE HCL, DIPHENHYDRAMINE HYDROCHLORIDE
ERGOLOID MESYLATES, ERGOLOID MESYLATES
FOLIC ACID, FOLIC ACID
HYDRALAZINE HCL, HYDRALAZINE HYDROCHLORIDE
HYDROCHLOROTHIAZIDE, HYDROCHLOROTHIAZIDE
HYDROXYZINE PAMOATE, HYDROXYZINE PAMOATE
IMIPRAMINE HCL, IMIPRAMINE HYDROCHLORIDE
LO-TROL, ATROPINE SULFATE
MECLIZINE HCL, MECLIZINE HYDROCHLORIDE
MEPROBAMATE, MEPROBAMATE
PAPA-DEINE #3, ACETAMINOPHEN
PAPA-DEINE #4, ACETAMINOPHEN
PREDNISONE, PREDNISONE
PROCAINAMIDE HCL, PROCAINAMIDE HYDROCHLORIDE
QUINIDINE SULFATE, QUINIDINE SULFATE
SPIRONOLACTONE, SPIRONOLACTONE
SPIRONOLACTONE W/ HYDROCHLOROTHIAZIDE, HYDROCHLOROTHIAZIDE
SULFINPYRAZONE, SULFINPYRAZONE
TOLBUTAMIDE, TOLBUTAMIDE
TRIHEXYPHENIDYL HCL, TRIHEXYPHENIDYL HYDROCHLORIDE

VESTAL LABS
* VESTAL LABORATORIES DIV CHEMED CORP
SEPTISOL, HEXACHLOROPHENE

VICKS
* VICKS HEALTH CARE DIV RICHARDSON VICKS INC
VICKS FORMULA 44, DIPHENHYDRAMINE HYDROCHLORIDE (OTC)

VINTAGE PHARMS
* VINTAGE PHARMACEUTICALS INC
ACETAMINOPHEN AND CODEINE PHOSPHATE, ACETAMINOPHEN
DOXYCYCLINE HYCLATE, DOXYCYCLINE HYCLATE
DOXYCYCLINE MONOHYDRATE, DOXYCYCLINE
FOLIC ACID, FOLIC ACID
HYDROCODONE BITARTRATE AND ACETAMINOPHEN, ACETAMINOPHEN
IBUPROFEN, IBUPROFEN
IBUPROFEN, IBUPROFEN (OTC)

VIRATEK
* VIRATEK INC
VIRAZOLE, RIBAVIRIN

VITARINE
* VITARINE PHARMACEUTICALS INC
ACETAMINOPHEN W/ CODEINE PHOSPHATE, ACETAMINOPHEN
AMPICILLIN, AMPICILLIN/AMPICILLIN TRIHYDRATE
BROMPHENIRAMINE MALEATE, BROMPHENIRAMINE MALEATE
CEPHALEXIN, CEPHALEXIN
CEPHRADINE, CEPHRADINE
CHLORPHENIRAMINE MALEATE, CHLORPHENIRAMINE MALEATE
CORTISONE ACETATE, CORTISONE ACETATE
CYPROHEPTADINE HCL, CYPROHEPTADINE HYDROCHLORIDE
DEXTROAMPHETAMINE SULFATE, DEXTROAMPHETAMINE SULFATE

APPENDIX B
PRODUCT NAME INDEX
LISTED BY APPLICANT *(continued)*

GLUTETHIMIDE, GLUTETHIMIDE
HYDRALAZINE HCL, HYDRALAZINE HYDROCHLORIDE
MECLOFENAMATE SODIUM, MECLOFENAMATE SODIUM
PENTOBARBITAL SODIUM, PENTOBARBITAL SODIUM
PHENDIMETRAZINE TARTRATE, PHENDIMETRAZINE TARTRATE
PHENTERMINE HCL, PHENTERMINE HYDROCHLORIDE
PREDNISOLONE, PREDNISOLONE
PREDNISONE, PREDNISONE
SECOBARBITAL SODIUM, SECOBARBITAL SODIUM
SERPIVITE, RESERPINE
SULFISOXAZOLE, SULFISOXAZOLE
TRIAMTERENE AND HYDROCHLOROTHIAZIDE, HYDROCHLOROTHIAZIDE
TRIPROLIDINE HCL, TRIPROLIDINE HYDROCHLORIDE
VITAMIN D, ERGOCALCIFEROL

VIVAN
* VIVAN PHARMACAL INC DIV ELLIS PHARMACEUTICAL CONSULTING IN
ALPHADERM, HYDROCORTISONE

W

WALLACE
* WALLACE LABORATORIES DIV CARTER WALLACE INC
AQUATENSEN, METHYCLOTHIAZIDE
BEPADIN, BEPRIDIL HYDROCHLORIDE
BUTICAPS, BUTABARBITAL SODIUM
BUTISOL SODIUM, BUTABARBITAL SODIUM
COLONAID, ATROPINE SULFATE
DEPEN 250, PENICILLAMINE
DIUTENSEN-R, METHYCLOTHIAZIDE
DORAL, QUAZEPAM
FELBATOL, FELBAMATE
HYZYD, ISONIAZID
LUFYLLIN, DYPHYLLINE
MYLAXEN, HEXAFLUORENIUM BROMIDE
NEOPASALATE, AMINOSALICYLATE SODIUM
RONDOMYCIN, METHACYCLINE HYDROCHLORIDE
SOMA, CARISOPRODOL
THYRO-BLOCK, POTASSIUM IODIDE (OTC)
UNITENSEN, CRYPTENAMINE ACETATES
UNITENSEN, CRYPTENAMINE TANNATES
VERTAVIS, VERATRUM VIRIDE
VOSOL, ACETIC ACID, GLACIAL
VOSOL HC, ACETIC ACID, GLACIAL
WAMPOCAP, NIACIN

WALLACE PHARMS
* WALLACE PHARMACEUTICALS DIV CARTER WALLACE INC
DORMATE, MEBUTAMATE
MEPROSPAN, MEPROBAMATE
MICRAININ, ASPIRIN
MILPREM-200, ESTROGENS, CONJUGATED
MILPREM-400, ESTROGENS, CONJUGATED
MILTOWN, MEPROBAMATE
SOMA COMPOUND, ASPIRIN
SOMA COMPOUND W/ CODEINE, ASPIRIN

WARNER CHILCOTT
* WARNER CHILCOTT DIV WARNER LAMBERT CO
ACETAMINOPHEN AND CODEINE PHOSPHATE, ACETAMINOPHEN
ACETAMINOPHEN W/ CODEINE PHOSPHATE, ACETAMINOPHEN
ALBUTEROL SULFATE, ALBUTEROL SULFATE
AMITRIL, AMITRIPTYLINE HYDROCHLORIDE
CARBAMAZEPINE, CARBAMAZEPINE
CHLORTHALIDONE, CHLORTHALIDONE
CLONIDINE HCL, CLONIDINE HYDROCHLORIDE
CLORAZEPATE DIPOTASSIUM, CLORAZEPATE DIPOTASSIUM
CYCLOPAR, TETRACYCLINE HYDROCHLORIDE
DIAZEPAM, DIAZEPAM
DOPAMINE HCL, DOPAMINE HYDROCHLORIDE
DOXYCYCLINE HYCLATE, DOXYCYCLINE HYCLATE
DURAQUIN, QUINIDINE GLUCONATE
ERYPAR, ERYTHROMYCIN STEARATE
FENOPROFEN CALCIUM, FENOPROFEN CALCIUM
FLURAZEPAM HCL, FLURAZEPAM HYDROCHLORIDE
FUROSEMIDE, FUROSEMIDE
HYDROCHLOROTHIAZIDE, HYDROCHLOROTHIAZIDE
KANAMYCIN SULFATE, KANAMYCIN SULFATE
LORAZEPAM, LORAZEPAM
MINOCYCLINE HCL, MINOCYCLINE HYDROCHLORIDE
PHENYTOIN SODIUM, PHENYTOIN SODIUM
PROCAINAMIDE HCL, PROCAINAMIDE HYDROCHLORIDE
PROPOXYPHENE HCL 65, PROPOXYPHENE HYDROCHLORIDE
PROPRANOLOL HCL, PROPRANOLOL HYDROCHLORIDE
PROPRANOLOL HCL AND HYDROCHLOROTHIAZIDE, HYDROCHLOROTHIAZIDE
QUINIDINE SULFATE, QUINIDINE SULFATE
SPIRONOLACTONE, SPIRONOLACTONE
SULINDAC, SULINDAC
TETRACYCLINE HCL, TETRACYCLINE HYDROCHLORIDE
VERAPAMIL HCL, VERAPAMIL HYDROCHLORIDE

WARNER WELLCOME
* WARNER WELLCOME CONSUMER HEALTH PRODUCTS
NIX, PERMETHRIN (OTC)
SUDAFED 12 HOUR, PSEUDOEPHEDRINE HYDROCHLORIDE (OTC)

WATSON LABS
* WATSON LABORATORIES INC
ALBUTEROL SULFATE, ALBUTEROL SULFATE
AMOXAPINE, AMOXAPINE
CARBIDOPA AND LEVODOPA, CARBIDOPA
CLORAZEPATE DIPOTASSIUM, CLORAZEPATE DIPOTASSIUM
CYCLOBENZAPRINE HCL, CYCLOBENZAPRINE HYDROCHLORIDE
ESTROPIPATE, ESTROPIPATE
ETHYNODIOL DIACETATE AND ETHINYL ESTRADIOL 1/35-21, ETHINYL ESTRADIOL
ETHYNODIOL DIACETATE AND ETHINYL ESTRADIOL 1/35-28, ETHINYL ESTRADIOL
ETHYNODIOL DIACETATE AND ETHINYL ESTRADIOL 1/50-21, ETHINYL ESTRADIOL
ETHYNODIOL DIACETATE AND ETHINYL ESTRADIOL 1/50-28, ETHINYL ESTRADIOL

APPENDIX B
PRODUCT NAME INDEX
LISTED BY APPLICANT *(continued)*

FENOPROFEN CALCIUM, FENOPROFEN CALCIUM
FUROSEMIDE, FUROSEMIDE
GUANABENZ ACETATE, GUANABENZ ACETATE
HYDROCODONE BITARTRATE AND ACETAMINOPHEN, ACETAMINOPHEN
INDOMETHACIN, INDOMETHACIN
LOPERAMIDE HCL, LOPERAMIDE HYDROCHLORIDE
LORAZEPAM, LORAZEPAM
LOXAPINE SUCCINATE, LOXAPINE SUCCINATE
MAPROTILINE HCL, MAPROTILINE HYDROCHLORIDE
METHYLDOPA AND HYDROCHLOROTHIAZIDE, HYDROCHLOROTHIAZIDE
METOCLOPRAMIDE HCL, METOCLOPRAMIDE HYDROCHLORIDE
METOPROLOL TARTRATE, METOPROLOL TARTRATE
NORETHINDRONE AND ETHINYL ESTRADIOL, ETHINYL ESTRADIOL
NORETHINDRONE AND ETHINYL ESTRADIOL (10/11), ETHINYL ESTRADIOL
NORETHINDRONE AND ETHINYL ESTRADIOL (7/14), ETHINYL ESTRADIO
NORETHINDRONE AND MESTRANOL, MESTRANOL
PROPRANOLOL HCL, PROPRANOLOL HYDROCHLORIDE
TRIAMTERENE AND HYDROCHLOROTHIAZIDE, HYDROCHLOROTHIAZIDE
VERAPAMIL HCL, VERAPAMIL HYDROCHLORIDE

WENDT
* WENDT LABORATORIES INC
NITROFURAZONE, NITROFURAZONE

WEST WARD PHARM
* WEST WARD PHARMACEUTICAL CORP
AMINOPHYLLINE, AMINOPHYLLINE
AMITRIPTYLINE HCL, AMITRIPTYLINE HYDROCHLORIDE
BUTALBITAL, ASPIRIN AND CAFFEINE, ASPIRIN
CHLORDIAZEPOXIDE HCL, CHLORDIAZEPOXIDE HYDROCHLORIDE
CHLOROQUINE PHOSPHATE, CHLOROQUINE PHOSPHATE
CHLOROTHIAZIDE, CHLOROTHIAZIDE
CHLOROTHIAZIDE AND RESERPINE, CHLOROTHIAZIDE
CHLORPHENIRAMINE MALEATE, CHLORPHENIRAMINE MALEATE
CHLORPROMAZINE HCL, CHLORPROMAZINE HYDROCHLORIDE
CORTISONE ACETATE, CORTISONE ACETATE
CYANOCOBALAMIN, CYANOCOBALAMIN
DIPHENHYDRAMINE HCL, DIPHENHYDRAMINE HYDROCHLORIDE
DIPHENOXYLATE HCL AND ATROPINE SULFATE, ATROPINE SULFATE
DOXYCYCLINE HYCLATE, DOXYCYCLINE HYCLATE
FLURAZEPAM HCL, FLURAZEPAM HYDROCHLORIDE
FOLIC ACID, FOLIC ACID
HYDRALAZINE HCL, HYDRALAZINE HYDROCHLORIDE
HYDROCHLOROTHIAZIDE, HYDROCHLOROTHIAZIDE
HYDROCORTISONE, HYDROCORTISONE
IMIPRAMINE HCL, IMIPRAMINE HYDROCHLORIDE
ISONIAZID, ISONIAZID
ISOSORBIDE DINITRATE, ISOSORBIDE DINITRATE
MEPROBAMATE, MEPROBAMATE
METHOCARBAMOL, METHOCARBAMOL
METHYLTESTOSTERONE, METHYLTESTOSTERONE
NIACIN, NIACIN
OXYTETRACYCLINE HCL, OXYTETRACYCLINE HYDROCHLORIDE
PREDNISOLONE, PREDNISOLONE
PREDNISONE, PREDNISONE
PROPOXYPHENE HCL, PROPOXYPHENE HYDROCHLORIDE
PROPYLTHIOURACIL, PROPYLTHIOURACIL
QUINIDINE SULFATE, QUINIDINE SULFATE
RESERPINE, RESERPINE
RESERPINE AND HYDROCHLOROTHIAZIDE-50, HYDROCHLOROTHIAZIDE
SODIUM BUTABARBITAL, BUTABARBITAL SODIUM
SODIUM SECOBARBITAL, SECOBARBITAL SODIUM
SULFISOXAZOLE, SULFISOXAZOLE
TETRACYCLINE HCL, TETRACYCLINE HYDROCHLORIDE
THIORIDAZINE HCL, THIORIDAZINE HYDROCHLORIDE
TRIPROLIDINE AND PSEUDOEPHEDRINE, PSEUDOEPHEDRINE HYDROCHLORIDE
VITAMIN A, VITAMIN A
VITAMIN A, VITAMIN A PALMITATE
VITAMIN D, ERGOCALCIFEROL

WESTWOOD SQUIBB
* WESTWOOD SQUIBB PHARMACEUTICALS INC
CAPITROL, CHLOROXINE
EURAX, CROTAMITON
EXELDERM, SULCONAZOLE NITRATE
FLEXICORT, HYDROCORTISONE
HALOG, HALCINONIDE
HALOG-E, HALCINONIDE
HALOTEX, HALOPROGIN
KENALOG, TRIAMCINOLONE ACETONIDE
KENALOG-H, TRIAMCINOLONE ACETONIDE
KENALOG-10, TRIAMCINOLONE ACETONIDE
KENALOG-40, TRIAMCINOLONE ACETONIDE
LAC-HYDRIN, AMMONIUM LACTATE
MYCOLOG-II, NYSTATIN
MYCOSTATIN, NYSTATIN
STATICIN, ERYTHROMYCIN
T-STAT, ERYTHROMYCIN
TACARYL, METHDILAZINE
TACARYL, METHDILAZINE HYDROCHLORIDE
ULTRAVATE, HALOBETASOL PROPIONATE
WESTCORT, HYDROCORTISONE VALERATE

WHARTON LABS
* WHARTON LABORATORIES INC DIV US ETHICALS
VITAMIN A, VITAMIN A PALMITATE

WHITBY
* WHITBY PHARMACEUTICALS INC
THEO-24, THEOPHYLLINE
THEOBID, THEOPHYLLINE
THEOBID JR., THEOPHYLLINE

WHITEHALL LABS
* WHITEHALL LABORATORIES INC DIV AMERICAN HOME PRODUCTS CORP
ADVIL, IBUPROFEN (OTC)
ADVIL COLD AND SINUS, IBUPROFEN (OTC)
BRONITIN MIST, EPINEPHRINE BITARTRATE (OTC)
CHILDREN'S ADVIL, IBUPROFEN
PRIMATENE MIST, EPINEPHRINE (OTC)
TODAY, NONOXYNOL-9 (OTC)

APPENDIX B
PRODUCT NAME INDEX
LISTED BY APPLICANT *(continued)*

WHITEWORTH TOWNE
* WHITEWORTH TOWNE PAULSEN INC
ACETAMINOPHEN W/ CODEINE PHOSPHATE, ACETAMINOPHEN
BUTABARBITAL SODIUM, BUTABARBITAL SODIUM
CORTISONE ACETATE, CORTISONE ACETATE
DEXAMETHASONE, DEXAMETHASONE
DIPHENHYDRAMINE HCL, DIPHENHYDRAMINE HYDROCHLORIDE
FOLIC ACID, FOLIC ACID
H.R.-50, HYDROCHLOROTHIAZIDE
HYDROCHLOROTHIAZIDE, HYDROCHLOROTHIAZIDE
HYDROCORTISONE, HYDROCORTISONE
ISONIAZID, ISONIAZID
MEPROBAMATE, MEPROBAMATE
NITROFURANTOIN, NITROFURANTOIN
PENTOBARBITAL SODIUM, PENTOBARBITAL SODIUM
PREDNISOLONE, PREDNISOLONE
PREDNISONE, PREDNISONE
PROMETHAZINE HCL, PROMETHAZINE HYDROCHLORIDE
PROPOXYPHENE HCL, PROPOXYPHENE HYDROCHLORIDE
QUINIDINE SULFATE, QUINIDINE SULFATE
RESERPINE, RESERPINE
SECOBARBITAL SODIUM, SECOBARBITAL SODIUM

WINTHROP
* WINTHROP PHARMACEUTICALS DIV STERLING DRUG INC
MIDOL, IBUPROFEN (OTC)
PHENYTOIN SODIUM, PHENYTOIN SODIUM
PROCAINAMIDE HCL, PROCAINAMIDE HYDROCHLORIDE

WOCKHARDT
* WOCKHARDT LTD
NIACIN, NIACIN

WYETH
* WYETH LABORATORIES INC
ISMO, ISOSORBIDE MONONITRATE

WYETH AYERST
* WYETH AYERST LABORATORIES INC
A.P.L., GONADOTROPIN, CHORIONIC
ANSOLYSEN, PENTOLINIUM TARTRATE
ANTABUSE, DISULFIRAM
ATIVAN, LORAZEPAM
ATROMID-S, CLOFIBRATE
AYGESTIN, NORETHINDRONE ACETATE
BICILLIN, PENICILLIN G BENZATHINE
BICILLIN C-R, PENICILLIN G BENZATHINE
BICILLIN C-R 900/300, PENICILLIN G BENZATHINE
BICILLIN L-A, PENICILLIN G BENZATHINE
CEFPIRAMIDE SODIUM, CEFPIRAMIDE SODIUM
CHLORPROMAZINE HCL, CHLORPROMAZINE HYDROCHLORIDE
CORDARONE, AMIODARONE HYDROCHLORIDE
CYANOCOBALAMIN, CYANOCOBALAMIN
CYCLAPEN-W, CYCLACILLIN
CYCRIN, MEDROXYPROGESTERONE ACETATE
DEXAMETHASONE SODIUM PHOSPHATE, DEXAMETHASONE SODIUM PHOSPHATE
DIGOXIN, DIGOXIN
DIMENHYDRINATE, DIMENHYDRINATE
DIMETANE-TEN, BROMPHENIRAMINE MALEATE
DIPHENHYDRAMINE HCL, DIPHENHYDRAMINE HYDROCHLORIDE
DIUCARDIN, HYDROFLUMETHIAZIDE
EFFEXOR, VENLAFAXINE HYDROCHLORIDE
EQUAGESIC, ASPIRIN
EQUANIL, MEPROBAMATE
ESTRADURIN, POLYESTRADIOL PHOSPHATE
ESTROGENIC SUBSTANCE, ESTRONE
FACTREL, GONADORELIN HYDROCHLORIDE
FLUOTHANE, HALOTHANE
FUROSEMIDE, FUROSEMIDE
GENTAMICIN SULFATE, GENTAMICIN SULFATE
GRISACTIN, GRISEOFULVIN, MICROCRYSTALLINE
GRISACTIN ULTRA, GRISEOFULVIN, ULTRAMICROCRYSTALLINE
HEPARIN LOCK FLUSH, HEPARIN SODIUM
HEPARIN SODIUM, HEPARIN SODIUM
HYDROXYZINE HCL, HYDROXYZINE HYDROCHLORIDE
INDERAL, PROPRANOLOL HYDROCHLORIDE
INDERAL LA, PROPRANOLOL HYDROCHLORIDE
INDERIDE LA 120/50, HYDROCHLOROTHIAZIDE
INDERIDE LA 160/50, HYDROCHLOROTHIAZIDE
INDERIDE LA 80/50, HYDROCHLOROTHIAZIDE
INDERIDE-40/25, HYDROCHLOROTHIAZIDE
INDERIDE-80/25, HYDROCHLOROTHIAZIDE
ISORDIL, ISOSORBIDE DINITRATE
LARGON, PROPIOMAZINE HYDROCHLORIDE
LIDOCAINE HCL, LIDOCAINE HYDROCHLORIDE
LO/OVRAL, ETHINYL ESTRADIOL
LO/OVRAL-28, ETHINYL ESTRADIOL
LODINE, ETODOLAC
MAZANOR, MAZINDOL
MEPERGAN, MEPERIDINE HYDROCHLORIDE
MEPERIDINE AND ATROPINE SULFATE, ATROPINE SULFATE
MEPERIDINE HCL, MEPERIDINE HYDROCHLORIDE
MYSOLINE, PRIMIDONE
NALOXONE, NALOXONE HYDROCHLORIDE
NORDETTE-21, ETHINYL ESTRADIOL
NORDETTE-28, ETHINYL ESTRADIOL
NORPLANT SYSTEM, LEVONORGESTREL
OMNIPEN (AMPICILLIN), AMPICILLIN/AMPICILLIN TRIHYDRATE
OMNIPEN-N, AMPICILLIN SODIUM
ORUDIS, KETOPROFEN
OVRAL, ETHINYL ESTRADIOL
OVRAL-28, ETHINYL ESTRADIOL
OVRETTE, NORGESTREL
OXYTOCIN, OXYTOCIN
PATHOCIL, DICLOXACILLIN SODIUM
PEN-VEE K, PENICILLIN V POTASSIUM
PENBRITIN, AMPICILLIN/AMPICILLIN TRIHYDRATE
PENBRITIN-S, AMPICILLIN SODIUM
PENICILLIN G POTASSIUM, PENICILLIN G POTASSIUM
PEPTAVLON, PENTAGASTRIN
PHENERGAN, PROMETHAZINE HYDROCHLORIDE
PHENERGAN FORTIS, PROMETHAZINE HYDROCHLORIDE
PHENERGAN PLAIN, PROMETHAZINE HYDROCHLORIDE
PHENERGAN VC, PHENYLEPHRINE HYDROCHLORIDE
PHENERGAN VC W/ CODEINE, CODEINE PHOSPHATE
PHENERGAN W/ CODEINE, CODEINE PHOSPHATE
PHENERGAN W/ DEXTROMETHORPHAN, DEXTROMETHORPHAN HYDROBROMIDE
PHOSPHOLINE IODIDE, ECHOTHIOPHATE IODIDE
PLEGINE, PHENDIMETRAZINE TARTRATE

APPENDIX B
PRODUCT NAME INDEX
LISTED BY APPLICANT *(continued)*

PMB 200, ESTROGENS, CONJUGATED
PMB 400, ESTROGENS, CONJUGATED
PRALIDOXIME CHLORIDE, PRALIDOXIME CHLORIDE
PREMARIN, ESTROGENS, CONJUGATED
PROCHLORPERAZINE EDISYLATE, PROCHLORPERAZINE EDISYLATE
PROKETAZINE, CARPHENAZINE MALEATE
PROTOPAM CHLORIDE, PRALIDOXIME CHLORIDE
ROBITET, TETRACYCLINE HYDROCHLORIDE
SECOBARBITAL SODIUM, SECOBARBITAL SODIUM
SECTRAL, ACEBUTOLOL HYDROCHLORIDE
SERAX, OXAZEPAM
SODIUM PENTOBARBITAL, PENTOBARBITAL SODIUM
SODIUM SECOBARBITAL, SECOBARBITAL SODIUM
SPARINE, PROMAZINE HYDROCHLORIDE
SULFOSE, TRISULFAPYRIMIDINES (SULFADIAZINE;SULFAMERAZINE;SULFAMETHAZINE)
SURMONTIL, TRIMIPRAMINE MALEATE
SYNALGOS-DC, ASPIRIN
SYNALGOS-DC-A, ACETAMINOPHEN
TETRACYCLINE HCL, TETRACYCLINE HYDROCHLORIDE
THIAMINE HCL, THIAMINE HYDROCHLORIDE
THIOSULFIL, SULFAMETHIZOLE
TRECATOR-SC, ETHIONAMIDE
TRIPHASIL-21, ETHINYL ESTRADIOL
TRIPHASIL-28, ETHINYL ESTRADIOL
UNIPEN, NAFCILLIN SODIUM
WYAMINE SULFATE, MEPHENTERMINE SULFATE
WYAMYCIN E, ERYTHROMYCIN ETHYLSUCCINATE
WYAMYCIN S, ERYTHROMYCIN STEARATE
WYCILLIN, PENICILLIN G PROCAINE
WYDASE, HYALURONIDASE
WYGESIC, ACETAMINOPHEN
WYMOX, AMOXICILLIN
WYTENSIN, GUANABENZ ACETATE

* WYETH AYERST RESEARCH
CERUBIDINE, DAUNORUBICIN HYDROCHLORIDE
ORUVAIL, KETOPROFEN

X

XTTRIUM
* XTTRIUM LABORATORIES INC
EXIDINE, CHLORHEXIDINE GLUCONATE (OTC)
TURGEX, HEXACHLOROPHENE

Y

YAMANOUCHI
* YAMANOUCHI EUROPE BV
LOCOID, HYDROCORTISONE BUTYRATE

YOSHITOMI
* YOSHITOMI PHARMACEUTICAL INDUSTRIES LTD
CEPHALEXIN, CEPHALEXIN

Z

ZENECA
* ZENECA INC
CEFOTAN, CEFOTETAN DISODIUM

* ZENECA LTD
DIPRIVAN, PROPOFOL
TENORETIC 100, ATENOLOL
TENORETIC 50, ATENOLOL
ZOLADEX, GOSERELIN ACETATE

* ZENECA PHARMACEUTICALS GROUP DIV ZENECA INC
CEFOTAN, CEFOTETAN DISODIUM
ELAVIL, AMITRIPTYLINE HYDROCHLORIDE
HIBICLENS, CHLORHEXIDINE GLUCONATE (OTC)
HIBISTAT, CHLORHEXIDINE GLUCONATE (OTC)
HIBITANE, CHLORHEXIDINE GLUCONATE (OTC)
NOLVADEX, TAMOXIFEN CITRATE
SORBITRATE, ISOSORBIDE DINITRATE
TENORMIN, ATENOLOL
ZESTORETIC 10-12.5, HYDROCHLOROTHIAZIDE
ZESTORETIC 20-12.5, HYDROCHLOROTHIAZIDE
ZESTORETIC 20-25, HYDROCHLOROTHIAZIDE
ZESTRIL, LISINOPRIL

ZENITH LABS
* ZENITH LABORATORIES INC
ACETAMINOPHEN AND CODEINE PHOSPHATE, ACETAMINOPHEN
ACETAMINOPHEN W/ CODEINE PHOSPHATE #3, ACETAMINOPHEN
ALPRAZOLAM, ALPRAZOLAM
AMPICILLIN, AMPICILLIN/AMPICILLIN TRIHYDRATE
BACLOFEN, BACLOFEN
BETHANECHOL CHLORIDE, BETHANECHOL CHLORIDE
BROMPHENIRAMINE MALEATE, BROMPHENIRAMINE MALEATE
BUTALBITAL COMPOUND, ASPIRIN
CEFADROXIL, CEFADROXIL/CEFADROXIL HEMIHYDRATE
CEPHALEXIN, CEPHALEXIN
CEPHRADINE, CEPHRADINE
CHLORAMPHENICOL, CHLORAMPHENICOL
CHLORDIAZEPOXIDE HCL, CHLORDIAZEPOXIDE HYDROCHLORIDE
CHLORPHENIRAMINE MALEATE, CHLORPHENIRAMINE MALEATE
CHLORPROMAZINE HCL, CHLORPROMAZINE HYDROCHLORIDE
CHLORPROPAMIDE, CHLORPROPAMIDE
CHLORTHALIDONE, CHLORTHALIDONE
CORTISONE ACETATE, CORTISONE ACETATE
CYPROHEPTADINE HCL, CYPROHEPTADINE HYDROCHLORIDE
DIAZEPAM, DIAZEPAM
DIPHENHYDRAMINE HCL, DIPHENHYDRAMINE HYDROCHLORIDE
DIPHENOXYLATE HCL W/ ATROPINE SULFATE, ATROPINE SULFATE
DISOPYRAMIDE PHOSPHATE, DISOPYRAMIDE PHOSPHATE
DOXYCYCLINE HYCLATE, DOXYCYCLINE HYCLATE
ERYTHROMYCIN ESTOLATE, ERYTHROMYCIN ESTOLATE
ERYTHROMYCIN STEARATE, ERYTHROMYCIN STEARATE
FENOPROFEN CALCIUM, FENOPROFEN CALCIUM
FOLIC ACID, FOLIC ACID
FUROSEMIDE, FUROSEMIDE
HYDRALAZINE HCL, HYDRALAZINE HYDROCHLORIDE
HYDRALAZINE HCL W/ HYDROCHLOROTHIAZIDE 100/50, HYDRALAZINE HYDROCHLORIDE

APPENDIX B
PRODUCT NAME INDEX
LISTED BY APPLICANT *(continued)*

HYDRALAZINE HCL W/ HYDROCHLOROTHIAZIDE 25/25, HYDRALAZINE HYDROCHLORIDE
HYDRALAZINE HCL W/ HYDROCHLOROTHIAZIDE 50/50, HYDRALAZINE HYDROCHLORIDE
HYDRALAZINE HCL, HYDROCHLOROTHIAZIDE AND RESERPINE, HYDRALAZINE HYDROCHLORIDE
HYDROCHLOROTHIAZIDE, HYDROCHLOROTHIAZIDE
HYDROCHLOROTHIAZIDE W/ RESERPINE, HYDROCHLOROTHIAZIDE
HYDROGENATED ERGOT ALKALOIDS, ERGOLOID MESYLATES
HYDROSERPINE PLUS (R-H-H), HYDRALAZINE HYDROCHLORIDE
HYDROXYZINE HCL, HYDROXYZINE HYDROCHLORIDE
HYDROXYZINE PAMOATE, HYDROXYZINE PAMOATE
IBUPROFEN, IBUPROFEN (OTC)
INDOMETHACIN, INDOMETHACIN
ISONIAZID, ISONIAZID
MECLIZINE HCL, MECLIZINE HYDROCHLORIDE
MEPROBAMATE, MEPROBAMATE
METHOCARBAMOL, METHOCARBAMOL
METHOCARBAMOL AND ASPIRIN, ASPIRIN
METHYCLOTHIAZIDE, METHYCLOTHIAZIDE
METHYLDOPA, METHYLDOPA
METHYLDOPA AND HYDROCHLOROTHIAZIDE, HYDROCHLOROTHIAZIDE
METRONIDAZOLE, METRONIDAZOLE
NIACIN, NIACIN
NITROFURANTOIN, NITROFURANTOIN
NITROFURANTOIN, NITROFURANTOIN, MACROCRYSTALLINE
OXAZEPAM, OXAZEPAM
PENICILLIN G POTASSIUM, PENICILLIN G POTASSIUM
PENICILLIN V POTASSIUM, PENICILLIN V POTASSIUM
PERPHENAZINE, PERPHENAZINE
PERPHENAZINE AND AMITRIPTYLINE HCL, AMITRIPTYLINE HYDROCHLORIDE
PHENDIMETRAZINE TARTRATE, PHENDIMETRAZINE TARTRATE
PHENTERMINE HCL, PHENTERMINE HYDROCHLORIDE
PHENYLBUTAZONE, PHENYLBUTAZONE
PINDOLOL, PINDOLOL
PRAZOSIN HCL, PRAZOSIN HYDROCHLORIDE
PREDNISOLONE, PREDNISOLONE
PREDNISONE, PREDNISONE
PROBENECID, PROBENECID
PROBENECID AND COLCHICINE, COLCHICINE
PROCAINAMIDE HCL, PROCAINAMIDE HYDROCHLORIDE
PROMETHAZINE HCL, PROMETHAZINE HYDROCHLORIDE
PROMPT PHENYTOIN SODIUM, PHENYTOIN SODIUM, PROMPT
PROPOXYPHENE COMPOUND 65, ASPIRIN
PROPOXYPHENE HCL, PROPOXYPHENE HYDROCHLORIDE
PROPOXYPHENE NAPSYLATE AND ACETAMINOPHEN, ACETAMINOPHEN
PROPRANOLOL HCL, PROPRANOLOL HYDROCHLORIDE
PROPRANOLOL HCL AND HYDROCHLOROTHIAZIDE, HYDROCHLOROTHIAZIDE
PROPYLTHIOURACIL, PROPYLTHIOURACIL
QUINIDINE SULFATE, QUINIDINE SULFATE
RAUWOLFIA SERPENTINA, RAUWOLFIA SERPENTINA
RESERPINE, RESERPINE
RESERPINE AND HYDROFLUMETHIAZIDE, HYDROFLUMETHIAZIDE
SECOBARBITAL SODIUM, SECOBARBITAL SODIUM
SODIUM BUTABARBITAL, BUTABARBITAL SODIUM
SODIUM PENTOBARBITAL, PENTOBARBITAL SODIUM
SPIRONOLACTONE, SPIRONOLACTONE
SPIRONOLACTONE W/ HYDROCHLOROTHIAZIDE, HYDROCHLOROTHIAZIDE
SULFINPYRAZONE, SULFINPYRAZONE
SULFISOXAZOLE, SULFISOXAZOLE
TETRACYCLINE HCL, TETRACYCLINE HYDROCHLORIDE
TETRAMED, TETRACYCLINE HYDROCHLORIDE
THIORIDAZINE HCL, THIORIDAZINE HYDROCHLORIDE
TOLAZAMIDE, TOLAZAMIDE
TOLBUTAMIDE, TOLBUTAMIDE
TRIAMCINOLONE, TRIAMCINOLONE
TRIFLUOPERAZINE HCL, TRIFLUOPERAZINE HYDROCHLORIDE
TRIPROLIDINE HCL AND PSEUDOEPHEDRINE HCL, PSEUDOEPHEDRINE HYDROCHLORIDE
VITAMIN A, VITAMIN A PALMITATE

1

1ST TX
* 1ST TEXAS PHARMACEUTICALS INC SUB SCHERER LABORATORIES INC
CODEINE, ASPIRIN, APAP FORMULA NO. 2, ACETAMINOPHEN
CODEINE, ASPIRIN, APAP FORMULA NO. 3, ACETAMINOPHEN
CODEINE, ASPIRIN, APAP FORMULA NO. 4, ACETAMINOPHEN
MEPROBAMATE, MEPROBAMATE
PREDNISONE, PREDNISONE
QUINIDINE SULFATE, QUINIDINE SULFATE

3

3M
* 3M
SCRUBTEAM SURGICAL SPONGEBRUSH, HEXACHLOROPHENE
* 3M MEDICAL PRODUCTS DIV
INSTANT MICROSPHERES, TECHNETIUM TC-99M ALBUMIN MICROSPHERES KIT
YTTERBIUM YB 169 DTPA, PENTETATE CALCIUM TRISODIUM YB-169
* 3M PHARMACEUTICALS INC
CALCIUM DISODIUM VERSENATE, EDETATE CALCIUM DISODIUM
CIRCANOL, ERGOLOID MESYLATES
DISIPAL, ORPHENADRINE HYDROCHLORIDE
DUO-MEDIHALER, ISOPROTERENOL HYDROCHLORIDE
ISOPROTERENOL HCL, ISOPROTERENOL HYDROCHLORIDE
LIPO-HEPIN, HEPARIN SODIUM

APPENDIX B
PRODUCT NAME INDEX
LISTED BY APPLICANT *(continued)*

MAXAIR, PIRBUTEROL ACETATE
MEDIHALER ERGOTAMINE, ERGOTAMINE TARTRATE
MEDIHALER-EPI, EPINEPHRINE BITARTRATE (OTC)
MEDIHALER-ISO, ISOPROTERENOL SULFATE
NORFLEX, ORPHENADRINE CITRATE
NORGESIC, ASPIRIN
NORGESIC FORTE, ASPIRIN
RAUWILOID, ALSEROXYLON
SODIUM VERSENATE, EDETATE DISODIUM
TAMBOCOR, FLECAINIDE ACETATE
TEPANIL, DIETHYLPROPION HYDROCHLORIDE
TEPANIL TEN-TAB, DIETHYLPROPION HYDROCHLORIDE
THEOLAIR, THEOPHYLLINE
THEOLAIR-SR, THEOPHYLLINE
ULO, CHLOPHEDIANOL HYDROCHLORIDE
UREX, METHENAMINE HIPPURATE
VERILOID, ALKAVERVIR

APPENDIX C
UNIFORM TERMS

DOSAGE FORMS

AEROSOL
AEROSOL, METERED
BAR, CHEWABLE
CAPSULE
CAPSULE, COATED PELLETS
CAPSULE, DELAYED REL PELLETS
CAPSULE, EXTENDED RELEASE
CAPSULE, LIQUID FILLED
CONCENTRATE
CREAM
CREAM, AUGMENTED
DRESSING
DROPS
ELIXIR
EMULSION
ENEMA
FILM, EXTENDED RELEASE
GAS
GEL
GRANULE
GRANULE, DELAYED RELEASE
GRANULE, EFFERVESCENT
GRANULE, FOR RECONSTITUTION
GRANULE, FOR RECONSTITUTION ER
GUM, CHEWING
IMPLANT
INJECTABLE
INSERT
INSERT, EXTENDED RELEASE
INTRAUTERINE DEVICE
JELLY
LIQUID
LOTION
LOTION, AUGMENTED
OIL
OINTMENT
OINTMENT, AUGMENTED
PASTE
PASTILLE
PELLET
POWDER
POWDER FOR RECONSTITUTION*
SHAMPOO
SOAP
SOLUTION
SOLUTION FOR SLUSH
SPONGE
SPRAY
SPRAY, METERED
SUPPOSITORY
SUSPENSION
SUSPENSION, EXTENDED RELEASE
SWAB
SYRUP
TABLET
TABLET, CHEWABLE
TABLET, COATED PARTICLES
TABLET, DELAYED RELEASE
TABLET, DISPERSABLE
TABLET, EXTENDED RELEASE
TAMPON
TAPE
TINCTURE
TROCHE/LOZENGE

ROUTES OF ADMINISTRATION

BUCCAL
DENTAL
ENDOCERVICAL
FOR RX COMPOUNDING
IMPLANTATION
INHALATION
INJECTION
INTRALYMPHATIC
INTRAPERITONEAL
INTRATHECAL
INTRATRACHEAL
INTRAUTERINE
INTRAVENOUS
INTRAVESICAL
IRRIGATION
NASAL
OPHTHALMIC
ORAL
ORAL-20
ORAL-21
ORAL-28
OTIC
PERFUSION, BILIARY
PERFUSION, CARDIAC
RECTAL
SPINAL
SUBLINGUAL
TOPICAL
TRANSDERMAL
URETERAL
URETHRAL
VAGINAL

ABBREVIATIONS

AMP	AMPULE
AMPICIL	AMPICILLIN
APPROX	APPROXIMATELY
BOT	BOTTLE
CI	CURIE
CSR	CAROTID SINUS REFLEX
CU	CLINICAL UNITS
DIPROP	DIPROPIONATE
EQ	EQUIVALENT TO
ELECT	ELECTROLYTE
ER	EXTENDED RELEASE
GM	GRAM
HBR	HYDROBROMIDE
HCL	HYDROCHLORIDE
HR	HOUR
INH	INHALATION
IU	INTERNATIONAL UNITS
KIU	KALLIKREN INHIBITOR UNITS
MCI	MILLICURIE
MEQ	MILLIEQUIVALENT
MG	MILLIGRAM
ML	MILLILITER
N/A	NOT APPLICABLE
REL	RELEASE
SQ CM	SQUARE CENTIMETER
UCI	MICROCURIE
UGM	MICROGRAM
UMOLAR	MICROMOLAR
USP	UNITED STATES PHARMACOPEIA

* FOR ORAL, OPHTHALMIC, INTRATRACHEAL OR INHALATION USE ONLY

PATENT AND EXCLUSIVITY INFORMATION ADDENDUM

This *Addendum* identifies drugs that qualify under the Drug Price Competition and Patent Term Restoration Act (1984 Amendments) for periods of exclusivity, during which abbreviated new drug applications (ANDAs) and applications described in Section 505(b)(2) of the Federal Food, Drug, and Cosmetic Act (the Act) for those drug products may, in some instances, not be submitted or made effective as described below, and provides patent information concerning the listed drug products. Those drugs that have qualified for Orphan Drug Exclusivity pursuant to Section 527 of the Act are also included in this *Addendum*. This section is arranged in alphabetical order by active ingredient name. For those drug products with multiple active ingredients, only the first active ingredient (in alphabetical order) will appear. For an explanation of the codes used in the *Addendum*, see the *Exclusivity Terms* page. Exclusivity prevents the submission or effective approval of ANDAs or applications described in Section 505(b)(2) of the Act. It does not prevent the submission or approval of a second full NDA. Applications qualifying for periods of exclusivity are:

(1) A new drug application approved between January 1, 1982 and September 24, 1984, for a drug product all active ingredients (including any ester or salt of the active ingredient) of which had never been approved in any other application under Section 505(b) of the Act. Approval of an ANDA or an application described in Section 505(b)(2) of the Act for the same drug may not be *made effective* for a period of *ten years* from the date of the approval of the original application.

(2) A new drug application approved after September 24, 1984, for a drug product all active ingredients (including any ester or salt of the active ingredient) of which had never been approved in any other new drug application under Section 505(b) of the Act. No subsequent ANDA or application described in Section 505(b)(2) of the Act for the same drug may be *submitted* for a period of *five years* from the date of approval of the original application, except that such an application may be *submitted* after *four years* if it contains a certification that a patent claiming the drug is invalid or will not be infringed by the product for which approval is sought.

(3) A new drug application approved after September 24, 1984, for a drug product containing an active ingredient (including any ester or salt of that active ingredient) that has been approved in an earlier new drug application and that includes reports of new clinical investigations (other than bioavailability studies). Such investigations must have been conducted or sponsored by the applicant and must have been essential to approval of the application. If these requirements are met, the approval of a subsequent ANDA or an application described in Section 505(b)(2) of the Act may not be *made effective* for the same drug or use, if for a new indication, before the expiration of *three years* from the date of approval of the original application. If an applicant has exclusivity for a new use or indication, this does not preclude the approval of an ANDA application or 505(b)(2) application for the drug product with indications not covered by the exclusivity.

(4) A supplement to a new drug application for a drug containing a previously approved active ingredient (including any ester or salt of the active ingredient) approved after September 24, 1984, that contains reports of new clinical investigations (other than bioavailability studies) essential to the approval of the supplement and conducted or sponsored by the applicant. The approval of a subsequent application for a change approved in the supplement may not be *made effective* for *three years* from the date of approval of the original supplement.

The Act requires that patent information must now be filed with all newly submitted drug applications, and that no NDA may be approved after September 24, 1984, without the submission of pertinent patent information to the Agency. The patent numbers and the expiration dates of appropriate patents claiming drug products that are the subject of approved applications will be published in this *Addendum* or in the monthly Cumulative Supplement to this publication. Patent information on unapproved applications or on patents beyond the scope of the Act (i.e., process or manufacturing patents) will not be published.

The patents that FDA regards as covered by the statutory provisions for submission of patent information are: patents that claim the active ingredient or ingredients; drug product patents, which include formulation/composition patents; and use patents for a particular approved indication or method of using the product. NDA holders or applicants amending or supplementing applications with formulation/composition patent information are asked to certify that the patent(s) is appropriate for publication and refers to an approved product or one for which approval is being sought. The Agency asks all applicants or application holders with use patents to provide information as to the approved indications or uses covered by such patents. This information will be included in the Cumulative Supplement to the List as it becomes available.

Title I of the 1984 Amendments does not apply to drug products submitted or approved under Section 507 of the Federal Food, Drug, and Cosmetic Act (antibiotic products). Therefore, (1) applicants submitting abbreviated applications for antibiotic products are not required to provide the patent certification statement that must be included in ANDAs, (2) antibiotic products are not eligible for exclusivity protection, and (3) holders of approved applications for antibiotic products need not submit the patent information as required of NDA application holders.

Since all parts of this publication are subject to changes, additions, or deletions, the *Addendum* must be used in conjunction with the most current Cumulative Supplement.

EXCLUSIVITY TERMS

DUE TO SPACE LIMITATIONS IN THE EXCLUSIVITY COLUMN, THE FOLLOWING ABBREVIATIONS HAVE BEEN DEVELOPED. PLEASE REFER BACK TO THIS PAGE FOR AN EXPLANATION OF THE EXCLUSIVITY ABBREVIATIONS FOUND IN THE ADDENDUM.

ABBREVIATIONS

D	NEW DOSING SCHEDULE (SEE REFERENCES, BELOW)
I	NEW INDICATION (SEE REFERENCES, BELOW)
NC	NEW COMBINATION
NCE	NEW CHEMICAL ENTITY
NDF	NEW DOSAGE FORM
NE	NEW ESTER OR SALT OF AN ACTIVE INGREDIENT
NP	NEW PRODUCT
NR	NEW ROUTE
NS	NEW STRENGTH
ODE	ORPHAN DRUG EXCLUSIVITY
PC	PATENT CHALLENGE
U	PATENT USE CODE (SEE REFERENCES, BELOW)

REFERENCES

NEW DOSING SCHEDULE

D-1	ONCE A DAY APPLICATION
D-2	ONCE DAILY DOSING
D-3	SEVEN DAYS/SEVEN DAYS/SEVEN DAYS DOSING SCHEDULE
D-4	SEVEN DAYS/FOURTEEN DAYS DOSING SCHEDULE
D-5	TEN DAYS/ELEVEN DAYS DOSING SCHEDULE
D-6	SEVEN DAYS/NINE DAYS/FIVE DAYS DOSING SCHEDULE
D-7	BID DOSING
D-8	INTRAVENOUS, EPIDURAL AND INTRATHECAL DOSING
D-9	NARCOTIC OVERDOSE IN ADULTS
D-10	NARCOTIC OVERDOSE IN CHILDREN
D-11	POSTOPERATIVE NARCOTIC DEPRESSION IN CHILDREN
D-12	BEDTIME DOSING OF 800 MG FOR TREATMENT OF ACTIVE DUODENAL ULCER
D-13	INCREASED MAXIMUM DAILY DOSAGE RECOMMENDATION
D-14	BEDTIME DOSING OF 800 MG FOR TREATMENT OF ACTIVE BENIGN GASTRIC ULCER
D-15	SINGLE DAILY DOSE OF 25 MG/37.5 MG
D-16	CONTINUOUS INTRAVENOUS INFUSION
D-17	400 MG EVERY 12 HOURS FOR THREE DAYS FOR UNCOMPLICATED URINARY TRACT INFECTIONS
D-18	LOWER RECOMMENDED STARTING DOSE GUIDELINES
D-19	BOLUS DOSING GUIDELINES
D-20	SINGLE 32 MG DOSE
D-21	ALTERNATIVE DOSAGE OF 300 MG ONCE DAILY AFTER THE EVENING MEAL
D-22	REDUCTION IN INFUSION TIME FROM 24 TO 4 HOURS FOR THE 60 MG DOSE
D-23	INCREASE MAXIMUM DOSE AND VARIATIONS IN THE DOSING REGIMEN
D-24	FOR OVARIAN CANCER THE RECOMMENDED REGIMEN IS 135 MG/M^2 OR 175 MG/M^2 INTRAVENOUSLY OVER THREE HOURS EVERY THREE WEEKS

REFERENCES

NEW INDICATION

I-1	DYSMENORRHEA
I-2	CHOLANGIOPANCREATOGRAPHY
I-3	INTRAVENOUS DIGITAL SUBTRACTION ANGIOGRAPHY
I-4	PERIPHERAL VENOGRAPHY (PHLEBOGRAPHY)
I-5	HYSTEROSALPINGOGRAPHY
I-6	TREATMENT OF JUVENILE ARTHRITIS
I-7	BIOPSY PROVEN MINIMAL CHANGE NEPHROTIC SYNDROME IN CHILDREN
I-8	ADULT INTRAVENOUS CONTRAST-ENHANCED COMPUTED TOMOGRAPHY OF THE HEAD AND BODY
I-9	PREVENTION OF POSTOPERATIVE NAUSEA AND VOMITING
I-10	PREVENTION OF POSTOPERATIVE DEEP VENOUS THROMBOSIS AND PULMONARY EMBOLISM IN TOTAL HIP REPLACEMENT SURGERY
I-11	RELIEF OF MILD TO MODERATE PAIN
I-12	TREATMENT OF CUTANEOUS CANDIDIASIS
I-13	URINARY TRACT INFECTION (UTI) PREVENTION FOR PERIODS UP TO FIVE MONTHS IN WOMEN WITH A HISTORY OF RECURRENT UTI
I-14	SEBORRHEIC DERMATITIS
I-15	PHOTOPHERESIS IN THE PALLIATIVE TREATMENT OF SKIN MANIFESTATIONS OF CUTANEOUS T-CELL LYMPHOMA IN PERSONS NOT RESPONSIVE TO OTHER TREATMENT
I-16	STIMULATE THE DEVELOPMENT OF MULTIPLE FOLLICLES/OOCYTES IN OVULATORY PATIENTS PARTICIPATING IN AN *IN VITRO* FERTILIZATION PROGRAM
I-17	MANAGEMENT OF CONGESTIVE HEART FAILURE
I-18	ENDOSCOPIC RETROGRADE PANCREATOGRAPHY
I-19	HERNIOGRAPHY
I-20	KNEE ARTHROGRAPHY

EXCLUSIVITY TERMS

NEW INDICATION (continued)

I-21 HIGH DOSE METHOTREXATE WITH LEUCOVORIN RESCUE IN COMBINATION WITH OTHER CHEMOTHERAPEUTIC AGENTS TO DELAY RECURRENCE IN PATIENTS WITH NONMETASTATIC OSTEOSARCOMA WHO HAVE UNDERGONE SURGICAL RESECTION OR AMPUTATION FOR THE PRIMARY TUMOR
I-22 RESCUE AFTER HIGH-DOSE METHOTREXATE THERAPY IN OSTEOSARCOMA
I-23 SHORT-TERM TREATMENT OF ACTIVE BENIGN GASTRIC ULCER
I-24 TREATMENT OF RHEUMATOID ARTHRITIS
I-25 ADULT INTRA-ARTERIAL DIGITAL SUBTRACTION ANGIOGRAPHY OF THE HEAD, NECK, ABDOMINAL, RENAL AND PERIPHERAL VESSELS
I-26 TREATMENT OF LIVER FLUKES
I-27 ADJUNCTIVE THERAPY TO DIET TO REDUCE THE RISK OF CORONARY ARTERY DISEASE
I-28 SELECTIVE ADULT VISCERAL ARTERIOGRAPHY
I-29 METASTATIC BREAST CANCER IN PREMENOPAUSAL WOMEN AS AN ALTERNATIVE TO OOPHORECTOMY OR OVARIAN IRRADIATION
I-30 TREATMENT OF TINEA PEDIS
I-31 CONTRAST ENHANCEMENT AGENT TO FACILITATE VISUALIZATION OF LESIONS IN THE SPINE AND ASSOCIATED TISSUES
I-32 PEDIATRIC MYELOGRAPHY
I-33 ORAL USE OF DILUTED OMNIPAQUE INJECTION IN ADULTS FOR CONTRAST ENHANCED COMPUTED TOMOGRAPHY OF THE ABDOMEN
I-34 ORAL USE IN ADULTS FOR PASS-THROUGH EXAMINATION OF THE GASTROINTESTINAL TRACT
I-35 PEDIATRIC CONTRAST ENHANCEMENT OF COMPUTED TOMOGRAPHIC HEAD IMAGING
I-36 ARTHROGRAPHY OF THE SHOULDER JOINTS IN ADULTS
I-37 RADIOGRAPHY OF THE TEMPOROMANDIBULAR JOINT IN ADULTS
I-38 CONTRAST ENHANCEMENT AGENT TO FACILITATE VISUALIZATION OF LESIONS OF THE CENTRAL NERVOUS SYSTEM IN CHILDREN (2 YEARS OF AGE AND OLDER)
I-39 TREATMENT OF ACUTE MYOCARDIAL INFARCTION
I-40 PRIMARY NOCTURNAL ENURESIS
I-41 MIGRAINE HEADACHE PROPHYLAXIS
I-42 HERPES ZOSTER
I-43 HERPES SIMPLEX ENCEPHALITIS
I-44 MAINTENANCE THERAPY IN HEALED DUODENAL ULCER PATIENTS AT DOSE OF 1 GRAM TWICE DAILY
I-45 ACUTE TREATMENT OF VARICELLA ZOSTER VIRUS
I-46 USE IN PEDIATRIC COMPUTED TOMOGRAPHIC HEAD AND BODY IMAGING
I-47 TREATMENT OF PEDIATRIC PATIENTS WITH SYMPTOMATIC HUMAN IMMUNODEFICIENCY VIRUS (HIV) DISEASE
I-48 PEDIATRIC ANGIOCARDIOGRAPHY
I-49 TREATMENT OF TRAVELERS' DIARRHEA DUE TO SUSCEPTIBLE STRAINS OF ENTEROTOXIGENIC ESCHERICHIA COLI
I-50 FOR USE IN WOMEN WITH AXILLARY NODE-NEGATIVE BREAST CANCER
I-51 TREATMENT OF PRIMARY DYSMENORRHEA AND FOR THE TREATMENT OF IDIOPATHIC HEAVY MENSTRUAL BLOOD LOSS.
I-52 PEDIATRIC EXCRETORY UROGRAPHY
I-53 TREATMENT OF PANIC DISORDER, WITH OR WITHOUT AGORAPHOBIA
I-54 RENAL CONCENTRATION CAPACITY TEST
I-55 HYPERTENSION
I-56 EROSIVE GASTROESOPHAGEAL REFLUX DISEASE
I-57 SHORT-TERM TREATMENT OF ACTIVE DUODENAL ULCER
I-58 INITIAL TREATMENT OF ADVANCED OVARIAN CARCINOMA IN COMBINATION WITH OTHER APPROVED CHEMOTHERAPEUTIC AGENTS
I-59 ENDOSCOPICALLY DIAGNOSED ESOPHAGITIS, INCLUDING EROSIVE AND ULCERATIVE ESOPHAGITIS, AND ASSOCIATED HEARTBURN DUE TO GASTROESOPHAGEAL REFLUX DISEASE
I-60 SINGLE APPLICATION TREATMENT OF HEAD LICE IN CHILDREN TWO MONTHS TO TWO YEARS IN AGE
I-61 FEMALE ADROGENETIC ALOPECIA
I-62 PREVENTION AND TREATMENT OF POSTMENOPAUSAL OSTEOPOROSIS
I-63 ONCE DAILY TREATMENT AS INITIAL THERAPY IN THE TREATMENT OF HYPERTENSION
I-64 PREVENTION OF SUPRAVENTRICULAR TACHYCARDIAS
I-65 PREVENTION OF UPPER GASTROINTESTINAL BLEEDING IN CRITICALLY ILL PATIENTS
I-66 UNCOMPLICATED GONORRHEA
I-67 TREATMENT OF ACUTE ASTHMATIC ATTACKS IN CHILDREN SIX YEARS OF AGE AND OLDER
I-68 CENTRAL PRECOCIOUS PUBERTY
I-69 SHORT-TERM TREATMENT OF PATIENTS WITH SYMPTOMS OF GASTROESOPHAGEAL REFLUX DISEASE (GERD), AND FOR THE SHORT TERM TREATMENT OF ESOPHAGITIS DUE TO GERD INCLUDING ULCERATIVE DISEASE DIAGNOSED BY ENDOSCOPY
I-70 USE IN COMBINATION WITH 5-FLUOROURACIL TO PROLONG SURVIVAL IN THE PALLIATIVE TREATMENT OF PATIENTS WITH ADVANCED COLORECTAL CANCER
I-71 VARICELLA INFECTIONS (CHICKENPOX)
I-72 PREVENTION OF CMV DISEASE IN TRANSPLANT PATIENTS AT RISK FOR CMV DISEASE
I-73 INITIATE AND MAINTAIN MONITORED ANESTHESIA CARE (MAC) SEDATION DURING DIAGNOSTIC PROCEDURES
I-74 INTRAVENOUS DIGITAL SUBTRACTION ANGIOGRAPHY
I-75 TREATMENT OF ENDOSCOPICALLY DIAGNOSED EROSIVE ESOPHAGITIS
I-76 PREVENTION OF OSTEOPOROSIS

EXCLUSIVITY TERMS

NEW INDICATION (continued)

I-77 DERMAL INFECTIONS-TINEA PEDIS, TINEA CORPORIS, TINEA CRURIS DUE TO EPIDERMOPHYTON FLOCCOSUM
I-78 CONTRAST ENHANCED COMPUTED TOMOGRAPHIC IMAGING OF THE HEAD AND BODY AND INTRAVENOUS EXCRETORY UROGRAPHY
I-79 MANAGEMENT OF CHRONIC STABLE ANGINA AND ANGINA DUE TO CORONARY ARTERY SPASM
I-80 DIAGNOSIS AND LOCALIZATION OF ISCHEMIA AND CORONARY HEART DISEASE
I-81 PROPHYLAXIS IN DESIGNATED IMMUNOCOMPROMISED CONDITIONS TO REDUCE THE INCIDENCE OF OROPHARYNGEAL CANDIDIASIS
I-82 TREATMENT OF TRAVELERS' DIARRHEA
I-83 ANGIOCARDIOGRAPHY, CONTRAST ENHANCED COMPUTED TOMOGRAPHIC IMAGING OF THE HEAD AND BODY, AND INTRAVENOUS EXCRETORY URUGRAPHY IN CHILDREN
I-84 INTRAOPERATIVE AND POSTOPERATIVE TACHYCARDIA AND/OR HYPERTENSION
I-85 TREATMENT OF ANOREXIA ASSOCIATED WITH WEIGHT LOSS IN PATIENTS WITH AIDS
I-86 TREATMENT OF SECONDARY CARNITINE DEFICIENCY
I-87 RENAL IMAGING AGENT FOR USE IN CHILDREN
I-88 MANAGEMENT OF ENDOMETRIOSIS
I-89 EPIDURAL USE IN LABOR AND DELIVERY AS AN ANALGESIC ADJUNCT TO BUPIVACAINE
I-90 INTENSIVE CARE UNIT SEDATION
I-91 MONOTHERAPY USE FOR HYPERTENSION
I-92 ADJUNCTIVE THERAPY IN THE MANAGEMENT OF HEART FAILURE
I-93 PREVENTION OF EXERCISE-INDUCED BRONCHOSPASM IN CHILDREN AGES 4-11 YEARS
I-94 USE WITH MRI IN ADULTS TO PROVIDE CONTRAST ENHANCEMENT AND FACILITATE VISUALIZATION OF LESIONS IN THE BODY [EXCLUDING THE HEART]
I-95 TREATMENT OF LEFT VENTRICULAR DYSFUNCTION FOLLOWING MYOCARDIAL INFARCTION
I-96 TREATMENT OF SYMPTOMATIC BENIGN PROSTATIC HYPERPLASIA
I-97 ORAL OR RECTAL USE IN CHILDREN FOR THE EXAMINATION OF THE GASTROINTESTINAL TRACT
I-98 TREATMENT OF CHILDREN WHO HAVE GROWTH FAILURE ASSOCIATED WITH CHRONIC RENAL INSUFFICIENCY
I-99 PEDIATRIC ANESTHESIA IN CHILDREN 3 YEARS AND OLDER
I-100 TO DECREASE THE INCIDENCE OF CANDIDIASIS IN PATIENTS UNDERGOING BONE MARROW TRANSPLANTATION WHO RECEIVE CYTOTOXIC CHEMOTHERAPY AND/OR RADIATION THERAPY
I-101 TREATMENT OF DIABETIC NEPHROPATHY IN PATIENTS WITH TYPE I INSULIN-DEPENDENT DIABETES MELLITUS AND RETINOPATHY
I-102 TREATMENT OF OBSESSIVE-COMPULSIVE DISORDER
I-103 PROPHYLAXIS AGAINST PNEUMOCYSTIS CARINII PNEUMONIA IN INDIVIDUALS WHO ARE IMMUNOCOMPROMISED AND CONSIDERED TO BE AT RISK OF DEVELOPING PNEUMOCYSTIS CARINII PNEUMONIA
I-104 TREATMENT OF PULMONARY AND EXTRAPULMONARY ASPERGILLOSIS IN PATIENTS WHO ARE INTOLERANT OF OR WHO ARE REFRACTORY TO AMPHOTERICIN B THERAPY
I-105 TREATMENT OF METASTATIC CARCINOMA OF THE BREAST AFTER FAILURE OF FIRST-LINE OR SUBSEQUENT CHEMOTHERAPY
I-106 TREATMENT OF ACROMEGALY
I-107 VAGINAL CANDIDIASIS
I-108 EXPANDED USE-FOR ICU PATIENTS UNDERGOING LONG-TERM INFUSION DURING MECHANICAL VENTILATION
I-109 TYPHOID FEVER

REFERENCES

PATENT USE CODE

U-1 PREVENTION OF PREGNANCY
U-2 TREATMENT OR PROPHYLAXIS OF ANGINA PECTORIS AND ARRHYTHMIA
U-3 TREATMENT OF HYPERTENSION
U-4 PROVIDING PREVENTION AND TREATMENT OF EMESIS AND NAUSEA IN MAMMALS
U-5 METHOD OF PRODUCING BRONCHODILATION
U-6 METHOD OF PRODUCING SYMPATHOMIMETIC EFFECTS
U-7 INCREASING CARDIAC CONTRACTILITY
U-8 ACUTE MYOCARDIAL INFARCTION
U-9 CONTROL OF EMESIS ASSOCIATED WITH ANY CANCER CHEMOTHERAPY AGENT
U-10 DIAGNOSTIC METHOD FOR DISTINGUISHING BETWEEN HYPOTHALMIC MALFUNCTIONS OR LESIONS IN HUMANS
U-11 TREATMENT OR PROPHYLAXIS OF CARDIAC DISORDERS
U-12 METHOD OF TREATING [A] HUMAN SUFFERING FROM DEPRESSION
U-13 A METHOD FOR TREATING ANXIETY IN A HUMAN SUBJECT IN NEED OF SUCH TREATMENT
U-14 ADJUNCTIVE THERAPY FOR THE PREVENTION AND TREATMENT OF HYPERAMMONEMIA IN THE CHRONIC MANAGEMENT OF PATIENTS WITH UREA CYCLE ENZYMOPATHIES
U-15 METHOD OF LOWERING INTRAOCULAR PRESSURE
U-16 USE IN LUNG SCANNING PROCEDURES
U-17 TREATMENT OF VENTRICULAR AND SUPRAVENTRICULAR ARRHYTHMIAS
U-18 METHOD FOR INHIBITING GASTRIC SECRETION IN MAMMALS
U-19 TREATMENT OF INFLAMMATION
U-20 A PROCESS FOR TREATING A PATIENT SUFFERING FROM PARKINSON'S SYNDROME AND IN NEED OF TREATMENT

EXCLUSIVITY TERMS

PATENT USE CODE (continued)

U-21 TREATMENT OF HUMANS SUFFERING UNDESIRED UROTOXIC SIDE EFFECTS CAUSED BY CYTOSTATICALLY ACTIVE ALKYLATING AGENTS
U-22 METHOD OF COMBATING PATHOLOGICALLY REDUCED CEREBRAL FUNCTIONS AND PERFORMANCE WEAKNESSES, CEREBRAL INSUFFICIENCY AND DISORDERS IN CEREBRAL CIRCULATION AND METABOLISM IN WARM-BLOODED ANIMALS
U-23 METHOD FOR TREATING PROSTATIC CARCINOMA COMPRISING ADMINISTERING FLUTAMIDE
U-24 METHOD FOR TREATING PROSTATE ADENOCARCINOMA COMPRISING ADMINISTERING AN ANTIANDROGEN INCLUDING FLUTAMIDE AND AN LHRH AGONIST
U-25 REDUCING CHOLESTEROL IN CHOLELITHIASIS PATIENTS
U-26 REDUCING CHOLESTEROL GALLSTONES AND/OR FRAGMENTS THEREOF
U-27 DISSOLVING CHOLESTEROL GALLSTONES AND/OR FRAGMENTS THEREOF
U-28 CEREBRAL, CORONARY, PERIPHERAL, VISCERAL AND RENAL ARTERIOGRAPHY, AORTOGRAPHY AND LEFT VENTRICULOGRAPHY
U-29 CT IMAGING OF THE HEAD AND BODY, AND INTRAVENOUS EXCRETORY UROGRAPHY
U-30 CEREBRAL ANGIOGRAPHY, AND VENOGRAPHY
U-31 INTRA-ARTERIAL DIGITAL SUBTRACTION ANGIOGRAPHY
U-32 PALLIATIVE TREATMENT OF PATIENTS WITH OVARIAN CARCINOMA RECURRENT AFTER PRIOR CHEMOTHERAPY, INCLUDING PATIENTS WHO HAVE BEEN PREVIOUSLY TREATED WITH CISPLATIN
U-33 TREATING VIRAL INFECTIONS IN A MAMMAL
U-34 TREATING VIRAL INFECTIONS IN A WARM-BLOODED ANIMAL
U-35 TREATING CYTOMEGALOVIRUS IN A HUMAN WITH AN INJECTABLE COMPOSITION
U-36 METHODS OF TREATING BACTERIAL ILLNESSES
U-37 METHOD OF TREATING GASTROINTESTINAL DISEASE
U-38 TREATMENT OF PAROXYSMAL SUPRAVENTRICULAR TACHYCARDIA
U-39 ANGINA PECTORIS
U-40 METHOD OF TREATMENT OF BURNS
U-41 METHOD OF TREATING CARDIAC ARRHYTHMIAS
U-42 ADJUVANT TREATMENT IN COMBINATION WITH FLUOROURACIL AFTER SURGICAL RESECTION IN PATIENTS WITH DUKES' STAGE C COLON CANCER.
U-43 MANAGEMENT OF CHRONIC PAIN IN PATIENTS REQUIRING OPIOID ANALGESIA
U-44 RELIEF OF NAUSEA AND VOMITING
U-45 TREATMENT OF INFLAMMATION AND ANALGESIA
U-46 TREATMENT OF PANIC DISORDER
U-47 STIMULATION OF THE RELEASE OF GROWTH HORMONE
U-48 ANALGESIA
U-49 SYMPTOMATIC CANCER-RELATED HYPERCALCEMIA
U-50 USE IN TREATING INFLAMMATORY DERMATOSES
U-51 BLOOD POOL IMAGING, INCLUDING CARDIAC FIRST PASS AND GATED EQUILIBRIUM IMAGING AND FOR DETECTION OF SITES OF GASTROINTESTINAL BLEEDING
U-52 TREATMENT OF ADULT AND PEDIATRIC PATIENTS (OVER SIX MONTHS OF AGE) WITH ADVANCED HIV INFECTION
U-53 HYPERCALCEMIA OF MALIGNANCY
U-54 REVERSAL AGENT OR ANTAGONIST OF NONDEPOLARIZING NEUROMUSCULAR BLOCKING AGENTS
U-55 TREATMENT OF PAIN
U-56 AID TO SMOKING CESSATION
U-57 OPHTHALMIC USE OF NORFLOXACIN
U-58 METHOD OF TREATING INFLAMMATORY INTESTINAL DISEASES
U-59 METHOD OF TREATING HYPERCHOLESTEROLEMIA
U-60 NASAL ADMINISTRATION OF BUTORPHANOL
U-61 CEREBRAL AND PERIPHERAL ARTERIOGRAPHY AND CT IMAGING OF THE HEAD
U-62 CORONARY ARTERIOGRAPHY, LEFT VENTRICULOGRAPHY, CT IMAGING OF THE BODY, INTRAVENOUS EXCRETORY UROGRAPHY, INTRAVENOUS DIGITAL SUBTRACTION ANGIOGRAPHY AND VENOGRAPHY
U-63 ISOPRENALINE ANTAGONISM ON THE HEART RATE OR BLOOD PRESSURE
U-64 TREATMENT OF VIRAL INFECTIONS
U-65 METHOD OF TREATMENT OF A PATIENT INFECTED WITH HIV
U-66 TRIPHASIC REGIMEN
U-67 METHOD OF INDUCING ANESTHESIA IN A WARM BLOODED ANIMAL
U-68 TREATMENT OF ACTINIC KERATOSIS
U-69 TREATMENT OF PNEUMOCYSTIS CARINII INFECTIONS
U-70 TREATMENT OF TRANSIENT INSOMNIA
U-71 METHOD OF TREATMENT OF HEART FAILURE
U-72 TREATMENT OF MIGRAINES
U-73 METHOD OF TREATING DISEASES OR INFECTIONS CAUSED BY MYCETES
U-74 METHOD OF PROVIDING HYPNOTIC EFFECT
U-75 RELIEF OF OCULAR ITCHING DUE TO SEASONAL ALLERGIC CONJUNCTIVITIS
U-76 USE TO IMAGE A SUBJECT WITH A MAGNETIC RESONANCE IMAGING SYSTEM
U-77 TREATMENT OF SYMPTOMS OF SEASONAL ALLERGIC RHINITIS
U-78 ULCERATIVE COLITIS
U-79 SYMPTOMATIC TREATMENT OF PATIENTS WITH NOCTURNAL HEARTBURN DUE TO GERD
U-80 METHOD OF TREATING OCULAR BACTERIAL INFECTIONS
U-81 RELIEF OF SYMPTOMS ASSOCIATED WITH SEASONAL ALLERGIC RHINITIS
U-82 TREATMENT FOR DEMENTIA IN PATIENTS WITH ALZHEIMER'S DISEASE

EXCLUSIVITY TERMS

PATENT USE CODE (continued)

U-83	TREATMENT OF SEIZURES
U-84	A METHOD OF BLOCKING THE UPTAKE OF MONOAMINES BY BRAIN NEURONS IN ANIMALS
U-85	NASAL TREATMENT OF SEASONAL AND PERENNIAL ALLERGIC RHINITIS SYMPTOMS
U-86	METHOD OF TREATMENT CERTAIN FORMS OF EPILEPSY
U-87	METHOD FOR NONINVASIVE ADMINISTRATION OF SEDATIVES, ANALGESICS, AND ANESTHETICS
U-88	TREATMENT OF MODERATE PLAQUE PSORIASIS
U-89	TREATMENT OR PROPHYLAXIS OF EMESIS
U-90	TREATMENT OF PSYCHOTIC DISORDERS
U-91	ALTERNATIVE THERAPY TO TRIMETHOPRIM-SULFAMETHOXAZOLE FOR TREATMENT OF MODERATE-TO-SEVERE PNEUMOCYSTIS CARINII PNEUMONIA IN IMMUNOCOMPROMISED AND AIDS PATIENTS
U-92	TREATMENT OF DIABETIC NEPHROPATHY IN PATIENTS WITH TYPE I INSULIN DEPENDENT DIABETES MELLITUS AND RETINOPATHY
U-93	USE AS AN ANTIHISTAMINE/DECONGESTANT
U-94	TREATMENT OF ADULTS WITH ADVANCED HIV INFECTION WHO ARE INTOLERANT OF APPROVED THERAPIES WITH PROVEN CLINICAL BENEFIT OR WHO HAVE EXPERIENCED SIGNIFICANT CLINICAL OR IMMUNOLOGIC DETERIORATION WHILE RECEIVING THESE THERAPIES OR FOR WHOM SUCH THERAPIES ARE CONTRAINDICATED
U-95	SHORT-TERM MANAGEMENT OF MODERATE PRURITUS IN ADULTS WITH ATOPIC DERMATITIS AND LICHEN SIMPLEX CHRONICUS

PRESCRIPTION AND OTC DRUG PRODUCT PATENT AND EXCLUSIVITY DATA

APPL/ PROD NUMBER	INGREDIENT NAME; TRADE NAME	PATENT NUMBER	PATENT EXPIRES	USE CODE	EX-CLUS CODE	EXCLUS EXPIRES
18458 001	ACETAMINOPHEN; TALACEN	4105659	AUG 08, 1995			
19872 001	ACETAMINOPHEN; TYLENOL				NDF	JUN 08, 1997
19806 001	ACRIVASTINE; SEMPREX-D	4650807	MAR 17, 2004	U-93		
		4501893	FEB 26, 2002		NC	MAR 25, 1997
18604 001	ACYCLOVIR; ZOVIRAX	4199574	APR 22, 1997			
18828 001	ACYCLOVIR; ZOVIRAX	4199574	APR 22, 1997		I-71	FEB 26, 1995
19909 001	ACYCLOVIR; ZOVIRAX	4199574	APR 22, 1997		I-71	FEB 26, 1995
20089 001	ACYCLOVIR; ZOVIRAX	4199574	APR 22, 1997		I-71	FEB 26, 1995
20089 002	ACYCLOVIR; ZOVIRAX	4199574	APR 22, 1997		I-71	FEB 26, 1995
18603 001	ACYCLOVIR SODIUM; ZOVIRAX	4199574	APR 22, 1997			
19937 002	ADENOSINE; ADENOCARD	4673563	JUN 16, 2004	U-38	NCE	OCT 30, 1994
18473 001	ALBUTEROL VENTOLIN				I-93	JUL 20, 1996
18062 001	ALBUTEROL SULFATE; PROVENTIL	4499108	FEB 12, 2002			
19489 001	ALBUTEROL SULFATE; VENTOLIN ROTACAPS				I-93	JUL 20, 1996
19604 001	ALBUTEROL SULFATE; VOLMAX	4851229	JUN 14, 2005			
		4777049	OCT 11, 2005			
		4751071	JUN 14, 2005			
19604 002	ALBUTEROL SULFATE; VOLMAX	4851229	JUN 14, 2005			
		4777049	OCT 11, 2005			
		4751071	JUN 14, 2005		NS	DEC 23, 1995
18702 001	ALCLOMETASONE DIPROPIONATE; ACLOVATE	4124707	NOV 07, 1995			
18707 001	ALCLOMETASONE DIPROPIONATE; ACLOVATE	4124707	NOV 07, 1995			
19353 001	ALFENTANIL HYDROCHLORIDE; ALFENTA	4167574	SEP 11, 1998			
20057 003	ALGLUCERASE; CEREDASE				NCE	APR 05, 1996
					ODE	APR 05, 1998
18276 001	ALPRAZOLAM; XANAX	4508726	APR 02, 2002	U-46		
18276 002	ALPRAZOLAM; XANAX	4508726	APR 02, 2002	U-46		
18276 003	ALPRAZOLAM; XANAX	4508726	APR 02, 2002	U-46		
18276 004	ALPRAZOLAM; XANAX	5061494	OCT 29, 2008			
		4508726	APR 02, 2002	U-46		
19926 001	ALTRETAMINE; HEXALEN				NCE	DEC 26, 1995
					ODE	DEC 26, 1997
18116 002	AMCINONIDE; CYCLOCORT	4158055	JUN 12, 1996	U-19		
18498 001	AMCINONIDE; CYCLOCORT	4158055	JUN 12, 1996	U-19		
19729 001	AMCINONIDE; CYCLOCORT	4158055	JUN 12, 1996	U-19		
18678 001	AMINO ACIDS; BRANCHAMIN 4%	4438144	MAR 20, 2001			
18684 001	AMINO ACIDS; BRANCHAMIN 4%	4438144	MAR 20, 2001			
74346 001	AMINOSALICYLIC ACID; PASER				ODE	JUN 30, 2001
19787 001	AMLODIPINE BESYLATE; NORVASC	4879303	NOV 07, 2006			
		4572909	AUG 01, 2006		NCE	JUL 31, 1997
19787 002	AMLODIPINE BESYLATE; NORVASC	4879303	NOV 07, 2006			
		4572909	AUG 01, 2006		NCE	JUL 31, 1997
19787 003	AMLODIPINE BESYLATE; NORVASC	4879303	NOV 07, 2006			
		452909	AUG 01, 2006		NCE	JUL 31, 1997
19155 001	AMMONIUM LACTATE; LAC-HYDRIN	4105783	OCT 26, 1995			

PRESCRIPTION AND OTC DRUG PRODUCT PATENT AND EXCLUSIVITY DATA *(continued)*

APPL/ PROD NUMBER	INGREDIENT NAME; TRADE NAME	PATENT NUMBER	PATENT EXPIRES	USE CODE	EX-CLUS CODE	EXCLUS EXPIRES
18700 001	AMRINONE LACTATE; INOCOR	4072746	JUL 31, 1998	U-7	NCE	JUL 31, 1994
19779 001	APRACLONIDINE HYDROCHLORIDE; IOPIDINE	4517199	MAY 14, 2002	U-15		
20258 001	APRACLONIDINE HYDROCHLORIDE; IOPIDINE	4517199	MAY 14, 2002	U-15	NS	JUL 30, 1996
20304 001	APROTININ BOVINE; TRASYLOL				NCE	DEC 29, 1998
					ODE	DEC 29, 2000
12365 005	ASPIRIN; SOMA COMPOUND	4534973	AUG 13, 2002			
12366 002	ASPIRIN; SOMA COMPOUND W/ CODEINE	4534974	AUG 13, 2002			
16891 001	ASPIRIN; TALWIN COMPOUND	4105659	AUG 08, 1995			
19402 001	ASTEMIZOLE; HISMANAL	4219559	AUG 26, 1999			
20259 001	ATOVAQUONE; MEPRON	5053432	OCT 01, 2008		ODE	NOV 20, 1999
		4981874	JAN 01, 2008	U-69	NCE	NOV 25, 1997
18831 001	ATRACURIUM BESYLATE; TRACRIUM	4179507	DEC 18, 1996		I-108	JUN 06, 1997
19677 001	ATROPINE SULFATE; ENLON-PLUS	4952586	AUG 28, 2007	U-54	NC	NOV 06, 1994
19678 001	ATROPINE SULFATE; ENLON-PLUS	4952586	AUG 28, 2007	U-54	NC	NOV 06, 1994
19459 001	AVOBENZONE; PHOTOPLEX	4387089	JUN 07, 2002			
20045 001	AVOBENZONE; SHADE UVAGUARD	4522807	JUN 11, 2002		NC	DEC 07, 1995
		4387089	JUN 07, 2002			
20075 001	BACLOFEN; LIORESAL				ODE	JUN 17, 1999
					NDF	JUN 17, 1995
20075 002	BACLOFEN; LIORESAL				ODE	JUN 17, 1999
					NDF	JUN 17, 1995
17573 001	BECLOMETHASONE DIPROPIONATE; VANCERIL	4414209	AUG 23, 1994			
		4364923	OCT 29, 1999			
		4225597	SEP 30, 1997			
18153 001	BECLOMETHASONE DIPROPIONATE; BECLOVENT	4414209	AUG 23, 1994			
		4364923	DEC 21, 1999			
18521 001	BECLOMETHASONE DIPROPIONATE; VANCENASE	4414209	AUG 23, 1994			
		4364923	OCT 29, 1999			
		4225597	SEP 30, 1997			
18584 001	BECLOMETHASONE DIPROPIONATE; BECONASE	4414209	AUG 23, 1994			
		4364923	DEC 21, 1999			
19851 001	BENAZEPRIL HYDROCHLORIDE; LOTENSIN	4410520	OCT 18, 2002		NCE	JUN 25, 1996
19851 002	BENAZEPRIL HYDROCHLORIDE; LOTENSIN	4410520	OCT 18, 2002		NCE	JUN 25, 1996
19851 003	BENAZEPRIL HYDROCHLORIDE; LOTENSIN	4410520	OCT 18, 2002		NCE	JUN 25, 1996
19851 004	BENAZEPRIL HYDROCHLORIDE; LOTENSIN	4410520	OCT 18, 2002		NCE	JUN 25, 1996
20033 001	BENAZEPRIL HYDROCHLORIDE; LOTENSIN HCT	4410520	OCT 18, 2002		NCE	JUN 25, 1996
					NC	MAY 19, 1995
20033 002	BENAZEPRIL HYDROCHLORIDE; LOTENSIN HCT	4410520	OCT 18, 2002		NCE	JUN 25, 1996
					NC	MAY 19, 1995
20033 003	BENAZEPRIL HYDROCHLORIDE; LOTENSIN HCT	4410520	OCT 18, 2002		NCE	JUN 25, 1996
					NC	MAY 19, 1995
20033 004	BENAZEPRIL HYDROCHLORIDE; LOTENSIN HCT	4410520	OCT 18, 2002		NCE	JUN 25, 1996
					NC	MAY 19, 1995
19001 001	BEPRIDIL HYDROCHLORIDE; BEPADIN	RE30577	JUN 08, 1995		NCE	DEC 28, 1995
19001 002	BEPRIDIL HYDROCHLORIDE; BEPADIN	RE30577	JUN 08, 1995		NCE	DEC 28, 1995
19001 003	BEPRIDIL HYDROCHLORIDE; BEPADIN	RE30577	JUN 08, 1995		NCE	DEC 28, 1995
19002 001	BEPRIDIL HYDROCHLORIDE; VASCOR	RE30577	JUN 08, 1995		NCE	DEC 28, 1995
19002 002	BEPRIDIL HYDROCHLORIDE; VASCOR	RE30577	JUN 08, 1995		NCE	DEC 28, 1995
19002 003	BEPRIDIL HYDROCHLORIDE; VASCOR	RE30577	JUN 08, 1995		NCE	DEC 28, 1995
20032 001	BERACTANT; SURVANTA	4397839	AUG 10, 2000		NCE	JUL 01, 1996
					ODE	JUL 01, 1998
18741 001	BETAMETHASONE DIPROPIONATE; DIPROLENE	4070462	JAN 24, 1995			
18827 001	BETAMETHASONE DIPROPIONATE; LOTRISONE	4298604	NOV 03, 1998			
19408 001	BETAMETHASONE DIPROPIONATE; DIPROLENE	4489070	DEC 18, 2001			
		4482539	NOV 03, 2001			
19555 001	BETAMETHASONE DIPROPIONATE; DIPROLENE AF	4489071	DEC 18, 2001			
19716 001	BETAMETHASONE DIPROPIONATE; DIPROLENE	4775529	OCT 04, 2005			
19270 001	BETAXOLOL HYDROCHLORIDE; BETOPTIC	4342783	AUG 03, 1999			
		4311708	JAN 19, 1999			
		4252984	AUG 30, 1999			
19507 001	BETAXOLOL HYDROCHLORIDE; KERLONE	4311708	JAN 19, 1999	U-3		
		4252984	AUG 30, 1999			
19507 002	BETAXOLOL HYDROCHLORIDE; KERLONE	4311708	JAN 19, 1999	U-3		
		4252984	AUG 30, 1999			
19807 001	BETAXOLOL HYDROCHLORIDE; KERLEDEX	4311708	JAN 19, 1999	U-3	NC	OCT 30, 1995
		4252984	AUG 30, 1999			
19807 002	BETAXOLOL HYDROCHLORIDE; KERLEDEX	4311708	JAN 19, 1999	U-3	NC	OCT 30, 1995
		4252984	AUG 30, 1999			

PRESCRIPTION AND OTC DRUG PRODUCT PATENT AND EXCLUSIVITY DATA *(continued)*

APPL/ PROD NUMBER	INGREDIENT NAME; TRADE NAME	PATENT NUMBER	PATENT EXPIRES	USE CODE	EX-CLUS CODE	EXCLUS EXPIRES
19845 001	BETAXOLOL HYDROCHLORIDE; BETOPTIC S	4911920	MAR 27, 2007			
		4342783	AUG 03, 1999			
		4311708	JAN 19, 1999			
		4252984	AUG 30, 1999			
19982 001	BISOPROLOL FUMARATE; ZEBETA	4258062	MAR 24, 2000	U-63	NCE	JUL 31, 1997
19982 002	BISOPROLOL FUMARATE; ZEBETA	4258062	MAR 24, 2000	U-63	NCE	JUL 31, 1997
20186 001	BISOPROLOL FUMARATE; ZIAC	4258062	MAR 24, 2000	U-63	NCE	JUL 31, 1997
					NC	FEB 26, 1996
20186 002	BISOPROLOL FUMARATE; ZIAC	4258062	MAR 24, 2000	U-63	NCE	JUL 31, 1997
					NC	FEB 26, 1996
20186 003	BISOPROLOL FUMARATE; ZIAC	4258062	MAR 24, 2000	U-63	NCE	JUL 31, 1997
					NC	FEB 26, 1996
18770 001	BITOLTEROL MESYLATE; TORNALATE	4336400	JUN 22, 1999	U-5		
		4336400	JUN 22, 1999	U-6		
		4138581	FEB 06, 1998			
19548 001	BITOLTEROL MESYLATE; TORNALATE	4336400	JUN 22, 1999	U-5		
		4138581	FEB 06, 1998		NDF	FEB 19, 1995
20233 001	BUDESONIDE; RHINOCORT				NCE	FEB 14, 1999
18644 001	BUPROPION HYDROCHLORIDE; WELLBUTRIN	4507323	MAR 26, 2002			
		4438138	MAR 20, 2001			
		4435449	MAR 06, 2001			
		4425363	JAN 10, 2001			
		4393078	JUL 12, 2000			
		4347257	AUG 31, 1999			
		3885046	MAY 20, 1994	U-12		
18644 002	BUPROPION HYDROCHLORIDE; WELLBUTRIN	4507323	MAR 26, 2002			
		4438138	MAR 20, 2001			
		4435449	MAR 06, 2001			
		4425363	JAN 10, 2001			
		4393078	JUL 12, 2000			
		4347257	AUG 31, 1999			
		3885046	MAY 20, 1994	U-12		
18644 003	BUPROPION HYDROCHLORIDE; WELLBUTRIN	4507323	MAR 26, 2002			
		4438138	MAR 20, 2001			
		4435449	MAR 06, 2001			
		4425363	JAN 10, 2001			
		4393078	JUL 12, 2000			
		4347257	AUG 31, 1999			
		3885046	MAY 20, 1994	U-12		
18731 001	BUSPIRONE HYDROCHLORIDE; BUSPAR	5015646	MAY 14, 2008	U-13		
		4182763	JAN 08, 1999			
18731 002	BUSPIRONE HYDROCHLORIDE; BUSPAR	5015646	MAY 14, 2008	U-13		
		4182763	JAN 08, 1999			
19215 001	BUTOCONAZOLE NITRATE; FEMSTAT	4078071	MAR 07, 1997			
19359 001	BUTOCONAZOLE NITRATE; FEMSTAT	4078071	MAR 07, 1997			
19890 001	BUTORPHANOL TARTRATE; STADOL	4464378	AUG 07, 2001	U-60	NDF	DEC 12, 1994
20273 001	CALCIPOTRIENE; DOVONEX	4866048	SEP 12, 2006	U-88	NCE	DEC 29, 1998
18470 001	CALCITONIN, HUMAN; CIBACALCIN	RE32347	JUN 30, 1998			
18044 001	CALCITRIOL; ROCALTROL	4391802	JUL 05, 2000			
		4341774	JUL 27, 1999			
		4225596	SEP 30, 1997			
18044 002	CALCITRIOL; ROCALTROL	4391802	JUL 05, 2000			
		4341774	JUL 27, 1999			
		4225596	SEP 30, 1997			
18874 001	CALCITRIOL; CALCIJEX	4308264	DEC 29, 1998			
18874 002	CALCITRIOL; CALCIJEX	4308264	DEC 29, 1998			
19976 001	CALCIUM ACETATE; PHOSLO	4870105	SEP 26, 2006		ODE	DEC 10, 1997
18469 001	CALCIUM CHLORIDE; BSS PLUS	4550022	OCT 29, 2002			
		4443432	APR 17, 2001			
18343 001	CAPTOPRIL; CAPOTEN	5238924	AUG 24, 2010	U-92	I-101	JAN 28, 1997
		4105776	AUG 08, 1995		I-95	SEP 23, 1996
18343 002	CAPTOPRIL; CAPOTEN	5238924	AUG 24, 2010	U-92	I-101	JAN 28, 1997
		4105776	AUG 08, 1995		I-95	SEP 23, 1996
18343 003	CAPTOPRIL; CAPOTEN	5238924	AUG 24, 2010	U-92	I-101	JAN 28, 1997
		4105776	AUG 08, 1995		I-95	SEP 23, 1996
18343 005	CAPTOPRIL; CAPOTEN	5238924	AUG 24, 2010	U-92	I-101	JAN 28, 1997
		4105776	AUG 08, 1995		I-95	SEP 23, 1996
18343 006	CAPTOPRIL; CAPOTEN	4105776	AUG 08, 1995		I-101	JAN 28, 1997
					I-95	SEP 23, 1996

PRESCRIPTION AND OTC DRUG PRODUCT PATENT AND EXCLUSIVITY DATA *(continued)*

APPL/ PROD NUMBER	INGREDIENT NAME; TRADE NAME	PATENT NUMBER	PATENT EXPIRES	USE CODE	EX-CLUS CODE	EXCLUS EXPIRES
18709 001	CAPTOPRIL; CAPOZIDE 25/15	4217347	AUG 12, 1997			
		4105776	AUG 08, 1995		I-63	OCT 24, 1994
18709 002	CAPTOPRIL; CAPOZIDE 25/25	4217347	AUG 12, 1997			
		4105776	AUG 08, 1995		I-63	OCT 24, 1994
18709 003	CAPTOPRIL; CAPOZIDE 50/25	4217347	AUG 12, 1997			
		4105776	AUG 08, 1995		I-63	OCT 24, 1994
18709 004	CAPTOPRIL; CAPOZIDE 50/15	4217347	AUG 12, 1997			
		4105776	AUG 08, 1995		I-63	OCT 24, 1994
16608 001	CARBAMAZEPINE; TEGRETOL	4409212	OCT 11, 2000			
18281 001	CARBAMAZEPINE; TEGRETOL	4409212	OCT 11, 2000			
18927 001	CARBAMAZEPINE; TEGRETOL	4409212	OCT 11, 2000			
19856 001	CARBIDOPA; SINEMET CR	4900755	MAY 23, 2006		NDF	MAY 30, 1994
		4832957	MAY 23, 2006			
19880 001	CARBOPLATIN; PARAPLATIN	4657927	APR 14, 2004	U-32	NCE	MAR 03, 1994
		4140707	AUG 25, 1998		I-58	JUL 05, 1994
19880 002	CARBOPLATIN; PARAPLATIN	4657927	APR 14, 2004	U-32	NCE	MAR 03, 1994
		4140707	AUG 25, 1998		I-58	JUL 05, 1994
19880 003	CARBOPLATIN; PARAPLATIN	4657927	APR 14, 2004	U-32	NCE	MAR 03, 1994
		4140707	AUG 25, 1998		I-58	JUL 05, 1994
18550 002	CARPROFEN; RIMADYL	3896145	JUL 22, 1994			
18550 003	CARPROFEN; RIMADYL	3896145	JUL 22, 1994			
19204 001	CARTEOLOL HYDROCHLORIDE; CARTROL	3910924	OCT 07, 1994			
19204 002	CARTEOLOL HYDROCHLORIDE; CARTROL	3910924	OCT 07, 1994			
19204 003	CARTEOLOL HYDROCHLORIDE; CARTROL	3910924	OCT 07, 1994			
19972 001	CARTEOLOL HYDROCHLORIDE; OPTIPRESS	4309432	JAN 05, 1999			
		3910924	OCT 07, 1994			
20044 001	CETYL ALCOHOL; EXOSURF NEONATAL	4826821	MAY 02, 2006		ODE	AUG 02, 1997
		4312860	NOV 23, 2001			
18050 001	CHLORPHENIRAMINE POLISTIREX; CORSYM	4221778	SEP 09, 1997			
18928 001	CHLORPHENIRAMINE POLISTIREX; PENNTUSS	4221778	SEP 09, 1997			
19111 001	CHLORPHENIRAMINE POLISTIREX; TUSSIONEX	4221778	SEP 09, 1997			
71621 001	CHOLESTYRAMINE; CHOLYBAR	4778676	OCT 18, 2005			
71739 001	CHOLESTYRAMINE; CHOLYBAR	4778676	OCT 18, 2005			
18663 001	CHYMOPAPAIN; CHYMODIACTIN	4439423	MAR 26, 2001			
18663 002	CHYMOPAPAIN; CHYMODIACTIN	4439423	MAR 26, 2001			
17920 002	CIMETIDINE; TAGAMET	4024271	MAY 17, 1994		I-56	MAR 07, 1994
17920 003	CIMETIDINE; TAGAMET	4024271	MAY 17, 1994		I-56	MAR 07, 1994
17920 004	CIMETIDINE; TAGAMET	4024271	MAY 17, 1994		I-56	MAR 07, 1994
17920 005	CIMETIDINE; TAGAMET	4024271	MAY 17, 1994		I-56	MAR 07, 1994
17924 001	CIMETIDINE HYDROCHLORIDE; TAGAMET	4024271	MAY 17, 1994			
					I-56	MAR 07, 1994
17939 002	CIMETIDINE HYDROCHLORIDE; TAGAMET	4024271	MAY 17, 1994		I-65	NOV 13, 1994
19434 001	CIMETIDINE HYDROCHLORIDE; TAGAMET HCL IN SODIUM CHLORIDE 0.9%	4024271	MAY 17, 1994			
19847 001	CIRPOFLOXACIN; CIPRO	4808583	FEB 28, 2006			
		4705789	NOV 10, 2004			
		4670444	OCT 01, 2002			
19857 001	CIPROFLOXACIN; CIPRO IN DEXTROSE 5%	4957922	SEP 18, 2007			
		4808583	FEB 28, 2006			
		4705789	NOV 10, 2004			
		4670444	OCT 01, 2002			
19858 001	CIPROFLOXACIN; CIPRO IN SODIUM CHLORIDE 0.9%	4957922	SEP 18, 2007			
		4808583	FEB 28, 2006			
		4705789	NOV 10, 2004			
		4670444	OCT 01, 2002			
19537 002	CIPROFLOXACIN HYDROCHLORIDE; CIPRO	4670444	OCT 01, 2002	U-36	I-66	JUL 21, 1997
					I-109	JUL 21, 1997
19537 003	CIPROFLOXACIN HYDROCHLORIDE; CIPRO	4670444	OCT 01, 2002	U-36	I-66	JUL 21, 1997
					I-109	JUL 21, 1997
19537 004	CIPROFLOXACIN HYDROCHLORIDE; CIPRO	4670444	OCT 01, 2002	U-36	I-66	JUL 21, 1997
					I-109	JUL 21, 1997
19992 001	CIPROFLOXACIN HYDROCHLORIDE; CILOXAN	4670444	OCT 01, 2002			
20210 001	CISAPRIDE MONOHYDRATE; PROPULSID	4962115	OCT 09, 2007	U-79	NCE	JUL 29, 1998
20210 002	CISAPRIDE MONOHYDRATE; PROPULSID	4962115	OCT 09, 2007	U-79	NCE	JUL 29, 1998
18057 001	CISPLATIN; PLATINOL	4177263	DEC 04, 1996			
18057 002	CISPLATIN; PLATINOL	4177263	DEC 04, 1996			
18057 003	CISPLATIN; PLATINOL-AQ	4310515	JAN 12, 1999			
		4177263	DEC 04, 1996			

PRESCRIPTION AND OTC DRUG PRODUCT PATENT AND EXCLUSIVITY DATA *(continued)*

APPL/ PROD NUMBER	INGREDIENT NAME; TRADE NAME	PATENT NUMBER	PATENT EXPIRES	USE CODE	EX-CLUS CODE	EXCLUS EXPIRES
18057 004	CISPLATIN; PLATINOL-AQ	4310515	JAN 12, 1999			
		4177263	DEC 04, 1996			
19481 001	CITRIC ACID; RENACIDIN				ODE	OCT 02, 1997
20229 001	CLADRIBINE; LEUSTATIN				NCE	FEB 26, 1998
					ODE	FEB 26, 2000
19906 001	CLOMIPRAMINE HYDROCHLORIDE; ANAFRANIL				NCE	DEC 29, 1994
19906 002	CLOMIPRAMINE HYDROCHLORIDE; ANAFRANIL				NCE	DEC 29, 1994
19906 003	CLOMIPRAMINE HYDROCHLORIDE; ANAFRANIL				NCE	DEC 29, 1994
18891 001	CLONIDINE; CATAPRES-TTS-1	4559222	DEC 17, 2002			
		4201211	MAY 06, 1997			
		4060084	JUN 28, 1994			
18891 002	CLONIDINE; CATAPRES-TTS-2	4559222	DEC 17, 2002			
		4201211	MAY 06, 1997			
		4060084	JUN 28, 1994			
18891 003	CLONIDINE; CATAPRES-TTS-3	4559222	DEC 17, 2002			
		4201211	MAY 06, 1997			
		4060084	JUN 28, 1994			
18713 001	CLOTRIMAZOLE; MYCELEX				I-81	SEP 29, 1995
19758 001	CLOZAPINE; CLOZARIL				NCE	SEP 26, 1994
19758 002	CLOZAPINE; CLOZARIL				NCE	SEP 26, 1994
17408 001	COPPER; CU-7	4040417	AUG 09, 1994			
18205 001	COPPER; TATUM-T	4040417	AUG 09, 1994			
18155 001	CROMOLYN SODIUM; OPTICROM	4053628	OCT 11, 1994			
18306 001	CROMOLYN SODIUM; NASALCROM	4053628	OCT 11, 1994			
18887 001	CROMOLYN SODIUM; INTAL	4405598	SEP 20, 2000			
19188 001	CROMOLYN SODIUM; GASTROCROM	4395421	JUL 26, 2000		ODE	DEC 22, 1996
12142 006	CYCLOPHOSPHAMIDE; LYOPHILIZED CYTOXAN	4537883	AUG 27, 2002			
12142 007	CYCLOPHOSPHAMIDE; LYOPHILIZED CYTOXAN	4537883	AUG 27, 2002			
12142 008	CYCLOPHOSPHAMIDE; LYOPHILIZED CYTOXAN	4537883	AUG 27, 2002			
12142 009	CYCLOPHOSPHAMIDE; LYOPHILIZED CYTOXAN	4537883	AUG 27, 2002			
12142 010	CYCLOPHOSPHAMIDE; LYOPHILIZED CYTOXAN	4537883	AUG 27, 2002			
20392 001	CYSTEAMINE BITARTRATE; CYSTAGON				NCE	AUG 15, 1999
					ODE	AUG 15, 2001
20392 002	CYSTEAMINE BITARTRATE; CYSTAGON				NCE	AUG 15, 1999
					ODE	AUG 15, 2001
19849 001	DAPIPRAZOLE HYDROCHLORIDE; REV-EYES	4252721	JAN 06, 2002		NCE	DEC 31, 1995
20118 001	DESFLURANE; SUPRANE	4762856	SEP 18, 2006	U-67	NCE	SEP 18, 1997
20355 001	DESMOPRESSIN ACETATE; DESMOPRESSIN ACETATE				NP	MAR 07, 1997
					ODE	MAR 07, 2001
20071 001	DESOGESTREL; DESOGEN	3927046	NOV 19, 1995		NC	DEC 10, 1995
20071 002	DESOGESTREL; DESOGEN	3927096	NOV 19, 1995		NC	DEC 10, 1995
20301 001	DESOGESTREL; ORTHO-CEPT	3927046	NOV 19, 1995		NC	DEC 10, 1995
20301 002	DESOGESTREL; ORTHO-CEPT	3927046	NOV 19, 1995		NC	DEC 10, 1995
18658 001	DEXTROMETHORPHAN POLISTIREX; DELSYM	4221778	SEP 09, 1997			
19082 001	DEZOCINE; DALGAN	4605671	AUG 12, 2003			
		4001331	JAN 04, 1996		NCE	DEC 29, 1994
19082 002	DEZOCINE; DALGAN	4605671	AUG 12, 2003			
		4001331	JAN 04, 1996		NCE	DEC 29, 1994
19082 003	DEZOCINE; DALGAN	4605671	AUG 12, 2003			
		4001331	JAN 04, 1996		NCE	DEC 29, 1994
19287 001	DIAZEPAM; DIZAC	RE32393	SEP 18, 1996		NDF	JUN 18, 1996
20142 001	DICLOFENAC POTASSIUM; CATAFLAM				NE	NOV 24, 1996
19201 002	DICLOFENAC POTASSIUM; CATAFLAM				NE	NOV 24, 1996
20037 001	DICLOFENAC SODIUM; VOLTAREN	4960799	OCT 02, 2007		NDF	MAR 28, 1994
20154 002	DIDANOSINE, VIDEX	4861759	AUG 29, 2006	U-52	NCE	OCT 09, 1996
					D-18	SEP 25, 1995
20154 003	DIDANOSINE, VIDEX	4861759	AUG 29, 2006	U-52	NCE	OCT 09, 1996
					D-18	SEP 25, 1995
20154 004	DIDANOSINE, VIDEX	4861759	AUG 29, 2006	U-52	NCE	OCT 09, 1996
					D-18	SEP 25, 1995
20154 005	DIDANOSINE, VIDEX	4861759	AUG 29, 2006	U-52	NCE	OCT 09, 1996
					D-18	SEP 25, 1995
20155 003	DIDANOSINE, VIDEX	4861759	AUG 29, 2006	U-52	NCE	OCT 09, 1996
					D-18	SEP 25, 1995
20155 004	DIDANOSINE, VIDEX	4861759	AUG 29, 2006	U-52	NCE	OCT 09, 1996
					D-18	SEP 25, 1995
20155 005	DIDANOSINE, VIDEX	4861759	AUG 29, 2006	U-52	NCE	OCT 09, 1996
					D-18	SEP 25, 1995

PRESCRIPTION AND OTC DRUG PRODUCT PATENT AND EXCLUSIVITY DATA *(continued)*

APPL/ PROD NUMBER	INGREDIENT NAME; TRADE NAME	PATENT NUMBER	PATENT EXPIRES	USE CODE	EX-CLUS CODE	EXCLUS EXPIRES
20155 006	DIDANOSINE, VIDEX	4861759	AUG 29, 2006	U-52	NCE	OCT 09, 1996
					D-18	SEP 25, 1995
20156 001	DIDANOSINE, VIDEX	4861759	AUG 29, 2006	U-52	NCE	OCT 09, 1996
					D-18	SEP 25, 1995
18118 001	DIGOXIN; LANOXICAPS	4088750	MAY 09, 1995			
18118 002	DIGOXIN; LANOXICAPS	4088750	MAY 09, 1995			
18118 003	DIGOXIN; LANOXICAPS	4088750	MAY 09, 1995			
18118 004	DIGOXIN; LANOXICAPS	4088750	MAY 09, 1995			
18885 001	DIHYDROERGOTAMINE MESYLATE; EMBOLEX	4451458	MAY 29, 2001			
		4402949	SEP 06, 2000			
18885 002	DIHYDROERGOTAMINE MESYLATE; EMBOLEX	4451458	MAY 29, 2001			
		4402949	SEP 06, 2000			
19471 001	DILTIAZEM HYDROCHLORIDE; CARDIZEM SR	4721619	JAN 26, 2005			
19471 002	DILTIAZEM HYDROCHLORIDE; CARDIZEM SR	4721619	JAN 26, 2005			
19471 003	DILTIAZEM HYDROCHLORIDE; CARDIZEM SR	4721619	JAN 26, 2005			
19471 004	DILTIAZEM HYDROCHLORIDE; CARDIZEM SR	4721619	JAN 26, 2005			
20027 001	DILTIAZEM HYDROCHLORIDE; CARDIZEM				NDF	OCT 24, 1994
20062 001	DILTIAZEM HYDROCHLORIDE; CARDIZEM CD	5286497	FEB 14, 2011			
		5002776	MAR 26, 2008		I-79	OCT 15, 1995
		4894240	JAN 16, 2007		NS	MAY 29, 1995
20062 002	DILTIAZEM HYDROCHLORIDE; CARDIZEM CD	5286497	FEB 14, 2011			
		5002776	MAR 26, 2008		I-79	OCT 15, 1995
		489420	JAN 16, 2007		NP	DEC 27, 1994
20062 003	DILTIAZEM HYDROCHLORIDE; CARDIZEM CD	5286497	FEB 14, 2011			
		5002776	MAR 26, 2008		I-79	OCT 15, 1995
		4894240	JAN 16, 2007		NP	DEC 27, 1994
20062 004	DILTIAZEM HYDROCHLORIDE; CARDIZEM CD	5286497	FEB 14, 2011			
		5002776	MAR 26, 2008		I-79	OCT 15, 1995
		4894240	JAN 16, 2007		NP	DEC 27, 1994
20092 001	DILTIAZEM HYDROCHLORIDE; DILACOR XR	4839177	JUN 13, 2006		NS	MAY 29, 1995
20092 002	DILTIAZEM HYDROCHLORIDE; DILACOR XR	4839177	JUN 13, 2006		NP	DEC 27, 1994
20092 003	DILTIAZEM HYDROCHLORIDE; DILACOR XR	4839177	JUN 13, 2006		NP	DEC 27, 1994
19617 001	DINOPROSTONE; PREPIDIL	4680312	JUL 14, 2004		NDF	DEC 09, 1995
18723 001	DIVALPROEX SODIUM; DEPAKOTE	5212326	JAN 29, 2008			
		4988731	JAN 29, 2008			
18723 002	DIVALPROEX SODIUM; DEPAKOTE	5212326	JAN 29, 2008			
		4988731	JAN 29, 2008			
18723 003	DIVALPROEX SODIUM; DEPAKOTE	5212326	JAN 29, 2008			
		4988731	JAN 29, 2008			
19680 001	DIVALPROEX SODIUM; DEPAKOTE	5212326	JAN 29, 2008			
		4988731	JAN 29, 2008			
19794 001	DIVALPROEX SODIUM; DEPAKOTE CP	5212326	JAN 29, 2008			
		4988731	JAN 29, 2008			
19794 002	DIVALPROEX SODIUM; DEPAKOTE CP	5212326	JAN 29, 2008			
		4988731	JAN 29, 2008			
19946 001	DOXACURIUM CHLORIDE; NUROMAX	4701460	MAR 06, 2005		NCE	MAR 07, 1996
19668 001	DOXAZOSIN MESYLATE; CARDURA	4188390	FEB 12, 1999		NCE	NOV 02, 1995
19668 002	DOXAZOSIN MESYLATE; CARDURA	4188390	FEB 12, 1999		NCE	NOV 02, 1995
19668 003	DOXAZOSIN MESYLATE; CARDURA	4188390	FEB 12, 1999		NCE	NOV 02, 1995
19668 004	DOXAZOSIN MESYLATE; CARDURA	4188390	FEB 12, 1999		NCE	NOV 02, 1995
20126 001	DOXEPIN HYDROCHLORIDE; ZONALON	4395420	JUL 26, 2000	U-95	NDF	APR 01, 1997
18651 001	DRONABINOL; MARINOL				I-85	DEC 22, 1995
					ODE	DEC 22, 1999
18651 002	DRONABINOL; MARINOL				I-85	DEC 22, 1995
					ODE	DEC 22, 1999
18651 003	DRONABINOL; MARINOL				I-85	DEC 22, 1995
					ODE	DEC 22, 1999
19879 002	EFLORNITHINE HYDROCHLORIDE; ORNIDYL	4413141	NOV 01, 2000		ODE	NOV 28, 1997
		4339151	AUG 16, 2000		NCE	NOV 28, 1995
18998 001	ENALAPRIL MALEATE; VASOTEC	4374829	FEB 22, 2000			
18998 002	ENALAPRIL MALEATE; VASOTEC	4374829	FEB 22, 2000			
18998 003	ENALAPRIL MALEATE; VASOTEC	4374829	FEB 22, 2000			
18998 005	ENALAPRIL MALEATE; VASOTEC	4374829	FEB 22, 2000			
19221 001	ENALAPRIL MALEATE; VASERETIC	4472380	SEP 18, 2001			
		4374829	FEB 22, 2000			
19309 001	ENALAPRILAT; VASOTEC	4374829	FEB 22, 2000			
18981 002	ENCAINIDE HYDROCHLORIDE; ENKAID	RE30811	DEC 20, 1996	U-17		
18981 003	ENCAINIDE HYDROCHLORIDE; ENKAID	RE30811	DEC 20, 1996	U-17		
18981 004	ENCAINIDE HYDROCHLORIDE; ENKAID	RE30811	DEC 20, 1996	U-17		

PRESCRIPTION AND OTC DRUG PRODUCT PATENT AND EXCLUSIVITY DATA *(continued)*

APPL/ PROD NUMBER	INGREDIENT NAME; TRADE NAME	PATENT NUMBER	PATENT EXPIRES	USE CODE	EX-CLUS CODE	EXCLUS EXPIRES
19616 004	ENOXACIN; PENETREX	4442101	APR 10, 2001			
		4359578	NOV 16, 1999		NCE	DEC 31, 1996
		4352803	OCT 05, 1999	U-36		
19616 005	ENOXACIN; PENETREX	4442101	APR 10, 2001			
		4359578	NOV 16, 1999		NCE	DEC 31, 1996
		4352803	OCT 05, 1999	U-36		
20164 001	ENOXAPARIN SODIUM; LOVENOX				NCE	MAR 29, 1998
18418 001	ERGOLOID MESYLATES; HYDERGINE	4138565	FEB 06, 1996			
18706 001	ERGOLOID MESYLATES; HYDERGINE LC	4366145	DEC 28, 1999			
19386 001	ESMOLOL HYDROCHLORIDE; BREVIBLOC	4593119	JUN 03, 2003		I-84	DEC 18, 1995
		4387103	JUN 07, 2000	U-11	D-19	DEC 18, 1995
19386 002	ESMOLOL HYDROCHLORIDE; BREVIBLOC	4593119	JUN 03, 2003		I-84	DEC 18, 1995
		4387103	JUN 07, 2000	U-11	D-19	DEC 18, 1995
19386 003	ESMOLOL HYDROCHLORIDE; BREVIBLOC	4387103	JUN 07, 2000	U-11		
19080 001	ESTAZOLAM; PROSOM	3987052	OCT 19, 1995		NCE	DEC 26, 1995
19080 002	ESTAZOLAM; PROSOM	3987052	OCT 19, 1995		NCE	DEC 26, 1995
19081 002	ESTRADIOL; ESTRADERM	4379454	APR 12, 2000		I-62	OCT 24, 1994
19081 003	ESTRADIOL; ESTRADERM	4379454	APR 12, 2000		I-62	OCT 24, 1994
81295 001	ESTRADIOL; ESTRACE				I-76	SEP 08, 1995
84499 001	ESTRADIOL; ESTRACE				I-76	SEP 08, 1995
84500 001	ESTRADIOL; ESTRACE				I-76	SEP 08, 1995
86069 001	ESTRADIOL; ESTRACE	4436738	MAR 13, 2001			
83220 001	ESTROPIPATE; OGEN .625				I-76	NOV 10, 1995
83220 002	ESTROPIPATE; OGEN 1.25				I-76	NOV 10, 1995
83220 003	ESTROPIPATE; OGEN 2.5				I-76	NOV 10, 1995
83220 004	ESTROPIPATE; OGEN 5				I-76	NOV 10, 1995
19357 001	ETHANOLAMINE OLEATE; ETHAMOLIN				ODE	DEC 22, 1995
18977 001	ETHINYL ESTRADIOL; TRI-NORINYL 21-DAY	4390531	JUN 28, 2000			
18977 002	ETHINYL ESTRADIOL; TRI-NORINYL 28-DAY	4390531	JUN 28, 2000			
18985 001	ETHINYL ESTRADIOL; ORTHO-NOVUM 7/7/7-21	4616006	OCT 07, 2003			
		4544554	JUL 23, 2002			
		4530839	JUL 23, 2002			
18985 002	ETHINYL ESTRADIOL; ORTHO-NOVUM 7/7/7-28	4616006	OCT 07, 2003			
		4544554	JUL 23, 2002			
		4530839	JUL 23, 2002			
19653 001	ETHINYL ESTRADIOL; ORTHO CYCLEN-21	4027019	MAY 31, 1996			
19653 002	ETHINYL ESTRADIOL; ORTHO CYCLEN-28	4027019	MAY 31, 1996			
19697 001	ETHINYL ESTRADIOL; ORTHO TRI-CYCLEN	4628051	OCT 01, 2002	U-66		
		4616006	OCT 07, 2003	U-66		
		4544554	JUL 23, 2002	U-66		
		4027019	MAY 31, 1996		NP	JUL 03, 1995
19697 002	ETHINYL ESTRADIOL; ORTHO TRI-CYCLEN	4628051	OCT 01, 2002	U-66		
		4616006	OCT 07, 2003	U-66		
		4544554	JUL 23, 2002	U-66		
		4027019	MAY 31, 1996		NP	JUL 03, 1995
17831 001	ETIDRONATE DISODIUM; DIDRONEL	4254114	MAR 03, 1998			
		4216211	AUG 05, 1997			
		4137309	JAN 30, 1996			
17831 002	ETIDRONATE DISODIUM; DIDRONEL	4254114	MAR 03, 1998			
		4216211	AUG 05, 1997			
		4137309	JAN 30, 1996			
19545 001	ETIDRONATE DISODIUM; DIDRONEL	4254114	MAR 03, 1998			
		4216211	AUG 05, 1997			
		4137309	JAN 30, 1996		ODE	APR 20, 1994
18922 002	ETODOLAC; LODINE	4076831	FEB 28, 1997	U-45	NCE	JAN 31, 1996
18922 003	ETODOLAC; LODINE	4076831	FEB 28, 1997	U-45	NCE	JAN 31, 1996
18922 004	ETODOLAC; LODINE	4076831	FEB 28, 1997	U-45	NCE	JAN 31, 1996
19369 001	ETRETINATE; TEGISON	4215215	JUL 29, 1999			
		4200647	APR 29, 1997			
19369 002	ETRETINATE; TEGISON	4215215	JUL 29, 1999			
		4200647	APR 29, 1997			
20363 002	FAMCICLOVIR; FAMVIR				NCE	JUN 29, 1999
19462 001	FAMOTIDINE; PEPCID	4283408	AUG 11, 2000		I-69	DEC 10, 1994
19462 002	FAMOTIDINE; PEPCID	4283408	AUG 11, 2000		I-69	DEC 10, 1994
19510 001	FAMOTIDINE; PEPCID	4283408	AUG 11, 2000			
19527 001	FAMOTIDINE; PEPCID	4283408	AUG 11, 2000		I-69	DEC 10, 1994
20189 001	FELBAMATE; FELBATOL	5082861	JAN 21, 2009	U-83	ODE	JUL 29, 1998
		4978680	DEC 18, 2007	U-83	NCE	JUL 29, 1998

PRESCRIPTION AND OTC DRUG PRODUCT PATENT AND EXCLUSIVITY DATA *(continued)*

APPL/ PROD NUMBER	INGREDIENT NAME; TRADE NAME	PATENT NUMBER	PATENT EXPIRES	USE CODE	EX-CLUS CODE	EXCLUS EXPIRES
20189 002	FELBAMATE; FELBATOL	5082861	JAN 21, 2009	U-83	ODE	JUL 29, 2000
		4978680	DEC 18, 2007	U-83	NCE	JUL 29, 1998
20189 003	FELBAMATE; FELBATOL	5082861	JAN 21, 2009	U-83	ODE	JUL 29, 2000
		4978680	DEC 18, 2007	U-83	NCE	JUL 29, 1998
19834 001	FELODIPINE; PLENDIL	4264611	APR 28, 1998		NCE	JUL 25, 1996
19834 002	FELODIPINE; PLENDIL	4264611	APR 28, 1998		NCE	JUL 25, 1996
19304 001	FENOFIBRATE; LIPIDIL	4058552	NOV 15, 1994		NCE	DEC 31, 1998
19813 001	FENTANYL; DURAGESIC	4588580	MAY 13, 2003	U-43		
		4060084	JUN 28, 1994	U-43		
19813 002	FENTANYL; DURAGESIC	4588580	MAY 13, 2003	U-43		
		4060084	JUN 28, 1994	U-43		
19813 003	FENTANYL; DURAGESIC	4588580	MAY 13, 2003	U-43		
		4060084	JUN 28, 1994	U-43		
19813 004	FENTANYL; DURAGESIC	4588580	MAY 13, 2003	U-43		
		4060084	JUN 28, 1994	U-43		
20195 001	FENTANYL CITRATE; FENTANYL	4671953	JUN 09, 2004	U-87	NDF	OCT 04, 1996
20195 002	FENTANYL CITRATE; FENTANYL	4671953	JUN 09, 2004	U-87	NDF	OCT 04, 1996
20195 003	FENTANYL CITRATE; FENTANYL	4671953	JUN 09, 2004	U-87	NDF	OCT 04, 1996
20180 001	FINASTERIDE; PROSCAR	4760071	JUL 26, 2005			
		4377584	MAR 22, 2000		NCE	JUN 19, 1997
18830 001	FLECAINIDE ACETATE; TAMBOCOR	4005209	JAN 25, 1996		I-64	OCT 23, 1994
18830 003	FLECAINIDE ACETATE; TAMBOCOR	4005209	JAN 25, 1996		I-64	OCT 23, 1994
18830 004	FLECAINIDE ACETATE; TAMBOCOR	4005209	JAN 25, 1996		I-64	OCT 23, 1994
19960 001	FLOSEQUINAN; MANOPLAX	4552884	NOV 12, 2002	U-71		
		4302460	NOV 24, 1998		NCE	DEC 30, 1997
19960 002	FLOSEQUINAN; MANOPLAX	4552884	NOV 12, 2002	U-71		
		4302460	NOV 24, 1998		NCE	DEC 30, 1997
19960 003	FLOSEQUINAN; MANOPLAX	4552884	NOV 12, 2002	U-71		
		4302460	NOV 24, 1998		NCE	DEC 30, 1997
19960 004	FLOSEQUINAN; MANOPLAX	4552884	NOV 12, 2002	U-71		
		4302460	NOV 24, 1998		NCE	DEC 30, 1997
19949 001	FLUCONAZOLE; DIFLUCAN	4416682	NOV 22, 2000		I-100	DEC 30, 1996
		4404216	OCT 16, 2003		NCE	JAN 29, 1995
19949 002	FLUCONAZOLE; DIFLUCAN	4416682	NOV 22, 2000		I-100	DEC 20, 1996
		4404216	OCT 16, 2003		NCE	JAN 29, 1995
19949 003	FLUCONAZOLE; DIFLUCAN	4416682	NOV 22, 2000		i-100	DEC 30, 1996
		4404216	OCT 16, 2003		NCE	JAN 29, 1995
19950 001	FLUCONAZOLE; DIFLUCAN	4416682	NOV 22, 2000		I-100	DEC 30, 1996
		4404216	OCT 16, 2003		NCE	JAN 29, 1995
20090 001	FLUCONAZOLE; DIFLUCAN	4416682	NOV 22, 2000			
		4404216	OCT 16, 2003		NCE	JAN 29, 1995
20090 002	FLUCONAZOLE; DIFLUCAN	4416682	NOV 22, 2000			
		4404216	OCT 16, 2003		NCE	JAN 29, 1995
20322 001	FLUCONAZOLE; DIFLUCAN	4552884	NOV 12, 2002		I-100	DEC 30, 1996
		4302460	NOV 24, 1998		NCE	JAN 29, 1995
					NS	JUN 30, 1997
					I-107	JUN 30, 1997
20038 001	FLUDARABINE PHOSPHATE; FLUDARA	4357324	NOV 02, 2001		NCE	APR 18, 1996
					ODE	APR 18, 1998
20073 001	FLUMAZENIL; ROMAZICON	4316839	MAR 03, 2003		NCE	DEC 20, 1996
16909 002	FLUOCINONIDE; LIDEX	4017615	APR 12, 1994			
18936 001	FLUOXETINE HYDROCHLORIDE; PROZAC	4626549	DEC 02, 2003	U-84		
		4314081	FEB 02, 2001			
		4194009	APR 19, 1994			
		4018895	APR 19, 1994	U-12	I-102	FEB 28, 1997
18936 006	FLUOXETINE HYDROCHLORIDE; PROZAC	4626549	DEC 02, 2003	U-84		
		4314081	FEB 02, 2001		I-102	FEB 28, 1997
		4194009	APR 19, 1994			
		4018895	APR 19, 1994	U-12		
20101 001	FLUOXETINE HYDROCHLORIDE; PROZAC	4626549	DEC 02, 2003	U-84		
		4314081	FEB 02, 2001		I-102	FEB 28, 1997
		4194009	APR 19, 1994			
		4194009	APR 19, 1994	U-12		
18554 001	FLUTAMIDE; EULEXIN	4472382	JAN 27, 2003	U-24		
		4329364	MAY 11, 2001	U-23	NCE	JAN 27, 1994
19957 001	FLUTICASONE PROPIONATE; CUTIVATE	4335121	MAR 16, 2002		NCE	DEC 14, 1995
19958 001	FLUTICASONE PROPIONATE; CUTIVATE	4335121	MAR 16, 2002		NCE	DEC 14, 1995
20261 001	FLUVASTATIN SODIUM; LESCOL				NCE	DEC 31, 1998
20261 002	FLUVASTATIN SODIUM; LESCOL				NCE	DEC 31, 1998

PRESCRIPTION AND OTC DRUG PRODUCT PATENT AND EXCLUSIVITY DATA *(continued)*

APPL/ PROD NUMBER	INGREDIENT NAME; TRADE NAME	PATENT NUMBER	PATENT EXPIRES	USE CODE	EX-CLUS CODE	EXCLUS EXPIRES
20068 001	FOSCARNET SODIUM; FOSCAVIR	4771041	JUL 29, 1997			
		4665062	JUL 29, 1997			
		4339445	JUL 29, 1997	U-64		
		4215113	JUN 06, 2000	U-64	NCE	SEP 27, 1996
19915 002	FOSINOPRIL SODIUM; MONOPRIL	4384123	MAY 17, 2000			
		4337201	JUN 29, 2001		NCE	MAY 16, 1996
19915 003	FOSINOPRIL SODIUM; MONOPRIL	4384123	MAY 17, 2000			
		4337201	JUN 29, 2001		NCE	MAY 16, 1996
20235 001	GABAPENTIN; NEURONTIN	4894476	JAN 16, 2007			
		4087544	MAY 02, 1995	U-86		
		4024175	MAY 17, 1994		NCE	DEC 30, 1998
20235 002	GABAPENTIN; NEURONTIN	4894476	JAN 16, 2007			
		4087544	MAY 02, 1995	U-86		
		4024175	MAY 17, 1994		NCE	DEC 30, 1998
20235 003	GABAPENTIN; NEURONTIN	4894476	JAN 16, 2007			
		4087544	MAY 02, 1995	U-86		
		4024175	MAY 17, 1994		NCE	DEC 30, 1998
20123 001	GADODIAMIDE; OMNISCAN	4687659	AUG 18, 2004	U-76	NCE	JAN 08, 1998
19596 001	GADOPENTETATE DIMEGLUMINE; MAGNEVIST	4963344	MAR 03, 2004			
		4957939	MAR 03, 2004		I-94	AUG 17, 1996
		4647447	MAR 03, 2004			
20131 001	GADOTERIDOL; PROHANCE	4885363	DEC 05, 2006		NCE	NOV 16, 1997
19961 002	GALLIUM NITRATE; GANITE	4529593	JAN 17, 2005	U-49	NCE	JAN 17, 1996
					ODE	JAN 17, 1998
19661 001	GANCICLOVIR SODIUM; CYTOVENE	4507305	OCT 19, 1999	U-35	I-72	MAY 15, 1995
		4423050	OCT 19, 1999	U-34		
		4355032	MAR 16, 2003	U-33	NCE	JUN 23, 1994
17783 001	GLIPIZIDE; GLUCOTROL				NCE	MAY 08, 1994
17783 002	GLIPIZIDE; GLUCOTROL				NCE	MAY 08, 1994
17783 003	GLIPIZIDE; GLUCOTROL				NCE	MAY 08, 1994
20329 001	GLIPIZIDE; GLUCOTROL XL				NDF	APR 26, 1997
20329 002	GLIPIZIDE; GLUCOTROL XL				NDF	APR 26, 1997
17498 001	GLYBURIDE; MICRONASE				NCE	MAY 01, 1994
17498 002	GLYBURIDE; MICRONASE				NCE	MAY 01, 1994
17498 003	GLYBURIDE; MICRONASE				NCE	MAY 01, 1994
17532 001	GLYBURIDE; DIABETA				NCE	MAY 01, 1994
17532 002	GLYBURIDE; DIABETA				NCE	MAY 01, 1994
17532 003	GLYBURIDE; DIABETA				NCE	MAY 01, 1994
20051 001	GLYBURIDE; GLYNASE	4916163	APR 10, 2007		NP	MAR 04, 1995
		4735805	APR 05, 2005		NCE	MAY 01, 1994
20051 002	GLYBURIDE; GLYNASE	4916163	APR 10, 2007		NP	MAR 04, 1995
		4735805	APR 05, 2005		NCE	MAY 01, 1994
20051 003	GLYBURIDE; GLYNASE	4916163	APR 10, 2007		NCE	MAY 01, 1994
		4735805	APR 05, 2005		NP	MAR 04, 1995
20051 004	GLYBURIDE; GLYNASE	4916163	APR 10, 2007		NCE	MAY 01, 1994
		4735805	APR 05, 2005		NP	MAR 04, 1995
20055 002	GLYBURIDE; GLUBATE				NP	MAR 04, 1995
					NCE	MAY 01, 1994
19726 001	GOSERELIN ACETATE; ZOLADEX	4100274	JUL 10, 1997		NCE	DEC 29, 1994
					I-88	FEB 02, 1996
20239 001	GRANISETRON HYDROCHLORIDE; KYTRIL	4886808	DEC 12, 2006	U-89	NCE	DEC 29, 1998
19032 001	GUANFACINE HYDROCHLORIDE; TENEX				I-91	MAY 11, 1996
19032 002	GUANFACINE HYDROCHLORIDE; TENEX				I-91	MAY 11, 1996
18234 001	HALCINONIDE; HALOG-E	4048310	SEP 13, 1994			
19967 001	HALOBETASOL PROPIONATE, ULTRAVATE	4619921	DEC 17, 2004		NCE	DEC 17, 1995
					D-1	DEC 31, 1994
19968 001	HALOBETASOL PROPIONATE; ULTRAVATE	4619921	DEC 17, 2004		NCE	DEC 17, 1995
					D-1	DEC 31, 1994
20250 001	HALOFANTRINE HYDROCHLORIDE; HALFAN				NCE	JUL 24, 1997
					ODE	JUL 24, 1999
19836 001	HISTRELIN ACETATE; SUPPRELIN	4244946	JAN 13, 1998		NCE	DEC 24, 1996
					ODE	DEC 24, 1998
19836 002	HISTRELIN ACETATE; SUPPRELIN	4244946	JAN 13, 1998		NCE	DEC 24, 1996
					ODE	DEC 24, 1998
19836 003	HISTRELIN ACETATE; SUPPRELIN	4244946	JAN 13, 1998		NCE	DEC 24, 1996
					ODE	DEC 24, 1998
18061 001	HYDROCHLOROTHIAZIDE; TIMOLIDE 10-25	4238485	DEC 09, 1997			
19046 001	HYDROCHLOROTHIAZIDE; NORMOZIDE	4066755	JAN 03, 1995			
		4012444	MAR 15, 1994		NCE	AUG 01, 1994

PRESCRIPTION AND OTC DRUG PRODUCT PATENT AND EXCLUSIVITY DATA *(continued)*

APPL/ PROD NUMBER	INGREDIENT NAME; TRADE NAME	PATENT NUMBER	PATENT EXPIRES	USE CODE	EX-CLUS CODE	EXCLUS EXPIRES
19046 002	HYDROCHLOROTHIAZIDE; NORMOZIDE	4066755	JAN 03, 1995			
		4012444	MAR 15, 1994		NCE	AUG 01, 1994
19046 003	HYDROCHLOROTHIAZIDE; NORMOZIDE	4066755	JAN 03, 1995			
		4012444	MAR 15, 1994		NCE	AUG 01, 1994
19046 004	HYDROCHLOROTHIAZIDE; NORMOZIDE	4066755	JAN 03, 1995			
		4012444	MAR 15, 1994		NCE	AUG 01, 1994
19059 001	HYDROCHLOROTHIAZIDE; INDERIDE LA 80/50	4138475	FEB 06, 1996			
19059 002	HYDROCHLOROTHIAZIDE; INDERIDE LA 120/50	4138475	FEB 06, 1996			
19059 003	HYDROCHLOROTHIAZIDE; INDERIDE LA 160/50	4138475	FEB 06, 1996			
19129 001	HYDROCHLOROTHIAZIDE; MAXZIDE	4444769	APR 24, 2001			
19129 003	HYDROCHLOROTHIAZIDE; MAXZIDE-25	4444769	APR 24, 2001			
19174 001	HYDROCHLOROTHIAZIDE; TRANDATE HCT	4066755	JAN 03, 1995			
		4012444	MAR 15, 1994		NCE	AUG 01, 1994
19174 002	HYDROCHLOROTHIAZIDE; TRANDATE HCT	4066755	JAN 03, 1995			
		4012444	MAR 15, 1994		NCE	AUG 01, 1994
19174 003	HYDROCHLOROTHIAZIDE; TRANDATE HCT	4066755	JAN 03, 1995			
		4012444	MAR 15, 1994		NCE	AUG 01, 1994
19174 004	HYDROCHLOROTHIAZIDE; TRANDATE HCT	4066755	JAN 03, 1995			
		4012444	MAR 15, 1994		NCE	AUG 01, 1994
19778 001	HYDROCHLOROTHIAZIDE; PRINZIDE 20-12.5	4472380	SEP 18, 2001			
		4374829	DEC 30, 2001			
19778 002	HYDROCHLOROTHIAZIDE; PRINZIDE 20-25	4472380	SEP 18, 2001			
		4374829	DEC 30, 2001			
19788 003	HYDROCHLOROTHIAZIDE; PRINZIDE 10-12.5	4472380	SEP 18, 2001			
		4374829	DEC 30, 2001	U-3	NS	NOV 18, 1996
19888 001	HYDROCHLOROTHIAZIDE; PRINZIDE 20-12.5	4472380	SEP 18, 2001			
		4374829	DEC 30, 2001	U-3		
19888 002	HYDROCHLOROTHIAZIDE; ZESTORETIC 20-25	4472380	SEP 18, 2001			
		4374829	DEC 30, 2001	U-3		
19888 003	HYDROCHLOROTHIAZIDE; ZESTORETIC 10-12.5	4472380	SEP 18, 2001			
		4374829	DEC 30, 2001	U-3		
19034 001	HYDROMORPHONE HYDROCHLORIDE; DILAUDID-HP				NCE	JAN 11, 1994
19891 001	HYDROMORPHONE HYDROCHLORIDE; DILAUDID				NCE	JAN 11, 1994
					NDF	DEC 07, 1995
19892 001	HYDROMORPHONE HYDROCHLORIDE; DILAUDID				NCE	JAN 11, 1994
					NDF	DEC 07, 1995
19261 001	HYDROXYAMPHETAMINE HYDROBROMIDE; PAREMYD				NC	JAN 30, 1995
19833 002	IBUPROFEN; CHILDREN'S ADVIL	4788220	NOV 29, 2005			
50661 001	IDARUBICIN HYDROCHLORIDE; IDAMYCIN				ODE	SEP 27, 1997
50661 002	IDARUBICIN HYDROCHLORIDE; IDAMYCIN				ODE	SEP 27, 1997
19763 001	IFOSFAMIDE; IFEX				ODE	DEC 30, 1995
19763 002	IFOSFAMIDE; IFEX				ODE	DEC 30, 1995
20367 001	IMIGLUCERASE; CEREZYME				NCE	MAY 23, 1999
					ODE	MAY 23, 2001
18538 002	INDAPAMIDE; LOZOL				NS	APR 29, 1996
19693 001	INDECAINIDE HYDROCHLORIDE; DECABID	4452745	JUN 05, 2003		NCE	DEC 29, 1994
		4389393	JUN 21, 2000			
		4382093	MAY 03, 2000			
		4197313	APR 08, 1997	U-41		
19693 002	INDECAINIDE HYDROCHLORIDE; DECABID	4452745	JUN 05, 2003		NCE	DEC 29, 1994
		4389393	JUN 21, 2000			
		4382093	MAY 03, 2000			
		4197313	APR 08, 1997	U-41		
19693 003	INDECAINIDE HYDROCHLORIDE; DECABID	4452745	JUN 05, 2003		NCE	DEC 29, 1994
		4389393	JUN 21, 2000			
		4382093	MAY 03, 2000			
		4197313	APR 08, 1997	U-41		
19044 001	INDIUM IN-111 OXYQUINOLINE; INDIUM IN-111 OXYQUINOLINE	4335095	JUN 15, 1999			
20314 001	INDIUM IN-111 PENTETREOTIDE KIT; OCTREOSCAN				NCE	JUN 02, 1999
18185 001	INDOMETHACIN; INDOCIN SR	4173626	NOV 06, 1996			
20100 001	INSULIN BIOSYNTHETIC HUMAN; HUMULIN 50/50				NP	APR 29, 1995
20084 001	IOBENGUANE SULFATE I 131; IOBENGUANE SULFATE I 131	4584187	APR 22, 2003		NCE	MAR 25, 1999
19432 001	IOFETAMINE HYDROCHLORIDE I-123; SPECTAMINE	4360511	NOV 23, 2001			

PRESCRIPTION AND OTC DRUG PRODUCT PATENT AND EXCLUSIVITY DATA *(continued)*

APPL/ PROD NUMBER	INGREDIENT NAME; TRADE NAME	PATENT NUMBER	PATENT EXPIRES	USE CODE	EX-CLUS CODE	EXCLUS EXPIRES
18956 001	IOHEXOL; OMNIPAQUE 180	4396597	JUL 14, 1998			
		4250113	DEC 26, 1999		I-97	JUL 13, 1996
		4021481	MAY 03, 1994		NR	JUL 13, 1996
18956 002	IOHEXOL; OMNIPAQUE 240	4396597	JUL 14, 1998			
		4250113	DEC 26, 1999			
		4021481	MAY 03, 1994			
18956 003	IOHEXOL; OMNIPAQUE 300	4396597	JUL 14, 1998			
		4250113	DEC 26, 1999			
		4021481	MAY 03, 1994			
18956 004	IOHEXOL; OMNIPAQUE 350	4396597	JUL 14, 1998			
		4250113	DEC 26, 1999			
		4021481	MAY 03, 1994			
18956 005	IOHEXOL; OMNIPAQUE 140	4396597	JUL 14, 1998			
		4250113	DEC 26, 1999			
		4021481	MAY 03, 1994			
18956 006	IOHEXOL; OMNIPAQUE 210	4396597	JUL 14, 1998			
		4250113	DEC 26, 1999			
		4021481	MAY 03, 1994			
18735 001	IOPAMIDOL; ISOVUE-M 200	4001323	JAN 04, 1996			
18735 002	IOPAMIDOL; ISOVUE-300	4001323	JAN 04, 1996			
18735 003	IOPAMIDOL; ISOVUE-370	4001323	JAN 04, 1996			
18735 004	IOPAMIDOL; ISOVUE-M 300	4001323	JAN 04, 1996			
18735 007	IOPAMIDOL; ISOVUE-250	4001323	JAN 04, 1996		NS	JUL 06, 1995
19580 001	IOTROLAN; OSMOVIST	4239747	DEC 16, 1999		NCE	DEC 07, 1994
19580 002	IOTROLAN; OSMOVIST	4239747	DEC 16, 1999		NCE	DEC 07, 1994
19710 001	IOVERSOL; OPTIRAY 320	4396598	OCT 26, 2002	U-28	NCE	
		4396598	OCT 26, 2002	U-29	I-83	DEC 11, 1995
19710 002	IOVERSOL; OPTIRAY 240	4396598	OCT 26, 2002	U-30	I-78	JUL 09, 1995
19710 003	IOVERSOL; OPTIRAY 160	4396598	OCT 26, 2002	U-31		
19710 004	IOVERSOL; OPTIRAY 300	4396598	OCT 26, 2002	U-61	NS	JAN 22, 1995
19710 005	IOVERSOL; OPTIRAY 350	4396598	OCT 26, 2002	U-62	NS	JAN 22, 1995
					I-74	JAN 22, 1995
					I-48	JUL 27, 1995
18905 002	IOXAGLATE MEGLUMINE; HEXABRIX	4094966	JUN 13, 1995			
		4065554	DEC 27, 1994			
		4065553	DEC 27, 1994			
		4014986	MAR 29, 1996			
20228 001	IPRATROPIUM BROMIDE; ATROVENT				NDF	SEP 29, 1996
50705 001	ISONIAZID; RIFATER				ODE	MAY 31, 2001
19091 001	ISOSORBIDE MONONITRATE; ISMO				NCE	DEC 30, 1996
20215 001	ISOSORBIDE MONONITRATE; MONOKET				NCE	DEC 30, 1996
20215 002	ISOSORBIDE MONONITRATE; MONOKET				NCE	DEC 30, 1996
					NS	JUN 30, 1996
20225 001	ISOSORBIDE MONONITRATE; IMDUR				NCE	DEC 30, 1996
					NDF	AUG 12, 1996
20225 002	ISOSORBIDE MONONITRATE; IMDUR				NCE	DEC 30, 1996
					NDF	AUG 12, 1996
18662 002	ISOTRETINOIN; ACCUTANE	4464394	AUG 07, 2001			
		4322438	MAR 30, 1999			
		4200647	APR 29, 1997			
18662 003	ISOTRETINOIN; ACCUTANE	4464394	AUG 07, 2001			
		4322438	MAR 30, 1999			
		4200647	APR 29, 1997			
18662 004	ISOTRETINOIN; ACCUTANE	4464394	AUG 07, 2001			
		4322438	MAR 30, 1999			
		4200647	APR 29, 1997			
19546 001	ISRADIPINE; DYNACIRC	4466972	AUG 21, 2003	U-3	NCE	DEC 20, 1995
19546 002	ISRADIPINE; DYNACIRC	4466972	AUG 21, 2003	U-3	NCE	DEC 20, 1995
20336 001	ISRADIPINE; DYNACIRC CR	5030456	JUL 09, 2008			
		4950486	AUG 21, 2007		NDF	JUN 01, 1997
		4946687	AUG 07, 2007		NCE	DEC 20, 1995
		4816263	MAR 28, 2006	U-3		
		4783337	SEP 16, 2003	U-3		
		4466972	AUG 21, 2003	U-3		

PRESCRIPTION AND OTC DRUG PRODUCT PATENT AND EXCLUSIVITY DATA *(continued)*

APPL/ PROD NUMBER	INGREDIENT NAME; TRADE NAME	PATENT NUMBER	PATENT EXPIRES	USE CODE	EX-CLUS CODE	EXCLUS EXPIRES
20336 002	ISRADIPINE; DYNACIRC CR	5030456	JUL 09, 2008			
		4950486	AUG 21, 2007		NDF	JUN 01, 1997
		4946687	AUG 07, 2007		NCE	DEC 20, 1995
		4816263	MAR 28, 2006	U-3		
		4783337	SEP 16, 2003	U-3		
		4466972	AUG 21, 2003	U-3		
20083 001	ITRACONAZOLE; SPORANOX	4267179	MAY 12, 1998		NCE	SEP 11, 1997
					I-104	MAR 29, 1997
18533 001	KETOCONAZOLE; NIZORAL	4335125	JUN 15, 1999			
19084 001	KETOCONAZOLE; NIZORAL	4335125	JUN 15, 1999		I-30	JAN 27, 1996
19576 001	KETOCONAZOLE; NIZORAL	4335125	JUN 15, 1999			
19648 001	KETOCONAZOLE; NIZORAL	4335125	JUN 15, 1999			
19927 001	KETOCONAZOLE; NIZORAL	4335125	JUN 15, 1999			
19816 001	KETOPROFEN; ORUVAIL				NDF	SEP 24, 1996
19645 001	KETOROLAC TROMETHAMINE; TORADOL	4089969	MAY 16, 1997	U-55	NDF	DEC 20, 1994
					NCE	NOV 30, 1994
19698 001	KETOROLAC TROMETHAMINE; TORADOL	4089969	MAY 16, 1997	U-55	NCE	NOV 30, 1994
19698 002	KETOROLAC TROMETHAMINE; TORADOL	4089969	MAY 16, 1997	U-55	NCE	NOV 30, 1994
19700 001	KETOROLAC TROMETHAMINE; ACULAR	5110493	MAY 05, 2009	U-75	NCE	NOV 30, 1994
		4454151	JUN 12, 2001	U-75	NCF	NOV 09, 1995
		4089969	MAY 16, 1997	U-75		
18686 001	LABETALOL HYDROCHLORIDE; NORMODYNE	4328213	MAY 04, 1999			
		4066755	JAN 03, 1995			
		4012444	AUG 2, 1998		NCE	AUG 01, 1994
18687 001	LABETALOL HYDROCHLORIDE; NORMODYNE	4066755	JAN 03, 1995			
		4012444	AUG 2, 1998		NCE	AUG 01, 1994
18687 002	LABETALOL HYDROCHLORIDE; NORMODYNE	4066755	JAN 03, 1995			
		4012444	AUG 2, 1998		NCE	AUG 01, 1994
18687 003	LABETALOL HYDROCHLORIDE; NORMODYNE	4066755	JAN 03, 1995			
		4012444	AUG 2, 1998		NCE	AUG 01, 1994
18687 004	LABETALOL HYDROCHLORIDE; NORMODYNE	4066755	JAN 03, 1995			
		4012444	AUG 2, 1998		NCE	AUG 01, 1994
18716 001	LABETALOL HYDROCHLORIDE; TRANDATE	4066755	JAN 03, 1995			
		4012444	AUG 2, 1998		NCE	AUG 01, 1994
18716 002	LABETALOL HYDROCHLORIDE; TRANDATE	4066755	JAN 03, 1995			
		4012444	AUG 2, 1998		NCE	AUG 01, 1994
18716 003	LABETALOL HYDROCHLORIDE; TRANDATE	4066755	JAN 03, 1995			
		4012444	AUG 02, 1998		NCE	AUG 01, 1994
18716 004	LABETALOL HYDROCHLORIDE; TRANDATE	4066755	JAN 03, 1995			
		4012444	AUG 02, 1998		NCE	AUG 01, 1994
19425 001	LABETALOL HYDROCHLORIDE; TRANDATE	4066755	JAN 03, 1995			
		4012444	AUG 02, 1998		NCE	AUG 01, 1994
08107 001	LEUCOVORIN CALCIUM; LEUCOVORIN CALCIUM				I-22	AUG 31, 1995
					ODE	DEC 12, 1998
					I-70	DEC 12, 1994
08107 002	LEUCOVORIN CALCIUM; LEUCOVORIN CALCIUM				ODE	AUG 31, 1995
					I-22	AUG 31, 1995
					ODE	DEC 12, 1998
					I-70	DEC 12, 1994
08107 003	LEUCOVORIN CALCIUM; LEUCOVORIN CALCIUM				ODE	AUG 31, 1995
					I-22	AUG 31, 1995
08107 004	LEUCOVORIN CALCIUM; LEUCOVORIN CALCIUM				ODE	AUG 31, 1995
					I-22	AUG 31, 1995
					ODE	DEC 12, 1998
					I-70	DEC 12, 1994
08107 005	LEUCOVORIN CALCIUM; LEUCOVORIN CALCIUM				ODE	AUG 31, 1995
					I-22	AUG 31, 1995
					ODE	DEC 12, 1998
					I-70	DEC 12, 1994
19010 001	LEUPROLIDE ACETATE; LUPRON	4005063	JAN 25, 1996			
19732 001	LEUPROLIDE ACETATE; LUPRON DEPOT	4917893	MAR 24, 2004			
		4849228	JUL 18, 2006			
		4728721	MAR 01, 2005			
		4677191	JUN 30, 2004			
		4652441	MAR 24, 2004			
		4005063	JAN 25, 1996			

PRESCRIPTION AND OTC DRUG PRODUCT PATENT AND EXCLUSIVITY DATA *(continued)*

APPL/ PROD NUMBER	INGREDIENT NAME; TRADE NAME	PATENT NUMBER	PATENT EXPIRES	USE CODE	EX-CLUS CODE	EXCLUS EXPIRES
20011 001	LEUPROLIDE ACETATE; LUPRON DEPOT	4917893	MAR 24, 2004			
		4849228	JUL 18, 2006			
		4728721	MAR 01, 2005			
		4677191	JUN 30, 2004			
		4652441	MAR 24, 2004			
		4005063	JAN 25, 1996			
20263 001	LEUPROLIDE ACETATE; LUPRON	4917893	MAR 24, 2004			
		4849228	JUL 18, 2006		NP	APR 16, 1996
		4728721	MAR 01, 2005			
		4677191	JUN 30, 2004			
		4652441	MAR 24, 2004			
		4005063	JAN 25, 1996		ODE	APR 16, 2000
20263 002	LEUPROLIDE ACETATE; LUPRON DEPOT-PED	4917893	MAR 24, 2004			
		4849228	JUL 18, 2006		NP	APR 16, 1996
		4728721	MAR 01, 2005			
		4677191	JUN 30, 2004			
		4652441	MAR 24, 2004			
		4005063	JAN 25, 1996		ODE	APR 16, 2000
20263 003	LEUPROLIDE ACETATE; LUPRON DEPOT-PED	4917893	MAR 24, 2004			
		4849228	JUL 18, 2006		NP	APR 16, 1996
		4728721	MAR 01, 2005			
		4677191	JUN 30, 2004			
		4652441	MAR 24, 2004			
		4005063	JAN 25, 1996		ODE	APR 16, 2000
20263 004	LEUPROLIDE ACETATE; LUPRON DEPOT-PED	4917893	MAR 24, 2004			
		4849228	JUL 18, 2006		NP	APR 16, 1996
		4728721	MAR 01, 2005			
		4677191	JUN 30, 2004			
		4652441	MAR 24, 2004			
		4005063	JAN 25, 1996		ODE	APR 16, 2000
20035 001	LEVAMISOLE HYDROCHLORIDE; ERGAMISOL	4584305	JUN 19, 2004	U-42	NCE	JUN 18, 1995
20219 001	LEVOCABASTINE HYDROCHLORIDE; LIVOSTIN	4369184	JAN 18, 2000		NCE	NOV 10, 1998
18948 001	LEVOCARNITINE; CARNITOR				I-86	DEC 16, 1995
					ODE	DEC 16, 1999
18948 002	LEVOCARNITINE; CARNITOR				I-86	DEC 16, 1995
					ODE	DEC 16, 1999
20182 001	LEVOCARNITINE; CARNITOR				I-86	DEC 16, 1995
					ODE	DEC 16, 1999
20315 001	LEVOMETHADYL ACETATE HYDROCHLORIDE;				NCE	JUL 09, 1998
	ORLAAM				ODE	JUL 09, 2000
19941 001	LIDOCAINE; EMLA	4562060	DEC 31, 2002			
		4529601	JUL 16, 2002		NC	DEC 30, 1995
20105 001	LIOTHYRONINE SODIUM; TRIOSTAT				NDF	DEC 31, 1994
					ODE	DEC 31, 1998
19558 001	LISINOPRIL; PRINIVIL	4374829	DEC 30, 2001		I-92	JUN 09, 1996
19558 002	LISINOPRIL; PRINIVIL	4374829	DEC 30, 2001		I-92	JUN 09, 1996
19558 003	LISINOPRIL; PRINIVIL	4374829	DEC 30, 2001		I-92	JUN 09, 1996
19558 004	LISINOPRIL; PRINIVIL	4374829	DEC 30, 2001		I-92	JUN 09, 1996
19558 006	LISINOPRIL; PRINIVIL	4374829	DEC 30, 2001		I-92	JUN 09, 1996
19777 001	LISINOPRIL; ZESTRIL	4374829	DEC 30, 2001		I-92	JUN 09, 1996
19777 002	LISINOPRIL; ZESTRIL	4374829	DEC 30, 2001		I-92	JUN 09, 1996
19777 003	LISINOPRIL; ZESTRIL	4374829	DEC 30, 2001		I-92	JUN 09, 1996
19777 004	LISINOPRIL; ZESTRIL	4374829	DEC 30, 2001		I-92	JUN 09, 1996
19777 005	LISINOPRIL; ZESTRIL	4374829	DEC 30, 2001		I-92	JUN 09, 1996
18027 001	LITHIUM CARBONATE; LITHOBID	4264573	APR 28, 1998			
20191 001	LODOXAMIDE TROMETHAMINE; ALOMIDE				NCE	SEP 23, 1998
					ODE	SEP 23, 2000
20013 001	LOMEFLOXACIN HYDROCHLORIDE; MAXAQUIN	4528287	MAY 05, 2005	U-36	NCE	FEB 21, 1997
19487 001	LOPERAMIDE HYDROCHLORIDE; IMODIUM A-D				I-82	NOV 23, 1995
19860 001	LOPERAMIDE HYDROCHLORIDE; IMODIUM A-D				I-82	NOV 23, 1995
19658 001	LORATADINE; CLARITIN	4282233	AUG 04, 1998	U-77	NCE	APR 12, 1998
18140 001	LORAZEPAM; ATIVAN	4017616	APR 12, 1994			
18140 002	LORAZEPAM; ATIVAN	4017616	APR 12, 1994			
19643 003	LOVASTATIN; MEVACOR	4231938	NOV 04, 1999			
19643 004	LOVASTATIN; MEVACOR	4231938	NOV 04, 1999			
17658 001	LOXAPINE HYDROCHLORIDE; LOXITANE C	4049809	SEP 20, 1994			
19940 001	MASOPROCOL; ACTINEX	5008294	APR 15, 2008	U-68		
		4695590	SEP 05, 2006		NCE	SEP 04, 1997

PRESCRIPTION AND OTC DRUG PRODUCT PATENT AND EXCLUSIVITY DATA *(continued)*

APPL/ PROD NUMBER	INGREDIENT NAME; TRADE NAME	PATENT NUMBER	PATENT EXPIRES	USE CODE	EX-CLUS CODE	EXCLUS EXPIRES
12541 002	MEDROXYPROGESTERONE ACETATE; DEPO-PROVERA	4038389	JUL 26, 1994			
12541 003	MEDROXYPROGESTERONE ACETATE; DEPO-PROVERA	4038389	JUL 26, 1994			
20246 001	MEDROXYPROGESTERONE ACETATE; DEPO-PROVERA				NP	OCT 29, 1995
19578 001	MEFLOQUINE HYDROCHLORIDE; MEFLOQUINE HCL				NCE	MAY 02, 1994
19591 001	MEFLOQUINE HYDROCHLORIDE; LARIAM				NCE	MAY 02, 1994
					ODE	MAY 02, 1996
20264 001	MEGESTROL ACETATE; MEGACE				ODE	SEP 10, 2000
					NDF	SEP 10, 1997
20207 001	MELPHALAN HYDROCHLORIDE; ALKERAN	4997651	MAR 05, 2008		ODE	NOV 18, 1999
19651 001	MESALAMINE; ASACOL				NDF	JAN 31, 1995
20049 001	MESALAMINE; PENTASA	4980173	DEC 25, 2007	U-78		
		4496553	JAN 29, 2002	U-78	NP	MAY 10, 1966
19884 001	MESNA; MESNEX	4220660	DEC 02, 1999	U-21	ODE	DEC 30, 1995
17659 001	METAPROTERENOL SULFATE; ALUPENT				I-67	NOV 14, 1994
11719 001	METHOTREXATE SODIUM; METHOTREXATE				ODE	APR 07, 1995
					I-21	APR 07, 1995
11719 003	METHOTREXATE SODIUM; METHOTREXATE				ODE	APR 07, 1995
					I-21	APR 07, 1995
11719 006	METHOTREXATE SODIUM; METHOTREXATE				ODE	APR 07, 1995
					I-21	APR 07, 1995
11719 007	METHOTREXATE SODIUM; METHOTREXATE LPF				ODE	APR 07, 1995
					I-21	APR 07, 1995
11719 009	METHOTREXATE SODIUM; METHOTREXATE				ODE	APR 07, 1995
					I-21	APR 07, 1995
19600 001	METHOXSALEN; OXSORALEN-ULTRA	4454152	JUN 12, 2001			
18389 001	METHYLDOPA; ALDOMET	4404193	SEP 13, 2000			
18029 001	METHYLPHENIDATE HYDROCHLORIDE; RITALIN-SR	4137300	JAN 30, 1996			
19907 001	METIPRANOLOL HYDROCHLOIDE; OPTIPRANOLOL				NCE	DEC 29, 1994
17862 001	METOCLOPRAMIDE HYDROCHLORIDE; REGLAN	4536386	AUG 20, 2002	U-9		
17862 004	METOCLOPRAMIDE HYDROCHLORIDE; REGLAN	4536386	AUG 20, 2002	U-9		
19532 001	METOLAZONE; MYKROX	4517179	MAY 14, 2002			
19786 003	METOPROLOL FUMARATE; LOPRESSOR	4892739	JAN 09, 2007			
19786 004	METOPROLOL FUMARATE; LOPRESSOR	4892739	JAN 09, 2007			
19962 001	METOPROLOL SUCCINATE; TOPROL XL				NE	JAN 10, 1995
19962 002	METOPROLOL SUCCINATE; TOPROL XL				NE	JAN 10, 1995
19962 003	METOPROLOL SUCCINATE; TOPROL XL				NE	JAN 10, 1995
19737 001	METRONIDAZOLE; METROGEL				ODE	NOV 22, 1995
20208 001	METRONIDAZOLE; METROGEL				NDF	AUG 17, 1995
18873 002	MEXILETINE HYDROCHLORIDE; MEXITIL	4031244	JUN 21, 1994			
		3954872	MAY 04, 1995			
18873 003	MEXILETINE HYDROCHLORIDE; MEXITIL	4031244	JUN 21, 1994			
		3954872	MAY 04, 1995			
18873 004	MEXILETINE HYDROCHLORIDE; MEXITIL	4031244	JUN 21, 1994			
		3954872	MAY 04, 1995			
18654 001	MIDAZOLAM HYDROCHLORIDE; VERSED	4280957	DEC 20, 1999			
18654 002	MIDAZOLAM HYDROCHLORIDE; VERSED	4280957	DEC 20, 1999			
20343 001	MILRINONE LACTATE; PRIMACOR IN DEXTROSE 5%	4313951	FEB 02, 2001			
20343 002	MILRINONE LACTATE; PRIMACOR IN DEXTROSE 5%	4313951	FEB 02, 2001			
20343 003	MILRINONE LACTATE; PRIMACOR IN DEXTROSE 5%	4313951	FEB 02, 2001			
19501 001	MINOXIDIL; ROGAINE	4596812	FEB 13, 1996		I-61	AUG 13, 1994
		4139619	FEB 13, 1996			
19268 001	MISOPROSTOL; CYTOTEC	4301146	NOV 17, 1998			
		3965143	JUN 22, 1995			
19297 001	MITOXANTRONE HYDROCHLORIDE; NOVANTRONE	4278689	JUL 14, 2000			
		4197249	APR 08, 1997			
		4138415	FEB 06, 1996		ODE	DEC 23, 1994
20098 001	MIVACURIUM CHLORIDE; MIVACRON	4761418	JAN 22, 2006		NCE	JAN 22, 1997
20098 002	MIVACURIUM CHLORIDE; MIVACRON IN DEXTROSE 5%	4761418	JAN 22, 2006		NCE	JAN 22, 1997
19543 001	MOMETASONE FUROATE; ELOCON	4472393	SEP 18, 2001			

PRESCRIPTION AND OTC DRUG PRODUCT PATENT AND EXCLUSIVITY DATA *(continued)*

APPL/ PROD NUMBER	INGREDIENT NAME; TRADE NAME	PATENT NUMBER	PATENT EXPIRES	USE CODE	EX-CLUS CODE	EXCLUS EXPIRES
19625 001	MOMETASONE FUROATE; ELOCON	4808610	FEB 28, 2006			
		4472393	SEP 18, 2001			
19796 001	MOMETASONE FUROATE; ELOCON	4775529	OCT 04, 2005			
		4472393	SEP 18, 2001			
19368 001	MONOCTANOIN; MOCTANIN	4205086	MAY 27, 1997			
19753 001	MORICIZINE HYDROCHLORIDE; ETHMOZINE	3864487	FEB 04, 1994		NCE	JUN 19, 1995
19753 002	MORICIZINE HYDROCHLORIDE; ETHMOZINE	3864487	FEB 04, 1994		NCE	JUN 19, 1995
19753 003	MORICIZINE HYDROCHLORIDE; ETHMOZINE	3864487	FEB 04, 1994		NCE	JUN 19, 1995
18565 003	MORPHINE SULFATE; INFUMORPH				ODE	JUL 19, 1998
18565 004	MORPHINE SULFATE; INFUMORPH				ODE	JUL 19, 1998
18677 001	NABILONE; CESAMET	4087545	MAY 02, 1997	U-4		
19583 001	NABUMETONE; RELAFEN	4420639	DEC 13, 2002		NCE	DEC 24, 1996
		4061779	DEC 06, 1994	U-19		
19583 002	NABUMETONE; RELAFEN	4420639	DEC 13, 2002		NCE	DEC 24, 1996
		4061779	DEC 06, 1994	U-19		
19886 001	NAFARELIN ACETATE; SYNAREL	4234571	NOV 18, 1999		NCE	FEB 13, 1995
					I-68	FEB 26, 1995
20109 001	NAFARELIN ACETATE; SYNAREL	4234571	NOV 18, 1997		NCE	FEB 13, 1995
					I-68	FEB 26, 1995
19356 001	NAFTIFINE HYDROCHLORIDE; NAFTIN	4282251	AUG 04, 2000			
19599 001	NAFTIFINE HYDROCHLORIDE; NAFTIN	4282251	AUG 04, 2000			
18733 001	NALOXONE HYDROCHLORIDE; TALWIN NX	4105659	AUG 08, 1995			
20065 001	NAPHAZOLINE HYDROCHLORIDE; OPCON-A				NC	JUN 08, 1997
20226 001	NAPHAZOLINE HYDROCHLORIDE; NAPHCON-A				NC	JUN 08, 1997
19660 001	NEDOCROMIL SODIUM; TILADE	4760072	JUL 26, 2005			
		4474787	OCT 02, 2001		NCE	DEC 30, 1997
19488 001	NICARDIPINE HYDROCHLORIDE; CARDENE	3985758	OCT 12, 1995			
19488 002	NICARDIPINE HYDROCHLORIDE; CARDENE	3985758	OCT 12, 1995			
19734 001	NICARDIPINE HYDROCHLORIDE; CARDENE	3985758	OCT 12, 1995		NDF	JAN 30, 1995
20005 001	NICARDIPINE HYDROCHLORIDE; CARDENE SR	3985758	OCT 12, 1995		NDF	FEB 21, 1995
20005 002	NICARDIPINE HYDROCHLORIDE; CARDENE SR	3985758	OCT 12, 1995		NDF	FEB 21, 1995
20005 003	NICARDIPINE HYDROCHLORIDE; CARDENE SR	3985758	OCT 12, 1995		NDF	FEB 21, 1995
19983 001	NICOTINE; PROSTEP	4946853	AUG 07, 2007	U-56	NS	JAN 28, 1995
19983 002	NICTOINE; PROSTEP	4946853	AUG 07, 2007	U-56	NS	JAN 28, 1995
20076 001	NICOTINE; HABITROL	5016652	MAY 21, 2008			
		4597961	JUL 01, 2003	U-56	NDF	NOV 07, 1994
20076 002	NICOTINE; HABITROL	5016652	MAY 21, 2008			
		4597961	JUL 01, 2003	U-56	NDF	NOV 07, 1994
20076 003	NICOTINE; HABITROL	5016652	MAY 21, 2008			
		4597961	JUL 01, 2003	U-56	NDF	NOV 07, 1994
20150 001	NICOTINE; NICOTROL	4915950	APR 10, 2007		NP	APR 22, 1995
20150 002	NICOTINE; NICOTROL	4915950	APR 10, 2007		NP	APR 22, 1995
20150 003	NICOTINE; NICOTROL	4915950	APR 10, 2007		NP	APR 22, 1995
20165 001	NICOTINE; NICODERM	5004610	APR 02, 2008		NDF	NOV 07, 1994
20165 002	NICOTINE; NICODERM	5004610	APR 02, 2008		NDF	NOV 07, 1994
20165 003	NICOTINE; NICODERM	5004610	APR 02, 2008		NDF	NOV 07, 1994
18612 001	NICOTINE POLACRILEX; NICORETTE				NCE	JAN 13, 1994
20066 001	NICOTINE POLACRILEX; NICORETTE DS				NP	JUN 08, 1995
					NCE	JAN 13, 1994
19684 001	NIFEDIPINE; PROCARDIA XL	4783337	SEP 16, 2003			
		4765989	SEP 16, 2003			
		4612008	SEP 16, 2003			
		4327725	MAY 04, 1997			
19684 002	NIFEDIPINE; PROCARDIA XL	4783337	SEP 16, 2003			
		4765989	SEP 16, 2003			
		4612008	SEP 16, 2003			
		4327725	MAY 04, 1997			
19684 003	NIFEDIPINE; PROCARDIA XL	4783337	SEP 16, 2003			
		4765989	SEP 16, 2003			
		4612008	SEP 16, 2003			
		4327725	MAY 04, 1997			
20198 001	NIFEDIPINE; ADALAT CC	4892741	JAN 09, 2007			
20198 002	NIFEDIPINE; ADALAT CC	4892741	JAN 09, 2007			
20198 003	NIFEDIPINE; ADALAT CC	4892741	JAN 09, 2007			
18869 001	NIMODIPINE; NIMOTOP	4406906	SEP 27, 2002	U-22		
20064 001	NITROFURANTOIN; MACROBID	4798725	JAN 17, 2006			
		4772473	SEP 20, 2005		NDF	DEC 24, 1994

PRESCRIPTION AND OTC DRUG PRODUCT PATENT AND EXCLUSIVITY DATA *(continued)*

APPL/ PROD NUMBER	INGREDIENT NAME; TRADE NAME	PATENT NUMBER	PATENT EXPIRES	USE CODE	EX-CLUS CODE	EXCLUS EXPIRES
19508 001	NIZATIDINE; AXID	4760075	MAY 03, 2000	U-18		
		4382090	MAY 03, 2000	U-18	I-59	JUL 26, 1994
		4375547	MAR 01, 2002		NCE	APR 12, 1993
19508 002	NIZATIDINE; AXID	4760075	MAY 03, 2000	U-18		
		4382090	MAY 03, 2000	U-18	I-59	JUL 26, 1994
		4375547	MAR 01, 2002			
18683 001	NONOXYNOL-9; TODAY	4393871	JUL 19, 2000			
19384 002	NORFLOXACIN; NOROXIN	4639458	JAN 27, 2004		I-66	NOV 26, 1994
		4146719	MAR 27, 1998		D-17	NOV 26, 1994
19757 001	NORFLOXACIN; CHIBROXIN	4551456	NOV 05, 2002	U-57		
		4146719	MAR 27, 1998		NDF	JUN 17, 1994
19667 001	OCTREOTIDE ACETATE; SANDOSTATIN	4395403	JUL 26, 2002		I-106	MAY 03, 1997
19667 002	OCTREOTIDE ACETATE; SANDOSTATIN	4395403	JUL 26, 2002		I-106	MAY 03, 1997
19667 003	OCTREOTIDE ACETATE; SANDOSTATIN	4395403	JUL 26, 2002		I-106	MAY 03, 1997
19667 004	OCTREOTIDE ACETATE; SANDOSTATIN	4395403	JUL 26, 2002		I-106	MAY 03, 1997
19667 005	OCTREOTIDE ACETATE; SANDOSTATIN	4395403	JUL 26, 2002		I-106	MAY 03, 1997
19735 001	OFLOXACIN; FLOXIN	4382892	MAY 10, 2000		NCE	DEC 28, 1995
19735 002	OFLOXACIN; FLOXIN	4382892	MAY 10, 2000		NCE	DEC 28, 1995
19735 003	OFLOXACIN, FLOXIN	4382892	MAY 10, 2000		NCE	DEC 28, 1995
19921 001	OFLOXACIN; OCUFLOX	4551456	NOV 5, 2002	U-80	NDF	JUL 30, 1996
		4382892	MAY 10, 2000			
20087 001	OFLOXACIN; FLOXIN IN DEXTROSE 5%	4382892	MAY 10, 2000		NCE	DEC 28, 1995
20087 002	OFLOXACIN; FLOXIN	4382892	MAY 10, 2000		NCE	DEC 28, 1995
20087 003	OFLOXACIN; FLOXIN	4382892	MAY 10, 2000		NCE	DEC 28, 1995
20087 004	OFLOXACIN; FLOXIN IN DEXTROSE 5%	4382892	MAY 10, 2000		NCE	DEC 28, 1995
20087 005	OFLOXACIN; FLOXIN IN DEXTROSE 5%	4382892	MAY 10, 2000		NCE	DEC 28, 1995
19715 001	OLSALAZINE SODIUM; DIPENTUM	4559330	AUG 04, 2004	U-58	NCE	JUL 31, 1995
19810 001	OMEPRAZOLE; PRILOSEC	4786505	NOV 22, 2005	U-37	NCE	SEP 14, 1994
		4255431	MAR 10, 2000		I-57	JUN 12, 1994
20007 001	ONDANSETRON HYDROCHLORIDE; ZOFRAN	4753789	JUN 28, 2005	U-44	NCE	JAN 04, 1996
		4695578	JAN 03, 2005		D-20	FEB 02, 1996
					I-9	AUG 13, 1996
20103 001	ONDANSETRON HYDROCHLORIDE; ZOFRAN	4753789	JUN 28, 2005	U-44	NDF	DEC 31, 1995
		4695578	JAN 03, 2005		NCE	JAN 04, 1996
20103 002	ONDANSETRON HYDROCHLORIDE; ZOFRAN	4753789	JUN 28, 2005	U-44	NDF	DEC 31, 1995
		4695578	JAN 03, 2005		NCE	JAN 04, 1996
18841 004	OXAPROZIN; DAYPRO				NCE	OCT 29, 1997
15539 002	OXAZEPAM; SERAX	4620974	NOV 04, 2003			
15539 004	OXAZEPAM; SERAX	4620974	NOV 04, 2003			
15539 006	OXAZEPAM; SERAX	4620974	NOV 04, 2003			
19828 001	OXICONAZOLE NITRATE; OXISTAT				I-77	SEP 30, 1995
20209 001	OXICONAZOLE NITRATE; OXISTAT				NP	SEP 30, 1995
					NCE	DEC 30, 1993
20262 001	PACLITAXEL; TAXOL				NCE	DEC 29, 1997
					I-105	APR 13, 1997
					D-24	JUN 22, 1997
20036 001	PAMIDRONATE DISODIUM; AREDIA	4711880	DEC 08, 2004		D-22	APR 15, 1997
		3962432	JUL 16, 1996	U-53	NCE	OCT 31, 1996
20036 003	PAMIDRONATE DISODIUM; AREDIA	4711880	DEC 08, 2004		D-22	APR 15, 1997
		3962432	JUL 16, 1996	U-53	NCE	OCT 31, 1996
20036 004	PAMIDRONATE DISODIUM; AREDIA	4711880	DEC 08, 2004		D-22	APR 15, 1997
		3962432	JUL 16, 1996	U-53	NCE	OCT 31, 1996
20031 001	PAROXETINE HYDROCHLORIDE; PAXIL				NCE	DEC 29, 1997
20031 002	PAROXETINE HYDROCHLORIDE; PAXIL				NCE	DEC 29, 1997
20031 003	PAROXETINE HYDROCHLORIDE; PAXIL				NCE	DEC 29, 1997
20031 004	PAROXETINE HYDROCHLORIDE; PAXIL				NCE	DEC 29, 1997
20031 005	PAROXETINE HYDROCHLORIDE; PAXIL				NCE	DEC 29, 1997
19818 001	PEGADEMASE BOVINE; ADAGEN	4179337	DEC 18, 1996		ODE	MAR 21, 1997
					NCE	MAR 21, 1995
19887 001	PENTAMIDINE ISETHIONATE; NEBUPENT				ODE	JUN 15, 1996
20122 001	PENTOSTATIN; NIPENT				ODE	OCT 11, 1998
					NCE	OCT 11, 1996
18631 001	PENTOXIFYLLINE; TRENTAL	4189469	FEB 02, 1997			
		3737433	APR 03, 1997		NCE	AUG 30, 1994
20091 001	PERFLUBRON; IMAGENT				NCE	AUG 13, 1998
20091 001	PERFLUBRON; IMAGENT				NCE	AUG 13, 1998
19385 001	PERGOLIDE MESYLATE; PERMAX	4797405	JAN 10, 2006			
		4180582	DEC 25, 1996	U-20		
		4166182	AUG 28, 1998			

PRESCRIPTION AND OTC DRUG PRODUCT PATENT AND EXCLUSIVITY DATA *(continued)*

APPL/ PROD NUMBER	INGREDIENT NAME; TRADE NAME	PATENT NUMBER	PATENT EXPIRES	USE CODE	EX-CLUS CODE	EXCLUS EXPIRES
19385 002	PERGOLIDE MESYLATE; PERMAX	4797405	JAN 10, 2006			
		4180582	DEC 25, 1996	U-20		
		4166182	AUG 28, 1998			
19385 003	PERGOLIDE MESYLATE; PERMAX	4797405	JAN 10, 2006			
		4180582	DEC 25, 1996	U-20		
		4166182	AUG 28, 1998			
20184 001	PERINDOPRIL ERBUMINE; ACEON	4508729	APR 02, 2002		NCE	DEC 30, 1998
20184 002	PERINDOPRIL ERBUMINE; ACEON	4508729	APR 02, 2002		NCE	DEC 30, 1998
20184 003	PERINDOPRIL ERBUMINE; ACEON	4508729	APR 02, 2002		NCE	DEC 30, 1998
19435 001	PERMETHRIN; NIX	4024163	MAY 17, 1996			
19855 001	PERMETHRIN; ELIMITE	4024163	MAY 17, 1996			
19918 001	PERMETHRIN; NIX	4024163	MAY 17, 1996		I-60	MAY 02, 1993
18796 001	PILOCARPINE HYDROCHLORIDE; PILOPINE HS	4271143	JUN 02, 1998			
20237 001	PILOCARPINE HYDROCHLORIDE; SALAGEN				ODE	MAR 22, 2001
					NDF	MAR 22, 1997
17473 001	PIMOZIDE; ORAP				NCE	JUL 31, 1994
19456 001	PINACIDIL; PINDAC	RE31244	NOV 08, 1996	U-3	NCE	DEC 28, 1994
19456 002	PINACIDIL; PINDAC	RE31244	NOV 08, 1996	U-3	NCE	DEC 28, 1994
19638 001	PIPECURONIUM BROMIDE; ARDUAN				NCE	JUN 26, 1995
19009 001	PIRBUTEROL ACETATE; MAXAIR	4175128	NOV 20, 1996			
20014 001	PIRBUTEROL ACETATE; MAXAIR	4664107	MAY 12, 2004			
19795 001	PODOFILOX; CONDYLOX				NCE	DEC 13, 1995
19797 001	POLYETHYLENE GLYCOL 3350; NULYTELY				NP	APR 22, 1994
17986 001	POLYTHIAZIDE; MINIZIDE	4130647	DEC 19, 1995			
17986 002	POLYTHIAZIDE; MINIZIDE	4130647	DEC 19, 1995			
17986 003	POLYTHIAZIDE; MINIZIDE	4130647	DEC 19, 1995			
17850 001	POTASSIUM CHLORIDE; KLOTRIX	4140756	FEB 20, 1996			
18238 001	POTASSIUM CHLORIDE; MICRO-K	4259315	MAR 31, 1998			
18238 002	POTASSIUM CHLORIDE; MICRO-K 10	4259315	MAR 31, 1998			
19561 003	POTASSIUM CHLORIDE; MICRO-K LS	4259315	MAR 31, 1998			
19898 002	PRAVASTATIN SODIUM; PRAVACHOL	4346227	AUG 24, 1999		NCE	OCT 31, 1996
19898 003	PRAVASTATIN SODIUM; PRAVACHOL	4346227	AUG 24, 1999		NCE	OCT 31, 1996
19898 004	PRAVASTATIN SODIUM; PRAVACHOL	4346227	AUG 24, 1999		NCE	OCT 31, 1996
18714 001	PRAZIQUANTEL; BILTRICIDE	4001411	JAN 04, 1994			
17442 001	PRAZOSIN HYDROCHLORIDE; MINIPRESS	4130647	DEC 19, 1995			
		4092315	MAY 30, 1995			
17442 002	PRAZOSIN HYDROCHLORIDE; MINIPRESS	4130647	DEC 19, 1995			
		4092315	MAY 30, 1995			
17442 003	PRAZOSIN HYDROCHLORIDE; MINIPRESS	4130647	DEC 19, 1995			
		4092315	MAY 30, 1995			
19775 001	PRAZOSIN HYDROCHLORIDE; MINIPRESS XL	5082668	SEP 16, 2003			
		4783337	SEP 16, 2003			
		4765989	SEP 16, 2003			
		4612008	SEP 16, 2003			
		4327725	MAY 04, 1999			
		4092315	MAY 30, 1995		NDF	JAN 29, 1995
19775 002	PRAZOSIN HYDROCHLORIDE; MINIPRESS XL	5082668	SEP 16, 2003			
		4783337	SEP 16, 2003			
		4765989	SEP 16, 2003			
		4612008	SEP 16, 2003			
		4327725	MAY 04, 1999			
		4092315	MAY 30, 1995		NDF	JAN 29, 1995
19568 001	PREDNICARBATE; DERMATOP	4242334	DEC 30, 1999	U-50	NE	SEP 23, 1994
20279 001	PREDNICARBATE; DERMATOP	4242334	DEC 30, 1999	U-50	NE	SEP 23, 1994
					NDF	OCT 29, 1996
19157 001	PREDNISOLONE SODIUM PHOSPHATE; PEDIAPRED	4448774	MAY 15, 2001			
87361 001	PROCAINAMIDE HYDROCHLORIDE; PRONESTYL-SR	4252786	FEB 24, 1998			
19151 001	PROPAFENONE HYDROCHLORIDE; RYTHMOL				NCE	NOV 27, 1994
19151 002	PROPAFENONE HYDROCHLORIDE; RYTHMOL				NCE	NOV 27, 1994
19627 001	PROPOFOL; DIPRIVAN	4798846	NOV 01, 1996		I-73	DEC 31, 1994
		4056635	NOV 01, 1996		NCE	OCT 02, 1994
					I-90	MAR 08, 1996
					I-99	OCT 26, 1996
18553 001	PROPRANOLOL HYDROCHLORIDE; INDERAL LA	4138475	FEB 06, 1996			
18553 002	PROPRANOLOL HYDROCHLORIDE; INDERAL LA	4138475	FEB 06, 1996			
18553 003	PROPRANOLOL HYDROCHLORIDE; INDERAL LA	4138475	FEB 06, 1996			
18553 004	PROPRANOLOL HYDROCHLORIDE; INDERAL LA	4138475	FEB 06, 1996			
19536 001	PROPRANOLOL HYDROCHLORIDE; INDERAL	4600708	JUL 15, 2003			

PRESCRIPTION AND OTC DRUG PRODUCT PATENT AND EXCLUSIVITY DATA *(continued)*

APPL/ PROD NUMBER	INGREDIENT NAME; TRADE NAME	PATENT NUMBER	PATENT EXPIRES	USE CODE	EX-CLUS CODE	EXCLUS EXPIRES
19664 001	PSEUDOEPHEDRINE HYDROCHLORIDE; SELDANE-D	4996061	FEB 26, 2008			
		4929605	MAY 29, 2007	U-81		
		4254129	MAR 03, 1998	U-81		
		3878217	APR 15, 1994		NC	AUG 19, 1994
20021 002	PSEUDOEPHEDRINE HYDROCHLORIDE;	4801461	MAY 05, 2004			
		4576604	MAR 18, 2003			
18708 001	QUAZEPAM; DORAL	3920818	NOV 18, 1994			
18708 003	QUAZEPAM; DORAL	3920818	NOV 18, 1994			
19885 001	QUINAPRIL HYDROCHLORIDE; ACCUPRIL	4743450	MAY 10, 2005		I-92	OCT 29, 1996
		4344949	AUG 17, 1999	U-3	NCE	NOV 19, 1996
19885 002	QUINAPRIL HYDROCHLORIDE; ACCUPRIL	4743450	MAY 10, 2005		I-92	OCT 29, 1996
		4344949	AUG 17, 1999	U-3	NCE	NOV 19, 1996
19885 003	QUINAPRIL HYDROCHLORIDE; ACCUPRIL	4743450	MAY 10, 2005		I-92	OCT 29, 1996
		4344949	AUG 17, 1999	U-3	NCE	NOV 19, 1996
19885 004	QUINAPRIL HYDROCHLORIDE; ACCUPRIL	4743450	MAY 10, 2005		I-92	OCT 29, 1996
		4344949	AUG 17, 1999	U-3	NCE	NOV 19, 1996
19901 001	RAMIPRIL; ALTACE	4587258	JAN 29, 2005		NCE	JAN 28, 1996
19901 002	RAMIPRIL; ALTACE	4587258	JAN 29, 2005		NCE	JAN 28, 1996
19901 003	RAMIPRIL; ALTACE	4587258	JAN 29, 2005		NCE	JAN 28, 1996
19901 004	RAMIPRIL; ALTACE	4587258	JAN 29, 2005		NCE	JAN 28, 1996
18703 001	RANITIDINE HYDROCHLORIDE; ZANTAC 150	4521431	JUN 04, 2002		I-75	MAY 19, 1995
		4128658	DEC 05, 1995		D-21	FEB 28, 1997
18703 002	RANITIDINE HYDROCHLORIDE; ZANTAC 300	4521431	JUN 04, 2002		I-75	MAY 19, 1995
		4128658	DEC 05, 1995		D-21	FEB 28, 1997
19090 001	RANITIDINE HYDROCHLORIDE; ZANTAC	4585790	APR 29, 2003			
		4521431	JUN 04, 2002			
		4128658	DEC 05, 1995			
19593 001	RANITIDINE HYDROCHLORIDE; ZANTAC	4585790	APR 29, 2003			
		4521431	JUN 04, 2002			
		4128658	DEC 05, 1995			
19675 001	RANITIDINE HYDROCHLORIDE; ZANTAC	4585790	APR 29, 2003			
		4521431	JUN 04, 2002		D-21	FEB 28, 1997
		4128658	DEC 05, 1995		I-75	MAY 19, 1995
20095 001	RANITIDINE HYDROCHLORIDE; ZANTAC 150	5028432	JUL 02, 2008			
		4521431	JUN 04, 2002		I-75	MAY 19, 1995
		4128658	DEC 05, 1995		D-21	FEB 28, 1997
20095 002	RANITIDINE HYDROCHLORIDE; ZANTAC 300	5028432	JUL 02, 2008			
		4521431	JUN 04, 2002		I-75	MAY 19, 1995
		4128658	DEC 05, 1995		D-21	FEB 28, 1997
20251 001	RANITIDINE HYDROCHLORIDE; ZANTAC 150	5102665	APR 07, 2009			
		4521431	JUN 04, 2002		I-75	MAY 19, 1995
		4128658	DEC 05, 1995		D-21	FEB 28, 1997
20251 002	RANITIDINE HYDROCHLORIDE; ZANTAC 150	5102665	APR 07, 2009			
		4521431	JUN 04, 2002		I-75	MAY 19, 1995
		4128658	DEC 05, 1995		D-21	FEB 28, 1997
18859 001	RIBAVIRIN; VIRAZOLE	4211771	JUL 08, 1999			
50689 001	RIFABUTIN; MYCOBUTIN				ODE	DEC 23, 1999
50627 001	RIFAMPIN; RIFADIN				ODE	MAY 25, 1996
19649 001	RIMANTADINE HYDROCHLORIDE; FLUMADINE				NCE	SEP 17, 1998
19650 001	RIMANTADINE HYDROCHLORIDE; FLUMADINE				NCE	SEP 17, 1998
20272 001	RISPERIDONE; RISPERDAL	4804663	FEB 14, 2006	U-90	NCE	DEC 29, 1998
20272 002	RISPERIDONE; RISPERDAL	4804663	FEB 14, 2006	U-90	NCE	DEC 29, 1998
20272 003	RISPERIDONE; RISPERDAL	4804663	FEB 14, 2006	U-90	NCE	DEC 29, 1998
20272 004	RISPERIDONE; RISPERDAL	4804663	FEB 14, 2006	U-90	NCE	DEC 29, 1998
20272 005	RISPERIDONE; RISPERDAL	4804663	FEB 14, 2006	U-90	NCE	DEC 29, 1998
20214 001	ROCURONIUM BROMIDE; ZEMURON (P/F)	4894369	JAN 16, 2007		NCE	MAR 17, 1999
20214 002	ROCURONIUM BROMIDE; ZEMURON	4894369	JAN 16, 2007		NCE	MAR 17, 1999
19414 001	RUBIDIUM CHLORIDE RB-82; CARDIOGEN-82	4400358	AUG 23, 2002		NCE	DEC 29, 1994
20236 001	SALMETEROL XINAFOATE; SEREVENT	4992474	FEB 12, 2008		NCE	FEB 04, 1999
17874 001	SCOPOLAMINE; TRANSDERM-SCOP	4436741	APR 14, 1998			
		4262003	APR 14, 1998			
		4031894	JUN 28, 1994			
19334 001	SELEGILINE HYDROCHLORIDE; ELDEPRYL				ODE	JUN 05, 1996
					NCE	JUN 05, 1994
19863 001	SERMORELIN ACETATE; GEREF	4703035	DEC 28, 2002	U-47	NCE	DEC 28, 1995
		4517181	MAY 14, 2002		NCE	DEC 28, 1995
19839 001	SERTRALINE HYDROCHLORIDE; ZOLOFT	5248699	SEP 28, 2010	U-12		
		4962128	OCT 09, 2007			
		4536518	DEC 31, 2005		NCE	DEC 30, 1996

PRESCRIPTION AND OTC DRUG PRODUCT PATENT AND EXCLUSIVITY DATA *(continued)*

APPL/ PROD NUMBER	INGREDIENT NAME; TRADE NAME	PATENT NUMBER	PATENT EXPIRES	USE CODE	EX-CLUS CODE	EXCLUS EXPIRES
19839 002	SERTRALINE HYDROCHLORIDE; ZOLOFT	5248699	SEP 28, 2010	U-12		
		4962128	OCT 09, 2007			
		4536518	DEC 31, 2005		NCE	DEC 30, 1996
19839 003	SERTRALINE HYDROCHLORIDE; ZOLOFT	5248699	SEP 28, 2010	U-12		
		4962128	OCT 09, 2007			
		4536518	DEC 31, 2005		NCE	DEC 30, 1996
19839 004	SERTRALINE HYDROCHLORIDE; ZOLOFT	5248699	SEP 28, 2010	U-12		
		4962128	OCT 09, 2007			
		4536518	DEC 31, 2005		NCE	DEC 30, 1996
19608 001	SILVER SULFADIAZINE; SILDIMAC	4563184	JAN 07, 2003			
19766 001	SIMVASTATIN; ZOCOR	4444784	DEC 24, 2005	U-59	NCE	DEC 23, 1996
19766 002	SIMVASTATIN; ZOCOR	4444784	DEC 24, 2005	U-59	NCE	DEC 23, 1996
19766 003	SIMVASTATIN; ZOCOR	4444784	DEC 24, 2005	U-59	NCE	DEC 23, 1996
19766 004	SIMVASTATIN; ZOCOR	4444784	DEC 24, 2005	U-59	NCE	DEC 23, 1996
19530 001	SODIUM BENZOATE; UCEPHAN	4284647	AUG 18, 2000	U-14	ODE	DEC 23, 1994
10929 001	SODIUM IODIDE, I-131; IODOTOPE	4349529	SEP 14, 1999			
10929 002	SODIUM IODIDE, I-131; IODOTOPE	4349529	SEP 14, 1999			
10929 003	SODIUM IODIDE, I-131; IODOTOPE	4349529	SEP 14, 1999			
20166 001	SODIUM THIOSULFATE; SODIUM THIOSULFATE				NCE	FEB 14, 1997
19107 001	SOMATREM; PROTROPIN	4658021	APR 14, 2004			
19640 001	SOMATROPIN, BIOSYNTHETIC; HUMATROPE				ODE	MAR 08, 1994
					D-23	APR 15, 1997
19640 004	SOMATROPIN, BIOSYNTHETIC; HUMATROPE				ODE	MAR 08, 1994
					D-23	APR 15, 1997
20168 001	SOMATROPIN, BIOSYNTHETIC; NUTROPIN				I-98	NOV 17, 1996
					ODE	NOV 17, 2000
20168 002	SOMATROPIN, BIOSYNTHETIC; NUTROPIN				I-98	NOV 17, 1996
					ODE	NOV 17, 2000
19865 001	SOTALOL HYDROCHLORIDE; BETAPACE				NCE	OCT 30, 1997
					ODE	OCT 30, 1999
19865 002	SOTALOL HYDROCHLORIDE; BETAPACE				NCE	OCT 30, 1997
					ODE	OCT 30, 1999
19865 003	SOTALOL HYDROCHLORIDE; BETAPACE				NCE	OCT 30, 1997
					ODE	OCT 30, 1999
19865 004	SOTALOL HYDROCHLORIDE; BETAPACE				NCE	OCT 30, 1997
					ODE	OCT 30, 1999
19865 005	SOTALOL HYDROCHLORIDE; BETAPACE				NCE	OCT 30, 1997
					ODE	OCT 30, 1999
20412 001	STAVUDINE; ZERIT	4978655	DEC 18, 2007	U-94	NCE	JUN 24, 1999
20412 002	STAVUDINE; ZERIT	4978655	DEC 18, 2007	U-94	NCE	JUN 24, 1999
20412 003	STAVUDINE; ZERIT	4978655	DEC 18, 2007	U-94	NCE	JUN 24, 1999
20412 004	STAVUDINE; ZERIT	4978655	DEC 18, 2007	U-94	NCE	JUN 24, 1999
20412 005	STAVUDINE; ZERIT	4978655	DEC 18, 2007	U-94	NCE	JUN 24, 1999
20134 001	STRONTIUM CHLORIDE, SR-89; METASTRON				NCE	JUN 18, 1998
19998 002	SUCCIMER; CHEMET				ODE	JAN 30, 1998
					NCE	JAN 30, 1996
19183 001	SUCRALFATE; CARAFATE				NDF	DEC 16, 1996
19050 001	SUFENTANIL CITRATE; SUFENTA				NR	MAR 19, 1996
					I-89	MAR 19, 1996
					NCE	MAY 04, 1994
18737 001	SULCONAZOLE NITRATE; EXELDERM	4055652	OCT 25, 1996			
18738 001	SULCONAZOLE NITRATE; EXELDERM	4055652	OCT 25, 1996			
17376 001	SULFAMETHOXAZOLE; SEPTRA	4209513	JUN 24, 1997		I-103	JAN 07, 1997
17376 002	SULFAMETHOXAZOLE; SEPTRA DS	4209513	JUN 24, 1997		I-103	JAN 07, 1997
17377 001	SULFAMETHOXAZOLE; BACTRIM				I-103	JAN 07, 1997
17377 002	SULFAMETHOXAZOLE; BACTRIM DS				I-103	JAN 07, 1997
17560 002	SULFAMETHOXAZOLE; BACTRIM PEDIATRIC				I-103	JAN 07, 1997
17598 001	SULFAMETHOXAZOLE; SEPTRA				I-103	JAN 07, 1997
17598 002	SULFAMETHOXAZOLE; SEPTRA GRAPE				I-103	JAN 07, 1997
20080 001	SUMATRIPTAN SUCCINATE; IMITREX	5037845	AUG 06, 2008	U-72	NCE	DEC 28, 1997
		4816470	MAR 28, 2006	U-72		
18217 001	SUPROFEN; SUPROL	4035376	JUL 12, 1996			
19387 001	SUPROFEN; PROFENAL	4559343	DEC 17, 2002			
		4035376	JUL 12, 1996			
20070 001	TACRINE HYDROCHLORIDE; COGNEX	4816456	MAR 28, 2006	U-82	NCE	SEP 09, 1998
20070 002	TACRINE HYDROCHLORIDE; COGNEX	4816456	MAR 28, 2006	U-82	NCE	SEP 09, 1998
20070 003	TACRINE HYDROCHLORIDE; COGNEX	4816456	MAR 28, 2006	U-82	NCE	SEP 09, 1998
20070 004	TACRINE HYDROCHLORIDE; COGNEX	4816456	MAR 28, 2006	U-82	NCE	SEP 09, 1998
17970 001	TAMOXIFEN CITRATE; NOLVADEX	4536516	AUG 20, 2002			

PRESCRIPTION AND OTC DRUG PRODUCT PATENT AND EXCLUSIVITY DATA *(continued)*

APPL/ PROD NUMBER	INGREDIENT NAME; TRADE NAME	PATENT NUMBER	PATENT EXPIRES	USE CODE	EX-CLUS CODE	EXCLUS EXPIRES
19829 001	TECHNETIUM TC-99M EXAMETAZIME KIT; CERETEC	4789736	DEC 06, 2005			
18489 001	TECHNETIUM TC-99M LIDOFENIN KIT; TECHNESCAN HIDA	RE31463	APR 12, 1994			
18963 001	TECHNETIUM TC-99M MEBROFENIN KIT; CHOLETEC	4418208	JAN 21, 2001			
18107 001	TECHNETIUM TC-99M MEDRONATE KIT; MDP-SQUIBB	4115541	SEP 19, 1995			
19882 001	TECHNETIUM TC-99M MERTIATIDE KIT; TECHNESCAN MAG3				NCE	JUN 15, 1995
					I-87	NOV 27, 1995
18321 001	TECHNETIUM TC-99M OXIDRONATE KIT; TECHNESCAN HDP	4497744	FEB 05, 2002			
		4432963	FEB 21, 2001			
		4247534	JAN 27, 1998			
		4233284	NOV 11, 1997			
19981 001	TECHNETIUM TC-99M RED BLOOD CELL KIT; ULTRATAG	4755375	JUL 05, 2005	U-51	NP	JUN 10, 1994
20063 001	TECHNETIUM TC-99M RED BLOOD CELL KIT; RBC-SCAN				NP	JUN 11, 1995
19785 001	TECHNETIUM TC-99M SESTAMIBI KIT; CARDIOLITE	4452774	SEP 09, 2004		NCE	DEC 21, 1995
					I-80	SEP 09, 1995
17339 001	TECHNETIUM TC-99M SODIUM PERTECHNETATE GENERATOR; MINITEC	4041317	AUG 09, 1994			
17944 001	TECHNETIUM TC-99M SUCCIMER KIT; MPI DMSA KIDNEY REAGENT	4233285	NOV 11, 1997			
		4208398	JUN 17, 1997			
19928 001	TECHNETIUM TC-99M TEBOROXIME KIT; CARDIOTEC	4705849	NOV 10, 2004		NCE	DEC 19, 1995
20043 003	TEMAFLOXACIN HYDROCHLORIDE; OMNIFLOX	4730000	JAN 30, 2006	U-36	NCE	JAN 30, 1997
20043 004	TEMAFLOXACIN HYDROCHLORIDE; OMNIFLOX	4730000	JAN 30, 2006	U-36	NCE	JAN 30, 1997
18163 003	TEMAZEPAM; RESTORIL	5211954	MAY 18, 2010			
		5030632	JUL 09, 2008	U-70	NS	OCT 25, 1994
20119 001	TENIPOSIDE; VUMON				NCE	JUL 14, 1997
					ODE	JUL 14, 1999
19057 001	TERAZOSIN HYDROCHLORIDE; HYTRIN	4251532	FEB 17, 2000	U-3	I-96	SEP 29, 1996
		4112097	SEP 05, 1995	U-3		
		4026894	MAY 31, 1994			
19057 002	TERAZOSIN HYDROCHLORIDE; HYTRIN	4251532	FEB 17, 2000	U-3	I-96	SEP 29, 1996
		4112097	SEP 05, 1995	U-3		
		4026894	MAY 31, 1994			
19057 003	TERAZOSIN HYDROCHLORIDE; HYTRIN	4251532	FEB 17, 2000	U-3	I-96	SEP 29, 1996
		4112097	SEP 05, 1995	U-3		
		4026894	MAY 31, 1994			
19057 004	TERAZOSIN HYDROCHLORIDE; HYTRIN	4251532	FEB 17, 2000	U-3	I-96	SEP 29, 1996
		4112097	SEP 05, 1995	U-3		
		4026894	MAY 31, 1994			
20223 001	TERAZOSIN HYDROCHLORIDE; HYTRIN	4251532	FEB 17, 2000			
		4112097	SEP 05, 1995			
		4026894	MAY 31, 1994		I-96	SEP 29, 1996
20223 002	TERAZOSIN HYDROCHLORIDE; HYTRIN	4251532	FEB 17, 2000			
		4112097	SEP 05, 1995			
		4026894	MAY 31, 1994		I-96	SEP 29, 1996
20223 003	TERAZOSIN HYDROCHLORIDE; HYTRIN	4251532	FEB 17, 2000			
		4112097	SEP 05, 1995			
		4026894	MAY 31, 1994		I-96	SEP 29, 1996
20223 004	TERAZOSIN HYDROCHLORIDE; HYTRIN	4251532	FEB 17, 2000			
		4112097	SEP 05, 1995			
		4026894	MAY 31, 1994		I-96	SEP 29, 1996
20192 001	TERBINAFINE HYDROCHLORIDE; LAMISIL	4775534	JUL 05, 2005	U-73	NCE	DEC 30, 1999
17466 001	TERBUTALINE SULFATE; BRICANYL	4011258	MAR 08, 1994			
17618 001	TERBUTALINE SULFATE; BRICANYL	4011258	MAR 08, 1994			
17618 002	TERBUTALINE SULFATE; BRICANYL	4011258	MAR 08, 1994			
17849 001	TERBUTALINE SULFATE; BRETHINE	4011258	MAR 08, 1994			
17849 002	TERBUTALINE SULFATE; BRETHINE	4011258	MAR 08, 1994			
18000 001	TERBUTALINE SULFATE; BRICANYL	4011258	MAR 08, 1994			
18571 001	TERBUTALINE SULFATE; BRETHINE	4011258	MAR 08, 1994			
18762 001	TERBUTALINE SULFATE; BRETHAIRE	4011258	MAR 08, 1994			
19579 001	TERCONAZOLE; TERAZOL 7	4358449	NOV 09, 2001			
19641 001	TERCONAZOLE; TERAZOL 3	4358449	NOV 09, 2001			

PRESCRIPTION AND OTC DRUG PRODUCT PATENT AND EXCLUSIVITY DATA *(continued)*

APPL/ PROD NUMBER	INGREDIENT NAME; TRADE NAME	PATENT NUMBER	PATENT EXPIRES	USE CODE	EX-CLUS CODE	EXCLUS EXPIRES
18949 001	TERFENADINE; SELDANE	4254129	MAR 03, 1998	U-81		
		3878217	APR 15, 1994			
19498 001	TERIPARATIDE ACETATE; PARATHAR				ODE	DEC 23, 1994
19762 001	TESTOSTERONE; TESTODERM	4867982	FEB 16, 2005			
		4725439	FEB 16, 2005			
		4704282	NOV 03, 2004		NDF	OCT 12, 1996
19762 002	TESTOSTERONE; TESTODERM	4867982	FEB 16, 2005			
		4725439	FEB 16, 2005			
		4704282	NOV 03, 2004		NDF	OCT 12, 1996
87563 001	THEOPHYLLINE; QUIBRON-T/SR	4465660	AUG 14, 2001			
19979 001	TICLOPIDINE HYDROCHLORIDE; TICLID	4591595	NOV 01, 2005			
		4051141	SEP 27, 1996		NCE	OCT 31, 1996
19979 002	TICLOPIDINE HYDROCHLORIDE; TICLID	4591592	NOV 01, 2005			
		4051141	SEP 27, 1996		NCE	OCT 31, 1996
18086 001	TIMOLOL MALEATE; TIMOPTIC	4195085	MAR 25, 1997			
18086 002	TIMOLOL MALEATE; TIMOPTIC	4195085	MAR 25, 1997			
19463 001	TIMOLOL MALEATE; TIMOPTIC IN OCUDOSE	4195085	MAR 25, 1997			
19463 002	TIMOLOL MALEATE; TIMOPTIC IN OCUDOSE	4195085	MAR 25, 1997			
20330 001	TIMOLOL MALEATE; TIMOPTIC-XE	4195085	MAR 25, 1997		NP	NOV 04, 1996
20330 002	TIMOLOL MALEATE; TIMOPTIC-XE	4861760	AUG 29, 2006			
		4195085	MAR 25, 1997		NP	NOV 04, 1996
18682 001	TIOCONAZOLE; TZ-3	4062966	DEC 13, 1994			
19355 001	TIOCONAZOLE; VAGISTAT-1	4062966	DEC 13, 1994			
19569 001	TIOPRONIN; TIOPRONIN				ODE	AUG 11, 1995
18257 001	TOCAINIDE HYDROCHLORIDE; TONOCARD	4237068	NOV 09, 1998			
		4218477	AUG 19, 1997			
18257 002	TOCAINIDE HYDROCHLORIDE; TONOCARD	4237068	NOV 09, 1998			
		4218477	AUG 19, 1997			
20136 001	TORSEMIDE; DEMADEX	4822807	APR 18, 2006			
		4018929	APR 19, 1994		NCE	AUG 23, 1998
		RE30633	APR 19, 1994			
20136 002	TORSEMIDE; DEMADEX	4822807	APR 18, 2006			
		4018929	APR 19, 1994		NCE	AUG 23, 1998
		RE30633	APR 19, 1994			
20136 003	TORSEMIDE; DEMADEX	4822807	APR 18, 2006			
		4018929	APR 19, 1994		NCE	AUG 23, 1998
		RE30633	APR 19, 1994			
20136 004	TORSEMIDE; DEMADEX	4822807	APR 18, 2006			
		4018929	APR 19, 1994		NCE	AUG 23, 1998
		RE30633	APR 19, 1994			
20137 002	TORSEMIDE; DEMADEX	4822807	APR 18, 2006			
		4018929	APR 19, 1994		NCE	AUG 23, 1998
20137 002	TORSEMIDE; DEMADEX	RE30633	APR 19, 1994			
18207 003	TRAZODONE HYDROCHLORIDE; DESYREL	4258027	MAR 24, 1998			
		4215104	JUL 29, 1997			
18207 004	TRAZODONE HYDROCHLORIDE; DESYREL	4258027	MAR 24, 1998			
		4215104	JUL 29, 1997			
17579 002	TRETINOIN; RETIN-A	4247547	JAN 27, 1998			
17955 001	TRETINOIN; RETIN-A	4247547	JAN 27, 1998			
19798 001	TRIAMCINOLONE ACETONIDE; NASACORT	476712	AUG 30, 2005	U-85	NR	JUL 11, 1994
86240 001	TRIAMCINOLONE ACETONIDE; KENALOG-H	4048310	SEP 13, 1994			
20326 001	TRIMETREXATE GLUCURONATE; NEUTREXIN	4694007	SEP 15, 2004	U-91	ODE	DEC 17, 2000
		4376858	MAR 15, 2000		NCE	DEC 17, 1998
19594 001	URSODIOL; ACTIGALL	RE30910	JAN 07, 1994	U-25		
		RE30910	JAN 07, 1994	U-26		
		RE30910	JAN 07, 1994	U-27		
19594 002	URSODIOL; ACTIGALL	RE30910	JAN 07, 1994	U-25		
		RE30910	JAN 07, 1994	U-26		
		RE30910	JAN 07, 1994	U-27		
18776 002	VECURONIUM BROMIDE; NORCURON	4297351	OCT 27, 1998			
		4237126	DEC 02, 1997		NCE	APR 30, 1994
18776 003	VECURONIUM BROMIDE; NORCURON	4297351	OCT 27, 1998			
		4237126	DEC 02, 1997		NCE	APR 30, 1994
20151 001	VENLAFAXINE HYDROCHLORIDE; EFFEXOR	4535186	AUG 13, 2002		NCE	DEC 28, 1998
20151 002	VENLAFAXINE HYDROCHLORIDE; EFFEXOR	4535186	AUG 13, 2002		NCE	DEC 28, 1998
20151 003	VENLAFAXINE HYDROCHLORIDE; EFFEXOR	4535186	AUG 13, 2002		NCE	DEC 28, 1998
20151 004	VENLAFAXINE HYDROCHLORIDE; EFFEXOR	4535186	AUG 13, 2002		NCE	DEC 28, 1998
20151 005	VENLAFAXINE HYDROCHLORIDE; EFFEXOR	4535186	AUG 13, 2002		NCE	DEC 28, 1998
20151 006	VENLAFAXINE HYDROCHLORIDE; EFFEXOR	4535186	AUG 13, 2002		NCE	DEC 28, 1998

PRESCRIPTION AND OTC DRUG PRODUCT
PATENT AND EXCLUSIVITY DATA *(continued)*

APPL/ PROD NUMBER	INGREDIENT NAME; TRADE NAME	PATENT NUMBER	PATENT EXPIRES	USE CODE	EX- CLUS CODE	EXCLUS EXPIRES
19614 001	VERAPAMIL HYDROCHLORIDE; VERELAN	4863742	SEP 05, 2006	U-3		
19614 002	VERAPAMIL HYDROCHLORIDE; VERELAN	4863742	SEP 05, 2006	U-3		
19614 003	VERAPAMIL HYDROCHLORIDE; VERELAN	4863742	SEP 05, 2006	U-3		
14103 003	VINCRISTINE SULFATE; ONCOVIN	4619935	OCT 28, 2003			
20199 001	ZALCITABINE; HIVID	5028595	JUL 02, 2008	U-65	NCE	JUN 19, 1997
		4879277	NOV 07, 2006	U-65	ODE	JUN 19, 1999
20199 002	ZALCITABINE; HIVID	5028595	JUL 02, 2008	U-65	NCE	JUN 19, 1997
		4879277	NOV 07, 2006	U-65	ODE	JUN 19, 1999
19655 001	ZIDOVUDINE; RETROVIR	4837208	FEB 09, 2005			
		4833130	FEB 09, 2005			
		4828838	FEB 09, 2005		ODE	MAR 19, 1994
		4724232	FEB 09, 2005			
19910 001	ZIDOVUDINE; RETROVIR	4837208	FEB 09, 2005			
		4833130	FEB 09, 2005		ODE	MAR 19, 1994
		4818538	FEB 09, 2005			
		4724232	FEB 09, 2005			
19951 001	ZIDOVUDINE; RETROVIR	4837208	FEB 09, 2005			
		4833130	FEB 09, 2005			
		4818538	FEB 09, 2005			
		4724232	FEB 09, 2005		ODE	MAR 19, 1994
19908 001	ZOLPIDEM TARTRATE; AMBIEN	4382938	MAY 10, 2000	U-74	NCE	DEC 16, 1997
19908 002	ZOLPIDEM TARTRATE; AMBIEN	4382938	MAY 10, 2000	U-74	NCE	DEC 16, 1997

DRUG PRODUCTS WITH APPROVAL UNDER SECTION 505 OF THE ACT ADMINISTERED BY THE CENTER FOR BIOLOGICS EVALUATION AND RESEARCH PATENT AND EXCLUSIVITY DATA

APPL/ PROD NUMBER	INGREDIENT NAME; TRADE NAME	PATENT NUMBER	PATENT EXPIRES	USE CODE	EX-CLUS CODE	EXCLUS EXPIRES
19862 001	INDIUM 111 CHLORIDE; INDICLOR				NCE	DEC 29, 1997
841207 001	PENTASTARCH 10% IN SODIUM CHLORIDE 0.9%; PENTASPAN				ODE	MAY 19, 1994
860909 001	PERFLUORODECALIN; FLUOSOL	3911138	OCT 07, 1994		NCE	DEC 26, 1994
		4252827	FEB 24, 1998			
900278 001	SATUMOMAB PENDETIDE; ONCOSCINT				ODE	DEC 29, 1999

II

Section II

LISTINGS OF B-RATED DRUGS AND "PRE-1938" PRODUCTS

Listing of B-Rated Drugs

Cumulative through the August Supplement to the 1994 "Orange Book"

The listing of "B-rated" drugs that follows has been extracted by the USPC from the "Orange Book" *(Approved Drug Products with Therapeutic Equivalence Evaluations)* listings. It is intended to provide a concise listing of drug products that the Food and Drug Administration (FDA) has approved but does not list as therapeutically equivalent. For each product with a "B" rating, the "Orange Book" entry for the entire dosage form of that particular drug substance is included so that practitioners will be able to readily determine whether there are other products available containing the same substance and in the same dosage form that are considered by FDA to be therapeutically equivalent.

The fact that a drug product is not listed in the "B listing" does not necessarily mean FDA considers it therapeutically equivalent to other products containing the same drug substance. For example, this listing is derived from the list of FDA-approved products and does not cover "grandfathered" (pre-1938) products that have not gone through the NDA process. Similarly, other products not specifically approved by FDA do not have therapeutic equivalency ratings assigned and do not appear in the "Orange Book."

The two-letter coding system for therapeutic equivalence evaluations used in the "Orange Book" is constructed to allow users to determine quickly whether FDA has evaluated a particular approved product as therapeutically equivalent to other pharmaceutically equivalent products (first letter) and to provide additional information on the basis of FDA's evaluations (second letter). The application and product numbers and final approval date have been omitted (because of space constraints). Please see the "Orange Book" section of this volume for the complete listings.

The two basic categories into which multisource drugs have been placed are indicated by the first letter as follows:

A—Drug products that FDA considers to be therapeutically equivalent to other pharmaceutically equivalent products, i.e., drug products for which:

(1) there are no known or suspected bioequivalence problems. These are designated **AA, AN, AO, AP,** or **AT,** depending on the dosage form; or

(2) actual or potential bioequivalence problems have been resolved with adequate *in vivo* and/or *in vitro* evidence supporting bioequivalence. These are designated **AB.**

B—Drug products that FDA at this time considers not to be therapeutically equivalent to other pharmaceutically equivalent products, i.e., drug products for which actual or potential bioequivalence problems have not been resolved by adequate evidence of bioequivalence. Often the problem is with specific dosage forms rather than with the active ingredients. These are designated BC, BD, BE, BN, BP, BR, BS, BT, BX, or B*.

Drug products designated with a **"B"** code fall under one of three main policies:

(1) the drug products contain active ingredients or are manufactured in dosage forms that have been identified by the Agency as having documented bioequivalence problems or a significant potential for such problems and for which no adequate studies demonstrating bioequivalence have been submitted to FDA; or

(2) the quality standards are inadequate or FDA has an insufficient basis to determine therapeutic equivalence; or.

(3) the drug products are under regulatory review.

The specific coding definitions and policies for the "B"sub-codes are as follows:

B*

Drug products requiring further FDA investigation and review to determine therapeutic equivalence

The code B* is assigned to products that were previously assigned an A or B code if FDA receives new information that raises a significant question regarding therapeutic equivalence that can be resolved only through further Agency investigation and/or review of data and information submitted by the applicant. The B* code signifies that the Agency will take no position regarding the therapeutic equivalence of the product until the Agency completes its investigation and review.

BC

Extended-release tablets, extended-release capsules, and extended-release injectables

An extended-release dosage form is defined by the official compendia as one that allows at least a twofold reduction in dosing frequency as compared to that drug presented as a conventional dosage form (e.g., as a solution or a prompt drug-releasing, conventional solid dosage form).

Although bioavailability studies have been conducted on these dosage forms, they are subject to bioavailability differences, primarily because firms developing extended-release products for the same active ingredient rarely employ the same formulation approach. FDA, therefore, does not consider different extended-release dosage forms containing the same active ingredient in equal strength to be therapeutically equivalent unless equivalence between individual products in both rate and extent has been specifically demonstrated through appropriate bioequivalence studies. Extended-release products for which such bioequivalence data have not been submitted are coded **BC**, while those for which such data are available have been coded **AB**.

BD

Active ingredients and dosage forms with documented bioequivalence problems

The **BD** code denotes products containing active ingredients with known bioequivalence problems and for which adequate studies have not been submitted to FDA demonstrating bioequivalence. Where studies showing bioequivalence have been submitted, the product has been coded **AB**.

BE

Delayed-release oral dosage forms

A delayed-release dosage form is defined by the official compendia as one that releases a drug (or drugs) at a time other than promptly after administration. Enteric-coated articles are delayed-release dosage forms.

Drug products in delayed-release dosage forms containing the same active ingredients are subject to significant differences in absorption. Unless otherwise specifically noted, the Agency considers different delayed-release products containing the same active ingredients as presenting a potential bioequivalence problem and codes these products **BE** in the absence of *in vivo* studies showing bioequivalence. If adequate *in vivo* studies have demonstrated the bioequivalence of specific delayed-release products, such products are coded **AB**.

BN

Products in aerosol-nebulizer drug delivery systems

This code applies to drug solutions or powders that are marketed only as a component of, or as compatible with, a specific drug delivery system. There may, for example, be significant differences in the dose of drug and particle size delivered by different products of this type. Therefore, the Agency does not consider different metered aerosol dosage forms containing the same active ingredient(s) in equal strengths to be therapeutically equivalent unless the drug products meet an appropriate bioequivalence standard.

BP

Active ingredients and dosage forms with potential bioequivalence problems

FDA's bioequivalence regulations (21 CFR 320.52) contain criteria and procedures for determining whether a specific active ingredient in a specific dosage form has a potential for causing a bioequivalence problem. It is FDA's policy to consider an ingredient meeting these criteria as having a potential bioequivalence problem even in the absence of positive data demonstrating inequivalence. Pharmaceutically equivalent products containing these ingredients in oral dosage forms are coded **BP** until adequate *in vivo* bioequivalence data are submitted.

Injectable suspensions containing an active ingredient suspended in an aqueous or oleaginous vehicle have also been coded **BP.** Injectable suspensions are subject to bioequivalence problems because differences in particle size, polymorphic structure of the suspended active ingredient, or the suspension formulation can significantly affect the rate of release and absorption. FDA does not consider pharmaceutical equivalents of these products bioequivalent without adequate evidence of bioequivalence.

BR

Suppositories or enemas that deliver drugs for systemic absorption

The absorption of active ingredients from suppositories or enemas that are intended to have a systemic effect (as distinct from suppositories administered for local effect) can vary significantly from product to product. Therefore, FDA considers pharmaceutically equivalent systemic suppositories or enemas bioequivalent only if *in vivo* evidence of bioequivalence is available. In those cases where *in vivo* evidence is available, the product is coded **AB.** If such evidence is not available, the products are coded **BR.**

BS

Products having drug standard deficiencies

If the drug standards for an active ingredient in a particular dosage form are found by FDA to be deficient so as to prevent an FDA evaluation of either pharmaceutical or therapeutic equivalence, all drug products containing that active ingredient in that dosage form are coded **BS.** For example, if the standards permit a wide variation in pharmacologically active components of the active ingredient such that pharmaceutical equivalence is in question, all products containing that active ingredient in that dosage form are coded **BS.**

BT

Topical products with bioequivalence issues

This code applies mainly to post-1962 dermatologic, ophthalmic, otic, rectal, and vaginal products for topical administration, including creams, ointments, gels, lotions, pastes, and sprays, as well as suppositories not intended for systemic drug absorption. Topical products evaluated as having acceptable performance, but that are not bioequivalent to other pharmaceutically equivalent products or that lack sufficient evidence of bioequivalence will be coded **BT.**

BX

Insufficient data

The code **BX** is assigned to specific drug products for which the data that has been reviewed by the Agency are insufficient to determine therapeutic equivalence under the policies stated in this document. In these situations, the drug products are presumed to be therapeutically inequivalent until the Agency has determined that there is adequate information to make a full evaluation of therapeutic equivalence.

LISTING OF B-RATED DRUGS

ALBUTEROL

AEROSOL, METERED; INHALATION

	PROVENTIL	
BN	SCHERING	0.09 MG/INH
	VENTOLIN	
BN	+ GLAXO	0.09 MG/INH

ALBUTEROL SULFATE

TABLET, EXTENDED RELEASE; ORAL

	PROVENTIL	
BC	SCHERING	EQ 4 MG BASE
	VOLMAX	
BC	+ MURO	EQ 4 MG BASE
	+	EQ 8 MG BASE

AMINOPHYLLINE

TABLET; ORAL

	AMINOPHYLLINE	
AB	GENEVA	100 MG
AB		200 MG
BD	HALSEY	100 MG
BD	PHOENIX LABS	100 MG
BD		200 MG
AB	RICHLYN	100 MG
AB		200 MG
AB	+ ROXANE	100 MG
AB	+	200 MG
AB	WEST WARD	100 MG
AB		200 MG

AMITRIPTYLINE HYDROCHLORIDE

TABLET; ORAL

	AMITRIPTYLINE HCL	
AB	BIOCRAFT	10 MG
AB		25 MG
AB		50 MG
AB		75 MG
AB		100 MG
BP	COPLEY	10 MG
BP		25 MG
BP		50 MG
BP		75 MG
BP		100 MG
BP		150 MG
AB	DANBURY PHARMA	10 MG
AB		25 MG
AB		50 MG
AB		75 MG
AB		100 MG
AB		150 MG
AB	GENEVA	10 MG
AB		25 MG
AB		50 MG
AB		75 MG
AB		100 MG
AB		150 MG

AMITRIPTYLINE HYDROCHLORIDE *(continued)*

TABLET; ORAL

	AMITRIPTYLINE HCL	
BP	HALSEY	10 MG
BP		25 MG
BP		50 MG
BP		75 MG
BP		100 MG
AB	MD PHARM	10 MG
AB		25 MG
AB		50 MG
AB		75 MG
AB		100 MG
AB		150 MG
AB	MUTUAL PHARM	10 MG
AB		25 MG
AB		50 MG
AB		75 MG
AB		100 MG
AB		150 MG
AB	MYLAN	10 MG
AB		25 MG
AB		50 MG
AB		75 MG
AB		100 MG
AB		150 MG
AB	PUREPAC	10 MG
AB		25 MG
AB		50 MG
AB		75 MG
AB		100 MG
AB	ROXANE	10 MG
AB		25 MG
AB		50 MG
AB		75 MG
AB		100 MG
AB		150 MG
AB	SIDMAK	10 MG
AB		25 MG
AB		50 MG
AB		75 MG
AB		100 MG
AB		150 MG
AB	SUPERPHARM	10 MG
AB		25 MG
AB		50 MG
AB		75 MG
AB		100 MG
	ELAVIL	
AB	ZENECA	10 MG
AB	+	25 MG
AB		50 MG
AB		75 MG
AB		100 MG
AB		150 MG
	ENDEP	
AB	ROCHE	10 MG
AB		25 MG
AB		50 MG
AB		75 MG
AB		100 MG
AB		150 MG

AMITRIPTYLINE HYDROCHLORIDE; PERPHENAZINE

TABLET; ORAL

	ETRAFON 2-10	
BP	SCHERING	10 MG;2 MG
	ETRAFON 2-25	
BP	SCHERING	25 MG;2 MG
	ETRAFON-A	
BP	SCHERING	10 MG;4 MG
	ETRAFON-FORTE	
BP	SCHERING	25 MG;4 MG
	PERPHENAZINE AND AMITRIPTYLINE HCL	
AB	BARR	10 MG;2 MG
AB		10 MG;4 MG
AB		25 MG;2 MG
AB		25 MG;4 MG
AB	DANBURY PHARMA	10 MG;2 MG
AB		10 MG;4 MG
AB		25 MG;2 MG
AB		25 MG;4 MG
AB		50 MG;4 MG
AB	GENEVA	10 MG;2 MG
AB		10 MG;4 MG
AB		25 MG;2 MG
AB		25 MG;4 MG
AB		50 MG;4 MG
AB	MYLAN	10 MG;2 MG
AB		10 MG;4 MG
AB		25 MG;2 MG
AB		25 MG;4 MG
AB		50 MG;4 MG
AB	ROYCE	10 MG;2 MG
AB		10 MG;4 MG
AB		25 MG;2 MG
AB		25 MG;4 MG
AB	ZENITH	10 MG;2 MG
AB		10 MG;4 MG
AB		25 MG;2 MG
AB		25 MG;4 MG
AB		50 MG;4 MG
	TRIAVIL 2-10	
AB	MSD	10 MG;2 MG
	TRIAVIL 2-25	
AB	MSD	25 MG;2 MG
	TRIAVIL 4-10	
AB	MSD	10 MG;4 MG
	TRIAVIL 4-25	
AB	+ MSD	25 MG;4 MG
	TRIAVIL 4-50	
AB	+ MSD	50 MG;4 MG

Listing of B-rated Drugs *(continued)*

BECLOMETHASONE DIPROPIONATE

AEROSOL, METERED; INHALATION

	BECLOVENT	
BN	GLAXO	0.042 MG/INH
	VANCERIL	
BN	+ SCHERING	0.042 MG/INH

AEROSOL, METERED; NASAL

	BECONASE	
BN	+ GLAXO	0.042 MG/INH
	VANCENASE	
BN	SCHERING	0.042 MG/INH

BECLOMETHASONE DIPROPIONATE MONOHYDRATE

SPRAY, METERED; NASAL

	BECONASE AQ	
BN	+ GLAXO	EQ 0.042 MG DIPROP/INH
	VANCENASE AQ	
BN	SCHERING	EQ 0.042 MG DIPROP/INH

CAFFEINE; ERGOTAMINE TARTRATE

SUPPOSITORY; RECTAL

	CAFERGOT	
BR	+ SANDOZ	100 MG;2 MG
	MIGERGOT	
BR	G AND W LABS	100 MG;2 MG

CHLOROTHIAZIDE; RESERPINE

TABLET; ORAL

	CHLOROTHIAZIDE AND RESERPINE	
BP	WEST WARD	250 MG;0.125 MG
BP		500 MG;0.125 MG
	CHLOROTHIAZIDE-RESERPINE	
BP	MYLAN	250 MG;0.125 MG
BP		500 MG;0.125 MG
	DIUPRES-250	
BP	MSD	250 MG;0.125 MG
	DIUPRES-500	
BP	+ MSD	500 MG;0.125 MG

CHLORPHENIRAMINE MALEATE; PHENYLPROPANOLAMINE HYDROCHLORIDE

CAPSULE, EXTENDED RELEASE; ORAL

	CHLORPHENIRAMINE MALEATE AND PHENYLPROPANOLAMINE HCL	
AB	GENEVA	12 MG;75 MG
	DRIZE	
BC	ASCHER	12 MG;75 MG
	ORNADE	
AB	+ SMITHKLINE BEECHAM	12 MG;75 MG

CHLORPROMAZINE HYDROCHLORIDE

TABLET; ORAL

	CHLORPROMAZINE HCL	
BP	GENEVA	10 MG
BP		25 MG
BP		50 MG
BP		100 MG
BP		200 MG
BP	KV	10 MG
BP		25 MG
BP		50 MG
BP		100 MG
BP		200 MG
BP	LEDERLE	10 MG
BP	PHARM BASICS	10 MG
BP		25 MG
BP		50 MG
BP		100 MG
BP		200 MG
BP	ZENITH	10 MG
BP		25 MG
BP		50 MG
BP		100 MG
BP		200 MG
	THORAZINE	
BP	+ SMITHKLINE BEECHAM	10 MG
BP		25 MG
BP		50 MG
BP	+	100 MG
BP		200 MG

CHLORTHALIDONE

TABLET; ORAL

	CHLORTHALIDONE	
AB	ABBOTT	25 MG
AB	BARR	25 MG
AB		50 MG
AB	CHELSEA	25 MG
AB	DANBURY PHARMA	25 MG
AB		25 MG
AB		50 MG
AB		50 MG
AB	EON LABS	50 MG
AB	GENEVA	25 MG
AB		50 MG
AB	KV	25 MG
AB		50 MG
AB	LEDERLE	25 MG
AB		50 MG
AB	MUTUAL PHARM	25 MG
AB		25 MG
AB		50 MG
AB		50 MG
AB	MYLAN	25 MG
AB		50 MG
AB	PHARM BASICS	25 MG

CHLORTHALIDONE *(continued)*

TABLET; ORAL

	CHLORTHALIDONE	
AB	PUREPAC	25 MG
AB		50 MG
AB	SIDMAK	25 MG
AB		50 MG
AB	SUPERPHARM	50 MG
AB	ZENITH	25 MG
AB		50 MG
AB		50 MG
	HYGROTON	
AB	RHONE POULENC RORER	25 MG
AB	+	50 MG
	THALITONE	
BX	HORUS	25 MG
	+	15 MG

CLOTRIMAZOLE

CREAM; TOPICAL

	CLOTRIMAZOLE	
AB	TARO	1%
	LOTRIMIN	
AB	+ SCHERING PLOUGH	1%
	MYCELEX	
BT	MILES	1%

COLCHICINE; PROBENECID

TABLET; ORAL

	COL-PROBENECID	
BP	DANBURY PHARMA	0.5 MG;500 MG
	COLBENEMID	
BP	+ MSD	0.5 MG;500 MG
	PROBENECID AND COLCHICINE	
BP	RICHLYN	0.5 MG;500 MG
BP	ZENITH	0.5 MG;500 MG

CORTICOTROPIN

INJECTABLE; INJECTION

	ACTH	
AP	PARKE DAVIS	40 UNITS/VIAL
	ACTHAR	
AP	RHONE POULENC RORER	40 UNITS/VIAL
	CORTICOTROPIN	
BC	ORGANICS	40 UNITS/ML
BC	+	80 UNITS/ML
AP	STERIS	40 UNITS/VIAL
	H.P. ACTHAR GEL	
BC	RHONE POULENC RORER	40 UNITS/ML
BC	+	80 UNITS/ML

Listing of B-rated Drugs *(continued)*

CORTISONE ACETATE
TABLET; ORAL
CORTISONE ACETATE
BP CHELSEA 25 MG
BP PUREPAC 25 MG
BP RICHLYN 25 MG
BP UPJOHN 25 MG
5 MG
10 MG
BP WEST WARD 25 MG
CORTONE
BP + MSD 25 MG

DESMOPRESSIN ACETATE
SOLUTION; NASAL
CONCENTRAID
BX FERRING 0.01%
DDAVP
BX + RHONE POULENC RORER 0.01%

DEXAMETHASONE
TABLET; ORAL
DECADRON
AB MSD 0.5 MG
AB + 0.75 MG
AB 1.5 MG
AB 4 MG
0.25 MG
BP + 6 MG
DEXAMETHASONE
BP DANBURY PHARMA 0.25 MG
BP 0.5 MG
BP 0.75 MG
BP 1.5 MG
BP PAR 0.25 MG
BP 0.5 MG
BP 0.75 MG
BP 1.5 MG
BP 4 MG
BP 6 MG
BP RICHLYN 0.75 MG
AB ROXANE 0.5 MG
AB 0.75 MG
AB 1.5 MG
AB 4 MG
BP 6 MG
1 MG
2 MG
DEXONE 0.5
BP SOLVAY 0.5 MG
DEXONE 0.75
BP SOLVAY 0.75 MG
DEXONE 1.5
BP SOLVAY 1.5 MG
DEXONE 4
BP SOLVAY 4 MG
HEXADROL
BP ORGANON 0.5 MG
BP 0.75 MG
BP 1.5 MG
BP 4 MG

DEXAMETHASONE ACETATE
INJECTABLE; INJECTION
DECADRON-LA
BP MERCK EQ 8 MG BASE/ML
DEXAMETHASONE ACETATE
BP STERIS EQ 8 MG BASE/ML
EQ 16 MG BASE/ML

DIETHYLPROPION HYDROCHLORIDE
TABLET, EXTENDED RELEASE; ORAL
TENUATE DOSPAN
BC + MERRELL DOW 75 MG
TEPANIL TEN-TAB
BC 3M 75 MG

DIETHYLSTILBESTROL
TABLET, DELAYED RELEASE; ORAL
BE + LILLY 1 MG
BE + 5 MG

DIFLORASONE DIACETATE
CREAM; TOPICAL
FLORONE
BX + UPJOHN 0.05%
PSORCON
BX DERMIK 0.05%

DILTIAZEM HYDROCHLORIDE
CAPSULE, EXTENDED RELEASE; ORAL
CARDIZEM CD
BC + CARDERM 120 MG
BC + 180 MG
BC + 240 MG
+ 300 MG
CARDIZEM SR
AB + MARION MERRELL DOW 60 MG
AB + 90 MG
AB + 120 MG
DILACOR XR
BC RHONE POULENC RORER 120 MG
BC 180 MG
BC 240 MG
DILTIAZEM HCL
AB PROGRAPHARM 60 MG
AB 90 MG
AB 120 MG

DISOPYRAMIDE PHOSPHATE
CAPSULE, EXTENDED-RELEASE; ORAL
DISOPYRAMIDE PHOSPHATE
B* KV EQ 100 MG BASE
AB EQ 150 MG BASE
NORPACE CR
AB SEARLE EQ 100 MG BASE
AB + EQ 150 MG BASE

DISULFIRAM
TABLET; ORAL
ANTABUSE
BX WYETH AYERST 250 MG
BX + 500 MG
DISULFIRAM
BX DANBURY PHARMA 250 MG
BX 500 MG
BX PAR 250 MG
BX 500 MG
BX SIDMAK 250 MG
BX 500 MG

DYPHYLLINE
TABLET; ORAL
DILOR
BP SAVAGE 200 MG
DILOR-400
BP SAVAGE 400 MG
LUFYLLIN
BP WALLACE 200 MG
BP 400 MG
NEOTHYLLINE
BP LEMMON 200 MG
BP + 400 MG

ESTROGENS, ESTERIFIED
TABLET; ORAL
ESTRATAB
BS SOLVAY 0.3 MG
BS + 0.625 MG
BS 1.25 MG
BS + 2.5 MG
MENEST
BS SMITHKLINE BEECHAM 0.3 MG
BS 0.625 MG
BS 1.25 MG
BS 2.5 MG

ESTRONE
INJECTABLE; INJECTION
ESTROGENIC SUBSTANCE
BP WYETH AYERST 2 MG/ML
ESTRONE
+ STERIS 5 MG/ML
NATURAL ESTROGENIC SUBSTANCE-ESTRONE
BP STERIS 2 MG/ML
THEELIN
BP + PARKE DAVIS 2 MG/ML

Listing of B-rated Drugs *(continued)*

FLUOXYMESTERONE

TABLET; ORAL

	FLUOXYMESTERONE	
BP	PHARM BASICS	10 MG
	HALOTESTIN	
BP	+ UPJOHN	10 MG
		2 MG
		5 MG

FLUPHENAZINE HYDROCHLORIDE

TABLET; ORAL

	FLUPHENAZINE HCL	
AB	GENEVA	1 MG
AB		2.5 MG
AB		5 MG
AB		10 MG
AB	MYLAN	1 MG
AB		2.5 MG
AB		5 MG
AB		10 MG
AB	PAR	1 MG
AB		2.5 MG
AB		5 MG
AB		10 MG
	PERMITIL	
BP	SCHERING	2.5 MG
BP		5 MG
BP		10 MG
	PROLIXIN	
AB	APOTHECON	1 MG
AB		2.5 MG
AB		5 MG
AB	+	10 MG

GALLIUM CITRATE, GA-67

INJECTABLE; INJECTION

	GALLIUM CITRATE GA 67	
BS	DUPONT	2 MCI/ML
BS	MALLINCKRODT	2 MCI/ML
	NEOSCAN	
BS	MEDI PHYSICS	2 MCI/ML

GLYBURIDE

TABLET; ORAL

	DIABETA	
BX	HOECHST ROUSSEL	1.25 MG
BX		2.5 MG
BX		5 MG
	GLYNASE	
		1.5 MG
	UPJOHN	3 MG
		4.5 MG
	+	6 MG
	MICRONASE	
BX	UPJOHN	1.25 MG
BX		2.5 MG
BX	+	5 MG

HYDRALAZINE HYDROCHLORIDE; HYDROCHLOROTHIAZIDE; RESERPINE

TABLET; ORAL

	CAM-AP-ES	
BP	CAMALL	25 MG;15 MG;0.1 MG
	HYDRALAZINE HCL, HYDROCHLOROTHIAZIDE AND RESERPINE	
BP	ZENITH	25 MG;15 MG;0.1 MG
	HYDROSERPINE PLUS (R-H-H)	
BP	ZENITH	25 MG;15 MG;0.1 MG
	RESERPINE, HYDRALAZINE HCL AND HYDROCHLOROTHIAZIDE	
BP	BARR	25 MG;15 MG;0.1 MG
BP	DANBURY PHARMA	25 MG;15 MG;0.1 MG
BP	SOLVAY	25 MG;15 MG;0.1 MG
	SER-AP-ES	
BP	+ CIBA	25 MG;15 MG;0.1 MG
	UNIPRES	
BP	SOLVAY	25 MG;15 MG;0.1 MG

HYDROCHLOROTHIAZIDE; RESERPINE

TABLET; ORAL

	HYDRO-RESERP	
BP	CAMALL	50 MG;0.125 MG
	HYDROCHLOROTHIAZIDE W/ RESERPINE	
BP	DANBURY PHARMA	25 MG;0.125 MG
BP		50 MG;0.125 MG
BP	ZENITH	25 MG;0.125 MG
BP		50 MG;0.125 MG
		25 MG;0.1 MG
		50 MG;0.1 MG
	HYDROPRES 25	
BP	MSD	25 MG;0.125 MG
	HYDROPRES 50	
BP	MSD	50 MG;0.125 MG
	RESERPINE AND HYDROCHLOROTHIAZIDE-50	
BP	WEST WARD	50 MG;0.125 MG

HYDROCHLOROTHIAZIDE; TRIAMTERENE

TABLET; ORAL

	MAXZIDE	
AB	+ MYLAN	50 MG;75 MG
	MAXZIDE-25	
AB	MYLAN	25 MG;37.5 MG
	TRIAMTERENE AND HYDROCHLOROTHIAZIDE	
AB	BARR	50 MG;75 MG
AB	DANBURY PHARMA	50 MG;75 MG
AB	GENEVA	50 MG;75 MG
AB		25 MG;37.5 MG
B*	PAR	50 MG;75 MG
AB	WATSON	50 MG;75 MG
AB	WATSON LABS	25 MG;37.5 MG

HYDROCORTISONE

TABLET; ORAL

	CORTEF	
BP	UPJOHN	10 MG
BP		20 MG
		5 MG
	HYDROCORTISONE	
BP	LANNETT	20 MG
BP	PUREPAC	10 MG
BP		20 MG
BP	RICHLYN	20 MG
BP	WEST WARD	20 MG
	HYDROCORTONE	
BP	MSD	10 MG
BP	+	20 MG

HYDROCORTISONE ACETATE

INJECTABLE; INJECTION

	HYDROCORTISONE ACETATE	
BP	AKORN	25 MG/ML
BP		50 MG/ML
BP	STERIS	25 MG/ML
BP		25 MG/ML
BP		50 MG/ML
	HYDROCORTONE	
BP	MSD	25 MG/ML
BP	+	50 MG/ML

HYDROCORTISONE ACETATE; PRAMOXINE HYDROCHLORIDE

AEROSOL; TOPICAL

	EPIFOAM	
BX	REED AND CARNRICK	1%;1%
	HYDROCORTISONE ACETATE 1% AND PRAMOXINE HCL 1%	
BX	COPLEY	1%;1%
	PROCTOFOAM HC	
BX	REED AND CARNRICK	1%;1%

HYDROFLUMETHIAZIDE; RESERPINE

TABLET; ORAL

	RESERPINE AND HYDROFLUMETHIAZIDE	
BP	PAR	50 MG;0.125 MG
BP	ZENITH	50 MG;0.125 MG
	SALUTENSIN	
BP	+ ROBERTS	50 MG;0.125 MG
	SALUTENSIN-DEMI	
	ROBERTS	25 MG;0.125 MG

Listing of B-rated Drugs *(continued)*

IBUPROFEN

SUSPENSION; ORAL

	CHILDREN'S ADVIL	
BX	WHITEHALL	100 MG/5 ML
	PEDIA PROFEN	
BX	+ MCNEIL	100 MG/5 ML
	RUFEN	
BX	BOOTS	100 MG/5 ML

IRON DEXTRAN

INJECTABLE; INJECTION

	INFED	
BP	+ SCHEIN PHARM	EQ 50 MG IRON/ML
	PROFERDEX	
BP	LOTUS	EQ 50 MG IRON/ML

ISOPROTERENOL HYDROCHLORIDE

AEROSOL, METERED; INHALATION

	ISOPROTERENOL HCL	
BN	BARRE	0.12 MG/INH
BN	+ 3M	0.12 MG/INH
	ISUPREL	
	+ STERLING WINTHROP	0.131 MG/INH

ISOSORBIDE DINITRATE

CAPSULE, EXTENDED RELEASE; ORAL

	DILATRATE-SR	
BC	REED AND CARNRICK	40 MG
	ISORDIL	
BC	+ WYETH AYERST	40 MG

LEUCOVORIN CALCIUM

TABLET; ORAL

	LEUCOVORIN CALCIUM	
AB	BARR	EQ 5 MG BASE
AB		EQ 25 MG BASE
AB	IMMUNEX	EQ 10 MG BASE
AB	+	EQ 15 MG BASE
BX		EQ 5 MG BASE

LEVODOPA

TABLET; ORAL

	DOPAR	
BD	ROBERTS	250 MG
BD		500 MG
	LARODOPA	
BD	ROCHE	250 MG
BD		500 MG
		100 MG

MAZINDOL

TABLET; ORAL

	MAZANOR	
BP	WYETH AYERST	1 MG
	SANOREX	
BP	SANDOZ	1 MG
	+	2 MG

MEDROXYPROGESTERONE ACETATE

TABLET; ORAL

	AMEN	
BP	CARNRICK	10 MG
	CURRETAB	
BP	SOLVAY	10 MG
	CYCRIN	
AB	WYETH AYERST	2.5 MG
AB		5 MG
AB		10 MG
	MEDROXYPROGESTERONE ACETATE	
BP	PHARM BASICS	10 MG
	PROVERA	
AB	UPJOHN	2.5 MG
AB		5 MG
AB	+	10 MG

METHYLPREDNISOLONE ACETATE

INJECTABLE; INJECTION

	DEPO-MEDROL	
BP	UPJOHN	20 MG/ML
BP		40 MG/ML
BP	+	80 MG/ML
	METHYLPREDNISOLONE ACETATE	
BP	AKORN	40 MG/ML
BP		80 MG/ML
BP	STERIS	20 MG/ML
BP		40 MG/ML
BP		80 MG/ML

METHYLTESTOSTERONE

CAPSULE; ORAL

	TESTRED	
BP	+ ICN	10 MG
	VIRILON	
BP	STAR PHARMS	10 MG

TABLET; BUCCAL/SUBLINGUAL

	METHYLTESTOSTERONE	
BP	+ LILLY	10 MG
BP	RICHLYN	10 MG

METHYLTESTOSTERONE *(continued)*

TABLET; ORAL

	ANDROID 10	
AB	ICN	10 MG
	ANDROID 25	
AB	ICN	25 MG
	METHYLTESTOSTERONE	
BP	LANNETT	10 MG
BP		25 MG
BP	LILLY	25 MG
BP	RICHLYN	10 MG
BP		25 MG
	ORETON METHYL	
BP	SCHERING	10 MG
BP	+	25 MG

MORPHINE SULFATE

TABLET, EXTENDED RELEASE; ORAL

	MS CONTIN	
BC	+ PURDUE FREDERICK	30 MG
BC	+	60 MG
BC	+	100 MG
	+	15 MG
	+	200 MG
	ORAMORPH SR	
BC	ROXANE	30 MG
BC		60 MG
BC		100 MG

NICOTINE

FILM, EXTENDED RELEASE; TRANSDERMAL

	HABITROL	
BC	+ BASEL PHARMS	7 MG/24 HR
BC	+	14 MG/24 HR
BC	+	21 MG/24 HR
	NICODERM	
BC	+ MARION MERRELL DOW	7 MG/24 HR
BC	+	14 MG/24 HR
BC	+	21 MG/24 HR
	NICOTROL	
	+ KABI	5 MG/16 HR
	+	10 MG/16 HR
	+	15 MG/16 HR
	PROSTEP	
	+ ELAN	11 MG/24 HR
	+	22 MG/24 HR

NIFEDIPINE

TABLET, EXTENDED RELEASE; ORAL

	ADALAT CC	
BC	MILES	30 MG
BC		60 MG
BC		90 MG
	PROCARDIA XL	
BC	+ PFIZER	30 MG
BC	+	60 MG
BC	+	90 MG

Listing of B-rated Drugs *(continued)*

NORTRIPTYLINE HYDROCHLORIDE

CAPSULE; ORAL

	AVENTYL HCL	
BD	LILLY	EQ 10 MG BASE
BD		EQ 25 MG BASE
	NORTRIPTYLINE HCL	
AB	DANBURY PHARMA	EQ 10 MG BASE
AB		EQ 25 MG BASE
AB		EQ 50 MG BASE
AB		EQ 75 MG BASE
AB	GENEVA	EQ 10 MG BASE
AB		EQ 25 MG BASE
AB		EQ 50 MG BASE
AB		EQ 75 MG BASE
AB	MYLAN	EQ 10 MG BASE
AB		EQ 25 MG BASE
AB		EQ 50 MG BASE
AB		EQ 75 MG BASE
	PAMELOR	
AB	SANDOZ	EQ 10 MG BASE
AB		EQ 25 MG BASE
AB		EQ 50 MG BASE
AB	+	EQ 75 MG BASE

PENICILLIN G BENZATHINE

INJECTABLE; INJECTION

	BICILLIN L-A	
BC	WYETH AYERST	600,000 UNITS/ML
	+	300,000 UNITS/ML
	PERMAPEN	
BC	PFIZER	600,000 UNITS/ML

PHENDIMETRAZINE TARTRATE

CAPSULE, EXTENDED RELEASE; ORAL

	PHENDIMETRAZINE TARTRATE	
BC	EON LABS	105 MG
BC	+ GENEVA	105 MG
BC	GRAHAM LABS	105 MG
BC		105 MG
BC		105 MG
BC		105 MG
BC		105 MG
BC		105 MG
BC		105 MG
	X-TROZINE L.A.	
BC	REXAR	105 MG

PHENYTOIN SODIUM, PROMPT

CAPSULE; ORAL

	PROMPT PHENYTOIN SODIUM	
BX	+ DANBURY PHARMA	100 MG
BX	ZENITH	100 MG

PHYTONADIONE

INJECTABLE; INJECTION

	AQUAMEPHYTON	
BP	MSD	1 MG/0.5 ML
BP	+	10 MG/ML
	KONAKION	
BP	ROCHE	1 MG/0.5 ML
BP		10 MG/ML
	PHYTONADIONE	
BP	INTL MEDICATION	1 MG/0.5 ML
	VITAMIN K1	
BP	ABBOTT	1 MG/0.5 ML
BP		10 MG/ML

POTASSIUM CHLORIDE

TABLET, EXTENDED RELEASE; ORAL

	K+10	
BC	ALRA	10 MEQ
	K+8	
AB	ALRA	8 MEQ
	K-DUR 10	
BC	SCHERING	10 MEQ
	K-DUR 20	
	SCHERING	20 MEQ
	K-TAB	
BC	+ ABBOTT	10 MEQ
	KAON CL	
	SAVAGE	6.7 MEQ
	KAON CL-10	
BC	SAVAGE	10 MEQ
	KLOR-CON	
AB	UPSHER SMITH	8 MEQ
BC		10 MEQ
	KLOTRIX	
BC	APOTHECON	10 MEQ
	POTASSIUM CHLORIDE	
BC	ABBOTT	8 MEQ
AB	COPLEY	8 MEQ
	SLOW-K	
AB	+ CIBA	8 MEQ
	TEN-K	
BC	CIBA	10 MEQ

PREDNISOLONE

TABLET; ORAL

	CORTALONE	
BX	HALSEY	1 MG
BX		2.5 MG
BX		5 MG
	PREDNISOLONE	
BX	CHELSEA	5 MG
BX	DANBURY PHARMA	5 MG
BX	EVERYLIFE	2.5 MG
BX		5 MG
BX	GENEVA	5 MG
BX	LANNETT	5 MG

PREDNISOLONE *(continued)*

TABLET; ORAL

	PREDNISOLONE	
BX	MARSHALL	2.5 MG
BX		5 MG
BX		5 MG
BX	PHOENIX LABS	5 MG
BX	PUREPAC	5 MG
BX	RICHLYN	5 MG
BX	ROXANE	5 MG
BX	SPERTI	1 MG
BX		2.5 MG
BX		5 MG
BX	ZENITH	5 MG

PREDNISOLONE TEBUTATE

INJECTABLE; INJECTION

	HYDELTRA-TBA	
BP	+ MSD	20 MG/ML
	PREDNISOLONE TEBUTATE	
BP	STERIS	20 MG/ML

PREDNISONE

TABLET; ORAL

	CORTAN	
BX	HALSEY	20 MG
	DELTASONE	
AB	UPJOHN	2.5 MG
AB		5 MG
AB		10 MG
AB		20 MG
AB	+	50 MG
	METICORTEN	
AB	+ SCHERING	1 MG
	ORASONE	
AB	SOLVAY	1 MG
AB		5 MG
AB		10 MG
AB		20 MG
AB		50 MG
	PREDNICEN-M	
AB	CENTRAL PHARMS	5 MG
	PREDNISONE	
AB	BARR	5 MG
AB		10 MG
AB		20 MG
AB	CHELSEA	5 MG
AB		10 MG
AB		20 MG
AB		50 MG
AB	DANBURY PHARMA	5 MG
AB		10 MG
AB		20 MG

Listing of B-rated Drugs *(continued)*

PREDNISONE *(continued)*

TABLET; ORAL

	PREDNISONE	
BX	EVERYLIFE	1 MG
BX		2.5 MG
BX		5 MG
AB	GENEVA	5 MG
AB		10 MG
AB		20 MG
AB		50 MG
AB	HALSEY	5 MG
AB	INTERPHARM	5 MG
AB		10 MG
AB		20 MG
BX	INWOOD	5 MG
BX	LANNETT	5 MG
BX		20 MG
BX	MARSHALL	5 MG
AB	MUTUAL PHARM	5 MG
AB		10 MG
AB		20 MG
BX	PHARMAVITE	5 MG
BX	PHOENIX LABS	5 MG
BX		20 MG
AB	PRIVATE FORM	5 MG
AB	PUREPAC	5 MG
AB		10 MG
AB		20 MG
AB	RICHLYN	5 MG
AB	ROXANE	1 MG
AB		2.5 MG
AB		5 MG
AB		10 MG
AB		20 MG
AB		50 MG
AB	SUPERPHARM	5 MG
AB		10 MG
AB		20 MG
AB	WEST WARD	5 MG
AB		10 MG
AB		20 MG
AB		50 MG
BX	ZENITH	5 MG
BX		10 MG

PROCAINAMIDE HYDROCHLORIDE

TABLET, EXTENDED RELEASE; ORAL

	PROCAINAMIDE HCL	
AB	COPLEY	500 MG
AB		750 MG
AB	DANBURY PHARMA	250 MG
AB		500 MG
AB		750 MG
AB	GENEVA	250 MG
AB		500 MG
AB		750 MG
AB	INVAMED	500 MG
AB	INWOOD	500 MG
AB	SIDMAK	250 MG
AB		500 MG

PROCAINAMIDE HYDROCHLORIDE *(continued)*

TABLET, EXTENDED RELEASE; ORAL

	PROCAN SR	
AB	PARKE DAVIS	250 MG
AB		500 MG
AB		750 MG
	+	1 GM
	PRONESTYL-SR	
BC	BRISTOL MYERS SQUIBB	500 MG

PROMETHAZINE HYDROCHLORIDE

SUPPOSITORY; RECTAL

	PHENERGAN	
BR	WYETH AYERST	25 MG
BR	+	50 MG
		12.5 MG
	PROMETHACON	
BR	POLYMEDICA	25 MG
BR		50 MG
	PROMETHEGAN	
BR	G AND W	50 MG

TABLET; ORAL

	PHENERGAN	
BP	WYETH AYERST	12.5 MG
BP		25 MG
BP	+	50 MG
	PROMETHAZINE HCL	
BP	DANBURY PHARMA	12.5 MG
BP		25 MG
BP		50 MG
BP	GENEVA	25 MG
BP		50 MG
BP	LANNETT	12.5 MG
BP		25 MG
BP		50 MG
BP	PRIVATE FORM	25 MG
BP	RICHLYN	25 MG
BP	ZENITH	12.5 MG
BP		25 MG

PROPYLTHIOURACIL

TABLET; ORAL

	PROPYLTHIOURACIL	
BD	BARR	50 MG
BD	HALSEY	50 MG
BD	+ LEDERLE	50 MG
BD	LILLY	50 MG
BD	PUREPAC	50 MG
BD	RICHLYN	50 MG
BD	WEST WARD	50 MG

QUINIDINE GLUCONATE

TABLET, EXTENDED RELEASE; ORAL

	QUINAGLUTE	
AB	+ BERLEX	324 MG
	QUINALAN	
BC	LANNETT	324 MG
	QUINIDINE GLUCONATE	
AB	DANBURY PHARMA	324 MG
AB	GENEVA	324 MG
AB	HALSEY	324 MG
AB	MUTUAL PHARM	324 MG

RAUWOLFIA SERPENTINA

TABLET; ORAL

	HIWOLFIA	
BP	BOWMAN	50 MG
	RAUDIXIN	
BP	APOTHECON	50 MG
BP	+	100 MG
	RAUVAL	
BP	VALE	50 MG
BP		100 MG
	RAUWOLFIA SERPENTINA	
BP	DANBURY PHARMA	50 MG
BP	HALSEY	50 MG
BP		100 MG
BP	RICHLYN	50 MG
BP		100 MG

RESERPINE

TABLET; ORAL

	RESERPINE	
BP	EON LABS	0.1 MG
BP		0.25 MG
BP	PUREPAC	0.1 MG
BP		0.25 MG
BP	RICHLYN	0.1 MG
BP		0.25 MG
	SERPALAN	
BP	LANNETT	0.1 MG
BP		0.25 MG
	SERPASIL	
BP	CIBA	0.1 MG
BP	+	0.25 MG
	SERPIVITE	
BP	VITARINE	0.25 MG

SOMATROPIN, BIOSYNTHETIC

INJECTABLE; INJECTION

	HUMATROPE	
BX	+ LILLY	5 MG/VIAL
	NUTROPIN	
BX	GENENTECH	5 MG/VIAL
	+	10 MG/VIAL

Listing of B-rated Drugs *(continued)*

TECHNETIUM TC-99M ALBUMIN AGGREGATED KIT

	INJECTABLE; INJECTION	
	AN-MAA	
BS	SORIN	N/A
	MACROTEC	
BS	BRACCO	N/A
	PULMOLITE	
BS	DUPONT	N/A
	TECHNESCAN MAA	
BS	MALLINCKRODT	N/A
	TECHNETIUM TC 99M ALBUMIN AGGREGATED KIT	
BS	MSD	N/A

TERBUTALINE SULFATE

	TABLET; ORAL	
	BRETHINE	
BP	GEIGY	2.5 MG
BP	+	5 MG
	BRICANYL	
BP	MERRELL DOW	2.5 MG
BP		5 MG

THEOPHYLLINE

	CAPSULE; ORAL	
	BRONKODYL	
BP	STERLING WINTHROP	100 MG
BP		200 MG
	ELIXOPHYLLIN	
BX	FOREST LABS	100 MG
BX	+	200 MG
	THEOPHYLLINE	
BP	KV	100 MG
BP		200 MG
	CAPSULE, EXTENDED RELEASE; ORAL	
	AEROLATE III	
	+ FLEMING	65 MG
	AEROLATE JR	
BC	FLEMING	130 MG
	AEROLATE SR	
BC	FLEMING	260 MG
	ELIXOPHYLLIN SR	
BC	FOREST LABS	125 MG
BC		250 MG
	SLO-BID	
BC	+ RHONE POULENC	50 MG
	RORER	
BC		75 MG
AB		100 MG
AB		125 MG
AB		200 MG
AB	+	300 MG
	SLO-PHYLLIN	
BC	RHONE POULENC	125 MG
	RORER	
BC		250 MG
		60 MG

THEOPHYLLINE *(continued)*

	CAPSULE, EXTENDED RELEASE; ORAL	
	SOMOPHYLLIN-CRT	
BC	GRAHAM LABS	50 MG
BC		100 MG
BC		200 MG
BC		250 MG
BC		300 MG
	THEO-DUR	
BC	KEY PHARMS	50 MG
BC		75 MG
BC		125 MG
BC		200 MG
	THEO-24	
BC	WHITBY	100 MG
BC		200 MG
BC		300 MG
		400 MG
	THEOCLEAR L.A.-130	
BC	+ CENTRAL PHARMS	130 MG
	THEOCLEAR L.A.-260	
BC	+ CENTRAL PHARMS	260 MG
	THEOPHYLLINE	
AB	INWOOD LABS	100 MG
AB		125 MG
AB		200 MG
AB		300 MG
	THEOVENT	
BC	SCHERING	125 MG
BC		250 MG
	TABLET, EXTENDED RELEASE; ORAL	
	LABID	
BC	+ P AND G	250 MG
	QUIBRON-T/SR	
BC	ROBERTS	300 MG
	SUSTAIRE	
BC	ROERIG	100 MG
BC		300 MG
	T-PHYL	
BC	PURDUE FREDERICK	200 MG
	THEO-DUR	
AB	+ KEY PHARMS	100 MG
AB	+	200 MG
AB	+	300 MG
AB	+	450 MG
	THEOCHRON	
AB	INWOOD	100 MG
AB		200 MG
AB		300 MG
	THEOLAIR-SR	
BC	3M	200 MG
BC		250 MG
BC		300 MG
	+	500 MG
	THEOPHYLLINE	
AB	SIDMAK	100 MG
AB		200 MG
AB		300 MG
AB		450 MG
	UNIPHYL	
	+ PURDUE FREDERICK	400 MG

TRIAMCINOLONE

	TABLET; ORAL	
	ARISTOCORT	
BP	LEDERLE	2 MG
BP		4 MG
BP	+	8 MG
		1 MG
	KENACORT	
BP	SQUIBB	4 MG
BP		8 MG
	TRIAMCINOLONE	
BP	DANBURY PHARMA	4 MG
BP	LEMMON	4 MG
BP	PUREPAC	2 MG
BP		4 MG
BP	RICHLYN	4 MG
BP	ROXANE	2 MG
BP		4 MG
BP		8 MG
BP	ZENITH	4 MG

TRIAMCINOLONE ACETONIDE

	INJECTABLE; INJECTION	
	KENALOG-10	
	+ WESTWOOD SQUIBB	10 MG/ML
	KENALOG-40	
BP	WESTWOOD SQUIBB	40 MG/ML
	TRIAMCINOLONE ACETONIDE	
	PARNELL	3 MG/ML
BP	STERIS	40 MG/ML

TRIAMCINOLONE DIACETATE

	INJECTABLE; INJECTION	
	ARISTOCORT	
BP	+ LEDERLE	25 MG/ML
BP	+	40 MG/ML
	TRIAMCINOLONE DIACETATE	
BP	AKORN	25 MG/ML
BP		40 MG/ML
BP	STERIS	40 MG/ML
BP		40 MG/ML

TRICHLORMETHIAZIDE

	TABLET; ORAL	
	METAHYDRIN	
BP	MERRELL DOW	2 MG
BP		4 MG
	NAQUA	
BP	SCHERING	2 MG
BP	+	4 MG
	TRICHLOREX	
BP	LANNETT	4 MG
BP		4 MG
	TRICHLORMAS	
BP	MAST	4 MG
	TRICHLORMETHIAZIDE	
BP	CAMALL	4 MG
BP	DANBURY PHARMA	2 MG
BP		4 MG
BP	PAR	2 MG
BP		4 MG
BP	RICHLYN	4 MG

Listing of "Pre-1938" Products

The Federal Food, Drug, and Cosmetic Act of 1938 required that drugs be shown to meet certain safety requirements prior to their being marketed. Drugs that were already being marketed at that time were "grandfathered" and were allowed to remain on the market without further regulatory approval if they were labeled with the same conditions of use. Many of these products remain on the market today. Because these products technically have never been *approved* by FDA, they do not appear in the listing of approved drug products with therapeutic equivalence evaluations (the "Orange Book").

The following listing identifies drug products that we believe are considered "pre-1938" or "grandfathered" and are still currently available. The list was developed by comparing an earlier general listing of frequently prescribed "pre-1938" drug entities developed by the U. S. Food and Drug Administration against current dosage form listings in the "Orange Book." The listing is not necessarily complete and represents our first attempt at incorporating such a list into *USP DI Update*. Comments are welcomed. Additions to or deletions from this list will be shown in future issues of *Update*. The listing of these products should not be interpreted as an attestation by USP as to their actual availability or the general recognition of safety and efficacy of the articles for medical or legal purposes or that a final determination has been made by the FDA.

Acetaminophen, Aspirin, Salicylamide, Codeine Phosphate, and Caffeine
- Tablets

Acetaminophen, Codeine Phosphate, and Caffeine
- Capsules
- Tablets

Amobarbital
- Tablets

Amobarbital Sodium
- Capsules
- Sterile

Amyl Nitrate
- Inhalant

Antipyrine and Benzocaine
- Solution, Otic

Aspirin and Codeine Phosphate
- Tablets

Chloral Hydrate
- Capsules
- Syrup
- Suppositories

Codeine and Calcium Iodide
- Syrup

Codeine Phosphate
- Injection
- Solution, Oral
- Tablets
- Tablets, Soluble

Codeine Sulfate
- Tablets
- Tablets, Soluble

Colchicine
- Injection
- Tablets

Digitoxin
- Tablets

Digoxin
- Elixir
- Tablets

Ephedrine Sulfate
- Capsules
- Injection
- Syrup

Ergonovine Maleate
- Injection
- Tablets

Ergotamine Tartrate
- Tablets

Erythrityl Tetranitrate
- Tablets

Hydrocodone Bitartrate
- Tablets

Hydrocodone Bitartrate, Aspirin, and Caffeine
- Tablets

Hydromorphone Hydrochloride
- Suppositories

Iodinated Glycerol
- Elixir
- Solution, Oral
- Tablets

Levothyroxine Sodium
- Injection
- for Injection
- Tablets

Meperidine Hydrochloride and Acetaminophen
- Tablets

Mephobarbital
- Tablets

Methenamine Mandelate
- for Solution, Oral
- Suspension, Oral
- Tablets
- Tablets (Enteric-coated)

Morphine Hydrochloride
- Suppositories

Morphine Sulfate
- Solution, Oral
- Tablets

Nitroglycerin
- Tablets (Sublingual)

Opium Alkaloids Hydrochlorides
- Injection

Opium Tincture

Oxycodone
- Tablets

Oxycodone Hydrochloride
- Solution, Oral

Paregoric

Pentaerythritol Tetranitrate
- Tablets

Phenazopyridine Hydrochloride
- Tablets

Phenobarbital
- Capsules
- Elixir
- Tablets

Phenobarbital Sodium
- Injection
- Sterile

Pilocarpine Hydrochloride
- Solution, Ophthalmic

Pilocarpine Nitrate
- Solution, Ophthalmic

Potassium Bicarbonate
- Effervescent Tablets for Oral Solution

Potassium Bicarbonate and Potassium Chloride
- for Effervescent Oral Solution
- Effervescent Tablets for Oral Solution

Potassium Bicarbonate and Potassium Citrate
- Effervescent Tablets for Oral Solution

Potassium Chloride
- Solution, Oral

Potassium Chloride, Potassium Bicarbonate, and Potassium Citrate
- Effervescent Tablets for Oral Solution

Potassium Gluconate
- Elixir
- Tablets

Potassium Gluconate and Potassium Chloride
- Solution, Oral
- for Solution, Oral

Potassium Gluconate and Potassium Citrate
- Solution, Oral

Potassium Iodide
- Solution, Oral
- Syrup
- Tablets (Enteric-coated)

Monobasic Potassium Phosphate
- Tablets for Oral Solution

Potassium Phosphates
- Capsules for Oral Solution
- for Solution, Oral

Potassium and Sodium Phosphates
- Capsules for Oral Solution
- for Solution, Oral
- Tablets for Oral Solution

Monobasic Potassium and Sodium Phosphates
- Tablets for Oral Solution

Quinacrine Hydrochloride
- Tablets

Quinine
- Capsules

Quinine Sulfate
- Tablets

Secobarbital Sodium and Amobarbital Sodium
- Capsules

Sodium Fluoride
- Solution, Oral
- Tablets

Thyroid
- Tablets
- Tablets, Enteric-coated

Trikates (Potassium Acetate, Potassium Bicarbonate, and Potassium Citrate)
- Solution, Oral

III

Section III

CHEMISTRY AND COMPENDIAL REQUIREMENTS

ACACIA

Description: Acacia NF—Practically odorless. Optical rotation varies depending on the source of Acacia. For example, specific rotation values, calculated on the anhydrous basis and determined on a 1.0% (w/v) solution, usually are between −25° and −35° for *Acacia senegal* and between +35° and +60° for *Acacia seyal*.

NF category: Emulsifying and/or solubilizing agent; suspending and/or viscosity-increasing agent; tablet binder.

Solubility: Acacia NF—Insoluble in alcohol.

NF requirements: Acacia NF—Preserve in tight containers. The dried gummy exudate from the stems and branches of *Acacia senegal* (Linné) Willdenow or of other related African species of *Acacia* (Fam. Leguminosae). Meets the requirements for Solubility and reaction, Botanic characteristics, Identification, Microbial limit, Water (not more than 15.0%), Total ash (not more than 4.0%), Acid-insoluble ash (not more than 0.5%), Insoluble residue, Arsenic (not more than 3 ppm), Lead (not more than 0.001%), Heavy metals (not more than 0.004%), Starch or dextrin, Tannin-bearing gums, and Organic volatile impurities.

ACEBUTOLOL

Chemical name: Acebutolol hydrochloride—Butanamide, *N*-[3-acetyl-4-[2-hydroxy-3-[(1-methylethyl)amino]propoxy]-phenyl]-, (±)-, monohydrochloride.

Molecular formula: Acebutolol hydrochloride—$C_{18}H_{28}N_2O_4 \cdot HCl$.

Molecular weight: Acebutolol hydrochloride—372.9.

Description: Acebutolol hydrochloride—White or slightly off-white powder. The melting point is 141–145 °C.

pKa: Acebutolol hydrochloride—Apparent in water: 9.4.

Solubility: Freely soluble in water; less soluble in alcohol.

Other characteristics: Lipid solubility—Low.

USP requirements:
Acebutolol Hydrochloride Capsules—Not in USP.
Acebutolol Hydrochloride Tablets—Not in USP.

ACENOCOUMAROL

Chemical name: 2*H*-1-Benzopyran-2-one, 4-hydroxy-3-[1-(4-nitrophenyl)-3-oxobutyl]-.

Molecular formula: $C_{19}H_{15}NO_6$.

Molecular weight: 353.33.

USP requirements: Acenocoumarol Tablets—Not in USP.

ACEPROMAZINE

Chemical name: Acepromazine maleate—Ethanone, 1-[10-[3-(dimethylamino)propyl]-10*H*-phenothiazin-2-yl]-, (*Z*)-2-butenedioate (1:1).

Molecular formula: Acepromazine maleate—$C_{19}H_{22}N_2OS \cdot C_4H_4O_4$.

Molecular weight: Acepromazine maleate—442.53.

Description: Acepromazine maleate—Yellow, odorless crystalline powder.

Solubility: Acepromazine maleate—Soluble 1 in 27 of water, 1 in 13 of alcohol, and 1 in 3 of chloroform; slightly soluble in ether.

USP requirements:

Acepromazine Maleate USP—Preserve in well-closed containers, protected from light. Label it to indicate that it is for veterinary use only. Contains not less than 98.0% and not more than 101.0% of acepromazine maleate, calculated on the anhydrous basis. Meets the requirements for Identification, Melting range (136–139 °C), pH (4.0–5.5, in a solution [1 in 100]), Water (not more than 1.0%), Residue on ignition (not more than 0.2%), and Related substances.

Acepromazine Maleate Injection USP—Preserve in single-dose or in multiple-dose containers, preferably of Type I glass, protected from light. A sterile solution of Acepromazine Maleate in Water for Injection. Label it to indicate that it is for veterinary use only. Contains the labeled amount, within ±10%. Meets the requirements for Identification, Sterility, pH (4.5–5.8), and Injections.

Acepromazine Maleate Tablets USP—Preserve in well-closed containers, protected from light. Label Tablets to indicate that they are for veterinary use only. Contain the labeled amount, within ±10%. Meet the requirement for Identification.

ACETAMINOPHEN

Chemical name: Acetamide, *N*-(4-hydroxyphenyl)-.

Molecular formula: $C_8H_9NO_2$.

Molecular weight: 151.16.

Description: Acetaminophen USP—White, odorless, crystalline powder.

Solubility: Acetaminophen USP—Soluble in boiling water and in 1 *N* sodium hydroxide; freely soluble in alcohol.

USP requirements:
Acetaminophen USP—Preserve in tight, light-resistant containers. Contains not less than 98.0% and not more than 101.0% of acetaminophen, calculated on the anhydrous basis. Meets the requirements for Identification, Melting

range (168–172 °C), Water (not more than 0.5%), Residue on ignition (not more than 0.1%), Chloride (not more than 0.014%), Sulfate (not more than 0.02%), Sulfide, Heavy metals (not more than 0.001%), Readily carbonizable substances, Free *p*-aminophenol (not more than 0.005%), *p*-Chloroacetanilide (not more than 0.001%), and Organic volatile impurities.

Acetaminophen Capsules USP—Preserve in tight containers. Contain the labeled amount, within ±10%. Meet the requirements for Identification, Dissolution (75% in 45 minutes in water in Apparatus 2 at 50 rpm), and Uniformity of dosage units.

Acetaminophen Oral Granules—Not in USP.

Acetaminophen Oral Powders—Not in USP.

Acetaminophen Oral Solution USP—Preserve in tight containers. Contains the labeled amount, within ±10%. Meets the requirements for Identification, pH (3.8–6.1), and Alcohol content (if present, the labeled amount, within −10% to +15%).

Acetaminophen Suppositories USP—Preserve in well-closed containers, at controlled room temperature or in a cool place. Contain the labeled amount, within ±10%. Meet the requirement for Identification.

Acetaminophen Oral Suspension USP—Preserve in tight containers. A suspension of acetaminophen in a suitable aqueous vehicle. Contains the labeled amount, within ±10%. Meets the requirements for Identification and pH (4.5–6.9).

Acetaminophen Tablets USP—Preserve in tight containers. Label Tablets that must be chewed to indicate that they are to be chewed before swallowing. Contain the labeled amount, within ±10%. Meet the requirements for Identification, Dissolution (80% in 30 minutes in phosphate buffer [pH 5.8] in Apparatus 2 at 50 rpm), and Uniformity of dosage units.

ACETAMINOPHEN AND ASPIRIN

For *Acetaminophen* and *Aspirin*—See individual listings for chemistry information.

USP requirements: Acetaminophen and Aspirin Tablets USP—Preserve in tight containers. Contain the labeled amounts, within ±10%. Meet the requirements for Identification, Dissolution (75% of each active ingredient in 45 minutes in water in Apparatus 2 at 50 rpm), Uniformity of dosage units, and Salicylic acid (not more than 3.0%).

ACETAMINOPHEN, ASPIRIN, AND CAFFEINE

For *Acetaminophen, Aspirin,* and *Caffeine*—See individual listings for chemistry information.

USP requirements:

Acetaminophen, Aspirin, and Caffeine Capsules USP—Preserve in tight containers. Contain the labeled amounts, within ±10%. Meet the requirements for Identification, Dissolution (75% of each active ingredient in 45 minutes in water in Apparatus 1 at 100 rpm), Uniformity of dosage units, and Salicylic acid (not more than 3.0%).

Acetaminophen, Aspirin, and Caffeine Oral Powders—Not in USP.

Acetaminophen, Aspirin, and Caffeine Tablets USP—Preserve in well-closed containers. Contain the labeled amounts, within ±10%. Meet the requirements for Identification, Dissolution (75% of each active ingredient in 60 minutes in water in Apparatus 2 at 100 rpm), Uniformity of dosage units, and Salicylic acid (not more than 3.0%).

BUFFERED ACETAMINOPHEN, ASPIRIN, AND CAFFEINE

Source: Caffeine—Coffee, tea, cola, and cocoa or chocolate. May also be synthesized from urea or dimethylurea.

Chemical group: Caffeine—Methylated xanthine.

Chemical name:

Acetaminophen—Acetamide, *N*-(4-hydroxyphenyl)-.
Aspirin—Benzoic acid, 2-(acetyloxy)-.
Caffeine—1*H*-Purine-2,6-dione, 3,7-dihydro-1,3,7-trimethyl-.
Calcium gluconate—D-Gluconic acid, calcium salt (2:1).
Aluminum hydroxide—Aluminum hydroxide.
Magnesium hydroxide—Magnesium hydroxide.

Molecular formula:

Acetaminophen—$C_8H_9NO_2$.
Aspirin—$C_9H_8O_4$.
Caffeine—$C_8H_{10}N_4O_2$ (anhydrous); $C_8H_{10}N_4O_2 \cdot H_2O$ (monohydrate).
Calcium gluconate—$C_{12}H_{22}CaO_{14}$.
Aluminum hydroxide—$Al(OH)_3$.
Magnesium hydroxide—$Mg(OH)_2$.

Molecular weight:

Acetaminophen—151.16.
Aspirin—180.16.
Caffeine—194.19 (anhydrous); 212.21 (monohydrate).
Calcium gluconate—430.38.
Aluminum hydroxide—78.00.
Magnesium hydroxide—58.32.

Description:

Acetaminophen USP—White, odorless, crystalline powder.

Aspirin USP—White crystals, commonly tabular or needle-like, or white, crystalline powder. Is odorless or has a faint odor. Is stable in dry air; in moist air it gradually hydrolyzes to salicylic and acetic acids.

Caffeine USP—White powder or white, glistening needles, usually matted together. Is odorless. Its solutions are neutral to litmus. The hydrate is efflorescent in air.

Calcium Gluconate USP—White, crystalline, odorless granules or powder. Is stable in air. Its solutions are neutral to litmus.

Aluminum Hydroxide Gel USP—White, viscous suspension, from which small amounts of clear liquid may separate on standing.

Dried Aluminum Hydroxide Gel USP—White, odorless, amorphous powder.

Magnesium Hydroxide USP—Bulky, white powder.

pKa: Aspirin—3.5

Solubility:

Acetaminophen USP—Soluble in boiling water and in 1 *N* sodium hydroxide; freely soluble in alcohol.

Aspirin USP—Slightly soluble in water; freely soluble in alcohol; soluble in chloroform and in ether; sparingly soluble in absolute ether.

Caffeine USP—Sparingly soluble in water and in alcohol; freely soluble in chloroform; slightly soluble in ether.

The aqueous solubility of caffeine is increased by organic acids or their alkali salts, such as citrates, benzoates, salicylates, or cinnamates, which dissociate to yield caffeine when dissolved in biological fluids.

Calcium Gluconate USP—Sparingly (and slowly) soluble in water; freely soluble in boiling water; insoluble in alcohol.

Dried Aluminum Hydroxide Gel USP—Insoluble in water and in alcohol; soluble in dilute mineral acids and in solutions of fixed alkali hydroxides.

Magnesium Hydroxide USP—Practically insoluble in water and in alcohol; soluble in dilute acids.

USP requirements: Buffered Acetaminophen, Aspirin, and Caffeine Tablets—Not in USP.

ACETAMINOPHEN, ASPIRIN, SALICYLAMIDE, AND ALUMINUM HYDROXIDE

For *Acetaminophen, Aspirin, Salicylamide,* and *Aluminum Hydroxide*—See individual listings for chemistry information.

USP requirements: Buffered Acetaminophen, Aspirin, and Salicylamide Tablets—Not in USP.

ACETAMINOPHEN, ASPIRIN, SALICYLAMIDE, AND CAFFEINE

For *Acetaminophen, Aspirin, Salicylamide,* and *Caffeine*—See individual listings for chemistry information.

USP requirements: Acetaminophen, Aspirin, Salicylamide, and Caffeine Tablets—Not in USP.

ACETAMINOPHEN, ASPIRIN, SALICYLAMIDE, CODEINE, AND CAFFEINE

For *Acetaminophen, Aspirin, Salicylamide, Codeine,* and *Caffeine*—See individual listings for chemistry information.

USP requirements: Acetaminophen, Aspirin, Salicylamide, Codeine Phosphate, and Caffeine Tablets—Not in USP.

ACETAMINOPHEN AND CAFFEINE

For *Acetaminophen* and *Caffeine*—See individual listings for chemistry information.

USP requirements:

Acetaminophen and Caffeine Capsules USP—Preserve in tight containers. Contain the labeled amounts, within ±10%. Meet the requirements for Identification, Dissolution (75% of each active ingredient in 45 minutes in water in Apparatus 1 at 100 rpm), and Uniformity of dosage units.

Acetaminophen and Caffeine Tablets USP—Preserve in tight containers. Contain the labeled amounts, within ±10%. Meet the requirements for Identification, Dissolution (75% of each active ingredient in 60 minutes in water in Apparatus 2 at 100 rpm), and Uniformity of dosage units.

ACETAMINOPHEN AND CALCIUM CARBONATE

For *Acetaminophen* and *Calcium Carbonate*—See individual listings for chemistry information.

USP requirements: Acetaminophen and Calcium Carbonate Tablets—Not in USP.

ACETAMINOPHEN, CALCIUM CARBONATE, MAGNESIUM CARBONATE, AND MAGNESIUM OXIDE

For *Acetaminophen, Calcium Carbonate, Magnesium Carbonate,* and *Magnesium Oxide*—See individual listings for chemistry information.

USP requirements: Acetaminophen, Calcium Carbonate, Magnesium Carbonate, and Magnesium Oxide Tablets—Not in USP.

ACETAMINOPHEN, CALCIUM CARBONATE, POTASSIUM AND SODIUM BICARBONATES, AND CITRIC ACID

For *Acetaminophen, Calcium Carbonate, Potassium Bicarbonate, Sodium Bicarbonate,* and *Citric Acid*—See individual listings for chemistry information.

USP requirements: Acetaminophen Effervescent Tablets for Oral Solution—Not in USP.

ACETAMINOPHEN AND CODEINE

For *Acetaminophen* and *Codeine*—See individual listings for chemistry information.

USP requirements:

Acetaminophen and Codeine Phosphate Capsules USP—Preserve in tight, light-resistant containers. Contain the labeled amounts, within ±10%. Meet the requirements for Identification, Dissolution (75% of each active ingredient in 30 minutes in 0.1 *N* hydrochloric acid in Apparatus 2 at 50 rpm), and Uniformity of dosage units.

Acetaminophen and Codeine Phosphate Oral Solution USP—Preserve in tight, light-resistant containers. Contains the labeled amounts, within ±10%. Meets the requirements for Identification, pH (4.0–6.1), and Alcohol content (if present, the labeled amount, within −10% to +20%).

Acetaminophen and Codeine Phosphate Oral Suspension USP—Preserve in tight, light-resistant containers. A suspension of Acetaminophen and Codeine Phosphate in a suitable aqueous vehicle. Contains the labeled amounts, within ±10%. Meets the requirements for Identification and pH (4.0–6.1).

Acetaminophen and Codeine Phosphate Tablets USP—Preserve in tight, light-resistant containers. Contain the labeled amounts, within ±10%. Meet the requirements for Identification, Dissolution (75% of each active ingredient in 45 minutes in 0.1 *N* hydrochloric acid in Apparatus 2 at 50 rpm), and Uniformity of dosage units.

ACETAMINOPHEN, CODEINE, AND CAFFEINE

For *Acetaminophen, Codeine,* and *Caffeine*—See individual listings for chemistry information.

USP requirements:

Acetaminophen, Codeine Phosphate, and Caffeine Capsules—Not in USP.

Acetaminophen, Codeine Phosphate, and Caffeine Tablets—Not in USP.

ACETAMINOPHEN AND DIPHENHYDRAMINE

For *Acetaminophen* and *Diphenhydramine*—See individual listings for chemistry information.

USP requirements: Acetaminophen and Diphenhydramine Citrate Tablets USP—Preserve in tight containers. Contain the labeled amounts, within ±10%. Meet the requirements for Identification, Dissolution (75% of each active ingredient in 45 minutes in water in Apparatus 2 at 50 rpm), and Uniformity of dosage units.

ACETAMINOPHEN AND PSEUDOEPHEDRINE

For *Acetaminophen* and *Pseudoephedrine*—See individual listings for chemistry information.

USP requirements:

Acetaminophen and Pseudoephedrine Hydrochloride Capsules—Not in USP.

Acetaminophen and Pseudoephedrine Hydrochloride Tablets USP—Preserve in tight containers. Contain the labeled amounts, within ±10%. Meet the requirements for Identification, Dissolution (75% of each active ingredient in 45 minutes in phosphate buffer [pH 5.8] in Apparatus 2 at 50 rpm), and Uniformity of dosage units.

ACETAMINOPHEN AND SALICYLAMIDE

For *Acetaminophen* and *Salicylamide*—See individual listings for chemistry information.

USP requirements: Acetaminophen and Salicylamide Capsules—Not in USP.

ACETAMINOPHEN, SALICYLAMIDE, AND CAFFEINE

For *Acetaminophen, Salicylamide,* and *Caffeine*—See individual listings for chemistry information.

USP requirements:
Acetaminophen, Salicylamide, and Caffeine Capsules—Not in USP.
Acetaminophen, Salicylamide, and Caffeine Tablets—Not in USP.

ACETAMINOPHEN, SODIUM BICARBONATE, AND CITRIC ACID

For *Acetaminophen, Sodium Bicarbonate,* and *Citric Acid*—See individual listings for chemistry information.

USP requirements: Acetaminophen for Effervescent Oral Solution USP—Preserve in tight containers. Contains, in each 100 grams, not less than 5.63 grams and not more than 6.88 grams of acetaminophen. Meets the requirements for Identification and Minimum fill (when packaged in multiple-unit containers) or Uniformity of dosage units (when packaged in single-unit containers).

ACETAZOLAMIDE

Chemical name:
Acetazolamide—Acetamide, *N*-[5-(aminosulfonyl)-1,3,4-thiadiazol-2-yl]-.
Acetazolamide sodium—Acetamide, *N*-[5-(aminosulfonyl)-1,3,4-thiadiazol-2-yl]-, monosodium salt.

Molecular formula:
Acetazolamide—$C_4H_6N_4O_3S_2$.
Acetazolamide sodium—$C_4H_5N_4NaO_3S_2$.

Molecular weight:
Acetazolamide—222.24.
Acetazolamide sodium—244.22.

Description:
Acetazolamide USP—White to faintly yellowish white, crystalline, odorless powder.
Sterile Acetazolamide Sodium USP—White solid, having the characteristic appearance of freeze-dried products.

Solubility: Acetazolamide USP—Very slightly soluble in water; sparingly soluble in practically boiling water; slightly soluble in alcohol.

USP requirements:
Acetazolamide USP—Preserve in well-closed containers. Contains not less than 98.0% and not more than 102.0% of acetazolamide, calculated on the anhydrous basis. Meets the requirements for Identification, Water (not more than 0.5%), Residue on ignition (not more than 0.1%), Chloride (not more than 0.014%), Sulfate (not more than 0.04%), Selenium (not more than 0.003%, a 200-mg specimen being used), Heavy metals (not more than 0.002%), Silver-reducing substances, Ordinary impurities, and Organic volatile impurities.
Acetazolamide Extended-release Capsules—Not in USP.
Acetazolamide Tablets USP—Preserve in well-closed containers. Contain the labeled amount, within ±5%. Meet the requirements for Identification, Dissolution (75% in 60 minutes in 0.1 *N* hydrochloric acid in Apparatus 1 at 100 rpm), and Uniformity of dosage units.
Sterile Acetazolamide Sodium USP—Preserve in Containers for Sterile Solids, preferably of Type III glass. It is prepared from Acetazolamide with the aid of Sodium Hydroxide. It is suitable for parenteral use. The contents of each container, when constituted as directed in the labeling, yields a solution containing an amount of acetazolamide sodium equivalent to the labeled amount of acetazolamide, within −5% to +10%. Meets the requirements for Completeness of solution, Constituted solution, Identification, Bacterial endotoxins, pH (9.0–10.0, in a freshly prepared solution [1 in 10]), Sterility tests, Uniformity of dosage units, and Labeling under Injections.

ACETIC ACID

Chemical name:
Acetic acid—Acetic acid.
Acetic acid, glacial—Acetic acid.

Molecular formula: Acetic acid, glacial—$C_2H_4O_2$.

Molecular weight: Acetic acid, glacial—60.05.

Description:
Acetic Acid NF—Clear, colorless liquid, having a strong, characteristic odor. Specific gravity is about 1.045.
NF category: Acidifying agent; buffering agent.
Glacial Acetic Acid USP—Clear, colorless liquid, having a pungent, characteristic odor. Boils at about 118 °C. Specific gravity is about 1.05.
NF category: Acidifying agent.

Solubility:
Acetic Acid NF—Miscible with water, with alcohol, and with glycerin.
Glacial Acetic Acid USP—Miscible with water, with alcohol, and with glycerin.

USP requirements:
Acetic Acid Irrigation USP—Preserve in single-dose containers, preferably of Type I or Type II glass. It may be packaged in suitable plastic containers. A sterile solution of Glacial Acetic Acid in Water for Injection. Contains, in each 100 mL, not less than 237.5 mg and not more than 262.5 mg of glacial acetic acid. Meets the requirements for Identification, Bacterial endotoxins, pH (2.8–3.4), and Injections (except that the container in which it is packaged may be designed to empty rapidly and may exceed 1000 mL in capacity).
Acetic Acid Otic Solution USP—Preserve in tight containers. A solution of Glacial Acetic Acid in a suitable nonaqueous solvent. Contains an amount of glacial acetic acid equivalent to the labeled amount, within −15% to +30%. Meets the requirements for Identification and pH (2.0–4.0, when diluted with an equal volume of water).
Glacial Acetic Acid USP—Preserve in tight containers. Contains not less than 99.5% and not more than 100.5%, by weight, of glacial acetic acid. Meets the requirements for Identification, Congealing temperature (not lower than 15.6 °C), Nonvolatile residue, Chloride, Sulfate, Heavy metals (not more than 5 ppm), and Readily oxidizable substances.

NF requirements: Acetic Acid NF—Preserve in tight containers. A solution. Contains not less than 36.0% and not more than 37.0%, by weight, of acetic acid. Meets the requirements for Identification, Nonvolatile residue (not more than 0.005%), Chloride, Sulfate, Heavy metals (not more than 0.001%), Readily oxidizable substances, and Organic volatile impurities.

ACETOHEXAMIDE

Chemical group: Sulfonylurea.

Chemical name: Benzenesulfonamide, 4-acetyl-*N*-[[(cyclohexylamino]carbonyl]-.

Molecular formula: $C_{15}H_{20}N_2O_4S$.

Molecular weight: 324.39.

Description: Acetohexamide USP—White, crystalline, practically odorless powder.

Solubility: Acetohexamide USP—Practically insoluble in water and in ether; soluble in pyridine and in dilute solutions of alkali hydroxides; slightly soluble in alcohol and in chloroform.

USP requirements:

Acetohexamide USP—Preserve in well-closed containers. Contains not less than 97.0% and not more than 101.0% of acetohexamide, calculated on the dried basis. Meets the requirements for Identification, Melting range (182.5–187 °C), Loss on drying (not more than 1.0%), Selenium (not more than 0.003%, a 200-mg specimen mixed with 200 mg of magnesium oxide being used), Residue on ignition (not more than 0.1%), Heavy metals (not more than 0.002%), and Organic volatile impurities.

Acetohexamide Tablets USP—Preserve in well-closed containers. Contain the labeled amount, within ±7%. Meet the requirements for Identification, Dissolution (50% in 60 minutes in phosphate buffer [pH 7.6] in Apparatus 1 at 100 rpm), and Uniformity of dosage units.

ACETOHYDROXAMIC ACID

Chemical name: Acetamide, *N*-hydroxy-.

Molecular formula: $C_2H_5NO_2$.

Molecular weight: 75.07.

Description: Acetohydroxamic Acid USP—White, slightly hygroscopic, crystalline powder. Melts, after drying at about 80 °C for 2 to 4 hours, at about 88 °C.

pKa: 9.32–9.4.

Solubility: Acetohydroxamic Acid USP—Freely soluble in water and in alcohol; very slightly soluble in chloroform.

Other characteristics: Chelates metals, especially iron.

USP requirements:

Acetohydroxamic Acid USP—Preserve in tight containers, and store in a cool, dry place. Dried over phosphorus pentoxide for 16 hours, contains not less than 98.0% and not more than 101.0% of acetohydroxamic acid. Meets the requirements for Completeness of solution, Color of solution (absorbance not greater than 0.050), Identification, Loss on drying (not more than 1.0%), Residue on ignition (not more than 0.1%), Heavy metals (not more than 0.002%), Hydroxylamine (not more than 0.5%), and Organic volatile impurities.

Acetohydroxamic Acid Tablets USP—Preserve in tight containers. Contain the labeled amount, within ±10%. Meet the requirements for Identification, Dissolution (85% in 30 minutes in water in Apparatus 1 at 100 rpm), Uniformity of dosage units, and Hydroxylamine (not more than 0.5%).

ACETONE

Chemical name: 2-Propanone.

Molecular formula: C_3H_6O.

Molecular weight: 58.08.

Description: Acetone NF—Transparent, colorless, mobile, volatile liquid, having a characteristic odor. A solution (1 in 2) is neutral to litmus.

NF category: Solvent.

Solubility: Acetone NF—Miscible with water, with alcohol, with ether, with chloroform, and with most volatile oils.

NF requirements: Acetone NF—Preserve in tight containers, remote from fire. Contains not less than 99.0% of acetone, calculated on the anhydrous basis. Meets the requirements for Identification, Specific gravity (not more than 0.789), Water (not more than 0.5%), Nonvolatile residue (not more than 0.004%), and Readily oxidizable substances.

Caution: Acetone is very flammable. Do not use where it may be ignited.

ACETOPHENAZINE

Chemical group: Piperazine phenothiazine.

Chemical name: Acetophenazine maleate—Ethanone, 1-[10-[3-[4-(2-hydroxyethyl)-1-piperazinyl]propyl]-10*H*-phenothiazin-2-yl]-, (*Z*) 2-butenedioate (1:2) (salt).

Molecular formula: Acetophenazine maleate—$C_{23}H_{29}N_3O_2S \cdot 2C_4H_4O_4$.

Molecular weight: Acetophenazine maleate—643.71.

Description: Acetophenazine Maleate USP—Fine, yellow powder. Melts at about 165 °C, with decomposition.

Solubility: Acetophenazine Maleate USP—Soluble in water; slightly soluble in acetone and in alcohol.

USP requirements:

Acetophenazine Maleate USP—Preserve in tight, light-resistant containers. Dried at 65 °C for 4 hours, contains not less than 97.0% and not more than 103.0% of acetophenazine maleate. Meets the requirements for Identification, Loss on drying (not more than 0.5%), Residue on ignition (not more than 0.1%), Ordinary impurities, and Organic volatile impurities.

Acetophenazine Maleate Tablets USP—Preserve in tight, light-resistant containers. Contain the labeled amount, within ±10%. Meet the requirements for Identification, Dissolution (75% in 45 minutes in 0.1 *N* hydrochloric acid in Apparatus 2 at 50 rpm), and Uniformity of dosage units.

ACETYLCHOLINE

Chemical name: Acetylcholine chloride—Ethanaminium, 2-(acetyloxy)-*N,N,N*-trimethyl-, chloride.

Molecular formula: Acetylcholine chloride—$C_7H_{16}ClNO_2$.

Molecular weight: Acetylcholine chloride—181.66.

Description: Acetylcholine Chloride USP—White or off-white crystals or crystalline powder.

Solubility: Acetylcholine Chloride USP—Very soluble in water; freely soluble in alcohol; insoluble in ether. Is decomposed by hot water and by alkalies.

USP requirements:

Acetylcholine Chloride USP—Preserve in tight containers. Contains not less than 98.0% and not more than 102.0% of acetylcholine chloride, calculated on the dried basis. Meets the requirements for Identification, Melting range (149–152 °C), Acidity, Loss on drying (not more than 1.0%), Residue on ignition (not more than 0.2%), Chloride content (19.3–19.8%, calculated on the dried basis), and Organic volatile impurities.

Acetylcholine Chloride for Ophthalmic Solution USP—Preserve in Containers for Sterile Solids. A sterile mixture of Acetylcholine Chloride with Mannitol or other suitable diluent, prepared by freeze-drying. Contains the labeled amount, within −10% to +15%. Meets the requirements for Constituted solution, Identification, Acidity, Water (not more than 1.0%), Sterility tests, and Uniformity of dosage units.

ACETYLCYSTEINE

Source: The N-acetyl derivative of the naturally occurring amino acid, L-cysteine.

Chemical name: L-Cysteine, *N*-acetyl-.

Molecular formula: $C_5H_9NO_3S$.

Molecular weight: 163.19.

Description: Acetylcysteine USP—White, crystalline powder, having a slight acetic odor.

Solubility: Acetylcysteine USP—Freely soluble in water and in alcohol; practically insoluble in chloroform and in ether.

USP requirements:

Acetylcysteine USP—Preserve in tight containers. Contains not less than 98.0% and not more than 102.0% of acetylcysteine, calculated on the dried basis. Meets the requirements for Identification, Melting range (104–110 °C), Specific rotation (+21° to +27°, calculated on the dried basis), pH (2.0–2.8, in a solution [1 in 100]), Loss on drying (not more than 1.0%), Residue on ignition (not more than 0.5%), Heavy metals (not more than 0.001%), and Organic volatile impurities.

Acetylcysteine Injection—Not in USP.

Acetylcysteine Solution USP—Preserve in single-unit or in multiple-unit tight containers that effectively exclude oxygen. A sterile solution of Acetylcysteine in water, prepared with the aid of Sodium Hydroxide. Contains the labeled amount, within ±10%. Meets the requirements for Identification, Sterility, and pH (6.0–7.5).

ACETYLCYSTEINE AND ISOPROTERENOL

For *Acetylcysteine* and *Isoproterenol*—See individual listings for chemistry information.

USP requirements: Acetylcysteine and Isoproterenol Hydrochloride Inhalation Solution USP—Preserve in single-dose or in multiple-dose containers, preferably of Type I glass, tightly closed with a glass or polyethylene closure. A sterile solution of Acetylcysteine and Isoproterenol Hydrochloride in water. The label indicates that the Inhalation Solution is not to be used if its color is pinkish or darker than slightly yellow or if it contains a precipitate. Contains the labeled amounts of acetylcysteine, within ±10%, and isoproterenol hydrochloride, within −10% to +15%. Meets the requirements for Color and clarity, Identification, Sterility, and pH (6.0–7.0).

ACRISORCIN

Chemical name: 1,3-Benzenediol, 4-hexyl-, compd. with 9-acridinamine (1:1).

Molecular formula: $C_{12}H_{18}O_2 \cdot C_{13}H_{10}N_2$.

Molecular weight: 388.51.

Description: Acrisorcin USP—Yellow, odorless powder. Melts at about 190 °C, with decomposition.

Solubility: Acrisorcin USP—Very slightly soluble in water and in ether; soluble in alcohol; slightly soluble in chloroform.

USP requirements:

Acrisorcin USP—Preserve in well-closed containers. Contains not less than 97.0% and not more than 101.0% of acrisorcin, calculated on the dried basis. Meets the requirements for Identification, Loss on drying (not more than 1.0%), and Residue on ignition (not more than 0.2%).

Acrisorcin Cream USP—Preserve in collapsible tubes or in tight containers. It is Acrisorcin in a suitable water-miscible base. Contains the labeled amount, within ±10%. Meets the requirements for Identification and Minimum fill.

ACRIVASTINE AND PSEUDOEPHEDRINE

Chemical name:

Acrivastine—2-Propenoic acid, 3-[6-[1-(4-methylphenyl)-3-(1-pyrrolidinyl)-1-propenyl]-2-pyridinyl]-, (*E,E*)-.

Pseudoephedrine hydrochloride—Benzenemethanol, alpha-[1-(methylamino)ethyl]-, [*S*-(*R**,*R**)]-, hydrochloride.

Molecular formula:

Acrivastine—$C_{22}H_{24}N_2O_2$.

Pseudoephedrine hydrochloride—$C_{10}H_{15}NO \cdot HCl$.

Molecular weight:

Acrivastine—348.44.

Pseudoephedrine hydrochloride—201.70.

Description: Pseudoephedrine Hydrochloride USP—Fine, white to off-white crystals or powder, having a faint characteristic odor.

Solubility: Pseudoephedrine Hydrochloride USP—Very soluble in water; freely soluble in alcohol; sparingly soluble in chloroform.

USP requirements: Acrivastine and Pseudoephedrine Hydrochloride Capsules—Not in USP.

ACYCLOVIR

Chemical group: Synthetic purine nucleoside analog.

Chemical name:

Acyclovir—6*H*-Purin-6-one, 2-amino-1,9-dihydro-9-[(2-hydroxyethoxy)methyl]-.

Acyclovir sodium—6*H*-Purin-6-one, 2-amino-1,9-dihydro-9-[(2-hydroxyethoxy)methyl]-, monosodium salt.

Molecular formula:

Acyclovir—$C_8H_{11}N_5O_3$.

Acyclovir sodium—$C_8H_{10}N_5NaO_3$.

Molecular weight:

Acyclovir—225.21.

Acyclovir sodium—247.19.

Description: Acyclovir USP—White to off-white crystalline powder. Melts at temperatures higher than 250 °C, with decomposition.

Solubility: Acyclovir USP—Soluble in 0.1 *N* hydrochloric acid; sparingly soluble in water; insoluble in alcohol.

USP requirements:

Acyclovir USP—Preserve in tight containers. Contains not less than 98.0% and not more than 101.0% of acyclovir,

calculated on the anhydrous basis. Meets the requirements for Identification, Water (not more than 6.0%), Ordinary impurities, and Organic volatile impurities.
Acyclovir Capsules—Not in USP.
Acyclovir Ointment—Not in USP.
Acyclovir Oral Suspension—Not in USP.
Acyclovir Tablets—Not in USP.
Sterile Acyclovir Sodium—Not in USP.

ADENINE

Chemical name: 1*H*-Purin-6-amine.

Molecular formula: $C_5H_5N_5$.

Molecular weight: 135.13.

Description: Adenine USP—White crystals or crystalline powder. Is odorless.

Solubility: Adenine USP—Very slightly soluble in water; sparingly soluble in boiling water; slightly soluble in alcohol; practically insoluble in ether and in chloroform.

USP requirements: Adenine USP—Preserve in well-closed containers. Contains not less than 98.0% and not more than 102.0% of adenine, calculated on the dried basis. Meets the requirements for Identification, Loss on drying (not more than 1.0%), Residue on ignition (not more than 0.1%), Heavy metals (not more than 0.001%), Organic impurities, Nitrogen content (50.2–53.4%, calculated on the dried basis), and Organic volatile impurities.

ADENOSINE

Chemical name: Adenosine.

Molecular formula: $C_{10}H_{13}N_5O_4$.

Molecular weight: 267.24.

Description: White crystalline powder.

Solubility: Soluble in water; practically insoluble in alcohol.

USP requirements: Adenosine Injection—Not in USP.

AGAR

Description: Agar NF—Odorless or has a slight odor.
NF category: Suspending and/or viscosity-increasing agent.

Solubility: Agar NF—Insoluble in cold water; soluble in boiling water.

NF requirements: Agar NF—The dried, hydrophilic, colloidal substance extracted from *Gelidium cartilagineum* (Linné) Gaillon (Fam. Gelidiaceae), *Gracilaria confervoides* (Linné) Greville (Fam. Sphaerococcaceae), and related red algae (Class Rhodophyceae). Meets the requirements for Botanic characteristics, Identification, Microbial limit, Water (not more than 20.0%), Total ash (not more than 6.5%, on a dry-weight basis), Acid-insoluble ash (not more than 0.5%, on a dry-weight basis), Foreign organic matter (not more than 1.0%), Foreign insoluble matter (not more than 1.0%), Arsenic (not more than 3 ppm), Lead (not more than 0.001%), Heavy metals (not more than 0.004%), Foreign starch, Gelatin, and Water absorption.

MEDICAL AIR

USP requirements: Medical Air USP—Preserve in cylinders or in a low pressure collecting tank. Containers used for Medical Air are not to be treated with any toxic, sleep-inducing, or narcosis-producing compounds, and are not to be treated with any compound that would be irritating to the respiratory tract when the Medical Air is used. (Notes: Reduce the container pressure by means of a regulator. Measure the gases with a gas volume meter downstream from the detector tube in order to minimize contamination or change of the specimens.) A natural or synthetic mixture of gases consisting largely of nitrogen and oxygen. Where it is piped directly from the collecting tank to the point of use, label each outlet "Medical Air." Contains not less than 19.5% and not more than 23.5%, by volume, of oxygen. Meets the requirements for Water and oil, Odor, Carbon dioxide (not more than 0.05%), Carbon monoxide (not more than 0.001%), Nitric oxide and nitrogen dioxide (not more than 2.5 ppm), and Sulfur dioxide (not more than 5 ppm).

ALANINE

Chemical name: L-Alanine.

Molecular formula: $C_3H_7NO_2$.

Molecular weight: 89.09.

Description: Alanine USP—White, odorless crystals or crystalline powder.

Solubility: Alanine USP—Freely soluble in water; slightly soluble in 80% alcohol; insoluble in ether.

USP requirements: Alanine USP—Preserve in well-closed containers. Contains not less than 98.5% and not more than 101.5% of alanine, as L-alanine, calculated on the dried basis. Meets the requirements for Identification, Specific rotation (+13.7° to +15.1°, calculated on the dried basis), pH (5.5–7.0 in a solution [1 in 20]), Loss on drying (not more than 0.2%), Residue on ignition (not more than 0.15%), Chloride (not more than 0.05%), Sulfate (not more than 0.03%), Arsenic (not more than 1.5 ppm), Iron (not more than 0.003%), Heavy metals (not more than 0.0015%), and Organic volatile impurities.

ALBENDAZOLE

Chemical name: Carbamic acid, [5-(propylthio)-1*H*-benzimidazol-2-yl]-, methyl ester.

Molecular formula: $C_{12}H_{15}N_3O_2S$.

Molecular weight: 265.33.

Description: Colorless crystals with a melting point of 208–210 °C.

USP requirements:
Albendazole USP—Preserve in well-closed containers. Contains not less than 98.0% and not more than 102.0% of albendazole, calculated on the dried basis. Meets the requirements for Identification, Loss on drying (not more than 0.5%), Residue on ignition (not more than 0.2%), and Chromatographic purity.
Albendazole Oral Suspension—Not in USP.
Albendazole Tablets—Not in USP.

ALBUMIN HUMAN

Description: Albumin Human USP—Practically odorless, moderately viscous, clear, brownish fluid.

USP requirements: Albumin Human USP—Preserve at the temperature indicated on the label. A sterile, non-pyrogenic preparation of serum albumin obtained by fractionating material (source blood, plasma, serum, or placentas) from healthy human donors, the source material being tested for the absence of hepatitis B surface antigen. It is made by a process that yields a product that is safe for intravenous use. Label it to state that it is not to be used if it is turbid and that it is to be used within 4 hours after the container is entered. Label it also to state the osmotic equivalent in terms of plasma, the sodium content, and the type of source material (venous plasma, placental plasma, or both) from which it was prepared. Label it also to indicate that additional fluids are needed when the 20-grams-per-100-mL or 25-grams-per-100-mL product is administered to a markedly dehydrated patient. Not less than 96% of its total protein is albumin. It is a solution containing, in each 100 mL, either 25 grams of serum albumin osmotically equivalent to 500 mL of normal human plasma, or 20 grams equivalent to 400 mL, or 5 grams equivalent to 100 mL, or 4 grams equivalent to 80 mL thereof, and contains not less than 93.75% and not more than 106.25% of the labeled amount in the case of the solution containing 4 grams in each 100 mL, and not less than 94.0% and not more than 106.0% of the labeled amount in the other cases. Contains no added antimicrobial agent, but may contain sodium acetyltryptophanate with or without sodium caprylate as a stabilizing agent. It has a sodium content of not less than 130 mEq per liter and not more than 160 mEq per liter. It has a heme content such that the absorbance of a solution, diluted to contain 1% of protein, in a 1-cm holding cell, measured at a wavelength of 403 nanometers, is not more than 0.25. Meets the requirements of the tests for heat stability and for pH, and for Expiration date (the expiration date is not later than 5 years after issue from manufacturer's cold storage [5 °C, 3 years] if labeling recommends storage between 2 and 10 °C; not later than 3 years after issue from manufacturer's cold storage [5 °C, 3 years] if labeling recommends storage at temperatures not higher than 37 °C; and not later than 10 years after date of manufacture if in a hermetically sealed metal container and labeling recommends storage between 2 and 10 °C). Conforms to the regulations of the U.S. Food and Drug Administration concerning biologics.

ALBUTEROL

Chemical name:
- Albuterol—1,3-Benzenedimethanol, alpha[1]-[[(1,1-dimethylethyl)amino]methyl]-4-hydroxy-.
- Albuterol sulfate—1,3-Benzenedimethanol, alpha[1]-[[(1,1-dimethylethyl)amino]methyl]-4-hydroxy-, sulfate (2:1) (salt).

Molecular formula:
- Albuterol—$C_{13}H_{21}NO_3$.
- Albuterol sulfate—$(C_{13}H_{21}NO_3)_2 \cdot H_2SO_4$.

Molecular weight:
- Albuterol—239.31.
- Albuterol sulfate—576.70.

Description:
- Albuterol USP—White, crystalline powder. Melts at about 156 °C.
- Albuterol Sulfate USP—White or practically white powder.

Solubility:
- Albuterol USP—Sparingly soluble in water; soluble in alcohol.
- Albuterol Sulfate USP—Freely soluble in water; slightly soluble in alcohol, in chloroform, and in ether.

USP requirements:
- Albuterol USP—Preserve in well-closed, light-resistant containers. Contains not less than 98.5% and not more than 101.0% of albuterol, calculated on the anhydrous basis. Meets the requirements for Identification, Water (not more than 0.5%), Residue on ignition (not more than 0.1%), and Chromatographic purity.
- Albuterol Inhalation Aerosol—Not in USP.
- Albuterol Tablets USP—Preserve in well-closed, light-resistant containers. Label Tablets to state both the content of the active moiety and the content of the salt used in formulating the article. Contain an amount of albuterol sulfate equivalent to the labeled amount of albuterol, within ±10%. Meet the requirements for Identification, Dissolution (80% in 30 minutes in water in Apparatus 2 at 50 rpm), Uniformity of dosage units, and Related substances.
- Albuterol Sulfate USP—Preserve in well-closed, light-resistant containers. Contains not less than 98.5% and not more than 101.0% of albuterol sulfate, calculated on the anhydrous basis. Meets the requirements for Identification, Water (not more than 0.5%), Residue on ignition (not more than 0.1%), Chromatographic purity, and Organic volatile impurities.
- Albuterol Sulfate for Inhalation—Not in USP.
- Albuterol Sulfate Injection—Not in USP.
- Albuterol Sulfate Inhalation Solution—Not in USP.
- Albuterol Sulfate Oral Solution—Not in USP.
- Albuterol Sulfate Syrup—Not in USP.
- Albuterol Sulfate Extended-release Tablets—Not in USP.

ALCLOMETASONE

Chemical name: Alclometasone dipropionate—Pregna-1,4-diene-3,20-dione, 7-chloro-11-hydroxy-16-methyl-17,21-bis(1-oxopropoxy)-, (7 alpha,11 beta,16 alpha)-.

Molecular formula: Alclometasone dipropionate—$C_{28}H_{37}ClO_7$.

Molecular weight: Alclometasone dipropionate—521.05.

Description: Alclometasone dipropionate—White powder.

Solubility: Alclometasone dipropionate—Insoluble in water; slightly soluble in propylene glycol; moderately soluble in hexylene glycol.

USP requirements:
- Alclometasone Dipropionate USP—Preserve in tight containers. Contains not less than 97.0% and not more than 102.0% of alclometasone dipropionate, calculated on the dried basis. Meets the requirements for Identification, Specific rotation (+21° to +25°, calculated on the dried basis), Loss on drying (not more than 0.5%), Residue on ignition (not more than 0.1%), Heavy metals (not more than 0.003%), and Chromatographic purity.
- Alclometasone Dipropionate Cream USP—Preserve in collapsible tubes or in tight containers. Contains the labeled amount, within ±10%, in a suitable cream base. Meets the requirements for Identification, Microbial limits, and Minimum fill.
- Alclometasone Dipropionate Ointment USP—Preserve in collapsible tubes or in tight containers. Contains the labeled amount, within ±10%, in a suitable ointment base. Meets the requirements for Identification, Microbial limits, and Minimum fill.

ALCOHOL

Chemical name: Ethanol.

Molecular formula: C_2H_6O.

Molecular weight: 46.07.

Description: Alcohol USP—Clear, colorless, mobile, volatile liquid. Has a characteristic odor. Is readily volatilized even at low temperatures, and boils at about 78 °C. Is flammable.

NF category: Solvent.

Solubility: Alcohol USP—Miscible with water and with practically all organic solvents.

USP requirements: Alcohol USP—Preserve in tight containers, remote from fire. Contains not less than 92.3% and not more than 93.8%, by weight, corresponding to not less than 94.9% and not more than 96.0%, by volume, at 15.56 °C, of alcohol. Meets the requirements for Identification, Specific gravity (0.812–0.816 at 15.56 °C, indicating 92.3%–93.8%, by weight, or 94.9–96.0%, by volume, of alcohol), Acidity, Nonvolatile residue, Water-insoluble substances, Aldehydes and other foreign organic substances, Amyl alcohol and nonvolatile, carbonizable substances, etc., Fusel oil constituents, Acetone and isopropyl alcohol, and Methanol.

DEHYDRATED ALCOHOL

Chemical name: Ethanol.

Molecular formula: C_2H_6O.

Molecular weight: 46.07.

Description: Dehydrated Alcohol USP—Clear, colorless, mobile, volatile liquid. Has a characteristic odor. Is readily volatilized even at low temperatures, and boils at about 78 °C. Is flammable.

Solubility: Dehydrated Alcohol USP— Miscible with water and with practically all organic solvents.

USP requirements:

Dehydrated Alcohol USP—Preserve in tight containers, remote from fire. Contains not less than 99.2%, by weight, corresponding to not less than 99.5%, by volume, of alcohol at 15.56 °C. Meets the requirements for Identification, Specific gravity (not more than 0.7964 at 15.56 °C, indicating not less than 99.2% of alcohol by weight), Acidity, Nonvolatile residue, Water-insoluble substances, Aldehydes and other foreign organic substances, Amyl alcohol and nonvolatile, carbonizable substances, Ultraviolet absorbance, Fusel oil constituents, Acetone and isopropyl alcohol, and Methanol.

Dehydrated Alcohol Injection USP—Preserve in single-dose containers, preferably of Type I glass. The container may contain an inert gas in the headspace. It is Dehydrated Alcohol suitable for parenteral use. Meets the requirements for Specific gravity (not more than 0.8035 at 15.56 °C, indicating not less than 96.8%, by weight, of alcohol) and Acidity, for Identification, Nonvolatile residue, Water-insoluble substances, Aldehydes and other foreign organic substances, Amyl alcohol and nonvolatile, carbonizable substances, Ultraviolet absorbance, Fusel oil constituents, Acetone and isopropyl alcohol, and Methanol under Dehydrated Alcohol, and for Injections.

DILUTED ALCOHOL

Description: Diluted Alcohol NF—Clear, colorless, mobile liquid, having a characteristic odor.

NF category: Solvent.

NF requirements: Diluted Alcohol NF—Preserve in tight containers, remote from fire. A mixture of Alcohol and water. Contains not less than 41.0% and not more than 42.0%, by weight, corresponding to not less than 48.4% and not more than 49.5%, by volume, at 15.56 °C, of alcohol.

Prepare Diluted Alcohol as follows: 500 mL of Alcohol and 500 mL of Purified Water. Measure the Alcohol and the Purified Water separately at the same temperature, and mix. If the water and the Alcohol and the resulting mixture are measured at 25 °C, the volume of the mixture will be about 970 mL.

Meets the requirements for Specific gravity (0.935–0.937 at 15.56 °C, indicating 41.0–42.0%, by weight, or 48.4–49.5%, by volume, of alcohol), and for the tests under Alcohol (allowance being made for the difference in alcohol concentration).

RUBBING ALCOHOL

Description: Rubbing Alcohol USP—Transparent, colorless, or colored as desired, mobile, volatile liquid. Has, in the absence of added odorous constituents, a characteristic odor. Is flammable.

USP requirements: Rubbing Alcohol USP—Preserve in tight containers, remote from fire. Rubbing Alcohol and all preparations under the classification of Rubbing Alcohols are manufactured in accordance with the requirements of the U.S. Treasury Department, Bureau of Alcohol, Tobacco, and Firearms, Formula 23-H (8 parts by volume of acetone, 1.5 parts by volume of methyl isobutyl ketone, and 100 parts by volume of ethyl alcohol) being used. Label it to indicate that it is flammable. Contains not less than 68.5% and not more than 71.5% by volume of dehydrated alcohol, the remainder consisting of water and the denaturants, with or without color additives, and perfume oils. Contains, in each 100 mL, not less than 355 mg of sucrose octaacetate or not less than 1.40 mg of denatonium benzoate. Meets the requirements for Specific gravity (0.8691–0.8771 at 15.56 °C), Nonvolatile residue, and Methanol. Complies with the requirements of the Bureau of Alcohol, Tobacco, and Firearms of the U.S. Treasury Department.

Note: Rubbing Alcohol is packaged, labeled, and sold in accordance with the regulations issued by the U.S. Treasury Department, Bureau of Alcohol, Tobacco, and Firearms.

ALCOHOL AND ACETONE

For *Alcohol* and *Acetone*—See individual listings for chemistry information.

USP requirements:

Alcohol and Acetone Detergent Lotion—Not in USP.
Alcohol and Acetone Pledgets—Not in USP.

ALCOHOL AND DEXTROSE

For *Alcohol* and *Dextrose*—See individual listings for chemistry information.

USP requirements: Alcohol in Dextrose Injection USP—Preserve in single-dose containers, preferably of Type I or Type II glass. A sterile solution of Alcohol and Dextrose in Water for Injection. The label states the total osmolarity of the solution expressed in mOsmol per liter. Contains the labeled amounts of alcohol, within ±10%, and dextrose, within ±5%. Meets the requirements for Identification, Bacterial endotoxins, pH (3.5–6.5), Heavy metals (not more than 0.0005*C*%, in which *C* is the labeled amount, in grams, of Dextrose per mL of Injection), 5-Hydroxymethylfurfural and related substances, and Injections.

ALCOHOL AND SULFUR

For *Alcohol* and *Sulfur*—See individual listings for chemistry information.

USP requirements:

Alcohol and Sulfur Gel—Not in USP.
Alcohol and Sulfur Lotion—Not in USP.

ALDESLEUKIN

Chemical group: Related to naturally occurring interleukins, which are lymphokines, a subgroup of the hormone-like glycoprotein growth factors also known as cytokines.

Chemical name: 2-133-Interleukin 2 (human reduced), 125-L-serine-.

Molecular formula: $C_{690}H_{1115}N_{177}O_{203}S_6$.

Molecular weight: 15,600.00 daltons.

USP requirements: Aldesleukin for Injection—Not in USP.

ALFACALCIDOL

Chemical name: (5*Z*,7*E*)-9,10-Secocholesta-5,7,10(19)-triene-1 alpha,3 beta-diol.

Molecular formula: $C_{27}H_{44}O_2$.

Molecular weight: 400.65.

USP requirements:
Alfacalcidol Capsules—Not in USP.
Alfacalcidol Oral Solution—Not in USP.

ALFENTANIL

Chemical group: Fentanyl derivative (anilinopiperidine-derivative opioid analgesics that are chemically related to anileridine and meperidine).

Chemical name: Alfentanil hydrochloride—Propanamide, *N*-[1-[2-(4-ethyl-4,5-dihydro-5-oxo-1*H*-tetrazol-1-yl)ethyl]-4-(methoxymethyl)-4-piperidinyl]-*N*-phenyl, monohydrochloride, monohydrate.

Molecular formula: Alfentanil hydrochloride—$C_{21}H_{32}N_6O_3 \cdot HCl \cdot H_2O$.

Molecular weight: Alfentanil hydrochloride—471.00.

pKa: 6.5.

Solubility: Alfentanil hydrochloride—Soluble in water.

Other characteristics: Partition coefficient (octanol:water)—Alfentanil hydrochloride: 130 at pH 7.4.

USP requirements: Alfentanil Hydrochloride Injection—Not in USP.

ALGINIC ACID

Description: Alginic Acid NF—White to yellowish white, fibrous powder. Odorless, or practically odorless.

NF category: Suspending and/or viscosity-increasing agent; tablet binder; tablet disintegrant.

Solubility: Alginic Acid NF—Insoluble in water and in organic solvents; soluble in alkaline solutions.

NF requirements: Alginic Acid NF—Preserve in well-closed containers. A hydrophilic colloidal carbohydrate extracted with dilute alkali from various species of brown seaweeds (Phaeophyceae). Meets the requirements for Identification, Microbial limits, pH (1.5–3.5, in a 3 in 100 dispersion in water), Loss on drying (not more than 15.0%), Ash (not more than 4.0%), Arsenic (not more than 3 ppm), Lead, Heavy metals (not more than 0.004%), and Acid value (not less than 230, calculated on the dried basis).

ALGLUCERASE

Source: Prepared from pooled human placental tissue of selected donors.

Chemical name: Glucosylceramidase (human placenta isoenzyme protein moiety reduced).

Molecular formula: $C_{2532}H_{3854}N_{672}O_{711}S_{16}$ (protein moiety).

Molecular weight: 59,300.

USP requirements: Alglucerase for Injection Concentrate—Not in USP.

ALLOPURINOL

Chemical group: A structural analogue of hypoxanthine.

Chemical name: 4*H*-Pyrazolo[3,4-*d*]pyrimidin-4-one, 1,5-dihydro-.

Molecular formula: $C_5H_4N_4O$.

Molecular weight: 136.11.

Description: Allopurinol USP—Fluffy white to off-white powder, having only a slight odor.

pKa: 10.2.

Solubility: Allopurinol USP—Very slightly soluble in water and in alcohol; soluble in solutions of potassium and sodium hydroxides; practically insoluble in chloroform and in ether.

USP requirements:
Allopurinol USP—Preserve in well-closed containers. Contains not less than 98.0% and not more than 101.0% of allopurinol, calculated on the dried basis. Meets the requirements for Identification, Loss on drying (not more than 0.5%), Chromatographic impurities, and Organic volatile impurities.
Allopurinol Tablets USP—Preserve in well-closed containers. Contain the labeled amount, within ±7%. Meet the requirements for Identification, Dissolution (75% in 45 minutes in 0.1 *N* hydrochloric acid in Apparatus 2 at 75 rpm), and Uniformity of dosage units.

ALMOND OIL

Description: Almond Oil NF—Clear, pale straw-colored or colorless, oily liquid. Remains clear at −10 °C, and does not congeal until cooled to almost −20 °C.

NF category: Flavors and perfumes; vehicle (oleaginous).

Solubility: Almond Oil NF—Slightly soluble in alcohol; miscible with ether, with chloroform, and with solvent hexane.

NF requirements: Almond Oil NF—Preserve in tight containers. The fixed oil obtained by expression from the kernels of varieties of *Prunus amygdalus* Batsch (Fam. Rosaceae). Meets the requirements for Specific gravity (0.910–0.915), Foreign kernel oils, Cottonseed oil, Sesame oil, Mineral oil and foreign fatty oils, Foreign oils, Free fatty acids, Iodine value (95–105), and Saponification value (190–200).

ALOE

Description: Aloe USP—Has a characteristic, somewhat sour and disagreeable, odor.

USP requirements: Aloe USP—The dried latex of the leaves of *Aloe barbadensis* Miller (*Aloe vera* Linné), known in commerce as Curaçao Aloe, or of *Aloe ferox* Miller and hybrids of this species with *Aloe africana* Miller and *Aloe spicata*

Baker, known in commerce as Cape Aloe (Fam. Liliaceae). Yields not less than 50.0% of water-soluble extractive. Meets the requirements for Botanic characteristics, Identification, Water (not more than 12.0%), Total ash (not more than 4.0%), and Alcohol-insoluble substances (not more than 10.0%).

ALPHA$_1$-PROTEINASE INHIBITOR, HUMAN

Source: Prepared from pooled human plasma of normal donors by modification and refinements of the cold ethanol method of Cohn.

Other characteristics: When alpha$_1$-PI is reconstituted, it has a pH of 6.6–7.4.

USP requirements: Alpha$_1$-proteinase Inhibitor, Human, for Injection—Not in USP.

ALPRAZOLAM

Chemical name: 4*H*-[1,2,4]Triazolo[4,3-*a*][1,4]benzodiazepine, 8-chloro-1-methyl-6-phenyl-.

Molecular formula: $C_{17}H_{13}ClN_4$.

Molecular weight: 308.77.

Description: Alprazolam USP—A white to off-white crystalline powder. Melts at about 225 °C.

Solubility: Alprazolam USP—Insoluble in water; slightly soluble in ethyl acetate; sparingly soluble in acetone; soluble in alcohol; freely soluble in chloroform.

USP requirements:

Alprazolam USP—Preserve in well-closed containers. Contains not less than 98.0% and not more than 102.0% of alprazolam. Meets the requirements for Identification, Loss on drying (not more than 0.5%), Residue on ignition (not more than 0.5%), Heavy metals (not more than 0.002%), and Chromatographic purity.

Caution: Care should be taken to prevent inhaling particles of Alprazolam and exposing the skin to it.

Alprazolam Oral Solution—Not in USP.

Alprazolam Tablets USP—Preserve in tight, light-resistant containers. Contain the labeled amount, within ±10%. Meet the requirements for Identification, Dissolution (80% in 30 minutes in Working buffer solution in Apparatus 1 at 100 rpm), and Uniformity of dosage units.

ALPROSTADIL

Chemical name: Prost-13-en-1-oic acid, 11,15-dihydroxy-9-oxo-, (11 alpha,13*E*,15*S*)-.

Molecular formula: $C_{20}H_{34}O_5$.

Molecular weight: 354.49.

Description: Alprostadil USP—A white to off-white, crystalline powder. Melts at about 110 °C.

pKa: 6.3 in 60% ethanol in water.

Solubility: Alprostadil USP—Soluble in water; freely soluble in alcohol; soluble in acetone; slightly soluble in ethyl acetate; very slightly soluble in chloroform and in ether.

USP requirements:

Alprostadil USP—Preserve in tight containers, in a refrigerator. Contains not less than 95.0% and not more than 105.0% of alprostadil, calculated on the anhydrous basis. Meets the requirements for Identification, Water (not more than 0.5%, using 0.5 grams), Residue on ignition (not more than 0.5%, using 0.3 grams), Prostaglandin A_1, prostaglandin B_1, and 13,14-dihydroprostaglandin E_1 (total not more than 0.5%), and Foreign prostaglandins (not more than 3.0% total and no single foreign prostaglandin greater than 2.0%).

Caution: Great care should be taken to prevent inhaling particles of Alprostadil and exposing the skin to it.

Alprostadil Injection USP—Preserve in single-dose containers, preferably of Type I glass. Store in a refrigerator. A sterile solution of Alprostadil in Dehydrated Alcohol. Contains the labeled amount, within −10% to +15%. Meets the requirements for Identification, Bacterial endotoxins, Sterility, Water (not more than 0.4%), and Injections.

ALTEPLASE

Source: An enzymatic glycoprotein composed of 527 amino acids. It is produced by recombinant DNA technology using the complementary DNA for natural human tissue-type plasminogen activator obtained from a human melanoma cell line.

Chemical name: Plasminogen activator (human tissue-type 2-chain form protein moiety).

Molecular formula: $C_{2569}H_{3894}N_{746}O_{781}S_{40}$.

Molecular weight: 59,008.71.

USP requirements:

Alteplase USP—Preserve in sealed containers in the frozen state at a temperature of −20 °C or below. A highly purified glycosylated serine protease with fibrin-binding properties and plasminogen-specific proteolytic activities. Produced by recombinant DNA synthesis in mammalian cell culture. Has a biological potency of not less than 90.0% and not more than 115.0% of the potency stated on the label, the potency being 580,000 USP Alteplase Units per mg of protein. The presence of host cell DNA and host cell protein impurities in Alteplase is process-specific; the limits of these impurities are determined by validated methods. Meets the requirements for Identification, Peptide mapping, Bacterial endotoxins, Chromatographic purity, Single-chain content, and Protein content.

Alteplase for Injection USP—Preserve in hermetic containers at a temperature between 2 and 30 °C, protected from light. A sterile lyophilized preparation of Alteplase. Its biological activity is not less tha 90% and not more than 115% of that stated on the label in USP Alteplase Units. Label it to state the biological activity in USP Alteplase Units per vial and the amount of protein per vial. Contains the total protein content stated on the label, within −5% to +11%. Meets the requirements for Constituted solution, Identification, Bacterial endotoxins, Safety, Sterility, Uniformity of dosage units, pH (7.1–7.5, in the solution constituted as directed in the labeling), Water (not more than 4.0%), Purity, Percent monomer, and Protein content.

Alteplase, Recombinant, for Injection—Not in USP.

ALTRETAMINE

Source: Synthetic s-triazine derivative.

Chemical name: 1,3,5-Triazine-2,4,6-triamine, *N,N,N′,N′,N″,N″*-hexamethyl-.

Molecular formula: $C_9H_{18}N_6$.

Molecular weight: 210.28.

Description: White, crystalline powder, with a melting point of 172 °C ±1 °C.

Solubility: Practically insoluble in water, but increasingly soluble at pH 3 and below.

USP requirements: Altretamine Capsules—Not in USP.

ALUM

Chemical name:
Ammonium alum—Sulfuric acid, aluminum ammonium salt (2:1:1), dodecahydrate.
Potassium alum—Sulfuric acid, aluminum potassium salt (2:1:1), dodecahydrate.

Molecular formula:
Ammonium alum—$AlNH_4(SO_4)_2 \cdot 12H_2O$.
Potassium alum—$AlK(SO_4)_2 \cdot 12H_2O$.

Molecular weight:
Ammonium alum—453.32.
Potassium alum—474.38.

Description:
Ammonium Alum USP—Large, colorless crystals, crystalline fragments, or white powder. Is odorless. Its solutions are acid to litmus.
Potassium Alum USP—Large, colorless crystals, crystalline fragments, or white powder. Is odorless. Its solutions are acid to litmus.

Solubility:
Ammonium Alum USP—Freely soluble in water; very soluble in boiling water; freely but slowly soluble in glycerin; insoluble in alcohol.
Potassium Alum USP—Freely soluble in water; very soluble in boiling water; freely but slowly soluble in glycerin; insoluble in alcohol.

USP requirements:
Ammonium Alum USP—Contains not less than 99.0% and not more than 100.5% of ammonium alum, calculated on the dried basis. Meets the requirements for Identification, Loss on drying (45.0–48.0%), Alkalies and alkaline earths (not more than 0.5%), Arsenic (not more than 3 ppm), Heavy metals (not more than 0.002%), and Iron.
Potassium Alum USP—Preserve in well-closed containers. Contains not less than 99.0% and not more than 100.5% of potassium alum, calculated on the dried basis. Meets the requirements for Identification, Loss on drying (43.0–46.0%), Arsenic (not more than 3 ppm), Heavy metals (not more than 0.002%), and Iron.

ALUMINA AND MAGNESIA

For *Alumina* (Aluminum Hydroxide) and *Magnesia* (Magnesium Hydroxide)—See individual listings for chemistry information.

USP requirements:
Alumina and Magnesia Oral Suspension USP—Preserve in tight containers, and avoid freezing. A mixture containing Aluminum Hydroxide and Magnesium Hydroxide. Oral Suspension may be labeled to state the aluminum hydroxide content in terms of the equivalent amount of dried aluminum hydroxide gel, on the basis that each mg of dried gel is equivalent to 0.765 mg of aluminum hydroxide. Contains the equivalent of the labeled amounts of aluminum hydroxide and magnesium hydroxide, within ±10%. Meets the requirements for Identification, Microbial limits, Acid-neutralizing capacity, pH (7.3–8.5), Chloride (not more than 0.14%), and Sulfate (not more than 0.1%), and for Arsenic and Heavy metals under Aluminum Hydroxide Gel.
Alumina and Magnesia Tablets USP—Preserve in well-closed containers. Tablets prepared with the use of Dried Aluminum Hydroxide Gel may be labeled to state the aluminum hydroxide content in terms of the equivalent amount of dried aluminum hydroxide gel, on the basis that each mg of dried gel is equivalent to 0.765 mg of aluminum hydroxide. Contain the equivalent of the labeled amounts of aluminum hydroxide and magnesium hydroxide, within ±10%. Meet the requirements for Identification, Disintegration (10 minutes, in simulated gastric fluid TS), Uniformity of dosage units, and Acid-neutralizing capacity.

ALUMINA, MAGNESIA, AND CALCIUM CARBONATE

For *Alumina* (Aluminum Hydroxide), *Magnesia* (Magnesium Hydroxide), and *Calcium Carbonate*—See individual listings for chemistry information.

USP requirements:
Alumina, Magnesia, and Calcium Carbonate Oral Suspension USP—Preserve in tight containers, and avoid freezing. Oral Suspension may be labeled to state the aluminum hydroxide content in terms of the equivalent amount of dried aluminum hydroxide gel, on the basis that each mg of dried gel is equivalent to 0.765 mg of aluminum hydroxide. Contains the labeled amounts of aluminum hydroxide, magnesium hydroxide, and calcium carbonate, within ±10%. Meets the requirements for Identification, Microbial limits, pH (7.5–8.5), Chloride (not more than 0.14%), Sulfate (not more than 0.1%), and Acid-neutralizing capacity, and for Arsenic and Heavy metals under Aluminum Hydroxide Gel.
Alumina, Magnesia, and Calcium Carbonate Tablets USP—Preserve in well-closed containers. Label the Tablets to indicate that they are to be chewed before being swallowed. Tablets prepared with the use of Dried Aluminum Hydroxide Gel may be labeled to state the aluminum hydroxide content in terms of the equivalent amount of dried aluminum hydroxide gel, on the basis that each mg of dried gel is equivalent to 0.765 mg of aluminum hydroxide. Contain the labeled amounts of aluminum hydroxide, magnesium hydroxide, and calcium carbonate, within ±10%. Meet the requirements for Identification, Disintegration (45 minutes), Uniformity of dosage units, and Acid-neutralizing capacity.

ALUMINA, MAGNESIA, CALCIUM CARBONATE, AND SIMETHICONE

For *Alumina* (Aluminum Hydroxide), *Magnesia* (Magnesium Hydroxide), *Calcium Carbonate,* and *Simethicone*—See individual listings for chemistry information.

USP requirements: Alumina, Magnesia, Calcium Carbonate, and Simethicone Tablets USP—Preserve in well-closed containers. The labeling indicates that Tablets are to be chewed before swallowing. Label Tablets to state the sodium content, if it is greater than 5 mg per Tablet. Contain the equivalent of the labeled amounts of aluminum hydroxide and magnesium hydroxide, within ±10%, the labeled amount of calcium carbonate, within ±10%, and an amount of polydimethylsiloxane equivalent to the labeled amount of simethicone, within ±15%. Meet the requirements for Identification, Uniformity of dosage units, Acid-neutralizing capacity, Defoaming activity (not more than 45 seconds), Microbial limits, and Sodium content (not more than 5 mg per Tablet; where labeled as containing more than 5 mg per Tablet, not more than +10% of the labeled amount).

ALUMINA, MAGNESIA, AND SIMETHICONE

For *Alumina* (Aluminum Hydroxide), *Magnesia* (Magnesium Hydroxide), and *Simethicone*—See individual listings for chemistry information.

USP requirements:

Alumina, Magnesia, and Simethicone Oral Suspension USP—Preserve in tight containers, and avoid freezing. Oral Suspension may be labeled to state the aluminum hydroxide content in terms of the equivalent amount of dried aluminum hydroxide gel, on the basis that each mg of dried gel is equivalent to 0.765 mg of aluminum hydroxide. Label it to state the sodium content if it is greater than 1 mg per mL. Contains the equivalent of the labeled amounts of aluminum hydroxide and magnesium hydroxide, within −10% to +15%. Contains an amount of polydimethylsiloxane equivalent to the labeled amount of simethicone, within ±15%. Meets the requirements for Identification, Microbial limits, Acid-neutralizing capacity, pH (7.0–8.6), Defoaming activity (not more than 45 seconds), and Sodium.

Alumina, Magnesia, and Simethicone Tablets USP—Preserve in well-closed containers. Label Tablets to indicate that they are to be chewed before being swallowed. Label Tablets to state the sodium content if it is greater than 5 mg per Tablet. Tablets may be labeled to state the aluminum hydroxide content in terms of the equivalent amount of dried aluminum hydroxide gel, on the basis that each mg of dried gel is equivalent to 0.765 mg of aluminum hydroxide. Contain the equivalent of the labeled amounts of aluminum hydroxide and magnesium hydroxide, within −10% to +15%. Contain an amount of polydimethylsiloxane equivalent to the labeled amount of simethicone, within ±15%. Meet the requirements for Identification, Uniformity of dosage units, Acid-neutralizing capacity, Defoaming activity (not more than 45 seconds), and Sodium.

ALUMINA AND MAGNESIUM CARBONATE

For *Alumina* (Aluminum Hydroxide) and *Magnesium Carbonate*—See individual listings for chemistry information.

USP requirements:

Alumina and Magnesium Carbonate Oral Suspension USP—Preserve in tight containers, and avoid freezing. Contains the equivalent of the labeled amounts of aluminum hydroxide and magnesium carbonate, within ±10%. Meets the requirements for Identification, Microbial limits, pH (7.5–9.5), and Acid-neutralizing capacity.

Alumina and Magnesium Carbonate Tablets USP—Preserve in tight containers. Contain the equivalent of the labeled amounts of aluminum hydroxide and magnesium carbonate, within ±10%. Meet the requirements for Identification, Disintegration (10 minutes, in simulated gastric fluid TS), Uniformity of dosage units, and Acid-neutralizing capacity.

ALUMINA, MAGNESIUM CARBONATE, AND MAGNESIUM OXIDE

For *Alumina* (Aluminum Hydroxide), *Magnesium Carbonate,* and *Magnesium Oxide*—See individual listings for chemistry information.

USP requirements: Alumina, Magnesium Carbonate, and Magnesium Oxide Tablets USP—Preserve in tight containers. Contain the equivalent of the labeled amounts of aluminum hydroxide and magnesium carbonate, within ±10%. Contain the labeled amount of magnesium oxide, within ±15%. Meet the requirements for Identification, Disintegration (10 minutes, in simulated gastric fluid TS), Uniformity of dosage units, and Acid-neutralizing capacity.

ALUMINA AND MAGNESIUM TRISILICATE

For *Alumina* (Aluminum Hydroxide) and *Magnesium Trisilicate*—See individual listings for chemistry information.

USP requirements:

Alumina and Magnesium Trisilicate Oral Suspension USP—Preserve in tight containers. Contains the equivalent of the labeled amount of aluminum hydroxide, within ±10%, and the labeled amount of magnesium trisilicate, within ±10%. Meets the requirements for Identification, Acid-neutralizing capacity, and pH (7.5–8.5).

Alumina and Magnesium Trisilicate Tablets USP—Preserve in well-closed containers. Tablets prepared with the use of Dried Aluminum Hydroxide Gel may be labeled to state the aluminum hydroxide content in terms of the equivalent amount of dried aluminum hydroxide gel, on the basis that each mg of dried gel is equivalent to 0.765 mg of aluminum hydroxide. Tablets intended for the temporary relief of heartburn (acid indigestion) due to acid reflux are so labeled. Tablets that must be chewed before swallowing are so labeled. Contain the equivalent of the labeled amount of aluminum hydroxide, within ±10%, and the labeled amount of magnesium trisilicate, within ±10%. Meet the requirements for Identification, Disintegration (10 minutes, in simulated gastric fluid TS [Note: Tablets that must be chewed before swallowing are exempt from this requirement]), Uniformity of dosage units, Acid-neutralizing capacity (Note: Tablets labeled for the temporary relief of heartburn [acid indigestion] due to acid reflux are exempt from this requirement), Foam (where Tablets are labeled for the temporary relief of heartburn [acid indigestion] due to acid reflux, thickness of foam not less than 10 mm), and pH (where Tablets are labeled for the temporary relief of heartburn [acid indigestion] due to acid reflux, not less than 4.5).

ALUMINA, MAGNESIUM TRISILICATE, AND SODIUM BICARBONATE

For *Alumina* (Aluminum Hydroxide), *Magnesium Trisilicate,* and *Sodium Bicarbonate*—See individual listings for chemistry information.

USP requirements: Alumina, Magnesium Trisilicate, and Sodium Bicarbonate Chewable Tablets—Not in USP.

ALUMINUM ACETATE

Chemical name: Acetic acid, aluminum salt.

Molecular formula: $C_6H_9AlO_6$.

Molecular weight: 204.12.

Description: Aluminum Acetate Topical Solution USP—Clear, colorless liquid having a faint odor of acetic acid. Specific gravity is about 1.02.

USP requirements: Aluminum Acetate Topical Solution USP—Preserve in tight containers. Yields, from each 100 mL, not less than 1.20 grams and not more than 1.45 grams of aluminum oxide, and not less than 4.24 grams and not more than 5.12 grams of acetic acid, corresponding to not less than 4.8 grams and not more than 5.8 grams of aluminum acetate. May be stabilized by the addition of not more than 0.6% of Boric Acid.

Prepare Aluminum Acetate Topical Solution as follows: 545 mL of Aluminum Subacetate Topical Solution, 15 mL of Glacial Acetic Acid, and a sufficient quantity of Purified Water to make 1000 mL. Add the Glacial Acetic Acid to the Aluminum Subacetate Topical Solution and sufficient Water to make 1000 mL. Mix, and filter, if necessary.

Meets the requirements for Identification, pH (3.6–4.4), Limit of boric acid, and Heavy metals (not more than 0.001%).

Note: Dispense only clear Aluminum Acetate Topical Solution.

BASIC ALUMINUM CARBONATE

Source: Combination of aluminum hydroxide and aluminum carbonate.

Description: Dried basic aluminum carbonate gel—White powder.

Solubility: Dried basic aluminum carbonate gel—Insoluble in water and in alcohol.

USP requirements:
Basic Aluminum Carbonate Gel (Oral Suspension)—Not in USP.
Dried Basic Aluminum Carbonate Gel Capsules—Not in USP.
Dried Basic Aluminum Carbonate Gel Tablets—Not in USP.

ALUMINUM CHLORIDE

Chemical name: Aluminum chloride, hexahydrate.

Molecular formula: $AlCl_3 \cdot 6H_2O$.

Molecular weight: 241.43.

Description: Aluminum Chloride USP—White, or yellowish white, deliquescent, crystalline powder. Is practically odorless. Its solutions are acid to litmus.

Solubility: Aluminum Chloride USP—Very soluble in water; freely soluble in alcohol; soluble in glycerin.

USP requirements: Aluminum Chloride USP—Preserve in tight containers. Contains not less than 95.0% and not more than 102.0% of aluminum chloride, calculated on the anhydrous basis. Meets the requirements for Identification, Water (42.0–48.0%), Sulfate, Alkalies and alkaline earths (not more than 0.5%), Arsenic (not more than 8 ppm), Heavy metals (not more than 0.002%), and Iron (not more than 0.001%).

ALUMINUM HYDROXIDE

Source: An amorphous form of aluminum hydroxide in which there is a partial substitution of carbonate for hydroxide.

Chemical name: Aluminum hydroxide.

Molecular formula: $Al(OH)_3$.

Molecular weight: 78.00.

Description:
Aluminum Hydroxide Gel USP—White, viscous suspension, from which small amounts of clear liquid may separate on standing.
Dried Aluminum Hydroxide Gel USP—White, odorless, amorphous powder.

Solubility: Dried Aluminum Hydroxide Gel USP—Insoluble in water and in alcohol; soluble in dilute mineral acids and in solutions of fixed alkali hydroxides.

USP requirements:
Aluminum Hydroxide Gel USP—Preserve in tight containers, and avoid freezing. A suspension of amorphous aluminum hydroxide in which there is a partial substitution of carbonate for hydroxide. Contains the equivalent of the labeled amount of aluminum hydroxide, within ±10%. Meets the requirements for Identification, Microbial limits, Acid-neutralizing capacity, pH (5.5–8.0), Chloride, Sulfate, Arsenic (not more than 0.001%, based on the aluminum hydroxide content), and Heavy metals (not more than 0.0083%, based on the aluminum hydroxide content).

Dried Aluminum Hydroxide Gel USP—Preserve in tight containers. An amorphous form of aluminum hydroxide in which there is a partial substitution of carbonate for hydroxide. Where the quantity of dried aluminum hydroxide gel equivalent is stated in the labeling of any preparation, this shall be understood to be on the basis that each mg of dried gel is equivalent to 0.765 mg of aluminum hydroxide. Contains the equivalent of not less than 76.5% of aluminum hydroxide, and may contain varying quantities of basic aluminum carbonate and bicarbonate. Meets the requirements for Identification, Acid-neutralizing capacity, pH (not more than 10.0, in an aqueous dispersion [1 in 25]), Chloride (not more than 0.85%), Sulfate (not more than 0.6%), Arsenic (not more than 8 ppm), and Heavy metals (not more than 0.006%).

Dried Aluminum Hydroxide Gel Capsules USP—Preserve in well-closed containers. Capsules may be labeled to state the aluminum hydroxide content in terms of the equivalent amount of dried aluminum hydroxide gel, on the basis that each mg of dried gel is equivalent to 0.765 mg of aluminum hydroxide. Contain the labeled amount, within ±10%. Meet the requirements for Identification, Disintegration (10 minutes, in simulated gastric fluid TS), Uniformity of dosage units, and Acid-neutralizing capacity.

Dried Aluminum Hydroxide Gel Tablets USP—Preserve in well-closed containers. Tablets may be labeled to state the aluminum hydroxide content in terms of the equivalent amount of dried aluminum hydroxide gel, on the basis that each mg of dried gel is equivalent to 0.765 mg of aluminum hydroxide. Contain the labeled amount, within ±10%. Meet the requirements for Identification, Disintegration (10 minutes, in simulated gastric fluid TS), Uniformity of dosage units, and Acid-neutralizing capacity.

ALUMINUM MONOSTEARATE

Chemical name: Aluminum, dihydroxy(octadecanoato-*O*-).

Molecular formula: $C_{18}H_{37}AlO_4$.

Molecular weight: 344.47.

Description: Aluminum Monostearate NF—Fine, white to yellowish white bulky powder, having a faint, characteristic odor.

NF category: Suspending and/or viscosity-increasing agent.

Solubility: Aluminum Monostearate NF—Insoluble in water, in alcohol, and in ether.

NF requirements: Aluminum Monostearate NF—Preserve in well-closed containers. A compound of aluminum with a mixture of solid organic acids obtained from fats, consisting chiefly of variable proportions of aluminum monostearate and aluminum monopalmitate. Contains the equivalent of not less than 14.5% and not more than 16.5% of aluminum oxide. Meets the requirements for Identification, Loss on drying (not more than 2.0%), Arsenic (not more than 4 ppm), and Heavy metals (not more than 0.005%).

ALUMINUM PHOSPHATE

Chemical name: Phosphoric acid, aluminum salt (1:1).

Molecular formula: $AlPO_4$.

Molecular weight: 121.95.

Description: Aluminum Phosphate Gel USP—White, viscous suspension from which small amounts of water separate on standing.

USP requirements: Aluminum Phosphate Gel USP—Preserve in tight containers. A water suspension. Contains not less than 4.0% and not more than 5.0% (w/w) of aluminum phosphate. Meets the requirements for Identification, pH (6.0–7.2), Chloride (not more than 0.16%), Soluble phosphate (not more than 0.30%), Sulfate (not more than 0.05%), Arsenic (not more than 0.6 ppm), and Heavy metals (not more than 5 ppm).

ALUMINUM SUBACETATE

Chemical name: Aluminum, bis(acetato-*O*)hydroxy-.

Molecular formula: $C_4H_7AlO_5$.

Molecular weight: 162.08.

Description: Aluminum Subacetate Topical Solution USP—Clear, colorless or faintly yellow liquid, having an odor of acetic acid and an acid reaction to litmus. Gradually becomes turbid on standing, through separation of a more basic salt.

USP requirements: Aluminum Subacetate Topical Solution USP—Preserve in tight containers. Yields, from each 100 mL, not less than 2.30 grams and not more than 2.60 grams of aluminum oxide, and not less than 5.43 grams and not more than 6.13 grams of acetic acid. May be stabilized by the addition of not more than 0.9% of boric acid.

Aluminum Subacetate Topical Solution may be prepared as follows: 145 grams of Aluminum Sulfate, 160 mL of Acetic Acid, 70 grams of Precipitated Calcium Carbonate, and a sufficient quantity of Purified Water to make 1000 mL. Dissolve the Aluminum Sulfate in 600 mL of cold water, filter the solution, and add the Precipitated Calcium Carbonate gradually, in several portions, with constant stirring. Then slowly add the Acetic Acid, mix, and set the mixture aside for 24 hours. Filter the product with the aid of vacuum if necessary, returning the first portion of the filtrate to the funnel. Wash the magma on the filter with small portions of cold water, until the total filtrate measures 1000 mL.

Meets the requirements for Identification, pH (3.8–4.6), and Limit of boric acid.

ALUMINUM SULFATE

Chemical name: Sulfuric acid, aluminum salt (3:2), hydrate.

Molecular formula: $Al_2(SO_4)_3 \cdot xH_2O$.

Molecular weight: 342.14 (anhydrous).

Description: Aluminum Sulfate USP—White, crystalline powder, shining plates, or crystalline fragments. Is stable in air. Is odorless.

Solubility: Aluminum Sulfate USP—Freely soluble in water; insoluble in alcohol.

USP requirements: Aluminum Sulfate USP—Preserve in well-closed containers. Contains not less than 54.0% and not more than 59.0% of anhydrous aluminum sulfate. Contains a varying amount of water of crystallization. Meets the requirements for Identification, pH (not less than 2.9, in a solution [1 in 20]), Water (41.0–46.0%), Alkalies and alkaline earths (not more than 0.4%), Ammonium salts, Arsenic (not more than 3 ppm), Heavy metals (not more than 0.004%), and Iron.

AMANTADINE

Chemical name: Amantadine hydrochloride—Tricyclo[3.3.1.1^{3,7}]decan-1-amine, hydrochloride.

Molecular formula: Amantadine hydrochloride—$C_{10}H_{17}N \cdot HCl$.

Molecular weight: Amantadine hydrochloride—187.71.

Description: Amantadine Hydrochloride USP—White or practically white, crystalline powder.

Solubility: Amantadine Hydrochloride USP—Freely soluble in water; soluble in alcohol and in chloroform.

USP requirements:

Amantadine Hydrochloride USP—Preserve in well-closed containers. Contains not less than 98.5% and not more than 101.5% of amantadine hydrochloride. Meets the requirements for Clarity and color of solution, Identification, pH (3.0–5.5, in a solution [1 in 5]), Heavy metals (not more than 0.001%), and Organic volatile impurities.

Amantadine Hydrochloride Capsules USP—Preserve in tight containers. Contain the labeled amount, within ±5%. Meet the requirements for Identification, Dissolution (75% in 45 minutes in water in Apparatus 1 at 100 rpm), and Uniformity of dosage units.

Amantadine Hydrochloride Syrup USP—Preserve in tight containers. Contains the labeled amount, within ±5%. Meets the requirement for Identification.

AMBENONIUM

Source: Quaternary ammonium compound.

Chemical name: Ambenonium chloride—Benzenemethanaminium, *N,N'*-[(1,2-dioxo-1,2-ethanediyl)bis(imino-2,1-ethanediyl)]bis[2-chloro-*N,N*-diethyl-, dichloride.

Molecular formula: Ambenonium chloride—$C_{28}H_{42}Cl_4N_4O_2$.

Molecular weight: Ambenonium chloride—608.48.

Description: Ambenonium chloride—White, odorless powder; melting point 196–199 °C.

Solubility: Ambenonium chloride—Soluble in water and in alcohol; slightly soluble in chloroform; practically insoluble in acetone and in ether.

USP requirements: Ambenonium Chloride Tablets—Not in USP.

AMCINONIDE

Chemical name: Pregna-1,4-diene-3,20-dione, 21-(acetyloxy)-16,17-[cyclopentylidenebis(oxy)]-9-fluoro-11-hydroxy-, (11 beta,16 alpha)-.

Molecular formula: $C_{28}H_{35}FO_7$.

Molecular weight: 502.58.

Description: White to cream colored crystalline powder, having not more than a slight odor. Its melting point range is 248–252 °C.

USP requirements:

Amcinonide USP—Preserve in well-closed containers. Contains not less than 97.0% and not more than 102.0% of amcinonide, calculated on the dried basis. Meets the requirements for Identification, Specific rotation (+89.4° to +94.0°, calculated on the dried basis), Loss on drying (not more than 1.0%), and Heavy metals (not more than 0.002%).

Amcinonide Cream USP—Preserve in tight containers. It is Amcinonide in a suitable cream base. Contains the labeled amount, within −10% to +15%. Meets the requirements for Identification, Microbial limits, Minimum fill, and pH (3.5–5.2).
Amcinonide Lotion—Not in USP.
Amcinonide Ointment USP—Preserve in tight containers. It is Amcinonide in a suitable ointment base. Contains the labeled amount, within −10% to +15%. Meets the requirements for Identification, Microbial limits, and Minimum fill.

AMDINOCILLIN

Chemical name: 4-Thia-1-azabicyclo[3.2.0]heptane-2-carboxylic acid, 6-[[(hexahydro-1*H*-azepin-1-yl)methylene]amino]-3,3-dimethyl-7-oxo-, [2*S*-(2 alpha,5 alpha,6 beta)]-.

Molecular formula:
Amdinocillin—$C_{15}H_{23}N_3O_3S$.
Amdinocillin pivoxil hydrochloride—$C_{21}H_{34}ClN_3O_5S$.

Molecular weight: 325.43.

Description:
Sterile Amdinocillin USP—White to off-white crystalline powder. Melts at 141–143 °C, with decomposition.
Amdinocillin pivoxil hydrochloride—Melting point 172–173 °C.

Solubility: Sterile Amdinocillin USP—Freely soluble in water and in methanol.

USP requirements:
Sterile Amdinocillin USP—Preserve in Containers for Sterile Solids. It is amdinocillin suitable for parenteral use. Contains not less than 950 mcg and not more than 1050 mcg per mg, calculated on the anhydrous basis and, where packaged for dispensing, contains the labeled amount, within −10% to +20%. Meets the requirements for Constituted solution, Identification, Crystallinity, Bacterial endotoxins, Sterility, pH (4.0–6.2, in a solution [1 in 10]), Water (not more than 0.5%), Particulate matter, and Hexamethyleneimine, for Uniformity of dosage units, and for Labeling under Injections.
Amdinocillin Pivoxil Hydrochloride Tablets—Not in USP.

AMIKACIN

Source: Semi-synthetic; derived from kanamycin.

Chemical group: Aminoglycoside.

Chemical name:
Amikacin—D-Streptamine, *O*-3-amino-3-deoxy-alpha-D-glucopyranosyl-(1→6)-*O*-[6-amino-6-deoxy-alpha-D-glucopyranosyl-(1→4)]-N^1-(4-amino-2-hydroxy-1-oxobutyl)-2-deoxy-, (*S*)-.
Amikacin sulfate—D-Streptamine, *O*-3-amino-3-deoxy-alpha-D-glucopyranosyl-(1→6)-*O*-[6-amino-6-deoxy-alpha-D-glucopyranosyl-(1→4)]-N^1-(4-amino-2-hydroxy-1-oxobutyl)-2-deoxy-, (*S*)-, sulfate (1:2 or 1:1.8) (salt).

Molecular formula:
Amikacin—$C_{22}H_{43}N_5O_{13}$.
Amikacin sulfate—$C_{22}H_{43}N_5O_{13} \cdot 2H_2SO_4$ or $C_{22}H_{43}N_5O_{13} \cdot 1.8\ H_2SO_4$.

Molecular weight:
Amikacin—585.61.
Amikacin sulfate 2 H_2O—781.76.
Amikacin sulfate 1.8 H_2O—762.14.

Description:
Amikacin USP—White, crystalline powder.
Amikacin Sulfate USP—White, crystalline powder.
Amikacin sulfate injection—Sterile, colorless to light straw colored solution. It has a pH adjusted to 4.5 with sulfuric acid.

Solubility:
Amikacin USP—Sparingly soluble in water.
Amikacin Sulfate USP—Freely soluble in water.

USP requirements:
Amikacin USP—Preserve in tight containers. Has a potency of not less than 900 mcg of amikacin per mg, calculated on the anhydrous basis. Meets the requirements for Identification, Specific rotation (+97° to +105°, calculated on the anhydrous basis), Crystallinity, pH (9.5–11.5, in a solution containing 10 mg per mL), Water (not more than 8.5%), and Residue on ignition (not more than 1.0%).
Amikacin Sulfate USP—Preserve in tight containers. Label it to indicate whether its molar ratio of amikacin to hydrogen sulfate is 1:2 or 1:1.8. Amikacin Sulfate having a molar ratio of amikacin to hydrogen sulfate of 1:2 contains an amount of amikacin sulfate equivalent to not less than 674 mcg and not more than 786 mcg of amikacin per mg, calculated on the dried basis. Amikacin Sulfate having a molar ratio of amikacin to hydrogen sulfate of 1:1.8 contains an amount of amikacin sulfate equivalent to not less than 691 mcg and not more than 806 mcg of amikacin per mg, calculated on the dried basis. Meets the requirements for Identification, Specific rotation (+76° to +84°, calculated on the dried basis), Crystallinity, pH (2.0–4.0 [1:2 salt], or 6.0–7.3 [1:1.8 salt], in a solution containing 10 mg per mL), Loss on drying (not more than 13.0%), and Residue on ignition (not more than 1.0%).
Amikacin Sulfate Injection USP—Preserve in single-dose or in multiple-dose containers, preferably of Type I or Type III glass. A sterile solution of Amikacin Sulfate in Water for Injection, or of Amikacin in Water for Injection prepared with the aid of Sulfuric Acid. Contains an amount of amikacin sulfate equivalent to the labeled amount of amikacin, within −10% to +20%. Meets the requirements for Identification, Bacterial endotoxins, pH (3.5–5.5), Particulate matter, and Injections.

AMILORIDE

Chemical name: Amiloride hydrochloride—Pyrazinecarboxamide, 3,5-diamino-*N*-(aminoiminomethyl)-6-chloro-, monohydrochloride dihydrate.

Molecular formula: Amiloride hydrochloride—$C_6H_8ClN_7O \cdot HCl \cdot 2H_2O$.

Molecular weight: Amiloride hydrochloride—302.12.

Description: Amiloride Hydrochloride USP—Yellow to greenish yellow, odorless or practically odorless powder.

pKa: 8.7.

Solubility: Amiloride Hydrochloride USP—Slightly soluble in water; insoluble in ether, in ethyl acetate, in acetone, and in chloroform; freely soluble in dimethylsulfoxide; sparingly soluble in methanol.

USP requirements:
Amiloride Hydrochloride USP—Preserve in well-closed containers. Contains not less than 98.0% and not more than 101.0% of amiloride hydrochloride, calculated on the dried basis. Meets the requirements for Identification, Acidity, Loss on drying (11.0–13.0%), Residue on ignition (not

more than 0.1%), Heavy metals (not more than 0.002%), Chromatographic purity, and Organic volatile impurities.

Amiloride Hydrochloride Tablets USP—Preserve in well-closed containers. Contain the labeled amount, within ±10%. Meet the requirements for Identification, Dissolution (80% in 30 minutes in 0.1 *N* hydrochloric acid in Apparatus 2 at 50 rpm), and Uniformity of dosage units.

AMILORIDE AND HYDROCHLOROTHIAZIDE

For *Amiloride* and *Hydrochlorothiazide*—See individual listings for chemistry information.

USP requirements: Amiloride Hydrochloride and Hydrochlorothiazide Tablets USP—Preserve in well-closed containers. Contain the labeled amounts, within ±10%. Meet the requirements for Identification, Dissolution (80% of amiloride hydrochloride and 75% of hydrochlorothiazide in 30 minutes in 0.1 *N* hydrochloric acid in Apparatus 2 at 50 rpm), 4-Amino-6-chloro-1,3-benzenedisulfonamide (not more than 1.0%), and Uniformity of dosage units.

AMINOBENZOATE POTASSIUM

Molecular formula: $C_7H_6KNO_2$.

Molecular weight: 175.23.

Description: Aminobenzoate Potassium USP—White crystalline powder. The pH of a 1 in 100 solution in water is about 7.

Solubility: Aminobenzoate Potassium USP—Very soluble in water; soluble in alcohol; practically insoluble in ether.

USP requirements:

Aminobenzoate Potassium USP—Preserve in well-closed containers. Contains not less than 98.5% and not more than 101.0% of aminobenzoate potassium, calculated on the dried basis. Meets the requirements for Identification, pH (8.0–9.0, in a solution [1 in 20]), Loss on drying (not more than 1.0%), Chloride (not more than 0.02%), Sulfate (not more than 0.02%), Heavy metals (not more than 0.002%), and Volatile diazotizable substances (not more than 0.002%, as *p*-toluidine).

Aminobenzoate Potassium Capsules USP—Preserve in well-closed containers. Contain the labeled amount, within ±10%. Meet the requirements for Identification, Dissolution (75% in 45 minutes in water in Apparatus 1 at 100 rpm), and Uniformity of dosage units.

Aminobenzoate Potassium for Oral Solution USP—Preserve in tight containers. Contains the labeled amount, within ±10%. Meets the requirements for Identification, pH (7.0–9.0, in a solution [1 in 10]), Minimum fill (multiple-unit containers), and Uniformity of dosage units (single-unit containers).

Aminobenzoate Potassium Tablets USP—Preserve in well-closed containers. Contain the labeled amount, within ±10%. Meet the requirements for Identification, Dissolution (75% in 45 minutes in water in Apparatus 1 at 100 rpm), and Uniformity of dosage units.

AMINOBENZOATE SODIUM

Molecular formula: $C_7H_6NNaO_2$.

Molecular weight: 159.12.

USP requirements: Aminobenzoate Sodium USP—Preserve in well-closed containers. Contains not less than 98.5% and not more than 101.0% of aminobenzoate sodium, calculated on the dried basis. Meets the requirements for Identification, pH (8.0–9.0, in a solution [1 in 20]), Loss on drying (not more than 1.0%), Chloride (not more than 0.02%), Sulfate (not more than 0.02%), Heavy metals (not more than 0.002%), and Volatile diazotizable substances (not more than 0.002%, as *p*-toluidine).

AMINOBENZOIC ACID

Chemical name: Benzoic acid, 4-amino.

Molecular formula: $C_7H_7NO_2$.

Molecular weight: 137.14.

Description:

Aminobenzoic Acid USP—White or slightly yellow, odorless crystals or crystalline powder. Discolors on exposure to air or light.

Aminobenzoic Acid Topical Solution USP—Straw-colored solution having the odor of alcohol.

Solubility: Aminobenzoic Acid USP—Slightly soluble in water and in chloroform; freely soluble in alcohol and in solutions of alkali hydroxides and carbonates; sparingly soluble in ether.

USP requirements:

Aminobenzoic Acid USP—Preserve in tight, light-resistant containers. Contains not less than 98.5% and not more than 101.5% of aminobenzoic acid, calculated on the dried basis. Meets the requirements for Identification, Melting range (186–189 °C), Loss on drying (not more than 0.2%), Residue on ignition (not more than 0.1%), Heavy metals (not more than 0.002%), Volatile diazotizable substances (not more than 0.002%, as *p*-toluidine), and Ordinary impurities.

Aminobenzoic Acid Gel USP—Preserve in tight, light-resistant containers. Contains the labeled amount, within ±10%. Meets the requirements for Identification, Minimum fill, pH (4.0–6.0), and Alcohol content (42.3–54.0% [w/w]).

Aminobenzoic Acid Topical Solution USP—Preserve in tight, light-resistant containers. Contains, in each mL, not less than 45 mg and not more than 55 mg of aminobenzoic acid. Meets the requirements for Identification, Specific gravity (0.895–0.905), and Alcohol content (65–75%).

AMINOCAPROIC ACID

Chemical name: Hexanoic acid, 6-amino-.

Molecular formula: $C_6H_{13}NO_2$.

Molecular weight: 131.17.

Description: Aminocaproic Acid USP—Fine, white, crystalline powder. Is odorless, or practically odorless. Its solutions are neutral to litmus. Melts at about 205 °C.

Solubility: Aminocaproic Acid USP—Freely soluble in water, in acids, and in alkalies; slightly soluble in methanol and in alcohol; practically insoluble in chloroform and in ether.

USP requirements:

Aminocaproic Acid USP—Preserve in tight containers. Contains not less than 98.5% and not more than 100.5% of aminocaproic acid, calculated on the anhydrous basis. Meets the requirements for Identification, Water (not more than 0.5%), Residue on ignition (not more than 0.1%), and Heavy metals (not more than 0.002%).

Aminocaproic Acid Injection USP—Preserve in single-dose or in multiple-dose containers, preferably of Type I glass. A sterile solution of Aminocaproic Acid in Water for Injection. Contains the labeled amount, within −5% to

+7.5%. Meets the requirements for Identification, Bacterial endotoxins, pH (6.0–7.6), and Injections.

Aminocaproic Acid Syrup USP—Preserve in tight containers. Contains the labeled amount, within −5% to +15%. Meets the requirements for Identification and pH (6.1–6.6).

Aminocaproic Acid Tablets USP—Preserve in tight containers. Contain the labeled amount, within ±5%. Meet the requirements for Identification, Dissolution (75% in 45 minutes in water in Apparatus 1 at 100 rpm), and Uniformity of dosage units.

AMINOGLUTETHIMIDE

Chemical name: 2,6-Piperidinedione, 3-(4-aminophenyl)-3-ethyl-.

Molecular formula: $C_{13}H_{16}N_2O_2$.

Molecular weight: 232.28.

Description: Aminoglutethimide USP—Fine, white, or creamy white, crystalline powder.

Solubility: Aminoglutethimide USP—Very slightly soluble in water; readily soluble in most organic solvents. Forms water-soluble salts with strong acids.

USP requirements:

Aminoglutethimide USP—Preserve in well-closed containers. Contains not less than 98.0% and not more than 102.0% of aminoglutethimide, calculated on the dried basis. Meets the requirements for Identification, pH (6.2–7.3, in a 1 in 1000 solution in dilute methanol [1 in 20]), Loss on drying (not more than 0.5%), Residue on ignition (not more than 0.1%), Heavy metals (not more than 0.001%), Sulfate, Chromatographic purity and limit of *m*-aminoglutethimide (not more than 1.0% total impurities, other than *m*-aminoglutethimide), Azo-aminoglutethimide (not more than 0.03%), and Organic volatile impurities.

Aminoglutethimide Tablets USP—Preserve in tight, light-resistant containers. Contain the labeled amount, within ±10%. Meet the requirements for Identification, Dissolution (70% in 30 minutes in dilute hydrochloric acid [7 in 1000] in Apparatus 1 at 100 rpm), Uniformity of dosage units, and Chromatographic purity (not more than 2.0% total impurities, other than *m*-aminoglutethimide).

AMINOHIPPURATE SODIUM

Chemical name: Glycine, *N*-(4-aminobenzoyl)-, monosodium salt.

Molecular formula: $C_9H_9N_2NaO_3$.

Molecular weight: 216.17.

Solubility: Soluble in water.

USP requirements: Aminohippurate Sodium Injection USP—Preserve in single-dose or in multiple-dose containers, preferably of Type I glass. A sterile solution of Aminohippuric Acid in Water for Injection prepared with the aid of Sodium Hydroxide. Contains the labeled amount, within ±5%. Meets the requirements for Identification, Bacterial endotoxins, pH (6.7–7.6), and Injections.

AMINOHIPPURIC ACID

Chemical name: Glycine, *N*-(4-aminobenzoyl)-.

Molecular formula: $C_9H_{10}N_2O_3$.

Molecular weight: 194.19.

Description: Aminohippuric Acid USP—White, crystalline powder. Discolors on exposure to light. Melts at about 195 °C, with decomposition.

Solubility: Aminohippuric Acid USP—Sparingly soluble in water and in alcohol; freely soluble in alkaline solutions, with some decomposition, and in diluted hydrochloric acid; very slightly soluble in carbon tetrachloride, in chloroform, and in ether.

USP requirements: Aminohippuric Acid USP—Preserve in tight, light-resistant containers. Contains not less than 98.0% and not more than 100.5% of aminohippuric acid, calculated on the dried basis. Meets the requirements for Identification, Loss on drying (not more than 0.25%), Residue on ignition (not more than 0.25%), and Heavy metals (not more than 0.001%).

AMINOPHYLLINE

Source: The ethylenediamine salt of theophylline.

Chemical name: 1*H*-Purine-2,6-dione, 3,7-dihydro-1,3-dimethyl-, compd. with 1,2-ethanediamine (2:1).

Molecular formula: $C_{16}H_{24}N_{10}O_4$.

Molecular weight: 420.43.

Description:

Aminophylline USP—White or slightly yellowish granules or powder, having a slight ammoniacal odor. Upon exposure to air, it gradually loses ethylenediamine and absorbs carbon dioxide with the liberation of free theophylline. Its solutions are alkaline to litmus.

Aminophylline Tablets USP—May have a faint ammoniacal odor.

Solubility: Aminophylline USP—One gram dissolves in 25 mL of water to give a clear solution; one gram dissolved in 5 mL of water crystallizes upon standing, but redissolves when a small amount of ethylenediamine is added. Insoluble in alcohol and in ether.

USP requirements:

Aminophylline USP—Preserve in tight containers. It is anhydrous or contains not more than two molecules of water of hydration. Label it to indicate whether it is anhydrous or hydrous, and also to state the content of anhydrous theophylline. Contains not less than 84.0% and not more than 87.4% of anhydrous theophylline, calculated on the anhydrous basis. Meets the requirements for Identification, Water (not more than 0.75% for the anhydrous form and not more than 7.9% for the hydrous form), Residue on ignition (not more than 0.15%), Ethylenediamine content (157–175 mg per gram of theophylline), and Organic volatile impurities.

Aminophylline Enema USP—Preserve in single-dose or in multiple-dose containers. An aqueous solution of Aminophylline, prepared with the aid of Ethylenediamine. Label the Enema to state the content of anhydrous theophylline. Contains an amount of aminophylline equivalent to the labeled amount of anhydrous theophylline, within ±10%. Aminophylline Enema may contain an excess of ethylenediamine, but no other substance may be added for the purpose of pH adjustment. Meets the requirements for Identification, pH (9.0–9.5), and Ethylenediamine content (218–267 mg per gram of anhydrous theophylline).

Aminophylline Injection USP—Preserve in single-dose containers from which carbon dioxide has been excluded, preferably of Type I glass, protected from light. A sterile solution of Aminophylline in Water for Injection, or a sterile solution of Theophylline in Water for Injection prepared with the aid of Ethylenediamine. Label the Injection to state the content of anhydrous theophylline. Contains, in each mL, an amount of aminophylline equivalent to the labeled amount of anhydrous theophylline, within ±7%. Aminophylline Injection may contain an excess of Ethylenediamine, but no other substance may be added for the purpose of pH adjustment. Meets the requirements for Identification, Bacterial endotoxins, pH (8.6–9.0), Particulate matter, Injections, and Ethylenediamine content (166–192 mg per gram of anhydrous theophylline).

Note: Do not use the Injection if crystals have separated.

Aminophylline Oral Solution USP—Preserve in tight containers. An aqueous solution of Aminophylline, prepared with the aid of Ethylenediamine. Label the Oral Solution to state the content of anhydrous theophylline. Contains an amount of aminophylline equivalent to the labeled amount of anhydrous theophylline, within ±10%. Aminophylline Oral Solution may contain an excess of ethylenediamine, but no other substance may be added for the purpose of pH adjustment. Meets the requirements for Identification, pH (8.5–9.7), and Ethylenediamine content (176–283 mg per gram of anhydrous theophylline).

Aminophylline Suppositories USP—Preserve in well-closed containers, in a cold place. Label the Suppositories to state the content of anhydrous theophylline. Contain an amount of aminophylline equivalent to the labeled amount of anhydrous theophylline, within ±10%. Meet the requirements for Identification and Ethylenediamine content (152–190 mg per gram of anhydrous theophylline).

Aminophylline Tablets USP—Preserve in tight containers. Label the Tablets to state the content of anhydrous theophylline. Contain an amount of aminophylline equivalent to the labeled amount of anhydrous theophylline, within ±7%. Meet the requirements for Identification, Disintegration (30 minutes, for enteric-coated tablets), Dissolution (75% in 45 minutes in water in Apparatus 2 at 50 rpm, for uncoated oı plain coated tablets), Uniformity of dosage units, and Ethylenediamine content (152–178 mg per gram of anhydrous theophylline).

Note: The ammoniacal odor present in the vapor space above Aminophylline Tablets is often quite strong, especially when bottles having suitably tight closures are newly opened. This is due to ethylenediamine vapor pressure build-up, a natural condition in the case of aminophylline.

Aminophylline Extended-release Tablets—Not in USP.

AMINOPHYLLINE AND SODIUM CHLORIDE

For *Aminophylline* and *Sodium Chloride*—See individual listings for chemistry information.

USP requirements: Aminophylline and Sodium Chloride Injection—Not in USP.

AMINOSALICYLATE SODIUM

Chemical name: Benzoic acid, 4-amino-2-hydroxy-, monosodium salt, dihydrate.

Molecular formula: $C_7H_6NNaO_3 \cdot 2H_2O$.

Molecular weight: 211.15.

Description: Aminosalicylate Sodium USP—White to cream-colored, crystalline powder. Is practically odorless. Its solutions decompose slowly and darken in color.

Solubility: Aminosalicylate Sodium USP—Freely soluble in water; sparingly soluble in alcohol; very slightly soluble in ether and in chloroform.

USP requirements:

Aminosalicylate Sodium USP—Preserve in tight, light-resistant containers, protected from excessive heat. Contains not less than 98.0% and not more than 101.0% of aminosalicylate sodium, calculated on the anhydrous basis. Meets the requirements for Clarity and color of solution, Identification, pH (6.5–8.5, in a solution [1 in 50]), Water (16.0–18.0%), Chloride (not more than 0.042%), Heavy metals (not more than 0.003%), *m*-Aminophenol (not more than 0.25%), Hydrogen sulfide, sulfur dioxide, and amyl alcohol, and Organic volatile impurities.

Note: Prepare solutions of Aminosalicylate Sodium within 24 hours of administration. Under no circumstances use a solution if its color is darker than that of a freshly prepared solution.

Aminosalicylate Sodium Tablets USP—Preserve in tight, light-resistant containers, protected from excessive heat. Contain the labeled amount, within ±5%. Meet the requirements for Identification, Dissolution (75% in 45 minutes in water in Apparatus 1 at 100 rpm), Uniformity of dosage units, and *m*-Aminophenol (not more than 1.0%).

AMINOSALICYLIC ACID

Chemical name: Benzoic acid, 4-amino-2-hydroxy-.

Molecular formula: $C_7H_7NO_3$.

Molecular weight: 153.14.

Description: Aminosalicylic Acid USP—White or practically white, bulky powder, that darkens on exposure to light and to air. Is odorless, or has a slight acetous odor.

Solubility: Aminosalicylic Acid USP—Slightly soluble in water and in ether; soluble in alcohol.

USP requirements:

Aminosalicylic Acid USP—Preserve in tight, light-resistant containers, at a temperature not exceeding 30 °C. Contains not less than 98.5% and not more than 100.5% of aminosalicylic acid, calculated on the anhydrous basis. Meets the requirements for Clarity and color of solution, Identification, pH (3.0–3.7, in a saturated solution), Water (not more than 0.5%), Residue on ignition (not more than 0.2%), Chloride (not more than 0.042%), Heavy metals (not more than 0.003%), *m*-Aminophenol (not more than 0.25%), and Hydrogen sulfide, sulfur dioxide, and amyl alcohol.

Note: Under no circumstances use a solution prepared from Aminosalicylic Acid if its color is darker than that of a freshly prepared solution.

Aminosalicylic Acid Tablets USP—Preserve in tight, light-resistant containers, at a temperature not exceeding 30 °C. Contain the labeled amount, within ±5%. Meet the requirements for Identification, Dissolution (75% in 45 minutes in phosphate buffer [pH 7.5] in Apparatus 1 at 100 rpm), Uniformity of dosage units, and *m*-Aminophenol (not more than 1.0%).

AMIODARONE

Chemical group: Benzofuran derivative.

Chemical name: Amiodarone hydrochloride—2-Butyl-3-benzofuranyl 4-[2-(diethylamino)-ethoxy]-3-5-diiodophenyl ketone, hydrochloride.

Molecular formula: Amiodarone hydrochloride—$C_{25}H_{29}I_2NO_3 \cdot HCl$.

Molecular weight: Amiodarone hydrochloride—681.8.

Description: Amiodarone hydrochloride—White to cream-colored crystalline powder.

pKa: 6.6.

Solubility: Amiodarone hydrochloride—Slightly soluble in water; soluble in alcohol; freely soluble in chloroform.

Other characteristics: Amiodarone hydrochloride—Contains 37.3% iodine by weight; highly lipophilic.

USP requirements: Amiodarone Hydrochloride Tablets—Not in USP.

AMITRIPTYLINE

Chemical group: Dibenzocycloheptadiene derivative.

Chemical name: Amitriptyline hydrochloride—1-Propanamine, 3-(10,11-dihydro-5*H*-dibenzo[*a,d*]cyclohepten-5-ylidene)-*N,N*-dimethyl-, hydrochloride.

Molecular formula: Amitriptyline hydrochloride—$C_{20}H_{23}N \cdot HCl$.

Molecular weight: Amitriptyline hydrochloride—313.87.

Description: Amitriptyline Hydrochloride USP—White or practically white, odorless or practically odorless, crystalline powder or small crystals.

pKa: Amitriptyline hydrochloride—9.4.

Solubility:

Amitriptyline Hydrochloride USP—Freely soluble in water, in alcohol, in chloroform, and in methanol; insoluble in ether.

Amitriptyline pamoate—Almost completely insoluble in water.

Other characteristics: Tertiary amine.

USP requirements:

Amitriptyline Hydrochloride USP—Preserve in well-closed containers. Contains not less than 99.0% and not more than 100.5% of amitriptyline hydrochloride, calculated on the dried basis. Meets the requirements for Identification, Melting range (195–199 °C), pH (5.0–6.0, in a solution [1 in 100]), Loss on drying (not more than 0.5%), Residue on ignition (not more than 0.1%), Heavy metals (not more than 0.001%), Chromatographic purity, and Organic volatile impurities.

Amitriptyline Hydrochloride Injection USP—Preserve in single-dose or in multiple-dose containers, preferably of Type I glass. A sterile solution of Amitriptyline Hydrochloride in Water for Injection. Contains the labeled amount, within ±10%. Meets the requirements for Identification, Pyrogen, pH (4.0–6.0), and Injections.

Amitriptyline Hydrochloride Tablets USP—Preserve in well-closed containers. Contain the labeled amount, within ±10%. Meet the requirements for Identification, Dissolution (75% in 45 minutes in 0.1 *N* hydrochloric acid in Apparatus 1 at 100 rpm), and Uniformity of dosage units.

Amitriptyline Pamoate Syrup—Not in USP.

AMLODIPINE

Chemical name: Amlodipine besylate—3,5-Pyridinedicarboxylic acid, 2-[(2-aminoethoxy)methyl]-4-(2-chlorophenyl)-1,4-dihydro-6-methyl-, 3-ethyl 5-methyl ester, (±)-, monobenzenesulfonate.

Molecular formula: Amlodipine besylate—$C_{20}H_{25}ClN_2O_5 \cdot C_6H_6O_3S$.

Molecular weight: Amlodipine besylate—567.05.

Description: Amlodipine besylate—White crystalline powder.

Solubility: Amlodipine besylate—Slightly soluble in water; sparingly soluble in ethanol.

USP requirements: Amlodipine Besylate Tablets—Not in USP.

STRONG AMMONIA SOLUTION

Chemical name: Ammonia.

Molecular formula: NH_3.

Molecular weight: 17.03.

Description: Strong Ammonia Solution NF—Clear, colorless liquid, having an exceedingly pungent, characteristic odor. Specific gravity is about 0.90.

NF category: Alkalizing agent.

NF requirements: Strong Ammonia Solution NF—Preserve in tight containers at a temperature not above 25 °C. A solution of ammonia containing not less than 27.0% and not more than 31.0% (w/w) of ammonia. On exposure to air it loses ammonia rapidly. Meets the requirements for Identification, Nonvolatile residue (not more than 0.05%), Heavy metals (not more than 0.0013%), and Readily oxidizable substances.

Caution: Use care in handling Strong Ammonia Solution because of the caustic nature of the Solution and the irritating properties of its vapor. Cool the container well before opening, and cover the closure with a cloth or similar material while opening. Do not taste Strong Ammonia Solution, and avoid inhalation of its vapor.

AROMATIC AMMONIA SPIRIT

Description: Aromatic Ammonia Spirit USP—Practically colorless liquid when recently prepared, but gradually acquiring a yellow color on standing. Has an aromatic and pungent odor, and is affected by light. Specific gravity is about 0.90.

USP requirements: Aromatic Ammonia Spirit USP—Preserve in tight, light-resistant containers, at a temperature not exceeding 30 °C. A hydroalcoholic solution that contains, in each 100 mL, not less than 1.7 grams and not more than 2.1 grams of total ammonia, and Ammonium Carbonate corresponding to not less than 3.5 grams and not more than 4.5 grams. Meets the requirement for Alcohol content (62.0–68.0%).

AMMONIO METHACRYLATE COPOLYMER

Description: Ammonio Methacrylate Copolymer NF—Colorless, clear to white-opaque granules with a faint amine-like odor.

NF category: Coating agent.

Solubility: Ammonio Methacrylate Copolymer NF—Soluble to freely soluble in methanol, in alcohol, and in isopropyl alcohol, each of which contains small amounts of water; soluble to freely soluble in acetone, in ethyl acetate, and in methylene chloride. The solutions are clear to slightly cloudy. Insoluble in petroleum ether and in water.

NF requirements: Ammonio Methacrylate Copolymer NF—Preserve in tight containers at a temperature not exceeding 30 °C. A fully polymerized copolymer of acrylic and methacrylic acid esters with a low content of quaternary ammonium groups. It is available in two types, which differ in content of ammonio methacrylate units. Label it to state whether it is Type A or B. Meets the requirements for Identification, Viscosity, Loss on drying (not more than 3.0%), Residue on ignition (not more than 0.1%), Arsenic (not more than 2 ppm), Heavy metals (not more than 0.002%), and Monomers (not more than 0.15% of each monomer).

AMMONIUM CARBONATE

Chemical name: Carbonic acid, monoammonium salt, mixt. with ammonium carbamate.

Molecular formula: Ammonium carbonate (normal)—$(NH_4)_2CO_3$.

Molecular weight: Ammonium carbonate (normal)—96.09.

Description: Ammonium Carbonate NF—White powder, or hard, white or translucent masses, having a strong odor of ammonia without empyreuma. Its solutions are alkaline to litmus. On exposure to air, it loses ammonia and carbon dioxide, becoming opaque, and is finally converted to friable porous lumps or a white powder of ammonium bicarbonate.

NF category: Alkalizing agent; buffering agent.

Solubility: Ammonium Carbonate NF—Freely soluble in water, but decomposed by hot water.

NF requirements: Ammonium Carbonate NF—Preserve in tight, light-resistant containers, at a temperature not above 30 °C. Consists of ammonium bicarbonate and ammonium carbamate in varying proportions. Yields not less than 30.0% and not more than 34.0% of ammonia. Meets the requirements for Identification, Residue on ignition (not more than 0.1%), Chloride (not more than 0.0035%), Sulfate (not more than 0.005%), and Heavy metals (not more than 0.001%).

AMMONIUM CHLORIDE

Chemical name: Ammonium chloride.

Molecular formula: NH_4Cl.

Molecular weight: 53.49.

Description: Ammonium Chloride USP—Colorless crystals or white, fine or coarse, crystalline powder. Is somewhat hygroscopic.

Solubility: Ammonium Chloride USP—Freely soluble in water and in glycerin, and even more so in boiling water; sparingly soluble in alcohol.

USP requirements:

Ammonium Chloride USP—Preserve in tight containers. Contains not less than 99.5% and not more than 100.5% of ammonium chloride, calculated on the dried basis. Meets the requirements for Identification, pH (4.6–6.0, in a solution [1 in 20]), Loss on drying (not more than 0.5%), Residue on ignition (not more than 0.1%), Thiocyanate, and Heavy metals (not more than 0.001%).

Ammonium Chloride Injection USP—Preserve in single-dose or in multiple-dose containers, preferably of Type I or Type II glass. A sterile solution of Ammonium Chloride in Water for Injection. The label states the content of ammonium chloride in terms of weight and of milliequivalents in a given volume. The label states also the total osmolar concentration in mOsmol per liter or per mL. The label states that the Injection is not for direct injection but is to be diluted with Sodium Chloride Injection to the appropriate strength before use. Contains the labeled amount, within ±5%. Hydrochloric acid may be added to adjust the pH. Meets the requirements for Identification, Bacterial endotoxins, pH (4.0–6.0, in a concentration of not more than 100 mg of ammonium chloride per mL), Particulate matter, Chloride content (63.0–70.3% of the labeled amount of ammonium chloride), and Injections.

Ammonium Chloride Delayed-release Tablets USP—Preserve in tight containers. Contain the labeled amount, within ±6%. Ammonium Chloride Delayed-release Tablets are enteric-coated. Meet the requirements for Identification, Disintegration (2 hours, determined as directed for Enteric-coated Tablets), and Thiocyanate.

AMMONIUM MOLYBDATE

Chemical name: Molybdate ($Mo_7O_{24}^{6-}$), hexaammonium, tetrahydrate.

Molecular formula: $(NH_4)_6Mo_7O_{24}\cdot 4H_2O$.

Molecular weight: 1235.86.

Description: Ammonium Molybdate USP—Colorless or slightly greenish or yellowish crystals.

Solubility: Ammonium Molybdate USP—Soluble in water; practically insoluble in alcohol.

USP requirements:

Ammonium Molybdate USP—Preserve in tight containers. Contains not less than 99.3% and not more than 101.8% of ammonium molybdate. Meets the requirements for Identification, Insoluble substances (not more than 0.005%), Chloride (not more than 0.002%), Nitrate, Sulfate (not more than 0.02%), Arsenate, phosphate, and silicate, Phosphate (not more than 5 ppm), Magnesium and alkali salts (not more than 0.02%), and Heavy metals (not more than 0.001%).

Ammonium Molybdate Injection USP—Preserve in single-dose or in multiple-dose containers, preferably of Type I or Type II glass. A sterile solution of Ammonium Molybdate in Water for Injection. Label the Injection to indicate that it is to be diluted to the appropriate strength with Sterile Water for Injection or other suitable fluid prior to administration. Contains an amount of ammonium molybdate equivalent to the labeled amount of molybdenum, within ±15%. Meets the requirements for Identification, Pyrogen, pH (3.0–6.0), Particulate matter, and Injections.

AMMONIUM PHOSPHATE

Chemical name: Phosphoric acid, diammonium salt.

Molecular formula: $(NH_4)_2HPO_4$.

Molecular weight: 132.06.

Description: Ammonium Phosphate NF—Colorless or white granules or powder.

NF category: Buffering agent.

Solubility: Ammonium Phosphate NF—Freely soluble in water; practically insoluble in acetone and in alcohol.

NF requirements: Ammonium Phosphate NF—Preserve in tight containers. Contains not less than 96.0% and not more than 102.0% of ammonium phosphate. Meets the requirements for Identification, pH (7.6–8.2, in a solution [1 in 100]), Chloride (not more than 0.03%), Sulfate (not more than 0.15%), Arsenic (not more than 3 ppm), and Heavy metals (not more than 0.001%).

AMOBARBITAL

Chemical name:
Amobarbital—2,4,6(1*H*,3*H*,5*H*)-Pyrimidinetrione, 5-ethyl-5-(3-methylbutyl)-.
Amobarbital sodium—2,4,6(1*H*,3*H*,5*H*)-Pyrimidinetrione, 5-ethyl-5-(3-methylbutyl)-, monosodium salt.

Molecular formula:
Amobarbital—$C_{11}H_{18}N_2O_3$.
Amobarbital sodium—$C_{11}H_{17}N_2NaO_3$.

Molecular weight:
Amobarbital—226.28.
Amobarbital sodium—248.26.

Description:
Amobarbital USP—White, odorless, crystalline powder. Its saturated solution has a pH of about 5.6, determined potentiometrically.
Amobarbital Sodium USP—White, friable, granular powder. Is odorless and hygroscopic. Its solutions decompose on standing, heat accelerating the decomposition.

Solubility:
Amobarbital USP—Very slightly soluble in water; freely soluble in alcohol and in ether; soluble in chloroform and in solutions of fixed alkali hydroxides and carbonates.
Amobarbital Sodium USP—Very soluble in water; soluble in alcohol; practically insoluble in ether and in chloroform.

USP requirements:
Amobarbital USP—Preserve in well-closed containers. Contains not less than 98.5% and not more than 101.0% of amobarbital, calculated on the dried basis. Meets the requirements for Identification, Melting range (156–161 °C, the range between beginning and end of melting not more than 3 °C), Loss on drying (not more than 1.0%), Residue on ignition (not more than 0.1%), and Organic volatile impurities.
Amobarbital Tablets USP—Preserve in well-closed containers. Contain the labeled amount, within ± 10%. Meet the requirements for Identification, Dissolution (70% in 30 minutes in phosphate buffer [pH 7.6] in Apparatus 1 at 100 rpm), and Uniformity of dosage units.
Amobarbital Sodium USP—Preserve in tight containers. Contains not less than 98.5% and not more than 100.5% of amobarbital sodium, calculated on the dried basis. Meets the requirements for Completeness of solution, Identification, pH (9.6–10.4), Loss on drying (not more than 2.0%), Heavy metals (not more than 0.003%), and Organic volatile impurities.
Amobarbital Sodium Capsules USP—Preserve in tight containers. Contain the labeled amount, within ± 10%. Meet the requirements for Identification, Dissolution (75% in 60 minutes in water in Apparatus 1 at 100 rpm), and Uniformity of dosage units.
Sterile Amobarbital Sodium USP—Preserve in Containers for Sterile Solids. It is Amobarbital Sodium suitable for parenteral use. Meets the requirements for Constituted solution, Bacterial endotoxins, and Loss on drying (not more than 1.0%), for Identification tests, Completeness of solution, pH, and Heavy metals under Amobarbital Sodium, and for Sterility tests, Uniformity of dosage units, and Labeling under Injections.

AMODIAQUINE

Chemical name:
Amodiaquine—Phenol, 4-[(7-chloro-4-quinolinyl)amino]-2-[(diethylamino)methyl]-.
Amodiaquine hydrochloride—Phenol, 4-[(7-chloro-4-quinolinyl)amino]-2-[(diethylamino)methyl]-, dihydrochloride, dihydrate.

Molecular formula:
Amodiaquine—$C_{20}H_{22}ClN_3O$.
Amodiaquine hydrochloride—$C_{20}H_{22}ClN_3O \cdot 2HCl \cdot 2H_2O$.

Molecular weight:
Amodiaquine—355.87.
Amodiaquine hydrochloride—464.82.

Description:
Amodiaquine USP—Very pale yellow to light tan-yellow, odorless powder.
Amodiaquine Hydrochloride USP—Yellow, crystalline powder. Is odorless.

Solubility:
Amodiaquine USP—Practically insoluble in water; sparingly soluble in 1.0 *N* hydrochloric acid; slightly soluble in alcohol.
Amodiaquine Hydrochoride USP—Soluble in water; sparingly soluble in alcohol; very slightly soluble in chloroform and in ether.

USP requirements:
Amodiaquine USP—Preserve in tight containers. Contains not less than 97.0% and not more than 103.0% of amodiaquine, calculated on the anhydrous basis. Meets the requirements for Identification, Water (not more than 0.5%), Residue on ignition (not more than 0.2%), Chromatographic purity, and Organic volatile impurities.
Amodiaquine Hydrochloride USP—Preserve in tight containers. Contains not less than 97.0% and not more than 103.0% of amodiaquine hydrochloride, calculated on the anhydrous basis. Meets the requirements for Completeness of solution, Identification, Water (7.0–9.0%), Residue on ignition (not more than 0.2%), Chromatographic purity, and Organic volatile impurities.
Amodiaquine Hydrochloride Tablets USP—Preserve in tight containers. Contain an amount of amodiaquine hydrochloride equivalent to the labeled amount of amodiaquine, within ±7%. Meet the requirements for Identification, Dissolution (75% in 30 minutes in water in Apparatus 2 at 50 rpm), and Uniformity of dosage units.

AMOXAPINE

Chemical group: Dibenzoxazepine.

Chemical name: Dibenz[*b,f*][1,4]oxazepine, 2-chloro-11-(1-piperazinyl)-.

Molecular formula: $C_{17}H_{16}ClN_3O$.

Molecular weight: 313.79.

Description: Amoxapine USP—White to yellowish crystalline powder.

pKa: 7.6 (apparent).

Solubility: Amoxapine USP—Freely soluble in chloroform; soluble in tetrahydrofuran; sparingly soluble in methanol and in toluene; slightly soluble in acetone; practically insoluble in water.

Other characteristics: Secondary amine.

USP requirements:
Amoxapine USP—Preserve in tight containers. Contains not less than 98.5% and not more than 101.0% of amoxapine, calculated on the dried basis. Meets the requirements for Identification, Melting range (177–181 °C), Loss on

drying (not more than 0.5%), Residue on ignition (not more than 0.1%), and Chromatographic purity.

Amoxapine Tablets USP—Preserve in well-closed containers. Contain the labeled amount, within ± 10%. Meet the requirements for Identification and Uniformity of dosage units.

AMOXICILLIN

Source: Semisynthetic derivative of ampicillin.

Chemical group: Semisynthetic penicillin.

Chemical name: 4-Thia-1-azabicyclo[3.2.0]heptane-2-carboxylic acid, 6-[[amino(4-hydroxyphenyl)acetyl]amino]-3,3-dimethyl-7-oxo-, trihydrate[2*S*-[2 alpha,5 alpha,6 beta(*S**)]]-.

Molecular formula: $C_{16}H_{19}N_3O_5S \cdot 3H_2O$.

Molecular weight: 419.45.

Description: Amoxicillin USP—White, practically odorless, crystalline powder.

Solubility: Amoxicillin USP—Slightly soluble in water and in methanol; insoluble in carbon tetrachloride and in chloroform.

USP requirements:

Amoxicillin USP—Preserve in tight containers, at controlled room temperature. Label it to indicate that it is to be used in the manufacture of nonparenteral drugs only. Contains not less than 90.0% of amoxicillin, calculated on the anhydrous basis. Has a potency equivalent to not less than 900 mcg and not more than 1050 mcg of amoxicillin per mg, calculated on the anhydrous basis. Meets the requirements for Identification, Crystallinity, pH (3.5–6.0, in a solution containing 2 mg per mL), Water (11.5–14.5%), and Dimethylaniline.

Amoxicillin Capsules USP—Preserve in tight containers, at controlled room temperature. Contain the labeled amount, within −10% to +20%. Meet the requirements for Identification, Dissolution (80% in 90 minutes in water in Apparatus 1 at 100 rpm), Uniformity of dosage units, and Water (not more than 14.5%).

Amoxicillin Intramammary Infusion USP—Preserve in well-closed disposable syringes. A suspension of Amoxicillin in a suitable vegetable oil vehicle. Label it to indicate that it is intended for veterinary use only. Contains the labeled amount, within −10% to +20%. Contains a suitable dispersing agent and preservative. Meets the requirements for Identification and Water (not more than 1.0%).

Sterile Amoxicillin USP—Preserve in Containers for Sterile Solids. It is Amoxicillin suitable for parenteral use. Label it to indicate that it is intended for veterinary use only. Has a potency equivalent to not less than 900 mcg and not more than 1050 mcg of amoxicillin per mg, calculated on the anhydrous basis. Meets the requirements for Bacterial endotoxins and Sterility, and for Identification test, Crystallinity, pH, Water, and Dimethylaniline under Amoxicillin.

Sterile Amoxicillin for Suspension USP—Preserve in Containers for Sterile Solids. A sterile mixture of Amoxicillin and one or more suitable buffers, preservatives, stabilizers, and suspending agents. Label it to indicate that it is for veterinary use only. Contains the labeled amount, within −10% to +20%. Meets the requirements for Identification, Bacterial endotoxins, Sterility, pH (5.0–7.0, in the suspension constituted as directed in the labeling), and Water (11.0–14.0%).

Amoxicillin Oral Suspension USP—Preserve in multiple-dose containers equipped with a suitable dosing pump. A suspension of Amoxicillin in Soybean Oil. Label it to indicate that it is for veterinary use only. Contains the labeled amount, within −10% to +20%. Meets the requirements for Identification and Water (not more than 2.0%).

Amoxicillin for Oral Suspension USP—Preserve in tight containers, at controlled room temperature. Contains the labeled amount, within −10% to +20%. Contains one or more suitable buffers, colors, flavors, preservatives, stabilizers, sweeteners, and suspending agents. Meets the requirements for Identification, pH (5.0–7.5 in the suspension constituted as directed in the labeling), Water (not more than 3.0%), Deliverable volume (multiple-unit containers), and Uniformity of dosage units (single-unit containers).

Amoxicillin Tablets USP—Preserve in tight containers, at controlled room temperature. Label chewable Tablets to indicate that they are to be chewed before swallowing. Label film-coated Tablets or Tablets having a diameter of greater than 15 mm to indicate that they are intended for veterinary use only. Contain the labeled amount, within −10% to +20%. Meet the requirements for Identification, Disintegration (30 minutes, in simulated gastric fluid TS [chewable Tablets and Tablets having a diameter of greater than 15 mm are exempt]), and Water (not more than 6.0%, not more than 7.0% for film-coated Tablets, not more than 7.5% for Tablets having a diameter greater than 15 mm).

AMOXICILLIN AND CLAVULANATE

For *Amoxicillin* and *Clavulanate*—See individual listings for chemistry information.

USP requirements:

Amoxicillin and Clavulanate Potassium for Oral Suspension USP—Preserve in tight containers, at controlled room temperature. Contains the labeled amount of amoxicillin, within −10% to +20%, and an amount of clavulanate potassium equivalent to the labeled amount of clavulanic acid, within −10% to +25%. Contains one or more suitable buffers, colors, flavors, preservatives, stabilizers, sweeteners, and suspending agents. Meets the requirements for Identification, pH (4.8–6.6, in the suspension constituted as directed in the labeling), and Water (not more than 7.5%, where the label indicates that after constitution as directed, the suspension contains 25 mg of amoxicillin per mL; not more than 8.5%, where the label indicates that after constitution as directed, the suspension contains 50 mg of amoxicillin per mL).

Amoxicillin and Clavulanate Potassium Tablets USP—Preserve in tight containers. Label chewable Tablets to include the word "chewable" in juxtaposition to the official name. The labeling indicates that chewable Tablets may be chewed before being swallowed or may be swallowed whole. Tablets intended for veterinary use only are so labeled. Contain the labeled amount of amoxicillin, within −10% to +20%, and an amount of clavulanate potassium equivalent to the labeled amount of clavulanic acid, within −10% to +20%. Meet the requirements for Identification, Disintegration (for Tablets labeled for veterinary use only, 30 minutes, in simulated gastric fluid TS), Dissolution (85% in 30 minutes in water in Apparatus 2 at 75 rpm [Note: Tablets labeled for veterinary use only are exempt from this requirement]), Uniformity of dosage units, and Water (not more than 6.0% where the Tablets are labeled as being chewable; not more than 7.0% where the labeled amount of amoxicillin in each Tablet is 250 mg or less; not more than 10.0% where the labeled amount of amoxicillin in each Tablets is greater than 250 mg).

AMPHETAMINE

Chemical name: Amphetamine sulfate—Benzeneethanamine, alpha-methyl-, sulfate (2:1), (±)-.

Molecular formula: Amphetamine sulfate—$(C_9H_{13}N)_2 \cdot H_2SO_4$.

Molecular weight: Amphetamine sulfate—368.49.

Description: Amphetamine Sulfate USP—White, odorless, crystalline powder. Its solutions are acid to litmus, having a pH of 5 to 6.

Solubility: Amphetamine Sulfate USP—Freely soluble in water; slightly soluble in alcohol; practically insoluble in ether.

USP requirements:

Amphetamine Sulfate USP—Preserve in well-closed containers. Dried at 105 °C for 2 hours, contains not less than 98.0% and not more than 100.5% of amphetamine sulfate. Meets the requirements for Identification, Loss on drying (not more than 1.0%), Residue on ignition (not more than 0.2%), Dextroamphetamine, Ordinary impurities, and Organic volatile impurities.

Amphetamine Sulfate Tablets USP—Preserve in well-closed containers. Contain the labeled amount, within ±7%. Meet the requirements for Identification, Dissolution (75% in 45 minutes in water in Apparatus 1 at 100 rpm), and Uniformity of dosage units.

AMPHETAMINE AND DEXTROAMPHETAMINE

USP requirements: Amphetamine and Dextroamphetamine Resin Complex Capsules—Not in USP.

AMPHOTERICIN B

Source: Derived from a strain of *Streptomyces nodosus.*

Chemical name: Amphotericin B.

Molecular formula: $C_{47}H_{73}NO_{17}$.

Molecular weight: 924.09.

Description: Amphotericin B USP—Yellow to orange powder; odorless or practically so.

Solubility:

Amphotericin B USP—Insoluble in water, in anhydrous alcohol, in ether, and in toluene; soluble in dimethylformamide, in dimethyl sulfoxide, and in propylene glycol; slightly soluble in methanol.

Amphotericin B for Injection USP—It yields a colloidal dispersion in water.

Other characteristics: Solubilized by the addition of sodium desoxycholate, which yields a colloidal dispersion in water after reconstitution.

USP requirements:

Amphotericin B USP—Preserve in tight, light-resistant containers, in a cold place. Label it to state whether it is intended for use in preparing dermatological and oral dosage forms or parenteral dosage forms. Has a potency of not less than 750 mcg of amphotericin B per mg, calculated on the dried basis. Meets the requirements for Identification, Loss on drying (not more than 5.0%), Residue on ignition (not more than 0.5% [Note: Amphotericin B intended for use in preparing dermatological creams, lotions, and ointments, and oral suspensions and capsules, yields not more than 3.0%]), and Amphotericin A (not more than 5.0%, calculated on the dried basis [Note: Amphotericin B intended for use in preparing dermatological creams, lotions, and ointments, and oral suspensions and capsules, contains not more than 15% of amphotericin A, calculated on the dried basis]).

Amphotericin B Cream USP—Preserve in collapsible tubes, or in other well-closed containers. Contains the labeled amount, within −10% to +25%. Meets the requirement for Minimum fill.

Amphotericin B for Injection USP—Preserve in Containers for Sterile Solids, in a refrigerator and protected from light. A sterile complex of amphotericin B and deoxycholate sodium and one or more suitable buffers. Label it to indicate that it is intended for use by intravenous infusion to hospitalized patients only, and that the solution should be protected from light during administration. Contains the labeled amount, within −10% to +20%. Meets the requirements for Bacterial endotoxins, Sterility, pH (7.2–8.0, in an aqueous solution containing 10 mg of amphotericin B per mL), and Loss on drying (not more than 8.0%), and for Uniformity of dosage units and Labeling under Injections.

Amphotericin B Lotion USP—Preserve in well-closed containers. Contains the labeled amount, within −10% to +25%. Meets the requirements for Minimum fill and pH (5.0–7.0).

Amphotericin B Ointment USP—Preserve in collapsible tubes, or in other well-closed containers. It is Amphotericin B in a suitable ointment base. Contains the labeled amount, within −10% to +25%. Meets the requirements for Minimum fill and Water (not more than 1.0%).

AMPICILLIN

Source: Semisynthetic penicillin.

Chemical name:

Ampicillin—4-Thia-1-azabicyclo[3.2.0]heptane-2-carboxylic acid, 6-[(aminophenylacetyl)amino]-3,3-dimethyl-7-oxo-, [2*S*-[2 alpha,5 alpha,6 beta(*S**)]]-.

Ampicillin sodium—4-Thia-1-azabicyclo[3.2.0]heptane-2-carboxylic acid, 6-[(aminophenylacetyl)amino]-3,3-dimethyl-7-oxo-, monosodium salt, [2*S*-[2 alpha,5 alpha,6 beta(*S**)]]-.

Molecular formula:

Ampicillin—$C_{16}H_{19}N_3O_4S$.

Ampicillin sodium—$C_{16}H_{18}N_3NaO_4S$.

Molecular weight:

Ampicillin—349.40.

Ampicillin sodium—371.39.

Description:

Ampicillin USP—White, practically odorless, crystalline powder.

Sterile Ampicillin Sodium USP—White to off-white, odorless or practically odorless, crystalline powder. Is hygroscopic.

Solubility:

Ampicillin USP—Slightly soluble in water and in methanol; insoluble in carbon tetrachloride and in chloroform.

Sterile Ampicillin Sodium USP—Very soluble in water and in isotonic sodium chloride and dextrose solutions.

USP requirements:

Ampicillin USP—Preserve in tight containers. It is anhydrous or contains three molecules of water of hydration. Label it to indicate whether it is anhydrous or is the trihydrate. Where the quantity of ampicillin is indicated in the labeling of any preparation containing Ampicillin, this shall be understood to be in terms of anhydrous ampicillin. Contains not less than 900 mcg and not more than 1050 mcg of ampicillin per mg, calculated on the anhydrous basis. Meets the requirements for Identification, Crystallinity, pH (3.5–6.0, in a solution containing 10 mg per mL), Loss on drying (not more than 2.0% for anhydrous; 12.0–15.0% for trihydrate), and Dimethylaniline.

Ampicillin Boluses USP—Preserve in tight containers. Label Boluses to indicate that they are for veterinary use only. Contain an amount of ampicillin (as the trihydrate) equivalent to the labeled amount of ampicillin, within −10% to +20%. Meet the requirements for Identification, Uniformity of dosage units, and Loss on drying (not more than 5.0%).

Ampicillin Capsules USP—Preserve in tight containers. Label Capsules to indicate whether the ampicillin therein is in the anhydrous form or is the trihydrate. Contain an amount of ampicillin (anhydrous or as the trihydrate) equivalent to the labeled amount of ampicillin, within −10% to +20%. Meet the requirements for Identification, Dissolution (75% in 45 minutes in water in Apparatus 1 at 100 rpm), Uniformity of dosage units, and Loss on drying (not more than 4.0% for the anhydrous and 10.0–15.0% for the trihydrate).

Ampicillin Soluble Powder USP—Preserve in tight containers. A dry mixture of Ampicillin (as the trihydrate) and one or more suitable diluents and stabilizing agents. Label it to indicate that it is for veterinary use only. Contains an amount of ampicillin (as the trihydrate) equivalent to the labeled amount of ampicillin, within −10% to +20%. Meets the requirements for Identification, pH (3.5–6.0, in an aqueous solution containing the equivalent of 20 mg of ampicillin per mL), and Water (not more than 5.0%).

Sterile Ampicillin USP—Preserve in Containers for Sterile Solids. It is the trihydrate form of Ampicillin suitable for parenteral use. Label it to indicate that it is the trihydrate. Where the quantity of ampicillin is indicated in the labeling of any preparation containing Sterile Ampicillin, this shall be understood to be in terms of anhydrous ampicillin. Contains not less than 900 mcg and not more than 1050 mcg of ampicillin per mg, calculated on the dried basis. Meets the requirements for Bacterial endotoxins, Sterility, and Loss on drying (12.0–15.0%), and for Identification test, pH, Dimethylaniline, and Crystallinity under Ampicillin.

Sterile Ampicillin Suspension USP—Preserve in single-dose or in multiple-dose containers, preferably of Type I glass. A sterile suspension of Ampicillin in a suitable oil vehicle. Label it to indicate that it is for veterinary use only. Contains an amount of ampicillin (as the trihydrate) equivalent to the labeled amount of ampicillin, within −10% to +20%. Meets the requirements for Identification, Sterility, and Water (not more than 4.0%).

Sterile Ampicillin for Suspension USP—Preserve in Containers for Sterile Solids. A dry mixture of Ampicillin (as the trihydrate) and one or more suitable buffers, preservatives, stabilizers, and suspending agents. Contains an amount of ampicillin (as the trihydrate) equivalent to the labeled amount of ampicillin, within −10% to +20%. Meets the requirements for Identification, Bacterial endotoxins, pH (5.0–7.0, in the suspension constituted as directed in the labeling), and Loss on drying (11.4–14.0%), and for Sterility under Sterile Ampicillin Suspension, Uniformity of dosage units, and Labeling under Injections.

Ampicillin for Oral Suspension USP—Preserve in tight containers. Label it to indicate whether the ampicillin therein is in the anhydrous form or is the trihydrate. Contains an amount of ampicillin (anhydrous or as the trihydrate) equivalent to the labeled amount of ampicillin, within −10% to +20%, when constituted as directed. Contains one or more suitable buffers, colors, flavors, preservatives, and sweetening ingredients. Meets the requirements for Identification, pH (5.0–7.5 in the suspension constituted as directed in the labeling), Water (not more than 2.5%; not more than 5.0% if it contains ampicillin trihydrate and contains the equivalent of 100 mg of ampicillin per mL when constituted as directed in the labeling), Deliverable volume (multiple-unit containers), and Uniformity of dosage units (single-unit containers).

Ampicillin Tablets USP—Preserve in tight containers. Label Tablets to indicate whether the ampicillin therein is in the anhydrous form or is the trihydrate. Label chewable Tablets to indicate that they are to be chewed before being swallowed. Tablets intended for veterinary use only are so labeled. Contain an amount of Ampicillin (anhydrous form or trihydrate form) equivalent to the labeled amount of ampicillin, within −10% to +20%. Meet the requirements for Identification, Dissolution (75% in 45 minutes in water in Apparatus 1 at 100 rpm), Uniformity of dosage units, Loss on drying (where the Tablets contain anhydrous ampicillin, not more than 4.0% for powder from nonchewable Tablets and not more than 3.0% for powder from chewable Tablets; where the Tablets contain ampicillin as the trihydrate, not more than 13.0% for powder from Tablets for veterinary use), and Water (where chewable Tablets contain ampicillin trihydrate, not more than 5.0%; where nonchewable Tablets contain ampicillin trihydrate, 9.5–12.0%).

Sterile Ampicillin Sodium USP—Preserve in Containers for Sterile Solids. Protect the constituted solution from freezing. Contains an amount of ampicillin sodium equivalent to not less than 845 mcg and not more than 988 mcg of ampicillin per mg, calculated on the anhydrous basis and, where packaged for dispensing, contains an amount of ampicillin sodium equivalent to the labeled amount of ampicillin within −10% to +15%. Meets the requirements for Constituted solution, Identification, Crystallinity (Note: Sterile Ampicillin Sodium in the freeze-dried form is exempt from this requirement), Bacterial endotoxins, pH (8.0–10.0, in a solution containing 10.0 mg of ampicillin per mL), Water (not more than 2.0%), Particulate matter, Dimethylaniline, and Methylene chloride (not more than 0.2%), and for Sterility tests, Uniformity of dosage units, and Labeling under Injections.

AMPICILLIN AND PROBENECID

For *Ampicillin* and *Probenecid*—See individual listings for chemistry information.

USP requirements:

Ampicillin and Probenecid Capsules USP—Preserve in tight containers. Contain an amount of ampicillin (as the trihydrate) equivalent to the labeled amount of ampicillin, within −10% to +20%, and the labeled amount of probenecid, within ±10%. Meet the requirements for Loss on drying (8.5–13.0%) and Uniformity of dosage units.

Ampicillin and Probenecid for Oral Suspension USP—Preserve in tight, unit-dose containers. Contains an amount of ampicillin (as the trihydrate) equivalent to the labeled amount of ampicillin, within −10% to +20%, and the labeled amount of probenecid, within ±10%. Contains one or more suitable colors, flavors, and suspending agents. Meets the requirements for pH (5.0–7.5, in the suspension constituted as directed in the labeling), Water (not more than 5.0%), Deliverable volume (for solid packaged in multiple-unit containers), and Uniformity of dosage units (for solid packaged in single-unit containers).

AMPICILLIN AND SULBACTAM

For *Ampicillin* and *Sulbactam*—See individual listings for chemistry information.

USP requirements: Sterile Ampicillin Sodium and Sulbactam Sodium USP—Preserve in Containers for Sterile Solids. A sterile, dry mixture of Sterile Ampicillin Sodium and Sterile Sulbactam Sodium. Contains amounts of ampicillin sodium and sulbactam sodium equivalent to the labeled amounts of ampicillin and sulbactam, within −10% to +15%, the labeled amounts representing proportions of ampicillin to sulbactam of 2:1. Contains not less than 563 mcg of ampicillin and 280 mcg of sulbactam per mg, calculated on the anhydrous basis. Meets the requirements for Constituted solution, Identification, Bacterial endotoxins, Sterility, pH (8.0–10.0, in a solution containing 10 mg of ampicillin and 5 mg of sulbactam per mL), Water (not more than 2.0%), and Particulate matter, and for Uniformity of dosage units and Labeling under Injections.

AMPROLIUM

Chemical group: Vitamin B_1 or thiamine structural analog.

Chemical name: 1-[(4-Amino-2-propyl-5-pyrimidinyl)methyl]-2-methylpyridinium chloride monohydrochloride.

Molecular formula: $C_{14}H_{19}ClN_4 \cdot HCl$.

Molecular weight: 315.25.

Description: Amprolium USP—White to light yellow powder.

Solubility: Amprolium USP—Freely soluble in water, in methanol, in alcohol, and in dimethylformamide; sparingly soluble in dehydrated alcohol; practically insoluble in isopropyl alcohol, in butyl alcohol, and in acetone.

USP requirements:

Amprolium USP—Preserve in well-closed containers. Label it to indicate that it is for veterinary use only. Contains not less than 97.0% and not more than 101.0% of amprolium, calculated on the dried basis. Meets the requirements for Identification and Loss on drying (not more than 1.0%).

Amprolium Soluble Powder USP—Preserve in tight containers. Label it to indicate that it is for veterinary use only. Contains the labeled amount, within ±5%. Meets the requirement for Identification.

Amprolium Oral Solution USP—Preserve in tight containers. Label it to indicate that it is for veterinary use only. Contains the labeled amount, within ±7%. Meets the requirements for Identification and pH (2.5–3.0).

AMRINONE

Chemical name: Amrinone lactate—5-Amino[3,4′-bipyridin]-6(1*H*)-one 2-hydroxypropanate.

Molecular formula: $C_{10}H_9N_3O$.

Molecular weight: 187.20.

Description: Pale yellow crystalline compound.

Solubility: Solubilities in water at pH 4.1, 6.0, and 8.0 are 25, 0.9, and 0.7 mg per mL, respectively.

USP requirements: Amrinone Lactate Injection—Not in USP.

AMSACRINE

Chemical name: Methanesulfonamide, *N*-[4-(9-acridinylamino)-3-methoxyphenyl]-.

Molecular formula: $C_{21}H_{19}N_3O_3S$.

Molecular weight: 393.46.

USP requirements: Amsacrine Injection—Not in USP.

AMYLENE HYDRATE

Chemical name: 2-Butanol, 2-methyl-.

Molecular formula: $C_5H_{12}O$.

Molecular weight: 88.15.

Description: Amylene Hydrate NF—Clear, colorless liquid, having a camphoraceous odor. Its solutions are neutral to litmus.

NF category: Solvent.

Solubility: Amylene Hydrate NF—Freely soluble in water; miscible with alcohol, with chloroform, with ether, and with glycerin.

NF requirements: Amylene Hydrate NF—Preserve in tight containers. Contains not less than 99.0% and not more than 100.0% of amylene hydrate. Meets the requirements for Identification, Specific gravity (0.803–0.807), Distilling range (97–103 °C), Water (not more than 0.5%), Nonvolatile residue (not more than 0.02%), Heavy metals (not more than 0.0005%), Readily oxidizable substances, Aldehyde, and Organic volatile impurities.

AMYL NITRITE

Chemical group: Mixture of nitrous acid, 2-methylbutyl ester, and nitrous acid, 3-methylbutyl ester.

Molecular formula: $C_5H_{11}NO_2$.

Molecular weight: 117.15.

Description: Amyl Nitrite USP—Clear, yellowish liquid, having a peculiar, ethereal, fruity odor. Is volatile even at low temperatures, and is flammable. Boils at about 96 °C.

Solubility: Amyl Nitrite USP—Practically insoluble in water. Miscible with alcohol and with ether.

USP requirements:

Amyl Nitrite USP—Preserve in tight containers, and store in a cool place, protected from light. A mixture of the nitrite esters of 3-methyl-1-butanol and 2-methyl-1-butanol. Contains not less than 85.0% and not more than 103.0% of amyl nitrite. Meets the requirements for Identification, Specific gravity (0.870–0.876), Acidity, Nonvolatile residue (not more than 0.02%), Total nitrites (not less than 97.0%), and Organic volatile impurities.

Caution: Amyl Nitrite is very flammable. Do not use where it may be ignited.

Amyl Nitrite Inhalant USP—Preserve in tight, unit-dose glass containers, wrapped loosely in gauze or other suitable material, and store in a cool place, protected from light. Contains a mixture of the nitrite esters of 3-methyl-1-butanol and 2-methyl-1-butanol. Contains the labeled amount, within −20% to +5%. Contains a suitable stabilizer. Meets the requirements for Specific gravity (0.870–0.880) and Total nitrites (not less than 95.0%), and for Identification tests and Acidity under Amyl Nitrite.

Caution: Amyl Nitrite Inhalant is very flammable. Do not use where it may be ignited.

ANETHOLE

Chemical name: Benzene, 1-methoxy-4-(1-propenyl)-, (*E*)-.

Molecular formula: $C_{10}H_{12}O$.

Molecular weight: 148.20.

Description: Anethole NF—Colorless or faintly yellow liquid at or above 23 °C. Has the aromatic odor of anise. Affected by light.

NF category: Flavors and perfumes.

Solubility: Anethole NF—Very slightly soluble in water; freely soluble in alcohol; readily miscible with ether and with chloroform.

NF requirements: Anethole NF—Preserve in tight, light-resistant containers. Obtained from Anise Oil and other sources, or is prepared synthetically. Label it to indicate whether it is obtained from natural sources or is prepared synthetically. Meets the requirements for Specific gravity (0.983–0.988), Congealing temperature (not less than 20 °C), Distilling range (231–237 °C), Angular rotation (−0.15° to +0.15°), Refractive index (1.557–1.561), Heavy metals (not more than 0.004%), Aldehydes and ketones, Phenols, and Organic volatile impurities.

ANILERIDINE

Chemical name:

Anileridine—4-Piperidinecarboxylic acid, 1-[2-(4-aminophenyl)ethyl]-4-phenyl-, ethyl ester.

Anileridine hydrochloride—4-Piperidinecarboxylic acid, 1-[2-(4-aminophenyl)ethyl]-4-phenyl-, ethyl ester, dihydrochloride.

Molecular formula:

Anileridine—$C_{22}H_{28}N_2O_2$.

Anileridine hydrochloride—$C_{22}H_{28}N_2O_2 \cdot 2HCl$.

Molecular weight:

Anileridine—352.48.

Anileridine hydrochloride—425.40.

Description:

Anileridine USP—White to yellowish white, odorless to practically odorless, crystalline powder. Is oxidized on exposure to air and light, becoming darker in color. It exhibits polymorphism, and of two crystalline forms observed, one melts at about 80 °C and the other at about 89 °C.

Anileridine Hydrochloride USP—White or nearly white, odorless, crystalline powder. Is stable in air. Melts at about 270 °C, with decomposition.

Solubility:

Anileridine USP—Very slightly soluble in water; freely soluble in alcohol and in chloroform; soluble in ether although it may show turbidity.

Anileridine Hydrochloride USP—Freely soluble in water; sparingly soluble in alcohol; practically insoluble in ether and in chloroform.

USP requirements:

Anileridine USP—Preserve in tight, light-resistant containers. Contains not less than 98.5% and not more than 101.0% of anileridine, calculated on the anhydrous basis. Meets the requirements for Identification, Water (not more than 1.0%), Residue on ignition (not more than 0.1%), and Chloride (not more than 0.040%).

Anileridine Injection USP—Preserve in single-dose or in multiple-dose containers, preferably of Type I glass, protected from light. A sterile solution of Anileridine in Water for Injection, prepared with the aid of Phosphoric Acid. Contains the labeled amount, as the phosphate, within −10% to +15%. Meets the requirements for Identification, Bacterial endotoxins, pH (4.5–5.0), and Injections.

Anileridine Hydrochloride USP—Preserve in tight, light-resistant containers. Contains not less than 96.0% and not more than 102.0% of anileridine hydrochloride, calculated on the dried basis. Meets the requirements for Identification, pH (2.5–3.0, in a solution [1 in 20]), Loss on drying (not more than 1.0%), Residue on ignition (not more than 0.1%), and Chloride content (16.0–17.2%).

Anileridine Hydrochloride Tablets USP—Preserve in tight, light-resistant containers. Contain an amount of anileridine hydrochloride equivalent to the labeled amount of anileridine, within ±5%. Meet the requirements for Identification, Dissolution (65% in 45 minutes in 0.1 *N* hydrochloric acid in Apparatus 1 at 100 rpm), and Uniformity of dosage units.

ANISINDIONE

Chemical group: Indandione derivative.

Chemical name: 2-(*p*-Methoxyphenyl)indane-1,3-dione.

Molecular formula: $C_{16}H_{12}O_3$.

Molecular weight: 252.27.

Description: White or off-white, crystalline powder.

Solubility: Practically insoluble in water.

USP requirements: Anisindione Tablets—Not in USP.

ANISOTROPINE

Chemical group: Quaternary ammonium salt.

Chemical name: Anisotropine methylbromide—8-Azoniabicyclo[3.2.1]octane, 8,8-dimethyl-3-[(1-oxo-2-propylpentyl)-oxy]-, bromide, *endo*-.

Molecular formula: Anisotropine methylbromide—$C_{17}H_{32}BrNO_2$.

Molecular weight: Anisotropine methylbromide—362.35.

Description: Anisotropine methylbromide—White, glistening powder.

Solubility: Anisotropine methylbromide—Soluble in water; sparingly soluble in alcohol.

USP requirements: Anisotropine Methylbromide Tablets—Not in USP.

ANISTREPLASE

Source: Prepared in vitro by acylating human plasma–derived, purified, heat-treated lys-plasminogen and purified streptokinase from group C beta-hemolytic streptococci.

Chemical name: Anistreplase.

Molecular weight: 131,000 daltons.

USP requirements: Anistreplase for Injection—Not in USP.

ANTAZOLINE

Chemical name: Antazoline phosphate—1*H*-Imidazole-2-methanamine, 4,5-dihydro-*N*-phenyl-*N*-(phenylmethyl)-, phosphate (1:1).

Molecular formula: Antazoline phosphate—$C_{17}H_{19}N_3 \cdot H_3PO_4$.

Molecular weight: Antazoline phosphate—363.35.

Description: Antazoline Phosphate USP—White to off-white, crystalline powder.

Solubility: Antazoline Phosphate USP—Soluble in water; sparingly soluble in methanol; practically insoluble in ether.

USP requirements: Antazoline Phosphate USP—Preserve in tight containers. Contains not less than 98.0% and not more than 101.0% of antazoline phosphate, calculated on the dried basis. Meets the requirements for Identification, Melting range (194–198 °C, with decomposition), pH (4.0–5.0, in a solution [1 in 50]), Loss on drying (not more than 0.5%), and Chromatographic purity.

ANTHRALIN

Chemical name: 9(10*H*)-Anthracenone, 1,8-dihydroxy-.

Molecular formula: $C_{14}H_{10}O_3$.

Molecular weight: 226.23.

Description: Anthralin USP—Yellowish brown, crystalline powder. Is odorless.

Solubility: Anthralin USP—Insoluble in water; soluble in chloroform, in acetone, and in solutions of alkali hydroxides; slightly soluble in alcohol, in ether, and in glacial acetic acid.

USP requirements:

Anthralin USP—Preserve in tight containers in a cool place. Protect from light. Contains not less than 97.0% and not more than 102.0% of anthralin, calculated on the dried basis. Meets the requirements for Identification, Melting range (178–181 °C), Acidity or alkalinity, Loss on drying (not more than 0.5%), Residue on ignition (not more than 0.1%), Chloride, and Sulfate.

Anthralin Cream USP—Preserve in tight containers, in a cool place. Protect from light. It is Anthralin in an aqueous (oil-in-water) or oily (water-in-oil) cream vehicle. Label it to indicate whether the cream vehicle is aqueous or oily. If labeled to contain more than 0.1% of anthralin, contains the labeled amount, within −10% to +15%; if labeled to contain 0.1% or less of anthralin, contains the labeled amount, within −10% to +30%.

Anthralin Ointment USP—Preserve in tight containers, in a cool place. Protect from light. It is Anthralin in a petrolatum or other oleaginous vehicle. If labeled to contain more than 0.1% of anthralin, contains the labeled amount, within −10% to +15%; if labeled to contain 0.1% or less of anthralin, contains the labeled amount, within −10% to +30%.

ANTICOAGULANT CITRATE DEXTROSE

Description: Anticoagulant Citrate Dextrose Solution USP—Clear, colorless, odorless liquid. Is dextrorotatory.

USP requirements: Anticoagulant Citrate Dextrose Solution USP—Preserve in single-dose containers, of colorless, transparent, Type I or Type II glass, or of a suitable plastic material. A sterile solution of Citric Acid, Sodium Citrate, and Dextrose in Water for Injection. Label it to indicate the number of mL of Solution required per 100 mL of whole blood or the number of mL of Solution required per volume of whole blood to be collected. Contains in each 1000 mL of Solution A, not less than 20.59 grams and not more than 22.75 grams of Total Citrate, expressed as citric acid, anhydrous, and not less than 23.28 grams and not more than 25.73 grams of Dextrose, and not less than 4.90 grams and not more than 5.42 grams of Sodium. Contains in each 1000 mL of Solution B, not less than 12.37 grams and not more than 13.67 grams of Total Citrate, expressed as citric acid, anhydrous, and not less than 13.96 grams and not more than 15.44 grams of Dextrose, and not less than 2.94 grams and not more than 3.25 grams of Sodium. Contains no antimicrobial agents.

Prepare Anticoagulant Citrate Dextrose Solution as follows: Solution A—7.3 grams of Citric Acid (anhydrous), 22.0 grams of Sodium Citrate (dihydrate), 24.5 grams of Dextrose (monohydrate), and a sufficient quantity of Water for Injection, to make 1000 mL. Solution B—4.4 grams of Citric Acid (anhydrous), 13.2 grams of Sodium Citrate (dihydrate), 14.7 grams of Dextrose (monohydrate), and a sufficient quantity of Water for Injection, to make 1000 mL. Dissolve the ingredients, and mix. Filter the solution until clear, place immediately in suitable containers, and sterilize. If desired, 8 grams and 4.8 grams of monohydrated citric acid may be used instead of the indicated, respective amounts of anhydrous citric acid; 19.3 grams and 11.6 grams of anhydrous sodium citrate may be used instead of the indicated, respective amounts of dihydrated sodium citrate; and 22.3 grams and 13.4 grams of anhydrous dextrose may be used instead of the indicated, respective amounts of monohydrated dextrose.

Meets the requirements for Identification, Bacterial endotoxins, pH (4.5–5.5), Chloride (not more than 0.0035%), and Injections.

ANTICOAGULANT CITRATE PHOSPHATE DEXTROSE

Description: Anticoagulant Citrate Phosphate Dextrose Solution USP—Clear, colorless to slightly yellow, odorless liquid. Is dextrorotatory.

USP requirements: Anticoagulant Citrate Phosphate Dextrose Solution USP—Preserve in single-dose containers, of colorless, transparent, Type I or Type II glass, or of a suitable plastic material. A sterile solution of Citric Acid, Sodium Citrate, Monobasic Sodium Phosphate, and Dextrose in Water for Injection. Label it to indicate the number of mL of Solution required per 100 mL of whole blood or the number of mL of Solution required per volume of whole blood to be collected. Contains, in each 1000 mL, not less than 2.11 grams and not more than 2.33 grams of monobasic sodium phosphate; not less than 24.22 grams and not more than 26.78 grams of dextrose; not less than 19.16 grams and not more than 21.18 grams of total citrate, expressed as citric acid, anhydrous; and not less than 6.21 grams and not more than 6.86 grams of Sodium. Contains no antimicrobial agents.

Prepare Anticoagulant Citrate Phosphate Dextrose Solution as follows: 2.99 grams of Citric Acid (anhydrous), 26.3 grams of Sodium Citrate (dihydrate), 2.22 grams of Monobasic Sodium Phosphate (monohydrate), 25.5 grams of Dextrose (monohydrate), and a sufficient quantity of Water for Injection, to make 1000 mL. Dissolve the ingredients, and mix. Filter the solution until clear, place immediately in suitable containers, and sterilize. If desired, 3.27 grams of monohydrated citric acid may be used instead of the indicated amount of anhydrous citric acid; 23.06 grams of anhydrous sodium citrate may be used instead of the indicated amount of dihydrated sodium citrate; 1.93 grams of anhydrous monobasic sodium phosphate may be used instead of the indicated amount of monohydrated monobasic sodium phosphate; and 23.2 grams of anhydrous dextrose may be used instead of the indicated amount of monohydrated dextrose.

Meets the requirements for Identification, Bacterial endotoxins, pH (5.0–6.0), Chloride (not more than 0.0035%), and Injections.

ANTICOAGULANT CITRATE PHOSPHATE DEXTROSE ADENINE

USP requirements: Anticoagulant Citrate Phosphate Dextrose Adenine Solution USP—Preserve in single-dose containers, of colorless, transparent, Type I or Type II glass, or of a suitable plastic material. A sterile solution of Citric Acid, Sodium Citrate, Monobasic Sodium Phosphate, Dextrose, and Adenine in Water for Injection. Label it to indicate the number of mL of solution required per 100 mL of whole blood or the number of mL of solution required per volume of whole blood to be collected. Contains, in each 1000 mL, not less than 2.11 grams and not more than 2.33 grams of monobasic sodium phosphate; not less than 30.30 grams and not more than 33.50 grams of dextrose; not less than 19.16 grams and not more than 21.18 grams of total citrate, expressed as citric acid, anhydrous; not less than 6.21 grams and not more than 6.86 grams of sodium; and not less than 0.247 grams and not more than 0.303 grams of adenine. Contains no antimicrobial agents.

Prepare Anticoagulant Citrate Phosphate Dextrose Adenine Solution as follows: 2.99 grams of Citric Acid (anhydrous), 26.3 grams of Sodium Citrate (dihydrate), 2.22 grams of Monobasic Sodium Phosphate (monohydrate), 31.9 grams of Dextrose (monohydrate), 0.275 grams of Adenine, and a sufficient quantity of Water for Injection, to make 1000 mL. Dissolve the ingredients, and mix. Filter the solution until clear, place immediately in suitable containers, and sterilize. If desired, 3.27 grams of monohydrated citric acid may be used instead of the indicated amount of anhydrous citric acid; 23.06 grams of anhydrous sodium citrate may be used instead of the indicated amount of dihydrated sodium citrate; 1.93 grams of anhydrous monobasic sodium phosphate may be used instead of the indicated amount of monohydrated monobasic sodium phosphate; and 29.0 grams of anhydrous dextrose may be used instead of the indicated amount of monohydrated dextrose.

Meets the requirements for Bacterial endotoxins, pH (5.0–6.0), Chloride (not more than 0.0035%), and Injections.

ANTICOAGULANT HEPARIN

USP requirements: Anticoagulant Heparin Solution USP—Preserve in single-dose containers, of colorless, transparent, Type I or Type II glass, or of a suitable plastic material. A sterile solution of Heparin Sodium in Sodium Chloride Injection. Its potency is within ±10% of the potency stated on the label in terms of USP Heparin Units. Label it in terms of USP Heparin Units, and to indicate the number of mL of Solution required per 100 mL of whole blood. Contains not less than 0.85% and not more than 0.95% of sodium chloride. Contains no antimicrobial agents.

Prepare Anticoagulant Heparin Solution as follows: 75,000 Units of Heparin Sodium and a sufficient quantity of Sodium Chloride Injection to make 1000 mL. Add the Heparin Sodium, in solid form or in solution, to the Sodium Chloride Injection, mix, filter if necessary, and sterilize.

Meets the requirements for Bacterial endotoxins, pH (5.0–7.5), and Injections.

ANTICOAGULANT SODIUM CITRATE

Description: Anticoagulant Sodium Citrate Solution USP—Clear and colorless liquid.

USP requirements: Anticoagulant Sodium Citrate Solution USP—Preserve in single-dose containers, preferably of Type I or Type II glass. A sterile solution of Sodium Citrate in Water for Injection. Contains, in each 100 mL, not less than 3.80 grams and not more than 4.20 grams of sodium citrate, dihydrate. Contains no antimicrobial agents.

Prepare Anticoagulant Sodium Citrate Solution as follows: 40 grams of Sodium Citrate (dihydrate) and a sufficient quantity of Water for Injection, to make 1000 mL. Dissolve the Sodium Citrate in sufficient Water for Injection to make 1000 mL, and filter until clear. Place the solution in suitable containers, and sterilize.

Note: Anhydrous sodium citrate (35.1 grams) may be used instead of the dihydrate.

Meets the requirements for Identification, pH (6.4–7.5), Bacterial endotoxins, and Injections.

ANTIHEMOPHILIC FACTOR

Description: Antihemophilic Factor USP—White or yellowish powder. On constitution is opalescent with a slight blue tinge or is a yellowish liquid.

USP requirements:

Antihemophilic Factor USP—Preserve in hermetic containers, in a refrigerator, unless otherwise indicated. A sterile, freeze-dried powder containing the Factor VIII fraction prepared from units of human venous plasma that have been tested for the absence of hepatitis B surface antigen, obtained from whole-blood donors and pooled. May contain Heparin Sodium or Sodium Citrate. Label it to state that it is to be used within 4 hours after constitution, that it is for intravenous administration, and that a filter is to be used in the administration equipment. Meets the requirements of the test for potency, by comparison with the U.S. Standard Antihemophilic Factor (Factor VIII) or with a working reference that has been calibrated with it, in containing ±20% of the potency stated on the label, the stated potency being not less than 100 Antihemophilic Factor Units per gram of protein. Meets the requirements of the test for Pyrogen, the test dose being 10 Antihemophilic Factor Units per kg, and for Expiration date (not later than 2 years from date of manufacture, within which time it may be stored at room temperature and used within 6 months of the time of such storage). Conforms to the regulations of the U.S. Food and Drug Administration concerning biologics.

Antihemophilic Factor (Porcine) for Injection—Not in USP.

Antihemophilic Factor (Recombinant) for Injection—Not in USP.

CRYOPRECIPITATED ANTIHEMOPHILIC FACTOR

Description: Cryoprecipitated Antihemophilic Factor USP—Yellowish frozen solid. On thawing becomes a very viscous, yellow, gummy liquid.

USP requirements: Cryoprecipitated Antihemophilic Factor USP—Preserve in hermetic containers at a temperature of −18 °C or lower. A sterile, frozen concentrate of human antihemophilic factor prepared from the Factor VIII–rich cryoprotein fraction of human venous plasma obtained from suitable whole-blood donors from a single unit of plasma derived from whole blood or by plasmapheresis, collected and processed in a closed system. Contains no preservative. Label it to indicate the ABO blood group designation and the identification number of the donor from whom the source material was obtained. Label it also with the type and result of a serologic test for syphilis, or to indicate that it was nonreactive in such test; with the type and result of a test for hepatitis B surface antigen, or to indicate that it was nonreactive in such test; with a warning not to use it if there is evidence of breakage or thawing; with instructions to thaw it before use to a temperature between 20 and 37 °C, after which it is to be stored at room temperature and used as soon as possible but within 6 hours after thawing; to state that it is to be used within 4 hours after the container is entered; and to state that it is for intravenous administration, and that a filter is to be used in the administration equipment. Meets the requirements of the test for potency by comparison with the U.S. Standard Antihemophilic Factor (Factor VIII) or with a working reference that has been calibrated with it, in having an average potency of not less than 80 Antihemophilic Factor Units per container, made at intervals of not more than 1 month during the dating period. Meets the requirement for Expiration date (not later than 1 year from the date of collection of source material). Conforms to the regulations of the U.S. Food and Drug Administration concerning biologics.

ANTIMONY

Chemical name:
Antimony potassium tartrate—Antimonate(2-), bis[mu-[2,3-dihydroxybutanedioato(4-)-O^1,O^2:O^3,O^4]]-di-, dipotassium, trihydrate, stereoisomer.
Antimony sodium tartrate—Antimonate(2-), bis[mu-[2,3-dihydroxybutanedioato(4-)-O^1,O^2:O^3,O^4]]di-, disodium, stereoisomer.

Molecular formula:
Antimony potassium tartrate—$C_8H_4K_2O_{12}Sb_2 \cdot 3H_2O$.
Antimony sodium tartrate—$C_8H_4Na_2O_{12}Sb_2$.

Molecular weight:
Antimony potassium tartrate—667.85.
Antimony sodium tartrate—581.59.

Description:
Antimony Potassium Tartrate USP—Colorless, odorless, transparent crystals, or white powder. The crystals effloresce upon exposure to air and do not readily rehydrate even on exposure to high humidity. Its solutions are acid to litmus.
Antimony Sodium Tartrate USP—Colorless, odorless, transparent crystals, or white powder. The crystals effloresce upon exposure to air.

Solubility:
Antimony Potassium Tartrate USP—Freely soluble in boiling water; soluble in water and in glycerin; insoluble in alcohol.
Antimony Sodium Tartrate USP—Freely soluble in water; insoluble in alcohol.

USP requirements:
Antimony Potassium Tartrate USP—Preserve in well-closed containers. Contains not less than 99.0% and not more than 103.0% of antimony potassium tartrate. Meets the requirements for Completeness of solution, Identification, Lead (not more than 0.002%), Acidity or alkalinity, Loss on drying (not more than 2.7%), and Arsenic (not more than 0.015%).
Antimony Sodium Tartrate USP—Preserve in well-closed containers. Contains not less than 98.0% and not more than 101.0% of antimony sodium tartrate, calculated on the dried basis. Meets the requirements for Identification, Acidity or alkalinity, Loss on drying (not more than 6.0%), Arsenic (not more than 8 ppm), and Lead (not more than 0.002%).

ANTIPYRINE

Chemical name: 1,2-Dihydro-1,5-dimethyl-2-phenyl-3*H*-pyrazol-3-one.

Molecular formula: $C_{11}H_{12}N_2O$.

Molecular weight: 188.23.

Description: Antipyrine USP—Colorless crystals, or white, crystalline powder. Is odorless. Its solutions are neutral to litmus.

Solubility: Antipyrine USP—Very soluble in water; freely soluble in alcohol and in chloroform; sparingly soluble in ether.

USP requirements: Antipyrine USP—Preserve in tight containers. Contains not less than 99.0% and not more than 100.5% of antipyrine, calculated on the dried basis. Meets the requirements for Completeness and color of solution, Identification, Melting range (110–112.5 °C), Loss on drying (not more than 1.0%), Residue on ignition (not more than 0.15%), Heavy metals (not more than 0.002%), and Ordinary impurities.

ANTIPYRINE AND BENZOCAINE

For *Antipyrine* and *Benzocaine*—See individual listings for chemistry information.

USP requirements: Antipyrine and Benzocaine Otic Solution USP—Preserve in tight, light-resistant containers. A solution of Antipyrine and Benzocaine in Glycerin. Contains the labeled amounts, within ±10%. Meets the requirements for Identification and Water (not more than 1.0%).
Note: In the preparation of this Otic Solution, use Glycerin that has a low water content, in order that the Otic Solution may comply with the *Water* limit. This may be ensured by using Glycerin having a specific gravity of not less than 1.2607, corresponding to a concentration of 99.5%.

ANTIPYRINE, BENZOCAINE, AND PHENYLEPHRINE

For *Antipyrine, Benzocaine,* and *Phenylephrine*—See individual listings for chemistry information.

USP requirements: Antipyrine, Benzocaine, and Phenylephrine Hydrochloride Otic Solution USP—Preserve in tight, light-resistant containers. A solution of Antipyrine, Benzocaine, and Phenylephrine Hydrochloride in a suitable nonaqueous solvent. Contains the labeled amounts, within ±10%. Meets the requirement for Identification.

ANTIRABIES SERUM

Description: Antirabies Serum USP—Transparent or slightly opalescent liquid, faint brownish, yellowish, or greenish in color, and practically odorless or having a slight odor because of the antimicrobial agent.

USP requirements: Antirabies Serum USP—Preserve at a temperature between 2 and 8 °C. A sterile, non-pyrogenic solution containing antiviral substances obtained from the blood serum or plasma of a healthy animal, usually the horse, that has been immunized against rabies by means of vaccine. Its potency is determined in mice using the Serum Neutralization Test (SNT) or, in cell culture using the Rapid Fluorescent Focus Inhibition Test (RFFIT) in comparison with the U.S. Standard Rabies Immune Globulin. The CVS strain of rabies virus (mouse-adapted or cell culture adapted) is used as the challenge strain. Label it to indicate the species of animal in which it was prepared. Contains a suitable antimicrobial agent. Meets the requirement for Expiration date (not later than 2 years after date of issue from manufacturer's cold storage [5 °C, 1 year; or 0 °C, 2 years]). Conforms to the regulations of the U.S. Food and Drug Administration concerning biologics.

ANTITHROMBIN III (HUMAN)

Source: Obtained from human plasma.

Chemical group: A glycoprotein.

Molecular weight: 58,000.

Description: Sterile, white powder.

Other characteristics: Antithrombin III (Human) for Injection—Has a pH of 6.5–7.5 after reconstitution.

USP requirements: Antithrombin III (Human) for Injection—Not in USP.

ANTIVENIN (CROTALIDAE) POLYVALENT

Description: Antivenin (Crotalidae) Polyvalent USP—Solid exhibiting the characteristic structure of a freeze-dried solid; light cream in color.

USP requirements: Antivenin (Crotalidae) Polyvalent USP—Preserve in single-dose containers, and avoid exposure to excessive heat. A sterile, non-pyrogenic preparation derived by drying a frozen solution of specific venom-neutralizing globulins obtained from the serum of healthy horses immunized against venoms of four species of pit vipers, *Crotalus atrox, Crotalus adamanteus, Crotalus durissus terrificus,* and *Bothrops atrox* (Fam. Crotalidae). It is standardized by biological assay on mice, in terms of one dose of antivenin neutralizing the venoms in not less than the number of mouse LD_{50} stated, of *Crotalus atrox* (Western diamondback), 180; *Crotalus durissus terrificus* (South American rattlesnake), 1320; and *Bothrops atrox* (South American fer de lance), 780. Label it to indicate the species of snakes against which the Antivenin is to be used, and to state that it was prepared from horse serum. When constituted as specified in the labeling, it is opalescent and contains not more than 20.0% of solids, determined by drying 1 mL at 105 °C to constant weight (±1 mg). Meets the requirements for general safety and Expiration date (for Antivenin containing a 10% excess of potency, not more than 5 years after date of issue from manufacturer's cold storage [5 °C, 1 year; or 0 °C, 2 years]). Conforms to the regulations of the U.S. Food and Drug Administration concerning biologics.

ANTIVENIN (LATRODECTUS MACTANS)

USP requirements: Antivenin (Latrodectus mactans) USP—Preserve in single-dose containers, and avoid exposure to excessive heat. The sterile, non-pyrogenic preparation derived by drying a frozen solution of specific venom-neutralizing globulins obtained from the serum of healthy horses immunized against venom of black widow spiders (*Latrodectus mactans*). It is standardized by biological assay on mice, in terms of one dose of antivenin neutralizing the venom of *Latrodectus mactans* in not less than 6000 mouse LD_{50}. Label it to indicate the species of spider against which the Antivenin is to be used, that it is not intended to protect against bites from other spider species, and to state that it was prepared in the horse. Thimerosal 1:10,000 is added as a preservative. When constituted as specified in the labeling, it is opalescent and contains not more than 20.0% of solids. Meets the requirement for Expiration date (for Antivenin containing a 10% excess of potency, not more than 5 years after date of issue from manufacturer's cold storage [5 °C, 1 year; or 0 °C, 2 years]). Conforms to the regulations of the U.S. Food and Drug Administration concerning biologics.

ANTIVENIN (MICRURUS FULVIUS)

Description: Antivenin (Micrurus Fulvius) USP—Solid exhibiting the characteristic structure of a freeze-dried solid; light cream in color.

USP requirements: Antivenin (Micrurus Fulvius) USP—Preserve in single-dose containers, and avoid exposure to excessive heat. The sterile, non-pyrogenic preparation derived by drying a frozen solution of specific venom-neutralizing globulins obtained from the serum of healthy horses immunized against venom of the Eastern Coral snake (*Micrurus fulvius*). It is standardized by biological assay on mice, in terms of one dose of antivenin neutralizing the venom of *Micrurus fulvius* in not less than 250 mouse LD_{50}. Label it to indicate the species of snake against which the Antivenin is to be used, and to state that it was prepared in the horse. When constituted as specified in the labeling, it is opalescent and contains not more than 20.0% of solids, determined by drying 1 mL at 105 °C to constant weight (±1 mg). Meets the requirements for general safety and Expiration date (for Antivenin containing a 10% excess of potency, not more than 5 years after date of issue from manufacturer's cold storage [5 °C, 1 year; or 0 °C, 2 years]). Conforms to the regulations of the U.S. Food and Drug Administration concerning biologics.

APOMORPHINE

Chemical name: Apomorphine hydrochloride—4*H*-Dibenzo-[*de,g*]quinoline-10,11-diol, 5,6,6a,7-tetrahydro-6-methyl-, hydrochloride, hemihydrate, (*R*)-.

Molecular formula: Apomorphine hydrochloride—$C_{17}H_{17}NO_2 \cdot HCl \cdot \frac{1}{2}H_2O$.

Molecular weight: Apomorphine hydrochloride—312.80.

Description: Apomorphine Hydrochloride USP—Minute, white or grayish white, glistening crystals or white powder. Is odorless. It gradually acquires a green color on exposure to light and to air. Its solutions are neutral to litmus.

Solubility: Apomorphine Hydrochloride USP—Sparingly soluble in water and in alcohol; soluble in water at 80 °C; very slightly soluble in chloroform and in ether.

USP requirements:

Apomorphine Hydrochloride USP—Preserve in small, tight, light-resistant containers. Containers from which Apomorphine Hydrochloride is to be taken for immediate use in compounding prescriptions contain not more than 350 mg. Contains not less than 98.5% and not more than 100.5% of apomorphine hydrochloride, calculated on the dried basis. Meets the requirements for Color of solution, Identification, Specific rotation (−60.5° to −63.0°, calculated on the dried basis), Loss on drying (2.0–3.5%), Residue on ignition (not more than 0.1%), Decomposition products, and Ordinary impurities.

Apomorphine Hydrochloride Tablets USP—Preserve in tight, light-resistant containers. Contain the labeled amount, within ±10%. Meet the requirements for Color of solution, Identification, Disintegration (15 minutes), and Uniformity of dosage units.

APRACLONIDINE

Chemical name: Apraclonidine hydrochloride—1,4-Benzenediamine, 2,6-dichloro-N^1-2-imidazolidinylidene-, monohydrochloride.

Molecular formula: Apraclonidine hydrochloride—$C_9H_{10}Cl_2N_4 \cdot HCl$.

Molecular weight: Apraclonidine hydrochloride—281.57.

Description: Apraclonidine Hydrochloride USP—White to off-white, odorless to practically odorless powder.

pKa: Apraclonidine hydrochloride—9.22.

Solubility: Apraclonidine Hydrochloride USP—Soluble in methanol; sparingly soluble in water and in alcohol; insoluble in chloroform, in ethyl acetate, and in hexanes.

USP requirements:
Apraclonidine Ophthalmic Solution USP—Preserve in tight, light-resistant containers. A sterile, aqueous solution of Apraclonidine Hydrochloride. Contains an amount of apraclonidine hydrochloride equivalent to the labeled amount of apraclonidine, within −10% to +15%. Meets the requirements for Identification, Sterility, and pH (4.4–7.8).
Apraclonidine Hydrochloride USP—Preserve in tight, light-resistant containers. Contains not less than 98.0% and not more than 102.0% of apraclonidine hydrochloride, calculated on the dried basis. Meets the requirements for Identification, pH (5.0–7.0, in a solution [1 in 100]), Loss on drying (not more than 1.0%), Residue on ignition (not more than 0.1%), Heavy metals (not more than 0.002%), and Chromatographic purity.

APROBARBITAL

Chemical name: 5-Allyl-5-isopropylbarbituric acid.

Molecular formula: $C_{10}H_{14}N_2O_3$.

Molecular weight: 210.23.

Description: White crystalline powder.

Solubility: Slightly soluble in water; soluble in alcohol.

USP requirements: Aprobarbital Elixir—Not in USP.

APROTININ

Source: Single-chain polypeptide derived from bovine tissues, consisting of 58 amino-acid residues.

Chemical name: Trypsin inhibitor, pancreatic basic.

Molecular formula: $C_{284}H_{432}N_{84}O_{79}S_7$.

Molecular weight: 6511.49.

Description: A clear colorless solution or an almost white hygroscopic powder.

Solubility: The solid is soluble in water and in solutions isotonic with blood; practically insoluble in organic solvents.

USP requirements: Aprotinin Injection—Not in USP.

ARGININE

Chemical name:
Arginine—L-Arginine.
Arginine hydrochloride—L-Arginine monohydrochloride.

Molecular formula:
Arginine—$C_6H_{14}N_4O_2$.
Arginine hydrochloride—$C_6H_{14}N_4O_2 \cdot HCl$.

Molecular weight:
Arginine—174.20.
Arginine hydrochloride—210.66.

Description:
Arginine USP—White, practically odorless crystals.
Arginine Hydrochloride USP—White crystals or crystalline powder, practically odorless.

Solubility:
Arginine USP—Freely soluble in water; sparingly soluble in alcohol; insoluble in ether.
Arginine Hydrochloride USP—Freely soluble in water.

USP requirements:
Arginine USP—Preserve in well-closed containers. Contains not less than 98.5% and not more than 101.5% of arginine, as L-arginine, calculated on the dried basis. Meets the requirements for Identification, Specific rotation (+26.2° to +27.6°, calculated on the dried basis), Loss on drying (not more than 0.5%), Residue on ignition (not more than 0.3%), Chloride (not more than 0.05%), Sulfate (not more than 0.03%), Arsenic (not more than 1.5 ppm), Iron (not more than 0.003%), Heavy metals (not more than 0.0015%), and Organic volatile impurities.
Arginine Hydrochloride USP—Preserve in well-closed containers. Contains not less than 98.5% and not more than 101.5% of arginine hydrochloride, calculated on the dried basis. Meets the requirements for Identification, Specific rotation (+21.4° to +23.6°, calculated on the dried basis), Loss on drying (not more than 0.2%), Residue on ignition (not more than 0.1%), Sulfate (not more than 0.03%), Arsenic (not more than 1.5 ppm), Chloride content (16.5–17.1%), Heavy metals (not more than 0.002%), and Organic volatile impurities.
Arginine Hydrochloride Injection USP—Preserve in single-dose containers, preferably of Type II glass. A sterile solution of Arginine Hydrochloride in Water for Injection. The label states the total osmolar concentration in mOsmol per liter. Where the contents are less than 100 mL, or where the label states that the Injection is not for direct injection but is to be diluted before use, the label alternatively may state the total osmolar concentration in mOsmol per mL. Contains not less than 9.5% and not more than 10.5% of arginine hydrochloride. Contains no antimicrobial agents. Meets the requirements for Identification, Bacterial endotoxins, pH (5.0–6.5), and Injections.
Note: The chloride ion content of Arginine Hydrochloride Injection is approximately 475 mEq per liter.

AROMATIC ELIXIR

Description: Aromatic Elixir NF—NF category: Flavored and/or sweetened vehicle.

NF requirements: Aromatic Elixir NF—Preserve in tight containers.
Prepare Aromatic Elixir as follows: Suitable essential oil(s), 375 mL of Syrup, 30 grams of Talc, and a sufficient quantity of Alcohol and Purified Water to make 1000 mL. Dissolve the oil(s) in Alcohol to make 250 mL. To this solution add the Syrup in several portions, agitating vigorously after each addition, and afterwards add, in the same manner, the required quantity of Purified Water. Mix the Talc with the liquid, and filter through a filter wetted with Diluted Alcohol, returning the filtrate until a clear liquid is obtained.
Meets the requirements for Alcohol content (21.0–23.0%) and Organic volatile impurities.

ARTICAINE AND EPINEPHRINE

Chemical name:
Articaine hydrochloride—Methyl 4-methyl-3-(2-propylaminopropionamido)thiophene-2-carboxylate hydrochloride.
Epinephrine—1,2-Benzenediol, 4-[1-hydroxy-2-(methylamino)ethyl]-, (*R*)-.

Molecular formula:
Articaine hydrochloride—$C_{13}H_{20}N_2O_3S \cdot HCl$.
Epinephrine—$C_9H_{13}NO_3$.

Molecular weight:
Articaine hydrochloride—320.8.
Epinephrine—183.21.

Description: Epinephrine USP—White to practically white, odorless, microcrystalline powder or granules, gradually darkening on exposure to light and air. With acids, it forms salts that are readily soluble in water, and the base may be recovered by the addition of ammonia water or alkali carbonates. Its solutions are alkaline to litmus.

Solubility: Epinephrine USP—Very slightly soluble in water and in alcohol; insoluble in ether, in chloroform, and in fixed and volatile oils.

USP requirements: Articaine Hydrochloride and Epinephrine Injection—Not in USP.

ASCORBIC ACID

Chemical name: L-Ascorbic acid.

Molecular formula: $C_6H_8O_6$.

Molecular weight: 176.13.

Description: Ascorbic Acid USP—White or slightly yellow crystals or powder. On exposure to light it gradually darkens. In the dry state, is reasonably stable in air, but in solution rapidly oxidizes. Melts at about 190 °C.
NF category: Antioxidant.

pKa: 4.2 and 11.6.

Solubility: Ascorbic Acid USP—Freely soluble in water; sparingly soluble in alcohol; insoluble in chloroform and in ether.

USP requirements:
Ascorbic Acid USP—Preserve in tight, light-resistant containers. Contains not less than 99.0% and not more than 100.5% of ascorbic acid. Meets the requirements for Identification, Specific rotation (+20.5° to +21.5°), Residue on ignition (not more than 0.1%), Heavy metals (not more than 0.002%), and Organic volatile impurities.
Ascorbic Acid Extended-release Capsules—Not in USP.
Ascorbic Acid Injection USP—Preserve in light-resistant, single-dose containers, preferably of Type I or Type II glass. A sterile solution, in Water for Injection, of Ascorbic Acid prepared with the aid of Sodium Hydroxide, Sodium Carbonate, or Sodium Bicarbonate. In addition to meeting the requirements for Labeling under Injections, fused-seal containers of the Injection in concentrations of 250 mg per mL and greater are labeled to indicate that since pressure may develop on long storage, precautions should be taken to wrap the container in a protective covering while it is being opened. Contains the labeled amount, within ±10%. Meets the requirements for Identification, Bacterial endotoxins, pH (5.5–7.0), Oxalate, and Injections.
Ascorbic Acid Oral Solution USP—Preserve in tight, light-resistant containers. A solution of Ascorbic Acid in a hydroxylic organic solvent or an aqueous mixture thereof. Label Oral Solution that contains alcohol to state the alcohol content. Contains the labeled amount, within ±10%. Meets requirements for Identification and Alcohol content (90–110% of the labeled amount).
Ascorbic Acid Syrup—Not in USP.
Ascorbic Acid Tablets USP—Preserve in tight, light-resistant containers. Contain the labeled amount, within ±10%. Meet requirements for Identification, Disintegration (30 minutes), and Uniformity of dosage units.
Ascorbic Acid Effervescent Tablets—Not in USP.
Ascorbic Acid Extended-release Tablets—Not in USP.

ASCORBYL PALMITATE

Chemical name: L-Ascorbic acid, 6-hexadecanoate.

Molecular formula: $C_{22}H_{38}O_7$.

Molecular weight: 414.54.

Description: Ascorbyl Palmitate NF—White to yellowish white powder, having a characteristic odor.
NF category: Antioxidant.

Solubility: Ascorbyl Palmitate NF—Very slightly soluble in water and in vegetable oils; soluble in alcohol.

NF requirements: Ascorbyl Palmitate NF—Preserve in tight containers, in a cool, dry place. Contains not less than 95.0% and not more than 100.5% of ascorbyl palmitate, calculated on the dried basis. Meets the requirements for Identification, Melting range (107–117 °C), Specific rotation (+21° to +24°, calculated on the dried basis), Loss on drying (not more than 2.0%), Residue on ignition (not more than 0.1%), and Heavy metals (not more than 0.001%).

ASPARAGINASE

Source: Commercially available asparaginase is a high molecular weight enzyme derived from *Escherichia coli*.

Chemical name: Asparaginase.

Description: White, crystalline powder; slightly hygroscopic.

Solubility: Freely soluble in water; practically insoluble in methanol, in acetone, and in chloroform.

Other characteristics: Enzyme active at pH 6.5–8.0.

USP requirements: Asparaginase for Injection—Not in USP.

ASPARTAME

Chemical Name: L-Phenylalanine, *N*-L-alpha-aspartyl-, 1-methyl ester.

Molecular formula: $C_{14}H_{18}N_2O_5$.

Molecular weight: 294.31.

Description: Aspartame NF—White, odorless, crystalline powder. Melts at about 246 °C. The pH of an 8 in 1000 solution is about 5.
NF category: Sweetening agent.

Solubility: Aspartame NF—Sparingly soluble in water; slightly soluble in alcohol.

NF requirements: Aspartame NF—Preserve in well-closed containers. Contains not less than 98.0% and not more than 102.0% of aspartame, calculated on the dried basis. Meets the requirements for Identification, Transmittance, Specific rotation (+14.5° to +16.5°, calculated on the dried basis), Loss on drying (not more than 4.5%), Residue on ignition (not more than 0.2%), Arsenic (not more than 3 ppm), Heavy metals (not more than 0.001%), Other related substances, 5-Benzyl-3,6-dioxo-2-piperazineacetic acid, and Organic volatile impurities.

ASPIRIN

Chemical name: Benzoic acid, 2-(acetyloxy)-.

Molecular formula: $C_9H_8O_4$.

Molecular weight: 180.16.

Description: Aspirin USP—White crystals, commonly tabular or needle-like, or white, crystalline powder. Is odorless or has a faint odor. Is stable in dry air; in moist air it gradually hydrolyzes to salicylic and acetic acids.

pKa: 3.5.

Solubility: Aspirin USP—Slightly soluble in water; freely soluble in alcohol; soluble in chloroform and in ether; sparingly soluble in absolute ether.

USP requirements:

Aspirin USP—Preserve in tight containers. Contains not less than 99.5% and not more than 100.5% of aspirin, calculated on the dried basis. Meets the requirements for Identification, Loss on drying (not more than 0.5%), Residue on ignition (not more than 0.05%), Chloride (not more than 0.014%), Sulfate (not more than 0.04%), Non-aspirin salicylates (not more than 0.1%), Heavy metals (not more than 0.001%), Readily carbonizable substances, Substances insoluble in sodium carbonate TS, and Organic volatile impurities.

Aspirin Capsules USP—Preserve in tight containers. Contain the labeled amount, within ±7%. Meet the requirements for Identification, Dissolution (80% in 30 minutes in 0.05 *M* acetate buffer [pH 4.5 ±0.05] in Apparatus 1 at 100 rpm), Uniformity of dosage units, and Free salicylic acid (not more than 0.75%, calculated on the labeled aspirin content).

Note: Capsules that are enteric-coated or the contents of which are enteric-coated meet the requirements for Aspirin Delayed-release Capsules USP.

Aspirin Delayed-release Capsules USP—Preserve in tight containers. The label indicates that Aspirin Delayed-release Capsules or the contents thereof are enteric-coated. Contain the labeled amount, within ±7%. Meet the requirements for Identification, Drug release, Uniformity of dosage units, and Free salicylic acid (not more than 3.0%).

Aspirin Suppositories USP—Preserve in well-closed containers, in a cool place. Contain the labeled amount, within ±10%. Meet the requirements for Identification and Non-aspirin salicylates (not more than 3.0%).

Aspirin Tablets USP—Preserve in tight containers. Preserve flavored or sweetened Tablets of 81-mg size or smaller in containers holding not more than 36 Tablets each. Contain the labeled amount, within ±10%. Tablets of larger than 81-mg size contain no sweeteners or other flavors. Meet the requirements for Identification, Dissolution (80% in 30 minutes in 0.05 *M* acetate buffer [pH 4.5 ±0.05] in Apparatus 1 at 50 rpm), Uniformity of dosage units, and Free salicylic acid (not more than 0.3% for uncoated tablets or not more than 3.0% for coated tablets).

Note: Tablets that are enteric-coated meet the requirements for Aspirin Delayed-release Tablets USP.

Aspirin Chewing Gum Tablets—Not in USP.

Aspirin Delayed-release Tablets USP—Preserve in tight containers. The label indicates that Aspirin Delayed-release Tablets are enteric-coated. Contain the labeled amount, within ±5%. Meet the requirements for Identification, Drug release, Uniformity of dosage units, and Free salicylic acid (not more than 3.0%).

Aspirin Dispersible Tablets—Not in USP.

Aspirin Extended-release Tablets USP—Preserve in tight containers. Label to indicate the Drug release test with which the product complies. Contain the labeled amount, within ±5%. Meet the requirements for Identification, Drug release, Uniformity of dosage units, and Free salicylic acid (not more than 3.0%).

BUFFERED ASPIRIN

Chemical name: Aspirin—Benzoic acid, 2-(acetyloxy)-.

Molecular formula: Aspirin—$C_9H_8O_4$.

Molecular weight: Aspirin—180.16.

Description: Aspirin USP—White crystals, commonly tabular or needle-like, or white, crystalline powder. Is odorless or has a faint odor. Is stable in dry air; in moist air it gradually hydrolyzes to salicylic and acetic acids.

pKa: Aspirin—3.5.

Solubility: Aspirin USP—Slightly soluble in water; freely soluble in alcohol; soluble in chloroform and in ether; sparingly soluble in absolute ether.

USP requirements: Buffered Aspirin Tablets USP—Preserve in tight containers. Contain Aspirin and suitable buffering agents. Contain the labeled amount of aspirin, within ±10%. Meet the requirements for Identification, Dissolution (80% in 30 minutes in 0.05 *M* acetate buffer [pH 4.5 ±0.05] in Apparatus 2 at 75 rpm), Uniformity of dosage units, Acid-neutralizing capacity, and Free salicylic acid limit (not more than 3.0%).

ASPIRIN, ALUMINA, AND MAGNESIA

For *Aspirin, Alumina* (Aluminum Hydroxide), and *Magnesia* (Magnesium Hydroxide)—See individual listings for chemistry information.

USP requirements: Aspirin, Alumina, and Magnesia Tablets USP—Preserve in tight containers. Contain the labeled amount of aspirin, within ±10%, and amounts of alumina and magnesia equivalent to the labeled amounts of aluminum hydroxide and magnesium hydroxide, within ±10%. Meet the requirements for Identification, Dissolution (75% of labeled amount of aspirin in 45 minutes in 0.05 *M* acetate buffer [pH 4.5 ±0.05] in Apparatus 2 at 75 rpm), Uniformity of dosage units, Acid-neutralizing capacity, and Free salicylic acid limit (not more than 3.0%).

ASPIRIN, ALUMINA, AND MAGNESIUM OXIDE

For *Aspirin, Alumina* (Aluminum Hydroxide), and *Magnesium Oxide*—See individual listings for chemistry information.

USP requirements: Aspirin, Alumina, and Magnesium Oxide Tablets USP—Preserve in tight containers. Contain the labeled amounts of aspirin and magnesium oxide, within ±10%, and an amount of alumina equivalent to the labeled amount of aluminum hydroxide, within ±10%. Meet the requirements for Identification, Dissolution (75% of labeled amount of aspirin in 45 minutes in 0.05 *M* acetate buffer [pH 4.5 ±0.05] in Apparatus 2 at 75 rpm), Uniformity of dosage units, Acid-neutralizing capacity, and Free salicylic acid limit (not more than 3.0%).

ASPIRIN AND CAFFEINE

For *Aspirin* and *Caffeine*—See individual listings for chemistry information.

USP requirements:

Aspirin and Caffeine Capsules—Not in USP.

Aspirin and Caffeine Tablets—Not in USP.

BUFFERED ASPIRIN AND CAFFEINE

Source: Caffeine—Coffee, tea, cola, and cocoa or chocolate. May also be synthesized from urea or dimethylurea.

Chemical group: Caffeine—Methylated xanthine.

Chemical name:
Aspirin—Benzoic acid, 2-(acetyloxy)-.
Caffeine—1*H*-Purine-2,6-dione, 3,7-dihydro-1,3,7-trimethyl-.

Molecular formula:
Aspirin—$C_9H_8O_4$.
Caffeine—$C_8H_{10}N_4O_2$ (anhydrous); $C_8H_{10}N_4O_2 \cdot H_2O$ (monohydrate).

Molecular weight:
Aspirin—180.16.
Caffeine—194.19 (anhydrous); 212.21 (monohydrate).

Description:
Aspirin USP—White crystals, commonly tabular or needle-like, or white, crystalline powder. Is odorless or has a faint odor. Is stable in dry air; in moist air it gradually hydrolyzes to salicylic and acetic acids.
Caffeine USP—White powder or white, glistening needles, usually matted together. Is odorless. Its solutions are neutral to litmus. The hydrate is efflorescent in air.

pKa: Aspirin—3.5.

Solubility:
Aspirin USP—Slightly soluble in water; freely soluble in alcohol; soluble in chloroform and in ether; sparingly soluble in absolute ether.
Caffeine USP—Sparingly soluble in water and in alcohol; freely soluble in chloroform; slightly soluble in ether.
The aqueous solubility of caffeine is increased by organic acids or their alkali salts, such as citrates, benzoates, salicylates, or cinnamates, which dissociate to yield caffeine when dissolved in biological fluids.

USP requirements: Buffered Aspirin and Caffeine Tablets—Not in USP.

ASPIRIN, CAFFEINE, AND DIHYDROCODEINE

For *Aspirin, Caffeine,* and *Dihydrocodeine*—See individual listings for chemistry information.

USP requirements: Aspirin, Caffeine, and Dihydrocodeine Bitartrate Capsules USP—Preserve in tight containers. Contain the labeled amounts, within ±10%. Meet the requirements for Identification, Dissolution (75% of each active ingredient in 45 minutes in 0.05 *M* acetate buffer [pH 4.50 ±0.05] in Apparatus 1 at 50 rpm), Uniformity of dosage units, and Limit of salicylic acid (not more than 3.0%).

ASPIRIN AND CODEINE

For *Aspirin* and *Codeine*—See individual listings for chemistry information.

USP requirements: Aspirin and Codeine Phosphate Tablets USP—Preserve in well-closed, light-resistant containers. Contain the labeled amounts of aspirin and codeine phosphate hemihydrate, within ±10%. Meet the requirements for Identification, Dissolution (75% of each active ingredient in 30 minutes in 0.05 *M* acetate buffer [pH 4.5 ±0.05] in Apparatus 2 at 75 rpm), Uniformity of dosage units, and Limit of free salicylic acid (not more than 3.0%).

ASPIRIN, CODEINE, ALUMINA, AND MAGNESIA

For *Aspirin, Codeine, Alumina* (Aluminum Hydroxide), and *Magnesia* (Magnesium Hydroxide)—See individual listings for chemistry information.

USP requirements: Aspirin, Codeine Phosphate, Alumina, and Magnesia Tablets USP—Preserve in well-closed, light-resistant containers. Contain the labeled amounts of aspirin and codeine phosphate hemihydrate, within ±10%, and amounts of alumina and magnesia equivalent to the labeled amounts of aluminum hydroxide and magnesium hydroxide, within ±10%. Meets the requirements for Identification, Dissolution (75% of the labeled amounts of aspirin and codeine phosphate hemihydrate in 30 minutes in 0.05 *M* acetate buffer [pH 4.50 ±0.05] in Apparatus 2 at 75 rpm), Uniformity of dosage units, Acid-neutralizing capacity, and Limit of free salicylic acid (not more than 3.0%).

ASPIRIN, CODEINE, AND CAFFEINE

For *Aspirin, Codeine,* and *Caffeine*—See individual listings for chemistry information.

USP requirements:
Aspirin, Codeine Phosphate, and Caffeine Capsules USP—Preserve in well-closed, light-resistant containers. Contain the labeled amounts of aspirin, codeine phosphate hemihydrate, and caffeine, within ±10%. Meet the requirements for Identification, Uniformity of dosage units, and Salicylic acid (not more than 3.0%).
Aspirin, Codeine Phosphate, and Caffeine Tablets USP—Preserve in well-closed, light-resistant containers. Contain the labeled amounts of aspirin, codeine phosphate hemihydrate, and caffeine, within ±10%. Meet the requirements for Identification, Uniformity of dosage units, and Salicylic acid (not more than 3.0%).

ASPIRIN, CODEINE, CAFFEINE, ALUMINA, AND MAGNESIA

For *Aspirin, Codeine, Caffeine, Alumina* (Aluminum Hydroxide), and *Magnesia* (Magnesium Hydroxide)—See individual listings for chemistry information.

USP requirements: Aspirin, Codeine Phosphate, Caffeine, Alumina, and Magnesia Tablets—Not in USP.

ASPIRIN, SODIUM BICARBONATE, AND CITRIC ACID

For *Aspirin, Sodium Bicarbonate,* and *Citric Acid*—See individual listings for chemistry information.

USP requirements: Aspirin Effervescent Tablets for Oral Solution USP—Preserve in tight containers. Contain Aspirin and an effervescent mixture of a suitable organic acid and an alkali metal bicarbonate and/or carbonate. Contain the labeled amount of aspirin, within ±10%. Meet the requirements for Identification, Solution time (within 5 minutes in water at 17.5 ±2.5 °C), Uniformity of dosage units, Acid-neutralizing capacity, and Free salicylate (not more than 8.0%).

ASTEMIZOLE

Chemical name: 1*H*-Benzimidazol-2-amine, 1-[(4-fluorophenyl)-methyl]-*N*-[1-[2-(4-methoxyphenyl)ethyl]-4-piperidinyl]-.

Molecular formula: $C_{28}H_{31}FN_4O$.

Molecular weight: 458.58.

Description: White to almost white powder. It has a melting point of 173–177 °C.

Solubility: Insoluble in water; soluble in chloroform and in methanol; slightly soluble in ethanol.

USP requirements:
Astemizole Oral Suspension—Not in USP.
Astemizole Tablets—Not in USP.

ATENOLOL

Chemical name: Benzeneacetamide, 4-[2-hydroxy-3-[(1-methylethyl)amino]propoxy]-.

Molecular formula: $C_{14}H_{22}N_2O_3$.

Molecular weight: 266.34.

Description: White or almost white powder. Melting point 152–155 °C.

Solubility: Sparingly soluble in water; soluble in dehydrated alcohol; slightly soluble in methylene chloride; practically insoluble in ether.

Other characteristics: Lipid solubility—Very low (log partition coefficient for octanol/water is 0.23).

USP requirements:
Atenolol Injection—Not in USP.
Atenolol Tablets—Not in USP.

ATENOLOL AND CHLORTHALIDONE

For *Atenolol* and *Chlorthalidone*—See individual listings for chemistry information.

USP requirements: Atenolol and Chlorthalidone Tablets—Not in USP.

ATOVAQUONE

Chemical name: 1,4-Naphthalenedione, 2-[4-(4-chlorophenyl)-cyclohexyl]-3-hydroxy-, *trans*-.

Molecular formula: $C_{22}H_{19}ClO_3$.

Molecular weight: 366.84.

Description: Yellow crystalline solid.

Solubility: Practically insoluble in water.

USP requirements: Atovaquone Tablets—Not in USP.

ATRACURIUM

Chemical name: Atracurium besylate—Isoquinolinium, 2,2′-[1,5-pentanediylbis[oxy(3-oxo-3,1-propanediyl)]]bis[1-[(3,4-dimethoxyphenyl)methyl]-1,2,3,4-tetrahydro-6,7-dimethoxy-2-methyl-, dibenzenesulfonate.

Molecular formula: Atracurium besylate—$C_{65}H_{82}N_2O_{18}S_2$.

Molecular weight: Atracurium besylate—1243.49.

Description: Atracurium besylate injection—Sterile, non-pyrogenic aqueous solution. The pH is adjusted to 3.25–3.65 with benzenesulfonic acid.

USP requirements: Atracurium Besylate Injection—Not in USP.

ATROPINE

Source: An alkaloid that may be extracted from belladonna root and hyoscyamine or may be produced synthetically.

Chemical group: Natural tertiary amine.

Chemical name:
Atropine—Benzeneacetic acid, alpha-(hydroxymethyl)-8-methyl-8-azabicyclo[3.2.1]oct-3-yl ester, *endo*-(±)-.
Atropine sulfate—Benzeneacetic acid, alpha-(hydroxymethyl)-, 8-methyl-8-azabicyclo[3.2.1]oct-3-yl ester, *endo*-(±)-, sulfate (2:1) (salt), monohydrate.

Molecular formula:
Atropine—$C_{17}H_{23}NO_3$.
Atropine sulfate—$(C_{17}H_{23}NO_3)_2 \cdot H_2SO_4 \cdot H_2O$.

Molecular weight:
Atropine—289.37.
Atropine sulfate—694.84.

Description:
Atropine USP—White crystals, usually needle-like, or white, crystalline powder. Its saturated solution is alkaline to phenolphthalein TS. Is optically inactive, but usually contains some levorotatory hyoscyamine.
Atropine Sulfate USP—Colorless crystals, or white, crystalline powder. Odorless; effloresces in dry air; is slowly affected by light.

Solubility:
Atropine USP—Slightly soluble in water, and sparingly soluble in water at 80 °C; freely soluble in alcohol and in chloroform; soluble in glycerin and in ether.
Atropine Sulfate USP—Very soluble in water; freely soluble in alcohol and even more so in boiling alcohol; freely soluble in glycerin.

USP requirements:
Atropine USP—Preserve in tight, light-resistant containers. Contains not less than 99.0% and not more than 100.5% of atropine, calculated on the anhydrous basis. Meets the requirements for Identification, Melting range (114–118 °C), Optical rotation (−0.70° to +0.05° [limit of hyoscyamine]), Water (not more than 0.2%), Residue on ignition (not more than 0.1%), Readily carbonizable substances, Foreign alkaloids and other impurities, and Organic volatile impurities.

Caution: Handle Atropine with exceptional care, since it is highly potent.

Atropine Sulfate USP—Preserve in tight containers. Contains not less than 98.5% and not more than 101.0% of atropine sulfate, calculated on the anhydrous basis. Meets the requirements for Identification, Melting temperature (not lower than 187 °C, determined after drying at 120 °C for 4 hours), Optical rotation (−0.60° to +0.05° [limit of hyoscyamine]), Acidity, Water (not more than 4.0%), Residue on ignition (not more than 0.2%), Other alkaloids, and Organic volatile impurities.

Caution: Handle Atropine Sulfate with exceptional care, since it is highly potent.

Atropine Sulfate Injection USP—Preserve in single-dose or in multiple-dose containers, preferably of Type I glass. A sterile solution of Atropine Sulfate in Water for Injection. Contains the labeled amount, within ±7%. Meets the requirements for Identification, Bacterial endotoxins, pH (3.0–6.5), and Injections.

Atropine Sulfate Ophthalmic Ointment USP—Preserve in collapsible ophthalmic ointment tubes. It is Atropine Sulfate in a suitable ophthalmic ointment base. Contains the labeled amount, within ±10%. It is sterile. Meets the requirements for Identification, Sterility, and Metal particles.

Atropine Sulfate Ophthalmic Solution USP—Preserve in tight containers. A sterile, aqueous solution of Atropine Sulfate. Contains the labeled amount, within ±7%. Meets the requirements for Identification, Sterility, and pH (3.5–6.0).

Atropine Sulfate Tablets USP—Preserve in well-closed containers. Contain the labeled amount, within ±10%. Meet the requirements for Identification, Disintegration (15 minutes), and Uniformity of dosage units.
Atropine Sulfate Soluble Tablets—Not in USP.

ATROPINE, HYOSCYAMINE, METHENAMINE, METHYLENE BLUE, PHENYL SALICYLATE, AND BENZOIC ACID

Chemical name:
Atropine sulfate—Benzeneacetic acid, alpha-(hydroxymethyl)-, 8-methyl-8-azabicyclo[3.2.1]oct-3-yl ester, *endo*-(±)-, sulfate (2:1) (salt), monohydrate.
Hyoscyamine—Benzeneacetic acid, alpha-(hydroxymethyl)-, 8-methyl-8-azabicyclo[3.2.1]oct-3-yl ester, [3(*S*)-*endo*]-.
Methenamine—1,3,5,7-Tetraazatricyclo[3.3.1.1^{3,7}]decane.
Methylene blue—Phenothiazin-5-ium, 3,7-bis(dimethylamino)-, chloride, trihydrate.
Phenyl salicylate—2-Hydroxybenzoic acid phenyl ester.
Benzoic acid—Benzoic acid.

Molecular formula:
Atropine sulfate—$(C_{17}H_{23}NO_3)_2 \cdot H_2SO_4 \cdot H_2O$.
Hyoscyamine—$C_{17}H_{23}NO_3$.
Methenamine—$C_6H_{12}N_4$.
Methylene blue—$C_{16}H_{18}ClN_3S \cdot 3H_2O$.
Phenyl salicylate—$C_{13}H_{10}O_3$.
Benzoic acid—$C_7H_6O_2$.

Molecular weight:
Atropine sulfate—694.84.
Hyoscyamine—289.37.
Methenamine—140.19.
Methylene blue—373.90.
Phenyl salicylate—214.21.
Benzoic acid—122.12.

Description:
Atropine Sulfate USP—Colorless crystals, or white, crystalline powder. Odorless; effloresces in dry air; is slowly affected by light.
Hyoscyamine USP—White, crystalline powder. Is affected by light. Its solutions are alkaline to litmus.
Methenamine USP—Colorless, lustrous crystals or white, crystalline powder. Is practically odorless. When brought into contact with fire, it readily ignites, burning with a smokeless flame. It sublimes at about 260 °C, without melting. Its solutions are alkaline to litmus.
Methylene Blue USP—Dark green crystals or crystalline powder having a bronze-like luster. Is odorless or practically so, and is stable in air. Its solutions in water and in alcohol are deep blue in color.
Phenyl salicylate—White crystals with a melting point of 40–43 °C.
Benzoic Acid USP—White crystals, scales, or needles. Has a slight odor, usually suggesting benzaldehyde or benzoin. Somewhat volatile at moderately warm temperatures. Freely volatile in steam.
NF category: Antimicrobial preservative.

Solubility:
Atropine Sulfate USP—Very soluble in water; freely soluble in alcohol and even more so in boiling alcohol; freely soluble in glycerin.
Hyoscyamine USP—Slightly soluble in water; freely soluble in alcohol, in chloroform, and in dilute acids; sparingly soluble in ether.
Methenamine USP—Freely soluble in water; soluble in alcohol and in chloroform.
Methylene Blue USP—Soluble in water and in chloroform; sparingly soluble in alcohol.
Phenyl salicylate—Very slightly soluble in water; freely soluble in alcohol.
Benzoic Acid USP—Slightly soluble in water; freely soluble in alcohol, in chloroform, and in ether.

USP requirements: Atropine Sulfate, Hyoscyamine, Methenamine, Methylene Blue, Phenyl Salicylate, and Benzoic Acid Tablets—Not in USP.

ATROPINE, HYOSCYAMINE, SCOPOLAMINE, AND PHENOBARBITAL

For *Atropine, Hyoscyamine, Scopolamine,* and *Phenobarbital*—See individual listings for chemistry information.

USP requirements:
Atropine Sulfate, Hyoscyamine Sulfate (or Hyoscyamine Hydrobromide), Scopolamine Hydrobromide, and Phenobarbital Capsules—Not in USP.
Atropine Sulfate, Hyoscyamine Sulfate (or Hyoscyamine Hydrobromide), Scopolamine Hydrobromide, and Phenobarbital Elixir—Not in USP.
Atropine Sulfate, Hyoscyamine Sulfate (or Hyoscyamine Hydrobromide), Scopolamine Hydrobromide, and Phenobarbital Tablets—Not in USP.
Atropine Sulfate, Hyoscyamine Sulfate, Scopolamine Hydrobromide, and Phenobarbital Chewable Tablets—Not in USP.
Atropine Sulfate, Hyoscyamine Sulfate, Scopolamine Hydrobromide, and Phenobarbital Extended-release Tablets—Not in USP.

ATROPINE AND PHENOBARBITAL

For *Atropine* and *Phenobarbital*—See individual listings for chemistry information.

USP requirements:
Atropine Sulfate and Phenobarbital Capsules—Not in USP.
Atropine Sulfate and Phenobarbital Elixir—Not in USP.
Atropine Sulfate and Phenobarbital Tablets—Not in USP.

ATTAPULGITE

Description:
Activated Attapulgite USP—Cream-colored, micronized, non-swelling powder, free from gritty particles. The high heat treatment used in its preparation causes it to yield only moderately viscous aqueous suspensions, its dispersion consisting mainly of particle groups.
NF category: Suspending and/or viscosity-increasing agent.
Colloidal Activated Attapulgite USP—Cream-colored, micronized, non-swelling powder, free from gritty particles. Yields viscous aqueous suspensions, as a result of dispersion into its constituent ultimate particles.
NF category: Suspending and/or viscosity-increasing agent.

Solubility:
Activated Attapulgite USP—Insoluble in water.
Colloidal Activated Attapulgite USP—Insoluble in water.

USP requirements:
Activated Attapulgite USP—Preserve in well-closed containers. A highly heat-treated, processed, native magnesium aluminum silicate. Meets the requirements for Identification, Loss on drying (not more than 4.0%), Volatile matter (3.0–7.5%, on the dried basis), Loss on ignition (4.0–12.0%), Acid-soluble matter (not more than 25%), and Powder fineness, and for Microbial limit, pH, Carbonate, Arsenic and Lead, and Adsorptive capacity under Colloidal Activated Attapulgite.

Colloidal Activated Attapulgite USP—Preserve in well-closed containers. A purified native magnesium aluminum silicate. Meets the requirements for Identification, Microbial limit, pH (7.0–9.5), Loss on drying (5.0–17.0%), Volatile matter (7.5–12.5%, on the dried basis), Loss on ignition (17.0–27.0%), Acid-soluble matter (not more than 15%), Carbonate, Arsenic and Lead (not more than 2 ppm for arsenic and not more than 0.001% for lead), Powder fineness, and Adsorptive capacity.

Attapulgite Oral Suspension—Not in USP.

Attapulgite Tablets—Not in USP.

Attapulgite Chewable Tablets—Not in USP.

AURANOFIN

Chemical name: Gold, (2,3,4,6-tetra-*O*-acetyl-1-thio-beta-D-glucopyranosato-*S*)(triethylphosphine)-.

Molecular formula: $C_{20}H_{34}AuO_9PS$.

Molecular weight: 678.48.

Description: White, odorless, crystalline powder.

Solubility: Very slightly soluble in water; soluble in alcohol.

USP requirements: Auranofin Capsules—Not in USP.

AUROTHIOGLUCOSE

Chemical name: Gold, (1-thio-D-glucopyranosato)-.

Molecular formula: $C_6H_{11}AuO_5S$.

Molecular weight: 392.18.

Description: Aurothioglucose USP—Yellow, odorless or practically odorless powder. Is stable in air. An aqueous solution is unstable on long standing. The pH of its 1 in 100 solution is about 6.3.

Solubility: Aurothioglucose USP—Freely soluble in water; practically insoluble in acetone, in alcohol, in chloroform, and in ether.

USP requirements:

Aurothioglucose USP—Preserve in tight, light-resistant containers. Contains not less than 95.0% and not more than 105.0% of aurothioglucose, calculated on the dried basis. It is stabilized by the addition of a small amount of Sodium Acetate. Meets the requirements for Identification, Specific rotation (+65° to +75°, calculated on the dried basis), and Loss on drying (not more than 1.0%).

Sterile Aurothioglucose Suspension USP—Preserve in single-dose or in multiple-dose containers, preferably of Type I glass. Protect from light. A sterile suspension of Aurothioglucose in a suitable vegetable oil. Contains the labeled amount, within ±10%. Meets the requirements for Identification and Injections.

AZAPERONE

Chemical name: 1-Butanone, 1-(4-fluorophenyl)-4-[4-(2-pyridinyl)-1-piperazinyl]-.

Molecular formula: $C_{19}H_{22}FN_3O$.

Molecular weight: 327.40.

Description: White to yellowish-white microcrystalline powder. Melting point 90–95 °C.

Solubility: Practically insoluble in water; soluble 1 in 29 of alcohol, 1 in 4 of chloroform, and 1 in 31 of ether.

USP requirements:

Azaperone USP—Preserve in well-closed containers, protected from light. Label it to indicate that it is for veterinary use only. Contains not less than 98.0% and not more than 102.0% of azaperone, calculated on the dried basis. Meets the requirements for Identification, Melting range (92–95 °C), Loss on drying (not more than 0.5%), Residue on ignition (not more than 0.1%), and Chromatographic purity.

Azaperone Injection USP—Preserve in single-dose or in multiple-dose containers, preferably of Type I glass, protected from light. A sterile solution of Azaperone in Water for Injection, prepared with the aid of Tartaric Acid. Label it to indicate that it is for veterinary use only. Contains the labeled amount, within ±10%. Meets the requirements for Identification, pH (4.0–5.6), and Injections.

AZATADINE

Chemical group: Piperidine derivative.

Chemical name: Azatadine maleate—5*H*-Benzo[5,6]cyclohepta[1,2-*b*]pyridine, 6,11-dihydro-11-(1-methyl-4-piperidinylidene)-, (*Z*)-2-butenedioate (1:2).

Molecular formula: Azatadine maleate—$C_{20}H_{22}N_2 \cdot 2C_4H_4O_4$.

Molecular weight: Azatadine maleate—522.55.

Description: Azatadine Maleate USP—White to light cream-colored, odorless powder. Melts at about 153 °C.

pKa: 9.3.

Solubility: Azatadine Maleate USP—Freely soluble in water, in alcohol, in chloroform, and in methanol; practically insoluble in ether.

USP requirements:

Azatadine Maleate USP—Preserve in well-closed containers. Contains not less than 98.0% and not more than 102.0% of azatadine maleate, calculated on the dried basis. Meets the requirements for Identification, Loss on drying (not more than 1.0%), Residue on ignition (not more than 0.1%), and Chromatographic purity.

Azatadine Maleate Tablets USP—Preserve in well-closed containers. Contain the labeled amount, within ±10%. Meet the requirements for Identification, Dissolution (80% in 30 minutes in 0.1 *N* hydrochloric acid in Apparatus 2 at 50 rpm), and Uniformity of dosage units.

AZATADINE AND PSEUDOEPHEDRINE

For *Azatadine* and *Pseudoephedrine*—See individual listings for chemistry information.

USP requirements: Azatadine Maleate and Pseudoephedrine Sulfate Extended-release Tablets—Not in USP.

AZATHIOPRINE

Chemical name: 1*H*-Purine, 6-[(1-methyl-4-nitro-1*H*-imidazol-5-yl)thio]-.

Molecular formula: $C_9H_7N_7O_2S$.

Molecular weight: 277.26.

Description:

Azathioprine USP—Pale yellow, odorless powder.

Azathioprine Sodium for Injection USP—Bright yellow, hygroscopic, amorphous mass or cake.

Solubility: Azathioprine USP—Insoluble in water; soluble in dilute solutions of alkali hydroxides; sparingly soluble in dilute mineral acids; very slightly soluble in alcohol and in chloroform.

USP requirements:

Azathioprine USP—Preserve in tight, light-resistant containers. Contains not less than 98.0% and not more than 101.5% of azathioprine, calculated on the dried basis. Meets the requirements for Identification, Acidity or alkalinity, Loss on drying (not more than 1.0%), Residue on ignition (not more than 0.1%), Limit of mercaptopurine, and Organic volatile impurities.

Azathioprine Tablets USP—Protect from light. Contain the labeled amount, within ±7%. Meet the requirements for Identification, Dissolution (65% in 45 minutes in water in Apparatus 2 at 50 rpm), and Uniformity of dosage units.

Azathioprine Sodium for Injection USP—Preserve in Containers for Sterile Solids, at controlled room temperature. A sterile solid prepared by the freeze-drying of an aqueous solution of Azathioprine and Sodium Hydroxide. Contains the labeled amount, within ±7%. Meets the requirements for Completeness of solution, Identification, Bacterial endotoxins, pH (9.8–11.0), Water (not more than 7.0%), and Limit of mercaptopurine, and for Injections and Uniformity of dosage units.

AZITHROMYCIN

Chemical name: 1-Oxa-6-azacyclopentadecan-15-one, 13-[(2,6-dideoxy-3-*C*-methyl-3-*O*-methyl-alpha-L-*ribo*-hexopyranosyl)oxy]-2-ethyl-3,4,10-trihydroxy-3,5,6,8,10,12,14-heptamethyl-11-[[3,4,6-trideoxy-3-(dimethylamino)-beta-D-*xylo*-hexopyranosyl]oxy]-, [2*R*-(2*R**,3*S**,4*R**,5*R**,8*R**,10*R**,11*R**,12*S**,13*S**,14*R**)]-.

Molecular formula: $C_{38}H_{72}N_2O_{12}$ (anhydrous); $C_{38}H_{72}N_2O_{12} \cdot 2H_2O$ (dihydrate).

Molecular weight: 749.00 (anhydrous); 785.0 (dihydrate).

Description: White crystalline powder (for the dihydrate).

USP requirements:

Azithromycin USP—Preserve in tight containers. Contains the equivalent of not less than 945 mcg and not more than 1030 mcg of azithromycin per mg, calculated on the anhydrous basis. Meets the requirements for Identification, Specific rotation (−45° to −49°, calculated on the anhydrous basis), Crystallinity, pH (9.0–11.0), Water (4.0–5.0%), Residue on ignition (not more than 0.3%), and Heavy metals (not more than 0.0025%).

Azithromycin Capsules USP—Preserve in well-closed containers. Contain the equivalent of the labeled amount of azithromycin, within ±10%. Meet the requirements for Identification, Dissolution (75% in 45 minutes in sodium phosphate buffer [pH 6.0] in Apparatus 2 at 100 rpm), Uniformity of dosage units, and Water (not more than 5.0%).

AZLOCILLIN

Chemical name: Azlocillin sodium—4-Thia-1-azabicyclo-[3.2.0]heptane-2-carboxylic acid, 3,3-dimethyl-7-oxo-6-[[[[(2-oxo-1-imidazolidinyl)carbonyl]amino]phenylacetyl]amino]-, monosodium salt, [2*S*-[2 alpha,5 alpha,6 beta(*S**)]]-.

Molecular formula: Azlocillin sodium—$C_{20}H_{22}N_5NaO_6S$.

Molecular weight: Azlocillin sodium—483.47.

Description: Sterile Azlocillin Sodium USP—White to pale yellow powder.

Solubility: Sterile Azlocillin Sodium USP—Freely soluble in water; soluble in methanol and in dimethylformamide; slightly soluble in alcohol and in isopropyl alcohol.

USP requirements: Sterile Azlocillin Sodium USP—Preserve in Containers for Sterile Solids. It is azlocillin sodium suitable for parenteral use. It has a potency equivalent to not less than 859 mcg and not more than 1000 mcg of azlocillin per mg, calculated on the anhydrous basis, and, where packaged for dispensing, contains an amount of azlocillin sodium equivalent to the labeled amount of azlocillin, within −10% to +15%. Meets the requirements for Constituted solution, Identification, Specific rotation (+170° to +200°), Bacterial endotoxins, Sterility, pH (6.0–8.0, in a solution containing the equivalent of 100 mg of azlocillin per mL), Water (not more than 2.5%), and Particulate matter, for Uniformity of dosage units, and for Labeling under Injections.

AZTREONAM

Chemical group: Monobactams (*mono*cyclic *bac*terially produced beta-lac*tams*).

Chemical name: Propanoic acid, 2-[[[1-(2-amino-4-thiazolyl)-2-[(2-methyl-4-oxo-1-sulfo-3-azetidinyl)amino]-2-oxoethylidene]amino]oxy]-2-methyl-, [2*S*-[2 alpha,3 beta(*Z*)]]-.

Molecular formula: $C_{13}H_{17}N_5O_8S_2$.

Molecular weight: 435.43.

Description: Aztreonam USP—White, odorless, crystalline powder.

Solubility: Aztreonam USP—Soluble in dimethylformamide and in dimethyl sulfoxide; slightly soluble in methanol; very slightly soluble in dehydrated alcohol; practically insoluble in ethyl acetate, in chloroform, and in toluene.

Other characteristics: pH of aqueous solutions—4.5 to 7.5.

USP requirements:

Aztreonam USP—Preserve in tight containers. Contains not less than 90.0% and not more than 105.0% of aztreonam. Meets the requirements for Identification, Water (not more than 2.0%), Residue on ignition (not more than 0.1%), and Heavy metals (not more than 0.003%).

Aztreonam Injection USP—Preserve in Containers for Sterile Solids. Maintain in the frozen state. A sterile solution of Aztreonam and Arginine and a suitable osmolality adjusting substance in Water for Injection. It meets the requirements for Labeling under Injections. The label states that it is to be thawed just prior to use, describes conditions for proper storage of the resultant solution, and directs that the solution is not to be refrozen. Contains the labeled amount of aztreonam, within −10% to +20%. Meets the requirements for Identification, Pyrogen, Sterility, pH (4.5–7.5), and Particulate matter.

Aztreonam for Injection USP—Preserve in Containers for Sterile Solids. A dry mixture of Sterile Aztreonam and Arginine. Contains not less than 90.0% and not more than 105.0% of aztreonam, calculated on the anhydrous and arginine-free basis. Each container contains the labeled amount, within −10% to +20%. Meets the requirements for Constituted solution, Identification, Bacterial endotoxins, Sterility, pH (4.5–7.5, in a solution containing 100 mg of aztreonam per mL), Water (not more than 2.0%), Particulate matter, and Content of arginine, and for Uniformity of dosage units and Labeling under Injections.

Sterile Aztreonam USP—Preserve in Containers for Sterile Solids. It is Aztreonam suitable for parenteral use. Contains the labeled amount, within −10% to +5%. Meets the requirements for Bacterial endotoxins and Sterility, and for Identification test, Water, Residue on ignition, and Heavy metals under Aztreonam.

BACAMPICILLIN

Chemical group: A semi-synthetic penicillin, an analogue of ampicillin.

Chemical name: Bacampicillin hydrochloride—4-Thia-1-azabicyclo[3.2.0]heptane-2-carboxylic acid, 6-[(aminophenylacetyl)amino]-3,3-dimethyl-7-oxo-, 1-[(ethoxycarbonyl)oxy]ethyl ester, monohydrochloride, [2*S*-[2 alpha,5 alpha,6 beta-(*S**)]]-.

Molecular formula: Bacampicillin hydrochloride—$C_{21}H_{27}N_3O_7S \cdot HCl$.

Molecular weight: Bacampicillin hydrochloride—501.98.

Description: Bacampicillin Hydrochloride USP—White or practically white powder. Is hygroscopic.

Solubility: Bacampicillin Hydrochloride USP—Soluble in methylene chloride and in water; freely soluble in alcohol and in chloroform; very slightly soluble in ether.

USP requirements:

Bacampicillin Hydrochloride USP—Preserve in tight containers. Has a potency of not less than 623 mcg and not more than 727 mcg of ampicillin per mg. Meets the requirements for Identification, pH (3.0–4.5, in a solution containing 20 mg per mL), Water (not more than 1.0%), and Dimethylaniline.

Bacampicillin Hydrochloride for Oral Suspension USP—Preserve in tight containers. Contains an amount of bacampicillin hydrochloride equivalent to the labeled amount of ampicillin, when constituted as directed, within −10% to +25%. Contains one or more suitable buffers, colors, flavors, suspending agents, and sweetening ingredients. Meets the requirements for Identification, pH (6.5–8.0, in the suspension constituted as directed in the labeling), Loss on drying (not more than 2.0%), Uniformity of dosage units (single-unit containers), and Deliverable volume (multiple-unit containers).

Bacampicillin Hydrochloride Tablets USP—Preserve in tight containers. Contain an amount of bacampicillin hydrochloride equivalent to the labeled amount of ampicillin, within −10% to +25%. Meet the requirements for Identification, Dissolution (85% in 30 minutes in water in Apparatus 2 at 75 rpm), Uniformity of dosage units, and Water (not more than 2.5%).

BACILLUS CALMETTE-GUÉRIN (BCG) VACCINE

Source: Obtained from a live culture of the bacillus Calmette-Guérin strain of *Mycobacterium tuberculosis* var. *bovis*. Commercially available strains (which are substrains of the Pasteur Institute strain) include the Armand-Frappier, Connaught, Glaxo, and Tice substrains.

Description: BCG Vaccine USP—White to creamy white, dried mass, having the characteristic texture of material dried in the frozen state.

USP requirements:

BCG Live (Connaught Strain)—Not USP.

BCG Vaccine USP (Tice Strain)—Preserve in hermetic containers, preferably of Type I glass, at a temperature between 2 and 8 °C. A dried, living culture of the bacillus Calmette-Guérin strain of *Mycobacterium tuberculosis* var. *bovis*, grown in a suitable medium from a seed strain of known history that has been maintained to preserve its capacity for conferring immunity. Contains an amount of viable bacteria such that inoculation, in the recommended dose, of tuberculin-negative persons results in an acceptable tuberculin conversion rate. It is free from other organisms, and contains a suitable stabilizer. Contains no antimicrobial agent. Meets the requirement for expiration date (not later than 6 months after date of issue, or not later than 1 year after date of issue if stored at a temperature below 5° C). Conforms to the regulations of the U.S. Food and Drug Administration concerning biologics.

Note: Use the Vaccine immediately after its constitution, and discard any unused portion after 2 hours.

BCG Vaccine for Injection—Not in USP.

BACITRACIN

Chemical name:

Bacitracin—Bacitracin.

Bacitracin zinc—Bacitracins, zinc complex.

Description:

Bacitracin USP—White to pale buff powder, odorless or having a slight odor. Is hygroscopic. Its solutions deteriorate rapidly at room temperature. Is precipitated from its solutions and is inactivated by salts of many of the heavy metals.

Sterile Bacitracin USP—White to pale buff powder, odorless or having a slight odor. Is hygroscopic. Its solutions deteriorate rapidly at room temperature. May be amorphous when prepared by freeze-drying. Is precipitated from its solutions and is inactivated by salts of many of the heavy metals.

Bacitracin Zinc USP—White to pale tan powder, odorless or having a slight odor. Is hygroscopic.

Solubility:

Bacitracin USP—Freely soluble in water; soluble in alcohol, in methanol, and in glacial acetic acid, the solution in the organic solvents usually showing some insoluble residue; insoluble in acetone, in chloroform, and in ether.

Sterile Bacitracin USP—Freely soluble in water; soluble in alcohol, in methanol, and in glacial acetic acid, the solution in the organic solvents usually showing some insoluble residue; insoluble in acetone, in chloroform, and in ether.

Bacitracin Zinc USP—Sparingly soluble in water.

USP requirements:

Bacitracin USP—Preserve in tight containers, and store in a cool place. A polypeptide produced by the growth of an organism of the *licheniformis* group of *Bacillus subtilis* (Fam. Bacillaceae). Where it is packaged for prescription compounding, label it to indicate that it is not sterile and that the potency cannot be assured for longer than 60 days after opening, and to state the number of Bacitracin Units per milligram. Has a potency of not less than 40 Bacitracin Units per mg. Meets the requirements for Identification, pH (5.5–7.5, in a solution containing 10,000 Bacitracin Units per mL), and Loss on drying (not more than 5.0%).

Bacitracin Ointment USP—Preserve in well-closed containers containing not more than 60 grams, unless labeled solely for hospital use, preferably at controlled room temperature. It is Bacitracin in an anhydrous ointment base. Contains the labeled amount, within −10% to +40%. Meets the requirements for Identification, Minimum fill, and Water (not more than 0.5%).

Bacitracin Ophthalmic Ointment USP—Preserve in collapsible ophthalmic ointment tubes. A sterile preparation of Bacitracin in an anhydrous ointment base. Contains the labeled amount, within −10% to +40%. Meets the requirements for Identification, Sterility, Water (not more than 0.5%), and Metal particles.

Sterile Bacitracin USP—Preserve in Containers for Sterile Solids, and store in a cool place. Has a potency of not less than 50 Bacitracin Units per mg. In addition, where packaged for dispensing, contains the labeled amount, within −10% to +15%. Meets the requirements for Constituted solution, Bacterial endotoxins, Sterility, Residue on ignition (not more than 3.0%), and Heavy metals (not more than 0.003%), and for Identification test, pH, and Loss on drying under Bacitracin. Where packaged for dispensing, meets the requirements for Injections and Uniformity of dosage units. Where intended for use in preparing sterile ophthalmic dosage forms, it is exempt from the requirements for Bacterial endotoxins, Residue on ignition, and Heavy metals.

Soluble Bacitracin Methylene Disalicylate USP—Preserve in well-closed containers. A mixture of bacitracin methylene disalicylate and Sodium Bicarbonate. Label it to indicate that it is for veterinary use only. Has a potency of not less than 8 Bacitracin Units per mg, calculated on the dried basis. Meets the requirements for Loss on drying (not more than 8.5%) and pH (8.0–9.5, in a solution containing 25 mg of specimen per mL).

Bacitracin Methylene Disalicylate Soluble Powder USP—Preserve in tight containers. Label it to indicate that it is for veterinary use only. Label it to state the content of bacitracin in terms of grams per pound, each gram of bacitracin being equivalent to 42,000 Bacitracin Units. Contains an amount of bacitracin methylene disalicylate equivalent to the labeled amount of Bacitracin, within −10% to +20%. Meets the requirements for Loss on drying (not more than 8.5%) and pH (8.0–9.5, in a solution containing 50 mg of specimen per mL).

Bacitracin Zinc USP—Preserve in tight containers, and store in a cool place. The zinc salt of a kind of bacitracin or a mixture of two or more such salts. Label it to indicate that it is to be used in the manufacture of nonparenteral drugs only. Where it is packaged for prescription compounding, label it to indicate that it is not sterile and that the potency cannot be assured for longer than 60 days after opening, and to state the number of Bacitracin Units per mg. Has a potency of not less than 40 Bacitracin Units per mg. Contains not less than 2.0% and not more than 10.0% of zinc, calculated on the dried basis. Meets the requirements for Identification, pH (6.0–7.5, in a [saturated] solution containing approximately 100 mg per mL), Loss on drying (not more than 5.0%), and Zinc content.

Bacitracin Zinc Ointment USP—Preserve in well-closed containers containing not more than 60 grams, unless labeled solely for hospital use, preferably at controlled room temperature. It is Bacitracin Zinc in an anhydrous ointment base. Contains an amount of bacitracin zinc equivalent to the labeled amount of bacitracin, within −10% to +40%. Meets the requirements for Identification, Minimum fill, and Water (not more than 0.5%).

Bacitracin Zinc Soluble Powder USP—Preserve in tight containers. A mixture of bacitracin zinc and zinc proteinates. Label it to indicate that it is for veterinary use only. Label it to state the content of bacitracin in terms of grams per pound, each gram of bacitracin being equivalent to 42,000 Bacitracin Units. Contains an amount of bacitracin zinc equivalent to the labeled amount of bacitracin, within −10% to +20%. Meets the requirements for Loss on drying (not more than 5.0%) and Zinc content (not more than 2.0 grams of Zinc for each 42,000 Bacitracin Units).

Sterile Bacitracin Zinc USP—Preserve in Containers for Sterile Solids. It is Bacitracin Zinc suitable for use in the manufacture of sterile topical dosage forms. Label it to indicate that it is to be used in the manufacture of topical drugs only. Has a potency of not less than 40 Bacitracin Units per mg. Meets the requirements for Sterility, and for Identification test, pH, Loss on drying, and Zinc content under Bacitracin Zinc.

BACITRACIN AND POLYMYXIN B

For *Bacitracin* and *Polymyxin B*—See individual listings for chemistry information.

USP requirements:

Bacitracin and Polymyxin B Sulfate Topical Aerosol USP—Preserve in pressurized containers, and avoid exposure to excessive heat. A suspension of Bacitracin and Polymyxin B Sulfate in a suitable vehicle, packaged in a pressurized container with a suitable inert propellant. Contains the labeled amount of bacitracin, within −10% to +30%, and an amount of polymyxin B sulfate equivalent to the labeled amount of polymyxin B, within −10% to +30%. May contain a suitable local anesthetic. Meets the requirements for Identification and Water (not more than 0.5%), and for Leak testing and Pressure testing under Aerosols.

Bacitracin Zinc and Polymyxin B Sulfate Ointment USP—Preserve in well-closed, light-resistant containers. Contains amounts of bacitracin zinc and polymyxin B sulfate equivalent to the labeled amounts of bacitracin and polymyxin B, within −10% to +30%. May contain a suitable local anesthetic. Meets the requirements for Identification, Minimum fill, and Water (not more than 0.5%).

Bacitracin Zinc and Polymyxin B Sulfate Ophthalmic Ointment USP—Preserve in collapsible ophthalmic ointment tubes. Contains amounts of bacitracin zinc and polymyxin B sulfate equivalent to the labeled amounts of bacitracin and polymyxin B, within −10% to +30%. Meets the requirements for Identification, Sterility, Minimum fill, Water (not more than 0.5%), and Metal particles.

BACLOFEN

Chemical name: Butanoic acid, 4-amino-3-(4-chlorophenyl)-.

Molecular formula: $C_{10}H_{12}ClNO_2$.

Molecular weight: 213.66.

Description: Baclofen USP—White to off-white, crystalline powder. Is odorless or practically so.

Solubility: Baclofen USP—Slightly soluble in water; very slightly soluble in methanol; insoluble in chloroform.

USP requirements:

Baclofen USP—Preserve in tight containers. Contains not less than 99.0% and not more than 101.0% of baclofen, calculated on the anhydrous basis. Meets the requirements for Identification, Water (not more than 3.0%), Residue on ignition (not more than 0.3%), Heavy metals (not more than 0.001%), Related compounds, and Organic volatile impurities.

Baclofen Injection—Not in USP.

Baclofen Tablets USP—Preserve in well-closed containers. Contain the labeled amount, within ±10%. Meet the requirements for Identification, Dissolution (75% in 30 minutes in 0.1 *N* hydrochloric acid in Apparatus 2 at 50 rpm), Limit of 4-(4-Chlorophenyl)-2-pyrrolidinone (not more than 4.0%), and Uniformity of dosage units.

ADHESIVE BANDAGE

Description: Adhesive Bandage USP—The compress of Adhesive Bandage is substantially free from loose threads or ravelings. The adhesive strip may be perforated, and the back may be coated with a water-repellent film.

USP requirements: Adhesive Bandage USP—Package Adhesive Bandage that does not exceed 15 cm (6 inches) in width individually in such manner that sterility is maintained until the individual package is opened. Package individual packages in a second protective container. Adhesive Bandage consists of a compress of four layers of Type I Absorbent Gauze, or other suitable material, affixed to a film or fabric coated with a pressure-sensitive adhesive substance. It is sterile. The adhesive surface is protected by a suitable removable covering. The label of the second protective container bears a statement that the contents may not be sterile if the individual package has been damaged or previously opened, and it bears the names of any added antimicrobial agents. Each individual package is labeled to indicate the dimensions of the compress and the name of the manufacturer, packer, or distributor, and each protective container indicates also the address of the manufacturer, packer, or distributor. Meets the requirement for Sterility.

GAUZE BANDAGE

Description: Gauze Bandage USP—One continuous piece, tightly rolled, in various widths and lengths and substantially free from loose threads and ravelings.

USP requirements: Gauze Bandage USP—Gauze Bandage that has been rendered sterile is so packaged that the sterility of the contents of the package is maintained until the package is opened for use. It is Type I Absorbent Gauze. Its length is not less than 98.0% of that declared on the label, and its average width is not more than 1.6 mm less than the declared width. Contains no dye or other additives. The width and length of the Bandage and the number of pieces contained, and the name of the manufacturer, packer, or distributor, are stated on the package. The designation "non-sterilized" or "not sterilized" appears prominently on the package unless the Gauze Bandage has been rendered sterile, in which case it may be labeled to indicate that it is sterile and that the contents may not be sterile if the package bears evidence of damage or if the package has been previously opened.

Note: Before determining the thread count, dimensions, and weight, hold the Bandage, unrolled for not less than 4 hours in a standard atmosphere of 65 ±2% relative humidity at 21 ±1.1 °C (70 ±2 °F).

Meets the requirements for Thread count (not more than 3 threads per inch allowed in either warp or filling, provided that the combined variations do not exceed 5 threads per square inch), Width (average of 5 measurements not more than 1.6 mm [$^1/_{16}$ inch] less than labeled width), Length (not less than 98.0% of labeled length), Weight (calculated weight in grams per 0.894 square meter is not less than 39.2 grams), Absorbency (complete submersion of entire bandage roll takes place in not more than 30 seconds), and Sterility, and for Ignited residue, Acid or alkali, and Dextrin or starch, in water extract, Residue on ignition, Fatty matter, and Alcohol-soluble dyes under Absorbent Gauze.

BARIUM HYDROXIDE LIME

Description: Barium Hydroxide Lime USP—White or grayish white granules. May have a color if an indicator has been added.

NF category: Sorbent, carbon dioxide.

USP requirements: Barium Hydroxide Lime USP—Preserve in tight containers. A mixture of barium hydroxide octahydrate and Calcium Hydroxide. May contain also Potassium Hydroxide and may contain an indicator that is inert toward anesthetic gases such as Ether, Cyclopropane, and Nitrous Oxide, and that changes color when the Barium Hydroxide Lime no longer can absorb carbon dioxide. If an indicator has been added, the name and color change of such indicator are stated on the container label. The container label indicates also the mesh size in terms of standard mesh sieve sizes. Meets the requirements for Identification, Size of granules, Loss on drying (11.0–16.0%), Hardness, and Carbon dioxide absorbency (not less than 19.0%).

Caution: Since Barium Hydroxide Lime contains a soluble form of barium, it is toxic if swallowed.

BARIUM SULFATE

Chemical name: Sulfuric acid, barium salt (1:1).

Molecular formula: $BaSO_4$.

Molecular weight: 233.39.

Description:
Barium Sulfate USP—Fine, white, odorless, bulky powder, free from grittiness.
Barium Sulfate for Suspension USP—White or colored, bulky or granular powder.

Solubility: Barium Sulfate USP—Practically insoluble in water, in organic solvents, and in solutions of acids and of alkalies.

USP requirements:
Barium Sulfate USP—Preserve in well-closed containers. Contains not less than 97.5% and not more than 100.5% of barium sulfate. Meets the requirements for Identification, Bulkiness, Acidity or alkalinity, Sulfide (not more than 0.5 ppm), Acid-soluble substances (not more than 0.3%), Soluble barium salts, Arsenic (not more than 0.8 ppm), and Heavy metals (not more than 0.001%).
Barium Sulfate Suspension—Not in USP.
Barium Sulfate Oral Suspension—Not in USP.
Barium Sulfate for Suspension USP—Preserve in well-closed containers. A dry mixture of Barium Sulfate and one or more suitable dispersing and/or suspending agents. Contains the labeled amount, within −10%. Meets the requirements for Identification, pH (4.0–10.0, in a 60% [w/w] aqueous suspension), Loss on drying (not more than 1.0%), and Heavy metals (not more than 0.001%), and for Sulfide and Arsenic under Barium Sulfate.
Barium Sulfate Rectal Suspension—Not in USP.
Barium Sulfate Tablets—Not in USP.

BECLOMETHASONE

Chemical name:
Beclomethasone dipropionate—Pregna-1,4-diene-3,20-dione, 9-chloro-11-hydroxy-16-methyl-17,21-bis(1-oxopropoxy)-, (11 beta,16 beta)-.
Beclomethasone dipropionate, monohydrate—9-Chloro-11 beta, 17,21-trihydroxy-16 beta-methylpregna-1,4-diene-3,20-dione 17,21-dipropionate, monohydrate.

Molecular formula:
Beclomethasone dipropionate—$C_{28}H_{37}ClO_7$.
Beclomethasone dipropionate monohydrate—$C_{28}H_{37}ClO_7 \cdot H_2O$.

Molecular weight:
Beclomethasone dipropionate—521.05.
Beclomethasone dipropionate monohydrate—539.06.

Description:
Beclomethasone Dipropionate USP—White to cream white, odorless powder.
Beclomethasone dipropionate monohydrate—White to creamy white, odorless powder.

Solubility:
Beclomethasone Dipropionate USP—Very slightly soluble in water; very soluble in chloroform; freely soluble in acetone and in alcohol.
Beclomethasone dipropionate monohydrate—Very slightly soluble in water; very soluble in chloroform; freely soluble in acetone and in alcohol.

USP requirements:
Beclomethasone Dipropionate USP—Preserve in well-closed containers. It is anhydrous or contains one molecule of water of hydration. Contains not less than 97.0% and not more than 103.0% of beclomethasone dipropionate, calculated on the dried basis. Meets the requirements for Identification, Specific rotation (+88° to +94°, calculated on the dried basis), Loss on drying (not more than 0.5% for the anhydrous and 2.8–3.8% for the monohydrate), and Residue on ignition (not more than 0.1%).
Beclomethasone Dipropionate Inhalation Aerosol—Not in USP.
Beclomethasone Dipropionate Nasal Aerosol—Not in USP.
Beclomethasone Dipropionate Cream—Not in USP.
Beclomethasone Dipropionate for Inhalation—Not in USP.
Beclomethasone Dipropionate Lotion—Not in USP.
Beclomethasone Dipropionate Ointment—Not in USP.
Beclomethasone Dipropionate Powder for Inhalation—Not in USP.
Beclomethasone Dipropionate Monohydrate Nasal Spray—Not in USP.

BELLADONNA

Source: The naturally occurring belladonna alkaloids are found in various solanaceous plants. Belladonna leaf is derived from the dried leaf and flowering or fruiting top of *Atropa belladonna* Linné (Fam. Solanaceae). The active alkaloids of belladonna include *l*-hyoscyamine (which racemizes to atropine on extraction) and scopolamine.

Description: Belladonna Leaf USP—When moistened, its odor is slight, somewhat tobacco-like.

USP requirements:
Belladonna Extract USP—Preserve in tight containers, at a temperature not exceeding 30 °C. Contains, in each 100 grams, not less than 1.15 grams and not more than 1.35 grams of the alkaloids of belladonna leaf.
Belladonna Extract Tablets USP—Preserve in tight, light-resistant containers. Contain the labeled amount of the alkaloids of belladonna leaf, within ±10%. Meet the requirements for Identification, Disintegration (30 minutes), and Uniformity of dosage units.
Belladonna Leaf USP—Preserve in well-closed containers and avoid long exposure to direct sunlight. Preserve powdered Belladonna Leaf in light-resistant containers. Consists of the dried leaf and flowering or fruiting top of *Atropa belladonna* Linné or of its variety *acuminata* Royle ex Lindley (Fam. Solanaceae). Yields not less than 0.35% of the alkaloids of belladonna leaf. Meets the requirements for Botanic characteristics, Acid-insoluble ash (not more than 3.0%), and Belladonna stems (proportion of belladonna stems over 10 mm in diameter not more than 3.0%).
Belladonna Tincture USP—Preserve in tight, light-resistant containers, and avoid exposure to direct sunlight and to excessive heat. Yields, from each 100 mL, not less than 27 mg and not more than 33 mg of the alkaloids of the belladonna leaf. Meets the requirement for Alcohol content (65.0–70.0%).

BELLADONNA AND BUTABARBITAL

For *Belladonna* and *Butabarbital*—See individual listings for chemistry information.

USP requirements:
Belladonna Extract and Butabarbital Sodium Elixir—Not in USP.
Belladonna Extract and Butabarbital Sodium Tablets—Not in USP.

BELLADONNA AND PHENOBARBITAL

For *Belladonna* and *Phenobarbital*—See individual listings for chemistry information.

USP requirements: Belladonna Extract and Phenobarbital Tablets—Not in USP.

BENAZEPRIL

Chemical name: Benazepril hydrochloride—1*H*-1-Benzazepine-1-acetic acid, 3-[[1-(ethoxycarbonyl)-3-phenylpropyl]-amino]-2,3,4,5-tetrahydro-2-oxo-, monohydrochloride, [*S*-(*R**,*R**)]-.

Molecular formula: Benazepril hydrochloride—$C_{24}H_{28}N_2O_5 \cdot HCl$.

Molecular weight: Benazepril hydrochloride—460.96.

Description: Benazepril hydrochloride—White to off-white crystalline powder.

Solubility: Benazepril hydrochloride—Soluble in water, in ethanol, and in methanol.

USP requirements: Benazepril Hydrochloride Tablets—Not in USP.

BENDROFLUMETHIAZIDE

Chemical name: 2*H*-1,2,4-Benzothiadiazine-7-sulfonamide, 3,4-dihydro-3-(phenylmethyl)-6-(trifluoromethyl)-, 1,1-dioxide-.

Molecular formula: $C_{15}H_{14}F_3N_3O_4S_2$.

Molecular weight: 421.41.

Description: Bendroflumethiazide USP—White to cream-colored, finely divided, crystalline powder. Is odorless or has a slight odor. Melts at about 220 °C.

pKa: 8.5.

Solubility: Bendroflumethiazide USP—Practically insoluble in water; freely soluble in alcohol and in acetone.

USP requirements:
Bendroflumethiazide USP—Preserve in tight containers. Contains not less than 98.0% and not more than 102.0% of bendroflumethiazide, calculated on the anhydrous basis. Meets the requirements for Identification, Water (not more than 0.5%), Residue on ignition (not more than 0.2%), Heavy metals (not more than 0.002%), Selenium (not more than 0.003%), Limit of 2,4-disulfamyl-5-trifluoromethylaniline (not more than 1.5%), and Organic volatile impurities.
Bendroflumethiazide Tablets USP—Preserve in tight containers. Contain the labeled amount, within ±10%. Meet the requirements for Identification, Dissolution (75% in 45 minutes in 0.1 *N* hydrochloric acid in Apparatus 2 at 50 rpm), and Uniformity of dosage units.

BENOXINATE

Chemical name: Benoxinate hydrochloride—Benzoic acid, 4-amino-3-butoxy-, 2-(diethylamino)ethyl ester, monohydrochloride.

Molecular formula: Benoxinate hydrochloride—$C_{17}H_{28}N_2O_3 \cdot HCl$.

Molecular weight: Benoxinate hydrochloride—344.88.

Description: Benoxinate Hydrochloride USP—White, or slightly off-white, crystals or crystalline powder. Is odorless, or has a slight characteristic odor. Its solutions are neutral to litmus, and it melts at about 158 °C.

Solubility: Benoxinate Hydrochloride USP—Very soluble in water; freely soluble in chloroform and in alcohol; insoluble in ether.

USP requirements:

Benoxinate Hydrochloride USP—Preserve in well-closed containers. Contains not less than 98.5% and not more than 101.5% of benoxinate hydrochloride, calculated on the dried basis. Meets the requirements for Identification, pH (5.0–6.0, in a solution [1 in 100]), Loss on drying (not more than 1.0%), Residue on ignition (not more than 0.2%), and Ordinary impurities.

Benoxinate Hydrochloride Ophthalmic Solution USP—Preserve in tight containers. A sterile solution of Benoxinate Hydrochloride in water. Contains the labeled amount, within ±5%. Meets the requirements for Identification, Sterility, and pH (3.0–6.0).

BENTIROMIDE

Chemical group: Synthetic peptide that contains a *p*-aminobenzoic acid (PABA) moiety as a marker.

Chemical name: Benzoic acid, 4-[[2-(benzoylamino)-3-(4-hydroxyphenyl)-1-oxopropyl]amino]-, (*S*)-.

Molecular formula: $C_{23}H_{20}N_2O_5$.

Molecular weight: 404.42.

Description: White to off-white, practically odorless powder.

pKa: 5.4.

Solubility: Practically insoluble in water, in dilute acid, and in ether; sparingly soluble in ethanol; freely soluble in dilute alkali.

USP requirements: Bentiromide Oral Solution—Not in USP.

BENTONITE

Chemical name: Bentonite.

Description:

Bentonite NF—Very fine, odorless, pale buff or cream-colored to grayish powder, free from grit. It is hygroscopic.

NF category: Suspending and/or viscosity-increasing agent.

Purified Bentonite NF—Odorless, fine (micronized) powder or small flakes that are creamy when viewed on their flat surfaces and tan to brown when viewed on their edges.

NF category: Suspending and/or viscosity-increasing agent.

Bentonite Magma NF—NF category: Suspending and/or viscosity-increasing agent.

Solubility:

Bentonite NF—Insoluble in water, but swells to approximately twelve times its volume when added to water. Insoluble in, and does not swell in, organic solvents.

Purified Bentonite NF—Insoluble in water and in alcohol. Swells when added to water or glycerin.

NF requirements:

Bentonite NF—Preserve in tight containers. A native, colloidal, hydrated aluminum silicate. Label it to indicate that absorption of atmospheric moisture should be avoided following the opening of the original package, preferably by storage of the remainder of the contents in a tight container. Meets the requirements for Identification, Microbial limit, pH (9.5–10.5), Loss on drying (5.0–8.0%), Arsenic (not more than 5 ppm), Lead (not more than 0.004%), Gel formation, Swelling power, and Fineness of powder.

Purified Bentonite NF—Preserve in tight containers. A colloidal montmorillonite that has been processed to remove grit and non-swellable ore components. Meets the requirements for Identification, Viscosity (40–200 centipoises), Microbial limits, pH (9.0–10.0, in a suspension [5 in 100] in water), Acid demand (pH not more than 4.0), Loss on drying (not more than 8.0%), Arsenic (not more than 3 ppm), and Lead (not more than 0.0015%).

Bentonite Magma NF—Preserve in tight containers.

Prepare Bentonite Magma as follows: 50 grams of Bentonite and a sufficient quantity of Purified Water to make 1000 grams. Sprinkle the Bentonite, in portions, upon 800 grams of hot purified water, allowing each portion to become thoroughly wetted without stirring. Allow it to stand with occasional stirring for 24 hours. Stir until a uniform magma is obtained, add Purified Water to make 1000 grams, and mix. The Magma may be prepared also by mechanical means such as by use of a blender, as follows: Place about 500 grams of Purified Water in the blender, and while the machine is running, add the Bentonite. Add Purified Water to make up to about 1000 grams or up to the operating capacity of the blender. Blend the mixture for 5 to 10 minutes, add Purified Water to make 1000 grams, and mix.

Meets the requirement for Microbial limit.

BENZALDEHYDE

Chemical name: Benzaldehyde.

Molecular formula: C_7H_6O.

Molecular weight: 106.12.

Description:

Benzaldehyde NF—Colorless, strongly refractive liquid, having an odor resembling that of bitter almond oil. Is affected by light.

NF category: Flavors and perfumes.

Compound Benzaldehyde Elixir NF—NF category: Flavored and/or sweetened vehicle.

Solubility: Benzaldehyde NF—Slightly soluble in water; miscible with alcohol, with ether, and with fixed and volatile oils.

NF requirements:

Benzaldehyde NF—Preserve in well-filled, tight, light-resistant containers. Contains not less than 98.0% and not more than 100.5% of benzaldehyde. Meets the requirements for Specific gravity (1.041–1.046 at 25 °C), Refractive index (1.544–1.546 at 20 °C), Hydrocyanic acid, Chlorinated compounds, Nitrobenzene, and Organic volatile impurities.

Compound Benzaldehyde Elixir NF—Preserve in tight, light-resistant containers. Contains 0.05% Benzaldehyde in a suitably flavored and sweetened hydroalcoholic vehicle. Meets the requirements for Alcohol content (3.0–5.0%) and Organic volatile impurities.

BENZALKONIUM CHLORIDE

Chemical name: Ammonium, alkyldimethyl(phenylmethyl)-, chloride.

Description:

Benzalkonium Chloride NF—White or yellowish white, thick gel or gelatinous pieces. Usually has a mild, aromatic odor. Its aqueous solution foams strongly when shaken, and usually is slightly alkaline.

NF category: Antimicrobial preservative; wetting and/or solubilizing agent.

Benzalkonium Chloride Solution NF—Clear liquid; colorless or slightly yellow unless a color has been added. It has an aromatic odor.

NF category: Antimicrobial preservative.

Solubility: Benzalkonium Chloride NF—Very soluble in water and in alcohol. Anhydrous form slightly soluble in ether.

USP requirements: Benzalkonium Chloride Vaginal Suppositories—Not in USP.

NF requirements:

Benzalkonium Chloride NF—Preserve in tight containers. A mixture of alkylbenzyldimethylammonium chlorides, the composition of which is restricted within certain limits. Meets the requirements for Identification, Water (not more than 15.0%), Residue on ignition (not more than 2.0%), Water-insoluble matter, Foreign amines, and Ratio of alkyl components.

Benzalkonium Chloride Solution NF—Preserve in tight containers, and prevent contact with metals. Contains the labeled amount, within ±5%, in concentrations of 1.0% or more; and contains the labeled amount, within ±7%, in concentrations of less than 1.0%. May contain a suitable coloring agent and may contain not more than 10% of alcohol. Meets the requirements for Identification, Microbial limit, Alcohol (if present, 95.0–105.0% of labeled amount), and Foreign amines.

Caution: Mixing Benzalkonium Chloride Solution with ordinary soaps and with anionic detergents may decrease or destroy the bacteriostatic activity of the Solution.

BENZETHONIUM

Chemical name: Benzethonium chloride—Benzenemethanaminium, *N,N*-dimethyl-*N*-[2-[2-[4-(1,1,3,3-tetramethylbutyl)phenoxy]ethoxy]ethyl]-, chloride.

Molecular formula: Benzethonium chloride—$C_{27}H_{42}ClNO_2$.

Molecular weight: Benzethonium chloride—448.09.

Description:

Benzethonium Chloride USP—White crystals, having a mild odor. Its solution (1 in 100) is slightly alkaline to litmus.

NF category: Antimicrobial preservative; wetting and/or solubilizing agent.

Benzethonium Chloride Solution USP—Odorless, clear liquid, slightly alkaline to litmus.

Benzethonium Chloride Tincture USP—Clear liquid, having the characteristic odor of acetone and of alcohol.

Solubility: Benzethonium Chloride USP—Soluble in water, in alcohol, and in chloroform; slightly soluble in ether.

USP requirements:

Benzethonium Chloride USP—Preserve in tight, light-resistant containers. Contains not less than 97.0% and not more than 103.0% of benzethonium chloride, calculated on the dried basis. Meets the requirements for Identification, Melting range (158–163 °C), Loss on drying (not more than 5.0%), Residue on ignition (not more than 0.1%), and Ammonium compounds.

Benzethonium Chloride Topical Solution USP—Preserve in tight, light-resistant containers. Contains the labeled amount, within ±5%. Meets the requirements for Identification, Oxidizing substances, and Nitrites.

Benzethonium Chloride Tincture USP—Preserve in tight, light-resistant containers. Contains, in each 100 mL, not less than 190 mg and not more than 210 mg of benzethonium chloride.

Prepare Benzethonium Chloride Tincture as follows: 2 grams of Benzethonium Chloride, 685 mL of Alcohol, 100 mL of Acetone, and a sufficient quantity of Purified Water to make 1000 mL. Dissolve the Benzethonium Chloride in a mixture of the Alcohol and the Acetone. Add sufficient Purified Water to make 1000 mL.

Meets the requirements for Identification, Specific gravity (0.868–0.876), and Alcohol and acetone content (62.0–68.0% of alcohol, and 9.0–11.0% of acetone).

Note: Benzethonium Chloride Tincture may be colored by the addition of any suitable color or combination of colors certified by the FDA for use in drugs.

BENZOCAINE

Chemical group: Ester of para-aminobenzoic acid (PABA).

Chemical name: Benzoic acid, 4-amino-, ethyl ester.

Molecular formula: $C_9H_{11}NO_2$.

Molecular weight: 165.19.

Description: Benzocaine USP—Small, white crystals or white, crystalline powder. Is odorless and is stable in air.

Solubility: Benzocaine USP—Very slightly soluble in water; freely soluble in alcohol, in chloroform, and in ether; sparingly soluble in almond oil and in olive oil; dissolves in dilute acids.

USP requirements:

Benzocaine USP—Preserve in well-closed containers. Dried over phosphorus pentoxide for 3 hours, contains not less than 98.0% and not more than 101.0% of benzocaine. Meets the requirements for Identification, Melting range (88–92 °C, the range between beginning and end of melting not more than 2 °C), Reaction, Loss on drying (not more than 1.0%), Residue on ignition (not more than 0.1%), Chloride, Heavy metals (not more than 0.001%), Readily carbonizable substances, and Ordinary impurities (not more than 1%).

Benzocaine Topical Aerosol USP (Solution)—Preserve in pressurized containers, and avoid exposure to excessive heat. A solution of Benzocaine in a pressurized container. Contains the labeled amount, within ±10%. Meets the requirements for Identification and for Leak testing under Aerosols.

Benzocaine Cream USP—Preserve in tight containers, protected from light, and avoid prolonged exposure to temperatures exceeding 30 °C. Contains the labeled amount, within ±10%, in a suitable cream base. Meets the requirements for Identification, Microbial limits, and Minimum fill.

Benzocaine Gel—Not in USP.
Benzocaine Jelly—Not in USP.
Benzocaine Lozenges—Not in USP.
Benzocaine Ointment USP—Preserve in tight containers, protected from light, and avoid prolonged exposure to temperatures exceeding 30 °C. Contains the labeled amount, within ± 10%, in a suitable ointment base. Meets the requirements for Identification, Microbial limits, and Minimum fill.
Benzocaine Dental Paste—Not in USP.
Benzocaine Otic Solution USP—Preserve in tight, light resistant containers. Contains the labeled amount, within ± 10%. Meets the requirements for Identification and Microbial limits.
Benzocaine Topical Solution USP—Preserve in tight containers, protected from light, and avoid prolonged exposure to temperatures exceeding 30 °C. A solution of Benzocaine in a suitable solvent. Contains the labeled amount, within ± 10%. Contains a suitable antimicrobial agent. Meets the requirements for Identification and Microbial limits.

BENZOCAINE, BUTAMBEN, AND TETRACAINE

For *Benzocaine, Butamben,* and *Tetracaine*—See individual listings for chemistry information.

USP requirements:
Benzocaine, Butamben, and Tetracaine Hydrochloride Topical Aerosol USP—Preserve in pressurized containers, and avoid exposure to excessive heat. It is Benzocaine, Butamben, and Tetracaine Hydrochloride Topical Solution packaged in a pressurized container with a suitable inert propellant. Contains the labeled amounts, within ± 10%. Meets the requirements for Identification and for Leak testing and Pressure testing under Aerosols.
Benzocaine, Butamben, and Tetracaine Hydrochloride Gel USP—Preserve in tight containers, and avoid freezing. It is Benzocaine, Butamben, and Tetracaine Hydrochloride in a suitable gel base. Contains the labeled amounts, within ± 10%. Meets the requirements for Identification and Minimum fill.
Benzocaine, Butamben, and Tetracaine Hydrochloride Ointment USP—Preserve in tight containers, and avoid freezing. It is Benzocaine, Butamben, and Tetracaine Hydrochloride in a suitable ointment base. Contains the labeled amounts, within ± 10%. Meets the requirements for Identification and Minimum fill.
Benzocaine, Butamben, and Tetracaine Hydrochloride Topical Solution USP—Preserve in tight containers, and avoid freezing. Contains the labeled amounts, within ± 10%. Meets the requirements for Identification and Minimum fill.

BENZOCAINE AND MENTHOL

For *Benzocaine* and *Menthol*—See individual listings for chemistry information.

USP requirements:
Benzocaine and Menthol Lotion—Not in USP.
Benzocaine and Menthol Topical Aerosol Solution—Not in USP.

BENZOIC ACID

Chemical name: Benzoic acid.

Molecular formula: $C_7H_6O_2$.

Molecular weight: 122.12.

Description: Benzoic Acid USP—White crystals, scales, or needles. Has a slight odor, usually suggesting benzaldehyde or benzoin. Somewhat volatile at moderately warm temperatures. Freely volatile in steam.

NF category: Antimicrobial preservative.

Solubility: Benzoic Acid USP—Slightly soluble in water; freely soluble in alcohol, in chloroform, and in ether.

USP requirements: Benzoic Acid USP—Preserve in well-closed containers. Contains not less than 99.5% and not more than 100.5% of benzoic acid, calculated on the anhydrous basis. Meets the requirements for Identification, Congealing range (121–123 °C), Water (not more than 0.7%), Residue on ignition (not more than 0.05%), Arsenic (not more than 3 ppm), Heavy metals (not more than 0.001%), Readily carbonizable substances, and Readily oxidizable substances.

BENZOIC AND SALICYLIC ACIDS

For *Benzoic Acid* and *Salicylic Acid*—See individual listings for chemistry information.

USP requirements: Benzoic and Salicylic Acids Ointment USP—Preserve in well-closed containers, and avoid exposure to temperatures exceeding 30 °C. It is Benzoic Acid and Salicylic Acid, present in a ratio of about 2 to 1, in a suitable ointment base. Label Ointment to indicate the concentrations of Benzoic Acid and Salicylic Acid and to indicate whether the ointment base is water-soluble or water-insoluble. Contains the labeled amounts, within ± 10%. Meets the requirements for Identification and Minimum fill.

BENZOIN

Description: Benzoin USP—Sumatra Benzoin has an aromatic and balsamic odor. When heated it does not emit a pinaceous odor. When Sumatra Benzoin is digested with boiling water, the odor suggests cinnamates or storax. Siam Benzoin has an agreeable, balsamic, vanilla-like odor.

USP requirements:
Benzoin USP—Preserve in well-closed containers. The balsamic resin obtained from *Styrax benzoin* Dryander or *Styrax paralleloneurus* Perkins, known in commerce as Sumatra Benzoin, or from *Styrax tonkinensis* (Pièrre) Craib ex Hartwich, or other species of the Section *Anthostyrax* of the genus *Styrax*, known in commerce as Siam Benzoin (Fam. Styraceae). Label it to indicate whether it is Sumatra Benzoin or Siam Benzoin. Sumatra Benzoin yields not less than 75.0% of alcohol-soluble extractive, and Siam Benzoin yields not less than 90.0% of alcohol-soluble extractive. Meets the requirements for Botanic characteristics, Identification, Benzoic acid (not less than 6.0% for Sumatra Benzoin and not less than 12.0% for Siam Benzoin), Acid-insoluble ash (not more than 1.0% for Sumatra Benzoin and not more than 0.5% for Siam Benzoin), and Foreign organic matter (not more than 1.0% for Siam Benzoin).
Compound Benzoin Tincture USP—Preserve in tight, light-resistant containers, and avoid exposure to direct sunlight and to excessive heat. Label it to indicate that it is flammable.

Prepare Compound Benzoin Tincture as follows: 100 grams of Benzoin, in moderately coarse powder, 20 grams of Aloe, in moderately coarse powder, 80 grams of Storax, and 40 grams of Tolu Balsam to make 1000 mL. Prepare a Tincture by Process M, using alcohol as the menstruum.

Meets the requirements for Specific gravity (0.870–0.885), Alcohol content (74.0–80.0%), and Nonvolatile residue.

BENZONATATE

Chemical name: Benzoic acid, 4-(butylamino)-, 2,5,8,11,14,17,-20,23,26-nonaoxaoctacos-28-yl ester.

Molecular formula: $C_{30}H_{53}NO_{11}$ (average).

Molecular weight: 603.00 (average).

Description: Benzonatate USP—Clear, pale yellow, viscous liquid, having a faint, characteristic odor.

Solubility: Benzonatate USP—Miscible with water in all proportions. Freely soluble in chloroform and in alcohol.

USP requirements:
Benzonatate USP—Preserve in tight, light-resistant containers. Contains not less than 95.0% and not more than 105.0% of benzonatate. Meets the requirements for Identification, Refractive index (1.509–1.511 at 20 °C), Water (not more than 0.3%), Residue on ignition (not more than 0.1%), Arsenic (not more than 1.5 ppm), Chloride (not more than 0.0035%), Sulfate (not more than 0.04%), Heavy metals (not more than 0.001%), and Organic volatile impurities.
Benzonatate Capsules USP—Preserve in tight, light-resistant containers. Contain the labeled amount, within ±10%. Meet the requirements for Identification and Uniformity of dosage units.

BENZOYL PEROXIDE

Chemical name: Dibenzoyl peroxide.

Molecular formula: $C_{14}H_{10}O_4$ (anhydrous).

Molecular weight: 242.23 (anhydrous).

Description:
Hydrous Benzoyl Peroxide USP—White, granular powder, having a characteristic odor.
Benzoyl Peroxide Gel USP—A soft, white gel, having a characteristic odor.
Benzoyl Peroxide Lotion USP—White, viscous, creamy lotion, having a characteristic odor.

Solubility: Hydrous Benzoyl Peroxide USP—Sparingly soluble in water and in alcohol; soluble in acetone, in chloroform, and in ether.

USP requirements:
Hydrous Benzoyl Peroxide USP—Store in the original container, at room temperature. (Note: Do not transfer Hydrous Benzoyl Peroxide to metal or glass containers fitted with friction tops. Do not return unused material to its original container, but destroy it by treatment with sodium hydroxide solution [1 in 10] until addition of a crystal of potassium iodide results in no release of free iodine.) Contains not less than 65.0% and not more than 82.0% of anhydrous benzoyl peroxide. Contains about 26% of water for the purpose of reducing flammability and shock sensitivity. Meets the requirements for Identification and Chromatographic purity.

Caution: Hydrous Benzoyl Peroxide may explode at temperatures higher than 60 °C or cause fires in the presence of reducing substances. Store it in the original container, treated to reduce static charges.

Benzoyl Peroxide Cleansing Bar—Not in USP.
Benzoyl Peroxide Cream—Not in USP.
Benzoyl Peroxide Gel USP—Preserve in tight containers. It is benzoyl peroxide in a suitable gel base. Contains the labeled amount, within −10% to +25%. Meets the requirements for Identification, pH (3.5–6.0), and Related substances.
Benzoyl Peroxide Lotion USP—Preserve in tight containers. It is benzoyl peroxide in a suitable lotion base. Contains the labeled amount, within ±10%. Meets the requirements for Identification, pH (2.8–6.6), and Related substances.
Benzoyl Peroxide Cleansing Lotion—Not in USP.
Benzoyl Peroxide Facial Mask—Not in USP.
Benzoyl Peroxide Stick—Not in USP.

BENZPHETAMINE

Chemical group: Phenethylamine (amphetamine-like).

Chemical name: Benzphetamine hydrochloride—(+)-*N*-Benzyl-*N*,alpha-dimethylphenethylamine hydrochloride.

Molecular formula: Benzphetamine hydrochloride—$C_{17}H_{21}N \cdot HCl$.

Molecular weight: Benzphetamine hydrochloride—275.82.

Description: Benzphetamine hydrochloride—White crystalline powder.

Solubility: Benzphetamine hydrochloride—Readily soluble in water and in 95% ethanol.

USP requirements: Benzphetamine Hydrochloride Tablets—Not in USP.

BENZTHIAZIDE

Chemical name: 2*H*-1,2,4-Benzothiadiazine-7-sulfonamide, 6-chloro-3-[[(phenylmethyl)thio]methyl]-, 1,1-dioxide.

Molecular formula: $C_{15}H_{14}ClN_3O_4S_3$.

Molecular weight: 431.93.

Description: Benzthiazide USP—White, crystalline powder, having a characteristic odor. Melts at about 240 °C.

Solubility: Benzthiazide USP—Practically insoluble in water; freely soluble in dimethylformamide and in solutions of fixed alkali hydroxides; slightly soluble in acetone; practically insoluble in ether and in chloroform.

USP requirements:
Benzthiazide USP—Preserve in tight containers. Contains not less than 98.0% and not more than 101.5% of benzthiazide, calculated on the dried basis. Meets the requirements for Identification, Loss on drying (not more than 1.0%), Residue on ignition (not more than 0.2%), Selenium (not more than 0.003%), Heavy metals (not more than 0.0025%), Diazotizable substances (not more than 1.0%), and Organic volatile impurities.
Benzthiazide Tablets USP—Preserve in tight containers. Contain the labeled amount, within ±10%. Meet the requirements for Identification, Disintegration (15 minutes, the use of disks being omitted), and Uniformity of dosage units.

BENZTROPINE

Chemical group: Synthetic tertiary amine.

Chemical name: Benztropine mesylate—8-Azabicyclo[3.2.1]-octane, 3-(diphenylmethoxy)-, *endo*, methanesulfonate.

Molecular formula: Benztropine mesylate—$C_{21}H_{25}NO \cdot CH_4O_3S$.

Molecular weight: Benztropine mesylate—403.54.

Description: Benztropine Mesylate USP—White, slightly hygroscopic, crystalline powder.

Solubility: Benztropine Mesylate USP—Very soluble in water; freely soluble in alcohol; very slightly soluble in ether.

USP requirements:

Benztropine Mesylate USP—Preserve in tight containers. Contains not less than 98.0% and not more than 100.5% of benztropine mesylate, calculated on the dried basis. Meets the requirements for Identification, Melting range (141–145 °C), Loss on drying (not more than 5.0%), Residue on ignition (not more than 0.1%), and Organic volatile impurities.

Benztropine Mesylate Injection USP—Preserve in single-dose or in multiple-dose containers, preferably of Type I glass. A sterile solution of Benztropine Mesylate in Water for Injection. Contains the labeled amount, within ± 10%. Meets the requirements for Identification, Bacterial endotoxins, pH (5.0–8.0), and Injections.

Benztropine Mesylate Tablets USP—Preserve in well-closed containers. Contain the labeled amount, within ± 10%. Meet the requirements for Identification, Dissolution (80% in 30 minutes in 0.1 *N* hydrochloric acid in Apparatus 2 at 50 rpm), and Uniformity of dosage units.

BENZYDAMINE

Chemical name: Benzydamine hydrochloride—1-Propanamine, *N,N*-dimethyl-3-[[1-(phenylmethyl)-1*H*-indazol-3-yl]oxy]-, monohydrochloride.

Molecular formula: Benzydamine hydrochloride—$C_{19}H_{23}N_3O \cdot HCl$.

Molecular weight: Benzydamine hydrochloride—345.87.

Description: Benzydamine hydrochloride—Melting point 160 °C.

Solubility: Benzydamine hydrochloride—Very soluble in water; rather soluble in ethanol, in chloroform, and in *n*-butanol.

USP requirements: Benzydamine Hydrochloride Oral Topical Solution—Not in USP.

BENZYL ALCOHOL

Chemical name: Benzenemethanol.

Molecular formula: C_7H_8O.

Molecular weight: 108.14.

Description: Benzyl Alcohol NF—Colorless liquid, having a faint, aromatic odor. Boils at about 206 °C, without decomposition. It is neutral to litmus.

NF category: Antimicrobial preservative.

Solubility: Benzyl Alcohol NF—Sparingly soluble in water; freely soluble in 50% alcohol. Miscible with alcohol, with ether, and with chloroform.

NF requirements: Benzyl Alcohol NF—Preserve in tight containers, and prevent exposure to light. Contains not less than 97.0% and not more than 100.5% of benzyl alcohol. Meets the requirements for Identification, Specific gravity (1.042–1.047), Refractive index (1.539–1.541 at 20 °C), Residue on ignition (not more than 0.005%), Acidity, Nonvolatile residue, Halogenated compounds and halides (0.03% as chlorine), Benzaldehyde (not more than 0.20%), and Organic volatile impurities.

BENZYL BENZOATE

Chemical name: Benzoic acid, phenylmethyl ester.

Molecular formula: $C_{14}H_{12}O_2$.

Molecular weight: 212.25.

Description: Benzyl Benzoate USP—Clear, colorless, oily liquid having a slight aromatic odor.

NF category: Solvent.

Solubility: Benzyl Benzoate USP—Practically insoluble in water and in glycerin; miscible with alcohol, with ether, and with chloroform.

USP requirements:

Benzyl Benzoate USP—Preserve in tight, well-filled, light-resistant containers, and avoid exposure to excessive heat. Contains not less than 99.0% and not more than 100.5% of benzyl benzoate. Meets the requirements for Identification, Specific gravity (1.116–1.120), Congealing temperature (not lower than 18.0 °C), Refractive index (1.568–1.570 at 20 °C), Aldehyde, Acidity, and Organic volatile impurities.

Benzyl Benzoate Lotion USP—Preserve in tight containers. Contains not less than 26.0% and not more than 30.0% (w/w) of benzyl benzoate.

Prepare Benzyl Benzoate Lotion as follows: 250 mL of Benzyl Benzoate, 5 grams of Triethanolamine, 20 grams of Oleic Acid, and 750 mL of Purified Water to make about 1000 mL. Mix the Triethanolamine with the Oleic Acid, add the Benzyl Benzoate, and mix. Transfer the mixture to a suitable container of about 2000-mL capacity, add 250 mL of Purified Water, and shake the mixture thoroughly. Finally add the remaining Purified Water, and again shake thoroughly.

Meets the requirement for pH (8.5–9.2).

BENZYLPENICILLOYL POLYLYSINE

USP requirements:

Benzylpenicilloyl Polylysine Concentrate USP—Preserve in tight containers. Has a molar concentration of benzylpenicilloyl moiety of not less than 0.0125 *M* and not more than 0.020 *M*. Contains one or more suitable buffers. Meets the requirements for pH (6.5–8.5, the undiluted Concentrate being used), Penicillenate (not more than 0.00020 *M*) and penamaldate (not more than 0.00060 *M*), and Benzylpenicilloyl substitution (50–70%).

Benzylpenicilloyl Polylysine Injection USP—Preserve in single-dose or in multiple-dose containers, preferably of Type I glass, in a refrigerator. Has a molar concentration of benzylpenicilloyl moiety of not less than 5.4×10^{-5} *M* and not more than 7.0×10^{-5} *M*. Contains one or more suitable buffers. Meets the requirements for Bacterial endotoxins, Sterility, and pH (6.5–8.5).

BEPRIDIL

Chemical name: Bepridil hydrochloride—1-Pyrrolideneethanamine, beta-[(2-methylpropoxy)methyl]-*N*-phenyl-*N*-(phenylmethyl)-, monohydrochloride, monohydrate.

Molecular formula: Bepridil hydrochloride—$C_{24}H_{34}N_2O \cdot HCl \cdot H_2O$.

Molecular weight: Bepridil hydrochloride—421.02.

Description: Bepridil hydrochloride—White to off-white, crystalline powder.

Solubility: Bepridil hydrochloride—Slightly soluble in water; very soluble in ethanol, in methanol, and in chloroform; freely soluble in acetone.

USP requirements: Bepridil Hydrochloride Tablets—Not in USP.

BERACTANT

Source: A natural bovine lung extract containing phospholipids, neutral lipids, fatty acids, and surfactant-associated proteins to which colfosceril palmitate (dipalmitoylphosphatidylcholine), palmitic acid, and tripalmitin are added to standardize the composition and to mimic surface-tension lowering properties of natural lung surfactant.

Chemical name: Beractant.

USP requirements: Beractant Intratracheal Suspension—Not in USP.

BETA CAROTENE

Chemical name: Beta,beta-carotene.

Molecular formula: $C_{40}H_{56}$.

Molecular weight: 536.88.

Description: Beta Carotene USP—Red or reddish brown to violet-brown crystals or crystalline powder.

Solubility: Beta Carotene USP—Insoluble in water and in acids and alkalies; soluble in carbon disulfide, and in chloroform; sparingly soluble in ether, in solvent hexane, and in vegetable oils; practically insoluble in methanol and in alcohol.

USP requirements:

Beta Carotene USP—Preserve in tight, light-resistant containers. Contains not less than 96.0% and not more than 101.0% of beta carotene. Meets the requirements for Identification, Melting range (176–182 °C, with decomposition), Loss on drying (not more than 0.2%), Residue on ignition (not more than 0.2%, 2 grams of specimen being used), Heavy metals (not more than 0.001%), and Arsenic (not more than 3 ppm).

Beta Carotene Capsules USP—Preserve in tight, light-resistant containers. Contain the labeled amount, within −10% to +25%. Meet the requirements for Identification and Uniformity of dosage units.

Beta Carotene Tablets—Not in USP.

BETA CYCLODEXTRIN

Description: Beta Cyclodextrin NF—White, practically odorless, fine crystalline powder.

NF category: Sequestering agent.

Solubility: Beta Cyclodextrin NF—Sparingly soluble in water.

NF requirements: Beta Cyclodextrin NF—Preserve in tight containers. A nonreducing cyclic compound composed of 7 alpha-(1-4) linked D-glucopyranosyl units. Contains not less than 98.0% and not more than 101.0% of beta cyclodextrin, calculated on the anhydrous basis. Meets the requirements for Color and clarity of solution, Identification, Specific rotation (+160° to +164°, calculated on the anhydrous basis), Microbial limits, Water (not more than 14.0%), Residue on ignition (not more than 0.1%), Heavy metals (not more than 5 ppm), and Reducing substances (not more than 1.0%).

BETAINE

Chemical name: Betaine hydrochloride—Methanaminium, 1-carboxy-*N,N,N*-trimethyl-, chloride.

Molecular formula: Betaine hydrochloride—$C_5H_{11}NO_2 \cdot HCl$.

Molecular weight: Betaine hydrochloride—153.61.

Solubility: Betaine hydrochloride—Soluble in water (64.7 grams/100 mL) and in ethanol (5.0 grams/100 mL) at 25 °C; practically insoluble in chloroform and in ether.

USP requirements: Betaine Hydrochloride USP—Preserve in well-closed containers. Contains not less than 98.0% and not more than 100.5% of betaine hydrochloride, calculated on the anhydrous basis. Meets the requirements for Identification, pH (0.8–1.2, in a solution [1 in 4]), Water (not more than 0.5%), Residue on ignition (not more than 0.1%), Arsenic (not more than 2 ppm), and Heavy metals (not more than 0.001%).

BETAMETHASONE

Chemical name:

Betamethasone—Pregna-1,4-diene-3,20-dione, 9-fluoro-11,17,21-trihydroxy-16-methyl-, (11 beta,16 beta)-.

Betamethasone acetate—Pregna-1,4-diene-3,20-dione, 9-fluoro-11,17-dihydroxy-16-methyl-21-(acetyloxy)-, (11 beta,16 beta)-.

Betamethasone benzoate—Pregna-1,4-diene-3,20-dione, 17-(benzoyloxy)-9-fluoro-11,21-dihydroxy-16-methyl-, (11 beta,16 beta)-.

Betamethasone dipropionate—Pregna-1,4-diene-3,20-dione, 9-fluoro-11-hydroxy-16-methyl-17,21-bis(1-oxopropoxy)-, (11 beta,16 beta).

Betamethasone sodium phosphate—Pregna-1,4-diene-3,20-dione, 9-fluoro-11,17-dihydroxy-16-methyl-21-(phosphonooxy)-, disodium salt, (11 beta,16 beta)-.

Betamethasone valerate—Pregna-1,4-diene-3,20-dione, 9-fluoro-11,21-dihydroxy-16-methyl-17-[(1-oxopentyl)oxy]-, (11 beta,16 beta)-.

Molecular formula:

Betamethasone—$C_{22}H_{29}FO_5$.

Betamethasone acetate—$C_{24}H_{31}FO_6$.

Betamethasone benzoate—$C_{29}H_{33}FO_6$.

Betamethasone dipropionate—$C_{28}H_{37}FO_7$.

Betamethasone sodium phosphate—$C_{22}H_{28}FNa_2O_8P$.

Betamethasone valerate—$C_{27}H_{37}FO_6$.

Molecular weight:

Betamethasone—392.47.

Betamethasone acetate—434.50.

Betamethasone benzoate—496.58.

Betamethasone dipropionate—504.60.

Betamethasone sodium phosphate—516.41.

Betamethasone valerate—476.59.

Description:

Betamethasone USP—White to practically white, odorless, crystalline powder. Melts at about 240 °C, with some decomposition.

Betamethasone Acetate USP—White to creamy white, odorless powder. Sinters and resolidifies at about 165 °C, and remelts at about 200 or 220 °C, with decomposition.

Betamethasone Benzoate USP—White to practically white, practically odorless powder. Melts at about 220 °C, with decomposition.

Betamethasone Dipropionate USP—White to cream-white, odorless powder.

Betamethasone Sodium Phosphate USP—White to practically white, odorless powder. Is hygroscopic.

Betamethasone Valerate USP—White to practically white, odorless powder. Melts at about 190 °C, with decomposition.

Solubility:

Betamethasone USP—Insoluble in water; sparingly soluble in acetone, in alcohol, in dioxane, and in methanol; very slightly soluble in chloroform and in ether.

Betamethasone Acetate USP—Practically insoluble in water; freely soluble in acetone; soluble in alcohol and in chloroform.
Betamethasone Benzoate USP—Insoluble in water; soluble in alcohol, in methanol, and in chloroform.
Betamethasone Dipropionate USP—Insoluble in water; freely soluble in acetone and in chloroform; sparingly soluble in alcohol.
Betamethasone Sodium Phosphate USP—Freely soluble in water and in methanol; practically insoluble in acetone and in chloroform.
Betamethasone Valerate USP—Practically insoluble in water; freely soluble in acetone and in chloroform; soluble in alcohol; slightly soluble in ether.

USP requirements:
Betamethasone USP—Preserve in well-closed containers. Contains not less than 97.0% and not more than 103.0% of betamethasone, calculated on the dried basis. Meets the requirements for Identification, Specific rotation (+112° to +120°, calculated on the dried basis), Loss on drying (not more than 1.0%), Residue on ignition (not more than 0.2%), Ordinary impurities, and Organic volatile impurities.
Betamethasone Cream USP—Preserve in collapsible tubes or in tight containers. Contains the labeled amount, within −10% to +15%, in a suitable cream base. Meets the requirements for Identification, Microbial limits, and Minimum fill.
Betamethasone Syrup USP—Preserve in well-closed containers. Contains the labeled amount, within −10% to +15%. Meets the requirement for Identification.
Betamethasone Tablets USP—Preserve in well-closed containers. Contain the labeled amount, within ±10%. Meet the requirements for Identification, Dissolution (75% in 45 minutes in water in Apparatus 2 at 50 rpm), and Uniformity of dosage units.
Betamethasone Effervescent Tablets—Not in USP.
Betamethasone Acetate USP—Preserve in tight containers. Contains not less than 97.0% and not more than 103.0% of betamethasone acetate, calculated on the anhydrous basis. Meets the requirements for Identification, Specific rotation (+120° to +128°, calculated on the anhydrous basis), Water (not more than 4.0%), Residue on ignition (not more than 0.2%), and Ordinary impurities.
Betamethasone Benzoate USP—Preserve in tight containers. Contains not less than 98.0% and not more than 102.0% of betamethasone benzoate, calculated on the dried basis. Meets the requirements for Identification, Specific rotation (+60° to +66°, calculated on the dried basis), Loss on drying (not more than 0.5%), and Related steroids.
Betamethasone Benzoate Cream—Not in USP.
Betamethasone Benzoate Gel USP—Preserve in collapsible tubes or tight containers. Contains an amount of betamethasone benzoate equivalent to the labeled amount of betamethasone, within ±10%. Meets the requirements for Identification, Microbial limits, and Minimum fill.
Betamethasone Benzoate Lotion—Not in USP.
Betamethasone Dipropionate USP—Preserve in well-closed containers. Contains not less than 97.0% and not more than 103.0% of betamethasone dipropionate, calculated on the dried basis. Meets the requirements for Identification, Specific rotation (+63° to +70°, calculated on the dried basis), Loss on drying (not more than 1.0%), Residue on ignition (not more than 0.2%), and Ordinary impurities.
Betamethasone Dipropionate Topical Aerosol USP—Preserve in tight, pressurized containers, and avoid exposure to excessive heat. A solution, in suitable propellants in a pressurized container. Contains an amount of betamethasone dipropionate equivalent to the labeled amount of betamethasone, within ±10%. Meets the requirements for Identification, and for Leak testing and Pressure testing under Aerosols.
Betamethasone Dipropionate Cream USP—Preserve in collapsible tubes or in tight containers. Contains an amount of betamethasone dipropionate equivalent to the labeled amount of betamethasone, within ±10%, in a suitable cream base. Meets the requirements for Identification and Minimum fill.
Betamethasone Dipropionate Augmented Cream—Not in USP.
Betamethasone Dipropionate Gel—Not in USP.
Betamethasone Dipropionate Lotion USP—Preserve in tight containers. Contains an amount of betamethasone dipropionate equivalent to the labeled amount of betamethasone, within ±10%, in a suitable lotion base. Meets the requirements for Identification and Minimum fill.
Betamethasone Dipropionate Augmented Lotion—Not in USP.
Betamethasone Dipropionate Ointment USP—Preserve in collapsible tubes or in well-closed containers. Contains an amount of betamethasone dipropionate equivalent to the labeled amount of betamethasone, within ±10%, in a suitable ointment base. Meets the requirements for Identification and Minimum fill.
Betamethasone Dipropionate Augmented Ointment—Not in USP.
Betamethasone Disodium Phosphate Enema—Not in USP.
Betamethasone Disodium Phosphate Dental Pellets—Not in USP.
Betamethasone Sodium Phosphate USP—Preserve in tight containers. Contains not less than 97.0% and not more than 103.0% of betamethasone sodium phosphate, calculated on the anhydrous basis. Meets the requirements for Identification, Specific rotation (+99° to +105°, calculated on the anhydrous basis), Water (not more than 10.0%), Phosphate ions (not more than 1.0%), and Limit of free betamethasone (not more than 1.0%).
Betamethasone Sodium Phosphate Injection USP—Preserve in single-dose or in multiple-dose containers, preferably of Type I glass. A sterile solution of Betamethasone Sodium Phosphate in Water for Injection. Contains an amount of betamethasone sodium phosphate equivalent to the labeled amount of betamethasone, within ±10%. Meets the requirements for Identification, Bacterial endotoxins, pH (8.0–9.0), Particulate matter, and Injections.
Betamethasone Sodium Phosphate Ophthalmic/Otic Solution—Not in USP.
Betamethasone Sodium Phosphate Extended-release Tablets—Not in USP.
Sterile Betamethasone Sodium Phosphate and Betamethasone Acetate Suspension USP—Preserve in multiple-dose containers, preferably of Type I glass. A sterile preparation of Betamethasone Sodium Phosphate in solution and Betamethasone Acetate in suspension in Water for Injection. Contains an amount of betamethasone sodium phosphate equivalent to the labeled amount of betamethasone, within −10% to +15%, and the labeled amount of betamethasone acetate, within −10% to +15%. Meets the requirements for Identification, Bacterial endotoxins, pH (6.8–7.2), and Injections.
Betamethasone Valerate USP—Preserve in tight containers. Contains not less than 97.0% and not more than 103.0% of betamethasone valerate, calculated on the dried basis. Meets the requirements for Identification, Specific rotation (+75° to +82°, calculated on the dried basis), Loss on drying (not more than 0.5%), and Residue on ignition (not more than 0.2%).
Betamethasone Valerate Cream USP—Preserve in collapsible tubes or in tight containers. Contains an amount of

betamethasone valerate equivalent to the labeled amount of betamethasone, within ±10%, in a suitable cream base. Meets the requirements for Identification, Microbial limits, and Minimum fill.

Betamethasone Valerate Lotion USP—Preserve in tight, light-resistant containers, and store at controlled room temperature. Contains an amount of betamethasone valerate equivalent to the labeled amount of betamethasone, within −5% to +15%. Meets the requirements for Identification, Microbial limits, pH (4.0–6.0), and Minimum fill.

Betamethasone Valerate Ointment USP—Preserve in collapsible tubes or in tight containers, and avoid exposure to excessive heat. Contains an amount of betamethasone valerate equivalent to the labeled amount of betamethasone, within ±10%, in a suitable ointment base. Meets the requirements for Identification, Microbial limits, and Minimum fill.

BETAXOLOL

Chemical name: Betaxolol hydrochloride—2-Propanol, 1-[4-[2-(cyclopropylmethoxy)ethyl]phenoxy]-3-[(1-methylethyl)-amino]-, hydrochloride, (±)-.

Molecular formula: Betaxolol hydrochloride—$C_{18}H_{29}NO_3 \cdot HCl$.

Molecular weight: Betaxolol hydrochloride—343.89.

Description: Betaxolol Hydrochloride USP—White, crystalline powder.

pKa: 9.4.

Solubility: Betaxolol Hydrochloride USP—Freely soluble in water, in alcohol, in chloroform, and in methanol.

USP requirements:

Betaxolol Ophthalmic Solution USP—Preserve in tight containers. A sterile, aqueous, isotonic solution of Betaxolol Hydrochloride. Label Ophthalmic Solution to state both the content of the betaxolol active moiety and the content of the salt used in formulating the article. Contains a suitable antimicrobial preservative. Contains an amount of betaxolol hydrochloride equivalent to the labeled amount of betaxolol, within ±10%. Meets the requirements for Identification, Sterility, and pH (4.0–8.0).

Betaxolol Tablets USP—Preserve in tight containers. Label Tablets to state both the content of the betaxolol active moiety and the content of betaxolol hydrochloride used in formulating them. Contain an amount of Betaxolol Hydrochloride equivalent to the labeled amount of betaxolol hydrochloride, within ±10%. Meet the requirements for Identification, Dissolution (80% in 30 minutes in water in Apparatus 2 at 50 rpm), and Uniformity of dosage units.

Betaxolol Hydrochloride USP—Preserve in tight containers. Contains not less than 98.5% and not more than 101.5% of betaxolol hydrochloride, calculated on the dried basis. Meets the requirements for Identification, Melting range (113–117 °C), pH (4.5–6.5, in a solution [1 in 50]), Loss on drying (not more than 1.0%), Residue on ignition (not more than 0.1%), Heavy metals (not more than 0.002%), and Chromatographic purity.

Betaxolol Hydrochloride Ophthalmic Suspension—Not in USP.

BETAXOLOL AND CHLORTHALIDONE

For *Betaxolol* and *Chlorthalidone*—See individual listings for chemistry information.

USP requirements: Betaxolol Hydrochloride and Chlorthalidone Tablets—Not in USP.

BETHANECHOL

Chemical group: Synthetic ester structurally related to acetylcholine.

Chemical name: Bethanechol chloride—1-Propanaminium, 2-[(aminocarbonyl)oxy]-*N,N,N*-trimethyl-, chloride.

Molecular formula: Bethanechol chloride—$C_7H_{17}ClN_2O_2$.

Molecular weight: Bethanechol chloride—196.68.

Description: Bethanechol Chloride USP—Colorless or white crystals or white, crystalline powder, usually having a slight, amine-like odor. Is hygroscopic. Exhibits polymorphism, and of two crystalline forms observed, one melts at about 211 °C and the other melts at about 219 °C.

Solubility: Bethanechol Chloride USP—Freely soluble in water and in alcohol; insoluble in chloroform and in ether.

USP requirements:

Bethanechol Chloride USP—Preserve in tight containers. Contains not less than 98.0% and not more than 101.5% of bethanechol chloride, calculated on the dried basis. Meets the requirements for Identification, pH (5.5–6.5, in a solution [1 in 100]), Loss on drying (not more than 1.0%), Residue on ignition (not more than 0.1%), Chloride content (17.7–18.3%), Heavy metals (not more than 0.003%), and Organic volatile impurities.

Bethanechol Chloride Injection USP—Preserve in single-dose containers, preferably of Type I glass. A sterile solution of Bethanechol Chloride in Water for Injection. Contains the labeled amount, within ±5%. Meets the requirements for Identification, Bacterial endotoxins, pH (5.5–7.5), and Injections.

Bethanechol Chloride Tablets USP—Preserve in tight containers. Contain the labeled amount, within ±10%. Meet the requirements for Identification, Dissolution (80% in 30 minutes in 0.1 *N* hydrochloric acid in Apparatus 2 at 50 rpm), and Uniformity of dosage units.

BIOLOGICAL INDICATOR FOR DRY-HEAT STERILIZATION, PAPER STRIP

USP requirements: Biological Indicator for Dry-heat Sterilization, Paper Strip USP—Preserve in the original package under the conditions recommended on the label, and protect from light, toxic substances, excessive heat, and moisture. A preparation of viable spores made from a culture derived from a specified strain of *Bacillus subtilis* subspecies ***niger***, on a suitable grade of paper carrier, individually packaged in a suitable container readily penetrable by dry heat, and characterized for predictable resistance to dry-heat sterilization. Label it to state that it is a Biological Indicator for Dry-heat Sterilization on a paper carrier, to indicate its D value, the method used to determine such D value, i.e., by spore count or fraction negative procedure after graded exposures to the sterilization conditions, survival time and kill time under the sterilization conditions stated on the label, its particular viable spore count, with a statement that such count has been determined after preliminary heat treatment, and its recommended storage conditions. State in the labeling the size of the paper carrier, the strain and ATCC number from which the spores were derived, and instructions for spore recovery and for its safe disposal. Indicate in the labeling that the stated D value is reproducible only under the exact conditions under which it was determined, that the user would not necessarily obtain the same result, and that the user would need to determine its suitability for the particular use. The packaged Biological Indicator for Dry-heat Sterilization, Paper Strip, has a particular labeled spore count per carrier of not less than 10^4 and not more than 10^9 spores.

When labeled for and subjected to dry-heat sterilization conditions at a particular temperature, it has a survival time and kill time appropriate to the labeled spore count and to the decimal reduction value (D value, in minutes) of the preparation, specified by: Survival time (in minutes) = not less than (labeled D value) × (log_{10} labeled spore count per carrier − 2); and Kill time (in minutes) = not more than (labeled D value) × (log_{10} labeled spore count per carrier + 4). Meets the requirements for Expiration date (not less than 18 months from the date of manufacture, the date of manufacture being the date on which the first determination of the total viable population was made), Identification, Resistance performance tests, Purity, and Stability.

Note: See Biological Indicators in *USP/NF* for directives on selection of suitable indicators and on their applicability for different sterilization cycles, and for the characteristics of the basic or prototype article.

BIOLOGICAL INDICATOR FOR ETHYLENE OXIDE STERILIZATION, PAPER STRIP

USP requirements: Biological Indicator for Ethylene Oxide Sterilization, Paper Strip USP—Preserve in the original package under the conditions recommended on the label, and protect it from light, toxic substances, excessive heat, and moisture. A preparation of viable spores made from a culture derived from a specified strain of *Bacillus subtilis* subspecies *niger*, on a suitable grade of paper carrier, individually packaged in a suitable container readily penetrable by ethylene oxide sterilizing gas mixture, and characterized for predictable resistance to sterilization with such gas. Label it to state that it is a Biological Indicator for Ethylene Oxide Sterilization on a paper carrier, to indicate its D value, the method used to determine such D value, i.e., by spore count or fraction negative procedure after graded exposures to the sterilization conditions, survival time and kill time under the sterilization conditions stated on the label, its particular viable spore count, with a statement that such count has been determined after preliminary heat treatment, and its recommended storage conditions. State in the labeling the size of the paper carrier, the strain and ATCC number from which the spores were derived, and instructions for spore recovery and for its safe disposal. Indicate in the labeling that the stated D value is reproducible only under the exact conditions under which it was determined, that the user would not necessarily obtain the same result and that the user would need to determine its suitability for the particular use. The packaged Biological Indicator for Ethylene Oxide Sterilization, Paper Strip, has a particular labeled spore count per carrier of not less than 10^4 and not more than 10^9 spores. Where labeled for and subjected to particular ethylene oxide sterilization conditions of a gaseous mixture, temperature, and relative humidity, it has a survival time and kill time appropriate to the labeled spore count and to the decimal reduction value (D value, in minutes) of the preparation, specified by: Survival time (in minutes) = not less than (labeled D value) × (log_{10} labeled spore count per carrier − 2); and Kill time (in minutes) = not more than (labeled D value) × (log_{10} labeled spore count per carrier + 4). Meets the requirements for Expiration date (not less than 18 months from the date of manufacture, the date of manufacture being the date on which the first determination of the total viable population was made), Identification, Resistance performance tests, Purity, and Stability.

Note: See Biological Indicators in *USP/NF* for directives on selection of suitable indicators and on their applicability for different sterilization cycles, and for the characteristics of the basic or prototype article.

BIOLOGICAL INDICATOR FOR STEAM STERILIZATION, PAPER STRIP

USP requirements: Biological Indicator for Steam Sterilization, Paper Strip USP—Preserve in the original package under the conditions recommended on the label, and protect it from light, toxic substances, excessive heat, and moisture. A preparation of viable spores made from a culture derived from a specified strain of *Bacillus stearothermophilus*, on a suitable grade of paper carrier, individually packaged in a suitable container readily penetrable by steam, and characterized for predictable resistance to steam sterilization. Label it to state that it is a Biological Indicator for Steam Sterilization on a paper carrier, to indicate its D value, the method used to determine such D value, i.e., by spore count or fraction negative procedure after graded exposures to the sterilization conditions, survival time and kill time under the sterilization conditions stated on the label, its particular viable spore count, with a statement that such count has been determined after preliminary heat treatment, and its recommended storage conditions. State in the labeling the size of the paper carrier, the strain and ATCC number from which the spores were derived, and instructions for spore recovery and for its safe disposal. Indicate in the labeling that the stated D value is reproducible only under the exact conditions under which it was determined, that the user would not necessarily obtain the same result, and that the user would need to determine its suitability for the particular use. The packaged Biological Indicator for Steam Sterilization, Paper Strip, has a particular labeled spore count per carrier of not less than 10^4 and not more than 10^9 spores. When labeled for and subjected to steam sterilization conditions at a particular temperature, it has a survival time and kill time appropriate to the labeled spore count and to the decimal reduction value (D value, in minutes) of the preparation, specified by: Survival time (in minutes) = not less than (labeled D value) × (log_{10} labeled spore count per carrier − 2); and Kill time (in minutes) = not more than (labeled D value) × (log_{10} labeled spore count per carrier + 4). Meets the requirements for Expiration date (not less than 18 months from the date of manufacture, the date of manufacture being the date on which the first determination of the total viable population was made), Identification, Resistance performance tests, Purity, and Stability.

Note: See Biological Indicators in *USP/NF* for directives on selection of suitable indicators and on their applicability for different sterilization cycles, and for the characteristics of the basic or prototype article.

BIOTIN

Chemical name: 1*H*-Thieno[3,4-*d*]imidazole-4-pentanoic acid, hexahydro-2-oxo-, [3a*S*-(3a alpha,4 beta,6a alpha)]-.

Molecular formula: $C_{10}H_{16}N_2O_3S$.

Molecular weight: 244.31.

Description: Biotin USP—Practically white, crystalline powder.

Solubility: Biotin USP—Very slightly soluble in water and in alcohol; insoluble in other common organic solvents.

USP requirements:

Biotin USP—Store in tight containers. Contains not less than 97.5% and not more than 100.5% of biotin. Meets the requirements for Identification, Specific rotation (+89° to +93°), and Organic volatile impurities.

Biotin Capsules—Not in USP.

Biotin Tablets—Not in USP.

BIPERIDEN

Chemical group: Synthetic tertiary amine.

Chemical name:
Biperiden—1-Piperidinepropanol, alpha-bicyclo[2.2.1]hept-5-en-2-yl-alpha-phenyl-.
Biperiden hydrochloride—1-Piperidinepropanol, alpha-bicyclo[2.2.1]hept-5-en-2-yl-alpha-phenyl-, hydrochloride.
Biperiden lactate—1-Piperidinepropanol, alpha-bicyclo-[2.2.1]-hept-5-en-2-yl-alpha-phenyl-, compd. with 2-hydroxypropanoic acid (1:1).

Molecular formula:
Biperiden—$C_{21}H_{29}NO$.
Biperiden hydrochloride—$C_{21}H_{29}NO \cdot HCl$.
Biperiden lactate—$C_{21}H_{29}NO \cdot C_3H_6O_3$.

Molecular weight:
Biperiden—311.47.
Biperiden hydrochloride—347.93.
Biperiden lactate—401.55.

Description:
Biperiden USP—White, practically odorless, crystalline powder.
Biperiden Hydrochloride USP—White, practically odorless, crystalline powder. Melts at about 275 °C, with decomposition. Is optically inactive.

Solubility:
Biperiden USP—Practically insoluble in water; freely soluble in chloroform; sparingly soluble in alcohol.
Biperiden Hydrochloride USP—Slightly soluble in water, in ether, in alcohol, and in chloroform; sparingly soluble in methanol.

USP requirements:
Biperiden USP—Preserve in well-closed, light-resistant containers. Contains not less than 98.0% and not more than 101.0% of biperiden, calculated on the dried basis. Meets the requirements for Identification, Melting range (112–116 °C), Loss on drying (not more than 1.0%), Residue on ignition (not more than 0.1%), Ordinary impurities, and Organic volatile impurities.
Biperiden Hydrochloride USP—Preserve in well-closed, light-resistant containers. Contains not less than 98.0% and not more than 101.0% of biperiden hydrochloride, calculated on the dried basis. Meets the requirements for Identification, Loss on drying (not more than 0.5%), and Ordinary impurities.
Biperiden Hydrochloride Tablets USP—Preserve in tight containers. Contain the labeled amount, within ±7%. Meet the requirements for Identification, Dissolution (75% in 45 minutes in 0.1 *N* hydrochloric acid in Apparatus 2 at 50 rpm), and Uniformity of dosage units.
Biperiden Lactate Injection USP—Preserve in single-dose containers, preferably of Type I glass, protected from light. A sterile solution of biperiden lactate in Water for Injection, prepared from Biperiden with the aid of Lactic Acid. Contains the labeled amount, within ±5%. Meets the requirements for Identification, Bacterial endotoxins, pH (4.8–5.8), and Injections.

BISACODYL

Chemical group: Diphenylmethane derivatives.

Chemical name:
Bisacodyl—Phenol, 4,4′-(2-pyridinylmethylene)bis-, diacetate (ester).
Bisacodyl tannex—Phenol, 4,4′-(2-pyridinylmethylene)bis-, diacetate (ester), complex with tannic acid.

Molecular formula: $C_{22}H_{19}NO_4$.

Molecular weight: 361.40.

Description:
Bisacodyl USP—White to off-white, crystalline powder, in which the number of particles having a longest diameter smaller than 50 micrometers predominate.
Bisacodyl tannex—Light tan, microcrystalline powder.

Solubility:
Bisacodyl USP—Practically insoluble in water; soluble in chloroform; sparingly soluble in alcohol and in methanol; slightly soluble in ether.
Bisacodyl tannex—Very soluble in water and in alcohol.

USP requirements:
Bisacodyl USP—Preserve in well-closed containers. Contains not less than 98.0% and not more than 101.0% of bisacodyl, calculated on the dried basis. Meets the requirements for Identification, Melting range (131–135 °C), Loss on drying (not more than 0.5%), Residue on ignition (not more than 0.1%), and Heavy metals (not more than 0.001%).
Caution: Avoid inhalation and contact with the eyes, skin, and mucous membranes.
Bisacodyl Rectal Solution—Not in USP.
Bisacodyl Suppositories USP—Preserve in well-closed containers at a temperature not exceeding 30 °C. Contain the labeled amount, within ±10%. Meet the requirement for Identification.
Bisacodyl Tablets USP—Preserve in well-closed containers at a temperature not exceeding 30 °C. Label Tablets to indicate that they are enteric-coated. Contain the labeled amount, within ±10%. Bisacodyl Tablets are enteric-coated. Meet the requirements for Identification, Disintegration (tablets do not disintegrate after 1 hour of agitation in simulated gastric fluid TS, but then disintegrate within 45 minutes in simulated intestinal fluid TS), and Uniformity of dosage units.
Bisacodyl Tannex Powder for Rectal Solution—Not in USP.

BISACODYL AND DOCUSATE

For *Bisacodyl* and *Docusate*—See individual listings for chemistry information.

USP requirements: Bisacodyl and Docusate Sodium Tablets—Not in USP.

BISMUTH

Chemical name:
Bismuth subgallate—Gallic acid bismuth basic salt.
Bismuth subnitrate—Bismuth hydroxide nitrate oxide ($Bi_5O(OH)_9(NO_3)_4$).
Bismuth subsalicylate—(2-Hydroxybenzoato-O^1)-oxobismuth.

Molecular formula:
Bismuth subgallate—$C_7H_5BiO_6$.
Bismuth subnitrate—$Bi_5O(OH)_9(NO_3)_4$.
Bismuth subsalicylate—$C_7H_5BiO_4$.

Molecular weight:
Bismuth subgallate—394.09.
Bismuth subnitrate—1461.99.
Bismuth subsalicylate—362.09.

Description:
Bismuth Subgallate USP—Amorphous, bright yellow powder. Odorless. Stable in air, but affected by light.

Bismuth Subnitrate USP—White, slightly hygroscopic powder.

Solubility:
Bismuth Subgallate USP—Dissolves readily with decomposition in warm, moderately dilute hydrochloric, nitric, or sulfuric acid; readily dissolved by solutions of alkali hydroxides, forming a clear, yellow liquid, which rapidly assumes a deep red color. Practically insoluble in water, in alcohol, in chloroform, and in ether; insoluble in very dilute mineral acids.
Bismuth Subnitrate USP—Practically insoluble in water and in alcohol; readily dissolved by hydrochloric acid or by nitric acid.
Bismuth subsalicylate—Practically insoluble in water or in alcohol; soluble in alkali; decomposed by hot water.

USP requirements:
Bismuth Subgallate USP—Preserve in tight, light-resistant containers. A basic salt. When dried at 105 °C for 3 hours, contains an amount of bismuth subgallate equivalent to not less than 52.0% and not more than 57.0% of bismuth trioxide. Meets the requirements for Identification, Loss on drying (not more than 7.0%), Nitrate, Alkalies and alkaline earths (not more than 0.5%), Arsenic (not more than 7.5 ppm), Copper, Lead, and Silver, and Free gallic acid (not more than 0.5%).
Bismuth Subnitrate USP—Preserve in well-closed containers. A basic salt. Contains an amount of bismuth subnitrate equivalent to not less than 79.0% of bismuth trioxide, calculated on the dried basis. Meets the requirements for Identification, Loss on drying (not more than 3.0%), Carbonate, Chloride (not more than 0.035%), Sulfate, Alkalies and alkaline earths (not more than 0.5%), Ammonium salts, Arsenic (not more than 8 ppm), Copper, Lead, and Silver.
Bismuth Subsalicylate Oral Suspension—Not in USP.
Bismuth Subsalicylate Chewable Tablets—Not in USP.

MILK OF BISMUTH

Description: Milk of Bismuth USP—Thick, white, opaque suspension that separates on standing. Is odorless.

Solubility: Milk of Bismuth USP—Miscible with water and with alcohol.

USP requirements: Milk of Bismuth USP—Preserve in tight containers, and protect from freezing. Contains bismuth hydroxide and bismuth subcarbonate in suspension in water, and yields not less than 5.2% and not more than 5.8% (w/w) of bismuth trioxide.

Prepare Milk of Bismuth as follows: 80 grams of Bismuth Subnitrate, 120 mL of Nitric Acid, 10 grams of Ammonium Carbonate, and a sufficient quantity of Strong Ammonia Solution and of Purified Water, to make 1000 mL. Mix the Bismuth Subnitrate with 60 mL of Purified Water and 60 mL of the Nitric Acid in a suitable container, and agitate, warming gently until solution is effected. Pour this solution, with constant stirring, into 5000 mL of Purified Water containing 60 mL of the Nitric Acid. Dilute 160 mL of Strong Ammonia Solution with 4300 mL of Purified Water in a glazed or glass vessel of at least 12,000-mL capacity. Dissolve the Ammonium Carbonate in this solution, and then pour the bismuth solution quickly into it with constant stirring. Add sufficient 6 *N* ammonium hydroxide, if necessary, to render the mixture distinctly alkaline, allow to stand until the precipitate has settled, then pour or siphon off the supernatant liquid, and wash the precipitate twice with Purified Water, by decantation. Transfer the magma to a strainer of close texture, so as to provide continuous washing with Purified Water, the outlet tube being elevated to prevent the surface of the magma from becoming dry. When the washings no longer yield a pink color with phenolphthalein TS, drain the moist preparation, transfer to a graduated vessel, add sufficient Purified Water to make 1000 mL, and mix.

Note: This method of preparation may be varied, provided the product meets the requirements.

Meets the requirements for Identification, Microbial limits, Water-soluble substances (not more than 0.1%), Alkalies and alkaline earths (not more than 0.3%), Arsenic (not more than 0.8 ppm), and Lead.

BISOPROLOL

Chemical name: Bisoprolol fumarate—2-Propanol, 1-[4-[[2-(1-methylethoxy)ethoxy]methyl]phenoxy]-3-[(1-methylethyl)-amino]-, (±)-, (*E*)-2-butenedioate (2:1) (salt).

Molecular formula: Bisoprolol fumarate—$(C_{18}H_{31}NO_4)_2 \cdot C_4H_4O_4$.

Molecular weight: Bisoprolol fumarate—766.97.

USP requirements: Bisoprolol Fumarate Tablets—Not in USP.

BITOLTEROL

Chemical name: Bitolterol mesylate—Benzoic acid, 4-methyl-, 4-[2-[(1,1-dimethylethyl)amino]-1-hydroxyethyl]-1,2-phenylene ester methanesulfonate (salt).

Molecular formula: Bitolterol mesylate—$C_{28}H_{31}NO_5 \cdot CH_4O_3S$.

Molecular weight: Bitolterol mesylate—557.66.

Description: Bitolterol mesylate—White to off-white, crystalline powder.

Solubility: Bitolterol mesylate—Sparingly soluble to soluble in water; freely soluble in alcohol.

USP requirements: Bitolterol Mesylate Inhalation Aerosol—Not in USP.

BLEOMYCIN

Source: A mixture of glycopeptide antibiotics isolated from a strain of *Streptomyces verticillus* and converted into sulfates.

Chemical name: Bleomycin sulfate—Bleomycin sulfate (salt).

Description: Sterile Bleomycin Sulfate USP—Cream-colored, amorphous powder.

Solubility: Sterile Bleomycin Sulfate USP—Very soluble in water.

Other characteristics: Inactivated in vitro by agents containing sulfhydryl groups, hydrogen peroxide, and ascorbic acid.

USP requirements: Sterile Bleomycin Sulfate USP—Preserve in Containers for Sterile Solids. The sulfate salt of bleomycin, a mixture of basic cytotoxic glycopeptides produced by the growth of *Streptomyces verticillus*, or produced by other means. Contains not less than 1.5 Bleomycin Units and not more than 2.0 Bleomycin Units per mg and, where packaged for dispensing, contains an amount of bleomycin sulfate equivalent to the labeled amount of bleomycin, within −10% to +20%. Meets the requirements for Constituted solution, Identification, Depressor substances, Bacterial endotoxins, Sterility, pH (4.5–6.0, in a solution containing 10 Bleomycin Units per mL), Loss on drying (not more than 6.0%), Content of bleomycins, and Copper (not more than 0.1%), and, where packaged for dispensing, for Uniformity of dosage units and Labeling under Injections.

ANTI-A BLOOD GROUPING SERUM

Description: Anti-A Blood Grouping Serum USP—Liquid Serum is a clear or slightly opalescent fluid unless artificially colored blue. Dried Serum is light yellow to deep cream color, unless artificially colored as indicated for liquid Serum. The liquid Serum may develop slight turbidity on storage. The dried Serum may show slight turbidity upon reconstitution for use.

USP requirements: Anti-A Blood Grouping Serum USP—Preserve at a temperature between 2 and 8 °C. A sterile, liquid or dried preparation containing the particular blood group antibodies derived from high-titered blood plasma or serum of human subjects, with or without stimulation by the injection of Blood Group Specific Substance A (or AB). Agglutinates human red cells containing A-antigens, i.e., blood groups A and AB (including subgroups A_1, A_2, A_1B, and A_2B but not necessarily weaker subgroups). Contains a suitable antimicrobial preservative. Label it to state that the source material was not reactive for hepatitis B surface antigen, but that no known test method offers assurance that products derived from human blood will not transmit hepatitis. Label it also to state that it is for in-vitro diagnostic use. (Note: The labeling is in black lettering imprinted on paper that is white or is colored completely or in part to match the specified blue color standard.) Meets the requirements of the tests for potency, specificity, and avidity. All fresh or frozen red blood cell suspensions used for these tests are prepared under specified conditions and meet specified criteria. Meets the requirement for Expiration date (for liquid Serum, not later than 1 year, and for dried Serum, not later than 5 years after date of issue from manufacturer's cold storage [5 °C, 1 year; or 0 °C, 2 years], provided that the expiration date for dried Serum is not later than 1 year after constitution). Conforms to the regulations of the U.S. Food and Drug Administration concerning biologics.

ANTI-B BLOOD GROUPING SERUM

Description: Anti-B Blood Grouping Serum USP—Liquid Serum is a clear or slightly opalescent fluid unless artificially colored yellow. Dried Serum is light yellow to deep cream color, unless artificially colored as indicated for liquid Serum. The liquid Serum may develop a slight turbidity on storage. The dried Serum may show slight turbidity upon reconstitution for use.

USP requirements: Anti-B Blood Grouping Serum USP—Preserve at a temperature between 2 and 8 °C. A sterile, liquid or dried preparation containing the particular blood group antibodies derived from high-titered blood plasma or serum of human subjects, with or without stimulation by the injection of Blood Group Specific Substance B (or AB). Agglutinates human red cells containing B-antigens, i.e., blood groups B and AB (including subgroups A_1B and A_2B). Contains a suitable antimicrobial preservative. Label it to state that the source material was not reactive for hepatitis B surface antigen, but that no known test method offers assurance that products derived from human blood will not transmit hepatitis. Label it also to state that it is for in-vitro diagnostic use. (Note: The labeling is in black lettering imprinted on paper that is white or is colored completely or in part to match the specified yellow color standard.) Meets the requirements of the tests for potency, specificity, and avidity. All fresh or frozen red blood cell suspensions used for these tests are prepared under specified conditions and meet specified criteria. Meets the requirement for Expiration date (for liquid Serum, not later than 1 year, and for dried Serum, not later than 5 years after date of issue from manufacturer's cold storage [5 °C, 1 year; or 0 °C, 2 years], provided that the expiration date for dried Serum is not later than 1 year after constitution). Conforms to the regulations of the U.S. Food and Drug Administration concerning biologics.

BLOOD GROUPING SERUMS

USP requirements: Blood Grouping Serums USP—Preserve at a temperature between 2 and 8 °C. Each serum is a sterile, liquid or dried preparation containing one or more of the particular blood group antibodies derived from high-titered blood plasma or serum of human subjects, with or without stimulation by the injection of red cells or other substances, or of animals after stimulation by substances that cause such antibody production. Causes either directly, or indirectly by the antiglobulin test, the visible agglutination of human red cells containing the particular antigen(s) for which it is specific. Contains a suitable antimicrobial preservative. Label each to state the source of the product if other than human and, if of human origin, to state that the source material was not reactive for hepatitis B surface antigen, but that no known test method offers assurance that products derived from human blood will not transmit hepatitis. Label each also to state that it is for in-vitro diagnostic use. Meets the requirements of the tests for potency, specificity, and avidity. All fresh or frozen red blood cell suspensions used for these tests are prepared under specified conditions and meet specified criteria. Meets the requirement for Expiration date (for liquid Serum, not later than 1 year, and for dried Serum, not later than 5 years after date of issue from manufacturer's cold storage [5 °C, 1 year; or 0 °C, 2 years], provided that the expiration date for dried Serum is not later than 1 year after constitution). Blood Grouping Serums conform to the regulations of the U.S. Food and Drug Administration concerning biologics.

Note: This monograph deals with those Blood Grouping Serums for which there are no individual monographs and which are not routinely used or required for the testing of blood or blood products for transfusion.

BLOOD GROUPING SERUMS ANTI-D, ANTI-C, ANTI-E, ANTI-c, ANTI-e

Description: Blood Grouping Serums Anti-D, Anti-C, Anti-E, Anti-c, Anti-e USP—The liquid Serums are clear, slightly yellowish fluids, that may develop slight turbidity on storage. The dried Serums are light yellow to deep cream color.

USP requirements: Blood Grouping Serums Anti-D, Anti-C, Anti-E, Anti-c, Anti-e USP—Preserve at a temperature between 2 and 8 °C. They are sterile, liquid or dried preparations derived from the blood plasma or serum of human subjects who have developed specific Rh antibodies. They are free from agglutinins for the A or B antigens and from alloantibodies other than those for which claims are made in the labeling. Contain a suitable antimicrobial preservative. Liquid serums are not artificially colored. Label each to state that the source material was not reactive for hepatitis B surface antigen, but that no known test method offers assurance that products derived from human blood will not transmit hepatitis. Label each to state that it is for in-vitro diagnostic use. Meet the requirements of the tests for potency, avidity, and specificity. All fresh or frozen red blood cell suspensions used for these tests are prepared under specified conditions and meet specified criteria. Meet the requirement for Expiration date (for liquid Serums, not later than 1 year, and for dried Serums, not later than 5 years, after date of issue from manufacturer's cold storage [5 °C, 1 year; or 0 °C, 2 years], provided that the expiration date for dried Serums is not later than 1 year after constitution). Conform to the regulations of the U.S. Food and Drug Administration concerning biologics.

LEUKOCYTE TYPING SERUM

USP requirements: Leukocyte Typing Serum USP—Preserve at the temperature recommended by the manufacturer. A dried or liquid preparation of serum derived from plasma or blood obtained from animals or from human donors containing an antibody or antibodies for identification of leukocyte antigens. Label it to state the source of the product if other than human and, if of human origin, to state either that the source material was found reactive for hepatitis B surface antigen and that the product may transmit hepatitis, or that the source material was not reactive for hepatitis B surface antigen but that no known test method offers assurance that products derived from human blood will not transmit hepatitis. Label it also to include the name of the specific antibody or antibodies present and the requirements for potency in relation to the antigen(s) of the corresponding specificity with which it complies; the permissible limits of error for specificity reactions with which it complies; the name of the test method or methods recommended for the product; and a statement that it is for in-vitro diagnostic use. Provide with the package enclosure the following: adequate directions for performing the tests, including a description of all recommended test methods; descriptions of all supplementary reagents, including one of a suitable complement source; description of precautions in use, including a warning against exposure of the product to carbon dioxide; a caution statement to the effect that more than one antiserum is to be used for each specificity, that the antiserum is not to be diluted, and that cross-reacting antigens exist; and directions for constitution of the product, including instructions for the use, storage, and labeling of the constituted product. Meets the requirements of the test for potency and for specificity. Meets the requirement for Expiration date (for dried Serum, not later than 2 years after date of issue from manufacturer's cold storage [5 °C, 1 year; or 0 °C, 2 years] and for liquid Serum not later than 1 year after such issue [5 °C, 1 year]). Conforms to the regulations of the U.S. Food and Drug Administration concerning biologics.

BLOOD GROUP SPECIFIC SUBSTANCES A, B, AND AB

Description: Blood Group Specific Substances A, B, and AB USP—Clear solution that may have a slight odor because of the preservative.

USP requirements: Blood Group Specific Substances A, B, and AB USP—Preserve in single-dose containers, each containing a volume of not more than 1 mL consisting of a solution containing not more than 1.25 mg of Blood Group Specific Substance powder, at a temperature between 2 and 8 °C. Dispense it in the unopened container in which it was placed by the manufacturer. A sterile, pyrogen-free, nonanaphylactic isotonic solution of the polysaccharide-amino acid complexes that are capable of neutralizing the anti-A and the anti-B isoagglutinins of group O blood, and are used in the immunization of plasma donors for the production of in-vitro diagnostic reagents. Contains no added preservative. Blood Group Specific Substance A is prepared from hog stomach (gastric mucin), and Blood Group Specific Substances B and AB are prepared from horse stomach (gastric mucosa). Has a total nitrogen content of not more than 8%, calculated on the moisture- and ash-free basis. Label it to state that it was derived from porcine or equine stomachs, whichever is applicable, and that it contains a single dose consisting of the stated content of dry weight of powder dissolved in the stated volume of product. Label it also to state the route of administration, and to state that it is not to be administered intravenously nor to fertile women. Label Blood Group Specific Substance B with a warning that it may contain immunogenic A activity. Meets the requirements of the test for potency (including identity). Meets the requirements for Expiration date (not more than 2 years after date of issue from manufacturer's cold storage [5 °C, 1 year; or 0 °C, 2 years]), pH (6.0–6.8), and of the tests for safety and for anaphylaxis. Conforms to the regulations of the U.S. Food and Drug Administration concerning biologics.

RED BLOOD CELLS

Description: Red Blood Cells USP—Dark red in color when packed. May show a slight creamy layer on the surface and a small supernatant layer of yellow or opalescent plasma. Also supplied in deep-frozen form with added cryophylactic substance to extend storage time.

USP requirements: Red Blood Cells USP—Preserve in a hermetic container, which is of colorless, transparent, sterile, pyrogen-free Type I or Type II glass, or of a suitable plastic material in which it was placed by the processor. Store if unfrozen at a temperature between 1 and 6 °C, held constant within a 2 °C range except during shipment when the temperature may be between 1 and 10 °C, and store if for extended manufacturers' storage in frozen form at −65 °C or colder. The container of Red Blood Cells is accompanied by a securely attached smaller container holding an original pilot sample of blood taken from the donor at the same time as the whole human blood, or a pilot sample of Red Blood Cells removed at the time of its preparation. It is the remaining red blood cells of whole human blood that have been collected from suitable whole blood donors, and from which plasma has been removed. Red Blood Cells may be prepared at any time during the dating period of the whole blood from which it is derived, by centrifuging or undisturbed sedimentation for the separation of plasma and cells, not later than 21 days after the blood has been drawn, except that when acid citrate dextrose adenine solution has been used as the anticoagulant, such preparation may be made within 35 days therefrom. Contains a portion of the plasma sufficient to ensure optional cell preservation or contains a cryophylactic substance if it is for extended manufacturers' storage at −65 °C or colder. In addition to labeling requirements of Whole Blood applicable to this product, label it to indicate the approved variation to which it conforms, such as "Frozen," or "Deglycerolized." Label it also with the instruction to use a filter in the administration equipment. Meets the requirement for Expiration date (for unfrozen Red Blood Cells, not later than that of the whole human blood from which it is derived if plasma has not been removed, except that if the hermetic seal of the container is broken during preparation, the expiration date is not later than 24 hours after the seal is broken; for frozen Red Blood Cells, not later than 3 years after the date of collection of the source blood when stored at −65 °C or colder and not later than 24 hours after removal from −65 °C storage provided it is then stored at the temperature for unfrozen Red Blood Cells). Conforms to the regulations of the U.S. Food and Drug Administration concerning biologics.

WHOLE BLOOD

Description: Whole Blood USP—Deep red, opaque liquid from which the corpuscles readily settle upon standing for 24 to 48 hours, leaving a clear, yellowish or pinkish supernatant layer of plasma.

USP requirements: Whole Blood USP—Preserve in the container into which it was originally drawn. Use pyrogen-free, sterile containers of colorless, transparent, Type I or Type II glass, or of a suitable plastic material. The container is provided with a hermetic contamination-proof closure. Accessory equipment supplied with the blood is sterile and pyrogen-free. Store at a temperature between 1 and 6 °C held constant within a 2 °C range, except during shipment, when the temperature may be between 1 and 10 °C. The container of Whole Blood is accompanied by at least one securely attached smaller container holding an original pilot sample of blood, for test purposes, taken at the same time from the same donor, with the same anticoagulant. Both containers bear the donor's identification symbol or number. It is blood that has been collected from suitable whole blood human donors under rigid aseptic precautions, for transfusion to human recipients. Contains citrate ion (acid citrate dextrose or citrate phosphate dextrose or citrate phosphate dextrose with adenine) or Heparin Sodium as an anticoagulant. May consist of blood from which the antihemophilic factor has been removed, in which case it is termed "Modified." Label it to indicate the donor classification, quantity and kind of anticoagulant used and the corresponding volume of blood, the designation of ABO blood group and Rh factors, and in the case of Group O blood, whether or not isoagglutinin titers or other tests for exclusion of specified Group O bloods were performed and to indicate any group classification of the blood resulting therefrom. If an ABO blood group color scheme is used, the labeling color used shall be: Group A (yellow), Group B (pink), Group O (blue), and Group AB (white). Label it also with the type and result of a serologic test for syphilis, or to indicate that it was non-reactive in such test; and with the type and result of a test for hepatitis B surface antigen, or to indicate that it was non-reactive in such test. If it has been issued prior to determination of test results, label it also with a warning not to use it until the test results have been received and to specify that a cross-match be performed. Where applicable, label it as "Modified," and indicate that antihemophilic factor has been removed and that it should not be used for patients requiring that factor. Meets the requirements of tests made on a pilot sample in non-reacting in a serologic test for syphilis; for ABO blood group designation; and for classification in regard to Rh type, including those tests specified for variants and other related factors. Containers of Whole Blood shall not be entered for sterility testing prior to use of the blood for transfusion. (Note: Whole Blood may be issued prior to the results of testing, under the specified provisions.) Meets the requirement for Expiration date (not later than 21 days after the date of bleeding the donor, if it contains anticoagulant citrate dextrose solution or anticoagulant citrate phosphate dextrose solution, as the anticoagulant; or not later than 35 days if it contains anticoagulant citrate phosphate dextrose adenine solution as the anticoagulant; or not later than 48 hours after date of bleeding the donor, if it contains heparin ion as the anticoagulant). Conforms to the regulations of the U.S. Food and Drug Administration concerning biologics.

BORIC ACID

Chemical name: Boric acid (H_3BO_3).

Molecular formula: H_3BO_3.

Molecular weight: 61.83.

Description: Boric Acid NF—Colorless, odorless scales of a somewhat pearly luster, or crystals, or white powder that is slightly unctuous to the touch. Stable in air.

NF category: Buffering agent.

Solubility: Boric Acid NF—Soluble in water and in alcohol; freely soluble in glycerin, in boiling water, and in boiling alcohol.

NF requirements: Boric Acid NF—Preserve in well-closed containers. Label the container with a warning that it is not for internal use. Contains not less than 99.5% and not more than 100.5% of boric acid, calculated on the dried basis. Meets the requirements for Solubility in alcohol, Completeness of solution, Identification, Loss on drying (not more than 0.5%), Arsenic (not more than 8 ppm), and Heavy metals (not more than 0.002%).

BOTULINUM TOXIN TYPE A

Source: Produced from a culture of the Hall strain of *Clostridium botulinum* grown in a medium containing N-Z amine and yeast extract.

USP requirements: Botulinum Toxin Type A for Injection—Not in USP.

BOTULISM ANTITOXIN

Description: Botulism Antitoxin USP—Transparent or slightly opalescent liquid, practically colorless, and practically odorless or having an odor because of the antimicrobial agent.

USP requirements: Botulism Antitoxin USP—Preserve in single-dose containers only, at a temperature between 2 and 8 °C. A sterile, non-pyrogenic solution of the refined and concentrated antitoxic antibodies, chiefly globulins, obtained from the blood of healthy horses that have been immunized against the toxins produced by the type A and type B and/or type E strains of *Clostridium botulinum*. Label it to state that it was prepared from horse blood. Its potency is determined with the U.S. Standard Botulism Antitoxin of the relevant type, tested by neutralizing activity in mice of the corresponding U.S. Control Botulism Test Toxin. Contains not more than 20.0% of solids, and contains a suitable antimicrobial agent. Meets the requirement for Expiration date (for Antitoxin containing a 20% excess of potency, not later than 5 years after date of issue from manufacturer's cold storage [5 °C, 1 year; or 0 °C, 2 years]). Conforms to the regulations of the U.S. Food and Drug Administration concerning biologics.

BRETYLIUM

Chemical group: Quaternary ammonium compound.

Chemical name: Bretylium tosylate—Benzenemethanaminium, 2-bromo-*N*-ethyl-*N*,*N*-dimethyl-, salt with 4-methylbenzenesulfonic acid (1:1).

Molecular formula: Bretylium tosylate—$C_{18}H_{24}BrNO_3S$.

Molecular weight: Bretylium tosylate—414.36.

Description: Bretylium tosylate—White, crystalline powder.

Solubility: Bretylium tosylate—Freely soluble in water and in alcohol.

USP requirements: Bretylium Tosylate Injection—Not in USP.

BRETYLIUM AND DEXTROSE

For *Bretylium* and *Dextrose*—See individual listings for chemistry information.

USP requirements: Bretylium Tosylate in 5% Dextrose Injection—Not in USP.

BROMAZEPAM

Chemical name: 2*H*-1,4-Benzodiazepin-2-one, 7-bromo-1,3-dihydro-5-(2-pyridinyl)-.

Molecular formula: $C_{14}H_{10}BrN_3O$.

Molecular weight: 316.16.

USP requirements: Bromazepam Tablets—Not in USP.

BROMOCRIPTINE

Source: An ergot derivative.

Chemical name: Bromocriptine mesylate—Ergotaman-3′,6′,18-trione, 2-bromo-12′-hydroxy-2′-(1-methylethyl)-5′-(2-methylpropyl)-, monomethanesulfonate (salt), (5′ alpha)-.

Molecular formula: Bromocriptine mesylate—$C_{32}H_{40}BrN_5O_5 \cdot CH_4SO_3$.

Molecular weight: Bromocriptine mesylate—750.70.

Description: Bromocriptine Mesylate USP—White or slightly colored, fine crystalline powder; odorless or having a weak, characteristic odor.

Solubility: Bromocriptine mesylate—Practically insoluble in water; sparingly soluble in methylene chloride; soluble in alcohol; freely soluble in methyl alcohol.

USP requirements:

Bromocriptine Mesylate USP—Preserve in tight, light-resistant containers, in a cold place. Contains not less than 98.0% and not more than 102.0% of bromocriptine mesylate, calculated on the dried basis. Meets the requirements for Identification, Color of solution, Specific rotation (+95° to +105°, calculated on the dried basis), Loss on drying (not more than 4.0%), Residue on ignition (not more than 0.1%), Heavy metals (not more than 0.002%), Related substances (not more than 1.0%), Methanesulfonic acid content (12.5–13.4%, calculated on the dried basis), and Organic volatile impurities.

Bromocriptine Mesylate Capsules USP—Preserve in tight, light-resistant containers. Contain an amount of bromocriptine mesylate equivalent to the labeled amount of bromocriptine, within ±10%. Meet the requirements for Identification, Related substances (not more than 5.0%), and Uniformity of dosage units.

Bromocriptine Mesylate Tablets USP—Preserve in tight, light-resistant containers. Contain an amount of bromocriptine mesylate equivalent to the labeled amount of bromocriptine, within ±10%. Meet the requirements for Identification, Related substances (not more than 5.0%), Dissolution (80% in 60 minutes in 0.1 *N* hydrochloric acid in Apparatus 1 at 120 rpm), and Uniformity of dosage units.

BROMODIPHENHYDRAMINE

Chemical name: Bromodiphenhydramine hydrochloride—Ethanamine, 2-[(4-bromophenyl)phenylmethoxy]-*N,N*-dimethyl-, hydrochloride.

Molecular formula: Bromodiphenhydramine hydrochloride—$C_{17}H_{20}BrNO \cdot HCl$.

Molecular weight: Bromodiphenhydramine hydrochloride—370.72.

Description: Bromodiphenhydramine Hydrochloride USP—White to pale buff, crystalline powder, having no more than a faint odor.

Solubility: Bromodiphenhydramine Hydrochloride USP—Freely soluble in water and in alcohol; soluble in isopropyl alcohol; insoluble in ether and in solvent hexane.

USP requirements:

Bromodiphenhydramine Hydrochloride USP—Preserve in tight containers. Contains not less than 98.0% and not more than 101.0% of bromodiphenhydramine hydrochloride, calculated on the dried basis. Meets the requirements for Identification, Melting range (148–152 °C), Loss on drying (not more than 0.5%), and Organic volatile impurities.

Bromodiphenhydramine Hydrochloride Capsules USP—Preserve in tight containers. Contain the labeled amount, within ±7%. Meet the requirements for Identification, Dissolution (75% in 45 minutes in water in Apparatus 1 at 100 rpm), and Uniformity of dosage units.

Bromodiphenhydramine Hydrochloride Elixir USP—Preserve in tight, light-resistant containers. Contains the labeled amount, within ±7%. Meets the requirements for Identification and Alcohol content (12.0–15.0%).

BROMODIPHENHYDRAMINE AND CODEINE

For *Bromodiphenhydramine* and *Codeine*—See individual listings for chemistry information.

USP requirements: Bromodiphenhydramine Hydrochloride and Codeine Phosphate Syrup—Not in USP.

BROMODIPHENHYDRAMINE, DIPHENHYDRAMINE, CODEINE, AMMONIUM CHLORIDE, AND POTASSIUM GUAIACOLSULFONATE

For *Bromodiphenhydramine, Diphenhydramine, Codeine, Ammonium Chloride,* and *Potassium Guaiacolsulfonate*—See individual listings for chemistry information.

USP requirements: Bromodiphenhydramine Hydrochloride, Diphenhydramine Hydrochloride, Codeine Phosphate, Ammonium Chloride, and Potassium Guaiacolsulfonate Oral Solution—Not in USP.

BROMPHENIRAMINE

Chemical group: Propylamine derivative (alkylamine).

Chemical name: Brompheniramine maleate—2-Pyridinepropanamine, gamma-(4-bromophenyl)-*N,N*-dimethyl-, (*Z*)-butenedioate (1:1).

Molecular formula: Brompheniramine maleate—$C_{16}H_{19}BrN_2 \cdot C_4H_4O_4$.

Molecular weight: Brompheniramine maleate—435.32.

Description: Brompheniramine Maleate USP—White, odorless, crystalline powder.

pKa: 3.59 and 9.12.

Solubility: Brompheniramine Maleate USP—Freely soluble in water; soluble in alcohol and in chloroform; slightly soluble in ether.

USP requirements:

Brompheniramine Maleate USP—Preserve in tight, light-resistant containers. Dried at 105 °C for 3 hours, contains not less than 98.0% and not more than 100.5% of brompheniramine maleate. Meets the requirements for Identification, Melting range (130–135 °C), pH (4.0–5.0, in a solution [1 in 100]), Loss on drying (not more than 0.5%), Residue on ignition (not more than 0.2%), Related compounds, and Organic volatile impurities.

Brompheniramine Maleate Elixir USP—Preserve in well-closed, light-resistant containers. Contains the labeled amount, within ±5%. Meets the requirements for Identification, pH (2.5–3.5), and Alcohol content (2.7–3.3%).
Brompheniramine Maleate Injection USP—Preserve in single-dose or in multiple-dose containers, preferably of Type I glass, protected from light. A sterile solution of Brompheniramine Maleate in Water for Injection. Contains the labeled amount, within ±10%. Meets the requirements for Identification, Bacterial endotoxins, pH (6.3–7.3), and Injections.
Brompheniramine Maleate Tablets USP—Preserve in tight containers. Contain the labeled amount, within ±5%. Meet the requirements for Identification, Dissolution (75% in 45 minutes in water in Apparatus 1 at 100 rpm), and Uniformity of dosage units.
Brompheniramine Maleate Extended-release Tablets—Not in USP.

BROMPHENIRAMINE AND PHENYLEPHRINE

For *Brompheniramine* and *Phenylephrine*—See individual listings for chemistry information.

USP requirements:
Brompheniramine Maleate and Phenylephrine Hydrochloride Elixir—Not in USP.
Brompheniramine Maleate and Phenylephrine Hydrochloride Tablets—Not in USP.

BROMPHENIRAMINE, PHENYLEPHRINE, AND PHENYLPROPANOLAMINE

For *Brompheniramine, Phenylephrine,* and *Phenylpropanolamine*—See individual listings for chemistry information.

USP requirements:
Brompheniramine Maleate, Phenylephrine Hydrochloride, and Phenylpropanolamine Hydrochloride Elixir—Not in USP.
Brompheniramine Maleate, Phenylephrine Hydrochloride, and Phenylpropanolamine Hydrochloride Oral Solution—Not in USP.
Brompheniramine Maleate, Phenylephrine Hydrochloride, and Phenylpropanolamine Hydrochloride Tablets—Not in USP.
Brompheniramine Maleate, Phenylephrine Hydrochloride, and Phenylpropanolamine Hydrochloride Extended-release Tablets—Not in USP.

BROMPHENIRAMINE, PHENYLEPHRINE, PHENYLPROPANOLAMINE, AND ACETAMINOPHEN

For *Brompheniramine, Phenylephrine, Phenylpropanolamine,* and *Acetaminophen*—See individual listings for chemistry information.

USP requirements:
Brompheniramine Maleate, Phenylephrine Hydrochloride, Phenylpropanolamine Hydrochloride, and Acetaminophen Oral Solution—Not in USP.
Brompheniramine Maleate, Phenylephrine Hydrochloride, Phenylpropanolamine Hydrochloride, and Acetaminophen Tablets—Not in USP.

BROMPHENIRAMINE, PHENYLEPHRINE, PHENYLPROPANOLAMINE, AND CODEINE

For *Brompheniramine, Phenylephrine, Phenylpropanolamine,* and *Codeine*—See individual listings for chemistry information.

USP requirements: Brompheniramine Maleate, Phenylephrine Hydrochloride, Phenylpropanolamine Hydrochloride, and Codeine Phosphate Tablets—Not in USP.

BROMPHENIRAMINE, PHENYLEPHRINE, PHENYLPROPANOLAMINE, CODEINE, AND GUAIFENESIN

For *Brompheniramine, Phenylephrine, Phenylpropanolamine, Codeine,* and *Guaifenesin*—See individual listings for chemistry information.

USP requirements: Brompheniramine Maleate, Phenylephrine Hydrochloride, Phenylpropanolamine Hydrochloride, Codeine Phosphate, and Guaifenesin Syrup—Not in USP.

BROMPHENIRAMINE, PHENYLEPHRINE, PHENYLPROPANOLAMINE, AND DEXTROMETHORPHAN

For *Brompheniramine, Phenylephrine, Phenylpropanolamine,* and *Dextromethorphan*—See individual listings for chemistry information.

USP requirements:
Brompheniramine Maleate, Phenylephrine Hydrochloride, Phenylpropanolamine Hydrochloride, and Dextromethorphan Hydrobromide Elixir—Not in USP.
Brompheniramine Maleate, Phenylephrine Hydrochloride, Phenylpropanolamine Hydrochloride, and Dextromethorphan Hydrobromide Tablets—Not in USP.

BROMPHENIRAMINE, PHENYLEPHRINE, PHENYLPROPANOLAMINE, AND GUAIFENESIN

For *Brompheniramine, Phenylephrine, Phenylpropanolamine,* and *Guaifenesin*—See individual listings for chemistry information.

USP requirements: Brompheniramine Maleate, Phenylephrine Hydrochloride, Phenylpropanolamine Hydrochloride, and Guaifenesin Syrup—Not in USP.

BROMPHENIRAMINE, PHENYLEPHRINE, PHENYLPROPANOLAMINE, HYDROCODONE, AND GUAIFENESIN

For *Brompheniramine, Phenylephrine, Phenylpropanolamine, Hydrocodone,* and *Guaifenesin*—See individual listings for chemistry information.

USP requirements: Brompheniramine Maleate, Phenylephrine Hydrochloride, Phenylpropanolamine Hydrochloride, Hydrocodone Bitartrate, and Guaifenesin Oral Solution—Not in USP.

BROMPHENIRAMINE AND PHENYLPROPANOLAMINE

For *Brompheniramine* and *Phenylpropanolamine*—See individual listings for chemistry information.

USP requirements:
Brompheniramine Maleate and Phenylpropanolamine Hydrochloride Capsules—Not in USP.
Brompheniramine Maleate and Phenylpropanolamine Hydrochloride Elixir—Not in USP.
Brompheniramine Maleate and Phenylpropanolamine Hydrochloride Tablets—Not in USP.
Brompheniramine Maleate and Phenylpropanolamine Hydrochloride Chewable Tablets—Not in USP.
Brompheniramine Maleate and Phenylpropanolamine Hydrochloride Extended-release Tablets—Not in USP.

BROMPHENIRAMINE, PHENYLPROPANOLAMINE, AND ACETAMINOPHEN

For *Brompheniramine, Phenylpropanolamine,* and *Acetaminophen*—See individual listings for chemistry information.

USP requirements: Brompheniramine Maleate, Phenylpropanolamine Hydrochloride, and Acetaminophen Tablets—Not in USP.

BROMPHENIRAMINE, PHENYLPROPANOLAMINE, AND ASPIRIN

Chemical group: Brompheniramine—Propylamine derivative (alkylamine).

Chemical name:
Brompheniramine maleate—2-Pyridinepropanamine, gamma-(4-bromophenyl)-*N,N*-dimethyl-, (*Z*)-butenedioate (1:1).
Aspirin—Benzoic acid, 2-(acetyloxy)-.

Molecular formula:
Brompheniramine maleate—$C_{16}H_{19}BrN_2 \cdot C_4H_4O_4$.
Aspirin—$C_9H_8O_4$.

Molecular weight:
Brompheniramine maleate—435.32.
Aspirin—180.16.

Description:
Brompheniramine Maleate USP—White, odorless, crystalline powder.
Aspirin USP—White crystals, commonly tabular or needle-like, or white, crystalline powder. Is odorless or has a faint odor. Is stable in dry air; in moist air it gradually hydrolyzes to salicylic and acetic acids.

pKa:
Brompheniramine—3.59 and 9.12.
Aspirin—3.5.

Solubility:
Brompheniramine Maleate USP—Freely soluble in water; soluble in alcohol and in chloroform; slightly soluble in ether.
Aspirin USP—Slightly soluble in water; freely soluble in alcohol; soluble in chloroform and in ether; sparingly soluble in absolute ether.

USP requirements: Brompheniramine Maleate, Phenylpropanolamine Bitartrate, and Aspirin Effervescent Tablets—Not in USP.

BROMPHENIRAMINE, PHENYLPROPANOLAMINE, AND CODEINE

For *Brompheniramine, Phenylpropanolamine,* and *Codeine*—See individual listings for chemistry information.

USP requirements: Brompheniramine Maleate, Phenylpropanolamine Hydrochloride, and Codeine Phosphate Syrup—Not in USP.

BROMPHENIRAMINE, PHENYLPROPANOLAMINE, AND DEXTROMETHORPHAN

For *Brompheniramine, Phenylpropanolamine,* and *Dextromethorphan*—See individual listings for chemistry information.

USP requirements: Brompheniramine Maleate, Phenylpropanolamine Hydrochloride, and Dextromethorphan Hydrobromide Syrup—Not in USP.

BROMPHENIRAMINE, PHENYLTOLOXAMINE, AND PHENYLEPHRINE

Chemical group:
Brompheniramine—Propylamine derivative (alkylamine).
Phenyltoloxamine citrate—Ethanolamine derivative.

Chemical name:
Brompheniramine maleate—2-Pyridinepropanamine, gamma-(4-bromophenyl)-*N,N*-dimethyl-, (*Z*)-butenedioate (1:1).
Phenyltoloxamine citrate—2-(2-Benzylphenoxy)-*N,N*-dimethylethylamine dihydrogen citrate.
Phenylephrine hydrochloride—Benzenemethanol, 3-hydroxy-alpha-[(methylamino)methyl]-, hydrochloride.

Molecular formula:
Brompheniramine maleate—$C_{16}H_{19}BrN_2 \cdot C_4H_4O_4$.
Phenyltoloxamine citrate—$C_{17}H_{21}NO \cdot C_6H_8O_7$.
Phenylephrine hydrochloride—$C_9H_{13}NO_2 \cdot HCl$.

Molecular weight:
Brompheniramine maleate—435.32.
Phenyltoloxamine citrate—447.5.
Phenylephrine hydrochloride—203.67.

Description:
Brompheniramine Maleate USP—White, odorless, crystalline powder.
Phenyltoloxamine citrate—It has a melting point of 138–140 °C.
Phenylephrine Hydrochloride USP—White or practically white, odorless crystals.

pKa: Brompheniramine maleate—3.59 and 9.12.

Solubility:
Brompheniramine Maleate USP—Freely soluble in water; soluble in alcohol and in chloroform; slightly soluble in ether.
Phenyltoloxamine citrate—Soluble in water.
Phenylephrine Hydrochloride USP—Freely soluble in water and in alcohol.

USP requirements: Brompheniramine Maleate, Phenyltoloxamine Citrate, and Phenylephrine Hydrochloride Extended-release Capsules—Not in USP.

BROMPHENIRAMINE, PHENYLTOLOXAMINE, PSEUDOEPHEDRINE, AND ATROPINE

Source: Atropine—An alkaloid that may be extracted from belladonna root and hyoscyamine or may be produced synthetically.

Chemical group:
Brompheniramine—Propylamine derivative (alkylamine).
Phenyltoloxamine citrate—Ethanolamine derivative.
Atropine—Natural tertiary amine.

Chemical name:
Brompheniramine maleate—2-Pyridinepropanamine, gamma-(4-bromophenyl)-*N,N*-dimethyl-, (*Z*)-butenedioate (1:1).
Phenyltoloxamine citrate—2-(2-Benzylphenoxy)-*N,N*-dimethylethylamine dihydrogen citrate.
Pseudoephedrine hydrochloride—Benzenemethanol, alpha-[1-(methylamino)ethyl]-, [*S*-(*R**,*R**)]-, hydrochloride.
Atropine sulfate—Benzeneacetic acid, alpha-(hydroxymethyl)-, 8-methyl-8-azabicyclo[3.2.1]oct-3-yl ester, *endo*-(±)-, sulfate (2:1) (salt), monohydrate.

Molecular formula:
Brompheniramine maleate—$C_{16}H_{19}BrN_2 \cdot C_4H_4O_4$.
Phenyltoloxamine citrate—$C_{17}H_{21}NO \cdot C_6H_8O_7$.
Pseudoephedrine hydrochloride—$C_{10}H_{15}NO \cdot HCl$.
Atropine sulfate—$(C_{17}H_{23}NO_3)_2 \cdot H_2SO_4 \cdot H_2O$.

Molecular weight:
Brompheniramine maleate—435.32.
Phenyltoloxamine citrate—447.5.
Pseudoephedrine hydrochloride—201.70.
Atropine sulfate—694.84.

Description:
Brompheniramine Maleate USP—White, odorless, crystalline powder.
Phenyltoloxamine citrate—It has a melting point of 138–140 °C.

Pseudoephedrine Hydrochloride USP—Fine, white to off-white crystals or powder, having a faint characteristic odor.
Atropine Sulfate USP—Colorless crystals, or white, crystalline powder. Odorless; effloresces in dry air; is slowly affected by light.

pKa: Brompheniramine maleate—3.59 and 9.12.

Solubility:
Brompheniramine Maleate USP—Freely soluble in water; soluble in alcohol and in chloroform; slightly soluble in ether.
Phenyltoloxamine citrate—Soluble in water.
Pseudoephedrine Hydrochloride USP—Very soluble in water; freely soluble in alcohol; sparingly soluble in chloroform.
Atropine Sulfate USP—Very soluble in water; freely soluble in alcohol and even more so in boiling alcohol; freely soluble in glycerin.

USP requirements: Brompheniramine Maleate, Phenyltoloxamine Citrate, Pseudoephedrine Hydrochloride, and Atropine Sulfate Extended-release Tablets—Not in USP.

BROMPHENIRAMINE AND PSEUDOEPHEDRINE

For *Brompheniramine* and *Pseudoephedrine*—See individual listings for chemistry information.

USP Requirements:
Brompheniramine Maleate and Pseudoephedrine Hydrochloride Extended-release Capsules—Not in USP.
Brompheniramine Maleate and Pseudoephedrine Hydrochloride Syrup—Not in USP.
Brompheniramine Maleate and Pseudoephedrine Hydrochloride Tablets—Not in USP.
Brompheniramine Maleate and Pseudoephedrine Sulfate Syrup USP—Contains the labeled amounts of brompheniramine maleate and pseudoephedrine sulfate, within ±10%. Meets the requirement for Identification.

BROMPHENIRAMINE, PSEUDOEPHEDRINE, AND ACETAMINOPHEN

For *Brompheniramine, Pseudoephedrine,* and *Acetaminophen*—See individual listings for chemistry information.

USP requirements: Brompheniramine Maleate, Pseudoephedrine Hydrochloride, and Acetaminophen Tablets—Not in USP.

BROMPHENIRAMINE, PSEUDOEPHEDRINE, AND DEXTROMETHORPHAN

For *Brompheniramine, Pseudoephedrine,* and *Dextromethorphan*—See individual listings for chemistry information.

USP requirements: Brompheniramine Maleate, Pseudoephedrine Hydrochloride, and Dextromethorphan Hydrobromide Syrup—Not in USP.

BUCLIZINE

Chemical group: Piperazine derivative.

Chemical name: Buclizine hydrochloride—Piperazine, 1-[(4-chlorophenyl)phenylmethyl]-4-[[4-(1,1-dimethylethyl)-phenyl]methyl]-, dihydrochloride.

Molecular formula: Buclizine hydrochloride—$C_{28}H_{33}ClN_2 \cdot 2HCl$.

Molecular weight: Buclizine hydrochloride—505.96.

Description: Buclizine hydrochloride—White, crystalline powder.

Solubility: Buclizine hydrochloride—Slightly soluble in water; insoluble in the usual organic solvents.

USP requirements: Buclizine Hydrochloride Chewable Tablets—Not in USP.

BUDESONIDE

Chemical name: Pregna-1,4-diene-3,20-dione, 16,17-butylidenebis(oxy)-11,21-dihydroxy-, [11 beta,16 alpha(17*R*)], and 16 alpha,17-[(*S*)-Butylidenebis(oxy)]-11 beta,21-dihydroxy-pregna-1,4-diene-3,20-dione.

Molecular formula: $C_{25}H_{34}O_6$.

Molecular weight: 430.54.

Description: White to off-white crystalline powder. Melts at 224–231.5 °C with decomposition.

Solubility: Freely soluble in chloroform; sparingly soluble in ethanol; practically insoluble in water and in heptane.

USP requirements:
Budesonide Inhalation Aerosol—Not in USP.
Budesonide Nasal Powder—Not in USP.
Budesonide Nasal Solution—Not in USP.

BUFEXAMAC

Chemical name: 2-(*p*-Butoxyphenyl)-acetohydroxamic acid.

Molecular formula: $C_{12}H_{17}NO_3$.

Molecular weight: 223.27.

Description: Melting point 153–155 °C.

Solubility: Practically insoluble in water.

USP requirements:
Bufexamac Cream—Not in USP.
Bufexamac Ointment—Not in USP.

BUMETANIDE

Chemical name: Benzoic acid, 3-(aminosulfonyl)-5-(butylamino)-4-phenoxy-.

Molecular formula: $C_{17}H_{20}N_2O_5S$.

Molecular weight: 364.42.

Description: Bumetanide USP—Practically white powder.

Solubility: Bumetanide USP—Slightly soluble in water; soluble in alkaline solutions.

USP requirements:
Bumetanide USP—Preserve in tight, light-resistant containers. Contains not less than 98.0% and not more than 102.0% of bumetanide, calculated on the dried basis. Meets the requirements for Identification, Loss on drying (not more than 0.5%), Residue on ignition (not more than 0.1%), Heavy metals (not more than 0.002%), and Chromatographic purity.
Bumetanide Injection USP—Preserve in single-dose or in multiple-dose containers, preferably of Type I glass, protected from light. A sterile solution of Bumetanide in Water for Injection, prepared with the aid of Sodium Hydroxide. Contains the labeled amount, within ±10%. Meets the requirements for Identification, Bacterial

endotoxins, pH (6.8–7.8), Chromatographic purity, and Injections.

Bumetanide Tablets USP—Preserve in tight, light-resistant containers. Contain the labeled amount, within ±10%. Meet the requirements for Identification, Dissolution (85% in 30 minutes in water in Apparatus 2 at 50 rpm), Chromatographic purity, and Uniformity of dosage units.

BUPIVACAINE

Chemical group: Amide.

Chemical name: Bupivacaine hydrochloride—2-Piperidinecarboxamide, 1-butyl-*N*-(2,6-dimethylphenyl)-, monohydrochloride, monohydrate.

Molecular formula: Bupivacaine hydrochloride—$C_{18}H_{28}N_2O \cdot HCl$ (anhydrous); $C_{18}H_{28}N_2O \cdot HCl \cdot H_2O$ (monohydrate).

Molecular weight: Bupivacaine hydrochloride—324.89 (anhydrous); 342.91 (monohydrate).

Description:

Bupivacaine Hydrochloride USP—White, odorless, crystalline powder. Melts at about 248 °C, with decomposition.

Bupivacaine Hydrochloride Injection USP—Clear, colorless solution.

pKa: 8.1.

Solubility: Bupivacaine Hydrochloride USP—Freely soluble in water and in alcohol; slightly soluble in chloroform and in acetone.

USP requirements:

Bupivacaine Hydrochloride USP—Preserve in well-closed containers. Contains not less than 98.5% and not more than 101.5% of bupivacaine hydrochloride, calculated on the anhydrous basis. Meets the requirements for Identification, pH (4.5–6.0, in a solution [1 in 100]), Water (4.0–6.0%), Residue on ignition (not more than 0.1%), Heavy metals (not more than 0.001%), Residual solvents (not more than 2.0%), and Chromatographic purity.

Bupivacaine Hydrochloride Injection USP—Preserve in single-dose or in multiple-dose containers, preferably of Type I glass. Injection labeled to contain 0.5% or less of bupivacaine hydrochloride may be packaged in 50-mL multiple-dose containers. A sterile solution of Bupivacaine Hydrochloride in Water for Injection. Contains the labeled amount, within ±7%. Meets the requirements for Identification, Bacterial endotoxins, pH (4.0–6.5), and Injections.

BUPIVACAINE AND DEXTROSE

For *Bupivacaine* and *Dextrose*—See individual listings for chemistry information.

USP requirements: Bupivacaine in Dextrose Injection USP—Preserve in single-dose containers, preferably of Type I glass. A sterile solution of Bupivacaine Hydrochloride and Dextrose in Water for Injection. Contains an amount of bupivacaine equivalent to the labeled amount of anhydrous bupivacaine hydrochloride and the labeled amount of dextrose, within ±7%. Contains no preservative. Meets the requirements for Identification, Bacterial endotoxins, and Injections.

BUPIVACAINE AND EPINEPHRINE

For *Bupivacaine* and *Epinephrine*—See individual listings for chemistry information.

USP requirements: Bupivacaine and Epinephrine Injection USP—Preserve in single-dose or in multiple-dose containers, preferably of Type I glass, protected from light. Injection labeled to contain 0.5% or less of bupivacaine hydrochloride may be packaged in 50-mL multiple-dose containers. A sterile solution of Bupivacaine Hydrochloride and Epinephrine or Epinephrine Bitartrate in Water for Injection. The content of epinephrine does not exceed 0.001% (1 in 100,000). The label indicates that the Injection is not to be used if its color is pinkish or darker than slightly yellow or if it contains a precipitate. Contains the labeled amount of bupivacaine hydrochloride, within ±7%, and the equivalent of the labeled amount of epinephrine, within −10% to +15%. Meets the requirements for Identification, Color and clarity, Bacterial endotoxins, pH (3.3–5.5), and Injections.

BUPRENORPHINE

Chemical group: Thebaine derivative.

Chemical name: Buprenorphine hydrochloride—6,14-Ethenomorphinan-7-methanol, 17-(cyclopropylmethyl)-alpha-(1,1-dimethylethyl)-4,5-epoxy-18,19-dihydro-3-hydroxy-6-methoxy-alpha-methyl-, hydrochloride, [5 alpha,7 alpha (*S*)]-.

Molecular formula: Buprenorphine hydrochloride—$C_{29}H_{41}NO_4 \cdot HCl$.

Molecular weight: Buprenorphine hydrochloride—504.11.

Description: Buprenorphine hydrochloride—White powder.

pKa: 8.42 and 9.92.

Solubility: Buprenorphine hydrochloride—Limited solubility in water.

Other characteristics: Weakly acidic; highly lipophilic.

USP requirements: Buprenorphine Hydrochloride Injection—Not in USP.

BUPROPION

Chemical group: Phenylaminoketone. Chemically unrelated to tricyclic, tetracyclic, or other antidepressants; structure closely resembles diethylpropion; related to phenylethylamines.

Chemical name: Bupropion hydrochloride—1-Propanone, 1-(3-chlorophenyl)-2-[(1,1-dimethylethyl)amino]-, hydrochloride, (±)-.

Molecular formula: Bupropion hydrochloride—$C_{13}H_{18}ClNO \cdot HCl$.

Molecular weight: Bupropion hydrochloride—276.21.

Description: White crystalline powder.

Solubility: Highly soluble in water.

USP requirements: Bupropion Hydrochloride Tablets—Not in USP.

BUSERELIN

Chemical name: Buserelin acetate—Luteinizing hormone-releasing factor (pig), 6-[*O*-(1,1-dimethylethyl)-D-serine]-9-(*N*-ethyl-L-prolinamide)-10-deglycinamide-, monoacetate (salt).

Molecular formula: Buserelin acetate—$C_{60}H_{86}N_{16}O_{13} \cdot C_2H_4O_2$.

Molecular weight: Buserelin acetate—1299.49.

Description: Buserelin acetate—Amorphous, white substance.

Solubility: Buserelin acetate—Freely soluble in water and in dilute acids.

Other characteristics: Buserelin acetate—Weak base.

USP requirements:
Buserelin Acetate Injection—Not in USP.
Buserelin Acetate Nasal Solution—Not in USP.

BUSPIRONE

Chemical group: Azaspirodecanedione. Not chemically related to benzodiazepines, barbiturates, or other sedative/antianxiety agents.

Chemical name: Buspirone hydrochloride—8-Azaspiro[4,5]-decane-7,9-dione, 8-[4-[4-(2-pyrimidinyl)-1-piperazinyl]-butyl]-, monohydrochloride.

Molecular formula: Buspirone hydrochloride—$C_{21}H_{31}N_5O_2 \cdot HCl$.

Molecular weight: Buspirone hydrochloride—421.97.

Description: Buspirone Hydrochloride USP—White crystalline powder.

Solubility: Buspirone Hydrochloride USP—Very soluble in water; freely soluble in methanol and in methylene chloride; sparingly soluble in ethanol and in acetonitrile; very slightly soluble in ethyl acetate; practically insoluble in hexanes.

Other characteristics: A fat-soluble, dibasic heterocyclic compound.

USP requirements:
Buspirone Hydrochloride USP—Preserve in tight, light-resistant containers, at controlled room temperature. Contains not less than 97.5% and not more than 102.5% of buspirone hydrochloride, calculated on the dried basis. Meets the requirements for Identification, Water (not more than 0.5%), Residue on ignition (not more than 0.5%), Heavy metals (not more than 0.002%), and Chloride content (8.0–8.8%).
Buspirone Hydrochloride Tablets—Not in USP.

BUSULFAN

Chemical name: 1,4-Butanediol, dimethanesulfonate.

Molecular formula: $C_6H_{14}O_6S_2$.

Molecular weight: 246.29.

Description: Busulfan USP—White, crystalline powder.

Solubility: Busulfan USP—Very slightly soluble in water; sparingly soluble in acetone; slightly soluble in alcohol.

USP requirements:
Busulfan USP—Preserve in tight containers. The label bears a warning that great care should be taken to prevent inhaling particles of Busulfan and exposing the skin to it. Contains not less than 98.0% and not more than 100.5% of busulfan, calculated on the dried basis. Meets the requirements for Identification, Melting range (115–118 °C), Loss on drying (not more than 2.0%), Residue on ignition (not more than 0.1%), and Organic volatile impurities.
Busulfan Tablets USP—Preserve in well-closed containers. Contain the labeled amount, within ±7%. Meet the requirements for Identification, Disintegration (30 minutes, the use of disks being omitted), and Uniformity of dosage units.

BUTABARBITAL

Chemical name:
Butabarbital—2,4,6(1*H*,3*H*,5*H*)-Pyrimidinetrione, 5-ethyl-5-(1-methylpropyl)-.
Butabarbital sodium—2,4,6(1*H*,3*H*,5*H*)-Pyrimidinetrione, 5-ethyl-5-(1-methylpropyl)-, monosodium salt.

Molecular formula:
Butabarbital—$C_{10}H_{16}N_2O_3$.
Butabarbital sodium—$C_{10}H_{15}N_2NaO_3$.

Molecular weight:
Butabarbital—212.25.
Butabarbital sodium—234.23.

Description:
Butabarbital USP—White, odorless, crystalline powder.
Butabarbital Sodium USP—White powder.

Solubility:
Butabarbital USP—Very slightly soluble in water; soluble in alcohol, in chloroform, in ether, and in solutions of alkali hydroxides and carbonates.
Butabarbital Sodium USP—Freely soluble in water and in alcohol; practically insoluble in absolute ether.

USP requirements:
Butabarbital USP—Preserve in tight containers. Contains not less than 98.5% and not more than 101.0% of butabarbital, calculated on the dried basis. Meets the requirements for Identification, Melting range (164–167 °C), Loss on drying (not more than 1.0%), Residue on ignition (not more than 0.1%), Chromatographic purity, and Organic volatile impurities.
Butabarbital Sodium USP—Preserve in tight containers. Contains not less than 98.2% and not more than 100.5% of butabarbital sodium, calculated on the dried basis. Meets the requirements for Completeness of solution, Identification, pH (10.0–11.2), Loss on drying (not more than 5.0%), Heavy metals (not more than 0.003%), Chromatographic purity, and Organic volatile impurities.
Butabarbital Sodium Capsules USP—Preserve in well-closed containers. Contain the labeled amount, within ±10%. Meet the requirements for Identification, Dissolution (75% in 45 minutes in water in Apparatus 1 at 100 rpm), and Uniformity of dosage units.
Butabarbital Sodium Elixir USP—Preserve in tight containers. Contains the labeled amount, within ±10%. Meets the requirements for Identification and Alcohol content (95.0–115.0% of labeled amount).
Butabarbital Sodium Tablets USP—Preserve in well-closed containers. Contain the labeled amount, within ±10%. Meet the requirements for Identification, Dissolution (75% in 45 minutes in water in Apparatus 1 at 100 rpm), and Uniformity of dosage units.

BUTACAINE

Chemical group: Ester, aminobenzoic acid (PABA)–derivative.

Chemical name: 3-(Dibutylamino)-1-propanol, 4-aminobenzoate.

Molecular formula: $C_{18}H_{30}N_2O_2$.

Molecular weight: 306.44.

USP requirements: Butacaine Dental Ointment—Not in USP.

BUTALBITAL

Chemical name: 2,4,6(1*H*,3*H*,5*H*)-Pyrimidinetrione, 5-(2-methylpropyl)-5-(2-propenyl)-.

Molecular formula: $C_{11}H_{16}N_2O_3$.

Molecular weight: 224.26.

Description: Butalbital USP—White, crystalline, odorless powder. Is stable in air. Its saturated solution is acid to litmus.

Solubility: Butalbital USP—Freely soluble in alcohol, in ether, and in chloroform; slightly soluble in cold water; soluble in boiling water, and in solutions of fixed alkalies and alkali carbonates.

USP requirements: Butalbital USP—Preserve in well-closed containers. Contains not less than 98.0% and not more than 102.0% of butalbital, calculated on the dried basis. Meets the requirements for Identification, Melting range (138–141 °C), Loss on drying (not more than 0.2%), Residue on ignition (not more than 0.1%), Heavy metals (not more than 0.002%), Chromatographic purity, and Organic volatile impurities.

BUTALBITAL AND ACETAMINOPHEN

For *Butalbital* and *Acetaminophen*—See individual listings for chemistry information.

USP requirements:
Butalbital and Acetaminophen Capsules—Not in USP.
Butalbital and Acetaminophen Tablets—Not in USP.

BUTALBITAL, ACETAMINOPHEN, AND CAFFEINE

For *Butalbital, Acetaminophen,* and *Caffeine*—See individual listings for chemistry information.

USP requirements:
Butalbital, Acetaminophen, and Caffeine Capsules USP—Preserve in tight containers. Contain the labeled amounts, within ±10%. Meet the requirements for Identification, Dissolution (80% of each active ingredient in 60 minutes in water in Apparatus 1 at 100 rpm), and Uniformity of dosage units.
Butalbital, Acetaminophen, and Caffeine Tablets USP—Preserve in tight containers. Contain the labeled amounts, within ±10%. Meet the requirements for Identification, Dissolution (80% of each active ingredient in 30 minutes in water in Apparatus 2 at 50 rpm), and Uniformity of dosage units.

BUTALBITAL AND ASPIRIN

For *Butalbital* and *Aspirin*—See individual listings for chemistry information.

USP requirements: Butalbital and Aspirin Tablets USP—Preserve in tight containers. Contain the labeled amounts, within ±10%. Meet the requirements for Identification, Dissolution (75% of each active ingredient in 60 minutes in water in Apparatus 1 at 100 rpm), Uniformity of dosage units, and Limit of free salicylic acid (not more than 3.0%).

BUTALBITAL, ASPIRIN, AND CAFFEINE

For *Butalbital, Aspirin,* and *Caffeine*—See individual listings for chemistry information.

USP requirements:
Butalbital, Aspirin, and Caffeine Capsules USP—Preserve in tight containers. Contain the labeled amounts, within ±10%. Meet the requirements for Identification, Uniformity of dosage units, and Free salicylic acid (not more than 2.5%).
Butalbital, Aspirin, and Caffeine Tablets USP—Preserve in tight containers. Contain the labeled amounts, within ±10%. Meet the requirements for Identification, Uniformity of dosage units, and Free salicylic acid (not more than 3.0%).

BUTALBITAL, ASPIRIN, CAFFEINE, AND CODEINE

For *Butalbital, Aspirin, Caffeine,* and *Codeine*—See individual listings for chemistry information.

USP requirements:
Butalbital, Aspirin, Caffeine, and Codeine Phosphate Capsules USP—Preserve in tight, light-resistant containers. Contain the labeled amounts, within ±10%. Meet the requirements for Identification, Dissolution (75% of each active ingredient in 60 minutes in water in Apparatus 2 at 50 rpm), Uniformity of dosage units, and Free salicylic acid (not more than 2.5%).
Butalbital, Aspirin, Caffeine, and Codeine Phosphate Tablets—Not in USP.

BUTAMBEN

Chemical group: Ester, aminobenzoic acid (PABA)–derivative.

Chemical name:
Butamben—Benzoic acid, 4-amino-, butyl ester.
Butamben picrate—Benzoic acid, 4-amino-, butyl ester, compound with 2,4,6-trinitrophenol (2:1).

Molecular formula:
Butamben—$C_{11}H_{15}NO_2$.
Butamben picrate—$(C_{11}H_{15}NO_2)_2 \cdot C_6H_3N_3O_7$.

Molecular weight:
Butamben—193.25.
Butamben picrate—615.60.

Description:
Butamben USP—White, crystalline powder. Is odorless.
Butamben picrate—Yellow powder; melting point 109–110 °C.

Solubility:
Butamben USP—Very slightly soluble in water; soluble in dilute acids, in alcohol, in chloroform, in ether, and in fixed oils. Is slowly hydrolyzed when boiled with water.
Butamben picrate—Soluble in alcohol, in chloroform, and in ether; soluble in water (1 gram/2000 mL).

USP requirements:
Butamben USP—Preserve in well-closed containers. Dried over phosphorus pentoxide for 3 hours, contains not less than 98.0% and not more than 101.0% of butamben. Meets the requirements for Completeness and color of solution, Identification, Melting range (57–59 °C), Reaction, Loss on drying (not more than 1.0%), Residue on ignition (not more than 0.2%), Chloride, and Heavy metals (not more than 0.001%).
Butamben Picrate Ointment—Not in USP.

BUTANE

Chemical name: *n*-Butane.

Molecular formula: C_4H_{10}.

Molecular weight: 58.12.

Description: Butane NF—Colorless, flammable gas (boiling temperature is about –0.5 °C). Vapor pressure at 21 °C is about 1620 mm of mercury (17 psig).
NF category: Aerosol propellant.

Solubility: Butane NF—One volume of water dissolves 0.15 volume, and 1 volume of alcohol dissolves 18 volumes at 17 °C and 770 mm; 1 volume of ether or chloroform at 17 °C dissolves 25 or 30 volumes, respectively.

NF requirements: Butane NF—Preserve in tight cylinders, and prevent exposure to excessive heat. Contains not less than 97.0% of *n*-butane. Meets the requirements for Identification, Water (not more than 0.001%), High-boiling residues (not more than 5 ppm), Acidity of residue, and Sulfur compounds.

Caution: Butane is highly flammable and explosive.

BUTOCONAZOLE

Chemical name: Butoconazole nitrate—1*H*-Imidazole, 1-[4-(4-chlorophenyl)-2-[(2,6-dichlorophenyl)thio]butyl]-, mononitrate, (±)-.

Molecular formula: Butoconazole nitrate—$C_{19}H_{17}Cl_3N_2S \cdot HNO_3$.

Molecular weight: Butoconazole nitrate—474.79.

Description: Butoconazole Nitrate USP—White to off-white, crystalline powder. Melts at about 160 °C.

Solubility: Butoconazole Nitrate USP—Practically insoluble in water; very slightly soluble in ethyl acetate; slightly soluble in acetonitrile, in acetone, in dichloromethane, and in tetrahydrofuran; sparingly soluble in methanol.

USP requirements:

Butoconazole Nitrate USP—Preserve in well-closed, light-resistant containers. Contains not less than 98.0% and not more than 102.0% of butoconazole nitrate, calculated on the dried basis. Meets the requirements for Identification, Loss on drying (not more than 1.0%), Residue on ignition (not more than 0.1%), and Ordinary impurities.

Butoconazole Nitrate Cream USP—Preserve in collapsible tubes or in tight containers. Avoid excessive heat and avoid freezing. It is Butoconazole Nitrate in a suitable cream base. Cream that is intended for use as a vaginal preparation may be labeled Butoconazole Nitrate Vaginal Cream. Contains the labeled amount, within ±10%. Meets the requirements for Identification and Minimum fill.

Butoconazole Nitrate Vaginal Suppositories—Not in USP.

BUTORPHANOL

Chemical name: Butorphanol tartrate—Morphinan-3,14-diol, 17-(cyclobutylmethyl)-, (–)-, [*S*-(*R**,*R**)]-2,3-dihydroxybutanedioate (1:1) (salt).

Molecular formula: Butorphanol tartrate—$C_{21}H_{29}NO_2 \cdot C_4H_6O_6$.

Molecular weight: Butorphanol tartrate—477.55.

Description: Butorphanol Tartrate USP—White powder. Its solutions are slightly acidic. Melts between 217 °C and 219 °C, with decomposition.

Solubility: Butorphanol Tartrate USP—Sparingly soluble in water; slightly soluble in methanol; insoluble in alcohol, in chloroform, in ethyl acetate, in ethyl ether, and in hexane; soluble in dilute acids.

USP requirements:

Butorphanol Tartrate USP—Preserve in tight containers. Contains not less than 98.0% and not more than 102.0% of butorphanol tartrate, calculated on the anhydrous basis. Meets the requirements for Identification, Specific rotation (−60° to −66°, calculated on the anhydrous basis), Water (not more than 2.0%), Residue on ignition (not more than 0.1%), Heavy metals (not more than 0.003%), and Chromatographic purity.

Butorphanol Tartrate Injection USP—Preserve in single-dose or in multiple-dose containers, preferably of Type I glass, protected from light. A sterile solution of Butorphanol Tartrate in Water for Injection. Contains the labeled amount, within ±10%. Meets the requirements for Identification, Bacterial endotoxins, pH (3.0–5.5), and Injections.

Butorphanol Tartrate Nasal Solution—Not in USP.

BUTYL ALCOHOL

Molecular formula: $C_4H_{10}O$.

Molecular weight: 74.12.

Description: Butyl Alcohol NF—Clear, colorless, mobile liquid, having a characteristic, penetrating vinous odor.

NF category: Solvent.

Solubility: Butyl Alcohol NF—Soluble in water. Miscible with alcohol, with ether, and with many other organic solvents.

NF requirements: Butyl Alcohol NF—Preserve in tight containers, and prevent exposure to excessive heat. It is *n*-butyl alcohol. Meets the requirements for Specific gravity (0.807–0.809), Distilling range (distils within a range of 1.5 °C, including 117.7 °C), Acidity, Water (not more than 0.1%), Nonvolatile residue (not more than 0.004%), Aldehydes, and Butyl ether (not more than 0.2%).

BUTYLATED HYDROXYANISOLE

Chemical name: Phenol, (1,1-dimethylethyl)-4-methoxy.

Molecular formula: $C_{11}H_{16}O_2$.

Molecular weight: 180.25.

Description: Butylated Hydroxyanisole NF—White or slightly yellow, waxy solid, having a faint, characteristic odor.

NF category: Antioxidant.

Solubility: Butylated Hydroxyanisole NF—Insoluble in water; freely soluble in alcohol, in propylene glycol, in chloroform, and in ether.

NF requirements: Butylated Hydroxyanisole NF—Preserve in well-closed containers. Contains not less than 98.5% of butylated hydroxyanisole. Meets the requirements for Identification, Residue on ignition (not more than 0.01%, determined on a 10-gram specimen), Arsenic (not more than 3 ppm), Heavy metals (not more than 0.001%), and Organic volatile impurities.

BUTYLATED HYDROXYTOLUENE

Chemical name: Phenol, 2,6-bis(1,1-dimethylethyl)-4-methyl-.

Molecular formula: $C_{15}H_{24}O$.

Molecular weight: 220.35.

Description: Butylated Hydroxytoluene NF—White, crystalline solid, having a faint characteristic odor.

NF category: Antioxidant.

Solubility: Butylated Hydroxytoluene NF—Insoluble in water and in propylene glycol; freely soluble in alcohol, in chloroform, and in ether.

NF requirements: Butylated Hydroxytoluene NF—Preserve in well-closed containers. Contains not less than 99.0% of butylated hydroxytoluene. Meets the requirements for Identification, Congealing temperature (not less than 69.2 °C, corresponding to not less than 99.0% of butylated hydroxytoluene), Residue on ignition (not more than 0.002%), Arsenic (not more than 3 ppm), and Heavy metals (not more than 0.001%).

BUTYLPARABEN

Chemical name: Benzoic acid, 4-hydroxy-, butyl ester.

Molecular formula: $C_{11}H_{14}O_3$.

Molecular weight: 194.23.

Description: Butylparaben NF—Small, colorless crystals or white powder.
NF category: Antimicrobial preservative.

Solubility: Butylparaben NF—Very slightly soluble in water and in glycerin; freely soluble in acetone, in alcohol, in ether, and in propylene glycol.

NF requirements: Butylparaben NF—Preserve in well-closed containers. Contains not less than 99.0% and not more than 100.5% of butylparaben, calculated on the dried basis. Meets the requirements for Identification, Melting range (68–72 °C), Acidity, Loss on drying (not more than 0.5%), and Residue on ignition (not more than 0.05%).

CAFFEINE

Source: Coffee, tea, cola, and cocoa or chocolate. May also be synthesized from urea or dimethylurea.

Chemical group: Methylated xanthine.

Chemical name: *1H*-Purine-2,6-dione, 3,7-dihydro-1,3,7-trimethyl-.

Molecular formula: $C_8H_{10}N_4O_2$ (anhydrous); $C_8H_{10}N_4O_2 \cdot H_2O$ (monohydrate).

Molecular weight: 194.19 (anhydrous); 212.21 (monohydrate).

Description: Caffeine USP—White powder or white, glistening needles, usually matted together. Is odorless. Its solutions are neutral to litmus. The hydrate is efflorescent in air.

Solubility: Caffeine USP—Sparingly soluble in water and in alcohol; freely soluble in chloroform; slightly soluble in ether. The aqueous solubility of caffeine is increased by organic acids or their alkali salts, such as citrates, benzoates, salicylates, or cinnamates, which dissociate to yield caffeine when dissolved in biological fluids.

USP requirements:
Caffeine USP—Preserve hydrous Caffeine in tight containers. Preserve anhydrous Caffeine in well-closed containers. It is anhydrous or contains one molecule of water of hydration. Label it to indicate whether it is anhydrous or hydrous. Contains not less than 98.5% and not more than 101.0% of caffeine, calculated on the anhydrous basis. Meets the requirements for Identification, Melting range (235–237.5 °C), Water (not more than 0.5% for anhydrous and not more than 8.5% for hydrous), Residue on ignition (not more than 0.1%), Arsenic (not more than 3 ppm), Heavy metals (not more than 0.001%), Readily carbonizable substances, Other alkaloids, and Organic volatile impurities.
Caffeine Extended-release Capsules—Not in USP.
Caffeine Tablets—Not in USP.

CITRATED CAFFEINE

Source: Caffeine—Coffee, tea, cola, and cocoa or chocolate. May also be synthesized from urea or dimethylurea.

Chemical group: Caffeine—Methylated xanthine.

Chemical name:
Caffeine—*1H*-Purine-2,6-dione, 3,7-dihydro-1,3,7-trimethyl-.
Citric acid—1,2,3-Propanetricarboxylic acid, 2-hydroxy-.

Molecular formula:
Caffeine—$C_8H_{10}N_4O_2$ (anhydrous); $C_8H_{10}N_4O_2 \cdot H_2O$ (monohydrate).
Citric acid—$C_6H_8O_7$ (anhydrous); $C_6H_8O_7 \cdot H_2O$ (monohydrate).

Molecular weight:
Caffeine—194.19 (anhydrous); 212.21 (monohydrate).
Citric acid—192.13 (anhydrous); 210.14 (monohydrate).

Description:
Caffeine USP—White powder or white, glistening needles, usually matted together. Is odorless. Its solutions are neutral to litmus. The hydrate is efflorescent in air.
Citric Acid USP—Colorless, translucent crystals, or white, granular to fine crystalline powder. Odorless or practically odorless. The hydrous form is efflorescent in dry air.
NF category: Acidifying agent; buffering agent.

Solubility:
Caffeine USP—Sparingly soluble in water and in alcohol; freely soluble in chloroform; slightly soluble in ether. The aqueous solubility of caffeine is increased by organic acids or their alkali salts, such as citrates, benzoates, salicylates, or cinnamates, which dissociate to yield caffeine when dissolved in biological fluids.
Citric Acid USP—Very soluble in water; freely soluble in alcohol; sparingly soluble in ether.

USP requirements:
Citrated Caffeine Injection—Not in USP.
Citrated Caffeine Solution—Not in USP.
Citrated Caffeine Tablets—Not in USP.

CAFFEINE AND SODIUM BENZOATE

For *Caffeine* and *Sodium Benzoate*—See individual listings for chemistry information.

USP requirements: Caffeine and Sodium Benzoate Injection USP—Preserve in single-dose containers, preferably of Type I glass. A sterile solution of Caffeine and Sodium Benzoate in Water for Injection. Contains an amount of anhydrous caffeine equivalent to 45–52.0%, and an amount of sodium benzoate equivalent to 47.55–55.5%, of the labeled amounts of caffeine and sodium benzoate. Meets the requirements for Identification, Bacterial endotoxins, pH (6.5–8.5), and Injections.

CALAMINE

Chemical name: Iron oxide (Fe_2O_3), mixture with zinc oxide.

Description: Calamine USP—Pink, odorless, fine powder.

Solubility: Calamine USP—Insoluble in water; practically completely soluble in mineral acids.

USP requirements:
Calamine USP—Preserve in well-closed containers. It is Zinc Oxide with a small proportion of ferric oxide. Contains, after ignition, not less than 98.0% and not more than

100.5% of zinc oxide. Meets the requirements for Identification, Microbial limits, Loss on ignition (not more than 2.0%), Acid-insoluble substances (not more than 2.0%), Alkaline substances, Arsenic (not more than 8 ppm), Calcium, Calcium or magnesium, and Lead.

Calamine Lotion USP—Preserve in tight containers.

Prepare Calamine Lotion as follows: 80 grams of Calamine, 80 grams of Zinc Oxide, 20 mL of Glycerin, 250 mL of Bentonite Magma, and a sufficient quantity of Calcium Hydroxide Topical Solution to make 1000 mL. Dilute the Bentonite Magma with an equal volume of Calcium Hydroxide Topical Solution. Mix the powders intimately with the Glycerin and about 100 mL of the diluted magma, triturating until a smooth, uniform paste is formed. Gradually incorporate the remainder of the diluted magma. Finally add enough Calcium Hydroxide Solution to make 1000 mL, and shake well. If a more viscous consistency in the Lotion is desired, the quantity of Bentonite Magma may be increased to not more than 400 mL.

Meets the requirement for Microbial limits.

Note: Shake Calamine Lotion well before dispensing.

PHENOLATED CALAMINE

Chemical name: Calamine—Iron oxide (Fe_2O_3), mixture with zinc oxide.

Description:

Calamine USP—Pink, odorless, fine powder.

Liquefied Phenol USP—Colorless to pink liquid, which may develop a red tint upon exposure to air or light. Has a characteristic, somewhat aromatic odor. It whitens and cauterizes the skin and mucous membranes. Specific gravity is about 1.065.

Solubility:

Calamine USP—Insoluble in water; practically completely soluble in mineral acids.

Liquefied Phenol USP—Miscible with alcohol, with ether, and with glycerin. A mixture of equal volumes of Liquefied Phenol and glycerin is miscible with water.

USP requirements: Phenolated Calamine Lotion USP—Preserve in tight containers.

Prepare Phenolated Calamine Lotion as follows: 10 mL of Liquefied Phenol and 990 mL of Calamine Lotion, to make 1000 mL. Mix the ingredients.

Note: Shake Phenolated Calamine Lotion well before dispensing.

CALCIFEDIOL

Chemical name: 9,10-Secocholesta-5,7,10(19)-triene-3,25-diol monohydrate, (3 beta,5*Z*,7*E*)-.

Molecular formula: $C_{27}H_{44}O_2 \cdot H_2O$.

Molecular weight: 418.66.

Description: A white powder. It has a melting point of about 105 °C.

Solubility: Practically insoluble in water; soluble in organic solvents.

USP requirements:

Calcifediol USP—Preserve in tight, light-resistant containers at controlled room temperature. Contains not less than 97.0% and not more than 103.0% of calcifediol. Meets the requirements for Identification, Water (3.8–5.0%, determined on a 0.2-gram specimen), and Organic volatile impurities.

Calcifediol Capsules USP—Preserve in tight, light-resistant containers. Contain the labeled amount, within −10% to +20%. Meet the requirements for Identification, Disintegration (30 minutes), and Uniformity of dosage units.

CALCIPOTRIENE

Chemical group: Vitamin D derivative.

Chemical name: 9,10-Secochola-5,7,10(19),22-tetraene-1,3,24-triol, 24-cyclopropyl-, (1 alpha,3 beta,5*Z*,7*E*,22*E*,24*S*)-.

Molecular formula: $C_{27}H_{40}O_3$.

Molecular weight: 412.61.

USP requirements: Calcipotriene Topical Ointment—Not in USP.

CALCITONIN

Source:

Calcitonin-human—A synthetic polypeptide hormone of 32 amino acids in the same linear sequence found in naturally occurring human calcitonin and differing from salmon calcitonin at 16 of the amino acid sites.

Calcitonin-salmon—A synthetic polypeptide hormone of 32 amino acids in the same linear sequence found in calcitonin of salmon origin.

Molecular formula:

Calcitonin-human—$C_{151}H_{226}N_{40}O_{45}S_3 \cdot 3HCl$.

Calcitonin-salmon—$C_{145}H_{240}N_{44}O_{48}S_2$.

Molecular weight:

Calcitonin-human—3527.20.

Calcitonin-salmon—3431.88.

Description:

Calcitonin-human—White to off-white amorphous powder.

Calcitonin-salmon—White or almost white, light powder.

Solubility:

Calcitonin-human—Soluble in water, in physiological salt solution, in dilute acid, and in dilute base; sparingly soluble in methanol; practically insoluble in chloroform.

Calcitonin-salmon—Freely soluble in water.

USP requirements:

Calcitonin-Human for Injection—Not in USP.

Calcitonin-Salmon Injection—Not in USP.

CALCITRIOL

Chemical name: 9,10-Secocholesta-5,7,10(19)-triene-1,3,25-triol, (1 alpha,3 beta,5*Z*,7*E*)-.

Molecular formula: $C_{27}H_{44}O_3$.

Molecular weight: 416.64.

Description: A practically white crystalline compound with a melting range of 111–115 °C.

Solubility: Insoluble in water; soluble in organic solvents.

USP requirements:

Calcitriol Capsules—Not in USP.

Calcitriol Injection—Not in USP.

CALCIUM ACETATE

Chemical name: Acetic acid, calcium salt.

Molecular formula: $C_4H_6CaO_4$.

Molecular weight: 158.17.

Description: Calcium Acetate USP—White, odorless or almost odorless, hygroscopic crystalline powder. When heated to above 160 °C, it decomposes to calcium carbonate and acetone.

Solubility: Calcium Acetate USP—Freely soluble in water; slightly soluble in methanol; practically insoluble in acetone and in dehydrated alcohol.

USP requirements:

Calcium Acetate USP—Preserve in tight containers. Where Calcium Acetate is intended for use in hemodialysis or peritoneal dialysis it is so labeled. Contains not less than 99.0% and not more than 100.5% of calcium acetate, calculated on the anhydrous basis. Meets the requirements for Identification, pH (6.3–9.6, in a solution [1 in 20]), Water (not more than 7.0%), Fluoride (not more than 0.005%), Arsenic (not more than 3 ppm), Heavy metals (not more than 0.0025%), Lead (not more than 0.001%), Chloride (not more than 0.05%), Sulfate (not more than 0.06%), Nitrate, Readily oxidizable substances, Aluminum (not more than 2 ppm), Barium (not more than 0.005%), Magnesium (not more than 0.05%), Potassium (not more than 0.05%), Sodium (not more than 0.5%), Strontium (not more than 0.05%), and Organic volatile impurities.

Calcium Acetate Tablets—Not in USP.

CALCIUM ASCORBATE

Chemical name: Ascorbic acid calcium salt.

Molecular formula: $C_{12}H_{14}CaO_{12} \cdot 2H_2O$.

Molecular weight: 426.35.

Description: Calcium Ascorbate USP—White to slightly yellow, practically odorless powder.

Solubility: Calcium Ascorbate USP—Freely soluble in water (approximately 50 grams per 100 mL); slightly soluble in alcohol; insoluble in ether.

USP requirements: Calcium Ascorbate USP—Preserve in tight, light-resistant containers. Contains not less than 98.0% and not more than 101.0% of calcium ascorbate calculated on as-is basis. Meets the requirements for Identification, Specific rotation (+95° to +97°), pH (6.8–7.4, in a solution [1 in 10]), Loss on drying (not more than 0.1%), Arsenic (not more than 0.003%), Fluoride (not more than 10 ppm), and Heavy metals (not more than 0.001%).

CALCIUM CARBONATE

Chemical name: Carbonic acid, calcium salt (1:1).

Molecular formula: $CaCO_3$.

Molecular weight: 100.09.

Description: Calcium Carbonate USP—Fine, white, odorless, microcrystalline powder. Is stable in air.

NF category: Tablet and/or capsule diluent.

Solubility: Calcium Carbonate USP—Practically insoluble in water. Its solubility in water is increased by the presence of any ammonium salt or of carbon dioxide. The presence of any alkali hydroxide reduces its solubility. Insoluble in alcohol. Dissolves with effervescence in 1 *N* acetic acid, in 3 *N* hydrochloric acid, and 2 *N* nitric acid.

USP requirements:

Calcium Carbonate USP—Preserve in well-closed containers. When dried at 200 °C for 4 hours, contains an amount of calcium equivalent to not less than 98.0% and not more than 100.5% of calcium carbonate. Meets the requirements for Identification, Loss on drying (not more than 2.0%), Acid-insoluble substances (not more than 0.2%), Fluoride (not more than 0.005%), Arsenic (not more than 3 ppm), Barium, Lead (not more than 3 ppm), Iron (not more than 0.1%), Mercury (not more than 0.5 ppm), Heavy metals (not more than 0.002%), and Magnesium and alkali salts (not more than 1.0%).

Calcium Carbonate Capsules—Not in USP.

Calcium Carbonate Chewing Gum—Not in USP.

Calcium Carbonate Oral Suspension USP—Preserve in tight containers, and avoid freezing. Contains the labeled amount, within ±10%. Meets the requirements for Identification, Microbial limits, and pH (7.5–8.7), and for Fluoride, Arsenic, Lead, and Heavy metals under Calcium Carbonate.

Calcium Carbonate Tablets USP—Preserve in well-closed containers. Contain the labeled amount, within ±7.5%. Meet the requirements for Identification, Disintegration (10 minutes, where Tablets are labeled solely for antacid use), Dissolution (75% in 30 minutes in 0.1 *N* hydrochloric acid in Apparatus 2 at 75 rpm, for Tablets labeled for any indication other than, or in addition to, antacid use), Uniformity of dosage units, and Acid-neutralizing capacity.

Calcium Carbonate (Oyster-shell derived) Tablets—Not in USP.

Calcium Carbonate (Oyster-shell derived) Chewable Tablets—Not in USP.

CALCIUM CARBONATE AND MAGNESIA

For *Calcium Carbonate* and *Magnesia* (Magnesium Hydroxide)—See individual listings for chemistry information.

USP requirements: Calcium Carbonate and Magnesia Tablets USP—Preserve in well-closed containers. Label the Tablets to indicate that they are to be chewed before being swallowed. Contain the labeled amount of calcium carbonate, within ±10%, and an amount of magnesia equivalent to the labeled amount of magnesium hydroxide, within ±10%. Meet the requirements for Identification, Disintegration (30 minutes, simulated gastric fluid TS being used as the test medium), Uniformity of dosage units, and Acid-neutralizing capacity.

CALCIUM CARBONATE, MAGNESIA, AND SIMETHICONE

For *Calcium Carbonate, Magnesia* (Magnesium Hydroxide), and *Simethicone*—See individual listings for chemistry information.

USP requirements: Calcium Carbonate, Magnesia, and Simethicone Tablets USP—Preserve in well-closed containers. Label it to indicate that Tablets are to be chewed before swallowing. Label Tablets to state the sodium content, in mg per Tablet, if it is greater than 5 mg per Tablet. Contain the labeled amount of calcium carbonate, within ±10%, an amount of magnesia equivalent to the labeled amount of magnesium hydroxide, within ±10%, and an amount of polydimethylsiloxane equivalent to the labeled amount of simethicone, within ±15%. Meet the requirements for Identification, Uniformity of dosage units, Acid-neutralizing capacity, Defoaming activity (not more than 45 seconds), and Sodium content (if so labeled, each tablet contains not more than the number of mg of sodium stated on the label).

CALCIUM AND MAGNESIUM CARBONATES

For *Calcium Carbonate* and *Magnesium Carbonate*—See individual listings for chemistry information.

USP requirements:
Calcium and Magnesium Carbonates Oral Suspension—Not in USP.
Calcium and Magnesium Carbonates Tablets USP—Preserve in well-closed containers. Contain the labeled amount of calcium carbonate, within ±10%, and the labeled amount of magnesium carbonate, within ±15%. Meet the requirements for Identification, Disintegration (10 minutes in simulated gastric fluid TS), Uniformity of dosage units, and Acid-neutralizing capacity.

CALCIUM AND MAGNESIUM CARBONATES AND MAGNESIUM OXIDE

For *Calcium Carbonate, Magnesium Carbonate,* and *Magnesium Oxide*—See individual listings for chemistry information.

USP requirements: Calcium and Magnesium Carbonates and Magnesium Oxide Tablets—Not in USP.

CALCIUM CARBONATE AND SIMETHICONE

For *Calcium Carbonate* and *Simethicone*—See individual listings for chemistry information.

USP requirements:
Calcium Carbonate and Simethicone Oral Suspension—Not in USP.
Calcium Carbonate and Simethicone Chewable Tablets—Not in USP.

CALCIUM CHLORIDE

Chemical name: Calcium chloride, dihydrate.

Molecular formula: $CaCl_2 \cdot 2H_2O$.

Molecular weight: 147.02.

Description: Calcium Chloride USP—White, hard, odorless fragments or granules; deliquescent.
NF category: Desiccant.

Solubility: Calcium Chloride USP—Freely soluble in water, in alcohol, and in boiling alcohol; very soluble in boiling water.

USP requirements:
Calcium Chloride USP—Preserve in tight containers. Where Calcium Chloride is intended for use in hemodialysis, it is so labeled. Contains an amount of anhydrous calcium chloride equivalent to not less than 99.0% and not more than 107.0% of calcium chloride dihydrate. Meets the requirements for Identification, pH (4.5–9.2, in a solution [1 in 20]), Arsenic (not more than 3 ppm), Heavy metals (not more than 0.001%), Iron, aluminum, and phosphate, Magnesium and alkali salts (not more than 1.0%), Aluminum (where it is labeled for use in hemodialysis, not more than 1 ppm), and Organic volatile impurities.
Calcium Chloride Injection USP—Preserve in single-dose containers, preferably of Type I glass. A sterile solution of Calcium Chloride in Water for Injection. The label states the total osmolar concentration in mOsmol per liter. Where the contents are less than 100 mL, or where the label states that the Injection is not for direct injection but is to be diluted before use, the label alternatively may state the total osmolar concentration in mOsmol per mL. Contains the labeled amount, within ±5%. Meets the requirements for Identification, Bacterial endotoxins, pH (5.5–7.5 in the undiluted Injection), Particulate matter, and Injections.

CALCIUM CITRATE

Chemical name: 1,2,3-Propanetricarboxylic acid, 2-hydroxy-, calcium salt (2:3), tetrahydrate.

Molecular formula: $C_{12}H_{10}Ca_3O_{14} \cdot 4H_2O$.

Molecular weight: 570.50.

Description: Calcium Citrate USP—White, odorless, crystalline powder.

Solubility: Calcium Citrate USP—Slightly soluble in water; freely soluble in diluted 3 *N* hydrochloric acid and in diluted 2 *N* nitric acid; insoluble in alcohol.

USP requirements:
Calcium Citrate USP—Preserve in well-closed containers. Contains four molecules of water of hydration. When dried at 150 °C to constant weight, contains not less than 97.5% and not more than 100.5% of anhydrous calcium citrate. Meets the requirements for Identification, Loss on drying (10.0–13.3%), Arsenic (not more than 3 ppm), Fluoride (not more than 0.003%), Acid-insoluble substances (not more than 0.2%), Lead (not more than 0.001%), and Heavy metals (not more than 0.002%).
Calcium Citrate Tablets—Not in USP.
Calcium Citrate Effervescent Tablets—Not in USP.

CALCIUM GLUBIONATE

Chemical name: Calcium, (4-*O*-beta-D-galactopyranosyl-D-gluconato-O[1])(D-gluconato-O[1])-, monohydrate.

Molecular formula: $C_{18}H_{32}CaO_{19} \cdot H_2O$.

Molecular weight: 610.54.

USP requirements:
Calcium Glubionate Injection—Not in USP.
Calcium Glubionate Syrup USP—Preserve in tight containers, at a temperature not exceeding 30 °C, and avoid freezing. A solution containing equimolar amounts of Calcium Gluconate and Calcium Lactobionate or with Calcium Lactobionate predominating. Contains an amount of calcium glubionate equivalent to the labeled amount of calcium, within ±5%. Meets the requirements for Identification and pH (3.4–4.5).

CALCIUM GLUCEPTATE

Chemical name: Glucoheptonic acid, calcium salt (2:1).

Molecular formula: $C_{14}H_{26}CaO_{16}$.

Molecular weight: 490.43.

Description: Calcium Gluceptate USP—White to faintly yellow, amorphous powder. Is stable in air, but the hydrous forms may lose part of their water of hydration on standing.

Solubility: Calcium Gluceptate USP—Freely soluble in water; insoluble in alcohol and in many other organic solvents.

USP requirements:
Calcium Gluceptate USP—Preserve in well-closed containers. It is anhydrous or contains varying amounts of water of hydration. Consists of the calcium salt of the alpha epimer of glucoheptonic acid or of a mixture of the alpha and beta epimers of glucoheptonic acid. Label it to indicate whether it is hydrous or anhydrous; if hydrous,

label it to indicate also the degree of hydration. Contains not less than 95.0% and not more than 102.0% of calcium gluceptate, calculated on the dried basis. Meets the requirements for Identification, pH (6.0–8.0, in a solution [1 in 10]), Loss on drying (not more than 1.0% for anhydrous, not more than 6.9% for $2H_2O$, and not more than 11.4% for $3\frac{1}{2}H_2O$), Chloride (not more than 0.07%), Sulfate (not more than 0.05%), Arsenic (not more than 1 ppm), Heavy metals (not more than 0.002%), Reducing sugars, and Organic volatile impurities.

Calcium Gluceptate Injection USP—Preserve in tight, single-dose containers, preferably of Type I or Type II glass. A sterile solution of Calcium Gluceptate in Water for Injection. The label states the total osmolar concentration in mOsmol per liter. Where the contents are less than 100 mL, or where the label states that the Injection is not for direct injection but is to be diluted before use, the label alternatively may state the total osmolar concentration in mOsm per mL. Contains an amount of calcium gluceptate equivalent to the labeled amount of calcium, within ±5%. Meets the requirements for Identification, Bacterial endotoxins, pH (5.6–7.0), Particulate matter, and Injections.

CALCIUM GLUCEPTATE AND CALCIUM GLUCONATE

For *Calcium Gluceptate* and *Calcium Gluconate*—See individual listings for chemistry information.

USP requirements: Calcium Gluceptate and Calcium Gluconate Oral Solution—Not in USP.

CALCIUM GLUCONATE

Chemical name: D-Gluconic acid, calcium salt (2:1).

Molecular formula: $C_{12}H_{22}CaO_{14}$.

Molecular weight: 430.38.

Description: Calcium Gluconate USP—White, crystalline, odorless granules or powder. Is stable in air. Its solutions are neutral to litmus.

Solubility: Calcium Gluconate USP—Sparingly (and slowly) soluble in water; freely soluble in boiling water; insoluble in alcohol.

USP requirements:

Calcium Gluconate USP—Preserve in well-closed containers. It is anhydrous or contains one molecule of water of hydration. Label it to indicate whether it is anhydrous or is the monohydrate. Where the quantity of calcium gluconate is indicated in the labeling of any preparation containing Calcium Gluconate, this shall be understood to be in terms of anhydrous calcium gluconate. Calcium Gluconate intended for use in preparing injectable dosage forms is so labeled. Calcium Gluconate not intended for use in preparing injectable dosage forms is so labeled; in addition, it may be labeled also as intended for use in preparing oral dosage forms. The anhydrous form contains not less than 98.0% and not more than 102.0% of calcium gluconate, calculated on the dried basis. The monohydrate form contains not less than 99.0% and not more than 101.0% of calcium gluconate (monohydrate) where labeled as intended for use in preparing injectable dosage forms, and not less than 98.5% and not more than 102.0% of calcium gluconate (monohydrate) where labeled as not intended for use in preparing injectable dosage forms. Meets the requirements for Identification, Loss on drying (for the anhydrous, not more than 3.0%; for the monohydrate, where labeled as intended for use in preparing injectable dosage forms, not more than 1.0% and where labeled as not intended for use in preparing injectable dosage forms, not more than 2.0%), Chloride (not more than 0.005%, and where labeled as not intended for use in preparation of injectable dosage forms, not more than 0.07%), Sulfate (not more than 0.005%, and where labeled as not intended for use in preparation of injectable dosage forms, not more than 0.05%), Arsenic (not more than 3 ppm), Heavy metals (not more than 0.001% [Note: Where Calcium Gluconate is labeled as not intended for use in preparation of injectable dosage forms, not more than 0.002%]), Reducing substances (not more than 1.0%), Magnesium and alkali metals (not more than 0.4% [Note: Calcium Gluconate labeled as not intended for use in preparing injectable dosage forms is exempt from this requirement]), Iron (not more than 5 ppm [Note: Calcium Gluconate labeled as not intended for use in preparation of injectable dosage forms is exempt from this requirement]), Phosphate (0.01% [Note: Calcium Gluconate labeled as not intended for use in preparation of injectable dosage forms is exempt from this requirement]), Oxalate (not more than 0.01% [Note: Calcium Gluconate labeled as not intended for use in preparation of injectable dosage forms is exempt from this requirement]), and Organic volatile impurities.

Calcium Gluconate Injection USP—Preserve in single-dose containers, preferably of Type I glass. A sterile solution of Calcium Gluconate in Water for Injection. Label the Injection to indicate its content, if any, of added calcium salts, calculated as percentage of calcium in the Injection. The label states the total osmolar concentration in mOsmol per liter. Where the contents are less than 100 mL, or where the label states that the Injection is not for direct injection but is to be diluted before use, the label alternatively may state the total osmolar concentration in mOsmol per mL. Contains an amount of calcium gluconate equivalent to the labeled amount of calcium, within ±5%. The calcium is in the form of calcium gluconate, except that a small amount may be replaced with an equal amount of calcium in the form of Calcium Saccharate, or other suitable calcium salts, for the purpose of stabilization. It may require warming before use if crystallization has occurred. Meets the requirements for Identification, Bacterial endotoxins, pH (6.0–8.2), Particulate matter, and Injections.

Note: If crystallization has occurred, warming may dissolve the precipitate. The Injection must be clear at the time of use.

Calcium Gluconate Tablets USP—Preserve in well-closed containers. Contain the labeled amount, within ±5%. Meet the requirements for Identification, Dissolution (75% in 45 minutes in water in Apparatus 2 at 50 rpm), and Uniformity of dosage units.

CALCIUM GLYCEROPHOSPHATE AND CALCIUM LACTATE

Chemical name:

Calcium glycerophosphate—1,2,3-Propanetriol, mono-(dihydrogen phosphate) calcium salt (1:1).

Calcium lactate—Propanoic acid, 2-hydroxy-, calcium salt (2:1), hydrate.

Molecular formula:

Calcium glycerophosphate—$C_3H_7CaO_6P$.

Calcium lactate—$C_6H_{10}CaO_6 \cdot 5H_2O$ (pentahydrate); $C_6H_{10}CaO_6$ (anhydrous).

Molecular weight:

Calcium glycerophosphate—210.15.

Calcium lactate—308.30 (pentahydrate); 218.22 (anhydrous).

Description:
Calcium glycerophosphate—Fine, odorless, slightly hygroscopic powder.
Calcium Lactate USP—White, practically odorless granules or powder. The pentahydrate is somewhat efflorescent and at 120 °C becomes anhydrous.

Solubility:
Calcium glycerophosphate—Soluble in about 50 parts of water; almost insoluble in alcohol and in boiling water.
Calcium Lactate USP—The pentahydrate is soluble in water; practically insoluble in alcohol.

USP requirements: Calcium Glycerophosphate and Calcium Lactate Injection—Not in USP.

CALCIUM HYDROXIDE

Chemical name: Calcium hydroxide.

Molecular formula: $Ca(OH)_2$.

Molecular weight: 74.09.

Description:
Calcium Hydroxide USP—White powder.
Calcium Hydroxide Solution USP—Clear, colorless liquid. Is alkaline to litmus.

Solubility: Calcium Hydroxide USP—Slightly soluble in water; soluble in glycerin and in syrup; very slightly soluble in boiling water; insoluble in alcohol.

USP requirements:
Calcium Hydroxide USP—Preserve in tight containers. Contains not less than 95.0% and not more than 100.5% of calcium hydroxide. Meets the requirements for Identification, Acid-insoluble substances (not more than 0.5%), Carbonate, Arsenic (not more than 3 ppm), Heavy metals (not more than 0.004%), and Magnesium and alkali salts (not more than 4.8%).
Calcium Hydroxide Topical Solution USP—Preserve in well-filled, tight containers, at a temperature not exceeding 25 °C. A solution containing, in each 100 mL, not less than 140 mg of Calcium Hydroxide.

Prepare Calcium Hydroxide Topical Solution as follows: 3 grams of Calcium Hydroxide and 1000 mL of Purified Water. Add the Calcium Hydroxide to 1000 mL of cool Purified Water, and agitate the mixture vigorously and repeatedly during 1 hour. Allow the excess calcium hydroxide to settle. Dispense only the clear, supernatant liquid.

Meets the requirements for Identification and Alkalies and their carbonates.

Note: The solubility of calcium hydroxide varies with the temperature at which the solution is stored, being about 170 mg per 100 mL at 15 °C, and less at a higher temperature. The official concentration is based upon a temperature of 25 °C. The undissolved portion of the mixture is not suitable for preparing additional quantities of Calcium Hydroxide Topical Solution.

CALCIUM LACTATE

Chemical name: Propanoic acid, 2-hydroxy-, calcium salt (2:1), hydrate.

Molecular formula: $C_6H_{10}CaO_6 \cdot 5H_2O$ (pentahydrate); $C_6H_{10}CaO_6$ (anhydrous).

Molecular weight: 308.30 (pentahydrate); 218.22 (anhydrous).

Description: Calcium Lactate USP—White, practically odorless granules or powder. The pentahydrate is somewhat efflorescent and at 120 °C becomes anhydrous.

Solubility: Calcium Lactate USP—The pentahydrate is soluble in water; practically insoluble in alcohol.

USP requirements:
Calcium Lactate USP—Preserve in tight containers. The label indicates whether it is the dried form or is hydrous; if the latter, the label indicates the degree of hydration. Where the quantity of Calcium Lactate is indicated in the labeling of any preparation containing Calcium Lactate, this shall be understood to be in terms of calcium lactate pentahydrate. Contains not less than 98.0% and not more than 101.0% of calcium lactate, calculated on the dried basis. Meets the requirements for Identification, Acidity, Loss on drying (22.0–27.0% for pentahydrate, 15.0–20.0% for trihydrate, 5.0–8.0% for monohydrate, and not more than 3.0% for dried form), Heavy metals (not more than 0.002%), Magnesium and alkali salts (not more than 1.0%), Volatile fatty acid, and Organic volatile impurities.
Calcium Lactate Tablets USP—Preserve in tight containers. The quantity of calcium lactate stated in the labeling is in terms of calcium lactate pentahydrate. Contain the labeled amount, within ±6%. Meet the requirements for Identification, Dissolution (75% in 45 minutes in water in Apparatus 1 at 100 rpm), and Uniformity of dosage units.

Note: An equivalent amount of Calcium Lactate with less water of hydration may be used in place of calcium lactate pentahydrate in preparing Calcium Lactate Tablets.

CALCIUM LACTATE-GLUCONATE AND CALCIUM CARBONATE

Chemical name: Calcium carbonate—Carbonic acid, calcium salt (1:1).

Molecular formula: Calcium carbonate—$CaCO_3$.

Molecular weight: Calcium carbonate—100.09.

Description: Calcium Carbonate USP—Fine, white, odorless, microcrystalline powder. Is stable in air.

NF category: Tablet and/or capsule diluent.

Solubility: Calcium Carbonate USP—Practically insoluble in water. Its solubility in water is increased by the presence of any ammonium salt or of carbon dioxide. The presence of any alkali hydroxide reduces its solubility. Insoluble in alcohol. Dissolves with effervescence in 1 *N* acetic acid, in 3 *N* hydrochloric acid, and 2 *N* nitric acid.

USP requirements: Calcium Lactate-Gluconate and Calcium Carbonate Effervescent Tablets—Not in USP.

CALCIUM LACTOBIONATE

Chemical name: D-Gluconic acid, 4-*O*-beta-D-galactopyranosyl-, calcium salt (2:1), dihydrate.

Molecular formula: $C_{24}H_{42}CaO_{24} \cdot 2H_2O$.

Molecular weight: 790.69.

USP requirements: Calcium Lactobionate USP—Preserve in well-closed containers. Contains not less than 96.0% and not more than 102.0% of calcium lactobionate. Meets the requirements for Identification, Specific rotation (+22.0° to

+26.5°), pH (5.4–7.4, in a solution [1 in 20]), Halides (not more than 0.04%), Sulfate (not more than 0.05%), Arsenic (not more than 3 ppm), Heavy metals (not more than 0.002%), Reducing substances (not more than 1.0%), and Organic volatile impurities.

CALCIUM LEVULINATE

Chemical name: Pentanoic acid, 4-oxo-, calcium salt (2:1), dihydrate.

Molecular formula: $C_{10}H_{14}CaO_6 \cdot 2H_2O$.

Molecular weight: 306.33.

Description: Calcium Levulinate USP—White, crystalline or amorphous, powder, having a faint odor suggestive of burnt sugar.

Solubility: Calcium Levulinate USP—Freely soluble in water; slightly soluble in alcohol; insoluble in ether and in chloroform.

USP requirements:

Calcium Levulinate USP—Preserve in well-closed containers. Contains not less than 97.5% and not more than 100.5% of calcium levulinate, calculated on the dried basis. Meets the requirements for Identification, Melting range (119–125 °C), pH 7.0–8.5, in a solution [1 in 10]), Loss on drying (10.5–12.0%), Chloride (not more than 0.07%), Sulfate (not more than 0.05%), Arsenic (not more than 3 ppm), Heavy metals (not more than 0.002%), Reducing sugars, and Organic volatile impurities.

Calcium Levulinate Injection USP—Preserve in single-dose containers, preferably of Type I glass. A sterile solution of Calcium Levulinate in Water for Injection. The label states the total osmolar concentration in mOsmol per liter. Where the contents are less than 100 mL, or where the label states that the Injection is not for direct injection but is to be diluted before use, the label alternatively may state the total osmolar concentration in mOsmol per mL. Contains the labeled amount, within ±5%. Meets the requirements for Identification, Bacterial endotoxins, pH (6.0–8.0), Particulate matter, and Injections.

CALCIUM PANTOTHENATE

Chemical name: Beta-alanine, *N*-(2,4-dihydroxy-3,3-dimethyl-1-oxobutyl)-, calcium salt (2:1), (*R*)-.

Molecular formula: $C_{18}H_{32}CaN_2O_{10}$.

Molecular weight: 476.54.

Description: Calcium Pantothenate USP—Slightly hygroscopic, white powder. Odorless.

Solubility: Calcium Pantothenate USP—Freely soluble in water; soluble in glycerin; practically insoluble in alcohol, in chloroform, and in ether.

USP requirements:

Calcium Pantothenate USP—Preserve in tight containers. The calcium salt of the dextrorotatory isomer of pantothenic acid. Contains not less than 5.7% and not more than 6.0% of nitrogen, and not less than 8.2% and not more than 8.6% of calcium, both calculated on the dried basis. Meets the requirements for Identification, Specific rotation (+25.0° to +27.5°, calculated on the dried basis), Alkalinity, Loss on drying (not more than 5.0%), Heavy metals (not more than 0.002%), Ordinary impurities (not more than 1.0%), Nitrogen content, Calcium content, and Organic volatile impurities.

Calcium Pantothenate Tablets USP—Preserve in tight containers. Label Tablets to indicate the content of dextrorotatory calcium pantothenate. Contain the labeled amount of the dextrorotatory isomer of Calcium Pantothenate, within −5% to +15%. Meet the requirements for Identification, Disintegration (30 minutes), Uniformity of dosage units, and Calcium content.

RACEMIC CALCIUM PANTOTHENATE

Chemical name: Beta-alanine, *N*-(2,4-dihydroxy-3,3-dimethyl-1-oxobutyl)-, calcium salt (2:1), (±)-.

Molecular formula: $C_{18}H_{32}CaN_2O_{10}$.

Molecular weight: 476.54.

Description: Racemic Calcium Pantothenate USP—White, slightly hygroscopic powder, having a faint, characteristic odor. Is stable in air. Its solutions are neutral or alkaline to litmus. Is optically inactive.

Solubility: Racemic Calcium Pantothenate USP—Freely soluble in water; soluble in glycerin; practically insoluble in alcohol, in chloroform, and in ether.

USP requirements: Racemic Calcium Pantothenate USP—Preserve in tight containers. A mixture of the calcium salts of the dextrorotatory and levorotatory isomers of pantothenic acid. Label preparations containing it in terms of the equivalent amount of dextrorotatory calcium pantothenate. Contains not less than 5.7% and not more than 6.0% of nitrogen, and not less than 8.2% and not more than 8.6% of calcium, both calculated on the dried basis. Meets the requirements for Specific rotation (−0.05° to +0.05°, calculated on the dried basis), Alkalinity, and Organic volatile impurities, and for Identification tests, Loss on drying, Heavy metals, Nitrogen content, and Calcium content under Calcium Pantothenate.

Note: The physiological activity of Racemic Calcium Pantothenate is approximately one-half that of Calcium Pantothenate.

DIBASIC CALCIUM PHOSPHATE

Chemical name: Phosphoric acid, calcium salt (1:1).

Molecular formula: $CaHPO_4$ (anhydrous); $CaHPO_4 \cdot 2H_2O$ (dihydrate).

Molecular weight: 136.06 (anhydrous); 172.09 (dihydrate).

Description: Dibasic Calcium Phosphate USP—White, odorless powder; stable in air.

NF category: Tablet and/or capsule diluent.

Solubility: Dibasic Calcium Phosphate USP—Practically insoluble in water; soluble in 3 *N* hydrochloric acid and in 2 *N* nitric acid; insoluble in alcohol.

USP requirements:

Dibasic Calcium Phosphate USP—Preserve in well-closed containers. It is anhydrous or contains two molecules of water of hydration. Label it to indicate whether it is anhydrous or the dihydrate. Contains not less than 98.0% and not more than 105.0% of anhydrous calcium phosphate or of dibasic calcium phosphate dihydrate. Meets the requirements for Identification, Loss on ignition (6.6–8.5% for anhydrous Dibasic Calcium Phosphate and 24.5–26.5% for dihydrate form of Dibasic Calcium Phosphate), Acid-insoluble substances (not more than 0.2%), Carbonate, Chloride (not more than 0.25%), Fluoride (not more than 0.005%), Sulfate (not more than 0.5%), Arsenic (not more than 3 ppm), Barium, and Heavy metals (not more than 0.003%).

Dibasic Calcium Phosphate Tablets USP—Preserve in well-closed containers. The quantity of dibasic calcium phosphate stated in the labeling is in terms of Dibasic Calcium Phosphate dihydrate. Contain the labeled amount, within ±7.5%. Meet the requirements for Identification, Disintegration (30 minutes), and Uniformity of dosage units.

Note: An equivalent amount of Dibasic Calcium Phosphate with less water of hydration may be used in place of Dibasic Calcium Phosphate dihydrate in preparing Dibasic Calcium Phosphate Tablets.

TRIBASIC CALCIUM PHOSPHATE

Chemical name: Calcium hydroxide phosphate.

Molecular formula: $Ca_5(OH)(PO_4)_3$.

Molecular weight: 502.32.

Description: Tribasic Calcium Phosphate NF—White, odorless, powder. Is stable in air.

NF category: Tablet and/or capsule diluent.

Solubility: Tribasic Calcium Phosphate NF—Practically insoluble in water; readily soluble in 3 *N* hydrochloric acid and in 2 *N* nitric acid; insoluble in alcohol.

USP requirements: Tribasic Calcium Phosphate Tablets—Not in USP.

NF requirements: Tribasic Calcium Phosphate NF—Preserve in well-closed containers. A variable mixture of calcium phosphates having the approximate composition $10CaO \cdot 3P_2O_5 \cdot H_2O$. Contains an amount of tribasic calcium phosphate equivalent to not less than 34.0% and not more than 40.0% of calcium. Meets the requirements for Identification, Loss on ignition (not more than 8.0%), Water-soluble substances (not more than 0.5%), Acid-insoluble substances (not more than 0.2%), Carbonate, Chloride (not more than 0.14%), Fluoride (not more than 0.0075%), Nitrate, Sulfate (not more than 0.8%), Arsenic (not more than 3 ppm), Barium, Dibasic salt and calcium oxide, and Heavy metals (not more than 0.003%).

CALCIUM POLYCARBOPHIL

Chemical name: Calcium polycarbophil.

Description: Calcium Polycarbophil USP—White to creamy white powder.

Solubility: Calcium Polycarbophil USP—Insoluble in water, in dilute acids, in dilute alkalies, and in common organic solvents.

USP requirements:

Calcium Polycarbophil USP—Preserve in tight containers. The calcium salt of polyacrylic acid cross-linked with divinyl glycol. Meets the requirements for Identification, Loss on drying (not more than 10.0%), Absorbing power, and Calcium content (18.0–22.0%, calculated on the dried basis).

Calcium Polycarbophil Tablets—Not in USP.

Calcium Polycarbophil Chewable Tablets—Not in USP.

CALCIUM SACCHARATE

Chemical name: D-Glucaric acid, calcium salt (1:1) tetrahydrate.

Molecular formula: $C_6H_8CaO_8 \cdot 4H_2O$.

Molecular weight: 320.27.

Description: Calcium Saccharate USP—White, odorless, crystalline powder.

Solubility: Calcium Saccharate USP—Very slightly soluble in cold water; slightly soluble in boiling water; very slightly soluble in alcohol; practically insoluble in ether and in chloroform; soluble in dilute mineral acids and in solutions of calcium gluconate.

USP requirements: Calcium Saccharate USP—Preserve in well-closed containers. The calcium salt of D-saccharic acid. Contains not less than 98.5% and not more than 102.0% of calcium saccharate. Meets the requirements for Identification, Specific rotation (+18.5° to +22.5°), Arsenic (not more than 3 ppm), Chloride (not more than 0.07%), Sulfate (not more than 0.12%), Heavy metals (not more than 0.002%), and Sucrose and reducing sugars.

CALCIUM SILICATE

Molecular formula:

Calcium metasilicate—$CaSiO_3$.
Calcium diorthosilicate—Ca_2SiO_4.
Calcium trisilicate—Ca_3SiO_5.

Molecular weight:

Calcium metasilicate—116.2.
Calcium diorthosilicate—172.2.
Calcium trisilicate—228.3.

Description: Calcium Silicate NF—White to off-white, free-flowing powder that remains so after absorbing relatively large amounts of water or other liquids.

NF category: Glidant and/or anticaking agent.

Solubility: Calcium Silicate NF—Insoluble in water. Forms a gel with mineral acids.

NF requirements: Calcium Silicate NF—Preserve in well-closed containers. A compound of calcium oxide and silicon dioxide. Contains not less than 25.0% of calcium oxide and not less than 45.0% of silicon dioxide. Meets the requirements for Identification, pH (8.4–10.2, determined in a well-mixed aqueous suspension [1 in 20]), Loss on ignition (not more than 20.0%), Fluoride (not more than 10 ppm), Arsenic (not more than 3 ppm), Lead (not more than 0.001%), Heavy metals (not more than 0.004%), Ratio of calcium oxide to silicon dioxide (quotient 1.65–2.65), and Sum of calcium oxide, silicon dioxide, and Loss on ignition (sum of percentages of three tests not less than 90.0%).

CALCIUM STEARATE

Chemical name: Octadecanoic acid, calcium salt.

Molecular formula: $C_{36}H_{70}CaO_4$.

Molecular weight: 607.00.

Description: Calcium Stearate NF—Fine, white to yellowish white, bulky powder having a slight, characteristic odor. Is unctuous, and is free from grittiness.

NF category: Tablet and/or capsule lubricant.

Solubility: Calcium Stearate NF—Insoluble in water, in alcohol, and in ether.

NF requirements: Calcium Stearate NF—Preserve in well-closed containers. A compound of calcium with a mixture of solid organic acids obtained from fats, consisting chiefly of variable proportions of calcium stearate and calcium palmitate. Contains the equivalent of not less than 9.0% and not more than 10.5% of calcium oxide. Meets the requirements for Identification, Loss on drying (not more than 4.0%), Arsenic (not more than 3 ppm), and Heavy metals (not more than 0.001%).

CALCIUM SULFATE

Chemical name: Sulfuric acid, calcium salt (1:1).

Molecular formula: $CaSO_4$.

Molecular weight: 136.14.

Description: Calcium Sulfate NF—Fine, white to slightly yellow-white, odorless powder.

NF category: Desiccant; tablet and/or capsule diluent.

Solubility: Calcium Sulfate NF—Slightly soluble in water; soluble in 3 *N* hydrochloric acid.

NF requirements: Calcium Sulfate NF—Preserve in well-closed containers. It is anhydrous or contains two molecules of water of hydration. Label it to indicate whether it is anhydrous or the dihydrate. Contains not less than 98.0% and not more than 101.0% of calcium sulfate, calculated on the dried basis. Meets the requirements for Identification, Loss on drying (not more than 1.5% for anhydrous and 19.0–23.0% for dihydrate), Iron (not more than 0.01%), and Heavy metals (not more than 0.001%).

CALCIUM UNDECYLENATE

Chemical name: 10-Undecenoic acid, calcium(2+) salt.

Molecular formula: $C_{22}H_{38}O_4Ca$.

Molecular weight: 406.62.

USP requirements: Calcium Undecylenate USP—Preserve in well-closed containers. Contains not less than 98.0% and not more than 102.0% of calcium undecylenate, calculated on the dried basis. Meets the requirements for Identification, Loss on drying (2.0–5.7%), Particle size, and Free undecylenic acid (not more than 0.1%).

CAMPHOR

Chemical name: Bicyclo[2.2.1]heptane-2-one, 1,7,7-trimethyl-.

Molecular formula: $C_{10}H_{16}O$.

Molecular weight: 152.24.

Description: Camphor USP—Colorless or white crystals, granules, or crystalline masses; or colorless to white, translucent, tough masses. Has a penetrating, characteristic odor. Specific gravity is about 0.99. Slowly volatilizes at ordinary temperatures.

Solubility: Camphor USP—Slightly soluble in water; very soluble in alcohol, in chloroform, and in ether; freely soluble in carbon disulfide, in solvent hexane, and in fixed and volatile oils.

USP requirements:

Camphor USP—Preserve in tight containers, and avoid exposure to excessive heat. A ketone obtained from *Cinnamomum camphora* (Linné) Nees et Ebermaier (Fam. Lauraceae) (Natural Camphor) or produced synthetically (Synthetic Camphor). Label it to indicate whether it is obtained from natural sources or is prepared synthetically. Meets the requirements for Melting range (174–179 °C), Specific rotation (+41° to +43° for natural Camphor), Water, Nonvolatile residue (not more than 0.05%), and Halogens (not more than 0.035%).

Camphor Spirit USP—Preserve in tight containers. An alcohol solution containing, in each 100 mL, not less than 9.0 grams and not more than 11.0 grams of camphor.

Prepare Camphor Spirit as follows: 100 grams of Camphor and a sufficient quantity of alcohol to make 1000 mL. Dissolve the camphor in about 800 mL of the alcohol, and add alcohol to make 1000 mL. Filter, if necessary.

Meets the requirement for Alcohol content (80.0–87.0%, the dilution to approximately 2% alcohol being made with methanol instead of with water).

CANDICIDIN

Chemical name: Candicidin.

Description: Candicidin USP—Yellow to brown powder.

Solubility: Candicidin USP—Sparingly soluble in water; very slightly soluble in alcohol, in acetone, and in butyl alcohol.

USP requirements:

Candicidin USP—Preserve in tight containers, in a refrigerator. A substance produced by the growth of *Streptomyces griseus* Waksman et Henrici (Fam. Streptomycetaceae). Has a potency of not less than 1000 mcg per mg, calculated on the dried basis. Meets the requirements for Identification, pH (8.0–10.0, in an aqueous suspension containing 10 mg per mL), and Loss on drying (not more than 4.0%).

Candicidin Ointment USP—Preserve in well-closed containers, in a refrigerator. Contains the labeled amount, within −10% to +40%. Meets the requirements for Minimum fill and Water (not more than 0.1%).

Candicidin Vaginal Tablets USP—Preserve in tight containers, in a refrigerator. Contain the labeled amount, within −10% to +50%. Meet the requirements for Disintegration (30 minutes) and Loss on drying (not more than 1.0%).

CAPREOMYCIN

Source: A complex of four microbiologically active components derived from *Streptomyces capreolus*.

Chemical name: Capreomycin sulfate.

Description: Sterile Capreomycin Sulfate USP—White to practically white, amorphous powder.

Solubility: Sterile Capreomycin Sulfate USP—Freely soluble in water; practically insoluble in most organic solvents.

USP requirements: Sterile Capreomycin Sulfate USP—Preserve in Containers for Sterile Solids. The constituted solution may be stored for 48 hours at room temperature, and up to 14 days in a refrigerator. The disulfate salt of capreomycin, a polypeptide mixture produced by the growth of *Streptomyces capreolus*, suitable for parenteral use. Has a potency equivalent to not less than 700 mcg and not more than 1050 mcg of capreomycin per mg and, where packaged for dispensing, contains an amount of capreomycin sulfate equivalent to the labeled amount of capreomycin, within −10% to +15%. Meets the requirements for Constituted solution, Identification, Depressor substances, Bacterial endotoxins, pH (4.5–7.5, in a solution containing 30 mg per mL [or, where packaged for dispensing, in the solution constituted as directed in the labeling]), Loss on drying (not more than 10.0%), Residue on ignition (not more than 3.0%), Heavy metals (not more than 0.003%), Capreomycin I content (not less than 90.0%), and Injections.

CAPSAICIN

Source: Naturally occurring substance derived from plants of the Solanaceae family.

Chemical name: Trans-8-methyl-*N*-vanillyl-6-nonenamide.

Molecular formula: $C_{18}H_{27}NO_3$.

Molecular weight: 305.4.

Description: White, crystalline powder.

Solubility: Practically insoluble in water; very soluble in alcohol, in ether, and in chloroform.

USP requirements: Capsaicin Cream—Not in USP.

CAPTOPRIL

Chemical name: L-Proline, 1-[(2*S*)-3-mercapto-2-methyl-1-oxopropyl]-.

Molecular formula: $C_9H_{15}NO_3S$.

Molecular weight: 217.28.

Description: Captopril USP—White to off-white, crystalline powder, which may have a characteristic, sulfide-like odor. Melts in the range of 104–110 °C.

pKa: 3.7 and 9.8 (apparent).

Solubility: Captopril USP—Freely soluble in water, in methanol, in alcohol, and in chloroform.

USP requirements:

Captopril USP—Preserve in tight containers. Contains not less than 97.5% and not more than 102.0% of captopril, calculated on the dried basis. Meets the requirements for Identification, Specific rotation (−125° to −134°, calculated on the dried basis, determined in a solution in absolute alcohol containing 10 mg per mL), Loss on drying (not more than 1.0%), Residue on ignition (not more than 0.2%), Heavy metals (not more than 0.003%), Related substances (not more than 0.1%), and Organic volatile impurities.

Captopril Tablets USP—Preserve in tight containers. Contain the labeled amount, within ±10%. Meet the requirements for Identification, Dissolution (80% in 20 minutes in 0.1 *N* hydrochloric acid in Apparatus 1 at 50 rpm), Related substance (not more than 3.0%), and Uniformity of dosage units.

CAPTOPRIL AND HYDROCHLOROTHIAZIDE

For *Captopril* and *Hydrochlorothiazide*—See individual listings for chemistry information.

USP requirements: Captopril and Hydrochlorothiazide Tablets—Not in USP.

CARAMEL

Description: Caramel NF—Thick, dark brown liquid having the characteristic odor of burnt sugar. One part dissolved in 1000 parts of water yields a clear solution having a distinct yellowish orange color. The color of the solution is not changed and no precipitate is formed after exposure to sunlight for 6 hours. When spread in a thin layer on a glass plate, it appears homogeneous, reddish brown, and transparent.

NF category: Color.

Solubility: Caramel NF—Miscible with water. Soluble in dilute alcohol up to 55% (v/v). Immiscible with ether, with chloroform, with acetone, and with solvent hexane.

NF requirements: Caramel NF—Preserve in tight containers. A concentrated solution of the product obtained by heating sugar or glucose until the sweet taste is destroyed and a uniform dark brown mass results, a small amount of alkali or of alkaline carbonate or a trace of mineral acid being added while heating. Meets the requirements for Specific gravity (not less than 1.30), Purity, Microbial limits, Ash (not more than 8.0%), Arsenic (not more than 3 ppm), and Lead (not more than 10 ppm).

Note: Where included in articles for coloring purposes, Caramel complies with the regulations of the U.S. Food and Drug Administration concerning color additives.

CARBACHOL

Chemical name: Ethanaminium, 2-[(aminocarbonyl)oxy]-*N,N,N*-trimethyl-, chloride.

Molecular formula: $C_6H_{15}ClN_2O_2$.

Molecular weight: 182.65.

Description: White or faintly yellow hygroscopic crystals or crystalline powder; odorless or with a faint amine-like odor. Its solutions in water are neutral to litmus.

Solubility: Soluble 1 in 1 of water and 1 in 50 of alcohol; practically insoluble in chloroform and in ether.

USP requirements:

Carbachol USP—Preserve in tight containers. Contains not less than 99.0% and not more than 101.0% of carbachol, calculated on the dried basis. Meets the requirements for Identification, Melting range (200–204 °C, with some decomposition), Loss on drying (not more than 2.0%), Residue on ignition (not more than 0.1%), and Ordinary impurities.

Carbachol Intraocular Solution USP—Preserve in tight containers, at controlled room temperature, and protect from freezing. A sterile solution of Carbachol in an aqueous medium. Label it to indicate that it is for single-dose intraocular use only, and that the unused portion is to be discarded. Contains the labeled amount, within −10% to +15%. Contains no preservatives or antimicrobial agents. Meets the requirements for Identification, Sterility, and pH (5.0–7.5).

Carbachol Ophthalmic Solution USP—Preserve in tight containers. A sterile solution of Carbachol in an isotonic, aqueous medium. Contains the labeled amount, within ±5%. Meets the requirements for Identification, Sterility, and pH (5.0–7.0).

CARBAMAZEPINE

Chemical group: Tricyclic iminostilbene derivative. Structurally resembles the psychoactive agents imipramine, chlorpromazine, and maprotiline; shares some structural features with the anticonvulsant agents phenytoin, clonazepam, and phenobarbital.

Chemical name: 5*H*-Dibenz[*b,f*]azepine-5-carboxamide.

Molecular formula: $C_{15}H_{12}N_2O$.

Molecular weight: 236.27.

Description: Carbamazepine USP—White to off-white powder.

pKa: 7.

Solubility: Carbamazepine USP—Practically insoluble in water; soluble in alcohol and in acetone.

USP requirements:
Carbamazepine USP—Preserve in tight containers. Contains not less than 98.0% and not more than 102.0% of carbamazepine, calculated on the dried basis. Meets the requirements for Identification, X-ray diffraction, Acidity, Alkalinity, Loss on drying (not more than 0.5%), Residue on ignition (not more than 0.1%), Chloride (not more than 0.014%), Heavy metals (not more than 0.001%), Chromatographic purity, and Organic volatile impurities.
Carbamazepine Oral Suspension USP—Preserve in tight, light-resistant containers, protected from freezing and from excessive heat. Contains the labeled amount, within ±10%. Meets the requirements for Identification and Microbial limits.
Carbamazepine Tablets USP—Preserve in tight containers, preferably of glass. Dispense Carbamazepine Tablets in a container labeled "Store in a dry place. Protect from moisture." Contain the labeled amount, within ±8%. Meet the requirements for Identification, Dissolution (75% in 60 minutes in water containing 1% sodium lauryl sulfate in Apparatus 2 at 75 rpm), Water (not more than 5.0%), and Uniformity of dosage units.
Carbamazepine Extended-release Tablets—Not in USP.

CARBAMIDE PEROXIDE

Chemical name: Urea, compd. with hydrogen peroxide (1:1).

Molecular formula: $CH_6N_2O_3$.

Molecular weight: 94.07.

Description: Carbamide Peroxide Topical Solution USP—Clear, colorless, viscous liquid, having a characteristic odor.

USP requirements:
Carbamide Peroxide USP—Preserve in tight, light-resistant containers, and avoid exposure to excessive heat. Contains not less than 96.0% and not more than 102.0% of carbamide peroxide. Meets the requirements for Identification and Organic volatile impurities.
Carbamide Peroxide Topical Solution USP—Preserve in tight, light-resistant containers, and avoid exposure to excessive heat. A solution in anhydrous glycerin of Carbamide Peroxide or of carbamide peroxide prepared from hydrogen peroxide and Urea. Contains the labeled amount, by weight, within −22% to +10%. Meets the requirements for Identification, Specific gravity (1.245–1.272), and pH (4.0–7.5).

CARBENICILLIN

Chemical name:
Carbenicillin disodium—4-Thia-1-azabicyclo[3.2.0]heptane-2-carboxylic acid, 6-[(carboxyphenylacetyl)amino]-3,3-dimethyl-7-oxo, disodium salt, [6*S*-(2 alpha,5 alpha,6 beta)]-.
Carbenicillin indanyl sodium—4-Thia-1-azabicyclo[3.2.0]-heptane-2-carboxylic acid, 6-[[3-[(2,3-dihydro-1*H*-inden-5-yl)-oxy]-1,3-dioxo-2-phenylpropyl]amino]-3,3-dimethyl-7-oxo-, monosodium salt, [2*S*-(2 alpha,5 alpha,6 beta)]-.

Molecular formula:
Carbenicillin disodium—$C_{17}H_{16}N_2Na_2O_6S$.
Carbenicillin indanyl sodium—$C_{26}H_{25}N_2NaO_6S$.

Molecular weight:
Carbenicillin disodium—422.36.
Carbenicillin indanyl sodium—516.54.

Description:
Sterile Carbenicillin Disodium USP—White to off-white, crystalline powder.
Carbenicillin Indanyl Sodium USP—White to off-white powder.

Solubility:
Sterile Carbenicillin Disodium USP—Freely soluble in water; soluble in alcohol; practically insoluble in chloroform and in ether.
Carbenicillin Indanyl Sodium USP—Soluble in water and in alcohol.

USP requirements:
Sterile Carbenicillin Disodium USP—Preserve in Containers for Sterile Solids. Has a potency equivalent to not less than 770 mcg of carbenicillin per mg, calculated on the anhydrous basis and, where packaged for dispensing, contains an amount of carbenicillin disodium equivalent to the labeled amount of carbenicillin, within −10% to +20%. Meets the requirements for Constituted solution, Identification, Bacterial endotoxins, Sterility, pH (6.5–8.0, in a solution containing 10 mg of carbenicillin per mL [or, where packaged for dispensing, in the solution constituted as directed in the labeling]), Water (not more than 6.0%), and Particulate matter, for Uniformity of dosage units, and for Constituted solutions and Labeling under Injections.
Carbenicillin Indanyl Sodium USP—Preserve in tight containers. For periods up to 18 months, store at controlled room temperature. Has a potency equivalent to not less than 630 mcg and not more then 769 mcg of carbenicillin per mg, calculated on the anhydrous basis. Meets the requirements for Identification, pH (5.0–8.0, in a solution containing 100 mg per mL), and Water (not more than 2.0%).
Carbenicillin Indanyl Sodium Tablets USP—Preserve in tight containers. Contain an amount of carbenicillin indanyl sodium equivalent to the labeled amount of carbenicillin, within −10% to +20%. Meet the requirements for Identification, Dissolution (75% in 45 minutes in water in Apparatus 1 at 100 rpm), Uniformity of dosage units, and Water (not more than 2.0%).

CARBIDOPA

Chemical group: Hydrazine analog of levodopa; inhibitor of aromatic amino acid decarboxylation.

Chemical name: Benzenepropanoic acid, alpha-hydrazino-3,4-dihydroxy-alpha-methyl-, monohydrate, (*S*).

Molecular formula: $C_{10}H_{14}N_2O_4 \cdot H_2O$.

Molecular weight: 244.25.

Description: Carbidopa USP—White to creamy white, odorless or practically odorless, powder.

Solubility: Carbidopa USP—Slightly soluble in water; freely soluble in 3 *N* hydrochloric acid; slightly soluble in methanol; practically insoluble in alcohol, in acetone, in chloroform, and in ether.

USP requirements: Carbidopa USP—Preserve in well-closed, light-resistant containers. Contains not less than 98.0% and not more than 101.0% of carbidopa. Meets the requirements for Identification, Specific rotation (−21.0° to −23.5°, calculated as the monohydrate), Loss on drying (6.9–7.9%), Residue on ignition (not more than 0.1%), Heavy metals (not more than 0.001%), and Methyldopa and 3-*O*-methylcarbidopa (not more than 0.5%).

CARBIDOPA AND LEVODOPA

For *Carbidopa* and *Levodopa*—See individual listings for chemistry information.

USP requirements:

Carbidopa and Levodopa Tablets USP—Preserve in well-closed, light-resistant containers. Contain the labeled amounts, within ±10%. Meet the requirements for Identification, Dissolution (80% of each active ingredient in 30 minutes in 0.1 *N* hydrochloric acid in Apparatus 1 at 50 rpm), and Uniformity of dosage units.

Carbidopa and Levodopa Extended-release Tablets—Not in USP.

CARBINOXAMINE

Chemical group: Ethanolamine derivative.

Chemical name: Carbinoxamine maleate—Ethanamine, 2-[(4-chlorophenyl)-2-pyridinylmethoxy]-*N*,*N*-dimethyl-, (*Z*)-2-butenedioate (1:1).

Molecular formula: Carbinoxamine maleate—$C_{16}H_{19}ClN_2O \cdot C_4H_4O_4$.

Molecular weight: Carbinoxamine maleate—406.87.

Description: Carbinoxamine Maleate USP—White, odorless, crystalline powder.

pKa: Carbinoxamine maleate—8.1.

Solubility: Carbinoxamine Maleate USP—Very soluble in water; freely soluble in alcohol and in chloroform; very slightly soluble in ether.

USP requirements:

Carbinoxamine Maleate USP—Preserve in tight, light-resistant containers. Dried at 105 °C for 2 hours, contains not less than 98.0% and not more than 102.0% of carbinoxamine maleate. Meets the requirements for Identification, Melting range (116–121 °C, determined after drying), pH (4.6–5.1, in a solution [1 in 100]), Loss on drying (not more than 0.5%), Residue on ignition (not more than 0.1%), Ordinary impurities, and Organic volatile impurities.

Carbinoxamine Maleate Tablets USP—Preserve in tight, light-resistant containers. Contain the labeled amount, within ±7%. Meet the requirements for Identification, Dissolution (75% in 45 minutes in water in Apparatus 2 at 50 rpm), and Uniformity of dosage units.

CARBINOXAMINE AND PSEUDOEPHEDRINE

For *Carbinoxamine* and *Pseudoephedrine*—See individual listings for chemistry information.

USP requirements:

Carbinoxamine Maleate and Pseudoephedrine Hydrochloride Oral Solution—Not in USP.

Carbinoxamine Maleate and Pseudoephedrine Hydrochloride Syrup—Not in USP.

Carbinoxamine Maleate and Pseudoephedrine Hydrochloride Tablets—Not in USP.

Carbinoxamine Maleate and Pseudoephedrine Hydrochloride Extended-release Tablets—Not in USP.

CARBINOXAMINE, PSEUDOEPHEDRINE, AND DEXTROMETHORPHAN

For *Carbinoxamine, Pseudoephedrine,* and *Dextromethorphan*—See individual listings for chemistry information.

USP requirements:

Carbinoxamine Maleate, Pseudoephedrine Hydrochloride, and Dextromethorphan Hydrobromide Oral Solution—Not in USP.

Carbinoxamine Maleate, Pseudoephedrine Hydrochloride, and Dextromethorphan Hydrobromide Syrup—Not in USP.

CARBINOXAMINE, PSEUDOEPHEDRINE, AND GUAIFENESIN

For *Carbinoxamine, Pseudoephedrine,* and *Guaifenesin*—See individual listings for chemistry information.

USP requirements:

Carbinoxamine Maleate, Pseudoephedrine Hydrochloride, and Guaifenesin Capsules—Not in USP.

Carbinoxamine Maleate, Pseudoephedrine Hydrochloride, and Guaifenesin Oral Solution—Not in USP.

CARBOL-FUCHSIN

For *Basic Fuchsin, Phenol, Resorcinol, Acetone,* and *Alcohol*—See individual listings for chemistry information.

Description: Carbol-Fuchsin Topical Solution USP—Dark purple liquid, which appears purplish red when spread in a thin film.

USP requirements: Carbol-Fuchsin Topical Solution USP—Preserve in tight, light-resistant containers.

Prepare Carbol-Fuchsin Topical Solution as follows: 3 grams of Basic Fuchsin, 45 grams of Phenol, 100 grams of Resorcinol, 50 mL of Acetone, 100 mL of Alcohol, and a sufficient quantity of Purified Water, to make 1000 mL. Dissolve the Basic Fuchsin in a mixture of the Acetone and Alcohol, and add to this solution the Phenol and Resorcinol previously dissolved in 725 mL of Purified Water. Then add sufficient Purified Water to make the product measure 1000 mL, and mix.

Meets the requirements for Specific gravity (0.990–1.050) and Alcohol content (7.0–10.0%).

CARBOMER

Chemical name:

Carbomer 910—Polymer of 2-propenoic acid, cross-linked with allyl ethers of pentaerythritol.

Carbomer 934—Polymer of 2-propenoic acid, cross-linked with allyl ethers of sucrose.

Carbomer 934P—Polymer of 2-propenoic acid, cross-linked with allyl ethers of sucrose or pentaerythritol.

Carbomer 940—Polymer of 2-propenoic acid, cross-linked with allyl ethers of pentaerythritol.

Carbomer 941—Polymer of 2-propenoic acid, cross-linked with allyl ethers of pentaerythritol.

Molecular weight:

Carbomer 910—Approximately 750,000.

Carbomer 934—Approximately 3,000,000.

Carbomer 934P—Approximately 3,000,000.

Carbomer 941—Approximately 1,250,000.

Description: Carbomer 910 NF; Carbomer 934 NF; Carbomer 934P NF; Carbomer 940 NF; Carbomer 941 NF; Carbomer 1342 NF—White, fluffy powder, having a slight, characteristic odor. Hygroscopic. The pH of a 1 in 100 dispersion is about 3.

NF category: Suspending and/or viscosity-increasing agent.

Solubility: Carbomer 910 NF; Carbomer 934 NF; Carbomer 934P NF; Carbomer 940 NF; Carbomer 941 NF; Carbomer 1342 NF—When neutralized with alkali hydroxides or with amines, it dissolves in water, in alcohol, and in glycerin.

NF requirements:

Carbomer 910 NF—Preserve in tight containers. A high molecular weight polymer of acrylic acid cross-linked with allyl ethers of pentaerythritol. Label it to indicate that it is not intended for internal use. Previously dried in vacuum at 80 °C for 1 hour, contains not less than 56.0% and not more than 68.0% of carboxylic acid groups. Meets the requirements for Viscosity (3000–7000 centipoises for neutralized 1.0% aqueous dispersion) and Benzene (not more than 0.5%), and for Identification, Loss on drying, and Heavy metals under Carbomer 934P.

Carbomer 934 NF—Preserve in tight containers. A high molecular weight polymer of acrylic acid cross-linked with allyl ethers of sucrose. Label it to indicate that it is not intended for internal use. Previously dried in vacuum at 80 °C for 1 hour, contains not less than 56.0% and not more than 68.0% of carboxylic acid groups. Meets the requirements for Viscosity (30,500–39,400 centipoises for neutralized 0.5% aqueous dispersion) and Benzene (not more than 0.5%), and for Identification, Loss on drying, and Heavy metals under Carbomer 934P.

Carbomer 934P NF—Preserve in tight containers. A high molecular weight polymer of acrylic acid cross-linked with allyl ethers of sucrose or pentaerythritol. Previously dried in vacuum at 80 °C for 1 hour, contains not less than 56.0% and not more than 68.0% of carboxylic acid groups. Meets the requirements for Identification, Viscosity (29,400–39,400 centipoises for neutralized 0.5% aqueous dispersion), Loss on drying (not more than 2.0%), Heavy metals (not more than 0.002%), and Benzene (not more than 0.01% of the weight of specimen taken).

Carbomer 940 NF—Preserve in tight containers. A high molecular weight polymer of acrylic acid cross-linked with allyl ethers of pentaerythritol. Label it to indicate that it is not intended for internal use. Previously dried in vacuum at 80 °C for 1 hour, contains not less than 56.0% and not more than 68.0% of carboxylic acid groups. Meets the requirements for Viscosity (40,000–60,000 centipoises for neutralized 0.5% aqueous dispersion) and Benzene (not more than 0.5%), and for Identification, Loss on drying, and Heavy metals under Carbomer 934P.

Carbomer 941 NF—Preserve in tight containers. A high molecular weight polymer of acrylic acid cross-linked with allyl ethers of pentaerythritol. Label it to indicate that it is not intended for internal use. Previously dried in vacuum at 80 °C for 1 hour, contains not less than 56.0% and not more than 68.0% of carboxylic acid groups. Meets the requirements for Viscosity (4,000–11,000 centipoises for neutralized 0.5% aqueous dispersion) and Benzene (not more than 0.5%), and for Identification, Loss on drying, and Heavy metals under Carbomer 934P.

Carbomer 1342 NF—Preserve in tight containers. A high molecular weight copolymer of acrylic acid and a long chain alkyl methacrylate cross-linked with allyl ethers of pentaerythritol. Label it to indicate that it is not intended for internal use. Previously dried in vacuum at 80 °C for 1 hour, contains not less than 52.0% and not more than 62.0% of carboxylic acid groups. Meets the requirements for Viscosity (9,500–26,500 centipoises for neutralized 1.0% aqueous dispersion) and Benzene (not more than 0.2%), and for Identification, Loss on drying, and Heavy metals under Carbomer 934P.

CARBON DIOXIDE

Chemical name: Carbon dioxide.

Molecular formula: CO_2.

Molecular weight: 44.01.

Description: Carbon Dioxide USP—Odorless, colorless gas. Its solutions are acid to litmus. One liter at 0 °C and at a pressure of 760 mm of mercury weighs 1.977 grams.
NF category: Air displacement.

Solubility: Carbon Dioxide USP—One volume dissolves in about 1 volume of water.

USP requirements: Carbon Dioxide USP—Preserve in cylinders. Contains not less than 99.0%, by volume, of carbon dioxide. Meets the requirements for Identification, Carbon monoxide (not more than 0.001%), Hydrogen sulfide (not more than 1 ppm), Nitric oxide (not more than 2.5 ppm), Nitrogen dioxide (not more than 2.5 ppm), Ammonia (not more than 0.0025%), Sulfur dioxide (not more than 5 ppm), and Water (not more than 150 mg per cubic meter).

CARBON TETRACHLORIDE

Chemical name: Methane, tetrachloro-.

Molecular formula: CCl_4.

Molecular weight: 153.82.

Description: Carbon Tetrachloride NF—Clear, colorless, mobile liquid, having a characteristic ethereal odor resembling that of chloroform.
NF category: Solvent.

Solubility: Carbon Tetrachloride NF—Practically insoluble in water. Miscible with alcohol, with ether, with chloroform, with solvent hexane, and with fixed and volatile oils.

NF requirements: Carbon Tetrachloride NF—Preserve in tight, light-resistant containers, at a temperature not exceeding 30 °C. Contains not less than 99.0% and not more than 100.5% of carbon tetrachloride. Meets the requirements for Specific gravity (1.588–1.590, indicating 99.0–100.5% of carbon tetrachloride), Distilling range (76.0–78.0 °C), Acidity, Nonvolatile residue (not more than 0.002%), Chloride and free chlorine, Readily carbonizable substances, and Carbon disulfide.

Caution: Avoid contact; vapor and liquid are poisonous. Care should be taken not to vaporize Carbon Tetrachloride in the presence of a flame because of the production of harmful gases (mainly phosgene).

CARBOPLATIN

Chemical group: A platinum coordination compound.

Chemical name: Platinum, diammine[1,1-cyclobutanedicarboxylato(2-)*O,O'*]-, (*SP*-4-2).

Molecular formula: $C_6H_{12}N_2O_4Pt$.

Molecular weight: 371.25.

Description: White to off-white crystalline powder.

Solubility: Soluble in water at a rate of approximately 14 mg per mL; virtually insoluble in ethanol, in acetone, and in dimethylacetamide.

Other characteristics: pH of a 1% solution is 5–7.

USP requirements:
Carboplatin Injection—Not in USP.
Carboplatin for Injection—Not in USP.

CARBOPROST

Source: Carboprost tromethamine—The tromethamine salt of the (15*S*)-15 methyl analogue of naturally occurring prostaglandin $F_{2\text{-alpha}}$.

Chemical name: Carboprost tromethamine—Prosta-5,13-dien-1-oic acid, 9,11,15-trihydroxy-15-methyl-, (5*Z*,9 alpha,11 alpha,13*E*,15*S*)-, compound with 2-amino-2-(hydroxymethyl)-1,3-propanediol (1:1).

Molecular formula: Carboprost tromethamine—$C_{21}H_{36}O_5 \cdot C_4H_{11}NO_3$.

Molecular weight: Carboprost tromethamine—489.65.

Description: Carboprost tromethamine—White to slightly off-white crystalline powder. It has a melting point between 95 and 105 °C, depending on the rate of heating.

Solubility: Carboprost tromethamine—Dissolves readily in water at room temperature at a concentration greater than 75 mg per mL.

USP requirements:

Carboprost Tromethamine USP—Preserve in well-closed containers, in a freezer. Contains not less than 95.0% and not more than 105.0% of carboprost tromethamine, calculated on the dried basis. Meets the requirements for Identification, Specific rotation (+18° to +24°, calculated on the dried basis), Loss on drying (not more than 1.0%), Residue on ignition (not more than 0.5%), and Limit of 15*R*-epimer and 5-*trans* isomer (not more than 3.0%).

Caution: Great care should be taken to prevent inhaling particles of Carboprost Tromethamine and exposing the skin to it.

Carboprost Tromethamine Injection USP—Preserve in single-dose or in multiple-dose containers, preferably of Type I glass, in a refrigerator. A sterile solution of Carboprost Tromethamine in aqueous solution, which may contain also benzyl alcohol, sodium chloride, and tromethamine. Contains an amount of carboprost tromethamine equivalent to the labeled amount of carboprost, within ± 10%. Meets the requirements for Identification, Bacterial endotoxins, pH (7.0–8.0), and Injections.

CARBOXYMETHYLCELLULOSE

Chemical group: Semisynthetic hydrophilic derivative of cellulose.

Chemical name:

Carboxymethylcellulose calcium—Cellulose, carboxymethyl ether, calcium salt.

Carboxymethylcellulose sodium (carmellose)—Cellulose, carboxymethyl ether, sodium salt.

Description:

Carboxymethylcellulose Calcium NF—White to yellowish white powder. Is hygroscopic. The pH of the suspension, obtained by shaking 1 gram with 100 mL of water, is between 4.5 and 6.0.

NF category: Suspending and/or viscosity-increasing agent.

Carboxymethylcellulose Sodium USP—White to cream-colored powder or granules. The powder is hygroscopic.

NF category: Coating agent; suspending and/or viscosity-increasing agent; tablet binder.

Carboxymethylcellulose Sodium 12 NF—White to cream-colored powder or granules. The powder is hygroscopic.

NF category: Suspending and/or viscosity-increasing agent.

Solubility:

Carboxymethylcellulose Calcium NF—Practically insoluble in alcohol, in acetone, in ether, and in chloroform. It swells with water to form a suspension.

Carboxymethylcellulose Sodium USP—Is easily dispersed in water to form colloidal solutions. Insoluble in alcohol, in ether, and in most other organic solvents.

Carboxymethylcellulose Sodium 12 NF—Is easily dispersed in water to form colloidal solutions. Insoluble in alcohol, in ether, and in most other organic solvents.

USP requirements:

Carboxymethylcellulose Ophthalmic Solution—Not in USP.

Carboxymethylcellulose Sodium USP—Preserve in tight containers. The sodium salt of a polycarboxymethyl ether of cellulose. Label it to indicate the viscosity in solutions of stated concentrations. Contains not less than 6.5% and not more than 9.5% of sodium, calculated on the dried basis. Meets the requirements for Identification, pH (6.5–8.5 in a solution [1 in 100]), Viscosity, Loss on drying (not more than 10.0%), and Heavy metals (not more than 0.004%).

Carboxymethylcellulose Sodium Paste USP—Preserve in well-closed containers, and avoid prolonged exposure to temperatures exceeding 30 °C. Contains not less than 16.0% and not more than 17.0% of carboxymethylcellulose sodium. Meets the requirements for Identification, Microbial limits, Loss on drying (not more than 2.0%), Heavy metals (not more than 0.005%), and Consistency.

Carboxymethylcellulose Sodium Tablets USP—Preserve in tight containers. Contain an amount of sodium equivalent to not less than 6.5% and not more than 9.5% of the labeled amount of carboxymethylcellulose sodium. Meet the requirements for Identification, Disintegration (2 hours), and Uniformity of dosage units.

NF requirements:

Carboxymethylcellulose Calcium NF—Preserve in tight containers. The calcium salt of a polycarboxymethyl ether of cellulose. Meets the requirements for Identification, Alkalinity, Loss on drying (not more than 10.0%), Residue on ignition (10.0–20.0%), Chloride (not more than 0.36%), Silicate (not more than 1.5%), Sulfate (not more than 0.96%), Arsenic (not more than 0.001%), Heavy metals (not more than 0.002%), and Starch.

Carboxymethylcellulose Sodium 12 NF—Preserve in tight containers. The sodium salt of a polycarboxymethyl ether of cellulose. Label it to indicate the viscosity in solutions of stated concentrations of either 1% (w/w) or 2% (w/w). Its degree of substitution is not less than 1.15 and not more than 1.45, corresponding to a sodium content of not less than 10.5% and not more than 12.0%, calculated on the dried basis. Meets the requirements for Identification, Viscosity, pH (6.5–8.5, in a solution [1 in 100]), Loss on drying (not more than 10.0%), Heavy metals (not more than 0.004%), Sodium chloride and Sodium glycolate (not more than 0.5%), and Degree of substitution.

CARBOXYMETHYLCELLULOSE, CASANTHRANOL, AND DOCUSATE

For *Carboxymethylcellulose, Casanthranol,* and *Docusate*—See individual listings for chemistry information.

USP requirements: Carboxymethylcellulose Sodium, Casanthranol, and Docusate Sodium Capsules—Not in USP.

CARBOXYMETHYLCELLULOSE AND DOCUSATE

For *Carboxymethylcellulose* and *Docusate*—See individual listings for chemistry information.

USP requirements: Carboxymethylcellulose Sodium and Docusate Sodium Capsules—Not in USP.

CARISOPRODOL

Chemical name: 2-Methyl-2-propyl-1,3-propanediol carbamate isopropylcarbamate.

Molecular formula: $C_{12}H_{24}N_2O_4$.

Molecular weight: 260.33.

Description: Carisoprodol USP—White, crystalline powder, having a mild, characteristic odor.

Solubility: Carisoprodol USP—Very slightly soluble in water; freely soluble in alcohol, in chloroform, and in acetone.

USP requirements:

Carisoprodol USP—Preserve in tight containers. Contains not less than 98.0% and not more than 102.0% of carisoprodol, calculated on the dried basis. Meets the requirements for Identification, Melting range (91–94 °C), Loss on drying (not more than 0.5%), Heavy metals (not more than 0.001%), Meprobamate (not more than 0.5%), and Organic volatile impurities.

Carisoprodol Tablets USP—Preserve in well-closed containers. Contain the labeled amount, within ±10%. Meet the requirements for Identification, Dissolution (80% in 60 minutes in 0.05 *M* phosphate buffer [pH 6.9] containing 5 units of alpha-amylase per mL in Apparatus 2 at 75 rpm), and Uniformity of dosage units.

CARISOPRODOL AND ASPIRIN

For *Carisoprodol* and *Aspirin*—See individual listings for chemistry information.

USP requirements: Carisoprodol and Aspirin Tablets USP—Preserve in well-closed containers. Contain the labeled amounts, within ±10%. Meet the requirements for Identification, Dissolution (75% of each active ingredient in 45 minutes in water in Apparatus 2 at 75 rpm), Uniformity of dosage units, and Limit of free salicylic acid (not more than 3.0%).

CARISOPRODOL, ASPIRIN, AND CODEINE

For *Carisoprodol, Aspirin,* and *Codeine*—See individual listings for chemistry information.

USP requirements: Carisoprodol, Aspirin, and Codeine Phosphate Tablets USP—Preserve in well-closed containers. Contain the labeled amounts, within ±10%. Meet the requirements for Identification, Dissolution (75% of each active ingredient in 45 minutes in water in Apparatus 2 at 75 rpm), Uniformity of dosage units, and Limit of free salicylic acid (not more than 3.0%).

CARMUSTINE

Chemical name: Urea, *N,N′*-bis(2-chloroethyl)-*N*-nitroso-.

Molecular formula: $C_5H_9Cl_2N_3O_2$.

Molecular weight: 214.05.

Description: Lyophilized pale yellow flakes or congealed mass.

Solubility: Highly soluble in alcohol and lipids; poorly soluble in water.

USP requirements: Carmustine for Injection—Not in USP.

CARPHENAZINE

Chemical name: Carphenazine maleate—1-Propanone, 1-[10-[3-[4-(2-hydroxyethyl)-1-piperazinyl]propyl]-10*H*-phenothiazin-2-yl]-, (*Z*)-2-butenedioate (1:2).

Molecular formula: Carphenazine maleate—$C_{24}H_{31}N_3O_2S \cdot 2C_4H_4O_4$.

Molecular weight: Carphenazine maleate—657.74.

Description: Carphenazine Maleate USP—Yellow, finely divided powder. Is odorless, or has a slight odor.

Solubility: Carphenazine Maleate USP—Slightly soluble in water and in alcohol; practically insoluble in ether.

USP requirements:

Carphenazine Maleate USP—Preserve in tight, light-resistant containers. Contains not less than 98.0% and not more than 102.0% of carphenazine maleate, calculated on the anhydrous basis. Meets the requirements for Identification, Melting range (176–185 °C, with decomposition, the range between beginning and end of melting not more than 3 °C), pH (2.5–3.5, in a suspension [1 in 100]), Water (not more than 1.0%), Residue on ignition (not more than 0.2%), Heavy metals (not more than 0.0025%), and Ordinary impurities.

Carphenazine Maleate Oral Solution USP—Preserve in tight, light-resistant containers. Contains the labeled amount, within −5% to +10%. Meets the requirements for Identification and pH (5.8–6.8).

CARRAGEENAN

Chemical name: Carrageenan.

Description: Carrageenan NF—Yellowish or tan to white, coarse to fine powder. Practically odorless.

NF category: Suspending and/or viscosity-increasing agent.

Solubility: Carrageenan NF—Soluble in water at a temperature of about 80 °C, forming a viscous, clear or slightly opalescent solution that flows readily. Disperses in water more readily if first moistened with alcohol, glycerin, or a saturated solution of sucrose in water.

NF requirements: Carrageenan NF—Preserve in tight containers, preferably in a cool place. The hydrocolloid obtained by extraction with water or aqueous alkali from some members of the class *Rhodophyceae* (red seaweeds). Consists chiefly of potassium, sodium, calcium, magnesium, and ammonium sulfate esters of galactose and 3,6-anhydrogalactose copolymers, which are subclassified by slight structural differences. The ester sulfate content for Carrageenan is 18 to 40%. In addition, contains inorganic salts that originate from the seaweed and from the process of recovery from the extract. Meets the requirements for Identification, Solubility in water (not more than 30 mL of water required to dissolve 1 gram at 80 °C), Viscosity (not less than 5 centipoises at 75 °C), Microbial limits, Loss on drying (not more than 12.5%), Acid-insoluble matter (not more than 2.0% of Carrageenan taken), Total ash (not more than 35.0%), Arsenic (not more than 3 ppm), Lead (not more than 0.001%), and Heavy metals (not more than 0.004%).

CARTEOLOL

Chemical name: Carteolol hydrochloride—2(1*H*)-Quinolinone, 5-[3-[(1,1-dimethylethyl)amino]-2-hydroxypropoxy]-3,4-dihydro-, monohydrochloride.

Molecular formula: Carteolol hydrochloride—$C_{16}H_{24}N_2O_3 \cdot HCl$.

Molecular weight: Carteolol hydrochloride—328.84.

Description: Carteolol hydrochloride—White crystalline powder.

pKa: 9.74.

Solubility: Carteolol hydrochloride—Soluble in water; slightly soluble in ethanol.

Other characteristics: Lipid solubility—Low.

USP requirements:
Carteolol Hydrochloride Ophthalmic Solution—Not in USP.
Carteolol Hydrochloride Tablets—Not in USP.

CASANTHRANOL

Source: A purified mixture of the anthranol glycosides derived from *Cascara sagrada.*

Chemical group: Anthraquinones.

Description: Casanthranol USP—Light tan to brown, amorphous, hygroscopic powder.

Solubility: Casanthranol USP—Freely soluble in water, with some residue; partially soluble in methanol and in hot isopropyl alcohol; practically insoluble in acetone.

USP requirements:
Casanthranol USP—Preserve in tight, light-resistant containers, at a temperature not exceeding 30 °C. Obtained from Cascara Sagrada. Contains in each 100 grams not less than 20.0 grams of total hydroxyanthracene derivatives, calculated on the dried basis, calculated as cascaroside A. Not less than 80.0% of the total hydroxyanthracene derivatives consists of cascarosides, calculated as cascaroside A. Meets the requirements for Loss on drying (not more than 10.0%), Residue on ignition (not more than 4.0%), and Heavy metals (not more than 0.0025%).
Casanthranol Syrup—Not in USP.

CASANTHRANOL AND DOCUSATE

For *Casanthranol* and *Docusate*—See individual listings for chemistry information.

USP requirements:
Casanthranol and Docusate Potassium Capsules—Not in USP.
Casanthranol and Docusate Sodium Capsules—Not in USP.
Casanthranol and Docusate Sodium Syrup—Not in USP.
Casanthranol and Docusate Sodium Tablets—Not in USP.

CASCARA SAGRADA

Source: Dried bark of *Rhamnus purshiana* (buckthorn tree); main active principles are cascarosides A and B (glycosides of barbaloin) and cascarosides C and D (glycosides of chrysaloin).

Chemical group: Anthraquinones.

Description: Cascara Sagrada USP—Has a distinct odor.

USP requirements:
Cascara Sagrada USP—The dried bark of *Rhamnus purshiana* De Candolle (Fam. Rhamnaceae). Yields not less than 7.0% of total hydroxyanthracene derivatives, calculated as cascaroside A, and calculated on the dried basis. Not less than 60% of the total hydroxyanthracene derivatives consists of cascarosides, calculated as cascaroside A. Meets the requirements for Botanic characteristics, Identification, Water (not more than 12.0%), and Foreign organic matter (not more than 4.0%).

Note: Collect Cascara Sagrada not less than one year prior to use.

Cascara Sagrada Extract USP—Preserve in tight, light-resistant containers, at a temperature not exceeding 30 °C. Contains, in each 100 grams, not less than 10.0 grams and not more than 12.0 grams of hydroxyanthracene derivatives, of which not less than 50.0% consists of cascarosides, both calculated as cascaroside A.

Prepare Cascara Sagrada Extract as follows: Mix 900 grams of Cascara Sagrada, in coarse powder, with 4000 mL of boiling water, and macerate the mixture for 3 hours. Then transfer it to a percolator, allow it to drain, exhaust it by percolation, using boiling water as the menstruum, and collect about 5000 mL of percolate. Evaporate the percolate to dryness, reduce the extract to a fine powder, and, after assaying, add sufficient starch, dried at 100 °C, or other inert, non-toxic diluents to make the product contain, in each 100 grams, 11 grams of hydroxyanthracene derivatives. Mix the powders, and pass the Extract through a number 60 sieve.

Cascara Tablets USP—Preserve in tight containers; if the Tablets are coated, well-closed containers may be used. They are prepared from Cascara Sagrada Extract. Contain an amount of hydroxyanthracene derivatives, calculated as cascaroside A, not less than 9.35% and not more than 12.65% of the labeled amount of Cascara Sagrada Extract. Not less than 50% of the hydroxyanthracene derivatives are cascarosides, calculated as cascaroside A. Meet the requirements for Disintegration (60 minutes) and Uniformity of dosage units.

Cascara Sagrada Fluidextract USP—Preserve in tight, light-resistant containers, and avoid exposure to direct sunlight and to excessive heat.

Prepare Cascara Sagrada Fluidextract as follows: To 1000 grams of coarsely ground Cascara Sagrada add 3000 mL of boiling water, mix, and allow to macerate in a suitable percolator for 2 hours. Allow the percolation to proceed at a moderate rate, gradually adding boiling water until the drug is practically exhausted of its active principles. Evaporate the percolate on a water bath or in a vacuum still to not more than 800 mL, cool, add 200 mL of alcohol and, if necessary, add sufficient water to make the product measure 1000 mL. Mix.

Meets the requirement for Alcohol content (18.0–20.0%).

Aromatic Cascara Fluidextract USP—Preserve in tight, light-resistant containers and avoid exposure to direct sunlight and to excessive heat.

Prepare Aromatic Cascara Fluidextract as follows: 1000 grams of Cascara Sagrada, in very coarse powder, 120 grams of Magnesium Oxide, Suitable sweetening agent(s), Suitable essential oils(s), Suitable flavoring agent(s), 200 mL of Alcohol, and a sufficient quantity of Purified Water, to make 1000 mL. Mix the Cascara Sagrada with the Magnesium Oxide, moisten it uniformly with 2000 mL of boiling water, and set it aside in a shallow container for 48 hours, stirring it occasionally. Pack it in a percolator, and percolate with boiling water until the drug is exhausted. Evaporate the percolate, at a temperature not exceeding 100 °C, to 750 mL, and at once dissolve in it the flavoring agent(s). When the liquid has cooled, add the Alcohol, in which the sweetening agent(s) and oils have been dissolved, add sufficient water to make the Aromatic Fluidextract measure 1000 mL, and mix.

Meets the requirement for Alcohol content (18.0–20.0%).

CASCARA SAGRADA AND ALOE

For *Cascara Sagrada* and *Aloe*—See individual listings for chemistry information.

USP requirements: Cascara Sagrada and Aloe Tablets—Not in USP.

CASCARA SAGRADA AND PHENOLPHTHALEIN

For *Cascara Sagrada* and *Phenolphthalein*—See individual listings for chemistry information.

USP requirements: Cascara Sagrada Extract and Phenolphthalein Tablets—Not in USP.

CASTOR OIL

Chemical group: Glycerides.

Description:
Castor Oil USP—Pale yellowish or almost colorless, transparent, viscid liquid. It has a faint, mild odor; it is free from foreign and rancid odor.
NF category: Plasticizer.
Hydrogenated Castor Oil NF—White, crystalline wax.
NF category: Stiffening agent.

Solubility:
Castor Oil USP—Soluble in alcohol; miscible with dehydrated alcohol, with glacial acetic acid, with chloroform, and with ether.
Hydrogenated Castor Oil NF—Insoluble in water and in most common organic solvents.

USP requirements:
Castor Oil USP—Preserve in tight containers, and avoid exposure to excessive heat. The fixed oil obtained from the seed of *Ricinus communis* Linné (Fam. Euphorbiaceae). Contains no added substances. Meets the requirements for Specific gravity (0.957–0.961), Distinction from most other fixed oils, Heavy metals (not more than 0.001%), Free fatty acids, Hydroxyl value (160–168), Iodine value (83–88), and Saponification value (176–182).
Aromatic Castor Oil USP—Preserve in tight containers. It is Castor Oil containing suitable flavoring agents. Contains the labeled amount, within −5%. Meets the requirement for Alcohol content (not more than 4.0%).
Castor Oil Capsules USP—Preserve in tight containers, preferably at controlled room temperature. Contain the labeled amount, within ±10%, calculated from the tests for Weight variation and Specific gravity. Meet the requirements for Identification and Uniformity of dosage units, and for Specific gravity, Hydroxyl value, Iodine value, and Saponification value under Castor Oil.
Castor Oil Emulsion USP—Preserve in tight containers. Contains the labeled amount, within −10% to +20%. Meets the requirement for Identification.

NF requirements: Hydrogenated Castor Oil NF—Preserve in tight containers, and avoid exposure to excessive heat. It is refined, bleached, hydrogenated, and deodorized Castor Oil, consisting mainly of the triglyceride of hydroxystearic acid. Meets the requirements for Melting range (85–88 °C), Heavy metals (not more than 0.001%), Free fatty acids, Hydroxyl value (154–162), Iodine value (not more than 5), and Saponification value (176–182).

CEFACLOR

Chemical name: 5-Thia-1-azabicyclo[4.2.0]oct-2-ene-2-carboxylic acid, 7-[(aminophenylacetyl)amino]-3-chloro-8-oxo-, monohydrate, [6*R*-[6 alpha,7 beta(*R**)]]-.

Molecular formula: $C_{15}H_{14}ClN_3O_4S \cdot H_2O$.

Molecular weight: 385.82.

Description: Cefaclor USP—White to off-white, crystalline powder.

Solubility: Cefaclor USP—Soluble in water; practically insoluble in methanol and in chloroform.

Other characteristics: A 2.5% aqueous suspension has a pH of 3.0–4.5.

USP requirements:
Cefaclor USP—Preserve in tight containers. Has a potency of not less than 860 mcg and not more than 1050 mcg of anhydrous cefaclor per mg. Meets the requirements for Identification, Crystallinity, pH (3.0–4.5, in an aqueous suspension containing 25 mg per mL), and Water (3.0–6.5%).
Cefaclor Capsules USP—Preserve in tight containers. Contain the equivalent of the labeled amount of anhydrous cefaclor, within −10% to +20%. Meet the requirements for Identification, Dissolution (80% in 30 minutes in water in Apparatus 2 at 50 rpm), Uniformity of dosage units, and Water (not more than 8.0%).
Cefaclor for Oral Suspension USP—Preserve in tight containers. A dry mixture of Cefaclor and one or more suitable buffers, colors, diluents, and flavors. Contains the equivalent of the labeled amount of anhydrous cefaclor, within −10% to +20%. Meets the requirements for Identification, pH (2.5–5.0, in the suspension constituted as directed in the labeling), Uniformity of dosage units (solid packaged in single-unit containers), Deliverable volume (solid packaged in multiple-unit containers), and Water (not more than 2.0%).

CEFADROXIL

Chemical name: 5-Thia-1-azabicyclo[4.2.0]oct-2-ene-2-carboxylic acid, 7-[[amino(4-hydroxyphenyl)acetyl]amino]-3-methyl-8-oxo-, monohydrate, [6*R*-[6 alpha,7 beta(*R**)]]-.

Molecular formula: $C_{16}H_{17}N_3O_5S \cdot H_2O$.

Molecular weight: 381.40; 372.39 (hemihydrate); 363.39 (anhydrous).

Description: Cefadroxil USP—White to off-white, crystalline powder.

Solubility: Cefadroxil USP—Slightly soluble in water; practically insoluble in alcohol, in chloroform, and in ether.

Other characteristics: Acid-stable.

USP requirements:
Cefadroxil USP—Preserve in tight containers. The hemihydrate form is so labeled. Has a potency equivalent to not less than 950 mcg and not more than 1050 mcg of cefadroxil per mg, calculated on the anhydrous basis. Meets the requirements for Identification, Specific rotation (+165.0° to +178.0°, calculated on the anhydrous basis), Crystallinity, pH (4.0–6.0, in a suspension containing 50 mg per mL), Water (4.2–6.0%, except that where it is labeled as being in the hemihydrate form it is 2.4–4.5%), Chromatographic purity, and Dimethylaniline.
Cefadroxil Capsules USP—Preserve in tight containers. The Capsules prepared using the hemihydrate form of Cefadroxil are so labeled. Contain the equivalent of the labeled amount of anhydrous cefadroxil, within −10% to +20%. Meet the requirements for Identification, Dissolution (75% in 45 minutes in water in Apparatus 1 at 100 rpm), Uniformity of dosage units, and Water (not more than 7.0%).
Cefadroxil for Oral Suspension USP—Preserve in tight containers. A dry mixture of Cefadroxil and one or more suitable buffers, colors, diluents, and flavors. Contains

the equivalent of the labeled amount of anhydrous cefadroxil, within −10% to +20%. Meets the requirements for Identification, pH (4.5–6.0, in the suspension constituted as directed in the labeling), Uniformity of dosage units (solid packaged in single-unit containers), Deliverable volume (solid packaged in multiple-unit containers), and Water (not more than 2.0%).

Cefadroxil Tablets USP—Preserve in tight containers. The Tablets prepared using the hemihydrate form of Cefadroxil are so labeled. Contain the labeled amount of anhydrous cefadroxil, within −10% to +20%. Meet the requirements for Identification, Dissolution (75% in 30 minutes in water in Apparatus 2 at 50 rpm), Uniformity of dosage units, and Water (not more than 8.0%).

CEFAMANDOLE

Chemical name:

Cefamandole nafate—5-Thia-1-azabicyclo[4.2.0]oct-2-ene-2-carboxylic acid, 7-[[(formyloxy)phenylacetyl]amino]-3-[[(1-methyl-1*H*-tetrazol-5-yl)thio]methyl]-8-oxo-, monosodium salt, [6*R*-[6 alpha,7 beta(*R**)]].

Cefamandole sodium—5-Thia-1-azabicyclo[4.2.0]oct-2-ene-2-carboxylic acid, 7-[(hydroxyphenylacetyl)amino]-3-[[(1-methyl-1*H*-tetrazol-5-yl)thio]methyl]-8-oxo-, [6*R*-[6 alpha,7 beta(*R**)]]-, monosodium salt.

Molecular formula:

Cefamandole nafate—$C_{19}H_{17}N_6NaO_6S_2$.

Cefamandole sodium—$C_{18}H_{17}N_6NaO_5S_2$.

Molecular weight:

Cefamandole nafate—512.49.

Cefamandole sodium—484.48.

Description:

Sterile Cefamandole Nafate USP—White, odorless, crystalline solid.

Cefamandole nafate for injection—After addition of diluent, cefamandole nafate rapidly hydrolyzes to cefamandole. Solutions of cefamandole nafate range from light yellow to amber, depending on concentration and diluent used.

Cefamandole Sodium USP—White to light yellowish-white, odorless crystalline powder.

Solubility:

Sterile Cefamandole Nafate USP—Soluble in water and in methanol; practically insoluble in ether, in chloroform, and in cyclohexane.

Cefamandole Sodium USP—Freely soluble in water and in dimethylformamide; soluble in methanol; slightly soluble in dehydrated alcohol; very slightly soluble in acetone.

Other characteristics: Cefamandole nafate—The pH of freshly reconstituted solutions usually ranges from 6.0 to 8.5.

USP requirements:

Cefamandole Nafate for Injection USP—Preserve in Containers for Sterile Solids. A sterile mixture of Sterile Cefamandole Nafate or cefamandole nafate and one or more suitable buffers. Has a potency equivalent to not less than 810 mcg and not more than 1000 mcg of cefamandole per mg, calculated on the anhydrous and sodium carbonate-free basis. Contains an amount of cefamandole nafate equivalent to the labeled amount of cefamandole, within −10% to +15%. Meets the requirements for Constituted solution, Identification, Bacterial endotoxins, Sterility, pH (6.0–8.0, determined after 30 minutes in a solution containing 100 mg per mL), Water (not more than 3.0%), and Particulate matter, and for Uniformity of dosage units and Injections.

Sterile Cefamandole Nafate USP—Preserve in Containers for Sterile Solids. It is Cefamandole Nafate suitable for parenteral use. Has a potency equivalent to not less than 810 mcg and not more than 1000 mcg of cefamandole per mg, calculated on the anhydrous basis. Meets the requirements for Identification, Bacterial endotoxins, Sterility, pH (3.5–7.0, in a solution containing 100 mg per mL), and Water (not more than 2.0%).

Cefamandole Sodium for Injection USP—Preserve in Containers for Sterile Solids. A sterile mixture of Sterile Cefamandole Sodium and one or more suitable buffers. Contains an amount of cefamandole sodium equivalent to the labeled amount of cefamandole, within −10% to +15%. Meets the requirements for Constituted solution, Identification, Bacterial endotoxins, Sterility, pH (6.0–8.5, in a solution containing 100 mg of cefamandole per mL), Water (not more than 3.0%), and Particulate matter, and for Uniformity of dosage units and Labeling under Injections.

Sterile Cefamandole Sodium USP—Preserve in Containers for Sterile Solids. Has a potency equivalent to not less than 860 mcg and not more than 1000 mcg of cefamandole per mg, calculated on the anhydrous basis. Meets the requirements for Identification, Bacterial endotoxins, Sterility, pH (3.5–7.0, in a solution [1 in 10]), Water (not more than 3.0%), and Particulate matter.

CEFAZOLIN

Chemical name:

Cefazolin—5-Thia-1-azabicyclo[4.2.0]oct-2-ene-2-carboxylic acid, 3-[[(5-methyl-1,3,4-thiadiazol-2-yl)thio]methyl]-8-oxo-7-[[1*H*-tetrazol-1-yl)acetyl]amino]-(6*R-trans*).

Cefazolin sodium—5-Thia-1-azabicyclo[4.2.0]oct-2-ene-2-carboxylic acid, 3-[[(5-methyl-1,3,4-thiadiazol-2-yl)thio]-methyl]-8-oxo-7-[[(1*H*-tetrazol-1-yl)acetyl]amino]-, monosodium salt (6*R-trans*)-.

Molecular formula:

Cefazolin—$C_{14}H_{14}N_8O_4S_3$.

Cefazolin sodium—$C_{14}H_{13}N_8NaO_4S_3$.

Molecular weight:

Cefazolin—454.50.

Cefazolin sodium—476.48.

Description:

Cefazolin USP—White to slightly off-white, odorless, crystalline powder. Melts at about 198 to 200 °C, with decomposition.

Cefazolin sodium—White to off-white, almost odorless, crystalline powder.

Sterile Cefazolin Sodium USP—White to off-white, practically odorless, crystalline powder, or white to off-white solid having the characteristic appearance of products prepared by freeze-drying.

Solubility:

Cefazolin USP—Soluble in dimethylformamide and in pyridine; sparingly soluble in acetone; slightly soluble in alcohol, in methanol, and in water; very slightly soluble in ethyl acetate, in isopropyl alcohol, and in methyl isobutyl ketone; practically insoluble in chloroform, in ether, and in methylene chloride.

Cefazolin sodium—Freely soluble in water, in 0.9% sodium chloride solution, and in glucose solutions; very slightly soluble in alcohol; practically insoluble in ether and in chloroform.

Sterile Cefazolin Sodium USP—Freely soluble in water, in saline TS, and in dextrose solutions; very slightly soluble in alcohol; practically insoluble in chloroform and in ether.

Other characteristics: Cefazolin sodium—A 10% solution in water has a pH of 4.5 to 6.0.

USP requirements:

Cefazolin USP—Preserve in tight containers. Contains not less than 950 mcg and not more than 1030 mcg of cefazolin per mg, calculated on the anhydrous basis. Meets the requirements for Identification, Water (not more than 2.0%), and Heavy metals (not more than 0.002%).

Cefazolin Sodium Injection USP—Preserve in Containers for Injections. Maintain in the frozen state. A sterile solution of Cefazolin and Sodium Bicarbonate in a diluent containing one or more suitable tonicity-adjusting agents. It meets the requirements for Labeling under Injections. The label states that it is to be thawed just prior to use, describes conditions for proper storage of the resultant solution, and directs that the solution is not to be refrozen. Contains an amount of cefazolin sodium equivalent to the labeled amount of cefazolin, within −10% to +15%. Meets the requirements for Identification, Bacterial endotoxins, Sterility, pH (4.5–7.0), and Particulate matter.

Sterile Cefazolin Sodium USP—Preserve in Containers for Sterile Solids. Has a potency equivalent to not less than 850 mcg and not more than 1050 mcg of cefazolin per mg, calculated on the anhydrous basis, and, where packaged for dispensing, contains an amount of cefazolin sodium equivalent to the labeled amount of cefazolin, within −10% to +15%. Meets the requirements for Constituted solution, Identification, Specific rotation (−24° to −10°), Bacterial endotoxins, Sterility, pH (4.0–6.0, in a solution containing 100 mg of cefazolin per mL), Water (not more than 6.0%), and Particulate matter, and for Uniformity of dosage units and Labeling under Injections.

CEFIXIME

Chemical name: 5-Thia-1-azabicyclo[4.2.0]oct-2-ene-2-carboxylic acid, 7-[[(2-amino-4-thiazolyl)[(carboxymethoxy)imino]-acetyl]amino]-3-ethenyl-8-oxo-, trihydrate, [6*R*-[6 alpha,7 beta(*Z*)]]-.

Molecular formula: $C_{16}H_{15}N_5O_7S_2 \cdot 3H_2O$.

Molecular weight: 507.49.

Description: Cefixime USP—White to light yellow, crystalline powder.

Solubility: Cefixime USP—Freely soluble in methanol; soluble in glycerin and in propylene glycol; sparingly soluble in acetone; slightly soluble in alcohol; very slightly soluble in 70% sorbitol and in octanol; practically insoluble in ether, in ethyl acetate, in hexane, and in water.

USP requirements:

Cefixime USP—Preserve in tight containers. Label to indicate that it is the trihydrate form. Where the quantity of cefixime is indicated in the labeling of any preparation containing Cefixime, this shall be understood to be in terms of anhydrous cefixime. Contains the equivalent of not less than 950 mcg and not more than 1030 mcg of cefixime per mg, calculated on the anhydrous basis. Meets the requirements for Identification, Specific rotation (−75° to −88°, calculated on the anhydrous basis), Crystallinity, pH (2.6–4.1, in a solution containing the equivalent of 0.7 mg of cefixime per mL), and Water (9.0–12.0%).

Cefixime for Oral Suspension USP—Preserve in tight containers. A dry mixture of Cefixime and one or more suitable diluents, flavors, preservatives, and suspending agents. Label it to indicate that the cefixime contained therein is in the trihydrate form. Contains the labeled amount of anhydrous cefixime, within −10% to +20%, per mL when constituted as directed in the labeling. Meets the requirements for Identification, Uniformity of dosage units (solid packaged in single-unit containers), Deliverable volume (solid packaged in multiple-unit containers), pH (2.5–4.5, in the suspension constituted as directed in the labeling), and Water (not more than 2.0%).

Cefixime Tablets USP—Preserve in tight containers. Label Tablets to indicate that the cefixime contained therein is in the trihydrate form. Contain the labeled amount of anhydrous cefixime, within ±10%. Meet the requirements for Identification, Dissolution (75% in 45 minutes in 0.05 *M* potassium phosphate buffer [pH 7.2] in Apparatus 1 at 100 rpm), Uniformity of dosage units, and Water (not more than 10.0%).

CEFMENOXIME

Chemical name: Cefmenoxime hydrochloride—5-Thia-1-azabicyclo[4.2.0]oct-2-ene-2-carboxylic acid, 7-[[(2-amino-4-thiazolyl)(methoxyimino)acetyl]amino]-3-[[(1-methyl-1*H*-tetrazol-5-yl)thio]methyl]-8-oxo-, hydrochloride (2:1), [6*R*-[6 alpha,7 beta(*Z*)]]-.

Molecular formula: Cefmenoxime hydrochloride—$(C_{16}H_{17}N_9O_5S_3)_2 \cdot HCl$.

Molecular weight: Cefmenoxime hydrochloride—1059.56.

Description: Sterile Cefmenoxime Hydrochloride USP—White to light orange-yellow crystals or crystalline powder.

Solubility: Sterile Cefmenoxime Hydrochloride USP—Very slightly soluble in water; freely soluble in formamide; slightly soluble in methanol; practically insoluble in dehydrated alcohol and in ether.

USP requirements:

Cefmenoxime for Injection USP—Preserve in Containers for Sterile Solids. A sterile mixture of Sterile Cefmenoxime Hydrochloride and Sodium Carbonate. Contains not less than 869 mcg and not more than 1015 mcg of cefmenoxime per mg, calculated on the dried and sodium carbonate-free basis, and the labeled amount of cefmenoxime, within −10% to +15%. Meets the requirements for Identification, Pyrogen, Sterility, pH (6.4–7.9, in a solution containing the equivalent of 100 mg of cefmenoxime per mL), Loss on drying (not more than 1.5%), Particulate matter, and Sodium carbonate content.

Sterile Cefmenoxime Hydrochloride USP—Preserve in Containers for Sterile Solids. It is Cefmenoxime Hydrochloride suitable for parenteral use. Contains the equivalent of not less than 869 mcg and not more than 1015 mcg of cefmenoxime per mg, calculated on the anhydrous basis. Meets the requirements for Identification, Crystallinity, Pyrogen, Sterility, and Water (not more than 1.5%).

CEFMETAZOLE

Chemical name: Cefmetazole sodium—5-Thia-1-azabicyclo-[4.2.0]oct-2-ene-2-carboxylic acid, 7-[[[(cyanomethyl)thio]-acetyl]amino]-7-methoxy-3-[[(1-methyl-1*H*-tetrazol-5-yl)-thio]methyl]-8-oxo-, monosodium salt, (6*R*-*cis*)-.

Molecular formula: Cefmetazole sodium—$C_{15}H_{16}N_7NaO_5S_3$.

Molecular weight: Cefmetazole sodium—493.51.

Description: Sterile Cefmetazole Sodium USP—White solid having the characteristic appearance of products prepared by freeze-drying.

Solubility: Sterile Cefmetazole Sodium USP—Very soluble in water and in methanol; soluble in acetone; practically insoluble in chloroform.

USP requirements:
Sterile Cefmetazole Sodium USP—Preserve in Containers for Sterile Solids. Contains the equivalent of not less than 860 mcg and not more than 1003 mcg of cefmetazole per mg, calculated on the anhydrous basis. In addition, where packaged for dispensing, contains an amount of cefmetazole sodium equivalent to the labeled amount of cefmetazole, within −10% to +20%. Meets the requirements for Identification, Bacterial endotoxins, Sterility, pH (4.2–6.2, in a solution [1 in 10]), Water (not more than 0.5%), and Particulate matter, for Uniformity of dosage units, and for Labeling under Injections.
Cefmetazole Sodium for Injection—Not in USP.

CEFONICID

Chemical name: Cefonicid sodium—5-Thia-1-azabicyclo[4.2.0]-oct-2-ene-2-carboxylic acid, 7-[(hydroxyphenylacetyl)amino]-8-oxo-3-[[[1-(sulfomethyl)-1*H*-tetrazol-5-yl]thio]methyl]-disodium salt, [6*R*-[6 alpha,7 beta(*R**)]].

Molecular formula: Cefonicid sodium—$C_{18}H_{16}N_6Na_2O_8S_3$.

Molecular weight: Cefonicid sodium—586.52.

Description: Sterile Cefonicid Sodium USP—White to off-white solid having the characteristic appearance of products prepared by freeze-drying.

Solubility: Sterile Cefonicid Sodium USP—Freely soluble in water, in 0.9% sodium chloride solution, and in 5% dextrose solution; soluble in methanol; very slightly soluble in dehydrated alcohol.

USP requirements: Sterile Cefonicid Sodium USP—Preserve in Containers for Sterile Solids. It is cefonicid sodium suitable for parenteral use. Contains the equivalent of not less than 832 mcg and not more than 970 mcg of cefonicid per mg, calculated on the anhydrous basis, and, where packaged for dispensing, contains an amount of cefonicid sodium equivalent to the labeled amount of cefonicid, within −10% to +20%. Meets the requirements for Constituted solution, Identification, Bacterial endotoxins, Sterility, Specific rotation (−37° to −47°, calculated on the anhydrous basis), pH (3.5–6.5, in a solution [1 in 20]), Water (not more than 5.0%), and Particulate matter, for Uniformity of dosage units, and for Labeling under Injections.

CEFOPERAZONE

Chemical name: Cefoperazone sodium—5-Thia-1-azabicyclo-[4.2.0]oct-2-ene-2-carboxylic acid, 7-[[[[(4-ethyl-2,3-dioxo-1-piperazinyl)carbonyl]amino](4-hydroxyphenyl)acetyl]amino]-3-[[(1-methyl-1*H*-tetrazol-5-yl)thio]methyl]-8-oxo, monosodium salt, [6*R*-[6 alpha,7 beta(*R**)]]-.

Molecular formula: Cefoperazone sodium—$C_{25}H_{26}N_9NaO_8S_2$.

Molecular weight: Cefoperazone sodium—667.65.

Description:
Cefoperazone Sodium USP—White to pale buff crystalline powder.
Sterile Cefoperazone Sodium USP—White to pale buff, crystalline powder or white to pale buff solid having the characteristic appearance of products prepared by freeze-drying.

Solubility:
Cefoperazone Sodium USP—Freely soluble in water and in methanol; slightly soluble in dehydrated alcohol; insoluble in acetone, in ethyl acetate, and in ether.
Sterile Cefoperazone Sodium USP—Freely soluble in water, in sodium chloride solution, and in dextrose solution.

USP requirements:
Cefoperazone Sodium USP—Preserve in tight containers. Contains the equivalent of not less than 870 mcg and not more than 1015 mcg of cefoperazone per mg, calculated on the anhydrous basis. Meets the requirements for Identification, Crystallinity (Note: Cefoperazone Sodium in the freeze-dried form is exempt from this requirement), pH (4.5–6.5, in a solution [1 in 4]), and Water (not more than 5.0%, except that where it is in the freeze-dried form, the limit is not more than 2.0%).
Cefoperazone Sodium Injection USP—Preserve in Containers for Injections. Maintain in the frozen state. A sterile solution of Cefoperazone Sodium and a suitable osmolality-adjusting substance in Water for Injection. Meets the requirements for Labeling under Injections. The label states that it is to be thawed just prior to use, describes conditions for proper storage of the resultant solution, and directs that the solution is not to be refrozen. Contains an amount of cefoperazone sodium equivalent to the labeled amount of cefoperazone, within −10% to +20%. Meets the requirements for Identification, Pyrogen, Sterility, pH (4.5–6.5), and Particulate matter.
Sterile Cefoperazone Sodium USP—Preserve in Containers for Sterile Solids. It is Cefoperazone Sodium suitable for parenteral use. Contains the equivalent of not less than 870 mcg and not more than 1015 mcg of cefoperazone per mg, calculated on the anhydrous basis, and, where packaged for dispensing, contains an amount of cefoperazone sodium equivalent to the labeled amount of cefoperazone, within −10% to +20%. Meets the requirements for Constituted solution, Identification, Crystallinity (Note: Sterile Cefoperazone Sodium packaged for dispensing in the freeze-dried form is exempt from this requirement), Bacterial endotoxins, Sterility, pH (4.5–6.5 in a solution [1 in 4]), Water (not more than 5.0%; where packaged for dispensing in the freeze-dried form, not more than 2.0%), and Particulate matter, for Uniformity of dosage units, and for Labeling under Injections.

CEFORANIDE

Chemical name: 5-Thia-1-azabicyclo[4.2.0]oct-2-ene-2-carboxylic acid, 7-[[[2-(aminomethyl)phenyl]acetyl]amino]-3-[[[1-(carboxymethyl)-1*H*-tetrazol-5-yl]thio]methyl]-8-oxo-, (6*R*-*trans*)-.

Molecular formula: $C_{20}H_{21}N_7O_6S_2$.

Molecular weight: 519.55.

Description:
Ceforanide for injection—Solutions of ceforanide range in color from light yellow to amber depending on the concentration and diluent used.
Sterile Ceforanide USP—White to off-white powder.

Solubility: Sterile Ceforanide USP—Practically insoluble in water, in methanol, in chloroform, and in ether; very soluble in 1 *N* sodium hydroxide.

Other characteristics: Ceforanide for injection—The pH of the solution ranges from 5.5 to 8.5.

USP requirements:
Ceforanide for Injection USP—Preserve in Containers for Sterile Solids. A sterile mixture of Sterile Ceforanide and L-Lysine. Contains not less than 900 mcg and not more than 1050 mcg of ceforanide per mg on the L-Lysine-free basis, and the labeled amount, within −10% to +15%. Meets the requirements for Identification, Bacterial endotoxins, Sterility, pH (5.5–8.5, constituted as directed in the labeling), Water (not more than 3.0%), Particulate

matter, and L-Lysine content, for Uniformity of dosage units, and for Labeling under Injections.

Sterile Ceforanide USP—Preserve in Containers for Sterile Solids. It is ceforanide suitable for parenteral use. Contains not less than 900 mcg and not more than 1050 mcg of ceforanide per mg. Meets the requirements for Identification, Bacterial endotoxins, Sterility, pH (2.5–4.5, in a suspension containing 50 mg per mL), and Water (not more than 5.0%).

CEFOTAXIME

Chemical name: Cefotaxime sodium—5-Thia-1-azabicyclo-[4.2.0]oct-2-ene-2-carboxylic acid, 3-[(acetyloxy)methyl]-7-[[(2-amino-4-thiazolyl)(methoxyimino)acetyl]amino]-8-oxo-, monosodium salt, [6*R*-[6 alpha,7 beta(*Z*)]]-.

Molecular formula: Cefotaxime sodium—$C_{16}H_{16}N_5NaO_7S_2$.

Molecular weight: Cefotaxime sodium—477.44.

Description:

Cefotaxime Sodium USP—Off-white to pale yellow crystalline powder.

Cefotaxime sodium injection—Solutions of cefotaxime sodium range from very pale yellow to light amber depending on the concentration and the diluent used.

Solubility: Cefotaxime Sodium USP—Freely soluble in water; practically insoluble in organic solvents.

Other characteristics: Cefotaxime sodium injection—Has a pH of 5.0–7.5.

USP requirements:

Cefotaxime Sodium USP—Preserve in tight containers. Contains the equivalent of not less than 855 mcg and not more than 1002 mcg of cefotaxime per mg, calculated on the anhydrous basis. Meets the requirements for Identification, pH (4.5–6.5, in a solution [1 in 10]), and Water (not more than 6.0%).

Cefotaxime Sodium Injection USP—Preserve in single-dose containers. Maintain in the frozen state. A sterile solution of Cefotaxime Sodium in Water for Injection. Contains one or more suitable buffers. It meets the requirements for Labeling under Injections. The label states that it is to be thawed just prior to use, describes conditions for proper storage of the resultant solution, and directs that the solution is not to be refrozen. Contains an amount of cefotaxime sodium equivalent to the labeled amount of cefotaxime, within ±10%. Meets the requirements for Identification, Bacterial endotoxins, Sterility, pH (5.0–7.5), and Particulate matter.

Sterile Cefotaxime Sodium USP—Preserve in Containers for Sterile Solids. It is Cefotaxime Sodium suitable for parenteral use. Contains the equivalent of not less than 855 mcg and not more than 1002 mcg of cefotaxime per mg, calculated on the anhydrous basis, and, where packaged for dispensing, contains an amount of cefotaxime sodium equivalent to the labeled amount of cefotaxime, within ±10%. Meets the requirements for Constituted solution, Bacterial endotoxins, Sterility, and Particulate matter, and for Identification tests, pH, and Water under Cefotaxime Sodium. In addition, where packaged for dispensing, it meets the requirements for Uniformity of dosage units and for Labeling under Injections.

CEFOTETAN

Chemical name: Cefotetan disodium—5-Thia-1-azabicyclo[4.2.0]-oct-2-ene-2-carboxylic acid, 7-[[[4-(2-amino-1-carboxy-2-oxoethylidene)-1,3-dithietan-2-yl]carbonyl]amino]-7-methoxy-3-[[(1-methyl-1*H*-tetrazol-5-yl)thio]methyl]-8-oxo-, disodium salt, [6*R*-(6 alpha,7 alpha)]-.

Molecular formula: Cefotetan disodium—$C_{17}H_{15}N_7Na_2O_8S_4$.

Molecular weight: Cefotetan disodium—619.57.

Description:

Cefotetan disodium—White to pale yellow powder.

Cefotetan disodium injection—Solution varies from colorless to yellow, depending on the concentration.

Solubility: Cefotetan disodium—Very soluble in water.

Other characteristics: Cefotetan disodium—The pH of freshly reconstituted solutions is usually between 4.5 and 6.5.

USP requirements: Sterile Cefotetan Disodium USP—Preserve in Containers for Sterile Solids. It is Cefotetan Disodium suitable for parenteral use. Contains the equivalent of not less than 830 mcg and not more than 970 mcg of cefotetan per mg, calculated on the anhydrous basis, and, where packaged for dispensing, contains an amount of cefotetan disodium equivalent to the labeled amount of cefotetan, within −10% to +20%. Meets the requirements for Constituted solution, Identification, Bacterial endotoxins, Sterility, pH (4.0–6.5, in a solution [1 in 10]), Water (not more than 1.5%), and Particulate matter, for Uniformity of dosage units, and for Labeling under Injections.

CEFOTIAM

Chemical name: Cefotiam hydrochloride—5-Thia-1-azabicyclo[4.2.0]oct-2-ene-2-carboxylic acid, 7-[[(2-amino-4-thiazolyl)acetyl]-amino]-3-[[[1-[2-(dimethylamino)ethyl]-1*H*-tetrazol-5-yl]thio]methyl]-8-oxo, hydrochloride, (6*R-trans*)-.

Molecular formula: Cefotiam hydrochloride—$C_{18}H_{23}N_9O_4S_3 \cdot 2HCl$.

Molecular weight: Cefotiam hydrochloride—598.54.

Description: Cefotiam hydrochloride—White to light yellow crystals.

Solubility: Cefotiam hydrochloride—Soluble in methanol; slightly soluble in ethanol.

USP requirements:

Cefotiam for Injection USP—Preserve in Containers for Sterile Solids. A sterile mixture of Sterile Cefotiam Hydrochloride and Sodium Carbonate. Contains not less than 790 mcg and not more than 925 mcg of cefotiam per mg, calculated on the dried and sodium carbonate-free basis, and the labeled amount of cefotiam, within −10% to +20%. Meets the requirements for Identification, Pyrogen, Sterility, pH (5.7–7.2, in a solution containing the equivalent of 100 mg of cefotiam per mL), Loss on drying (not more than 6.0%), Particulate matter, and Sodium carbonate content.

Sterile Cefotiam Hydrochloride USP—Preserve in Containers for Sterile Solids. It is cefotiam hydrochloride suitable for parenteral use. Contains the equivalent of not less than 790 mcg and not more than 925 mcg of cefotiam per mg, calculated on the anhydrous basis. Meets the requirements for Identification, Crystallinity, Pyrogen, Sterility, and Water (not more than 7.0%).

CEFOXITIN

Source: Cefoxitin sodium—Semisynthetic cephamycin derived from cephamycin C, produced by *Streptomyces lactamdurans*.

Chemical name: Cefoxitin sodium—5-Thia-1-azabicyclo[4.2.0]-oct-2-ene-2-carboxylic acid, 3-[[(aminocarbonyl)oxy]-methyl]-7-methoxy-8-oxo-7-[(2-thienylacetyl)amino]-, sodium salt, (6*R-cis*)-.

Molecular formula: Cefoxitin sodium—$C_{16}H_{16}N_3NaO_7S_2$.

Molecular weight: Cefoxitin sodium—449.43.

Description: Sterile Cefoxitin Sodium USP—White to off-white, granules or powder, having a slight characteristic odor. Is somewhat hygroscopic.

Solubility: Sterile Cefoxitin Sodium USP—Very soluble in water; soluble in methanol; sparingly soluble in dimethylformamide; slightly soluble in acetone; insoluble in ether and in chloroform.

USP requirements:

Cefoxitin Sodium USP—Preserve in tight containers. Contains the equivalent of not less than 927 mcg and not more than 970 mcg of cefoxitin per mg, corresponding to not less than 97.5% and not more than 102.0% of cefoxitin sodium, calculated on the anhydrous and acetone- and methanol-free basis. Meets the requirements for Identification, Specific rotation (+206° to +214°, calculated on the anhydrous and acetone- and methanol-free basis), Crystallinity, pH (4.2–7.0, in a solution containing 100 mg per mL), Water (not more than 1.0%), Heavy metals (not more than 0.002%), and Acetone and methanol (not more than 0.7% of acetone and 0.1% of methanol).

Cefoxitin Sodium Injection USP—Preserve in Containers for Injections. Maintain in the frozen state. A sterile solution of Cefoxitin Sodium and one or more suitable buffer substances in Water for Injection. Contains Dextrose or Sodium Chloride as a tonicity-adjusting agent. Meets the requirements for Labeling under Injections. The label states that it is to be thawed just prior to use, describes conditions for proper storage of the resultant solution, and directs that the solution is not to be refrozen. Contains an amount of cefoxitin sodium equivalent to the labeled amount of cefoxitin, within −10% to +20%. Meets the requirements for Identification, Bacterial endotoxins, Sterility, pH (4.5–8.0), and Particulate matter.

Sterile Cefoxitin Sodium USP—Preserve in Containers for Sterile Solids. Contains the equivalent of not less than 927 mcg and not more than 970 mcg of cefoxitin per mg, corresponding to not less than 97.5% and not more than 102.0% of cefoxitin sodium, calculated on the anhydrous and acetone- and methanol-free basis, and, where packaged for dispensing, contains an amount of cefoxitin sodium equivalent to the labeled amount of cefoxitin, within −10% to +20%. Meets the requirements for Constituted solution, Bacterial endotoxins, Sterility, and Particulate matter, and for Identification tests, Specific rotation, Crystallinity, pH, Water, Heavy metals, and Acetone and methanol under Cefoxitin Sodium. In addition, where packaged for dispensing, meets the requirements for Uniformity of dosage units and for Labeling under Injections.

CEFPIRAMIDE

Chemical name: 5-Thia-1-azabicyclo[4.2.0]oct-2-ene-2-carboxylic acid, 7-[[[[(4-hydroxy-6-methyl-3-pyridinyl)-carbonyl]amino](4-hydroxyphenyl)acetyl]amino]-3-[[(1-methyl-1*H*-tetrazol-5-yl)thio]methyl]-8-oxo-, [6*R*-[6 alpha,7 beta(*R**)]]-.

Molecular formula: $C_{25}H_{24}N_8O_7S_2$.

Molecular weight: 612.63.

Description: Yellow crystals. Melting point is 213–215 °C.

USP requirements:

Cefpiramide USP—Preserve in tight containers. Contains the equivalent of not less than 974 mcg and not more than 1026 mcg of cefpiramide per mg, calculated on the anhydrous basis. Meets the requirements for Identification, Specific rotation (−100° to −112°, calculated on the anhydrous basis), Crystallinity, pH (3.0–5.0, in a suspension [1 in 200]), Water (not more than 9.0%), and Related substances (not more than 2.0%).

Cefpiramide for Injection USP—Preserve in Containers for Sterile Solids. A sterile mixture of Cefpiramide, Sodium Benzoate, and other buffers and preservatives. Contains not less than 754 mcg and not more than 924 mcg of cefpiramide per mg, calculated on the anhydrous basis, and where packaged for dispensing contains the labeled amount, within −10% to +20%. Meets the requirements for Identification, Pyrogen, Sterility, pH (6.0–8.0, in a solution containing the equivalent of 100 mg of cefpiramide per mL), Water (not more than 3.0%), and Particulate matter.

CEFPODOXIME

Chemical name: Cefpodoxime proxetil—5-Thia-1-azabicyclo-[4.2.0]oct-2-ene-2-carboxylic acid, 7-[[(2-amino-4-thiazolyl)-(methoxyimino)acetyl]amino]-3-(methoxymethyl)-8-oxo-, 1-[[(1-methylethoxy)carbonyl]oxy]ethyl ester, [6*R*-[6 alpha,7 beta(*Z*)]]-.

Molecular formula: Cefpodoxime proxetil—$C_{21}H_{27}N_5O_9S_2$.

Molecular weight: Cefpodoxime proxetil—557.59.

USP requirements:

Cefpodoxime Proxetil for Oral Suspension—Not in USP.

Cefpodoxime Proxetil Tablets—Not in USP.

CEFPROZIL

Chemical name: 5-Thia-1-azabicyclo[4.2.0]oct-2-ene-2-carboxylic acid, 7-[[amino(4-hydroxyphenyl)acetyl]amino]-8-oxo-3-(1-propenyl)-, monohydrate, [6*R*-[6 alpha,7 beta(*R**)]]-.

Molecular formula: $C_{18}H_{19}N_3O_5S \cdot H_2O$.

Molecular weight: 407.44.

Description: White to yellowish powder.

USP requirements:

Cefprozil USP—Preserve in tight containers. Contains not less than 900 mcg and not more than 1050 mcg of cefprozil per mg, calculated on the anhydrous basis. Meets the requirements for Identification, Crystallinity, pH (3.5–6.5, in a solution containing 5 mg per mL), Water (3.5–6.5%), and Cefprozil (*E*)-isomer ratio (0.06–0.11).

Cefprozil Oral Suspension—Not in USP.

Cefprozil for Oral Suspension USP—Preserve in tight containers. A dry mixture of Cefprozil and one or more suitable buffers, flavors, preservatives, suspending agents, and sweeteners. Contains the labeled amount, within −10% to +20%. Meets the requirements for Identification, Uniformity of dosage units, pH (4.0–6.0, in the Oral Suspension constituted as directed in the labeling), and Water (not more than 3.0%).

Cefprozil Tablets USP—Preserve in tight containers. Contain the labeled amount, within −10% to +20%. Meet the requirements for Identification, Dissolution (75% in 45 minutes in water in Apparatus 1 at 100 rpm), Uniformity of dosage units, and Water (not more than 7.0%).

CEFTAZIDIME

Chemical name: Pyridinium, 1-[[7-[[(2-amino-4-thiazolyl)[(1-carboxy-1-methylethoxy)imino]acetyl]amino]-2-carboxy-8-oxo-5-thia-1-azabicyclo[4.2.0]oct-2-en-3-yl]methyl]-, hydroxide, inner salt, pentahydrate, [6*R*-[6 alpha,7 beta(*Z*)]]-.

Molecular formula: $C_{22}H_{22}N_6O_7S_2 \cdot 5H_2O$.

Molecular weight: 636.65.

Description:
Ceftazidime USP—White to cream-colored, crystalline powder.
Ceftazidime for injection—Solutions of ceftazidime range in color from light yellow to amber, depending upon the diluent and volume used.

Solubility: Ceftazidime USP—Soluble in alkali and in dimethyl sulfoxide; slightly soluble in dimethylformamide, in methanol, and in water; insoluble in acetone, in alcohol, in chloroform, in dioxane, in ether, in ethyl acetate, and in toluene.

Other characteristics: Ceftazidime for injection—The pH of freshly constituted solutions usually ranges from 5 to 8.

USP requirements:
Ceftazidime USP—Preserve in tight containers. Contains not less than 95.0% and not more than 102.0% of ceftazidime, calculated on the dried basis. Meets the requirements for Identification, Crystallinity, pH (3.0–4.0, in a solution containing 5 mg per mL), Loss on drying (13.0–15.0%), and High molecular weight ceftazidime polymer (not more than 0.05%).
Ceftazidime Injection USP—Preserve in Containers for Injections. Maintain in the frozen state. A sterile isoosmotic solution of Ceftazidime in Water for Injection. It meets the requirements for Labeling under Injections. The label states that it is to be thawed just prior to use, describes conditions for proper storage of the resultant solution, and directs that the solution is not to be refrozen. Contains one or more suitable buffers and a tonicity-adjusting agent. Contains an amount equivalent to the labeled amount of anhydrous ceftazidime, within −10% to +20%. Meets the requirements for Identification, Pyrogen, Sterility, pH (5.0–7.5), and Particulate matter.
Ceftazidime for Injection USP—Preserve in Containers for Sterile Solids, protected from light. A sterile mixture of Sterile Ceftazidime and Sodium Carbonate or Arginine. Contains not less than 90.0% and not more than 105.0% of ceftazidime, on the dried and sodium carbonate– or arginine–free basis, and contains an amount equivalent to the labeled amount of anhydrous ceftazidine, within −10% to +20%. Meets the requirements for Identification, Bacterial endotoxins, Sterility, pH (5.0–7.5, in a solution constituted in the sealed container, taking care to relieve the pressure inside the container during constitution, containing 100 mg of ceftazidime per mL), Loss on drying (not more than 13.5%), Particulate matter, Sodium carbonate (where present), High molecular weight ceftazidime polymer (not more than 0.4%), and Content of arginine (where present), and for Uniformity of dosage units and Labeling under Injections.
Sterile Ceftazidime USP—Preserve in Containers for Sterile Solids, protected from light. It is ceftazidime pentahydrate suitable for parenteral use. Contains not less than 95.0% and not more than 102.0% of ceftazidime, calculated on the dried basis. Meets the requirements for Bacterial endotoxins and Sterility, and for Identification test, Crystallinity, pH, Loss on drying, and High molecular weight ceftazidime polymer under Ceftazidime. In addition, where packaged for dispensing, meets the requirements for Uniformity of dosage units and for Labeling under Injections.

CEFTIZOXIME

Chemical name: Ceftizoxime sodium—5-Thia-1-azabicyclo-[4.2.0]oct-2-ene-2-carboxylic acid, 7-[[(2,3-dihydro-2-imino-4-thiazolyl)(methoxyimino)acetyl]amino]-8-oxomonosodium salt, [6*R*-[6 alpha,7 beta(*Z*)]]-.

Molecular formula: Ceftizoxime sodium—$C_{13}H_{12}N_5NaO_5S_2$.

Molecular weight: Ceftizoxime sodium—405.38.

Description:
Ceftizoxime Sodium USP—White to pale yellow crystalline powder.
Sterile ceftizoxime sodium—White to pale yellow crystalline powder.

Solubility: Ceftizoxime Sodium USP—Freely soluble in water.

Other characteristics: Ceftizoxime sodium—A 10% solution in water has a pH of 6 to 8.

USP requirements:
Ceftizoxime Sodium USP—Preserve in tight containers. Contains the equivalent of not less than 850 mcg and not more than 995 mcg of ceftizoxime per mg, calculated on the anhydrous basis. Meets the requirements for Identification, Crystallinity, pH (6.0–8.0, in a solution [1 in 10]), and Water (not more than 8.5%).
Ceftizoxime Sodium Injection USP—Preserve in Containers for Injections. Maintain in the frozen state. A sterile solution of Ceftizoxime Sodium in a diluent containing one or more tonicity-adjusting agents in Water for Injection. It meets the requirements for Labeling under Injections. The label states that it is to be thawed just prior to use, describes conditions for proper storage of the resultant solution, and directs that the solution is not to be refrozen. Contains an amount of ceftizoxime sodium equivalent to the labeled amount of ceftizoxime, within −10% to +15%. Meets the requirements for Identification, Bacterial endotoxins, Sterility, pH (5.5–8.0), and Particulate matter.
Sterile Ceftizoxime Sodium USP—Preserve in Containers for Sterile Solids. It is ceftizoxime sodium suitable for parenteral use. Contains the equivalent of not less than 850 mcg and not more than 995 mcg of ceftizoxime per mg, calculated on the anhydrous basis, and, where packaged for dispensing, contains an amount of ceftizoxime sodium equivalent to the labeled amount of ceftizoxime, within −10% to +15%. Meets the requirements for Constituted solution, Identification, Crystallinity, Bacterial endotoxins, Sterility, pH (6.0–8.0 in a solution [1 in 10]), Water (not more than 8.5%), and Particulate matter, for Uniformity of dosage units, and for Labeling under Injections.

CEFTRIAXONE

Chemical name: Ceftriaxone sodium—5-Thia-1-azabicyclo-[4.2.0]oct-2-ene-2-carboxylic acid, 7-[[(2-amino-4-thiazolyl)-(methoxyimino)acetyl]amino]-8-oxo-3-[[(1,2,5,6-tetrahydro-2-methyl-5,6-dioxo-1,2,4-triazin-3-yl)thio]methyl]-, disodium salt, [6*R*-[6 alpha,7 beta(*Z*)]]-, hydrate (2:7).

Molecular formula: Ceftriaxone sodium—$C_{18}H_{16}N_8Na_2O_7S_3$ (anhydrous).

Molecular weight: Ceftriaxone sodium—598.53 (anhydrous).

Description:
Ceftriaxone sodium—White to yellowish-orange crystalline powder.
Ceftriaxone injection—The color of ceftriaxone sodium solution ranges from light yellow to amber, depending on the length of storage and the concentration and diluent used.
Sterile Ceftriaxone Sodium USP—White to yellowish-orange crystalline powder.

Solubility:
Ceftriaxone sodium—Readily soluble in water; sparingly soluble in methanol; very slightly soluble in alcohol.

Sterile Ceftriaxone Sodium USP—Freely soluble in water; sparingly soluble in methanol; very slightly soluble in alcohol.

USP requirements:

Ceftriaxone Sodium USP—Preserve in tight containers. Contains the equivalent of not less than 795 mcg of ceftriaxone per mg, calculated on the anhydrous basis. Meets the requirements for Identification, Crystallinity, pH (6.0–8.0 in a solution [1 in 10]), and Water (8.0–11.0%).

Ceftriaxone Sodium Injection USP—Preserve in Containers for Injections. Maintain in the frozen state. A sterile solution of Ceftriaxone Sodium in a diluent containing one or more tonicity-adjusting agents in Water for Injection. It meets the requirements for Labeling under Injections. The label states that it is to be thawed just prior to use, describes conditions for proper storage of the resultant solution, and directs that the solution is not to be refrozen. Contains an amount of ceftriaxone sodium equivalent to the labeled amount of ceftriaxone, within −10% to +15%. Meets the requirements for Identification, Bacterial endotoxins, Sterility, pH (6.0–8.0), and Particulate matter.

Sterile Ceftriaxone Sodium USP—Preserve in Containers for Sterile Solids. It is Ceftriaxone Sodium suitable for parenteral use. Where it is not packaged for dispensing, contains the equivalent of not less than 795 mcg of ceftriaxone per mg, calculated on the anhydrous basis. Where it is packaged for dispensing, contains the equivalent of not less than 776 mcg of ceftriaxone per mg, calculated on the anhydrous basis, and contains an amount of ceftriaxone sodium equivalent to the labeled amount of ceftriaxone, within −10% to +15%. Meets the requirements for Constituted solution, Bacterial endotoxins, Sterility, and Particulate matter, and for Identification tests, Crystallinity, pH, and Water under Ceftriaxone Sodium. In addition, where packaged for dispensing, meets the requirements for Uniformity of dosage units and for Labeling under Injections.

CEFUROXIME

Chemical name:

Cefuroxime axetil—5-Thia-1-azabicyclo[4.2.0]oct-2-ene-2-carboxylic acid, 3-[[(aminocarbonyl)oxy]methyl]-7-[[2-furanyl(methoxyimino)acetyl]amino]-8-oxo-, 1-(acetyloxy)ethyl ester, [6*R*-[6 alpha,7 beta(*Z*)]]-.

Cefuroxime sodium—5-Thia-1-azabicyclo[4.2.0]oct-2-ene-2-carboxylic acid, 3-[[(aminocarbonyl)oxy]methyl]-7-[[2-furanyl(methoxyimino)acetyl]amino]-8-oxo-, monosodium salt [6*R*-[6 alpha,7 beta(*Z*)]]-.

Molecular formula:

Cefuroxime axetil—$C_{20}H_{22}N_4O_{10}S$.

Cefuroxime sodium—$C_{16}H_{15}N_4NaO_8S$.

Molecular weight:

Cefuroxime axetil—510.48.

Cefuroxime sodium—446.37.

Description:

Cefuroxime Axetil USP—White to almost white amorphous powder.

Cefuroxime sodium—White to faintly yellow crystalline powder.

Sterile Cefuroxime Sodium USP—White or faintly yellow powder.

Sterile cefuroxime sodium for injection—Solutions range from light yellow to amber, depending on the concentration and the diluent used.

Solubility:

Cefuroxime Axetil USP—Slightly soluble in dehydrated alcohol, in ether, and in water; soluble in acetone, in chloroform, in ethyl acetate, and in methanol.

Cefuroxime sodium—Soluble in water; sparingly soluble in ethanol; insoluble in chloroform, in toluene, in ether, in ethyl acetate, and in acetone.

Sterile Cefuroxime Sodium USP—Soluble in water; sparingly soluble in alcohol; insoluble in chloroform, in toluene, in ether, in ethyl acetate, and in acetone.

Other characteristics: Sterile cefuroxime sodium for injection—The pH of freshly reconstituted solutions usually ranges from 6.0 to 8.5.

USP requirements:

Cefuroxime Axetil USP—Preserve in tight containers. A mixture of the amorphous diastereoisomers of cefuroxime axetil. Contains the equivalent of not less than 745 mcg and not more than 875 mcg of cefuroxime per mg, calculated on the anhydrous basis. Meets the requirements for Identification, Crystallinity, Water (not more than 1.5%), and Diastereoisomer ratio (0.48–0.55).

Cefuroxime Axetil Tablets USP—Preserve in well-closed containers. Contain an amount of cefuroxime axetil equivalent to the labeled amount of cefuroxime, within ±10%. Meet the requirements for Identification, Dissolution (60% in 15 minutes, 75% in 45 minutes in 0.07 *N* hydrochloric acid in Apparatus 2 at 55 rpm), Uniformity of dosage units, and Water (not more than 6.0%).

Cefuroxime Sodium USP—Preserve in tight containers. Contains the equivalent of not less than 855 mcg and not more than 1000 mcg of cefuroxime, calculated on the anhydrous basis. Meets the requirements for Identification, pH (6.0–8.5, in a solution [1 in 10]), and Water (not more than 3.5%).

Cefuroxime Sodium Injection USP—Preserve in Containers for Injections. Maintain in the frozen state. A sterile iso-osmotic solution of Cefuroxime Sodium in Water for Injection. Contains one or more suitable buffers and a tonicity-adjusting agent. It meets the requirements for Labeling under Injections. The label states that it is to be thawed just prior to use, describes conditions for proper storage of the resultant solution, and directs that the solution is not to be refrozen. Contains an amount of cefuroxime sodium equivalent to the labeled amount of cefuroxime, within −10% to +20%. Meets the requirements for Identification, Pyrogen, Sterility, pH (5.0–7.5), and Particulate matter, and for Uniformity of dosage units and Labeling under Injections.

Sterile Cefuroxime Sodium USP—Preserve in Containers for Sterile Solids. It is Cefuroxime Sodium suitable for parenteral use. Contains the equivalent of not less than 855 mcg and not more than 1000 mcg of cefuroxime per mg, calculated on the anhydrous basis, and, where packaged for dispensing, contains an amount of cefuroxime sodium equivalent to the labeled amount of cefuroxime, within −10% to +20%. Meets the requirements for Constituted solution, Bacterial endotoxins, Sterility, and Particulate matter, and for Identification tests, pH, and Water under Cefuroxime Sodium. In addition, where packaged for dispensing, meets the requirements for Uniformity of dosage units and for Labeling under Injections.

CELLULOSE ACETATE

Chemical name: Cellulose acetate.

Description: Cellulose Acetate NF—Fine, white powder or free-flowing pellets. Available in a range of viscosities and acetyl contents.

NF category: Coating agent; polymer membrane, insoluble.

Solubility: Cellulose Acetate NF—High viscosity, which reflects high molecular weight, decreases solubility slightly. High acetyl content cellulose acetates generally have more limited solubility in commonly used organic solvents than low acetyl content cellulose acetates, but are more soluble in methylene chloride. All acetyl content cellulose acetates are insoluble in alcohol and in water; soluble in dioxane and in dimethylformamide.

NF requirements: Cellulose Acetate NF—Preserve in well-closed containers. It is partially or completely acetylated cellulose. Label it to indicate the percentage content of acetyl. Contains not less than 29.0% and not more than 44.8%, by weight, of acetyl groups. Its acetyl content is not less than 90.0% and not more than 110.0% of that indicated on the label. Meets the requirements for Identification, Loss on drying (not more than 5.0%), Residue on ignition (not more than 0.1%), Heavy metals (not more than 0.001%), Free acid (not more than 0.1%, on the dried basis), and Acetyl content.

CELLULOSE ACETATE PHTHALATE

Chemical name: Cellulose, acetate, 1,2-benzenedicarboxylate.

Description: Cellulose Acetate Phthalate NF—Free-flowing, white powder. It may have a slight odor of acetic acid.

NF category: Coating agent.

Solubility: Cellulose Acetate Phthalate NF—Insoluble in water and in alcohol; soluble in acetone and in dioxane.

NF requirements: Cellulose Acetate Phthalate NF—Preserve in tight containers. A reaction product of phthalic anhydride and a partial acetate ester of cellulose. Contains not less than 21.5% and not more than 26.0% of acetyl groups and not less than 30.0% and not more than 36.0% of phthalyl groups, calculated on the anhydrous, acid-free basis. Meets the requirements for Identification, Viscosity (45–90 centipoises), Water (not more than 5.0%), Residue on ignition (not more than 0.1%), Free acid (not more than 6.0%), Phthalyl content, and Acetyl content.

MICROCRYSTALLINE CELLULOSE

Chemical name: Cellulose.

Description: Microcrystalline Cellulose NF—Fine, white, odorless, crystalline powder. It consists of free-flowing, nonfibrous particles that may be compressed into self-binding tablets which disintegrate rapidly in water.

NF category: Tablet binder; tablet disintegrant; tablet and/or capsule diluent.

Solubility: Microcrystalline Cellulose NF—Insoluble in water, in dilute acids, and in most organic solvents; practically insoluble in sodium hydroxide solution (1 in 20).

NF requirements: Microcrystalline Cellulose NF—Preserve in tight containers. A purified, partially depolymerized cellulose prepared by treating alpha cellulose, obtained as a pulp from fibrous plant material, with mineral acids. Contains an amount of microcrystalline cellulose equivalent to not less than 97.0% and not more than 102.0% of cellulose, calculated on the dried basis. Meets the requirements for Identification, pH (5.5–7.0 for the grades of Microcrystalline Cellulose that have a sieve fraction greater than 5% retained on the 37-micrometer screen, and 5.0–7.0 for the grades with less than 5% retained on the 37-micrometer screen), Loss on drying (not more than 5.0%), Residue on ignition (not more than 0.05%), Water-soluble substances (not more than 0.16% of residue obtained for the grades that have a sieve fraction more than 5% retention on the 37-micrometer screen; not more than 0.24% of residue obtained for the grades that have a sieve fraction not more than 5% retention on the 37-micrometer screen), Heavy metals (not more than 0.001%), Starch, and Organic volatile impurities.

MICROCRYSTALLINE CELLULOSE AND CARBOXYMETHYLCELLULOSE SODIUM

Chemical name:

Microcrystalline cellulose—Cellulose.

Carboxymethylcellulose sodium—Cellulose, carboxymethyl ether, sodium salt.

Description: Microcrystalline Cellulose and Carboxymethylcellulose Sodium NF—Odorless, white to off-white, coarse to fine powder.

NF category: Suspending and/or viscosity-increasing agent.

Solubility: Microcrystalline Cellulose and Carboxymethylcellulose Sodium NF—Swells in water, producing, when dispersed, a white, opaque dispersion or gel. Insoluble in organic solvents and in dilute acids.

NF requirements: Microcrystalline Cellulose and Carboxymethylcellulose Sodium NF—Preserve in tight containers. Store in a dry place, and avoid exposure to excessive heat. A colloid-forming, attrited mixture of Microcrystalline Cellulose and Carboxymethylcellulose Sodium. Label it to indicate the percentage content of carboxymethylcellulose sodium and the viscosity of the dispersion in water of the designated weight percentage composition. Contains not less than 75.0% and not more than 125.0% of the labeled amount of carboxymethylcellulose sodium, calculated on the dried basis. The viscosity of its aqueous dispersion of percent by weight stated on the label is 60.0 to 140.0% of that stated on the label in centipoises. Meets the requirements for Identification, Viscosity, pH (6.0–8.0), Loss on drying (not more than 8.0%), Residue on ignition (not more than 5.0%), and Heavy metals (not more than 0.001%).

OXIDIZED CELLULOSE

Description: Oxidized Cellulose USP—In the form of gauze or lint. Is slightly off-white in color, and has a slight, charred odor.

Solubility: Oxidized Cellulose USP—Insoluble in water and in acids; soluble in dilute alkalies.

USP requirements: Oxidized Cellulose USP—Preserve in Containers for Sterile Solids, protected from direct sunlight. Store in a cold place. The package bears a statement to the effect that the sterility of Oxidized Cellulose cannot be guaranteed if the package bears evidence of damage, or if the package has been previously opened. Oxidized Cellulose meets the requirements for Labeling under Injections. Contains not less than 16.0% and not more than 24.0% of carboxyl groups, calculated on the dried basis. It is sterile. Meets the requirements for Identification, Sterility, Loss on drying (not more than 15.0%), Residue on ignition (not more than 0.15%), Nitrogen as nitrate or nitrite (not more than 0.5%), and Formaldehyde (not more than 0.5%).

OXIDIZED REGENERATED CELLULOSE

Description: Oxidized Regenerated Cellulose USP—A knit fabric, usually in the form of sterile strips. Slightly off-white, having a slight odor.

Solubility: Oxidized Regenerated Cellulose USP—Insoluble in water and in dilute acids; soluble in dilute alkalies.

USP requirements: Oxidized Regenerated Cellulose USP—Preserve in Containers for Sterile Solids, protected from direct sunlight. Store at controlled room temperature. The package bears a statement to the effect that the sterility of Oxidized Regenerated Cellulose cannot be guaranteed if the package bears evidence of damage, or if the package has been previously opened. Oxidized Regenerated Cellulose meets the requirements for Labeling under Injections. Contains not less than 18.0% and not more than 24.0% of carboxyl groups, calculated on the dried basis. It is sterile. Meets the requirements for Identification, Sterility, Loss on drying (not more than 15%), Residue on ignition (not more than 0.15%), Nitrogen content (not more than 0.5%), and Formaldehyde (not more than 0.5%).

POWDERED CELLULOSE

Description: Powdered Cellulose NF—White, odorless substance, consisting of fibrous particles. Exhibits degrees of fineness ranging from a free-flowing dense powder to a coarse, fluffy, non-flowing material.

NF category: Filtering aid sorbent; tablet and/or capsule diluent.

Solubility: Powdered Cellulose NF—Insoluble in water, in dilute acids, and in nearly all organic solvents; slightly soluble in sodium hydroxide solution (1 in 20).

NF requirements: Powdered Cellulose NF—Preserve in well-closed containers. A purified, mechanically disintegrated cellulose prepared by processing alpha cellulose obtained as a pulp from fibrous plant materials. Contains not less than 97.0% and not more than 102.0% of cellulose, calculated on the dried basis. Meets the requirements for Identification, pH (5.0–7.5), Loss on drying (not more than 7.0%), Residue on ignition (not more than 0.3%, calculated on the dried basis), Water-soluble substances (not more than 1.5%), Heavy metals (not more than 0.001%), Starch, and Organic volatile impurities.

CELLULOSE SODIUM PHOSPHATE

Source: An insoluble, nonabsorbable ion-exchange resin made by phosphorylation of cellulose.

Chemical name: Cellulose, dihydrogen phosphate, disodium salt.

Description: Cellulose Sodium Phosphate USP—Free-flowing cream-colored, odorless powder.

Solubility: Cellulose Sodium Phosphate USP—Insoluble in water, in dilute acids, and in most organic solvents.

Other characteristics: Exchanges sodium for calcium and other polyvalent cations. Inorganic phosphate content is approximately 34%; sodium content is approximately 11%.

USP requirements: Cellulose Sodium Phosphate USP—Preserve in well-closed containers. It is prepared by phosphorylation of alpha cellulose. Has an inorganic bound phosphate content of not less than 31.0% and not more than 36.0%, calculated on the dried basis. Meets the requirements for pH (6.0–9.0, for the filtrate), Loss on drying (not more than 10.0%), Nitrogen (not more than 1.0%), Heavy metals (not more than 0.004%), Calcium binding capacity (not less than 1.8 mmol per gram), Sodium content (9.5–13.0%), Free phosphate (not more than 3.5%, calculated on the dried basis), and Inorganic bound phosphate.

CEPHALEXIN

Chemical name:

Cephalexin—5-Thia-1-azabicyclo[4.2.0]oct-2-ene-2-carboxylic acid, 7-[(aminophenylacetyl)amino]-3-methyl-8-oxo-, monohydrate [6*R*-[6 alpha,7 beta(*R**)]]-.

Cephalexin hydrochloride—5-Thia-1-azabicyclo[4.2.0]oct-2-ene-2-carboxylic acid, 7-[(aminophenylacetyl)amino]-3-methyl-8-oxo-, monohydrochloride, monohydrate, [6*R*-[6 alpha,7 beta(*R**)]]-.

Molecular formula:

Cephalexin—$C_{16}H_{17}N_3O_4S \cdot H_2O$.

Cephalexin hydrochloride—$C_{16}H_{17}N_3O_4S \cdot HCl \cdot H_2O$.

Molecular weight:

Cephalexin—365.40.

Cephalexin hydrochloride—401.86.

Description:

Cephalexin USP—White to off-white, crystalline powder.

Cephalexin Hydrochloride USP—White to off-white crystalline powder.

Solubility:

Cephalexin USP—Slightly soluble in water; practically insoluble in alcohol, in chloroform, and in ether.

Cephalexin Hydrochloride USP—Soluble to the extent of 10 mg per mL in water, in acetone, in acetonitrile, in alcohol, in dimethylformamide, and in methanol; practically insoluble in chloroform, in ether, in ethyl acetate, and in isopropyl alcohol.

Other characteristics: A zwitterion (contains both a basic and an acidic group); isoelectric point of cephalexin in water is approximately 4.5 to 5.

USP requirements:

Cephalexin USP—Preserve in tight containers. Has a potency of not less than 950 mcg and not more than 1010 mcg of cephalexin per mg, calculated on the anhydrous basis. Meets the requirements for Identification, Specific rotation (+149° to +158°, calculated on the anhydrous basis), Crystallinity, pH (3.0–5.5, in an aqueous suspension containing 50 mg per mL), Water (4.0–8.0%), Related compounds (not more than 5.0%), and Dimethylaniline.

Cephalexin Capsules USP—Preserve in tight containers. Contain an amount of cephalexin equivalent to the labeled amount of anhydrous cephalexin, within −10% to +20%. Meet the requirements for Identification, Dissolution (75% in 45 minutes in water in Apparatus 1 at 100 rpm), Uniformity of dosage units, and Water (not more than 10.0%).

Cephalexin for Oral Suspension USP—Preserve in tight containers. A dry mixture of Cephalexin and one or more suitable buffers, colors, diluents, and flavors. Contains an amount of cephalexin equivalent to the labeled amount of anhydrous cephalexin per mL when constituted as directed in the labeling, within −10% to +20%. Meets the requirements for Identification, Uniformity of dosage units (solid packaged in single-unit containers), pH (3.0–6.0, in the suspension constituted as directed in the labeling), Water (not more than 2.0%), and Deliverable volume (solid packaged in multiple-unit containers).

Cephalexin Tablets USP—Preserve in tight containers. They are prepared from Cephalexin or Cephalexin Hydrochloride. The label states whether the Tablets contain Cephalexin or Cephalexin Hydrochloride. Contain the equivalent of the labeled amount of anhydrous cephalexin, within −10% to +20%. Meet the requirements for Identification, Dissolution (75% in 45 minutes in water in Apparatus 1 at 150 rpm where Tablets contain cephalexin hydrochloride and 100 rpm where Tablets contain cephalexin), Uniformity of dosage units, and Water (not more than 9.0% where Tablets contain cephalexin; not more than 8.0% where Tablets contain cephalexin hydrochloride).

Cephalexin Hydrochloride USP—Preserve in tight containers. Contains the equivalent of not less than 800 mcg and not more than 880 mcg of anhydrous cephalexin per mg. Meets the requirements for Identification, Crystallinity, pH (1.5–3.0, in a solution containing 10 mg per mL), Water (3.0–6.5%), Related compounds (not more than 5.0%), and Dimethylaniline.

CEPHALOTHIN

Source: Cephalosporanic acid nucleus derived from cephalosporin C, produced by the fungus *Cephalosporium*.

Chemical name: Cephalothin sodium—5-Thia-1-azabicyclo-[4.2.0]oct-2-ene-2-carboxylic acid, 3-[(acetyloxy)methyl]-8-oxo-7-[(2-thienylacetyl)amino]-, monosodium salt, (6*R-trans*)-.

Molecular formula: Cephalothin sodium—$C_{16}H_{15}N_2NaO_6S_2$.

Molecular weight: Cephalothin sodium—418.41.

Description: Sterile Cephalothin Sodium USP—White to off-white, practically odorless, crystalline powder.

Solubility: Sterile Cephalothin Sodium USP—Freely soluble in water, in saline TS, and in dextrose solutions; insoluble in most organic solvents.

Other characteristics: Cephalothin sodium for injection—Contains 30 mg of sodium bicarbonate per gram of cephalothin sodium. Since free cephalothin acid does not form within the pH range produced by the addition of sodium bicarbonate, solubility and freezability are thereby enhanced.

USP requirements:

Cephalothin Sodium USP—Preserve in tight containers. Contains the equivalent of not less than 850 mcg of cephalothin per mg, calculated on the dried basis. Meets the requirements for Identification, Specific rotation (+124° to +134°, calculated on the dried basis), Crystallinity, Bacterial endotoxins, pH (4.5–7.0, in a solution containing 250 mg per mL, or, where packaged for dispensing, in the solution constituted as directed in the labeling), and Loss on drying (not more than 1.5%).

Cephalothin Sodium Injection USP—Preserve in Containers for Injections. Maintain in the frozen state. A sterile solution of Cephalothin Sodium, or Sterile Cephalothin Sodium, in Water for Injection. Meets the requirements for Labeling under Injections. The label states that it is to be thawed just prior to use, describes conditions for proper storage of the resultant solution, and directs that the solution is not to be refrozen. Contains an amount of cephalothin sodium equivalent to the labeled amount of cephalothin, within −10% to +15%. Meets the requirements for Bacterial endotoxins, pH (6.0–8.5), and Particulate matter, for Identification test A under Cephalothin Sodium, and for Sterility under Sterile Cephalothin Sodium.

Cephalothin Sodium for Injection USP—Preserve in Containers for Sterile Solids. A sterile mixture of Sterile Cephalothin Sodium or cephalothin sodium and one or more suitable buffers. Has a potency equivalent to not less than 850 mcg of cephalothin per mg, calculated on the dried and sodium bicarbonate-free basis, and, where packaged for dispensing, contains an amount of cephalothin sodium equivalent to the labeled amount of cephalothin, within −10% to +15%. Meets the requirements for Constituted solution, Specific rotation (+124° to +134°, calculated on the dried and sodium bicarbonate-free basis), Bacterial endotoxins, pH (6.0–8.5, in the solution constituted as directed in the labeling), and Particulate matter, for Identification test A and Loss on drying under Cephalothin Sodium, for Sterility under Sterile Cephalothin Sodium, and for Uniformity of dosage units and Labeling under Injections.

Sterile Cephalothin Sodium USP—Preserve in Containers for Sterile Solids. It is cephalothin sodium suitable for parenteral use. Has a potency equivalent to not less than 850 mcg of cephalothin per mg, calculated on the dried basis. In addition, where packaged for dispensing, contains an amount of cephalothin sodium equivalent to the labeled amount of cephalothin, within −10% to +15%. Meets the requirements for Constituted solution, Bacterial endotoxins, Sterility, pH (4.5–7.0, in a solution containing 250 mg per mL, or, where packaged for dispensing, in the solution constituted as directed in the labeling), and Particulate matter, and for Identification tests, Specific rotation, Crystallinity, and Loss on drying under Cephalothin Sodium. In addition, where packaged for dispensing, meets the requirements for Injections and for Uniformity of dosage units.

CEPHAPIRIN

Chemical name: Cephapirin sodium—5-Thia-1-azabicyclo-[4.2.0]oct-2-ene-2-carboxylic acid, 3-[(acetyloxy)methyl]-8-oxo-7-[[(4-pyridylthio)acetyl]amino]-, monosodium salt, [6*R-trans*]-.

Molecular formula: Cephapirin sodium—$C_{17}H_{16}N_3NaO_6S_2$.

Molecular weight: Cephapirin sodium—445.44.

Description: Sterile Cephapirin Sodium USP—White to off-white crystalline powder, odorless or having a slight odor.

Solubility: Sterile Cephapirin Sodium USP—Very soluble in water; insoluble in most organic solvents.

USP requirements: Sterile Cephapirin Sodium USP—Preserve in Containers for Sterile Solids. Has a potency equivalent to not less than 855 mcg and not more than 1000 mcg of cephapirin per mg, and, where packaged for dispensing, contains an amount of cephapirin sodium equivalent to the labeled amount of cephapirin, within −10% to +15%. Meets the requirements for Constituted solution, Identification, Crystallinity, Bacterial endotoxins, Sterility, pH (6.5–8.5, in a solution containing 10 mg of cephapirin per mL), Water (not more than 2.0%), Particulate matter, and for Uniformity of dosage units and Labeling under Injections.

CEPHRADINE

Chemical name: 5-Thia-1-azabicyclo[4.2.0]oct-2-ene-2-carboxylic acid, 7-[(amino-1,4-cyclohexadien-1-ylacetyl)amino]-3-methyl-8-oxo-, [6*R*-[6 alpha,7 beta(*R**)]]-.

Molecular formula: $C_{16}H_{19}N_3O_4S$.

Molecular weight: 349.40.

Description: Cephradine USP—White to off-white, crystalline powder.

Solubility: Cephradine USP—Sparingly soluble in water; very slightly soluble in alcohol and in chloroform; practically insoluble in ether.

USP requirements:

Cephradine USP—Preserve in tight containers. Where it is the dihydrate form, the label so indicates. Where the quantity of cephradine is indicated in the labeling of any preparation containing Cephradine, this shall be understood to be in terms of anhydrous cephradine. Has a potency of not less than 900 mcg and not more than 1050 mcg of cephradine per mg, calculated on the anhydrous basis. Meets the requirements for Identification, Crystallinity, pH (3.5–6.0, in a solution containing 10 mg per mL), Water (not more than 6.0%, except that if it is the dihydrate form, the limit is 8.5–10.5%), and Cephalexin (not more than 5.0%, calculated on the anhydrous basis).

Cephradine Capsules USP—Preserve in tight containers. The quantity of cephradine stated in the labeling is in terms of anhydrous cephradine. Contain the labeled amount, within −10% to +20%. Meet the requirements for Identification, Dissolution (75% in 45 minutes in 0.12 *N* hydrochloric acid in Apparatus 1 at 100 rpm), Uniformity of dosage units, and Loss on drying (not more than 7.0%).

Cephradine for Injection USP—Preserve in Containers for Sterile Solids. A dry mixture of Cephradine and one or more suitable buffers and solubilizers. Contains the labeled amount, within −10% to +15%. Meets the requirements for Identification, Bacterial endotoxins, pH (8.0–9.6, in a solution containing 10 mg per mL), Loss on drying (not more than 5.0%), and Particulate matter, for Sterility under Sterile Cephradine, and for Uniformity of dosage units and Labeling under Injections.

Cephradine for Oral Suspension USP—Preserve in tight containers. A dry mixture of Cephradine and one or more suitable buffers, colors, diluents, and flavors. Contains the labeled amount, within −10% to +25%. Meets the requirements for Identification, Uniformity of dosage units (solid packaged in single-unit containers), pH (3.5–6.0, in the suspension constituted as directed in the labeling), Water (not more than 1.5%), and Deliverable volume (solid packaged in multiple-unit containers).

Sterile Cephradine USP—Preserve in Containers for Sterile Solids. Has a potency of not less than 900 mcg and not more than 1050 mcg of cephradine per mg, calculated on the anhydrous basis, and, where packaged for dispensing, contains the labeled amount, within −10% to +15%. Meets the requirements for Constituted solution, Bacterial endotoxins, and Sterility, for Identification test, pH, Water, Crystallinity, and Cephalexin under Cephradine, and for Uniformity of dosage units and Labeling under Injections.

Cephradine Tablets USP—Preserve in tight containers. Contain the labeled amount, within −10% to +20%. Meet the requirements for Identification, Dissolution (85% in 60 minutes in 0.12 *N* hydrochloric acid in Apparatus 2 at 75 rpm), Uniformity of dosage units, and Water (not more than 6.0%).

CETIRIZINE

Chemical name: Cetirizine hydrochloride—Acetic acid, [2-[4-[(4-chlorophenyl)phenylmethyl]-1-piperazinyl]ethoxy]-, dihydrochloride, (±)-.

Molecular formula: Cetirizine hydrochloride—$C_{21}H_{25}ClN_2O_3 \cdot 2HCl$.

Molecular weight: Cetirizine hydrochloride—461.82.

Description: Cetirizine hydrochloride—Melting point 225 °C.

USP requirements: Cetirizine Hydrochloride Tablets—Not in USP.

CETOSTEARYL ALCOHOL

Description: Cetostearyl Alcohol NF—Unctuous, white flakes or granules having a faint, characteristic odor.

NF category: Stiffening agent.

Solubility: Cetostearyl Alcohol NF—Insoluble in water; soluble in alcohol and in ether.

NF requirements: Cetostearyl Alcohol NF—Preserve in well-closed containers. Contains not less than 40.0% of stearyl alcohol, and the sum of the stearyl alcohol content and the cetyl alcohol content is not less than 90.0%. Meets the requirements for Identification, Melting range (48–55 °C), Acid value (not more than 2), Iodine value (not more than 4), and Hydroxyl value (208–228).

CETYL ALCOHOL

Chemical name: 1-Hexadecanol.

Molecular formula: $C_{16}H_{34}O$.

Molecular weight: 242.45.

Description: Cetyl Alcohol NF—Unctuous, white flakes, granules, cubes, or castings. Has a faint characteristic odor. Usually melts in the range between 45–50 °C.

NF category: Stiffening agent.

Solubility: Cetyl Alcohol NF—Insoluble in water; soluble in alcohol and in ether, the solubility increasing with an increase in temperature.

NF requirements: Cetyl Alcohol NF—Preserve in well-closed containers. Contains not less than 90.0% of cetyl alcohol, the remainder consisting chiefly of related alcohols. Meets the requirements for Identification, Acid value (not more than 2), Iodine value (not more than 5), and Hydroxyl value (218–238).

CETYL ESTERS WAX

Description: Cetyl Esters Wax NF—White to off-white, somewhat translucent flakes, having a crystalline structure and a pearly luster when caked. It has a faint odor and has a specific gravity of about 0.83 at 50 °C.

NF category: Stiffening agent.

Solubility: Cetyl Esters Wax NF—Insoluble in water; soluble in boiling alcohol, in ether, in chloroform, and in fixed and volatile oils; slightly soluble in cold solvent hexane; practically insoluble in cold alcohol.

NF requirements: Cetyl Esters Wax NF—Preserve in well-closed containers in a dry place, and prevent exposure to excessive heat. A mixture consisting primarily of esters of saturated fatty alcohols and saturated fatty acids. Meets the requirements for Melting range (43–47 °C), Acid value (not more than 5), Iodine value (not more than 1), Saponification value (109–120), and Paraffin and free acids.

CETYLPYRIDINIUM

Chemical name: Cetylpyridinium chloride—Pyridinium, 1-hexadecyl-, chloride, monohydrate.

Molecular formula: Cetylpyridinium chloride—$C_{21}H_{38}ClN \cdot H_2O$.

Molecular weight: Cetylpyridinium chloride—358.01.

Description:

Cetylpyridinium Chloride USP—White powder, having a slight, characteristic odor.

NF category: Antimicrobial preservative; wetting and/or solubilizing agent.

Cetylpyridinium Chloride Topical Solution USP—Clear liquid. Is colorless unless a color has been added; has an aromatic odor.

Solubility: Cetylpyridinium Chloride USP—Very soluble in water, in alcohol, and in chloroform; slightly soluble in ether.

USP requirements:
Cetylpyridinium Chloride USP—Preserve in well-closed containers. Contains not less than 99.0% and not more than 102.0% of cetylpyridinium chloride, calculated on the anhydrous basis. Meets the requirements for Identification, Melting range (80–84 °C), Acidity, Water (4.5–5.5%), Residue on ignition (not more than 0.2%, calculated on the anhydrous basis), Heavy metals (not more than 0.002%), Pyridine, and Organic volatile impurities.
Cetylpyridinium Chloride Lozenges USP—Preserve in well-closed containers. Contain the labeled amount, within −10% to +25%, in a suitable molded base. Meet the requirement for Identification.
Cetylpyridinium Chloride Topical Solution USP—Preserve in tight containers. Contains the labeled amount, within ±5%. Meets the requirement for Identification.

ACTIVATED CHARCOAL

Source: Carbon residue derived from heating organic material in the absence of oxygen.

Description: Activated Charcoal USP—Fine, black, odorless powder, free from gritty matter.
NF category: Sorbent.

Solubility: Practically insoluble in all usual solvents.

USP requirements:
Activated Charcoal USP—Preserve in well-closed containers. The residue from the destructive distillation of various organic materials, treated to increase its adsorptive power. Meets the requirements for Microbial limits, Reaction (neutral to litmus), Loss on drying (not more than 15.0%), Residue on ignition (not more than 4.0%), Acid-soluble substances (not more than 3.5%), Chloride (not more than 0.2%), Sulfate (not more than 0.2%), Sulfide, Cyanogen compounds, Heavy metals (not more than 0.005%), Uncarbonized constituents, and Adsorptive power.
Activated Charcoal Capsules—Not in USP.
Activated Charcoal Oral Suspension—Not in USP.
Activated Charcoal Tablets—Not in USP.

ACTIVATED CHARCOAL AND SORBITOL

For *Activated Charcoal* and *Sorbitol*—See individual listings for chemistry information.

USP requirements: Activated Charcoal and Sorbitol Oral Suspension—Not in USP.

CHENODIOL

Source: Chenodeoxycholic acid, a naturally occurring human bile acid.

Chemical name: Cholan-24-oic acid, 3,7-dihydroxy-, (3 alpha,-5 beta,7 alpha)-.

Molecular formula: $C_{24}H_{40}O_4$.

Molecular weight: 392.58.

Description: White powder consisting of crystalline and amorphous particles.

Solubility: Practically insoluble in water; freely soluble in methanol, in acetone, and in acetic acid.

USP requirements: Chenodiol Tablets—Not in USP.

CHLOPHEDIANOL

Chemical name: Chlophedianol hydrochloride—Benzenemethanol, 2-chloro-alpha-[2-(dimethylamino)ethyl]-alpha-phenyl-, hydrochloride.

Molecular formula: Chlophedianol hydrochloride—$C_{17}H_{20}ClNO \cdot HCl$.

Molecular weight: Chlophedianol hydrochloride—326.26.

Description: Chlophedianol hydrochloride—White, crystalline powder. Melting point 190–191 °C.

Solubility: Chlophedianol hydrochloride—Freely soluble in water, in methanol, and in ethanol. Sparingly soluble in ether and in ethyl acetate.

USP requirements: Chlophedianol Hydrochloride Syrup—Not in USP.

CHLORAL HYDRATE

Chemical name: 1,1-Ethanediol, 2,2,2-trichloro-.

Molecular formula: $C_2H_3Cl_3O_2$.

Molecular weight: 165.40.

Description: Chloral Hydrate USP—Colorless, transparent, or white crystals having an aromatic, penetrating, and slightly acrid odor. Melts at about 55 °C, and slowly volatilizes when exposed to air.

Solubility: Chloral Hydrate USP—Very soluble in water and in olive oil; freely soluble in alcohol, in chloroform, and in ether.

USP requirements:
Chloral Hydrate USP—Preserve in tight containers. Contains not less than 99.5% and not more than 102.5% of chloral hydrate. Meets the requirements for Identification, Acidity, Residue on ignition (not more than 0.1%), Chloride (not more than 0.007%), Readily carbonizable substances, and Organic volatile impurities.
Chloral Hydrate Capsules USP—Preserve in tight containers, preferably at controlled room temperature. Contain the labeled amount, within −5% to +10%. Meet the requirements for Identification and Uniformity of dosage units.
Chloral Hydrate Suppositories—Not in USP.
Chloral Hydrate Syrup USP—Preserve in tight, light-resistant containers. Contains the labeled amount, within −5% to +10%. Meets the requirement for Identification.

CHLORAMBUCIL

Chemical name: Benzenebutanoic acid, 4-[bis(2-chloroethyl)-amino]-.

Molecular formula: $C_{14}H_{19}Cl_2NO_2$.

Molecular weight: 304.22.

Description: Chlorambucil USP—Off-white, slightly granular powder.

pKa: 5.8.

Solubility: Chlorambucil USP—Very slightly soluble in water; freely soluble in acetone; soluble in dilute alkali.

USP requirements:
Chlorambucil USP—Preserve in tight, light-resistant containers. Contains not less than 98.0% and not more than

101.0% of chlorambucil, calculated on the anhydrous basis. Meets the requirements for Identification, Melting range (65–69 °C), Water (not more than 0.5%), and Organic volatile impurities.

Caution: Great care should be taken to prevent inhaling particles of Chlorambucil and exposing the skin to it.

Chlorambucil Tablets USP—Preserve coated Tablets in well-closed containers; preserve uncoated Tablets in well-closed, light-resistant containers. Contain the labeled amount, within −15% to +10%. Meet the requirements for Identification, Disintegration (15 minutes, the use of disks being omitted), and Uniformity of dosage units.

CHLORAMPHENICOL

Source: Originally derived from *Streptomyces venezuelae.*

Chemical name:

Chloramphenicol—Acetamide, 2,2-dichloro-*N*-[2-hydroxy-1-(hydroxymethyl)-2-(4-nitrophenyl)ethyl]-, [*R*-(*R**,*R**)]-.

Chloramphenicol palmitate—Hexadecanoic acid, 2-[(2,2-dichloroacetyl)amino]-3-hydroxy-3-(4-nitrophenyl) propyl ester, [*R*-(*R**,*R**)]-.

Molecular formula:

Chloramphenicol—$C_{11}H_{12}Cl_2N_2O_5$.

Chloramphenicol palmitate—$C_{27}H_{42}Cl_2N_2O_6$.

Chloramphenicol sodium succinate—$C_{15}H_{15}Cl_2N_2NaO_8$.

Molecular weight:

Chloramphenicol—323.13.

Chloramphenicol palmitate—561.55.

Chloramphenicol sodium succinate—445.19.

Description:

Chloramphenicol USP—Fine, white to grayish white or yellowish white, needle-like crystals or elongated plates. Its solutions are practically neutral to litmus. Is reasonably stable in neutral or moderately acid solutions. Its alcohol solution is dextrorotatory and its ethyl acetate solution is levorotatory.

Chloramphenicol Palmitate USP—Fine, white, unctuous, crystalline powder, having a faint odor.

Sterile Chloramphenicol Sodium Succinate USP—Light yellow powder.

Solubility:

Chloramphenicol USP—Slightly soluble in water; freely soluble in alcohol, in propylene glycol, in acetone, and in ethyl acetate.

Chloramphenicol Palmitate USP—Insoluble in water; freely soluble in acetone and in chloroform; soluble in ether; sparingly soluble in alcohol; very slightly soluble in solvent hexane.

Sterile Chloramphenicol Sodium Succinate USP—Freely soluble in water and in alcohol.

USP requirements:

Chloramphenicol USP—Preserve in tight containers. Contains not less than 97.0% and not more than 103.0% of chloramphenicol. Meets the requirements for Identification, Melting range (149–153 °C), Specific rotation (+17.0° to +20.0°), Crystallinity, pH (4.5–7.5, in an aqueous suspension containing 25 mg per mL), and Chromatographic purity.

Chloramphenicol Capsules USP—Preserve in tight containers. Contain the labeled amount, within −10% to +20%. Meet the requirements for Identification, Dissolution (85% in 30 minutes in 0.1 *N* hydrochloric acid in Apparatus 1 at 100 rpm), and Uniformity of dosage units.

Chloramphenicol Cream USP—Preserve in collapsible tubes or in tight containers. Contains the labeled amount, within −10% to +30%. Meets the requirements for Identification and Minimum fill.

Chloramphenicol Injection USP—Preserve in single-dose or in multiple-dose containers. A sterile solution of Chloramphenicol in one or more suitable solvents. Label it to indicate that it is for veterinary use only. Contains the labeled amount, within −10% to +15%. Meets the requirements for Identification, Bacterial endotoxins, Sterility, pH (5.0–8.0, in a solution diluted with water [1:1]), and Injections.

Chloramphenicol Ophthalmic Ointment USP—Preserve in collapsible ophthalmic ointment tubes. Contains the labeled amount, within −10% to +30%. Meets the requirements for Identification, Sterility, Minimum fill, and Metal particles.

Chloramphenicol Ophthalmic Solution USP—Preserve in tight containers, and store in a refrigerator until dispensed. The containers or individual cartons are sealed and tamper-proof so that sterility is assured at time of first use. A sterile solution of Chloramphenicol. The labeling states that there is a 21-day beyond-use period after dispensing. Contains the labeled amount, within −10% to +30%. Meets the requirements for Identification, Sterility, and pH (7.0–7.5, except that in the case of Ophthalmic Solution that is unbuffered or is labeled for veterinary use it is 3.0–6.0).

Chloramphenicol for Ophthalmic Solution USP—Preserve in tight containers. A sterile, dry mixture of Chloramphenicol with or without one or more suitable buffers, diluents, and preservatives. If packaged in combination with a container of solvent, label it with a warning that it is not for injection. Contains the labeled amount, within −10% to +30%, when constituted as directed. Meets the requirements for Identification, Sterility, and pH (7.1–7.5, in an aqueous solution containing 5 mg of chloramphenicol per mL).

Chloramphenicol Oral Solution USP—Preserve in tight containers. A solution of Chloramphenicol in a suitable solvent. Label it to indicate that it is for veterinary use only and that it is not to be used in animals raised for food production. Contains the labeled amount, within −10% to +20%. Contains one or more suitable buffers and preservatives. Meets the requirements for Identification and pH (5.0–8.5, when diluted with an equal volume of water).

Chloramphenicol Otic Solution USP—Preserve in tight containers. A sterile solution of Chloramphenicol in a suitable solvent. Contains the labeled amount, within −10% to +30%. Meets the requirements for Identification, Sterility, pH (4.0–8.0, when diluted with an equal volume of water), and Water (not more than 2.0%).

Sterile Chloramphenicol USP—Preserve in Containers for Sterile Solids. It is Chloramphenicol suitable for parenteral use. Contains not less than 97.0% and not more than 103.0% of chloramphenicol. Meets the requirements for Bacterial endotoxins and Sterility, and for Identification test, Melting range, Specific rotation, pH, and Crystallinity under Chloramphenicol.

Chloramphenicol Tablets USP—Preserve in tight containers. Label Tablets to indicate that they are for veterinary use only and are not to be used in animals raised for food production. Contain the labeled amount, within −10% to +20%. Meet the requirements for Identification, Disintegration (60 minutes), and Uniformity of dosage units.

Chloramphenicol Palmitate USP—Preserve in tight containers. Has a potency equivalent to not less than 555 mcg and not more than 595 mcg of chloramphenicol per mg. Meets the requirements for Identification, Melting range (87–95 °C), Specific rotation (+21° to+25°), Crystallinity, Loss on drying (not more than 0.5%), Acidity, and Free chloramphenicol.

Chloramphenicol Palmitate Oral Suspension USP—Preserve in tight, light-resistant containers. Contains an amount of chloramphenicol palmitate equivalent to the labeled amount of chloramphenicol, within −10% to +20%. Contains one or more suitable buffers, colors, flavors, preservatives, and suspending agents. Meets the requirements for Identification, Uniformity of dosage units (suspension packaged in single-unit containers), pH (4.5–7.0), Polymorph A, and Deliverable volume (suspension packaged in multiple-unit containers).

Sterile Chloramphenicol Sodium Succinate USP—Preserve in Containers for Sterile Solids. Has a potency equivalent to not less than 650 mcg and not more than 765 mcg of chloramphenicol per mg, and, where packaged for dispensing and constituted as directed in the labeling, contains an amount of chloramphenicol sodium succinate equivalent to the labeled amount of chloramphenicol, within −10% to +15%. Meets the requirements for Identification, Specific rotation (+5.0° to +8.0°, calculated on the anhydrous basis), Bacterial endotoxins, Sterility, pH (6.4–7.0, in a solution containing the equivalent of 250 mg of chloramphenicol per mL), Water (not more than 5.0%), Particulate matter, and Free chloramphenicol (not more than 2.0%).

CHLORAMPHENICOL AND HYDROCORTISONE

For *Chloramphenicol* and *Hydrocortisone*—See individual listings for chemistry information.

USP requirements: Chloramphenicol and Hydrocortisone Acetate for Ophthalmic Suspension USP—A sterile, dry mixture of Chloramphenicol and Hydrocortisone Acetate with or without one or more suitable buffers, diluents, and preservatives. If packaged in combination with a container of solvent, label it with a warning that it is not for injection. Contains the labeled amounts of chloramphenicol, within −10% to +30%, and hydrocortisone acetate, within −10% to +15%, when constituted as directed. Meets the requirements for Identification, Sterility, and pH (7.1–7.5, in an aqueous suspension containing 5 mg of chloramphenicol per mL).

CHLORAMPHENICOL AND POLYMYXIN B

For *Chloramphenicol* and *Polymyxin B*—See individual listings for chemistry information.

USP requirements: Chloramphenicol and Polymyxin B Sulfate Ophthalmic Ointment USP—Preserve in collapsible ophthalmic ointment tubes. Contains the labeled amount of chloramphenicol, within −10% to +20%, and an amount of polymyxin B sulfate equivalent to the labeled amount of polymyxin B, within −10% to +25%. Meets the requirements for Identification, Sterility, and Metal particles.

CHLORAMPHENICOL, POLYMYXIN B, AND HYDROCORTISONE

For *Chloramphenicol, Polymyxin B,* and *Hydrocortisone*—See individual listings for chemistry information.

USP requirements: Chloramphenicol, Polymyxin B Sulfate, and Hydrocortisone Acetate Ophthalmic Ointment USP—Preserve in collapsible ophthalmic ointment tubes. Contains the labeled amount of chloramphenicol, within −10% to +20%, an amount of polymyxin B sulfate equivalent to the labeled amount of polymyxin B, within −10% to +25%, and the labeled amount of hydrocortisone acetate, within −10% to +15%. Meets the requirements for Identification, Sterility, Minimum fill, and Metal particles.

CHLORAMPHENICOL AND PREDNISOLONE

For *Chloramphenicol* and *Prednisolone*—See individual listings for chemistry information.

USP requirements: Chloramphenicol and Prednisolone Ophthalmic Ointment USP—Preserve in collapsible ophthalmic ointment tubes. Contains the labeled amounts of chloramphenicol, within −10% to +30%, and prednisolone, within −10% to +15%. Meets the requirements for Identification, Sterility, Minimum fill, and Metal particles.

CHLORDIAZEPOXIDE

Chemical name:
Chlordiazepoxide—3*H*-1,4-Benzodiazepin-2-amine, 7-chloro-*N*-methyl-5-phenyl, 4-oxide.
Chlordiazepoxide hydrochloride—3*H*-1,4-Benzodiazepin-2-amine, 7-chloro-*N*-methyl-5-phenyl-, 4-oxide, monohydrochloride.

Molecular formula:
Chlordiazepoxide—$C_{16}H_{14}ClN_3O$.
Chlordiazepoxide hydrochloride—$C_{16}H_{14}ClN_3O \cdot HCl$.

Molecular weight:
Chlordiazepoxide—299.76.
Chlordiazepoxide hydrochloride—336.22.

Description:
Chlordiazepoxide USP—Yellow, practically odorless, crystalline powder. Is sensitive to sunlight. Melts at about 240 °C.
Chlordiazepoxide Hydrochloride USP—White or practically white, odorless, crystalline powder. Is affected by sunlight.
Sterile Chlordiazepoxide Hydrochloride USP—White or practically white, odorless, crystalline powder. Is affected by sunlight.

Solubility:
Chlordiazepoxide USP—Insoluble in water; sparingly soluble in chloroform and in alcohol.
Chlordiazepoxide Hydrochloride USP—Soluble in water and in alcohol; insoluble in solvent hexane.
Sterile Chlordiazepoxide Hydrochloride USP—Soluble in water and in alcohol; insoluble in solvent hexane.

USP requirements:
Chlordiazepoxide USP—Preserve in tight, light-resistant containers. Contains not less than 98.0% and not more than 102.0% of chlordiazepoxide, calculated on the dried basis. Meets the requirements for Identification, Loss on drying (not more than 0.3%), Residue on ignition (not more than 0.1%), Heavy metals (not more than 0.002%), and Related compounds.

Chlordiazepoxide Tablets USP—Preserve in tight, light-resistant containers. Contain the labeled amount, within ±10%. Meet the requirements for Identification, Dissolution (85% in 30 minutes in simulated gastric fluid TS, prepared without pepsin, in Apparatus 1 at 100 rpm), Uniformity of dosage units, and Related compounds.

Chlordiazepoxide Hydrochloride USP—Preserve in tight, light-resistant containers. Contains not less than 98.0% and not more than 102.0% of chlordiazepoxide hydrochloride, calculated on the dried basis. Meets the requirements for Identification, Melting range (212–218 °C, with decomposition), Loss on drying (not more than 0.5%), Residue on ignition (not more than 0.1%), Heavy metals (not more than 0.002%), Related compounds, and Organic volatile impurities.

Chlordiazepoxide Hydrochloride Capsules USP—Preserve in tight, light-resistant containers. Contain the labeled amount, within ±10%. Meet the requirements for Identification, Dissolution (85% in 30 minutes in water in Apparatus 1 at 100 rpm), Uniformity of dosage units, and Related compounds.

Sterile Chlordiazepoxide Hydrochloride USP—Preserve in Containers for Sterile Solids, protected from light. It is Chlordiazepoxide Hydrochloride suitable for parenteral use. Meets the requirements for Completeness of solution, Constituted solution, Bacterial endotoxins, pH (2.5–3.5, in a solution [1 in 100]), for Identification tests, Loss on drying and Heavy metals under Chlordiazepoxide Hydrochloride, for Related compounds under Chlordiazepoxide, and for Sterility tests, Uniformity of dosage units, and Labeling under Injections.

CHLORDIAZEPOXIDE AND AMITRIPTYLINE

For *Chlordiazepoxide* and *Amitriptyline*—See individual listings for chemistry information.

USP requirements: Chlordiazepoxide and Amitriptyline Hydrochloride Tablets USP—Preserve in tight, light-resistant containers. Contain the labeled amount of chlordiazepoxide, within ±10%, and an amount of amitriptyline hydrochloride equivalent to the labeled amount of amitriptyline, within ±10%. Meet the requirements for Identification, Dissolution (85% of chlordiazepoxide and an amount of amitriptyline hydrochloride equivalent to not less than 85% of amitriptyline in 30 minutes in simulated gastric fluid TS, prepared without pepsin, in Apparatus 1 at 100 rpm), Uniformity of dosage units, and Related compounds.

CHLORDIAZEPOXIDE AND CLIDINIUM

For *Chlordiazepoxide* and *Clidinium*—See individual listings for chemistry information.

USP requirements: Chlordiazepoxide Hydrochloride and Clidinium Bromide Capsules USP—Preserve in tight, light-resistant containers. Contain the labeled amounts of chlordiazepoxide hydrochloride and clidinium bromide, within ±10%. Meet the requirements for Identification, Dissolution (75% of each active ingredient in 30 minutes in water in Apparatus 1 at 100 rpm), Uniformity of dosage units, and Related compounds.

CHLORHEXIDINE

Chemical group: Chlorhexidine gluconate—Bis-biguanide.

Chemical name: Chlorhexidine gluconate—2,4,11,13-Tetraazatetradecanediimidamide, *N,N''*-bis(4-chlorophenyl)-3,12-diimino-, di-D-gluconate.

Molecular formula: Chlorhexidine gluconate—$C_{22}H_{30}Cl_2N_{10} \cdot 2C_6H_{12}O_7$.

Molecular weight: Chlorhexidine gluconate—897.77.

Other characteristics: Chlorhexidine gluconate—A 5% v/v dilution in water has a pH of 5.5 to 7.0.

USP requirements: Chlorhexidine Gluconate Oral Rinse—Not in USP.

CHLORMEZANONE

Chemical group: A substituted metathiazanone compound.

Chemical name: 2-(*p*-Chlorophenyl)tetrahydro-3-methyl-4*H*-1,3-thiazin-4-one 1,1-dioxide.

Molecular formula: $C_{11}H_{12}ClNO_3S$.

Molecular weight: 273.73.

Description: A white, crystalline powder with a faint characteristic odor.

Solubility: Soluble in water (less than 0.25% w/v) and in alcohol.

USP requirements: Chlormezanone Tablets—Not in USP.

CHLOROBUTANOL

Chemical name: 2-Propanol, 1,1,1-trichloro-2-methyl-.

Molecular formula: $C_4H_7Cl_3O$ (anhydrous).

Molecular weight: 177.46 (anhydrous).

Description: Chlorobutanol NF—Colorless to white crystals, having a characteristic, somewhat camphoraceous, odor. The anhydrous form melts at about 95 °C, and the hydrous form melts at about 76 °C.

NF category: Antimicrobial preservative.

Solubility: Chlorobutanol NF—Slightly soluble in water; freely soluble in alcohol, in ether, in chloroform, and in volatile oils; soluble in glycerin.

NF requirements: Chlorobutanol NF—Preserve in tight containers. It is anhydrous or contains not more than one-half molecule of water of hydration. Label it to indicate whether it is anhydrous or hydrous. Contains not less than 98.0% and not more than 100.5% of chlorobutanol, calculated on the anhydrous basis. Meets the requirements for Identification, Reaction, Water (for anhydrous, not more than 1.0%; for hydrous, not more than 6.0%), and Chloride (not more than 0.07%).

CHLOROCRESOL

Chemical name: Phenol, 4-chloro-3-methyl-.

Molecular formula: C_7H_7ClO.

Molecular weight: 142.58.

Description: Chlorocresol NF—Colorless or practically colorless crystals or crystalline powder, having a characteristic, nontarry odor. Volatile in steam.

NF category: Antimicrobial preservative.

Solubility: Chlorocresol NF—Slightly soluble in water and more soluble in hot water; very soluble in alcohol; soluble in ether, in terpenes, in fixed oils, and in solutions of alkali hydroxides.

NF requirements: Chlorocresol NF—Preserve in tight, light-resistant containers. Contains not less than 99.0% and not more than 101.0% of chlorocresol. Meets the requirements for Completeness of solution, Identification, Melting range (63–66 °C), and Nonvolatile residue (not more than 0.1%).

CHLOROFORM

Chemical name: Methane, trichloro-.

Molecular formula: $CHCl_3$.

Molecular weight: 119.38.

Description: Chloroform NF—Clear, colorless, mobile liquid, having a characteristic, ethereal odor. It is not flammable, but its heated vapor burns with a green flame. Boils at about 61 °C. Affected by light.

NF category: Solvent.

Solubility: Chloroform NF—Slightly soluble in water. Miscible with alcohol, with ether, with solvent hexane, and with fixed and volatile oils.

NF requirements: Chloroform NF—Preserve in tight, light-resistant containers, at a temperature not exceeding 30 °C. Contains not less than 99.0% and not more than 99.5% of chloroform, the remainder consisting of alcohol. Meets the requirements for Specific gravity (1.476–1.480), Nonvolatile residue (not more than 0.002%), Free chlorine, Readily carbonizable substances, Chlorinated decomposition products and chloride, Acid and phosgene, and Aldehyde and ketone.

Caution: Care should be taken not to vaporize Chloroform in the presence of a flame, because of the production of harmful gases.

CHLOROPROCAINE

Chemical group: Ester, aminobenzoic acid (PABA)-derivative.

Chemical name: Chloroprocaine hydrochloride—Benzoic acid, 4-amino-2-chloro-, 2-(diethylamino)ethyl ester, monohydrochloride.

Molecular formula: Chloroprocaine hydrochloride—$C_{13}H_{19}ClN_2O_2 \cdot HCl$.

Molecular weight: Chloroprocaine hydrochloride—307.22.

Description: Chloroprocaine Hydrochloride USP—White, crystalline powder. Is odorless, and is stable in air. Its solutions are acid to litmus.

pKa: 9.0.

Solubility: Chloroprocaine Hydrochloride USP—Soluble in water; slightly soluble in alcohol; very slightly soluble in chloroform; practically insoluble in ether.

USP requirements:

Chloroprocaine Hydrochloride USP—Preserve in well-closed containers. Contains not less than 98.0% and not more than 102.0% of chloroprocaine hydrochloride, calculated on the dried basis. Meets the requirements for Identification, Melting range (173–176 °C), Acidity, Loss on drying (not more than 1.0%), Residue on ignition (not more than 0.2%), and Related substances (not more than 0.625%).

Chloroprocaine Hydrochloride Injection USP—Preserve in single-dose or in multiple-dose containers, preferably of Type I glass. A sterile solution of Chloroprocaine Hydrochloride in Water for Injection. Contains the labeled amount, within ±5%. Meets the requirements for Identification, pH (2.7–4.0), Related substances (not more than 3.0%), and Injections.

CHLOROQUINE

Chemical name:

Chloroquine—1,4-Pentanediamine, *N*⁴-(7-chloro-4-quinolinyl)-*N*¹,*N*¹-diethyl.

Chloroquine hydrochloride—1,4-Pentanediamine, N^4-(7-chloro-4-quinolinyl)-N^1,N^1-diethyl-, dihydrochloride.

Chloroquine phosphate—1,4-Pentanediamine, N^4-(7-chloro-4-quinolinyl)-N^1,N^1-diethyl-, phosphate (1:2).

Molecular formula:

Chloroquine—$C_{18}H_{26}ClN_3$.

Chloroquine hydrochloride—$C_{18}H_{26}ClN_3 \cdot 2HCl$.

Chloroquine phosphate—$C_{18}H_{26}ClN_3 \cdot 2H_3PO_4$.

Molecular weight:

Chloroquine—319.88.

Chloroquine hydrochloride—392.80.

Chloroquine phosphate—515.87.

Description:

Chloroquine USP—White or slightly yellow, crystalline powder. Is odorless.

Chloroquine Hydrochloride Injection USP—Colorless liquid.

Chloroquine Phosphate USP—White, crystalline powder. Is odorless and is discolored slowly on exposure to light. Its solutions have a pH of about 4.5. Exists in two polymorphic forms, one melting between 193 °C and 195 °C and the other between 210 °C and 215 °C; mixture of the forms melts between 193 °C and 215 °C.

Solubility:

Chloroquine USP—Very slightly soluble in water; soluble in dilute acids, in chloroform, and in ether.

Chloroquine Phosphate USP—Freely soluble in water; practically insoluble in alcohol, in chloroform, and in ether.

USP requirements:

Chloroquine USP—Preserve in well-closed containers. Contains not less than 98.0% and not more than 102.0% of chloroquine, calculated on the dried basis. Meets the requirements for Identification, Melting range (87–92 °C), Loss on drying (not more than 2.0%), Residue on ignition (not more than 0.2%), and Organic volatile impurities.

Chloroquine Hydrochloride Injection USP—Preserve in single-dose containers, preferably of Type I glass. A sterile solution of Chloroquine in Water for Injection prepared with the aid of Hydrochloric Acid. Contains, in each mL, not less than 47.5 mg and not more than 52.5 mg of chloroquine hydrochloride. Meets the requirements for Identification, Bacterial endotoxins, pH (5.5–6.5), and Injections.

Chloroquine Phosphate USP—Preserve in well-closed containers. Contains not less than 98.0% and not more than 102.0% of chloroquine phosphate, calculated on the dried basis. Meets the requirements for Identification, Loss on drying (not more than 2.0%), and Organic volatile impurities.

Chloroquine Phosphate Tablets USP—Preserve in well-closed containers. Contain the labeled amount, within ±7%. Meet the requirements for Identification, Dissolution (75% in 45 minutes in water in Apparatus 2 at 100 rpm), and Uniformity of dosage units.

CHLOROTHIAZIDE

Chemical name:

Chlorothiazide—2*H*-1,2,4-Benzothiadiazine-7-sulfonamide, 6-chloro-, 1,1-dioxide.

Chlorothiazide sodium—2*H*-1,2,4-Benzothiadiazine-7-sulfonamide, 6-chloro-, 1,1-dioxide, monosodium salt.

Molecular formula:

Chlorothiazide—$C_7H_6ClN_3O_4S_2$.

Chlorothiazide sodium—$C_7H_5ClN_3NaO_4S_2$.

Molecular weight:

Chlorothiazide—295.72.

Chlorothiazide sodium—317.70.

Description:

Chlorothiazide USP—White or practically white, crystalline, odorless powder. Melts at about 340 °C, with decomposition.

Chlorothiazide sodium—White powder.

pKa: 6.7 and 9.5.

Solubility:
Chlorothiazide USP—Very slightly soluble in water; freely soluble in dimethylformamide and in dimethyl sulfoxide; slightly soluble in methanol and in pyridine; practically insoluble in ether and in chloroform.
Chlorothiazide sodium—Very soluble in water and in alcohol.

USP requirements:
Chlorothiazide USP—Preserve in well-closed containers. Contains not less than 98.0% and not more than 102.0% of chlorothiazide, calculated on the dried basis. Meets the requirements for Identification, Loss on drying (not more than 1.0%), Residue on ignition (not more than 0.1%), Chloride (not more than 0.05%), Selenium (not more than 0.003%), Heavy metals (not more than 0.001%), 4-Amino-6-chloro-1,3-benzenedisulfonamide (not more than 1.0%), and Organic volatile impurities.
Chlorothiazide Oral Suspension USP—Preserve in tight containers. Contains the labeled amount, within ±10%. Meets the requirements for Identification and pH (3.2–4.0).
Chlorothiazide Tablets USP—Preserve in well-closed containers. Contain the labeled amount, within ±10%. Meet the requirements for Identification, Dissolution (75% in 60 minutes in 0.05 *M* phosphate buffer [pH 8.0] in Apparatus 2 at 75 rpm), and Uniformity of dosage units.
Chlorothiazide Sodium for Injection USP—Preserve in Containers for Sterile Solids. A sterile, freeze-dried mixture of Chlorothiazide Sodium (prepared by the neutralization of Chlorothiazide with the aid of Sodium Hydroxide) and Mannitol. Contains an amount of chlorothiazide sodium equivalent to the labeled amount of chlorothiazide, within ±7%. Meets the requirements for Constituted solution, Identification, Bacterial endotoxins, pH (9.2–10.0, in a solution prepared as directed in the labeling), Uniformity of dosage units, and Injections.

CHLOROTRIANISENE

Chemical name: Benzene, 1,1′,1″-(1-chloro-1-ethenyl-2-ylidene)-tris[4-methoxy]-.

Molecular formula: $C_{23}H_{21}ClO_3$.

Molecular weight: 380.87.

Description: Small, white crystals or crystalline powder. It is odorless.

Solubility: Very slightly soluble in water; slightly soluble in alcohol.

USP requirements:
Chlorotrianisene USP—Preserve in tight containers. Dried in vacuum at 60 °C for 6 hours, contains not less than 97.0% and not more than 103.0% of chlorotrianisene. Meets the requirements for Identification, Loss on drying (not more than 1.0%), Residue on ignition (not more than 1.0%), Heavy metals (not more than 0.002%), Volatile related compounds (not more than 1.0%), and Organic volatile impurities.
Chlorotrianisene Capsules USP—Preserve in well-closed containers, protected from excessive heat, cold, and moisture. Label Chlorotrianisene Capsules to indicate the vehicle used in the Capsules. Contain the labeled amount, within ±7%. Meet the requirements for Identification and Uniformity of dosage units.

CHLOROXINE

Chemical name: 8-Quinolinol, 5,7-dichloro-.

Molecular formula: $C_9H_5Cl_2NO$.

Molecular weight: 214.05.

Description: Melting point 179–180 °C.

Solubility: Soluble in acetone; slightly soluble in cold alcohol and in acetic acid; readily soluble in sodium and potassium hydroxides and in acids, forming yellow solutions.

USP requirements: Chloroxine Lotion Shampoo—Not in USP.

CHLOROXYLENOL

Chemical name: Phenol, 4-chloro-3,5-dimethyl-.

Molecular formula: C_8H_9ClO.

Molecular weight: 156.61.

Description: Chloroxylenol USP—White crystals or crystalline powder, having a characteristic odor. Volatile in steam.

Solubility: Chloroxylenol USP—Very slightly soluble in water; freely soluble in alcohol, in ether, in terpenes, in fixed oils, and in solutions of alkali hydroxides.

USP requirements: Chloroxylenol USP—Preserve in well-closed containers. Contains not less than 98.5% of chloroxylenol. Meets the requirements for Identification, Melting range (114–116 °C), Residue on ignition (not more than 0.1%), Iron (not more than 0.01%), Water (not more than 0.5%), and Chromatographic purity.

CHLORPHENESIN

Chemical name: Chlorphenesin carbamate—1,2-Propanediol, 3-(4-chlorophenoxy)-, 1-carbamate.

Molecular formula: Chlorphenesin carbamate—$C_{10}H_{12}ClNO_4$.

Molecular weight: Chlorphenesin carbamate—245.66.

Description: Chlorphenesin carbamate—White to off-white crystalline solid.

Solubility: Chlorphenesin carbamate—Almost insoluble in cold water or in cyclohexane; fairly readily soluble in dioxane; readily soluble in ethyl acetate, in 95.0% ethanol, and in acetone.

USP requirements: Chlorphenesin Carbamate Tablets—Not in USP.

CHLORPHENIRAMINE

Chemical group: Chlorpheniramine maleate—Alkylamine derivative.

Chemical name: Chlorpheniramine maleate—2-Pyridinepropanamine, gamma-(4-chlorophenyl)-*N,N*-dimethyl-, (*Z*)-2-butenedioate (1:1).

Molecular formula: Chlorpheniramine maleate—$C_{16}H_{19}ClN_2 \cdot C_4H_4O_4$.

Molecular weight: Chlorpheniramine maleate—390.87.

Description: Chlorpheniramine Maleate USP—White, odorless, crystalline powder. Its solutions have a pH between 4 and 5.

pKa: 9.2.

Solubility: Chlorpheniramine Maleate USP—Freely soluble in water; soluble in alcohol and in chloroform; slightly soluble in ether.

USP requirements:
Chlorpheniramine Maleate USP—Preserve in tight, light-resistant containers. Contains not less than 98.0% and not

more than 100.5% of chlorpheniramine maleate, calculated on the dried basis. Meets the requirements for Identification, Melting range (130–135 °C), Loss on drying (not more than 0.5%), Residue on ignition (not more than 0.2%), Related compounds, and Organic volatile impurities.

Chlorpheniramine Maleate Extended-release Capsules USP—Preserve in tight containers. Label the Capsules to indicate the Drug Release Test with which the product complies. Contain the labeled amount, within ±10%. Meet the requirements for Identification, Drug release, and Uniformity of dosage units.

Chlorpheniramine Maleate Injection USP—Preserve in single-dose or in multiple-dose containers, preferably of Type I glass, protected from light. A sterile solution of Chlorpheniramine Maleate in Water for Injection. Contains the labeled amount, within ±10%. Meets the requirements for Identification, Bacterial endotoxins, pH (4.0–5.2), and Injections.

Chlorpheniramine Maleate Syrup USP—Preserve in tight, light-resistant containers. Contains the labeled amount, within ±10%. Meets the requirements for Identification and Alcohol content (6.0–8.0%).

Chlorpheniramine Maleate Tablets USP—Preserve in tight containers. Contain the labeled amount, within ±7%. Meet the requirements for Identification, Dissolution (75% in 45 minutes in water in Apparatus 2 at 50 rpm), and Uniformity of dosage units.

Chlorpheniramine Maleate Extended-release Tablets—Not in USP.

CHLORPHENIRAMINE, CODEINE, ASPIRIN, AND CAFFEINE

For *Chlorpheniramine, Codeine, Aspirin,* and *Caffeine*—See individual listings for chemistry information.

USP requirements: Chlorpheniramine Maleate, Codeine Phosphate, Aspirin, and Caffeine Tablets—Not in USP.

CHLORPHENIRAMINE, CODEINE, AND GUAIFENESIN

For *Chlorpheniramine, Codeine,* and *Guaifenesin*—See individual listings for chemistry information.

USP requirements: Chlorpheniramine Maleate, Codeine Phosphate, and Guaifenesin Syrup—Not in USP.

CHLORPHENIRAMINE AND DEXTROMETHORPHAN

For *Chlorpheniramine* and *Dextromethorphan*—See individual listings for chemistry information.

USP requirements: Chlorpheniramine Maleate and Dextromethorphan Hydrobromide Oral Solution—Not in USP.

CHLORPHENIRAMINE, DEXTROMETHORPHAN, AND ACETAMINOPHEN

For *Chlorpheniramine, Dextromethorphan,* and *Acetaminophen*—See individual listings for chemistry information.

USP requirements: Chlorpheniramine Maleate, Dextromethorphan Hydrobromide, and Acetaminophen Capsules—Not in USP.

CHLORPHENIRAMINE, EPHEDRINE, AND GUAIFENESIN

For *Chlorpheniramine, Ephedrine,* and *Guaifenesin*—See individual listings for chemistry information.

USP requirements: Chlorpheniramine Maleate, Ephedrine Sulfate, and Guaifenesin Oral Solution—Not in USP.

CHLORPHENIRAMINE, EPHEDRINE, PHENYLEPHRINE, AND CARBETAPENTANE

Description: Chlorpheniramine tannate—Light tan to buff or yellowish-tan, amorphous, fine powder having not more than a slight characteristic odor.

Solubility: Chlorpheniramine tannate—Slightly soluble in water at 25 °C.

USP requirements:

Chlorpheniramine Tannate, Ephedrine Tannate, Phenylephrine Tannate, and Carbetapentane Tannate Oral Suspension—Not in USP.

Chlorpheniramine Tannate, Ephedrine Tannate, Phenylephrine Tannate, and Carbetapentane Tannate Tablets—Not in USP.

CHLORPHENIRAMINE, EPHEDRINE, PHENYLEPHRINE, DEXTROMETHORPHAN, AMMONIUM CHLORIDE, AND IPECAC

For *Chlorpheniramine, Ephedrine, Phenylephrine, Dextromethorphan, Ammonium Chloride,* and *Ipecac*—See individual listings for chemistry information.

USP requirements: Chlorpheniramine Maleate, Ephedrine Hydrochloride, Phenylephrine Hydrochloride, Dextromethorphan Hydrobromide, Ammonium Chloride, and Ipecac Fluidextract Syrup—Not in USP.

CHLORPHENIRAMINE AND HYDROCODONE

For *Chlorpheniramine* and *Hydrocodone*—See individual listings for chemistry information.

USP requirements: Chlorpheniramine Maleate and Hydrocodone Bitartrate Oral Suspension—Not in USP.

CHLORPHENIRAMINE, PHENINDAMINE, PHENYLEPHRINE, DEXTROMETHORPHAN, ACETAMINOPHEN, SALICYLAMIDE, CAFFEINE, AND ASCORBIC ACID

For *Chlorpheniramine, Phenindamine, Phenylephrine, Dextromethorphan, Acetaminophen, Salicylamide, Caffeine,* and *Ascorbic Acid*—See individual listings for chemistry information.

USP requirements: Chlorpheniramine Maleate, Phenindamine Tartrate, Phenylephrine Hydrochloride, Dextromethorphan Hydrobromide, Acetaminophen, Salicylamide, Caffeine, and Ascorbic Acid Tablets—Not in USP.

CHLORPHENIRAMINE, PHENINDAMINE, AND PHENYLPROPANOLAMINE

For *Chlorpheniramine, Phenindamine,* and *Phenylpropanolamine*—See individual listings for chemistry information.

USP requirements: Chlorpheniramine Maleate, Phenindamine Tartrate, and Phenylpropanolamine Hydrochloride Extended-release Tablets—Not in USP.

CHLORPHENIRAMINE, PHENINDAMINE, PYRILAMINE, PHENYLEPHRINE, HYDROCODONE, AND AMMONIUM CHLORIDE

For *Chlorpheniramine, Phenindamine, Pyrilamine, Phenylephrine, Hydrocodone,* and *Ammonium Chloride*—See individual listings for chemistry information.

USP requirements: Chlorpheniramine Maleate, Phenindamine Tartrate, Pyrilamine Maleate, Phenylephrine Hydrochloride, Hydrocodone Bitartrate, and Ammonium Chloride Syrup—Not in USP.

CHLORPHENIRAMINE, PHENIRAMINE, PYRILAMINE, PHENYLEPHRINE, HYDROCODONE, SALICYLAMIDE, CAFFEINE, AND ASCORBIC ACID

Source: Caffeine—Coffee, tea, cola, and cocoa or chocolate. May also be synthesized from urea or dimethylurea.

Chemical group:
Chlorpheniramine maleate—Alkylamine derivative.
Pheniramine—Alkylamine.
Pyrilamine—Ethylenediamine derivative.
Caffeine—Methylated xanthine.

Chemical name:
Chlorpheniramine maleate—2-Pyridinepropanamine, gamma-(4-chlorophenyl)-*N*,N-dimethyl-, (*Z*)-2-butenedioate (1:1).
Pheniramine maleate—2-[alpha-[2-Dimethylaminoethyl]-benzyl]pyridine bimaleate.
Pyrilamine maleate—1,2-Ethanediamine, *N*-[(4-methoxyphenyl)methyl]-*N'*,*N'*-dimethyl-*N*-2-pyridinyl-, (*Z*)-2-butenedioate (1:1).
Phenylephrine hydrochloride—Benzenemethanol, 3-hydroxy-alpha-[(methylamino)methyl]-, hydrochloride.
Hydrocodone bitartrate—Morphinan-6-one, 4,5-epoxy-3-methoxy-17-methyl-, (5 alpha)-, [*R*-(*R**,*R**)]-2,3-dihydroxybutanedioate (1:1), hydrate (2:5).
Salicylamide—Benzamide, 2-hydroxy-.
Caffeine—1*H*-Purine-2,6-dione, 3,7-dihydro-1,3,7-trimethyl-.
Ascorbic acid—L-Ascorbic acid.

Molecular formula:
Chlorpheniramine maleate—$C_{16}H_{19}ClN_2 \cdot C_4H_4O_4$.
Pheniramine maleate—$C_{16}H_{20}N_2 \cdot C_4H_4O_4$.
Pyrilamine maleate—$C_{17}H_{23}N_3O \cdot C_4H_4O_4$.
Phenylephrine hydrochloride—$C_9H_{13}NO_2 \cdot HCl$.
Hydrocodone bitartrate—$C_{18}H_{21}NO_3 \cdot C_4H_6O_6 \cdot 2\frac{1}{2}H_2O$ (hydrate); $C_{18}H_{21}NO_3 \cdot C_4H_6O_6$ (anhydrous).
Salicylamide—$C_7H_7NO_2$.
Caffeine (anhydrous)—$C_8H_{10}N_4O_2$.
Ascorbic acid—$C_6H_8O_6$.

Molecular weight:
Chlorpheniramine maleate—390.87.
Pheniramine maleate—356.42.
Pyrilamine maleate—401.46.
Phenylephrine hydrochloride—203.67.
Hydrocodone bitartrate—494.50 (hydrate); 449.46 (anhydrous).
Salicylamide—137.14.
Caffeine (anhydrous)—194.19.
Ascorbic acid—176.13.

Description:
Chlorpheniramine Maleate USP—White, odorless, crystalline powder. Its solutions have a pH between 4 and 5.
Pheniramine maleate—White or almost white crystalline powder, odorless or with a slight odor.
Pyrilamine Maleate USP—White, crystalline powder, usually having a faint odor. Its solutions are acid to litmus.
Phenylephrine Hydrochloride USP—White or practically white, odorless crystals.
Hydrocodone Bitartrate USP—Fine, white crystals or a crystalline powder. Is affected by light.
Salicylamide USP—White, practically odorless, crystalline powder.
Caffeine USP—White powder, or white, glistening needles, usually matted together. Is odorless. Its solutions are neutral to litmus. The hydrate is efflorescent in air.
Ascorbic Acid USP—White or slightly yellow crystals or powder. On exposure to light it gradually darkens. In the dry state, is reasonably stable in air, but in solution rapidly oxidizes. Melts at about 190 °C.

NF category: Antioxidant.

pKa:
Chlorpheniramine—9.2.
Ascorbic acid—4.2 and 11.6.

Solubility:
Chlorpheniramine Maleate USP—Freely soluble in water; soluble in alcohol and in chloroform; slightly soluble in ether.
Pheniramine maleate—Soluble 1 in 0.3 of water, 1 in 2.5 of alcohol, and 1 in 1.5 of chloroform; very slightly soluble in ether.
Pyrilamine Maleate USP—Very soluble in water; freely soluble in alcohol and in chloroform; slightly soluble in ether.
Phenylephrine Hydrochloride USP—Freely soluble in water and in alcohol.
Hydrocodone Bitartrate USP—Soluble in water; slightly soluble in alcohol; insoluble in ether and in chloroform.
Salicylamide USP—Slightly soluble in water and in chloroform; soluble in alcohol and in propylene glycol; freely soluble in ether and in solutions of alkalies.
Caffeine USP—Sparingly soluble in water and in alcohol; freely soluble in chloroform; slightly soluble in ether.

The aqueous solubility of caffeine is increased by organic acids or their alkali salts, such as citrates, benzoates, salicylates, or cinnamates, which dissociate to yield caffeine when dissolved in biological fluids.

Ascorbic Acid USP—Freely soluble in water; sparingly soluble in alcohol; insoluble in chloroform and in ether.

USP requirements: Chlorpheniramine Maleate, Pheniramine Maleate, Pyrilamine Maleate, Phenylephrine Hydrochloride, Hydrocodone Bitartrate, Salicylamide, Caffeine, and Ascorbic Acid Capsules—Not in USP.

CHLORPHENIRAMINE AND PHENYLEPHRINE

For *Chlorpheniramine* and *Phenylephrine*—See individual listings for chemistry information.

USP requirements:
Chlorpheniramine Maleate and Phenylephrine Hydrochloride Extended-release Capsules—Not in USP.
Chlorpheniramine Maleate and Phenylephrine Hydrochloride Elixir—Not in USP.
Chlorpheniramine Maleate and Phenylephrine Hydrochloride Oral Solution—Not in USP.
Chlorpheniramine Maleate and Phenylephrine Hydrochloride Syrup—Not in USP.
Chlorpheniramine Maleate and Phenylephrine Hydrochloride Tablets—Not in USP.
Chlorpheniramine Maleate and Phenylephrine Hydrochloride Chewable Tablets—Not in USP.

CHLORPHENIRAMINE, PHENYLEPHRINE, AND ACETAMINOPHEN

For *Chlorpheniramine, Phenylephrine,* and *Acetaminophen*—See individual listings for chemistry information.

USP requirements: Chlorpheniramine Maleate, Phenylephrine Hydrochloride, and Acetaminophen Tablets—Not in USP.

CHLORPHENIRAMINE, PHENYLEPHRINE, ACETAMINOPHEN, AND CAFFEINE

For *Chlorpheniramine, Phenylephrine, Acetaminophen,* and *Caffeine*—See individual listings for chemistry information.

USP requirements: Chlorpheniramine Maleate, Phenylephrine Hydrochloride, Acetaminophen, and Caffeine Tablets—Not in USP.

CHLORPHENIRAMINE, PHENYLEPHRINE, ACETAMINOPHEN, AND SALICYLAMIDE

For *Chlorpheniramine, Phenylephrine, Acetaminophen,* and *Salicylamide*—See individual listings for chemistry information.

USP requirements:
Chlorpheniramine Maleate, Phenylephrine Hydrochloride, Acetaminophen, and Salicylamide Capsules—Not in USP.
Chlorpheniramine Maleate, Phenylephrine Hydrochloride, Acetaminophen, and Salicylamide Tablets—Not in USP.

CHLORPHENIRAMINE, PHENYLEPHRINE, ACETAMINOPHEN, SALICYLAMIDE, AND CAFFEINE

For *Chlorpheniramine, Phenylephrine, Acetaminophen, Salicylamide,* and *Caffeine*—See individual listings for chemistry information.

USP requirements: Chlorpheniramine Maleate, Phenylephrine Hydrochloride, Acetaminophen, Salicylamide, and Caffeine Capsules—Not in USP.

CHLORPHENIRAMINE, PHENYLEPHRINE, CODEINE, AND AMMONIUM CHLORIDE

For *Chlorpheniramine, Phenylephrine, Codeine,* and *Ammonium Chloride*—See individual listings for chemistry information.

USP requirements: Chlorpheniramine Maleate, Phenylephrine Hydrochloride, Codeine Phosphate, and Ammonium Chloride Oral Solution—Not in USP.

CHLORPHENIRAMINE, PHENYLEPHRINE, CODEINE, AMMONIUM CHLORIDE, POTASSIUM GUAIACOLSULFONATE, AND SODIUM CITRATE

For *Chlorpheniramine, Phenylephrine, Codeine, Ammonium Chloride, Potassium Guaiacolsulfonate,* and *Sodium Citrate*—See individual listings for chemistry information.

USP requirements: Chlorpheniramine Maleate, Phenylephrine Hydrochloride, Codeine Phosphate, Ammonium Chloride, Potassium Guaiacolsulfonate, and Sodium Citrate Oral Solution—Not in USP.

CHLORPHENIRAMINE, PHENYLEPHRINE, CODEINE, AND POTASSIUM IODIDE

For *Chlorpheniramine, Phenylephrine, Codeine,* and *Potassium Iodide*—See individual listings for chemistry information.

USP requirements: Chlorpheniramine Maleate, Phenylephrine Hydrochloride, Codeine Phosphate, and Potassium Iodide Syrup—Not in USP.

CHLORPHENIRAMINE, PHENYLEPHRINE, AND DEXTROMETHORPHAN

For *Chlorpheniramine, Phenylephrine,* and *Dextromethorphan*—See individual listings for chemistry information.

USP requirements:
Chlorpheniramine Maleate, Phenylephrine Hydrochloride, and Dextromethorphan Hydrobromide Oral Solution—Not in USP.
Chlorpheniramine Maleate, Phenylephrine Hydrochloride, and Dextromethorphan Hydrobromide Tablets—Not in USP.

CHLORPHENIRAMINE, PHENYLEPHRINE, DEXTROMETHORPHAN, ACETAMINOPHEN, AND SALICYLAMIDE

For *Chlorpheniramine, Phenylephrine, Dextromethorphan, Acetaminophen,* and *Salicylamide*—See individual listings for chemistry information.

USP requirements: Chlorpheniramine Maleate, Phenylephrine Hydrochloride, Dextromethorphan Hydrobromide, Acetaminophen, and Salicylamide Tablets—Not in USP.

CHLORPHENIRAMINE, PHENYLEPHRINE, DEXTROMETHORPHAN, AND GUAIFENESIN

For *Chlorpheniramine, Phenylephrine, Dextromethorphan,* and *Guaifenesin*—See individual listings for chemistry information.

USP requirements: Chlorpheniramine Maleate, Phenylephrine Hydrochloride, Dextromethorphan Hydrobromide, and Guaifenesin Syrup—Not in USP.

CHLORPHENIRAMINE, PHENYLEPHRINE, DEXTROMETHORPHAN, GUAIFENESIN, AND AMMONIUM CHLORIDE

For *Chlorpheniramine, Phenylephrine, Dextromethorphan, Guaifenesin,* and *Ammonium Chloride*—See individual listings for chemistry information.

USP requirements: Chlorpheniramine Maleate, Phenylephrine Hydrochloride, Dextromethorphan Hydrobromide, Guaifenesin, and Ammonium Chloride Oral Solution—Not in USP.

CHLORPHENIRAMINE, PHENYLEPHRINE, AND GUAIFENESIN

For *Chlorpheniramine, Phenylephrine,* and *Guaifenesin*—See individual listings for chemistry information.

USP requirements: Chlorpheniramine Maleate, Phenylephrine Hydrochloride, and Guaifenesin Oral Solution—Not in USP.

CHLORPHENIRAMINE, PHENYLEPHRINE, AND HYDROCODONE

For *Chlorpheniramine, Phenylephrine,* and *Hydrocodone*—See individual listings for chemistry information.

USP requirements:
Chlorpheniramine Maleate, Phenylephrine Hydrochloride, and Hydrocodone Bitartrate Oral Solution—Not in USP.
Chlorpheniramine Maleate, Phenylephrine Hydrochloride, and Hydrocodone Bitartrate Syrup—Not in USP.

CHLORPHENIRAMINE, PHENYLEPHRINE, HYDROCODONE, ACETAMINOPHEN, AND CAFFEINE

For *Chlorpheniramine, Phenylephrine, Hydrocodone, Acetaminophen,* and *Caffeine*—See individual listings for chemistry information.

USP requirements: Chlorpheniramine Maleate, Phenylephrine Hydrochloride, Hydrocodone Bitartrate, Acetaminophen, and Caffeine Tablets—Not in USP.

CHLORPHENIRAMINE, PHENYLEPHRINE, AND METHSCOPOLAMINE

Chemical group: Chlorpheniramine maleate—Alkylamine derivative.

Chemical name:
Chlorpheniramine maleate—2-Pyridinepropanamine, gamma-(4-chlorophenyl)-*N,N*-dimethyl-, (*Z*)-2-butenedioate (1:1).
Phenylephrine hydrochloride—Benzenemethanol, 3-hydroxy-alpha-[(methylamino)methyl]-, hydrochloride.
Methscopolamine nitrate—(−)-(1*S*,3*s*,5*R*,6*R*,7*S*)-6,7-Epoxy-8-methyl-3-[(*S*)-tropoyloxy]tropanium nitrate.

Molecular formula:
Chlorpheniramine maleate—$C_{16}H_{19}ClN_2 \cdot C_4H_4O_4$.

Phenylephrine hydrochloride—$C_9H_{13}NO_2 \cdot HCl$.
Methscopolamine nitrate—$C_{18}H_{24}N_2O_7$.

Molecular weight:
Chlorpheniramine maleate—390.87.
Phenylephrine hydrochloride—203.67.
Methscopolamine nitrate—380.4.

Description:
Chlorpheniramine Maleate USP—White, odorless, crystalline powder. Its solutions have a pH between 4 and 5.
Phenylephrine Hydrochloride USP—White or practically white, odorless crystals.

Solubility:
Chlorpheniramine Maleate USP—Freely soluble in water; soluble in alcohol and in chloroform; slightly soluble in ether.
Phenylephrine Hydrochloride USP—Freely soluble in water and in alcohol.

USP requirements:
Chlorpheniramine Maleate, Phenylephrine Hydrochoride, and Methscopolamine Nitrate Extended-release Capsules—Not in USP.
Chlorpheniramine Maleate, Phenylephrine Hydrochoride, and Methscopolamine Nitrate Syrup—Not in USP.
Chlorpheniramine Maleate, Phenylephrine Hydrochoride, and Methscopolamine Nitrate Tablets—Not in USP.
Chlorpheniramine Maleate, Phenylephrine Hydrochoride, and Methscopolamine Nitrate Chewable Tablets—Not in USP.
Chlorpheniramine Maleate, Phenylephrine Hydrochoride, and Methscopolamine Nitrate Extended-release Tablets—Not in USP.

CHLORPHENIRAMINE, PHENYLEPHRINE, AND PHENYLPROPANOLAMINE

For *Chlorpheniramine, Phenylephrine,* and *Phenylpropanolamine*—See individual listings for chemistry information.

USP requirements:
Chlorpheniramine Maleate, Phenylephrine Hydrochloride, and Phenylpropanolamine Hydrochloride Extended-release Capsules—Not in USP.
Chlorpheniramine Maleate, Phenylephrine Hydrochloride, and Phenylpropanolamine Hydrochloride Tablets—Not in USP.

CHLORPHENIRAMINE, PHENYLEPHRINE, PHENYLPROPANOLAMINE, ATROPINE, HYOSCYAMINE, AND SCOPOLAMINE

For *Chlorpheniramine, Phenylephrine, Phenylpropanolamine, Atropine, Hyoscyamine,* and *Scopolamine*—See individual listings for chemistry information.

USP requirements: Chlorpheniramine Maleate, Phenylephrine Hydrochloride, Phenylpropanolamine Hydrochloride, Atropine Sulfate, Hyoscyamine Sulfate, and Scopolamine Bromide Extended-release Tablets—Not in USP.

CHLORPHENIRAMINE, PHENYLEPHRINE, PHENYLPROPANOLAMINE, CARBETAPENTANE, AND POTASSIUM GUAIACOLSULFONATE

Chemical group:
Chlorpheniramine maleate—Alkylamine derivative.
Phenylpropanolamine hydrochloride—Synthetic phenylisopropanolamine.

Chemical name:
Chlorpheniramine maleate—2-Pyridinepropanamine, gamma-(4-chlorophenyl)-*N,N*-dimethyl-, (*Z*)-2-butenedioate (1:1).
Phenylephrine hydrochloride—Benzenemethanol, 3-hydroxy-alpha-[(methylamino)methyl]-, hydrochloride.
Phenylpropanolamine hydrochloride—Benzenemethanol, alpha-(1-aminoethyl)-, hydrochloride, (R^*,S^*)-, (±).
Carbetapentane citrate—2-[2-(Diethylamino)ethoxy]ethyl 1-phenylcyclopentanecarboxylate citrate (1:1).
Potassium guaiacolsulfonate—Benzenesulfonic acid, hydroxymethoxy-, monopotassium salt, hemihydrate.

Molecular formula:
Chlorpheniramine maleate—$C_{16}H_{19}ClN_2 \cdot C_4H_4O_4$.
Phenylephrine hydrochloride—$C_9H_{13}NO_2 \cdot HCl$.
Phenylpropanolamine hydrochloride—$C_9H_{13}NO \cdot HCl$.
Carbetapentane citrate—$C_{20}H_{31}NO_3 \cdot C_6H_8O_7$.
Potassium guaiacolsulfonate—$C_7H_7KO_5S \cdot \frac{1}{2}H_2O$.

Molecular weight:
Chlorpheniramine maleate—390.87.
Phenylephrine hydrochloride—203.67.
Phenylpropanolamine hydrochloride—187.67.
Carbetapentane citrate—525.60.
Potassium guaiacolsulfonate—251.30.

Description:
Chlorpheniramine Maleate USP—White, odorless, crystalline powder. Its solutions have a pH between 4 and 5.
Phenylephrine Hydrochloride USP—White or practically white, odorless crystals.
Phenylpropanolamine Hydrochloride USP—White, crystalline powder, having a slight aromatic odor. Is affected by light.
Potassium guaiacolsulfonate—White, odorless crystals or crystalline powder. Gradually turns pink on exposure to air and light.

pKa:
Chlorpheniramine—9.2.
Phenylpropanolamine hydrochloride—9.

Solubility:
Chlorpheniramine Maleate USP—Freely soluble in water; soluble in alcohol and in chloroform; slightly soluble in ether.
Phenylephrine Hydrochloride USP—Freely soluble in water and in alcohol.
Phenylpropanolamine Hydrochloride USP—Freely soluble in water and in alcohol; insoluble in ether.
Potassium guaiacolsulfonate—Soluble in 7.5 parts water; almost insoluble in alcohol; insoluble in ether.

USP requirements:
Chlorpheniramine Maleate, Phenylephrine Hydrochloride, Phenylpropanolamine Hydrochloride, Carbetapentane Citrate, and Potassium Guaiacolsulfonate Capsules—Not in USP.
Chlorpheniramine Maleate, Phenylephrine Hydrochloride, Phenylpropanolamine Hydrochloride, Carbetapentane Citrate, and Potassium Guaiacolsulfonate Syrup—Not in USP.

CHLORPHENIRAMINE, PHENYLEPHRINE, PHENYLPROPANOLAMINE, AND CODEINE

For *Chlorpheniramine, Phenylephrine, Phenylpropanolamine,* and *Codeine*—See individual listings for chemistry information.

USP requirements: Chlorpheniramine Maleate, Phenylephrine Hydrochloride, Phenylpropanolamine Hydrochloride, and Codeine Phosphate Syrup—Not in USP.

CHLORPHENIRAMINE, PHENYLEPHRINE, PHENYLPROPANOLAMINE, AND DEXTROMETHORPHAN

For *Chlorpheniramine, Phenylephrine, Phenylpropanolamine,* and *Dextromethorphan*—See individual listings for chemistry information.

USP requirements: Chlorpheniramine Maleate, Phenylephrine Hydrochloride, Phenylpropanolamine Hydrochloride, and Dextromethorphan Hydrobromide Syrup—Not in USP.

CHLORPHENIRAMINE, PHENYLEPHRINE, PHENYLPROPANOLAMINE, DEXTROMETHORPHAN, GUAIFENESIN, AND ACETAMINOPHEN

For *Chlorpheniramine, Phenylephrine, Phenylpropanolamine, Dextromethorphan, Guaifenesin,* and *Acetaminophen*—See individual listings for chemistry information.

USP requirements:

Chlorpheniramine Maleate, Phenylephrine Hydrochloride, Phenylpropanolamine Hydrochloride, Dextromethorphan Hydrobromide, Guaifenesin, and Acetaminophen Syrup—Not in USP.

Chlorpheniramine Maleate, Phenylephrine Hydrochloride, Phenylpropanolamine Hydrochloride, Dextromethorphan Hydrobromide, Guaifenesin, and Acetaminophen Tablets—Not in USP.

CHLORPHENIRAMINE, PHENYLEPHRINE, PHENYLPROPANOLAMINE, AND DIHYDROCODEINE

For *Chlorpheniramine, Phenylephrine, Phenylpropanolamine,* and *Dihydrocodeine*—See individual listings for chemistry information.

USP requirements: Chlorpheniramine Maleate, Phenylephrine Hydrochloride, Phenylpropanolamine Hydrochloride, and Dihydrocodeine Bitartrate Syrup—Not in USP.

CHLORPHENIRAMINE AND PHENYLPROPANOLAMINE

Chemical group:

Chlorpheniramine maleate—Alkylamine derivative.

Phenylpropanolamine hydrochloride—Synthetic phenylisopropanolamine.

Chemical name:

Chlorpheniramine maleate—2-Pyridinepropanamine, gamma-(4-chlorophenyl)-*N,N*-dimethyl-, (*Z*)-2-butenedioate (1:1).

Chlorpheniramine polistirex—Benzene, diethenyl-, polymer with ethenylbenzene, sulfonated, complex with gamma-(4-chlorophenyl)-*N,N*-dimethyl-2-pyridinepropanamine.

Phenylpropanolamine hydrochloride—Benzenemethanol, alpha-(1-aminoethyl)-, hydrochloride, (*R**,*S**)-, (±).

Phenylpropanolamine polistirex—Benzene, diethenyl-, polymer with ethenylbenzene, sulfonated, complex with (±)-(*R**,*S**)-alpha-(1-aminoethyl)benzenemethanol.

Molecular formula:

Chlorpheniramine maleate—$C_{16}H_{19}ClN_2 \cdot C_4H_4O_4$.

Phenylpropanolamine hydrochloride—$C_9H_{13}NO \cdot HCl$.

Molecular weight:

Chlorpheniramine maleate—390.87.

Phenylpropanolamine hydrochloride—187.67.

Description:

Chlorpheniramine Maleate USP—White, odorless, crystalline powder. Its solutions have a pH between 4 and 5.

Phenylpropanolamine Hydrochloride USP—White, crystalline powder, having a slight aromatic odor. Is affected by light.

pKa:

Chlorpheniramine—9.2.

Phenylpropanolamine hydrochloride—9.

Solubility:

Chlorpheniramine Maleate USP—Freely soluble in water; soluble in alcohol and in chloroform; slightly soluble in ether.

Phenylpropanolamine Hydrochloride USP—Freely soluble in water and in alcohol; insoluble in ether.

USP requirements:

Chlorpheniramine Maleate and Phenylpropanolamine Hydrochloride Extended-release Capsules—Not in USP.

Chlorpheniramine Maleate and Phenylpropanolamine Hydrochloride Granules—Not in USP.

Chlorpheniramine Maleate and Phenylpropanolamine Hydrochloride Oral Solution—Not in USP.

Chlorpheniramine Maleate and Phenylpropanolamine Hydrochloride Syrup—Not in USP.

Chlorpheniramine Maleate and Phenylpropanolamine Hydrochloride Tablets—Not in USP.

Chlorpheniramine Maleate and Phenylpropanolamine Hydrochloride Chewable Tablets—Not in USP.

Chlorpheniramine Maleate and Phenylpropanolamine Hydrochloride Extended-release Tablets—Not in USP.

Chlorpheniramine and Phenylpropanolamine Polistirexes Extended-release Oral Suspension—Not in USP.

CHLORPHENIRAMINE, PHENYLPROPANOLAMINE, AND ACETAMINOPHEN

For *Chlorpheniramine, Phenylpropanolamine,* and *Acetaminophen*—See individual listings for chemistry information.

USP requirements:

Chlorpheniramine Maleate, Phenylpropanolamine Hydrochloride, and Acetaminophen Capsules—Not in USP.

Chlorpheniramine Maleate, Phenylpropanolamine Hydrochloride, and Acetaminophen Tablets—Not in USP.

Chlorpheniramine Maleate, Phenylpropanolamine Hydrochloride, and Acetaminophen Chewable Tablets—Not in USP.

Chlorpheniramine Maleate, Phenylpropanolamine Hydrochloride, and Acetaminophen Effervescent Tablets—Not in USP.

Chlorpheniramine Maleate, Phenylpropanolamine Hydrochloride, and Acetaminophen Extended-release Tablets—Not in USP.

CHLORPHENIRAMINE, PHENYLPROPANOLAMINE, ACETAMINOPHEN, AND CAFFEINE

For *Chlorpheniramine, Phenylpropanolamine, Acetaminophen,* and *Caffeine*—See individual listings for chemistry information.

USP requirements: Chlorpheniramine Maleate, Phenylpropanolamine Hydrochloride, Acetaminophen, and Caffeine Tablets—Not in USP.

CHLORPHENIRAMINE, PHENYLPROPANOLAMINE, AND ASPIRIN

Chemical group:

Chlorpheniramine maleate—Alkylamine derivative.

Phenylpropanolamine hydrochloride—Synthetic phenylisopropanolamine.

Chemical name:

Chlorpheniramine maleate—2-Pyridinepropanamine, gamma-(4-chlorophenyl)-*N,N*-dimethyl-, (*Z*)-2-butenedioate (1:1).

Phenylpropanolamine hydrochloride—Benzenemethanol, alpha-(1-aminoethyl)-, hydrochloride, (R^*,S^*)-, ($\pm$).
Aspirin—Benzoic acid, 2-(acetyloxy)-.

Molecular formula:
Chlorpheniramine maleate—$C_{16}H_{19}ClN_2 \cdot C_4H_4O_4$.
Phenylpropanolamine hydrochloride—$C_9H_{13}NO \cdot HCl$.
Aspirin—$C_9H_8O_4$.

Molecular weight:
Chlorpheniramine maleate—390.87.
Phenylpropanolamine hydrochloride—187.67.
Aspirin—180.16.

Description:
Chlorpheniramine Maleate USP—White, odorless, crystalline powder. Its solutions have a pH between 4 and 5.
Phenylpropanolamine Hydrochloride USP—White, crystalline powder, having a slight aromatic odor. Is affected by light.
Aspirin USP—White crystals, commonly tabular or needle-like, or white, crystalline powder. Is odorless or has a faint odor. Is stable in dry air; in moist air it gradually hydrolyzes to salicylic and acetic acids.

pKa:
Chlorpheniramine—9.2.
Phenylpropanolamine hydrochloride—9.
Aspirin—3.5.

Solubility:
Chlorpheniramine Maleate USP—Freely soluble in water; soluble in alcohol and in chloroform; slightly soluble in ether.
Phenylpropanolamine Hydrochloride USP—Freely soluble in water and in alcohol; insoluble in ether.
Aspirin USP—Slightly soluble in water; freely soluble in alcohol; soluble in chloroform and in ether; sparingly soluble in absolute ether.

USP requirements:
Chlorpheniramine Maleate, Phenylpropanolamine Bitartrate, and Aspirin Tablets—Not in USP.
Chlorpheniramine Maleate, Phenylpropanolamine Hydrochloride, and Aspirin for Oral Solution—Not in USP.
Chlorpheniramine Maleate, Phenylpropanolamine Hydrochloride, and Aspirin Tablets—Not in USP.

CHLORPHENIRAMINE, PHENYLPROPANOLAMINE, ASPIRIN, AND CAFFEINE

For *Chlorpheniramine, Phenylpropanolamine, Aspirin,* and *Caffeine*—See individual listings for chemistry information.

USP requirements:
Chlorpheniramine Maleate, Phenylpropanolamine Hydrochloride, Aspirin, and Caffeine Capsules—Not in USP.
Chlorpheniramine Maleate, Phenylpropanolamine Hydrochloride, Aspirin, and Caffeine Tablets—Not in USP.

CHLORPHENIRAMINE, PHENYLPROPANOLAMINE, AND CARAMIPHEN

Chemical group:
Chlorpheniramine maleate—Alkylamine derivative.
Phenylpropanolamine hydrochloride—Synthetic phenylisopropanolamine.

Chemical name:
Chlorpheniramine maleate—2-Pyridinepropanamine, gamma-(4-chlorophenyl)-*N,N*-dimethyl-, (*Z*)-2-butenedioate (1:1).
Phenylpropanolamine hydrochloride—Benzenemethanol, alpha-(1-aminoethyl)-, hydrochloride, (R^*,S^*)-, ($\pm$).
Caramiphen edisylate—1-Phenylcyclopentane-1-carboxylic acid, 2-diethylaminoethyl ester, 1,2-ethanedisulfonate (2:1).

Molecular formula:
Chlorpheniramine maleate—$C_{16}H_{19}ClN_2 \cdot C_4H_4O_4$.
Phenylpropanolamine hydrochloride—$C_9H_{13}NO \cdot HCl$.
Caramiphen edisylate—$(C_{18}H_{27}NO_2)_2 \cdot C_2H_6O_6S_2$.

Molecular weight:
Chlorpheniramine maleate—390.87.
Phenylpropanolamine hydrochloride—187.67.
Caramiphen edisylate—769.03.

Description:
Chlorpheniramine Maleate USP—White, odorless, crystalline powder. Its solutions have a pH between 4 and 5.
Phenylpropanolamine Hydrochloride USP—White, crystalline powder, having a slight aromatic odor. Is affected by light.
Caramiphen edisylate—Off-white crystals. Melting point 115–116 °C.

pKa:
Chlorpheniramine—9.2.
Phenylpropanolamine hydrochloride—9.

Solubility:
Chlorpheniramine Maleate USP—Freely soluble in water; soluble in alcohol and in chloroform; slightly soluble in ether.
Phenylpropanolamine Hydrochloride USP—Freely soluble in water and in alcohol; insoluble in ether.
Caramiphen edisylate—One gram dissolves in about 2 mL of water; soluble in alcohol.

USP requirements: Chlorpheniramine Maleate, Phenylpropanolamine Hydrochloride, and Caramiphen Edisylate Extended-release Capsules—Not in USP.

CHLORPHENIRAMINE, PHENYLPROPANOLAMINE, CODEINE, GUAIFENESIN, AND ACETAMINOPHEN

For *Chlorpheniramine, Phenylpropanolamine, Codeine, Guaifenesin,* and *Acetaminophen*—See individual listings for chemistry information.

USP requirements:
Chlorpheniramine Maleate, Phenylpropanolamine Hydrochloride, Codeine Phosphate, Guaifenesin, and Acetaminophen Syrup—Not in USP.
Chlorpheniramine Maleate, Phenylpropanolamine Hydrochloride, Codeine Phosphate, Guaifenesin, and Acetaminophen Tablets—Not in USP.

CHLORPHENIRAMINE, PHENYLPROPANOLAMINE, AND DEXTROMETHORPHAN

For *Chlorpheniramine, Phenylpropanolamine,* and *Dextromethorphan*—See individual listings for chemistry information.

USP requirements:
Chlorpheniramine Maleate, Phenylpropanolamine Hydrochloride, and Dextromethorphan Hydrobromide Oral Gel—Not in USP.
Chlorpheniramine Maleate, Phenylpropanolamine Hydrochloride, and Dextromethorphan Hydrobromide Granules—Not in USP.
Chlorpheniramine Maleate, Phenylpropanolamine Hydrochloride, and Dextromethorphan Hydrobromide Oral Solution—Not in USP.
Chlorpheniramine Maleate, Phenylpropanolamine Hydrochloride, and Dextromethorphan Hydrobromide Syrup—Not in USP.

Chlorpheniramine Maleate, Phenylpropanolamine Hydrochloride, and Dextromethorphan Hydrobromide Tablets—Not in USP.

CHLORPHENIRAMINE, PHENYLPROPANOLAMINE, DEXTROMETHORPHAN, AND ACETAMINOPHEN

For *Chlorpheniramine, Phenylpropanolamine, Dextromethorphan,* and *Acetaminophen*—See individual listings for chemistry information.

USP requirements:
Chlorpheniramine Maleate, Phenylpropanolamine Hydrochloride, Dextromethorphan Hydrobromide, and Acetaminophen Capsules—Not in USP.
Chlorpheniramine Maleate, Phenylpropanolamine Hydrochloride, Dextromethorphan Hydrobromide, and Acetaminophen Oral Solution—Not in USP.
Chlorpheniramine Maleate, Phenylpropanolamine Hydrochloride, Dextromethorphan Hydrobromide, and Acetaminophen Tablets—Not in USP.

CHLORPHENIRAMINE, PHENYLPROPANOLAMINE, DEXTROMETHORPHAN, ACETAMINOPHEN, AND CAFFEINE

For *Chlorpheniramine, Phenylpropanolamine, Dextromethorphan, Acetaminophen,* and *Caffeine*—See individual listings for chemistry information.

USP requirements: Chlorpheniramine Maleate, Phenylpropanolamine Hydrochloride, Dextromethorphan Hydrobromide, Acetaminophen, and Caffeine Capsules—Not in USP.

CHLORPHENIRAMINE, PHENYLPROPANOLAMINE, DEXTROMETHORPHAN, AND AMMONIUM CHLORIDE

For *Chlorpheniramine, Phenylpropanolamine, Dextromethorphan,* and *Ammonium Chloride*—See individual listings for chemistry information.

USP requirements: Chlorpheniramine Maleate, Phenylpropanolamine Hydrochloride, Dextromethorphan Hydrobromide, and Ammonium Chloride Syrup—Not in USP.

CHLORPHENIRAMINE, PHENYLPROPANOLAMINE, AND GUAIFENESIN

For *Chlorpheniramine, Phenylpropanolamine,* and *Guaifenesin*—See individual listings for chemistry information.

USP requirements: Chlorpheniramine Maleate, Phenylpropanolamine Hydrochloride, and Guaifenesin Oral Solution—Not in USP.

CHLORPHENIRAMINE, PHENYLPROPANOLAMINE, GUAIFENESIN, SODIUM CITRATE, AND CITRIC ACID

For *Chlorpheniramine, Phenylpropanolamine, Guaifenesin, Sodium Citrate* and *Citric Acid*—See individual listings for chemistry information.

USP requirements: Chlorpheniramine Maleate, Phenylpropanolamine Hydrochloride, Guaifenesin, Sodium Citrate, and Citric Acid Oral Solution—Not in USP.

CHLORPHENIRAMINE, PHENYLPROPANOLAMINE, HYDROCODONE, GUAIFENESIN, AND SALICYLAMIDE

For *Chlorpheniramine, Phenylpropanolamine, Hydrocodone, Guaifenesin,* and *Salicylamide*—See individual listings for chemistry information.

USP requirements: Chlorpheniramine Maleate, Phenylpropanolamine Hydrochloride, Hydrocodone Bitartrate, Guaifenesin, and Salicylamide Tablets—Not in USP.

CHLORPHENIRAMINE, PHENYLPROPANOLAMINE, AND METHSCOPOLAMINE

Chemical group:
Chlorpheniramine maleate—Alkylamine derivative.
Phenylpropanolamine hydrochloride—Synthetic phenylisopropanolamine.

Chemical name:
Chlorpheniramine maleate—2-Pyridinepropanamine, gamma-(4-chlorophenyl)-*N*,*N*-dimethyl-, (*Z*)-2-butenedioate (1:1).
Phenylpropanolamine hydrochloride—Benzenemethanol, alpha-(1-aminoethyl)-, hydrochloride, (R^*,S^*)-, (±).
Methscopolamine nitrate—(–)-(1*S*,3*s*,5*R*,6*R*,7*S*)-6,7-Epoxy-8-methyl-3-[(*S*)-tropoyloxy]tropanium nitrate.

Molecular formula:
Chlorpheniramine maleate—$C_{16}H_{19}ClN_2 \cdot C_4H_4O_4$.
Phenylpropanolamine hydrochloride—$C_9H_{13}NO \cdot HCl$.
Methscopolamine nitrate—$C_{18}H_{24}N_2O_7$.

Molecular weight:
Chlorpheniramine maleate—390.87.
Phenylpropanolamine hydrochloride—187.67.
Methscopolamine nitrate—380.4.

Description:
Chlorpheniramine Maleate USP—White, odorless, crystalline powder. Its solutions have a pH between 4 and 5.
Phenylpropanolamine Hydrochloride USP—White, crystalline powder, having a slight aromatic odor. Is affected by light.

pKa: Phenylpropanolamine hydrochloride—9.

Solubility:
Chlorpheniramine Maleate USP—Freely soluble in water; soluble in alcohol and in chloroform; slightly soluble in ether.
Phenylpropanolamine Hydrochloride USP—Freely soluble in water and in alcohol; insoluble in ether.

USP requirements: Chlorpheniramine Maleate, Phenylpropanolamine Hydrochoride, and Methscopolamine Nitrate Extended-release Capsules—Not in USP.

CHLORPHENIRAMINE, PHENYLTOLOXAMINE, EPHEDRINE, CODEINE, AND GUAIACOL

Chemical name: Guaiacol carbonate—Carbonic acid bis(2-methoxyphenyl) ester; guaiacol carbonic acid neutral ester; carbonic acid guaiacol ether.

Molecular formula: Guaiacol carbonate—$C_{15}H_{14}O_5$.

Molecular weight: Guaiacol carbonate—274.26.

Description: Guaiacol carbonate—Odorless needles from ethanol. It has a melting point of 88.1 °C.

Solubility: Guaiacol carbonate—Practically insoluble in water; soluble in ethanol, in chloroform, and in ether; slightly soluble in liquid fatty acids.

USP requirements: Chlorpheniramine, Phenyltoloxamine, Ephedrine, Codeine, and Guaiacol Carbonate Oral Suspension—Not in USP.

CHLORPHENIRAMINE, PHENYLTOLOXAMINE, AND PHENYLEPHRINE

Chemical group:
Chlorpheniramine maleate—Alkylamine derivative.
Phenyltoloxamine citrate—Ethanolamine derivative.

Chemical name:

Chlorpheniramine maleate—2-Pyridinepropanamine, gamma-(4-chlorophenyl)-*N,N*-dimethyl-, (*Z*)-2-butenedioate (1:1).

Phenyltoloxamine citrate—2-(2-Benzylphenoxy)-*NN*-dimethylethylamine dihydrogen citrate.

Phenylephrine hydrochloride—Benzenemethanol, 3-hydroxy-alpha-[(methylamino)methyl]-, hydrochloride.

Molecular formula:

Chlorpheniramine maleate—$C_{16}H_{19}ClN_2 \cdot C_4H_4O_4$.

Phenyltoloxamine citrate—$C_{17}H_{21}NO \cdot C_6H_8O_7$.

Phenylephrine hydrochloride—$C_9H_{13}NO_2 \cdot HCl$.

Molecular weight:

Chlorpheniramine maleate—390.87.

Phenyltoloxamine citrate—447.5.

Phenylephrine hydrochloride—203.67.

Description:

Chlorpheniramine Maleate USP—White, odorless, crystalline powder. Its solutions have a pH between 4 and 5.

Phenyltoloxamine citrate—It has a melting point of 138–140 °C.

Phenylephrine Hydrochloride USP—White or practically white, odorless crystals.

pKa: Chlorpheniramine—9.2.

Solubility:

Chlorpheniramine Maleate USP—Freely soluble in water; soluble in alcohol and in chloroform; slightly soluble in ether.

Phenyltoloxamine citrate—Soluble in water.

Phenylephrine Hydrochloride USP—Freely soluble in water and in alcohol.

USP requirements:

Chlorpheniramine Maleate, Phenyltoloxamine Citrate, and Phenylephrine Hydrochloride Extended-release Capsules—Not in USP.

Chlorpheniramine Maleate, Phenyltoloxamine Citrate, and Phenylephrine Hydrochloride Tablets—Not in USP.

CHLORPHENIRAMINE, PHENYLTOLOXAMINE, PHENYLEPHRINE, AND PHENYLPROPANOLAMINE

Chemical group:

Chlorpheniramine maleate—Alkylamine derivative.

Phenyltoloxamine citrate—Ethanolamine derivative.

Phenylpropanolamine hydrochloride—Synthetic phenylisopropanolamine.

Chemical name:

Chlorpheniramine maleate—2-Pyridinepropanamine, gamma-(4-chlorophenyl)-*N,N*-dimethyl-, (*Z*)-2-butenedioate (1:1).

Phenyltoloxamine citrate—2-(2-Benzylphenoxy)-*NN*-dimethylethylamine dihydrogen citrate.

Phenylephrine hydrochloride—Benzenemethanol, 3-hydroxy-alpha-[(methylamino)methyl]-, hydrochloride.

Phenylpropanolamine hydrochloride—Benzenemethanol, alpha-(1-aminoethyl)-, hydrochloride, (*R**,*S**)-, (±).

Molecular formula:

Chlorpheniramine maleate—$C_{16}H_{19}ClN_2 \cdot C_4H_4O_4$.

Phenyltoloxamine citrate—$C_{17}H_{21}NO \cdot C_6H_8O_7$.

Phenylephrine hydrochloride—$C_9H_{13}NO_2 \cdot HCl$.

Phenylpropanolamine hydrochloride—$C_9H_{13}NO \cdot HCl$.

Molecular weight:

Chlorpheniramine maleate—390.87.

Phenyltoloxamine citrate—447.5.

Phenylephrine hydrochloride—203.67.

Phenylpropanolamine hydrochloride—187.67.

Description:

Chlorpheniramine Maleate USP—White, odorless, crystalline powder. Its solutions have a pH between 4 and 5.

Phenyltoloxamine citrate—It has a melting point of 138–140 °C.

Phenylephrine Hydrochloride USP—White or practically white, odorless crystals.

Phenylpropanolamine Hydrochloride USP—White, crystalline powder, having a slight aromatic odor. Is affected by light.

pKa:

Chlorpheniramine—9.2.

Phenylpropanolamine hydrochloride—9.

Solubility:

Chlorpheniramine Maleate USP—Freely soluble in water; soluble in alcohol and in chloroform; slightly soluble in ether.

Phenyltoloxamine citrate—Soluble in water.

Phenylephrine Hydrochloride USP—Freely soluble in water and in alcohol.

Phenylpropanolamine Hydrochloride USP—Freely soluble in water and in alcohol; insoluble in ether.

USP requirements:

Chlorpheniramine Maleate, Phenyltoloxamine Citrate, Phenylephrine Hydrochloride, and Phenylpropanolamine Hydrochloride Extended-release Capsules—Not in USP.

Chlorpheniramine Maleate, Phenyltoloxamine Citrate, Phenylephrine Hydrochloride, and Phenylpropanolamine Hydrochloride Oral Solution—Not in USP.

Chlorpheniramine Maleate, Phenyltoloxamine Citrate, Phenylephrine Hydrochloride, and Phenylpropanolamine Hydrochloride Syrup—Not in USP.

Chlorpheniramine Maleate, Phenyltoloxamine Citrate, Phenylephrine Hydrochloride, and Phenylpropanolamine Hydrochloride Extended-release Tablets—Not in USP.

CHLORPHENIRAMINE, PHENYLTOLOXAMINE, PHENYLPROPANOLAMINE, AND ACETAMINOPHEN

Chemical group:

Chlorpheniramine maleate—Alkylamine derivative.

Phenylpropanolamine hydrochloride—Synthetic phenylisopropanolamine.

Chemical name:

Chlorpheniramine maleate—2-Pyridinepropanamine, gamma-(4-chlorophenyl)-*N,N*-dimethyl-, (*Z*)-2-butenedioate (1:1).

Phenyltoloxamine dihydrogen citrate—2-(2-Benzylphenoxy)-*NN*-dimethylethylamine dihydrogen citrate.

Phenylpropanolamine hydrochloride—Benzenemethanol, alpha-(1-aminoethyl)-, hydrochloride, (*R**,*S**)-, (±).

Acetaminophen—Acetamide, *N*-(4-hydroxyphenyl)-.

Molecular formula:

Chlorpheniramine maleate—$C_{16}H_{19}ClN_2 \cdot C_4H_4O_4$.

Phenyltoloxamine dihydrogen citrate—$C_{17}H_{21}NO \cdot C_6H_8O_7$.

Phenylpropanolamine hydrochloride—$C_9H_{13}NO \cdot HCl$.

Acetaminophen—$C_8H_9NO_2$.

Molecular weight:

Chlorpheniramine maleate—390.87.

Phenyltoloxamine dihydrogen citrate—447.5.

Phenylpropanolamine hydrochloride—187.67.

Acetaminophen—151.16.

Description:
Chlorpheniramine Maleate USP—White, odorless, crystalline powder. Its solutions have a pH between 4 and 5.
Phenyltoloxamine dihydrogen citrate—It has a melting point of 138–140 °C.
Phenylpropanolamine Hydrochloride USP—White, crystalline powder, having a slight aromatic odor. Is affected by light.
Acetaminophen USP—White, odorless, crystalline powder.

pKa:
Chlorpheniramine—9.2.
Phenylpropanolamine hydrochloride—9.

Solubility:
Chlorpheniramine Maleate USP—Freely soluble in water; soluble in alcohol and in chloroform; slightly soluble in ether.
Phenyltoloxamine dihydrogen citrate—Soluble in water.
Phenylpropanolamine Hydrochloride USP—Freely soluble in water and in alcohol; insoluble in ether.
Acetaminophen USP—Soluble in boiling water and in 1 *N* sodium hydroxide; freely soluble in alcohol.

USP requirements: Chlorpheniramine Maleate, Phenyltoloxamine Dihydrogen Citrate, Phenylpropanolamine Hydrochloride, and Acetaminophen Capsules—Not in USP.

CHLORPHENIRAMINE, PHENYLTOLOXAMINE, PHENYLPROPANOLAMINE, DEXTROMETHORPHAN, AND GUAIFENESIN

Source: Dextromethorphan—Methylated dextroisomer of levorphanol.

Chemical group:
Chlorpheniramine maleate—Alkylamine derivative.
Phenylpropanolamine hydrochloride—Synthetic phenylisopropanolamine.
Dextromethorphan—Nonopioid, morphinan-derivative.

Chemical name:
Chlorpheniramine maleate—2-Pyridinepropanamine, gamma-(4-chlorophenyl)-*N*,*N*-dimethyl-, (*Z*)-2-butenedioate (1:1).
Phenyltoloxamine citrate—2-(2-Benzylphenoxy)-*NN*-dimethylethylamine dihydrogen citrate.
Phenylpropanolamine hydrochloride—Benzenemethanol, alpha-(1-aminoethyl)-, hydrochloride, (*R**,*S**)-, (±).
Dextromethorphan hydrobromide—Morphinan, 3-methoxy-17-methyl-, (9 alpha,13 alpha,14 alpha)-, hydrobromide, monohydrate.
Guaifenesin—1,2-Propanediol, 3-(2-methoxyphenoxy)-.

Molecular formula:
Chlorpheniramine maleate—$C_{16}H_{19}ClN_2 \cdot C_4H_4O_4$.
Phenyltoloxamine citrate—$C_{17}H_{21}NO \cdot C_6H_8O_7$.
Phenylpropanolamine hydrochloride—$C_9H_{13}NO \cdot HCl$.
Dextromethorphan hydrobromide—$C_{18}H_{25}NO \cdot HBr \cdot H_2O$.
Guaifenesin—$C_{10}H_{14}O_4$.

Molecular weight:
Chlorpheniramine maleate—390.87.
Phenyltoloxamine citrate—447.5.
Phenylpropanolamine hydrochloride—187.67.
Dextromethorphan hydrobromide—370.33.
Guaifenesin—198.22.

Description:
Chlorpheniramine Maleate USP—White, odorless, crystalline powder. Its solutions have a pH between 4 and 5.
Phenyltoloxamine citrate—It has a melting point of 138–140 °C.
Phenylpropanolamine Hydrochloride USP—White, crystalline powder, having a slight aromatic odor. Is affected by light.
Dextromethorphan Hydrobromide USP—Practically white crystals or crystalline powder, having a faint odor. Melts at about 126 °C, with decomposition.
Guaifenesin USP—White to slightly gray, crystalline powder. May have a slight characteristic odor.

pKa:
Chlorpheniramine—9.2.
Phenylpropanolamine hydrochloride—9.

Solubility:
Chlorpheniramine Maleate USP—Freely soluble in water; soluble in alcohol and in chloroform; slightly soluble in ether.
Phenyltoloxamine citrate—Soluble in water.
Phenylpropanolamine Hydrochloride USP—Freely soluble in water and in alcohol; insoluble in ether.
Dextromethorphan Hydrobromide USP—Sparingly soluble in water; freely soluble in alcohol and in chloroform; insoluble in ether.
Guaifenesin USP—Soluble in water, in alcohol, in chloroform, in glycerin, and in propylene glycol.

USP requirements: Chlorpheniramine Maleate, Phenyltoloxamine Citrate, Phenylpropanolamine Hydrochloride, Dextromethorphan Hydrobromide, and Guaifenesin Syrup—Not in USP.

CHLORPHENIRAMINE AND PSEUDOEPHEDRINE

For *Chlorpheniramine* and *Pseudoephedrine*—See individual listings for chemistry information.

USP requirements:
Chlorpheniramine Maleate and Pseudoephedrine Hydrochloride Capsules—Not in USP.
Chlorpheniramine Maleate and Pseudoephedrine Hydrochloride Extended-release Capsules—Not in USP.
Chlorpheniramine Maleate and Pseudoephedrine Hydrochloride Oral Solution—Not in USP.
Chlorpheniramine Maleate and Pseudoephedrine Sulfate Tablets—Not in USP.
Chlorpheniramine Maleate and Pseudoephedrine Sulfate Extended-release Tablets—Not in USP.

CHLORPHENIRAMINE, PSEUDOEPHEDRINE, AND ACETAMINOPHEN

For *Chlorpheniramine, Pseudoephedrine,* and *Acetaminophen*—See individual listings for chemistry information.

USP requirements:
Chlorpheniramine Maleate, Pseudoephedrine Hydrochloride, and Acetaminophen Capsules—Not in USP.
Chlorpheniramine Maleate, Pseudoephedrine Hydrochloride, and Acetaminophen Oral Solution—Not in USP.
Chlorpheniramine Maleate, Pseudoephedrine Hydrochloride, and Acetaminophen for Oral Solution—Not in USP.
Chlorpheniramine Maleate, Pseudoephedrine Hydrochloride, and Acetaminophen Tablets—Not in USP.
Chlorpheniramine Maleate, Pseudoephedrine Hydrochloride, and Acetaminophen Chewable Tablets—Not in USP.

CHLORPHENIRAMINE, PSEUDOEPHEDRINE, AND CODEINE

For *Chlorpheniramine, Pseudoephedrine,* and *Codeine*—See individual listings for chemistry information.

USP requirements:
Chlorpheniramine Maleate, Pseudoephedrine Hydrochloride, and Codeine Phosphate Elixir—Not in USP.

Chlorpheniramine Maleate, Pseudoephedrine Hydrochloride, and Codeine Phosphate Oral Solution—Not in USP.

CHLORPHENIRAMINE, PSEUDOEPHEDRINE, AND DEXTROMETHORPHAN

For *Chlorpheniramine, Pseudoephedrine,* and *Dextromethorphan*—See individual listings for chemistry information.

USP requirements:
Chlorpheniramine Maleate, Pseudoephedrine Hydrochloride, and Dextromethorphan Hydrobromide Oral Solution—Not in USP.
Chlorpheniramine Maleate, Pseudoephedrine Hydrochloride, and Dextromethorphan Hydrobromide Syrup—Not in USP.
Chlorpheniramine Maleate, Pseudoephedrine Hydrochloride, and Dextromethorphan Hydrobromide Chewable Tablets—Not in USP.

CHLORPHENIRAMINE, PSEUDOEPHEDRINE, DEXTROMETHORPHAN, AND ACETAMINOPHEN

For *Chlorpheniramine, Pseudoephedrine, Dextromethorphan,* and *Acetaminophen*—See individual listings for chemistry information.

USP requirements:
Chlorpheniramine Maleate, Pseudoephedrine Hydrochloride, Dextromethorphan Hydrobromide, and Acetaminophen Capsules—Not in USP.
Chlorpheniramine Maleate, Pseudoephedrine Hydrochloride, Dextromethorphan Hydrobromide, and Acetaminophen Oral Solution—Not in USP.
Chlorpheniramine Maleate, Pseudoephedrine Hydrochloride, Dextromethorphan Hydrobromide, and Acetaminophen for Oral Solution—Not in USP.
Chlorpheniramine Maleate, Pseudoephedrine Hydrochloride, Dextromethorphan Hydrobromide, and Acetaminophen Tablets—Not in USP.

CHLORPHENIRAMINE, PSEUDOEPHEDRINE, DEXTROMETHORPHAN, GUAIFENESIN, AND ASPIRIN

For *Chlorpheniramine, Pseudoephedrine, Dextromethorphan, Guaifenesin,* and *Aspirin*—See individual listings for chemistry information.

USP requirements: Chlorpheniramine Maleate, Pseudoephedrine Hydrochloride, Dextromethorphan Hydrobromide, Guaifenesin, and Aspirin Tablets—Not in USP.

CHLORPHENIRAMINE, PSEUDOEPHEDRINE, AND GUAIFENESIN

For *Chlorpheniramine, Pseudoephedrine,* and *Guaifenesin*—See individual listings for chemistry information.

USP requirements: Chlorpheniramine Maleate, Pseudoephedrine Hydrochloride, and Guaifenesin Extended-release Tablets—Not in USP.

CHLORPHENIRAMINE, PSEUDOEPHEDRINE, AND HYDROCODONE

For *Chlorpheniramine, Pseudoephedrine,* and *Hydrocodone*—See individual listings for chemistry information.

USP requirements: Chlorpheniramine Maleate, Pseudoephedrine Hydrochloride, and Hydrocodone Bitartrate Oral Solution—Not in USP.

CHLORPHENIRAMINE, PYRILAMINE, AND PHENYLEPHRINE

Chemical group: Chlorpheniramine maleate—Alkylamine derivative.

Description: Chlorpheniramine tannate—Light tan to buff or yellowish-tan, amorphous, fine powder having not more than a slight characteristic odor.

Solubility: Chlorpheniramine tannate—Slightly soluble in water at 25 °C.

USP requirements:
Chlorpheniramine Tannate, Pyrilamine Tannate, and Phenylephrine Tannate Oral Suspension—Not in USP.
Chlorpheniramine Tannate, Pyrilamine Tannate, and Phenylephrine Tannate Tablets—Not in USP.
Chlorpheniramine Tannate, Pyrilamine Tannate, and Phenylephrine Tannate Extended-release Tablets—Not in USP.

CHLORPHENIRAMINE, PYRILAMINE, PHENYLEPHRINE, AND ACETAMINOPHEN

For *Chlorpheniramine, Pyrilamine, Phenylephrine,* and *Acetaminophen*—See individual listings for chemistry information.

USP requirements: Chlorpheniramine Maleate, Pyrilamine Maleate, Phenylephrine Hydrochloride, and Acetaminophen Tablets—Not in USP.

CHLORPHENIRAMINE, PYRILAMINE, PHENYLEPHRINE, AND PHENYLPROPANOLAMINE

For *Chlorpheniramine, Pyrilamine, Phenylephrine,* and *Phenylpropanolamine*—See individual listings for chemistry information.

USP requirements: Chlorpheniramine Maleate, Pyrilamine Maleate, Phenylephrine Hydrochloride, and Phenylpropanolamine Hydrochloride Tablets—Not in USP.

CHLORPHENIRAMINE, PYRILAMINE, PHENYLEPHRINE, PHENYLPROPANOLAMINE, AND ACETAMINOPHEN

For *Chlorpheniramine, Pyrilamine, Phenylephrine, Phenylpropanolamine,* and *Acetaminophen*—See individual listings for chemistry information.

USP requirements: Chlorpheniramine Maleate, Pyrilamine Maleate, Phenylephrine Hydrochloride, Phenylpropanolamine Hydrochloride, and Acetaminophen Tablets—Not in USP.

CHLORPROMAZINE

Chemical group: Aliphatic phenothiazine.

Chemical name:
Chlorpromazine—10*H*-Phenothiazine-10-propanamine, 2-chloro-*N,N*-dimethyl-.
Chlorpromazine hydrochloride—10*H*-Phenothiazine-10-propanamine, 2-chloro-*N,N*-dimethyl-, monohydrochloride.

Molecular formula:
Chlorpromazine—$C_{17}H_{19}ClN_2S$.
Chlorpromazine hydrochloride—$C_{17}H_{19}ClN_2S \cdot HCl$.

Molecular weight:
Chlorpromazine—318.86.
Chlorpromazine hydrochloride—355.33.

Description:
Chlorpromazine USP—White, crystalline solid, having an amine-like odor. Darkens on prolonged exposure to light. Melts at about 60 °C.

Chlorpromazine Hydrochloride USP—White or slightly creamy white, odorless, crystalline powder. Darkens on prolonged exposure to light.

Solubility:
Chlorpromazine USP—Practically insoluble in water and in dilute alkali hydroxides; freely soluble in alcohol, in chloroform, in ether, and in dilute mineral acids.
Chlorpromazine Hydrochloride USP—Very soluble in water; freely soluble in alcohol and in chloroform; insoluble in ether.

USP requirements:
Chlorpromazine USP—Preserve in tight, light-resistant containers. Contains not less than 98.0% and not more than 101.0% of chlorpromazine, calculated on the dried basis. Meets the requirements for Identification, Loss on drying (not more than 1.0%), Other alkylated phenothiazines, and Organic volatile impurities.
Chlorpromazine Suppositories USP—Preserve in well-closed, light-resistant containers, at controlled room temperature. Contain the labeled amount, within ±10%. Meet the requirements for Identification and Other alkylated phenothiazines.
Chlorpromazine Hydrochloride USP—Preserve in tight, light-resistant containers. Contains not less than 98.0% and not more than 101.5% of chlorpromazine hydrochloride, calculated on the dried basis. Meets the requirements for Identification, Melting range (195–198 °C), Loss on drying (not more than 0.5%), Residue on ignition (not more than 0.1%), Other alkylated phenothiazines, and Organic volatile impurities.
Chlorpromazine Hydrochloride Extended-release Capsules—Not in USP.
Chlorpromazine Hydrochloride Oral Concentrate USP—Preserve in tight, light-resistant containers. Label it to indicate that it must be diluted prior to administration. Contains the labeled amount, within ±10%. Meets the requirements for Identification, Microbial limits, pH (2.3–4.1), and Chlorpromazine sulfoxide.
Chlorpromazine Hydrochloride Injection USP—Preserve in single-dose or in multiple-dose containers, preferably of Type I glass, protected from light. A sterile solution of Chlorpromazine Hydrochloride in Water for Injection. Contains, in each mL, not less than 23.75 mg and not more than 26.25 mg of chlorpromazine hydrochloride. Meets the requirements for Identification, Bacterial endotoxins, pH (3.4–5.4), Injections, and Chlorpromazine sulfoxide.
Chlorpromazine Hydrochloride Syrup USP—Preserve in tight, light-resistant containers. Contains, in each 100 mL, not less than 190 mg and not more than 210 mg of chlorpromazine hydrochloride. Meets the requirement for Identification and Chlorpromazine sulfoxide.
Chlorpromazine Hydrochloride Tablets USP—Preserve in well-closed, light-resistant containers. Contain the labeled amount, within ±5%. Meet the requirements for Identification, Dissolution (80% in 30 minutes in 0.1 *N* hydrochloric acid in Apparatus 1 at 50 rpm), Uniformity of dosage units, and Other alkylated phenothiazines.

CHLORPROPAMIDE

Chemical group: Sulfonylurea.

Chemical name: Benzenesulfonamide, 4-chloro-*N*-[(propylamino)carbonyl]-.

Molecular formula: $C_{10}H_{13}ClN_2O_3S$.

Molecular weight: 276.74.

Description: Chlorpropamide USP—White, crystalline powder, having a slight odor.

pKa: 4.8.

Solubility: Chlorpropamide USP—Practically insoluble in water; soluble in alcohol; sparingly soluble in chloroform.

USP requirements:
Chlorpropamide USP—Preserve in well-closed containers. Contains not less than 97.0% and not more than 103.0% of chlorpropamide, calculated on the dried basis. Meets the requirements for Identification, Melting range (126–129 °C), Loss on drying (not more than 1.0%), Selenium (not more than 0.003%), Heavy metals (not more than 0.003%), and Residue on ignition (not more than 0.4%).
Chlorpropamide Tablets USP—Preserve in well-closed containers. Contain the labeled amount, within ±10%. Meet the requirements for Identification, Dissolution (75% in 60 minutes in water in Apparatus 2 at 50 rpm), and Uniformity of dosage units.

CHLORPROTHIXENE

Chemical group: Thioxanthene derivative with general properties similar to those of the phenothiazine.

Chemical name: 1-Propanamine, 3-(2-chloro-9*H*-thioxanthen-9-ylidene)-*N*,*N*-dimethyl-, (*Z*)-.

Molecular formula: $C_{18}H_{18}ClNS$.

Molecular weight: 315.86.

Description: Chlorprothixene USP—Yellow, crystalline powder, having a slight amine-like odor.

Solubility: Chlorprothixene USP—Practically insoluble in water; soluble in alcohol and in ether; freely soluble in chloroform.

USP requirements:
Chlorprothixene USP—Preserve in tight, light-resistant containers. Contains not less than 99.0% and not more than 101.0% of chlorprothixene, calculated on the dried basis. Meets the requirements for Identification, Melting range (96.5–101.5 °C), Loss on drying (not more than 0.1%), Residue on ignition (not more than 0.1%), Heavy metals (not more than 0.002%), Limit of (*E*)-chlorprothixene [(*E*)-2-chloro-*N*,*N*-dimethylthioxanthene-Delta$^{9, gamma}$-propylamine (not more than 3.0%), and Organic volatile impurities.
Chlorprothixene Injection USP—Preserve in single-dose, low-actinic containers, protected from light. A sterile solution of Chlorprothixene in Water for Injection, prepared with the aid of Hydrochloric Acid. Contains the labeled amount, within ±5%. Meets the requirements for Identification, Bacterial endotoxins, pH (3.0–4.0), and Injections.
Chlorprothixene Oral Suspension USP—Preserve in tight, light-resistant containers. Contains the labeled amount, within ±10%. Meets the requirements for Identification and pH (3.5–4.5).
Chlorprothixene Tablets USP—Preserve in well-closed, light-resistant containers. Contain the labeled amount, within ±7%. Meet the requirements for Identification, Dissolution (75% in 30 minutes in 0.1 *N* hydrochloric acid in Apparatus 1 at 100 rpm), and Uniformity of dosage units.

CHLORTETRACYCLINE

Chemical name: Chlortetracycline hydrochloride—2-Naphthacenecarboxamide, 7-chloro-4-(dimethylamino)-1,4,4a,5,5a,-6,11,12a-octahydro-3,6,10,12,12a-pentahydroxy-6-methyl-1,11-dioxo-, monohydrochloride [4*S*-(4 alpha,4a alpha,5a alpha,6 beta,12a alpha)]-.

Molecular formula: Chlortetracycline hydrochloride—$C_{22}H_{23}ClN_2O_8 \cdot HCl$.

Molecular weight: Chlortetracycline hydrochloride—515.35.

Description: Chlortetracycline Hydrochloride USP—Yellow, crystalline powder. Is odorless. Is stable in air, but is slowly affected by light.

Solubility: Chlortetracycline Hydrochloride USP—Sparingly soluble in water; soluble in solutions of alkali hydroxides and carbonates; slightly soluble in alcohol; practically insoluble in acetone, in chloroform, in dioxane, and in ether.

USP requirements:

Chlortetracycline Bisulfate USP—Preserve in tight, light-resistant containers. Label it to indicate that it is intended for veterinary use only. Has a potency equivalent to not less than 760 mcg of chlortetracycline hydrochloride per mg, calculated on the dried and butyl alcohol-free basis. Meets the requirements for Identification, Crystallinity, Loss on drying (not more than 2.0%), Sulfate content (not less than 15.0%, calculated on the dried and butyl alcohol-free basis), and Butyl alcohol (not more than 15.0%).

Chlortetracycline Hydrochloride USP—Preserve in tight, light-resistant containers. Has a potency of not less than 900 mcg of chlortetracycline hydrochloride per mg. Meets the requirements for Identification, Specific rotation (−235° to −250°, calculated on the dried basis), Crystallinity, pH (2.3–3.3, in a solution containing 10 mg per mL), and Loss on drying (not more than 2.0%).

Note: Chlortetracycline Hydrochloride labeled solely for use in preparing oral veterinary dosage forms has a potency of not less than 820 mcg of chlortetracycline hydrochloride per mg.

Chlortetracycline Hydrochloride Capsules USP—Preserve in tight, light-resistant containers. Contain the labeled amount, within −10% to +20%. Meet the requirements for Identification, Dissolution (75% in 45 minutes in water in Apparatus 2 at 75 rpm), Uniformity of dosage units, and Loss on drying (not more than 1.0%).

Chlortetracycline Hydrochloride Ointment USP—Preserve in collapsible tubes or in well-closed, light-resistant containers. Contains the labeled amount, within −10% to +25%, in a suitable ointment base. Meets the requirements for Water (not more than 0.5%) and Minimum fill.

Chlortetracycline Hydrochloride Ophthalmic Ointment USP—Preserve in collapsible ophthalmic ointment tubes. Contains the labeled amount, within −10% to +25%. Meets the requirements for Sterility, Minimum fill, Water (not more than 0.5%), and Metal particles.

Chlortetracycline Hydrochloride Soluble Powder USP—Preserve in tight containers, protected from light. Label it to indicate that it is intended for oral veterinary use only. Contains the labeled amount, within −10% to +25%. Meets the requirement for Loss on drying (not more than 2.0%).

Sterile Chlortetracycline Hydrochloride USP—Preserve in Containers for Sterile Solids. It is Chlortetracycline Hydrochloride suitable for parenteral use. Has a potency of not less than 900 mcg of chlortetracycline hydrochloride per mg. Meets the requirements for Depressor substances, Bacterial endotoxins, and Sterility, and for Identification tests, pH, Specific rotation, Loss on drying, and Crystallinity under Chlortetracycline Hydrochloride.

Chlortetracycline Hydrochloride Tablets USP—Preserve in tight containers, protected from light. Label Tablets to indicate that they are intended for veterinary use only. Contain the labeled amount, within −10% to +20%. Meet the requirements for Identification, Disintegration (1 hour, with simulated gastric fluid TS being used as the test medium instead of water), Uniformity of dosage units, and Water (not more than 3.0%, or where the Tablets have a diameter of greater than 15 mm, not more than 6.0%).

CHLORTETRACYCLINE AND SULFAMETHAZINE

USP requirements: Chlortetracycline and Sulfamethazine Bisulfates Soluble Powder USP—Preserve in tight, light-resistant containers. A dry mixture of Chlortetracycline Bisulfate and Sulfamethazine Bisulfate and one or more suitable buffers and diluents. Label it to indicate that it is intended for veterinary use only. Contains amounts of chlortetracycline and sulfamethazine bisulfates equivalent to the labeled amounts of chlortetracycline hydrochloride and sulfamethazine, within −15% to +25%. Meets the requirement for Loss on drying (not more than 2.0%).

CHLORTHALIDONE

Chemical name: Benzenesulfonamide, 2-chloro-5-(2,3-dihydro-1-hydroxy-3-oxo-1*H*-isoindol-1-yl)-.

Molecular formula: $C_{14}H_{11}ClN_2O_4S$.

Molecular weight: 338.77.

Description: Chlorthalidone USP—White to yellowish white, crystalline powder. Melts at a temperature above 215 °C, with decomposition.

pKa: 9.4.

Solubility: Chlorthalidone USP—Practically insoluble in water, in ether, and in chloroform; soluble in methanol; slightly soluble in alcohol.

USP requirements:

Chlorthalidone USP—Preserve in well-closed containers. Contains not less than 98.0% and not more than 102.0% of chlorthalidone, calculated on the dried basis. Meets the requirements for Identification, Loss on drying (not more than 0.4%), Residue on ignition (not more than 0.1%), Chloride (not more than 0.035%), Heavy metals (not more than 0.001%), and Limit of 4′-chloro-3′-sulfamoyl-2-benzophenone carboxylic acid (CCA) (not more than 1.0%).

Chlorthalidone Tablets USP—Preserve in well-closed containers. Contain the labeled amount, within ±8%. Meet the requirements for Identification, Dissolution (50% in 60 minutes in water in Apparatus 2 at 100 rpm), and Uniformity of dosage units.

CHLORZOXAZONE

Chemical name: 2(3*H*)-Benzoxazolone, 5-chloro-.

Molecular formula: $C_7H_4ClNO_2$.

Molecular weight: 169.57.

Description: Chlorzoxazone USP—White or practically white, practically odorless, crystalline powder.

Solubility: Chlorzoxazone USP—Slightly soluble in water; sparingly soluble in alcohol, in isopropyl alcohol, and in methanol; soluble in solutions of alkali hydroxides and ammonia.

USP requirements:

Chlorzoxazone USP—Preserve in tight containers. Contains not less than 98.0% and not more than 102.0% of chlorzoxazone, calculated on the dried basis. Meets the requirements for Identification, Melting range (189–194 °C), Loss on drying (not more than 0.5%), Heavy metals (not more than 0.002%), Residue on ignition (not more than 0.15%), Chromatographic impurities, Chlorine content (20.6–21.2%, calculated on the dried basis), and Organic volatile impurities.

Chlorzoxazone Tablets USP—Preserve in tight containers. Contain the labeled amount, within ±10%. Meet the requirements for Identification, Dissolution (75% in 60 minutes in phosphate buffer [pH 8.0] in Apparatus 2 at 75 rpm), and Uniformity of dosage units.

CHLORZOXAZONE AND ACETAMINOPHEN

For *Chlorzoxazone* and *Acetaminophen*—See individual listings for chemistry information.

USP requirements: Chlorzoxazone and Acetaminophen Tablets—Not in USP.

CHOLECALCIFEROL

Chemical name: 9,10-Secocholesta-5,7,10(19)-trien-3-ol, (3 beta,-5*Z*,7*E*)-.

Molecular formula: $C_{27}H_{44}O$.

Molecular weight: 384.64.

Description: Cholecalciferol USP—White, odorless crystals. Is affected by air and by light. Melts at about 85 °C.

Solubility: Cholecalciferol USP—Insoluble in water; soluble in alcohol, in chloroform, and in fatty oils.

USP requirements: Cholecalciferol USP—Preserve in hermetically sealed containers under nitrogen, in a cool place and protected from light. Contains not less than 97.0% and not more than 103.0% of cholecalciferol. Meets the requirements for Identification and Specific rotation (+105° to +112°).

CHOLERA VACCINE

Description: Cholera Vaccine USP—Practically water-clear liquid to milky suspension, nearly odorless or having a faint odor because of the antimicrobial agent.

USP requirements: Cholera Vaccine USP—Preserve at a temperature between 2 and 8 °C. A sterile suspension, in Sodium Chloride Injection or other suitable diluent, of killed cholera vibrios (*Vibrio cholerae*) of a strain or strains selected for high antigenic efficiency, shown to yield a vaccine not less potent than vaccines prepared from Inaba strain 35A3 and Ogawa strain 41. Prepared from equal portions of suspensions of cholera vibrios of the Inaba and Ogawa strains. Label it to state that it is to be well shaken before use and that it is not to be frozen. Has a labeled potency of 8 units per serotype per mL. Its potency, determined by the specific mouse potency test based on the U.S. Standard Cholera Vaccines for the respective serotypes, is not less than 4.4 units per serotype per mL. Contains a suitable antimicrobial agent. Meets the requirements of the specific mouse toxicity test and of the test for nitrogen content, and for Expiration date (not later than 18 months after date of issue from manufacturer's cold storage [5 °C, 1 year]). Conforms to the regulations of the U.S. Food and Drug Administration concerning biologics.

CHOLESTEROL

Chemical name: Cholest-5-en-3-ol, (3 beta)-.

Molecular formula: $C_{27}H_{46}O$.

Molecular weight: 386.66.

Description: Cholesterol NF—White or faintly yellow, practically odorless, pearly leaflets, needles, powder, or granules. Acquires a yellow to pale tan color on prolonged exposure to light.

NF category: Emulsifying and/or solubilizing agent.

Solubility: Cholesterol NF—Insoluble in water; soluble in acetone, in chloroform, in dioxane, in ether, in ethyl acetate, in solvent hexane, and in vegetable oils; sparingly soluble in dehydrated alcohol; slightly (and slowly) soluble in alcohol.

NF requirements: Cholesterol NF—Preserve in well-closed, light-resistant containers. A steroid alcohol used as an emulsifying agent. Meets the requirements for Solubility in alcohol, Identification, Melting range (147–150 °C), Specific rotation (−34° to −38°), Acidity, Loss on drying (not more than 0.3%), and Residue on ignition (not more than 0.1%).

CHOLESTYRAMINE

Chemical name: Cholestyramine resin—Cholestyramine.

Description: Cholestyramine Resin USP—White to buff-colored, hygroscopic, fine powder. Is odorless or has not more than a slight amine-like odor.

Solubility: Cholestyramine Resin USP—Insoluble in water, in alcohol, in chloroform, and in ether.

USP requirements:

Cholestyramine Resin USP—Preserve in tight containers. A strongly basic anion-exchange resin in the chloride form, consisting of styrene-divinylbenzene copolymer with quaternary ammonium functional groups. Each gram exchanges not less than 1.8 grams and not more than 2.2 grams of sodium glycocholate, calculated on the dried basis. Meets the requirements for Identification, pH (4.0–6.0, in a slurry [1 in 100]), Loss on drying (not more than 12.0%), Residue on ignition (not more than 0.1%), Heavy metals (not more than 0.002%), Dialyzable quaternary amines, Chloride content (13.0–17.0%, calculated on the dried basis), and Exchange capacity.

Cholestyramine Chewable Bar—Not in USP.

Cholestyramine for Oral Suspension USP—Preserve in tight containers. A mixture of Cholestyramine Resin with suitable excipients and coloring and flavoring agents. Contains the labeled amount of dried cholestyramine resin, within ±15%. Meets the requirements for Identification, Uniformity of dosage units, and Loss on drying (not more than 12.0%).

CHOLINE SALICYLATE

Chemical name: (2-Hydroxyethyl)trimethylammonium salicylate.

Molecular formula: $C_{12}H_{19}NO_4$.

Molecular weight: 241.29.

Description: White, hygroscopic solid with a melting point of about 50 °C.

Solubility: Freely soluble in water; soluble in most hydrophilic solvents; insoluble in organic solvents.

USP requirements: Choline Salicylate Oral Solution—Not in USP.

CHOLINE SALICYLATE AND CETYL-DIMETHYL-BENZYL-AMMONIUM CHLORIDE

Chemical name: Choline salicylate—(2-Hydroxyethyl)trimethylammonium salicylate.

Molecular formula: Choline salicylate—$C_{12}H_{19}NO_4$.

Molecular weight: Choline salicylate—241.29.

Description: Choline salicylate—White, hygroscopic solid with a melting point of about 50 °C.

Solubility: Choline salicylate—Freely soluble in water; soluble in most hydrophilic solvents; insoluble in organic solvents.

USP requirements: Choline Salicylate and Cetyl-dimethyl-benzyl-ammonium Chloride Gel—Not in USP.

CHOLINE AND MAGNESIUM SALICYLATES

For *Choline Salicylate* and *Magnesium Salicylate*—See individual listings for chemistry information.

USP requirements:

Choline and Magnesium Salicylates Oral Solution—Not in USP.

Choline and Magnesium Salicylates Tablets—Not in USP.

SODIUM CHROMATE Cr 51

Chemical name: Chromic acid ($H_2{}^{51}CrO_4$), disodium salt.

Molecular formula: $Na_2{}^{51}CrO_4$.

Description: Sodium Chromate Cr 51 Injection USP—Clear, slightly yellow solution.

USP requirements: Sodium Chromate Cr 51 Injection USP—Preserve in single-dose or in multiple-dose containers. A sterile solution of radioactive chromium (^{51}Cr) processed in the form of sodium chromate in Water for Injection. For those uses where an isotonic solution is required, Sodium Chloride may be added in appropriate amounts. Chromium 51 is produced by the neutron bombardment of enriched chromium 50. Label it to include the following, in addition to the information specified for Labeling under Injections: the time and date of calibration; the amount of sodium chromate expressed in mcg per mL; the amount of ^{51}Cr as sodium chromate expressed as total megabecquerels (or millicuries) and as megabecquerels (or millicuries) per mL at the time of calibration; a statement to indicate whether the contents are intended for diagnostic or therapeutic use; the expiration date; and the statement, "Caution—Radioactive Material." The labeling indicates that in making dosage calculations, correction is to be made for radioactive decay and the quantity of chromium, and also indicates that the radioactive half-life of ^{51}Cr is 27.8 days. Contains the labeled amount of ^{51}Cr, within ±10%, as sodium chromate expressed in megabecquerels (or millicuries) per mL at the time indicated in the labeling. The sodium chromate content is not less than 90.0% and not more than 110.0% of the labeled amount. The specific activity is not less than 370 megabecquerels (10 millicuries) per mg of sodium chromate at the end of the expiry period. Other chemical forms of radioactivity do not exceed 10.0% of the total radioactivity. Meets the requirements for Radionuclide identification, Bacterial endotoxins, pH (7.5–8.5), Radiochemical purity, and Injections (except that it is not subject to the recommendation on Volume in Container).

CHROMIC CHLORIDE

Chemical name: Chromium chloride ($CrCl_3$) hexahydrate.

Molecular formula: $CrCl_3 \cdot 6H_2O$.

Molecular weight: 266.45.

Description: Chromic Chloride USP—Dark green, odorless, slightly deliquescent crystals.

Solubility: Chromic Chloride USP—Soluble in water and in alcohol; slightly soluble in acetone; practically insoluble in ether.

USP requirements:

Chromic Chloride USP—Preserve in tight containers. Contains not less than 98.0% and not more than 101.0% of chromic chloride. Meets the requirements for Identification, Insoluble matter (not more than 0.01%), Substances not precipitated by ammonium hydroxide (not more than 0.20% as sulfate), Sulfate (not more than 0.01%), and Iron (not more than 0.01%).

Chromic Chloride Injection USP—Preserve in single-dose or in multiple-dose containers, preferably of Type I or Type II glass. A sterile solution of Chromic Chloride in Water for Injection. Label the Injection to indicate that it is to be diluted to the appropriate strength with Sterile Water for Injection or other suitable fluid prior to administration. Contains an amount of chromic chloride equivalent to the labeled amount of chromium, within ±10%. Meets the requirements for Identification, Bacterial endotoxins, pH (1.5–2.5), and Injections.

CHROMIUM

Molecular formula: Cr.

Molecular weight: 52 (elemental).

Description: Steel-gray, lustrous metal. Melting point 1900 °C.

USP requirements: Chromium Tablets—Not in USP.

CHYMOPAPAIN

Source: A proteolytic enzyme isolated from the crude latex of *Carica papaya*, differing from papain in electrophoretic mobility, solubility, and substrate specificity.

Chemical name: Chymopapain.

Molecular weight: Approximately 27,000.

USP requirements: Chymopapain for Injection—Not in USP.

CHYMOTRYPSIN

Chemical name: Chymotrypsin.

Description: Chymotrypsin USP—White to yellowish white, crystalline or amorphous, odorless, powder.

Solubility: Chymotrypsin USP—An amount equivalent to 100,000 USP Units is soluble in 10 mL of water and in 10 mL of saline TS.

USP requirements:

Chymotrypsin USP—Preserve in tight containers, and avoid exposure to excessive heat. A proteolytic enzyme crystallized from an extract of the pancreas gland of the ox, *Bos taurus* Linné (Fam. Bovidae). Contains not less than 1000 USP Chymotrypsin Units in each mg, calculated on the dried basis, and not less than 90.0% and not more than 110.0% of the labeled potency, as determined by the *Assay*. Meets the requirements for Microbial limits, Loss on drying (not more than 5.0%), Residue on ignition (not more than 2.5%), and Trypsin (not more than 1.0%).

Chymotrypsin for Ophthalmic Solution USP—Preserve in single-dose containers, preferably of Type I glass, and avoid exposure to excessive heat. It is sterile Chymotrypsin. When constituted as directed in the labeling, yields a solution containing the labeled potency, within ±20%. Meets the requirements for Completeness of solution,

Identification, pH (4.3–8.7, in the solution constituted as directed in the labeling), and Uniformity of dosage units, for the test for Trypsin under Chymotrypsin, and for Sterility tests.

CICLOPIROX

Chemical group: Synthetic pyridinone derivative; chemically unrelated to the imidazole.

Chemical name: Ciclopirox olamine—2(1*H*)-Pyridinone, 6-cyclohexyl-1-hydroxy-4-methyl-, compd. with 2-aminoethanol (1:1).

Molecular formula: Ciclopirox olamine—$C_{12}H_{17}NO_2 \cdot C_2H_7NO$.

Molecular weight: Ciclopirox olamine—268.36.

Description: Ciclopirox olamine—White to pale yellow crystalline powder.

Solubility: Ciclopirox olamine—Soluble in methanol.

Other characteristics: Ciclopirox olamine—1% cream has a pH of 7.

USP requirements:

Ciclopirox Olamine USP—Preserve in well-closed containers. Contains not less than 98.0% and not more than 102.0% of ciclopirox olamine, calculated on the dried basis. Meets the requirements for Identification, Loss on drying (not more than 1.5%), Residue on ignition (not more than 0.1%), Heavy metals (not more than 0.002%), pH (8.0–9.0, in a solution [1 in 100]), and Monoethanolamine content (223–230 mg per gram of ciclopirox olamine, calculated on the anhydrous basis).

Ciclopirox Olamine Cream USP—Preserve in collapsible tubes, at controlled room temperature. Contains the labeled amount, within ±10%. Meets the requirements for Identification, Minimum fill, pH (5.0–8.0), and Benzyl alcohol content (if present, within ±10% of claimed amount).

Ciclopirox Olamine Lotion—Not in USP.

Ciclopirox Olamine Topical Suspension USP—Preserve in tight containers. Contains the labeled amount, within ±10%. Meets the requirements for Identification, Minimum fill, pH (5.0–8.0), and Benzyl alcohol content (if present, within ±10% of claimed amount).

CILASTATIN

Chemical name: Cilastatin sodium—2-Heptenoic acid, 7-[(2-amino-2-carboxyethyl)thio]-2-[[(2,2-dimethylcyclopropyl)carbonyl]amino]-, monosodium salt, [*R*-[*R**,*S**(*Z*)]]-.

Molecular formula: Cilastatin sodium—$C_{16}H_{25}N_2NaO_5S$.

Molecular weight: Cilastatin sodium—380.43.

Description: Cilastatin Sodium USP—White to tan-colored powder.

Solubility: Cilastatin Sodium USP—Soluble in water and in methanol.

USP requirements: Sterile Cilastatin Sodium USP—Preserve in Containers for Sterile Solids, and store in a cold place. It is cilastatin sodium suitable for parenteral use. Contains not less than 98.0% and not more than 101.5% of cilastatin sodium, calculated on the anhydrous and solvent-free basis. Meets the requirements for Identification, Bacterial endotoxins, Sterility, pH (6.5–7.5, in a solution [1 in 100]), Specific rotation (+41.5° to +44.5°, calculated on the anhydrous and solvent-free basis), Water (not more than 2.0%), Heavy metals (not more than 0.002%), Solvents (not more than 1.0% of acetone, 0.5% of methanol, and 0.4% of mesityl oxide), and Chromatographic purity.

CIMETIDINE

Chemical group: Imidazole derivative of histamine.

Chemical name:

Cimetidine—Guanidine, *N″*-cyano-*N*-methyl-*N′*-[2-[[(5-methyl-1*H*-imidazol-4-yl)methyl]thio]ethyl]-.

Cimetidine hydrochloride—Guanidine, *N″*-cyano-*N*-methyl-*N′*-[2-[[(5-methyl-1*H*-imidazol-4-yl)methyl]thio]ethyl]-, monohydrochloride.

Molecular formula:

Cimetidine—$C_{10}H_{16}N_6S$.

Cimetidine hydrochloride—$C_{10}H_{16}N_6S \cdot HCl$.

Molecular weight:

Cimetidine—252.34.

Cimetidine hydrochloride—288.80.

Description:

Cimetidine USP—White to off-white, crystalline powder; odorless, or having a slight mercaptan odor.

Cimetidine hydrochloride—White crystalline powder.

pKa:

Cimetidine—6.8.

Cimetidine hydrochloride—7.11.

Solubility:

Cimetidine USP—Soluble in alcohol and in polyethylene glycol 400; freely soluble in methanol; sparingly soluble in isopropyl alcohol; slightly soluble in water and in chloroform; practically insoluble in ether.

Cimetidine hydrochloride—Freely soluble in water; soluble in alcohol; very slightly soluble in chloroform; and practically insoluble in ether.

USP requirements:

Cimetidine USP—Preserve in tight, light-resistant containers. Contains not less than 98.0% and not more than 102.0% of cimetidine, calculated on the dried basis. Meets the requirements for Identification, Melting range (139–144 °C), Loss on drying (not more than 1.0%), Residue on ignition (not more than 0.2%), Heavy metals (not more than 0.002%), and Chromatographic purity.

Cimetidine Tablets USP—Preserve in tight, light-resistant containers, at controlled room temperature. Contain the labeled amount, within ±10%. Meet the requirements for Identification, Dissolution (75% in 15 minutes in water in Apparatus 1 at 100 rpm), and Uniformity of dosage units.

Cimetidine Hydrochloride Injection—Not in USP.

Cimetidine Hydrochloride Oral Solution—Not in USP.

CINOXACIN

Chemical group: Similar in chemical structure to nalidixic acid and oxolinic acid.

Chemical name: [1,3]Dioxolo[4,5-*g*]cinnoline-3-carboxylic acid, 1-ethyl-1,4-dihydro-4-oxo-.

Molecular formula: $C_{12}H_{10}N_2O_5$.

Molecular weight: 262.22.

Description: Cinoxacin USP—White to yellowish white, crystalline solid. Is odorless.

Solubility: Cinoxacin USP—Insoluble in water and in most common organic solvents; soluble in alkaline solution.

USP requirements:

Cinoxacin USP—Preserve in tight containers. Contains not less than 97.0% and not more than 102.0% of cinoxacin, calculated on the dried basis. Meets the requirements for Identification, Loss on drying (not more than 1.0%), and Related substances (not more than 1.0%).

Cinoxacin Capsules USP—Preserve in well-closed containers. Contain the labeled amount, within ± 10%. Meet the requirements for Identification, Dissolution (60% in 30 minutes in phosphate buffer [pH 6.5] in Apparatus 1 at 100 rpm), and Uniformity of dosage units.

CINOXATE

Chemical name: Propenoic acid, 3-(4-methoxyphenyl)-, 2-ethoxyethyl ester.

Molecular formula: $C_{14}H_{18}O_4$.

Molecular weight: 250.29.

Description: Cinoxate USP—Slightly yellow, practically odorless, viscous liquid.

Solubility: Cinoxate USP—Very slightly soluble in water; slightly soluble in glycerin; soluble in propylene glycol. Miscible with alcohol and with vegetable oils.

USP requirements:

Cinoxate USP—Preserve in tight, light-resistant containers. Contains not less than 98.0% and not more than 101.0% of cinoxate. Meets the requirements for Identification, Specific gravity (1.100–1.105), Refractive index (1.564–1.569), and Acidity.

Cinoxate Lotion USP—Preserve in tight, light-resistant containers. It is Cinoxate in a suitable hydroalcoholic vehicle. Contains the labeled amount, within ± 10%. Meets the requirements for Identification, pH (5.4–6.4), and Alcohol content (47–57%).

CIPROFLOXACIN

Chemical group: Fluoroquinolone derivative; structurally related to cinoxacin, nalidixic acid, norfloxacin, and other quinolones.

Chemical name:

Ciprofloxacin—3-Quinolinecarboxylic acid, 1-cyclopropyl-6-fluoro-1,4-dihydro-4-oxo-7-(1-piperazinyl)-.

Ciprofloxacin hydrochloride—3-Quinolinecarboxylic acid, 1-cyclopropyl-6-fluoro-1,4-dihydro-4-oxo-7-(1-piperazinyl)-, monohydrochloride, monohydrate.

Molecular formula:

Ciprofloxacin—$C_{17}H_{18}FN_3O_3$.

Ciprofloxacin hydrochloride—$C_{17}H_{18}FN_3O_3 \cdot HCl \cdot H_2O$.

Molecular weight:

Ciprofloxacin—331.35.

Ciprofloxacin hydrochloride—385.82.

Description: Ciprofloxacin Hydrochloride USP—Faintly yellowish to light yellow crystals.

Solubility: Ciprofloxacin Hydrochloride USP—Sparingly soluble in water; slightly soluble in acetic acid and in methanol; very slightly soluble in dehydrated alcohol; practically insoluble in acetone, in acetonitrile, in ethyl acetate, in hexane, and in methylene chloride.

USP requirements:

Ciprofloxacin USP—Preserve in tight, light-resistant containers. Contains not less than 98.0% and not more than 102.0% of ciprofloxacin, calculated on the dried basis. Meets the requirements for Clarity of solution, Identification, Loss on drying (not more than 1.0%), Chloride (not more than 0.02%), Sulfate (not more than 0.04%), Residue on ignition (not more than 0.1%), Heavy metals (not more than 0.002%), Fluoroquinolonic acid, and Chromatographic purity.

Ciprofloxacin Injection USP—Preserve in single-dose containers, preferably of Type I glass, in a cool place or at controlled room temperature. Avoid freezing and exposure to light. A sterile solution of Ciprofloxacin in 5% Dextrose Injection or in 0.9% Sodium Chloride Injection prepared with the aid of Lactic Acid. The label indicates whether the vehicle is 5% Dextrose Injection or 0.9% Sodium Chloride Injection. Contains the labeled amount, within ± 10%. Meets the requirements for Identification, Pyrogen, Sterility, pH (3.5–4.6), Particulate matter, Limit of ciprofloxacin ethylenediamine analog (not more than 0.5%), Lactic acid content (0.288–0.352 mg per mg of ciprofloxacin claimed on label), Dextrose content (if present), Sodium chloride content (if present), and Volume in Container under Injections.

Ciprofloxacin for Injection—Not in USP.

Ciprofloxacin Ophthalmic Solution USP—Preserve in tight containers protected from light, at room temperature. A sterile, aqueous solution of Ciprofloxacin Hydrochloride. Contains the labeled amount, within ± 10%. Meets the requirements for Identification, Sterility, and pH (3.5–5.5).

Ciprofloxacin Tablets USP—Preserve in well-closed containers. Contain an amount of ciprofloxacin hydrochloride equivalent to the labeled amount of ciprofloxacin, within ± 10%. Meet the requirements for Identification, Dissolution (80% in 30 minutes in water in Apparatus 2 at 50 rpm), and Uniformity of dosage units.

Ciprofloxacin Hydrochloride USP—Preserve in tight, light-resistant containers. Contains not less than 98.0% and not more than 102.0% of ciprofloxacin hydrochloride, calculated on the anhydrous basis. Meets the requirements for Identification, pH (3.0–4.5, in a solution [1 in 40]), Water (4.7–6.7%), Residue on ignition (not more than 0.1%), Sulfate (not more than 0.04%), Heavy metals (not more than 0.002%), Limit of fluoroquinolonic acid (not more than 0.2%), and Chromatographic purity.

CISAPRIDE

Chemical name: Benzamide, 4-amino-5-chloro-*N*-[1-[3-(4-fluorophenoxy)propyl]-3-methoxy-4-piperidinyl]-2-methoxy-, *cis*-.

Molecular formula: $C_{23}H_{29}ClFN_3O_4$.

Molecular weight: 465.95.

Description: White to slightly beige odorless powder.

Solubility: Practically insoluble in water; sparingly soluble in methanol; soluble in acetone.

USP requirements:

Cisapride Oral Suspension—Not in USP.

Cisapride Tablets—Not in USP.

CISPLATIN

Chemical group: A heavy metal complex.

Chemical name: Platinum, diamminedichloro-, (*SP*-4-2)-.

Molecular formula: $Cl_2H_6N_2Pt$.

Molecular weight: 300.05.

Description: White lyophilized powder. It has a melting point of 207 °C.

Solubility: Soluble in water or saline at 1 mg per mL and in dimethylformamide at 24 mg per mL.

USP requirements:

Cisplatin USP—Preserve in tight containers. Protect from light. Contains not less than 98.0% and not more than 102.0% of cisplatin, calculated on the anhydrous basis. Meets the requirements for Identification, Crystallinity, Water (not more than 1.0%), UV purity ratio, Platinum content (64.42–65.22%, on the anhydrous basis), Trichloroammineplatinate (not more than 1.0%), and Transplatin (not more than 2.0%).

Caution: Cisplatin is potentially cytotoxic. Great care should be taken to prevent inhaling particles and exposing the skin to it.

Cisplatin Injection—Not in USP.

Cisplatin for Injection USP—Preserve in Containers for Sterile Solids. Protect from light. A sterile, lyophilized mixture of Cisplatin, Mannitol, and Sodium Chloride. Contains the labeled amount, within ±10%. Meets the requirements for Identification, Constituted solution, Bacterial endotoxins, Sterility, pH (3.5–6.2, in the solution constituted as directed in the labeling, using Sterile Water for Injection), Water (not more than 2.0%), Uniformity of dosage units, Trichloroammineplatinate (not more than 1.0%), and Transplatin (not more than 2.0%), and for Labeling under Injections.

Caution: Cisplatin is potentially cytotoxic. Great care should be taken in handling the powder and preparing solutions.

CITRIC ACID

Chemical name: 1,2,3-Propanetricarboxylic acid, 2-hydroxy-.

Molecular formula: $C_6H_8O_7$ (anhydrous); $C_6H_8O_7 \cdot H_2O$ (monohydrate).

Molecular weight: 192.13 (anhydrous); 210.14 (monohydrate).

Description: Citric Acid USP—Colorless, translucent crystals, or white, granular to fine crystalline powder. Odorless or practically odorless. The hydrous form is efflorescent in dry air.

NF category: Acidifying agent; buffering agent.

Solubility: Citric Acid USP—Very soluble in water; freely soluble in alcohol; sparingly soluble in ether.

USP requirements: Citric Acid USP—Preserve in tight containers. It is anhydrous or contains one molecule of water of hydration. Label it to indicate whether it is anhydrous or hydrous. Contains not less than 99.5% and not more than 100.5% of citric acid, calculated on the anhydrous basis. Meets the requirements for Identification, Water (not more than 0.5% for anhydrous form and not more than 8.8% for hydrous form), Residue on ignition (not more than 0.05%), Oxalate, Sulfate, Arsenic (not more than 3 ppm), Heavy metals (not more than 0.001%), Readily carbonizable substances, and Organic volatile impurities.

CITRIC ACID AND D-GLUCONIC ACID

Chemical name: Citric acid—1,2,3-Propanetricarboxylic acid, 2-hydroxy-.

Molecular formula:

Citric acid—$C_6H_8O_7$ (anhydrous); $C_6H_8O_7 \cdot H_2O$ (monohydrate).

D-Gluconic acid—$C_6H_{12}O_7$.

Molecular weight:

Citric acid—192.13 (anhydrous); 210.14 (monohydrate).

D-Gluconic acid—196.16.

Description:

Citric Acid USP—Colorless, translucent crystals, or white, granular to fine crystalline powder. Odorless or practically odorless. The hydrous form is efflorescent in dry air.

NF category: Acidifying agent; buffering agent.

D-Gluconic acid—Melting point 131 °C.

Solubility:

Citric Acid USP—Very soluble in water; freely soluble in alcohol; sparingly soluble in ether.

D-Gluconic acid—Freely soluble in water; slightly soluble in alcohol; insoluble in ether and most other organic solvents.

USP requirements: Citric Acid and D-Gluconic Acid for Topical Solution—Not in USP.

CITRIC ACID, GLUCONO-DELTA-LACTONE, AND MAGNESIUM CARBONATE

Chemical name:

Citric acid—1,2,3-Propanetricarboxylic acid, 2-hydroxy-.

Magnesium carbonate—Carbonic acid, magnesium salt, basic; or, Carbonic acid, magnesium salt (1:1), hydrate.

Molecular formula:

Citric acid—$C_6H_8O_7$ (anhydrous); $C_6H_8O_7 \cdot H_2O$ (monohydrate).

Glucono-delta-lactone—$C_6H_{10}O_6$.

Magnesium carbonate—$MgCO_3 \cdot H_2O$.

Magnesium carbonate, basic (approx.)—$(MgCO_3)_4 \cdot Mg(OH)_2 \cdot 5H_2O$.

Molecular weight:

Citric acid—192.13 (anhydrous); 210.14 (monohydrate).

Glucono-delta-lactone—178.14.

Magnesium carbonate—102.33.

Magnesium carbonate, basic (approx.)—485.65.

Description:

Citric Acid USP—Colorless, translucent crystals, or white, granular to fine crystalline powder. Odorless or practically odorless. The hydrous form is efflorescent in dry air.

NF category: Acidifying agent; buffering agent.

Magnesium Carbonate USP—Light, white, friable masses or bulky, white powder. Is odorless, and is stable in air.

Solubility:

Citric Acid USP—Very soluble in water; freely soluble in alcohol; sparingly soluble in ether.

Glucono-delta-lactone—Soluble in water (59 grams/100 mL); insoluble in ether.

Magnesium Carbonate USP—Practically insoluble in water; to which, however, it imparts a slightly alkaline reaction; insoluble in alcohol, but is dissolved by dilute acids with effervescence.

USP requirements: Citric Acid, Glucono-delta-lactone, and Magnesium Carbonate Solution—Not in USP.

CITRIC ACID, MAGNESIUM OXIDE, AND SODIUM CARBONATE

For *Citric Acid, Magnesium Oxide,* and *Sodium Carbonate*—See individual listings for chemistry information.

USP requirements: Citric Acid, Magnesium Oxide, and Sodium Carbonate Irrigation USP—Preserve in single-dose containers, preferably of Type I or Type II glass. A sterile solution of Citric Acid, Magnesium Oxide, and Sodium Carbonate in Water for Injection. Contains an amount of citric acid equivalent to the labeled amount of citric acid (as the monohydrate), within ±5%, and the labeled amounts of magnesium oxide and sodium carbonate, within ±5%. Meets the requirements for Identification, Bacterial endotoxins, pH (3.8–4.2), and Injections (except that the container may be designed to empty rapidly, and may exceed 1000 mL in capacity).

CLADRIBINE

Chemical name: 2-Chloro-2′-deoxyadenosine.

Molecular formula: $C_{10}H_{12}ClN_5O_3$.

Molecular weight: 285.7.

USP requirements: Cladribine Injection—Not in USP.

CLARITHROMYCIN

Chemical name: Erythromycin, 6-*O*-methyl-.

Molecular formula: $C_{38}H_{69}NO_{13}$.

Molecular weight: 747.96.

Description: White to off-white crystalline powder.

Solubility: Soluble in acetone; slightly soluble in methanol, in ethanol, and in acetonitrile; practically insoluble in water.

USP requirements:
Clarithromycin USP—Preserve in tight containers. Contains not less than 960 mcg and not more than 1040 mcg of clarithromycin, calculated on the anhydrous basis. Meets the requirements for Identification, Specific rotation (−89° to −95°, calculated on the anhydrous basis), Crystallinity, pH (7.5–10.0, determined in a 1 in 500 suspension of it in a mixture of water and methanol [19:1]), Water (not more than 2.0%), Residue on ignition (not more than 0.3%), and Heavy metals (not more than 0.002%).
Clarithromycin Oral Suspension—Not in USP.
Clarithromycin Tablets USP—Preserve in tight containers. Contain the labeled amount, within ±10%. Meet the requirements for Identification, Dissolution (80% in 30 minutes in 0.1 *M* Sodium acetate buffer in Apparatus 2 at 50 rpm), Uniformity of dosage units, and Loss on drying (not more than 6.0%).

CLAVULANATE

Chemical name:
Clavulanate potassium—4-Oxa-1-azabicyclo[3.2.0]heptane-2-carboxylic acid, 3-(2-hydroxyethylidene)-7-oxo-, monopotassium salt, [2*R*-(2 alpha,3*Z*,5 alpha)]-.
Clavulanic acid—(*Z*)-(2*R*,5*R*)-3-(2-Hydroxyethylidene)-7-oxo-4-oxa-1-azabicyclo[3.2.0]heptane-2-carboxylic acid.

Molecular formula:
Clavulanate potassium—$C_8H_8KNO_5$.
Clavulanic acid—$C_8H_9NO_5$.

Molecular weight:
Clavulanate potassium—237.25.
Clavulanic acid—199.16.

Description: Clavulanate Potassium USP—White to off-white powder. Is moisture-sensitive.

Solubility: Clavulanate Potassium USP—Freely soluble in water, but stability in aqueous solution is not good, optimum stability at a pH of 6.0 to 6.3; soluble in methanol, with decomposition.

USP requirements:
Clavulanate Potassium USP—Preserve in tight containers. Contains an amount of clavulanate potassium equivalent to not less than 75.5% and not more than 92.0% of clavulanic acid, calculated on the anhydrous basis. Meets the requirements for Identification, pH (5.5–8.0, in a solution [1 in 100]), Water (not more than 1.5%), and Clavam-2-carboxylate potassium (not more than 0.01%).
Sterile Clavulanate Potassium USP—Preserve in Containers for Sterile Solids. It is clavulanate potassium suitable for parenteral use. Contains an amount of clavulanate potassium equivalent to not less than 75.5% and not more than 92.0% of clavulanic acid, calculated on the anhydrous basis. Meets the requirements for Pyrogen and Sterility, and for Identification tests, pH, Water, and Clavam-2-carboxylate potassium under Clavulanate Potassium.

CLEMASTINE

Chemical group: Ethanolamine derivative.

Chemical name: Clemastine fumarate—Pyrrolidine, 2-[2-[1-(4-chlorophenyl)-1-phenylethoxy]ethyl]-1-methyl-, [*R*-(*R**,*R**)]-, (*E*)-2-butenedioate (1:1).

Molecular formula: Clemastine fumarate—$C_{21}H_{26}ClNO \cdot C_4H_4O_4$.

Molecular weight: Clemastine fumarate—459.97.

Description: Clemastine Fumarate USP—Colorless to faintly yellow, odorless, crystalline powder. Its solutions are acid to litmus.

Solubility: Clemastine Fumarate USP—Very slightly soluble in water; slightly soluble in methanol; very slightly soluble in chloroform.

USP requirements:
Clemastine Fumarate USP—Preserve in tight, light-resistant containers, at a temperature not exceeding 25 °C. Contains not less than 98.0% and not more than 102.0% of clemastine fumarate, calculated on the dried basis. Meets the requirements for Clarity and color of solution, Identification, Specific rotation (+15.0° to 18.0°, calculated on the dried basis), pH (3.2–4.2, in a suspension [1 in 10]), Loss on drying (not more than 0.5%), Heavy metals (not more than 0.002%), and Chromatographic purity.
Clemastine Fumarate Syrup—Not in USP.
Clemastine Fumarate Tablets USP—Preserve in well-closed containers. Contain the labeled amount, within ±10%. Meet the requirements for Identification, Dissolution (75% in 30 minutes in citrate buffer [pH 4.0] in Apparatus 2 at 50 rpm), and Uniformity of dosage units.

CLEMASTINE AND PHENYLPROPANOLAMINE

For *Clemastine* and *Phenylpropanolamine*—See individual listings for chemistry information.

USP requirements: Clemastine Fumarate and Phenylpropanolamine Hydrochloride Extended-release Tablets—Not in USP.

CLIDINIUM

Chemical group: Quaternary ammonium compound.

Chemical name: Clidinium bromide—1-Azoniabicyclo[2.2.2]-octane, 3-[(hydroxydiphenylacetyl)oxy]-1-methyl-, bromide.

Molecular formula: Clidinium bromide—$C_{22}H_{26}BrNO_3$.

Molecular weight: Clidinium bromide—432.36.

Description: Clidinium Bromide USP—White to nearly white, practically odorless, crystalline powder. Is optically inactive. Melts at about 242 °C.

Solubility: Clidinium Bromide USP—Soluble in water and in alcohol; slightly soluble in ether.

USP requirements:

Clidinium Bromide USP—Preserve in tight, light-resistant containers. Contains not less than 99.0% and not more than 100.5% of clidinium bromide, calculated on the dried basis. Meets the requirements for Identification, Loss on drying (not more than 0.5%), Residue on ignition (not more than 0.1%), Heavy metals (not more than 0.002%), Related compounds, and Organic volatile impurities.

Clidinium Bromide Capsules USP—Preserve in tight, light-resistant containers. Contain the labeled amount, within ±10%. Meet the requirements for Identification, Dissolution (80% in 15 minutes in 0.1 *N* hydrochloric acid in Apparatus 1 at 100 rpm), Uniformity of dosage units, and Related compounds.

CLINDAMYCIN

Source: 7(*S*)-Chloro derivative of lincomycin.

Chemical name:

Clindamycin hydrochloride—L-*threo*-alpha-D-*galacto*-Octopyranoside, methyl 7-chloro-6,7,8-trideoxy-6-[[(1-methyl-4-propyl-2-pyrrolidinyl)carbonyl]amino]-1-thio-, (2*S*-*trans*)-, monohydrochloride.

Clindamycin palmitate hydrochloride—L-*threo*-alpha-D-*galacto*-Octopyranoside, methyl 7-chloro-6,7,8-trideoxy-6-[[(1-methyl-4-propyl-2-pyrrolidinyl)carbonyl]amino]-1-thio-2-hexadecanoate, monohydrochloride, (2*S*-*trans*)-.

Clindamycin phosphate—L-*threo*-alpha-D-*galacto*-Octopyranoside, methyl 7-chloro-6,7,8-trideoxy-6-[[(1-methyl-4-propyl-2-pyrrolidinyl)carbonyl]amino]-1-thio-, 2-(dihydrogen phosphate), (2*S*-*trans*)-.

Molecular formula:

Clindamycin hydrochloride—$C_{18}H_{33}ClN_2O_5S \cdot HCl$.

Clindamycin palmitate hydrochloride—$C_{34}H_{63}ClN_2O_6S \cdot HCl$.

Clindamycin phosphate—$C_{18}H_{34}ClN_2O_8PS$.

Molecular weight:

Clindamycin hydrochloride—461.44.

Clindamycin palmitate hydrochloride—699.86.

Clindamycin phosphate—504.96.

Description:

Clindamycin Hydrochloride USP—White or practically white, crystalline powder. Is odorless or has a faint mercaptan-like odor. Is stable in the presence of air and light. Its solutions are acidic and are dextrorotatory.

Clindamycin Palmitate Hydrochloride USP—White to off-white amorphous powder, having a characteristic odor.

Clindamycin Phosphate USP—White to off-white, hygroscopic, crystalline powder. Is odorless or practically odorless.

Solubility:

Clindamycin Hydrochloride USP—Freely soluble in water, in dimethylformamide, and in methanol; soluble in alcohol; practically insoluble in acetone.

Clindamycin Palmitate Hydrochloride USP—Very soluble in ethyl acetate and in dimethylformamide; freely soluble in water, in ether, in chloroform, and in alcohol.

Clindamycin Phosphate USP—Freely soluble in water; slightly soluble in dehydrated alcohol; very slightly soluble in acetone; practically insoluble in chloroform and in ether.

USP requirements:

Clindamycin Hydrochloride USP—Preserve in tight containers. It is the hydrated hydrochloride salt of clindamycin, a substance produced by the chlorination of lincomycin. Has a potency equivalent to not less than 800 mcg of clindamycin per mg. Meets the requirements for Identification, Crystallinity, pH (3.0–5.5, in a solution containing 100 mg per mL), and Water (3.0–6.0%).

Clindamycin Hydrochloride Capsules USP—Preserve in tight containers. Contain an amount of clindamycin hydrochloride equivalent to the labeled amount of clindamycin, within −10% to +20%. Meet the requirements for Identification, Dissolution (80% in 30 minutes in water in Apparatus 1 at 100 rpm), Uniformity of dosage units, and Water (not more than 7.0%).

Clindamycin Palmitate Hydrochloride USP—Preserve in tight containers. Has a potency equivalent to not less than 540 mcg of clindamycin per mg. Meets the requirements for Identification, pH (2.8–3.8, in a solution containing 10 mg per mL), Water (not more than 3.0%), and Residue on ignition (not more than 0.5%).

Clindamycin Palmitate Hydrochloride for Oral Solution USP—Preserve in tight containers. A dry mixture of Clindamycin Palmitate Hydrochloride and one or more suitable buffers, colors, diluents, flavors, and preservatives. Contains an amount of clindamycin palmitate hydrochloride equivalent to the labeled amount of clindamycin (15 mg per mL when constituted as directed in the labeling), within −10% to +20%. Meets the requirements for Uniformity of dosage units (solid packaged in single-unit containers), pH (2.5–5.0, in the solution constituted as directed in the labeling), Water (not more than 3.0%), and Deliverable volume (solid packaged in multiple-unit containers).

Clindamycin Phosphate USP—Preserve in tight containers. Has a potency equivalent to not less than 758 mcg of clindamycin per mg, calculated on the anhydrous basis. Meets the requirements for Identification, Crystallinity, pH (3.5–4.5, in a solution containing 10 mg per mL), and Water (not more than 6.0%), and for Bacterial endotoxins and Depressor substances under Sterile Clindamycin Phosphate (for Clindamycin Phosphate intended for use in making Clindamycin Phosphate Injection).

Clindamycin Phosphate Vaginal Cream—Not in USP.

Clindamycin Phosphate Gel USP—Preserve in tight containers. Contains an amount of clindamycin phosphate equivalent to the labeled amount of clindamycin, within ±10%. Meets the requirements for Identification, Minimum fill, and pH (4.5–6.5).

Clindamycin Phosphate Injection USP—Preserve in single-dose or in multiple-dose containers, preferably of Type I glass, or in suitable plastic containers. A sterile solution of Sterile Clindamycin Phosphate or Clindamycin Phosphate in Water for Injection with one or more suitable preservatives, sequestering agents, or tonicity-adjusting agents. It meets the requirement for Labeling under Injections. Where it is maintained in the frozen state, the label states that it is to be thawed just prior to use, describes the conditions for proper storage of the resultant solution, and directs that the solution is not to be refrozen. Contains an amount of clindamycin phosphate equivalent to the labeled amount of clindamycin, within −10% to +20%. Meets the requirements for Identification, Bacterial endotoxins, pH (5.5–7.0), Particulate matter, and Injections.

Clindamycin Phosphate Topical Solution USP—Preserve in tight containers. Contains an amount of clindamycin phosphate equivalent to the labeled amount of clindamycin, within ±10%. Meets the requirements for Identification and pH (4.0–7.0).

Clindamycin Phosphate Topical Suspension USP—Preserve in tight containers. Contains an amount of clindamycin phosphate equivalent to the labeled amount of clindamycin, within ±10%. Meets the requirements for Identification, Minimum fill, and pH (4.5–6.5).

Sterile Clindamycin Phosphate USP—Preserve in Containers for Sterile Solids. It is Clindamycin Phosphate suitable for parenteral use. Has a potency equivalent to not less than 758 mcg of clindamycin per mg, calculated on the anhydrous basis. Meets the requirements for Depressor substances, Bacterial endotoxins, and Sterility, and for Identification test, pH, Water, and Crystallinity under Clindamycin Phosphate.

CLIOQUINOL

Chemical name: 8-Quinolinol, 5-chloro-7-iodo-.

Molecular formula: C_9H_5ClINO.

Molecular weight: 305.50.

Description: Clioquinol USP—Voluminous, spongy, yellowish white to brownish yellow powder, having a slight, characteristic odor. Darkens on exposure to light. Melts at about 180 °C, with decomposition.

Solubility: Clioquinol USP—Practically insoluble in water and in alcohol; soluble in hot ethyl acetate and in hot glacial acetic acid.

USP requirements:

Clioquinol USP—Preserve in tight, light-resistant containers. Dried over phosphorus pentoxide for 5 hours, contains not less than 93.0% and not more than 100.5% of clioquinol (the 5-chloro-7-iodo-8-quinolinol isomer). Meets the requirements for Identification, Loss on drying (not more than 0.5%), Residue on ignition (not more than 0.5%), and Free iodine and iodide.

Clioquinol Cream USP—Preserve in collapsible tubes or tight, light-resistant containers. Contains the labeled amount, within ±10%, in a suitable cream base. Meets the requirement for Identification.

Clioquinol Ointment USP—Preserve in collapsible tubes or tight, light-resistant containers. Contains the labeled amount, within ±10%, in a suitable ointment base. Meets the requirement for Identification.

Compound Clioquinol Topical Powder USP—Preserve in well-closed, light-resistant containers. Contains not less than 22.5% and not more than 27.5% of clioquinol.

Prepare Compound Clioquinol Powder as follows: 250 grams of Clioquinol, 25 grams of Lactic Acid, 200 grams of Zinc Stearate, and 525 grams of Lactose to make 1000 grams. Mix the Lactic Acid with the Lactose, then add the Clioquinol and the Zinc Stearate, and mix.

Meets the requirement for Identification.

CLIOQUINOL AND FLUMETHASONE

For *Clioquinol* and *Flumethasone*—See individual listings for chemistry information.

USP requirements:

Clioquinol and Flumethasone Pivalate Cream—Not in USP.

Clioquinol and Flumethasone Pivalate Ointment—Not in USP.

Clioquinol and Flumethasone Pivalate Otic Solution—Not in USP.

CLIOQUINOL AND HYDROCORTISONE

For *Clioquinol* and *Hydrocortisone*—See individual listings for chemistry information.

USP requirements:

Clioquinol and Hydrocortisone Cream USP—Preserve in collapsible tubes or in tight, light-resistant containers. Contains the labeled amounts, within ±10%, in a suitable cream base. Meets the requirements for Identification and Minimum fill.

Clioquinol and Hydrocortisone Lotion—Not in USP.

Clioquinol and Hydrocortisone Ointment USP—Preserve in collapsible tubes or in tight, light-resistant containers. Contains the labeled amounts, within ±10%, in a suitable ointment base. Meets the requirements for Identification and Minimum fill.

CLOBAZAM

Chemical name: 1*H*-1,5-Benzodiazepine-2,4(3*H*,5*H*)-dione, 7-chloro-1-methyl-5-phenyl-.

Molecular formula: $C_{16}H_{13}ClN_2O_2$.

Molecular weight: 300.74.

Description: White, odorless, crystalline powder. Melting range of 182 ±3 °C.

Solubility: Soluble in chloroform and in methanol; very slightly soluble in water.

USP requirements: Clobazam Tablets—Not in USP.

CLOBETASOL

Chemical name: Clobetasol propionate—Pregna-1,4-diene-3,20-dione, 21-chloro-9-fluoro-11-hydroxy-16-methyl-17-(1-oxopropoxy)-, (11 beta,16 beta)-.

Molecular formula: Clobetasol propionate—$C_{25}H_{32}ClFO_5$.

Molecular weight: Clobetasol propionate—466.98.

Description: Clobetasol propionate—White to cream-colored crystalline powder.

Solubility: Clobetasol propionate—Insoluble in water.

USP requirements:

Clobetasol Propionate Cream—Not in USP.

Clobetasol Propionate Ointment—Not in USP.

Clobetasol Propionate Solution—Not in USP.

CLOBETASONE

Chemical name: Clobetasone butyrate—Pregna-1,4-diene-3,11,-20-trione, 21-chloro-9-fluoro-16-methyl-17-(1-oxobutoxy)-, (16 beta)-.

Molecular formula: Clobetasone butyrate—$C_{26}H_{32}ClFO_5$.

Molecular weight: Clobetasone butyrate—478.99.

Description: Clobetasone butyrate—White to cream-colored crystalline powder.

USP requirements:

Clobetasone Butyrate Cream—Not in USP.

Clobetasone Butyrate Ointment—Not in USP.

CLOCORTOLONE

Chemical name: Clocortolone pivalate—Pregna-1,4-diene-3,20-dione, 9-chloro-21-(2,2-dimethyl-1-oxopropoxy)-6-fluoro-11-hydroxy-16-methyl-, (6 alpha,11 beta,16 alpha)-.

Molecular formula: Clocortolone pivalate—$C_{27}H_{36}ClFO_5$.

Molecular weight: Clocortolone pivalate—495.03.

Description: Clocortolone Pivalate USP—White to yellowish white, odorless powder. Melts at about 230 °C, with decomposition.

Solubility: Clocortolone Pivalate USP—Freely soluble in chloroform and in dioxane; soluble in acetone; sparingly soluble in alcohol; slightly soluble in ether.

USP requirements:
Clocortolone Pivalate USP—Preserve in tight, light-resistant containers. Contains not less than 97.0% and not more than 103.0% of clocortolone pivalate, calculated on the dried basis. Meets the requirements for Color and clarity of solution, Identification, Specific rotation (+125° to +135°, calculated on the dried basis), Loss on drying (not more than 1.0%), Residue on ignition (not more than 0.2%), and Chromatographic impurities.
Clocortolone Pivalate Cream USP—Preserve in collapsible tubes or in tight, light-resistant containers. Contains the labeled amount, within ± 10%, in a suitable cream base. Meets the requirements for Identification, Minimum fill, pH (5.0–7.0, in a 1 in 10 aqueous dispersion), and Particle size determination (no particle more than 50 microns when measured in the longitudinal axis).

CLOFAZIMINE

Chemical group: Substituted iminophenazine dye.

Chemical name: 2-Phenazinamine, *N*,5-bis(4-chlorophenyl)-3,5-dihydro-3-[(1-methylethyl)imino]-.

Molecular formula: $C_{27}H_{22}Cl_2N_4$.

Molecular weight: 473.40.

Description: Clofazimine USP—Dark red crystals. Melts at about 217 °C, with decomposition.

Solubility: Clofazimine USP—Practically insoluble in water; soluble in chloroform; sparingly soluble in alcohol, in acetone, and in ethyl acetate.

Other characteristics: Highly lipophilic.

USP requirements:
Clofazimine USP—Preserve in tight, light-resistant containers, at room temperature. Contains not less than 98.5% and not more than 101.5% of clofazimine, calculated on the dried basis. Meets the requirements for Identification, Loss on drying (not more than 0.5%), Residue on ignition (not more than 0.1%), and Chromatographic purity.
Clofazimine Capsules USP—Preserve in well-closed containers. Contain the labeled amount, within ± 10%. Meet the requirements for Identification, Disintegration (15 minutes, in simulated gastric fluid TS), Uniformity of dosage units, and Chromatographic purity.

CLOFIBRATE

Chemical name: Propanoic acid, 2-(4-chlorophenoxy)-2-methyl-, ethyl ester.

Molecular formula: $C_{12}H_{15}ClO_3$.

Molecular weight: 242.70.

Description: Clofibrate USP—Colorless to pale yellow liquid having a characteristic odor.

Solubility: Clofibrate USP—Insoluble in water; soluble in acetone, in alcohol, and in chloroform.

USP requirements:
Clofibrate USP—Preserve in tight, light-resistant containers. Contains not less than 97.0% and not more than 103.0% of clofibrate, calculated on the anhydrous basis. Meets the requirements for Identification, Refractive index (1.500–1.505, at 20 °C), Acidity, Water (not more than 0.2%), Chromatographic impurities, *p*-Chlorophenol (not more than 0.003%), and Organic volatile impurities.
Clofibrate Capsules USP—Preserve in well-closed, light-resistant containers. Contain the labeled amount, within ± 10%. Meet the requirements for Identification, Dissolution (75% in 180 minutes in sodium lauryl sulfate solution [5 in 100] in Apparatus 2 at 75 rpm), and Uniformity of dosage units.

CLOMIPHENE

Chemical name: Clomiphene citrate—Ethanamine, 2-[4-(2-chloro-1,2-diphenylethenyl)phenoxy]-*N,N*-diethyl-, 2-hydroxy-1,2,3-propanetricarboxylate (1:1).

Molecular formula: Clomiphene citrate—$C_{26}H_{28}ClNO \cdot C_6H_8O_7$.

Molecular weight: Clomiphene citrate—598.09.

Description: Clomiphene Citrate USP—White to pale yellow, essentially odorless powder.

Solubility: Clomiphene Citrate USP—Slightly soluble in water and in chloroform; freely soluble in methanol; sparingly soluble in alcohol; insoluble in ether.

USP requirements:
Clomiphene Citrate USP—Preserve in well-closed containers. Contains not less than 98.0% and not more than 102.0% of a mixture of the (*E*)- and (*Z*)- geometric isomers of clomiphene citrate, calculated on the anhydrous basis. Contains not less than 30.0% and not more than 50.0% of the *Z*-isomer, [(*Z*)-2-[4-(2-chloro-1,2-diphenylethenyl)phenoxy]-*N,N*-diethylethanamine 2-hydroxy-1,2,3-propanetricarboxylate (1:1). Meets the requirements for Identification, Water (not more than 1.0%), Heavy metals (not more than 0.002%), *Z*-isomer (30.0–50.0%), Limit of related compounds (not more than 1.0% of any single extraneous volatile substance and not more than 2.0% of total extraneous volatile substances), and Organic volatile impurities.
Clomiphene Citrate Tablets USP—Preserve in well-closed containers, protected from light. Contain the labeled amount, within ± 7%. Meet the requirements for Identification, Dissolution (75% in 60 minutes in water in Apparatus 1 at 100 rpm), and Uniformity of dosage units.

CLOMIPRAMINE

Chemical group: Dibenzazepine.

Chemical name: Clomipramine hydrochloride—5*H*-Dibenz[*b,f*]-azepine-5-propanamine, 3-chloro-10,11-dihydro-*N,N*-dimethyl-, monohydrochloride.

Molecular formula: Clomipramine hydrochloride—$C_{19}H_{23}ClN_2 \cdot HCl$.

Molecular weight: Clomipramine hydrochloride—351.32.

Description: Clomipramine hydrochloride—White to off-white crystalline powder.

Solubility: Clomipramine hydrochloride—Freely soluble in water, in methanol, and in methylene chloride; insoluble in ethyl ether and in hexane.

Other characteristics: Clomipramine hydrochloride—A 10% solution in water has a pH of 3.5–5.0.

USP requirements:
Clomipramine Hydrochloride Capsules—Not in USP.
Clomipramine Hydrochloride Tablets—Not in USP.

CLONAZEPAM

Chemical name: 2*H*-1,4-Benzodiazepin-2-one, 5-(2-chlorophenyl)-1,3-dihydro-7-nitro-.

Molecular formula: $C_{15}H_{10}ClN_3O_3$.

Molecular weight: 315.72.

Description: Clonazepam USP—Light yellow powder, having a faint odor. Melts at about 239 °C.

Solubility: Clonazepam USP—Insoluble in water; sparingly soluble in acetone and in chloroform; slightly soluble in alcohol and in ether.

USP requirements:
Clonazepam USP—Preserve in tight, light-resistant containers, at room temperature. Contains not less than 99.0% and not more than 101.0% of clonazepam, calculated on the dried basis. Meets the requirements for Identification, Loss on drying (not more than 0.5%), Residue on ignition (not more than 0.1%), Heavy metals (not more than 0.002%), Related compounds, and Organic volatile impurities.
Clonazepam Tablets USP—Preserve in tight, light-resistant containers, at room temperature. Contain the labeled amount, within ±10%. Meet the requirements for Identification, Dissolution (80% in 60 minutes in degassed water in Apparatus 2 at 100 rpm), Uniformity of dosage units, and Related compounds.

CLONIDINE

Chemical name:
Clonidine—Benzenamine, 2,6-dichloro-*N*-2-imidazolidinylidene-.
Clonidine hydrochloride—Benzenamine, 2,6-dichloro-*N*-2-imidazolidinylidene-, monohydrochloride.

Molecular formula:
Clonidine—$C_9H_9Cl_2N_3$.
Clonidine hydrochloride—$C_9H_9Cl_2N_3 \cdot HCl$.

Molecular weight:
Clonidine—230.10.
Clonidine hydrochloride—266.56.

Description: Clonidine hydrochloride—Odorless, white, crystalline substance.

Solubility: Clonidine hydrochloride—Soluble in water and in alcohol; practically insoluble in chloroform and in ether.

Other characteristics: Clonidine hydrochloride—The pH of a 10% aqueous solution is between 3 and 5.

USP requirements:
Clonidine Transdermal System—Not in USP.
Clonidine Hydrochloride USP—Preserve in tight containers. Contains not less than 98.5% and not more than 101.0% of clonidine hydrochloride, calculated on the dried basis. Meets the requirements for Identification, pH (3.5–5.5, in a solution [1 in 20]), Loss on drying (not more than 0.5%), Residue on ignition (not more than 0.1%), and Chromatographic purity.
Clonidine Hydrochloride Tablets USP—Preserve in well-closed containers. Contain the labeled amount, within ±10%. Meet the requirements for Identification, Dissolution (75% in 30 minutes in water in Apparatus 2 at 50 rpm), and Uniformity of dosage units.

CLONIDINE AND CHLORTHALIDONE

For *Clonidine* and *Chlorthalidone*—See individual listings for chemistry information.

USP requirements: Clonidine Hydrochloride and Chlorthalidone Tablets USP—Preserve in well-closed containers. Contain the labeled amounts, within ±10%. Meet the requirements for Identification, Dissolution (80% of clonidine hydrochloride and 50% of chlorthalidone in 60 minutes in water in Apparatus 2 at 100 rpm), and Uniformity of dosage units.

CLORAZEPATE

Chemical name: Clorazepate dipotassium—1*H*-1,4-Benzodiazepine-3-carboxylic acid, 7-chloro-2,3-dihydro-2-oxo-5-phenyl-, potassium salt compd. with potassium hydroxide (1:1).

Molecular formula: Clorazepate dipotassium—$C_{16}H_{11}ClK_2N_2O_4$.

Molecular weight: Clorazepate dipotassium—408.92.

Description: Clorazepate Dipotassium USP—Light yellow, crystalline powder. Darkens on exposure to light.

Solubility: Clorazepate Dipotassium USP—Soluble in water but, upon standing, may precipitate from the solution; slightly soluble in alcohol and in isopropyl alcohol; practically insoluble in acetone, in chloroform, in ether, and in methylene chloride.

USP requirements:
Clorazepate Dipotassium USP—Preserve under nitrogen in tight, light-resistant containers. Contains not less than 98.5% and not more than 101.5% of clorazepate dipotassium, calculated on the dried basis. Meets the requirements for Identification, Loss on drying (not more than 0.5%), Heavy metals (not more than 0.002%), Related compounds (not more than 1.0%), and Organic volatile impurities.
Clorazepate Dipotassium Capsules—Not in USP.
Clorazepate Dipotassium Tablets—Not in USP.

CLORSULON

Chemical name: 1,3-Benzenedisulfonamide, 4-amino-6-(trichloroethenyl)-.

Molecular formula: $C_8H_8Cl_3N_3O_4S_2$.

Molecular weight: 380.65.

Description: Clorsulon USP—White to off-white powder.

Solubility: Clorsulon USP—Slightly soluble in water; freely soluble in acetonitrile and in methanol; very slightly soluble in methylene chloride.

USP requirements: Clorsulon USP—Preserve in well-closed containers. Label it to indicate that it is for veterinary use only. Contains not less than 98.0% and not more than 101.0% of clorsulon, calculated on the dried basis. Meets the requirements for Identification, Melting range (197–203 °C), Loss on drying (not more than 0.5%), Residue on ignition (not more than 0.1%), Heavy metals (not more than 0.003%), and Chromatographic purity.

CLOTRIMAZOLE

Chemical name: 1*H*-Imidazole, 1-[(2-chlorophenyl)diphenylmethyl]-.

Molecular formula: $C_{22}H_{17}ClN_2$.

Molecular weight: 344.84.

Description: Clotrimazole USP—White to pale yellow, crystalline powder. Melts at about 142 °C, with decomposition.

Solubility: Clotrimazole USP—Practically insoluble in water; freely soluble in methanol, in acetone, in chloroform, and in alcohol.

USP requirements:

Clotrimazole USP—Preserve in tight containers. Contains not less than 98.0% and not more than 102.0% of clotrimazole, calculated on the dried basis. Meets the requirements for Identification, Loss on drying (not more than 0.5%), Residue on ignition (not more than 0.1%), Heavy metals (not more than 0.001%), Imidazole (not more than 0.5%), and (*o*-Chlorophenyl)diphenylmethanol (not more than 0.5%).

Clotrimazole Cream USP—Preserve in collapsible tubes or in tight containers, at a temperature between 2 and 30 °C. Cream that is intended for use as a vaginal preparation may be labeled Clotrimazole Vaginal Cream. Contains the labeled amount, within ±10%. Meets the requirement for Identification.

Clotrimazole Lotion USP—Preserve in tight containers, at a temperature between 2 and 30 °C. Contains the labeled amount, within ±10%. Meets the requirements for Identification, pH (5.0–7.0), Microbial limits, and (*o*-Chlorophenyl)diphenylmethanol (not more than 5%).

Clotrimazole Lozenges—Not in USP.

Clotrimazole Topical Solution USP—Preserve in tight containers, at a temperature between 2 and 30 °C. A solution of Clotrimazole in a suitable nonaqueous, hydrophilic solvent. Contains the labeled amount, within −10% to +15%. Meets the requirement for Identification.

Clotrimazole Vaginal Tablets USP—Preserve in well-closed containers. Contain the labeled amount, within ±10%. Meet the requirements for Identification, Disintegration (20 minutes), and Uniformity of dosage units.

CLOTRIMAZOLE AND BETAMETHASONE

For *Clotrimazole* and *Betamethasone*—See individual listings for chemistry information.

USP requirements: Clotrimazole and Betamethasone Dipropionate Cream USP—Preserve in collapsible tubes or in tight containers. Contains the labeled amount of clotrimazole, within ±10%, and an amount of betamethasone dipropionate equivalent to the labeled amount of betamethasone, within ±10%, in a suitable cream base. Meets the requirements for Identification, Microbial limits, Minimum fill, and Limit of (*o*-chlorophenyl)diphenylmethanol (not more than 5.0% of labeled amount of clotrimazole in the Cream).

CLOXACILLIN

Chemical name:

Cloxacillin benzathine—4-Thia-1-azabicyclo[3.2.0]heptane-2-carboxylic acid, 6-[[[3-(2-chlorophenyl)-5-methyl-4-isoxazolyl]carbonyl]amino]-3,3-dimethyl-7-oxo-, [2*S*-(2 alpha,5 alpha,6 beta)]-, compd. with *N,N'*bis(phenylmethyl)-1,2-ethanediamine (2:1).

Cloxacillin sodium—4-Thia-1-azabicyclo[3.2.0]heptane-2-carboxylic acid, 6-[[[3-(2-chlorophenyl)-5-methyl-4-isoxazolyl]carbonyl]amino]-3,3-dimethyl-7-oxo-, monosodium salt, monohydrate, [2*S*-(2 alpha,5 alpha,6 beta)]-.

Molecular formula:

Cloxacillin benzathine—$(C_{19}H_{18}ClN_3O_5S)_2 \cdot C_{16}H_{20}N_2$.

Cloxacillin sodium—$C_{19}H_{17}ClN_3NaO_5S \cdot H_2O$.

Molecular weight:

Cloxacillin benzathine—1112.11.

Cloxacillin sodium—475.88.

Description:

Cloxacillin Benzathine USP—White or almost white, almost odorless, crystals or crystalline powder.

Cloxacillin Sodium USP—White, odorless, crystalline powder.

Solubility:

Cloxacillin Benzathine USP—Slightly soluble in water, in alcohol, and in isopropyl alcohol; soluble in chloroform and in methanol; sparingly soluble in acetone.

Cloxacillin Sodium USP—Freely soluble in water; soluble in alcohol; slightly soluble in chloroform.

USP requirements:

Cloxacillin Benzathine USP—Preserve in tight containers. Label it to indicate that it is for veterinary use only. Has a potency equivalent to not less than 704 mcg and not more than 821 mcg of cloxacillin per mg, calculated on the anhydrous basis. Meets the requirements for Identification, Crystallinity, pH (3.0–6.5, in a suspension containing 10 mg per mL), and Water (not more than 5.0%).

Cloxacillin Benzathine Intramammary Infusion USP—Preserve in disposable syringes that are well-closed containers, except that where the Infusion is labeled as sterile, the individual syringes or cartons are sealed and tamperproof so that sterility is assured at time of use. A suspension of Cloxacillin Benzathine or Sterile Cloxacillin Benzathine in a suitable oil vehicle. Label it to indicate that it is for veterinary use only. Infusion that is sterile may be so labeled. Contains an amount of cloxacillin benzathine equivalent to the labeled amount of cloxacillin, within −10% to +20%. Meets the requirements for Identification, Sterility (where labeled as being sterile), and Water (not more than 1.0%).

Sterile Cloxacillin Benzathine USP—Preserve in tight containers. Label it to indicate that it is for veterinary use only. Has a potency equivalent to not less than 704 mcg and not more than 821 mcg of cloxacillin per mg, calculated on the anhydrous basis. Meets the requirements for Sterility and for Identification, Crystallinity, pH, and Water under Cloxacillin Benzathine.

Cloxacillin Sodium USP—Preserve in tight containers, at a temperature not exceeding 25 °C. Contains the equivalent of not less than 825 mcg of cloxacillin per mg. Meets the requirements for Identification, Crystallinity, pH (4.5–7.5, in a solution containing 10 mg per mL), Water (3.0–5.0%), and Dimethylaniline.

Cloxacillin Sodium Capsules USP—Preserve in tight containers. Contain an amount of cloxacillin sodium equivalent to the labeled amount of cloxacillin, within −10% to +20%. Meet the requirements for Dissolution (75% in 45 minutes in water in Apparatus 1 at 100 rpm), Uniformity of dosage units, and Water (not more than 5.0%).

Cloxacillin Sodium Intramammary Infusion USP—Preserve in disposable syringes that are well-closed containers, except that where the Infusion is labeled as sterile, the individual syringes or cartons are sealed and tamperproof so that sterility is assured at time of use. A suspension of Sterile Cloxacillin Sodium in a suitable natural or chemically modified vegetable oil vehicle with a suitable dispersing agent. Label it to indicate that it is for veterinary use only. Infusion that is sterile may be so labeled. Contains an amount of cloxacillin sodium equivalent to the labeled amount of cloxacillin, within −10% to +20%.

Meets the requirements for Identification, Sterility, and Water (not more than 1.0%).

Cloxacillin Sodium Injection—Not in USP.

Cloxacillin Sodium for Oral Solution USP—Preserve in tight containers. A dry mixture of Cloxacillin Sodium and one or more suitable buffers, colors, flavors, and preservatives. Contains an amount of cloxacillin sodium equivalent to the labeled amount of cloxacillin, within -10% to $+20\%$. Meets the requirements for pH (5.0–7.5, in the solution constituted as directed in the labeling), Water (not more than 1.0%), Uniformity of dosage units (solid packaged in single-unit containers), and Deliverable volume (multiple-unit containers).

Sterile Cloxacillin Sodium USP—Preserve in tight containers. Label it to indicate that it is for veterinary use only. Contains an amount of cloxacillin sodium equivalent to not less than 825 mcg of cloxacillin per mg. Meets the requirements for Bacterial endotoxins and Sterility, and for Identification tests, Crystallinity, pH, Water, and Dimethylaniline under Cloxacillin Sodium.

CLOZAPINE

Chemical name: 5*H*-Dibenzo[*b*,*e*][1,4]diazepine, 8-chloro-11-(4-methyl-1-piperazinyl)-.

Molecular formula: $C_{18}H_{19}ClN_4$.

Molecular weight: 326.83.

Description: Yellow, crystalline powder.

Solubility: Very slightly soluble in water.

USP requirements: Clozapine Tablets—Not in USP.

COAL TAR

Description: Coal Tar USP—Nearly black, viscous liquid, heavier than water, having a characteristic, naphthalene-like odor.

Solubility: Coal Tar USP—Slightly soluble in water, to which it imparts its characteristic odor and a faintly alkaline reaction. Partially soluble in acetone, in alcohol, in carbon disulfide, in chloroform, in ether, in methanol, and in solvent hexane.

USP requirements:

Coal Tar USP—Preserve in tight containers. The tar obtained as a by-product during the destructive distillation of bituminous coal at temperatures in the range of 900 to 1100 °C. May be processed further either by extraction with alcohol and suitable dispersing agents and maceration times or by fractional distillation with or without the use of suitable solvents. Meets the requirement for Residue on ignition (not more than 2.0%, from 100 mg).

Coal Tar Cleansing Bar—Not in USP.

Coal Tar Cream—Not in USP.

Coal Tar Gel—Not in USP.

Coal Tar Lotion—Not in USP.

Coal Tar Ointment USP—Preserve in tight containers.

Prepare Coal Tar Ointment as follows: 10 grams of Coal Tar, 5 grams of Polysorbate 80, and 985 grams of Zinc Oxide Paste to make 1000 grams. Blend the Coal Tar with the Polysorbate 80, and incorporate the mixture with the Zinc Oxide Paste.

Coal Tar Shampoo—Not in USP.

Coal Tar Topical Solution USP—Preserve in tight containers.

Prepare Coal Tar Topical Solution as follows: 200 grams of Coal Tar, 50 grams of Polysorbate 80, and a sufficient quantity of Alcohol, to make 1000 mL. Mix the Coal Tar with 500 grams of washed sand, and add the Polysorbate 80 and 700 mL of Alcohol. Macerate the mixture for 7 days in a closed vessel with frequent agitation. Filter, and rinse the vessel and the filter with sufficient Alcohol to make the product measure 1000 mL.

Meets the requirement for Alcohol content (81.0–86.0%).

Coal Tar Topical Suspension—Not in USP.

CYANOCOBALAMIN Co 57

Chemical name: Vitamin B_{12}-^{57}*Co*.

Molecular formula: $C_{63}H_{88}{}^{57}CoN_{14}O_{14}P$.

Description:

Cyanocobalamin Co 57 Capsules USP—May contain a small amount of solid or solids, or may appear empty.

Cyanocobalamin Co 57 Oral Solution USP—Clear, colorless to pink solution.

USP requirements:

Cyanocobalamin Co 57 Capsules USP—Preserve in well-closed, light-resistant containers. Contain Cyanocobalamin in which a portion of the molecules contain radioactive cobalt (^{57}Co) in the molecular structure. Label Capsules to include the following: the date of calibration; the amount of cyanocobalamin expressed in mcg per Capsule; the amount of ^{57}Co as cyanocobalamin expressed in megabecquerels (or microcuries) per Capsule at the time of calibration; the expiration date; and the statement, "Caution—Radioactive Material." The labeling indicates that in making dosage calculations, correction is to be made for radioactive decay, and also indicates that the radioactive half-life of ^{57}Co is 270.9 days. Contain the labeled amount of ^{57}Co, within $\pm 10\%$, as cyanocobalamin expressed in megabecquerels (or microcuries) at the time indicated in the labeling. Contain the labeled amount of cyanocobalamin, within $\pm 10\%$. The specific activity is not less than 0.02 megabecquerel (0.5 microcurie) per mcg of cyanocobalamin. Meet the requirements for Radionuclide identification, Uniformity of dosage units, Radiochemical purity, and Cyanocobalamin content.

Cyanocobalamin Co 57 Oral Solution USP—Preserve in tight containers, and protect from light. A solution suitable for oral administration, containing Cyanocobalamin in which a portion of the molecules contain radioactive cobalt (^{57}Co) in the molecular structure. Label it to include the following: the date of calibration; the amount of ^{57}Co as cyanocobalamin expressed as total megabecquerels (or microcuries) and as megabecquerels (or microcuries) per mL at the time of calibration; the amount of cyanocobalamin expressed in mcg per mL; the name and quantity of the added preservative; the expiration date; and the statement, "Caution—Radioactive Material." The labeling indicates that in making dosage calculations, correction is to be made for radioactive decay, and also indicates that the radioactive half-life of ^{57}Co is 270.9 days, and directs that the Oral Solution be protected from light. Contains the labeled amount of ^{57}Co, within $\pm 10\%$, as cyanocobalamin expressed in megabecquerels (or microcuries) per mL at the time indicated in the labeling. Contains the labeled amount of cyanocobalamin, within $\pm 10\%$. The specific activity is not less than 0.02 megabecquerel (0.5 microcurie) per mcg of cyanocobalamin. Contains a suitable antimicrobial agent. Meets the requirements for Radionuclide identification, pH (4.0–5.5), Radiochemical purity (not less than 95.0%), and Cyanocobalamin content.

CYANOCOBALAMIN Co 60

Chemical name: Vitamin B_{12}-^{60}*Co*.

Molecular formula: $C_{63}H_{88}{}^{60}CoN_{14}O_{14}P$.

Description:
Cyanocobalamin Co 60 Capsules USP—Capsules may contain a small, rectangular solid, or may appear empty.
Cyanocobalamin Co 60 Oral Solution USP—Clear, colorless to pink solution.

USP requirements:
Cyanocobalamin Co 60 Capsules USP—Preserve in well-closed, light-resistant containers. Contain Cyanocobalamin in which a portion of the molecules contain radioactive cobalt (^{60}Co) in the molecular structure. Label Capsules to include the following: the date of calibration; the amount of cyanocobalamin expressed in mcg per Capsule; the amount of ^{60}Co as cyanocobalamin expressed in megabecquerels (or microcuries) per Capsule on the date of calibration; the expiration date; and the statement, "Caution—Radioactive Material." The labeling indicates that in making dosage calculations, correction is to be made for radioactive decay, and also indicates that the radioactive half-life of ^{60}Co is 5.27 years. Contain the labeled amount of ^{60}Co, within ±10%, as cyanocobalamin expressed in megabecquerels (or microcuries) on the date indicated in the labeling. Contain the labeled amount of cyanocobalamin, within ±10%. The specific activity is not less than 0.02 megabecquerel (0.5 microcurie) per mcg of cyanocobalamin. Meet the requirements for Radionuclide identification, Uniformity of dosage units, and Cyanocobalamin content.
Cyanocobalamin Co 60 Oral Solution USP—Preserve in single-dose or in multiple-dose containers, protected from light. A solution suitable for oral administration, containing Cyanocobalamin in which a portion of the molecules contain radioactive cobalt (^{60}Co) in the molecular structure. Label it to include the following: the date of calibration; the amount of ^{60}Co as cyanocobalamin expressed as total megabecquerels (or microcuries) and as megabecquerels (or microcuries) per mL on the date of calibration; the amount of cyanocobalamin expressed in mcg per mL; the name and quantity of the added preservative; the expiration date; and the statement, "Caution—Radioactive Material." The labeling indicates that in making dosage calculations, correction is to be made for radioactive decay, and also indicates that the radioactive half-life of ^{60}Co is 5.27 years. Contains the labeled amount of ^{60}Co, within ±10%, as cyanocobalamin expressed in megabecquerels (or microcuries) per mL on the date indicated in the labeling. Contains the labeled amount of cyanocobalamin per mL, within ±10%. The amount of cobalt 60 as cyanocobalamin is not more than 0.04 megabecquerel (1 microcurie) per mL. The specific activity is not less than 0.02 megabecquerel (0.5 microcurie) per mcg of cyanocobalamin. Contains a suitable antimicrobial agent. Meets the requirements for Radionuclide identification, pH (4.0–5.5), Radiochemical purity, and Cyanocobalamin content.

COCAINE

Source: An alkaloid obtained from the leaves of *Erythroxylum coca* and other species of *Erythroxylum*.

Chemical name:
Cocaine—8-Azabicyclo[3.2.1]octane-2-carboxylic acid, 3-(benzoyloxy)-8-methyl-, methyl ester, [1*R*-(*exo,exo*)]-.
Cocaine hydrochloride—8-Azabicyclo[3.2.1]octane-2-carboxylic acid, 3-(benzoyloxy)-8-methyl-, methyl ester, hydrochloride, [1*R*-(*exo,exo*)]-.

Molecular formula:
Cocaine—$C_{17}H_{21}NO_4$.
Cocaine hydrochloride—$C_{17}H_{21}NO_4 \cdot HCl$.

Molecular weight:
Cocaine—303.36.
Cocaine hydrochloride—339.82.

Description:
Cocaine USP—Colorless to white crystals or white, crystalline powder. Is levorotatory in 3 *N* hydrochloric acid solution. Its saturated solution is alkaline to litmus.
Cocaine Hydrochloride USP—Colorless crystals or white, crystalline powder.

Solubility:
Cocaine USP—Slightly soluble in water; very soluble in warm alcohol; freely soluble in alcohol, in chloroform, and in ether; soluble in olive oil; sparingly soluble in mineral oil.
Cocaine Hydrochloride USP—Very soluble in water; freely soluble in alcohol; soluble in chloroform and in glycerin; insoluble in ether.

USP requirements:
Cocaine USP—Preserve in well-closed, light-resistant containers. Dried over phosphorus pentoxide for 3 hours, contains not less than 99.0% and not more than 101.0% of cocaine. Meets the requirements for Identification, Melting range (96–98 °C), Loss on drying (not more than 1.0%), Residue on ignition (not more than 0.1%), Readily carbonizable substances, Cinnamyl-cocaine and other reducing substances, and Isoatropyl-cocaine.
Cocaine Hydrochloride USP—Preserve in well-closed, light-resistant containers. Contains not less than 99.0% and not more than 101.0% of cocaine hydrochloride, calculated on the dried basis. Meets the requirements for Identification, Specific rotation (−71° to −73°), Acidity, Loss on drying (not more than 1.0%), Residue on ignition (not more than 0.1%), Readily carbonizable substances, Cinnamyl-cocaine and other reducing substances, and Isoatropyl-cocaine.
Cocaine Hydrochloride Topical Solution—Not in USP.
Cocaine Hydrochloride Viscous Topical Solution—Not in USP.
Cocaine Hydrochloride Tablets for Topical Solution USP—Preserve in well-closed, light-resistant containers. Contain the labeled amount, within ±9%. Meet the requirements for Identification, Disintegration (15 minutes), and Uniformity of dosage units.

COCCIDIOIDIN

Description: Coccidioidin USP—Clear, practically colorless or amber-colored liquid.

USP requirements: Coccidioidin USP—Preserve at a temperature between 2 and 8 °C. A sterile solution containing the antigens obtained from the by-products of mycelial growth or from the spherules of the fungus *Coccidioides immitis*. Contains a suitable antimicrobial agent. Label it to state that any dilutions made of the product should be stored in a refrigerator and used within 24 hours. Label it also to state that a separate syringe and needle shall be used for each individual injection. Has a potency such that the 1:100 dilution is bioequivalent to the U.S. Reference Coccidioidin 1:100. Meets the requirement for Expiration date (not later than 3 years after date of issue from manufacturer's cold storage [5 °C, 1 year] for the mycelial product and not later than 18 months after date of issue from manufacturer's cold storage [5 °C, 18 months] for the spherule-derived product). Conforms to the regulations of the U.S. Food and Drug Administration concerning biologics.

COCOA BUTTER

Description: Cocoa Butter NF—Yellowish white solid, having a faint, agreeable odor. Usually brittle at temperatures below 25 °C.

NF category: Suppository base.

Solubility: Cocoa Butter NF—Freely soluble in ether and in chloroform; soluble in boiling dehydrated alcohol; slightly soluble in alcohol.

NF requirements: Cocoa Butter NF—Preserve in well-closed containers. The fat obtained from the seed of *Theobroma cacao* Linné (Fam. Sterculiaceae). Meets the requirements for Melting range (clear melting point 31–35 °C), Refractive index (1.454–1.459 at 40 °C), Fatty acid composition, Free fatty acids, Iodine value (33–42), and Saponification value (188–198).

CODEINE

Chemical name:

Codeine—Morphinan-6-ol, 7,8-didehydro-4,5-epoxy-3-methoxy-17-methyl-, monohydrate, (5 alpha,6 alpha)-.

Codeine phosphate—Morphinan-6-ol, 7,8-didehydro-4,5-epoxy-3-methoxy-17-methyl-, (5 alpha,6 alpha)-, phosphate (1:1) (salt), hemihydrate.

Codeine polistirex—Benzene, diethenyl-, polymer with ethenylbenzene, sulfonated, complex with (5 alpha,6 alpha)-7,8-didehydro-4,5-epoxy-3-methoxy-17-methylmorphinan-6-ol.

Codeine sulfate—Morphinan-6-ol, 7,8-didehydro-4,5-epoxy-3-methoxy-17-methyl-, (5 alpha,6 alpha)-, sulfate (2:1) (salt), trihydrate.

Molecular formula:

Codeine—$C_{18}H_{21}NO_3 \cdot H_2O$ (monohydrate); $C_{18}H_{21}NO_3$ (anhydrous).

Codeine phosphate—$C_{18}H_{21}NO_3 \cdot H_3PO_4 \cdot \frac{1}{2}H_2O$ (hemihydrate); $C_{18}H_{21}NO_3 \cdot H_3PO_4$ (anhydrous).

Codeine sulfate—$(C_{18}H_{21}NO_3)_2 \cdot H_2SO_4 \cdot 3H_2O$ (trihydrate); $(C_{18}H_{21}NO_3)_2 \cdot H_2SO_4$ (anhydrous).

Molecular weight:

Codeine—317.38 (monohydrate); 299.37 (anhydrous).

Codeine phosphate—406.37 (hemihydrate); 397.36 (anhydrous).

Codeine sulfate—750.86 (trihydrate); 696.81 (anhydrous).

Description:

Codeine USP—Colorless or white crystals or white, crystalline powder. Effloresces slowly in dry air, and is affected by light. In acid or alcohol solutions it is levorotatory. Its saturated solution is alkaline to litmus.

Codeine Phosphate USP—Fine, white, needle-shaped crystals, or white, crystalline powder. Odorless. Is affected by light. Its solutions are acid to litmus.

Codeine Sulfate USP—White crystals, usually needle-like, or white, crystalline powder. Is affected by light.

Solubility:

Codeine USP—Slightly soluble in water; very soluble in chloroform; freely soluble in alcohol; sparingly soluble in ether. When heated in an amount of water insufficient for complete solution, it melts to oily drops which crystallize on cooling.

Codeine Phosphate USP—Freely soluble in water; very soluble in hot water; slightly soluble in alcohol but more so in boiling alcohol.

Codeine Sulfate USP—Soluble in water; freely soluble in water at 80 °C; very slightly soluble in alcohol; insoluble in chloroform and in ether.

USP requirements:

Codeine USP—Preserve in tight, light-resistant containers. Dried at 80 °C for 4 hours, contains not less than 98.5% and not more than 100.5% of anhydrous codeine. Meets the requirements for Identification, Melting range (154–158 °C, the range between beginning and end of melting not more than 2 °C), Loss on drying (not more than 6.0%), Residue on ignition (not more than 0.1%), Readily carbonizable substances, Chromatographic purity, and Morphine.

Codeine Phosphate USP—Preserve in tight, light-resistant containers. Contains not less than 99.0% and not more than 101.5% of codeine phosphate, calculated on the anhydrous basis. Meets the requirements for Identification, Acidity, Water (not more than 3.0%), Chloride, Sulfate, Morphine, and Chromatographic purity.

Codeine Phosphate Injection USP—Preserve in single-dose or in multiple-dose containers, preferably of Type I glass, protected from light. A sterile solution of Codeine Phosphate in Water for Injection. Contains the labeled amount of codeine phosphate (as the hemihydrate), within ±7%. Meets the requirements for Identification, Bacterial endotoxins, pH (3.0–6.0), Morphine, and Injections.

Note: Do not use the Injection if it is more than slightly discolored or contains a precipitate.

Codeine Phosphate Oral Solution—Not in USP.

Codeine Phosphate Tablets USP—Preserve in well-closed, light-resistant containers. Contain the labeled amount of codeine phosphate (as the hemihydrate), within ±7%. Meet the requirements for Identification, Dissolution (75% in 45 minutes in water in Apparatus 2 at 50 rpm), Uniformity of dosage units, and Morphine.

Codeine Phosphate Soluble Tablets—Not in USP.

Codeine Sulfate USP—Preserve in tight, light-resistant containers. Dried at 105 °C for 3 hours, contains not less than 98.5% and not more than 100.5% of anhydrous codeine sulfate. Meets the requirements for Identification, Specific rotation (−112.5° to −115.0°, calculated on the dried basis), Acidity, Water (6.0–7.5%), Residue on ignition (not more than 0.1%), Readily carbonizable substances, Chromatographic purity, and Morphine.

Codeine Sulfate Tablets USP—Preserve in well-closed containers. Contain the labeled amount of codeine sulfate (as the trihydrate), within ±7%. Meet the requirements for Identification, Dissolution (75% in 45 minutes in water in Apparatus 1 at 100 rpm), and Uniformity of dosage units.

Codeine Sulfate Soluble Tablets—Not in USP.

CODEINE AND CALCIUM IODIDE

Chemical name: Codeine—Morphinan-6-ol, 7,8-didehydro-4,5-epoxy-3-methoxy-17-methyl-, monohydrate, (5 alpha,6 alpha)-.

Molecular formula:

Codeine—$C_{18}H_{21}NO_3 \cdot H_2O$.

Calcium iodide—CaI_2.

Molecular weight:

Codeine—317.38.

Calcium iodide—293.9.

Description:

Codeine USP—Colorless or white crystals or white, crystalline powder. It effloresces slowly in dry air, and is affected by light. In acid or alcohol solutions it is levorotatory. Its saturated solution is alkaline to litmus.

Calcium iodide—Very hygroscopic. Aqueous solution is neutral or slightly alkaline.

Solubility:

Codeine USP—Slightly soluble in water; very soluble in chloroform; freely soluble in alcohol; sparingly soluble in ether. When heated in an amount of water insufficient for complete solution, it melts to oily drops which crystallize on cooling.

Calcium iodide—Very soluble in water, in methanol, in ethanol, and in acetone; practically insoluble in ether and in dioxane.

USP requirements: Codeine and Calcium Iodide Syrup—Not in USP.

CODEINE AND IODINATED GLYCEROL

For *Codeine* and *Iodinated Glycerol*—See individual listings for chemistry information.

USP requirements: Codeine Phosphate and Iodinated Glycerol Oral Solution—Not in USP.

COD LIVER OIL

Description: Cod Liver Oil USP—Thin, oily liquid, having a characteristic, slightly fishy but not rancid odor.

Solubility: Cod Liver Oil USP—Slightly soluble in alcohol; freely soluble in ether, in chloroform, in carbon disulfide, and in ethyl acetate.

USP requirements: Cod Liver Oil USP—Preserve in tight containers. It may be bottled or otherwise packaged in containers from which air has been expelled by the production of a vacuum or by an inert gas. The partially destearinated fixed oil obtained from fresh livers of *Gadus morrhua* Linné and other species of Fam. Gadidae. The vitamin A potency and vitamin D potency, when designated on the label, are expressed in USP Units per gram of oil. The potencies may be expressed also in metric units, on the basis that 1 USP Vitamin A Unit = 0.3 mcg and 40 USP Vitamin D Units = 1 mcg. Contains, in each gram, not less than 255 mcg (850 USP Units) of vitamin A and not less than 2.125 mcg (85 USP Units) of vitamin D. Meets the requirements for Identification for vitamin A, Specific gravity (0.918–0.927), Color, Nondestearinated cod liver oil, Unsaponifiable matter (not more than 1.30%), Acid value, Iodine value (145–180), and Saponification value (180–192).

COLCHICINE

Chemical name: Acetamide, *N*-(5,6,7,9-tetrahydro-1,2,3,10-tetramethoxy-9-oxobenzo[*a*]heptalen-7-yl)-, (*S*)-.

Molecular formula: $C_{22}H_{25}NO_6$.

Molecular weight: 399.44.

Description: Colchicine USP—Pale yellow to pale greenish yellow, amorphous scales, or powder or crystalline powder. Is odorless or nearly so, and darkens on exposure to light.

pKa: 12.35.

Solubility: Colchicine USP—Soluble in water; freely soluble in alcohol and in chloroform; slightly soluble in ether.

USP requirements:

Colchicine USP—Preserve in tight, light-resistant containers. An alkaloid obtained from various species of *Colchicum*. Contains not less than 94.0% and not more than 101.0% of colchicine, calculated on the anhydrous, solvent-free basis. Meets the requirements for Identification, Specific rotation (−240° to −250°, calculated on the anhydrous and solvent-free basis), Water (not more than 2.0%), Colchiceine, Limit of ethyl acetate (not more than 8.0%), Chromatographic purity, and Organic volatile impurities.

Caution: Colchicine is extremely poisonous.

Colchicine Injection USP—Preserve in single-dose containers, preferably of Type I glass, protected from light. A sterile solution of Colchicine in Water for Injection, prepared from Colchicine with the aid of Sodium Hydroxide. Contains the labeled amount, within ±10%. Meets the requirements for Identification, Bacterial endotoxins, pH (6.0–7.2, in a solution of Injection containing 1.0 mg of potassium chloride in each mL), and Injections.

Caution: Colchicine is extremely poisonous.

Colchicine Tablets USP—Preserve in well-closed, light-resistant containers. Contain the labeled amount, within ±10%. Meet the requirements for Identification, Dissolution (75% in 30 minutes in water in Apparatus 1 at 100 rpm), and Uniformity of dosage units.

COLESTIPOL

Chemical group: An anion-exchange resin.

Chemical name: Colestipol hydrochloride—Colestipol hydrochloride. Copolymer of diethylenetriamine and 1-chloro-2,3-epoxypropane, hydrochloride (with approximately 1 out of 5 amine nitrogens protonated).

Description: Colestipol Hydrochloride USP—Yellow to orange beads.

Solubility: Colestipol Hydrochloride USP—Swells but does not dissolve in water or dilute aqueous solutions of acid or alkali. Insoluble in the common organic solvents.

USP requirements:

Colestipol Hydrochloride USP—Preserve in tight containers. An insoluble, high molecular weight basic anion-exchange copolymer of diethylenetriamine and 1-chloro-2,3-epoxypropane with approximately one out of five amino nitrogens protonated. Each gram binds not less than 1.1 mEq and not more than 1.6 mEq of sodium cholate, calculated as cholate binding capacity. Meets the requirements for Identification, pH (6.0–7.5), Loss on drying (not more than 1.0%), Residue on ignition (not more than 0.3%), Heavy metals (not more than 0.002%), Chloride content (6.5–9.0%, calculated on the dried basis), Water absorption (3.3–5.3 grams of water per gram), Cholate binding capacity (1.1–1.6 mEq per gram), Water-soluble substances (not more than 0.5%), and Colestipol exchange capacity (9.0–11.0 mEq of sodium hydroxide per gram).

Colestipol Hydrochloride for Oral Suspension USP—Preserve in tight, single-dose or multiple-dose containers. A mixture of Colestipol Hydrochloride with a suitable flow-promoting agent. Each gram binds not less than 1.1 mEq and not more than 1.6 mEq of sodium cholate, calculated as the cholate binding capacity. Meets the requirements for Minimum fill and Water-soluble substances (not more than 0.5%), and for Cholate binding capacity, Identification, Water absorption, and pH under Colestipol Hydrochloride.

COLFOSCERIL, CETYL ALCOHOL, AND TYLOXAPOL

Chemical name:

Colfosceril palmitate—3,5,9-Trioxa-4-phosphapentacosan-1-aminium, 4-hydroxy-*N*,*N*,*N*-trimethyl-10-oxo-7-[(1-oxohexadecyl)oxy]-, hydroxide, inner salt, 4-oxide, (*R*)-.

Cetyl alcohol—1-Hexadecanol.

Tyloxapol—Phenol, 4-(1,1,3,3-tetramethylbutyl)-, polymer with formaldehyde and oxirane.

Molecular formula:
Colfosceril palmitate—$C_{40}H_{80}NO_8P$.
Cetyl alcohol—$C_{16}H_{34}O$.

Molecular weight:
Colfosceril palmitate—734.05.
Cetyl alcohol—242.45.

Description:
Cetyl Alcohol NF—Unctuous, white flakes, granules, cubes, or castings. Has a faint characteristic odor. Usually melts in the range between 45–50 °C.
NF category: Stiffening agent.
Tyloxapol USP—Viscous, amber liquid, having a slight, aromatic odor. May exhibit a slight turbidity.
NF category: Wetting and/or solubilizing agent.

Solubility:
Cetyl Alcohol NF—Insoluble in water; soluble in alcohol and in ether, the solubility increasing with an increase in temperature.
Tyloxapol USP—Slowly but freely miscible with water. Soluble in glacial acetic acid, in toluene, in carbon tetrachloride, in chloroform, and in carbon disulfide.

USP requirements: Colfosceril Palmitate, Cetyl Alcohol, and Tyloxapol for Intratracheal Suspension—Not in USP.

COLISTIMETHATE

Chemical name: Colistimethate sodium—Colistimethate sodium.

Molecular formula: $C_{58}H_{105}N_{16}Na_5O_{28}S_5$ (colistin A component); $C_{57}H_{103}N_{16}Na_5O_{28}S_5$ (colistin B component).

Molecular weight: 1749.81 (colistin A component); 1735.78 (colistin B component).

Description: Sterile Colistimethate Sodium USP—White to slightly yellow, odorless, fine powder.

Solubility: Sterile Colistimethate Sodium USP—Freely soluble in water; soluble in methanol; insoluble in acetone and in ether.

USP requirements: Sterile Colistimethate Sodium USP—Preserve in Containers for Sterile Solids. It is colistimethate sodium suitable for parenteral use. Has a potency equivalent to not less than 390 mcg of colistin per mg, and, where packaged for dispensing, contains an amount of colistimethate sodium equivalent to the labeled amount of colistin, within −10% to +20%. Meets the requirements for Constituted solution, Identification, Bacterial endotoxins, Sterility, pH (6.5–8.5, in a solution containing 10 mg per mL), Loss on drying (not more than 7.0%), Heavy metals (not more than 0.003%), and Free colistin. Where packaged for dispensing, meets the requirements for Uniformity of dosage units and for Constituted solutions and Labeling under Injections.

COLISTIN

Chemical name: Colistin sulfate—Colistin, sulfate.

Molecular formula:
Sulfate, Colistin A component—$C_{53}H_{100}N_{16}O_{13} \cdot 2\frac{1}{2}H_2SO_4$.
Sulfate, Colistin B component—$C_{52}H_{98}N_{16}O_{13} \cdot 2\frac{1}{2}H_2SO_4$.

Molecular weight:
Sulfate, Colistin A component—1414.65.
Sulfate, Colistin B component—1400.63.

Description: Colistin Sulfate USP—White to slightly yellow, odorless, fine powder.

Solubility: Colistin Sulfate USP—Freely soluble in water; slightly soluble in methanol; insoluble in acetone and in ether.

USP requirements:
Colistin Sulfate USP—Preserve in tight containers. The sulfate salt of an antibacterial substance produced by the growth of *Bacillus polymyxa* var. *colistinus*. Has a potency equivalent to not less than 500 mcg of colistin per mg. Meets the requirements for Identification, pH (4.0–7.0, in a solution containing 10 mg per mL), and Loss on drying (not more than 7.0%).
Colistin Sulfate for Oral Suspension USP—Preserve in tight containers, protected from light. A dry mixture of Colistin Sulfate with or without one or more suitable buffers, colors, diluents, dispersants, and flavors. Contains an amount of colistin sulfate equivalent to the labeled amount of colistin, within −10% to +20%. Meets the requirements for Uniformity of dosage units (solid packaged in single-unit containers), Deliverable volume (solid packaged in multiple-unit containers), pH (5.0–6.0, in the suspension constituted as directed in the labeling), and Loss on drying (not more than 3.0%).

COLISTIN, NEOMYCIN, AND HYDROCORTISONE

For *Colistin, Neomycin,* and *Hydrocortisone*—See individual listings for chemistry information.

USP requirements: Colistin and Neomycin Sulfates and Hydrocortisone Acetate Otic Suspension USP—Preserve in tight containers. A sterile suspension. Contains an amount of colistin sulfate equivalent to the labeled amount of colistin, within −10% to +35%, an amount of neomycin sulfate equivalent to the labeled amount of neomycin, within −10% to +25%, and the labeled amount of hydrocortisone acetate, within ±10%. Contains one or more suitable buffers, detergents, dispersants, and preservatives. Meets the requirements for Sterility and pH (4.8–5.2).
Note: Where Colistin and Neomycin Sulfates and Hydrocortisone Acetate Otic Suspension is prescribed, without reference to the quantity of colistin, neomycin, or hydrocortisone acetate contained therein, a product containing 3.0 mg of colistin, 3.3 mg of neomycin, and 10 mg of hydrocortisone acetate per mL shall be dispensed.

COLLODION

USP requirements: Collodion USP—Preserve in tight containers, at a temperature not exceeding 30 °C, remote from fire. The label bears a caution statement to the effect that Collodion is highly flammable. Contains not less than 5.0%, by weight, of pyroxylin.
Prepare Collodion as follows: 40 grams of Pyroxylin, 750 mL of Ether, and 250 mL of Alcohol to make about 1000 mL. Add the Alcohol and Ether to the Pyroxylin contained in a suitable container, and insert the stopper into the container well. Shake the mixture occasionally until the Pyroxylin is dissolved.
Meets the requirements for Identification, Specific gravity (0.765–0.775), Acidity, and Alcohol content (22.0–26.0%).
Caution: Collodion is highly flammable.

FLEXIBLE COLLODION

Description: Flexible Collodion USP—Clear, or slightly opalescent, viscous liquid. Is colorless or slightly yellow, and has the odor of ether. The strong odor of camphor becomes noticeable as the ether evaporates.

USP requirements: Flexible Collodion USP—Preserve in tight containers, at a temperature not exceeding 30 °C, remote from fire. The label bears a caution statement to the effect that Flexible Collodion is highly flammable.

Prepare Flexible Collodion as follows: 20 grams of Camphor, 30 grams of Castor Oil, and a sufficient quantity of Collodion, to make 1000 grams. Weigh the ingredients, successively, into a dry, tared bottle, insert the stopper in the bottle, and shake the mixture until the camphor is dissolved.

Meets the requirements for Identification, Specific gravity (0.770–0.790), and Alcohol content (21.0–25.0%).

COLLOIDAL OATMEAL

USP requirements: Colloidal Oatmeal USP—Preserve in well-closed containers. The powder resulting from the grinding and further processing of whole oat grain meeting U.S. Standards for Number 1 or Number 2 oats. Meets the requirements for Identification, Viscosity, Microbial limits, Loss on drying (not more than 10%), Total ash (not more than 2.5% on the dried basis), Fat content (not less than 3%), and Nitrogen content (not less than 2.0%).

COPPER

Chemical name: Copper gluconate—Copper, bis (D-gluconato-O^1,O^2)-.

Molecular formula: Copper gluconate—$C_{12}H_{22}CuO_{14}$.

Molecular weight: Copper gluconate—453.84.

USP requirements:

Copper Gluconate USP—Preserve in well-closed containers. Contains not less than 98.0% and not more than 102.0% of copper gluconate. Meets the requirements for Identification, Chloride (not more than 0.07%), Sulfate (not more than 0.05%), Arsenic (not more than 3 ppm), Lead (not more than 0.0025%), and Reducing substances (not more than 1.0%).

Copper Gluconate Tablets—Not in USP.

CORN OIL

Description: Corn Oil NF—Clear, light yellow, oily liquid, having a faint, characteristic odor.

NF category: Solvent; vehicle (oleaginous).

Solubility: Corn Oil NF—Slightly soluble in alcohol; miscible with ether, with chloroform, and with solvent hexane.

NF requirements: Corn Oil NF—Preserve in tight, light-resistant containers, and avoid exposure to excessive heat. The refined fixed oil obtained from the embryo of *Zea mays* Linné (Fam. Gramineae). Meets the requirements for Specific gravity (0.914–0.921), Heavy metals (not more than 0.001%), Cottonseed oil, Fatty acid composition, Free fatty acids, Iodine value (102–130), Saponification value (187–193), Unsaponifiable matter (not more than 1.5%), and Organic volatile impurities.

CORTICOTROPIN

Chemical name:

Corticotropin—Corticotropin.

Corticotropin, repository—Corticotropin.

Corticotropin zinc hydroxide—Corticotropin zinc hydroxide.

Description:

Corticotropin Injection USP—Colorless or light straw-colored liquid.

Corticotropin for Injection USP—White or practically white, soluble, amorphous solid having the characteristic appearance of substances prepared by freeze-drying.

Repository Corticotropin Injection USP—Colorless or light straw-colored liquid, which may be quite viscid at room temperature. Is odorless or has an odor of an antimicrobial agent.

Sterile Corticotropin Zinc Hydroxide Suspension USP—Flocculent, white, aqueous suspension, free from large particles following moderate shaking.

USP requirements:

Corticotropin Injection USP—Preserve in single-dose or in multiple-dose containers, preferably of Type I glass. Store in a cold place. A sterile solution, in a suitable diluent, of the material containing the polypeptide hormone having the property of increasing the rate of secretion of adrenal corticosteroids, which is obtained from the anterior lobe of the pituitary of mammals used for food by man. If the labeling of Corticotropin Injection recommends intravenous administration, include specific information on dosage. Its potency is within −20% to +25% of the potency stated on the label in USP Corticotropin Units. Meets the requirements for Vasopressin activity, Bacterial endotoxins, pH (3.0–7.0), Particulate matter, and Injections.

Corticotropin for Injection USP—Preserve in Containers for Sterile Solids. A sterile, dry material containing the polypeptide hormone having the property of increasing the rate of secretion of adrenal corticosteroids, which is obtained from the anterior lobe of the pituitary of mammals used for food by man. If the labeling of Corticotropin for Injection recommends intravenous administration, include specific information on dosage. Its potency is within −20% to +25% of the potency stated on the label in USP Corticotropin Units. Meets the requirements for Vasopressin activity, Bacterial endotoxins, pH (2.5–6.0, in a solution constituted as directed in the labeling supplied by the manufacturer), and Particulate matter, and for Sterility tests, Uniformity of dosage units, Constituted solutions and Labeling under Injections.

Repository Corticotropin Injection USP—Preserve in single-dose or in multiple-dose containers, preferably of Type I glass. It is corticotropin in a solution of partially hydrolyzed gelatin. Its potency is within −20% to +25% of the potency stated on the label in USP Corticotropin Units. Meets the requirements for Bacterial endotoxins, for Vasopressin activity and pH under Corticotropin Injection, and for Injections.

Sterile Corticotropin Zinc Hydroxide Suspension USP—Preserve in single-dose or in multiple-dose containers, preferably of Type I glass. Store at controlled room temperature. A sterile suspension of corticotropin adsorbed on zinc hydroxide. Label it to indicate that it is not recommended for intravenous use and that the suspension is to be well shaken before use. The container label and the package label state the potency in USP Corticotropin Units in each mL. Its potency is within −20% to +25% of the potency stated on the label in USP Corticotropin Units. Contains not less than 1800 mcg and not more than 2200 mcg of zinc, and not less than 604 mcg and not more than 776 mcg of anhydrous dibasic sodium phosphate, for each 40 USP Corticotropin Units. Meets the requirements for Bacterial endotoxins, pH (7.5–8.5), Zinc, Anhydrous dibasic sodium phosphate, and Injections.

CORTISONE

Chemical name: Cortisone acetate—Pregn-4-ene-3,11,20-trione, 21-(acetyloxy)-17-hydroxy-.

Molecular formula: Cortisone acetate—$C_{23}H_{30}O_6$.

Molecular weight: Cortisone acetate—402.49.

Description: Cortisone Acetate USP—White or practically white, odorless, crystalline powder. Is stable in air. Melts at about 240 °C, with some decomposition.

Solubility: Cortisone Acetate USP—Insoluble in water; freely soluble in chloroform; soluble in dioxane; sparingly soluble in acetone; slightly soluble in alcohol.

USP requirements:

Cortisone Acetate USP—Preserve in well-closed containers. Contains not less than 97.0% and not more than 102.0% of cortisone acetate, calculated on the dried basis. Meets the requirements for Identification, Specific rotation (+208° to +217°, calculated on the dried basis), Loss on drying (not more than 1.0%), Residue on ignition (negligible, from 100 mg), and Ordinary impurities.

Sterile Cortisone Acetate Suspension USP—Preserve in single-dose or in multiple-dose containers, preferably of Type I glass. A sterile suspension of Cortisone Acetate in a suitable aqueous medium. Contains the labeled amount, within ±10%. Meets the requirements for Identification, pH (5.0–7.0), and Injections.

Cortisone Acetate Tablets USP—Preserve in well-closed containers. Contain the labeled amount, within ±10%. Meet the requirements for Identification, Dissolution (60% in 30 minutes in a mixture of isopropyl alcohol and dilute hydrochloric acid [1 in 100] in Apparatus 1 at 100 rpm), and Uniformity of dosage units.

COSYNTROPIN

Source: Synthetic polypeptide identical to the first 24 of the 39 amino acids of corticotropin.

Chemical name: Alpha$^{1\text{-}24}$-Corticotropin.

Molecular formula: $C_{136}H_{210}N_{40}O_{31}S$.

Molecular weight: 2933.47.

Description: White to off-white lyophilized mixture.

Solubility: Soluble in water.

USP requirements: Cosyntropin for Injection—Not in USP.

PURIFIED COTTON

Description: Purified Cotton USP—White, soft, fine filament-like hairs appearing under the microscope as hollow, flattened and twisted bands, striate and slightly thickened at the edges. Is practically odorless.

Solubility: Purified Cotton USP—Insoluble in ordinary solvents; soluble in ammoniated cupric oxide TS.

USP requirements: Purified Cotton USP—Package it in rolls of not more than 500 grams of a continuous lap, with a light-weight paper running under the entire lap, the paper being of such width that it may be folded over the edges of the lap to a distance of at least 25 millimeters, the two together being tightly and evenly rolled, and enclosed and sealed in a well-closed container. It may be packaged also in other types of containers if these are so constructed that the sterility of the product is maintained. The hair of the seed of cultivated varieties of *Gossypium hirsutum* Linné, or of other species of *Gossypium* (Fam. Malvaceae), freed from adhering impurities, deprived of fatty matter, bleached, and sterilized in its final container. Its label bears a statement to the effect that the sterility cannot be guaranteed if the package bears evidence of damage or if the package has been opened previously. Meets the requirements for Alkalinity or acidity, Residue on ignition (not more than 0.20%), Water-soluble substances (not more than 0.35%), Fatty matter (not more than 0.7%), Dyes, Other foreign matter, Fiber length and Absorbency (not less than 60% of fibers, by weight, are 12.5 millimeters or greater in length and not more than 10% of fibers, by weight, are 6.25 millimeters or less in length; retains not less than 24 times its weight of water), and Sterility.

COTTONSEED OIL

Description: Cottonseed Oil NF—Pale yellow, oily liquid. It is odorless or nearly so. At temperatures below 10 °C particles of solid fat may separate from the Oil, and at about 0 to −5 °C, the oil becomes a solid or nearly so.

NF category: Solvent; oleaginous vehicle.

Solubility: Cottonseed Oil NF—Slightly soluble in alcohol. Miscible with ether, with chloroform, with solvent hexane, and with carbon disulfide.

NF requirements: Cottonseed Oil NF—Preserve in tight, light-resistant containers, and avoid exposure to excessive heat. The refined fixed oil obtained from the seed of cultivated plants of various varieties of *Gossypium hirsutum* Linné or of other species of *Gossypium* (Fam. Malvaceae). Meets the requirements for Identification, Specific gravity (0.915–0.921), Heavy metals (not more than 0.001%), Solidification range of the fatty acids (31–35 °C), Free fatty acids, Iodine value (109–120), Saponification value (190–198), and Organic volatile impurities.

CREATININE

Molecular formula: $C_4H_7N_3O$.

Molecular weight: 113.12.

Description: Creatinine NF—White crystals or crystalline powder. Is odorless.

NF category: Bulking agent for freeze-drying.

Solubility: Creatinine NF—Soluble in water; slightly soluble in alcohol; practically insoluble in acetone, in ether, and in chloroform.

NF requirements: Creatinine NF—Preserve in well-closed containers. Contains not less than 98.5% and not more than 102.0% of creatinine, as Creatinine, calculated on the dried basis. Meets the requirements for Identification, Loss on drying (not more than 3.0%), Residue on ignition (not more than 0.2%), and Heavy metals (not more than 0.001%).

CRESOL

Chemical name: Phenol, methyl-.

Molecular formula: C_7H_8O.

Molecular weight: 108.14.

Description: Cresol NF—Colorless, or yellowish to brownish yellow, or pinkish, highly refractive liquid, becoming darker with age and on exposure to light. It has a phenol-like, sometimes empyreumatic odor. A saturated solution of it is neutral or only slightly acid to litmus.

NF category: Antimicrobial preservative.

Solubility: Cresol NF—Sparingly soluble in water, usually forming a cloudy solution; dissolves in solutions of fixed alkali hydroxides. Miscible with alcohol, with ether, and with glycerin.

NF requirements: Cresol NF—Preserve in tight, light-resistant containers. A mixture of isomeric cresols obtained from coal tar or from petroleum. Meets the requirements for Identification, Specific gravity (1.030–1.038), Distilling range (195–205 °C, not less than 90.0% distils), Hydrocarbons, and Phenol (not more than 5.0%).

CROMOLYN

Chemical name: Cromolyn sodium—4*H*-1-Benzopyran-2-carboxylic acid, 5,5′-[(2-hydroxy-1,3-propanediyl)bis(oxy)]bis-[4-oxo-, disodium salt].

Molecular formula: Cromolyn sodium—$C_{23}H_{14}Na_2O_{11}$.

Molecular weight: Cromolyn sodium—512.34.

Description:
Cromolyn Sodium USP—White, odorless, crystalline powder. Is hygroscopic.
Cromolyn Sodium for Inhalation USP—White to creamy white, odorless, hygroscopic, and very finely divided powder.

Solubility: Cromolyn Sodium USP—Soluble in water; insoluble in alcohol and in chloroform.

USP requirements:
Cromolyn Sodium USP—Preserve in tight containers. Contains not less than 98.0% and not more than 101.0% of cromolyn sodium, calculated on the dried basis. Meets the requirements for Identification, Acidity or alkalinity, Water (not more than 10.0%), Related compounds, Oxalate, and Organic volatile impurities.
Cromolyn Sodium Capsules—Not in USP.
Cromolyn Sodium Inhalation Solution USP—Preserve in single-unit, double-ended glass ampuls or in low-density polyethylene ampuls. A sterile, aqueous solution of Cromolyn Sodium. The label indicates that the Inhalation Solution is not to be used if it contains a precipitate. Contains the labeled amount, within ±10%. Meets the requirements for Identification, Related compounds, pH (4.0–7.0), Sterility, and Uniformity of dosage units.
Cromolyn Sodium Inhalation Aerosol—Not in USP.
Cromolyn Sodium for Inhalation USP (Capsules)—Preserve in tight, light-resistant containers. Avoid excessive heat. A mixture of equal parts of Lactose and Cromolyn Sodium contained in a hard gelatin capsule. Contains the labeled amount, within −5% to +25%. Meets the requirements for Identification and Uniformity of dosage units.
Cromolyn Sodium for Nasal Insufflation—Not in USP.
Cromolyn Sodium Nasal Solution USP—Preserve in tight, light-resistant containers. An aqueous solution of Cromolyn Sodium. Contains the labeled amount, within ±10%. Meets the requirements for Identification, pH (4.0–7.0), and Related compounds.
Cromolyn Sodium Ophthalmic Solution USP—Preserve in tight, light-resistant, single-dose or multiple-dose containers. Ophthalmic Solution that is packaged in multiple-dose containers contains a suitable antimicrobial agent. A sterile, aqueous solution of Cromolyn Sodium. Contains the labeled amount, within ±10%. Meets the requirements for Identification, Sterility, pH (4.0–7.0), and Related compounds.

CROSCARMELLOSE SODIUM

Description: Croscarmellose Sodium NF—White, free-flowing powder.
NF category: Tablet disintegrant.

Solubility: Croscarmellose Sodium NF—Partially soluble in water; insoluble in alcohol, in ether, and in other organic solvents.

NF requirements: Croscarmellose Sodium NF—Preserve in tight containers. A cross-linked polymer of carboxymethylcellulose sodium. Meets the requirements for Identification, pH (5.0–7.0), Loss on drying (not more than 10.0%), Heavy metals (not more than 0.001%), Sodium chloride and sodium glycolate (not more than 0.5%), Degree of substitution (0.60–0.85, calculated on the dried basis), Content of water-soluble material (1.0–10.0%), and Settling volume.

CROSPOVIDONE

Chemical name: 2-Pyrrolidinone, 1-ethenyl-, homopolymer.

Molecular formula: $(C_6H_9NO)_n$.

Description: Crospovidone NF—White to creamy-white, hygroscopic powder, having a faint odor.
NF category: Tablet disintegrant.

Solubility: Crospovidone NF—Insoluble in water and in ordinary organic solvents.

NF requirements: Crospovidone NF—Preserve in tight containers. A water-insoluble synthetic, cross-linked homopolymer of *N*-vinyl-2-pyrrolidinone. Contains not less than 11.0% and not more than 12.8% of nitrogen, calculated on the anhydrous basis. Meets the requirements for Identification, pH (5.0–8.0, in an aqueous suspension [1 in 100]), Water (not more than 5.0%), Residue on ignition (not more than 0.4%), Water-soluble substances (not more than 1.5%), Heavy metals (not more than 0.001%), Vinylpyrrolidinone (not more than 0.1%), and Nitrogen content.

CROTAMITON

Chemical name: 2-Butenamide, *N*-ethyl-*N*-(2-methylphenyl)-.

Molecular formula: $C_{13}H_{17}NO$.

Molecular weight: 203.28.

Description: Crotamiton USP—Colorless to slightly yellowish oil, having a faint amine-like odor.

Solubility: Crotamiton USP—Soluble in alcohol and in methanol.

USP requirements:
Crotamiton USP—Preserve in tight, light-resistant containers. A mixture of *cis* and *trans* isomers containing not less than 97.0% and not more than 103.0% of crotamiton. Meets the requirements for Identification, Specific gravity (1.008–1.011 at 20 °C), Refractive index (1.540–1.543 at 20 °C), Residue on ignition (not more than 0.1%), and Bound halogen.
Crotamiton Cream USP—Preserve in collapsible tubes or in tight, light-resistant containers. Contains the labeled amount, within ±7%. Meets the requirements for Identification and Minimum fill.
Crotamiton Lotion—Not in USP.

CUPRIC CHLORIDE

Chemical name: Copper chloride ($CuCl_2$) dihydrate.

Molecular formula: $CuCl_2 \cdot 2H_2O$.

Molecular weight: 170.48.

Description: Cupric Chloride USP—Bluish green, deliquescent crystals.

Solubility: Cupric Chloride USP—Freely soluble in water; soluble in alcohol; slightly soluble in ether.

USP requirements:

Cupric Chloride USP—Preserve in tight containers. Contains not less than 99.0% and not more than 100.5% of cupric chloride, calculated on the dried basis. Meets the requirements for Identification, Loss on drying (20.9–21.4%), Insoluble matter (not more than 0.01%), Sulfate (not more than 0.005%), Substances not precipitated by hydrogen sulfide (not more than 0.1%), Iron, Other metals, and Organic volatile impurities.

Cupric Chloride Injection USP—Preserve in single-dose or in multiple-dose containers, preferably of Type I or Type II glass. A sterile solution of Cupric Chloride in Water for Injection. Label the Injection to indicate that it is to be diluted to the appropriate strength with Sterile Water for Injection or other suitable fluid prior to administration. Contains an amount of cupric chloride equivalent to the labeled amount of copper, within ±5%. Meets the requirements for Identification, Bacterial endotoxins, pH (1.5–2.5), Particulate matter, and Injections.

CUPRIC SULFATE

Chemical name: Sulfuric acid, copper(2+) salt (1:1), pentahydrate.

Molecular formula: $CuSO_4 \cdot 5H_2O$.

Molecular weight: 249.68.

Description: Cupric Sulfate USP—Deep blue, triclinic crystals or blue, crystalline granules or powder. It effloresces slowly in dry air. Its solutions are acid to litmus.

Solubility: Cupric Sulfate USP—Freely soluble in water and in glycerin; very soluble in boiling water; slightly soluble in alcohol.

USP requirements:

Cupric Sulfate USP—Preserve in tight containers. Dried at 250 °C to constant weight, contains not less than 98.5% and not more than 100.5% of cupric sulfate. Meets the requirements for Identification, Loss on drying (33.0–36.5%), Alkalies and alkaline earths (not more than 0.3%), Substances not precipitated by hydrogen sulfide (not more than 0.3%), and Organic volatile impurities.

Cupric Sulfate Injection USP—Preserve in single-dose or in multiple-dose containers, preferably of Type I or Type II glass. A sterile solution of Cupric Sulfate in Water for Injection. Label the Injection to indicate that it is to be diluted to the appropriate strength with Sterile Water for Injection or other suitable fluid prior to administration. Contains an amount of cupric sulfate equivalent to the labeled amount of copper, within ±5%. Meets the requirements for Identification, Bacterial endotoxins, pH (2.0–3.5), Particulate matter, and Injections.

CYANOCOBALAMIN

Chemical name: Vitamin B_{12}.

Molecular formula: $C_{63}H_{88}CoN_{14}O_{14}P$.

Molecular weight: 1355.38.

Description: Cyanocobalamin USP—Dark red crystals or amorphous or crystalline red powder. In the anhydrous form, it is very hygroscopic and when exposed to air it may absorb about 12% of water.

Solubility: Cyanocobalamin USP—Sparingly soluble in water; soluble in alcohol; insoluble in acetone, in chloroform, and in ether.

USP requirements:

Cyanocobalamin USP—Preserve in tight, light-resistant containers. Contains not less than 96.0% and not more than 100.5% of cyanocobalamin, calculated on the dried basis. Meets the requirements for Identification, Loss on drying (not more than 12.0%), and Pseudo cyanocobalamin.

Cyanocobalamin Injection USP—Preserve in light-resistant, single-dose or multiple-dose containers, preferably of Type I glass. A sterile solution of Cyanocobalamin in Water for Injection, or in Water for Injection rendered isotonic by the addition of Sodium Chloride. Contains the labeled amount of anhydrous cyanocobalamin, within −5% to +15%. Meets the requirements for Identification, Bacterial endotoxins, pH (4.5–7.0), and Injections.

Cyanocobalamin Tablets—Not in USP.

CYCLACILLIN

Chemical name: 4-Thia-1-azabicyclo[3.2.0]heptane-2-carboxylic acid, 6-[[(1-aminocyclohexyl)carbonyl]amino]-3,3-dimethyl-7-oxo-, [2*S*-(2 alpha,5 alpha,6 beta)]-.

Molecular formula: $C_{15}H_{23}N_3O_4S$.

Molecular weight: 341.43.

Description: White, crystalline, anhydrous powder.

Solubility: Sparingly soluble in water.

USP requirements:

Cyclacillin USP—Preserve in tight containers. Contains not less than 90.0% of cyclacillin, calculated on the anhydrous basis. Has a potency of not less than 900 mcg and not more than 1050 mcg of cyclacillin per mg. Meets the requirements for Identification, Crystallinity, pH (4.0–6.5, in a solution containing 10 mg per mL), Water (not more than 1.0%), Concordance (not more than 6.0%), and Content of cyclacillin.

Cyclacillin for Oral Suspension USP—Preserve in tight containers. A dry mixture of Cyclacillin with one or more suitable buffers, colors, flavors, preservatives, sweeteners, and suspending agents. Contains the labeled amount, within −10% to +20%. Meets the requirements for Identification, Uniformity of dosage units (solid packaged in single-unit containers), Deliverable volume (multiple-unit containers), pH (4.5–6.5, in the suspension constituted as directed in the labeling), and Water (not more than 1.5%).

Cyclacillin Tablets USP—Preserve in tight containers. Contain the labeled amount, within −10% to +20%. Meet the requirements for Identification, Dissolution (75% in 45 minutes in water in Apparatus 2 at 50 rpm), and Water (not more than 5.0%).

CYCLANDELATE

Chemical name: 3,3,5-Trimethylcyclohexanol alpha-phenyl-alpha-hydroxyacetate.

Molecular formula: $C_{17}H_{24}O_3$.

Molecular weight: 276.37.

Description: White, amorphous powder having a faint menthol-like odor.

Solubility: Slightly soluble in water; highly soluble in ethyl alcohol and in organic solvents.

USP requirements:

Cyclandelate Capsules—Not in USP.

Cyclandelate Tablets—Not in USP.

CYCLIZINE

Chemical group: Piperazine derivative.

Chemical name:
Cyclizine—Piperazine, 1-(diphenylmethyl)-4-methyl-.
Cyclizine hydrochloride—Piperazine, 1-(diphenylmethyl)-4-methyl-, monohydrochloride.
Cyclizine lactate—Piperazine, 1-(diphenylmethyl)-4-methyl-, mono(2-hydroxypropanoate).

Molecular formula:
Cyclizine—$C_{18}H_{22}N_2$.
Cyclizine hydrochloride—$C_{18}H_{22}N_2 \cdot HCl$.
Cyclizine lactate—$C_{18}H_{22}N_2 \cdot C_3H_6O_3$.

Molecular weight:
Cyclizine—266.39.
Cyclizine hydrochloride—302.85.
Cyclizine lactate—356.46.

Description:
Cyclizine USP—White, or creamy white, crystalline, practically odorless powder.
Cyclizine Hydrochloride USP—White, crystalline powder or small, colorless crystals. Is odorless or nearly so. Melts indistinctly at about 285 °C, with decomposition.

pka: 7.7.

Solubility:
Cyclizine USP—Slightly soluble in water; soluble in alcohol and in chloroform.
Cyclizine Hydrochloride USP—Slightly soluble in water and in alcohol; sparingly soluble in chloroform; insoluble in ether.

USP requirements:
Cyclizine USP—Preserve in tight, light-resistant containers. Contains not less than 98.0% and not more than 100.5% of cyclizine, calculated on the anhydrous basis. Meets the requirements for Clarity and color of solution, Identification, Melting range (106–109 °C), pH (7.6–8.6, in a saturated solution), Water (not more than 1.0%), Residue on ignition (not more than 0.1%), Chloride (not more than 0.014%), Ordinary impurities, and Organic volatile impurities.
Cyclizine Hydrochloride USP—Preserve in tight, light-resistant containers. Contains not less than 98.0% and not more than 100.5% of cyclizine hydrochloride, calculated on the dried basis. Meets the requirements for Identification, pH (4.5–5.5, determined potentiometrically in a 1 in 50 solution), Loss on drying (not more than 1.0%), Residue on ignition (not more than 0.2%), and Ordinary impurities.
Cyclizine Hydrochloride Tablets USP—Preserve in tight, light-resistant containers. Contain the labeled amount, within ±7%. Meet the requirements for Identification, Dissolution (75% in 45 minutes in water in Apparatus 2 at 50 rpm), and Uniformity of dosage units.
Cyclizine Lactate Injection USP—Preserve in single-dose containers, preferably of Type I glass, protected from light. A sterile solution of cyclizine lactate in Water for Injection, prepared from Cyclizine with the aid of Lactic Acid. Contains the labeled amount, within ±5%. Meets the requirements for Identification, pH (3.2–4.7), and Injections.

CYCLOBENZAPRINE

Chemical name: Cyclobenzaprine hydrochloride—1-Propanamine, 3-(5*H*-dibenzo[*a*,*d*]cyclohepten-5-ylidene)-*N*,*N*-dimethyl-, hydrochloride.

Molecular formula: Cyclobenzaprine hydrochloride—$C_{20}H_{21}N \cdot HCl$.

Molecular weight: Cyclobenzaprine hydrochloride—311.85.

Description: Cyclobenzaprine Hydrochloride USP—White to off-white, odorless, crystalline powder.

pKa: 8.47 at 25 °C.

Solubility: Cyclobenzaprine Hydrochloride USP—Freely soluble in water, in alcohol, and in methanol; sparingly soluble in isopropanol; slightly soluble in chloroform and in methylene chloride; insoluble in hydrocarbons.

USP requirements:
Cyclobenzaprine Hydrochloride USP—Preserve in well-closed containers. Contains not less than 99.0% and not more than 101.0% of cyclobenzaprine hydrochloride, calculated on the dried basis. Meets the requirements for Identification, Melting range (215–219 °C, not more than 2 °C range between beginning and end of melting), Loss on drying (not more than 1.0%), Residue on ignition (not more than 0.1%), Heavy metals (not more than 0.001%), and Chromatographic purity.
Cyclobenzaprine Hydrochloride Tablets USP—Preserve in well-closed containers. Contain the labeled amount, within ±10%. Meet the requirements for Identification, Dissolution (75% in 30 minutes in 0.1 *N* hydrochloric acid in Apparatus 1 at 50 rpm), and Uniformity of dosage units.

CYCLOMETHICONE

Chemical name: Cyclopolydimethylsiloxane.

Molecular formula: $(C_2H_6OSi)_n$.

Description: Cyclomethicone NF—NF category: Water repelling agent.

NF requirements: Cyclomethicone NF—Preserve in tight containers. A fully methylated cyclic siloxane containing repeating units of the formula $[-(CH_3)_2SiO-]_n$, in which *n* is 4, 5, or 6, or a mixture of them. Label it to state, as part of the official title, the *n*-value of the Cyclomethicone. Where it is a mixture of 2 or 3 such cyclic siloxanes, the label states the *n*-value and percentage of each in the mixture. Contains not less than 98.0% of cyclomethicone, calculated as the sum of cyclomethicone 4, cyclomethicone 5, and cyclomethicone 6, and not less than 95.0% and not more than 105.0% of the labeled amount of any one or more of the individual cyclomethicone components. Meets the requirements for Identification and Nonvolatile residue (not more than 0.15% [w/w]).

CYCLOPENTOLATE

Chemical name: Cyclopentolate hydrochloride—Benzeneacetic acid, alpha-(1-hydroxycyclopentyl)-, 2-(dimethylamino)ethyl ester, hydrochloride.

Molecular formula: Cyclopentolate hydrochloride—$C_{17}H_{25}NO_3 \cdot HCl$.

Molecular weight: Cyclopentolate hydrochloride—327.85.

Description: Cyclopentolate Hydrochloride USP—White, crystalline powder, which upon standing develops a characteristic odor. Its solutions are acid to litmus. Melts at about 138 °C, the melt appearing opaque.

Solubility: Cyclopentolate Hydrochloride USP—Very soluble in water; freely soluble in alcohol; insoluble in ether.

USP requirements:

Cyclopentolate Hydrochloride USP—Preserve in tight containers, and store in a cold place. Contains not less than 98.0% and not more than 102.0% of cyclopentolate hydrochloride, calculated on the dried basis. Meets the requirements for Identification, pH (4.5–5.5, in a solution [1 in 100]), Loss on drying (not more than 0.5%), Residue on ignition (not more than 0.05%), and Chromatographic purity.

Cyclopentolate Hydrochloride Ophthalmic Solution USP—Preserve in tight containers, and store at controlled room temperature. A sterile, aqueous solution of Cyclopentolate Hydrochloride. Contains the labeled amount, within ±10%. Meets the requirements for Identification, Sterility, and pH (3.0–5.5).

CYCLOPHOSPHAMIDE

Chemical name: 2*H*-1,3,2-Oxazaphosphorin-2-amine, *N,N*-bis(2-chloroethyl)tetrahydro-, 2-oxide, monohydrate.

Molecular formula: $C_7H_{15}Cl_2N_2O_2P \cdot H_2O$.

Molecular weight: 279.10.

Description: Cyclophosphamide USP—White, crystalline powder. Liquefies upon loss of its water of crystallization.

Solubility: Cyclophosphamide USP—Soluble in water and in alcohol.

USP requirements:

Cyclophosphamide USP—Preserve in tight containers, at a temperature between 2 and 30 °C. Contains not less than 97.0% and not more than 103.0% of cyclophosphamide, calculated on the anhydrous basis. Meets the requirements for Identification, pH (3.9–7.1, in a solution [1 in 100]), Water (5.7–6.8%), and Heavy metals (not more than 0.002%).

Caution: Great care should be taken in handling Cyclophosphamide, as it is a potent cytotoxic agent.

Cyclophosphamide for Injection USP—Preserve in Containers for Sterile Solids. Storage at a temperature not exceeding 25 °C is recommended. It will withstand brief exposure to temperatures up to 30 °C, but is to be protected from temperatures above 30 °C. A sterile mixture of Cyclophosphamide with or without a suitable diluent. Contains the labeled amount of anhydrous cyclophosphamide, within ±10%. Meets the requirements for Constituted solution, Identification, Bacterial endotoxins, and pH (3.0–9.0, the range not exceeding 3 pH units), and for Sterility tests, Uniformity of dosage units, and Labeling under Injections.

Cyclophosphamide Oral Solution—Not in USP.

Cyclophosphamide Tablets USP—Preserve in tight containers. Storage at a temperature not exceeding 25 °C is recommended. Tablets will withstand brief exposure to temperatures up to 30 °C, but are to be protected from temperatures above 30 °C. Contain an amount of cyclophosphamide equivalent to the labeled amount of anhydrous cyclophosphamide, within ±10%. Meet the requirements for Identification, Disintegration (30 minutes, determined as directed under Uncoated Tablets), and Uniformity of dosage units.

CYCLOPROPANE

Chemical name: Cyclopropane.

Molecular formula: C_3H_6.

Molecular weight: 42.08.

Description: Cyclopropane USP—Colorless gas having a characteristic odor. One liter at a pressure of 760 millimeters and a temperature of 0 °C weighs about 1.88 grams.

Solubility: Cyclopropane USP—One volume dissolves in about 2.7 volumes of water at 15 °C. Freely soluble in alcohol; soluble in fixed oils.

USP requirements: Cyclopropane USP—Preserve in cylinders. The label bears a warning that cyclopropane is highly flammable and is not to be used where it may be ignited. Contains not less than 99.0%, by volume, of cyclopropane. Meets the requirements for Acidity or alkalinity, Carbon dioxide (not more than 0.03%), Halogens (not more than 0.02% as chloride), and Propylene, allene, and other unsaturated hydrocarbons.

Caution: Cyclopropane is highly flammable. Do not use where it may be ignited.

CYCLOSERINE

Source: Produced by a strain of *Streptomyces orchidaceus*; has also been synthesized.

Chemical name: 3-Isoxazolidinone, 4-amino-, (*R*)-.

Molecular formula: $C_3H_6N_2O_2$.

Molecular weight: 102.09.

Description: Cycloserine USP—White to pale yellow, crystalline powder. Is odorless or has a faint odor. Is hygroscopic and deteriorates upon absorbing water. Its solutions are dextrorotatory.

Solubility: Cycloserine USP—Freely soluble in water.

Other characteristics: Stable in alkaline solution, but rapidly destroyed at neutral or acid pH.

USP requirements:

Cycloserine USP—Preserve in tight containers. Has a potency of not less than 900 mcg of cycloserine per mg. Meets the requirements for Identification, Specific rotation (108° to 114°), Crystallinity, pH (5.5–6.5, in a solution [1 in 10]), Loss on drying (not more than 1.0%), Residue on ignition (not more than 0.5%), and Condensation products.

Cycloserine Capsules USP—Preserve in tight containers. Contain the labeled amount, within −10% to +20%. Meet the requirements for Identification, Dissolution (75% in 45 minutes in water in Apparatus 1 at 100 rpm), Uniformity of dosage units, and Loss on drying (not more than 1.0%).

CYCLOSPORINE

Chemical name: Cyclosporin A.

Molecular formula: $C_{62}H_{111}N_{11}O_{12}$.

Molecular weight: 1202.63.

Description: White or off-white finely crystalline powder with a weak characteristic odor.

Solubility: Soluble in methanol, in ethanol, in acetone, in ether, and in chloroform; slightly soluble in water and in saturated hydrocarbons.

Other characteristics: Lipophilic; hydrophobic.

USP requirements:

Cyclosporine USP—Preserve in tight, light-resistant containers. Contains not less than 975 mcg and not more than 1020 mcg of cyclosporine per mg, calculated on the dried basis. Meets the requirements for Identification, Loss on drying (not more than 2.0%), and Heavy metals (not more than 0.002%).

Cyclosporine Capsules USP—Preserve in tight containers. Contain a solution of Cyclosporine in a suitable vehicle. Contain the labeled amount, within ±10%. Meet the requirements for Identification and Disintegration (30 minutes, as directed for Uncoated Tablets).

Cyclosporine Concentrate for Injection USP—Preserve in single-dose or in multiple-dose containers. A sterile solution of Cyclosporine in a suitable vehicle. Label it to indicate that it is to be diluted with a suitable parenteral vehicle prior to intravenous infusion. Contains the labeled amount, within ±10%. Meets the requirements for Identification, Bacterial endotoxins, Sterility, and Alcohol content (where present, the labeled amount, within ±20%).

Cyclosporine Oral Solution USP—Preserve in tight containers. A solution of Cyclosporine in a suitable vehicle. Contains the labeled amount, within ±10%. Meets the requirements for Identification and Alcohol content (where present, the labeled amount, within ±20%).

CYCLOTHIAZIDE

Chemical name: *2H*-1,2,4-Benzothiadiazine-7-sulfonamide, 3-bicyclo[2.2.1]hept-5-en-2-yl-6-chloro-3,4-dihydro-, 1,1-dioxide.

Molecular formula: $C_{14}H_{16}ClN_3O_4S_2$.

Molecular weight: 389.87.

Description: White, crystalline solid. It has a melting point of approximately 220 °C.

pKa: 10.7 in water.

Solubility: Moderately soluble in hot ethyl alcohol and in hot dilute alcohol; very soluble in cold ethyl acetate (an ethyl acetate solvate is formed); relatively insoluble in ether and in chloroform.

USP requirements:

Cyclothiazide USP—Preserve in well-closed containers. Contains not less than 98.0% and not more than 102.0% of cyclothiazide, calculated on the anhydrous basis. Meets the requirements for Identification, Melting range (217–225 °C, not more than 4 °C range between beginning and end of melting), Water (not more than 1.0%), Residue on ignition (not more than 0.2%), Selenium (not more than 0.003%), Diazotizable substances (not more than 1.0%), and Organic volatile impurities.

Cyclothiazide Tablets USP—Preserve in well-closed containers. Contain the labeled amount, within ±10%. Meet the requirements for Identification, Dissolution (70% in 60 minutes in water in Apparatus 2 at 50 rpm), and Uniformity of dosage units.

CYPROHEPTADINE

Chemical group: Piperidine derivative.

Chemical name: Cyproheptadine hydrochloride—Piperidine,4-(*5H*-dibenzo[*a,d*]-cyclohepten-5-ylidene)-1-methyl-, hydrochloride, sesquihydrate.

Molecular formula: Cyproheptadine hydrochloride—$C_{21}H_{21}N \cdot HCl \cdot 1\frac{1}{2}H_2O$.

Molecular weight: Cyproheptadine hydrochloride—350.89.

Description: Cyproheptadine Hydrochloride USP—White to slightly yellow, odorless or practically odorless, crystalline powder.

pKa: 9.3.

Solubility: Cyproheptadine Hydrochloride USP—Slightly soluble in water; freely soluble in methanol; soluble in chloroform; sparingly soluble in alcohol; practically insoluble in ether.

USP requirements:

Cyproheptadine Hydrochloride USP—Preserve in well-closed containers. Previously dried, contains not less than 98.5% and not more than 100.5% of cyproheptadine hydrochloride. Meets the requirements for Identification, Acidity, Loss on drying (7.0–9.0%), Residue on ignition (not more than 0.1%), Heavy metals (not more than 0.003%), and Organic volatile impurities.

Cyproheptadine Hydrochloride Syrup USP—Preserve in tight containers. Contains the labeled amount, within ±10%. Meets the requirements for Identification and pH (3.5–4.5).

Cyproheptadine Hydrochloride Tablets USP—Preserve in well-closed containers. Contain the labeled amount, within ±10%. Meet the requirements for Identification, Dissolution (80% in 30 minutes in 0.1 *N* hydrochloric acid in Apparatus 2 at 50 rpm), and Uniformity of dosage units.

CYPROTERONE

Chemical name: Cyproterone acetate—*3'H*-Cyclopropa[1,2]pregna-1,4,6-triene-3,20-dione, 17-(acetyloxy)-6-chloro-1,2-dihydro-, (1 beta,2 beta)-.

Molecular formula: Cyproterone acetate—$C_{24}H_{29}ClO_4$.

Molecular weight: Cyproterone acetate—416.94.

Description: Cyproterone acetate—White crystals melting at about 200 °C.

USP requirements:

Cyproterone Acetate Injection—Not in USP.

Cyproterone Acetate Tablets—Not in USP.

CYSTEINE

Chemical name: Cysteine hydrochloride—L-Cysteine hydrochloride monohydrate.

Molecular formula: Cysteine hydrochloride—$C_3H_7NO_2S \cdot HCl \cdot H_2O$.

Molecular weight: Cysteine hydrochloride—175.63.

Description: Cysteine Hydrochloride USP—White crystals or crystalline powder.

Solubility: Cysteine Hydrochloride USP—Soluble in water, in alcohol, and in acetone.

USP requirements:

Cysteine Hydrochloride USP—Preserve in well-closed containers. Contains not less than 98.5% and not more than 101.5% of cysteine hydrochloride, as L-cysteine hydrochloride, calculated on the dried basis. Meets the requirements for Identification, Specific rotation (+5.7° to +6.8°, calculated on the dried basis), Loss on drying (8.0–12.0%), Residue on ignition (not more than 0.4%), Sulfate (not more than 0.03%), Arsenic (not more than 1.5 ppm), Iron (not more than 0.003%), Heavy metals (not more than 0.0015%), Chloride content (19.8–20.8%), and Organic volatile impurities.

Cysteine Hydrochloride Injection USP—Preserve in single-dose or in multiple-dose containers, preferably of Type I glass. A sterile solution of Cysteine Hydrochloride in

Water for Injection. Contains the labeled amount, within ±15%. Meets the requirements for Identification, Bacterial endotoxins, pH (1.0–2.5), Heavy metals (not more than 2 ppm), and Injections.

CYTARABINE

Chemical name: 2(1*H*)-Pyrimidinone, 4-amino-1-beta-D-arabinofuranosyl-.

Molecular formula: $C_9H_{13}N_3O_5$.

Molecular weight: 243.22.

Description: Cytarabine USP—Odorless, white to off-white, crystalline powder.

pKa: 4.35.

Solubility: Cytarabine USP—Freely soluble in water; slightly soluble in alcohol and in chloroform.

USP requirements:

Cytarabine USP—Preserve in well-closed, light-resistant containers. Contains not less than 95.0% and not more than 105.0% of cytarabine, calculated on the dried basis. Meets the requirements for Identification, Specific rotation (+154° to +160°, calculated on the dried basis), Loss on drying (not more than 1.0%), Residue on ignition (not more than 0.5%), Heavy metals (not more than 0.001%), and Related substances (not more than 0.5%).

Sterile Cytarabine USP—Preserve in Containers for Sterile Solids. It is Cytarabine suitable for parenteral use. Contains the labeled amount, within ±10%. Meets the requirements for Constituted solution, Identification, pH (4.0–6.0, in a solution containing the equivalent of 10 mg of cytarabine per mL), Water (not more than 3.0%), and Bacterial endotoxins, and for Sterility tests, Uniformity of dosage units, and Labeling under Injections. The drug substance in the vial meets the requirements for Cytarabine.

DACARBAZINE

Chemical name: 1*H*-Imidazole-4-carboxamide, 5-(3,3-dimethyl-1-triazenyl)-.

Molecular formula: $C_6H_{10}N_6O$.

Molecular weight: 182.19.

Description: Colorless to ivory colored solid which is light sensitive.

pKa: 4.42.

Solubility: Slightly soluble in water and in alcohol.

USP requirements:

Dacarbazine USP—Preserve in tight, light-resistant containers, in a refrigerator. Contains not less than 97.0% and not more than 102.0% of dacarbazine. Meets the requirements for Identification, Residue on ignition (not more than 0.1%), and Related compounds.

Caution: Great care should be taken in handling Dacarbazine, as it is a potent cytotoxic agent.

Dacarbazine for Injection USP—Preserve in single-dose or multiple-dose Containers for Sterile Solids, preferably of Type I glass, protected from light. A sterile, freeze-dried mixture of Dacarbazine and suitable buffers or diluents. Contains the labeled amount, within ±10%. Meets the requirements for Completeness of solution, Constituted solution, Identification, Bacterial endotoxins, pH (3.0–4.0), Water (not more than 1.5%), and Limit of 2-azahypoxanthine (not more than 1.0%), and for Sterility tests, Uniformity of dosage units, and Labeling under Injections.

Caution: Great care should be taken to prevent inhaling particles of Dacarbazine for Injection and exposing the skin to it.

DACTINOMYCIN

Source: An actinomycin derived from a mixture of actinomycins produced by *Streptomyces parvullus.*

Chemical name: Actinomycin D. Specific stereoisomer of *N,N'*-[(2-amino-4,6-dimethyl-3-oxo-3*H*-phenoxazine-1,9-diyl)bis-[carbonylimino(2-hydroxypropylidene)carbonyliminoisobutylidenecarbonyl-1,2-pyrrolidinediylcarbonyl(methylimino)methylenecarbonyl]]bis[*N*-methyl-L-valine] dilactone.

Molecular formula: $C_{62}H_{86}N_{12}O_{16}$.

Molecular weight: 1255.44.

Description: Dactinomycin USP—Bright red, crystalline powder. Is somewhat hygroscopic and is affected by light and heat.

Solubility: Dactinomycin USP—Soluble in water at 10 °C and slightly soluble in water at 37 °C; freely soluble in alcohol; very slightly soluble in ether.

USP requirements:

Dactinomycin USP—Preserve in tight containers, protected from light and excessive heat. Contains not less than 950 mcg and not more than 1030 mcg of dactinomycin per mg, calculated on the dried basis. Meets the requirements for Identification, Specific rotation (−292° to −317°, calculated on the dried basis), Crystallinity, Bacterial endotoxins, and Loss on drying (not more than 5.0%).

Caution: Great care should be taken to prevent inhaling particles of Dactinomycin and exposing the skin to it.

Dactinomycin for Injection USP—Preserve in light-resistant Containers for Sterile Solids. A sterile mixture of Dactinomycin and Mannitol. Label it to include the statement, "Protect from light." Contains the labeled amount, within −10% to +20%, the labeled amount being 0.5 mg in each container. Meets the requirements for Constituted solution, Identification, Bacterial endotoxins, Sterility, pH (5.5–7.5, in the solution constituted as directed in the labeling), Loss on drying (not more than 4.0%), and Injections.

Caution: Great care should be taken to prevent inhaling particles of Dactinomycin and exposing the skin to it.

DANAZOL

Chemical name: Pregna-2,4-dien-20-yno[2,3-*d*]isoxazol-17-ol,(17 alpha)-.

Molecular formula: $C_{22}H_{27}NO_2$.

Molecular weight: 337.46.

Description: Danazol USP—White to pale yellow, crystalline powder. Melts at about 225 °C, with some decomposition.

Solubility: Danazol USP—Practically insoluble or insoluble in water and in hexane; freely soluble in chloroform; soluble in acetone; sparingly soluble in alcohol; slightly soluble in ether.

USP requirements:
Danazol USP—Preserve in tight, light-resistant containers. Contains not less than 97.0% and not more than 102.0% of danazol, calculated on the dried basis. Meets the requirements for Identification, Specific rotation (+21° to +27°, calculated on the dried basis), Loss on drying (not more than 2.0%), Chromatographic impurities, and Organic volatile impurities.
Danazol Capsules USP—Preserve in well-closed containers. Contain the labeled amount, within ±10%. Meet the requirements for Identification, Dissolution (65% in 30 minutes in isopropyl alcohol in 0.1 *N* hydrochloric acid [4 in 10] in Apparatus 2 at 80 rpm), and Uniformity of dosage units.

DANTHRON AND DOCUSATE

Chemical group:
Danthron—Anthraquinones.
Docusate—Surfactants, anionic.

Chemical name:
Danthron—9,10-Anthracenedione, 1,8-dihydroxy-.
Docusate sodium—Butanedioic acid, sulfo-, 1,4-bis(2-ethylhexyl) ester, sodium salt.

Molecular formula:
Danthron—$C_{14}H_8O_4$.
Docusate sodium—$C_{20}H_{37}NaO_7S$.

Molecular weight:
Danthron—240.22.
Docusate sodium—444.56.

Description:
Danthron—Orange, odorless or almost odorless, crystalline powder.
Docusate Sodium USP—White, wax-like, plastic solid, having a characteristic odor suggestive of octyl alcohol, but no odor of other solvents.
NF category: Wetting and/or solubilizing agent.

Solubility:
Danthron—Practically insoluble in water; very slightly soluble in alcohol; soluble in chloroform; slightly soluble in ether; dissolves in solutions of alkali hydroxides.
Docusate Sodium USP—Sparingly soluble in water; very soluble in solvent hexane; freely soluble in alcohol and in glycerin.

USP requirements:
Danthron and Docusate Sodium Capsules—Not in USP.
Danthron and Docusate Sodium Tablets—Not in USP.

DANTROLENE

Chemical name: Dantrolene sodium—2,4-Imidazolidinedione, 1-[[[5-(4-nitrophenyl)-2-furanyl]methylene]amino]-, sodium salt, hydrate (2:7).

Molecular formula: Dantrolene sodium—$C_{14}H_9N_4NaO_5 \cdot 3\frac{1}{2}H_2O$.

Molecular weight: Dantrolene sodium—399.29.

Description: Dantrolene sodium—Orange powder.

Solubility: Dantrolene sodium—Slightly soluble in water, but due to its slightly acidic nature the solubility increases somewhat in alkaline solution.

USP requirements:
Dantrolene Sodium Capsules—Not in USP.
Dantrolene Sodium for Injection—Not in USP.

DAPIPRAZOLE

Chemical name: Dapiprazole hydrochloride—1,2,4-Triazolo-[4,3-*a*]pyridine, 5,6,7,8-tetrahydro-3-[2-[4-(2-methylphenyl)-1-piperazinyl]ethyl]-, monohydrochloride.

Molecular formula: Dapiprazole hydrochloride—$C_{19}H_{27}N_5 \cdot HCl$.

Molecular weight: Dapiprazole hydrochloride—361.92.

Description: Dapiprazole hydrochloride—Sterile, white, lyophilized powder.

Solubility: Dapiprazole hydrochloride—Soluble in water.

USP requirements: Dapiprazole Hydrochloride for Ophthalmic Solution—Not in USP.

DAPSONE

Chemical group: Sulfone.

Chemical name: Benzenamine, 4,4′-sulfonylbis-.

Molecular formula: $C_{12}H_{12}N_2O_2S$.

Molecular weight: 248.30.

Description: Dapsone USP—White or creamy white, crystalline powder. Is odorless.

Solubility: Dapsone USP—Very slightly soluble in water; freely soluble in alcohol; soluble in acetone and in dilute mineral acids.

USP requirements:
Dapsone USP—Preserve in well-closed, light-resistant containers. Contains not less than 99.0% and not more than 101.0% of dapsone, calculated on the dried basis. Meets the requirements for Identification, Melting range (175–181 °C), Loss on drying (not more than 1.5%), Residue on ignition (not more than 0.1%), Selenium (not more than 0.003%), Chromatographic purity, and Organic volatile impurities.
Dapsone Tablets USP—Preserve in well-closed, light-resistant containers. Contain the labeled amount, within ±7.5%. Meet the requirements for Identification, Dissolution (75% in 60 minutes in dilute hydrochloric acid [2 in 100] in Apparatus 1 at 100 rpm), and Uniformity of dosage units.

DAUNORUBICIN

Source: Daunorubicin hydrochloride—An anthracycline produced by *Streptomyces coeruleorubidus or S. peucetius.*

Chemical name: Daunorubicin hydrochloride—5,12-Naphthacenedione, 8-acetyl-10-[(3-amino-2,3,6-trideoxy-alpha-L-*lyxo*-hexopyranosyl)]oxy]-7,8,9,10-tetrahydro-6,8,11-trihydroxy-1-methoxy-, (8*S-cis*)-, hydrochloride.

Molecular formula: Daunorubicin hydrochloride—$C_{27}H_{29}NO_{10} \cdot HCl$.

Molecular weight: Daunorubicin hydrochloride—563.99.

Description: Daunorubicin Hydrochloride USP—Orange-red, crystalline, hygroscopic powder.

pKa: Daunorubicin hydrochloride—10.3.

Solubility: Daunorubicin Hydrochloride USP—Freely soluble in water and in methanol; slightly soluble in alcohol; very slightly soluble in chloroform; practically insoluble in acetone.

USP requirements:

Daunorubicin Hydrochloride USP—Preserve in tight containers, protected from light and excessive heat. Has a potency equivalent to not less than 842 mcg and not more than 1030 mcg of daunorubicin per mg. Meets the requirements for Identification, Crystallinity, pH (4.5–6.5, in a solution containing 5 mg per mL), and Water (not more than 3.0%).

Caution: Great care should be taken to prevent inhaling particles of daunorubicin hydrochloride and exposing the skin to it.

Daunorubicin Hydrochloride for Injection USP—Preserve in light-resistant Containers for Sterile Solids. A sterile mixture of Daunorubicin Hydrochloride and Mannitol. Contains an amount of daunorubicin hydrochloride equivalent to the labeled amount of daunorubicin, within −10% to +15%. Meets the requirements for Constituted solution, Identification, Depressor substances, Bacterial endotoxins, pH (4.5–6.5, in the solution constituted as directed in the labeling), Water (not more than 3.0%), and Injections.

DEBRISOQUINE

Chemical name: Debrisoquine sulfate—2(1*H*)-Isoquinolinecarboximidamide, 3,4-dihydro-, sulfate (2:1).

Molecular formula: Debrisoquine sulfate—$(C_{10}H_{13}N_2)_2 \cdot H_2SO_4$.

Molecular weight: Debrisoquine sulfate—448.54.

Description: Debrisoquine sulfate—White odorless or almost odorless crystalline powder.

Solubility: Debrisoquine sulfate—Soluble 1 in 40 of water; very slightly soluble in alcohol; almost insoluble in chloroform and in ether.

USP requirements: Debrisoquine Sulfate Tablets—Not in USP.

DECOQUINATE

Chemical name: 3-Quinolinecarboxylic acid, 6-(decyloxy)-7-ethoxy-4-hydroxy-, ethyl ester.

Molecular formula: $C_{24}H_{35}NO_5$.

Molecular weight: 417.55.

Description: Cream to buff-colored, odorless or almost odorless, microcrystalline powder.

Solubility: Insoluble in water; practically insoluble in alcohol; very slightly soluble in chloroform and in ether.

USP requirements:

Decoquinate USP—Preserve in tight containers. Label it to indicate that it is for veterinary use only. Contains not less than 99.0% and not more than 101.0% of decoquinate, calculated on the dried basis. Meets the requirements for Identification, Loss on drying (not more than 0.5%), Residue on ignition (not more than 0.1%), and Ordinary impurities.

Decoquinate Premix USP—Preserve in well-closed containers. Label it to indicate that it is for veterinary use only. Contains the labeled amount, within ±10%, the labeled amount being between 1 gram and 10 grams per 100 grams of Premix. Meets the requirement for Identification.

DEFEROXAMINE

Source: Isolated as the iron chelate from *Streptomyces pilosus* and treated chemically to obtain the metal-free ligand.

Chemical name: Deferoxamine mesylate—Butanediamide, *N'*-[5-[[4-[[5-(acetylhydroxyamino)pentyl]amino]-1,4-dioxobutyl]hydroxyamino]pentyl]-*N*-(5-aminopentyl)-*N*-hydroxy-, monomethanesulfonate.

Molecular formula: Deferoxamine mesylate—$C_{25}H_{48}N_6O_8 \cdot CH_4O_3S$.

Molecular weight: Deferoxamine mesylate—656.79.

Description: Deferoxamine Mesylate USP—White to off-white powder.

Solubility: Deferoxamine Mesylate USP—Freely soluble in water; slightly soluble in methanol.

USP requirements:

Deferoxamine Mesylate USP—Preserve in tight containers. Contains not less than 98.0% and not more than 102.0% of deferoxamine mesylate, calculated on the anhydrous basis. Meets the requirements for Identification, pH (4.0–6.0, in a solution [1 in 100]), Water (not more than 2.0%), Residue on ignition (not more than 0.1%), Chloride (not more than 0.012%), Sulfate (not more than 0.04%), and Heavy metals (not more than 0.001%).

Sterile Deferoxamine Mesylate USP—Preserve in single-dose or in multiple-dose containers, preferably of Type I glass. It is Deferoxamine Mesylate suitable for parenteral use. Contains the labeled amount, within ±10%. Meets the requirements for Constituted solution, Identification, pH (4.0–6.0, in a solution [1 in 100]), Bacterial endotoxins, Water (not more than 1.5%), Injections, and Uniformity of dosage units.

DEHYDROACETIC ACID

Chemical name: 2*H*-Pyran-2,4(3*H*)-dione, 3-acetyl-6-methyl-.

Molecular formula: $C_8H_8O_4$.

Molecular weight: 168.15.

Description: Dehydroacetic Acid NF—White or nearly white, crystalline powder. Odorless or practically odorless.

NF category: Antimicrobial preservative.

Solubility: Dehydroacetic Acid NF—Very slightly soluble in water, freely soluble in acetone; soluble in aqueous solutions of fixed alkalies; sparingly soluble in alcohol.

NF requirements: Dehydroacetic Acid NF—Preserve in well-closed containers. Contains not less than 98.0% and not more than 100.5% of dehydroacetic acid, calculated on the anhydrous basis. Meets the requirements for Identification, Melting range (109–111 °C), Water (not more than 1.0%), Residue on ignition (not more than 0.1%), Arsenic (not more than 3 ppm), Heavy metals (not more than 0.001%), and Organic volatile impurities.

DEHYDROCHOLIC ACID

Source: Oxidized bile acid produced from the main constituent of ox bile, cholic acid.

Chemical name: Cholan-24-oic acid, 3,7,12-trioxo-, (5 beta)-.

Molecular formula: $C_{24}H_{34}O_5$.

Molecular weight: 402.53.

Description: Dehydrocholic Acid USP—White, fluffy, odorless powder.

Solubility: Dehydrocholic Acid USP—Practically insoluble in water; soluble in glacial acetic acid and in solutions of alkali hydroxides and carbonates; slightly soluble in alcohol and in ether; sparingly soluble in chloroform (the solutions in alcohol and in chloroform usually are slightly turbid).

USP requirements:
Dehydrocholic Acid USP—Preserve in well-closed containers. Contains not less than 98.5% and not more than 101.0% of dehydrocholic acid, calculated on the dried basis. Dehydrocholic Acid for parenteral use melts between 237 and 242 °C. Meets the requirements for Identification, Melting range (231–242 °C, not more than 3 °C between beginning and end of melting), Specific rotation (+29.0° to +32.5°, calculated on the dried basis), Microbial limit, Loss on drying (not more than 1.0%), Residue on ignition (not more than 0.3%), Odor on boiling, Barium, Heavy metals (not more than 0.002%), and Organic volatile impurities.
Dehydrocholic Acid Tablets USP—Preserve in well-closed containers. Contain the labeled amount, within ±6%. Meet the requirements for Identification, Microbial limit, Disintegration (30 minutes), and Uniformity of dosage units.

DEHYDROCHOLIC ACID AND DOCUSATE

For *Dehydrocholic Acid* and *Docusate*—See individual listings for chemistry information.

USP requirements:
Dehydrocholic Acid and Docusate Sodium Capsules—Not in USP.
Dehydrocholic Acid and Docusate Sodium Tablets—Not in USP.

DEHYDROCHOLIC ACID, DOCUSATE, AND PHENOLPHTHALEIN

For *Dehydrocholic Acid, Docusate,* and *Phenolphthalein*—See individual listings for chemistry information.

USP requirements: Dehydrocholic Acid, Docusate Sodium, and Phenolphthalein Capsules—Not in USP.

DEMECARIUM

Chemical name: Demecarium bromide—Benzenaminium, 3,3′-[1,10-decanediylbis[(methylimino)carbonyloxy]]bis[*N,N,N*-trimethyl-, dibromide.

Molecular formula: Demecarium bromide—$C_{32}H_{52}Br_2N_4O_4$.

Molecular weight: Demecarium bromide—716.60.

Description: Demecarium Bromide USP—White or slightly yellow, slightly hygroscopic, crystalline powder.

Solubility: Demecarium Bromide USP—Freely soluble in water and in alcohol; soluble in ether; sparingly soluble in acetone.

USP requirements:
Demecarium Bromide USP—Preserve in tight, light-resistant containers. Contains not less than 95.0% and not more than 100.5% of demecarium bromide, calculated on the anhydrous basis. Meets the requirements for Identification, pH (5.0–7.0, in a solution [1 in 100]), Water (not more than 2.0%), Residue on ignition (not more than 0.1%), Heavy metals (not more than 0.002%), and *m*-Trimethylammoniophenol bromide.
Demecarium Bromide Ophthalmic Solution USP—Preserve in tight, light-resistant containers. A sterile, aqueous solution of Demecarium Bromide. Contains the labeled amount, within ±8%. Contains a suitable antimicrobial agent. Meets the requirements for Identification and Sterility.

DEMECLOCYCLINE

Chemical name:
Demeclocycline—2-Naphthacenecarboxamide, 7-chloro-4-(dimethylamino)-1,4,4a,5,5a,6,11,12a-octahydro-3,6,10,-12,12a-pentahydroxy-1,11-dioxo-, [4*S*-(4 alpha,4a alpha,5a alpha,6 beta,12a alpha)]-.
Demeclocycline hydrochloride—2-Naphthacenecarboxamide, 7-chloro-4-(dimethylamino)-1,4,4a,5,5a,6,11,12a-octahydro-3,6,10,12,12a-pentahydroxy-1,11-dioxo-, monohydrochloride, [4*S*-(4 alpha,4a alpha,5a alpha,6 beta,12a alpha)]-.

Molecular formula:
Demeclocycline—$C_{21}H_{21}ClN_2O_8$.
Demeclocycline hydrochloride—$C_{21}H_{21}ClN_2O_8 \cdot HCl$.

Molecular weight:
Demeclocycline—464.86.
Demeclocycline hydrochloride—501.32.

Description:
Demeclocycline USP—Yellow, crystalline odorless powder.
Demeclocycline Hydrochloride USP—Yellow, crystalline, odorless powder.

Solubility:
Demeclocycline USP—Sparingly soluble in water; soluble in alcohol. Dissolves readily in 3 *N* hydrochloric acid and in alkaline solutions.
Demeclocycline Hydrochloride USP—Sparingly soluble in water and in solutions of alkali hydroxides and carbonates; slightly soluble in alcohol; practically insoluble in acetone and in chloroform.

USP requirements:
Demeclocycline USP—Preserve in tight, light-resistant containers. Has a potency equivalent to not less than 970 mcg of demeclocycline hydrochloride per mg, calculated on the anhydrous basis. Meets the requirements for Identification, Crystallinity, pH (4.0–5.5, in a solution containing 10 mg per mL), and Water (4.3–6.7%).
Demeclocycline Oral Suspension USP—Preserve in tight containers, protected from light. Contains an amount of demeclocycline equivalent to the labeled amount of demeclocycline hydrochloride, within −10% to +25%. Meets the requirements for Identification and pH (4.0–5.8).
Demeclocycline Hydrochloride USP—Preserve in tight, light-resistant containers. Has a potency of not less than 900 mcg of demeclocycline hydrochloride per mg, calculated on the dried basis. Meets the requirements for Identification, Crystallinity, pH (2.0–3.0, in a solution containing 10 mg per mL), and Loss on drying (not more than 2.0%).
Demeclocycline Hydrochloride Capsules USP—Preserve in tight, light-resistant containers. Contain the labeled amount, within −10% to +25%. Meet the requirements for Identification, Dissolution (75% in 45 minutes in water in Apparatus 2 at 75 rpm), Uniformity of dosage units, and Loss on drying (not more than 2.0%; not more than 8.0% if the Capsules contain starch).
Demeclocycline Hydrochloride Tablets USP—Preserve in tight, light-resistant containers. Contain the labeled amount, within −10% to +25%. Meet the requirements for Identification, Dissolution (75% in 45 minutes in water

in Apparatus 2 at 75 rpm), Uniformity of dosage units, and Loss on drying (not more than 2.0%).

DEMECLOCYCLINE AND NYSTATIN

For *Demeclocycline* and *Nystatin*—See individual listings for chemistry information.

USP requirements:

Demeclocycline Hydrochloride and Nystatin Capsules USP—Preserve in tight, light-resistant containers. Contain the labeled amounts of demeclocycline hydrochloride, within −10% to +25%, and USP Nystatin Units, within −10% to +35%. Meet the requirements for Identification, Dissolution (75% of the labeled amount of demeclocycline hydrochloride in 45 minutes in water in Apparatus 2 at 75 rpm), and Loss on drying (not more than 5.0%).

Demeclocycline Hydrochloride and Nystatin Tablets USP—Preserve in tight, light-resistant containers. Contain the labeled amounts of demeclocycline hydrochloride, within −10% to +25%, and USP Nystatin Units, within −10% to +35%. Meet the requirements for Identification, Dissolution (75% of the labeled amount of demeclocycline hydrochloride in 45 minutes in water in Apparatus 2 at 75 rpm), and Loss on drying (not more than 4.0%).

DENATONIUM BENZOATE

Chemical name: Benzenemethanaminium, *N*-[2-[(2,6-dimethylphenyl)amino]-2-oxoethyl]-*N*,*N*-diethyl-, benzoate, monohydrate.

Molecular formula: $C_{28}H_{34}N_2O_3 \cdot H_2O$ (hydrous).

Molecular weight: 464.60 (hydrous); 446.59 (anhydrous).

Description: Denatonium Benzoate NF—NF category: Alcohol denaturant.

Solubility: Denatonium Benzoate NF—Freely soluble in water and in alcohol; very soluble in chloroform and in methanol; very slightly soluble in ether.

NF requirements: Denatonium Benzoate NF—Preserve in tight containers. Dried at 105 °C for 2 hours, contains one molecule of water of hydration, or is anhydrous. Label it to indicate whether it is hydrous or anhydrous. When dried at 105 °C for 2 hours, contains not less than 99.5% and not more than 101.0% of denatonium benzoate. Meets the requirements for Identification, Melting range (163–170 °C), pH (6.5–7.5, in a solution [3 in 100]), Loss on drying (not more than 1.0%), Residue on ignition (not more than 0.1%), and Chloride (not more than 0.2%).

DESERPIDINE

Source: Alkaloid from *Rauwolfia canescens*.

Chemical name: Methyl 17 alpha-methoxy-18 beta-[(3,4,5-trimethoxybenzoyl)oxy]-3 beta,20 alpha-yohimban-16 beta-carboxylate.

Molecular formula: $C_{32}H_{38}N_2O_8$.

Molecular weight: 578.66.

Description: White to light yellow, crystalline powder.

pKa: 5.67.

Solubility: Insoluble in water; slightly soluble in alcohol.

USP requirements: Deserpidine Tablets—Not in USP.

DESERPIDINE AND HYDROCHLOROTHIAZIDE

For *Deserpidine* and *Hydrochlorothiazide*—See individual listings for chemistry information.

USP requirements: Deserpidine and Hydrochlorothiazide Tablets—Not in USP.

DESERPIDINE AND METHYCLOTHIAZIDE

For *Deserpidine* and *Methyclothiazide*—See individual listings for chemistry information.

USP requirements: Deserpidine and Methyclothiazide Tablets—Not in USP.

DESFLURANE

Chemical name: Ethane, 2-(difluoromethoxy)-1,1,1,2-tetrafluoro-, (±)-.

Molecular formula: $C_3H_2F_6O$.

Molecular weight: 168.04.

USP requirements: Desflurane—Not in USP.

DESIPRAMINE

Chemical group: Dibenzazepine; secondary amine.

Chemical name: Desipramine hydrochloride—5*H*-Dibenz[*b*,*f*]azepine-5-propanamine, 10,11-dihydro-*N*-methyl-, monohydrochloride.

Molecular formula: Desipramine hydrochloride—$C_{18}H_{22}N_2 \cdot HCl$.

Molecular weight: Desipramine hydrochloride—302.85.

Description: Desipramine Hydrochloride USP—White to off-white, crystalline powder. Melts at about 213 °C.

pKa: 1.5 and 10.2.

Solubility: Desipramine Hydrochloride USP—Soluble in water and in alcohol; freely soluble in methanol and in chloroform; insoluble in ether.

USP requirements:

Desipramine Hydrochloride USP—Preserve in tight containers. Dried in vacuum at 105 °C for 2 hours, contains not less than 98.0% and not more than 100.5% of desipramine hydrochloride. Meets the requirements for Identification, Loss on drying (not more than 0.5%), Residue on ignition (not more than 0.1%), Heavy metals (not more than 0.001%), Iminodibenzyl, and Organic volatile impurities.

Desipramine Hydrochloride Capsules USP—Preserve in tight containers. Contain the labeled amount, within ±8%. Meet the requirements for Identification, Dissolution (75% in 45 minutes in water in Apparatus 1 at 100 rpm), and Uniformity of dosage units.

Desipramine Hydrochloride Tablets USP—Preserve in tight containers. Contain the labeled amount, within ±5%. Meet the requirements for Identification, Dissolution (75% in 60 minutes in 0.1 *N* hydrochloric acid in Apparatus 2 at 50 rpm), and Uniformity of dosage units.

DESLANOSIDE

Source: Obtained naturally from *Digitalis lanata* or may be produced synthetically.

Chemical name: Card-20(22)-enolide, 3-[(*O*-beta-D-glucopyranosyl-(1→4)-*O*-2,6-dideoxy-beta-D-*ribo*-hexopyranosyl-(1→4)-*O*-2,6-dideoxy-beta-D-*ribo*-hexopyranosyl-(1→4)-2,6-dideoxy-beta-D-*ribo*-hexopyranosyl)oxy]-12,14-dihydroxy-, (3 beta,5 beta,12 beta)-.

Molecular formula: $C_{47}H_{74}O_{19}$.

Molecular weight: 943.09.

Description: Hygroscopic white crystals or crystalline powder.

Solubility: Practically insoluble in water, in chloroform, and in ether; very slightly soluble in alcohol.

USP requirements:
Deslanoside USP—Preserve in tight, light-resistant containers. Contains not less than 95.0% and not more than 103.0% of deslanoside, calculated on the dried basis. Meets the requirements for Identification, Specific rotation (+7.0° to +8.5°, calculated on the dried basis), Loss on drying (not more than 5.0%), and Residue on ignition (not more than 0.2%).
Deslanoside Injection USP—Preserve in single-dose containers, preferably of Type I glass. A sterile solution of Deslanoside in a suitable solvent. Contains the labeled amount, within ±10%. Meets the requirements for Identification, pH (5.5–7.0), and Injections.

DESMOPRESSIN

Chemical group: Synthetic polypeptide structurally related to the posterior pituitary hormone arginine vasopressin (antidiuretic hormone).

Chemical name: Desmopressin acetate—Vasopressin, 1-(3-mercaptopropanoic acid)-8-D-arginine-, monoacetate (salt), trihydrate.

Molecular formula: Desmopressin acetate—$C_{48}H_{68}N_{14}O_{14}S_2 \cdot 3H_2O$.

Molecular weight: Desmopressin acetate—1183.32.

USP requirements:
Desmopressin Acetate Injection—Not in USP.
Desmopressin Acetate Nasal Solution—Not in USP.

DESOGESTREL AND ETHINYL ESTRADIOL

Chemical name:
Desogestrel—18,19-Dinorpregn-4-en-20-yn-17-ol, 13-ethyl-11-methylene-, (17 alpha)-.
Ethinyl estradiol—19-Norpregna-1,3,5(10)-trien-20-yne-3,17-diol, (17 alpha)-.

Molecular formula:
Desogestrel—$C_{22}H_{30}O$.
Ethinyl estradiol—$C_{20}H_{24}O_2$.

Molecular weight:
Desogestrel—310.48.
Ethinyl estradiol—296.41.

Description:
Desogestrel—Melting point 109–110 °C.
Ethinyl Estradiol USP—White to creamy white, odorless, crystalline powder.

Solubility: Ethinyl Estradiol USP—Insoluble in water; soluble in alcohol, in chloroform, in ether, in vegetable oils, and in solutions of fixed alkali hydroxides.

USP requirements: Desogestrel and Ethinyl Estradiol Tablets—Not in USP.

DESONIDE

Chemical name: Pregna-1,4-diene-3,20-dione, 11,21-dihydroxy-16,17-[(1-methylethylidene)bis(oxy)]-, (11 beta,16 alpha)-.

Molecular formula: $C_{24}H_{32}O_6$.

Molecular weight: 416.51.

Description: Small plates of white to off-white, odorless powder.

Solubility: Insoluble in water.

USP requirements:
Desonide Cream—Not in USP.
Desonide Lotion—Not in USP.
Desonide Ointment—Not in USP.

DESONIDE AND ACETIC ACID

For *Desonide* and *Acetic Acid*—See individual listings for chemistry information.

USP requirements: Desonide and Acetic Acid Otic Solution—Not in USP.

DESOXIMETASONE

Chemical name: Pregna-1,4-diene-3,20-dione, 9-fluoro-11,21-dihydroxy-16-methyl-, (11 beta,16 alpha)-.

Molecular formula: $C_{22}H_{29}FO_4$.

Molecular weight: 376.47.

Description: Desoximetasone USP—White to practically white, odorless, crystalline powder.

Solubility: Desoximetasone USP—Insoluble in water; freely soluble in alcohol, in acetone, and in chloroform.

USP requirements:
Desoximetasone USP—Preserve in well-closed containers. Contains not less than 97.0% and not more than 103.0% of desoximetasone, calculated on the dried basis. Meets the requirements for Identification, Melting range (206–218 °C, not more than 4 °C between beginning and end of melting), Specific rotation (+107° to +112°, calculated on the dried basis), Loss on drying (not more than 1.0%), Residue on ignition (not more than 0.2%), and Heavy metals (not more than 0.002%).
Desoximetasone Cream USP—Preserve in collapsible tubes, at controlled room temperature. It is Desoximetasone in an emollient cream base. Contains the labeled amount, within ±10%. Meets the requirements for Identification, Minimum fill, and pH (4.0–8.0).
Desoximetasone Gel USP—Preserve in collapsible tubes, at controlled room temperature. Contains the labeled amount, within ±10%. Meets the requirements for Identification, Minimum fill, and Alcohol content (18.0–24.0% [w/w]).
Desoximetasone Ointment USP—Preserve in collapsible tubes, at controlled room temperature. Contains the labeled amount, within ±10%. Meets the requirements for Identification and Minimum fill.

DESOXYCORTICOSTERONE

Chemical name:
Desoxycorticosterone acetate—Pregn-4-ene-3,20-dione, 21-(acetyloxy)-.
Desoxycorticosterone pivalate—Pregn-4-ene-3,20-dione, 21-(2,2-dimethyl-1-oxopropoxy)-.

Molecular formula:
Desoxycorticosterone acetate—$C_{23}H_{32}O_4$.
Desoxycorticosterone pivalate—$C_{26}H_{38}O_4$.

Molecular weight:
Desoxycorticosterone acetate—372.50.
Desoxycorticosterone pivalate—414.59.

Description:

Desoxycorticosterone Acetate USP—White or creamy white, crystalline powder. Is odorless, and is stable in air.

Desoxycorticosterone Pivalate USP—White or creamy white, crystalline powder. Is odorless, and is stable in air.

Solubility:

Desoxycorticosterone Acetate USP—Practically insoluble in water; sparingly soluble in alcohol, in acetone, and in dioxane; slightly soluble in vegetable oils.

Desoxycorticosterone Pivalate USP—Practically insoluble in water; soluble in dioxane; sparingly soluble in acetone; slightly soluble in alcohol, in methanol, in ether, and in vegetable oils.

USP requirements:

Desoxycorticosterone Acetate USP—Preserve in well-closed, light-resistant containers. Contains not less than 97.0% and not more than 103.0% of desoxycorticosterone acetate, calculated on the dried basis. Meets the requirements for Identification, Melting range (155–161 °C), Specific rotation (+171° to +179°), and Loss on drying (not more than 0.5%).

Desoxycorticosterone Acetate Injection USP—Preserve in single-dose or in multiple-dose containers, preferably of Type I or Type III glass, protected from light. A sterile solution of Desoxycorticosterone Acetate in vegetable oil. Contains the labeled amount, within −10% to +15%. Meets the requirements for Identification, Bacterial endotoxins, and Injections.

Desoxycorticosterone Acetate Pellets USP—Preserve in tight containers suitable for maintaining sterile contents, holding one pellet each. Sterile pellets composed of Desoxycorticosterone Acetate in compressed form, without the presence of any binder, diluent, or excipient. Contain the labeled amount, within ±3%. Meet the requirements for Identification, Solubility in alcohol, Melting range (155–161 °C), Specific rotation (+171° to +179°), Sterility, and Weight variation (average weight of 5 Pellets 95–105% of labeled weight; each Pellet weighs 90–110% of labeled weight).

Desoxycorticosterone Pivalate USP—Preserve in well-closed, light-resistant containers. Contains not less than 97.0% and not more than 103.0% of desoxycorticosterone pivalate, calculated on the dried basis. Meets the requirements for Identification, Melting range (200–206 °C), Specific rotation (+155° to +163°, calculated on the dried basis), and Loss on drying (not more than 0.5%).

Sterile Desoxycorticosterone Pivalate Suspension USP—Preserve in single-dose or in multiple-dose containers, preferably of Type I glass, protected from light. A sterile suspension of Desoxycorticosterone Pivalate in an aqueous medium. Contains the labeled amount, within ±10%. Meets the requirements for Identification, Bacterial endotoxins, pH (5.0–7.0), and Injections.

DEXAMETHASONE

Chemical name:

Dexamethasone—Pregna-1,4-diene-3,20-dione, 9-fluoro-11,17,21-trihydroxy-16-methyl-, (11 beta,16 alpha)-.

Dexamethasone acetate—Pregna-1,4-diene-3,20-dione, 21-(acetyloxy)-9-fluoro-11,17-dihydroxy-16-methyl, monohydrate, (11 beta,16 alpha)-.

Dexamethasone sodium phosphate—Pregna-1,4-diene-3,20-dione, 9-fluoro-11,17-dihydroxy-16-methyl-21-(phosphonooxy)-, disodium salt, (11 beta,16 alpha)-.

Molecular formula:

Dexamethasone—$C_{22}H_{29}FO_5$.

Dexamethasone acetate—$C_{24}H_{31}FO_6$ (anhydrous); $C_{24}H_{31}FO_6 \cdot H_2O$ (monohydrate).

Dexamethasone sodium phosphate—$C_{22}H_{28}FNa_2O_8P$.

Molecular weight:

Dexamethasone—392.47.

Dexamethasone acetate—434.50 (anhydrous); 452.52 (monohydrate).

Dexamethasone sodium phosphate—516.41.

Description:

Dexamethasone USP—White to practically white, odorless, crystalline powder. Is stable in air. Melts at about 250 °C, with some decomposition.

Dexamethasone Acetate USP—Clear, white to off-white, odorless powder.

Dexamethasone Sodium Phosphate USP— White or slightly yellow, crystalline powder. Is odorless or has a slight odor of alcohol, and is exceedingly hygroscopic.

Solubility:

Dexamethasone USP—Practically insoluble in water; sparingly soluble in acetone, in alcohol, in dioxane, and in methanol; slightly soluble in chloroform; very slightly soluble in ether.

Dexamethasone Acetate USP—Practically insoluble in water; freely soluble in methanol, in acetone, and in dioxane.

Dexamethasone Sodium Phosphate USP—Freely soluble in water; slightly soluble in alcohol; very slightly soluble in dioxane; insoluble in chloroform and in ether.

USP requirements:

Dexamethasone USP—Preserve in well-closed containers. Contains not less than 97.0% and not more than 102.0% of dexamethasone, calculated on the dried basis. Meets the requirements for Identification, Specific rotation (+72° to +80°, calculated on the dried basis), Loss on drying (not more than 0.5%), Residue on ignition (not more than 0.2% from 250 mg), and Ordinary impurities.

Dexamethasone Topical Aerosol USP—Preserve in pressurized containers, and avoid exposure to excessive heat. It is Dexamethasone in a suitable lotion base mixed with suitable propellants in a pressurized container. Delivers the labeled amount, within −10% to +20%. Meets the requirements for Identification and Microbial limits, and for Leak testing and Pressure testing under Aerosols.

Dexamethasone Elixir USP—Preserve in tight containers. Contains the labeled amount, within ±10%. Meets the requirements for Identification and Alcohol content (3.8–5.7%, *n*-propyl alcohol being used as the internal standard).

Dexamethasone Gel USP—Preserve in collapsible tubes. Keep tightly closed. Avoid exposure to temperatures exceeding 30 °C. Contains the labeled amount, within ±10%. Meets the requirements for Identification and Minimum fill.

Dexamethasone Ophthalmic Ointment—Not in USP.

Dexamethasone Oral Solution—Not in USP.

Dexamethasone Ophthalmic Suspension USP—Preserve in tight containers. A sterile, aqueous suspension of dexamethasone containing a suitable antimicrobial preservative. Contains the labeled amount, within ±10%. Meets the requirements for Identification, Sterility, and pH (5.0–6.0).

Dexamethasone Tablets USP—Preserve in well-closed containers. Contain the labeled amount, within ±10%. Meet the requirements for Identification, Dissolution (70% in 45 minutes in dilute hydrochloric acid [1 in 100] in Apparatus 1 at 100 rpm), and Uniformity of dosage units.

Dexamethasone Acetate USP—Preserve in well-closed containers. Contains one molecule of water of hydration or is anhydrous. Label it to indicate whether it is hydrous or anhydrous. Contains not less than 97.0% and not more than 102.0% of dexamethasone acetate, calculated on the dried basis. Meets the requirements for Identification, Specific rotation (+82° to +88°, calculated on the dried basis), Loss on drying (3.5–4.5% for the hydrous; not more than 0.4% for the anhydrous), Residue on ignition (not more than 0.1%), Heavy metals (not more than 0.002%), and Organic volatile impurities.

Sterile Dexamethasone Acetate Suspension USP—Preserve in single-dose or in multiple-dose containers, preferably of Type I glass. A sterile suspension of Dexamethasone Acetate in Water for Injection. Contains an amount of dexamethasone acetate monohydrate equivalent to the labeled amount of dexamethasone, within ±10%. Meets the requirements for Identification, Bacterial endotoxins, pH (5.0–7.5), and Injections.

Dexamethasone Sodium Phosphate USP—Preserve in tight containers. Contains not less than 97.0% and not more than 102.0% of dexamethasone sodium phosphate, calculated on the water-free and alcohol-free basis. Meets the requirements for Identification, Specific rotation (+74° to +82°, calculated on the water-free and alcohol-free basis), pH (7.5–10.5, in a solution [1 in 100]), Water (sum of percentages of water content and of alcohol content not more than 16.0%), Alcohol (not more than 8.0%), Phosphate ions (not more than 1.0%), and Free dexamethasone (not more than 1.0%).

Dexamethasone Sodium Phosphate Inhalation Aerosol USP—Preserve in tight, pressurized containers, and avoid exposure to excessive heat. A suspension, in suitable propellants and alcohol, in a pressurized container, of dexamethasone sodium phosphate. Contains an amount of dexamethasone sodium phosphate equivalent to the labeled amount of dexamethasone phosphate, within ±10%. Delivers the labeled dose of dexamethasone phosphate, within ±20% per metered spray. Meets the requirements for Identification and Alcohol content (1.7–2.3%), for Leak testing and Pressure testing under Aerosols, and for Unit spray content (not less than 80.0% and not more than 120.0% of the labeled amount of dexamethasone phosphate is delivered per spray).

Dexamethasone Sodium Phosphate Nasal Aerosol—Not in USP.

Dexamethasone Sodium Phosphate Cream USP—Preserve in collapsible tubes or in tight containers. Contains an amount of dexamethasone sodium phosphate equivalent to the labeled amount of dexamethasone phosphate, within −10% to +15%. Meets the requirements for Identification, Microbial limits, and Minimum fill.

Dexamethasone Sodium Phosphate Injection USP—Preserve in single-dose or in multiple-dose containers, preferably of Type I glass, protected from light. A sterile solution of Dexamethasone Sodium Phosphate in Water for Injection. Contains an amount of dexamethasone sodium phosphate equivalent to the labeled amount of dexamethasone phosphate, within −10% to +15%, present as the disodium salt. Meets the requirements for Identification, Bacterial endotoxins, pH (7.0–8.5), and Injections.

Dexamethasone Sodium Phosphate Ophthalmic Ointment USP—Preserve in collapsible ophthalmic ointment tubes. A sterile ointment. Contains an amount of dexamethasone sodium phosphate equivalent to the labeled amount of dexamethasone phosphate, within −10% to +15%. Meets the requirements for Identification, Minimum fill, Sterility, and Metal particles.

Dexamethasone Sodium Phosphate Ophthalmic Solution USP—Preserve in tight, light-resistant containers. A sterile, aqueous solution of Dexamethasone Sodium Phosphate. Contains an amount of dexamethasone sodium phosphate equivalent to the labeled amount of dexamethasone phosphate, within −10% to +15%. Meets the requirements for Identification, pH (6.6–7.8), and Sterility.

DEXBROMPHENIRAMINE

Chemical group: Propylamine derivative (alkylamine).

Chemical name: Dexbrompheniramine maleate—2-Pyridinepropanamine, gamma-(4-bromophenyl)-*N,N*-dimethyl-, (*S*)-, (*Z*)-2-butenedioate (1:1).

Molecular formula: Dexbrompheniramine maleate—$C_{16}H_{19}BrN_2 \cdot C_4H_4O_4$.

Molecular weight: Dexbrompheniramine maleate—435.32.

Description: Dexbrompheniramine Maleate USP—White, odorless, crystalline powder. Exists in two polymorphic forms, one melting between 106 and 107 °C and the other between 112 and 113 °C. Mixtures of the forms may melt between 105 and 113 °C. The pH of a solution (1 in 100) is about 5.

Solubility: Dexbrompheniramine Maleate USP—Freely soluble in water; soluble in alcohol and in chloroform.

USP requirements: Dexbrompheniramine Maleate USP—Preserve in tight, light-resistant containers. Contains not less than 98.0% and not more than 100.5% of dexbrompheniramine maleate, calculated on the dried basis. Meets the requirements for Identification, Specific rotation (+35.0° to +38.5°, calculated on the dried basis), Loss on drying (not more than 0.5%), Residue on ignition (not more than 0.2%), Related compounds (not more than 2.0%), and Organic volatile impurities.

DEXBROMPHENIRAMINE AND PSEUDOEPHEDRINE

For *Dexbrompheniramine* and *Pseudoephedrine*—See individual listings for chemistry information.

USP requirements:

Dexbrompheniramine Maleate and Pseudoephedrine Sulfate Extended-release Capsules—Not in USP.

Dexbrompheniramine Maleate and Pseudoephedrine Sulfate Syrup—Not in USP.

Dexbrompheniramine Maleate and Pseudoephedrine Sulfate Tablets—Not in USP.

Dexbrompheniramine Maleate and Pseudoephedrine Sulfate Extended-release Tablets—Not in USP.

DEXBROMPHENIRAMINE, PSEUDOEPHEDRINE, AND ACETAMINOPHEN

For *Dexbrompheniramine, Pseudoephedrine,* and *Acetaminophen*—See individual listings for chemistry information.

USP requirements: Dexbrompheniramine Maleate, Pseudoephedrine Sulfate, and Acetaminophen Extended-release Tablets—Not in USP.

DEXCHLORPHENIRAMINE

Chemical group: Propylamine derivative (alkylamine).

Chemical name: Dexchlorpheniramine maleate—2-Pyridinepropanamine, gamma-(4-chlorophenyl)-*N,N*-dimethyl-, (*S*)-, (*Z*)-2-butenedioate (1:1).

Molecular formula: Dexchlorpheniramine maleate—$C_{16}H_{19}ClN_2 \cdot C_4H_4O_4$.

Molecular weight: Dexchlorpheniramine maleate—390.87.

Description: Dexchlorpheniramine Maleate USP—White, odorless, crystalline powder.

Solubility: Dexchlorpheniramine Maleate USP—Freely soluble in water; soluble in alcohol and in chloroform; slightly soluble in ether.

USP requirements:

Dexchlorpheniramine Maleate USP—Preserve in tight, light-resistant containers. Dried at 65 °C for 4 hours, contains not less than 98.0% and not more than 100.5% of dexchlorpheniramine maleate. Meets the requirements for Identification, Melting range (110–115 °C), Specific rotation (+39.5° to +43.0°, calculated on the dried basis), pH (4.0–5.0, in a solution [1 in 100]), Loss on drying (not more than 0.5%), Residue on ignition (not more than 0.2%), Related compounds (not more than 2.0%), and Organic volatile impurities.

Dexchlorpheniramine Maleate Syrup USP—Preserve in tight, light-resistant containers. Contains the labeled amount, within ±10%. Meets the requirements for Identification and Alcohol content (5.0–7.0%).

Dexchlorpheniramine Maleate Tablets USP—Preserve in tight containers. Contain the labeled amount, within ±10%. Meet the requirements for Identification, Dissolution (75% in 45 minutes in water in Apparatus 2 at 50 rpm), and Uniformity of dosage units.

Dexchlorpheniramine Maleate Extended-release Tablets—Not in USP.

DEXCHLORPHENIRAMINE, PSEUDOEPHEDRINE, AND GUAIFENESIN

For *Dexchlorpheniramine, Pseudoephedrine,* and *Guaifenesin*—See individual listings for chemistry information.

USP requirements: Dexchlorpheniramine Maleate, Pseudoephedrine Sulfate, and Guaifenesin Oral Solution—Not in USP.

DEXPANTHENOL

Chemical name: Butanamide, 2,4-dihydroxy-*N*-(3-hydroxypropyl)-3,3-dimethyl-, (*R*)-.

Molecular formula: $C_9H_{19}NO_4$.

Molecular weight: 205.25.

Description: Dexpanthenol USP—Clear, viscous, somewhat hygroscopic liquid, having a slight, characteristic odor. Some crystallization may occur on standing.

Solubility: Dexpanthenol USP—Freely soluble in water, in alcohol, in methanol, and in propylene glycol; soluble in chloroform and in ether; slightly soluble in glycerin.

USP requirements:

Dexpanthenol USP—Preserve in tight containers. Contains not less than 98.0% and not more than 102.0% of dexpanthenol, calculated on the anhydrous basis. Meets the requirements for Identification, Specific rotation (+29.0° to +31.5°, calculated on the anhydrous basis), Refractive index (1.495–1.502 at 20 °C), Water (not more than 1.0%), Residue on ignition (not more than 0.1%), and Aminopropanol (not more than 1.0%).

Dexpanthenol Preparation USP—Preserve in tight containers. Contains not less than 94.5% and not more than 98.5% of dexpanthenol, and not less than 2.7% and not more than 4.2% of pantolactone, both calculated on the anhydrous basis. Meets the requirements for Identification, Specific rotation (+27.5° to +30.0°, calculated on the anhydrous basis), and Pantolactone, and for Refractive index, Water, Residue on ignition, and Aminopropanol under Dexpanthenol.

DEXTRATES

Description: Dextrates NF—Free-flowing, porous, white, odorless, spherical granules consisting of aggregates of microcrystals. May be compressed directly into self-binding tablets.

NF category: Sweetening agent; tablet and/or capsule diluent.

Solubility: Dextrates NF—Freely soluble in water; heating increases its solubility in water; soluble in dilute acids and alkalies and in basic organic solvents such as pyridine; insoluble in the common organic solvents.

NF requirements: Dextrates NF—Preserve in well-closed containers in a cool, dry place. A purified mixture of saccharides resulting from the controlled enzymatic hydrolysis of starch. Label it to state whether it is anhydrous or hydrated. Contains dextrose equivalent to not less than 93.0% and not more than 99.0%, calculated on the dried basis. Meets the requirements for pH (3.8–5.8, determined in a 1 in 5 solution in carbon dioxide-free water), Loss on drying (not more than 2.0% for the anhydrous; 7.8–9.2% for the hydrated form), Residue on ignition (not more than 0.1%), Heavy metals (not more than 5 ppm), Dextrose equivalent, and Organic volatile impurities.

DEXTRIN

Description: Dextrin NF—Free-flowing, white, yellow, or brown powder.

NF category: Suspending and/or viscosity-increasing agent; tablet binder; tablet and/or capsule diluent.

Solubility: Dextrin NF—Its solubility in water varies; it is usually very soluble, but often contains an insoluble portion.

NF requirements: Dextrin NF—Preserve in well-closed containers. Starch or partially hydrolyzed starch, modified by heating in a dry state, with or without acids, alkalies, or pH control agents. Meets the requirements for Botanic characteristics, Identification, Loss on drying (not more than 13.0%), Acidity, Residue on ignition (not more than 0.5%), Chloride (not more than 0.2%), Arsenic (not more than 3 ppm), Heavy metals (not more than 0.004%), Protein, Reducing sugars, and Organic volatile impurities.

DEXTROAMPHETAMINE

Chemical name: Dextroamphetamine sulfate—Benzeneethanamine, alpha-methyl-, (*S*)-, sulfate (2:1).

Molecular formula: Dextroamphetamine sulfate—$(C_9H_{13}N)_2 \cdot H_2SO_4$.

Molecular weight: Dextroamphetamine sulfate—368.49.

Description: Dextroamphetamine Sulfate USP—White, odorless, crystalline powder.

Solubility: Dextroamphetamine Sulfate USP—Soluble in water; slightly soluble in alcohol; insoluble in ether.

USP requirements:

Dextroamphetamine Sulfate USP—Preserve in well-closed containers. The dextrorotatory isomer of amphetamine sulfate. Contains not less than 98.0% and not more than 101.0% of amphetamine sulfate, calculated on the dried basis. Meets the requirements for Identification, Specific rotation (+20° to +23.5°, calculated on the dried basis), pH (5.0–6.0, in a solution [1 in 20]), Loss on drying (not more than 1.0%), Residue on ignition (not more than 0.1%), Ordinary impurities, and Organic volatile impurities.

Dextroamphetamine Sulfate Capsules USP—Preserve in tight containers. Contain the labeled amount, within ±10%. Meet the requirements for Identification, Dissolution (75% in 45 minutes in water in Apparatus 1 at 100 rpm), and Uniformity of dosage units.

Dextroamphetamine Sulfate Extended-release Capsules—Not in USP.

Dextroamphetamine Sulfate Elixir USP—Preserve in tight, light-resistant containers. Contains, in each 100 mL, not less than 90.0 mg and not more than 110.0 mg of dextroamphetamine sulfate. Meets the requirements for Identification, Alcohol content (9.0–11.0%), and Isomeric purity.

Dextroamphetamine Sulfate Tablets USP—Preserve in well-closed containers. Contain the labeled amount, within ±7%. Meet the requirements for Identification, Dissolution (75% in 45 minutes in water in Apparatus 1 at 100 rpm), Uniformity of dosage units, and Isomeric purity.

DEXTROMETHORPHAN

Source: Methylated dextroisomer of levorphanol.

Chemical group: Synthetic derivative of morphine.

Chemical name:

Dextromethorphan—Morphinan, 3-methoxy-17-methyl-, (9 alpha,13 alpha,14 alpha)-.

Dextromethorphan hydrobromide—Morphinan, 3-methoxy-17-methyl-, (9 alpha,13 alpha,14 alpha)-, hydrobromide, monohydrate.

Dextromethorphan polistirex—Benzene, diethenyl-, polymer with ethenylbenzene, sulfonated, complex with (9 alpha,13 alpha,14 alpha)-3-methoxy-17-methylmorphinan.

Molecular formula:

Dextromethorphan—$C_{18}H_{25}NO$.

Dextromethorphan hydrobromide—$C_{18}H_{25}NO \cdot HBr \cdot H_2O$.

Molecular weight:

Dextromethorphan—271.40.

Dextromethorphan hydrobromide—370.33.

Description:

Dextromethorphan USP—Practically white to slightly yellow, odorless, crystalline powder. Eleven mg of Dextromethorphan is equivalent to 15 mg of dextromethorphan hydrobromide monohydrate.

Dextromethorphan Hydrobromide USP—Practically white crystals or crystalline powder, having a faint odor. Melts at about 126 °C, with decomposition.

Solubility:

Dextromethorphan USP—Practically insoluble in water; freely soluble in chloroform.

Dextromethorphan Hydrobromide USP—Sparingly soluble in water; freely soluble in alcohol and in chloroform; insoluble in ether.

USP requirements:

Dextromethorphan USP—Preserve in tight containers. Contains not less than 98.0% and not more than 101.0% of dextromethorphan, calculated on the anhydrous basis. Meets the requirements for Identification, Melting range (109.5–112.5 °C), Specific rotation, Water (not more than 0.5%), Residue on ignition (not more than 0.1%), Heavy metals (not more than 0.002%), Dimethylaniline (not more than 0.001%), and Phenolic compounds.

Dextromethorphan Hydrobromide USP—Preserve in tight containers. Contains not less than 98.0% and not more than 102.0% of dextromethorphan hydrobromide, calculated on the anhydrous basis. Meets the requirements for Identification, Specific rotation, pH (5.2–6.5, in a solution [1 in 100]), Water (3.5–5.5%), Residue on ignition (not more than 0.1%), *N,N*-Dimethylaniline (not more than 0.001%), and Phenolic compounds.

Dextromethorphan Hydrobromide Capsules—Not in USP.

Dextromethorphan Hydrobromide Lozenges—Not in USP.

Dextromethorphan Hydrobromide Oral Solution—Not in USP.

Dextromethorphan Hydrobromide Syrup USP—Preserve in tight, light-resistant containers. Contains the labeled amount, within ±5%. Meets the requirement for Identification.

Dextromethorphan Hydrobromide Chewable Tablets—Not in USP.

Dextromethorphan Polistirex Extended-release Oral Suspension—Not in USP.

DEXTROMETHORPHAN AND ACETAMINOPHEN

For *Dextromethorphan* and *Acetaminophen*—See individual listings for chemistry information.

USP requirements: Dextromethorphan Hydrobromide and Acetaminophen Oral Solution—Not in USP.

DEXTROMETHORPHAN AND GUAIFENESIN

For *Dextromethorphan* and *Guaifenesin*—See individual listings for chemistry information.

USP requirements:

Dextromethorphan Hydrobromide and Guaifenesin Capsules—Not in USP.

Dextromethorphan Hydrobromide and Guaifenesin Oral Gel—Not in USP.

Dextromethorphan Hydrobromide and Guaifenesin Oral Solution—Not in USP.

Dextromethorphan Hydrobromide and Guaifenesin Syrup—Not in USP.

Dextromethorphan Hydrobromide and Guaifenesin Tablets—Not in USP.

DEXTROMETHORPHAN, GUAIFENESIN, POTASSIUM CITRATE, AND CITRIC ACID

For *Dextromethorphan, Guaifenesin, Potassium Citrate,* and *Citric Acid*—See individual listings for chemistry information.

USP requirements: Dextromethorphan Hydrobromide, Guaifenesin, Potassium Citrate, and Citric Acid Syrup—Not in USP.

DEXTROMETHORPHAN AND IODINATED GLYCEROL

For *Dextromethorphan* and *Iodinated Glycerol*—See individual listings for chemistry information.

USP requirements: Dextromethorphan Hydrobromide and Iodinated Glycerol Oral Solution—Not in USP.

DEXTROSE

Chemical name: D-Glucose, monohydrate.

Molecular formula: $C_6H_{12}O_6 \cdot H_2O$ (monohydrate); $C_6H_{12}O_6$ (anhydrous).

Molecular weight: 198.17 (monohydrate); 180.16 (anhydrous).

Description: Dextrose USP—Colorless crystals or white, crystalline or granular powder. Is odorless.

NF category: Sweetening agent; tonicity agent.

Solubility: Dextrose USP—Freely soluble in water; very soluble in boiling water; soluble in boiling alcohol; slightly soluble in alcohol.

USP requirements:
Dextrose USP—Preserve in well-closed containers. A sugar usually obtained by the hydrolysis of Starch. Contains one molecule of water of hydration or is anhydrous. Label it to indicate whether it is hydrous or anhydrous. Meets the requirements for Identification, Color of solution, Specific rotation (+52.6° to +53.2°, calculated on the anhydrous basis), Acidity, Water (7.5–9.5% for the hydrous form; not more than 0.5% for the anhydrous form), Residue on ignition (not more than 0.1%), Chloride (not more than 0.018%), Sulfate (not more than 0.025%), Arsenic (not more than 1 ppm), Heavy metals (not more than 5 ppm), Dextrin, and Soluble starch, sulfites.
Dextrose Injection USP—Preserve in single-dose glass or plastic containers. Glass containers are preferably of Type I or Type II glass. A sterile solution of Dextrose in Water for Injection. The label states the total osmolar concentration in mOsmol per liter. Where the contents are less than 100 mL, or where the label states that the Injection is not for direct injection but is to be diluted before use, the label alternatively may state the total osmolar concentration in mOsmol per mL. Contains the labeled amount of dextrose monohydrate, within ±5%. Contains no antimicrobial agents. Meets the requirements for Identification, Bacterial endotoxins, pH (3.2–6.5), Particulate matter, Heavy metals (not more than 0.0005*C*%), 5-Hydroxymethylfurfural and related substances, and Injections.

DEXTROSE AND ELECTROLYTES

For *Calcium Chloride, Citric Acid, Dextrose, Dibasic Sodium Phosphate, Magnesium Chloride, Potassium Chloride, Potassium Citrate, Sodium Chloride,* and *Sodium Citrate*—See individual listings for chemistry information.

USP requirements: Dextrose and Electrolytes Solution—Not in USP.

DEXTROSE EXCIPIENT

Description: Dextrose Excipient NF—Colorless crystals or white, crystalline or granular powder. Is odorless.
NF category: Sweetening agent; tablet and/or capsule diluent.

Solubility: Dextrose Excipient NF—Freely soluble in water; very soluble in boiling water; sparingly soluble in boiling alcohol; slightly soluble in alcohol.

NF requirements: Dextrose Excipient NF—Preserve in well-closed containers. A sugar usually obtained by hydrolysis of starch. Contains one molecule of water of hydration. Label it to indicate that it is not intended for parenteral use. Meets the requirements for Specific rotation (+52.5° to +53.5°, calculated on anhydrous basis), Water (7.5–9.5%), and Organic volatile impurities, and for Identification test, Color of solution, Acidity, Residue on ignition, Chloride, Sulfate, Arsenic, Heavy metals, Dextrin, and Soluble starch, sulfites under Dextrose.

DEXTROSE AND SODIUM CHLORIDE

For *Dextrose* and *Sodium Chloride*—See individual listings for chemistry information.

USP requirements: Dextrose and Sodium Chloride Injection USP—Preserve in single-dose glass or plastic containers. Glass containers are preferably of Type I or Type II glass. A sterile solution of Dextrose and Sodium Chloride in Water for Injection. The label states the total osmolar concentration in mOsmol per liter. Where the contents are less than 100 mL, or where the label states that the Injection is not for direct injection but is to be diluted before use, the label alternatively may state the total osmolar concentration in mOsmol per mL. Contains the labeled amounts, within ±5%. Contains no antimicrobial agents. Meets the requirements for Identification, Bacterial endotoxins, pH (3.5–6.5, determined on a portion diluted with water, if necessary, to a concentration of not more than 5% of dextrose), 5-Hydroxymethylfurfural and related substances, and Injections.

DEXTROTHYROXINE

Chemical name: Dextrothyroxine sodium—D-Tyrosine, *O*-(4-hydroxy-3,5-diiodophenyl)-3,5-diiodo-, monosodium salt hydrate.

Molecular formula: Dextrothyroxine sodium—$C_{15}H_{10}I_4NNaO_4 \cdot xH_2O$.

Molecular weight: Dextrothyroxine sodium—798.86 (anhydrous).

Description: Dextrothyroxine sodium—Light yellow to buff-colored, odorless powder which may assume a slight pink color on exposure to light.

Solubility: Dextrothyroxine sodium—Soluble 1 in 700 of water and 1 in 300 of alcohol; soluble in solutions of alkali hydroxides and in hot solutions of alkali carbonates; practically insoluble in acetone, in chloroform, and in ether.

USP requirements: Dextrothyroxine Sodium Tablets—Not in USP.

DEZOCINE

Chemical group: An opioid agonist/antagonist analgesic of the aminotetralin series.

Chemical name: 5,11-Methanobenzocyclodecen-3-ol, 13-amino-5,6,7,8,9,10,11,12-octahydro-5-methyl-, (5 alpha,11 alpha,-13*S**)-, (−)-.

Molecular formula: $C_{16}H_{23}NO$.

Molecular weight: 245.36.

Other characteristics: *n*-Octanol:Water partition coefficient—1.7.

USP requirements: Dezocine Injection—Not in USP.

DIACETYLATED MONOGLYCERIDES

Description: Diacetylated Monoglycerides NF—Clear liquid.
NF category: Plasticizer.

Solubility: Diacetylated Monoglycerides NF—Very soluble in 80% (w/w) aqueous alcohol, in vegetable oils, and in mineral oils; sparingly soluble in 70% alcohol.

NF requirements: Diacetylated Monoglycerides NF—Preserve in tight, light-resistant containers. Glycerin esterified with edible fat-forming fatty acids and acetic acid. May be prepared by the interesterification of edible oils with triacetin in the presence of catalytic agents, followed by molecular distillation, or by the direct acetylation of edible monoglycerides with acetic anhydride without the use of catalyst or molecular distillation. Meets the requirements for Identification, Residue on ignition (not more than 0.1%), Arsenic (not more than 3 ppm), Heavy metals (not more than 0.001%), Acid value (not more than 3), Hydroxyl value (not more than 15), and Saponification value (365–385).

DIATRIZOATE AND IODIPAMIDE

For *Diatrizoates* and *Iodipamide*—See individual listings for chemistry information.

USP requirements: Diatrizoate Meglumine and Iodipamide Meglumine Injection—Not in USP.

DIATRIZOATES

Chemical group: Ionic, monomeric, triiodinated benzoic acid derivative.

Chemical name:
Diatrizoate meglumine—Benzoic acid, 3,5-bis(acetylamino)-2,4,6-triiodo-, compd. with 1-deoxy-1-(methylamino)-D-glucitol (1:1).
Diatrizoate sodium—Benzoic acid, 3,5-bis(acetylamino)-2,4,6-triiodo-, monosodium salt.

Molecular formula:
Diatrizoate meglumine—$C_{11}H_9I_3N_2O_4 \cdot C_7H_{17}NO_5$.
Diatrizoate sodium—$C_{11}H_8I_3N_2NaO_4$.

Molecular weight:
Diatrizoate meglumine—809.13.
Diatrizoate sodium—635.90.

Description:
Diatrizoate Meglumine USP—White, odorless powder.
Diatrizoate Meglumine Injection USP—Clear, colorless to pale yellow, slightly viscous liquid.
Diatrizoate Meglumine and Diatrizoate Sodium Injection USP—Clear, colorless to pale yellow, slightly viscous liquid. May crystallize at room temperature or below.
Diatrizoate Sodium USP—White, odorless powder.
Diatrizoate Sodium Injection USP—Clear, colorless to pale yellow, slightly viscous liquid.
Diatrizoate Sodium Solution USP—Clear, pale yellow to light brown liquid.

Solubility:
Diatrizoate Meglumine USP—Freely soluble in water.
Diatrizoate Sodium USP—Soluble in water; slightly soluble in alcohol; practically insoluble in acetone and in ether.

Other characteristics: High osmolality.

USP requirements:
Diatrizoate Meglumine USP—Preserve in well-closed containers. Contains not less than 98.0% and not more than 102.0% of diatrizoate meglumine, calculated on the dried basis. Meets the requirements for Identification, Specific rotation (−5.65° to −6.37°, calculated on the dried basis), Loss on drying (not more than 1.0%), Residue on ignition (not more than 0.1%), Free aromatic amine, Iodine and iodide (0.02% iodide), and Heavy metals (not more than 0.002%).

Diatrizoate Meglumine Injection USP—Preserve Injection intended for intravascular injection either in single-dose containers, preferably of Type I or Type III glass, protected from light or, where intended for administration with a pressure injector through a suitable transfer connection, in similar glass 500-mL or 1000-mL bottles, protected from light. Injection packaged for other than intravascular use may be packaged in 100-mL multiple-dose containers, preferably of Type I or Type III glass, protected from light. A sterile solution of Diatrizoate Meglumine in Water for Injection, or a sterile solution of Diatrizoic Acid in Water for Injection prepared with the aid of Meglumine. Label containers of Injection intended for intravascular injection, where packaged in single-dose containers, to direct the user to discard any unused portion remaining in the container or, where packaged in bulk bottles to state, "Bulk Container—only for sterile filling of pressure injectors," to state that it contains no antimicrobial preservatives, and to direct the user to discard any unused portion remaining in the container after 6 hours. Indicate also in the labeling of bulk bottles that a pressure injector is to be charged with a dose just prior to administration of the Injection. Label containers of Injection intended for other than intravascular injection to show that the contents are not intended for intravascular injection. Contains the labeled amount, within ±5%. Diatrizoate Meglumine Injection intended for intravascular use contains no antimicrobial agents. Meets the requirements for Identification, Bacterial endotoxins, pH (6.0–7.7), Free aromatic amine, Iodine and iodide (0.02% iodide), Heavy metals (not more than 0.002%), Meglumine content (22.9–25.3% of the labeled amount of diatrizoate meglumine), and Injections.

Diatrizoate Meglumine and Diatrizoate Sodium Injection USP—Preserve either in single-dose containers, preferably of Type I or Type III glass, protected from light or, where intended for administration with a pressure injector through a suitable transfer connection, in similar glass 500-mL or 1000-mL bottles, protected from light. A sterile solution of Diatrizoate Meglumine and Diatrizoate Sodium in Water for Injection, or a sterile solution of Diatrizoic Acid in Water for Injection prepared with the aid of Sodium Hydroxide and Meglumine. Label containers of Injection intended for intravascular injection, where packaged in single-dose containers, to direct the user to discard any unused portion remaining in the container or, where packaged in bulk bottles to state, "Bulk Container—only for sterile filling of pressure injectors," to state that it contains no antimicrobial preservatives, and to direct the user to discard any unused portion remaining in the container after 6 hours. Indicate also in the labeling of bulk bottles that a pressure injector is to be charged with a dose just prior to administration of the Injection. Label containers of Injection intended for other than intravascular injection to show that the contents are not intended for intravascular injection. Contains the labeled amounts of diatrizoate meglumine and iodine, within ±5%. Diatrizoate Meglumine and Diatrizoate Sodium Injection intended for intravascular use contains no antimicrobial agents. Meets the requirements for Identification, Bacterial endotoxins, pH (6.0–7.7), Free aromatic amine, Iodine and iodide (0.02% iodide), Heavy metals (not more than 0.002%), and Injections.

Diatrizoate Meglumine and Diatrizoate Sodium Solution USP—Preserve in tight, light-resistant containers. A solution of Diatrizoic Acid in Purified Water prepared with the aid of Meglumine and Sodium Hydroxide. Label the container to indicate that the contents are not intended for parenteral use. Contains the labeled amounts of diatrizoate meglumine and iodine, within ±5%. Meets the requirements for Identification, pH (6.0–7.6), and Iodine and iodide (0.02% iodide).

Diatrizoate Sodium USP—Preserve in well-closed containers. Contains not less than 98.0% and not more than 102.0% of diatrizoate sodium, calculated on the anhydrous basis. Meets the requirements for Identification, Water (not more than 10.0%), Free aromatic amine, Iodine and iodide (0.02% iodide), and Heavy metals (not more than 0.002%).

Diatrizoate Sodium Injection USP—Preserve Injection intended for intravascular injection in single-dose containers, preferably of Type I or Type III glass, protected from light. Injection intended for other than intravascular use may be packaged in 100-mL multiple-dose containers, preferably of Type I or Type III glass, protected from light. A sterile solution of Diatrizoate Sodium in Water for Injection, or a sterile solution of Diatrizoic Acid in Water for Injection prepared with the aid of Sodium Hydroxide. Label containers of Injection intended for intravascular injection to direct the user to discard any unused portion remaining in the container. Label containers of Injection intended for other than intravascular injection to show that the contents are not intended for intravascular injection. Contains the labeled amount, within ±5%. Diatrizoate Sodium Injection intended for intravascular use contains no antimicrobial agents. Meets the requirements for Identification, Bacterial endotoxins, pH (6.0–7.7), Free aromatic amine, Iodine and iodide (0.02% iodide), Heavy metals (not more than 0.002%), and Injections.

Diatrizoate Sodium Solution USP—Preserve in tight, light-resistant containers. A solution of Diatrizoate Sodium in Purified Water, or a solution of Diatrizoic Acid in Purified Water prepared with the aid of Sodium Hydroxide. Label the container to indicate that the contents are not intended for parenteral use. Contains the labeled amount, within ±5%. Meets the requirements for Identification, pH (4.5–7.5), and Iodine and iodide (0.02% iodide).

Diatrizoate Sodium for Solution—Not in USP.

DIATRIZOIC ACID

Chemical name: Benzoic acid, 3,5-bis(acetylamino)-2,4,6-triiodo-.

Molecular formula: $C_{11}H_9I_3N_2O_4$.

Molecular weight: 613.92.

Description: Diatrizoic Acid USP—White, odorless powder.

Solubility: Diatrizoic Acid USP—Very slightly soluble in water and in alcohol; soluble in dimethylformamide and in alkali hydroxide solutions.

USP requirements: Diatrizoic Acid USP—Preserve in well-closed containers. It is anhydrous or contains two molecules of water of hydration. Label it to indicate whether it is anhydrous or hydrous. Contains not less than 98.0% and not more than 102.0% of diatrizoic acid, calculated on the anhydrous basis. Meets the requirements for Identification, Water (not more than 1.0% for the anhydrous form; 4.5–7.0% for the hydrous form), Residue on ignition (not more than 0.1%), Free aromatic amine, Iodine and iodide (0.02% iodide), and Heavy metals (not more than 0.002%).

DIAZEPAM

Chemical name: *2H*-1,4-Benzodiazepin-2-one, 7-chloro-1,3-dihydro-1-methyl-5-phenyl-.

Molecular formula: $C_{16}H_{13}ClN_2O$.

Molecular weight: 284.75.

Description: Diazepam USP—Off-white to yellow, practically odorless, crystalline powder.

Solubility: Diazepam USP—Practically insoluble in water; freely soluble in chloroform; soluble in alcohol.

USP requirements:

Diazepam USP—Preserve in tight, light-resistant containers. Contains not less than 98.5% and not more than 101.0% of diazepam, calculated on the dried basis. Meets the requirements for Identification, Melting range (131–135 °C), Loss on drying (not more than 0.5%), Residue on ignition (not more than 0.1%), Heavy metals (not more than 0.002%), Related compounds, and Organic volatile impurities.

Diazepam Capsules USP—Preserve in tight, light-resistant containers. Contain the labeled amount, within ±10%. Meet the requirements for Identification, Dissolution (85% in 45 minutes in 0.1 *N* hydrochloric acid in Apparatus 1 at 100 rpm), and Uniformity of dosage units.

Diazepam Extended-release Capsules USP—Preserve in tight, light-resistant containers. Contain the labeled amount, within ±10%. Meet the requirements for Identification, Drug release (15–27% in 0.042*D* hours, 49–66% in 0.167*D* hours, 76–96% in 0.333*D* hours, and 85–115% in 0.500*D* hours in simulated gastric fluid TS, prepared without enzymes, in Apparatus 1 at 100 rpm), and Uniformity of dosage units.

Sterile Diazepam Emulsion—Not in USP.

Diazepam Injection USP—Preserve in single-dose or in multiple-dose containers, preferably of Type I glass, protected from light. A sterile solution of Diazepam in a suitable medium. Contains the labeled amount, within ±10%. Meets the requirements for Identification, Bacterial endotoxins, pH (6.2–6.9), and Injections.

Diazepam Oral Solution—Not in USP.

Diazepam for Rectal Solution—Not in USP.

Diazepam Tablets USP—Preserve in tight, light-resistant containers. Contain the labeled amount, within ±10%. Meet the requirements for Identification, Dissolution (85% in 30 minutes in 0.1 *N* hydrochloric acid in Apparatus 1 at 100 rpm), and Uniformity of dosage units.

DIAZOXIDE

Chemical group: A nondiuretic benzothiadiazine derivative.

Chemical name: *2H*-1,2,4-Benzothiadiazine, 7-chloro-3-methyl-, 1,1-dioxide.

Molecular formula: $C_8H_7ClN_2O_2S$.

Molecular weight: 230.67.

Description: Diazoxide USP—White or cream-white crystals or crystalline powder.

pKa: 8.5.

Solubility: Diazoxide USP—Practically insoluble to sparingly soluble in water and in most organic solvents; very soluble in strong alkaline solutions; freely soluble in dimethylformamide.

USP requirements:

Diazoxide USP—Preserve in well-closed containers. Contains not less than 97.0% and not more than 102.0% of diazoxide, calculated on the dried basis. Meets the requirements for Identification, Loss on drying (not more than 0.5%), and Residue on ignition (not more than 0.1%).

Diazoxide Capsules USP—Preserve in well-closed containers. Contain the labeled amount, within ±10%. Meet the requirements for Identification, Dissolution (75% in 45 minutes in phosphate buffer [pH 7.6] in Apparatus 1 at 100 rpm), and Uniformity of dosage units.

Diazoxide Injection USP—Preserve in single-dose containers, preferably of Type I glass, protected from light. A sterile solution of Diazoxide in Water for Injection, prepared with the aid of Sodium Hydroxide. Contains the labeled amount, within ±10%. Meets the requirements for Identification, Bacterial endotoxins, pH (11.2–11.9), and Injections.

Diazoxide Oral Suspension USP—Preserve in tight, light-resistant containers. Contains the labeled amount, within ±10%. Meets the requirement for Identification.

DIBUCAINE

Chemical group: Amide.

Chemical name:
Dibucaine—4-Quinolinecarboxamide, 2-butoxy-*N*-[2-(diethylamino)ethyl]-.
Dibucaine hydrochloride—4-Quinolinecarboxamide, 2-butoxy-*N*-[2-(diethylamino)ethyl]-, monohydrochloride.

Molecular formula:
Dibucaine—$C_{20}H_{29}N_3O_2$.
Dibucaine hydrochloride—$C_{20}H_{29}N_3O_2 \cdot HCl$.

Molecular weight:
Dibucaine—343.47.
Dibucaine hydrochloride—379.93.

Description:
Dibucaine USP—White to off-white powder, having a slight, characteristic odor. Darkens on exposure to light.
Dibucaine Hydrochloride USP—Colorless or white to off-white crystals or white to off-white, crystalline powder. Is odorless, is somewhat hygroscopic, and darkens on exposure to light. Its solutions have a pH of about 5.5.

pKa: 8.8.

Solubility:
Dibucaine USP—Slightly soluble in water; soluble in 1 *N* hydrochloric acid and in ether.
Dibucaine Hydrochloride USP—Freely soluble in water, in alcohol, in acetone, and in chloroform.

USP requirements:
Dibucaine USP—Preserve in tight, light-resistant containers. Contains not less than 97.0% and not more than 100.5% of dibucaine, calculated on the dried basis. Meets the requirements for Identification, Melting range (62.5–66.0 °C, determined after drying), Loss on drying (not more than 1.0%), Residue on ignition (not more than 0.2%), and Chromatographic purity.
Dibucaine Cream USP—Preserve in collapsible tubes or in tight, light-resistant containers. Contains the labeled amount, within ±10%, in a suitable cream base. Meets the requirements for Identification, Microbial limits, and Minimum fill.
Dibucaine Ointment USP—Preserve in collapsible tubes or in tight, light-resistant containers. Contains the labeled amount, within ±10%, in a suitable ointment base. Meets the requirements for Identification, Microbial limits, and Minimum fill.
Dibucaine Hydrochloride USP—Preserve in tight, light-resistant containers. Contains not less than 97.0% and not more than 100.5% of dibucaine hydrochloride, calculated on the dried basis. Meets the requirements for Identification, Loss on drying (not more than 2.0%), Residue on ignition (not more than 0.1%), and Chromatographic purity.
Dibucaine Hydrochloride Injection—Preserve in single-dose or in multiple-dose containers, preferably of Type I glass, and protect from light. A sterile solution of Dibucaine Hydrochloride in Water for Injection. Contains the labeled amount, within ±5%. Meets the requirements for Identification, Bacterial endotoxins, pH (4.5–7.0), Particulate matter, and Injections.

DIBUTYL SEBACATE

Description: Dibutyl Sebacate NF—Colorless, oily liquid of very mild odor.

NF category: Plasticizer.

Solubility: Dibutyl Sebacate NF—Soluble in alcohol, in isopropyl alcohol, and in mineral oil; very slightly soluble in propylene glycol; practically insoluble in water and in glycerin.

NF requirements: Dibutyl Sebacate NF—Preserve in tight containers. Consists of esters of *n*-butyl alcohol and saturated dibasic acids, principally sebacic acid. Contains not less than 92.0% of dibutyl sebacate. Meets the requirements for Specific gravity (0.935–0.939 at 20 °C), Refractive index (1.429–1.441), Acid value (not more than 0.1), and Saponification value (352–357).

DICHLORALPHENAZONE

Source: A complex of chloral hydrate and phenazone.

Molecular formula: $C_{15}H_{18}Cl_6N_2O_5$.

Molecular weight: 519.04.

Description: Dichloralphenazone USP—White, microcrystalline powder. Has a slight odor characteristic of chloral hydrate. Decomposed by dilute alkali, liberating chloroform.

Solubility: Dichloralphenazone USP—Freely soluble in water, in alcohol, and in chloroform; soluble in dilute acids.

USP requirements: Dichloralphenazone USP—Preserve in well-closed containers. Contains not less than 97.0% and not more than 100.5% of dichloralphenazone, determined by both *Assay* procedures. Meets the requirements for Identification, Melting range (64–67 °C), Residue on ignition (not more than 0.1%), and Heavy metals (not more than 0.00%1).

DICHLORODIFLUOROMETHANE

Chemical name: Methane, dichlorodifluoro-.

Molecular formula: CCl_2F_2.

Molecular weight: 120.91.

Description: Dichlorodifluoromethane NF—Clear, colorless gas having a faint ethereal odor. Its vapor pressure at 25 °C is about 4880 mm of mercury (80 psig).

NF category: Aerosol propellant.

NF requirements: Dichlorodifluoromethane NF—Preserve in tight cylinders, and avoid exposure to excessive heat. Meets the requirements for Identification, Boiling temperature (approximately −30 °C), Water (not more than 0.001%), High-boiling residues (not more than 0.01%), and Inorganic chlorides.

DICHLOROTETRAFLUOROETHANE

Chemical name: Ethane, 1,2-dichloro-1,1,2,2-tetrafluoro-.

Molecular formula: $C_2Cl_2F_4$.

Molecular weight: 170.92.

Description: Dichlorotetrafluoroethane NF—Clear, colorless gas having a faint ethereal odor. Its vapor pressure at 25 °C is about 1620 mm of mercury (17 psig). Usually contains between 6% and 10% of its isomer, 1,1-dichloro-1,2,2,2-tetrafluoro ethane.

NF category: Aerosol propellant.

NF requirements: Dichlorotetrafluoroethane NF—Preserve in tight cylinders and avoid exposure to excessive heat. Meets the requirements for Identification, Boiling temperature (approximately 4 °C), Water (not more than 0.001%), High-boiling residues (not more than 0.01%), and Inorganic chlorides.

DICHLORPHENAMIDE

Chemical name: 1,3-Benzenedisulfonamide, 4,5-dichloro-.

Molecular formula: $C_6H_6Cl_2N_2O_4S_2$.

Molecular weight: 305.15.

Description: White or practically white, crystalline compound.

Solubility: Very slightly soluble in water; soluble in dilute solutions of sodium carbonate and sodium hydroxide.

USP requirements:

Dichlorphenamide USP—Preserve in well-closed containers. Contains not less than 98.0% and not more than 101.0% of dichlorphenamide, calculated on the dried basis. Meets the requirements for Identification, Melting range (236.5–240 °C), Loss on drying (not more than 1.0%), Residue on ignition (not more than 0.2%), Chloride (not more than 0.20%), Selenium (not more than 0.003%), Heavy metals (not more than 0.001%), and Organic volatile impurities.

Dichlorphenamide Tablets USP—Preserve in well-closed containers. Contain the labeled amount, within ±8%. Meet the requirements for Identification, Dissolution (80% in 60 minutes in 0.1 *M* phosphate buffer [pH 8.0] in Apparatus 2 at 75 rpm), and Uniformity of dosage units.

DICLOFENAC

Chemical group: Phenylacetic acid derivative.

Chemical name:

Diclofenac potassium—Benzeneacetic acid, 2-[(2,6-dichlorophenyl)amino]-, monopotassium salt.

Diclofenac sodium—Benzeneacetic acid, 2-[(2,6-dichlorophenyl)amino]-, monosodium salt.

Molecular formula:

Diclofenac potassium—$C_{14}H_{10}Cl_2KNO_2$.

Diclofenac sodium—$C_{14}H_{10}Cl_2NNaO_2$.

Molecular weight:

Diclofenac potassium—334.24.

Diclofenac sodium—318.13.

Description: Diclofenac sodium—Faintly yellow-white to light beige, virtually odorless, slightly hygroscopic, crystalline powder.

Solubility: Diclofenac sodium—Freely soluble in methanol; sparingly soluble in water; very slightly soluble in acetonitrile; insoluble in chloroform and in 0.1 *N* hydrochloric acid.

USP requirements:

Diclofenac Delayed-release Tablets—Not in USP.
Diclofenac Potassium Tablets—Not in USP.
Diclofenac Sodium Ophthalmic Solution—Not in USP.
Diclofenac Sodium Suppositories—Not in USP.
Diclofenac Sodium Delayed-release Tablets—Not in USP.
Diclofenac Sodium Extended-release Tablets—Not in USP.

DICLOXACILLIN

Chemical name: Dicloxacillin sodium—4-Thia-1-azabicyclo[3.2.0]heptane-2-carboxylic acid, 6-[[[3-(2,6-dichlorophenyl)-5-methyl-4-isoxazolyl]carbonyl]amino]-3,3-dimethyl-7-oxo-, monosodium salt, monohydrate, [2*S*-(2 alpha,5 alpha,6 beta)]-.

Molecular formula: Dicloxacillin sodium—$C_{19}H_{16}Cl_2N_3NaO_5S \cdot H_2O$.

Molecular weight: Dicloxacillin sodium—510.32.

Description: Dicloxacillin Sodium USP—White to off-white, crystalline powder.

Solubility: Dicloxacillin Sodium USP—Freely soluble in water.

USP requirements:

Dicloxacillin Sodium USP—Preserve in tight containers. Contains an amount of dicloxacillin sodium equivalent to not less than 850 mcg of dicloxacillin per mg. Meets the requirements for Identification, Crystallinity, pH (4.5–7.5, in a solution containing 10 mg per mL), Water (3.0–5.0%), and Dimethylaniline.

Dicloxacillin Sodium Capsules USP—Preserve in tight containers. Contain an amount of dicloxacillin sodium equivalent to the labeled amount of dicloxacillin, within −10% to +20%. Meet the requirements for Identification, Dissolution (75% in 45 minutes in water in Apparatus 1 at 100 rpm), Uniformity of dosage units, and Water (not more than 5.0%).

Sterile Dicloxacillin Sodium USP—Preserve in Containers for Sterile Solids. It is Dicloxacillin Sodium suitable for parenteral use. Contains an amount of dicloxacillin sodium equivalent to not less than 850 mcg of dicloxacillin per mg, and, where packaged for dispensing, contains an amount of dicloxacillin sodium equivalent to the labeled amount of dicloxacillin, within −10% to +20%. Meets the requirements for Constituted solution, Bacterial endotoxins, Sterility, pH (4.5–7.5, in a solution containing 10 mg per mL or, where packaged for dispensing, in the solution constituted as directed in the labeling), and Particulate matter, for Identification tests, Water, Dimethylaniline, and Crystallinity under Dicloxacillin Sodium, and for Uniformity of dosage units and Labeling under Injections.

Dicloxacillin Sodium for Oral Suspension USP—Preserve in tight containers. A dry mixture of Dicloxacillin Sodium and one or more suitable buffers, colors, flavors, and preservatives. Contains an amount of dicloxacillin sodium equivalent to the labeled amount of dicloxacillin, within −10% to +20%. Meets the requirements for Identification, pH (4.5–7.5, in the suspension constituted as directed in the labeling), Water (not more than 2.0%), Uniformity of dosage units (solid packaged in single-unit containers), and Deliverable volume (solid packaged in multiple-unit containers).

DICUMAROL

Chemical group: Coumarin derivative.

Chemical name: 2*H*-1-Benzopyran-2-one], 3,3′-Methylenebis[4-hydroxy-.

Molecular formula: $C_{19}H_{12}O_6$.

Molecular weight: 336.30.

Description: Dicumarol USP—White or creamy white, crystalline powder, having a faint, pleasant odor. Melts at about 290 °C.

Solubility: Dicumarol USP—Practically insoluble in water, in alcohol, and in ether; readily soluble in solutions of fixed alkali hydroxides; slightly soluble in chloroform.

USP requirements:

Dicumarol USP—Preserve in well-closed containers. Contains not less than 98.5% and not more than 101.0% of dicumarol, calculated on the dried basis. Meets the requirements for Identification, Acidity, Loss on drying (not more than 0.5%), Residue on ignition (not more than 0.25%), and Ordinary impurities.

Dicumarol Tablets USP—Preserve in well-closed containers. Label Tablets to state that Dicumarol Tablets may not be interchangeable with Dicumarol Capsules without retitration of the patient. Contain the labeled amount, within ±10%. Meet the requirements for Identification, Dissolution (60% in 30 minutes in 0.1 *M* tris buffer in Apparatus 1 at 100 rpm), and Uniformity of dosage units.

DICYCLOMINE

Chemical group: Synthetic tertiary amine.

Chemical name: Dicyclomine hydrochloride—[Bicyclohexyl]-1-carboxylic acid, 2-(diethylamino)ethyl ester, hydrochloride.

Molecular formula: Dicyclomine hydrochloride—$C_{19}H_{35}NO_2 \cdot HCl$.

Molecular weight: Dicyclomine hydrochloride—345.95.

Description:

Dicyclomine Hydrochloride USP—Fine, white, crystalline powder. Is practically odorless.

Dicyclomine Hydrochloride Injection USP—Colorless solution, which may have the odor of a preservative.

pKa: Dicyclomine hydrochloride—9.0.

Solubility: Dicyclomine Hydrochloride USP—Soluble in water; freely soluble in alcohol and in chloroform; very slightly soluble in ether.

USP requirements:

Dicyclomine Hydrochloride USP—Preserve in well-closed containers. Contains not less than 99.0% and not more than 102.0% of dicyclomine hydrochloride, calculated on the dried basis. Meets the requirements for Identification, Melting range (169–174 °C), pH (5.0–5.5, in a solution [1 in 100]), Readily carbonizable substances, and Organic volatile impurities.

Dicyclomine Hydrochloride Capsules USP—Preserve in well-closed containers. Contain the labeled amount, within ±7%. Meet the requirements for Identification, Dissolution (75% in 45 minutes in 0.01 *N* hydrochloric acid in Apparatus 2 at 50 rpm), and Uniformity of dosage units.

Dicyclomine Hydrochloride Injection USP—Preserve in single-dose or in multiple-dose containers, preferably of Type I glass. A sterile, isotonic solution of Dicyclomine Hydrochloride in Water for Injection. Contains the labeled amount, within ±7%. Meets the requirements for Identification, Bacterial endotoxins, and Injections.

Dicyclomine Hydrochloride Syrup USP—Preserve in tight containers. Contains the labeled amount, within ±5%. Meets the requirement for Identification.

Dicyclomine Hydrochloride Tablets USP—Preserve in well-closed containers. Contain the labeled amount, within ±7%. Meet the requirements for Identification, Dissolution (75% in 45 minutes in 0.01 *N* hydrochloric acid in Apparatus 2 at 50 rpm), and Uniformity of dosage units.

Dicyclomine Hydrochloride Extended-release Tablets—Not in USP.

DIDANOSINE

Chemical name: Inosine, 2′,3′-dideoxy-.

Molecular formula: $C_{10}H_{12}N_4O_3$.

Molecular weight: 236.23.

Description: White, crystalline powder. Unstable in acidic solutions.

Solubility: Aqueous solubility at 25 °C and pH of approximately 6 is 27.3 mg per mL.

USP requirements:

Buffered Didanosine for Oral Solution—Not in USP.

Didanosine for Buffered Oral Suspension—Not in USP.

Didanosine Tablets—Not in USP.

DIENESTROL

Chemical name: Phenol, 4,4′-(1,2-diethylidene-1,2-ethanediyl)-bis-, (*E,E*)-.

Molecular formula: $C_{18}H_{18}O_2$.

Molecular weight: 266.34.

Description: Dienestrol USP—Colorless, white or practically white, needle-like crystals, or white or practically white, crystalline powder. Is odorless.

Solubility: Dienestrol USP—Practically insoluble in water; soluble in alcohol, in acetone, in ether, in methanol, in propylene glycol, and in solutions of alkali hydroxides; slightly soluble in chloroform and in fatty oils.

USP requirements:

Dienestrol USP—Preserve in well-closed containers. Contains not less than 98.0% and not more than 100.5% of dienestrol, calculated on the dried basis. Meets the requirements for Identification, Melting range (227–234 °C, not more than 3 °C between beginning and end of melting), Loss on drying (not more than 0.5%), and Residue on ignition (not more than 0.2%).

Dienestrol Cream USP—Preserve in collapsible tubes or in tight containers. It is Dienestrol in a suitable water-miscible base. Contains the labeled amount, within ±10%. Meets the requirements for Identification and Minimum fill.

DIETHANOLAMINE

Chemical name: Ethanol, 2,2′-iminobis-.

Molecular formula: $C_4H_{11}NO_2$.

Molecular weight: 105.14.

Description: Diethanolamine NF—White or clear, colorless crystals, deliquescing in moist air; or colorless liquid.

NF category: Alkalizing agent; emulsifying and/or solubilizing agent.

Solubility: Diethanolamine NF—Miscible with water, with alcohol, with acetone, with chloroform, and with glycerin. Slightly soluble to insoluble in ether and in petroleum ether.

NF requirements: Diethanolamine NF—Preserve in tight, light-resistant containers. A mixture of ethanolamines, consisting largely of diethanolamine. Contains not less than 98.5% and not more than 101.0% of ethanolamines, calculated on the anhydrous basis as diethanolamine. Meets the requirements for Identification, Refractive index (1.473–1.476, at 30 °C), Water (not more than 0.15%), and Triethanolamine (not more than 1.0%).

DIETHYLAMINE SALICYLATE

Molecular formula: $C_{11}H_{17}NO_3$.

Molecular weight: 211.3.

Description: White or almost white, odorless or almost odorless crystals.

Solubility: Soluble 1 in less than 1 of water, 1 in 2 of alcohol, and 1 in 1.5 of chloroform.

USP requirements: Diethylamine Salicylate Cream—Not in USP.

DIETHYLCARBAMAZINE

Chemical group: Piperazine derivative.

Chemical name: Diethylcarbamazine citrate—1-Piperazinecarboxamide, *N,N*-diethyl-4-methyl-, 2-hydroxy-1,2,3-propanetricarboxylate.

Molecular formula: Diethylcarbamazine citrate—$C_{10}H_{21}N_3O \cdot C_6H_8O_7$.

Molecular weight: Diethylcarbamazine citrate—391.42.

Description: Diethylcarbamazine Citrate USP—White, crystalline powder. Melts at about 136 °C, with decomposition. Is odorless or has a slight odor; is slightly hygroscopic.

Solubility: Diethylcarbamazine Citrate USP—Very soluble in water; sparingly soluble in alcohol; practically insoluble in acetone, in chloroform, and in ether.

USP requirements:

Diethylcarbamazine Citrate USP—Preserve in tight containers. Contains not less than 98.0% and not more than 100.5% of diethylcarbamazine citrate, calculated on the anhydrous basis. Meets the requirements for Identification, Water (not more than 0.5%), Residue on ignition (not more than 0.1%), Heavy metals (not more than 0.002%), and Ordinary impurities.

Diethylcarbamazine Citrate Tablets USP—Preserve in tight containers. Contain the labeled amount, within ±5%. Meet the requirements for Identification, Disintegration (for Tablets labeled solely for veterinary use: 30 minutes), Dissolution (75% in 45 minutes in water in Apparatus 2 at 50 rpm), and Uniformity of dosage units.

Note: Diethylcarbamazine Citrate Tablets labeled solely for veterinary use are exempt from the requirements of the test for *Dissolution*.

DIETHYL PHTHALATE

Chemical name: 1,2-Benzenedicarboxylic acid, diethyl ester.

Molecular formula: $C_{12}H_{14}O_4$.

Molecular weight: 222.24.

Description: Diethyl Phthalate NF—Colorless, practically odorless, oily liquid.

NF category: Plasticizer.

Solubility: Diethyl Phthalate NF—Insoluble in water. Miscible with alcohol, with ether, and with other usual organic solvents.

NF requirements: Diethyl Phthalate NF—Preserve in tight containers. Contains not less than 98.0% and not more than 102.0% of diethyl phthalate, calculated on the anhydrous basis. Meets the requirements for Identification, Specific gravity (1.118–1.122, at 20 °C), Refractive index (1.500–1.505, at 20 °C), Acidity, Water (not more than 0.2%), and Residue on ignition (not more than 0.02%).

Caution: Avoid contact.

DIETHYLPROPION

Chemical group: Phenethylamine.

Chemical name: Diethylpropion hydrochloride—1-Propanone, 2-(diethylamino)-1-phenyl-, hydrochloride.

Molecular formula: Diethylpropion hydrochloride—$C_{13}H_{19}NO \cdot HCl$.

Molecular weight: Diethylpropion hydrochloride—241.76.

Description: Diethylpropion Hydrochloride USP—White to off-white, fine crystalline powder. Is odorless, or has a slight characteristic odor. It melts at about 175 °C, with decomposition.

Solubility: Diethylpropion Hydrochloride USP—Freely soluble in water, in chloroform, and in alcohol; practically insoluble in ether.

USP requirements:

Diethylpropion Hydrochloride USP—Preserve in well-closed, light-resistant containers. The label indicates whether it contains tartaric acid as a stabilizer. Contains not less than 97.0% and not more than 103.0% of diethylpropion hydrochloride, calculated on the anhydrous basis. Meets the requirements for Identification, Water (not more than 0.5%), Secondary amines (not more than 0.5%), Free bromine, Hydrobromic acid and bromide, Chromatographic purity, and Organic volatile impurities.

Diethylpropion Hydrochloride Extended-release Capsules—Not in USP.

Diethylpropion Hydrochloride Tablets USP—Preserve in well-closed containers. Contain the labeled amount, within ±10%. Meet the requirements for Identification, Dissolution (75% in 45 minutes in water in Apparatus 2 at 50 rpm), and Uniformity of dosage units.

Diethylpropion Hydrochloride Extended-release Tablets—Not in USP.

DIETHYLSTILBESTROL

Chemical name:

Diethylstilbestrol—Phenol 4,4′-(1,2-diethyl-1,2-ethenediyl)bis-, (*E*)-.

Diethylstilbestrol diphosphate—Phenol, 4,4′-(1,2-diethyl-1,2-ethenediyl)bis-, bis(dihydrogen phosphate), (*E*)-.

Molecular formula:

Diethylstilbestrol—$C_{18}H_{20}O_2$.

Diethylstilbestrol diphosphate—$C_{18}H_{22}O_8P_2$.

Molecular weight:

Diethylstilbestrol—268.36.

Diethylstilbestrol diphosphate—428.32.

Description:

Diethylstilbestrol USP—White, odorless, crystalline powder.

Diethylstilbestrol Diphosphate USP—Off-white, odorless, crystalline powder.

Diethylstilbestrol Diphosphate Injection USP—Colorless to light, straw-colored liquid.

Solubility:

Diethylstilbestrol USP—Practically insoluble in water; soluble in alcohol, in chloroform, in ether, in fatty oils, and in dilute alkali hydroxides.

Diethylstilbestrol Diphosphate USP—Sparingly soluble in water; soluble in alcohol and in dilute alkali.

USP requirements:

Diethylstilbestrol USP—Preserve in tight, light-resistant containers. Contains not less than 97.0% and not more than 100.5% of diethylstilbestrol, calculated on the dried basis. Meets the requirements for Identification, Melting range (169–175 °C, not more than 4 °C between beginning and end of melting), Acidity and alkalinity, Loss on drying (not more than 0.5%), Residue on ignition (not more than 0.05%), and Organic volatile impurities.

Diethylstilbestrol Injection USP—Preserve in light-resistant, single-dose or multiple-dose containers, preferably of Type I glass. A sterile solution of Diethylstilbestrol in a suitable vegetable oil. Contains the labeled amount, within ±10%. Meets the requirements for Identification, Bacterial endotoxins, and Injections.

Diethylstilbestrol Tablets USP—Preserve in well-closed containers. Contain the labeled amount, within ±10%. Meet the requirements for Identification, Disintegration (30 minutes), and Uniformity of dosage units.

Diethylstilbestrol Diphosphate USP—Preserve in tight containers, at a temperature not exceeding 21 °C. Contains not less than 95.0% and not more than 101.0% of diethylstilbestrol diphosphate, calculated on the dried basis. Meets the requirements for Identification, Loss on drying (not more than 1.0%), Chloride (not more than 1.5%), Free diethylstilbestrol (not more than 0.15%), Diethylstilbestrol monophosphate (not more than 1.5%), Pyridine, and Organic volatile impurities.

Diethylstilbestrol Diphosphate Injection USP—Preserve in single-dose or in multiple-dose containers. A sterile, buffered solution of Diethylstilbestrol Diphosphate. Contains not less than 45.0 mg and not more than 55.0 mg of diethylstilbestrol diphosphate in each mL. Meets the requirements for Identification, Bacterial endotoxins, pH (9.0–10.5), Free diethylstilbestrol (not more than 0.2 mg per mL of Injection), Diethylstilbestrol monophosphate (not more than 2.0 mg per mL of Injection), and Injections.

Diethylstilbestrol Diphosphate Tablets—Not in USP.

DIETHYLSTILBESTROL AND METHYLTESTOSTERONE

For *Diethylstilbestrol* and *Methyltestosterone*—See individual listings for chemistry information.

USP requirements: Diethylstilbestrol and Methyltestosterone Tablets—Not in USP.

DIETHYLTOLUAMIDE

Chemical name: Benzamide, *N,N*-diethyl-3-methyl-.

Molecular formula: $C_{12}H_{17}NO$.

Molecular weight: 191.27.

Description: Diethyltoluamide USP—Colorless liquid, having a faint, pleasant odor. Boils at about 111 °C under a pressure of 1 mm of mercury.

Solubility: Diethyltoluamide USP—Practically insoluble in water and in glycerin. Miscible with alcohol, with isopropyl alcohol, with ether, with chloroform, and with carbon disulfide.

USP requirements:

Diethyltoluamide USP—Preserve in tight containers. Contains not less than 95.0% and not more than 103.0% of the *meta*-isomer of diethyltoluamide, calculated on the anhydrous basis. Meets the requirements for Identification, Specific gravity (0.996–1.002), Refractive index (1.520–1.524), Acidity, and Water (not more than 0.5%).

Diethyltoluamide Topical Solution USP—Preserve in tight containers. A solution of Diethyltoluamide in Alcohol or Isopropyl Alcohol. Contains the labeled amount of the meta isomer of diethyltoluamide, within ±8%. If it contains Alcohol, contains the labeled amount of alcohol, within ±5%. Meets the requirements for Identification and Alcohol content (if present, 29.0–89.0%).

DIFENOXIN AND ATROPINE

Source: Atropine—An alkaloid that may be extracted from belladonna root and hyoscyamine or may be produced synthetically.

Chemical group:

Atropine—Natural tertiary amine.

Difenoxin—Diphenoxylic acid, principal active metabolite of diphenoxylate.

Chemical name:

Atropine sulfate—Benzeneacetic acid, alpha-(hydroxymethyl)-, 8-methyl-8-azabicyclo[3.2.1]oct-3-yl ester, *endo*-(±)-, sulfate (2:1) (salt), monohydrate.

Difenoxin hydrochloride—1-(3-Cyano-3,3-diphenylpropyl)-4-phenyl-4-piperidinecarboxylic acid monohydrochloride.

Molecular formula:

Atropine sulfate—$(C_{17}H_{23}NO_3)_2 \cdot H_2SO_4 \cdot H_2O$.

Difenoxin hydrochloride—$C_{28}H_{28}N_2O_2 \cdot HCl$.

Molecular weight:

Atropine sulfate—694.84.

Difenoxin hydrochloride—461.0.

Description:

Atropine Sulfate USP—Colorless crystals, or white, crystalline powder. Odorless; effloresces in dry air; is slowly affected by light.

Difenoxin hydrochloride—White amorphous powder. It has a melting point of 290 °C.

Solubility:

Atropine Sulfate USP—Very soluble in water; freely soluble in alcohol and even more so in boiling alcohol; freely soluble in glycerin.

Difenoxin hydrochloride—Very slightly soluble in water; sparingly soluble in chloroform, in tetrahydrofuran, in dimethylacetamide, and in dimethyl sulfoxide.

USP requirements: Difenoxin Hydrochloride and Atropine Sulfate Tablets—Not in USP.

DIFLORASONE

Chemical name: Diflorasone diacetate—Pregna-1,4-diene-3,20-dione, 17,21-bis(acetyloxy)-6,9-difluoro-11-hydroxy-16-methyl-, (6 alpha,11 beta,16 beta)-.

Molecular formula: Diflorasone diacetate—$C_{26}H_{32}F_2O_7$.

Molecular weight: Diflorasone diacetate—494.53.

Description: Diflorasone Diacetate USP—White to pale yellow, crystalline powder.

Solubility: Diflorasone Diacetate USP—Insoluble in water; soluble in methanol and in acetone; sparingly soluble in ethyl acetate; slightly soluble in toluene; very slightly soluble in ether.

USP requirements:

Diflorasone Diacetate USP—Preserve in tight containers. Contains not less than 97.0% and not more than 103.0% of diflorasone diacetate, calculated on the dried basis. Meets the requirements for Identification, Specific rotation (+58° to +68°), Loss on drying (not more than 0.5%), and Residue on ignition (not more than 0.5%).

Diflorasone Diacetate Cream USP—Preserve in collapsible tubes, preferably at controlled room temperature. Contains the labeled amount, within ±10%. Meets the requirements for Identification, Microbial limits, and Minimum fill.

Diflorasone Diacetate Ointment USP—Preserve in collapsible tubes, preferably at controlled room temperature. Contains the labeled amount, within ±10%. Meets the requirements for Identification, Microbial limits, and Minimum fill.

DIFLUCORTOLONE

Chemical name: Diflucortolone valerate—6 alpha,9 alpha-Difluoro-11 beta,21-dihydroxy-16 alpha-methylpregna-1,4-diene-3,20-dione 21-valerate.

Molecular formula: Diflucortolone valerate—$C_{27}H_{36}F_2O_5$.

Molecular weight: Diflucortolone valerate—478.6.

Description: Diflucortolone valerate—Melting point 200–205 °C.

Solubility: Diflucortolone valerate—Soluble in chloroform; slightly soluble in methyl alcohol; practically insoluble in ether.

USP requirements:
Diflucortolone Valerate Cream—Not in USP.
Diflucortolone Valerate Ointment—Not in USP.

DIFLUNISAL

Chemical group: Salicylic acid derivative. However, diflunisal is not metabolized to salicylic acid in vivo.

Chemical name: [1,1′-Biphenyl]-3-carboxylic acid, 2′,4′-difluoro-4-hydroxy-.

Molecular formula: $C_{13}H_8F_2O_3$.

Molecular weight: 250.20.

Description: Diflunisal USP—White to off-white, practically odorless powder.

pKa: 3.3.

Solubility: Diflunisal USP—Freely soluble in alcohol and in methanol; soluble in acetone and in ethyl acetate; slightly soluble in chloroform, in carbon tetrachloride, and in methylene chloride; insoluble in hexane and in water.

USP requirements:
Diflunisal USP—Preserve in well-closed containers. Contains not less than 98.0% and not more than 101.5% of diflunisal, calculated on the dried basis. Meets the requirements for Identification, Loss on drying (not more than 0.3%), Residue on ignition (not more than 0.1%), Heavy metals (not more than 0.001%), Chromatographic purity, and Organic volatile impurities.
Diflunisal Tablets USP—Preserve in well-closed containers. Contain the labeled amount, within ±10%. Meet the requirements for Identification, Dissolution (80% in 30 minutes in 0.1 *M* Tris buffer [pH 7.2] in Apparatus 2 at 50 rpm), and Uniformity of dosage units.

DIGITALIS

USP requirements:
Digitalis USP—Preserve in containers that protect it from absorbing moisture. Digitalis labeled to indicate that it is to be used only in the manufacture of glycosides is exempt from the moisture and storage requirements. The dried leaf of *Digitalis purpurea* Linné (Fam Scrophulariaceae). The potency of Digitalis is such that, when assayed as directed, 100 mg is equivalent to not less than 1 USP Digitalis Unit. (One Digitalis Unit represents the potency of 100 mg of USP Digitalis RS.) Meets the requirements for Botanic characteristics, Acid-insoluble ash (not more than 5.0%), Foreign organic matter (not more than 2.0%), and Water (not more than 6.0%).
Note: When Digitalis is prescribed, Powdered Digitalis is to be dispensed.
Powdered Digitalis USP—Preserve in tight, light-resistant containers. A package of suitable desiccant may be enclosed in the container. It is Digitalis dried at a temperature not exceeding 60 °C, reduced to a fine or a very fine powder, and adjusted, if necessary to conform to the official potency by admixture with sufficient Lactose, Starch or exhausted marc of digitalis, or with Powdered Digitalis having either a lower or a higher potency. The potency of Powdered Digitalis is such that, when assayed as directed, 100 mg is equivalent to 1 USP Digitalis Unit. (One Digitalis Unit represents the potency of 100 mg of USP Digitalis RS.) Meets the requirements for Identification, Microbial limit, Acid-insoluble ash (not more than 5.0%), and Water (not more than 5.0%).
Digitalis Capsules USP—Preserve in tight containers. Contain an amount of Powdered Digitalis equivalent to the labeled potency, within −15% to +20%. Meet the requirements for Microbial limit and Uniformity of dosage units.
Digitalis Tablets USP—Preserve in tight containers. Contain an amount of Powdered Digitalis equivalent to the labeled potency, within −15% to +20%. Meet the requirements for Disintegration (30 minutes), Microbial limit, and Uniformity of dosage units.

DIGITOXIN

Chemical name: Card-20(22)-enolide, 3-[(*O*-2,6-dideoxy-beta-D-*ribo*-hexopyranosyl-(1→4)-*O*-2,6-dideoxy-beta-D-*ribo*-hexopyranosyl-(1→4)-2,6-dideoxy-beta-D-*ribo*-hexopyranosyl)oxy]-14-hydroxy, (3 beta,5 beta)-.

Molecular formula: $C_{41}H_{64}O_{13}$.

Molecular weight: 764.95.

Description: Digitoxin USP—White or pale buff, odorless, microcrystalline powder.

Solubility: Digitoxin USP—Practically insoluble in water; sparingly soluble in chloroform; slightly soluble in alcohol; very slightly soluble in ether.

USP requirements:
Digitoxin USP—Preserve in tight containers. A cardiotonic glycoside obtained from *Digitalis purpurea* Linné, *Digitalis lanata* Ehrhart (Fam. Scrophulariaceae), and other suitable species of *Digitalis*. Contains not less than 92.0% and not more than 103.0% of digitoxin, calculated on the dried basis. Meets the requirements for Identification, Loss on drying (not more than 1.5%), and Residue on ignition.
Caution: Handle Digitoxin with exceptional care since it is highly potent.
Digitoxin Injection USP—Preserve in single-dose or in multiple-dose containers, preferably of Type I glass, protected from light. A sterile solution of Digitoxin in 5 to 50% (v/v) of alcohol, and may contain Glycerin or other suitable solubilizing agents. Contains the labeled amount, within ±10%. Meets the requirements for Identification, Bacterial endotoxins, Alcohol content (90.0–110.0% of labeled percentage of alcohol), and Injections.
Digitoxin Tablets USP—Preserve in well-closed containers. Contain the labeled amount, within ±10%. Meet the requirements for Identification, Dissolution (60% dissolved

in 30 minutes and 85% dissolved in 60 minutes in dilute hydrochloric acid [3 in 500] in Apparatus 1 at 120 ±5 rpm), and Uniformity of dosage units.

Note: Avoid the use of strongly adsorbing substances, such as bentonite, in the manufacture of Digitoxin Tablets.

DIGOXIN

Source: Obtained naturally from *Digitalis lanata* or may be produced synthetically.

Chemical name: Card-20(22)-enolide, 3-[(*O*-2,6-dideoxy-beta-D-*ribo*-hexopyranosyl-(1→4)-*O*-2,6-dideoxy-beta-D-*ribo*-hexopyranosyl-(1→4)-2,6-dideoxy-beta-D-*ribo*-hexopyranosyl)oxy]-12,14-dihydroxy-, (3 beta,5 beta,12 beta)-.

Molecular formula: $C_{41}H_{64}O_{14}$.

Molecular weight: 780.95.

Description: Digoxin USP—Clear to white, odorless crystals or white, odorless crystalline powder.

Solubility: Digoxin USP—Practically insoluble in water and in ether; freely soluble in pyridine; slightly soluble in diluted alcohol and in chloroform.

USP requirements:

Digoxin USP—Preserve in tight containers. A cardiotonic glycoside obtained from the leaves of *Digitalis lanata* Ehrhart (Fam. Scrophulariaceae). Contains not less than 95.0% and not more than 101.0% of digoxin, calculated on the dried basis. Meets the requirements for Identification, Loss on drying (not more than 1.0%), Residue on ignition (not more than 0.5%), and Related glycosides (not more than 3.0%).

Caution: Handle Digoxin with exceptional care, since it is extremely poisonous.

Digoxin Capsules—Not in USP.

Digoxin Elixir USP—Preserve in tight containers, and avoid exposure to excessive heat. Contains, in each 100 mL, not less than 4.50 mg and not more than 5.25 mg of digoxin. Meets the requirements for Identification and Alcohol content (9.0–11.5%).

Digoxin Injection USP—Preserve in single-dose containers, preferably of Type I glass. Avoid exposure to excessive heat. A sterile solution of Digoxin in Water for Injection and Alcohol or other suitable solvents. Contains the labeled amount, within −10% to +5%. Meets the requirements for Identification, Bacterial endotoxins, Alcohol content (9.0–11.0%), and Injections.

Digoxin Tablets USP—Preserve in tight containers. Contain the labeled amount, within −10% to +5%. Meet the requirements for Identification, Dissolution (65% for not fewer than eleven-twelfths of the Tablets tested, and 55% for any individual Tablet, in 60 minutes in 0.1 *N* hydrochloric acid in Apparatus 1 at 120 rpm), and Uniformity of dosage units.

DIGOXIN IMMUNE FAB (OVINE)

Source: Produced by a process involving immunization of sheep with digoxin that has been coupled as a hapten to human serum albumin, to stimulate production of digoxin-specific antibodies. After papain digestion of the antibody, digoxin-specific antigen binding (Fab) fragments (molecular weight 50,000 daltons) are isolated and purified by affinity chromatography.

Molecular weight: 50,000.

Description: Sterile, lyophilized powder.

USP requirements: Digoxin Immune Fab (Ovine) for Injection—Not in USP.

DIHYDROCODEINE

Chemical name: Dihydrocodeine bitartrate—Morphinan-6-ol, 4,5-epoxy-3-methoxy-17-methyl-, (5 alpha,6 alpha)-2,3-dihydroxybutanedioate (1:1) (salt).

Molecular formula: Dihydrocodeine bitartrate—$C_{18}H_{23}NO_3 \cdot C_4H_6O_6$.

Molecular weight: Dihydrocodeine bitartrate—451.47.

Description: Dihydrocodeine bitartrate—Odorless, or almost odorless, colorless crystals or white crystalline powder.

Solubility: Dihydrocodeine bitartrate—Soluble 1 in 4.5 of water; sparingly soluble in alcohol; practically insoluble in ether.

USP requirements: Dihydrocodeine Bitartrate USP—Preserve in tight containers. Contains not less than 98.5% and not more than 100.5% of dihydrocodeine bitartrate, calculated on the dried basis. Meets the requirements for Identification, Melting range (186–190 °C, not more than 2.5 °C between beginning and end of melting), Specific rotation (−72° to −75°, calculated on the dried basis), pH (3.2–4.2, in a solution [1 in 10]), Loss on drying (not more than 0.5%), Residue on ignition (not more than 0.1%), Ammonium salts, and Ordinary impurities.

DIHYDROCODEINE, ACETAMINOPHEN, AND CAFFEINE

For *Dihydrocodeine, Acetaminophen,* and *Caffeine*—See individual listings for chemistry information.

USP requirements: Dihydrocodeine Bitartrate, Acetaminophen, and Caffeine Capsules—Not in USP.

DIHYDROERGOTAMINE

Chemical name: Dihydroergotamine mesylate—Ergotoman-3′,6′,18-trione,9,10-dihydro-12′-hydroxy-2′-methyl-5′-(phenylmethyl)-, (5′ alpha)-, monomethanesulfonate (salt).

Molecular formula: Dihydroergotamine mesylate—$C_{33}H_{37}N_5O_5 \cdot CH_4O_3S$.

Molecular weight: Dihydroergotamine mesylate—679.79.

Description: Dihydroergotamine Mesylate USP—White to slightly yellowish powder, or off-white to faintly red powder, having a faint odor.

pKa: 6.75.

Solubility: Dihydroergotamine Mesylate USP—Slightly soluble in water and in chloroform; soluble in alcohol.

USP requirements:

Dihydroergotamine Mesylate USP—Preserve in well-closed, light-resistant containers. Contains not less than 97.0% and not more than 103.0% of dihydroergotamine mesylate, calculated on the dried basis. Meets the requirements for Identification, Specific rotation (−16.7° to −22.7°, calculated on the dried basis), pH (4.4–5.4, in a solution [1 in 1000]), Loss on drying (not more than 4.0%), and Related alkaloids (not more than 2.0%).

Dihydroergotamine Mesylate Injection USP—Preserve in single-dose containers, preferably of Type I glass, protected from light. A sterile solution of Dihydroergotamine Mesylate in Water for Injection. Contains the labeled amount, within ±10%. Meets the requirements for Identification, Bacterial endotoxins, pH (3.4–4.9), and Injections.

DIHYDROERGOTAMINE, HEPARIN, AND LIDOCAINE

For *Dihydroergotamine, Heparin,* and *Lidocaine*—See individual listings for chemistry information.

USP requirements: Dihydroergotamine Mesylate, Heparin Sodium, and Lidocaine Hydrochloride Injection USP—Preserve in single-dose or in multiple-dose containers, preferably of Type I glass. A sterile solution of Dihydroergotamine Mesylate, Heparin Sodium, and Lidocaine Hydrochloride in Water for Injection. Contains the labeled amounts of dihydroergotamine mesylate and lidocaine hydrochloride, within ±10%, and exhibits the labeled potency of heparin, within ±10%, stated on the label in terms of USP Heparin Units. Meets the requirements for Identification, Bacterial endotoxins, pH (5.0–6.5, determined on a portion diluted with an equal volume of potassium nitrate solution [1 in 100]), and Injections.

Note: Heparin Units are consistently established on the basis of the Assay set forth in *USP/NF,* independently of International Units, and the respective units are not equivalent.

DIHYDROSTREPTOMYCIN

Chemical name: Dihydrostreptomycin sulfate—Dihydrostreptomycinium sulfate(2:3)(salt).

Molecular formula: Dihydrostreptomycin sulfate—$(C_{21}H_{41}N_7O_{12})_2 \cdot 3H_2SO_4$.

Molecular weight: Dihydrostreptomycin sulfate—1461.41.

Description: Dihydrostreptomycin Sulfate USP—White or almost white, amorphous or crystalline powder. Amorphous form is hygroscopic.

Solubility: Dihydrostreptomycin Sulfate USP—Freely soluble in water; practically insoluble in acetone, in chloroform, and in methanol.

USP requirements:

Dihydrostreptomycin Sulfate USP—Preserve in tight containers. Label it to indicate that it is intended for veterinary use only. If it is crystalline, it may be so labeled. If it is intended solely for oral use, it is so labeled. Has a potency equivalent to not less than 650 mcg of dihydrostreptomycin per mg, except that if it is labeled as being crystalline, has a potency equivalent to not less than 725 mcg of dihydrostreptomycin per mg, or if it is labeled as being solely for oral use, has a potency equivalent to not less than 450 mcg of dihydrostreptomyin per mg. Meets the requirements for Identification, Crystallinity, pH (4.5–7.0, in a solution containing 200 mg of dihydrostreptomycin per mL; 3.0–7.0, if it is labeled as being solely for oral use), Loss on drying (not more than 5.0%; not more than 14.0% if it is labeled as being solely for oral use), and Streptomycin (not more than 3.0%; not more than 1.0% if it is labeled as being crystalline; not more than 5.0% if it is labeled as being solely for oral use).

Dihydrostreptomycin Sulfate Boluses USP—Preserve in tight containers. Label Boluses to indicate that they are intended for veterinary use only. Contain an amount of dihydrostreptomycin sulfate equivalent to the labeled amount of dihydrostreptomycin, within −15% to +20%. Meet the requirement for Loss on drying (not more than 10.0%).

Dihydrostreptomycin Sulfate Injection USP—Preserve in single-dose or in multiple-dose containers. Label it to indicate that it is intended for veterinary use only. Contains an amount of dihydrostreptomycin sulfate equivalent to the labeled amount of dihydrostreptomycin, within −10% to +20%. Contains one or more suitable preservatives. Meets the requirements for Identification, Depressor substances, Bacterial endotoxins, Sterility, and pH (5.0–8.0).

Sterile Dihydrostreptomycin Sulfate USP—Preserve in Containers for Sterile Solids. It is Dihydrostreptomycin Sulfate suitable for parenteral use. Label it to indicate that it is intended for veterinary use only. If it is crystalline, it may be so labeled. Has a potency equivalent to not less than 650 mcg of dihydrostreptomycin per mg, except that if it is labeled as being crystalline, has a potency equivalent to not less than 725 mcg of dihydrostreptomycin per mg. Meets the requirements for Depressor substances, Bacterial endotoxins, and Sterility, and for Identification tests, Crystallinity, pH, Loss on drying, and Streptomycin under Dihydrostreptomycin Sulfate.

DIHYDROTACHYSTEROL

Chemical name: 9,10-Secoergosta-5,7,22-trien-3-ol, (3 beta,-5*E*,7*E*,10 alpha,22*E*)-.

Molecular formula: $C_{28}H_{46}O$.

Molecular weight: 398.67.

Description: Dihydrotachysterol USP—Colorless or white, odorless crystals, or white, odorless, crystalline powder.

Solubility: Dihydrotachysterol USP—Practically insoluble in water; soluble in alcohol; freely soluble in ether and in chloroform; sparingly soluble in vegetable oils.

USP requirements:

Dihydrotachysterol USP—Preserve in light-resistant, hermetic glass containers from which air has been displaced by an inert gas. Contains not less than 97.0% and not more than 103.0% of dihydrotachysterol. Meets the requirements for Identification, Specific rotation (+100° to +103°), and Residue on ignition (not more than 0.1%).

Dihydrotachysterol Capsules USP—Preserve in well-closed, light-resistant containers. Contain a solution of Dihydrotachysterol in a suitable vegetable oil. Contain the labeled amount, within ±10%. Meet the requirements for Identification and Uniformity of dosage units.

Dihydrotachysterol Oral Solution USP—Preserve in tight, light-resistant glass containers. Contains the labeled amount, within ±10%. Meets the requirement for Identification.

Dihydrotachysterol Tablets USP—Preserve in well-closed, light-resistant containers. Contain the labeled amount, within ±10%. Meet the requirements for Identification, Disintegration (10 minutes), and Uniformity of dosage units.

DIHYDROXYALUMINUM AMINOACETATE

Source: A basic salt of aluminum and glycine.

Chemical name: Aluminum, (glycinato-*N,O*)dihydroxy-, hydrate.

Molecular formula: $C_2H_6AlNO_4$ (anhydrous).

Molecular weight: 135.06 (anhydrous).

Description:

Dihydroxyaluminum Aminoacetate USP—White, odorless powder.

Dihydroxyaluminum Aminoacetate Magma USP—White, viscous suspension, from which small amounts of water may separate on standing.

Solubility: Dihydroxyaluminum Aminoacetate USP—Insoluble in water and in organic solvents; soluble in dilute mineral acids and in solutions of fixed alkalies.

USP requirements:

Dihydroxyaluminum Aminoacetate USP—Preserve in well-closed containers. Yields not less than 94.0% and not more than 102.0% of dihydroxyaluminum aminoacetate, calculated on the dried basis. Meets the requirements for Identification, pH (6.5–7.5, in a suspension of 1 gram of it, finely powdered, in 25 mL of water), Loss on drying (not more than 14.5%), Mercury (not more than 1 ppm), Isopropyl alcohol, and Nitrogen (9.90–10.60%).

Dihydroxyaluminum Aminoacetate Capsules USP—Preserve in well-closed containers. Contain the labeled amount, within ±10%. Meet the requirements for Identification, Disintegration (10 minutes, in simulated gastric fluid TS), Uniformity of dosage units, Acid-neutralizing capacity, and pH (6.5–7.5, in a suspension of Capsule powder equivalent to about 1 gram of dihydroxyaluminum aminoacetate in 25 mL of water).

Dihydroxyaluminum Aminoacetate Magma USP—Preserve in tight containers, and protect from freezing. A suspension that contains the labeled amount, within ±10%. Meets the requirements for Identification, Microbial limits, Acid-neutralizing capacity, and pH (6.5–7.5, in a dilution in water, equivalent to about 1 gram of dihydroxyaluminum aminoacetate in 25 mL).

Dihydroxyaluminum Aminoacetate Tablets USP—Preserve in well-closed containers. Contain the labeled amount, within ±10%. Meet the requirements for Identification, Disintegration (10 minutes in simulated gastric fluid TS), Acid-neutralizing capacity, pH (6.5–7.5, in a suspension of ground Tablet powder in water, equivalent to about 1 gram of dihydroxyaluminum aminoacetate in 25 mL of water), and Uniformity of dosage units.

DIHYDROXYALUMINUM SODIUM CARBONATE

Chemical name: Aluminum, [carbonato(1-)-*O*]dihydroxy-, monosodium salt.

Molecular formula: $NaAl(OH)_2CO_3$.

Molecular weight: 144.00.

Description: Dihydroxyaluminum Sodium Carbonate USP—Fine, white, odorless powder.

Solubility: Dihydroxyaluminum Sodium Carbonate USP—Practically insoluble in water and in organic solvents; soluble in dilute mineral acids with the evolution of carbon dioxide.

USP requirements:

Dihydroxyaluminum Sodium Carbonate USP—Preserve in tight containers. Contains not less than 98.3% and not more than 107.9% of dihydroxyaluminum sodium carbonate, calculated on the dried basis. Meets the requirements for Identification, pH (9.9–10.2 in a suspension [1 in 25]), Loss on drying (not more than 14.5%), Acid-neutralizing capacity, Isopropyl alcohol (not more than 1.0%), Sodium content (15.2–16.8%), and Mercury (not more than 1 ppm).

Dihydroxyaluminum Sodium Carbonate Tablets USP—Preserve in well-closed containers. Label the Tablets to indicate that they are to be chewed before swallowing. Contain the labeled amount, within ±10%. Meet the requirements for Identification, Acid-neutralizing capacity, and Uniformity of dosage units.

DIISOPROPANOLAMINE

Chemical name: 2-Propanol, 1,1′-iminobis-.

Molecular formula: $C_6H_{15}NO_2$.

Molecular weight: 133.19.

Description: Diisopropanolamine NF—NF category: Alkalizing agent.

NF requirements: Diisopropanolamine NF—Preserve in tight, light-resistant containers. A mixture of isopropanolamines, consisting largely of diisopropanolamine. Contains not less than 98.0% and not more than 102.0% of isopropanolamines, calculated on the anhydrous basis. Meets the requirements for Identification, Water (not more than 0.50%), Triisopropanolamine (not more than 1.0%), and Organic volatile impurities.

DILTIAZEM

Chemical name: Diltiazem hydrochloride—1,5-Benzothiazepin-4(5*H*)one, 3-(acetyloxy)-5-[2-(dimethylamino)ethyl]-2,3-dihydro-2-(4-methoxyphenyl)-, monohydrochloride, (+)-*cis*-.

Molecular formula: Diltiazem hydrochloride—$C_{22}H_{26}N_2O_4S \cdot HCl$.

Molecular weight: Diltiazem hydrochloride—450.99.

Description: Diltiazem Hydrochloride USP— White, odorless, crystalline powder or small crystals. Melts at about 210 °C, with decomposition.

Solubility: Diltiazem Hydrochloride USP—Freely soluble in chloroform, in formic acid, in methanol, and in water; sparingly soluble in dehydrated alcohol; insoluble in ether.

USP requirements:

Diltiazem Hydrochloride USP—Preserve in tight, light-resistant containers. Contains not less than 98.5% and not more than 101.5% of diltiazem hydrochloride, calculated on the dried basis. Meets the requirements for Identification, Specific rotation (+110° to +116°), Loss on drying (not more than 0.5%), Residue on ignition (not more than 0.1%), Heavy metals (not more than 20 ppm), Related compounds, and Organic volatile impurities.

Diltiazem Hydrochloride Extended-release Capsules USP—Preserve in tight containers. Contain the labeled amount, within ±10%. Meet the requirements for Identification and Uniformity of dosage units.

Diltiazem Hydrochloride Injection—Not in USP.

Diltiazem Hydrochloride Tablets USP—Preserve in tight, light-resistant containers. Contain the labeled amount, within ±10%. Meet the requirements for Identification, Dissolution (60% in 30 minutes and 80% in 3 hours in water in Apparatus 2 at 100 rpm), and Uniformity of dosage units.

DIMENHYDRINATE

Chemical group: Ethanolamine derivative.

Chemical name: 1*H*-Purine-2,6-dione, 8-chloro-3,7-dihydro-1,3-dimethyl-, compd. with 2-(diphenylmethoxy)-*N,N*-dimethylethanamine (1:1).

Molecular formula: $C_{17}H_{21}NO \cdot C_7H_7ClN_4O_2$.

Molecular weight: 469.97.

Description: Dimenhydrinate USP—White, crystalline, odorless powder.

Solubility: Dimenhydrinate USP—Slightly soluble in water; freely soluble in alcohol and in chloroform; sparingly soluble in ether.

USP requirements:

Dimenhydrinate USP—Preserve in well-closed containers. Contains not less than 53.0% and not more than 55.5% of diphenhydramine, and not less than 44.0% and not more than 47.0% of 8-chlorotheophylline, calculated on the dried basis. Meets the requirements for Identification, Melting range (102–107 °C), Loss on drying (not more than 0.5%), Residue on ignition (not more than 0.3%), Chloride, Bromide and iodide, and Organic volatile impurities.

Dimenhydrinate Capsules—Not in USP.

Dimenhydrinate Extended-release Capsules—Not in USP.

Dimenhydrinate Elixir—Not in USP.

Dimenhydrinate Injection USP—Preserve in single-dose or in multiple-dose containers, preferably of Type I or Type III glass. A solution of Dimenhydrinate in a mixture of Propylene Glycol and water. Contains the labeled amount, within ±5%. Meets the requirements for Identification, pH (6.4–7.2), Content of 8-chlorotheophylline, and Injections.

Dimenhydrinate Suppositories—Not in USP.

Dimenhydrinate Syrup USP—Preserve in tight containers. Contains the labeled amount, within ±10%. Meets the requirements for Identification, Alcohol content (4.0–6.0%), and Content of 8-chlorotheophylline.

Dimenhydrinate Tablets USP—Preserve in well-closed containers. Contain the labeled amount, within ±10%. Meet the requirements for Identification, Dissolution (75% in 45 minutes in water in Apparatus 2 at 50 rpm), Uniformity of dosage units, and Content of 8-chlorotheophylline.

DIMERCAPROL

Chemical group: Dithiol.

Chemical name: 1-Propanol, 2,3-dimercapto.

Molecular formula: $C_3H_8OS_2$.

Molecular weight: 124.22.

Description:

Dimercaprol USP—Colorless or practically colorless liquid, having a disagreeable, mercaptan-like odor.

Dimercaprol Injection USP—Yellow, viscous solution having a pungent, disagreeable odor. Specific gravity is about 0.978.

Solubility: Dimercaprol USP—Soluble in water, in alcohol, in benzyl benzoate, and in methanol.

USP requirements:

Dimercaprol USP—Preserve in tight containers, in a cold place. Contains not less than 97.0% and not more than 100.5% of dimercaprol, and not more than 1.5% of 1,2,3-trimercaptopropane. Meets the requirements for Specific gravity (1.242–1.244), Distilling range (66–68 °C, under a pressure of 0.2 mm of mercury), Refractive index (1.567–1.573), and 1,2,3-Trimercaptopropane and related impurities (not more than 1.5% of 1,2,3-trimercaptopropane).

Dimercaprol Injection USP—Preserve in single-dose or in multiple-dose containers, preferably of Type I or Type III glass. A sterile solution of Dimercaprol in a mixture of Benzyl Benzoate and vegetable oil. Contains, in each 100 grams, not less than 9.0 grams and not more than 11.0 grams of dimercaprol. Meets the requirements for 1,2,3-Trimercaptopropane and related impurities and Injections (except that at times it may be turbid or contain small amounts of flocculent material).

DIMETHICONE

Chemical name: Dimethicone.

Description: Dimethicone NF—Clear, colorless, odorless liquid. NF category: Antifoaming agent; water repelling agent.

Solubility: Dimethicone NF—Insoluble in water, in methanol, in alcohol, and in acetone; very slightly soluble in isopropyl alcohol; soluble in chlorinated hydrocarbons, in toluene, in xylene, in *n*-hexane, in petroleum spirits, in ether, and in amyl acetate.

NF requirements: Dimethicone NF—Preserve in tight containers. A mixture of fully methylated linear siloxane polymers containing repeating units of the formula $[-(CH_3)_2SiO-]_n$, stabilized with trimethylsiloxy end-blocking units of the formula $[(CH_3)_3SiO-]$, wherein *n* has an average value such that the corresponding nominal viscosity is in a discrete range between 20 and 12,500 centistokes. Label it to indicate its nominal viscosity value. Dimethicone intended for use in coating containers that come in contact with articles for parenteral use is so labeled. Contains not less than 97.0% and not more than 103.0% of polydimethylsiloxane. The requirements for viscosity, specific gravity, refractive index, and loss on heating differ for the several types of Dimethicone. Meets the requirements for Identification, Specific gravity, Viscosity, Refractive index, Acidity, Loss on heating, and Heavy metals (not more than 0.001%). Additionally, Dimethicone intended for use in coating containers that come in contact with articles for parenteral use meets the requirements for Pyrogen and Biological suitability.

DIMETHYL SULFOXIDE

Chemical name: Methane, sulfinylbis-.

Molecular formula: C_2H_6OS.

Molecular weight: 78.13.

Description: Dimethyl Sulfoxide USP—Clear, colorless, odorless, hygroscopic liquid. Melts at about 18.4 °C. Boils at about 189 °C.

Solubility: Dimethyl Sulfoxide USP—Soluble in water; practically insoluble in acetone, in alcohol, in chloroform, and in ether.

USP requirements:

Dimethyl Sulfoxide USP—Preserve in tight, light-resistant containers. Contains not less than 99.9% of dimethyl sulfoxide. Meets the requirements for Identification, Specific gravity (1.095–1.097), Congealing temperature (18.3 °C), Refractive index (1.4755–1.4775), Water (not more than 0.1%), Acidity, Nonvolatile residue, Ultraviolet absorbance, Substances darkened by potassium hydroxide, and Dimethyl sulfone.

Dimethyl Sulfoxide Irrigation USP—Preserve in single-dose containers, and store at controlled room temperature, protected from strong light. A sterile solution of Dimethyl Sulfoxide in Water for Injection. Label it to indicate prominently that it is not intended for injection. Contains the labeled amount, within ±5%. Meets the requirements for Identification, Bacterial endotoxins, Sterility, and pH (5.0–7.0, when diluted with water to obtain a solution containing 50 mg of dimethyl sulfoxide per mL).

Dimethyl Sulfoxide Solution—Not in USP.

DINOPROST

Source: Dinoprost tromethamine—The tromethamine salt of naturally occurring prostaglandin $F_{2\text{-alpha}}$.

Chemical name: Dinoprost tromethamine—Prosta-5,13-dien-1-oic acid, 9,11,15-trihydroxy-, (5*Z*,9 alpha,11 alpha,13*E*,-15*S*)-, compd. with 2-amino-2-(hydroxymethyl)-1,3-propanediol (1:1).

Molecular formula: Dinoprost tromethamine—$C_{20}H_{34}O_5 \cdot C_4H_{11}NO_3$.

Molecular weight: Dinoprost tromethamine—475.62.

Description: Dinoprost Tromethamine USP—White to off-white, crystalline powder.

Solubility: Dinoprost Tromethamine USP—Very soluble in water; freely soluble in dimethylformamide; soluble in methanol; slightly soluble in chloroform.

USP requirements:

Dinoprost Tromethamine USP—Preserve in tight containers. Contains not less than 95.0% and not more than 105.0% of dinoprost tromethamine, calculated on the dried basis. Meets the requirements for Identification, Specific rotation (+19° to +26°, calculated on the dried basis), Loss on drying (not more than 1.0%), Residue on ignition (not more than 0.5%), and Limit of 5,6-*trans* Isomer and 15-*R* epimer (not more than 1.5%).

Caution: Great care should be taken to prevent inhaling particles of Dinoprost Tromethamine and exposing the skin to it.

Dinoprost Tromethamine Injection USP—Preserve in single-dose or in multiple-dose containers, preferably of Type I glass. A sterile solution of Dinoprost Tromethamine in Water for Injection. Contains an amount of dinoprost tromethamine equivalent to the labeled amount of dinoprost, within ±10%. Meets the requirements for Identification, Bacterial endotoxins, pH (7.0–9.0), and Injections, and for Sterility tests.

DINOPROSTONE

Source: The naturally occurring prostaglandin E_2.

Chemical name: Prosta-5,13-dien-1-oic acid, 11,15-dihydroxy-9-oxo-, (5*Z*,11 alpha,13*E*,15*S*)-.

Molecular formula: $C_{20}H_{32}O_5$.

Molecular weight: 352.47.

Description: White crystalline powder. Melting point 64–71 °C.

Solubility: Soluble in ethanol and in 25% ethanol in water; soluble in water to the extent of 130 mg/100 mL.

USP requirements:

Dinoprostone Cervical Gel—Not in USP.
Dinoprostone Vaginal Gel—Not in USP.
Dinoprostone Vaginal Suppositories—Not in USP.

DIOXYBENZONE

Chemical name: Methanone, (2-hydroxy-4-methoxyphenyl)(2-hydroxyphenyl)-.

Molecular formula: $C_{14}H_{12}O_4$.

Molecular weight: 244.25.

Description: Dioxybenzone USP—Yellow powder.

Solubility: Dioxybenzone USP—Practically insoluble in water; freely soluble in alcohol and in toluene.

USP requirements: Dioxybenzone USP—Preserve in tight, light-resistant containers. Contains not less than 97.0% and not more than 103.0% of dioxybenzone, calculated on the dried basis. Meets the requirements for Identification, Congealing temperature (not lower than 68.0 °C), and Loss on drying (not more than 2.0%).

DIOXYBENZONE AND OXYBENZONE

For *Dioxybenzone* and *Oxybenzone*—See individual listings for chemistry information.

USP requirements: Dioxybenzone and Oxybenzone Cream USP—Preserve in tight containers. A mixture of approximately equal parts of Dioxybenzone and Oxybenzone in a suitable cream base. Contains, in each 100 grams, not less than 2.7 grams and not more than 3.3 grams each of dioxybenzone and oxybenzone. Meets the requirements for Identification and Minimum fill.

DIPERODON

Chemical name: 1,2-Propanediol, 3-(1-piperidinyl)-, bis(phenylcarbamate) (ester), monohydrate.

Molecular formula: $C_{22}H_{27}N_3O_4 \cdot H_2O$.

Molecular weight: 415.49.

Description: Diperodon USP—White to cream-colored powder having a characteristic odor.

Solubility: Diperodon USP—Insoluble in water.

USP requirements:

Diperodon USP—Preserve in well-closed containers. Contains not less than 98.0% and not more than 102.0% of diperodon, calculated on the anhydrous basis. Meets the requirements for Identification, Water (3.5–5.0%), Residue on ignition (not more than 0.1%), Chloride (not more than 0.1%), and Heavy metals (not more than 0.002%).

Diperodon Ointment USP—Preserve in collapsible tubes or in tight containers. Contains an amount of diperodon equivalent to the labeled amount of anhydrous diperodon, within ±10%, in a suitable ointment base. Meets the requirements for Identification and Minimum fill.

DIPHEMANIL

Chemical name: Diphemanil methylsulfate—Piperidinium, 4-(diphenylmethylene)-1,1-dimethyl-, methyl sulfate.

Molecular formula: Diphemanil methylsulfate—$C_{21}H_{27}NO_4S$.

Molecular weight Diphemanil methylsulfate—389.51.

Description: Diphemanil Methylsulfate USP—White or nearly white, crystalline solid, having a a faint characteristic odor. Is stable to heat and to light, and is somewhat hygroscopic.

Solubility: Diphemanil Methylsulfate USP—Sparingly soluble in water, in alcohol, and in chloroform.

USP requirements:

Diphemanil Methylsulfate USP—Preserve in tight containers. Contains not less than 97.0% and not more than 103.0% of diphemanil methylsulfate, calculated on the dried basis. Meets the requirements for Identification, Melting range (189–196 °C), Loss on drying (not more than 0.5%), Residue on ignition (not more than 0.1%), Heavy metals (not more than 0.002%), and Ordinary impurities.

Diphemanil Methylsulfate Tablets USP—Preserve in tight containers. Contain the labeled amount, within ±7.5%. Meet the requirements for Identification, Dissolution (80% in 30 minutes in water in Apparatus 1 at 100 rpm), and Uniformity of dosage units.

DIPHENHYDRAMINE

Chemical group: Ethanolamine derivative.

Chemical name:

Diphenhydramine citrate—Ethanamine, 2-(diphenylmethoxy)-*N,N*-dimethyl-, 2-hydroxy-1,2,3-propanetricarboxylate (1:1).

Diphenhydramine hydrochloride—Ethanamine, 2-(diphenylmethoxy)-*N,N*-dimethyl-, hydrochloride.

Molecular formula:

Diphenhydramine citrate—$C_{17}H_{21}NO \cdot C_6H_8O_7$.

Diphenhydramine hydrochloride—$C_{17}H_{21}NO \cdot HCl$.

Molecular weight:

Diphenhydramine citrate—447.49.

Diphenhydramine hydrochloride—291.82.

Description: Diphenhydramine Hydrochloride USP—White, odorless, crystalline powder. Slowly darkens on exposure to light. Its solutions are practically neutral to litmus.

pKa: 9.

Solubility: Diphenhydramine Hydrochloride USP—Freely soluble in water, in alcohol, and in chloroform; sparingly soluble in acetone; very slightly soluble in ether.

USP requirements:

Diphenhydramine Citrate USP—Preserve in tight, light-resistant containers. Contains not less than 98.0% and not more than 100.5% of diphenhydramine citrate, calculated on the dried basis. Meets the requirements for Identification, Melting range (146–150 °C, range between beginning and end of melting not more than 2 °C), Loss on drying (not more than 0.5%), Residue on ignition (not more than 0.1%), and Organic volatile impurities.

Diphenhydramine Hydrochloride USP—Preserve in tight, light-resistant containers. Contains not less than 98.0% and not more than 102.0% of diphenhydramine hydrochloride, calculated on the dried basis. Meets the requirements for Identification, Melting range (167–172 °C), Loss on drying (not more than 0.5%), Residue on ignition (not more than 0.1%), and Organic volatile impurities.

Diphenhydramine Hydrochloride Capsules USP—Preserve in tight containers. Contain the labeled amount, within ±10%. Meet the requirements for Identification, Dissolution (75% in 45 minutes in water in Apparatus 1 at 100 rpm), and Uniformity of dosage units.

Diphenhydramine Hydrochloride Elixir USP—Preserve in tight, light-resistant containers. Contains the labeled amount, within ±10%. Meets the requirements for Identification and Alcohol content (the labeled amount, within ±10%).

Diphenhydramine Hydrochloride Injection USP—Preserve in single-dose or in multiple-dose containers, preferably of Type I glass, protected from light. A sterile solution of Diphenhydramine Hydrochloride in Water for Injection. Contains the labeled amount, within ±10%. Meets the requirements for Identification, Bacterial endotoxins, pH (4.0–6.5), and Injections.

Diphenhydramine Hydrochloride Syrup—Not in USP.

Diphenyhydramine Hydrochloride Tablets—Not in USP.

DIPHENHYDRAMINE, CODEINE, AND AMMONIUM CHLORIDE

For *Diphenhydramine, Codeine,* and *Ammonium Chloride*—See individual listings for chemistry information.

USP requirements: Diphenhydramine Hydrochloride, Codeine Phosphate, and Ammonium Chloride Syrup—Not in USP.

DIPHENHYDRAMINE, DEXTROMETHORPHAN, AND AMMONIUM CHLORIDE

For *Diphenhydramine, Dextromethorphan,* and *Ammonium Chloride*—See individual listings for chemistry information.

USP requirements: Diphenhydramine Hydrochloride, Dextromethorphan Hydrobromide, and Ammonium Chloride Syrup—Not in USP.

DIPHENHYDRAMINE, PHENYLPROPANOLAMINE, AND ASPIRIN

Chemical group:

Diphenhydramine—Ethanolamine derivative.

Phenylpropanolamine—A synthetic phenylisopropanolamine.

Chemical name:

Diphenhydramine citrate—Ethanamine, 2-(diphenylmethoxy)-*N,N*-dimethyl-, 2-hydroxy-1,2,3-propanetricarboxylate (1:1).

Aspirin—Benzoic acid, 2-(acetyloxy)-.

Molecular formula:

Diphenhydramine citrate—$C_{17}H_{21}NO \cdot C_6H_8O_7$.

Aspirin—$C_9H_8O_4$.

Molecular weight:

Diphenhydramine citrate—447.49.

Aspirin—180.16.

Description: Aspirin USP—White crystals, commonly tabular or needle-like, or white, crystalline powder. Is odorless or has a faint odor. Is stable in dry air; in moist air it gradually hydrolyzes to salicylic and acetic acids.

pKa:

Diphenhydramine—9.

Aspirin—3.5.

Solubility: Aspirin USP—Slightly soluble in water; freely soluble in alcohol; soluble in chloroform and in ether; sparingly soluble in absolute ether.

USP requirements: Diphenhydramine Citrate, Phenylpropanolamine Bitartrate, and Aspirin Tablets—Not in USP.

DIPHENHYDRAMINE AND PSEUDOEPHEDRINE

For *Diphenhydramine* and *Pseudoephedrine*—See individual listings for chemistry information.

USP requirements:

Diphenhydramine and Pseudoephedrine Capsules USP—Preserve in tight containers. Label Capsules to state both the contents of the active moieties and the contents of the salts used in formulating the article. Contain the labeled amounts of diphenhydramine hydrochloride and pseudoephedrine hydrochloride, within ±10%. Meet the requirements for Identification, Dissolution (75% of each active ingredient in 30 minutes in water in Apparatus 1 at 100 rpm), Uniformity of dosage units, and Related compounds (sum of amounts of benzhydrol and benzophenone not more than 2% [w/w] of diphenhydramine hydrochloride).

Diphenhydramine and Pseudoephedrine Hydrochlorides Oral Solution—Not in USP.
Diphenhydramine and Pseudoephedrine Hydrochlorides Tablets—Not in USP.

DIPHENHYDRAMINE, PSEUDOEPHEDRINE, AND ACETAMINOPHEN

For *Diphenhydramine, Pseudoephedrine,* and *Acetaminophen*—See individual listings for chemistry information.

USP requirements:
Diphenhydramine Hydrochloride, Pseudoephedrine Hydrochloride, and Acetaminophen Oral Solution—Not in USP.
Diphenhydramine Hydrochloride, Pseudoephedrine Hydrochloride, and Acetaminophen Tablets—Not in USP.

DIPHENHYDRAMINE, PSEUDOEPHEDRINE, DEXTROMETHORPHAN, AND ACETAMINOPHEN

For *Diphenhydramine, Pseudoephedrine, Dextromethorphan,* and *Acetaminophen*—See individual listings for chemistry information.

USP requirements:
Diphenhydramine Hydrochloride, Pseudoephedrine Hydrochloride, Dextromethorphan Hydrobromide, and Acetaminophen Capsules—Not in USP.
Diphenhydramine Hydrochloride, Pseudoephedrine Hydrochloride, Dextromethorphan Hydrobromide, and Acetaminophen Oral Solution—Not in USP.
Diphenhydramine Hydrochloride, Pseudoephedrine Hydrochloride, Dextromethorphan Hydrobromide, and Acetaminophen Tablets—Not in USP.

DIPHENIDOL

Chemical name: Diphenidol hydrochloride—1-Piperidinebutanol, alpha,alpha-diphenyl, hydrochloride.

Molecular formula: Diphenidol hydrochloride—$C_{21}H_{27}NO \cdot HCl$.

Molecular weight: Diphenidol hydrochloride—345.91.

Description: Diphenidol hydrochloride—Melting point 212–214 °C.

Solubility: Diphenidol hydrochloride—Freely soluble in methanol; soluble in water and in chloroform; practically insoluble in ether.

USP requirements: Diphenidol Hydrochloride Tablets—Not in USP.

DIPHENOXYLATE

Chemical group: Diphenoxylate hydrochloride—Similar in structure to meperidine.

Chemical name: Diphenoxylate hydrochloride—4-Piperidinecarboxylic acid, 1-(3-cyano-3,3-diphenylpropyl)-4-phenyl-, ethyl ester, monohydrochloride.

Molecular formula: Diphenoxylate hydrochloride—$C_{30}H_{32}N_2O_2 \cdot HCl$.

Molecular weight: Diphenoxylate hydrochloride—489.06.

Description: Diphenoxylate Hydrochloride USP—White, odorless, crystalline powder. Its saturated solution has a pH of about 3.3.

Solubility: Diphenoxylate Hydrochloride USP—Slightly soluble in water and in isopropanol; freely soluble in chloroform; soluble in methanol; sparingly soluble in alcohol and in acetone; practically insoluble in ether and in solvent hexane.

USP requirements: Diphenoxylate Hydrochloride USP—Preserve in well-closed containers. Contains not less than 98.0% and not more than 102.0% of diphenoxylate hydrochloride, calculated on the dried basis. Meets the requirements for Identification, Melting range (220–226 °C), Loss on drying (not more than 0.5%), and Ordinary impurities.

DIPHENOXYLATE AND ATROPINE

For *Diphenoxylate* and *Atropine*—See individual listings for chemistry information.

USP requirements:
Diphenoxylate Hydrochloride and Atropine Sulfate Oral Solution USP—Preserve in tight, light-resistant containers. Contains the labeled amount of diphenoxylate hydrochloride, within ±7%, and the labeled amount of atropine sulfate, within ±20%. Meets the requirements for Identification, pH (3.0–4.3, determined in a dilution of the Oral Solution with an equal volume of water), and Alcohol content (13.5–16.5%).
Diphenoxylate Hydrochloride and Atropine Sulfate Tablets USP—Preserve in well-closed, light-resistant containers. Contain the labeled amount of diphenoxylate hydrochloride, within ±5%, and the labeled amount of atropine sulfate, within ±20%. Meet the requirements for Identification, Dissolution (75% of the labeled amount of diphenoxylate hydrochloride in 45 minutes in 0.2 *M* acetic acid in Apparatus 1 at 150 rpm), and Uniformity of dosage units.

DIPHENYLPYRALINE, PHENYLEPHRINE, AND CODEINE

Chemical group: Diphenylpyraline hydrochloride—Piperidine derivative.

Chemical name:
Diphenylpyraline hydrochloride—Piperidine, 4-(diphenylmethoxy)-1-methyl-, hydrochloride.
Phenylephrine hydrochloride—Benzenemethanol, 3-hydroxy-alpha-[(methylamino)methyl]-, hydrochloride.
Codeine phosphate—Morphinan-6-ol, 7,8-didehydro-4,5-epoxy-3-methoxy-17-methyl-, (5 alpha,6 alpha)-, phosphate (1:1) (salt), hemihydrate.

Molecular formula:
Diphenylpyraline hydrochloride—$C_{19}H_{23}NO \cdot HCl$.
Phenylephrine hydrochloride—$C_9H_{13}NO_2 \cdot HCl$.
Codeine phosphate—$C_{18}H_{21}NO_3 \cdot H_3PO_4 \cdot ½H_2O$ (hemihydrate); $C_{18}H_{21}NO_3 \cdot H_3PO_4$ (anhydrous).

Molecular weight:
Diphenylpyraline hydrochloride—317.86.
Phenylephrine hydrochloride—203.67.
Codeine phosphate—406.37 (hemihydrate); 397.36 (anhydrous).

Description:
Diphenylpyraline hydrochloride—White or almost white, odorless or almost odorless powder.
Phenylephrine Hydrochloride USP—White or practically white, odorless crystals.
Codeine Phosphate USP—Fine, white, needle-shaped crystals, or white, crystalline powder. Odorless. Is affected by light. Its solutions are acid to litmus.

Solubility:
Diphenylpyraline hydrochloride—Soluble 1 in 1 of water, 1 in 3 of alcohol, and 1 in 2 of chloroform; practically insoluble in ether.
Phenylephrine Hydrochloride USP—Freely soluble in water and in alcohol.

Codeine Phosphate USP—Freely soluble in water; very soluble in hot water; slightly soluble in alcohol but more so in boiling alcohol.

USP requirements: Diphenylpyraline Hydrochloride, Phenylephrine Hydrochloride, and Codeine Phosphate Oral Solution—Not in USP.

DIPHENYLPYRALINE, PHENYLEPHRINE, AND DEXTROMETHORPHAN

Source: Dextromethorphan—Methylated dextroisomer of levorphanol.

Chemical group:
Diphenylpyraline hydrochloride—Piperidine derivative.
Dextromethorphan—Synthetic derivative of morphine.

Chemical name:
Diphenylpyraline hydrochloride—Piperidine, 4-(diphenylmethoxy)-1-methyl-, hydrochloride.
Phenylephrine hydrochloride—Benzenemethanol, 3-hydroxy-alpha-[(methylamino)methyl]-, hydrochloride.
Dextromethorphan hydrobromide—Morphinan, 3-methoxy-17-methyl-, (9 alpha,13 alpha,14 alpha)-, hydrobromide, monohydrate.

Molecular formula:
Diphenylpyraline hydrochloride—$C_{19}H_{23}NO \cdot HCl$.
Phenylephrine hydrochloride—$C_9H_{13}NO_2 \cdot HCl$.
Dextromethorphan hydrobromide—$C_{18}H_{25}NO \cdot HBr \cdot H_2O$.

Molecular weight:
Diphenylpyraline hydrochloride—317.86.
Phenylephrine hydrochloride—203.67.
Dextromethorphan hydrobromide—370.33.

Description:
Diphenylpyraline hydrochloride—White or almost white, odorless or almost odorless powder.
Phenylephrine Hydrochloride USP—White or practically white, odorless crystals.
Dextromethorphan Hydrobromide USP—Practically white crystals or crystalline powder, having a faint odor. Melts at about 126 °C, with decomposition.

Solubility:
Diphenylpyraline hydrochloride—Soluble 1 in 1 of water, 1 in 3 of alcohol, and 1 in 2 of chloroform; practically insoluble in ether.
Phenylephrine Hydrochloride USP—Freely soluble in water and in alcohol.
Dextromethorphan Hydrobromide USP—Sparingly soluble in water; freely soluble in alcohol and in chloroform; insoluble in ether.

USP requirements: Diphenylpyraline Hydrochloride, Phenylephrine Hydrochloride, and Dextromethorphan Hydrobromide Syrup—Not in USP.

DIPHENYLPYRALINE, PHENYLEPHRINE, AND HYDROCODONE

Chemical group: Diphenylpyraline hydrochloride—Piperidine derivative.

Chemical name:
Diphenylpyraline hydrochloride—Piperidine, 4-(diphenylmethoxy)-1-methyl-, hydrochloride.
Phenylephrine hydrochloride—Benzenemethanol, 3-hydroxy-alpha-[(methylamino)methyl]-, hydrochloride.
Hydrocodone bitartrate—Morphinan-6-one, 4,5-epoxy-3-methoxy-17-methyl-, (5 alpha)-, [*R*-(*R**,*R**)]-2,3-dihydroxybutanedioate (1:1), hydrate (2:5).

Molecular formula:
Diphenylpyraline hydrochloride—$C_{19}H_{23}NO \cdot HCl$.
Phenylephrine hydrochloride—$C_9H_{13}NO_2 \cdot HCl$.
Hydrocodone bitartrate—$C_{18}H_{21}NO_3 \cdot C_4H_6O_6 \cdot 2\frac{1}{2}H_2O$ (hydrate); $C_{18}H_{21}NO_3 \cdot C_4H_6O_6$ (anhydrous).

Molecular weight:
Diphenylpyraline hydrochloride—317.86.
Phenylephrine hydrochloride—203.67.
Hydrocodone bitartrate—494.50 (hydrate); 449.46 (anhydrous).

Description:
Diphenylpyraline hydrochloride—White or almost white, odorless or almost odorless powder.
Phenylephrine Hydrochloride USP—White or practically white, odorless crystals.
Hydrocodone Bitartrate USP—Fine, white crystals or a crystalline powder. Is affected by light.

Solubility:
Diphenylpyraline hydrochloride—Soluble 1 in 1 of water, 1 in 3 of alcohol, and 1 in 2 of chloroform; practically insoluble in ether.
Phenylephrine Hydrochloride USP—Freely soluble in water and in alcohol.
Hydrocodone Bitartrate USP—Soluble in water; slightly soluble in alcohol; insoluble in ether and in chloroform.

USP requirements:
Diphenylpyraline Hydrochloride, Phenylephrine Hydrochloride, and Hydrocodone Bitartrate Oral Solution—Not in USP.
Diphenylpyraline Hydrochloride, Phenylephrine Hydrochloride, and Hydrocodone Bitartrate Syrup—Not in USP.

DIPHENYLPYRALINE, PHENYLEPHRINE, HYDROCODONE, AND GUAIFENESIN

Chemical group: Diphenylpyraline hydrochloride—Piperidine derivative.

Chemical name:
Diphenylpyraline hydrochloride—Piperidine, 4-(diphenylmethoxy)-1-methyl-, hydrochloride.
Phenylephrine hydrochloride—Benzenemethanol, 3-hydroxy-alpha-[(methylamino)methyl]-, hydrochloride.
Hydrocodone bitartrate—Morphinan-6-one, 4,5-epoxy-3-methoxy-17-methyl-, (5 alpha)-, [*R*-(*R**,*R**)]-2,3-dihydroxybutanedioate (1:1), hydrate (2:5).
Guaifenesin—1,2-Propanediol, 3-(2-methoxyphenoxy)-.

Molecular formula:
Diphenylpyraline hydrochloride—$C_{19}H_{23}NO \cdot HCl$.
Phenylephrine hydrochloride—$C_9H_{13}NO_2 \cdot HCl$.
Hydrocodone bitartrate—$C_{18}H_{21}NO_3 \cdot C_4H_6O_6 \cdot 2\frac{1}{2}H_2O$ (hydrate); $C_{18}H_{21}NO_3 \cdot C_4H_6O_6$ (anhydrous).
Guaifenesin—$C_{10}H_{14}O_4$.

Molecular weight:
Diphenylpyraline hydrochloride—317.86.
Phenylephrine hydrochloride—203.67.
Hydrocodone bitartrate—494.50 (hydrate); 449.46 (anhydrous).
Guaifenesin—198.22.

Description:
Diphenylpyraline hydrochloride—White or almost white, odorless or almost odorless powder.
Phenylephrine Hydrochloride USP—White or practically white, odorless crystals.
Hydrocodone Bitartrate USP—Fine, white crystals or a crystalline powder. Is affected by light.

Guaifenesin USP—White to slightly gray, crystalline powder. May have a slight characteristic odor.

Solubility:
Diphenylpyraline hydrochloride—Soluble 1 in 1 of water, 1 in 3 of alcohol, and 1 in 2 of chloroform; practically insoluble in ether.
Phenylephrine Hydrochloride USP—Freely soluble in water and in alcohol.
Hydrocodone Bitartrate USP—Soluble in water; slightly soluble in alcohol; insoluble in ether and in chloroform.
Guaifenesin USP—Soluble in water, in alcohol, in chloroform, in glycerin, and in propylene glycol.

USP requirements: Diphenylpyraline Hydrochloride, Phenylephrine Hydrochloride, Hydrocodone Bitartrate, and Guaifenesin Oral Solution—Not in USP.

DIPHTHERIA ANTITOXIN

Description: Diphtheria Antitoxin USP—Transparent or slightly opalescent liquid, practically colorless, and practically odorless or having an odor because of the preservative.

USP requirements: Diphtheria Antitoxin USP—Preserve at a temperature between 2 and 8 °C. A sterile, non-pyrogenic solution of the refined and concentrated proteins, chiefly globulins, containing antitoxic antibodies obtained from the blood serum or plasma of healthy horses that have been immunized against diphtheria toxin or toxoid. Label it to state that it was prepared from horse serum or plasma. Has a potency of not less than 500 antitoxin units per mL based on the U.S. Standard Diphtheria Antitoxin, and a diphtheria test toxin, tested in guinea pigs. Contains not more than 20.0% of solids. Meets the requirement for Expiration date (for Antitoxin containing a 20% excess of potency, not later than 5 years after date of issue from manufacturer's cold storage). Conforms to the regulations of the U.S. Food and Drug Administration concerning biologics.

DIPHTHERIA AND TETANUS TOXOIDS AND ACELLULAR PERTUSSIS VACCINE ADSORBED

Source: Acellular pertussis vaccine components are isolated from culture fluids of Phase 1 *Bordetella pertussis* grown in a modified Stainer-Scholte medium. After purification by salt precipitation, ultracentrifugation, and ultrafiltration, pertussis toxin (PT) and filamentous hemagglutinin (FHA) are combined to obtain a 1:1 ratio and treated with formaldehyde to inactivate PT.

Corynebacterium diphtheriae cultures are grown in a modified Mueller and Miller medium. *Clostridium tetani* cultures are grown in a peptone-based medium. Both toxins are detoxified with formaldehyde. The detoxified materials are then separately purified by serial ammonium sulfate fractionation and diafiltration.

The toxoids are adsorbed using aluminum potassium sulfate (alum). The adsorbed diphtheria and tetanus toxoids are combined with acellular pertussis concentrate, and diluted to a final volume using sterile phosphate-buffered physiological saline.

USP requirements: Diphtheria and Tetanus Toxoids and Acellular Pertussis Vaccine Adsorbed—Not in USP.

DIPHTHERIA TOXIN FOR SCHICK TEST

Description: Diphtheria Toxin for Schick Test USP—Transparent liquid.

USP requirements: Diphtheria Toxin for Schick Test USP—Preserve at a temperature between 2 and 8 °C. A sterile solution of the diluted, standardized toxic products of growth of the diphtheria bacillus (*Corynebacterium diphtheriae*) of which the parent toxin contains not less than 400 MLD (minimum lethal doses) per mL or 400,000 MRD (minimum skin reaction doses) per mL in guinea pigs. Potency is determined in terms of the U.S. Standard Diphtheria Toxin for Schick Test, tested in guinea pigs. Meets the requirement for Expiration date (not later than 1 year after date of issue from manufacturer's cold storage [5 °C, 1 year]). Conforms to the regulations of the U.S. Food and Drug Administration concerning biologics.

DIPHTHERIA TOXOID

Description: Diphtheria Toxoid USP—Clear, brownish yellow, or slightly turbid liquid, free from evident clumps or particles, having a faint, characteristic odor.

USP requirements: Diphtheria Toxoid USP—Preserve at a temperature between 2 and 8 °C. A sterile solution of the formaldehyde-treated products of growth of the diphtheria bacillus (*Corynebacterium diphtheriae*). Label it to state that it is not to be frozen. Meets the requirements of the specific guinea pig potency and detoxification tests. Contains not more than 0.02% of residual free formaldehyde. Contains a preservative other than a phenoloid compound. Meets the requirement for Expiration date (not later than 2 years after date of issue from manufacturer's cold storage [5 °C, 1 year]). Conforms to the regulations of the U.S. Food and Drug Administration concerning biologics.

DIPHTHERIA TOXOID ADSORBED

Description: Diphtheria Toxoid Adsorbed USP—White, slightly gray, or slightly pink suspension, free from evident clumps after shaking.

USP requirements: Diphtheria Toxoid Adsorbed USP—Preserve at a temperature between 2 and 8 °C. A sterile preparation of plain diphtheria toxoid that meets all of the requirements for that product with the exception of those for antigenicity, and that has been precipitated or adsorbed by alum, aluminum hydroxide, or aluminum phosphate adjuvants. Label it to state that it is to be well shaken before use and that it is not to be frozen. Meets the requirements of the specific guinea pig antigenicity test in the production of not less than 2 units of antitoxin per mL based on the U.S. Standard Diphtheria Antitoxin and a diphtheria test toxin. Meets the requirements of the specific guinea pig detoxification test. Meets the requirements for Expiration date (not later than 2 years after date of issue from manufacturer's cold storage [5 °C, 1 year]) and Aluminum content (not more than 0.85 mg per single injection, determined by analysis, or not more than 1.14 mg calculated on the basis of the amount of aluminum compound added). Conforms to the regulations of the U.S. Food and Drug Administration concerning biologics.

DIPHTHERIA AND TETANUS TOXOIDS

Description: Diphtheria and Tetanus Toxoids USP—Clear, colorless to brownish yellow or very slightly turbid liquid, free from evident clumps or particles, having a characteristic odor.

USP requirements: Diphtheria and Tetanus Toxoids USP—Preserve at a temperature between 2 and 8 °C. A sterile solution prepared by mixing suitable quantities of fluid diphtheria toxoid and fluid tetanus toxoid. Label it to state that it is not to be frozen. The antigenicity or potency and the proportions of the toxoids are such as to provide an immunizing dose of each toxoid in the total dosage prescribed in the labeling, and each component meets the requirements for those products. Contains not more than 0.02% of residual free formaldehyde. Meets the requirement for Expiration date (not later than 2 years after date of issue from manufacturer's cold storage [5 °C, 1 year]). Conforms to the regulations of the U.S. Food and Drug Administration concerning biologics.

DIPHTHERIA AND TETANUS TOXOIDS ADSORBED

Description: Diphtheria and Tetanus Toxoids Adsorbed USP—Turbid, and white, slightly gray, or slightly pink suspension, free from evident clumps after shaking.

USP requirements: Diphtheria and Tetanus Toxoids Adsorbed USP—Preserve at a temperature between 2 and 8 °C. A sterile suspension prepared by mixing suitable quantities of plain or adsorbed diphtheria toxoid and plain or adsorbed tetanus toxoid, and an aluminum adsorbing agent if plain toxoids are used. Label it to state that it is to be well shaken before use and that it is not to be frozen. The antigenicity or potency and the proportions of the toxoids are such as to provide an immunizing dose of each toxoid in the total dosage prescribed in the labeling, and each component meets the requirements for those products. Contains not more than 0.02% of residual free formaldehyde. Meets the requirement for Expiration date (not later than 2 years after date of issue from manufacturer's cold storage [5 °C, 1 year]). Conforms to the regulations of the U.S. Food and Drug Administration concerning biologics.

DIPHTHERIA AND TETANUS TOXOIDS AND PERTUSSIS VACCINE

Description: Diphtheria and Tetanus Toxoids and Pertussis Vaccine USP—More or less turbid, whitish to light yellowish or brownish liquid, free from evident clumps after shaking, having a faint odor because of the toxoid components, the antimicrobial agent, or both.

USP requirements: Diphtheria and Tetanus Toxoids and Pertussis Vaccine USP—Preserve at a temperature between 2 and 8 °C. A sterile suspension prepared by mixing suitable quantities of pertussis vaccine component of killed pertussis bacilli (*Bordetella pertussis*), or a fraction of this organism, fluid diphtheria toxoid, and fluid tetanus toxoid. Label it to state that it is to be well shaken before use and that it is not to be frozen. The antigenicity or potency and the proportions of the components are such as to provide an immunizing dose of each product in the total dosage prescribed in the labeling, and each component meets the requirements for those products. Meets the requirement for Expiration date (not later than 18 months after date of issue from manufacturer's cold storage [5 °C, 1 year]). Conforms to the regulations of the U.S. Food and Drug Administration concerning biologics.

DIPHTHERIA AND TETANUS TOXOIDS AND PERTUSSIS VACCINE ADSORBED

Source: Diphtheria, tetanus toxoids, and pertussis vaccine consists of a mixture of the detoxified toxins (toxoids) of diphtheria and tetanus and inactivated *B. pertussis* bacteria that have been adsorbed onto an aluminum salt.

Description: Diphtheria and Tetanus Toxoids and Pertussis Vaccine Adsorbed USP—Markedly turbid, whitish liquid, free from evident clumps after shaking; nearly odorless or having a faint odor because of the preservative.

USP requirements: Diphtheria and Tetanus Toxoids and Pertussis Vaccine Adsorbed USP—Preserve at a temperature between 2 and 8 °C. A sterile suspension prepared by mixing suitable quantities of plain or adsorbed diphtheria toxoid, plain or adsorbed tetanus toxoid, plain or adsorbed pertussis vaccine, and an aluminum adsorbing agent if plain antigen components are used. Label it to state that it is to be well shaken before use and that it is not to be frozen. The antigenicity or potency and the proportions of the components are such as to provide an immunizing dose of each product in the total dosage prescribed in the labeling, and each component meets the requirements for those products. Meets the requirement for Expiration date (not later than 18 months after date of issue from manufacturer's cold storage [5 °C, 1 year]). Conforms to the regulations of the U.S. Food and Drug Administration concerning biologics.

DIPHTHERIA AND TETANUS TOXOIDS AND PERTUSSIS VACCINE ADSORBED AND HAEMOPHILUS B CONJUGATE VACCINE

Source: Diphtheria and tetanus toxoids are derived from *Corynebacterium diphtheriae* and *Clostridium tetani*, respectively.

Pertussis Vaccine is prepared by growing Phase I *Bordetella pertussis* in a modified Cohen-Wheeler broth containing acid hydrolysate of casein.

The oligosaccharides for the Haemophilus b conjugate component are derived from highly purified capsular polysaccharide, polyribosylribitol phosphate, isolated from *Haemophilus influenzae* type b grown in a chemically defined medium.

USP requirements: Diphtheria and Tetanus Toxoids and Pertussis Vaccine Adsorbed and Haemophilus b Conjugate Vaccine (diphtheria CRM_{197} protein conjugate)—Not in USP.

DIPIVEFRIN

Source: Formed by the diesterification of epinephrine and pivalic acid.

Chemical name: Dipivefrin hydrochloride—Propanoic acid, 2,2-dimethyl-, 4-[1-hydroxy-2-(methylamino)ethyl]-1,2-phenylene ester, hydrochloride, (±)-.

Molecular formula: Dipivefrin hydrochloride—$C_{19}H_{29}NO_5 \cdot HCl$.

Molecular weight: Dipivefrin hydrochloride—387.90.

Description: Dipivefrin Hydrochloride USP—White, crystalline powder or small crystals, having a faint odor.

Solubility: Dipivefrin Hydrochloride USP—Very soluble in water.

USP requirements:

Dipivefrin Hydrochloride USP—Preserve in tight containers. Contains not less than 98.5% and not more than 101.5% of dipivefrin hydrochloride, calculated on the dried basis. Meets the requirements for Identification, Melting range (155–165 °C, range between beginning and end of melting not more than 2 °C), Loss on drying (not more than 1.0%), Residue on ignition (not more than 0.3%), Heavy metals (not more than 0.0015%), and Iron (not more than 5 ppm).

Dipivefrin Hydrochloride Ophthalmic Solution USP—Preserve in tight, light-resistant containers. A sterile, aqueous solution of Dipivefrin Hydrochloride. Contains the labeled amount, within −10% to +15%. Contains a suitable antimicrobial agent. Meets the requirements for Identification, Sterility, and pH (2.5–3.5).

DIPYRIDAMOLE

Chemical name: Ethanol, 2,2′,2″,2‴-[(4,8-di-1-piperidinylpyrimido[5,4-*d*]pyrimidine-2,6-diyl)dinitrilo]tetrakis-.

Molecular formula: $C_{24}H_{40}N_8O_4$.

Molecular weight: 504.63.

Description: Dipyridamole USP—Intensely yellow, crystalline powder or needles.

Solubility: Dipyridamole USP—Very soluble in methanol, in alcohol, and in chloroform; slightly soluble in water; very slightly soluble in acetone and in ethyl acetate.

USP requirements:

Dipyridamole USP—Preserve in tight, light-resistant containers. Contains not less than 98.0% and not more than 102.0% of dipyridamole, calculated on the dried basis. Meets the requirements for Identification, Melting range (162–168 °C, range between beginning and end of melting not more than 2 °C), Loss on drying (not more than 0.2%), Chloride, Residue on ignition (not more than 0.1%), Heavy metals (not more than 0.001%), and Chromatographic purity.

Dipyridamole Injection—Not in USP.

Dipyridamole Tablets USP—Preserve in tight, light-resistant containers. Contain the labeled amount, within ±10%. Meet the requirements for Identification, Dissolution (70% in 30 minutes in 0.1 *N* hydrochloric acid in Apparatus 2 at 50 rpm), and Uniformity of dosage units.

DIPYRIDAMOLE AND ASPIRIN

For *Dipyridamole* and *Aspirin*—See individual listings for chemistry information.

USP requirements: Dipyridamole and Aspirin Capsules—Not in USP.

DISOPYRAMIDE

Chemical name:

Disopyramide—2-Pyridineacetamide, alpha-[2-[bis(1-methylethyl)amino]ethyl]-alpha-phenyl-.

Disopyramide phosphate—2-Pyridineacetamide, alpha-[2-[bis(1-methylethyl)amino]ethyl]-alpha-phenyl-, phosphate (1:1).

Molecular formula:

Disopyramide—$C_{21}H_{29}N_3O$.

Disopyramide phosphate—$C_{21}H_{29}N_3O \cdot H_3PO_4$.

Molecular weight:

Disopyramide—339.48.

Disopyramide phosphate—437.48.

Description:

Disopyramide—White, odorless or almost odorless powder.

Disopyramide Phosphate USP—White or practically white, odorless powder. Melts at about 205 °C, with decomposition.

pKa: 10.4.

Solubility:

Disopyramide—Slightly soluble in water; soluble 1 in 10 of alcohol, 1 in 5 of chloroform, and 1 in 5 of ether.

Disopyramide Phosphate USP—Freely soluble in water; slightly soluble in alcohol; practically insoluble in chloroform and in ether.

Other characteristics: Chloroform: water partition coefficient—3.1 at pH 7.2.

USP requirements:

Disopyramide Capsules—Not in USP.

Disopyramide Injection—Not in USP.

Disopyramide Phosphate USP—Preserve in tight, light-resistant containers. Contains not less than 98.0% and not more than 102.0% of disopyramide phosphate, calculated on the dried basis. Meets the requirements for Identification, pH (4.0–5.0 in a solution [1 in 20]), Loss on drying (not more than 0.5%), Heavy metals (not more than 0.002%), Chromatographic purity, and Organic volatile impurities.

Disopyramide Phosphate Capsules USP—Preserve in well-closed containers. Contain an amount of Disopyramide Phosphate equivalent to the labeled amount of disopyramide, within ±10%. Meet the requirements for Identification, Dissolution (80% in 20 minutes in water in Apparatus 2 at 50 rpm), and Uniformity of dosage units.

Disopyramide Phosphate Extended-release Capsules USP—Preserve in well-closed containers. Contain an amount of Disopyramide Phosphate equivalent to the labeled amount of disopyramide, within ±10%. Meet the requirements for Identification, Drug release (5–25% in 0.083*D* hours, 17–43% in 0.167*D* hours, 50–80% in 0.417*D* hours, and not less than 85% in 1.000*D* hours in 0.1 *M* phosphate buffer [pH 2.5] in Apparatus 1 at 100 rpm), and Uniformity of dosage units.

Disopyramide Phosphate Extended-release Tablets—Not in USP.

DISULFIRAM

Chemical name: Thioperoxydicarbonic diamide $[(H_2N)C(S)]_2S_2$, tetraethyl-.

Molecular formula: $C_{10}H_{20}N_2S_4$.

Molecular weight: 296.52.

Description: Disulfiram USP—White to off-white, odorless, crystalline powder.

Solubility: Disulfiram USP—Very slightly soluble in water; soluble in acetone, in alcohol, in carbon disulfide, and in chloroform.

USP requirements:

Disulfiram USP—Preserve in tight, light-resistant containers. Contains not less than 98.0% and not more than 102.0% of disulfiram. Meets the requirements for Identification, Melting range (69–72 °C), Residue on ignition (not more than 0.1%), Selenium (not more than 0.003%), and Organic volatile impurities.

Disulfiram Tablets USP—Preserve in tight, light-resistant containers. Contain the labeled amount, within ±10%. Meet the requirements for Identification, Disintegration (15 minutes, the use of disks being omitted), and Uniformity of dosage units.

DIVALPROEX SODIUM

Chemical name: Pentanoic acid, 2-propyl-, sodium salt (2:1).

Molecular formula: $C_{16}H_{31}NaO_4$.

Molecular weight: 310.41.

Description: White powder, having a characteristic odor.

Solubility: Insoluble in water; very soluble in alcohol.

USP requirements:

Divalproex Sodium Delayed-release Capsules—Not in USP.

Divalproex Sodium Delayed-release Tablets—Not in USP.

DOBUTAMINE

Chemical group: A synthetic catecholamine.

Chemical name: Dobutamine hydrochloride—1,2-Benzenediol, 4-[2-[[3-(4-hydroxyphenyl)-1-methylpropyl]amino]ethyl]-, hydrochloride, (±)-.

Molecular formula: Dobutamine hydrochloride—$C_{18}H_{23}NO_3 \cdot HCl$.

Molecular weight: Dobutamine hydrochloride—337.85.

Description: Dobutamine Hydrochloride USP—White to practically white, crystalline powder.

pKa: 9.4.

Solubility: Dobutamine Hydrochloride USP—Sparingly soluble in water and in methanol; soluble in alcohol and in pyridine.

USP requirements:

Dobutamine Hydrochloride USP—Preserve in tight containers, and store at controlled room temperature. Contains not less than 97.0% and not more than 103.0% of dobutamine hydrochloride, calculated on the anhydrous basis. Meets the requirements for Identification, Water (not more than 1.0%), Residue on ignition (not more than 0.2%), and Heavy metals (not more than 0.003%).

Caution: Great care should be taken to prevent inhaling particles of Dobutamine Hydrochloride and exposing the skin to it. Protect the eyes.

Dobutamine Hydrochloride Injection—Not in USP.

Dobutamine Hydrochloride for Injection USP—Preserve in Containers for Sterile Solids, at controlled room temperature. A sterile mixture of Dobutamine Hydrochloride with suitable diluents. Contains an amount of dobutamine hydrochloride equivalent to the labeled amount of dobutamine, within ± 10%. Meets the requirements for Constituted solution, Identification, Bacterial endotoxins, Uniformity of dosage units, pH (2.5–5.5), Particulate matter, and Injections.

Caution: Great care should be taken to prevent inhaling particles of Dobutamine Hydrochloride for Injection and exposing the skin to it. Protect the eyes.

DOCUSATE

Chemical group: Anionic surfactants.

Chemical name:

Docusate calcium—Butanedioic acid, sulfo-, 1,4-bis(2-ethylhexyl) ester, calcium salt.

Docusate potassium—Butanedioic acid, sulfo-, 1,4-bis(2-ethylhexyl) ester, potassium salt.

Docusate sodium—Butanedioic acid, sulfo-, 1,4-bis(2-ethylhexyl) ester, sodium salt.

Molecular formula:

Docusate calcium—$C_{40}H_{74}CaO_{14}S_2$.

Docusate potassium—$C_{20}H_{37}KO_7S$.

Docusate sodium—$C_{20}H_{37}NaO_7S$.

Molecular weight:

Docusate calcium—883.22.

Docusate potassium—460.67.

Docusate sodium—444.56.

Description:

Docusate Calcium USP—White, amorphous solid, having the characteristic odor of octyl alcohol. It is free of the odor of other solvents.

Docusate Potassium USP—White, amorphous solid, having a characteristic odor suggestive of octyl alcohol.

Docusate Sodium USP—White, wax-like, plastic solid, having a characteristic odor suggestive of octyl alcohol, but no odor of other solvents.

NF category: Wetting and/or solubilizing agent.

Solubility:

Docusate Calcium USP—Very slightly soluble in water; very soluble in alcohol, in polyethylene glycol 400, and in corn oil.

Docusate Potassium USP—Sparingly soluble in water; very soluble in solvent hexane; soluble in alcohol and in glycerin.

Docusate Sodium USP—Sparingly soluble in water; very soluble in solvent hexane; freely soluble in alcohol and in glycerin.

USP requirements:

Docusate Calcium USP—Preserve in well-closed containers. Contains not less than 91.0% and not more than 100.5% of docusate calcium, calculated on the anhydrous basis. Meets the requirements for Clarity of solution, Identification, Water (not more than 2.0%), Residue on ignition (14.5–16.5%, calculated on the anhydrous basis), Arsenic (not more than 2 ppm), Heavy metals (not more than 0.001%), and Bis(2-ethylhexyl) maleate (not more than 0.4%).

Docusate Calcium Capsules USP—Preserve in tight containers, and store at controlled room temperature in a dry place. Contain the labeled amount, within ±15%. Meet the requirements for Identification and Uniformity of dosage units.

Docusate Potassium USP—Preserve in well-closed containers. Contains not less than 95.0% and not more than 100.5% of docusate potassium, calculated on the dried basis. Meets the requirements for Identification, Loss on drying (not more than 3.0%), Residue on ignition (18.0–20.0%, calculated on the dried basis), Arsenic (not more than 2 ppm), Heavy metals (not more than 0.001%), and Bis(2-ethylhexyl) maleate (not more than 0.4%).

Docusate Potassium Capsules USP—Preserve in tight containers, and store at controlled room temperature. Contain the labeled amount, within ±10%. Meet the requirements for Identification and Uniformity of dosage units.

Docusate Sodium USP—Preserve in well-closed containers. Contains not less than 99.0% and not more than 100.5% of docusate sodium, calculated on the anhydrous basis. Meets the requirements for Clarity of solution, Identification, Water (not more than 2.0%), Residue on ignition (15.5–16.5%, calculated on anhydrous basis), Arsenic (not more than 3 ppm), Heavy metals (not more than 0.001%), and Bis(2-ethylhexyl) maleate (not more than 0.4%).

Docusate Sodium Capsules USP—Preserve in tight containers, and store at controlled room temperature. Contain the labeled amount, within ±10%. Meet the requirements for Identification and Uniformity of dosage units.

Docusate Sodium Solution USP (Oral)—Preserve in tight containers. Contains the labeled amount, within ±10%. Meets the requirements for Identification and pH (4.5–6.9).

Docusate Sodium Rectal Solution—Not in USP.

Docusate Sodium Syrup USP—Preserve in tight, light-resistant containers. Contains the labeled amount, within ±10%. Meets the requirements for Identification and pH (5.5–6.5).

Docusate Sodium Tablets USP—Preserve in well-closed containers. Contain the labeled amount, within ±10%. Meet the requirements for Identification, Disintegration (1 hour, simulated gastric fluid TS being substituted for water in the test for Uncoated Tablets), and Uniformity of dosage units.

DOCUSATE AND PHENOLPHTHALEIN

For *Docusate* and *Phenolphthalein*—See individual listings for chemistry information.

USP requirements:
Docusate Calcium and Phenolphthalein Capsules—Not in USP.
Docusate Sodium and Phenolphthalein Capsules—Not in USP.
Docusate Sodium and Phenolphthalein Tablets—Not in USP.
Docusate Sodium and Phenolphthalein Chewable Tablets—Not in USP.

DOMPERIDONE

Chemical name: 2*H*-Benzimidazol-2-one, 5-chloro-1-[1-[3-(2,3-dihydro-2-oxo-1*H*-benzimidazol-1-yl)propyl]-4-piperidinyl]-1,3-dihydro-.

Molecular formula: $C_{22}H_{24}ClN_5O_2$.

Molecular weight: 425.92.

USP requirements: Domperidone Tablets—Not in USP.

DOPAMINE

Chemical group: A naturally occurring biochemical catecholamine precursor of norepinephrine.

Chemical name: Dopamine hydrochloride—1,2-Benzenediol, 4-(2-aminoethyl)-, hydrochloride.

Molecular formula: Dopamine hydrochloride—$C_8H_{11}NO_2 \cdot HCl$.

Molecular weight: Dopamine hydrochloride—189.64.

Description: Dopamine Hydrochloride USP—White to off-white, crystalline powder. May have a slight odor of hydrochloric acid. Melts at about 240 °C, with decomposition.

Solubility: Dopamine Hydrochloride USP—Freely soluble in water, in methanol, and in aqueous solutions of alkali hydroxides; insoluble in ether and in chloroform.

USP requirements:
Dopamine Hydrochloride USP—Preserve in tight containers. Contains not less than 98.0% and not more than 102.0% of dopamine hydrochloride, calculated on the dried basis. Meets the requirements for Clarity and color of solution, Identification, pH (3.0–5.5, in a solution [1 in 25]), Loss on drying (not more than 0.5%), Residue on ignition (not more than 0.1%), Heavy metals (not more than 0.002%), Sulfate, Readily carbonizable substances, and Chromatographic purity.
Dopamine Hydrochloride Injection USP—Preserve in single-dose containers of Type I glass. A sterile solution of Dopamine Hydrochloride in Water for Injection. May contain a suitable antioxidant. Label it to indicate that the Injection is to be diluted with a suitable parenteral vehicle prior to intravenous infusion. Contains the labeled amount, within ±5%. Meets the requirements for Identification, Bacterial endotoxins, pH (2.5–5.0), Particulate matter, and Injections.
Note: Do not use the Injection if it is darker than slightly yellow or discolored in any other way.

DOPAMINE AND DEXTROSE

For *Dopamine* and *Dextrose*—See individual listings for chemistry information.

USP requirements: Dopamine Hydrochloride and Dextrose Injection USP—Preserve in single-dose glass or plastic containers. Glass containers are preferably of Type I or Type II glass. A sterile solution of Dopamine Hydrochloride and Dextrose in Water for Injection. The label states the total osmolar concentration in mOsmol per liter. Where the contents are less than 100 mL, or where the label states that the Injection is not for direct injection but is to be diluted before use, the label alternatively may state the total osmolar concentration in mOsm per mL. Contains the labeled amounts, within ±5%. Meets the requirements for Identification, Bacterial endotoxins, pH (2.5–4.5), Particulate matter, and Injections.
Note: Do not use the Injection if it is darker than slightly yellow or discolored in any other way.

DORNASE ALFA

Source: Produced by genetically engineered Chinese Hamster Ovary (CHO) cells containing DNA encoding for the native human protein, deoxyribonuclease I (DNase). The product is purified by tangential flow filtration and column chromatography. The purified glycoprotein contains 260 amino acids with an approximate molecular weight of 37,000 daltons. The primary amino acid sequence is identical to that of the native human enzyme.

USP requirements: Dornase Alfa Recombinant Inhalation Solution—Not in USP.

DOXACURIUM

Chemical name: Doxacurium chloride—Isoquinolinium, 2,2′-[(1,4-dioxo-1,4-butanediyl)bis(oxy-3,1-propanediyl)]-bis[1,2,3,4-tetrahydro-6,7,8-trimethoxy-2-methyl-1-[(3,4,5-trimethoxyphenyl)-methyl]-, dichloride, [1 alpha,2 beta(1′*S**,-2′*R**)]-, mixture with (±)-[1 alpha,2 beta(1′*R**,2′*S**)]-2,2′-[(1,4-dioxo-1,4-butanediyl)bis(oxy-3,1-propanediyl)]bis-[1,2,3,4-tetrahydro-6,7,8-trimethoxy-2-methyl-1-[(3,4,5-trimethoxyphenyl)methyl]isoquinolinium] dichloride.

Molecular formula: Doxacurium chloride—$C_{56}H_{78}Cl_2N_2O_{16}$.

Molecular weight: Doxacurium chloride—1106.15.

Description: Doxacurium chloride injection—Sterile, nonpyrogenic aqueous solution.

Other characteristics:
Doxacurium chloride—N-octanol:water partition coefficient: 0.
Doxacurium chloride injection—pH 3.9–5.0.

USP requirements: Doxacurium Chloride Injection—Not in USP.

DOXAPRAM

Chemical name: Doxapram hydrochloride—2-Pyrrolidinone, 1-ethyl-4-[2-(4-morpholinyl)ethyl]-3,3-diphenyl-, monohydrochloride, monohydrate.

Molecular formula: Doxapram hydrochloride—$C_{24}H_{30}N_2O_2 \cdot HCl \cdot H_2O$.

Molecular weight: Doxapram hydrochloride—432.99.

Description: Doxapram Hydrochloride USP—White to off-white, odorless, crystalline powder. Melts at about 220 °C.

Solubility: Doxapram Hydrochloride USP—Soluble in water and in chloroform; sparingly soluble in alcohol; practically insoluble in ether.

USP requirements:
Doxapram Hydrochloride USP—Preserve in tight containers. Dried at 105 °C for 2 hours, contains not less

than 98.0% and not more than 100.5% of doxapram hydrochloride. Meets the requirements for Identification, pH (3.5–5.0, in a solution [1 in 100]), Loss on drying (3.0–4.5%), Residue on ignition (not more than 0.3%), Arsenic (not more than 5 ppm), Heavy metals (not more than 0.002%), and Chromatographic purity.

Doxapram Hydrochloride Injection USP—Preserve in single-dose or in multiple-dose containers, preferably of Type I glass. A sterile solution of Doxapram Hydrochloride in Water for Injection. Contains the labeled amount, within ±10%. Meets the requirements for Identification, Bacterial endotoxins, pH (3.5–5.0), and Injections.

DOXAZOSIN

Chemical name: Doxazosin mesylate—Piperazine, 1-(4-amino-6,7-dimethoxy-2-quinazolinyl)-4-[(2,3-dihydro-1,4-benzodioxin-2-yl)carbonyl]-, monomethanesulfonate.

Molecular formula: Doxazosin mesylate—$C_{23}H_{25}N_5O_5 \cdot CH_4O_3S$.

Molecular weight: Doxazosin mesylate—547.58.

Description: Doxazosin mesylate—White to off-white crystalline solid of uniform appearance. Melting point 273.7 °C.

Solubility: Doxazosin mesylate—Freely soluble in dimethylsulfoxide; soluble in dimethylformamide; slightly soluble in methanol, in ethanol, and in water (0.8% w/v at 25 °C); very slightly soluble in acetone and in methylene chloride.

USP requirements: Doxazosin Mesylate Tablets—Not in USP.

DOXEPIN

Chemical group: Doxepin hydrochloride—Dibenzoxepin derivative.

Chemical name: Doxepin hydrochloride—1-Propanamine, 3-dibenz[*b,e*]oxepin-11(6*H*)ylidene-*N,N*-dimethyl-, hydrochloride.

Molecular formula: Doxepin hydrochloride—$C_{19}H_{21}NO \cdot HCl$.

Molecular weight: Doxepin hydrochloride—315.84.

Description: Doxepin hydrochloride—White, crystalline solid.

pKa: Doxepin hydrochloride—8.0.

Solubility: Doxepin hydrochloride—Readily soluble in water, in lower alcohols, and in chloroform.

Other characteristics: Tertiary amine.

USP requirements:

Doxepin Hydrochloride USP—Preserve in well-closed containers. An (*E*) and (*Z*) geometric isomer mixture. Contains the equivalent of not less than 98.0% and not more than 102.0% of doxepin, calculated on the dried basis. Contains not less than 13.6% and not more than 18.1% of the (*Z*)-isomer, and not less than 81.4% and not more than 88.2% of the (*E*)-isomer. Meets the requirements for Identification, Melting range (185–191 °C), Loss on drying (not more than 0.5%), Residue on ignition (not more than 0.2%), Heavy metals (not more than 0.002%), Chloride content (10.9–11.6%), and Organic volatile impurities.

Doxepin Hydrochloride Capsules USP—Preserve in well-closed containers. Contain an amount of doxepin hydrochloride equivalent to the labeled amount of doxepin, within ±10%. Meet the requirements for Identification, Dissolution (80% in 30 minutes in water in Apparatus 1 at 50 rpm), Uniformity of dosage units, and Water (not more than 9.0%).

Doxepin Hydrochloride Oral Solution USP—Preserve in tight, light-resistant containers. Label it to indicate that it is to be diluted with water or other suitable fluid to approximately 120 mL, just prior to administration. Contains an amount of doxepin hydrochloride equivalent to the labeled amount of doxepin, within ±10%. Meets the requirements for Identification and pH (4.0–7.0).

DOXORUBICIN

Source: An anthracycline glycoside obtained from *Streptomyces peucetius* var. *caesius*.

Chemical name: Doxorubicin hydrochloride—5,12-Naphthacenedione, 10-[(3-amino-2,3,6-trideoxy-alpha-L-*lyxo*-hexopyranosyl)oxy]-7,8,9,10-tetrahydro-6,8,11-trihydroxy-8-(hydroxylacetyl)-1-methoxy-, hydrochloride (8*S*-*cis*)-.

Molecular formula: Doxorubicin hydrochloride—$C_{27}H_{29}NO_{11} \cdot HCl$.

Molecular weight: Doxorubicin hydrochloride—579.99.

Description: Doxorubicin Hydrochloride USP—Red-orange, hygroscopic, crystalline powder.

Solubility: Doxorubicin Hydrochloride USP—Soluble in water, in isotonic sodium chloride solution, and in methanol; practically insoluble in chloroform, in ether, and in other organic solvents.

Other characteristics: Unstable in solutions with a pH less than 3 or greater than 7.

USP requirements:

Doxorubicin Hydrochloride USP—Preserve in tight containers. Contains not less than 98.0% and not more than 102.0% of doxorubicin hydrochloride, calculated on the anhydrous, solvent-free basis. Meets the requirements for Identification, Crystallinity, Depressor substances, pH (4.0–5.5, in a solution containing 5 mg per mL), Water (not more than 4.0%), Chromatographic purity, and Limit of solvent residues (as acetone and alcohol, not more than 0.5% of acetone and total of acetone and alcohol not more than 2.5%).

Caution: Great care should be taken to prevent inhaling particles of doxorubicin hydrochloride and exposing the skin to it.

Doxorubicin Hydrochloride Injection USP—Preserve in single-dose or in multiple-dose containers, preferably of Type I glass, protected from light. Store in a refrigerator. Injection may be packaged in multiple-dose containers not exceeding 100 mL in volume. A sterile solution of Doxorubicin Hydrochloride in Sterile Water for Injection made isoosmotic with Sodium Chloride, Dextrose, or other suitable added substances. Contains the labeled amount, within −10% to +15%. Meets the requirements for Identification, Bacterial endotoxins, Sterility, pH (2.5–4.5), and Injections.

Doxorubicin Hydrochloride for Injection USP—Preserve in Containers for Sterile Solids, except that multiple-dose containers may provide for the withdrawal of not more than 100 mL when constituted as directed in the labeling. A sterile mixture of Doxorubicin Hydrochloride and Lactose. Contains the labeled amount, within −10% to +15%. Meets the requirements for Constituted solution, Bacterial endotoxins, Sterility, pH (4.5–6.5, in the solution constituted as directed in the labeling, except that water is used as the diluent), Water (not more than 4.0%), for Identification under Doxorubicin Hydrochloride, and for Uniformity of dosage units and Labeling under Injections.

Caution: Great care should be taken to prevent inhaling particles of Doxorubicin Hydrochloride and exposing the skin to it.

DOXYCYCLINE

Chemical name:

Doxycycline—2-Naphthacenecarboxamide, 4-(dimethylamino) - 1,4,4a,5,5a,6,11,12a - octahydro - 3,5,10,12,12a - pentahydroxy-6-methyl-1,11-dioxo-, [4*S*-(4alpha,4aalpha,5 alpha,5a alpha,6 alpha,12a alpha)]-, monohydrate.

Doxycycline hyclate—2-Naphthacenecarboxamide, 4-(dimethylamino)-1, 4, 4a, 5, 5a, 6, 11, 12a-octahydro-3, 5, 10, 12, 12a-pentahydroxy-6-methyl-1, 11-dioxo-, monohydrochloride, compd. with ethanol (2:1), monohydrate, [4*S*-(4 alpha,4a alpha,5 alpha,5a alpha,6 alpha,12a alpha)]-.

Molecular formula:

Doxycycline—$C_{22}H_{24}N_2O_8 \cdot H_2O$.

Doxycycline hyclate—$(C_{22}H_{24}N_2O_8 \cdot HCl)_2 \cdot C_2H_6O \cdot H_2O$.

Molecular weight:

Doxycycline—462.46.

Doxycycline hyclate—1025.89.

Description:

Doxycycline USP—Yellow, crystalline powder.

Doxycycline Hyclate USP—Yellow, crystalline powder.

Solubility:

Doxycycline USP—Very slightly soluble in water; freely soluble in dilute acid and in alkali hydroxide solutions; sparingly soluble in alcohol; practically insoluble in chloroform and in ether.

Doxycycline Hyclate USP—Soluble in water and in solutions of alkali hydroxides and carbonates; slightly soluble in alcohol; practically insoluble in chloroform and in ether.

USP requirements:

Doxycycline USP—Preserve in tight, light-resistant containers. Has a potency equivalent to not less than 880 mcg and not more than 980 mcg of doxycycline per mg. Meets the requirements for Identification, Crystallinity, pH (5.0–6.5, in an aqueous suspension containing 10 mg per mL), and Water (3.6–4.6%).

Doxycycline Capsules USP—Preserve in tight, light-resistant containers. Contain the labeled amount, within −10% to +20%. Meet the requirements for Identification, Dissolution (85% in 60 minutes in water in Apparatus 2 at 75 rpm), Uniformity of dosage units, and Water (not more than 5.5%).

Doxycycline for Oral Suspension USP—Preserve in tight, light-resistant containers. Contains one or more suitable buffers, colors, diluents, flavors, and preservatives. Contains the labeled amount, within −10% to +25% when constituted as directed. Meets the requirements for Identification, pH (5.0–6.5, in the suspension constituted as directed in the labeling), Deliverable volume, Water (not more than 3.0%), and Uniformity of dosage units (single-unit containers).

Doxycycline Calcium Oral Suspension USP—Preserve in tight, light-resistant containers. Prepared from Doxycycline Hyclate, and contains one or more suitable buffers, colors, diluents, flavors, and preservatives. Contains an amount of doxycycline calcium equivalent to the labeled amount of doxycycline, within −10% to +25%. Meets the requirements for Identification, pH (6.5–8.0), Deliverable volume, and Uniformity of dosage units (single-unit containers).

Doxycycline Hyclate USP—Preserve in tight containers, protected from light. Has a potency equivalent to not less than 800 mcg and not more than 920 mcg of doxycycline per mg. Meets the requirements for Identification, Crystallinity, pH (2.0–3.0, in a solution containing 10 mg of doxycycline per mL), and Water (1.4–2.75%).

Doxycycline Hyclate Capsules USP—Preserve in tight, light-resistant containers. Contain an amount of doxycycline hyclate equivalent to the labeled amount of doxycycline, within −10% to +20%. Meet the requirements for Identification, Dissolution (80% in 30 minutes in water in Apparatus 2 at 75 rpm), Uniformity of dosage units, and Water (not more than 5.0%).

Doxycycline Hyclate Delayed-release Capsules USP—Preserve in tight, light-resistant containers. The label indicates that the contents of the Delayed-release Capsules are enteric-coated. Contain an amount of doxycycline hyclate equivalent to the labeled amount of doxycycline, within −10% to +20%. Meet the requirements for Identification, Drug release (Acid stage: 50% [Level 1 and Level 2] in 20 minutes in 0.06 *N* hydrochloric acid in Apparatus 1 at 50 rpm; Buffer stage: 85% in 30 minutes in neutralized phthalate buffer [pH 5.5] in Apparatus 1 at 50 rpm), Uniformity of dosage units, and Water (not more than 5.0%).

Doxycycline Hyclate for Injection USP—Preserve in Containers for Sterile Solids, protected from light. A sterile, dry mixture of Doxycycline Hyclate and a suitable buffer or a sterile-filtered and lyophilized mixture of Doxycycline Hyclate and a suitable buffer. Contains an amount of doxycycline hyclate equivalent to the labeled amount of doxycycline, within −10% to +20%. Meets the requirements for Constituted solution, Identification, Depressor substances, Bacterial endotoxins, Sterility, pH (1.8–3.3, in the solution constituted as directed in the labeling), Loss on drying (for article containing added substances not more than 2.0% and for article containing no added substances not more than 4.0%), and Particulate matter.

Sterile Doxycycline Hyclate USP—Preserve in Containers for Sterile Solids, protected from light. It is Doxycycline Hyclate suitable for parenteral use. Has a potency equivalent to not less than 800 mcg and not more than 920 mcg of doxycycline per mg. Meets the requirements for Depressor substances, Bacterial endotoxins, and Sterility, and for Identification test, pH, Water, and Crystallinity under Doxycycline Hyclate.

Doxycycline Hyclate Tablets USP—Preserve in tight, light-resistant containers. Contain an amount of doxycycline hyclate equivalent to the labeled amount of doxycycline, within −10% to +20%. Meet the requirements for Identification, Dissolution (85% in 90 minutes in water in Apparatus 2 at 75 rpm), Uniformity of dosage units, and Water (not more than 5.0%).

DOXYLAMINE

Chemical group: Doxylamine succinate—Ethanolamine derivative.

Chemical name: Doxylamine succinate—Ethanamine, *N,N*-dimethyl-2-[1-phenyl-1-(2-pyridinyl)ethoxy]-, butanedioate (1:1).

Molecular formula: Doxylamine succinate—$C_{17}H_{22}N_2O \cdot C_4H_6O_4$.

Molecular weight: Doxylamine succinate—388.46.

Description: Doxylamine Succinate USP—White or creamy white powder, having a characteristic odor.

pKa: Doxylamine succinate—5.8 and 9.3.

Solubility: Doxylamine Succinate USP—Very soluble in water and in alcohol; freely soluble in chloroform; very slightly soluble in ether.

USP requirements:
Doxylamine Succinate USP—Preserve in well-closed, light-resistant containers. Contains not less than 98.0% and not more than 101.0% of doxylamine succinate, calculated on the dried basis. Meets the requirements for Identification, Melting range (103–108 °C, the range between beginning and end of melting not more than 3 °C), Loss on drying (not more than 0.5%), Residue on ignition (not more than 0.1%), Volatile related compounds, and Organic volatile impurities.
Doxylamine Succinate Syrup USP—Preserve in tight, light-resistant containers. Contains the labeled amount, within ±8%. Meets the requirement for Identification.
Doxylamine Succinate Tablets USP—Preserve in well-closed, light-resistant containers. Contain the labeled amount, within ±8%. Meet the requirements for Identification, Dissolution (80% in 30 minutes in 0.1 *N* hydrochloric acid in Apparatus 2 at 50 rpm), and Uniformity of dosage units.

DOXYLAMINE, PSEUDOEPHEDRINE, DEXTROMETHORPHAN, AND ACETAMINOPHEN

For *Doxylamine, Pseudoephedrine, Dextromethorphan,* and *Acetaminophen*—See individual listings for chemistry information.

USP requirements:
Doxylamine Succinate, Pseudoephedrine Hydrochloride, Dextromethorphan Hydrobromide, and Acetaminophen Oral Solution—Not in USP.
Doxylamine Succinate, Pseudoephedrine Hydrochloride, Dextromethorphan Hydrobromide, and Acetaminophen for Oral Solution—Not in USP.

DRONABINOL

Chemical group: A cannabinoid; synthetic form of one of the major active substances in *Cannabis sativa* L. (marijuana).

Chemical name: 6*H*-Dibenzo[*b,d*]pyran-1-ol, 6a,7,8,10a-tetrahydro-6,6,9-trimethyl-3-pentyl-, (6a*R-trans*)-.

Molecular formula: $C_{21}H_{30}O_2$.

Molecular weight: 314.47.

Description: Viscous, oily liquid.

Solubility: Insoluble in water; soluble in 1 part of alcohol or acetone, 3 parts of glycerol; soluble in fixed oils.

USP requirements:
Dronabinol USP—Preserve in tight, light-resistant glass containers in inert atmosphere. Store in a cool place. It is Delta^9-tetrahydrocannabinol. Contains not less than 95.0% of dronabinol. Meets the requirements for Identification and Limit of Delta^8-tetrahydrocannabinol (not more than 2.0%).
Dronabinol Capsules USP—Preserve in well-closed, light-resistant containers, in a cool place. Contain dronabinol in sesame oil. Contain the labeled amount, within ±10%. Meet the requirements for Identification and Uniformity of dosage units.

DROPERIDOL

Chemical name: 2*H*-Benzimidazol-2-one, 1-[1-[4-(4-fluorophenyl)-4-oxobutyl]-1,2,3,6-tetrahydro-4-pyridinyl]-1,3-dihydro-.

Molecular formula: $C_{22}H_{22}FN_3O_2$.

Molecular weight: 379.43.

Description: Droperidol USP—White to light tan, amorphous or microcrystalline powder.

Solubility: Droperidol USP—Practically insoluble in water; freely soluble in chloroform; slightly soluble in alcohol and in ether.

USP requirements:
Droperidol USP—Preserve in tight, light-resistant containers, under nitrogen, in a cool place. Dried in vacuum at 70 °C for 4 hours, contains not less than 98.0% and not more than 102.0% of droperidol. Meets the requirements for Identification, Melting range (147–150 °C), Loss on drying (not more than 5.0%), Residue on ignition (not more than 0.2%), Heavy metals (not more than 0.002%), and 4,4′-Bis[1,2,3,6-tetrahydro-4-(2-oxo-1-benzimidazolinyl)-1-pyridyl]butyrophenone (not more than 1.5%).
Droperidol Injection USP—Preserve in single-dose or in multiple-dose containers, preferably of Type I glass, protected from light. A sterile solution of Droperidol in Water for Injection, prepared with the aid of Lactic Acid. Contains the labeled amount of droperidol, as the lactate, within ±10%. Meets the requirements for Identification, Bacterial endotoxins, pH (3.0–3.8), Related substances, and Injections.

ABSORBABLE DUSTING POWDER

Description: Absorbable Dusting Powder USP—White, odorless powder.

USP requirements: Absorbable Dusting Powder USP—Preserve in well-closed containers. It may be preserved in sealed paper packets. An absorbable powder prepared by processing cornstarch and intended for use as a lubricant for surgical gloves. Contains not more than 2.0% of magnesium oxide. Meets the requirements for Identification, Stability to autoclaving, Sedimentation, pH (10.0–10.8, in a 1 in 10 suspension), Loss on drying (not more than 12%), Residue on ignition (not more than 3.0%), and Heavy metals (not more than 0.001%).

DYCLONINE

Chemical name: Dyclonine hydrochloride—1-Propanone, 1-(4-butoxyphenyl)-3-(1-piperidinyl)-, hydrochloride.

Molecular formula: Dyclonine hydrochloride—$C_{18}H_{27}NO_2 \cdot HCl$.

Molecular weight: Dyclonine hydrochloride—325.88.

Description: Dyclonine Hydrochloride USP—White crystals or white crystalline powder, which may have a slight odor.

Solubility: Dyclonine Hydrochloride USP—Soluble in water, in acetone, in alcohol, and in chloroform.

USP requirements:
Dyclonine Hydrochloride USP—Preserve in tight, light-resistant containers. Contains not less than 98.0% and not more than 102.0% of dyclonine hydrochloride, calculated on the dried basis. Meets the requirements for Identification, Melting range (173–178 °C), pH (4.0–7.0, in a solution [1 in 100]), Loss on drying (not more than 1.0%), and Residue on ignition (not more than 0.2%).
Dyclonine Hydrochloride Gel USP—Preserve in collapsible, opaque plastic tubes or in tight, light-resistant glass containers. (Note: Do not use aluminum or tin tubes.) Contains the labeled amount, within ±10%. Meets the requirements for Identification and pH (2.0–4.0).
Dyclonine Hydrochloride Lozenges—Not in USP.
Dyclonine Hydrochloride Oral Topical Solution—Not in USP.

Dyclonine Hydrochloride Topical Solution USP—Preserve in tight, light-resistant containers. A sterile, aqueous solution of Dyclonine Hydrochloride. Contains the labeled amount, within ±8%. Meets the requirements for Identification, Sterility, and pH (3.0–5.0).

DYDROGESTERONE

Chemical name: Pregna-4,6-diene-3,20-dione, (9 beta,10 alpha)-.

Molecular formula: $C_{21}H_{28}O_2$.

Molecular weight: 312.45.

Description: Dydrogesterone USP—White to pale yellow, crystalline powder.

Solubility: Dydrogesterone USP—Practically insoluble in water; sparingly soluble in alcohol.

USP requirements:

Dydrogesterone USP—Preserve in well-closed containers. Contains not less than 98.0% and not more than 102.0% of dydrogesterone, calculated on the dried basis. Meets the requirements for Identification, Melting range (167–171 °C), Specific rotation (−442° to −462°, calculated on the dried basis), Loss on drying (not more than 0.5%), Residue on ignition (not more than 0.1%), Heavy metals (not more than 0.002%), and Related substances.

Dydrogesterone Tablets USP—Preserve in well-closed containers. Contain the labeled amount, within ±10%. Meet the requirements for Identification, Dissolution (75% in 45 minutes in water:isopropyl alcohol [89:11] in Apparatus 2 at 100 rpm), and Uniformity of dosage units.

DYPHYLLINE

Source: A chemical derivative of theophylline, but not a theophylline salt as are the other agents.

Chemical name: *1H*-Purine-2,6-dione, 7-(2,3-dihydroxypropyl)-3,7-dihydro-1,3-dimethyl-.

Molecular formula: $C_{10}H_{14}N_4O_4$.

Molecular weight: 254.25.

Description: Dyphylline USP—White, odorless, amorphous or crystalline solid.

Solubility: Dyphylline USP—Freely soluble in water; sparingly soluble in alcohol and in chloroform; practically insoluble in ether.

USP requirements:

Dyphylline USP—Preserve in tight containers. Contains not less than 98.0% and not more than 102.0% of dyphylline, calculated on the dried basis. Meets the requirements for Identification, Melting range (160–164 °C), pH (5.0–7.5, in a solution [1 in 100]), Loss on drying (not more than 0.5%), Residue on ignition (not more than 0.15%), Chloride (not more than 0.035%), Sulfate (not more than 0.010%), Heavy metals (not more than 0.002%), Limit of theophylline, Related substances, and Organic volatile impurities.

Dyphylline Elixir USP—Preserve in tight containers. Contains the labeled amount, within ±10%. Meets the requirements for Identification and Alcohol content (±10% of labeled amount).

Dyphylline Injection USP—Preserve in single-dose or in multiple-dose containers, preferably of Type I glass, protected from light. To avoid precipitation, store at a temperature of not below 15 °C, but avoid excessive heat. Label it to indicate that the Injection is not to be used if crystals have separated. Contains the labeled amount, within ±10%. Meets the requirements for Identification, Bacterial endotoxins, pH (5.0–8.0), and Injections.

Dyphylline Oral Solution—Not in USP.

Dyphylline Tablets USP—Preserve in tight containers. Contain the labeled amount, within ±10%. Meet the requirements for Identification, Dissolution (75% in 45 minutes in water in Apparatus 1 at 100 rpm), and Uniformity of dosage units.

DYPHYLLINE AND GUAIFENESIN

For *Dyphylline* and *Guaifenesin*—See individual listings for chemistry information.

USP requirements:

Dyphylline and Guaifenesin Elixir USP—Preserve in tight containers. Contains the labeled amounts, within ±10%. Meets the requirements for Identification, pH (5.0–7.0), and Alcohol content (within ±10% of labeled amount).

Dyphylline and Guaifenesin Tablets USP—Preserve in tight containers. Contain the labeled amounts, within ±10%. Meet the requirements for Identification, Dissolution (75% of each active ingredient in 45 minutes in water in Apparatus 1 at 100 rpm), and Uniformity of dosage units.

ECHOTHIOPHATE

Chemical name: Echothiophate iodide—Ethanaminium, 2-[(diethoxyphosphinyl)thio]-*N*,*N*,*N*-trimethyl-, iodide.

Molecular formula: Echothiophate iodide—$C_9H_{23}INO_3PS$.

Molecular weight: Echothiophate iodide—383.22.

Description:

Echothiophate Iodide USP—White, crystalline, hygroscopic solid having a slight mercaptan-like odor. Its solutions have a pH of about 4.

Echothiophate Iodide for Ophthalmic Solution USP—White, amorphous powder.

Solubility: Echothiophate Iodide USP—Freely soluble in water and in methanol; soluble in dehydrated alcohol; practically insoluble in other organic solvents.

USP requirements:

Echothiophate Iodide USP—Preserve in tight, light-resistant containers, preferably at a temperature below 0 °C. Contains not less than 95.0% and not more than 100.5% of echothiophate iodide, calculated on the dried basis. Meets the requirements for Identification and Loss on drying (not more than 1.0%).

Echothiophate Iodide for Ophthalmic Solution USP—Preserve in tight containers, preferably of Type I glass, at controlled room temperature. It is sterile Echothiophate Iodide. Contains the labeled amount, within −5% to +15%. Meets the requirements for Completeness of solution, Identification, Sterility, and Water (not more than 2.0%).

ECONAZOLE

Chemical group: Synthetic imidazole derivative, differing structurally from miconazole.

Chemical name: Econazole nitrate—*1H*-Imidazole, 1-[2-[(4-chlorophenyl)methoxy]-2-(2,4-dichlorophenyl)ethyl]-, mononitrate, (±)-.

Molecular formula: Econazole nitrate—$C_{18}H_{15}Cl_3N_2O \cdot HNO_3$.

Molecular weight: Econazole nitrate—444.70.

Description: Econazole Nitrate USP—White or practically white, crystalline powder, having not more than a slight odor.

Solubility: Econazole Nitrate USP—Very slightly soluble in water and in ether; slightly soluble in alcohol; sparingly soluble in chloroform; soluble in methanol.

USP requirements:

Econazole Nitrate USP—Preserve in well-closed containers, protected from light. Contains not less than 98.5% and not more than 101.0% of econazole nitrate, calculated on the dried basis. Meets the requirements for Identification, Melting range (162–166 °C, with decomposition), Loss on drying (not more than 0.5%), Residue on ignition (not more than 0.1%), and Chromatographic purity.

Econazole Nitrate Cream—Not in USP.

Econazole Nitrate Vaginal Suppositories—Not in USP.

EDETATE CALCIUM DISODIUM

Chemical name: Calciate(2-), [[*N,N'*-1,2-ethanediylbis[*N*-(carboxymethyl)glycinato]](4-)-*N,N',O,O',O^N,O^{N'}*], disodium, hydrate, (*OC*-6-21)-.

Molecular formula: $C_{10}H_{12}CaN_2Na_2O_8$ (anhydrous).

Molecular weight: 374.27 (anhydrous).

Description: Edetate Calcium Disodium USP—White, crystalline granules or white, crystalline powder; odorless; slightly hygroscopic; stable in air.

Solubility: Edetate Calcium Disodium USP—Freely soluble in water.

USP requirements:

Edetate Calcium Disodium USP—Preserve in tight containers. A mixture of the dihydrate and trihydrate of calcium disodium ethylenediaminetetraacetate (predominantly the dihydrate). Contains not less than 97.0% and not more than 102.0% of edetate calcium disodium, calculated on the anhydrous basis. Meets the requirements for Identification, pH (6.5–8.0, in a solution [1 in 5]), Water (not more than 13.0%), Heavy metals (not more than 0.002%), Magnesium-chelating substances, and Nitrilotriacetic acid.

Edetate Calcium Disodium Injection USP—Preserve in single-dose containers, preferably of Type I glass. A sterile solution of Edetate Calcium Disodium in Water for Injection. Contains, in each mL, not less than 180 mg and not more than 220 mg of edetate calcium disodium. Meets the requirements for Identification, Bacterial endotoxins, pH (6.5–8.0), Particulate matter, and Injections.

EDETATE DISODIUM

Chemical group: The disodium salt of ethylenediamine tetraacetic acid (EDTA).

Chemical name: Glycine, *N,N'*-1,2-ethanediylbis[*N*-(carboxymethyl)-, disodium salt, dihydrate.

Molecular formula: $C_{10}H_{14}N_2Na_2O_8 \cdot 2H_2O$.

Molecular weight: 372.24.

Description: Edetate Disodium USP—White, crystalline powder.

NF category: Chelating agent; complexing agent.

Solubility: Edetate Disodium USP—Soluble in water.

USP requirements:

Edetate Disodium USP—Preserve in well-closed containers. Contains not less than 99.0% and not more than 101.0% of edetate disodium, calculated on the dried basis. Meets the requirements for Identification, pH (4.0–6.0, in a solution [1 in 20]), Loss on drying (8.7–11.4%), Calcium, Heavy metals (not more than 0.005%), and Nitrilotriacetic acid.

Edetate Disodium Injection USP—Preserve in single-dose containers, preferably of Type I glass. A sterile solution of Edetate Disodium in Water for Injection, which as a result of pH adjustment, contains varying amounts of the disodium and trisodium salts. Contains the labeled amount, within ±10%. Meets requirements for Identification, Bacterial endotoxins, pH (6.5–7.5), and Injections.

Edetate Disodium Ophthalmic Solution—Not in USP.

EDETIC ACID

Chemical name: Glycine, *N,N'*-1,2-ethanediylbis[*N*-(carboxymethyl)-.

Molecular formula: $C_{10}H_{16}N_2O_8$.

Molecular weight: 292.25.

Description: Edetic Acid NF—White, crystalline powder. Melts above 220 °C, with decomposition.

NF category: Chelating agent; complexing agent.

Solubility: Edetic Acid NF—Very slightly soluble in water; soluble in solutions of alkali hydroxides.

NF requirements: Edetic Acid NF—Preserve in well-closed containers. Contains not less than 98.0% and not more than 100.5% of edetic acid. Meets the requirements for Identification, Residue on ignition (not more than 0.2%), Heavy metals (not more than 0.003%), Nitrilotriacetic acid, and Iron (not more than 0.005%).

EDROPHONIUM

Chemical group: Synthetic quaternary ammonium compound.

Chemical name: Edrophonium chloride—Benzenaminium, *N*-ethyl-3-hydroxy-*N,N*-dimethyl-, chloride.

Molecular formula: Edrophonium chloride—$C_{10}H_{16}ClNO$.

Molecular weight: Edrophonium chloride—201.70.

Description: Edrophonium Chloride USP—White, odorless, crystalline powder. Its solution (1 in 10) is practically colorless.

Solubility: Edrophonium Chloride USP—Very soluble in water; freely soluble in alcohol; insoluble in chloroform and in ether.

USP requirements:

Edrophonium Chloride USP—Preserve in well-closed containers. Contains not less than 98.0% and not more than 100.5% of edrophonium chloride, calculated on the dried basis. Meets the requirements for Identification, Melting range (165–170 °C, with decomposition), pH (4.0–5.0, in a solution [1 in 10]), Loss on drying (not more than 0.5%), Residue on ignition (not more than 0.1%), Heavy metals (not more than 0.002%), and Dimethylaminophenol.

Edrophonium Chloride Injection USP—Preserve in single-dose or in multiple-dose containers, preferably of Type I glass. A sterile solution of Edrophonium Chloride in Water for Injection. Label Injection in multiple-dose containers to indicate an expiration date of not later than 3 years after date of manufacture, and label Injection in single-dose containers to indicate an expiration date of not later than 4 years after the date of manufacture. Contains the labeled amount, within ±5%. Meets the requirements for

Identification, Bacterial endotoxins, pH (5.0–5.8), and Injections.

EDROPHONIUM AND ATROPINE

For *Edrophonium* and *Atropine*—See individual listings for chemistry information.

USP requirements: Edrophonium Chloride and Atropine Sulfate Injection—Not in USP.

EFLORNITHINE

Chemical name: Eflornithine hydrochloride—DL-Ornithine, 2-(difluoromethyl)-, monohydrochloride, monohydrate.

Molecular formula: Eflornithine hydrochloride—$C_6H_{12}F_2N_2O_2 \cdot HCl \cdot H_2O$.

Molecular weight: Eflornithine hydrochloride—236.65.

Description: Eflornithine hydrochloride—White to off-white, odorless, crystalline powder.

Solubility: Eflornithine hydrochloride—Freely soluble in water and sparingly soluble in ethanol.

USP requirements: Eflornithine Hydrochloride Concentrate for Injection—Not in USP.

MULTIPLE ELECTROLYTES

USP requirements:

Multiple Electrolytes Injection Type 1 USP—Preserve in single-dose glass or plastic containers. Glass containers are preferably of Type I or Type II glass. A sterile solution of suitable salts in Water for Injection to provide sodium, potassium, magnesium, and chloride ions. In addition, the salts may provide ions of acetate, or acetate and gluconate, or acetate, gluconate, and phosphate. The label states the content of each electrolyte in terms of milliequivalents in a given volume. The label states the total osmolar concentration in mOsmol per liter. When the contents are less than 100 mL, the label alternatively may state the total osmolar concentration in mOsmol per mL. Contains the labeled amounts of sodium, potassium, magnesium, chloride, acetate, gluconate, and phosphate, within ±10%. Contains no antimicrobial agents. Meets the requirements for Identification, Bacterial endotoxins, pH (4.0–8.0), and Injections.

Multiple Electrolytes Injection Type 2 USP—Preserve in single-dose glass or plastic containers. Glass containers are preferably of Type I or Type II glass. A sterile solution of suitable salts in Water for Injection to provide sodium, potassium, calcium, magnesium, and chloride ions. In addition, the salts may provide ions of either acetate and citrate, or acetate and lactate. The label states the content of each electrolyte in terms of milliequivalents in a given volume. The label states the total osmolar concentration in mOsmol per liter. When the contents are less than 100 mL, the label alternatively may state the total osmolar concentration in mOsmol per mL. Contains the labeled amounts of sodium, potassium, magnesium, calcium, chloride, acetate, citrate, and lactate, within ±10%. Contains no antimicrobial agents. Meets the requirements for Identification, Bacterial endotoxins, pH (4.0–8.0), and Injections.

MULTIPLE ELECTROLYTES AND DEXTROSE

USP requirements:

Multiple Electrolytes and Dextrose Injection Type 1 USP—Preserve in single-dose glass or plastic containers. Glass containers are preferably of Type I or Type II glass. A sterile solution of Dextrose and suitable salts in Water for Injection to provide sodium, potassium, magnesium, and chloride ions. In addition, the salts may provide ions of acetate, or acetate and gluconate, or acetate and phosphate, or phosphate and lactate, or phosphate and sulfate. The label states the content of each electrolyte in terms of milliequivalents in a given volume. The label states the total osmolar concentration in mOsmol per liter. When the contents are less than 100 mL, the label alternatively may state the total osmolar concentration in mOsmol per mL. Contains the labeled amounts of sodium, potassium, magnesium, acetate, gluconate, phosphate, lactate, and sulfate, within ±10%, the labeled amount of chloride, within −10% to +20%, and the labeled amount of dextrose, within −10% to +5%. Contains no antimicrobial agents. Meets the requirements for Identification, Bacterial endotoxins, pH (4.0–6.5), and Injections.

Multiple Electrolytes and Dextrose Injection Type 2 USP—Preserve in single-dose glass or plastic containers. Glass containers are preferably of Type I or Type II glass. A sterile solution of Dextrose and suitable salts in Water for Injection to provide sodium, potassium, magnesium, calcium, and chloride ions. In addition, the salts may provide ions of acetate, or acetate and citrate, or acetate and lactate, or gluconate and sulfate. The label states the content of each electrolyte in terms of milliequivalents in a given volume. The label states the total osmolar concentration in mOsmol per liter. When the contents are less than 100 mL, the label alternatively may state the total osmolar concentration in mOsmol per mL. Contains the labeled amounts of sodium, potassium, magnesium, calcium, acetate, citrate, lactate, gluconate, and sulfate, within ±10%, the labeled amount of chloride, within −10% to +20%, and the labeled amount of dextrose, within −10% to +5%. Contains no antimicrobial agents. Meets the requirements for Identification, Bacterial endotoxins, pH (4.0–6.5), and Injections.

Multiple Electrolytes and Dextrose Injection Type 3 USP—Preserve in single-dose glass or plastic containers. Glass containers are preferably of Type I or Type II glass. A sterile solution of Dextrose and suitable salts in Water for Injection to provide sodium, potassium, and chloride ions. In addition, the salts may provide ions of ammonium, or acetate and phosphate, or phosphate and lactate. The label states the content of each electrolyte in terms of milliequivalents in a given volume. The label states the total osmolar concentration in mOsmol per liter. When the contents are less than 100 mL, the label alternatively may state the total osmolar concentration in mOsmol per mL. Contains the labeled amounts of sodium, potassium, ammonium, acetate, phosphate, and lactate, within ±10%, the labeled amount of chloride, within −10% to +20%, and the labeled amount of dextrose, within −10% to +5%. Contains no antimicrobial agents. Meets the requirements for Identification, Bacterial endotoxins, pH (4.0–6.5), and Injections.

Multiple Electrolytes and Dextrose Injection Type 4 USP—Preserve in single-dose glass or plastic containers. Glass containers are preferably of Type I or Type II glass. A sterile solution of Dextrose and suitable salts in Water for Injection to provide sodium, magnesium, calcium, chloride, gluconate, and sulfate ions. The label states the content of each electrolyte in terms of milliequivalents in a given volume. The label states the total osmolar concentration in mOsmol per liter. When the contents are less than 100 mL, the label alternatively may state the total osmolar concentration in mOsmol per mL. Contains the labeled amounts of sodium, magnesium, calcium, gluconate, and sulfate, within ±10%, the labeled amount of chloride, within −10% to +20%, and the labeled amount of dextrose, within −10% to +5%. Contains no antimicrobial agents. Meets the requirements for Identification, Bacterial endotoxins, pH (4.2–5.2), and Injections.

MULTIPLE ELECTROLYTES AND INVERT SUGAR

USP requirements:

Multiple Electrolytes and Invert Sugar Injection Type 1 USP—Preserve in single-dose glass or plastic containers. Glass containers are preferably of Type I or Type II glass. A sterile solution of a mixture of equal amounts of Dextrose and Fructose, or an equivalent solution produced by the hydrolysis of Sucrose, and suitable salts in Water for Injection to provide sodium, potassium, magnesium, chloride, phosphate, and lactate ions. The label states the content of each electrolyte in terms of milliequivalents in a given volume. The label states the total osmolar concentration in mOsmol per liter. When the contents are less than 100 mL, the label alternatively may state the total osmolar concentration in mOsmol per mL. Contains the labeled amounts of sodium, potassium, magnesium, phosphate, lactate, and invert sugar, within ±10%, and the labeled amount of chloride, within −10% to +20%. Contains no antimicrobial agents. Meets the requirements for Identification, Pyrogen, pH (3.0–6.0), Completeness of inversion, and Injections.

Multiple Electrolytes and Invert Sugar Injection Type 2 USP—Preserve in single-dose glass or plastic containers. Glass containers are preferably of Type I or Type II glass. A sterile solution of a mixture of equal amounts of Dextrose and Fructose, or an equivalent solution produced by the hydrolysis of Sucrose, and suitable salts in Water for Injection to provide sodium, potassium, magnesium, calcium, chloride, and lactate ions. The label states the content of each electrolyte in terms of milliequivalents in a given volume. The label states the total osmolar concentration in mOsmol per liter. When the contents are less than 100 mL, the label alternatively may state the total osmolar concentration in mOsmol per mL. Contains the labeled amounts of sodium, potassium, magnesium, calcium, lactate, and invert sugar, within ±10%, and the labeled amount of chloride, within −10% to +20%. Contains no antimicrobial agents. Meets the requirements for Identification, Pyrogen, pH (4.5–6.0), Completeness of inversion, and Injections.

Multiple Electrolytes and Invert Sugar Injection Type 3 USP—Preserve in single-dose glass or plastic containers. Glass containers are preferably of Type I or Type II glass. A sterile solution of a mixture of equal amounts of Dextrose and Fructose, or an equivalent solution produced by the hydrolysis of Sucrose, and suitable salts in Water for Injection to provide sodium, potassium, chloride, and ammonium ions. The label states the content of each electrolyte in terms of milliequivalents in a given volume. The label states the total osmolar concentration in mOsmol per liter. When the contents are less than 100 mL, the label alternatively may state the total osmolar concentration in mOsmol per mL. Contains the labeled amounts of sodium, potassium, ammonium, and invert sugar, within ±10%, and the labeled amount of chloride, within −10% to +20%. Contains no antimicrobial agents. Meets the requirements for Identification, Pyrogen, pH (3.0–5.5), Completeness of inversion, and Injections.

TRACE ELEMENTS

For *Zinc Chloride, Zinc Sulfate, Cupric Chloride, Cupric Sulfate, Chromic Chloride, Manganese Chloride, Magnesium Sulfate, Selenious Acid, Sodium Iodide,* and *Ammonium Molybdate*—See individual listings for chemistry information.

USP requirements: Trace Elements Injection USP—Preserve in single-dose or in multiple-dose containers, preferably of Type I or Type II glass. A sterile solution in Water for Injection of two or more of the following: Zinc Chloride or Zinc Sulfate, Cupric Chloride or Cupric Sulfate, Chromic Chloride, Manganese Chloride or Manganese Sulfate, Selenious Acid, Sodium Iodide, and Ammonium Molybdate. Label the Injection to specify that it is to be diluted to the appropriate strength with Sterile Water for Injection or other suitable fluid prior to administration. The label shows by an appropriate number juxtaposed to the official name, the number of trace elements contained in the Injection according to the following: zinc and copper (2), and then cumulatively, chromium (3), manganese (4), selenium (5), iodine (6), and molybdenum (7). Other combinations are indicated separately by citing the number of trace elements contained in each followed by an asterisk that is repeated with the list of labeled ingredients. Label the Injection for its contents of zinc chloride ($ZnCl_2$), zinc sulfate ($ZnSO_4 \cdot 7H_2O$), cupric chloride ($CuCl_2$), cupric sulfate ($CuSO_4$), chromic chloride ($CrCl_2$), manganese chloride ($MnCl_2$), manganese sulfate ($MnSO_4$), selenious acid (H_2SeO_3), sodium iodide (NaI), and ammonium molybdate [$(NH_4)Mo_7 \cdot 4H_2O$], and for elemental zinc (Zn), copper (Cu), chromium (Cr), manganese (Mn), selenium (Se), iodine (I), and molybdenum (Mo), as appropriate in relation to the ingredients claimed to be present. Contains the labeled amounts of zinc (Zn), copper (Cu), chromium (Cr), manganese (Mn), selenium (Se), iodine (I), and molybdenum (Mo), within ±10%. Meets the requirements for Identification, Pyrogen, pH (1.5–3.5), Particulate matter, and Injection.

EMETINE

Chemical name: Emetine hydrochloride—Emetan, 6′,7′,10,11-tetramethoxy-, dihydrochloride.

Molecular formula: Emetine hydrochloride—$C_{29}H_{40}N_2O_4 \cdot 2HCl$.

Molecular weight: Emetine hydrochloride—553.57.

Description: Emetine Hydrochloride USP—White or very slightly yellowish, odorless, crystalline powder. Affected by light.

Solubility: Emetine Hydrochloride USP—Freely soluble in water and in alcohol.

USP requirements:

Emetine Hydrochloride USP—Preserve in tight, light-resistant containers. The hydrochloride of an alkaloid obtained from Ipecac, or prepared by methylation of cephaeline, or prepared synthetically. Contains not less than 98.0% and not more than 101.5% of emetine hydrochloride, calculated on the anhydrous basis. Meets the requirements for Identification, Water (15.0–19.0%), Residue on ignition (not more than 0.2%), Acidity, and Cephaeline.

Emetine Hydrochloride Injection USP—Preserve in single-dose, light-resistant containers, preferably of Type I glass. A sterile solution of Emetine Hydrochloride in Water for Injection. Contains an amount of anhydrous emetine hydrochloride equivalent to the labeled amount of emetine hydrochloride, within −16% to −6%. Meets the requirements for Identification, Bacterial endotoxins, pH (3.0–5.0), Cephaeline, and Injections.

ENALAPRIL

Chemical name: Enalapril maleate—L-Proline, 1-[*N*-[1-(ethoxycarbonyl)-3-phenylpropyl]-L-alanyl]-, (*S*)-, (*Z*)-2-butenedioate (1:1).

Molecular formula: Enalapril maleate—$C_{20}H_{28}N_2O_5 \cdot C_4H_4O_4$.

Molecular weight: Enalapril maleate—492.53.

Description: Enalapril Maleate USP—Off-white, crystalline powder. Melts at about 144 °C.

Solubility: Enalapril Maleate USP—Practically insoluble in nonpolar organic solvents; slightly soluble in semipolar organic solvents; sparingly soluble in water; soluble in alcohol; freely soluble in methanol and in dimethylformamide.

USP requirements:

Enalapril Maleate USP—Preserve in well-closed containers. Contains not less than 98.0% and not more than 102.0% of enalapril maleate, calculated on the dried basis. Meets the requirements for Identification, Specific rotation (−41.0° to −43.5°, calculated on the dried basis), Loss on drying (not more than 1.0%), Residue on ignition (not more than 0.2%), Heavy metals (not more than 0.001%), and Organic volatile impurities.

Enalapril Maleate Tablets USP—Preserve in well-closed containers. Contain the labeled amount, within ±10%. Meet the requirements for Identification, Dissolution (80% in 30 minutes in water in Apparatus 2 at 50 rpm), Uniformity of dosage units, and Related substances (not more than 5.0%).

ENALAPRIL AND HYDROCHLOROTHIAZIDE

For *Enalapril* and *Hydrochlorothiazide*—See individual listings for chemistry information.

USP requirements: Enalapril Maleate and Hydrochlorothiazide Tablets—Not in USP.

ENALAPRILAT

Chemical name: L-Proline, 1-[*N*-(1-carboxy-3-phenylpropyl)-L-alanyl]-, dihydrate, (*S*)-.

Molecular formula: $C_{18}H_{24}N_2O_5 \cdot 2H_2O$.

Molecular weight: 384.43.

Description: Enalaprilat USP—White to nearly white, hygroscopic, crystalline powder.

Solubility: Enalaprilat USP—Sparingly soluble in methanol and in dimethylformamide; slightly soluble in water and in isopropyl alcohol; very slightly soluble in acetone, in alcohol, and in hexane; practically insoluble in acetonitrile and in chloroform.

USP requirements:

Enalaprilat USP—Preserve in well-closed containers. Contains not less than 98.0% and not more than 101.0% of enalaprilat, calculated on the anhydrous basis. Meets the requirements for Identification, Specific rotation (−53.0° to −56.0°, calculated on the anhydrous basis), Water (7.0–11.0%), Residue on ignition (not more than 0.2%), and Heavy metals (not more than 0.002%).

Enalaprilat Injection—Not in USP.

ENCAINIDE

Chemical name: Encainide hydrochloride—Benzamide, 4-methoxy-*N*-[2-[2-(1-methyl-2-piperidinyl)ethyl]phenyl]-, monohydrochloride, (±)-.

Molecular formula: Encainide hydrochloride—$C_{22}H_{28}N_2O_2 \cdot HCl$.

Molecular weight: Encainide hydrochloride—388.94.

Description: White solid.

Solubility: Freely soluble in water; slightly soluble in ethanol; insoluble in heptane.

USP requirements: Encainide Hydrochloride Capsules—Not in USP.

ENFLURANE

Chemical name: Ethane, 2-chloro-1-(difluoromethoxy)-1,1,2-trifluoro-.

Molecular formula: $C_3H_2ClF_5O$.

Molecular weight: 184.49.

Description: Enflurane USP—Clear, colorless, stable, volatile liquid, having a mild, sweet odor. Is non-flammable.

Solubility: Enflurane USP—Slightly soluble in water; miscible with organic solvents, fats, and oils.

Other characteristics:

Blood-to-Gas partition coefficient—1.91 at 37 °C.

Oil-to-Gas partition coefficient—98.5 at 37 °C.

USP requirements: Enflurane USP—Preserve in tight, light-resistant containers, and avoid exposure to excessive heat. Contains not less than 99.9% and not more than 100.0% of enflurane. Meets the requirements for Identification, Specific gravity (1.516–1.519), Distilling range (55.5–57.5 °C, a correction factor of 0.041 °C per mm being applied as necessary), Refractive index (1.3020–1.3038 at 20 °C), Acidity or alkalinity, Water (not more than 0.14%), Nonvolatile residue, Chloride, and Fluoride ions (not more than 10 mcg per mL).

ENOXACIN

Chemical name: 1,8-Naphthyridine-3-carboxylic acid, 1-ethyl-6-fluoro-1,4-dihydro-4-oxo-7-(1-piperazinyl)-.

Molecular formula: $C_{15}H_{17}FN_4O_3$.

Molecular weight: 320.32.

Description: Ivory to slightly yellow powder. In dilute aqueous solution, unstable in strong sunlight.

USP requirements: Enoxacin Tablets—Not in USP.

ENOXAPARIN

Source: Obtained by alkaline degradation of heparin benzyl ester derived from porcine intestinal mucosa.

Molecular weight: 4500 (average).

USP requirements: Enoxaparin Injection—Not in USP.

ENTERAL NUTRITION FORMULA

USP requirements:

Blenderized Enteral Nutrition Formula Oral Solution—Not in USP.

Disease-specific Enteral Nutrition Formula Oral Solution—Not in USP.

Disease-specific Enteral Nutrition Formula for Oral Solution—Not in USP.

Fiber-containing Enteral Nutrition Formula Oral Solution—Not in USP.

Milk-based Enteral Nutrition Formula Oral Solution—Not in USP.

Milk-based Enteral Nutrition Formula for Oral Solution—Not in USP.
Modular Enteral Nutrition Formula Oral Powder—Not in USP.
Modular Enteral Nutrition Formula Oral Solution—Not in USP.
Monomeric Enteral Nutrition Formula Oral Solution—Not in USP.
Monomeric Enteral Nutrition Formula for Oral Solution—Not in USP.
Polymeric Enteral Nutrition Formula Oral Solution—Not in USP.
Polymeric Enteral Nutrition Formula for Oral Solution—Not in USP.

EPHEDRINE

Chemical name:
Ephedrine—Benzenemethanol, alpha-[1-(methylamino)-ethyl]-, [*R*-(*R**,*S**)]-.
Ephedrine hydrochloride—Benzenemethanol, alpha-[1-(methylamino)ethyl]-, hydrochloride, [*R*-(*R**,*S**)]-.
Ephedrine sulfate—Benzenemethanol, alpha-[1-(methylamino)ethyl]-, [*R*-(*R**,*S**)]-, sulfate (2:1) (salt).

Molecular formula:
Ephedrine—$C_{10}H_{15}NO$ (anhydrous); $C_{10}H_{15}NO \cdot ½H_2O$ (hemihydrate).
Ephedrine hydrochloride—$C_{10}H_{15}NO \cdot HCl$.
Ephedrine sulfate—$(C_{10}H_{15}NO)_2 \cdot H_2SO_4$.

Molecular weight:
Ephedrine—165.24 (anhydrous); 174.24 (hemihydrate).
Ephedrine hydrochloride—201.70.
Ephedrine sulfate—428.54.

Description:
Ephedrine USP—Unctuous, practically colorless solid or white crystals or granules. Gradually decomposes on exposure to light. Melts between 33 and 40 °C, the variability of the melting point being the result of differences in the moisture content, anhydrous Ephedrine having a lower melting point than the hemihydrate of Ephedrine. Its solutions are alkaline to litmus.
Ephedrine Hydrochloride USP—Fine, white, odorless crystals or powder. Is affected by light.
Ephedrine Sulfate USP—Fine, white, odorless crystals or powder. Darkens on exposure to light.
Ephedrine Sulfate Nasal Solution USP—Clear, colorless solution. Is neutral or slightly acid to litmus.

Solubility:
Ephedrine USP—Soluble in water, in alcohol, in chloroform, and in ether; moderately and slowly soluble in mineral oil, the solution becoming turbid if the Ephedrine contains more than about 1% of water.
Ephedrine Hydrochloride USP—Freely soluble in water; soluble in alcohol; insoluble in ether.
Ephedrine Sulfate USP—Freely soluble in water; sparingly soluble in alcohol.

USP requirements:
Ephedrine USP—Preserve in tight, light-resistant containers, in a cold place. It is anhydrous or contains not more than one-half molecule of water of hydration. Label it to indicate whether it is hydrous or anhydrous. Where the quantity of Ephedrine is indicated in the labeling of any preparation containing Ephedrine, this shall be understood to be in terms of anhydrous Ephedrine. Contains not less than 98.5% and not more than 100.5% of ephedrine, calculated on the anhydrous basis. Meets the requirements for Identification, Specific rotation (−33.0° to −35.5°), Water (4.5–5.5% for hydrated Ephedrine; not more than 0.5% for anhydrous Ephedrine), Residue on ignition (not more than 0.1%), Chloride (not more than 0.030%), Sulfate, Ordinary impurities, and Organic volatile impurities.
Ephedrine Hydrochloride USP—Preserve in well-closed, light-resistant containers. Contains not less than 98.0% and not more than 100.5% of ephedrine hydrochloride, calculated on the dried basis. Meets the requirements for Identification, Melting range (217–220 °C), Specific rotation (−33.0° to −35.5°, calculated on the dried basis), Acidity or alkalinity, Loss on drying (not more than 0.5%), Residue on ignition (not more than 0.1%), Sulfate, and Organic volatile impurities.
Ephedrine Sulfate USP—Preserve in well-closed, light-resistant containers. Contains not less than 98.0% and not more than 101.0% of ephedrine sulfate, calculated on the dried basis. Meets the requirements for Identification, Specific rotation (−30.5° to −32.5°, calculated on the dried basis), Acidity or alkalinity, Loss on drying (not more than 0.5%), Residue on ignition (not more than 0.1%), Chloride (not more than 0.14%), Ordinary impurities, and Organic volatile impurities.
Ephedrine Sulfate Capsules USP—Preserve in tight, light-resistant containers. Contain the labeled amount, within ±8%. Meet the requirements for Identification, Dissolution (80% in 30 minutes in water in Apparatus 1 at 100 rpm), and Uniformity of dosage units.
Ephedrine Sulfate Injection USP—Preserve in single-dose or in multiple-dose, light-resistant containers, preferably of Type I glass. A sterile solution of Ephedrine Sulfate in Water for Injection. Contains the labeled amount, within ±5%. Meets the requirements for Identification, Bacterial endotoxins, pH (4.5–7.0), and Injections.
Ephedrine Sulfate Nasal Solution USP—Preserve in tight, light-resistant containers. Contains the labeled amount, within ±7%. Meets the requirements for Identification and Microbial limits.
Ephedrine Sulfate Syrup USP—Preserve in tight, light-resistant containers, and avoid exposure to excessive heat. Contains, in each 100 mL, not less than 360 mg and not more than 440 mg of ephedrine sulfate. Meets the requirements for Identification and Alcohol content (2.0–4.0%).
Ephedrine Sulfate Tablets USP—Preserve in well-closed containers. Contain the labeled amount, within ±7%. Meet the requirements for Identification, Dissolution (75% in 45 minutes in water in Apparatus 2 at 50 rpm), and Uniformity of dosage units.

EPHEDRINE AND GUAIFENESIN

For *Ephedrine* and *Guaifenesin*—See individual listings for chemistry information.

USP requirements:
Ephedrine Hydrochloride and Guaifenesin Capsules—Not in USP.
Ephedrine Hydrochloride and Guaifenesin Syrup—Not in USP.

EPHEDRINE AND PHENOBARBITAL

For *Ephedrine* and *Phenobarbital*—See individual listings for chemistry information.

USP requirements: Ephedrine Sulfate and Phenobarbital Capsules USP—Preserve in well-closed containers. Contain the labeled amounts, within ±9%. Meet the requirements for Identification, Dissolution (75% of each active ingredient in 45 minutes in water in Apparatus 1 at 100 rpm), and Uniformity of dosage units.

EPHEDRINE AND POTASSIUM IODIDE

For *Ephedrine* and *Potassium Iodide*—See individual listings for chemistry information.

USP requirements: Ephedrine Hydrochloride and Potassium Iodide Syrup—Not in USP.

EPINEPHRINE

Chemical name:
Epinephrine—1,2-Benzenediol, 4-[1-hydroxy-2-(methylamino)-ethyl]-, (*R*)-.
Epinephrine bitartrate—1,2-Benzenediol, 4-[1-hydroxy-2-(methylamino)ethyl]-, (*R*)-, [*R*-(*R**,*R**)]-2,3-dihydroxy-butanedioate (1:1) (salt).

Molecular formula:
Epinephrine—$C_9H_{13}NO_3$.
Epinephrine bitartrate—$C_9H_{13}NO_3 \cdot C_4H_6O_6$.

Molecular weight:
Epinephrine—183.21.
Epinephrine bitartrate—333.30.

Description:
Epinephrine USP—White to practically white, odorless, microcrystalline powder or granules, gradually darkening on exposure to light and air. With acids, it forms salts that are readily soluble in water, and the base may be recovered by the addition of ammonia water or alkali carbonates. Its solutions are alkaline to litmus.
Epinephrine Injection USP—Practically colorless, slightly acid liquid. Gradually turns dark on exposure to light and to air.
Epinephrine Inhalation Solution USP—Practically colorless, slightly acid liquid. Gradually turns dark on exposure to light and air.
Epinephrine Nasal Solution USP—Nearly colorless, slightly acid liquid. Gradually turns dark on exposure to light and air.
Epinephrine Ophthalmic Solution USP—Colorless to faint yellow solution. Gradually turns dark on exposure to light and air.
Epinephrine Bitartrate USP—White, or grayish white or light brownish gray, odorless, crystalline powder. Slowly darkens on exposure to air and light. Its solutions are acid to litmus, having a pH of about 3.5.
Epinephrine Bitartrate for Ophthalmic Solution USP—White to off-white solid.

Solubility:
Epinephrine USP—Very slightly soluble in water and in alcohol; insoluble in ether, in chloroform, and in fixed and volatile oils.
Epinephrine Bitartrate USP—Freely soluble in water; slightly soluble in alcohol; practically insoluble in chloroform and in ether.

USP requirements:
Epinephrine USP—Preserve in tight, light-resistant containers. Contains not less than 97.0% and not more than 100.5% of epinephrine, calculated on the dried basis. Meets the requirements for Identification, Specific rotation (−50.0° to −53.5°, calculated on the dried basis), Loss on drying (not more than 2.0%), Residue on ignition (negligible, from 100 mg), Adrenalone, and Limit of norepinephrine (not more than 4.0%).
Epinephrine Inhalation Aerosol USP—Preserve in small, nonreactive, light-resistant aerosol containers equipped with metered-dose valves and provided with oral inhalation actuators. A solution of Epinephrine in propellants and Alcohol prepared with the aid of mineral acid in a pressurized container. Contains the labeled amount within −10% to +15%, and delivers the labeled dose per inhalation, within ±25%, through an oral inhalation actuator. Meets the requirements for Identification and Unit spray content, and for Leak testing under Aerosols.
Epinephrine Injection USP—Preserve in single-dose or in multiple-dose, light-resistant containers, preferably of Type I glass. A sterile solution of Epinephrine in Water for Injection prepared with the aid of Hydrochloric acid. The label indicates that the Injection is not to be used if its color is pinkish or darker than slightly yellow or if it contains a precipitate. Contains the labeled amount, within −10% to +15%. Meets the requirements for Color and clarity, Identification, Bacterial endotoxins, pH (2.2–5.0), Total acidity, and Injections.
Epinephrine Inhalation Solution USP—Preserve in small, well-filled, tight, light-resistant containers. A solution of Epinephrine in Purified Water prepared with the aid of Hydrochloric Acid. The label indicates that the Inhalation Solution is not to be used if its color is pinkish or darker than slightly yellow or if it contains a precipitate. Contains, in each 100 mL, not less than 0.9 grams and not more than 1.15 grams of epinephrine. Meets the requirements for Color and clarity and Identification.
Epinephrine Nasal Solution USP—Preserve in small, well-filled, tight, light-resistant containers. A solution of Epinephrine in Purified Water prepared with the aid of Hydrochloric Acid. The label indicates that the Nasal Solution is not to be used if its color is pinkish or darker than slightly yellow or if it contains a precipitate. Contains, in each 100 mL, not less than 90 mg and not more than 115 mg of epinephrine. Meets the requirements for Color and clarity and Identification.
Epinephrine Ophthalmic Solution USP—Preserve in tight, light-resistant containers. A sterile, aqueous solution of Epinephrine prepared with the aid of Hydrochloric Acid. The label indicates that the Ophthalmic Solution is not to be used if its color is pinkish or darker than slightly yellow or if it contains a precipitate. Contains the labeled amount, within −10% to +15%. Contains a suitable antibacterial agent. Meets the requirements for Color and clarity, Identification, Sterility, and pH (2.2–4.5).
Sterile Epinephrine Suspension—Not in USP.
Sterile Epinephrine Oil Suspension USP—Preserve in single-dose, light-resistant containers, preferably of Type I or Type III glass. A sterile suspension of Epinephrine in a suitable vegetable oil. Contains, in each mL, not less than 1.8 mg and not more than 2.4 mg of epinephrine. Meets the requirement for Injections.
Epinephrine Bitartrate USP—Preserve in tight, light-resistant containers. Contains not less than 97.0% and not more than 102.0% of epinephrine bitartrate, calculated on the dried basis. Meets the requirements for Identification, Melting range (147–152 °C, with decomposition), Loss on drying (not more than 0.5%), Residue on ignition (negligible, from 100 mg), Adrenalone, and Limit of norepinephrine bitartrate (not more than 4.0%).
Epinephrine Bitartrate Inhalation Aerosol USP—Preserve in small, nonreactive, light-resistant aerosol containers equipped with metered-dose valves and provided with oral inhalation actuators. A suspension of microfine Epinephrine Bitartrate in propellants in a pressurized container. Contains the labeled amount, within ±10%, and delivers the labeled dose per inhalation, within ±25%, through an oral inhalation actuator. Meets the requirements for Identification, Unit spray content, and Particle size, and for Leak testing under Aerosols.
Epinephrine Bitartrate Ophthalmic Solution USP—Preserve in small, well-filled, tight, light-resistant containers. A sterile, buffered, aqueous solution of Epinephrine Bitartrate. The label indicates that the Ophthalmic Solution

is not to be used if its color is pinkish or darker than slightly yellow or if it contains a precipitate. Contains an amount of epinephrine bitartrate equivalent to the labeled amount of epinephrine, within −10% to +15%. Contains a suitable antibacterial agent. Meets the requirements for Color and clarity and pH (3.0–3.8), and for Identification test for Epinephrine Nasal Solution and Sterility tests.

Epinephrine Bitartrate for Ophthalmic Solution USP—Preserve in Containers for Sterile Solids. A sterile, dry mixture of Epinephrine Bitartrate and suitable antioxidants, prepared by freeze-drying. Contains an amount of epinephrine bitartrate equivalent to the labeled amount of epinephrine, within ±10%. Meets the requirements for Completeness of solution and Constituted solution, for Identification test under Epinephrine Nasal Solution, and for Sterility tests and Uniformity of dosage units.

EPINEPHRYL BORATE

Chemical name: 1,3,2-Benzodioxaborole-5-methanol, 2-hydroxy-alpha-[(methylamino)methyl]-, (*R*)-.

Molecular formula: $C_9H_{12}BNO_4$.

Molecular weight: 209.01.

Description: Epinephryl Borate Ophthalmic Solution USP—Clear, pale yellow liquid, gradually darkening on exposure to light and to air.

USP requirements: Epinephryl Borate Ophthalmic Solution USP—Preserve in small, well-filled, tight, light-resistant containers. A sterile solution in water of Epinephrine as a borate complex. The label indicates that the Ophthalmic Solution is not to be used if its color is pinkish or darker than slightly yellow or if it contains a precipitate. Contains an amount of epinephryl borate equivalent to the labeled amount of epinephrine, within −10% to +15%. Contains a suitable antibacterial agent and one or more suitable preservatives and buffering agents. Meets the requirements for Color and clarity, Identification, Sterility, and pH (5.5–7.6).

EPIRUBICIN

Chemical name: Epirubicin hydrochloride—5,12-Naphthacenedione, 10-[(3-amino-2,3,6-trideoxy-alpha-L-*arabino*-hexopyranosyl)oxy]-7,8,9,10-tetrahydro-6,8,11-trihydroxy-8-(hydroxyacetyl)-1-methoxy-, hydrochloride, (8*S*-*cis*)-.

Molecular formula: Epirubicin hydrochloride—$C_{27}H_{29}NO_{11} \cdot HCl$.

Molecular weight: Epirubicin hydrochloride—579.99.

Description: Epirubicin hydrochloride—Red-orange crystals with a melting point of 185 °C.

USP requirements: Epirubicin Hydrochloride for Injection—Not in USP.

EPITETRACYCLINE

Chemical name: Epitetracycline hydrochloride—2-Naphthacenecarboxamide, 4-(dimethylamino)-1,4,4a,5,5a,6,11,12a-octahydro-3,6,10,12,12a-pentahydroxy-6-methyl-1,11-dioxo, monohydrochloride, 4-epimer [4*S*-(4 alpha,4a alpha,5a alpha,6 beta,12a alpha)]-.

Molecular formula: Epitetracycline hydrochloride—$C_{22}H_{24}N_2O_8 \cdot HCl$.

Molecular weight: Epitetracycline hydrochloride—480.90.

USP requirements: Epitetracycline Hydrochloride USP—Preserve in tight, light-resistant containers. Contains not less than 70.0% of epitetracycline hydrochloride. Meets the requirements for pH (2.3–4.0, in a solution containing 10 mg per mL), Loss on drying (not more than 6.0%), and 4-Epianhydrotetracycline (not more than 2.0%).

EPOETIN ALFA

Chemical name: 1-165-Erythropoietin (human clone lambdaHEPOFL13 protein moiety), glycoform alpha.

Molecular formula: $C_{809}H_{1301}N_{229}O_{240}S_5$ (amino acid sequence).

Molecular weight: 30,400.00 ±400.

USP requirements: Epoetin Alfa, Recombinant, Injection—Not in USP.

EQUILIN

Chemical name: Estra-1,3,5(10),7-tetraen-17-one, 3-hydroxy-.

Molecular formula: $C_{18}H_{20}O_2$.

Molecular weight: 268.36.

Description: Melting point 238–240 °C.

Solubility: Soluble in alcohol, in dioxane, in acetone, in ethyl acetate, and in other organic solvents; sparingly soluble in water.

USP requirements: Equilin USP—Preserve in tight, light-resistant containers. Contains not less than 97.0% and not more than 103.0% of equilin, calculated on the dried basis. Meets the requirements for Identification, Specific rotation (+300° to +316°, calculated on the dried basis), Loss on drying (not more than 0.5%), and Residue on ignition (not more than 0.5%).

ERGOCALCIFEROL

Chemical name: 9,10-Secoergosta-5,7,10(19),22-tetraen-3-ol, (3 beta,5*Z*,7*E*,22*E*)-.

Molecular formula: $C_{28}H_{44}O$.

Molecular weight: 396.66.

Description:

Ergocalciferol USP—White, odorless crystals. Is affected by air and by light.

Ergocalciferol Oral Solution USP—Clear liquid having the characteristics of the solvent used in preparing the Solution.

Solubility: Ergocalciferol USP—Insoluble in water; soluble in alcohol, in chloroform, in ether, and in fatty oils.

USP requirements:

Ergocalciferol USP—Preserve in hermetically sealed containers under nitrogen, in a cool place and protected from light. Contains not less than 97.0% and not more than 103.0% of ergocalciferol. Meets the requirements for Identification, Melting range (115–119 °C), Specific rotation (+103° to +106°), Reducing substances, and Organic volatile impurities.

Ergocalciferol Capsules USP—Preserve in tight, light-resistant containers. Usually consist of an edible vegetable oil solution of Ergocalciferol, encapsulated with Gelatin. Label the Capsules to indicate the content of ergocalciferol in mg. The activity may be expressed also in terms of USP Units, on the basis that 40 USP Vitamin D Units

= 1 mcg. Contain the labeled amount, within +20%. Meet the requirement for Uniformity of dosage units.

Ergocalciferol Injection—Not in USP.

Ergocalciferol Oral Solution USP—Preserve in tight, light-resistant containers. A solution of Ergocalciferol in an edible vegetable oil, in Polysorbate 80, or in Propylene Glycol. Label the Oral Solution to indicate the concentration of ergocalciferol in mg. The activity may be expressed also in terms of USP Units, on the basis that 40 USP Vitamin D Units = 1 mcg. Contains the labeled amount, within +20%.

Ergocalciferol Tablets USP—Preserve in tight, light-resistant containers. Label the Tablets to indicate the content of ergocalciferol in mg. The activity may be expressed also in terms of USP Units, on the basis that 40 USP Vitamin D Units = 1 mcg. Contain the labeled amount, within +20%. Meet the requirements for Identification, Disintegration (30 minutes), and Uniformity of dosage units.

ERGOLOID MESYLATES

Chemical name: Ergotaman-3′,6′,18-trione, 9,10-dihydro-12′-hydroxy-2′,5′-bis(1-methylethyl)-, (5′ alpha,10 alpha)-, monomethanesulfonate (salt) mixture with 9,10 alpha-dihydro-12′-hydroxy-2′-(1-methylethyl)-5′alpha-(phenylmethyl)ergotaman-3′,6′,18-trione monomethanesulfonate (salt), 9,10 alpha-dihydro-12′-hydroxy-2′-(1-methylethyl)-5′alpha-(2-methylpropyl)ergotaman-3′,6′,18-trione monomethanesulfonate (salt), and 9,10 alpha-dihydro-12′-hydroxy-2′-(1-methylethyl)-5′alpha-(1-methylpropyl)ergotaman-3′,6′,18-trione monomethanesulfonate (salt).

Molecular formula:
Dihydroergocornine mesylate—$C_{31}H_{41}N_5O_5 \cdot CH_4O_3S$.
Dihydroergocristine mesylate—$C_{35}H_{41}N_5O_5 \cdot CH_4O_3S$.
Dihydro-alpha-ergocryptine mesylate—$C_{32}H_{43}N_5O_5 \cdot CH_4O_3S$.
Dihydro-beta-ergocryptine mesylate—$C_{32}H_{43}N_5O_5 \cdot CH_4O_3S$.

Molecular weight:
Dihydroergocornine mesylate—659.80.
Dihydroergocristine mesylate—707.84.
Dihydro-alpha-ergocryptine mesylate—673.82.
Dihydro-beta-ergocryptine mesylate—673.82.

Description: Ergoloid Mesylates USP—White to off-white, microcrystalline or amorphous, practically odorless powder.

Solubility: Ergoloid Mesylates USP—Slightly soluble in water; soluble in methanol and in alcohol; sparingly soluble in acetone.

USP requirements:

Ergoloid Mesylates USP—Preserve in tight, light-resistant containers. A mixture of the methanesulfonate salts of the three hydrogenated alkaloids, dihydroergocristine, dihydroergocornine, and dihydroergocryptine, in an approximate weight ratio of 1:1:1. Contains not less than 97.0% and not more than 103.0% of the alkaloid methanesulfonate mixture, calculated on the anhydrous basis, and not less than 30.3% and not more than 36.3% of the methanesulfonate salt of each of the individual alkaloids. Dihydroergocryptine mesylate exists as a mixture of *alpha-* and *beta-* isomers. The ratio of *alpha-* to *beta-* isomers is not less than 1.5:1.0 and not more than 2.5:1.0. Meets the requirements for Identification, Specific rotation (+11.0° to +15.0°, calculated on the anhydrous basis), pH (4.2–5.2, in a solution [1 in 200]), Water (not more than 5.0%), Ergotamine, and Non-hydrogenated alkaloids.

Ergoloid Mesylates Capsules—Not in USP.

Ergoloid Mesylates Oral Solution USP—Preserve in tight, light-resistant containers at a temperature not exceeding 30 °C. Contains the labeled amount, within ±10%, consisting of not less than 30.3% and not more than 36.3% of the methanesulfonate salt of each of the individual alkaloids (dihydroergocristine, dihydroergocornine, and dihydroergocryptine); the ratio of *alpha-* to *beta-*dihydroergocryptine mesylate is not less than 1.5:1.0 and not more than 2.5:1.0. Meets the requirements for Identification and Alcohol content (within ±10% of the labeled amount).

Ergoloid Mesylates Tablets USP—Preserve in tight, light-resistant containers. Label Tablets to indicate whether they are intended for sublingual administration or for swallowing. Contain the labeled amount, within ±10%, consisting of not less than 30.3% and not more than 36.3% of the methanesulfonate salt of each of the individual alkaloids (dihydroergocristine, dihydroergocornine, and dihydroergocryptine); the ratio of *alpha-* to *beta-*dihydroergocryptine mesylate is not less than 1.5:1.0 and not more than 2.5:1.0. Meet the requirements for Identification, Disintegration (15 minutes, for Tablets intended for sublingual use), Dissolution (75% in 30 minutes in water in Apparatus 2 at 50 rpm, for Tablets intended to be swallowed), and Uniformity of dosage units.

ERGONOVINE

Chemical group: Ergot alkaloid.

Chemical name: Ergonovine maleate—Ergoline-8-carboxamide, 9,10-didehydro-*N*-(2-hydroxy-1-methylethyl)-6-methyl-, [8 beta(*S*)]-, (*Z*)-2-butenedioate (1:1) (salt).

Molecular formula: Ergonovine maleate—$C_{19}H_{23}N_3O_2 \cdot C_4H_4O_4$.

Molecular weight: Ergonovine maleate—441.48.

Description: Ergonovine Maleate USP—White to grayish white or faintly yellow, odorless, microcrystalline powder. Darkens with age and on exposure to light.

Solubility: Ergonovine Maleate USP—Sparingly soluble in water; slightly soluble in alcohol; insoluble in ether and in chloroform.

USP requirements:

Ergonovine Maleate USP—Preserve in tight, light-resistant containers, in a cold place. Contains not less than 97.0% and not more than 103.0% of ergonovine maleate, calculated on the dried basis. Meets the requirements for Identification, Specific rotation (+51° to +56°, calculated on the dried basis), Loss on drying (not more than 2.0%), and Related alkaloids.

Ergonovine Maleate Injection USP—Preserve in single-dose, light-resistant containers, preferably of Type I glass, and store in a cold place. A sterile solution of Ergonovine Maleate in Water for Injection. Contains the labeled amount, within ±10%. Meets the requirements for Identification, Bacterial endotoxins, pH (2.7–3.5), Related alkaloids, and Injections.

Ergonovine Maleate Tablets USP—Preserve in well-closed containers. Contain the labeled amount, within ±10%. Meet the requirements for Identification, Dissolution (75% in 45 minutes in water in Apparatus 1 at 100 rpm), Uniformity of dosage units, and Related alkaloids.

ERGOTAMINE

Chemical name: Ergotamine tartrate—Ergotaman-3′,6′,18-trione, 12′-hydroxy-2′-methyl-5′-(phenylmethyl)-, (5′alpha)-, [*R*-(*R**,*R**)]-2,3-dihydroxybutanedioate (2:1) (salt).

Molecular formula: Ergotamine tartrate—$(C_{33}H_{35}N_5O_5)_2 \cdot C_4H_6O_6$.

Molecular weight: Ergotamine tartrate—1313.43.

Description: Ergotamine Tartrate USP—Colorless crystals or white to yellowish white, crystalline powder. Is odorless. Melts at about 180 °C, with decomposition.

Solubility: Ergotamine Tartrate USP—One gram dissolves in about 3200 mL of water; in the presence of a slight excess of tartaric acid, 1 gram dissolves in about 500 mL of water. Slightly soluble in alcohol.

USP requirements:

Ergotamine Tartrate USP—Preserve in well-closed, light-resistant containers in a cold place. Contains not less than 97.0% and not more than 100.5% of ergotamine tartrate, calculated on the dried basis. Meets the requirements for Identification, Specific rotation of ergotamine base (−155° to −165°), Loss on drying (not more than 5.0%), and Related alkaloids.

Ergotamine Tartrate Inhalation Aerosol USP—Preserve in small, non-reactive, light-resistant aerosol containers equipped with metered-dose valves and provided with oral inhalation actuators. A suspension of microfine Ergotamine Tartrate in propellants in a pressurized container. Contains the labeled amount, within ±10%, and delivers within ±25% of the labeled amount per inhalation, through an oral inhalation actuator. Meets the requirements for Identification, Unit spray content, and Particle size, and for Leak testing under Aerosols.

Ergotamine Tartrate Injection USP—Preserve in single-dose, light-resistant containers, preferably of Type I glass. A sterile solution of Ergotamine Tartrate and the tartrates of its epimer, ergotaminine, and of other related alkaloids, in Water for Injection to which Tartaric Acid or suitable stabilizers have been added. The total alkaloid content, in each mL, is not less than 450 mcg and not more than 550 mcg. The content of ergotamine tartrate is not less than 52.0% and not more than 74.0% of the content of total alkaloid; the content of ergotaminine tartrate is not more than 45.0% of the content of total alkaloid. Meets the requirements for Bacterial endotoxins, pH (3.5–4.0) and Injections.

Ergotamine Tartrate Tablets USP—Preserve in well-closed, light-resistant containers. Label Tablets to indicate whether they are intended for sublingual administration or for swallowing. Contain the labeled amount, within ±10%. Meet the requirements for Identification, Disintegration (5 minutes, for Tablets intended for sublingual use), Dissolution (75% in 30 minutes in tartaric acid solution [1 in 100] in Apparatus 2 at 75 rpm, for Tablets intended to be swallowed), and Uniformity of dosage units.

ERGOTAMINE, BELLADONNA ALKALOIDS, AND PHENOBARBITAL

For *Ergotamine, Belladonna Alkaloids* (Atropine, Belladonna, Hyoscyamine, and Scopolamine), and *Phenobarbital*—See individual listings for chemistry information.

USP requirements:

Ergotamine Tartrate, Belladonna Alkaloids, and Phenobarbital Sodium Tablets—Not in USP.

Ergotamine Tartrate, Belladonna Alkaloids, and Phenobarbital Sodium Extended-release Tablets—Not in USP.

ERGOTAMINE AND CAFFEINE

For *Ergotamine* and *Caffeine*—See individual listings for chemistry information.

USP requirements:

Ergotamine Tartrate and Caffeine Suppositories USP—Preserve in tight containers at a temperature not above 25 °C. Do not expose unwrapped Suppositories to sunlight. Contain the labeled amounts, within ±10%. Meet the requirement for Identification.

Ergotamine Tartrate and Caffeine Tablets USP—Preserve in well-closed, light-resistant containers. Contain the labeled amounts, within ±10%. Meet the requirements for Identification, Dissolution (70% of ergotamine tartrate and 75% of caffeine in 30 minutes in tartaric acid solution [1 in 100] in Apparatus 2 at 75 rpm), and Uniformity of dosage units.

ERGOTAMINE, CAFFEINE, AND BELLADONNA ALKALOIDS

For *Ergotamine, Caffeine,* and *Belladonna Alkaloids* (Atropine, Belladonna, Hyoscyamine, and Scopolamine)—See individual listings for chemistry information.

USP requirements:

Ergotamine Tartrate, Caffeine, and Belladonna Alkaloids Suppositories—Not in USP.

Ergotamine Tartrate, Caffeine, and Belladonna Alkaloids Tablets—Not in USP.

ERGOTAMINE, CAFFEINE, BELLADONNA ALKALOIDS, AND PENTOBARBITAL

For *Ergotamine, Caffeine, Belladonna Alkaloids* (Anisotropine, Atropine, Belladonna, Hyoscyamine, Methscopolamine, and Scopolamine), and *Pentobarbital*—See individual listings for chemistry information.

USP requirements:

Ergotamine Tartrate, Caffeine, Belladonna Alkaloids, and Pentobarbital Suppositories—Not in USP.

Ergotamine Tartrate, Caffeine, Belladonna Alkaloids, and Pentobarbital Sodium Tablets—Not in USP.

ERGOTAMINE, CAFFEINE, AND CYCLIZINE

For *Ergotamine, Caffeine,* and *Cyclizine*—See individual listings for chemistry information.

USP requirements: Ergotamine Tartrate, Caffeine, and Cyclizine Hydrochloride Tablets—Not in USP.

ERGOTAMINE, CAFFEINE, AND DIMENHYDRINATE

For *Ergotamine, Caffeine,* and *Dimenhydrinate*—See individual listings for chemistry information.

USP requirements: Ergotamine Tartrate, Caffeine, and Dimenhydrinate Capsules—Not in USP.

ERGOTAMINE, CAFFEINE, AND DIPHENHYDRAMINE

For *Ergotamine, Caffeine,* and *Diphenhydramine*—See individual listings for chemistry information.

USP requirements: Ergotamine Tartrate, Caffeine, and Diphenhydramine Hydrochloride Capsules—Not in USP.

ERYTHRITYL TETRANITRATE

Chemical name: 1,2,3,4-Butanetetrol, tetranitrate, (*R**, *S**)-.

Molecular formula: $C_4H_6N_4O_{12}$.

Molecular weight: 302.11.

Description: Diluted Erythrityl Tetranitrate USP—White powder, having a slight odor of nitric oxides.

Solubility: Undiluted erythrityl tetranitrate—Practically insoluble in water; soluble in acetone, in acetonitrile, and in alcohol.

USP requirements:

Diluted Erythrityl Tetranitrate USP—Preserve in tight containers, and avoid exposure to excessive heat. A dry mixture of erythrityl tetranitrate with lactose or other suitable inert excipients to permit safe handling and compliance with U.S. Interstate Commerce Commission regulations pertaining to interstate shipment. Contains not less than 90.0% and not more than 110.0% of labeled amount of erythrityl tetranitrate. Meets the requirement for Identification.

Caution: Undiluted erythrityl tetranitrate is a powerful explosive, and proper precautions must be taken in handling. It can be exploded by percussion or by excessive heat. Only extremely small amounts should be isolated.

Erythrityl Tetranitrate Tablets USP—Preserve in tight containers, and avoid exposure to excessive heat. Erythrityl Tetranitrate Tablets are prepared from Diluted Erythrityl Tetranitrate. Contain the labeled amount of erythrityl tetranitrate, within ±10%. Meet the requirements for Identification, Disintegration (10 minutes), and Uniformity of dosage units.

Caution: Undiluted erythrityl tetranitrate is a powerful explosive, and proper precautions must be taken in handling. It can be exploded by percussion or by excessive heat. Only extremely small amounts should be isolated.

ERYTHROMYCIN

Source: Produced from a strain of *Streptomyces erythraeus.*

Chemical group: Macrolide group of antibiotics.

Chemical name:

Erythromycin—Erythromycin.

Erythromycin estolate—Erythromycin, 2′-propanoate, dodecyl sulfate (salt).

Erythromycin ethylsuccinate—Erythromycin 2′-(ethyl butanedioate).

Erythromycin gluceptate—Erythromycin monoglucoheptonate (salt).

Erythromycin lactobionate—Erythromycin mono(4-*O*-beta-D-galactopyranosyl-D-gluconate) (salt).

Erythromycin stearate—Erythromycin octadecanoate (salt).

Molecular formula:

Erythromycin—$C_{37}H_{67}NO_{13}$.

Erythromycin estolate—$C_{40}H_{71}NO_{14} \cdot C_{12}H_{26}O_4S$.

Erythromycin ethylsuccinate—$C_{43}H_{75}NO_{16}$.

Erythromycin gluceptate—$C_{37}H_{67}NO_{13} \cdot C_7H_{14}O_8$.

Erythromycin lactobionate—$C_{37}H_{67}NO_{13} \cdot C_{12}H_{22}O_{12}$.

Erythromycin stearate—$C_{37}H_{67}NO_{13} \cdot C_{18}H_{36}O_2$.

Molecular weight:

Erythromycin—733.94.

Erythromycin estolate—1056.40.

Erythromycin ethylsuccinate—862.07.

Erythromycin gluceptate—960.12.

Erythromycin lactobionate—1092.24.

Erythromycin stearate—1018.42.

Description:

Erythromycin USP—White or slightly yellow, crystalline powder. Is odorless or practically odorless.

Erythromycin Estolate USP—White, crystalline powder. Is odorless or practically odorless.

Erythromycin Ethylsuccinate USP—White or slightly yellow crystalline powder. Is odorless or practically odorless.

Sterile Erythromycin Gluceptate USP—White powder. Is odorless or practically odorless, and is slightly hygroscopic. Its solution (1 in 20) is neutral or slightly acid.

Erythromycin Lactobionate for Injection USP—White or slightly yellow crystals or powder, having a faint odor. Its solution (1 in 20) is neutral or slightly alkaline.

Erythromycin Stearate USP—White or slightly yellow crystals or powder. Is odorless or may have a slight, earthy odor.

Solubility:

Erythromycin USP—Slightly soluble in water; soluble in alcohol, in chloroform, and in ether.

Erythromycin Estolate USP—Soluble in alcohol, in acetone, and in chloroform; practically insoluble in water.

Erythromycin Ethylsuccinate USP—Very slightly soluble in water; freely soluble in alcohol, in chloroform, and in polyethylene glycol 400.

Sterile Erythromycin Gluceptate USP—Freely soluble in water, in alcohol, and in methanol; slightly soluble in acetone and in chloroform; practically insoluble in ether.

Erythromycin Lactobionate for Injection USP—Freely soluble in water, in alcohol, and in methanol; slightly soluble in acetone and in chloroform; practically insoluble in ether.

Erythromycin Stearate USP—Practically insoluble in water; soluble in alcohol, in chloroform, in methanol, and in ether.

USP requirements:

Erythromycin USP—Preserve in tight containers. Contains not less than 850 mcg of erythromycin, calculated on the anhydrous basis. Meets the requirements for Identification, Specific rotation (−71° to −78°, calculated on the anhydrous basis), Crystallinity, pH (8.0–10.5), Water (not more than 10.0%), and Residue on ignition (not more than 2.0%).

Erythromycin Delayed-release Capsules USP—Preserve in tight containers. Contain the labeled amount, within −10% to +15%. Meet the requirements for Identification, Drug release (Method B: 80% in 60 minutes for Acid stage and 60 minutes for Buffer stage in Apparatus 1 at 50 rpm), and Water (not more than 7.5%).

Erythromycin Topical Gel USP—Preserve in tight containers. It is Erythromycin in a suitable gel vehicle. Contains the labeled amount, within −10% to +25%. Meets the requirements for Identification and Minimum fill.

Erythromycin Ointment USP—Preserve in collapsible tubes or in other tight containers, preferably at controlled room temperature. It is Erythromycin in a suitable ointment base. Contains the labeled amount, within −10% to +25%. Meets the requirements for Identification, Minimum fill, and Water (not more than 1.0%).

Erythromycin Ophthalmic Ointment USP—Preserve in collapsible ophthalmic ointment tubes. A sterile preparation of Erythromycin in a suitable ointment base. Contains the labeled amount, within −10% to +20%. Meets the requirements for Identification, Sterility, Minimum fill, and Metal particles, and for Water under Erythromycin Ointment.

Erythromycin Pledgets USP—Preserve in tight containers. Suitable absorbent pads impregnated with Erythromycin Topical Solution. Label Pledgets to indicate that each Pledget is to be used once and then discarded. Label Pledgets also to indicate the volume, in mL, of Erythromycin Topical Solution contained in each Pledget, and the concentration, in mg of erythromycin per mL, of the Erythromycin Topical Solution. Contain not less than 90% of the labeled volume of Erythromycin Topical Solution. The Erythromycin Topical Solution expressed from Erythromycin Pledgets meets the requirements for Identification, Water, and Alcohol content under Erythromycin Topical Solution.

Erythromycin Topical Solution USP—Preserve in tight containers. A solution of Erythromycin in a suitable vehicle.

Contains the labeled amount, within −10% to +25%. Meets the requirements for Identification, Water (not more than 8.0% [20 mg per mL]; not more than 5.0% [15 mg per mL]; or not more than 2.0% [acetone-containing solutions]), and Alcohol content (within ±7.5% of the labeled amount).

Erythromycin Tablets USP—Preserve in tight containers. Contain the labeled amount, within −10% to +20%. Meet the requirements for Identification, Dissolution (70% in 60 minutes in 0.05 *M* phosphate buffer [pH 6.8] in Apparatus 2 at 50 rpm), Uniformity of dosage units, and Loss on drying (not more than 5.0%).

Note: Tablets that are enteric-coated meet the requirements for Erythromycin Delayed-release Tablets.

Erythromycin Delayed-release Tablets USP—Preserve in tight containers. The label indicates that Erythromycin Delayed-release Tablets are enteric-coated. Contain the labeled amount, within −10% to +20%. Meet the requirements for Identification, Drug Release (Method B: 75% in 60 minutes for Acid stage and 60 minutes for Buffer stage in Apparatus 1 at 100 rpm), Uniformity of dosage units, and Water (not more than 6.0%).

Erythromycin Estolate USP—Preserve in tight containers. Has a potency equivalent to not less than 600 mcg of erythromycin per mg, calculated on the anhydrous basis. Meets the requirements for Identification, Crystallinity, pH (4.5–7.0, in an aqueous suspension containing 10 mg per mL), Water (not more than 4.0%), and Free erythromycin.

Erythromycin Estolate Capsules USP—Preserve in tight containers. Contain an amount of erythromycin estolate equivalent to the labeled amount of erythromycin, within −10% to +15%. Meet the requirements for Identification, Uniformity of dosage units, and Water (not more than 5.0%).

Erythromycin Estolate Oral Suspension USP—Preserve in tight containers, in a cold place. Contains one or more suitable buffers, colors, diluents, dispersants, and flavors. Contains an amount of erythromycin estolate equivalent to the labeled amount of erythromycin, within −10% to +15%. Meets the requirements for Identification, Deliverable volume, pH (3.5–6.5), and Uniformity of dosage units (single-unit containers).

Erythromycin Estolate for Oral Suspension USP—Preserve in tight containers. A dry mixture of Erythromycin Estolate with one or more suitable buffers, colors, diluents, dispersants, and flavors. Contains an amount of erythromycin estolate equivalent to the labeled amount of erythromycin, within −10% to +15%. Meets the requirements for Identification, pH (5.0–7.0 [if pediatric drops, between 5.0 and 5.5], in the suspension constituted as directed in the labeling), Deliverable volume, Uniformity of dosage units, and Water (not more than 2.0%).

Erythromycin Estolate Tablets USP—Preserve in tight containers. Label Tablets to indicate whether they are to be chewed before swallowing. Contain an amount of erythromycin estolate equivalent to the labeled amount of erythromycin, within −10% to +20% (+15%, if chewable). Meet the requirements for Identification, Disintegration (30 minutes [Note: Chewable tablets are exempt from this requirement]), Uniformity of dosage units, and Water (not more than 5.0%; if chewable, not more than 4.0%).

Erythromycin Ethylsuccinate USP—Preserve in tight containers. Erythromycin Ethylsuccinate that is noncrystalline is labeled to indicate that it is amorphous. Any preparation containing the amorphous form of Erythromycin Ethylsuccinate is so labeled. Has a potency equivalent to not less than 765 mcg of erythromycin per mg, calculated on the anhydrous basis. Meets the requirements for Identification, Crystallinity (except that when it is labeled as being in the amorphous state it does not meet the requirements), pH (6.0–8.5, in a 1% aqueous suspension), X-ray diffraction, Water (not more than 3.0%), and Residue on ignition (not more than 1.0%).

Erythromycin Ethylsuccinate Injection USP—Preserve in single-dose or in multiple-dose containers, preferably of Type I glass. A sterile solution of Erythromycin Ethylsuccinate in Polyethylene Glycol 400, containing 2% of butylaminobenzoate and a suitable preservative. Contains an amount of erythromycin ethylsuccinate equivalent to the labeled amount of erythromycin, within −10% to +15%. Meets the requirements for Sterility, Water (not more than 1.5%), and Injections.

Erythromycin Ethylsuccinate Oral Suspension USP—Preserve in tight containers, and store in a cold place. A suspension of Erythromycin Ethylsuccinate containing one or more suitable buffers, colors, dispersants, flavors, and preservatives. Contains an amount of erythromycin ethylsuccinate equivalent to the labeled amount of erythromycin, within −10% to +20%. Meets the requirements for Identification, pH (6.5–8.5), Deliverable volume, and Uniformity of dosage units (single-unit containers).

Erythromycin Ethylsuccinate for Oral Suspension USP—Preserve in tight containers. A dry mixture of Erythromycin Ethylsuccinate with one or more suitable buffers, colors, diluents, dispersants, and flavors. Contains an amount of erythromycin ethylsuccinate equivalent to the labeled amount of erythromycin, within −10% to +20%. Meets the requirements for Identification, pH (7.0–9.0, in the suspension constituted as directed in the labeling), Loss on drying (not more than 1.0%), Deliverable volume, and Uniformity of dosage units (single-unit containers).

Erythromycin Ethylsuccinate Tablets USP—Preserve in tight containers. Label chewable Tablets to indicate that they are to be chewed before swallowing. Contain an amount of erythromycin ethylsuccinate equivalent to the labeled amount of erythromycin, within −10% to +20%. Meet the requirements for Identification, Dissolution (75% in 45 minutes in 0.1 *N* hydrochloric acid in Apparatus 2 at 50 rpm), Uniformity of dosage units, Loss on drying (not more than 4.0% [Note: Chewable Tablets are exempt from this requirement]), and Water (Chewable Tablets only, not more than 5.0%).

Sterile Erythromycin Ethylsuccinate USP—Preserve in Containers for Sterile Solids. It is Erythromycin Ethylsuccinate suitable for parenteral use. Has a potency equivalent to not less than 765 mcg of erythromycin per mg, calculated on the anhydrous basis. Meets the requirements for Sterility and Heavy metals (not more than 0.002%), and for Identification test, pH, Water, Residue on ignition, and Crystallinity under Erythromycin Ethylsuccinate.

Sterile Erythromycin Gluceptate USP—Preserve in Containers for Sterile Solids. It is Erythromycin Gluceptate suitable for parenteral use. Has a potency equivalent to not less than 600 mcg of erythromycin per mg, calculated on the anhydrous basis. In addition, where packaged for dispensing, contains an amount of erythromycin gluceptate equivalent to the labeled amount of erythromycin, within −10% to +15%. Meets the requirements for Identification, Bacterial endotoxins, Sterility, pH (6.0–8.0, in a solution containing 25 mg per mL), Water (not more than 5.0%), and Particulate matter, and, where packaged for dispensing, Uniformity of dosage units, Constituted solutions, and Labeling under Injections.

Erythromycin Lactobionate for Injection USP—Preserve in Containers for Sterile Solids. A sterile, dry mixture of erythromycin lactobionate and a suitable preservative. Contains an amount of erythromycin lactobionate equivalent to the labeled amount of erythromycin, within −10%

to +20%. Meets the requirements for Constituted solution, Identification, Bacterial endotoxins, pH (6.5–7.5, in a solution containing the equivalent of 50 mg of erythromycin per mL), Water (not more than 5.0%), Particulate matter, and Heavy metals (not more than 0.005%), and for Injections.

Sterile Erythromycin Lactobionate USP—Preserve in Containers for Sterile Solids. Has a potency equivalent to not less than 525 mcg of erythromycin per mg, calculated on the anhydrous basis, and where packaged for dispensing, contains an amount of erythromycin lactobionate equivalent to the labeled amount of erythromycin, within −10% to +20%. Meets the requirements for Identification, Bacterial endotoxins, Sterility, pH (6.5–7.5, in a solution containing the equivalent of 50 mg of erythromycin per mL), Water (not more than 5.0%), Particulate matter, Residue on ignition (not more than 2.0%), and Heavy metals (not more than 0.005%), and where packaged for dispensing, for Uniformity of dosage units and for Constituted solutions and Labeling under Injections.

Erythromycin Stearate USP—Preserve in tight containers. The stearic acid salt of Erythromycin, with an excess of Stearic Acid. Has a potency equivalent to not less than 550 mcg of erythromycin per mg, calculated on the anhydrous basis. Meets the requirements for Identification, Crystallinity, pH (6.0–11.0, in a 1% aqueous suspension), Water (not more than 4.0%), and Residue on ignition (not more than 1.0%).

Erythromycin Stearate Oral Suspension—Not in USP.

Erythromycin Stearate for Oral Suspension USP—Preserve in tight containers. A dry mixture of Erythromycin Stearate with one or more suitable buffers, colors, diluents, dispersants, and flavors. Contains an amount of erythromycin stearate equivalent to the labeled amount of erythromycin, within −10% to +20%. Meets the requirements for Identification, pH (6.0–9.0, in the suspension constituted as directed in the labeling), Water (not more than 2.0%), Deliverable volume, and Uniformity of dosage units.

Erythromycin Stearate Tablets USP—Preserve in tight containers. Contain an amount of erythromycin stearate equivalent to the labeled amount of erythromycin, within −10% to +20%. Meet the requirements for Identification, Dissolution (75% in 120 minutes in monobasic sodium phosphate buffer in Apparatus 2 at 100 rpm), Uniformity of dosage units, and Loss on drying (not more than 5.0%).

ERYTHROMYCIN AND BENZOYL PEROXIDE

For *Erythromycin* and *Benzoyl Peroxide*—See individual listings for chemistry information.

USP requirements: Erythromycin and Benzoyl Peroxide Topical Gel USP—Before mixing, preserve the Erythromycin and the vehicle containing benzoyl peroxide in separate, tight containers. After mixing, preserve the mixture in tight containers. A mixture of Erythromycin in a suitable gel vehicle containing benzoyl peroxide and one or more suitable dispersants, stabilizers, and wetting agents. Contains the labeled amounts, within −10% to +25%. Meets the requirements for Identification, Benzoyl peroxide related substances, and Minimum fill.

ERYTHROMYCIN AND SULFISOXAZOLE

For *Erythromycin* and *Sulfisoxazole*—See individual listings for chemistry information.

USP requirements:

Erythromycin Estolate and Sulfisoxazole Acetyl Oral Suspension USP—Preserve in tight containers. Contains an amount of erythromycin estolate equivalent to the labeled amount of erythromycin, within −10% to +20%, and an amount of sulfisoxazole acetyl equivalent to the labeled amount of sulfisoxazole, within −10% to +15%. Contains one or more suitable buffers, colors, diluents, emulsifiers, flavors, preservatives, and suspending agents. Meets the requirements for Identification, Uniformity of dosage units (single-unit containers), Deliverable volume, and pH (3.5–6.5).

Erythromycin Ethylsuccinate and Sulfisoxazole Acetyl for Oral Suspension USP—Preserve in tight containers. A dry mixture of Erythromycin Ethylsuccinate and Sulfisoxazole Acetyl with one or more suitable buffers, colors, flavors, surfactants, and suspending agents. Contains an amount of erythromycin ethylsuccinate equivalent to the labeled amount of erythromycin, within −10% to +20%, and an amount of sulfisoxazole acetyl equivalent to the labeled amount of sulfisoxazole, within −10% to +15%. Meets the requirements for Identification, pH (5.0–7.0, in the suspension constituted as directed in the labeling), Loss on drying (not more than 1.0%), Deliverable volume, and Uniformity of dosage units (single-unit containers).

Note: Where Erythromycin Ethylsuccinate and Sulfisoxazole Acetyl for Oral Suspension is prescribed, without reference to the quantity of erythromycin or sulfisoxazole contained therein, a product containing 40 mg of erythromycin and 120 mg of sulfisoxazole per mL when constituted as directed in the labeling shall be dispensed.

ERYTHROSINE

Chemical name: Erythrosine sodium—Spiro[isobenzofuran-1(3*H*),9′-[9*H*]-xanthen]-3-one, 3′,6′-dihydroxy-2′,4′,5′,7′-tetraiodo-, disodium salt, monohydrate.

Molecular formula: Erythrosine sodium—$C_{20}H_6I_4Na_2O_5 \cdot H_2O$.

Molecular weight: Erythrosine sodium—897.88.

Description: Erythrosine Sodium USP—Red or brownish red, odorless powder. Dissolves in water to form a bluish red solution that shows no fluorescence in ordinary light. Hygroscopic.

Solubility: Erythrosine Sodium USP—Soluble in water, in glycerin, and in propylene glycol; sparingly soluble in alcohol; insoluble in fats and in oils.

USP requirements:

Erythrosine Sodium USP—Preserve in tight containers. A dye consisting principally of the monohydrate of 2′,4′,5′,7′-tetraiodofluorescein disodium salt, with smaller amounts of lower iodinated fluoresceins. Contains not less than 87.0% of dye, calculated as erythrosine sodium. Meets the requirements for volatile matter, chlorides and sulfates, water-insoluble matter, unhalogenated intermediates, sodium iodide, triiodoresorcinol, 2-(2′,4′-dihydroxy-3′,5′-diiodobenzoyl)benzoic acid, monoiodofluoresceins, lead, arsenic, and other requirements of the U.S. Food and Drug Administration concerning Erythrosine Sodium. Conforms to the regulations of the U.S. FDA concerning certified dyes.

Erythrosine Sodium Topical Solution USP—Preserve in tight, light-resistant containers. A solution of Erythrosine Sodium in Purified Water. Contains the labeled amount, within ±10%, calculated as hydrous erythrosine sodium. Contains one or more suitable flavoring and preservative agents. Meets the requirements for Identification and pH (6.8–8.0).

Erythrosine Sodium Soluble Tablets USP—Preserve in tight, moisture-resistant, light-resistant containers. Contain the labeled amount, within ±10%, calculated as hydrous erythrosine sodium. Meet the requirements for Identification and Uniformity of dosage units.

ESMOLOL

Chemical name: Esmolol hydrochloride—Benzenepropanoic acid, 4-[2-hydroxy-3-[(1-methylethyl)amino]propoxy]-, methyl ester, hydrochloride, (±)-.

Molecular formula: Esmolol hydrochloride—$C_{16}H_{25}NO_4 \cdot HCl$.

Molecular weight: Esmolol hydrochloride—331.84.

Description: Esmolol hydrochloride—White to off-white crystalline powder; injection is clear, colorless to light yellow.

Solubility: Esmolol hydrochloride—Very soluble in water; freely soluble in alcohol.

Other characteristics: Esmolol hydrochloride—Partition coefficient: Octanol/water at pH 7.0 is 0.42.

USP requirements: Esmolol Hydrochloride Injection—Not in USP.

ESTAZOLAM

Chemical group: A triazolobenzodiazepine derivative.

Chemical name: 4*H*-[1,2,4]Triazolo[4,3-*a*][1,4]benzodiazepine, 8-chloro-6-phenyl-.

Molecular formula: $C_{16}H_{11}ClN_4$.

Molecular weight: 294.74.

Description: Fine, white, odorless powder.

Solubility: Soluble in alcohol; practically insoluble in water.

USP requirements: Estazolam Tablets—Not in USP.

ESTRADIOL

Chemical name:

Estradiol—Estra-1,3,5(10)-triene-3,17-diol, (17 beta)-.

Estradiol cypionate—Estra-1,3,5(10)-triene-3,17-diol, (17 beta)-, 17-cyclopentanepropanoate.

Estradiol valerate—Estra-1,3,5(10)-triene-3,17-diol(17 beta)-, 17-pentanoate.

Molecular formula:

Estradiol—$C_{18}H_{24}O_2$.

Estradiol cypionate—$C_{26}H_{36}O_3$.

Estradiol valerate—$C_{23}H_{32}O_3$.

Molecular weight:

Estradiol—272.39.

Estradiol cypionate—396.57.

Estradiol valerate—356.51.

Description:

Estradiol USP—White or creamy white, small crystals or crystalline powder. Is odorless, and is stable in air. Is hygroscopic.

Estradiol Cypionate USP—White to practically white, crystalline powder. Is odorless or has a slight odor.

Estradiol Valerate USP—White, crystalline powder. Is usually odorless but may have a faint, fatty odor.

Solubility:

Estradiol USP—Practically insoluble in water; soluble in alcohol, in acetone, in dioxane, in chloroform, and in solutions of fixed alkali hydroxides; sparingly soluble in vegetable oils.

Estradiol Cypionate USP—Insoluble in water; soluble in alcohol, in acetone, in chloroform, and in dioxane; sparingly soluble in vegetable oils.

Estradiol Valerate USP—Practically insoluble in water; soluble in castor oil, in methanol, in benzyl benzoate, and in dioxane; sparingly soluble in sesame oil and in peanut oil.

USP requirements:

Estradiol USP—Preserve in tight, light-resistant containers. Contains not less than 97.0% and not more than 103.0% of estradiol, calculated on the anhydrous basis. Meets the requirements for Identification, Melting range (173–179 °C), Specific rotation (+76° to +83°, calculated on the anhydrous basis), and Water (not more than 3.5%).

Estradiol Vaginal Cream USP—Preserve in collapsible tubes or in tight containers. Contains the labeled amount, within ±10% in a suitable cream base. Meets the requirements for Identification, Microbial limits, Minimum fill, and pH (3.5–6.5).

Estradiol Pellets USP—Preserve in tight containers, suitable for maintaining sterile contents, that hold 1 Pellet each. Sterile pellets composed of Estradiol in compressed form, without the presence of any binder, diluent, or excipient. Contain the labeled amount, within ±3%. Meet the requirements for Solubility in chloroform and Weight variation (for 5 pellets, average weight within ±5% of labeled weight; for each pellet, within ±10% of labeled weight), and for the requirements under Estradiol and under Sterility tests.

Sterile Estradiol Suspension USP—Preserve in single-dose or in multiple-dose containers, preferably of Type I glass. A sterile suspension of Estradiol in Water for Injection. Contains the labeled amount, within ±10%. Meets the requirements for Identification, Bacterial endotoxins, Uniformity of dosage units, and Injections.

Estradiol Tablets USP—Preserve in tight, light-resistant containers. Contain the labeled amount, within −10% to +15%. Meet the requirements for Identification, Dissolution (75% in 60 minutes in 0.3% sodium lauryl sulfate in water in Apparatus 2 at 100 rpm), and Uniformity of dosage units.

Estradiol Transdermal System—Not in USP.

Estradiol Cypionate USP—Preserve in tight, light-resistant containers. Contains not less than 97.0% and not more than 103.0% of estradiol cypionate, calculated on the dried basis. Meets the requirements for Identification, Melting range (149–153 °C), Specific rotation (+39° to +44°, calculated on the dried basis), Loss on drying (not more than 1.0%), and Residue on ignition (not more than 0.2%).

Estradiol Cypionate Injection USP—Preserve in single-dose or in multiple-dose, light-resistant containers, preferably of Type I glass. A sterile solution of Estradiol Cypionate in a suitable oil. Contains the labeled amount, within ±10%. Meets the requirements for Identification and Injections.

Estradiol Valerate USP—Preserve in tight, light-resistant containers. Contains not less than 98.0% and not more than 102.0% of estradiol valerate, calculated on the dried basis. Meets the requirements for Identification, Melting range (143–150 °C), Specific rotation (+41° to +47°), Water (not more than 0.1%), Limit of estradiol (not more than 1.0%), Free acid (not more than 0.5%), and Ordinary impurities.

Estradiol Valerate Injection USP—Preserve in single-dose or in multiple-dose, light-resistant containers, preferably of Type I or Type III glass. A sterile solution of Estradiol Valerate in a suitable vegetable oil. Contains the labeled amount, within −10% to +15%. Meets the requirements for Identification, Limit of estradiol (not more than 3.0%), and Injections.

ESTRAMUSTINE

Chemical name: Estramustine phosphate sodium—Estra-1,3,5-(10)-triene-3,17-diol (17 beta)-, 3-[bis(2-chloroethyl)carbamate] 17-(dihydrogen phosphate), disodium salt.

Molecular formula: Estramustine phosphate sodium—$C_{23}H_{30}Cl_2NNa_2O_6P$.

Molecular weight: Estramustine phosphate sodium—564.35.

Description: Estramustine phosphate sodium—Off-white powder.

Solubility: Estramustine phosphate sodium—Readily soluble in water.

USP requirements: Estramustine Phosphate Sodium Capsules—Not in USP.

ESTRIOL

Chemical name: Estra-1,3,5(10)-triene-3,16,17-triol, (16 alpha,-17 beta)-.

Molecular formula: $C_{18}H_{24}O_3$.

Molecular weight: 288.39.

Description: Estriol USP—White to practically white, odorless, crystalline powder. Melts at about 280 °C.

Solubility: Estriol USP—Insoluble in water; sparingly soluble in alcohol; soluble in acetone, in chloroform, in dioxane, in ether, and in vegetable oils.

USP requirements: Estriol USP—Preserve in tight containers. Contains not less than 97.0% and not more than 102.0% of estriol, calculated on the dried basis. Meets the requirements for Identification, Specific rotation (+54° to +62°, calculated on the dried basis), Loss on drying (not more than 0.5%), Residue on ignition (not more than 0.1%), and Chromatographic impurities.

CONJUGATED ESTROGENS

Description: Conjugated Estrogens USP—Conjugated estrogens obtained from natural sources is a buff-colored, amorphous powder, odorless or having a slight, characteristic odor. The synthetic form is a white to light buff, crystalline or amorphous powder, odorless or having a slight odor.

USP requirements:

Conjugated Estrogens USP—Preserve in tight containers. A mixture of sodium estrone sulfate and sodium equilin sulfate, derived wholly or in part from equine urine or synthetically from Estrone and Equilin. Contains other conjugated estrogenic substances of the type excreted by pregnant mares. A dispersion of the estrogenic substances on a suitable powdered diluent. Label it to state the content of Conjugated Estrogens on a weight to weight basis. Contains not less than 52.5% and not more than 61.5% of sodium estrone sulfate and not less than 22.5% and not more than 30.5% of sodium equilin sulfate, and the total of sodium estrone sulfate and sodium equilin sulfate is not less than 79.5% of the labeled content of Conjugated Estrogens. Contains as concomitant components as sodium sulfate conjugates not less than 13.5% and not more than 19.5% of 17 alpha-dihydroequilin, not less than 2.5% and not more than 9.5% of 17 alpha-estradiol, and not less than 0.5% and not more than 4.0% of 17 beta-dihydroequilin, of the labeled content of Conjugated Estrogens. Meets the requirements for Identification, Concomitant components, Signal impurities, Limits of 17 beta-estradiol and Delta^{8,9}-dehydroestrone, Free steroids (not more than 1.3%), and Organic volatile impurities.

Conjugated Estrogens Vaginal Cream—Not in USP.

Conjugated Estrogens for Injection—Not in USP.

Conjugated Estrogens Tablets USP—Preserve in well-closed containers. Contain the labeled amount of conjugated estrogens as the total of sodium estrone sulfate and sodium equilin sulfate, within −27% to −5%. The ratio of sodium equilin sulfate to sodium estrone sulfate is not less than 0.35 and not more than 0.65. Meet the requirements for Identification, Dissolution (75% in 1 hour in simulated gastric fluid TS, without pepsin, in a modified Disintegration basket assembly), and Uniformity of dosage units.

CONJUGATED ESTROGENS AND METHYLTESTOSTERONE

For *Conjugated Estrogens* and *Methyltestosterone*—See individual listings for chemistry information.

USP requirements: Conjugated Estrogens and Methyltestosterone Tablets—Not in USP.

ESTERIFIED ESTROGENS

Description: Esterified Estrogens USP—White or buff-colored, amorphous powder, odorless or having a slight, characteristic odor.

USP requirements:

Esterified Estrogens USP—Preserve in tight containers. A mixture of the sodium salts of the sulfate esters of the estrogenic substances, principally estrone. A dispersion of the estrogenic substances on a suitable powdered diluent. Label it to state the content of Esterified Estrogens on a weight to weight basis. The content of total esterified estrogens is not less than 90.0% and not more than 110.0% of the labeled amount. Contains not less than 75.0% and not more than 85.0% of sodium estrone sulfate, and not less than 6.0% and not more than 15.0% of sodium equilin sulfate, in such proportion that the total of these two components is not less than 90.0% of the labeled amount of esterified estrogens. Meets the requirements for Identification, Free steroids (not more than 3.0%), and Organic volatile impurities.

Esterified Estrogens Tablets USP—Preserve in well-closed containers. Contain the labeled amount of esterified estrogens as the total of sodium estrone sulfate and sodium equilin sulfate, within −10% to +15%. The ratio of sodium equilin sulfate to sodium estrone sulfate is not less than 0.071 and not more than 0.20. Meet the requirements for Identification, Disintegration (60 minutes), and Uniformity of dosage units.

ESTERIFIED ESTROGENS AND METHYLTESTOSTERONE

For *Esterified Estrogens* and *Methyltestosterone*—See individual listings for chemistry information.

USP requirements: Esterified Estrogens and Methyltestosterone Tablets—Not in USP.

ESTRONE

Chemical name: Estra-1,3,5(10)-trien-17-one, 3-hydroxy-.

Molecular formula: $C_{18}H_{22}O_2$.

Molecular weight: 270.37.

Description: Estrone USP—Small, white crystals or white to creamy white, crystalline powder. Is odorless, and is stable in air. Melts at about 260 °C.

Solubility: Estrone USP—Practically insoluble in water; soluble in alcohol, in acetone, in dioxane, and in vegetable oils; slightly soluble in solutions of fixed alkali hydroxides.

USP requirements:

Estrone USP—Preserve in tight, light-resistant containers. Contains not less than 97.0% and not more than 103.0% of estrone, calculated on the dried basis. Meets the requirements for Clarity of solution, Identification, Specific rotation (+158° to +165°), Loss on drying (not more than 0.5%), Residue on ignition (not more than 0.5%), Equilenin and equilin, and Ordinary impurities.

Estrone Vaginal Cream—Not in USP.

Estrone Injection USP—Preserve in single-dose or in multiple-dose containers, preferably of Type I glass. A sterile solution of Estrone in a suitable oil. Contains the labeled amount, within −10% to +15%. Meets the requirements for Identification and Injections.

Estrone Vaginal Suppositories—Not in USP.

Sterile Estrone Suspension USP—Preserve in single-dose or in multiple-dose containers, preferably of Type I glass. A sterile suspension of Estrone in Water for Injection. Contains the labeled amount, within −10% to +15%. Meets the requirements for Identification, Bacterial endotoxins, Uniformity of dosage units, and Injections.

ESTROPIPATE

Chemical name: Estra-1,3,5(10)-trien-17-one, 3-(sulfooxy)-, compd. with piperazine (1:1).

Molecular formula: $C_{18}H_{22}O_5S \cdot C_4H_{10}N_2$.

Molecular weight: 436.57.

Description: Estropipate USP—White to yellowish white, fine crystalline powder. Is odorless, or may have a slight odor. Melts at about 190 °C to a light brown, viscous liquid which solidifies, on further heating, and finally melts at about 245 °C, with decomposition.

Solubility: Estropipate USP—Very slightly soluble in water, in alcohol, in chloroform, and in ether; soluble in warm water.

USP requirements:

Estropipate USP—Preserve in tight containers. Contains not less than 97.0% and not more than 103.0% of estropipate, calculated on the dried basis. Meets the requirements for Identification, Loss on drying (not more than 1.0%), Residue on ignition (not more than 0.5%), Free estrone (not more than 2.0%), and Organic volatile impurities.

Estropipate Vaginal Cream USP—Preserve in collapsible tubes. Contains the labeled amount, within −10% to +20%, in a suitable cream base. Meets the requirements for Identification and Minimum fill.

Estropipate Tablets USP—Preserve in well-closed containers. Contain the labeled amount, within ±10%. Meet the requirements for Identification, Dissolution (75% in 60 minutes in water in Apparatus 2 at 75 rpm), and Uniformity of dosage units.

ETHACRYNATE SODIUM

Chemical name: Acetic acid, [2,3-dichloro-4-(2-methylene-1-oxobutyl)phenoxy]-, sodium salt.

Molecular formula: $C_{13}H_{11}Cl_2NaO_4$.

Molecular weight: 325.12.

Description: Ethacrynate sodium for injection—White, crystalline powder or plug.

Solubility: Soluble in water at 25 °C to the extent of about 7%.

USP requirements: Ethacrynate Sodium for Injection USP—Preserve in Containers for Sterile Solids. A sterile, freeze-dried powder prepared by the neutralization of Ethacrynic Acid with the aid of Sodium Hydroxide. Label it to indicate that it was prepared by freeze-drying, having been filled into its container in the form of a true solution. Contains an amount of ethacrynate sodium equivalent to the labeled amount of ethacrynic acid, within ±10%. Meets the requirements for Constituted solution, Identification, Bacterial endotoxins, pH (6.3–7.7), and for Sterility tests, Uniformity of dosage units, and Labeling under Injections.

ETHACRYNIC ACID

Chemical name: Acetic acid, [2,3-dichloro-4-(2-methylene-1-oxobutyl)phenoxy]-.

Molecular formula: $C_{13}H_{12}Cl_2O_4$.

Molecular weight: 303.14.

Description: Ethacrynic Acid USP—White or practically white, odorless or practically odorless, crystalline powder.

pKa: 3.5.

Solubility: Ethacrynic Acid USP—Very slightly soluble in water; freely soluble in alcohol, in chloroform, and in ether.

USP requirements:

Ethacrynic Acid USP—Preserve in well-closed containers. Contains not less than 97.0% and not more than 102.0% of ethacrynic acid, calculated on the dried basis. Meets the requirements for Identification, Loss on drying (not more than 0.25%), Residue on ignition (not more than 0.1%), Toluene extractives (not more than 2.0%), Equivalent weight (294–309, on the dried basis), Heavy metals (not more than 0.001%), and Organic volatile impurities.

Caution: Use care in handling Ethacrynic Acid, since it irritates the skin, eyes, and mucous membranes.

Ethacrynic Acid Oral Solution—Not in USP.

Ethacrynic Acid Tablets USP—Preserve in well-closed containers. Contain the labeled amount, within ±10%. Meet the requirements for Identification, Dissolution (75% in 45 minutes in 0.1 *M* phosphate buffer [pH 8.0] in Apparatus 2 at 50 rpm), and Uniformity of dosage units.

ETHAMBUTOL

Chemical name: Ethambutol hydrochloride—1-Butanol, 2,2′-(1,2-ethanediyldiimino)bis-, dihydrochloride, [*S*-(*R**,*R**)]-.

Molecular formula: Ethambutol hydrochloride—$C_{10}H_{24}N_2O_2 \cdot 2HCl$.

Molecular weight: Ethambutol hydrochloride—277.23.

Description: Ethambutol Hydrochloride USP—White, crystalline powder.

Solubility: Ethambutol Hydrochloride USP—Freely soluble in water; soluble in alcohol and in methanol; slightly soluble in ether and in chloroform.

USP requirements:

Ethambutol Hydrochloride USP—Preserve in well-closed containers. Contains not less than 98.0% and not more than 100.5% of ethambutol hydrochloride, calculated on the dried basis. Meets the requirements for Identification, Specific rotation (+6.0° to +6.7°, calculated on the dried basis), Loss on drying (not more than 0.5%), Heavy metals (not more than 0.002%), Aminobutanol (not more than 1.0%), and Organic volatile impurities.

Ethambutol Hydrochloride Tablets USP—Preserve in well-closed containers. Contain the labeled amount, within ±5%. Meet the requirements for Identification, Dissolution (75% in 45 minutes in water in Apparatus 1 at 100 rpm), Uniformity of dosage units, and Aminobutanol (not more than 1.0%).

ETHANOLAMINE

Chemical name: Ethanolamine oleate—9-Octadecenoic acid (*Z*)-, compound with 2-aminoethanol (1:1).

Molecular formula: Ethanolamine oleate—$C_{18}H_{34}O_2 \cdot C_2H_7NO$.

Molecular weight: Ethanolamine oleate—343.55.

USP requirements: Ethanolamine Oleate Injection—Not in USP.

ETHCHLORVYNOL

Chemical name: 1-Penten-4-yn-3-ol, 1-chloro-3-ethyl-.

Molecular formula: C_7H_9ClO.

Molecular weight: 144.60.

Description: Ethchlorvynol USP—Colorless to yellow, slightly viscous liquid, having a characteristic pungent odor. Darkens on exposure to light and to air.

Solubility: Ethchlorvynol USP—Immiscible with water; miscible with most organic solvents.

USP requirements:

Ethchlorvynol USP—Preserve in tight, light-resistant glass or polyethylene containers, using polyethylene-lined closures. Contains not less than 98.0% and not more than 100.0% of *E*-ethchlorvynol, calculated on the anhydrous basis. Meets the requirements for Identification, Refractive index (1.476–1.480), Acidity, Water (not more than 0.2%), and Chromatographic purity.

Ethchlorvynol Capsules USP—Preserve in tight, light-resistant containers. Contain the labeled amount of *E*-ethchlorvynol, within ±10%. Meet the requirements for Identification and Uniformity of dosage units.

ETHER

Chemical name: Ethane, 1,1′-oxybis-.

Molecular formula: $C_4H_{10}O$.

Molecular weight: 74.12.

Description: Ether USP—Colorless, mobile, volatile liquid, having a characteristic odor. Is slowly oxidized by the action of air and light, with the formation of peroxides. Boils at about 35 °C.

Solubility: Ether USP—Soluble in water. Miscible with alcohol, with chloroform, with solvent hexane, and with fixed and volatile oils.

USP requirements: Ether USP—Preserve in partly filled, tight, light-resistant containers, at a temperature not exceeding 30 °C, remote from fire. Where Ether is intended for anesthetic use, the label so states. Contains not less than 96.0% and not more than 98.0% of ether, the remainder consisting of alcohol and water. Meets the requirements for Specific gravity (0.713–0.716 [indicating 96.0–98.0% of ether]), Acidity, Water (not more than 0.5%, except where labeled as intended for anesthetic use, contains not more than 0.2%), Nonvolatile residue (not more than 0.003%), Foreign odor, Aldehyde, Peroxide (not more than 0.3 ppm), and Low-boiling hydrocarbons.

Caution: Ether is highly volatile and flammable. Its vapor, when mixed with air and ignited, may explode.

Note: Ether to be used for anesthesia must be preserved in tight containers of not more than 3-kg capacity, and is not to be used for anesthesia if it has been removed from the original container longer than 24 hours. Ether to be used for anesthesia may, however, be shipped in larger containers for repackaging in containers as directed above, provided the ether at the time of repackaging meets the requirements of the tests in *USP/NF*.

ETHINAMATE

Chemical name: Cyclohexanol, 1-ethynyl-, carbamate.

Molecular formula: $C_9H_{13}NO_2$.

Molecular weight: 167.21.

Description: Ethinamate USP—White, essentially odorless powder. Its saturated aqueous solution has a pH of about 6.5.

Solubility: Ethinamate USP—Slightly soluble in water; freely soluble in alcohol, in chloroform, and in ether.

USP requirements:

Ethinamate USP—Preserve in tight containers. Dried in vacuum at 50 °C for 4 hours, contains not less than 98.0% and not more than 100.5% of ethinamate, calculated on the dried basis. Meets the requirements for Identification, Melting range (94–98 °C), Loss on drying (not more than 1.0%), and Residue on ignition (not more than 0.2%).

Ethinamate Capsules USP—Preserve in tight containers. Contain the labeled amount, within ±10%. Meet the requirements for Identification, Dissolution (75% in 45 minutes in water in Apparatus 2 at 50 rpm), and Uniformity of dosage units.

ETHINYL ESTRADIOL

Chemical name: 19-Norpregna-1,3,5(10)-trien-20-yne-3,17-diol, (17 alpha)-.

Molecular formula: $C_{20}H_{24}O_2$.

Molecular weight: 296.41.

Description: Ethinyl Estradiol USP—White to creamy white, odorless, crystalline powder.

Solubility: Ethinyl Estradiol USP—Insoluble in water; soluble in alcohol, in chloroform, in ether, in vegetable oils, and in solutions of fixed alkali hydroxides.

USP requirements:

Ethinyl Estradiol USP—Preserve in tight, non-metallic, light-resistant containers. Contains not less than 97.0% and not more than 102.0% of ethinyl estradiol, calculated on the dried basis. Meets the requirements for Completeness of solution, Identification, Melting range (180–186 °C; in a polymorphic modification, 142–146 °C), Specific rotation (−28.0° to −29.5°, calculated on the dried basis), and Loss on drying (not more than 0.5%).

Ethinyl Estradiol Tablets USP—Preserve in well-closed containers. Contain the labeled amount, within −10% to +15%. Meet the requirements for Identification, Disintegration (30 minutes), and Uniformity of dosage units.

ETHIODIZED OIL

Description: Ethiodized Oil Injection USP—Straw-colored to amber-colored, oily liquid. May possess an alliaceous odor.

Solubility: Ethiodized Oil Injection USP—Insoluble in water; soluble in acetone, in chloroform, in ether, and in solvent hexane.

USP requirements: Ethiodized Oil Injection USP—Preserve in well-filled, light-resistant, single-dose or multiple-dose containers. An iodine addition product of the ethyl ester of the fatty acids of poppyseed oil, containing not less than 35.2% and not more than 38.9% of organically combined iodine. It is sterile. Meets the requirements for Identification, Specific gravity (1.280–1.293, at 15 °C), Viscosity (50–100 centipoises, at 15 °C), Sterility, Acidity, and Free iodine.

ETHIONAMIDE

Chemical group: Synthetic derivative of isonicotinic acid.

Chemical name: 4-Pyridinecarbothioamide, 2-ethyl-.

Molecular formula: $C_8H_{10}N_2S$.

Molecular weight: 166.24.

Description: Ethionamide USP—Bright yellow powder, having a faint to moderate sulfide-like odor.

Solubility: Ethionamide USP—Slightly soluble in water, in chloroform, and in ether; soluble in methanol; sparingly soluble in alcohol and in propylene glycol.

USP requirements:

Ethionamide USP—Preserve in tight containers. Contains not less than 98.0% and not more than 102.0% of ethionamide, calculated on the anhydrous basis. Meets the requirements for Identification, Melting range (158–164 °C), pH (6.0–7.0, in a 1 in 100 slurry in water), Water (not more than 2.0%), Residue on ignition (not more than 0.2%), Selenium (not more than 0.003%), and Organic volatile impurities.

Ethionamide Tablets USP—Preserve in tight containers. Contain the labeled amount, within −5% to +10%. Meet the requirements for Identification, Disintegration (15 minutes, the use of disks being omitted), and Uniformity of dosage units.

ETHOPROPAZINE

Chemical group: Phenothiazine derivative.

Chemical name: Ethopropazine hydrochloride—10*H*-Phenothiazine-10-ethanamine, *N*,*N*-diethyl-alpha-methyl-, monohydrochloride.

Molecular formula: Ethopropazine hydrochloride—$C_{19}H_{24}N_2S \cdot HCl$.

Molecular weight: Ethopropazine hydrochloride—348.93.

Description: Ethopropazine Hydrochloride USP—White or slightly off-white, odorless, crystalline powder. Melts at about 210 °C, with decomposition.

Solubility: Ethopropazine Hydrochloride USP—Soluble in water at 40 °C; slightly soluble in water at 20 °C; soluble in alcohol and in chloroform; sparingly soluble in acetone; insoluble in ether.

USP requirements:

Ethopropazine Hydrochloride USP—Preserve in tight, light-resistant containers. Contains not less than 98.0% and not more than 101.5% of ethopropazine hydrochloride, calculated on the dried basis. Meets the requirements for Identification, Loss on drying (not more than 0.5%), Heavy metals (not more than 0.002%), Ordinary impurities, and Organic volatile impurities.

Ethopropazine Hydrochloride Tablets USP—Preserve in well-closed containers, protected from light. Contain the labeled amount, within ±10%. Meet the requirements for Identification, Dissolution (75% in 45 minutes in 0.1 *N* hydrochloric acid in Apparatus 1 at 100 rpm), Uniformity of dosage units, and Other alkylated phenothiazines.

ETHOSUXIMIDE

Chemical name: 2,5-Pyrrolidinedione, 3-ethyl-3-methyl-.

Molecular formula: $C_7H_{11}NO_2$.

Molecular weight: 141.17.

Description: Ethosuximide USP—White to off-white, crystalline powder or waxy solid, having a characteristic odor.

Solubility: Ethosuximide USP—Freely soluble in water and in chloroform; very soluble in alcohol and in ether; very slightly soluble in solvent hexane.

USP requirements:

Ethosuximide USP—Preserve in tight containers. Contains not less than 98.0% and not more than 101.0% of ethosuximide, calculated on the anhydrous basis. Meets the requirements for Identification, Melting range (47–52 °C), Water (not more than 0.5%), Residue on ignition (not more than 0.5%), Cyanide, 2-Ethyl-2-methylsuccinic anhydride and other impurities, and Organic volatile impurities.

Ethosuximide Capsules USP—Preserve in tight containers. Contain the labeled amount, within ±7%, as a solution in Polyethylene Glycol 400 or other suitable solvent. Meet the requirements for Identification and Uniformity of dosage units.

Ethosuximide Syrup—Not in USP.

ETHOTOIN

Chemical group: Related to the barbiturates in chemical structure, but having a five-membered ring.

Chemical name: 3-Ethyl-5-phenylimidazolidin-2,4-dione.

Molecular formula: $C_{11}H_{12}N_2O_2$.

Molecular weight: 204.23.

Description: Ethotoin USP—White, crystalline powder.

Solubility: Ethotoin USP—Insoluble in water; freely soluble in dehydrated alcohol and in chloroform; soluble in ether.

USP requirements:

Ethotoin USP—Preserve in tight containers. Contains not less than 97.5% and not more than 102.0% of ethotoin, calculated on the dried basis. Meets the requirements for Identification, Loss on drying (not more than 1.0%), Residue on ignition (not more than 0.1%), Chloride (not more than 0.014%), Heavy metals (not more than 0.002%), 5-Phenylhydantoin and related compounds (not more than 1.0%), and Organic volatile impurities.

Ethotoin Tablets USP—Preserve in tight containers. Contain the labeled amount, within ±10%. Meet the requirements for Identification, Dissolution (80% in 60 minutes in 0.1 *N* hydrochloric acid in Apparatus 2 at 100 rpm), and Uniformity of dosage units.

ETHYL ACETATE

Chemical name: Acetic acid, ethyl ester.

Molecular formula: $C_4H_8O_2$.

Molecular weight: 88.11.

Description: Ethyl Acetate NF—Transparent, colorless liquid, having a fragrant, refreshing, slightly acetous odor.

NF category: Flavors and perfumes; solvent.

Solubility: Ethyl Acetate NF—Soluble in water; miscible with alcohol, with ether, with fixed oils, and with volatile oils.

NF requirements: Ethyl Acetate NF—Preserve in tight containers, and avoid exposure to excessive heat. Contains not less than 99.0% and not more than 100.5% of ethyl acetate. Meets the requirements for Identification, Specific gravity (0.894–0.898), Acidity, Nonvolatile residue (not more than 0.02%), Readily carbonizable substances, Methyl compounds, Chromatographic purity, and Organic volatile impurities.

ETHYLCELLULOSE

Chemical name: Cellulose, ethyl ester.

Description: Ethylcellulose NF—Free-flowing, white to light tan powder. It forms films that have a refractive index of about 1.47. Its aqueous suspensions are neutral to litmus.

NF category: Coating agent; tablet binder.

Solubility: Ethylcellulose NF—Insoluble in water, in glycerin, and in propylene glycol. Ethylcellulose containing less than 46.5% of ethoxy groups is freely soluble in tetrahydrofuran, in methyl acetate, in chloroform, and in mixtures of aromatic hydrocarbons with alcohol. Ethylcellulose containing not less than 46.5% of ethoxy groups is freely soluble in alcohol, in methanol, in toluene, in chloroform, and in ethyl acetate.

NF requirements:

Ethylcellulose NF—Preserve in well-closed containers. An ethyl ether of cellulose. Label it to indicate its viscosity (under the conditions specified herein), and its ethoxy content. When dried at 105 °C for 2 hours, contains not less than 44.0% and not more than 51.0% of ethoxy ($-OC_2H_5$) groups. Meets the requirements for Identification, Viscosity, Loss on drying (not more than 3.0%), Residue on ignition (not more than 0.4%), Arsenic (not more than 3 ppm), Lead (not more than 10 ppm), and Heavy metals (not more than 40 ppm).

Ethylcellulose Aqueous Dispersion NF—Preserve in tight containers, and protect from freezing. A colloidal dispersion of Ethylcellulose in water. The labeling states the ethoxy content of the Ethylcellulose and the percentage of Ethylcellulose. Contains the labeled amount of Ethylcellulose, within ±10%. Contains suitable amounts of Cetyl Alcohol and Sodium Lauryl Sulfate, which assist in the formation and stabilization of the dispersion. Meets the requirements for Identification, Viscosity (not more than 150 centipoises), pH (4.0–7.0), Loss on drying (not more than 71.0%), Heavy metals (not more than 0.001%), and Organic volatile impurities.

ETHYL CHLORIDE

Chemical name: Ethane, chloro-.

Molecular formula: C_2H_5Cl.

Molecular weight: 64.51.

Description: Ethyl Chloride USP—Colorless, mobile, very volatile liquid at low temperatures or under pressure, having a characteristic, ethereal odor. Boils between 12–13 °C, and its specific gravity at 0 °C is about 0.921. When liberated at room temperature from its sealed container, it vaporizes immediately. Burns with a smoky, greenish flame, producing hydrogen chloride.

Solubility: Ethyl Chloride USP—Slightly soluble in water; freely soluble in alcohol and in ether.

USP requirements: Ethyl Chloride USP—Preserve in tight containers, preferably hermetically sealed, and remote from fire. Contains not less than 99.5% and not more than 100.5% of ethyl chloride. Meets the requirements for Reaction, Alcohol, Nonvolatile residue and odor, and Chloride.

ETHYLENEDIAMINE

Chemical name: 1,2-Ethanediamine.

Molecular formula: $C_2H_8N_2$.

Molecular weight: 60.10.

Description: Ethylenediamine USP—Clear, colorless or only slightly yellow liquid, having an ammonia-like odor and a strong alkaline reaction.

Solubility: Ethylenediamine USP—Miscible with water and with alcohol.

USP requirements: Ethylenediamine USP—Preserve in well-filled, tight, glass containers. Contains not less than 98.0% and not more than 100.5%, by weight, of ethylenediamine. Meets the requirements for Identification, Heavy metals (not more than 0.002%), and Organic volatile impurities.

Caution: Use care in handling Ethylenediamine because of its caustic nature and the irritating properties of its vapor.

Note: Ethylenediamine is strongly alkaline and may readily absorb carbon dioxide from the air to form a nonvolatile carbonate. Protect Ethylenediamine against undue exposure to the atmosphere.

ETHYLNOREPINEPHRINE

Chemical name: Ethylnorepinephrine hydrochloride—1,2-Benzenediol, 4-(2-amino-1-hydroxybutyl)-, hydrochloride.

Molecular formula: Ethylnorepinephrine hydrochloride—$C_{10}H_{15}NO_3 \cdot HCl$.

Molecular weight: Ethylnorepinephrine hydrochloride—233.69.

Description: Ethylnorepinephrine Hydrochloride USP—White to practically white, crystalline powder, which gradually darkens on exposure to light. Melts at about 190 °C, with decomposition.

Solubility: Ethylnorepinephrine Hydrochloride USP—Soluble in water and in alcohol; practically insoluble in ether.

USP requirements:

Ethylnorepinephrine Hydrochloride USP—Preserve in well-closed, light-resistant containers. Contains not less than 98.0% and not more than 101.0% of ethylnorepinephrine hydrochloride, calculated on the dried basis. Meets the requirements for Identification, Loss on drying (not more than 1.0%), Residue on ignition (not more than 0.1%), Sulfate (not more than 0.2%), and Ordinary impurities.

Ethylnorepinephrine Hydrochloride Injection USP—Preserve in single-dose or in multiple-dose, light-resistant containers, preferably of Type I glass. A sterile solution of

Ethylnorepinephrine Hydrochloride in Water for Injection. Contains the labeled amount, within −10% to +15%. Meets the requirements for Identification, Bacterial endotoxins, pH (2.5–5.0), and Injections.

Note: Do not use the Injection if it is brown or contains a precipitate.

ETHYL OLEATE

Chemical name: 9-Octadecenoic acid, (*Z*)-, ethyl ester.

Molecular formula: $C_{20}H_{38}O_2$.

Molecular weight: 310.52.

Description: Ethyl Oleate NF—Mobile, practically colorless liquid.

NF category: Vehicle (oleaginous).

Solubility: Ethyl Oleate NF—Insoluble in water; miscible with vegetable oils, with mineral oil, with alcohol, and with most organic solvents.

NF requirements: Ethyl Oleate NF—Preserve in tight, light-resistant containers. Consists of esters of ethyl alcohol and high molecular weight fatty acids, principally oleic acid. Meets the requirements for Specific gravity (0.866–0.874 at 20 °C), Viscosity (not less than 5.15 centipoises), Refractive index (1.443–1.450), Acid value (not more than 0.5), Iodine value (75–85), and Saponification value (177–188).

ETHYLPARABEN

Chemical name: Benzoic acid, 4-hydroxy-, ethyl ester.

Molecular formula: $C_9H_{10}O_3$.

Molecular weight: 166.18.

Description: Ethylparaben NF—Small, colorless crystals or white powder.

NF category: Antimicrobial preservative.

Solubility: Ethylparaben NF—Slightly soluble in water and in glycerin; freely soluble in acetone, in alcohol, in ether, and in propylene glycol.

NF requirements: Ethylparaben NF—Preserve in well-closed containers. Contains not less than 99.0% and not more than 100.5% of ethylparaben, calculated on the dried basis. Meets the requirements for Identification and Melting range (115–118 °C), and for Acidity, Loss on drying, Residue on ignition under Butylparaben, and Organic volatile impurities.

ETHYL VANILLIN

Chemical name: Benzaldehyde, 3-ethoxy-4-hydroxy-.

Molecular formula: $C_9H_{10}O_3$.

Molecular weight: 166.18.

Description: Ethyl Vanillin NF—Fine, white or slightly yellowish crystals. Its odor is similar to the odor of vanillin. It is affected by light. Its solutions are acid to litmus.

NF category: Flavors and perfumes.

Solubility: Ethyl Vanillin NF—Sparingly soluble in water at 50 °C; freely soluble in alcohol, in chloroform, in ether, and in solutions of alkali hydroxides.

NF requirements: Ethyl Vanillin NF—Preserve in tight, light-resistant containers. Dried over phosphorus pentoxide for 4 hours, contains not less than 98.0% and not more than 101.0% of ethyl vanillin. Meets the requirements for Identification, Melting range (76–78 °C), Loss on drying (not more than 1.0%), and Residue on ignition (not more than 0.1%).

ETHYNODIOL DIACETATE

Chemical name: 19-Norpregn-4-en-20-yne-3,17-diol, diacetate, (3 beta,17 alpha)-.

Molecular formula: $C_{24}H_{32}O_4$.

Molecular weight: 384.52.

Description: Ethynodiol Diacetate USP—White, odorless, crystalline powder. Is stable in air.

Solubility: Ethynodiol Diacetate USP—Insoluble in water; very soluble in chloroform; freely soluble in ether; soluble in alcohol; sparingly soluble in fixed oils.

USP requirements: Ethynodiol Diacetate USP—Preserve in well-closed, light-resistant containers. Contains not less than 97.0% and not more than 102.0% of ethynodiol diacetate. Meets the requirements for Identification, Specific rotation (−70° to −76°), Limit of conjugated diene, and Chromatographic purity.

ETHYNODIOL DIACETATE AND ETHINYL ESTRADIOL

For *Ethynodiol Diacetate* and *Ethinyl Estradiol*—See individual listings for chemistry information.

USP requirements: Ethynodiol Diacetate and Ethinyl Estradiol Tablets USP—Preserve in well-closed containers. Contain the labeled amount of ethynodiol diacetate, within ±7%, and the labeled amount of ethinyl estradiol, within ±10%. Meet the requirements for Identification, Disintegration (15 minutes, the use of disks being omitted), and Uniformity of dosage units.

ETHYNODIOL DIACETATE AND MESTRANOL

For *Ethynodiol Diacetate* and *Mestranol*—See individual listings for chemistry information.

USP requirements: Ethynodiol Diacetate and Mestranol Tablets USP—Preserve in well-closed containers. Contain the labeled amounts, within ±10%. Meet the requirements for Identification, Disintegration (15 minutes, the use of disks being omitted), and Uniformity of dosage units.

ETIDOCAINE

Chemical group: Amide.

Chemical name: Etidocaine hydrochloride—Butanamide, *N*-(2,6-dimethylphenyl)-2-(ethylpropylamine)-, monohydrochloride.

Molecular formula: Etidocaine hydrochloride—$C_{17}H_{28}N_2O \cdot HCl$.

Molecular weight: Etidocaine hydrochloride—312.88.

Description: Etidocaine hydrochloride—White, crystalline powder.

pKa: 7.74.

Solubility: Etidocaine hydrochloride—Soluble in water; freely soluble in alcohol.

USP requirements: Etidocaine Hydrochloride Injection—Not in USP.

ETIDOCAINE AND EPINEPHRINE

For *Etidocaine* and *Epinephrine*—See individual listings for chemistry information.

USP requirements: Etidocaine Hydrochloride and Epinephrine Injection—Not in USP.

ETIDRONATE

Source: Synthetic analogue of inorganic pyrophosphate.

Chemical group: Diphosphonate.

Chemical name: Etidronate disodium—Phosphonic acid, (1-hydroxyethylidene)bis-, disodium salt.

Molecular formula: Etidronate disodium—$C_2H_6Na_2O_7P_2$.

Molecular weight: Etidronate disodium—249.99.

Description: Etidronate disodium—White powder.

Solubility: Etidronate disodium—Highly soluble in water.

USP requirements:

Etidronate Disodium USP—Preserve in tight containers. Contains not less than 97.0% and not more than 101.0% of etidronate disodium, calculated on the anhydrous basis. Meets the requirements for Identification, pH (4.2–5.2, in a solution [1 in 100]), Water (not more than 5.0%), Heavy metals, Phosphite (not more than 1.0%), and Organic volatile impurities.

Etidronate Disodium Injection—Not in USP.

Etidronate Disodium Tablets USP—Preserve in tight containers. Contain the labeled amount, within ±10%. Meet the requirements for Identification, Dissolution (70% in 30 minutes in water in Apparatus 1 at 100 rpm), and Uniformity of dosage units.

ETODOLAC

Chemical name: Pyrano[3,4-*b*]indole-1-acetic acid, 1,8-diethyl-1,3,4,9-tetrahydro-.

Molecular formula: $C_{17}H_{21}NO_3$.

Molecular weight: 287.36.

Description: White, crystalline compound.

pKa: 4.65.

Solubility: Insoluble in water; soluble in alcohols, in chloroform, in dimethyl sulfoxide, and in aqueous polyethylene glycol.

Other characteristics: N-octanol:water partition coefficient 11.4 at pH 7.4.

USP requirements: Etodolac Capsules—Not in USP.

ETOMIDATE

Chemical name: 1*H*-Imidazole-5-carboxylic acid, 1-(1-phenylethyl)-, ethyl ester, (+)-.

Molecular formula: $C_{14}H_{16}N_2O_2$.

Molecular weight: 244.29.

Description: A white or yellowish crystalline or amorphous powder. Melting point about 67 °C.

Solubility: Soluble in water at 25 °C (0.0045 mg/100 mL), in chloroform, in methanol, in ethanol, in propylene glycol, and in acetone.

USP requirements: Etomidate Injection—Not in USP.

ETOPOSIDE

Source: A semisynthetic podophyllotoxin of the mandrake plant. Also known as VP-16 or VP-16-213.

Chemical name: Furo[3′,4′:6,7]naphtho[2,3-*d*]-1,3-dioxol-6(5a*H*)-one-, 9-[(4,6-*O*-ethylidene-beta-D-glucopyranosyl)oxy]5,8,8a,-9-tetrahydro-5-(4-hydroxy-3,5-dimethoxyphenyl), [5*R*-[5 alpha,5a beta,8a alpha,9 beta(*R**)]]-.

Molecular formula: $C_{29}H_{32}O_{13}$.

Molecular weight: 588.57.

Description: Etoposide USP—Fine, white to off-white, crystalline powder.

Solubility: Etoposide USP—Very slightly soluble in water; slightly soluble in alcohol, in chloroform, in ethyl acetate, and in methylene chloride; sparingly soluble in methanol.

Other characteristics: Lipophilic.

USP requirements:

Etoposide USP—Preserve in tight, light-resistant containers. Contains not less than 95.0% and not more than 105.0% of etoposide, calculated on the dried basis. Meets the requirements for Identification, Specific rotation (−110° to −118°), Loss on drying (not more than 3.0%), Residue on ignition (not more than 0.1%), Heavy metals (not more than 0.002%), and Related compounds.

Caution: Etoposide is potentially cytotoxic. Great care should be taken to prevent inhaling particles and exposing the skin to it.

Etoposide Capsules USP—Preserve in tight containers in a cold place. Do not freeze. Contain the labeled amount, within ±10%. Meet the requirements for Identification, Uniformity of dosage units, and Related compounds.

Caution: Etoposide is potentially cytotoxic. Great care should be taken to prevent inhaling particles of Etoposide and exposing the skin to it.

Etoposide Injection—Not in USP.

ETRETINATE

Source: Ethyl ester of an aromatic analog of retinoic acid.

Chemical group: Related to both retinoic acid and retinol (vitamin A).

Chemical name: 2,4,6,8-Nonatetraenoic acid, 9-(4-methoxy-2,3,6-trimethylphenyl)-, ethyl ester, (*all-E-*).

Molecular formula: $C_{23}H_{30}O_3$.

Molecular weight: 354.49.

Description: Greenish-yellow to yellow powder.

Solubility: Insoluble in water.

Other characteristics: Both etretinate and its pharmacologically active metabolite, acetretin (etretin), have an all-*trans* structure.

USP requirements: Etretinate Capsules—Not in USP.

EUCATROPINE

Chemical name: Eucatropine hydrochloride—Benzeneacetic acid, alpha-hydroxy-, 1,2,2,6-tetramethyl-4-piperidinyl ester hydrochloride.

Molecular formula: Eucatropine hydrochloride—$C_{17}H_{25}NO_3 \cdot HCl$.

Molecular weight: Eucatropine hydrochloride—327.85.

Description: Eucatropine Hydrochloride USP—White, granular, odorless powder. Its solutions are neutral to litmus.

Solubility: Eucatropine Hydrochloride USP—Very soluble in water; freely soluble in alcohol and in chloroform; insoluble in ether.

USP requirements:

Eucatropine Hydrochloride USP—Preserve in tight, light-resistant containers. Contains not less than 99.0% and not more than 100.5% of eucatropine hydrochloride, calculated on the dried basis. Meets the requirements for Identification, Melting range (183–186 °C), Loss on drying (not more than 0.5%), Residue on ignition (not more than 0.1%), and Organic volatile impurities.

Eucatropine Hydrochloride Ophthalmic Solution USP—Preserve in tight containers. A sterile, isotonic, aqueous solution of Eucatropine Hydrochloride. Contains the labeled amount, within ±5%. Meets the requirements for Identification, Sterility, and pH (4.0–5.0).

EUGENOL

Chemical name: Phenol, 2-methoxy-4-(2-propenyl)-.

Molecular formula: $C_{10}H_{12}O_2$.

Molecular weight: 164.20.

Description: Eugenol USP—Colorless or pale yellow liquid, having a strongly aromatic odor of clove. Upon exposure to air, it darkens and thickens. Is optically inactive.

Solubility: Eugenol USP—Slightly soluble in water. Miscible with alcohol, with chloroform, with ether, and with fixed oils.

USP requirements: Eugenol USP—Preserve in tight, light-resistant containers. Obtained from Clove Oil and from other sources. Meets the requirements for Solubility in 70% alcohol (1 volume dissolves in 2 volumes of 70% alcohol), Specific gravity (1.064–1.070), Distilling range (not less than 95% at 250–255 °C), Refractive index (1.540–1.542 at 20 °C), Heavy metals (not more than 0.004%), Hydrocarbons, and Phenol.

EVANS BLUE

Chemical name: 1,3-Naphthalenedisulfonic acid, 6,6′-[(3,3′-dimethyl[1,1′-biphenyl]-4,4′-diyl)bis(azo)]bis[4-amino-5-hydroxy]-, tetrasodium salt.

Molecular formula: $C_{34}H_{24}N_6Na_4O_{14}S_4$.

Molecular weight: 960.80.

Description: Evans Blue USP—Green, bluish green, or brown, odorless powder.

Solubility: Evans Blue USP—Very soluble in water; very slightly soluble in alcohol; practically insoluble in carbon tetrachloride, in chloroform, and in ether.

USP requirements:

Evans Blue USP—Preserve in tight containers. Contains not less than 95.0% and not more than 105.0% of Evans blue, calculated on the dried basis. Meets the requirements for Identification, Loss on drying (not more than 15.0%), Insoluble substances, Acetate, Chloride, and Heavy metals (not more than 0.007%).

Evans Blue Injection USP—Preserve in single-dose containers, preferably of Type I glass. A sterile solution of Evans Blue in Water for Injection. Contains, in each mL, not less than 4.30 mg and not more than 4.75 mg of Evans Blue. Meets the requirements for Identification, Bacterial endotoxins, pH (5.5–7.5), and Injections.

FACTOR IX COMPLEX

USP requirements: Factor IX Complex USP—Preserve in hermetic containers in a refrigerator. A sterile, freeze-dried powder consisting of partially purified Factor IX fraction, as well as concentrated Factors II, VII, and X fractions, of venous plasma obtained from healthy human donors. Contains no preservative. Label it with a warning that it is to be used within 4 hours after constitution, and to state that it is for intravenous administration and that a filter is to be used in the administration equipment. Meets the requirements of the test for potency in having within ±20% of the potency stated on the label in Factor IX Units by comparison with the U.S. Factor IX Standard or with a working reference that has been calibrated with it. Meets the requirement for Expiration date (not later than 2 years from the date of manufacture). Conforms to the regulations of the U.S. Food and Drug Administration concerning biologics.

FAMOTIDINE

Chemical group: Thiazole derivative of histamine.

Chemical name: Propanimidamide, *N′*-(aminosulfonyl)-3-[[[2-[(diaminomethylene)amino]-4-thiazolyl]methyl]thio]-.

Molecular formula: $C_8H_{15}N_7O_2S_3$.

Molecular weight: 337.43.

Description: Famotidine USP—White to pale yellowish-white crystalline powder. Sensitive to light.

Solubility: Famotidine USP—Freely soluble in dimethylformamide and in glacial acetic acid; slightly soluble in methanol; very slightly soluble in water; practically insoluble in acetone, in alcohol, in chloroform, in ether, and in ethyl acetate.

USP requirements:

Famotidine USP—Preserve in well-closed containers, protected from light. Contains not less than 98.5% and not more than 101.0% of famotidine, calculated on the dried basis. Meets the requirements for Identification, Loss on drying (not more than 0.5%), Residue on ignition (not more than 0.1%), Heavy metals (not more than 0.001%), Chromatographic purity, and Organic volatile impurities.

Famotidine Injection—Not in USP.

Famotidine for Oral Suspension—Not in USP.

Famotidine Tablets USP—Preserve in well-closed, light-resistant containers. Contain the labeled amount, within ±10%. Meet the requirements for Identification, Dissolution (75% in 30 minutes in 0.1 *M* phosphate buffer [pH 4.5] in Apparatus 2 at 50 rpm), and Uniformity of dosage units.

HARD FAT

Description: Hard Fat NF—White mass; almost odorless and free from rancid odor; greasy to the touch. On warming, melts to give a colorless or slightly yellowish liquid. When the molten material is shaken with an equal quantity of hot water, a white emulsion is formed.

NF category: Stiffening agent; suppository base.

Solubility: Hard Fat NF—Practically insoluble in water; freely soluble in ether; slightly soluble in alcohol.

NF requirements: Hard Fat NF—Preserve in tight containers at a temperature that is 5 °C or more below the melting range stated in the labeling. A mixture of glycerides of saturated fatty acids. The labeling includes a melting range, which is not greater than 4 °C and which is between 27 and 44 °C. Meets the requirements for Melting range, Residue on ignition (not more than 0.05%), Acid value (not more than 1.0), Iodine value (not more than 7.0), Saponification value (215–255), Hydroxyl value (not more than 70), Unsaponifiable matter (not more than 3.0%), and Alkaline impurities.

FAT EMULSIONS

Source:
Egg phosphatides—A mixture of naturally occurring phospholipids which are isolated from the egg yolk.
Safflower oil—Refined fixed oil obtained from seeds of the safflower, or false (bastard) saffron, *Carthamus tinctorius* (Compositae).
Soybean oil—Obtained from soybeans by solvent extraction using petroleum hydrocarbons or, to a lesser extent, by expression using continuous screw press operations.

Chemical name:
Glycerin—1,2,3-Propanetriol.
Linoleic acid—(*Z,Z*)-9,12-Octadecadienoic acid.
Linolenic acid—(*Z,Z,Z*)-9,12,15-Octadecatrienoic acid.
Oleic acid—9-Octadecenoic acid, (*Z*)-.
Palmitic acid—Hexadecanoic acid.
Stearic acid—Octadecanoic acid.

Molecular formula:
Glycerin—$C_3H_8O_3$.
Linoleic acid—$C_{18}H_{32}O_2$.
Linolenic acid—$C_{18}H_{30}O_2$.
Oleic acid—$C_{18}H_{34}O_2$.
Palmitic acid—$C_{16}H_{32}O_2$.
Stearic acid—$C_{18}H_{36}O_2$.

Molecular weight:
Glycerin—92.09.
Linoleic acid—280.44.
Linolenic acid—278.42.
Oleic acid—282.47.
Palmitic acid—256.42.
Stearic acid—284.47.

Description:
Glycerin USP—Clear, colorless, syrupy liquid. Has not more than a slight characteristic odor, which is neither harsh nor disagreeable. Is hygroscopic. Its solutions are neutral to litmus.
NF category: Humectant; plasticizer; solvent; tonicity agent.
Linoleic acid—Colorless oil; easily oxidized by air; cannot be distilled without decomposition.
Linolenic acid—Colorless liquid.
Oleic Acid NF—Colorless to pale yellow, oily liquid when freshly prepared, but on exposure to air it gradually absorbs oxygen and darkens. It has a characteristic, lard-like odor. When strongly heated in air, it is decomposed with the production of acrid vapors.
NF category: Emulsifying and/or solubilizing agent.
Palmitic acid—White crystalline scales. Melting point 63–64 °C.
Safflower oil—Thickens and becomes rancid on prolonged exposure to air.
Soybean Oil USP—Clear, pale yellow, oily liquid having a characteristic odor.
NF category: Oleaginous vehicle.
Stearic Acid NF—Hard, white or faintly yellowish, somewhat glossy and crystalline solid, or white or yellowish white powder. Slight odor, suggesting tallow.
NF category: Emulsifying and/or solubilizing agent; tablet and/or capsule lubricant.

Solubility:
Glycerin USP—Miscible with water and with alcohol. Insoluble in chloroform, in ether, and in fixed and volatile oils.
Linoleic acid—Freely soluble in ether; soluble in absolute alcohol. One mL dissolves in 10 mL petroleum ether. Miscible with dimethylformamide, with fat solvents, and with oils.
Linolenic acid—Insoluble in water; soluble in organic solvents.
Oleic Acid NF—Practically insoluble in water. Miscible with alcohol, with chloroform, with ether, and with fixed and volatile oils.
Palmitic acid—Insoluble in water; sparingly soluble in cold alcohol or in petroleum ether; freely soluble in hot alcohol, in ether, in propyl alcohol, and in chloroform.
Safflower oil—Soluble in the usual oil and fat solvents.
Soybean Oil USP—Insoluble in water; miscible with ether and with chloroform.
Stearic Acid NF—Practically insoluble in water; freely soluble in chloroform and in ether; soluble in alcohol.

USP requirements: Fat Emulsions Injection—Not in USP.

FELBAMATE

Chemical name: 1,3-Propanediol, 2-phenyl-, dicarbamate.

Molecular formula: $C_{11}H_{14}N_2O_4$.

Molecular weight: 238.24.

Description: White to off-white crystalline powder with a characteristic odor.

Solubility: Very slightly soluble in water; slightly soluble in ethanol; sparingly soluble in methanol; freely soluble in dimethyl sulfoxide.

USP requirements:
Felbamate Oral Suspension—Not in USP.
Felbamate Tablets—Not in USP.

FELODIPINE

Chemical group: Dihydropyridine derivative.

Chemical name: 3,5-Pyridinedicarboxylic acid, 4-(2,3-dichlorophenyl)-1,4-dihydro-2,6-dimethyl-, ethyl methyl ester, (±)-.

Molecular formula: $C_{18}H_{19}Cl_2NO_4$.

Molecular weight: 384.26.

Description: Slightly yellowish, crystalline powder.

Solubility: Insoluble in water; freely soluble in dichloromethane and in ethanol.

USP requirements: Felodipine Extended-release Tablets—Not in USP.

FENFLURAMINE

Chemical group: Phenethylamine.

Chemical name: Fenfluramine hydrochloride—Benzeneethanamine, *N*-ethyl-alpha-methyl-3-(trifluoromethyl)-, hydrochloride.

Molecular formula: Fenfluramine hydrochloride—$C_{12}H_{16}F_3N \cdot HCl$.

Molecular weight: Fenfluramine hydrochloride—267.72.

Description: Fenfluramine hydrochloride—White, odorless, or almost odorless, crystalline powder.

Solubility: Fenfluramine hydrochloride—Soluble 1 in 20 of water, 1 in 10 of alcohol, and 1 in 10 of chloroform; practically insoluble in ether.

USP requirements:
Fenfluramine Hydrochloride Extended-release Capsules—Not in USP.
Fenfluramine Hydrochloride Tablets—Not in USP.
Fenfluramine Hydrochloride Extended-release Tablets—Not in USP.

FENOPROFEN

Chemical group: Fenoprofen calcium—Arylacetic acid derivative.

Chemical name: Fenoprofen calcium—Benzeneacetic acid, alpha-methyl-3-phenoxy-, calcium salt dihydrate, (±)-.

Molecular formula: Fenoprofen calcium—$C_{30}H_{26}CaO_6 \cdot 2H_2O$.

Molecular weight: Fenoprofen calcium—558.64.

Description: Fenoprofen Calcium USP—White, crystalline powder.

pKa: Fenoprofen calcium—4.5 at 25 °C.

Solubility: Fenoprofen Calcium USP—Slightly soluble in *n*-hexanol, in methanol, and in water; practically insoluble in chloroform.

USP requirements:
Fenoprofen Calcium USP—Preserve in tight containers. Contains not less than 97.0% and not more than 103.0% of fenoprofen calcium, calculated on the anhydrous basis. Meets the requirements for Identification, Water (5.0–8.0%), Heavy metals (not more than 0.001%), Chromatographic purity, Calcium content, and Organic volatile impurities.
Fenoprofen Calcium Capsules USP—Preserve in well-closed containers. Contain an amount of fenoprofen calcium equivalent to the labeled amount of fenoprofen, within ±10%. Meet the requirements for Identification, Dissolution (75% in 60 minutes in phosphate buffer [pH 7.0] in Apparatus 1 [10-mesh basket] at 100 rpm), and Uniformity of dosage units.
Fenoprofen Calcium Tablets USP—Preserve in well-closed containers. Contain an amount of fenoprofen calcium equivalent to the labeled amount of fenoprofen, within ±10%. Meet the requirements for Identification, Dissolution (75% in 60 minutes in phosphate buffer [pH 7.0] in Apparatus 1 [10-mesh basket] at 100 rpm), and Uniformity of dosage units.

FENOTEROL

Chemical name: Fenoterol hydrobromide—1,3-Benzenediol, 5-[1-hydroxy-2-[[2-(4-hydroxyphenyl)-1-methylethyl]amino]-ethyl]-, hydrobromide.

Molecular formula: Fenoterol hydrobromide—$C_{17}H_{21}NO_4 \cdot HBr$.

Molecular weight: Fenoterol hydrobromide—384.28.

Description: Fenoterol hydrobromide—White, odorless, crystalline powder. Melting point approximately 230 °C.

Solubility: Fenoterol hydrobromide—Soluble in water and in alcohol; practically insoluble in chloroform.

USP requirements:
Fenoterol Hydrobromide Inhalation Aerosol—Not in USP.
Fenoterol Hydrobromide Inhalation Solution—Not in USP.
Fenoterol Hydrobromide Tablets—Not in USP.

FENTANYL

Chemical group: Fentanyl derivatives are anilinopiperidine-derivative opioid analgesics and are chemically related to anileridine and meperidine.

Chemical name:
Fentanyl—*N*-phenyl-*N*-(1-2-phenylethyl-4-piperidyl) propanamide.
Fentanyl citrate—Propanamide, *N*-phenyl-*N*-[1-(2-phenylethyl)-4-piperidinyl]-, 2-hydroxy-1,2,3-propanetricarboxylate (1:1).

Molecular formula:
Fentanyl—$C_{22}H_{28}N_2O$.
Fentanyl citrate—$C_{22}H_{28}N_2O \cdot C_6H_8O_7$.

Molecular weight:
Fentanyl—336.5.
Fentanyl citrate—528.60.

Description: Fentanyl Citrate USP—White, crystalline powder or white, glistening crystals. Melts at about 150 °C, with decomposition.

pKa: 8.4.

Solubility: Fentanyl Citrate USP—Sparingly soluble in water; soluble in methanol; slightly soluble in chloroform.

Other characteristics: Fentanyl citrate—Partition coefficient (octanol:water): 816 at pH 7.4.

USP requirements:
Fentanyl Transdermal Systems—Not in USP.
Fentanyl Citrate USP—Preserve in well-closed, light-resistant containers. Contains not less than 98.0% and not more than 102.0% of fentanyl citrate, calculated on the dried basis. Meets the requirements for Identification, Loss on drying (not more than 0.5%), Residue on ignition (not more than 0.5%), Heavy metals (not more than 0.002%), and Ordinary impurities.
Caution: Great care should be taken to prevent inhaling particles of Fentanyl Citrate and exposing the skin to it.
Fentanyl Citrate Injection USP—Preserve in single-dose containers, preferably of Type I glass, protected from light. A sterile solution of Fentanyl Citrate in Water for Injection. Contains an amount of fentanyl citrate equivalent to the labeled amount of fentanyl, present as the citrate, within ±10%. Meets the requirements for Identification, Bacterial endotoxins, pH (4.0–7.5), and Injections.

FERRIC OXIDE

Molecular formula: Fe_2O_3.

Molecular weight: 159.69.

Description: Ferric Oxide NF—Powder exhibiting two basic colors (red and yellow) or other shades produced on blending the basic colors.
NF category: Color.

Solubility: Ferric Oxide NF—Insoluble in water and in organic solvents; dissolves in hydrochloric acid upon warming, a small amount of insoluble residue usually remaining.

NF requirements: Ferric Oxide NF—Preserve in well-closed containers. Contains not less than 97.0% and not more than 100.5% of ferric oxide, calculated on the ignited basis. (Note: The U.S. Food and Drug Administration requires that not more than 3 ppm arsenic, not more than 10 ppm lead, and not more than 3 ppm mercury be present [21 CFR 73.1200].) Meets the requirements for Identification, Water-soluble substances (not more than 1.0%), Acid-insoluble substances (not more than 0.1%), and Organic colors and lakes.

FERROUS FUMARATE

Chemical name: 2-Butenedioic acid, (*E*)-, iron(2+) salt.

Molecular formula: $C_4H_2FeO_4$.

Molecular weight: 169.90.

Description: Ferrous Fumarate USP—Reddish orange to red-brown, odorless powder. May contain soft lumps that produce a yellow streak when crushed.

Solubility: Ferrous Fumarate USP—Slightly soluble in water; very slightly soluble in alcohol. Its solubility in dilute hydrochloric acid is limited by the separation of fumaric acid.

USP requirements:

Ferrous Fumarate USP—Preserve in well-closed containers. Contains not less than 97.0% and not more than 101.0% of ferrous fumarate, calculated on the dried basis. Meets the requirements for Identification, Loss on drying (not more than 1.5%), Sulfate (not more than 0.2%), Arsenic (not more than 3 ppm), Ferric iron (not more than 2.0%), Lead (not more than 0.001%), and Mercury (not more than 3 ppm).

Ferrous Fumarate Capsules—Not in USP.

Ferrous Fumarate Extended-release Capsules—Not in USP.

Ferrous Fumarate Oral Solution—Not in USP.

Ferrous Fumarate Oral Suspension—Not in USP.

Ferrous Fumarate Tablets USP—Preserve in tight containers. Label Tablets in terms of ferrous fumarate and in terms of elemental iron. Contain the labeled amount, within −5% to +10%. Meet the requirements for Identification, Disintegration (30 minutes), and Uniformity of dosage units.

FERROUS FUMARATE AND DOCUSATE

For *Ferrous Fumarate* and *Docusate*—See individual listings for chemistry information.

USP requirements: Ferrous Fumarate and Docusate Sodium Extended-release Tablets USP—Preserve in well-closed containers. Label Tablets in terms of the content of ferrous fumarate and in terms of the content of elemental iron. Contain the labeled amount of ferrous fumarate, within ±10%, and the labeled amount of docusate sodium, within −10% to +15%. Meet the requirement for Uniformity of dosage units.

FERROUS GLUCONATE

Chemical name: D-Gluconic acid, iron(2+) salt (2:1), dihydrate.

Molecular formula: $C_{12}H_{22}FeO_{14} \cdot 2H_2O$.

Molecular weight: 482.18.

Description: Ferrous Gluconate USP—Yellowish gray or pale greenish yellow, fine powder or granules, having a slight odor resembling that of burned sugar. Its solution (1 in 20) is acid to litmus.

Solubility: Ferrous Gluconate USP—Soluble in water, with slight heating; practically insoluble in alcohol.

USP requirements:

Ferrous Gluconate USP—Preserve in tight containers. Contains not less than 97.0% and not more than 102.0% of ferrous gluconate, calculated on the dried basis. Meets the requirements for Identification, Loss on drying (6.5–10.0%), Chloride (not more than 0.07%), Sulfate (not more than 0.1%), Oxalic acid, Arsenic (not more than 3 ppm), Ferric iron (not more than 2.0%), Lead (not more than 0.001%), Mercury (not more than 3 ppm), Reducing sugars, and Organic volatile impurities.

Ferrous Gluconate Capsules USP—Preserve in tight containers. Label Capsules in terms of the content of ferrous gluconate and in terms of the content of elemental iron. Contain the labeled amount, within ±7%. Meet the requirements for Identification, Dissolution (75% in 45 minutes in 0.1 *N* hydrochloric acid in Apparatus 1 at 100 rpm), and Uniformity of dosage units.

Ferrous Gluconate Elixir USP—Preserve in tight, light-resistant containers. Label Elixir in terms of the content of ferrous gluconate and in terms of the content of elemental iron. Contains the labeled amount, within ±6%. Meets the requirements for Identification, pH (3.4–3.8), and Alcohol content (6.3–7.7%).

Ferrous Gluconate Syrup—Not in USP.

Ferrous Gluconate Tablets USP—Preserve in tight containers. Label Tablets in terms of the content of ferrous gluconate and in terms of the content of elemental iron. Contain the labeled amount, within ±7%. Meet the requirements for Identification, Dissolution (80% in 80 minutes in simulated gastric fluid TS in Apparatus 2 at 150 rpm), and Uniformity of dosage units.

FERROUS SULFATE

Chemical name:

Ferrous sulfate—Sulfuric acid, iron(2+) salt (1:1), heptahydrate.

Ferrous sulfate, dried—Sulfuric acid, iron(2+) salt (1:1), hydrate.

Molecular formula:

Ferrous sulfate—$FeSO_4 \cdot 7H_2O$.

Ferrous sulfate, dried—$FeSO_4 \cdot xH_2O$.

Molecular weight:

Ferrous sulfate—278.01.

Ferrous sulfate, dried—151.90.

Description:

Ferrous Sulfate USP—Pale, bluish green crystals or granules. Is odorless and efflorescent in dry air. Oxidizes readily in moist air to form brownish yellow basic ferric sulfate. Its solution (1 in 10) is acid to litmus, having a pH of about 3.7.

Dried Ferrous Sulfate USP—Grayish white to buff-colored powder, consisting primarily of $FeSO_4 \cdot H_2O$ with varying amounts of $FeSO_4 \cdot 4H_2O$.

Solubility:

Ferrous Sulfate USP—Freely soluble in water; very soluble in boiling water; insoluble in alcohol.

Dried Ferrous Sulfate USP—Slowly soluble in water; insoluble in alcohol.

USP requirements:

Ferrous Sulfate USP—Preserve in tight containers. Label it to indicate that it is not to be used if it is coated with brownish-yellow basic ferric sulfate. Contains an amount of anhydrous ferrous sulfate equivalent to not less than

99.5% and not more than 104.5% of ferrous sulfate heptahydrate. Meets the requirements for Identification, Arsenic (not more than 3 ppm), Lead (not more than 0.001%), Mercury (not more than 3 ppm), and Organic volatile impurities.

Ferrous Sulfate (Dried) Capsules—Not in USP.

Ferrous Sulfate Extended-release Capsules—Not in USP.

Ferrous Sulfate Elixir—Not in USP.

Ferrous Sulfate Oral Solution USP—Preserve in tight, light-resistant containers. Label Oral Solution in terms of the content of ferrous sulfate and in terms of the content of elemental iron. Contains the labeled amount, within ±6%. Meets the requirements for Identification and pH (1.8–5.3).

Ferrous Sulfate Syrup USP—Preserve in tight containers. Label Syrup in terms of the content of ferrous sulfate and in terms of the content of elemental iron. Contains, in each 100 mL, not less than 3.75 grams and not more than 4.25 grams of Ferrous Sulfate, equivalent to not less than 0.75 grams and not more than 0.85 grams of elemental iron.

Prepare Ferrous Sulfate Syrup as follows: 40 grams of Ferrous Sulfate, 2.1 grams of Citric Acid, hydrous, 2 mL of Peppermint Spirit, 825 grams of Sucrose, and a sufficient quantity of Purified Water, to make 1000 mL. Dissolve the Ferrous Sulfate, the Citric Acid, the Peppermint Spirit, and 200 grams of the Sucrose in 450 mL of Purified Water, and filter the solution until clear. Dissolve the remainder of the Sucrose in the clear filtrate, and add Purified Water to make 1000 mL. Mix, and filter, if necessary, through a pledget of cotton.

Meets the requirement for Identification.

Ferrous Sulfate Tablets USP—Preserve in tight containers. Label Tablets in terms of ferrous sulfate and in terms of elemental iron. Contain the labeled amount, within −5% to +10%. Meet the requirements for Identification, Disintegration (30 minutes), and Uniformity of dosage units.

Note: An equivalent amount of Dried Ferrous Sulfate may be used in place of ferrous sulfate heptahydrate in preparing Ferrous Sulfate Tablets.

Ferrous Sulfate Enteric-coated Tablets—Not in USP.

Ferrous Sulfate Extended-release Tablets—Not in USP.

Ferrous Sulfate (Dried) Extended-release Tablets—Not in USP.

Dried Ferrous Sulfate USP—Preserve in well-closed containers. Contains not less than 86.0% and not more than 89.0% of anhydrous ferrous sulfate. Meets the requirements for Identification, Insoluble substances (not more than 0.05%), Arsenic (not more than 3 ppm), Lead (not more than 0.001%), and Mercury (not more than 3 ppm).

FILGRASTIM

Chemical name: Colony-stimulating factor (human clone 1034), *N*-L-methionyl-.

Molecular formula: $C_{845}H_{1339}N_{223}O_{243}S_9$.

Molecular weight: 18,800.00 daltons.

USP requirements: Filgrastim Injection—Not in USP.

FINASTERIDE

Chemical name: 4-Azaandrost-1-ene-17-carboxamide, *N*-(1,1-dimethylethyl)-3-oxo, (5 alpha,17 beta)-.

Molecular formula: $C_{23}H_{36}N_2O_2$.

Molecular weight: 372.55.

Description: White, crystalline powder with a melting point near 250 °C.

Solubility: Freely soluble in chloroform and in lower alcohol solvents; practically insoluble in water.

USP requirements: Finasteride Tablets—Not in USP.

FLAVOXATE

Chemical name: Flavoxate hydrochloride—4*H*-1-Benzopyran-8-carboxylic acid, 3-methyl-4-oxo-2-phenyl-, 2-(1-piperidinyl)-ethyl ester, hydrochloride.

Molecular formula: Flavoxate hydrochloride—$C_{24}H_{25}NO_4 \cdot HCl$.

Molecular weight: Flavoxate hydrochloride—427.93.

Description: Flavoxate hydrochloride—Off-white, crystalline powder. Melts at about 230 °C, with decomposition.

Solubility: Flavoxate hydrochloride—One gram dissolves in 6 mL water or in 500 mL alcohol.

USP requirements: Flavoxate Hydrochloride Tablets—Not in USP.

FLECAINIDE

Chemical name: Flecainide acetate—Benzamide, *N*-(2-piperidinylmethyl)-2,5-bis(2,2,2-trifluoroethoxy)-, monoacetate.

Molecular formula: Flecainide acetate—$C_{17}H_{20}F_6N_2O_3 \cdot C_2H_4O_2$.

Molecular weight: Flecainide acetate—474.40.

Description: Flecainide acetate—White crystalline substance.

pKa: Flecainide acetate—9.3.

Solubility: Flecainide acetate—Aqueous: 48.4 mg per mL at 37 °C.

USP requirements: Flecainide Acetate Tablets—Not in USP.

FLOCTAFENINE

Chemical name: Benzoic acid, 2-[[8-(trifluoromethyl)-4-quinolinyl]amino]-, 2,3-dihydroxypropyl ester.

Molecular formula: $C_{20}H_{17}F_3N_2O_4$.

Molecular weight: 406.36.

Description: Melting point 179–180 °C.

Solubility: Soluble in alcohol and in acetone; very slightly soluble in ether, in chloroform, and in methylene chloride; insoluble in water.

USP requirements: Floctafenine Tablets—Not in USP.

FLOXURIDINE

Chemical group: A fluorinated pyrimidine derivative.

Chemical name: Uridine, 2′-deoxy-5-fluoro-.

Molecular formula: $C_9H_{11}FN_2O_5$.

Molecular weight: 246.20.

Description: White to off-white odorless solid.

Solubility: Freely soluble in water; soluble in alcohol.

Other characteristics: Hydrophilic.

USP requirements:
Floxuridine USP—Preserve in tight, light-resistant containers. Contains not less than 98.5% and not more than 101.0% of floxuridine, calculated on the dried basis. Meets the requirements for Identification, Melting range (149–153 °C), Specific rotation (+36° to +39°, calculated on the dried basis), Loss on drying (not more than 0.2%), Residue on ignition (not more than 0.1%), Fluoride ions (not more than 0.05%), and Heavy metals (not more than 0.002%).
Sterile Floxuridine USP—Preserve in Containers for Sterile Solids, as described under Injections, protected from light. Store containers of constituted Sterile Floxuridine under refrigeration for not more than 2 weeks. It is lyophilized Floxuridine suitable for intraarterial infusion. Contains the labeled amount, within ±10%. Meets the requirements for Constituted solution, Identification, Pyrogen, Uniformity of dosage units, pH (4.0–5.5 in a solution [1 in 50]), and Injections (Sterile Solids).

FLUCLOXACILLIN

Molecular formula: Flucloxacillin sodium—$C_{19}H_{16}ClFN_3NaO_5S \cdot H_2O$.

Molecular weight: Flucloxacillin sodium—493.9.

Description: Flucloxacillin sodium—White or almost white crystalline hygroscopic powder.

Solubility: Flucloxacillin sodium—Soluble 1 in 1 of water and 1 in 2 of methyl alcohol; soluble in alcohol.

USP requirements:
Flucloxacillin Sodium Capsules—Not in USP.
Flucloxacillin Sodium for Oral Solution—Not in USP.

FLUCONAZOLE

Chemical name: 1*H*-1,2,4-Triazole-1-ethanol, alpha-(2,4-difluorophenyl)-alpha-(1*H*-1,2,4-triazol-1-ylmethyl)-.

Molecular formula: $C_{13}H_{12}F_2N_6O$.

Molecular weight: 306.27.

Description: White crystalline solid.

Solubility: Slightly soluble in water and in saline.

USP requirements:
Fluconazole Injection—Not in USP.
Fluconazole Tablets—Not in USP.

FLUCYTOSINE

Chemical group: Fluorinated pyrimidine derivative; chemically related to fluorouracil and floxuridine.

Chemical name: Cytosine, 5-fluoro-.

Molecular formula: $C_4H_4FN_3O$.

Molecular weight: 129.09.

Description: Flucytosine USP—White to off-white, crystalline powder. Is odorless or has a slight odor.

Solubility: Flucytosine USP—Sparingly soluble in water; slightly soluble in alcohol; practically insoluble in chloroform and in ether.

USP requirements:
Flucytosine USP—Preserve in tight, light-resistant containers. Contains not less than 98.5% and not more than 101.0% of flucytosine, calculated on the dried basis. Meets the requirements for Identification, Loss on drying (not more than 1.5%), Residue on ignition (not more than 0.1%), Heavy metals (not more than 0.002%), Fluoride ions (not more than 0.05%), Fluorouracil (not more than 0.1%), and Organic volatile impurities.
Flucytosine Capsules USP—Preserve in tight, light-resistant containers. Contain the labeled amount, within ±10%. Meet the requirements for Identification, Dissolution (75% in 45 minutes in water in Apparatus 2 at 100 rpm), and Uniformity of dosage units.

FLUDARABINE

Chemical name: Fludarabine phosphate—9*H*-Purin-6-amine, 2-fluoro-9-(5-*O*-phosphono-beta-D-arabinofuranosyl)-.

Molecular formula: Fludarabine phosphate—$C_{10}H_{13}FN_5O_7P$.

Molecular weight: Fludarabine phosphate—365.21.

USP requirements: Fludarabine Phosphate for Injection—Not in USP.

FLUDROCORTISONE

Chemical name: Fludrocortisone acetate—Pregn-4-ene-3,20-dione, 21-(acetyloxy)-9-fluoro-11,17-dihydroxy-, (11 beta)-.

Molecular formula: Fludrocortisone acetate—$C_{23}H_{31}FO_6$.

Molecular weight: Fludrocortisone acetate—422.49.

Description: Fludrocortisone Acetate USP—White to pale yellow crystals or crystalline powder. Is odorless or practically odorless. Is hygroscopic.

Solubility: Fludrocortisone Acetate USP—Insoluble in water; slightly soluble in ether; sparingly soluble in alcohol and in chloroform.

USP requirements:
Fludrocortisone Acetate USP—Preserve in well-closed containers, protected from light. Contains not less than 97.0% and not more than 103.0% of fludrocortisone acetate, calculated on the dried basis. Meets the requirements for Identification, Specific rotation (+126° to +138°, calculated on the dried basis), Loss on drying (not more than 3.0%), Residue on ignition (not more than 0.1%), and Chromatographic impurities.
Fludrocortisone Acetate Tablets USP—Preserve in well-closed containers. Contain the labeled amount, within ±10%. Meet the requirements for Identification, Disintegration (30 minutes), and Uniformity of dosage units.

FLUMAZENIL

Chemical name: 4*H*-Imidazo[1,5-alpha][1,4]benzodiazepine-3-carboxylic acid, 8-fluoro-5,6-dihydro-5-methyl-6-oxo-, ethyl ester.

Molecular formula: $C_{15}H_{14}FN_3O_3$.

Molecular weight: 303.29.

Description: White to off-white crystalline compound.

Solubility: Insoluble in water; slightly soluble in acidic aqueous solutions.

Other characteristics: Octanol:buffer partition coefficient—14 to 1 at pH 7.4.

USP requirements: Flumazenil Injection—Not in USP.

FLUMETHASONE

Chemical name: Flumethasone pivalate—Pregna-1,4-diene-3,20-dione, 21-(2,2-dimethyl-1-oxopropoxy)-6,9-difluoro-11,17-dihydroxy-16-methyl-, (6 alpha,11 beta,16 alpha)-.

Molecular formula: Flumethasone pivalate—$C_{27}H_{36}F_2O_6$.

Molecular weight: Flumethasone pivalate—494.58.

Description: Flumethasone Pivalate USP—White to off-white, crystalline powder.

Solubility: Flumethasone Pivalate USP—Insoluble in water; slightly soluble in methanol; very slightly soluble in chloroform and in methylene chloride.

USP requirements:
Flumethasone Pivalate USP—Preserve in tight, light-resistant containers. Contains not less than 97.0% and not more than 103.0% of flumethasone pivalate, calculated on the dried basis. Meets the requirements for Identification, Specific rotation (+71° to +82°, calculated on the dried basis), Loss on drying (not more than 1.0%), and Chromatographic impurities.
Flumethasone Pivalate Cream USP—Preserve in collapsible tubes. Contains the labeled amount, within ±10%, in a suitable cream base. Meets the requirements for Identification, Microbial limits, and Minimum fill.
Flumethasone Pivalate Ointment—Not in USP.

FLUNARIZINE

Chemical name: Flunarizine hydrochloride—Piperazine, 1-[bis(4-fluorophenyl)methyl]-4-(3-phenyl-2-propenyl)-, dihydrochloride, (*E*)-.

Molecular formula: Flunarizine hydrochloride—$C_{26}H_{26}F_2N_2 \cdot 2HCl$.

Molecular weight: Flunarizine hydrochloride—477.42.

Description: White to pale cream colored powder.

Solubility: Soluble in dimethylsulfoxide, in polyethylene glycol (PEG) 400, in propylene glycol, in *N,N*-dimethylformamide, and in methanol; poorly soluble in water and in ethanol (0.1–1.0%).

USP requirements: Flunarizine Hydrochloride Capsules—Not in USP.

FLUNISOLIDE

Chemical name: Pregna-1,4-diene-3,20-dione, 6-fluoro-11,21-dihydroxy-16,17-[(1-methylethylidene)bis(oxy)]-, hemihydrate, (6 alpha,11 beta,16 alpha)-.

Molecular formula: $C_{24}H_{31}FO_6 \cdot ½H_2O$.

Molecular weight: 443.51; 434.51 (anhydrous).

Description: Flunisolide USP—White to creamy-white, crystalline powder. Melts at about 245 °C, with decomposition.

Solubility: Flunisolide USP—Practically insoluble in water; soluble in acetone; sparingly soluble in chloroform; slightly soluble in methanol.

USP requirements:
Flunisolide USP—Preserve in well-closed containers. Contains not less than 97.0% and not more than 102.0% of flunisolide, calculated on the anhydrous basis. Meets the requirements for Identification, Specific rotation (+103° to +111°, calculated on the dried basis), Loss on drying (not more than 1.0%), Water (not more than 1.0% for the anhydrous form and 1.8–2.5% for the hemihydrate form [determined on a dried specimen]), Residue on ignition (not more than 0.1% from 250 mg), Chromatographic impurities, and Organic volatile impurities.
Flunisolide Inhalation Aerosol—Not in USP.
Flunisolide Nasal Solution USP—Preserve in tight containers, protected from light, at controlled room temperature. An aqueous, buffered solution of Flunisolide. It is supplied in a form suitable for nasal administration. Contains the labeled amount, within ±10%. Meets the requirements for Identification, pH (4.5–6.0), and Quantity delivered per spray (17–33 mcg).

FLUOCINOLONE

Chemical name: Fluocinolone acetonide—Pregna-1,4-diene-3,20-dione, 6,9-difluoro-11,21-dihydroxy-16,17-[(1-methylethylidene)bis(oxy)]-, (6 alpha,11 beta,16 alpha)-.

Molecular formula: Fluocinolone acetonide—$C_{24}H_{30}F_2O_6$ (anhydrous); $C_{24}H_{30}F_2O_6 \cdot 2H_2O$ (dihydrate).

Molecular weight: Fluocinolone acetonide—452.50 (anhydrous); 488.53 (dihydrate).

Description: Fluocinolone Acetonide USP—White or practically white, odorless, crystalline powder. Is stable in air. Melts at about 270 °C, with decomposition.

Solubility: Fluocinolone Acetonide USP—Insoluble in water; soluble in methanol; slightly soluble in ether and in chloroform.

USP requirements:
Fluocinolone Acetonide USP—Preserve in well-closed containers. It is anhydrous or contains two molecules of water of hydration. Label it to indicate whether it is anhydrous or hydrous. Contains not less than 97.0% and not more than 102.0% of fluocinolone acetonide, calculated on the dried basis. Meets the requirements for Identification, Specific rotation (+98° to +108°, calculated on the dried basis), and Loss on drying (not more than 8.5%).
Fluocinolone Acetonide Cream USP—Preserve in collapsible tubes or in tight containers. Contains the labeled amount, within ±10%. Meets the requirements for Identification, Microbial limits, and Minimum fill.
Fluocinolone Acetonide Ointment USP—Preserve in collapsible tubes or in tight containers. Contains the labeled amount, within ±10%. Meets the requirements for Identification, Microbial limits, and Minimum fill.
Fluocinolone Acetonide Topical Solution USP—Preserve in tight containers. Contains the labeled amount, within ±10%. Meets the requirements for Identification and Microbial limits.

FLUOCINONIDE

Chemical name: Pregna-1,4-diene-3,20-dione, 21-(acetyloxy)-6,9-difluoro-11-hydroxy-16,17-[(1-methylethylidene)bis(oxy)]-, (6 alpha,11 beta,16 alpha)-.

Molecular formula: $C_{26}H_{32}F_2O_7$.

Molecular weight: 494.53.

Description: Fluocinonide USP—White to cream-colored, crystalline powder, having not more than a slight odor.

Solubility: Fluocinonide USP—Practically insoluble in water; sparingly soluble in acetone and in chloroform; slightly soluble in alcohol, in methanol, and in dioxane; very slightly soluble in ether.

USP requirements:

Fluocinonide USP—Preserve in well-closed containers. Contains not less than 97.0% and not more than 103.0% of fluocinonide, calculated on the dried basis. Meets the requirements for Identification, Specific rotation (+81° to +89°, calculated on the dried basis), Loss on drying (not more than 1.0%), Residue on ignition (negligible, from 100 mg), and Chromatographic purity.

Fluocinonide Cream USP—Preserve in collapsible tubes or in tight containers. Contains the labeled amount, within ±10%. Meets the requirements for Identification, Microbial limits, and Minimum fill.

Fluocinonide Gel USP—Preserve in collapsible tubes or in tight containers. Contains the labeled amount, within ±10%. Meets the requirements for Identification and Minimum fill.

Fluocinonide Ointment USP—Preserve in collapsible tubes or in tight containers. Contains the labeled amount, within ±10%. Meets the requirements for Identification and Minimum fill.

Fluocinonide Topical Solution USP—Preserve in tight containers. Contains the labeled amount, within ±10%. Meets the requirements for Identification, Alcohol content (28.4–39.0%), and Minimum fill.

FLUOCINONIDE, PROCINONIDE, AND CIPROCINONIDE

Chemical name:

Fluocinonide—Pregna-1,4-diene-3,20-dione, 21-(acetyloxy)-6,9-difluoro-11-hydroxy-16,17-[(1-methylethylidene)bis(oxy)]-, (6 alpha,11 beta,16 alpha)-.

Procinonide—Pregna-1,4-diene-3,20-dione, 6,9-difluoro-11-hydroxy-16,17-[(1-methylethylidene)bis(oxy)]-21-(1-oxopropoxy)-, (6 alpha,11 beta,16 alpha)-.

Ciprocinonide—Pregna-1,4-diene-3,20-dione, 21-[(cyclopropylcarbonyl)oxy]-6,9-difluoro-11-hydroxy-16,17-[(1-methylethylidene)bis(oxy)]-, (6 alpha,11 beta,16 alpha)-.

Molecular formula:

Fluocinonide—$C_{26}H_{32}F_2O_7$.
Procinonide—$C_{27}H_{34}F_2O_7$.
Ciprocinonide—$C_{28}H_{34}F_2O_7$.

Molecular weight:

Fluocinonide—494.53.
Procinonide—508.56.
Ciprocinonide—520.57.

Description: Fluocinonide USP—White to cream-colored, crystalline powder, having not more than a slight odor.

Solubility: Fluocinonide USP—Practically insoluble in water; sparingly soluble in acetone and in chloroform; slightly soluble in alcohol, in methanol, and in dioxane; very slightly soluble in ether.

USP requirements: Fluocinonide, Procinonide, and Ciprocinonide Cream—Not in USP.

FLUORESCEIN

Chemical name:

Fluorescein—Spiro[isobenzofuran-1(3*H*),9′-[9*H*]xanthen]-3-one,3′6′-dihydroxy-.

Fluorescein sodium—Spiro[isobenzofuran-1(3*H*),9′-[9*H*]-xanthene]-3-one, 3′6′-dihydroxy, disodium salt.

Molecular formula:

Fluorescein—$C_{20}H_{12}O_5$.
Fluorescein sodium—$C_{20}H_{10}Na_2O_5$.

Molecular weight:

Fluorescein—332.31.
Fluorescein sodium—376.28.

Description:

Fluorescein USP—Yellowish red to red, odorless powder.

Fluorescein Sodium USP—Orange-red, hygroscopic, odorless powder.

Fluorescein Sodium Ophthalmic Strip USP—Each Strip is a dry, white piece of paper, one end of which is rounded and is uniformly orange-red in color because of the fluorescein sodium impregnated in the paper.

Solubility:

Fluorescein USP—Insoluble in water; soluble in dilute alkali hydroxides.

Fluorescein Sodium USP—Freely soluble in water; sparingly soluble in alcohol.

USP requirements:

Fluorescein USP—Preserve in tight containers. Contains not less than 97.0% and not more than 102.0% of fluorescein, calculated on the anhydrous basis. Meets the requirements for Identification, Water (not more than 1.0%), Zinc, and Acriflavine.

Fluorescein Injection USP—Preserve in single-dose containers, preferably of Type I glass. A sterile solution, in Water for Injection, of Fluorescein prepared with the aid of Sodium Hydroxide. Contains an amount of fluorescein equivalent to the labeled amount of fluorescein sodium, within ±10%. Meets the requirements for Identification, Pyrogen, pH (8.0–9.8), and Injections.

Fluorescein Sodium USP—Preserve in tight containers. Contains not less than 90.0% and not more than 102.0% of fluorescein sodium, calculated on the anhydrous basis. Meets the requirements for Identification, Water (not more than 17.0%), Zinc, and Acriflavine.

Fluorescein Sodium Ophthalmic Strips USP—Package not more than 2 Strips in a single-unit container in such manner as to maintain sterility until the package is opened. Package individual packages in a second protective container. The label of the second protective container bears a statement that the contents may not be sterile if the individual package has been damaged or previously opened. The label states the amount of fluorescein sodium in each Strip. Contain the labeled amount, within +60%. Meet the requirements for Identification, Sterility, and Content uniformity (85.0–175.0% of labeled amount).

FLUORESCEIN AND BENOXINATE

For *Fluorescein* and *Benoxinate*—See individual listings for chemistry information.

USP requirements: Fluorescein Sodium and Benoxinate Hydrochloride Ophthalmic Solution USP—Preserve in tight, light-resistant containers. A sterile aqueous solution of Fluorescein Sodium and Benoxinate Hydrochloride. Contains the labeled amounts, within −10% to +20%. Contains a suitable preservative. Meets the requirements for Identification, Sterility, and pH (4.3–5.3).

FLUORESCEIN AND PROPARACAINE

For *Fluorescein* and *Proparacaine*—See individual listings for chemistry information.

USP requirements: Fluorescein Sodium and Proparacaine Hydrochloride Ophthalmic Solution USP—Preserve in tight, light-resistant containers, preferably of Type I amber glass, and store in a refrigerator. A sterile aqueous solution of Fluorescein Sodium and Proparacaine Hydrochloride. Label it to state that it is to be stored in a refrigerator before and after the container is opened. Contains the labeled amounts, within ±10%. Contains a suitable preservative. Meets the requirements for Identification, Sterility, and pH (4.0–5.2).

FLUDEOXYGLUCOSE F 18

Source: Different methods are being used in the various clinical facilities for the on-site production of FDG injection. It can be prepared either by the electrophilic reaction of ^{18}F-enriched fluorine gas with 3,4,6-tri-O-acetyl-D-glucal or by the nucleophilic reaction of ^{18}F-labeled acetylhypofluorite with suitably protected D-mannopyranose. The fluorinated product is hydrolyzed with acid to give a mixture of 2-fluoro-2-deoxy-D-glucose and 2-fluoro-2-deoxy-D-mannose. Subsequently, it is purified by column chromatography and dissolved in an appropriate solvent, most commonly 0.9% saline.

Chemical group: D-glucose analog.

Chemical name: Alpha-D-glucopyranose, 2-deoxy-2-(fluoro-^{18}F)-.

Molecular formula: $C_6H_{11}{}^{18}FO_5$.

Molecular weight: 182.

pKa: None between pH 1–13.

Solubility: Very soluble in water.

Other characteristics: Partition coefficient—Hydrocarbon: water (<0.001).

USP requirements: Fludeoxyglucose F 18 Injection USP—Preserve in single-dose or in multiple-dose containers that are adequately shielded. A sterile, isotonic aqueous solution, suitable for intravenous administration, of 2-deoxy-2-[^{18}F]fluoro-D-glucose in which a portion of the molecules are labeled with radioactive ^{18}F. Label it to include the following, in addition to the information specified for Labeling under Injection: the time and date of calibration; the amount of ^{18}F as fludeoxyglucose expressed as total MBq (or millicurie) per mL, at the time of calibration; the expiration date; the name and quantity of any added preservative or stabilizer; and the statement, "Caution, Radioactive Material." The labeling indicates that in making dosage calculations, correction is to be made for radioactive decay. The radioactive half-life of ^{18}F is 110 minutes. The label indicates "Do not use if cloudy or if it contains particulate matter." Contains the labeled amount of ^{18}F, within ±10%, expressed in MBq (or millicurie) per mL at the time indicated in the labeling. It has a Specific activity of not less than 37×10^3 MBq (1 curie) per mmol. Meets the requirements for Radionuclide identification, Bacterial endotoxins, pH (4.5–8.5), Radiochemical purity, Isomeric purity, Radionuclidic purity, Chemical purity, and Injections (except that the Injection may be distributed or dispensed prior to completion of the test for Sterility, the latter test being started on the day following final manufacture, and except that it is not subject to the recommendation on Volume in Container).

FLUORODOPA F 18

Chemical name: L-Tyrosine, 2-(fluoro-^{18}F)-5-hydroxy-.

Molecular formula: $C_9H_{10}{}^{18}FNO_4$.

USP requirements: Fluorodopa F 18 Injection USP—Preserve in single-dose or in multiple-dose containers that are adequately shielded. A sterile, isotonic aqueous solution, suitable for intravenous administration of 6-[^{18}F]fluorolevodopa in which a portion of the molecules are labeled with radioactive ^{18}F. Label it to include the following, in addition to the information specified for Labeling under Injections: the time and date of calibration; the amount of ^{18}F as fluorodopa expressed as total megabecquerels (MBq or millicuries) per mL, at time of calibration; the expiration date; the name and quantity of any added preservative or stabilizer; and the statement "Caution—Radioactive Material." The labeling indicates that in making dosage calculations correction is to be made for radioactive decay. The radioactive half-life of ^{18}F is 110 minutes. The label indicates "Do not use if cloudy or if it contains particulate matter." Contains the labeled amount of ^{18}F expressed in megabecquerels (MBq or millicuries) per mL at the time indicated in the labeling, within ±10%. Meets the requirements for Specific activity (not less than 3.7×10^3 MBq [100 millicuries] per mmol), Radionuclide identification, Bacterial endotoxins, pH (4.0–5.0), Radiochemical purity, Radionuclidic purity, Chemical purity, Enantiomeric purity, and Injections (except that the Injection may be distributed or dispensed prior to completion of the test for Sterility, the latter test being started on the day following final manufacture, and except that it is not subject to the recommendation of Volume in Container).

FLUOROMETHOLONE

Chemical name:
Fluorometholone—Pregna-1,4-diene-3,20-dione, 9-fluoro-11,17-dihydroxy-6-methyl-, (6 alpha,11 beta)-.
Fluorometholone acetate—Pregna-1,4-diene-3,20-dione, 17-(acetyloxy)-9-fluoro-11-hydroxy-6-methyl-, (6 alpha,11 beta)-.

Molecular formula:
Fluorometholone—$C_{22}H_{29}FO_4$.
Fluorometholone acetate—$C_{24}H_{31}FO_5$.

Molecular weight:
Fluorometholone—376.47.
Fluorometholone acetate—418.51.

Description: Fluorometholone USP—White to yellowish white, odorless, crystalline powder. Melts at about 280 °C, with some decomposition.

Solubility: Fluorometholone USP—Practically insoluble in water; slightly soluble in alcohol; very slightly soluble in chloroform and in ether.

USP requirements:
Fluorometholone USP—Preserve in tight, light-resistant containers. Contains not less than 97.0% and not more than 103.0% of fluorometholone, calculated on the dried basis. Meets the requirements for Identification, Specific rotation (+52° to +60°, calculated on the dried basis), Loss on drying (not more than 1.0%), and Residue on ignition (not more than 0.2%).
Fluorometholone Cream USP—Preserve in collapsible tubes. Contains the labeled amount, within ±10%. Meets the requirements for Identification, Microbial limits, and Minimum fill.
Fluorometholone Ophthalmic Ointment—Not in USP.
Fluorometholone Ophthalmic Suspension USP—Preserve in tight containers. A sterile suspension of Fluorometholone in a suitable aqueous medium. Contains the labeled amount, within ±10%. Meets the requirements for Identification, Sterility, and pH (6.0–7.5).
Fluorometholone Acetate Ophthalmic Suspension—Not in USP.

FLUOROURACIL

Chemical name: 2,4(1*H*,3*H*)-Pyrimidinedione, 5-fluoro-.

Molecular formula: $C_4H_3FN_2O_2$.

Molecular weight: 130.08.

Description: Fluorouracil USP—White to practically white, practically odorless, crystalline powder. Decomposes at about 282 °C.

pKa: 8.0 and 13.0.

Solubility: Fluorouracil USP—Sparingly soluble in water; slightly soluble in alcohol; practically insoluble in chloroform and in ether.

USP requirements:

Fluorouracil USP—Preserve in tight, light-resistant containers. Contains not less than 98.5% and not more than 101.0% of fluorouracil, calculated on the dried basis. Meets the requirements for Identification, Loss on drying (not more than 0.5%), Residue on ignition (not more than 0.1%), Heavy metals (not more than 0.002%), and Fluorine content (13.9–15.0%).

Caution: Great care should be taken to prevent inhaling particles of Fluorouracil and exposing the skin to it.

Fluorouracil Cream USP—Preserve in tight containers, at controlled room temperature. Contains the labeled amount, within ±10%. Meets the requirements for Identification, Microbial limits, and Minimum fill.

Fluorouracil Injection USP—Preserve in single-dose containers, preferably of Type I glass, at controlled room temperature. Avoid freezing and exposure to light. A sterile solution of Fluorouracil in Water for Injection, prepared with the aid of Sodium Hydroxide. Label it to indicate the expiration date, which is not more than 24 months after date of manufacture. Contains, in each mL, not less than 45 mg and not more than 55 mg of fluorouracil. Meets the requirements for Identification, Bacterial endotoxins, pH (8.6–9.4), and Injections.

Note: If a precipitate is formed as a result of exposure to low temperatures, redissolve it by heating to 60 °C with vigorous shaking, and allow to cool to body temperature prior to use.

Fluorouracil Topical Solution USP—Preserve in tight containers, at controlled room temperature. Contains the labeled amount, within ±10%. Meets the requirements for Identification and Microbial limits.

FLUOXETINE

Chemical group: Cyclic, propylamine derivative. Chemically unrelated to tricyclic, tetracyclic, or other available antidepressants.

Chemical name:

Fluoxetine—Benzenepropanamine, *N*-methyl-gamma-[4-(trifluoromethyl)phenoxy]-, (±)-.

Fluoxetine hydrochloride—Benzenepropanamine, *N*-methyl-gamma-[4-(trifluoromethyl)phenoxy]-, hydrochloride, (±)-.

Molecular formula:

Fluoxetine—$C_{17}H_{18}F_3NO$.

Fluoxetine hydrochloride—$C_{17}H_{18}F_3NO \cdot HCl$.

Molecular weight:

Fluoxetine—309.33.

Fluoxetine hydrochloride—345.79.

Description: Fluoxetine hydrochloride—White to off-white crystalline solid.

Solubility: Fluoxetine hydrochloride—Soluble in water.

USP requirements:

Fluoxetine Capsules—Not in USP.

Fluoxetine Hydrochloride Capsules—Not in USP.

Fluoxetine Hydrochloride Oral Solution—Not in USP.

FLUOXYMESTERONE

Chemical group: Synthetic androgen; halogenated derivative of 17-alpha-methyltestosterone.

Chemical name: Androst-4-en-3-one, 9-fluoro-11,17-dihydroxy-17-methyl-, (11 beta,17 beta)-.

Molecular formula: $C_{20}H_{29}FO_3$.

Molecular weight: 336.45.

Description: Fluoxymesterone USP—White or practically white, odorless, crystalline powder. Melts at about 240 °C, with some decomposition.

Solubility: Fluoxymesterone USP—Practically insoluble in water; sparingly soluble in alcohol; slightly soluble in chloroform.

USP requirements:

Fluoxymesterone USP—Preserve in well-closed containers, protected from light. Contains not less than 97.0% and not more than 102.0% of fluoxymesterone, calculated on the dried basis. Meets the requirements for Identification, Specific rotation (+104° to +112°, calculated on the dried basis), Loss on drying (not more than 1.0%), Ordinary impurities, and Organic volatile impurities.

Fluoxymesterone Tablets USP—Preserve in well-closed containers, protected from light. Contain the labeled amount, within ±10%. Meet the requirements for Identification, Dissolution (70% in 60 minutes in 0.1 *N* hydrochloric acid in Apparatus 2 at 75 rpm), and Uniformity of dosage units.

FLUOXYMESTERONE AND ETHINYL ESTRADIOL

For *Fluoxymesterone* and *Ethinyl Estradiol*—See individual listings for chemistry information.

USP requirements: Fluoxymesterone and Ethinyl Estradiol Tablets—Not in USP.

FLUPENTHIXOL

Chemical group: Thioxanthene.

Chemical name:

Flupenthixol decanoate—Cis-2-trifluoromethyl-9-(3-(4-(2-hydroxyethyl)-1-piperazinyl)-propylidene)-thioxanthene decanoate acid ester.

Flupenthixol dihydrochloride—2-Trifluoromethyl-9-(3-(4-(2-hydroxyethyl)-1-piperazinyl)-propylidene)-thioxanthene dihydrochloride.

Molecular formula:

Flupenthixol decanoate—$C_{33}H_{43}F_3N_2O_2S$.

Flupenthixol dihydrochloride—$C_{23}H_{25}F_3N_2OS \cdot 2HCl$.

Molecular weight:

Flupenthixol decanoate—588.8.

Flupenthixol dihydrochloride—507.4.

Description:

Flupenthixol decanoate—Yellow oil with a slight odor.

Flupenthixol dihydrochloride—White or yellowish white powder.

Solubility:

Flupenthixol decanoate—Very slightly soluble in water; soluble in alcohol; freely soluble in chloroform and in ether.

Flupenthixol dihydrochloride—Soluble in water and in alcohol.

Other characteristics: Structurally and pharmacologically similar to the piperazine phenothiazines, which are acetophenazine, fluphenazine, perphenazine, prochlorperazine, and trifluoperazine.

USP requirements:
Flupenthixol Decanoate Injection—Not in USP.
Flupenthixol Dihydrochloride Tablets—Not in USP.

FLUPHENAZINE

Chemical group: Trifluoromethyl phenothiazine derivative.

Chemical name:
Fluphenazine decanoate—2-{4-[3-(2-Trifluoromethylphenothiazin-10-yl)propyl]-piperazin-1-yl}ethyl decanoate.
Fluphenazine enanthate—Heptanoic acid, 2-[4-[3-[2-(trifluoromethyl)-10*H*-phenothiazin-10-yl]propyl]-1-piperazinyl]ethyl ester.
Fluphenazine hydrochloride—1-Piperazineethanol, 4-[3-[2-(trifluoromethyl)-10*H*-phenothiazin-10-yl]propyl]-, dihydrochloride.

Molecular formula:
Fluphenazine decanoate—$C_{32}H_{44}F_3N_3O_2S$.
Fluphenazine enanthate—$C_{29}H_{38}F_3N_3O_2S$.
Fluphenazine hydrochloride—$C_{22}H_{26}F_3N_3OS \cdot 2HCl$.

Molecular weight:
Fluphenazine decanoate—591.8.
Fluphenazine enanthate—549.69.
Fluphenazine hydrochloride—510.45.

Description:
Fluphenazine decanoate—Pale yellow viscous liquid or a yellow crystalline oily solid with a faint ester-like odor.
Fluphenazine Enanthate USP—Pale yellow to yellow-orange, clear to slightly turbid, viscous liquid, having a characteristic odor; unstable in strong light, but stable to air at room temperature.
Fluphenazine Hydrochloride USP—White or nearly white, odorless, crystalline powder; melts, within a range of 5°, at a temperature above 225 °C.

Solubility:
Fluphenazine decanoate—Practically insoluble in water; miscible with dehydrated alcohol, with chloroform, and with ether; soluble in fixed oils.
Fluphenazine Enanthate USP—Insoluble in water; freely soluble in alcohol, in chloroform, and in ether.
Fluphenazine Hydrochloride USP—Freely soluble in water; slightly soluble in acetone, in alcohol, and in chloroform; practically insoluble in ether.

USP requirements:
Fluphenazine Decanoate USP—Preserve in tight, light-resistant containers. Contains not less than 98.0% and not more than 102.0% of fluphenazine decanoate, calculated on the dried basis. Meets the requirements for Identification, Loss on drying (not more than 1.0%), Residue on ignition (not more than 0.2%), and Ordinary impurities.
Fluphenazine Decanoate Injection USP—Preserve in single-dose or in multiple-dose containers, of Type I glass, protected from light. A sterile solution of Fluphenazine Decanoate in a suitable vegetable oil. Contains the labeled amount, within −10% to +15%. Meets the requirements for Identification, Chromatographic purity, and Injections.
Fluphenazine Enanthate USP—Preserve in tight, light-resistant containers. Contains not less than 97.0% and not more than 103.0% of fluphenazine enanthate, calculated on the dried basis. Meets the requirements for Identification, Loss on drying (not more than 1.0%), Residue on ignition (not more than 0.2%), Heavy metals (not more than 0.003%), and Ordinary impurities.
Fluphenazine Enanthate Injection USP—Preserve in single-dose or in multiple-dose containers, preferably of Type I or Type III glass, protected from light. A sterile solution of Fluphenazine Enanthate in a suitable vegetable oil. Contains the labeled amount, within ±10%. Meets the requirements for Identification and Injections.
Fluphenazine Hydrochloride USP—Preserve in tight, light-resistant containers. Contains not less than 97.0% and not more than 103.0% of fluphenazine hydrochloride, calculated on the dried basis. Meets the requirements for Identification, Loss on drying (not more than 1%), Residue on ignition (not more than 0.5%), Heavy metals (not more than 0.003%), Ordinary impurities, and Organic volatile impurities.
Fluphenazine Hydrochloride Elixir USP—Preserve in tight containers, protected from light. Contains the labeled amount, within ±10%. Meets the requirements for Identification, pH (5.3–5.8), and Alcohol content (13.5–15.0%).
Fluphenazine Hydrochloride Injection USP—Preserve in single-dose or in multiple-dose containers, preferably of Type I glass, protected from light. A sterile solution of Fluphenazine Hydrochloride in Water for Injection. Contains the labeled amount, within −5% to +10%. Meets the requirements for Identification, Bacterial endotoxins, pH (4.8–5.2), and Injections.
Fluphenazine Hydrochloride Oral Solution USP—Preserve in tight containers, protected from light. An aqueous solution of Fluphenazine Hydrochloride. Contains the labeled amount, within ±10%. Label it to indicate that it is to be diluted to appropriate strength with water or other suitable fluid prior to administration. Meets the requirements for Identification, pH (4.0–5.0), and Alcohol content (within ±10% of the labeled amount, the labeled amount being not more than 15.0%).
Fluphenazine Hydrochloride Tablets USP—Preserve in tight, light-resistant containers. Contain the labeled amount, within ±10%. Meet the requirements for Identification, Dissolution (75% in 45 minutes in 0.1 *N* hydrochloric acid in Apparatus 1 at 100 rpm), and Uniformity of dosage units.

FLURANDRENOLIDE

Chemical name: Pregn-4-ene-3,20-dione, 6-fluoro-11,21-dihydroxy-16,17-[(1-methylethylidene)bis(oxy)]-, (6 alpha,11 beta,16 alpha)-.

Molecular formula: $C_{24}H_{33}FO_6$.

Molecular weight: 436.52.

Description: Flurandrenolide USP—White to off-white, fluffy, crystalline powder. Is odorless.

Solubility: Flurandrenolide USP—Practically insoluble in water and in ether; freely soluble in chloroform; soluble in methanol; sparingly soluble in alcohol.

USP requirements:
Flurandrenolide USP—Preserve in tight containers in a cold place, protected from light. Contains not less than 97.0% and not more than 102.0% of flurandrenolide, calculated on the dried basis. Meets the requirements for Identification, Specific rotation (+145° to +153°, calculated on the dried basis), Loss on drying (not more than 1.0%), and Ordinary impurities.
Flurandrenolide Cream USP—Preserve in tight containers, protected from light. Contains the labeled amount, within ±10%. Meets the requirements for Identification, Microbial limits, and Minimum fill.

Flurandrenolide Lotion USP—Preserve in tight containers, protected from heat, light, and freezing. Contains the labeled amount, within ±10%. Meets the requirements for Identification, Microbial limits, pH (3.5–6.0), and Minimum fill.

Flurandrenolide Ointment USP—Preserve in tight containers, protected from light. Contains the labeled amount, within ±10%. Meets the requirements for Identification, Microbial limits, and Minimum fill.

Flurandrenolide Tape USP—Preserve at controlled room temperature. A non-porous, pliable, adhesive-type tape having Flurandrenolide impregnated in the adhesive material, the adhesive material on one side being transported on a removable, protective slit-paper liner. Contains the labeled amount, within −20% to +25%. Meets the requirements for Identification and Microbial limits.

FLURAZEPAM

Chemical name:

Flurazepam hydrochloride—2*H*-1,4-Benzodiazepin-2-one, 7-chloro-1-[2-(diethylamino)ethyl]-5-(2-fluorophenyl)-1,3-dihydro-, dihydrochloride.

Flurazepam monohydrochloride—7-Chloro-1-(2-diethylaminoethyl)-5-(2-fluorophenyl)-1,3-dihydro-1,4-benzodiazepin-2-one hydrochloride.

Molecular formula:

Flurazepam hydrochloride—$C_{21}H_{23}ClFN_3O \cdot 2HCl$.

Flurazepam monohydrochloride—$C_{21}H_{23}ClFN_3O \cdot HCl$.

Molecular weight:

Flurazepam hydrochloride—460.81.

Flurazepam monohydrochloride—424.4.

Description:

Flurazepam Hydrochloride USP—Off-white to yellow, crystalline powder. Is odorless, or has a slight odor, and its solutions are acid to litmus. Melts at about 212 °C, with decomposition.

Flurazepam monohydrochloride—White or almost white, odorless or almost odorless crystalline powder.

Solubility:

Flurazepam Hydrochloride USP—Freely soluble in water and in alcohol; slightly soluble in isopropyl alcohol and in chloroform.

Flurazepam monohydrochloride—Very soluble in water; freely soluble in alcohol; practically insoluble in ether.

USP requirements:

Flurazepam Hydrochloride USP—Preserve in tight, light-resistant containers. Contains not less than 99.0% and not more than 101.0% of flurazepam hydrochloride, calculated on the dried basis. Meets the requirements for Identification, Loss on drying (not more than 1.5%), Residue on ignition (not more than 0.1%), Heavy metals (not more than 0.002%), Limit of fluoride ion (not more than 0.05%), Related compounds, and Organic volatile impurities.

Flurazepam Hydrochloride Capsules USP—Preserve in tight, light-resistant containers. Contain the labeled amount, within ±10%. Meet the requirements for Identification, Dissolution (75% in 20 minutes in 0.1 *N* hydrochloric acid in Apparatus 1 at 100 rpm), and Uniformity of dosage units.

Flurazepam Monohydrochloride Tablets—Not in USP.

FLURBIPROFEN

Chemical group: A phenylalkanoic acid derivative chemically related to fenoprofen, ibuprofen, ketoprofen, naproxen, and tiaprofenic acid.

Chemical name:

Flurbiprofen—[1,1′-Biphenyl]-4-acetic acid, 2-fluoro-alpha-methyl-, (±)-.

Flurbiprofen sodium—[1,1′-Biphenyl]-4-acetic acid, 2-fluoro-alpha-methyl, sodium salt dihydrate, (±)-.

Molecular formula:

Flurbiprofen—$C_{15}H_{13}FO_2$.

Flurbiprofen sodium—$C_{15}H_{12}FNaO_2 \cdot 2H_2O$.

Molecular weight:

Flurbiprofen—244.27.

Flurbiprofen sodium—302.28.

Description: White or slightly yellow crystalline powder.

pKa: 4.22.

Solubility: Slightly soluble in water at pH 7.0; readily soluble in most polar solvents.

Other characteristics: Acidic.

USP requirements:

Flurbiprofen USP—Preserve in tight containers. Contains not less than 99.0% and not more than 100.5% of flurbiprofen, calculated on the dried basis. Meets the requirements for Identification, Melting range (114–117 °C), Loss on drying (not more than 0.5%), Residue on ignition (not more than 0.1%), Heavy metals (not more than 0.001%), and Related compounds.

Flurbiprofen Extended-release Capsules—Not in USP.

Flurbiprofen Tablets USP—Preserve in well-closed containers. Contain the labeled amount, within ±10%. Meet the requirements for Identification, Dissolution (75% in 45 minutes in phosphate buffer [pH 7.2] in Apparatus 2 at 50 rpm), and Uniformity of dosage units.

Flurbiprofen Sodium USP—Preserve in well-closed containers. Contains not less than 98.5% and not more than 101.5% of flurbiprofen sodium. Meets the requirements for Identification, Specific rotation (−0.45° to +0.45°, calculated on the dried basis), Loss on drying (11.3–12.5%), Heavy metals (not more than 0.001%), Limit of 2-(4-biphenylyl)propionic acid (not more than 1.5%), and Organic volatile impurities.

Flurbiprofen Sodium Ophthalmic Solution USP—Preserve in tight containers. Contains the labeled amount, within ±10%. Meets the requirements for Identification, pH (6.0–7.0), Antimicrobial preservatives—Effectiveness, and Sterility.

FLUSPIRILENE

Chemical name: 1,3,8-Triazaspiro[4.5]decan-4-one, 8-[4,4-bis(4-fluorophenyl)butyl]-1-phenyl-.

Molecular formula: $C_{29}H_{31}F_2N_3O$.

Molecular weight: 475.58.

Description: White to yellowish amorphous or crystalline solid with a melting point of 187.5–190 °C.

Solubility: Soluble in water (0.015–0.020 mg/mL).

USP requirements: Fluspirilene Injection—Not in USP.

FLUTAMIDE

Chemical name: Propanamide, 2-methyl-*N*-[4-nitro-3-(trifluoromethyl)phenyl]-.

Molecular formula: $C_{11}H_{11}F_3N_2O_3$.

Molecular weight: 276.22.

Description: Buff to yellow powder.

Solubility: Practically insoluble in water.

USP requirements:
Flutamide Capsules—Not in USP.
Flutamide Tablets—Not in USP.

FLUTICASONE

Chemical name: Fluticasone proprionate—Androsta-1,4-diene-17-carbothioic acid, 6,9-difluoro-11-hydroxy-16-methyl-3-oxo-17-(1-oxopropoxy)-, (6 alpha,11 beta,16 alpha,17 alpha)-*S*-(fluoromethyl) ester.

Molecular formula: Fluticasone propionate—$C_{25}H_{31}F_3O_5S$.

Molecular weight: Fluticasone propionate—500.57.

Description: Fluticasone propionate—White to off-white powder.

Solubility: Fluticasone propionate—Insoluble in water.

USP requirements:
Fluticasone Propionate Cream—Not in USP.
Fluticasone Propionate Ointment—Not in USP.

FOLIC ACID

Chemical name: L-Glutamic acid, *N*-[4-[[(2-amino-1,4-dihydro-4-oxo-6-pteridinyl)methyl]amino]benzoyl]-.

Molecular formula: $C_{19}H_{19}N_7O_6$.

Molecular weight: 441.40.

Description:
Folic Acid USP—Yellow, yellow-brownish, or yellowish orange, odorless, crystalline powder.
Folic Acid Injection USP—Clear, yellow to orange-yellow, alkaline liquid.

Solubility: Folic Acid USP—Very slightly soluble in water; insoluble in alcohol, in acetone, in chloroform, and in ether; readily dissolves in dilute solutions of alkali hydroxides and carbonates, and is soluble in hot, 3 *N* hydrochloric acid and in hot, 2 *N* sulfuric acid. Soluble in hydrochloric acid and in sulfuric acid, yielding very pale yellow solutions.

USP requirements:
Folic Acid USP—Preserve in well-closed, light-resistant containers. Contains not less than 95.0% and not more than 102.0% of folic acid, calculated on the anhydrous basis. Meets the requirements for Identification, Water (not more than 8.5%), Residue on ignition (not more than 0.3%), and Organic volatile impurities.
Folic Acid Injection USP—Preserve in single-dose or in multiple-dose containers, preferably of Type I glass, protected from light. A sterile solution of Folic Acid in Water for Injection prepared with the aid of Sodium Hydroxide or Sodium Carbonate. Contains the labeled amount, within −5% to +10%. Meets the requirements for Identification, Bacterial endotoxins, pH (8.0–11.0), and Injections.
Folic Acid Tablets USP—Preserve in well-closed containers. Contain the labeled amount, within −10% to +15%. Meet the requirements for Identification, Disintegration (30 minutes), and Uniformity of dosage units.

FORMALDEHYDE

Chemical name: Formaldehyde solution—Formaldehyde.

Molecular formula: Formaldehyde solution—CH_2O.

Molecular weight: Formaldehyde solution—30.03.

Description: Formaldehyde Solution USP—Clear, colorless or practically colorless liquid, having a pungent odor. The vapor from it irritates the mucous membrane of the throat and nose. On long standing, especially in the cold, it may become cloudy because of the separation of paraformaldehyde. This cloudiness disappears when the solution is warmed.

Solubility: Formaldehyde Solution USP—Miscible with water and with alcohol.

USP requirements: Formaldehyde Solution USP—Preserve in tight containers, preferably at a temperature not below 15 °C. The label of bulk containers of Formaldehyde Solution directs the drug repackager to demonstrate compliance with the USP *Assay* limit for formaldehyde of not less than 37.0%, by weight, immediately prior to repackaging. In bulk containers, contains not less than 37.0%, by weight, of formaldehyde, with methanol added to prevent polymerization. In small containers (4 liters or less), contains not less than 36.5%, by weight, of formaldehyde, with methanol present to prevent polymerization. Meets the requirements for Identification and Acidity.

FOSCARNET

Chemical group: Pyrophosphate analog.

Chemical name: Foscarnet sodium—Phosphinecarboxylic acid, dihydroxy-, oxide, trisodium salt.

Molecular formula:
Foscarnet sodium—CNa_3O_5P.
Foscarnet sodium hexahydrate—$Na_3CO_5P \cdot 6H_2O$.

Molecular weight:
Foscarnet sodium—191.95.
Foscarnet sodium hexahydrate—300.1.

Description:
Foscarnet sodium—White, crystalline powder.
Foscarnet sodium injection—Clear and colorless solution.

Solubility: Foscarnet sodium—Soluble in water at pH 7 and 25 °C (about 5% w/w).

Other characteristics: Foscarnet sodium injection—pH is 7.4.

USP requirements: Foscarnet Sodium Injection—Not in USP.

FOSINOPRIL

Chemical name: Fosinopril sodium—L-Proline, 4-cyclohexyl-1-[[[2-methyl-1-(1-oxopropoxy)propoxy](4-phenylbutyl)phosphinyl]acetyl]-, sodium salt, *trans*-.

Molecular formula: Fosinopril sodium—$C_{30}H_{45}NNaO_7P$.

Molecular weight: Fosinopril sodium—585.65.

Description: Fosinopril sodium—White to off-white crystalline powder.

Solubility: Fosinopril sodium—Soluble in water (100 mg/mL), in methanol, and in ethanol; slightly soluble in hexane.

USP requirements: Fosinopril Sodium Tablets—Not in USP.

FRAMYCETIN

Source: Produced by certain strains of *Streptomyces fradiae* or *Streptomyces decaris*.

Chemical name: 2-Deoxy-4-*O*-(2,6-diamino-2,6-dideoxy-alpha-D-glucopyranosyl)-5-*O*-[3-*O*-(2,6-diamino-2,6-dideoxy-beta-L-idopyranosyl)-beta-D-ribofuranosyl]streptamine sulfate.

Molecular formula: Framycetin sulfate—$C_{23}H_{46}N_6O_{13} \cdot 3H_2SO_4$.

Molecular weight: Framycetin sulfate—908.9.

Description: Framycetin sulfate—White or yellowish-white, odorless or almost odorless, hygroscopic powder.

Solubility: Framycetin sulfate—Soluble 1 in 1 of water; very slightly soluble in alcohol; practically insoluble in acetone, in chloroform, and in ether.

USP requirements:
Framycetin Sulfate Impregnated Gauze—Not in USP.
Framycetin Sulfate Ophthalmic Ointment—Not in USP.
Framycetin Sulfate Ophthalmic Solution—Not in USP.

FRAMYCETIN AND GRAMICIDIN

For *Framycetin* and *Gramicidin*—See individual listings for chemistry information.

USP requirements: Framycetin Sulfate and Gramicidin Ointment—Not in USP.

FRAMYCETIN, GRAMICIDIN, AND DEXAMETHASONE

For *Framycetin, Gramicidin,* and *Dexamethasone*—See individual listings for chemistry information.

USP requirements:
Framycetin Sulfate, Gramicidin, and Dexamethasone Ophthalmic Ointment—Not in USP.
Framycetin Sulfate, Gramicidin, and Dexamethasone Otic Ointment—Not in USP.
Framycetin Sulfate, Gramicidin, and Dexamethasone Ophthalmic Solution—Not in USP.
Framycetin Sulfate, Gramicidin, and Dexamethasone Otic Solution—Not in USP.

FRUCTOSE

Chemical name: D-Fructose.

Molecular formula: $C_6H_{12}O_6$.

Molecular weight: 180.16.

Description: Fructose USP—Colorless crystals or white crystalline powder. Odorless.

NF category: Sweetening agent; tablet and/or capsule diluent.

Solubility: Fructose USP—Freely soluble in water; soluble in alcohol and in methanol.

USP requirements:
Fructose USP—Preserve in well-closed containers. Dried in vacuum at 70 °C for 4 hours, contains not less than 98.0% and not more than 102.0% of fructose. Meets the requirements for Identification, Color of solution, Acidity, Loss on drying (not more than 0.5%), Residue on ignition (not more than 0.5%), Chloride (not more than 0.018%), Sulfate (not more than 0.025%), Arsenic (not more than 1 ppm), Calcium and magnesium (as calcium) (not more than 0.005% calcium), Heavy metals (not more than 5 ppm), and Hydroxymethylfurfural.
Fructose Injection USP—Preserve in single-dose containers, preferably of Type I or Type II glass. A sterile solution of Fructose in Water for Injection. The label states the total osmolar concentration in mOsmol per liter. Where the contents are less than 100 mL, or where the label states that the Injection is not for direct injection but is to be diluted before use, the label alternatively may state the total osmolar concentration in mOsmol per mL. Contains the labeled amount, within ±5%. Contains no antimicrobial agents. Meets the requirements for Identification, Bacterial endotoxins, pH (3.0–6.0), Heavy metals (not more than 5 ppm), Hydroxymethylfurfural, and Injections.

FRUCTOSE, DEXTROSE, AND PHOSPHORIC ACID

For *Fructose, Dextrose,* and *Phosphoric Acid*—See individual listings for chemistry information.

USP requirements: Fructose, Dextrose, and Phosphoric Acid Oral Solution—Not in USP.

FRUCTOSE AND SODIUM CHLORIDE

For *Fructose* and *Sodium Chloride*—See individual listings for chemistry information.

USP requirements: Fructose and Sodium Chloride Injection USP—Preserve in single-dose containers, preferably of Type I or Type II glass. A sterile solution of Fructose and Sodium Chloride in Water for Injection. The label states the total osmolar concentration in mOsmol per liter. Where the contents are less than 100 mL, or where the label states that the Injection is not for direct injection but is to be diluted before use, the label alternatively may state the total osmolar concentration in mOsmol per mL. Contains the labeled amounts of fructose and sodium chloride, within ±5%. Contains no antimicrobial agents. Meets the requirements for Identification, Bacterial endotoxins, pH (3.0–6.0), Heavy metals (not more than 5 ppm), Hydroxymethylfurfural, and Injections.

BASIC FUCHSIN

Chemical name: Benzenamine, 4-[(4-aminophenyl)(4-imino-2,5-cyclohexadien-1-ylidene)methyl]-2-methyl-, monohydrochloride.

Description: Basic Fuchsin USP—Dark green powder or greenish glistening crystalline fragments, having a bronze-like luster and not more than a faint odor.

Solubility: Basic Fuchsin USP—Soluble in water, in alcohol, and in amyl alcohol; insoluble in ether.

USP requirements: Basic Fuchsin USP—Preserve in well-closed containers. A mixture of rosaniline and pararosaniline hydrochlorides. Contains the equivalent of not less than 88.0% of rosaniline hydrochloride, calculated on the dried basis. Meets the requirements for Identification, Loss on drying (not more than 5.0%), Residue on ignition (not more than 0.3%), Alcohol-insoluble substances (not more than 1.0%), Arsenic (not more than 8 ppm), and Lead (not more than 30 ppm).

FUMARIC ACID

Chemical name: 2-Butenedioic acid, [*E*]-.

Molecular formula: $C_4H_4O_4$.

Molecular weight: 116.07.

Description: Fumaric Acid NF—White, odorless granules or crystalline powder.

NF category: Acidifying agent.

Solubility: Fumaric Acid NF—Soluble in alcohol; slightly soluble in water and in ether; very slightly soluble in chloroform.

NF requirements: Fumaric Acid NF—Preserve in well-closed containers. Contains not less than 99.5% and not more than 100.5% of fumaric acid, calculated on the anhydrous basis. Meets the requirements for Identification, Water (0.5%), Residue on ignition (not more than 0.1%), Heavy metals (not more than 0.001%), Maleic acid (not more than 0.1%), and Organic volatile impurities.

FURAZOLIDONE

Chemical group: Nitrofuran.

Chemical name: 2-Oxazolidinone, 3-[[(5-nitro-2-furanyl)methylene]amino]-.

Molecular formula: $C_8H_7N_3O_5$.

Molecular weight: 225.16.

Description: Furazolidone USP—Yellow, odorless, crystalline powder.

Solubility: Furazolidone USP—Practically insoluble in water, in alcohol, and in carbon tetrachloride.

USP requirements:
Furazolidone USP—Preserve in tight, light-resistant containers, and avoid exposure to direct sunlight. Contains not less than 97.0% and not more than 103.0% of furazolidone, calculated on the dried basis. Meets the requirements for Identification, Loss on drying (not more than 1.0%), and Residue on ignition (not more than 0.5%).
Furazolidone Oral Suspension USP—Preserve in tight, light-resistant containers, and avoid exposure to excessive heat. A suspension of Furazolidone in a suitable aqueous vehicle. Contains the labeled amount, within ±10%. Meets the requirements for Identification and pH (6.0–8.5).
Furazolidone Tablets USP—Preserve in tight, light-resistant containers, and avoid exposure to excessive heat. Contain the labeled amount, within ±10%. Meet the requirements for Identification and Uniformity of dosage units.

FUROSEMIDE

Chemical name: Benzoic acid, 5-(aminosulfonyl)-4-chloro-2-[(2-furanylmethyl)amino]-.

Molecular formula: $C_{12}H_{11}ClN_2O_5S$.

Molecular weight: 330.74.

Description:
Furosemide USP—White to slightly yellow, odorless, crystalline powder.
Furosemide Injection USP—Clear, colorless solution.

pKa: 3.9.

Solubility: Furosemide USP—Practically insoluble in water; freely soluble in acetone, in dimethylformamide, and in solutions of alkali hydroxides; soluble in methanol; sparingly soluble in alcohol; slightly soluble in ether; very slightly soluble in chloroform.

USP requirements:
Furosemide USP—Preserve in well-closed, light-resistant containers. Contains not less than 98.0% and not more than 101.0% of furosemide, calculated on the dried basis. Meets the requirements for Identification, Loss on drying (not more than 1.0%), Residue on ignition (not more than 0.1%), Heavy metals (not more than 0.002%), Related compounds, and Organic volatile impurities.
Furosemide Injection USP—Store in single-dose or in multiple-dose, light-resistant containers, of Type I glass. A sterile solution of Furosemide in Water for Injection prepared with the aid of Sodium Hydroxide or, where intended solely for veterinary use, Diethanolamine. Injection intended solely for veterinary use is so labeled. Contains the labeled amount, within ±10%. Meets the requirements for Identification, Bacterial endotoxins, pH (8.0–9.3 or, where labeled as intended solely for veterinary use, 7.0–7.8), Particulate matter, Limit of 4-chloro-5-sulfamoylanthranilic acid, and Injections.
Furosemide Oral Solution—Not in USP.
Furosemide Tablets USP—Preserve in well-closed, light-resistant containers. Tablets intended solely for veterinary use are so labeled. Contain the labeled amount, within ±10%. Meet the requirements for Identification, Dissolution (80.0% in 60 minutes in phosphate buffer [pH 5.8] in Apparatus 2 at 50 rpm; where Tablets are labeled as intended for veterinary use only, use 65 rpm), Uniformity of dosage units, and 4-Chloro-5-sulfamoylanthranilic acid (not more than 0.8%).

FUSIDIC ACID

Chemical name: 29-Nordammara-17(20),24-dien-21-oic acid, 16-(acetyloxy)-3,11-dihydroxy-, (3 alpha,4 alpha,8 alpha,9 beta,11 alpha,13 alpha,14 beta,16 beta,17*Z*)-.

Molecular formula: $C_{31}H_{48}O_6$.

Molecular weight: 516.72.

Description: White crystalline powder.

Solubility: Practically insoluble in water; soluble 1 in 5 of alcohol, 1 in 4 of chloroform, and 1 in 60 of ether.

USP requirements:
Fusidic Acid Cream—Not in USP.
Fusidic Acid Impregnated Gauze—Not in USP.
Fusidic Acid for Injection—Not in USP.
Fusidic Acid Ointment—Not in USP.
Fusidic Acid Oral Suspension—Not in USP.
Fusidic Acid Tablets—Not in USP.

GABAPENTIN

Chemical name: Cyclohexaneacetic acid, 1-(aminomethyl)-.

Molecular formula: $C_9H_{17}NO_2$.

Molecular weight: 171.24.

Description: White to off-white crystalline solid.

Solubility: Freely soluble in water and in both basic and acidic aqueous solutions.

USP requirements: Gabapentin Capsules—Not in USP.

GADODIAMIDE

Chemical name: [5,8-Bis(carboxymethyl)-11-[2-(methylamino)-2-oxoethyl]-3-oxo-2,5,8,11-tetraazatridecan-13-oato(3-)-$N^5,N^8,N^{11},O^3,O^5,O^{11},O^{13}$]gadolinium.

Molecular formula: $C_{16}H_{26}GdN_5O_8$.

Molecular weight: 573.66 (anhydrous).

Description: Gadodiamide injection—Sterile, clear, colorless to slightly yellow, aqueous solution.

USP requirements: Gadodiamide Injection—Not in USP.

GADOPENTETATE

Chemical name: Gadopentetate dimeglumine—Gadolinate(2−), [*N*,*N*-bis[2-[bis(carboxymethyl)amino]ethyl]glycinato(5−)]-, dihydrogen, compd. with 1-deoxy-1-(methylamino)-D-glucitol (1:2).

Molecular formula: Gadopentetate dimeglumine—$C_{14}H_{20}GdN_3O_{10} \cdot 2C_7H_{17}NO_5$.

Molecular weight: Gadopentetate dimeglumine—938.01.

Description: Gadopentetate dimeglumine injection—Clear, colorless to slightly yellow aqueous solution, with a pH of 6.5–8.0.

Solubility: Gadopentetate dimeglumine—Freely soluble in water.

USP requirements: Gadopentetate Dimeglumine Injection—Not in USP.

GADOTERIDOL

Chemical name: Gadolinium, [10-(2-hydroxypropyl)-1,4,7,10-tetraazacyclododecane-1,4,7-triacetato(3-)-N^1,N^4,N^7,N^{10},-O^1,O^4,O^7,O^{10}]-.

Molecular formula: $C_{17}H_{29}GdN_4O_7$.

Molecular weight: 558.69.

USP requirements: Gadoteridol Injection—Not in USP.

GALLAMINE

Chemical name: Gallamine triethiodide—Ethanaminium, 2,2′,2″-[1,2,3-benzenetriyltris(oxy)]tris[*N*,*N*,*N*-triethyl]-, triiodide.

Molecular formula: Gallamine triethiodide—$C_{30}H_{60}I_3N_3O_3$.

Molecular weight: Gallamine triethiodide—891.54.

Description: Gallamine Triethiodide USP—White, odorless, amorphous powder. Is hygroscopic.

Solubility: Gallamine Triethiodide USP—Very soluble in water; sparingly soluble in alcohol; very slightly soluble in chloroform.

USP requirements:

Gallamine Triethiodide USP—Preserve in tight containers, protected from light. Contains not less than 98.0% and not more than 101.0% of gallamine triethiodide, calculated on the dried basis. Meets the requirements for Clarity and color of solution, Identification, pH (5.3–7.0, in a solution [1 in 50]), Loss on drying (not more than 1.5%), Residue on ignition (not more than 0.1%), and Heavy metals (not more than 0.002%).

Gallamine Triethiodide Injection USP—Preserve in single-dose or in multiple-dose containers, preferably of Type I glass, protected from light. A sterile solution of Gallamine Triethiodide in Water for Injection. Contains the labeled amount, within ±5%. Meets the requirements for Identification, Bacterial endotoxins, pH (6.5–7.5), and Injections.

GALLIUM CITRATE Ga 67

Chemical name: 1,2,3-Propanetricarboxylic acid, 2-hydroxy-, gallium-^{67}*Ga* (1:1) salt.

Molecular formula: $C_6H_5{}^{67}GaO_7$.

USP requirements: Gallium Citrate Ga 67 Injection USP—Preserve in single-dose or in multiple-dose containers. A sterile aqueous solution of radioactive, essentially carrier-free, gallium citrate Ga 67 suitable for intravenous administration. Label it to include the following, in addition to the information specified for Labeling under Injections: the time and date of calibration; the amount of ^{67}Ga as labeled gallium citrate expressed as total megabecquerels (or microcuries or millicuries) and concentration as megabecquerels (or microcuries or millicuries) per mL at the time of calibration; the expiration date and time; and the statement, "Caution—Radioactive Material." The labeling indicates that in making dosage calculations, correction is to be made for radioactive decay, and also indicates that the radioactive half-life of ^{67}Ga is 78.26 hours. Contains the labeled amount of ^{67}Ga as citrate, within ±10%, expressed in megabecquerels (or microcuries or millicuries) per mL at the time indicated in the labeling. Meets the requirements for Bacterial endotoxins, pH (4.5–8.0), Radiochemical purity, Radionuclide identification, Radionuclidic purity, and Injections (except that the Injection may be distributed or dispensed prior to completion of the test for Sterility, the latter test being started on the day of manufacture, and except that it is not subject to the recommendation of Volume in Container).

GALLIUM NITRATE

Chemical name: Nitric acid, gallium salt, nonahydrate.

Molecular formula: $GaN_3O_9 \cdot 9H_2O$.

Molecular weight: 417.88.

Description:

Gallium nitrate—White, slightly hygroscopic, crystalline powder (nonahydrate).

Gallium nitrate injection—Clear, colorless, odorless, sterile solution.

USP requirements: Gallium Nitrate Injection—Not in USP.

GANCICLOVIR

Chemical name: Ganciclovir sodium—6*H*-Purin-6-one, 2-amino-1,9-dihydro-9-[[2-hydroxy-1-(hydroxymethyl)ethoxy]methyl]-, monosodium salt.

Molecular formula: Ganciclovir sodium—$C_9H_{12}N_5NaO_4$.

Molecular weight: Ganciclovir sodium—277.22.

Description: White lyophilized powder.

pKa: 2.2 and 9.4.

Solubility: Aqueous solubility greater than 50 mg/mL at 25 °C.

USP requirements: Sterile Ganciclovir Sodium—Not in USP.

ABSORBENT GAUZE

USP requirements: Absorbent Gauze USP—Preserve in well-closed containers. Absorbent Gauze that has been rendered sterile is so packaged that the sterility of the contents of the package is maintained until the package is opened for use. It is cotton, or a mixture of cotton and not more than 53.0%, by weight, of rayon, and is in the form of a plain woven cloth conforming to the standards set forth in *USP/NF*. Absorbent Gauze that has been rendered sterile is packaged to protect it from contamination. Its type or thread count, length, and width, and the number of pieces contained, are stated on the container, and the designation "non-sterilized" or "not sterilized" appears prominently thereon unless the Gauze has been rendered sterile, in which case it may be labeled to indicate that it is sterile. The package label of sterile Gauze indicates that the contents may not be sterile if the package bears evidence of damage or has been previously opened. The name of the manufacturer, packer, or distributor is stated on the package. Meets the requirements for General characteristics, Thread count, Length (not less than 98.0% of that stated on label), Width (average of three measurements is within 1.6 mm of width stated on label), Weight, Absorbency (complete submersion takes place in not more than 30 seconds), Sterility, Dried and ignited residue, Acid or alkali, and Dextrin or starch, in water extract, Residue on ignition, Fatty matter, Alcohol-soluble dyes, and Cotton and rayon content.

Note: Condition all Absorbent Gauze for not less than 4 hours in a standard atmosphere of 65 ±2% relative humidity at 21 ±1.1 °C (70 ±2 °F), before determining the weight, thread count, and absorbency. Remove the Absorbent Gauze from its wrappings before placing it in the conditioning atmosphere, and if it is in the form of bolts or rolls, cut the quantity necessary for the various tests from the piece, excluding the first two and the last two meters when the total quantity of Gauze available so permits.

PETROLATUM GAUZE

USP requirements: Petrolatum Gauze USP—Each Petrolatum Gauze unit is so packaged individually that the sterility of the unit is maintained until the package is opened for use. It is Absorbent Gauze saturated with White Petrolatum. The package label bears a statement to the effect that the sterility of the Petrolatum Gauze cannot be guaranteed if the package bears evidence of damage or has been opened previously. The package label states the width, length, and type or thread count of the Gauze. The weight of the petrolatum in the gauze is not less than 70.0% and not more than 80.0% of the weight of petrolatum gauze. Petrolatum Gauze is sterile. May be prepared by adding, under aseptic conditions, molten, sterile, White Petrolatum to dry, sterile, Absorbent Gauze, previously cut to size, in the ratio of 60 grams of petrolatum to each 20 grams of gauze. Meets the requirements for Sterility, of tests under White Petrolatum, and of tests for Thread count, Length, Width, and Weight under Absorbent Gauze.

GELATIN

Description: Gelatin NF—Sheets, flakes, or shreds, or coarse to fine powder. Faintly yellow or amber in color, the color varying in depth according to the particle size. It has a slight, characteristic, bouillon-like odor in solution. Stable in air when dry, but subject to microbic decomposition when moist or in solution. Gelatin has any suitable strength that is designated by Bloom Gelometer number. Type A Gelatin exhibits an isoelectric point between pH 7 and pH 9, and Type B Gelatin exhibits an isoelectric point between pH 4.7 and pH 5.2.

NF category: Coating agent; suspending and/or viscosity-increasing agent; tablet binder.

Solubility: Gelatin NF—Insoluble in cold water, but swells and softens when immersed in it, gradually absorbing from 5 to 10 times its own weight of water. Soluble in hot water, in 6 *N* acetic acid, and in a hot mixture of glycerin and water. Insoluble in alcohol, in chloroform, in ether, and in fixed and volatile oils.

NF requirements: Gelatin NF—Preserve in well-closed containers in a dry place. A product obtained by the partial hydrolysis of collagen derived from the skin, white connective tissue, and bones of animals. Gelatin derived from an acid-treated precursor is known as Type A, and Gelatin derived from an alkali-treated precursor is known as Type B. Gelatin, where being used in the manufacture of capsules, or for the coating of tablets, may be colored with a certified color, may contain not more than 0.15% of sulfur dioxide, and may contain a suitable concentration of sodium lauryl sulfate and suitable antimicrobial agents. Meets the requirements for Identification, Microbial limits, Residue on ignition (not more than 2.0%), Odor and water-insoluble substances, Sulfur dioxide, Arsenic (not more than 0.8 ppm), and Heavy metals (not more than 0.005%).

ABSORBABLE GELATIN

Description:

Absorbable Gelatin Film USP—Light amber, transparent, pliable film which becomes rubbery when moistened.

Absorbable Gelatin Sponge USP—Light, nearly white, non-elastic, tough, porous, hydrophilic solid.

Solubility:

Absorbable Gelatin Film USP—Insoluble in water.

Absorbable Gelatin Sponge USP—Insoluble in water.

USP requirements:

Absorbable Gelatin Film USP—Preserve in hermetically sealed or other suitable container in such manner that the sterility of the product is maintained until the container is opened for use. It is Gelatin in the form of a sterile, absorbable, water-insoluble film. The package bears a statement to the effect that the sterility of Absorbable Gelatin Film cannot be guaranteed if the package bears evidence of damage, or if the package has been previously opened. Meets the requirements for Sterility, Residue on ignition (not more than 2.0%), and Proteolytic digest (average time of 3 proteolytic digest determinations, 4–8 hours).

Absorbable Gelatin Sponge USP—Preserve in a hermetically sealed or other suitable container in such manner that the sterility of the product is maintained until the container is opened for use. It is Gelatin in the form of a sterile, absorbable, water-insoluble sponge. The package bears a statement to the effect that the sterility of Absorbable Gelatin Sponge cannot be guaranteed if the package bears evidence of damage, or if the package has been previously opened. Meets the requirements for Sterility, Residue on ignition (not more than 2.0%), Digestibility (average digestion time of 3 determinations not more than 75 minutes), and Water absorption (not less than 35 times its weight of water).

GEMFIBROZIL

Chemical name: Pentanoic acid, 5-(2,5-dimethylphenoxy)-2,2-dimethyl-.

Molecular formula: $C_{15}H_{22}O_3$.

Molecular weight: 250.34.

Description: Gemfibrozil USP—White, waxy, crystalline solid.

Solubility: Gemfibrozil USP—Practically insoluble in water; soluble in alcohol, in methanol, and in chloroform.

USP requirements:

Gemfibrozil USP—Preserve in tight containers. Contains not less than 98.0% and not more than 102.0% of gemfibrozil, calculated on the dried basis. Meets the requirements for Identification, Melting range (58–61 °C), Water (not more than 0.25%), Heavy metals (not more than 0.002%), Chromatographic purity, and Organic volatile impurities.

Gemfibrozil Capsules USP—Preserve in tight containers. Contain the labeled amount, within ±10%. Meet the requirements for Identification, Dissolution (80% in 45 minutes in 0.2 *M* phosphate buffer [pH 7.5] in Apparatus 2 at 50 rpm), and Uniformity of dosage units.

Gemfibrozil Tablets USP—Preserve in tight containers. Contain the labeled amount, within ±10%. Meet the requirements for Identification, Dissolution (80% in 30 minutes in 0.2 *M* phosphate buffer [pH 7.5] in Apparatus 2 at 50 rpm), and Uniformity of dosage units.

GENTAMICIN

Chemical group: Aminoglycosides.

Chemical name: Gentamicin sulfate—Gentamicin sulfate (salt).

Description:

Gentamicin Sulfate USP—White to buff powder.

Gentamicin Sulfate Injection USP—Clear, slightly yellow solution, having a faint odor.

Solubility: Gentamicin Sulfate USP—Freely soluble in water; insoluble in alcohol, in acetone, in chloroform, and in ether.

USP requirements:

Gentamicin Sulfate USP—Preserve in tight containers. The sulfate salt, or a mixture of such salts, of the antibiotic substances produced by the growth of *Micromonospora purpurea*. Has a potency equivalent to not less than 590 mcg of gentamicin per mg, calculated on the dried basis. Meets the requirements for Identification, Specific rotation (+107° to +121°, calculated on the dried basis), pH (3.5–5.5, in a solution [1 in 25]), Loss on drying (not more than 18.0%), Residue on ignition (not more than 1.0%), Methanol (not more than 1.0%), and Content of gentamicins.

Gentamicin Sulfate Cream USP—Preserve in collapsible tubes or in other tight containers, and avoid exposure to excessive heat. Contains an amount of gentamicin sulfate equivalent to the labeled amount of gentamicin, within −10% to +35%. Meets the requirements for Identification and Minimum fill.

Gentamicin Sulfate Injection USP—Preserve in single-dose or in multiple-dose containers, preferably of Type I glass. A sterile solution of Gentamicin Sulfate in Water for Injection. May contain suitable buffers, preservatives, and sequestering agents, unless it is intended for intrathecal use, in which case it contains only suitable tonicity agents. Contains an amount of gentamicin sulfate equivalent to the labeled amount of gentamicin, within −10% to +25%. Meets the requirements for Identification, Bacterial endotoxins, pH (3.0–5.5), Particulate matter, and Injections.

Gentamicin Sulfate Ointment USP—Preserve in collapsible tubes or in other tight containers, and avoid exposure to excessive heat. Contains an amount of gentamicin sulfate equivalent to the labeled amount of gentamicin, within −10% to +35%. Meets the requirements for Identification, Minimum fill, and Water (not more than 1.0%).

Gentamicin Sulfate Ophthalmic Ointment USP—Preserve in collapsible ophthalmic ointment tubes, and avoid exposure to excessive heat. Contains an amount of gentamicin sulfate equivalent to the labeled amount of gentamicin, within −10% to +35%. Meets the requirements for Identification, Sterility, Minimum fill, and Metal particles, and for Water under Gentamicin Sulfate Ointment.

Gentamicin Sulfate Ophthalmic Solution USP—Preserve in tight containers, and avoid exposure to excessive heat. A sterile, buffered solution of Gentamicin Sulfate with preservatives. Contains an amount of gentamicin sulfate equivalent to the labeled amount of gentamicin, within −10% to +35%. Meets the requirements for pH (6.5–7.5) and for Identification test under Gentamicin Sulfate Injection and Sterility tests.

Gentamicin Sulfate Otic Solution—Not in USP.

Sterile Gentamicin Sulfate USP—Preserve in Containers for Sterile Solids. It is Gentamicin Sulfate suitable for parenteral use. Has a potency equivalent to not less than 590 mcg of gentamicin per mg, calculated on the dried basis. Meets the requirements for Bacterial endotoxins and Sterility, and for Identification tests, Specific rotation, pH, Loss on drying, Methanol, and Content of gentamicins under Gentamicin Sulfate.

GENTAMICIN AND PREDNISOLONE

For *Gentamicin* and *Prednisolone*—See individual listings for chemistry information.

USP requirements:

Gentamicin and Prednisolone Acetate Ophthalmic Ointment USP—Preserve in collapsible ophthalmic ointment tubes, and avoid exposure to excessive heat. Contains the equivalent of the labeled amount of gentamicin, within −10% to +20%, and the labeled amount of prednisolone acetate, within ±10%. Meets the requirements for Identification, Sterility, Minimum fill, Water (not more than 2.0%), and Metal particles.

Gentamicin and Prednisolone Acetate Ophthalmic Suspension USP—Preserve in tight containers. A sterile aqueous suspension containing Gentamicin Sulfate and Prednisolone Acetate. Contains the equivalent of the labeled amount of gentamicin, within −10% to +30%, and the labeled amount of prednisolone acetate, within ±10%. Meets the requirements for Identification, Sterility, and pH (5.4–6.6).

GENTAMICIN AND SODIUM CHLORIDE

For *Gentamicin* and *Sodium Chloride*—See individual listings for chemistry information.

USP requirements: Gentamicin Sulfate in Sodium Chloride Injection—Not in USP.

GENTIAN VIOLET

Chemical name: Methanaminium, *N*-[4-[bis[4-(dimethylamino)-phenyl]methylene]-2,5-cyclohexadien-1-ylidene]-*N*-methyl-, chloride.

Molecular formula: $C_{25}H_{30}ClN_3$.

Molecular weight: 407.99.

Description:

Gentian Violet USP—Dark green powder or greenish, glistening pieces having a metallic luster, and having not more than a faint odor.

Gentian Violet Cream USP—Dark purple, water-washable cream.

Gentian Violet Topical Solution USP—Purple liquid, having a slight odor of alcohol. A dilution (1 in 100), viewed downward through 1 cm of depth, is deep purple in color.

Solubility: Gentian Violet USP—Sparingly soluble in water; soluble in alcohol, in glycerin, and in chloroform; insoluble in ether.

USP requirements:

Gentian Violet USP—Preserve in well-closed containers. Contains not less than 96.0% and not more than 100.5% of gentian violet, calculated on the anhydrous basis. Meets the requirements for Identification, Water (not more than 7.5%), Residue on ignition (not more than 1.5%), Alcohol-insoluble substances (not more than 1.0%), Arsenic (not more than 0.001%), Lead (not more than 0.003%), Zinc, and Chromatographic purity.

Gentian Violet Cream USP—Preserve in collapsible tubes, or in other tight containers, and avoid exposure to excessive heat. It is Gentian Violet in a suitable cream base. Contains, in each 100 grams, not less than 1.20 grams and not more than 1.60 grams of gentian violet, calculated as hexamethylpararosaniline chloride. Meets the requirements for Identification and Minimum fill.

Gentian Violet Topical Solution USP—Preserve in tight containers. Contains, in each 100 mL, not less than 0.95 gram and not more than 1.05 grams of gentian violet, calculated as hexamethylpararosaniline chloride. Meets the requirements for Identification, Solution of residue in alcohol, and Alcohol content (8.0–10.0%).

Gentian Violet Vaginal Tampons—Not in USP.

GENTISIC ACID ETHANOLAMIDE

Molecular formula: $C_9H_{11}NO_4$.

Molecular weight: 197.19.

Description: Gentisic Acid Ethanolamide NF—White to tan powder. Melts at about 149 °C.

NF category: Complexing agent.

Solubility: Gentisic Acid Ethanolamide NF—Sparingly soluble in water; freely soluble in acetone, in methanol, and in alcohol; very slightly soluble in ether; practically insoluble in chloroform.

NF requirements: Gentisic Acid Ethanolamide NF—Preserve in well-closed containers. Contains not less than 99.0% and not more than 100.5% of gentisic acid ethanolamide, calculated on the dried basis. Meets the requirements for Identification, Loss on drying (not more than 0.5%), Residue on ignition (not more than 0.1%), Chloride (not more than 0.01%), Sulfate (not more than 0.02%), Heavy metals (not more than 0.001%), Chromatographic impurities, and Organic volatile impurities.

PHARMACEUTICAL GLAZE

Description: Pharmaceutical Glaze NF—NF category: Coating agent.

NF requirements: Pharmaceutical Glaze NF—Preserve in tight, lined metal or plastic containers, protected from excessive heat, preferably at a temperature below 25 °C. A specially denatured alcoholic solution of Shellac containing between 20.0 and 57.0% of anhydrous shellac, and is made with either anhydrous alcohol or alcohol containing 5% of water by volume. The solvent is a specially denatured alcohol approved for glaze manufacturing by the Internal Revenue Service. Label it to indicate the shellac type and concentration, the composition of the solvent, and the quantity of titanium dioxide, if present. Where titanium dioxide or waxes are present, the label states that the Glaze requires mixing before use. Meets the requirements for Identification, Arsenic, Heavy metals, and Rosin under Shellac, Acid value under Shellac, and Wax under Shellac.

GLIPIZIDE

Chemical group: Sulfonylurea.

Chemical name: Pyrazinecarboxamide, *N*-[2-[4-[[[(cyclohexylamino)carbonyl]amino]sulfonyl]phenyl]ethyl]-5-methyl-.

Molecular formula: $C_{21}H_{27}N_5O_4S$.

Molecular weight: 445.54.

Description: Whitish, odorless powder.

pKa: 5.9.

Solubility: Insoluble in water and in alcohols; soluble in 0.1 *N* sodium hydroxide; freely soluble in dimethylformamide.

USP requirements:

Glipizide USP—Preserve in tight containers. Contains not less than 98.0% and not more than 102.0% of glipizide, calculated on the dried basis. Meets the requirements for Identification, Loss on drying (not more than 1.0%), Residue on ignition (not more than 0.4%), Heavy metals (not more than 0.005%), and Ordinary impurities.

Glipizide Tablets—Not in USP.

ANTI-HUMAN GLOBULIN SERUM

USP requirements: Anti-Human Globulin Serum USP—Preserve at a temperature between 2 and 8 °C. A sterile, liquid preparation of serum produced by immunizing lower animals such as rabbits or goats with human serum or plasma, or with selected human plasma proteins. It is free from agglutinins and from hemolysins to non-sensitized human red cells of all blood groups. Contains a suitable antimicrobial preservative. Label it to state the animal source of the product. Label it also to state the specific antibody activities present; to state the application for which the reagent is intended; to include a cautionary statement that it does not contain antibodies to immunoglobulins or that it does not contain antibodies to complement components, wherever and whichever is applicable; and to state that it is for in-vitro diagnostic use. (Note: The lettering on the label of the general-purpose polyspecific reagent is black on a white background. The label of all other Anti-Human Globulin Serum containers is in white lettering on a black background.) Anti-Human Globulin Serums containing Anti-IgG meet the requirements of the test for potency, in parallel with the U.S. Reference Anti-Human Globulin (Anti-IgG) Serum (at a 1:4 dilution) when tested with red cells suspended in isotonic saline sensitized with decreasing amounts of non-agglutinating Anti-D (Anti-Rh_o) serum, and with cells sensitized in the same manner with an immunoglobulin IgG Anti-Fy^a serum of similar potency. Anti-Human Globulin Serum containing one or more Anti-complement components meets the requirements of the tests for potency in giving a 2+ agglutination reaction (i.e., agglutinated cells dislodged into many small clumps of equal size) by the low-ionic sucrose or sucrose-trypsin procedures when tested as recommended in the labeling. Anti-Human Globulin Serum containing Anti-3Cd activity meets the requirements for stability, by potency testing of representative lots every 3 months during the dating period. Meets the requirement for Expiration date (not later than 1 year after the date of issue from manufacturer's cold storage [5 °C, 1 year; or 0 °C, 2 years]). Conforms to the regulations of the U.S. Food and Drug Administration concerning biologics.

IMMUNE GLOBULIN

Description: Immune Globulin USP—Transparent or slightly opalescent liquid, either colorless or of a brownish color due to denatured hemoglobin. Practically odorless. May develop a slight, granular deposit during storage.

USP requirements:

Immune Globulin USP—Preserve at a temperature between 2 and 8 °C. A sterile, non-pyrogenic solution of globulins that contains many antibodies normally present in adult human blood, prepared by pooling approximately equal amounts of material (source blood, plasma, serum, or placentas) from not less than 1000 donors. Label it to state that passive immunization with Immune Globulin modifies hepatitis A, prevents or modifies measles, and provides replacement therapy in persons having hypo- or agammaglobulinemia, that it is not standardized with respect to antibody titers against hepatitis B surface antigen and that it should be used for prophylaxis of viral hepatitis type B only when the specific Immune Globulin is not available, that it may be of benefit in women who have been exposed to rubella in the first trimester of pregnancy but who would not consider a therapeutic abortion, and that it may be used in immunosuppressed patients for passive immunization against varicella if the specific Immune Globulin is not available. Label it also to state that it is not indicated for routine prophylaxis or treatment of rubella, poliomyelitis or mumps, or for allergy or asthma in patients who have normal levels of immunoglobulin, that the plasma units from which it has been derived have been tested and found non-reactive for hepatitis B surface antigen, and that it should not be administered intravenously but be given intramuscularly, preferably in the gluteal region. Contains not less than 15 grams and not more than 18 grams of protein per 100 mL, not less than 90.0% of which is gamma globulin. Contains 0.3 *M* glycine as a stabilizing agent and contains a suitable preservative. Has a potency of component antibodies of diphtheria antitoxin based on the U.S. Standard Diphtheria Antitoxin and a diphtheria test toxin, tested in guinea pigs (not less than 2 antitoxin units per mL), and antibodies for measles and poliovirus. Meets the requirements of the tests for heat stability in absence of gelation on heating, and for pH. Meets the requirement for Expiration date (not later than 3 years after date of issue from manufacturer's cold storage [5 °C, 3 years]). Conforms to the regulations of the U.S. Food and Drug Administration concerning biologics.

Immune Globulin Intravenous (Human) Injection—Not in USP.

Immune Globulin Intravenous (Human) for Injection—Not in USP.

RH_o (D) IMMUNE GLOBULIN

Description: RH_o (D) Immune Globulin USP—Transparent or slightly opalescent liquid. Practically colorless and practically odorless. May develop a slight, granular deposit during storage.

USP requirements: RH_o (D) Immune Globulin USP—Preserve at a temperature between 2 and 8 °C. A sterile, non-pyrogenic solution of globulins derived from human blood plasma containing antibody to the erythrocyte factor Rh_o (D). Contains not less than 10 grams and not more than 18 grams of protein per 100 mL, not less than 90.0% of which is gamma globulin. Has a potency, determined by a suitable method, not less than that of the U.S. Reference Rh_o (D) Immune Globulin. Contains 0.3 *M* glycine as a stabilizing agent and contains a suitable preservative. Meets the requirement for Expiration date (not later than 6 months from the date of issue from manufacturer's cold storage, or not later than 1 year from the date of manufacture, as indicated on the label). Conforms to the regulations of the U.S. Food and Drug Administration concerning biologics.

GLUCAGON

Chemical name: Glucagon (pig).

Molecular formula: $C_{153}H_{225}N_{43}O_{49}S$.

Molecular weight: 3482.79.

Description:

Glucagon USP—Fine, white or faintly colored, crystalline powder. Is practically odorless.

Glucagon for Injection USP—White, odorless powder.

Solubility: Glucagon USP—Soluble in dilute alkali and acid solutions; insoluble in most organic solvents.

Other characteristics: A single-chain polypeptide containing 29 amino acid residues. Chemically unrelated to insulin. One USP Unit of glucagon is equivalent to 1 International Unit of glucagon and also to about 1 mg of glucagon.

USP requirements:

Glucagon USP—Preserve in tight, glass containers, under nitrogen, in a refrigerator. A polypeptide hormone, which has the property of increasing the concentration of glucose in the blood. Obtained from porcine and bovine pancreas glands. Meets the requirements for Water (not more than 10.0%), Residue on ignition (not more than 2.5%), Nitrogen content (16.0–18.5%, calculated on the anhydrous basis), and Zinc content (not more than 0.05%).

Glucagon for Injection USP—Preserve in Containers for Sterile Solids. Preserve the accompanying solvent in single-dose or in multiple-dose containers, preferably of Type I glass. A mixture of the hydrochloride of Glucagon with one or more suitable, dry diluents. Contains the labeled amount, within −20% to +25%. Meets the requirements for Constituted solution and pH (2.5–3.0) and Clarity of solution, for Sterility tests and Labeling under Injections, and for Uniformity of dosage units.

GLUCONOLACTONE

Chemical name: D-Gluconic acid delta-lactone.

Molecular formula: $C_6H_{10}O_6$.

Molecular weight: 178.14.

Description: Gluconolactone USP—Fine, white, practically odorless, crystalline powder.

Solubility: Gluconolactone USP—Freely soluble in water; sparingly soluble in alcohol; insoluble in ether.

USP requirements: Gluconolactone USP—Preserve in well-closed containers. Contains not less than 99.0% and not more than 101.0% of gluconolactone. Meets the requirements for Identification, Melting range (151–155 °C), Arsenic (not more than 3 ppm), Lead (not more than 0.001%), Heavy metals (not more than 0.002%), and Reducing substances.

GLUCOSE ENZYMATIC TEST STRIP

USP requirements: Glucose Enzymatic Test Strip USP—Preserve in the original container, in a dry place, at controlled room temperature. Consists of the enzymes glucose oxidase and horseradish peroxidase, a suitable substrate for the reaction of hydrogen peroxide catalyzed by peroxidase, and other inactive ingredients impregnated and dried on filter paper. When tested in human urine containing known glucose concentrations, it reacts in the specified times to produce colors corresponding to the color chart provided. Meets the requirements for Identification and Calibration.

LIQUID GLUCOSE

Description: Liquid Glucose NF—Colorless or yellowish, thick, syrupy liquid. Odorless or nearly odorless.

NF category: Tablet binder.

Solubility: Liquid Glucose NF—Miscible with water; sparingly soluble in alcohol.

NF requirements: Liquid Glucose NF—Preserve in tight containers. A product obtained by the incomplete hydrolysis of starch. Consists chiefly of dextrose, dextrins, maltose, and water. Meets the requirements for Identification, Acidity, Water (not more than 21.0%), Residue on ignition (not more than 0.5%), Sulfite, Arsenic (not more than 1 ppm), Heavy metals (not more than 0.001%), Starch, and Organic volatile impurities.

GLUTARAL

Chemical name: Pentanedial.

Molecular formula: $C_5H_8O_2$.

Molecular weight: 100.12.

Description: Glutaral Concentrate USP—Clear, colorless or faintly yellow liquid, having a characteristic, irritating odor.

USP requirements: Glutaral Concentrate USP—Preserve in tight containers, protected from light, and avoid exposure to excessive heat. A solution of glutaraldehyde in Purified Water. Contains the labeled amount, within +4%, the labeled amount being 50.0 grams of glutaral per 100.0 grams of Concentrate. Meets the requirements for Clarity of solution, Identification, Specific gravity (1.128 to 1.135 at 20 °C/20 °C), Acidity (not more than 0.4% of acid (w/w), calculated as acetic acid), pH (3.7–4.5), and Heavy metals (not more than 0.001%).

NF requirements: Glutaral Disinfectant Solution NF—Preserve in tight, light-resistant containers, and avoid exposure to excessive heat. Contains, by weight, the labeled amount of glutaral, within +10%. Meets the requirements for Identification and pH (2.7–3.7).

GLUTETHIMIDE

Chemical name: 2,6-Piperidinedione, 3-ethyl-3-phenyl-.

Molecular formula: $C_{13}H_{15}NO_2$.

Molecular weight: 217.27.

Description: Glutethimide USP—White, crystalline powder. Its saturated solution is acid to litmus.

Solubility: Glutethimide USP—Practically insoluble in water; freely soluble in ethyl acetate, in acetone, in ether, and in chloroform; soluble in alcohol and in methanol.

USP requirements:

Glutethimide USP—Preserve in well-closed containers. Dried over phosphorus pentoxide at 45 °C to constant weight, contains not less than 98.0% and not more than 102.0% of glutethimide. Meets the requirements for Identification, Melting range (86–89 °C), Loss on drying (not more than 1.0%), Residue on ignition (not more than 0.1%), and Chromatographic purity.

Glutethimide Capsules USP—Preserve in well-closed containers. Contain the labeled amount, within ±5%. Meet the requirements for Identification, Dissolution (75% in 45 minutes in water in Apparatus 1 at 100 rpm), and Uniformity of dosage units.

Glutethimide Tablets USP—Preserve in well-closed containers. Contain the labeled amount, within ±10%. Meet the requirements for Identification, Dissolution (70% in 60 minutes in water in Apparatus 2 at 50 rpm), and Uniformity of dosage units.

GLYBURIDE

Chemical group: Sulfonylurea.

Chemical name: Benzamide, 5-chloro-*N*-[2-[4-[[[(cyclohexylamino)carbonyl]amino]sulfonyl]phenyl]ethyl]-2-methoxy-.

Molecular formula: $C_{23}H_{28}ClN_3O_5S$.

Molecular weight: 494.01.

Description: White, crystalline compound.

pKa: 5.3.

Solubility: Practically insoluble in water and in ether; slightly soluble in alcohol and in methyl alcohol.

USP requirements:

Glyburide USP—Preserve in tight containers. Contains not less than 98.0% and not more than 102.0% of glyburide, calculated on the dried basis. Meets the requirements for Identification, Loss on drying (not more than 1.0%), Residue on ignition (not more than 0.5%), Heavy metals (not more than 0.002%), and Chromatographic purity.

Glyburide Tablets—Not in USP.

GLYCERIN

Chemical name: 1,2,3-Propanetriol.

Molecular formula: $C_3H_8O_3$.

Molecular weight: 92.09.

Description: Glycerin USP—Clear, colorless, syrupy liquid. Has not more than a slight characteristic odor, which is neither harsh nor disagreeable. Is hygroscopic. Its solutions are neutral to litmus.

NF category: Humectant; plasticizer; solvent; tonicity agent.

Solubility: Glycerin USP—Miscible with water and with alcohol. Insoluble in chloroform, in ether, and in fixed and volatile oils.

USP requirements:

Glycerin USP—Preserve in tight containers. Contains not less than 95.0% and not more than 101.0% of glycerin. Meets the requirements for Identification, Specific gravity (not less than 1.249), Color, Residue on ignition (not more than 0.01%), Chloride (not more than 0.001%), Sulfate (not more than 0.002%), Arsenic (not more than 1.5 ppm), Heavy metals (not more than 5 ppm), Chlorinated compounds (not more than 0.003% of chlorine), Fatty acids and esters, and Organic volatile impurities.

Glycerin Ophthalmic Solution USP—Preserve in tight containers of glass or plastic, containing not more than 15 mL, protected from light. The container or individual carton is sealed and tamper-proof so that sterility is assured at time of first use. A sterile, anhydrous solution of Glycerin, containing the labeled amount, within −1.5%. (Note: In the preparation of this Ophthalmic Solution, use Glycerin that has a low water content, in order that the Ophthalmic Solution may comply with the Water limit. This may be ensured by using Glycerin having a specific gravity of not less than 1.2607, corresponding to a concentration of 99.5%.) Meets the requirements for Identification, Sterility, pH (4.5–7.5), and Water (not more than 1.0%).

Note: Do not use the Ophthalmic Solution if it contains crystals, or if it is cloudy or discolored or contains a precipitate.

Glycerin Oral Solution USP—Preserve in tight containers. Contains the labeled amount, within ±5%. Meets the requirements for Identification and pH (5.5–7.5).

Glycerin Rectal Solution—Not in USP.

Glycerin Suppositories USP—Preserve in well-closed containers. Contain Glycerin solidified with Sodium Stearate. Contain the labeled amount, by weight, of glycerin, within −25% to −10%. Meet the requirements for Identification and Water (not more than 15.0%).

GLYCERYL BEHENATE

Description: Glyceryl Behenate NF—Fine powder, having a faint odor. Melts at about 70 °C.

NF category: Tablet and/or capsule lubricant.

Solubility: Glyceryl Behenate NF—Practically insoluble in water and in alcohol; soluble in chloroform.

NF requirements: Glyceryl Behenate NF—Preserve in tight containers, at a temperature not higher than 35 °C. A mixture of glycerides of fatty acids, mainly behenic acid. Meets the requirements for Identification, Residue on ignition (not more than 0.1%), Heavy metals (not more than 0.001%), Acid value (not more than 4), Iodine value (not more than 3), Saponification value (145–165), 1-Monoglycerides (12.0–18.0%), and Free glycerin (not more than 1.0%).

GLYCERYL MONOSTEARATE

Chemical name: Octadecanoic acid, monoester with 1,2,3-propanetriol.

Molecular formula: $C_{21}H_{42}O_4$.

Molecular weight: 358.56.

Description: Glyceryl Monostearate NF—White, wax-like solid, or white, wax-like beads or flakes. Slight agreeable fatty odor. Affected by light.

NF category: Emulsifying and/or solubilizing agent.

Solubility: Glyceryl Monostearate NF—Dissolves in hot organic solvents such as alcohol, mineral or fixed oils, ether, and acetone. Insoluble in water, but it may be dispersed in hot water with the aid of a small amount of soap or other suitable surface-active agent.

NF requirements: Glyceryl Monostearate NF—Preserve in tight, light-resistant containers. Contains not less than 90.0% of monoglycerides of saturated fatty acids, chiefly glyceryl monostearate and glyceryl monopalmitate. Meets the requirements for Melting range (not less than 55 °C), Residue on ignition (not more than 0.5%), Arsenic (not more than 3 ppm), Heavy metals (not more than 0.001%), Acid value (not more than 6), Iodine value (not more than 3), Saponification value (155–165), Hydroxyl value (300–330), and Free glycerin (not more than 1.2%).

GLYCINE

Chemical name: Glycine.

Molecular formula: $C_2H_5NO_2$.

Molecular weight: 75.07.

Description: Glycine USP—White, odorless, crystalline powder. Its solutions are acid to litmus.

Solubility: Glycine USP—Freely soluble in water; very slightly soluble in alcohol and in ether.

USP requirements:

Glycine USP—Preserve in well-closed containers. Contains not less than 98.5% and not more than 101.5% of glycine, calculated on the dried basis. Meets the requirements for Identification, Loss on drying (not more than 0.2%), Residue on ignition (not more than 0.1%), Chloride (not more than 0.007%), Sulfate (not more than 0.0065%), Heavy metals (not more than 0.002%), Readily carbonizable substances, Hydrolyzable substances, and Organic volatile impurities.

Glycine Irrigation USP—Preserve in single-dose containers, preferably of Type I or Type II glass. A sterile solution of Glycine in Water for Injection. Contains the labeled amount, within ±5%. Meets the requirements for Identification, Bacterial endotoxins, pH (4.5–6.5), and Injections (except the container in which the solution is packaged may be designed to empty rapidly and may exceed 1000 mL in capacity).

GLYCOPYRROLATE

Chemical group: Quaternary ammonium compound.

Chemical name: Pyrrolidinium, 3-[(cyclopentylhydroxyphenylacetyl)oxy]-1,1-dimethyl-, bromide.

Molecular formula: $C_{19}H_{28}BrNO_3$.

Molecular weight: 398.34.

Description: Glycopyrrolate USP—White, odorless, crystalline powder.

Solubility: Glycopyrrolate USP—Soluble in water and in alcohol; practically insoluble in chloroform and in ether.

USP requirements:

Glycopyrrolate USP—Preserve in tight containers. Dried at 105 °C for 3 hours, contains not less than 98.0% and not more than 100.5% of glycopyrrolate. Meets the requirements for Identification, Melting range (193–198 °C, the range between beginning and end of melting not more than 2 °C), Loss on drying (not more than 0.5%), Residue on ignition (not more than 0.3%), and Ordinary impurities.

Glycopyrrolate Injection USP—Preserve in single-dose or in multiple-dose containers, preferably of Type I glass. A sterile solution of Glycopyrrolate in Water for Injection. Contains the labeled amount, within ±7%. Meets the requirements for Identification, Bacterial endotoxins, pH (2.0–3.0), and Injections.

Glycopyrrolate Tablets USP—Preserve in tight containers. Contain the labeled amount, within ±7%. Meet the requirements for Identification, Dissolution (75% in 45 minutes in water in Apparatus 1 at 100 rpm), and Uniformity of dosage units.

GOLD SODIUM THIOMALATE

Chemical name: Butanedioic acid, mercapto-, monogold(1+) sodium salt.

Molecular formula: $C_4H_3AuNa_2O_4S$ + $C_4H_4AuNaO_4S$.

Molecular weight: 758.16.

Description: Gold sodium thiomalate—White to yellowish white, odorless or practically odorless, lumpy solid.

Solubility: Gold sodium thiomalate—Very soluble in water; insoluble in alcohol, in ether, and in most organic solvents.

USP requirements:

Gold Sodium Thiomalate USP—Preserve in tight, light-resistant containers. A mixture of the mono- and di-sodium salts of gold thiomalic acid. Contains not less than 44.8% and not more than 49.6% of gold. Contains not less than

49.0% and not more than 52.5% of gold, on a dry, glycerin-free basis. Meets the requirements for Identification, pH (5.8–6.5, in a solution [1 in 10]), Loss on drying (not more than 8.0%), and Glycerin (not more than 5.5%).

Gold Sodium Thiomalate Injection USP—Preserve in single-dose or in multiple-dose containers, preferably of Type I glass, protected from light. A sterile solution of Gold Sodium Thiomalate in Water for Injection. Contains the labeled amount, within ±5%. Meets the requirements for Identification, pH (5.8–6.5), and Injections.

GONADORELIN

Source: A gonad stimulating principle (luteinizing hormone-releasing factor). Source of this compound may be sheep, pig, or other species, or it could be synthetic.

Chemical name:
Gonadorelin acetate—5-Oxo-L-prolyl-L-histidyl-L-tryptophyl-L-seryl-L-tyrosylglycyl-L-leucyl-L-arginyl-L-prolylglycinamide acetate (salt) hydrate.
Gonadorelin hydrochloride—5-Oxo-L-prolyl-L-histidyl-L-tryptophyl-L-seryl-L-tyrosyl-glycyl-L-leucyl-L-arginyl-L-prolylglycinamide hydrochloride.

Molecular formula:
Gonadorelin acetate—$C_{55}H_{75}N_{17}O_{13} \cdot xC_2H_4O_2 \cdot yH_2O$.
Gonadorelin hydrochloride—$C_{55}H_{75}N_{17}O_{13} \cdot xHCl$.
Note: Gonadorelin acetate is $C_{55}H_{75}N_{17}O_{13}$ as the diacetate (as the tetrahydrate) or a mixture of monoacetate and diacetate hydrates. Gonadorelin hydrochloride is $C_{55}H_{75}N_{17}O_{13}$ as the monohydrochloride or the dihydrochloride or as a mixture of these.

Molecular weight: 1182.33.

Description: White powder. Hygroscopic and moisture-sensitive.

Solubility: Soluble in alcohol and in water.

USP requirements:
Gonadorelin Acetate for Injection—Not in USP.
Gonadorelin Hydrochloride for Injection—Not in USP.

CHORIONIC GONADOTROPIN

Description:
Chorionic Gonadotropin USP—White or practically white, amorphous powder.
Chorionic Gonadotropin for Injection USP—White or practically white, amorphous solid having the characteristic appearance of substances prepared by freeze-drying.

Solubility: Chorionic Gonadotropin USP—Freely soluble in water.

USP requirements:
Chorionic Gonadotropin USP—Preserve in tight containers, preferably of Type I glass, in a refrigerator. A gonad-stimulating polypeptide hormone obtained from the urine of pregnant women. Its potency is not less than 1500 USP Chorionic Gonadotropin Units in each mg, and not less than 80.0% and not more than 125.0% of the potency stated on the label. Meets the requirements for Bacterial endotoxins, Acute toxicity, Water (not more than 5.0%), and Estrogenic activity.
Chorionic Gonadotropin for Injection USP—Preserve in Containers for Sterile Solids. A sterile, dry mixture of Chorionic Gonadotropin with suitable diluents and buffers. Label it to indicate the expiration date. Contains the labeled amount in USP Chorionic Gonadotropin Units, within −20% to +25%. Meets the requirements for Constituted solution, Bacterial endotoxins, pH (6.0–8.0), Estrogenic activity, and Uniformity of dosage units, and for Sterility tests and Labeling under Injections.

GOSERELIN

Source: Goserelin acetate—Synthetic decapeptide analog of luteinizing hormone-releasing hormone (LHRH).

Chemical name: Goserelin acetate—L-pyroglutamyl-L-histidyl-L-tryptophyl-L-seryl-L-tyrosyl-D-(0-tert-butyl)seryl-L-leucyl-L-arginyl-L-prolyl-azaglycine amide acetate.

Molecular formula: Goserelin acetate—$C_{61}H_{87}N_{18}O_{16}$.

Molecular weight: Goserelin acetate—1328.

Description: Goserelin acetate—Off-white powder.

Solubility: Goserelin acetate—Freely soluble in glacial acetic acid; soluble in water, in 0.1 *M* hydrochloric acid, in 0.1 *M* sodium hydroxide, in dimethylformamide, and in dimethyl sulfoxide; practically insoluble in acetone, in chloroform, and in ether.

USP requirements: Goserelin Acetate Implants—Not in USP.

GRAMICIDIN

Chemical name: Gramicidin.

Description: Gramicidin USP—White or practically white, odorless, crystalline powder.

Solubility: Gramicidin USP—Insoluble in water; soluble in alcohol.

USP requirements: Gramicidin USP—Preserve in tight containers. An antibacterial substance produced by the growth of *Bacillus brevis* Dubos (Fam. Bacillaceae). May be obtained from tyrothricin. Has a potency of not less than 900 mcg of gramicidin per mg, calculated on the dried basis. Meets the requirements for Identification, Melting temperature (not less than 229 °C, determined after drying), Crystallinity, Loss on drying (not more than 3.0%), and Residue on ignition (not more than 1.0%).

GRANISETRON

Chemical name: 1*H*-Indazole-3-carboxamide, 1-methyl-*N*-(9-methyl-9-azabicyclo[3.3.1]non-3-yl)-, *endo*-.

Molecular formula: $C_{18}H_{24}N_4O$.

Molecular weight: 312.41.

USP requirements: Granisetron Injection—Not in USP.

GREEN SOAP

Description: Green Soap USP—Soft, unctuous, yellowish white to brownish or greenish yellow, transparent to translucent mass. Has a slight, characteristic odor, often suggesting the oil from which it was prepared. Its solution (1 in 20) is alkaline to bromothymol blue TS.

USP requirements:
Green Soap USP—Preserve in well-closed containers. A potassium soap made by the saponification of suitable vegetable oils, excluding coconut oil and palm kernel oil, without the removal of glycerin.

Green Soap may be prepared as follows: 380 grams of the Vegetable Oil, 20 grams of Oleic Acid, 91.7 grams of Potassium Hydroxide (total alkali 85%), 50 mL of Glycerin, and a sufficient quantity of Purified Water to make about 1000 grams. Mix the oil and the Oleic Acid, and heat the mixture to about 80 °C. Dissolve the Potassium Hydroxide in a mixture of the Glycerin and 100 mL of Purified Water, and add the solution, while it is still hot, to the hot oil. Stir the mixture vigorously until emulsified, then heat while continuing the stirring, until the mixture is homogeneous and a test portion will dissolve to give a clear solution in hot water. Add hot purified water to make the product weigh 1000 grams, continuing the stirring until the Soap is homogeneous.

Meets the requirements for Water (not more than 52.0%), Alcohol-insoluble substances (not more than 3.0%), Free alkali hydroxides (not more than 0.25% of potassium hydroxide), Alkali carbonates (0.35%, as potassium carbonate), Unsaponified matter, and Characteristics of the liberated fatty acids.

Green Soap Tincture USP—Preserve in tight containers.

Prepare Green Soap Tincture as follows: 650 grams of Green Soap, Suitable essential oil(s), 316 mL of Alcohol, and a sufficient quantity of Purified Water to make 1000 mL. Mix the oil(s) and Alcohol, dissolve in this the Green Soap by stirring or by agitation, set the solution aside for 24 hours, filter through paper, and add water to make 1000 mL.

Meets the requirements for Identification, pH (9.5–11.5), and Alcohol content (28.0–32.0%).

GRISEOFULVIN

Source: Derived from a species of *Penicillium*.

Chemical name: Spiro[benzofuran-2(3*H*),1′-[2]cyclohexene]-3,4′-dione, 7-chloro-2′,4,6-trimethoxy-6′-methyl-, (1′*S*-*trans*)-.

Molecular formula: $C_{17}H_{17}ClO_6$.

Molecular weight: 352.77.

Description: Griseofulvin USP—White to creamy white, odorless powder, in which particles of the order of 4 micrometers in diameter predominate.

Solubility: Griseofulvin USP—Very slightly soluble in water; soluble in acetone, in dimethylformamide, and in chloroform; sparingly soluble in alcohol.

USP requirements:

Griseofulvin USP—Preserve in tight containers. Has a potency of not less than 900 mcg of griseofulvin per mg. Meets the requirements for Identification, Melting range (217–224 °C), Specific rotation (+348° to +364°), Crystallinity, Loss on drying (not more than 1.0%), Residue on ignition (not more than 0.2%), Heavy metals (not more than 0.0025%), Specific surface area (1.3–1.7 square meters per gram), and Organic volatile impurities.

Griseofulvin Capsules USP (Microsize)—Preserve in tight containers. The label indicates that the griseofulvin contained is known as griseofulvin (microsize). Contain the labeled amount, within −10% to +15%. Meet the requirements for Identification, Dissolution (80% in 30 minutes in water containing 5.4 mg of sodium lauryl sulfate per mL in Apparatus 2 at 100 rpm), Uniformity of dosage units, and Loss on drying (not more than 1.0%).

Griseofulvin Oral Suspension USP (Microsize)—Preserve in tight containers. Contains one or more suitable colors, diluents, flavors, preservatives, and wetting agents. The label indicates that the griseofulvin contained is known as griseofulvin (microsize). Contains the labeled amount, within −10% to +15%. Meets the requirements for Identification, pH (5.5–7.5), Deliverable volume (multiple-unit containers), and Uniformity of dosage units (single-unit containers).

Griseofulvin Tablets USP (Microsize)—Preserve in tight containers. The label indicates that the griseofulvin contained is known as griseofulvin (microsize). Contain the labeled amount, within −10% to +15%. Meet the requirements for Identification, Dissolution (75% in 90 minutes in water containing 40.0 mg of sodium lauryl sulfate per mL in Apparatus 2 at 75 rpm), Uniformity of dosage units, and Loss on drying (not more than 5.0%).

Ultramicrosize Griseofulvin Tablets USP—Preserve in well-closed containers. Composed of ultramicrosize crystals of Griseofulvin dispersed in Polyethylene Glycol 6000 or dispersed by other suitable means. Contain the labeled amount, within −10% to +15%. Meet the requirements for Identification, Dissolution (85% in 60 minutes in water containing 5.4 mg of sodium lauryl sulfate per mL in Apparatus 2 at 100 rpm), Uniformity of dosage units, and Loss on drying (not more than 5.0%).

GUAIFENESIN

Chemical name: 1,2-Propanediol, 3-(2-methoxyphenoxy)-.

Molecular formula: $C_{10}H_{14}O_4$.

Molecular weight: 198.22.

Description: Guaifenesin USP—White to slightly gray, crystalline powder. May have a slight characteristic odor.

Solubility: Guaifenesin USP—Soluble in water, in alcohol, in chloroform, in glycerin, and in propylene glycol.

USP requirements:

Guaifenesin USP—Preserve in tight containers. Contains not less than 98.0% and not more than 102.0% of guaifenesin, calculated on the dried basis. Meets the requirements for Identification, Melting range (78–82 °C, the range between beginning and end of melting not more than 3 °C), pH (5.0–7.0, in a solution [1 in 100]), Loss on drying (not more than 0.5%), Heavy metals (not more than 0.0025%), Related substances (not more than 1.0%), Free guaiacol, and Organic volatile impurities.

Guaifenesin Capsules USP—Preserve in tight containers. Contain the labeled amount, within ±10%. Meet the requirements for Identification, Dissolution (75% in 45 minutes in water in Apparatus 1 at 100 rpm), and Uniformity of dosage units.

Guaifenesin Extended-release Capsules—Not in USP.

Guaifenesin Oral Solution—Not in USP.

Guaifenesin Syrup USP—Preserve in tight containers. Contains the labeled amount, within ±5%. Meets the requirements for Identification, pH (2.3–3.0), and Alcohol content (if present, within −10% to +15% of labeled amount).

Guaifenesin Tablets USP—Preserve in tight containers. Contain the labeled amount, within ±10%. Meet the requirements for Identification, Dissolution (75% in 45 minutes in water in Apparatus 2 at 50 rpm), and Uniformity of dosage units.

Guaifenesin Extended-release Tablets—Not in USP.

GUAIFENESIN AND CODEINE

For *Guaifenesin* and *Codeine*—See individual listings for chemistry information.

USP requirements:

Guaifenesin and Codeine Phosphate Oral Solution—Not in USP.

Guaifenesin and Codeine Phosphate Syrup USP—Preserve in tight, light-resistant containers, at controlled room temperature. Contains the labeled amounts, within ±10%. Meets the requirements for Identification, pH (2.3–3.0 if it contains alcohol; 5.0–5.5 if it does not contain alcohol), and Alcohol content (if present, within −10% to +15% of labeled amount).

GUANABENZ

Chemical name: Guanabenz acetate—Hydrazinecarboximidamide, 2-[(2,6-dichlorophenyl)methylene]-, monoacetate.

Molecular formula: Guanabenz acetate—$C_8H_8Cl_2N_4 \cdot C_2H_4O_2$.

Molecular weight: Guanabenz acetate—291.14.

Description: Guanabenz Acetate USP—White or almost white powder having not more than a slight odor.

Solubility: Guanabenz Acetate USP—Sparingly soluble in water and in 0.1 *N* hydrochloric acid; soluble in alcohol and in propylene glycol.

USP requirements:

Guanabenz Acetate USP—Preserve in tight, light-resistant containers. Contains not less than 98.0% and not more than 101.5% of guanabenz acetate. Meets the requirements for Identification, pH (5.5–7.0, in a solution [7 in 1000]), Loss on drying (not more than 1.0%), Residue on ignition (not more than 0.2%), Limit of 2,6-dichlorobenzaldehyde, Chromatographic purity, and Organic volatile impurities.

Guanabenz Acetate Tablets USP—Preserve in tight, light-resistant containers. Contain an amount of guanabenz acetate equivalent to the labeled amount of guanabenz, within ±10%. Meet the requirements for Identification, Dissolution (75% in 60 minutes in water in Apparatus 2 at 50 rpm), Uniformity of dosage units, and Chromatographic purity.

GUANADREL

Chemical name: Guanadrel sulfate—Guanidine (1,4-dioxaspiro-[4.5]dec-2-ylmethyl)-, sulfate (2:1).

Molecular formula: Guanadrel sulfate—$(C_{10}H_{19}N_3O_2)_2 \cdot H_2SO_4$.

Molecular weight: Guanadrel sulfate—524.63.

Description: Guanadrel Sulfate USP—White to off-white, crystalline powder. Melts at about 235 °C, with decomposition.

Solubility: Guanadrel Sulfate USP—Soluble in water; sparingly soluble in methanol; slightly soluble in alcohol and in acetone.

USP requirements:

Guanadrel Sulfate USP—Preserve in well-closed containers. Contains not less than 97.0% and not more than 103.0% of guanadrel sulfate, calculated on the dried basis. Meets the requirements for Identification, Loss on drying (not more than 0.5%), Residue on ignition (not more than 0.5%), Heavy metals (not more than 0.002%), and Organic volatile impurities.

Guanadrel Sulfate Tablets USP—Preserve in tight, light-resistant containers. Contain the labeled amount, within ±10%. Meet the requirements for Identification, Dissolution (70% in 20 minutes in Working buffer solution in Apparatus 2 at 50 rpm), and Uniformity of dosage units.

GUANETHIDINE

Chemical name:

Guanethidine monosulfate—Guanidine, [2-(hexahydro-1(2*H*)-azocinyl)ethyl]-, sulfate (1:1).

Guanethidine sulfate—Guanidine, [2-(hexahydro-1(2*H*)-azocinyl)ethyl]-, sulfate (2:1).

Molecular formula:

Guanethidine monosulfate—$C_{10}H_{22}N_4 \cdot H_2SO_4$.

Guanethidine sulfate—$(C_{10}H_{22}N_4)_2 \cdot H_2SO_4$.

Molecular weight:

Guanethidine monosulfate—296.38.

Guanethidine sulfate—494.70.

Description: Guanethidine Monosulfate USP—White to off-white, crystalline powder.

pKa: 9.0 and 12.0.

Solubility: Guanethidine Monosulfate USP—Very soluble in water; sparingly soluble in alcohol; practically insoluble in chloroform.

USP requirements:

Guanethidine Monosulfate USP—Preserve in well-closed containers. Contains not less than 97.0% and not more than 103.0% of guanethidine monosulfate, calculated on the dried basis. Meets the requirements for Identification, pH (4.7–5.7, in a solution containing 20 mg per mL), Loss on drying (not more than 0.5%), Residue on ignition (not more than 0.2%), Heavy metals (not more than 0.001%), and Organic volatile impurities.

Guanethidine Monosulfate Tablets USP—Preserve in well-closed containers. Contain an amount of guanethidine monosulfate equivalent to the labeled amount of guanethidine sulfate, within ±10%. Meet the requirements for Identification, Dissolution (75% in 45 minutes in water in Apparatus 1 at 100 rpm), and Uniformity of dosage units.

GUANETHIDINE AND HYDROCHLOROTHIAZIDE

For *Guanethidine* and *Hydrochlorothiazide*—See individual listings for chemistry information.

USP requirements: Guanethidine Monosulfate and Hydrochlorothiazide Tablets—Not in USP.

GUANFACINE

Chemical name: Guanfacine hydrochloride—Benzeneacetamide, *N*-(aminoiminomethyl)-2,6-dichloro-, monohydrochloride.

Molecular formula: Guanfacine hydrochloride—$C_9H_9Cl_2N_3O \cdot HCl$.

Molecular weight: Guanfacine hydrochloride—282.56.

Description: Guanfacine hydrochloride—White to off-white powder.

Solubility: Guanfacine hydrochloride—Sparingly soluble in water and in alcohol; slightly soluble in acetone.

USP requirements: Guanfacine Hydrochloride Tablets—Not in USP.

GUAR GUM

Description: Guar Gum NF—White to yellowish white, practically odorless powder.

NF category: Suspending and/or viscosity-increasing agent; tablet binder.

Solubility: Guar Gum NF—Dispersible in hot or cold water, forming a colloidal solution.

NF requirements: Guar Gum NF—Preserve in well-closed containers. A gum obtained from the ground endosperms of *Cyamopsis tetragonolobus* (Linné) Taub. (Fam. Leguminosae). Consists chiefly of a high molecular weight hydrocolloidal polysaccharide composed of galactan and mannan units combined through glycosidic linkages, which may be described chemically as a galactomannan. Meets the requirements for Identification, Loss on drying (not more than 15.0%), Ash (not more than 1.5%), Acid-insoluble matter (not more than 7.0%), Arsenic (not more than 3 ppm), Lead (not more than 0.001%), Heavy metals (not more than 0.002%), Protein (not more than 10.0%), Starch, and Galactomannans (not less than 66.0%).

GUTTA PERCHA

Source: *Trans* isomer of rubber prepared from the exudate of various trees of the genus *Palaquium*, Fam. *Sapotaceae*.

Description: Gutta Percha USP—Lumps or blocks of variable size; externally brown or grayish brown to grayish white in color; internally reddish yellow or reddish gray and having a laminated or fibrous appearance. Is flexible but only slightly elastic. Has a slight, characteristic odor.

Solubility: Gutta Percha USP—Insoluble in water; about 90% soluble in chloroform; partly soluble in carbon disulfide and in turpentine oil.

USP requirements: Gutta Percha USP—Preserve under water in well-closed containers, protected from light. The coagulated, dried, purified latex of the trees of the genera *Palaquium* and *Payena* and most commonly *Palaquium gutta* (Hooker) Baillon (Fam. Sapotaceae). Meets the requirement for Residue on ignition (not more than 1.7%).

HAEMOPHILUS B CONJUGATE VACCINE

Source: Purified capsular polysaccharide, a polymer of ribose, ribitol, and phosphate (PRP), from the bacterium *Haemophilus influenzae* type b (Hib). It has been conjugated in one of the following ways—For the diphtheria toxoid conjugate, the polysaccharide has been conjugated to the diphtheria toxoid via a 6-carbon linker molecule; for the diphtheria CRM_{197} protein conjugate, the oligosaccharide has been derived from the polysaccharide and has been bound directly to CRM_{197} (a nontoxic variant of diphtheria toxin) by reductive amination; for the meningococcal protein conjugate, the polysaccharide has been covalently bound to an outer membrane protein complex (OMPC) of the B11 strain of *Neisseria meningitidis* serogroup B; and for the tetanus protein conjugate, the polysaccharide has been covalently bound to tetanus toxoid protein.

USP requirements:
- Haemophilus b Conjugate Vaccine (HbOC—Diphtheria CRM_{197} Protein Conjugate) Injection—Not in USP.
- Haemophilus b Conjugate Vaccine (PRP-D—Diphtheria Toxoid Conjugate) Injection—Not in USP.
- Haemophilus b Conjugate Vaccine (PRP-OMP—Meningococcal Protein Conjugate) Injection—Not in USP.
- Haemophilus b Conjugate Vaccine (PRP-T—Tetanus Protein Conjugate) Injection—Not in USP.
- Haemophilus b Conjugate Vaccine (with tetanus protein conjugate) Injection—Not in USP.

HAEMOPHILUS B POLYSACCHARIDE VACCINE

Source: Purified capsular polysaccharide, a polymer of ribose, ribitol, and phosphate (PRP), from the bacterium *Haemophilus influenzae* type b (Hib).

USP requirements: Haemophilus b Polysaccharide Vaccine for Injection—Not in USP.

HALAZEPAM

Chemical name: 2*H*-1,4-Benzodiazepin-2-one, 7-chloro-1,3-dihydro-5-phenyl-1-(2,2,2-trifluoroethyl)-.

Molecular formula: $C_{17}H_{12}ClF_3N_2O$.

Molecular weight: 352.74.

Description: Halazepam USP—Fine, white to light cream-colored powder. Melts at about 165 °C.

Solubility: Halazepam USP—Freely soluble in chloroform; soluble in methanol; very slightly soluble in water.

USP requirements:
- Halazepam USP—Preserve in well-closed containers. Contains not less than 98.5% and not more than 101.0% of halazepam, calculated on the dried basis. Meets the requirements for Identification, Loss on drying (not more than 1.0%), Residue on ignition (not more than 0.2%), Heavy metals (not more than 0.002%), Related compounds, and Organic volatile impurities.
- Halazepam Tablets USP—Preserve in well-closed containers. Contain the labeled amount, within ±10%. Meet the requirements for Identification, Dissolution (75% in 30 minutes in 0.1 *N* hydrochloric acid in Apparatus 1 at 100 rpm), and Uniformity of dosage units.

HALAZONE

Chemical name: Benzoic acid, 4-[(dichloroamino)sulfonyl]-.

Molecular formula: $C_7H_5Cl_2NO_4S$.

Molecular weight: 270.09.

Description: Halazone USP—White, crystalline powder, having a characteristic chlorine-like odor. Affected by light. Melts at about 194 °C, with decomposition.

Solubility:
- Halazone USP—Very slightly soluble in water and in chloroform; soluble in glacial acetic acid. Dissolves in solutions of alkali hydroxides and carbonates with the formation of a salt.
- Halazone Tablets for Solution USP—Soluble in water.

USP requirements:
- Halazone USP—Preserve in tight, light-resistant containers. Contains not less than 91.5% and not more than 100.5% of halazone, calculated on the dried basis. Meets the requirements for Identification, Loss on drying (not more than 0.5%), and Readily carbonizable substances.
- Halazone Tablets for Solution USP—Preserve in tight, light-resistant containers. Label Tablets to indicate that they are not intended to be swallowed. Contain the labeled amount, within −10% to +35%. Meet the requirements for Identification, Disintegration (10 minutes), Uniformity of dosage units, and pH (not less than 7.0, in a solution of 1 Tablet, containing 4 mg of halazone, in 200 mL of water).

HALCINONIDE

Chemical name: Pregn-4-ene-3,20-dione, 21-chloro-9-fluoro-11-hydroxy-16,17-[(1-methylethylidene)bis(oxy)]-, (11 beta,16 alpha)-.

Molecular formula: $C_{24}H_{32}ClFO_5$.

Molecular weight: 454.97.

Description: Halcinonide USP—White to off-white, odorless, crystalline powder.

Solubility: Halcinonide USP—Soluble in acetone and in chloroform; slightly soluble in alcohol and in ethyl ether; insoluble in water and in hexanes.

USP requirements:
Halcinonide USP—Preserve in well-closed containers. Contains not less than 97.0% and not more than 102.0% of halcinonide. Meets the requirements for Identification, Specific rotation (+150° to +160°), Loss on drying (not more than 1.0%), Residue on ignition (not more than 0.2%), and Chromatographic purity.
Halcinonide Cream USP—Preserve in well-closed containers. It is Halcinonide in a suitable cream base. Contains the labeled amount, within ±10%. Meets the requirements for Identification, Microbial limits, and Minimum fill.
Halcinonide Ointment USP—Preserve in well-closed containers. It is Halcinonide in a suitable ointment base. Contains the labeled amount, within ±10%. Meets the requirements for Identification, Microbial limits, and Minimum fill.
Halcinonide Topical Solution USP—Preserve in well-closed containers. It is Halcinonide in a suitable aqueous vehicle. Contains the labeled amount, within ±10%. Meets the requirements for Identification and Microbial limits.

HALOBETASOL

Chemical name: Halobetasol propionate—Pregna-1,4-diene-3,20-dione, 21-chloro-6,9-difluoro-11-hydroxy-16-methyl-17-(1-oxopropoxy)-, (6 alpha,11 beta,16 beta)-.

Molecular formula: Halobetasol propionate—$C_{25}H_{31}ClF_2O_5$.

Molecular weight: Halobetasol propionate—484.97.

Description: Halobetasol propionate—White crystalline powder.

Solubility: Halobetasol propionate—Insoluble in water.

USP requirements:
Halobetasol Propionate Cream—Not in USP.
Halobetasol Propionate Ointment—Not in USP.

HALOFANTRINE

Chemical name: Halofantrine hydrochloride—9-Phenanthrenemethanol, 1,3-dichloro-alpha-[2-(dibutylamino)ethyl]-6-(trifluoromethyl)-, hydrochloride.

Molecular formula: Halofantrine hydrochloride—$C_{26}H_{30}Cl_2F_3NO \cdot HCl$.

Molecular weight: Halofantrine hydrochloride—536.89.

USP requirements:
Halofantrine Hydrochloride Oral Suspension—Not in USP.
Halofantrine Hydrochloride Tablets—Not in USP.

HALOPERIDOL

Chemical group: A butyrophenone derivative.

Chemical name:
Haloperidol—1-Butanone, 4-[4-(4-chlorophenyl)-4-hydroxy-1-piperidinyl]-1-(4-fluorophenyl)-.
Haloperidol decanoate—Decanoic acid, 4-(4-chlorophenyl)-1-[4-(4-fluorophenyl)-4-oxobutyl]-4-piperidinyl ester.

Molecular formula:
Haloperidol—$C_{21}H_{23}ClFNO_2$.
Haloperidol decanoate—$C_{31}H_{41}ClFNO_3$.

Molecular weight:
Haloperidol—375.87.
Haloperidol decanoate—530.12.

Description: Haloperidol USP—White to faintly yellowish, amorphous or microcrystalline powder. Its saturated solution is neutral to litmus.

Solubility:
Haloperidol USP—Practically insoluble in water; soluble in chloroform; sparingly soluble in alcohol; slightly soluble in ether.
Haloperidol decanoate—Practically insoluble in water; soluble in most organic solvents.

USP requirements:
Haloperidol USP—Preserve in tight, light-resistant containers. Contains not less than 98.0% and not more than 102.0% of haloperidol, calculated on the dried basis. Meets the requirements for Identification, Melting range (147–152 °C), Loss on drying (not more than 0.5%), Residue on ignition (not more than 0.1%), 4,4′-Bis[4-(*p*-chlorophenyl)-4-hydroxypiperidino]butyrophenone, and Organic volatile impurities.
Haloperidol Injection USP—Preserve in single-dose or in multiple-dose containers, preferably of Type I glass, protected from light. A sterile solution of Haloperidol in Water for Injection, prepared with the aid of Lactic Acid. Contains the labeled amount, within ±10%. Meets the requirements for Identification, Bacterial endotoxins, pH (3.0–3.8), and Injections.
Haloperidol Oral Solution USP—Preserve in tight, light-resistant containers. A solution of Haloperidol in Water, prepared with the aid of Lactic Acid. Contains the labeled amount, within ±10%. Meets the requirements for Identification and pH (2.75–3.75).
Haloperidol Tablets USP—Preserve in tight, light-resistant containers. Contain the labeled amount, within ±10%. Meet the requirements for Identification, Dissolution (80% in 60 minutes in simulated gastric fluid TS, without the enzyme, in Apparatus 1 at 100 rpm), and Uniformity of dosage units.
Haloperidol Decanoate Injection—Not in USP.

HALOPROGIN

Chemical name: Benzene, 1,2,4-trichloro-5-[(3-iodo-2-propynyl)-oxy]-.

Molecular formula: $C_9H_4Cl_3IO$.

Molecular weight: 361.39.

Description: White or pale yellow crystals. Melting point is about 113–114 °C.

Solubility: Very slightly soluble in water; easily soluble in methanol and in ethanol.

USP requirements:
Haloprogin USP—Preserve in tight, light-resistant containers. Contains not less than 95.0% and not more than 102.0% of haloprogin, calculated on the dried basis. Meets the requirements for Identification, Melting range (110–114 °C), Acidity, Loss on drying (not more than 0.5%), Residue on ignition (not more than 0.1%), and Heavy metals (not more than 0.005%).
Haloprogin Cream USP—Preserve in tight, light-resistant containers, at controlled room temperature. Contains the

labeled amount, within ±10%. Meets the requirements for Identification, Microbial limits, Minimum fill, and Water (not more than 3.0%).

Haloprogin Topical Solution USP—Preserve in tight, light-resistant containers, at controlled room temperature. Contains the labeled amount, within ±10%. Meets the requirements for Identification, Specific gravity (0.838–0.852), and Alcohol (within ±5% of the labeled amount).

HALOTHANE

Chemical name: Ethane, 2-bromo-2-chloro-1,1,1-trifluoro-.

Molecular formula: $C_2HBrClF_3$.

Molecular weight: 197.38.

Description: Halothane USP—Colorless, mobile, nonflammable, heavy liquid, having a characteristic odor resembling that of chloroform.

Solubility: Halothane USP—Slightly soluble in water; miscible with alcohol, with chloroform, with ether, and with fixed oils.

Other characteristics:
Blood/gas coefficient—2.5 at 37 °C.
Olive oil/water coefficient—220 at 37 °C.

USP requirements: Halothane USP—Preserve in tight, light-resistant containers, preferably of Type NP glass, and avoid exposure to excessive heat. Dispense it only in the original container. Contains 0.008% to 0.012% of thymol, by weight, as a stabilizer. Meets the requirements for Identification, Specific gravity (1.872–1.877 at 20 °C), Distilling range (not less than 95% within a 1° range between 49 and 51 °C; not less than 100% between 49 and 51 °C, a correction factor of 0.040 °C per mm being applied as necessary), Refractive index (1.369–1.371 at 20 °C), Acidity or alkalinity, Water (not more than 0.03%), Nonvolatile residue (not more than 1 mg per 50 mL), Chloride and bromide, Thymol content, and Chromatographic purity.

HELIUM

Chemical name: Helium.

Molecular formula: He.

Molecular weight: 4.00.

Description: Helium USP—Colorless, odorless gas, which is not combustible and does not support combustion. At 0 °C and at a pressure of 760 mm of mercury, 1000 mL of the gas weighs about 180 mg.

Solubility: Helium USP—Very slightly soluble in water.

USP requirements: Helium USP—Preserve in cylinders. Contains not less than 99.0%, by volume, of helium. Meets the requirements for Identification, Odor, Carbon monoxide (not more than 0.001%), and Air (not more than 1.0%).

HEMIN

Chemical name: Chloro[7,12-diethenyl-3,8,13,17-tetramethyl-21*H*,23*H*-porphine-2,18-dipropanoato(2-)-N^{21},N^{22},N^{23},N^{24}]-iron.

Molecular formula: $C_{34}H_{32}ClFeN_4O_4$.

Molecular weight: 651.96.

Description: Polychromatic crystals (usually brownish to blue) which do not melt under 300 °C.

Solubility: Freely soluble in dilute base through conversion to hematin by replacement of the chlorine atom by hydroxyl; sparingly soluble in alcohol; insoluble in water.

USP requirements: Hemin for Injection—Not in USP.

HEPARIN

Description:
Heparin calcium—White or almost white, moderately hygroscopic powder.
Heparin Sodium USP—White or pale-colored, amorphous powder. Is odorless or practically so, and is hygroscopic.

Solubility:
Heparin calcium—Soluble 1 in less than 5 of water.
Heparin Sodium USP—Soluble in water.

Other characteristics: Highly acidic.

USP requirements:

Heparin Lock Flush Solution USP—Preserve in single-dose pre-filled syringes or containers, or in multiple-dose containers, preferably of Type I glass. A sterile preparation of Heparin Sodium Injection with sufficient Sodium Chloride to make it isotonic with blood. Label it to indicate the volume of the total contents, and to indicate the potency in terms of USP Heparin Units only per mL, except that single unit-dose containers may be labeled additionally to indicate the single unit-dose volume and the total number of USP Heparin Units in the contents. Where it is labeled with total content, the label states clearly that the entire contents are to be used or, if not, any remaining portion is to be discarded. Label it to indicate the organ and species from which the heparin sodium is derived. The label states also that the Solution is intended for maintenance of patency of intravenous injection devices only, and that it is not to be used for anticoagulant therapy. The label states also that in the case of Solution having a concentration of 10 USP Heparin Units per mL, it may alter, and that in the case of higher concentrations it will alter, the results of blood coagulation tests. Exhibits the labeled potency, within −10% to +20%, stated in terms of USP Heparin Units. Contains not more than 1.00% of sodium chloride. Meets the requirements for Bacterial endotoxins, pH (5.0–7.5), and Particulate matter, and for Injections.

Heparin Calcium USP—Preserve in tight containers. The calcium salt of forms of a sulfated glycosaminoglycan of mixed mucopolysaccharide nature varying in molecular weights. Present in mammalian tissues and usually obtained from the intestinal mucosa or other suitable tissues of domestic mammals used for food by man. Composed of polymers of alternating derivatives of D-glycosamine (N-sulfated or N-acetylated) and uronic acid (L-iduronic acid or D-glucuronic acid) joined by glycosidic linkages, the components being liberated in varying proportions on complete hydrolysis. A mixture of active principles some of which have the property of prolonging the clotting time of blood mainly through the formation of a complex with the plasma protein Anti-thrombin to potentiate the inactivation of Thrombin and to inhibit other coagulation proteases such as Activated Factor X in the clotting sequence. Label it to indicate the organ and species from which it is derived. The potency of heparin calcium, calculated on the dried basis, is not less than 140 USP Heparin Units in each mg, and not less than 90.0% and not more than 110.0% of the potency stated on the label. Heparin Calcium is essentially free from sodium. Meets the requirements for Identification, Bacterial endotoxins, pH (5.0–7.5, in a solution [1 in 100]), Loss on drying (not more than 5%), Residue on ignition (28.0–41.0%), Nitrogen content (1.3–2.5%, calculated on the dried basis), Protein, Heavy metals (not more than 0.003%), and Anti-factor X_a activity.

Note: USP Heparin Units are consistently established on the basis of the Assay set forth in *USP/NF*, independently of International Units, and the respective units are not equivalent. The USP Units for Anti-factor X_a activity are defined by the USP Heparin Sodium Reference Standard.

Heparin Calcium Injection USP—Preserve in single-dose or in multiple-dose containers, preferably of Type I glass. A sterile solution of Heparin Calcium in Water for Injection. Label it to indicate the volume of the total contents and the potency in terms of USP Heparin Units only per mL, except that single unit-dose containers may be labeled additionally to indicate the single unit-dose volume and the total number of USP Heparin Units in the contents. Where it is labeled with total content, the label states also that the entire contents are to be used or, if not, any remaining portion is to be discarded. Label it to indicate also the organ and species from which it is derived. Exhibits the labeled potency, within ± 10%, stated in terms of USP Heparin Units. Meets the requirements for Bacterial endotoxins, pH (5.0–7.5), Particulate matter, Injections, and Anti-factor X_a activity.

Note: USP Heparin Units are consistently established on the basis of the Assay set forth in *USP/NF*, independently of International Units, and the respective units are not equivalent. The USP Units for Anti-factor X_a activity are defined by the USP Heparin Sodium Reference Standard.

Heparin Sodium USP—Preserve in tight containers, and store below 40 °C, preferably between 15 and 30 °C, unless otherwise specified by the manufacturer. The sodium salt of a sulfated glycosaminoglycan of mixed mucopolysaccharides varying in molecular weights. Present in mammalian tissues and usually obtained from the intestinal mucosa or other suitable tissues of domestic mammals used for food by man. Composed of polymers of alternating derivatives of D-glycosamine (N-sulfated or N-acetylated) and uronic acid (L-iduronic acid or D-glucuronic acid) joined by glycosidic linkages, the components being liberated in varying proportions on complete hydrolysis. A mixture of active principles some of which have the property of prolonging the clotting time of blood mainly through the formation of a complex with the plasma protein Anti-thrombin III to potentiate the inactivation of Thrombin and to inhibit other coagulation proteases such as Activated Factor X in the clotting sequence. Label it to indicate the organ and species from which it is derived. The potency of heparin sodium, calculated on the dried basis, is not less than 140 USP Heparin Units in each mg, and not less than 90.0% and not more than 110.0% of the potency stated on the label. Meets the requirements for Identification, Bacterial endotoxins, pH (5.0–7.5, in a solution [1 in 100]), Loss on drying (not more than 5%), Residue on ignition (28.0–41.0%), Nitrogen content (1.3–2.5%, calculated on the dried basis), Protein, Heavy metals (not more than 0.003%), and Anti-factor X_a activity.

Note: USP Heparin Units are consistently established on the basis of the Assay set forth in *USP/NF*, independently of International Units, and the respective units are not equivalent. The USP Units for Anti-factor X_a activity are defined by the USP Heparin Sodium Reference Standard.

Heparin Sodium Injection USP—Preserve in single-dose or in multiple-dose containers, preferably of Type I glass. A sterile solution of Heparin Sodium in Water for Injection. Label it to indicate the volume of the total contents and the potency in terms of USP Heparin Units only per mL, except that single unit-dose containers may be labeled additionally to indicate the single unit-dose volume and the total number of USP Heparin Units in the contents. Where it is labeled with total content, the label states also that the entire contents are to be used or, if not, any remaining portion is to be discarded. Label it to indicate also the organ and species from which it is derived. Exhibits the labeled potency, within ± 10%, stated in terms of USP Heparin Units. Meets the requirements for Bacterial endotoxins, pH (5.0–7.5), Particulate matter, Anti-factor X_a activity, and Injections.

Note: USP Heparin Units are consistently established on the basis of the Assay set forth in *USP/NF*, independently of International Units, and the respective units are not equivalent. The USP Units for Anti-factor X_a activity are defined by the USP Heparin Sodium Reference Standard.

HEPARIN AND DEXTROSE

For *Heparin* and *Dextrose*—See individual listings for chemistry information.

USP requirements: Heparin Sodium in Dextrose Injection—Not in USP.

HEPARIN AND SODIUM CHLORIDE

For *Heparin* and *Sodium Chloride*—See individual listings for chemistry information.

USP requirements: Heparin Sodium in Sodium Chloride Injection—Not in USP.

HEPATITIS B IMMUNE GLOBULIN

USP requirements: Hepatitis B Immune Globulin USP—Preserve at a temperature between 2 and 8 °C. A sterile, nonpyrogenic solution free from turbidity, consisting of globulins derived from the blood plasma of human donors who have high titers of antibodies against hepatitis B surface antigen. Label it to state that it is not for intravenous injection. Contains not less than 10.0 grams and not more than 18.0 grams of protein per 100 mL, of which not less than 80% is monomeric immunoglobulin G, having no ultracentrifugally detectable fragments, nor aggregates having a sedimentation coefficient greater than 12S. Contains 0.3 *M* glycine as a stabilizing agent, and contains a suitable preservative. Has a potency per mL not less than that of the U.S. Reference Hepatitis B Immune Globulin tested by an approved radioimmunoassay for the detection and measurement of antibody to hepatitis B surface antigen. Has a pH between 6.4 and 7.2, measured in a solution diluted to contain 1% of protein with 0.15 *M* sodium chloride. Meets the requirements of the test for heat stability and for Expiration date (not later than 1 year after the date of manufacture, such date being that of the first valid potency test of the product). Conforms to the regulations of the U.S. Food and Drug Administration concerning biologics.

HEPATITIS B VACCINE RECOMBINANT

Source:

A non-infectious subunit viral vaccine derived from hepatitis B surface antigen (HBsAg) produced in yeast cells. A portion of the hepatitis B virus gene, coding for HBsAg, is cloned into yeast, and the vaccine for hepatitis B is produced from cultures of this recombinant yeast strain according to methods developed in the Merck Research Laboratories.

The antigen is harvested and purified from fermentation cultures of a recombinant strain of the teast *Saccharomyces cerevisiae* containing the gene for the *adw* subtype of HBsAg.

USP requirements: Hepatitis B Vaccine Recombinant Sterile Suspension—Not in USP.

HEPATITIS B VIRUS VACCINE INACTIVATED

USP requirements: Hepatitis B Virus Vaccine Inactivated USP—Preserve at a temperature between 2 and 8 °C. A sterile preparation consisting of a suspension of particles of Hepatitis B surface antigen (HBsAg) isolated from the plasma of HBsAg carriers; treated with pepsin at pH 2, 8 *M* urea, and 1:4000 formalin so as to inactivate any hepatitis B virus and any representative viruses from all known virus groups that may be present; purified by ultracentrifugation and biochemical procedures and standardized to a concentration of 35 mcg to 55 mcg of Lowry (HBsAg) protein per mL. The preparation is adsorbed on aluminum hydroxide and diluted to a concentration of 20 mcg Lowry protein per mL or other appropriate concentration, depending on the intended use. Label it to state the content of HBsAg protein per recommended dose. Label it also to state that it is to be shaken before use and that it is not to be frozen. Contains not more than 0.62 mg of aluminum per mL and not more than 0.02% of residual free formaldehyde. Contains thimerosal as a preservative. Meets the requirements for potency in animal tests using mice and by a quantitative parallel line radioimmunoassay, of tests for pyrogen, for general safety, and for Expiration date (not later than 3 years from the date of manufacture, the date of manufacture being the date on which the last valid potency test was initiated).

HETACILLIN

Chemical name:

Hetacillin—4-Thia-1-azabicyclo[3.2.0]heptane-2-carboxylic acid, 6-(2,2-dimethyl-5-oxo-4-phenyl-1-imidazolidinyl)-3,3-dimethyl-7-oxo-, [2*S*-[2 alpha,5 alpha,6 beta(S*)]]-.

Hetacillin potassium—4-Thia-1-azabicyclo[3.2.0]heptane-2-carboxylic acid, 6-(2,2-dimethyl-5-oxo-4-phenyl-1-imidazolidinyl)-3,3-dimethyl-7-oxo-, monopotassium salt, [2*S*-[2 alpha,5 alpha,6 beta(S*)]]-.

Molecular formula:

Hetacillin—$C_{19}H_{23}N_3O_4S$.

Hetacillin potassium—$C_{19}H_{22}KN_3O_4S$.

Molecular weight:

Hetacillin—389.47.

Hetacillin potassium—427.56.

Description:

Hetacillin USP—White to off-white, crystalline powder.

Hetacillin Potassium USP—White to light buff, crystalline powder.

Solubility:

Hetacillin USP—Practically insoluble in water and in most organic solvents; soluble in dilute sodium hydroxide solution and in methanol.

Hetacillin Potassium USP—Freely soluble in water; soluble in alcohol.

USP requirements:

Hetacillin USP—Preserve in tight containers. Has a potency equivalent to not less than 810 mcg of ampicillin per mg. Meets the requirements for Identification, Crystallinity, pH (2.5–5.5, in a suspension containing 10 mg per mL), Water (not more than 1.0%), and Hetacillin content (90.0–105.0%).

Hetacillin for Oral Suspension USP—Preserve in tight containers. Contains an amount of hetacillin equivalent to the labeled amount of ampicillin, within −10% to +20%. Contains one or more suitable colors, flavors, preservatives, sweeteners, and suspending agents. Meets the requirements for Identification, pH (2.0–5.0, in the suspension constituted as directed in the labeling), Water (not more than 2.0%), Deliverable volume, and Uniformity of dosage units (for solid packaged in single-unit containers).

Hetacillin Tablets USP—Preserve in tight containers. Label Tablets to indicate that they are to be chewed before swallowing. Contain an amount of hetacillin equivalent to the labeled amount of ampicillin, within −10% to +20%. Meet the requirements for Identification, Dissolution (75% in 45 minutes in 0.05 *M* phosphate buffer [pH 7.6] in Apparatus 2 at 50 rpm), Uniformity of dosage units, and Water (not more than 2.0%).

Hetacillin Potassium USP—Preserve in tight containers. Has a potency equivalent to not less than 735 mcg of ampicillin per mg. Meets the requirements for Identification, Crystallinity, pH (7.0–9.0, in a solution containing 10 mg per mL), Water (not more than 1.0%), and Hetacillin content (82.0–95.5%).

Hetacillin Potassium Capsules USP—Preserve in tight containers. Contain an amount of hetacillin potassium equivalent to the labeled amount of ampicillin, within −10% to +20%. Meet the requirements for Identification, Dissolution (75% in 45 minutes in water in Apparatus 1 at 100 rpm), Uniformity of dosage units, and Water (not more than 3.0%).

Hetacillin Potassium Intramammary Infusion USP—Preserve in suitable, well-closed, disposable syringes. A suspension of Hetacillin Potassium in a Peanut Oil vehicle with a suitable dispersing agent. Label it to indicate that it is for veterinary use only. Contains an amount of hetacillin potassium equivalent to the labeled amount of ampicillin, within −10% to +20%. Meets the requirements for Identification and Water (not more than 1.0%).

Sterile Hetacillin Potassium USP—Preserve in Containers for Sterile Solids. It is Hetacillin Potassium suitable for parenteral use. Contains an amount of hetacillin potassium equivalent to the labeled amount of ampicillin, within −10% to +20%. Meets the requirements for Bacterial endotoxins, Sterility, pH (7.0–9.0, in the solution constituted as directed in the labeling), for Identification tests, pH, Water, Crystallinity, and Hetacillin content under Hetacillin Potassium, and for Uniformity of dosage units and Labeling under Injections.

Hetacillin Potassium Oral Suspension USP—Preserve in tight containers. It is Hetacillin Potassium suspended in a suitable nonaqueous vehicle. Label it to indicate that it is for veterinary use only. Contains an amount of hetacillin potassium equivalent to the labeled amount of ampicillin, within −10% to +20%. Contains one or more suitable colors, flavors, and gelling agents. Meets the requirements for Identification, Deliverable volume, Uniformity of dosage units (for suspension packaged in single-unit containers), pH (7.0–9.0), and Water (not more than 1.0%).

Hetacillin Potassium Tablets USP—Preserve in tight containers. Label Tablets to indicate that they are for veterinary use only. Contain an amount of hetacillin potassium equivalent to the labeled amount of ampicillin, within −10% to +20%. Meet the requirements for Identification, Disintegration (30 minutes), and Water (not more than 5.0%).

HEXACHLOROPHENE

Chemical name: Phenol, 2,2′-methylenebis[3,4,6-trichloro-.

Molecular formula: $C_{13}H_6Cl_6O_2$.

Molecular weight: 406.91.

Description:

Hexachlorophene USP—White to light tan, crystalline powder. Odorless, or has only a slight, phenolic odor.

Hexachlorophene Liquid Soap USP—Clear, amber-colored liquid, having a slight, characteristic odor. Its solution (1 in 20) is clear and has an alkaline reaction.

Solubility: Hexachlorophene USP—Insoluble in water; freely soluble in acetone, in alcohol, and in ether; soluble in chloroform and in dilute solutions of fixed alkali hydroxides.

USP requirements:

Hexachlorophene USP—Preserve in tight, light-resistant containers. Contains not less than 98.0% and not more than 100.5% of hexachlorophene, calculated on the dried basis. Meets the requirements for Identification, Melting range (161–167 °C), Loss on drying (not more than 1.0%), Residue on ignition (not more than 0.1%), and 2,3,7,8-Tetrachlorodibenzo-*p*-dioxin (not more than 1 ppb).

Hexachlorophene Cleansing Emulsion USP—Preserve in tight, light-resistant, non-metallic containers. It is Hexachlorophene in a suitable aqueous vehicle. Contains the labeled amount, within ±10%. Contains no coloring agents. Meets the requirements for Identification, Microbial limits, and pH (5.0–6.0).

Hexachlorophene Liquid Soap USP—Preserve in tight, light-resistant containers. A solution of Hexachlorophene in a 10.0 to 13.0% solution of a potassium soap. Solutions of higher concentrations of hexachlorophene and potassium soap, in which the ratios of these components are consistent with the official limits, may be labeled "For the preparation of Hexachlorophene Liquid Soap, USP," provided that the label indicates also that the soap is a concentrate, and provided that directions are given for dilution to the official strength. Contains, in each 100 grams, not less than 225 mg and not more than 260 mg of hexachlorophene. Meets the requirements for Identification, Microbial limits, Water (86.5–90.0% by weight of the portion of Soap taken), Alcohol-insoluble substances (not more than 3.0%), Free alkali hydroxides (not more than 0.05% of potassium hydroxide), and Alkali carbonates (not more than 0.35% of potassium carbonate).

Note: The inclusion of non-ionic detergents in Hexachlorophene Liquid Soap in amounts greater than 8% on a total weight basis may decrease the bacteriostatic activity of the Soap.

HEXYLCAINE

Chemical name: Hexylcaine hydrochloride—2-Propanol, 1-(cyclohexylamino)-, benzoate (ester), hydrochloride.

Molecular formula: Hexylcaine hydrochloride—$C_{16}H_{23}NO_2 \cdot HCl$.

Molecular weight: Hexylcaine hydrochloride—297.83.

Description:

Hexylcaine Hydrochloride USP—White powder, having not more than a slight, aromatic odor.

Hexylcaine Hydrochloride Topical Solution USP—Clear, colorless solution of Hexylcaine Hydrochloride in water.

Solubility: Hexylcaine Hydrochloride USP—Soluble in water; freely soluble in alcohol and in chloroform; practically insoluble in ether.

USP requirements:

Hexylcaine Hydrochloride USP—Preserve in tight containers. Dried in vacuum over phosphorus pentoxide for 4 hours, contains not less than 98.0% and not more than 102.0% of hexylcaine hydrochloride. Meets the requirements for Identification, Melting range (182–184 °C), pH (4.0–6.0, in a solution [1 in 20]), Acidity, Loss on drying (not more than 0.2%), Residue on ignition (not more than 0.1%), and Heavy metals (not more than 0.003%).

Hexylcaine Hydrochloride Topical Solution USP—Preserve in tight containers. Contains the labeled amount, within ±7%. Meets the requirements for Identification and pH (3.0–5.0).

HEXYLENE GLYCOL

Chemical name: 2,4-Pentanediol, 2-methyl-.

Molecular formula: $C_6H_{14}O_2$.

Molecular weight: 118.18.

Description: Hexylene Glycol NF—Clear, colorless, viscous liquid. Absorbs moisture when exposed to moist air.

NF category: Humectant; solvent.

Solubility: Hexylene Glycol NF—Miscible with water and with many organic solvents, including alcohol, ether, chloroform, acetone, and hexanes.

NF requirements: Hexylene Glycol NF—Preserve in tight containers. Hexylene Glycol is 2-methyl-2,4-pentanediol. Meets the requirements for Identification, Specific gravity (0.917–0.923), Refractive index (1.424–1.430), Acidity, and Water (not more than 0.5%).

HEXYLRESORCINOL

Chemical name: 1,3-Benzenediol, 4-hexyl-.

Molecular formula: $C_{12}H_{18}O_2$.

Molecular weight: 194.27.

Description: White or almost white needles, crystalline powder, plates, or plate aggregates composed of needle masses with a pungent odor. Acquires a brownish-pink tint on exposure to light and air. Melting point 66–68 °C.

Solubility: Very slightly soluble in water; freely soluble in alcohol, in chloroform, in ether, in glycerol, and in fixed oils; practically insoluble in petroleum spirit.

USP requirements:

Hexylresorcinol USP—Preserve in tight, light-resistant containers. Dried over silica gel for 4 hours, contains not less than 98.0% and not more than 100.5% of hexylresorcinol. Meets the requirements for Identification, Melting range (62–67 °C), Acidity, Residue on ignition (not more than 0.1%), Mercury (not more than 3 ppm), and Resorcinol and other phenols.

Caution: Hexylresorcinol is irritating to the oral mucosa and respiratory tract and to the skin, and its solution in alcohol has vesicant properties.

Hexylresorcinol Lozenges USP—Preserve in well-closed containers. Contain the labeled amount, within ±10%. Meet the requirements for Identification and Uniformity of dosage units.

HISTAMINE

Chemical name: Histamine phosphate—1*H*-Imidazole-4-ethanamine, phosphate (1:2).

Molecular formula: Histamine phosphate—$C_5H_9N_3 \cdot 2H_3PO_4$.

Molecular weight: Histamine phosphate—307.14.

Description: Histamine Phosphate USP—Colorless, odorless, long prismatic crystals. Is stable in air but is affected by light. Its solutions are acid to litmus.

Solubility: Histamine Phosphate USP—Freely soluble in water.

USP requirements:

Histamine Phosphate USP—Preserve in tight, light-resistant containers. Contains not less than 98.0% and not more than 101.0% of histamine phosphate, calculated on the dried basis. Meets the requirements for Identification and Loss on drying (not more than 3.0%).

Histamine Phosphate Injection USP—Preserve in single-dose or in multiple-dose containers, preferably of Type I glass, protected from light. A sterile solution of Histamine Phosphate in Water for Injection. Contains the labeled amount, within ±10%. Meets the requirements for Identification, Bacterial endotoxins, pH (3.0–6.0), and Injections.

HISTIDINE

Chemical name: L-Histidine.

Molecular formula: $C_6H_9N_3O_2$.

Molecular weight: 155.16.

Description: Histidine USP—White, odorless crystals.

Solubility: Histidine USP—Soluble in water; very slightly soluble in alcohol; insoluble in ether.

USP requirements: Histidine USP—Preserve in well-closed containers. Contains not less than 98.5% and not more than 101.5% of histidine, calculated on the dried basis. Meets the requirements for Identification, Specific rotation (+12.6° to +14.0°, calculated on the dried basis), pH (7.0–8.5, in a solution [1 in 50]), Loss on drying (not more than 0.2%), Residue on ignition (not more than 0.4%), Chloride (not more than 0.05%), Sulfate (not more than 0.03%), Arsenic (not more than 1.5 ppm), Iron (not more than 0.003%), and Heavy metals (not more than 0.0015%).

HISTOPLASMIN

Description: Histoplasmin USP—Clear, red liquid.

Solubility: Histoplasmin USP—Miscible with water.

USP requirements: Histoplasmin USP—Preserve at a temperature between 2 and 8 °C. A clear, colorless, sterile solution containing standardized culture filtrates of *Histoplasma capsulatum* grown on liquid synthetic medium. Label it to state that only the diluent supplied is to be used for making dilutions, and that it is not to be injected other than intradermally. Label it also to state that a separate syringe and needle shall be used for each individual injection. Has a potency of the 1:100 dilution equivalent to and determined in terms of the Histoplasmin Reference diluted 1:100 tested in guinea pigs. Meets the requirement for Expiration date (not later than 2 years after date of issue from manufacturer's cold storage [5 °C, 1 year]). Conforms to the regulations of the U.S. Food and Drug Administration concerning biologics.

HISTRELIN

Chemical name: Luteinizing hormone-releasing factor (pig), 6-[1-(phenylmethyl)-D-histidine]-9-(*N*-ethyl-L-prolinamide)-10-deglycinamide-.

Molecular formula: $C_{66}H_{86}N_{18}O_{12}$.

Molecular weight: 1323.52.

USP requirements: Histrelin Injection—Not in USP.

HOMATROPINE

Source: Semisynthetic tertiary amine derivative of mandelic acid and tropine.

Chemical group: Homatropine methylbromide—Semisynthetic quaternary ammonium compound.

Chemical name:

Homatropine hydrobromide—Benzeneacetic acid, alpha-hydroxy-, 8-methyl-8-azabicyclo[3.2.1]oct-3-yl ester, hydrobromide, *endo*-(±)-.

Homatropine methylbromide—8-Azoniabicyclo[3.2.1]octane, 3-[(hydroxyphenylacetyl)oxy]-8,8-dimethyl-, bromide, *endo*-.

Molecular formula:

Homatropine hydrobromide—$C_{16}H_{21}NO_3 \cdot HBr$.

Homatropine methylbromide—$C_{17}H_{24}BrNO_3$.

Molecular weight:

Homatropine hydrobromide—356.26.

Homatropine methylbromide—370.29.

Description:

Homatropine Hydrobromide USP—White crystals, or white, crystalline powder. Is affected by light.

Homatropine Methylbromide USP—White, odorless powder. Slowly darkens on exposure to light. Melts at about 190 °C.

Solubility:

Homatropine Hydrobromide USP—Freely soluble in water; sparingly soluble in alcohol; slightly soluble in chloroform; insoluble in ether.

Homatropine Methylbromide USP—Very soluble in water; freely soluble in alcohol and in acetone containing about 20% of water; practically insoluble in ether and in acetone.

USP requirements:

Homatropine Hydrobromide USP—Preserve in tight, light-resistant containers. Contains not less than 98.5% and not more than 100.5% of homatropine hydrobromide, calculated on the dried basis. Meets the requirements for Identification, Melting range (214–217 °C, with slight decomposition), pH (5.7–7.0, in a solution [1 in 50]), Loss on drying (not more than 1.5%), and Residue on ignition (not more than 0.25%).

Homatropine Hydrobromide Ophthalmic Solution USP—Preserve in tight containers. A sterile, buffered, aqueous solution of Homatropine Hydrobromide. Contains the labeled amount, within ±5%. Meets the requirements for Identification, Sterility, and pH (2.5–5.0).

Homatropine Methylbromide USP—Preserve in tight, light-resistant containers. Contains not less than 98.5% and not more than 100.5% of homatropine methylbromide, calculated on the dried basis. Meets the requirements for Identification, pH (4.5–6.5, in a solution [1 in 100]), Loss on drying (not more than 0.5%), Residue on ignition (not more than 0.2%), Homatropine, atropine, and other solanaceous alkaloids, and Organic volatile impurities.

Homatropine Methylbromide Tablets USP—Preserve in tight, light-resistant containers. Contain the labeled amount, within ±10%. Meet the requirements for Identification, Dissolution (75% in 45 minutes in water in Apparatus 2 at 50 rpm), and Uniformity of dosage units.

HYALURONIDASE

Description: White or yellowish-white powder.

Solubility: Very soluble in water; practically insoluble in alcohol, in acetone, and in ether.

USP requirements:

Hyaluronidase Injection USP—Preserve in single-dose or in multiple-dose containers, preferably of Type I glass, in a refrigerator. A sterile solution of dry, soluble enzyme product, prepared from mammalian testes and capable of hydrolyzing mucopolysaccharides of the type of hyaluronic acid, in Water for Injection. Contains the labeled amount of USP Hyaluronidase Units, within −10%. Contains not more than 0.25 mcg of tyrosine for each USP Hyaluronidase Unit. Meets the requirements for Tyrosine (not more than 0.25 mcg for each USP Hyaluronidase Unit), Bacterial endotoxins, pH (6.4–7.4), and Injections.

Hyaluronidase for Injection USP—Preserve in Containers for Sterile Solids, preferably of Type I or Type III glass, at controlled room temperature. A sterile, dry, soluble, enzyme product prepared from mammalian testes and capable of hydrolyzing mucopolysaccharides of the type of hyaluronic acid. Its potency, in USP Hyaluronidase Units, is not less than the labeled potency. Contains not more than 0.25 mcg of tyrosine for each USP Hyaluronidase Unit. Meets the requirements for Tyrosine (not more than 0.25 mcg for each USP Hyaluronidase Unit), Bacterial endotoxins, and Sterility.

HYDRALAZINE

Chemical name: Hydralazine hydrochloride—Phthalazine, 1-hydrazino-, monohydrochloride.

Molecular formula: Hydralazine hydrochloride—$C_8H_8N_4 \cdot HCl$.

Molecular weight: Hydralazine hydrochloride—196.64.

Description: Hydralazine Hydrochloride USP—White to off-white, odorless, crystalline powder. Melts at about 275 °C, with decomposition.

pKa: Hydralazine hydrochloride—7.3.

Solubility: Hydralazine Hydrochloride USP—Soluble in water; slightly soluble in alcohol; very slightly soluble in ether.

USP requirements:

Hydralazine Hydrochloride USP—Preserve in tight containers. Contains not less than 98.0% and not more than 102.0% of hydralazine hydrochloride, calculated on the dried basis. Meets the requirements for Identification, pH (3.5–4.2, in a solution [1 in 50]), Loss on drying (not more than 0.5%), Residue on ignition (not more than 0.1%), Water-insoluble substances (not more than 0.5%), Heavy metals (not more than 0.002%), Limit of hydrazine (not more than 0.001%), Chromatographic purity, and Organic volatile impurities.

Hydralazine Hydrochloride Injection USP—Preserve in single-dose or in multiple-dose containers, preferably of Type I glass. A sterile solution of Hydralazine Hydrochloride in Water for Injection. Contains the labeled amount, within ±5%. Meets the requirements for Identification, Bacterial endotoxins, pH (3.4–4.4), Particulate matter, and Injections.

Hydralazine Hydrochloride Tablets USP—Preserve in tight, light-resistant containers. Contain the labeled amount, within ±10%. Meet the requirements for Identification, Dissolution (60% in 30 minutes in 0.1 *N* hydrochloric acid in Apparatus 1 at 100 rpm), and Uniformity of dosage units.

HYDRALAZINE AND HYDROCHLOROTHIAZIDE

For *Hydralazine* and *Hydrochlorothiazide*—See individual listings for chemistry information.

USP requirements:

Hydralazine Hydrochloride and Hydrochlorothiazide Capsules—Not in USP.

Hydralazine Hydrochloride and Hydrochlorothiazide Tablets—Not in USP.

HYDROCHLORIC ACID

Chemical name: Hydrochloric acid.

Molecular formula: HCl.

Molecular weight: 36.46.

Description: Hydrochloric Acid NF—Colorless, fuming liquid, having a pungent odor. It ceases to fume when it is diluted with 2 volumes of water. Specific gravity is about 1.18.

NF category: Acidifying agent.

NF requirements: Hydrochloric Acid NF—Preserve in tight containers. Contains not less than 36.5% and not more than 38.0%, by weight, of hydrochloric acid. Meets the requirements for Identification, Residue on ignition (not more than 0.008%), Bromide or iodide, Free bromine or chlorine, Sulfate, and Sulfite, Arsenic (not more than 1 ppm), and Heavy metals (not more than 5 ppm).

DILUTED HYDROCHLORIC ACID

Description: Diluted Hydrochloric Acid NF—Colorless, odorless liquid. Specific gravity is about 1.05.

NF category: Acidifying agent.

NF requirements: Diluted Hydrochloric Acid NF—Preserve in tight containers. Contains, in each 100 mL, not less than 9.5 grams and not more than 10.5 grams of hydrochloric acid.

Diluted Hydrochloric Acid may be prepared as follows: 226 mL of Hydrochloric Acid and a sufficient quantity of Purified Water to make 1000 mL. Mix the ingredients.

Meets the requirements for Identification, Residue on ignition, Sulfate, Sulfite, Arsenic (not more than 0.6 ppm), Heavy metals (not more than 5 ppm), and Free bromine or chlorine.

HYDROCHLOROTHIAZIDE

Chemical name: 2*H*-1,2,4-Benzothiadiazine-7-sulfonamide, 6-chloro-3,4-dihydro-, 1,1-dioxide.

Molecular formula: $C_7H_8ClN_3O_4S_2$.

Molecular weight: 297.73.

Description: Hydrochlorothiazide USP—White or practically white, practically odorless, crystalline powder.

pKa: 7.9 and 9.2.

Solubility: Hydrochlorothiazide USP—Slightly soluble in water; freely soluble in sodium hydroxide solution, in *n*-butylamine, and in dimethylformamide; sparingly soluble in methanol; insoluble in ether, in chloroform, and in dilute mineral acids.

USP requirements:
Hydrochlorothiazide USP—Preserve in well-closed containers. Contains not less than 98.0% and not more than 102.0% of hydrochlorothiazide, calculated on the dried basis. Meets the requirements for Identification, Loss on drying (not more than 1.0%), Residue on ignition (not more than 0.1%), Chloride (not more than 0.07%), Selenium (not more than 0.003%), Heavy metals (not more than 0.001%), 4-Amino-6-chloro-1,3-benzenedisulfonamide (not more than 1.0%), and Organic volatile impurities.
Hydrochlorothiazide Oral Solution—Not in USP.
Hydrochlorothiazide Tablets USP—Preserve in well-closed containers. Contain the labeled amount, within ±10%. Meet the requirements for Identification, Dissolution (60% in 60 minutes in 0.1 *N* hydrochloric acid in Apparatus 1 at 100 rpm), Uniformity of dosage units, and 4-Amino-6-chloro-1,3-benzenedisulfonamide.

HYDROCODONE

Chemical name: Hydrocodone bitartrate—Morphinan-6-one, 4,5-epoxy-3-methoxy-17-methyl-, (5 alpha)-, [*R*-(*R**,*R**)]-2,3-dihydroxybutanedioate (1:1), hydrate (2:5).

Molecular formula: Hydrocodone bitartrate—$C_{18}H_{21}NO_3 \cdot C_4H_6O_6 \cdot 2\frac{1}{2}H_2O$ (hydrate); $C_{18}H_{21}NO_3 \cdot C_4H_6O_6$ (anhydrous).

Molecular weight: Hydrocodone bitartrate—494.50 (hydrate); 449.46 (anhydrous).

Description: Hydrocodone Bitartrate USP—Fine, white crystals or a crystalline powder. Is affected by light.

Solubility: Hydrocodone Bitartrate USP—Soluble in water; slightly soluble in alcohol; insoluble in ether and in chloroform.

USP requirements:
Hydrocodone Bitartrate USP—Preserve in tight, light-resistant containers. Dried in vacuum at 105 °C for 2 hours, contains not less than 98.0% and not more than 102.0% of hydrocodone bitartrate. Meets the requirements for Identification, Specific rotation (−79° to −84°), pH (3.2–3.8, in a solution [1 in 50]), Loss on drying (7.5–12.0%), Residue on ignition (not more than 0.1%), Chloride, Ordinary impurities, and Organic volatile impurities.
Hydrocodone Bitartrate Syrup—Not in USP.
Hydrocodone Bitartrate Tablets USP—Preserve in tight, light-resistant containers. Contain the labeled amount, within ±10%. Meet the requirements for Identification, Dissolution (75% in 45 minutes in water in Apparatus 2 at 50 rpm), and Uniformity of dosage units.

HYDROCODONE AND ACETAMINOPHEN

For *Hydrocodone* and *Acetaminophen*—See individual listings for chemistry information.

USP requirements:
Hydrocodone Bitartrate and Acetaminophen Capsules—Not in USP.
Hydrocodone Bitartrate and Acetaminophen Oral Solution—Not in USP.
Hydrocodone Bitartrate and Acetaminophen Tablets USP—Preserve in tight, light-resistant containers. Contain the labeled amounts, within ±10%. Meet the requirements for Identification, Dissolution (80% of each active ingredient in 30 minutes in phosphate buffer [pH 5.8 ±0.05] in Apparatus 2 at 50 rpm), and Uniformity of dosage units.

HYDROCODONE AND ASPIRIN

For *Hydrocodone* and *Aspirin*—See individual listings for chemistry information.

USP requirements: Hydrocodone Bitartrate and Aspirin Tablets—Not in USP.

HYDROCODONE, ASPIRIN, AND CAFFEINE

For *Hydrocodone, Aspirin,* and *Caffeine*—See individual listings for chemistry information.

USP requirements: Hydrocodone Bitartrate, Aspirin, and Caffeine Tablets—Not in USP.

HYDROCODONE AND GUAIFENESIN

For *Hydrocodone* and *Guaifenesin*—See individual listings for chemistry information.

USP requirements:
Hydrocodone Bitartrate and Guaifenesin Oral Solution—Not in USP.
Hydrocodone Bitartrate and Guaifenesin Syrup—Not in USP.
Hydrocodone Bitartrate and Guaifenesin Tablets—Not in USP.

HYDROCODONE AND HOMATROPINE

For *Hydrocodone* and *Homatropine*—See individual listings for chemistry information.

USP requirements:
Hydrocodone Bitartrate and Homatropine Methylbromide Syrup—Not in USP.
Hydrocodone Bitartrate and Homatropine Methylbromide Tablets—Not in USP.

HYDROCODONE AND POTASSIUM GUAIACOLSULFONATE

For *Hydrocodone* and *Potassium Guaiacolsulfonate*—See individual listings for chemistry information.

USP requirements: Hydrocodone Bitartrate and Potassium Guaiacolsulfonate Syrup—Not in USP.

HYDROCORTISONE

Chemical name:
Hydrocortisone—Pregn-4-ene-3,20-dione, 11,17,21,trihydroxy-, (11 beta)-.
Hydrocortisone acetate—Pregn-4-ene-3,20-dione, 21-(acetyloxy)-11,17-dihydroxy-, (11 beta)-.
Hydrocortisone butyrate—Pregn-4-ene-3,20-dione, 11,21-dihydroxy-17-(1-oxobutoxy)-, (11 beta)-.
Hydrocortisone cypionate—Pregn-4-ene-3,20-dione, 21-(3-cyclopentyl-1-oxopropoxy)-11,17-dihydroxy-, (11 beta)-.
Hydrocortisone hemisuccinate—Pregn-4-ene-3,20-dione, 21-(3-carboxy-1-oxopropoxy)-11,17-dihydroxy-, (11 beta)-, monohydrate.
Hydrocortisone sodium phosphate—Pregn-4-ene-3,20-dione, 11,17-dihydroxy-21-(phosphonooxy)-, disodium salt, (11 beta)-.
Hydrocortisone sodium succinate—Pregn-4-ene-3,20-dione, 21-(3-carboxy-1-oxopropoxy)-11,17-dihydroxy-, monosodium salt, (11 beta)-.

Hydrocortisone valerate—Pregn-4-ene-3,20-dione, 11,21-dihydroxy-17-[(1-oxopentyl)oxy]-, (11 beta)-.

Molecular formula:
Hydrocortisone—$C_{21}H_{30}O_5$.
Hydrocortisone acetate—$C_{23}H_{32}O_6$.
Hydrocortisone butyrate—$C_{25}H_{36}O_6$.
Hydrocortisone cypionate—$C_{29}H_{42}O_6$.
Hydrocortisone hemisuccinate—$C_{25}H_{34}O_8 \cdot H_2O$.
Hydrocortisone sodium phosphate—$C_{21}H_{29}Na_2O_8P$.
Hydrocortisone sodium succinate—$C_{25}H_{33}NaO_8$.
Hydrocortisone valerate—$C_{26}H_{38}O_6$.

Molecular weight:
Hydrocortisone—362.47.
Hydrocortisone acetate—404.50.
Hydrocortisone butyrate—432.56.
Hydrocortisone cypionate—486.65.
Hydrocortisone hemisuccinate—480.56.
Hydrocortisone sodium phosphate—486.41.
Hydrocortisone sodium succinate—484.52.
Hydrocortisone valerate—446.58.

Description:
Hydrocortisone USP—White to practically white, odorless, crystalline powder. Melts at about 215 °C, with decomposition.
Hydrocortisone Acetate USP—White to practically white, odorless, crystalline powder. Melts at about 200 °C, with decomposition.
Hydrocortisone Butyrate USP—White to practically white, practically odorless, crystalline powder.
Hydrocortisone Cypionate USP—White to practically white crystalline powder. Is odorless, or has a slight odor.
Hydrocortisone Sodium Phosphate USP—White to light yellow, odorless or practically odorless, powder. Is exceedingly hygroscopic.
Hydrocortisone Sodium Succinate USP—White or nearly white, odorless, hygroscopic, amorphous solid.

Solubility:
Hydrocortisone USP—Very slightly soluble in water and in ether; sparingly soluble in acetone and in alcohol; slightly soluble in chloroform.
Hydrocortisone Acetate USP—Insoluble in water; slightly soluble in alcohol and in chloroform.
Hydrocortisone Butyrate USP—Practically insoluble in water; slightly soluble in ether; soluble in methanol, in alcohol, and in acetone; freely soluble in chloroform.
Hydrocortisone Cypionate USP—Insoluble in water; very soluble in chloroform; soluble in alcohol; slightly soluble in ether.
Hydrocortisone Sodium Phosphate USP—Freely soluble in water; slightly soluble in alcohol; practically insoluble in chloroform, in dioxane, and in ether.
Hydrocortisone Sodium Succinate USP—Very soluble in water and in alcohol; very slightly soluble in acetone; insoluble in chloroform.

USP requirements:
Hydrocortisone USP—Preserve in well-closed containers. Contains not less than 97.0% and not more than 102.0% of hydrocortisone, calculated on the dried basis. Meets the requirements for Identification, Specific rotation (+150° to +156°, calculated on the dried basis), Loss on drying (not more than 1.0%), Residue on ignition (negligible, from 100 mg), Chromatographic purity, and Organic volatile impurities.
Hydrocortisone Cream USP—Preserve in tight containers. It is Hydrocortisone in a suitable cream base. Contains the labeled amount, within ±10%. Meets the requirements for Identification, Microbial limits, and Minimum fill.
Hydrocortisone Enema USP—Preserve in tight containers. Contains the labeled amount, within ±10%. Meets the requirements for Identification and pH (5.5–7.0).
Hydrocortisone Gel USP—Preserve in tight containers. It is Hydrocortisone in a suitable hydroalcoholic gel base. Contains the labeled amount, within ±10%. Meets the requirements for Identification and Minimum fill.
Hydrocortisone Lotion USP—Preserve in tight containers. It is Hydrocortisone in a suitable aqueous vehicle. Contains the labeled amount, within ±10%. Meets the requirements for Identification, Microbial limits, and Minimum fill.
Hydrocortisone Ointment USP—Preserve in well-closed containers. It is Hydrocortisone in a suitable ointment base. Contains the labeled amount, within ±10%. Meets the requirements for Identification, Microbial limits, and Minimum fill.
Hydrocortisone Rectal Ointment—Not in USP.
Hydrocortisone Topical Solution—Not in USP.
Hydrocortisone Suppositories—Not in USP.
Sterile Hydrocortisone Suspension USP—Preserve in single-dose or in multiple-dose containers, preferably of Type I glass. A sterile suspension of Hydrocortisone in Water for Injection. Contains the labeled amount, within ±10%. Meets the requirements for Identification, Bacterial endotoxins, pH (5.0–7.0), and Injections.
Hydrocortisone Tablets USP—Preserve in well-closed containers. Contain the labeled amount, within ±10%. Meet the requirements for Identification, Dissolution (70% in 30 minutes in water in Apparatus 2 at 50 rpm), and Uniformity of dosage units.
Hydrocortisone Acetate USP—Preserve in well-closed containers. Contains not less than 97.0% and not more than 102.0% of hydrocortisone acetate, calculated on the dried basis. Meets the requirements for Identification, Specific rotation (+158° to +165°, calculated on the dried basis), Loss on drying (not more than 1.0%), Residue on ignition (negligible, from 100 mg), and Ordinary impurities.
Hydrocortisone Acetate Rectal Aerosol (Foam)—Not in USP.
Hydrocortisone Acetate Topical Aerosol (Foam)—Not in USP.
Hydrocortisone Acetate Cream USP—Preserve in well-closed containers. It is Hydrocortisone Acetate in a suitable cream base. Contains the labeled amount, within ±10%. Meets the requirements for Identification, Microbial limits, and Minimum fill.
Hydrocortisone Acetate Lotion USP—Preserve in tight containers. It is Hydrocortisone Acetate in a suitable aqueous vehicle. Contains the labeled amount, within ±10%. Meets the requirements for Identification and Minimum fill.
Hydrocortisone Acetate Ointment USP—Preserve in well-closed containers. It is Hydrocortisone Acetate in a suitable ointment base. Contains the labeled amount, within ±10%. Meets the requirements for Identification, Microbial limits, and Minimum fill.
Hydrocortisone Acetate Ophthalmic Ointment USP—Preserve in collapsible ophthalmic ointment tubes. It is Hydrocortisone Acetate in a suitable ophthalmic ointment base. It is sterile. Contains the labeled amount of total steroids, calculated as hydrocortisone acetate, within ±10%. Meets the requirements for Identification, Sterility, Minimum fill, and Particulate matter.
Hydrocortisone Acetate Dental Paste—Not in USP.
Hydrocortisone Acetate Suppositories—Not in USP.
Hydrocortisone Acetate Ophthalmic Suspension USP—Preserve in tight containers. A sterile suspension of Hydrocortisone Acetate in an aqueous medium containing a suitable antimicrobial agent. Contains the labeled amount of total steroids, calculated as Hydrocortisone Acetate, within ±10%. Meets the requirements for Identification, Sterility, and pH (6.0–8.0).

Sterile Hydrocortisone Acetate Suspension USP—Preserve in single-dose or in multiple-dose containers, preferably of Type I glass. A sterile suspension of Hydrocortisone Acetate in a suitable aqueous medium. Contains the labeled amount of total steroids, calculated as hydrocortisone acetate, within ±10%. Meets the requirements for Identification, pH (5.0–7.0), and Injections.

Hydrocortisone Butyrate USP—Preserve in well-closed containers. Contains not less than 97.0% and not more than 102.0% of hydrocortisone butyrate, calculated on the dried basis. Meets the requirements for Clarity of solution, Identification, Melting range (197–208 °C, with decomposition, the range between beginning and end of melting not more than 4 °C), Specific rotation (+47° to +54°, calculated on the dried basis), Loss on drying (not more than 1.0%), and Hydrocortisone 21-butyrate and other related impurities.

Hydrocortisone Butyrate Cream USP—Preserve in well-closed containers. It is Hydrocortisone Butyrate in a suitable cream base. Contains the labeled amount, within ±10%. Meets the requirements for Identification, pH (3.5–4.5), Microbial limits, and Minimum fill.

Hydrocortisone Butyrate Ointment—Not in USP.

Hydrocortisone Cypionate USP—Preserve in tight containers, and store in a cold place, protected from light. Contains not less than 97.0% and not more than 103.0% of hydrocortisone cypionate, calculated on the dried basis. Meets the requirements for Identification, Specific rotation (+142° to +152°, calculated on the dried basis), Loss on drying (not more than 1.0%), Residue on ignition (not more than 0.2%), and Ordinary impurities.

Hydrocortisone Cypionate Oral Suspension USP—Preserve in tight, light-resistant containers. Contains an amount of hydrocortisone cypionate equivalent to the labeled amount of hydrocortisone, within ±10%. Meets the requirements for Identification and pH (2.8–3.2).

Hydrocortisone Hemisuccinate USP—Preserve in tight containers. Contains not less than 97.0% and not more than 103.0% of hydrocortisone hemisuccinate, calculated on the dried basis. Contains one molecule of water of hydration or is anhydrous. Meets the requirements for Identification, Specific rotation (+124° to +134°, calculated on the dried basis), Loss on drying (not more than 1.0% for the anhydrous form and not more than 4.0% for the hydrous form), and Residue on ignition (not more than 0.1%).

Hydrocortisone Sodium Phosphate USP—Preserve in tight containers. Contains not less than 96.0% and not more than 102.0% of hydrocortisone sodium phosphate, calculated on the dried basis. Meets the requirements for Identification, Phosphate ions (not more than 1.0%), Chloride (not more than 1.00% as sodium chloride), Specific rotation, pH, and Free hydrocortisone (+121° to +129°, calculated on the dried basis, for specific rotation, and 7.5–10.5 for pH), Loss on drying (not more than 5.0%), Heavy metals (not more than 0.004%), and Organic volatile impurities.

Hydrocortisone Sodium Phosphate Injection USP—Preserve in single-dose or in multiple-dose containers, preferably of Type I glass. A sterile, buffered solution of Hydrocortisone Sodium Phosphate in Water for Injection. Contains an amount of hydrocortisone sodium phosphate equivalent to the labeled amount of hydrocortisone, within −10% to +15%. Meets the requirements for Identification, Bacterial endotoxins, pH (7.5–8.5), Particulate matter, and Injections.

Hydrocortisone Sodium Succinate USP—Preserve in tight, light-resistant containers. Contains not less than 97.0% and not more than 102.0% of total steroids, calculated as hydrocortisone sodium succinate, on the dried basis. Meets the requirements for Identification, Specific rotation (+135° to +145°, calculated on the dried basis), Loss on drying (not more than 2.0%), and Sodium content (4.60–4.84%, calculated on the dried basis).

Hydrocortisone Sodium Succinate for Injection USP—Preserve in Containers for Sterile Solids. A sterile mixture of Hydrocortisone Sodium Succinate and suitable buffers. It may be prepared from Hydrocortisone Sodium Succinate, or from Hydrocortisone Hemisuccinate with the aid of Sodium Hydroxide or Sodium Carbonate. Label it to indicate that the constituted solution prepared from Hydrocortisone Sodium Succinate for Injection is suitable for use only if it is clear, and that the solution is to be discarded after 3 days. Label it to indicate that it was prepared by freeze-drying, having been filled into its container in the form of a true solution. Contains an amount of hydrocortisone sodium succinate equivalent to the labeled amount of hydrocortisone, within ±10%, in single-compartment containers, or in the volume of solution designated on the label of containers that are constructed to hold in separate compartments the Hydrocortisone Sodium Succinate for Injection and a solvent. Meets the requirements for Constituted solution, Identification, Bacterial endotoxins, pH (7.0–8.0 in a solution containing the equivalent of 50 mg of hydrocortisone per mL), Loss on drying (not more than 2.0%), Particulate matter, and Free hydrocortisone (not more than 6.7%), and for Sterility tests, Uniformity of dosage units, and Labeling under Injections.

Hydrocortisone Valerate USP—Preserve in well-closed containers. Contains not less than 97.0% and not more than 102.0% of hydrocortisone valerate, calculated on the dried basis. Meets the requirements for Identification, Specific rotation (37° to 43°, calculated on the dried basis), and Loss on drying (not more than 1.0%).

Hydrocortisone Valerate Cream USP—Preserve in well-closed containers. It is Hydrocortisone Valerate in a suitable cream base. Contains the labeled amount, within ±10%. Meets the requirements for Identification and Minimum fill.

Hydrocortisone Valerate Ointment—Not in USP.

HYDROCORTISONE AND ACETIC ACID

For *Hydrocortisone* and *Acetic Acid*—See individual listings for chemistry information.

USP requirements: Hydrocortisone and Acetic Acid Otic Solution USP—Preserve in tight, light-resistant containers. A solution of Hydrocortisone and Glacial Acetic Acid in a suitable nonaqueous solvent. Contains the labeled amount of hydrocortisone, within −10% to +20%, and the labeled amount of acetic acid, within −15% to +30%. Meets the requirements for Identification and pH (2.0–4.0, when diluted with an equal volume of water).

HYDROCORTISONE AND UREA

For *Hydrocortisone* and *Urea*—See individual listings for chemistry information.

USP requirements: Hydrocortisone and Urea Cream—Not in USP.

HYDROFLUMETHIAZIDE

Chemical name: 2*H*-1,2,4-Benzothiadiazine-7-sulfonamide, 3,4-dihydro-6-(trifluoromethyl)-, 1,1-dioxide.

Molecular formula: $C_8H_8F_3N_3O_4S_2$.

Molecular weight: 331.28.

Description: Hydroflumethiazide USP—White to cream-colored, finely divided, odorless, crystalline powder.

pKa: 8.9 and 10.7.

Solubility: Hydroflumethiazide USP—Very slightly soluble in water; freely soluble in acetone; soluble in alcohol.

USP requirements:
Hydroflumethiazide USP—Preserve in tight containers. Contains not less than 98.0% and not more than 102.0% of hydroflumethiazide, calculated on the anhydrous basis. Meets the requirements for Identification, Melting range (270–275 °C), pH (4.5–7.5, in a 1 in 100 dispersion in water), Water (not more than 1.0%), Residue on ignition (not more than 1.0%), Heavy metals (not more than 0.002%), Selenium (not more than 0.003%), Diazotizable substances (not more than 1.0%), and Organic volatile impurities.
Hydroflumethiazide Tablets USP—Preserve in tight containers. Contain the labeled amount, within ±5%. Meet the requirements for Identification, Dissolution (80% in 60 minutes in dilute hydrochloric acid [1 in 100] in Apparatus 2 at 50 rpm), and Uniformity of dosage units.

HYDROGEN PEROXIDE

Chemical name: Hydrogen peroxide.

Molecular formula: H_2O_2.

Molecular weight: 34.01.

Description:
Hydrogen Peroxide Concentrate USP—Clear, colorless liquid. Acid to litmus. Slowly decomposes, and is affected by light.
Hydrogen Peroxide Solution USP—Clear, colorless liquid, odorless or having an odor resembling that of ozone. Acid to litmus. Rapidly decomposes when in contact with many oxidizing as well as reducing substances. When rapidly heated, it may decompose suddenly. Affected by light. Specific gravity is about 1.01.

USP requirements:
Hydrogen Peroxide Concentrate USP—Preserve in partially-filled containers having a small vent in the closure, and store in a cool place. Label it to indicate the name and amount of any added preservative. Contains not less than 29.0% and not more than 32.0%, by weight, of hydrogen peroxide. Contains not more than 0.05% of a suitable preservative or preservatives. Meets the requirements for Acidity and Chloride (not more than 0.005%), and for Identification test, Nonvolatile residue, Heavy metals, and Limit of preservative under Hydrogen Peroxide Topical Solution.
Caution: Hydrogen Peroxide Concentrate is a strong oxidant.
Hydrogen Peroxide Topical Solution USP—Preserve in tight, light-resistant containers, at controlled room temperature. Contains, in each 100 mL, not less than 2.5 grams and not more than 3.5 grams of Hydrogen Peroxide. Contains not more than 0.05% of a suitable preservative or preservatives. Meets the requirements for Identification, Acidity, Nonvolatile residue, Barium, Heavy metals (not more than 5 ppm), and Limit of preservative (not more than 0.05%).

HYDROMORPHONE

Chemical name: Hydromorphone hydrochloride—Morphinan-6-one, 4,5-epoxy-3-hydroxy-17-methyl-, hydrochloride, (5 alpha)-.

Molecular formula: Hydromorphone hydrochloride—$C_{17}H_{19}NO_3 \cdot HCl$.

Molecular weight: Hydromorphone hydrochloride—321.80.

Description: Hydromorphone Hydrochloride USP—Fine, white or practically white, odorless, crystalline powder. Is affected by light.

Solubility: Hydromorphone Hydrochloride USP—Freely soluble in water; sparingly soluble in alcohol; practically insoluble in ether.

USP requirements:
Hydromorphone Hydrochloride USP—Preserve in tight, light-resistant containers. Dried at 105 °C for 2 hours, contains not less than 98.0% and not more than 101.0% of hydromorphone hydrochloride. Meets the requirements for Identification, Specific rotation (−136° to −139°, calculated on the dried basis), Loss on drying (not more than 1.5%), Residue on ignition (not more than 0.3%), Sulfate, Ordinary impurities, and Organic volatile impurities.
Hydromorphone Hydrochloride Injection USP—Preserve in single-dose or in multiple-dose containers, preferably of Type I glass, protected from light. A sterile solution of Hydromorphone Hydrochloride in Water for Injection. Contains the labeled amount, within ±5%. Meets the requirements for Identification, Bacterial endotoxins, pH (3.5–5.5), and Injections.
Hydromorphone Hydrochloride Suppositories—Not in USP.
Hydromorphone Hydrochloride Tablets USP—Preserve in tight, light-resistant containers. Contain the labeled amount, within ±10%. Meet the requirements for Identification, Dissolution (75% in 45 minutes in water in Apparatus 2 at 50 rpm), and Uniformity of dosage units.

HYDROMORPHONE AND GUAIFENESIN

For *Hydromorphone* and *Guaifenesin*—See individual listings for chemistry information.

USP requirements: Hydromorphone Hydrochloride and Guaifenesin Syrup—Not in USP.

HYDROQUINONE

Chemical name: 1,4-Benzenediol.

Molecular formula: $C_6H_6O_2$.

Molecular weight: 110.11.

Description: Hydroquinone USP—Fine white needles. Darkens upon exposure to light and to air.

Solubility: Hydroquinone USP—Freely soluble in water, in alcohol, and in ether.

USP requirements:
Hydroquinone USP—Preserve in tight, light-resistant containers. Contains not less than 99.0% and not more than 100.5% of hydroquinone, calculated on the anhydrous basis. Meets the requirements for Identification, Melting range (172–174 °C), Water (not more than 0.5%), Residue on ignition (not more than 0.5%), and Organic volatile impurities.
Hydroquinone Cream USP—Preserve in well-closed, light-resistant containers. Contains the labeled amount, within ±6%. Meets the requirements for Identification and Minimum fill.
Hydroquinone Topical Solution USP—Preserve in tight, light-resistant containers. Contains the labeled amount, within

−5% to +10%. Meets the requirements for Identification and pH (3.0–4.2).

HYDROXOCOBALAMIN

Chemical name: Cobinamide, dihydroxide, dihydrogen phosphate (ester), mono(inner salt), 3′-ester with 5,6-dimethyl-1-alpha-D-ribofuranosyl-1*H*-benzimidazole.

Molecular formula: $C_{62}H_{89}CoN_{13}O_{15}P$.

Molecular weight: 1346.37.

Description: Hydroxocobalamin USP—Dark red crystals or red crystalline powder. Is odorless, or has not more than a slight acetone odor. The anhydrous form is very hygroscopic.

Solubility: Hydroxocobalamin USP—Sparingly soluble in water, in alcohol, and in methanol; practically insoluble in acetone, in ether, and in chloroform.

USP requirements:

Hydroxocobalamin USP—Preserve in tight, light-resistant containers, and store in a cool place. Contains not less than 95.0% and not more than 102.0% of hydroxocobalamin, calculated on the dried basis. Meets the requirements for Identification, pH (8.0–10.0, in a solution [2 in 100]), Loss on drying (14.0–18.0%), pH-dependent cobalamins (95.0–102.0%), and Cyanocobalamin (not more than 5.0%, calculated on the dried basis).

Hydroxocobalamin Injection USP—Preserve in single-dose or in multiple-dose containers, preferably of Type I glass, protected from light. A sterile solution of Hydroxocobalamin in Water for Injection. Contains the labeled amount, within −5% to +15%. Meets the requirements for Identification, Bacterial endotoxins, pH (3.5–5.0), and Injections.

HYDROXYAMPHETAMINE

Chemical name: Hydroxyamphetamine hydrobromide—Phenol, 4-(2-aminopropyl)-, hydrobromide.

Molecular formula: Hydroxyamphetamine hydrobromide—$C_9H_{13}NO \cdot HBr$.

Molecular weight: Hydroxyamphetamine hydrobromide—232.12.

Description: Hydroxyamphetamine Hydrobromide USP—White, crystalline powder. Its solutions are slightly acid to litmus, having a pH of about 5.

Solubility: Hydroxyamphetamine Hydrobromide USP—Freely soluble in water and in alcohol; slightly soluble in chloroform; practically insoluble in ether.

USP requirements:

Hydroxyamphetamine Hydrobromide USP—Preserve in well-closed, light-resistant containers. Contains not less than 98.0% and not more than 101.5% of hydroxyamphetamine hydrobromide, calculated on the dried basis. Meets the requirements for Identification, Melting range (189–192 °C), Loss on drying (not more than 0.5%), Residue on ignition (not more than 0.1%), Bromide content (33.6–35.2%, calculated on the dried basis), and Ordinary impurities.

Hydroxyamphetamine Hydrobromide Ophthalmic Solution USP—Preserve in tight, light-resistant containers. A sterile, buffered, aqueous solution of Hydroxyamphetamine Hydrobromide. Contains the labeled amount, within ±5%. Contains a suitable antimicrobial agent. Meets the requirements for Identification, Sterility, and pH (4.2–6.0).

HYDROXYCHLOROQUINE

Chemical name: Hydroxychloroquine sulfate—Ethanol, 2-[[4-[(7-chloro-4-quinolinyl)amino]pentyl]ethylamino]-, sulfate (1:1) salt.

Molecular formula: Hydroxychloroquine sulfate—$C_{18}H_{26}ClN_3O \cdot H_2SO_4$.

Molecular weight: Hydroxychloroquine sulfate—433.95.

Description: Hydroxychloroquine Sulfate USP—White or practically white, crystalline powder. Is odorless. Its solutions have a pH of about 4.5. Exists in two forms, the usual form melting at about 240 °C and the other form melting at about 198 °C.

Solubility: Hydroxychloroquine Sulfate USP—Freely soluble in water; practically insoluble in alcohol, in chloroform, and in ether.

USP requirements:

Hydroxychloroquine Sulfate USP—Preserve in well-closed, light-resistant containers. Contains not less than 98.0% and not more than 102.0% of hydroxychloroquine sulfate, calculated on the dried basis. Meets the requirements for Identification, Loss on drying (not more than 2.0%), Ordinary impurities, and Organic volatile impurities.

Hydroxychloroquine Sulfate Tablets USP—Preserve in tight, light-resistant containers. Contain the labeled amount, within ±7%. Meet the requirements for Identification, Dissolution (70% in 60 minutes in water in Apparatus 2 at 100 rpm), and Uniformity of dosage units.

HYDROXYETHYL CELLULOSE

Chemical name: Cellulose, 2-hydroxyethyl ether.

Description: Hydroxyethyl Cellulose NF—White to light tan, practically odorless, hygroscopic powder.

NF category: Suspending and/or viscosity-increasing agent.

Solubility: Hydroxyethyl Cellulose NF—Soluble in hot water and in cold water, giving a colloidal solution; practically insoluble in alcohol and in most organic solvents.

NF requirements: Hydroxyethyl Cellulose NF—Preserve in well-closed containers. A partially substituted poly(hydroxyethyl) ether of cellulose. It is available in several grades, varying in viscosity and degree of substitution, and some grades are modified to improve their dispersion in water. The labeling indicates its viscosity, under specified conditions, in aqueous solution. The indicated viscosity may be in the form of a range encompassing 50% to 150% of the average value. Meets the requirements for Identification, Viscosity (not less than 50% and not more than 150% of the labeled viscosity, where stated as a single value, or it is between the maximum and minimum values, where stated as a range of viscosities), pH (6.0–8.5, in a solution [1 in 100]), Loss on drying (not more than 10.0%), Residue on ignition (not more than 5.0%), Lead (not more than 0.001%), Arsenic (not more than 3 ppm), Heavy metals (not more than 0.004%), and Organic volatile impurities.

HYDROXYPROGESTERONE

Chemical name: Hydroxyprogesterone caproate—Pregn-4-ene-3,20-dione, 17-[(1-oxohexyl)oxy]-.

Molecular formula: Hydroxyprogesterone caproate—$C_{27}H_{40}O_4$.

Molecular weight: Hydroxyprogesterone caproate—428.61.

Description: Hydroxyprogesterone Caproate USP—White or creamy white, crystalline powder. Is odorless or has a slight odor.

Solubility: Hydroxyprogesterone Caproate USP—Insoluble in water; soluble in ether.

USP requirements:

Hydroxyprogesterone Caproate USP—Preserve in well-closed, light-resistant containers. Contains not less than 97.0% and not more than 103.0% of hydroxyprogesterone caproate, calculated on the anhydrous basis. Meets the requirements for Identification, Melting range (120–124 °C), Specific rotation (+58° to +64°, calculated on the anhydrous basis), Water (not more than 0.1%), Free *n*-caproic acid, and Ordinary impurities.

Hydroxyprogesterone Caproate Injection USP—Preserve in single-dose or in multiple-dose containers, preferably of Type I or Type III glass. A sterile solution of Hydroxyprogesterone Caproate in a suitable vegetable oil. Contains the labeled amount, within ±10%. Meets the requirements for Identification, Water (not more than 0.2%), and Injections.

HYDROXYPROPYL CELLULOSE

Chemical name: Cellulose, 2-hydroxypropyl ether.

Description: Hydroxypropyl Cellulose NF—White to cream-colored, practically odorless, granular solid or powder. Is hygroscopic after drying.

NF category: Coating agent; suspending and/or viscosity-increasing agent.

Solubility: Hydroxypropyl Cellulose NF—Soluble in cold water, in alcohol, in chloroform, and in propylene glycol, giving a colloidal solution; insoluble in hot water.

USP requirements: Hydroxypropyl Cellulose Ocular System USP—Preserve in single-dose containers, at a temperature not exceeding 30 °C. Contains the labeled amount, within ±15%. Contains no other substance. It is sterile. Meets the requirements for Identification, Sterility, and Weight variation.

NF requirements: Hydroxypropyl Cellulose NF—Store in well-closed containers. A partially substituted poly(hydroxypropyl) ether of cellulose. Label it to indicate the viscosity in an aqueous solution of stated concentration and temperature. The indicated viscosity may be in the form of a range encompassing 50% to 150% of the average value. When dried at 105 °C for 3 hours, contains not more than 80.5% of hydroxypropoxy groups. Meets the requirements for Identification, Apparent viscosity, pH (5.0–8.0, in a solution [1 in 100]), Loss on drying (not more than 5.0%), Residue on ignition (except for silica, not more than 0.2%), Arsenic (not more than 3 ppm), Lead (not more than 0.001%), Heavy metals (not more than 0.004%), and Organic volatile impurities.

LOW-SUBSTITUTED HYDROXYPROPYL CELLULOSE

Description: Low-Substituted Hydroxypropyl Cellulose NF—White to yellowish white, practically odorless, fibrous or granular powder. Is hygroscopic. The pH of the suspension, obtained by shaking 1.0 gram with 100 mL of water, is between 5.0 and 7.5.

NF category: Tablet disintegrant and/or tablet binder.

Solubility: Low-Substituted Hydroxypropyl Cellulose NF—Practically insoluble in ethanol and in ether. Dissolves in a solution of sodium hydroxide (1 in 10), and produces a viscous solution. Swells in water, in sodium carbonate TS, and in 2 *N* hydrochloric acid.

NF requirements: Low-Substituted Hydroxypropyl Cellulose NF—Preserve in tight containers. A low-substituted hydroxypropyl ether of cellulose. When dried at 105 °C for 1 hour, contains not less than 5.0% and not more than 16.0% of hydroxypropoxy groups ($-OCH_2CHOHCH_3$). Meets the requirements for Identification, Loss on drying (not more than 5.0%), Residue on ignition (not more than 0.5%), Chloride (not more than 0.36%), Arsenic (not more than 2 ppm), and Heavy metals (not more than 0.001%).

HYDROXYPROPYL METHYLCELLULOSE

Chemical name: Cellulose, 2-hydroxypropyl methyl ether.

Description: Hydroxypropyl Methylcellulose USP—White to slightly off-white, fibrous or granular powder. Swells in water and produces a clear to opalescent, viscous, colloidal mixture.

NF category: Coating agent; suspending and/or viscosity-increasing agent; tablet binder.

Solubility: Hydroxypropyl Methylcellulose USP—Insoluble in dehydrated alcohol, in ether, and in chloroform.

USP requirements:

Hydroxypropyl Methylcellulose USP—Preserve in well-closed containers. A propylene glycol ether of methylcellulose. Label it to indicate its substitution type and its viscosity type (viscosity of a solution [1 in 50]). When dried at 105 °C for 2 hours, contains methoxy and hydroxypropoxy groups conforming to the limits for the 4 substitution types for methoxy and hydroxypropoxy contents. Meets the requirements for Identification, Apparent viscosity, Loss on drying (not more than 5.0%), Residue on ignition (not more than 1.5% for labeled viscosity of greater than 50 centipoises, 3% for labeled viscosity of 50 centipoises or less, or 5% of all labeled viscosities), Arsenic (not more than 3 ppm), and Heavy metals (not more than 0.001%).

Hydroxypropyl Methylcellulose Ophthalmic Solution USP—Preserve in tight containers. A sterile solution of Hydroxypropyl Methylcellulose. Contains the labeled amount, within ±15%. Meets the requirements for Identification, Sterility, and pH (6.0–7.8).

Hydroxypropyl Methylcellulose Injection—Not in USP.

HYDROXYPROPYL METHYLCELLULOSE PHTHALATE

Description: Hydroxypropyl Methylcellulose Phthalate NF—White powder or granules. Is odorless.

NF category: Coating agent.

Solubility: Hydroxypropyl Methylcellulose Phthalate NF—Practically insoluble in water, in dehydrated alcohol, and in hexane. Produces a viscous solution in a mixture of methanol and dichloromethane (1:1), or in a mixture of dehydrated alcohol and acetone (1:1). Dissolves in 1 *N* sodium hydroxide.

NF requirements: Hydroxypropyl Methylcellulose Phthalate NF—Preserve in well-closed containers. A monophthalic acid ester of hydroxypropyl methylcellulose. Label it to indicate its substitution type and its viscosity. When dried at 105 °C for 1 hour, contains methoxy, hydroxypropoxy, and phthalyl groups conforming to the limits for the 2 substitution types for methoxy, hydroxypropxy, and phthalyl. Meets the requirements for Clarity and color of solution, Identification, Viscosity (80–120% of that indicated by the label), Loss on drying (not more than 5.0%), Residue on ignition (not more than 0.20%), Chloride (not more than 0.07%), Arsenic (not more than 2 ppm), Heavy metals (not more than 0.001%), Free phthalic acid (not more than 1.0%), Phthalyl content, and Methoxy and hydroxypropoxy contents.

HYDROXYSTILBAMIDINE

Chemical name: Hydroxystilbamidine isethionate—Benzenecarboximidamide, 4-[2-[4-(aminoiminomethyl)phenyl]-ethenyl]-3-hydroxy-, bis(2-hydroxyethanesulfonate) (salt).

Molecular formula: Hydroxystilbamidine isethionate—$C_{16}H_{16}N_4O \cdot 2C_2H_6O_4S$.

Molecular weight: Hydroxystilbamidine isethionate—532.58.

Description:

Hydroxystilbamidine Isethionate USP—Yellow, fine, odorless, crystalline powder. Is stable in air but decomposes upon exposure to light. Melts at about 280 °C.

Sterile Hydroxystilbamidine Isethionate USP—Yellow, fine, odorless, crystalline powder. Is stable in air, but decomposes upon exposure to light. Melts at about 280 °C.

Solubility:

Hydroxystilbamidine Isethionate USP—Soluble in water; slightly soluble in alcohol; insoluble in ether.

Sterile Hydroxystilbamidine Isethionate USP—Soluble in water; slightly soluble in alcohol; insoluble in ether.

USP requirements:

Hydroxystilbamidine Isethionate USP—Preserve in tight, light-resistant containers. Contains not less than 95.0% and not more than 105.0% of hydroxystilbamidine isethionate, calculated on the dried basis. Meets the requirements for Identification, pH (4.0–5.5, in a solution [1 in 100]), Loss on drying (not more than 1.0%), Residue on ignition (not more than 0.1%), Selenium (not more than 0.003%), and Heavy metals (not more than 0.001%).

Sterile Hydroxystilbamidine Isethionate USP—Preserve in light-resistant Containers for Sterile Solids. It is Hydroxystilbamidine Isethionate suitable for parenteral use. Meets the requirements for Completeness of solution, Constituted solution, and Bacterial endotoxins, for Identification tests, pH, Loss on drying, Residue on ignition, Selenium, and Heavy metals under Hydroxystilbamidine Isethionate, and for Sterility tests, Uniformity of dosage units, and Labeling under Injections.

HYDROXYUREA

Chemical name: Urea, hydroxy-.

Molecular formula: $CH_4N_2O_2$.

Molecular weight: 76.05.

Description: Hydroxyurea USP—White to off-white powder. Is somewhat hygroscopic, decomposing in the presence of moisture. Melts at a temperature exceeding 133 °C, with decomposition.

Solubility: Hydroxyurea USP—Freely soluble in water and in hot alcohol.

USP requirements:

Hydroxyurea USP—Preserve in tight containers, in a dry atmosphere. Contains not less than 97.0% and not more than 103.0% of hydroxyurea, calculated on the dried basis. Meets the requirements for Identification, Loss on drying (not more than 1.0%), Residue on ignition (not more than 0.50%), Heavy metals (not more than 0.003%), Urea and related compounds, and Organic volatile impurities.

Hydroxyurea Capsules USP—Preserve in tight containers, in a dry atmosphere. Contain the labeled amount, within ±10%. Meet the requirements for Identification and Uniformity of dosage units.

HYDROXYZINE

Chemical group: Piperazine derivative.

Chemical name:

Hydroxyzine hydrochloride—Ethanol, 2-[2-[4-[(4-chlorophenyl)phenylmethyl]-1-piperazinyl]ethoxy]-, dihydrochloride.

Hydroxyzine pamoate—Ethanol, 2-[2-[4-[(4-chlorophenyl)-phenylmethyl]-1-piperazinyl]ethoxy]-, compd. with 4,4′-methylenebis[3-hydroxy-2-naphthalenecarboxylic acid] (1:1).

Molecular formula:

Hydroxyzine hydrochloride—$C_{21}H_{27}ClN_2O_2 \cdot 2HCl$.

Hydroxyzine pamoate—$C_{21}H_{27}ClN_2O_2 \cdot C_{23}H_{16}O_6$.

Molecular weight:

Hydroxyzine hydrochloride—447.83.

Hydroxyzine pamoate—763.29.

Description:

Hydroxyzine Hydrochloride USP—White, odorless powder. Melts at about 200 °C, with decomposition.

Hydroxyzine Pamoate USP—Light yellow, practically odorless powder.

pKa: Hydroxyzine hydrochloride—2.6 and 7.

Solubility:

Hydroxyzine Hydrochloride USP—Very soluble in water; soluble in chloroform; slightly soluble in acetone; practically insoluble in ether.

Hydroxyzine Pamoate USP—Practically insoluble in water and in methanol; freely soluble in dimethylformamide.

USP requirements:

Hydroxyzine Hydrochloride USP—Preserve in tight containers. Contains not less than 98.0% and not more than 100.5% of hydroxyzine hydrochloride, calculated on the dried basis. Meets the requirements for Identification, Loss on drying (not more than 5.0%), Residue on ignition (not more than 0.5%), Heavy metals (not more than 0.002%), Chromatographic purity, and Organic volatile impurities.

Hydroxyzine Hydrochloride Capsules—Not in USP.

Hydroxyzine Hydrochloride Injection USP—Preserve in single-dose or in multiple-dose containers, protected from light. A sterile solution of Hydroxyzine Hydrochloride in Water for Injection. Contains the labeled amount, within ±10%. Meets the requirements for Identification, Bacterial endotoxins, pH (3.5–6.0), Limit of 4-chlorobenzophenone (not more than 0.2%), and Injections.

Hydroxyzine Hydrochloride Syrup USP—Preserve in tight, light-resistant containers. Contains the labeled amount, within ±10%. Meets the requirement for Identification.

Hydroxyzine Hydrochloride Tablets USP—Preserve in tight containers. Contain the labeled amount, within ±10%. Meet the requirements for Identification, Dissolution (75% in 45 minutes in water in a modified basket-rack assembly as directed for Uncoated tablets under Disintegration), and Uniformity of dosage units.

Hydroxyzine Pamoate USP—Preserve in tight containers. Contains not less than 97.0% and not more than 102.0% of hydroxyzine pamoate, calculated on the anhydrous basis. Meets the requirements for Identification, Water (not more than 5.0%), Residue on ignition (not more than

0.5%), Heavy metals (not more than 0.005%), Pamoic acid content (49.4–51.9%, calculated on the anhydrous basis), and Organic volatile impurities.

Hydroxyzine Pamoate Capsules USP—Preserve in well-closed containers. Contain an amount of hydroxyzine pamoate equivalent to the labeled amount of hydroxyzine hydrochloride, within ±10%. Meet the requirements for Identification, Dissolution (75% in 60 minutes in 0.1 *N* hydrochloric acid in Apparatus 2 at 50 rpm), and Uniformity of dosage units.

Hydroxyzine Pamoate Oral Suspension USP—Preserve in tight, light-resistant containers. Contains an amount of hydroxyzine pamoate equivalent to the labeled amount of hydroxyzine hydrochloride, within ±10%. Meets the requirements for Identification and pH (4.5–7.0).

HYOSCYAMINE

Source: The levo-isomer of atropine; the major active alkaloid of belladonna.

Chemical group: Natural tertiary amine.

Chemical name:

Hyoscyamine—Benzeneacetic acid, alpha-(hydroxymethyl)-, 8-methyl-8-azabicyclo[3.2.1]oct-3-yl ester, [3(*S*)-*endo*]-.

Hyoscyamine hydrobromide—Benzeneacetic acid, alpha-(hydroxymethyl)-, 8-methyl-8-azabicyclo[3.2.1]oct-3-yl ester, hydrobromide [3(*S*)-*endo*]-.

Hyoscyamine sulfate—Benzeneacetic acid, alpha-(hydroxymethyl)-, 8-methyl-8-azabicyclo[3.2.1]oct-3-yl ester, [3(*S*)-*endo*]-, sulfate (2:1), dihydrate.

Molecular formula:

Hyoscyamine—$C_{17}H_{23}NO_3$.

Hyoscyamine hydrobromide—$C_{17}H_{23}NO_3 \cdot HBr$.

Hyoscyamine sulfate—$(C_{17}H_{23}NO_3)_2 \cdot H_2SO_4 \cdot 2H_2O$.

Molecular weight:

Hyoscyamine—289.37.

Hyoscyamine hydrobromide—370.29.

Hyoscyamine sulfate—712.85.

Description:

Hyoscyamine USP—White, crystalline powder. Is affected by light. Its solutions are alkaline to litmus.

Hyoscyamine Hydrobromide USP—White, odorless crystals or crystalline powder. The pH of a solution (1 in 20) is about 5.4. Is affected by light.

Hyoscyamine Sulfate USP—White, odorless crystals or crystalline powder. Is deliquescent and is affected by light. The pH of a solution (1 in 100) is about 5.3.

Solubility:

Hyoscyamine USP—Slightly soluble in water; freely soluble in alcohol, in chloroform, and in dilute acids; sparingly soluble in ether.

Hyoscyamine Hydrobromide USP—Freely soluble in water, in alcohol, and in chloroform; very slightly soluble in ether.

Hyoscyamine Sulfate USP—Very soluble in water; freely soluble in alcohol; practically insoluble in ether.

USP requirements:

Hyoscyamine USP—Preserve in tight, light-resistant containers. Contains not less than 98.0% and not more than 101.0% of hyoscyamine, calculated on the dried basis. Meets the requirements for Identification, Melting range (106–109 °C), Specific rotation (−20° to −23°, calculated on the dried basis), Loss on drying (not more than 0.2%), Residue on ignition (not more than 0.1%), Foreign alkaloids and other impurities.

Caution: Handle Hyoscyamine with exceptional care, since it is highly potent.

Hyoscyamine Tablets USP—Preserve in well-closed, light-resistant containers. Contain the labeled amount, within ±10%. Meet the requirements for Identification, Disintegration (30 minutes, the use of disks being omitted), and Uniformity of dosage units.

Hyoscyamine Hydrobromide USP—Preserve in tight, light-resistant containers. Contains not less than 98.5% and not more than 100.5% of hyoscyamine hydrobromide, calculated on the dried basis. Meets the requirements for Identification, Melting range (not less than 149 °C), Specific rotation (not less than −24°, calculated on the dried basis), Loss on drying (not more than 1.0%), Residue on ignition (not more than 0.2%), and Other alkaloids.

Caution: Handle Hyoscyamine Hydrobromide with exceptional care, since it is highly potent.

Hyoscyamine Sulfate USP—Preserve in tight, light-resistant containers. Contains not less than 98.5% and not more than 100.5% of hyoscyamine sulfate, calculated on the dried basis. Meets the requirements for Identification, Melting range (not less than 200 °C), Specific rotation (not less than −24°, calculated on the dried basis), Loss on drying (2.0–5.5%), Residue on ignition (not more than 0.2%), Readily carbonizable substances, Other alkaloids, and Organic volatile impurities.

Caution: Handle Hyoscyamine Sulfate with exceptional care, since it is highly potent.

Hyoscyamine Sulfate Extended-release Capsules—Not in USP.

Hyoscyamine Sulfate Elixir USP—Preserve in tight, light-resistant containers, at controlled room temperature. Contains the labeled amount, within ±10%. Meets the requirements for Identification, pH (3.0–6.5), and Alcohol content (within ±10% of labeled amount).

Hyoscyamine Sulfate Injection USP—Preserve in single-dose or in multiple-dose containers, preferably of Type I glass, at controlled room temperature. A sterile solution of Hyoscyamine Sulfate in Water for Injection. Contains the labeled amount, within ±7%. Meets the requirements for Identification, Bacterial endotoxins, pH (3.0–6.5), and Injections.

Hyoscyamine Sulfate Oral Solution USP—Preserve in tight, light-resistant containers, at controlled room temperature. Contains the labeled amount, within ±10%. Meets the requirements for Identification and pH (3.0–6.5).

Hyoscyamine Sulfate Tablets USP—Preserve in tight, light-resistant containers. Contain the labeled amount, within ±10%. Meet the requirements for Identification, Disintegration (15 minutes), and Uniformity of dosage units.

HYOSCYAMINE AND PHENOBARBITAL

For *Hyoscyamine* and *Phenobarbital*—See individual listings for chemistry information.

USP requirements:

Hyoscyamine Sulfate and Phenobarbital Elixir—Not in USP.

Hyoscyamine Sulfate and Phenobarbital Oral Solution—Not in USP.

Hyoscyamine Sulfate and Phenobarbital Tablets—Not in USP.

HYPOPHOSPHOROUS ACID

Chemical name: Phosphinic acid.

Molecular formula: H_3PO_2.

Molecular weight: 66.00.

Description: Hypophosphorous Acid NF—Colorless or slightly yellow, odorless liquid. Specific gravity is about 1.13.

NF category: Antioxidant.

NF requirements: Hypophosphorous Acid NF—Preserve in tight containers. Contains not less than 30.0% and not more than 32.0% of hypophosphorous acid. Meets the requirements for Identification, Arsenic, Barium, and Oxalate (not more than 1.5 ppm arsenic), and Heavy metals (not more than 0.002%).

IBUPROFEN

Chemical group: Propionic acid derivative.

Chemical name: Benzeneacetic acid, alpha-methyl-4-(2-methylpropyl), (±)-.

Molecular formula: $C_{13}H_{18}O_2$.

Molecular weight: 206.28.

Description: Ibuprofen USP—White to off-white, crystalline powder, having a slight, characteristic odor.

pKa: 5.2 (apparent).

Solubility: Ibuprofen USP—Practically insoluble in water; very soluble in alcohol, in methanol, in acetone, and in chloroform; slightly soluble in ethyl acetate.

USP requirements:

Ibuprofen USP—Preserve in tight containers. Contains not less than 97.0% and not more than 103.0% of ibuprofen, calculated on the anhydrous basis. Meets the requirements for Identification, Water (not more than 1.0%), Residue on ignition (not more than 0.5%), Heavy metals (not more than 0.002%), Chromatographic purity, and Organic volatile impurities.

Ibuprofen Capsules—Not in USP.

Ibuprofen Oral Suspension—Not in USP.

Ibuprofen Tablets USP—Preserve in well-closed containers. Contain the labeled amount, within ±10%. Meet the requirements for Identification, Dissolution (70% in 30 minutes in phosphate buffer [pH 7.2] in Apparatus 1 at 150 rpm), Uniformity of dosage units, and Water (not more than 5.0%).

ICHTHAMMOL

Chemical name: Ichthammol.

Description: Ichthammol USP—Reddish brown to brownish black, viscous fluid, having a strong, characteristic, empyreumatic odor.

Solubility: Ichthammol USP—Miscible with water, with glycerin, and with fixed oils and fats. Partially soluble in alcohol and in ether.

USP requirements:

Ichthammol USP—Preserve in well-closed containers. Obtained by the destructive distillation of certain bituminous schists, sulfonation of the distillate, and neutralization of the product with ammonia. Yields not less than 2.5% of ammonia and not less than 10.0% of total sulfur. Meets the requirements for Identification, Loss on drying (not more than 50.0%), Residue on ignition (not more than 0.5%), and Limit for ammonium sulfate (not more than 8.0%).

Ichthammol Ointment USP—Preserve in collapsible tubes or in tight containers, and avoid prolonged exposure to temperatures exceeding 30 °C. Contains an amount of Ichthammol equivalent to not less than 0.25% of ammonia.

Prepare Ichthammol Ointment as follows: 100 grams of Ichthammol, 100 grams of Lanolin, 800 grams of Petrolatum, to make 1000 grams. Thoroughly incorporate the Ichthammol with the Lanolin, and combine this mixture with the Petrolatum.

IDARUBICIN

Chemical name: Idarubicin hydrochloride—5,12-Naphthacenedione, 9-acetyl-7-[(3-amino-2,3,6-trideoxy-alpha-L-*lyxo*-hexopyranosyl)oxy]-7,8,9,10-tetrahydro-6,9,11-trihydroxy-hydrochloride, (7*S*-*cis*)-.

Molecular formula: Idarubicin hydrochloride—$C_{26}H_{27}NO_9 \cdot HCl$.

Molecular weight: Idarubicin hydrochloride—533.96.

USP requirements:

Idarubicin Hydrochloride USP—Preserve in tight containers. Contains not less than 960 mcg and not more than 1030 mcg of idarubicin hydrochloride per mg, calculated on the anhydrous basis. Meets the requirements for Identification, Crystallinity, pH (5.0–6.5, in a solution containing 5 mg per mL), Water (not more than 5.0%), and Chromatographic purity.

Caution: Great care should be taken to prevent inhaling particles of Idarubicin Hydrochloride and exposing the skin to it.

Idarubicin Hydrochloride for Injection USP—Preserve in Containers for Sterile Solids. A sterile mixture of Idarubicin Hydrochloride and Lactose. Contains the labeled amount, within ±10%. Meets the requirements for Constituted solution, Identification, Bacterial endotoxins, Sterility, pH (5.0–7.0, in a solution constituted as directed in the labeling, water being used as the diluent), and Water (not more than 4.0%), and for Uniformity of dosage units and Labeling under Injections.

Caution: Great care should be taken to prevent inhaling particles of Idarubicin Hydrochloride and exposing the skin to it.

IDOXURIDINE

Chemical group: An antimetabolite of thymidine.

Chemical name: Uridine, 2′-deoxy-5-iodo-.

Molecular formula: $C_9H_{11}IN_2O_5$.

Molecular weight: 354.10.

Description: Idoxuridine USP—White, crystalline, practically odorless powder.

Solubility: Idoxuridine USP—Slightly soluble in water and in alcohol; practically insoluble in chloroform and in ether.

USP requirements:

Idoxuridine USP—Preserve in tight, light-resistant containers. Contains not less than 98.0% and not more than 101.0% of idoxuridine, calculated on the dried basis. Meets the requirements for Identification and Loss on drying (not more than 1.0%).

Idoxuridine Ophthalmic Ointment USP—Preserve in collapsible ophthalmic ointment tubes in a cool place. It is Idoxuridine in a Petrolatum base. It is sterile. Contains 0.45% to 0.55% of idoxuridine. Meets the requirements for Identification, Sterility, and Metal particles.

Idoxuridine Ophthalmic Solution USP—Preserve in tight, light-resistant containers in a cold place. A sterile, aqueous solution of Idoxuridine. Contains 0.09% to 0.11% of idoxuridine. Meets the requirements for Identification, Sterility, and pH (4.5–7.0).

IFOSFAMIDE

Chemical name: 2*H*-1,3,2-Oxazaphosphorin-2-amine, *N*,3-bis(2-chloroethyl)tetrahydro-, 2-oxide.

Molecular formula: $C_7H_{15}Cl_2N_2O_2P$.

Molecular weight: 261.09.

Description: Ifosfamide USP—White, crystalline powder. Melts at about 40 °C.

Solubility: Ifosfamide USP—Freely soluble in water; very soluble in alcohol, in ethyl acetate, in isopropyl alcohol, in methanol, and in methylene chloride; very slightly soluble in hexanes.

USP requirements:

Ifosfamide USP—Preserve in tight containers at a temperature not exceeding 25 °C. Contains not less than 98.0% and not more than 102.0% of ifosfamide. Meets the requirements for Identification, pH (4.0–7.0 in a solution [1 in 10]), Water (not more than 0.3%), Heavy metals (not more than 0.002%), Ionic chloride (not more than 0.018%), Chloroform-insoluble phosphorus (not more than 0.0415%), and Limit of 2-chloroethylamine hydrochloride (not more than 0.25%).

Caution: Great care should be taken in handling Ifosfamide, as it is a potent cytotoxic agent and suspected carcinogen.

Sterile Ifosfamide USP—Preserve in Containers for Sterile Solids, at controlled room temperature. It is Ifosfamide suitable for parenteral use. Contains the labeled amount, within ± 10%. Meets the requirements for Identification, Bacterial endotoxins, pH (4.0–7.0), and Water (not more than 0.3%), and for Sterility tests, Uniformity of dosage units, and Labeling under Injections.

Caution: Great care should be taken in handling Ifosfamide, as it is a potent cytotoxic agent and suspected carcinogen.

IMIDUREA

Chemical name: *N,N″*-Methylenebis[*N′*-[3-(hydroxymethyl)-2,5-dioxo-4-imidazolidinyl]urea].

Molecular formula: $C_{11}H_{16}N_8O_8$.

Molecular weight: 388.30.

Description: Imidurea NF—White, odorless powder.

Solubility: Imidurea NF—Soluble in water and in glycerin; sparingly soluble in propylene glycol; insoluble in most organic solvents.

NF requirements: Imidurea NF—Preserve in tight containers. Contains not less than 26.0% and not more than 28.0% of nitrogen, calculated on the dried basis. Meets the requirements for Color and clarity of solution, Identification, pH (6.0–7.5, in a solution [1 in 100]), Loss on drying (not more than 3.0%), Residue on ignition (not more than 3.0%), Heavy metals (not more than 0.001%), Nitrogen content, and Organic volatile impurities.

IMIPENEM

Source: Derivative of thienamycin, produced by the soil organism *Streptomyces cattleya*.

Chemical group: A carbapenem, which is a subclass of the beta-lactams.

Chemical name: 1-Azabicyclo[3.2.0]hept-2-ene-2-carboxylic acid, 6-(1-hydroxyethyl)-3-[[2-[(iminomethyl)amino]ethyl]thio]-7-oxo-, monohydrate, [5*R*-[5 alpha,6 alpha(*R**)]]-.

Molecular formula: $C_{12}H_{17}N_3O_4S \cdot H_2O$.

Molecular weight: 317.36.

Description: Imipenem USP—White to tan-colored crystalline powder.

Solubility: Imipenem USP—Sparingly soluble in water; slightly soluble in methanol.

USP requirements: Sterile Imipenem USP—Preserve in Containers for Sterile Solids, and store in a cold place. It is imipenem suitable for parenteral use. Contains the equivalent of not less than 98.0% and not more than 101.0% of imipenem monohydrate. Meets the requirements for Identification, Specific rotation (+84° to +89°, calculated on the dried basis), Crystallinity, Bacterial endotoxins, Sterility, Loss on drying (5.0–8.0%), Residue on ignition (not more than 0.2%), Heavy metals (not more than 0.002%), and Solvents (not more than 0.25%).

IMIPENEM AND CILASTATIN

For *Imipenem* and *Cilastatin*—See individual listings for chemistry information.

USP requirements:

Imipenem and Cilastatin Sodium for Injection USP—Preserve in Containers for Sterile Solids and store in a cold place. A sterile mixture of Sterile Imipenem, Sterile Cilastatin Sodium, and Sodium Bicarbonate. Contains the equivalent of not less than 400 mcg per mg of imipenem and not less than 400 mcg per mg of cilastatin. In addition, contains the labeled amount of imipenem and an amount of cilastatin sodium equivalent to the labeled amount of cilastatin, within −10% to +15%. Meets the requirements for Constituted solution, Identification, Pyrogen, Sterility, pH (6.5–8.5, when constituted as directed in the labeling), Loss on drying (not more than 3.5%), and Particulate matter.

Imipenem and Cilastatin Sodium for Suspension—Not in USP.

Sterile Imipenem and Cilastatin Sodium USP—Preserve in Containers for Sterile Solids and store in a cold place. A sterile mixture of Sterile Imipenem and Sterile Cilastatin Sodium. Contains the equivalent of not less than 400 mcg per mg of imipenem and not less than 400 mcg per mg of cilastatin. In addition, contains the labeled amount of imipenem and an amount of cilastatin sodium equivalent to the labeled amount of cilastatin, within −10% to +15%. Meets the requirements for Constituted solution, Identification, Pyrogen, Sterility, pH (6.0–7.5, when constituted as directed in the labeling), Loss on drying (not more than 3.5%), and Particulate matter.

IMIPRAMINE

Chemical group: Dibenzazepine.

Chemical name:

Imipramine hydrochloride—5*H*-Dibenz[*b,f*]azepine-5-propanamine, 10,11-dihydro-*N,N*-dimethyl-, monohydrochloride.

Imipramine pamoate—5-(3-[Dimethylamino)propyl]-10,11-dihydro-5*H*-dibenz[*b,f*]azepine 4,4′-methylenebis-(3-hydroxy-2-naphthoate)(2:1).

Molecular formula:

Imipramine hydrochloride—$C_{19}H_{24}N_2 \cdot HCl$.

Imipramine pamoate—$(C_{19}H_{24}N_2)_2 \cdot C_{23}H_{16}O_6$.

Molecular weight:
Imipramine hydrochloride—316.87.
Imipramine pamoate—949.21.

Description:
Imipramine Hydrochloride USP—White to off-white, odorless or practically odorless, crystalline powder.
Imipramine pamoate—Fine, yellow, odorless powder.

pKa: Imipramine hydrochloride—9.5.

Solubility:
Imipramine Hydrochloride USP—Freely soluble in water and in alcohol; soluble in acetone; insoluble in ether.
Imipramine pamoate—Soluble in ethanol, in acetone, in ether, in chloroform, and in carbon tetrachloride. Insoluble in water.

USP requirements:
Imipramine Hydrochloride USP—Preserve in tight containers. Contains not less than 98.0% and not more than 102.0% of imipramine hydrochloride, calculated on the dried basis. Meets the requirements for Identification, Melting range (170–174 °C), Loss on drying (not more than 0.5%), Residue on ignition (not more than 0.1%), Heavy metals (not more than 0.001%), Iminodibenzyl, and Organic volatile impurities.
Imipramine Hydrochloride Injection USP—Preserve in single-dose containers, preferably of Type I glass. A sterile solution of Imipramine Hydrochloride in Water for Injection. Contains, in each mL, not less than 11.5 mg and not more than 13.5 mg of imipramine hydrochloride. Meets the requirements for Identification, Bacterial endotoxins, pH (4.0–5.0), and Injections.
Imipramine Hydrochloride Tablets USP—Preserve in tight containers. Contain the labeled amount, within ±7%. Meet the requirements for Identification, Dissolution (75% in 45 minutes in 0.1 *N* hydrochloric acid in Apparatus 1 at 100 rpm), and Uniformity of dosage units.
Imipramine Pamoate Capsules—Not in USP.

INDAPAMIDE

Chemical name: Benzamide, 3-(aminosulfonyl)-4-chloro-*N*-(2,3-dihydro-2-methyl-1*H*-indol-1-yl)-.

Molecular formula: $C_{16}H_{16}ClN_3O_3S$.

Molecular weight: 365.83.

Description: Indapamide USP—White to off-white crystalline powder. Melts between 167 and 170 °C.

Solubility: Indapamide USP—Soluble in methanol, in alcohol, in acetonitrile, in glacial acetic acid, and in ethyl acetate; very slightly soluble in ether and in chloroform; practically insoluble in water.

USP requirements:
Indapamide USP—Preserve in well-closed containers. Contains not less than 98.0% and not more than 101.0% of indapamide, calculated on the dried basis. Meets the requirements for Identification, Loss on drying (not more than 3.0%), Residue on ignition (not more than 0.1%), Chromatographic purity, and Organic volatile impurities.
Indapamide Tablets USP—Preserve in well-closed containers. Contain the labeled amount, within ±10%. Meet the requirements for Identification, Dissolution (75% in 60 minutes in simulated gastric fluid TS [without enzyme] in Apparatus 1 at 100 rpm), and Uniformity of dosage units.

INDIGOTINDISULFONATE

Chemical name: Indigotindisulfonate sodium—1*H*-Indole-5-sulfonic acid, 2-(1,3-dihydro-3-oxo-5-sulfo-2*H*-indol-2-ylidene)-2,3-dihydro-3-oxo-, disodium salt.

Molecular formula: Indigotindisulfonate sodium—$C_{16}H_8N_2Na_2O_8S_2$.

Molecular weight: Indigotindisulfonate sodium—466.35.

Description: Indigotindisulfonate Sodium USP—Dusky, purplish blue powder, or blue granules having a coppery luster. Affected by light. Its solutions have a blue or bluish purple color.

Solubility: Indigotindisulfonate Sodium USP—Slightly soluble in water and in alcohol; practically insoluble in most other organic solvents.

USP requirements:
Indigotindisulfonate Sodium USP—Preserve in tight, light-resistant containers. Contains not less than 96.0% and not more than 102.0% of sodium indigotinsulfonates, calculated on the dried basis as indigotindisulfonate sodium. Meets the requirements for Identification, Loss on drying (not more than 5.0%), Water-insoluble substances, Arsenic (not more than 8 ppm), Lead (not more than 0.001%), and Sulfur content (13.0–14.0%, calculated on the dried basis).
Indigotindisulfonate Sodium Injection USP—Preserve in single-dose, light-resistant containers, preferably of Type I glass. A sterile solution of Indigotindisulfonate Sodium in Water for Injection. Contains the labeled amount, within −10% to +5%. Meets the requirements for Identification, Bacterial endotoxins, pH (3.0–6.5), and Injections.

INDIUM In 111 OXYQUINOLINE

Source: Saturated (1:3) complex of indium and oxyquinoline (oxine), a chelating agent.

Chemical name: Indium-^{111}*In*, tris(8-quinolinolato-N^1,O^8)-.

Molecular formula: $C_{27}H_{18}{}^{111}InN_3O_3$.

Molecular weight: 543.46.

USP requirements: Indium In 111 Oxyquinoline Solution USP—Preserve in single-unit containers at a temperature between 15 and 25 °C. A sterile, nonpyrogenic, isotonic aqueous solution suitable for the radiolabeling of blood cells, especially leukocytes and platelets, containing radioactive indium (^{111}In) in the form of a complex with 8-hydroxyquinoline, the latter being present in excess. Label it to contain the following, in addition to the information specified for Labeling under Injections: the time and date of calibration; the amount of ^{111}In as the 8-hydroxyquinoline complex expressed as total megabecquerels (or millicuries) and concentration as megabecquerels (or millicuries) per mL on the date and time of calibration; the expiration date; the statement, "Not for direct administration. Use only for radiolabeling of leucocytes in vitro. Administer radiolabeled cells subsequently by intravenous injection;" and the statement, "Caution—Radioactive Material." The labeling indicates that in making dosage calculations, correction is to be made for radioactive decay, and also indicates that the radioactive half-life of ^{111}In is 67.9 hours. Contains the labeled amount of ^{111}In, within ±10%, as the 8-hydroxyquinoline complex expressed as megabecquerels (or millicuries) per mL at the time indicated in the labeling. Other chemical forms of radioactivity do not exceed 10.0% of the total radioactivity. Meets the requirements for Specific activity (not less than 1.85 gigabecquerels [50 millicuries] per mcg of indium), Pyrogen, pH (6.5–7.5),

Radionuclide identification, Radiochemical purity, and Radionuclidic purity.

INDIUM In 111 PENTETATE

USP requirements: Indium In 111 Pentetate Injection USP—Preserve in single-dose containers. A sterile, isotonic solution suitable for intrathecal administration, containing radioactive indium (^{111}In) in the form of a chelate of pentetic acid. Label it to include the following, in addition to the information specified for Labeling under Injections: the time and date of calibration; the amount of ^{111}In as labeled pentetic acid complex expressed as total megabecquerels (or millicuries or microcuries) and concentration as megabecquerels (or microcuries or millicuries) per mL on the date and time of calibration; the expiration date; and the statement, "Caution—Radioactive Material." The labeling indicates that in making dosage calculations, correction is to be made for radioactive decay, and also indicates that the radioactive half-life of ^{111}In is 2.83 days. Contains the labeled amount of ^{111}In, within ±10%, as pentetic acid complex expressed in megabecquerels (or microcuries or millicuries) per mL at the time indicated in the labeling. Other chemical forms of radioactivity do not exceed 10.0% of the total radioactivity. Meets the requirements for Bacterial endotoxins, pH (7.0–8.0), Radionuclide identification, Radiochemical purity (not less than 90.0%), Radionuclidic purity, and Injections (except that the Injection may be distributed or dispensed prior to completion of the test for Sterility, the latter test being started on the day of final manufacture, and except that it is not subject to the recommendation on Volume in Container).

INDIUM IN 111 PENTETREOTIDE

Chemical name: Pentetreotide—*N*-[2-[[2-[Bis(carboxymethyl)-amino]ethyl](carboxymethyl)amino]ethyl]-*N*-(carboxymethyl)glycyl-D-phenylalanyl-L-cysteinyl-L-phenylalanyl-D-tryptophyl-L-lysyl-L-threonyl-*N*-[(1*R*,2*R*)-2-hydroxy-1-(hydroxymethyl)propyl]-L-cysteinamide cyclic (3→8)-disulfide.

Molecular formula: Pentetreotide—$C_{63}H_{87}N_{13}O_{19}S_2$.

Molecular weight: Pentetreotide—1394.60.

USP requirements: Indium In 111 Pentetreotide Injection—Not in USP.

INDIUM IN 111 SATUMOMAB PENDETIDE

Source: The monoclonal antibody B72.3 is site-specifically labeled with ^{111}In using the linker-chelator glycyl-tyrosyl-(N,epsilon-diethylenetriaminepentaacetic acid)-lysine (GYK-DTPA). This involves conjugating B72.3 with a linker-chelator complex at oxidized carbohydrate sites on the constant region of the antibody.

Chemical name: Immunoglobulin G 1 (mouse monoclonal B72.3 anti-human glycoprotein TAG-72), disulfide with mouse monoclonal B72.3 light chain, dimer, N^6-[*N*-[2-[[2-[bis-(carboxymethyl)amino]ethyl](carboxymethyl)amino]ethyl]-*N*-(carboxymethyl)glycyl]-N^2-(*N*-glycyl-L-tyrosyl)-L-lysine conjugate, indium-^{111}*In* chelate.

USP requirements: Indium In 111 Satumomab Pendetide Injection—Not in USP.

INDOCYANINE GREEN

Chemical name: 1*H*-Benz[*e*]indolium, 2-[7-[1,3-dihydro-1,1-dimethyl-3-(4-sulfobutyl)-2*H*-benz[*e*]indol-2-ylidene]-1,3,5-heptatrienyl]-1,1-dimethyl-3-(4-sulfobutyl)-, hydroxide, inner salt, sodium salt.

Molecular formula: $C_{43}H_{47}N_2NaO_6S_2$.

Molecular weight: 774.97.

Description:

Indocyanine Green USP—Olive-brown, dark green, blue-green, dark blue, or black powder. Odorless, or has a slight odor. Its solutions are deep emerald-green in color. The pH of a solution (1 in 200) is about 6. Its aqueous solutions are stable for about 8 hours.

Sterile Indocyanine Green USP—Olive-brown, dark green, blue-green, dark blue, or black powder. Odorless, or has a slight odor. Its solutions are deep emerald-green in color. The pH of a solution (1 in 200) is about 6. Its aqueous solutions are stable for about 8 hours.

Solubility: Indocyanine Green USP—Soluble in water and in methanol; practically insoluble in most other organic solvents.

USP requirements:

Indocyanine Green USP—Preserve in well-closed containers. Contains not less than 94.0% and not more than 105.0% of indocyanine green, calculated on the dried basis. Contains not more than 5.0% of sodium iodide, calculated on the dried basis. Meets the requirements for Identification, Loss on drying (not more than 6.0%), Arsenic (not more than 8 ppm), Lead (not more than 0.001%), and Sodium iodide (not more than 5.0%, calculated on the dried basis).

Sterile Indocyanine Green USP—Preserve in Containers for Sterile Solids. It is Indocyanine Green suitable for parenteral use. Contains the labeled amount, within ±10%. Meets the requirements for Constituted solution, Bacterial endotoxins, pH (5.5–6.5, in a solution [1 in 200]), and Content variation, for Identification tests, Arsenic, Lead, and Sodium iodide under Indocyanine Green, for Sterility tests, and for Labeling under Injections.

INDOMETHACIN

Chemical group: An indoleacetic acid derivative structurally related to the pyrroleacetic acid derivative sulindac.

Chemical name:

Indomethacin—1*H*-Indole-3-acetic acid, 1-(4-chlorobenzoyl)-5-methoxy-2-methyl-.

Indomethacin sodium—1*H*-Indole-3-acetic acid, 1-(4-chlorobenzoyl)-5-methoxy-2-methyl-, sodium salt, trihydrate.

Molecular formula:

Indomethacin—$C_{19}H_{16}ClNO_4$.

Indomethacin sodium (trihydrate)—$C_{19}H_{15}ClNNaO_4 \cdot 3H_2O$.

Molecular weight:

Indomethacin—357.79.

Indomethacin sodium (trihydrate)—433.82.

Description: Indomethacin USP—Pale yellow to yellow-tan, crystalline powder, having not more than a slight odor. Is sensitive to light. Melts at about 162 °C. Exhibits polymorphism.

pKa: 4.5.

Solubility: Indomethacin USP—Practically insoluble in water; sparingly soluble in alcohol, in chloroform, and in ether.

USP requirements:

Indomethacin USP—Preserve in well-closed, light-resistant containers. Contains not less than 98.0% and not more than 101.0% of indomethacin, calculated on the dried basis. Meets the requirements for Identification, Loss on drying (not more than 0.5%), Residue on ignition (not more than 0.2%), and Heavy metals (not more than 0.002%).

Indomethacin Capsules USP—Preserve in well-closed containers. Contain the labeled amount, within ±10%. Meet the requirements for Identification, Dissolution (80% in 20 minutes in 1 volume of phosphate buffer [pH 7.2] mixed with 4 volumes of water in Apparatus 1 at 100 rpm), and Uniformity of dosage units.

Indomethacin Extended-release Capsules USP—Preserve in well-closed containers. Label it to indicate the Drug Release test with which the product complies. Contain the labeled amount, within ±10%. Meet the requirements for Identification, Drug release, Uniformity of dosage units, and Limit of 4-Chlorobenzoic acid (not more than 0.44%).

Indomethacin Suppositories USP—Preserve in well-closed containers, at controlled room temperature. Contain the labeled amount, within ±10%. Meet the requirements for Identification, Dissolution (75% in 60 minutes in 0.1 *M* phosphate buffer [pH 7.2] in Apparatus 2 at 50 rpm), and Uniformity of dosage units.

Indomethacin Ophthalmic Suspension—Not in USP

Indomethacin Oral Suspension USP—Preserve in tight, light-resistant containers. Contains the labeled amount, within ±10%. Meets the requirements for Identification, Dissolution (80% in 20 minutes in 0.01 *M* phosphate buffer [pH 7.2] in Apparatus 2 at 50 rpm), pH (3.0–5.0), 4-Chlorobenzoic acid (not more than 0.44%), and Sorbic acid content (where present, within ±20% of labeled amount).

Indomethacin Sodium USP—Preserve in well-closed, light-resistant containers. Contains not less than 98.0% and not more than 101.0% of indomethacin sodium, calculated on the dried basis. Meets the requirements for Identification, Loss on drying (11.5–13.5%), Heavy metals (not more than 0.002%), Residual solvent (not more than 0.1%), and Chromatographic purity.

Sterile Indomethacin Sodium USP—Preserve in Containers for Sterile Solids. Contains the equivalent of the labeled amount of indomethacin, within ±10%. Meets the requirements for Constituted solution, Identification, Pyrogen, pH (6.0–7.5, in a 1 in 2000 solution), Particulate matter, and Limit of 4-chlorobenzoic acid, and for Sterility tests, Uniformity of dosage units, and Labeling under Injections.

INFANT FORMULA

USP requirements:

Hypoallergenic Infant Formula Oral Concentrate—Not in USP.

Hypoallergenic Infant Formula Oral Solution—Not in USP.

Hypoallergenic Infant Formula for Oral Solution—Not in USP.

Milk-based Infant Formula Oral Concentrate—Not in USP.

Milk-based Infant Formula Oral Powder—Not in USP.

Milk-based Infant Formula Oral Solution—Not in USP.

Milk-based Infant Formula for Oral Solution—Not in USP.

Soy-based Infant Formula Oral Concentrate—Not in USP.

Soy-based Infant Formula Oral Solution—Not in USP.

Soy-based Infant Formula for Oral Solution—Not in USP.

INFLUENZA VIRUS VACCINE

Source: Influenza vaccine is available as either a whole-virus or split-virus preparation. The vaccine is prepared from highly purified, egg-grown influenza viruses that have been inactivated to yield a whole-virus preparation. The split-virus vaccine is produced by chemically treating a whole-virus preparation to cause inactivation and disruption of a significant proportion of the virus into smaller subunit particles called subvirions. The preparation is then refined to remove the unwanted substances.

Description: Influenza Virus Vaccine USP—Slightly turbid liquid or suspension, which may have a slight yellow or reddish tinge and may have an odor because of the preservative.

Note: The Canadian product is more likely to be bluish.

Other characteristics: The viral antigen content of both the whole-virus vaccine and the split-virus vaccine has been standardized by immunodiffusion tests, according to current U.S. Public Health Service requirements. Each 0.5 mL dose contains the proportions and not less than the microgram amounts of hemagglutinin antigens (mcg HA) representative of the specific components recommended for the present year's vaccine.

USP requirements: Influenza Virus Vaccine USP—Preserve at a temperature between 2 and 8 °C. A sterile, aqueous suspension of suitably inactivated influenza virus types A and B, either individually or combined, or virus sub-units prepared from the extra-embryonic fluid of influenza virus–infected chicken embryo. Label it to state that it is to be shaken before use and that it is not to be frozen. Label it also to state that it was prepared in embryonated chicken eggs. The strains of influenza virus used in the preparation of this Vaccine are those designated by the U.S. Government's Expert Committee on Influenza and recommended by the Surgeon General of the U.S. Public Health Service. Influenza Virus Vaccine has a composition of such strains and a content of virus antigen of each, designated for the particular season, of not less than the specified weight (in micrograms) of influenza virus hemagglutinin determined in specific radial-immunodiffusion tests relative to the U.S. Reference Influenza Virus Vaccine. If formalin is used for inactivation, it contains not more than 0.02% of residual free formaldehyde. Meets the requirements for Expiration date (not later than 18 months after date of issue from manufacturer's cold storage [5 °C, 1 year]). Conforms to the regulations of the U.S. Food and Drug Administration concerning biologics.

INSULIN

Chemical name:

Insulin—Insulin (ox), 8^{A}-L-threonine-10^{A}-L-isoleucine-.

Insulin zinc—Insulin zinc.

Protamine zinc insulin—Insulin protamine zinc.

Molecular formula:

Insulin—$C_{256}H_{381}N_{65}O_{76}S_6$ (pork); $C_{254}H_{377}H_{65}O_{75}S_6$ (beef).

Insulin Human—$C_{257}H_{383}N_{65}O_{77}S_6$.

Molecular weight:

Insulin—5777.59 (pork); 5733.54 (beef).

Insulin Human—5807.62.

Description:

Insulin USP—White or practically white crystals.

Insulin Injection USP—The Injection containing, in each mL, not more than 100 USP Units is a clear, colorless or almost colorless liquid; the Injection containing, in each mL, 500 Units may be straw-colored. Contains between 0.1% and 0.25% (w/v) of either phenol or cresol. Contains between 1.4% and 1.8% (w/v) of glycerin.

Insulin Zinc Suspension USP—Practically colorless suspension of a mixture of characteristic crystals predominantly between 10 micrometers and 40 micrometers in maximum dimension and many particles that have no uniform shape and do not exceed 2 micrometers in maximum dimension. Contains between 0.15% and 0.17% (w/v) of sodium acetate, between 0.65% and 0.75% (w/v) of sodium chloride, and between 0.09% and 0.11% (w/v) of methylparaben.

Isophane Insulin Suspension USP—White suspension of rod-shaped crystals, free from large aggregates of crystals following moderate agitation. Contains either (1) between 1.4% and 1.8% (w/v) of glycerin, between 0.15% and 0.17% (w/v) of metacresol, and between 0.06% and 0.07% (w/v) of phenol, or (2) between 1.4% and 1.8% (w/v) of glycerin and between 0.20% and 0.25% (w/v) of phenol. Contains between 0.15% and 0.25% (w/v) of dibasic sodium phosphate. When examined microscopically, the insoluble matter in the Suspension is crystalline, and contains not more than traces of amorphous material.

Extended Insulin Zinc Suspension USP—Practically colorless suspension of a mixture of characteristic crystals the maximum dimension of which is predominantly between 10 micrometers and 40 micrometers. Contains between 0.15% and 0.17% (w/v) of sodium acetate, between 0.65% and 0.75% (w/v) of sodium chloride, and between 0.09% and 0.11% (w/v) of methylparaben.

Prompt Insulin Zinc Suspension USP—Practically colorless suspension of particles that have no uniform shape and the maximum dimension of which does not exceed 2 micrometers. Contains between 0.15% and 0.17% (w/v) of sodium acetate, between 0.65% and 0.75% (w/v) of sodium chloride, and between 0.09% and 0.11% (w/v) of methylparaben.

Protamine Zinc Insulin Suspension USP—White or practically white suspension, free from large particles following moderate agitation. Contains between 1.4% and 1.8% (w/v) of glycerin, and either between 0.18% and 0.22% (w/v) of cresol or between 0.22% and 0.28% (w/v) of phenol. Contains between 0.15% and 0.25% (w/v) of dibasic sodium phosphate, and between 1.0 mg and 1.5 mg of protamine for each 100 USP Insulin Units.

Solubility: Insulin USP—Soluble in solutions of dilute acids and alkalies.

USP requirements:

Insulin USP—Preserve in tight containers, protected from light, in a cold place. A protein, obtained from the pancreas of healthy bovine and porcine animals used for food by man, that affects the metabolism of glucose. Label it to indicate the one or more animal species to which it is related, as porcine, as bovine, or as a mixture of porcine and bovine. Where it is highly purified, label it as such. Its biological potency, determined by *Assay A* and calculated on the dried basis, is not less than 26.0 USP Insulin Units in each mg. Meets the requirements for Identification, Microbial limits, Bacterial endotoxins, Loss on drying (not more than 10.0%), Residue on ignition (not more than 2.5%, calculated on the dried basis), Nitrogen content (14.5–16.5%, calculated on the dried basis), Zinc content (not more than 1.08%, calculated on the dried basis), Proinsulin content (not more than 10 ppm), and High molecular weight protein (not more than 1.0%).

Insulin Injection USP—Preserve in a refrigerator. Avoid freezing. Dispense it in the unopened, multiple-dose container in which it was placed by the manufacturer. The container for Insulin Injection, up to 100 USP Units in each mL, is of approximately 10-mL capacity and contains not less than 10 mL of the Injection, and the container for Insulin Injection, 500 USP Units per mL, is of approximately 20-mL capacity and contains not less than 20 mL of the Injection. A sterile, acidified or neutral solution of Insulin. The Injection container label and package label state the potency in USP Insulin Units in each mL, based on the results of *Assay A,* and the expiration date, which is not later than 24 months after the immediate container was filled. If the Injection is prepared from neutral solution, the word "neutral" appears on the label. Label it to indicate the one or more animal species to which it is related, as porcine, as bovine, or as a mixture of porcine and bovine. Where it is highly purified, label it as such. Label it to state that it is to be stored in a refrigerator and that freezing is to be avoided. It has a biological potency, determined by *Assay A,* of ±5% of the potency stated on the label, expressed in USP Insulin Units, the potency being 40, 100, or 500 USP Insulin Units in each mL. Meets the requirements for Identification, Bacterial endotoxins, Sterility, pH (2.5–3.5 for acidified and 7.0–7.8 for neutral), Particulate matter, Residue on ignition, Nitrogen content (not more than 0.7 mg for each 100 USP Insulin Units), Zinc content (10–40 mcg for each 100 USP Insulin Units), and Injections, and, where highly purified, for Proinsulin content and High molecular weight protein.

Insulin Human USP—Preserve in tight containers, in a cold place. A protein corresponding to the active principle elaborated in the human pancreas that affects the metabolism of carbohydrate (particularly glucose), fat, and protein. Derived by enzymatic modification of insulin from pork pancreas in order to change its amino acid sequence appropriately, or produced by microbial synthesis. Its potency, determined chromatographically and calculated on the dried basis, is not less than 27.5 USP Insulin Human Units in each mg. Meets the requirements for Identification, Microbial limits, Biological potency (not less than 26.0 USP Insulin Human Units in each mg, calculated on the dried basis), Bacterial endotoxins, Loss on drying (not more than 10.0%), Residue on ignition (not more than 2.5%, calculated on the dried basis), Nitrogen content (14.5–16.5%, calculated on the dried basis), Zinc content (not more than 1.08%, calculated on the dried basis), Proinsulin content (not more than 10 ppm), Pancreatic polypeptide content (not more than 1 ppm), High molecular weight protein, and Content of desamido insulin and other insulin-related substances.

Insulin Human Injection USP—Preserve in a refrigerator and avoid freezing. The container for Insulin Human Injection, 40 or 100 USP Units in each mL, is of approximately 10-mL capacity and contains not less than 10 mL of the Injection, and the container for Insulin Human Injection, 500 USP Units per mL, is of approximately 20-mL capacity and contains not less than 20 mL of the Injection. A sterile solution of Insulin Human in Water for Injection. The Injection container label and package label state the potency in USP Insulin Human Units in each mL on the basis of the results of the *Assay,* and the expiration date, which is not later than 24 months after the immediate container was filled. The labeling states also that it has been prepared either with Insulin Human derived by enzyme modification of pork pancreas Insulin or with Insulin Human obtained from microbial synthesis, whichever is applicable. Label it to state that it is to be stored in a refrigerator and that freezing is to be avoided. It has a potency, determined chromatographically, of ±5% of the potency stated on the label, expressed in USP Insulin Human Units in each mL. Meets the requirements for Identification, Bacterial endotoxins, Sterility, Biological potency (labeled potency ±5%), pH (7.0–7.8), Particulate matter, Nitrogen content (not more than 0.7 mg for each 100 USP Insulin Human Units), Zinc content (10–40 mcg for each 100 USP Insulin Human Units), and Injections, and for High molecular weight protein, and, where derived from pork pancreas insulin, for Proinsulin content, and Pancreatic polypeptide content under Insulin Human.

Buffered Insulin Human Injection—Not in USP.

Insulin Injection and Isophane Insulin, Human Semi-synthetic Injection—Not in USP.

Isophane Insulin Suspension USP—Preserve in a refrigerator. Avoid freezing. Dispense it in the unopened, multiple-dose container in which it was placed by the manufacturer. The container is of approximately 10-mL capacity and contains not less than 10 mL of the Suspension. A sterile suspension of zinc-insulin crystals and Protamine Sulfate in buffered Water for Injection, combined in a manner such that the solid phase of the suspension consists of crystals composed of insulin, protamine, and zinc. The Protamine Sulfate is prepared from the sperm or from the mature testes of fish belonging to the genus *Oncorhynchus* Suckley, or *Salmo* Linné (Fam. Salmonidae). Label it to indicate the one or more animal species to which it is related, as porcine, as bovine, or as a mixture of porcine and bovine. Where it is highly purified, label it as such. The Suspension container label states that the Suspension is to be shaken carefully before use. The container label and the package label state the potency in USP Insulin Units in each mL, and the expiration date, which is not later than 24 months after the immediate container was filled. Label it to state that it is to be stored in a refrigerator and that freezing is to be avoided. Each mL of Isophane Insulin Suspension is prepared from sufficient insulin to provide 40, 80, or 100 USP Insulin Units of insulin activity. Meets the requirements for Identification, Bacterial endotoxins, Sterility, pH (7.0–7.8), Nitrogen content (not more than 0.85 mg for each 100 USP Insulin Units), Zinc content (0.01–0.04 mg for each 100 USP Insulin Units), and Biological activity of the supernatant liquid.

Isophane Insulin, Human, Suspension—Not in USP.

Isophane Insulin Suspension and Insulin Injection—Not in USP.

Isophane Insulin, Human, Suspension and Insulin Human Injection—Not in USP.

Insulin Zinc Suspension USP—Preserve in a refrigerator. Avoid freezing. Dispense it in the unopened, multiple-dose container in which it was placed by the manufacturer. The container is of approximately 10-mL capacity and contains not less than 10 mL of the Suspension. A sterile suspension of Insulin in buffered Water for Injection, modified by the addition of Zinc Chloride in a manner such that the solid phase of the suspension consists of a mixture of crystalline and amorphous insulin in a ratio of approximately 7 parts of crystals to 3 parts of amorphous material. Label it to indicate the one or more animal species to which it is related, as porcine, as bovine, or as a mixture of porcine and bovine. Where it is highly purified, label it as such. The Suspension container label states that the Suspension is to be shaken carefully before use. The container label and the package label state the potency in USP Insulin Units in each mL, and the expiration date, which is not later than 24 months after the immediate container was filled. Label it to state that it is to be stored in a refrigerator and that freezing is to be avoided. Each mL of Insulin Zinc Suspension is prepared from sufficient insulin to provide 40, 80, or 100 USP Insulin Units of insulin activity. Meets the requirements for Identification, Bacterial endotoxins, Sterility, pH (7.0–7.8), Nitrogen content (not more than 0.70 mg for each 100 USP Insulin Units), Zinc content (0.12–0.25 mg for each 100 USP Insulin Units), Zinc in the supernatant liquid, and Insulin not extracted by buffered acetone solution.

Insulin Zinc, Human, Suspension—Not in USP.

Extended Insulin Zinc Suspension USP—Preserve in a refrigerator. Avoid freezing. Dispense it in the unopened multiple-dose container in which it was placed by the manufacturer. The container is of approximately 10-mL capacity and contains not less than 10 mL of the Suspension. A sterile suspension of Insulin in buffered Water for Injection, modified by the addition of Zinc Chloride in a manner such that the solid phase of the suspension is predominantly crystalline. Label it to indicate the one or more animal species to which it is related, as porcine, as bovine, or as a mixture of porcine and bovine. Its container label states that the Suspension is to be shaken carefully before use. Its container label and its package label state the potency in USP Insulin Units in each mL, and the expiration date, which is not later than 24 months after the immediate container was filled. Label it to state that it is to be stored in a refrigerator and that freezing is to be avoided. In its preparation, sufficient insulin is used to provide 40, 80, or 100 USP Insulin Units for each mL of the Suspension. Meets the requirements for Identification, Bacterial endotoxins, Sterility, pH (7.0–7.8), Nitrogen content (not more than 0.70 mg for each 100 USP Insulin Units), Zinc content (0.12–0.25 mg for each 100 USP Insulin Units), Zinc in the supernatant liquid, and Insulin not extracted by buffered acetone solution.

Extended Insulin Zinc, Human, Suspension—Not in USP.

Prompt Insulin Zinc Suspension USP—Preserve in a refrigerator. Avoid freezing. Dispense it in the unopened, multiple-dose container in which it was placed by the manufacturer. The container is of approximately 10-mL capacity and contains not less than 10 mL of the Suspension. A sterile suspension of Insulin in buffered Water for Injection, modified by the addition of Zinc Chloride in a manner such that the solid phase of the suspension is amorphous. Label it to indicate the one or more animal species to which it is related, as porcine, as bovine, or as a mixture of porcine and bovine. Its container label states that the Suspension is to be shaken carefully before use. Its container label and its package label state the potency in USP Insulin Units in each mL, and the expiration date, which is not later than 24 months after the immediate container was filled. Label it to state that it is to be stored in a refrigerator and that freezing is to be avoided. In its preparation, sufficient insulin is used to provide 40, 80, or 100 USP Insulin Units for each mL of the Suspension. Meets the requirements for Identification, Bacterial endotoxins, Sterility, pH (7.0–7.8), Nitrogen content (not more than 0.70 mg for each 100 USP Insulin Units), Zinc content (0.12–0.25 mg for each 100 USP Insulin Units), Zinc in the supernatant liquid, and Insulin not extracted by buffered acetone solution.

Protamine Zinc Insulin Suspension USP—Preserve in a refrigerator. Avoid freezing. Dispense it in the unopened, multiple-dose container in which it was placed by the manufacturer. The container is of approximately 10-mL capacity and contains not less than 10 mL of the Suspension. A sterile suspension of Insulin in buffered Water for Injection modified by the addition of Zinc Chloride and Protamine Sulfate. The Protamine Sulfate is prepared from the sperm or from the mature testes of fish belonging to the genus *Oncorhynchus* Suckley, or *Salmo* Linné (Fam. Salmonidae), and conforms to the regulations of the U.S. Food and Drug Administration. Label it to indicate the one or more animal species to which it is related, as porcine, as bovine, or as a mixture of porcine and bovine. Where it is highly purified, label it as such. The Suspension container label states that the Suspension is to be shaken carefully before use. The container label and package label state the potency in USP Insulin Units in each mL, and the expiration date, which is not later than 24 months after the immediate container was filled. Label it to state that it is to be stored in a refrigerator and that freezing is to be avoided. In the preparation of

Protamine Zinc Insulin Suspension, the amount of insulin used is sufficient to provide 40, 80, or 100 USP Insulin Units for each mL of the Suspension. Meets the requirements for Identification, Bacterial endotoxins, Sterility, pH (7.1–7.4), Nitrogen content (not more than 1.25 mg for each 100 USP Insulin Units), Zinc content (0.15–0.25 mg for each 100 USP Insulin Units), and Biological reaction.

INTERFERON ALFA

Source:
Interferon Alfa-2a, recombinant—Synthetic. A protein chain of 165 amino acids produced by a recombinant DNA process involving genetically engineered *Escherichia coli.* Recombinant interferon alfa-2a has a lysine group at position 23. Purification procedure for recombinant interferon alfa-2a includes affinity chromatography using a murine monoclonal antibody.
Interferon Alfa-2b, recombinant—Synthetic. A protein chain of 165 amino acids produced by a recombinant DNA process involving genetically engineered *Escherichia coli.* Recombinant interferon alfa-2b has an arginine group at position 23. Purification of recombinant interferon alfa-2b is done by proprietary methods.
Interferon Alfa-n1 (lns)—A highly purified blend of natural human alpha interferons, obtained from human lymphoblastoid cells following induction with Sendai virus.
Interferon Alfa-n3—A protein chain of approximately 166 amino acids. Manufactured from pooled units of human leukocytes that have been induced by incomplete infection with an avian virus (Sendai virus) to produce interferon alfa-n3. The manufacturing process includes immunoaffinity chromatography with a murine monoclonal antibody, acidification (pH 2) for 5 days at 4 °C, and gel filtration chromatography.

Chemical group: Related to naturally occurring alfa interferons. Interferons are produced and secreted by cells in response to viral infections or various synthetic and biologic inducers; alfa interferons are produced mainly by leukocytes.

Chemical name:
Interferon Alfa-2a—Interferon alphaA (human leukocyte protein moiety reduced).
Interferon Alfa-2b—Interferon alpha2b (human leukocyte clone Hif-SN206 protein moiety reduced).
Interferon Alfa-n1—alpha-Interferons.
Interferon Alfa-n3—Interferons, alpha-.

Molecular formula:
Interferon Alfa-2a—$C_{860}H_{1353}N_{227}O_{255}S_9$.
Interferon Alfa-2b—$C_{860}H_{1353}N_{229}O_{255}S_9$.

Molecular weight:
Interferon Alfa-2a—19,241.11.
Interferon Alfa-2b—19,269.12.

Solubility: Water-soluble.

USP requirements:
Interferon Alfa-2a, Recombinant, Injection—Not in USP.
Interferon Alfa-2a, Recombinant, for Injection—Not in USP.
Interferon Alfa-2b, Recombinant, for Injection—Not in USP.
Interferon Alfa-n1 (lns) Injection—Not in USP.
Interferon Alfa-n3 Injection—Not in USP.

INTERFERON BETA

Source: Interferon beta-1b—Manufactured by bacterial fermentation of a strain of *Escherichia coli* that bears a genetically engineered plasmid containing the gene for human interferon $beta_{ser17}$.

Molecular weight: Interferon beta-1b—18,500 daltons (approximate).

USP requirements: Interferon Beta-1b for Injection—Not in USP.

INTERFERON GAMMA

Chemical name: Interferon gamma-1b—1-139-Interferon gamma (human lymphocyte protein moiety reduced), N^2-L-methionyl-.

Molecular formula: Interferon gamma-1b—$C_{734}H_{1166}N_{204}O_{216}S_5$.

Molecular weight: Interferon gamma-1b—16,464.87.

Description: Interferon gamma-1b injection—Sterile, clear, colorless solution.

USP requirements: Interferon Gamma-1b, Recombinant, Injection—Not in USP.

INULIN

Source: A polysaccharide obtained from the tubers of *Dahlia variabilis, Helianthus tuberosus,* and other genera of the family Compositae.

Chemical name: Inulin.

Molecular formula: $C_6H_{11}O_5(C_6H_{10}O_5)_nOH$.

Description: Inulin USP—White, friable, chalk-like, amorphous, odorless powder.

Solubility: Inulin USP—Soluble in hot water; slightly soluble in cold water and in organic solvents.

Other characteristics: Hygroscopic.

USP requirements:
Inulin USP—Preserve in well-closed containers. A polysaccharide which, on hydrolysis, yields mainly fructose. Contains not less than 94.0% and not more than 102.0% of inulin, calculated on the dried basis. Meets the requirements for Completeness of solution, Specific rotation (−32° to −40°, calculated on the dried basis), Microbial limits, Loss on drying (not more than 10.0%), Residue on ignition (not more than 0.05%), Calcium (not more than 0.10%), pH, Chloride, Sulfate, Iron, and Reducing sugars (4.5–7.0 for pH and not more than 0.014% for chloride), Heavy metals (not more than 5 ppm), and Free fructose (not more than 2.0%).
Inulin Injection—Not in USP.

INULIN AND SODIUM CHLORIDE

For *Inulin* and *Sodium Chloride*—See individual listings for chemistry information.

USP requirements: Inulin in Sodium Chloride Injection USP—Preserve in single-dose containers, preferably of Type I or Type II glass. A sterile solution, which may be supersaturated, of Inulin and Sodium Chloride in Water for Injection. May require heating before use if crystallization has occurred. Contains the labeled amounts of inulin, within ± 10%, and sodium chloride, within ± 5%. Contains no antimicrobial agents. Meets the requirements for Clarity, Bacterial endotoxins, pH (5.0–7.0), Free fructose (2.2 mg per mL), and Injections.

IOBENGUANE SULFATE I 131

USP requirements: Iobenguane Sulfate I 131 Injection—Not in USP.

IOCETAMIC ACID

Chemical group: Ionic, triiodinated benzoic acid derivative.

Chemical name: Propanoic acid, 3-[acetyl(3-amino-2,4,6-triiodophenyl)amino]-2-methyl-.

Molecular formula: $C_{12}H_{13}I_3N_2O_3$.

Molecular weight: 613.96.

Description: White to light cream-colored powder. Melting point 224–225 °C.

pKa: 4.1 and 4.25.

Solubility: Practically insoluble in water; very slightly soluble in ether and in ethanol; slightly soluble in acetone and in chloroform.

USP requirements:
Iocetamic Acid USP—Preserve in well-closed containers. Contains not less than 98.0% and not more than 102.0% of iocetamic acid, calculated on the dried basis. Meets the requirements for Identification, Loss on drying (not more than 1.0%), Residue on ignition (not more than 0.1%), Iodide (not more than 0.005%), and Heavy metals (not more than 0.002%).
Iocetamic Acid Tablets USP—Preserve in tight containers. Contain the labeled amount, within ±10%. Meet the requirements for Identification, Dissolution (35% in 30 minutes and 50% in 60 minutes in simulated intestinal fluid TS, prepared without pancreatin, in Apparatus 1 at 150 rpm), and Uniformity of dosage units.

IODINATED GLYCEROL

Chemical group: An isomeric mixture formed by the interaction of iodine and glycerol, the active ingredient thought to be iodopropylidene glycerol; contains about 50% of organically bound iodine.

Chemical name: 1,3-Dioxolane-4-methanol, 2-(1-iodoethyl)-.

Molecular formula: $C_6H_{11}IO_3$.

Molecular weight: 258.06.

Description: Viscous, amber liquid stable in acid media, including gastric juice, which contains virtually no inorganic iodide and no free iodine.

Solubility: Miscible with water, with alcohol, and with glycerin; soluble in ether, in chloroform, in isobutyl alcohol, in methyl acetate, in ethyl acetate, in methyl formate, and in tetrahydrofuran.

USP requirements:
Iodinated Glycerol Elixir—Not in USP.
Iodinated Glycerol Oral Solution—Not in USP.
Iodinated Glycerol Tablets—Not in USP.

IODINATED I 125 ALBUMIN

Description: Iodinated I 125 Albumin Injection USP—Clear, colorless to slightly yellow solution. Upon standing, both the Albumin and the glass container may darken as a result of the effects of the radiation.

USP requirements: Iodinated I 125 Albumin Injection USP—Preserve in single-dose or multiple-dose containers, at a temperature between 2 and 8 °C. A sterile, buffered, isotonic solution containing normal human albumin adjusted to provide not more than 37 MBq (or 1 millicurie) of radioactivity per mL. Derived by mild iodination of normal human albumin with the use of radioactive iodine (^{125}I) to introduce not more than one gram-atom of iodine for each gram-molecule (60,000 grams) of albumin. Label it to include the following, in addition to the information specified for Labeling under Injections: the date of calibration; the amount of ^{125}I as iodinated albumin, expressed as total megabecquerels (or microcuries or millicuries), and concentration as megabecquerels (or microcuries or millicuries) per mL on the date of calibration; the expiration date; and the statement, "Caution—Radioactive Material." The labeling indicates that in making dosage calculations, correction is to be made for radioactive decay, and also indicates that the radioactive half-life of ^{125}I is 60 days. Contains the labeled amount of ^{125}I, within ±5%, as iodinated albumin, expressed in megabecquerels (or microcuries or in millicuries) per mL at the time indicated in the labeling. Other forms of radioactivity do not exceed 3% of the total radioactivity. Its production and distribution are subject to federal regulations. Meets the requirements for Radionuclide identification, Bacterial endotoxins, pH (7.0–8.5), Radiochemical purity (not less than 97.0%), and for Biologics and Injections (except that it is not subject to the recommendation on Volume in Container and meets all other applicable requirements of the U.S. Food and Drug Administration).

IOTHALAMATE SODIUM I 125

Chemical name: Benzoic acid, 3-(acetylamino)diiodoiodo-^{125}I-5-[(methylamino)carbonyl]-, monosodium salt.

Molecular formula: $C_{11}H_8{}^{125}I_3N_2NaO_4$.

USP requirements: Iothalamate Sodium I 125 Injection USP—Preserve in single-dose or in multiple-dose containers that are adequately shielded. A sterile solution of Iothalamic Acid in Water for Injection prepared with the aid of Sodium Bicarbonate. A portion of the molecules contain radioactive iodine (^{125}I) in the molecular structure. Label it to include the following, in addition to the information specified for Labeling under Injections: the time and date of calibration; the amount of ^{125}I as iothalamate sodium expressed as total megabecquerels (or microcuries or millicuries equivalent) per mL at the time of calibration; the expiration date; and the statement "Caution—Radioactive Material." The labeling indicates that in making dosage calculations, correction is to be made for radioactive decay, and also indicates that the radioactive half-life of ^{125}I is 60 days. Contains the concentration of Iothalamate Sodium and the labeled amount of ^{125}I as Iothalamate Sodium, within ±10%, expressed in kilobecquerels (or in microcuries) per mL at the time indicated in the labeling. Other chemical forms of radioactivity do not exceed 2.0% of the total radioactivity. Meets the requirements for Bacterial endotoxins, pH (7.0–8.5), Radionuclide identification, and Radiochemical purity, and for Injections (except that it is not subject to the recommendation in Volume in Container).

IODINATED I 131 ALBUMIN

Description:
Iodinated I 131 Albumin Injection USP—Clear, colorless to slightly yellow solution. Upon standing, both the albumin and the glass container may darken as a result of the effects of the radiation.
Iodinated I 131 Albumin Aggregated Injection USP—Dilute suspension of white to faintly yellow particles, which may settle on standing. The glass container may darken on standing, as a result of the effects of the radiation.

USP requirements:
Iodinated I 131 Albumin Injection USP—A sterile, buffered, isotonic solution containing normal human albumin

adjusted to provide not more than 37 MBq (1 millicurie) of radioactivity per mL. Derived by mild iodination of normal human albumin with the use of radioactive iodine (^{131}I) to introduce not more than one gram-atom of iodine for each gram-molecule (60,000 grams) of albumin. Label it to include the following, in addition to the information specified for Labeling under Injections: the date of calibration; the amount of ^{131}I as iodinated albumin expressed as total megabecquerels (or millicuries or microcuries), and concentration as megabecquerels (or millicuries or microcuries) per mL on the date of calibration; the expiration date; and the statement, "Caution—Radioactive Material." The labeling indicates that in making dosage calculations, correction is to be made for radioactive decay, and also indicates that the radioactive half-life of ^{131}I is 8.08 days. Contains the labeled amount of ^{131}I, within ±5%, as iodinated albumin, expressed in megabecquerels (or millicuries or microcuries) per mL at the time indicated in the labeling. Other forms of radioactivity do not exceed 3% of the total radioactivity. Its production and distribution are subject to federal regulations. Meets the requirements for Radionuclide identification, for Packaging and storage, Bacterial endotoxins, pH (7.0–8.5), and Radiochemical purity under Iodinated I 125 Albumin Injection USP, and for Biologics and Injections (except that it is not subject to the recommendation on Volume in Container and meets all other applicable requirements of the U.S. Food and Drug Administration.

Iodinated I 131 Albumin Aggregated Injection USP—Preserve in single-dose or in multiple-dose containers, at a temperature between 2 and 8 °C. A sterile aqueous suspension of Albumin Human that has been iodinated with ^{131}I and denatured to produce aggregates of controlled particle size. Label it to include the following, in addition to the information specified for Labeling under Injections: the time and date of calibration; the amount of ^{131}I as aggregated albumin expressed as total megabecquerels (or microcuries or millicuries) and as aggregated albumin in mg per mL on the date of calibration; the expiration date; and the statement, "Caution—Radioactive Material." The labeling indicates that in making dosage calculations, correction is to be made for radioactive decay, and also indicates that the radioactive half-life of ^{131}I is 8.08 days; in addition, the labeling states that it is not to be used if clumping of the albumin is observed and directs that the container be agitated before the contents are withdrawn into a syringe. Each mL of the suspension contains not less than 300 mcg and not more than 3.0 mg of aggregated albumin with a specific activity of not less than 7.4 megabecquerels (200 microcuries) per mg and not more than 44.4 megabecquerels (1.2 millicuries) per mg of aggregated albumin. Contains the labeled amount of ^{131}I, within ±5%, as aggregated albumin, expressed in megabecquerels (or microcuries) per mL or megabecquerels (or millicuries) per mL at the time indicated in the labeling. Other chemical forms of radioactivity do not exceed 6% of the total radioactivity. Its production and distribution are subject to federal regulations. Meets the requirements for Radionuclide identification and pH (5.0–6.0), for Biologics and Injections (except that it is not subject to the recommendation on Volume in Container), and for Particle size, Bacterial endotoxins, and Radiochemical purity under Technetium Tc 99m Albumin Aggregated Injection (except that in the test for Radiochemical purity, not more than 6% of the radioactivity is found in the supernaturant liquid following centrifugation).

IODINE

Chemical name: Iodine.

Molecular formula: I.

Molecular weight: 126.90.

Description:

Iodine USP—Heavy, grayish black plates or granules, having a metallic luster and a characteristic odor.

Iodine Topical Solution USP—Transparent, reddish brown liquid, having the odor of iodine.

Iodine Tincture USP—Transparent liquid having a reddish brown color and the odor of iodine and of alcohol.

Solubility: Iodine USP—Very slightly soluble in water; freely soluble in carbon disulfide, in chloroform, in carbon tetrachloride, and in ether; soluble in alcohol and in solutions of iodides; sparingly soluble in glycerin.

USP requirements:

Iodine USP—Preserve in tight containers. Contains not less than 99.8% and not more than 100.5% of iodine. Meets the requirements for Identification, Nonvolatile residue (not more than 0.05%), and Chloride or bromide (not more than 0.028% as chloride).

Iodine Topical Solution USP—Preserve in tight, light-resistant containers, at a temperature not exceeding 35 °C. Contains, in each 100 mL, not less than 1.8 grams and not more than 2.2 grams of iodine, and not less than 2.1 grams and not more than 2.6 grams of sodium iodide.

Prepare Iodine Topical Solution as follows: 20 grams of Iodine, 24 grams of Sodium Iodide, and a sufficient quantity of Purified Water to make 1000 mL. Dissolve the Iodine and the Sodium Iodide in 50 mL of Purified Water, then add Purified Water to make 1000 mL.

Meets the requirement for Identification.

Iodine Tincture USP—Preserve in tight containers. Contains, in each 100 mL, not less than 1.8 grams and not more than 2.2 grams of iodine, and not less than 2.1 grams and not more than 2.6 grams of sodium iodide.

Iodine Tincture may be prepared by dissolving 20 grams of iodine and 24 grams of Sodium Iodide in 500 mL of Alcohol and then adding Purified Water to make the product measure 1000 mL.

Meets the requirements for Identification and Alcohol content (44.0–50.0%).

STRONG IODINE

Chemical name:

Iodine—Iodine.

Potassium iodide—Potassium iodide.

Molecular formula:

Iodine—I.

Potassium Iodide—KI.

Molecular weight:

Iodine—126.90.

Potassium Iodide—166.00.

Description:

Iodine USP—Heavy, grayish black plates or granules, having a metallic luster and a characteristic odor.

Strong Iodine Solution USP—Transparent liquid having a deep brown color and having the odor of iodine.

Potassium Iodide USP—Hexahedral crystals, either transparent and colorless or somewhat opaque and white, or a white, granular powder. Is slightly hygroscopic. Its solutions are neutral or alkaline to litmus.

Solubility:

Iodine USP—Very slightly soluble in water; freely soluble in carbon disulfide, in chloroform, in carbon tetrachloride, and in ether; soluble in alcohol and in solutions of iodides; sparingly soluble in glycerin.

Potassium Iodide USP—Very soluble in water and even more soluble in boiling water; freely soluble in glycerin; soluble in alcohol.

USP requirements:

Strong Iodine Solution USP—Preserve in tight containers, preferably at a temperature not exceeding 35 °C. Contains, in each 100 mL, not less than 4.5 grams and not more than 5.5 grams of iodine, and not less than 9.5 grams and not more than 10.5 grams of potassium iodide.

Strong Iodine Solution may be prepared by dissolving 50 grams of Iodine and 100 grams of Potassium Iodide in 100 mL of Purified Water, then adding Purified Water to make the product measure 1000 mL.

Meets the requirement for Identification.

Strong Iodine Tincture USP—Preserve in tight, light-resistant containers. Contains, in each 100 mL, not less than 6.8 grams and not more than 7.5 grams of iodine, and not less than 4.7 grams and not more than 5.5 grams of potassium iodide.

Strong Iodine Tincture may be prepared by dissolving 50 grams of Potassium Iodide in 50 mL of Purified Water, adding 70 grams of Iodine, and agitating until solution is effected, and then adding Alcohol to make the product measure 1000 mL.

Meets the requirements for Identification and Alcohol content (82.5–88.5%).

IODOHIPPURATE SODIUM I 123

Chemical name: Glycine, *N*-[2-(iodo-^{123}I)benzoyl]-, monosodium salt.

Molecular formula: $C_9H_7{}^{123}INNaO_3$.

USP requirements: Iodohippurate Sodium I 123 Injection USP—Preserve in single-dose or in multiple-dose containers that are adequately shielded. A sterile, aqueous solution containing *o*-iodohippurate sodium in which a portion of the molecules contain radioactive iodine (^{123}I) in the molecular structure. Label it to include the following, in addition to the information specified for Labeling under Injections: the time and date of calibration; the amount of I 123 as iodohippurate sodium expressed as total megabecquerels (or microcuries or millicuries) per mL at the time of calibration; the name and quantity of any added preservative or stabilizer; the expiration time; and the statement, "Caution—Radioactive Material." The labeling indicates that in making dosage calculations, correction is to be made for radioactive decay, and also indicates that the radioactive half-life of I 123 is 13.2 hours. Contains the labeled amount of I 123, within ±10%, as iodohippurate sodium expressed in megabecquerels (or microcuries or millicuries) per mL at the time indicated in the labeling. Contains the labeled amount of *o*-iodohippuric acid, within ±10%. Other chemical forms of radioactivity do not exceed 3.0% of total radioactivity. Meets the requirements for Radionuclide identification, Bacterial endotoxins, pH (7.0–8.5), Radionuclidic purity (not less than 85%), Radiochemical purity, Biological distribution, and Injections (except that the Injection may be distributed or dispensed prior to completion of the test for Sterility, the latter test being started on the day of final manufacture, and except that it is not subject to the recommendation on Volume in Container).

IODOHIPPURATE SODIUM I 131

Chemical name: Glycine, *N*-[2-(iodo-^{131}I)benzoyl]-, monosodium salt.

Molecular formula: $C_9H_7{}^{131}INNaO_3$.

Description: Iodohippurate Sodium 131 Injection USP—Clear, colorless solution. Upon standing, both the Injection and the glass container may darken as a result of the effects of the radiation.

USP requirements: Iodohippurate Sodium I 131 Injection USP—Preserve in single-dose or in multiple-dose containers. A sterile solution containing *o*-iodohippurate sodium in which a portion of the molecules contain radioactive iodine (^{131}I) in the molecular structure. Label it to include the following, in addition to the information specified for Labeling under Injections: the time and date of calibration; the amount of ^{131}I as iodohippurate sodium expressed as total megabecquerels (or microcuries or millicuries) and as megabecquerels (or microcuries or millicuries) per mL at the time of calibration; the expiration date; and the statement, "Caution—Radioactive Material." The labeling indicates that in making dosage calculations, correction is to be made for radioactive decay, and also indicates that the radioactive half-life of ^{131}I is 8.08 days. Contains the labeled amount of ^{131}I, within ±10%, as iodohippurate sodium expressed in megabecquerels (or microcuries or millicuries) per mL at the time indicated in the labeling. Other chemical forms of radioactivity do not exceed 3.0% of the total radioactivity. Meets the requirements for Radionuclide identification, Bacterial endotoxins, pH (7.0–8.5), Radiochemical purity, and Injections (except that the Injection may be distributed or dispensed prior to the completion of the test for Sterility, the latter test being started on the day of final manufacture and except that it is not subject to the recommendation on Volume in Container).

SODIUM IODIDE I 123

Molecular formula: $Na^{123}I$.

Description:

Sodium Iodide I 123 Capsules USP—Capsules may contain a small amount of solid or solids, or may appear empty.

Sodium Iodide I 123 Solution USP—Clear, colorless solution. Upon standing, both the Solution and the glass container may darken as a result of the effects of the radiation.

USP requirements:

Sodium Iodide I 123 Capsules USP—Preserve in well-closed containers that are adequately shielded. Contain radioactive iodine (^{123}I) processed in the form of Sodium Iodide obtained from the bombardment of enriched tellurium 124 with protons or of enriched tellurium 122 with deuterons or by the decay of xenon 123 in such manner that it is carrier-free. Label Capsules to include the following: the name of the Capsules; the name, address, and batch or lot number of the manufacturer; the time and date of calibration; the amount of ^{123}I as iodide expressed in megabecquerels (or microcuries or millicuries) per Capsule at the time of calibration; the name and quantity of any added preservative or stabilizer; a statement indicating that the Capsules are for oral use only; the expiration date and time; and the statement, "Caution—Radioactive Material." The labeling indicates that in making dosage calculations, correction is to be made for radioactive decay, and also indicates that the radioactive half-life of ^{123}I is 13.2 hours. Contain the labeled amount of ^{123}I, within ±10%, as iodide expressed in megabecquerels (or microcuries or millicuries) at the time indicated in the labeling. Other chemical forms of radioactivity do not exceed 5% of the total radioactivity. Meet the requirements for Radionuclide identification, Uniformity of dosage units, Radionuclidic purity (not less than 85.0%), and Radiochemical purity.

Sodium Iodide I 123 Solution USP—Preserve in single-dose or in multiple-dose containers that previously have been treated to prevent adsorption, if necessary. A solution, suitable for oral or for intravenous administration, containing radioactive iodine (^{123}I) processed in the form of Sodium Iodide, obtained from the bombardment of enriched tellurium 124 with protons or of enriched tellurium 122 with deuterons, or by the decay of xenon 123 in such manner that it is carrier-free. Label it to include the following: the time and date of calibration; the amount of ^{123}I as iodide expressed as total megabecquerels (or microcuries or millicuries) per mL at the time of calibration; the name and quantity of any added preservative or stabilizer; a statement indicating whether the contents are intended for oral or for intravenous use; the expiration date and time; and the statement, "Caution—Radioactive Material." The labeling indicates that in making dosage calculations, correction is to be made for radioactive decay, and also indicates that the radioactive half-life of ^{123}I is 13.2 hours. Contains the labeled amount of ^{123}I, within ±10%, as iodide expressed in megabecquerels (or microcuries or in millicuries) per mL at the time indicated in the labeling. Other chemical forms of radioactivity do not exceed 5% of the total radioactivity. Meets the requirements for Radionuclide identification, Radionuclidic purity (not less than 85.0%), Bacterial endotoxins, pH (7.5–9.0), Radiochemical purity, and Injections (if for intravenous use, except that it may be distributed or dispensed prior to completion of the test for Sterility, the latter test being started on the day of final manufacture, and except that it is not subject to the recommendation on Volume in Container).

SODIUM IODIDE I 125

Chemical name: Sodium iodide ($Na^{125}I$).

Molecular formula: $Na^{125}I$.

Description: Sodium Iodide I 125 Solution USP—Clear, colorless solution. Upon standing, both the Solution and the glass container may darken as a result of the effects of the radiation.

USP requirements:

Sodium Iodide I 125 Capsules USP—Preserve in well-closed containers that are adequately shielded. Contain radioactive iodine (^{125}I) processed in the form of Sodium Iodide in such manner that it is carrier-free. Label Capsules to include the following: the date of calibration; the amount of ^{125}I as iodide expressed as total megabecquerels (or microcuries or millicuries) at the time of calibration; the name and quantity of any added preservative or stabilizer; a statement indicating that the Capsules are for oral use only; the expiration date; and the statement, "Caution—Radioactive Material." The labeling indicates that in making dosage calculations, correction is to be made for radioactive decay, and also indicates that the radioactive half-life of ^{125}I is 60 days. Contain the labeled amount of ^{125}I, within ±10%, as iodide expressed in megabecquerels (or microcuries or in millicuries) at the time indicated in the labeling. Other chemical forms of radioactivity do not exceed 5% of the total radioactivity. Meet the requirements for Radionuclide identification, Uniformity of dosage units, and Radiochemical purity.

Sodium Iodide I 125 Solution USP—Preserve in single-dose or in multiple-dose containers that previously have been treated to prevent adsorption. A solution suitable for either oral or intravenous administration, containing radioactive iodine (^{125}I) processed in the form of sodium iodide from the neutron bombardment of xenon gas in such a manner that it is essentially carrier-free. Label it to include the following: the name of the Solution; the name, address, and batch or lot number of the manufacturer; the date of calibration; the amount of ^{125}I as iodide expressed as total megabecquerels (or microcuries or millicuries) and as megabecquerels (or microcuries or millicuries) per mL at the time of calibration; the name and quantity of any added preservative or stabilizer; a statement of the intended use, whether oral or intravenous; a statement of whether diagnostic or therapeutic; the expiration date; and the statement, "Caution—Radioactive Material." The labeling indicates that in making dosage calculations, correction is to be made for radioactive decay, and also indicates that the radioactive half-life of ^{125}I is 60 days. Contains the labeled amount of ^{125}I, within ±15%, as iodide expressed in megabecquerels (or microcuries or in millicuries) per mL at the time indicated in the labeling. Other chemical forms of radioactivity do not exceed 5% of the total radioactivity. Meets the requirements for Radionuclide identification, Bacterial endotoxins, pH (7.5–9.0), Radiochemical purity, and Injections (for solution intended for intravenous use, except that it is not subject to the recommendation on Volume in Container).

SODIUM IODIDE I 131

Chemical name: Sodium iodide ($Na^{131}I$).

Molecular formula: $Na^{131}I$.

Description:

Sodium Iodide I 131 Capsules USP—May contain a small amount of solid or solids, or may appear empty.

Sodium Iodide I 131 Solution USP—Clear, colorless solution. Upon standing, both the Solution and the glass container may darken as a result of the effects of the radiation.

USP requirements:

Sodium Iodide I 131 Capsules USP—Preserve in well-closed containers. Contain radioactive iodine (^{131}I) processed in the form of Sodium Iodide from products of uranium fission or the neutron bombardment of tellurium in such a manner that it is essentially carrier-free and contains only minute amounts of naturally occurring iodine 127. Label Capsules to include the following: the date of calibration; the amount of ^{131}I as iodide expressed in megabecquerels (or microcuries or in millicuries) per Capsule at the time of calibration; a statement of whether the contents are intended for diagnostic or therapeutic use; the expiration date; and the statement, "Caution—Radioactive Material." The labeling indicates that in making dosage calculations, correction is to be made for radioactive decay, and also indicates that the radioactive half-life of ^{131}I is 8.08 days. Contain the labeled amount of ^{131}I, within ±10%, as iodide expressed in megabecquerels (or microcuries or in millicuries) at the time indicated in the labeling. Other chemical forms of radioactivity do not exceed 5% of the total radioactivity. Meet the requirements for Radionuclide identification, Uniformity of dosage units, and Radiochemical purity.

Sodium Iodide I 131 Solution USP—Preserve in single-dose or in multiple-dose containers that previously have been treated to prevent adsorption. A solution suitable for either oral or intravenous administration, containing radioactive iodine (^{131}I) processed in the form of Sodium Iodide from the products of uranium fission or the neutron bombardment of tellurium in such a manner that it is essentially carrier-free and contains only minute amounts of naturally occurring iodine 127. Label it to include the following: the time and date of calibration; the amount of ^{131}I as iodide expressed as total megabecquerels (or microcuries or millicuries) and as megabecquerels (or microcuries or millicuries) per mL at the time of calibration; the name and quantity of any added preservative or stabilizer; a statement of the intended use, whether oral or intravenous; a statement of whether the contents are intended for diagnostic or therapeutic use; the expiration date; and the statement, "Caution—Radioactive Material." The labeling indicates that in making dosage calculations, correction is to be made for radioactive decay, and also indicates that the radioactive half-life of ^{131}I is 8.08 days. Contains the labeled amount of ^{131}I, within ±10%, as iodide expressed in megabecquerels (or microcuries or in millicuries) per mL at the time indicated in the labeling. Other chemical forms of radioactivity do not exceed 5% of the total radioactivity. Meets the requirements for Radionuclide identification, Bacterial endotoxins (if intended for intravenous use), pH (7.5–9.0), Radiochemical purity, and Injections (if for intravenous use, except that the Solution may be distributed or dispensed prior to completion of the test for Sterility, the latter test being started on the day of final manufacture, and except that it is not subject to the recommendation on Volume in Container).

ROSE BENGAL SODIUM I 131

Chemical name: Spiro[isobenzofuran-1(3*H*),9′-[9*H*]-xanthene]-3-one, 4,5,6,7-tetrachloro-3′,6′-dihydroxy-2′,4′,5′,7′-tetraiodo-, disodium salt, labeled with iodine-131.

Molecular formula: $C_{20}H_2Cl_4{}^{131}I_4Na_2O_5$.

Description: Sodium Rose Bengal I 131 Injection USP—Clear, deep-red solution.

USP requirements: Rose Bengal Sodium I 131 Injection USP—Preserve in single-dose or in multiple-dose containers. A sterile solution containing rose bengal sodium in which a portion of the molecules contain radioactive iodine (^{131}I) in the molecular structure. Label it to include the following, in addition to the information specified for Labeling under Injections: the time and date of calibration; the amount of ^{131}I as rose bengal sodium expressed as total megabecquerels (or microcuries or millicuries) and as megabecquerels (or microcuries or millicuries) per mL on the date of calibration; the expiration date; and the statement, "Caution—Radioactive Material." The labeling indicates that in making dosage calculations, correction is to be made for radioactive decay, and also indicates that the radioactive half-life of ^{131}I is 8.08 days. Contains the labeled amount of ^{131}I, within ±10%, as rose bengal sodium expressed in megabecquerels (or microcuries or millicuries) per mL at the time indicated in the labeling. Contains the labeled amount of rose bengal sodium, within ±10%. Other chemical forms of radioactivity do not exceed 10% of the total radioactivity. Meets the requirements for Radionuclide identification, Bacterial endotoxins, pH (7.0–8.5), Radiochemical purity, and Injections (except that the Injection may be distributed or dispensed prior to the completion of the test for Sterility, the latter test being started on the day of final manufacture, and except that it is not subject to the recommendation on Volume in Container).

IODIPAMIDE

Chemical group: Ionic, dimeric, triiodinated benzoic acid derivative.

Chemical name:
- Iodipamide—Benzoic acid, 3,3′-[(1,6-dioxo-1,6-hexanediyl)diimino]bis[2,4,6-triiodo-.
- Iodipamide meglumine—Benzoic acid, 3,3′-[(1,6-dioxo-1,6-hexanediyl)diimino]bis[2,4,6-triiodo-, compd. with 1-deoxy-1-(methylamino)-D-glucitol (1:2).

Molecular formula:
- Iodipamide—$C_{20}H_{14}I_6N_2O_6$.
- Iodipamide meglumine—$C_{20}H_{14}I_6N_2O_6 \cdot 2C_7H_{17}NO_5$.

Molecular weight:
- Iodipamide—1139.77.
- Iodipamide meglumine—1530.20.

Description:
- Iodipamide USP—White, practically odorless, crystalline powder.
- Iodipamide Meglumine Injection USP—Clear, colorless to pale yellow, slightly viscous liquid.

Solubility: Iodipamide USP—Very slightly soluble in water, in chloroform, and in ether; slightly soluble in alcohol.

USP requirements:
- Iodipamide USP—Preserve in well-closed containers. Contains not less than 98.0% and not more than 102.0% of iodipamide, calculated on the anhydrous basis. Meets the requirements for Identification, Water (not more than 1.0%), Residue on ignition (not more than 0.1%), and Free aromatic amine, and for Iodine and iodide and Heavy metals under Diatrizoic Acid.
- Iodipamide Meglumine Injection USP—Preserve in single-dose containers, preferably of Type I or Type III glass, protected from light. A sterile solution of Iodipamide in Water for Injection, prepared with the aid of Meglumine. Label containers of Injection intended for intravascular injection to direct the user to discard any unused portion remaining in the container. Label containers of Injection intended for other than intravascular injection to show that the contents are not intended for intravascular injection. Contains the labeled amount, within ±5%. Iodipamide Meglumine Injection intended for intravascular use contains no antimicrobial agents. Meets the requirements for Identification, Bacterial endotoxins, pH (6.5–7.7), Free aromatic amine, and Meglumine content (24.2–26.8% of the labeled amount of iodipamide meglumine), for the tests for Iodine and iodide and Heavy metals under Diatrizoate Meglumine Injection, and for Injections.

IODOQUINOL

Chemical group: Halogenated 8-hydroxyquinoline.

Chemical name: 8-Quinolinol, 5,7-diiodo-.

Molecular formula: $C_9H_5I_2NO$.

Molecular weight: 396.95.

Description: Iodoquinol USP—Light yellowish to tan, microcrystalline powder not readily wetted by water. Is odorless or has a faint odor; is stable in air. Melts with decomposition.

Solubility: Iodoquinol USP—Practically insoluble in water; sparingly soluble in alcohol and in ether.

USP requirements:
- Iodoquinol USP—Preserve in well-closed containers. Contains not less than 96.0% and not more than 100.5% of

iodoquinol, calculated on the dried basis. Meets the requirements for Identification, Loss on drying (not more than 0.5%), Residue on ignition (not more than 0.5%), and Free iodine and iodide.

Iodoquinol Tablets USP—Preserve in well-closed containers. Contain the labeled amount, within ±5%. Meet the requirements for Identification, Disintegration (1 hour), Uniformity of dosage units, and Soluble iodides.

IOFETAMINE I 123

Chemical name: Iofetamine hydrochloride I 123—Benzeneethanamine, 4-(iodo-^{123}I)-alpha-methyl-*N*-(1-methylethyl)-, hydrochloride, (±)-.

Molecular formula: Iofetamine hydrochloride I 123—$C_{12}H_{18}{}^{123}IN \cdot HCl$.

Molecular weight: Iofetamine hydrochloride I 123—335.74.

Description: Iofetamine hydrochloride I 123—Melting point 156–158 °C.

USP requirements: Iofetamine Hydrochloride I 123 Injection—Not in USP.

IOHEXOL

Chemical group: Non-ionic, monomeric, triiodinated benzoic acid derivative.

Chemical name: 1,3-Benzenedicarboxamide, 5-[acetyl(2,3-dihydroxypropyl)amino]-*N,N'*-bis(2,3-dihydroxypropyl)-2,4,6-triiodo.

Molecular formula: $C_{19}H_{26}I_3N_3O_9$.

Molecular weight: 821.14.

Description:

Iohexol USP—White to off-white, hygroscopic, odorless powder.

Iohexol Injection USP—Clear, colorless to pale yellow liquid.

Solubility: Iohexol USP—Very soluble in water and in methanol; practically insoluble or insoluble in ether and in chloroform.

Other characteristics: Low osmolality. The osmolality of iohexol injection with iodine concentrations of 180, 240, 300, and 350 mg per mL is 408, 520, 672, and 844 mOsmol per kg of water, respectively.

USP requirements:

Iohexol USP—Preserve in well-closed, light-resistant containers. Contains not less than 98.0% and not more than 102.0% of iohexol, calculated on the anhydrous basis. Meets the requirements for Identification, Specific rotation (−0.5° to +0.5°), Water (not more than 4.0%), Free aromatic amine, Free iodine, Free iodide, Ionic compounds (not more than 0.05% as sodium chloride), Heavy metals (not more than 0.002%), Limit of methanol, isopropyl alcohol, and methoxyethanol (not more than 0.005% of methanol and not more than 0.010% each of isopropyl alcohol and methoxyethanol), Limit of 3-chloro-1,2-propanediol (not more than 0.010%), Chromatographic purity, and Limit of *O*-alkylated compounds (not more than 0.6%).

Iohexol Injection USP—Preserve Injection intended for intravascular or intrathecal use in single-dose containers of Type I glass, protected from light. A sterile solution of Iohexol in Water for Injection. Label containers of Injection to direct the user to discard any unused portion. The labeling states also that it is not to be used if it is discolored or contains a precipitate. Contains the labeled amount of Iohexol as organically bound iodine, within ±5%. Iohexol Injection intended for intravascular or intrathecal use contains no antimicrobial agents. Meets the requirements for Identification, Bacterial endotoxins, pH (6.8–7.7), Free iodide (not more than 0.02%, based on the content of iohexol), and Injections, and for Heavy metals and Chromatographic purity under Iohexol.

IOPAMIDOL

Chemical group: A nonionic contrast medium.

Chemical name: 1,3-Benzenedicarboxamide, *N,N'*-bis[2-hydroxy-1-(hydroxymethyl)ethyl]-5-[(2-hydroxy-1-oxopropyl)amino]-2,4,6-triiodo-, (*S*)-.

Molecular formula: $C_{17}H_{22}I_3N_3O_8$.

Molecular weight: 777.09.

Description: Iopamidol USP—Practically odorless, white to off-white powder.

Solubility: Iopamidol USP—Very soluble in water; sparingly soluble in methanol; practically insoluble in alcohol and in chloroform.

Other characteristics: Low osmolality. The osmolality of iopamidol injection with iodine concentrations of 200, 300, and 370 mg per mL is 413, 616, and 796 mOsmol per kg of water, respectively.

USP requirements:

Iopamidol USP—Preserve in well-closed, light-resistant containers. Contains not less than 98.0% and not more than 101.0% of iopamidol, calculated on the dried basis. Meets the requirements for Identification, Specific rotation (−4.6° to −5.2°, calculated on the dried basis), Loss on drying (not more than 0.5%), Residue on ignition (not more than 0.1%), Free aromatic amine, Free iodine, Free iodide, Free acid or alkali, Heavy metals (not more than 0.001%), and Chromatographic purity.

Iopamidol Injection USP—Preserve Injection intended for intravascular or intrathecal use in single-dose containers, preferably of Type I glass, and protected from light. A sterile solution of Iopamidol in Water for Injection. Label containers of Injection to direct the user to discard any unused portion remaining in the container and to check for the presence of particulate matter before using. Contains the labeled amount, within ±5%. Iopamidol Injection intended for intravascular or intrathecal use contains no antimicrobial agents. Meets the requirements for Identification, Bacterial endotoxins, pH (6.5–7.5), Free aromatic amine, Free iodine, Free iodide (not more than 0.04 mg of iodide per mL), and Injections.

IOPANOIC ACID

Chemical group: Ionic, triiodinated benzoic acid derivative.

Chemical name: Benzenepropanoic acid, 3-amino-alpha-ethyl-2,4,6-triiodo-.

Molecular formula: $C_{11}H_{12}I_3NO_2$.

Molecular weight: 570.94.

Description: Iopanoic Acid USP—Cream-colored powder. Has a faint, characteristic odor. Affected by light.

pKa: 4.8.

Solubility: Iopanoic Acid USP—Insoluble in water; soluble in alcohol, in chloroform, and in ether; soluble in solutions of alkali hydroxides and carbonates.

USP requirements:
Iopanoic Acid USP—Preserve in tight, light-resistant containers. Contains an amount of iodine equivalent to not less than 97.0% and not more than 101.0% of iopanoic acid, calculated on the dried basis. Meets the requirements for Identification, Melting range (152–158 °C, with decomposition), Loss on drying (not more than 1.0%), Residue on ignition (not more than 0.1%), Free iodine, Halide ions, and Heavy metals (not more than 0.002%).
Iopanoic Acid Tablets USP—Preserve in tight, light-resistant containers. Contain the labeled amount, within ±5%. Meet the requirements for Identification, Disintegration (30 minutes), Uniformity of dosage units, and Halide ions.

IOPHENDYLATE

Chemical group: Ionic organic iodine compound.

Chemical name: Benzenedecanoic acid, iodo-iota-methyl-, ethyl ester.

Molecular formula: $C_{19}H_{29}IO_2$.

Molecular weight: 416.34.

Description:
Iophendylate USP—Colorless to pale yellow, viscous liquid, the color darkening on long exposure to air. Is odorless or has a faintly ethereal odor.
Iophendylate Injection USP—Colorless to pale yellow, viscous liquid, the color darkening on long exposure to air. Is odorless or has a faintly ethereal odor.

Solubility:
Iophendylate USP—Very slightly soluble in water; freely soluble in alcohol, in chloroform, and in ether.
Iophendylate Injection USP—Very slightly soluble in water; freely soluble in alcohol, in chloroform, and in ether.

Other characteristics: Iophendylate injection—Immiscible with CSF; high specific gravity in relation to that of CSF.

USP requirements:
Iophendylate USP—Preserve in tight, light-resistant containers. A mixture of isomers of ethyl iodophenylundecanoate, consisting chiefly of ethyl 10-(iodophenyl)-undecanoate. Contains not less than 98.0% and not more than 102.0% of iophendylate. Meets the requirements for Identification, Specific gravity (1.248–1.257), Refractive index (1.524–1.526), Residue on ignition (not more than 0.1%), Free acids, Free iodine, and Saponification value (132–142).
Iophendylate Injection USP—Preserve in single-dose containers, preferably of Type I glass, protected from light. It is sterile Iophendylate. Contains the labeled amount, within ±2%. Meets the requirements for Bacterial endotoxins, for Identification, Specific gravity, Refractive index, Residue on ignition, Free acids, Free iodine, and Saponification value under Iophendylate, and for Injections.

IOTHALAMATE

Chemical group: Ionic, monomeric, triiodinated benzoic acid derivative.

Chemical name:
Iothalamate meglumine—Benzoic acid, 3-(acetylamino)-2,4,6-triiodo-5-[(methylamino)carbonyl]-, compd. with 1-deoxy-1-(methylamino)-D-glucitol (1:1).
Iothalamate sodium—Benzoic acid, 3-(acetylamino)-2,4,6-triiodo-5-[(methylamino)carbonyl]-, monosodium salt.

Molecular formula:
Iothalamate meglumine—$C_{11}H_9I_3N_2O_4 \cdot C_7H_{17}NO_5$.
Iothalamate sodium—$C_{11}H_8I_3N_2NaO_4$.

Molecular weight:
Iothalamate meglumine—809.13.
Iothalamate sodium—635.90.

Description:
Iothalamate Meglumine Injection USP—Clear, colorless to pale yellow, slightly viscous liquid.
Iothalamate Meglumine and Iothalamate Sodium Injection USP—Clear, colorless to pale yellow, slightly viscous liquid.
Iothalamate Sodium Injection USP—Clear, colorless to pale yellow, slightly viscous liquid.

USP requirements:
Iothalamate Meglumine Injection USP—Preserve in single-dose containers, preferably of Type I glass, protected from light. A sterile solution of Iothalamic Acid in Water for Injection, prepared with the aid of Meglumine. Label containers of Injection intended for intravascular injection to direct the user to discard any unused portion remaining in the container. Label containers of Injection intended for other than intravascular injection to show that the contents are not intended for intravascular injection. Contains the labeled amount, within ±5%. Iothalamate Meglumine Injection intended for intravascular use contains no antimicrobial agents. Meets the requirements for Identification, Bacterial endotoxins, pH (6.5–7.7), Free aromatic amine, Iodine and iodide, Heavy metals (not more than 0.002%), Meglumine content (22.9% to 25.3% of the labeled amount of iothalamate meglumine), and Injections.
Iothalamate Meglumine and Iothalamate Sodium Injection USP—Preserve in single-dose containers, preferably of Type I glass, protected from light. A sterile solution of Iothalamic Acid in Water for Injection, prepared with the aid of Meglumine and Sodium Hydroxide. Label containers of Injection intended for intravascular injection to direct the user to discard any unused portion remaining in the container. Label containers of Injection intended for other than intravascular use to show that the contents are not intended for intravascular injection. Contains the labeled amounts of iothalamate meglumine and iothalamate sodium, within ±5%. Iothalamate Meglumine and Iothalamate Sodium Injection intended for intravascular use contains no antimicrobial agents. Meets the requirements for Identification, Bacterial endotoxins, pH (6.5–7.7), Free aromatic amine, Iodine and iodide (not more than 0.02% iodide), Heavy metals (not more than 0.002%), and Injections.
Iothalamate Sodium Injection USP—Preserve in single-dose containers, preferably of Type I glass, protected from light. A sterile solution of Iothalamic Acid in Water for Injection prepared with the aid of Sodium Hydroxide. Label containers of the Injection intended for intravascular injection to direct the user to discard any unused portion remaining in the container. Label containers of the Injection intended for other than intravascular injection to show that the contents are not intended for intravascular injection. Contains the labeled amount, within ±5%. Iothalamate Sodium Injection intended for intravascular use contains no antimicrobial agents. Meets the requirements for Identification, Bacterial endotoxins, pH (6.5–7.7), Free aromatic amine, Iodine and iodide (not more than 0.02% of iodide), Heavy metals (not more than 0.002%), and Injections.

IOTHALAMIC ACID

Chemical name: Benzoic acid, 3-(acetylamino)-2,4,6-triiodo-5-[(methylamino)carbonyl]-.

Molecular formula: $C_{11}H_9I_3N_2O_4$.

Molecular weight: 613.92.

Description: Iothalamic Acid USP—White, odorless powder.

Solubility: Iothalamic Acid USP—Slightly soluble in water and in alcohol; soluble in solutions of alkali hydroxides.

USP requirements: Iothalamic Acid USP—Preserve in well-closed containers. Contains not less than 98.0% and not more than 102.0% of iothalamic acid, calculated on the anhydrous basis. Meets the requirements for Identification, Water (not more than 1.0%), Residue on ignition (not more than 0.1%), Free aromatic amine, Iodine and iodide, and Heavy metals (not more than 0.002%).

IOVERSOL

Chemical name: 1,3-Benzenedicarboxamide, *N,N'*-bis(2,3-dihydroxypropyl)-5-[(hydroxyacetyl)(2-hydroxyethyl)amino]-2,4,6-triiodo-.

Molecular formula: $C_{18}H_{24}I_3N_3O_9$.

Molecular weight: 807.12.

USP requirements: Ioversol Injection—Not in USP.

IOXAGLATE

Chemical group: Ionic, dimeric, contrast agent; benzoic acid salt.

Chemical name:
Ioxaglate meglumine—Benzoic acid, 3-[[[[3-(acetylmethylamino)-2,4,6-triiodo-5-[(methylamino)carbonyl]benzoyl]amino]acetyl]amino]-5-[[(2-hydroxyethyl)amino]carbonyl]-2,4,6-triiodo-, compound with 1-deoxy-1-(methylamino)-D-glucitol (1:1).
Ioxaglate sodium—Benzoic acid, 3-[[[[3-(acetylmethylamino)-2,4,6-triiodo-5-[(methylamino)carbonyl]benzoyl]amino]acetyl]amino]-5-[[(2-hydroxyethyl)amino]carbonyl]-2,4,6-triiodo-, sodium salt.

Molecular formula:
Ioxaglate meglumine—$C_{24}H_{21}I_6N_5O_8 \cdot C_7H_{17}NO_5$.
Ioxaglate sodium—$C_{24}H_{20}I_6N_5NaO_8$.

Molecular weight:
Ioxaglate meglumine—1464.10.
Ioxaglate sodium—1290.87.

Solubility: Soluble in water.

USP requirements: Ioxaglate Meglumine and Ioxaglate Sodium Injection—Not in USP.

IPECAC

Description: Powdered Ipecac USP—Pale brown, weak yellow, or light olive-gray powder.

USP requirements:
Ipecac USP—Consists of the dried rhizome and roots of *Cephaëlis acuminata* Karsten, or of *Cephaëlis ipecacuanha* (Brotero) A. Richard (Fam. Rubiaceae). Yields not less than 2.0% of the total ether-soluble alkaloids of ipecac. Its content of emetine and cephaeline together is not less than 90.0% of the amount of the total ether-soluble alkaloids. The content of cephaeline varies from an amount equal to, to an amount not more than 2.5 times, the content of emetine. Meets the requirements for Botanic characteristics, Overground stems (not more than 5%), and Foreign organic matter (not more than 2.0%).

Powdered Ipecac USP—Preserve in tight containers. It is Ipecac reduced to a fine or a very fine powder and adjusted to a potency of not less than 1.9% and not more than 2.1% of the total ether-soluble alkaloids of ipecac, by the addition of exhausted marc of ipecac or of other suitable inert diluent or by the addition of powdered ipecac of either a lower or a higher potency. The content of emetine and cephaeline together is not less than 90.0% of the total amount of the ether-soluble alkaloids. The content of cephaeline varies from an amount equal to, to an amount not more than 2.5 times, the content of emetine. Meets the requirement for Botanic characteristics.

Ipecac Syrup USP—Preserve in tight containers, preferably at a temperature not exceeding 25 °C. Containers intended for sale to the public without prescription contain not more than 30 mL of Ipecac Syrup USP. Contains, in each 100 mL, not less than 123 mg and not more than 157 mg of the total ether-soluble alkaloids of ipecac. The content of emetine and cephaeline together is not less than 90.0% of the amount of the total ether-soluble alkaloids. The content of cephaeline varies from an amount equal to, to an amount not more than 2.5 times, the content of emetine.

Prepare Ipecac Syrup as follows: 70 grams of Powdered Ipecac, 100 mL of Glycerin, and a sufficient quantity of Syrup to make 1000 mL. Exhaust the powdered Ipecac by percolation, using a mixture of 3 volumes of alcohol and 1 volume of water as the menstruum, macerating for 72 hours, and percolating slowly. Reduce the entire percolate to a volume of 70 mL by evaporation at a temperature not exceeding 60 °C and preferably in vacuum, and add 140 mL of water. Allow the mixture to stand overnight, filter, and wash the residue on the filter with water. Evaporate the filtrate and washings to 40 mL, and to this add 2.5 mL of hydrochloric acid and 20 mL of alcohol, mix, and filter. Wash the filter with a mixture of 30 volumes of alcohol, 3.5 volumes of hydrochloric acid, and 66.5 volumes of water, using a volume sufficient to produce 70 mL of the filtrate. Add 100 mL of Glycerin and enough Syrup to make the product measure 1000 mL, and mix.

Meets the requirements for Microbial limits and Alcohol content (1.0–2.5%).

IPODATE

Chemical group: Triiodinated benzoic acid derivative.

Chemical name:
Ipodate calcium—Benzenepropanoic acid, 3-[[(dimethylamino)methylene]amino]-2,4,6-triiodo-, calcium salt.
Ipodate sodium—Benzenepropanoic acid, 3-[[(dimethylamino)methylene]amino]-2,4,6-triiodo-, sodium salt.

Molecular formula:
Ipodate calcium—$C_{24}H_{24}CaI_6N_4O_4$.
Ipodate sodium—$C_{12}H_{12}I_3N_2NaO_2$.

Molecular weight:
Ipodate calcium—1233.99.
Ipodate sodium—619.94.

Description:
Ipodate Calcium USP—White to off-white, odorless, fine, crystalline powder.

Ipodate Sodium USP—White to off-white, odorless, fine, crystalline powder.

Solubility:
Ipodate Calcium USP—Slightly soluble in water, in alcohol, in chloroform, and in methanol.
Ipodate Sodium USP—Freely soluble in water, in alcohol, and in methanol; very slightly soluble in chloroform.

USP requirements:
Ipodate Calcium USP—Preserve in tight containers. Contains not less than 97.5% and not more than 102.5% of ipodate calcium, calculated on the anhydrous basis. Meets the requirements for Identification, Water (not more than 3.5%), Iodide or iodine, and Heavy metals (not more than 0.003%).
Ipodate Calcium for Oral Suspension USP—Preserve in well-closed containers. A dry mixture of Ipodate Calcium and one or more suitable suspending, dispersing, and flavoring agents. Contains the labeled amount, within ±15%. Meets the requirements for Identification and Minimum fill.
Ipodate Sodium USP—Preserve in tight containers. Contains not less than 97.5% and not more than 102.5% of ipodate sodium, calculated on the dried basis. Meets the requirements for Identification, Loss on drying (not more than 0.5%), Iodide or iodine, and Heavy metals (not more than 0.003%).
Ipodate Sodium Capsules USP—Preserve in tight containers. Contain the labeled amount, within ±10%. Meet the requirements for Identification and Uniformity of dosage units.

IPRATROPIUM

Source: A synthetic quaternary ammonium derivative of atropine.

Chemical name: Ipratropium bromide—8-Azoniabicyclo[3.2.1]octane, 3-(3-hydroxy-1-oxo-2-phenylpropoxy)-8-methyl-8-(1-methylethyl)-, bromide, monohydrate(*endo,syn*)-, (±)-.

Molecular formula: Ipratropium bromide—$C_{20}H_{30}BrNO_3 \cdot H_2O$.

Molecular weight: Ipratropium bromide—430.38.

Description: Ipratropium bromide—A white, crystalline substance.

Solubility: Ipratropium bromide—Freely soluble in water and in lower alcohols; insoluble in lipophilic solvents such as chloroform, ether, and fluorocarbons. Has a low lipid solubility.

Other characteristics: Ipratropium bromide—Fairly stable in neutral solutions and in acid solutions; rapidly hydrolyzed in alkaline solutions.

USP requirements:
Ipratropium Bromide Inhalation Aerosol—Not in USP.
Ipratropium Bromide Nasal Inhalation—Not in USP.
Ipratropium Bromide Inhalation Solution—Not in USP.

FERROUS CITRATE Fe 59

Chemical name: 1,2,3-Propanetricarboxylic acid, 2-hydroxy-, iron(2+)-^{59}*Fe* salt.

Molecular formula: $C_{12}H_{10}{}^{59}Fe_3O_{14}$.

USP requirements: Ferrous Citrate Fe 59 Injection USP—Preserve in single-dose or in multiple-dose containers. A sterile solution of radioactive iron (^{59}Fe) in the ferrous state and complexed with citrate ion in Water for Injection. Iron 59 is produced by the neutron bombardment of iron 58. Label it to include the following, in addition to the information specified for Labeling under Injections: the date of calibration; the amount of ^{59}Fe as ferrous citrate expressed as total megabecquerels (or millicuries) and concentration as megabecquerels (or millicuries) per mL on the date of calibration; the expiration date; and the statement, "Caution—Radioactive Material." The labeling indicates that correction is to be made for radioactive decay, and also indicates that the radioactive half-life of ^{59}Fe is 44.6 days. Contains the labeled amount of ^{59}Fe, within ±10%, expressed in megabecquerels (or microcuries or millicuries) per mL at the time indicated in the labeling. Its specific activity is not less than 185 megabecquerels (5 millicuries) per mg of ferrous citrate on the date of manufacture. Meets the requirements for Radionuclide identification, Bacterial endotoxins, pH (5.0–7.0), and Injections (not subject to the recommendation on Volume in Container).

IRON DEXTRAN

Chemical name: A complex of ferric oxyhydroxide and a low-molecular weight dextran derivative.

Description: Iron Dextran Injection USP—Dark brown, slightly viscous liquid.

USP requirements: Iron Dextran Injection USP—Preserve in single-dose or in multiple-dose containers, preferably of Type I or Type II glass. A sterile, colloidal solution of ferric hydroxide in complex with partially hydrolyzed Dextran of low molecular weight, in Water for Injection. Contains the labeled amount of iron, within ±5%. Meets the requirements for Identification, Bacterial endotoxins, Acute toxicity, Absorption from injection site, pH (5.2–6.5), Nonvolatile residue, Chloride content, Phenol content (not more than 0.5% as a preservative), and Injections.

IRON-POLYSACCHARIDE

Source: A complex of ferric iron and a low-molecular weight polysaccharide.

Description: Polysaccharide-iron complex—An amorphous brown powder.

Solubility: Polysaccharide-iron complex—Very soluble in water; insoluble in alcohol.

USP requirements:
Iron-Polysaccharide Capsules—Not in USP.
Iron-Polysaccharide Elixir—Not in USP.
Iron-Polysaccharide Tablets—Not in USP.

IRON SORBITEX

Source: A sterile, colloidal solution of a complex of trivalent iron, sorbitol, and citric acid, stabilized with dextrin and sorbitol.

Chemical name: Iron sorbitex.

Molecular weight: Average of complex less than 5000.

Description: Iron Sorbitex Injection USP—Clear liquid, having a dark brown color.

USP requirements:
Iron Sorbitex Injection USP—Preserve in single-dose containers, preferably of Type I glass. A sterile solution of a complex of iron, Sorbitol, and Citric Acid that is stabilized with the aid of Dextrin and an excess of Sorbitol. Label it to indicate its expiration date, which is not more than 24 months after date of manufacture. Contains an amount of iron sorbitex equivalent to the labeled amount

of iron, within −6% to +4%. Meets the requirements for Identification, Specific gravity (1.17–1.19 at 20 °C), Viscosity (8–13 centipoises, determined at 20 °C with a capillary tube viscometer), Bacterial endotoxins, pH (7.2–7.9), Ferrous iron (not more than 8.5 mg per mL), and Injections.
Iron Sorbitol Injection—Not in USP.

ISOBUTANE

Molecular formula: C_4H_{10}.

Molecular weight: 58.12.

Description: Isobutane NF—Colorless, flammable gas (boiling temperature is about −11 °C). Vapor pressure at 21 °C is about 2950 mm of mercury (31 psig).
NF category: Aerosol propellant.

NF requirements: Isobutane NF—Preserve in tight cylinders and prevent exposure to excessive heat. Contains not less than 95.0% of isobutane. Meets the requirements for Identification, Water (not more than 0.001%), High-boiling residues (not more than 5 ppm), Acidity of residue, and Sulfur compounds.
Caution: Isobutane is highly flammable and explosive.

ISOCARBOXAZID

Chemical group: Hydrazine derivative, structurally similar to amphetamine.

Chemical name: 3-Isoxazolecarboxylic acid, 5-methyl-, 2-(phenylmethyl)hydrazide.

Molecular formula: $C_{12}H_{13}N_3O_2$.

Molecular weight: 231.25.

Description: Isocarboxazid USP—White, or practically white, crystalline powder, having a slight characteristic odor.

Solubility: Isocarboxazid USP—Slightly soluble in water; very soluble in chloroform; soluble in alcohol.

USP requirements:
Isocarboxazid USP—Preserve in well-closed containers. Contains not less than 98.5% and not more than 100.5% of isocarboxazid, calculated on the dried basis. Meets the requirements for Identification, Melting range (105–108 °C), Loss on drying (not more than 0.3%), Residue on ignition (not more than 0.1%), Chloride (not more than 0.02%), Limit of methyl 5-methyl-3-isoxazolecarboxylate and 1-benzyl-3-methyl-5-aminopyrazole, and Organic volatile impurities.
Isocarboxazid Tablets USP—Preserve in well-closed, light-resistant containers. Contain the labeled amount, within ±5%. Meet the requirements for Identification, Dissolution (80% in 45 minutes in 0.1 *N* hydrochloric acid in Apparatus 2 at 50 rpm), and Uniformity of dosage units.

ISOETHARINE

Chemical name:
Isoetharine hydrochloride—1,2-Benzenediol, 4-[1-hydroxy-2-[(1-methylethyl)amino]butyl]-, hydrochloride.
Isoetharine mesylate—1,2-Benzenediol, 4-[1-hydroxy-2-[(1-methylethyl)amino]butyl]-, methanesulfonate (salt).

Molecular formula:
Isoetharine hydrochloride—$C_{13}H_{21}NO_3 \cdot HCl$.
Isoetharine mesylate—$C_{13}H_{21}NO_3 \cdot CH_4O_3S$.

Molecular weight:
Isoetharine hydrochloride—275.78.
Isoetharine mesylate—335.42.

Description:
Isoetharine Inhalation Solution USP—Colorless or slightly yellow, slightly acid liquid, gradually turning dark on exposure to air and light.
Isoetharine Hydrochloride USP—White to off-white, odorless, crystalline solid. Melts between 196 and 208 °C, with decomposition.
Isoetharine Mesylate USP—White or practically white, odorless crystals.

Solubility:
Isoetharine Hydrochloride USP—Soluble in water; sparingly soluble in alcohol; practically insoluble in ether.
Isoetharine Mesylate USP—Freely soluble in water; soluble in alcohol; practically insoluble in acetone and in ether.

USP requirements:
Isoetharine Inhalation Solution USP—Preserve in small, tight containers that are well-filled or otherwise protected from oxidation. Protect from light. A solution of Isoetharine Hydrochloride in Purified Water. The label indicates that the Inhalation Solution is not to be used if its color is pinkish or darker than slightly yellow or if it contains a precipitate. Contains the labeled amount of isoetharine hydrochloride, within ±8%. Meets the requirements for Color and clarity, Identification, and pH (2.5–5.5).
Isoetharine Hydrochloride USP—Preserve in tight containers. Contains not less than 97.0% and not more than 102.0% of isoetharine hydrochloride, calculated on the dried basis. Meets the requirements for Identification, pH (4.0–5.6, in a solution [1 in 100]), Loss on drying (not more than 1.0%), and Aromatic ketones.
Isoetharine Mesylate USP—Preserve in tight containers. Contains not less than 97.0% and not more than 102.0% of isoetharine mesylate, calculated on the dried basis. Meets the requirements for Identification, Melting range (162–168 °C), pH (4.5–5.5, in a solution [1 in 100]), Loss on drying (not more than 1.0%), and Keto precursor.
Isoetharine Mesylate Inhalation Aerosol USP—Preserve in small, nonreactive, light-resistant, aerosol containers equipped with metered-dose valves and provided with oral inhalation actuators. A solution of Isoetharine Mesylate in Alcohol in an inert propellant base. Contains the labeled amount within ±10%, and delivers the labeled dose per inhalation, within ±25%, through an oral inhalation actuator. Meets the requirements for Identification, Alcohol content (25.9–35.0% [w/w]), and Unit spray content, and for Leak testing under Aerosols.

ISOFLURANE

Chemical name: Ethane, 2-chloro-2-(difluoromethoxy)-1,1,1-trifluoro-.

Molecular formula: $C_3H_2ClF_5O$.

Molecular weight: 184.49.

Description: Isoflurane USP—Clear, colorless, volatile liquid, having a slight odor. Boils at about 49 °C.

Solubility: Isoflurane USP—Insoluble in water; miscible with common organic solvents and with fats and oils.

Other characteristics:
Blood-to-Gas partition coefficient at 37 °C—1.43.
Oil-to-Gas partition coefficient at 37 °C—90.8.

USP requirements: Isoflurane USP—Preserve in tight, light-resistant containers. Contains not less than 99.0% and not more than 101.0% of isoflurane, calculated on the anhydrous basis. Meets the requirements for Identification, Refractive index (1.2990–1.3005 at 20 °C), Water (not more than 0.14%), Chloride (not more than 0.001%), Nonvolatile residue (not more than 0.02%), and Fluoride (not more than 0.001%).

ISOFLUROPHATE

Chemical name: Phosphorofluoridic acid, bis(1-methylethyl) ester.

Molecular formula: $C_6H_{14}FO_3P$.

Molecular weight: 184.15.

Description: Isoflurophate USP—Clear, colorless or faintly yellow, liquid. Its vapor is extremely irritating to the eye and mucous membranes. Is decomposed by moisture, with the formation of hydrogen fluoride. Specific gravity is about 1.05.

Solubility: Isoflurophate USP—Sparingly soluble in water; soluble in alcohol and in vegetable oils.

USP requirements:

Isoflurophate USP—Preserve in glass, fuse-sealed containers, or in other suitable sealed containers, in a cool place. Label it to indicate that in the handling of Isoflurophate in open containers, the eyes, nose, and mouth are to be protected with a suitable mask, and contact with the skin is to be avoided. Contains not less than 95.0% of isoflurophate. Meets the requirements for Identification, Acidity (not more than 0.01%), and Ionic fluorine (not more than 0.15%).

Isoflurophate Ophthalmic Ointment USP—Preserve in collapsible ophthalmic ointment tubes. Label it to indicate the expiration date, which is not later than 2 years after date of manufacture. Contains not less than 0.0225% and not more than 0.0275% of isoflurophate, in a suitable anhydrous ointment base. It is sterile. Meets the requirements for Identification, Irritation, Sterility, Minimum fill, Water (not more than 0.03%), and Metal particles.

ISOLEUCINE

Chemical name: L-Isoleucine.

Molecular formula: $C_6H_{13}NO_2$.

Molecular weight: 131.17.

Description: Isoleucine USP—White, practically odorless crystals.

Solubility: Isoleucine USP—Soluble in water; slightly soluble in hot alcohol; insoluble in ether.

USP requirements: Isoleucine USP—Preserve in well-closed containers. Contains not less than 98.5% and not more than 101.5% of isoleucine, as L-isoleucine, calculated on the dried basis. Meets the requirements for Identification, Specific rotation (+38.9° to +41.8°, calculated on the dried basis), pH (5.5–7.0, in a solution [1 in 100]), Loss on drying (not more than 0.3%), Residue on ignition (not more than 0.3%), Chloride (not more than 0.05%), Sulfate (not more than 0.03%), Arsenic (not more than 1.5 ppm), Iron (not more than 0.003%), Heavy metals (not more than 0.0015%), and Organic volatile impurities.

ISOMETHEPTENE

Chemical name: Isometheptene mucate—Isometheptene, galactarate (2:1) (salt).

Molecular formula: Isometheptene mucate—$(C_9H_{19}N)_2 \cdot C_6H_{10}O_8$.

Molecular weight: Isometheptene mucate—492.65.

Description: Isometheptene Mucate USP—White, crystalline powder.

Solubility: Isometheptene Mucate USP—Freely soluble in water; soluble in alcohol; practically insoluble in chloroform and in ether.

USP requirements: Isometheptene Mucate USP—Preserve in well-closed containers. Contains not less than 99.0% and not more than 103.0% of isometheptene mucate, calculated on the dried basis. Meets the requirements for Identification, pH (6.0–7.5, in a solution [1 in 20]), Loss on drying (not more than 1.0%), and Residue on ignition (not more than 0.1%).

ISOMETHEPTENE, DICHLORALPHENAZONE, AND ACETAMINOPHEN

For *Isometheptene, Dichloralphenazone,* and *Acetaminophen*—See individual listings for chemistry information.

USP requirements: Isometheptene Mucate, Dichloralphenazone, and Acetaminophen Capsules USP—Preserve in well-closed containers. Contain the labeled amounts of isometheptene mucate and dichloralphenazone, within −15% to +10%, and the labeled amount of acetaminophen, within ±10%. Meet the requirements for Identification, Dissolution (65% of each active ingredient in 60 minutes in water in Apparatus 1 at 100 rpm), and Uniformity of dosage units.

ISONIAZID

Chemical group: Hydrazide derivative of isonicotinic acid.

Chemical name: 4-Pyridinecarboxylic acid, hydrazide.

Molecular formula: $C_6H_7N_3O$.

Molecular weight: 137.14.

Description:

Isoniazid USP—Colorless or white crystals or white, crystalline powder. Is odorless and is slowly affected by exposure to air and to light.

Isoniazid Injection USP—Clear, colorless to faintly greenish yellow liquid. Gradually darkens on exposure to air and to light. Tends to crystallize at low temperatures.

Solubility: Isoniazid USP—Freely soluble in water; sparingly soluble in alcohol; slightly soluble in chloroform and in ether.

USP requirements:

Isoniazid USP—Preserve in tight, light-resistant containers. Contains not less than 98.0% and not more than 102.0% of isoniazid, calculated on the dried basis. Meets the requirements for Identification, Melting range (170–173 °C), pH (6.0–7.5, in a solution [1 in 10]), Loss on drying (not more than 1.0%), Residue on ignition (not more than 0.2%), Heavy metals (not more than 0.002%), and Organic volatile impurities.

Isoniazid Injection USP—Preserve in single-dose or in multiple-dose containers, preferably of Type I glass, protected from light. A sterile solution of Isoniazid in Water for Injection. Its package label states that if crystallization has occurred, the Injection should be warmed to redissolve the crystals prior to use. Contains the labeled amount, within ±10%. Meets the requirements for Identification, Bacterial endotoxins, pH (6.0–7.0), and for Injections.

Isoniazid Syrup USP—Preserve in tight, light-resistant containers. Contains, in each 100 mL, not less than 0.93 gram and not more than 1.10 grams of isoniazid. Meets the requirement for Identification.

Isoniazid Tablets USP—Preserve in well-closed, light-resistant containers. Contain the labeled amount, within ± 10%. Meet the requirements for Identification, Dissolution (80% in 45 minutes in 0.1 *N* hydrochloric acid in Apparatus 1 at 100 rpm), and Uniformity of dosage units.

ISOPROPAMIDE

Chemical group: Quaternary ammonium compound, synthetic.

Chemical name: Isopropamide iodide—Benzenepropanaminium, gamma-(aminocarbonyl)-*N*-methyl-*N,N*-bis(1-methylethyl)-gamma-phenyl-, iodide.

Molecular formula: Isopropamide iodide—$C_{23}H_{33}IN_2O$.

Molecular weight: Isopropamide iodide—480.43.

Description: Isopropamide Iodide USP—White to pale yellow, crystalline powder.

Solubility: Isopropamide Iodide USP—Sparingly soluble in water; freely soluble in chloroform and in alcohol; very slightly soluble in ether.

USP requirements:

Isopropamide Iodide USP—Preserve in well-closed, light-resistant containers. Dried in vacuum at 60 °C for 2 hours, contains not less than 98.0% and not more than 101.0% of isopropamide iodide. Meets the requirements for Identification, Loss on drying (not more than 1.0%), Residue on ignition (not more than 0.5%), Heavy metals (not more than 0.002%), Ordinary impurities, and Organic volatile impurities.

Isopropamide Iodide Tablets USP—Preserve in well-closed containers. Contain an amount of isopropamide iodide equivalent to the labeled amount of isopropamide, within ± 7%. Meet the requirements for Identification, Dissolution (70% in 60 minutes in water in Apparatus 2 at 100 rpm), and Uniformity of dosage units.

ISOPROPYL ALCOHOL

Chemical name: 2-Propanol.

Molecular formula: C_3H_8O.

Molecular weight: 60.10.

Description: Isopropyl Alcohol USP—Transparent, colorless, mobile, volatile liquid, having a characteristic odor. Is flammable.

NF category: Solvent.

Solubility: Isopropyl Alcohol USP—Miscible with water, with alcohol, with ether, and with chloroform.

USP requirements: Isopropyl Alcohol USP—Preserve in tight containers, remote from heat. Contains not less than 99.0% of isopropyl alcohol. Meets the requirements for Identification, Specific gravity (0.783–0.787), Refractive index (1.376–1.378 at 20 °C), Acidity, and Nonvolatile residue (not more than 0.005%).

AZEOTROPIC ISOPROPYL ALCOHOL

Description: Azeotropic Isopropyl Alcohol USP—Transparent, colorless, mobile, volatile liquid, having a characteristic odor. Is flammable.

Solubility: Azeotropic Isopropyl Alcohol USP—Miscible with water, with alcohol, with ether, and with chloroform.

USP requirements: Azeotropic Isopropyl Alcohol USP—Preserve in tight containers, remote from heat. Contains not less than 91.0% and not more than 93.0% of isopropyl alcohol, by volume, the remainder consisting of water. Meets the requirements for Identification, Specific gravity (0.815–0.810, indicating 91.0–93.0% by volume of isopropyl alcohol), Refractive index (1.376–1.378 at 20 °C), Acidity, Nonvolatile residue (not more than 0.005%), and Volatile impurities.

ISOPROPYL MYRISTATE

Chemical name: Tetradecanoic acid, 1-methylethyl ester.

Molecular formula: $C_{17}H_{34}O_2$.

Molecular weight: 270.46.

Description: Isopropyl Myristate NF—Clear, practically colorless, oily liquid. It is practically odorless and congeals at about 5 °C.

NF category: Oleaginous vehicle.

Solubility: Isopropyl Myristate NF—Insoluble in water, in glycerin, and in propylene glycol; freely soluble in 90% alcohol; miscible with most organic solvents and with fixed oils.

NF requirements: Isopropyl Myristate NF—Preserve in tight, light-resistant containers. Consists of esters of isopropyl alcohol and saturated high molecular weight fatty acids, principally myristic acid. Contains not less than 90.0% of isopropyl myristate. Meets the requirements for Identification, Specific gravity (0.846–0.854), Refractive index (1.432–1.436 at 20 °C), Residue on ignition (not more than 0.1%), Acid value (not more than 1), Saponification value (202–212), and Iodine value (not more than 1).

ISOPROPYL PALMITATE

Chemical name: Hexadecanoic acid, 1-methylethyl ester.

Molecular formula: $C_{19}H_{38}O_2$.

Molecular weight: 298.51.

Description: Isopropyl Palmitate NF—Colorless, mobile liquid having a very slight odor.

NF category: Oleaginous vehicle.

Solubility: Isopropyl Palmitate NF—Soluble in acetone, in castor oil, in chloroform, in cottonseed oil, in ethyl acetate, in alcohol, and in mineral oil; insoluble in water, in glycerin, and in propylene glycol.

NF requirements: Isopropyl Palmitate NF—Preserve in tight, light-resistant containers. Consists of esters of isopropyl alcohol and saturated high molecular weight fatty acids. Contains not less than 90.0% of isopropyl palmitate. Meets the requirements for Identification, Specific gravity (0.850–0.855), Refractive index (1.435–1.438), Residue on ignition (not more than 0.1%), Acid value (not more than 1), Iodine value (not more than 1), and Saponification value (183–193).

ISOPROPYL RUBBING ALCOHOL

USP requirements: Isopropyl Rubbing Alcohol USP—Preserve in tight containers, remote from heat. Label it to indicate that it is flammable. Contains not less than 68.0% and not more than 72.0% of isopropyl alcohol, by volume, the remainder consisting of water, with or without suitable stabilizers, perfume oils, and color additives certified by the U.S. Food and Drug Administration for use in drugs. Meets the requirements for Specific gravity (0.872–0.883 at 20 °C), Acidity, and Nonvolatile residue (not more than 0.01%).

ISOPROTERENOL

Chemical name:

Isoproterenol hydrochloride—1,2-Benzenediol, 4-[1-hydroxy-2-[(1-methylethyl)amino]ethyl]-, hydrochloride.

Isoproterenol sulfate—1,2-Benzenediol, 4-[1-hydroxy-2-[(methylethyl)amino]ethyl]-, sulfate (2:1) (salt), dihydrate.

Molecular formula:

Isoproterenol hydrochloride—$C_{11}H_{17}NO_3 \cdot HCl$.

Isoproterenol sulfate—$(C_{11}H_{17}NO_3)_2 \cdot H_2SO_4 \cdot 2H_2O$.

Molecular weight:

Isoproterenol hydrochloride—247.72.

Isoproterenol sulfate—556.63.

Description:

Isoproterenol Inhalation Solution USP—Colorless or practically colorless, slightly acid liquid, gradually turning dark on exposure to air and to light.

Isoproterenol Hydrochloride USP—White to practically white, odorless, crystalline powder. Gradually darkens on exposure to air and to light. Its solutions become pink to brownish pink on standing exposed to air, and almost immediately so when rendered alkaline. Its solution (1 in 100) has a pH of about 5.

Isoproterenol Hydrochloride Injection USP—Colorless or practically colorless liquid, gradually turning dark on exposure to air and to light.

Isoproterenol Sulfate USP—White to practically white, odorless, crystalline powder. It gradually darkens on exposure to air and to light. Its solutions become pink to brownish pink on standing exposed to air, doing so almost immediately when rendered alkaline. A solution (1 in 100) has a pH of about 5.

Solubility:

Isoproterenol Hydrochloride USP—Freely soluble in water; sparingly soluble in alcohol and less soluble in dehydrated alcohol; insoluble in chloroform and in ether.

Isoproterenol Sulfate USP—Freely soluble in water; very slightly soluble in alcohol and in ether.

USP requirements:

Isoproterenol Inhalation Solution USP—Preserve in small, tight containers that are well-filled or otherwise protected from oxidation. Protect from light. Label it to indicate that the Inhalation Solution is not to be used if its color is pinkish or darker than slightly yellow or if it contains a precipitate. A solution of Isoproterenol Hydrochloride in Purified Water. It may contain Sodium Chloride. Contains the labeled amount of isoproterenol hydrochloride, within −10% to +15%. Meets the requirements for Color and clarity, Identification, and pH (2.5–5.5).

Isoproterenol Hydrochloride USP—Preserve in tight, light-resistant containers. Contains not less than 97.0% and not more than 101.5% of isoproterenol hydrochloride, calculated on the dried basis. Meets the requirements for Identification, Melting range (165–170 °C), Loss on drying (not more than 1.0%), Residue on ignition (not more than 0.2%), Sulfate (not more than 0.2%), Isoproterenone, Chloride content (13.9–14.6%, calculated on the dried basis), and Organic volatile impurities.

Isoproterenol Hydrochloride Inhalation Aerosol USP—Preserve in small, nonreactive, light-resistant aerosol containers equipped with metered-dose valves and provided with oral inhalation actuators. A solution of Isoproterenol Hydrochloride in Alcohol in an inert propellant base. Contains the labeled amount within −10% to +15%, and delivers the labeled dose per inhalation, within ±25%, through an oral inhalation actuator. Meets the requirements for Identification, Alcohol content (28.5–38.5% [w/w]), and Unit spray content, and for Leak testing under Aerosols.

Isoproterenol Hydrochloride Injection USP—Preserve in single-dose containers, preferably of Type I glass, protected from light. Label it to indicate that the Injection is not to be used if its color is pinkish or darker than slightly yellow or if it contains a precipitate. A sterile solution of Isoproterenol Hydrochloride in Water for Injection. Contains the labeled amount, within −10% to +15%. Meets the requirements for Color and clarity, Identification, Bacterial endotoxins, pH (2.5–4.5), Particulate matter, and Injections.

Isoproterenol Hydrochloride Tablets USP—Preserve in well-closed, light-resistant containers. Contain the labeled amount, within ±7%. Meet the requirements for Identification, Dissolution (75% in 45 minutes in water in Apparatus 2 at 50 rpm), and Uniformity of dosage units.

Isoproterenol Sulfate USP—Preserve in tight, light-resistant containers. Contains not less than 97.0% and not more than 103.0% of isoproterenol sulfate, calculated on the anhydrous basis. Meets the requirements for Identification, Water (not more than 7.0%), Residue on ignition (not more than 0.2%), Chloride (not more than 0.14%), Isoproterenone, and Organic volatile impurities.

Isoproterenol Sulfate Inhalation Aerosol USP—Preserve in small, nonreactive, light-resistant aerosol containers equipped with metered-dose valves and provided with oral inhalation actuators. A suspension of microfine Isoproterenol Sulfate in fluorochlorohydrocarbon propellants in a pressurized container. Contains the labeled amount within ±10%, and delivers the labeled dose per inhalation, within ±25%, through an oral inhalation actuator. Meets the requirements for Identification, Microbial limits, Unit spray content, and Particle size, and for Leak testing under Aerosols.

Isoproterenol Sulfate Inhalation Solution USP—Store in small, tight containers that are well-filled or otherwise protected from oxidation. Protect from light. A solution of Isoproterenol Sulfate in Purified Water. Label it to indicate that the Inhalation Solution is not to be used if its color is pinkish or darker than slightly yellow or if it contains a precipitate. Contains the labeled amount, within −10% to +15%. Meets the requirements for Color and clarity and Identification.

ISOPROTERENOL AND PHENYLEPHRINE

Chemical name:

Isoproterenol hydrochloride—1,2-Benzenediol, 4-[1-hydroxy-2-[(1-methylethyl)amino]ethyl]-, hydrochloride.

Phenylephrine hydrochloride—Benzenemethanol, 3-hydroxy-alpha-[(methylamino)methyl]-, hydrochloride.

Molecular formula:

Isoproterenol hydrochloride—$C_{11}H_{17}NO_3 \cdot HCl$.

Phenylephrine bitartrate—$C_9H_{13}NO_2 \cdot C_4H_6O_6$.

Phenylephrine hydrochloride—$C_9H_{13}NO_2 \cdot HCl$.

Molecular weight:

Isoproterenol hydrochloride—247.72.

Phenylephrine bitartrate—317.29.

Phenylephrine hydrochloride—203.67.

Description:

Isoproterenol Hydrochloride USP—White to practically white, odorless, crystalline powder. Gradually darkens on exposure to air and to light. Its solutions become pink to brownish pink on standing exposed to air, and almost immediately so when rendered alkaline. Its solution (1 in 100) has a pH of about 5.

Phenylephrine bitartrate—White, crystalline powder.

Phenylephrine Hydrochloride USP—White or practically white, odorless crystals.

Solubility:

Isoproterenol Hydrochloride USP—Freely soluble in water; sparingly soluble in alcohol and less soluble in dehydrated alcohol; insoluble in chloroform and in ether.

Phenylephrine bitartrate—Soluble in water; insoluble in alcohol.

Phenylephrine Hydrochloride USP—Freely soluble in water and in alcohol.

USP requirements:

Isoproterenol Hydrochloride and Phenylephrine Bitartrate Inhalation Aerosol USP—Preserve in small, non-reactive, light-resistant aerosol containers equipped with metered-dose valves and provided with oral inhalation actuators. A suspension of microfine Isoproterenol Hydrochloride and Phenylephrine Bitartrate in suitable propellants in a pressurized container. Contains the labeled amounts of isoproterenol hydrochloride and phenylephrine bitartrate within ±10%, and delivers the labeled dose per inhalation, within ±25%, through an oral inhalation actuator. Meets the requirements for Identification, Unit spray content, and Particle size, and for Leak testing under Aerosols.

Isoproterenol Hydrochloride and Phenylephrine Hydrochloride Inhalation Aerosol—Not in USP.

ISOSORBIDE

Chemical name:

Isosorbide—D-Glucitol, 1,4:3,6-dianhydro.

Isosorbide dinitrate—D-Glucitol, 1,4:3,6-dianhydro-, dinitrate.

Isosorbide mononitrate—D-Glucitol, 1,4:3,6-dianhydro-, 5-nitrate.

Molecular formula:

Isosorbide—$C_6H_{10}O_4$.

Isosorbide dinitrate—$C_6H_8N_2O_8$.

Isosorbide mononitrate—$C_6H_9NO_6$.

Molecular weight:

Isosorbide—146.14.

Isosorbide dinitrate—236.14.

Isosorbide mononitrate—191.14.

Description:

Isosorbide Concentrate USP—Colorless to slightly yellow liquid.

Diluted Isosorbide Dinitrate USP—Ivory-white, odorless powder. (Note: Undiluted isosorbide dinitrate occurs as white, crystalline rosettes.)

Solubility:

Isosorbide Concentrate USP—Soluble in water and in alcohol.

Undiluted isosorbide dinitrate—Very slightly soluble in water; very soluble in acetone; freely soluble in chloroform; sparingly soluble in alcohol.

USP requirements:

Isosorbide Concentrate USP—Preserve in tight, light-resistant containers. An aqueous solution. Contains, in each 100 grams, not less than 70.0 grams and not more than 80.0 grams of isosorbide. Meets the requirements for Identification, Specific rotation (+44.5° to +47.0°, calculated on the anhydrous basis), Water (24.0–26.0%), Residue on ignition (not more than 0.01%), Arsenic (not more than 1 ppm, calculated on the anhydrous basis), Heavy metals (not more than 5 ppm, calculated on the anhydrous basis), Periodate consumption, Acid value (not more than 0.5, calculated on the anhydrous basis), and Methyl ethyl ketone (not more than 0.05 mg per mL).

Isosorbide Oral Solution USP—Preserve in tight containers. Contains the labeled amount, within ±10%. Meets the requirements for Identification and pH (3.2–3.8).

Diluted Isosorbide Dinitrate USP—Preserve in tight containers. A dry mixture of isosorbide dinitrate with Lactose, Mannitol, or suitable inert excipients to permit safe handling. Contains the labeled amount of isosorbide dinitrate, within ±5%. Usually contains approximately 25% of isosorbide dinitrate. Meets the requirements for Identification, Loss on drying (not more than 1.0%), and Heavy metals (not more than 0.001%).

Caution: Exercise proper precautions in handling undiluted isosorbide dinitrate, which is a powerful explosive and can be exploded by percussion or excessive heat. Only exceedingly small amounts should be isolated.

Isosorbide Dinitrate Capsules—Not in USP.

Isosorbide Dinitrate Extended-release Capsules USP—Preserve in well-closed containers. Contain the labeled amount, within ±10%. Meet the requirements for Identification and Uniformity of dosage units.

Isosorbide Dinitrate Tablets USP—Preserve in well-closed containers. Contain the labeled amount, within ±10%. Meet the requirements for Identification, Dissolution (70% in 45 minutes in water in Apparatus 2 at 75 rpm), and Uniformity of dosage units.

Isosorbide Dinitrate Chewable Tablets USP—Preserve in well-closed containers. Contain the labeled amount, within ±10%. Meet the requirements for Identification and Uniformity of dosage units.

Isosorbide Dinitrate Extended-release Tablets USP—Preserve in well-closed containers. Contain the labeled amount, within ±10%. Meet the requirements for Identification and Uniformity of dosage units.

Isosorbide Dinitrate Sublingual Tablets USP—Preserve in well-closed containers. Contain the labeled amount, within ±10%. Meet the requirements for Identification, Disintegration (2 minutes), Dissolution (50% in 15 minutes and 70% in 30 minutes in water in Apparatus 2 at 50 rpm), and Uniformity of dosage units.

Isosorbide Mononitrate Tablets—Not in USP.

ISOTRETINOIN

Chemical group: Vitamin A derivative (retinoid).

Chemical name: Retinoic acid, 13-*cis*-.

Molecular formula: $C_{20}H_{28}O_2$.

Molecular weight: 300.44.

Description: Isotretinoin USP—Yellow crystals.

Solubility: Isotretinoin USP—Practically insoluble in water; soluble in chloroform; sparingly soluble in alcohol, in isopropyl alcohol, and in polyethylene glycol 400.

USP requirements:

Isotretinoin USP—Preserve in tight containers, under an atmosphere of an inert gas, protected from light. Contains not less than 98.0% and not more than 102.0% of isotretinoin, calculated on the dried basis. Meets the requirements for Identification, Loss on drying (not more than 0.5%), Residue on ignition (not more than 0.1%), Heavy metals (not more than 0.002%), Limit of tretinoin (not more than 1.0%), and Organic volatile impurities.

Isotretinoin Capsules—Not in USP.

Isotretinoin Gel—Not in USP.

ISOXSUPRINE

Chemical name: Isoxsuprine hydrochloride—Benzenemethanol, 4-hydroxy-alpha-[1-[(1-methyl-2-phenoxyethyl)amino]ethyl]-, hydrochloride, stereoisomer.

Molecular formula: Isoxsuprine hydrochloride—$C_{18}H_{23}NO_3 \cdot HCl$.

Molecular weight: Isoxsuprine hydrochloride—337.85.

Description: Isoxsuprine Hydrochloride USP—White, odorless, crystalline powder. Melts, with decomposition, at about 200 °C.

Solubility: Isoxsuprine Hydrochloride USP—Slightly soluble in water; sparingly soluble in alcohol.

USP requirements:
Isoxsuprine Hydrochloride USP—Preserve in tight containers. Contains not less than 97.0% and not more than 103.0% of isoxsuprine hydrochloride, calculated on the dried basis. Meets the requirements for Identification, pH (4.5–6.0, in a solution [1 in 100]), Loss on drying (not more than 0.5%), Residue on ignition (not more than 0.2%), Heavy metals (not more than 0.002%), Related compounds (not more than 2.0%), and Organic volatile impurities.
Isoxsuprine Hydrochloride Injection USP—Preserve in single-dose or in multiple-dose containers, preferably of Type I glass. A sterile solution of Isoxsuprine Hydrochloride in Water for Injection. Contains the labeled amount, within ±5%. Meets the requirements for Identification, Bacterial endotoxins, pH (4.9–6.0), and Injections.
Isoxsuprine Hydrochloride Tablets USP—Preserve in tight containers. Contain the labeled amount, within ±7%. Meet the requirements for Identification, Dissolution (75% in 45 minutes in water in Apparatus 1 at 100 rpm), and Uniformity of dosage units.

ISRADIPINE

Chemical name: 3,5-Pyridinedicarboxylic acid, 4-(4-benzofurazanyl)-1,4-dihydro-2,6-dimethyl-, methyl 1-methylethyl ester, (±)-.

Molecular formula: $C_{19}H_{21}N_3O_5$.

Molecular weight: 371.39.

Description: Yellow, fine crystalline powder. Is odorless or has a faint characteristic odor.

Solubility: Practically insoluble in water; soluble in ethanol; freely soluble in acetone, in chloroform, and in methylene chloride.

USP requirements: Isradipine Capsules—Not in USP.

ITRACONAZOLE

Chemical name: 3*H*-1,2,4-Triazol-3-one, 4-[4-[4-[4-[[2-(2,4-dichlorophenyl)-2-(1*H*-1,2,4-triazol-1-ylmethyl)-1,3-dioxolan-4-yl]methoxy]phenyl]-1-piperazinyl]phenyl]-2,4-dihydro-2-(1-methylpropyl)-.

Molecular formula: $C_{35}H_{38}Cl_2N_8O_4$.

Molecular weight: 705.64.

Description: White to slightly yellowish powder.

pKa: 3.70.

Solubility: Insoluble in water at pH 1–12; very slightly soluble in alcohols; freely soluble in dichloromethane.

Other characteristics: Log (n-octanol/water partition coefficient)—5.66 at pH 8.1.

USP requirements: Itraconazole Capsules—Not in USP.

IVERMECTIN

Source: Semisynthetic macrocyclic lactone produced by the actinomycete *Streptomyces avermitilis*.

Chemical group: Avermectins.

Other characteristics: A mixture of Ivermectin component B_{1a} and Ivermectin component B_{1b}.

USP requirements: Ivermectin Tablets—Not in USP.

JAPANESE ENCEPHALITIS VIRUS VACCINE INACTIVATED

Source: Prepared by inoculating mice intracerebrally with Japanese encephalitis (JE) virus, "Nakayama-NIH" strain, manufactured by The Research Foundation for Microbial Diseases of Osaka University. Infected brains are harvested and homogenized in phosphate buffer saline, pH 8.0. The homogenate is centrifuged and the supernatant inactivated with formaldehyde, then processed to yield a partially purified, inactivated virus suspension. This is further purified by ultra-centrifugation through 40 w/v% sucrose.

USP requirements: Japanese Encephalitis Virus Vaccine Inactivated for Injection—Not in USP.

JUNIPER TAR

Description: Juniper Tar USP—Dark brown, clear, thick liquid, having a tarry odor.

Solubility: Juniper Tar USP—Very slightly soluble in water; partially soluble in solvent hexane. One volume dissolves in 9 volumes of alcohol. Dissolves in 3 volumes of ether, leaving only a slight, flocculent residue. Miscible with amyl alcohol, with chloroform, and with glacial acetic acid.

USP requirements: Juniper Tar USP—Preserve in tight, light-resistant containers, and avoid exposure to excessive heat. The empyreumatic volatile oil obtained from the woody portions of *Juniperus oxycedrus* Linné (Fam. Pinaceae). Meets the requirements for Identification, Specific gravity (0.950–1.055), Reaction, and Rosin or rosin oils.

KANAMYCIN

Source: Derived from *Streptomyces kanamyceticus*.

Chemical group: Aminoglycosides.

Chemical name: Kanamycin sulfate—D-Streptamine, *O*-3-amino-3-deoxy-alpha-D-glucopyranosyl(1→6)-*O*-[6-amino-6-deoxy-alpha-D-glucopyranosyl(1→4)]-2-deoxy-, sulfate (1:1) (salt).

Molecular formula: Kanamycin sulfate—$C_{18}H_{36}N_4O_{11} \cdot H_2SO_4$.

Molecular weight: Kanamycin sulfate—582.58.

Description: Kanamycin Sulfate USP—White, odorless, crystalline powder.

Solubility: Kanamycin Sulfate USP—Freely soluble in water; insoluble in acetone and in ethyl acetate.

USP requirements:
Kanamycin Sulfate USP—Preserve in tight containers. Has a potency equivalent to not less than 750 mcg of kanamycin per mg, calculated on the dried basis. Meets the

requirements for Identification, Crystallinity, pH (6.5–8.5, in a solution [1 in 100]), Loss on drying (not more than 4.0%), Residue on ignition (not more than 1.0%), and Chromatographic purity.

Kanamycin Sulfate Capsules USP—Preserve in tight containers. Contain an amount of kanamycin sulfate equivalent to the labeled amount of kanamycin, within −10% to +15%. Meet the requirements for Identification, Dissolution (75% in 45 minutes in 0.1 *N* hydrochloric acid in Apparatus 1 at 100 rpm), and Loss on drying (not more than 4.0%).

Kanamycin Sulfate Injection USP—Preserve in single-dose or in multiple-dose containers preferably of Type I or Type III glass. Contains suitable buffers and preservatives. Contains an amount of kanamycin sulfate equivalent to the labeled amount of kanamycin, within −10% to +15%. Meets the requirements for Identification, Bacterial endotoxins, Sterility, pH (3.5–5.0), and Particulate matter.

Sterile Kanamycin Sulfate USP—Preserve in Containers for Sterile Solids. It is Kanamycin Sulfate suitable for parenteral use. Has a potency equivalent to not less than 750 mcg of kanamycin per mg, calculated on the dried basis. Meets the requirements for Bacterial endotoxins and Sterility and for Identification tests, pH, Loss on drying, Residue on ignition, Crystallinity, and Chromatographic purity under Kanamycin Sulfate.

KAOLIN

Description: Kaolin USP—Soft, white or yellowish white powder or lumps. When moistened with water, it assumes a darker color and develops a marked clay-like odor.

NF category: Tablet and/or capsule diluent.

Solubility: Kaolin USP—Insoluble in water, in cold, dilute acids, and in solutions of alkali hydroxides.

USP requirements: Kaolin USP—Preserve in well-closed containers. A native hydrated aluminum silicate, powdered and freed from gritty particles by elutriation. Meets the requirements for Identification, Microbial limits, Loss on ignition (not more than 15.0%), Acid-soluble substances (not more than 2.0%), Carbonate, Iron, and Lead (not more than 0.001%).

KAOLIN AND PECTIN

For *Kaolin* and *Pectin*—See individual listings for chemistry information.

USP requirements: Kaolin and Pectin Oral Suspension—Not in USP.

KAOLIN, PECTIN, HYOSCYAMINE, ATROPINE, SCOPOLAMINE, AND OPIUM

For *Kaolin, Pectin, Hyoscyamine, Atropine, Scopolamine,* and *Opium*—See individual listings for chemistry information.

USP requirements: Kaolin, Pectin, Hyoscyamine Sulfate, Atropine Sulfate, Scopolamine Hydrobromide, and Opium Oral Suspension—Not in USP.

KAOLIN, PECTIN, AND PAREGORIC

For *Kaolin, Pectin,* and *Paregoric*—See individual listings for chemistry information.

USP requirements: Kaolin, Pectin, and Paregoric Oral Suspension—Not in USP.

KETAMINE

Chemical name: Ketamine hydrochloride—Cyclohexanone, 2-(2-chlorophenyl)-2-(methylamino)-, hydrochloride.

Molecular formula: Ketamine hydrochloride—$C_{13}H_{16}ClNO \cdot HCl$.

Molecular weight: Ketamine hydrochloride—274.19.

Description: Ketamine Hydrochloride USP—White, crystalline powder, having a slight, characteristic odor.

Solubility: Ketamine Hydrochloride USP—Freely soluble in water and in methanol; soluble in alcohol; sparingly soluble in chloroform.

USP requirements:

Ketamine Hydrochloride USP—Preserve in well-closed containers. Contains not less than 98.5% and not more than 101.0% of ketamine hydrochloride. Meets the requirements for Clarity and color of solution, Identification, Melting range (258–261 °C), pH (3.5–4.1, in a solution [1 in 10]), Residue on ignition (not more than 0.1%), Heavy metals (not more than 0.002%), Foreign amines, and Chromatographic purity.

Ketamine Hydrochloride Injection USP—Preserve in single-dose or in multiple-dose containers, preferably of Type I glass, protected from light and heat. A sterile solution of Ketamine Hydrochloride in Water for Injection. Contains an amount of ketamine hydrochloride equivalent to the labeled amount of ketamine, within ±5%. Meets the requirements for Identification, Bacterial endotoxins, pH (3.5–5.5), and Injections.

KETAZOLAM

Chemical name: 4*H*-[1,3]-Oxazino[3,2-*d*][1,4]benzodiazepine-4,7(6*H*)-dione, 11-chloro-8,12b-dihydro-2,8-dimethyl-.

Molecular formula: $C_{20}H_{17}ClN_2O_3$.

Molecular weight: 368.82.

Description: Melting point 182–183.5 °C.

USP requirements: Ketazolam Capsules—Not in USP.

KETOCONAZOLE

Chemical group: Imidazoles.

Chemical name: Piperazine, 1-acetyl-4-[4-[[2-(2,4-dichlorophenyl)-2-(1*H*-imidazol-1-ylmethyl)-1,3-dioxolan-4-yl]methoxy]phenyl]-, *cis*-.

Molecular formula: $C_{26}H_{28}Cl_2N_4O_4$.

Molecular weight: 531.44.

Description: Almost white to slightly beige powder.

Solubility: Freely soluble in chloroform, in methanol, and in diluted hydrochloric acid; sparingly soluble in isopropyl alcohol and in acetone; practically insoluble in water.

Other characteristics: Weakly dibasic; requires acidity for dissolution and absorption.

USP requirements:

Ketoconazole USP—Preserve in well-closed containers. Contains not less than 98.0% and not more than 102.0% of ketoconazole, calculated on the dried basis. Meets the requirements for Identification, Melting range (148–152 °C), Specific rotation (−1° to +1°, at 20 °C, calculated on the dried basis), Loss on drying (not more than 0.5%),

Residue on ignition (not more than 0.1% from 2 grams), Heavy metals (not more than 0.002%), and Chromatographic purity.
Ketoconazole Cream—Not in USP.
Ketoconazole Shampoo—Not in USP.
Ketoconazole Oral Suspension—Not in USP.
Ketoconazole Tablets USP—Preserve in well-closed containers. Contain the labeled amount, within ± 10%. Meet the requirements for Identification, Disintegration (10 minutes), and Uniformity of dosage units.

KETOPROFEN

Chemical group: Propionic acid derivative.

Chemical name: Benzeneacetic acid, 3-benzoyl-alpha-methyl-.

Molecular formula: $C_{16}H_{14}O_3$.

Molecular weight: 254.29.

Description: White or off-white, odorless, nonhygroscopic, fine to granular powder. Melts at about 95 °C.

Solubility: Freely soluble in ethanol, in chloroform, in acetone, and in ether; soluble in strong alkali; practically insoluble in water at 20 °C.

Other characteristics: Highly lipophilic.

USP requirements:
Ketoprofen Capsules—Not in USP.
Ketoprofen Delayed-release Capsules—Not in USP.
Ketoprofen Extended-release Capsules—Not in USP.
Ketoprofen Suppositories—Not in USP.
Ketoprofen Delayed-release Tablets—Not in USP.
Ketoprofen Extended-release Tablets—Not in USP.

KETOROLAC

Chemical name: Ketorolac tromethamine—1*H*-Pyrrolizine-1-carboxylic acid, 5-benzoyl-2,3-dihydro, (±)-, compound with 2-amino-2-(hydroxymethyl)-1,3-propanediol (1:1).

Molecular formula: Ketorolac tromethamine—$C_{19}H_{24}N_2O_6$.

Molecular weight: Ketorolac tromethamine—376.41.

Description:
Ketorolac tromethamine—Off-white crystalline powder.
Ketorolac tromethamine injection—Clear and slightly yellow in color.

pKa: Ketorolac tromethamine—3.54.

Solubility: Ketorolac tromethamine—Soluble in water.

Other characteristics: Ketorolac tromethamine—*n*-Octanol: water partition coefficient: 0.26.

USP requirements:
Ketorolac Tromethamine Injection—Not in USP.
Ketorolac Tromethamine Ophthalmic Solution—Not in USP.
Ketorolac Tromethamine Tablets—Not in USP.

KETOTIFEN

Chemical name: Ketotifen fumarate—10*H*-Benzo[4,5]cyclohepta[1,2-*b*]thiophen-10-one, 4,9-dihydro-4-(1-methyl-4-piperidinylidene)-, (*E*)-2-butenedioate (1:1).

Molecular formula: Ketotifen fumarate—$C_{19}H_{19}NOS \cdot C_4H_4O_4$.

Molecular weight: Ketotifen fumarate—425.50.

Description: Ketotifen fumarate—Fine crystalline, yellowish-gray powder.

Solubility: Ketotifen fumarate—Readily soluble in water.

USP requirements:
Ketotifen Fumarate Syrup—Not in USP.
Ketotifen Fumarate Tablets—Not in USP.

KRYPTON Kr 81m

Chemical name: Krypton, isotope of mass 81 (metastable).

Molecular formula: Kr 81m.

USP requirements: Krypton Kr 81m USP—The generator column is enclosed in a lead container. The unit is stored at room temperature. A gas suitable only for inhalation in diagnostic studies, and is obtained from a generator that contains rubidium 81 adsorbed on an immobilized suitable column support. Rubidium 81 decays with a half-life of 4.58 hours and forms its radioactive daughter ^{81m}Kr, which is eluted from the generator by passage of humidified oxygen or air through the column. Rubidium 81 is produced in an accelerator by proton bombardment of Kr 82. Other radioisotopes of rubidium are produced and are present on the generator column. These other radioisotopes do not decay to ^{81m}Kr. The labeling indicates the name and address of the manufacturer, the name of the generator, the quantity of ^{81}Rb at the date and time of calibration, and the statement, "Caution—Radioactive Material." The labeling indicates that in making dosage calculations, correction is to be made for radioactive decay, and also indicates that the radioactive half-life of ^{81m}Kr is 13.1 seconds. The column contains the labeled amount of Rb 81, within ±10%, at the date and time indicated in the labeling, and on elution yields not less than 80.0% of ^{81m}Kr. Meets the requirements for Radionuclide identification and Radionuclidic purity.

LABETALOL

Chemical name: Labetalol hydrochloride—Benzamide, 2-hydroxy-5-[1-hydroxy-2-[(1-methyl-3-phenylpropyl)amino]ethyl]-, monohydrochloride.

Molecular formula: Labetalol hydrochloride—$C_{19}H_{24}N_2O_3 \cdot HCl$.

Molecular weight: Labetalol hydrochloride—364.87.

Description: Labetalol Hydrochloride USP—White to off-white powder. Melts at about 180 °C, with decomposition.

pKa: 9.45.

Solubility: Labetalol Hydrochloride USP—Soluble in water and in alcohol; insoluble in ether and in chloroform.

Other characteristics: Lipid solubility—Low.

USP requirements:
Labetalol Hydrochloride USP—Preserve in tight, light-resistant containers. Contains not less than 97.5% and not more than 101.0% of labetalol hydrochloride, calculated on the dried basis. Meets the requirements for Identification, pH (4.0–5.0, in a solution [1 in 100]), Loss on drying (not more than 1.0%), Residue on ignition (not more than 0.1%), Heavy metals (not more than 0.002%), Chromatographic purity, Diastereoisomer ratio, and Organic volatile impurities.
Labetalol Hydrochloride Injection USP—Preserve in single-dose containers, or in multiple-dose containers not exceeding 60 mL in volume, preferably of Type I glass, at a temperature between 2 and 30 °C. Avoid freezing and

exposure to light. A sterile solution of Labetalol Hydrochloride in Water for Injection. Contains the labeled amount, within ±10%. Meets the requirements for Identification, Bacterial endotoxins, pH (3.0–4.5), and Injections.

Labetalol Hydrochloride Tablets USP—Preserve in tight, light-resistant containers, at a temperature between 2 and 30 °C. Contain the labeled amount, within ±10%. Meet the requirements for Identification, Dissolution (80% in 45 minutes in water in Apparatus 2 at 50 rpm), and Uniformity of dosage units.

LABETALOL AND HYDROCHLOROTHIAZIDE

For *Labetalol* and *Hydrochlorothiazide*—See individual listings for chemistry information.

USP requirements: Labetalol Hydrochloride and Hydrochlorothiazide Tablets—Not in USP.

LACTIC ACID

Chemical name: Propanoic acid, 2-hydroxy-.

Molecular formula: $C_3H_6O_3$.

Molecular weight: 90.08.

Description: Lactic Acid USP—Colorless or yellowish, practically odorless, syrupy liquid. Is hygroscopic. When it is concentrated by boiling, lactic acid lactate is formed. Specific gravity is about 1.20.

NF category: Buffering agent.

Solubility: Lactic Acid USP—Miscible with water, with alcohol, and with ether. Insoluble in chloroform.

USP requirements: Lactic Acid USP—Preserve in tight containers. A mixture of lactic acid and lactic acid lactate equivalent to a total of not less than 85.0% and not more than 90.0%, by weight, of lactic acid. Obtained by the lactic fermentation of sugars or prepared synthetically. Lactic Acid obtained by fermentation of sugars is levorotatory, while that prepared synthetically is racemic. (Note: Lactic Acid prepared by fermentation becomes dextrorotatory on dilution, which hydrolyzes L(–) lactic acid lactate to L(+) lactic acid.) Label it to indicate whether it is levorotatory or racemic. Meets the requirements for Identification, Specific rotation (−0.05° to +0.05°, for racemic Lactic Acid), Residue on ignition (not more than 0.05%), Sugars, Chloride, Citric, oxalic, phosphoric, or tartaric acid, Sulfate, Heavy metals (not more than 0.001%), and Readily carbonizable substances.

ANHYDROUS LACTOSE

Chemical name: D-Glucose, 4-*O*-beta-D-galactopyranosyl-.

Molecular formula: $C_{12}H_{22}O_{11}$.

Molecular weight: 342.30.

Description: Anhydrous Lactose NF—White or almost white powder.

NF category: Tablet and/or capsule diluent.

Solubility: Anhydrous Lactose NF—Freely soluble in water; practically insoluble in alcohol.

NF requirements: Anhydrous Lactose NF—It is primarily beta lactose or a mixture of alpha and beta lactose. Where the labeling indicates the relative quantities of alpha and beta lactose, determine compliance using Content of alpha and beta forms. Meets the requirements for Identification, Loss on drying (not more than 0.5%), Water (not more than 1.0%), and Content of alpha and beta forms, and for Packaging and storage, Labeling, Clarity and color of solution, Specific rotation, Microbial limits, Acidity or alkalinity, Residue on ignition, Heavy metals, Organic volatile impurities, and Protein and light-absorbing impurities under Lactose Monohydrate.

LACTOSE MONOHYDRATE

Chemical name: D-Glucose, 4-*O*-beta-D-galactopyranosyl-, monohydrate.

Molecular formula: $C_{12}H_{22}O_{11} \cdot H_2O$.

Molecular weight: 360.31.

Description: Lactose Monohydrate NF—White, free-flowing powder.

NF category: Tablet and/or capsule diluent.

Solubility: Lactose Monohydrate NF—Freely but slowly soluble in water; practically insoluble in alcohol.

NF requirements: Lactose Monohydrate NF—Preserve in tight containers. A natural disaccharide, obtained from milk, which consists of one glucose and one galactose moiety. (Note: Lactose Monohydrate may be modified as to its physical characteristics. May contain varying proportions of amorphous lactose.) Where there is a labeling claim regarding particle size distribution, the labeling indicates the d_{10}, d_{50}, and d_{90} values and the range for each. For modified Lactose Monohydrate, also label it to indicate the method of modification. Meets the requirements for Clarity and color of solution, Identification, Specific rotation (+54.4° to +55.9°, calculated on the anhydrous basis at 20 °C), Microbial limits, Acidity or alkalinity, Loss on drying (not more than 0.5% for the monohydrate form and not more than 1.0% for the modified monohydrate form), Water (4.5–5.5%), Residue on ignition (not more than 0.1%), Heavy metals (not more than 5 ppm), Organic volatile impurities, and Protein and light-absorbing impurities.

LACTULOSE

Chemical name: D-Fructose, 4-*O*-beta-D-galactopyranosyl-.

Molecular formula: $C_{12}H_{22}O_{11}$.

Molecular weight: 342.30.

Description: Lactulose Concentrate USP—Colorless to amber syrupy liquid, which may exhibit some precipitation and darkening upon standing.

Solubility: Lactulose Concentrate USP—Miscible with water.

USP requirements:

Lactulose Concentrate USP—Preserve in tight containers, preferably at a temperature between 2 and 30 °C. Avoid subfreezing temperatures. A solution of sugars prepared from Lactose. Consists principally of lactulose together with minor quantities of lactose and galactose, and traces of other related sugars and water. Contains the labeled amount, within ±5%. Contains no added substances. Meets the requirements for Identification, Refractive index (not less than 1.451, at 20 °C), Residue on ignition (not more than 0.1%), and Limit of related substances.

Lactulose Solution USP—Preserve in tight containers, preferably at a temperature between 2 and 30 °C. Avoid subfreezing temperatures. A solution in water prepared from Lactulose Concentrate. Contains the labeled amount, within ±10%. Meets the requirements for Microbial limits and pH (3.0–7.0, after 15 minutes of contact with the electrodes), and for Identification tests and Limit of related substances under Lactulose Concentrate.

LANOLIN

Description: Lanolin USP—Yellow, tenacious, unctuous mass, having a slight characteristic odor.

NF category: Ointment base.

Solubility: Lanolin USP—Insoluble in water, but mixes without separation with about twice its weight of water. Sparingly soluble in cold alcohol; more soluble in hot alcohol; freely soluble in ether and in chloroform.

USP requirements: Lanolin USP—Preserve in well-closed containers, preferably at controlled room temperature. The purified, wax-like substance from the wool of sheep, *Ovis aries* Linné (Fam. Bovidae), that has been cleaned, decolorized, and deodorized. The label states that it is not to be used undiluted. Contains not more than 0.25% of water. May contain not more than 0.02% of a suitable antioxidant. Meets the requirements for Melting range (38–44 °C), Acidity, Alkalinity, Water (not more than 0.25%), Residue on ignition (not more than 0.1%), Water-soluble acids and alkalies, Water-soluble oxidizable substances, Chloride (not more than 0.035%), Ammonia, Iodine value (18–36), Petrolatum, and Foreign substances (not more than 10 ppm of any individual specified residue and not more than 40 ppm for total of all specified residues).

LANOLIN ALCOHOLS

Description: Lanolin Alcohols NF—Hard, waxy, amber solid, having a characteristic odor.

NF category: Emulsifying and/or solubilizing agent.

Solubility: Lanolin Alcohols NF—Insoluble in water; slightly soluble in alcohol; freely soluble in chloroform, in ether, and in petroleum ether.

NF requirements: Lanolin Alcohols NF—Preserve in well-closed, light-resistant containers, preferably at controlled room temperature. A mixture of aliphatic alcohols, triterpenoid alcohols, and sterols, obtained by the hydrolysis of Lanolin. Contains not less than 30.0% of cholesterol. Meets the requirements for Identification, Melting range (not below 56 °C), Acidity and alkalinity, Loss on drying (not more than 0.5%), Residue on ignition (not more than 0.15%), Copper (not more than 5 ppm), Acid value (not more than 2), and Saponifaction value (not more than 12).

MODIFIED LANOLIN

USP requirements: Modified Lanolin USP—Preserve in tight, preferably rust-proof containers, preferably at controlled room temperature. The purified wax-like substance from the wool of sheep, *Ovis aries* Linné (Fam. Bovidae), that has been processed to reduce the contents of free lanolin alcohols and detergent and pesticide residues. Contains not more than 0.25% of water. May contain not more than 0.02% of a suitable antioxidant. Meets the requirements for Acidity, Alkalinity, Water (not more than 0.25%), Water-soluble acids and alkalies, Ammonia, Limit of free lanolin alcohols (not more than 6%), Foreign substances (not more than 3 ppm for total specified residues and not more than 1 ppm for individual specified residue), and Petrolatum.

LECITHIN

Description: Lecithin NF—The consistency of both natural grades and refined grades of lecithin may vary from plastic to fluid, depending upon free fatty acid and oil content, and upon the presence or absence of other diluents. Its color varies from light yellow to brown, depending on the source, on crop variations, and on whether it is bleached or unbleached. Odorless, or has a characteristic, slight, nutlike odor.

NF category: Emulsifying and/or solubilizing agent.

Solubility: Lecithin NF—Partially soluble in water, but it readily hydrates to form emulsions. The oil-free phosphatides are soluble in fatty acids, but are practically insoluble in fixed oils. When all phosphatide fractions are present, lecithin is partially soluble in alcohol and practically insoluble in acetone.

NF requirements: Lecithin NF—Preserve in well-closed containers. A complex mixture of acetone-insoluble phosphatides, which consist chiefly of phosphatidyl choline, phosphatidyl ethanolamine, phosphatidyl serine, and phosphatidyl inositol, combined with various amounts of other substances such as triglycerides, fatty acids, and carbohydrates, as separated from the crude vegetable oil source. Contains not less than 50.0% of Acetone-insoluble matter. Meets the requirements for Water (not more than 1.5%), Arsenic (not more than 3 ppm), Lead (not more than 0.001%), Heavy metals (not more than 0.004%), Acid value, Hexane-insoluble matter (not more than 0.3%), and Acetone-insoluble matter.

LEUCINE

Chemical name: L-Leucine.

Molecular formula: $C_6H_{13}NO_2$.

Molecular weight: 131.17.

Description: Leucine USP—White, practically odorless crystals.

Solubility: Leucine USP—Sparingly soluble in water; insoluble in ether.

USP requirements: Leucine USP—Preserve in well-closed containers. Contains not less than 98.5% and not more than 101.5% of leucine, as L-leucine, calculated on the dried basis. Meets the requirements for Identification, Specific rotation (+14.9° to +17.3°, calculated on the dried basis), pH (5.5–7.0, in a solution [1 in 100]), Loss on drying (not more than 0.2%), Residue on ignition (not more than 0.4%), Chloride (not more than 0.05%), Sulfate (not more than 0.03%), Arsenic (not more than 1.5 ppm), Iron (not more than 0.003%), Heavy metals (not more than 0.0015%), and Organic volatile impurities.

LEUCOVORIN

Chemical name: Leucovorin calcium—L-Glutamic acid, *N*-[4-[[(2-amino-5-formyl-1,4,5,6,7,8-hexahydro-4-oxo-6-pteridinyl)methyl]amino]benzoyl]-, calcium salt (1:1).

Molecular formula: Leucovorin calcium—$C_{20}H_{21}CaN_7O_7$.

Molecular weight: Leucovorin calcium—511.51.

Description:

Leucovorin Calcium USP—Yellowish white or yellow, odorless powder.

Leucovorin Calcium Injection USP—Clear, yellowish solution.

pKa: Leucovorin calcium—3.8, 4.8, and 10.4.

Solubility: Leucovorin Calcium USP—Very soluble in water; practically insoluble in alcohol.

USP requirements:
Leucovorin Calcium USP—Preserve in well-closed, light-resistant containers. Contains not less than 95.0% and not more than 105.0% of leucovorin calcium, calculated on the anhydrous basis. Meets the requirements for Identification, Water (not more than 17.0%), and Heavy metals (not more than 0.005%).
Leucovorin Calcium Injection USP—Preserve in single-dose, light-resistant containers, preferably of Type I glass. A sterile solution of Leucovorin Calcium in Water for Injection. Contains an amount of leucovorin calcium equivalent to the labeled amount of leucovorin, within −10% to +20%. Meets the requirements for Identification, Bacterial endotoxins, pH (6.5–8.5), and Injections.
Leucovorin Calcium for Injection—Not in USP.
Leucovorin Calcium Tablets USP—Preserve in well-closed containers, protected from light, at controlled room temperature. Contain an amount of leucovorin calcium equivalent to the labeled amount of leucovorin, within ±10%. Meet the requirements for Identification, Dissolution (75% in 30 minutes in water in Apparatus 2 at 50 rpm), Uniformity of dosage units, and Chromatographic purity.

LEUPROLIDE

Source: Luteinizing hormone–releasing hormone analog.

Chemical name: Leuprolide acetate—Luteinizing hormone–releasing factor (pig), 6-D-leucine-9-(*N*-ethyl-L-prolinamide)-10-deglycinamide-, monoacetate (salt).

Molecular formula: Leuprolide acetate—$C_{59}H_{84}N_{16}O_{12} \cdot C_2H_4O_2$.

Molecular weight: Leuprolide acetate—1269.47.

Description: Leuprolide acetate—White to off-white powder.

Solubility: Leuprolide acetate—Solubility greater than 250 mg/mL in water and greater than 1 g/mL in alcohol at 25 °C.

USP requirements:
Leuprolide Acetate Injection—Not in USP.
Leuprolide Acetate for Injection—Not in USP.

LEVAMISOLE

Chemical name: Levamisole hydrochloride—Imidazo[2,1-*b*]thiazole, 2,3,5,6-tetrahydro-6-phenyl-, monohydrochloride, (*S*)-.

Molecular formula: Levamisole hydrochloride—$C_{11}H_{12}N_2S \cdot HCl$.

Molecular weight: Levamisole hydrochloride—240.75.

Description: Levamisole Hydrochloride USP—White or almost white crystalline powder.

Solubility: Levamisole Hydrochloride USP—Freely soluble in water; soluble in alcohol; slightly soluble in methylene chloride; practically insoluble in ether.

USP requirements:
Levamisole Hydrochloride USP—Preserve in well-closed containers, protected from light. Contains not less than 98.5% and not more than 101.0% of levamisole hydrochloride, calculated on the dried basis. Meets the requirements for Completeness of solution, Color of solution, Identification, Melting range (226–231 °C), Light absorption, pH (3.0–4.5, in a solution [1 in 20]), Loss on drying (not more than 0.5%), Specific rotation (−121.5° to −128.0°, calculated on the dried basis), Heavy metals (not more than 0.001%), Residue on ignition (not more than 0.1%), and Chromatographic purity.
Levamisole Hydrochloride Tablets USP—Preserve in well-closed containers. Label Tablets to state both the content of the active moiety and the content of the salt used in formulating the article. Contain an amount of levamisole hydrochloride equivalent to the labeled amount of levamisole, within ±10%. Meet the requirements for Identification, Dissolution (75% in 45 minutes in water in Apparatus 2 at 50 rpm), Uniformity of dosage units, and Chromatographic purity.

LEVOBUNOLOL

Chemical name: Levobunolol hydrochloride—1(2*H*)-Naphthalenone, 5-[3-[(1,1-dimethylethyl)amino]-2-hydroxypropoxy]-3,4-dihydro-, hydrochloride, (−)-.

Molecular formula: Levobunolol hydrochloride—$C_{17}H_{25}NO_3 \cdot HCl$.

Molecular weight: Levobunolol hydrochloride—327.85.

Description: Levobunolol hydrochloride—White, crystalline, odorless powder.

pKa: Levobunolol hydrochloride—9.4.

Solubility: Levobunolol hydrochloride—Solubility of 300 mg/mL in water and 24 mg/mL in alcohol at 25 °C.

USP requirements:
Levobunolol Hydrochloride USP—Preserve in well-closed containers. Contains not less than 98.5% and not more than 101.0% of levobunolol hydrochloride, calculated on the dried basis. Meets the requirements for Identification, Specific rotation (−19° to −20°, calculated on the dried basis), Melting range (206–211 °C, within a range of 3 °C, determined after drying), pH (4.5–6.5, in a solution [1 in 20]), Loss on drying (not more than 0.5%), and Residue on ignition (not more than 0.1%).
Levobunolol Hydrochloride Ophthalmic Solution USP—Preserve in tight containers. Contains the labeled amount, within ±10%. Meets the requirements for Identification, pH (5.5–7.5), Antimicrobial preservatives—Effectiveness, and Sterility.

LEVOCABASTINE

Chemical name: Levocabastine hydrochloride—4-Piperidinecarboxylic acid, 1-[4-cyano-4-(4-fluorophenyl)cyclohexyl]-3-methyl-4-phenyl-, monohydrochloride, (–)-[1(*cis*),3 alpha,4 beta]-.

Molecular formula: Levocabastine hydrochloride—$C_{26}H_{29}FN_2O_2 \cdot HCl$.

Molecular weight: Levocabastine hydrochloride—456.99.

Description: Levocabastine hydrochloride—White to almost white powder with a melting temperature of less than 300 °C.

pKa: Levocabastine hydrochloride—3.1 and 9.7.

Solubility: Levocabastine hydrochloride—Freely soluble in dimethylsulfoxide; soluble in *N,N*-dimethylformamide and in methanol; slightly soluble in propylene glycol, in polyethylene glycol, and in ethanol. In aqueous medium the solubility is a function of pH, with minimum solubility at pH 4.1 to 9.8.

Other characteristics: Levocabastine hydrochloride—Log-partition coefficient (*n*-octanol/aqueous buffer at pH 8.0): 1.82.

USP requirements:
Levocabastine Hydrochloride Nasal Suspension—Not in USP.

Levocabastine Hydrochloride Ophthalmic Suspension—Not in USP.

LEVOCARNITINE

Source: Naturally occurring amino acid derivative.

Chemical name: 1-Propanaminium, 3-carboxy-2-hydroxy-*N,N,N*-trimethyl-, hydroxide, inner salt, (*R*)-.

Molecular formula: $C_7H_{15}NO_3$.

Molecular weight: 161.20.

Description: Levocarnitine USP—White, odorless crystals or crystalline powder. Hygroscopic.

Solubility: Levocarnitine USP—Freely soluble in water and in hot alcohol; practically insoluble in acetone and in ether.

USP requirements:

Levocarnitine USP—Preserve in tight containers. Contains not less than 97.0% and not more than 103.0% of levocarnitine, calculated on the anhydrous basis. Meets the requirements for Identification, Specific rotation (−29° to −32°, calculated on the anhydrous basis), pH (5.5–9.5, in a solution [1 in 20]), Water content (not more than 4.0%), Residue on ignition (not more than 0.5%), Chloride (not more than 0.4%), Arsenic (not more than 2 ppm), Potassium (not more than 0.2%), Sodium (not more than 0.1%), and Heavy metals (not more than 0.002%).

Levocarnitine Capsules—Not in USP.

Levocarnitine Injection—Not in USP.

Levocarnitine Oral Solution USP—Preserve in tight containers. A solution of Levocarnitine in water. Contains suitable antimicrobial agents. Contains the labeled amount, within ±10%. Meets the requirements for Identification and pH (4.0–6.0).

Levocarnitine Tablets USP—Preserve in tight containers. Contain the labeled amount, within ±10%. Meet the requirements for Identification and Uniformity of dosage units.

LEVODOPA

Chemical group: L-Dihydroxyphenylalanine; precursor of dopamine.

Chemical name: L-Tyrosine, 3-hydroxy-.

Molecular formula: $C_9H_{11}NO_4$.

Molecular weight: 197.19.

Description: Levodopa USP—White to off-white, odorless, crystalline powder. In the presence of moisture, is rapidly oxidized by atmospheric oxygen and darkens.

Solubility: Levodopa USP—Slightly soluble in water; freely soluble in 3 *N* hydrochloric acid; insoluble in alcohol.

USP requirements:

Levodopa USP—Preserve in tight, light-resistant containers, in a dry place, and prevent exposure to excessive heat. Contains not less than 99.0% and not more than 100.5% of levodopa, calculated on the dried basis. Meets the requirements for Identification, Specific rotation (−160° to −167°), Loss on drying (not more than 0.5%), Residue on ignition (not more than 0.1%), Heavy metals (not more than 0.002%), Related compounds, and Organic volatile impurities.

Levodopa Capsules USP—Preserve in tight, light-resistant containers, in a dry place, and prevent exposure to excessive heat. Contain the labeled amount, within ±10%. Meet the requirements for Identification, Dissolution (75% in 30 minutes in 0.1 *N* hydrochloric acid in Apparatus 1 at 100 rpm), Related compounds, and Uniformity of dosage units.

Levodopa Tablets USP—Preserve in tight, light-resistant containers, in a dry place, and prevent exposure to excessive heat. Contain the labeled amount, within ±10%. Meet the requirements for Identification, Dissolution (75% in 30 minutes in 0.1 *N* hydrochloric acid in Apparatus 1 at 100 rpm), Related compounds, and Uniformity of dosage units.

LEVODOPA AND BENSERAZIDE

Chemical group: Levodopa—L-Dihydroxyphenylalanine; precursor of dopamine.

Chemical name:

Levodopa—L-Tyrosine, 3-hydroxy-.

Benserazide—DL-Serine, 2-[(2,3,4-trihydroxyphenyl)methyl]-hydrazide.

Molecular formula:

Levodopa—$C_9H_{11}NO_4$.

Benserazide—$C_{10}H_{15}N_3O_5$.

Molecular weight:

Levodopa—197.19.

Benserazide—257.25.

Description:

Levodopa USP—White to off-white, odorless, crystalline powder. In the presence of moisture, is rapidly oxidized by atmospheric oxygen and darkens.

Benserazide—Unstable in a neutral, alkaline, or strongly acidic medium.

Solubility:

Levodopa USP—Slightly soluble in water; freely soluble in 3 *N* hydrochloric acid; insoluble in alcohol.

Benserazide—Highly soluble in water.

USP requirements: Levodopa and Benserazide Capsules—Not in USP.

LEVONORDEFRIN

Chemical name: 1,2-Benzenediol, 4-(2-amino-1-hydroxypropyl)-, [*R*-(*R**,*S**)]-.

Molecular formula: $C_9H_{13}NO_3$.

Molecular weight: 183.21.

Description: Levonordefrin USP—White to buff-colored, odorless, crystalline solid. Melts at about 210 °C.

Solubility: Levonordefrin USP—Practically insoluble in water; freely soluble in aqueous solutions of mineral acids; slightly soluble in acetone, in chloroform, in alcohol, and in ether.

USP requirements: Levonordefrin USP—Preserve in well-closed containers. Dried in vacuum at 60 °C for 15 hours, contains not less than 98.0% and not more than 102.0% of levonordefrin. Meets the requirements for Identification, Specific rotation (−28° to −31°), Loss on drying (not more than 1.0%), Residue on ignition (not more than 0.2%), and Chromatographic impurities.

LEVONORGESTREL

Chemical name: 18,19-Dinorpregn-4-en-20-yn-3-one, 13-ethyl-17-hydroxy-, (17 alpha)-(−)-.

Molecular formula: $C_{21}H_{28}O_2$.

Molecular weight: 312.45.

Description: Levonorgestrel USP—White or practically white, odorless powder.

Solubility: Levonorgestrel USP—Practically insoluble in water; soluble in chloroform; slightly soluble in alcohol.

USP requirements:
Levonorgestrel USP—Preserve in well-closed, light-resistant containers. Contains not less than 98.0% and not more than 102.0% of levonorgestrel, calculated on the dried basis. Meets the requirements for Identification, Melting range (232–239 °C, the range between beginning and end of melting not more than 4 °C), Specific rotation (−30° to −35°, calculated on the dried basis), Loss on drying (not more than 0.5%), Residue on ignition (not more than 0.3%), Ethynyl group (7.81–8.18%), and Chromatographic impurities.
Levonorgestrel Implants—Not in USP.

LEVONORGESTREL AND ETHINYL ESTRADIOL

For *Levonorgestrel* and *Ethinyl Estradiol*—See individual listings for chemistry information.

USP requirements: Levonorgestrel and Ethinyl Estradiol Tablets USP—Preserve in well-closed containers. Contain the labeled amounts, within ±10%. Meet the requirements for Identification, Dissolution (for uncoated tablets, 60% of levonorgestrel in 30 minutes and 75% of ethinyl estradiol in 60 minutes; for sugar-coated tablets, 60% of levonorgestrel in 60 minutes and 60% of ethinyl estradiol in 60 minutes; both, in polysorbate 80 [5 ppm] in Water in Apparatus 2 at 75 rpm), and Uniformity of dosage units.

LEVOPROPOXYPHENE

Chemical name: Levopropoxyphene napsylate—Benzeneethanol, alpha-[2-(dimethylamino)-1-methylethyl]-alpha-phenyl-, propanoate (ester), [*R*-(*R**,*S**)]-, compd. with 2-naphthalenesulfonic acid (1:1), monohydrate.

Molecular formula: Levopropoxyphene napsylate—$C_{22}H_{29}NO_2 \cdot C_{10}H_8O_3S \cdot H_2O$.

Molecular weight: Levopropoxyphene napsylate—565.72.

Description: Levopropoxyphene Napsylate USP—White powder, having essentially no odor.

Solubility: Levopropoxyphene Napsylate USP—Very slightly soluble in water; soluble in methanol, in alcohol, in chloroform, and in acetone.

USP requirements:
Levopropoxyphene Napsylate USP—Preserve in tight containers. Contains not less than 97.0% and not more than 103.0% of levopropoxyphene napsylate, calculated on the anhydrous basis. Meets the requirements for Identification, Melting range (158–165 °C, the range between beginning and end of melting not more than 4 °C), Specific rotation (−35° to −43°), Water (not more than 5.0%), Residue on ignition (not more than 0.5%), Heavy metals (not more than 0.003%), and Related compounds (not more than 0.60%).
Levopropoxyphene Napsylate Capsules USP—Preserve in tight containers. Contain an amount of levopropoxyphene napsylate equivalent to the labeled amount of levopropoxyphene, within ±10%. Meet the requirements for Identification, Dissolution (75% in 60 minutes in acetate buffer [pH 4.5] in Apparatus 1 at 100 rpm) and Uniformity of dosage units.
Levopropoxyphene Napsylate Oral Suspension USP—Preserve in tight containers, protected from light. Avoid freezing. Contains an amount of levopropoxyphene napsylate equivalent to the labeled amount of levopropoxyphene, within ±10%. Meets the requirements for Identification and Alcohol content (0.5–1.5%).

LEVORPHANOL

Chemical name: Levorphanol tartrate—Morphinan-3-ol, 17-methyl-, [*R*-(*R**,*R**)]-2,3-dihydroxybutanedioate (1:1) (salt), dihydrate.

Molecular formula: Levorphanol tartrate—$C_{17}H_{23}NO \cdot C_4H_6O_6 \cdot 2H_2O$ (dihydrate); $C_{17}H_{23}NO \cdot C_4H_6O_6$ (anhydrous).

Molecular weight: Levorphanol tartrate—443.49 (dihydrate); 407.46 (anhydrous).

Description: Levorphanol Tartrate USP—Practically white, odorless, crystalline powder. Melts, in a sealed tube, at about 110 °C, with decomposition.

Solubility: Levorphanol Tartrate USP—Sparingly soluble in water; slightly soluble in alcohol; insoluble in chloroform and in ether.

USP requirements:
Levorphanol Tartrate USP—Preserve in well-closed containers. Contains not less than 99.0% and not more than 101.0% of levorphanol tartrate, calculated on the anhydrous basis. Meets the requirements for Identification, Specific rotation (−14.7° to −16.3°, calculated on the anhydrous basis), Water (7.0–9.0%), Residue on ignition (not more than 0.1%), and Ordinary impurities.
Levorphanol Tartrate Injection USP—Preserve in single-dose or in multiple-dose containers, preferably of Type I glass. A sterile solution of Levorphanol Tartrate in Water for Injection. Contains the labeled amount, within ±7%. Meets the requirements for Identification, Bacterial endotoxins, pH (4.1–4.5), and Injections.
Levorphanol Tartrate Tablets USP—Preserve in well-closed containers. Contain the labeled amount, within ±7%. Meet the requirements for Identification, Dissolution (75% in 30 minutes in water in Apparatus 2 at 50 rpm), and Uniformity of dosage units.

LEVOTHYROXINE

Chemical name: Levothyroxine sodium—L-Tyrosine, *O*-(4-hydroxy-3,5-diiodophenyl)-3,5-diiodo-, monosodium salt, hydrate.

Molecular formula: Levothyroxine sodium—$C_{15}H_{10}I_4NNaO_4 \cdot xH_2O$.

Molecular weight: Levothyroxine sodium—798.86 (anhydrous).

Description: Levothyroxine Sodium USP—Light yellow to buff-colored, odorless, hygroscopic powder. Is stable in dry air but may assume a slight pink color upon exposure to light. The pH of a saturated solution is about 8.9.

Solubility: Levothyroxine Sodium USP—Very slightly soluble in water; soluble in solutions of alkali hydroxides and in hot solutions of alkali carbonates; slightly soluble in alcohol; insoluble in acetone, in chloroform, and in ether.

USP requirements:
Levothyroxine Sodium USP—Preserve in tight containers, protected from light. The sodium salt of the levo isomer of thyroxine, an active physiological principle obtained

from the thyroid gland of domesticated animals used for food by man or prepared synthetically. Contains not less than 97.0% and not more than 103.0% of levothyroxine sodium, calculated on the anhydrous basis. Meets the requirements for Identification, Specific rotation (−5° to −6°), Water (not more than 11.0%), Soluble halides (not more than 0.7% as chloride), and Liothyronine sodium (not more than 2.0%).

Levothyroxine Sodium Injection—Not in USP.

Levothyroxine Sodium for Injection—Not in USP.

Levothyroxine Sodium Oral Powder USP—Preserve in tight, light-resistant containers. Contains the labeled amount, within ±10%. Meets the requirement for Loss on drying (not more than 2.0%).

Levothyroxine Sodium Tablets USP—Preserve in tight, light-resistant containers. Contain the labeled amount, within ±10%. Meet the requirements for Identification, Dissolution (55% in 80 minutes in 0.05 *M* phosphate buffer [pH 7.4] in Apparatus 2 at 100 rpm), Uniformity of dosage units, Soluble halides (not more than 7.1%), and Liothyronine sodium (not more than 2.0%).

LIDOCAINE

Chemical group: Amide.

Chemical name:

Lidocaine—Acetamide, 2-(diethylamino)-*N*-(2,6-dimethylphenyl)-.

Lidocaine hydrochloride—Acetamide, 2-(diethylamino)-*N*-(2,6-dimethylphenyl)-, monohydrochloride, monohydrate.

Molecular formula:

Lidocaine—$C_{14}H_{22}N_2O$.

Lidocaine hydrochloride—$C_{14}H_{22}N_2O \cdot HCl \cdot H_2O$.

Molecular weight:

Lidocaine—234.34.

Lidocaine hydrochloride—288.82.

Description:

Lidocaine USP—White or slightly yellow, crystalline powder. Has a characteristic odor and is stable in air.

Lidocaine Hydrochloride USP—White, odorless, crystalline powder.

pKa:

Lidocaine—7.9.

Lidocaine hydrochloride—7.86.

Solubility:

Lidocaine USP—Practically insoluble in water; very soluble in alcohol and in chloroform; freely soluble in ether; dissolves in oils.

Lidocaine Hydrochloride USP—Very soluble in water and in alcohol; soluble in chloroform; insoluble in ether.

USP requirements:

Lidocaine USP—Preserve in well-closed containers. Contains not less than 97.5% and not more than 102.5% of lidocaine. Meets the requirements for Identification, Melting range (66–69 °C), Residue on ignition (not more than 0.1%), Sulfate, Chloride (not more than 0.0035%), and Heavy metals (not more than 0.002%).

Lidocaine Topical Aerosol USP (Solution)—Preserve in nonreactive aerosol containers equipped with metered-dose valves. A solution of Lidocaine in a suitable flavored vehicle with suitable propellants in a pressurized container equipped with a metering valve. Contains the labeled amount, within ±10%, and delivers within ±15% of the labeled amount per actuation. Meets the requirements for Identification and Microbial limits, and for Leak Testing under Aerosols.

Lidocaine Ointment USP—Preserve in tight containers. It is Lidocaine in a suitable hydrophilic ointment base. Contains the labeled amount, within ±5%. Meets the requirements for Identification, Microbial limits, and Minimum fill.

Lidocaine Oral Topical Solution USP—Preserve in tight containers. Contains the labeled amount, within ±5%. Contains a suitable flavor. Meets the requirement for Identification.

Lidocaine Hydrochloride USP—Preserve in well-closed containers. Contains not less than 97.5% and not more than 102.5% of lidocaine hydrochloride, calculated on the anhydrous basis. Meets the requirements for Identification, Melting range (74–79 °C), Water (5.0–7.0%), Residue on ignition (not more than 0.1%), Sulfate, and Heavy metals (not more than 0.002%).

Lidocaine Hydrochloride Injection USP—Preserve in single-dose or in multiple-dose containers, preferably of Type I glass. A sterile solution of Lidocaine Hydrochloride in Water for Injection, or a sterile solution prepared from Lidocaine with the aid of Hydrochloric Acid in Water for Injection. Injection may be packaged in 50-mL multiple-dose containers. Injections that are of such concentration that they are not intended for direct injection into tissues are labeled to indicate that they are to be diluted prior to administration. Contains the labeled amount, within ±5%. Meets the requirements for Identification, Bacterial endotoxins, pH (5.0–7.0), Particulate matter, and Injections.

Lidocaine Hydrochloride Jelly USP—Preserve in tight containers. It is Lidocaine Hydrochloride in a suitable, water-soluble, sterile, viscous base. Contains the labeled amount, within ±5%. Meets the requirements for Identification, Sterility, Minimum fill, and pH (6.0–7.0).

Lidocaine Hydrochloride Ointment—Not in USP.

Lidocaine Hydrochloride Topical Solution USP—Preserve in tight containers. Contains the labeled amount, within ±5%. Meets the requirements for Identification and pH (5.0–7.0).

Lidocaine Hydrochloride Oral Topical Solution USP—Preserve in tight containers. Contains the labeled amount, within ±5%. Contains a suitable flavor and/or sweetening agent. Meets the requirements for Identification and pH (5.0–7.0).

Sterile Lidocaine Hydrochloride USP—Preserve in Containers for Sterile Solids. It is Lidocaine Hydrochloride suitable for parenteral use. Contains the labeled amount, within ±5%. Meets the requirements for Bacterial endotoxins, for Identification test, Melting range, Water, Residue on ignition, Sulfate, and Heavy metals under Lidocaine Hydrochloride, for Sterility tests, Uniformity of dosage units, and Constituted solutions, and for Labeling under Injections.

LIDOCAINE AND DEXTROSE

For *Lidocaine* and *Dextrose*—See individual listings for chemistry information.

USP requirements: Lidocaine Hydrochloride and Dextrose Injection USP—Preserve in single-dose containers of Type I or Type II glass, or of a suitable plastic material. A sterile solution of Lidocaine Hydrochloride and Dextrose in Water for Injection. Contains the labeled amounts, within ±5%. Meets the requirements for Identification, Bacterial endotoxins, pH (3.0–7.0), and Injections.

LIDOCAINE AND EPINEPHRINE

For *Lidocaine* and *Epinephrine*—See individual listings for chemistry information.

USP requirements: Lidocaine and Epinephrine Injection USP—Preserve in single-dose or in multiple-dose, light-resistant containers, preferably of Type I glass. A sterile solution prepared from Lidocaine Hydrochloride and Epinephrine with the aid of Hydrochloric Acid in Water for Injection, or a sterile solution prepared from Lidocaine and Epinephrine with the aid of Hydrochloric Acid in Water for Injection, or a sterile solution of Lidocaine Hydrochloride and Epinephrine Bitartrate in Water for Injection. The content of epinephrine does not exceed 0.002% (1 in 50,000). The label indicates that the Injection is not to be used if its color is pinkish or darker than slightly yellow or if it contains a precipitate. Contains the equivalent of the labeled amount of lidocaine hydrochloride, within ±5%, and the equivalent of the labeled amount of epinephrine, within −10% to +15%. Meets the requirements for Color and clarity, Bacterial endotoxins, and pH (3.3–5.5), for Identification test under Lidocaine Hydrochloride Injection, and for Injections.

LIDOCAINE AND PRILOCAINE

For *Lidocaine* and *Prilocaine*—See individual listings for chemistry information.

USP requirements: Lidocaine and Prilocaine Cream—Not in USP.

LIME

Chemical name: Calcium oxide.

Molecular formula: CaO.

Molecular weight: 56.08.

Description: Lime USP—Hard, white or grayish white masses or granules, or white or grayish white powder. Is odorless.

Solubility: Lime USP—Slightly soluble in water; very slightly soluble in boiling water.

USP requirements: Lime USP—Preserve in tight containers. When freshly ignited to constant weight, contains not less than 95.0% of lime. Meets the requirements for Identification, Loss on ignition (not more than 10.0%), Insoluble substances (not more than 1.0%), Carbonate, Magnesium and alkali salts, and Organic volatile impurities.

SULFURATED LIME

Source: Mixture of sublimed sulfur, lime, and water resulting in formation of calcium pentasulfide and calcium thiosulfate.

Description: Sulfurated lime solution—Clear orange liquid with a slight odor of hydrogen sulfide.

USP requirements:
Sulfurated Lime Mask—Not in USP.
Sulfurated Lime Topical Solution—Not in USP.

LINCOMYCIN

Source: Produced by the growth of a member of the *lincolnensis* group of *Streptomyces lincolnensis* (Fam. *Streptomycetaceae*).

Chemical name: Lincomycin hydrochloride—D-*erythro*-alpha-D-*galacto*-Octopyranoside, methyl 6,8-dideoxy-6-[[(1-methyl-4-propyl-2-pyrrolidinyl)carbonyl]amino]-1-thio-, monohydrochloride, monohydrate, (2*S*-*trans*)-.

Molecular formula: Lincomycin hydrochloride—$C_{18}H_{34}N_2O_6S \cdot HCl \cdot H_2O$.

Molecular weight: Lincomycin hydrochloride—461.01.

Description:
Lincomycin Hydrochloride USP—White or practically white, crystalline powder. Is odorless or has a faint odor. Is stable in the presence of air and light. Its solutions are acid and are dextrorotatory.
Lincomycin Hydrochloride Injection USP—Clear, colorless to slightly yellow solution, having a slight odor.

Solubility: Lincomycin Hydrochloride USP—Freely soluble in water; soluble in dimethylformamide; very slightly soluble in acetone.

USP requirements:
Lincomycin Hydrochloride USP—Preserve in tight containers. Has a potency equivalent to not less than 790 mcg of lincomycin per mg. Meets the requirements for Identification, Specific rotation (+135° to +150°, calculated on the anhydrous basis), Crystallinity, pH (3.0–5.5, in a solution [1 in 10]), Water (3.0–6.0%), and Lincomycin B, and for Bacterial endotoxins and Depressor substances under Sterile Lincomycin Hydrochloride for Lincomycin Hydrochloride intended for use in making Lincomycin Hydrochloride Injection.
Lincomycin Hydrochloride Capsules USP—Preserve in tight containers. Contain an amount of lincomycin hydrochloride equivalent to the labeled amount of lincomycin, within −10% to +20%. Meet the requirements for Dissolution (75% in 45 minutes in water in Apparatus 1 at 100 rpm), Uniformity of dosage units, and Water (not more than 7.0%).
Lincomycin Hydrochloride Injection USP—Preserve in single-dose or in multiple-dose containers, preferably of Type I glass. A sterile solution of Lincomycin Hydrochloride in Water for Injection. Contains benzyl alcohol as a preservative. Contains an amount of lincomycin hydrochloride equivalent to the labeled amount of lincomycin, within −10% to +20%. Meets the requirements for Sterility, Bacterial endotoxins, pH (3.0–5.5), Particulate matter, and Injections.
Sterile Lincomycin Hydrochloride USP—Preserve in Containers for Sterile Solids. It is Lincomycin Hydrochloride suitable for parenteral use. Has a potency equivalent to not less than 790 mcg of lincomycin per mg. Meets the requirements for Depressor substances, Bacterial endotoxins, and Sterility, and for Identification test, Specific rotation, pH, Water, Crystallinity, and Lincomycin B under Lincomycin Hydrochloride.
Lincomycin Hydrochloride Syrup USP—Preserve in tight containers. Contains an amount of Lincomycin Hydrochloride equivalent to the labeled amount of lincomycin, within −10% to +20%, and one or more suitable colors, flavors, preservatives, and sweeteners in water. Meets the requirements for pH (3–5.5), Deliverable volume (for syrup packaged in multiple-unit containers), and Uniformity of dosage units (for syrup packaged in single-unit containers).

LINDANE

Chemical name: Cyclohexane, 1,2,3,4,5,6-hexachloro-, (1 alpha,2 alpha,3 beta,4 alpha,5 alpha,6 beta)-.

Molecular formula: $C_6H_6Cl_6$.

Molecular weight: 290.83.

Description: Lindane USP—White, crystalline powder, having a slight, musty odor.

Solubility: Lindane USP—Practically insoluble in water; freely soluble in chloroform; soluble in dehydrated alcohol; sparingly soluble in ether; slightly soluble in ethylene glycol.

USP requirements:

Lindane USP—Preserve in well-closed containers. The gamma isomer of hexachlorocyclohexane. Contains not less than 99.0% and not more than 100.5% of lindane. Meets the requirements for Identification, Congealing temperature (not less than 112 °C), Water (not more than 0.5%), and Chloride ion.

Lindane Cream USP—Preserve in tight containers. It is Lindane in a suitable cream base. Contains the labeled amount, within ± 10%. Meets the requirements for Identification and pH (8.0–9.0, in a 1 in 5 dilution).

Lindane Lotion USP—Preserve in tight containers. It is Lindane in a suitable aqueous vehicle. Contains the labeled amount, within ± 10%. Meets the requirements for Identification and pH (6.5–8.5).

Lindane Shampoo USP—Preserve in tight containers. It is Lindane in a suitable vehicle. Contains the labeled amount, within ± 10%. Meets the requirements for Identification and pH (6.2–7.0).

LIOTHYRONINE

Chemical name: Liothyronine sodium—L-Tyrosine, *O*-(4-hydroxy-3-iodophenyl)-3,5-diiodo-, monosodium salt.

Molecular formula: Liothyronine sodium—$C_{15}H_{11}I_3NNaO_4$.

Molecular weight: Liothyronine sodium—672.96.

Description: Liothyronine Sodium USP—Light tan, odorless, crystalline powder.

Solubility: Liothyronine Sodium USP—Very slightly soluble in water; slightly soluble in alcohol; practically insoluble in most other organic solvents.

USP requirements:

Liothyronine Sodium USP—Preserve in tight containers. The sodium salt of L-3,3′,5-triiodothyronine. Contains not less than 95.0% and not more than 101.0% of liothyronine sodium, calculated on the dried basis. Meets the requirements for Identification, Specific rotation (+18° to +22°, calculated on the dried basis), Loss on drying (not more than 4.0%), Inorganic iodide, Chloride content (not more than 1.2%), Sodium content (2.9–4.0%), and Levothyroxine sodium (not more than 5.0%).

Liothyronine Sodium Injection—Not in USP.

Liothyronine Sodium Tablets USP—Preserve in tight containers. Contain an amount of liothyronine sodium equivalent to the labeled amount of liothyronine, within ± 10%. Meet the requirements for Identification, Disintegration (30 minutes), and Uniformity of dosage units.

LIOTRIX

Source: A mixture of liothyronine sodium and levothyroxine sodium, in a ratio of 1:1 in terms of biological activity, or in a ratio of 1:4 in terms of weight.

Chemical name: L-Tyrosine, *O*-(4-hydroxy-3,5-diiodophenyl)-3,5-diiodo-, monosodium salt, hydrate, mixt. with *O*-(4-hydroxy-3-iodophenyl)-3,5-diiodo-L-tyrosine monosodium salt.

USP requirements: Liotrix Tablets USP—Preserve in tight containers. Contain the labeled amounts of levothyroxine sodium and liothyronine sodium, within ± 10%. Meet the requirements for Identification, Disintegration (30 minutes), and Uniformity of dosage units.

LISINOPRIL

Chemical name: L-Proline, 1-[N^2-(1-carboxy-3-phenylpropyl)-L-lysyl]-, dihydrate, (*S*)-.

Molecular formula: $C_{21}H_{31}N_3O_5 \cdot 2H_2O$.

Molecular weight: 441.52.

Description: Lisinopril USP—White, crystalline powder. Melts at about 160 °C, with decomposition.

Solubility: Lisinopril USP—Soluble in water; sparingly soluble in methanol; practically insoluble in alcohol, in acetone, in acetonitrile, and in chloroform.

USP requirements:

Lisinopril USP—Preserve in well-closed containers. Contains not less than 98.0% and not more than 102.0% of lisinopril, calculated on the anhydrous basis. Meets the requirements for Identification, Specific rotation (−115.3° to −122.5°, calculated on the anhydrous basis), Water (8.0–9.5%), Residue on ignition (not more than 0.1%), and Heavy metals (not more than 0.001%).

Lisinopril Tablets USP—Preserve in tight containers. Contain the labeled amount, within ± 10%. Meet the requirements for Identification, Dissolution (80% in 30 minutes in 0.1 *N* hydrochloric acid in Apparatus 2 at 50 rpm), Uniformity of dosage units, and Related compounds.

LISINOPRIL AND HYDROCHLOROTHIAZIDE

For *Lisinopril* and *Hydrochlorothiazide*—See individual listings for chemistry information.

USP requirements: Lisinopril and Hydrochlorothiazide Tablets—Not in USP.

LITHIUM

Chemical name:

Lithium carbonate—Carbonic acid, dilithium salt.

Lithium citrate—1,2,3-Propanetricarboxylic acid, 2-hydroxy-trilithium salt tetrahydrate.

Lithium hydroxide—Lithium hydroxide monohydrate.

Molecular formula:

Lithium carbonate—Li_2CO_3.

Lithium citrate—$C_6H_5Li_3O_7 \cdot 4H_2O$.

Lithium hydroxide—$LiOH \cdot H_2O$.

Molecular weight:

Lithium carbonate—73.89.

Lithium citrate—281.99.

Lithium hydroxide—41.96.

Description:

Lithium Carbonate USP—White, granular, odorless powder.

Lithium Citrate USP—White, odorless, deliquescent powder or granules.

Lithium hydroxide—Small crystals.

Solubility:

Lithium Carbonate USP—Sparingly soluble in water; very slightly soluble in alcohol. Dissolves, with effervescence, in dilute mineral acids.

Lithium Citrate USP—Freely soluble in water; slightly soluble in alcohol.

Lithium hydroxide—Solubility in water (w/w) at 0 °C: 10.7%, at 20 °C: 10.9%, and at 100 °C: 14.8%; slightly soluble in alcohol.

Other characteristics: A monovalent cation; salts share some chemical characteristics with salts of sodium and potassium.

USP requirements:

Lithium Carbonate USP—Preserve in well-closed containers. Contains not less than 99.0% of lithium carbonate, calculated on the dried basis. Meets the requirements for Identification, Reaction, Loss on drying (not more than 1.0%), Insoluble substances, Chloride (not more than

0.07%), Sulfate (not more than 0.1%), Aluminum and iron, Arsenic (not more than 8 ppm), Calcium, Sodium (not more than 0.1%), Heavy metals (not more than 0.002%), and Organic volatile impurities.

Lithium Carbonate Capsules USP—Preserve in well-closed containers. Contain the labeled amount, within ±5%. Meet the requirements for Identification, Dissolution (60% in 30 minutes in water in Apparatus 1 at 100 rpm), and Uniformity of dosage units.

Lithium Carbonate Slow-release Capsules—Not in USP.

Lithium Carbonate Tablets USP—Preserve in well-closed containers. Contain the labeled amount, within ±5%. Meet the requirements for Identification, Dissolution (60% in 30 minutes in water in Apparatus 1 at 100 rpm), and Uniformity of dosage units.

Lithium Carbonate Extended-release Tablets USP—Preserve in well-closed containers. Contain the labeled amount, within ±10%. Meet the requirements for Identification and Uniformity of dosage units.

Lithium Citrate USP—Preserve in tight containers. Contains not less than 98.0% and not more than 102.0% of lithium citrate, calculated on the anhydrous basis. Meets the requirements for Identification, pH (7.0–10.0, in a solution [1 in 20]), Water (24.0–28.0%), Carbonate, Arsenic (not more than 5 ppm), Heavy metals (not more than 0.001%), and Organic volatile impurities.

Lithium Citrate Syrup USP—Preserve in tight containers. It is prepared from Lithium Citrate or Lithium Hydroxide to which an excess of Citric Acid has been added. Contains an amount of lithium citrate equivalent to the labeled amount of lithium, within ±10%. Meets the requirements for Identification and pH (4.0–5.0).

Lithium Hydroxide USP—Preserve in tight containers. Contains not less than 98.0% and not more than 102.0% of lithium hydroxide, calculated on the anhydrous basis. Meets the requirements for Identification, Water (41.0–43.5%), Carbonate, Sulfate (not more than 0.05%), Arsenic (not more than 5 ppm), Calcium, Heavy metals (not more than 0.002%), Lithium content (28.4–29.1%), and Organic volatile impurities.

Caution: Exercise great care in handling Lithium Hydroxide, as it rapidly destroys tissues.

LODOXAMIDE

Chemical name: Lodoxamide tromethamine—Acetic acid, 2,2′-[(2-chloro-5-cyano-1,3-phenylene)diimino]bis[2-oxo-, compound with 2-amino-2-(hydroxymethyl)-1,3-propanediol (1:2).

Molecular formula: Lodoxamide tromethamine—$C_{11}H_6ClN_3O_6 \cdot 2C_4H_{11}NO_3$.

Molecular weight: Lodoxamide tromethamine—553.91.

Description: Lodoxamide tromethamine—White, crystalline powder.

Solubility: Lodoxamide tromethamine—Soluble in water.

USP requirements: Lodoxamide Tromethamine Ophthalmic Solution—Not in USP.

LOMEFLOXACIN

Chemical name: Lomefloxacin hydrochloride—3-Quinolinecarboxylic acid, 1-ethyl-6,8-difluoro-1,4-dihydro-7-(3-methyl-1-piperazinyl)-4-oxo, monohydrochloride, (±)-.

Molecular formula: Lomefloxacin hydrochloride—$C_{17}H_{19}F_2N_3O_3 \cdot HCl$.

Molecular weight: Lomefloxacin hydrochloride—387.81.

Description: Lomefloxacin hydrochloride—White to pale yellow powder. Stable to heat and moisture but sensitive to light in dilute aqueous solution.

Solubility: Lomefloxacin hydrochloride—Slightly soluble in water; practically insoluble in alcohol.

USP requirements: Lomefloxacin Hydrochloride Tablets—Not in USP.

LOMUSTINE

Chemical name: Urea, *N*-(2-chloroethyl)-*N′*-cyclohexyl-*N*-nitroso-.

Molecular formula: $C_9H_{16}ClN_3O_2$.

Molecular weight: 233.70.

Description: Yellow powder.

Solubility: Soluble in 10% ethanol and in absolute alcohol; relatively insoluble in water; highly soluble in lipids.

USP requirements: Lomustine Capsules—Not in USP.

LOPERAMIDE

Source: Synthetic piperidine derivative.

Chemical group: Opiate agonist.

Chemical name: Loperamide hydrochloride—1-Piperidinebutanamide, 4-(4-chlorophenyl)-4-hydroxy-*N,N*-dimethyl-alpha,alpha-diphenyl-, monohydrochloride.

Molecular formula: Loperamide hydrochloride—$C_{29}H_{33}ClN_2O_2 \cdot HCl$.

Molecular weight: Loperamide hydrochloride—513.51.

Description: Loperamide Hydrochloride USP—White to slightly yellow powder. Melts at about 225 °C, with some decomposition.

pKa: Loperamide hydrochloride—8.6.

Solubility: Loperamide Hydrochloride USP—Freely soluble in methanol, in isopropyl alcohol, and in chloroform; slightly soluble in water and in dilute acids.

USP requirements:

Loperamide Hydrochloride USP—Preserve in well-closed containers. Contains not less than 98.0% and not more than 102.0% of loperamide hydrochloride, calculated on the dried basis. Meets the requirements for Identification, Loss on drying (not more than 0.5%), Residue on ignition (not more than 0.2%), Heavy metals (not more than 0.002%), Chromatographic purity, and Chloride content (13.52–14.20%).

Loperamide Hydrochloride Capsules USP—Preserve in well-closed containers. Contain the labeled amount, within ±10%. Meet the requirements for Identification, Dissolution (70% in 30 minutes in acetate buffer [pH 4.7] in Apparatus 1 at 100 rpm), and Uniformity of dosage units.

Loperamide Hydrochloride Oral Solution—Not in USP.

Loperamide Hydrochloride Tablets USP—Preserve in well-closed, light-resistant containers. Contain the labeled amount, within ±10%. Meet the requirements for Identification, Dissolution (80% in 30 minutes in 0.1 *N* hydrochloric acid in Apparatus 2 at 50 rpm), and Uniformity of dosage units.

LORACARBEF

Chemical name: 1-Azabicyclo[4.2.0]oct-2-ene-2-carboxylic acid, 7-[(aminophenylacetyl)amino]-3-chloro-8-oxo-, monohydrate, [6*R*-[6 alpha,7 beta(*R**)]]-.

Molecular formula: $C_{16}H_{16}ClN_3O_4 \cdot H_2O$.

Molecular weight: 367.79.

Description: White crystalline compound.

USP requirements:

Loracarbef USP—Preserve in tight containers. Contains not less than 960 mcg and not more than 1020 mcg of anhydrous loracarbef per mg, calculated on the anhydrous basis. Meets the requirements for Identification, Specific rotation (+27° to +33°, calculated on the anhydrous basis), Crystallinity, pH (3.5–5.5, in a suspension [1 in 10]), and Water (3.5–6.0%).

Loracarbef Capsules USP—Preserve in well-closed containers. Contain the labeled amount of anhydrous loracarbef, within ±10%. Meet the requirements for Identification, Dissolution (75% in 30 minutes in water in Apparatus 2 at 50 rpm), Uniformity of dosage units, and Water (not more than 8.5%).

Loracarbef for Oral Suspension USP—Preserve in tight containers. A dry mixture of Loracarbef and one or more suitable suspending agents, preservatives, coloring agents, antifoaming agents, flavorings, and sweeteners. Contains the labeled amount of anhydrous loracarbef, within −10% to +15%. Meets the requirements for Identification, Uniformity of dosage units, Deliverable volume, pH (3.5–6.0, in the Oral Suspension constituted as directed in the labeling), and Water (not more than 2.0%).

LORATADINE

Chemical name: 1-Piperidinecarboxylic acid, 4-(8-chloro-5,6-dihydro-11*H*-benzo[5,6]cyclohepta[1,2-*b*]pyridin-11-ylidene)-, ethyl ester.

Molecular formula: $C_{22}H_{23}ClN_2O_2$.

Molecular weight: 382.89.

Description: Melting point 134–136 °C.

USP requirements: Loratadine Tablets—Not in USP.

LORATADINE AND PSEUDOEPHEDRINE

For *Loratadine* and *Pseudoephedrine*—See individual listings for chemistry information.

USP requirements: Loratadine and Pseudoephedrine Tablets—Not in USP.

LORAZEPAM

Chemical name: 2*H*-1,4-Benzodiazepin-2-one, 7-chloro-5-(2-chlorophenyl)-1,3-dihydro-3-hydroxy-.

Molecular formula: $C_{15}H_{10}Cl_2N_2O_2$.

Molecular weight: 321.16.

Description: Lorazepam USP—White or practically white, practically odorless powder.

Solubility: Lorazepam USP—Insoluble in water; sparingly soluble in alcohol; slightly soluble in chloroform.

USP requirements:

Lorazepam USP—Preserve in tight, light-resistant containers. Contains not less than 98.0% and not more than 102.0% of lorazepam, calculated on the dried basis. Meets the requirements for Identification, Loss on drying (not more than 0.5%), Residue on ignition (not more than 0.3%), Heavy metals (not more than 0.002%), and Related compounds.

Lorazepam Injection USP—Preserve in a single-dose or in multiple-dose containers, preferably of Type I glass, protected from light. A sterile solution of Lorazepam in a suitable medium. Contains the labeled amount, within ±10%. Meets the requirements for Identification, Bacterial endotoxins, Related compounds, and Injections.

Lorazepam Oral Concentrate USP—Preserve in well-closed, light-resistant containers. Contains the labeled amount, within ±10%. Meets the requirements for Identification and Related compounds.

Lorazepam Oral Solution—Not in USP.

Lorazepam Tablets USP—Preserve in tight, light-resistant containers. Contain the labeled amount, within ±10%. Meet the requirements for Identification, Dissolution (60% in 30 minutes and 80% in 60 minutes in water in Apparatus 1 at 100 rpm), Uniformity of dosage units, and Related compounds.

Lorazepam Sublingual Tablets—Not in USP.

LOVASTATIN

Source: Isolated from a strain of *Aspergillus terreus*.

Chemical name: Butanoic acid, 2-methyl-, 1,2,3,7,8,8a-hexahydro-3,7-dimethyl-8-[2-(tetrahydro-4-hydroxy-6-oxo-2*H*-pyran-2-yl)ethyl]-1-naphthalenyl ester, [1*S*-[1 alpha(*R**), 3 alpha,7 beta,8 beta(2*S**,4*S**)8a beta]]-.

Molecular formula: $C_{24}H_{36}O_5$.

Molecular weight: 404.55.

Description: Lovastatin USP—White to off-white, crystalline powder.

Solubility: Lovastatin USP—Freely soluble in choroform; soluble in acetone, in acetonitrile, and in methanol; sparingly soluble in alcohol; practically insoluble in hexane; insoluble in water.

USP requirements:

Lovastatin USP—Preserve in well-closed containers under nitrogen in a cold place. Contains not less than 98.5% and not more than 101.0% of lovastatin, calculated on the dried basis. Meets the requirements for Identification, Specific rotation (+324° to +338°, calculated on the dried basis), Loss on drying (not more than 0.3%), Residue on ignition (not more than 0.2%), Heavy metals (not more than 0.002%), and Chromatographic purity.

Lovastatin Tablets USP—Preserve in well-closed light-resistant containers. Protect from light and store in a cool place or at controlled room temperature. Contain the labeled amount, within ±10%. Meet the requirements for Identification, Dissolution (80% in 30 minutes in buffer solution:*n*-propyl alcohol [2:1] in Apparatus 2 at 50 rpm), and Uniformity of dosage units.

LOXAPINE

Chemical group: A tricyclic dibenzoxazepine derivative.

Chemical name:

Loxapine—Dibenz[*b,f*][1,4]oxazepine, 2-chloro-11-(4-methyl-1-piperazinyl)-.

Loxapine succinate—Butanedioic acid, compd. with 2-chloro-11-(4-methyl-1-piperazinyl)dibenz[*b,f*][1,4]oxazepine (1:1).

Molecular formula:
Loxapine—$C_{18}H_{18}ClN_3O$.
Loxapine hydrochloride—$C_{18}H_{18}ClN_3O \cdot HCl$.
Loxapine succinate—$C_{18}H_{18}ClN_3O \cdot C_4H_6O_4$.

Molecular weight:
Loxapine—327.81.
Loxapine hydrochloride—364.3.
Loxapine succinate—445.90.

Description: Loxapine Succinate USP—White to yellowish, crystalline powder. Is odorless.

pKa: 6.6.

Solubility: Loxapine succinate—Slightly soluble in water and in alcohol.

USP requirements:
Loxapine Capsules USP—Preserve in tight containers. Contain an amount of loxapine succinate equivalent to the labeled amount of loxapine, within ±10%. Label Capsules to state both the content of the active moiety and the content of the salt used in formulating the article. Meet the requirements for Identification, Dissolution (75% in 45 minutes in water in Apparatus 1 at 100 rpm), and Uniformity of dosage units.
Loxapine Hydrochloride Injection—Not in USP.
Loxapine Hydrochloride Oral Solution—Not in USP.
Loxapine Succinate USP—Preserve in tight containers. Contains not less than 98.5% and not more than 101.0% of loxapine succinate, calculated on the dried basis. Meets the requirements for Identification, Melting range (150–153 °C), Loss on drying (not more than 0.5%), Residue on ignition (not more than 0.1%), Heavy metals (not more than 0.002%), Chromatographic purity, and Organic volatile impurities.
Loxapine Succinate Tablets—Not in USP.

LYPRESSIN

Source: A synthetic vasopressin analog.

Chemical name: Vasopressin, 8-L-lysine-.

Molecular formula: $C_{46}H_{65}N_{13}O_{12}S_2$.

Molecular weight: 1056.22.

Description: Hygroscopic, crystalline powder.

Solubility: Freely soluble in water.

USP requirements: Lypressin Nasal Solution USP—Preserve in containers suitable for administering the contents by spraying into the nasal cavities in a controlled individualized dosage. A solution, in a suitable diluent, of the polypeptide hormone, prepared synthetically and free from foreign proteins, which has the properties of causing the contraction of vascular and other smooth muscle and of producing antidiuresis, and which is present in the posterior lobe of the pituitary of healthy pigs. Contains suitable preservatives, and is packaged in a form suitable for nasal administration so that the required dose can be controlled as required. Label it to indicate that it is for intranasal administration only. Label it also to state that the package insert should be consulted for instructions to regulate the dosage according to symptoms. Each mL possesses a pressor activity of the labeled activity of USP Posterior Pituitary Units, within −15% to +20%. Meets the requirements for Oxytocic activity and pH (3.0–4.3).

LYSINE

Chemical name:
Lysine acetate—L-Lysine monoacetate.
Lysine hydrochloride—L-Lysine monohydrochloride.

Molecular formula:
Lysine acetate—$C_6H_{14}N_2O_2 \cdot C_2H_4O_2$.
Lysine hydrochloride—$C_6H_{14}N_2O_2 \cdot HCl$.

Molecular weight:
Lysine acetate—206.24.
Lysine hydrochloride—182.65.

Description:
Lysine Acetate USP—White, odorless crystals or crystalline powder.
Lysine Hydrochloride USP—White, odorless powder.

Solubility:
Lysine Acetate USP—Freely soluble in water.
Lysine Hydrochloride USP—Freely soluble in water.

USP requirements:
Lysine Acetate USP—Preserve in well-closed containers. Contains not less than 98.0% and not more than 102.0% of lysine acetate, as L-lysine acetate, calculated on the dried basis. Meets the requirements for Identification, Specific rotation (+8.0° to +10.0°, calculated on the dried basis), Loss on drying (not more than 0.2%), Residue on ignition (not more than 0.4%), Chloride (not more than 0.05%), Sulfate (not more than 0.03%), Arsenic (not more than 1.5 ppm), Iron (not more than 0.003%), Heavy metals (not more than 0.0015%), and Organic volatile impurities.
Lysine Hydrochloride USP—Preserve in well-closed containers. Contains not less than 98.5% and not more than 101.5% of lysine hydrochloride, as L-lysine hydrochloride, calculated on the dried basis. Meets the requirements for Identification, Specific rotation (+20.4° to +21.4°, calculated on the dried basis), Loss on drying (not more than 0.4%), Residue on ignition (not more than 0.1%), Chloride (19.0–19.6%), Sulfate (not more than 0.03%), Arsenic (not more than 1.5 ppm), Iron (not more than 0.003%), Heavy metals (not more than 0.0015%), and Organic volatile impurities.

MAFENIDE

Chemical group: Methylated sulfonamide.

Chemical name: Mafenide acetate—Benzenesulfonamide, 4-(aminomethyl)-, monoacetate.

Molecular formula: Mafenide acetate—$C_7H_{10}N_2O_2S \cdot C_2H_4O_2$.

Molecular weight: Mafenide acetate—246.28.

Description: Mafenide Acetate USP—White, crystalline powder.

Solubility: Mafenide Acetate USP—Freely soluble in water.

Other characteristics: Sulfonamides have certain chemical similarities to some goitrogens, diuretics (acetazolamide and thiazides), and oral antidiabetic agents.

USP requirements:
Mafenide Acetate USP—Preserve in tight, light-resistant containers. Contains not less than 98.0% and not more than 102.0% of mafenide acetate, calculated on the dried basis. Meets the requirements for Identification, Melting range (162–171 °C, the range between beginning and end of melting not more than 4 °C), pH (6.4–6.8, in a solution [1 in 10]), Loss on drying (not more than 1.0%), Residue

on ignition (not more than 0.2%), Selenium (not more than 0.003%), Heavy metals (not more than 0.002%), Chromatographic purity, and Organic volatile impurities.

Mafenide Acetate Cream USP—Preserve in tight, light-resistant containers, and avoid exposure to excessive heat. It is Mafenide Acetate in a water-miscible, oil-in-water cream base, containing suitable preservatives. Contains an amount of mafenide acetate equivalent to the labeled amount of mafenide, within ±10%. Meets the requirement for Identification.

MAGALDRATE

Source: A combination of aluminum and magnesium hydroxides and sulfate.

Chemical name: Aluminum magnesium hydroxide sulfate.

Molecular formula: $Al_5Mg_{10}(OH)_{31}(SO_4)_2 \cdot xH_2O$.

Molecular weight: 1097.38 (anhydrous, approx.).

Description: Magaldrate USP—White, odorless, crystalline powder.

Solubility: Magaldrate USP—Insoluble in water and in alcohol; soluble in dilute solutions of mineral acids.

USP requirements:

Magaldrate USP—Preserve in well-closed containers. A chemical combination of aluminum and magnesium hydroxides and sulfate, corresponding approximately to the formula: $Al_5Mg_{10}(OH)_{31}(SO_4)_2 \cdot xH_2O$. Contains the equivalent of not less than 90.0% and not more than 105.0% of magaldrate, calculated on the dried basis. Meets the requirements for Identification, Microbial limit, Loss on drying (10.0–20.0%), Soluble chloride (not more than 3.5%), Soluble sulfate (not more than 1.9%), Sodium (not more than 0.11%), Arsenic (not more than 8 ppm), Heavy metals (not more than 0.006%), Magnesium hydroxide content (49.2–66.6%, calculated on the dried basis), Aluminum hydroxide content (32.1–45.9%, calculated on the dried basis), Sulfate content (16.0–21.0%, calculated on the dried basis), and Organic volatile impurities.

Magaldrate Oral Suspension USP—Preserve in tight containers. Contains the labeled amount, within ±10%. Meets the requirements for Identification, Microbial limits, Acid-neutralizing capacity, Magnesium hydroxide content (492–666 mg per gram of labeled amount of magaldrate), and Aluminum hydroxide content (321–459 mg per gram of labeled amount of magaldrate), and for Arsenic and Heavy metals under Magaldrate.

Magaldrate Tablets USP—Preserve in well-closed containers. Label Tablets to indicate whether they are to be swallowed or to be chewed. Contain the labeled amount, within ±10%. Meet the requirements for Identification, Microbial limit, Disintegration (2 minutes, for Magaldrate Tablets labeled to be swallowed), Uniformity of dosage units, Acid-neutralizing capacity, Magnesium hydroxide content (492–666 mg per gram of labeled amount of magaldrate), and Aluminum hydroxide content (321–459 mg per gram of labeled amount of magaldrate).

MAGALDRATE AND SIMETHICONE

For *Magaldrate* and *Simethicone*—See individual listings for chemistry information.

USP requirements:

Magaldrate and Simethicone Oral Suspension USP—Preserve in tight containers, and keep from freezing. Contains the labeled amount of magaldrate, within ±10%. Contains an amount of polydimethylsiloxane equivalent to the labeled amount of simethicone, within ±15%. Meets the requirements for Identification, Acid-neutralizing capacity, Defoaming activity, Microbial limits, Magnesium hydroxide content (492–666 mg per gram of labeled amount of magaldrate), and Aluminum hydroxide content (321–459 mg per gram of labeled amount of magaldrate), and for Arsenic and Heavy metals under Magaldrate.

Magaldrate and Simethicone Tablets USP—Preserve in well-closed containers. Label Tablets to indicate that they are to be chewed before being swallowed. Contain the labeled amount of magaldrate, within ±10%. Contain an amount of polydimethylsiloxane equivalent to the labeled amount of simethicone, within ±15%. Meet the requirements for Identification, Microbial limit, Uniformity of dosage units, Acid-neutralizing capacity, Magnesium hydroxide content (492–666 mg per gram of labeled amount of magaldrate), and Aluminum hydroxide content (321–459 mg per gram of labeled amount of magaldrate).

MAGNESIUM ALUMINUM SILICATE

Description: Magnesium Aluminum Silicate NF—Odorless, fine (micronized) powder or small flakes that are creamy when viewed on their flat surfaces and tan to brown when viewed on their edges.

NF category: Suspending and/or viscosity-increasing agent.

Solubility: Magnesium Aluminum Silicate NF—Insoluble in water and in alcohol. Swells when added to water or glycerin.

NF requirements: Magnesium Aluminum Silicate NF—Preserve in tight containers. A blend of colloidal montmorillonite and saponite that has been processed to remove grit and non-swellable ore components. It is available in 4 types that differ in requirements for viscosity and ratio of aluminum content to magnesium content. Label it to indicate its type. Meets the requirements for Identification, Viscosity, Microbial limits, pH (9.0–10.0, in a suspension [5 in 100] in water), Acid demand (pH not more than 4.0), Loss on drying (not more than 8.0%), Arsenic (not more than 3 ppm), and Lead.

MAGNESIUM CARBONATE

Chemical name: Carbonic acid, magnesium salt, basic; or, Carbonic acid, magnesium salt (1:1), hydrate.

Molecular formula:

Magnesium carbonate—$MgCO_3 \cdot H_2O$.

Magnesium carbonate, basic (approx.)—$(MgCO_3)_4 \cdot Mg(OH)_2 \cdot 5H_2O$.

Molecular weight:

Magnesium carbonate—102.33.

Magnesium carbonate, basic (approx.)—485.65.

Description: Magnesium Carbonate USP—Light, white, friable masses or bulky, white powder. Is odorless, and is stable in air.

Solubility: Magnesium Carbonate USP—Practically insoluble in water; to which, however, it imparts a slightly alkaline reaction; insoluble in alcohol, but is dissolved by dilute acids with effervescence.

USP requirements: Magnesium Carbonate USP—Preserve in well-closed containers. A basic hydrated magnesium carbonate or a normal hydrated magnesium carbonate. Contains the equivalent of not less than 40.0% and not more than 43.5% of magnesium oxide. Meets the requirements for Identification, Microbial limit, Soluble salts (not more than 1.0%), Acid-insoluble substances (not more than 0.05%), Arsenic (not more than 4 ppm), Calcium (not more than 0.45%), Heavy metals (not more than 0.003%), and Iron (not more than 0.02%).

MAGNESIUM CARBONATE AND SODIUM BICARBONATE

For *Magnesium Carbonate* and *Sodium Bicarbonate*—See individual listings for chemistry information.

USP requirements: Magnesium Carbonate and Sodium Bicarbonate for Oral Suspension USP—Preserve in tight containers. Contains the labeled amounts, within ± 10%. Meets the requirements for Identification, Acid-neutralizing capacity, and Minimum fill.

MAGNESIUM CHLORIDE

Chemical name: Magnesium chloride, hexahydrate.

Molecular formula: $MgCl_2 \cdot 6H_2O$.

Molecular weight: 203.30.

Description: Magnesium Chloride USP—Colorless, odorless, deliquescent flakes or crystals, which lose water when heated to 100 °C and lose hydrochloric acid when heated to 110 °C.

Solubility: Magnesium Chloride USP—Very soluble in water; freely soluble in alcohol.

USP requirements:

Magnesium Chloride USP—Preserve in tight containers. Where Magnesium Chloride is intended for use in hemodialysis, it is so labeled. Contains not less than 98.0% and not more than 101.0% of magnesium chloride. Meets the requirements for Identification, pH (4.5–7.0, in a 1 in 20 solution in carbon dioxide-free water), Insoluble matter (not more than 0.005%), Sulfate (not more than 0.005%), Arsenic (not more than 3 ppm), Aluminum (where it is labeled as intended for use in hemodialysis, not more than 1 ppm), Barium, Calcium (not more than 0.01%), Potassium, Heavy metals (not more than 0.001%), and Organic volatile impurities.

Magnesium Chloride Injection—Not in USP.

Magnesium Chloride Tablets—Not in USP.

MAGNESIUM CITRATE

Chemical name: 1,2,3-Propanetricarboxylic acid, hydroxy-, magnesium salt (2:3).

Molecular formula: $C_{12}H_{10}Mg_3O_{14}$.

Molecular weight: 451.12.

Description: Magnesium Citrate Oral Solution USP—Colorless to slightly yellow, clear, effervescent liquid.

USP requirements: Magnesium Citrate Oral Solution USP—Preserve at controlled room temperature or in a cool place, in bottles containing not less than 200 mL. A sterilized or pasteurized solution. Contains, in each 100 mL, not less than 7.59 grams of anhydrous citric acid and an amount of magnesium citrate equivalent to not less than 1.55 grams and not more than 1.9 grams of magnesium oxide.

Prepare Magnesium Citrate Oral Solution as follows: 15 grams of Magnesium Carbonate, 27.4 grams of Anhydrous Citric Acid, 60 mL of Syrup, 5 grams of Talc, 0.1 mL of Lemon Oil, 2.5 grams of Potassium Bicarbonate, and a sufficient quantity of Purified Water to make 350 mL. Dissolve the anhydrous Citric Acid in 150 mL of hot Purified Water in a suitable dish, slowly add the Magnesium Carbonate, previously mixed with 100 mL of Purified Water, and stir until it is dissolved. Then add the Syrup, heat the mixed liquids to the boiling point, immediately add the Lemon Oil, previously triturated with the Talc, and filter the mixture, while hot, into a strong bottle (previously rinsed with boiling Purified Water) of suitable capacity. Add boiled Purified Water to make the product measure 350 mL. Use Purified Cotton as a stopper for the bottle, allow to cool, add the Potassium Bicarbonate, and immediately insert the stopper in the bottle securely. Finally, shake the solution occasionally until the Potassium Bicarbonate is dissolved, cap the bottle, and sterilize or pasteurize the solution.

Note: An amount (30 grams) of citric acid containing 1 molecule of water of hydration, equivalent to 27.4 grams of anhydrous citric acid, may be used in the foregoing formula. In this process the 2.5 grams of potassium bicarbonate may be replaced by 2.1 grams of sodium bicarbonate, preferably in tablet form. The Oral Solution may be further carbonated by the use of carbon dioxide under pressure.

Meets the requirements for Identification, Chloride (not more than 0.01%), Sulfate (not more than 0.015%), and Tartaric acid.

MAGNESIUM GLUCEPTATE

Molecular formula: $C_{14}H_{26}MgO_{16}$.

Molecular weight: 474.7.

USP requirements: Magnesium Gluceptate Oral Solution—Not in USP.

MAGNESIUM GLUCONATE

Chemical name: D-Gluconic acid, magnesium salt (2:1), hydrate.

Molecular formula: $C_{12}H_{22}MgO_{14}$ (anhydrous); $C_{12}H_{22}MgO_{14} \cdot 2H_2O$ (dihydrate).

Molecular weight: 414.60 (anhydrous); 450.63 (dihydrate).

Description: Magnesium Gluconate USP—Colorless crystals or white powder or granules. Odorless.

Solubility: Magnesium Gluconate USP—Freely soluble in water; very slightly soluble in alcohol; insoluble in ether.

USP requirements:

Magnesium Gluconate USP—Preserve in well-closed containers. Contains not less than 98.0% and not more than 102.0% of magnesium gluconate, calculated on the anhydrous basis. Meets the requirements for Identification, pH (6.0–7.8, in a solution [1 in 20]), Water (3.0–12.0%), Chloride (not more than 0.05%), Sulfate (not more than 0.05%), Arsenic (not more than 3 ppm), Heavy metals (not more than 0.002%), Reducing substances (not more than 1.0%), and Organic volatile impurities.

Magnesium Gluconate Tablets USP—Preserve in well-closed containers. Contain the labeled amount, within ± 5%. Meet the requirements for Identification, Dissolution (80% in 30 minutes in water in Apparatus 2 at 50 rpm), and Uniformity of dosage units.

MAGNESIUM HYDROXIDE

Chemical name: Magnesium hydroxide.

Molecular formula: $Mg(OH)_2$.

Molecular weight: 58.32.

Description: Magnesium Hydroxide USP—Bulky, white powder.

Solubility: Magnesium Hydroxide USP—Practically insoluble in water and in alcohol; soluble in dilute acids.

USP requirements:

Magnesium Hydroxide USP—Preserve in tight containers. Dried at 105 °C for 2 hours, contains not less than 95.0% and not more than 100.5% of magnesium hydroxide. Meets the requirements for Identification, Microbial limit, Loss on drying (not more than 2.0%), Loss on ignition (30.0–33.0%), Soluble salts, Carbonate, Arsenic (not more than 3 ppm), Calcium (not more than 0.7%), Heavy metals (not more than 0.004%), and Lead (not more than 0.001%).

Magnesia Tablets USP—Preserve in well-closed containers. Contain an amount of magnesia equivalent to the labeled amount of magnesium hydroxide, within ±7%. Meet the requirements for Identification, Disintegration (10 minutes, simulated gastric fluid TS), Acid-neutralizing capacity, and Uniformity of dosage units.

Milk of Magnesia USP—Preserve in tight containers, preferably at a temperature not exceeding 35 °C. Avoid freezing. A suspension of Magnesium Hydroxide. Double- or Triple-strength Milk of Magnesia is so labeled, or may be labeled as 2X or 3X Concentrated Milk of Magnesia, respectively. Milk of Magnesia, Double-strength Milk of Magnesia, and Triple-strength Milk of Magnesia contain an amount of magnesia equivalent to the labeled amount of magnesium hydroxide, within −10% to +15%, the labeled amount being 80, 160, and 240 mg of magnesium hydroxide per mL, respectively. Meets the requirements for Identification, Acid-neutralizing capacity, Microbial limits, Soluble alkalies, Soluble salts, Carbonate and acid-insoluble matter, Arsenic (not more than $2/W$ ppm, W being the weight, in grams, of specimen taken), Calcium (not more than 0.07%), and Heavy metals (not more than $20/W$ ppm, the W being the weight, in grams, of specimen taken).

Magnesium Hydroxide Paste USP—Preserve in tight containers. An aqueous paste of magnesium hydroxide, each 100 grams of which contains not less than 29.0 grams and not more than 33.0 grams of magnesium hydroxide. Meets the requirements for Identification, Microbial limits, Soluble alkalies, Soluble salts (not more than 12 mg from 1.67 grams of Paste), Carbonate and acid-insoluble matter, Arsenic (not more than 0.6 ppm, based on amount of diluted Paste taken), Calcium (not more than 0.7% based on the magnesium hydroxide content), and Heavy metals (not more than 5 ppm, based on amount of diluted Paste taken).

MAGNESIUM HYDROXIDE AND MINERAL OIL

For *Magnesium Hydroxide* and *Mineral Oil*—See individual listings for chemistry information.

USP requirements: Milk of Magnesia and Mineral Oil Emulsion—Not in USP.

MAGNESIUM HYDROXIDE, MINERAL OIL, AND GLYCERIN

For *Magnesium Hydroxide, Mineral Oil,* and *Glycerin*—See individual listings for chemistry information.

USP requirements: Milk of Magnesia, Mineral Oil, and Glycerin Emulsion—Not in USP.

MAGNESIUM LACTATE

Chemical name: 2-Hydroxypropanoic acid magnesium salt.

Molecular formula: $C_6H_{10}MgO_6$.

Molecular weight: 202.4.

USP requirements: Magnesium Lactate Extended-release Tablets—Not in USP.

MAGNESIUM OXIDE

Chemical name: Magnesium oxide.

Molecular formula: MgO.

Molecular weight: 40.30.

Description: Magnesium Oxide USP—Very bulky, white powder known as Light Magnesium Oxide or relatively dense, white powder known as Heavy Magnesium Oxide. Five grams of Light Magnesium Oxide occupies a volume of approximately 40 to 50 mL, while 5 grams of Heavy Magnesium Oxide occupies a volume of approximately 10 to 20 mL.

Solubility: Magnesium Oxide USP—Practically insoluble in water; soluble in dilute acids; insoluble in alcohol.

USP requirements:

Magnesium Oxide USP—Preserve in tight containers. Label it to indicate whether it is Light Magnesium Oxide or Heavy Magnesium Oxide. After ignition, contains not less than 96.0% and not more than 100.5% of magnesium oxide. Meets the requirements for Identification, Loss on ignition (not more than 10.0%), Free alkali and soluble salts (not more than 2.0%), Acid-insoluble substances (not more than 0.1%), Arsenic (not more than 3 ppm), Calcium (not more than 1.1%), Heavy metals (not more than 0.004%), and Iron (not more than 0.05%).

Magnesium Oxide Capsules USP—Preserve in well-closed containers. Contain the labeled amount, within ±10%. Meet the requirements for Identification, Disintegration (10 minutes in simulated gastric fluid TS), Acid-neutralizing capacity, and Uniformity of dosage units.

Magnesium Oxide Tablets USP—Preserve in well-closed containers. Contain the labeled amount, within ±10%. Meet the requirements for Disintegration (with disks; 10 minutes in simulated gastric fluid TS), Acid-neutralizing capacity (where Tablets are labeled as intended for antacid use), and Uniformity of dosage units, and for Identification test under Magnesium Oxide Capsules.

MAGNESIUM PHOSPHATE

Chemical name: Phosphoric acid, magnesium salt (2:3), pentahydrate.

Molecular formula: $Mg_3(PO_4)_2 \cdot 5H_2O$.

Molecular weight: 352.93.

Description: Magnesium Phosphate USP—White, odorless powder.

Solubility: Magnesium Phosphate USP—Almost insoluble in water; readily soluble in diluted mineral acids.

USP requirements: Magnesium Phosphate USP—Preserve in well-closed containers. Ignited at 425 °C to constant weight, contains not less than 98.0% and not more than 101.5% of magnesium phosphate. Meets the requirements for Identification, Microbial limit, Loss on ignition (20.0–27.0%), Acid-insoluble substances (not more than 0.2%), Soluble substances (not more than 1.5%), Carbonate, Chloride (not more than 0.14%), Nitrate, Sulfate (not more than 0.6%), Arsenic (not more than 3 ppm), Barium, Calcium, Heavy metals (not more than 0.003%), Dibasic salt and magnesium oxide, and Lead (not more than 5 ppm).

MAGNESIUM PIDOLATE

Molecular formula: $(C_5H_6NO_3)_2Mg$.

Molecular weight: 280.5.

USP requirements: Magnesium Pidolate for Oral Solution—Not in USP.

MAGNESIUM SALICYLATE

Chemical name: Magnesium, bis(2-hydroxybenzoato-O^1,O^2)-, tetrahydrate.

Molecular formula: $C_{14}H_{10}MgO_6 \cdot 4H_2O$ (tetrahydrate); $C_{14}H_{10}MgO_6$ (anhydrous).

Molecular weight: 370.60 (tetrahydrate); 298.53 (anhydrous).

Description: White, odorless, efflorescent, crystalline powder.

Solubility: Soluble in 13 parts water; soluble in alcohol.

USP requirements:

Magnesium Salicylate USP—Store in tight containers. Contains not less than 98.0% and not more than 103.0% of magnesium salicylate. Meets the requirements for Identification, Water (17.5–21.0%), Heavy metals (not more than 0.004%), Magnesium content (6.3–6.7%), and Organic volatile impurities.

Magnesium Salicylate Tablets USP—Preserve in tight containers. Contain an amount of magnesium salicylate tetrahydrate equivalent to the labeled amount of anhydrous magnesium salicylate, within ±5%. Meet the requirements for Identification, Dissolution (80% in 120 minutes in water in Apparatus 2 at 50 rpm), and Uniformity of dosage units.

MAGNESIUM SILICATE

Description: Magnesium Silicate NF—Fine, white, odorless powder, free from grittiness.

NF category: Glidant and/or anticaking agent.

Solubility: Magnesium Silicate NF—Insoluble in water and in alcohol. Readily decomposed by mineral acids.

NF requirements: Magnesium Silicate NF—Preserve in well-closed containers. A compound of magnesium oxide and silicon dioxide. Contains not less than 15.0% of magnesium oxide and not less than 67.0% of silicon dioxide, calculated on the ignited basis. Meets the requirements for Identification, pH (7.0–10.8, determined in a well-mixed aqueous suspension [1 in 10]), Loss on drying (not more than 15.0%), Loss on ignition (not more than 15%), Soluble salts (not more than 3.0%), Fluoride (not more than 10 ppm), Free alkali, Arsenic (not more than 3 ppm), Lead (not more than 0.001%), Ratio of silicon dioxide to magnesium oxide (quotient 2.50–4.50), Heavy metals (not more than 0.004%), and Organic volatile impurities.

MAGNESIUM STEARATE

Chemical name: Octadecanoic acid, magnesium salt.

Molecular formula: $C_{36}H_{70}MgO_4$.

Molecular weight: 591.25.

Description: Magnesium Stearate NF—Fine, white, bulky powder, having a faint, characteristic odor. It is unctuous, adheres readily to the skin, and is free from grittiness.

NF category: Tablet and/or capsule lubricant.

Solubility: Magnesium Stearate NF—Insoluble in water, in alcohol, and in ether.

NF requirements: Magnesium Stearate NF—Preserve in tight containers. A compound of magnesium with a mixture of solid organic acids, consisting chiefly of variable proportions of magnesium stearate and magnesium palmitate. The fatty acids are derived from edible sources. Contains not less than 4.0% and not more than 5.0% of Magnesium, calculated on the dried basis. Meets the requirements for Identification, Microbial limits, Acidity or alkalinity, Loss on drying (not more than 6.0%), Limit of chloride (not more than 0.1%), Limit of sulfate (not more than 1.0%), Lead (not more than 0.001%), Organic volatile impurities, and Relative content of stearic acid and palmitic acid.

MAGNESIUM SULFATE

Chemical name: Sulfuric acid magnesium salt (1:1), heptahydrate.

Molecular formula: $MgSO_4 \cdot 7H_2O$.

Molecular weight: 246.47.

Description: Magnesium Sulfate USP—Small, colorless crystals, usually needle-like. It effloresces in warm, dry air.

Solubility: Magnesium Sulfate USP—Freely soluble in water; freely (and slowly) soluble in glycerin; very soluble in boiling water; sparingly soluble in alcohol.

USP requirements:

Magnesium Sulfate USP (Crystals)—Preserve in well-closed containers. The label states whether it is the monohydrate, the dried form, or the heptahydrate. Magnesium Sulfate intended for use in preparing parenteral dosage forms is so labeled. Magnesium Sulfate not intended for use in preparing parenteral dosage forms is so labeled; in addition, it may be labeled also as intended for use in preparing nonparenteral dosage forms. When rendered anhydrous by ignition, contains not less than 99.0% and not more than 100.5% of magnesium sulfate. Meets the requirements for Identification, pH (5.0–9.2, in a solution [1 in 20]), Loss on ignition (monohydrate, 13.0–16.0%; dried form, 22.0–28.0%; heptahydrate, 40.0–52.0%), Chloride (not more than 0.014%), Arsenic (not more than 3 ppm), Heavy metals (not more than 0.001%), Selenium (not more than 0.003%), Iron (not more than 0.002%, when intended for use in preparing nonparenteral dosage forms; not more than 0.5 ppm, when intended for use in preparing parenteral dosage forms), and Organic volatile impurities.

Magnesium Sulfate Injection USP—Preserve in single-dose or in multiple-dose containers, preferably of Type I glass. A sterile solution of Magnesium Sulfate in Water for Injection. The label states the total osmolar concentration in mOsmol per liter. Where the contents are less than 100 mL, or where the label states that the Injection is not for direct injection but is to be diluted before use, the label alternatively may state the total osmolar concentration in mOsmol per mL. Contains the labeled amount, within ±7%. Meets the requirements for Identification, Bacterial endotoxins, pH (5.5–7.0 in a 5% solution), Particulate matter, and Injections.

Magnesium Sulfate Tablets—Not in USP.

MAGNESIUM TRISILICATE

Chemical name: Silicic acid ($H_4Si_3O_8$), magnesium salt (1:2), hydrate.

Molecular formula: $2MgO \cdot 3SiO_2 \cdot xH_2O$ (hydrate); $Mg_2Si_3O_8$ (anhydrous).

Molecular weight: 260.86 (anhydrous).

Description: Magnesium Trisilicate USP—Fine, white, odorless powder, free from grittiness.

Solubility: Magnesium Trisilicate USP—Insoluble in water and in alcohol. Is readily decomposed by mineral acids.

USP requirements:

Magnesium Trisilicate USP—Preserve in well-closed containers. A compound of Magnesium Oxide and silicon dioxide with varying proportions of water. Contains not less than 20.0% of magnesium oxide and not less than 45.0% of silicon dioxide. Meets the requirements for Identification, Water (17.0–34.0%), Soluble salts (not more than 1.5%), Chloride (not more than 0.055%), Sulfate (not more than 0.5%), Free alkali, Arsenic (not more than 8 ppm), Heavy metals (not more than 0.003%), Acid-consuming capacity, and Ratio of silicon dioxide to magnesium oxide (quotient 2.10–2.37).

Magnesium Trisilicate Tablets USP—Preserve in well-closed containers. Contain the labeled amount, within ±10%. Meet the requirements for Identification, Disintegration (10 minutes, in simulated gastric fluid TS), Acid-neutralizing capacity, and Uniformity of dosage units.

MAGNESIUM TRISILICATE, ALUMINA, AND MAGNESIA

For *Magnesium Trisilicate, Alumina* (Aluminum Hydroxide), and *Magnesia* (Magnesium Hydroxide)—See individual listings for chemistry information.

USP requirements:

Magnesium Trisilicate, Alumina, and Magnesia Oral Suspension—Not in USP.

Magnesium Trisilicate, Alumina, and Magnesia Chewable Tablets—Not in USP.

MALATHION

Chemical name: Butanedioic acid, [(dimethoxyphosphinothioyl)-thio]-, diethyl ester.

Molecular formula: $C_{10}H_{19}O_6PS_2$.

Molecular weight: 330.35.

Description: Malathion USP—Yellow to deep brown liquid, having a characteristic odor. Congeals at about 2.9 °C.

Solubility: Malathion USP—Slightly soluble in water. Miscible with alcohols, with esters, with ketones, with ethers, with aromatic and alkylated aromatic hydrocarbons, and with vegetable oils.

USP requirements:

Malathion USP—Preserve in tight, light-resistant containers. Contains not less than 98.0% and not more than 102.0% of malathion. Meets the requirements for Identification, Specific gravity (1.220–1.240), Water (not more than 0.1%), and Isomalathion (not more than 0.3%).

Malathion Lotion USP—Preserve in tight, glass containers. It is Malathion in a suitable isopropyl alcohol vehicle. The labeling states the percentage (v/v) of isopropyl alcohol in the Lotion. Contains the labeled amount, within ±10%. Meets the requirements for Identification and Isopropyl alcohol content (within ±10% of labeled amount).

MALIC ACID

Chemical name: Hydroxybutanedioic acid.

Molecular formula: $C_4H_6O_5$.

Molecular weight: 134.09.

Description: Malic Acid NF—White, or practically white, crystalline powder or granules. Melts at about 130 °C.

NF category: Acidifying agent.

Solubility: Malic Acid NF—Very soluble in water; freely soluble in alcohol.

NF requirements: Malic Acid NF—Preserve in well-closed containers. Contains not less than 99.0% and not more than 100.5% of malic acid. Meets the requirements for Identification, Specific rotation (−0.10° to +0.10°), Residue on ignition (not more than 0.1%), Water-insoluble substances (not more than 0.1%), Heavy metals (not more than 0.002%), Fumaric and maleic acids (not more than 1.0% of fumaric acid; not more than 0.05% of maleic acid), and Organic volatile impurities.

MALTITOL SOLUTION

NF requirements: Maltitol Solution NF—Preserve in tight containers. A water solution of a hydrogenated, partially hydrolyzed starch. Contains, on the anhydrous basis, not less than 50.0% of D-maltitol (w/w), and not more than 16.0% of D-sorbitol (w/w). Meets the requirements for Identification, Water (not more than 30.0%), Residue on ignition (not more than 0.1%), Chloride (not more than 0.005%), Sulfate (not more than 0.010%), Arsenic (not more than 2.5 ppm), Heavy metals (not more than 0.001%), and Reducing sugars.

MALTODEXTRIN

Description: Maltodextrin NF—White, hygroscopic powder or granules.

NF category: Tablet and/or capsule diluent; coating agent; tablet binder; viscosity-increasing agent.

Solubility: Maltodextrin NF—Freely soluble or readily dispersible in water; slightly soluble to insoluble in anhydrous alcohol.

NF requirements: Maltodextrin NF—Preserve in tight containers, or in well-closed containers at a temperature not exceeding 30 °C and a relative humidity not exceeding 50%. A nonsweet, nutritive saccharide mixture of polymers that consist of D-glucose units, with a Dextrose Equivalent less than 20. Prepared by the partial hydrolysis of a food grade starch with suitable acids and/or enzymes. May be physically modified to improve its physical and functional characteristics. Meets the requirements for Microbial limits, pH (4.0–7.0, in a 1 in 5 solution in carbon dioxide-free water), Loss on drying (not more than 6.0%), Residue on ignition (not more than 0.5%), Heavy metals (not more than 5 ppm), Protein (not more than 0.1%), Sulfur dioxide (not more than 0.004%), and Dextrose equivalent (less than 20).

MALT SOUP EXTRACT

Source: Obtained from the grain of one or more varieties of barley; contains 73% maltose, 12% other polymeric carbohydrates, 7% protein, 1.5% potassium, and small amounts of calcium, magnesium, phosphorus, and vitamins.

USP requirements:

Malt Soup Extract Powder—Not in USP.

Malt Soup Extract Oral Solution—Not in USP.

Malt Soup Extract Tablets—Not in USP.

MALT SOUP EXTRACT AND PSYLLIUM

For *Malt Soup Extract* and *Psyllium*—See individual listings for chemistry information.

USP requirements: Malt Soup Extract and Psyllium Powder—Not in USP.

MANGANESE

Chemical name:
Manganese chloride—Manganese chloride ($MnCl_2$) tetrahydrate.
Manganese gluconate—Bis(D-gluconato-O^1,O^2)manganese.
Manganese sulfate—Sulfuric acid, manganese(2+) salt (1:1) monohydrate.

Molecular formula:
Manganese chloride—$MnCl_2 \cdot 4H_2O$.
Manganese gluconate—$C_{12}H_{22}MnO_{14}$.
Manganese sulfate—$MnSO_4 \cdot H_2O$.

Molecular weight:
Manganese chloride—197.91.
Manganese gluconate—445.24.
Manganese sulfate—169.01.

Description:
Manganese Chloride USP—Large, irregular, pink, odorless, translucent crystals.
Manganese Sulfate USP—Pale red, slightly efflorescent crystals, or purple, odorless powder.

Solubility:
Manganese Chloride USP—Soluble in water and in alcohol; insoluble in ether.
Manganese Sulfate USP—Soluble in water; insoluble in alcohol.

USP requirements:
Manganese Chloride USP—Preserve in tight containers. Contains not less than 98.0% and not more than 101.0% of manganese chloride, calculated on the dried basis. Meets the requirements for Identification, Loss on drying (36.0–38.5%), pH (3.5–6.0), Insoluble matter (not more than 0.005%), Sulfate (not more than 0.005%), Substances not precipitated by ammonium sulfide (not more than 0.2% as sulfate), Heavy metals (not more than 5 ppm), Iron (not more than 5 ppm), Zinc, and Organic volatile impurities.
Manganese Chloride Injection USP—Preserve in single-dose or in multiple-dose containers, preferably of Type I or Type II glass. A sterile solution of Manganese Chloride in Water for Injection. Label the Injection to indicate that it is to be diluted to the appropriate strength with Sterile Water for Injection or other suitable fluid prior to administration. Contains an amount of manganese chloride equivalent to the labeled amount of manganese, within ±5%. Meets the requirements for Identification, Bacterial endotoxins, pH (1.5–2.5), Particulate matter, and Injections.
Manganese Gluconate USP—Preserve in well-closed containers. It is dried or contains two molecules of water of hydration. The label indicates whether it is the dried or the dihydrate form. Contains not less than 98.0% and not more than 102.0% of manganese gluconate, calculated on the anhydrous basis. Meets the requirements for Identification, Water (3.0–9.0% where labeled as the dried form and 6.0–9.0% where labeled as the dihydrate), Chloride (not more than 0.05%), Sulfate (not more than 0.2%), Arsenic (not more than 3 ppm), Reducing substances (not more than 1.0%), Heavy metals (not more than 0.004%), Lead (not more than 0.001%), and Organic volatile impurities.
Manganese Gluconate Tablets—Not in USP.
Manganese Sulfate USP—Preserve in tight containers. Contains not less than 98.0% and not more than 102.0% of manganese sulfate. Meets the requirements for Identification, Loss on ignition (10.0–13.0%), Substances not precipitated by ammonium sulfide (not more than 0.5%), and Organic volatile impurities.
Manganese Sulfate Injection USP—Preserve in single-dose or in multiple-dose containers, preferably of Type I or Type II glass. A sterile solution of Manganese Sulfate in Water for Injection. Label the Injection to indicate that it is to be diluted to the appropriate strength with Sterile Water for Injection or other suitable fluid prior to administration. Contains an amount of manganese sulfate equivalent to the labeled amount of manganese, within ±5%. Meets the requirements for Identification, Bacterial endotoxins, pH (2.0–3.5), Particulate matter, and Injections.

MANNITOL

Chemical name: D-Mannitol.

Molecular formula: $C_6H_{14}O_6$.

Molecular weight: 182.17.

Description: Mannitol USP—White, crystalline powder or free-flowing granules. Is odorless.
NF category: Sweetening agent; tablet and/or capsule diluent; tonicity agent; bulking agent for freeze-drying.

Solubility: Mannitol USP—Freely soluble in water; soluble in alkaline solutions; slightly soluble in pyridine; very slightly soluble in alcohol; practically insoluble in ether.

USP requirements:
Mannitol USP—Preserve in well-closed containers. Contains not less than 96.0% and not more than 101.5% of mannitol, calculated on the dried basis. Meets the requirements for Identification, Melting range (165–169 °C), Specific rotation (+137° to +145°), Acidity, Loss on drying (not more than 0.3%), Chloride (not more than 0.007%), Sulfate (not more than 0.01%), Arsenic (not more than 1 ppm), and Reducing sugars.
Mannitol Injection USP—Preserve in single-dose glass or plastic containers. Glass containers are preferably of Type I or Type II glass. A sterile solution, which may be supersaturated, of Mannitol in Water for Injection. Contains no antimicrobial agents. May require warming or autoclaving before use if crystallization has occurred. The label states the total osmolar concentration in mOsmol per liter. Where the contents are less than 100 mL, or where the label states that the Injection is not for direct injection but is to be diluted before use, the label alternatively may state the total osmolar concentration in mOsmol per mL. Contains the labeled amount, within ±5%. Meets the requirements for Identification, Specific rotation, Bacterial endotoxins, pH (4.5–7.0), Particulate matter, and Injections.

MANNITOL AND SODIUM CHLORIDE

For *Mannitol* and *Sodium Chloride*—See individual listings for chemistry information.

USP requirements: Mannitol in Sodium Chloride Injection USP—A sterile solution of Mannitol and Sodium Chloride in Water for Injection. The label states the total osmolar concentration in mOsmol per liter. Where the contents are less than 100 mL, or where the label states that the Injection is not for direct injection but is to be diluted before use, the label alternatively may state the total osmolar concentration in mOsmol per mL. Contains the labeled amounts, within ±5%. Contains no antimicrobial agents. Meets the requirements for Identification, Bacterial endotoxins, and pH (4.5–7.0), for Packaging and storage under Mannitol Injection, and for Injections.

MAPROTILINE

Chemical group: Dibenzo-bicyclo-octadiene.

Chemical name: Maprotiline hydrochloride—9,10-Ethanoanthracene-9(10*H*)-propanamine, *N*-methyl-, hydrochloride.

Molecular formula: Maprotiline hydrochloride—$C_{20}H_{23}N \cdot HCl$.

Molecular weight: Maprotiline hydrochloride—313.87.

Description: Maprotiline Hydrochloride USP—Fine, white to off-white, crystalline powder. Is practically odorless.

Solubility: Maprotiline Hydrochloride USP—Freely soluble in methanol and in chloroform; slightly soluble in water; practically insoluble in isooctane.

USP requirements:

Maprotiline Hydrochloride USP—Preserve in tight containers. Contains not less than 99.0% and not more than 101.0% of maprotiline hydrochloride, calculated on the dried basis. Meets the requirements for Identification, Loss on drying (not more than 1.0%), Residue on ignition (not more than 0.1%), Heavy metals (not more than 0.001%), Chromatographic purity, and Organic volatile impurities.

Maprotiline Hydrochloride Tablets USP—Preserve in well-closed containers. Contain the labeled amount, within ±10%. Meet the requirements for Identification, Dissolution (75% in 60 minutes in dilute hydrochloric acid [7 in 1000] in Apparatus 2 at 50 rpm), and Uniformity of dosage units.

MASOPROCOL

Chemical name: 1,2-Benzenediol, 4,4′-(2,3-dimethyl-1,4-butanediyl)bis-, (*R**,*S**)-.

Molecular formula: $C_{18}H_{22}O_4$.

Molecular weight: 302.37.

Description: White to off-white crystalline powder.

USP requirements: Masoprocol Cream—Not in USP.

MAZINDOL

Chemical group: Imidazoisoindole.

Chemical name: 3*H*-Imidazo[2,1-*a*]isoindol-5-ol, 5-(4-chlorophenyl)-2,5-dihydro-.

Molecular formula: $C_{16}H_{13}ClN_2O$.

Molecular weight: 284.75.

Description: Mazindol USP—White to off-white, crystalline powder, having not more than a faint odor.

Solubility: Mazindol USP—Insoluble in water; slightly soluble in methanol and in chloroform.

USP requirements:

Mazindol USP—Preserve in tight containers. Contains not less than 98.0% and not more than 102.0% of mazindol, calculated on the dried basis. Meets the requirements for Clarity and color of solution, Identification, Loss on drying (not more than 0.5%), Residue on ignition (not more than 0.1%), Heavy metals (not more than 0.002%), Sulfate (not more than 0.04%), and Chromatographic purity.

Mazindol Tablets USP—Preserve in tight containers, at a temperature not exceeding 25 °C. Contain the labeled amount, within ±10%. Meet the requirements for Identification, Dissolution (60% in 60 minutes in 0.1 *N* hydrochloric acid in Apparatus 2 at 50 rpm), and Uniformity of dosage units.

MEASLES AND MUMPS VIRUS VACCINE LIVE

Description: Measles and Mumps Virus Vaccine Live USP—Solid having the characteristic appearance of substances dried from the frozen state. The Vaccine is to be constituted with a suitable diluent just prior to use. Constituted vaccine undergoes loss of potency on exposure to sunlight.

USP requirements: Measles and Mumps Virus Vaccine Live USP—Preserve in single-dose containers, or in light-resistant, multiple-dose containers, at a temperature between 2 and 8 °C. Multiple-dose containers for 50 doses are adapted for use only in jet injectors, and those for 10 doses for use by jet or syringe injection. A bacterially sterile preparation of a combination of live measles virus and live mumps virus such that each component is prepared in conformity with and meets the requirements for Measles Virus Vaccine Live and for Mumps Virus Vaccine Live, whichever is applicable. Each component provides an immunizing dose and meets the requirements of the corresponding Virus Vaccine in the total dosage prescribed in the labeling. Label the Vaccine in multiple-dose containers to indicate that the contents are intended solely for use by jet injector or for use by either jet or syringe injection, whichever is applicable. Label the Vaccine in single-dose containers, if such containers are not light-resistant, to state that it should be protected from sunlight. Label it also to state that constituted Vaccine should be discarded if not used within 8 hours. Meets the requirement for Expiration date (1 to 2 years, depending on the manufacturer's data, after date of issue from manufacturer's cold storage [−20 °C, 1 year]). Conforms to the regulations of the U.S. Food and Drug Administration concerning biologics.

MEASLES, MUMPS, AND RUBELLA VIRUS VACCINE LIVE

Description: Measles, Mumps, and Rubella Virus Vaccine Live USP—Solid having the characteristic appearance of substances dried from the frozen state. The Vaccine is to be constituted with a suitable diluent just prior to use. Constituted vaccine undergoes loss of potency on exposure to sunlight.

USP requirements: Measles, Mumps, and Rubella Virus Vaccine Live USP—Preserve in single-dose containers, or in light-resistant, multiple-dose containers, at a temperature between 2 and 8 °C. Multiple-dose containers for 50 doses are adapted for use only in jet injectors, and those for 10 doses for use by jet or syringe injection. A bacterially sterile preparation of a combination of live measles virus, live mumps virus, and live rubella virus such that each component is prepared in conformity with and meets the requirements for Measles Virus Vaccine Live, for Mumps Virus Vaccine Live, and for Rubella Virus Vaccine Live, whichever is applicable. Each component provides an immunizing dose and meets the requirements of the corresponding Virus Vaccine in the total dosage prescribed in the labeling. Label the Vaccine in multiple-dose containers to indicate that the contents are intended solely for use by jet injector or for use by either jet or syringe injection, whichever is applicable. Label the Vaccine in single-dose containers, if such containers are not light-resistant, to state that it should be protected from sunlight. Label it also to state that constituted Vaccine should be discarded if not used within 8 hours. Meets the requirement for Expiration date (1 to 2 years, depending on the manufacturer's data, after date of issue from manufacturer's cold storage [−20 °C, 1 year]). Conforms to the regulations of the U.S. Food and Drug Administration concerning biologics.

MEASLES AND RUBELLA VIRUS VACCINE LIVE

Description: Measles and Rubella Virus Vaccine Live USP—Solid having the characteristic appearance of substances dried from the frozen state. The Vaccine is to be constituted with a suitable diluent just prior to use. Constituted vaccine undergoes loss of potency on exposure to sunlight.

USP requirements: Measles and Rubella Virus Vaccine Live USP—Preserve in single-dose containers, or in light-resistant, multiple-dose containers, at a temperature between 2 and 8 °C. Multiple-dose containers for 50 doses are adapted for use only in jet injectors, and those for 10 doses for use by jet or syringe injection. A bacterially sterile preparation of a combination of live measles virus and live rubella virus such that each component is prepared in conformity with and meets the requirements for Measles Virus Vaccine Live and for Rubella Virus Vaccine Live, whichever is applicable. Each component provides an immunizing dose and meets the requirements of the corresponding Virus Vaccine in the total dosage prescribed in the labeling. Label the Vaccine in multiple-dose containers to indicate that the contents are intended solely for use by jet injector or for use by either jet or syringe injection, whichever is applicable. Label the Vaccine in single-dose containers, if such containers are not light-resistant, to state that it should be protected from sunlight. Label it also to state that constituted Vaccine should be discarded if not used within 8 hours. Meets the requirement for Expiration date (1 to 2 years, depending on the manufacturer's data, after date of issue from manufacturer's cold storage [−20 °C, 1 year]). Conforms to the regulations of the U.S. Food and Drug Administration concerning biologics.

MEASLES VIRUS VACCINE LIVE

Source: The currently available vaccine in the U.S. (*Attenuvax*, MSD) contains a lyophilized preparation of a more attenuated line of live measles virus derived from Enders' attenuated Edmonston strain. Further modification of the virus was achieved by multiple passage of Edmonston virus in cell cultures of chick embryo at low temperature. *Attenuvax*, Morson (UK) and Measles Virus Vaccine, Live Attenuated (Dried), Connaught (Canada) brands of live measles virus vaccine also contain the Enders' attenuated Edmonston strain.

Description: Measles Virus Vaccine Live USP—Solid having the characteristic appearance of substances dried from the frozen state. Undergoes loss of potency on exposure to sunlight. The Vaccine is to be constituted with a suitable diluent just prior to use.

Other characteristics: Slightly acidic, pH 6.2 to 6.6.

USP requirements: Measles Virus Vaccine Live USP—Preserve in single-dose containers, or in light-resistant, multiple-dose containers, at a temperature between 2 and 8 °C. Multiple-dose containers for 50 doses are adapted for use only in jet injectors, and those for 10 doses for use by jet or syringe injection. A bacterially sterile preparation of live virus derived from a strain of measles virus tested for neurovirulence in monkeys, for safety, and for immunogenicity, free from all demonstrable viable microbial agents except unavoidable bacteriophage, and found suitable for human immunization. The strain is grown for purposes of vaccine production on chicken embryo primary cell tissue cultures derived from pathogen-free flocks, meets the requirements of the specific safety tests in adult and suckling mice; the requirements of the tests in monkey kidney, chicken embryo and human tissue cell cultures and embryonated eggs; and the requirements of the tests for absence of *Mycobacterium tuberculosis* and of avian leucosis, unless the production cultures were derived from certified avian leucosis-free sources and the control fluids were tested for avian leucosis. The strain cultures are treated to remove all intact tissue cells. The Vaccine meets the requirements of the specific tissue culture test for live virus titer, in a single immunizing dose, of not less than the equivalent of 1000 $TCID_{50}$ (quantity of virus estimated to infect 50% of inoculated cultures × 1000) when tested in parallel with the U.S. Reference Measles Virus, Live Attenuated. Label the Vaccine in multiple-dose containers to indicate that the contents are intended solely for use by jet injector or for use by either jet or syringe injection, whichever is applicable. Label the Vaccine in single-dose containers, if such containers are not light-resistant, to state that it should be protected from sunlight. Label it also to state that constituted Vaccine should be discarded if not used within 8 hours. Meets the requirement for Expiration date (1 to 2 years, depending on the manufacturer's data, after date of issue from manufacturer's cold storage [−20 °C, 1 year]). Conforms to the regulations of the U.S. Food and Drug Administration concerning biologics.

MEBENDAZOLE

Chemical group: Benzimidazole carbamate derivative.

Chemical name: Carbamic acid, (5-benzoyl-1*H*-benzimidazol-2-yl)-, methyl ester.

Molecular formula: $C_{16}H_{13}N_3O_3$.

Molecular weight: 295.30.

Description: Mebendazole USP—White to slightly yellow powder. Is almost odorless. Melts at about 290 °C.

Solubility: Mebendazole USP—Practically insoluble in water, in dilute solutions of mineral acids, in alcohol, in ether, and in chloroform; freely soluble in formic acid.

USP requirements:

Mebendazole USP—Preserve in well-closed containers. Contains not less than 98.0% and not more than 102.0% of mebendazole, calculated on the dried basis. Meets the requirements for Identification, Loss on drying (not more than 0.5%), Residue on ignition (not more than 0.1%), Heavy metals (not more than 0.002%), and Chromatographic purity.

Mebendazole Tablets USP—Preserve in well-closed containers. Contain the labeled amount, within ±10%. Meet the requirements for Identification, Disintegration (10 minutes), and Uniformity of dosage units.

MEBROFENIN

Chemical name: Glycine, *N*-[2-[(3-bromo-2,4,6-trimethylphenyl)-amino]-2-oxoethyl]-*N*-(carboxymethyl)-.

Molecular formula: $C_{15}H_{19}BrN_2O_5$.

Molecular weight: 387.23.

USP requirements: Mebrofenin USP—Preserve in tight containers. Contains not less than 97.0% and not more than 101.0% of mebrofenin, calculated on the dried basis. Meets the requirements for Identification, Melting range (185–200 °C, the range between beginning and end of melting not more than 4 °C), Loss on drying (not more than 0.3%), Residue on ignition (not more than 0.1%), Heavy metals (not more than 0.003%), Limit of nitrilotriacetic acid (not more than 0.1%), and Chromatographic purity.

MECAMYLAMINE

Chemical name: Mecamylamine hydrochloride—Bicyclo[2.2.1]-heptan-2-amine, *N*,2,3,3-tetramethyl-, hydrochloride.

Molecular formula: Mecamylamine hydrochloride—$C_{11}H_{21}N \cdot HCl$.

Molecular weight: Mecamylamine hydrochloride—203.76.

Description: Mecamylamine hydrochloride—White, odorless or practically odorless, crystalline powder. Melts at about 245 °C, with decomposition.

pKa: Mecamylamine hydrochloride—11.2.

Solubility: Mecamylamine hydrochloride—Freely soluble in water and in chloroform; soluble in isopropyl alcohol; practically insoluble in ether.

USP requirements:

Mecamylamine Hydrochloride USP—Preserve in tight containers. Contains not less than 95.0% and not more than 100.5% of mecamylamine hydrochloride, calculated on the dried basis. Meets the requirements for Identification, Acidity, Loss on drying (not more than 1.0%), Residue on ignition (not more than 0.5%), Heavy metals (not more than 0.005%), Organic volatile impurities, and Chloride content (17.0–17.8%).

Mecamylamine Hydrochloride Tablets USP—Preserve in well-closed containers. Contain the labeled amount, within ±10%. Meet the requirements for Identification, Dissolution (75% in 30 minutes in water in Apparatus 2 at 50 rpm), and Uniformity of dosage units.

MECHLORETHAMINE

Chemical name: Mechlorethamine hydrochloride—Ethanamine, 2-chloro-*N*-(2-chloroethyl)-*N*-methyl-, hydrochloride.

Molecular formula: Mechlorethamine hydrochloride—$C_5H_{11}Cl_2N \cdot HCl$.

Molecular weight: Mechlorethamine hydrochloride—192.52.

Description: Mechlorethamine Hydrochloride USP—White, crystalline powder. Is hygroscopic.

pKa: Mechlorethamine hydrochloride—6.1.

Solubility: Mechlorethamine hydrochloride—Very soluble in water; soluble in alcohol.

USP requirements:

Mechlorethamine Hydrochloride USP—Preserve in tight, light-resistant containers. The label bears a warning that great care should be taken to prevent inhaling particles of Mechlorethamine Hydrochloride and exposing the skin to it. Contains not less than 97.5% and not more than 100.5% of mechlorethamine hydrochloride, calculated on the anhydrous basis. Meets the requirements for Identification, Melting range (108–111 °C), pH (3.0–5.0, in a solution [1 in 500]), Water (not more than 0.4%), and Ionic chloride content (18.0–19.3%).

Mechlorethamine Hydrochloride for Injection USP—Preserve in Containers for Sterile Solids. A sterile mixture of Mechlorethamine Hydrochloride with Sodium Chloride or other suitable diluent. The label bears a warning that great care should be taken to prevent inhaling particles of Mechlorethamine Hydrochloride for Injection and exposing the skin to it. Contains the labeled amount, within ±10%. Meets the requirements for Labeling under Injections, Completeness of solution, Constituted solution, Identification, Bacterial endotoxins, pH (3.0–5.0, in a solution [1 in 50]), Water (not more than 1.0%), and Particulate matter, and for Sterility tests and Uniformity of dosage units.

Mechlorethamine Hydrochloride Ointment—Not in USP.

Mechlorethamine Hydrochloride Topical Solution—Not in USP.

MECLIZINE

Chemical group: Piperazine derivative.

Chemical name: Meclizine hydrochloride—Piperazine, 1-[(4-chlorophenyl)phenylmethyl]-4-[(3-methylphenyl)methyl]-, dihydrochloride, monohydrate.

Molecular formula: Meclizine hydrochloride—$C_{25}H_{27}ClN_2 \cdot 2HCl \cdot H_2O$.

Molecular weight: Meclizine hydrochloride—481.89.

Description: Meclizine Hydrochloride USP—White or slightly yellowish, crystalline powder. Has a slight odor.

Solubility: Meclizine Hydrochloride USP—Practically insoluble in water and in ether; freely soluble in chloroform, in pyridine, and in acid-alcohol-water mixtures; slightly soluble in dilute acids and in alcohol.

USP requirements:

Meclizine Hydrochloride USP—Preserve in tight containers. Contains not less than 97.0% and not more than 100.5% of meclizine hydrochloride, calculated on the anhydrous basis. Meets the requirements for Identification, Water (not more than 5.0%), Residue on ignition (not more than 0.1%), and Chromatographic purity.

Meclizine Hydrochloride Capsules—Not in USP.

Meclizine Hydrochloride Tablets USP—Preserve in well-closed containers. Contain the labeled amount, within −5% to +10%. Meet the requirements for Identification, Dissolution (75% in 45 minutes in 0.1 *N* hydrochloric acid in Apparatus 1 at 100 rpm), and Uniformity of dosage units.

MECLOCYCLINE

Chemical name: Meclocycline sulfosalicylate—2-Naphthacenecarboxamide, 7-chloro-4-(dimethylamino)-1,4,4a,5,5a,6,-11,12a-octahydro-3,5,10,12,12a-pentahydroxy-6-methylene-1,11-dioxo-, [4*S*-(4 alpha,4a alpha,5 alpha,5a alpha,12a alpha)]-, mono(2-hydroxy-5-sulfobenzoate) (salt).

Molecular formula: Meclocycline sulfosalicylate—$C_{22}H_{21}ClN_2O_8 \cdot C_7H_6O_6S$.

Molecular weight: Meclocycline sulfosalicylate—695.05.

Description: Meclocycline sulfosalicylate—Yellow, crystalline powder.

USP requirements:

Meclocycline Sulfosalicylate USP—Preserve in tight containers, protected from light. Has a potency equivalent to not less than 620 mcg of meclocycline per mg. Meets the requirements for Identification, Crystallinity, pH (2.5–3.5, in a solution containing 10 mg per mL), and Water (not more than 4.0%).

Meclocycline Sulfosalicylate Cream USP—Preserve in tight containers, protected from light. Contains an amount of meclocycline sulfosalicylate equivalent to the labeled amount of meclocycline, within −10% to +25%. Meets the requirement for Minimum fill.

MECLOFENAMATE

Chemical group: Fenamate derivative.

Chemical name: Meclofenamate sodium—Benzoic acid, 2-[(2,6-dichloro-3-methylphenyl)amino]-, monosodium salt, monohydrate.

Molecular formula: Meclofenamate sodium—$C_{14}H_{10}Cl_2NNaO_2 \cdot H_2O$.

Molecular weight: Meclofenamate sodium—336.15.

Description: Meclofenamate Sodium USP—White to creamy white, odorless to almost odorless, crystalline powder.

Solubility: Meclofenamate Sodium USP—Soluble in methanol; slightly soluble in chloroform; practically insoluble in ether. Freely soluble in water, the solution sometimes being somewhat turbid due to partial hydrolysis and absorption of carbon dioxide; the solution is clear above pH 11.5.

USP requirements:

Meclofenamate Sodium USP—Preserve in tight, light-resistant containers. Contains not less than 97.0% and not more than 103.0% of meclofenamate sodium, calculated on the anhydrous basis. Meets the requirements for Identification, Water (4.8–5.8%), Copper, Chromatographic purity, and Organic volatile impurities.

Meclofenamate Sodium Capsules USP—Preserve in tight, light-resistant containers. Contain an amount of meclofenamate sodium equivalent to the labeled amount of meclofenamic acid, within ±10%. Meet the requirements for Identification, Dissolution (75% in 45 minutes in 0.05 *M* phosphate buffer [pH 8.0] in Apparatus 2 at 50 rpm), and Uniformity of dosage units.

MEDROXYPROGESTERONE

Chemical name: Medroxyprogesterone acetate—Pregn-4-ene-3,20-dione, 17-(acetyloxy)-6-methyl-, (6 alpha)-.

Molecular formula: Medroxyprogesterone acetate—$C_{24}H_{34}O_4$.

Molecular weight: Medroxyprogesterone acetate—386.53.

Description: Medroxyprogesterone Acetate USP—White to off-white, odorless, crystalline powder. Melts at about 205 °C. Is stable in air.

Solubility: Medroxyprogesterone Acetate USP—Insoluble in water; freely soluble in chloroform; soluble in acetone and in dioxane; sparingly soluble in alcohol and in methanol; slightly soluble in ether.

USP requirements:

Medroxyprogesterone Acetate USP—Preserve in tight, light-resistant containers. Contains not less than 97.0% and not more than 103.0% of medroxyprogesterone acetate, calculated on the dried basis. Meets the requirements for Identification, Specific rotation (+45° to +51°, calculated on the dried basis), and Loss on drying (not more than 1.0%).

Sterile Medroxyprogesterone Acetate Suspension USP—Preserve in single-dose or in multiple-dose containers, preferably of Type I glass. A sterile suspension of Medroxyprogesterone Acetate in a suitable aqueous medium. Contains the labeled amount, within ±10%. Meets the requirements for Identification, pH (3.0–7.0), and Injections.

Medroxyprogesterone Acetate Tablets USP—Preserve in well-closed containers. Contain the labeled amount, within ±7%. Meet the requirements for Identification, Dissolution (50% in 45 minutes in 0.5% sodium lauryl sulfate in Apparatus 2 at 50 rpm), and Uniformity of dosage units.

MEDRYSONE

Chemical name: Pregn-4-ene-3,20-dione, 11-hydroxy-6-methyl-, (6 alpha,11 beta)-.

Molecular formula: $C_{22}H_{32}O_3$.

Molecular weight: 344.49.

Description: Medrysone USP—White to off-white, crystalline powder. Is odorless or may have a slight odor. Melts at about 158 °C, with decomposition.

Solubility: Medrysone USP—Sparingly soluble in water; soluble in methylene chloride and in chloroform.

USP requirements:

Medrysone USP—Preserve in well-closed containers. Contains not less than 97.0% and not more than 103.0% of medrysone, calculated on the dried basis. Meets the requirements for Identification, Specific rotation (+186° to +194°, calculated on the dried basis), Loss on drying (not more than 3.0%), and Ordinary impurities.

Medrysone Ophthalmic Suspension USP—Preserve in tight, light-resistant containers. A sterile suspension of Medrysone in a buffered aqueous medium containing a suitable antimicrobial agent and preservative. Contains the labeled amount, within −10% to +15%. Meets the requirements for Identification, Sterility, and pH (6.2–7.5).

MEFENAMIC ACID

Chemical group: Fenamate derivative.

Chemical name: Benzoic acid, 2-[(2,3-dimethylphenyl)amino]-.

Molecular formula: $C_{15}H_{15}NO_2$.

Molecular weight: 241.29.

Description: Mefenamic Acid USP—White to off-white, crystalline powder. Melts at about 230 °C, with decomposition.

pKa: 4.2.

Solubility: Mefenamic Acid USP—Soluble in solutions of alkali hydroxides; sparingly soluble in chloroform; slightly soluble in alcohol and in methanol; practically insoluble in water.

USP requirements:

Mefenamic Acid USP—Preserve in tight, light-resistant containers. Contains not less than 98.0% and not more than 102.0% of mefenamic acid, calculated on the dried basis. Meets the requirements for Identification, Loss on drying (not more than 1.0%), Residue on ignition (not more than 0.1%), Heavy metals (not more than 0.002%), and Ordinary impurities.

Mefenamic Acid Capsules USP—Preserve in tight containers. Contain the labeled amount, within ±10%. Meet the requirements for Identification and Uniformity of dosage units.

MEFLOQUINE

Chemical name: Mefloquine hydrochloride—4-Quinolinemethanol, alpha-2-piperidinyl-2,8-bis(trifluoromethyl)-, monohydrochloride, (R^*,S^*)-(±)-.

Molecular formula: Mefloquine hydrochloride—$C_{17}H_{16}F_6N_2O \cdot HCl$.

Molecular weight: Mefloquine hydrochloride—414.78.

Description: Mefloquine hydrochloride—White to almost white crystalline compound.

Solubility: Mefloquine hydrochloride—Slightly soluble in water.

USP requirements: Mefloquine Hydrochloride Tablets—Not in USP.

MEGESTROL

Chemical name: Megestrol acetate—Pregna-4,6-diene-3,20-dione, 17-(acetyloxy)-6-methyl-.

Molecular formula: Megestrol acetate—$C_{24}H_{32}O_4$.

Molecular weight: Megestrol acetate—384.52.

Description: Megestrol Acetate USP—White to creamy white, essentially odorless, crystalline powder. Is unstable under aqueous conditions at pH 7 or above.

Solubility: Megestrol Acetate USP—Insoluble in water; sparingly soluble in alcohol; slightly soluble in ether and in fixed oils; soluble in acetone; very soluble in chloroform.

USP requirements:

Megestrol Acetate USP—Preserve in well-closed containers, protected from light. Contains not less than 97.0% and not more than 103.0% of megestrol acetate, calculated on the anhydrous basis. Meets the requirements for Completeness of solution, Identification, Melting range (213–220 °C, the range between beginning and end of melting not more than 3 °C), Specific rotation (+8.8° to +12.0°, calculated on the anhydrous basis), Water (not more than 0.5%), Residue on ignition (not more than 0.2%), and Heavy metals (not more than 0.002%).

Megestrol Acetate Suspension—Not in USP.

Megestrol Acetate Tablets USP—Preserve in well-closed containers. Contain the labeled amount, within ±7%. Meet the requirements for Identification, Dissolution (75% in 60 minutes in 1% sodium lauryl sulfate in Apparatus 2 at 100 rpm), and Uniformity of dosage units.

MEGLUMINE

Chemical name: D-Glucitol, 1-deoxy-1-(methylamino)-.

Molecular formula: $C_7H_{17}NO_5$.

Molecular weight: 195.22.

Description: Meglumine USP—White to faintly yellowish white, odorless crystals or powder.

Solubility: Meglumine USP—Freely soluble in water; sparingly soluble in alcohol.

USP requirements: Meglumine USP—Preserve in well-closed containers. Contains not less than 99.0% and not more than 100.5% of meglumine, calculated on the dried basis. Meets the requirements for Identification, Melting range (128–132 °C), Specific rotation (−15.7° to −17.3°), Loss on drying (not more than 1.0%), Residue on ignition (not more than 0.1%), Absence of reducing substances, and Heavy metals (not more than 0.002%).

MELPHALAN

Chemical name: L-Phenylalanine, 4-[bis(2-chloroethyl)amino]-.

Molecular formula: $C_{13}H_{18}Cl_2N_2O_2$.

Molecular weight: 305.20.

Description: Melphalan USP—Off-white to buff powder, having a faint odor. Melts at about 180 °C, with decomposition.

Solubility: Melphalan USP—Practically insoluble in water, in chloroform, and in ether; soluble in dilute mineral acids; slightly soluble in alcohol and in methanol.

USP requirements:

Melphalan USP—Preserve in tight, light-resistant, glass containers. Contains not less than 93.0% and not more than 100.5% of melphalan, calculated on the dried and ionizable chlorine-free basis. Meets the requirements for Identification, Specific rotation (−30° to −36°, calculated on the dried basis), Loss on drying (not more than 7.0%), Residue on ignition (not more than 0.3%), Ionizable chlorine, and Nitrogen content (8.90–9.45%).

Caution: Handle Melphalan with exceptional care since it is a highly potent agent.

Melphalan Tablets USP—Preserve in well-closed, light-resistant, glass containers. Contain the labeled amount, within ±10%. Meet the requirements for Identification, Disintegration (15 minutes), and Uniformity of dosage units.

Melphalan Hydrochloride for Injection—Not in USP.

MENADIOL

Chemical name: Menadiol sodium diphosphate—1,4-Naphthalenediol, 2-methyl-, bis(dihydrogen phosphate), tetrasodium salt, hexahydrate.

Molecular formula: Menadiol sodium diphosphate—$C_{11}H_8Na_4O_8P_2 \cdot 6H_2O$.

Molecular weight: Menadiol sodium diphosphate—530.18.

Description: Menadiol Sodium Diphosphate USP—White to pink powder, having a characteristic odor. Is hygroscopic. Its solutions are neutral or slightly alkaline to litmus, having a pH of about 8.

Solubility: Menadiol Sodium Diphosphate USP—Very soluble in water; insoluble in alcohol.

USP requirements:

Menadiol Sodium Diphosphate USP—Preserve in tight, light-resistant containers, and store in a cold place. Contains not less than 97.5% and not more than 102.0% of menadiol sodium diphosphate, calculated on the anhydrous basis. Meets the requirements for Identification and Water (19.0–21.5%).

Menadiol Sodium Diphosphate Injection USP—Preserve in single-dose, light-resistant containers, preferably of Type I glass. A sterile solution of Menadiol Sodium Diphosphate in Water for Injection. Contains the labeled amount, within −5% to +10%. Meets the requirements for Identification, Bacterial endotoxins, pH (7.5–8.5), and Injections.

Menadiol Sodium Diphosphate Tablets USP—Preserve in well-closed, light-resistant containers. Contain the labeled amount, within −5% to +10%. Meet the requirements for Identification, Dissolution (75% in 30 minutes in 0.1 *N* hydrochloric acid in Apparatus 1 at 100 rpm), and Uniformity of dosage units.

MENADIONE

Chemical name: 1,4-Naphthalenedione, 2-methyl.

Molecular formula: $C_{11}H_8O_2$.

Molecular weight: 172.18.

Description: Menadione USP—Bright yellow, crystalline, practically odorless powder. Affected by sunlight.

Solubility: Menadione USP—Practically insoluble in water; soluble in vegetable oils; sparingly soluble in chloroform and in alcohol.

USP requirements:

Menadione USP—Preserve in well-closed, light-resistant containers. Contains not less than 98.5% and not more than 101.0% of menadione, calculated on the dried basis. Meets the requirements for Identification, Melting range (105–107 °C), Loss on drying (not more than 0.3%), Residue on ignition (not more than 0.1%), and Ordinary impurities.

Caution: Menadione powder is irritating to the respiratory tract and to the skin, and a solution of it in alcohol is a vesicant.

Menadione Injection USP—Preserve in single-dose or in multiple-dose containers, preferably of Type I glass. A sterile solution of Menadione in oil. Contains the labeled amount, within −10% to +20%. Meets the requirements for Bacterial endotoxins and Injections.

MENINGOCOCCAL POLYSACCHARIDE VACCINE

Source: The vaccine currently available in the U.S. and Canada contains a freeze-dried preparation of the group-specific polysaccharide antigens from *Neisseria meningitidis*, Group A, Group C, Group Y, and Group W-135.

USP requirements:

Meningococcal Polysaccharide Vaccine for Injection—Not in USP.

Meningococcal Polysaccharide Vaccine Group A USP—Preserve in multiple-dose containers for subcutaneous or jet injection at a temperature between 2 and 8 °C. (Note: Use the constituted vaccine immediately after its constitution, or if stored in a refrigerator within 8 hours after constitution.) A sterile preparation of the group-specific polysaccharide antigen from *Neisseria meningitidis*, Group A, consisting of a polymer of *N*-acetyl mannosamine phosphate. Contains 50 mcg of isolated product and 2.5 to 5 mg of lactose as a stabilizer per 0.5-mL dose, when constituted as directed. The constituting fluid is Bacteriostatic Sodium Chloride Injection in which the antimicrobial agent is Thimerosal in a suitable concentration. Meets the requirements of the tests for potency, and for Expiration date (not later than 18 months after date of issue from manufacturer's cold storage [−20 °C, 6 months]). Conforms to the regulations of the U.S. Food and Drug Administration concerning biologics.

Meningococcal Polysaccharide Vaccine Groups A and C Combined USP—Preserve in multiple-dose containers for subcutaneous or jet injection at a temperature between 2 and 8 °C. (Note: Use the constituted vaccine immediately after its constitution, or if stored in a refrigerator within 8 hours after constitution.) A sterile preparation consisting of Meningococcal Polysaccharide Group A and C specific antigens. Contains 50 mcg of each isolated product and 2.5 to 5 mg of lactose as a stabilizer per 0.5-mL dose, when constituted as directed. The constituting fluid is Bacteriostatic Sodium Chloride Injection in which the antimicrobial agent is Thimerosal in a suitable concentration. Each component meets the requirements for antigenicity or potency, and for Expiration date (not later than 18 months after date of issue from manufacturer's cold storage [−20 °C, 6 months]). Conforms to the regulations of the U.S. Food and Drug Administration concerning biologics.

Meningococcal Polysaccharide Vaccine Group C USP—Preserve in multiple-dose containers for subcutaneous or jet injection at a temperature between 2 and 8 °C. (Note: Use the constituted vaccine immediately after its constitution, or if stored in a refrigerator within 8 hours after constitution.) A sterile preparation of the group-specific polysaccharide antigen from *Neisseria meningitidis*, Group C, consisting of a polymer of sialic acid. Contains 50 mcg of isolated product and 2.5 to 5 mg of lactose as a stabilizer per 0.5-mL dose, when constituted as directed. The constituting fluid is Bacteriostatic Sodium Chloride Injection in which the antimicrobial agent is Thimerosal in a suitable concentration. Meets the requirements of the tests for potency, and for Expiration date (not later than 18 months after date of issue from manufacturer's cold storage [−20 °C, 6 months]). Conforms to the regulations of the U.S. Food and Drug Administration concerning biologics.

MENOTROPINS

Source: Extracted from urine of postmenopausal women.

Chemical name: Follicle stimulating hormone.

USP requirements:

Menotropins USP—Preserve in tight containers, preferably of Type I glass, in a refrigerator. An extract of human postmenopausal urine containing both follicle-stimulating hormone and luteinizing hormone, having the property in females of stimulating growth and maturation of ovarian follicles and the properties in males of maintaining and stimulating testicular interstitial cells (Leydig tissue) related to testosterone production and of being responsible for the full development and maturation of spermatozoa in the seminiferous tubules. Has a potency of not less than 40 USP Follicle-stimulating Hormone Units and not less than 40 USP Luteinizing Hormone Units per mg, and contains each of the hormone potencies stated on the label, within −20% to +25%. The ratio of units of Follicle-stimulating Hormone to units of Luteinizing Hormone is approximately 1. Meets the requirements for Bacterial endotoxins, Safety, and Water (not more than 5.0%).

Menotropins for Injection USP—Preserve in Containers for Sterile Solids. A sterile, freeze-dried mixture of menotropins and suitable excipients. Contains labeled potencies of Follicle-stimulating Hormone and Luteinizing Hormone, within −20% to +25%. Meets the requirements for Constituted solution, Bacterial endotoxins, and pH (6.0–7.0, in the solution constituted as directed in the labeling), and for Sterility tests, Uniformity of dosage units, and Labeling under Injections.

MENTHOL

Chemical name: Cyclohexanol, 5-methyl-2-(1-methylethyl)-.

Molecular formula: $C_{10}H_{20}O$.

Molecular weight: 156.27.

Description: Menthol USP—Colorless, hexagonal crystals, usually needle-like, or in fused masses, or crystalline powder. It has a pleasant, peppermint-like odor.

NF category: Flavors and perfumes.

Solubility: Menthol USP—Slightly soluble in water; very soluble in alcohol, in chloroform, in ether, and in solvent hexane; freely soluble in glacial acetic acid, in mineral oil, and in fixed and volatile oils.

USP requirements: Menthol USP—Preserve in tight containers, preferably at controlled room temperature. An alcohol obtained from diverse mint oils or prepared synthetically. Menthol may be levorotatory (*l*-Menthol), from natural or synthetic sources, or racemic (*dl*-Menthol). Label it to indicate whether it is levorotatory or racemic. Meets the requirements for Identification, Melting range of *l*-Menthol (41–44 °C), Congealing range of *dl*-Menthol, Specific rotation (−45° to −51° for *l*-Menthol; −2° to +2° for *dl*-Menthol), Nonvolatile residue (not more than 0.05%), Readily oxidizable substances in *dl*-Menthol, Chromatographic purity, and Organic volatile impurities.

MEPENZOLATE

Chemical group: Quaternary ammonium compound.

Chemical name: Mepenzolate bromide—Piperidinium, 3-[(hydroxydiphenylacetyl)oxy]-1,1-dimethyl-, bromide.

Molecular formula: Mepenzolate bromide—$C_{21}H_{26}BrNO_3$.

Molecular weight: Mepenzolate bromide—420.35.

Description: Mepenzolate bromide—White or light cream-colored powder.

Solubility: Mepenzolate bromide—Slightly soluble in water and in chloroform; freely soluble in methanol; practically insoluble in ether.

USP requirements:

Mepenzolate Bromide USP—Preserve in tight containers. Contains not less than 98.0% and not more than 101.0% of mepenzolate bromide, calculated on the dried basis. Meets the requirements for Identification, Loss on drying (not more than 0.5%), Residue on ignition (not more than 0.2%), Heavy metals (not more than 0.002%), Organic volatile impurities, and Bromide content (18.60–19.40%).

Mepenzolate Bromide Syrup USP—Preserve in tight, light-resistant containers. Contains the labeled amount, within ±7%. Meets the requirement for Identification.

Mepenzolate Bromide Tablets USP—Preserve in well-closed containers. Contain the labeled amount, within ±7%. Meet the requirements for Identification, Disintegration (30 minutes), and Uniformity of dosage units.

MEPERIDINE

Chemical name: Meperidine hydrochloride—4-Piperidinecarboxylic acid, 1-methyl-4-phenyl-, ethyl ester, hydrochloride.

Molecular formula: Meperidine hydrochloride—$C_{15}H_{21}NO_2 \cdot HCl$.

Molecular weight: Meperidine hydrochloride—283.80.

Description: Meperidine Hydrochloride USP—Fine, white, crystalline, odorless powder. The pH of a solution (1 in 20) is about 5.

Solubility: Meperidine Hydrochloride USP—Very soluble in water; soluble in alcohol; sparingly soluble in ether.

USP requirements:

Meperidine Hydrochloride USP—Preserve in well-closed, light-resistant containers. Contains not less than 98.0% and not more than 102.0% of meperidine hydrochloride, calculated on the dried basis. Meets the requirements for Identification, Melting range (186–189 °C), Loss on drying (not more than 1.0%), Residue on ignition (not more than 0.1%), Chloride content (12.2–12.7%), Chromatographic purity, and Organic volatile impurities.

Meperidine Hydrochloride Injection USP—Preserve in single-dose or in multiple-dose containers, preferably of Type I glass. A sterile solution of Meperidine Hydrochloride in Water for Injection. Contains the labeled amount, within ±5%. Meets the requirements for Identification, Bacterial endotoxins, pH (3.5–6.0), and Injections.

Meperidine Hydrochloride Syrup USP—Preserve in tight, light-resistant containers. Contains the labeled amount, within ±5%. Meets the requirements for Identification and pH (3.5–4.1).

Meperidine Hydrochloride Tablets USP—Preserve in well-closed, light-resistant containers. Contain the labeled amount, within ±5%. Meet the requirements for Identification, Dissolution (75% in 45 minutes in water in Apparatus 1 at 100 rpm), and Uniformity of dosage units.

MEPERIDINE AND ACETAMINOPHEN

For *Meperidine* and *Acetaminophen*—See individual listings for chemistry information.

USP requirements: Meperidine Hydrochloride and Acetaminophen Tablets—Not in USP.

MEPHENTERMINE

Chemical group: Structurally similar to methamphetamine.

Chemical name: Mephentermine sulfate—Benzeneethanamine, *N*,alpha,alpha-trimethyl-, sulfate (2:1).

Molecular formula: Mephentermine sulfate—$(C_{11}H_{17}N)_2 \cdot H_2SO_4$.

Molecular weight: Mephentermine sulfate—424.60.

Description: Mephentermine Sulfate USP—White, odorless crystals or crystalline powder. Its solutions are slightly acid to litmus, having a pH of about 6.

pKa: 10.11.

Solubility: Mephentermine Sulfate USP—Soluble in water; slightly soluble in alcohol; insoluble in chloroform.

USP requirements:

Mephentermine Sulfate USP—Preserve in well-closed, light-resistant containers. It is anhydrous or contains two molecules of water of hydration. Label it to indicate whether it is anhydrous or hydrous. Contains not less than 98.0% and not more than 102.0% of mephentermine sulfate, calculated on the anhydrous basis. Meets the requirements for Identification, Water (not more than 0.2% for the anhydrous and 6.8–8.8% for the hydrated form), Residue on ignition (not more than 0.1%), and Chromatographic purity.

Mephentermine Sulfate Injection USP—Preserve in single-dose or in multiple-dose containers, preferably of Type I glass. A sterile solution of Mephentermine Sulfate in Water for Injection. Contains an amount of mephentermine sulfate equivalent to the labeled amount of mephentermine, within ±5%. Meets the requirements for Identification, Bacterial endotoxins, pH (4.0–6.5), Particulate matter, and Injections.

MEPHENYTOIN

Chemical group: Related to the barbiturates in chemical structure, but having a five-membered ring.

Chemical name: 2,4-Imidazolidinedione, 5-ethyl-3-methyl-5-phenyl-.

Molecular formula: $C_{12}H_{14}N_2O_2$.

Molecular weight: 218.25.

Description: Mephenytoin USP—White, crystalline powder.

Solubility: Mephenytoin USP—Very slightly soluble in water; freely soluble in chloroform; soluble in alcohol and in aqueous solutions of alkali hydroxides; sparingly soluble in ether.

USP requirements:

Mephenytoin USP—Preserve in well-closed containers. Contains not less than 98.0% and not more than 102.0% of mephenytoin, calculated on the dried basis. Meets the requirements for Identification, Melting range (136–140 °C), Loss on drying (not more than 1.0%), Residue on ignition (not more than 0.1%), Heavy metals (not more than 0.002%), Chromatographic purity, Ordinary impurities, and Organic volatile impurities.

Mephenytoin Tablets USP—Preserve in well-closed containers. Contain the labeled amount, within ±10%. Meet the requirements for Dissolution (70% in 60 minutes in water in Apparatus 2 at 75 rpm), and Uniformity of dosage units.

MEPHOBARBITAL

Chemical name: 2,4,6(1*H*,3*H*,5*H*)-Pyrimidinetrione, 5-ethyl-1-methyl-5-phenyl-.

Molecular formula: $C_{13}H_{14}N_2O_3$.

Molecular weight: 246.27.

Description: Mephobarbital USP—White, odorless, crystalline powder. Its saturated solution is acid to litmus.

Solubility: Mephobarbital USP—Slightly soluble in water, in alcohol, and in ether; soluble in chloroform and in solutions of fixed alkali hydroxides and carbonates.

USP requirements:

Mephobarbital USP—Preserve in well-closed containers. Contains not less than 98.0% and not more than 100.5% of mephobarbital, calculated on the dried basis. Meets the requirements for Identification, Melting range (176–181 °C), Loss on drying (not more than 1.0%), and Residue on ignition (not more than 0.1%).

Mephobarbital Tablets USP—Preserve in well-closed containers. Contain the labeled amount, within −5% to +10%. Meet the requirements for Identification, Dissolution (70% in 75 minutes in alkaline borate buffer [pH 10.0] in Apparatus 2 at 75 rpm), and Uniformity of dosage units.

MEPIVACAINE

Chemical group: Amide.

Chemical name: Mepivacaine hydrochloride—2-Piperidinecarboxamide, *N*-(2,6-dimethylphenyl)-1-methyl-, monohydrochloride.

Molecular formula: Mepivacaine hydrochloride—$C_{15}H_{22}N_2O \cdot HCl$.

Molecular weight: Mepivacaine hydrochloride—282.81.

Description: Mepivacaine Hydrochloride USP—White, odorless, crystalline solid. The pH of a solution (1 in 50) is about 4.5.

pKa: Mepivacaine hydrochloride—7.6 and 7.8.

Solubility: Mepivacaine Hydrochloride USP—Freely soluble in water and in methanol; very slightly soluble in chloroform; practically insoluble in ether.

USP requirements:

Mepivacaine Hydrochloride USP—Preserve in well-closed containers. Contains not less than 98.0% and not more than 102.0% of mepivacaine hydrochloride, calculated on the dried basis. Meets the requirements for Identification, Loss on drying (not more than 1.0%), Residue on ignition (not more than 0.1%), and Chromatographic purity.

Mepivacaine Hydrochloride Injection USP—Preserve in single-dose or in multiple-dose containers, preferably of Type I glass. Injection labeled to contain 2% or less of mepivacaine hydrochloride may be packaged in 50-mL multiple-dose containers. A sterile solution of Mepivacaine Hydrochloride in Water for Injection. Contains the labeled amount, within ±5%. Meets the requirements for Identification, Bacterial endotoxins, pH (4.5–6.8), and Injections.

MEPIVACAINE AND LEVONORDEFRIN

For *Mepivacaine* and *Levonordefrin*—See individual listings for chemistry information.

USP requirements: Mepivacaine Hydrochloride and Levonordefrin Injection USP—Preserve in single-dose or in multiple-dose containers, preferably of Type I glass. A sterile solution of Mepivacaine Hydrochloride and Levonordefrin in Water for Injection.The label indicates that the Injection is not to be used if its color is pinkish or darker than slightly yellow or if it contains a precipitate. Contains the labeled amount of mepivacaine hydrochloride, within ±5%, and the labeled amount of levonordefrin, within ±10%. Meets the requirements for Color and clarity, Identification, Bacterial endotoxins, pH (3.3–5.5), and Injections.

MEPREDNISONE

Chemical name: Pregna-1,4-diene-3,11,20-trione, 17,21-dihydroxy-16-methyl-, (16 beta)-.

Molecular formula: $C_{22}H_{28}O_5$.

Molecular weight: 372.46.

Description: Melting point 200–205°C.

USP requirements: Meprednisone USP—Preserve in tight, light-resistant containers, and avoid exposure to excessive heat. Contains not less than 97.5% and not more than 102.5% of meprednisone, calculated on the dried basis. Meets the requirements for Identification, Specific rotation (+180° to +188°, calculated on the dried basis), Loss on drying (not more than 1.0%), and Residue on ignition (not more than 0.1%).

MEPROBAMATE

Chemical group: A carbamate derivative.

Chemical name: 1,3-Propanediol, 2-methyl-2-propyl-, dicarbamate.

Molecular formula: $C_9H_{18}N_2O_4$.

Molecular weight: 218.25.

Description: Meprobamate USP—White powder, having a characteristic odor.

Solubility: Meprobamate USP—Slightly soluble in water; freely soluble in acetone and in alcohol; sparingly soluble in ether.

USP requirements:

Meprobamate USP—Preserve in tight containers. Contains not less than 97.0% and not more than 101.0% of meprobamate, calculated on the dried basis. Meets the requirements for Identification, Melting range (103–107

°C, the range between beginning and end of melting not more than 2 °C), Loss on drying (not more than 0.5%), Chromatographic purity, Methyl carbamate (not more than 0.5%), and Organic volatile impurities.
Meprobamate Extended-release Capsules—Not in USP.
Meprobamate Oral Suspension USP—Preserve in tight containers. Contains the labeled amount, within −5% to +10%. Meets the requirement for Identification.
Meprobamate Tablets USP—Preserve in well-closed containers. Contain the labeled amount, within ±10%. Meet the requirements for Identification, Dissolution (75% in 30 minutes in deaerated water in Apparatus 1 at 100 rpm), and Uniformity of dosage units.

MEPROBAMATE AND ASPIRIN

For *Meprobamate* and *Aspirin*—See individual listings for chemistry information.

USP requirements: Meprobamate and Aspirin Tablets—Not in USP.

MEPRYLCAINE

Chemical name: Meprylcaine hydrochloride—1-Propanol-2-methyl-2-(propylamino)-, benzoate (ester), hydrochloride.

Molecular formula: Meprylcaine hydrochloride—$C_{14}H_{21}NO_2 \cdot HCl$.

Molecular weight: Meprylcaine hydrochloride—271.79.

Description: Meprylcaine Hydrochloride USP—White, odorless, crystalline solid. The pH of a solution (1 in 50) is about 5.7.

Solubility: Meprylcaine Hydrochloride USP—Freely soluble in water, in alcohol, and in chloroform; slightly soluble in acetone.

USP requirements: Meprylcaine Hydrochloride USP—Preserve in well-closed containers. Contains not less than 98.5% and not more than 101.5% of meprylcaine hydrochloride, calculated on the dried basis. Meets the requirements for Identification, Melting range (150–153 °C), Loss on drying (not more than 0.5%), and Residue on ignition (not more than 0.1%).

MEPRYLCAINE AND EPINEPHRINE

For *Meprylcaine* and *Epinephrine*—See individual listings for chemistry information.

USP requirements: Meprylcaine Hydrochloride and Epinephrine Injection USP—Preserve in single-dose containers, preferably of Type I glass, protected from light. A sterile solution of Meprylcaine Hydrochloride and Epinephrine in Water for Injection. The label indicates that the Injection is not to be used if its color is pinkish or darker than slightly yellow or if it contains a precipitate. Contains the labeled amounts of meprylcaine hydrochloride, within ±10%, and epinephrine, within −5% to +10%. Meets the requirements for Color and clarity, Identification, Bacterial endotoxins, and Injections.

MERCAPTOPURINE

Chemical name: 6*H*-Purine-6-thione, 1,7-dihydro-, monohydrate.

Molecular formula: $C_5H_4N_4S \cdot H_2O$.

Molecular weight: 170.19.

Description: Mercaptopurine USP—Yellow, odorless or practically odorless, crystalline powder. Melts at a temperature exceeding 308 °C, with decomposition.

pKa: 7.77 and 11.17.

Solubility: Mercaptopurine USP—Insoluble in water, in acetone, and in ether; soluble in hot alcohol and in dilute alkali solutions; slightly soluble in 2 *N* sulfuric acid.

USP requirements:
Mercaptopurine USP—Preserve in well-closed containers. Contains not less than 97.0% and not more than 102.0% of mercaptopurine, calculated on the anhydrous basis. Meets the requirements for Identification, Water (not more than 12.0%), Phosphorus, and Organic volatile impurities.
Mercaptopurine Tablets USP—Preserve in well-closed containers. Contain the labeled amount, within −7% to +10%. Meet the requirements for Identification, Disintegration (30 minutes), and Uniformity of dosage units.

AMMONIATED MERCURY

Chemical name: Mercury amide chloride.

Molecular formula: $Hg(NH_2)Cl$.

Molecular weight: 252.07.

Description: Ammoniated Mercury USP—White, pulverulent pieces or white, amorphous powder. Is odorless, and is stable in air, but darkens on exposure to light.

Solubility: Ammoniated Mercury USP—Insoluble in water, and in alcohol; readily soluble in warm hydrochloric, nitric, and acetic acids.

USP requirements:
Ammoniated Mercury USP—Preserve in well-closed, light-resistant containers. Contains not less than 98.0% and not more than 100.5% of ammoniated mercury. Meets the requirements for Identification, Residue on ignition (not more than 0.2%), and Mercurous compounds (not more than 0.2%).
Ammoniated Mercury Ointment USP—Preserve in collapsible tubes or in well-closed, light-resistant containers. Contains the labeled amount, within ±10%, in a suitable oleaginous ointment base. Meets the requirements for Identification and Minimum fill.
Ammoniated Mercury Ophthalmic Ointment USP—Preserve in collapsible ophthalmic ointment tubes. A sterile ointment. Contains the labeled amount, within ±10%, in a suitable oleaginous ointment base. Meets the requirements for Sterility, Metal particles, and Identification tests, and for Minimum fill under Ammoniated Mercury Ointment.

MESALAMINE

Chemical group: The active moiety of the prodrug sulfasalazine, which belongs to the salicylate and sulfonamide groups.

Chemical name: Benzoic acid, 5-amino-2-hydroxy-.

Molecular formula: $C_7H_7NO_3$.

Molecular weight: 153.14.

Description: Mesalamine USP—Light tan to pink colored needle-shaped crystals. Color may darken on exposure to air. Odorless or may have a slight characteristic odor.

Solubility: Mesalamine USP—Slightly soluble in water; very slightly soluble in methanol, in dehydrated alcohol, and in acetone; practically insoluble in *n*-butyl alcohol, in chloroform, in ether, in ethyl acetate, in *n*-hexane, in methylene chloride, and in *n*-propyl alcohol; soluble in dilute hydrochloric acid and in dilute alkali hydroxides.

USP requirements:
Mesalamine Delayed-release Capsules—Not in USP.
Mesalamine Suppositories—Not in USP.
Mesalamine Rectal Suspension—Not in USP.
Mesalamine Delayed-release Tablets—Not in USP.

MESNA

Chemical name: Ethanesulfonic acid, 2-mercapto-, monosodium salt.

Molecular formula: $C_2H_5NaO_3S_2$.

Molecular weight: 164.17.

Description: Mesna injection—Clear and colorless solution, with a pH of 6.5–8.5.

USP requirements: Mesna Injection—Not in USP.

MESORIDAZINE

Chemical group: Mesoridazine besylate—Salt of a metabolite of thioridazine, a phenothiazine derivative.

Chemical name: Mesoridazine besylate—10*H*-Phenothiazine, 10-[2-(1-methyl-2-piperidinyl)ethyl]-2-(methylsulfinyl)-, monobenzenesulfonate.

Molecular formula: Mesoridazine besylate—$C_{21}H_{26}N_2OS_2 \cdot C_6H_6O_3S$.

Molecular weight: Mesoridazine besylate—544.74.

Description: Mesoridazine Besylate USP—White to pale yellowish powder, having not more than a faint odor. Melts at about 178 °C, with decomposition.

Solubility: Mesoridazine Besylate USP—Freely soluble in water, in chloroform, and in methanol.

USP requirements:
Mesoridazine Besylate USP—Preserve in tight, light-resistant containers. Contains not less than 98.0% and not more than 102.0% of mesoridazine besylate, calculated on the dried basis. Meets the requirements for Identification, pH (4.2–5.7, in a freshly prepared solution [1 in 100]), Loss on drying (not more than 0.5%), Residue on ignition (not more than 0.2%), Heavy metals (not more than 0.002%), Selenium (not more than 0.003%), Ordinary impurities, and Organic volatile impurities.
Mesoridazine Besylate Injection USP—Preserve in single-dose containers, preferably of Type I glass, protected from light. A sterile solution of Mesoridazine Besylate in Water for Injection. Contains an amount of mesoridazine besylate equivalent to the labeled amount of mesoridazine, within ±10%. Meets the requirements for Identification, Bacterial endotoxins, pH (4.0–5.0), and Injections.
Mesoridazine Besylate Oral Solution USP—Preserve in tight, light-resistant containers, at a temperature not exceeding 25 °C. Contains an amount of mesoridazine besylate equivalent to the labeled amount of mesoridazine, within ±10%. Label it to indicate that it is to be diluted to the appropriate strength with water or other suitable fluid prior to administration. Meets the requirements for Identification and Alcohol content (0.25–1.0%).
Mesoridazine Besylate Tablets USP—Preserve in well-closed, light-resistant containers. Preserve Tablets having an opaque coating in well-closed containers. Contain an amount of mesoridazine besylate equivalent to the labeled amount of mesoridazine, within ±10%. Meet the requirements for Identification, Dissolution (80% in 60 minutes in 0.1 *N* hydrochloric acid in Apparatus 2 at 100 rpm), and Uniformity of dosage units.

MESTRANOL

Chemical name: 19-Norpregna-1,3,5(10)-trien-20-yn-17-ol, 3-methoxy-, (17 alpha)-.

Molecular formula: $C_{21}H_{26}O_2$.

Molecular weight: 310.44.

Description: Mestranol USP—White to creamy white, odorless, crystalline powder.

Solubility: Mestranol USP—Insoluble in water; freely soluble in chloroform; soluble in dioxane; sparingly soluble in dehydrated alcohol; slightly soluble in methanol.

USP requirements: Mestranol USP—Preserve in well-closed, light-resistant containers. Contains not less than 97.0% and not more than 102.0% of mestranol, calculated on the dried basis. Meets the requirements for Identification, Melting range (146–154 °C, the range between beginning and end of melting not more than 4 °C), Specific rotation (+2° to +8°), and Loss on drying (not more than 1.0%).

METAPROTERENOL

Chemical name: Metaproterenol sulfate—1,3-Benzenediol, 5-[1-hydroxy-2-[(1-methylethyl)amino]ethyl]-, sulfate (2:1) (salt).

Molecular formula: Metaproterenol sulfate—$(C_{11}H_{17}NO_3)_2 \cdot H_2SO_4$.

Molecular weight: Metaproterenol sulfate—520.60.

Description: Metaproterenol Sulfate USP—White to off-white, crystalline powder.

Solubility: Metaproterenol Sulfate USP—Freely soluble in water.

USP requirements:
Metaproterenol Sulfate USP—Preserve in tight, light-resistant containers. Contains not less than 98.0% and not more than 102.0% of metaproterenol sulfate, calculated on the anhydrous, isopropyl alcohol-free, and methanol-free basis. Meets the requirements for Identification, pH (4.0–5.5, in a solution containing 100 mg per mL), Water (not more than 2.0%), Residue on ignition (not more than 0.1%), Heavy metals (not more than 0.001%), Iron (not more than 5 ppm), Metaproterenone sulfate (not more than 0.1%), Isopropyl alcohol and methanol (not more than 0.3% of isopropyl alcohol and not more than 0.1% of methanol), and Organic volatile impurities.
Metaproterenol Sulfate Inhalation Aerosol USP—Preserve in small, nonreactive, light-resistant aerosol containers equipped with metered-dose valves and provided with oral inhalation actuators. A suspension of microfine Metaproterenol Sulfate in fluorochlorohydrocarbon propellants in a pressurized container. Contains the labeled amount within ±10%, and delivers the labeled dose per inhalation, within ±25%, through an oral inhalation actuator. Meets the requirements for Identification, Unit spray content, Particle size, and Water (not more than 0.075%), and for Leak testing under Aerosols.
Metaproterenol Sulfate Inhalation Solution USP—Store in small, tight containers that are well-filled or otherwise protected from oxidation. Protect from light. A solution of Metaproterenol Sulfate in Purified Water. Label it to

indicate that the Inhalation Solution is not to be used if its color is pinkish or darker than slightly yellow or if it contains a precipitate. Contains the labeled amount, within ±10%. Meets the requirements for Color and clarity, Identification, and pH (2.8–4.0).

Metaproterenol Sulfate Syrup USP—Preserve in tight, light-resistant containers. Contains the labeled amount, within ±10%. Meets the requirements for Identification and pH (2.5–4.0, in a solution obtained by mixing 1 volume of Syrup and 4 volumes of water).

Metaproterenol Sulfate Tablets USP—Preserve in well-closed, light-resistant containers. Contain the labeled amount, within ±8%. Meet the requirements for Identification, Dissolution (70% in 30 minutes in water in Apparatus 2 at 50 rpm), and Uniformity of dosage units.

METARAMINOL

Chemical name: Metaraminol bitartrate—Benzenemethanol, alpha-(1-aminoethyl)-3-hydroxy-, [*R*-(*R**,*S**)]-, [*R*-(*R**,*R**)]-2,3-dihydroxybutanedioate (1:1) (salt).

Molecular formula: Metaraminol bitartrate—$C_9H_{13}NO_2 \cdot C_4H_6O_6$.

Molecular weight: Metaraminol bitartrate—317.30.

Description: Metaraminol bitartrate—White, practically odorless, crystalline powder.

Solubility: Metaraminol bitartrate—Freely soluble in water; slightly soluble in alcohol; practically insoluble in chloroform and in ether.

USP requirements:

Metaraminol Bitartrate USP—Preserve in well-closed containers. Contains not less than 99.0% and not more than 100.5% of metaraminol bitartrate, calculated on the dried basis. Meets the requirements for Identification, Melting range (171–175 °C), Specific rotation (−31.5° to −33.5°, calculated on the dried basis), pH (3.2–3.5, in a solution [1 in 20]), Loss on drying (not more than 1.0%), Residue on ignition (not more than 0.1%), and Heavy metals (not more than 0.002%).

Metaraminol Bitartrate Injection USP—Preserve in single-dose or in multiple-dose containers, preferably of Type I glass, protected from light. A sterile solution of Metaraminol Bitartrate in Water for Injection. Contains, in each mL, an amount of metaraminol bitartrate equivalent to not less than 9.0 mg and not more than 11.0 mg of metaraminol. Meets the requirements for Identification, Bacterial endotoxins, pH (3.2–4.5), Particulate matter, and Injections.

METAXALONE

Chemical name: 2-Oxazolidinone, 5-[(3,5-dimethylphenoxy)-methyl]-.

Molecular formula: $C_{12}H_{15}NO_3$.

Molecular weight: 221.26.

Description: White, crystalline powder. Melts at about 123 °C.

Solubility: Very slightly soluble in water; soluble in alcohol; freely soluble in chloroform.

USP requirements: Metaxalone Tablets—Not in USP.

METFORMIN

Chemical name: Metformin hydrochloride—1,1-Dimethylbiguanide hydrochloride.

Molecular formula: Metformin hydrochloride—$C_4H_{11}N_5 \cdot HCl$.

Molecular weight: Metformin hydrochloride—165.6.

Description: Metformin hydrochloride—White, odorless or almost odorless, hygroscopic, crystalline powder.

Solubility: Metformin hydrochloride—Soluble 1 in 2 of water; slightly soluble in alcohol; practically insoluble in chloroform and in ether.

USP requirements: Metformin Hydrochloride Tablets—Not in USP.

METHACHOLINE

Chemical name: Methacholine chloride—1-Propanaminium, 2-(acetyloxy)-*N*,*N*,*N*-trimethyl-, chloride.

Molecular formula: Methacholine chloride—$C_8H_{18}ClNO_2$.

Molecular weight: Methacholine chloride—195.69.

Description: Methacholine Chloride USP—Colorless or white crystals, or white, crystalline powder. Is odorless or has a slight odor, and is very hygroscopic. Its solutions are neutral to litmus.

Solubility: Methacholine Chloride USP—Very soluble in water; freely soluble in alcohol and in chloroform.

USP requirements:

Methacholine Chloride USP—Preserve in tight containers. Dried at 105 °C for 4 hours, contains not less than 98.0% and not more than 101.0% of methacholine chloride. Meets the requirements for Identification, Melting range (170–173 °C), Loss on drying (not more than 1.5%), Residue on ignition (not more than 0.1%), Acetylcholine chloride, and Heavy metals (not more than 0.002%).

Methacholine Chloride for Inhalation—Not in USP.

METHACRYLIC ACID COPOLYMER

Description: Methacrylic Acid Copolymer NF—White powder, having a faint characteristic odor.

NF category: Coating agent.

Solubility: Methacrylic Acid Copolymer NF—The polymer is insoluble in water, in diluted acids, in simulated gastric fluid TS, and in buffer solutions of up to pH 5; soluble in diluted alkali, in simulated intestinal fluid TS, and in buffer solutions of pH 7 and above. The solubility between pH 5.5 and pH 7 depends on the content of methacrylic acid units in the copolymer. Soluble to freely soluble in methanol, in alcohol, in isopropyl alcohol, and in acetone, each of which contains not less than 3% of water.

NF requirements: Methacrylic Acid Copolymer NF—Preserve in tight containers. A fully polymerized copolymer of methacrylic acid and an acrylic or methacrylic ester. It is available in 3 types, which differ in content of methacrylic acid units and viscosity. Label it to state whether it is Type A, B, or C. Meets the requirements for Identification, Viscosity, Loss on drying (not more than 5.0%), Residue on ignition (not more than 0.1% for Types A and B; not more than 0.4% for Type C), Arsenic (not more than 2 ppm), Heavy metals (not more than 0.002%), Monomers (not more than 0.3%), and Organic volatile impurities.

METHACYCLINE

Chemical name: Methacycline hydrochloride—2-Naphthacenecarboxamide, 4-(dimethylamino)-1,4,4a,5,5a,6,11,12a-octahydro-3,5,10,12,12a-pentahydroxy-6-methylene-1,11-dioxo-, monohydrochloride, [4*S*-(4 alpha,4a alpha,5 alpha,5a alpha,12a alpha)]-.

Molecular formula: Methacycline hydrochloride—$C_{22}H_{22}N_2O_8 \cdot HCl$.

Molecular weight: Methacycline hydrochloride—478.89.

Description: Methacycline Hydrochloride USP—Yellow to dark yellow, crystalline powder.

Solubility: Methacycline Hydrochloride USP—Soluble in water.

USP requirements:
Methacycline Hydrochloride USP—Preserve in tight, light-resistant containers. Has a potency equivalent to not less than 832 mcg of methacycline per mg. Meets the requirements for Identification, Crystallinity, pH (2.0–3.0, in a solution containing 10 mg of methacycline per mL), and Water (not more than 2.0%).
Methacycline Hydrochloride Capsules USP—Preserve in tight, light-resistant containers. Contain an amount of methacycline hydrochloride equivalent to the labeled amount of methacycline, within −10% to +20%. Meet the requirements for Identification, Dissolution (70% in 60 minutes in water in Apparatus 1 at 100 rpm), Uniformity of dosage units, and Water (not more than 7.5%).
Methacycline Hydrochloride Oral Suspension USP—Preserve in tight, light-resistant containers. Contains an amount of methacycline hydrochloride equivalent to the labeled amount of methacycline, within −10% to +25%. Contains one or more suitable and harmless buffers, colors, diluents, dispersants, flavors, and preservatives. Meets the requirements for Identification, pH (6.5–8.0), Deliverable volume (for Suspension packaged in multiple-unit containers), and Uniformity of dosage units (for Suspension packaged in single-unit containers).

METHADONE

Chemical name: Methadone hydrochloride—3-Heptanone, 6-(dimethylamino)-4,4-diphenyl-, hydrochloride.

Molecular formula: Methadone hydrochloride—$C_{21}H_{27}NO \cdot HCl$.

Molecular weight: Methadone hydrochloride—345.91.

Description:
Methadone Hydrochloride USP—Colorless crystals or white, crystalline, odorless powder.
Methadone Hydrochloride Oral Concentrate USP—Clear to slightly hazy, syrupy liquid.

Solubility: Methadone Hydrochloride USP—Soluble in water; freely soluble in alcohol and in chloroform; practically insoluble in ether and in glycerin.

USP requirements:
Methadone Hydrochloride USP—Preserve in tight, light-resistant containers. Contains not less than 98.5% and not more than 100.5% of methadone hydrochloride, calculated on the dried basis. Meets the requirements for Identification, pH (4.5–6.5, in a solution [1 in 100]), Loss on drying (not more than 0.3%), Residue on ignition (not more than 0.1%), Ordinary impurities, and Organic volatile impurities.
Methadone Hydrochloride Oral Concentrate USP—Preserve in tight containers, protected from light, at controlled room temperature. Label it to indicate that it is to be diluted with water or other liquid to 30 mL or more prior to administration. Contains, in each mL, not less than 9.0 mg and not more than 11.0 mg of methadone hydrochloride. Contains a suitable preservative. Meets the requirements for Identification and pH (1.0–6.0).
Methadone Hydrochloride Injection USP—Preserve in single-dose or in multiple-dose, light-resistant containers, preferably of Type I glass. A sterile solution of Methadone Hydrochloride in Water for Injection. Contains, in each mL, not less than 9.5 mg and not more than 10.5 mg of methadone hydrochloride. Meets the requirements for Identification, Bacterial endotoxins, pH (3.0–6.5), and Injections.
Methadone Hydrochloride Oral Solution USP—Preserve in tight containers, protected from light, at controlled room temperature. Contains the labeled amount, within ±10%. Meets the requirements for Identification, pH (1.0–4.0), and Alcohol content (7.0–9.0%).
Methadone Hydrochloride Tablets USP—Preserve in well-closed containers. Label Tablets that are not intended for oral administration as intact Tablets to state that they are dispersible tablets or to indicate that they are intended for dispersion in a liquid prior to oral administration of the prescribed dose. Contain the labeled amount, within ±7%. Meet the requirements for Identification, Disintegration (for dispersible Tablets, 15 minutes, the use of disks being omitted), Dissolution (for Tablets intended to be swallowed, 75% in 45 minutes in water in Apparatus 1 at 100 rpm), and Uniformity of dosage units.

METHAMPHETAMINE

Chemical name: Methamphetamine hydrochloride—(+)-*N*,-alpha-Dimethylphenethylamine hydrochloride.

Molecular formula: Methamphetamine hydrochloride—$C_{10}H_{15}N \cdot HCl$.

Molecular weight: Methamphetamine hydrochloride—185.70.

Description: Methamphetamine Hydrochloride USP—White crystals or white, crystalline powder. Is odorless or practically so. Its solutions have a pH of about 6.

Solubility: Methamphetamine Hydrochloride USP—Freely soluble in water, in alcohol, and in chloroform; very slightly soluble in absolute ether.

USP requirements:
Methamphetamine Hydrochloride USP—Preserve in tight, light-resistant containers. Contains not less than 98.5% and not more than 100.5% of methamphetamine hydrochloride, calculated on the dried basis. Meets the requirements for Identification, Melting range (171–175 °C), Specific rotation (+16° to +19°), Loss on drying (not more than 0.5%), Residue on ignition (not more than 0.1%), Ordinary impurities, and Organic volatile impurities.
Methamphetamine Hydrochloride Tablets USP—Preserve in tight, light-resistant containers. Contain the labeled amount, within ±10%. Meet the requirements for Identification, Dissolution (75% in 45 minutes in water in Apparatus 2 at 50 rpm), and Uniformity of dosage units.
Methamphetamine Hydrochloride Extended-release Tablets—Not in USP.

METHANTHELINE

Chemical group: Quaternary ammonium compound.

Chemical name: Methantheline bromide—Ethanaminium, *N,N*-diethyl-*N*-methyl-2-[(9*H*-xanthen-9-ylcarbonyl)oxy]-, bromide.

Molecular formula: Methantheline bromide—$C_{21}H_{26}BrNO_3$.

Molecular weight: Methantheline bromide—420.35.

Description:
Methantheline Bromide USP—White or nearly white, practically odorless powder. Its solutions have a pH of about 5.

Sterile Methantheline Bromide USP—White or nearly white, practically odorless powder. Its solutions have a pH of about 5.

Solubility:
Methantheline Bromide USP—Very soluble in water; freely soluble in alcohol and in chloroform; practically insoluble in ether. Its water solution decomposes on standing.
Sterile Methantheline Bromide USP—Very soluble in water; freely soluble in alcohol and in chloroform; practically insoluble in ether. Its water solution decomposes on standing.

USP requirements:
Methantheline Bromide USP—Preserve in well-closed containers. Contains not less than 98.0% and not more than 102.0% of methantheline bromide, calculated on the dried basis. Meets the requirements for Identification, Melting range (171–177 °C), Loss on drying (not more than 0.5%), Residue on ignition (not more than 0.2%), and Organic volatile impurities.
Methantheline Bromide Tablets USP—Preserve in well-closed containers. Contain the labeled amount, within ±5%. Meet the requirements for Identification, Dissolution (75% in 45 minutes in water in Apparatus 2 at 50 rpm), and Uniformity of dosage units.
Sterile Methantheline Bromide USP—Preserve in Containers for Sterile Solids. Contains the labeled amount, within ±2%, calculated on the dried basis. Meets the requirements for Completeness of solution, Constituted solution, Pyrogen, and Uniformity of dosage units, for Identification tests, Melting range, Loss on drying, and Residue on ignition under Methantheline Bromide, and for Sterility tests and Labeling under Injections.

METHARBITAL

Chemical name: 2,4,6(1*H*,3*H*,5*H*)-Pyrimidinetrione, 5,5-diethyl-1-methyl-.

Molecular formula: $C_9H_{14}N_2O_3$.

Molecular weight: 198.22.

Description: Metharbital USP—White to nearly white, crystalline powder, having a faint aromatic odor. The pH of a saturated solution is about 6.

Solubility: Metharbital USP—Slightly soluble in water; soluble in alcohol; sparingly soluble in ether.

USP requirements:
Metharbital USP—Preserve in tight containers. Dried at 105 °C for 4 hours, contains not less than 98.0% and not more than 102.0% of metharbital. Meets the requirements for Identification, Melting range (151–155 °C), Water (not more than 1.0%), Residue on ignition (not more than 0.1%), and Organic volatile impurities.
Metharbital Tablets USP—Preserve in tight containers. Contain the labeled amount, within ±5%. Meet the requirements for Identification, Dissolution (75% in 45 minutes in water in Apparatus 1 at 100 rpm), and Uniformity of dosage units.

METHAZOLAMIDE

Chemical name: Acetamide, *N*-[5-(aminosulfonyl)-3-methyl-1,3,4-thiadiazol-2(3*H*)-ylidene]-.

Molecular formula: $C_5H_8N_4O_3S_2$.

Molecular weight: 236.26.

Description: Methazolamide USP—White or faintly yellow, crystalline powder having a slight odor. Melts at about 213 °C.

Solubility: Methazolamide USP—Very slightly soluble in water and in alcohol; soluble in dimethylformamide; slightly soluble in acetone.

USP requirements:
Methazolamide USP—Preserve in well-closed, light-resistant containers. Contains not less than 96.0% and not more than 100.5% of methazolamide, calculated on the dried basis. Meets the requirements for Identification, Loss on drying (not more than 0.5%), Residue on ignition (not more than 0.1%), Selenium (not more than 0.003%), Heavy metals (not more than 0.002%), and Organic volatile impurities.
Methazolamide Tablets USP—Preserve in well-closed containers. Contain the labeled amount, within ±5%. Meet the requirements for Identification, Dissolution (75% in 45 minutes in acetate buffer [pH 4.5] in Apparatus 2 at 100 rpm), and Uniformity of dosage units.

METHDILAZINE

Chemical name:
Methdilazine—10*H*-Phenothiazine, 10-[(1-methyl-3-pyrrolidinyl)methyl]-.
Methdilazine hydrochloride—10*H*-Phenothiazine, 10-[(1-methyl-3-pyrrolidinyl)methyl]-, monohydrochloride.

Molecular formula:
Methdilazine—$C_{18}H_{20}N_2S$.
Methdilazine hydrochloride—$C_{18}H_{20}N_2S \cdot HCl$.

Molecular weight:
Methdilazine—296.43.
Methdilazine hydrochloride—332.89.

Description:
Methdilazine USP—Light tan, crystalline powder, having a characteristic odor.
Methdilazine Hydrochloride USP—Light tan, crystalline powder, having a slight, characteristic odor.

Solubility:
Methdilazine USP—Practically insoluble in water; freely soluble in 3 *N* hydrochloric acid; soluble in alcohol and in chloroform.
Methdilazine Hydrochloride USP—Freely soluble in water, in alcohol, and in chloroform.

USP requirements:
Methdilazine USP—Preserve in tight, light-resistant containers. Contains not less than 97.0% and not more than 103.0% of methdilazine, calculated on the dried basis. Meets the requirements for Identification, Melting range (83–88 °C, the range between beginning and end of melting not more than 2 °C), Loss on drying (not more than 1.0%), Residue on ignition (not more than 0.5%), Selenium (not more than 0.003%), Heavy metals (not more than 0.002%), and Organic volatile impurities.
Methdilazine Tablets USP—Preserve in tight, light-resistant containers. Contains the labeled amount, within ±7%. Meets the requirements for Identification, Disintegration (30 minutes), and Uniformity of dosage units.
Methdilazine Hydrochloride USP—Preserve in tight, light-resistant containers. Contains not less than 97.0% and not more than 103.0% of methdilazine hydrochloride, calculated on the dried basis. Meets the requirements for Identification, Melting range (184–190 °C), pH (4.8–6.0, in a solution [1 in 100]), Loss on drying (not more than

1.0%), Residue on ignition (not more than 0.5%), Heavy metals (not more than 0.002%), Selenium (not more than 0.003%), Ordinary impurities, and Organic volatile impurities.

Methdilazine Hydrochloride Syrup USP—Preserve in tight, light-resistant containers. Contains the labeled amount, within ±7%. Meets the requirements for Identification, pH (3.3–4.1), and Alcohol content (6.5–7.5%).

Methdilazine Hydrochloride Tablets USP—Preserve in tight, light-resistant containers. Contain the labeled amount, within ±7%. Meet the requirements for Identification, Dissolution (75% in 45 minutes in water in Apparatus 1 at 100 rpm), and Uniformity of dosage units.

METHENAMINE

Chemical name:

Methenamine—1,3,5,7-Tetraazatricyclo[$3.3.1.1^{3,7}$]decane.

Methenamine hippurate—Glycine, *N*-benzoyl, compd. with 1,3,5,7-tetraazatricyclo[$3.3.1.1^{3,7}$]decane (1:1).

Methenamine mandelate—Benzeneacetic acid, alpha-hydroxy-, compd. with 1,3,5,7-tetraazatricyclo[$3.3.1.1^{3,7}$]-decane (1:1).

Molecular formula:

Methenamine—$C_6H_{12}N_4$.

Methenamine hippurate—$C_6H_{12}N_4 \cdot C_9H_9NO_3$.

Methenamine mandelate—$C_6H_{12}N_4 \cdot C_8H_8O_3$.

Molecular weight:

Methenamine—140.19.

Methenamine hippurate—319.36.

Methenamine mandelate—292.34.

Description:

Methenamine USP—Colorless, lustrous crystals or white, crystalline powder. Is practically odorless. When brought into contact with fire, it readily ignites, burning with a smokeless flame. It sublimes at about 260 °C, without melting. Its solutions are alkaline to litmus.

Methenamine hippurate—White, crystalline powder.

Methenamine Mandelate USP—White crystalline powder. Is practically odorless. Its solutions have a pH of about 4. Melts at about 127 °C, with decomposition.

Solubility:

Methenamine USP—Freely soluble in water; soluble in alcohol and in chloroform.

Methenamine hippurate—Freely soluble in water and in alcohol.

Methenamine Mandelate USP—Very soluble in water; soluble in alcohol and in chloroform; slightly soluble in ether.

USP requirements:

Methenamine USP—Preserve in well-closed containers. Dried over phosphorus pentoxide for 4 hours, contains not less than 99.0% and not more than 100.5% of methenamine. Meets the requirements for Identification, Loss on drying (not more than 2.0%), Residue on ignition (not more than 0.1%), Chloride (not more than 0.014%), Sulfate, Ammonium salts, Heavy metals (not more than 0.001%), and Organic volatile impurities.

Methenamine Elixir USP—Preserve in tight containers. Contains the labeled amount, within ±10%. Meets the requirements for Identification and Alcohol content (the labeled amount, within ±10%).

Methenamine Tablets USP—Preserve in well-closed containers. Contain the labeled amount, within ±5%. Meet the requirements for Identification, Dissolution (75% in 45 minutes in water in Apparatus 1 at 100 rpm), and Uniformity of dosage units.

Methenamine Hippurate USP—Preserve in well-closed containers. Dried in vacuum at 60 °C for 1 hour, contains not less than 95.5% and not more than 102.0% of methenamine hippurate, and contains not less than 54.0% and not more than 58.0% of hippuric acid. Meets the requirements for Identification, Loss on drying (not more than 1.0%), Residue on ignition (not more than 0.1%), Sulfate, Heavy metals (not more than 0.0015%), Hippuric acid content, and Organic volatile impurities.

Methenamine Hippurate Tablets USP—Preserve in well-closed containers. Contain the labeled amount, within ±5%. Meet the requirements for Identification, Disintegration (30 minutes), and Uniformity of dosage units.

Methenamine Mandelate USP—Preserve in well-closed containers. Contains not less than 95.5% and not more than 102.0% of methenamine mandelate, and contains not less than 50.0% and and not more than 53.0% of mandelic acid, calculated on the dried basis. Meets the requirements for Identification, Loss on drying (not more than 1.5%), Residue on ignition (not more than 0.1%), Chloride (not more than 0.01%), Sulfate, Heavy metals (not more than 0.0015%), Mandelic acid content, and Organic volatile impurities.

Methenamine Mandelate for Oral Solution USP—Preserve in well-closed containers. Label Methenamine Mandelate for Oral Solution that contains insoluble ingredients to indicate that the aqueous constituted Oral Solution contains dissolved methenamine mandelate but may remain turbid because of the presence of added substances. Contains the labeled amount, within ±10%. Meets the requirements for Identification, pH (4.0–4.5 in a mixture of 1 gram with 30 mL of water), and Water (not more than 0.5%).

Methenamine Mandelate Oral Suspension USP—Preserve in tight containers. It is Methenamine Mandelate suspended in vegetable oil. Contains the labeled amount, within ±10%. Meets the requirements for Identification and Water (not more than 0.1%).

Methenamine Mandelate Tablets USP—Preserve in well-closed containers. Contain the labeled amount, within ±5%. Meet the requirements for Identification, Disintegration (for enteric-coated Tablets, 2 hours and 30 minutes), Dissolution (for uncoated or plain coated Tablets, 75% in 45 minutes in water in Apparatus 1 at 100 rpm), and Uniformity of dosage units.

METHENAMINE AND MONOBASIC SODIUM PHOSPHATE

For *Methenamine* and *Monobasic Sodium Phosphate*—See individual listings for chemistry information.

USP requirements: Methenamine and Monobasic Sodium Phosphate Tablets USP—Preserve in tight containers. Contain the labeled amounts, within ±7.5%. Meet the requirements for Identification, Dissolution (75% of labeled amount of methenamine in 45 minutes in water in Apparatus 1 at 100 rpm), Uniformity of dosage units, and Ammonium salts.

METHICILLIN

Chemical name: Methicillin sodium—4-Thia-1-azabicyclo[3.2.0]-heptane-2-carboxylic acid, 6-[(2,6-dimethoxybenzoyl)amino]-3,3-dimethyl-7-oxo-, monosodium salt, monohydrate, [2*S*-(2 alpha,5 alpha,6 beta)]-.

Molecular formula: Methicillin sodium—$C_{17}H_{19}N_2NaO_6S \cdot H_2O$.

Molecular weight: Methicillin sodium—420.41.

Description:

Methicillin Sodium for Injection USP—Fine, white, crystalline powder, odorless or having a slight odor.

Sterile Methicillin Sodium USP—Fine, white, crystalline powder, odorless or having a slight odor.

Solubility:
Methicillin Sodium for Injection USP—Freely soluble in water, in methanol, and in pyridine; slightly soluble in propyl and amyl alcohols, in chloroform, and in ethylene chloride; insoluble in acetone and in ether.
Sterile Methicillin Sodium USP—Freely soluble in water, in methanol, and in pyridine; slightly soluble in propyl and amyl alcohols, in chloroform, and in ethylene chloride; insoluble in acetone and in ether.

USP requirements:
Methicillin Sodium for Injection USP—Preserve in Containers for Sterile Solids, at controlled room temperature. A sterile mixture of Sterile Methicillin Sodium and Sodium Citrate. Contains an amount of methicillin sodium equivalent to the labeled amount of methicillin, within −10% to +15%. Meets the requirements for Constituted solution, Identification, Bacterial endotoxins, Sterility, pH (6.0–8.5, in a solution containing 10 mg per mL), Water (not more than 6.0%), and Particulate matter, and for Uniformity of dosage units and Labeling under Injections.
Sterile Methicillin Sodium USP—Preserve in Containers for Sterile Solids, at controlled room temperature. It is Methicillin Sodium for parenteral use. Has a potency equivalent to not less than 815 mcg of methicillin per mg. Meets the requirements for Identification, Crystallinity, Bacterial endotoxins, Sterility, pH (5.0–7.5, in a solution containing 10 mg per mL), and Water (3.0–6.0%).

METHIMAZOLE

Chemical group: Thioimidazole derivative.

Chemical name: 2*H*-Imidazole-2-thione, 1,3-dihydro-1-methyl-.

Molecular formula: $C_4H_6N_2S$.

Molecular weight: 114.17.

Description: Methimazole USP—White to pale buff, crystalline powder, having a faint, characteristic odor. It solutions are practically neutral to litmus.

Solubility: Methimazole USP—Freely soluble in water, in alcohol, and in chloroform; slightly soluble in ether.

USP requirements:
Methimazole USP—Preserve in well-closed, light-resistant containers. Contains not less than 98.0% and not more than 101.0% of methimazole, calculated on the dried basis. Meets the requirements for Identification, Melting range (143–146 °C), Loss on drying (not more than 0.5%), Residue on ignition (not more than 0.1%), Selenium (not more than 0.003%), Ordinary impurities, and Organic volatile impurities.
Methimazole Suppositories—Not in USP.
Methimazole Tablets USP—Preserve in well-closed, light-resistant containers. Contain the labeled amount, within ±6%. Meet the requirements for Identification, Dissolution (80% in 30 minutes in water in Apparatus 1 at 100 rpm), and Uniformity of dosage units.

METHIONINE

Chemical name: L-Methionine.

Molecular formula: $C_5H_{11}NO_2S$.

Molecular weight: 149.21.

Description: Methionine USP—White crystals, having a characteristic odor.

Solubility: Methionine USP—Soluble in water, in warm dilute alcohol, and in dilute mineral acids; insoluble in ether, in absolute alcohol, and in acetone (L-form).

USP requirements: Methionine USP—Preserve in well-closed containers. Contains not less than 98.5% and not more than 101.5% of methionine, as L-methionine, calculated on the dried basis. Meets the requirements for Identification, Specific rotation (+21.9° to +24.1°, calculated on the dried basis), pH (5.6–6.1 in a solution [1 in 100]), Loss on drying (not more than 0.3%), Residue on ignition (not more than 0.4%), Chloride (not more than 0.05%), Sulfate (not more than 0.03%), Arsenic (not more than 1.5 ppm), Iron (not more than 0.003%), Heavy metals (not more than 0.0015%), and Organic volatile impurities.

METHOCARBAMOL

Chemical name: 1,2-Propanediol, 3-(2-methoxyphenoxy)-, 1-carbamate.

Molecular formula: $C_{11}H_{15}NO_5$.

Molecular weight: 241.24.

Description: Methocarbamol USP—White powder, odorless, or having a slight characteristic odor. Melts at about 94 °C, or, if previously ground to a fine powder, melts at about 90 °C.

Solubility: Methocarbamol USP—Sparingly soluble in water and in chloroform; soluble in alcohol only with heating; insoluble in *n*-hexane.

USP requirements:
Methocarbamol USP—Preserve in tight containers. Contains not less than 98.5% and not more than 101.5% of methocarbamol, calculated on the dried basis. Meets the requirements for Identification, Loss on drying (not more than 0.5%), Residue on ignition (not more than 0.1%), Heavy metals (not more than 0.002%), Related impurities (not more than 2.0%), and Organic volatile impurities.
Methocarbamol Injection USP—Preserve in single-dose containers, preferably of Type I glass. A sterile solution of Methocarbamol in an aqueous solution of Polyethylene Glycol 300. Contains the labeled amount, within ±5%. Meets the requirements for Identification, Bacterial endotoxins, pH (3.5–6.0), Particulate matter under Small-volume Injections, Aldehydes (not more than 0.01%, as formaldehyde), and Injections.
Methocarbamol Tablets USP—Preserve in tight containers. Contain the labeled amount, within ±5%. Meet the requirements for Identification, Dissolution (75% in 45 minutes in water in Apparatus 2 at 50 rpm), and Uniformity of dosage units.

METHOHEXITAL

Chemical group: Methohexital sodium—A methylated oxybarbiturate; differs chemically from the established barbiturate anesthetics in that it contains no sulfur.

Chemical name:
Methohexital—2,4,6(1*H*,3*H*,5*H*)-Pyrimidinetrione, 1-methyl-5-(1-methyl-2-pentynyl)-5-(2-propenyl)-, (±)-.
Methohexital sodium—2,4,6(1*H*,3*H*,5*H*)-Pyrimidinetrione, 1-methyl-5-(1-methyl-2-pentynyl)-5-(2-propenyl)-, (±)-, monosodium salt.

Molecular formula:
Methohexital—$C_{14}H_{18}N_2O_3$.
Methohexital sodium—$C_{14}H_{17}N_2NaO_3$.

Molecular weight:
Methohexital—262.31.
Methohexital sodium—284.29.

Description:
Methohexital USP—White to faintly yellowish white, crystalline odorless powder.
Methohexital Sodium for Injection USP—White to off-white hygroscopic powder. Is essentially odorless.

Solubility:
Methohexital USP—Very slightly soluble in water; slightly soluble in alcohol, in chloroform, and in dilute alkalies.
Methohexital sodium—Freely soluble in water.

Other characteristics:
Methohexital sodium—75% un-ionized at pH 7.4.
Methohexital sodium for injection—A 1% solution in sterile water has a pH of 10 to 11; a 0.2% solution in 5% dextrose has a pH of 9.5 to 10.5.

USP requirements:
Methohexital USP—Preserve in well-closed containers. Contains not less than 98.0% and not more than 101.0% of methohexital, calculated on the anhydrous basis. Meets the requirements for Identification, Melting range (92–96 °C, but the range between beginning and end of melting not more than 3 °C), Water (not more than 2.0%), Chloride (not more than 0.03%), Heavy metals (not more than 0.001%), and Ordinary impurities.
Methohexital Sodium for Injection USP—Preserve in Containers for Sterile Solids. A freeze-dried, sterile mixture of methohexital sodium and anhydrous Sodium Carbonate as a buffer, prepared from an aqueous solution of Methohexital, Sodium Hydroxide, and Sodium Carbonate. Contains the labeled amount, within ±10%. Meets the requirements for Completeness of solution, Constituted solution, Identification, Uniformity of dosage units, Bacterial endotoxins, pH (10.6–11.6), Loss on drying (not more than 2.0%), Heavy metals (not more than 0.001%), and Injections.
Methohexital Sodium for Rectal Solution—Not in USP.

METHOTREXATE

Chemical name: L-Glutamic acid, *N*-[4-[[(2,4-diamino-6-pteridinyl)methyl]methylamino]benzoyl]-.

Molecular formula: $C_{20}H_{22}N_8O_5$.

Molecular weight: 454.45.

Description: Methotrexate USP—Orange-brown, or yellow, crystalline powder.

Solubility: Methotrexate USP—Practically insoluble in water, in alcohol, in chloroform, and in ether; freely soluble in dilute solutions of alkali hydroxides and carbonates; slightly soluble in 6 *N* hydrochloric acid.

USP requirements:
Methotrexate USP—Preserve in tight, light-resistant containers. A mixture of 4-amino-10-methylfolic acid and closely related compounds. Contains not less than 98.0% and not more than 102.0% of methotrexate, calculated on the anhydrous basis. Meets the requirements for Identification, Specific rotation (+19° to +24°, calculated on the anhydrous basis), Water (not more than 12.0%), Residue on ignition (not more than 0.1%), Chromatographic purity, and Organic volatile impurities.
Caution: Great care should be taken to prevent inhaling particles of Methotrexate and exposing the skin to it.
Methotrexate Injection USP—Preserve in single-dose or in multiple-dose containers, preferably of Type I glass, protected from light. A sterile solution of Methotrexate in Water for Injection prepared with the aid of Sodium Hydroxide. Contains the labeled amount of methotrexate, within ±10%. Meets the requirements for Identification, Pyrogen, and pH (7.0–9.0), and for Injections.
Methotrexate for Injection USP—Preserve in Containers for Sterile Solids, protected from light. A sterile, freeze-dried preparation of methotrexate sodium with or without suitable added substances, buffers, and/or diluents. Contains the labeled amount of methotrexate, within −5% to +15%. Meets the requirements for Constituted solution, Identification, Bacterial endotoxins, and pH (7.0–9.0 in a solution constituted as directed in the labeling, except that water is used as the diluent), and for Labeling under Injections, Sterility tests and Uniformity of dosage units.
Caution: Great care should be taken to prevent inhaling particles of methotrexate sodium and exposing the skin to it.
Methotrexate Tablets USP—Preserve in well-closed containers. Contain the labeled amount, within ±10%. Meet the requirements for Identification, Dissolution (75% in 45 minutes in 0.1 *N* hydrochloric acid in Apparatus 2 at 50 rpm), and Uniformity of dosage units.

METHOTRIMEPRAZINE

Chemical group: Phenothiazine derivative.

Chemical name: 10*H*-Phenothiazine-10-propanamine, 2-methoxy-*N,N*,beta-trimethyl-, (–)-.

Molecular formula:
Methotrimeprazine—$C_{19}H_{24}N_2OS$.
Methotrimeprazine hydrochloride—$C_{19}H_{24}N_2OS \cdot HCl$.
Methotrimeprazine maleate—$C_{19}H_{24}N_2OS \cdot C_4H_4O_4$.

Molecular weight:
Methotrimeprazine—328.47.
Methotrimeprazine hydrochloride—364.9.
Methotrimeprazine maleate—444.5.

Description:
Methotrimeprazine USP—Fine, white, practically odorless, crystalline powder. Melts at about 126 °C.
Methotrimeprazine hydrochloride—White or slightly yellow, slightly hygroscopic crystalline powder. It deteriorates on exposure to air and light.

Solubility:
Methotrimeprazine USP—Practically insoluble in water; freely soluble in chloroform and in ether; sparingly soluble in methanol; sparingly soluble in alcohol at 25 °C; freely soluble in boiling alcohol.
Methotrimeprazine hydrochloride—Freely soluble in water, in alcohol, and in chloroform; practically insoluble in ether.
Methotrimeprazine maleate—Sparingly soluble in water and in ethanol.

USP requirements:
Methotrimeprazine USP—Preserve in well-closed, light-resistant containers. Contains not less than 98.0% and not more than 101.0% of methotrimeprazine, calculated on the dried basis. Meets the requirements for Identification, Specific rotation (−15° to −18°, calculated on the dried basis), Loss on drying (not more than 0.5%), and Selenium (not more than 0.003%).
Methotrimeprazine Injection USP—Preserve in single-dose or in multiple-dose containers, preferably of Type I glass, protected from light. A sterile solution of Methotrimeprazine in Water for Injection, prepared with the aid of

hydrochloric acid. Contains the labeled amount, as the hydrochloride, within ±10%. Meets the requirements for Identification, Bacterial endotoxins, pH (3.0–5.0), and Injections.

Methotrimeprazine Hydrochloride Oral Solution—Not in USP.

Methotrimeprazine Hydrochloride Syrup—Not in USP.

Methotrimeprazine Maleate Tablets—Not in USP.

METHOXAMINE

Chemical name: Methoxamine hydrochloride—Benzenemethanol, alpha-(1-aminoethyl)-2,5-dimethoxy-, hydrochloride.

Molecular formula: Methoxamine hydrochloride—$C_{11}H_{17}NO_3 \cdot HCl$.

Molecular weight: Methoxamine hydrochloride—247.72.

Description: Methoxamine Hydrochloride USP—Colorless or white, plate-like crystals or white, crystalline powder. Is odorless or has only a slight odor. Its solutions have a pH of about 5.

Solubility: Methoxamine Hydrochloride USP—Freely soluble in water; soluble in alcohol; practically insoluble in chloroform and in ether.

USP requirements:

Methoxamine Hydrochloride USP—Preserve in well-closed, light-resistant containers. Contains not less than 98.0% and not more than 100.5% of methoxamine hydrochloride, calculated on the dried basis. Meets the requirements for Identification, Melting range (214–219 °C), Loss on drying (not more than 1.0%), Residue on ignition (not more than 0.2%), and Chloride content (14.1–14.5%, calculated on the dried basis).

Methoxamine Hydrochloride Injection USP—Preserve in single-dose or in multiple-dose containers, preferably of Type I glass, and protect from light. Contains the labeled amount, within ±7%. Meets the requirements for Identification, Bacterial endotoxins, pH (3.0–5.0), and Injections.

METHOXSALEN

Chemical name: 7*H*-Furo[3,2-*g*][1]benzopyran-7-one, 9-methoxy-.

Molecular formula: $C_{12}H_8O_4$.

Molecular weight: 216.19.

Description:

Methoxsalen USP—White to cream-colored, fluffy, needle-like crystals. Is odorless.

Methoxsalen Topical Solution USP—Clear, colorless liquid.

Solubility: Methoxsalen USP—Practically insoluble in water; freely soluble in chloroform; soluble in boiling alcohol, in acetone, in acetic acid, and in propylene glycol; sparingly soluble in boiling water and in ether.

USP requirements:

Methoxsalen USP—Preserve in well-closed, light-resistant containers. Contains not less than 98.0% and not more than 102.0% of methoxsalen, calculated on the anhydrous basis. Meets the requirements for Identification, Melting range (143–148 °C), Water (not more than 0.5%), Residue on ignition (not more than 0.1%), Heavy metals (not more than 0.002%), Chromatographic impurities, and Organic volatile impurities.

Caution: Avoid contact with the skin.

Methoxsalen Capsules USP—Preserve in tight, light-resistant containers. Label the Capsules to state that Methoxsalen Hard Gelatin Capsules may not be interchangeable with Methoxsalen Soft Gelatin Capsules without retitration of the patient. Contain the labeled amount, within ±10%. Meet the requirements for Identification, Dissolution (75% in 45 minutes in water in Apparatus 2 at 50 rpm for Soft Gelatin Capsules and 75% in 90 minutes in water in Apparatus 1 at 150 rpm for Hard Gelatin Capsules), and Uniformity of dosage units.

Methoxsalen Topical Solution USP—Store in tight, light-resistant containers. A solution of Methoxsalen in a suitable vehicle. Contains not less than 9.2 mg and not more than 10.8 mg of methoxsalen per mL. Meets the requirements for Identification and Alcohol content (66.5–77.0%).

METHOXYFLURANE

Chemical name: Ethane, 2,2-dichloro-1,1-difluoro-1-methoxy-.

Molecular formula: $C_3H_4Cl_2F_2O$.

Molecular weight: 164.97.

Description: Methoxyflurane USP—Clear, practically colorless, mobile liquid, having a characteristic odor. Boils at about 105 °C.

Solubility: Methoxyflurane USP—Miscible with alcohol, with acetone, with chloroform, with ether, and with fixed oils.

Other characteristics:

Blood-to-Gas (mean range) partition coefficient at 37 °C—10.20 to 14.06.

Oil-to-Gas partition coefficient at 37 °C—825.

USP requirements: Methoxyflurane USP—Preserve in tight, light-resistant containers, and avoid exposure to excessive heat. Contains not less than 99.9% and not more than 100.0% of methoxyflurane. Meets the requirements for Identification, Specific gravity (1.420–1.425), Nonvolatile residue (not more than 1 mg per 50 mL), Acidity, Water (not more than 0.1%), and Foreign odor.

METHSCOPOLAMINE

Source: Quaternary ammonium derivative of scopolamine.

Chemical name: Methscopolamine bromide—3-Oxa-9-azoniatricyclo[3.3.1.0^{2,4}]nonane, 7-(3-hydroxy-1-oxo-2-phenylpropoxy)-9,9-dimethyl-, bromide, [7(*S*)-(1 alpha,2 beta,4 beta,5 alpha,7 beta)]-.

Molecular formula: Methscopolamine bromide—$C_{18}H_{24}BrNO_4$.

Molecular weight: Methscopolamine bromide—398.30.

Description: Methscopolamine Bromide USP—White crystals or white, odorless, crystalline powder. Melts at about 225 °C, with decomposition.

Solubility: Methscopolamine Bromide USP—Freely soluble in water; slightly soluble in alcohol; insoluble in acetone and in chloroform.

USP requirements:

Methscopolamine Bromide USP—Preserve in tight, light-resistant containers. Contains not less than 97.0% and not more than 103.0% of methscopolamine bromide, calculated on the dried basis. Meets the requirements for Identification, Specific rotation (−21° to −25°, calculated on the dried basis), Loss on drying (not more than 2.0%), Residue on ignition (not more than 0.1%), and Organic volatile impurities.

Methscopolamine Bromide Tablets USP—Preserve in tight containers. Contain the labeled amount, within ±7%. Meet the requirements for Identification, Disintegration (15 minutes), and Uniformity of dosage units.

METHSUXIMIDE

Chemical name: 2,5-Pyrrolidinedione, 1,3-dimethyl-3-phenyl-.

Molecular formula: $C_{12}H_{13}NO_2$.

Molecular weight: 203.24.

Description: Methsuximide USP—White to grayish white, crystalline powder. Is odorless, or has not more than a slight odor.

Solubility: Methsuximide USP—Slightly soluble in hot water; very soluble in chloroform; freely soluble in alcohol and in ether.

USP requirements:

Methsuximide USP—Preserve in tight containers. Contains not less than 97.0% and not more than 103.0% of methsuximide, calculated on the dried basis. Meets the requirements for Identification, Melting range (50–56 °C), Loss on drying (not more than 0.5%), Residue on ignition (not more than 0.2%), Cyanide, Ordinary impurities, and Organic volatile impurities.

Methsuximide Capsules USP—Preserve in tight containers, and avoid exposure to excessive heat. Contain the labeled amount, within ±8%. Meet the requirements for Identification, Dissolution (75% in 120 minutes in water in Apparatus 1 at 100 rpm), and Uniformity of dosage units.

METHYCLOTHIAZIDE

Chemical name: 2*H*-1,2,4-Benzothiadiazine-7-sulfonamide, 6-chloro-3-(chloromethyl)-3,4-dihydro-2-methyl-, 1,1-dioxide.

Molecular formula: $C_9H_{11}Cl_2N_3O_4S_2$.

Molecular weight: 360.23.

Description: Methyclothiazide USP—White or practically white, crystalline powder. Is odorless, or has a slight odor.

pKa: 9.4.

Solubility: Methyclothiazide USP—Very slightly soluble in water and in chloroform; freely soluble in acetone and in pyridine; sparingly soluble in methanol; slightly soluble in alcohol.

USP requirements:

Methyclothiazide USP—Preserve in well-closed containers. Contains not less than 97.0% and not more than 102.0% of methyclothiazide, calculated on the dried basis. Meets the requirements for Identification, Loss on drying (not more than 0.5%), Residue on ignition (not more than 0.2%), Chloride (not more than 0.02%), Selenium (not more than 0.003%), Heavy metals (not more than 0.002%), and Diazotizable substances (not more than 1.0%).

Methyclothiazide Tablets USP—Preserve in well-closed containers. Contain the labeled amount, within ±10%. Meet the requirements for Identification, Dissolution (70% in 60 minutes in 0.1 *N* hydrochloric acid in Apparatus 2 at 50 rpm), and Uniformity of dosage units.

METHYL ALCOHOL

Chemical name: Methanol.

Molecular formula: CH_4O.

Molecular weight: 32.04.

Description: Methyl Alcohol NF—Clear, colorless liquid, having a characteristic odor. Is flammable.

NF category: Solvent.

Solubility: Methyl Alcohol NF—Miscible with water, with alcohol, with ether, and with most other organic solvents.

NF requirements: Methyl Alcohol NF—Preserve in tight containers, remote from heat, sparks, and open flames. Contains not less than 99.5% of methyl alcohol. Meets the requirements for Identification, Acidity, Alkalinity (as ammonia, not more than 3 ppm), Water (not more than 0.1%), Nonvolatile residue (not more than 0.001% [w/w]), Readily carbonizable substances, Readily oxidizable substances, Acetone and aldehydes (as acetone, not more than 0.003%), and Organic volatile impurities.

Caution: Methyl Alcohol is poisonous.

METHYLBENZETHONIUM

Chemical name: Methylbenzethonium chloride—Benzenemethanaminium, *N,N*-dimethyl-*N*-[2-[2-[methyl-4-(1,1,3,3-tetramethylbutyl)phenoxy]ethoxy]ethyl]-, chloride, monohydrate.

Molecular formula: Methylbenzethonium chloride—$C_{28}H_{44}ClNO_2 \cdot H_2O$.

Molecular weight: Methylbenzethonium chloride—480.13.

Description: Methylbenzethonium Chloride USP—White, hygroscopic crystals, having a mild odor. Its solutions are neutral or slightly alkaline to litmus.

Solubility: Methylbenzethonium Chloride USP—Very soluble in water, in alcohol, and in ether; practically insoluble in chloroform.

USP requirements:

Methylbenzethonium Chloride USP—Preserve in tight containers. Contains not less than 97.0% and not more than 103.0% of methylbenzethonium chloride, calculated on the dried basis. Meets the requirements for Identification, Melting range (159–163 °C, the specimen having been previously dried), Loss on drying (not more than 5.0%), Residue on ignition (not more than 0.1%), and Ammonia.

Methylbenzethonium Chloride Lotion USP—Preserve in tight containers. An emulsion containing the labeled amount, within ±10%. Meets the requirements for Identification and pH (5.2–6.0).

Methylbenzethonium Chloride Ointment USP—Preserve in collapsible tubes or in tight containers. Contains the labeled amount, within ±10%. Meets the requirements for Identification and pH (5.0–7.0, in a dispersion of it in carbon dioxide-free water [1 in 100]).

Methylbenzethonium Chloride Topical Powder USP—Preserve in well-closed containers. Contains the labeled amount, within ±15%, in a suitable fine powder base, free from grittiness. Meets the requirements for Identification, pH (9.0–10.5, in a dispersion of it in carbon dioxide-free water [1 in 100]), and Powder fineness (not less than 99% of it passes through a No. 200 sieve).

METHYLCELLULOSE

Chemical group: Semisynthetic hydrophilic derivative of cellulose.

Chemical name: Cellulose, methyl ether.

Description: Methylcellulose USP—White, fibrous powder or granules. Its aqueous suspensions are neutral to litmus. It swells in water and produces a clear to opalescent, viscous colloidal suspension.

NF category: Coating agent; suspending and/or viscosity-increasing agent; tablet binder.

Solubility: Methylcellulose USP—Insoluble in alcohol, in ether, and in chloroform; soluble in glacial acetic acid and in a mixture of equal volumes of alcohol and chloroform.

USP requirements:
Methylcellulose Capsules—Not in USP.
Methylcellulose USP (Granules or Powder)—Preserve in well-closed containers. A methyl ether of cellulose. When dried at 105 °C for 2 hours, contains not less than 27.5% and not more than 31.5% of methoxy (OCH_3) groups. Label it to indicate its viscosity type (viscosity of a solution [1 in 50]). Meets the requirements for Identification, Apparent viscosity (within ±20% of labeled viscosity when 100 centipoises or less, within −25% to +40% of labeled viscosity when greater than 100 centipoises), Loss on drying (not more than 5.0%), Residue on ignition (not more than 1.5%), Arsenic (not more than 3 ppm), Heavy metals (not more than 0.001%), and Organic volatile impurities.
Methylcellulose Ophthalmic Solution USP—Preserve in tight containers. A sterile solution of Methylcellulose. Contains the labeled amount, within ±15%. Meets the requirements for Identification, Sterility, and pH (6.0–7.8).
Methylcellulose Oral Solution USP—Preserve in tight, light-resistant containers, and avoid exposure to direct sunlight and to excessive heat. Avoid freezing. A flavored solution of Methylcellulose. Contains the labeled amount, within ±15%. Meets the requirements for Identification, Microbial limits, and Alcohol content (3.5–6.5%).
Methylcellulose Tablets USP—Preserve in well-closed containers. Contain the labeled amount, within ±10%. Meet the requirements for Identification, Disintegration (30 minutes), and Uniformity of dosage units.

METHYLDOPA

Chemical name:
Methyldopa—L-Tyrosine, 3-hydroxy-alpha-methyl-, sesquihydrate.
Methyldopate hydrochloride—L-Tyrosine, 3-hydroxy-alpha-methyl-, ethyl ester, hydrochloride.

Molecular formula:
Methyldopa—$C_{10}H_{13}NO_4 \cdot 1\frac{1}{2}H_2O$.
Methyldopate hydrochloride—$C_{12}H_{17}NO_4 \cdot HCl$.

Molecular weight:
Methyldopa—238.24.
Methyldopate hydrochloride—275.73.

Description:
Methyldopa USP—White to yellowish white, odorless, fine powder, which may contain friable lumps.
Methyldopate Hydrochloride USP—White or practically white, odorless or practically odorless, crystalline powder.

Solubility:
Methyldopa USP—Sparingly soluble in water; very soluble in 3 *N* hydrochloric acid; slightly soluble in alcohol; practically insoluble in ether.
Methyldopate Hydrochloride USP—Freely soluble in water, in alcohol, and in methanol; slightly soluble in chloroform; practically insoluble in ether.

USP requirements:
Methyldopa USP—Preserve in well-closed, light-resistant containers. Contains not less than 98.0% and not more than 101.0% of methyldopa, calculated on the anhydrous basis. Meets the requirements for Identification, Specific rotation (−25° to −28°, calculated on the anhydrous basis), Acidity, Water (10.0–13.0%), Residue on ignition (not more than 0.1%), Heavy metals (not more than 0.001%), 3-*O*-Methylmethyldopa, and Organic volatile impurities.
Methyldopa Oral Suspension USP—Preserve in tight, light-resistant containers, at a temperature not exceeding 26 °C. An aqueous suspension of Methyldopa. Contains one or more suitable flavors, wetting agents, and preservatives. Contains the labeled amount, within ±10%. Meets the requirements for Identification, pH (3.0–5.0; 3.2–3.8 if sucrose is present), and Limit of methyldopa-glucose reaction product (if sucrose is present).
Methyldopa Tablets USP—Preserve in well-closed containers. Contain the labeled amount, within ±10%. Meet the requirements for Identification, Dissolution (80% in 20 minutes in 0.1 *N* hydrochloric acid in Apparatus 2 at 50 rpm), and Uniformity of dosage units.
Methyldopate Hydrochloride USP—Preserve in well-closed containers. Contains not less than 98.0% and not more than 101.0% of methyldopate hydrochloride, calculated on the dried basis. Meets the requirements for Identification, Specific rotation (−13.5° to −14.9°, calculated on the dried basis), pH (3.0–5.0, in a solution [1 in 100]), Loss on drying (not more than 0.5%), Residue on ignition (not more than 0.1%), and Heavy metals (not more than 0.001%).
Methyldopate Hydrochloride Injection USP—Preserve in single-dose containers, preferably of Type I glass. A sterile solution of Methyldopate Hydrochloride in Water for Injection. Contains the labeled amount, within ±10%. Meets the requirements for Identification, Bacterial endotoxins, pH (3.0–4.2), Particulate matter, and Injections.

METHYLDOPA AND CHLOROTHIAZIDE

For *Methyldopa* and *Chlorothiazide*—See individual listings for chemistry information.

USP requirements: Methyldopa and Chlorothiazide Tablets USP—Preserve in well-closed containers. Contain the labeled amounts, within ±10%. Meet the requirements for Identification, Dissolution (80% of methyldopa in 30 minutes in 0.1 *N* hydrochloric acid in Apparatus 2 at 75 rpm; and 75% of chlorothiazide in 60 minutes in 0.05 *M* phosphate buffer [pH 8.0] in Apparatus 2 at 75 rpm), and Uniformity of dosage units.

METHYLDOPA AND HYDROCHLOROTHIAZIDE

For *Methyldopa* and *Hydrochlorothiazide*—See individual listings for chemistry information.

USP requirements: Methyldopa and Hydrochlorothiazide Tablets USP—Preserve in well-closed containers. Contain the labeled amounts, within ±10%. Meet the requirements for Identification, Dissolution (80% of methyldopa in 30 minutes and 80% of hydrochlorothiazide in 60 minutes in 0.1 *N* hydrochloric acid in Apparatus 2 at 50 rpm), and Uniformity of dosage units.

METHYLENE BLUE

Chemical name: Phenothiazin-5-ium, 3,7-bis(dimethylamino)-, chloride, trihydrate.

Molecular formula: $C_{16}H_{18}ClN_3S \cdot 3H_2O$.

Molecular weight: 373.90.

Description: Methylene Blue USP—Dark green crystals or crystalline powder having a bronze-like luster. Odorless or practically so. Stable in air. Its solutions in water and in alcohol are deep blue in color.

Solubility: Methylene Blue USP—Soluble in water and in chloroform; sparingly soluble in alcohol.

USP requirements:

Methylene Blue USP—Preserve in well-closed containers. Contains not less than 98.0% and not more than 103.0% of methylene blue, calculated on the dried basis. Meets the requirements for Identification, Loss on drying (8.0–18.0%), Residue on ignition (not more than 1.2%), Arsenic (not more than 8 ppm), Copper or zinc (not more than 0.02% of copper), Chromatographic purity, and Organic volatile impurities.

Methylene Blue Injection USP—Preserve in single-dose containers, preferably of Type I glass. A sterile solution of Methylene Blue in Water for Injection. Contains, in each mL, not less than 9.5 mg and not more than 10.5 mg of methylene blue. Meets the requirements for Identification, Bacterial endotoxins, pH (3.0–4.5), and Injections.

METHYLENE CHLORIDE

Chemical name: Methane, dichloro-.

Molecular formula: CH_2Cl_2.

Molecular weight: 84.93.

Description: Methylene Chloride NF—Clear, colorless, mobile liquid, having an odor resembling that of chloroform.

NF category: Solvent.

Solubility: Methylene Chloride NF—Miscible with alcohol, with ether, and with fixed and volatile oils.

NF requirements: Methylene Chloride NF—Preserve in tight containers. Contains not less than 99.0% of methylene chloride. Meets the requirements for Identification, Specific gravity (1.318–1.322), Distilling range (39.5–40.5 °C), Water (not more than 0.02%), Hydrogen chloride, Nonvolatile residue (not more than 0.002%), Heavy metals (not more than 1 ppm), and Free chlorine.

Caution: Perform all steps involving evaporation of methylene chloride in a well-ventilated fume hood.

METHYLERGONOVINE

Chemical group: Semi-synthetic ergot alkaloid.

Chemical name: Methylergonovine maleate—Ergoline-8-carboxamide, 9,10-didehydro-*N*-[1-(hydroxymethyl)propyl]-6-methyl-, [8 beta(*S*)]-, (*Z*)-2-butenedioate (1:1) (salt).

Molecular formula: Methylergonovine maleate—$C_{20}H_{25}N_3O_2 \cdot C_4H_4O_4$.

Molecular weight: Methylergonovine maleate—455.51.

Description: Methylergonovine Maleate USP—White to pinkish tan, microcrystalline powder. Is odorless.

Solubility: Methylergonovine Maleate USP—Slightly soluble in water and in alcohol; very slightly soluble in chloroform and in ether.

USP requirements:

Methylergonovine Maleate USP—Preserve in tight, light-resistant containers, and store in a cold place. Contains not less than 97.0% and not more than 103.0% of methylergonovine maleate, calculated on the dried basis. Meets the requirements for Identification, Specific rotation (+44° to +50°, calculated on the dried basis), pH (4.4–5.2, in a solution [1 in 5000]), Loss on drying (not more than 2.0%), Residue on ignition (not more than 0.1%), and Related alkaloids.

Methylergonovine Maleate Injection USP—Preserve in single-dose, light-resistant containers, preferably of Type I glass. A sterile solution of Methylergonovine Maleate in Water for Injection. Contains, in each mL, the labeled amount, within ±10%. Meets the requirements for Identification, Bacterial endotoxins, pH (2.7–3.5), Related alkaloids, and Injections.

Methylergonovine Maleate Tablets USP—Preserve in tight, light-resistant containers. Contain the labeled amount, within ±10%. Meet the requirements for Identification, Dissolution (70% in 30 minutes in tartaric acid solution [1 in 200] in Apparatus 2 at 100 rpm), Uniformity of dosage units, and Related alkaloids.

METHYL ISOBUTYL KETONE

Chemical name: 2-Pentanone, 4-methyl-.

Molecular formula: $C_6H_{12}O$.

Molecular weight: 100.16.

Description: Methyl Isobutyl Ketone NF—Transparent, colorless, mobile, volatile liquid, having a faint ketonic and camphoraceous odor.

NF category: Alcohol denaturant; solvent.

Solubility: Methyl Isobutyl Ketone NF—Slightly soluble in water; miscible with alcohol and with ether.

NF requirements: Methyl Isobutyl Ketone NF—Preserve in tight containers. Contains not less than 99.0% of methyl isobutyl ketone. Meets the requirements for Identification, Specific gravity (not more than 0.799), Distilling range (114–117 °C), Acidity, and Nonvolatile residue (not more than 0.008%).

METHYLPARABEN

Chemical name:

Methylparaben—Benzoic acid, 4-hydroxy-, methyl ester.

Methylparaben sodium—Benzoic acid, 4-hydroxy-, methyl ester, sodium salt.

Molecular formula:

Methylparaben—$C_8H_8O_3$.

Methylparaben sodium—$C_8H_7NaO_3$.

Molecular weight:

Methylparaben—152.15.

Methylparaben sodium—174.13.

Description:

Methylparaben NF—Small, colorless crystals, or white, crystalline powder. It is odorless, or has a faint, characteristic odor.

NF category: Antimicrobial preservative.

Methylparaben Sodium NF—White, hygroscopic powder.

NF category: Antimicrobial preservative.

Solubility:

Methylparaben NF—Slightly soluble in water and in carbon tetrachloride; freely soluble in alcohol and in ether.

Methylparaben Sodium NF—Freely soluble in water; sparingly soluble in alcohol; insoluble in fixed oils.

NF requirements:

Methylparaben NF—Preserve in well-closed containers. Contains not less than 99.0% and not more than 100.5%

of methylparaben, calculated on the dried basis. Meets the requirements for Identification and Melting range (125–128 °C), and for Acidity, Loss on drying, and Residue on ignition under Butylparaben.

Methylparaben Sodium NF—Preserve in tight containers. Contains not less than 98.5% and not more than 101.5% of methylparaben sodium. Meets the requirements for Completeness of solution, Identification, pH (9.5–10.5, in a solution [1 in 1000]), Water (not more than 5.0%), Chloride (not more than 0.035%), Sulfate (not more than 0.12%), and Organic volatile impurities.

METHYLPHENIDATE

Chemical name: Methylphenidate hydrochloride—2-Piperidineacetic acid, alpha-phenyl-, methyl ester, hydrochloride, (*R*,R**)-(±)-.

Molecular formula: Methylphenidate hydrochloride—$C_{14}H_{19}NO_2 \cdot HCl$.

Molecular weight: Methylphenidate hydrochloride—269.77.

Description: Methylphenidate Hydrochloride USP—White, odorless, fine, crystalline powder. Its solutions are acid to litmus.

Solubility: Methylphenidate Hydrochloride USP—Freely soluble in water and in methanol; soluble in alcohol; slightly soluble in chloroform and in acetone.

USP requirements:

Methylphenidate Hydrochloride USP—Preserve in well-closed containers. Contains not less than 98.0% and not more than 100.5% of methylphenidate hydrochloride, calculated on the dried basis. Meets the requirements for Identification, Loss on drying (not more than 0.5%), Residue on ignition (not more than 0.1%), Heavy metals (not more than 0.001%), Limit of erythro [(*R*,S**)] isomer, Limit of alpha-phenyl-2-piperidineacetic acid hydrochloride, and Organic volatile impurities.

Methylphenidate Hydrochloride Tablets USP—Preserve in tight containers. Contain the labeled amount, within ±7%. Meet the requirements for Identification, Dissolution (75% in 45 minutes in water in Apparatus 1 at 100 rpm), and Uniformity of dosage units.

Methylphenidate Hydrochloride Extended-release Tablets USP—Preserve in tight containers. Contain the labeled amount, within ±10%. Meet the requirements for Identification, Drug release (20 to 50% in 0.125*D* hours, 35 to 70% in 0.250*D* hours, 53 to 83% in 0.438*D* hours, 70 to 95% in 0.625*D* hours, not less than 80% in 0.875*D* hours, in water in Apparatus 2 at 50 rpm), and Uniformity of dosage units.

METHYLPREDNISOLONE

Chemical name:

Methylprednisolone—Pregna-1,4-diene-3,20-dione, 11,17,21-trihydroxy-6-methyl-, (6 alpha,11 beta)-.

Methylprednisolone acetate—Pregna-1,4-diene-3,20-dione, 21-(acetyloxy)-11,17-dihydroxy-6-methyl-, (6 alpha,11 beta)-.

Methylprednisolone hemisuccinate—Pregna-1,4-diene-3,20-dione, 21-(3-carboxy-1-oxopropoxy)-11,17-dihydroxy-6-methyl-, (6 alpha,11 beta)-.

Methylprednisolone sodium succinate—Pregna-1,4-diene-3,20-dione, 21-(3-carboxy-1-oxopropoxy)-11,17-dihydroxy-6-methyl-, monosodium salt, (6 alpha,11 beta)-.

Molecular formula:

Methylprednisolone—$C_{22}H_{30}O_5$.
Methylprednisolone acetate—$C_{24}H_{32}O_6$.
Methylprednisolone hemisuccinate—$C_{26}H_{34}O_8$.
Methylprednisolone sodium succinate—$C_{26}H_{33}NaO_8$.

Molecular weight:

Methylprednisolone—374.48.
Methylprednisolone acetate—416.51.
Methylprednisolone hemisuccinate—474.55.
Methylprednisolone sodium succinate—496.53.

Description:

Methylprednisolone USP—White to practically white, odorless, crystalline powder. Melts at about 240 °C, with some decomposition.

Methylprednisolone Acetate USP—White or practically white, odorless, crystalline powder. Melts at about 225 °C, with some decomposition.

Methylprednisolone Hemisuccinate USP—White or nearly white, odorless or nearly odorless, hygroscopic solid.

Methylprednisolone Sodium Succinate USP—White or nearly white, odorless, hygroscopic, amorphous solid.

Solubility:

Methylprednisolone USP—Practically insoluble in water; sparingly soluble in alcohol, in dioxane, and in methanol; slightly soluble in acetone and in chloroform; very slightly soluble in ether.

Methylprednisolone Acetate USP—Practically insoluble in water; soluble in dioxane; sparingly soluble in acetone, in alcohol, in chloroform, and in methanol; slightly soluble in ether.

Methylprednisolone Hemisuccinate USP—Very slightly soluble in water; freely soluble in alcohol; soluble in acetone.

Methylprednisolone Sodium Succinate USP—Very soluble in water and in alcohol; very slightly soluble in acetone; insoluble in chloroform.

USP requirements:

Methylprednisolone USP—Preserve in tight, light-resistant containers. Contains not less than 97.0% and not more than 103.0% of methylprednisolone, calculated on the dried basis. Meets the requirements for Identification, Specific rotation (+79° to +86°, calculated on the dried basis), Loss on drying (not more than 1.0%), Residue on ignition (not more than 0.2%), and Ordinary impurities.

Methylprednisolone Tablets USP—Preserve in tight containers. Contain the labeled amount, within ±7.5%. Meet the requirements for Identification, Dissolution (50% in 30 minutes in water in Apparatus 1 at 100 rpm), and Uniformity of dosage units.

Methylprednisolone Acetate USP—Preserve in tight, light-resistant containers. Contains not less than 97.0% and not more than 103.0% of methylprednisolone acetate, calculated on the dried basis. Meets the requirements for Identification, Specific rotation (+97° to +105°, calculated on the dried basis), Loss on drying (not more than 1.0%), and Residue on ignition (not more than 0.2%).

Methylprednisolone Acetate Cream USP—Preserve in collapsible tubes or in tight containers, protected from light. Contains the labeled amount, within ±10%. Meets the requirements for Identification and Minimum fill.

Methylprednisolone Acetate for Enema USP—Preserve in well-closed containers. A dry mixture of Methylprednisolone Acetate with one or more suitable excipients. Contains the labeled amount, within ±10%. Meets the requirements for Identification and Uniformity of dosage units.

Sterile Methylprednisolone Acetate Suspension USP—Preserve in single-dose or in multiple-dose containers, preferably of Type I glass. A sterile suspension of Methylprednisolone Acetate in a suitable aqueous medium. Contains the labeled amount, within ±10%. Meets the requirements for Identification, Uniformity of dosage units, pH (3.5–7.0), Particle size (not less than 99% are less than 20 micrometers in length [measured on longest axis] and not less than 75% are less than 10 micrometers in length, using 400x magnification), and Injections.

Methylprednisolone Hemisuccinate USP—Preserve in tight containers. Contains not less than 97.0% and not more than 103.0% of methylprednisolone hemisuccinate, calculated on the dried basis. Meets the requirements for Identification, Specific rotation (+87° to +95°, calculated on the dried basis), Loss on drying (not more than 1.0%), and Residue on ignition (not more than 0.2%).

Methylprednisolone Sodium Succinate USP—Preserve in tight, light-resistant containers. Contains not less than 97.0% and not more than 103.0% of methylprednisolone sodium succinate, calculated on the dried basis. Meets the requirements for Identification, Specific rotation (+96° to +104°, calculated on the dried basis), Loss on drying (not more than 3.0%), and Sodium content (4.49–4.77%, calculated on the dried basis).

Methylprednisolone Sodium Succinate for Injection USP—Preserve in Containers for Sterile Solids. A sterile mixture of Methylprednisolone Sodium Succinate with suitable buffers. May be prepared from Methylprednisolone Sodium Succinate or from Methylprednisolone Hemisuccinate with the aid of Sodium Hydroxide or Sodium Carbonate. Contains an amount of methylprednisolone sodium succinate equivalent to the labeled amount of methylprednisolone, within ± 10%, in the volume of constituted solution designated on the label. Meets the requirements for Constituted solution, Identification, Bacterial endotoxins, pH (7.0–8.0, in a solution containing about 50 mg of methylprednisolone sodium succinate per mL), Loss on drying (not more than 2.0%), Particulate matter, and Free methylprednisolone (not more than 6.6% of labeled amount of methylprednisolone), and for Sterility tests, Uniformity of dosage units, and Labeling under Injections.

METHYL SALICYLATE

Chemical name: Benzoic acid, 2-hydroxy-, methyl ester.

Molecular formula: $C_8H_8O_3$.

Molecular weight: 152.15.

Description: Methyl Salicylate NF—Colorless, yellowish, or reddish liquid, having the characteristic odor of wintergreen. It boils between 219 and 224 °C, with some decomposition.
NF category: Flavors and perfumes.

Solubility: Methyl Salicylate NF—Slightly soluble in water; soluble in alcohol and in glacial acetic acid.

NF requirements: Methyl Salicylate NF—Preserve in tight containers. It is produced synthetically or is obtained by maceration and subsequent distillation with steam from the leaves of *Gaultheria procumbens* Linné (Fam. Ericaceae) or from the bark of *Betula lenta* Linné (Fam. Betulaceae). Label it to indicate whether it was made synthetically or distilled from either of the plants mentioned above. Contains not less than 98.0% and not more than 100.5% of methyl salicylate. Meets the requirements for Solubility in 70% alcohol (if it is synthetic, one volume dissolves in 7 volumes of 70% alcohol; if it is natural, one volume dissolves in 7 volumes of 70% alcohol, the solution having not more than a slight cloudiness), Identification, Specific gravity (for the synthetic, 1.180–1.185; for the natural, 1.176–1.182), Angular rotation, Refractive index (1.535–1.538 at 20 °C), and Heavy metals (not more than 0.004%).

METHYLTESTOSTERONE

Chemical group: Synthetic derivative of testosterone.

Chemical name: Androst-4-en-3-one, 17-hydroxy-17-methyl-, (17 beta)-.

Molecular formula: $C_{20}H_{30}O_2$.

Molecular weight: 302.46.

Description: Methyltestosterone USP—White or creamy white crystals or crystalline powder. Is odorless and is stable in air, but is slightly hygroscopic. Is affected by light.

Solubility: Methyltestosterone USP—Practically insoluble in water; soluble in alcohol, in methanol, in ether, and in other organic solvents; sparingly soluble in vegetable oils.

USP requirements:

Methyltestosterone USP—Preserve in well-closed, light-resistant containers. Contains not less than 97.0% and not more than 103.0% of methyltestosterone, calculated on the dried basis. Meets the requirements for Identification, Melting range (162–167 °C), Specific rotation (+79° to +85°, calculated on the dried basis), Loss on drying (not more than 2.0%), and Chromatographic purity.

Methyltestosterone Capsules USP—Preserve in well-closed containers. Contain the labeled amount, within ± 10%. Meet the requirements for Identification, Dissolution (60% in 30 minutes in water in Apparatus 1 at 100 rpm), and Uniformity of dosage units.

Methyltestosterone Tablets USP—Preserve in well-closed containers. Contain the labeled amount, within ± 10%. Meet the requirements for Identification, Disintegration (30 minutes. Tablets intended for buccal administration meet the requirements for Buccal Tablets), and Uniformity of dosage units.

METHYPRYLON

Chemical name: 2,4-Piperidinedione, 3,3-diethyl-5-methyl-.

Molecular formula: $C_{10}H_{17}NO_2$.

Molecular weight: 183.25.

Description: Methyprylon USP—White, or practically white, crystalline powder, having a slight, characteristic odor.

Solubility: Methyprylon USP—Soluble in water; freely soluble in alcohol, in chloroform, and in ether.

USP requirements:

Methyprylon USP—Preserve in well-closed, light-resistant containers. Contains not less than 98.0% and not more than 101.0% of methyprylon, calculated on the dried basis. Meets the requirements for Identification, Melting range (74.0–77.5 °C), Loss on drying (not more than 1.0%), Residue on ignition (not more than 0.1%), Ordinary impurities, and Organic volatile impurities.

Methyprylon Capsules USP—Preserve in tight, light-resistant containers. Contain the labeled amount, within ± 10%. Meet the requirements for Identification, Dissolution (75% in 45 minutes in water in Apparatus 1 at 100 rpm), and Uniformity of dosage units.

Methyprylon Tablets USP—Preserve in tight, light-resistant containers. Contain the labeled amount, within ± 5%. Meet the requirements for Identification, Dissolution (75% in 45 minutes in water in Apparatus 1 at 100 rpm), and Uniformity of dosage units.

METHYSERGIDE

Chemical name: Methysergide maleate—Ergoline-8-carboxamide, 9,10-didehydro-*N*-[1-(hydroxymethyl)propyl]-1,6-dimethyl-, (8 beta)-, (*Z*)-2-butenedioate (1:1) (salt).

Molecular formula: Methysergide maleate—$C_{21}H_{27}N_3O_2 \cdot C_4H_4O_4$.

Molecular weight: Methysergide maleate—469.54.

Description: Methysergide Maleate USP—White to yellowish white or reddish white, crystalline powder. Is odorless or has not more than a slight odor.

Solubility: Methysergide Maleate USP—Slightly soluble in water and in alcohol; very slightly soluble in chloroform; practically insoluble in ether.

USP requirements:

Methysergide Maleate USP—Preserve in tight, light-resistant containers, in a cold place. Contains not less than 97.0% and not more than 103.0% of methysergide maleate, calculated on the dried basis. Meets the requirements for Identification, Specific rotation (+35° to +45°, calculated on the dried basis), pH (3.7–4.7, in a 1 in 500 solution in carbon dioxide-free water), Loss on drying (not more than 7.0%), and Ordinary impurities.

Methysergide Maleate Tablets USP—Preserve in tight containers. Contain the labeled amount, within ±10%. Meet the requirements for Identification, Dissolution (70% in 30 minutes in tartaric acid solution [1 in 200] in Apparatus 2 at 100 rpm), and Uniformity of dosage units.

METIPRANOLOL

Chemical name: Phenol, 4-[2-hydroxy-3-[(1-methylethyl)amino]propoxy]-2,3,6-trimethyl-, (±)-, 1-acetate.

Molecular formula: $C_{17}H_{27}NO_4$.

Molecular weight: 309.41.

Description: White, odorless, crystalline powder.

Solubility: Metipranolol hydrochloride—Soluble in water.

USP requirements: Metipranolol Hydrochloride Ophthalmic Solution—Not in USP.

METOCLOPRAMIDE

Source: *p*-Aminobenzoic acid derivative, structurally related to procainamide.

Chemical name: Metoclopramide hydrochloride—Benzamide, 4-amino-5-chloro-*N*-[2-(diethylamino)ethyl]-2-methoxy-, monohydrochloride, monohydrate.

Molecular formula: Metoclopramide hydrochloride—$C_{14}H_{22}ClN_3O_2 \cdot HCl \cdot H_2O$.

Molecular weight: Metoclopramide hydrochloride—354.28.

Description: Metoclopramide Hydrochloride USP—White or practically white, crystalline, odorless or practically odorless powder.

pKa: Metoclopramide hydrochloride—0.6 and 9.3.

Solubility: Metoclopramide Hydrochloride USP—Very soluble in water; freely soluble in alcohol; sparingly soluble in chloroform; practically insoluble in ether.

USP requirements:

Metoclopramide Injection USP—Preserve in single-dose or in multiple-dose containers, preferably of Type I glass, protected from light. (Note: Injection containing an antioxidant agent does not require protection from light.) A sterile solution of Metoclopramide Hydrochloride in Water for Injection. Contains the labeled amount, within ±10%. Meets the requirements for Identification, Bacterial endotoxins, pH (2.5–6.5), Particulate matter, and Injections.

Metoclopramide Oral Solution USP—Store in tight, light-resistant containers at controlled room temperature. Protect from freezing. Contains an amount of Metoclopramide Hydrochloride equivalent to the labeled amount of metoclopramide, within ±10%. Meets the requirements for Identification and pH (2.0–5.5).

Metoclopramide Tablets USP—Preserve in tight, light-resistant containers. Contain an amount of metoclopramide hydrochloride equivalent to the labeled amount of metoclopramide, within ±10%. Meet the requirements for Identification, Dissolution (75% in 30 minutes in water in Apparatus 1 at 50 rpm), and Uniformity of dosage units.

Metoclopromide Hydrochloride USP—Preserve in tight, light-resistant containers. Contains not less than 98.0% and not more than 101.0% of metoclopromide hydrochloride, calculated on the anhydrous basis. Meets the requirements for Identification, Water (4.5–6.0%), Residue on ignition (not more than 0.1%), Chromatographic purity, and Organic volatile impurities.

Metoclopramide Hydrochloride Syrup—Not in USP.

METOCURINE

Chemical name: Metocurine iodide—Tubocuraranium, 6,6′,7′,12′-tetramethoxy-2,2,2′,2′-tetramethyl-, diiodide.

Molecular formula: Metocurine iodide—$C_{40}H_{48}I_2N_2O_6$.

Molecular weight: Metocurine iodide—906.64.

Description: Metocurine Iodide USP—White or pale yellow, crystalline powder.

Solubility: Metocurine Iodide USP—Slightly soluble in water, in 3 *N* hydrochloric acid, and in dilute solutions of sodium hydroxide; very slightly soluble in alcohol; practically insoluble in chloroform and in ether.

USP requirements:

Metocurine Iodide USP—Preserve in tight containers. Contains not less than 95.0% and not more than 105.0% of metocurine iodide, calculated on the anhydrous basis. Meets the requirements for Identification, Specific rotation (+148° to +158°, calculated on the anhydrous basis), Water (not more than 7.0%), and Related substances.

Caution: Handle Metocurine Iodide with exceptional care since it is a highly potent skeletal muscle relaxant.

Metocurine Iodide Injection USP—Preserve in single-dose or in multiple-dose containers, preferably of Type I glass. Phenol, 0.5%, or some other suitable bacteriostatic substance, is added to the Injection in multiple-dose containers. A sterile solution of Metocurine Iodide in isotonic sodium chloride solution. Contains the labeled amount, within ±7%. Meets the requirements for Identification, Bacterial endotoxins, and Injections.

METOLAZONE

Chemical name: 6-Quinazolinesulfonamide, 7-chloro-1,2,3,4-tetrahydro-2-methyl-3-(2-methylphenyl)-4-oxo.

Molecular formula: $C_{16}H_{16}ClN_3O_3S$.

Molecular weight: 365.83.

Description: Colorless, odorless crystalline powder; is light-sensitive.

pKa: 9.72.

Solubility: Sparingly soluble in water; more soluble in plasma, in blood, in alkali, and in organic solvents.

USP requirements:
Metolazone USP—Preserve in tight, light-resistant containers. Contains not less than 97.0% and not more than 102.0% of metolazone, calculated on the dried basis. Meets the requirements for Identification, Loss on drying (not more than 1.0%), Residue on ignition (not more than 0.1%), Heavy metals (not more than 0.0015%), and Chromatographic purity.
Metolazone Tablets USP—Preserve in tight, light-resistant containers. Contain the labeled amount, within ±10%. Meet the requirements for Identification and Uniformity of dosage units.
Extended Metolazone Tablets—Not in USP.
Prompt Metolazone Tablets—Not in USP.

METOPROLOL

Chemical name:
Metoprolol fumarate—2-Propanol, 1-[4-(2-methoxyethyl)-phenoxy]-3-[(1-methylethyl)amino]-, (±)-, (*E*)-2-butenedioate (2:1) (salt).
Metoprolol succinate—2-Propanol, 1-[4-(2-methoxyethyl)-phenoxy]-3-[(1-methylethyl)amino]-, (±)-, butanedioate (2:1) (salt).
Metoprolol tartrate—2-Propanol, 1-[4-(2-methoxyethyl)-phenoxy]-3-[(1-methylethyl)amino]-, (±)-, [*R*-(*R**,*R**)]-2,3-dihydroxybutanedioate (2:1) (salt).

Molecular formula:
Metoprolol fumarate—$(C_{15}H_{25}NO_3)_2 \cdot C_4H_4O_4$.
Metoprolol succinate—$(C_{15}H_{25}NO_3)_2 \cdot C_4H_6O_4$.
Metoprolol tartrate—$(C_{15}H_{25}NO_3)_2 \cdot C_4H_6O_6$.

Molecular weight:
Metoprolol fumarate—650.81.
Metoprolol succinate—652.83.
Metoprolol tartrate—684.82.

Description:
Metoprolol succinate—White, crystalline powder.
Metoprolol Tartrate USP—White, crystalline powder.

pKa: Metoprolol tartrate—9.68.

Solubility:
Metoprolol succinate—Freely soluble in water; soluble in methanol; sparingly soluble in ethanol; slightly soluble in dichloromethane and in 2-propanol; practically insoluble in ethyl-acetate, in acetone, in diethylether, and in heptane.
Metoprolol Tartrate USP—Very soluble in water; freely soluble in methylene chloride, in chloroform, and in alcohol; slightly soluble in acetone; insoluble in ether.

Other characteristics: Lipid solubility—Moderate.

USP requirements:
Metoprolol Fumarate USP—Preserve in tight, light-resistant containers. Contains not less than 99.0% and not more than 100.5% of metoprolol fumarate, calculated on the dried basis. Meets the requirements for Identification, Melting range (145–148 °C), pH (5.5–6.5, in a solution [1 in 10]), Loss on drying (not more than 0.5%), Residue on ignition (not more than 0.1%), Heavy metals (not more than 0.001%), Organic volatile impurities, and Chromatographic purity.
Metoprolol Succinate Extended-release Tablets—Not in USP.
Metoprolol Tartrate USP—Preserve in tight, light-resistant containers. Contains not less than 99.0% and not more than 101.0% of metoprolol tartrate, calculated on the dried basis. Meets the requirements for Identification, Specific rotation (+6.5° to +10.5°), pH (6.0–7.0, in a solution [1 in 10]), Loss on drying (not more than 0.5%), Residue on ignition (not more than 0.1%), Heavy metals (not more than 0.001%), Chromatographic purity, and Organic volatile impurities.
Metoprolol Tartrate Injection USP—Preserve in single-dose, light-resistant containers, preferably of Type I or Type II glass. A sterile solution of Metoprolol Tartrate in Water for Injection. Contains Sodium Chloride as a tonicity-adjusting agent. Contains the labeled amount, within ±10%. Meets the requirements for Identification, Bacterial endotoxins, pH (5.0–8.0), Sterility, and Injections.
Metoprolol Tartrate Tablets USP—Preserve in tight, light-resistant containers. Contain the labeled amount, within ±10%. Meet the requirements for Identification, Dissolution (75% in 30 minutes in simulated gastric fluid TS [without enzyme] in Apparatus 1 at 100 rpm), and Uniformity of dosage units.
Metoprolol Tartrate Extended-release Tablets—Not in USP.

METOPROLOL AND HYDROCHLOROTHIAZIDE

For *Metoprolol* and *Hydrochlorothiazide*—See individual listings for chemistry information.

USP requirements: Metoprolol Tartrate and Hydrochlorothiazide Tablets USP—Preserve in tight, light-resistant containers. Contain the labeled amounts, within ±10%. Meet the requirements for Identification, Dissolution (80% of each active ingredient in 30 minutes in simulated gastric fluid TS [without enzyme] in Apparatus 1 at 100 rpm), Uniformity of dosage units, and Diazotizable substances (not more than 1.0%).

METRIZAMIDE

Chemical group: Non-ionic, monomeric, triiodinated benzoic acid derivative.

Chemical name: D-Glucose, 2-[[3-(acetylamino)-5-(acetylmethylamino)-2,4,6-triiodobenzoyl]amino]-2-deoxy-.

Molecular formula: $C_{18}H_{22}I_3N_3O_8$.

Molecular weight: 789.10.

Description: White crystals.

Solubility: Very soluble in water (50% w/v) at room temperature.

Other characteristics: Low osmolality. The osmolality of metrizamide injection with iodine concentrations of 200 and 300 mg per mL is 340 and 484 mOsmol per kg of water, respectively.

USP requirements: Metrizamide for Injection—Not in USP.

METRONIDAZOLE

Chemical group: Nitroimidazoles.

Chemical name:
Metronidazole—1*H*-Imidazole-1-ethanol, 2-methyl-5-nitro-.
Metronidazole hydrochloride—1*H*-Imidazole-1-ethanol, 2-methyl-5-nitro-, hydrochloride.

Molecular formula:
Metronidazole—$C_6H_9N_3O_3$.
Metronidazole hydrochloride—$C_6H_9N_3O_3 \cdot HCl$.

Molecular weight:
Metronidazole—171.16.
Metronidazole hydrochloride—207.62.

Description: Metronidazole USP—White to pale yellow, odorless crystals or crystalline powder. Is stable in air, but darkens on exposure to light.

Solubility: Metronidazole USP—Sparingly soluble in water and in alcohol; slightly soluble in ether and in chloroform.

USP requirements:
Metronidazole USP—Preserve in well-closed, light-resistant containers. Contains not less than 99.0% and not more than 101.0% of metronidazole, calculated on the dried basis. Meets the requirements for Identification, Melting range (159–163 °C), Loss on drying (not more than 0.5%), Residue on ignition (not more than 0.1%), Heavy metals (not more than 0.005%), Non-basic substances, and Chromatographic purity.
Metronidazole Capsules—Not in USP.
Metronidazole Vaginal Cream—Not in USP.
Metronidazole Gel USP—Preserve in laminated collapsible tubes at controlled room temperature. Contains the labeled amount, within ±10%. Meets the requirements for Identification, pH (4.0–6.5), and Minimum fill.
Metronidazole Topical Gel—Not in USP.
Metronidazole Vaginal Gel—Not in USP.
Metronidazole Injection USP—Preserve in single-dose containers of Type I or Type II glass, or in suitable plastic containers, protected from light. A sterile, isotonic, buffered solution of Metronidazole in Water for Injection. Contains the labeled amount, within ±10%. Meets the requirements for Identification, Bacterial endotoxins, pH (4.5–7.0), Particulate matter, and Injections.
Metronidazole Vaginal Inserts—Not in USP.
Metronidazole Vaginal Suppositories—Not in USP.
Metronidazole Tablets USP—Preserve in well-closed, light-resistant containers. Contain the labeled amount, within ±10%. Meet the requirements for Identification, Dissolution (85% in 60 minutes in 0.1 *N* hydrochloric acid in Apparatus 1 at 100 rpm), and Uniformity of dosage units.
Metronidazole Hydrochloride for Injection—Not in USP.

METRONIDAZOLE AND NYSTATIN

For *Metronidazole* and *Nystatin*—See individual listings for chemistry information.

USP requirements:
Metronidazole and Nystatin Vaginal Cream—Not in USP.
Metronidazole and Nystatin Vaginal Suppositories—Not in USP.
Metronidazole and Nystatin Vaginal Tablets—Not in USP.

METYRAPONE

Chemical name: 1-Propanone, 2-methyl-1,2-di-3-pyridinyl-.

Molecular formula: $C_{14}H_{14}N_2O$.

Molecular weight: 226.28.

Description: Metyrapone USP—White to light amber, fine, crystalline powder, having a characteristic odor. Darkens on exposure to light.

Solubility: Metyrapone USP—Sparingly soluble in water; soluble in methanol and in chloroform. It forms water-soluble salts with acids.

USP requirements:
Metyrapone USP—Preserve in tight containers, protected from heat and light. Contains not less than 98.0% and not more than 102.0% of metyrapone, calculated on the dried basis. Meets the requirements for Identification, Loss on drying (not more than 0.5%), Heavy metals (not more than 0.001%), Residue on ignition (not more than 0.1%), and Chromatographic purity.
Metyrapone Tablets USP—Preserve in tight, light-resistant containers, and avoid exposure to excessive heat. Contain the labeled amount, within ±5%. Meet the requirements for Identification, Dissolution (60% in 45 minutes in 0.1 *N* hydrochloric acid in Apparatus 1 at 100 rpm), and Uniformity of dosage units.

METYROSINE

Chemical name: L-Tyrosine, alpha-methyl-, (−)-.

Molecular formula: $C_{10}H_{13}NO_3$.

Molecular weight: 195.22.

Description: White, crystalline compound.

pKa: 2.7 and 10.1.

Solubility: Very slightly soluble in water, in acetone, and in methanol; soluble in acidic aqueous solutions; soluble in alkaline aqueous solutions, but is subject to oxidative degradation in them; insoluble in chloroform.

USP requirements:
Metyrosine USP—Preserve in well-closed containers. Contains not less than 98.6% and not more than 101.0% of metyrosine, calculated on the dried basis. Meets the requirements for Identification, Specific rotation (+185° to +195°, calculated on the dried basis), Loss on drying (not more than 1.0%), Residue on ignition (not more than 0.1%), Heavy metals (not more than 0.003%), and Chromatographic purity.
Metyrosine Capsules USP—Preserve in well-closed containers. Contain the labeled amount, within ±10%. Meet the requirements for Identification, Dissolution (75% in 60 minutes in 0.1 *N* hydrochloric acid in Apparatus 1 at 100 rpm), and Uniformity of dosage units.

MEXILETINE

Chemical name: Mexiletine hydrochloride—2-Propanamine, 1-(2,6-dimethylphenoxy)-, hydrochloride.

Molecular formula: Mexiletine hydrochloride—$C_{11}H_{17}NO \cdot HCl$.

Molecular weight: Mexiletine hydrochloride—215.72.

Description: Mexiletine hydrochloride—White to off-white crystalline powder.

pKa: 9.2.

Solubility: Mexiletine hydrochloride—Freely soluble in water and in alcohol.

USP requirements:
Mexiletine Hydrochloride USP—Preserve in tight containers. Contains not less than 98.0% and not more than 102.0% of mexiletine hydrochloride, calculated on the dried basis. Meets the requirements for Identification, Chromatographic purity, pH (3.5–5.5, in a solution [1 in 10]), Loss on drying (not more than 0.5%), Residue on ignition (not more than 0.1%), Heavy metals (not more than 0.001%), and Organic volatile impurities.
Mexiletine Hydrochloride Capsules USP—Preserve in tight containers. Contain the labeled amount, within ±10%.

Meet the requirements for Identification, Dissolution (80% in 30 minutes in water in Apparatus 2 at 50 rpm), Uniformity of dosage units, and Chromatographic purity.

MEZLOCILLIN

Chemical name: Mezlocillin sodium—4-Thia-1-azabicyclo-[3.2.0]heptane-2-carboxylic acid, 3,3-dimethyl-6-[[[[[3-(methylsulfonyl)-2-oxo-1-imidazolidinyl]carbonyl]amino]phenylacetyl]amino]-7-oxo-, monosodium salt, [2*S*-[2 alpha,5 alpha,6 beta(*S**)]].

Molecular formula: Mezlocillin sodium—$C_{21}H_{24}NaN_5O_8S_2$.

Molecular weight: Mezlocillin sodium—561.56.

Description: Sterile Mezlocillin Sodium USP—White to pale yellow, crystalline powder.

Solubility: Sterile Mezlocillin Sodium USP—Freely soluble in water.

USP requirements: Sterile Mezlocillin Sodium USP—Preserve in Containers for Sterile Solids. It is mezlocillin sodium suitable for parenteral use. Contains an amount of mezlocillin sodium equivalent to not less than 838 mcg and not more than 978 mcg of mezlocillin per mg, calculated on the anhydrous basis and, where packaged for dispensing, contains an amount of mezlocillin sodium equivalent to the labeled amount of mezlocillin within −10% to +15%. Meets the requirements for Constituted solution, Identification, Specific rotation (+175° to +195°, calculated on the anhydrous basis), Bacterial endotoxins, Sterility, pH (4.5–8.0, in a solution [1 in 10]), Water (not more than 6.0%), and Particulate matter, and for Uniformity of dosage units and Labeling under Injections.

MICONAZOLE

Chemical group: Imidazoles.

Chemical name:
Miconazole—1*H*-Imidazole, 1-[2-(2,4-dichlorophenyl)-2-[(2,4-dichlorophenyl)methoxy]ethyl]-.
Miconazole nitrate—1*H*-Imidazole, 1-[2-(2,4-dichlorophenyl)-2-[(2,4-dichlorophenyl)methoxy]ethyl]-, mononitrate.

Molecular formula:
Miconazole—$C_{18}H_{14}Cl_4N_2O$.
Miconazole nitrate—$C_{18}H_{14}Cl_4N_2O \cdot HNO_3$.

Molecular weight:
Miconazole—416.13.
Miconazole nitrate—479.15.

Description:
Miconazole USP—White to pale cream powder. Melts in the range of 78 °C to 82 °C.
Miconazole Nitrate USP—White or practically white, crystalline powder, having not more than a slight odor. Melts in the range of 178 °C to 183 °C, with decomposition.

Solubility:
Miconazole USP—Insoluble in water; soluble in ether; freely soluble in alcohol, in methanol, in isopropyl alcohol, in acetone, in propylene glycol, in chloroform, and in dimethylformamide.
Miconazole Nitrate USP—Insoluble in ether; very slightly soluble in water and in isopropyl alcohol; slightly soluble in alcohol, in chloroform, and in propylene glycol; sparingly soluble in methanol; soluble in dimethylformamide; freely soluble in dimethylsulfoxide.

USP requirements:
Miconazole USP—Preserve in well-closed containers, protected from light. Contains not less than 98.0% and not more than 102.0% of miconazole, calculated on the dried basis. Meets the requirements for Identification, Loss on drying (not more than 0.5%), Residue on ignition (not more than 0.2%), and Chromatographic purity.
Miconazole Injection USP—Preserve in single-dose containers, preferably of Type I glass, at controlled room temperature. A sterile solution of Miconazole in Water for Injection. Contains the labeled amount, within ± 10%. Meets the requirements for Identification, Bacterial endotoxins, pH (3.7–5.7), Particulate matter, and Injections.
Miconazole Nitrate USP—Preserve in well-closed containers, protected from light. Contains not less than 98.0% and not more than 102.0% of miconazole nitrate, calculated on the dried basis. Meets the requirements for Identification, Loss on drying (not more than 0.5%), Residue on ignition (not more than 0.2%), Chromatographic purity, and Ordinary impurities.
Miconazole Nitrate Topical Aerosol Powder—Not in USP.
Miconazole Nitrate Topical Aerosol Solution—Not in USP.
Miconazole Nitrate Cream USP—Preserve in collapsible tubes or in tight containers. Contains the labeled amount, within ± 10%. Meets the requirements for Identification and Minimum fill.
Miconazole Nitrate Vaginal Cream—Not in USP.
Miconazole Nitrate Lotion—Not in USP.
Miconazole Nitrate Topical Powder USP—Preserve in well-closed containers. Contains the labeled amount, within ± 10%. Meets the requirements for Identification, Microbial limits, and Minimum fill.
Miconazole Nitrate Vaginal Suppositories USP—Preserve in tight containers, at controlled room temperature. Contain the labeled amount, within ± 10%. Meet the requirement for Identification.
Miconazole Nitrate Vaginal Tampons—Not in USP.

MIDAZOLAM

Chemical group: Benzodiazepine.

Chemical name: Midazolam hydrochloride—4*H*-Imidazo[1,5-*a*][1,4]benzodiazepine, 8-chloro-6-(2-fluorophenyl)-1-methyl-, monohydrochloride.

Molecular formula: Midazolam hydrochloride—$C_{18}H_{13}ClFN_3 \cdot HCl$.

Molecular weight: Midazolam hydrochloride—362.23.

Description: White to light yellow crystalline compound.

pKa: 6.0.

Solubility: Midazolam hydrochloride—Soluble in aqueous solutions. At physiologic pH, midazolam becomes highly lipophilic, and is one of the most lipid soluble of the benzodiazepines.

Other characteristics: Midazolam hydrochloride injection—An aqueous solution with an acidic pH of approximately 3.

USP requirements: Midazolam Hydrohcloride Injection—Not in USP.

MILRINONE

Chemical name: Milrinone lactate—1,6-Dihydro-2-methyl-6-oxo-[3,4′-bipyridine]-5-carbonitrile lactate.

Molecular formula: $C_{12}H_9N_3O$.

Molecular weight: 211.22.

Description: Off-white to tan crystalline compound.

Solubility: Slightly soluble in methanol; very slightly soluble in chloroform and in water.

USP requirements: Milrinone Lactate Injection—Not in USP.

MINERAL OIL

Source: Complex mixture of hydrocarbons derived from crude petroleum; aromatic amines and unsaturated hydrocarbons are removed when refined for human use, leaving various saturated hydrocarbons behind.

Description: Mineral Oil USP—Colorless, transparent, oily liquid, free, or practically free from fluorescence. Is odorless when cold, and develops not more than a faint odor of petroleum when heated.

NF category: Solvent; vehicle (oleaginous).

Solubility: Mineral Oil USP—Insoluble in water and in alcohol; soluble in volatile oils. Miscible with most fixed oils, but not with castor oil.

USP requirements:

Mineral Oil USP—Preserve in tight containers. A mixture of liquid hydrocarbons obtained from petroleum. Label it to indicate the name of any substance added as a stabilizer. Meets the requirements for Specific gravity (0.845–0.905), Viscosity (not less than 34.5 centistokes at 40.0 °C), Neutrality, Readily carbonizable substances, Limit of polynuclear compounds, and Solid paraffin.

Mineral Oil Emulsion USP—Preserve in tight containers.

Prepare Mineral Oil Emulsion as follows: 500 mL of Mineral Oil, 125 grams of Acacia in very fine powder, 100 mL of Syrup, 40 mg of Vanillin, 60 mL of Alcohol, and a sufficient quantity of Purified Water to make 1000 mL. Mix the Mineral Oil with the Powdered Acacia in a dry mortar, add 250 mL of Purified Water all at once, and emulsify the mixture. Then add, in divided portions, triturating after each addition, a mixture of the Syrup, 50 mL of Purified Water, and the Vanillin dissolved in the alcohol. Finally add Purified Water to make the product measure 1000 mL, and mix. The Vanillin may be replaced by not more than 1% of any other official flavoring substance or any mixture of official flavoring substances. Sixty mL of sweet orange peel tincture or 2 grams of benzoic acid may be used as a preservative in place of Alcohol.

Meets the requirement for Alcohol content (4.0–6.0%).

Mineral Oil Enema USP—Preserve in tight, single-unit containers. It is Mineral Oil that has been suitably packaged. Meets the requirements for Specific gravity (0.845–0.905), Viscosity (not less than 34.5 centistokes at 40.0 °C), and Neutrality.

Mineral Oil Gel—Not in USP.

Mineral Oil Oral Suspension—Not in USP.

LIGHT MINERAL OIL

Description: Light Mineral Oil NF—Colorless, transparent, oily liquid, free, or practically free, from fluorescence. Odorless when cold, and develops not more than a faint odor of petroleum when heated.

NF category: Tablet and/or capsule lubricant; vehicle (oleaginous).

Solubility: Light Mineral Oil NF—Insoluble in water and in alcohol; soluble in volatile oils. Miscible with most fixed oils, but not with castor oil.

USP requirements: Topical Light Mineral Oil USP—Preserve in tight containers. It is Light Mineral Oil that has been suitably packaged. Label it to indicate the name of any substance added as a stabilizer, and label packages intended for direct use by the public to indicate that it is not intended for internal use. Meets the requirements for Specific gravity (0.818–0.880) and Viscosity (not more than 33.5 centistokes at 40 °C), and for Neutrality and Solid paraffin under Mineral Oil.

NF requirements: Light Mineral Oil NF—Preserve in tight containers. A mixture of liquid hydrocarbons obtained from petroleum. Label it to indicate the name of any substance added as a stabilizer, and label packages intended for direct use by the public to indicate that it is not intended for internal use. Meets the requirements for Specific gravity (0.818–0.880) and Viscosity (not more than 33.5 centistokes at 40 °C), and for Neutrality, Readily carbonizable substances, Limit of polynuclear compounds, and Solid paraffin under Mineral Oil.

MINERAL OIL AND CASCARA SAGRADA

For *Mineral Oil* and *Cascara Sagrada*—See individual listings for chemistry information.

USP requirements: Mineral Oil and Cascara Sagrada Extract Emulsion—Not in USP.

MINERAL OIL, GLYCERIN, AND PHENOLPHTHALEIN

For *Mineral Oil, Glycerin,* and *Phenolphthalein*—See individual listings for chemistry information.

USP requirements: Mineral Oil, Glycerin, and Phenolphthalein Emulsion—Not in USP.

MINERAL OIL AND PHENOLPHTHALEIN

For *Mineral Oil* and *Phenolphthalein*—See individual listings for chemistry information.

USP requirements:

Mineral Oil and Phenolphthalein Emulsion—Not in USP.

Mineral Oil and Phenolphthalein Oral Suspension—Not in USP.

MINERALS

USP requirements:

Minerals Capsules USP—Preserve in tight, light-resistant containers. Contain two or more minerals derived from substances generally recognized as safe, furnishing two or more of the following elements in ionic form: calcium, chromium, copper, fluorine, iodine, iron, magnesium, manganese, molybdenum, phosphorus, potassium, selenium, and zinc. The label states that the product is Minerals Capsules. The label states also the salt form of the mineral used as the source of each element. Where more than one *Assay* method is given for a particular mineral, the labeling states with which *Assay* method the product complies only if *Method 1* is not used. Contain the labeled amounts of calcium, copper, iron, magnesium, manganese, phosphorus, potassium, and zinc, within −10% to +25%, and the labeled amounts of chromium, fluorine, iodine, molybdenum, and selenium, within −10% to +100%. Contain no vitamins or any other minerals for which nutritional value is claimed. May contain other labeled added substances in amounts that are unobjectionable. Meet the requirements for Disintegration, Weight variation, and Microbial limits.

Minerals Tablets USP—Preserve in tight, light-resistant containers. Contain two or more minerals derived from substances generally recognized as safe, furnishing two or more of the following elements in ionic form: calcium, chromium, copper, fluorine, iodine, iron, magnesium, manganese, molybdenum, phosphorus, potassium, selenium, and zinc. The label states that the product is Minerals Tablets. The label states also the salt form of the mineral used as the source of each element. Where more than one *Assay* method is given for a particular mineral, the labeling states with which *Assay* method the product complies only if *Method 1* is not used. Contain the labeled amounts of calcium, copper, iron, magnesium, manganese, phosphorus, potassium, and zinc, within −10% to +25%, and the labeled amounts of chromium, fluorine, iodine, molybdenum, and selenium, within −10% to +100%. Contain no vitamins or any other minerals for which nutritional value is claimed. May contain other labeled added substances in amounts that are unobjectionable. Meet the requirements for Disintegration, Weight variation, and Microbial limits.

MINOCYCLINE

Chemical name: Minocycline hydrochloride—2-Naphthacenecarboxamide, 4,7-bis(dimethylamino)-1,4,4a,5,5a,6,11,12a-octahydro-3,10,12,12a-tetrahydroxy-1,11-dioxo-, monohydrochloride, [4*S*-(4 alpha,4a alpha,5a alpha,12a alpha)]-.

Molecular formula: Minocycline hydrochloride—$C_{23}H_{27}N_3O_7 \cdot HCl$.

Molecular weight: Minocycline hydrochloride—493.94.

Description: Minocycline Hydrochloride USP—Yellow, crystalline powder.

Solubility: Minocycline Hydrochloride USP—Soluble in water and in solutions of alkali hydroxides and carbonates; slightly soluble in alcohol; practically insoluble in chloroform and in ether.

USP requirements:

Minocycline Hydrochloride USP—Preserve in tight containers, protected from light. Contains the equivalent of not less than 890 mcg and not more than 950 mcg of minocycline per mg, calculated on the anhydrous basis. Meets the requirements for Identification, Crystallinity, pH (3.5–4.5, in a solution containing the equivalent of 10 mg of minocycline per mL), Water (4.3–8.0%), Residue on ignition (not more than 0.15%), Heavy metals (not more than 0.005%), and Chromatographic purity.

Minocycline Hydrochloride Capsules USP—Preserve in tight, light-resistant containers. Contain an amount of minocycline hydrochloride equivalent to the labeled amount of minocycline, within −10% to +15%. Meet the requirements for Identification, Dissolution (75% in 45 minutes in water in Apparatus 2 at 50 rpm), Uniformity of dosage units, and Water (not more than 12.0%).

Sterile Minocycline Hydrochloride USP—Preserve in Containers for Sterile Solids, protected from light. It is sterile, freeze-dried Minocycline Hydrochloride suitable for parenteral use. Contains an amount of minocycline hydrochloride equivalent to the labeled amount of minocycline, within −10% to +20%. Meets the requirements for Constituted solution, Identification, Depressor substances, Bacterial endotoxins, pH (2.0–3.5, in a solution containing the equivalent of 10 mg of minocycline per mL), Water (not more than 3.0%), Particulate matter, and Epiminocycline (not more than 6.0%), and for Sterility tests, Uniformity of dosage units, and Labeling under Injections.

Minocycline Hydrochloride Oral Suspension USP—Preserve in tight, light-resistant containers. Contains one or more suitable diluents, flavors, preservatives, and wetting agents in an aqueous vehicle. Contains an amount of minocycline hydrochloride equivalent to the labeled amount of minocycline, within −10% to +30%. Meets the requirements for Identification, pH (7.0–9.0), Deliverable volume (multiple-unit containers), and Uniformity of dosage units (single-unit containers).

Minocycline Hydrochloride Tablets USP—Preserve in tight, light-resistant containers. Contain an amount of minocycline hydrochloride equivalent to the labeled amount of minocycline, within −10% to +15%. Meet the requirements for Identification, Dissolution (75% in 45 minutes in water in Apparatus 2 at 50 rpm), Uniformity of dosage units, and Water (not more than 12.0%).

MINOXIDIL

Chemical name: 2,4-Pyrimidinediamine, 6-(1-piperidinyl)-, 3-oxide.

Molecular formula: $C_9H_{15}N_5O$.

Molecular weight: 209.25.

Description:

Minoxidil USP—White to off-white, crystalline powder. Melts in the approximate range of between 248 and 268 °C, with decomposition.

Minoxidil topical solution—Clear, colorless to slightly yellow solution.

pKa: 4.61.

Solubility: Minoxidil USP—Soluble in alcohol and in propylene glycol; sparingly soluble in methanol; slightly soluble in water; practically insoluble in chloroform, in acetone, in ethyl acetate, and in hexane.

USP requirements:

Minoxidil USP—Preserve in well-closed containers. Contains not less than 97.0% and not more than 103.0% of minoxidil, calculated on the dried basis. Meets the requirements for Identification, Loss on drying (not more than 0.5%), Residue on ignition (not more than 0.5%), Heavy metals (not more than 0.002%), and Chromatographic purity.

Minoxidil Topical Solution—Not in USP.

Minoxidil Tablets USP—Preserve in tight containers. Contain the labeled amount, within ±10%. Meet the requirements for Identification, Dissolution (50% in 15 minutes in phosphate buffer [pH 7.2] in Apparatus 1 at 75 rpm), and Uniformity of dosage units.

MISOPROSTOL

Chemical group: Synthetic prostaglandin E_1 analog.

Chemical name: Prost-13-en-1-oic acid, 11,16-dihydroxy-16-methyl-9-oxo-, methyl ester, (11 alpha,13*E*)-(±)-.

Molecular formula: $C_{22}H_{38}O_5$.

Molecular weight: 382.54.

Description: Light yellow, viscous liquid with a musty odor.

Solubility: Soluble in water.

USP requirements: Misoprostol Tablets—Not in USP.

MITOMYCIN

Source: Isolated from the broth of *Streptomyces caespitosus.*

Chemical name: Azirino[2′,3′:3,4]pyrrolo[1,2-*a*]indole-4,7-dione, 6-amino-8-[[(aminocarbonyl)oxy]methyl]-1,1a,2,8,8a,8b-hexahydro-8a-methoxy-5-methyl-, [1a*R*-(1a alpha,8 beta,8a alpha,8b alpha)]-.

Molecular formula: $C_{15}H_{18}N_4O_5$.

Molecular weight: 334.33.

Description: Mitomycin USP—Blue-violet, crystalline powder.

Solubility: Mitomycin USP—Slightly soluble in water; soluble in acetone, in methanol, in butyl acetate, and in cyclohexanone.

USP requirements:

Mitomycin USP—Preserve in tight, light-resistant containers. Has a potency of not less than 970 mcg of mitomycin per mg. Meets the requirements for Identification, Crystallinity, pH (6.0–7.5, in an aqueous suspension containing 5 mg per mL), and Water (not more than 2.5%).

Mitomycin for Injection USP—Preserve in Containers for Sterile Solids, protected from light. A dry mixture of Mitomycin and Mannitol. Contains the labeled amount, within −10% to +20%. Meets the requirements for Constituted solution, Identification, Depressor substances, Bacterial endotoxins, Sterility, pH (6.0–8.0, in the solution constituted as directed in the labeling), Water (not more than 5.0%), and Injections.

MITOTANE

Chemical name: Benzene, 1-chloro-2-[2,2-dichloro-1-(4-chlorophenyl)ethyl]-.

Molecular formula: $C_{14}H_{10}Cl_4$.

Molecular weight: 320.05.

Description: Mitotane USP—White, crystalline powder, having a slight aromatic odor.

Solubility: Mitotane USP—Practically insoluble in water; soluble in alcohol, in ether, in solvent hexane, and in fixed oils and fats.

USP requirements:

Mitotane USP—Preserve in tight, light-resistant containers. Contains not less than 97.0% and not more than 103.0% of mitotane, calculated on the dried basis. Meets the requirements for Identification, Melting range (75–81 °C), Loss on drying (not more than 0.5%), Residue on ignition (not more than 0.5%), and Organic volatile impurities.

Caution: Handle Mitotane with exceptional care, since it is a highly potent agent.

Mitotane Tablets USP—Preserve in tight, light-resistant containers. Contain the labeled amount, within ±10%. Meet the requirements for Identification, Disintegration (15 minutes, the use of disks being omitted), and Uniformity of dosage units.

MITOXANTRONE

Chemical group: Synthetic anthracenedione.

Chemical name: Mitoxantrone hydrochloride—9,10-Anthracenedione, 1,4-dihydroxy-5,8-bis-[[2-[(2-hydroxyethyl)amino]ethyl]amino]-, dihydrochloride.

Molecular formula: Mitoxantrone hydrochloride—$C_{22}H_{28}N_4O_6 \cdot 2HCl$.

Molecular weight: Mitoxantrone hydrochloride—517.41.

Description:

Mitoxantrone Hydrochloride USP—Dark blue powder.

Mitoxantrone hydrochloride concentrate for injection—Dark blue aqueous solution.

Solubility: Mitoxantrone Hydrochloride USP—Sparingly soluble in water; slightly soluble in methanol; practically insoluble in acetone, in acetonitrile, and in chloroform.

USP requirements:

Mitoxantrone Hydrochloride USP—Preserve in tight containers. Contains not less than 97.0% and not more than 102.0% of mitoxantrone hydrochloride, calculated on the anhydrous basis. Meets the requirements for Identification, Water (not more than 6.0%), Alcohol (not more than 1.5%), Heavy metals (not more than 0.002%), and Chromatographic purity.

Mitoxantrone for Injection Concentrate USP—Preserve in single-dose containers, preferably of Type I glass. A sterile solution of Mitoxantrone Hydrochloride in Water for Injection. Label Concentrate to state both the content of the active moiety and the name of the salt used in formulating the article. Label Concentrate to indicate that it is to be diluted to appropriate strength with water or other suitable fluid prior to administration. Contains the equivalent of the labeled amount of mitoxantrone, within −10% to +5%. Meets the requirements for Identification, Bacterial endotoxins, Sterility, pH (3.0–4.5), and Chromatographic purity, and for Injections.

MIVACURIUM

Chemical name: Mivacurium chloride—Isoquinolinium, 2,2′-[(1,8-dioxo-4-octene-1,8-diyl)bis(oxy-3,1-propanediyl)]bis-[1,2,3,4-tetrahydro-6,7-dimethoxy-2-methyl-1-[(3,4,5-trimethoxyphenyl)methyl]-, dichloride, [*R*-[*R**,*R**-(*E*)]]-.

Molecular formula: Mivacurium chloride—$C_{58}H_{80}Cl_2N_2O_{14}$.

Molecular weight: Mivacurium chloride—1100.18.

USP requirements: Mivacurium Chloride Injection—Not in USP.

MIVACURIUM AND DEXTROSE

For *Mivacurium* and *Dextrose*—See individual listings for chemistry information.

USP requirements: Mivacurium Chloride in Dextrose Injection—Not in USP.

MOLINDONE

Chemical group: Dihydroindolone.

Chemical name: Molindone hydrochloride—4*H*-Indol-4-one, 3-ethyl-1,5,6,7-tetrahydro-2-methyl-5-(4-morpholinylmethyl)-, monohydrochloride.

Molecular formula: Molindone hydrochloride—$C_{16}H_{24}N_2O_2 \cdot HCl$.

Molecular weight: Molindone hydrochloride—312.84.

Description: Molindone hydrochloride—White, crystalline powder.

pKa: 6.94.

Solubility: Molindone hydrochloride—Freely soluble in water and in alcohol.

USP requirements:

Molindone Hydrochloride USP—Preserve in tight, light-resistant containers. Contains not less than 98.0% and not more than 101.5% of molindone hydrochloride, calculated on the anhydrous basis. Meets the requirements for Identification, pH (4.0–5.0, in a solution [1 in 100]), Water (not more than 0.5%), Residue on ignition (not more than 0.25%), Heavy metals (not more than 0.003%), and Chromatographic purity.

Molindone Hydrochloride Oral Solution—Not in USP.

Molindone Hydrochloride Tablets USP—Preserve in tight, light-resistant containers. Contain the labeled amount, within ±10%. Meet the requirements for Identification and Uniformity of dosage units.

MOMETASONE

Chemical name: Mometasone furoate—Pregna-1,4-diene-3,20-dione, 9,21-dichloro-17-[(2-furanylcarbonyl)oxy]-11-hydroxy-16-methyl-, (11 beta,16 alpha)-.

Molecular formula: Mometasone furoate—$C_{27}H_{30}Cl_2O_6$.

Molecular weight: Mometasone furoate—521.44.

Description: Mometasone furoate—White to off-white powder.

Solubility: Mometasone furoate—Practically insoluble in water; slightly soluble in octanol; moderately soluble in ethyl alcohol.

USP requirements:

Mometasone Furoate Cream—Not in USP.

Mometasone Furoate Lotion—Not in USP.

Mometasone Furoate Ointment—Not in USP.

MONOBENZONE

Chemical name: Phenol, 4-(phenylmethoxy)-.

Molecular formula: $C_{13}H_{12}O_2$.

Molecular weight: 200.24.

Description: Monobenzone USP—White, odorless, crystalline powder.

Solubility:

Monobenzone USP—Practically insoluble in water; soluble in alcohol, in chloroform, in ether, and in acetone.

Monobenzone Ointment USP—Dispersible with, but not soluble in, water.

USP requirements:

Monobenzone USP—Preserve in tight, light-resistant containers, and avoid exposure to temperatures above 30 °C. Dried at 105° C for 3 hours, contains not less than 98.0% and not more than 102.0% of monobenzone. Meets the requirements for Identification, Melting range (117–120 °C), Loss on drying (not more than 1.0%), Residue on ignition (not more than 0.5%), and Organic volatile impurities.

Monobenzone Cream USP—Preserve in tight containers, and avoid exposure to temperatures above 30 °C. Contains the labeled amount, within ±6%. Meets the requirement for Identification.

MONO- AND DI-ACETYLATED MONOGLYCERIDES

Description: Mono- and Di-acetylated Monoglycerides NF—White to pale yellow waxy solid, melting at about 45 °C.

NF category: Plasticizer.

Solubility: Mono- and Di-acetylated Monoglycerides NF—Soluble in ether and in chloroform; slightly soluble in carbon disulfide; insoluble in water.

NF requirements: Mono- and Di-acetylated Monoglycerides NF—Preserve in tight, light-resistant containers. It is glycerin esterified with edible fat-forming fatty acids and acetic acid. May be prepared by the inter-esterification of edible oils with triacetin or a mixture of triacetin and glycerin, in the presence of catalytic agents, followed by molecular distillation, or by direct acetylation of edible monoglycerides and diglycerides with acetic anhydride with or without the use of catalysts or molecular distillation. Meets the requirements for Identification, Residue on ignition (not more than 0.5%), Arsenic (not more than 3 ppm), Heavy metals (not more than 0.001%), Acid value (not more than 3), Hydroxyl value (133–152), Saponification value (279–292), Free glycerin (not more than 1.5%), and Organic volatile impurities.

MONO- AND DI-GLYCERIDES

Description: Mono- and Di-glycerides NF—Varies in consistency from yellow liquids through ivory-colored plastics to hard ivory-colored solids having a bland odor.

NF category: Emulsifying and/or solubilizing agent.

Solubility: Mono- and Di-glycerides NF—Insoluble in water; soluble in alcohol, in ethyl acetate, in chloroform, and in other chlorinated hydrocarbons.

NF requirements: Mono- and Di-glycerides NF—Preserve in tight, light-resistant containers. A mixture of glycerol mono- and di-esters, with minor amounts of tri-esters, of fatty acids from edible oils. Contains not less than 40.0% of monoglycerides. The labeling indicates the monoglyceride content, hydroxyl value, iodine value, saponification value, and the name and quantity of any stabilizers. The monoglyceride content is within ±10% of the value indicated in the labeling. Meets the requirements for Residue on ignition (not more than 0.1%), Arsenic (not more than 3 ppm), Heavy metals (not more than 0.001%), Acid value (not more than 4), Hydroxyl value (within ±10.0% of value indicated in labeling), Iodine value (within ±10.0% of value indicated in labeling), Saponification value (within ±10% of value indicated in labeling), Free glycerin (not more than 7.0%), and Organic volatile impurities.

MONOETHANOLAMINE

Chemical name: Ethanol, 2-amino-.

Molecular formula: C_2H_7NO.

Molecular weight: 61.08.

Description: Monoethanolamine NF—Clear, colorless, moderately viscous liquid, having a distinctly ammoniacal odor.

NF category: Emulsifying and/or solubilizing agent (adjunct).

Solubility: Monoethanolamine NF—Miscible with water, with acetone, with alcohol, with glycerin, and with chloroform. Immiscible with ether, with solvent hexane, and with fixed oils, although it dissolves in many essential oils.

NF requirements: Monoethanolamine NF—Preserve in tight, light-resistant containers. Contains not less than 98.0% and not more than 100.5%, by weight, of monoethanolamine. Meets the requirements for Specific gravity (1.013–1.016), Distilling range (not less than 95% distils at 167–173 °C), Residue on ignition (not more than 0.1%), and Organic volatile impurities.

MONOOCTANOIN

Source: A semisynthetic mixture of glycerol esters, containing 80–85% of glyceryl mono-octanoate, 10–15% of glyceryl mono-decanoate and glyceryl di-octanoate, and a maximum of 2.5% of free glycerol.

Chemical group: Mono- and diglycerides of medium chain length fatty acids.

Chemical name: Octanoic acid monoester with 1,2,3-propanetriol.

USP requirements: Monooctanoin Irrigation—Not in USP.

MONOSODIUM GLUTAMATE

Molecular formula: $C_5H_8NNaO_4 \cdot H_2O$.

Molecular weight: 187.13.

Description: Monosodium Glutamate NF—White, practically odorless, free-flowing crystals or crystalline powder.
NF category: Flavors and perfumes.

Solubility: Monosodium Glutamate NF—Freely soluble in water; sparingly soluble in alcohol.

NF requirements: Monosodium Glutamate NF—Preserve in tight containers. Contains not less than 99.0% and not more than 100.5% of monosodium glutamate. Meets the requirements for Clarity and color of solution, Identification, Specific rotation (+24.8° to +25.3° at 20 °C), pH (6.7–7.2, in a solution [1 in 20]), Loss on drying (not more than 0.5%), Chloride (not more than 0.25%), Arsenic (not more than 3 ppm), Lead (not more than 10 ppm), Heavy metals (not more than 0.002%), and Organic volatile impurities.

MONOTHIOGLYCEROL

Chemical name: 1,2-Propanediol, 3-mercapto-.

Molecular formula: $C_3H_8O_2S$.

Molecular weight: 108.16.

Description: Monothioglycerol NF—Colorless or pale yellow viscous liquid, having a slight sulfidic odor. Hygroscopic.
NF category: Antioxidant.

Solubility: Monothioglycerol NF—Miscible with alcohol. Freely soluble in water; insoluble in ether.

NF requirements: Monothioglycerol NF—Preserve in tight containers. Contains not less than 97.0% and not more than 101.0% of monothioglycerol, calculated on the anhydrous basis. Meets the requirements for Specific gravity (1.241–1.250), Refractive index (1.521–1.526), pH (3.5–7.0, in a solution [1 in 10]), Water (not more than 5.0%), Residue on ignition (not more than 0.1%), Selenium (not more than 0.003%), Heavy metals (not more than 0.002%), and Organic volatile impurities.

MORICIZINE

Chemical name: Moricizine hydrochloride—10-(3-morpholinopropionyl) phenothiazine-2-carbamic acid ethyl ester hydrochloride.

Molecular formula: Moricizine hydrochloride—$C_{22}H_{25}N_3O_4S \cdot HCl$.

Molecular weight: Moricizine hydrochloride—464.

Description: Moricizine hydrochloride—White to tan crystalline powder.

pKa: Moricizine hydrochloride—6.4 (weak base).

Solubility: Moricizine hydrochloride—Freely soluble in water.

USP requirements: Moricizine Hydrochloride Tablets—Not in USP.

MORPHINE

Chemical name:
Morphine hydrochloride—Morphinan-3,6-diol, 7,8-didehydro-4,5-epoxy-17-methyl, (5 alpha,6 alpha)-, hydrochloride (1:1) (salt), trihydrate.
Morphine sulfate—Morphinan-3,6-diol, 7,8-didehydro-4,5-epoxy-17-methyl, (5 alpha,6 alpha)-, sulfate (2:1) (salt), pentahydrate.

Molecular formula:
Morphine hydrochloride—$C_{17}H_{19}NO_3 \cdot HCl \cdot 3H_2O$.
Morphine sulfate—$(C_{17}H_{19}NO_3)_2 \cdot H_2SO_4 \cdot 5H_2O$ (pentahydrate); $(C_{17}H_{19}NO_3)_2 \cdot H_2SO_4$ (anhydrous).

Molecular weight:
Morphine hydrochloride—375.8.
Morphine sulfate—758.84 (pentahydrate); 668.76 (anhydrous).

Description:
Morphine hydrochloride—Colorless, silky crystals, cubical masses, or a white or almost white, crystalline powder.
Morphine Sulfate USP—White, feathery, silky crystals, cubical masses of crystals, or white, crystalline powder. Is odorless, and when exposed to air it gradually loses water of hydration. Darkens on prolonged exposure to light.

Solubility:
Morphine hydrochloride—Soluble 1 in 24 of water and 1 in 10 of boiling alcohol (90%); practically insoluble in chloroform and in ether.
Morphine Sulfate USP—Soluble in water; freely soluble in hot water; slightly soluble in alcohol but more so in hot alcohol; insoluble in chloroform and in ether.

USP requirements:
Morphine Hydrochloride Suppositories—Not in USP.
Morphine Hydrochloride Syrup—Not in USP.
Morphine Hydrochloride Tablets—Not in USP.
Morphine Hydrochloride Extended-release Tablets—Not in USP.
Morphine Sulfate USP—Preserve in tight, light-resistant containers. Contains not less than 98.0% and not more than 102.0% of morphine sulfate, calculated on the anhydrous basis. Meets the requirements for Identification, Specific rotation (−107° to −109.5°, calculated on the anhydrous basis), Acidity, Water (10.4–13.4%), Residue on ignition (not more than 0.1%, from 500 mg), Chloride, Ammonium salts, Foreign alkaloids, and Organic volatile impurities.
Morphine Sulfate Injection USP—Preserve in single-dose or in multiple-dose containers, preferably of Type I glass, protected from light. Preserve Injection labeled "Preservative-free" in single-dose containers. A sterile solution of Morphine Sulfate in Water for Injection. Label it to state that the Injection is not to be used if it is darker than pale yellow, if it is discolored in any other way, or if it contains a precipitate. Injection containing no antioxidant or antimicrobial agents prominently bears on its label the words "Preservative-free" and includes, in its labeling, its routes of administration and the statement that it is not to be heat-sterilized. Injection containing antioxidant or antimicrobial agents includes in its labeling its routes of administration and the statement that it is

not for intrathecal or epidural use. Contains the labeled amount, within ±10%. Injection intended for intramuscular or intravenous administration may contain sodium chloride as a tonicity-adjusting agent, and suitable antioxidants and antimicrobial agents. Injection intended for intrathecal or epidural use may contain sodium chloride as a tonicity-adjusting agent, but contains no other added substances. Meets the requirements for Identification, Bacterial endotoxins, pH (2.5–6.5), Particulate matter, Injections, and Labeling under Injections.

Morphine Sulfate Oral Solution—Not in USP.
Morphine Sulfate Sterile Solution (Preservative-free)—Not in USP.
Morphine Sulfate Suppositories—Not in USP.
Morphine Sulfate Syrup—Not in USP.
Morphine Sulfate Tablets—Not in USP.
Morphine Sulfate Extended-release Tablets—Not in USP.
Morphine Sulfate Soluble Tablets—Not in USP.

MORRHUATE SODIUM

Description: Pale-yellowish, granular powder with a slight fishy odor.

Solubility: Soluble in water and in alcohol.

USP requirements: Morrhuate Sodium Injection USP—Preserve in single-dose or in multiple-dose containers, preferably of Type I glass. May be packaged in 50-mL multiple-dose containers. A sterile solution of the sodium salts of the fatty acids of Cod Liver Oil. Contains, in each mL, not less than 46.5 mg and not more than 53.5 mg of morrhuate sodium. Meets the requirements for Identification, Bacterial endotoxins, Acidity and alkalinity, Iodine value of the fatty acids (not less than 130), and Injections (except that at times it may show a slight turbidity or precipitate).

Note: Morrhuate Sodium Injection may show a separation of solid matter on standing. Do not use the material if such solid does not dissolve completely upon warming.

MOXALACTAM

Source: Semisynthetic 1-oxa-beta-lactam antibiotic structurally related to cephalosporins, cephamycins, and penicillins.

Chemical name: Moxalactam disodium—5-Oxa-1-azabicyclo-[4.2.0]oct-2-ene-2-carboxylic acid, 7-[[carboxy(4-hydroxyphenyl)acetyl]amino]-7-methoxy-3-[[(1-methyl-1*H*-tetrazol-5-yl)thio]methyl]-8-oxo-, disodium salt.

Molecular formula: Moxalactam disodium—$C_{20}H_{18}N_6Na_2O_9S$.

Molecular weight: Moxalactam disodium—564.44.

Description: Moxalactam disodium—White to off-white powder with a faint characteristic odor.

Solubility: Moxalactam disodium—Very soluble in water.

USP requirements: Moxalactam Disodium for Injection USP—Preserve in Containers for Sterile Solids. A sterile mixture of moxalactam disodium and Mannitol. The mixture has a potency equivalent to not less than 722 mcg of moxalactam per mg. Contains an amount of moxalactam disodium equivalent to the labeled amount of moxalactam, within −10% to +20%. Meets the requirements for Constituted solution, Identification, Bacterial endotoxins, Sterility, pH (4.5–7.0 in a solution [1 in 10]), Water (not more than 3.0%), Particulate matter, and Isomer ratio (response ratio of R-isomer to S-isomer 0.8–1.4), and for Uniformity of dosage units and Labeling under Injections.

MUMPS SKIN TEST ANTIGEN

Description: Mumps Skin Test Antigen USP—Slightly turbid liquid.

USP requirements: Mumps Skin Test Antigen USP—Preserve at a temperature between 2 and 8 °C. A sterile suspension of formaldehyde-inactivated mumps virus prepared from the extra-embryonic fluids of the mumps virus–infected chicken embryo, concentrated and purified by differential centrifugation, and diluted with isotonic sodium chloride solution. Label it to state that it was prepared in embryonated chicken eggs and that a separate syringe and needle are to be used for each individual injection. Contains not less than 20 complement-fixing units in each mL. Contains approximately 0.006 *M* glycine as a stabilizing agent, and contains a preservative. Meets the requirement for Expiration date (not later than 18 months after date of manufacture or date of issue from manufacturer's cold storage [5 °C, 1 year]). Conforms to the regulations of the U.S. Food and Drug Administration concerning biologics.

MUMPS VIRUS VACCINE LIVE

Source: The vaccine currently available in the U.S. (*Mumpsvax*, MSD) contains a lyophilized preparation of the Jeryl Lynn (B level) strain of mumps virus. This virus was adapted to and propagated in cell cultures of chick embryo free of avian leukosis virus and other adventitious agents. *Mumpsvax*, MSD (Canada) and Morson (U.K.) brands of mumps virus vaccine live, also contain the Jeryl Lynn strain of mumps virus.

Description: Mumps Virus Vaccine Live USP—Solid having the characteristic appearance of substances dried from the frozen state. The vaccine is to be constituted with a suitable diluent just prior to use. Constituted vaccine undergoes loss of potency on exposure to sunlight.

USP requirements: Mumps Virus Vaccine Live USP—Preserve in single-dose containers, or in light-resistant, multiple-dose containers, at a temperature between 2 and 8 °C. Multiple-dose containers for 50 doses are adapted for use only in jet injectors, and those for 10 doses for use by jet or syringe injection. A bacterially sterile preparation of live virus derived from a strain of mumps virus tested for neurovirulence in monkeys, and for immunogenicity, free from all demonstrable viable microbial agents except unavoidable bacteriophage, and found suitable for human immunization. The strain is grown for the purpose of vaccine production on chicken embryo primary cell tissue cultures derived from pathogen-free flocks, meets the requirements of the specific safety tests in adult and suckling mice; the requirements of the tests in monkey kidney, chicken embryo and human tissue cell cultures and embryonated eggs; and the requirements of the tests for absence of *Mycobacterium tuberculosis* and of avian leucosis, unless the production cultures were derived from certified avian leucosis-free sources and the control fluids were tested for avian leucosis. The strain cultures are treated to remove all intact tissue cells. The Vaccine meets the requirements of the specific tissue culture test for live virus titer, in a single immunizing dose, of not less than the equivalent of 5000 $TCID_{50}$ (quantity of virus estimated to infect 50% of inoculated cultures × 5000) when tested in parallel with the U.S. Reference Mumps Virus, Live. Label the Vaccine in multiple-dose containers to indicate that the contents are intended solely for use by jet injector or for use by either jet or syringe injection, whichever is applicable. Label the Vaccine in single-dose containers, if such containers are not light-resistant, to state that it should be protected from sunlight. Label it also to state that constituted Vaccine should be discarded if not used within 8 hours. Meets the requirement for Expiration date (1 to 2 years, depending on the manufacturer's data, after date of issue from manufacturer's cold storage [−20 °C, 1 year]). Conforms to the regulations of the U.S. Food and Drug Administration concerning biologics.

MUPIROCIN

Source: Produced by fermentation of *Pseudomonas fluorescens*.

Chemical name: Nonanoic acid, 9-[[3-methyl-1-oxo-4-[tetrahydro-3,4-dihydroxy-5-[[3-(2-hydroxy-1-methylpropyl)oxiranyl]methyl]2*H*-pyran-2-yl]-2-butenyl]oxy]-, [2*S*-[2 alpha(*E*), 3 beta,4 beta,5 alpha[2*R**,3*R**(1*R**,2*R**)]]]-.

Molecular formula: $C_{26}H_{44}O_9$.

Molecular weight: 500.63.

Description: Mupirocin USP—White to off-white, crystalline solid.

Solubility: Mupirocin USP—Freely soluble in acetone, in chloroform, in dehydrated alcohol, and in methanol; slightly soluble in ether; very slightly soluble in water.

USP requirements:
Mupirocin USP—Preserve in tight containers. Contains not less than 920 mcg and not more than 1020 mcg of mupirocin per mg, calculated on the anhydrous basis. Meets the requirements for Identification, Crystallinity, pH (3.5–4.5, in a saturated aqueous solution), and Water (not more than 1.0%).
Mupirocin Ointment USP—Preserve in collapsible tubes or in well-closed containers. Contains the labeled amount, within ±10%. Meets the requirements for Identification and Minimum fill.

MUROMONAB-CD3

Source: Produced by a process involving fusion of mouse myeloma cells to lymphocytes from immunized animals to produce a hybridoma which secretes antigen-specific antibodies (murine monoclonal antibodies). Muromonab-CD3 is a biochemically purified $IgG_{2\ alpha}$ immunoglobulin with a heavy chain of approximately 50,000 daltons and a light chain of approximately 25,000 daltons.

USP requirements: Muromonab-CD3 Injection—Not in USP.

MYRISTYL ALCOHOL

Molecular formula: $C_{14}H_{30}O$.

Molecular weight: 214.39.

Description: Myristyl Alcohol NF—White wax-like mass.
NF category: Oleaginous vehicle.

Solubility: Myristyl Alcohol NF—Soluble in ether; slightly soluble in alcohol; insoluble in water.

NF requirements: Myristyl Alcohol NF—Preserve in well-closed containers. Contains not less than 90.0% of myristyl alcohol, the remainder consisting chiefly of related alcohols. Meets the requirements for Identification, Melting range (36–40 °C), Acid value (not more than 2), Iodine value (not more than 1), Hydroxyl value (250–267), and Organic volatile impurities.

NABILONE

Chemical group: Synthetic cannabinoid. Resembles the cannabinols but is not a tetrahydrocannabinol.

Chemical name: 9*H*-Dibenzo[*b,d*]pyran-9-one, 3-(1,1-dimethylheptyl)-6,6a,7,8,10,10a-hexahydro-1-hydroxy-6,6-dimethyl-, *trans*-, (±)-.

Molecular formula: $C_{24}H_{36}O_3$.

Molecular weight: 372.55.

Description: White, polymorphic crystalline powder.

Solubility: In aqueous media, solubility less than 0.5 mg/L.

USP requirements: Nabilone Capsules—Not in USP.

NABUMETONE

Chemical name: 2-Butanone, 4-(6-methoxy-2-naphthalenyl)-.

Molecular formula: $C_{15}H_{16}O_2$.

Molecular weight: 228.29.

Description: White to off-white crystalline substance.

Solubility: Practically insoluble in water; soluble in alcohol and in most organic solvents.

Other characteristics: N-octanol:phosphate buffer partition coefficient—2400 at pH 7.4.

USP requirements: Nabumetone Tablets—Not in USP.

NADOLOL

Chemical name: 2,3-Naphthalenediol, 5-[3-[(1,1-dimethylethyl)amino]-2-hydroxypropoxy]-1,2,3,4-tetrahydro-, *cis*-.

Molecular formula: $C_{17}H_{27}NO_4$.

Molecular weight: 309.41.

Description: Nadolol USP—White to off-white, practically odorless, crystalline powder.

pKa: 9.67.

Solubility: Nadolol USP—Freely soluble in alcohol and in methanol; slightly soluble in chloroform, in methylene chloride, in isopropyl alcohol, and in water; insoluble in acetone, in ether, in hexane, and in trichloroethane.

Other characteristics: Lipid solubility—Low.

USP requirements:
Nadolol USP—Preserve in well-closed containers. Contains not less than 98.0% and not more than 101.5% of nadolol, calculated on the dried basis. Meets the requirements for Identification, Loss on drying (not more than 2.0%), Residue on ignition (not more than 0.1%), Heavy metals (not more than 0.003%), Racemate composition, Chromatographic purity, and Organic volatile impurities.
Nadolol Tablets USP—Preserve in tight containers. Contain the labeled amount, within ±10%. Meet the requirements for Identification, Dissolution (80% in 50 minutes in 0.1 *N* hydrochloric acid in Apparatus 1 at 100 rpm), and Uniformity of dosage units.

NADOLOL AND BENDROFLUMETHIAZIDE

For *Nadolol* and *Bendroflumethiazide*—See individual listings for chemistry information.

USP requirements: Nadolol and Bendroflumethiazide Tablets USP—Preserve in tight containers. Contain the labeled amounts, within ±10%. Meet the requirements for Identification, Dissolution (80% of each active ingredient in 30 minutes in 0.1 *N* hydrochloric acid in Apparatus 2 at 50 rpm), and Uniformity of dosage units.

NAFARELIN

Source: Nafarelin acetate—Synthetic analog of the naturally occurring gonadotropin releasing hormone (GnRH).

Chemical name: Nafarelin acetate—Luteinizing hormone-releasing factor (pig), 6-[3-(2-naphthalenyl)-D-alanine]-, acetate (salt), hydrate.

Molecular formula: Nafarelin acetate—$C_{66}H_{83}N_{17}O_{13} \cdot xC_2H_4O_2 \cdot yH_2O$.

Description: Nafarelin acetate—Fine white to off-white amorphous powder.

Solubility: Nafarelin acetate—Slightly soluble in water; slightly soluble in 0.02 *M* phosphate buffer (pH 7.58), in methanol, and in ethanol; practically insoluble in acetonitrite and in dichloromethane.

USP requirements: Nafarelin Acetate Nasal Solution—Not in USP.

NAFCILLIN

Chemical name: Nafcillin sodium—4-Thia-1-azabicyclo[3.2.0]-heptane-2-carboxylic acid, 6-[[(2-ethoxy-1-naphthalenyl)-carbonyl]amino]-3,3-dimethyl-7-oxo-, monosodium salt, monohydrate, [2*S*-(2 alpha,5 alpha,6 beta)].

Molecular formula: Nafcillin sodium—$C_{21}H_{21}N_2NaO_5S \cdot H_2O$.

Molecular weight: Nafcillin sodium—454.47.

Description:

Nafcillin Sodium USP—White to yellowish white powder, having not more than a slight characteristic odor.

Nafcillin Sodium for Injection USP—White to yellowish white powder, having not more than a slight characteristic odor.

Solubility:

Nafcillin Sodium USP—Freely soluble in water and in chloroform; soluble in alcohol.

Nafcillin Sodium for Injection USP—Freely soluble in water and in chloroform; soluble in alcohol.

USP requirements:

Nafcillin Sodium USP—Preserve in tight containers. Has a potency equivalent to not less than 820 mcg of nafcillin per mg. Meets the requirements for Identification, Crystallinity, pH (5.0–7.0, in a solution containing 30 mg per mL), and Water (3.5–5.3%).

Nafcillin Sodium Capsules USP—Preserve in tight containers. Contain an amount of nafcillin sodium equivalent to the labeled amount of nafcillin, within −10% to +20%. Meet the requirements for Dissolution (75% in 45 minutes in water in Apparatus 1 at 100 rpm), Uniformity of dosage units, and Water (not more than 5.0%).

Nafcillin Sodium Injection USP—Preserve in Containers for Injections. Maintain in the frozen state. A sterile isoosmotic solution of Nafcillin Sodium and one or more buffer substances in Water for Injection. Contains dextrose as a tonicity-adjusting agent. The label states that it is to be thawed just prior to use, describes conditions for proper storage of the resultant solution, and directs that the solution is not to be refrozen. Contains an amount of nafcillin sodium equivalent to the labeled amount of nafcillin, within −10% to +20%. Contains no antimicrobial preservatives. Meets the requirements for Identification, Pyrogen, Sterility, pH (6.0–8.5), Particulate matter, and Labeling under Injections.

Nafcillin Sodium for Injection USP—Preserve in Containers for Sterile Solids. A sterile, dry mixture of Nafcillin Sodium and a suitable buffer. Contains an amount of nafcillin sodium equivalent to the labeled amount of nafcillin, within −10% to +20%. Meets the requirements for Constituted solution, Identification, Bacterial endotoxins, Sterility, pH (6.0–8.5, in the solution constituted as directed in the labeling), Water (3.5–5.3%), and Particulate matter, and for Uniformity of dosage units and Labeling under Injections.

Nafcillin Sodium for Oral Solution USP—Preserve in tight containers. Contains an amount of nafcillin sodium equivalent to the labeled amount of nafcillin, within −10% to +20%. Contains one or more suitable buffers, colors, diluents, dispersants, flavors, and preservatives. Meets the requirements for pH (5.5–7.5, in the solution constituted as directed in the labeling), Water (not more than 5.0%), Uniformity of dosage units (single-unit containers), and Deliverable volume (multiple-unit containers).

Sterile Nafcillin Sodium USP—Preserve in Containers for Sterile Solids. It is Nafcillin Sodium suitable for parenteral use. Has a potency equivalent to not less than 820 mcg of nafcillin per mg. Meets the requirements for Bacterial endotoxins and Sterility, and for Identification tests, pH, Water, and Crystallinity under Nafcillin Sodium.

Nafcillin Sodium Tablets USP—Preserve in tight, light-resistant containers. Contain an amount of nafcillin sodium equivalent to the labeled amount of nafcillin, within −10% to +20%. Meet the requirements for Dissolution (75% in 45 minutes in pH 4.0 buffer in Apparatus 2 at 50 rpm), Uniformity of dosage units, and Water (not more than 5.0%).

NAFTIFINE

Chemical group: Allylamine derivative.

Chemical name: Naftifine hydrochloride—1-Naphthalenemethanamine, *N*-methyl-*N*-(3-phenyl-2-propenyl)-, hydrochloride, (*E*)-.

Molecular formula: Naftifine hydrochloride—$C_{21}H_{21}N \cdot HCl$.

Molecular weight: Naftifine hydrochloride—323.87.

Description: Naftifine hydrochloride—White to yellow, fine, crystalline powder.

Solubility: Naftifine hydrochloride—0.68 mg/mL in water and 3.4 mg/mL in alcohol at 25 °C.

USP requirements:

Naftifine Hydrochloride Gel—Not in USP.

Naftifine Hydrochloride Cream—Not in USP.

NALBUPHINE

Chemical name: Nalbuphine hydrochloride—Morphinan-3,6,14-triol, 17-(cyclobutylmethyl)-4,5-epoxy-, hydrochloride, (5 alpha,6 alpha)-.

Molecular formula: Nalbuphine hydrochloride—$C_{21}H_{27}NO_4 \cdot HCl$.

Molecular weight: Nalbuphine hydrochloride—393.91.

Description: Nalbuphine hydrochloride—White to slightly off-white powder.

Solubility: Nalbuphine hydrochloride—Soluble in water; slightly soluble in alcohol.

USP requirements: Nalbuphine Hydrochloride Injection—Not in USP.

NALIDIXIC ACID

Chemical group: Closely related chemically to cinoxacin.

Chemical name: 1,8-Naphthyridine-3-carboxylic acid, 1-ethyl-1,4-dihydro-7-methyl-4-oxo-.

Molecular formula: $C_{12}H_{12}N_2O_3$.

Molecular weight: 232.24.

Description: Nalidixic Acid USP—White to very pale yellow, odorless, crystalline powder.

Solubility: Nalidixic Acid USP—Soluble in chloroform, in methylene chloride, and in solutions of fixed alkali hydroxides and carbonates; slightly soluble in acetone, in alcohol, in methanol, and in toluene; very slightly soluble in ether and in water.

USP requirements:

Nalidixic Acid USP—Preserve in tight containers. Contains not less than 99.0% and not more than 101.0% of nalidixic acid, calculated on the dried basis. Meets the requirements for Identification, Melting range (225–231 °C), Loss on drying (not more than 0.5%), Residue on ignition (not more than 0.1%), Heavy metals (not more than 0.002%), and Chromatographic purity.

Nalidixic Acid Oral Suspension USP—Preserve in tight containers. Contains the labeled amount, within ±5%, in a suitable aqueous vehicle. Meets the requirement for Identification.

Nalidixic Acid Tablets USP—Preserve in tight containers. Contain the labeled amount, within ±7%. Meet the requirements for Identification, Dissolution (80% in 30 minutes in pH 8.60 buffer in Apparatus 2 at 60 rpm), and Uniformity of dosage units.

NALORPHINE

Chemical name: Nalorphine hydrochloride—Morphinan-3,6-diol, 7,8-didehydro-4,5-epoxy-17-(2-propenyl)-(5 alpha,6 alpha)-, hydrochloride.

Molecular formula: Nalorphine hydrochloride—$C_{19}H_{21}NO_3 \cdot HCl$.

Molecular weight: Nalorphine hydrochloride—347.84.

Description: Nalorphine hydrochloride—White or practically white, odorless, crystalline powder, slowly darkening on exposure to air and light. Melting point about 261 °C.

Solubility: Nalorphine hydrochloride—1 gram in about 8 mL of water or about 35 mL of alcohol; insoluble in chloroform or in ether; soluble in diluted alkali hydroxide solution.

USP requirements:

Nalorphine Hydrochloride USP—Preserve in tight, light-resistant containers. Contains not less than 97.0% and not more than 103.0% of nalorphine hydrochloride, calculated on the dried basis. Meets the requirements for Identification, Specific rotation (−122° to −125°, calculated on the dried basis), Loss on drying (not more than 0.5%), and Residue on ignition (not more than 0.1%).

Nalorphine Hydrochloride Injection USP—Preserve in single-dose or in multiple-dose containers, preferably of Type I glass. A suitably buffered, sterile solution of Nalorphine Hydrochloride in Water for Injection. Contains the labeled amount, within ±10%. Meets the requirements for Identification, Bacterial endotoxins, pH (6.0–7.5), and Injections.

NALOXONE

Chemical name: Naloxone hydrochloride—Morphinan-6-one, 4,5-epoxy-3,14-dihydroxy-17-(2-propenyl)-, hydrochloride, (5 alpha)-.

Molecular formula: Naloxone hydrochloride—$C_{19}H_{21}NO_4 \cdot HCl$.

Molecular weight: Naloxone hydrochloride—363.84.

Description:

Naloxone Hydrochloride USP—White to slightly off-white powder. Its aqueous solution is acidic.

Naloxone Hydrochloride Injection USP—Clear, colorless liquid.

Solubility: Naloxone Hydrochloride USP—Soluble in water, in dilute acids, and in strong alkali; slightly soluble in alcohol; practically insoluble in ether and in chloroform.

USP requirements:

Naloxone Hydrochloride USP—Preserve in tight, light-resistant containers. It is anhydrous or contains two molecules of water of hydration. Contains not less than 98.0% and not more than 100.5% of naloxone hydrochloride, calculated on the dried basis. Meets the requirements for Identification, Specific rotation (−170° to −181°, calculated on the dried basis), Loss on drying (not more than 0.5% for the anhydrous form and not more than 11.0% for the hydrous form), Noroxymorphone hydrochloride and other impurities, and Chloride content (9.54–9.94%, calculated on the dried basis).

Naloxone Hydrochloride Injection USP—Preserve in single-dose or in multiple-dose containers of Type I glass, protected from light. A sterile, isotonic solution of Naloxone Hydrochloride in Water for Injection. Contains the labeled amount, within ±10%. Meets the requirements for Identification, Bacterial endotoxins, pH (3.0–4.5), and Injections.

NALTREXONE

Chemical group: A synthetic congener of oxymorphone; technically a thebaine derivative; also chemically related to the opioid antagonist naloxone.

Chemical name: Naltrexone hydrochloride—(5*R*)-9a-Cyclopropylmethyl-3,14-dihydroxy-4,5-epoxymorphinan-6-one hydrochloride.

Molecular formula: Naltrexone hydrochloride—$C_{20}H_{23}NO_4 \cdot HCl$.

Molecular weight: Naltrexone hydrochloride—377.9.

Description: Naltrexone hydrochloride—White, crystalline compound.

Solubility: Naltrexone hydrochloride—Soluble in water to the extent of about 100 mg per mL.

USP requirements: Naltrexone Hydrochloride Tablets—Not in USP.

NANDROLONE

Chemical name:

Nandrolone decanoate—Estr-4-en-3-one, 17-[(1-oxodecyl)-oxy]-, (17 beta)-.

Nandrolone phenpropionate—Estr-4-en-3-one, 17-(1-oxo-3-phenylpropoxy)-, (17 beta)-.

Molecular formula:

Nandrolone decanoate—$C_{28}H_{44}O_3$.

Nandrolone phenpropionate—$C_{27}H_{34}O_3$.

Molecular weight:
Nandrolone decanoate—428.66.
Nandrolone phenpropionate—406.57.

Description:
Nandrolone Decanoate USP—Fine, white to creamy white, crystalline powder. Is odorless, or may have a slight odor.
Nandrolone phenpropionate—Fine, white to creamy white, crystalline powder, having a slight, characteristic odor.

Solubility:
Nandrolone Decanoate USP—Practically insoluble in water; soluble in chloroform, in alcohol, in acetone, and in vegetable oils.
Nandrolone phenpropionate—Practically insoluble in water; soluble in alcohol, in chloroform, in dioxane, and in vegetable oils.

USP requirements:
Nandrolone Decanoate USP—Preserve in tight, light-resistant containers, and store in a refrigerator. Contains not less than 97.0% and not more than 103.0% of nandrolone decanoate, calculated on the dried basis. Meets the requirements for Completeness and clarity of solution, Identification, Melting range (33–37 °C), Specific rotation (+32° to +36°), Loss on drying (not more than 0.5%), and Organic volatile impurities.
Nandrolone Decanoate Injection USP—Preserve in single-dose or in multiple-dose containers, preferably of Type I glass, protected from light. A sterile solution of Nandrolone Decanoate in Sesame Oil, with a suitable preservative. Contains the labeled amount, within ±10%. Meets the requirements for Identification, Nandrolone (not more than 1.0%), and Injections.
Nandrolone Phenpropionate USP—Preserve in tight, light-resistant containers. Contains not less than 97.0% and not more than 103.0% of nandrolone phenpropionate, calculated on the dried basis. Meets the requirements for Identification, Melting range (95–99 °C), Specific rotation (+48° to +51°, calculated on the dried basis), Loss on drying (not more than 0.5%), and Organic volatile impurities.
Nandrolone Phenpropionate Injection USP—Preserve in single-dose or in multiple-dose containers, preferably of Type I glass, protected from light. A sterile solution of Nandrolone Phenpropionate in a suitable oil. Contains the labeled amount, within ±10%. Meets the requirements for Identification, Nandrolone, and Injections.

NAPHAZOLINE

Chemical name: Naphazoline hydrochloride—1*H*-Imidazole, 4,5-dihydro-2-(1-naphthalenylmethyl)-, monohydrochloride.

Molecular formula: Naphazoline hydrochloride—$C_{14}H_{14}N_2 \cdot HCl$.

Molecular weight: Naphazoline hydrochloride—246.74.

Description: Naphazoline Hydrochloride USP—White, crystalline powder. Is odorless. Melts at a temperature of about 255 °C, with decomposition.

Solubility: Naphazoline Hydrochloride USP—Freely soluble in water and in alcohol; very slightly soluble in chloroform; practically insoluble in ether.

USP requirements:
Naphazoline Hydrochloride USP—Preserve in tight, light-resistant containers. Contains not less than 98.0% and not more than 100.5% of naphazoline hydrochloride, calculated on the dried basis. Meets the requirements for Identification, pH (5.0–6.6, in a 1 in 100 solution in carbon dioxide-free water), Loss on drying (not more than 0.5%), Residue on ignition (not more than 0.2%), and Ordinary impurities.
Naphazoline Hydrochloride Nasal Solution USP—Preserve in tight, light-resistant containers. A solution of Naphazoline Hydrochloride in water adjusted to a suitable pH and tonicity. Contains the labeled amount, within ±10%. Meets the requirement for Identification.
Naphazoline Hydrochloride Ophthalmic Solution USP—Preserve in tight containers. A sterile, buffered solution of Naphazoline Hydrochloride in water adjusted to a suitable tonicity. Contains the labeled amount, within −10% to +15%. Contains a suitable preservative. Meets the requirements for Identification, Sterility, and pH (5.5–7.0).

NAPROXEN

Chemical group: Propionic acid derivative.

Chemical name:
Naproxen—2-Naphthaleneacetic acid, 6-methoxy-alpha-methyl-, (+)-.
Naproxen sodium—2-Naphthaleneacetic acid, 6-methoxy-alpha-methyl-, sodium salt, (−)-.

Molecular formula:
Naproxen—$C_{14}H_{14}O_3$.
Naproxen sodium—$C_{14}H_{13}NaO_3$.

Molecular weight:
Naproxen—230.26.
Naproxen sodium—252.25.

Description:
Naproxen USP—White to off-white, practically odorless, crystalline powder.
Naproxen Sodium USP—White to creamy crystalline powder. Melts at about 255 °C, with decomposition.

pKa: 4.15 (apparent).

Solubility:
Naproxen USP—Practically insoluble in water; freely soluble in chloroform and in dehydrated alcohol; soluble in alcohol; sparingly soluble in ether.
Naproxen Sodium USP—Soluble in water and in methanol; sparingly soluble in alcohol; very slightly soluble in acetone; practically insoluble in chloroform and in toluene.

USP requirements:
Naproxen USP—Preserve in tight containers. Contains not less than 98.5% and not more than 101.5% of naproxen, calculated on the dried basis. Meets the requirements for Identification, Specific rotation (+63.0° to +68.5°, calculated on the dried basis), Loss on drying (not more than 0.5%), Heavy metals (not more than 0.002%), Chromatographic purity, and Organic volatile impurities.
Naproxen Suppositories—Not in USP.
Naproxen Oral Suspension USP—Preserve in tight, light-resistant containers. Store at room temperature. Contains the labeled amount, within ±10%. Meets the requirements for Identification and pH (2.2–3.7).
Naproxen Tablets USP—Preserve in well-closed containers. Contain the labeled amount, within ±10%. Meet the requirements for Identification, Dissolution (80% in 45 minutes in 0.1 *M* phosphate buffer [pH 7.4] in Apparatus 2 at 50 rpm), and Uniformity of dosage units.
Naproxen Extended-release Tablets—Not in USP.
Naproxen Sodium USP—Preserve in tight containers. Contains not less than 98.0% and not more than 102.0% of naproxen sodium, calculated on the dried basis. Meets

the requirements for Identification, Specific rotation (−17.0° to −15.3°, calculated on the dried basis), Loss on drying (not more than 1.0%), Heavy metals (not more than 0.002%), Chromatographic purity, Free naproxen, and Organic volatile impurities.

Naproxen Sodium Tablets USP—Preserve in well-closed containers. Contain the labeled amount, within ±10%. Meet the requirements for Identification, Dissolution (70% in 45 minutes in 0.1 *M* phosphate buffer [pH 7.4] in Apparatus 2 at 50 rpm), and Uniformity of dosage units.

NATAMYCIN

Source: Derived from *Streptomyces natalensis.*

Chemical group: Tetraene polyene antifungal.

Chemical name: Pimaricin.

Molecular formula: $C_{33}H_{47}NO_{13}$.

Molecular weight: 665.74.

Description: Natamycin USP—Off-white to cream-colored powder, which may contain up to 3 moles of water.

Solubility: Natamycin USP—Practically insoluble in water; slightly soluble in methanol; soluble in glacial acetic acid and in dimethylformamide.

USP requirements:

Natamycin USP—Preserve in tight, light-resistant containers. Contains not less than 90.0% and not more than 102.0% of natamycin, calculated on the anhydrous basis. Meets the requirements for Identification, Crystallinity, pH (5.0–7.5, in an aqueous suspension containing 10 mg per mL), and Water (6.0–9.0%).

Natamycin Ophthalmic Suspension USP—Preserve in tight, light-resistant containers. The containers or individual cartons are sealed and tamper-proof so that sterility is assured at time of first use. A sterile suspension of Natamycin in a suitable aqueous vehicle. Contains one or more suitable preservatives. Contains the labeled amount, within −10% to +25%. Meets the requirements for Identification, Sterility, and pH (5.0–7.5).

NEDOCROMIL

Chemical group: Nedocromil sodium—Pyranoquinoline.

Chemical name: Nedocromil sodium—4*H*-Pyrano[3,2-*g*]quinoline-2,8-dicarboxylic acid, 9-ethyl-6,9-dihydro-4,6-dioxo-10-propyl, disodium salt.

Molecular formula: Nedocromil sodium—$C_{19}H_{15}NNa_2O_7$.

Molecular weight: Nedocromil sodium—415.31.

Description: Nedocromil sodium—Yellow powder. Melting point over 300 °C with decomposition.

Solubility: Nedocromil sodium—Soluble in water. Greater than 26 mg/mL at 24 °C in aqueous buffer at pH 4.4–7.4.

USP requirements: Nedocromil Sodium Inhalation Aerosol—Not in USP.

NEOMYCIN

Chemical group: Aminoglycosides.

Chemical name: Neomycin sulfate.

Description: Neomycin Sulfate USP—White to slightly yellow powder, or cryodesiccated solid. Is odorless or practically so and is hygroscopic. Its solutions are dextrorotatory.

Solubility: Neomycin Sulfate USP—Freely soluble in water; very slightly soluble in alcohol; insoluble in acetone, in chloroform, and in ether.

USP requirements:

Neomycin Sulfate USP—Preserve in tight, light-resistant containers. The sulfate salt of a kind of neomycin, an antibacterial substance produced by the growth of *Streptomyces fradiae* Waksman (Fam. Streptomycetaceae), or a mixture of two or more such salts. Has a potency equivalent to not less than 600 mcg of neomycin per mg, calculated on the dried basis. Meets the requirements for Identification, pH (5.0–7.5, in a solution containing 33 mg of neomycin per mL), and Loss on drying (not more than 8.0%), and for Sterility (for Neomycin Sulfate intended for use in making ophthalmic ointments).

Neomycin Sulfate Cream USP—Preserve in well-closed containers, preferably at controlled room temperature. Contains an amount of neomycin sulfate equivalent to the labeled amount of neomycin, within −10% to +35%. Meets the requirements for Identification and Minimum fill.

Neomycin Sulfate Ointment USP—Preserve in well-closed containers, preferably at controlled room temperature. Contains an amount of neomycin sulfate equivalent to the labeled amount of neomycin, within −10% to +35%. Meets the requirements for Identification, Minimum fill, and Water (not more than 1.0%).

Neomycin Sulfate Ophthalmic Ointment USP—Preserve in collapsible ophthalmic ointment tubes. A sterile preparation of Neomycin Sulfate in a suitable ointment base. Contains an amount of neomycin sulfate equivalent to the labeled amount of neomycin, within −10% to +35%. Meets the requirements for Identification, Sterility, Minimum fill, Water (not more than 1.0%), and Metal particles.

Neomycin Sulfate Oral Solution USP—Preserve in tight, light-resistant containers, preferably at controlled room temperature. Contains an amount of neomycin sulfate equivalent to the labeled amount of neomycin, within −10% to +25%. Meets the requirements for Identification and pH (5.0–7.5).

Sterile Neomycin Sulfate USP—Preserve in Containers for Sterile Solids. It is Neomycin Sulfate suitable for parenteral use. Contains an amount of neomycin sulfate equivalent to not less than 600 mcg of neomycin per mg, calculated on the dried basis and, where packaged for dispensing, contains an amount of neomycin sulfate equivalent to the labeled amount of neomycin within −10% to +20%. Meets the requirements for Bacterial endotoxins and Sterility, and for Identification tests, pH, and Loss on drying under Neomycin Sulfate. Where packaged for dispensing, it meets also the requirements for Uniformity of dosage units and Labeling under Injections. Where intended for use in preparing sterile ophthalmic dosage forms, it is exempt from the requirements for Bacterial endotoxins.

Neomycin Sulfate Tablets USP—Preserve in tight containers. Contain an amount of neomycin sulfate equivalent to the labeled amount of neomycin, within −10% to +25%. Meet the requirements for Identification, Disintegration (60 minutes), Uniformity of dosage units, and Loss on drying (not more than 10.0%).

NEOMYCIN AND BACITRACIN

For *Neomycin* and *Bacitracin*—See individual listings for chemistry information.

USP requirements:

Neomycin Sulfate and Bacitracin Ointment USP—Preserve in tight, light-resistant containers, preferably at controlled room temperature. Contains amounts of neomycin sulfate and bacitracin equivalent to the labeled amounts of neomycin and bacitracin, within −10% to +30%. Meets the requirements for Identification, Minimum fill, and Water (not more than 0.5%).

Neomycin Sulfate and Bacitracin Zinc Ointment USP—Preserve in collapsible tubes or in well-closed containers. Contains amounts of neomycin sulfate and bacitracin zinc equivalent to the labeled amounts of neomycin and bacitracin, within −10% to +30%. Meets the requirements for Identification, Minimum fill, and Water (not more than 0.5%).

NEOMYCIN AND DEXAMETHASONE

For *Neomycin* and *Dexamethasone*—See individual listings for chemistry information.

USP requirements:

Neomycin Sulfate and Dexamethasone Sodium Phosphate Cream USP—Preserve in collapsible tubes or in tight containers. Contains an amount of neomycin sulfate equivalent to the labeled amount of neomycin, within −10% to +35%, and an amount of dexamethasone sodium phosphate equivalent to the labeled amount of dexamethasone phosphate, within ±10%. Meets the requirements for Identification and Minimum fill.

Neomycin Sulfate and Dexamethasone Sodium Phosphate Ophthalmic Ointment USP—Preserve in collapsible ophthalmic ointment tubes. A sterile ointment containing Neomycin Sulfate and Dexamethasone Sodium Phosphate. Contains an amount of neomycin sulfate equivalent to the labeled amount of neomycin, within −10% to +35%, and an amount of dexamethasone sodium phosphate equivalent to the labeled amount of dexamethasone phosphate, within ±10%. Meets the requirements for Identification, Sterility, Minimum fill, Water (not more than 1.0%), and Metal particles.

Note: Where Neomycin Sulfate and Dexamethasone Sodium Phosphate Ophthalmic Ointment is prescribed without reference to the quantity of neomycin or dexamethasone phosphate contained therein, a product containing 3.5 mg of neomycin and 0.5 mg of dexamethasone phosphate per gram shall be dispensed.

Neomycin Sulfate and Dexamethasone Sodium Phosphate Ophthalmic Solution USP—Preserve in tight, light-resistant containers, and avoid exposure to excessive heat. A sterile, aqueous solution of Neomycin Sulfate and Dexamethasone Sodium Phosphate. Contains an amount of neomycin sulfate equivalent to the labeled amount of neomycin, within −10% to +30%, and an amount of dexamethasone sodium phosphate equivalent to the labeled amount of dexamethasone phosphate, within −10% to +15%. Meets the requirements for Identification, Sterility, and pH (6.0–8.0).

Note: Where Neomycin Sulfate and Dexamethasone Sodium Phosphate Ophthalmic Solution is prescribed, without reference to the amount of neomycin or dexamethasone phosphate contained therein, a product containing 3.5 mg of neomycin and 1.0 mg of dexamethasone phosphate per mL shall be dispensed.

NEOMYCIN AND FLUOCINOLONE

For *Neomycin* and *Fluocinolone*—See individual listings for chemistry information.

USP requirements: Neomycin Sulfate and Fluocinolone Acetonide Cream USP—Preserve in collapsible tubes or in tight containers. Contains an amount of neomycin sulfate equivalent to the labeled amount of neomycin, within −10% to +35%, and the labeled amount of fluocinolone acetonide, within ±10%. Meets the requirements for Identification and Minimum fill.

NEOMYCIN AND FLUOROMETHOLONE

For *Neomycin* and *Fluorometholone*—See individual listings for chemistry information.

USP requirements: Neomycin Sulfate and Fluorometholone Ointment USP—Preserve in collapsible tubes or in well-closed containers. Contains an amount of neomycin sulfate equivalent to the labeled amount of neomycin, within −10% to +35%, and the labeled amount of fluorometholone, within ±10%. Meets the requirements for Identification, Minimum fill, and Water (not more than 1.0%).

NEOMYCIN AND FLURANDRENOLIDE

For *Neomycin* and *Flurandrenolide*—See individual listings for chemistry information.

USP requirements:

Neomycin Sulfate and Flurandrenolide Cream USP—Preserve in collapsible tubes or in tight containers, protected from light. Contains an amount of neomycin sulfate equivalent to the labeled amount of neomycin, within −10% to +35%, and the labeled amount of flurandrenolide, within ±10%. Meets the requirements for Identification and Minimum fill.

Neomycin Sulfate and Flurandrenolide Lotion USP—Preserve in tight containers, protected from light. Contains an amount of neomycin sulfate equivalent to the labeled amount of neomycin, within −10% to +30%, and the labeled amount of flurandrenolide, within ±10%. Meets the requirements for Identification, Microbial limits, and Minimum fill.

Neomycin Sulfate and Flurandrenolide Ointment USP—Preserve in collapsible tubes or in tight containers, protected from light. Contains an amount of neomycin sulfate equivalent to the labeled amount of neomycin, within −10% to +35%, and the labeled amount of flurandrenolide, within ±10%. Meets the requirements for Identification, Minimum fill, and Water (not more than 1.0%).

NEOMYCIN AND GRAMICIDIN

For *Neomycin* and *Gramicidin*—See individual listings for chemistry information.

USP requirements: Neomycin Sulfate and Gramicidin Ointment USP—Preserve in collapsible tubes or in well-closed containers. Contains amounts of neomycin sulfate and gramicidin equivalent to the labeled amounts of neomycin and gramicidin, within −10% to +40%. Meets the requirements for Identification, Minimum fill, and Water (not more than 1.0%).

NEOMYCIN AND HYDROCORTISONE

For *Neomycin* and *Hydrocortisone*—See individual listings for chemistry information.

USP requirements:

Neomycin Sulfate and Hydrocortisone Cream USP—Preserve in collapsible tubes or in well-closed containers. Contains an amount of neomycin sulfate equivalent to the labeled amount of neomycin, within −10% to +35%, and the labeled amount of hydrocortisone, within ±10%. Meets the requirements for Identification and Minimum fill.

Neomycin Sulfate and Hydrocortisone Ointment USP—Preserve in collapsible tubes or in well-closed containers. Contains an amount of neomycin sulfate equivalent to the labeled amount of neomycin, within −10% to +35%, and the labeled amount of hydrocortisone, within ±10%. Meets the requirements for Identification, Minimum fill, and Water (not more than 1.0%).

Neomycin Sulfate and Hydrocortisone Otic Suspension USP—Preserve in tight, light-resistant containers. A sterile suspension. Contains an amount of neomycin sulfate equivalent to the labeled amount of neomycin, within −10% to +30%, and the labeled amount of hydrocortisone, within ±10%. Contains Acetic Acid. Meets the requirements for Sterility and pH (4.5–6.0).

Note: Where Neomycin Sulfate and Hydrocortisone Otic Suspension is prescribed, without reference to the quantity of neomycin or hydrocortisone contained therein, a product containing 3.5 mg of neomycin and 10 mg of hydrocortisone per mL shall be dispensed.

Neomycin Sulfate and Hydrocortisone Acetate Cream USP—Preserve in well-closed containers. Contains an amount of neomycin sulfate equivalent to the labeled amount of neomycin, within −10% to +35%, and the labeled amount of hydrocortisone acetate, within ±10%. Meets the requirements for Identification and Minimum fill.

Neomycin Sulfate and Hydrocortisone Acetate Lotion USP—Preserve in well-closed containers. Contains an amount of neomycin sulfate equivalent to the labeled amount of neomycin, within −10% to +30%, and the labeled amount of hydrocortisone acetate, within ±10%. Meets the requirements for Identification and Minimum fill.

Neomycin Sulfate and Hydrocortisone Acetate Ointment USP—Preserve in collapsible tubes or in well-closed containers. Contains an amount of neomycin sulfate equivalent to the labeled amount of neomycin, within −10% to +35%, and the labeled amount of hydrocortisone acetate, within ±10%. Meets the requirements for Identification, Minimum fill, and Water (not more than 1.0%).

Neomycin Sulfate and Hydrocortisone Acetate Ophthalmic Ointment USP—Preserve in collapsible ophthalmic ointment tubes. Contains an amount of neomycin sulfate equivalent to the labeled amount of neomycin, within −10% to +35%, and the labeled amount of hydrocortisone acetate, within ±10%. Meets the requirements for Identification, Sterility, Minimum fill, Water (not more than 1.0%), and Metal particles.

Neomycin Sulfate and Hydrocortisone Acetate Ophthalmic Suspension USP—Preserve in tight containers. The containers or individual cartons are sealed and tamper-proof so that sterility is assured at time of first use. A sterile, aqueous suspension. Contains an amount of neomycin sulfate equivalent to the labeled amount of neomycin, within −10% to +30%, and the labeled amount of hydrocortisone acetate, within ±10%. Meets the requirements for Identification, Sterility, and pH (5.5–7.5).

NEOMYCIN AND METHYLPREDNISOLONE

For *Neomycin* and *Methylprednisolone*—See individual listings for chemistry information.

USP requirements: Neomycin Sulfate and Methylprednisolone Acetate Cream USP—Preserve in collapsible tubes or in tight containers, protected from light. Contains an amount of neomycin sulfate equivalent to the labeled amount of neomycin, within −10% to +35%, and the labeled amount of methylprednisolone acetate, within ±10%. Meets the requirements for Identification and Minimum fill.

NEOMYCIN AND POLYMYXIN B

For *Neomycin* and *Polymyxin B*—See individual listings for chemistry information.

USP requirements:

Neomycin and Polymyxin B Sulfates Cream USP—Preserve in well-closed containers, preferably at controlled room temperature. Contains amounts of neomycin sulfate and polymyxin B sulfate equivalent to the labeled amounts of neomycin and polymyxin B, within −10% to +30%. May contain a suitable local anesthetic. Meets the requirements for Identification and Minimum fill.

Neomycin and Polymyxin B Sulfates Ophthalmic Ointment USP—Preserve in collapsible ophthalmic ointment tubes. A sterile ointment containing Neomycin Sulfate and Polymyxin B Sulfate. Contains amounts of neomycin sulfate and polymyxin B sulfate equivalent to the labeled amounts of neomycin and polymyxin B, within −10% to +30%. Meets the requirements for Identification, Sterility, Minimum fill, Water (not more than 0.5%), and Metal particles.

Neomycin and Polymyxin B Sulfates Solution for Irrigation USP—Preserve in tight containers. A sterile, aqueous solution. Label it to indicate that it is to be diluted for use in a urinary bladder irrigation and is not intended for injection. Contains amounts of neomycin sulfate and polymyxin B sulfate equivalent to the labeled amounts of neomycin and polymyxin B, within −10% to +30%. Meets the requirements for Identification, Sterility, and pH (4.5–6.0).

Neomycin and Polymyxin B Sulfates Ophthalmic Solution USP—Preserve in tight containers, and avoid exposure to excessive heat. Contains amounts of neomycin sulfate and polymyxin B sulfate equivalent to the labeled amounts of neomycin and polymyxin B, within −10% to +30%. Meets the requirements for Identification, Sterility, and pH (5.0–7.0).

NEOMYCIN, POLYMYXIN B, AND BACITRACIN

For *Neomycin, Polymyxin B,* and *Bacitracin*—See individual listings for chemistry information.

USP requirements:

Neomycin and Polymyxin B Sulfates and Bacitracin Ointment USP—Preserve in tight, light-resistant containers, preferably at controlled room temperature. Contains amounts of neomycin sulfate, polymyxin B sulfate, and bacitracin equivalent to the labeled amounts of neomycin, polymyxin B, and bacitracin, within −10% to +30%. May contain a suitable local anesthetic. Meets the requirements for Identification, Minimum fill, and Water (not more than 0.5%).

Neomycin and Polymyxin B Sulfates and Bacitracin Ophthalmic Ointment USP—Preserve in collapsible ophthalmic ointment tubes. A sterile ointment containing Neomycin Sulfate, Polymyxin B Sulfate, and Bacitracin. Contains amounts of neomycin sulfate, polymyxin B sulfate, and bacitracin equivalent to the labeled amounts of neomycin, polymyxin B, and bacitracin, within −10% to +40%. Meets the requirements for Identification, Sterility, Minimum fill, Water (not more than 0.5%), and Metal particles.

Neomycin and Polymyxin B Sulfates and Bacitracin Zinc Ointment USP—Preserve in well-closed containers, preferably at controlled room temperature. Contains amounts of neomycin sulfate, polymyxin B sulfate, and bacitracin zinc equivalent to the labeled amounts of neomycin, polymyxin B, and bacitracin, within −10% to +30%. May contain a suitable local anesthetic. Meets the requirements for Identification, Minimum fill, and Water (not more than 0.5%).

Neomycin and Polymyxin B Sulfates and Bacitracin Zinc Ophthalmic Ointment USP—Preserve in collapsible ophthalmic ointment tubes. Contains amounts of neomycin sulfate, polymyxin B sulfate, and bacitracin zinc equivalent to the labeled amounts of neomycin, polymyxin B, and bacitracin, within −10% to +40%. Meets the requirements for Identification, Sterility, Minimum fill, Water (not more than 0.5%), and Metal particles.

NEOMYCIN, POLYMYXIN B, BACITRACIN, AND HYDROCORTISONE

For *Neomycin, Polymyxin B, Bacitracin,* and *Hydrocortisone*—See individual listings for chemistry information.

USP requirements:

Neomycin and Polymyxin B Sulfates, Bacitracin, and Hydrocortisone Acetate Ointment USP—Preserve in collapsible tubes or in well-closed containers. Contains amounts of neomycin sulfate, polymyxin B sulfate, and bacitracin equivalent to the labeled amounts of neomycin, polymyxin B, and bacitracin, within −10% to +30%, and the labeled amount of hydrocortisone acetate, within ±10%, in a suitable ointment base. Meets the requirements for Identification, Minimum fill, and Water (not more than 0.5%).

Neomycin and Polymyxin B Sulfates, Bacitracin, and Hydrocortisone Acetate Ophthalmic Ointment USP—Preserve in collapsible ophthalmic ointment tubes. Contains amounts of neomycin sulfate, polymyxin B sulfate, and bacitracin equivalent to the labeled amounts of neomycin, polymyxin B, and bacitracin, within −10% to +40%, and the labeled amount of hydrocortisone acetate, within ±10%, in a suitable ointment base. Meets the requirements for Identification, Sterility, Minimum fill, Water (not more than 0.5%), and Metal particles.

Neomycin and Polymyxin B Sulfates, Bacitracin Zinc, and Hydrocortisone Ointment USP—Preserve in well-closed containers, preferably at controlled room temperature. Contains amounts of neomycin sulfate, polymyxin B sulfate, and bacitracin zinc equivalent to the labeled amounts of neomycin, polymyxin B, and bacitracin, within −10% to +30%, and the labeled amount of hydrocortisone, within ±10%. Meets the requirements for Identification, Minimum fill, and Water (not more than 0.5%).

Neomycin and Polymyxin B Sulfates, Bacitracin Zinc, and Hydrocortisone Ophthalmic Ointment USP—Preserve in collapsible ophthalmic ointment tubes. A sterile ointment containing Neomycin Sulfate, Polymyxin B Sulfate, Bacitracin Zinc, and Hydrocortisone. Contains amounts of neomycin sulfate, polymyxin B sulfate, and bacitracin zinc equivalent to the labeled amounts of neomycin, polymyxin B, and bacitracin, within −10% to +40%, and the labeled amount of hydrocortisone, within ±10%. Meets the requirements for Identification, Sterility, Minimum fill, Water (not more than 0.5%), and Metal particles.

Neomycin and Polymyxin B Sulfates, Bacitracin Zinc, and Hydrocortisone Acetate Ophthalmic Ointment USP—Preserve in collapsible ophthalmic ointment tubes. A sterile ointment containing Neomycin Sulfate, Polymyxin B Sulfate, Bacitracin Zinc, and Hydrocortisone Acetate. Contains amounts of neomycin sulfate, polymyxin B sulfate, and bacitracin zinc equivalent to the labeled amounts of neomycin, polymyxin B, and bacitracin, within −10% to +40%, and the labeled amount of hydrocortisone acetate, within ±10%. Meets the requirements for Identification, Sterility, Minimum fill, Water (not more than 0.5%), and Metal particles.

NEOMYCIN, POLYMYXIN B, BACITRACIN, AND LIDOCAINE

For *Neomycin, Polymyxin B, Bacitracin,* and *Lidocaine*—See individual listings for chemistry information.

USP requirements:

Neomycin and Polymyxin B Sulfates, Bacitracin, and Lidocaine Ointment USP—Preserve in well-closed containers, preferably at controlled room temperature. Contains amounts of neomycin sulfate, polymyxin B sulfate, and bacitracin equivalent to the labeled amounts of neomycin, polymyxin B, and bacitracin, within −10% to +30%, and the labeled amount of lidocaine, within ±10%. Meets the requirements for Identification, Minimum fill, and Water (not more than 0.5%).

Neomycin and Polymyxin B Sulfates, Bacitracin Zinc, and Lidocaine Ointment USP—Preserve in well-closed containers, preferably at controlled room temperature. Contains amounts of neomycin sulfate, polymyxin B sulfate, and bacitracin zinc equivalent to the labeled amounts of neomycin, polymyxin B, and bacitracin, within −10% to +30%, and the labeled amount of lidocaine, within ±10%. Meets the requirements for Identification, Minimum fill, and Water (not more than 0.5%).

NEOMYCIN, POLYMYXIN B, AND DEXAMETHASONE

For *Neomycin, Polymyxin B,* and *Dexamethasone*—See individual listings for chemistry information.

USP requirements:

Neomycin and Polymyxin B Sulfates and Dexamethasone Ophthalmic Ointment USP—Preserve in collapsible ophthalmic ointment tubes. Contains amounts of neomycin sulfate and polymyxin B sulfate equivalent to the labeled amounts of neomycin and polymyxin B, within −10% to +30%, and the labeled amount of dexamethasone, within ±10%. Meets the requirements for Identification, Sterility, Minimum fill, Water (not more than 0.5%), and Metal particles.

Neomycin and Polymyxin B Sulfates and Dexamethasone Ophthalmic Suspension USP—Preserve in tight, light-resistant containers in a cool place or at controlled room temperature. The containers or individual cartons are sealed and tamper-proof so that sterility is assured at time of first use. Contains amounts of neomycin sulfate and polymyxin B sulfate equivalent to the labeled amounts of neomycin and polymyxin B, within −10% to +30%, and the labeled amount of dexamethasone, within ±10%. Meets the requirements for Identification, Sterility, and pH (3.5–6.0).

NEOMYCIN, POLYMYXIN B, AND GRAMICIDIN

For *Neomycin, Polymyxin B,* and *Gramicidin*—See individual listings for chemistry information.

USP requirements:

Neomycin and Polymyxin B Sulfates and Gramicidin Cream USP—Preserve in collapsible tubes or in well-closed containers. Contains amounts of neomycin sulfate, polymyxin B sulfate, and gramicidin equivalent to the labeled amounts of neomycin, polymyxin B, and gramicidin, within −10% to +30%. Meets the requirement for Minimum fill.

Neomycin and Polymyxin B Sulfates and Gramicidin Ophthalmic Solution USP—Preserve in tight containers. The containers or individual cartons are sealed and tamper-proof so that sterility is assured at time of first use. A sterile, isotonic aqueous solution of Neomycin Sulfate, Polymyxin B Sulfate, and Gramicidin. Contains amounts of neomycin sulfate, polymyxin B sulfate, and gramicidin equivalent to the labeled amounts of neomycin, polymyxin B, and gramicidin, within −10% to +30%. Meets the requirements for Identification, Sterility, and pH (4.7–6.0).

NEOMYCIN, POLYMYXIN B, GRAMICIDIN, AND HYDROCORTISONE

For *Neomycin, Polymyxin B, Gramicidin,* and *Hydrocortisone*—See individual listings for chemistry information.

USP requirements: Neomycin and Polymyxin B Sulfates, Gramicidin, and Hydrocortisone Acetate Cream USP—Preserve in well-closed containers. Contains amounts of neomycin sulfate, polymyxin B sulfate, and gramicidin equivalent to the labeled amounts of neomycin, polymyxin B, and gramicidin, within −10% to +30%, and the labeled amount of hydrocortisone acetate, within ±10%. Meets the requirement for Minimum fill.

NEOMYCIN, POLYMYXIN B, AND HYDROCORTISONE

For *Neomycin, Polymyxin B,* and *Hydrocortisone*—See individual listings for chemistry information.

USP requirements:

Neomycin and Polymyxin B Sulfates and Hydrocortisone Otic Solution USP—Preserve in tight, light-resistant containers. The containers or individual cartons are sealed and tamper-proof so that sterility is assured at time of first use. A sterile solution containing Neomycin Sulfate, Polymyxin B Sulfate, and Hydrocortisone. Contains amounts of neomycin sulfate and polymyxin B sulfate equivalent to the labeled amounts of neomycin and polymyxin B, within −10% to +30%. Contains the labeled amount of hydrocortisone, within ±10%. Meets the requirements for Sterility and pH (2.0–4.5).

Neomycin and Polymyxin B Sulfates and Hydrocortisone Ophthalmic Suspension USP—Preserve in tight containers. The containers or individual cartons are sealed and tamper-proof so that sterility is assured at time of first use. A sterile, aqueous suspension of Neomycin Sulfate, Polymyxin B Sulfate, and Hydrocortisone. Contains amounts of neomycin sulfate and polymyxin B sulfate equivalent to the labeled amounts of neomycin and polymyxin B, within −10% to +30%. Contains the labeled amount of hydrocortisone, within ±10%. Meets the requirements for Identification, Sterility, and pH (4.1–7.0).

Neomycin and Polymyxin B Sulfates and Hydrocortisone Otic Suspension USP—Preserve in tight, light-resistant containers. The containers or individual cartons are sealed and tamper-proof so that sterility is assured at time of first use. A sterile suspension containing Neomycin Sulfate, Polymyxin B Sulfate, and Hydrocortisone. Contains amounts of neomycin sulfate and polymyxin B sulfate equivalent to the labeled amounts of neomycin and polymyxin B, within −10% to +30%. Contains the labeled amount of hydrocortisone, within ±10%. Meets the requirements for Identification, Sterility, and pH (3.0–7.0).

Neomycin and Polymyxin B Sulfates and Hydrocortisone Acetate Cream USP—Preserve in well-closed containers. Contains amounts of neomycin sulfate and polymyxin B sulfate equivalent to the labeled amounts of neomycin and polymyxin B, within −10% to +30%. Contains the labeled amount of hydrocortisone acetate, within ±10%. Meets the requirements for Identification and Minimum fill.

Neomycin and Polymyxin B Sulfates and Hydrocortisone Acetate Ophthalmic Suspension USP—Preserve in tight containers. The containers or individual cartons are sealed and tamper-proof so that sterility is assured at time of first use. A sterile suspension of Hydrocortisone Acetate in an aqueous solution of Neomycin Sulfate and Polymyxin B Sulfate. Contains amounts of neomycin sulfate and polymyxin B sulfate equivalent to the labeled amounts of neomycin and polymyxin B, within −10% to +25%. Contains the labeled amount of hydrocortisone acetate, within ±10%. Meets the requirements for Sterility and pH (5.0–7.0).

NEOMYCIN, POLYMYXIN B, AND LIDOCAINE

For *Neomycin, Polymyxin B,* and *Lidocaine*—See individual listings for chemistry information.

USP requirements: Neomycin and Polymyxin B Sulfates and Lidocaine Cream USP—Preserve in well-closed containers, preferably at controlled room temperature. Contains the equivalent of the labeled amounts of neomycin and polymyxin B, within −10% to +30%, and the labeled amount of lidocaine, within ±10%. Meets the requirements for Identification and Minimum fill.

NEOMYCIN, POLYMYXIN B, AND PREDNISOLONE

For *Neomycin, Polymyxin B,* and *Prednisolone*—See individual listings for chemistry information.

USP requirements: Neomycin and Polymyxin B Sulfates and Prednisolone Acetate Ophthalmic Suspension USP—Preserve in tight containers. The containers or individual cartons are sealed and tamper-proof so that sterility is assured at time of first use. A sterile suspension of Prednisolone Acetate in an aqueous solution of Neomycin Sulfate and Polymyxin B Sulfate. Contains amounts of neomycin sulfate and polymyxin B sulfate equivalent to the labeled amounts of neomycin and polymyxin B, within −10% to +25%, and the labeled amount of prednisolone acetate, within ±10%. Meets the requirements for Identification, Sterility, and pH (5.0–7.0).

NEOMYCIN AND PREDNISOLONE

For *Neomycin* and *Prednisolone*—See individual listings for chemistry information.

USP requirements:

Neomycin Sulfate and Prednisolone Acetate Ointment USP—Preserve in collapsible tubes or in tight containers, protected from light. Contains an amount of neomycin sulfate equivalent to the labeled amount of neomycin, within −10% to +35%, and the labeled amount of prednisolone acetate, within ±10%. Meets the requirements for Identification, Minimum fill, and Water (not more than 1.0%).

Neomycin Sulfate and Prednisolone Acetate Ophthalmic Ointment USP—Preserve in collapsible ophthalmic ointment tubes. A sterile ointment containing Neomycin Sulfate and Prednisolone Acetate. Contains an amount of neomycin sulfate equivalent to the labeled amount of neomycin, within −10% to +35%, and the labeled amount of prednisolone acetate, within ±10%. Meets the requirements for Identification, Sterility, Minimum fill, Water (not more than 1.0%), and Metal particles.

Neomycin Sulfate and Prednisolone Acetate Ophthalmic Suspension USP—Preserve in tight containers. The containers or individual cartons are sealed and tamper-proof so that sterility is assured at time of first use. Contains an amount of neomycin sulfate equivalent to the labeled amount of neomycin, within −10% to +30%, and the labeled amount of prednisolone acetate, within ±10%. Meets the requirements for Identification, Sterility, and pH (5.5–7.5).

Neomycin Sulfate and Prednisolone Sodium Phosphate Ophthalmic Ointment USP—Preserve in collapsible ophthalmic ointment tubes. A sterile ointment containing Neomycin Sulfate and Prednisolone Sodium Phosphate. Contains amounts of neomycin sulfate and prednisolone sodium phosphate equivalent to the labeled amounts of neomycin, within −10% to +35%, and prednisolone phosphate, within −10% to +15%. Meets the requirements for Identification, Sterility, Minimum fill, Water (not more than 1.0%), and Metal particles.

Note: Where Neomycin Sulfate and Prednisolone Sodium Phosphate Ophthalmic Ointment is prescribed without reference to the quantity of neomycin or prednisolone phosphate contained therein, a product containing 3.5 mg of neomycin and 2.5 mg of prednisolone phosphate per gram shall be dispensed.

NEOMYCIN, SULFACETAMIDE, AND PREDNISOLONE

For *Neomycin, Sulfacetamide,* and *Prednisolone*—See individual listings for chemistry information.

USP requirements: Neomycin Sulfate, Sulfacetamide Sodium, and Prednisolone Acetate Ophthalmic Ointment USP—Preserve in collapsible ophthalmic ointment tubes. Contains an amount of neomycin sulfate equivalent to the labeled amount of neomycin, within −10% to +35%, and the labeled amounts of sulfacetamide sodium and prednisolone acetate, within ±10%. Meets the requirements for Identification, Sterility, Minimum fill, and Metal particles.

NEOMYCIN AND TRIAMCINOLONE

For *Neomycin* and *Triamcinolone*—See individual listings for chemistry information.

USP requirements:

Neomycin Sulfate and Triamcinolone Acetonide Cream USP—Preserve in collapsible tubes or in tight containers. Contains an amount of neomycin sulfate equivalent to the labeled amount of neomycin, within −10% to +35%, and the labeled amount of triamcinolone acetonide, within ±10%. Meets the requirements for Identification and Minimum fill.

Neomycin Sulfate and Triamcinolone Acetonide Ophthalmic Ointment USP—Preserve in collapsible ophthalmic ointment tubes. Contains an amount of neomycin sulfate equivalent to the labeled amount of neomycin, within −10% to +35%, and the labeled amount of triamcinolone acetonide, within ±10%. Meets the requirements for Identification, Sterility, Minimum fill, Water (not more than 1.0%), and Metal particles.

NEOSTIGMINE

Chemical name:

Neostigmine bromide—Benzenaminium, 3-[[(dimethylamino)carbonyl]oxy]-*N,N,N*-trimethyl-, bromide.

Neostigmine methylsulfate—Benzenaminium, 3-[[(dimethylamino)carbonyl]oxy]-*N,N,N*-trimethyl-, methyl sulfate.

Molecular formula:

Neostigmine bromide—$C_{12}H_{19}BrN_2O_2$.

Neostigmine methylsulfate—$C_{13}H_{22}N_2O_6S$.

Molecular weight:

Neostigmine bromide—303.20.

Neostigmine methylsulfate—334.39.

Description:

Neostigmine bromide—White, crystalline powder. Odorless. Its solutions are neutral to litmus.

Neostigmine methylsulfate—White, crystalline powder. Odorless. Its solutions are neutral to litmus.

Solubility

Neostigmine bromide—Very soluble in water; soluble in alcohol; practically insoluble in ether.

Neostigmine methylsulfate—Very soluble in water; soluble in alcohol.

USP requirements:

Neostigmine Bromide USP—Preserve in tight containers. Contains not less than 98.0% and not more than 102.0% of neostigmine bromide, calculated on the dried basis. Meets the requirements for Identification, Melting range (171–176 °C, with decomposition), Loss on drying (not more than 2.0%), Residue on ignition (not more than 0.15%), and Sulfate.

Neostigmine Bromide Tablets USP—Preserve in tight containers. Contain the labeled amount, within ±7%. Meet the requirements for Identification, Dissolution (75% in 45 minutes in water in Apparatus 2 at 50 rpm), and Uniformity of dosage units.

Neostigmine Methylsulfate USP—Preserve in tight containers. Contains not less than 98.0% and not more than 102.0% of neostigmine methylsulfate, calculated on the dried basis. Meets the requirements for Identification, Melting range (144–149 °C), Loss on drying (not more than 1.0%), Residue on ignition (not more than 0.1%), Chloride, and Sulfate ion.

Neostigmine Methylsulfate Injection USP—Preserve in single-dose or in multiple-dose containers, protected from light. A sterile solution of Neostigmine Methylsulfate in Water for Injection. Contains the labeled amount, within ±10%. Meets the requirements for Identification, pH (5.0–6.5), and Injections.

NETILMICIN

Source: Semi-synthetic derivative of sisomicin.

Chemical name: Netilmicin sulfate—D-Streptamine, *O*-3-deoxy-4-*C*-methyl-3-(methylamino)-beta-L-arabinopyranosyl-(1→6)-*O*-[2,6-diamino-2,3,4,6-tetradeoxy-alpha-D-*glycero*-hex-4-enopyranosyl-(1→4)]-2-deoxy-N^1-ethyl-, sulfate (2:5) (salt).

Molecular formula: Netilmicin sulfate—$(C_{21}H_{41}N_5O_7)_2 \cdot 5H_2SO_4$.

Molecular weight: Netilmicin sulfate—1441.54.

Description: Netilmicin sulfate—White- to buff-colored powder.

Solubility: Netilmicin sulfate—Readily soluble in water.

USP requirements:

Netilmicin Sulfate USP—Preserve in tight containers. Has a potency equivalent to not less than 595 mcg of netilmicin per mg, calculated on the dried basis. Meets the requirements for Identification, Specific rotation (+88° to +96°, calculated on the dried basis), pH (3.5–5.5, in a solution containing 40 mg of netilmicin per mL), Loss on drying (not more than 15.0%), and Residue on ignition (not more than 1.0%).

Netilmicin Sulfate Injection USP—Preserve in single-dose or in multiple-dose containers, preferably of Type I glass. A sterile solution of Netilmicin Sulfate in Water for Injection. Contains an amount of netilmicin sulfate equivalent to the labeled amount of netilmicin, within −10% to +15%. Meets the requirements for Identification, Bacterial endotoxins, Sterility, pH (3.5–6.0), Particulate matter, and Injections.

NIACIN

Chemical name: 3-Pyridinecarboxylic acid.

Molecular formula: $C_6H_5NO_2$.

Molecular weight: 123.11.

Description: Niacin USP—White crystals or crystalline powder. Is odorless, or has a slight odor. Melts at about 235 °C.

pKa: 4.85.

Solubility: Niacin USP—Sparingly soluble in water; freely soluble in boiling water, in boiling alcohol, and in solutions of alkali hydroxides and carbonates; practically insoluble in ether.

USP requirements:

Niacin USP—Preserve in well-closed containers. Contains not less than 99.0% and not more than 101.0% of niacin, calculated on the dried basis. Meets the requirements for Identification, Loss on drying (not more than 1.0%), Residue on ignition (not more than 0.1%), Chloride (not more than 0.02%), Sulfate (not more than 0.02%), Heavy metals (not more than 0.002%), Ordinary impurities, and Organic volatile impurities.

Niacin Extended-release Capsules—Not in USP.

Niacin Injection USP—Preserve in single-dose or in multiple-dose containers, preferably of Type I glass. A sterile solution of Niacin and niacin sodium in Water for Injection, made with the aid of Sodium Carbonate or Sodium Hydroxide. Contains the labeled amount, within −5% to +10%. Meets the requirements for Identification, Bacterial endotoxins, pH (4.0–6.0), and Injections.

Niacin Oral Solution—Not in USP.

Niacin Tablets USP—Preserve in well-closed containers. Contain the labeled amount, within ±10%. Meet the requirements for Identification, Disintegration (30 minutes), and Uniformity of dosage units.

Niacin Extended-release Tablets—Not in USP.

NIACINAMIDE

Chemical name: 3-Pyridinecarboxamide.

Molecular formula: $C_6H_6N_2O$.

Molecular weight: 122.13.

Description: Niacinamide USP—White, crystalline powder. Is odorless or practically so. Its solutions are neutral to litmus.

pKa: 0.5 and 3.35.

Solubility: Niacinamide USP—Freely soluble in water and in alcohol; soluble in glycerin.

USP requirements:

Niacinamide USP—Preserve in tight containers. Contains not less than 98.5% and not more than 101.5% of niacinamide, calculated on the dried basis. Meets the requirements for Identification, Melting range (128–131 °C), Loss on drying (not more than 0.5%), Residue on ignition (not more than 0.1%), Heavy metals (not more than 0.003%), Readily carbonizable substances, and Organic volatile impurities.

Niacinamide Capsules—Not in USP.

Niacinamide Gel—Not in USP.

Niacinamide Injection USP—Preserve in single-dose or in multiple-dose containers, preferably of Type I glass. A sterile solution of Niacinamide in Water for Injection. Contains the labeled amount, within −5% to +10%. Meets the requirements for Identification, Bacterial endotoxins, pH (5.0–7.0), and Injections.

Niacinamide Tablets USP—Preserve in tight containers. Contain the labeled amount, within ±10%. Meet the requirements for Identification, Disintegration (30 minutes), and Uniformity of dosage units.

NICARDIPINE

Chemical name: Nicardipine hydrochloride—3,5-Pyridinedicarboxylic acid, 1,4-dihydro-2,6-dimethyl-4-(3-nitrophenyl)-, methyl 2-[methyl(phenylmethyl)amino]ethyl ester, monohydrochloride.

Molecular formula: Nicardipine hydrochloride—$C_{26}H_{29}N_3O_6 \cdot HCl$.

Molecular weight: Nicardipine hydrochloride—515.99.

Description: Nicardipine hydrochloride—Greenish-yellow, odorless, crystalline powder. Melts at about 169 °C.

Solubility: Nicardipine hydrochloride—Freely soluble in chloroform, in methanol, and in glacial acetic acid; sparingly soluble in anhydrous ethanol; slightly soluble in n-butanol, in water, in 0.01 *M* potassium dihydrogen phosphate, in acetone, and in dioxane; very slightly soluble in ethyl acetate; practically insoluble in ether and in hexane.

USP requirements: Nicardipine Hydrochloride Capsules —Not in USP.

NICLOSAMIDE

Chemical group: Derivative of salicylanilide.

Chemical name: Benzamide, 5-chloro-*N*-(2-chloro-4-nitrophenyl)-2-hydroxy-.

Molecular formula: $C_{13}H_8Cl_2N_2O_4$.

Molecular weight: 327.12.

Description: Pale yellow crystals with a melting point of 225–230 °C.

Solubility: Practically insoluble in water; sparingly soluble in ethanol, in chloroform, and in ether.

USP requirements: Niclosamide Chewable Tablets—Not in USP.

NICOTINE

Chemical name:

Nicotine—(*S*)-3-(1-methyl-2-pyrrolidinyl)pyridine.

Nicotine polacrilex—2-Propenoic acid, 2-methyl-, polymer with diethenylbenzene, complex with (*S*)-3-(1-methyl-2-pyrrolidinyl)pyridine.

Molecular formula:

Nicotine—$C_{10}H_{14}N_2$.

Nicotine polacrilex—$[(C_4H_6O_2)_x(C_{10}H_{10})_y](C_{10}H_{14}N_2)$.

Molecular weight: 162.23.

Description: Colorless to pale yellow, strongly alkaline, oily, volatile, hygroscopic liquid; has a characteristic pungent odor; turns brown on exposure to air or light.

Solubility: Freely soluble in water.

USP requirements:

Nicotine Transdermal Systems—Not in USP.

Nicotine Polacrilex Chewing Gum Tablets—Not in USP.

NICOTINYL ALCOHOL

Molecular formula: Nicotinyl alcohol tartrate—$C_6H_7NO \cdot C_4H_6O_6$.

Molecular weight: Nicotinyl alcohol tartrate—259.2.

Description: Nicotinyl alcohol tartrate—White or almost white, odorless or almost odorless, crystalline powder.

Solubility: Nicotinyl alcohol tartrate—Freely soluble in water; slightly soluble in alcohol; practically insoluble in chloroform and in ether.

USP requirements: Nicotinyl Alcohol Tartrate Extended-release Tablets—Not in USP.

NIFEDIPINE

Chemical name: 3,5-Pyridinedicarboxylic acid, 1,4-dihydro-2,6-dimethyl-4-(2-nitrophenyl)-, dimethyl ester.

Molecular formula: $C_{17}H_{18}N_2O_6$.

Molecular weight: 346.34.

Description: Nifedipine USP—Yellow powder; affected by exposure to light.

Solubility: Nifedipine USP—Practically insoluble in water; freely soluble in acetone.

USP requirements:
Nifedipine USP—Preserve in tight, light-resistant containers. Contains not less than 98.0% and not more than 102.0% of nifedipine, calculated on the dried basis. Meets the requirements for Identification, Melting range (171–175 °C), Loss on drying (not more than 0.5%), Residue on ignition (not more than 0.1%), Heavy metals (not more than 0.001%), Perchloric acid titration, Chloride and sulfate, Related compounds, and Organic volatile impurities.
Nifedipine Capsules USP—Preserve in tight, light-resistant containers at a temperature between 15 and 25 °C. Contain the labeled amount, within ± 10%. Meet the requirements for Identification, Dissolution (80% in 20 minutes in simulated gastric fluid TS [without pepsin] in Apparatus 2 at 50 rpm), Uniformity of dosage units, and Related compounds.
Nifedipine Tablets—Not in USP.
Nifedipine Extended-release Tablets—Not in USP.

NILUTAMIDE

Chemical name: 5,5-Dimethyl-3-(alpha,alpha,alpha-trifluoro-4-nitro-*m*-tolyl)hydantoin.

Molecular formula: $C_{12}H_{10}F_3N_3O_4$.

Molecular weight: 317.22.

Description: White to off-white powder. Melts between 153–156 °C.

Solubility: Soluble in ethyl acetate, in acetone, in chloroform, in ethyl alcohol, in dichloromethane, and in methanol; slightly soluble in water (less than 0.1% w/v) at 25 °C.

USP requirements: Nilutamide Tablets—Not in USP.

NIMODIPINE

Chemical name: 3,5-Pyridinedicarboxylic acid, 1,4-dihydro-2,6-dimethyl-4-(3-nitrophenyl)-, 2-methoxyethyl 1-methylethyl ester.

Molecular formula: $C_{21}H_{26}N_2O_7$.

Molecular weight: 418.45.

Description: Yellow crystalline substance.

Solubility: Practically insoluble in water.

USP requirements: Nimodipine Capsules—Not in USP.

NITRAZEPAM

Chemical name: 2*H*-1,4-Benzodiazepin-2-one, 1,3-dihydro-7-nitro-5-phenyl-.

Molecular formula: $C_{15}H_{11}N_3O_3$.

Molecular weight: 281.27.

Description: Yellow, crystalline powder.

Solubility: Practically insoluble in water; slightly soluble in alcohol and in ether; sparingly soluble in chloroform.

USP requirements: Nitrazepam Tablets—Not in USP.

NITRIC ACID

Chemical name: Nitric acid.

Molecular formula: HNO_3.

Molecular weight: 63.01.

Description: Nitric Acid NF—Highly corrosive, fuming liquid, having a characteristic, highly irritating odor. Stains animal tissue yellow. Boils at about 120 °C. Specific gravity is about 1.41.
NF category: Acidifying agent.

NF requirements: Nitric Acid NF—Preserve in tight containers. Contains not less than 69.0% and not more than 71.0%, by weight, of nitric acid. Meets the requirements for Clarity and color, Identification, Residue on ignition (not more than 5 ppm), Chloride (not more than 0.5 ppm), Sulfate (not more than 1 ppm), Arsenic (not more than 0.01 ppm), Iron (not more than 0.2 ppm), and Heavy metals (not more than 0.2 ppm).
Caution: Avoid contact since Nitric Acid rapidly destroys tissues.

NITROFURANTOIN

Chemical group: Nitrofuran derivative.

Chemical name: 2,4-Imidazolidenedione, 1-[[(5-nitro-2-furanyl)-methylene]amino]-.

Molecular formula: $C_8H_6N_4O_5$.

Molecular weight: 238.16.

Description: Nitrofurantoin USP—Lemon-yellow, odorless crystals or fine powder.

Solubility: Nitrofurantoin USP—Very slightly soluble in water and in alcohol; soluble in dimethylformamide.

USP requirements:
Nitrofurantoin USP—Preserve in tight, light-resistant containers. It is anhydrous or contains one molecule of water of hydration. Label it to indicate whether it is anhydrous or hydrous. Contains not less than 98.0% and not more than 102.0% of nitrofurantoin, calculated on the anhydrous basis. Meets the requirements for Identification, Water (not more than 1.0% for the anhydrous form and 6.5–7.5% for the hydrous form), Nitrofurfural diacetate (not more than 1.0%), and Nitrofurazone.

Caution: Nitrofurantoin and solutions of it are discolored by alkali and by exposure to light, and are decomposed upon contact with metals other than stainless steel and aluminum.

Nitrofurantoin Capsules USP—Preserve in tight, light-resistant containers. Contain the labeled amount, within ±10%. Meet the requirements for Identification, Uniformity of dosage units, and Nitrofurazone (not more than 0.01%).

Nitrofurantoin Extended-release Capsules—Not in USP.

Nitrofurantoin Oral Suspension USP—Preserve in tight, light-resistant containers. A suspension of Nitrofurantoin in a suitable, aqueous vehicle. Contains, in each 100 mL, not less than 460 mg and not more than 540 mg of nitrofurantoin. Meets the requirements for Identification, pH (4.5–6.5), and Limit of *N*-(aminocarbonyl)-*N*-[([5-nitro-2-furanyl]methylene)amino]glycine.

Nitrofurantoin Tablets USP—Preserve in tight, light-resistant containers. Contain the labeled amount, within ±10%. Meet the requirements for Identification, Dissolution (25% in 60 minutes and 85% in 120 minutes in phosphate buffer [pH 7.2] in Apparatus 1 at 100 rpm), Uniformity of dosage units, and Nitrofurazone (not more than 0.01%).

NITROFURAZONE

Chemical name: Hydrazinecarboxamide, 2-[(5-nitro-2-furanyl)-methylene]-.

Molecular formula: $C_6H_6N_4O_4$.

Molecular weight: 198.14.

Description:

Nitrofurazone USP—Lemon yellow, odorless, crystalline powder. Darkens slowly on exposure to light. Melts at about 236 °C, with decomposition.

Nitrofurazone Cream USP—Yellow, opaque cream.

Nitrofurazone Ointment USP—Yellow, opaque, and has ointment-like consistency.

Nitrofurazone Topical Solution USP—Light yellow, clear, somewhat viscous liquid, having a faint, characteristic odor.

Solubility:

Nitrofurazone USP—Very slightly soluble in alcohol and in water; soluble in dimethylformamide; slightly soluble in propylene glycol and in polyethylene glycol mixtures; practically insoluble in chloroform and in ether.

Nitrofurazone Cream USP—Miscible with water.

Nitrofurazone Ointment USP—Miscible with water.

Nitrofurazone Topical Solution USP—Miscible with water.

USP requirements:

Nitrofurazone USP—Preserve in tight, light-resistant containers, and avoid exposure to direct sunlight and to excessive heat. Dried at 105 °C for 1 hour, contains not less than 98.0% and not more than 102.0% of nitrofurazone. Meets the requirements for Identification, pH (5.0–7.5), Loss on drying (not more than 0.5%), Residue on ignition (not more than 0.1%), Ordinary impurities, and Limit of 5-nitro-2-furfuraldazine.

Note: Avoid exposing solutions of nitrofurazone at all times to direct sunlight, excessive heat, strong fluorescent lighting, and alkaline materials.

Nitrofurazone Cream USP—Preserve in tight, light-resistant containers. Avoid exposure to direct sunlight, strong fluorescent lighting, and excessive heat. It is Nitrofurazone in a suitable, emulsified water-miscible base. Contains the labeled amount, within ±10%. Meets the requirements for Identification and Minimum fill.

Note: Avoid exposure at all times to direct sunlight, excessive heat, strong fluorescent lighting, and alkaline materials.

Nitrofurazone Ointment USP—Preserve in tight, light-resistant containers. Avoid exposure to direct sunlight, strong fluorescent lighting, and excessive heat. It is Nitrofurazone in a suitable water-miscible base. Contains the labeled amount, within ±10%. Meets the requirements for Completeness of solution and Identification.

Nitrofurazone Topical Solution USP—Preserve in tight, light-resistant containers. Avoid exposure to direct sunlight and excessive heat. Contains the labeled amount, within ±5% (w/w). Meets the requirement for Identification.

Note: Avoid exposure at all times to direct sunlight, excessive heat, and alkaline materials.

NITROGEN

Chemical name: Nitrogen.

Molecular formula: N_2.

Molecular weight: 28.01.

Description: Nitrogen NF—Colorless, odorless gas. It is nonflammable and does not support combustion. One liter at 0 °C and at a pressure of 760 mm of mercury weighs about 1.251 grams.

NF category: Air displacement.

Solubility: Nitrogen NF—One volume dissolves in about 65 volumes of water and in about 9 volumes of alcohol at 20 °C and at a pressure of 760 mm of mercury.

NF requirements: Nitrogen NF—Preserve in cylinders. Contains not less than 99.0%, by volume, of nitrogen. Meets the requirements for Identification, Odor, Carbon monoxide (not more than 0.001%), and Oxygen (not more than 1.0%).

NITROGEN 97 PERCENT

NF requirements: Nitrogen 97 Percent NF—Preserve in cylinders or in a low-pressure collecting tank. It is Nitrogen produced from air by physical separation methods. Where it is piped directly from the collecting tank to the point of use, label each outlet "Nitrogen 97 Percent." Contains not less than 97.0%, by volume, of nitrogen. Meets the requirements for Identification, Odor, Carbon dioxide (not more than 0.03%), Carbon monoxide (not more than 0.001%), Nitric oxide and nitrogen dioxide (not more than 2.5 ppm), Sulfur dioxide (not more than 5 ppm), and Oxygen (not more than 3.0%).

AMMONIA N 13

Source: Different methods are being used in the various clinical facilities for the on-site production of $^{13}NH_3$. It can be produced by irradiation of ^{16}O-water with protons and subsequent reduction using De Varda's alloy or titanium (III) salts. The resultant $^{13}NH_3$ is collected as the ammonium ion in saline solution.

Chemical name: Ammonia-^{13}N.

Molecular formula: $H_3{}^{13}N$.

USP requirements: Ammonia N 13 Injection USP—Preserve in single-dose or in multiple-dose containers that are adequately shielded. A sterile, aqueous solution, suitable for intravenous administration, of $^{13}NH_3$ in which a portion of the molecules are labeled with radioactive ^{13}N. Label it to include the following, in addition to the information specified for Labeling under Injections: the time and date of calibration; the amount of ^{13}N as ammonia expressed as total megabecquerels (or millicuries) per mL, at time of calibration; the expiration time and date; the name and quantity of any added preservative or stabilizer; and the statement "Caution—Radioactive Material." The labeling indicates that in making dosage calculations correction is to be made for radioactive decay and also indicates that the radioactive half-life of ^{13}N is 9.96 minutes. The label indicates "Do not use if cloudy or if it contains particulate matter." Contains the labeled amount of ^{13}N expressed in megabecquerels (or millicuries) per mL, within ±10%, at the time indicated in the labeling. Meets the requirements for Specific activity (not less than 37×10^4 megabecquerels [10 curies] per mmol), Radionuclide identification, Bacterial endotoxins, pH (4.5–8.5), Radiochemical purity, Radionuclidic purity, Chemical purity, and Injections (except that the Injection may be distributed or dispensed prior to completion of the test for Sterility, the latter test being started on the day following final manufacture, and except that it is not subject to the recommendation in Volume in Container).

NITROGLYCERIN

Chemical name: 1,2,3-Propanetriol, trinitrate.

Molecular formula: $C_3H_5N_3O_9$.

Molecular weight: 227.09.

Description: Diluted Nitroglycerin USP—White, odorless powder, when diluted with lactose. When diluted with propylene glycol or alcohol, it is a clear, colorless, or pale yellow liquid. (Note: Undiluted nitroglycerin is a white to pale yellow, thick, flammable, explosive liquid.)

Solubility: Undiluted nitroglycerin—Slightly soluble in water; soluble in methanol, in alcohol, in carbon disulfide, in acetone, in ethyl ether, in ethyl acetate, in glacial acetic acid, in toluene, in phenol, in chloroform, and in methylene chloride.

USP requirements:

Diluted Nitroglycerin USP—Preserve in tight, light-resistant containers, and prevent exposure to excessive heat. A mixture of nitroglycerin with lactose, dextrose, alcohol, propylene glycol, or other suitable inert excipient to permit safe handling. Contains the labeled amount of nitroglycerin, within ±10%. Usually contains approximately 10% of nitroglycerin. Meets the requirements for Identification and Chromatographic purity.

Caution: Exercise proper precautions in handling undiluted nitroglycerin, since it is a powerful explosive and can be exploded by percussion or excessive heat. Only exceedingly small amounts should be isolated.

Nitroglycerin Lingual Aerosol—Not in USP.

Nitroglycerin Extended-release Capsules—Not in USP.

Nitroglycerin Injection USP—Preserve in single-dose or in multiple-dose containers, preferably of Type I or Type II glass. A sterile solution prepared from Diluted Nitroglycerin; the solvent may contain Alcohol, Propylene Glycol, and Water for Injection. Where necessary, label it to indicate that it is to be diluted before use. Contains the labeled amount, within ±10%. Meets the requirements for Identification, Bacterial endotoxins, pH (3.0–6.5), Alcohol content (labeled amount, within ±10%), Particulate matter, and Injections.

Nitroglycerin Ointment USP—Preserve in tight containers. It is Diluted Nitroglycerin in a suitable ointment base. Label multiple-dose containers with a direction to close tightly, immediately after each use. Contains the labeled amount, within −10% to +15%. Meets the requirements for Identification, Minimum fill, and Homogeneity (within ±10% of mean value).

Nitroglycerin Transdermal Systems—Not in USP.

Nitroglycerin Tablets USP (Sublingual)—Preserve in tight containers, preferably of glass, at controlled room temperature. Each container holds not more than 100 Tablets. The labeling indicates that the Tablets are for sublingual use, and the label directs that the Tablets be dispensed in the original, unopened container, labeled with the following statement directed to the patient. "Warning: to prevent loss of potency, keep these tablets in the original container or in a supplemental Nitroglycerin container specifically labeled as being suitable for Nitroglycerin Tablets. Close tightly immediately after each use." Contain the labeled amount, within −10% to +15%. Meet the requirements for Identification, Disintegration (2 minutes), and Uniformity of dosage units.

Nitroglycerin Extended-release Tablets—Not in USP.

Nitroglycerin Extended-release Buccal Tablets—Not in USP.

NITROMERSOL

Chemical name: 7-Oxa-8-mercurabicyclo[4.2.0]octa-1,3,5-triene, 5-methyl-2-nitro.

Molecular formula: $C_7H_5HgNO_3$.

Molecular weight: 351.71.

Description:

Nitromersol USP—Brownish yellow to yellow granules or brownish yellow to yellow powder. Odorless. Affected by light.

Nitromersol Topical Solution USP—Clear, reddish orange solution. Affected by light.

Solubility: Nitromersol USP—Very slightly soluble in water, in alcohol, in acetone, and in ether; soluble in solutions of alkalies and of ammonia by opening of the anhydride ring and the formation of a salt.

USP requirements:

Nitromersol USP—Preserve in tight, light-resistant containers. Dried at 105 °C for 2 hours, contains not less than 98.0% and not more than 100.5% of nitromersol. Meets the requirements for Identification, Loss on drying (not more than 1.0%), Residue on ignition (not more than 0.1%), Mercury ions, Alkali-insoluble substances (not more than 0.1%), and Uncombined nitrocresol (not more than 1%).

Nitromersol Topical Solution USP—Preserve in tight, light-resistant containers. Yields, from each 100 mL, not less than 180.0 mg and not more than 220.0 mg of Nitromersol.

Prepare Nitromersol Topical Solution as follows: 2 grams of Nitromersol, 0.4 gram of Sodium Hydroxide, 4.25 grams of Sodium Carbonate, monohydrate, and a sufficient quantity of Purified Water to make 1000 mL. Dissolve the Sodium Hydroxide and the monohydrated Sodium Carbonate in 50 mL of Purified Water, add the Nitromersol, and stir until dissolved. Gradually add Purified Water to make 1000 mL.

Meets the requirements for Identification, Specific gravity (1.005–1.010), and Mercury ions.

Note: Prepare dilutions of Nitromersol Topical Solution as needed, since they tend to precipitate on standing.

NITROUS OXIDE

Chemical name: Nitrogen oxide (N_2O).

Molecular formula: N_2O.

Molecular weight: 44.01.

Description: Nitrous Oxide USP—Colorless gas, without appreciable odor. One liter at 0 °C and at a pressure of 760 mm of mercury weighs about 1.97 grams.

Solubility: Nitrous Oxide USP—One volume dissolves in about 1.4 volumes of water at 20 °C and at a pressure of 760 mm of mercury; freely soluble in alcohol; soluble in ether and in oils.

Other characteristics:
Blood-to-Gas partition coefficient at 37 °C—0.47.
Oil-to-Gas partition coefficient at 37 °C—1.4.

USP requirements: Nitrous Oxide USP—Preserve in cylinders. Contains not less than 99%, by volume, of nitrous oxide. Meets the requirements for Identification, Carbon monoxide (not more than 0.001%), Nitric oxide (not more than 1 ppm), Nitrogen dioxide (not more than 1 ppm), Halogens (not more than 1 ppm), Carbon dioxide (not more than 0.03%), Ammonia (not more than 0.0025%), Water (not more than 150 mg per cubic meter), and Air (not more than 1.0%).

NIZATIDINE

Chemical name: 1,1-Ethenediamine, *N*-[2-[[[2-[(dimethylamino)-methyl]-4-thiazolyl]methyl]thio]ethyl]-*N'*-methyl-2-nitro-.

Molecular formula: $C_{12}H_{21}N_5O_2S_2$.

Molecular weight: 331.45.

Description: Off-white to buff crystalline solid.

Solubility: Soluble in water.

USP requirements:
Nizatidine USP—Preserve in tight, light-resistant containers. Contains not less than 98.0% and not more than 101.0% of nizatidine, calculated on the dried basis. Meets the requirements for Identification, Loss on drying (not more than 1.0%), Residue on ignition (not more than 0.1%), Heavy metals (not more than 0.001%), and Chromatographic purity.
Nizatidine Capsules USP—Preserve in tight, light-resistant containers. Store at controlled room temperature. Contain the labeled amount, within ± 10%. Meet the requirements for Identification, Dissolution (75% in 30 minutes in water in Apparatus 2 at 50 rpm), Uniformity of dosage units, and Chromatographic purity.

NONOXYNOL 9

Chemical name: Poly(oxy-1,2-ethanediyl), alpha-(4-nonyl-phenyl)-omega-hydroxy-.

Molecular formula: $C_{15}H_{24}O(C_2H_4O)_n$ (n = approximately 9).

Description: Nonoxynol 9 USP—Clear, colorless to light yellow viscous liquid.
NF category: Wetting and/or solubilizing agent.

Solubility: Nonoxynol 9 USP—Soluble in water, in alcohol, and in corn oil.

USP requirements:
Nonoxynol 9 USP—Preserve in tight containers. An anhydrous liquid mixture consisting chiefly of mono-nonylphenyl ethers of polyethylene glycols corresponding to the formula $C_9H_{19}C_6H_4(OCH_2CH_2)_nOH$, in which the average value of n is about 9. Contains not less than 90.0% and not more than 110.0% of nonoxynol 9. Meets the requirements for Identification, Acid value (not more than 0.2), Water (not more than 0.5%), Polyethylene glycol (not more than 1.6%), Cloud point (52–56 °C), Free ethylene oxide (not more than 5 ppm), Dioxane, and Organic volatile impurities.
Nonoxynol 9 Vaginal Cream—Not in USP.
Nonoxynol 9 Vaginal Film—Not in USP.
Nonoxynol 9 Vaginal Foam—Not in USP.
Nonoxynol 9 Vaginal Gel—Not in USP.
Nonoxynol 9 Vaginal Jelly—Not in USP.
Nonoxynol 9 Vaginal Sponge—Not in USP.
Nonoxynol 9 Vaginal Suppositories—Not in USP.

NONOXYNOL 10

Chemical name: Poly(oxy-1,2-ethanediyl), alpha-(4-nonyl-phenyl)-omega-hydroxy-.

Description: Nonoxynol 10 NF—Colorless to light amber viscous liquid, having an aromatic odor.
NF category: Wetting and/or solubilizing agent.

Solubility: Nonoxynol 10 NF—Soluble in polar organic solvents and in water.

NF requirements: Nonoxynol 10 NF—Preserve in tight containers. An anhydrous liquid mixture consisting chiefly of monononylphenyl ethers of polyethylene glycols corresponding to the formula $C_9H_{19}C_6H_4(OCH_2CH_2)_nOH$, in which the average value of n is about 10. The labeling includes a cloud point range which is not greater than 6 °C and which is between 52 ° and 67 °C. Meets the requirements for Identification, Water (not more than 0.5%), Residue on ignition (not more than 0.4%), Arsenic (not more than 2 ppm), Heavy metals (not more than 0.002%), Hydroxyl value (81–97), Cloud point, and Organic volatile impurities.

NOREPINEPHRINE

Chemical group: A primary amine, differing from epinephrine by the absence of a methyl group on the nitrogen atom.

Chemical name: Norepinephrine bitartrate—1,2-Benzenediol, 4-(2-amino-1-hydroxyethyl)-, (*R*)-[*R*-(*R**,*R**)]-2,3-dihydroxy-butanedioate (1:1) (salt), monohydrate.

Molecular formula: Norepinephrine bitartrate—$C_8H_{11}NO_3 \cdot C_4H_6O_6 \cdot H_2O$.

Molecular weight: Norepinephrine bitartrate—337.28.

Description:
Norepinephrine Bitartrate USP—White or faintly gray, odorless, crystalline powder. Slowly darkens on exposure to air and light. Its solutions are acid to litmus, having a pH of about 3.5. Melts between 98 and 104 °C, without previous drying of the specimen, the melt being turbid.
Norepinephrine Bitartrate Injection USP— Colorless or practically colorless liquid, gradually turning dark on exposure to air and light.

Solubility: Norepinephrine Bitartrate USP—Freely soluble in water; slightly soluble in alcohol; practically insoluble in chloroform and in ether.

USP requirements:
Norepinephrine Bitartrate USP—Preserve in tight, light-resistant containers. Contains not less than 97.0% and not more than 102.0% of norepinephrine bitartrate, calculated on the anhydrous basis. Meets the requirements for Identification, Specific rotation (−10° to −12°, calculated on the anhydrous basis), Water (4.5–5.8%), Residue on ignition (negligible, from 200 mg), and Arterenone.
Norepinephrine Bitartrate Injection USP—Preserve in single-dose, light-resistant containers, preferably of Type I

glass. A sterile solution of Norepinephrine Bitartrate in Water for Injection. Label the Injection in terms of mg of norepinephrine per mL, and, where necessary, label it to indicate that it must be diluted prior to use. The label indicates that the Injection is not to be used if its color is pinkish or darker than slightly yellow or if it contains a precipitate. Contains an amount of norepinephrine bitartrate equivalent to the labeled amount of norepinephrine, within −10% to +15%. Meets the requirements for Color and clarity, Identification, Bacterial endotoxins, pH (3.0–4.5), Particulate matter, and Injections.

NORETHINDRONE

Chemical name:
Norethindrone—19-Norpregn-4-en-20-yn-3-one, 17-hydroxy-, (17 alpha)-.
Norethindrone acetate—19-Norpregn-4-en-20-yn-3-one, 17-(acetyloxy)-, (17 alpha).

Molecular formula:
Norethindrone—$C_{20}H_{26}O_2$.
Norethindrone acetate—$C_{22}H_{28}O_3$.

Molecular weight:
Norethindrone—298.43.
Norethindrone acetate—340.46.

Description:
Norethindrone USP—White to creamy white, odorless, crystalline powder. Is stable in air.
Norethindrone Acetate USP—White to creamy white, odorless, crystalline powder.

Solubility:
Norethindrone USP—Practically insoluble in water; soluble in chloroform and in dioxane; sparingly soluble in alcohol; slightly soluble in ether.
Norethindrone Acetate USP—Practically insoluble in water; very soluble in chloroform; freely soluble in dioxane; soluble in ether and in alcohol.

USP requirements:
Norethindrone USP—Preserve in well-closed containers. Contains not less than 97.0% and not more than 102.0% of norethindrone, calculated on the dried basis. Meets the requirements for Completeness of solution, Identification, Melting range (202–208 °C), Specific rotation (−30° to −38°), Loss on drying (not more than 0.5%), Chromatographic impurities, and Ethynyl group (8.18–8.43%).
Norethindrone Tablets USP—Preserve in well-closed containers. Contain the labeled amount, within ±10%. Meet the requirements for Identification, Disintegration (15 minutes, the use of disks being omitted), and Uniformity of dosage units.
Norethindrone Acetate USP—Preserve in well-closed containers. Contains not less than 97.0% and not more than 103.0% of norethindrone acetate, calculated on the dried basis. Meets the requirements for Completeness of solution, Identification, Specific rotation (−32° to −38°, calculated on the dried basis), Loss on drying (not more than 0.5%), Chromatographic impurities, and Ethynyl group (7.13–7.57%).
Norethindrone Acetate Tablets USP— Preserve in well-closed containers. Contain the labeled amount, within ±10%. Meet the requirements for Identification, Dissolution (70% in 60 minutes in dilute hydrochloric acid [1 in 100] containing 0.02% of sodium lauryl sulfate in Apparatus 1 at 100 rpm), and Uniformity of dosage units.

NORETHINDRONE AND ETHINYL ESTRADIOL

For *Norethindrone* and *Ethinyl Estradiol*—See individual listings for chemistry information.

USP requirements:
Norethindrone and Ethinyl Estradiol Tablets USP—Preserve in well-closed containers. Contain the labeled amounts of norethindrone and ethinyl estradiol, within ±10%. Meet the requirements for Identification, Dissolution (75% of each active ingredient in 60 minutes in 0.09% sodium lauryl sulfate in 0.1 *N* hydrochloric acid in Apparatus 2 at 75 rpm), and Uniformity of dosage units.
Norethindrone Acetate and Ethinyl Estradiol Tablets USP—Preserve in well-closed containers. Contain the labeled amount of norethindrone acetate, within ±10%, and the labeled amount of ethinyl estradiol, within ±12%. Meet the requirements for Identification, Disintegration (20 minutes, the use of disks being omitted), and Uniformity of dosage units.

NORETHINDRONE AND MESTRANOL

For *Norethindrone* and *Mestranol*—See individual listings for chemistry information.

USP requirements: Norethindrone and Mestranol Tablets USP—Preserve in well-closed containers. Contain the labeled amounts of norethindrone and mestranol, within ±10%. Meet the requirements for Identification, Dissolution (75% of each active ingredient in 60 minutes in 0.09% sodium lauryl sulfate in 0.1 *N* hydrochloric acid in Apparatus 2 at 75 rpm), and Uniformity of dosage units.

NORETHYNODREL

Chemical name: 19-Norpregn-5(10)-en-20-yn-3-one, 17-hydroxy-, (17 alpha)-.

Molecular formula: $C_{20}H_{26}O_2$.

Molecular weight: 298.43.

Description: Norethynodrel USP—White or practically white, odorless, crystalline powder. Melts at about 175 °C, over a range of about 3 C°. Is stable in air.

Solubility: Norethynodrel USP—Very slightly soluble in water and in solvent hexane; freely soluble in chloroform; soluble in acetone; sparingly soluble in alcohol.

USP requirements: Norethynodrel USP—Preserve in well-closed containers. Contains not less than 97.0% and not more than 101.0% of norethynodrel. Meets the requirements for Identification, Specific rotation (+119° to +125°), Ethynyl group (8.18–8.43%), Limit of norethindrone, Ordinary impurities, and Organic volatile impurities.

NORFLOXACIN

Chemical group: Fluoroquinolone derivative; structurally related to nalidixic acid.

Chemical name: 3-Quinolinecarboxylic acid, 1-ethyl-6-fluoro-1,4-dihydro-4-oxo-7-(1-piperazinyl)-.

Molecular formula: $C_{16}H_{18}FN_3O_3$.

Molecular weight: 319.34.

Description: Norfloxacin USP—White to pale yellow crystalline powder. Sensitive to light and moisture.

Solubility: Norfloxacin USP—Slightly soluble in acetone, in water, and in alcohol; freely soluble in acetic acid; sparingly soluble in chloroform; very slightly soluble in methanol and in ethyl acetate; insoluble in ether.

USP requirements:
Norfloxacin USP—Preserve in tight, light-resistant containers. Contains not less than 99.0% and not more than 101.0% of norfloxacin, calculated on the dried basis. Meets the requirements for Identification, Loss on drying (not more than 1.0%), Residue on ignition (not more than 0.1%, a platinum crucible being used), Heavy metals (not more than 0.0015%), and Chromatographic purity.
Norfloxacin Ophthalmic Solution—Not in USP.
Norfloxacin Tablets USP—Preserve in well-closed containers. Contain the labeled amount, within ±10%. Meet the requirements for Identification, Dissolution (80% in 30 minutes in pH 4.0 buffer in Apparatus 2 at 50 rpm), and Uniformity of dosage units.

NORGESTIMATE AND ETHINYL ESTRADIOL

Chemical name:
Norgestimate—18,19-Dinor-17-pregn-4-en-20-yn-3-one, 17-(acetyloxy)-13-ethyl-, oxime, (17 alpha)-(+)-.
Ethinyl estradiol—19-Norpregna-1,3,5(10)-trien-20-yne-3,17-diol, (17 alpha)-.

Molecular formula:
Norgestimate—$C_{23}H_{31}NO_3$.
Ethinyl estradiol—$C_{20}H_{24}O_2$.

Molecular weight:
Norgestimate—369.50.
Ethinyl estradiol—296.41.

Description:
Norgestimate—White to off-white fine granular powder. Melting and decomposition begin at 221 °C.
Ethinyl Estradiol USP—White to creamy white, odorless, crystalline powder.

Solubility:
Norgestimate—Insoluble in distilled water and in heptane; sparingly soluble in methanol, in ethanol, in octanol, and in acetonitrile; freely to very soluble in methylene chloride; slightly soluble in sesame oil.
Ethinyl Estradiol USP—Insoluble in water; soluble in alcohol, in chloroform, in ether, in vegetable oils, and in solutions of fixed alkali hydroxides.

USP requirements: Norgestimate and Ethinyl Estradiol Tablets—Not in USP.

NORGESTREL

Chemical name: 18,19-Dinorpregn-4-en-20-yn-3-one, 13-ethyl-17-hydroxy-, (17 alpha)-(±)-.

Molecular formula: $C_{21}H_{28}O_2$.

Molecular weight: 312.45.

Description: Norgestrel USP—White or practically white, practically odorless, crystalline powder.

Solubility: Norgestrel USP—Insoluble in water; freely soluble in chloroform; sparingly soluble in alcohol.

USP requirements:
Norgestrel USP—Preserve in well-closed containers. Contains not less than 98.0% and not more than 102.0% of norgestrel, calculated on the dried basis. Meets the requirements for Identification, Melting range (205–212 °C, the range between beginning and end of melting not more than 4 °C), Optical rotation (−0.1° to +0.1°), Loss on drying (not more than 0.5%), Residue on ignition (not more than 0.3%), Chromatographic impurities, and Ethynyl group (7.81–8.18%).
Norgestrel Tablets USP—Preserve in well-closed containers. Contain the labeled amount, within ±10%. Meet the requirements for Identification, Disintegration (15 minutes, the use of disks being omitted), and Uniformity of dosage units.

NORGESTREL AND ETHINYL ESTRADIOL

For *Norgestrel* and *Ethinyl Estradiol*—See individual listings for chemistry information.

USP requirements: Norgestrel and Ethinyl Estradiol Tablets USP—Preserve in well-closed containers. Contain the labeled amounts, within ±10%. Meet the requirements for Identification, Disintegration (15 minutes, the use of disks being omitted), and Uniformity of dosage units.

NORTRIPTYLINE

Chemical group: Dibenzocycloheptadiene.

Chemical name: Nortriptyline hydrochloride—1-Propanamine, 3-(10,11-dihydro-5*H*-dibenzo[*a,d*]cyclohepten-5-ylidene)-*N*-methyl-, hydrochloride.

Molecular formula: Nortriptyline hydrochloride—$C_{19}H_{21}N \cdot HCl$.

Molecular weight: Nortriptyline hydrochloride—299.84.

Description: Nortriptyline Hydrochloride USP—White to off-white powder, having a slight, characteristic odor. Its solution (1 in 100) has a pH of about 5.

pKa: Nortriptyline hydrochloride—9.73.

Solubility: Nortriptyline Hydrochloride USP—Soluble in water and in chloroform; sparingly soluble in methanol; practically insoluble in ether and in most other organic solvents.

USP requirements:
Nortriptyline Hydrochloride USP—Preserve in tight, light-resistant containers. Contains not less than 97.0% and not more than 101.5% of nortriptyline hydrochloride, calculated on the dried basis. Meets the requirements for Identification, Melting range (215–220 °C, the range between beginning and end of melting not more than 3 °C), Loss on drying (not more than 0.5%), Residue on ignition (not more than 0.1%), Heavy metals (not more than 0.001%), and Organic volatile impurities.
Nortriptyline Hydrochloride Capsules USP—Preserve in tight containers. Contain an amount of nortriptyline hydrochloride equivalent to the labeled amount of nortriptyline, within ±10%. Meet the requirements for Identification, Dissolution (70% in 30 minutes in water in Apparatus 1 at 100 rpm), and Uniformity of dosage units.
Nortriptyline Hydrochloride Oral Solution USP—Preserve in tight, light-resistant containers. Contains an amount of nortriptyline hydrochloride equivalent to the labeled amount of nortriptyline, within ±10%. Meets the requirements for Identification, pH (2.5–4.0), and Alcohol content (3.0–5.0%).

NOSCAPINE

Chemical name: 1(3*H*)-Isobenzofuranone, 6,7-dimethoxy-3-(5,6,7,8-tetrahydro-4-methoxy-6-methyl-1,3-dioxolo[4,5-*g*]isoquinolin-5-yl), [*S*-(*R**,*S**)]-.

Molecular formula: $C_{22}H_{23}NO_7$.

Molecular weight: 413.43.

Description: Noscapine USP—Fine, white or practically white, crystalline powder.

Solubility: Noscapine USP—Freely soluble in chloroform; soluble in acetone; slightly soluble in alcohol and in ether; practically insoluble in water.

USP requirements: Noscapine USP—Preserve in well-closed containers. Contains not less than 99.0% and not more than 100.5% of noscapine, calculated on the anhydrous basis. Meets the requirements for Identification, Melting range (174–176 °C), Specific rotation (+42° to +48°, calculated on the anhydrous basis), Water (not more than 1.0%), Residue on ignition (not more than 0.1%), Chloride (not more than 0.02%), Morphine, and Ordinary impurities.

NOVOBIOCIN

Chemical name:
Novobiocin calcium—Benzamide, *N*-[7-[[3-*O*-(aminocarbonyl)-6-deoxy-5-*C*-methyl-4-*O*-methyl-beta-L-*lyxo*-hexopyranosyl]oxy]-4-hydroxy-8-methyl-2-oxo-2*H*-1-benzopyran-3-yl]-4-hydroxy-3-(3-methyl-2-butenyl)-, calcium salt (2:1).
Novobiocin sodium—Benzamide, *N*-[7-[[3-*O*-(aminocarbonyl)-6-deoxy-5-*C*-methyl-4-*O*-methyl beta-L-*lyxo*-hexopyranosyl]oxy]-4-hydroxy-8-methyl-2-oxo-2*H*-1-benzopyran-3-yl]-4-hydroxy-3-(3-methyl-2-butenyl)-, monosodium salt.

Molecular formula:
Novobiocin calcium—$C_{62}H_{70}CaN_4O_{22}$.
Novobiocin sodium—$C_{31}H_{35}N_2NaO_{11}$.

Molecular weight:
Novobiocin calcium—1263.33.
Novobiocin sodium—634.62.

Description:
Novobiocin Calcium USP—White or yellowish-white, odorless, crystalline powder.
Novobiocin Sodium USP—White or yellowish-white, odorless, hygroscopic crystalline powder.

Solubility:
Novobiocin Calcium USP—Slightly soluble in water and in ether; freely soluble in alcohol and in methanol; sparingly soluble in acetone and in butyl acetate; very slightly soluble in chloroform.
Novobiocin Sodium USP—Freely soluble in water, in alcohol, in methanol, in glycerin, and in propylene glycol; slightly soluble in butyl acetate; practically insoluble in acetone, in chloroform, and in ether.

USP requirements:
Novobiocin Calcium USP—Preserve in tight containers. Has a potency equivalent to not less than 840 mcg of novobiocin per mg, calculated on the dried basis. Meets the requirements for Identification, Specific rotation (−50° to −58°, calculated on the dried basis), Crystallinity, pH (6.5–8.5, in a saturated aqueous suspension containing 25 mg per mL), and Loss on drying (not more than 10.0%).
Novobiocin Calcium Oral Suspension USP—Preserve in tight, light-resistant containers. It is prepared from Novobiocin Calcium or Novobiocin Sodium reacted with a suitable calcium salt, and it contains one or more suitable buffers, colors, diluents, flavors, and preservatives. Contains an amount of novobiocin calcium or novobiocin sodium equivalent to the labeled amount of novobiocin, within −10% to +20%. Meets the requirements for Identification, pH (6.0–7.5), Deliverable volume (multiple-unit containers), and Uniformity of dosage units (single-unit containers).
Novobiocin Sodium USP—Preserve in tight containers. Has a potency equivalent to not less than 850 mcg of novobiocin per mg, calculated on the dried basis. Meets the requirements for Identification, Specific rotation (−50° to −58°, calculated on the dried basis), Crystallinity, pH (6.5–8.5, in a solution containing 25 mg per mL), Loss on drying (not more than 6.0%), and Residue on ignition (10.5–12.0%).
Novobiocin Sodium Capsules USP—Preserve in tight, light-resistant containers. Contain an amount of novobiocin sodium equivalent to the labeled amount of novobiocin, within −10% to +20%. Meet the requirements for Identification and Loss on drying (not more than 6.0%).
Novobiocin Sodium Intramammary Infusion USP—Preserve in disposable syringes that are well-closed containers. A suspension of Novobiocin Sodium in a suitable vegetable oil vehicle. Contains suitable preservative and suspending agents. Label it to indicate that it is for veterinary use only. Contains an amount of novobiocin sodium equivalent to the labeled amount of novobiocin, within −10% to +25%. Meets the requirement for Water (not more than 1.0%).

NYLIDRIN

Chemical name: Nylidrin hydrochloride—Benzenemethanol, 4-hydroxy-alpha-[1-[(1-methyl-3-phenylpropyl)amino]ethyl]-, hydrochloride.

Molecular formula: Nylidrin hydrochloride—$C_{19}H_{25}NO_2 \cdot HCl$.

Molecular weight: Nylidrin hydrochloride—335.87.

Description: Nylidrin Hydrochloride USP—White, odorless, crystalline powder.

Solubility: Nylidrin Hydrochloride USP—Sparingly soluble in water and in alcohol; slightly soluble in chloroform and in ether.

USP requirements:
Nylidrin Hydrochloride USP—Preserve in tight containers. Contains not less than 98.0% and not more than 102.0% of nylidrin hydrochloride, calculated on the dried basis. Meets the requirements for Identification, pH (4.5–6.5, in a solution [1 in 100]), Loss on drying (not more than 0.5%), and Residue on ignition (not more than 0.5%).
Nylidrin Hydrochloride Injection USP—Preserve in single-dose or in multiple-dose containers, preferably of Type I glass. A sterile solution of Nylidrin Hydrochloride in Water for Injection. Contains the labeled amount, within ±5%. Meets the requirements for Identification and Injections.
Nylidrin Hydrochloride Tablets USP—Preserve in tight containers. Contain the labeled amount, within ±7%. Meet the requirements for Identification, Dissolution (75% in 30 minutes in water in Apparatus 1 at 100 rpm), and Uniformity of dosage units.

NYSTATIN

Source: Derived from *Streptomyces noursei*.

Chemical name: Nystatin.

Description: Nystatin USP—Yellow to light tan powder, having an odor suggestive of cereals. Is hygroscopic, and is affected by long exposure to light, heat, and air.

Solubility: Nystatin USP—Very slightly soluble in water; slightly to sparingly soluble in alcohol, in methanol, in *n*-propyl alcohol, and in *n*-butyl alcohol; insoluble in chloroform and in ether.

USP requirements:

Nystatin USP—Preserve in tight, light-resistant containers. A substance, or a mixture of two or more substances, produced by the growth of *Streptomyces noursei* Brown et al. (Fam. Streptomycetaceae). Where packaged for use in the extemporaneous preparation of oral suspensions, the label so states. Has a potency of not less than 4400 USP Nystatin Units per mg, or, where intended for use in the extemporaneous preparation of oral suspensions, not less than 5000 USP Nystatin Units per mg. Meets the requirements for Identification, Suspendibility (where packaged for use in the extemporaneous preparation of oral suspensions), Crystallinity, pH (6.5–8.0, in a 3% aqueous suspension), and Loss on drying (not more than 5.0%).

Nystatin Cream USP—Preserve in collapsible tubes, or in other tight containers, and avoid exposure to excessive heat. Contains the labeled amount of USP Nystatin Units, within −10% to +30%. Meets the requirement for Minimum fill.

Nystatin Vaginal Cream—Not in USP.

Nystatin Lotion USP—Preserve in tight containers, at controlled room temperature. Contains the labeled amount of USP Nystatin Units, within −10% to +40%. Meets the requirement for pH (5.5–7.5).

Nystatin Lozenges USP—Preserve in tight, light-resistant containers. Contain the labeled amount of USP Nystatin Units, within −10% to +25%. Meet the requirements for Disintegration (90 minutes, determined as set forth under Uncoated Tablets) and pH (5.0–7.5).

Nystatin Ointment USP—Preserve in well-closed containers, preferably at controlled room temperature. Contains the labeled amount of USP Nystatin Units, within −10% to +30%. Meets the requirements for Minimum fill and Water (not more than 0.5%).

Nystatin Topical Powder USP—Preserve in well-closed containers. A dry powder composed of Nystatin and Talc. Contains the labeled amount of USP Nystatin Units, within −10% to +30%. Meets the requirement for Loss on drying (not more than 2.0%).

Nystatin Vaginal Suppositories USP—Preserve in tight, light-resistant containers, at controlled room temperature. Contain the labeled amount of USP Nystatin Units, within −10% to +30%. Meet the requirement for Water (not more than 1.5%).

Nystatin Oral Suspension USP—Preserve in tight, light-resistant containers. Contains suitable dispersants, flavors, preservatives, and suspending agents. Contains the labeled amount of USP Nystatin Units, within −10% to +30%. Meets the requirements for pH (4.5–6.0; or 5.3–7.5 if it contains glycerin), Uniformity of dosage units (single-unit containers), and Deliverable volume (multiple-dose units).

Nystatin for Oral Suspension USP—Preserve in tight containers. A dry mixture of Nystatin with one or more suitable colors, diluents, suspending agents, flavors, and preservatives. Contains the labeled amount of USP Nystatin Units, within −10% to +40%. Meets the requirements for pH (4.9–5.5, in the suspension constituted as directed in the labeling) and Water (not more than 7.0%).

Nystatin Tablets USP—Preserve in tight, light-resistant containers. Label the Tablets to indicate that they are intended for oral use only (as distinguished from Vaginal Tablets). Contain the labeled amount of USP Nystatin Units, within −10% to +30%. Meet the requirements for Disintegration (120 minutes for plain-coated) and Loss on drying (not more than 5.0% for plain-coated; not more than 8.0% for film-coated).

Nystatin Vaginal Tablets USP—Preserve in tight, light-resistant containers and, where so specified in the labeling, in a refrigerator. Tablets composed of Nystatin with suitable binders, diluents and lubricants. Contain the labeled amount of USP Nystatin Units, within −10% to +40%. Meet the requirements for Disintegration (60 minutes) and Loss on drying (not more than 5.0%).

NYSTATIN AND CLIOQUINOL

For *Nystatin* and *Clioquinol*—See individual listings for chemistry information.

USP requirements: Nystatin and Clioquinol Ointment USP—Preserve in collapsible tubes or in tight, light-resistant containers, at controlled room temperature. Contains the labeled amount of USP Nystatin Units, within −10% to +40%, and the labeled amount of clioquinol, within ±10%. Meets the requirements for Identification, Minimum fill, and Water (not more than 0.5%).

NYSTATIN, NEOMYCIN, GRAMICIDIN, AND TRIAMCINOLONE

For *Nystatin, Neomycin, Gramicidin,* and *Triamcinolone*—See individual listings for chemistry information.

USP requirements:

Nystatin, Neomycin Sulfate, Gramicidin, and Triamcinolone Acetonide Cream USP—Preserve in tight containers. Contains amounts of nystatin, neomycin sulfate, and gramicidin equivalent to the labeled amounts of nystatin, neomycin, and gramicidin, within −10% to +40%, and the labeled amount of triamcinolone acetonide, within ±10%. Meets the requirements for Identification and Minimum fill.

Nystatin, Neomycin Sulfate, Gramicidin, and Triamcinolone Acetonide Ointment USP—Preserve in tight containers. Contains amounts of nystatin, neomycin sulfate, and gramicidin equivalent to the labeled amounts of nystatin, neomycin, and gramicidin, within −10% to +40%, and the labeled amount of triamcinolone acetonide, within ±10%. Meets the requirements for Identification, Water (not more than 0.5%), and Minimum fill.

NYSTATIN, NEOMYCIN, THIOSTREPTON, AND TRIAMCINOLONE

For *Nystatin, Neomycin, Thiostrepton,* and *Triamcinolone*—See individual listings for chemistry information.

USP requirements:

Nystatin, Neomycin Sulfate, Thiostrepton, and Triamcinolone Acetonide Cream USP—Preserve in tight containers. Label it to indicate that it is for veterinary use only. Contains the labeled amounts of nystatin and thiostrepton, within −10% to +30%, an amount of neomycin sulfate equivalent to the labeled amount of neomycin, within −10% to +30%, and the labeled amount of triamcinolone acetonide, within ±10%. Meets the requirements for Identification and Minimum fill.

Nystatin, Neomycin Sulfate, Thiostrepton, and Triamcinolone Acetonide Ointment USP—Preserve in tight containers. Label it to indicate that it is for veterinary use only. Contains the labeled amounts of nystatin and thiostrepton, within −10% to +30%, an amount of neomycin sulfate equivalent to the labeled amount of neomycin, within −10% to +30%, and the labeled amount of triamcinolone acetonide, within ±10%. Meets the requirements for Identification and Minimum fill.

NYSTATIN AND TRIAMCINOLONE

For *Nystatin* and *Triamcinolone*—See individual listings for chemistry information.

USP requirements:

Nystatin and Triamcinolone Acetonide Cream USP—Preserve in tight containers. Contains the labeled amount of

USP Nystatin Units, within −10% to +40%, and the labeled amount of triamcinolone acetonide, within ±10%. Meets the requirements for Identification and Minimum fill.

Nystatin and Triamcinolone Acetonide Ointment USP—Preserve in tight containers. Contains the labeled amount of USP Nystatin Units, within −10% to +40%, and the labeled amount of triamcinolone acetonide, within ±10%. Meets the requirements for Identification, Minimum fill, and Water (not more than 0.5%).

OCTOXYNOL 9

Chemical name: Poly(oxy-1,2-ethanediyl), alpha-(octylphenyl)-omega-hydroxy-.

Molecular formula: $C_{34}H_{62}O_{11}$ (average).

Molecular weight: 647.00 (average).

Description: Octoxynol 9 NF—Clear, pale yellow, viscous liquid, having a faint odor.

NF category: Wetting and/or solubilizing agent.

Solubility: Octoxynol 9 NF—Miscible with water, with alcohol, and with acetone; soluble in toluene; practically insoluble in solvent hexane.

USP requirements:
Octoxynol 9 Vaginal Cream—Not in USP.
Octoxynol 9 Vaginal Jelly—Not in USP.

NF requirements: Octoxynol 9 NF—Preserve in tight containers. An anhydrous liquid mixture consisting chiefly of monooctylphenyl ethers of polyethylene glycols, corresponding to the formula $C_8H_{17}C_6H_4(OCH_2CH_2)_nOH$, in which the average value of n is 9. Meets the requirements for Identification, Water (not more than 0.5%), Residue on ignition (not more than 0.4%), Arsenic (not more than 2 ppm), Heavy metals (not more than 0.002%), Hydroxyl value (85–101), Cloud point (63–69 °C), Free ethylene oxide (not more than 5 ppm), and Dioxane.

OCTREOTIDE

Source: Synthetic octapeptide analog of somatostatin.

Chemical name: Octreotide acetate—L-Cysteinamide, D-phenylalanyl-L-cysteinyl-L-phenylalanyl-D-tryptophyl-L-lysyl-L-threonyl-*N*-[2-hydroxy-1-(hydroxymethyl)propyl]-, cyclic (2→7)-disulfide, [*R*-(*R**,*R**)]-, acetate (salt).

Molecular formula: Octreotide acetate—$C_{49}H_{66}N_{10}O_{10}S_2 \cdot xC_2H_4O_2$.

Description: Octreotide acetate injection—Clear sterile solution.

USP requirements: Octreotide Acetate Injection—Not in USP.

OCTYLDODECANOL

Molecular formula: $C_{20}H_{42}O$.

Molecular weight: 298.55.

Description: Octyldodecanol NF—Clear, water-white, free-flowing liquid.

NF category: Oleaginous vehicle.

Solubility: Octyldodecanol NF—Insoluble in water; soluble in alcohol and in ether.

NF requirements: Octyldodecanol NF—Preserve in tight containers. Contains not less than 90.0% of 2-octyldodecanol, the remainder consisting chiefly of related alcohols. Meets the requirements for Identification, Acid value (not more than 0.5), Iodine value (not more than 8), Hydroxyl value (175–190), Saponification value (not more than 5), and Organic volatile impurities.

OFLOXACIN

Chemical name: 7*H*-Pyrido[1,2,3-*de*]-1,4-benzoxazine-6-carboxylic acid, 9-fluoro-2,3-dihydro-3-methyl-10-(4-methyl-1-piperazinyl)-7-oxo-, (±)-.

Molecular formula: $C_{18}H_{20}FN_3O_4$.

Molecular weight: 361.37.

Description: Cream to pale yellow crystalline powder.

Solubility: At room temperature, aqueous solubility 60 mg/mL at pH 2–5, 4 mg/mL at pH 7, and 303 mg/mL at pH 9.8.

USP requirements:
Ofloxacin Injection—Not in USP.
Ofloxacin Ophthalmic Solution—Not in USP.
Ofloxacin Tablets—Not in USP.

OFLOXACIN AND DEXTROSE

For *Ofloxacin* and *Dextrose*—See individual listings for chemistry information.

USP requirements: Ofloxacin in Dextrose Injection—Not in USP.

BLAND LUBRICATING OPHTHALMIC OINTMENT

USP requirements: Bland Lubricating Ophthalmic Ointment USP—Preserve in suitable collapsible ophthalmic ointment tubes. A sterile ointment of white petrolatum and mineral oil. May contain Lanolin, Modified Lanolin, or Lanolin Alcohols. Meets the requirements for Appearance, Color, Sterility, Homogeneity, Acidity or alkalinity, and Metal particles.

HYDROPHILIC OINTMENT

Description: Hydrophilic Ointment USP—NF category: Ointment base.

USP requirements: Hydrophilic Ointment USP—Preserve in tight containers.

Prepare Hydrophilic Ointment as follows: 0.25 gram of Methylparaben, 0.15 gram of Propylparaben, 10 grams of Sodium Lauryl Sulfate, 120 grams of Propylene Glycol, 250 grams of Stearyl Alcohol, 250 grams of White Petrolatum, and 370 grams of Purified Water, to make about 1000 grams. Melt the Stearyl Alcohol and the White Petrolatum on a steam bath, and warm to about 75 °C. Add the other ingredients, previously dissolved in the water and warmed to 75 °C, and stir the mixture until it congeals.

WHITE OINTMENT

Description: White Ointment USP—NF category: Ointment base.

USP requirements: White Ointment USP—Preserve in well-closed containers.

Prepare White Ointment as follows: 50 grams of White Wax and 950 grams of White Petrolatum, to make 1000 grams. Melt the White Wax in a suitable dish on a water bath, add the White Petrolatum, warm until liquefied, then discontinue the heating, and stir the mixture until it begins to congeal.

YELLOW OINTMENT

Description: Yellow Ointment USP—NF category: Ointment base.

USP requirements: Yellow Ointment USP—Preserve in well-closed containers.

Prepare Yellow Ointment as follows: 50 grams of Yellow Wax and 950 grams of Petrolatum, to make 1000 grams. Melt the Yellow Wax in a suitable dish on a steam bath, add the Petrolatum, warm until liquefied, then discontinue the heating, and stir the mixture until it begins to congeal.

OLEIC ACID

Chemical name: 9-Octadecenoic acid, (*Z*)-.

Molecular formula: $C_{18}H_{34}O_2$.

Molecular weight: 282.47.

Description: Oleic Acid NF—Colorless to pale yellow, oily liquid when freshly prepared, but on exposure to air it gradually absorbs oxygen and darkens. It has a characteristic, lard-like odor. When strongly heated in air, it is decomposed with the production of acrid vapors.

NF category: Emulsifying and/or solubilizing agent.

Solubility: Oleic Acid NF—Practically insoluble in water. Miscible with alcohol, with chloroform, with ether, and with fixed and volatile oils.

NF requirements: Oleic Acid NF—Preserve in tight containers. It is manufactured from fats and oils derived from edible sources, and consists chiefly of (*Z*)-9-octadecenoic acid [$CH_3(CH_2)_7CH{:}CH(CH_2)_7COOH$]. If it is for external use only, the labeling so indicates. Meets the requirements for Specific gravity (0.889–0.895), Congealing temperature (not above 10 °C), Residue on ignition (not more than 0.01% [about]), Mineral acids, Neutral fat or mineral oil, Acid value (196–204), and Iodine value (85–95).

Note: Oleic Acid labeled solely for external use is exempt from the requirement that it be prepared from edible sources.

OLEOVITAMIN A AND D

Description:

Oleovitamin A and D USP—Yellow to red, oily liquid, practically odorless or having a fish-like odor, and having no rancid odor. It is a clear liquid at temperatures exceeding 65 °C, and may crystallize on cooling. Unstable in air and in light.

Oleovitamin A and D Capsules USP—The oil contained in Oleovitamin A and D Capsules is a yellow to red, oily liquid, practically odorless or having a fish-like odor, and having no rancid odor. Is a clear liquid at temperatures exceeding 65 °C, and may crystallize on cooling. Is unstable in air and in light.

Solubility: Oleovitamin A and D USP—Insoluble in water and in glycerin; very soluble in ether and in chloroform; soluble in dehydrated alcohol and in vegetable oils.

USP requirements:

Oleovitamin A and D USP—Preserve in tight containers, protected from light and air, preferably under an atmosphere of an inert gas. Store in a dry place. A solution of vitamin A and vitamin D in fish liver oil or in an edible vegetable oil. The vitamin D is present as ergocalciferol or cholecalciferol obtained by the activation of ergosterol or 7-dehydrocholesterol or from natural sources. Label it to indicate the content of vitamin A in mg per gram. The vitamin A content may also be expressed in USP Vitamin A Units per gram. Label it to show whether it contains ergocalciferol, cholecalciferol, or vitamin D from a natural source. Label it to indicate also the vitamin D content in mcg per gram. Its vitamin D content may be expressed also in USP Vitamin D Units per gram. Contains not less than 90.0% of the labeled amounts of vitamins A and D. Meets the requirement for Organic volatile impurities.

Oleovitamin A and D Capsules USP—Preserve in tight, light-resistant containers. Store in a dry place. Label the Capsules to indicate the content, in mg, of vitamin A in each capsule. The vitamin A content in each capsule may be expressed also in USP Vitamin A Units. Label the Capsules to show whether they contain ergocalciferol, cholecalciferol, or vitamin D from a natural source. Label the Capsules to indicate also the vitamin D content, in mcg, in each capsule. The vitamin D content may be expressed also in USP Vitamin D Units in each capsule. Contain the labeled amounts of vitamins A and D, within −10%. The oil in Oleovitamin A and D Capsules conforms to the definition for Oleovitamin A and D.

OLEYL ALCOHOL

Chemical name: 9-Octadecen-1-ol, (*Z*)-.

Molecular formula: $C_{18}H_{36}O$.

Molecular weight: 268.48.

Description: Oleyl Alcohol NF—Clear, colorless to light yellow, oily liquid. Has a faint characteristic odor.

NF category: Emulsifying and/or solubilizing agent (stabilizer).

Solubility: Oleyl Alcohol NF—Insoluble in water; soluble in alcohol, in ether, in isopropyl alcohol, and in light mineral oil.

NF requirements: Oleyl Alcohol NF—Preserve in well-filled, tight containers, and store at controlled room temperature. A mixture of unsaturated and saturated high molecular weight fatty alcohols consisting chiefly of oleyl alcohol. Meets the requirements for Cloud point (not above 10 °C), Refractive index (1.458–1.460), Acid value (not more than 1), Hydroxyl value (205–215), and Iodine value (85–95).

OLIVE OIL

Description: Olive Oil NF—Pale yellow, or light greenish yellow, oily liquid, having a slight characteristic odor.

NF category: Oleaginous vehicle.

Solubility: Olive Oil NF—Slightly soluble in alcohol. Miscible with ether, with chloroform, and with carbon disulfide.

NF requirements: Olive Oil NF—Preserve in tight containers and prevent exposure to excessive heat. The fixed oil obtained from the ripe fruit of *Olea europaea* Linné (Fam. Oleaceae). Meets the requirements for Specific gravity (0.910–0.915), Heavy metals (not more than 0.001%), Cottonseed oil, Peanut oil, Sesame oil, Teaseed oil, Solidification range of fatty acids (17–26 °C), Free fatty acids, Iodine value (79–88), and Saponification value (190–195).

OLSALAZINE

Chemical name: Olsalazine sodium—Benzoic acid, 3,3′-azobis[6-hydroxy-, disodium salt.

Molecular formula: Olsalazine sodium—$C_{14}H_8N_2Na_2O_6$.

Molecular weight: Olsalazine sodium—346.21.

Description: Olsalazine sodium—Yellow crystalline powder; melts with decomposition at 240 °C.

Solubility: Olsalazine sodium—Soluble in water and in dimethyl sulfoxide; practically insoluble in ethanol, in chloroform, and in ether.

USP requirements: Olsalazine Sodium Capsules—Not in USP.

OMEPRAZOLE

Chemical group: Substituted benzimidazole.

Chemical name: 1*H*-Benzimidazole, 5-methoxy-2-[[(4-methoxy-3,5-dimethyl-2-pyridinyl) methyl]sulfinyl]-.

Molecular formula: $C_{17}H_{19}N_3O_3S$.

Molecular weight: 345.42.

Description: White to off-white crystalline powder.

pKa: 4 and 8.8.

Solubility: Freely soluble in ethanol and in methanol; slightly soluble in acetone and in isopropanol; very slightly soluble in water.

Other characteristics: The stability of omeprazole is a function of pH; omeprazole is rapidly degraded in acid media, but has acceptable stability under alkaline conditions.

USP requirements: Omeprazole Delayed-release Capsules—Not in USP.

ONDANSETRON

Chemical name: Ondansetron hydrochloride—4*H*-Carbazol-4-one, 1,2,3,9-tetrahydro-9-methyl-3-[(2-methyl-1*H*-imidazol-1-yl)methyl]-, monohydrochloride, (±)-, dihydrate.

Molecular formula: Ondansetron hydrochloride—$C_{18}H_{19}N_3O \cdot HCl \cdot 2H_2O$.

Molecular weight: Ondansetron hydrochloride—365.86.

Description: Ondansetron hydrochloride—White to off-white powder.

Solubility: Ondansetron hydrochloride—Soluble in water and in normal saline.

USP requirements:
Ondansetron Hydrochloride Injection—Not in USP.
Ondansetron Hydrochloride Tablets—Not in USP.

OPIUM

Description:
Opium USP—Has a very characteristic odor.
Powdered Opium USP—Light brown or moderately yellowish brown powder.

USP requirements:
Opium USP—The air-dried milky exudate obtained by incising the unripe capsules of *Papaver somniferum* Linné or its variety *album* De Candolle (Fam. Papaveraceae). Yields not less than 9.5% of anhydrous morphine. Meets the requirement for Botanic characteristics.

Powdered Opium USP—Preserve in well-closed containers. It is Opium dried at a temperature not exceeding 70 °C, and reduced to a very fine powder. Yields not less than 10.0% and not more than 10.5% of anhydrous morphine. Meets the requirement for Botanic characteristics.

Opium Tincture USP (Laudanum)—Preserve in tight, light-resistant containers, and avoid exposure to direct sunlight and to excessive heat. Contains, in each 100 mL, not less than 0.90 gram and not more than 1.10 grams of anhydrous morphine.

Opium Tincture may be prepared as follows: Place 100 grams of granulated or sliced Opium in a suitable vessel. (Note: Do not use Powdered Opium.) Add 500 mL of boiling water, and allow to stand, with frequent stirring, for 24 hours. Transfer the mixture to a percolator, allow it to drain, percolate with water as the menstruum to complete extraction, and evaporate the percolate to a volume of 400 mL. Boil actively for not less than 15 minutes, and allow to stand overnight. Heat the mixture to 80 °C, add 50 grams of paraffin, and heat until the paraffin is melted. Beat the mixture thoroughly, and cool. Remove the paraffin, and filter the concentrate, washing the paraffin and the filter with sufficient water to make the filtrate measure 750 mL. Add 188 mL of alcohol to the filtrate, mix, and assay a 10-mL portion of the resulting solution as directed. Dilute the remaining solution with a mixture of 1 volume of alcohol and 4 volumes of water to obtain a Tincture containing 1 gram of anhydrous morphine in each 100 mL. Mix.

Meets the requirement for Alcohol content (17.0–21.0%).

Opium Alkaloids Hydrochlorides Injection—Not in USP.

ORANGE FLOWER OIL

Description: Orange Flower Oil NF—Pale yellow, slightly fluorescent liquid, which becomes reddish brown on exposure to light and air. Has a distinctive, fragrant odor, similar to that of orange blossoms. May become turbid or solid at low temperatures. Neutral to litmus.

NF category: Flavors and perfumes.

NF requirements: Orange Flower Oil NF—Preserve in tight, light-resistant containers. The volatile oil distilled from the fresh flowers of *Citrus aurantium* Linné (Fam. Rutaceae). Meets the requirements for Solubility in alcohol (miscible with an equal volume of alcohol and with about 2 volumes of 80% alcohol, the solution becoming cloudy on the further addition of 80% alcohol), Identification, Specific gravity (0.863–0.880), Angular rotation (+1.5° to +9.1°, in a 100-mm tube), and Heavy metals (not more than 0.004%).

ORPHENADRINE

Chemical name:
Orphenadrine citrate—Ethanamine, *N,N*-dimethyl-2-[(2-methylphenyl)phenylmethoxy]-, 2-hydroxy-1,2,3-propanetricarboxylate (1:1).
Orphenadrine hydrochloride—2-Dimethylaminoethyl 2-methylbenzhydryl ether hydrochloride.

Molecular formula:
Orphenadrine citrate—$C_{18}H_{23}NO \cdot C_6H_8O_7$.
Orphenadrine hydrochloride—$C_{18}H_{23}NO \cdot HCl$.

Molecular weight:
Orphenadrine citrate—461.51.
Orphenadrine hydrochloride—305.83.

Description:
Orphenadrine Citrate USP—White, practically odorless, crystalline powder.
Orphenadrine hydrochloride—White or almost white, odorless or almost odorless, crystalline powder.

Solubility:

Orphenadrine Citrate USP—Sparingly soluble in water; slightly soluble in alcohol; insoluble in chloroform and in ether.

Orphenadrine hydrochloride—Soluble 1 in 1 of water and of alcohol and 1 in 2 of chloroform; practically insoluble in ether.

USP requirements:

Orphenadrine Citrate USP—Preserve in tight, light-resistant containers. Contains not less than 98.0% and not more than 101.5% of orphenadrine citrate, calculated on the dried basis. Meets the requirements for Clarity and color of solution, Identification, Melting range (134–138 °C), Loss on drying (not more than 0.5%), Residue on ignition (not more than 0.1%), Chromatographic purity, Isomer content (not more than 3.0%), and Organic volatile impurities.

Orphenadrine Citrate Injection USP—Preserve in single-dose or in multiple-dose containers, preferably of Type I glass, protected from light. A sterile solution of Orphenadrine Citrate in Water for Injection, prepared with the aid of Sodium Hydroxide. Contains the labeled amount, within ±7%. Meets the requirements for Identification, Bacterial endotoxins, pH (5.0–6.0), and Injections.

Orphenadrine Citrate Extended-release Tablets—Not in USP.

Orphenadrine Hydrochloride Tablets—Not in USP.

ORPHENADRINE, ASPIRIN, AND CAFFEINE

For *Orphenadrine, Aspirin,* and *Caffeine*—See individual listings for chemistry information.

USP requirements: Orphenadrine Citrate, Aspirin, and Caffeine Tablets—Not in USP.

OXACILLIN

Chemical name: Oxacillin sodium—4-Thia-1-azabicyclo[3.2.0]-heptane-2-carboxylic acid, 3,3-dimethyl-6-[[(5-methyl-3-phenyl-4-isoxazolyl)carbonyl]amino]-7-oxo-, monosodium salt, monohydrate, [2*S*-(2 alpha,5 alpha,6 beta)]-.

Molecular formula: Oxacillin sodium—$C_{19}H_{18}N_3NaO_5S \cdot H_2O$.

Molecular weight: Oxacillin sodium—441.43.

Description:

Oxacillin Sodium USP—Fine, white, crystalline powder, odorless or having a slight odor.

Oxacillin Sodium for Injection USP—Fine, white, crystalline powder, odorless or having a slight odor.

Solubility:

Oxacillin Sodium USP—Freely soluble in water, in methanol, and in dimethylsulfoxide; slightly soluble in absolute alcohol, in chloroform, in pyridine, and in methyl acetate; insoluble in ethyl acetate, in ether, and in ethylene chloride.

Oxacillin Sodium for Injection USP—Freely soluble in water, in methanol, and in dimethylsulfoxide; slightly soluble in absolute alcohol, in chloroform, in pyridine, and in methyl acetate; insoluble in ethyl acetate, in ether, and in ethylene chloride.

USP requirements:

Oxacillin Sodium USP—Preserve in tight containers, at controlled room temperature. Contains the equivalent of not less than 815 mcg and not more than 950 mcg of oxacillin per mg. Meets the requirements for Identification, Crystallinity, pH (4.5–7.5, in a solution containing 30 mg per mL), and Water (3.5–5.0%).

Oxacillin Sodium Capsules USP—Preserve in tight containers, at controlled room temperature. Contain an amount of oxacillin sodium equivalent to the labeled amount of oxacillin, within −10% to +20%. Meet the requirements for Identification, Dissolution (75% in 45 minutes in water in Apparatus 1 at 100 rpm), Uniformity of dosage units, and Water (not more than 6.0%).

Oxacillin Sodium Injection USP—Preserve in Containers for Injections. Maintain in the frozen state. A sterile isoosmotic solution of Oxacillin Sodium in Water for Injection. Contains dextrose as a tonicity-adjusting agent and one or more suitable buffer substances. Contains no preservatives. The label states that it is to be thawed just prior to use, describes conditions for proper storage of the resultant solution, and directs that the solution is not to be refrozen. Contains an amount of oxacillin sodium equivalent to the labeled amount of oxacillin, within −10% to +15%. Meets the requirements for Identification, Pyrogen, Sterility, pH (6.0–8.5), Particulate matter, and Labeling under Injections.

Oxacillin Sodium for Injection USP—Preserve in Containers for Sterile Solids, at controlled room temperature. A sterile, dry mixture of Oxacillin Sodium and one or more suitable buffers. Contains an amount of oxacillin sodium equivalent to the labeled amount of oxacillin, within −10% to +15%. Meets the requirements for Constituted solution, Identification, Bacterial endotoxins, Sterility, Uniformity of dosage units, pH (6.0–8.5, in a solution containing 30 mg per mL), Water (not more than 6.0%), and Particulate matter.

Oxacillin Sodium for Oral Solution USP—Preserve in tight containers, at controlled room temperature. Contains one or more suitable buffers, colors, flavors, preservatives, and stabilizers. Contains an amount of oxacillin sodium equivalent to the labeled amount of oxacillin, within −10% to +20%. Meets the requirements for Identification, pH (5.0–7.5, in the solution constituted as directed in the labeling), Water (not more than 1.0%), Uniformity of dosage units (single-unit containers), and Deliverable volume (multiple-unit containers).

Sterile Oxacillin Sodium USP—Preserve in Containers for Sterile Solids. It is Oxacillin Sodium suitable for parenteral use. Contains an amount of oxacillin sodium equivalent to not less than 815 mcg and not more than 950 mcg of oxacillin per mg. Meets the requirements for Bacterial endotoxins and Sterility, and for Identification tests, pH, Water, and Crystallinity under Oxacillin Sodium.

OXAMNIQUINE

Chemical group: Tetrahydroquinoline derivative.

Chemical name: 6-Quinolinemethanol, 1,2,3,4-tetrahydro-2-[[(1-methylethyl)amino]methyl]-7-nitro-.

Molecular formula: $C_{14}H_{21}N_3O_3$.

Molecular weight: 279.34.

Description: Oxamniquine USP—Yellow-orange crystalline solid.

Solubility: Oxamniquine USP—Sparingly soluble in water; soluble in methanol, in chloroform, and in acetone.

USP requirements:

Oxamniquine USP—Preserve in well-closed containers. Contains not less than 97.0% and not more than 103.0% of oxamniquine, calculated on the anhydrous basis. Meets the requirements for Identification, Melting range (145–152 °C), Specific rotation (−4° to +4°), pH (8.0–10.0 in a suspension [1 in 100]), Water (not more than 1.0%),

Residue on ignition (not more than 0.2%, determined on a 2.0-gram test specimen), Iron (not more than 0.005%), Alcohol, Methyl isobutyl ketone, Heavy metals (not more than 0.005%), and Related compounds.

Oxamniquine Capsules USP—Preserve in tight containers. Contain the labeled amount, within ±10%. Meet the requirements for Identification, Dissolution (70% in 60 minutes in 0.1 *N* hydrochloric acid in Apparatus 2 at 50 rpm), and Uniformity of dosage units.

OXANDROLONE

Chemical group: 17-alpha alkylated anabolic steroid.

Chemical name: 2-Oxaandrostan-3-one, 17-hydroxy-17-methyl-, (5 alpha,17 beta)-.

Molecular formula: $C_{19}H_{30}O_3$.

Molecular weight: 306.45.

Description: Oxandrolone USP—White, odorless, crystalline powder. Is stable in air, but darkens on exposure to light. Melts at about 225 °C.

Solubility: Oxandrolone USP—Practically insoluble in water; freely soluble in chloroform; sparingly soluble in alcohol and in acetone.

USP requirements:

Oxandrolone USP—Preserve in well-closed, light-resistant containers. Contains not less than 97.0% and not more than 100.5% of oxandrolone, calculated on the dried basis. Meets the requirements for Identification, Specific rotation (−18° to −24°, calculated on the dried basis), Loss on drying (not more than 1.0%), Residue on ignition (not more than 0.2%), Ordinary impurities, and Organic volatile impurities.

Oxandrolone Tablets USP—Preserve in tight, light-resistant containers. Contain the labeled amount, within ±8%. Meet the requirements for Identification, Disintegration (15 minutes), and Uniformity of dosage units.

OXAPROZIN

Chemical name: 2-Oxazolepropanoic acid, 4,5-diphenyl-.

Molecular formula: $C_{18}H_{15}NO_3$.

Molecular weight: 293.32.

Description: White to off-white powder with a slight odor and a melting point of 162–163 °C.

pKa: 4.3 in water.

Solubility: Slightly soluble in alcohol; insoluble in water.

Other characteristics: Octanol/water partition coefficient—4.8 at physiologic pH (7.4).

USP requirements: Oxaprozin Tablets—Not in USP.

OXAZEPAM

Chemical name: 2*H*-1,4-Benzodiazepin-2-one, 7-chloro-1,3-dihydro-3-hydroxy-5-phenyl-.

Molecular formula: $C_{15}H_{11}ClN_2O_2$.

Molecular weight: 286.72.

Description: Oxazepam USP—Creamy white to pale yellow powder. Is practically odorless.

Solubility: Oxazepam USP—Practically insoluble in water; slightly soluble in alcohol and in chloroform; very slightly soluble in ether.

USP requirements:

Oxazepam USP—Preserve in well-closed containers. Contains not less than 98.0% and not more than 102.0% of oxazepam, calculated on the dried basis. Meets the requirements for Identification, pH (4.8–7.0, in an aqueous suspension [1 in 50]), Loss on drying (not more than 2.0%), Residue on ignition (not more than 0.3%), and Organic volatile impurities.

Oxazepam Capsules USP—Preserve in well-closed containers. Contain the labeled amount, within ±10%. Meet the requirements for Identification, Dissolution (75% in 60 minutes in 0.1 *N* hydrochloric acid in Apparatus 2 at 75 rpm), and Uniformity of dosage units.

Oxazepam Tablets USP—Preserve in well-closed containers. Contain the labeled amount, within ±10%. Meet the requirements for Identification, Dissolution (80% in 60 minutes in 0.1 *N* hydrochloric acid in Apparatus 2 at 50 rpm), and Uniformity of dosage units.

OXICONAZOLE

Chemical name: Oxiconazole nitrate—Ethanone, 1-(2,4-dichlorophenyl)-2-(1*H*-imidazol-1-yl)-, *O*-[(2,4-dichlorophenyl)-methyl]oxime, (*Z*)-, mononitrate.

Molecular formula: Oxiconazole nitrate—$C_{18}H_{13}Cl_4N_3O \cdot HNO_3$.

Molecular weight: Oxiconazole nitrate—492.15.

Description: Oxiconazole nitrate—Nearly white crystalline powder.

Solubility: Oxiconazole nitrate—Soluble in methanol; sparingly soluble in ethanol, in chloroform, and in acetone; very slightly soluble in water.

USP requirements:

Oxiconazole Nitrate Cream—Not in USP.

Oxiconazole Nitrate Lotion—Not in USP.

OXPRENOLOL

Chemical name: Oxprenolol hydrochloride—2-Propanol, 1-(*o*-allyloxyphenoxy)-3-isopropylamino-, hydrochloride.

Molecular formula: Oxprenolol hydrochloride—$C_{15}H_{23}NO_3 \cdot HCl$.

Molecular weight: Oxprenolol hydrochloride—301.82.

Description: Oxprenolol Hydrochloride USP—White, crystalline powder.

Solubility: Oxprenolol Hydrochloride USP—Freely soluble in alcohol, in chloroform, and in water; sparingly soluble in acetone; practically insoluble in ether.

Other characteristics: Lipid solubility—Moderate.

USP requirements:

Oxprenolol Hydrochloride USP—Preserve in well-closed containers. Contains not less than 98.5% and not more than 101.0% of oxprenolol hydrochloride, calculated on the dried basis. Meets the requirements for Clarity of solution, Identification, pH (4.0–6.0, in a solution [1 in 10]), Loss on drying (not more than 0.5%), Residue on ignition (not more than 0.1%), Heavy metals (not more than 0.001%), Chromatographic purity, and Organic volatile impurities.

Oxprenolol Hydrochloride Tablets USP—Preserve in well-closed, light-resistant containers. Contain the labeled amount, within ±10%. Meet the requirements for Identification, Dissolution (80% in 30 minutes in 0.1 *N* hydrochloric acid in Apparatus 1 at 100 rpm), and Uniformity of dosage units.

Oxprenolol Hydrochloride Extended-release Tablets USP—Preserve in well-closed, light-resistant containers. Contain the labeled amount, within ±10%. Meet the requirements for Identification, Drug release (15–45% in 1 hour in 0.1 *N* hydrochloric acid, 30–60% in 1 hour in Dissolution medium, 50–80% in 3 hours in Dissolution medium, and not less than 75% in 7 hours in Dissolution medium, in Apparatus 1 at 100 rpm, the Dissolution medium being simulated intestinal fluid TS without enzyme), and Uniformity of dosage units.

OXTRIPHYLLINE

Source: The choline salt of theophylline.

Chemical name: Ethanaminium, 2-hydroxy-*N,N,N*-trimethyl-, salt with 3,7-dihydro-1,3-dimethyl-1*H*-purine-2,6-dione.

Molecular formula: $C_{12}H_{21}N_5O_3$.

Molecular weight: 283.33.

Description: Oxtriphylline USP—White, crystalline powder, having an amine-like odor. A solution (1 in 100) has a pH of about 10.3.

Solubility: Oxtriphylline USP—Freely soluble in water and in alcohol; very slightly soluble in chloroform.

USP requirements:

Oxtriphylline USP—Preserve in tight containers. Contains not less than 61.7% and not more than 65.5% of anhydrous theophylline, calculated on the dried basis. Meets the requirements for Identification, Melting range (185–189 °C), Loss on drying (not more than 1.0%), Residue on ignition (not more than 0.3%), Chloride (not more than 0.02%), Ordinary impurities, Choline content, and Organic volatile impurities.

Oxtriphylline Oral Solution USP—Preserve in tight containers. Label Oral Solution to state both the content of oxtriphylline and the content of anhydrous theophylline. Contains an amount of oxtriphylline equivalent to the labeled amount of anhydrous theophylline, within ±10%. Meets the requirements for Identification, pH (6.4–9.0), and Alcohol content (if present, within −10% to +15% of labeled amount, the labeled amount being not more than 20.0%).

Oxtriphylline Syrup—Not in USP.

Oxtriphylline Tablets—Not in USP.

Oxtriphylline Delayed-release Tablets USP—Preserve in tight containers. Label Delayed-release Tablets to state both the content of oxtriphylline and the content of anhydrous theophylline. The label indicates that Oxtriphylline Delayed-release Tablets are enteric-coated. Contain an amount of oxtriphylline equivalent to the labeled amount of anhydrous theophylline, within ±10%. Meet the requirements for Identification, Disintegration, and Uniformity of dosage units.

Oxtriphylline Extended-release Tablets USP—Preserve in tight containers. Label Extended-release Tablets to state both the content of oxtriphylline and the content of anhydrous theophylline. Contain an amount of oxtriphylline equivalent to the labeled amount of anhydrous theophylline, within ±10%. Meet the requirements for Identification and Uniformity of dosage units.

OXTRIPHYLLINE AND GUAIFENESIN

For *Oxtriphylline* and *Guaifenesin*—See individual listings for chemistry information.

USP requirements:

Oxtriphylline and Guaifenesin Elixir—Not in USP.

Oxtriphylline and Guaifenesin Tablets—Not in USP.

OXYBENZONE

Chemical name: Methanone, (2-hydroxy-4-methoxyphenyl)-phenyl-.

Molecular formula: $C_{14}H_{12}O_3$.

Molecular weight: 228.25.

Description: Oxybenzone USP—Pale yellow powder.

Solubility: Oxybenzone USP—Practically insoluble in water; freely soluble in alcohol and in toluene.

USP requirements: Oxybenzone USP—Preserve in tight, light-resistant containers. Contains not less than 97.0% and not more than 103.0% of oxybenzone, calculated on the dried basis. Meets the requirements for Identification, Congealing temperature (not lower than 62.0 °C), and Loss on drying (not more than 2.0%).

OXYBUTYNIN

Chemical group: Synthetic tertiary amine.

Chemical name: Oxybutynin chloride—Benzeneacetic acid, alpha-cyclohexyl-alpha-hydroxy-, 4-(diethylamino)-2-butynyl ester hydrochloride.

Molecular formula: Oxybutynin chloride—$C_{22}H_{31}NO_3 \cdot HCl$.

Molecular weight: Oxybutynin chloride—393.95.

Description: Oxybutynin Chloride USP—White, crystalline, practically odorless powder.

pKa: Oxybutynin chloride—6.96.

Solubility: Oxybutynin Chloride USP—Freely soluble in water and in alcohol; very soluble in methanol and in chloroform; soluble in acetone; slightly soluble in ether; very slightly soluble in hexane.

USP requirements:

Oxybutynin Chloride USP—Preserve in well-closed containers. Contains not less than 97.0% and not more than 101.0% of oxybutynin chloride, calculated on the dried basis. Meets the requirements for Identification, Melting range (124–129 °C), Loss on drying (not more than 3%), Residue on ignition (not more than 0.1%), Heavy metals (not more than 0.002%), Chromatographic purity, Chloride content (8–10%), and Organic volatile impurities.

Oxybutynin Chloride Syrup USP—Preserve in tight, light-resistant containers. Contains the labeled amount, within ±10%. Meets the requirement for Identification.

Oxybutynin Chloride Tablets USP—Preserve in tight, light-resistant containers. Contain the labeled amount, within ±10%. Meet the requirements for Identification, Dissolution (80% in 30 minutes in water in Apparatus 2 at 50 rpm), and Uniformity of dosage units.

OXYCODONE

Chemical name:

Oxycodone hydrochloride—Morphinan-6-one, 4,5-epoxy-14-hydroxy-3-methoxy-17-methyl-, hydrochloride, (5 alpha)-.

Oxycodone terephthalate—Morphinan-6-one, 4,5-epoxy-14-hydroxy-3-methoxy-17-methyl-, 1,4-benzenedicarboxylate (2:1) salt), (5 alpha).

Molecular formula:
Oxycodone hydrochloride—$C_{18}H_{21}NO_4 \cdot HCl$.
Oxycodone terephthalate—$(C_{18}H_{21}NO_4)_2 \cdot C_8H_6O_4$.

Molecular weight:
Oxycodone hydrochloride—351.83.
Oxycodone terephthalate—796.88.

Description: Oxycodone Hydrochloride USP—White to off-white, hygroscopic crystals or powder. Is odorless.

Solubility: Oxycodone Hydrochloride USP—Soluble in water; slightly soluble in alcohol.

USP requirements:
Oxycodone Hydrochloride USP—Preserve in tight containers. Contains not less than 97.0% and not more than 103.0% of oxycodone hydrochloride, calculated on the dried basis. Meets the requirements for Identification, Specific rotation (−137° to −149°), Loss on drying (not more than 7.0%), Residue on ignition (not more than 0.05%), Related compounds, and Chloride content (9.8–10.4%, calculated on the dried basis).
Oxycodone Hydrochloride Oral Solution USP—Preserve in tight, light-resistant containers. Contains the labeled amount, within ±10%. Meets the requirements for Identification, pH (1.4–4.0), and Alcohol content (7.0–9.0%).
Oxycodone Hydrochloride Suppositories—Not in USP.
Oxycodone Hydrochloride Tablets USP—Preserve in tight, light-resistant containers. Contain the labeled amount, within ±10%. Meet the requirements for Identification, Dissolution (70% in 45 minutes in water in Apparatus 2 at 50 rpm), and Uniformity of dosage units.
Oxycodone Terephthalate USP—Preserve in tight containers. Contains not less than 97.0% and not more than 103.0% of oxycodone terephthalate, calculated on the dried basis. Meets the requirements for Identification, Loss on drying (not more than 1.5%), Residue on ignition (not more than 1%), Related compounds, and Terephthalic acid content (20.2–21.5%, calculated on the dried basis).

OXYCODONE AND ACETAMINOPHEN

For *Oxycodone* and *Acetaminophen*—See individual listings for chemistry information.

USP requirements:
Oxycodone and Acetaminophen Capsules USP—Preserve in tight, light-resistant containers. Contain Oxycodone Hydrochloride and Acetaminophen, or Oxycodone Hydrochloride, Oxycodone Terephthalate, and Acetaminophen. Label Capsules to indicate whether they contain Oxycodone Hydrochloride or Oxycodone Hydrochloride and Oxycodone Terephthalate. Capsules may be labeled to indicate the total content of oxycodone equivalent. Each mg of oxycodone hydrochloride or oxycodone terephthalate is equivalent to 0.8963 mg or 0.7915 mg of oxycodone, respectively. Contain the labeled amounts of oxycodone hydrochloride or oxycodone hydrochloride and oxycodone terephthalate, calculated as total oxycodone, and the labeled amount of acetaminophen, within ±10%. Meet the requirements for Identification, Dissolution (75% of each active ingredient in 45 minutes in 0.1 *N* hydrochloric acid in Apparatus 2 at 50 rpm), and Uniformity of dosage units.
Oxycodone and Acetaminophen Oral Solution—Not in USP.
Oxycodone and Acetaminophen Tablets USP—Preserve in tight, light-resistant containers. Contain Oxycodone Hydrochloride and Acetaminophen. Tablets may be labeled to indicate the content of oxycodone hydrochloride equivalent. Each mg of oxycodone is equivalent to 1.116 mg of oxycodone hydrochloride. Contain the labeled amounts of oxycodone and acetaminophen, within ±10%. Meet the requirements for Identification, Dissolution (75% of each active ingredient in 45 minutes in 0.1 *N* hydrochloric acid in Apparatus 2 at 50 rpm), and Uniformity of dosage units.

OXYCODONE AND ASPIRIN

For *Oxycodone* and *Aspirin*—See individual listings for chemistry information.

USP requirements: Oxycodone and Aspirin Tablets USP—Preserve in tight, light-resistant containers. Contain Oxycodone Hydrochloride and Aspirin, or Oxycodone Hydrochloride, Oxycodone Terephthalate, and Aspirin. Label Tablets to state both the content of the oxycodone active moiety and the content or contents of the salt or salts of oxycodone used in formulating the article. Contain the labeled amount of oxycodone, within ±7%, and the labeled amount of aspirin, within ±10%. Meet the requirements for Identification, Dissolution (80% of oxycodone and 75% of aspirin in 30 minutes in 0.05 *M* acetate buffer [pH 4.50] in Apparatus 1 at 50 rpm), Uniformity of dosage units, and Salicylic acid (not more than 3.0%).

OXYGEN

Chemical name: Oxygen.

Molecular formula: O_2.

Molecular weight: 32.00.

Description: Oxygen USP—Colorless, odorless gas, which supports combustion more energetically than does air. One liter at 0 °C and at a pressure of 760 mm of mercury weighs about 1.429 grams.

Solubility: Oxygen USP—One volume dissolves in about 32 volumes of water and in about 7 volumes of alcohol at 20 °C and at a pressure of 760 mm of mercury.

USP requirements: Oxygen USP—Preserve in cylinders or in a pressurized storage tank. Containers used for Oxygen must not be treated with any toxic, sleep-inducing, or narcosis-producing compounds, and must not be treated with any compound that will be irritating to the respiratory tract when the Oxygen is used. Label it to indicate whether or not it has been produced by the air-liquefaction process. Where it is piped directly from the cylinder or storage tank to the point of use, label each outlet "Oxygen." Contains not less than 99.0%, by volume, of oxygen. (Note: Oxygen that is produced by the air-liquefaction process is exempt from the requirements of the tests for Carbon dioxide and Carbon monoxide.) Meets the requirements for Identification, Odor, Carbon dioxide (not more than 0.03%), and Carbon monoxide (not more than 0.001%).

OXYGEN 93 PERCENT

USP requirements: Oxygen 93 Percent USP—Preserve in cylinders or in a low pressure collecting tank. Containers used for Oxygen 93 Percent must not be treated with any toxic, sleep-inducing, or narcosis-producing compounds, and must not be treated with any compound that will be irritating to the respiratory tract when the Oxygen 93 Percent is used. It is Oxygen produced from air by the molecular sieve process. Where it is piped directly from the collecting tank to the point of use, label each outlet "Oxygen 93 Percent."

Contains not less than 90.0% and not more than 96.0%, by volume, of oxygen, the remainder consisting mostly of argon and nitrogen. Meets the requirements for Identification, Odor, Carbon dioxide (not more than 0.03%), and Carbon monoxide (not more than 0.001%).

WATER O 15

Chemical name: Water-^{15}O.

Molecular formula: $H_2{}^{15}O$.

USP requirements: Water O 15 Injection USP—Preserve in a single-dose container that is adequately shielded. A sterile solution of Water O 15 in isotonic Sodium Chloride Injection in which a portion of the molecules are labeled with radioactive ^{15}O. Label container to include the following, in addition to the information specified for Labeling under Injections: the time and date of calibration; the amount of ^{15}O as water expressed as megabecquerels (or millicuries) per mL, at time of calibration; total activity at time of calibration; the expiration time and date; the name and quantity of any added preservative or stabilizer; and the statement "Caution—Radioactive Material." The labeling indicates that in making dosage calculations, correction is to be made for radioactive decay and also indicates that the radioactive half-life of ^{15}O is 123 seconds. The label indicates "Do not use if cloudy or if it contains particulate matter." Contains the labeled amount of ^{15}O, within ±10%, expressed in megabecquerels (or millicuries) per mL at the time indicated in the labeling. Meets the requirements for Specific activity, Identification, Radionuclide identification, Bacterial endotoxins, Sterility, pH (4.5–8.0), Particulate matter, Radiochemical purity, Radionuclidic purity, and Heavy metals (not more than 5 ppm), and for Injections (except that the Injection may be distributed or dispensed prior to completion of the test for Sterility, the latter test being started on the day of final manufacture, and except that it is not subject to the recommendation for Volume in Container under Injections).

OXYMETAZOLINE

Source: Prepared from (4-*tert*-butyl-2,6-dimethyl-3-hydroxyphenyl)acetonitrile and ethylenediamine.

Chemical name: Oxymetazoline hydrochloride—Phenol, 3-[(4,5-dihydro-1*H*-imidazol-2-yl)methyl]-6-(1,1-dimethylethyl)-2,4-dimethyl-, monohydrochloride.

Molecular formula: Oxymetazoline hydrochloride—$C_{16}H_{24}N_2O \cdot HCl$.

Molecular weight: Oxymetazoline hydrochloride—296.84.

Description: Oxymetazoline Hydrochloride USP—White to practically white, fine crystalline powder. Is hygroscopic. Melts at about 300 °C, with decomposition.

Solubility: Oxymetazoline Hydrochloride USP—Soluble in water and in alcohol; practically insoluble in chloroform and in ether.

USP requirements:

Oxymetazoline Hydrochloride USP—Preserve in tight containers. Contains not less than 98.5% and not more than 101.5% of oxymetazoline hydrochloride, calculated on the dried basis. Meets the requirements for Identification, pH (4.0–6.5, in a solution [1 in 20]), Loss on drying (not more than 1.0%), Residue on ignition (not more than 0.1%), and Heavy metals (not more than 0.001%).

Oxymetazoline Hydrochloride Nasal Solution USP—Preserve in tight containers. A solution of Oxymetazoline Hydrochloride in water adjusted to a suitable tonicity. Contains the labeled amount, within ±10%. Meets the requirements for Identification and pH (4.0–6.5).

Oxymetazoline Hydrochloride Ophthalmic Solution USP—Preserve in tight containers. A sterile, buffered solution of Oxymetazoline Hydrochloride in water adjusted to a suitable tonicity. Contains the labeled amount, within ±10%. Contains a suitable preservative. Meets the requirements for Identification, Sterility, and pH (5.8–6.8).

OXYMETHOLONE

Chemical group: 17-alpha alkylated anabolic steroid.

Chemical name: Androstan-3-one, 17-hydroxy-2-(hydroxymethylene)-17-methyl-, (5 alpha,17 beta)-.

Molecular formula: $C_{21}H_{32}O_3$.

Molecular weight: 332.48.

Description: Oxymetholone USP—White to creamy white, crystalline powder. Is odorless, and is stable in air.

Solubility: Oxymetholone USP—Practically insoluble in water; freely soluble in chloroform; soluble in dioxane; sparingly soluble in alcohol; slightly soluble in ether.

USP requirements:

Oxymetholone USP—Preserve in well-closed containers. Contains not less than 97.0% and not more than 103.0% of oxymetholone, calculated on the dried basis. Meets the requirements for Completeness of solution, Identification, Melting range (172–180 °C), Specific rotation (+34° to +38°, calculated on the dried basis), Loss on drying (not more than 1.0%), and Organic volatile impurities.

Oxymetholone Tablets USP—Preserve in well-closed containers. Contain the labeled amount, within ±10%. Meet the requirements for Identification, Dissolution (75% in 45 minutes in 0.05 *M* alkaline borate buffer [pH 8.5] in Apparatus 1 at 100 rpm), and Uniformity of dosage units.

OXYMORPHONE

Chemical name: Oxymorphone hydrochloride—Morphinan-6-one, 4,5-epoxy-3,14-dihydroxy-17-methyl-, hydrochloride, (5 alpha)-.

Molecular formula: Oxymorphone hydrochloride—$C_{17}H_{19}NO_4 \cdot HCl$.

Molecular weight: Oxymorphone hydrochloride—337.80.

Description: Oxymorphone Hydrochloride USP—White or slightly off-white, odorless powder. Darkens on exposure to light. Its aqueous solutions are slightly acidic.

Solubility: Oxymorphone Hydrochloride USP—Freely soluble in water; sparingly soluble in alcohol and in ether.

USP requirements:

Oxymorphone Hydrochloride USP—Preserve in tight, light-resistant containers. Contains not less than 97.0% and not more than 102.0% of oxymorphone hydrochloride, calculated on the dried basis. Meets the requirements for Identification, Specific rotation (−145° to −155°, calculated on the dried basis), Acidity, Loss on drying (not more than 8.0%), Residue on ignition (not more than 0.3%), Ordinary impurities, Chloride content (10.2–10.8%, calculated on the dried basis), and Nonphenolic substances

Oxymorphone Hydrochloride Injection USP—Preserve in single-dose or in multiple-dose containers of Type I glass, protected from light. A sterile solution of Oxymorphone

Hydrochloride in Water for Injection. Contains the labeled amount, within ±7%. Meets the requirements for Identification, Bacterial endotoxins, pH (2.7–4.5), and Injections.

Oxymorphone Hydrochloride Suppositories USP—Preserve in well-closed containers, and store in a refrigerator. Contain the labeled amount, within ±7%. Meet the requirement for Identification.

OXYPHENBUTAZONE

Chemical name: 3,5-Pyrazolidinedione, 4-butyl-1-(4-hydroxyphenyl)-2-phenyl-, monohydrate.

Molecular formula: $C_{19}H_{20}N_2O_3 \cdot H_2O$.

Molecular weight: 342.39.

Description: Oxyphenbutazone USP—White to yellowish white, odorless, crystalline powder. Melts over a wide range between about 85 and 100 °C.

Solubility: Oxyphenbutazone USP—Very slightly soluble in water; soluble in alcohol; freely soluble in acetone and in ether.

USP requirements:

Oxyphenbutazone USP—Preserve in tight containers. Contains not less than 98.0% and not more than 100.5% of oxyphenbutazone, calculated on the anhydrous basis. Meets the requirements for Identification, Water (5.0–6.0%), Residue on ignition (not more than 0.1%), Chloride, and Chromatographic purity.

Oxyphenbutazone Tablets USP—Preserve in tight containers. Contain the labeled amount, within ±6%. Meet the requirements for Identification, Dissolution (60% in 30 minutes in phosphate buffer [pH 7.5] in Apparatus 1 at 100 rpm), and Uniformity of dosage units.

OXYPHENCYCLIMINE

Chemical group: Tertiary amine.

Chemical name: Oxyphencyclimine hydrochloride—Benzeneacetic acid, alpha-cyclohexyl-alpha-hydroxy-, (1,4,5,6-tetrahydro-1-methyl-2-pyrimidinyl)methyl ester monohydrochloride.

Molecular formula: Oxyphencyclimine hydrochloride—$C_{20}H_{28}N_2O_3 \cdot HCl$.

Molecular weight: Oxyphencyclimine hydrochloride—380.91.

Description: Oxyphencyclimine Hydrochloride USP—White, odorless, crystalline powder. Melts at about 234 °C.

Solubility: Oxyphencyclimine Hydrochloride USP—Sparingly soluble in water; soluble in methanol; slightly soluble in chloroform.

USP requirements:

Oxyphencyclimine Hydrochloride USP—Preserve in tight containers. Dried in vacuum at 60 °C for 2.5 hours, contains not less than 98.0% and not more than 101.0% of oxyphencyclimine hydrochloride. Meets the requirements for Identification, Loss on drying (not more than 2.0%), Residue on ignition (not more than 0.2%), and Heavy metals (not more than 0.005%).

Oxyphencyclimine Hydrochloride Tablets USP—Preserve in tight containers. Contain the labeled amount, within ±10%. Meet the requirements for Identification, Dissolution (75% in 45 minutes in water in Apparatus 1 at 100 rpm), and Uniformity of dosage units.

OXYQUINOLINE SULFATE

Chemical name: 8-Quinolinol sulfate (2:1) (salt).

Molecular formula: $(C_9H_7NO)_2 \cdot H_2SO_4$.

Molecular weight: 388.39.

Description: Oxyquinoline Sulfate NF—Yellow powder. Melts at about 185 °C.

NF category: Complexing agent.

Solubility: Oxyquinoline Sulfate NF—Very soluble in water; freely soluble in methanol; slightly soluble in alcohol; practically insoluble in acetone and in ether.

NF requirements: Oxyquinoline Sulfate NF—Preserve in well-closed containers. It is 8-hydroxyquinoline sulfate. Contains not less than 97.0% and not more than 101.0% of oxyquinoline sulfate, calculated on the anhydrous basis. Meets the requirements for Identification, Water (4.0–6.0%), Residue on ignition (not more than 0.3%), Arsenic (not more than 3 ppm), Heavy metals (not more than 0.004%), and Organic volatile impurities.

OXYTETRACYCLINE

Chemical name:

Oxytetracycline—2-Naphthacenecarboxamide, 4-(dimethylamino)-1,4,4a,5,5a,6,11,12a-octahydro-3,5,6,10,12,-12a-hexahydroxy-6-methyl-1,11-dioxo-, [4*S*-(4 alpha,4a alpha,5 alpha,5a alpha,6 beta,12a alpha)]-, dihydrate.

Oxytetracycline calcium—2-Naphthacenecarboxamide, 4-(dimethylamino)-1,4,4a,5,5a,6,11,12a-octahydro-3,5,6,10,-12,12a-hexahydroxy-6-methyl-1,11-dioxo-, calcium salt, [4*S*-(4 alpha,4a alpha,5 alpha,5a alpha,6 beta,12a alpha)]-.

Oxytetracycline hydrochloride—2-Naphthacenecarboxamide, 4-(dimethylamino)-1,4,4a,5,5a,6,11,12a-octahydro-3,5,6,10,12,12a-hexahydroxy-6-methyl-1,11-dioxo-, monohydrochloride, [4*S*-(4 alpha,4a alpha,5 alpha,5a alpha,6 beta,12a alpha)]-.

Molecular formula:

Oxytetracycline—$C_{22}H_{24}N_2O_9 \cdot 2H_2O$.
Oxytetracycline calcium—$C_{44}H_{46}CaN_4O_{18}$.
Oxytetracycline hydrochloride—$C_{22}H_{24}N_2O_9 \cdot HCl$.

Molecular weight:

Oxytetracycline—496.47.
Oxytetracycline calcium—958.95.
Oxytetracycline hydrochloride—496.90.

Description:

Oxytetracycline USP—Pale yellow to tan, odorless, crystalline powder. Is stable in air, but exposure to strong sunlight causes it to darken. It loses potency in solutions of pH below 2, and is rapidly destroyed by alkali hydroxide solutions.

Oxytetracycline Calcium USP—Yellow to light brown, crystalline powder.

Oxytetracycline Hydrochloride USP—Yellow, odorless, crystalline powder. Is hygroscopic. Decomposes at a temperature exceeding 180 °C, and exposure to strong sunlight or to temperatures exceeding 90 °C in moist air causes it to darken. Its potency is diminished in solutions having a pH below 2, and is rapidly destroyed by alkali hydroxide solutions.

Solubility:

Oxytetracycline USP—Very slightly soluble in water; freely soluble in 3 *N* hydrochloric acid and in alkaline solutions; sparingly soluble in alcohol.

Oxytetracycline Calcium USP—Insoluble in water.

Oxytetracycline Hydrochloride USP—Freely soluble in water, but crystals of oxytetracycline base separate as a result of partial hydrolysis of the hydrochloride. Sparingly soluble in alcohol and in methanol, and even less soluble in dehydrated alcohol; insoluble in chloroform and in ether.

USP requirements:

Oxytetracycline USP—Preserve in tight, light-resistant containers. Has a potency equivalent to not less than 832 mcg of oxytetracycline per mg. Meets the requirements for Identification, Crystallinity, pH (4.5–7.0, in an aqueous suspension containing 10 mg per mL), and Water (6.0–9.0%).

Oxytetracycline Injection USP—Preserve in single-dose or in multiple-dose containers, protected from light. A sterile solution of Oxytetracycline with or without one or more suitable anesthetics, antioxidants, buffers, complexing agents, preservatives, and solvents. Contains the labeled amount, within −10% to +20%. Meets the requirements for Identification, Depressor substances, Bacterial endotoxins, Sterility, and pH (8.0–9.0).

Sterile Oxytetracycline USP—Preserve in Containers for Sterile Solids, protected from light. It is Oxytetracycline suitable for parenteral use. Has a potency of not less than 832 mcg of oxytetracycline per mg. Meets the requirements for Depressor substances, Bacterial endotoxins, and Sterility, and for Identification tests, pH, Water, and Crystallinity under Oxytetracycline.

Oxytetracycline Tablets USP—Preserve in tight, light-resistant containers. Contain the labeled amount, within −10% to +20%. Meet the requirements for Identification, Dissolution (75% in 45 minutes in 0.1 *N* hydrochloric acid in Apparatus 1 at 100 rpm), Uniformity of dosage units, and Water (not more than 7.5%).

Oxytetracycline Calcium USP—Preserve in tight, light-resistant containers, and store in a cool place. Has a potency equivalent to not less than 865 mcg of oxytetracycline per mg, calculated on the anhydrous basis. Meets the requirements for Identification, Crystallinity, pH (6.0–8.0, in an aqueous suspension containing 25 mg per mL), Water (8.0–14.0%), and Calcium content (3.85–4.35%, calculated on the anhydrous basis).

Oxytetracycline Calcium Oral Suspension USP—Preserve in tight, light-resistant containers. Contains an amount of oxytetracycline calcium equivalent to the labeled amount of oxytetracycline, within −10% to +20%. Contains one or more suitable buffers, colors, flavors, preservatives, stabilizers, and suspending agents. Meets the requirements for Identification, pH (5.0–8.0), Deliverable volume (for Suspension packaged in multiple-unit containers), and Uniformity of dosage units (for Suspension packaged in single-unit containers).

Oxytetracycline Hydrochloride USP—Preserve in tight, light-resistant containers. Has a potency equivalent to not less than 835 mcg of oxytetracycline per mg, calculated on the dried basis. Meets the requirements for Identification, Crystallinity, pH (2.0–3.0, in a solution containing 10 mg per mL), and Loss on drying (not more than 2.0%).

Oxytetracycline Hydrochloride Capsules USP—Preserve in tight, light-resistant containers. Contain an amount of oxytetracycline hydrochloride equivalent to the labeled amount of oxytetracycline, within −10% to +20%. Meet the requirements for Identification, Dissolution (80% in 60 minutes in water in Apparatus 2 at 75 rpm), Uniformity of dosage units, and Loss on drying (not more than 5.0%).

Oxytetracycline Hydrochloride for Injection USP—Preserve in Containers for Sterile Solids, protected from light. A sterile dry mixture of Sterile Oxytetracycline Hydrochloride and a suitable buffer. Contains an amount of oxytetracycline hydrochloride equivalent to the labeled amount of oxytetracycline, within −10% to +15%. Meets the requirements for Constituted solution, Bacterial endotoxins, pH (1.8–2.8, in a solution containing 25 mg per mL), Loss on drying (not more than 3.0%), and Particulate matter, for Identification test B under Oxytetracycline Hydrochloride, for Depressor substances and Sterility under Sterile Oxytetracycline Hydrochloride, and for Uniformity of dosage units and Labeling under Injections.

Sterile Oxytetracycline Hydrochloride USP—Preserve in Containers for Sterile Solids, protected from light. It is Oxytetracycline Hydrochloride suitable for parenteral use. Has a potency equivalent to not less than 835 mcg of oxytetracycline per mg, calculated on the dried basis. Meets the requirements for Depressor substances, Bacterial endotoxins, and Sterility, and for Identification tests, pH, Loss on drying, and Crystallinity under Oxytetracycline Hydrochloride.

OXYTETRACYCLINE AND HYDROCORTISONE

For *Oxytetracycline* and *Hydrocortisone*—See individual listings for chemistry information.

USP requirements:

Oxytetracycline Hydrochloride and Hydrocortisone Ointment USP—Preserve in collapsible tubes or in well-closed, light-resistant containers. Contains an amount of oxytetracycline hydrochloride equivalent to the labeled amount of oxytetracycline, within −10% to +15%, and the labeled amount of hydrocortisone, within ±10%. Meets the requirements for Minimum fill and Water (not more than 1.0%).

Oxytetracycline Hydrochloride and Hydrocortisone Acetate Ophthalmic Suspension USP—Preserve in tight, light-resistant containers. The containers are sealed and tamper-proof so that sterility is assured at time of first use. A sterile suspension of Oxytetracycline Hydrochloride and Hydrocortisone Acetate in a suitable oil vehicle with one or more suitable suspending agents. Contains an amount of oxytetracycline hydrochloride equivalent to the labeled amount of oxytetracycline, within −10% to +15%, and the labeled amount of hydrocortisone acetate, within ±10%. Meets the requirements for Sterility and Water (not more than 1.0%).

OXYTETRACYCLINE AND NYSTATIN

For *Oxytetracycline* and *Nystatin*—See individual listings for chemistry information.

USP requirements:

Oxytetracycline and Nystatin Capsules USP—Preserve in tight, light-resistant containers. Contain the labeled amount of oxytetracycline, within −10% to +20%, and the labeled amount of USP Nystatin Units, within −10% to +35%. Meet the requirements for Identification, Dissolution (75% of oxytetracycline in 45 minutes in 0.1 *N* hydrochloric acid in Apparatus 1 at 100 rpm), Uniformity of dosage units, and Water (not more than 7.5%).

Oxytetracycline and Nystatin for Oral Suspension USP—Preserve in tight, light-resistant containers, at controlled room temperature. A dry mixture of Oxytetracycline and Nystatin with one or more suitable buffers, colors, diluents, flavors, suspending agents, and preservatives. When constituted as directed in the labeling, contains the labeled amount of oxytetracycline, within −10% to +20%, and the labeled amount of USP Nystatin Units, within −10% to +35%. Meets the requirements for Identification, pH (4.5–7.5, in the suspension constituted as directed in the labeling), Water (not more than 2.0%), Deliverable volume (for solid packaged in multiple-unit containers), and Uniformity of dosage units (for solid packaged in single-unit containers).

OXYTETRACYCLINE, PHENAZOPYRIDINE, AND SULFAMETHIZOLE

For *Oxytetracycline, Phenazopyridine,* and *Sulfamethizole*—See individual listings for chemistry information.

USP requirements: Oxytetracycline and Phenazopyridine Hydrochlorides and Sulfamethizole Capsules USP—Preserve in tight, light-resistant containers. Contain an amount of oxytetracycline hydrochloride equivalent to the labeled amount of oxytetracycline, within −10% to +20%, and the labeled amounts of phenazopyridine hydrochloride, within −10% to +15%, and sulfamethizole, within ±10%. Meet the requirements for Uniformity of dosage units and Loss on drying (not more than 5.0%).

OXYTETRACYCLINE AND POLYMYXIN B

For *Oxytetracycline* and *Polymyxin B*—See individual listings for chemistry information.

USP requirements:

Oxytetracycline Hydrochloride and Polymyxin B Sulfate Ointment USP—Preserve in collapsible tubes or in well-closed, light-resistant containers. Contains amounts of oxytetracycline hydrochloride and polymyxin B sulfate equivalent to the labeled amounts of oxytetracycline, within −10% to +20%, and polymyxin B, within −10% to +25%. Meets the requirements for Minimum fill and Water (not more than 1.0%).

Oxytetracycline Hydrochloride and Polymyxin B Sulfate Ophthalmic Ointment USP—Preserve in collapsible ophthalmic ointment tubes. A sterile ointment containing Oxytetracycline Hydrochloride and Polymyxin B Sulfate. Contains amounts of oxytetracycline hydrochloride and polymyxin B sulfate equivalent to the labeled amounts of oxytetracycline, within −10% to +20%, and polymyxin B, within −10% to +25%. Meets the requirements for Sterility, Minimum fill, Water (not more than 1.0%), and Metal particles.

Oxytetracycline Hydrochloride and Polymyxin B Sulfate Topical Powder USP—Preserve in well-closed containers. Contains amounts of oxytetracycline hydrochloride and polymyxin B sulfate equivalent to the labeled amounts of oxytetracycline and polymyxin B, within −10% to +20%, in a suitable fine powder base. Meets the requirements for Minimum fill and Loss on drying (not more than 2.0%).

Oxytetracycline Hydrochloride and Polymyxin B Sulfate Vaginal Tablets USP—Preserve in well-closed containers. Contain amounts of oxytetracycline hydrochloride and polymyxin B sulfate equivalent to the labeled amounts of oxytetracycline and polymyxin B, within −10% to +20%. Meet the requirement for Loss on drying (not more than 3.0%).

OXYTOCIN

Chemical name: Oxytocin.

Molecular formula: $C_{43}H_{66}N_{12}O_{12}S_2$.

Molecular weight: 1007.19.

Description: White powder.

Solubility: Soluble in water.

USP requirements:

Oxytocin Injection USP—Preserve in single-dose or in multiple-dose containers, preferably of Type I glass. Do not freeze. A sterile solution, in a suitable diluent, of material containing the polypeptide hormone having the property of causing the contraction of uterine, vascular, and other smooth muscle, which is prepared by synthesis or obtained from the posterior lobe of the pituitary of healthy, domestic animals used for food by man. Each mL of Oxytocin Injection possesses an oxytocic activity of that stated on the label in USP Posterior Pituitary Units, within −15% to +20%. Meets the requirements for pH (2.5–4.5), Particulate matter, Pressor activity, and Injections.

Oxytocin Nasal Solution USP—Preserve in containers suitable for administering the contents by spraying into the nasal cavities with the patient in the upright position, or for instillation in drop form. A solution, in a suitable diluent, of the polypeptide hormone, prepared synthetically, which has the property of causing the contraction of uterine, vascular, and other smooth muscle, and which is present in the posterior lobe of the pituitary of healthy, domestic animals used for food by man. Label it to indicate that it is for intranasal administration only. Contains suitable preservatives, and is packaged in a form suitable for nasal administration. Each mL of Oxytocin Nasal Solution possesses an oxytocic activity of that stated on the label in USP Posterior Pituitary Units, within −15% to +20%. Meets the requirements for pH (3.7–4.3) and Pressor activity.

PACLITAXEL

Chemical name: (2a*R*,4*S*,4a*S*,6*R*,9*S*,11*S*,12*S*,12a*R*,12b*S*)-1,2a,-3,4,4a,6,9,10,11,12,12a,12b-Dodecahydro-4,6,9,11,12,12b-hexahydroxy-4a,8,13,13-tetramethyl-7,11-methano-5*H*-cyclodeca[3,4]benz[1,2-*b*]oxet-5-one 6,12b-diacetate 12-benzoate, 9-ester with (2*R*,3*S*)-*N*-benzoyl-3-phenylisoserine.

Molecular formula: $C_{47}H_{51}NO_{14}$.

Molecular weight: 853.92.

Description: White to off-white crystalline powder. Melts at around 216–217 °C.

Solubility: Insoluble in water.

Other characteristics: Highly lipophilic.

USP requirements: Paclitaxel Concentrate for Injection—Not in USP.

PADIMATE O

Chemical name: Benzoic acid, 4-(dimethylamino)-, 2-ethylhexyl ester.

Molecular formula: $C_{17}H_{27}NO_2$.

Molecular weight: 277.41.

Description: Padimate O USP—Light yellow, mobile liquid having a faint, aromatic odor.

Solubility: Padimate O USP—Practically insoluble in water; soluble in alcohol, in isopropyl alcohol, and in mineral oil; practically insoluble in glycerin and in propylene glycol.

USP requirements:

Padimate O USP—Preserve in tight, light-resistant containers. Contains not less than 97.0% and not more than 103.8% of padimate O. Meets the requirements for Identification, Specific gravity (0.990–1.000), Refractive index (1.5390–1.5430), Acid value (not more than 1.0), Saponification value (195–215), and Chromatographic purity.

Padimate O Lotion USP—Preserve in tight, light-resistant containers. Contains the labeled amount, within ±10%. Meets the requirement for Identification.

PAMIDRONATE

Chemical name: Pamidronate disodium—Phosphonic acid, (3-amino-1-hydroxypropylidene)bis-, disodium salt, pentahydrate.

Molecular formula: Pamidronate disodium—$C_3H_9NNa_2O_7P_2 \cdot 5H_2O$.

Molecular weight: Pamidronate disodium—369.11.

Description: Pamidronate disodium—White to practically white powder.

Solubility: Pamidronate disodium—Soluble in water and in 2 *N* sodium hydroxide; sparingly soluble in 0.1 *N* hydrochloric acid and in 0.1 *N* acetic acid; practically insoluble in organic solvents.

USP requirements:
Pamidronate Disodium Injection—Not in USP.
Pamidronate Disodium for Injection—Not in USP.

PANCREATIN

Chemical name: Pancreatin.

Description: Pancreatin USP—Cream-colored, amorphous powder, having a faint, characteristic, but not offensive odor. It hydrolyzes fats to glycerol and fatty acids, changes protein into proteoses and derived substances, and converts starch into dextrins and sugars. Its greatest activities are in neutral or faintly alkaline media; more than traces of mineral acids or large amounts of alkali hydroxides make it inert. An excess of alkali carbonate also inhibits its action.

USP requirements:
Pancreatin USP—Preserve in tight containers, at a temperature not exceeding 30 °C. A substance containing enzymes, principally amylase, lipase, and protease, obtained from the pancreas of the hog, *Sus scrofa* Linné var. *domesticus* Gray (Fam. Suidae) or of the ox, *Bos taurus* Linné (Fam. Bovidae). Contains, in each mg, not less than 25 USP Units of amylase activity, not less than 2.0 USP Units of lipase activity, and not less than 25 USP Units of protease activity. Pancreatin of a higher digestive power may be labeled as a whole-number multiple of the three minimun activities or may be diluted by admixture with lactose, or with sucrose containing not more than 3.25% of starch, or with pancreatin of lower digestive power. Meets the requirements for Microbial limit, Loss on drying (not more than 5.0%), and Fat.

Note: One USP Unit of amylase activity is contained in the amount of pancreatin that decomposes starch at an initial rate such that one microequivalent of glucosidic linkage is hydrolyzed per minute under the conditions of the *Assay for amylase activity*. One USP Unit of lipase activity is contained in the amount of pancreatin that liberates 1.0 microequivalent of acid per minute at a pH of 9.0 and 37 °C under the conditions of the *Assay for lipase activity*. One USP Unit of protease activity is contained in the amount of pancreatin that digests 1.0 mg of casein under the conditions of the *Assay for protease activity*.

Pancreatin Capsules USP—Preserve in tight containers, preferably at a temperature not exceeding 30 °C. Label Capsules to indicate minimum pancreatin fat digestive power; i.e., single strength, double strength, triple strength. Contain the labeled amount, within −10%. Meet the requirement for Microbial limit.

Pancreatin Tablets USP—Preserve in tight containers, preferably at a temperature not exceeding 30 °C. Label Tablets to indicate minimum pancreatin fat digestive power; i.e., single strength, double strength, triple strength. Contain the labeled amount, within −10%. Meet the requirements for Microbial limit and Disintegration (60 minutes).

PANCREATIN, PEPSIN, BILE SALTS, HYOSCYAMINE, ATROPINE, SCOPOLAMINE, AND PHENOBARBITAL

Source: Pancreatin—Obtained from pancreas of the hog, *Sus scrofa* Linné var. *domesticus* Gray (Fam. Suidae) or of the ox, *Bos taurus* Linné (Fam. Bovidae).

Chemical name:
Hyoscyamine sulfate—Benzeneacetic acid, alpha-(hydroxymethyl)-, 8-methyl-8-azabicyclo[3.2.1]oct-3-yl ester, [3(*S*)-*endo*]-, sulfate (2:1), dihydrate.
Atropine sulfate—Benzeneacetic acid, alpha-(hydroxymethyl)-, 8-methyl-8-azabicyclo[3.2.1]oct-3-yl ester, *endo*-(±)-, sulfate (2:1) (salt), monohydrate.
Scopolamine hydrobromide—Benzeneacetic acid, alpha-(hydroxymethyl)-, 9-methyl-3-oxa-9-azatricyclo[$3.3.1.0^{2,4}$]non-7-yl ester, hydrobromide, trihydrate, [7(*S*)-(1 alpha,2 beta,4 beta,5 alpha,7 beta)]-.
Phenobarbital—2,4,6(1*H*,3*H*,5*H*)-Pyrimidinetrione, 5-ethyl-5-phenyl-.

Molecular formula:
Hyoscyamine sulfate—$(C_{17}H_{23}NO_3)_2 \cdot H_2SO_4 \cdot 2H_2O$.
Atropine sulfate—$(C_{17}H_{23}NO_3)_2 \cdot H_2SO_4 \cdot H_2O$.
Scopolamine hydrobromide—$C_{17}H_{21}NO_4 \cdot HBr \cdot 3H_2O$.
Phenobarbital—$C_{12}H_{12}N_2O_3$.

Molecular weight:
Hyoscyamine sulfate—712.85.
Atropine sulfate—694.84.
Scopolamine hydrobromide—438.32.
Phenobarbital—232.24.

Description:
Pancreatin USP—Cream-colored, amorphous powder, having a faint, characteristic, but not offensive odor. It hydrolyzes fats to glycerol and fatty acids, changes protein into proteoses and derived substances, and converts starch into dextrins and sugars. Its greatest activities are in neutral or faintly alkaline media; more than traces of mineral acids or large amounts of alkali hydroxides make it inert. An excess of alkali carbonate also inhibits its action.
Hyoscyamine Sulfate USP—White, odorless crystals or crystalline powder. Is deliquescent and is affected by light. The pH of a solution (1 in 100) is about 5.3.
Atropine Sulfate USP—Colorless crystals, or white, crystalline powder. Odorless; effloresces in dry air; is slowly affected by light.
Scopolamine Hydrobromide USP—Colorless or white crystals or white, granular powder. Is odorless, and slightly efflorescent in dry air.
Phenobarbital USP—White, odorless, glistening, small crystals, or white, crystalline powder, which may exhibit polymorphism. Is stable in air. Its saturated solution has a pH of about 5.

pKa:
Atropine—9.8.
Scopolamine—7.55 (23 °C)–7.81 (25 °C).

Solubility:
Hyoscyamine Sulfate USP—Very soluble in water; freely soluble in alcohol; practically insoluble in ether.

Atropine Sulfate USP—Very soluble in water; freely soluble in alcohol and even more so in boiling alcohol; freely soluble in glycerin.

Scopolamine Hydrobromide USP—Freely soluble in water; soluble in alcohol; slightly soluble in chloroform; insoluble in ether.

Phenobarbital USP—Very slightly soluble in water; soluble in alcohol, in ether, and in solutions of fixed alkali hydroxides and carbonates; sparingly soluble in chloroform.

USP requirements: Pancreatin, Pepsin, Bile Salts, Hyoscyamine Sulfate, Atropine Sulfate, Scopolamine Hydrobromide, and Phenobarbital Tablets—Not in USP.

PANCRELIPASE

Chemical name: Lipase, triacylglycerol.

Description:

Pancrelipase USP—Cream-colored, amorphous powder, having a faint, characteristic, but not offensive odor. It hydrolyzes fats to glycerol and fatty acids, changes protein into proteoses and derived substances, and converts starch into dextrins and sugars. Its greatest activities are in neutral or faintly alkaline media; more than traces of mineral acids or large amounts of alkali hydroxides make it inert. An excess of alkali carbonate also inhibits its action.

Pancrelipase Capsules USP—The contents of the Capsules conform to the Description under Pancrelipase, except that the odor may vary with the flavoring agent used.

USP requirements:

Pancrelipase USP—Preserve in tight containers, preferably at a temperature not exceeding 25 °C. A substance containing enzymes, principally lipase, with amylase and protease, obtained from the pancreas of the hog, *Sus scrofa* Linné var. *domesticus* Gray (Fam. Suidae). Label it to indicate lipase activity in USP Units. Contains, in each mg, not less than 24 USP Units of lipase activity, not less than 100 USP Units of amylase activity, and not less than 100 USP Units of protease activity. Meets the requirements for Microbial limits, Loss on drying (not more than 5.0%), and Fat (not more than 5.0%).

Note: One USP Unit of amylase activity is contained in the amount of pancrelipase that decomposes starch at an initial rate such that one microequivalent of glucosidic linkage is hydrolyzed per minute under the conditions of the *Assay for amylase activity*. One USP Unit of lipase activity is contained in the amount of pancrelipase that liberates 1.0 microequivalent of acid per minute at pH 9.0 and 37 °C under the conditions of the *Assay for lipase activity*. One USP Unit of protease activity is contained in the amount of pancrelipase that digests 1.0 mg of casein under the conditions of the *Assay for protease activity*.

Pancrelipase Capsules USP—Preserve in tight containers, preferably with a desiccant, at a temperature not exceeding 25 °C. Label Capsules to indicate lipase activity in USP Units. Contain an amount of pancrelipase equivalent to the labeled lipase activity, within −10% to +25%, expressed in USP Units, the labeled activity being not less than 8000 USP Units per capsule. They contain, in each capsule, the pancrelipase equivalent of not less than 30,000 USP Units of amylase activity, and not less than 30,000 USP Units of protease activity. Meet the requirements for Microbial limits and Loss on drying (not more than 5.0%).

Pancrelipase Delayed-release Capsules—Not in USP.

Pancrelipase Powder—Not in USP.

Pancrelipase Tablets USP—Preserve in tight containers, preferably with a desiccant, at a temperature not exceeding 25 °C. Label Tablets to indicate the lipase activity in USP Units. Contain an amount of pancrelipase equivalent to the labeled lipase activity, within −10% to +25%, expressed in USP Units, the labeled activity being not less than 8000 USP Units per Tablet. They contain, in each Tablet, the pancrelipase equivalent of not less than 30,000 USP Units of amylase activity, and not less than 30,000 USP Units of protease activity. Meet the requirements for Microbial limits, Disintegration (75 minutes), and Loss on drying (not more than 5.0%).

PANCURONIUM

Chemical name: Pancuronium bromide—Piperidinium, 1,1′-[(2 beta,3 alpha,5 alpha,16 beta,17 beta)-3,17-bis(acetyloxy)-androstane-2,16-diyl]bis[1-methyl]-, dibromide.

Molecular formula: Pancuronium bromide—$C_{35}H_{60}Br_2N_2O_4$.

Molecular weight: Pancuronium bromide—732.68.

Description: Pancuronium bromide—White or almost white, hygroscopic crystalline powder.

Solubility: Pancuronium bromide—Freely or very soluble in water; freely soluble in alcohol and in chloroform; practically insoluble in ether.

USP requirements: Pancuronium Bromide Injection—Not in USP.

PANTHENOL

Chemical name: Butanamide, 2,4-dihydroxy-*N*-(3-hydroxypropyl)-3,3-dimethyl-, (±)-.

Molecular formula: $C_9H_{19}NO_4$.

Molecular weight: 205.25.

Description: Panthenol USP—White to creamy white, crystalline powder having a slight, characteristic odor.

Solubility: Panthenol USP—Freely soluble in water, in alcohol, and in propylene glycol; soluble in chloroform and in ether; slightly soluble in glycerin.

USP requirements: Panthenol USP—Preserve in tight containers. A racemic mixture of the dextrorotatory and levorotatory isomers of panthenol. Contains not less than 99.0% and not more than 102.0% of panthenol, calculated on the dried basis. Meets the requirements for Identification, Melting range (64.5–68.5 °C), Specific rotation (−0.05° to +0.05°, calculated on the dried basis), Loss on drying (not more than 0.5%), Residue on ignition (not more than 0.1%), Aminopropanol (not more than 0.10%), and Organic volatile impurities.

PANTOTHENIC ACID

Chemical name: (+)-(*R*)-3-(2,4-Dihydroxy-3,3-dimethylbutyramido)propionic acid.

Molecular formula: $C_9H_{17}NO_5$.

Molecular weight: 219.2.

Description: Unstable, viscous oil. Extremely hygroscopic.

Solubility: Freely soluble in water, in ethyl acetate, in dioxane, and in glacial acetic acid; moderately soluble in ether and in amyl alcohol; practically insoluble in chloroform.

USP requirements: Pantothenic Acid Tablets—Not in USP.

PAPAIN

Description: Papain USP—White to light tan, amorphous powder.

Solubility: Papain USP—Soluble in water, the solution being colorless to light yellow and more or less opalescent; practically insoluble in alcohol, in chloroform, and in ether.

USP requirements:

Papain USP—Preserve in tight, light-resistant containers, in a cool place. A purified proteolytic substance derived from *Carica papaya* Linné (Fam. Caricaceae). Papain, when assayed as directed in *USP/NF,* contains not less than 6000 Units per mg. Papain of a higher digestive power may be reduced to the official standard by admixture with papain of lower activity, lactose, or other suitable diluents. One USP Unit of Papain activity is the activity that releases the equivalent of 1 mcg of tyrosine from a specified casein substrate under the conditions of the *Assay,* using the enzyme concentration that liberates 40 mcg of tyrosine per mL of test solution. Meets the requirements for pH (4.8–6.2, in a solution [1 in 50]) and Loss on drying (not more than 7.0%).

Papain Tablets for Topical Solution USP—Preserve in tight, light-resistant containers in a cool place. Contain not less than 100.0% of the labeled potency. Meet the requirements for Completeness of solution, Microbial limits, Disintegration (not more than 15 minutes at 23 ±2 °C), and pH (6.9–8.0, determined in a solution of 1 Tablet in 10 mL).

PAPAVERINE

Chemical name: Papaverine hydrochloride—Isoquinoline, 1-[(3,4-dimethoxyphenyl)methyl]-6,7-dimethoxy-, hydrochloride.

Molecular formula: Papaverine hydrochloride—$C_{20}H_{21}NO_4 \cdot HCl$.

Molecular weight: Papaverine hydrochloride—375.85.

Description: Papaverine Hydrochloride USP—White crystals or white, crystalline powder. Odorless. Optically inactive. Its solutions are acid to litmus. Melts at about 220 °C, with decomposition.

Solubility: Papaverine Hydrochloride USP—Soluble in water and in chloroform; slightly soluble in alcohol; practically insoluble in ether.

USP requirements:

Papaverine Hydrochloride USP—Preserve in tight, light-resistant containers. Contains not less than 98.5% and not more than 100.5% of papaverine hydrochloride, calculated on the dried basis. Meets the requirements for Completeness of solution, Identification, pH (3.0–4.5, in a solution [1 in 50]), Loss on drying (not more than 0.5%), Residue on ignition (not more than 0.1%), and Cryptopine, thebaine, or other organic impurities.

Papaverine Hydrochloride Extended-release Capsules—Not in USP.

Papaverine Hydrochloride Injection USP—Preserve in single-dose or in multiple-dose containers, preferably of Type I glass. A sterile solution of Papaverine Hydrochloride in Water for Injection. Contains the labeled amount, within ±5%. Meets the requirements for Identification, Bacterial endotoxins, pH (not less than 3.0), and Injections.

Papaverine Hydrochloride Tablets USP—Preserve in tight containers. Contain the labeled amount, within ±7%. Meet the requirements for Identification, Dissolution (80% in 30 minutes in water in Apparatus 1 at 100 rpm), and Uniformity of dosage units.

PARACHLOROPHENOL

Chemical name: Phenol, 4-chloro-.

Molecular formula: C_6H_5ClO.

Molecular weight: 128.56.

Description: Parachlorophenol USP—White or pink crystals having a characteristic phenolic odor. When undiluted, it whitens and cauterizes the skin and mucous membranes. Melts at about 42 °C.

Solubility: Parachlorophenol USP—Sparingly soluble in water and in liquid petrolatum; very soluble in alcohol, in glycerin, in chloroform, in ether, and in fixed and volatile oils; soluble in petrolatum.

USP requirements: Parachlorophenol USP—Preserve in tight, light-resistant containers. Contains not less than 99.0% and not more than 100.5% of parachlorophenol. Meets the requirements for Clarity and reaction of solution, Identification, Congealing temperature (42–44 °C), Nonvolatile residue (not more than 0.1%), and Chloride.

CAMPHORATED PARACHLOROPHENOL

Chemical name:

Camphor—Bicyclo[2.2.1]heptane-2-one, 1,7,7-trimethyl-.
Parachlorophenol—Phenol, 4-chloro-.

Molecular formula:

Camphor—$C_{10}H_{16}O$.
Parachlorophenol—C_6H_5ClO.

Molecular weight:

Camphor—152.24.
Parachlorophenol—128.56.

Description:

Camphor USP—Colorless or white crystals, granules, or crystalline masses; or colorless to white, translucent, tough masses. Has a penetrating, characteristic odor. Specific gravity is about 0.99. Slowly volatilizes at ordinary temperatures.

Parachlorophenol USP—White or pink crystals having a characteristic phenolic odor. When undiluted, it whitens and cauterizes the skin and mucous membranes. Melts at about 42 °C.

Solubility:

Camphor USP—Slightly soluble in water; very soluble in alcohol, in chloroform, and in ether; freely soluble in carbon disulfide, in solvent hexane, and in fixed and volatile oils.

Parachlorophenol USP—Sparingly soluble in water and in liquid petrolatum; very soluble in alcohol, in glycerin, in chloroform, in ether, and in fixed and volatile oils; soluble in petrolatum.

USP requirements: Camphorated Parachlorophenol USP—Preserve in tight, light-resistant containers. A triturated mixture. Contains not less than 33.0% and not more than 37.0% of parachlorophenol and not less than 63.0% and not more than 67.0% of camphor. The sum of the percentages of parachlorophenol and camphor is not less than 97.0% and not more than 103.0%.

PARAFFIN

Description: Paraffin NF—Colorless or white, more or less translucent mass showing a crystalline structure. Odorless. Slightly greasy to the touch.

NF category: Stiffening agent.

Solubility: Paraffin NF—Insoluble in water and in alcohol; freely soluble in chloroform, in ether, in volatile oils, and in most warm fixed oils; slightly soluble in dehydrated alcohol.

NF requirements: Paraffin NF—Preserve in well-closed containers, and avoid exposure to excessive heat. A purified mixture of solid hydrocarbons obtained from petroleum. Meets the requirements for Identification, Congealing range (47–65 °C), Reaction, and Readily carbonizable substances.

SYNTHETIC PARAFFIN

Description: Synthetic Paraffin NF—Very hard, white, practically odorless wax. Contains mostly long-chain, unbranched, saturated hydrocarbons, with a small amount of branched hydrocarbons. Is represented by the formula C_nH_{2n+2}, in which n may range from 20 to about 100. The average molecular weight may range from 400 to 1400.

NF category: Stiffening agent.

Solubility: Synthetic Paraffin NF—Insoluble in water; very slightly soluble in aliphatic, oxygenated, and halogenated hydrocarbon solvents; slightly soluble in aromatic and normal paraffinic solvents.

NF requirements: Synthetic Paraffin NF—Preserve in well-closed containers. Synthesized by the Fischer-Tropsch process from carbon monoxide and hydrogen, which are catalytically converted to a mixture of paraffin hydrocarbons; the lower molecular weight fractions are removed by distillation, and the residue is hydrogenated and further treated by percolation through activated charcoal. This mixture may be fractionated into its components by a solvent separation method, using a suitable synthetic isoparaffinic petroleum hydrocarbon solvent. The labeling indicates its congealing temperature, viscosity, and needle penetration range under specified conditions. Meets the requirements for Identification, Absorptivity (not more than 0.01), Heavy metals (not more than 0.002%), and Oil content (not more than 0.5%).

PARALDEHYDE

Chemical name: 1,3,5-Trioxane, 2,4,6-trimethyl-.

Molecular formula: $C_6H_{12}O_3$.

Molecular weight: 132.16.

Description: Paraldehyde USP—Colorless, transparent liquid. Has a strong, characteristic but not unpleasant or pungent odor. Specific gravity is about 0.99.

Solubility: Paraldehyde USP—Soluble in water, but less soluble in boiling water. Miscible with alcohol, with chloroform, with ether, and with volatile oils.

USP requirements:

Paraldehyde USP—Preserve in well-filled, tight, light-resistant containers, preferably of Type I or Type II glass, holding not more than 30 mL, at a temperature not exceeding 25 °C. Paraldehyde may be shipped in bulk containers holding a minimum of 22.5 kg (50 lb) to commercial drug repackagers only. The label of all containers of Paraldehyde, including those dispensed by the pharmacist, includes a statement directing the user to discard the unused contents of any container that has been opened for more than 24 hours. (Note: The label of bulk containers of Paraldehyde directs the commercial drug repackager to demonstrate compliance with the USP purity tests for Paraldehyde immediately prior to repackaging, and not to repackage from a container that has been opened longer than 24 hours.) Meets the requirements for Identification, Congealing temperature (not lower than 11 °C), Distilling range (120–126 °C), Acidity (not more than 0.5% as acetic acid), Nonvolatile residue (not more than 0.06%), Chloride, Sulfate, and Acetaldehyde (not more than 0.4%).

Note: Paraldehyde is subject to oxidation to form acetic acid. It may contain a suitable stabilizer.

Sterile Paraldehyde—Not in USP.

PARAMETHADIONE

Chemical group: Oxazolidinedione.

Chemical name: 2,4-Oxazolidinedione, 5-ethyl-3,5-dimethyl-.

Molecular formula: $C_7H_{11}NO_3$.

Molecular weight: 157.17.

Description: Paramethadione USP—Clear, colorless liquid. May have an aromatic odor. A solution (1 in 40) has a pH of about 6.

Solubility: Paramethadione USP—Sparingly soluble in water; freely soluble in alcohol, in chloroform, and in ether.

USP requirements:

Paramethadione USP—Preserve in tight containers. Contains not less than 98.0% and not more than 100.5% of paramethadione. Meets the requirements for Identification, Refractive index (1.449–1.501), Residue on ignition (not more than 0.1%), Urethane (not more than 5 ppm), Ordinary impurities, and Organic volatile impurities.

Paramethadione Capsules USP—Preserve in tight containers. Contain the labeled amount, within ±10%. Meet the requirements for Identification and Uniformity of dosage units.

Paramethadione Oral Solution USP—Preserve in tight, light-resistant containers. A solution of Paramethadione in dilute Alcohol. Contains, in each mL, not less than 282 mg and not more than 318 mg of paramethadione. Meets the requirements for Identification and Alcohol content (62.0–68.0%).

PARAMETHASONE

Chemical name: Paramethasone acetate—Pregna-1,4-diene-3,20-dione, 21-(acetyloxy)-6-fluoro-11,17-dihydroxy-16-methyl-, (6 alpha,11 beta,16 alpha)-.

Molecular formula: Paramethasone acetate—$C_{24}H_{31}FO_6$.

Molecular weight: Paramethasone acetate—434.50.

Description: Paramethasone Acetate USP—Fluffy, white to creamy white, odorless, crystalline powder. Melts at about 240 °C, with decomposition.

Solubility: Paramethasone Acetate USP—Insoluble in water; soluble in chloroform, in ether, and in methanol.

USP requirements:

Paramethasone Acetate USP—Preserve in tight containers. Contains not less than 95.0% and not more than 101.0% of paramethasone acetate, calculated on the dried basis. Meets the requirements for Identification, Specific rotation (+67° to +77°, calculated on the dried basis), X-ray diffraction, and Loss on drying (not more than 1.0%).

Paramethasone Acetate Tablets USP—Preserve in well-closed containers. Contain the labeled amount, within ±15%. Meet the requirements for Identification, Disintegration (15 minutes, the use of disks being omitted), and Uniformity of dosage units.

PAREGORIC

USP requirements: Paregoric USP—Preserve in tight, light-resistant containers, and avoid exposure to direct sunlight and to excessive heat. Yields, from each 100 mL, not less than 35 mg and not more than 45 mg of anhydrous morphine.

Paregoric may be prepared as follows: 4.3 grams of Powdered Opium, Suitable essential oil(s), 3.8 grams of Benzoic Acid, 900 mL of Diluted Alcohol, and 38 mL of Glycerin to make about 950 mL. Macerate for 5 days the Powdered Opium, Benzoic Acid, and essential oil(s), with occasional agitation, in a mixture of 900 mL of Diluted Alcohol and 38 mL of Glycerin. Then filter, and pass enough Diluted Alcohol through the filter to obtain 950 mL of total filtrate. Assay a portion of this filtrate as directed, and dilute the remainder with a sufficient quantity of Diluted Alcohol containing, in each 100 mL, 400 mg of Benzoic Acid, 4 mL of Glycerin, and sufficient essential oil(s) to yield a solution containing, in each 100 mL, 40 mg of anhydrous morphine.

Meets the requirement for Alcohol content (43.0–47.0%).

Note: Paregoric may be prepared also by using Opium or Opium Tincture instead of Powdered Opium, the anhydrous morphine content being adjusted to 40 mg in each 100 mL and the alcohol content being adjusted to 45%.

PARGYLINE

Chemical name: Pargyline hydrochloride—Benzenemethanamine, *N*-methyl-*N*-2-propynyl-, hydrochloride.

Molecular formula: Pargyline hydrochloride—$C_{11}H_{13}N \cdot HCl$.

Molecular weight: Pargyline hydrochloride—195.69.

Description: Pargyline Hydrochloride USP—White or practically white, crystalline powder, having a slight odor. Sublimes slowly at elevated temperatures.

Solubility: Pargyline Hydrochloride USP—Very soluble in water; freely soluble in alcohol and in chloroform; very slightly soluble in acetone.

USP requirements:

Pargyline Hydrochloride USP—Preserve in tight containers. Contains not less than 98.0% and not more than 101.0% of pargyline hydrochloride, calculated on the anhydrous basis. Meets the requirements for Identification, Melting range (158–162 °C), Water (not more than 1.0%), Residue on ignition (not more than 0.2%), Heavy metals (not more than 0.002%), Ordinary impurities, and Organic volatile impurities.

Pargyline Hydrochloride Tablets USP—Preserve in well-closed containers. Contain the labeled amount, within ±10%. Meet the requirements for Identification, Dissolution (70% in 60 minutes in phosphate buffer [pH 6.0] in Apparatus 2 at 100 rpm), and Uniformity of dosage units.

PAROMOMYCIN

Chemical name: Paromomycin sulfate—D-Streptamine, *O*-2-amino-2-deoxy-alpha-D-glucopyranosyl-(1→4)-*O*-[*O*-2,6-diamino-2,6-dideoxy-beta-L-idopyranosyl-(1→3)-beta-D-ribofuranosyl-(1→5)]-2-deoxy-, sulfate (salt).

Molecular formula: Paromomycin sulfate—$C_{23}H_{45}N_5O_{14} \cdot xH_2SO_4$.

Molecular weight: 615.64.

Description: Paromomycin Sulfate USP—Creamy white to light yellow powder. Odorless or practically so. Very hygroscopic.

Solubility: Paromomycin Sulfate USP—Very soluble in water; insoluble in alcohol, in chloroform, and in ether.

USP requirements:

Paromomycin Sulfate USP—Preserve in tight containers. The sulfate salt of an antibiotic substance or substances produced by the growth of *Streptomyces rimosus* var. *paromomycinus*, or a mixture of two or more such salts. Has a potency equivalent to not less than 675 mcg of paromomycin per mg, calculated on the dried basis. Meets the requirements for Identification, Specific rotation (+50° to +55°, calculated on the anhydrous basis), pH (5.0–7.5, in a solution [3 in 100]), Loss on drying (not more than 5.0%), and Residue on ignition (not more than 2.0%).

Paromomycin Sulfate Capsules USP—Preserve in tight containers. Contain an amount of paromomycin sulfate equivalent to the labeled amount of paromomycin, within −10% to +25%. Meet the requirements for Identification, Disintegration (15 minutes, the use of disks being omitted), Uniformity of dosage units, and Loss on drying (not more than 7.0%).

Paromomycin Sulfate Syrup USP—Preserve in tight containers. Contains an amount of paromomycin sulfate equivalent to the labeled amount of paromomycin, within −10% to +30%. Meets the requirements for pH (7.5–8.5), Deliverable volume (multiple-unit containers), and Uniformity of dosage units (single-unit containers).

PAROXETINE

Chemical name: Paroxetine hydrochloride—(–)-*trans*-5-(4-*p*-Fluorophenyl-3-piperidylmethoxy)-1,3-benzodioxole hydrochloride.

Molecular formula: Paroxetine hydrochloride—$C_{19}H_{20}FNO_3 \cdot HCl$.

Molecular weight: Paroxetine hydrochloride—365.8.

Description: Paroxetine hydrochloride—Odorless, off-white powder, having a melting point range of 120–138 °C.

Solubility: Paroxetine hydrochloride—Soluble in water (5.4 mg/mL).

USP requirements: Paroxetine Hydrochloride Tablets—Not in USP.

PEANUT OIL

Description: Peanut Oil NF—Colorless or pale yellow oily liquid. May have a characteristic, nutty odor.

NF category: Solvent; vehicle (oleaginous).

Solubility: Peanut Oil NF—Very slightly soluble in alcohol. Miscible with ether, with chloroform, and with carbon disulfide.

NF requirements: Peanut Oil NF—Preserve in tight, light-resistant containers, and prevent exposure to excessive heat. The refined fixed oil obtained from the seed kernels of one or more of the cultivated varieties of *Arachis hypogaea* Linné (Fam. Leguminosae). Meets the requirements for Identification, Specific gravity (0.912–0.920), Refractive index (1.462–1.464 at 40 °C), Heavy metals (not more than 0.001%), Cottonseed oil, Rancidity, Solidification range of fatty acids (26–33 °C), Free fatty acids, Iodine value (84–100), Saponification value (185–195), and Unsaponifiable matter (not more than 1.5%).

PECTIN

Chemical name: Pectin.

Description: Pectin USP—Coarse or fine powder, yellowish white in color, almost odorless.

NF category: Suspending and/or viscosity-increasing agent.

Solubility: Pectin USP—Almost completely soluble in 20 parts of water, forming a viscous, opalescent, colloidal solution that flows readily and is acid to litmus. Is practically insoluble in alcohol or in diluted alcohol and in other organic solvents. Pectin dissolves in water more readily if first moistened with alcohol, glycerin, or simple syrup, or if first mixed with 3 or more parts of sucrose.

USP requirements: Pectin USP—Preserve in tight containers. A purified carbohydrate product obtained from the dilute acid extract of the inner portion of the rind of citrus fruits or from apple pomace. Consists chiefly of partially methoxylated polygalacturonic acids. Label it to indicate whether it is of apple or of citrus origin. Pectin yields not less than 6.7% of methoxy groups and not less than 74.0% of galacturonic acid, calculated on the dried basis. Meets the requirements for Identification, Microbial limit, Loss on drying (not more than 10.0%), Arsenic (not more than 3 ppm), Lead, and Sugars and organic acids.

Note: Commercial pectin for the production of jellied food products is standardized to the convenient "150 jelly grade" by addition of dextrose or other sugars, and sometimes contains sodium citrate or other buffer salts. This monograph refers to the pure pectin to which no such additions have been made.

PEG 3350 AND ELECTROLYTES

For *Polyethylene Glycol, Sodium Bicarbonate, Sodium Chloride, Sodium Sulfate,* and *Potassium Chloride*—See individual listings for chemistry information.

USP requirements:

PEG 3350 and Electrolytes for Oral Solution USP—Preserve in tight containers. A mixture of Polyethylene Glycol 3350, Sodium Bicarbonate, Sodium Chloride, Sodium Sulfate (anhydrous), and Potassium Chloride. When constituted as directed in the labeling it contains the labeled amounts of polyethylene glycol 3350, potassium, sodium, bicarbonate, chloride, and sulfate, within ±10%, the labeled amounts per liter being 10 mmol (10 mEq) of potassium, 125 mmol (125 mEq) of sodium, 20 mmol (20 mEq) of bicarbonate, 35 mmol (35 mEq) of chloride, and 40 mmol (80 mEq) of sulfate. Meets the requirements for Completeness of solution, Identification, pH (7.5–9.5, in the solution prepared as directed in the labeling), Uniformity of dosage units, and Osmolarity (235–304 mOsmol, in the solution prepared as directed in the labeling).

Polyethylene Glycol 3350 and Electrolytes Oral Solution—Not in USP.

PEGADEMASE

Source: Pegademase bovine—A conjugate of numerous strands of monomethoxypolyethylene glycol (PEG), covalently attached to the enzyme adenosine deaminase (ADA); ADA used in the manufacture of pegademase bovine injection is derived from bovine intestine.

Chemical name: Pegademase bovine—Deaminase, adenosine, cattle, reaction product with succinic anhydride, esters with polyethylene glycol, mono-Me ether.

Description: Pegademase bovine injection—Clear, colorless solution; pH 7.2–7.4.

USP requirements: Pegademase Bovine Injection—Not in USP.

PEGASPARGASE

Chemical name: Pegaspargase.

Molecular weight: 460,000.

USP requirements: Pegaspargase Injection—Not in USP.

PEMOLINE

Chemical group: Oxazolidine.

Chemical name: 4(5*H*)-Oxazolone, 2-amino-5-phenyl-.

Molecular formula: $C_9H_8N_2O_2$.

Molecular weight: 176.17.

Description: White, odorless powder.

Solubility: Relatively insoluble (less than 1 mg/mL) in water, in chloroform, in ether, and in acetone; solubility in 95% ethyl alcohol 2.2 mg/mL.

USP requirements:

Pemoline Tablets—Not in USP.
Pemoline Chewable Tablets—Not in USP.

PENBUTOLOL

Chemical name: Penbutolol sulfate—2-Propanol, 1-(2-cyclopentylphenoxy)-3-[(1,1-dimethylethyl)amino]-, (*S*)-, sulfate (2:1) (salt).

Molecular formula: Penbutolol sulfate—$(C_{18}H_{29}NO_2)_2 \cdot H_2SO_4$.

Molecular weight: Penbutolol sulfate—680.94.

Description: White, odorless, crystalline powder.

pKa: 9.3.

Solubility: Soluble in methanol, in ethanol, and in chloroform.

Other characteristics: Lipid solubility—Moderate.

USP requirements: Penbutolol Sulfate Tablets—Not in USP.

PENICILLAMINE

Chemical name: D-Valine, 3-mercapto-.

Molecular formula: $C_5H_{11}NO_2S$.

Molecular weight: 149.21.

Description: Penicillamine USP—White or practically white, crystalline powder, having a slight, characteristic odor.

Solubility: Penicillamine USP—Freely soluble in water; slightly soluble in alcohol; insoluble in chloroform and in ether.

USP requirements:

Penicillamine USP—Preserve in tight containers. Contains not less than 97.0% and not more than 100.5% of penicillamine, calculated on the dried basis. Meets the requirements for Identification, Specific rotation (−60.5° to −64.5°, calculated on the dried basis), pH (4.5–5.5, in a solution [1 in 100]), Loss on drying (not more than 0.5%), Residue on ignition (not more than 0.1%), Heavy metals (not more than 0.002%), Limit of penicillin activity, Mercury (not more than 0.002%), and Penicillamine disulfide (not more than 1.0%).

Penicillamine Capsules USP—Preserve in tight containers. Contain the labeled amount, within ±10%. Meet the requirements for Identification, Dissolution (80% in 30 minutes in 0.1 *N* hydrochloric acid in Apparatus 1 at 100 rpm), Uniformity of dosage units, Water (not more than 7.5%), and Penicillamine disulfide (not more than 2.0%).

Penicillamine Tablets USP—Preserve in tight containers. Contain the labeled amount, within ±10%. Meet the requirements for Identification, Dissolution (60% in 60 minutes in 0.5% disodium EDTA in Apparatus 1 at 150 rpm), Uniformity of dosage units, Loss on drying (not more than 3.0%), and Penicillamine disulfide (not more than 3.0%).

PENICILLIN G

Chemical name:

Penicillin G benzathine—4-Thia-1-azabicyclo[3.2.0]heptane-2-carboxylic acid, 3,3-dimethyl-7-oxo-6-[(phenylacetyl)-amino]-, [2*S*-(2 alpha,5 alpha,6 beta)]-, compd. with *N,N'*-bis(phenylmethyl)-1,2-ethanediamine (2:1), tetrahydrate.

Penicillin G potassium—4-Thia-1-azabicyclo[3.2.0]heptane-2-carboxylic acid, 3,3-dimethyl-7-oxo-6-[(phenylacetyl)amino]-, monopotassium salt, [2*S*-(2 alpha,5 alpha,6 beta)]-.

Penicillin G procaine—4-Thia-1-azabicyclo[3.2.0]heptane-2-carboxylic acid, 3,3-dimethyl-7-oxo-6-[(phenylacetyl)amino]-, [2*S*-(2 alpha,5 alpha,6 beta)]-, compd. with 2-(diethylamino)ethyl 4-aminobenzoate (1:1) monohydrate.

Penicillin G sodium (sterile)—4-Thia-1-azabicyclo-[3.2.0]heptane-2-carboxylic acid, 3,3-dimethyl-7-oxo-6-[(phenylacetyl)amino]-, [2*S*-(2 alpha,5 alpha,6 beta)]-, monosodium salt.

Molecular formula:

Penicillin G benzathine—$(C_{16}H_{18}N_2O_4S)_2 \cdot C_{16}H_{20}N_2 \cdot 4H_2O$.
Penicillin G potassium—$C_{16}H_{17}KN_2O_4S$.
Penicillin G procaine—$C_{16}H_{18}N_2O_4S \cdot C_{13}H_{20}N_2O_2 \cdot H_2O$.
Penicillin G sodium—$C_{16}H_{17}N_2NaO_4S$.

Molecular weight:

Penicillin G benzathine—981.19.
Penicillin G potassium—372.48.
Penicillin G procaine—588.72.
Penicillin G sodium—356.37.

Description:

Penicillin G Benzathine USP—White, odorless, crystalline powder.

Sterile Penicillin G Potassium USP—Colorless or white crystals, or white, crystalline powder. Is odorless or practically so, and is moderately hygroscopic. Its solutions are dextrorotatory. Its solutions retain substantially full potency for several days at temperatures below 15 °C, but are rapidly inactivated by acids, alkali hydroxides, glycerin, and oxidizing agents.

Sterile Penicillin G Procaine USP—White crystals or white, very fine, microcrystalline powder. Is odorless or practically odorless, and is relatively stable in air. Its solutions are dextrorotatory. Is rapidly inactivated by acids, by alkali hydroxides, and by oxidizing agents.

Sterile Penicillin G Sodium USP—Colorless or white crystals or white to slightly yellow, crystalline powder. Is odorless or practically odorless, and is moderately hygroscopic. Its solutions are dextrorotatory. Is relatively stable in air, but is inactivated by prolonged heating at about 100 °C, especially in the presence of moisture. Its solutions lose potency fairly rapidly at room temperature, but retain substantially full potency for several days at temperatures below 15 °C. Its solutions are rapidly inactivated by acids, alkali hydroxides, oxidizing agents, and penicillinase.

Solubility:

Penicillin G Benzathine USP—Very slightly soluble in water; sparingly soluble in alcohol.

Sterile Penicillin G Potassium USP—Very soluble in water, in saline TS, and in dextrose solutions; sparingly soluble in alcohol.

Sterile Penicillin G Procaine USP—Slightly soluble in water; soluble in alcohol and in chloroform.

USP requirements:

Penicillin G Benzathine USP—Preserve in tight containers. Has a potency of not less than 1090 Penicillin G Units and not more than 1272 Penicillin G Units per mg. Meets the requirements for Identification, Crystallinity, pH (4.0–6.5), Water (5.0–8.0%), Penicillin G content (61.3–71.6%), and Benzathine content (24.0–27.0%, calculated on the anhydrous basis).

Sterile Penicillin G Benzathine USP—Preserve in Containers for Sterile Solids. It is Penicillin G Benzathine suitable for parenteral use. Has a potency of not less than 1090 and not more than 1272 Penicillin G Units per mg. Meets the requirements for Bacterial endotoxins and Sterility, and for Identification test, pH, Water, Crystallinity, Penicillin G content, and Benzathine content under Penicillin G Benzathine.

Penicillin G Benzathine Oral Suspension USP—Preserve in tight containers. Contains an amount of penicillin G benzathine equivalent to the labeled amount of penicillin G, within −10% to +20%. Contains one or more suitable buffers, colors, dispersants, flavors, and preservatives. Meets the requirements for Identification, pH (6.0–7.0), Uniformity of dosage units (single-unit containers), and Deliverable volume (multiple-unit containers).

Sterile Penicillin G Benzathine Suspension USP—Preserve in single-dose or in multiple-dose containers, preferably of Type I or Type II glass, in a refrigerator. A sterile suspension of Sterile Penicillin G Benzathine in Water for Injection with one or more suitable buffers, dispersants, preservatives, and suspending agents. Contains an amount of penicillin G benzathine equivalent to the labeled amount of penicillin G, within −10% to +15%. Meets the requirements for Identification, Bacterial endotoxins, Sterility, pH (5.0–7.5), and Injections.

Penicillin G Benzathine Tablets USP—Preserve in tight containers. Contain an amount of penicillin G benzathine equivalent to the labeled amount of penicillin G, within −10% to +20%. Meet the requirements for Identification, Disintegration (60 minutes in simulated gastric fluid TS), Uniformity of dosage units, and Water (not more than 8.0%).

Sterile Penicillin G Benzathine and Penicillin G Procaine Suspension USP—Preserve in single-dose or in multiple-dose containers, preferably of Type I or Type III glass. A sterile suspension of Sterile Penicillin G Benzathine and Sterile Penicillin G Procaine in Water for Injection. Contains the labeled amounts, within −10% to +15%. Meets the requirements for Identification and pH (5.0–7.5), for Pyrogen and Sterility under Sterile Penicillin G Procaine Suspension, and for Injections.

Penicillin G Potassium USP—Preserve in tight containers. Has a potency of not less than 1440 Penicillin G Units and not more than 1680 Penicillin G Units per mg. Meets the requirements for Identification, Crystallinity, pH (5.0–7.5, in a solution containing 60 mg per mL), Loss on drying (not more than 1.5%), and Penicillin G content (80.8–94.3%).

Penicillin G Potassium Capsules USP—Preserve in tight containers. Contain the labeled number of Penicillin G Units, within −10% to +20%. Meet the requirements for Identification, Dissolution (75% in 45 minutes in phosphate buffer [pH 6.0] in Apparatus 1 at 100 rpm), Uniformity of dosage units, and Loss on drying (not more than 1.5%).

Penicillin G Potassium Injection USP—Preserve in single-dose containers. Maintain in the frozen state. A sterile isoosmotic solution of Penicillin G Potassium in Water for Injection. Contains one or more suitable buffers and a tonicity-adjusting agent. The label states that it is to be thawed just prior to use, describes conditions for proper storage of the resultant solution, and directs that the solution is not to be refrozen. Contains the labeled number of Penicillin G Units, within −10% to +15%. Meets the requirements for Identification, Bacterial endotoxins, Sterility, pH (5.5–8.0), Particulate matter, and Labeling under Injections.

Penicillin G Potassium for Injection USP—Preserve in Containers for Sterile Solids. A sterile, dry mixture of Penicillin G Potassium with not less than 4.0% and not more than 5.0% of Sodium Citrate, of which not more than 0.15% may be replaced by Citric Acid. Has a potency of not less than 1355 and not more than 1595 Penicillin G Units per mg and, where packaged for dispensing, contains the labeled number of Penicillin G Units within −10% to +20%. Meets the requirements for Constituted solution, Identification, Crystallinity, Bacterial endotoxins, Sterility, pH (6.0–8.5, in a solution containing 60 mg per mL or, where packaged for dispensing, in the solution constituted as directed in the labeling), Loss on drying (not more than 1.5%), Particulate matter, and Penicillin G content (76.3–89.8%), and for Uniformity of dosage units, and Labeling under Injections.

Penicillin G Potassium for Oral Solution USP—Preserve in tight containers. A dry mixture of Penicillin G Potassium and one or more suitable buffers, colors, diluents, flavors, and preservatives. Contains the labeled number of Penicillin G Units when constituted as directed in the labeling, within −10% to +30%. Meets the requirements for Identification, pH (5.5–7.5, in the solution constituted as directed in the labeling), Water (not more than 1.0%), Uniformity of dosage units (single-unit containers), and Deliverable volume (multiple-unit containers).

Sterile Penicillin G Potassium USP—Preserve in Containers for Sterile Solids. It is Penicillin G Potassium suitable for parenteral use. Has a potency of not less than 1440 Penicillin G Units and not more than 1680 Penicillin G Units per mg and, where packaged for dispensing, contains the labeled number of Penicillin G Units, within −10% to +15%. Meets the requirements for Constituted solution, Bacterial endotoxins, Sterility, and Particulate matter, for Identification tests, pH (5.0–7.5, in a solution containing 60 mg per mL), Loss on drying (not more than 1.5%), Crystallinity, and Penicillin G content (80.8–94.3%) under Penicillin G Potassium, and for Uniformity of dosage units and Labeling under Injections.

Penicillin G Potassium Tablets USP—Preserve in tight containers. Contain the labeled number of Penicillin G Units, within −10% to +20%. Meet the requirements for Identification, Dissolution (70% in 60 minutes in phosphate buffer [pH 6.0] in Apparatus 2 at 75 rpm), Uniformity of dosage units, and Loss on drying (not more than 1.0%).

Penicillin G Potassium Tablets for Oral Solution USP—Preserve in tight containers. Contain the labeled number of Penicillin G Units, within −10% to +20%. Meet the requirements for Identification and Loss on drying (not more than 1.0%), and for Uniformity of dosage units under Penicillin G Potassium Tablets.

Penicillin G Procaine Intramammary Infusion USP—Preserve in well-closed disposable syringes. A suspension of Penicillin G Procaine in a suitable vegetable oil vehicle. Label it to indicate that it is for veterinary use only. Contains an amount of penicillin G procaine equivalent to the labeled amount of penicillin G, within −10% to +15%. Meets the requirements for Identification and Water (not more than 1.4%).

Sterile Penicillin G Procaine USP—Preserve in Containers for Sterile Solids. It is penicillin G procaine suitable for parenteral use. Has a potency of not less than 900 Penicillin G Units and not more than 1050 Penicillin G Units per mg. Meets the requirements for Identification, Crystallinity, Bacterial endotoxins, Sterility, pH (5.0–7.5, in a [saturated] solution containing about 300 mg per mL), Water (2.8–4.2%), and Penicillin G and procaine contents (37.5–43.0%).

Sterile Penicillin G Procaine Suspension USP—Preserve in single-dose or in multiple-dose containers, preferably of Type I or Type III glass, in a refrigerator. A sterile suspension of Sterile Penicillin G Procaine in Water for Injection and contains one or more suitable buffers, dispersants, or suspending agents, and a suitable preservative. It may contain procaine hydrochloride in a concentration not exceeding 2.0%. Contains an amount of penicillin G procaine equivalent to the labeled amount of penicillin G, within −10% to +15%, the labeled amount being not less than 300,000 Penicillin G Units per mL or per container. Meets the requirements for Identification, Pyrogen, Sterility, pH (5.0–7.5), and for Injections.

Sterile Penicillin G Procaine for Suspension USP—Preserve in single-dose or in multiple-dose containers, preferably of Type I or Type III glass. A sterile mixture of Sterile Penicillin G Procaine and one or more suitable buffers, dispersants, or suspending agents, and preservatives. Contains an amount of penicillin G procaine equivalent to the labeled amount of penicillin G, within −10% to +15%, the labeled amount being not less than 300,000 Penicillin G Units per container or per mL of constituted Suspension. Meets the requirements for Identification, pH (5.0–7.5, when constituted as directed in the labeling), and Water (2.8–4.2%), for Pyrogen and Sterility under Sterile Penicillin G Procaine Suspension, and for Injections and Uniformity of dosage units.

Penicillin G Sodium for Injection USP—Preserve in Containers for Sterile Solids. A sterile mixture of penicillin G sodium with not less than 4.0% and not more than 5.0% of Sodium Citrate, of which not more than 0.15% may be replaced by Citric Acid. Has a potency of not less than 1420 Penicillin G Units and not more than 1667 Penicillin G Units per mg and, where packaged for dispensing, contains an amount of penicillin G sodium equivalent to the labeled amount of penicillin G, within −10% to +20%. Meets the requirements for Constituted solution, Identification, Crystallinity, Bacterial endotoxins, pH (6.0–7.5, in a solution containing 60 mg per mL), Loss on drying (not more than 1.5%), Particulate matter, and Penicillin G content (80.0–93.8%), for Sterility under Sterile Penicillin G Sodium, and for Uniformity of dosage units and Labeling under Injections.

Note: It contains 2.0 mEq of sodium per million Penicillin G Units.

Sterile Penicillin G Sodium USP—Preserve in containers for Sterile Solids. It is penicillin G sodium suitable for parenteral use. Has a potency of not less than 1500 Penicillin G Units and not more than 1750 Penicillin G Units per mg. In addition, where packaged for dispensing, contains an amount of penicillin G sodium equivalent to the labeled amount of penicillin G, within −10% to +15%. Meets the requirements for Constituted solution, Identification, Crystallinity, Bacterial endotoxins, Sterility, pH

(5.0–7.5, in a solution containing 60 mg per mL), Loss on drying (not more than 1.5%), Particulate matter, and Penicillin G content (84.5–98.5%), and for Uniformity of dosage units and Labeling under Injections.

PENICILLIN G AND ALUMINUM STEARATE

Chemical name:
Penicillin G procaine—4-Thia-1-azabicyclo[3.2.0]heptane-2-carboxylic acid, 3,3-dimethyl-7-oxo-6-[(phenylacetyl)-amino]-,[2*S*-(2alpha,5alpha,6beta]-,compd.with2-(diethyl-amino)ethyl 4-aminobenzoate (1:1) monohydrate.
Aluminum stearate—Octadecanoic acid aluminum salt.

Molecular formula:
Penicillin G procaine—$C_{16}H_{18}N_2O_4S \cdot C_{13}H_{20}N_2O_2 \cdot H_2O$.
Aluminum stearate—$C_{54}H_{105}AlO_6$.

Molecular weight:
Penicillin G procaine—588.72.
Aluminum stearate—877.35.

Description: Aluminum stearate—Melting point 117–120 °C.

Solubility: Aluminum stearate—Practically insoluble in water; when freshly made, soluble in alcohol, in oil turpentine, and in mineral oils.

USP requirements: Sterile Penicillin G Procaine with Aluminum Stearate Suspension USP—Preserve in single-dose or in multiple-dose containers, preferably of Type I or Type III glass. A sterile suspension of Sterile Penicillin G Procaine in a refined vegetable oil with one or more suitable dispersants and hardening agents. Contains an amount of penicillin G procaine equivalent to the labeled amount of penicillin G, within −10% to +15%. Meets the requirements for Bacterial endotoxins, Sterility, Water (not more than 1.4%), and Injections.

PENICILLIN G AND DIHYDROSTREPTOMYCIN

For *Penicillin G* and *Dihydrostreptomycin*—See individual listings for chemistry information.

USP requirements:
Penicillin G Procaine and Dihydrostreptomycin Sulfate Intramammary Infusion USP—Preserve in well-closed, disposable syringes. A suspension of Penicillin G Procaine and Dihydrostreptomycin Sulfate in a suitable vegetable oil vehicle. Label it to indicate that it is intended for veterinary use only. Contains amounts of penicillin G procaine and dihydrostreptomycin sulfate equivalent to the labeled amounts of Penicillin G Units and dihydrostreptomycin, within −10% to +20%. Meets the requirements for Identification and Water (not more than 1.4%).
Sterile Penicillin G Procaine and Dihydrostreptomycin Sulfate Suspension USP—Preserve in single-dose or in multiple-dose, tight containers. A sterile suspension of Sterile Penicillin G Procaine in a solution of Dihydrostreptomycin Sulfate in Water for Injection, and contains one or more suitable buffers, preservatives, and dispersing or suspending agents. May contain Procaine Hydrochloride in a concentration not exceeding 2.0%. Label it to indicate that it is intended for veterinary use only. Contains amounts of penicillin G procaine and dihydrostreptomycin sulfate equivalent to the labeled amounts of Penicillin G Units and dihydrostreptomycin, within −10% to +15%. Meets the requirements for Identification, Pyrogen, Sterility, and pH (5.0–8.0).

PENICILLIN G, DIHYDROSTREPTOMYCIN, CHLORPHENIRAMINE, AND DEXAMETHASONE

For *Penicillin G, Dihydrostreptomycin, Chlorpheniramine,* and *Dexamethasone*—See individual listings for chemistry information.

USP requirements: Sterile Penicillin G Procaine, Dihydrostreptomycin Sulfate, Chlorpheniramine Maleate, and Dexamethasone Suspension USP—Preserve in single-dose or in multiple-dose, tight containers, in a cool place. A sterile suspension of Sterile Penicillin G Procaine and Dexamethasone in a solution of Sterile Dihydrostreptomycin Sulfate and Chlorpheniramine Maleate in Water for Injection. Label it to indicate that it is intended for veterinary use only. Contains one or more suitable buffers, preservatives, and dispersing or suspending agents. May contain Procaine Hydrochloride in a concentration not exceeding 2.0%. Contains amounts of penicillin G procaine and dihydrostreptomycin sulfate equivalent to the labeled amounts of Penicillin G Units and dihydrostreptomycin, within −10% to +15%. Contains the labeled amounts of chlorpheniramine maleate and dexamethasone, within ±10%. Meets the requirements for Identification, Bacterial endotoxins, and pH (5.0–6.0), for Sterility under Sterile Penicillin G Procaine and Dihydrostreptomycin Sulfate Suspension, and for Injections.

PENICILLIN G, DIHYDROSTREPTOMYCIN, AND PREDNISOLONE

For *Penicillin G, Dihydrostreptomycin,* and *Prednisolone*—See individual listings for chemistry information.

USP requirements: Sterile Penicillin G Procaine, Dihydrostreptomycin Sulfate, and Prednisolone Suspension USP—Preserve in single-dose or in multiple-dose, tight containers. A sterile suspension of Sterile Penicillin G Procaine and Prednisolone in a solution of Sterile Dihydrostreptomycin Sulfate in Water for Injection. Contains one or more suitable buffers, dispersants, preservatives, and suspending agents. Label it to indicate that it is intended for veterinary use only, and is not to be used in animals to be slaughtered for human consumption. Contains amounts of penicillin G procaine and dihydrostreptomycin sulfate equivalent to the labeled number of Penicillin G Units, within −10% to +15%, and the labeled amount of dihydrostreptomycin, within −10% to +15%. Contains the labeled amount of prednisolone, within ±10%. Meets the requirements for Identification and Bacterial endotoxins, and for Sterility and pH under Sterile Penicillin G Procaine and Dihydrostreptomycin Sulfate Suspension.

PENICILLIN G, NEOMYCIN, POLYMYXIN B, AND HYDROCORTISONE

For *Penicillin G, Neomycin, Polymyxin B,* and *Hydrocortisone*—See individual listings for chemistry information.

USP requirements: Penicillin G Procaine, Neomycin and Polymyxin B Sulfates, and Hydrocortisone Acetate Topical Suspension USP—Preserve in well-closed containers. A suspension of Penicillin G Procaine, Neomycin Sulfate, Polymyxin B Sulfate, and Hydrocortisone Acetate in Peanut Oil or Sesame Oil. Label it to indicate that it is intended for veterinary use only. Contains amounts of penicillin G procaine, neomycin sulfate, and polymyxin B sulfate equivalent to the labeled amounts of Penicillin G Units, neomycin, and polymyxin B Units, within −10% to +40%. Contains the labeled amount of hydrocortisone acetate, within ±10%. Meets the requirement for Water (not more than 1.0%).

PENICILLIN G AND NOVOBIOCIN

For *Penicillin G* and *Novobiocin*—See individual listings for chemistry information.

USP requirements: Penicillin G Procaine and Novobiocin Sodium Intramammary Infusion USP—Preserve in disposable syringes that are well-closed containers. A suspension of Penicillin G Procaine and Novobiocin Sodium in a suitable vegetable oil vehicle. Contains a suitable preservative and suspending agent. Label it to indicate that it is for veterinary use only. Contains amounts of penicillin G procaine and novobiocin sodium equivalent to the labeled amounts of Penicillin G Units and novobiocin, within −10% to +25%. Meets the requirement for Water (not more than 1.0%).

PENICILLIN V

Chemical name:
Penicillin V—4-Thia-1-azabicyclo[3.2.0]heptane-2-carboxylic acid, 3,3-dimethyl-7-oxo-6-[(phenoxyacetyl)amino]-, [2*S*-(2 alpha,5 alpha,6 beta)]-.
Penicillin V benzathine—4-Thia-1-azabicyclo[3.2.0]heptane-2-carboxylic acid, 3,3-dimethyl-7-oxo-6-[(phenoxyacetyl)-amino]-, [2*S*-(2 alpha,5 alpha,6 beta)]-, compd. with *N,N'*-bis(phenylmethyl)-1,2-ethanediamine (2:1).
Penicillin V potassium—4-Thia-1-azabicyclo[3.2.0]heptane-2-carboxylic acid, 3,3-dimethyl-7-oxo-6-[(phenoxyacetyl)amino]-, monopotassium salt, [2*S*-(2 alpha,5 alpha,6 beta)]-.

Molecular formula:
Penicillin V—$C_{16}H_{18}N_2O_5S$.
Penicillin V benzathine—$(C_{16}H_{18}N_2O_5S)_2 \cdot C_{16}H_{20}N_2$.
Penicillin V potassium—$C_{16}H_{17}KN_2O_5S$.

Molecular weight:
Penicillin V—350.39.
Penicillin V benzathine—941.13.
Penicillin V potassium—388.48.

Description:
Penicillin V USP—White, odorless, crystalline powder.
Penicillin V Benzathine USP—Practically white powder, having a characteristic odor.
Penicillin V Potassium USP—White, odorless, crystalline powder.

Solubility:
Penicillin V USP—Very slightly soluble in water; freely soluble in alcohol and in acetone; insoluble in fixed oils.
Penicillin V Benzathine USP—Very slightly soluble in water; slightly soluble in alcohol and in ether; sparingly soluble in chloroform.
Penicillin V Potassium USP—Very soluble in water; slightly soluble in alcohol; insoluble in acetone.

USP requirements:
Penicillin V USP—Preserve in tight containers. Label it to indicate that it is to be used in the manufacture of nonparenteral drugs only. Has a potency of not less than 1525 and not more than 1780 Penicillin V Units per mg. Meets the requirements for Identification, Crystallinity, pH (2.5–4.0, in a suspension containing 30 mg per mL), Water (not more than 2.0%), and Phenoxyacetic acid (not more than 0.5%).
Penicillin V for Oral Suspension USP—Preserve in tight containers. A dry mixture of Penicillin V with or without one or more suitable buffers, colors, flavors, and suspending agents. It may be labeled in terms of the weight of penicillin V contained therein, in addition to or instead of Units, on the basis that 1600 Penicillin V Units are equivalent to 1 mg of penicillin V. Contains the labeled number of Penicillin V Units, within −10% to +20%, when constituted as directed. Meets the requirements for Identification, Uniformity of dosage units (single-unit containers), Deliverable volume (multiple-unit containers), pH (2.0–4.0, in the suspension constituted as directed in the labeling), and Water (not more than 1.0%).
Penicillin V Tablets USP—Preserve in tight containers. Tablets may be labeled in terms of the weight of penicillin V contained therein, in addition to or instead of Units, on the basis that 1600 Penicillin V Units are equivalent to 1 mg of penicillin V. Contain the labeled number of Penicillin V Units, within −10% to +20%. Meet the requirements for Identification, Dissolution (75% in 45 minutes in water in Apparatus 2 at 50 rpm), Uniformity of dosage units, and Water (not more than 3.0%).
Penicillin V Benzathine USP—Preserve in tight containers. Has a potency of not less than 1060 and not more than 1240 Penicillin V Units per mg. Meets the requirements for Crystallinity, pH (4.0–6.5, in a suspension containing about 30 mg per mL), Water (5.0–8.0%), and Penicillin V content (62.3–72.5%).
Penicillin V Benazthine Oral Suspension USP—Preserve in tight containers, and store in a refrigerator. It may be labeled in terms of the weight of penicillin V contained therein, in addition to or instead of Units, on the basis that 1600 Penicillin V Units are equivalent to 1 mg of penicillin V. Contains the labeled number of Penicillin V Units, within −10% to +20%. Contains one or more suitable buffers, colors, dispersants, flavors, and preservatives. Meets the requirements for Uniformity of dosage units (single-unit containers), Deliverable volume (multiple-unit containers), and pH (6.0–7.0).
Penicillin V Potassium USP—Preserve in tight containers. Label it to indicate that it is to be used in the manufacture of nonparenteral drugs only. Has a potency of not less than 1380 and not more than 1610 Penicillin V Units per mg. Meets the requirements for Identification, Crystallinity, pH (4.0–7.5, in a solution containing 30 mg per mL), Loss on drying (not more than 1.5%), and Phenoxyacetic acid (not more than 0.5%).
Penicillin V Potassium for Oral Solution USP—Preserve in tight containers. A dry mixture of Penicillin V Potassium with or without one or more suitable buffers, colors, flavors, preservatives, and suspending agents. It may be labeled in terms of the weight of penicillin V contained therein, in addition to or instead of Units, on the basis that 1600 Penicillin V Units are equivalent to 1 mg of penicillin V. Contains the labeled number of Penicillin V Units, within −10% to +35%, when constituted as directed. Meets the requirements for Identification, pH (5.0–7.5, when constituted as directed in the labeling), Water (not more than 1.0%), Uniformity of dosage units (single-unit containers), and Deliverable volume (multiple-unit containers).
Penicillin V Potassium Tablets USP—Preserve in tight containers. Label chewable Tablets to indicate that they are to be chewed before swallowing. Tablets may be labeled in terms of the weight of penicillin V contained therein, in addition to or instead of Units, on the basis that 1600 Penicillin V Units are equivalent to 1 mg of penicillin V. Contain the labeled number of Penicillin V Units, within −10% to +20%. Meet the requirements for Identification, Dissolution (75% in 45 minutes in phosphate buffer [pH 6.0] in Apparatus 2 at 50 rpm), Uniformity of dosage units, and Loss on drying (not more than 1.5%).

PENTAERYTHRITOL TETRANITRATE

Chemical name: 1,3-Propanediol, 2,2-bis[(nitrooxy) methyl]-, dinitrate (ester).

Molecular formula: $C_5H_8N_4O_{12}$.

Molecular weight: 316.14.

Description: Diluted Pentaerythritol Tetranitrate USP—White to ivory-colored powder, having a faint, mild odor.

Solubility: Undiluted pentaerythritol tetranitrate—Soluble in acetone; slightly soluble in alcohol and in ether; practically insoluble in water.

USP requirements:

Diluted Pentaerythritol Tetranitrate USP—Preserve in tight containers, and prevent exposure to excessive heat. A dry mixture of pentaerythritol tetranitrate with Lactose or Mannitol or other suitable inert excipients, to permit safe handling and compliance with U.S. Interstate Commerce Commission regulations pertaining to interstate shipment. Contains the labeled amount of pentaerythritol tetranitrate, within ±5%. Meets the requirements for Identification and Organic volatile impurities.

Caution: Undiluted pentaerythritol tetranitrate is a powerful explosive; take proper precautions in handling. It can be exploded by percussion or by excessive heat. Only exceedingly small amounts should be isolated.

Pentaerythritol Tetranitrate Extended-release Capsules—Not in USP.

Pentaerythritol Tetranitrate Tablets USP—Preserve in tight containers. Prepared from Diluted Pentaerythritol Tetranitrate. Contain the labeled amount of Diluted Pentaerythritol Tetranitrate, within ±7%. Meet the requirements for Identification, Disintegration (10 minutes), and Uniformity of dosage units.

Caution: Undiluted pentaerythritol tetranitrate is a powerful explosive; take proper precautions in handling. It can be exploded by percussion or by excessive heat. Only exceedingly small amounts should be isolated.

Pentaerythritol Tetranitrate Extended-release Tablets—Not in USP.

PENTAGASTRIN

Chemical name: L-Phenylalaninamide, *N*-[(1,1-dimethylethoxy)carbonyl]-beta-alanyl-L-tryptophyl-L-methionyl-L-alpha-aspartyl-.

Molecular formula: $C_{37}H_{49}N_7O_9S$.

Molecular weight: 767.90.

Description: Colorless crystalline solid.

Solubility: Soluble in dimethylformamide and in dimethylsulfoxide; almost insoluble in water, in ethanol, in ether, in chloroform, and in ethyl acetate.

USP requirements: Pentagastrin Injection—Not in USP.

PENTAMIDINE

Chemical group: Diamidine derivative, related to hydroxystilbamidine.

Chemical name: Pentamidine isethionate—4,4′-diamidinodiphenoxypentane di-(beta-hydroxyethanesulfonate).

Molecular formula: Pentamidine isethionate—$C_{19}H_{24}N_4O_2 \cdot 2C_2H_6O_4S$.

Molecular weight: Pentamidine isethionate—592.68.

Description: Pentamidine isethionate—White crystalline powder.

Solubility: Pentamidine isethionate—Soluble in water and in glycerin; insoluble in acetone, in chloroform, and in ether.

USP requirements:

Pentamidine Isethionate for Inhalation Solution—Not in USP.

Sterile Pentamidine Isethionate—Not in USP.

PENTASTARCH AND SODIUM CHLORIDE

Source: Pentastarch—A starch composed of more than 90% amylopectin that has been etherified to the extent that an average of 4 to 5 of the OH groups present in every 10 D-glucopyranose units of the starch polymer have been converted to OCH_2CH_2OH groups.

Chemical name:

Pentastarch—Starch 2-hydroxyethyl ether.

Sodium chloride—Sodium chloride.

Molecular formula: Sodium chloride—NaCl.

Molecular weight:

Pentastarch—Average approximately 264,000 with a range of 150,000 to 350,000 and with 80% of the polymers falling between 10,000 and 2,000,000.

Sodium chloride—58.44.

Description:

Pentastarch in sodium chloride injection—Clear, pale yellow to amber solution.

Sodium Chloride USP—Colorless, cubic crystals or white crystalline powder.

NF category: Tonicity agent.

Solubility: Sodium Chloride USP—Freely soluble in water; and slightly more soluble in boiling water; soluble in glycerin; slightly soluble in alcohol.

USP requirements: Pentastarch in Sodium Chloride Injection—Not in USP.

PENTAZOCINE

Chemical name:

Pentazocine—2,6-Methano-3-benzazocin-8-ol, 1,2,3,4,5,6-hexahydro-6,11-dimethyl-3-(3-methyl-2-butenyl)-, (2 alpha,6 alpha,11*R**)-.

Pentazocine hydrochloride—2,6-Methano-3-benzazocin-8-ol, 1,2,3,4,5,6-hexahydro-6,11-dimethyl-3-(3-methyl-2-butenyl)-, hydrochloride, (2 alpha,6 alpha,11*R**)-.

Pentazocine lactate—2,6-Methano-3-benzazocin-8-ol, 1,2,-3,4,5,6-hexahydro-6,11-dimethyl-3-(3-methyl-2-butenyl)-, (2 alpha,6 alpha,11*R**)-, compd. with 2-hydroxypropanoic acid (1:1).

Molecular formula:

Pentazocine—$C_{19}H_{27}NO$.

Pentazocine hydrochloride—$C_{19}H_{27}NO \cdot HCl$.

Pentazocine lactate—$C_{19}H_{27}NO \cdot C_3H_6O_3$.

Molecular weight:

Pentazocine—285.43.

Pentazocine hydrochloride—321.89.

Pentazocine lactate—375.51.

Description:

Pentazocine USP—White or very pale, tan-colored powder.

Pentazocine Hydrochloride USP—White, crystalline powder. It exhibits polymorphism, one form melting at about 254 °C and the other at about 218 °C.

Pentazocine lactate—White, crystalline substance.

Solubility:

Pentazocine USP—Practically insoluble in water; freely soluble in chloroform; soluble in alcohol, in acetone, and in ether; sparingly soluble in ethyl acetate.

Pentazocine Hydrochloride USP—Freely soluble in chloroform; soluble in alcohol; sparingly soluble in water; very slightly soluble in acetone and in ether.

Pentazocine lactate—Soluble in acidic aqueous solutions.

USP requirements:

Pentazocine USP—Preserve in tight, light-resistant containers. Contains not less than 98.0% and not more than 101.5% of pentazocine, calculated on the dried basis. Meets the requirements for Identification, Melting range (147–158 °C, with slight darkening), Loss on drying (not more than 1.0%), Residue on ignition (not more than 0.2%), and Ordinary impurities.

Pentazocine Hydrochloride USP—Preserve in tight, light-resistant containers. Contains not less than 98.0% and not more than 102.0% of pentazocine hydrochloride, calculated on the dried basis. Meets the requirements for Identification, Loss on drying (not more than 1.0%), Residue on ignition (not more than 0.2%), and Ordinary impurities.

Pentazocine Hydrochloride Tablets USP—Preserve in tight, light-resistant containers. Contain an amount of pentazocine hydrochloride equivalent to the labeled amount of pentazocine, within ±10%. Meet the requirements for Identification, Dissolution (75% in 45 minutes in water in Apparatus 2 at 50 rpm), and Uniformity of dosage units.

Pentazocine Lactate Injection USP—Preserve in single-dose or in multiple-dose containers, preferably of Type I glass. A sterile solution of pentazocine lactate in Water for Injection, prepared from Pentazocine with the aid of Lactic Acid. Contains an amount of pentazocine lactate equivalent to the labeled amount of pentazocine, within ±5%. Meets the requirements for Identification, Bacterial endotoxins, pH (4.0–5.0), and Injections.

PENTAZOCINE AND ACETAMINOPHEN

For *Pentazocine* and *Acetaminophen*—See individual listings for chemistry information.

USP requirements: Pentazocine Hydrochloride and Acetaminophen Tablets—Not in USP.

PENTAZOCINE AND ASPIRIN

For *Pentazocine* and *Aspirin*—See individual listings for chemistry information.

USP requirements: Pentazocine Hydrochloride and Aspirin Tablets USP—Preserve in tight, light-resistant containers. Contain an amount of pentazocine hydrochloride equivalent to the labeled amount of pentazocine, within ±10%, and the labeled amount of aspirin, within ±10%. Meet the requirements for Identification, Non-aspirin salicylates (not more than 3.0%), Dissolution (80% of pentazocine and 70% of aspirin in 30 minutes in water in Apparatus 1 at 80 rpm), and Uniformity of dosage units.

PENTAZOCINE AND NALOXONE

For *Pentazocine* and *Naloxone*—See individual listings for chemistry information.

USP requirements: Pentazocine and Naloxone Hydrochlorides Tablets USP—Preserve in tight, light-resistant containers. Contain amounts of pentazocine hydrochloride and naloxone hydrochloride equivalent to the labeled amounts of pentazocine and naloxone, within ±10%. Meet the requirements for Identification, Dissolution (75% of pentazocine in 45 minutes in water in Apparatus 2 at 50 rpm), and Uniformity of dosage units.

PENTETIC ACID

Chemical name: Glycine, *N,N*-bis[2-[bis(carboxymethyl)amino]-ethyl]-.

Molecular formula: $C_{14}H_{23}N_3O_{10}$.

Molecular weight: 393.35.

USP requirements: Pentetic Acid USP—Preserve in well-closed containers. Contains not less than 98.0% and not more than 100.5% of pentetic acid. Meets the requirements for Identification, Melting range (215–225 °C), Residue on ignition (not more than 0.2%), Heavy metals (not more than 0.005%), Limit of nitrilotriacetic acid (not more than 0.1%), and Iron (not more than 0.01%).

PENTOBARBITAL

Chemical name:

Pentobarbital—2,4,6(1*H*,3*H*,5*H*)-Pyrimidinetrione, 5-ethyl-5-(1-methylbutyl)-.

Pentobarbital sodium—2,4,6(1*H*,3*H*,5*H*)-Pyrimidinetrione, 5-ethyl-5-(1-methylbutyl), monosodium salt.

Molecular formula:

Pentobarbital—$C_{11}H_{18}N_2O_3$.

Pentobarbital sodium—$C_{11}H_{17}N_2NaO_3$.

Molecular weight:

Pentobarbital—226.28.

Pentobarbital sodium—248.26.

Description:

Pentobarbital USP—White to practically white, fine, practically odorless powder. May occur in a polymorphic form that melts at about 116 °C. This form gradually reverts to the more stable higher-melting form upon being heated at about 110 °C.

Pentobarbital Sodium USP—White, crystalline granules or white powder. Is odorless or has a slight characteristic odor. Its solutions decompose on standing, heat accelerating the decomposition.

Solubility:

Pentobarbital USP—Very slightly soluble in water and in carbon tetrachloride; very soluble in alcohol, in methanol, in ether, in chloroform, and in acetone.

Pentobarbital Sodium USP—Very soluble in water; freely soluble in alcohol; practically insoluble in ether.

USP requirements:

Pentobarbital USP—Preserve in tight containers. Contains not less than 98.5% and not more than 101.0% of pentobarbital, calculated on the dried basis. Meets the requirements for Identification, Melting range (127–133 °C), Loss on drying (not more than 1.0%), Isomer content, Residue on ignition (not more than 0.1%), Heavy metals (not more than 0.002%), and Organic volatile impurities.

Pentobarbital Elixir USP—Preserve in tight containers. Contains the labeled amount, within ±7.5%. Meets the requirements for Identification and Alcohol content (16.0–20.0%).

Pentobarbital Sodium USP—Preserve in tight containers. Contains not less than 98.5% and not more than 101.0% of pentobarbital sodium, calculated on the dried basis. Meets the requirements for Completeness of solution, Identification, pH (9.8–11.0, in the solution prepared in the test for Completeness of solution), Loss on drying (not more than 3.5%), Isomer content, Heavy metals (not more than 0.003%), and Organic volatile impurities.

Pentobarbital Sodium Capsules USP—Preserve in tight containers. Contain the labeled amount, within ±7.5%. Meet the requirements for Identification, Dissolution (75% in 45 minutes in water in Apparatus 1 at 100 rpm), and Uniformity of dosage units.

Pentobarbital Sodium Injection USP—Preserve in single-dose or in multiple-dose containers, preferably of Type I glass. The Injection may be packaged in 50-mL containers. A sterile solution of Pentobarbital Sodium in a suitable solvent. Pentobarbital may be substituted for the equivalent amount of Pentobarbital Sodium, for adjustment of the pH. The label indicates that the Injection is not to be used if it contains a precipitate. Contains the equivalent of the labeled amount, within ±8%. Meets the requirements for Identification, Bacterial endotoxins, pH (9.0–10.5), and Injections.

Pentobarbital Sodium Suppositories—Not in USP.

PENTOSTATIN

Chemical name: Imidazo[4,5-*d*][1,3]diazepin-8-ol, 3-(2-deoxy-beta-D-*erythro*-pentofuranosyl)-3,6,7,8-tetrahydro-, (*R*)-.

Molecular formula: $C_{11}H_{16}N_4O_4$.

Molecular weight: 268.27.

Description: White to off-white solid.

Solubility: Freely soluble in distilled water.

USP requirements: Pentostatin for Injection—Not in USP.

PENTOXIFYLLINE

Chemical group: A trisubstituted xanthine derivative.

Chemical name: 1*H*-purine-2,6-dione, 3,7-dihydro-3,7-dimethyl-1-(5-oxohexyl)-.

Molecular formula: $C_{13}H_{18}N_4O_3$.

Molecular weight: 278.31.

Description: Odorless, colorless, crystalline powder. Melts at 101–106 °C.

Solubility: Soluble in water and in ethanol; sparingly soluble in toluene.

USP requirements: Pentoxifylline Extended-release Tablets—Not in USP.

PEPPERMINT

Description: Peppermint NF—Has an aromatic, characteristic odor.

NF category: Flavors and perfumes.

NF requirements: Peppermint NF—Consists of the dried leaf and flowering top of *Mentha piperita* Linné (Fam. Labiatae). Meets the requirements for Stems and other foreign organic matter and Botanic characteristics.

PEPPERMINT OIL

Description: Peppermint Oil NF—Colorless or pale yellow liquid, having a strong, penetrating, characteristic odor.

NF category: Flavors and perfumes.

NF requirements: Peppermint Oil NF—Preserve in tight containers, and prevent exposure to excessive heat. The volatile oil distilled with steam from the fresh overground parts of the flowering plant of *Mentha piperita* Linné (Fam. Labiatae), rectified by distillation and neither partially nor wholly dementholized. Yields not less than 5.0% of esters, calculated as menthyl acetate, and not less than 50.0% of total menthol, free and as esters. Meets the requirements for Solubility in 70% alcohol (one volume dissolves in 3 volumes of 70% alcohol, with not more than slight opalescence), Identification, Specific gravity (0.896–0.908), Angular rotation (−18° to −32° in a 100-mm tube), Refractive index (1.459–1.465 at 20 °C), Heavy metals (not more than 0.004%), and Dimethyl sulfide.

PEPPERMINT SPIRIT

Description: Peppermint Spirit USP—NF category: Flavors and perfumes.

USP requirements: Peppermint Spirit USP—Preserve in tight containers, protected from light. Contains, in each 100 mL, not less than 9.0 mL and not more than 11.0 mL of peppermint oil.

Prepare Peppermint Spirit as follows: 100 mL of Peppermint Oil, 10 grams of Peppermint, in coarse powder, and a sufficient quantity of Alcohol to make 1000 mL. Macerate the peppermint leaves, freed as much as possible from stems and coarsely powdered, for 1 hour in 500 mL of purified water, and then strongly express them. Add the moist, macerated leaves to 900 mL of alcohol, and allow the mixture to stand for 6 hours with frequent agitation. Filter, and to the filtrate add the oil and add alcohol to make the product measure 1000 mL.

Meets the requirement for Alcohol content (79.0–85.0%).

PEPPERMINT WATER

Description: Peppermint Water NF—NF category: Flavored and/or sweetened vehicle.

NF requirements: Peppermint Water NF—Preserve in tight containers. A clear, saturated solution of Peppermint Oil in Purified Water, prepared by one of the processes described under *Aromatic Waters*. Meets the requirement for Organic volatile impurities.

PERFLUBRON

Chemical name: Octane, 1-bromo-1,1,2,2,3,3,4,4,5,5,6,6,7,7,8,8,8-heptadecafluoro-.

Molecular formula: C_8BrF_{17}.

Molecular weight: 498.96.

Description: Clear, colorless liquid with a boiling point of 143 °C at one atmosphere.

Solubility: Not miscible with water.

USP requirements: Perflubron Oral Solution—Not in USP.

PERFLUOROCHEMICAL EMULSION

Molecular formula:
Perfluorodecalin—$C_{10}F_{18}$.
Perfluorotri-n-propylamine—$C_9F_{21}N$.

Description: Stable emulsion of synthetic perfluorochemicals (perfluorodecalin, perfluorotri-n-propylamine) in Water for Injection. Also contains Poloxamer 188 (a nonionic surfactant which is a polyoxyethylene [160]-polyoxypropylene [30] glycol block copolymer), glycerin, egg yolk phospholipids (a mixture of naturally occurring phospholipids isolated from egg yolk), dextrose (a naturally occurring sugar), and the potassium salt of oleic acid (a naturally occurring fatty acid), plus electrolytes in physiologic concentrations.

Other characteristics:
Osmolarity—Approximately 410 mOsmol per liter.
Mean particle diameter—Less than 270 nanometers as determined by laser light scattering spectrophotometry. The

content of particles greater than 400 nanometers is less than 10%.
pH—After preparation for administration: 7.3.
Solubility of oxygen—At 37 °C and at partial pressure of oxygen (pO_2) of 760 mm Hg: 7 volume %. Increases with decreasing temperature; at 10 °C and pO_2 of 760 mm Hg, is 9 volume %.
Solubility of carbon dioxide—At 37 °C and at partial pressure of carbon dioxide (pCO_2) of 760 mm Hg: 66 volume %.
Viscosity—Less viscous than whole blood at 37 °C and physiological shear rates.

USP requirements: Perfluorochemical Emulsion for Injection—Not in USP.

PERGOLIDE

Source: Ergot derivative.

Chemical name: Pergolide mesylate—Ergoline, 8-[(methylthio)methyl]-6-propyl-, monomethanesulfonate, (8 beta)-.

Molecular formula: Pergolide mesylate—$C_{19}H_{26}N_2S \cdot CH_4O_3S$.

Molecular weight: Pergolide mesylate—410.59.

Description: Pergolide mesylate—Off-white crystals; melting point about 225 °C.

USP requirements: Pergolide Mesylate Tablets—Not in USP.

PERICYAZINE

Chemical group: Piperidine.

Chemical name: 10-[3-(4-Hydroxypiperidino)propyl]phenothiazine-2-carbonitrile.

Molecular formula: $C_{21}H_{23}N_3OS$.

Molecular weight: 365.49.

Description: A yellow almost odorless powder. Melts at 115 °C.

Solubility: Practically insoluble in water; soluble in alcohol and in acetone; freely soluble in chloroform; slightly soluble in ether.

USP requirements:
Pericyazine Capsules—Not in USP.
Pericyazine Oral Solution—Not in USP.

PERMETHRIN

Source: A mixture of the *cis* and *trans* isomers of a synthetic pyrethroid. Permethrin is the first pyrethroid formulated for human use.

Chemical name: Cyclopropanecarboxylic acid, 3-(2,2-dichloroethenyl)-2,2-dimethyl-, (3-phenoxyphenyl)methyl ester.

Molecular formula: $C_{21}H_{20}Cl_2O_3$.

Molecular weight: 391.29.

Description: A yellow to light orange-brown, low-melting solid or viscous liquid.

Solubility: Practically insoluble in water; soluble in nonpolar organic solvents.

USP requirements:
Permethrin Cream—Not in USP.
Permethrin Lotion—Not in USP.

PERPHENAZINE

Chemical group: Piperazinyl phenothiazine.

Chemical name: Piperazineethanol, 4-[3-(2-chloro-10*H*-phenothiazin-10-yl)propyl]-.

Molecular formula: $C_{21}H_{26}ClN_3OS$.

Molecular weight: 403.97.

Description: Perphenazine USP—White to creamy white, odorless powder.

Solubility: Perphenazine USP—Practically insoluble in water; freely soluble in alcohol and in chloroform; soluble in acetone.

USP requirements:
Perphenazine USP—Preserve in tight, light-resistant containers. Contains not less than 98.0% and not more than 102.0% of perphenazine, calculated on the dried basis. Meets the requirements for Clarity and color of solution, Identification, Melting range (94–100 °C), Loss on drying (not more than 0.5%), Residue on ignition (not more than 0.1%), Ordinary impurities, and Organic volatile impurities.
Perphenazine Injection USP—Preserve in single-dose or in multiple-dose containers, preferably of Type I glass, protected from light. A sterile solution of Perphenazine in Water for Injection, prepared with the aid of Citric Acid. Contains the labeled amount, as the citrate, within ±10%. Meets the requirements for Identification, Bacterial endotoxins, pH (4.2–5.6), and Injections.
Perphenazine Oral Solution USP—Preserve in well-closed, light-resistant containers. Contains the labeled amount, within ±10%. Meets the requirements for Identification and Perphenazine sulfoxide (not more than 5.0%).
Perphenazine Syrup USP—Preserve in well-closed, light-resistant containers. Contains the labeled amount, within ±10%. Meets the requirement for Identification.
Perphenazine Tablets USP—Preserve in tight, light-resistant containers. Contain the labeled amount, within ±10%. Meet the requirements for Identification, Dissolution (75% in 45 minutes in 0.1 *N* hydrochloric acid in Apparatus 2 at 50 rpm), and Uniformity of dosage units.

PERPHENAZINE AND AMITRIPTYLINE

For *Perphenazine* and *Amitriptyline*—See individual listings for chemistry information.

USP requirements: Perphenazine and Amitriptyline Hydrochloride Tablets USP—Preserve in well-closed containers. Contain the labeled amounts, within ±10%. Meet the requirements for Identification, Dissolution (75% of each active ingredient in 60 minutes in 0.1 *N* hydrochloric acid in Apparatus 2 at 50 rpm), and Uniformity of dosage units.

PERSIC OIL

Description: Persic Oil NF—Clear, pale straw-colored or colorless oily liquid. Is almost odorless. Is not turbid at temperatures exceeding 15 °C.
NF category: Vehicle (oleaginous).

Solubility: Persic Oil NF—Slightly soluble in alcohol. Miscible with ether, with chloroform, and with solvent hexane.

NF requirements: Persic Oil NF—Preserve in tight containers. The oil expressed from the kernels of varieties of *Prunus armeniaca* Linné (Apricot Kernel Oil), or from the kernels of varieties of *Prunus persica* Sieb. et Zucc. (Peach Kernel Oil) (Fam. Rosaceae). Label it to indicate whether it was derived from apricot kernels or from peach kernels. Meets the requirements for Specific gravity (0.910–0.923), Heavy metals (not more than 0.004%), Mineral oil, Cottonseed oil, Sesame oil, Free fatty acids, Iodine value (90–108), and Saponification value (185–195).

PERTUSSIS IMMUNE GLOBULIN

Description: Pertussis Immune Globulin USP—Transparent or slightly opalescent liquid, practically colorless, free from turbidity or particles, and practically odorless. May develop a slight, granular deposit during storage. Is standardized for agglutinating activity with the U.S. Standard Antipertussis Serum.

USP requirements: Pertussis Immune Globulin USP—Preserve at a temperature between 2 and 8 °C. A sterile, non-pyrogenic solution of globulins derived from the blood plasma of adult human donors who have been immunized with pertussis vaccine such that each 1.25 mL contains not less than the amount of immune globulin to be equivalent to 25 mL of human hyperimmune serum. Contains a suitable preservative. Label it to state that it is not intended for intravenous injection. Meets the requirement for Expiration date (not later than 3 years after date of issue from manufacturer's cold storage [5 °C, 3 years]). Conforms to the regulations of the U.S. Food and Drug Administration concerning biologics.

PERTUSSIS VACCINE

Description: Pertussis Vaccine USP—More or less turbid, whitish liquid. Practically odorless, or having a faint odor because of the antimicrobial agent.

USP requirements: Pertussis Vaccine USP—Preserve at a temperature between 2 and 8 °C. A sterile bacterial fraction or suspension of killed pertussis bacilli (*Bordetella pertussis*) of a strain or strains selected for high antigenic efficiency. Label it to state that it is to be well shaken before use and that it is not to be frozen. Has a potency determined by the specific mouse potency test based on the U.S. Standard Pertussis Vaccine, and a pertussis challenge, of 12 protective units per total immunizing dose, and, in the case of whole bacterial vaccine, such dose contains not more than 60 opacity units. Contains a preservative. Meets the requirements of the specific mouse toxicity test and for Expiration date (not later than 18 months after date of issue from manufacturer's cold storage [5 °C, 1 year]). Conforms to the regulations of the U.S. Food and Drug Administration concerning biologics.

PERTUSSIS VACCINE ADSORBED

Description: Pertussis Vaccine Adsorbed USP—Markedly turbid, whitish liquid. Substantially odorless, or has a faint odor because of the antimicrobial agent.

USP requirements: Pertussis Vaccine Adsorbed USP—Preserve at a temperature between 2 and 8 °C, and avoid freezing. A sterile bacterial fraction or suspension, in a suitable diluent, of killed pertussis bacilli (*Bordetella pertussis*) of a strain or strains selected for high antigenic efficiency precipitated or adsorbed by the addition of aluminum hydroxide or aluminum phosphate, and re-suspended. Label it to state that it is to be well shaken before use and that it is not to be frozen. Has a potency determined by the specific mouse potency test based on the U.S. Standard Pertussis Vaccine, and a pertussis challenge, of 12 protective units per total immunizing dose, and, in the case of whole bacterial vaccine, such dose contains not more than 48 opacity units. Contains a preservative. Meets the requirements of the specific mouse toxicity test and for Expiration date (not later than 18 months after date of issue from manufacturer's cold storage [5 °C, 1 year]). Conforms to the regulations of the U.S. Food and Drug Administration concerning biologics.

PETROLATUM

Description: Petrolatum USP—Unctuous, yellowish to light amber mass, having not more than a slight fluorescence, even after being melted. It is transparent in thin layers. Free or practically free from odor.

NF category: Ointment base.

Solubility: Petrolatum USP—Insoluble in water; freely soluble in carbon disulfide, in chloroform, and in turpentine oil; soluble in ether, in solvent hexane, and in most fixed and volatile oils; practically insoluble in cold alcohol and hot alcohol and in cold dehydrated alcohol.

USP requirements: Petrolatum USP—Preserve in well-closed containers. A purified mixture of semisolid hydrocarbons obtained from petroleum. Label it to indicate the name and proportion of any added stabilizer. Meets the requirements for Specific gravity (0.815–0.880 at 60 °C), Melting range (38–60 °C), Consistency (value of 100–300), Alkalinity, Acidity, Residue on ignition (not more than 0.1%), Organic acids, Fixed oils, fats, and rosin, and Color.

HYDROPHILIC PETROLATUM

Description: Hydrophilic Petrolatum USP—NF category: Ointment base.

USP requirements: Hydrophilic Petrolatum USP—Prepare Hydrophilic Petrolatum as follows: 30 grams of Cholesterol, 30 grams of Stearyl Alcohol, 80 grams of White Wax, and 860 grams of White Petrolatum to make 1000 grams. Melt the Stearyl Alcohol and White Wax together on a steam bath, then add the Cholesterol, and stir until completely dissolved. Add the White Petrolatum, and mix. Remove from the bath, and stir until the mixture congeals.

WHITE PETROLATUM

Description: White Petrolatum USP—White or faintly yellowish, unctuous mass, transparent in thin layers even after cooling to 0 °C.

NF category: Ointment base.

Solubility: White Petrolatum USP—Insoluble in water; slightly soluble in cold or hot alcohol, and in cold dehydrated alcohol; freely soluble in carbon disulfide and in chloroform; soluble in ether, in solvent hexane, and in most fixed and volatile oils.

USP requirements: White Petrolatum USP—Preserve in well-closed containers. A purified mixture of semisolid hydrocarbons obtained from petroleum, and wholly or nearly decolorized. Label it to indicate the name and proportion of any added stabilizer. Meets the requirements for Residue on ignition (not more than 0.05%) and Color, and for Specific gravity, Melting range, Consistency, Alkalinity, Acidity, Organic acids, and Fixed oils, fats, and rosin under Petrolatum.

PHENACEMIDE

Chemical group: Substituted acetylurea derivative.

Chemical name: Benzeneacetamide, *N*-(aminocarbonyl)-.

Molecular formula: $C_9H_{10}N_2O_2$.

Molecular weight: 178.19.

Description: Phenacemide USP—White to practically white, fine crystalline powder. Is odorless, or practically odorless, and melts at about 213 °C.

Solubility: Phenacemide USP—Very slightly soluble in water, in alcohol, in chloroform, and in ether; slightly soluble in acetone and in methanol.

USP requirements:
Phenacemide USP—Preserve in tight containers. Contains not less than 98.0% and not more than 100.5% of phenacemide, calculated on the dried basis. Meets the requirements for Identification, Loss on drying (not more than 1.0%), Residue on ignition (not more than 0.1%), Heavy metals (not more than 0.002%), Ordinary impurities, and Organic volatile impurities.
Phenacemide Tablets USP—Preserve in well-closed containers. Contain the labeled amount, within ±5%. Meet the requirements for Identification, Dissolution (35% in 60 minutes in 0.1 *N* hydrochloric acid in Apparatus 2 at 100 rpm), and Uniformity of dosage units.

PHENAZOPYRIDINE

Chemical name: Phenazopyridine hydrochloride—2,6-Pyridinediamine, 3-(phenylazo)-, monohydrochloride.

Molecular formula: Phenazopyridine hydrochloride—$C_{11}H_{11}N_5 \cdot HCl$.

Molecular weight: Phenazopyridine hydrochloride—249.70.

Description: Phenazopyridine Hydrochloride USP—Light or dark red to dark violet, crystalline powder. Is odorless, or has a slight odor. Melts at about 235 °C, with decomposition.

Solubility: Phenazopyridine Hydrochloride USP—Slightly soluble in water, in alcohol, and in chloroform.

USP requirements:
Phenazopyridine Hydrochloride USP—Preserve in tight containers. Contains not less than 99.0% and not more than 101.0% of phenazopyridine hydrochloride, calculated on the dried basis. Meets the requirements for Identification, Loss on drying (not more than 1.0%), Residue on ignition (not more than 0.2%), Water-insoluble substances (not more than 0.1%), Heavy metals (not more than 0.002%), and Ordinary impurities.
Phenazopyridine Hydrochloride Tablets USP—Preserve in tight containers. Contain the labeled amount, within ±5%. Meet the requirements for Identification, Dissolution (75% in 45 minutes in water in Apparatus 2 at 50 rpm), and Uniformity of dosage units.

PHENDIMETRAZINE

Chemical group: Morpholine.

Chemical name: Phendimetrazine tartrate—Morpholine, 3,4-dimethyl-2-phenyl-, (2*S-trans*)-, [*R*-(*R**,*R**)]-2,3-dihydroxybutanedioate (1:1).

Molecular formula: Phendimetrazine tartrate—$C_{12}H_{17}NO \cdot C_4H_6O_6$.

Molecular weight: Phendimetrazine tartrate—341.36.

Description: Phendimetrazine Tartrate USP—White, odorless, crystalline powder.

Solubility: Phendimetrazine Tartrate USP—Freely soluble in water; sparingly soluble in warm alcohol; insoluble in chloroform, in acetone, and in ether. Phendimetrazine base is extracted by organic solvents from alkaline solution.

USP requirements:
Phendimetrazine Tartrate USP—Preserve in tight containers. Contains not less than 98.0% and not more than 102.0% of phendimetrazine tartrate, calculated on the dried basis. Meets the requirements for Identification, Melting range (182–188 °C, with decomposition, the range between beginning and end of melting not more than 3 °C), Specific rotation (32° to 36°, calculated on the dried basis), pH (3.0–4.0, in a solution [1 in 40]), Loss on drying (not more than 0.5%), Residue on ignition (not more than 0.1%), Chloride (not more than 0.035%), Sulfate (not more than 0.01%), Heavy metals (not more than 0.001%), Chromatographic purity, L-*erythro* isomer (not more than 0.1%), and Organic volatile impurities.
Phendimetrazine Tartrate Capsules USP—Preserve in tight containers. Contain the labeled amount, within ±5%. Meet the requirements for Identification and Uniformity of dosage units.
Phendimetrazine Tartrate Extended-release Capsules—Not in USP.
Phendimetrazine Tartrate Tablets USP—Preserve in well-closed containers. Contain the labeled amount, within ±10%. Meet the requirements for Identification, Dissolution (60% in 45 minutes in water in Apparatus 1 at 100 rpm), and Uniformity of dosage units.
Phendimetrazine Tartrate Extended-release Tablets—Not in USP.

PHENELZINE

Chemical group: Hydrazine derivative.

Chemical name: Phenelzine sulfate—Hydrazine, (2-phenylethyl)-, sulfate (1:1).

Molecular formula: Phenelzine sulfate—$C_8H_{12}N_2 \cdot H_2SO_4$.

Molecular weight: Phenelzine sulfate—234.27.

Description: Phenelzine Sulfate USP—White to yellowish white powder, having a characteristic odor.

Solubility: Phenelzine Sulfate USP—Freely soluble in water; practically insoluble in alcohol, in chloroform, and in ether.

USP requirements:
Phenelzine Sulfate USP—Preserve in tight containers, protected from heat and light. Contains not less than 97.0% and not more than 100.5% of phenelzine sulfate, calculated on the dried basis. Meets the requirements for Identification, Melting range (164–168 °C), pH (1.4–1.9, in a solution [1 in 100]), Loss on drying (not more than 1.0%), Heavy metals (not more than 0.002%), Ordinary impurities, and Organic volatile impurities.
Phenelzine Sulfate Tablets USP—Preserve in tight containers, protected from heat and light. Contain an amount of phenelzine sulfate equivalent to the labeled amount of phenelzine, within ±5%. Meet the requirements for Identification, Disintegration (1 hour), and Uniformity of dosage units.

PHENINDAMINE

Chemical group: Piperidine derivative.

Chemical name: Phenindamine tartrate—2,3,4,9-Tetrahydro-2-methyl-9-phenyl-1*H*-indeno[2,1-*c*]pyridine.

Molecular formula: Phenindamine tartrate—$C_{19}H_{19}N \cdot C_4H_6O_6$.

Molecular weight: Phenindamine tartrate—411.45.

Description: Phenindamine tartrate—White or almost white, odorless or almost odorless, voluminous powder. A 1% solution in water has a pH of 3.4 to 3.9.

Solubility: Phenindamine tartrate—Soluble 1 in 70 of water; slightly soluble in alcohol; practically insoluble in chloroform and in ether.

USP requirements: Phenindamime Tartrate Tablets—Not in USP.

PHENINDAMINE, HYDROCODONE, AND GUAIFENESIN

For *Phenindamine, Hydrocodone,* and *Guaifenesin*—See individual listings for chemistry information.

USP requirements: Phenindamine Tartrate, Hydrocodone Bitartrate, and Guaifenesin Tablets—Not in USP.

PHENINDIONE

Chemical name: 1*H*-Indene-1,3(2*H*)-dione, 2-phenyl-.

Molecular formula: $C_{15}H_{10}O_2$.

Molecular weight: 222.24.

Description: Phenindione USP—Creamy white to pale yellow, almost odorless crystals or crystalline powder.

Solubility: Phenindione USP—Very slightly soluble in water; freely soluble in chloroform; slightly soluble in alcohol and in ether.

USP requirements:
Phenindione USP—Preserve in well-closed containers. Contains not less than 98.0% and not more than 100.5% of phenindione, calculated on the dried basis. Meets the requirements for Identification, Melting range (148–151 °C), Loss on drying (not more than 1.0%), Residue on ignition (not more than 0.2%), Heavy metals (not more than 0.002%), Ordinary impurities, and Organic volatile impurities.
Phenindione Tablets USP—Preserve in well-closed containers. Contain the labeled amount, within ±10%. Meet the requirements for Identification, Dissolution (85% in 45 minutes in phosphate buffer [pH 8.0] in Apparatus 1 at 100 rpm), and Uniformity of dosage units.

PHENIRAMINE, CODEINE, AND GUAIFENESIN

Chemical group: Pheniramine—Alkylamine derivative.

Chemical name:
Pheniramine maleate—2-[alpha-[2-Dimethylaminoethyl]-benzyl]pyridine bimaleate.
Codeine phosphate—Morphinan-6-ol, 7,8-didehydro-4,5-epoxy-3-methoxy-17-methyl-, (5 alpha,6 alpha)-, phosphate (1:1) (salt), hemihydrate.
Guaifenesin—1,2-Propanediol, 3-(2-methoxyphenoxy)-.

Molecular formula:
Pheniramine maleate—$C_{16}H_{20}N_2 \cdot C_4H_4O_4$.
Codeine phosphate—$C_{18}H_{21}NO_3 \cdot H_3PO_4 \cdot \frac{1}{2}H_2O$ (hemihydrate); $C_{18}H_{21}NO_3 \cdot H_3PO_4$ (anhydrous).
Guaifenesin—$C_{10}H_{14}O_4$.

Molecular weight:
Pheniramine maleate—356.42.
Codeine phosphate—406.37 (hemihydrate); 397.36 (anhydrous).
Guaifenesin—198.22.

Description:
Pheniramine maleate—White or almost white, crystalline powder, odorless or with a slight odor.
Codeine Phosphate USP—Fine, white, needle-shaped crystals, or white, crystalline powder. Is odorless, and is affected by light. Its solutions are acid to litmus.
Guaifenesin USP—White to slightly gray, crystalline powder. May have a slight characteristic odor.

Solubility:
Pheniramine maleate—Soluble 1 in 0.3 of water, 1 in 2.5 of alcohol, and 1 in 1.5 of chloroform; very slightly soluble in ether.
Codeine Phosphate USP—Freely soluble in water; very soluble in hot water; slightly soluble in alcohol but more so in boiling alcohol.
Guaifenesin USP—Soluble in water, in alcohol, in chloroform, in glycerin, and in propylene glycol.

USP requirements: Pheniramine Maleate, Codeine Phosphate, and Guaifenesin Syrup—Not in USP.

PHENIRAMINE, PHENYLEPHRINE, CODEINE, SODIUM CITRATE, SODIUM SALICYLATE, AND CAFFEINE

Source: Caffeine—Coffee, tea, cola, and cocoa or chocolate. May also be synthesized from urea or dimethylurea.

Chemical group:
Pheniramine—Alkylamine derivative.
Caffeine—Methylated xanthine.

Chemical name:
Pheniramine maleate—2-[alpha-[2-Dimethylaminoethyl]-benzyl]pyridine bimaleate.
Phenylephrine hydrochloride—Benzenemethanol, 3-hydroxy-alpha-[(methylamino)methyl]-, hydrochloride.
Codeine phosphate—Morphinan-6-ol, 7,8-didehydro-4,5-epoxy-3-methoxy-17-methyl-, (5 alpha,6 alpha)-, phosphate (1:1) (salt), hemihydrate.
Sodium citrate—1,2,3-Propanetricarboxylic acid, 2-hydroxy-, trisodium salt.
Sodium salicylate—Benzoic acid, 2-hydroxy-, monosodium salt.
Caffeine—1*H*-Purine-2,6-dione, 3,7-dihydro-1,3,7-trimethyl-.
Citric Acid—1,2,3-Propanetricarboxylic acid, 2-hydroxy-.

Molecular formula:
Pheniramine maleate—$C_{16}H_{20}N_2 \cdot C_4H_4O_4$.
Phenylephrine hydrochloride—$C_9H_{13}NO_2 \cdot HCl$.
Codeine phosphate—$C_{18}H_{21}NO_3 \cdot H_3PO_4 \cdot \frac{1}{2}H_2O$ (hemihydrate); $C_{18}H_{21}NO_3 \cdot H_3PO_4$ (anhydrous).
Sodium citrate—$C_6H_5Na_3O_7$.
Sodium salicylate—$C_7H_5NaO_3$.
Caffeine—$C_8H_{10}N_4O_2$ (anhydrous); $C_8H_{10}N_4O_2 \cdot H_2O$ (monohydrate).
Citric acid—$C_6H_8O_7$ (anhydrous); $C_6H_8O_7 \cdot H_2O$ (monohydrate).

Molecular weight:
Pheniramine maleate—356.42.
Phenylephrine hydrochloride—203.67.
Codeine phosphate—406.37 (hemihydrate); 397.36 (anhydrous).
Sodium citrate—258.07 (anhydrous).
Sodium salicylate—160.10.
Caffeine—194.19 (anhydrous); 212.21 (monohydrate).
Citric acid—192.13 (anhydrous); 210.14 (monohydrate).

Description:
Pheniramine maleate—White or almost white, crystalline powder, odorless or with a slight odor.
Phenylephrine Hydrochloride USP—White or practically white, odorless crystals.

Codeine Phosphate USP—Fine, white, needle-shaped crystals, or white, crystalline powder. Is odorless, and is affected by light. Its solutions are acid to litmus.

Sodium Citrate USP—Colorless crystals or white, crystalline powder.

NF category: Buffering agent.

Sodium Salicylate USP—Amorphous or microcrystalline powder or scales. Is colorless, or has not more than a faint, pink tinge. Is odorless, or has a faint, characteristic odor, and is affected by light. A freshly made solution (1 in 10) is neutral or acid to litmus.

Caffeine USP—White powder or white, glistening needles, usually matted together. Is odorless. Its solutions are neutral to litmus. The hydrate is efflorescent in air.

Citric Acid USP—Colorless, translucent crystals, or white, granular to fine crystalline powder. Odorless or practically odorless. The hydrous form is efflorescent in dry air.

NF category: Acidifying agent; buffering agent.

Solubility:

Pheniramine maleate—Soluble 1 in 0.3 of water, 1 in 2.5 of alcohol, and 1 in 1.5 of chloroform; very slightly soluble in ether.

Phenylephrine Hydrochloride USP—Freely soluble in water and in alcohol.

Codeine Phosphate USP—Freely soluble in water; very soluble in hot water; slightly soluble in alcohol but more so in boiling alcohol.

Sodium Citrate USP—Hydrous form freely soluble in water and very soluble in boiling water; insoluble in alcohol.

Sodium Salicylate USP—Freely (and slowly) soluble in water and in glycerin; very soluble in boiling water and in boiling alcohol; slowly soluble in alcohol.

Caffeine USP—Sparingly soluble in water and in alcohol; freely soluble in chloroform; slightly soluble in ether.

The aqueous solubility of caffeine is increased by organic acids or their alkali salts, such as citrates, benzoates, salicylates, or cinnamates, which dissociate to yield caffeine when dissolved in biological fluids.

Citric Acid USP—Very soluble in water; freely soluble in alcohol; sparingly soluble in ether.

USP requirements: Pheniramine Maleate, Phenylephrine Hydrochloride, Codeine Phosphate, Sodium Citrate, Sodium Salicylate, and Caffeine Citrate Syrup—Not in USP.

PHENIRAMINE, PHENYLEPHRINE, SODIUM SALICYLATE, AND CAFFEINE

Source: Caffeine—Coffee, tea, cola, and cocoa or chocolate. May also be synthesized from urea or dimethylurea.

Chemical group:

Pheniramine—Alkylamine derivative.

Caffeine—Methylated xanthine.

Chemical name:

Pheniramine maleate—2-[alpha-[2-Dimethylaminoethyl]-benzyl]pyridine bimaleate.

Phenylephrine hydrochloride—Benzenemethanol, 3-hydroxy-alpha-[(methylamino)methyl]-, hydrochloride.

Sodium salicylate—Benzoic acid, 2-hydroxy-, monosodium salt.

Caffeine—1*H*-Purine-2,6-dione, 3,7-dihydro-1,3,7-trimethyl-.

Citric Acid—1,2,3-Propanetricarboxylic acid, 2-hydroxy-.

Molecular formula:

Pheniramine maleate—$C_{16}H_{20}N_2 \cdot C_4H_4O_4$.

Phenylephrine hydrochloride—$C_9H_{13}NO_2 \cdot HCl$.

Sodium salicylate—$C_7H_5NaO_3$.

Caffeine—$C_8H_{10}N_4O_2$ (anhydrous); $C_8H_{10}N_4O_2 \cdot H_2O$ (monohydrate).

Citric acid—$C_6H_8O_7$ (anhydrous); $C_6H_8O_7 \cdot H_2O$ (monohydrate).

Molecular weight:

Pheniramine maleate—356.42.

Phenylephrine hydrochloride—203.67.

Sodium salicylate—160.10.

Caffeine—194.19 (anhydrous); 212.21 (monohydrate).

Citric acid—192.13 (anhydrous); 210.14 (monohydrate).

Description:

Pheniramine maleate—White or almost white, crystalline powder, odorless or with a slight odor.

Phenylephrine Hydrochloride USP—White or practically white, odorless crystals.

Sodium Salicylate USP—Amorphous or microcrystalline powder or scales. Is colorless, or has not more than a faint, pink tinge. Is odorless, or has a faint, characteristic odor, and is affected by light. A freshly made solution (1 in 10) is neutral or acid to litmus.

Caffeine USP—White powder or white, glistening needles, usually matted together. Is odorless. Its solutions are neutral to litmus. The hydrate is efflorescent in air.

Citric Acid USP—Colorless, translucent crystals, or white, granular to fine crystalline powder. Odorless or practically odorless. The hydrous form is efflorescent in dry air.

NF category: Acidifying agent; buffering agent.

Solubility:

Pheniramine maleate—Soluble 1 in 0.3 of water, 1 in 2.5 of alcohol, and 1 in 1.5 of chloroform; very slightly soluble in ether.

Phenylephrine Hydrochloride USP—Freely soluble in water and in alcohol.

Sodium Salicylate USP—Freely (and slowly) soluble in water and in glycerin; very soluble in boiling water and in boiling alcohol; slowly soluble in alcohol.

Caffeine USP—Sparingly soluble in water and in alcohol; freely soluble in chloroform; slightly soluble in ether.

The aqueous solubility of caffeine is increased by organic acids or their alkali salts, such as citrates, benzoates, salicylates, or cinnamates, which dissociate to yield caffeine when dissolved in biological fluids.

Citric Acid USP—Very soluble in water; freely soluble in alcohol; sparingly soluble in ether.

USP requirements: Pheniramine Maleate, Phenylephrine Hydrochloride, Sodium Salicylate, and Caffeine Citrate Oral Solution—Not in USP.

PHENIRAMINE, PHENYLTOLOXAMINE, PYRILAMINE, AND PHENYLPROPANOLAMINE

Chemical group:

Pheniramine—Alkylamine derivative.

Phenyltoloxamine citrate—Ethanolamine derivative.

Pyrilamine—Ethylenediamine derivative.

Chemical name:

Pheniramine maleate—2-[alpha-[2-Dimethylaminoethyl]benzyl]pyridine bimaleate.

Phenyltoloxamine citrate—2-(2-Benzylphenoxy)-*N*,*N*-dimethylethylamine dihydrogen citrate.

Pyrilamine maleate—1,2-Ethanediamine, *N*-[(4-methoxyphenyl)methyl]-*N*′,*N*′-dimethyl-*N*-2-pyridinyl-, (*Z*)-2-butenedioate (1:1).

Phenylpropanolamine hydrochloride—Benzenemethanol, alpha-(1-aminoethyl)-, hydrochloride, (*R**,*S**)-, (±).

Molecular formula:
Pheniramine maleate—$C_{16}H_{20}N_2 \cdot C_4H_4O_4$.
Phenyltoloxamine citrate—$C_{17}H_{21}NO \cdot C_6H_8O_7$.
Pyrilamine maleate—$C_{17}H_{23}N_3O \cdot C_4H_4O_4$.
Phenylpropanolamine hydrochloride—$C_9H_{13}NO \cdot HCl$.

Molecular weight:
Pheniramine maleate—356.42.
Phenyltoloxamine citrate—447.5.
Pyrilamine maleate—401.46.
Phenylpropanolamine hydrochloride—187.67.

Description:
Pheniramine maleate—White or almost white, crystalline powder, odorless or with a slight odor.
Pyrilamine Maleate USP—White, crystalline powder, usually having a faint odor. Its solutions are acid to litmus.
Phenyltoloxamine citrate—It has a melting point of 138–140 °C.
Phenylpropanolamine Hydrochloride USP—White, crystalline powder, having a slight aromatic odor. Affected by light.

pKa: Phenylpropanolamine hydrochloride—9.

Solubility:
Pheniramine maleate—Soluble 1 in 0.3 of water, 1 in 2.5 of alcohol, and 1 in 1.5 of chloroform; very slightly soluble in ether.
Pyrilamine Maleate USP—Very soluble in water; freely soluble in alcohol and in chloroform; slightly soluble in ether.
Phenyltoloxamine citrate—Soluble in water.
Phenylpropanolamine Hydrochloride USP—Freely soluble in water and in alcohol; insoluble in ether.

USP requirements:
Pheniramine Maleate, Phenyltoloxamine Citrate, Pyrilamine Maleate, and Phenylpropanolamine Hydrochloride Extended-release Capsules—Not in USP.
Pheniramine Maleate, Phenyltoloxamine Citrate, Pyrilamine Maleate, and Phenylpropanolamine Hydrochloride Elixir—Not in USP.

PHENIRAMINE, PYRILAMINE, HYDROCODONE, POTASSIUM CITRATE, AND ASCORBIC ACID

Chemical group:
Pheniramine—Alkylamine derivative.
Pyrilamine—Ethylenediamine derivative.

Chemical name:
Pheniramine maleate—2-[alpha-[2-Dimethylaminoethyl]-benzyl]pyridine bimaleate.
Pyrilamine maleate—1,2-Ethanediamine, *N*-[(4-methoxyphenyl) methyl]-*N'*,*N'*-dimethyl-*N*-2-pyridinyl-, (*Z*)-2-butenedioate (1:1).
Hydrocodone bitartrate—Morphinan-6-one, 4,5-epoxy-3-methoxy-17-methyl-, (5 alpha)-, [*R*-(*R**,*R**)]-2,3-dihydroxybutanedioate (1:1), hydrate (2:5).
Potassium citrate—1,2,3-Propanetricarboxylic acid, 2-hydroxy-, tripotassium salt, monohydrate.
Ascorbic acid—L-Ascorbic acid.

Molecular formula:
Pheniramine maleate—$C_{16}H_{20}N_2 \cdot C_4H_4O_4$.
Pyrilamine maleate—$C_{17}H_{23}N_3O \cdot C_4H_4O_4$.
Hydrocodone bitartrate—$C_{18}H_{21}NO_3 \cdot C_4H_6O_6 \cdot 2\frac{1}{2}H_2O$ (hydrate); $C_{18}H_{21}NO_3 \cdot C_4H_6O_6$ (anhydrous).
Potassium citrate—$C_6H_5K_3O_7 \cdot H_2O$.
Ascorbic acid—$C_6H_8O_6$.

Molecular weight:
Pheniramine maleate—356.42.
Pyrilamine maleate—401.46.
Hydrocodone bitartrate—494.50 (hydrate); 449.46 (anhydrous).
Potassium citrate—324.41.
Ascorbic acid—176.13.

Description:
Pheniramine maleate—White or almost white, crystalline powder, odorless or with a slight odor.
Pyrilamine Maleate USP—White, crystalline powder, usually having a faint odor. Its solutions are acid to litmus.
Hydrocodone Bitartrate USP—Fine, white crystals or a crystalline powder. Is affected by light.
Potassium Citrate USP—Transparent crystals or white, granular powder. Is odorless and is deliquescent when exposed to moist air.
Ascorbic Acid USP—White or slightly yellow crystals or powder. On exposure to light it gradually darkens. In the dry state, is reasonably stable in air, but in solution rapidly oxidizes. Melts at about 190 °C.
NF category: Antioxidant.

Solubility:
Pheniramine maleate—Soluble 1 in 0.3 of water, 1 in 2.5 of alcohol, and 1 in 1.5 of chloroform; very slightly soluble in ether.
Pyrilamine Maleate USP—Very soluble in water; freely soluble in alcohol and in chloroform; slightly soluble in ether.
Hydrocodone Bitartrate USP—Soluble in water; slightly soluble in alcohol; insoluble in ether and in chloroform.
Potassium Citrate USP—Freely soluble in water; almost insoluble in alcohol.
Ascorbic Acid USP—Freely soluble in water; sparingly soluble in alcohol; insoluble in chloroform and in ether.

USP requirements: Pheniramine Maleate, Pyrilamine Maleate, Hydrocodone Bitartrate, Potassium Citrate, and Ascorbic Acid Syrup—Not in USP.

PHENIRAMINE, PYRILAMINE, PHENYLEPHRINE, PHENYLPROPANOLAMINE, AND HYDROCODONE

Chemical group:
Pheniramine—Alkylamine derivative.
Pyrilamine—Ethylenediamine derivative.

Chemical name:
Pheniramine maleate—2-[alpha-[2-Dimethylaminoethyl]-benzyl]pyridine bimaleate.
Pyrilamine maleate—1,2-Ethanediamine, *N*-[(4-methoxyphenyl)methyl]-*N'*,*N'*-dimethyl-*N*-2-pyridinyl-, (*Z*)-2-butenedioate (1:1).
Phenylephrine hydrochloride—Benzenemethanol, 3-hydroxy-alpha-[(methylamino)methyl]-, hydrochloride.
Phenylpropanolamine hydrochloride—Benzenemethanol, alpha-(1-aminoethyl)-, hydrochloride, (*R**,*S**)-, (±).
Hydrocodone bitartrate—Morphinan-6-one, 4,5-epoxy-3-methoxy-17-methyl-, (5 alpha)-, [*R*-(*R**,*R**)]-2,3-dihydroxybutanedioate (1:1), hydrate (2:5).

Molecular formula:
Pheniramine maleate—$C_{16}H_{20}N_2 \cdot C_4H_4O_4$.
Pyrilamine maleate—$C_{17}H_{23}N_3O \cdot C_4H_4O_4$.
Phenylephrine hydrochloride—$C_9H_{13}NO_2 \cdot HCl$.
Phenylpropanolamine hydrochloride—$C_9H_{13}NO \cdot HCl$.
Hydrocodone bitartrate—$C_{18}H_{21}NO_3 \cdot C_4H_6O_6 \cdot 2\frac{1}{2}H_2O$ (hydrate); $C_{18}H_{21}NO_3 \cdot C_4H_6O_6$ (anhydrous).

Molecular weight:
Pheniramine maleate—356.42.
Pyrilamine maleate—401.46.
Phenylephrine hydrochloride—203.67.

Phenylpropanolamine hydrochloride—187.67.
Hydrocodone bitartrate—494.50 (hydrate); 449.46 (anhydrous).

Description:
Pheniramine maleate—White or almost white, crystalline powder, odorless or with a slight odor.
Pyrilamine Maleate USP—White, crystalline powder, usually having a faint odor. Its solutions are acid to litmus.
Phenylephrine Hydrochloride USP—White or practically white, odorless crystals.
Phenylpropanolamine Hydrochloride USP—White, crystalline powder, having a slight aromatic odor. Is affected by light.
Hydrocodone Bitartrate USP—Fine, white crystals or a crystalline powder. Is affected by light.

pKa: Phenylpropanolamine hydrochloride—9.

Solubility:
Pheniramine maleate—Soluble 1 in 0.3 of water, 1 in 2.5 of alcohol, and 1 in 1.5 of chloroform; very slightly soluble in ether.
Pyrilamine Maleate USP—Very soluble in water; freely soluble in alcohol and in chloroform; slightly soluble in ether.
Phenylephrine Hydrochloride USP—Freely soluble in water and in alcohol.
Phenylpropanolamine Hydrochloride USP—Freely soluble in water and in alcohol; insoluble in ether.
Hydrocodone Bitartrate USP—Soluble in water; slightly soluble in alcohol; insoluble in ether and in chloroform.

USP requirements: Pheniramine Maleate, Pyrilamine Maleate, Phenylephrine Hydrochloride, Phenylpropanolamine Hydrochloride, and Hydrocodone Bitartrate Oral Solution—Not in USP.

PHENIRAMINE, PYRILAMINE, AND PHENYLPROPANOLAMINE

Chemical group:
Pheniramine—Alkylamine derivative.
Pyrilamine—Ethylenediamine derivative.

Chemical name:
Pheniramine maleate—2-[alpha-[2-Dimethylaminoethyl]-benzyl]pyridine bimaleate.
Pyrilamine maleate—1,2-Ethanediamine, *N*-[(4-methoxyphenyl)methyl]-*N*′,*N*′-dimethyl-*N*-2-pyridinyl-, (*Z*)-2-butenedioate (1:1).
Phenylpropanolamine hydrochloride—Benzenemethanol, alpha-(1-aminoethyl)-, hydrochloride, (*R**,*S**)-, (±).

Molecular formula:
Pheniramine maleate—$C_{16}H_{20}N_2 \cdot C_4H_4O_4$.
Pyrilamine maleate—$C_{17}H_{23}N_3O \cdot C_4H_4O_4$.
Phenylpropanolamine hydrochloride—$C_9H_{13}NO \cdot HCl$.

Molecular weight:
Pheniramine maleate—356.42.
Pyrilamine maleate—401.46.
Phenylpropanolamine hydrochloride—187.67.

Description:
Pheniramine maleate—White or almost white, crystalline powder, odorless or with a slight odor.
Pyrilamine Maleate USP—White, crystalline powder, usually having a faint odor. Its solutions are acid to litmus.
Phenylpropanolamine Hydrochloride USP—White, crystalline powder, having a slight aromatic odor. Affected by light.

pKa: Phenylpropanolamine hydrochloride—9.

Solubility:
Pheniramine maleate—Soluble 1 in 0.3 of water, 1 in 2.5 of alcohol, and 1 in 1.5 of chloroform; very slightly soluble in ether.
Pyrilamine Maleate USP—Very soluble in water; freely soluble in alcohol and in chloroform; slightly soluble in ether.
Phenylpropanolamine Hydrochloride USP—Freely soluble in water and in alcohol; insoluble in ether.

USP requirements:
Pheniramine Maleate, Pyrilamine Maleate, and Phenylpropanolamine Hydrochloride Oral Solution—Not in USP.
Pheniramine Maleate, Pyrilamine Maleate, and Phenylpropanolamine Hydrochloride Extended-release Tablets—Not in USP.

PHENIRAMINE, PYRILAMINE, PHENYLPROPANOLAMINE, AND ASPIRIN

Chemical group:
Pheniramine—Alkylamine derivative.
Pyrilamine—Ethylenediamine derivative.

Chemical name:
Pheniramine maleate—2-[alpha-[2-Dimethylaminoethyl]-benzyl]pyridine bimaleate.
Pyrilamine maleate—1,2-Ethanediamine, *N*-[(4-methoxyphenyl)methyl]-*N*′,*N*′-dimethyl-*N*-2-pyridinyl-, (*Z*)-2-butenedioate (1:1).
Phenylpropanolamine hydrochloride—Benzenemethanol, alpha-(1-aminoethyl)-, hydrochloride, (*R**,*S**)-, (±).
Aspirin—Benzoic acid, 2-(acetyloxy)-.

Molecular formula:
Pheniramine maleate—$C_{16}H_{20}N_2 \cdot C_4H_4O_4$.
Pyrilamine maleate—$C_{17}H_{23}N_3O \cdot C_4H_4O_4$.
Phenylpropanolamine hydrochloride—$C_9H_{13}NO \cdot HCl$.
Aspirin—$C_9H_8O_4$.

Molecular weight:
Pheniramine maleate—356.42.
Pyrilamine maleate—401.46.
Phenylpropanolamine hydrochloride—187.67.
Aspirin—180.16.

Description:
Pheniramine maleate—White or almost white, crystalline powder, odorless or with a slight odor.
Pyrilamine Maleate USP—White, crystalline powder, usually having a faint odor. Its solutions are acid to litmus.
Phenylpropanolamine Hydrochloride USP—White, crystalline powder, having a slight aromatic odor. Affected by light.
Aspirin USP—White crystals, commonly tabular or needle-like, or white, crystalline powder. Is odorless or has a faint odor. Is stable in dry air; in moist air it gradually hydrolyzes to salicylic and acetic acids.

pKa:
Phenylpropanolamine hydrochloride—9.
Aspirin—3.5.

Solubility:
Pheniramine maleate—Soluble 1 in 0.3 of water, 1 in 2.5 of alcohol, and 1 in 1.5 of chloroform; very slightly soluble in ether.
Pyrilamine Maleate USP—Very soluble in water; freely soluble in alcohol and in chloroform; slightly soluble in ether.
Phenylpropanolamine Hydrochloride USP—Freely soluble in water and in alcohol; insoluble in ether.
Aspirin USP—Slightly soluble in water; freely soluble in alcohol; soluble in chloroform and in ether; sparingly soluble in absolute ether.

USP requirements: Pheniramine Maleate, Pyrilamine Maleate, Phenylpropanolamine Hydrochloride, and Aspirin Tablets—Not in USP.

PHENIRAMINE, PYRILAMINE, PHENYLPROPANOLAMINE, AND CODEINE

Chemical group:
Pheniramine—Alkylamine derivative.
Pyrilamine—Ethylenediamine derivative.

Chemical name:
Pheniramine maleate—2-[alpha-[2-Dimethylaminoethyl]-benzyl]pyridine bimaleate.
Pyrilamine maleate—1,2-Ethanediamine, *N*-[(4-methoxyphenyl)methyl]-*N'*,*N'*-dimethyl-*N*-2-pyridinyl-, (*Z*)-2-butenedioate (1:1).
Phenylpropanolamine hydrochloride—Benzenemethanol, alpha-(1-aminoethyl)-, hydrochloride, (*R**,*S**)-, (±).
Codeine phosphate—Morphinan-6-ol, 7,8-didehydro-4,5-epoxy-3-methoxy-17-methyl-, (5 alpha,6 alpha)-, phosphate (1:1) (salt), hemihydrate.

Molecular formula:
Pheniramine maleate—$C_{16}H_{20}N_2 \cdot C_4H_4O_4$.
Pyrilamine maleate—$C_{17}H_{23}N_3O \cdot C_4H_4O_4$.
Phenylpropanolamine hydrochloride—$C_9H_{13}NO \cdot HCl$.
Codeine phosphate—$C_{18}H_{21}NO_3 \cdot H_3PO_4 \cdot ½H_2O$ (hemihydrate); $C_{18}H_{21}NO_3 \cdot H_3PO_4$ (anhydrous).

Molecular weight:
Pheniramine maleate—356.42.
Pyrilamine maleate—401.46.
Phenylpropanolamine hydrochloride—187.67.
Codeine phosphate—406.37 (hemihydrate); 397.36 (anhydrous).

Description:
Pheniramine maleate—White or almost white, crystalline powder, odorless or with a slight odor.
Pyrilamine Maleate USP—White, crystalline powder, usually having a faint odor. Its solutions are acid to litmus.
Phenylpropanolamine Hydrochloride USP—White, crystalline powder, having a slight aromatic odor. Affected by light.
Codeine Phosphate USP—Fine, white, needle-shaped crystals, or white, crystalline powder. Is odorless, and is affected by light. Its solutions are acid to litmus.

pKa: Phenylpropanolamine hydrochloride—9.

Solubility:
Pheniramine maleate—Soluble 1 in 0.3 of water, 1 in 2.5 of alcohol, and 1 in 1.5 of chloroform; very slightly soluble in ether.
Pyrilamine Maleate USP—Very soluble in water; freely soluble in alcohol and in chloroform; slightly soluble in ether.
Phenylpropanolamine Hydrochloride USP—Freely soluble in water and in alcohol; insoluble in ether.
Codeine Phosphate USP—Freely soluble in water; very soluble in hot water; slightly soluble in alcohol but more so in boiling alcohol.

USP requirements: Pheniramine Maleate, Pyrilamine Maleate, Phenylpropanolamine Hydrochloride and Codeine Phosphate Syrup—Not in USP.

PHENIRAMINE, PYRILAMINE, PHENYLPROPANOLAMINE, CODEINE, ACETAMINOPHEN, AND CAFFEINE

Source: Caffeine—Coffee, tea, cola, and cocoa or chocolate. May also be synthesized from urea or dimethylurea.

Chemical group:
Pheniramine—Alkylamine derivative.
Pyrilamine—Ethylenediamine derivative.
Caffeine—Methylated xanthine.

Chemical name:
Pheniramine maleate—2-[alpha-[2-Dimethylaminoethyl]-benzyl]pyridine bimaleate.
Pyrilamine maleate—1,2-Ethanediamine, *N*-[(4-methoxyphenyl)methyl]-*N'*,*N'*-dimethyl-*N*-2-pyridinyl-, (*Z*)-2-butenedioate (1:1).
Phenylpropanolamine hydrochloride—Benzenemethanol, alpha-(1-aminoethyl)-, hydrochloride, (*R**,*S**)-, (±).
Codeine phosphate—Morphinan-6-ol, 7,8-didehydro-4,5-epoxy-3-methoxy-17-methyl-, (5 alpha,6 alpha)-, phosphate (1:1) (salt), hemihydrate.
Acetaminophen—Acetamide, *N*-(4-hydroxyphenyl)-.
Caffeine—1*H*-Purine-2,6-dione, 3,7-dihydro-1,3,7-trimethyl-.

Molecular formula:
Pheniramine maleate—$C_{16}H_{20}N_2 \cdot C_4H_4O_4$.
Pyrilamine maleate—$C_{17}H_{23}N_3O \cdot C_4H_4O_4$.
Phenylpropanolamine hydrochloride—$C_9H_{13}NO \cdot HCl$.
Codeine phosphate—$C_{18}H_{21}NO_3 \cdot H_3PO_4 \cdot ½H_2O$ (hemihydrate); $C_{18}H_{21}NO_3 \cdot H_3PO_4$ (anhydrous).
Acetaminophen—$C_8H_9NO_2$.
Caffeine—$C_8H_{10}N_4O_2$ (anhydrous); $C_8H_{10}N_4O_2 \cdot H_2O$ (monohydrate).

Molecular weight:
Pheniramine maleate—356.42.
Pyrilamine maleate—401.46.
Phenylpropanolamine hydrochloride—187.67.
Codeine phosphate—406.37 (hemihydrate); 397.36 (anhydrous).
Acetaminophen—151.16.
Caffeine—194.19 (anhydrous); 212.21 (monohydrate).

Description:
Pheniramine maleate—White or almost white, crystalline powder, odorless or with a slight odor.
Pyrilamine Maleate USP—White, crystalline powder, usually having a faint odor. Its solutions are acid to litmus.
Phenylpropanolamine Hydrochloride USP—White, crystalline powder, having a slight aromatic odor. Is affected by light.
Codeine Phosphate USP—Fine, white, needle-shaped crystals, or white, crystalline powder. Is odorless, and is affected by light. Its solutions are acid to litmus.
Acetaminophen USP—White, odorless, crystalline powder.
Caffeine USP—White powder, or white, glistening needles, usually matted together. Is odorless. Its solutions are neutral to litmus. The hydrate is efflorescent in air.

pKa: Phenylpropanolamine hydrochloride—9.

Solubility:
Pheniramine maleate—Soluble 1 in 0.3 of water, 1 in 2.5 of alcohol, and 1 in 1.5 of chloroform; very slightly soluble in ether.
Pyrilamine Maleate USP—Very soluble in water; freely soluble in alcohol and in chloroform; slightly soluble in ether.
Phenylpropanolamine Hydrochloride USP—Freely soluble in water and in alcohol; insoluble in ether.
Codeine Phosphate USP—Freely soluble in water; very soluble in hot water; slightly soluble in alcohol but more so in boiling alcohol.
Acetaminophen USP—Soluble in boiling water and in 1 *N* sodium hydroxide; freely soluble in alcohol.
Caffeine USP—Sparingly soluble in water and in alcohol; freely soluble in chloroform; slightly soluble in ether.
The aqueous solubility of caffeine is increased by organic acids or their alkali salts, such as citrates, benzoates, salicylates, or cinnamates, which dissociate to yield caffeine when dissolved in biological fluids.

USP requirements: Pheniramine Maleate, Pyrilamine Maleate, Phenylpropanolamine Hydrochloride, Codeine Phosphate, Acetaminophen, and Caffeine Tablets—Not in USP.

PHENIRAMINE, PYRILAMINE, PHENYLPROPANOLAMINE, AND DEXTROMETHORPHAN

Source: Dextromethorphan—Methylated dextroisomer of levorphanol.

Chemical group:
- Pheniramine—Alkylamine derivative.
- Pyrilamine—Ethylenediamine derivative.
- Dextromethorphan—Synthetic derivative of morphine.

Chemical name:
- Pheniramine maleate—2-[alpha-[2-Dimethylaminoethyl]-benzyl]pyridine bimaleate.
- Pyrilamine maleate—1,2-Ethanediamine, *N*-[(4-methoxyphenyl)methyl]-*N′*,*N′*-dimethyl-*N*-2-pyridinyl-, (*Z*)-2-butenedioate (1:1).
- Phenylpropanolamine hydrochloride—Benzenemethanol, alpha-(1-aminoethyl)-, hydrochloride, (*R**,*S**)-, (±).
- Dextromethorphan hydrobromide—Morphinan, 3-methoxy-17-methyl-, (9 alpha,13 alpha,14 alpha)-, hydrobromide, monohydrate.

Molecular formula:
- Pheniramine maleate—$C_{16}H_{20}N_2 \cdot C_4H_4O_4$.
- Pyrilamine maleate—$C_{17}H_{23}N_3O \cdot C_4H_4O_4$.
- Phenylpropanolamine hydrochloride—$C_9H_{13}NO \cdot HCl$.
- Dextromethorphan hydrobromide—$C_{18}H_{25}NO \cdot HBr \cdot H_2O$.

Molecular weight:
- Pheniramine maleate—356.42.
- Pyrilamine maleate—401.46.
- Phenylpropanolamine hydrochloride—187.67.
- Dextromethorphan hydrobromide—370.33.

Description:
- Pheniramine maleate—White or almost white, crystalline powder, odorless or with a slight odor.
- Pyrilamine Maleate USP—White, crystalline powder, usually having a faint odor. Its solutions are acid to litmus.
- Phenylpropanolamine Hydrochloride USP—White, crystalline powder, having a slight aromatic odor. Is affected by light.
- Dextromethorphan Hydrobromide USP—Practically white crystals or crystalline powder, having a faint odor. Melts at about 126 °C, with decomposition.

pKa: Phenylpropanolamine hydrochloride—9.

Solubility:
- Pheniramine maleate—Soluble 1 in 0.3 of water, 1 in 2.5 of alcohol, and 1 in 1.5 of chloroform; very slightly soluble in ether.
- Pyrilamine Maleate USP—Very soluble in water; freely soluble in alcohol and in chloroform; slightly soluble in ether.
- Phenylpropanolamine Hydrochloride USP—Freely soluble in water and in alcohol; insoluble in ether.
- Dextromethorphan Hydrobromide USP—Sparingly soluble in water; freely soluble in alcohol and in chloroform; insoluble in ether.

USP requirements: Pheniramine Maleate, Pyrilamine Maleate, Phenylpropanolamine Hydrochloride, and Dextromethorphan Hydrobromide Syrup—Not in USP.

PHENIRAMINE, PYRILAMINE, PHENYLPROPANOLAMINE, DEXTROMETHORPHAN, AND AMMONIUM CHLORIDE

Source: Dextromethorphan—Methylated dextroisomer of levorphanol.

Chemical group:
- Pheniramine—Alkylamine derivative.
- Pyrilamine—Ethylenediamine derivative.
- Dextromethorphan—Synthetic derivative of morphine.

Chemical name:
- Pheniramine maleate—2-[alpha-[2-Dimethylaminoethyl]-benzyl]pyridine bimaleate.
- Pyrilamine maleate—1,2-Ethanediamine, *N*-[(4-methoxyphenyl)methyl]-*N′*,*N′*-dimethyl-*N*-2-pyridinyl-, (*Z*)-2-butenedioate (1:1).
- Phenylpropanolamine hydrochloride—Benzenemethanol, alpha-(1-aminoethyl)-, hydrochloride, (*R**,*S**)-, (±).
- Dextromethorphan hydrobromide—Morphinan, 3-methoxy-17-methyl-, (9 alpha,13 alpha,14 alpha)-, hydrobromide, monohydrate.
- Ammonium chloride—Ammonium chloride.

Molecular formula:
- Pheniramine maleate—$C_{16}H_{20}N_2 \cdot C_4H_4O_4$.
- Pyrilamine maleate—$C_{17}H_{23}N_3O \cdot C_4H_4O_4$.
- Phenylpropanolamine hydrochloride—$C_9H_{13}NO \cdot HCl$.
- Dextromethorphan hydrobromide—$C_{18}H_{25}NO \cdot HBr \cdot H_2O$.
- Ammonium chloride—NH_4Cl.

Molecular weight:
- Pheniramine maleate—356.42.
- Pyrilamine maleate—401.46.
- Phenylpropanolamine hydrochloride—187.67.
- Dextromethorphan hydrobromide—370.33.
- Ammonium chloride—53.49.

Description:
- Pheniramine maleate—White or almost white, crystalline powder, odorless or with a slight odor.
- Pyrilamine Maleate USP—White, crystalline powder, usually having a faint odor. Its solutions are acid to litmus.
- Phenylpropanolamine Hydrochloride USP—White, crystalline powder, having a slight aromatic odor. Is affected by light.
- Dextromethorphan Hydrobromide USP—Practically white crystals or crystalline powder, having a faint odor. Melts at about 126 °C, with decomposition.
- Ammonium Chloride USP—Colorless crystals or white, fine or coarse, crystalline powder. Is somewhat hygroscopic.

pKa: Phenylpropanolamine hydrochloride—9.

Solubility:
- Pheniramine maleate—Soluble 1 in 0.3 of water, 1 in 2.5 of alcohol, and 1 in 1.5 of chloroform; very slightly soluble in ether.
- Pyrilamine Maleate USP—Very soluble in water; freely soluble in alcohol and in chloroform; slightly soluble in ether.
- Phenylpropanolamine Hydrochloride USP—Freely soluble in water and in alcohol; insoluble in ether.
- Dextromethorphan Hydrobromide USP—Sparingly soluble in water; freely soluble in alcohol and in chloroform; insoluble in ether.
- Ammonium Chloride USP—Freely soluble in water and in glycerin, and even more so in boiling water; sparingly soluble in alcohol.

USP requirements: Pheniramine Maleate, Pyrilamine Maleate, Phenylpropanolamine Hydrochloride, Dextromethorphan Hydrobromide, and Ammonium Chloride Syrup—Not in USP.

PHENIRAMINE, PYRILAMINE, PHENYLPROPANOLAMINE, DEXTROMETHORPHAN, AND GUAIFENESIN

Source: Dextromethorphan—Methylated dextroisomer of levorphanol.

Chemical group:
Pheniramine—Alkylamine derivative.
Pyrilamine—Ethylenediamine derivative.
Dextromethorphan—Synthetic derivative of morphine.

Chemical name:
Pheniramine maleate—2-[alpha-[2-Dimethylaminoethyl]-benzyl]pyridine bimaleate.
Pyrilamine maleate—1,2-Ethanediamine, *N*-[(4-methoxyphenyl)methyl]-*N′*,*N′*-dimethyl-*N*-2-pyridinyl-, (*Z*)-2-butenedioate (1:1).
Phenylpropanolamine hydrochloride—Benzenemethanol, alpha-(1-aminoethyl)-, hydrochloride, (*R**,*S**)-, (±).
Dextromethorphan hydrobromide—Morphinan, 3-methoxy-17-methyl-, (9 alpha,13 alpha,14 alpha)-, hydrobromide, monohydrate.
Guaifenesin—1,2-Propanediol, 3-(2-methoxyphenoxy)-.

Molecular formula:
Pheniramine maleate—$C_{16}H_{20}N_2 \cdot C_4H_4O_4$.
Pyrilamine maleate—$C_{17}H_{23}N_3O \cdot C_4H_4O_4$.
Phenylpropanolamine hydrochloride—$C_9H_{13}NO \cdot HCl$.
Dextromethorphan hydrobromide—$C_{18}H_{25}NO \cdot HBr \cdot H_2O$.
Guaifenesin—$C_{10}H_{14}O_4$.

Molecular weight:
Pheniramine maleate—356.42.
Pyrilamine maleate—401.46.
Phenylpropanolamine hydrochloride—187.67.
Dextromethorphan hydrobromide—370.33.
Guaifenesin—198.22.

Description:
Pheniramine maleate—White or almost white, crystalline powder, odorless or with a slight odor.
Pyrilamine Maleate USP—White, crystalline powder, usually having a faint odor. Its solutions are acid to litmus.
Phenylpropanolamine Hydrochloride USP—White, crystalline powder, having a slight aromatic odor. Is affected by light.
Dextromethorphan Hydrobromide USP—Practically white crystals or crystalline powder, having a faint odor. Melts at about 126 °C, with decomposition.
Guaifenesin USP—White to slightly gray, crystalline powder. May have a slight characteristic odor.

pKa: Phenylpropanolamine hydrochloride—9.

Solubility:
Pheniramine maleate—Soluble 1 in 0.3 of water, 1 in 2.5 of alcohol, and 1 in 1.5 of chloroform; very slightly soluble in ether.
Pyrilamine Maleate USP—Very soluble in water; freely soluble in alcohol and in chloroform; slightly soluble in ether.
Phenylpropanolamine Hydrochloride USP—Freely soluble in water and in alcohol; insoluble in ether.
Dextromethorphan Hydrobromide USP—Sparingly soluble in water; freely soluble in alcohol and in chloroform; insoluble in ether.
Guaifenesin USP—Soluble in water, in alcohol, in chloroform, in glycerin, and in propylene glycol.

USP requirements: Pheniramine Maleate, Pyrilamine Maleate, Phenylpropanolamine Hydrochloride, Dextromethorphan Hydrobromide, and Guaifenesin Oral Solution—Not in USP.

PHENIRAMINE, PYRILAMINE, PHENYLPROPANOLAMINE, AND GUAIFENESIN

Chemical group:
Pheniramine—Alkylamine derivative.
Pyrilamine—Ethylenediamine derivative.

Chemical name:
Pheniramine maleate—2-[alpha-[2-Dimethylaminoethyl]-benzyl]pyridine bimaleate.
Pyrilamine maleate—1,2-Ethanediamine, *N*-[(4-methoxyphenyl)methyl]-*N′*,*N′*-dimethyl-*N*-2-pyridinyl-, (*Z*)-2-butenedioate (1:1).
Phenylpropanolamine hydrochloride—Benzenemethanol, alpha-(1-aminoethyl)-, hydrochloride, (*R**,*S**)-, (±).
Guaifenesin—1,2-Propanediol, 3-(2-methoxyphenoxy)-.

Molecular formula:
Pheniramine maleate—$C_{16}H_{20}N_2 \cdot C_4H_4O_4$.
Pyrilamine maleate—$C_{17}H_{23}N_3O \cdot C_4H_4O_4$.
Phenylpropanolamine hydrochloride—$C_9H_{13}NO \cdot HCl$.
Guaifenesin—$C_{10}H_{14}O_4$.

Molecular weight:
Pheniramine maleate—356.42.
Pyrilamine maleate—401.46.
Phenylpropanolamine hydrochloride—187.67.
Guaifenesin—198.22.

Description:
Pheniramine maleate—White or almost white, crystalline powder, odorless or with a slight odor.
Pyrilamine Maleate USP—White, crystalline powder, usually having a faint odor. Its solutions are acid to litmus.
Phenylpropanolamine Hydrochloride USP—White, crystalline powder, having a slight aromatic odor. Is affected by light.
Guaifenesin USP—White to slightly gray, crystalline powder. May have a slight characteristic odor.

pKa: Phenylpropanolamine hydrochloride—9.

Solubility:
Pheniramine maleate—Soluble 1 in 0.3 of water, 1 in 2.5 of alcohol, and 1 in 1.5 of chloroform; very slightly soluble in ether.
Pyrilamine Maleate USP—Very soluble in water; freely soluble in alcohol and in chloroform; slightly soluble in ether.
Phenylpropanolamine Hydrochloride USP—Freely soluble in water and in alcohol; insoluble in ether.
Guaifenesin USP—Soluble in water, in alcohol, in chloroform, in glycerin, and in propylene glycol.

USP requirements: Pheniramine Maleate, Pyrilamine Maleate, Phenylpropanolamine Hydrochloride, and Guaifenesin Oral Solution—Not in USP.

PHENIRAMINE, PYRILAMINE, PHENYLPROPANOLAMINE, AND HYDROCODONE

Chemical group:
Pheniramine—Alkylamine derivative.
Pyrilamine—Ethylenediamine derivative.

Chemical name:
Pheniramine maleate—2-[alpha-[2-Dimethylaminoethyl]-benzyl]pyridine bimaleate.
Pyrilamine maleate—1,2-Ethanediamine, *N*-[(4-methoxyphenyl)methyl]-*N′*,*N′*-dimethyl-*N*-2-pyridinyl-, (*Z*)-2-butenedioate (1:1).
Phenylpropanolamine hydrochloride—Benzenemethanol, alpha-(1-aminoethyl)-, hydrochloride, (*R**,*S**)-, (±).

Hydrocodone bitartrate—Morphinan-6-one, 4,5-epoxy-3-methoxy-17-methyl-, (5 alpha)-, [*R*-(*R**,*R**)]-2,3-dihydroxybutanedioate (1:1), hydrate (2:5).

Molecular formula:
Pheniramine maleate—$C_{16}H_{20}N_2 \cdot C_4H_4O_4$.
Pyrilamine maleate—$C_{17}H_{23}N_3O \cdot C_4H_4O_4$.
Phenylpropanolamine hydrochloride—$C_9H_{13}NO \cdot HCl$.
Hydrocodone bitartrate—$C_{18}H_{21}NO_3 \cdot C_4H_6O_6 \cdot 2½H_2O$ (hydrate); $C_{18}H_{21}NO_3 \cdot C_4H_6O_6$ (anhydrous).

Molecular weight:
Pheniramine maleate—356.42.
Pyrilamine maleate—401.46.
Phenylpropanolamine hydrochloride—187.67.
Hydrocodone bitartrate—494.50 (hydrate); 449.46 (anhydrous).

Description:
Pheniramine maleate—White or almost white, crystalline powder, odorless or with a slight odor.
Pyrilamine Maleate USP—White, crystalline powder, usually having a faint odor. Its solutions are acid to litmus.
Phenylpropanolamine Hydrochloride USP—White, crystalline powder, having a slight aromatic odor. Is affected by light.
Hydrocodone Bitartrate USP—Fine, white crystals or a crystalline powder. Is affected by light.

pKa: Phenylpropanolamine hydrochloride—9.

Solubility:
Pheniramine maleate—Soluble 1 in 0.3 of water, 1 in 2.5 of alcohol, and 1 in 1.5 of chloroform; very slightly soluble in ether.
Pyrilamine Maleate USP—Very soluble in water; freely soluble in alcohol and in chloroform; slightly soluble in ether.
Phenylpropanolamine Hydrochloride USP—Freely soluble in water and in alcohol; insoluble in ether.
Hydrocodone Bitartrate USP—Soluble in water; slightly soluble in alcohol; insoluble in ether and in chloroform.

USP requirements: Pheniramine Maleate, Pyrilamine Maleate, Phenylpropanolamine Hydrochloride, and Hydrocodone Bitartrate Oral Solution—Not in USP.

PHENIRAMINE, PYRILAMINE, PHENYLPROPANOLAMINE, HYDROCODONE, AND GUAIFENESIN

Chemical group:
Pheniramine—Alkylamine derivative.
Pyrilamine—Ethylenediamine derivative.

Chemical name:
Pheniramine maleate—2-[alpha-[2-Dimethylaminoethyl]-benzyl]pyridine bimaleate.
Pyrilamine maleate—1,2-Ethanediamine, *N*-[(4-methoxyphenyl)methyl]-*N'*,*N'*-dimethyl-*N*-2-pyridinyl-, (*Z*)-2-butenedioate (1:1).
Phenylpropanolamine hydrochloride—Benzenemethanol, alpha-(1-aminoethyl)-, hydrochloride, (*R**,*S**)-, (±).
Hydrocodone bitartrate—Morphinan-6-one, 4,5-epoxy-3-methoxy-17-methyl-, (5 alpha)-, [*R*-(*R**,*R**)]-2,3-dihydroxybutanedioate (1:1), hydrate (2:5).
Guaifenesin—1,2-Propanediol, 3-(2-methoxyphenoxy)-.

Molecular formula:
Pheniramine maleate—$C_{16}H_{20}N_2 \cdot C_4H_4O_4$.
Pyrilamine maleate—$C_{17}H_{23}N_3O \cdot C_4H_4O_4$.
Phenylpropanolamine hydrochloride—$C_9H_{13}NO \cdot HCl$.
Hydrocodone bitartrate—$C_{18}H_{21}NO_3 \cdot C_4H_6O_6 \cdot 2½H_2O$ (hydrate); $C_{18}H_{21}NO_3 \cdot C_4H_6O_6$ (anhydrous).
Guaifenesin—$C_{10}H_{14}O_4$.

Molecular weight:
Pheniramine maleate—356.42.
Pyrilamine maleate—401.46.
Phenylpropanolamine hydrochloride—187.67.
Hydrocodone bitartrate—494.50 (hydrate); 449.46 (anhydrous).
Guaifenesin—198.22.

Description:
Pheniramine maleate—White or almost white, crystalline powder, odorless or with a slight odor.
Pyrilamine Maleate USP—White, crystalline powder, usually having a faint odor. Its solutions are acid to litmus.
Phenylpropanolamine Hydrochloride USP—White, crystalline powder, having a slight aromatic odor. Is affected by light.
Hydrocodone Bitartrate USP—Fine, white crystals or a crystalline powder. Is affected by light.
Guaifenesin USP—White to slightly gray, crystalline powder. May have a slight characteristic odor.

pKa: Phenylpropanolamine hydrochloride—9.

Solubility:
Pheniramine maleate—Soluble 1 in 0.3 of water, 1 in 2.5 of alcohol, and 1 in 1.5 of chloroform; very slightly soluble in ether.
Pyrilamine Maleate USP—Very soluble in water; freely soluble in alcohol and in chloroform; slightly soluble in ether.
Phenylpropanolamine Hydrochloride USP—Freely soluble in water and in alcohol; insoluble in ether.
Hydrocodone Bitartrate USP—Soluble in water; slightly soluble in alcohol; insoluble in ether and in chloroform.
Guaifenesin USP—Soluble in water, in alcohol, in chloroform, in glycerin, and in propylene glycol.

USP requirements: Pheniramine Maleate, Pyrilamine Maleate, Phenylpropanolamine Hydrochloride, Hydrocodone Bitartrate, and Guaifenesin Oral Solution—Not in USP.

PHENMETRAZINE

Chemical group: Morpholine.

Chemical name: Phenmetrazine hydrochloride—Morpholine, 3-methyl-2-phenyl-, hydrochloride.

Molecular formula: Phenmetrazine hydrochloride—$C_{11}H_{15}NO \cdot HCl$.

Molecular weight: Phenmetrazine hydrochloride—213.71.

Description: Phenmetrazine Hydrochloride USP—White to off-white, crystalline powder.

Solubility: Phenmetrazine Hydrochloride USP—Very soluble in water; freely soluble in alcohol and in chloroform.

USP requirements:
Phenmetrazine Hydrochloride USP—Preserve in tight containers. Dried at 105 °C for 2 hours, contains not less than 98.0% and not more than 102.0% of phenmetrazine hydrochloride. Meets the requirements for Identification, Melting range (172–182 °C, the range between beginning and end of melting not more than 3 °C), pH (4.5–5.5, in a solution [1 in 40]), Loss on drying (not more than 0.5%), Residue on ignition (not more than 0.1%), Sulfate (not more than 0.01%), Chloride content (16.3–17.0%), Heavy metals (not more than 0.001%), Ordinary impurities, and Organic volatile impurities.
Phenmetrazine Hydrochloride Tablets USP—Preserve in tight containers. Contain the labeled amount, within ±7%.

Meet the requirements for Identification, Dissolution (75% in 45 minutes in water in Apparatus 2 at 50 rpm), and Uniformity of dosage units.

PHENOBARBITAL

Chemical name:
Phenobarbital—2,4,6(1*H*,3*H*,5*H*)-Pyrimidinetrione, 5-ethyl-5-phenyl-.
Phenobarbital sodium—2,4,6(1*H*,3*H*,5*H*)-Pyrimidinetrione, 5-ethyl-5-phenyl-, monosodium salt.

Molecular formula:
Phenobarbital—$C_{12}H_{12}N_2O_3$.
Phenobarbital sodium—$C_{12}H_{11}N_2NaO_3$.

Molecular weight:
Phenobarbital—232.24.
Phenobarbital sodium—254.22.

Description:
Phenobarbital USP—White, odorless, glistening, small crystals, or white, crystalline powder, which may exhibit polymorphism. Is stable in air. Its saturated solution has a pH of about 5.
Phenobarbital Sodium USP—Flaky crystals, or white, crystalline granules, or white powder. Is odorless and is hygroscopic. Its solutions are alkaline to phenolphthalein TS, and decompose on standing.

Solubility:
Phenobarbital USP—Very slightly soluble in water; soluble in alcohol, in ether, and in solutions of fixed alkali hydroxides and carbonates; sparingly soluble in chloroform.
Phenobarbital Sodium USP—Very soluble in water; soluble in alcohol; practically insoluble in ether and in chloroform.

USP requirements:
Phenobarbital USP—Preserve in well-closed containers. Contains not less than 98.0% and not more than 101.0% of phenobarbital, calculated on the dried basis. Meets the requirements for Identification, Melting range (174–178 °C, the range between beginning and end of melting not more than 2 °C), Loss on drying (not more than 1.0%), Residue on ignition (not more than 0.15%), and Organic volatile impurities.
Phenobarbital Capsules—Not in USP.
Phenobarbital Elixir USP—Preserve in tight, light-resistant containers. Contains the labeled amount, within ±10%. Meets the requirements for Identification and Alcohol content (12.0–15.0%).
Phenobarbital Tablets USP—Preserve in well-closed containers. Contain the labeled amount, within ±10%. Meet the requirements for Identification, Dissolution (75% in 45 minutes in water in Apparatus 2 at 50 rpm), and Uniformity of dosage units.
Phenobarbital Sodium USP—Preserve in tight containers. Contains not less than 98.5% and not more than 101.0% of phenobarbital sodium, calculated on the dried basis. Meets the requirements for Completeness of solution, Identification, pH (9.2–10.2, in the solution prepared in the test for Completeness of solution), Loss on drying (not more than 7.0%), Heavy metals (not more than 0.003%), and Organic volatile impurities.
Phenobarbital Sodium Injection USP—Preserve in single-dose or in multiple-dose containers, preferably of Type I glass. A sterile solution of Phenobarbital Sodium in a suitable solvent. Phenobarbital may be substituted for the equivalent amount of Phenobarbital Sodium, for adjustment of the pH. The label indicates that the Injection is not to be used if it contains a precipitate. Contains the labeled amount, within −10% to +5%. Meets the requirements for Identification, Bacterial endotoxins, pH (9.2–10.2), and Injections.
Sterile Phenobarbital Sodium USP—Preserve in Containers for Sterile Solids. It is Phenobarbital Sodium suitable for parenteral use. Meets the requirements for Constituted solution and Bacterial endotoxins, for Identification tests, Completeness of solution, pH (9.2–10.2), Loss on drying (not more than 7.0%), and Heavy metals (not more than 0.003%) under Phenobarbital Sodium, and for Sterility tests, Uniformity of dosage units, and Labeling under Injections.

PHENOBARBITAL, ASPIRIN, AND CODEINE

For *Phenobarbital, Aspirin* (ASA), and *Codeine*—See individual listings for chemistry information.

USP requirements: Phenobarbital, ASA, and Codeine Phosphate Capsules—Not in USP.

PHENOL

Chemical name: Phenol.

Molecular formula: C_6H_6O.

Molecular weight: 94.11.

Description: Phenol USP—Colorless to light pink, interlaced or separate, needleshaped crystals, or white to light pink, crystalline mass. It has a characteristic odor. Liquefied by warming, and by the addition of 10% of water. Boils at about 182 °C, and its vapor is flammable. Gradually darkens on exposure to light and air.
NF category: Antimicrobial preservative.

Solubility: Phenol USP—Soluble in water. Very soluble in alcohol, in glycerin, in chloroform, in ether, and in fixed and volatile oils; sparingly soluble in mineral oil.

USP requirements: Phenol USP—Preserve in tight, light-resistant containers. Label it to indicate the name and amount of any substance added as a stabilizer. Contains not less than 99.0% and not more than 100.5% of phenol, calculated on the anhydrous basis. Meets the requirements for Clarity of solution and reaction, Identification, Congealing temperature (not lower than 39 °C), Water (not more than 0.5%), Nonvolatile residue (not more than 0.05%), and Organic volatile impurities.
Caution: Avoid contact with skin, since serious burns may result.

LIQUEFIED PHENOL

Description: Liquefied Phenol USP—Colorless to pink liquid, which may develop a red tint upon exposure to air or light. Has a characteristic, somewhat aromatic odor. It whitens and cauterizes the skin and mucous membranes. Specific gravity is about 1.065.

Solubility: Liquefied Phenol USP—Miscible with alcohol, with ether, and with glycerin. A mixture of equal volumes of Liquefied Phenol and glycerin is miscible with water.

USP requirements: Liquefied Phenol USP—Preserve in tight, light-resistant containers. It is Phenol maintained in a liquid condition by the presence of about 10% of water. Label it to indicate the name and amount of any substance added as a stabilizer. Contains not less than 89.0% by weight of phenol. Meets the requirements for Distilling range (not higher than

182.5 °C) and Organic volatile impurities, and for Identifications tests, Clarity of solution and reaction, and Nonvolatile residue under Phenol.

Caution: Avoid contact with skin, since serious burns may result.

Note: When phenol is to be mixed with a fixed oil, mineral oil, or white petrolatum, use crystalline Phenol, not Liquefied Phenol.

PHENOLPHTHALEIN

Chemical group: Diphenylmethane derivative.

Chemical name: 1(3*H*)-Isobenzofuranone, 3,3-bis(4-hydroxyphenyl)-.

Molecular formula: $C_{20}H_{14}O_4$.

Molecular weight: 318.33.

Description: Phenolphthalein USP—White or faintly yellowish white, crystalline powder. Is odorless, and is stable in air.

Solubility: Phenolphthalein USP—Practically insoluble in water; soluble in alcohol; sparingly soluble in ether.

USP requirements:

Phenolphthalein USP—Preserve in well-closed containers. Contains not less than 98.0% and not more than 101.0% of phenolphthalein, calculated on the dried basis. Meets the requirements for Color of solution, Identification, Melting temperature (not lower than 258 °C), Loss on drying (not more than 1.0%), Residue on ignition (not more than 0.1%), Arsenic (not more than 8 ppm), Heavy metals (not more than 0.0015%), Fluoran, Chromatographic impurities, and Organic volatile impurities.

Phenolphthalein Chewing Gum—Not in USP.

Phenolphthalein Tablets USP—Preserve in tight containers. Where Tablets contain Yellow Phenolphthalein, the labeling so indicates. Contain the labeled amount, within ±10%. Meet the requirements for Identification, Disintegration (30 minutes), and Uniformity of dosage units.

Phenolphthalein Wafers—Not in USP.

YELLOW PHENOLPHTHALEIN

USP requirements: Yellow Phenolphthalein USP—Preserve in well-closed containers. Contains not less than 93.0% and not more than 100.0% of phenolphthalein, calculated on the dried basis. Meets the requirements for Color of solution, Melting temperature (not lower than 255 °C), and Chromatographic impurities, and for Identification tests, Loss on drying, Residue on ignition, Arsenic, and Heavy metals under Phenolphthalein.

PHENOLSULFONPHTHALEIN

Chemical name: Phenol, 4,4′-(3*H*-2,1-benzoxathiol-3-ylidene)bis-, (*S*,*S*-dioxide).

Molecular formula: $C_{19}H_{14}O_5S$.

Molecular weight: 354.38.

Description: Bright to dark red, odorless, crystalline powder.

pKa: 7.9.

Solubility: Very slightly soluble in water; slightly soluble in alcohol.

USP requirements: Phenolsulfonphthalein Injection—Not in USP.

PHENOXYBENZAMINE

Chemical name: Phenoxybenzamine hydrochloride—Benzenemethanamine, *N*-(2-chloroethyl)-*N*-(1-methyl-2-phenoxyethyl)-, hydrochloride.

Molecular formula: Phenoxybenzamine hydrochloride—$C_{18}H_{22}ClNO \cdot HCl$.

Molecular weight: Phenoxybenzamine hydrochloride—340.29.

Description: Phenoxybenzamine hydrochloride—Colorless, crystalline powder. Melting point is 136 to 141 °C.

pKa: Phenoxybenzamine hydrochloride—4.4.

Solubility: Phenoxybenzamine hydrochloride—Soluble in water, in alcohol, and in chloroform; insoluble in ether.

USP requirements:

Phenoxybenzamine Hydrochloride USP—Preserve in well-closed containers. Contains not less than 98.0% and not more than 101.0% of phenoxybenzamine hydrochloride, calculated on the dried basis. Meets the requirements for Identification, Melting range (136–141 °C), Loss on drying (not more than 0.5%), Ordinary impurities, and Organic volatile impurities.

Phenoxybenzamine Hydrochloride Capsules USP—Preserve in well-closed containers. Contain the labeled amount, within ±10%. Meet the requirements for Identification, Dissolution (75% in 45 minutes in 0.1 *N* hydrochloric acid in Apparatus 1 at 100 rpm), and Uniformity of dosage units.

PHENPROCOUMON

Chemical name: 2*H*-1-Benzopyran-2-one, 4-hydroxy-3-(1-phenylpropyl)-.

Molecular formula: $C_{18}H_{16}O_3$.

Molecular weight: 280.32.

Description: Phenprocoumon USP—Fine, white, crystalline powder. Odorless, or has a slight odor.

Solubility: Phenprocoumon USP—Practically insoluble in water; soluble in chloroform, in methanol, and in solutions of alkali hydroxides.

USP requirements:

Phenprocoumon USP—Preserve in well-closed containers. Contains not less than 98.0% and not more than 101.0% of phenprocoumon, calculated on the dried basis. Meets the requirements for Identification, Melting range (177–181 °C), Acidity, Loss on drying (not more than 0.5%), Residue on ignition (not more than 0.1%), Salicylic acid (not more than 0.1%), and Organic volatile impurities.

Phenprocoumon Tablets USP—Preserve in well-closed containers. Contain the labeled amount, within ±10%. Meet the requirements for Identification, Dissolution (75% in 45 minutes in water in Apparatus 2 at 50 rpm), and Uniformity of dosage units.

PHENSUXIMIDE

Chemical name: 2,5-Pyrrolidinedione, 1-methyl-3-phenyl-.

Molecular formula: $C_{11}H_{11}NO_2$.

Molecular weight: 189.21.

Description: Phensuximide USP—White to off-white crystalline powder. Is odorless, or has not more than a slight odor.

Solubility: Phensuximide USP—Slightly soluble in water; very soluble in chloroform; soluble in alcohol.

USP requirements:

Phensuximide USP—Preserve in tight containers. Contains not less than 97.0% and not more than 103.0% of phensuximide, calculated on the anhydrous basis. Meets the requirements for Identification, Melting range (68–74 °C), Water (not more than 1.0%), Residue on ignition (not more than 0.5%), Cyanide, Ordinary impurities, and Organic volatile impurities.

Phensuximide Capsules USP—Preserve in tight containers. Contain the labeled amount, within ±7%. Meet the requirements for Identification, Dissolution (75% in 120 minutes in water in Apparatus 1 at 100 rpm), and Uniformity of dosage units.

PHENTERMINE

Chemical group: Phenethylamine.

Chemical name: Phentermine hydrochloride—Benzeneethanamine, alpha,alpha-dimethyl-, hydrochloride.

Molecular formula: Phentermine hydrochloride—$C_{10}H_{15}N \cdot HCl$.

Molecular weight: Phentermine hydrochloride—185.70.

Description:

Phentermine Hydrochloride USP—White, odorless, hygroscopic, crystalline powder.

Phentermine resin—Coarse granular substance.

Solubility:

Phentermine Hydrochloride USP—Soluble in water and in the lower alcohols; slightly soluble in chloroform; insoluble in ether.

Phentermine resin—Practically insoluble in water.

USP requirements:

Phentermine Hydrochloride USP—Preserve in tight containers. Contains not less than 98.0% and not more than 101.0% of phentermine hydrochloride, calculated on the dried basis. Meets the requirements for Identification, Melting range (202–205 °C), pH (5.0–6.0, in a solution [1 in 50]), Loss on drying (not more than 2.0%), Residue on ignition (not more than 0.1%), Chromatographic purity, and Organic volatile impurities.

Phentermine Hydrochloride Capsules USP—Preserve in tight containers. Contain the labeled amount, within ±10%. Meet the requirements for Identification, Dissolution (75% in 45 minutes in water in Apparatus 2 at 50 rpm), and Uniformity of dosage units.

Phentermine Hydrochloride Tablets USP—Preserve in tight containers. Contain the labeled amount, within ±10%. Meet the requirements for Identification, Dissolution (75% in 45 minutes in water in Apparatus 2 at 50 rpm), and Uniformity of dosage units.

Phentermine Resin Capsules—Not in USP.

PHENTOLAMINE

Chemical name: Phentolamine mesylate—Phenol, 3-[[(4,5-dihydro-1*H*-imidazol-2-yl)methyl](4-methylphenyl)amino]-, monomethanesulfonate (salt).

Molecular formula: Phentolamine mesylate—$C_{17}H_{19}N_3O \cdot CH_4O_3S$.

Molecular weight: Phentolamine mesylate—377.46.

Description: Phentolamine Mesylate USP—White or off-white, odorless, crystalline powder. Its solutions are acid to litmus, having a pH of about 5, and slowly deteriorate. Melts at about 178 °C.

Solubility: Phentolamine Mesylate USP—Freely soluble in water and in alcohol; slightly soluble in chloroform.

USP requirements:

Phentolamine Mesylate USP—Preserve in tight, light-resistant containers. Contains not less than 98.0% and not more than 102.0% of phentolamine mesylate, calculated on the dried basis. Meets the requirements for Identification, Loss on drying (not more than 0.5%), Residue on ignition (not more than 0.1%), Sulfate (not more than 0.2%), and Chromatographic purity.

Phentolamine Mesylate for Injection USP—Preserve in Containers for Sterile Solids. It is sterile Phentolamine Mesylate or a sterile mixture of Phentolamine Mesylate with a suitable buffer or suitable diluents. Contains the labeled amount, within ±10%. Meets the requirements for Constituted solution, Identification, Uniformity of dosage units, Bacterial endotoxins, and pH (4.5–6.5 in a freshly prepared solution of 1 in 100), and for Sterility tests and Labeling under Injections.

PHENYLALANINE

Chemical name: L-Phenylalanine.

Molecular formula: $C_9H_{11}NO_2$.

Molecular weight: 165.19.

Description: Phenylalanine USP—White, odorless crystals.

Solubility: Phenylalanine USP—Sparingly soluble in water; very slightly soluble in methanol, in alcohol, and in dilute mineral acids.

USP requirements: Phenylalanine USP—Preserve in well-closed containers. Contains not less than 98.5% and not more than 101.5% of phenylalanine, calculated on the dried basis. Meets the requirements for Identification, Specific rotation (−32.7° to −34.7°, calculated on the dried basis), pH (5.4–6.0, in a solution [1 in 100]), Loss on drying (not more than 0.3%), Residue on ignition (not more than 0.4%), Chloride (not more than 0.05%), Sulfate (not more than 0.03%), Arsenic (not more than 1.5 ppm), Iron (not more than 0.003%), Heavy metals (not more than 0.0015%), and Organic volatile impurities.

PHENYLBUTAZONE

Chemical group: Pyrazole derivative.

Chemical name: 3,5-Pyrazolidinedione, 4-butyl-1,2-diphenyl-.

Molecular formula: $C_{19}H_{20}N_2O_2$.

Molecular weight: 308.38.

Description: Phenylbutazone USP—White to off-white, odorless, crystalline powder.

Solubility: Phenylbutazone USP—Very slightly soluble in water; freely soluble in acetone and in ether; soluble in alcohol.

USP requirements:

Phenylbutazone USP—Preserve in tight containers. Contains not less than 98.0% and not more than 100.5% of phenylbutazone, calculated on the dried basis. Meets the requirements for Identification, Melting range (104–107 °C), Loss on drying (not more than 0.5%), Residue on ignition (not more than 0.1%), Chloride (not more than 0.007%), Sulfate (not more than 0.01%), Heavy metals (not more than 0.001%), and Organic volatile impurities.

Phenylbutazone Capsules USP—Preserve in tight containers. Contain the labeled amount, within ±10%. Meet the requirements for Identification, Dissolution (60% in 30 minutes in phosphate buffer [pH 7.5] in Apparatus 1 at 100 rpm), and Uniformity of dosage units.

Phenylbutazone Tablets USP—Preserve in tight containers. Contain the labeled amount, within ±7%. Meet the requirements for Identification, Dissolution (60% in 30 minutes in simulated intestinal fluid TS [without the enzyme] in Apparatus 1 at 100 rpm), and Uniformity of dosage units.

Phenylbutazone Delayed-release Tablets—Not in USP.

BUFFERED PHENYLBUTAZONE

Chemical group: Phenylbutazone—Pyrazole derivative.

Chemical name:

Phenylbutazone—3,5-Pyrazolidinedione, 4-butyl-1,2-diphenyl-.

Magnesium trisilicate—Silicic acid ($H_4Si_3O_8$), magnesium salt (1:2), hydrate.

Molecular formula:

Phenylbutazone—$C_{19}H_{20}N_2O_2$.

Magnesium trisilicate—$2MgO \cdot 3SiO_2 \cdot xH_2O$ (hydrate); $Mg_2Si_3O_8$ (anhydrous).

Molecular weight:

Phenylbutazone—308.38.

Magnesium trisilicate—260.86 (anhydrous).

Description:

Phenylbutazone USP—White to off-white, odorless, crystalline powder.

Magnesium Trisilicate USP—Fine, white, odorless powder, free from grittiness.

Dried Aluminum Hydroxide Gel USP—White, odorless, amorphous powder.

Solubility:

Phenylbutazone USP—Very slightly soluble in water; freely soluble in acetone and in ether; soluble in alcohol.

Magnesium Trisilicate USP—Insoluble in water and in alcohol. Is readily decomposed by mineral acids.

Dried Aluminum Hydroxide Gel USP—Insoluble in water and in alcohol; soluble in dilute mineral acids and in solutions of fixed alkali hydroxides.

USP requirements: Buffered Phenylbutazone Tablets—Not in USP.

PHENYLEPHRINE

Chemical name: Phenylephrine hydrochloride—Benzenemethanol, 3-hydroxy-alpha-[(methylamino)methyl]-, hydrochloride.

Molecular formula: Phenylephrine hydrochloride—$C_9H_{13}NO_2 \cdot HCl$.

Molecular weight: Phenylephrine hydrochloride—203.67.

Description:

Phenylephrine Hydrochloride USP—White or practically white, odorless crystals.

Phenylephrine Hydrochloride Nasal Solution USP—Clear, colorless or slightly yellow, odorless liquid. Is neutral or acid to litmus.

Phenylephrine Hydrochloride Ophthalmic Solution USP—Clear, colorless or slightly yellow liquid, depending on the concentration.

Solubility: Phenylephrine Hydrochloride USP—Freely soluble in water and in alcohol.

USP requirements:

Phenylephrine Hydrochloride USP—Preserve in tight, light-resistant containers. Contains not less than 97.5% and not more than 102.5% of phenylephrine hydrochloride, calculated on the dried basis. Meets the requirements for Identification, Melting range (140–145 °C), Specific rotation (−42° to −47.5°, calculated on the dried basis), Loss on drying (not more than 1.0%), Residue on ignition (not more than 0.2%), Sulfate (not more than 0.20%), Ketones, Chromatographic purity, and Chloride content (17.0–17.7%, calculated on the dried basis).

Phenylephrine Hydrochloride Injection USP—Preserve in single-dose or in multiple-dose containers, preferably of Type I glass, protected from light. A sterile solution of Phenylephrine Hydrochloride in Water for Injection. Contains the labeled amount, within −10% to +15%. Meets the requirements for Identification, Bacterial endotoxins, pH (3.0–6.5), and Injections.

Phenylephrine Hydrochloride Nasal Jelly USP—Preserve in tight containers. Contains the labeled amount, within ±10%. Meets the requirements for Identification and Minimum fill.

Phenylephrine Hydrochloride Nasal Solution USP—Preserve in tight, light-resistant containers. Contains the labeled amount, within −10% to +15%. Meets the requirement for Identification.

Phenylephrine Hydrochloride Ophthalmic Solution USP—Preserve in tight, light-resistant containers of not more than 15-mL size. A sterile, aqueous solution of Phenylephrine Hydrochloride. Contains the labeled amount, within −10% to +15%. Meets the requirements for Identification, Sterility, and pH (4.0–7.5 for buffered Ophthalmic Solution; 3.0–4.5 for unbuffered Ophthalmic Solution).

PHENYLEPHRINE AND ACETAMINOPHEN

For *Phenylephrine* and *Acetaminophen*—See individual listings for chemistry information.

USP requirements:

Phenylephrine Hydrochloride and Acetaminophen for Oral Solution—Not in USP.

Phenylephrine Hydrochloride and Acetaminophen Chewable Tablets—Not in USP.

PHENYLEPHRINE AND DEXTROMETHORPHAN

For *Phenylephrine* and *Dextromethorphan*—See individual listings for chemistry information.

USP requirements: Phenylephrine Hydrochloride and Dextromethorphan Hydrobromide Oral Suspension—Not in USP.

PHENYLEPHRINE, DEXTROMETHORPHAN, AND GUAIFENESIN

For *Phenylephrine, Dextromethorphan,* and *Guaifenesin*—See individual listings for chemistry information.

USP requirements: Phenylephrine Hydrochloride, Dextromethorphan Hydrobromide, and Guaifenesin Syrup—Not in USP.

PHENYLEPHRINE, DEXTROMETHORPHAN, GUAIFENESIN, AND ACETAMINOPHEN

For *Phenylephrine, Dextromethorphan, Guaifenesin,* and *Acetaminophen*—See individual listings for chemistry information.

USP requirements: Phenylephrine Hydrochloride, Dextromethorphan Hydrobromide, Guaifenesin, and Acetaminophen Tablets—Not in USP.

PHENYLEPHRINE, GUAIFENESIN, ACETAMINOPHEN, SALICYLAMIDE, AND CAFFEINE

For *Phenylephrine, Guaifenesin, Acetaminophen, Salicylamide,* and *Caffeine*—See individual listings for chemistry information.

USP requirements: Phenylephrine Hydrochloride, Guaifenesin, Acetaminophen, Salicylamide, and Caffeine Tablets—Not in USP.

PHENYLEPHRINE, HYDROCODONE, AND GUAIFENESIN

For *Phenylephrine, Hydrocodone,* and *Guaifenesin*—See individual listings for chemistry information.

USP requirements: Phenylephrine Hydrochloride, Hydrocodone Bitartrate, and Guaifenesin Syrup—Not in USP.

PHENYLEPHRINE, PHENYLPROPANOLAMINE, AND GUAIFENESIN

For *Phenylephrine, Phenylpropanolamine,* and *Guaifenesin*—See individual listings for chemistry information.

USP requirements:

Phenylephrine Hydrochloride, Phenylpropanolamine Hydrochloride, and Guaifenesin Capsules—Not in USP.

Phenylephrine Hydrochloride, Phenylpropanolamine Hydrochloride, and Guaifenesin Oral Solution—Not in USP.

Phenylephrine Hydrochloride, Phenylpropanolamine Hydrochloride, and Guaifenesin Tablets—Not in USP.

PHENYLETHYL ALCOHOL

Chemical name: Benzeneethanol.

Molecular formula: $C_8H_{10}O$.

Molecular weight: 122.17.

Description: Phenylethyl Alcohol USP—Colorless liquid, having a rose-like odor.

NF category: Antimicrobial preservative.

Solubility: Phenylethyl Alcohol USP—Sparingly soluble in water; very soluble in alcohol, in fixed oils, in glycerin, and in propylene glycol; slightly soluble in mineral oil.

USP requirements: Phenylethyl Alcohol USP—Preserve in tight, light-resistant containers, and store in a cool, dry place. Meets the requirements for Identification, Specific gravity (1.017–1.020), Refractive index (1.531–1.534 at 20 °C), Residue on ignition (not more than 0.005%), Chlorinated compounds, and Aldehyde.

PHENYLMERCURIC ACETATE

Chemical name: Mercury, (acetato-*O*)phenyl-.

Molecular formula: $C_8H_8HgO_2$.

Molecular weight: 336.74.

Description: Phenylmercuric Acetate NF—White to creamy white crystalline powder, or small, white prisms or leaflets. Odorless.

NF category: Antimicrobial preservative.

Solubility: Phenylmercuric Acetate NF—Slightly soluble in water; soluble in alcohol and in acetone.

NF requirements: Phenylmercuric Acetate NF—Preserve in tight, light-resistant containers. Contains not less than 98.0% and not more than 100.5% of phenylmercuric acetate. Meets the requirements for Identification, Melting range (149–153 °C), Residue on ignition (not more than 0.2%), Mercuric salts and heavy metals, and Polymercurated benzene compounds (not more than 1.5%).

PHENYLMERCURIC NITRATE

Chemical name: Mercury, (nitrato-*O*)phenyl-.

Molecular formula: $C_6H_5HgNO_3$.

Molecular weight: 339.70.

Description: Phenylmercuric Nitrate NF—White, crystalline powder. Affected by light. Its saturated solution is acid to litmus.

NF category: Antimicrobial preservative.

Solubility: Phenylmercuric Nitrate NF—Very slightly soluble in water; slightly soluble in alcohol and in glycerin. It is more soluble in the presence of either nitric acid or alkali hydroxides.

NF requirements: Phenylmercuric Nitrate NF—Preserve in tight, light-resistant containers. A mixture of phenylmercuric nitrate and phenylmercuric hydroxide containing not less than 87.0% and not more than 87.9% of phenylmercuric ion, and not less than 62.75% and not more than 63.50% of mercury. Meets the requirements for Identification, Residue on ignition (not more than 0.1%), and Mercury ions.

PHENYLPROPANOLAMINE

Chemical group: Phenylpropanolamine hydrochloride—Synthetic phenylisopropanolamine.

Chemical name: Phenylpropanolamine hydrochloride—Benzenemethanol, alpha-(1-aminoethyl)-, hydrochloride, (*R**,*S**)-, (±).

Molecular formula: Phenylpropanolamine hydrochloride—$C_9H_{13}NO \cdot HCl$.

Molecular weight: Phenylpropanolamine hydrochloride—187.67.

Description: Phenylpropanolamine Hydrochloride USP—White, crystalline powder, having a slight aromatic odor. Is affected by light.

pKa: Phenylpropanolamine hydrochloride—9.

Solubility: Phenylpropanolamine Hydrochloride USP—Freely soluble in water and in alcohol; insoluble in ether.

Other characteristics: Similar in structure and action to ephedrine but with less central nervous system (CNS) stimulation.

USP requirements:

Phenylpropanolamine Hydrochloride USP—Preserve in tight, light-resistant containers. Contains not less than 98.0% and not more than 101.0% of phenylpropanolamine hydrochloride, calculated on the dried basis. Meets the requirements for Identification, Melting range (191–196 °C), pH (4.2–5.5, in a solution [3 in 100]), Loss on drying (not more than 0.5%), Residue on ignition (not more than 0.1%), alpha-Aminopropiophenone hydrochloride, Amphetamine hydrochloride (not more than 0.001%), Heavy metals (not more than 0.002%), and Organic volatile impurities.

Phenylpropanolamine Hydrochloride Capsules—Not in USP.

Phenylpropanolamine Hydrochloride Extended-release Capsules USP—Preserve in tight, light-resistant containers. Label Capsules to indicate the Drug Release Test with which the product complies. Contain the labeled amount, within ± 10%. Meet the requirements for Identification, Drug release (15–45% in 3 hours, 40–70% in 6 hours, and not less than 70% in 12 hours in water in Apparatus 1 at 100 rpm for Drug Release Test 1; 5–30% in 1 hour, 30–65% in 3 hours, and not less than 70% in 6 hours in 0.1 *N* hydrochloric acid for 1 hour and in phosphate buffer [pH 6.8 ±0.05] for 5 hours in Apparatus 1 at 200 rpm for Drug Release Test 2), and Uniformity of dosage units.

Phenylpropanolamine Hydrochloride Tablets—Not in USP.

Phenylpropanolamine Hydrochloride Extended-release Tablets USP—Preserve in tight, light-resistant containers. The labeling states the in-vitro Drug release test conditions of times and tolerances, as directed under Drug release. Contain the labeled amount, within ±10%. Meet the requirements for Identification, Drug release, and Uniformity of dosage units.

Phenylpropanolamine Hydrochloride Chewing Gum Tablets—Not in USP.

PHENYLPROPANOLAMINE AND ACETAMINOPHEN

For *Phenylpropanolamine* and *Acetaminophen*—See individual listings for chemistry information.

USP requirements:

Phenylpropanolamine Hydrochloride and Acetaminophen Capsules—Not in USP.

Phenylpropanolamine Hydrochloride and Acetaminophen Oral Solution—Not in USP.

Phenylpropanolamine Hydrochloride and Acetaminophen Tablets—Not in USP.

Phenylpropanolamine Hydrochloride and Acetaminophen Chewable Tablets—Not in USP.

PHENYLPROPANOLAMINE, ACETAMINOPHEN, AND ASPIRIN

For *Phenylpropanolamine, Acetaminophen,* and *Aspirin*—See individual listings for chemistry information.

USP requirements: Phenylpropanolamine Hydrochloride, Acetaminophen, and Aspirin Capsules—Not in USP.

PHENYLPROPANOLAMINE, ACETAMINOPHEN, ASPIRIN, AND CAFFEINE

For *Phenylpropanolamine, Acetaminophen, Aspirin,* and *Caffeine*—See individual listings for chemistry information.

USP requirements: Phenylpropanolamine Hydrochloride, Acetaminophen, Aspirin, and Caffeine Capsules—Not in USP.

PHENYLPROPANOLAMINE, ACETAMINOPHEN, SALICYLAMIDE, AND CAFFEINE

For *Phenylpropanolamine, Acetaminophen, Salicylamide,* and *Caffeine*—See individual listings for chemistry information.

USP requirements: Phenylpropanolamine Hydrochloride, Acetaminophen, Salicylamide, and Caffeine Capsules—Not in USP.

PHENYLPROPANOLAMINE AND ASPIRIN

For *Phenylpropanolamine* and *Aspirin*—See individual listings for chemistry information.

USP requirements: Phenylpropanolamine Hydrochloride and Aspirin for Oral Solution—Not in USP.

PHENYLPROPANOLAMINE AND CARAMIPHEN

Chemical name:

Phenylpropanolamine hydrochloride—Benzenemethanol, alpha-(1-aminoethyl)-, hydrochloride, (*R**,*S**)-, (±).

Caramiphen edisylate—1-Phenylcyclopentane-1-carboxylic acid, 2-diethylaminoethyl ester, 1,2-ethanedisulfonate (2:1).

Molecular formula:

Phenylpropanolamine hydrochloride—$C_9H_{13}NO \cdot HCl$.

Caramiphen edisylate—$(C_{18}H_{27}NO_2)_2 \cdot C_2H_6O_6S_2$.

Molecular weight:

Phenylpropanolamine hydrochloride—187.67.

Caramiphen edisylate—769.03.

Description:

Phenylpropanolamine Hydrochloride USP—White, crystalline powder, having a slight aromatic odor. Is affected by light.

Caramiphen edisylate—Off-white crystals with a melting point of 115–116 °C.

pKa: Phenylpropanolamine hydrochloride—9.

Solubility:

Phenylpropanolamine Hydrochloride USP—Freely soluble in water and in alcohol; insoluble in ether.

Caramiphen edisylate—1 gram dissolves in about 2 mL of water; soluble in alcohol.

USP requirements:

Phenylpropanolamine Hydrochloride and Caramiphen Edisylate Extended-release Capsules—Not in USP.

Phenylpropanolamine Hydrochloride and Caramiphen Edisylate Oral Solution—Not in USP.

PHENYLPROPANOLAMINE, CODEINE, AND GUAIFENESIN

For *Phenylpropanolamine, Codeine,* and *Guaifenesin*—See individual listings for chemistry information.

USP requirements:

Phenylpropanolamine Hydrochloride, Codeine Phosphate, and Guaifenesin Oral Solution—Not in USP.

Phenylpropanolamine Hydrochloride, Codeine Phosphate, and Guaifenesin Oral Suspension—Not in USP.

Phenylpropanolamine Hydrochloride, Codeine Phosphate, and Guaifenesin Syrup—Not in USP.

PHENYLPROPANOLAMINE AND DEXTROMETHORPHAN

For *Phenylpropanolamine* and *Dextromethorphan*—See individual listings for chemistry information.

USP requirements:

Phenylpropanolamine Hydrochloride and Dextromethorphan Hydrobromide Oral Gel—Not in USP.

Phenylpropanolamine Hydrochloride and Dextromethorphan Hydrobromide Granules—Not in USP.

Phenylpropanolamine Hydrochloride and Dextromethorphan Hydrobromide Lozenges—Not in USP.

Phenylpropanolamine Hydrochloride and Dextromethorphan Hydrobromide Oral Solution—Not in USP.

Phenylpropanolamine Hydrochloride and Dextromethorphan Hydrobromide Syrup—Not in USP.

PHENYLPROPANOLAMINE, DEXTROMETHORPHAN, AND ACETAMINOPHEN

For *Phenylpropanolamine, Dextromethorphan,* and *Acetaminophen*—See individual listings for chemistry information.

USP requirements:

Phenylpropanolamine Hydrochloride, Dextromethorphan Hydrobromide, and Acetaminophen Oral Solution—Not in USP.

Phenylpropanolamine Hydrochloride, Dextromethorphan Hydrobromide, and Acetaminophen Tablets—Not in USP.

PHENYLPROPANOLAMINE, DEXTROMETHORPHAN, AND GUAIFENESIN

For *Phenylpropanolanine, Dextromethorphan,* and *Guaifenesin*—See individual listings for chemistry information.

USP requirements:
Phenylpropanolamine Hydrochloride, Dextromethorphan Hydrobromide, and Guaifenesin Oral Solution—Not in USP.
Phenylpropanolamine Hydrochloride, Dextromethorphan Hydrobromide, and Guaifenesin Syrup—Not in USP.

PHENYLPROPANOLAMINE AND GUAIFENESIN

For *Phenylpropanolamine* and *Guaifenesin*—See individual listings for chemistry information.

USP requirements:
Phenylpropanolamine Hydrochloride and Guaifenesin Extended-release Capsules—Not in USP.
Phenylpropanolamine Hydrochloride and Guaifenesin Granules—Not in USP.
Phenylpropanolamine Hydrochloride and Guaifenesin Oral Solution—Not in USP.
Phenylpropanolamine Hydrochloride and Guaifenesin Syrup—Not in USP.
Phenylpropanolamine Hydrochloride and Guaifenesin Tablets—Not in USP.
Phenylpropanolamine Hydrochloride and Guaifenesin Extended-release Tablets—Not in USP.

PHENYLPROPANOLAMINE AND HYDROCODONE

For *Phenylpropanolamine* and *Hydrocodone*—See individual listings for chemistry information.

USP requirements:
Phenylpropanolamine Hydrochloride and Hydrocodone Bitartrate Oral Solution—Not in USP.
Phenylpropanolamine Hydrochloride and Hydrocodone Bitartrate Syrup—Not in USP.

PHENYLTOLOXAMINE AND HYDROCODONE

Chemical name: Hydrocodone polistirex—Benzene, diethenyl-, polymer with ethenylbenzene, sulfonated, complex with (5 alpha)-4,5-epoxy-3-methoxy-17-methylmorphinan-6-one.

USP requirements:
Phenyltoloxamine and Hydrocodone Polistirexes Capsules—Not in USP.
Phenyltoloxamine and Hydrocodone Polistirexes Oral Suspension—Not in USP.

PHENYLTOLOXAMINE, PHENYLPROPANOLAMINE, AND ACETAMINOPHEN

Chemical name:
Phenyltoloxamine citrate—2-(2-Benzylphenoxy)-*N,N*-dimethylethylamine dihydrogen citrate.
Phenylpropanolamine hydrochloride—Benzenemethanol, alpha-(1-aminoethyl)-, hydrochloride, (*R**,*S**)-, (±).
Acetaminophen—Acetamide, *N*-(4-hydroxyphenyl)-.

Molecular formula:
Phenyltoloxamine citrate—$C_{17}H_{21}NO \cdot C_6H_8O_7$.
Phenylpropanolamine hydrochloride—$C_9H_{13}NO \cdot HCl$.
Acetaminophen—$C_8H_9NO_2$.

Molecular weight:
Phenyltoloxamine citrate—447.5.
Phenylpropanolamine hydrochloride—187.67.
Acetaminophen—151.16.

Description:
Phenyltoloxamine citrate—It has a melting point of 138–140 °C.
Phenylpropanolamine Hydrochloride USP—White, crystalline powder, having a slight aromatic odor. Affected by light.
Acetaminophen USP—White, odorless, crystalline powder.

pKa: Phenylpropanolamine hydrochloride—9.

Solubility:
Phenyltoloxamine citrate—Soluble in water.
Phenylpropanolamine Hydrochloride USP—Freely soluble in water and in alcohol; insoluble in ether.
Acetaminophen USP—Soluble in boiling water and in 1 *N* sodium hydroxide; freely soluble in alcohol.

USP requirements: Phenyltoloxamine Citrate, Phenylpropanolamine Hydrochloride, and Acetaminophen Extended-release Tablets—Not in USP.

PHENYTOIN

Chemical group: Related to the barbiturates in chemical structure, but has a five-membered ring.

Chemical name:
Phenytoin—2,4-Imidazolidinedione, 5,5-diphenyl-.
Phenytoin sodium—2,4-Imidazolidinedione, 5,5-diphenyl-, monosodium salt.

Molecular formula:
Phenytoin—$C_{15}H_{12}N_2O_2$.
Phenytoin sodium—$C_{15}H_{11}N_2NaO_2$.

Molecular weight:
Phenytoin—252.27.
Phenytoin sodium—274.25.

Description:
Phenytoin USP—White, odorless powder. Melts at about 295 °C.
Phenytoin Sodium USP—White, odorless powder. Is somewhat hygroscopic and on exposure to air gradually absorbs carbon dioxide.

pKa: 8.06–8.33 (apparent).

Solubility:
Phenytoin USP—Practically insoluble in water; soluble in hot alcohol; slightly soluble in cold alcohol, in chloroform, and in ether.
Phenytoin Sodium USP—Freely soluble in water, the solution usually being somewhat turbid due to partial hydrolysis and absorption of carbon dioxide. Soluble in alcohol; practically insoluble in ether and in chloroform.

USP requirements:
Phenytoin USP—Preserve in tight containers. Contains not less than 98.5% and not more than 100.5% of phenytoin, calculated on the dried basis. Meets the requirements for Clarity and color of solution, Identification, Loss on drying (not more than 1.0%), Heavy metals (not more than 0.002%), Benzophenone (not more than 0.1%), and Organic volatile impurities.
Phenytoin Oral Suspension USP—Preserve in tight containers. Avoid freezing. It is Phenytoin suspended in a suitable medium. Contains the labeled amount, within ±10%. Meets the requirement for Identification.

Phenytoin Tablets USP—Preserve in well-closed containers. Label the Tablets to indicate that they are to be chewed. Contain the labeled amount, within ±7%. Meet the requirements for Identification and Uniformity of dosage units.

Phenytoin Sodium USP—Preserve in tight containers. Contains not less than 98.0% and not more than 102.0% of phenytoin sodium, calculated on the dried basis. Meets the requirements for Clarity and color of solution, Identification, Loss on drying (not more than 2.5%), Heavy metals (not more than 0.002%), Limit of benzophenone (not more than 0.1%), and Organic volatile impurities.

Extended Phenytoin Sodium Capsules USP—Preserve in tight containers. Contain the labeled amount, within ±5%. Meet the requirements for Identification, Dissolution (not more than 40% in 30 minutes, 55% in 60 minutes, and not less than 70% in 120 minutes in water in Apparatus 1 at 50 rpm), and Uniformity of dosage units.

Prompt Phenytoin Sodium Capsules USP—Preserve in tight containers. Label Prompt Phenytoin Sodium Capsules with the statement, "Not for once-a-day dosing," printed immediately under the official name, in a bold and contrasting color and/or enclosed within a box. Contain the labeled amount, within ±7%. Meet the requirements for Identification, Dissolution (85% in 30 minutes in water in Apparatus 1 at 50 rpm), and Uniformity of dosage units.

Phenytoin Sodium Injection USP—Preserve in single-dose or in multiple-dose containers, preferably of Type I glass, at controlled room temperature. A sterile solution of Phenytoin Sodium with Propylene Glycol and Alcohol in Water for Injection. Contains the labeled amount, within ±10%. Meets the requirements for Identification, Bacterial endotoxins, pH (10.0–12.3), Alcohol and propylene glycol content (9–11% alcohol; 37–43% propylene glycol), Particulate matter, and Injections.

Note: Do not use the Injection if it is hazy or contains a precipitate.

CHROMIC PHOSPHATE P 32

Chemical name: Phosphoric-^{32}P acid, chromium(3+) salt (1:1).

Molecular formula: $Cr^{32}PO_4$.

Description: Chromic phosphate P 32 suspension—Grayish-green to brownish-green suspension.

USP requirements: Chromic Phosphate P 32 Suspension USP—Preserve in single-dose or in multiple-dose containers. A sterile, aqueous suspension of radioactive chromic phosphate P 32 in a 30% Dextrose solution suitable for intraperitoneal, intrapleural, or interstitial administration. Label it to include the following, in addition to the information specified for Labeling under Injections: the time and date of calibration; the amount of ^{32}P as labeled chromic phosphate expressed as total megabecquerels (or millicuries) and concentration as megabecquerels (or millicuries) per mL at the time of calibration; the expiration date; and the statements, "Caution—Radioactive Material," and "For intracavitary use only." The labeling indicates that in making dosage calculations, correction is to be made for radioactive decay, and also indicates that the radioactive half-life of ^{32}P is 14.3 days. Contains the labeled amount, within ±10%, of ^{32}P as chromic phosphate expressed in megabecquerels (or millicuries) per mL at the time indicated in the labeling. Other chemical forms of radioactivity do not exceed 5.0% of the total radioactivity. Meets the requirements for Radionuclide identification, Bacterial endotoxins, pH (3.0–5.0), Radiochemical purity, and Injections (except that the Suspension may be distributed or dispensed prior to the completion of the test for Sterility, the latter test being started on the day of final manufacture, and except that it is not subject to the recommendations on Volume in Container).

SODIUM PHOSPHATE P 32

Chemical name: Phosphoric-^{32}P acid, disodium salt.

Description: Sodium Phosphate P 32 Solution USP—Clear, colorless solution. Upon standing, both the solution and the glass container may darken as a result of the effects of the radiation.

USP requirements: Sodium Phosphate P 32 Solution USP—Preserve in single-dose or in multiple-dose containers that previously have been treated to prevent adsorption. A solution suitable for either oral or intravenous administration, containing radioactive phosphorus processed in the form of Dibasic Sodium Phosphate from the neutron bombardment of elemental sulfur. Label it to include the following: the time and date of calibration; the amount of ^{32}P as phosphate expressed in total megabecquerels (or microcuries or millicuries) and in megabecquerels (or microcuries or in millicuries) per mL at the time of calibration; the name and quantity of any added preservative or stabilizer; a statement of the intended use, whether oral or intravenous; a statement of whether the contents are intended for diagnostic or therapeutic use; the expiration date; and the statements, "Caution—Radioactive Material" and "Not for intracavitary use." The labeling indicates that in making dosage calculations, correction is to be made for radioactive decay, and also indicates that the radioactive half-life of ^{32}P is 14.3 days. Contains the labeled amount of ^{32}P, within ±10%, as phosphate expressed in megabecquerels (or microcuries or millicuries) per mL at the time indicated in the labeling. Other chemical forms of radioactivity are absent. Meets the requirements for Radionuclide identification, Bacterial endotoxins, pH (5.0–6.0), Radiochemical purity, and Injections (if for intravenous use, except that the Solution may be distributed or dispensed prior to completion of the test for Sterility, the latter test being started on the day of final manufacture, and except that it is not subject to the recommendation on Volume in Container).

PHOSPHORIC ACID

Chemical name: Phosphoric acid.

Molecular formula: H_3PO_4.

Molecular weight: 98.00.

Description: Phosphoric Acid NF—Colorless, odorless liquid of syrupy consistency. Specific gravity is about 1.71.

NF category: Acidifying agent; buffering agent.

Solubility: Phosphoric Acid NF—Miscible with water and with alcohol.

NF requirements: Phosphoric Acid NF—Preserve in tight containers. Contains not less than 85.0% and not more than 88.0%, by weight, of phosphoric acid. Meets the requirements for Identification, Nitrate, Phosphorous or hypophosphorous acid, Sulfate, Arsenic (not more than 3 ppm), Alkali phosphates, and Heavy metals (not more than 0.001%).

Caution: Avoid contact, as Phosphoric Acid rapidly destroys tissues.

DILUTED PHOSPHORIC ACID

Description: Diluted Phosphoric Acid NF—Clear, colorless, odorless liquid. Specific gravity is about 1.057.

NF category: Acidifying agent.

NF requirements: Diluted Phosphoric Acid NF—Preserve in tight containers. Contains, in each 100 mL, not less than 9.5 grams and not more than 10.5 grams of phosphoric acid.

Prepare Diluted Phosphoric Acid as follows: 69 mL of Phosphoric Acid and a sufficient quantity of Purified Water to make 1000 mL. Mix the ingredients.

Meets the requirements for Alkali phosphates, Arsenic (not more than 1.5 ppm), and Heavy metals (not more than 5 ppm), and for Identification test, Nitrate, Phosphorous or hypophosphorous acid, and Sulfate under Phosphoric Acid.

PHYSOSTIGMINE

Source: Derivative of Calabar bean.

Chemical name:
Physostigmine—Pyrrolo[2,3-*b*]indol-5-ol, 1,2,3,3a,8,8a-hexahydro-1,3a,8-trimethyl-, methylcarbamate (ester), (3a*S*-*cis*).
Physostigmine salicylate—Pyrrolo[2,3-*b*]indol-5-ol, 1,2,3,3a,8,8a-hexahydro-1,3a,8-trimethyl-, methylcarbamate (ester), (3a*S*-*cis*)-, mono(2-hydroxybenzoate).
Physostigmine sulfate—Pyrrolo[2,3-*b*]indol-5-ol, 1,2,3,3a,8,8a-hexahydro-1,3a,8-trimethyl-, methylcarbamate (ester), (3a*S*-*cis*)-, sulfate (2:1).

Molecular formula:
Physostigmine—$C_{15}H_{21}N_3O_2$.
Physostigmine salicylate—$C_{15}H_{21}N_3O_2 \cdot C_7H_6O_3$.
Physostigmine sulfate—$(C_{15}H_{21}N_3O_2)_2 \cdot H_2SO_4$.

Molecular weight:
Physostigmine—275.35.
Physostigmine salicylate—413.47.
Physostigmine sulfate—648.77.

Description:
Physostigmine USP—White, odorless, microcrystalline powder. Acquires a red tint when exposed to heat, light, air, or contact with traces of metals. Melts at a temperature not lower than 103 °C.
Physostigmine Salicylate USP—White, shining, odorless crystals or white powder. Acquires a red tint when exposed to heat, light, air, or contact with traces of metals for long periods. Melts at about 184 °C.
Physostigmine Sulfate USP—White, odorless, microcrystalline powder. Is deliquescent in moist air and acquires a red tint when exposed to heat, light, air, or contact with traces of metals for long periods. Melts at about 143 °C.

Solubility:
Physostigmine USP—Slightly soluble in water; very soluble in chloroform and in dichloromethane; freely soluble in alcohol; soluble in fixed oils.
Physostigmine Salicylate USP—Sparingly soluble in water; freely soluble in chloroform; soluble in alcohol; slightly soluble in ether.
Physostigmine Sulfate USP—Freely soluble in water; very soluble in alcohol; very slightly soluble in ether.

USP requirements:
Physostigmine USP—Preserve in tight, light-resistant containers. An alkaloid usually obtained from the dried ripe seed of *Physostigma venenosum* Balfour (Fam. Leguminosae). Contains not less than 97.0% and not more than 102.0% of physostigmine, calculated on the dried basis. Meets the requirements for Identification, Specific rotation (−236° to −246°, calculated on the dried basis), Loss on drying (not more than 1.0%), Residue on ignition (negligible, from 100 mg), and Readily carbonizable substances.
Physostigmine Salicylate USP—Preserve in tight, light-resistant containers. Contains not less than 97.0% and not more than 102.0% of physostigmine salicylate, calculated on the dried basis. Meets the requirements for Identification, Specific rotation (−91° to −94°, calculated on the dried basis), Loss on drying (not more than 1.0%), Residue on ignition (negligible, from 100 mg), Sulfate, and Readily carbonizable substances.
Physostigmine Salicylate Injection USP—Preserve in single-dose containers, preferably of Type I glass, protected from light. A sterile solution of Physostigmine Salicylate in Water for Injection. Contains the labeled amount, within ±10%. Meets the requirements for Identification, Bacterial endotoxins, pH (3.5–5.0), and Injections.

Note: Do not use the Injection if it is more than slightly discolored.

Physostigmine Salicylate Ophthalmic Solution USP—Preserve in tight, light-resistant containers. A sterile aqueous solution of Physostigmine Salicylate. Contains the labeled amount, within ±10%. Meets the requirements for Identification, Sterility, and pH (2.0–4.0).
Physostigmine Sulfate USP—Preserve in tight, light-resistant containers. Contains not less than 97.0% and not more than 102.0% of physostigmine sulfate, calculated on the dried basis. Meets the requirements for Identification, Specific rotation (−116° to −120°, calculated on the dried basis), Loss on drying (not more than 1.0%), Residue on ignition (negligible, from 100 mg), and Readily carbonizable substances.
Physostigmine Sulfate Ophthalmic Ointment USP—Preserve in collapsible ophthalmic ointment tubes. Contains the labeled amount, within ±10%. It is sterile. Meets the requirements for Identification, Sterility, and Metal particles.

PHYTONADIONE

Chemical name: 1,4-Naphthalenedione, 2-methyl-3-(3,7,11,15-tetramethyl-2-hexadecenyl)-, [*R*-[*R**,*R**-(*E*)]]-.

Molecular formula: $C_{31}H_{46}O_2$.

Molecular weight: 450.71.

Description: Phytonadione USP—Clear, yellow to amber, very viscous, odorless or practically odorless liquid, having a specific gravity of about 0.967. Is stable in air, but decomposes on exposure to sunlight.

Solubility: Phytonadione USP—Insoluble in water; soluble in dehydrated alcohol, in chloroform, in ether, and in vegetable oils; slightly soluble in alcohol.

USP requirements:
Phytonadione USP—Preserve in tight, light-resistant containers. A mixture of *E* and *Z* isomers. Contains not less than 97.0% and not more than 103.0% of phytonadione. Contains not more than 21.0% of the *Z* isomer. Meets the requirements for Identification, Refractive index (1.523–1.526), Reaction, Menadione, and *Z* isomer content.
Phytonadione Injection USP—Preserve in single-dose or in multiple-dose containers, preferably of Type I glass, protected from light. A sterile, aqueous dispersion of Phytonadione. Contains the labeled amount, within ±10%. Contains suitable solubilizing and/or dispersing agents. Meets the requirements for Identification, Bacterial endotoxins, pH (3.5–7.0), and Injections.
Phytonadione Tablets USP—Preserve in well-closed, light-resistant containers. Contain the labeled amount, within ±10%. Meet the requirements for Identification, Disintegration (30 minutes), and Uniformity of dosage units.

PILOCARPINE

Chemical name:

Pilocarpine—2(3*H*)-Furanone, 3-ethyldihydro-4-[(1-methyl-1*H*-imidazol-5-yl)methyl]-, (3*S*-*cis*)-.

Pilocarpine hydrochloride—2(3*H*)-Furanone, 3-ethyldihydro-4-[(1-methyl-1*H*-imidazol-5-yl)methyl]-, monohydrochloride, (3*S*-*cis*)-.

Pilocarpine nitrate—2(3*H*)-Furanone, 3-ethyldihydro-4-[(1-methyl-1*H*-imidazol-5-yl)methyl]-, (3*S*-*cis*)-, mononitrate.

Molecular formula:

Pilocarpine—$C_{11}H_{16}N_2O_2$.

Pilocarpine hydrochloride—$C_{11}H_{16}N_2O_2 \cdot HCl$.

Pilocarpine nitrate—$C_{11}H_{16}N_2O_2 \cdot HNO_3$.

Molecular weight:

Pilocarpine—208.26.

Pilocarpine hydrochloride—244.72.

Pilocarpine nitrate—271.27.

Description:

Pilocarpine USP—A viscous, oily liquid, or crystals melting at about 34 °C. Exceedingly hygroscopic.

Pilocarpine Hydrochloride USP—Colorless, translucent, odorless crystals. Is hygroscopic and is affected by light. Its solutions are acid to litmus.

Pilocarpine Nitrate USP—Shining, white crystals. Is stable in air but is affected by light. Its solutions are acid to litmus.

Solubility:

Pilocarpine USP—Soluble in water, in alcohol, and in chloroform; practically insoluble in petroleum ether; sparingly soluble in ether.

Pilocarpine Hydrochloride USP—Very soluble in water; freely soluble in alcohol; slightly soluble in chloroform; insoluble in ether.

Pilocarpine Nitrate USP—Freely soluble in water; sparingly soluble in alcohol; insoluble in chloroform and in ether.

USP requirements:

Pilocarpine USP—Preserve in tight, light-resistant containers, in a cold place. Contains not less than 95.0% and not more than 100.5% of pilocarpine, calculated on the anhydrous basis. Meets the requirements for Identification, Specific rotation (+102° to +107°, calculated on the anhydrous basis), Refractive index (1.5170–1.5210 at 25 °C), Water (not more than 0.5%), Sulfate (not more than 0.004%), Nitrate, and Related substances (not more than 5.0%).

Pilocarpine Ocular System USP—Preserve in single-dose containers, in a cold place. It is sterile. Contains the labeled amount, within ±15%. Meets the requirements for Identification, Sterility, Uniformity of dosage units (for capsules), and Drug release pattern.

Pilocarpine Hydrochloride USP—Preserve in tight, light-resistant containers. Contains not less than 98.5% and not more than 101.0% of pilocarpine hydrochloride, calculated on the dried basis. Meets the requirements for Identification, Melting range (199–205 °C, the range between beginning and end of melting not more than 3 °C), Specific rotation (+88.5° to 91.5°, calculated on the dried basis), Loss on drying (not more than 3.0%), Readily carbonizable substances, Other alkaloids, and Ordinary impurities.

Pilocarpine Hydrochloride Ophthalmic Gel—Not in USP.

Pilocarpine Hydrochloride Ophthalmic Solution USP—Preserve in tight containers. A sterile, buffered, aqueous solution of Pilocarpine Hydrochloride. Contains the labeled amount, within ±10%. Meets the requirements for Identification, Sterility, and pH (3.5–5.5).

Pilocarpine Hydrochloride Tablets—Not in USP.

Pilocarpine Nitrate USP—Preserve in tight, light-resistant containers. Contains not less than 98.5% and not more than 101.0% of pilocarpine nitrate, calculated on the dried basis. Meets the requirements for Identification, Melting range (171–176 °C, with decomposition, the range between beginning and end of melting not more than 3 °C), Specific rotation (+79.5° to +82.5°, calculated on the dried basis), Loss on drying (not more than 2.0%), Chloride, Readily carbonizable substances, and Other alkaloids.

Pilocarpine Nitrate Ophthalmic Solution USP—Preserve in tight, light-resistant containers. A sterile, buffered aqueous solution of Pilocarpine Nitrate. Contains the labeled amount, within ±10%. Meets the requirements for Identification, Sterility, and pH (4.0–5.5).

PIMOZIDE

Chemical group: A diphenylbutylpiperidine derivative.

Chemical name: 2*H*-Benzimidazol-2-one, 1-[1-[4,4-bis(4-fluorophenyl)butyl]-4-piperidinyl]-1,3-dihydro-.

Molecular formula: $C_{28}H_{29}F_2N_3O$.

Molecular weight: 461.55.

Description: Pimozide USP—White, crystalline powder.

Solubility: Pimozide USP—Insoluble in water; slightly soluble in ether and in alcohol; freely soluble in chloroform.

USP requirements:

Pimozide USP—Preserve in tight, light-resistant containers. Contains not less than 98.0% and not more than 102.0% of pimozide, calculated on the dried basis. Meets the requirements for Identification, Melting range (214–218 °C), Loss on drying (not more than 0.5%), Residue on ignition (not more than 0.2%), Heavy metals (not more than 0.002%), Ordinary impurities, and Organic volatile impurities.

Pimozide Tablets USP—Preserve in tight, light-resistant containers. Contain the labeled amount, within ±10%. Meet the requirements for Identification, Dissolution (80% in 45 minutes in 0.1 *N* hydrochloric acid in Apparatus 2 at 50 rpm), and Uniformity of dosage units.

PINDOLOL

Chemical name: 2-Propanol, 1-(1*H*-indol-4-yloxy)-3-[(1-methylethyl)amino]-.

Molecular formula: $C_{14}H_{20}N_2O_2$.

Molecular weight: 248.33.

Description: Pindolol USP—White to off-white, crystalline powder, having a faint odor.

Solubility: Pindolol USP—Practically insoluble in water; slightly soluble in methanol; very slightly soluble in chloroform.

Other characteristics: Lipid solubility—Moderate.

USP requirements:

Pindolol USP—Preserve in well-closed containers, protected from light. Contains not less than 98.5% and not more than 101.0% of pindolol, calculated on the dried basis. Meets the requirements for Identification, Melting range (169–173 °C, the range between beginning and end of melting not more than 3 °C), Loss on drying (not more than 0.5%), Residue on ignition (not more than 0.1%), Heavy metals (not more than 0.002%), Chromatographic purity, and Organic volatile impurities.

Pindolol Tablets USP—Preserve in well-closed containers, protected from light. Contain the labeled amount, within ±10%. Meet the requirements for Identification, Dissolution (80% in 15 minutes in 0.1 *N* hydrochloric acid in Apparatus 2 at 50 rpm), Uniformity of dosage units, and Chromatographic purity.

PINDOLOL AND HYDROCHLOROTHIAZIDE

For *Pindolol* and *Hydrochlorothiazide*—See individual listings for chemistry information.

USP requirements: Pindolol and Hydrochlorothiazide Tablets—Not in USP.

PIPECURONIUM

Chemical name: Pipecuronium bromide—Piperazinium, 4,4′-[(2 beta,3 alpha,5 alpha,16 beta,17 beta)-3,17-bis(acetyloxy)-androstane-2,16-diyl]bis[1,1-dimethyl-, dibromide, dihydrate.

Molecular formula: Pipecuronium bromide—$C_{35}H_{62}Br_2N_4O_4 \cdot 2H_2O$.

Molecular weight: Pipecuronium bromide—798.74.

Description: Pipecuronium bromide—Melting point 262–264 °C.

USP requirements: Pipecuronium Bromide for Injection—Not in USP.

PIPERACETAZINE

Chemical name: Ethanone, 1-[10-[3-[4-(2-hydroxyethyl)-1-piperidinyl]propyl]-10*H*-phenothiazin-2-yl]-.

Molecular formula: $C_{24}H_{30}N_2O_2S$.

Molecular weight: 410.57.

Description: Piperacetazine USP—Yellow, granular powder.

Solubility: Piperacetazine USP—Practically insoluble in water; freely soluble in chloroform; soluble in alcohol and in dilute hydrochloric acid.

USP requirements:

Piperacetazine USP—Preserve in tight, light-resistant containers. Contains not less than 98.0% and not more than 101.5% of piperacetazine, calculated on the dried basis. Meets the requirements for Identification, Melting range (102–106 °C), Loss on drying (not more than 1.0%), Residue on ignition (not more than 0.1%), Heavy metals (not more than 0.002%), Ordinary impurities, and Organic volatile impurities.

Piperacetazine Tablets USP—Preserve in well-closed, light-resistant containers. Contain the labeled amount, within ±7%. Meet the requirements for Identification, Dissolution (75% in 45 minutes in 0.1 *N* hydrochloric acid in Apparatus 1 at 100 rpm), and Uniformity of dosage units.

PIPERACILLIN

Chemical name: Piperacillin sodium—4-Thia-1-azabicyclo-[3.2.0]heptane-2-carboxylic acid, 6-[[[[(4-ethyl-2,3-dioxo-1-piperazinyl)carbonyl]amino]phenylacetyl]amino]-3,3-dimethyl-7-oxo-, monosodium salt, [2*S*-[2 alpha,5 alpha,6 beta(*S**)]].

Molecular formula: Piperacillin sodium—$C_{23}H_{26}N_5NaO_7S$.

Molecular weight: Piperacillin sodium—539.54.

Description: Sterile Piperacillin Sodium USP—White to off-white solid having the characteristic appearance of products prepared by freeze-drying.

Solubility: Sterile Piperacillin Sodium USP—Freely soluble in water and in alcohol.

USP requirements: Sterile Piperacillin Sodium USP—Preserve in Containers for Sterile Solids. It is piperacillin sodium suitable for parenteral use. Has a potency equivalent to not less than 863 mcg and not more than 1007 mcg of piperacillin per mg, calculated on the anhydrous basis and, where packaged for dispensing, contains an amount of piperacillin sodium equivalent to the labeled amount of piperacillin within −10% to +20%. Meets the requirements for Constituted solution, Identification, Bacterial endotoxins, Sterility, pH (5.5–7.5, in a solution containing 400 mg per mL), Water (not more than 1.0%), and Particulate matter, and for Uniformity of dosage units and Labeling under Injections.

PIPERACILLIN AND TAZOBACTAM

Chemical group: Tazobactam—A penicillanic acid sulphone derivative similar to sulbactam.

Chemical name:

Piperacillin sodium—4-Thia-1-azabicyclo[3.2.0]heptane-2-carboxylic acid, 6-[[[[(4-ethyl-2,3-dioxo-1-piperazinyl)-carbonyl]amino]phenylacetyl]amino]-3,3-dimethyl-7-oxo-, monosodium salt, [2*S*-[2 alpha,5 alpha,6 beta(*S**)]].

Tazobactam sodium—4-Thia-1-azabicyclo[3.2.0]heptane-2-carboxylic acid, 3-methyl-7-oxo-3-(1*H*-1,2,3-triazol-1-ylmethyl)-, 4,4-dioxide, sodium salt, [2*S*-(2 alpha,3 beta,5 alpha)]-.

Molecular formula:

Piperacillin sodium—$C_{23}H_{26}N_5NaO_7S$.

Tazobactam sodium—$C_{10}H_{11}N_4NaO_5S$.

Molecular weight:

Piperacillin sodium—539.54.

Tazobactam sodium—322.27.

Description: Sterile Piperacillin Sodium USP—White to off-white solid having the characteristic appearance of products prepared by freeze-drying.

Solubility: Sterile Piperacillin Sodium USP—Freely soluble in water and in alcohol.

USP requirements: Sterile Piperacillin Sodium and Tazobactam Sodium Injection—Not in USP.

PIPERAZINE

Chemical name:

Piperazine—Piperazine.

Piperazine adipate—Hexanedioic acid compd. with piperazine (1:1).

Piperazine citrate—Piperazine, 2-hydroxy-1,2,3-propanetricarboxylate (3:2), hydrate.

Molecular formula:

Piperazine—$C_4H_{10}N_2$.

Piperazine adipate—$C_4H_{10}N_2 \cdot C_6H_{10}O_4$.

Piperazine citrate—$(C_4H_{10}H_2)_3 \cdot 2C_6H_8O_7$ (anhydrous).

Molecular weight:

Piperazine—86.14.

Piperazine adipate—232.3.

Piperazine citrate (anhydrous)—642.66.

Description:

Piperazine USP—White to slightly off-white lumps or flakes, having an ammoniacal odor.

Piperazine adipate—White, crystalline powder.
Piperazine Citrate USP—White, crystalline powder, having not more than a slight odor. Its solution (1 in 10) has a pH of about 5.

Solubility:
Piperazine USP—Soluble in water and in alcohol; insoluble in ether.
Piperazine adipate—Soluble 1 in 18 of water; practically insoluble in alcohol.
Piperazine Citrate USP—Soluble in water; insoluble in alcohol and in ether.

USP requirements:
Piperazine USP—Preserve in tight containers, protected from light. Contains not less than 98.0% and not more than 101.0% of piperazine, calculated on the anhydrous basis. Meets the requirements for Color of solution, Identification, Melting range (109–113 °C), Water (not more than 2.0%), and Primary amines and ammonia (not more than 0.7%).
Piperazine Adipate Granules for Oral Solution—Not in USP.
Piperazine Adipate Oral Suspension—Not in USP.
Piperazine Citrate USP—Preserve in well-closed containers. Contains not less than 98.0% and not more than 100.5% of piperazine citrate, calculated on the anhydrous basis. Meets the requirements for Identification, Water (not more than 12.0%), and Primary amines and ammonia (not more than 0.7%).
Piperazine Citrate Syrup USP—Preserve in tight containers. Prepared from Piperazine Citrate or from Piperazine to which an equivalent amount of Citric Acid is added. Contains an amount of piperazine citrate equivalent to the labeled amount of piperazine hexahydrate, within ±7%. Meets the requirement for Identification.
Piperazine Citrate Tablets USP—Preserve in tight containers. Contain an amount of piperazine citrate equivalent to the labeled amount of piperazine hexahydrate, within ±7%. Meet the requirements for Identification, Dissolution (75% in 45 minutes in water in Apparatus 2 at 50 rpm), and Uniformity of dosage units.

PIPOBROMAN

Chemical name: Piperazine, 1,4-bis(3-bromo-1-oxopropyl)-.

Molecular formula: $C_{10}H_{16}Br_2N_2O_2$.

Molecular weight: 356.06.

Description: Pipobroman USP—White, or practically white, crystalline powder, having a slightly sharp, fruity odor.

Solubility: Pipobroman USP—Slightly soluble in water; freely soluble in chloroform; soluble in acetone; sparingly soluble in alcohol; very slightly soluble in ether.

USP requirements:
Pipobroman USP—Preserve in well-closed containers. Contains not less than 98.0% and not more than 101.5% of pipobroman, calculated on the dried basis. Meets the requirements for Identification, Melting range (101–105 °C), Loss on drying (not more than 1.0%), Residue on ignition (not more than 0.5%), Free bromide (not more than 0.50%), Heavy metals (not more than 0.002%), and Organic volatile impurities.
Caution: Handle Pipobroman with exceptional care since it is a highly potent agent.
Pipobroman Tablets USP—Preserve in well-closed containers. Contain the labeled amount, within ±10%. Meet the requirements for Identification, Disintegration (45 minutes, the use of disks being omitted), and Uniformity of dosage units.

PIPOTIAZINE

Chemical group: Piperidine phenothiazine.

Chemical name: Pipotiazine palmitate—Hexadecanoic acid, 2-[1-[3-[2-[(dimethylamino)sulfonyl]-10*H*-phenothiazin-10-yl]propyl]-4-piperidinyl]ethyl ester.

Molecular formula: Pipotiazine palmitate—$C_{40}H_{63}N_3O_4S_2$.

Molecular weight: Pipotiazine palmitate—714.08.

USP requirements: Pipotiazine Palmitate Injection—Not in USP.

PIRBUTEROL

Chemical name: Pirbuterol acetate—2,6-Pyridinedimethanol, alpha^6-[[(1,1-dimethylethyl)amino]methyl]-3-hydroxy-, monoacetate (salt).

Molecular formula: Pirbuterol acetate—$C_{12}H_{20}N_2O_3 \cdot C_2H_4O_2$.

Molecular weight: Pirbuterol acetate—300.35.

Description: Pirbuterol acetate—A white, crystalline powder.

Solubility: Pirbuterol acetate—Freely soluble in water.

USP requirements: Pirbuterol Acetate Inhalation Aerosol—Not in USP.

PIRENZEPINE

Chemical group: Synthetic tertiary amine.

Chemical name: Pirenzepine hydrochloride—6*H*-Pyrido[2,3-*b*][1,4]benzodiazepin-6-one, 5,11-dihydro-11-[(4-methyl-1-piperazinyl)acetyl]-, dihydrochloride.

Molecular formula: Pirenzepine hydrochloride—$C_{19}H_{21}N_5O_2 \cdot 2HCl$.

Molecular weight: Pirenzepine hydrochloride—424.33.

Solubility: Pirenzepine hydrochloride—Soluble in water; slightly soluble in methanol; practically insoluble in ether.

USP requirements: Pirenzepine Hydrochloride Tablets—Not in USP.

PIROXICAM

Chemical group: Oxicam derivative.

Chemical name: 2*H*-1,2-Benzothiazine-3-carboxamide, 4-hydroxy-2-methyl-*N*-2-pyridinyl-, 1,1-dioxide.

Molecular formula: $C_{15}H_{13}N_3O_4S$.

Molecular weight: 331.35.

Description: Piroxicam USP—Off-white to light tan or light yellow, odorless powder. Forms a monohydrate that is yellow.

pKa: 1.8 and 5.1.

Solubility: Piroxicam USP—Very slightly soluble in water, in dilute acids, and in most organic solvents; slightly soluble in alcohol and in aqueous alkaline solutions.

USP requirements:
Piroxicam USP—Preserve in tight, light-resistant containers. Contains not less than 97.0% and not more than 103.0% of piroxicam. Meets the requirements for Identification, Water (not more than 0.5%), Residue on ignition (not more than 0.3%), Heavy metals (not more than 0.005%), and Organic volatile impurities.

Piroxicam Capsules USP—Preserve in tight, light-resistant containers. Contain the labeled amount, within ±7.5%. Meet the requirements for Identification, Dissolution (75% in 45 minutes in simulated gastric fluid TS, prepared without pepsin, in Apparatus 1 at 50 rpm), Uniformity of dosage units, and Water (not more than 8.0%).
Piroxicam Suppositories—Not in USP.

POSTERIOR PITUITARY

USP requirements: Posterior Pituitary Injection USP—Preserve in single-dose or in multiple-dose containers, preferably of Type I glass. Do not freeze. A sterile solution, in a suitable diluent, of material containing the polypeptide hormones having the property of causing the contraction of uterine, vascular, and other smooth muscle, which is prepared from the posterior lobe of the pituitary body of healthy, domestic animals used for food by man. Each mL of Posterior Pituitary Injection possesses oxytocic and pressor activities of not less than 85.0% and not more than 120.0% of those stated on the label in USP Posterior Pituitary Units. Meets the requirements for Bacterial endotoxins, pH (2.5–4.5), and Injections.

PIVAMPICILLIN

Chemical name: Pivaloyloxymethyl (6*R*)-6(alpha-D-phenylglycylamino)penicillanate.

Molecular formula: $C_{22}H_{29}N_3O_6S$.

Molecular weight: 463.6.

USP requirements:
Pivampicillin for Oral Suspension—Not in USP.
Pivampicillin Tablets—Not in USP.

PIZOTYLINE

Chemical name: Pizotyline hydrogen malate—9,10-Dihydro-4-(1-methyl-4-piperidylidene)-4*H*-benzo[4,5]cycloheptal[1,2-*b*]thiophene hydrogen malate.

Molecular formula: Pizotyline hydrogen malate—$C_{19}H_{21}NS \cdot C_4H_6O_5$.

Molecular weight: Pizotyline hydrogen malate—429.5.

Description: Pizotyline hydrogen malate—White or slightly yellowish-white, odorless or almost odorless, crystalline powder.

Solubility: Pizotyline hydrogen malate—Very slightly soluble in water; slightly soluble in alcohol and in chloroform; sparingly soluble in methyl alcohol.

USP requirements: Pizotyline Hydrogen Malate Tablets—Not in USP.

PLAGUE VACCINE

Description: Plague Vaccine USP—Turbid, whitish liquid, practically odorless, or having a faint odor because of the preservative.

USP requirements: Plague Vaccine USP—Preserve at a temperature between 2 and 8 °C. A sterile suspension of plague bacilli (*Yersinia pestis*) of the 195/P strain grown on E medium, harvested and killed by the addition of formaldehyde. Its potency is determined with the specific mouse protection test on the basis of the U.S. Reference Plague Vaccine. Label it to state that it is to be well shaken before use and that it is not to be frozen. Meets the requirements of the specific mouse test for inactivation and for Expiration date (not later than 18 months after date of issue from manufacturer's cold storage [5 °C, 1 year]) and Potency test. Conforms to the regulations of the U.S. Food and Drug Administration concerning biologics.

PLANTAGO SEED

Description: Plantago Seed USP—All varieties are practically odorless.

USP requirements: Plantago Seed USP—Preserve in well-closed containers, secure against insect attack. The cleaned, dried, ripe seed of *Plantago psyllium* Linné, or of *Plantago indica* Linné (*Plantago arenaria* Waldstein et Kitaibel), known in commerce as Spanish or French Psyllium Seed; or of *Plantago ovata* Forskal, known in commerce as Blond Psyllium or Indian Plantago Seed (Fam. Plantaginaceae). Meets the requirements for Botanic characteristics, Water absorption, Total ash (not more than 4.0%), Acid-insoluble ash (not more than 1.0%), and Foreign organic matter (not more than 0.50%).

PLASMA PROTEIN FRACTION

USP requirements: Plasma Protein Fraction USP—Preserve at the temperature indicated on the label. A sterile preparation of serum albumin and globulin obtained by fractionating material (source blood, plasma, or serum) from healthy human donors, the source material being tested for the absence of hepatitis B surface antigen. Made by a process that yields a product having protein components of approved composition and sedimentation coefficient content. Label it to state that it is not to be used if it is turbid and that it is to be used within 4 hours after the container is entered. Label it also to state the osmotic equivalent in terms of plasma and the sodium content. Not less than 83% of its total protein is albumin and not more than 17% of its total protein consists of alpha and beta globulins. Not more than 1% of its total protein has the electrophoretic properties of gamma globulin. A solution containing, in each 100 mL, 5 grams of protein, and contains the labeled amount, within ±6%. Contains no added antimicrobial agent, but contains sodium acetyltryptophanate with or without sodium caprylate as a stabilizing agent. Has a sodium content of not less than 130 mEq per liter and not more than 160 mEq per liter and a potassium content of not more than 2 mEq per liter. Has a pH between 6.7 and 7.3, measured in a solution diluted to contain 1% of protein with 0.15 *M* sodium chloride. Meets the requirements of the test for heat stability and for Expiration date (minimum date not later than 5 years after issue from manufacturer's cold storage [5 °C, 1 year] if labeling recommends storage between 2 and 10 °C; not later than 3 years after issue from manufacturer's cold storage [5 °C, 1 year] if labeling recommends storage at temperatures not higher than 30 °C). Conforms to the regulations of the U.S. Food and Drug Administration concerning biologics.

PLATELET CONCENTRATE

USP requirements: Platelet Concentrate USP—Preserve in hermetic containers of colorless, transparent, sterile, pyrogen-free Type I or Type II glass, or of a suitable plastic material. Preserve at the temperature relevant to the volume of resuspension plasma, either between 20 and 24 °C or between 1 and 6 °C, the latter except during shipment, when the temperature may be between 1 and 10 °C. In addition to the labeling requirements of Whole Blood applicable to this product, label it to state the volume of original plasma present, the kind and volume of anticoagulant solution present in the original plasma, the blood group designation of the source blood, and the hour of expiration on the stated expiration date. Where labeled for storage at 20 to 24 °C, label it also to state that a continuous gentle agitation shall be maintained, or where labeled for storage at 1 to 6 °C, to state that such agitation is optional. Label it also with the type and result of a serologic test for syphilis, or to indicate that it was nonreactive in such test; with the type and result of a test for hepatitis B surface antigen, or to indicate that it was nonreactive in such test; with a warning that it is to be used as soon as possible but not more than 4 hours after entering the container; to state that a filter is to be used in the administration equipment; and to state that the instruction circular provided is to be consulted for directions for use. Contains the platelets taken from plasma obtained by whole blood collection, by plasmapheresis, or by plateletpheresis, from a single suitable human donor of whole blood; or from a plasmapheresis donor; or from a plateletpheresis donor who meets the criteria described in the product license application (in which case the collection procedure is as described therein), except where a licensed physician has determined that the recipient is to be transfused with the platelets from a specific donor (in which case the plateletpheresis procedure is performed under the supervision of a licensed physician who is aware of the health status of the donor and has certified that the donor's health permits such procedure). In all cases, the collection of source material is made by a single, uninterrupted venipuncture with minimal damage to and manipulation of the donor's tissue. Concentrate consists of such platelets suspended in a specified volume of the original plasma, the separation of plasma and resuspension of the platelets being done in a closed system, within 4 hours of collection of the whole blood or plasma. The separation of platelets is by a procedure shown to yield an unclumped product without visible hemolysis, with a content of not less than 5.5×10^{10} platelets per unit in not less than 75% of the units tested, and the volume of original plasma used for resuspension of the separated platelets is such that the product has a pH of not less than 6 during the storage period when kept at the selected storage temperature, the selected storage temperature and corresponding volume of resuspension plasma being either 30 to 50 mL of plasma for storage at 20 to 24 °C, or 20 to 30 mL of plasma for storage at 1 to 6 °C. Meets the aforementioned requirements for platelet count, pH, and actual plasma volume, when tested 72 hours after preparation, and for Expiration date (not more than 72 hours from the time of collection of the source material). Conforms to the regulations of the U.S. Food and Drug Administration concerning biologics.

PLICAMYCIN

Source: Antibiotic produced by *Streptomyces argillaceus, Streptomyces tanashiensis, and Streptomyces plicatus.*

Chemical name: Plicamycin.

Molecular formula: $C_{52}H_{76}O_{24}$.

Molecular weight: 1085.16.

Description: Plicamycin USP—Yellow, odorless, hygroscopic, crystalline powder.

Solubility: Plicamycin USP—Slightly soluble in water and in methanol; very slightly soluble in alcohol; freely soluble in ethyl acetate.

USP requirements:

Plicamycin USP—Preserve in tight, light-resistant containers, at a temperature between 2 and 8 °C. Has a potency of not less than 900 mcg of plicamycin per mg, calculated on the dried basis. Meets the requirements for Identification, Crystallinity, pH (4.5–5.5, in a solution containing 0.5 mg per mL), and Loss on drying (not more than 8.0%).

Plicamycin for Injection USP—Preserve in light-resistant Containers for Sterile Solids, at a temperature between 2 and 8 °C. A sterile, dry mixture of Plicamycin and Mannitol. Label it with the mandatory instruction to consult the professional information for dosage and warnings, and with the warning that it is intended for hospital use only, under the direct supervision of a physician. Contains the labeled amount, within ±10%. Meets the requirements for Constituted solution, Identification, Depressor substances, Bacterial endotoxins, Sterility, pH (5.0–7.5), and Water (not more than 2.0%).

PNEUMOCOCCAL VACCINE POLYVALENT

Source:

The currently available vaccines in the U.S. (*Pneumovax 23,* MSD, and *Pnu-Imune 23,* Lederle) contain a mixture of purified capsular polysaccharides from the 23 most prevalent pneumococcal types responsible for approximately 90% of serious pneumococcal disease. Each of the pneumococcal polysaccharide types is produced separately. The resultant 23 polysaccharides are separated from the cells, purified, and combined to give 25 mcg of each type per 0.5-mL dose of the final vaccine.

Pneumovax 23, MSD (Canada) brand of pneumococcal vaccine polyvalent, also contains 23 polysaccharides.

Other characteristics:

The U.S. nomenclature for these 23 types is: 1, 2, 3, 4, 5, 26, 51, 8, 9, 68, 34, 43, 12, 14, 54, 17, 56, 57, 19, 20, 22, 23, 70.

The Danish nomenclature for these 23 types is: 1, 2, 3, 4, 5, 6B, 7F, 8, 9N, 9V, 10A, 11A, 12F, 14, 15B, 17F, 18C, 19A, 19F, 20, 22F, 23F, 33F.

USP requirements: Pneumococcal Vaccine Polyvalent Injection—Not in USP.

PODOFILOX

Chemical name: Furo[3′,4′:6,7]naphtho[2,3-*d*]-1,3-dioxol-6(5a*H*)-one, 5,8,8a,9-tetrahydro-9-hydroxy-5-(3,4,5-trimethoxyphenyl)-, [5*R*-(5 alpha,5a beta,8a alpha,9 alpha)]-.

Molecular formula: $C_{22}H_{22}O_8$.

Molecular weight: 414.41.

Solubility: Soluble in alcohol; sparingly soluble in water.

USP requirements: Podofilox Solution—Not in USP.

PODOPHYLLUM

Source: Podophyllum resin—Dried resin from the roots and rhizomes of *Podophyllum peltatum* (mandrake or May apple plant), the North American variety; active constituents are lignans including podophyllotoxin (20%), alpha-peltatin (10%), and beta-peltatin (5%).

Description: Podophyllum Resin USP—Amorphous powder, varying in color from light brown to greenish yellow, turning darker when subjected to a temperature exceeding 25 °C or when exposed to light. Its alcohol solution is acid to moistened litmus paper.

Solubility: Podophyllum Resin USP—Soluble in alcohol with a slight opalescence; partially soluble in ether and in chloroform.

The major active constituent of podophyllum, podophyllotoxin, is lipid soluble.

USP requirements:

Podophyllum USP—Consists of the dried rhizomes and roots of *Podophyllum peltatum* Linné (Fam. Berberidaceae). Yields not less than 5.0% of podophyllum resin. Meets the requirements for Botanic characteristics, Indian podophyllum, Acid-insoluble ash (not more than 2.0%), and Foreign organic matter (not more than 2.0%).

Podophyllum Resin USP—Preserve in tight, light-resistant containers. The powdered mixture of resins extracted from Podophyllum by percolation with Alcohol and subsequent precipitation from the concentrated percolate upon addition to acidified water. Contains not less than 40.0% and not more than 50.0% of hexane-insoluble matter. Meets the requirements for Identification, Residue on ignition (not more than 1.5%), Distinction from resin of Indian podophyllum, and Hexane-insoluble matter.

Caution: Podophyllum Resin is highly irritating to the eye and to mucous membranes in general.

Podophyllum Resin Topical Solution USP—Preserve in tight, light-resistant containers. A solution in Alcohol consisting of Podophyllum Resin and an alcoholic extract of Benzoin. Contains, in each 100 mL, not less than 10 grams and not more than 13 grams of hexane-insoluble matter. Meets requirements for Identification and Alcohol content (69.0–72.0%).

Caution: Podophyllum Resin Topical Solution is highly irritating to the eye and to mucous membranes in general.

POLACRILIN POTASSIUM

Chemical name: 2-Propenoic acid, 2-methyl-, polymer with divinylbenzene, potassium salt.

Description: Polacrilin Potassium NF—White to off-white, free-flowing powder. It has a faint odor or is odorless.

NF category: Tablet disintegrant.

Solubility: Polacrilin Potassium NF—Insoluble in water and in most liquids.

NF requirements: Polacrilin Potassium NF—Preserve in well-closed containers. The potassium salt of a unifunctional low-cross-linked carboxylic cation-exchange resin prepared from methacrylic acid and divinylbenzene. When previously dried at 105 °C for 6 hours, contains not less than 20.6% and not more than 25.1% of potassium. Meets the requirements for Identification, Loss on drying (not more than 10.0%), Powder fineness, Arsenic (not more than 3 ppm), Iron (not more than 0.01%), Sodium (not more than 0.20%), and Heavy metals (not more than 0.002%).

POLIOVIRUS VACCINE

Source: Produced from a mixture of 3 types of attenuated polioviruses that have been propagated in monkey kidney cell culture.

Poliovirus vaccine inactivated (IPV) and Poliovirus vaccine inactivated enhanced potency (enhanced-potency IPV): The polioviruses are inactivated with formaldehyde.

Poliovirus vaccine live oral (OPV): Contains the live, attenuated polioviruses.

Description:

Poliovirus Vaccine Inactivated USP—Clear, reddish-tinged or yellowish liquid, that may have a slight odor because of the preservative.

Poliovirus Vaccine Live Oral USP—Generally frozen but, in liquid form, is clear and colorless, or may have a yellow or red tinge.

USP requirements:

Poliovirus Vaccine Inactivated USP (Injection)—Preserve at a temperature between 2 and 8 °C. A sterile aqueous suspension of inactivated poliomyelitis virus of Types 1, 2, and 3. Label it to state that it is to be well shaken before use. Label it also to state that it was prepared in monkey tissue cultures. The virus strains are grown separately in primary cell cultures of monkey kidney tissue, and from a virus suspension with a virus titer of not less than $10^{6.5}$ $TCID_{50}$ measured in comparison with the U.S. Reference Poliovirus of the corresponding type, are inactivated so as to reduce the virus titer by a factor of 10^{-8}, and after inactivation are combined in suitable proportions. No extraneous protein, capable of producing allergenic effects upon injection into human subjects, is added to the final virus production medium. If animal serum is used at any stage, its calculated concentration in the final medium does not exceed 1 part per million. Suitable antimicrobial agents may be used during the production. Meets the requirements of the specific monkey potency test by virus neutralizing antibody production, based on the U.S. Reference Poliovirus Antiserum, such that the ratio of the geometric mean titer of the group of monkey serums representing the vaccine to the mean titer value of the reference serum is not less than 1.29 for Type 1, 1.13 for Type 2, and 0.72 for Type 3. Meets the requirement for Expiration date (not later than 1 year after date of issue from manufacturer's cold storage [5 °C, 1 year]). Conforms to the regulations of the U.S. Food and Drug Administration concerning biologics.

Poliovirus Vaccine Inactivated Enhanced Potency (Injection)—Not in USP.

Poliovirus Vaccine Live Oral USP (Oral Solution)—Preserve in single-dose or in multiple-dose containers at a temperature that will maintain ice continuously in a solid state. Preserve thawed Vaccine at a temperature between 2 and 8 °C. A preparation of a combination of the three types of live, attenuated polioviruses derived from strains of virus tested for neurovirulence in monkeys in comparison with the U.S. Reference Attenuated Poliovirus, Type 1, for such tests, and for immunogenicity, free from all demonstrable viable microbial agents except unavoidable bacteriophage, and found suitable for human immunization. The strains are grown, for purposes of vaccine production, separately in primary cell cultures of monkey renal tissue. Label the Vaccine to state that it may be thawed and refrozen not more than 10 times, provided that the thawed material is kept refrigerated and the total cumulative duration of the thaw is not more than 24 hours. Label the Vaccine to state the type of tissue in which it was prepared and to state that it is not for injection. Meets the requirements of the specific monkey neurovirulence test in comparison with the Reference Attenuated Poliovirus, and the requirements of the specific in-vitro marker tests. The Vaccine meets the requirements of the specific tissue culture tests for live virus titer, in a single immunizing dose, of not less than $10^{5.4}$ to $10^{6.4}$ for Type 1, $10^{4.5}$ to $10^{5.5}$ for Type 2, and $10^{5.2}$ to $10^{6.2}$ for Type 3, using the U.S. Reference Poliovirus, Live, Attenuated of the corresponding type for correlation of such titers. The Vaccine is filtered to prevent possible inclusion of bacteria in the final product. Meets the requirement for Expiration date (not later than 1 year after date of issue from manufacturer's cold storage [−10 °C, 1 year]). Conforms to the regulations of the U.S. Food and Drug Administration concerning biologics.

POLOXAMER

Chemical group: Nonionic surfactants.

Chemical name: Oxirane, methyl-, polymer with oxirane.

Molecular formula: $HO(C_2H_4O)_a(C_3H_6O)_b(C_2H_4O)_aH$.

Molecular weight: Average—
Poloxamer 124: 2090–2360.
Poloxamer 188: 7680–9510.
Poloxamer 237: 6840–8830.
Poloxamer 338: 12700–17400.
Poloxamer 407: 9840–14600.

Description: Poloxamer NF—Poloxamer 124 is a colorless liquid, having a mild odor. When solidified, it melts at about 16 °C. Poloxamer 188 (melting at about 52 °C), Poloxamer 237 (melting at about 49 °C), Poloxamer 338 (melting at about 57 °C), and Poloxamer 407 (melting at about 56 °C), are white, prilled or cast solids, odorless, or having a very mild odor.
NF category: Emulsifying and/or solubilizing agent.

Solubility: Poloxamer NF—Poloxamer 124 is freely soluble in water, in alcohol, in isopropyl alcohol, in propylene glycol, and in xylene. Poloxamer 188 is freely soluble in water and in alcohol. Poloxamer 237 is freely soluble in water and in alcohol; sparingly soluble in isopropyl alcohol and in xylene. Poloxamer 338 is freely soluble in water and in alcohol; sparingly soluble in propylene glycol. Poloxamer 407 is freely soluble in water, in alcohol, and in isopropyl alcohol.

USP requirements: Poloxamer 188 Capsules—Not in USP.

NF requirements: Poloxamer NF—Preserve in tight containers. A synthetic block copolymer of ethylene oxide and propylene oxide. It is available in several types. Label it to state, as part of the official title, the Poloxamer number. Meets the requirements for Average molecular weight, Weight percent oxyethylene, pH (5.0–7.5, in a solution [1 in 40]), Unsaturation, Heavy metals (not more than 0.002%), Organic volatile impurities, and Free ethylene oxide, propylene oxide, and 1, 4-dioxane (not more than 5 ppm of each).

POLYACRYLAMIDE

Source: A homopolymer of acrylamide, made of long chains of carbon atoms which are commonly found in fatty acids, carotinoids, and natural rubber.

USP requirements: Polyacrylamide Injection—Not in USP.

POLYCARBOPHIL

Chemical name: Polycarbophil.

Description: Polycarbophil UPS—White to creamy white granules, having a characteristic, ester-like odor. Swells in water to a range of volumes, depending primarily on the pH.

Solubility: Polycarbophil USP—Insoluble in water, in dilute acids, in dilute alkalies, and in common organic solvents.

USP requirements: Polycarbophil USP—Preserve in tight containers. Polyacrylic acid cross-linked with divinyl glycol. Meets the requirements for Identification, pH (not more than 4.0), Loss on drying (not more than 1.5%), Residue on ignition (not more than 4.0%), Absorbing power, Limit of acrylic acid (not more than 0.3%), Limit of ethyl acetate (not more than 0.45%), and Organic volatile impurities.

POLYETHYLENE EXCIPIENT

Description: Polyethylene Excipient NF—White, translucent, partially crystalline and partially amorphous resin. Available in various grades and types, differing from one another in molecular weight, molecular weight distribution, degree of chain branching, and extent of crystallinity.
NF category: Stiffening agent.

Solubility: Polyethylene Excipient NF—Insoluble in water.

NF requirements: Polyethylene Excipient NF—Preserve in well-closed containers. A homopolymer produced by the direct polymerization of ethylene. Meets the requirements for Identification, Intrinsic viscosity in 1,2,3,4-tetrahydronaphthalene (not less than 0.126), Heavy metals (not more than 0.004%), and Volatile substances (not more than 0.5%).

POLYETHYLENE GLYCOL

Chemical name: Poly(oxy-1,2-ethanediyl, alpha-hydro-omega-hydroxy-.

Molecular formula: $H(OCH_2CH_2)_nOH$.

Description:
Polyethylene Glycol NF—Polyethylene Glycol is usually designated by a number that corresponds approximately to its average molecular weight. As the average molecular weight increases, the water solubility, vapor pressure, hygroscopicity, and solubility in organic solvents decrease, while congealing temperature, specific gravity, flash point, and viscosity increase. Liquid grades occur as clear to slightly hazy, colorless or practically colorless, slightly hygroscopic, viscous liquids, having a slight, characteristic odor, and a specific gravity at 25 °C of about 1.12. Solid grades occur as practically odorless white, waxy, plastic material having a consistency similar to beeswax, or as creamy white flakes, beads, or powders. The accompanying table states the approximate congealing temperatures that are characteristic of commonly available grades.

Nominal Molecular Weight Polyethylene Glycol	Approximate Congealing Temperature (°C)
300	−11
400	6
600	20
900	34
1000	38
1450	44
3350	56
4500	58
8000	60

NF category: Coating agent; plasticizer; solvent; suppository base; tablet and/or capsule lubricant.

Polyethylene Glycol Ointment NF—NF category: Ointment base.

Solubility: Polyethylene Glycol NF—Liquid grades are miscible with water; solid grades are freely soluble in water; and all are soluble in acetone, in alcohol, in chloroform, in ethylene glycol monoethyl ether, in ethyl acetate, and in toluene; all are insoluble in ether and in hexane.

NF requirements:
Polyethylene Glycol NF—Preserve in tight containers. An addition polymer of ethylene oxide and water, represented by the formula $H(OCH_2CH_2)_nOH$, in which *n* represents the average number of of oxyethylene groups. The average molecular weight is not less than 95.0% and not

more than 105.0% of the labeled nominal value if the labeled nominal value is below 1000; it is not less than 90.0% and not more than 110.0% of the labeled nominal value if the labeled nominal value is between 1000 and 7000; it is not less than 87.5% and not more than 112.5% of the labeled nominal value if the labeled nominal value is above 7000. Label it to state, as part of the official title, the average nominal molecular weight of the Polyethylene Glycol. Meets the requirements for Completeness and color of solution, Viscosity, Average molecular weight, pH (4.5–7.5), Residue on ignition (not more than 0.1%), Arsenic (not more than 3 ppm), Free ethylene oxide and 1, 4-dioxane (not more than 10 ppm of each), Limit of ethylene glycol and diethylene glycol (not more than 0.25%), Heavy metals (not more than 5 ppm), and Organic volatile impurities.

Polyethylene Glycol Ointment NF—Preserve in well-closed containers.

Prepare Polyethylene Glycol Oinment as follows: 400 grams of Polyethylene Glycol 3350 and 600 grams of Polyethylene Glycol 400 to make 1000 grams. Heat the two ingredients on a water bath to 65 °C. Allow to cool, and stir until congealed. If a firmer preparation is desired, replace up to 100 grams of the polyethylene glycol 400 with an equal amount of polyethylene glycol 3350.

Note: If 6% to 25% of an aqueous solution is to be incorporated in Polyethylene Glycol Ointment, replace 50 grams of the polyethylene glycol 3350 with an equal amount of stearyl alcohol.

POLYETHYLENE GLYCOL MONOMETHYL ETHER

Chemical name: Poly(oxy-1,2-ethanediyl), alpha-methyl-omega-hydroxy-.

Description: Polyethylene Glycol Monomethyl Ether NF—Polyethylene Glycol Monomethyl Ether is usually designated by a number that corresponds approximately to its average molecular weight. As the average molecular weight increases, the water solubility, vapor pressure, hygroscopicity, and solubility in organic solvents decrease, while congealing temperature, specific gravity, flash point, and viscosity increase. Liquid grades occur as clear to slightly hazy, colorless or practically colorless, slightly hygroscopic, viscous liquids, having a slight, characteristic odor, and a specific gravity at 25 °C of about 1.09–1.10. Solid grades occur as practically odorless, white, waxy, plastic material having a consistency similar to beeswax, or as creamy white flakes, beads, or powders. The accompanying table states the approximate congealing temperatures that are characteristic of commonly available grades.

Nominal Molecular Weight Polyethylene Glycol Monomethyl Ether	Approximate Congealing Temperature (°C)
350	−7
550	17
750	28
1000	35
2000	51
5000	59
8000	60
10000	61

NF category: Ointment base; solvent; plasticizer.

Solubility: Polyethylene Glycol Monomethyl Ether NF—Liquid grades are miscible with water; solid grades are freely soluble in water; and all are soluble in acetone, in alcohol, in chloroform, in ethylene glycol monoethyl ether, in ethyl acetate, and in toluene; all are insoluble in ether and in hexane.

NF requirements: Polyethylene Glycol Monomethyl Ether NF—Preserve in tight containers. An addition polymer of ethylene oxide and methanol, represented by the formula $CH_3(OCH_2CH_2)_nOH$, in which *n* represents the average number of oxyethylene groups. The average molecular weight is not less than 95.0% and not more than 105.0% of the labeled nominal value if the labeled nominal value is below 1000; it is not less than 90.0% and not more than 110.0% of the labeled nominal value if the labeled nominal value is between 1000 and 4750; it is not less than 87.5% and not more than 112.5% of the labeled nominal value if the labeled nominal value is above 4750. Label it to state, as part of the official title, the average nominal molecular weight of the Polyethylene Glycol Monomethyl Ether. Meets the requirements for Completeness and color of solution, Viscosity, Average molecular weight, pH (4.5–7.5), Residue on ignition (not more than 0.1%), Arsenic (not more than 3 ppm), Limit of ethylene glycol and diethylene glycol (not more than 0.25%), Heavy metals (not more than 5 ppm), Free ethylene oxide and 1,4-dioxane (not more than 10 ppm of each), and 2-Methoxyethanol (not more than 10 ppm).

POLYETHYLENE OXIDE

Description: Polyethylene Oxide NF—Polyethylene oxide resins are high molecular weight polymers having the common structure $(-O-CH_2CH_2-)_n$, in which *n*, the degree of polymerization, varies from about 2000 to over 100,000. Polyethylene oxide, being a polyether, strongly hydrogen, bonds with water. It is nonionic and undergoes salting-out effects associated with neutral molecules in solutions of high dielectric media. Salting-out effects manifest themselves in depressing the upper temperature limit of solubility, and in reducing the viscosity of both dilute and concentrated solutions of the polymers. All molecular weight grades are powdered or granular solids.

NF category: Suspending and/or viscosity-increasing agent; tablet binder.

Solubility: Polyethylene Oxide NF—Soluble in water, but, because of the high solution viscosities obtained (see table), solutions over 1% in water may be difficult to prepare.

Approximate Molecular Weight	Typical Solution Viscosity (cps), 25 °C 5% Solution	1% Solution
100,000	40	
200,000	100	
300,000	800	
400,000	3000	
600,000	6000	
900,000	15000	
4,000,000		3500
5,000,000		5500

The water solubility, hygroscopicity, solubility in organic solvents, and melting point do not vary in the specified molecular weight range. At room temperature polyethylene oxide is miscible with water in all proportions. At concentrations of about 20% polymer in water the solutions are nontacky, reversible, elastic gels. At higher concentrations, the solutions are tough, elastic materials with the water acting as a plasticizer. Polyethylene oxide is also freely soluble in acetonitrile, in ethylene dichloride, in trichloroethylene, and in methylene chloride. Heating may be required to obtain solutions in many other organic solvents. It is insoluble in aliphatic hydrocarbons, in ethylene glycol, in diethylene glycol, and in glycerol.

NF requirements: Polyethylene Oxide NF—Preserve in tight, light-resistant containers. A nonionic homopolymer of ethylene oxide, represented by the formula $(OCH_2CH_2)_n$, in which *n* represents the average number of oxyethylene groups. It is a white to off-white powder obtainable in several grades, varying in viscosity profile in an aqueous isopropyl alcohol solution. May contain not more than 3.0% of silicon dioxide. The labeling indicates its viscosity profile in aqueous isopropyl alcohol solution. Meets the requirements for Identification, Loss on drying (not more than 1.0%), Silicon dioxide and Non–silicon dioxide residue on ignition (not more than 2.0%), Arsenic (not more than 3 ppm), Heavy metals (not more than 0.001%), Free ethylene oxide (not more than 0.001%), and Organic volatile impurities.

POLYMYXIN B

Chemical group: Polypeptide.

Chemical name: Polymyxin B sulfate—Polymyxin B, sulfate.

Description: Polymyxin B Sulfate USP—White to buff-colored powder. Odorless or has a faint odor.

Solubility: Polymyxin B Sulfate USP—Freely soluble in water; slightly soluble in alcohol.

USP requirements:

Polymyxin B Sulfate USP—Preserve in tight, light-resistant containers. The sulfate salt of a kind of polymyxin, a substance produced by the growth of *Bacillus polymyxa* (Prazmowski) Migula (Fam. Bacillaceae), or a mixture of two or more such salts. Where packaged for prescription compounding, the label states the number of Polymyxin B Units in the container and per milligram, that it is not intended for manufacturing use, that it is not sterile, and that its potency cannot be assured for longer than 60 days after opening. Has a potency of not less than 6000 Polymyxin B Units per mg, calculated on the dried basis. Meets the requirements for Identification, pH (5.0–7.5, in a solution containing 5 mg per mL), and Loss on drying (not more than 7.0%), and for Residue on ignition under Sterile Polymyxin B Sulfate (if for prescription compounding).

Polymyxin B Sulfate for Ophthalmic Solution—Not in USP.

Sterile Polymyxin B Sulfate USP—Preserve in Containers for Sterile Solids, protected from light. It is Polymyxin B Sulfate suitable for parenteral use. Label it to indicate that where it is administered intramuscularly and/or intrathecally, it is to be given only to patients hospitalized so as to provide constant supervision by a physician. Has a potency of not less than 6000 Polymyxin B Units per mg, calculated on the dried basis. Contains, where packaged for dispensing, an amount of polymyxin B sulfate equivalent to the labeled amount of polymyxin B, within −10% to +20%. Meets the requirements for Constituted solution, Pyrogen, Sterility, Particulate matter, Residue on ignition (not more than 5.0%), and Heavy metals (not more than 0.01%), for Identification tests, pH, and Loss on drying under Polymyxin B Sulfate, and where packaged for dispensing, for Uniformity of dosage units and Labeling under Injections. Where intended for use in preparing sterile ophthalmic dosage forms, it is exempt from requirements for Pyrogen, Particulate matter, and Heavy metals.

POLYMYXIN B AND BACITRACIN

For *Polymyxin B* and *Bacitracin*—See individual listings for chemistry information.

USP requirements:

Polymyxin B Sulfate and Bacitracin Zinc Topical Aerosol USP—Preserve in pressurized containers, and avoid exposure to excessive heat. Contains amounts of polymyxin B sulfate and bacitracin zinc equivalent to the labeled amounts of polymyxin B and bacitracin, within −10% to +30%. Meets the requirements for Identification, Microbial limits, and Water (not more than 0.5%), and for Leak testing and Pressure testing under Aerosols.

Polymyxin B Sulfate and Bacitracin Zinc Topical Powder USP—Preserve in well-closed containers. Contains amounts of polymyxin B sulfate and bacitracin zinc equivalent to the labeled amounts of polymyxin B and bacitracin, within −10% to +30%. Meets the requirements for Microbial limits and Water (not more than 7.0%).

POLYMYXIN B AND HYDROCORTISONE

For *Polymyxin B* and *Hydrocortisone*—See individual listings for chemistry information.

USP requirements: Polymyxin B Sulfate and Hydrocortisone Otic Solution USP—Preserve in tight, light-resistant containers. A sterile solution. Contains an amount of polymyxin B sulfate equivalent to the labeled amount of polymyxin B, within −10% to +30%, and the labeled amount of hydrocortisone, within ±10%. Meets the requirements for Sterility and pH (3.0–5.0).

Note: Where Polymyxin B Sulfate and Hydrocortisone Otic Solution is prescribed, without reference to the quantity of polymyxin B or hydrocortisone contained therein, a product containing 10,000 Polymyxin B Units and 5 mg of hydrocortisone per mL shall be dispensed.

POLYOXYL 10 OLEYL ETHER

Chemical name: Polyoxy-1,2-ethanediyl, alpha-[(*Z*)-9-octadecenyl-omega-hydroxy-.

Description: Polyoxyl 10 Oleyl Ether NF—White, soft semisolid, or pale yellow liquid, having a bland odor.

NF category: Emulsifying and/or solubilizing agent; wetting and or solubilizing agent.

Solubility: Polyoxyl 10 Oleyl Ether NF—Soluble in water and in alcohol; dispersible in mineral oil and in propylene glycol, with possible separation on standing.

NF requirements: Polyoxyl 10 Oleyl Ether NF—Preserve in tight containers, in a cool place. A mixture of the monooleyl ethers of mixed polyoxyethylene diols, the average polymer length being equivalent to not less than 8.6 and not more than 10.4 oxyethylene units. Label it to indicate the names and proportions of any added stabilizers. Meets the requirements for Identification, Water (not more than 3.0%), Residue on ignition (not more than 0.4%), Arsenic (not more than 2 ppm), Heavy metals (not more than 0.002%), Acid value (not more than 1.0), Hydroxyl value (75–95), Iodine value (23–40), Saponification value (not more than 3), Free polyethylene glycols (not more than 7.5%), Free ethylene oxide (not more than 0.01%), Average polymer length, and Organic volatile impurities.

POLYOXYL 20 CETOSTEARYL ETHER

Description: Polyoxyl 20 Cetostearyl Ether NF—Cream-colored, waxy, unctuous mass, melting, when heated, to a clear, brownish yellow liquid.

NF category: Emulsifying and/or solubilizing agent; wetting and/or solubilizing agent.

Solubility: Polyoxyl 20 Cetostearyl Ether NF—Soluble in water, in alcohol, and in acetone; insoluble in solvent hexane.

NF requirements: Polyoxyl 20 Cetostearyl Ether NF—Preserve in tight containers in a cool place. A mixture of monocetostearyl (mixed hexadecyl and octadecyl) ethers of mixed polyoxyethylene diols, the average polymer length being equivalent to not less than 17.2 and not more than 25.0 oxyethylene units. Meets the requirements for Identification, pH (4.5–7.5, determined in a solution [1 in 10]), Water (not more than 1.0%), Residue on ignition (not more than 0.4%), Arsenic (not more than 2 ppm), Heavy metals (not more than 0.002%), Acid value (not more than 0.5%), Hydroxyl value (42–60), Saponification value (not more than 2), Free polyethylene glycols (not more than 7.5%), Free ethylene oxide (not more than 0.01%), Average polymer length, and Organic volatile impurities.

POLYOXYL 35 CASTOR OIL

Description: Polyoxyl 35 Castor Oil NF—Yellow, oily liquid, having a faint, characteristic odor.

NF category: Emulsifying and/or solubilizing agent; wetting and/or solubilizing agent.

Solubility: Polyoxyl 35 Castor Oil NF—Very soluble in water, producing a practically odorless and colorless solution; soluble in alcohol and in ethyl acetate; insoluble in mineral oils.

NF requirements: Polyoxyl 35 Castor Oil NF—Preserve in tight containers. Contains mainly the tri-ricinoleate ester of ethoxylated glycerol, with smaller amounts of polyethylene glycol ricinoleate and the corresponding free glycols. Results from the reaction of glycerol ricinoleate with about 35 moles of ethylene oxide. Meets the requirements for Identification, Specific gravity (1.05–1.06), Viscosity (650–850 centipoises at 25 °C), Water (not more than 3.0%), Residue on ignition (not more than 0.3%), Heavy metals (not more than 0.001%), Acid value (not more than 2.0), Hydroxyl value (65–80), Iodine value (25–35), Saponification value (60–75), and Organic volatile impurities.

POLYOXYL 40 HYDROGENATED CASTOR OIL

Description: Polyoxyl 40 Hydrogenated Castor Oil NF—White to yellowish paste or pasty liquid, having a faint odor.

NF category: Emulsifying and/or solubilizing agent; wetting and/or solubilizing agent.

Solubility: Polyoxyl 40 Hydrogenated Castor Oil NF—Very soluble in water, producing a practically odorless and colorless solution; soluble in alcohol and in ethyl acetate; insoluble in mineral oils.

NF requirements: Polyoxyl 40 Hydrogenated Castor Oil NF—Preserve in tight containers. Contains mainly the tri-hydroxystearate ester of ethoxylated glycerol, with smaller amounts of polyethylene glycol tri-hydroxystearate and of the corresponding free glycols. Results from the reaction of glycerol tri-hydroxystearate with about 40 to 45 moles of ethylene oxide. Meets the requirements for Identification, Congealing temperature (20–30 °C), Water (not more than 3.0%), Residue on ignition (not more than 0.3%), Heavy metals (not more than 0.001%), Acid value (not more than 2.0), Hydroxyl value (60–80), Iodine value (not more than 2.0), Saponification value (45–69), and Organic volatile impurities.

POLYOXYL 40 STEARATE

Chemical name: Poly(oxy-1,2-ethanediyl), alpha-hydro-omega-hydroxy-, octadecanoate.

Description: Polyoxyl 40 Stearate NF—Waxy, white to light tan solid. It is odorless or has a faint fat-like odor.

NF category: Emulsifying and/or solubilizing agent; wetting and/or solubilizing agent.

Solubility: Polyoxyl 40 Stearate NF—Soluble in water, in alcohol, in ether, and in acetone; insoluble in mineral oil and in vegetable oils.

NF requirements: Polyoxyl 40 Stearate NF—Preserve in tight containers. A mixture of the monoesters and diesters of Stearic Acid or Purified Stearic Acid with mixed polyoxyethylene diols, the average polymer length being about 40 oxyethylene units. Meets the requirements for Identification, Congealing temperature (37–47 °C), Water (not more than 3.0%), Arsenic (not more than 3 ppm), Heavy metals (not more than 0.001%), Acid value (not more than 2), Hydroxyl value (25–40), Saponification value (25–35), Free polyethylene glycols (17–27%), and Organic volatile impurities.

POLYOXYL 50 STEARATE

Chemical name: Poly(oxy-1,2-ethanediyl), alpha-(1-oxooctadecyl)-omega-hydroxy-.

Description: Polyoxyl 50 Stearate NF—Soft, cream-colored, waxy solid, having a faint, fat-like odor. Melts at about 45 °C.

NF category: Wetting and/or solubilizing agent.

Solubility: Polyoxyl 50 Stearate NF—Soluble in water and in isopropyl alcohol.

NF requirements: Polyoxyl 50 Stearate NF—Preserve in tight containers. A mixture of the monostearate and distearate esters of mixed polyoxyethylene diols and the corresponding free diols. The average polymer length is about 50 oxyethylene units. Meets the requirements for Identification, Free polyethylene glycols (17–27%), Acid value (not more than 2), Hydroxyl value (23–35), Saponification value (20–28), and Organic volatile impurities, and for Water, Arsenic, and Heavy metals under Polyoxyl 40 Stearate.

POLYSORBATE 20

Chemical name: Sorbitan, monododecanoate, poly(oxy-1,2-ethanediyl) derivs.

Molecular formula: $C_{58}H_{114}O_{26}$ (approximate).

Description: Polysorbate 20 NF—Lemon to amber liquid, having a faint characteristic odor.

NF category: Emulsifying and/or solubilizing agent; wetting and/or solubilizing agent.

Solubility: Polysorbate 20 NF—Soluble in water, in alcohol, in ethyl acetate, in methanol, and in dioxane; insoluble in mineral oil.

NF requirements: Polysorbate 20 NF—Preserve in tight containers. A laurate ester of sorbitol and its anhydrides copolymerized with approximately 20 moles of ethylene oxide for each mole of sorbitol and sorbitol anhydrides. Meets the requirements for Identification, Hydroxyl value (96–108), and Saponification value (40–50), and for Water, Residue on ignition, Arsenic, Heavy metals, and Acid value under Polysorbate 80.

POLYSORBATE 40

Chemical name: Sorbitan, monohexadecanoate, poly(oxy-1,2-ethanediyl) derivs.

Molecular formula: $C_{62}H_{122}O_{26}$ (approximate).

Description: Polysorbate 40 NF—Yellow liquid, having a faint, characteristic odor.

NF category: Emulsifying and/or solubilizing agent; wetting and/or solubilizing agent.

Solubility: Polysorbate 40 NF—Soluble in water and in alcohol; insoluble in mineral oil and in vegetable oils.

NF requirements: Polysorbate 40 NF—Preserve in tight containers. A palmitate ester of sorbitol and its anhydrides copolymerized with approximately 20 moles of ethylene oxide for each mole of sorbitol and sorbitol anhydrides. Meets the requirements for Identification, Hydroxyl value (89–105), and Saponification value (41–52), and for Water, Residue on ignition, Arsenic, Heavy metals, and Acid value under Polysorbate 80.

POLYSORBATE 60

Chemical name: Sorbitan, monooctadecanoate, poly(oxy-1,2-ethanediyl) derivs.

Molecular formula: $C_{64}H_{126}O_{26}$ (approximate).

Description: Polysorbate 60 NF—Lemon- to orange-colored, oily liquid or semi-gel, having a faint, characteristic odor.

NF category: Emulsifying and/or solubilizing agent; wetting and/or solubilizing agent.

Solubility: Polysorbate 60 NF—Soluble in water, in ethyl acetate, and in toluene; insoluble in mineral oil and in vegetable oils.

NF requirements: Polysorbate 60 NF—Preserve in tight containers. A mixture of stearate and palmitate esters of sorbitol and its anhydrides copolymerized with approximately 20 moles of ethylene oxide for each mole of sorbitol and sorbitol anhydrides. Meets the requirements for Identification, Hydroxyl value (81–96), and Saponification value (45–55), and for Water, Residue on ignition, Arsenic, Heavy metals, and Acid value under Polysorbate 80.

POLYSORBATE 80

Chemical name: Sorbitan, mono-9-octadecenoate, poly(oxy-1,2-ethanediyl) derivs., (*Z*)-.

Description: Polysorbate 80 NF—Lemon- to amber-colored, oily liquid, having a faint, characteristic odor.

NF category: Emulsifying and/or solubilizing agent; wetting and/or solubilizing agent.

Solubility: Polysorbate 80 NF—Very soluble in water, producing an odorless and practically colorless solution; soluble in alcohol and in ethyl acetate; insoluble in mineral oil.

NF requirements: Polysorbate 80 NF—Preserve in tight containers. An oleate ester of sorbitol and its anhydrides copolymerized with approximately 20 moles of ethylene oxide for each mole of sorbitol and sorbitol anhydrides. Meets the requirements for Identification, Specific gravity (1.06–1.09), Viscosity (300–500 centistokes when determined at 25 °C), Water (not more than 3.0%), Residue on ignition (not more than 0.25%), Arsenic (not more than 1 ppm), Heavy metals (not more than 0.001%), Acid value (2.2), Hydroxyl value (65–80), and Saponification value (45–55).

POLYTHIAZIDE

Chemical name: 2*H*-1,2,4-Benzothiadiazine-7-sulfonamide, 6-chloro-3,4-dihydro-2-methyl-3-[[(2,2,2-trifluoroethyl)thio]-methyl]-, 1,1-dioxide.

Molecular formula: $C_{11}H_{13}ClF_3N_3O_4S_3$.

Molecular weight: 439.87.

Description: Polythiazide USP—White, crystalline powder, having a characteristic odor.

Solubility: Polythiazide USP—Practically insoluble in water and in chloroform; soluble in methanol and in acetone.

USP requirements:

Polythiazide USP—Preserve in tight, light-resistant containers. Dried in vacuum for 2 hours, contains not less than 97.0% and not more than 101.0% of polythiazide. Meets the requirements for Identification, Melting range (207–217 °C, with decomposition), Loss on drying (not more than 1.0%), Residue on ignition (not more than 0.2%), Heavy metals (not more than 0.0025%), Selenium (not more than 0.003%), and Diazotizable substances (not more than 1.0%).

Polythiazide Tablets USP—Preserve in tight, light-resistant containers. Contain the labeled amount, within ±10%. Meet the requirements for Identification, Dissolution (50% in 90 minutes in dilute hydrochloric acid [1 in 100] in Apparatus 2 at 50 rpm), and Uniformity of dosage units.

POLYVINYL ACETATE PHTHALATE

Description: Polyvinyl Acetate Phthalate NF—Free-flowing, white powder. May have a slight odor of acetic acid.

NF category: Coating agent.

Solubility: Polyvinyl Acetate Phthalate NF—Insoluble in water, in methylene chloride, and in chloroform. Soluble in methanol and in alcohol.

NF requirements: Polyvinyl Acetate Phthalate NF—Preserve in tight containers. A reaction product of phthalic anhydride and partially hydrolyzed polyvinyl acetate. Contains not less than 55.0% and not more than 62.0% of phthalyl (*o*-carboxybenzoyl, $C_8H_5O_3$) groups, calculated on an anhydrous acid-free basis. Meets the requirements for Identification, Viscosity (7–11 centipoises, determined at 25 °C ±0.2 °C [apparent]), Water (not more than 5.0%), Residue on ignition (not more than 1.0%), Free phthalic acid (not more than 0.6%, on the anhydrous basis), Free acid other than phthalic (not more than 0.6%, on the anhydrous basis), and Phthalyl content.

POLYVINYL ALCOHOL

Chemical name: Ethenol, homopolymer.

Molecular formula: $(C_2H_4O)_n$.

Description: Polyvinyl Alcohol USP—White to cream-colored granules, or white to cream-colored powder. Is odorless.

NF category: Suspending and/or viscosity-increasing agent.

Solubility: Polyvinyl Alcohol USP—Freely soluble in water at room temperature. Solution may be effected more rapidly at somewhat higher temperatures.

USP requirements: Polyvinyl Alcohol USP—Preserve in well-closed containers. A water-soluble synthetic resin, represented by the formula: $(C_2H_4O)_n$, in which the average value of n lies between 500 and 5000. Prepared by 85 to 89% hydrolysis of polyvinyl acetate. The apparent viscosity, in centipoises, at 20 °C, of a solution containing 4 grams of Polyvinyl Alcohol in each 100 grams, is within ±15% of that stated on the label. Meets the requirements for Viscosity, pH (5.0–8.0, in a solution [1 in 25]), Loss on drying (not more than 5.0%), Residue on ignition (not more than 2.0%), Water-insoluble substances (not more than 0.1%), Degree of hydrolysis (85–89%), and Organic volatile impurities.

SULFURATED POTASH

Chemical name: Thiosulfuric acid, dipotassium salt, mixt. with potassium sulfide (K_2S_x).

Description: Sulfurated Potash USP—Irregular, liver-brown pieces when freshly made, changing to a greenish-yellow. Has an odor of hydrogen sulfide and decomposes on exposure to air. A solution (1 in 10) is light brown in color and is alkaline to litmus.

Solubility: Sulfurated Potash USP—Freely soluble in water, usually leaving a slight residue. Alcohol dissolves only the sulfides.

USP requirements: Sulfurated Potash USP—Preserve in tight containers. Containers from which it is to be taken for immediate use in compounding prescriptions contain not more than 120 grams. A mixture composed chiefly of potassium polysulfides and potassium thiosulfate. Contains not less than 12.8% of sulfur in combination as sulfide. Meets the requirement for Identification.

POTASSIUM ACETATE

Chemical name: Acetic acid, potassium salt.

Molecular formula: $C_2H_3KO_2$.

Molecular weight: 98.14.

Description: Potassium Acetate USP—Colorless, monoclinic crystals or white, crystalline powder. Is odorless, or has a faint acetous odor. Deliquesces on exposure to moist air.

Solubility: Potassium Acetate USP—Very soluble in water; freely soluble in alcohol.

USP requirements:

Potassium Acetate USP—Preserve in tight containers. Contains not less than 99.0% and not more than 100.5% of potassium acetate, calculated on the dried basis. Meets the requirements for Identification, pH (7.5–8.5, in a solution [1 in 20]), Loss on drying (not more than 1.0%), Arsenic (not more than 8 ppm), Heavy metals (not more than 0.002%), and Sodium (not more than 0.03%).

Potassium Acetate Injection USP—Preserve in single-dose or in multiple-dose containers, preferably of Type I or Type II glass. A sterile solution of Potassium Acetate in Water for Injection. The label states the potassium acetate content in terms of weight and of milliequivalents in a given volume. Label the Injection to indicate that it is to be diluted to appropriate strength with water or other suitable fluid prior to administration. The label states also the total osmolar concentration in mOsmol per liter. Where the contents are less than 100 mL, or where the label states that the Injection is not for direct injection but is to be diluted before use, the label alternatively may state the total osmolar concentration in mOsmol per mL. Contains the labeled amount, within ±5%. Meets the requirements for Identification, Bacterial endotoxins, pH (5.5–8.0, when diluted with water to 1.0% of potassium acetate), Particulate matter, and Injections.

POTASSIUM BENZOATE

Chemical name: Benzoic acid, potassium salt.

Molecular formula: $C_7H_5KO_2$.

Molecular weight: 160.21.

Description: Potassium Benzoate NF—White, odorless, or practically odorless, granular or crystalline powder. Stable in air.

NF category: Antimicrobial preservative.

Solubility: Potassium Benzoate NF—Freely soluble in water; sparingly soluble in alcohol and somewhat more soluble in 90% alcohol.

NF requirements: Potassium Benzoate NF—Preserve in well-closed containers. Contains not less than 99.0% and not more than 100.5% of potassium benzoate, calculated on the anhydrous basis. Meets the requirements for Identification, Alkalinity, Water (not more than 1.5%), Arsenic (not more than 3 ppm), Heavy metals (not more than 0.001%), and Organic volatile impurities.

POTASSIUM BICARBONATE

Chemical name: Carbonic acid, monopotassium salt.

Molecular formula: $KHCO_3$.

Molecular weight: 100.12.

Description: Potassium Bicarbonate USP—Colorless, transparent, monoclinic prisms or as a white, granular powder. Is odorless, and is stable in air. Its solutions are neutral or alkaline to phenolphthalein TS.

Solubility: Potassium Bicarbonate USP—Freely soluble in water; practically insoluble in alcohol.

USP requirements:

Potassium Bicarbonate USP—Preserve in well-closed containers. Contains not less than 99.5% and not more than 101.5% of potassium bicarbonate, calculated on the dried basis. Meets the requirements for Identification, Loss on drying (not more than 0.3%), Normal carbonate (not more than 2.5%), Heavy metals (not more than 0.001%), and Organic volatile impurities.

Potassium Bicarbonate Effervescent Tablets for Oral Solution USP—Preserve in tight containers, protected from excessive heat. The label states the potassium content in terms of weight and in terms of milliequivalents. Where Tablets are packaged in individual pouches, the label instructs the user not to open until the time of use. Contain an amount of potassium bicarbonate equivalent to the labeled amount of potassium, within ±10%. Meet the requirements for Identification and Uniformity of dosage units.

POTASSIUM BICARBONATE AND POTASSIUM CHLORIDE

For *Potassium Bicarbonate* and *Potassium Chloride*—See individual listings for chemistry information.

USP requirements:

Potassium Bicarbonate and Potassium Chloride for Effervescent Oral Solution USP—Preserve in tight containers, protected from excessive heat. The label states the potassium and chloride contents in terms of weight and in terms of milliequivalents. Where packaged in individual pouches, the label instructs the user not to open until the time of use. Contains amounts of potassium bicarbonate and potassium chloride equivalent to the labeled amounts of potassium and chloride, within ±10%. Meets the requirements for Identification, Uniformity of dosage units (single-unit containers), and Minimum fill (multiple-unit containers).

Potassium Bicarbonate and Potassium Chloride Effervescent Tablets for Oral Solution USP—Preserve in tight containers, protected from excessive heat. The label states the potassium and chloride contents in terms of weight and in terms of milliequivalents. Where Tablets are packaged in individual pouches, the label instructs the user not to open until the time of use. Contain amounts of potassium bicarbonate and potassium chloride equivalent to the labeled amounts of potassium and chloride, within ±10%. Meet the requirements for Identification and Uniformity of dosage units.

POTASSIUM BICARBONATE AND POTASSIUM CITRATE

For *Potassium Bicarbonate* and *Potassium Citrate*—See individual listings for chemistry information.

USP requirements: Potassium Bicarbonate and Potassium Citrate Effervescent Tablets for Oral Solution—Not in USP.

POTASSIUM AND SODIUM BICARBONATES AND CITRIC ACID

For *Potassium Bicarbonate, Sodium Bicarbonate,* and *Citric Acid*—See individual listings for chemistry information.

USP requirements: Potassium and Sodium Bicarbonates and Citric Acid Effervescent Tablets for Oral Solution USP—Preserve in tight containers. Label it to state the sodium content. The label states also that Tablets are to be dissolved in water before being taken. Contain the labeled amounts of potassium bicarbonate, sodium bicarbonate, and anhydrous citric acid, within ±10%. Meet the requirements for Identification and Acid-neutralizing capacity.

POTASSIUM BITARTRATE AND SODIUM BICARBONATE

Chemical name:
Potassium bitartrate—Potassium acid tartrate.
Sodium bicarbonate—Carbonic acid monosodium salt.

Molecular formula:
Potassium bitartrate—$C_4H_5KO_6$.
Sodium bicarbonate—$NaHCO_3$.

Molecular weight:
Potassium bitartrate—188.18.
Sodium bicarbonate 84.01.

Description:
Potassium bitartrate—Odorless, or almost odorless, colorless crystals or white crystalline powder.
Sodium Bicarbonate USP—White, crystalline powder. Is stable in dry air, but slowly decomposes in moist air. Its solutions, when freshly prepared with cold water, without shaking, are alkaline to litmus. The alkalinity increases as the solutions stand, as they are agitated, or as they are heated.
NF category: Alkalizing agent.

Solubility:
Potassium bitartrate—Soluble 1 in 190 of water and 1 in 16 of boiling water; practically insoluble in alcohol.
Sodium Bicarbonate USP—Soluble in water; insoluble in alcohol.

USP requirements: Potassium Bitartrate and Sodium Bicarbonate Suppositories—Not in USP.

POTASSIUM CARBONATE

Chemical name: Carbonic acid, dipotassium salt.

Molecular formula: K_2CO_3.

Molecular weight: 138.21.

Description: Hygroscopic, odorless granules or granular powder.

Solubility: Soluble in 1 part cold, 0.7 part boiling water; practically insoluble in alcohol.

USP requirements: Potassium Carbonate USP—Preserve in well-closed containers. Contains not less than 99.5% and not more than 100.5% of potassium carbonate, calculated on the dried basis. Meets the requirements for Identification, Loss on drying (not more than 0.5%), Insoluble substances, Arsenic (not more than 2 ppm), Heavy metals (not more than 0.0005%), and Organic volatile impurities.

POTASSIUM CHLORIDE

Chemical name: Potassium chloride.

Molecular formula: KCl.

Molecular weight: 74.55.

Description: Potassium Chloride USP—Colorless, elongated, prismatic, or cubical crystals, or white, granular powder. Is odorless and is stable in air. Its solutions are neutral to litmus.
NF category: Tonicity agent.

Solubility: Potassium Chloride USP—Freely soluble in water and even more soluble in boiling water; insoluble in alcohol.

USP requirements:
Potassium Chloride USP—Preserve in well-closed containers. Where Potassium Chloride is intended for use in hemodialysis, it is so labeled. Contains not less than 99.0% and not more than 100.5% of potassium chloride, calculated on the dried basis. Meets the requirements for Identification, Acidity or alkalinity, Loss on drying (not more than 1.0%), Iodide or bromide, Arsenic (not more than 3 ppm), Calcium and magnesium, Heavy metals (not more than 0.001%), Sodium, Aluminum (not more than 1 ppm), and Organic volatile impurities.
Potassium Chloride Extended-release Capsules USP—Preserve in tight containers at a temperature not exceeding 30 °C. Contain the labeled amount, within ±10%. Meet the requirements for Identification, Dissolution (not more than 35% of labeled amount in 2 hours in water in Apparatus 1 at 100 rpm), and Uniformity of dosage units.
Potassium Chloride for Injection Concentrate USP—Preserve in single-dose or in multiple-dose containers, preferably of Type I or Type II glass. A sterile solution of Potassium Chloride in Water for Injection. The label states the potassium chloride content in terms of weight and of milliequivalents in a given volume. Label the Concentrate to indicate that it is to be diluted to appropriate strength with water or other suitable fluid prior to administration. Immediately following the name, the label bears the boxed warning (in large letters): **Concentrate Must be Diluted Before Use.** The cap of the container and the overseal of the cap must be black and both bear the words: "Must be Diluted" in readily legible type, in a color that stands out from its background. Ampuls shall be identified by a black band or a series of black bands above the constriction. The label states also the total osmolar concentration in mOsmol per liter. Where the contents are less than 100 mL, the label alternatively may state the total osmolar concentration in mOsmol per mL. Contains the labeled amount, within ±5%. Meets the requirements for Identification, Pyrogen, pH (4.0–8.0), Particulate matter, and Injections.
Potassium Chloride Oral Solution USP—Preserve in tight containers. Contains the labeled amount, within ±5%. May contain alcohol. Meets the requirements for Identification and Alcohol content (within −10% to +15% of the labeled amount which is not more than 7.5%).

Potassium Chloride for Oral Solution USP—Preserve in tight containers. A dry mixture of Potassium Chloride and one or more suitable colors, diluents, and flavors. The label states the Potassium Chloride content in terms of weight and in terms of milliequivalents. Contains the labeled amount, within ±10%. Meets the requirements for Identification, Uniformity of dosage units (single-unit containers), and Minimum fill (multiple-unit containers).

Potassium Chloride for Oral Suspension—Not in USP.

Potassium Chloride Extended-release Tablets USP—Preserve in tight containers at a temperature not exceeding 30 °C. Contain the labeled amount, within ±10%. Meet the requirements for Identification, Dissolution (not more than 35% of labeled amount in 2 hours in water in Apparatus 2 at 50 rpm), and Uniformity of dosage units.

POTASSIUM CHLORIDE AND DEXTROSE

For *Potassium Chloride* and *Dextrose*—See individual listings for chemistry information.

USP requirements: Potassium Chloride in Dextrose Injection USP—Preserve in single-dose glass or plastic containers. Glass containers are preferably of Type I or Type II glass. A sterile solution of Potassium Chloride and Dextrose in Water for Injection. The label states the total osmolar concentration in mOsmol per liter. Where the contents are less than 100 mL, or where the label states that the Injection is not for direct injection but is to be diluted before use, the label alternatively may state the total osmolar concentration in mOsmol per mL. The content of potassium, in milliequivalents, is prominently displayed on the label. Contains the labeled amounts of potassium chloride, within −5% to +10%, and dextrose, within ±5%. Contains no antimicrobial agents. Meets the requirements for Identification, Bacterial endotoxins, pH (3.5–6.5, determined on a portion diluted with water, if necessary, to a concentration of not more than 5% of dextrose), 5-Hydroxymethylfurfural and related substances, and Injections, and for Heavy metals under Dextrose Injection.

POTASSIUM CHLORIDE, DEXTROSE, AND SODIUM CHLORIDE

For *Potassium Chloride, Dextrose,* and *Sodium Chloride*—See individual listings for chemistry information.

USP requirements: Potassium Chloride in Dextrose and Sodium Chloride Injection USP—Preserve in single-dose containers, preferably of Type I or Type II glass, or of a suitable plastic. A sterile solution of Potassuim Chloride, Dextrose, and Sodium Chloride in Water for Injection. The label states the potassium, sodium, and chloride contents in terms of milliequivalents in a given volume. The label states also the total osmolar concentration in mOsmol per liter. Where the contents are less than 100 mL, the label alternatively may state the total osmolar concentration in mOsmol per mL. Contains the equivalent of the labeled amounts of potassium and chloride, within −5% to +10%, and the equivalent of the labeled amounts of dextrose and sodium, within ±5%. Contains no antimicrobial agents. Meets the requirements for Identification, Bacterial endotoxins, pH (3.5–6.5), Heavy metals, 5-Hydroxymethylfurfural and related substances, and Injections.

POTASSIUM CHLORIDE, LACTATED RINGER'S, AND DEXTROSE

For *Potassium Chloride, Calcium Chloride, Sodium Chloride, Sodium Lactate,* and *Dextrose*—See individual listings for chemistry information.

USP requirements: Potassium Chloride in Lactated Ringer's and Dextrose Injection USP—Preserve in single-dose glass or plastic containers. Glass containers are preferably of Type I or Type II glass. A sterile solution of Calcium Chloride, Potassium Chloride, Sodium Chloride, and Sodium Lactate in Water for Injection. The label states the total osmolar concentration in mOsmol per liter. Where the contents are less than 100 mL, the label alternatively may state the total osmolar concentration in mOsmol per mL. The label includes also the warning: "Not for use in the treatment of lactic acidosis." Contains, in each 100 mL, not less than 285.0 mg and not more than 315.0 mg of sodium (as sodium chloride and sodium lactate), not less than 4.90 mg and not more than 6.00 mg of calcium (calcium, equivalent to not less than 18.0 mg and not more than 22.0 mg of hydrous calcium chloride), and not less than 231.0 mg and not more than 261.0 mg of lactate (lactate, equivalent to not less than 290.0 mg and not more than 330.0 mg of sodium lactate). Contains the labeled amounts of Potassium Chloride and dextrose, within ±5%, and the equivalent of the labeled amount of chloride (chloride, as sodium chloride, potassium chloride, and hydrous calcium chloride), within ±10%. Contains no antimicrobial agents. Meets the requirements for Identification, Bacterial endotoxins, pH (3.5–6.5), Heavy metals, 5-Hydroxymethylfurfural and related substances, and Injections.

POTASSIUM CHLORIDE, POTASSIUM BICARBONATE, AND POTASSIUM CITRATE

For *Potassium Chloride, Potassium Bicarbonate,* and *Potassium Citrate*—See individual listings for chemistry information.

USP requirements: Potassium Chloride, Potassium Bicarbonate, and Potassium Citrate Effervescent Tablets for Oral Solution USP—Preserve in tight containers, protected from excessive heat. The label states the potassium and chloride contents in terms of weight and in terms of milliequivalents. Where Tablets are packaged in individual pouches, the label instructs the user not to open until the time of use. Contain the equivalent of the labeled amounts of potassium and chloride, within ±10%. Meet the requirements for Identification and Uniformity of dosage units.

POTASSIUM CHLORIDE AND SODIUM CHLORIDE

For *Potassium Chloride* and *Sodium Chloride*—See individual listings for chemistry information.

USP requirements: Potassium Chloride in Sodium Chloride Injection USP—Preserve in single-dose containers, preferably of Type I or Type II glass, or of a suitable plastic. A sterile solution of Potassium Chloride and Sodium Chloride in Water for Injection. The label states the potassium, sodium, and chloride contents in terms of milliequivalents in a given volume. The label states also the total osmolar concentration in mOsmol per liter. Where the contents are less than 100 mL, the label may alternatively state the total osmolar concentration in mOsmol per mL. Contains the equivalent of the labeled amounts of potassium and chloride, within −5% to +10%, and the equivalent of the labeled amount of sodium, within ±5%. Contains no antimicrobial agents. Meets the requirements for Identification, Bacterial endotoxins, pH (3.5–6.5), Heavy metals, and Injections.

POTASSIUM CITRATE

Chemical name: 1,2,3-Propanetricarboxylic acid, 2-hydroxy-, tripotassium salt, monohydrate.

Molecular formula: $C_6H_5K_3O_7 \cdot H_2O$.

Molecular weight: 324.41.

Description: Potassium Citrate USP—Transparent crystals or white, granular powder. Is odorless and is deliquescent when exposed to moist air.

NF category: Buffering agent.

Solubility: Potassium Citrate USP—Freely soluble in water; almost insoluble in alcohol.

USP requirements:

Potassium Citrate USP—Preserve in tight containers. Contains not less than 99.0% and not more than 100.5% of potassium citrate, calculated on the dried basis. Meets the requirements for Identification, Alkalinity, Loss on drying (3.0–6.0%), Tartrate, Heavy metals (not more than 0.001%), and Organic volatile impurities.

Potassium Citrate Tablets—Not in USP.

Potassium Citrate Extended-release Tablets USP—Preserve in tight containers. Contain the labeled amount, within ±10%. Meet the requirements for Identification, Dissolution (not more than 45% in 30 minutes, not more than 60% in 1 hour, and not less than 80% in 3 hours, in water in Apparatus 2 at 50 rpm), Uniformity of dosage units, and Potassium content (36.4–40.2%).

POTASSIUM CITRATE AND CITRIC ACID

For *Potassium Citrate* and *Citric Acid*—See individual listings for chemistry information.

USP requirements:

Potassium Citrate and Citric Acid Oral Solution USP—Preserve in tight containers. A solution of Potassium Citrate and Citric Acid in a suitable aqueous medium. Contains, in each 100 mL, not less than 7.55 grams and not more than 8.35 grams of potassium; not less than 12.18 grams and not more than 13.46 grams of citrate, equivalent to not less than 20.9 grams and not more than 23.1 grams of potassium citrate monohydrate; and not less than 6.34 grams and not more than 7.02 grams of citric acid monohydrate. Meets the requirements for Identification and pH (4.9–5.4).

Note: The potassium ion content of Potassium Citrate and Citric Acid Oral Solution is approximately 2 mEq per mL.

Potassium Citrate and Citric Acid for Oral Solution—Not in USP.

POTASSIUM CITRATE AND SODIUM CITRATE

For *Potassium Citrate* and *Sodium Citrate*—See individual listings for chemistry information.

USP requirements: Potassium Citrate and Sodium Citrate Tablets—Not in USP.

POTASSIUM GLUCONATE

Chemical name: D-Gluconic acid, monopotassium salt.

Molecular formula: $C_6H_{11}KO_7$.

Molecular weight: 234.25.

Description: Potassium Gluconate USP—White to yellowish white, crystalline powder or granules. Is odorless and is stable in air. Its solutions are slightly alkaline to litmus.

Solubility: Potassium Gluconate USP—Freely soluble in water; practically insoluble in dehydrated alcohol, in ether, and in chloroform.

USP requirements:

Potassium Gluconate USP—Preserve in tight containers. It is anhydrous or contains one molecule of water of hydration. Label it to indicate whether it is anhydrous or the monohydrate. Contains not less than 97.0% and not more than 103.0% of potassium gluconate, calculated on the dried basis. Meets the requirements for Identification, Loss on drying (not more than 3.0% for the anhydrous form and 6.0–7.5% for the monohydrate form), Heavy metals (not more than 0.002%), Reducing substances (not more than 1.0%), and Organic volatile impurities.

Potassium Gluconate Elixir USP—Preserve in tight, light-resistant containers. Contains the labeled amount, within ±5%. Meets the requirements for Identification and Alcohol content (4.5–5.5%).

Potassium Gluconate Tablets USP—Preserve in tight containers. Contain the labeled amount, within ±5%. Meet the requirements for Identification, Dissolution (75% in 45 minutes in water in Apparatus 2 at 100 rpm), and Uniformity of dosage units.

POTASSIUM GLUCONATE AND POTASSIUM CHLORIDE

For *Potassium Gluconate* and *Potassium Chloride*—See individual listings for chemistry information.

USP requirements:

Potassium Gluconate and Potassium Chloride Oral Solution USP—Preserve in tight containers. A solution of Potassium Gluconate and Potassium Chloride in a suitable aqueous medium. Label it to state the potassium and chloride contents in terms of milliequivalents of each in a given volume of Oral Solution. Contains the equivalent of the labeled amounts of potassium and chloride, within ±10%. Meets the requirement for Identification.

Potassium Gluconate and Potassium Chloride for Oral Solution USP—Preserve in tight containers. A dry mixture of Potassium Gluconate and Potassium Chloride and one or more suitable colors, diluents, and flavors. Label it to state the potassium and chloride contents in terms of milliequivalents. Where packaged in unit-dose pouches, the label instructs the user not to open until the time of use. Contains the equivalent of the labeled amounts of potassium and chloride, within ±10%. Meets the requirements for Identification and Minimum fill.

POTASSIUM GLUCONATE AND POTASSIUM CITRATE

For *Potassium Gluconate* and *Potassium Citrate*—See individual listings for chemistry information.

USP requirements: Potassium Gluconate and Potassium Citrate Oral Solution USP—Preserve in tight containers. A solution of Potassium Gluconate and Potassium Citrate in a suitable aqueous medium. Label it to state the potassium content in terms of milliequivalents in a given volume of Oral Solution. Contains the equivalent of the labeled amount of potassium, within ±10%. Meets the requirement for Identification.

POTASSIUM GLUCONATE, POTASSIUM CITRATE, AND AMMONIUM CHLORIDE

For *Potassium Gluconate, Potassium Citrate,* and *Ammonium Chloride*—See individual listings for chemistry information.

USP requirements: Potassium Gluconate, Potassium Citrate, and Ammonium Chloride Oral Solution USP—Preserve in tight containers. A solution of Potassium Gluconate, Potassium Citrate, and Ammonium Chloride in a suitable aqueous medium. Label it to state the potassium and chloride contents in terms of milliequivalents of each in a given volume of Oral Solution. Contains the equivalent of the labeled amounts of potassium and chloride, within ±10%. Meets the requirement for Identification.

POTASSIUM GUAIACOLSULFONATE

Chemical name: Benzenesulfonic acid, hydroxymethoxy-, monopotassium salt, hemihydrate.

Molecular formula: $C_7H_7KO_5S \cdot \frac{1}{2}H_2O$.

Molecular weight: 251.30 (hemihydrate); 242.29 (anhydrous).

Description: White, odorless crystals or crystalline powder. Gradually turns pink on exposure to air and light.

Solubility: Soluble in 7.5 parts water; almost insoluble in alcohol; insoluble in ether.

USP requirements: Potassium Guaiacolsulfonate USP—Preserve in well-closed, light-resistant containers. Contains not less than 98.0% and not more than 102.0% of potassium guaiacolsulfonate, calculated on the anhydrous basis. Meets the requirements for Identification, Water (3.0–6.0%), Selenium (not more than 0.003%), Sulfate, and Heavy metals (not more than 0.002%).

POTASSIUM HYDROXIDE

Chemical name: Potassium hydroxide.

Molecular formula: KOH.

Molecular weight: 56.11.

Description: Potassium Hydroxide NF—White or practically white fused masses, or small pellets, or flakes, or sticks, or other forms. It is hard and brittle and shows a crystalline fracture. Exposed to air, it rapidly absorbs carbon dioxide and moisture, and deliquesces.

NF category: Alkalizing agent.

Solubility: Potassium Hydroxide NF—Freely soluble in water, in alcohol, and in glycerin; very soluble in boiling alcohol.

NF requirements: Potassium Hydroxide NF—Preserve in tight containers. Contains not less than 85.0% of total alkali, calculated as potassium hydroxide, including not more than 3.5% of anhydrous potassium carbonate. Meets the requirements for Identification, Insoluble substances, and Heavy metals (not more than 0.003%).

Caution: Exercise great care in handling Potassium Hydroxide, as it rapidly destroys tissues.

POTASSIUM IODIDE

Chemical group: Inorganic iodides.

Chemical name: Potassium iodide.

Molecular formula: KI.

Molecular weight: 166.00.

Description:

Potassium Iodide USP—Hexahedral crystals, either transparent and colorless or somewhat opaque and white, or a white, granular powder. Is slightly hygroscopic. Its solutions are neutral or alkaline to litmus.

Potassium Iodide Oral Solution USP—Clear, colorless, odorless liquid. Is neutral or alkaline to litmus. Specific gravity is about 1.70.

Solubility: Potassium Iodide USP—Very soluble in water and even more soluble in boiling water; freely soluble in glycerin; soluble in alcohol.

USP requirements:

Potassium Iodide USP—Preserve in well-closed containers. Contains not less than 99.0% and not more than 101.5% of potassium iodide, calculated on the dried basis. Meets the requirements for Identification, Alkalinity, Loss on drying (not more than 1.0%), Iodate (not more than 4 ppm), Nitrate, nitrite, and ammonia, Thiosulfate and barium, Heavy metals (not more than 0.001%), and Organic volatile impurities.

Potassium Iodide Oral Solution USP—Preserve in tight, light-resistant containers. Contains the labeled amount, within ±6%. Meets the requirement for Identification.

Note: If Potassium Iodide Oral Solution is not to be used within a short time, add 0.5 mg of sodium thiosulfate for each gram of potassium iodide. Crystals of potassium iodide may form in Potassium Iodide Oral Solution under normal conditions of storage, especially if refrigerated.

Potassium Iodide Syrup—Not in USP.

Potassium Iodide Tablets USP—Preserve in tight containers. Contain the labeled amount, within ±6% for Tablets of 300 mg or more; within ±7.5% for Tablets of less than 300 mg. Meet the requirements for Identification, Disintegration (for Enteric-coated Tablets, the tablets do not disintegrate after 1 hour of agitation in simulated gastric fluid TS, but they disintegrate within 90 minutes in simulated intestinal fluid TS), Dissolution (for uncoated Tablets, 75% in 15 minutes in water in Apparatus 2 at 50 rpm), and Uniformity of dosage units.

POTASSIUM METABISULFITE

Chemical name: Disulfurous acid, dipotassium salt.

Molecular formula: $K_2S_2O_5$.

Molecular weight: 222.31.

Description: Potassium Metabisulfite NF—White or colorless, free-flowing crystals, crystalline powder, or granules, usually having an odor of sulfur dioxide. Gradually oxidizes in air to the sulfate. Its solutions are acid to litmus.

NF category: Antioxidant.

Solubility: Potassium Metabisulfite NF—Soluble in water; insoluble in alcohol.

NF requirements: Potassium Metabisulfite NF—Preserve in well-fitted, tight containers, and avoid exposure to excessive heat. Contains an amount of potassium metabisulfite equivalent to not less than 51.8% and not more than 57.6% of sulfur dioxide. Meets the requirements for Identification, Arsenic (not more than 3 ppm), Iron (not more than 0.001%), Heavy metals (not more than 0.001%), and Organic volatile impurities.

POTASSIUM METAPHOSPHATE

Chemical name: Metaphosphoric acid (HPO_3), potassium salt.

Molecular formula: KPO_3.

Molecular weight: 118.07.

Description: Potassium Metaphosphate NF—White, odorless powder.

NF category: Buffering agent.

Solubility: Potassium Metaphosphate NF—Insoluble in water; soluble in dilute solutions of sodium salts.

NF requirements: Potassium Metaphosphate NF—Preserve in well-closed containers. A straight-chain polyphosphate, having a high degree of polymerization. Contains the equivalent of not less than 59.0% and not more than 61.0% of phosphorus pentoxide. Meets the requirements for Identification, Viscosity (6.5–15 centipoises), Fluoride (not more than 0.001%), Arsenic (not more than 3 ppm), Lead (not more than 5 ppm), and Heavy metals (not more than 0.002%).

POTASSIUM PERMANGANATE

Chemical name: Permanganic acid ($HMnO_4$), potassium salt.

Molecular formula: $KMnO_4$.

Molecular weight: 158.03.

Description: Potassium Permanganate USP—Dark purple crystals, almost opaque by transmitted light and of a blue metallic luster by reflected light. Its color is sometimes modified by a dark bronze-like appearance. Is stable in air.

Solubility: Potassium Permanganate USP—Soluble in water; freely soluble in boiling water.

USP requirements: Potassium Permanganate USP—Preserve in well-closed containers. Contains not less than 99.0% and not more than 100.5% of potassium permanganate, calculated on the dried basis. Meets the requirements for Identification, Loss on drying (not more than 0.5%), and Insoluble substances (not more than 0.2%).

Caution: Observe great care in handling Potassium Permanganate, as dangerous explosions may occur if it is brought into contact with organic or other readily oxidizable substances, either in solution or in the dry state.

DIBASIC POTASSIUM PHOSPHATE

Chemical name: Phosphoric acid, dipotassium salt.

Molecular formula: K_2HPO_4.

Molecular weight: 174.18.

Description: Dibasic Potassium Phosphate USP—Colorless or white, somewhat hygroscopic, granular powder. The pH of a solution (1 in 20) is about 8.5 to 9.6.

NF category: Buffering agent.

Solubility: Dibasic Potassium Phosphate USP—Freely soluble in water; very slightly soluble in alcohol.

USP requirements: Dibasic Potassium Phosphate USP—Preserve in well-closed containers. Contains not less than 98.0% and not more than 100.5% of dibasic potassium phosphate, calculated on the dried basis. Meets the requirements for Identification, pH (8.5–9.6, in a solution [1 in 20]), Loss on drying (not more than 1.0%), Insoluble substances (not more than 0.2%), Carbonate, Chloride (not more than 0.03%), Sulfate (not more than 0.1%), Fluoride (not more than 0.001%), Arsenic (not more than 3 ppm), Iron (not more than 0.003%), Sodium, Heavy metals (not more than 0.001%), and Monobasic or tribasic salt.

MONOBASIC POTASSIUM PHOSPHATE

Chemical name: Phosphoric acid, monopotassium salt.

Molecular formula: KH_2PO_4.

Molecular weight: 136.09.

Description: Monobasic Potassium Phosphate NF—Colorless crystals or white, granular or crystalline powder. Is odorless, and is stable in air. The pH of a solution (1 in 100) is about 4.5.

NF category: Buffering agent.

Solubility: Monobasic Potassium Phosphate NF—Freely soluble in water; practically insoluble in alcohol.

USP requirements: Monobasic Potassium Phosphate Tablets for Oral Solution—Not in USP.

NF requirements: Monobasic Potassium Phosphate NF—Preserve in tight containers. Dried at 105 °C for 4 hours, contains not less than 98.0% and not more than 100.5% of monobasic potassium phosphate. Meets the requirements for Identification, Loss on drying (not more than 1.0%), Insoluble substances (not more than 0.2%), Fluoride (not more than 0.001%), Arsenic (not more than 3 ppm), Heavy metals (not more than 0.002%), Lead (not more than 5 ppm), and Organic volatile impurities.

POTASSIUM PHOSPHATES

For *Monobasic Potassium Phosphate* and *Dibasic Potassium Phosphate*—See individual listings for chemistry information.

USP requirements:

Potassium Phosphates Capsules for Oral Solution—Not in USP.

Potassium Phosphates Injection USP—Preserve in single-dose containers, preferably of Type I glass. A sterile solution of Monobasic Potassium Phosphate and Dibasic Potassium Phosphate in Water for Injection. The label states the potassium content in terms of milliequivalents in a given volume, and states also the elemental phosphorus content in terms of millimoles in a given volume. Label the Injection to indicate that it is to be diluted to appropriate strength with water or other suitable fluid prior to administration, and that once opened any unused portion is to be discarded. The label states also the total osmolar concentration in mOsmol per liter. Where the contents are less than 100 mL, or where the label states that the Injection is not for direct injection but is to be diluted before use, the label alternatively may state the total osmolar concentration in mOsmol per mL. Contains the labeled amounts of monobasic potassium phosphate and dibasic potassium phosphate, within ±5%. Contains no bacteriostat or other preservative. Meets the requirements for Identification, Bacterial endotoxins, Particulate matter, and Injections.

Potassium Phosphates for Oral Solution—Not in USP.

POTASSIUM AND SODIUM PHOSPHATES

For *Dibasic Potassium Phosphate, Dibasic Sodium Phosphate, Monobasic Potassium Phosphate,* and *Monobasic Sodium Phosphate*—See individual listings for chemistry information.

USP requirements:

Potassium and Sodium Phosphates Capsules for Oral Solution—Not in USP.

Potassium and Sodium Phosphates for Oral Solution—Not in USP.

Potassium and Sodium Phosphates Tablets for Oral Solution—Not in USP.

MONOBASIC POTASSIUM AND SODIUM PHOSPHATES

For *Monobasic Potassium Phosphate* and *Monobasic Sodium Phosphate*—See individual listings for chemistry information.

USP requirements: Monobasic Potassium and Sodium Phosphates Tablets for Oral Solution—Not in USP.

POTASSIUM SODIUM TARTRATE

Chemical name: Butanedioic acid, 2,3-dihydroxy-, [*R*-(*R**,*R**)]-, monopotassium monosodium salt, tetrahydrate.

Molecular formula: $C_4H_4KNaO_6 \cdot 4H_2O$.

Molecular weight: 282.22 (tetrahydrate); 210.16 (anhydrous).

Description: Potassium Sodium Tartrate USP—Colorless crystals or white, crystalline powder. As it effloresces slightly in warm, dry air, the crystals are often coated with a white powder.

Solubility: Potassium Sodium Tartrate USP—Freely soluble in water; practically insoluble in alcohol.

USP requirements: Potassium Sodium Tartrate USP—Preserve in tight containers. Contains not less than 99.0% and not more than 102.0% of potassium sodium tartrate, calculated on the anhydrous basis. Meets the requirements for Identification, Alkalinity, Water (21.0–27.0%), Ammonia, and Heavy metals (not more than 0.001%).

POTASSIUM SORBATE

Chemical name: 2,4-Hexadienoic acid, (*E,E'*)- potassium salt.

Molecular formula: $C_6H_7KO_2$.

Molecular weight: 150.22.

Description: Potassium Sorbate NF—White crystals or powder, having a characteristic odor. Melts at about 270 °C, with decomposition.

NF category: Antimicrobial preservative.

Solubility: Potassium Sorbate NF—Freely soluble in water; soluble in alcohol.

NF requirements: Potassium Sorbate NF—Preserve in tight containers, protected from light, and avoid exposure to excessive heat. Contains not less than 98.0% and not more than 101.0% of potassium sorbate, calculated on the dried basis. Meets the requirements for Identification, Acidity or alkalinity, Loss on drying (not more than 1.0%), Heavy metals (not more than 0.001%), and Organic volatile impurities.

POVIDONE

Chemical name: 2-Pyrrolidinone, 1-ethenyl-, homopolymer.

Molecular formula: $(C_6H_9NO)_n$.

Description: Povidone USP—White to creamy white powder, having a faint odor. Is hygroscopic.

NF category: Suspending and/or viscosity-increasing agent; tablet binder.

Solubility: Povidone USP—Soluble in water, in alcohol, and in chloroform; insoluble in ether.

USP requirements: Povidone USP—Preserve in tight containers. A synthetic polymer consisting essentially of linear 1-vinyl-2-pyrrolidinone groups, the degree of polymerization of which results in polymers of various molecular weights. Characterized by its viscosity in aqueous solution, relative to that of water, expressed as a K-value, ranging from 10 to 120. Label it to state, as part of the official title, the K-value or K-value range of the Povidone. The K-value of Povidone having a nominal K-value of 15 or less is not less than 85.0% and not more than 115.0% of the nominal K-value, and the K-value of Povidone having a nominal K-value or nominal K-value range with an average of more than 15 is not less than 90.0% and not more than 108.0% of the nominal K-value or average of the nominal K-value range. Meets the requirements for Identification, pH (3.0–7.0, in a solution [1 in 20]), Water (not more than 5.0%), Residue on ignition (not more than 0.1%), Lead (not more than 10 ppm), Limit of aldehydes, Hydrazine (not more than 1 ppm), Vinylpyrrolidinone (not more than 0.2%), K-value, and Nitrogen content (11.5–12.8%, on the anhydrous basis).

POVIDONE-IODINE

Chemical name: 2-Pyrrolidinone, 1-ethenyl-, homopolymer, compd. with iodine.

Molecular formula: $(C_6H_9NO)_n \cdot xI$.

Description:

Povidone-Iodine USP—Yellowish brown, amorphous powder, having a slight characteristic odor. Its solution is acid to litmus.

Povidone-Iodine Topical Aerosol Solution USP—The liquid obtained from Povidone-Iodine Topical Aerosol Solution is transparent, having a reddish-brown color.

Solubility: Povidone-Iodine USP—Soluble in water and in alcohol; practically insoluble in chloroform, in carbon tetrachloride, in ether, in solvent hexane, and in acetone.

USP requirements:

Povidone-Iodine USP—Preserve in tight containers. A complex of Iodine with Povidone. Contains not less than 9.0% and not more than 12.0% of available iodine, calculated on the dried basis. Meets the requirements for Identification, Loss on drying (not more than 8.0%), Residue on ignition (negligible, from 2 grams), Iodide ion (not more than 6.6%, calculated on the dried basis), Heavy metals (not more than 0.002%), and Nitrogen content (9.5%–11.5%, calculated on the dried basis).

Povidone-Iodine Ointment USP—Preserve in tight containers. An emulsion, solution, or suspension of Povidone-Iodine in a suitable water-soluble ointment base. Contains an amount of povidone-iodine equivalent to the labeled amount of iodine, within −15% to +20%. Meets the requirements for Identification, Minimum fill, and pH (1.5–6.5, determined in a solution [1 in 20]).

Povidone-Iodine Topical Aerosol Solution USP—Preserve in pressurized containers, and avoid exposure to excessive heat. A solution of Povidone-Iodine under nitrogen in a pressurized container. Contains an amount of povidone-iodine equivalent to the labeled amount of iodine, within −15% to +20%. Meets the requirements for Identification and pH (not more than 6.0), and for Leak testing and Pressure testing under Aerosols.

Povidone-Iodine Cleansing Solution USP—Preserve in tight containers. A solution of Povidone-Iodine with one or more suitable surface-active agents. Contains an amount of povidone-iodine equivalent to the labeled amount of iodine, within −15% to +20%. Meets the requirements for Identification, pH (1.5–6.5), and Alcohol content (if present, within ±10% of labeled amount).

Povidone-Iodine Topical Solution USP—Preserve in tight containers. A solution of Povidone-Iodine. Contains the labeled amount of iodine, within −15% to +20%. Meets the requirements for Identification, pH (1.5–6.5), and Alcohol content (within ±10% of the labeled amount).

PRALIDOXIME

Chemical name: Pralidoxime chloride—Pyridinium, 2-[(hydroxyimino)methyl]-1-methyl-, chloride.

Molecular formula: Pralidoxime chloride—$C_7H_9ClN_2O$.

Molecular weight: Pralidoxime chloride—172.61.

Description:

Pralidoxime Chloride USP—White to pale-yellow, crystalline powder. Odorless and stable in air.

Sterile Pralidoxime Chloride USP—White to pale-yellow, crystalline powder. Odorless and stable in air.

Solubility:
Pralidoxime Chloride USP—Freely soluble in water.
Sterile Pralidoxime Chloride USP—Freely soluble in water.

USP requirements:
Pralidoxime Chloride USP—Preserve in well-closed containers. Contains not less than 97.0% and not more than 102.0% of pralidoxime chloride, calculated on the dried basis. Meets the requirements for Identification, Melting range (215–225 °C, with decomposition), Loss on drying (not more than 2.0%), Residue on ignition (not more than 0.5%), Heavy metals (not more than 0.002%), and Chloride content (20.2–20.8%, calculated on the dried basis).
Sterile Pralidoxime Chloride USP—Preserve in Containers for Sterile Solids. It is Pralidoxime Chloride suitable for parenteral use. Contains the labeled amount, within ±10%. Meets the requirements for Completeness of solution, Constituted solution, Bacterial endotoxins, and pH (3.5–4.5, in a solution [1 in 20]), for Identification tests, Loss on drying, and Heavy metals under Pralidoxime Chloride, and for Sterility tests, Uniformity of dosage units, and Labeling under Injections.
Pralidoxime Chloride Tablets USP—Preserve in well-closed containers. Contain the labeled amount, within ±5%. Meet the requirements for Identification, Dissolution (55% in 60 minutes in water in Apparatus 1 at 100 rpm), and Uniformity of dosage units.

PRAMOXINE

Chemical name:
Pramoxine—4-[3-(4-Butoxyphenoxy)propyl]morpholine.
Pramoxine hydrochloride—Morpholine, 4-[3-(4-butoxyphenoxy)propyl]-, hydrochloride.

Molecular formula:
Pramoxine—$C_{17}H_{27}NO_3$.
Pramoxine hydrochloride—$C_{17}H_{27}NO_3 \cdot HCl$.

Molecular weight:
Pramoxine—293.41.
Pramoxine hydrochloride—329.87.

Description: Pramoxine Hydrochloride USP—White to practically white, crystalline powder. May have a slight aromatic odor. The pH of a solution (1 in 100) is about 4.5.

Solubility: Pramoxine Hydrochloride USP—Freely soluble in water and in alcohol; soluble in chloroform; very slightly soluble in ether.

USP requirements:
Pramoxine Hydrochloride USP—Preserve in tight containers. Contains not less than 98.0% and not more than 100.5% of pramoxine hydrochloride, calculated on the dried basis. Meets the requirements for Identification, Melting range (170–174 °C), Loss on drying (not more than 1.0%), and Residue on ignition (not more than 0.1%).
Pramoxine Hydrochloride Cream USP—Preserve in tight containers. Contains the labeled amount, within ±10%, in a suitable water-miscible base. Meets the requirements for Identification, Microbial limits, and Minimum fill.
Pramoxine Hydrochloride Aerosol Foam—Not in USP.
Pramoxine Hydrochloride Jelly USP—Preserve in tight containers, preferably in collapsible tubes. Contains the labeled amount, within ±6%. Meets the requirements for Identification and Microbial limits.
Pramoxine Hydrochloride Lotion—Not in USP.
Pramoxine Hydrochloride Ointment—Not in USP.
Pramoxine and Pramoxine Hydrochloride Suppositories—Not in USP.

PRAMOXINE AND MENTHOL

For *Pramoxine* and *Menthol*—See individual listings for chemistry information.

USP requirements: Pramoxine Hydrochloride and Menthol Gel—Not in USP.

PRAVASTATIN

Chemical name: Pravastatin sodium—1-Naphthalene-heptanoic acid, 1,2,6,7,8,8a-hexahydro-beta,delta,6-trihydroxy-2-methyl-8-(2-methyl-1-oxobutoxy)-, monosodium salt, [1*S*-[1 alpha(beta*S**,delta*S**),2 alpha,6 alpha,8 beta(*R**),8a alpha]]-.

Molecular formula: Pravastatin sodium—$C_{23}H_{35}NaO_7$.

Molecular weight: Pravastatin sodium—446.52.

Description: Pravastatin sodium—Odorless, white to off-white, fine or crystalline powder.

Solubility: Pravastatin sodium—Soluble in methanol and in water; slightly soluble in isopropanol; practically insoluble in acetone, in acetonitrile, in chloroform, and in ether.

Other characteristics: Pravastatin sodium—Partition coefficient (octanol/water) 0.59 at pH 7.0.

USP requirements: Pravastatin Sodium Tablets—Not in USP.

PRAZEPAM

Chemical name: 2*H*-1,4-Benzodiazepin-2-one, 7-chloro-1-(cyclopropylmethyl)-1,3-dihydro-5-phenyl-.

Molecular formula: $C_{19}H_{17}ClN_2O$.

Molecular weight: 324.81.

Description: Prazepam USP—White to off-white crystalline powder.

Solubility: Prazepam USP—Freely soluble in acetone; soluble in dilute mineral acids, in alcohol, and in chloroform.

USP requirements:
Prazepam USP—Preserve in tight, light-resistant containers. Contains not less than 98.5% and not more than 101.0% of prazepam, calculated on the dried basis. Meets the requirements for Identification, Melting range (143–148 °C, the range between beginning and end of melting not more than 3 °C), Loss on drying (not more than 0.5%), Residue on ignition (not more than 0.1%), Heavy metals (not more than 0.002%), Related compounds, and Organic volatile impurities.
Prazepam Capsules USP—Preserve in tight, light-resistant containers. Contain the labeled amount, within ±10%. Meet the requirements for Identification, Dissolution (80% in 60 minutes in 0.1 *N* hydrochloric acid in Apparatus 1 at 50 rpm), and Uniformity of dosage units.
Prazepam Tablets USP—Preserve in tight, light-resistant containers. Contain the labeled amount, within ±10%. Meet the requirements for Identification, Dissolution (80% in 60 minutes in 0.1 *N* hydrochloric acid in Apparatus 1 at 50 rpm), and Uniformity of dosage units.

PRAZIQUANTEL

Chemical group: Pyrazinoisoquinoline derivative.

Chemical name: 4*H*-Pyrazino[2,1-*a*]isoquinolin-4-one, 2-(cyclohexylcarbonyl)-1,2,3,6,7,11b-hexahydro-.

Molecular formula: $C_{19}H_{24}N_2O_2$.

Molecular weight: 312.41.

Description: Praziquantel USP—White or practically white, crystalline powder; odorless or having a faint characteristic odor.

Solubility: Praziquantel USP—Very slightly soluble in water; freely soluble in alcohol and in chloroform.

Other characteristics: Hygroscopic.

USP requirements:

Praziquantel USP—Preserve in well-closed, light-resistant containers. Contains not less than 98.5% and not more than 101.0% of praziquantel, calculated on the dried basis. Meets the requirements for Identification, Melting range (136–142 °C), Loss on drying (not more than 0.5%), Residue on ignition (not more than 0.1%), Heavy metals (not more than 0.002%), Related compounds, and Phosphate.

Praziquantel Tablets USP—Preserve in tight containers. Contain the labeled amount, within ±10%. Meet the requirements for Identification, Dissolution (75% in 60 minutes in 0.1 *N* hydrochloric acid containing 2.0 mg of sodium lauryl sulfate per mL in Apparatus 2 at 50 rpm), and Uniformity of dosage units.

PRAZOSIN

Chemical name: Prazosin hydrochloride—Piperazine, 1-(4-amino-6,7-dimethoxy-2-quinazolinyl)-4-(2-furanylcarbonyl)-, monohydrochloride.

Molecular formula: Prazosin hydrochloride—$C_{19}H_{21}N_5O_4 \cdot HCl$.

Molecular weight: Prazosin hydrochloride—419.87.

Description: Prazosin Hydrochloride USP—White to tan powder.

pKa: 6.5 in 1:1 water-ethanol solution.

Solubility: Prazosin Hydrochloride USP—Slightly soluble in water, in methanol, in dimethylformamide, and in dimethylacetamide; very slightly soluble in alcohol; practically insoluble in chloroform and in acetone.

USP requirements:

Prazosin Hydrochloride USP—Preserve in tight, light-resistant containers. Label it to indicate whether it is anhydrous or is the polyhydrate. Contains not less than 97.0% and not more than 103.0% of prazosin hydrochloride, calculated on the anhydrous basis. Meets the requirements for Identification, Water (not more than 2.0% for the anhydrous form and 8.0–15.0% for the polyhydrate form), Residue on ignition (not more than 0.4%), Heavy metals (not more than 0.005%), Iron, Nickel, and Ordinary impurities.

Caution: Care should be taken to prevent inhaling particles of Prazosin Hydrochloride and to prevent its contacting any part of the body.

Prazosin Hydrochloride Capsules USP—Preserve in well-closed, light-resistant containers. Contain an amount of prazosin hydrochloride equivalent to the labeled amount of prazosin, within ±10%. Meet the requirements for Identification, Dissolution (75% in 60 minutes in 0.1 *N* hydrochloric acid containing 3% sodium lauryl sulfate in Apparatus 1 at 100 rpm), and Uniformity of dosage units.

Caution: Care should be taken to prevent inhaling particles of Prazosin Hydrochloride and to prevent its contacting any part of the body.

Prazosin Hydrochloride Tablets—Not in USP.

PRAZOSIN AND POLYTHIAZIDE

For *Prazosin* and *Polythiazide*—See individual listings for chemistry information.

USP requirements: Prazosin Hydrochloride and Polythiazide Capsules—Not in USP.

PREDNISOLONE

Chemical name:

Prednisolone—Pregna-1,4-diene-3,20-dione, 11,17,21-trihydroxy-, (11 beta)-.
Prednisolone acetate—Pregna-1,4-diene-3,20-dione, 21-(acetyloxy)-11,17-dihydroxy-, (11 beta)-.
Prednisolone hemisuccinate—Pregna-1,4-diene-3,20-dione, 21-(3-carboxy-1-oxopropoxy)-11,17-dihydroxy-, (11 beta)-.
Prednisolone sodium phosphate—Pregna-1,4-diene-3,20-dione, 11,17-dihydroxy-21-(phosphonooxy)-, disodium salt, (11 beta)-.
Prednisolone sodium succinate—Pregna-1,4-diene-3,20-dione, 21-(3-carboxyl-1-oxopropoxy)-11,17-dihydroxy-, monosodium salt, (11 beta)-.
Prednisolone tebutate—Pregna-1,4-diene-3,20-dione, 11,17-dihydroxy-21-[(3,3-dimethyl-1-oxobutyl)oxy]-, (11 beta)-.

Molecular formula:

Prednisolone—$C_{21}H_{28}O_5$.
Prednisolone acetate—$C_{23}H_{30}O_6$.
Prednisolone hemisuccinate—$C_{25}H_{32}O_8$.
Prednisolone sodium phosphate—$C_{21}H_{27}Na_2O_8P$.
Prednisolone sodium succinate—$C_{25}H_{31}NaO_8$.
Prednisolone tebutate—$C_{27}H_{38}O_6$.

Molecular weight:

Prednisolone—360.45.
Prednisolone acetate—402.49.
Prednisolone hemisuccinate—460.52.
Prednisolone sodium phosphate—484.39.
Prednisolone sodium succinate—482.51.
Prednisolone tebutate—458.60.

Description:

Prednisolone USP—White to practically white, odorless, crystalline powder. Melts at about 235 °C, with some decomposition.

Prednisolone Acetate USP—White to practically white, odorless, crystalline powder. Melts at about 235 °C, with some decomposition.

Prednisolone Hemisuccinate USP—Fine, creamy white powder with friable lumps; practically odorless. Melts at about 205 °C, with decomposition.

Prednisolone Sodium Phosphate USP—White or slightly yellow, friable granules or powder. Is odorless or has a slight odor. Is slightly hygroscopic.

Prednisolone Sodium Succinate for Injection USP—Creamy white powder with friable lumps, having a slight odor.

Prednisolone Tebutate USP—White to slightly yellow, free-flowing powder, which may show some soft lumps. Is odorless or has not more than a moderate, characteristic odor. Is hygroscopic.

Solubility:

Prednisolone USP—Very slightly soluble in water; soluble in methanol and in dioxane; sparingly soluble in acetone and in alcohol; slightly soluble in chloroform.

Prednisolone Acetate USP—Practically insoluble in water; slightly soluble in acetone, in alcohol, and in chloroform.

Prednisolone Hemisuccinate USP—Very slightly soluble in water; freely soluble in alcohol; soluble in acetone.

Prednisolone Sodium Phosphate USP—Freely soluble in water; soluble in methanol; slightly soluble in alcohol and in chloroform; very slightly soluble in acetone and in dioxane.

Prednisolone Tebutate USP—Very slightly soluble in water; freely soluble in chloroform and in dioxane; soluble in acetone; sparingly soluble in alcohol and in methanol.

USP requirements:

Prednisolone USP—Preserve in well-closed containers. It is anhydrous or contains one and one-half molecules of water of hydration. Label it to indicate whether it is anhydrous or hydrous. Contains not less than 97.0% and not more than 102.0% of prednisolone, calculated on the dried basis. Meets the requirements for Identification, Specific rotation (+97° to +103°, calculated on the dried basis), Loss on drying (not more than 1.0% for anhydrous Prednisolone and not more than 7.0% for hydrous Prednisolone), Residue on ignition (negligible, from 100 mg), Selenium (not more than 0.003%), and Ordinary impurities.

Prednisolone Cream USP—Preserve in collapsible tubes or in tight containers. Contains the labeled amount, within ±10%, in a suitable cream base. Meets the requirements for Identification and Minimum fill.

Prednisolone Syrup USP—Preserve in tight, light-resistant containers. Contains the labeled amount, within ±10%. Prednisolone Syrup may contain alcohol. Meets the requirements for Identification, pH (3.0–4.5), and Alcohol content (if present, within ±10% of labeled amount).

Prednisolone Tablets USP—Preserve in well-closed containers. Contain the labeled amount, within ±10%. Meet the requirements for Identification, Dissolution (70% in 30 minutes in water in Apparatus 2 at 50 rpm), and Uniformity of dosage units.

Prednisolone Acetate USP—Preserve in well-closed containers. Contains not less than 97.0% and not more than 102.0% of prednisolone acetate, calculated on the dried basis. Meets the requirements for Identification, Specific rotation (+112° to +119°, calculated on the dried basis), and Loss on drying (not more than 1.0%).

Prednisolone Acetate Ophthalmic Suspension USP—Preserve in tight containers. A sterile, aqueous suspension of prednisolone acetate containing a suitable antimicrobial preservative. Contains the labeled amount, within −10% to +15%. Meets the requirements for Identification, Sterility, and pH (5.0–6.0).

Sterile Prednisolone Acetate Suspension USP—Preserve in single-dose or in multiple-dose containers, preferably of Type I glass. A sterile suspension of Prednisolone Acetate in a suitable aqueous medium. Contains the labeled amount, within ±10%. Meets the requirements for Identification, pH (5.0–7.5), and Injections.

Sterile Prednisolone Acetate and Prednisolone Sodium Phosphate Suspension—Not in USP.

Prednisolone Hemisuccinate USP—Preserve in tight containers. Contains not less than 98.0% and not more than 102.0% of prednisolone hemisuccinate, calculated on the dried basis. Meets the requirements for Identification, Specific rotation (+99° to +104°, calculated on the dried basis), Loss on drying (not more than 0.5%), and Residue on ignition (negligible, from 100 mg).

Prednisolone Sodium Phosphate USP—Preserve in tight containers. Contains not less than 96.0% and not more than 102.0% of prednisolone sodium phosphate, calculated on the dried basis. Meets the requirements for Identification, Specific rotation (+95° to +102°, calculated on the dried basis), pH (7.5–10.5, in a solution [1 in 100]), Water (not more than 6.5%), Phosphate ions (not more than 1.0%), Free prednisolone (not more than 1.0%), and Selenium (not more than 0.003%).

Prednisolone Sodium Phosphate Injection USP—Preserve in single-dose or in multiple-dose containers, preferably of Type I glass, protected from light. A sterile solution of Prednisolone Sodium Phosphate in Water for Injection. Contains an amount of prednisolone sodium phosphate equivalent to the labeled amount of prednisolone phosphate, present as the disodium salt, within ±10%. Meets the requirements for Identification, Bacterial endotoxins, pH (7.0–8.0), Particulate matter, and Injections.

Prednisolone Sodium Phosphate Ophthalmic Solution USP—Preserve in tight, light-resistant containers. A sterile solution of Prednisolone Sodium Phosphate in a buffered, aqueous medium. Contains an amount of prednisolone sodium phosphate equivalent to the labeled amount of prednisolone phosphate, present as the disodium salt, within −10% to +15%. Meets the requirements for Identification, Sterility, and pH (6.2–8.2).

Prednisolone Sodium Phosphate Oral Solution—Not in USP.

Prednisolone Sodium Succinate for Injection USP—Preserve in Containers for Sterile Solids. It is sterile prednisolone sodium succinate prepared from Prednisolone Hemisuccinate with the aid of Sodium Hydroxide or Sodium Carbonate. Contains an amount of prednisolone sodium succinate equivalent to the labeled amount of prednisolone, within ±10%. Contains suitable buffers. Meets the requirements for Constituted solution, Identification, Bacterial endotoxins, pH (6.7–8.0, determined in the solution constituted as directed in the labeling), Loss on drying (not more than 2.0%), and Particulate matter, and for Sterility tests, Uniformity of dosage units, and Labeling under Injections.

Prednisolone Tebutate USP—Preserve in tight containers sealed under sterile nitrogen, in a cold place. Contains not less than 97.0% and not more than 103.0% of prednisolone tebutate, calculated on the dried basis. Meets the requirements for Identification, Specific rotation (+100° to +115°, calculated on the dried basis), Loss on drying (not more than 5.0%), Residue on ignition (not more than 0.1%), and Selenium (not more than 0.003%).

Sterile Prednisolone Tebutate Suspension USP—Preserve in single-dose or in multiple-dose containers, preferably of Type I glass. A sterile suspension of Prednisolone Tebutate in a suitable aqueous medium. Contains the labeled amount, within ±10%. Meets the requirements for Identification, Bacterial endotoxins, pH (6.0–8.0), and Injections.

PREDNISONE

Chemical name: Pregna-1,4-diene-3,11,20-trione, 17,21-dihydroxy-.

Molecular formula: $C_{21}H_{26}O_5$.

Molecular weight: 358.43.

Description: Prednisone USP—White to practically white, odorless, crystalline powder. Melts at about 230 °C, with some decomposition.

Solubility: Prednisone USP—Very slightly soluble in water; slightly soluble in alcohol, in chloroform, in dioxane, and in methanol.

USP requirements:

Prednisone USP—Preserve in well-closed containers. Contains not less than 97.0% and not more than 102.0% of prednisone, calculated on the dried basis. Meets the requirements for Identification, Specific rotation (+167°

to +175°, calculated on the dried basis), Loss on drying (not more than 1.0%), Residue on ignition (negligible, from 100 mg), and Ordinary impurities.

Prednisone Oral Solution USP—Preserve in tight containers. Contains the labeled amount, within ±10%. Meets the requirements for Identification, pH (2.6–4.0), and Alcohol content (4.0–6.0%).

Prednisone Syrup USP—Preserve in tight containers. Contains the labeled amount, within ±10%. Meets the requirements for Identification, Specific gravity (1.220–1.280 at 25 °C), pH (3.0–4.5), and Alcohol content (2.0–5.0%).

Prednisone Tablets USP—Preserve in well-closed containers. Contain the labeled amount, within ±10%. Meet the requirements for Identification, Dissolution (80% in 30 minutes in water in Apparatus 2 at 50 rpm), and Uniformity of dosage units.

PRILOCAINE

Chemical group: Amide.

Chemical name: Prilocaine hydrochloride—Propanamide, *N*-(2-methylphenyl)-2-(propylamino)-, monohydrochloride.

Molecular formula: Prilocaine hydrochloride—$C_{13}H_{20}N_2O \cdot HCl$.

Molecular weight: Prilocaine hydrochloride—256.78.

Description: Prilocaine Hydrochloride USP—White, odorless, crystalline powder.

pKa: Prilocaine hydrochloride—7.89.

Solubility: Prilocaine Hydrochloride USP—Freely soluble in water and in alcohol; slightly soluble in chloroform; very slightly soluble in acetone; practically insoluble in ether.

USP requirements:

Prilocaine Hydrochloride USP—Preserve in well-closed containers. Contains not less than 99.0% and not more than 101.0% of prilocaine hydrochloride, calculated on the dried basis. Meets the requirements for Identification, Melting range (166–169 °C), Loss on drying (not more than 0.3%), Residue on ignition (not more than 0.1%), and Heavy metals (not more than 0.002%).

Prilocaine Hydrochloride Injection USP—Preserve in single-dose or in multiple-dose containers, preferably of Type I glass. A sterile solution of Prilocaine Hydrochloride in Water for Injection. Contains the labeled amount, ±5%. Meets the requirements for Identification, Bacterial endotoxins, pH (6.0–7.0), and Injections.

PRILOCAINE AND EPINEPHRINE

For *Prilocaine* and *Epinephrine*—See individual listings for chemistry information.

USP requirements: Prilocaine and Epinephrine Injection USP—Preserve in single-dose or in multiple-dose, light-resistant containers, preferably of Type I glass. A sterile solution prepared from Prilocaine Hydrochloride and Epinephrine with the aid of Hydrochloric Acid in Water for Injection, or a sterile solution of Prilocaine Hydrochloride and Epinephrine Bitartrate in Water for Injection. The content of epinephrine does not exceed 0.002% (1 in 50,000). The label indicates that the Injection is not to be used if its color is pinkish or darker than slightly yellow or if it contains a precipitate. Contains the labeled amount of prilocaine hydrochloride, within ±5%, and the labeled amount of epinephrine, within −10% to +15%. Meets the requirements for Color and clarity, Identification, Bacterial endotoxins, pH (3.3–5.5), and Injections.

PRIMAQUINE

Chemical group: 8-Aminoquinolines.

Chemical name: Primaquine phosphate—1,4-Pentanediamine, N^4-(6-methoxy-8-quinolinyl)-, phosphate (1:2).

Molecular formula: Primaquine phosphate—$C_{15}H_{21}N_3O \cdot 2H_3PO_4$.

Molecular weight: Primaquine phosphate—455.34.

Description: Primaquine Phosphate USP—Orange-red, crystalline powder. Is odorless. Its solutions are acid to litmus. Melts at about 200 °C.

Solubility: Primaquine Phosphate USP—Soluble in water; insoluble in chloroform and in ether.

USP requirements:

Primaquine Phosphate USP—Preserve in well-closed, light-resistant containers. Contains not less than 98.0% and not more than 102.0% of primaquine phosphate, calculated on the dried basis. Meets the requirements for Identification, Loss on drying (not more than 1.0%), and Organic volatile impurities.

Primaquine Phosphate Tablets USP—Preserve in well-closed, light-resistant containers. Contain the labeled amount, within ±7%. Meet the requirements for Identification, Dissolution (75% in 60 minutes in simulated gastric fluid TS in Apparatus 2 at 100 rpm), and Uniformity of dosage units.

PRIMIDONE

Chemical group: A congener of phenobarbital in which the carbonyl oxygen of the urea moiety is replaced by two hydrogen atoms.

Chemical name: 4,6(1*H*,5*H*)-Pyrimidinedione, 5-ethyldihydro-5-phenyl-.

Molecular formula: $C_{12}H_{14}N_2O_2$.

Molecular weight: 218.26.

Description: Primidone USP—White, crystalline powder. Is odorless.

Solubility: Primidone USP—Very slightly soluble in water and in most organic solvents; slightly soluble in alcohol.

Other characteristics: Highly stable compound; no acidic properties, in contrast to its barbiturate analog.

USP requirements:

Primidone USP—Preserve in well-closed containers. Contains not less than 98.0% and not more than 102.0% of primidone, calculated on the dried basis. Meets the requirements for Identification, Melting range (279–284 °C), Loss on drying (not more than 0.5%), Residue on ignition (not more than 0.2%), Ordinary impurities, and Organic volatile impurities.

Primidone Oral Suspension USP—Preserve in tight, light-resistant containers. A suspension of Primidone in a suitable aqueous vehicle. Contains, in each 100 mL, not less than 4.5 grams and not more than 5.5 grams of primidone. Meets the requirements for Identification and pH (5.5–8.5).

Primidone Tablets USP—Preserve in well-closed containers. Tablets intended solely for veterinary use are so labeled. Contain the labeled amount, within ±5%. Meet the requirements for Identification, Disintegration (for Tablets labeled solely for veterinary use 30 minutes, disks being used), Dissolution ([Note: Tablets labeled solely for veterinary use are exempt from this requirement.] 75% in

60 minutes in water in Apparatus 2 at 50 rpm), and Uniformity of dosage units.

PROBENECID

Chemical name: Benzoic acid, 4-[(dipropylamino)sulfonyl]-.

Molecular formula: $C_{13}H_{19}NO_4S$.

Molecular weight: 285.36.

Description: Probenecid USP—White or practically white, fine, crystalline powder. Is practically odorless.

pKa: 3.4.

Solubility: Probenecid USP—Practically insoluble in water and in dilute acids; soluble in dilute alkali, in chloroform, in alcohol, and in acetone.

USP requirements:

Probenecid USP—Preserve in well-closed containers. Contains not less than 98.0% and not more than 101.0% of probenecid, calculated on the dried basis. Meets the requirements for Identification, Melting range (198–200 °C), Acidity, Loss on drying (not more than 0.5%), Residue on ignition (not more than 0.1%), Selenium (not more than 0.003%), Heavy metals (not more than 0.002%), Chromatographic purity, and Organic volatile impurities.

Probenecid Tablets USP—Preserve in well-closed containers. Contain the labeled amount, within ±7%. Meet the requirements for Identification, Dissolution (80% in 30 minutes in simulated intestinal fluid TS [pH 7.5 ±0.1], prepared without pancreatin, in Apparatus 2 at 50 rpm), and Uniformity of dosage units.

PROBENECID AND COLCHICINE

For *Probenecid* and *Colchicine*—See individual listings for chemistry information.

USP requirements: Probenecid and Colchicine Tablets USP—Preserve in well-closed, light-resistant containers. Contain the labeled amount of colchicine, within −10% to +15%, and the labeled amount of probenecid, within ±10%. Meet the requirements for Identification, Dissolution (80% of each active ingredient in 30 minutes in 0.05 *M* phosphate buffer [pH 7.5] in Apparatus 2 at 50 rpm), and Uniformity of dosage units.

PROBUCOL

Chemical name: Phenol, 4,4′-[(1-methylethylidene)bis(thio)]-bis[2,6-bis(1,1-dimethylethyl)-.

Molecular formula: $C_{31}H_{48}O_2S_2$.

Molecular weight: 516.84.

Description: Probucol USP—White to off-white, crystalline powder.

Solubility: Probucol USP—Insoluble in water; freely soluble in chloroform and in *n*-propyl alcohol; soluble in alcohol and in solvent hexane.

USP requirements:

Probucol USP—Preserve in well-closed, light-resistant containers. Contains not less than 98.0% and not more than 102.0% of probucol, calculated on the dried basis. Meets the requirements for Identification, Melting range (124–127 °C), Loss on drying (not more than 1.0%), Residue on ignition (not more than 0.1%), Heavy metals (not more than 0.002%), Related compounds, and Organic volatile impurities.

Probucol Tablets USP—Preserve in well-closed, light-resistant containers. Contain the labeled amount, within ±10%. Meet the requirements for Identification and Uniformity of dosage units.

PROCAINAMIDE

Chemical name: Procainamide hydrochloride—Benzamide, 4-amino-*N*-[2-(diethylamino)ethyl]-, monohydrochloride.

Molecular formula: Procainamide hydrochloride—$C_{13}H_{21}N_3O \cdot HCl$.

Molecular weight: Procainamide hydrochloride—271.79.

Description:

Procainamide Hydrochloride USP—White to tan, crystalline powder. Is odorless. Its solution (1 in 10) has a pH of 5.0–6.5.

Procainamide Hydrochloride Injection USP—Colorless, or having not more than a slight yellow color.

pKa: 9.23.

Solubility: Procainamide Hydrochloride USP—Very soluble in water; soluble in alcohol; slightly soluble in chloroform; very slightly soluble in ether.

USP requirements:

Procainamide Hydrochloride USP—Preserve in tight containers. Contains not less than 98.0% and not more than 102.0% of procainamide hydrochloride, calculated on the dried basis. Meets the requirements for Identification, Melting range (165–169 °C), Loss on drying (not more than 0.3%), Residue on ignition (not more than 0.1%), Heavy metals (not more than 0.002%), Free *p*-aminobenzoic acid, Ordinary impurities, and Organic volatile impurities.

Procainamide Hydrochloride Capsules USP—Preserve in tight containers. Contain the labeled amount, within ±5%. Meet the requirements for Identification, Dissolution (75% in 90 minutes in 0.1 *N* hydrochloric acid in Apparatus 2 at 50 rpm), and Uniformity of dosage units.

Procainamide Hydrochloride Injection USP—Preserve in single-dose or in multiple-dose containers, preferably of Type I glass. A sterile solution of Procainamide Hydrochloride in Water for Injection. Label it to indicate that the Injection is not to be used if it is darker than slightly yellow, or is discolored in any other way. Contains the labeled amount, within ±5%. Meets the requirements for Identification, Bacterial endotoxins, pH (4.0–6.0), Particulate matter, and Injections.

Procainamide Hydrochloride Tablets USP—Preserve in tight containers. Contain the labeled amount, within ±5%. Meet the requirements for Identification, Dissolution (80% in 75 minutes in 0.1 *N* hydrochloric acid in Apparatus 1 at 100 rpm), and Uniformity of dosage units.

Procainamide Hydrochloride Extended-release Tablets USP—Preserve in tight containers. The labeling indicates the Drug Release Test with which the product complies. Contain the labeled amount, within ±7%. Meet the requirements for Identification, Drug release, and Uniformity of dosage units.

PROCAINE

Chemical group: Ester.

Chemical name: Procaine hydrochloride—Benzoic acid, 4-amino-, 2-(diethylamino)ethyl ester, monohydrochloride.

Molecular formula: Procaine hydrochloride—$C_{13}H_{20}N_2O_2 \cdot HCl$.

Molecular weight: Procaine hydrochloride—272.77.

Description:
Procaine Hydrochloride USP—Small, white crystals or white, crystalline powder. Is odorless.
Procaine Hydrochloride Injection USP—Clear, colorless liquid.
Sterile Procaine Hydrochloride USP—Small, white crystals or white, crystalline powder. Is odorless.

pKa: Procaine hydrochloride—8.7.

Solubility:
Procaine Hydrochloride USP—Freely soluble in water; soluble in alcohol; slightly soluble in chloroform; practically insoluble in ether.
Sterile Procaine Hydrochloride USP—Freely soluble in water; soluble in alcohol; slightly soluble in chloroform; practically insoluble in ether.

USP requirements:
Procaine Hydrochloride USP—Preserve in well-closed containers. Contains not less than 99.0% and not more than 101.0% of procaine hydrochloride, calculated on the dried basis. Meets the requirements for Identification, Melting range (153–158 °C), Acidity, Loss on drying (not more than 1.0%), Residue on ignition (not more than 0.15%), Heavy metals (not more than 0.002%), and Chromatographic purity.
Procaine Hydrochloride Injection USP—Preserve in single-dose or in multiple-dose containers, preferably of Type I or Type II glass. The Injection may be packaged in 100-mL multiple-dose containers. A sterile solution of Procaine Hydrochloride in Water for Injection. Contains the labeled amount, within ±5%. Meets the requirements for Identification, Bacterial endotoxins, pH (3.0–5.5), Particulate matter, and Injections.
Sterile Procaine Hydrochloride USP—Preserve in Containers for Sterile Solids. Each package contains not more than 1 gram, and the container may be of such size as to permit solution within the container. It is Procaine Hydrochloride suitable for parenteral use. Meets the requirements for Completeness of solution, Constituted solution, Bacterial endotoxins, and Particulate matter, for Identification tests, Melting range, Acidity, and Loss on drying under Procaine Hydrochloride, and for Sterility tests, Uniformity of dosage units, and Labeling under Injections.

PROCAINE AND EPINEPHRINE

For *Procaine* and *Epinephrine*—See individual listings for chemistry information.

USP requirements: Procaine Hydrochloride and Epinephrine Injection USP—Preserve in single-dose or in multiple-dose, light-resistant containers, preferably of Type I or Type II glass. A sterile solution of Procaine Hydrochloride and epinephrine hydrochloride in Water for Injection. The content of epinephrine does not exceed 0.002% (1 in 50,000). The label indicates that the Injection is not to be used if its color is pinkish or darker than slightly yellow or if it contains a precipitate. Contains the labeled amounts of procaine hydrochloride, within ±5%, and epinephrine, within −10% to +15%. Meets the requirements for Color and clarity, Identification, Bacterial endotoxins, pH (3.0–5.5), Content of epinephrine, and Injections.

PROCAINE AND PHENYLEPHRINE

For *Procaine* and *Phenylephrine*—See individual listings for chemistry information.

USP requirements: Procaine and Phenylephrine Hydrochlorides Injection USP—Preserve in single-dose or in multiple-dose containers, preferably of Type I glass. A sterile solution of Procaine Hydrochloride and Phenylephrine Hydrochloride in Water for Injection. Contains the labeled amounts of procaine hydrochloride, within ±5%, and phenylephrine hydrochloride, within ±10%. Meets the requirements for Identification, Bacterial endotoxins, pH (3.0–5.5), and Injections.

PROCAINE, TETRACAINE, AND LEVONORDEFRIN

For *Procaine, Tetracaine,* and *Levonordefrin*—See individual listings for chemistry information.

USP requirements: Procaine and Tetracaine Hydrochlorides and Levonordefrin Injection USP—Preserve in single-dose or in multiple-dose containers, preferably of Type I glass. A sterile solution of Procaine Hydrochloride, Tetracaine Hydrochloride, and Levonordefrin in Water for Injection. The label indicates that the Injection is not to be used if its color is pinkish or darker than slightly yellow or if it contains a precipitate. Contains the labeled amounts of procaine hydrochloride and tetracaine hydrochloride, within ±5%, and levonordefrin, within ±10%. Meets the requirements for Color and clarity, Identification, Bacterial endotoxins, pH (3.5–5.0), and Injections.

PROCARBAZINE

Chemical name: Procarbazine hydrochloride—Benzamide, *N*-(1-methylethyl)-4-[(2-methylhydrazino)methyl]-, monohydrochloride.

Molecular formula: Procarbazine hydrochloride—$C_{12}H_{19}N_3O \cdot HCl$.

Molecular weight: Procarbazine hydrochloride—257.76.

Description: Procarbazine hydrochloride—White to pale yellow, crystalline powder.

Solubility: Procarbazine hydrochloride—Soluble but unstable in water or in aqueous solutions.

USP requirements:
Procarbazine Hydrochloride USP—Preserve in tight, light-resistant containers. Contains not less than 98.5% and not more than 100.5% of procarbazine hydrochloride. Meets the requirements for Identification, Residue on ignition (not more than 0.1%), Heavy metals (not more than 0.002%), and Organic volatile impurities.
Caution: Handle Procarbazine Hydrochloride with exceptional care, since it is a highly potent agent.
Procarbazine Hydrochloride Capsules USP—Preserve in tight, light-resistant containers. Contain the labeled amount, within ±10%. Meet the requirements for Identification, Dissolution (75% in 45 minutes in water in Apparatus 2 at 50 rpm), and Uniformity of dosage units.

PROCATEROL

Chemical name: Procaterol hydrochloride hemihydrate—8-hydroxy-5-[1-hydroxy-2[(1-methylethyl)amino]butyl]-2-(1*H*)quinolone, monohydrochloride, hemihydrate, racemic mixture of (±) (*R**,*S**) isomers.

Molecular formula: Procaterol hydrochloride hemihydrate—$C_{16}H_{22}N_2O_3 \cdot HCl \cdot \frac{1}{2}H_2O$.

Molecular weight: Procaterol hydrochloride hemihydrate—335.83.

Description: Procaterol hydrochloride hemihydrate—White to off-white powder, unstable to light.

Solubility: Procaterol hydrochloride hemihydrate—Soluble in water and in methanol; slightly soluble in ethanol; practically insoluble in acetone, in ether, in ethyl acetate, and in chloroform.

USP requirements: Procaterol Hydrochloride Hemihydrate Inhalation Aerosol—Not in USP.

PROCHLORPERAZINE

Chemical group: Phenothiazine derivative of piperazine group.

Chemical name:
Prochlorperazine—10*H*-Phenothiazine, 2-chloro-10-[3-(4-methyl-1-piperazinyl)propyl]-.
Prochlorperazine edisylate—10*H*-Phenothiazine, 2-chloro-10-[3-(4-methyl-1-piperazinyl)propyl]-, 1,2-ethanedisulfonate (1:1).
Prochlorperazine maleate—10*H*-Phenothiazine, 2-chloro-10-[3-(4-methyl-1-piperazinyl)propyl]-, (*Z*)-2-butenedioate (1:2).
Prochlorperazine mesylate—10*H*-Phenothiazine, 2-chloro-10-[3-(4-methyl-1-piperazinyl)propyl]-, dimethanesulphonate.

Molecular formula:
Prochlorperazine—$C_{20}H_{24}ClN_3S$.
Prochlorperazine edisylate—$C_{20}H_{24}ClN_3S \cdot C_2H_6O_6S_2$.
Prochlorperazine maleate—$C_{20}H_{24}ClN_3S \cdot 2C_4H_4O_4$.
Prochlorperazine mesylate—$C_{20}H_{24}ClN_3S \cdot 2CH_3SO_3H$.

Molecular weight:
Prochlorperazine—373.94.
Prochlorperazine edisylate—564.13.
Prochlorperazine maleate—606.09.
Prochlorperazine mesylate—566.1.

Description:
Prochlorperazine USP—Clear, pale yellow, viscous liquid. Is sensitive to light.
Prochlorperazine Edisylate USP—White to very light yellow, odorless, crystalline powder. Its solutions are acid to litmus.
Prochlorperazine Maleate USP—White or pale yellow, practically odorless, crystalline powder. Its saturated solution is acid to litmus.
Prochlorperazine mesylate—White or almost white, odorless or almost odorless, powder.

Solubility:
Prochlorperazine USP—Very slightly soluble in water; freely soluble in alcohol, in chloroform, and in ether.
Prochlorperazine Edisylate USP—Freely soluble in water; very slightly soluble in alcohol; insoluble in ether and in chloroform.
Prochlorperazine Maleate USP—Practically insoluble in water and in alcohol; slightly soluble in warm chloroform.
Prochlorperazine mesylate—Soluble 1 in less than 0.5 of water and 1 in 40 of alcohol; slightly soluble in chloroform; practically insoluble in ether.

USP requirements:
Prochlorperazine USP—Preserve in tight, light-resistant containers. Contains not less than 98.0% and not more than 101.0% of prochlorperazine. Meets the requirements for Identification, Residue on ignition (not more than 0.1%), and Ordinary impurities.
Prochlorperazine Suppositories USP—Preserve in tight containers at a temperature below 37 °C. Do not expose the unwrapped Suppositories to sunlight. Contain the labeled amount, within ±10%. Meet the requirement for Identification.
Prochlorperazine Edisylate USP—Preserve in tight, light-resistant containers. Contains not less than 98.0% and not more than 101.5% of prochlorperazine edisylate, calculated on the dried basis. Meets the requirements for Identification, Loss on drying (not more than 0.5%), Residue on ignition (not more than 0.1%), Selenium (not more than 0.003%), Ordinary impurities, and Organic volatile impurities.
Prochlorperazine Edisylate Injection USP—Preserve in single-dose or in multiple-dose containers, preferably of Type I glass, protected from light. A sterile solution of Prochlorperazine Edisylate in Water for Injection. Contains an amount of prochlorperazine edisylate equivalent to the labeled amount of prochlorperazine, within ±10%. Meets the requirements for Identification, Bacterial endotoxins, pH (4.2–6.2), and Injections.
Prochlorperazine Edisylate Oral Solution USP—Preserve in tight, light-resistant containers. Label it to indicate that it is to be diluted to appropriate strength with water or other suitable fluid prior to administration. Contains an amount of prochlorperazine edisylate equivalent to the labeled amount of prochlorperazine, within ±8%. Meets the requirement for Identification.
Prochlorperazine Edisylate Syrup USP—Preserve in tight, light-resistant containers. Contains, in each 100 mL, an amount of prochlorperazine edisylate equivalent to not less than 92.0 mg and not more than 108.0 mg of prochlorperazine. Meets the requirement for Identification.
Prochlorperazine Maleate USP—Preserve in tight, light-resistant containers. Contains not less than 98.0% and not more than 101.5% of prochlorperazine maleate, calculated on the dried basis. Meets the requirements for Identification, Loss on drying (not more than 0.5%), Residue on ignition (not more than 0.1%), Ordinary impurities, and Organic volatile impurities.
Prochlorperazine Maleate Extended-release Capsules—Not in USP.
Prochlorperazine Maleate Tablets USP—Preserve in well-closed containers, protected from light. Contain an amount of prochlorperazine maleate equivalent to the labeled amount of prochlorperazine, within ±5%. Meet the requirements for Identification, Dissolution (75% in 60 minutes in 0.1 *N* hydrochloric acid in Apparatus 2 at 75 rpm), and Uniformity of dosage units.
Prochlorperazine Mesylate Injection—Not in USP.
Prochlorperazine Mesylate Syrup—Not in USP.

PROCYCLIDINE

Chemical group: Synthetic tertiary amine.

Chemical name: Procyclidine hydrochloride—1-Pyrrolidinepropanol, alpha-cyclohexyl-alpha-phenyl-, hydrochloride.

Molecular formula: Procyclidine hydrochloride—$C_{19}H_{29}NO \cdot HCl$.

Molecular weight: Procyclidine hydrochloride—323.91.

Description: Procyclidine Hydrochloride USP—White, crystalline powder, having a moderate, characteristic odor. Melts at about 225 °C, with decomposition.

Solubility: Procyclidine Hydrochloride USP—Soluble in water and in alcohol; insoluble in ether and in acetone.

USP requirements:
Procyclidine Hydrochloride USP—Preserve in tight, light-resistant containers, and store in a dry place. Contains not less than 99.0% and not more than 101.0% of procyclidine hydrochloride, calculated on the dried basis. Meets the requirements for Identification, pH (5.0–6.5,

in a solution [1 in 100]), Loss on drying (not more than 0.5%), Residue on ignition (not more than 0.1%), Related compounds (not more than 4.0%), and Organic volatile impurities.

Procyclidine Hydrochloride Elixir—Not in USP.

Procyclidine Hydrochloride Tablets USP—Preserve in tight containers, and store in a dry place. Contain the labeled amount, within ±7%. Meet the requirements for Identification, Dissolution (75% in 45 minutes in water in Apparatus 2 at 50 rpm), Related compounds, and Uniformity of dosage units.

PROGESTERONE

Chemical name: Pregn-4-ene-3,20-dione.

Molecular formula: $C_{21}H_{30}O_2$.

Molecular weight: 314.47.

Description: Progesterone USP—White or creamy white, odorless, crystalline powder. Is stable in air.

Solubility: Progesterone USP—Practically insoluble in water; soluble in alcohol, in acetone, and in dioxane; sparingly soluble in vegetable oils.

USP requirements:

Progesterone USP—Preserve in tight, light-resistant containers. Contains not less than 97.0% and not more than 103.0% of progesterone, calculated on the dried basis. Meets the requirements for Identification, Melting range (126–131 °C; if existing in a polymorphic modification, melting at about 121 °C), Specific rotation (+175° to +183°, calculated on the dried basis), and Loss on drying (not more than 0.5%).

Progesterone Injection USP—Preserve in single-dose or in multiple-dose containers, preferably of Type I or Type III glass. A sterile solution of Progesterone in a suitable solvent. Contains the labeled amount, within ±10%. Meets the requirements for Identification and Injections.

Progesterone Rectal Suppositories—Not in USP.

Progesterone Vaginal Suppositories—Not in USP.

Sterile Progesterone Suspension USP—Preserve in single-dose or in multiple-dose containers, preferably of Type I glass. A sterile suspension of Progesterone in Water for Injection. Contains the labeled amount, within ±7%. Meets the requirements for Identification, pH (4.0–7.5), and Injections.

Progesterone Intrauterine Contraceptive System USP—Preserve in sealed, single-unit containers. Contains the labeled amount, within ±10%. It is sterile. Meets the requirements for Identification, Sterility, Uniformity of dosage units, Chromatographic impurities, and Drug-release pattern.

PROLINE

Chemical name: L-Proline.

Molecular formula: $C_5H_9NO_2$.

Molecular weight: 115.13.

Description: Proline USP—White, odorless crystals.

Solubility: Proline USP—Freely soluble in water and in absolute alcohol; insoluble in ether, in butanol, and in isopropanol.

USP requirements: Proline USP—Preserve in well-closed containers. Contains not less than 98.5% and not more than 101.5% of proline, as L-proline, calculated on the dried basis. Meets the requirements for Identification, Specific rotation (−83.7° to −85.7°, calculated on the dried basis), Loss on drying (not more than 0.4%), Residue on ignition (not more than 0.4%), Chloride (not more than 0.05%), Sulfate (not more than 0.03%), Arsenic (not more than 1.5 ppm), Iron (not more than 0.003%), Heavy metals (not more than 0.0015%), and Organic volatile impurities.

PROMAZINE

Chemical group: Phenothiazine.

Chemical name: Promazine hydrochloride—10*H*-Phenothiazine-10-propanamine, *N,N*-dimethyl-, monohydrochloride.

Molecular formula: Promazine hydrochloride—$C_{17}H_{20}N_2S \cdot HCl$.

Molecular weight: Promazine hydrochloride—320.88.

Description: Promazine Hydrochloride USP—White to slightly yellow, practically odorless, crystalline powder. It oxidizes upon prolonged exposure to air and acquires a blue or pink color.

Solubility: Promazine Hydrochloride USP—Freely soluble in water and in chloroform.

USP requirements:

Promazine Hydrochloride USP—Preserve in tight, light-resistant containers. Dried at 105 °C for 2 hours, contains not less than 98.0% and not more than 102.0% of promazine hydrochloride. Meets the requirements for Completeness and clarity of solution, Identification, Melting range (172–182 °C, the range between beginning and end of melting not more than 3 °C), pH (4.2–5.2, in a solution [1 in 20]), Loss on drying (not more than 0.5%), Residue on ignition (not more than 0.1%), Selenium (not more than 0.003%), Heavy metals (not more than 0.005%), Chromatographic purity, and Organic volatile impurities.

Promazine Hydrochloride Injection USP—Preserve in single-dose or in multiple-dose containers, preferably of Type I glass, protected from light. A sterile solution of Promazine Hydrochloride in Water for Injection. Contains the labeled amount, within −5% to +10%. Meets the requirements for Identification, Bacterial endotoxins, pH (4.0–5.5), and Injections.

Promazine Hydrochloride Oral Solution USP—Preserve in tight, light-resistant containers. Contains the labeled amount, within −5% to +10%. Meets the requirements for Identification and pH (5.0–5.5).

Promazine Hydrochloride Syrup USP—Preserve in tight, light-resistant containers. Contains the labeled amount, within −5% to +10%. Meets the requirement for Identification.

Promazine Hydrochloride Tablets USP—Preserve in tight, light-resistant containers. Contain the labeled amount, within −5% to +10%. Meet the requirements for Identification, Disintegration (30 minutes, with disks), and Uniformity of dosage units.

PROMETHAZINE

Chemical group: Phenothiazine derivative.

Chemical name: Promethazine hydrochloride—10*H*-Phenothiazine-10-ethanamine, *N,N*,alpha-trimethyl-, monohydrochloride.

Molecular formula: Promethazine hydrochloride—$C_{17}H_{20}N_2S \cdot HCl$.

Molecular weight: Promethazine hydrochloride—320.88.

Description: Promethazine Hydrochloride USP—White to faint yellow, practically odorless, crystalline powder. Slowly oxidizes, and acquires a blue color, on prolonged exposure to air.

pKa: Promethazine hydrochloride—9.1.

Solubility: Promethazine Hydrochloride USP—Very soluble in water, in hot dehydrated alcohol, and in chloroform; practically insoluble in ether, in acetone, and in ethyl acetate.

USP requirements:

Promethazine Hydrochloride USP—Preserve in tight, light-resistant containers. Contains not less than 97.0% and not more than 101.5% of promethazine hydrochloride, calculated on the dried basis. Meets the requirements for Completeness and clarity of solution, Identification, pH (4.0–5.0, in a solution [1 in 20]), Loss on drying (not more than 0.5%), Residue on ignition (not more than 0.1%), and Related substances.

Promethazine Hydrochloride Injection USP—Preserve in single-dose or in multiple-dose containers, preferably of Type I glass, protected from light. A sterile solution of Promethazine Hydrochloride in Water for Injection. Contains the labeled amount, within −5% to +10%. Meets the requirements for Identification, Bacterial endotoxins, pH (4.0–5.5), and Injections.

Promethazine Hydrochloride Suppositories USP—Preserve in tight, light-resistant containers, and store in a cold place. Contain the labeled amount, within −5% to +10%. Meet the requirement for Identification.

Promethazine Hydrochloride Syrup USP—Preserve in tight, light-resistant containers. Contains the labeled amount, within ±10%. Meets the requirement for Identification.

Promethazine Hydrochloride Tablets USP—Preserve in tight, light-resistant containers. Contain the labeled amount, within −5% to +10%. Meet the requirements for Identification, Dissolution (75% in 45 minutes in 0.1 *N* hydrochloric acid in Apparatus 1 at 100 rpm), and Uniformity of dosage units.

PROMETHAZINE AND CODEINE

For *Promethazine* and *Codeine*—See individual listings for chemistry information.

USP requirements: Promethazine Hydrochloride and Codeine Phosphate Syrup—Not in USP.

PROMETHAZINE AND DEXTROMETHORPHAN

For *Promethazine* and *Dextromethorphan*—See individual listings for chemistry information.

USP requirements: Promethazine Hydrochloride and Dextromethorphan Hydrobromide Syrup—Not in USP.

PROMETHAZINE AND PHENYLEPHRINE

For *Promethazine* and *Phenylephrine*—See individual listings for chemistry information.

USP requirements: Promethazine Hydrochloride and Phenylephrine Hydrochloride Syrup—Not in USP.

PROMETHAZINE, PHENYLEPHRINE, AND CODEINE

For *Promethazine, Phenylephrine,* and *Codeine*—See individual listings for chemistry information.

USP requirements: Promethazine Hydrochloride, Phenylephrine Hydrochloride, and Codeine Phosphate Syrup—Not in USP.

PROMETHAZINE AND PSEUDOEPHEDRINE

For *Promethazine* and *Pseudoephedrine*—See individual listings for chemistry information.

USP requirements: Promethazine Hydrochloride and Pseudoephedrine Hydrochloride Tablets—Not in USP.

PROPAFENONE

Chemical name: Propafenone hydrochloride—1-Propanone, 1-[2-[2-hydroxy-3-(propylamino)propoxy]phenyl]-3-phenyl-, hydrochloride.

Molecular formula: Propafenone hydrochloride—$C_{21}H_{27}NO_3 \cdot HCl$.

Molecular weight: Propafenone hydrochloride—377.91.

Description: Propafenone Hydrochloride USP—White powder.

Solubility: Propafenone Hydrochloride USP—Soluble in methanol and in hot water; slightly soluble in alcohol and in chloroform; very slightly soluble in acetone; insoluble in diethyl ether and in toluene.

USP requirements:

Propafenone Hydrochloride USP—Preserve in tight, light-resistant containers. Contains not less than 98.0% and not more than 102.0% of propafenone hydrochloride, calculated on the dried basis. Meets the requirements for Clarity of solution, Identification, Melting range (171–175 °C), pH (5.0–6.2), Loss on drying (not more than 0.5%), Residue on ignition (not more than 0.1%), Heavy metals (not more than 20 ppm), Limit of methanol and acetone (not more than 100 ppm of methanol and not more than 1000 ppm of acetone), and Chromatographic purity.

Propafenone Hydrochloride Tablets—Not in USP.

PROPANE

Molecular formula: C_3H_8.

Molecular weight: 44.10.

Description: Propane NF—Colorless, flammable gas (boiling temperature is about −42 °C). Vapor pressure at 21 °C is about 10290 mm of mercury (108 psig).

NF category: Aerosol propellant.

Solubility: Propane NF—One hundred volumes of water dissolves 6.5 volumes at 17.8 °C and 753 mm pressure; 100 volumes of anhydrous alcohol dissolves 790 volumes at 16.6 °C and 754 mm pressure; 100 volumes of ether dissolves 926 volumes at 16.6 °C and 757 mm pressure; 100 volumes of chloroform dissolves 1299 volumes at 21.6 °C and 757 mm pressure.

NF requirements: Propane NF—Preserve in tight cylinders, and prevent exposure to excessive heat. Contains not less than 98.0% of propane. Meets the requirements for Identification, Water (not more than 0.001%), High-boiling residues (not more than 5 ppm), Acidity of residue, and Sulfur compounds.

Caution: Propane is highly flammable and explosive.

PROPANTHELINE

Chemical group: Synthetic quaternary ammonium compound.

Chemical name: Propantheline bromide—2-Propanaminium, *N*-methyl-*N*-(1-methylethyl)-*N*-[2-[(9*H*-xanthen-9-ylcarbonyl)-oxy]ethyl]-, bromide.

Molecular formula: Propantheline bromide—$C_{23}H_{30}BrNO_3$.

Molecular weight: Propantheline bromide—448.40.

Description:
Propantheline Bromide USP—White or practically white crystals. Is odorless. Melts at about 160 °C, with decomposition.
Sterile Propantheline Bromide USP—White or practically white crystals. Is odorless.

Solubility:
Propantheline Bromide USP—Very soluble in water, in alcohol, and in chloroform; practically insoluble in ether.
Sterile Propantheline Bromide USP—Very soluble in water, in alcohol, and in chloroform; practically insoluble in ether.

USP requirements:
Propantheline Bromide USP—Preserve in well-closed containers. Contains not less than 98.0% and not more than 102.0% of propantheline bromide, calculated on the dried basis. Meets the requirements for Identification, Loss on drying (not more than 0.5%), Residue on ignition (not more than 0.1%), Related compounds (not more than 3.0%), Bromide content (17.5–18.2%, calculated on the dried basis), and Organic volatile impurities.
Sterile Propantheline Bromide USP—Preserve in Containers for Sterile Solids. It is Propantheline Bromide suitable for parenteral use. Meets the requirements for Completeness of solution, Constituted solution, and Bacterial endotoxins, for Identification tests, Loss on drying, Residue on ignition, Related compounds, and Bromide content under Propantheline Bromide, and for Sterility tests, Uniformity of dosage units, and Labeling under Injections.
Propantheline Bromide Tablets USP—Preserve in well-closed containers. Contain the labeled amount, within ±10%. Meet the requirements for Identification, Dissolution (75% in 45 minutes in Acetate buffer [pH 4.5 +0.05] in Apparatus 2 at 50 rpm), Related compounds, and Uniformity of dosage units.

PROPARACAINE

Chemical name: Proparacaine hydrochloride—Benzoic acid, 3-amino-4-propoxy, 2-(diethylamino)ethyl ester, monohydrochloride.

Molecular formula: Proparacaine hydrochloride—$C_{16}H_{26}N_2O_3 \cdot HCl$.

Molecular weight: Proparacaine hydrochloride—330.85.

Description:
Proparacaine Hydrochloride USP—White to off-white, or faintly buff-colored, odorless, crystalline powder. Its solutions are neutral to litmus.
Proparacaine Hydrochloride Ophthalmic Solution USP—Colorless or faint yellow solution.

Solubility: Proparacaine Hydrochloride USP—Soluble in water, in warm alcohol, and in methanol; insoluble in ether.

USP requirements:
Proparacaine Hydrochloride USP—Preserve in well-closed containers. Contains not less than 97.0% and not more than 103.0% of proparacaine hydrochloride, calculated on the dried basis. Meets the requirements for Identification, Melting range (178–185 °C, the range between beginning and end of melting not more than 2 °C), Loss on drying (not more than 0.5%), Residue on ignition (not more than 0.15%), and Ordinary impurities.
Proparacaine Hydrochloride Ophthalmic Solution USP—Preserve in tight, light-resistant containers. A sterile, aqueous solution of Proparacaine Hydrochloride. Label it to indicate that it is to be stored in a refrigerator after the container is opened. Contains the labeled amount, within −5% to +10%. Meets the requirements for Identification, Sterility, and pH (3.5–6.0).

PROPIOMAZINE

Chemical name: Propiomazine hydrochloride—1-Propanone, 1-[10-[2-(dimethylamino)propyl]-10*H*-phenothiazin-2-yl]-, monohydrochloride.

Molecular formula: Propiomazine hydrochloride—$C_{20}H_{24}N_2OS \cdot HCl$.

Molecular weight: Propiomazine hydrochloride—376.94.

Description: Propiomazine Hydrochloride USP—Yellow, practically odorless powder.

Solubility: Propiomazine Hydrochloride USP—Very soluble in water; freely soluble in alcohol.

USP requirements:
Propiomazine Hydrochloride USP—Preserve in tight, light-resistant containers. Contains not less than 98.0% and not more than 102.0% of propiomazine hydrochloride, calculated on the anhydrous basis. Meets the requirements for Identification, pH (4.6–5.6, in a solution [1 in 50]), Water (not more than 0.5%), and Residue on ignition (not more than 0.1%).
Propiomazine Hydrochloride Injection USP—Preserve in single-dose containers, preferably of Type I glass, at controlled room temperature, protected from light. A sterile solution of Propiomazine Hydrochloride in Water for Injection. Contains the labeled amount, within −5% to +10%. Meets the requirements for Identification, Bacterial endotoxins, pH (4.7–5.3), and Injections.
Note: Do not use the Injection if it is cloudy or contains a precipitate.

PROPIONIC ACID

Molecular formula: $C_3H_6O_2$.

Molecular weight: 74.08.

Description: Propionic Acid NF—Oily liquid, having a slight, pungent, rancid odor.
NF category: Acidifying agent.

Solubility: Propionic Acid NF—Miscible with water and with alcohol and with various other organic solvents.

NF requirements: Propionic Acid NF—Preserve in tight containers. Contains not less than 99.5% and not more than 100.5%, by weight, of propionic acid. Meets the requirements for Specific gravity (0.988–0.993), Distilling range (138.5–142.5 °C), Nonvolatile residue, Arsenic (not more than 3 ppm), Heavy metals (not more than 0.001%), Readily oxidizable substances, Aldehydes, and Organic volatile impurities.

PROPOFOL

Chemical group: Alkyl phenol.

Chemical name: Phenol, 2,6-bis(1-methylethyl).

Molecular formula: $C_{12}H_{18}O$.

Molecular weight: 178.27.

Description: Propofol exists as an oil at room temperature. Propofol injection is formulated as a white, oil-in-water emulsion and has a pH of 7–8.5.

Solubility: Very slightly soluble in water.

USP requirements: Propofol Injection—Not in USP.

PROPOXYCAINE

Chemical name: Propoxycaine hydrochloride—Benzoic acid, 4-amino-2-propoxy-, 2-(diethylamino)ethyl ester, monohydrochloride.

Molecular formula: Propoxycaine hydrochloride—$C_{16}H_{26}N_2O_3 \cdot HCl$.

Molecular weight: Propoxycaine hydrochloride—330.85.

Description: Propoxycaine Hydrochloride USP—White, odorless, crystalline solid which discolors on prolonged exposure to light and to air. The pH of a solution (1 in 50) is about 5.4.

Solubility: Propoxycaine Hydrochloride USP—Freely soluble in water; soluble in alcohol; sparingly soluble in ether; practically insoluble in acetone and in chloroform.

USP requirements: Propoxycaine Hydrochloride USP—Preserve in well-closed, light-resistant containers. Dried at 105 °C for 3 hours, contains not less than 98.0% and not more than 102.0% of propoxycaine hydrochloride. Meets the requirements for Identification, Melting range (146–151 °C), Loss on drying (not more than 0.5%), Residue on ignition (not more than 0.2%), and Chromatographic purity.

PROPOXYCAINE, PROCAINE, AND LEVONORDEFRIN

For *Propoxycaine, Procaine,* and *Levonordefrin*—See individual listings for chemistry information.

USP requirements: Propoxycaine and Procaine Hydrochlorides and Levonordefrin Injection USP—Preserve in single-dose containers, preferably of Type I glass. A sterile solution of Propoxycaine Hydrochloride, Procaine Hydrochloride, and Levonordefrin in Water for Injection. The label indicates that the Injection is not to be used if its color is pinkish or darker than slightly yellow or if it contains a precipitate. Contains the labeled amounts of propoxycaine hydrochloride and procaine hydrochloride, within ±5%, and the labeled amount of levonordefrin, within ±10%. Meets the requirements for Color and clarity, Identification, Bacterial endotoxins, pH (3.5–5.0), and Injections.

PROPOXYCAINE, PROCAINE, AND NOREPINEPHRINE

For *Propoxycaine, Procaine,* and *Norepinephrine*—See individual listings for chemistry information.

USP requirements: Propoxycaine and Procaine Hydrochlorides and Norepinephrine Bitartrate Injection USP—Preserve in single-dose or in multiple-dose containers, preferably of Type I glass. A sterile solution of Propoxycaine Hydrochloride, Procaine Hydrochloride, and Norepinephrine Bitartrate in Water for Injection. The label indicates that the Injection is not to be used if its color is pinkish or darker than slightly yellow or if it contains a precipitate. Contains the labeled amounts of propoxycaine hydrochloride and procaine hydrochloride, within ±5%, and an amount of norepinephrine bitartrate equivalent to the labeled amount of norepinephrine, within ±10%. Meets the requirements for Color and clarity, Identification, Bacterial endotoxins, pH (3.5–5.0), and Injections.

PROPOXYPHENE

Chemical name:

Propoxyphene hydrochloride—Benzeneethanol, alpha-[2-(dimethylamino)-1-methylethyl]-alpha-phenyl-, propanoate (ester), hydrochloride, [*S*-(*R**,*S**)]-.

Propoxyphene napsylate—Benzeneethanol, alpha-[2-(dimethylamino)-1-methylethyl]-alpha-phenyl-, propanoate (ester), [*S*-(*R**,*S**)]-, compd. with 2-naphthalenesulfonic acid (1:1), monohydrate.

Molecular formula:

Propoxyphene hydrochloride—$C_{22}H_{29}NO_2 \cdot HCl$.

Propoxyphene napsylate—$C_{22}H_{29}NO_2 \cdot C_{10}H_8O_3S \cdot H_2O$ (monohydrate); $C_{22}H_{29}NO_2 \cdot C_{10}H_8O_3S$ (anhydrous).

Molecular weight:

Propoxyphene hydrochloride—375.94.

Propoxyphene napsylate—565.72 (monohydrate); 547.71 (anhydrous).

Description:

Propoxyphene Hydrochloride USP—White, crystalline powder. Is odorless.

Propoxyphene Napsylate USP—White powder, having essentially no odor.

Solubility:

Propoxyphene Hydrochloride USP—Freely soluble in water; soluble in alcohol, in chloroform, and in acetone; practically insoluble in ether.

Propoxyphene Napsylate USP—Very slightly soluble in water; soluble in methanol, in alcohol, in chloroform, and in acetone.

USP requirements:

Propoxyphene Hydrochloride USP—Preserve in tight containers. Contains not less than 98.0% and not more than 101.0% of propoxyphene hydrochloride, calculated on the dried basis. Meets the requirements for Identification, Melting range (163.5–168.5 °C, the range between beginning and end of melting not more than 3 °C), Specific rotation (+52° to +57°, calculated on the dried basis), Loss on drying (not more than 1.0%), Related compounds (not more than 0.6%), and Organic volatile impurities.

Propoxyphene Hydrochloride Capsules USP—Preserve in tight containers. Contain the labeled amount, within ±7.5%. Meet the requirements for Identification, Dissolution (85% in 60 minutes in acetate buffer [pH 4.5] in Apparatus 1 at 100 rpm), and Uniformity of dosage units.

Propoxyphene Hydrochloride Tablets—Not in USP.

Propoxyphene Napsylate USP—Preserve in tight containers. Contains not less than 97.0% and not more than 103.0% of propoxyphene napsylate, calculated on the anhydrous basis. Meets the requirements for Identification, Melting range (158–165 °C, the range between beginning and end of melting not more than 4 °C, determined after drying at 105 ° C for 3 hours), Specific rotation (+35° to +43°), Water (2.5–5.0%), Residue on ignition (not more than 0.5%), Heavy metals (not more than 0.003%), Related compounds (not more than 0.6%), and Organic volatile impurities.

Propoxyphene Napsylate Capsules—Not in USP.

Propoxyphene Napsylate Oral Suspension USP—Preserve in tight containers, protected from light. Avoid freezing. Contains the labeled amount, within ±10%. Meets the requirements for Identification and Alcohol content (0.5–1.5%).

Propoxyphene Napsylate Tablets USP—Preserve in tight containers. Contain the labeled amount, within ±10%. Meet the requirements for Identification, Dissolution (75% in 60 minutes in acetate buffer [pH 4.5] in Apparatus 1 at 100 rpm), and Uniformity of dosage units.

PROPOXYPHENE AND ACETAMINOPHEN

For *Propoxyphene* and *Acetaminophen*—See individual listings for chemistry information.

USP requirements:

Propoxyphene Hydrochloride and Acetaminophen Capsules—Not in USP.

Propoxyphene Hydrochloride and Acetaminophen Tablets USP—Preserve in tight containers. Contain the labeled amounts, within ±10%. Meet the requirements for Identification, Dissolution (75% of propoxyphene hydrochloride in 30 minutes in acetate buffer [pH 4.5] in Apparatus 2 at 50 rpm), and Uniformity of dosage units (with respect to propoxyphene hydrochloride).

Propoxyphene Napsylate and Acetaminophen Tablets USP—Preserve in tight containers, at controlled room temperature. Contain the labeled amounts of propoxyphene napsylate and acetaminophen, within ±10%. Meet the requirements for Identification, Dissolution (75% of each active ingredient in 60 minutes in acetate buffer [pH 4.5] in Apparatus 1 at 100 rpm), and Uniformity of dosage units (with respect to propoxyphene napsylate and acetaminophen).

PROPOXYPHENE AND ASPIRIN

For *Propoxyphene* and *Aspirin*—See individual listings for chemistry information.

USP requirements:

Propoxyphene Hydrochloride and Aspirin Capsules—Not in USP.

Propoxyphene Napsylate and Aspirin Capsules—Not in USP.

Propoxyphene Napsylate and Aspirin Tablets USP—Preserve in tight containers, at controlled room temperature. Contain the labeled amounts, within ±10%. Meet the requirements for Identification, Dissolution (75% of each active ingredient in 60 minutes in acetate buffer [pH 4.5] in Apparatus 1 at 100 rpm), Uniformity of dosage units (with respect to propoxyphene napsylate), and Free salicylic acid (not more than 3.0%, calculated on the basis of labeled amount of aspirin).

PROPOXYPHENE, ASPIRIN, AND CAFFEINE

For *Propoxyphene, Aspirin,* and *Caffeine*—See individual listings for chemistry information.

USP requirements:

Propoxyphene Hydrochloride, Aspirin, and Caffeine Capsules USP—Preserve in tight containers at controlled room temperature. Contain the labeled amounts, within ±10%. Meet the requirements for Identification, Dissolution (75% of the aspirin and 85% of the propoxyphene hydrochloride in 60 minutes in acetate buffer [pH 4.5] in Apparatus 1 at 100 rpm), Free salicylic acid (not more than 3.0%, calculated on the basis of labeled amount of aspirin), and Uniformity of dosage units (with respect to propoxyphene hydrochloride and caffeine).

Note: Where Propoxyphene Hydrochloride, Aspirin, and Caffeine Capsules are prescribed, the quantity of propoxyphene hydrochloride is to be specified. Where the Capsules are prescribed without reference to the quantity of aspirin or caffeine contained therein, a product containing 389 mg of aspirin and 32.4 mg of caffeine shall be dispensed.

Propoxyphene Hydrochloride, Aspirin, and Caffeine Tablets—Not in USP.

Propoxyphene Napsylate, Aspirin, and Caffeine Capsules—Not in USP.

PROPRANOLOL

Chemical name: Propranolol hydrochloride—2-Propanol, 1-[(1-methylethyl)amino]-3-(1-naphthalenyloxy)-, hydrochloride.

Molecular formula: Propranolol hydrochloride—$C_{16}H_{21}NO_2 \cdot HCl$.

Molecular weight: Propranolol hydrochloride—295.81.

Description: Propranolol Hydrochloride USP—White to off-white, crystalline powder. Is odorless. Melts at about 164 °C.

Solubility: Propranolol Hydrochloride USP—Soluble in water and in alcohol; slightly soluble in chloroform; practically insoluble in ether.

Other characteristics: Lipid solubility—High.

USP requirements:

Propranolol Hydrochloride USP—Preserve in well-closed containers. Contains not less than 98.0% and not more than 101.5% of propranolol hydrochloride, calculated on the dried basis. Meets the requirements for Identification, Melting range (162–165 °C), Specific rotation (−1.0° to +1.0°, calculated on the dried basis), Loss on drying (not more than 0.5%), Residue on ignition (not more than 0.1%), and Organic volatile impurities.

Propranolol Hydrochloride Extended-release Capsules USP—Preserve in well-closed containers. The labeling states the Drug Release Test with which the product complies. Contain the labeled amount, within ±10%. Meet the requirements for Identification, Drug release (for Test 1: not more than 30% in 1.5 hours in buffer solution [pH 1.2 for the Acid stage], and 35–60% in 4 hours, 55–80% in 8 hours, 70–95% in 14 hours, and 81–110% in 24 hours in buffer solution [pH 6.8 for the Buffer stage] in Apparatus 1 at 100 rpm; for Test 2: not more than 20% in 1 hour in buffer solution [pH 1.2 for the Acid stage], and 20–45% in 3 hours, 45–80% in 6 hours, and not less than 80% in 12 hours in buffer solution [pH 7.5 for the Buffer stage] in Apparatus 1 at 50 rpm), and Uniformity of dosage units.

Propranolol Hydrochloride Injection USP—Preserve in single-dose, light-resistant containers, preferably of Type I glass. A sterile solution of Propranolol Hydrochloride in Water for Injection. Contains the labeled amount, within ±10%. Meets the requirements for Identification, Bacterial endotoxins, pH (2.8–4.0), and Injections.

Propranolol Hydrochloride Oral Solution—Not in USP.

Propranolol Hydrochloride Tablets USP—Preserve in well-closed, light-resistant containers. Contain the labeled amount, within ±10%. Meet the requirements for Identification, Dissolution (75% in 30 minutes in dilute hydrochloric acid [1 in 100] in Apparatus 1 at 100 rpm), and Uniformity of dosage units.

PROPRANOLOL AND HYDROCHLOROTHIAZIDE

For *Propranolol* and *Hydrochlorothiazide*—See individual listings for chemistry information.

USP requirements:

Propranolol Hydrochloride and Hydrochlorothiazide Extended-release Capsules USP—Preserve in well-closed containers. Contain the labeled amounts, within ±10%. Meet the requirements for Identification, Drug release (propranolol hydrochloride: not more than 30% in 0.0625 *D* hours in buffer solution [pH 1.5 for the Acid stage], 35–60% in 0.167 *D* hours, 55–80% in 0.333 *D* hours, 70–95% in 0.583 *D* hours, and 83–108% in 1.00 *D* hours in buffer solution [pH 6.8 for the Buffer stage]; hydrochlorothiazide: not less than 80% in 30 minutes in buffer solution [pH 1.5], in Apparatus 1 at 100 rpm), Related substance (not more than 1.0%), and Uniformity of dosage units.

Propranolol Hydrochloride and Hydrochlorothiazide Tablets USP—Preserve in well-closed containers. Contain the labeled amounts, within ± 10%. Meet the requirements for Identification, Dissolution (80% of each active ingredient in 30 minutes in 0.1 *N* hydrochloric acid in Apparatus 1 at 100 rpm), and Uniformity of dosage units.

PROPYLENE CARBONATE

Chemical name: 4-Methyl-1,3-dioxolan-2-one.

Molecular formula: $C_4H_6O_3$.

Molecular weight: 102.09.

Description: Propylene Carbonate NF—Clear, colorless, mobile liquid.

NF category: Solvent.

Solubility: Propylene Carbonate NF—Freely soluble in water; insoluble in hexane; miscible with alcohol and with chloroform.

NF requirements: Propylene Carbonate NF—Preserve in tight containers. Contains not less than 99.0% and not more than 100.5% of propylene carbonate. Meets the requirements for Identification, Specific gravity (1.203–1.210 at 20 °C), pH (6.0–7.5), Residue on ignition (not more than 0.01%), and Organic volatile impurities.

PROPYLENE GLYCOL

Chemical name: 1,2-Propanediol.

Molecular formula: $C_3H_8O_2$.

Molecular weight: 76.10.

Description: Propylene Glycol USP—Clear, colorless, viscous liquid. It is practically odorless. It absorbs moisture when exposed to moist air.

NF category: Humectant; plasticizer; solvent.

Solubility: Propylene Glycol USP—Miscible with water, with acetone, and with chloroform. Soluble in ether and will dissolve many essential oils, but is immiscible with fixed oils.

USP requirements: Propylene Glycol USP—Preserve in tight containers. Contains not less than 99.5% of propylene glycol. Meets the requirements for Identification, Specific gravity (1.035–1.037), Acidity, Water (not more than 0.2%), Residue on ignition, Chloride (not more than 0.007%), Sulfate (not more than 0.006%), Arsenic (not more than 3 ppm), Heavy metals (not more than 5 ppm), and Organic volatile impurities.

PROPYLENE GLYCOL ALGINATE

Description: Propylene Glycol Alginate NF—White to yellowish fibrous or granular powder. Practically odorless.

NF category: Suspending and/or viscosity-increasing agent.

Solubility: Propylene Glycol Alginate NF—Soluble in water, in solutions of dilute organic acids, and, depending on the degree of esterification, in hydroalcoholic mixtures containing up to 60% by weight of alcohol to form stable, viscous colloidal solutions at a pH of 3.

NF requirements: Propylene Glycol Alginate NF—Preserve in well-closed containers. A propylene glycol ester of alginic acid. Each gram yields not less than 0.16 and not more than 0.20 gram of carbon dioxide, calculated on the dried basis. Meets the requirements for Identification, Microbial limits, Loss on drying (not more than 20.0%), Ash (not more than 10.0%, calculated on the dried basis), Arsenic (not more than 3 ppm), Lead (not more than 0.001%), Heavy metals (not more than 0.004%), Free carboxyl groups, and Esterified carboxyl groups.

PROPYLENE GLYCOL DIACETATE

Molecular formula: $C_7H_{12}O_4$.

Molecular weight: 160.17.

Description: Propylene Glycol Diacetate NF—Clear, colorless liquid, having a mild, fruity odor.

NF category: Emulsifying and/or solubilizing agent.

Solubility: Propylene Glycol Diacetate NF—Soluble in water.

NF requirements: Propylene Glycol Diacetate NF—Preserve in tight containers, and avoid contact with metal. Contains not less than 98.0% and not more than 102.0% of propylene glycol diacetate. Meets the requirements for Identification, Specific gravity (1.040–1.060), Refractive index (1.4130–1.4150 at 20 °C), pH (4.0–6.0, in a solution [1 in 20]), Acetic acid (not more than 0.2%), Chromatographic purity, and Organic volatile impurities.

PROPYLENE GLYCOL MONOSTEARATE

Chemical name: Octadecanoic acid, monoester with 1,2-propanediol.

Molecular formula: $C_{21}H_{42}O_3$.

Molecular weight: 342.56.

Description: Propylene Glycol Monostearate NF—White, wax-like solid, or white, wax-like beads or flakes. It has a slight, agreeable, fatty odor.

NF category: Emulsifying and/or solubilizing agent.

Solubility: Propylene Glycol Monostearate NF—Insoluble in water, but may be dispersed in hot water with the aid of a small amount of soap or other suitable surface-active agent; soluble in organic solvents, such as alcohol, mineral or fixed oils, ether, and acetone.

NF requirements: Propylene Glycol Monostearate NF—Preserve in well-closed containers. A mixture of the propylene glycol mono- and di-esters of stearic and palmitic acids. Contains not less than 90.0% of monoesters of saturated fatty acids, chiefly propylene glycol monostearate and propylene glycol monopalmitate. Meets the requirements for Congealing temperature (not lower than 45 °C), Residue on ignition (not more than 0.5%), Acid value (not more than 4), Saponification value (155–165), Hydroxyl value (160–175), Iodine value (not more than 3), Free glycerin and propylene glycol, and Propylene glycol monoesters.

PROPYL GALLATE

Chemical name: Benzoic acid, 3,4,5-trihydroxy-, propyl ester.

Molecular formula: $C_{10}H_{12}O_5$.

Molecular weight: 212.20.

Description: Propyl Gallate NF—White, crystalline powder, having a very slight, characteristic odor.

NF category: Antioxidant.

Solubility: Propyl Gallate NF—Slightly soluble in water; freely soluble in alcohol.

NF requirements: Propyl Gallate NF—Preserve in tight containers, protected from light, and avoid contact with metals. Contains not less than 98.0% and not more than 102.0% of propyl gallate, calculated on the dried basis. Meets the requirements for Identification, Melting range (146–150 °C), Loss on drying (not more than 0.5%), Residue on ignition (not more than 0.1%), Heavy metals (not more than 0.001%), and Organic volatile impurities.

PROPYLHEXEDRINE

Chemical name: Cyclohexaneethanamine, *N*,alpha-dimethyl-, (±).

Molecular weight: $C_{10}H_{21}N$.

Molecular weight: 155.28.

Description: Propylhexedrine USP—Clear, colorless liquid, having a characteristic, amine-like odor. Volatilizes slowly at room temperature. Absorbs carbon dioxide from the air, and its solutions are alkaline to litmus. Boils at about 205 °C.

Solubility: Propylhexedrine USP—Very slightly soluble in water. Miscible with alcohol, with chloroform, and with ether.

USP requirements:

Propylhexedrine USP—Preserve in tight containers. Contains not less than 98.0% and not more than 101.0% of propylhexedrine. Meets the requirements for Identification and Specific gravity (0.848–0.852).

Propylhexedrine Inhalant USP—Preserve in tight containers (inhalers), and avoid exposure to excessive heat. Consists of cylindrical rolls of suitable fibrous material impregnated with Propylhexedrine, usually aromatized, and contained in a suitable inhaler. Inhaler contains the labeled amount, within −10% to +25%. Meets the requirement for Identification.

PROPYLIODONE

Chemical name: 1(4*H*)-Pyridineacetic acid, 3,5-diiodo-4-oxo-, propyl ester.

Molecular formula: $C_{10}H_{11}I_2NO_3$.

Molecular weight: 447.01.

Description: Propyliodone USP—White or almost white, crystalline powder. Odorless or has a faint odor.

Solubility: Propyliodone USP—Practically insoluble in water; soluble in acetone, in alcohol, and in ether.

USP requirements:

Propyliodone USP—Preserve in tight, light-resistant containers. Contains not less than 99.0% and not more than 101.0% of propyliodone, calculated on the dried basis. Meets the requirements for Identification, Melting range (187–190 °C), Acidity, Loss on drying (not more than 0.5%), Residue on ignition (not more than 0.1%), Iodine and iodide, and Heavy metals (not more than 0.002%).

Sterile Propyliodone Oil Suspension USP—Preserve in single-dose, light-resistant containers. A sterile suspension of Propyliodone in Peanut Oil. Contains not less than 57.0% and not more than 63.0% of propyliodone. Meets the requirements for Identification, Weight per mL (1.236–1.276 grams), Iodine and iodide, and Injections.

PROPYLPARABEN

Chemical name: Benzoic acid, 4-hydroxy-, propyl ester.

Molecular formula: $C_{10}H_{12}O_3$.

Molecular weight: 180.20.

Description: Propylparaben NF—Small, colorless crystals or white powder.

NF category: Antimicrobial preservative.

Solubility: Propylparaben NF—Very slightly soluble in water; freely soluble in alcohol and in ether; slightly soluble in boiling water.

NF requirements: Propylparaben NF—Preserve in well-closed containers. Contains not less than 99.0% and not more than 100.5% of propylparaben, calculated on the dried basis. Meets the requirements for Identification, Melting range (95–98 °C), and Organic volatile impurities, and for Acidity, Loss on drying, and Residue on ignition under Butylparaben.

PROPYLPARABEN SODIUM

Chemical name: Benzoic acid, 4-hydroxy-, propyl ester, sodium salt.

Molecular formula: $C_{10}H_{11}NaO_3$.

Molecular weight: 202.19.

Description: Propylparaben Sodium NF—White powder. It is odorless and hygroscopic.

NF category: Antimicrobial preservative.

Solubility: Propylparaben Sodium NF—Freely soluble in water; sparingly soluble in alcohol; insoluble in fixed oils.

NF requirements: Propylparaben Sodium NF—Preserve in tight containers. Contains not less than 98.5% and not more than 101.5% of propylparaben sodium, calculated on the anhydrous basis. Meets the requirements for Completeness of solution, Identification, pH (9.5–10.5, in a solution [1 in 1000]), Water (not more than 5.0%), Chloride (not more than 0.035%), Sulfate (not more than 0.12%), and Organic volatile impurities.

PROPYLTHIOURACIL

Chemical group: Thiourea derivative.

Chemical name: 4(1*H*)-Pyrimidinone, 2,3-dihydro-6-propyl-2-thioxo-.

Molecular formula: $C_7H_{10}N_2OS$.

Molecular weight: 170.23.

Description: Propylthiouracil USP—White, powdery, crystalline substance; starch-like in appearance and to the touch.

Solubility: Propylthiouracil USP—Slightly soluble in water; sparingly soluble in alcohol; slightly soluble in chloroform and in ether; soluble in ammonium hydroxide and in alkali hydroxides.

USP requirements:

Propylthiouracil USP—Preserve in well-closed, light-resistant containers. Contains not less than 98.0% and not more than 100.5% of propylthiouracil, calculated on the dried basis. Meets the requirements for Identification, Melting range (218–221 °C), Loss on drying (not more than 0.5%), Residue on ignition (not more than 0.1%), Selenium (not more than 0.003%), Heavy metals (not more than 0.002%), Ordinary impurities, and Organic volatile impurities.

Propylthiouracil Enema—Not in USP.

Propylthiouracil Suppositories—Not in USP.

Propylthiouracil Tablets USP—Preserve in well-closed containers. Contain the labeled amount, within ±7%. Meet the requirements for Identification, Dissolution (85% in 30 minutes in water in Apparatus 1 at 100 rpm), and Uniformity of dosage units.

PROTAMINE

Description:

Protamine Sulfate Injection USP—Colorless solution, which may have the odor of a preservative.

Protamine Sulfate for Injection USP—White, odorless powder, having the characteristic appearance of solids dried from the frozen state.

USP requirements:

Protamine Sulfate USP—Preserve in tight containers, in a refrigerator. A purified mixture of simple protein principles obtained from the sperm or testes of suitable species of fish, which has the property of neutralizing heparin. Each mg of Protamine Sulfate, calculated on the dried basis, neutralizes not less than 100 USP Heparin Units. Meets the requirements for Loss on drying (not more than 5%), Sulfate (16–22%, calculated on the dried basis), and Nitrogen content (22.5–25.5%, calculated on the dried basis).

Protamine Sulfate Injection USP—Preserve in single-dose containers, preferably of Type I glass. Store in a refrigerator. A sterile, isotonic solution of Protamine Sulfate. Label it to indicate the approximate neutralization capacity in USP Heparin Units. Contains the labeled amount, within −10% to +20%. Meets the requirements for Identification (tests for Sulfate), Bacterial endotoxins, and Injections.

Protamine Sulfate for Injection USP—Preserve in Containers for Sterile Solids. Preserve the accompanying solvent in single-dose or in multiple-dose containers, preferably of Type I glass. A sterile mixture of Protamine Sulfate with one or more suitable, dry diluents. Label it to indicate the approximate neutralization capacity in USP Heparin Units. Contains the labeled amount, within −10% to +20%. Meets the requirements for Constituted solution (under Injections at time of use), Bacterial endotoxins, pH and clarity of solution (6.5–7.5, and the solution is clear), and Uniformity of dosage units, and both the medication and the accompanying solvent meet the requirements for Sterility tests and Labeling under Injections.

PROTEIN HYDROLYSATE

Description: Protein Hydrolysate Injection USP—Yellowish to reddish amber, transparent liquid.

USP requirements: Protein Hydrolysate Injection USP—Preserve in single-dose containers, preferably of Type I or Type II glass, and avoid excessive heat. A sterile solution of amino acids and short-chain peptides which represent the approximate nutritive equivalent of the casein, lactalbumin, plasma, fibrin, or other suitable protein from which it is derived by acid, enzymatic, or other method of hydrolysis. May be modified by partial removal and restoration or addition of one or more amino acids. May contain alcohol, dextrose, or other carbohydrate suitable for intravenous infusion. Not less than 50.0% of the total nitrogen present is in the form of alpha-amino nitrogen. The label of the immediate container bears in a subtitle the name of the protein from which the hydrolysate has been derived and the word "modified" if one or more of the "essential" amino acids has been partially removed, restored, or added. The label bears a statement of the pH range; the name and percentage of any added other nutritive ingredient; the method of hydrolysis; the nature of the modification, if any, in amino acid content after hydrolysis; the percentage of each essential amino acid or its equivalent; the approximate protein equivalent, in grams per liter; the approximate number of calories per liter; the percentage of the total nitrogen in the form of alpha-amino nitrogen; and the quantity of the sodium and of the potassium ions present in each 100 mL of the Injection. Injection that contains not more than 30 mg of sodium per 100 mL may be labeled "Protein Hydrolysate Injection, Low Sodium," or by a similar title the approximate equivalent thereof. The label states the total osmolar concentration in mOsmol per liter. Where the contents are less than 100 mL, or where the label states that the Injection is not for direct injection but is to be diluted before use, the label may alternatively state the total osmolar concentration in mOsmol per mL. Meets the requirements for Non-antigenicity, Bacterial endotoxins, Biological adequacy (for Protein), pH (4.0–7.0, determined potentiometrically, but the variation from the pH range stated on the label is not greater than ±0.5 pH unit), Nitrogen content, alpha-Amino nitrogen, Potassium content, Sodium content, and Injections.

PROTIRELIN

Source: A synthetic tripeptide thought to be structurally identical to the naturally occurring thyrotropin-releasing hormone produced by the hypothalamus.

Chemical name: L-Prolinamide, 5-oxo-L-prolyl-L-histidyl-.

Molecular formula: $C_{16}H_{22}N_6O_4$.

Molecular weight: 362.39.

Description: Slightly yellowish hygroscopic powder.

Solubility: Very soluble in water and in methanol; soluble in isopropanol.

USP requirements: Protirelin Injection—Not in USP.

PROTRIPTYLINE

Chemical group: Dibenzocycloheptene derivative.

Chemical name: Protriptyline hydrochloride—5*H*-Dibenzo[*a,d*]cycloheptene-5-propanamine, *N*-methyl-, hydrochloride.

Molecular formula: Protriptyline hydrochloride—$C_{19}H_{21}N \cdot HCl$.

Molecular weight: Protriptyline hydrochloride—299.84.

Description: Protriptyline Hydrochloride USP—White to yellowish powder. Is odorless, or has not more than a slight odor. Melts at about 168 °C.

Solubility: Protriptyline Hydrochloride USP—Freely soluble in water, in alcohol, and in chloroform; practically insoluble in ether.

Other characteristics: Secondary amine.

USP requirements:

Protriptyline Hydrochloride USP—Preserve in well-closed containers. Contains not less than 99.0% and not more than 101.0% of protriptyline hydrochloride, calculated on the dried basis. Meets the requirements for Identification, pH (5.0–6.5, in a solution [1 in 100]), Loss on drying (not more than 0.3%), Residue on ignition (not more than 0.1%), Heavy metals (not more than 0.001%), and Organic volatile impurities.

Protriptyline Hydrochloride Tablets USP—Preserve in tight containers. Contain the labeled amount, within ±10%. Meet the requirements for Identification, Dissolution (75% in 45 minutes in water in Apparatus 1 at 100 rpm), and Uniformity of dosage units.

PSEUDOEPHEDRINE

Chemical name:
Pseudoephedrine hydrochloride—Benzenemethanol, alpha-[1-(methylamino)ethyl]-, [*S*-(*R**,*R**)]-, hydrochloride.
Pseudoephedrine sulfate—Benzenemethanol, alpha-[1-(methylamino)ethyl]-, [*S*-(*R**,*R**)]-, sulfate (2:1) (salt).

Molecular formula:
Pseudoephedrine hydrochloride—$C_{10}H_{15}NO \cdot HCl$.
Pseudoephedrine sulfate—$(C_{10}H_{15}NO)_2 \cdot H_2SO_4$.

Molecular weight:
Pseudoephedrine hydrochloride—201.70.
Pseudoephedrine sulfate—428.54.

Description:
Pseudoephedrine Hydrochloride USP—Fine, white to off-white crystals or powder, having a faint characteristic odor.
Pseudoephedrine Sulfate USP—White crystals or crystalline powder. Is odorless.

Solubility:
Pseudoephedrine Hydrochloride USP—Very soluble in water; freely soluble in alcohol; sparingly soluble in chloroform.
Pseudoephedrine Sulfate USP—Freely soluble in alcohol.

USP requirements:
Pseudoephedrine Hydrochloride USP—Preserve in tight, light-resistant containers. Contains not less than 98.0% and not more than 100.5% of pseudoephedrine hydrochloride, calculated on the dried basis. Meets the requirements for Identification, Melting range (182–186 °C, the range between beginning and end of melting not more than 2 °C), Specific rotation (+61.0° to +62.5°, calculated on the dried basis), pH (4.6–6.0, in a solution [1 in 20]), Loss on drying (not more than 0.5%), Residue on ignition (not more than 0.1%), and Organic volatile impurities.

Pseudoephedrine Hydrochloride Capsules—Not in USP.

Pseudoephedrine Hydrochloride Extended-release Capsules—Not in USP.

Pseudoephedrine Hydrochloride Oral Solution—Not in USP.

Pseudoephedrine Hydrochloride Syrup USP—Preserve in tight, light-resistant containers. Contains the labeled amount, within ±10%. Meets the requirements for Identification and Reaction (acid to litmus).

Pseudoephedrine Hydrochloride Tablets USP—Preserve in tight containers. Contain the labeled amount, within ±7%. Meet the requirements for Identification, Dissolution (75% in 45 minutes in water in Apparatus 2 at 50 rpm), and Uniformity of dosage units.

Pseudoephedrine Hydrochloride Extended-release Tablets—Not in USP.

Pseudoephedrine Sulfate USP—Preserve in tight, light-resistant containers. Contains not less than 98.0% and not more than 100.5% of pseudoephedrine sulfate, calculated on the dried basis. Meets the requirements for Identification, Melting range (174–179 °C, the range between beginning and end of melting not more than 2 °C), Specific rotation (+56.0° to +59.0°, calculated on the dried basis), pH (5.0–6.5, in a solution [1 in 20]), Loss on drying (not more than 2.0%), Residue on ignition (not more than 0.1%), Heavy metals, and Chloride (not more than 0.14%).

Pseudoephedrine Sulfate Tablets—Not in USP.

Pseudoephedrine Sulfate Extended-release Tablets—Not in USP.

PSEUDOEPHEDRINE, ACETAMINOPHEN, AND CAFFEINE

For *Pseudoephedrine, Acetaminophen,* and *Caffeine*—See individual listings for chemistry information.

USP requirements: Pseudoephedrine Hydrochloride, Acetaminophen, and Caffeine Capsules—Not in USP.

PSEUDOEPHEDRINE AND ASPIRIN

For *Pseudoephedrine* and *Aspirin*—See individual listings for chemistry information.

USP requirements: Pseudoephedrine Hydrochloride and Aspirin Tablets—Not in USP.

PSEUDOEPHEDRINE, ASPIRIN, AND CAFFEINE

For *Pseudoephedrine, Aspirin,* and *Caffeine*—See individual listings for chemistry information.

USP requirements: Pseudoephedrine Hydrochloride, Aspirin, and Caffeine Capsules—Not in USP.

PSEUDOEPHEDRINE AND CODEINE

For *Pseudoephedrine* and *Codeine*—See individual listings for chemistry information.

USP requirements:
Pseudoephedrine Hydrochloride and Codeine Phosphate Capsules—Not in USP.
Pseudoephedrine Hydrochloride and Codeine Phosphate Syrup—Not in USP.

PSEUDOEPHEDRINE, CODEINE, AND GUAIFENESIN

For *Pseudoephedrine, Codeine,* and *Guaifenesin*—See individual listings for chemistry information.

USP requirements:
Pseudoephedrine Hydrochloride, Codeine Phosphate, and Guaifenesin Oral Solution—Not in USP.
Pseudoephedrine Hydrochloride, Codeine Phosphate, and Guaifenesin Syrup—Not in USP.

PSEUDOEPHEDRINE AND DEXTROMETHORPHAN

For *Pseudoephedrine* and *Dextromethorphan*—See individual listings for chemistry information.

USP requirements:
Pseudoephedrine Hydrochloride and Dextromethorphan Hydrobromide Capsules—Not in USP.
Pseudoephedrine Hydrochloride and Dextromethorphan Hydrobromide Oral Solution—Not in USP.
Pseudoephedrine Hydrochloride and Dextromethorphan Hydrobromide Chewable Tablets—Not in USP.

PSEUDOEPHEDRINE, DEXTROMETHORPHAN, AND ACETAMINOPHEN

For *Pseudoephedrine, Dextromethorphan,* and *Acetaminophen*—See individual listings for chemistry information.

USP requirements:
Pseudoephedrine Hydrochloride, Dextromethorphan Hydrobromide, and Acetaminophen Oral Solution—Not in USP.

Pseudoephedrine Hydrochloride, Dextromethorphan Hydrobromide, and Acetaminophen for Oral Solution—Not in USP.
Pseudoephedrine Hydrochloride, Dextromethorphan Hydrobromide, and Acetaminophen Tablets—Not in USP.

PSEUDOEPHEDRINE, DEXTROMETHORPHAN, AND GUAIFENESIN

For *Pseudoephedrine, Dextromethorphan,* and *Guaifenesin*—See individual listings for chemistry information.

USP requirements:
Pseudoephedrine Hydrochloride, Dextromethorphan Hydrobromide, and Guaifenesin Capsules—Not in USP.
Pseudoephedrine Hydrochloride, Dextromethorphan Hydrobromide, and Guaifenesin Oral Solution—Not in USP.
Pseudoephedrine Hydrochloride, Dextromethorphan Hydrobromide, and Guaifenesin Syrup—Not in USP.
Pseudoephedrine Hydrochloride, Dextromethorphan Hydrobromide, and Guaifenesin Tablets—Not in USP.

PSEUDOEPHEDRINE, DEXTROMETHORPHAN, GUAIFENESIN, AND ACETAMINOPHEN

For *Pseudoephedrine, Dextromethorphan, Guaifenesin,* and *Acetaminophen*—See individual listings for chemistry information.

USP requirements:
Pseudoephedrine Hydrochloride, Dextromethorphan Hydrobromide, Guaifenesin, and Acetaminophen Capsules—Not in USP.
Pseudoephedrine Hydrochloride, Dextromethorphan Hydrobromide, Guaifenesin, and Acetaminophen Oral Solution—Not in USP.
Pseudoephedrine Hydrochloride, Dextromethorphan Hydrobromide, Guaifenesin, and Acetaminophen Tablets—Not in USP.

PSEUDOEPHEDRINE AND GUAIFENESIN

For *Pseudoephedrine* and *Guaifenesin*—See individual listings for chemistry information.

USP requirements:
Pseudoephedrine Hydrochloride and Guaifenesin Capsules—Not in USP.
Pseudoephedrine Hydrochloride and Guaifenesin Extended-release Capsules—Not in USP.
Pseudoephedrine Hydrochloride and Guaifenesin Oral Solution—Not in USP.
Pseudoephedrine Hydrochloride and Guaifenesin Syrup—Not in USP.
Pseudoephedrine Hydrochloride and Guaifenesin Tablets—Not in USP.
Pseudoephedrine Hydrochloride and Guaifenesin Extended-release Tablets—Not in USP.

PSEUDOEPHEDRINE AND HYDROCODONE

For *Pseudoephedrine* and *Hydrocodone*—See individual listings for chemistry information.

USP requirements:
Pseudoephedrine Hydrochloride and Hydrocodone Bitartrate Oral Solution—Not in USP.
Pseudoephedrine Hydrochloride and Hydrocodone Bitartrate Syrup—Not in USP.

PSEUDOEPHEDRINE, HYDROCODONE, AND GUAIFENESIN

For *Pseudoephedrine, Hydrocodone,* and *Guaifenesin*—See individual listings for chemistry information.

USP requirements:
Pseudoephedrine Hydrochloride, Hydrocodone Bitartrate, and Guaifenesin Elixir—Not in USP.
Pseudoephedrine Hydrochloride, Hydrocodone Bitartrate, and Guaifenesin Oral Solution—Not in USP.
Pseudoephedrine Hydrochloride, Hydrocodone Bitartrate, and Guaifenesin Syrup—Not in USP.
Pseudoephedrine Hydrochloride, Hydrocodone Bitartrate, and Guaifenesin Tablets—Not in USP.

PSEUDOEPHEDRINE AND IBUPROFEN

For *Pseudoephedrine* and *Ibuprofen*—See individual listings for chemistry information.

USP requirements: Pseudoephedrine Hydrochloride and Ibuprofen Tablets—Not in USP.

PSYLLIUM

Source: Psyllium seed—Cleaned, dried, ripe seed of *Plantago psyllium* and related species having a high content of hemicellulose mucilages.

USP requirements:
Psyllium Caramels—Not in USP.
Psyllium Granules—Not in USP.
Psyllium Powder—Not in USP.

PSYLLIUM HUSK

USP requirements: Psyllium Husk USP—Preserve in well-closed containers, secured against insect attack. The cleaned, dried seed coat (epidermis) separated by winnowing and thrashing from the seeds of *Plantago ovata* Forskal, known in commerce as Blond Psyllium or Indian Psyllium or Ispaghula, or from *Plantago psyllium* Linné or from *Plantago indica* Linné (*Plantago arenaria* Waldstein et Kitaibel) known in commerce as Spanish or French Psyllium (Fam. Plantaginaceae), in whole or in powdered form. Meets the requirements for Botanic characteristics, Identification, Microbial limits, Total ash (not more than 4.0%), Acid-insoluble ash (not more than 1.0%), Water (not more than 12.0%), Light extraneous matter (not more than 15%), Heavy extraneous matter (not more than 1.1%), Insect infestation, and Swell volume.

PSYLLIUM HYDROPHILIC MUCILLOID

Source: Obtained from the coating of *Plantago ovata*; contains about 50% hemicellulose.

Description: White to cream-colored, slightly granular powder with little or no odor.

USP requirements:
Psyllium Hydrophilic Mucilloid Granules—Not in USP.
Psyllium Hydrophilic Mucilloid Powder—Not in USP.
Psyllium Hydrophilic Mucilloid Effervescent Powder—Not in USP.
Psyllium Hydrophilic Mucilloid for Oral Suspension USP—Preserve in tight containers. A dry mixture of Psyllium Husk with suitable additives. Meets the requirements for Identification, Microbial limits, and Swell volume.
Psyllium Hydrophilic Mucilloid Wafers—Not in USP.

PSYLLIUM HYDROPHILIC MUCILLOID AND CARBOXYMETHYLCELLULOSE

For *Psyllium Hydrophilic Mucilloid* and *Carboxymethylcellulose*—See individual listings for chemistry information.

USP requirements: Psyllium Hydrophilic Mucilloid and Carboxymethylcellulose Sodium Granules—Not in USP.

PSYLLIUM HYDROPHILIC MUCILLOID AND SENNA

For *Psyllium Hydrophilic Mucilloid* and *Senna*—See individual listings for chemistry information.

USP requirements: Psyllium Hydrophilic Mucilloid and Senna Granules—Not in USP.

PSYLLIUM HYDROPHILIC MUCILLOID AND SENNOSIDES

For *Psyllium Hydrophilic Mucilloid* and *Sennosides*—See individual listings for chemistry information.

USP requirements: Psyllium Hydrophilic Mucilloid and Sennosides Powder—Not in USP.

PSYLLIUM AND SENNA

For *Psyllium* and *Senna*—See individual listings for chemistry information.

USP requirements: Psyllium and Senna Granules—Not in USP.

PUMICE

Description: Pumice USP—Very light, hard, rough, porous, grayish masses or gritty, grayish powder. Is odorless and stable in air.

Solubility: Pumice USP—Practically insoluble in water; is not attacked by acids.

USP requirements: Pumice USP—Preserve in well-closed containers. A substance of volcanic origin, consisting chiefly of complex silicates of aluminum, potassium, and sodium. Label powdered Pumice to indicate, in descriptive terms, the fineness of the powder. Powdered Pumice meets requirements for several sizes (Pumice Flour or Superfine Pumice, Fine Pumice, and Coarse Pumice). Meets the requirements for Water-soluble substances (not more than 0.20%), Acid-soluble substances (not more than 6.0%), and Iron.

PYRANTEL

Chemical name: Pyrantel pamoate—Pyrimidine, 1,4,5,6-tetrahydro-1-methyl-2-[2-(2-thienyl)ethenyl]-, (*E*)-, compd. with 4,4′-methylenebis[3-hydroxy-2-naphthalenecarboxylic acid] (1:1).

Molecular formula: Pyrantel pamoate—$C_{11}H_{14}N_2S \cdot C_{23}H_{16}O_6$.

Molecular weight: Pyrantel pamoate—594.68.

Description: Pyrantel Pamoate USP—Yellow to tan solid.

Solubility: Pyrantel Pamoate USP—Practically insoluble in water and in methanol; soluble in dimethylsulfoxide; slightly soluble in dimethylformamide.

USP requirements:

Pyrantel Pamoate USP—Preserve in well-closed, light-resistant containers. Contains not less than 97.0% and not more than 103.0% of pyrantel pamoate, calculated on the dried basis. Meets the requirements for Identification, Loss on drying (not more than 2.0%), Residue on ignition (not more than 0.5%), Heavy metals (not more than 0.005%), Iron (not more than 0.0075%), Related compounds, and Pamoic acid content (63.4–67.3%, calculated on the dried basis).

Pyrantel Pamoate Oral Suspension USP—Preserve in tight, light-resistant containers. A suspension of Pyrantel Pamoate in a suitable aqueous vehicle. Contains an amount of pyrantel pamoate equivalent to the labeled amount of pyrantel, within ±10%. Meets the requirements for Identification and pH (4.5–6.0).

Pyrantel Pamoate Tablets—Not in USP.

PYRAZINAMIDE

Source: Pyrazine derivative of nicotinamide.

Chemical name: Pyrazinecarboxamide.

Molecular formula: $C_5H_5N_3O$.

Molecular weight: 123.11.

Description: Pyrazinamide USP—White to practically white, odorless or practically odorless, crystalline powder.

Solubility: Pyrazinamide USP—Sparingly soluble in water; slightly soluble in alcohol, in ether, and in chloroform.

USP requirements:

Pyrazinamide USP—Preserve in well-closed containers. Contains not less than 99.0% and not more than 101.0% of pyrazinamide, calculated on the anhydrous basis. Meets the requirements for Identification, Melting range (188–191 °C), Water (not more than 0.5%), Residue on ignition (not more than 0.1%), Heavy metals (not more than 0.001%), and Organic volatile impurities.

Pyrazinamide Tablets USP—Preserve in well-closed containers. Contain the labeled amount, within ±7%. Meet the requirements for Identification, Dissolution (75% in 45 minutes in water in Apparatus 2 at 50 rpm), and Uniformity of dosage units.

PYRETHRINS AND PIPERONYL BUTOXIDE

Source:

Pyrethrins—Obtained from flowers of the pyrethrum plant, *Chrysanthemum cincerariaefolium*, which is related to the ragweed plant; esters formed by the combination of chrysanthenic and pyrethric acids and pyrethrolone, cinerolone, and jasmolone alcohols.

Piperonyl butoxide—Synthetic piperic acid derivative.

Chemical name: Piperonyl butoxide—5-[2-(2-Butoxyethoxy)-ethoxymethyl]-6-propyl-1,3-benzodioxole.

Molecular formula: Piperonyl butoxide—$C_{19}H_{30}O_5$.

Molecular weight: Piperonyl butoxide—338.44.

Description:

Pyrethrins—Viscous liquid.

Piperonyl butoxide—Yellow or pale brown oily liquid with a faint characteristic odor.

Solubility:

Pyrethrins—Practically insoluble in water; soluble in alcohol, in petroleum ether, in kerosene, in carbon tetrachloride, in ethylene dichloride, and in nitromethane.

Piperonyl butoxide—Very slightly soluble in water; miscible with alcohol, with chloroform, with ether, with petroleum oils, and with liquefied aerosol propellents.

USP requirements:

Pyrethrins and Piperonyl Butoxide Gel—Not in USP.

Pyrethrins and Piperonyl Butoxide Solution Shampoo—Not in USP.

Pyrethrins and Piperonyl Butoxide Topical Solution—Not in USP.

PYRETHRUM EXTRACT

Description: Pyrethrum Extract USP—Pale yellow liquid having a bland, flowery odor. *Pyrethrins I* denotes the group containing pyrethrin 1, cinerin 1, and jasmolin 1; *Pyrethrins*

II denotes the group containing pyrethrin 2, cinerin 2, and jasmolin 2.

Solubility: Pyrethrum Extract USP—Insoluble in water; soluble in mineral oil and in most organic solvents.

USP requirements: Pyrethrum Extract USP—Preserve in tight, light-resistant containers. A mixture of three naturally occurring, closely related insecticidal esters of chrysanthemic acid (Pyrethrins I) and three closely related esters of pyrethric acid (Pyrethrins II). Contains not less than 45.0% and not more than 55.0% of the sum of Pyrethrins I and Pyrethrins II in a mixture consisting of approximately 20–25% (w/w) light isoparaffins. The ratio of Pyrethrins I to Pyrethrins II in the Extract is not less than 0.8 and not more than 2.8. May also contain 3–5% butylated hydroxytoluene as an antioxidant and 23–25% phytochemical extracts containing triglyceride oils, terpenoids, and carotenoid plant colors. Contains no other added substances. Meets the requirement for Identification.

PYRIDOSTIGMINE

Source: Synthetic quaternary ammonium compound.

Chemical name: Pyridostigmine bromide—Pyridinium, 3-[[(dimethylamino)carbonyl]oxy]-1-methyl-, bromide.

Molecular formula: Pyridostigmine bromide—$C_9H_{13}BrN_2O_2$.

Molecular weight: Pyridostigmine bromide—261.12.

Description: Pyridostigmine Bromide USP—White or practically white, crystalline powder, having an agreeable, characteristic odor. Hygroscopic.

Solubility: Pyridostigmine Bromide USP—Freely soluble in water, in alcohol, and in chloroform; slightly soluble in solvent hexane; practically insoluble in ether.

USP requirements:

Pyridostigmine Bromide USP—Preserve in tight containers. Contains not less than 98.5% and not more than 100.5% of pyridostigmine bromide, calculated on the dried basis. Meets the requirements for Identification, Melting range (154–157 °C), Loss on drying (not more than 2.0%), Residue on ignition (not more than 0.1%), Ordinary impurities, and Organic volatile impurities.

Pyridostigmine Bromide Injection USP—Preserve in single-dose containers, preferably of Type I glass, protected from light. A sterile solution of Pyridostigmine Bromide in a suitable medium. Contains the labeled amount, within ±10%. Meets the requirements for Identification, Bacterial endotoxins, pH (4.5–5.5), and Injections.

Pyridostigmine Bromide Syrup USP—Preserve in tight, light-resistant containers. Contains, in each 100 mL, not less than 1.08 grams and not more than 1.32 grams of pyridostigmine bromide. Meets the requirement for Identification.

Pyridostigmine Bromide Tablets USP—Preserve in tight containers. Contain the labeled amount, within ±5%. Meet the requirements for Identification, Dissolution (75% in 45 minutes in water in Apparatus 2 at 50 rpm), and Uniformity of dosage units.

Pyridostigmine Bromide Extended-release Tablets—Not in USP.

PYRIDOXINE

Chemical name: Pyridoxine hydrochloride—3,4-Pyridinedimethanol, 5-hydroxy-6-methyl-, hydrochloride.

Molecular formula: Pyridoxine hydrochloride—$C_8H_{11}NO_3 \cdot HCl$.

Molecular weight: Pyridoxine hydrochloride—205.64.

Description: Pyridoxine Hydrochloride USP—White to practically white crystals or crystalline powder. Is stable in air, and is slowly affected by sunlight. Its solutions have a pH of about 3.

Solubility: Pyridoxine Hydrochloride USP—Freely soluble in water; slightly soluble in alcohol; insoluble in ether.

USP requirements:

Pyridoxine Hydrochloride USP—Preserve in tight, light-resistant containers. Contains not less than 98.0% and not more than 102.0% of pyridoxine hydrochloride, calculated on the dried basis. Meets the requirements for Identification, Loss on drying (not more than 0.5%), Residue on ignition (not more than 0.1%), Heavy metals (not more than 0.003%), Chloride content (16.9–17.6%, calculated on the dried basis), and Organic volatile impurities.

Pyridoxine Hydrochloride Extended-release Capsules—Not in USP.

Pyridoxine Hydrochloride Injection USP—Preserve in single-dose or in multiple-dose containers, preferably of Type I glass, protected from light. A sterile solution of Pyridoxine Hydrochloride in Water for Injection. Contains the labeled amount, within −5% to +15%. Meets the requirements for Identification, Bacterial endotoxins, pH (2.0–3.8), and Injections.

Pyridoxine Hydrochloride Tablets USP—Preserve in well-closed containers, protected from light. Contain the labeled amount, within −5% to +15%. Meet the requirements for Identification, Disintegration (30 minutes), and Uniformity of dosage units.

PYRILAMINE

Chemical group: Ethylenediamine derivative.

Chemical name: Pyrilamine maleate—1,2-Ethanediamine, *N*-[(4-methoxyphenyl)methyl]-*N′*,*N′*-dimethyl-*N*-2-pyridinyl-, (*Z*)-2-butenedioate (1:1).

Molecular formula: Pyrilamine maleate—$C_{17}H_{23}N_3O \cdot C_4H_4O_4$.

Molecular weight: Pyrilamine maleate—401.46.

Description: Pyrilamine Maleate USP—White, crystalline powder, usually having a faint odor. Its solutions are acid to litmus.

Solubility: Pyrilamine Maleate USP—Very soluble in water; freely soluble in alcohol and in chloroform; slightly soluble in ether.

USP requirements:

Pyrilamine Maleate USP—Preserve in tight, light-resistant containers. Dried in vacuum over phosphorus pentoxide for 5 hours, contains not less than 98.0% and not more than 100.5% of pyrilamine maleate. Meets the requirements for Identification, Melting range (99–103 °C), Loss on drying (not more than 0.5%), Residue on ignition (not more than 0.1%), Related substances, and Organic volatile impurities.

Pyrilamine Maleate Tablets USP—Preserve in well-closed containers. Contain the labeled amount, within ±7%. Meet the requirements for Identification, Dissolution (75% in 45 minutes in water in Apparatus 2 at 50 rpm), and Uniformity of dosage units.

PYRILAMINE, PHENYLEPHRINE, ASPIRIN, AND CAFFEINE

For *Pyrilamine, Phenylephrine, Aspirin,* and *Caffeine*—See individual listings for chemistry information.

USP requirements: Pyrilamine Maleate, Phenylephrine Hydrochloride, Aspirin, and Caffeine Tablets—Not in USP.

PYRILAMINE, PHENYLEPHRINE, AND CODEINE

For *Pyrilamine, Phenylephrine,* and *Codeine*—See individual listings for chemistry information.

USP requirements: Pyrilamine Maleate, Phenylephrine Hydrochloride, and Codeine Phosphate Syrup—Not in USP.

PYRILAMINE, PHENYLEPHRINE, AND DEXTROMETHORPHAN

For *Pyrilamine, Phenylephrine,* and *Dextromethorphan*—See individual listings for chemistry information.

USP requirements: Pyrilamine Maleate, Phenylephrine Hydrochloride, and Dextromethorphan Hydrobromide Oral Solution—Not in USP.

PYRILAMINE, PHENYLEPHRINE, DEXTROMETHORPHAN, AND ACETAMINOPHEN

For *Pyrilamine, Phenylephrine, Dextromethorphan,* and *Acetaminophen*—See individual listings for chemistry information.

USP requirements: Pyrilamine Maleate, Phenylephrine Hydrochloride, Dextromethorphan Hydrobromide, and Acetaminophen Oral Solution—Not in USP.

PYRILAMINE, PHENYLEPHRINE, AND HYDROCODONE

For *Pyrilamine, Phenylephrine,* and *Hydrocodone*—See individual listings for chemistry information.

USP requirements: Pyrilamine Maleate, Phenylephrine Hydrochloride, and Hydrocodone Bitartrate Syrup—Not in USP.

PYRILAMINE, PHENYLEPHRINE, HYDROCODONE, AND AMMONIUM CHLORIDE

For *Pyrilamine, Phenylephrine, Hydrocodone,* and *Ammonium Chloride*—See individual listings for chemistry information.

USP requirements: Pyrilamine Maleate, Phenylephrine Hydrochloride, Hydrocodone Bitartrate, and Ammonium Chloride Syrup—Not in USP.

PYRILAMINE, PHENYLPROPANOLAMINE, ACETAMINOPHEN, AND CAFFEINE

For *Pyrilamine, Phenylpropanolamine, Acetaminophen,* and *Caffeine*—See individual listings for chemistry information.

USP requirements: Pyrilamine Maleate, Phenylpropanolamine Hydrochloride, Acetaminophen, and Caffeine Tablets—Not in USP.

PYRILAMINE, PHENYLPROPANOLAMINE, DEXTROMETHORPHAN, GUAIFENESIN, POTASSIUM CITRATE, AND CITRIC ACID

For *Pyrilamine, Phenylpropanolamine, Dextromethorphan, Guaifenesin, Potassium Citrate,* and *Citric Acid*—See individual listings for chemistry information.

USP requirements: Pyrilamine Maleate, Phenylpropanolamine Hydrochloride, Dextromethorphan Hydrobromide, Guaifenesin, Potassium Citrate, and Citric Acid Syrup—Not in USP.

PYRILAMINE, PHENYLPROPANOLAMINE, DEXTROMETHORPHAN, AND SODIUM SALICYLATE

For *Pyrilamine, Phenylpropanolamine, Dextromethorphan,* and *Sodium Salicylate*—See individual listings for chemistry information.

USP requirements: Pyrilamine Maleate, Phenylpropanolamine Hydrochloride, Dextromethorphan Hydrobromide, and Sodium Salicylate Oral Solution—Not in USP.

PYRILAMINE, PSEUDOEPHEDRINE, DEXTROMETHORPHAN, AND ACETAMINOPHEN

For *Pyrilamine, Pseudoephedrine, Dextromethorphan,* and *Acetaminophen*—See individual listings for chemistry information.

USP requirements: Pyrilamine Maleate, Pseudoephedrine Hydrochloride, Dextromethorphan Hydrobromide, and Acetaminophen Oral Solution—Not in USP.

PYRIMETHAMINE

Chemical group: Structurally related to trimethoprim.

Chemical name: 2,4-Pyrimidinediamine, 5-(4-chlorophenyl)-6-ethyl-.

Molecular formula: $C_{12}H_{13}ClN_4$.

Molecular weight: 248.72.

Description: Pyrimethamine USP—White, odorless, crystalline powder.

Solubility: Pyrimethamine USP—Practically insoluble in water; slightly soluble in acetone, in alcohol, and in chloroform.

USP requirements:

Pyrimethamine USP—Preserve in tight, light-resistant containers. Contains not less than 99.0% and not more than 101.0% of pyrimethamine, calculated on the dried basis. Meets the requirements for Identification, Melting range (238–242 °C), Loss on drying (not more than 0.5%), Residue on ignition (not more than 0.1%), Ordinary impurities, and Organic volatile impurities.

Pyrimethamine Tablets USP—Preserve in tight, light-resistant containers. Contain the labeled amount, within ±7%. Meet the requirements for Identification, Dissolution (75% in 45 minutes in 0.1 *N* hydrochloric acid in Apparatus 2 at 50 rpm), and Uniformity of dosage units.

PYRITHIONE

Chemical name: Pyrithione zinc—Zinc, bis(1-hydroxy-2(1*H*)-pyridinethionato-*O,S*)-(T-4)-.

Molecular formula: Pyrithione zinc—$C_{10}H_8N_2O_2S_2Zn$.

Molecular weight: Pyrithione zinc—317.70.

Description: Pyrithione zinc—Off-white to gray colored powder with not more than a mild characteristic odor.

Solubility: Pyrithione zinc—Soluble in dimethylsulfoxide; practically insoluble in acetone, in alcohol, and in water.

USP requirements:

Pyrithione Zinc Bar Shampoo—Not in USP.
Pyrithione Zinc Cream Shampoo—Not in USP.
Pyrithione Zinc Lotion Shampoo—Not in USP.

PYROXYLIN

Chemical name: Cellulose, nitrate.

Description: White to light yellow cuboid granules or fibrous material resembling cotton wool but harsher to the touch and more powdery.

Solubility: Soluble in acetone and in glacial acetic acid.

USP requirements: Pyroxylin USP—Preserve loosely packed in cartons, protected from light. A product obtained by the action of a mixture of nitric and sulfuric acids on cotton, and consists chiefly of cellulose tetranitrate. The label bears a caution statement to the effect that Pyroxylin is highly flammable. Meets the requirements for Viscosity (110–147 poises), Residue on ignition (not more than 0.3%), Acidity and water-soluble substances, and Organic volatile impurities.

Note: Dry Pyroxylin is a light yellow, matted mass of filaments, resembling raw cotton in appearance, but harsh to the touch. *It is exceedingly flammable,* burning, when unconfined, very rapidly and with a luminous flame. When kept in well-closed bottles and exposed to light, it is decomposed with the evolution of nitrous vapors, leaving a carbonaceous residue. Pyroxylin available commercially is moistened with about 30% of alcohol or other suitable solvent. The alcohol or other solvent must be allowed to evaporate from the Pyroxylin to yield the dried substance described in *USP/NF*. Pyroxylin moistened with alcohol or other solvent may be used in these tests, provided the weight of test specimen taken corresponds to the specified amount of dry Pyroxylin.

PYRVINIUM

Chemical name: Pyrvinium pamoate—Quinolinium, 6-(dimethylamino)-2-[2-(2,5-dimethyl-1-phenyl-1*H*-pyrrol-3-yl)ethenyl]-1-methyl-, salt with 4,4′-methylenebis[3-hydroxy-2-naphthalenecarboxylic acid] (2:1).

Molecular formula: Pyrvinium pamoate—$C_{75}H_{70}N_6O_6$.

Molecular weight: Pyrvinium pamoate—1151.42.

Description:

Pyrvinium Pamoate USP—Bright orange or orange-red to practically black, crystalline powder.

Pyrvinium Pamoate Oral Suspension USP—Dark red, opaque suspension of essentially very fine, amorphous particles or aggregates, usually less than 10 micrometers in size. Larger particles, some of which may be crystals, up to 100 micrometers in size also may be present.

Solubility: Pyrvinium Pamoate USP—Practically insoluble in water and in ether; freely soluble in glacial acetic acid; slightly soluble in chloroform and in methoxyethanol; very slightly soluble in methanol.

USP requirements:

Pyrvinium Pamoate USP—Preserve in tight, light-resistant containers. Contains not less than 96.0% and not more than 104.0% of pyrvinium pamoate, calculated on the anhydrous basis. Meets the requirements for Identification, Water (not more than 6.0%), and Residue on ignition (not more than 0.5%).

Pyrvinium Pamoate Oral Suspension USP—Preserve in tight, light-resistant containers. Contains, in each 100 mL, an amount of pyrvinium pamoate equivalent to not less than 0.90 gram and not more than 1.10 grams of pyrvinium. Meets the requirements for Identification and pH (6.0–8.0).

Pyrvinium Pamoate Tablets USP—Preserve in tight, light-resistant containers. Contain an amount of pyrvinium pamoate equivalent to the labeled amount of pyrvinium, within ±8%. Meet the requirements for Identification, Disintegration (30 minutes), and Uniformity of dosage units.

QUAZEPAM

Chemical name: 2*H*-1,4-Benzodiazepine-2-thione, 7-chloro-5-(2-fluorophenyl)-1,3-dihydro-1-(2,2,2-trifluoroethyl)-.

Molecular formula: $C_{17}H_{11}ClF_4N_2S$.

Molecular weight: 386.79.

Description: White, crystalline compound.

Solubility: Soluble in ethanol; insoluble in water.

USP requirements: Quazepam Tablets—Not in USP.

QUINACRINE

Chemical group: Acridine derivative.

Chemical name: Quinacrine hydrochloride—1,4-Pentanediamine, N^4-(6-chloro-2-methoxy-9-acridinyl)-N^1,N^1-diethyl-, dihydrochloride, dihydrate.

Molecular formula: Quinacrine hydrochloride—$C_{23}H_{30}ClN_3O \cdot 2HCl \cdot 2H_2O$.

Molecular weight: Quinacrine hydrochloride—508.92.

Description: Quinacrine Hydrochloride USP—Bright yellow, crystalline powder. Is odorless. Its solution (1 in 100) has a pH of about 4.5. Melts at about 250 °C, with decomposition.

Solubility: Quinacrine Hydrochloride USP—Sparingly soluble in water; soluble in alcohol.

USP requirements:

Quinacrine Hydrochloride USP—Preserve in tight, light-resistant containers. Contains not less than 99.0% and not more than 101.0% of quinacrine hydrochloride, calculated on the anhydrous basis. Meets the requirements for Identification, Water (6.0–8.0%), Residue on ignition (not more than 0.1%), Ordinary impurities, and Organic volatile impurities.

Quinacrine Hydrochloride Tablets USP—Preserve in tight containers. Contain the labeled amount, within ±7%. Meet the requirements for Identification, Dissolution (75% in 45 minutes in water in Apparatus 2 at 50 rpm), and Uniformity of dosage units.

QUINAPRIL

Chemical name: Quinapril hydrochloride—3-Isoquinolinecarboxylic acid, 2-[2-[[1-(ethoxycarbonyl)-3-phenylpropyl]-amino]-1-oxopropyl]-1,2,3,4-tetrahydro-, monohydrochloride, [3*S*-[2[*R**(*R**)],3*R**]].

Molecular formula: Quinapril hydrochloride—$C_{25}H_{30}N_2O_5 \cdot HCl$.

Molecular weight: Quinapril hydrochloride—474.98.

Description: Quinapril hydrochloride—White to off-white amorphous powder.

Solubility: Quinapril hydrochloride—Freely soluble in aqueous solvents.

USP requirements: Quinapril Hydrochloride Tablets—Not in USP.

QUINESTROL

Chemical name: 19-Norpregna-1,3,5(10)-trien-20-yn-17-ol, 3-(cyclopentyloxy)-, (17 alpha)-.

Molecular formula: $C_{25}H_{32}O_2$.

Molecular weight: 364.53.

Description: Quinestrol USP—White, practically odorless powder.

Solubility: Quinestrol USP—Insoluble in water; soluble in alcohol, in chloroform, and in ether.

USP requirements:

Quinestrol USP—Preserve in well-closed containers. Contains not less than 98.0% and not more than 102.0% of quinestrol, calculated on the dried basis. Meets the requirements for Identification, Melting range (107–110.5 °C), Specific rotation (+3° to +5°, calculated on the dried basis), Loss on drying (not more than 0.5%), and Ordinary impurities.

Quinestrol Tablets USP—Preserve in well-closed containers. Contain the labeled amount, within ±10%. Meet the requirements for Identification, Dissolution (80% in 30 minutes in 0.29% sodium lauryl sulfate in Apparatus 2 at 50 rpm), and Uniformity of dosage units.

QUINETHAZONE

Chemical name: 6-Quinazolinesulfonamide, 7-chloro-2-ethyl-1,2,3,4-tetrahydro-4-oxo-.

Molecular formula: $C_{10}H_{12}ClN_3O_3S$.

Molecular weight: 289.74.

Description: Quinethazone USP—White to yellowish white, crystalline powder.

pKa: 9.3 and 10.7.

Solubility: Quinethazone USP—Very slightly soluble in water; freely soluble in solutions of alkali hydroxides and carbonates; sparingly soluble in pyridine; slightly soluble in alcohol.

USP requirements:

Quinethazone USP—Preserve in well-closed containers. Contains not less than 98.0% and not more than 102.0% of quinethazone, calculated on the dried basis. Meets the requirements for Identification, Loss on drying (not more than 1.0%), Residue on ignition (not more than 0.1%), Selenium (not more than 0.003%), Heavy metals (not more than 0.002%), and Organic volatile impurities.

Quinethazone Tablets USP—Preserve in tight containers. Contain the labeled amount, within ±7.5%. Meet the requirements for Identification, Disintegration (30 minutes), and Uniformity of dosage units.

QUINIDINE

Source: Quinidine polygalacturonate—A polymer of quinidine and polygalacturonic acid.

Chemical name:

Quinidine gluconate—Cinchonan-9-ol, 6′-methoxy-, (9*S*)-, mono-D-gluconate (salt).

Quinidine sulfate—Cinchonan-9-ol, 6′-methoxy-, (9*S*)-, sulfate (2:1) (salt), dihydrate.

Molecular formula:

Quinidine gluconate—$C_{20}H_{24}N_2O_2 \cdot C_6H_{12}O_7$.

Quinidine polygalacturonate—$(C_{20}H_{24}N_2O_2 \cdot C_6H_{10}O_7 \cdot H_2O)_x$.

Quinidine sulfate—$(C_{20}H_{24}N_2O_2)_2 \cdot H_2SO_4 \cdot 2H_2O$.

Molecular weight:

Quinidine gluconate—520.58.

Quinidine sulfate—782.95.

Description:

Quinidine Gluconate USP—White powder. Odorless.

Quinidine polygalacturonate—Creamy white, amorphous powder.

Quinidine Sulfate USP—Fine, needle-like, white crystals, frequently cohering in masses, or fine, white powder. Is odorless, and darkens on exposure to light. Its solutions are neutral or alkaline to litmus.

Solubility:

Quinidine Gluconate USP—Freely soluble in water; slightly soluble in alcohol.

Quinidine polygalacturonate—Sparingly soluble in water; freely soluble in hot 40% alcohol.

Quinidine Sulfate USP—Slightly soluble in water; soluble in alcohol and in chloroform; insoluble in ether.

USP requirements:

Quinidine Gluconate USP—Preserve in well-closed, light-resistant containers. The gluconate of an alkaloid that may be obtained from various species of *Cinchona* and their hybrids, or from *Remijia pedunculata* Flückiger (Fam. Rubiaceae), or prepared from quinine. Contains not less than 99.0% and not more than 100.5% of total alkaloid salt, calculated as quinidine gluconate, on the dried basis. Meets the requirements for Identification, Loss on drying (not more than 0.5%), Residue on ignition (not more than 0.15%), Heavy metals (not more than 0.001%), Chromatographic purity, Limit of dihydroquinidine gluconate, and Organic volatile impurities.

Quinidine Gluconate Injection USP—Preserve in single-dose or in multiple-dose containers, preferably of Type I glass. A sterile solution of Quinidine Gluconate in Water for Injection. Contains, in each mL, amounts of quinidine gluconate and dihydroquinidine gluconate totaling not less than 76 mg and not more than 84 mg of quinidine gluconate, calculated as quinidine gluconate. Meets the requirements for Identification, Bacterial endotoxins, Chromatographic purity, and Injections.

Quinidine Gluconate Tablets—Not in USP.

Quinidine Gluconate Extended-release Tablets USP—Preserve in well-closed, light-resistant containers. Contain amounts of quinidine gluconate and dihydroquinidine gluconate totaling the labeled amount of quinidine gluconate, calculated as quinidine gluconate, within ±10%. Meet the requirements for Identification, Chromatographic purity, and Uniformity of dosage units.

Quinidine Polygalacturonate Tablets—Not in USP.

Quinidine Sulfate USP—Preserve in well-closed, light-resistant containers. The sulfate of an alkaloid obtained from various species of *Cinchona* and their hybrids and from *Remijia pedunculata* Flückiger (Fam. Rubiaceae), or prepared from quinine. Contains not less than 99.0% and not more than 101.0% of total alkaloid salt, calculated as quinidine sulfate, on the anhydrous basis. Meets the requirements for Identification, Specific rotation (+275° to +288°, calculated on the anhydrous basis), Water (4.0–5.5%), Residue on ignition (not more than 0.1%), Heavy metals (not more than 0.001%), Chloroform-alcohol-insoluble substances (not more than 0.1%), Limit of dihydroquinidine sulfate, Chromatographic purity, and Organic volatile impurities.

Quinidine Sulfate Capsules USP—Preserve in tight, light-resistant containers. Contain amounts of quinidine sulfate and dihydroquinidine sulfate totaling the labeled amount of quinidine sulfate, calculated as quinidine sulfate, within ±10%. Meet the requirements for Identification, Dissolution (85% in 30 minutes in 0.1 *N* hydrochloric acid in Apparatus 1 at 100 rpm), Uniformity of dosage units, and Chromatographic purity.

Quinidine Sulfate Injection—Not in USP.

Quinidine Sulfate Tablets USP—Preserve in well-closed, light-resistant containers. Contain amounts of quinidine sulfate and dihydroquinidine sulfate totaling the labeled amount of quinidine sulfate, calculated as quinidine sulfate, within ±10%. Meet the requirements for Identification, Dissolution (85% in 30 minutes in 0.1 *N* hydrochloric acid in Apparatus 1 at 100 rpm), Uniformity of dosage units, and Chromatographic purity.

Quinidine Sulfate Extended-release Tablets USP—Preserve in well-closed, light-resistant containers. Contain amounts of quinidine sulfate and dihydroquinidine sulfate totaling the labeled amount of quinidine sulfate, calculated as quinidine sulfate, within ±10%. Meet the requirements for Identification, Drug release (20–50% in 1 hour, 43–73% in 4 hours, and not less than 70% in 12 hours in 0.1 *N* hydrochloric acid in Apparatus 1 at 100 rpm), Uniformity of dosage units, and Chromatographic purity.

QUININE

Chemical name: Quinine sulfate—Cinchonan-9-ol, 6′-methoxy-, (8 alpha,9*R*)-, sulfate (2:1) (salt), dihydrate.

Molecular formula: Quinine sulfate—$(C_{20}H_{24}N_2O_2)_2 \cdot H_2SO_4 \cdot 2H_2O$.

Molecular weight: Quinine sulfate—782.95.

Description: Quinine Sulfate USP—White, fine, needle-like crystals, usually lusterless, making a light and readily compressible mass. Is odorless. It darkens on exposure to light. Its saturated solution is neutral or alkaline to litmus.

Solubility: Quinine Sulfate USP—Slightly soluble in water, in alcohol, in chloroform, and in ether; freely soluble in alcohol at 80 °C, and in a mixture of 2 volumes of chloroform and 1 volume of dehydrated alcohol; sparingly soluble in water at 100 °C.

USP requirements:

Quinine Sulfate USP—Preserve in well-closed, light-resistant containers. The sulfate of an alkaloid obtained from the bark of species of *Cinchona*. Contains not less than 99.0% and not more than 101.0% of total alkaloid salt, calculated as quinine sulfate, on the dried basis. Meets the requirements for Identification, Specific rotation (−235° to −245°, calculated on the anhydrous basis), Water (4.0–5.5%), Residue on ignition (not more than 0.1%), Heavy metals (not more than 0.001%), Chloroform-alcohol-insoluble substances (not more than 0.1%), Chromatographic purity, and Dihydroquinine sulfate.

Quinine Sulfate Capsules USP—Preserve in tight containers. Contain amounts of quinine sulfate and dihydroquinine sulfate totaling the labeled amount of quinine sulfate, calculated as quinine sulfate dihydrate, within ±10%. Meet the requirements for Identification, Dissolution (75% in 45 minutes in 0.1 *N* hydrochloric acid in Apparatus 1 at 100 rpm), Uniformity of dosage units, and Chromatographic purity.

Quinine Sulfate Tablets USP—Preserve in well-closed containers. Contain amounts of quinine sulfate and dihydroquinine sulfate totaling the labeled amount of quinine sulfate, calculated as quinine sulfate dihydrate, within ±10%. Meet the requirements for Identification, Dissolution (75% in 45 minutes in 0.1 *N* hydrochloric acid in Apparatus 1 at 100 rpm), Uniformity of dosage units, and Chromatographic purity.

RABIES IMMUNE GLOBULIN

Description: Rabies Immune Globulin USP—Transparent or slightly opalescent liquid, practically colorless and practically odorless. May develop a slight, granular deposit during storage.

USP requirements: Rabies Immune Globulin USP—Preserve at a temperature between 2 and 8 °C. A sterile, non-pyrogenic, slightly opalescent solution consisting of globulins derived from blood plasma or serum that has been tested for the absence of hepatitis B surface antigen, derived from selected adult human donors who have been immunized with rabies vaccine and have developed high titers of rabies antibody. Label it to state that it is not for intravenous injection. Has a potency such that when labeled as 150 International Units (IU) per mL, it has a geometric mean lower limit (95% confidence) potency value of not less than 110 IU per mL, and proportionate lower limit potency values for other labeled potencies, based on the U.S. Standard Rabies Immune Globulin and using the CVS Virus challenge, by neutralization test in mice or tissue culture. Contains not less than 10 grams and not more than 18 grams of protein per 100 mL, of which not less than 80% is monomeric immunoglobilin G, having a sedimentation coefficient in the range of 6.0 to 7.5S, with no fragments having a sedimentation coefficient less than 6S and no aggregates having a sedimentation coefficient greater than 12S. Contains 0.3 *M* glycine as a stabilizing agent, and contains a suitable preservative. Has a pH of 6.4–7.2, measured in a solution diluted to contain 1% of protein with 0.15 *M* sodium chloride. Meets the requirements of the test for heat stability and for Expiration date (not later than 1 year after date of issue from manufacturer's cold storage [5 °C, 1 year]). Conforms to the regulations of the U.S. Food and Drug Administration concerning biologics.

RABIES VACCINE

Description: Rabies Vaccine USP—White to straw-colored, amorphous pellet, which may or may not become fragmented when shaken.

USP requirements: Rabies Vaccine USP—Preserve at a temperature between 2 and 8 °C. A sterile preparation, in dried or liquid form, of inactivated rabies virus harvested from inoculated diploid cell cultures. Label it to state that it contains rabies antigen equivalent to not less than 2.5 IU per dose and that it is intended for intramuscular injection only. The cell cultures are shown to consist of diploid cells by tests of karyology, to be non-tumorigenic by tests in hamsters treated with anti-lymphocytic serum (ALS), and to be free from extraneous agents by tests in animals or cell-culture systems. The harvested virus meets the requirements for identity by serological tests, for absence of infectivity by tests in mice or cell-culture systems, and for absence of extraneous agents by tests in animals or cell-culture systems. The Vaccine meets the requirements for absence of live virus by tests using a suitable virus amplification system involving inoculation and incubation of sensitive cell cultures for not less than 14 days followed by inoculation of the cell-culture fluid thereafter into not less than 20 adult mice. Has a potency of rabies antigen equivalent to not less than 2.5 International Units for Rabies Vaccine, per dose, determined with the specific mouse protection test using the U.S. Standard Rabies Vaccine. Meets the requirements for general safety and Expiration date (not later than 2 years after date of issue from manufacturer's cold storage [5 °C, 1 year]). Conforms to the regulations of the U.S. Food and Drug Administration concerning biologics.

RACEPINEPHRINE

Chemical name: 1,2-Benzenediol, 4-[1-hydroxy-2-(methylamino)ethyl]-, (±)-.

Molecular formula:

Racepinephrine—$C_9H_{13}NO_3$.

Racepinephrine hydrochloride—$C_9H_{13}NO_3 \cdot HCl$.

Molecular weight:

Racepinephrine—183.21.

Racepinephrine hydrochloride—219.67.

Description:
Racepinephrine USP—White to nearly white, crystalline, odorless powder, gradually darkening on exposure to light and air. With acids, it forms salts that are readily soluble in water, and the base may be recovered by the addition of ammonium hydroxide.
Racepinephrine Hydrochloride USP—Fine, white, odorless powder. Darkens on exposure to light and air. Its solutions are acid to litmus. Melts at about 157 °C.

Solubility:
Racepinephrine USP—Very slightly soluble in water and in alcohol; insoluble in ether, in chloroform, and in fixed and volatile oils.
Racepinephrine Hydrochloride USP—Freely soluble in water; sparingly soluble in alcohol.

USP requirements:
Racepinephrine USP—Preserve in tight, light-resistant containers. A racemic mixture of the enantiomorphs of epinephrine. Contains not less than 97.0% and not more than 102.0% of racepinephrine, calculated on the dried basis. Meets the requirements for Identification, Loss on drying (not more than 2.0%), Residue on ignition (not more than 0.5%), Specific rotation (−1° to +1°), Adrenalone, Limit of norepinephrine (not more than 4.0%), and Organic volatile impurities.
Racepinephrine Inhalation Solution USP—Preserve in tight, light-resistant containers. Do not freeze. A solution of Racepinephrine in Purified Water prepared with the aid of Hydrochloric Acid or of Racepinephrine Hydrochloride in Purified Water. The label indicates that the Inhalation Solution is not to be used if its color is pinkish or darker than slightly yellow or if it contains a precipitate. Contains the labeled amount, within ±10%. Meets the requirements for Color and clarity, Identification, and pH (2.0–3.5).
Racepinephrine Hydrochloride USP—Preserve in tight, light-resistant containers. A racemic mixture of the hydrochlorides of the enantiomorphs of epinephrine. Contains not less than 97.0% and not more than 102.0% of racepinephrine hydrochloride, calculated on the anhydrous basis. Meets the requirements for Identification, Water (not more than 0.5%), Specific rotation (−1° to +1°), Residue on ignition (not more than 0.5%), and Organic volatile impurities, and for Adrenalone and Limit of norepinephrine under Racepinephrine.

RAMIPRIL

Chemical name: Cyclopenta[*b*]pyrrole-2-carboxylic acid, 1-[2-[[1-(ethoxycarbonyl)-3-phenylpropyl]amino]-1-oxopropyl]-octahydro-, [2*S*-[1[*R**(*R**)],2 alpha,3a beta,6a beta]]-.

Molecular formula: $C_{23}H_{32}N_2O_5$.

Molecular weight: 416.52.

Description: White, crystalline substance. Melts between 105–112 °C.

Solubility: Soluble in polar organic solvents and in buffered aqueous solutions.

USP requirements: Ramipril Capsules—Not in USP.

RANITIDINE

Chemical group: Amino-alkyl furan derivative of histamine.

Chemical name:
Ranitidine—1,1-Ethenediamine, *N*-[2-[[[5-[(dimethylamino)-methyl]-2-furanyl]methyl]thio]ethyl]-*N′*-methyl-2-nitro-.
Ranitidine hydrochloride—1,1-Ethenediamine, *N*-[2-[[[5-[(dimethylamino)methyl]-2-furanyl]methyl]thio]ethyl]-*N′*-methyl-2-nitro-, monohydrochloride.

Molecular formula:
Ranitidine—$C_{13}H_{22}N_4O_3S$.
Ranitidine hydrochloride—$C_{13}H_{22}N_4O_3S \cdot HCl$.

Molecular weight:
Ranitidine—314.40.
Ranitidine hydrochloride—350.86.

Description: Ranitidine Hydrochloride USP—White to pale yellow, crystalline, practically odorless powder. Is sensitive to light and moisture. Melts at about 140 °C, with decomposition.

pKa: Ranitidine hydrochloride—8.2 and 2.7.

Solubility: Ranitidine Hydrochloride USP—Very soluble in water; moderately soluble in alcohol; and sparingly soluble in chloroform.

USP requirements:
Ranitidine Capsules—Not in USP.
Ranitidine Injection USP—Preserve in single-dose or in multiple-dose containers of Type I glass, protected from light. Store below 30 °C. Do not freeze. A sterile solution of Ranitidine Hydrochloride in Water for Injection. Label Injection to state both the content of the active moiety and the content of the salt used in formulating the article. Contain the labeled amount, within ±10%. Meets the requirements for Identification, Bacterial endotoxins, pH (6.7–7.3), Particulate matter, Chromatographic purity, and Injections.
Ranitidine Oral Solution USP—Preserve in tight, light-resistant containers. Store below 25 °C. Do not freeze. A solution of Ranitidine Hydrochloride in water. Label Oral Solution to state both the content of the active moiety and the content of the ranitidine salt used in formulating the article. Contains the equivalent of the labeled amount of ranitidine, within ±10%. Meets the requirements for Identification, Antimicrobial preservatives—effectiveness, Microbial limits, pH (6.7–7.5), and Chromatographic purity.
Ranitidine Tablets USP—Preserve in tight, light-resistant containers. Label Tablets to state both the content of the active moiety and the content of the salt used in formulating the article. Contain the labeled amount, within ±10%. Meet the requirements for Identification, Dissolution (80% in 45 minutes in water in Apparatus 2 at 50 rpm), Chromatographic purity, and Uniformity of dosage units.
Ranitidine Hydrochloride USP—Preserve in tight, light-resistant containers. Contains not less than 97.5% and not more than 102.0% of ranitidine hydrochloride, calculated on the dried basis. Meets the requirements for Identification, pH (4.5–6.0, in a solution [1 in 100]), Loss on drying (not more than 0.75%), Residue on ignition (not more than 0.1%), and Chromatographic purity.
Ranitidine Hydrochloride Syrup—Not in USP.

RANITIDINE AND SODIUM CHLORIDE

For *Ranitidine* and *Sodium Chloride*—See individual listings for chemistry information.

USP requirements: Ranitidine in Sodium Chloride Injection USP—Preserve in intact flexible containers meeting the general requirements in Containers, protected from light. Store at a temperature between 2 ° and 25 °C. Do not freeze. A sterile solution of Ranitidine Hydrochloride and Sodium Chloride in Water for Injection. Label Ranitidine in Sodium

Chloride Injection to state both the content of the active moiety and the content of the ranitidine salt used in formulating the article. Contains the labeled amounts of both ranitidine and sodium chloride, within ±10%. Meets the requirements for Identification, Bacterial endotoxins, pH (6.7–7.3), Chromatographic purity, and Injections.

RAUWOLFIA SERPENTINA

Description: Powdered rauwolfia serpentina—Light tan to light brown powder.

Solubility: Powdered rauwolfia serpentina—Slightly soluble in water; sparingly soluble in alcohol.

USP requirements:

Rauwolfia Serpentina USP—Preserve in well-closed containers, and store at controlled room temperature, in a dry place, secure against insect attack. The dried root of *Rauwolfia serpentina* (Linné) Bentham ex Kurz (Fam. Apocynaceae), sometimes having fragments of rhizome and aerial stem bases attached. Contains not less than 0.15% of reserpine-rescinnamine group alkaloids, calculated as reserpine. Meets the requirements for Botanic characteristics, Loss on drying (not more than 12.0%), Microbial limit, Acid-insoluble ash (not more than 2.0%), Stems and other foreign organic matter (not more than 2.0% of stems and not more than 3.0% of other foreign organic matter), and Chemical identification.

Powdered Rauwolfia Serpentina USP—Preserve in well-closed containers, and store at controlled room temperature, in a dry place, secure against insect attack. It is Rauwolfia Serpentina reduced to a fine or a very fine powder, and adjusted, if necessary, to conform to the requirements for reserpine-rescinnamine group alkaloids by admixture with lactose or starch or with a powdered rauwolfia serpentina containing a higher or lower content of these alkaloids. Contains not less than 0.15% and not more than 0.20% of reserpine-rescinnamine group alkaloids, calculated as reserpine. Meets the requirements for Identification, Microbial limit, and Acid-insoluble ash (not more than 2.0%).

Rauwolfia Serpentina Tablets USP—Preserve in tight, light-resistant containers. Contain an amount of reserpine-rescinnamine group alkaloids, calculated as reserpine, equivalent to not less than 0.15% and not more than 0.20% of the labeled amount of powdered rauwolfia serpentina. Meet the requirements for Identification, Microbial limit, Disintegration (1 hour, with disks using simulated gastric fluid TS, without enzyme), and Uniformity of dosage units.

RAUWOLFIA SERPENTINA AND BENDROFLUMETHIAZIDE

For *Rauwolfia Serpentina* and *Bendroflumethiazide*—See individual listings for chemistry information.

USP requirements: Rauwolfia Serpentina and Bendroflumethiazide Tablets—Not in USP.

PURIFIED RAYON

Description: Purified Rayon USP—White, lustrous or dull, fine, soft, filamentous fibers, appearing under the microscope as round, oval, or slightly flattened translucent rods, straight or crimped, striate and with serrate cross-sectional edges. Is practically odorless.

Solubility: Purified Rayon USP—Very soluble in ammoniated cupric oxide TS and in dilute sulfuric acid (3 in 5); insoluble in ordinary solvents.

USP requirements: Purified Rayon USP—A fibrous form of bleached, regenerated cellulose. May contain not more than 1.25% of titanium dioxide. Meets the requirements for Alkalinity or acidity, Residue on ignition (not more than 1.50%, from 5.0 grams), Acid-insoluble ash (not more than 1.25%), Water-soluble substances (not more than 1.0%), and Fiber length and absorbency, and for Dyes and Other foreign matter under Purified Cotton.

ORAL REHYDRATION SALTS

For *Dextrose, Potassium Chloride, Sodium Bicarbonate, Sodium Chloride,* and *Sodium Citrate*—See individual listings for chemistry information.

USP requirements: Oral Rehydration Salts USP (For Oral Solution)—Preserve in tight containers, and avoid exposure to temperatures in excess of 30 °C. The Sodium Bicarbonate or Sodium Citrate component may be omitted from the mixture and packaged in a separate, accompanying container. A dry mixture of Sodium Chloride, Potassium Chloride, Sodium Bicarbonate, and Dextrose (anhydrous). Alternatively, may contain Sodium Citrate (anhydrous or dihydrate) instead of Sodium Bicarbonate. May contain Dextrose (monohydrate) instead of Dextrose (anhydrous), provided that the Sodium Bicarbonate or Sodium Citrate is packaged in a separate, accompanying container. Contains the equivalent of the amounts of sodium, potassium, chloride, and bicarbonate or citrate, calculated from the labeled amounts of Sodium Chloride, Potassium Chloride, and Sodium Bicarbonate (or Sodium Citrate [anhydrous or dihydrate]), within ±10%. Contains the labeled amounts of anhydrous dextrose or dextrose monohydrate, within ±10%. The label indicates prominently whether Sodium Bicarbonate or Sodium Citrate is a component by the placement of the word "Bicarbonate" or "Citrate," as appropriate, in juxtaposition to the official title. The label states the name and quantity, in grams, of each component in each unit-dose container, or in a stated quantity, in grams, of Salts in a multiple-unit container. The label states the net weight in each container, and provides directions for constitution. Where packaged in individual unit-dose pouches, the label instructs the user not to open until the time of use. The label states also that any solution that remains unused 24 hours after constitution is to be discarded. Meets the requirements for Identification, Loss on drying (not more than 1.0%), Minimum fill, and pH (7.0–8.8, in the solution constituted as directed in labeling).

RESERPINE

Chemical source: A crystalline alkaloid derived from *Rauwolfia serpentina*.

Chemical name: Yohimban-16-carboxylic acid, 11,17-dimethoxy-18-[(3,4,5-trimethoxybenzoyl)oxy]-, methyl ester, (3 beta,16 beta,17 alpha,18 beta,20 alpha)-.

Molecular formula: $C_{33}H_{40}N_2O_9$.

Molecular weight: 608.69.

Description: Reserpine USP—White or pale buff to slightly yellowish, odorless, crystalline powder. Darkens slowly on exposure to light, but more rapidly when in solution.

pKa: 6.6.

Solubility: Reserpine USP—Insoluble in water; freely soluble in acetic acid and in chloroform; very slightly soluble in alcohol and in ether.

USP requirements:

Reserpine USP—Preserve in tight, light-resistant containers. Contains not less than 97.0% and not more than 101.0%

of reserpine, calculated on the dried basis. Meets the requirements for Identification, Loss on drying (not more than 0.5%), and Residue on ignition (not more than 0.1%).

Reserpine Elixir USP—Preserve in tight, light-resistant containers. Contains the labeled amount, within ±10%. Meets the requirements for Identification and Alcohol content (11.0–13.0%).

Reserpine Injection USP—Preserve in single-dose (or, if stabilizers are present, in multiple-dose), light-resistant containers, preferably of Type I glass. A sterile solution of Reserpine in Water for Injection, prepared with the aid of a suitable acid. Contains the labeled amount, within ±10%. Contains suitable antioxidants. Meets the requirements for Identification, Bacterial endotoxins, pH (3.0–4.0), Other alkaloids, and Injections.

Reserpine Tablets USP—Preserve in tight, light-resistant containers. Contain the labeled amount, within ±10%. Meet the requirements for Identification, Other alkaloids, Dissolution (75% in 45 minutes in 0.1 *N* acetic acid in Apparatus 1 at 100 rpm), and Uniformity of dosage units.

RESERPINE AND CHLOROTHIAZIDE

For *Reserpine* and *Chlorothiazide*—See individual listings for chemistry information.

USP requirements: Reserpine and Chlorothiazide Tablets USP—Preserve in tight, light-resistant containers. Contain the labeled amount of reserpine, within ±10%, and the labeled amount of chlorothiazide, within ±7%. Meet the requirements for Identification, Dissolution (75% of each active ingredient in 60 minutes in mixture of phosphate buffer [pH 8.0] and *n*-propyl alcohol [3:2] in Apparatus 2 at 75 rpm), and Uniformity of dosage units.

RESERPINE AND CHLORTHALIDONE

For *Reserpine* and *Chlorthalidone*—See individual listings for chemistry information.

USP requirements: Reserpine and Chlorthalidone Tablets—Not in USP.

RESERPINE, HYDRALAZINE, AND HYDROCHLOROTHIAZIDE

For *Reserpine, Hydralazine,* and *Hydrochlorothiazide*—See individual listings for chemistry information.

USP requirements: Reserpine, Hydralazine Hydrochloride, and Hydrochlorothiazide Tablets USP—Preserve in tight, light-resistant containers. Contain the labeled amount of reserpine, within ±10%, and the labeled amounts of hydralazine hydrochloride and hydrochlorothiazide, within ±7%. Meet the requirements for Identification, Disintegration (30 minutes), Uniformity of dosage units, and Diazotizable substances.

Note: Where Reserpine, Hydralazine Hydrochloride, and Hydrochlorothiazide Tablets are prescribed, without reference to the quantity of reserpine, hydralazine hydrochloride, or hydrochlorothiazide contained therein, a product containing 0.1 mg of reserpine, 25 mg of hydralazine hydrochloride, and 15 mg of hydrochlorothiazide shall be dispensed.

RESERPINE AND HYDROCHLOROTHIAZIDE

For *Reserpine* and *Hydrochlorothiazide*—See individual listings for chemistry information.

USP requirements: Reserpine and Hydrochlorothiazide Tablets USP—Preserve in tight, light-resistant containers. Contain the labeled amount of reserpine, within ±10%, and the labeled amount of hydrochlorothiazide, within ±7%. Meet the requirements for Identification, Dissolution (80% of reserpine in 45 minutes and 80% of hydrochlorothiazide in 60 minutes in mixture of 0.1 *N* hydrochloric acid and *n*-propyl alcohol [3:2] in Apparatus 2 at 50 rpm), Diazotizable substances, and Uniformity of dosage units.

RESERPINE AND HYDROFLUMETHIAZIDE

For *Reserpine* and *Hydroflumethiazide*—See individual listings for chemistry information.

USP requirements: Reserpine and Hydroflumethiazide Tablets—Not in USP.

RESERPINE AND METHYCLOTHIAZIDE

For *Reserpine* and *Methyclothiazide*—See individual listings for chemistry information.

USP requirements: Reserpine and Methyclothiazide Tablets—Not in USP.

RESERPINE AND POLYTHIAZIDE

For *Reserpine* and *Polythiazide*—See individual listings for chemistry information.

USP requirements: Reserpine and Polythiazide Tablets—Not in USP.

RESERPINE AND TRICHLORMETHIAZIDE

For *Reserpine* and *Trichlormethiazide*—See individual listings for chemistry information.

USP requirements: Reserpine and Trichlormethiazide Tablets—Not in USP.

RESORCINOL

Chemical name:
Resorcinol—1,3-Benzenediol.
Resorcinol monoacetate—1,3-Benzenediol, monoacetate.

Molecular formula:
Resorcinol—$C_6H_6O_2$.
Resorcinol monoacetate—$C_8H_8O_3$.

Molecular weight:
Resorcinol—110.11.
Resorcinol monoacetate—152.15.

Description:
Resorcinol USP—White, or practically white, needle-shaped crystals or powder. Has a faint, characteristic odor. Acquires a pink tint on exposure to light and air. Its solution (1 in 20) is neutral or acid to litmus.

Resorcinol Monoacetate USP—Viscous, pale yellow or amber liquid, having a faint characteristic odor. Boils at about 283 °C, with decomposition. Its saturated solution is acid to litmus.

Solubility:
Resorcinol USP—Freely soluble in water, in alcohol, in glycerin, and in ether; slightly soluble in chloroform.

Resorcinol Monoacetate USP—Sparingly soluble in water; soluble in alcohol and in most organic solvents.

USP requirements:
Resorcinol USP—Preserve in well-closed, light-resistant containers. Contains not less than 99.0% and not more than 100.5% of resorcinol, calculated on the dried basis. Meets

the requirements for Identification, Melting range (109–111 °C), Loss on drying (not more than 1.0%), Residue on ignition (not more than 0.05%), Phenol, Catechol, Ordinary impurities, and Organic volatile impurities.
Resorcinol Lotion—Not in USP.
Resorcinol Ointment—Not in USP.
Compound Resorcinol Ointment USP—Preserve in tight containers and avoid prolonged exposure to temperatures exceeding 30 °C.

Prepare Compound Resorcinol Ointment as follows: 60 grams of Resorcinol, 60 grams of Zinc Oxide, 60 grams of Bismuth Subnitrate, 20 grams of Juniper Tar, 100 grams of Yellow Wax, 290 grams of Petrolatum, 280 grams of Lanolin, and 130 grams of Glycerin, to make 1000 grams of Compound Resorcinol Ointment. Melt the Yellow Wax and the Lanolin in a dish on a steam bath. Triturate the Zinc Oxide and the Bismuth Subnitrate with the Petrolatum until smooth, and add it to the melted mixture. Dissolve the Resorcinol in the Glycerin, incorporate the solution with the warm mixture just prepared, then add the Juniper Tar, and stir the Ointment until it congeals.

Resorcinol Monoacetate USP—Preserve in tight, light-resistant containers. Meets the requirements for Identification, Specific gravity (1.203–1.207), Acidity, Loss on drying (not more than 2.5%), Residue on ignition (not more than 0.1%), and Organic volatile impurities.

RESORCINOL AND SULFUR

For *Resorcinol* and *Sulfur*—See individual listings for chemistry information.

USP requirements:
Resorcinol and Sulfur Cake—Not in USP.
Resorcinol and Sulfur Cream—Not in USP.
Resorcinol and Sulfur Gel—Not in USP.
Resorcinol and Sulfur Lotion USP—Preserve in tight containers. It is Resorcinol and Sulfur in a suitable hydroalcoholic vehicle. Contains the labeled amount of resorcinol, within ±10%, and the labeled amount of sulfur, within −5% to +10%. Meets the requirements for Identification and Alcohol content (within ±10% of labeled amount).
Resorcinol and Sulfur Stick—Not in USP.

RIBAVIRIN

Chemical group: A synthetic nucleoside; structurally related to inosine, guanosine, and xanthosine.

Chemical name: 1*H*-1,2,4-Triazole-3-carboxamide, 1-beta-D-ribofuranosyl-.

Molecular formula: $C_8H_{12}N_4O_5$.

Molecular weight: 244.21.

Description: Ribavirin USP—White, crystalline powder.

Solubility: Ribavirin USP—Freely soluble in water; slightly soluble in dehydrated alcohol.

USP requirements:
Ribavirin USP—Preserve in tight containers. Contains not less than 98.9% and not more than 101.5% of ribavirin, calculated on the dried basis. Meets the requirements for Identification, Specific rotation (−35.0° to −38.0°, calculated on the dried basis, determined at 20 °C), pH (4.0–6.5, in a solution [1 in 50]), Loss on drying (not more than 0.5%), Residue on ignition (not more than 0.25%), Heavy metals (not more than 0.001%), and Chromatographic purity.
Ribavirin for Injection—Not in USP.
Ribavirin for Inhalation Solution USP—Preserve in tight containers, in a dry place at controlled room temperature. A sterile, freeze-dried form of ribavirin. The labeling indicates that Ribavirin for Inhalation Solution must be constituted with a measured volume of Sterile Water for Injection or with Sterile Water for Inhalation containing no preservatives, and that the constituted solution is to be administered only by a small-particle aerosol generator. When constituted as directed in the labeling, the inhalation solution so obtained contains the labeled amount, within ±5%. Meets the requirements for Identification, Sterility, pH (4.0–6.5, in the solution constituted as directed in the labeling), and Chromatographic purity, and for Specific rotation, Loss on drying, Residue on ignition, and Heavy metals under Ribavirin.
Ribavirin for Oral Solution—Not in USP.

RIBOFLAVIN

Chemical name:
Riboflavin—Riboflavine.
Riboflavin 5′-phosphate sodium—Riboflavin 5′-(dihydrogen phosphate), monosodium salt, dihydrate.

Molecular formula:
Riboflavin—$C_{17}H_{20}N_4O_6$.
Riboflavin 5′-phosphate sodium—$C_{17}H_{20}N_4NaO_9P \cdot 2H_2O$.

Molecular weight:
Riboflavin—376.37.
Riboflavin 5′-phosphate sodium—514.36.

Description:
Riboflavin USP—Yellow to orange-yellow, crystalline powder having a slight odor. Melts at about 280 °C. Its saturated solution is neutral to litmus. When dry, it is not appreciably affected by diffused light, but when in solution, light induces quite rapid deterioration, especially in the presence of alkalies.
Riboflavin 5′-Phosphate Sodium USP—Fine, orange-yellow, crystalline powder, having a slight odor. When dry, it is not affected by diffused light, but when in solution, light induces deterioration rapidly. Is hygroscopic.

pKa: 10.2.

Solubility:
Riboflavin USP—Very slightly soluble in water, in alcohol, and in isotonic sodium chloride solution; soluble in dilute solutions of alkalies; insoluble in ether and in chloroform.
Riboflavin 5′-Phosphate Sodium USP—Sparingly soluble in water.

USP requirements:
Riboflavin USP—Preserve in tight, light-resistant containers. Contains not less than 98.0% and not more than 102.0% of riboflavin, calculated on the dried basis. Meets the requirements for Identification, Specific rotation (+56.5° to +59.5°, calculated on the dried basis), Loss on drying (not more than 1.5%), Residue on ignition (not more than 0.3%), and Lumiflavin.
Riboflavin Injection USP—Preserve in light-resistant, in single-dose or in multiple-dose containers, preferably of Type I glass. A sterile solution of Riboflavin in Water for Injection. Contains the labeled amount, within −5% to +20%. Meets the requirements for Identification, Bacterial endotoxins, pH (4.5–7.0), and Injections.
Riboflavin Tablets USP—Preserve in tight, light-resistant containers. Contain the labeled amount, within −5% to +15%. Meet the requirements for Disintegration (30 minutes) and Uniformity of dosage units.

Riboflavin 5′-Phosphate Sodium USP—Preserve in tight, light-resistant containers. Contains not less than the equivalent of 73.0% and not more than the equivalent of 79.0% of riboflavin, calculated on the dried basis. Meets the requirements for Identification, Specific rotation (+37.0° to +42.0°, calculated on the dried basis), pH (5.0–6.5, in a solution [1 in 100]), Loss on drying (not more than 7.5%), Residue on ignition (not more than 25.0%), Free phosphate, Free riboflavin and riboflavin diphosphates (not more than 6.0% of free riboflavin and not more than 6.0% of riboflavin diphosphates, as riboflavin, calculated on the dried basis), and Lumiflavin.

RICE SYRUP SOLIDS AND ELECTROLYTES

Chemical name:
Sodium chloride—Sodium chloride.
Potassium citrate—1,2,3-Propanetricarboxylic acid, 2-hydroxy-, tripotassium salt, monohydrate.
Sodium citrate—1,2,3-Propanetricarboxylic acid, 2-hydroxy-, trisodium salt.
Citric acid—1,2,3-Propanetricarboxylic acid, 2-hydroxy-.

Molecular formula:
Sodium chloride—NaCl.
Potassium citrate—$C_6H_5K_3O_7 \cdot H_2O$.
Sodium citrate—$C_6H_5Na_3O_7$.
Citric acid—$C_6H_8O_7$ (anhydrous); $C_6H_8O_7 \cdot H_2O$ (monohydrate).

Molecular weight:
Sodium chloride—58.44.
Potassium citrate—324.41.
Sodium citrate—258.07 (anhydrous).
Citric acid—192.13 (anhydrous); 210.14 (monohydrate).

Description:
Sodium Chloride USP—Colorless, cubic crystals or white crystalline powder.
NF category: Tonicity agent.
Potassium Citrate USP—Transparent crystals or white, granular powder. Is odorless and is deliquescent when exposed to moist air.
NF category: Buffering agent.
Sodium Citrate USP—Colorless crystals or white, crystalline powder.
NF category: Buffering agent.
Citric Acid USP—Colorless, translucent crystals, or white, granular to fine crystalline powder. Odorless or practically odorless. The hydrous form is efflorescent in dry air.
NF category: Acidifying agent; buffering agent.

Solubility:
Sodium Chloride USP—Freely soluble in water; and slightly more soluble in boiling water; soluble in glycerin; slightly soluble in alcohol.
Potassium Citrate USP—Freely soluble in water; almost insoluble in alcohol.
Sodium Citrate USP—Hydrous form freely soluble in water and very soluble in boiling water. Insoluble in alcohol.
Citric Acid USP—Very soluble in water; freely soluble in alcohol; sparingly soluble in ether.

USP requirements: Rice Syrup Solids and Electrolytes Solution—Not in USP.

RIFABUTIN

Chemical name: (9*S*,12*E*,14*S*,15*R*,16*S*,17*R*,18*R*,19*R*,20*S*,21*S*,-22*E*,24*Z*)-6,16,18,20-tetrahydroxy-1′-isobutyl-14-methoxy-7,9,15,17,19,21,25-heptamethyl-spiro[9,4-(epoxypentadeca-[1,11,13]trienimino)-2*H*-furo[2′,3′:7,8]naphth[1,2-*d*]imidazole-2,4′-piperidine]-5,10,26-(3*H*,9*H*)-trione-16-acetate.

Molecular formula: $C_{46}H_{62}N_4O_{11}$.

Molecular weight: 847.02.

Description: Red-violet powder.

Solubility: Soluble in chloroform and in methanol; sparingly soluble in ethanol; very slightly soluble in water (0.19 mg/mL).

USP requirements: Rifabutin Capsules—Not in USP.

RIFAMPIN

Source: Semisynthetic derivative of rifamycin B.

Chemical name: Rifamycin, 3-[[(4-methyl-1-piperazinyl)imino]-methyl]-.

Molecular formula: $C_{43}H_{58}N_4O_{12}$.

Molecular weight: 822.95.

Description: Rifampin USP—Red-brown, crystalline powder.

Solubility: Rifampin USP—Very slightly soluble in water; freely soluble in chloroform; soluble in ethyl acetate and in methanol.

USP requirements:
Rifampin USP—Preserve in tight, light-resistant containers, protected from excessive heat. Contains not less than 95.0% and not more than 103.0% of rifampin per mg, calculated on the dried basis. Meets the requirements for Identification, Crystallinity, pH (4.5–6.5, in a suspension [1 in 100]), Loss on drying (not more than 2.0%), and Related substances.
Rifampin Capsules USP—Preserve in tight, light-resistant containers, protected from excessive heat. Contain the labeled amount, within ±10%. Meet the requirements for Identification, Uniformity of dosage units, Dissolution (75% in 45 minutes in 0.1 *N* hydrochloric acid in Apparatus 1 at 50 rpm), and Loss on drying (not more than 3.0%).
Rifampin for Injection USP—Preserve in Containers for Sterile Solids. Contains the labeled amount, within −10% to +15%. Meets the requirements for Identification, Bacterial endotoxins, Sterility, pH (7.8–8.8, in a solution containing 60 mg of rifampin per mL), Water (not more than 1.0%), and Particulate matter.

RIFAMPIN AND ISONIAZID

For *Rifampin* and *Isoniazid*—See individual listings for chemistry information.

USP requirements: Rifampin and Isoniazid Capsules USP—Preserve in tight, light-resistant containers, and avoid exposure to excessive heat. Contain the labeled amount of rifampin, within −10% to +30%, and the labeled amount of isoniazid, within ±10%. Meet the requirement for Loss on drying (not more than 3.0%).
Note: Where Rifampin and Isoniazid Capsules are prescribed without reference to the quantity of rifampin or isoniazid contained therein, a product containing 300 mg of rifampin and 150 mg of isoniazid shall be dispensed.

RIMANTADINE

Chemical name: Rimantadine hydrochloride—Tricyclo-[3.3.1.1^{3,7}]-decane-1-methanamine, alpha-methyl-, hydrochloride.

Molecular formula: Rimantadine hydrochloride—$C_{12}H_{21}N \cdot HCl$.

Molecular weight: Rimantadine hydrochloride—215.77.

Description: Rimantadine hydrochloride—White to off-white crystalline powder.

Solubility: Rimantadine hydrochloride—Freely soluble in water (50 mg/mL at 20 °C).

USP requirements:
Rimantadine Hydrochloride Syrup—Not in USP.
Rimantadine Hydrochloride Tablets—Not in USP.

RINGER'S

For *Sodium Chloride, Potassium Chloride,* and *Calcium Chloride*—See individual listings for chemistry information.

USP requirements:
Ringer's Injection USP—Preserve in single-dose glass or plastic containers. Glass containers are preferably of Type I or Type II glass. A sterile solution of Sodium Chloride, Potassium Chloride, and Calcium Chloride in Water for Injection. The label states the total osmolar concentration in mOsmol per liter. Where the contents are less than 100 mL, the label alternatively may state the total osmolar concentration in mOsmol per mL. Contains, in each 100 mL, not less than 323.0 mg and not more than 354.0 mg of sodium (equivalent to not less than 820.0 mg and not more than 900.0 mg of sodium chloride); not less than 14.9 mg and not more than 16.5 mg of potassium (equivalent to not less than 28.5 mg and not more than 31.5 mg of potassium chloride); not less than 8.20 mg and not more than 9.80 mg of calcium (equivalent to not less than 30.0 mg and not more than 36.0 mg of calcium chloride dihydrate); and not less than 523.0 mg and not more than 580.0 mg of chloride (as sodium chloride, potassium chloride, and calcium chloride dihydrate). Contains no antimicrobial agents.

Prepare Ringer's Injection as follows: Combine 8.6 grams of Sodium Chloride, 0.3 grams of Potassium Chloride, 0.33 grams of Calcium Chloride, and a sufficient quantity of Water for Injection, to make 1000 mL. Dissolve the three salts in the Water for Injection, filter until clear, place in suitable containers, and sterilize.

Meets the requirements for Identification, Bacterial endotoxins, pH (5.0–7.5), Heavy metals (not more than 0.3 ppm), and Injections.

Note: The calcium, chloride, potassium, and sodium ion contents of Ringer's Injection are approximately 4.5, 156, 4, and 147.5 milliequivalents per liter, respectively.

Ringer's Irrigation USP—Preserve in single-dose glass or plastic containers. Glass containers are preferably of Type I or Type II glass. The container may be designed to empty rapidly and may contain a volume of more than 1 liter. It is Ringer's Injection that has been suitably packaged, and it contains no antimicrobial agents. The designation "not for injection" appears prominently on the label. Meets the requirements for Sterility and for Identification tests, pH, and Heavy metals under Ringer's Injection.

RINGER'S AND DEXTROSE

For *Sodium Chloride, Potassium Chloride, Calcium Chloride,* and *Dextrose*—See individual listings for chemistry information.

USP requirements: Ringer's and Dextrose Injection USP—Preserve in single-dose glass or plastic containers. Glass containers are preferably of Type I or Type II glass. A sterile solution of Sodium Chloride, Potassium Chloride, Calcium Chloride, and Dextrose in Water for Injection. The label states the total osmolar concentration in mOsmol per liter. Where the contents are less than 100 mL, the label alternatively may state the total osmolar concentration in mOsmol per mL. The label includes also the warning: "Not for use in the treatment of lactic acidosis." Contains, in each 100 mL, not less than 323.0 mg and not more than 354.0 mg of sodium (equivalent to not less than 820.0 mg and not more than 900.0 mg of sodium chloride), not less than 14.9 mg and not more than 16.5 mg of potassium (equivalent to not less than 28.5 mg and not more than 31.5 mg of potassium chloride), not less than 8.20 mg and not more than 9.80 mg of calcium (equivalent to not less than 30.0 mg and not more than 36.0 mg of calcium chloride dihydrate), and not less than 523.0 mg and not more than 608.5 mg of chloride (as sodium choride, potassium chloride, and calcium chloride dihydrate). Contains the labeled amount of dextrose, within ±5%. Contains no antimicrobial agents. Meets the requirements for Identification, Bacterial endotoxins, pH (3.5–6.5), 5-Hydroxymethylfurfural and related substances, Heavy metals, and Injections.

Note: The calcium, chloride, potassium, and sodium ion contents of Ringer's and Dextrose Injection are approximately 4.5, 156, 4, and 147.5 milliequivalents per liter, respectively.

LACTATED RINGER'S

For *Calcium Chloride, Potassium Chloride, Sodium Chloride,* and *Sodium Lactate*—See individual listings for chemistry information.

USP requirements: Lactated Ringer's Injection USP—Preserve in single-dose glass or plastic containers. Glass containers are preferably of Type I or Type II glass. A sterile solution of Calcium Chloride, Potassium Chloride, Sodium Chloride, and Sodium Lactate in Water for Injection. The label states the total osmolar concentration in mOsmol per liter. Where the contents are less than 100 mL, the label alternatively may state the total osmolar concentration in mOsmol per mL. The label includes also the warning: "Not for use in the treatment of lactic acidosis." Contains, in each 100 mL, not less than 285.0 mg and not more than 315.0 mg of sodium (as sodium chloride and sodium lactate), not less than 14.1 mg and not more than 17.3 mg of potassium (equivalent to not less than 27.0 mg and not more than 33.0 mg of potassium chloride), not less than 4.90 mg and not more than 6.00 mg of calcium (equivalent to not less than 18.0 mg and not more than 22.0 mg of calcium chloride dihydrate), not less than 368.0 mg and not more than 408.0 mg of chloride (as sodium chloride, potassium chloride, and calcium chloride dihydrate), and not less than 231.0 mg and not more than 261.0 mg of lactate (equivalent to not less than 290.0 mg and not more than 330.0 mg of sodium lactate). Contains no antimicrobial agents. Meets the requirements for Identification, Bacterial endotoxins, pH (6.0–7.5), Heavy metals (not more than 0.3 ppm), and Injections.

Note: The calcium, potassium, and sodium contents of Lactated Ringer's Injection are approximately 2.7, 4, and 130 milliequivalents per liter, respectively.

LACTATED RINGER'S AND DEXTROSE

For *Calcium Chloride, Potassium Chloride, Sodium Chloride, Sodium Lactate,* and *Dextrose*—See individual listings for chemistry information.

USP requirements:
Lactated Ringer's and Dextrose Injection USP—Preserve in single-dose glass or plastic containers. Glass containers are preferably of Type I or Type II glass. A sterile solution of Calcium Chloride, Potassium Chloride, Sodium Chloride, Sodium Lactate, and Dextrose in Water for Injection. The label states the total osmolar concentration in

mOsmol per liter. Where the contents are less than 100 mL, the label alternatively may state the total osmolar concentration in mOsmol per mL. The label includes also the warning: "Not for use in the treatment of lactic acidosis." Contains, in each 100 mL, not less than 285.0 mg and not more than 315.0 mg of sodium (as sodium chloride and sodium lactate), not less than 14.1 mg and not more than 17.3 mg of potassium (equivalent to not less than 27.0 mg and not more than 33.0 mg of potassium chloride), not less than 4.90 mg and not more than 6.00 mg of calcium (equivalent to not less than 18.0 mg and not more than 22.0 mg of calcium chloride dihydrate), not less than 368.0 mg and not more than 428.0 mg of chloride (as sodium chloride, potassium chloride, and calcium chloride dihydrate), and not less than 231.0 mg and not more than 261.0 mg of lactate (equivalent to not less than 290.0 mg and not more than 330.0 mg of sodium lactate). Contains the labeled amount of dextrose, within ±5%. Contains no antimicrobial agents. Meets the requirements for Identification, Bacterial endotoxins, pH (4.0–6.5), 5-Hydroxymethylfurfural and related substances, Heavy metals, and Injections.

Note: The calcium, potassium, and sodium contents of Lactated Ringer's and Dextrose Injection are approximately 2.7, 4, and 130 milliequivalents per liter, respectively.

Half-strength Lactated Ringer's and Dextrose Injection USP—Preserve in single-dose glass or plastic containers. Glass containers are preferably of Type I or Type II glass. A sterile solution of Calcium Chloride, Potassium Chloride, Sodium Chloride, Sodium Lactate, and Dextrose in Water for Injection. The label states the total osmolar concentration in mOsmol per liter. Where the contents are less than 100 mL, the label alternatively may state the total osmolar concentration in mOsmol per mL. The label includes also the warning: "Not for use in the treatment of lactic acidosis." Contains, in each 100 mL, not less than 142.5 mg and not more than 157.5 mg of sodium (as sodium chloride and sodium lactate), not less than 7.05 mg and not more than 8.65 mg of potassium (equivalent to not less than 13.5 mg and not more than 16.5 mg of potassium chloride), not less than 2.45 mg and not more than 3.00 mg of calcium (equivalent to not less than 9.0 mg and not more than 11.0 mg of calcium chloride dihydrate), not less than 184.0 mg and not more than 214.0 mg of chloride (as sodium chloride, potassium chloride, and calcium chloride dihydrate), and not less than 115.5 mg and not more than 130.5 mg of lactate (equivalent to not less than 145.0 mg and not more than 165.0 mg of sodium lactate). Contains the labeled amount of dextrose, within ±5%. Contains no antimicrobial agents. Meets the requirements for Identification, Bacterial endotoxins, pH (4.0–6.5), Heavy metals, 5-Hydroxymethylfurfural and related substances, and Injections.

Note: The calcium, potassium, and sodium contents of Half-strength Lactated Ringer's and Dextrose Injection are approximately 1.4, 2, and 65 milliequivalents per liter, respectively.

Modified Lactated Ringer's and Dextrose Injection USP—Preserve in single-dose glass or plastic containers. Glass containers are preferably of Type I or Type II glass. A sterile solution of Calcium Chloride, Potassium Chloride, Sodium Chloride, Sodium Lactate, and Dextrose in Water for Injection. The label states the total osmolar concentration in mOsmol per liter. Where the contents are less than 100 mL, the label alternatively may state the total osmolar concentration in mOsmol per mL. The label includes also the warning: "Not for use in the treatment of lactic acidosis." Contains, in each 100 mL, not less than 57.0 mg and not more than 63.0 mg of sodium (as sodium chloride and sodium lactate), not less than 2.82 mg and not more than 3.46 mg of potassium (equivalent to not less than 5.4 mg and not more than 6.6 mg of potassium chloride), not less than 0.98 mg and not more than 1.20 mg of calcium (equivalent to not less than 3.6 mg and not more than 4.4 mg of calcium chloride dihydrate), not less than 73.6 mg and not more than 85.6 mg of chloride (as sodium chloride, potassium chloride, and calcium chloride dihydrate), and not less than 46.2 mg and not more than 52.20 mg of lactate (equivalent to not less than 58.0 mg and not more than 66.0 mg of sodium lactate). Contains the labeled amount of dextrose, within ±5%. Contains no antimicrobial agents. Meets the requirements for Identification, Bacterial endotoxins, pH (4.0–6.5), Heavy metals, 5-Hydroxymethylfurfural and related substances, and Injections.

Note: The calcium, potassium, and sodium contents of Modified Lactated Ringer's and Dextrose Injection are approximately 0.5, 0.8, and 26 milliequivalents per liter, respectively.

RISPERIDONE

Chemical group: Benzisoxazole derivative.

Chemical name: 4*H*-Pyrido[1,2-*a*]pyrimidin-4-one, 3-[2-[4-(6-fluoro-1,2-benzisoxazol-3-yl)-1-piperidinyl]ethyl]-6,7,8,9-tetrahydro-2-methyl-.

Molecular formula: $C_{23}H_{27}FN_4O_2$.

Molecular weight: 410.49.

Description: Slightly beige to almost white powder. Melting point 169–173 °C.

Solubility: Practically insoluble in water (pH 8.7); freely soluble in dichloromethane; soluble in methanol and in 0.1 *N* hydrochloric acid.

USP requirements: Risperidone Tablets—Not in USP.

RITODRINE

Chemical name: Ritodrine hydrochloride—Benzenemethanol, 4-hydroxy-alpha-[1-[[2-(4-hydroxyphenyl)ethyl]amino]ethyl]-, hydrochloride, (*R**, *S**)-.

Molecular formula: Ritodrine hydrochloride—$C_{17}H_{21}NO_3 \cdot HCl$.

Molecular weight: Ritodrine hydrochloride—323.82.

Description: Ritodrine Hydrochloride USP—White to nearly white, odorless or practically odorless, crystalline powder. Melts at about 200 °C.

Solubility: Ritodrine Hydrochloride USP—Freely soluble in water and in alcohol; soluble in *n*-propyl alcohol; practically insoluble in ether.

USP requirements:

Ritodrine Hydrochloride USP—Preserve in tight containers. Contains not less than 97.0% and not more than 103.0% of ritodrine hydrochloride, calculated on the dried basis. Meets the requirements for Identification, pH (4.5–6.0, in a solution [1 in 50]), Loss on drying (not more than 1.0%), Residue on ignition (not more than 0.2%), Heavy metals (not more than 0.002%), Related compounds, and Organic volatile impurities.

Ritodrine Hydrochloride Injection USP—Preserve in single-dose containers, preferably of Type I glass. Store at room temperature, preferably below 30 °C. A sterile solution of Ritodrine Hydrochloride in Water for Injection. Contains the labeled amount, within ±10%. Meets the requirements for Identification, Bacterial endotoxins, pH (4.8–5.5), and Injections.

Ritodrine Hydrochloride Tablets USP—Preserve in tight containers. Store at room temperature, preferably below 30 °C. Contain the labeled amount, within ±10%. Meet the requirements for Identification, Dissolution (80% in 30 minutes in 0.1 *N* hydrochloric acid in Apparatus 2 at 50 rpm), and Uniformity of dosage units.

ROLITETRACYCLINE

Chemical name: 2-Naphthacenecarboxamide, 4-(dimethylamino)-1,4,4a,5,5a,6,11,12a-octahydro-3,6,10,12,12a-pentahydroxy-6-methyl-1,11-dioxo-*N*-(1-pyrrolidinylmethyl)-, [4*S*-(4 alpha,-4a alpha,5a alpha,6 beta,12a alpha)]-.

Molecular formula: $C_{27}H_{33}N_3O_8$.

Molecular weight: 527.57.

Description: Sterile Rolitetracycline USP—Light yellow, crystalline powder, having a characteristic, musty, amine-like odor.

Solubility: Sterile Rolitetracycline USP—Soluble in water and in acetone; slightly soluble in dehydrated alcohol; very slightly soluble in ether.

USP requirements:

Rolitetracycline for Injection USP—Preserve in Containers for Sterile Solids, protected from light. A sterile dry mixture of Sterile Rolitetracycline and one or more suitable buffers, and if intended for intramuscular use, one or more suitable anesthetics. Contains the labeled amount, within −10% to +15%. Meets the requirements for Constituted solution, Depressor substances (exempt from this requirement when intended for intramuscular use only), Bacterial endotoxins, Sterility, pH (3.0–4.5, in the solution constituted as directed in the labeling), and Loss on drying (not more than 5.0%).

Sterile Rolitetracycline USP—Preserve in Containers for Sterile Solids, protected from light. It is rolitetracycline suitable for parenteral use. Has a potency of not less than 900 mcg of rolitetracycline per mg, calculated on the anhydrous basis. Meets the requirements for Identification, Crystallinity, Depressor substances, Bacterial endotoxins, Sterility, pH (7–9, in a solution containing 10 mg per mL), and Water (not more than 3.0%).

ROSE OIL

Description: Rose Oil NF—Colorless or yellow liquid, having the characteristic odor of rose. At 25 °C it is a viscous liquid. Upon gradual cooling, it changes to a translucent, crystalline mass, easily liquefied by warming.

NF category: Flavors and perfumes.

NF requirements: Rose Oil NF—Preserve in well-filled, tight containers. A volatile oil distilled with steam from the fresh flowers of *Rosa gallica* Linné, *Rosa damascena* Miller, *Rosa alba* Linné, *Rosa centifolia* Linné, and varieties of these species (Fam. Rosaceae). Meets the requirements for Solubility test (1 mL is miscible with 1 mL of chloroform without turbidity. Add 20 mL of 90% alcohol to this mixture: the resulting liquid is neutral or acid to moistened litmus paper and, upon standing at 20 °C, deposits crystals within 5 minutes), Specific gravity (0.848–0.863 at 30 °C compared with water at 15 °C), Angular rotation (−1° to −4° when determined in a 100-mm tube), and Refractive index (1.457–1.463 at 30 °C).

ROSE WATER OINTMENT

Description: Rose Water Ointment USP—NF category: Ointment base.

USP requirements: Rose Water Ointment USP—Preserve in tight, light-resistant containers.

Prepare Rose Water Ointment as follows: 125 grams of Cetyl Esters Wax, 120 grams of White Wax, 560 grams of Almond Oil, 5 grams of Sodium Borate, 25 mL of Stronger Rose Water, 165 mL of Purified Water, and 200 microliters of Rose Oil, to make about 1000 grams of Rose Water Ointment. Reduce the cetyl esters wax and the white wax to small pieces, melt them on a steam bath, add the almond oil, and continue heating until the temperature of the mixture reaches 70 °C. Dissolve the sodium borate in the purified water and the stronger rose water, warmed to 70 °C, and gradually add the warm aqueous phase to the melted oil phase, stirring rapidly and continuously until it has cooled to about 45 °C. Then incorporate the rose oil.

Note: Rose Water Ointment is free from rancidity. If the Ointment has been chilled, warm it slightly before attempting to incorporate other ingredients.

STRONGER ROSE WATER

Description: Stronger Rose Water NF—Practically colorless and clear, having the pleasant odor of fresh rose blossoms. It is free from empyreuma, mustiness, and fungal growths.

NF category: Flavors and perfumes.

NF requirements: Stronger Rose Water NF—The odor of Stronger Rose Water is best preserved by allowing a limited access of fresh air to the container. A saturated solution of the odoriferous principles of the flowers of *Rosa centifolia* Linné (Fam. Rosaceae) prepared by distilling the fresh flowers with water and separating the excess volatile oil from the clear, water portion of the distillate. Meets the requirements for Reaction (neutral or acid to litmus), Residue on evaporation (not more than 0.015%), Heavy metals (not more than 2 ppm), and Organic volatile impurities.

Note: Stronger Rose Water, diluted with an equal volume of purified water, may be supplied when "Rose Water" is required.

RUBELLA AND MUMPS VIRUS VACCINE LIVE

Description: Rubella and Mumps Virus Vaccine Live USP—Solid having the characteristic appearance of substances dried from the frozen state. The Vaccine is to be constituted with a suitable diluent just prior to use. Constituted vaccine undergoes loss of potency on exposure to sunlight.

USP requirements: Rubella and Mumps Virus Vaccine Live USP—Preserve in single-dose containers, or in light-resistant, multiple-dose containers, at a temperature between 2 and 8 °C. Multiple-dose containers for 50 doses are adapted for use only in jet injectors, and those for 10 doses for use by jet or syringe injection. A bacterially sterile preparation of a combination of live rubella virus and live mumps virus such that each component is prepared in conformity with and meets the requirements for Rubella Virus Vaccine Live, and for Mumps Virus Vaccine Live, whichever is applicable. Label the Vaccine in multiple-dose containers to indicate that the contents are intended solely for use by jet injector or for use by either jet or syringe injection, whichever is applicable. Label the Vaccine in single-dose containers, if such containers are not light-resistant, to state that it should be protected from sunlight. Label it also to state that constituted Vaccine should be discarded if not used within 8 hours. Meets the requirement for Expiration date (1 to 2 years, depending on the manufacturer's data, after date of issue from manufacturer's cold storage [−20 °C, 1 year]). Conforms to the regulations of the U.S. Food and Drug Administration concerning biologics.

RUBELLA VIRUS VACCINE LIVE

Source:

The vaccine currently available in the U.S. contains a sterile, lyophilized preparation of live, attenuated Wistar Institute RA 27/3 strain of rubella virus. The virus is propagated in human diploid (WI-38) cell culture.

The vaccines currently available in Canada also contain the RA 27/3 strain of rubella virus.

Description: Rubella Virus Vaccine Live USP—Solid having the characteristic appearance of substances dried from the frozen state. Undergoes loss of potency on exposure to sunlight. The vaccine is to be constituted with a suitable diluent just prior to use.

Other characteristics: Slightly acidic, pH 6.2 to 6.6.

USP requirements: Rubella Virus Vaccine Live USP—Preserve in single-dose containers, or in light-resistant, multiple-dose containers, at a temperature between 2 and 8 °C. Multiple-dose containers for 50 doses are adapted for use only in jet injectors, and those for 10 doses for use by jet or syringe injection. A bacterially sterile preparation of live virus derived from a strain of rubella virus that has been tested for neurovirulence in monkeys, and for immunogenicity, that is free from all demonstrable viable microbial agents except unavoidable bacteriophage, and that has been found suitable for human immunization. The strain is grown, for purposes of vaccine production, on primary cell cultures of duck embryo tissue, derived from pathogen-free flocks, or on primary cell cultures of a designated strain of human tissue, provided that the same cell culture system is used as that in which the strain was tested. The strain meets the requirements of the specific safety tests in adult and suckling mice; and the requirements of the tests in monkey kidney, chicken embryo, and human tissue cell cultures and embryonated eggs. In the case of virus grown in duck embryo cell cultures, the strain meets the requirements of the test by inoculation of embryonated duck eggs, and of the tests for absence of *Mycobacterium tuberculosis* and of avian leucosis. In the case of virus grown in rabbit kidney cell cultures, the strain meets the requirements of the tests by inoculation of rabbits and guinea pigs, and of the tests for absence of *Mycobacterium tuberculosis* and of known adventitious agents of rabbits. In the case of virus grown in human tissue cell cultures, the strain meets the requirements of the specific safety tests and tests for absence of *Mycobacterium tuberculosis* or other adventitious agents tests by inoculation of rabbits and guinea pigs and the requirements for karyology and of the tests for absence of adventitious and other infective agents, including hemadsorption viruses and *Mycoplasma,* in human diploid cell cultures. The strain cultures are treated to remove all intact tissue cells. The Vaccine meets the requirements of the specific tissue culture test for live virus titer, in a single immunizing dose, of not less than the equivalent of 1000 $TCID_{50}$ (quantity of virus estimated to infect 50% of inoculated cultures × 1000) when tested in parallel with the U.S. Reference Rubella Virus, Live. Label the Vaccine in multiple-dose containers to indicate that the contents are intended solely for use by jet injector or for use by either jet or syringe injection, whichever is applicable. Label the Vaccine in single-dose containers, if such containers are not light-resistant, to state that it should be protected from sunlight. Label it also to state that constituted Vaccine should be discarded if not used within 8 hours. Meets the requirement for Expiration date (1 to 2 years, depending on the manufacturer's data, after date of issue from manufacturer's cold storage [−20 °C, 1 year]). Conforms to the regulations of the U.S. Food and Drug Administration concerning biologics.

RUBIDIUM RB 82

Chemical name: Rubidium chloride Rb 82—Rubidium chloride ($^{82}RbCl$).

Molecular formula: Rubidium chloride Rb 82—$Cl^{82}Rb$.

USP requirements: Rubidium Chloride Rb 82 Injection USP—Requirements for packaging, storage, and labeling do not apply; Rubidium Chloride Rb 82 Injection is obtained by elution from the generator and is administered by direct infusion. A sterile solution, suitable for intravenous administration. Contains the labeled amount of ^{82}Rb, within ±10%, expressed in megabecquerels (or in millicuries) per mL at the time indicated in the labeling. Obtained by elution from a strontium 82-rubidium 82 generator system. ^{82}Rb, with a half-life of 76 seconds, is a short-lived positron-emitting radionuclide formed by the radioactive decay of the parent nuclide ^{82}Sr. Strontium Sr 82 with a half-life of 25.5 days is produced by the proton irradiation of rubidium or spallation of molybdenum. The chemical form of the Injection is $^{82}RbCl$. (Note: Elute with additive-free Sodium Chloride Injection only. Discard the first 50 mL of the eluate each day the generator is eluted.) Meets the requirements for Bacterial endotoxins, Radionuclide identification, pH (4.0–8.0), Radionuclidic purity, and Chemical purity, and for Injections (except that the Injection may be distributed or dispensed prior to completion of the test for Sterility, the latter test being started on the day of final manufacture, and except that it is not subject to the recommendation for Volume in Container under Injections).

SACCHARIN

Chemical name:

Saccharin—1,2-Benzisothiazol-3(2*H*)-one, 1,1-dioxide.

Saccharin calcium—1,2-Benzisothiazol-3(2*H*)-one, 1,1-dioxide, calcium salt, hydrate (2:7).

Saccharin sodium—1,2-Benzisothiazol-3(2*H*)-one, 1,1-dioxide, sodium salt, dihydrate.

Molecular formula:

Saccharin—$C_7H_5NO_3S$.

Saccharin calcium—$C_{14}H_8CaN_2O_6S_2 \cdot 3\frac{1}{2}H_2O$.

Saccharin sodium—$C_7H_4NNaO_3S \cdot 2H_2O$.

Molecular weight:

Saccharin—183.18.

Saccharin calcium—467.48.

Saccharin sodium—241.19.

Description:

Saccharin NF—White crystals or white crystalline powder. Odorless or has a faint, aromatic odor. Its solutions are acid to litmus.

NF category: Sweetening agent.

Saccharin Calcium USP—White crystals or white, crystalline powder. Odorless or has a faint aromatic odor.

NF category: Sweetening agent.

Saccharin Sodium USP—White crystals or white crystalline powder. Odorless or has a faint aromatic odor. When in powdered form it usually contains about ⅓ the theoretical amount of water of hydration as a result of efflorescence.

NF category: Sweetening agent.

Solubility:
Saccharin NF—Slightly soluble in water, in chloroform, and in ether; soluble in boiling water; sparingly soluble in alcohol. Readily dissolved by dilute solutions of ammonia, by solutions of alkali hydroxides, and by solutions of alkali carbonates with the evolution of carbon dioxide.
Saccharin Calcium USP—Freely soluble in water.
Saccharin Sodium USP—Freely soluble in water; sparingly soluble in alcohol.

USP requirements:
Saccharin Calcium USP—Preserve in well-closed containers. Where the quantity of saccharin calcium is indicated in the labeling of any preparation containing Saccharin Calcium, this shall be expressed in terms of saccharin. Contains not less than 98.0% and not more than 101.0% of saccharin calcium, calculated on the anhydrous basis. Meets the requirements for Identification, Water (not more than 15.0%), Benzoate and salicylate, Arsenic (not more than 3 ppm), Selenium (not more than 0.003%), Toluenesulfonamides (not more than 0.0025%), Heavy metals (not more than 0.001%), Readily carbonizable substances, and Organic volatile impurities.
Saccharin Sodium USP—Preserve in well-closed containers. Where the quantity of saccharin sodium is indicated in the labeling of any preparation containing Saccharin Sodium, this shall be expressed in terms of saccharin. Contains not less than 98.0% and not more than 101.0% of saccharin sodium, calculated on the anhydrous basis. Meets the requirements for Identification, Alkalinity, Toluenesulfonamides (not more than 0.0025%), and Heavy metals (not more than 0.001%), and for Identification tests, Water, Benzoate and salicylate, Arsenic, Selenium, and Readily carbonizable substances under Saccharin Calcium.
Saccharin Sodium Oral Solution USP—Preserve in tight containers. Contains an amount of saccharin sodium equivalent to the labeled amount of saccharin, within ±5%. Meets the requirements for Identification and pH (3.0–5.0).
Saccharin Sodium Tablets USP—Preserve in well-closed containers. Contain an amount of saccharin sodium equivalent to the labeled amount of saccharin, within −5% to +10%. Meet the requirements for Completeness of solution, Identification, and Ammonium salts.

NF requirements: Saccharin NF—Preserve in well-closed containers. Contains not less than 98.0% and not more than 101.0% of saccharin, calculated on the dried basis. Meets the requirements for Identification, Melting range (226–230 °C), Loss on drying (not more than 1.0%), Residue on ignition (not more than 0.2%), Toluenesulfonamides (not more than 0.0025%), Arsenic (not more than 3 ppm), Selenium (not more than 0.003%), Heavy metals (not more than 0.001%), Readily carbonizable substances, Benzoic and salicylic acids, and Organic volatile impurities.

SAFFLOWER OIL

Description: Safflower Oil USP—Light yellow oil. Thickens and becomes rancid on prolonged exposure to air.
NF category: Vehicle (oleaginous).

Solubility: Safflower Oil USP—Insoluble in water. Miscible with ether and with chloroform.

USP requirements: Safflower Oil USP—Preserve in tight, light-resistant containers. The refined fixed oil obtained from the seed of *Carthamus tinctorius* Linné (Fam. Compositae). Meets the requirements for Fatty acid composition, Free fatty acids, Iodine value (135–150), Heavy metals (not more than 0.001%), Unsaponifiable matter (not more than 1.5%), and Peroxide (not more than 10.0).

SALICYLAMIDE

Chemical name: Benzamide, 2-hydroxy-.

Molecular formula: $C_7H_7NO_2$.

Molecular weight: 137.14.

Description: Salicylamide USP—White, practically odorless, crystalline powder.

Solubility: Salicylamide USP—Slightly soluble in water and in chloroform; soluble in alcohol and in propylene glycol; freely soluble in ether and in solutions of alkalies.

USP requirements: Salicylamide USP—Preserve in well-closed containers. Contains not less than 98.0% and not more than 102.0% of salicylamide, calculated on the anhydrous basis. Meets the requirements for Identification, Melting range (139–142 °C), Water (not more than 0.5%), Residue on ignition (not more than 0.1%), Heavy metals (not more than 0.001%), Chromatographic purity, and Organic volatile impurities.

SALICYLIC ACID

Chemical name: Benzoic acid, 2-hydroxy-.

Molecular formula: $C_7H_6O_3$.

Molecular weight: 138.12.

Description: Salicylic Acid USP—White crystals, usually in fine needles, or fluffy, white, crystalline powder. Is stable in air. The synthetic form is white and odorless. When prepared from natural methyl salicylate, it may have a slightly yellow or pink tint, and a faint, mint-like odor.

Solubility: Salicylic Acid USP—Slightly soluble in water; freely soluble in alcohol and in ether; soluble in boiling water; sparingly soluble in chloroform.

USP requirements:
Salicylic Acid USP—Preserve in well-closed containers. Contains not less than 99.5% and not more than 101.0% of salicylic acid, calculated on the dried basis. Meets the requirements for Identification, Melting range (158–161 °C), Loss on drying (not more than 0.5%), Residue on ignition (not more than 0.05%), Chloride (not more than 0.014%), Sulfate, Heavy metals, and Related compounds.
Salicylic Acid Collodion USP—Preserve in tight containers at controlled room temperature, remote from fire. Contains not less than 9.5% and not more than 11.5% of salicylic acid.
Prepare Salicylic Acid Collodion as follows: 100 grams of Salicylic Acid and a sufficient quantity of Flexible Collodion to make 1000 mL. Dissolve the Salicylic Acid in about 750 mL of Flexible Collodion, add sufficient of the latter to make the product measure 1000 mL, and mix.
Salicylic Acid Cream—Not in USP.
Salicylic Acid Topical Foam USP—Preserve in tight containers. Contains the labeled amount, within ±10%. Meets the requirements for Identification and pH (5.0–6.0).
Salicylic Acid Gel USP—Preserve in collapsible tubes or in tight containers, preferably at controlled room temperature. It is Salicylic Acid in a suitable viscous hydrophilic vehicle. Contains the labeled amount, within ±10%. Meets the requirements for Identification and Alcohol content (if present, within ±10% of labeled amount).

Salicylic Acid Lotion—Not in USP.
Salicylic Acid Ointment—Not in USP.
Salicylic Acid Pads—Not in USP.
Salicylic Acid Plaster USP—Preserve in well-closed containers, preferably at controlled room temperature. A uniform mixture of Salicylic Acid in a suitable base, spread on paper, cotton cloth, or other suitable backing material. The plaster mass contains the labeled amount, within ± 10%.
Salicylic Acid Shampoo—Not in USP.
Salicylic Acid Soap—Not in USP.
Salicylic Acid Topical Solution—Not in USP.

SALICYLIC ACID AND SULFUR

For *Salicylic Acid* and *Sulfur*—See individual listings for chemistry information.

USP requirements:
Salicylic Acid and Sulfur Cream—Not in USP.
Salicylic Acid and Sulfur Cleansing Cream—Not in USP.
Salicylic Acid and Sulfur Lotion—Not in USP.
Salicylic Acid and Sulfur Cleansing Lotion—Not in USP.
Salicylic Acid and Sulfur Cream Shampoo—Not in USP.
Salicylic Acid and Sulfur Lotion Shampoo—Not in USP.
Salicylic Acid and Sulfur Suspension Shampoo—Not in USP.
Salicylic Acid and Sulfur Bar Soap—Not in USP.
Salicylic Acid and Sulfur Cleansing Suspension—Not in USP.
Salicylic Acid and Sulfur Topical Suspension—Not in USP.

SALICYLIC ACID, SULFUR, AND COAL TAR

For *Salicylic Acid, Sulfur,* and *Coal Tar*—See individual listings for chemistry information.

USP requirements:
Salicylic Acid, Sulfur, and Coal Tar Cream Shampoo—Not in USP.
Salicylic Acid, Sulfur, and Coal Tar Lotion Shampoo—Not in USP.

SALMETEROL

Chemical name: Salmeterol xinafoate—1,3-Benzenedimethanol, 4-hydroxy-alpha[1]-[[[6-(4-phenylbutoxy)hexyl]amino]-methyl]-, (±)-, 1-hydroxy-2-naphthalenecarboxylate (salt).

Molecular formula: Salmeterol xinafoate—$C_{25}H_{37}NO_4 \cdot C_{11}H_8O_3$.

Molecular weight: Salmeterol xinafoate—603.76.

Description: Salmeterol xinafoate—White to off-white powder.

Solubility: Salmeterol xinafoate—Freely soluble in methanol; slightly soluble in ethanol, in chloroform, and in isopropanol; sparingly soluble in water.

USP requirements: Salmeterol Xinafoate Inhalation Aerosol—Not in USP.

SALSALATE

Chemical name: Benzoic acid, 2-hydroxy-, 2-carboxyphenyl ester.

Molecular formula: $C_{14}H_{10}O_5$.

Molecular weight: 258.23.

Description: Odorless or almost odorless, white or almost white powder.

Solubility: Very slightly soluble in water; soluble 1 in 6 of alcohol, 1 in 8 of chloroform, and 1 in 12 of ether.

USP requirements:
Salsalate USP—Preserve in tight containers. Contains not less than 98.0% and not more than 102.0% of total salicylates, expressed as the sum of the percentages of salsalate, salicylic acid, and trisalicylic acid, calculated on the dried basis. Meets the requirements for Identification, Loss on drying (not more than 0.5%), Residue on ignition (not more than 0.10%), Chloride (not more than 0.01%), Sulfate (not more than 0.05%), Heavy metals (not more than 0.001%), Dimethylaniline (not more than 0.01%), Isopropyl, ethyl, and methyl salicylates, Related substances (not more than 0.5% of salicylic acid and not more than 2.5% of trisalicylic acid), Chromatographic purity, and Organic volatile impurities.
Salsalate Capsules USP—Preserve in tight containers. Contain the labeled amount, within ± 10%. Meet the requirements for Identification, Disintegration (30 minutes, simulated gastric fluid TS [without pepsin] being used), Uniformity of dosage units, and Limit of salicylic acid (not more than 1.5%).
Salsalate Tablets USP—Preserve in tight containers. Contain the labeled amount, within ± 10%. Meet the requirements for Identification, Dissolution (70% in 60 minutes in 0.25 *M* phosphate buffer [pH 7.4] in Apparatus 2 at 50 rpm), Uniformity of dosage units, and Limit of salicylic acid (not more than 3.0%).

SARGRAMOSTIM

Source: A single chain, glycosylated polypeptide of 127 amino acid residues expressed from *Saccharomyces cerevisiae*.

Chemical name: Colony-stimulating factor 2 (human clone pHG_{25} protein moiety), 23-L-leucine-.

Molecular formula: $C_{639}H_{1002}N_{168}O_{196}S_8$ (protein moiety).

Molecular weight: 15,500–19,500 daltons.

Description: White, crystalline powder.

Solubility: In water, 500 mcg per mL.

USP requirements: Sargramostim for Injection—Not in USP.

SCHICK TEST CONTROL

Description: Schick Test Control USP—Transparent liquid.

USP requirements: Schick Test Control USP—Preserve at a temperature between 2 and 8 °C. It is Diphtheria Toxin for Schick Test that has been inactivated by heat for use as control for the Schick Test. Meets the requirements of the specific guinea pig test for detoxification by injection of not less than 2.0 mL into each of at least four guinea pigs. The animals are observed daily for 30 days and during this period show no evidence of diphtheria toxin poisoning (extensive necrosis, paralysis, or specific lethality). Meets the requirement for Expiration date (not later than 1 year after date of issue from manufacturer's cold storage [5 °C, 1 year]). Conforms to the regulations of the U.S. Food and Drug Administration concerning biologics.

SCOPOLAMINE

Chemical group: Natural tertiary amine.

Chemical name:
Scopolamine butylbromide—(–)-(1*S*,3*s*,5*R*,6*R*,7*S*,8*r*)-6,7-Epoxy-8-butyl-3-[(*S*)-tropoyloxy]tropanium bromide.

Scopolamine hydrobromide—Benzeneacetic acid, alpha-(hydroxymethyl)-, 9-methyl-3-oxa-9-azatricyclo-[3.3.1.0^{2,4}]-non-7-yl ester, hydrobromide, trihydrate, [7(*S*)-(1 alpha,2 beta,4 beta,5 alpha,7 beta)]-.

Molecular formula:
Scopolamine butylbromide—$C_{21}H_{30}BrNO_4$.
Scopolamine hydrobromide—$C_{17}H_{21}NO_4 \cdot HBr \cdot 3H_2O$.

Molecular weight:
Scopolamine butylbromide—440.4.
Scopolamine hydrobromide—438.32.

Description:
Scopolamine butylbromide—White or almost white, odorless or almost odorless, crystalline powder.
Scopolamine Hydrobromide USP—Colorless or white crystals or white, granular powder. Is odorless, and slightly efflorescent in dry air.

pKa: 7.55 (23 °C)–7.81 (25 °C).

Solubility:
Scopolamine butylbromide—Soluble 1 in 1 of water, 1 in 50 of alcohol, and 1 in 5 of chloroform.
Scopolamine Hydrobromide USP—Freely soluble in water; soluble in alcohol; slightly soluble in chloroform; insoluble in ether.

USP requirements:
Scopolamine Transdermal System—Not in USP.
Scopolamine Butylbromide Injection—Not in USP.
Scopolamine Butylbromide Suppositories—Not in USP.
Scopolamine Butylbromide Tablets—Not in USP.
Scopolamine Hydrobromide USP—Preserve in tight, light-resistant containers. Contains not less than 98.5% and not more than 102.0% of scopolamine hydrobromide, calculated on the anhydrous basis. Meets the requirements for Identification, Melting range (195–199 °C), Specific rotation (−24° to −26°, calculated on the anhydrous basis), pH (4.0–5.5, in a solution [1 in 20]), Water (not more than 13.0%), Residue on ignition (negligible, from 100 mg), Apoatropine, Other foreign alkaloids, and Organic volatile impurities.
Caution: Handle Scopolamine Hydrobromide with exceptional care, since it is highly potent.
Scopolamine Hydrobromide Injection USP—Preserve in light-resistant, single-dose or multiple-dose containers, preferably of Type I glass. A sterile solution of Scopolamine Hydrobromide in Water for Injection. Contains the labeled amount, within ±10%. Meets the requirements for Identification, Bacterial endotoxins, pH (3.5–6.5), and Injections.
Scopolamine Hydrobromide Ophthalmic Ointment USP—Preserve in collapsible ophthalmic ointment tubes. It is Scopolamine Hydrobromide in a suitable ophthalmic ointment base. It is sterile. Contains the labeled amount, within ±10%. Meets the requirements for Identification, Sterility, and Metal particles.
Scopolamine Hydrobromide Ophthalmic Solution USP—Preserve in tight containers. A sterile, buffered, aqueous solution of Scopolamine Hydrobromide. Contains the labeled amount, within ±10%. Meets the requirements for Identification, Sterility, and pH (4.0–6.0).
Scopolamine Hydrobromide Tablets USP—Preserve in tight, light-resistant containers. Contain the labeled amount of scopolamine hydrobromide, within ±10%. Meet the requirements for Identification, Disintegration (15 minutes, the use of disks being omitted), and Uniformity of dosage units.

SECOBARBITAL

Chemical name:
Secobarbital—2,4,6(1*H*,3*H*,5*H*)-Pyrimidinetrione, 5-(1-methylbutyl)-5-(2-propenyl)-.
Secobarbital sodium—2,4,6(1*H*,3*H*,5*H*)-Pyrimidinetrione, 5-(1-methylbutyl)-5-(2-propenyl)-, monosodium salt.

Molecular formula:
Secobarbital—$C_{12}H_{18}N_2O_3$.
Secobarbital sodium—$C_{12}H_{17}N_2NaO_3$.

Molecular weight:
Secobarbital—238.29.
Secobarbital sodium—260.27.

Description:
Secobarbital USP—White, amorphous or crystalline, odorless powder. Its saturated solution has a pH of about 5.6.
Secobarbital Sodium USP—White powder. Is odorless and is hygroscopic. Its solutions decompose on standing, heat accelerating the decomposition.

Solubility:
Secobarbital USP—Very slightly soluble in water; freely soluble in alcohol, in ether, and in solutions of fixed alkali hydroxides and carbonates; soluble in chloroform.
Secobarbital Sodium USP—Very soluble in water; soluble in alcohol; practically insoluble in ether.

USP requirements:
Secobarbital USP—Preserve in tight containers. Contains not less than 97.5% and not more than 100.5% of secobarbital, calculated on the dried basis. Meets the requirements for Identification, Loss on drying (not more than 1.0%), Residue on ignition (not more than 0.1%), Isomer content, and Organic volatile impurities.
Secobarbital Elixir USP—Preserve in tight containers. Contains, in each 100 mL, not less than 417 mg and not more than 461 mg of secobarbital, in a suitable, flavored vehicle. Meets the requirements for Identification and Alcohol content (10.0–14.0%).
Secobarbital Sodium USP—Preserve in tight containers. Contains not less than 98.5% and not more than 100.5% of secobarbital sodium, calculated on the dried basis. Meets the requirements for Completeness of solution, Identification, pH (9.7–10.5, in the solution prepared in the test for Completenesss of solution), Loss on drying (not more than 3.0%), Heavy metals (not more than 0.003%), Isomer content, and Organic volatile impurities.
Secobarbital Sodium Capsules USP—Preserve in tight containers. Contain the labeled amount, within ±7.5%. Meet the requirements for Identification, Dissolution (75% in 60 minutes in water in Apparatus 1 at 100 rpm), and Uniformity of dosage units.
Secobarbital Sodium Injection USP—Preserve in single-dose or in multiple-dose containers, preferably of Type I glass, protected from light, in a refrigerator. A sterile solution of Secobarbital Sodium in a suitable solvent. The label indicates that the Injection is not to be used if it contains a precipitate. Contains the labeled amount, within ±10%. Meets the requirements for Identification, Bacterial endotoxins, pH (9.0–10.5), and Injections.
Sterile Secobarbital Sodium USP—Preserve in Containers for Sterile Solids. It is Secobarbital Sodium suitable for parenteral use. Contains the labeled amount, within ±10%. Meets the requirements for Constituted solution and Bacterial endotoxins, for Identification tests, pH, Completeness of solution, Loss on drying, and Heavy metals under Secobarbital Sodium, and for Sterility tests, Uniformity of dosage units, and Labeling under Injections.

SECOBARBITAL AND AMOBARBITAL

For *Secobarbital* and *Amobarbital*—See individual listings for chemistry information.

USP requirements: Secobarbital Sodium and Amobarbital Sodium Capsules USP—Preserve in well-closed containers. Contain the labeled amounts, within ±10%. Meet the requirements for Identification, Dissolution (60% of each active ingredient in 60 minutes in water in Apparatus 1 at 100 rpm), and Uniformity of dosage units.

SELEGILINE

Chemical name: Selegiline hydrochloride—Benzeneethanamine, *N*,alpha-dimethyl-*N*-2-propynyl-, hydrochloride, (*R*)-.

Molecular formula: Selegiline hydrochloride—$C_{13}H_{17}N \cdot HCl$.

Molecular weight: Selegiline hydrochloride—223.75.

Description: Selegiline hydrochloride—White to near white, crystalline powder.

Solubility: Selegiline hydrochloride—Freely soluble in water, in chloroform, and in methanol.

USP requirements: Selegiline Hydrochloride Tablets—Not in USP.

SELENIOUS ACID

Chemical name: Selenium dioxide, monohydrated.

Molecular formula: H_2SeO_3.

Molecular weight: 128.97.

USP requirements:

Selenious Acid USP—Preserve in tight containers. Contains not less than 93.0% and not more than 101.0% of selenious acid. Meets the requirements for Identification, Residue on ignition (not more than 0.01%), Insoluble matter, Selenate and sulfate, and Organic volatile impurities.

Selenious Acid Injection USP—Preserve in single-dose or in multiple-dose containers, preferably of Type I or Type II glass. A sterile solution in Water for Injection of Selenious Acid or of selenium dissolved in nitric acid. Label the Injection to indicate that it is to be diluted to the appropriate strength with Sterile Water for Injection or other suitable fluid prior to administration. Contains an amount of selenious acid equivalent to the labeled amount of selenium, within ±5%. Meets the requirements for Identification, Bacterial endotoxins, pH (1.8–2.4), Particulate matter, and Injections.

SELENIUM

Molecular formula: Se.

Molecular weight: 78.96.

Description: Dark-red amorphous, or bluish black crystalline, powder.

Solubility: Insoluble in water; soluble in solutions of sodium and potassium hydroxides or sulfides.

USP requirements: Selenium Tablets—Not in USP.

SELENIUM SULFIDE

Chemical name: Selenium sulfide (SeS_2).

Molecular formula: SeS_2.

Molecular weight: 143.08.

Description: Selenium Sulfide USP—Reddish brown to bright orange powder, having not more than a faint odor.

Solubility: Selenium Sulfide USP—Practically insoluble in water and in organic solvents.

USP requirements:

Selenium Sulfide USP—Preserve in well-closed containers. Contains not less than 52.0% and not more than 55.5% of selenium. Meets the requirements for Identification, Residue on ignition (not more than 0.2%), and Soluble selenium compounds.

Selenium Sulfide Lotion USP—Preserve in tight containers. An aqueous, stabilized suspension of Selenium Sulfide. Contains the labeled amount, within ±10%. Contains suitable buffering and dispersing agents. Meets the requirements for Identification and pH (2.0–6.0).

Note: Where labeled for use as a shampoo, it contains a detergent. Where labeled for other uses, it may contain a detergent.

SELENOMETHIONINE SE 75

Chemical name: Butanoic acid, 2-amino-4-(methylseleno-^{75}*Se*)-, (*S*)-.

Molecular formula: $C_5H_{11}NO_2{}^{75}Se$.

Description: Selenomethionine Se 75 Injection USP—Clear, colorless to pale yellow liquid.

USP requirements: Selenomethionine Se 75 Injection USP—Preserve in single-dose or in multiple-dose containers, at a temperature between 2 and 8 °C, unless otherwise specified by the manufacturer. A sterile, aqueous solution of radioactive L-selenomethionine which is the analog of the essential amino acid, methionine, in which the sulfur atom is replaced by a selenium atom. Label it to include the following, in addition to the information specified for Labeling under Injections: the date of calibration; the amount of ^{75}Se as selenomethionine expressed as total megabecquerels (or microcuries or millicuries), and concentration as megabecquerels (or microcuries or millicuries) per mL at the time of calibration; the expiration date; and the statement, "Caution—Radioactive Material." The labeling indicates that in making dosage calculations, correction is to be made for radioactive decay, and also indicates that the radioactive half-life of ^{75}Se is 120 days. Contains the labeled amount of ^{75}Se, within ±10%, expressed in megabecquerels (or microcuries or millicuries) per mL at the time indicated in the labeling. Its specific activity is not less than 37.0 MBq (1.0 millicurie) per mg of selenium at the time of manufacture. Meets the requirements for Radionuclide identification, Bacterial endotoxins, pH (3.5–8.0), Radiochemical purity, and Injections (except that it is not subject to the recommendation on Volume in Container).

SENNA

Source: Dried leaflet of *Cassia acutifolia* or *Cassia angustifolia*; main active cathartic principles are sennosides A and B. Standardized senna concentrate is a dry powder from whole deseeded senna pod. Standardized extract of senna fruit is a liquid extract from whole senna pod.

Chemical group: Anthraquinones.

USP requirements:

Senna USP—Preserve against attack by insects and rodents. Consists of the dried leaflet of *Cassia acutifolia* Delile, known in commerce as Alexandria Senna, or of *Cassia angustifolia* Vahl, known in commerce as Tinnevelly

Senna (Fam. Leguminosae). Meets the requirements for Botanic characteristics, Identification, Senna stems, pods, or other foreign organic matter (not more than 2.0%), and Acid-insoluble ash (not more than 3.0%).

Senna Fluidextract USP—Preserve in tight, light-resistant containers, and avoid exposure to direct sunlight and excessive heat.

Prepare Senna Fluidextract as follows: Mix 1000 grams of Senna, in coarse powder, with a sufficient quantity (600 mL to 800 mL) of menstruum consisting of a mixture of 1 volume of alcohol and 2 volumes of water to make it evenly and distinctly damp. After 15 minutes, pack the mixture firmly into a suitable percolator, and cover the drug with additional menstruum. Macerate for 24 hours, then percolate at a moderate rate, adding fresh menstruum, until the drug is practically exhausted of its active principles. Reserve the first 800 mL of percolate, and use it to dissolve the residue from the additional percolate that has been concentrated to a soft extract at a temperature not to exceed 60 °C. Add water and alcohol to make the product measure 1000 mL, and mix.

Meets the requirement for Alcohol content (23.0–27.0%).

Senna Granules—Not in USP.
Senna Oral Solution—Not in USP.
Senna Suppositories—Not in USP.
Senna Syrup USP—Preserve in tight containers, at a temperature not exceeding 25 °C.

Prepare Senna Syrup as follows: 250 mL of Senna Fluidextract, Suitable essential oil(s), 635 grams of Sucrose, and a sufficient quantity of Purified Water to make 1000 mL. Mix the oil(s) with the Senna Fluidextract, and gradually add 330 mL of Purified Water. Allow the mixture to stand for 24 hours in a cool place, with occasional agitation, then filter, and pass enough Purified Water through the filter to obtain 580 mL of filtrate. Dissolve the Sucrose in this liquid, and add sufficient Purified Water to make the product measure 1000 mL. Mix, and strain.

Meets the requirement for Alcohol content (within ±10% of labeled amount).

Senna Tablets—Not in USP.

SENNA AND DOCUSATE

For *Senna* and *Docusate*—See individual listings for chemistry information.

USP requirements: Senna and Docusate Sodium Tablets—Not in USP.

SENNOSIDES

Chemical group: Anthraquinones.

Description: Sennosides USP—Brownish powder.

Solubility: Soluble 1 in 35 of water, 1 in 2100 of alcohol, 1 in 3700 of chloroform, and 1 in 6100 of ether.

USP requirements:

Sennosides USP—Preserve in well-closed containers. A partially purified natural complex of anthraquinone glucosides found in senna, isolated from *Cassia angustifolia* or *C. acutifolia* as calcium salts. Contains not less than 90.0% and not more than 110.0% of sennosides, calculated on the dried basis, or, if the sennosides is in higher concentration, not less than 90.0% and not more than 110.0% of the concentration indicated on the label. Meets the requirements for Identification, pH (6.3–7.3, in a solution [1 in 10]), Loss on drying (not more than 5.0%), Residue on ignition (5.0–8.0%), and Heavy metals (not more than 0.006%).

Sennosides Tablets USP—Preserve in well-closed containers. Contain the labeled amount, within ±10%. Meet the requirements for Identification, Dissolution (75% in 120 minutes in water in Apparatus 1 at 100 rpm), and Uniformity of dosage units.

SERINE

Chemical name: $C_3H_7NO_3$.

Molecular formula: L-Serine.

Molecular weight: 105.09.

Description: Serine USP—White, odorless crystals.

Solubility: Serine USP—Soluble in water; practically insoluble in absolute alcohol and in ether.

USP requirements: Serine USP—Preserve in well-closed containers. Contains not less than 98.5% and not more than 101.5% of serine, as L-serine, calculated on the dried basis. Meets the requirements for Identification, Specific rotation (+13.6° to +15.6°, calculated on the dried basis), Loss on drying (not more than 0.2%), Residue on ignition (not more than 0.1%), Chloride (not more than 0.05%), Sulfate (not more than 0.03%), Arsenic (not more than 1.5 ppm), Iron (not more than 0.003%), Heavy metals (not more than 0.0015%), and Organic volatile impurities.

SERMORELIN

Chemical name: Sermorelin acetate—Somatoliberin (human pancreatic islet), 29-L-argininamide-30-de-L-glutamine-31-de-L-glutamine-32-deglycine-33-de-L-glutamic acid-34-de-L-serine-35-de-L-asparagine-36-de-L-glutamine-37-de-L-glutamic acid-38-de-L-arginine-39-deglycine-40-de-L-alanine-41-de-L-arginine-42-de-L-alanine-43-de-L-arginine-44-de-L-leucinamide-, acetate (salt), hydrate.

Molecular formula: Sermorelin acetate—$C_{149}H_{246}N_{44}O_{42}S \cdot xC_2H_4O_2 \cdot yH_2O$.

USP requirements: Sermorelin Acetate Injection—Not in USP.

SERTRALINE

Chemical name: Sertraline hydrochloride—1-Naphthalenamine, 4-(3,4-dichlorophenyl)-1,2,3,4-tetrahydro-*N*-methyl-, hydrochloride, (1*S-cis*)-.

Molecular formula: Sertraline hydrochloride—$C_{17}H_{17}Cl_2N \cdot HCl$.

Molecular weight: Sertraline hydrochloride—342.70.

Description: Sertraline hydrochloride—White, crystalline powder.

Solubility: Sertraline hydrochloride—Slightly soluble in water and in isopropyl alcohol; sparingly soluble in ethanol.

USP requirements:

Sertraline Hydrochloride Capsules—Not in USP.
Sertraline Hydrochloride Tablets—Not in USP.

SESAME OIL

Description: Sesame Oil NF—Pale yellow, oily liquid. Practically odorless.

NF category: Solvent; vehicle (oleaginous).

Solubility: Sesame Oil NF—Slightly soluble in alcohol. Miscible with ether, with chloroform, with solvent hexane, and with carbon disulfide.

NF requirements: Sesame Oil NF—Preserve in tight, light-resistant containers, and prevent exposure to excessive heat. The refined fixed oil obtained from the seed of one or more cultivated varieties of *Sesamum indicum* Linné (Fam. Pedaliaceae). Meets the requirements for Identification, Specific gravity (0.916–0.921), Heavy metals (not more than 0.001%), Cottonseed oil, Solidification range of fatty acids (20–25 °C), Free fatty acids, Iodine value (103–116), Saponification value (188–195), and Unsaponifiable matter (not more than 1.5%).

SHELLAC

Description: Shellac NF—

Orange Shellac: Thin, hard, brittle, transparent, pale lemon-yellow to brownish orange flakes, having little or no odor.

Bleached Shellac: Opaque, amorphous cream to yellow granules or coarse powder, having little or no odor.

NF category: Coating agent.

Solubility: Shellac NF—Insoluble in water; very slowly soluble in alcohol, 85 to 95% (w/w); in ether, 13 to 15%; in petroleum ether, 2 to 6%; soluble in aqueous solutions of ethanolamines, alkalies, and borax; sparingly soluble in oil of turpentine.

NF requirements: Shellac NF—Preserve in well-closed containers, preferably in a cold place. Obtained by the purification of Lac, the resinous secretion of the insect *Laccifer Lacca Kerr* (Fam. Coccidae). Orange Shellac is produced either by a process of filtration in the molten state, or by hot solvent process, or both. Orange Shellac may retain most of its wax or be dewaxed, and may contain lesser amounts of the natural color than originally present. Bleached (White) Shellac is prepared by dissolving the Lac in aqueous sodium carbonate, bleaching the solution with sodium hypochlorite and precipitating the Bleached Shellac with 2 *N* sulfuric acid. Removal of the wax, by filtration, during the process results in Refined Bleached Shellac. Label it to indicate whether it is bleached or is orange, and whether it is dewaxed or wax-containing. Meets the requirements for Identification, Loss on drying, Arsenic (not more than 1.5 ppm), Heavy metals (not more than 0.001%), Acid value, Wax, and Rosin. Shellac conforms to the specifications in the accompanying table.

	Acid value (on dried basis)	Loss on drying	Wax
Orange Shellac	between 68 and 76	not more than 2.0%	not more than 5.5%
Dewaxed Orange Shellac	between 71 and 79	not more than 2.0%	not more than 0.2%
Regular Bleached Shellac	between 73 and 89	not more than 6.0%	not more than 5.5%
Refined Bleached Shellac	between 75 and 91	not more than 6.0%	not more than 0.2%

DENTAL-TYPE SILICA

Description: Dental-Type Silica NF—Fine, white, hygroscopic, odorless, amorphous powder, in which the diameter of the average particle ranges between 0.5 micrometer and 40 micrometers.

NF category: Glidant and/or anticaking agent; suspending and/or viscosity-increasing agent.

Solubility: Dental-Type Silica NF—Insoluble in water, in alcohol, and in acid (except hydrofluoric acid); soluble in hot solutions of alkali hydroxides.

NF requirements: Dental-Type Silica NF—Preserve in tight containers. Obtained from sodium silicate solution by destabilizing with acid in such a way as to yield very fine particles. The sum of the Assay value and the Sodium Sulfate content is not less than 98.0%. Label it to indicate the maximum percentage of Loss on drying. Meets the requirements for pH (4.0–8.5 in a slurry [1 in 20]), Loss on drying, and Sodium sulfate (not more than 4.0%), and for Loss on ignition, Chloride, Arsenic, and Heavy metals under Silicon Dioxide.

PURIFIED SILICEOUS EARTH

Description: Purified Siliceous Earth NF—Very fine, white, light gray, or pale buff mixture of amorphous powder and lesser amounts of crystalline polymorphs, including quartz and cristobalite. It is gritty, readily absorbs moisture, and retains about 4 times its weight of water without becoming fluid.

NF category: Filtering aid; sorbent.

Solubility: Purified Siliceous Earth NF—Insoluble in water, in acids, and in dilute solutions of alkali hydroxides.

NF requirements: Purified Siliceous Earth NF—Preserve in well-closed containers. A form of silica (SiO_2) consisting of the frustules and fragments of diatoms, purified by calcining. Meets the requirements for Loss on drying (not more than 0.5%), Loss on ignition (not more than 2.0%), Acid-soluble substances (not more than 2.0%), Water-soluble substances (not more than 0.2%), Leachable arsenic (not more than 0.001%), Leachable lead (not more than 0.001%), and Non-siliceous substances.

SILICON DIOXIDE

Molecular formula: SiO_2xH_2O.

Molecular weight: 60.08 (anhydrous).

Description: Silicon Dioxide NF—Fine, white, hygroscopic, odorless, amorphous powder, in which the diameter of the average particles ranges between 2 and 10 micrometers.

NF category: Desiccant; suspending and/or viscosity-increasing agent.

Solubility: Silicon Dioxide NF—Insoluble in water, in alcohol, and in other organic solvents; soluble in hot solutions of alkali hydroxides.

NF requirements: Silicon Dioxide NF—Preserve in tight containers, protected from moisture. Obtained by insolubilizing the dissolved silica in sodium silicate solution. Where obtained by addition of sodium silicate to a mineral acid, the product is termed silica gel; where obtained by the destabilization of a solution of sodium silicate in such manner as to yield very fine particles, the product is termed precipitated silica. Label it to state whether it is silica gel or precipitated silica. After ignition at 1000 °C for not less than 1 hour, contains not less than 99.0% of anhydrous silicon dioxide. Meets the requirements for Identification, pH (4–8, in a slurry [1 in 20]), Loss on drying (not more than 5.0%), Loss on ignition (not more than 8.5%), Chloride (not more than 0.1%), Sulfate (not more than 0.5%), Arsenic (not more than 3 ppm), and Heavy metals (not more than 0.003%).

COLLOIDAL SILICON DIOXIDE

Chemical name: Silica.

Molecular formula: SiO_2.

Molecular weight: 60.08.

Description: Colloidal Silicon Dioxide NF—Light, white, non-gritty powder of extremely fine particle size (about 15 nm).
NF category: Glidant and/or anticaking agent; suspending and/or viscosity-increasing agent.

Solubility: Colloidal Silicon Dioxide NF—Insoluble in water and in acid (except hydrofluoric); soluble in hot solutions of alkali hydroxides.

NF requirements: Colloidal Silicon Dioxide NF—Preserve in well-closed containers. A submicroscopic fumed silica prepared by the vapor-phase hydrolysis of a silicon compound. When ignited at 1000 °C for 2 hours, contains not less than 99.0% and not more than 100.5% of silicon dioxide. Meets the requirements for Identification, pH (3.5–4.4, in a 1 in 25 dispersion), Loss on drying (not more than 2.5%), Loss on ignition (not more than 2.0%), and Arsenic (not more than 8 ppm).

SILVER NITRATE

Chemical name: Nitric acid silver(1+) salt.

Molecular formula: $AgNO_3$.

Molecular weight: 169.87.

Description:
Silver Nitrate USP—Colorless or white crystals. The pH of its solutions is about 5.5. On exposure to light in the presence of organic matter, it becomes gray or grayish black.
Toughened Silver Nitrate USP—White, crystalline masses generally molded as pencils or cones. It breaks with a fibrous fracture. Its solutions are neutral to litmus. It becomes gray or grayish black upon exposure to light.

Solubility:
Silver Nitrate USP—Very soluble in water and even more so in boiling water; sparingly soluble in alcohol; freely soluble in boiling alcohol; slightly soluble in ether.
Toughened Silver Nitrate USP—Soluble in water to the extent of its nitrate content (there is always a residue of silver chloride). Partially soluble in alcohol; slightly soluble in ether.

USP requirements:
Silver Nitrate USP—Preserve in tight, light-resistant containers. Powdered and then dried in the dark over silica gel for 4 hours, contains not less than 99.8% and not more than 100.5% of silver nitrate. Meets the requirements for Clarity and color of solution, Identification, and Copper.
Silver Nitrate Ophthalmic Solution USP—Preserve it protected from light, in inert, collapsible capsules or in other suitable single-dose containers. A solution of Silver Nitrate in a water medium. The solution may be buffered by the addition of Sodium Acetate. Contains the labeled amount, within ±5%. Meets the requirements for Clarity and color of solution, Identification, Sterility, and pH (4.5–6.0).
Toughened Silver Nitrate USP—Preserve in tight, light-resistant containers. Contains not less than 94.5% of silver nitrate, the remainder consisting of silver chloride. Meets the requirements for Identification and Copper.

SIMETHICONE

Chemical name: Simethicone.

Description: Simethicone USP—Translucent, gray, viscous fluid.
NF category: Antifoaming agent; water-repelling agent.

Solubility: Simethicone USP—Insoluble in water and in alcohol. The liquid phase is soluble in chloroform and in ether, but silicon dioxide remains as a residue in these solvents.

USP requirements:
Simethicone USP—Preserve in tight containers. A mixture of fully methylated linear siloxane polymers containing repeating units of the formula $[-(CH_3)_2SiO-]_n$, stabilized with trimethylsiloxy end-blocking units of the formula $[(CH_3)_3SiO-]$, and silicon dioxide. Contains not less than 90.5% and not more than 99.0% of polydimethylsiloxane, and not less than 4.0% and not more than 7.0% of silicon dioxide. Meets the requirements for Identification, Loss on heating (not more than 18.0%), Heavy metals (not more than 0.001%), Defoaming activity (not more than 15 seconds), and Silicon dioxide content.
Simethicone Capsules USP—Preserve in well-closed containers. Contain an amount of polydimethylsiloxane equivalent to the labeled amount of simethicone, within ±15%. Meet the requirements for Identification, Disintegration (30 minutes), Uniformity of dosage units, and Defoaming activity.
Simethicone Emulsion USP—Preserve in tight containers. A water-dispersible form of Simethicone composed of Simethicone, suitable emulsifiers, preservatives, and water. Contains an amount of polydimethylsiloxane equivalent to the labeled amount of simethicone, within −15% to +10%. Meets the requirements for Identification, Microbial limit (total aerobic microbial count not more than 100 per gram), Heavy metals (not more than 0.001%), and Defoaming activity (not more than 15 seconds).
Simethicone Oral Suspension USP—Preserve in tight, light-resistant containers. A suspension of Simethicone in Water. Contains an amount of polydimethylsiloxane equivalent to the labeled amount of simethicone, within ±15%. Meets the requirements for Identification, pH (4.4–4.6), and Defoaming activity (not more than 45 seconds).
Simethicone Tablets USP—Preserve in well-closed containers. Contain an amount of polydimethylsiloxane equivalent to the labeled amount of simethicone, within ±15%. Meet the requirements for Identification, Disintegration (30 minutes), Defoaming activity, and Uniformity of dosage units.

SIMETHICONE, ALUMINA, CALCIUM CARBONATE, AND MAGNESIA

For *Simethicone, Alumina* (Aluminum Hydroxide), *Calcium Carbonate,* and *Magnesia* (Magnesium Hydroxide)—See individual listings for chemistry information.

USP requirements: Simethicone, Alumina, Calcium Carbonate, and Magnesia Chewable Tablets—Not in USP.

SIMETHICONE, ALUMINA, MAGNESIUM CARBONATE, AND MAGNESIA

For *Simethicone, Alumina* (Aluminum Hydroxide), *Magnesium Carbonate,* and *Magnesia* (Magnesium Hydroxide)—See individual listings for chemistry information.

USP requirements: Simethicone, Alumina, Magnesium Carbonate, and Magnesia Chewable Tablets—Not in USP.

SIMVASTATIN

Source: Derived synthetically from a fermentation product of *Aspergillus terreus*.

Chemical name: Butanoic acid, 2,2-dimethyl-, 1,2,3,7,8,8a-hexahydro-3,7-dimethyl-8-[2-(tetrahydro-4-hydroxy-6-oxo-2*H*-pyran-2-yl)ethyl]-1-naphthalenyl ester, [1*S*-[1 alpha,3 alpha,-7 beta,8 beta(2*S**,4*S**),8a beta]]-.

Molecular formula: $C_{25}H_{38}O_5$.

Molecular weight: 418.57.

Description: White to off-white, nonhygroscopic, crystalline powder.

Solubility: Practically insoluble in water; freely soluble in chloroform, in methanol, and in ethanol.

USP requirements: Simvastatin Tablets—Not in USP.

SISOMICIN

Chemical name: Sisomicin sulfate—D-Streptamine, (2*S*-*cis*)-4-*O*-[3-amino-6-(aminomethyl)-3,4-dihydro-2*H*-pyran-2-yl]-2-deoxy-6-*O*-[3-deoxy-4-*C*-methyl-3-(methylamino)-beta-L-arabinopyranosyl]-, sulfate (2:5) (salt).

Molecular formula: Sisomicin sulfate—$(C_{19}H_{37}N_5O_7)_2 \cdot 5H_2SO_4$.

Molecular weight: Sisomicin sulfate—1385.43.

USP requirements:

Sisomicin Sulfate USP—Preserve in tight containers. Has a potency equivalent to not less than 580 mg of sisomicin per mg, calculated on the dried basis. Meets the requirements for Identification, Specific rotation (+100° to +110°, calculated on the dried basis), pH (3.5–5.5, in a solution containing 40 mg of sisomicin per mL), Loss on drying (not more than 15.0%), and Residue on ignition (not more than 1.0%).

Sisomicin Sulfate Injection USP—Preserve in single-dose or in multiple-dose containers, preferably of Type I glass. A sterile solution of Sisomicin Sulfate in Water for Injection. Contains an amount of sisomicin sulfate equivalent to the labeled amount of sisomicin, within −10% to +20%. Meets the requirements for Identification, Bacterial endotoxins, pH (2.5–5.5), and Injections.

SMALLPOX VACCINE

Description: Smallpox Vaccine USP—Liquid vaccine is a turbid, whitish to greenish suspension, which may have a slight odor due to the antimicrobial agent. Dried vaccine is a yellow to grayish pellet, which may or may not become fragmented when shaken.

USP requirements: Smallpox Vaccine USP—Preserve and dispense in the containers in which it was placed by the manufacturer. Keep liquid Vaccine during storage and in shipment at a temperature below 0 °C. Keep dried Vaccine at a temperature between 2 and 8 °C. A suspension or solid containing the living virus of vaccinia of a strain of approved origin and manipulation, that has been grown in the skin of a vaccinated bovine calf. Label it to state that it contains not more than 200 microorganisms per mL in the case of Vaccine intended for multiple-puncture administration, or that it contains not more than 1 microorganism per 100 doses in the case of Vaccine intended for jet injection, unless it meets the requirements for sterility. In the case of Vaccine intended for jet injection, so state on the label. In the case of dried Vaccine, label it to state that after constitution it is to be well shaken before use. Label it also to state that it was prepared in the bovine calf. Meets the requirements of the specific potency test using embryonated chicken eggs in comparison with the U.S. Reference Smallpox Vaccine in the case of Vaccine intended for multiple-puncture administration or with such Reference Vaccine diluted (1:30) in the case of Vaccine intended for jet injection, and the requirements for the tests for absence of specific microorganisms. Meets the requirement for Expiration date (for liquid Vaccine, not later than 3 months after date of issue from manufacturer's cold storage [−10° C, 9 months as glycerinated or equivalent preparation]; for dried Vaccine, not later than 18 months after date of issue from manufacturer's cold storage [5 °C, 6 months]). Conforms to the regulations of the U.S. Food and Drug Administration concerning biologics.

SODA LIME

Description: Soda Lime NF—White or grayish white granules. It may have a color if an indicator has been added.

NF category: Sorbent, carbon dioxide.

NF requirements: Soda Lime NF—A mixture of Calcium Hydroxide and Sodium or Potassium Hydroxide or both. May contain an indicator that is inert toward anesthetic gases such as Ether, Cyclopropane, and Nitrous Oxide, and that changes color when the Soda Lime no longer can absorb Carbon Dioxide. Meets the requirements for Identification, Loss on drying (12.0–19.0%), Moisture absorption (increase in weight not more than 7.5%), Hardness, and Carbon dioxide absorbency (not less than 19.0%), and for Packaging and storage, Labeling, and Size of granules under Barium Hydroxide Lime.

SODIUM ACETATE

Chemical name: Acetic acid, sodium salt, trihydrate.

Molecular formula: $C_2H_3NaO_2 \cdot 3H_2O$ (trihydrate); $C_2H_3NaO_2$ (anhydrous).

Molecular weight: 136.08 (trihydrate); 82.03 (anhydrous).

Description: Sodium Acetate USP—Colorless, transparent crystals, or white, granular crystalline powder, or white flakes. It is odorless, or has a faint, acetous odor. Efflorescent in warm, dry air.

NF category: Buffering agent.

Solubility: Sodium Acetate USP—Very soluble in water; soluble in alcohol.

USP requirements:

Sodium Acetate USP—Preserve in tight containers. Contains three molecules of water of hydration, or is anhydrous. Contains not less than 99.0% and not more than 101.0% of sodium acetate, calculated on the dried basis. Label it to indicate whether it is the trihydrate or is anhydrous. Where Sodium Acetate is intended for use in hemodialysis, it is so labeled. Meets the requirements for Identification, pH (7.5–9.2, in a solution in carbon dioxide–free water containing the equivalent of 30 mg of anhydrous sodium acetate per mL), Loss on drying (38.0–41.0% for the hydrous, not more than 1.0% for the anhydrous), Insoluble matter (not more than 0.05%), Chloride (not more than 0.035%), Sulfate (not more than 0.005%), Arsenic (not more than 3 ppm), Calcium and magnesium, Potassium, Heavy metals (not more than 0.001%), Aluminum (not more than 0.2 ppm), and Organic volatile impurities.

Sodium Acetate Injection USP—Preserve in single-dose containers, preferably of Type I glass. A sterile solution of Sodium Acetate in Water for Injection. The label states the sodium acetate content in terms of weight and of milliequivalents in a given volume. Label the Injection to indicate that it is to be diluted to appropriate strength with water or other suitable fluid prior to administration. The label states also the total osmolar concentration in mOsmol per liter. Where the contents are less than 100 mL, or where the label states that the Injection is not for direct injection but is to be diluted before use, the label alternatively may state the total osmolar concentration in mOsmol per mL. Contains the labeled amount, within ±5%. Meets the requirements for Identification, Bacterial endotoxins, pH (6.0–7.0), Particulate matter, and Injections.

Sodium Acetate Solution USP—Preserve in tight containers. An aqueous solution of Sodium Acetate. Contains the labeled amount, within ±3% (w/w). Meets the requirements for Identification, pH (7.5–9.2, when diluted with carbon dioxide–free water to contain 5% of solids), Insoluble matter (not more than 0.005%), Chloride (not more than 0.035%), Sulfate (not more than 0.005%), Arsenic (not more than 3 ppm), Calcium and magnesium, Potassium, and Heavy metals (not more than 0.001%).

SODIUM ALGINATE

Chemical name: Alginic acid, sodium salt.

Description: Sodium Alginate NF—Practically odorless, coarse or fine powder, yellowish white in color.

NF category: Suspending and/or viscosity-increasing agent.

Solubility: Sodium Alginate NF—Soluble in water, forming a viscous, colloidal solution; insoluble in alcohol and in hydroalcoholic solutions in which the alcohol content is greater than about 30% by weight; insoluble in chloroform, in ether, and in acids when the pH of the resulting solution becomes lower than about 3.

NF requirements: Sodium Alginate NF—Preserve in tight containers. The purified carbohydrate product extracted from brown seaweeds by the use of dilute alkali. Consists chiefly of the sodium salt of Alginic Acid, a polyuronic acid composed of beta-D-mannuronic acid residues linked so that the carboxyl group of each unit is free while the aldehyde group is shielded by a glycosidic linkage. Contains not less than 90.8% and not more than 106.0% of sodium alginate of average equivalent weight 222.00, calculated on the dried basis. Meets the requirements for Identification, Microbial limits, Loss on drying (not more than 15.0%), Ash (18.0–24.0%), Arsenic (not more than 1.5 ppm), Lead (not more than 0.001%), and Heavy metals (not more than 0.004%).

SODIUM ASCORBATE

Chemical name: L-Ascorbic acid, monosodium salt.

Molecular formula: $C_6H_7NaO_6$.

Molecular weight: 198.11.

Description: Sodium Ascorbate USP—White or very faintly yellow crystals or crystalline powder. Is odorless or practically odorless. Is relatively stable in air. On exposure to light it gradually darkens.

Solubility: Sodium Ascorbate USP—Freely soluble in water; very slightly soluble in alcohol; insoluble in chloroform and in ether.

USP requirements:

Sodium Ascorbate USP—Preserve in tight, light-resistant containers. Contains not less than 99.0% and not more than 101.0% of sodium ascorbate, calculated on the dried basis. Meets the requirements for Identification, Specific rotation (+103° to +108°, calculated on the dried basis), pH (7.0–8.0, in a solution [1 in 10]), Loss on drying (not more than 0.25%), Heavy metals (not more than 0.002%), and Organic volatile impurities.

Sodium Ascorbate Injection—Not in USP.

SODIUM BENZOATE

Chemical name: Benzoic acid, sodium salt.

Molecular formula: $C_7H_5NaO_2$.

Molecular weight: 144.11.

Description: Sodium Benzoate NF—White, odorless or practically odorless, granular or crystalline powder. It is stable in air.

NF category: Antimicrobial preservative.

Solubility: Sodium Benzoate NF—Freely soluble in water; sparingly soluble in alcohol, and somewhat more soluble in 90% alcohol.

NF requirements: Sodium Benzoate NF—Preserve in well-closed containers. Contains not less than 99.0% and not more than 100.5% of sodium benzoate. Meets the requirements for Identification, Alkalinity, Water (not more than 1.5%), Arsenic (not more than 3 ppm), Heavy metals (not more than 0.001%), and Organic volatile impurities.

SODIUM BENZOATE AND SODIUM PHENYLACETATE

Chemical name:

Sodium benzoate—Benzoic acid, sodium salt.
Sodium phenylacetate—Benzeneacetic acid, sodium salt.

Molecular formula:

Sodium benzoate—$C_7H_5NaO_2$.
Sodium phenylacetate—$C_8H_7NaO_2$.

Molecular weight:

Sodium benzoate—144.11.
Sodium phenylacetate—158.13.

Description: Sodium Benzoate NF—White, odorless or practically odorless, granular or crystalline powder. It is stable in air.

NF category: Antimicrobial preservative.

Solubility: Sodium Benzoate NF—Freely soluble in water; sparingly soluble in alcohol, and somewhat more soluble in 90% alcohol.

Other characteristics: The pH of the undiluted sodium benzoate and sodium phenylacetate combination solution is approximately 6.0.

USP requirements: Sodium Benzoate and Sodium Phenylacetate Oral Solution—Not in USP.

SODIUM BICARBONATE

Chemical name: Carbonic acid monosodium salt.

Molecular formula: $NaHCO_3$.

Molecular weight: 84.01.

Description: Sodium Bicarbonate USP—White, crystalline powder. Is stable in dry air, but slowly decomposes in moist air. Its solutions, when freshly prepared with cold water, without shaking, are alkaline to litmus. The alkalinity increases as the solutions stand, as they are agitated, or as they are heated.

NF category: Alkalizing agent.

Solubility: Sodium Bicarbonate USP—Soluble in water; insoluble in alcohol.

USP requirements:

Sodium Bicarbonate USP—Preserve in well-closed containers. Contains not less than 99.0% and not more than 100.5% of sodium bicarbonate, calculated on the dried basis. Meets the requirements for Identification, Loss on drying (not more than 0.25%), Insoluble substances, Carbonate (where it is labeled as intended for use in hemodialysis, not more than 0.23%), Normal carbonate, Chloride (not more than 0.015%), Sulfate (not more than 0.015%), Ammonia, Aluminum (where it is labeled as intended for use in hemodialysis, not more than 2 ppm), Arsenic (not more than 2 ppm), Calcium and magnesium (where it is labeled as intended for use in hemodialysis, not more than 0.01% for calcium, and not more than 0.004% for magnesium), Copper (where it is labeled as intended for use in hemodialysis, not more than 1 ppm), Iron (where it is labeled as intended for use in hemodialysis, not more than 5 ppm), Heavy metals (not more than 5 ppm), Organics (where it is labeled as intended for use in hemodialysis, not more than 0.01%), and Organic volatile impurities.

Effervescent Sodium Bicarbonate—Not in USP.

Sodium Bicarbonate Injection USP—Preserve in single-dose containers, of Type I glass. A sterile solution of Sodium Bicarbonate in Water for Injection, the pH of which may be adjusted by means of Carbon Dioxide. The label states the total osmolar concentration in mOsmol per liter. Where the contents are less than 100 mL, or where the label states that the Injection is not for direct injection, but is to be diluted before use, the label alternatively may state the total osmolar concentration in mOsmol per mL. Contains the labeled amount, within ±5%. Meets the requirements for Identification, Bacterial endotoxins, pH (7.0–8.5), Particulate matter, and Injections.

Note: Do not use the Injection if it contains a precipitate.

Sodium Bicarbonate Oral Powder USP—Preserve in well-closed containers. Contains Sodium Bicarbonate and suitable added substances. Label Oral Powder to indicate that it is for oral use only. Contains not less than 98.5% and not more than 100.5% of sodium bicarbonate, calculated on the dried basis. Meets the requirements for Identification and Loss on drying under Sodium Bicarbonate.

Sodium Bicarbonate Tablets USP—Preserve in well-closed containers. Contain the labeled amount, within ±5%. Meet the requirements for Identification, Disintegration (30 minutes, simulated gastric fluid TS being substituted for water in the test), and Uniformity of dosage units.

SODIUM BORATE

Chemical name: Borax.

Molecular formula: $Na_2B_4O_7 \cdot 10H_2O$.

Molecular weight: 381.37.

Description: Sodium Borate NF—Colorless, transparent crystals or white, crystalline powder. It is odorless. Its solutions are alkaline to phenolphthalein TS. As it effloresces in warm, dry air, the crystals are often coated with white powder.

NF category: Alkalizing agent.

Solubility: Sodium Borate NF—Soluble in water; freely soluble in boiling water and in glycerin; insoluble in alcohol.

NF requirements: Sodium Borate NF—Preserve in tight containers. Contains an amount of anhydrous sodium borate equivalent to not less than 99.0% and not more than 105.0% of hydrous sodium borate. Meets the requirements for Identification, Carbonate and bicarbonate, Arsenic (not more than 8 ppm), Heavy metals (not more than 0.002%), and Organic volatile impurities.

SODIUM CARBONATE

Chemical name: Carbonic acid, disodium salt.

Molecular formula: Na_2CO_3 (anhydrous); $Na_2CO_3 \cdot H_2O$ (monohydrate).

Molecular weight: 105.99 (anhydrous); 124.00 (monohydrate).

Description: Sodium Carbonate NF—Colorless crystals, or white crystalline powder or granules. Stable in air under ordinary conditions. When exposed to air above 50 °C, the hydrous salt effloresces and, at 100 °C, becomes anhydrous.

NF category: Alkalizing agent.

Solubility: Sodium Carbonate NF—Freely soluble in water, but still more soluble in boiling water.

NF requirements: Sodium Carbonate NF—Preserve in well-closed containers. It is anhydrous or contains one molecule of water of hydration. Label it to indicate whether it is anhydrous or hydrous. Contains not less than 99.5% and not more than 100.5% of sodium carbonate, calculated on the anhydrous basis. Meets the requirements for Identification, Water (for the anhydrous form, not more than 0.5%; for the hydrous form, 12.0–15.0%), Arsenic (not more than 3 ppm), Heavy metals (not more than 0.001%), and Organic volatile impurities.

SODIUM CHLORIDE

Chemical name: Sodium chloride.

Molecular formula: NaCl.

Molecular weight: 58.44.

Description:

Sodium Chloride USP—Colorless, cubic crystals or white crystalline powder.

NF category: Tonicity agent.

Sodium Chloride Inhalation Solution USP—Clear, colorless solution.

Bacteriostatic Sodium Chloride Injection USP—Clear, colorless solution, odorless or having the odor of the bacteriostatic substance.

NF category: Vehicle (sterile).

Sodium Chloride Irrigation USP—Clear, colorless solution.

Solubility: Sodium Chloride USP—Freely soluble in water; and slightly more soluble in boiling water; soluble in glycerin; slightly soluble in alcohol.

USP requirements:

Sodium Chloride USP—Preserve in well-closed containers. Where Sodium Chloride is intended for use in hemodialysis, it is so labeled. Contains not less than 99.0% and not more than 101.0% of sodium chloride, calculated on the dried basis. Contains no added substance. Meets the requirements for Identification, Acidity or alkalinity, Loss on drying (not more than 0.5%), Arsenic (not more than 3 ppm), Barium, Iodide or bromide, Calcium and magnesium (not more than 0.005%), Iron (not more than 2 ppm), Sulfate (not more than 0.015%), Sodium ferrocyanide, Aluminum (where it is labeled as intended for use in hemodialysis, not more than 0.2 ppm), Heavy metals (not more than 5 ppm), and Organic volatile impurities.

Sodium Chloride Injection USP—Preserve in single-dose glass or plastic containers. Glass containers are preferably of Type I or Type II glass. A sterile solution of Sodium Chloride in Water for Injection. Contains no antimicrobial agents. The label states the total osmolar concentration in mOsmol per liter. Where the contents are less than 100 mL, or where the label states that the Injection is not for direct injection but is to be diluted before use, the label alternatively may state the total osmolar concentration in mOsmol per mL. Contains the labeled amount, within ±5%. Meets the requirements for Identification, Bacterial endotoxins, pH (4.5–7.0), Particulate matter, Iron (not more than 2 ppm), Heavy metals (not more than 0.001%, based on amount of sodium chloride), and Injections.

Bacteriostatic Sodium Chloride Injection USP—Preserve in single-dose or in multiple-dose containers, of not larger than 30-mL size, preferably of Type I or Type II glass. A sterile, isotonic solution of Sodium Chloride in Water for Injection, containing one or more suitable antimicrobial agents. Label it to indicate the name(s) and proportion(s) of the added antimicrobial agent(s). Label it also to include the statement, **"NOT FOR USE IN NEWBORNS"** in boldface capital letters, on the label immediately under the official name, printed in a contrasting color, preferably red. Alternatively, the statement may be placed prominently elsewhere on the label if the statement is enclosed within a box. Label it also to include the statement **"NOT FOR INHALATION."** Contains not less than 0.85% and not more than 0.95% of sodium chloride. Meets the requirements for Antimicrobial agent(s), Bacterial endotoxins, and Particulate matter, for Identification test, pH, Iron, and Heavy metals under Sodium Chloride Injection, and for Injections.

Note: Use Bacteriostatic Sodium Chloride Injection with due regard for the compatibility of the antimicrobial agent or agents it contains with the particular medicinal substance that is to be dissolved or diluted.

Sodium Chloride Irrigation USP—Preserve in single-dose glass or plastic containers. Glass containers are preferably of Type I or Type II glass. The container may be designed to empty rapidly and may contain a volume of more than 1 liter. It is Sodium Chloride Injection that has been suitably packaged, and it contains no antimicrobial agents. The designation "not for injection" appears prominently on the label. Contains the labeled amount, within ±5%. Meets the requirements for Identification, Bacterial endotoxins, and Sterility, and for pH, Iron, and Heavy metals under Sodium Chloride Injection.

Sodium Chloride Ophthalmic Ointment USP—Preserve in collapsible ophthalmic ointment tubes. It is Sodium Chloride in a suitable ophthalmic ointment base. Contains the labeled amount, within ±10%. Meets the requirements for Identification, Sterility, Minimum fill, and Particulate matter.

Sodium Chloride Inhalation Solution USP—Preserve in single-dose containers. A sterile solution of Sodium Chloride in water purified by distillation or by reverse osmosis and rendered sterile. Contains the labeled amount, within ±10%. Contains no antimicrobial agents or other added substances. Meets the requirements for Identification, Sterility, and pH (4.5–7.0).

Sodium Chloride Ophthalmic Solution USP—Preserve in tight containers. A sterile solution of Sodium Chloride. Contains the labeled amount, within ±10%. Contains a buffer. Meets the requirements for Identification, Sterility, and pH (6.0–8.0).

Sodium Chloride Tablets USP—Preserve in well-closed containers. Contain the labeled amount, within ±5%. Meet the requirements for Identification, Iodide or bromide, Barium, Calcium and magnesium, Disintegration (30 minutes), and Uniformity of dosage units.

Sodium Chloride Tablets for Solution USP—Composed of Sodium Chloride in compressed form, containing no added substance. Contain the labeled amount, within ±5%. Meet the requirements for Identification test, Packaging and storage, Iodide or bromide, Barium, Calcium and magnesium, Disintegration, and Uniformity of dosage units under Sodium Chloride Tablets.

SODIUM CHLORIDE AND DEXTROSE

For *Sodium Chloride* and *Dextrose*—See individual listings for chemistry information.

USP requirements: Sodium Chloride and Dextrose Tablets USP—Preserve in well-closed containers. Contain the labeled amounts, within ±7.5%. Meet the requirements for Identification, Disintegration (30 minutes), and Uniformity of dosage units.

SODIUM CITRATE

Chemical name: 1,2,3-Propanetricarboxylic acid, 2-hydroxy-, trisodium salt.

Molecular formula: $C_6H_5Na_3O_7$ (anhydrous); $C_6H_5Na_3O_7 \cdot 2H_2O$ (hydrous).

Molecular weight: 258.07 (anhydrous); 294.10 (hydrous).

Description: Sodium Citrate USP—Colorless crystals or white, crystalline powder.

NF category: Buffering agent.

Solubility: Sodium Citrate USP—Hydrous form freely soluble in water and very soluble in boiling water. Insoluble in alcohol.

USP requirements: Sodium Citrate USP—Preserve in tight containers. It is anhydrous or contains two molecules of water of hydration. Label it to indicate whether it is anhydrous or hydrous. Contains not less than 99.0% and not more than 100.5% of sodium citrate, calculated on the anhydrous basis. Meets the requirements for Identification, Alkalinity, Water (10.0–13.0% for the hydrous form, not more than 1.0% for the anhydrous form), Tartrate, and Heavy metals (not more than 0.001%).

SODIUM CITRATE AND CITRIC ACID

For *Sodium Citrate* and *Citric Acid*—See individual listings for chemistry information.

Description: Sodium Citrate and Citric Acid Oral Solution USP—Clear solution having the color of any added preservative or flavoring agents.

USP requirements: Sodium Citrate and Citric Acid Oral Solution USP—Preserve in tight containers. A solution of Sodium Citrate and Citric Acid in a suitable aqueous medium. Contains, in each 100 mL, not less than 2.23 grams and not more than 2.46 grams of sodium, and not less than 6.11 grams and not more than 6.75 grams of citrate, equivalent to not less than 9.5 grams and not more than 10.5 grams of sodium citrate dihydrate; and not less than 6.34 grams and not more than 7.02 grams of citric acid monohydrate. Meets the requirements for Identification and pH (4.0–4.4).

SODIUM DEHYDROACETATE

Chemical name: 2*H*-Pyran-2,4(3*H*)-dione, 3-acetyl-6-methyl-, monosodium salt.

Molecular formula: $C_8H_7NaO_4$.

Molecular weight: 190.13.

Description: Sodium Dehydroacetate NF—White or practically white odorless powder.

NF category: Antimicrobial preservative.

Solubility: Sodium Dehydroacetate NF—Freely soluble in water, in propylene glycol, and in glycerin.

NF requirements: Sodium Dehydroacetate NF—Preserve in well-closed containers. Contains not less than 98.0% and not more than 100.5% of sodium dehydroacetate, calculated on the anhydrous basis. Meets the requirements for Identification, Water (8.5–10.0%), Arsenic (not more than 3 ppm), Heavy metals (not more than 0.001%), and Organic volatile impurities.

SODIUM FLUORIDE

Chemical name: Sodium fluoride.

Molecular formula: NaF.

Molecular weight: 41.99.

Description: Sodium Fluoride USP—White, odorless powder.

Solubility: Sodium Fluoride USP—Soluble in water; insoluble in alcohol.

USP requirements:

Sodium Fluoride USP—Preserve in well-closed containers. Contains not less than 98.0% and not more than 102.0% of sodium fluoride, calculated on the dried basis. Meets the requirements for Identification, Acidity or alkalinity, Loss on drying (not more than 1.0%), Fluosilicate, Chloride (not more than 0.012%), Heavy metals (not more than 0.003%), and Organic volatile impurities.

Sodium Fluoride Oral Solution USP—Preserve in tight containers, plastic containers being used for Oral Solution having a pH below 7.5. Label Oral Solution in terms of the content of sodium fluoride (NaF) and in terms of the content of fluoride ion. Contains the labeled amount, within ±10%. Meets the requirement for Identification.

Sodium Fluoride Tablets USP—Preserve in tight containers. Label Tablets in terms of the content of sodium fluoride (NaF) and in terms of the content of fluoride ion. Tablets that are to be chewed may be labeled as Sodium Fluoride Chewable Tablets. Contain the labeled amount, within ±10%. Meet the requirements for Identification, Disintegration (15 minutes), and Uniformity of dosage units.

SODIUM FLUORIDE AND PHOSPHORIC ACID

For *Sodium Fluoride* and *Phosphoric Acid*—See individual listings for chemistry information.

USP requirements:

Sodium Fluoride and Phosphoric Acid Gel USP—Preserve in tight, plastic containers. Label Gel in terms of the content of sodium fluoride (NaF) and in terms of the content of fluoride ion. Contains the labeled amount of fluoride ion, within ±10%, in an aqueous medium containing a suitable viscosity-inducing agent. Meets the requirements for Identification, Viscosity (7,000–20,000 centipoises), and pH (3.0–4.0).

Sodium Fluoride and Phosphoric Acid Topical Solution USP—Preserve in tight, plastic containers. Label Topical Solution in terms of the content of sodium fluoride (NaF) and in terms of the content of fluoride ion. Contains the labeled amount of fluoride ion, within ±10%. Meets the requirements for Identification tests and pH under Sodium Fluoride and Phosphoric Acid Gel.

SODIUM FORMALDEHYDE SULFOXYLATE

Chemical name: Methanesulfinic acid, hydroxy-, monosodium salt.

Molecular formula: CH_3NaO_3S.

Molecular weight: 118.08.

Description: Sodium Formaldehyde Sulfoxylate NF—White crystals or hard white masses, having the characteristic odor of garlic.

NF category: Antioxidant.

Solubility: Sodium Formaldehyde Sulfoxylate NF—Freely soluble in water; slightly soluble in alcohol, in ether, and in chloroform.

NF requirements: Sodium Formaldehyde Sulfoxylate NF—Preserve in well-closed, light-resistant containers, and store at controlled room temperature. Contains an amount of sodium formaldehyde sulfoxylate equivalent to not less than 45.5% and not more than 54.5% of sulfur dioxide, calculated on the dried basis. Meets the requirements for Clarity and color of solution, Identification, Alkalinity, pH (9.5–10.5, in a solution [1 in 50]), Loss on drying (not more than 27.0%), Sulfide, Iron (not more than 0.0025%), Sodium sulfite (not more than 5.0%, calculated on the dried basis), and Organic volatile impurities.

SODIUM GLUCONATE

Chemical name: D-Gluconic acid, monosodium salt.

Molecular formula: $C_6H_{11}NaO_7$.

Molecular weight: 218.14.

Description: Crystals. Technical grade may have a pleasant odor.

Solubility: Soluble in water at 25 °C: 59 grams/100 mL; sparingly soluble in alcohol; insoluble in ether.

USP requirements: Sodium Gluconate USP—Preserve in well-closed containers. Contains not less than 98.0% and not more than 102.0% of sodium gluconate. Meets the requirements for Identification, Chloride (not more than 0.07%), Sulfate (not more than 0.05%), Arsenic (not more than 3 ppm), Lead (not more than 0.001%), Heavy metals (not more than 0.002%), and Reducing substances (not more than 0.5%).

SODIUM HYDROXIDE

Chemical name: Sodium hydroxide.

Molecular formula: NaOH.

Molecular weight: 40.00.

Description: Sodium Hydroxide NF—White or practically white, fused masses, in small pellets, in flakes, or sticks, and in other forms. It is hard and brittle and shows a crystalline fracture. Exposed to the air, it rapidly absorbs carbon dioxide and moisture.

NF category: Alkalizing agent.

Solubility: Sodium Hydroxide NF—Freely soluble in water and in alcohol.

NF requirements: Sodium Hydroxide NF—Preserve in tight containers. Contains not less than 95.0% and not more than 100.5% of total alkali, calculated as sodium hydroxide, including not more than 3.0% of anhydrous sodium carbonate. Meets the requirements for Identification, Insoluble substances and organic matter, Potassium, and Heavy metals (not more than 0.003%).

Caution: Exercise great care in handling Sodium Hydroxide, as it rapidly destroys tissues.

SODIUM HYPOCHLORITE

Chemical name: Hypochlorous acid, sodium salt.

Molecular formula: $NaClO$.

Molecular weight: 74.44.

Description: Sodium Hypochlorite Solution USP—Clear, pale greenish yellow liquid, having the odor of chlorine. Affected by light.

USP requirements: Sodium Hypochlorite Solution USP—Preserve in tight, light-resistant containers, at a temperature not exceeding 25 °C. Contains not less than 4.0% and not more than 6.0%, by weight, of sodium hypochlorite. Meets the requirement for Identification.

Caution: This solution is not suitable for application to wounds.

SODIUM IODIDE

Chemical name: Sodium iodide.

Molecular formula: NaI.

Molecular weight: 149.89.

Description: Sodium Iodide USP—Colorless, odorless crystals, or white, crystalline powder. Is deliquescent in moist air, and develops a brown tint upon decomposition.

Solubility: Sodium Iodide USP—Very soluble in water; freely soluble in alcohol and in glycerin.

USP requirements:

Sodium Iodide USP—Preserve in tight containers. Contains not less than 99.0% and not more than 101.5% of sodium iodide, calculated on the anhydrous basis. Meets the requirements for Identification, Alkalinity, Water (not more than 2.0%), Iodate, Nitrate, nitrite, and ammonia, Thiosulfate and barium, Potassium, Heavy metals (not more than 0.001%), and Organic volatile impurities.

Sodium Iodide Injection—Not in USP.

SODIUM LACTATE

Chemical name: Sodium lactate—Propanoic acid, 2-hydroxy-, monosodium salt.

Molecular formula: Sodium lactate—$C_3H_5NaO_3$.

Molecular weight: Sodium lactate—112.06.

Description: Sodium Lactate Solution USP—Clear, colorless or practically colorless, slightly viscous liquid, odorless, or having a slight, not unpleasant odor.

NF category: Buffering agent.

Solubility: Sodium Lactate Solution USP—Miscible with water.

USP requirements:

Sodium Lactate Injection USP—Preserve in single-dose glass or plastic containers. Glass containers are preferably of Type I or Type II glass. It is sterile Sodium Lactate Solution in Water for Injection, or a sterile solution of Lactic Acid in Water for Injection prepared with the aid of Sodium Hydroxide. The label states the total osmolar concentration in mOsmol per liter. Where the contents are less than 100 mL, or where the label states that the Injection is not for direct injection but is to be diluted before use, the label alternatively may state the total osmolar concentration in mOsmol per mL. The label includes also the warning: "Not for use in the treatment of lactic acidosis." Contains the labeled amount, within −5% to +10%. Meets the requirements for Identification, Bacterial endotoxins, pH (6.0–7.3, the Injection being diluted with water, if necessary, to approximately 0.16 *M* [20 mg per mL]), Particulate matter, Heavy metals (not more than 0.001%), and Injections.

Sodium Lactate Solution USP—Preserve in tight containers. An aqueous solution containing not less than 50.0%, by weight, of monosodium lactate. Label it to indicate its content of sodium lactate. Contains the labeled amount, within ±2%. Meets the requirements for Identification, pH (5.0–9.0), Chloride (not more than 0.05%), Citrate, oxalate, phosphate, or tartrate, Sulfate, Heavy metals (not more than 0.001%), Sugars, and Methanol and methyl esters.

SODIUM LAURYL SULFATE

Chemical name: Sulfuric acid monododecyl ester sodium salt.

Molecular formula: $C_{12}H_{25}NaO_4S$.

Molecular weight: 288.38.

Description: Sodium Lauryl Sulfate NF—Small, white or light yellow crystals having a slight characteristic odor.

NF category: Emulsifying and/or solubilizing agent; wetting and/or solubilizing agent.

Solubility: Sodium Lauryl Sulfate NF—Freely soluble in water, forming an opalescent solution.

NF requirements: Sodium Lauryl Sulfate NF—Preserve in well-closed containers. A mixture of sodium alkyl sulfates consisting chiefly of sodium lauryl sulfate [$CH_3(CH_2)_{10}$-CH_2OSO_3Na]. The combined content of sodium chloride and sodium sulfate is not more than 8.0%. Meets the requirements for Identification, Alkalinity, Arsenic (not more than 3 ppm), Heavy metals (not more than 0.002%), Sodium chloride, Sodium sulfate, Unsulfated alcohols, and Total alcohols.

SODIUM METABISULFITE

Chemical name: Disulfurous acid, disodium salt.

Molecular formula: $Na_2S_2O_5$.

Molecular weight: 190.10.

Description: Sodium Metabisulfite NF—White crystals or white to yellowish crystalline powder, having the odor of sulfur dioxide.

NF category: Antioxidant.

Solubility: Sodium Metabisulfite NF—Freely soluble in water and in glycerin; slightly soluble in alcohol.

NF requirements: Sodium Metabisulfite NF—Preserve in well-filled, tight containers, and avoid exposure to excessive heat. Contains an amount of sodium metabisulfite equivalent to not less than 65.0% and not more than 67.4% of sulfur dioxide. Meets the requirements for Identification, Chloride (not more than 0.05%), Thiosulfate (not more than 0.05%), Arsenic (not more than 3 ppm), Iron (not more than 0.002%), and Heavy metals (not more than 0.002%).

SODIUM MONOFLUOROPHOSPHATE

Chemical name: Phosphorofluoridic acid, disodium salt.

Molecular formula: Na_2PFO_3.

Molecular weight: 143.95.

Description: Sodium Monofluorophosphate USP—White to slightly gray, odorless powder.

Solubility: Sodium Monofluorophosphate USP—Freely soluble in water.

USP requirements: Sodium Monofluorophosphate USP—Preserve in well-closed containers. Contains not less than 91.7% and not more than 100.5% of sodium monofluorophosphate, calculated on the dried basis. Meets the requirements for Identification, pH (6.5–8.0, in a solution [1 in 50]), Loss on drying (not more than 0.2%), Arsenic (not more than 3 ppm), Limit of fluoride ion (not more than 1.2%), Heavy metals (not more than 0.005%), and Organic volatile impurities.

SODIUM NITRITE

Chemical name: Nitrous acid, sodium salt.

Molecular formula: $NaNO_2$.

Molecular weight: 69.00.

Description:

Sodium Nitrite USP—White to slightly yellow, granular powder, or white or practically white, opaque, fused masses or sticks. Deliquescent in air. Its solutions are alkaline to litmus.

Sodium Nitrite Injection USP—Clear, colorless liquid.

Solubility: Sodium Nitrite USP—Freely soluble in water; sparingly soluble in alcohol.

USP requirements:

Sodium Nitrite USP—Preserve in tight containers. Contains not less than 97.0% and not more than 101.0% of sodium nitrite, calculated on the dried basis. Meets the requirements for Identification, Loss on drying (not more than 0.25%), and Heavy metals (not more than 0.002%).

Sodium Nitrite Injection USP—Preserve in single-dose containers, of Type I glass. A sterile solution of Sodium Nitrite in Water for Injection. Contains the labeled amount, within ±5%. Meets the requirements for Identification, Pyrogen, pH (7.0–9.0), and Injections.

SODIUM NITROPRUSSIDE

Chemical name: Ferrate(2-), pentakis(cyano-*C*)nitrosyl-, disodium, dihydrate, (*OC*-6-22)-.

Molecular formula: $Na_2[Fe(CN)_5NO]\cdot 2H_2O$.

Molecular weight: 297.95.

Description:

Sodium Nitroprusside USP—Reddish brown, practically odorless, crystals or powder.

Sterile Sodium Nitroprusside USP—Reddish brown, practically odorless, crystals or powder.

Solubility:

Sodium Nitroprusside USP—Freely soluble in water; slightly soluble in alcohol; very slightly soluble in chloroform.

Sterile Sodium Nitroprusside USP—Freely soluble in water; slightly soluble in alcohol; very slightly soluble in chloroform.

USP requirements:

Sodium Nitroprusside USP—Preserve in tight, light-resistant containers. Contains not less than 99.0% of sodium nitroprusside. Meets the requirements for Identification, Water (9.0–15.0%), Insoluble substances (not more than 0.01%), Chloride (not more than 0.02%), Ferricyanide (not more than 0.02%), Ferrocyanide (not more than 0.02%), and Sulfate (not more than 0.01%).

Sterile Sodium Nitroprusside USP—Preserve protected from light in Containers for Sterile Solids. It is Sodium Nitroprusside suitable for parenteral use. Contains the labeled amount, within ±10%. Meets the requirements for Constituted solution, Identification, Bacterial endotoxins, and Water (not more than 15.0%), for Identification test under Sodium Nitroprusside, and for Sterility tests, Uniformity of dosage units, and Labeling under Injections.

DIBASIC SODIUM PHOSPHATE

Chemical name: Phosphoric acid, disodium salt, heptahydrate.

Molecular formula: $Na_2HPO_4\cdot 7H_2O$.

Molecular weight: 268.07.

Description:

Dibasic Sodium Phosphate USP (dried)—White powder that readily absorbs moisture.

NF category: Buffering agent.

Dibasic Sodium Phosphate USP (heptahydrate)—Colorless or white, granular or caked salt. Effloresces in warm, dry air. Its solutions are alkaline to phenolphthalein TS, a 0.1 *M* solution having a pH of about 9.

NF category: Buffering agent.

Solubility:

Dibasic Sodium Phosphate USP (dried)—Freely soluble in water; insoluble in alcohol.

Dibasic Sodium Phosphate USP (heptahydrate)—Freely soluble in water; very slightly soluble in alcohol.

USP requirements:

Dibasic Sodium Phosphate USP—Preserve in tight containers. It is dried or contains seven molecules of water of hydration. Label it to indicate whether it is dried or is the heptahydrate. Contains not less than 98.0% and not more than 100.5% of dibasic sodium phosphate, calculated on the dried basis. Meets the requirements for Identification, Loss on drying (not more than 5.0% for the dried form and 43.0–50.0% for the heptahydrate), Insoluble substances (not more than 0.4%), Chloride (not more than 0.06%), Sulfate (not more than 0.2%), Arsenic (not more than 16 ppm), and Heavy metals (not more than 0.002%).

Effervescent Sodium Phosphate Powder—Not in USP.

MONOBASIC SODIUM PHOSPHATE

Chemical name: Phosphoric acid, monosodium salt, monohydrate; phosphoric acid, monosodium salt, dihydrate.

Molecular formula: $NaH_2PO_4\cdot xH_2O$.

Molecular weight: 137.99 (monohydrate); 119.98 (anhydrous); 156.01 (dihydrate).

Description: Monobasic Sodium Phosphate USP—Colorless crystals or white, crystalline powder. Odorless and slightly deliquescent. Its solutions are acid to litmus and effervesce with sodium carbonate.

NF category: Buffering agent.

Solubility: Monobasic Sodium Phosphate USP—Freely soluble in water; practically insoluble in alcohol.

USP requirements: Monobasic Sodium Phosphate USP—Preserve in well-closed containers. Contains one or two molecules of water of hydration, or is anhydrous. Label it to indicate whether it is anhydrous or is the monohydrate or the dihydrate. Contains not less than 98.0% and not more than 103.0% of monobasic sodium phosphate, calculated on the anhydrous basis. Meets the requirements for Identification, pH (4.1–4.5, in a solution containing the equivalent of 1.0 gram of monobasic sodium phosphate [monohydrate] in 20 mL of water), Water (less than 2.0% for the anhydrous form, 10.0–15.0% for the monohydrate, 18.0–26.5% for the dihydrate), Insoluble substances (not more than 0.2%), Chloride (not more than 0.014%), Sulfate (not more than 0.15%), Aluminum, calcium, and related elements, Arsenic (not more than 8 ppm), Heavy metals (not more than 0.002%), and Organic volatile impurities.

SODIUM PHOSPHATES

For *Dibasic Sodium Phosphate* and *Monobasic Sodium Phosphate*—See individual listings for chemistry information.

USP requirements:

Sodium Phosphates Enema USP—Preserve in well-closed, single-unit containers. A solution of Dibasic Sodium Phosphate and Monobasic Sodium Phosphate, or Dibasic Sodium Phosphate and Phosphoric Acid, in Purified Water. Contains, in each 100 mL, not less than 5.7 grams and not more than 6.3 grams of dibasic sodium phosphate (heptahydrate), and not less than 15.2 grams and not more than 16.8 grams of monobasic sodium phosphate (monohydrate). Meets the requirements for Identification, Specific gravity (1.121–1.128), pH (5.0–5.8), Chloride (not more than 0.008%), Arsenic (not more than 2 ppm), and Heavy metals (not more than 0.001%).

Sodium Phosphates Injection USP—Preserve in single-dose containers, preferably of Type I glass. A sterile solution of Monobasic Sodium Phosphate and Dibasic Sodium Phosphate in Water for Injection. The label states the sodium content in terms of milliequivalents in a given volume, and states also the phosphorus content in terms of millimoles in a given volume. Label the Injection to indicate that it is to be diluted to appropriate strength with water or other suitable fluid prior to administration, and that once opened any unused portion is to be discarded. The label states also the total osmolar concentration in mOsmol per liter. Where the contents are less than 100 mL, or where the label states that the Injection is not for direct injection but is to be diluted before use, the label alternatively may state the total osmolar concentration in mOsmol per mL. Contains the labeled amounts of monobasic sodium phosphate and dibasic sodium phosphate, within ±5%. Contains no bacteriostat or other preservative. Meets the requirements for Identification, Bacterial endotoxins, Particulate matter, and Injections.

Sodium Phosphates Oral Solution USP—Preserve in tight containers. A solution of Dibasic Sodium Phosphate and Monobasic Sodium Phosphate, or Dibasic Sodium Phosphate and Phosphoric Acid, in Purified Water. Contains, in each 100 mL, not less than 17.1 grams and not more than 18.9 grams of dibasic sodium phosphate (heptahydrate), and not less than 45.6 grams and not more than 50.4 grams of monobasic sodium phosphate (monohydrate). Meets the requirements for Identification, pH (4.4–5.2), Chloride (not more than 0.01%), Arsenic (not more than 2 ppm), and Heavy metals (not more than 0.001%).

SODIUM POLYSTYRENE SULFONATE

Chemical name: Benzene, diethenyl-, polymer with ethenylbenzene, sulfonated, sodium salt.

Description: Sodium Polystyrene Sulfonate USP—Golden brown, fine powder. Is odorless.

Solubility: Sodium Polystyrene Sulfonate USP—Insoluble in water.

USP requirements:

Sodium Polystyrene Sulfonate USP (for Suspension)—Preserve in well-closed containers. A cation-exchange resin prepared in the sodium form. Sodium Polystyrene Sulfonate that is intended for preparing suspensions for oral or rectal administration may be labeled Sodium Polystyrene Sulfonate for Suspension. Each gram exchanges not less than 110 mg and not more than 135 mg of potassium, calculated on the anhydrous basis. Meets the requirements for Water (not more than 10.0%), Ammonia, Sodium content (9.4–11.5%, calculated on the anhydrous basis), and Potassium exchange capacity.

Sodium Polystyrene Sulfonate Suspension USP—Preserve in well-closed containers, protected from freezing and from excessive heat. A suspension of Sodium Polystyrene Sulfonate in an aqueous vehicle containing a suitable quantity of sorbitol. Label it to state the quantity of sorbitol in a given volume of Suspension. Contains the labeled amount of sorbitol, within ±10%. Each gram of the labeled amount of sodium polystyrene sulfonate exchanges not less than 110 mg and not more than 135 mg of potassium. Meets the requirements for Microbial limits, Sodium content (9.4–11.5%, based on the labeled amount) and Potassium exchange capacity.

SODIUM PROPIONATE

Chemical name: Propanoic acid, sodium salt, hydrate.

Molecular formula: $C_3H_5NaO_2 \cdot xH_2O$.

Molecular weight: 96.06 (anhydrous).

Description: Sodium Propionate NF—Colorless, transparent crystals or granular, crystalline powder. Odorless, or has a slight acetic-butyric odor. Deliquescent in moist air.

NF category: Antimicrobial preservative.

Solubility: Sodium Propionate NF—Very soluble in water; soluble in alcohol.

NF requirements: Sodium Propionate NF—Preserve in tight containers. Dried at 105 °C for 2 hours, contains not less than 99.0% and not more than 100.5% of anhydrous sodium propionate. Meets the requirements for Identification, Alkalinity, Water (not more than 1.0%), Arsenic (not more than 3 ppm), Heavy metals (not more than 0.001%), and Organic volatile impurities.

SODIUM SALICYLATE

Chemical name: Benzoic acid, 2-hydroxy-, monosodium salt.

Molecular formula: $C_7H_5NaO_3$.

Molecular weight: 160.10.

Description: Sodium Salicylate USP—Amorphous or microcrystalline powder or scales. Is colorless, or has not more than a faint, pink tinge. Is odorless, or has a faint, characteristic odor, and is affected by light. A freshly made solution (1 in 10) is neutral or acid to litmus.

Solubility: Sodium Salicylate USP—Freely (and slowly) soluble in water and in glycerin; very soluble in boiling water and in boiling alcohol; slowly soluble in alcohol.

USP requirements:

Sodium Salicylate USP—Preserve in well-closed, light-resistant containers. Contains not less than 99.5% and not more than 100.5% of sodium salicylate, calculated on the anhydrous basis. Meets the requirements for Identification, Water (not more than 0.5%), Sulfite or thiosulfate,

Heavy metals (not more than 0.002%), and Organic volatile impurities.

Sodium Salicylate Tablets USP—Preserve in well-closed containers. Contain the labeled amount, within ±5%. Meet the requirements for Identification, Dissolution (75% in 45 minutes in water in Apparatus 1 at 100 rpm), and Uniformity of dosage units.

Sodium Salicylate Delayed-release Tablets—Not in USP.

SODIUM STARCH GLYCOLATE

Chemical name: Starch carboxymethyl ether, sodium salt.

Description: Sodium Starch Glycolate NF—White, odorless, relatively free-flowing powder; available in several different viscosity grades. A 2% (w/v) dispersion in cold water settles, on standing, in the form of a highly hydrated layer.

NF category: Tablet disintegrant.

NF requirements: Sodium Starch Glycolate NF—Preserve in well-closed containers, preferably protected from wide variations in temperature and humidity, which may cause caking. The sodium salt of a carboxymethyl ether of starch. The labeling indicates the pH range. Contains not less than 2.8% and not more than 4.2% of sodium on the dried, alcohol-washed basis. May contain not more than 7.0% of Sodium Chloride. Meets the requirements for Identification, Microbial limits, pH (3.0–5.0 or 5.5–7.5), Loss on drying (not more than 10.0%), Iron (not more than 0.002%), Heavy metals (not more than 0.002%), and Sodium chloride.

SODIUM STEARATE

Chemical name: Octadecanoic acid, sodium salt.

Molecular formula: $C_{18}H_{35}NaO_2$.

Molecular weight: 306.46.

Description: Sodium Stearate NF—Fine, white powder, soapy to the touch, usually having a slight tallow-like odor. It is affected by light. Its solutions are alkaline to phenolphthalein TS.

NF category: Emulsifying and/or solubilizing agent.

Solubility: Sodium Stearate NF—Slowly soluble in cold water and in cold alcohol; readily soluble in hot water and in hot alcohol.

NF requirements: Sodium Stearate NF—Preserve in well-closed, light-resistant containers. A mixture of sodium stearate and sodium palmitate, which together constitute not less than 90.0% of the total content. The content of sodium stearate is not less than 40.0% of the total. Contains small amounts of the sodium salts of other fatty acids. Meets the requirements for Identification, Acidity, Loss on drying (not more than 5.0%), Alcohol-insoluble substances, Iodine value of fatty acids (not more than 4.0), Acid value of fatty acids (196–211), and Organic volatile impurities.

SODIUM STEARYL FUMARATE

Description: Sodium Stearyl Fumarate NF—Fine, white powder.

NF category: Tablet and/or capsule lubricant.

Solubility: Sodium Stearyl Fumarate NF—Slightly soluble in methanol; practically insoluble in water.

NF requirements: Sodium Stearyl Fumarate NF—Preserve in well-closed containers. Contains not less than 99.0% and not more than 101.5% of sodium stearyl fumarate. Meets the requirements for Identification, Water (not more than 5.0%), Arsenic (not more than 3 ppm), Lead (not more than 0.001%), Heavy metals (not more than 0.002%), Limit of sodium stearyl maleate and stearyl alcohol (not more than 0.25% of sodium stearyl maleate and not more than 0.5% of stearyl alcohol), and Saponification value (142.2–146.0, calculated on the anhydrous basis).

SODIUM SULFATE

Chemical name: Sulfuric acid disodium salt, decahydrate.

Molecular formula: $Na_2SO_4 \cdot 10H_2O$.

Molecular weight: 322.19.

Description: Sodium Sulfate USP—Large, colorless, odorless, transparent crystals, or granular powder. Effloresces rapidly in air, liquifies in its water of hydration at about 33 °C, and loses all of its water of hydration at about 100 °C.

Solubility: Sodium Sulfate USP—Freely soluble in water; soluble in glycerin; insoluble in alcohol.

USP requirements:

Sodium Sulfate USP—Preserve in tight containers, preferably at a temperature not exceeding 30 °C. Contains ten molecules of water of hydration, or is anhydrous. Label it to indicate whether it is the decahydrate or is anhydrous. Contains not less than 99.0% of sodium sulfate, calculated on the dried basis. Meets the requirements for Identification, Acidity or alkalinity, Loss on drying (51.0–57.0% for the decahydrate and not more than 0.5% for the anhydrous form), Chloride (not more than 0.02%), Arsenic (not more than 0.001%), and Heavy metals (not more than 0.001%).

Sodium Sulfate Injection USP—Preserve in single-dose containers, preferably of Type I glass. A sterile, concentrated solution of Sodium Sulfate in Water for Injection, which upon dilution is suitable for parenteral use. Label it to indicate that it is to be diluted before injection to render it isotonic (3.89% of sodium sulfate decahydrate). Contains the labeled amount, within ±5%. Meets the requirements for Identification, Pyrogen, pH (5.0–6.5), and Injections.

SODIUM THIOSULFATE

Chemical name: Thiosulfuric acid, disodium salt, pentahydrate.

Molecular formula: $Na_2S_2O_3 \cdot 5H_2O$.

Molecular weight: 248.17.

Description: Sodium Thiosulfate USP—Large, colorless crystals or coarse, crystalline powder. Is deliquescent in moist air and effloresces in dry air at temperatures exceeding 33 °C. Its solutions are neutral or faintly alkaline to litmus.

NF category: Antioxidant.

Solubility: Sodium Thiosulfate USP—Very soluble in water; insoluble in alcohol.

USP requirements:

Sodium Thiosulfate USP—Preserve in tight containers. Contains not less than 99.0% and not more than 100.5% of sodium thiosulfate, calculated on the anhydrous basis. Meets the requirements for Identification, Water (32.0–37.0%), Calcium, Arsenic (not more than 3 ppm), and Heavy metals (not more than 0.002%).

Sodium Thiosulfate Injection USP—Preserve in single-dose containers, of Type I glass. A sterile solution of Sodium

Thiosulfate in freshly boiled Water for Injection. Contains the labeled amount, within ±5%. Meets the requirements for Identification, Bacterial endotoxins, pH (6.0–9.5), and Injections.

SOMATREM

Source: Biosynthetic. A single polypeptide chain of 192 amino acids, one more (methionine) than naturally occurring human growth hormone, produced by a recombinant DNA process in *Escherichia coli*.

Chemical name: Somatotropin (human), *N*-L-methionyl-.

Molecular formula: $C_{995}H_{1537}N_{263}O_{301}S_8$.

Molecular weight: 22,256.21.

USP requirements: Somatrem for Injection—Not in USP.

SOMATROPIN

Source: Somatropin, recombinant—Biosynthetic, produced by a recombinant DNA process in *Escherichia coli*; same amino acid sequence as pituitary-derived somatropin. A single polypeptide chain of 191 amino acids.

Chemical name: Growth hormone (human).

Molecular formula: $C_{990}H_{1528}N_{262}O_{300}S_7$.

Molecular weight: 22,125.02.

USP requirements: Somatropin, Recombinant, for Injection—Not in USP.

SORBIC ACID

Chemical name: 2,4-Hexadienoic acid, (*E,E*)-.

Molecular formula: $C_6H_8O_2$.

Molecular weight: 112.13.

Description: Sorbic Acid NF—Free-flowing, white, crystalline powder, having a characteristic odor.

NF category: Antimicrobial preservative.

Solubility: Sorbic Acid NF—Slightly soluble in water; soluble in alcohol and in ether.

NF requirements: Sorbic Acid NF—Preserve in tight containers, protected from light, and avoid exposure to excessive heat. Contains not less than 99.0% and not more than 101.0% of sorbic acid, calculated on the anhydrous basis. Meets the requirements for Identification, Melting range (132–135 °C), Water (not more than 0.5%), Residue on ignition (not more than 0.2%), Heavy metals (not more than 0.001%), and Organic volatile impurities.

SORBITAN MONOLAURATE

Chemical name: Sorbitan, esters, monododecanoate.

Description: Sorbitan Monolaurate NF—Yellow to amber oily liquid, having a bland, characteristic odor.

NF category: Emulsifying and/or solubilizing agent; wetting and/or solubilizing agent.

Solubility: Sorbitan Monolaurate NF—Insoluble in water; soluble in mineral oil; slightly soluble in cottonseed oil and in ethyl acetate.

NF requirements: Sorbitan Monolaurate NF—Preserve in tight containers. A partial ester of lauric acid with Sorbitol and its mono- and dianhydrides. Yields, upon saponification, not less than 55.0% and not more than 63.0% of fatty acids, and not less than 39.0% and not more than 45.0% of polyols (w/w). Meets the requirements for Identification, Water (not more than 1.5%), Residue on ignition (not more than 0.5%), Heavy metals (not more than 0.001%), Acid value (not more than 8), Hydroxyl value (330–358), Saponification value (158–170), and Organic volatile impurities.

SORBITAN MONOOLEATE

Chemical name: Sorbitan esters, mono(*Z*)-9-octadecenoate.

Molecular formula: $C_{24}H_{44}O_6$ (approximate).

Description: Sorbitan Monooleate NF—Viscous, yellow to amber-colored, oily liquid, having a bland, characteristic odor.

NF category: Emulsifying and/or solubilizing agent; wetting and/or solubilizing agent.

Solubility: Sorbitan Monooleate NF—Insoluble in water and in propylene glycol. Miscible with mineral and vegetable oils.

NF requirements: Sorbitan Monooleate NF—Preserve in tight containers. A partial oleate ester of Sorbitol and its mono- and dianhydrides. Yields, upon saponification, not less than 72.0% and not more than 78.0% of fatty acids, and not less than 25.0% and not more than 31.0% of polyols (w/w). Meets the requirements for Identification, Water (not more than 1.0%), Residue on ignition (not more than 0.5%), Heavy metals (not more than 0.001%), Acid value (not more than 8), Hydroxyl value (190–215), Iodine value (62–76), and Saponification value (145–160).

SORBITAN MONOPALMITATE

Chemical name: Sorbitan, esters, monohexadecanoate.

Molecular formula: $C_{22}H_{42}O_6$ (approximate).

Description: Sorbitan Monopalmitate NF—Cream-colored, waxy solid, having a faint fatty odor.

NF category: Emulsifying and/or solubilizing agent; wetting and/or solubilizing agent.

Solubility: Sorbitan Monopalmitate NF—Insoluble in water; soluble in warm absolute alcohol; soluble, with haze, in warm peanut oil and in warm mineral oil.

NF requirements: Sorbitan Monopalmitate NF—Preserve in well-closed containers. A partial ester of palmitic acid with Sorbitol and its mono- and dianhydrides. Yields, upon saponification, not less than 63.0% and not more than 71.0% of fatty acids, and not less than 32.0% and not more than 38.0% of polyols (w/w). Meets the requirements for Identification, Water (not more than 1.5%), Residue on ignition (not more than 0.5%), Heavy metals (not more than 0.001%), Acid value (not more than 8), Hydroxyl value (275–305), and Saponification value (140–150).

SORBITAN MONOSTEARATE

Chemical name: Sorbitan, esters, monooctadecanoate.

Molecular formula: $C_{24}H_{46}O_6$ (approximate).

Description: Sorbitan Monostearate NF—Cream-colored to tan, hard, waxy solid, having a bland odor.

NF category: Emulsifying and/or solubilizing agent; wetting and/or solubilizing agent.

Solubility: Sorbitan Monostearate NF—Insoluble in cold water and in acetone; dispersible in warm water; soluble, with haze, above 50 °C in mineral oil and in ethyl acetate.

NF requirements: Sorbitan Monostearate NF—Preserve in well-closed containers. A partial ester of Stearic Acid with Sorbitol and its mono- and dianhydrides. Yields, upon saponification, not less than 68.0% and not more than 76.0% of fatty acids, and not less than 27.0% and not more than 34.0% of polyols (w/w). Meets the requirements for Identification, Water (not more than 1.5%), Residue on ignition (not more than 0.5%), Heavy metals (not more than 0.001%), Acid value (not more than 10), Hydroxyl value (235–260), and Saponification value (147–157).

SORBITAN SESQUIOLEATE

Chemical name: Sorbitan, esters, sesqui-9-octadecenoate, (*Z*)-.

Molecular formula: $C_{33}H_{60}O_{6.5}$ (approximate).

Description: Sorbitan Sesquioleate NF—Viscous, yellow to amber-colored, oily liquid.

NF category: Emulsifying and/or solubilizing agent; wetting and/or solubilizing agent.

Solubility: Sorbitan Sesquioleate NF—Insoluble in water and in propylene glycol; soluble in alcohol, in isopropyl alcohol, in cottonseed oil, and in mineral oil.

NF requirements: Sorbitan Sesquioleate NF—Preserve in tight containers. A partial oleate ester of Sorbitol and its mono- and dianhydrides. Yields, upon saponification, not less than 74.0% and not more than 80.0% of fatty acids, and not less than 22.0% and not more than 28.0% of polyols (w/w). Meets the requirements for Identification, Water (not more than 1.0%), Residue on ignition (not more than 1.4%), Heavy metals (not more than 0.001%), Acid value (not more than 14), Hydroxyl value (182–220), Iodine value (65–75), and Saponification value (143–165).

SORBITAN TRIOLEATE

Chemical name: Sorbitan, esters, tri-9-octadecenoate, (*Z,Z,Z*)-.

Molecular formula: $C_{60}H_{108}O_8$ (approximate).

Description: Sorbitan Trioleate NF—Yellow to amber-colored, oily liquid.

NF category: Emulsifying and/or solubilizing agent; wetting and/or solubilizing agent.

Solubility: Sorbitan Trioleate NF—Insoluble in water, in ethylene glycol, and in propylene glycol; soluble in methyl alcohol, in alcohol, in isopropyl alcohol, in corn oil, in cottonseed oil, and in mineral oil.

NF requirements: Sorbitan Trioleate NF—Preserve in tight containers. The triester of Oleic Acid and Sorbitol and its mono- and dianhydrides. Yields, upon saponification, not less than 85.5% and not more than 90.0% of fatty acids, and not less than 13.0% and not more than 19.0% of polyols (w/w). Meets the requirements for Identification, Water (not more than 0.7%), Residue on ignition (not more than 0.25%), Heavy metals (not more than 0.001%), Acid value (not more than 17), Hydroxyl value (50–75), Iodine value (77–85), and Saponification value (169–183).

SORBITOL

Chemical name: D-Glucitol.

Molecular formula: $C_6H_{14}O_6$.

Molecular weight: 182.17.

Description:

Sorbitol NF—White, hygroscopic powder, granules, or flakes.

NF category: Humectant; sweetening agent; tablet and/or capsule diluent.

Sorbitol Solution USP—Clear, colorless, syrupy liquid. Neutral to litmus.

NF category: Sweetening agent; vehicle (flavored and/or sweetened).

Solubility: Sorbitol NF—Very soluble in water; slightly soluble in alcohol, in methanol, and in acetic acid.

USP requirements: Sorbitol Solution USP—Preserve in tight containers. A water solution containing, in each 100.0 grams, not less than 64.0 grams of D–sorbitol. Meets the requirements for Identification, Specific gravity (not less than 1.285), Refractive index (1.455–1.465 at 20 °C), Water (28.5–31.5%), Residue on ignition (not more than 0.1%), Chloride (not more than 0.005%), Sulfate (not more than 0.010%), Arsenic (not more than 2.5 ppm), Heavy metals (not more than 0.001%), and Reducing sugars.

NF requirements: Sorbitol NF—Preserve in tight containers. Contains not less than 91.0% and not more than 100.5% of sorbitol, calculated on the anhydrous basis. May contain small amounts of other polyhydric alcohols. Meets the requirements for Identification, Water (not more than 1.0%), Residue on ignition (not more than 0.1%), Chloride (not more than 0.0050%), Sulfate (not more than 0.010%), Arsenic (not more than 3 ppm), Heavy metals (not more than 0.001%), Reducing sugars, and Total sugars.

SOTALOL

Chemical name: Sotalol hydrochloride—Methanesulfonamide, *N*-[4-[1-hydroxy-2-[(1-methylethyl)amino]ethyl]phenyl]-, monohydrochloride.

Molecular formula: Sotalol hydrochloride—$C_{12}H_{20}N_2O_3S \cdot HCl$.

Molecular weight: Sotalol hydrochloride—308.82.

Description: Sotalol hydrochloride—White, crystalline solid. Melting point 206.5–207 °C with decomposition.

Solubility: Sotalol hydrochloride—Freely soluble in water; slightly soluble in chloroform.

Other characteristics: Lipid solubility—Low.

USP requirements: Sotalol Hydrochloride Tablets—Not in USP.

SOYBEAN OIL

Description: Soybean Oil USP—Clear, pale yellow, oily liquid having a characteristic odor.

NF category: Vehicle (oleaginous).

Solubility: Soybean Oil USP—Insoluble in water. Miscible with ether and with chloroform.

USP requirements: Soybean Oil USP—Preserve in tight, light-resistant containers, and avoid exposure to excessive heat. The refined fixed oil obtained from the seeds of the soya plant *Glycine soja* (Fam. Leguminosae). Meets the requirements for Specific gravity (0.916–0.922), Refractive index (1.465–1.475), Heavy metals (not more than 0.001%), Free fatty acids, Fatty acid composition, Iodine value (120–141), Saponification value (180–200), Unsaponifiable matter (not more than 1.0%), Cottonseed oil, and Peroxide.

SPECTINOMYCIN

Source: Produced by a species of the soil microorganism *Streptomyces spectabilis.*

Chemical name: Spectinomycin hydrochloride—4*H*-Pyrano-[2,3-*b*][1,4]benzodioxin-4-one, decahydro-4a,7,9-trihydroxy-2-methyl-6,8-bis(methylamino)-, dihydrochloride, pentahydrate.

Molecular formula: Spectinomycin hydrochloride—$C_{14}H_{24}N_2O_7 \cdot 2HCl \cdot 5H_2O$.

Molecular weight: Spectinomycin hydrochloride—495.35.

Description: Sterile Spectinomycin Hydrochloride USP—White to pale-buff crystalline powder.

Solubility: Sterile Spectinomycin Hydrochloride USP—Freely soluble in water; practically insoluble in alcohol, in chloroform, and in ether.

USP requirements:

Sterile Spectinomycin Hydrochloride USP—Preserve in Containers for Sterile Solids. Has a potency equivalent to not less than 603 mcg of spectinomycin per mg. Meets the requirements for Identification, Crystallinity, Depressor substances, Bacterial endotoxins, Sterility, pH (3.8–5.6, in a solution containing 10 mg per mL [where packaged for dispensing, 4.0–7.0, in the solution constituted as directed in the labeling]), Water (16.0–20.0%), and Residue on ignition (not more than 1.0%).

Sterile Spectinomycin Hydrochloride for Suspension USP—Preserve in Containers for Sterile Solids. It is Sterile Spectinomycin Hydrochloride packaged for dispensing. Contains an amount of spectinomycin hydrochloride equivalent to the labeled amount of spectinomycin, within −10% to +20%. Conforms to the definition and meets the requirements for Identification test, Crystallinity, Bacterial endotoxins, Sterility, pH, Water, and Residue on ignition under Sterile Spectinomycin Hydrochloride, and for Uniformity of dosage units and Labeling under Injections.

SPIRONOLACTONE

Chemical name: Pregn-4-ene-21-carboxylic acid, 7-(acetylthio)-17-hydroxy-3-oxo-, gamma-lactone, (7 alpha,17 alpha)-.

Molecular formula: $C_{24}H_{32}O_4S$.

Molecular weight: 416.58.

Description: Spironolactone USP—Light cream-colored to light tan, crystalline powder. Has a faint to mild mercaptan-like odor; is stable in air.

Solubility: Spironolactone USP—Practically insoluble in water; freely soluble in chloroform; soluble in ethyl acetate and in alcohol; slightly soluble in methanol and in fixed oils.

USP requirements:

Spironolactone USP—Preserve in well-closed containers. Contains not less than 97.0% and not more than 103.0% of spironolactone, calculated on the dried basis. Meets the requirements for Identification, Melting range (198–207 °C, with decomposition), Specific rotation (−33° to −37°), Loss on drying (not more than 0.5%), Limit of mercapto compounds, Ordinary impurities, and Organic volatile impurities.

Spironolactone Tablets USP—Preserve in tight, light-resistant containers. Contain the labeled amount, within ±5%. Meet the requirements for Identification, Dissolution (75% in 60 minutes in 0.1 *N* hydrochloric acid containing 0.1% of sodium lauryl sulfate in Apparatus 2 at 75 rpm), and Uniformity of dosage units.

SPIRONOLACTONE AND HYDROCHLOROTHIAZIDE

For *Spironolactone* and *Hydrochlorothiazide*—See individual listings for chemistry information.

USP requirements: Spironolactone and Hydrochlorothiazide Tablets USP—Preserve in tight, light-resistant containers. Contain the labeled amounts, within ±10%. Meet the requirements for Identification, Dissolution (75% of each active ingredient in 60 minutes in 0.1 *N* hydrochloric acid containing 0.1% sodium lauryl sulfate in Apparatus 2 at 75 rpm), and Uniformity of dosage units.

SQUALANE

Chemical name: Tetracosane, 2,6,10,15,19,23-hexamethyl-.

Molecular formula: $C_{30}H_{62}$.

Molecular weight: 422.82.

Description: Squalane NF—Colorless, practically odorless transparent oil.

NF category: Ointment base; vehicle (oleaginous).

Solubility: Squalane NF—Insoluble in water; very slightly soluble in absolute alcohol; slightly soluble in acetone. Miscible with ether and with chloroform.

NF requirements: Squalane NF—Preserve in tight containers. A saturated hydrocarbon obtained by hydrogenation of squalene, an aliphatic triterpene occurring in some fish oils. Meets the requirements for Identification, Specific gravity (0.807–0.810 at 20 °C), Refractive index (1.4510–1.4525 at 20 °C), Residue on ignition (not more than 0.5%), Acid value (not more than 0.2), Iodine value (not more than 4), Saponification value (not more than 2), and Chromatographic purity.

STANNOUS FLUORIDE

Chemical name: Tin fluoride (SnF_2).

Molecular formula: SnF_2.

Molecular weight: 156.71.

Description: Stannous Fluoride USP—White, crystalline powder. Melts at about 213 °C.

Solubility: Stannous Fluoride USP—Freely soluble in water; practically insoluble in alcohol, in ether, and in chloroform.

USP requirements:

Stannous Fluoride USP—Preserve in well-closed containers. Contains not less than 71.2% of stannous tin, and not less than 22.3% and not more than 25.5% of fluoride, calculated on the dried basis. Meets the requirements for Identification, pH (2.8–3.5, in a freshly prepared 0.4% solution), Loss on drying (not more than 0.5%), Water-insoluble substances (not more than 0.2%), and Antimony (not more than 0.005%).

Stannous Fluoride Gel USP—Preserve in well-closed containers. Contains the labeled amount, within −5% to +15%, in a suitable medium containing a suitable viscosity-inducing agent. Meets the requirements for Identification, Viscosity (600–170,000 centipoises), pH (2.8–4.0, in a freshly prepared mixture with water [1:1]), and Stannous ion content (not less than 68.2% of the labeled amount of stannous fluoride).

Note: If Glycerin is used as the medium in the preparation of this Gel, use Glycerin that has a low water content, that is, Glycerin having a specific gravity of not less than 1.2607, corresponding to a concentration of 99.5%.

STANOZOLOL

Chemical group: 17-alpha alkylated anabolic steroid.

Chemical name: 2′*H*-Androst-2-eno[3,2-*c*]pyrazol-17-ol, 17-methyl-, (5 alpha,17 beta)-.

Molecular formula: $C_{21}H_{32}N_2O$.

Molecular weight: 328.50.

Description: Stanozolol USP—Odorless, crystalline powder, occurring in two forms: as needles, melting at about 155 °C, and as prisms, melting at about 235 °C.

Solubility: Stanozolol USP—Insoluble in water; soluble in dimethylformamide; sparingly soluble in alcohol and in chloroform; slightly soluble in ethyl acetate and in acetone.

USP requirements:

Stanozolol USP—Preserve in tight, light-resistant containers. Contains not less than 98.0% and not more than 100.5% of stanozolol, calculated on the dried basis. Meets the requirements for Identification, Specific rotation (+34° to +40°), Loss on drying (not more than 1.0%), Chromatographic purity, and Organic volatile impurities.

Stanozolol Tablets USP—Preserve in tight, light-resistant containers. Contain the labeled amount, within ±10%. Meet the requirements for Identification, Dissolution (75% in 45 minutes in 0.1 *N* hydrochloric acid in Apparatus 2 at 50 rpm), and Uniformity of dosage units.

STARCH

Chemical name: Starch.

Description: Starch NF—Irregular, angular, white masses or fine powder. Odorless.

NF category: Tablet and/or capsule diluent; tablet disintegrant.

Solubility: Starch NF—Insoluble in cold water and in alcohol.

NF requirements: Starch NF—Preserve in well-closed containers. Consists of the granules separated from the mature grain of corn (*Zea mays* Linné [Fam. Gramineae]) or of wheat (*Triticum aestivum* Linné [Fam. Gramineae]), or from tubers of the potato (*Solanum tuberosum* Linné [Fam. Solanaceae]) or of tapioca (*Manihot utilissima* Pehl [Fam. Euphorbi Aceae]). Label it to indicate the botanical source from which it was derived. Meets the requirements for Botanic characteristics, Identification, Microbial limits, pH (4.5–7.0 for Corn starch, Tapioca starch, and Wheat starch, and 5.0–8.0 for Potato starch), Loss on drying (not more than 14.0%), Residue on ignition (not more than 0.5%), Iron (not more than 0.002%), Oxidizing substances (not more than 0.002%), and Sulfur dioxide (not more than 0.008%).

Note: Starches obtained from different botanical sources may not have identical properties with respect to their use for specific pharmaceutical purposes, e.g., as a tablet-disintegrating agent. Therefore, types of starch should not be interchanged unless performance equivalency has been ascertained.

PREGELATINIZED STARCH

Description: Pregelatinized Starch NF—Moderately coarse to fine, white to off-white powder. Odorless.

NF category: Tablet binder; tablet and/or capsule diluent; tablet disintegrant.

Solubility: Pregelatinized Starch NF—Slightly soluble to soluble in cold water; insoluble in alcohol.

NF requirements: Pregelatinized Starch NF—Starch that has been chemically and/or mechanically processed to rupture all or part of the granules in the presence of water and subsequently dried. Some types of Pregelatinized Starch may be modified to render them compressible and flowable in character. Meets the requirements for pH (4.5–7.0, determined potentiometrically), Iron (not more than 0.002%), Oxidizing substances, Sulfur dioxide (not more than 0.008%), and Organic volatile impurities, and for Identification test B, Packaging and storage, Labeling, Microbial limits, Loss on drying, and Residue on ignition under Starch.

TOPICAL STARCH

USP requirements: Topical Starch USP—Preserve in well-closed containers. Consists of granules separated from the mature grain of corn (*Zea mays* Linné [Fam. Gramineae]). Meets the requirements for Botanic characteristics, Identification, Microbial limits, pH (4.5–7.0, determined potentiometrically), Loss on drying (not more than 14.0%), Residue on ignition (not more than 0.5%), Iron (not more than 0.001%), Oxidizing substances (not more than 0.018%), and Sulfur dioxide (not more than 0.008%).

STEARIC ACID

Chemical name: Octadecanoic acid.

Molecular formula: $C_{18}H_{36}O_2$.

Molecular weight: 284.48.

Description: Stearic Acid NF—Hard, white or faintly yellowish, somewhat glossy and crystalline solid, or white or yellowish-white powder. Slight odor, suggesting tallow.

NF category: Emulsifying and/or solubilizing agent; tablet and/or capsule lubricant.

Solubility: Stearic Acid NF—Practically insoluble in water; freely soluble in chloroform and in ether; soluble in alcohol.

NF requirements: Stearic Acid NF—Preserve in well-closed containers. Manufactured from fats and oils derived from edible sources and is a mixture of Stearic Acid and palmitic acid. The content of Stearic Acid is not less than 40.0%, and the sum of the two is not less than 90.0%. If it is for external use only, the labeling so indicates. Meets the requirements for Congealing temperature (not lower than 54 °C), Residue on ignition (not more than 0.1%), Heavy metals (not more than 0.001%), Mineral acid, Neutral fat or paraffin, Iodine value (not more than 4), and Organic volatile impurities.

Note: Stearic Acid labeled solely for external use is exempt from the requirement that it be prepared from edible sources.

PURIFIED STEARIC ACID

Description: Purified Stearic Acid NF—Hard, white or faintly yellowish, somewhat glossy and crystalline solid, or white or yellowish-white powder. Its odor is slight, suggesting tallow.

NF category: Tablet and/or capsule lubricant.

Solubility: Purified Stearic Acid NF—Practically insoluble in water; freely soluble in chloroform and in ether; soluble in alcohol.

NF requirements: Purified Stearic Acid NF—Preserve in well-closed containers. Manufactured from fats and oils derived from edible sources and is a mixture of Stearic Acid and palmitic acid, which together constitute not less than 96.0% of the total content. The content of Stearic Acid is not less than 90.0% of the total. If it is for external use only, the labeling so indicates. Meets the requirements for Congealing temperature (66–69 °C), Acid value (195–200), Iodine value (not more than 1.5), and Organic volatile impurities, and for Residue on ignition, Heavy metals, Mineral acid, and Neutral fat or paraffin under Stearic Acid.

Note: Purified Stearic Acid labeled solely for external use is exempt from the requirement that it be prepared from edible sources.

STEARYL ALCOHOL

Chemical name: 1-Octadecanol.

Molecular formula: $C_{18}H_{38}O$.

Molecular weight: 270.50.

Description: Stearyl Alcohol NF—Unctuous, white flakes or granules. Has a faint, characteristic odor.

NF category: Stiffening agent.

Solubility: Stearyl Alcohol NF—Insoluble in water; soluble in alcohol and in ether.

NF requirements: Stearyl Alcohol NF—Preserve in well-closed containers. Contains not less than 90.0% of stearyl alcohol, the remainder consisting chiefly of related alcohols. Meets the requirements for Identification, Melting range (55–60 °C), Acid value (not more than 2), Iodine value (not more than 2), and Hydroxyl value (195–220).

STORAX

Description: Storax USP—Semiliquid, grayish to grayish-brown, sticky, opaque mass depositing on standing a heavy dark brown layer (Levant Storax); or semisolid, sometimes a solid mass, softened by gently warming (American Storax). Is transparent in thin layers, has a characteristic odor, and is more dense than water.

Solubility: Storax USP—Insoluble in water; soluble, usually incompletely, in an equal weight of warm alcohol; soluble in acetone, in carbon disulfide, and in ether, some insoluble residue usually remaining.

USP requirements: Storax USP—Preserve in well-closed containers. A balsam obtained from the trunk of *Liquidambar orientalis* Miller, known in commerce as Levant Storax, or of *Liquidambar styraciflua* Linné, known in commerce as American Storax (Fam. Hamamelidaceae). Meets the requirements for Loss on drying (not more than 20.0%), Alcohol-insoluble substances (not more than 5.0%), Alcohol-soluble substances, and Acid value, Saponification value, Cinnamic acid (acid value 50–85 for Levant Storax and 36–85 for American Storax and saponification value 160–200).

STREPTOKINASE

Source: A protein obtained from culture filtrates of certain strains of *Streptococcus haemolyticus* group C.

Molecular weight: About 46,000 daltons.

Description: Hygroscopic white powder or friable solid.

Solubility: Freely soluble in water.

USP requirements: Streptokinase for Injection—Not in USP.

STREPTOMYCIN

Source: Derived from *Streptomyces griseus*.

Chemical name: Streptomycin sulfate—D-Streptamine, *O*-2-deoxy-2-(methylamino)-alpha-L-glucopyranosyl-(1→2)-*O*-5-deoxy-3-*C*-formyl-alpha-L-lyxofuranosyl-(1→4)-*N*,*N'*-bis(aminoiminomethyl)-, sulfate (2:3) (salt).

Molecular formula: Streptomycin sulfate—$(C_{21}H_{39}N_7O_{12})_2 \cdot 3H_2SO_4$.

Molecular weight: Streptomycin sulfate—1457.38.

Description:

Streptomycin Sulfate Injection USP—Clear, colorless to yellow, viscous liquid. Is odorless or has a slight odor.

Sterile Streptomycin Sulfate USP—White or practically white powder. Is odorless or has not more than a faint odor. Is hygroscopic, but is stable in air and on exposure to light. Its solutions are acid to practically neutral to litmus.

Solubility: Sterile Streptomycin Sulfate USP—Freely soluble in water; very slightly soluble in alcohol; practically insoluble in chloroform.

USP requirements:

Streptomycin Sulfate Injection USP—Preserve in single-dose or in multiple-dose containers, preferably of Type I glass. Contains an amount of streptomycin sulfate equivalent to the labeled amount of streptomycin, within −10% to +15%. Meets the requirements for Bacterial endotoxins and pH (5.0–8.0), for Identification test A, Depressor substances, and Sterility under Sterile Streptomycin Sulfate, and for Injections.

Sterile Streptomycin Sulfate USP—Preserve in Containers for Sterile Solids. Has a potency equivalent to not less than 650 mcg and not more than 850 mcg of streptomycin per mg and, where packaged for dispensing, contains an amount of streptomycin sulfate equivalent to the labeled amount of streptomycin, within −10% to +15%. Meets the requirements for Constituted solution, Identification, Depressor substances, Bacterial endotoxins, Sterility, pH (4.5–7.0, in a solution containing 200 mg of streptomycin per mL), and Loss on drying (not more than 5.0%), and for Uniformity of dosage units and Labeling under Injections.

STREPTOZOCIN

Chemical name: D-Glucopyranose, 2-deoxy-2-[[(methylnitrosoamino)carbonyl]amino]-.

Molecular formula: $C_8H_{15}N_3O_7$.

Molecular weight: 265.22.

Description: Ivory-colored crystalline powder.

Solubility: Very soluble in water or in physiological saline; soluble in alcohol.

USP requirements: Streptozocin for Injection—Not in USP.

SUCCIMER

Chemical name: Butanedioic acid, 2,3-dimercapto-, (***R****,***S****).-

Molecular formula: $C_4H_6O_4S_2$.

Molecular weight: 182.21.

Description: White, crystalline powder with an unpleasant, characteristic mercaptan odor.

USP requirements: Succimer Capsules—Not in USP.

SUCCINYLCHOLINE

Chemical name: Succinylcholine chloride—Ethanaminium, 2,2'-[(1,4-dioxo-1,4-butanediyl)bis(oxy)]bis[*N*,*N*,*N*-trimethyl-], dichloride.

Molecular formula: Succinylcholine chloride—$C_{14}H_{30}Cl_2N_2O_4$.

Molecular weight: Succinylcholine chloride—361.31.

Description:

Succinylcholine Chloride USP—White, odorless, crystalline powder. Its solutions have a pH of about 4. The dihydrate form melts at about 160 °C; the anhydrous form melts at about 190 °C, and is hygroscopic.

Sterile Succinylcholine Chloride USP—White, odorless, crystalline powder. Its solutions have a pH of about 4. The dihydrate form melts at about 160 °C; the anhydrous form melts at about 190 °C, and is hygroscopic.

Solubility:

Succinylcholine Chloride USP—Freely soluble in water; slightly soluble in alcohol and in chloroform; practically insoluble in ether.

Sterile Succinylcholine Chloride USP—Freely soluble in water; slightly soluble in alcohol and in chloroform; practically insoluble in ether.

USP requirements:

Succinylcholine Chloride USP—Preserve in tight containers. Usually contains approximately two molecules of water of hydration. Label it in terms of its anhydrous equivalent. Contains not less than 96.0% and not more than 102.0% of succinylcholine chloride, calculated on the anhydrous basis. Meets the requirements for Identification, Water (not more than 10.0%), Residue on ignition (not more than 0.2%), Limit of ammonium salts, Chromatographic purity, and Chloride content (19.3–19.8%).

Succinylcholine Chloride Injection USP—Preserve in single-dose or in multiple-dose containers, preferably of Type I or Type II glass, in a refrigerator. A sterile solution of Succinylcholine Chloride in a suitable aqueous vehicle. Label it to indicate, as its expiration date, the month and year not more than 2 years from the month during which the Injection was last assayed and released by the manufacturer. Contains an amount of succinylcholine chloride equivalent to the labeled amount of anhydrous succinylcholine chloride, within ±10%. Meets the requirements for Identification, Bacterial endotoxins, pH (3.0–4.5), and Injections.

Sterile Succinylcholine Chloride USP—Preserve in Containers for Sterile Solids. It is Succinylcholine Chloride suitable for parenteral use. Meets the requirements for Completeness of solution, Constituted solution, Bacterial endotoxins, and Chromatographic purity, for Identification, Water, Residue on ignition, Ammonium salts, and Chloride content under Succinylcholine Chloride, and for Sterility, Uniformity of dosage units, and Labeling under Injections.

SUCRALFATE

Chemical name: Alpha-D-glucopyranoside, beta-D-fructofuranosyl-, octakis(hydrogen sulfate), aluminum complex.

Molecular formula: $C_{12}H_mAl_{16}O_nS_8$.

Description: Whitish or white, odorless, amorphous powder.

Solubility: Soluble in dilute hydrochloric acid and in sodium hydroxide; practically insoluble in water, in boiling water, in ethanol, and in chloroform.

Other characteristics: Metal salt of a sulfated disaccharide.

USP requirements:

Sucralfate USP—Preserve in tight containers. The hydrous basic aluminum salt of sucrose octasulfate. Contains not less than the equivalent of 30.0% and not more than the equivalent of 38.0% of sucrose octasulfate. Meets the requirements for Clarity and color of solution, Identification, Chloride (not more than 0.50%), Arsenic (not more than 4 ppm), Heavy metals (not more than 0.002%), Limit of pyridine and 2-methylpyridine (not more than 0.05% of either), Related compounds, Aluminum content (15.5–18.5%, calculated on an "as is" basis), Acid neutralization equivalent, and Organic volatile impurities.

Sucralfate Oral Suspension–Not in USP.

Sucralfate Tablets USP—Preserve in tight containers. Contain the labeled amount, within ±10%, corresponding to not less than 30.6% and not more than 37.4% of sucrose octasulfate. Meet the requirements for Identification, Disintegration (15 minutes), Uniformity of dosage units, and Acid neutralization equivalent.

SUCROSE

Chemical name: Alpha-D-glucopyranoside, beta-D-fructofuranosyl-.

Molecular formula: $C_{12}H_{22}O_{11}$.

Molecular weight: 342.30.

Description: Sucrose NF—Colorless or white crystals, crystalline masses or blocks, or white crystalline powder. Odorless and stable in air. Its solutions are neutral to litmus.

NF category: Coating agent; sweetening agent; tablet and/or capsule diluent.

Solubility: Sucrose NF—Very soluble in water, and even more soluble in boiling water; slightly soluble in alcohol; insoluble in chloroform and in ether.

NF requirements: Sucrose NF—Preserve in well-closed containers. A sugar obtained from *Saccharum officinarum* Linné (Fam. Gramineae), *Beta vulgaris* Linné (Fam. Chenopodiaceae), and other sources. Contains no added substances. Meets the requirements for Specific rotation (not less than +65.9°), Residue on ignition (not more than 0.05%), Chloride (not more than 0.0035%), Sulfate (not more than 0.006%), Calcium, Heavy metals (not more than 5 ppm), Invert sugar, and Organic volatile impurities.

SUCROSE OCTAACETATE

Chemical name: Alpha-D-glucopyranoside, 1,3,4,6-tetra-*O*-acetyl-beta-D-fructofuranosyl, tetraacetate.

Molecular formula: $C_{28}H_{38}O_{19}$.

Molecular weight: 678.60.

Description: Sucrose Octaacetate NF—White, practically odorless powder. Hygroscopic.

NF category: Alcohol denaturant.

Solubility: Sucrose Octaacetate NF—Very slightly soluble in water; very soluble in methanol and in chloroform; soluble in alcohol and in ether.

NF requirements: Sucrose Octaacetate NF—Preserve in tight containers. Contains not less than 98.0% and not more than 100.5% of sucrose octaacetate, calculated on the anhydrous basis. Meets the requirements for Melting temperature (not lower than 78 °C), Acidity, Water (not more than 1.0%), and Residue on ignition (not more than 0.1%).

SUFENTANIL

Chemical group: Fentanyl derivatives are anilinopiperidine-derivative opioid analgesics and are chemically related to anileridine and meperidine.

Chemical name: Sufentanil citrate—Propanamide, *N*-[4-(methoxymethyl)-1-[2-(thienyl)ethyl]-4-piperidinyl]-*N*-phenyl-, 2-hydroxy-1,2,3-propanetricarboxylate (1:1).

Molecular formula: Sufentanil citrate—$C_{22}H_{30}N_2O_2S \cdot C_6H_8O_7$.

Molecular weight: Sufentanil citrate—578.68.

Description: Sufentanil Citrate USP—White powder. Melts between 133 and 140 °C.

pKa: Sufentanil citrate—8.01.

Solubility: Sufentanil Citrate USP—Soluble in water; freely soluble in methanol; sparingly soluble in acetone, in alcohol, and in chloroform.

Other characteristics: Log partition coefficient (*n*-octanol/aqueous buffer solution at pH 10.8)—3.95.

USP requirements:

Sufentanil Citrate USP—Preserve in well-closed containers. Contains not less than 98.0% and not more than 101.0% of sufentanil citrate, calculated on the dried basis. Meets the requirements for Identification, Loss on drying (not more than 0.5%), Heavy metals (not more than 0.002%), Limit of acetone (not more than 0.2%), and Chromatographic purity.

Caution: Handle Sufentanil Citrate with great care since it is a potent opioid analgesic. Great care should be taken to prevent inhaling particles of Sufentanil Citrate and exposing the skin to it.

Sufentanil Citrate Injection USP—Preserve in single-dose or in multiple-dose containers, preferably of Type I glass. A sterile solution of Sufentanil Citrate in Water for Injection. Contains an amount of sufentanil citrate equivalent to the labeled amount of sufentanil, within ±10%, as the citrate. Meets the requirements for Identification, Bacterial endotoxins, pH (3.5–6.0), Particulate matter, and Injections.

Caution: Handle Sufentanil Citrate Injection with great care since it is a potent opioid analgesic.

COMPRESSIBLE SUGAR

Description: Compressible Sugar NF—Practically white, crystalline, odorless powder. Stable in air.

NF category: Sweetening agent; tablet and/or capsule diluent.

Solubility: Compressible Sugar NF—The sucrose portion of Compressible Sugar is very soluble in water.

NF requirements: Compressible Sugar NF—Preserve in well-closed containers. Previously dried at 105 °C for 4 hours, contains not less than 95.0% and not more than 98.0% of sucrose. Meets the requirements for Identification, Microbial limits, Loss on drying (0.25–1.0%), Residue on ignition (not more than 0.1%), Chloride, Sulfate, Calcium, and Heavy metals (not more than 0.014% for chloride, not more than 0.010% for sulfate, and not more than 5 ppm for heavy metals).

CONFECTIONER'S SUGAR

Description: Confectioner's Sugar NF—Fine, white, odorless powder. Stable in air.

NF category: Sweetening agent; tablet and/or capsule diluent.

Solubility: Confectioner's Sugar NF—The sucrose portion of Confectioner's Sugar is soluble in cold water. Freely soluble in boiling water.

NF requirements: Confectioner's Sugar NF—Preserve in well-closed containers. It is Sucrose ground together with corn starch to a fine powder. Contains not less than 95.0% of sucrose, calculated on the dried basis. Meets the requirements for Identification, Specific rotation, Chloride, Calcium, Sulfate, and Heavy metals (not less than +62.6°, calculated on the dried basis, for specific rotation, not more than 0.014% for chloride, not more than 0.006% for sulfate, and not more than 5 ppm for heavy metals), Microbial limits, Loss on drying (not more than 1.0%), and Residue on ignition (not more than 0.08%).

INVERT SUGAR

USP requirements: Invert Sugar Injection USP—Preserve in single-dose containers, preferably of Type I or Type II glass, or of a suitable plastic material. A sterile solution of a mixture of equal amounts of Dextrose and Fructose in Water for Injection, or an equivalent sterile solution produced by the hydrolysis of Sucrose, in Water for Injection. The label states the total osmolar concentration in mOsmol per liter. Contains the labeled amount of fructose, within ±5%. Contains no antimicrobial agents. Meets the requirements for Identification, Bacterial endotoxins, pH (3.0–6.5), Chloride (not more than 0.012%), Heavy metals, Limit of 5-hydroxymethylfurfural and related substances, Completeness of inversion, and Injections.

Note: Invert Sugar Injection that is produced by mixing Dextrose and Fructose is exempt from the requirement of the test for Completeness of inversion.

SUGAR SPHERES

Description: Sugar Spheres NF—Hard, brittle, free-flowing, spherical masses ranging generally in size from 10- to 60-mesh. Usually white, but may be colored.

NF category: Vehicle (solid carrier).

Solubility: Sugar Spheres NF—Solubility in water varies according to the sugar-to-starch ratio.

NF requirements: Sugar Spheres NF—Preserve in well-closed containers. The label states the nominal particle size range. Contain not less than 62.5% and not more than 91.5% of sucrose, calculated on the dried basis, the remainder consisting chiefly of starch. Consist of approximately spherical particles of a labeled nominal size range. Meet the requirements for Identification and Specific rotation (+41° to +61°, calculated on the dried basis, for specific rotation), Microbial limits, Loss on drying (not more than 4.0%), Residue on ignition (not more than 0.25%), Particle size, and Heavy metals (not more than 5 ppm).

SULBACTAM

Chemical name: Sulbactam sodium—4-Thia-1-azabicyclo[3.2.0]-heptane-2-carboxylic acid, 3,3-dimethyl-7-oxo-, 4,4-dioxide, sodium salt, (2*S*-*cis*)-.

Molecular formula: Sulbactam sodium—$C_8H_{10}NNaO_5S$.

Molecular weight: Sulbactam sodium—255.22.

Description: Sterile Sulbactam Sodium USP—White to off-white crystalline powder.

Solubility: Sterile Sulbactam Sodium USP—Freely soluble in water and in dilute acid; sparingly soluble in acetone, in ethyl acetate, and in chloroform.

USP requirements: Sterile Sulbactam Sodium USP—Preserve in tight containers. It is sulbactam sodium suitable for parenteral use. Contains not less than 886 mcg and not more than 941 mcg of sulbactam, calculated on the anhydrous basis. Meets the requirements for Identification, Crystallinity, Pyrogen, Sterility, and Water (not more than 1.0%).

SULCONAZOLE

Chemical name: Sulconazole nitrate—1*H*-Imidazole, 1-[2-[[(4-chlorophenyl)methyl]thio]-2-(2,4-dichlorophenyl)ethyl]-, mononitrate, (±)-.

Molecular formula: Sulconazole nitrate—$C_{18}H_{15}Cl_3N_2S \cdot HNO_3$.

Molecular weight: Sulconazole nitrate—460.76.

Description: Sulconazole Nitrate USP—White to off-white, crystalline powder. Melts at about 130 °C, with decomposition.

Solubility: Sulconazole Nitrate USP—Very slightly soluble in water, in toluene, and in dioxane; slightly soluble in alcohol, in chloroform, in acetone, and in methylene chloride; sparingly soluble in methanol; freely soluble in pyridine.

USP requirements:

Sulconazole Nitrate USP—Preserve in well-closed containers, protected from light. Contains not less than 98.0% and not more than 102.0% of sulconazole nitrate, calculated on the dried basis. Meets the requirements for Identification, Loss on drying (not more than 1.0%), Residue on ignition (not more than 0.1%), and Ordinary impurities.

Sulconazole Nitrate Topical Cream—Not in USP.

Sulconazole Nitrate Topical Solution—Not in USP.

TRIPLE SULFA

For *Sulfathiazole, Sulfacetamide,* and *Sulfabenzamide*—See individual listings for chemistry information.

USP requirements:

Triple Sulfa Vaginal Cream USP—Preserve in well-closed, light-resistant containers, or in collapsible tubes. Contains the labeled amounts of sulfathiazole, sulfacetamide, and sulfabenzamide, within ±10%. Meets the requirements for Identification, Minimum fill, and pH (3.0–4.0).

Triple Sulfa Vaginal Tablets USP—Preserve in well-closed, light-resistant containers. Contain the labeled amounts of sulfathiazole, sulfacetamide, and sulfabenzamide, within ±10%. Meet the requirements for Identification, Disintegration (30 minutes), and Uniformity of dosage units.

SULFABENZAMIDE

Chemical name: Benzamide, *N*-[(4-aminophenyl)sulfonyl]-.

Molecular formula: $C_{13}H_{12}N_2O_3S$.

Molecular weight: 276.31.

Description: Sulfabenzamide USP—Fine, white, practically odorless powder.

Solubility: Sulfabenzamide USP—Insoluble in water and in ether; soluble in alcohol, in acetone, and in sodium hydroxide TS.

USP requirements: Sulfabenzamide USP—Preserve in well-closed, light-resistant containers. Contains not less than 99.0% and not more than 100.5% of sulfabenzamide, calculated on the dried basis. Meets the requirements for Color and clarity of solution, Identification, Melting range (180–184 °C), Loss on drying (not more than 0.5%), Selenium (not more than 0.001%), Heavy metals (not more than 0.002%), and Ordinary impurities.

SULFACETAMIDE

Chemical name:

Sulfacetamide—Acetamide, *N*-[(4-aminophenyl)sulfonyl]-.

Sulfacetamide sodium—Acetamide, *N*-[(4-aminophenyl)-sulfonyl]-, monosodium salt, monohydrate.

Molecular formula:

Sulfacetamide—$C_8H_{10}N_2O_3S$.

Sulfacetamide sodium—$C_8H_9N_2NaO_3S \cdot H_2O$.

Molecular weight:

Sulfacetamide—214.24.

Sulfacetamide sodium—254.24.

Description:

Sulfacetamide USP—White, crystalline, odorless powder. Its aqueous solutions are sensitive to light, and are unstable when acidic or strongly alkaline.

Sulfacetamide Sodium USP—White, crystalline powder. Is odorless.

Solubility:

Sulfacetamide USP—Slightly soluble in water and in ether; freely soluble in dilute mineral acids and in solutions of potassium and sodium hydroxides; soluble in alcohol; very slightly soluble in chloroform.

Sulfacetamide Sodium USP—Freely soluble in water; sparingly soluble in alcohol; practically insoluble in chloroform and in ether.

USP requirements:

Sulfacetamide USP—Preserve in well-closed, light-resistant containers. Contains not less than 99.0% and not more than 100.5% of sulfacetamide, calculated on the dried basis. Meets the requirements for Clarity and color of solution, Identification, Melting range (181–184 °C), Reaction (a solution [1 in 150] is acid to litmus), Loss on drying (not more than 0.5%), Residue on ignition (not more than 0.1%), Selenium (not more than 0.003%), Sulfate (not more than 0.04%), and Heavy metals (not more than 0.002%).

Sulfacetamide Sodium USP—Preserve in tight, light-resistant containers. Contains not less than 99.0% and not more than 100.5% of sulfacetamide sodium, calculated on the anhydrous basis. Meets the requirements for Identification, pH (8.0–9.5, in a solution [1 in 20]), Water (not more than 8.1%), Selenium (not more than 0.003%), Heavy metals (not more than 0.002%), and Ordinary impurities.

Sulfacetamide Sodium Ophthalmic Ointment USP— Preserve in collapsible ophthalmic ointment tubes. It is sterile. Contains the labeled amount, within ±10%. Meets the requirements for Identification, Sterility, and Metal particles.

Sulfacetamide Sodium Ophthalmic Solution USP—Preserve in tight, light-resistant containers, in a cool place. A sterile solution. Contains the labeled amount, within ±10%. Meets the requirements for Identification and Sterility.

SULFACETAMIDE AND PREDNISOLONE

For *Sulfacetamide* and *Prednisolone*—See individual listings for chemistry information.

USP requirements:

Sulfacetamide Sodium and Prednisolone Acetate Ophthalmic Ointment USP—Preserve in collapsible ophthalmic ointment tubes that are tamper-proof so that sterility is assured at time of first use. A sterile ointment. Contains the labeled amounts, within ±10%. Meets the requirements for Identification, Minimum fill, Sterility, and Metal particles.

Sulfacetamide Sodium and Prednisolone Acetate Ophthalmic Suspension USP—Preserve in tight containers. The containers or individual cartons are sealed and tamper-proof so that sterility is assured at time of first use. A sterile, aqueous suspension. Contains the labeled amounts, within ±10%. Meets the requirements for Identification, Sterility, and pH (6.0–7.4).

SULFACHLORPYRIDAZINE

Chemical name: N^1-(6-Chloro-3-pyridazinyl)sulfanilamide.

Molecular formula: $C_{10}H_9ClN_4O_2S$.

Molecular weight: 284.72.

USP requirements: Sulfachlorpyridazine USP—Preserve in well-closed, light-resistant containers. Label it to indicate that it is for veterinary use only. Contains not less than 97.0% and not more than 103.0% of sulfachlorpyridazine, calculated on the dried basis. Meets the requirements for Identification, Clarity and color of solution, Acidity, Loss on drying (not more than 0.5%), Residue on ignition (not more than 0.1%), and Heavy metals (not more than 0.002%).

SULFACYTINE

Chemical name: Benzenesulfonamide, 4-amino-*N*-(1-ethyl-1,2-dihydro-2-oxo-4-pyrimidinyl)-.

Molecular formula: $C_{12}H_{14}N_4O_3S$.

Molecular weight: 294.33.

Description: White to cream-colored crystalline powder. Melts at about 169 °C.

Solubility: Slightly soluble in water.

Other characteristics: Sulfonamides have certain chemical similarities to some goitrogens, diuretics (acetazolamide and thiazides), and oral antidiabetic agents.

USP requirements: Sulfacytine Tablets—Not in USP.

SULFADIAZINE

Chemical name:
Sulfadiazine—Benzenesulfonamide, 4-amino-*N*-2-pyrimidinyl-.
Sulfadiazine sodium—Benzenesulfonamide, 4-amino-*N*-2-pyrimidinyl-, monosodium salt.

Molecular formula:
Sulfadiazine—$C_{10}H_{10}N_4O_2S$.
Sulfadiazine sodium—$C_{10}H_9N_4NaO_2S$.

Molecular weight:
Sulfadiazine—250.28.
Sulfadiazine sodium—272.26.

Description
Sulfadiazine USP—White or slightly yellow powder. Odorless or nearly odorless and stable in air, but slowly darkens on exposure to light.
Sulfadiazine Sodium USP—White powder. On prolonged exposure to humid air it absorbs carbon dioxide with liberation of sulfadiazine and becomes incompletely soluble in water. Its solutions are alkaline to phenolphthalein. Affected by light.

Solubility:
Sulfadiazine USP—Practically insoluble in water; freely soluble in dilute mineral acids, in solutions of potassium and sodium hydroxides, and in ammonia TS; sparingly soluble in alcohol and in acetone; slightly soluble in human serum at 37 °C.
Sulfadiazine Sodium USP—Freely soluble in water; slightly soluble in alcohol.

USP requirements:
Sulfadiazine USP—Preserve in well-closed, light-resistant containers. Contains not less than 98.0% and not more than 102.0% of sulfadiazine, calculated on the dried basis. Meets the requirements for Clarity and color of solution, Identification, Acidity, Loss on drying (not more than 0.5%), Residue on ignition (not more than 0.1%), Selenium (not more than 0.003%), Heavy metals (not more than 0.002%), and Ordinary impurities.
Sulfadiazine Tablets USP—Preserve in well-closed, light-resistant containers. Contain the labeled amount, within ±5%. Meet the requirements for Identification, Dissolution (70% in 90 minutes in 0.1 *N* hydrochloric acid in Apparatus 2 at 75 rpm), and Uniformity of dosage units.
Sulfadiazine Sodium USP—Preserve in tight, light-resistant containers. Contains not less than 99.0% and not more than 100.5% of sulfadiazine sodium, calculated on the dried basis. Meets the requirements for Identification, Loss on drying (not more than 0.5%), Selenium (not more than 0.003%), and Heavy metals (not more than 0.002%).
Sulfadiazine Sodium Injection USP—Preserve in single-dose, light-resistant containers, of Type I glass. A sterile solution of Sulfadiazine Sodium in Water for Injection. Contains, in each mL, not less than 237.5 mg and not more than 262.5 mg of sulfadiazine sodium. Meets the requirements for Identification, Bacterial endotoxins, pH (8.5–10.5), Particulate matter, and Injections.

SILVER SULFADIAZINE

Chemical group: Metal sulfanilamide derivative.

Chemical name: Benzenesulfonamide, 4-amino-*N*-2-pyrimidinyl-, monosilver(1+) salt.

Molecular formula: $C_{10}H_9AgN_4O_2S$.

Molecular weight: 357.14.

Description: Silver Sulfadiazine USP—White to creamy-white, crystalline powder, odorless to having a slight odor. Is stable in air, but turns yellow on exposure to light.

Solubility: Silver Sulfadiazine USP—Slightly soluble in acetone; practically insoluble in alcohol, in chloroform, and in ether; freely soluble in 30% ammonium solution; decomposes in moderately strong mineral acids.

Other characteristics: Sulfonamides have certain chemical similarities to some goitrogens, diuretics (acetazolamide and thiazides), and oral antidiabetic agents.

USP requirements:
Silver Sulfadiazine USP—Preserve in well-closed, light-resistant containers. Contains not less than 98.0% and not more than 102.0% of silver sulfadiazine, calculated on the dried basis. Meets the requirements for Identification, Particle size, Loss on drying (not more than 0.5%), Limit of nitrate (not more than 0.1%), Chromatographic purity, and Silver content (29.3–30.5%).
Silver Sulfadiazine Cream USP—Preserve in collapsible tubes or in tight, light-resistant containers. Contains the labeled amount, within ±10%. Meets the requirements for Identification, Microbial limits, Minimum fill, and pH (4.0–7.0).

SULFADIAZINE AND TRIMETHOPRIM

For *Sulfadiazine* and *Trimethoprim*—See individual listings for chemistry information.

USP requirements:
Sulfadiazine and Trimethoprim Oral Suspension—Not in USP.
Sulfadiazine and Trimethoprim Tablets—Not in USP.

SULFADOXINE

Chemical name: Benzenesulfonamide, 4-amino-*N*-(5,6-dimethoxy-4-pyrimidinyl)-.

Molecular formula: $C_{12}H_{14}N_4O_4S$.

Molecular weight: 310.33.

Description: White or yellowish-white crystalline powder, melting at 197–200 °C.

Solubility: Very slightly soluble in water; slightly soluble in alcohol and in methyl alcohol; practically insoluble in ether. Dissolves in solutions of alkali hydroxides and in dilute mineral acids.

USP requirements: Sulfadoxine USP—Preserve in well-closed, light-resistant containers. Contains not less than 99.0% and not more than 101.0% of sulfadoxine, calculated on the dried basis. Meets the requirements for Identification, Melting range (197–200 °C), Loss on drying (not more than 0.5%), Residue on ignition (not more than 0.1%), Heavy metals (not more than 0.002%), and Chromatographic purity.

SULFADOXINE AND PYRIMETHAMINE

For *Sulfadoxine* and *Pyrimethamine*—See individual listings for chemistry information.

USP requirements: Sulfadoxine and Pyrimethamine Tablets USP—Preserve in well-closed, light-resistant containers. Contain the labeled amounts, within ±10%. Meet the requirements for Identification, Dissolution (60% of each active ingredient in 30 minutes in phosphate buffer [pH 6.8] in Apparatus 2 at 75 rpm), and Uniformity of dosage units.

SULFAMERAZINE

Chemical name: Benzenesulfonamide, 4-amino-*N*-(4-methyl-2-pyrimidinyl)-.

Molecular formula: $C_{11}H_{12}N_4O_2S$.

Molecular weight: 264.30.

Description: Sulfamerazine USP—White or faintly yellowish white crystals or powder. Odorless or practically odorless. Stable in air, but slowly darkens on exposure to light.

Solubility: Sulfamerazine USP—Very slightly soluble in water; sparingly soluble in acetone; slightly soluble in alcohol; very slightly soluble in ether and in chloroform.

USP requirements:
Sulfamerazine USP—Preserve in well-closed, light-resistant containers. Contains not less than 99.0% and not more than 100.5% of sulfamerazine, calculated on the dried basis. Meets the requirements for Clarity and color of solution, Identification, Melting range (234–239 °C), Acidity, Loss on drying (not more than 0.5%), Residue on ignition (not more than 0.1%), Selenium (not more than 0.003%), Heavy metals (not more than 0.002%), and Ordinary impurities.
Sulfamerazine Tablets USP—Preserve in well-closed containers. Contain the labeled amount, within ±5%. Meet the requirements for Identification, Dissolution (75% in 45 minutes in water in Apparatus 1 at 100 rpm), and Uniformity of dosage units.

SULFAMETHAZINE

Chemical name: Benzenesulfonamide, 4-amino-*N*-(4,6-dimethyl-2-pyrimidinyl)-.

Molecular formula: $C_{12}H_{14}N_4O_2S$.

Molecular weight: 278.33.

Description: Sulfamethazine USP—White to yellowish white powder, which may darken on exposure to light. Practically odorless.

Solubility: Sulfamethazine USP—Very slightly soluble in water and in ether; soluble in acetone; slightly soluble in alcohol.

USP requirements:
Sulfamethazine USP—Preserve in well-closed, light-resistant containers. Contains not less than 99.0% and not more than 100.5% of sulfamethazine, calculated on the dried basis. Meets the requirements for Clarity and color of solution, Identification, Melting range (197–200 °C), Acidity, Loss on drying (not more than 0.5%), Residue on ignition (not more than 0.1%), Selenium (not more than 0.003%), Heavy metals (not more than 0.002%), and Ordinary impurities.
Sulfamethazine Granulated USP—Preserve in well-closed containers. Contains Sulfamethazine mixed with suitable diluents, carriers, and inactive ingredients. Label it to indicate that it is for veterinary use only. Label it also to indicate that it is for manufacturing, processing, or repackaging. Meets the requirements for Identification, Loss on drying (not more than 10%), and Powder fineness.

SULFAMETHIZOLE

Chemical name: Benzenesulfonamide, 4-amino-*N*-(5-methyl-1,3,4-thiadiazol-2-yl)-.

Molecular formula: $C_9H_{10}N_4O_2S_2$.

Molecular weight: 270.32.

Description: Sulfamethizole USP—White crystals or powder. Practically odorless, and has no odor of hydrogen sulfide.

Solubility: Sulfamethizole USP—Very slightly soluble in water, in chloroform, and in ether; freely soluble in solutions of ammonium, potassium, and sodium hydroxides; soluble in dilute mineral acids and in acetone; sparingly soluble in alcohol.

USP requirements:
Sulfamethizole USP—Preserve in well-closed, light-resistant containers. Contains not less than 98.0% and not more than 101.0% of sulfamethizole, calculated on the dried basis. Meets the requirements for Clarity and color of solution, Identification, Melting range (208–212 °C), Acidity, Loss on drying (not more than 0.5%), Residue on ignition (not more than 0.1%), Chloride (not more than 0.014%), Sulfate (not more than 0.04%), Selenium (not more than 0.003%), Heavy metals (not more than 0.002%), and Ordinary impurities.
Sulfamethizole Oral Suspension USP—Preserve in tight, light-resistant containers. Contains the labeled amount, within ±10%, in a buffered aqueous suspension. Meets the requirement for Identification.

Sulfamethizole Tablets USP—Preserve in well-closed containers. Contain the labeled amount, within ±5%. Meet the requirements for Identification, Dissolution (75% in 30 minutes in 0.1 *N* hydrochloric acid in Apparatus 2 at 50 rpm), and Uniformity of dosage units.

SULFAMETHOXAZOLE

Chemical name: Benzenesulfonamide, 4-amino-*N*-(5-methyl-3-isoxazolyl)-.

Molecular formula: $C_{10}H_{11}N_3O_3S$.

Molecular weight: 253.28.

Description: Sulfamethoxazole USP—White to off-white, practically odorless, crystalline powder.

Solubility: Sulfamethoxazole USP—Practically insoluble in water, in ether, and in chloroform; freely soluble in acetone and in dilute solutions of sodium hydroxide; sparingly soluble in alcohol.

Other characteristics: Sulfonamides have certain chemical similarities to some goitrogens, diuretics (acetazolamide and thiazides), and oral antidiabetic agents.

USP requirements:

Sulfamethoxazole USP—Preserve in well-closed, light-resistant containers. Contains not less than 99.0% and not more than 101.0% of sulfamethoxazole, calculated on the dried basis. Meets the requirements for Identification, Melting range (168–172 °C), Loss on drying (not more than 0.5%), Residue on ignition (not more than 0.1%), Selenium (not more than 0.003%), and Sulfanilamide and sulfanilic acid.

Sulfamethoxazole Oral Suspension USP—Preserve in tight, light-resistant containers. Contains the labeled amount, within −5% to + 10%. Meets the requirement for Identification.

Sulfamethoxazole Tablets USP—Preserve in well-closed, light-resistant containers. Contain the labeled amount, within ±5%. Meet the requirements for Identification, Dissolution (50% in 20 minutes in dilute hydrochloric acid [7 in 100] in Apparatus 1 at 100 rpm), and Uniformity of dosage units.

SULFAMETHOXAZOLE AND PHENAZOPYRIDINE

For *Sulfamethoxazole* and *Phenazopyridine*—See individual listings for chemistry information.

USP requirements: Sulfamethoxazole and Phenazopyridine Hydrochloride Tablets—Not in USP.

SULFAMETHOXAZOLE AND TRIMETHOPRIM

For *Sulfamethoxazole* and *Trimethoprim*—See individual listings for chemistry information.

USP requirements:

Sulfamethoxazole and Trimethoprim for Injection Concentrate USP—Preserve in single-dose, light-resistant containers, preferably of Type I glass. Sulfamethoxazole and Trimethoprim for Injection Concentrate may be packaged in 50-mL multiple-dose containers. A sterile solution of Sulfamethoxazole and Trimethoprim in Water for Injection which, when diluted with Dextrose Injection, is suitable for intravenous infusion. Label it to indicate that it is to be diluted with 5% Dextrose Injection prior to administration. Contains the labeled amounts, within ±10%. Meets the requirements for Identification, Pyrogen, pH (9.5–10.5), Particulate matter, Related compounds, and Injections.

Sulfamethoxazole and Trimethoprim Oral Suspension USP—Preserve in tight, light-resistant containers. Contains the labeled amounts, within ±10%. Meets the requirements for Identification, pH (5.0–6.5), Alcohol content (not more than 0.5%), and Chromatographic purity.

Sulfamethoxazole and Trimethoprim Tablets USP—Preserve in well-closed, light-resistant containers. Contain the labeled amounts, within ±7%. Meet the requirements for Identification, Dissolution (70% of each active ingredient in 60 minutes in 0.1 *N* hydrochloric acid in Apparatus 2 at 75 rpm), and Uniformity of dosage units.

SULFANILAMIDE

Chemical name: *p*-Aminobenzenesulfonamide.

Molecular formula: $C_6H_8N_2O_2S$.

Molecular weight: 172.20.

Description: White, odorless, crystalline powder.

Solubility: Slightly soluble in water, in alcohol, in acetone, in glycerin, in propylene glycol, in hydrochloric acid, and in solutions of potassium and sodium hydroxide; practically insoluble in chloroform, in ether, and in petroleum ether.

USP requirements:

Sulfanilamide Vaginal Cream—Not in USP.

Sulfanilamide Vaginal Suppositories—Not in USP.

SULFANILAMIDE, AMINACRINE, AND ALLANTOIN

Chemical name:

Sulfanilamide—*p*-Aminobenzenesulfonamide.

Aminacrine hydrochloride—9-Acridinamine monohydrochloride.

Allantoin—Urea, (2,5-dioxo-4-imidazolidinyl)-.

Molecular formula:

Sulfanilamide—$C_6H_8N_2O_2S$.

Aminacrine hydrochloride—$C_{13}H_{10}N_2 \cdot HCl$.

Allantoin—$C_4H_6N_4O_3$.

Molecular weight:

Sulfanilamide—172.20.

Aminacrine hydrochloride—320.70.

Allantoin—158.12.

Description:

Sulfanilamide—White, odorless crystalline powder.

Aminacrine hydrochloride—Pale yellow, crystalline powder; highly fluorescent.

Allantoin—Colorless crystals, melting at 238 °C.

Solubility:

Sulfanilamide—Slightly soluble in water, in alcohol, in acetone, in glycerin, in propylene glycol, in hydrochloric acid, and in solutions of potassium and sodium hydroxide; practically insoluble in chloroform, in ether, and in petroleum ether.

Aminacrine hydrochloride—1 gram soluble in 300 mL of water and in 150 mL of alcohol; soluble in glycerin.

Allantoin—1 gram dissolves in 190 mL of water or in 500 mL of alcohol; nearly insoluble in ether.

USP requirements:

Sulfanilamide, Aminacrine Hydrochloride, and Allantoin Vaginal Cream—Not in USP.

Sulfanilamide, Aminacrine Hydrochloride, and Allantoin Vaginal Suppositories—Not in USP.

SULFAPYRIDINE

Chemical group: Sulfonamide.

Chemical name: Benzenesulfonamide, 4-amino-*N*-2-pyridinyl-.

Molecular formula: $C_{11}H_{11}N_3O_2S$.

Molecular weight: 249.29.

Description: Sulfapyridine USP—White or faintly yellowish white crystals, granules, or powder. Is odorless or practically odorless, and is stable in air, but slowly darkens on exposure to light.

Solubility: Sulfapyridine USP—Very slightly soluble in water; freely soluble in dilute mineral acids and in solutions of potassium and sodium hydroxides; sparingly soluble in acetone; slightly soluble in alcohol.

Other characteristics: Sulfonamides have certain chemical similarities to some goitrogens, diuretics (acetazolamide and thiazides), and oral hypoglycemic agents.

USP requirements:
Sulfapyridine USP—Preserve in well-closed, light-resistant containers. Contains not less than 99.0% and not more than 100.5% of sulfapyridine, calculated on the dried basis. Meets the requirements for Clarity and color of solution, Identification, Melting range (190–193 °C), Acidity, Loss on drying (not more than 0.5%), Residue on ignition (not more than 0.1%), Selenium (not more than 0.003%), Heavy metals (not more than 0.002%), and Organic volatile impurities.
Sulfapyridine Tablets USP—Preserve in well-closed, light-resistant containers. Contain the labeled amount, within ±5%. Meet the requirements for Identification, Dissolution (70% in 60 minutes in 0.1 *N* hydrochloric acid in Apparatus 2 at 50 rpm), and Uniformity of dosage units.

SULFAQUINOXALINE

Chemical name: N^1-2-Quinoxalinylsulfanilamide.

Molecular formula: $C_{14}H_{12}N_4O_2S$.

Molecular weight: 300.33.

Description: Yellow, odorless powder.

Solubility: Practically insoluble in water; very slightly soluble in alcohol; practically insoluble in ether; freely soluble in aqueous solutions of alkalis.

USP requirements: Sulfaquinoxaline USP—Preserve in well-closed containers, protected from light. Contains not less than 98.0% and not more than 101.0% of sulfaquinoxaline, calculated on the dried basis. Meets the requirements for Identification, Acidity, Loss on drying (not more than 1.0%), Residue on ignition (not more than 0.1%), Heavy metals (not more than 0.002%), and Related compounds.

SULFASALAZINE

Source: Synthesized by the diazotization of sulfapyridine and the coupling of the diazonium salt with salicylic acid.

Chemical name: Benzoic acid, 2-hydroxy-5-[[4-[(2-pyridinylamino)sulfonyl]phenyl]azo]-.

Molecular formula: $C_{18}H_{14}N_4O_5S$.

Molecular weight: 398.39.

Description: Sulfasalazine USP—Bright yellow or brownish yellow, odorless, fine powder. Melts at about 255 °C, with decomposition.

Solubility: Sulfasalazine USP—Very slightly soluble in alcohol; practically insoluble in water, in ether, and in chloroform; soluble in aqueous solutions of alkali hydroxides.

USP requirements:
Sulfasalazine USP—Preserve in tight, light-resistant containers. Contains not less than 97.0% and not more than 101.5% of sulfasalazine, calculated on the dried basis. Meets the requirements for Identification, Loss on drying (not more than 1.0%), Residue on ignition (not more than 0.5%), Chloride (not more than 0.014%), Sulfate (not more than 0.04%), Heavy metals (not more than 0.002%), Chromatographic purity, and Organic volatile impurities.
Sulfasalazine Oral Suspension—Not in USP.
Sulfasalazine Tablets USP—Preserve in well-closed containers. Contain the labeled amount, within ±5%. Meet the requirements for Identification, Disintegration (15 minutes, for Tablets that are enteric-coated), Dissolution (85% in 60 minutes in phosphate buffer [pH 7.5] in Apparatus 1 at 100 rpm), and Uniformity of dosage units.

SULFATHIAZOLE

Chemical name: Benzenesulfonamide, 4-amino-*N*-2-thiazolyl-.

Molecular formula: $C_9H_9N_3O_2S_2$.

Molecular weight: 255.31.

Description: Sulfathiazole USP—Fine, white or faintly yellowish white, practically odorless powder.

Solubility: Sulfathiazole USP—Very slightly soluble in water; soluble in acetone, in dilute mineral acids, in solutions of alkali hydroxides, and in 6 *N* ammonium hydroxide; slightly soluble in alcohol.

USP requirements: Sulfathiazole USP—Preserve in well-closed, light-resistant containers. Contains not less than 99.0% and not more than 100.5% of sulfathiazole, calculated on the dried basis. Meets the requirements for Identification, Melting range (200–204 °C), Acidity, Loss on drying (not more than 0.5%), Residue on ignition (not more than 0.1%), Chloride (not more than 0.014%), Sulfate (not more than 0.04%), Heavy metals (not more than 0.002%), and Ordinary impurities.

SULFINPYRAZONE

Chemical group: A pyrazole compound chemically related to phenylbutazone.

Chemical name: 3,5-Pyrazolidinedione, 1,2-diphenyl-4-[2-(phenylsulfinyl)ethyl]-.

Molecular formula: $C_{23}H_{20}N_2O_3S$.

Molecular weight: 404.48.

Description: Sulfinpyrazone USP—White to off-white powder.

pKa: 2.8.

Solubility: Sulfinpyrazone USP—Practically insoluble in water and in solvent hexane; soluble in alcohol and in acetone; sparingly soluble in dilute alkali.

USP requirements:
Sulfinpyrazone USP—Preserve in well-closed containers. Contains not less than 98.5% and not more than 101.5% of sulfinpyrazone, calculated on the dried basis. Meets the requirements for Solubility in acetone, Solubility in 0.50 *N* sodium hydroxide, Identification, Melting range (130.5–134.5 °C), Loss on drying (not more than 0.5%), Residue on ignition (not more than 0.1%), Heavy metals

(not more than 0.001%), Chromatographic purity, and Organic volatile impurities.

Sulfinpyrazone Capsules USP—Preserve in well-closed containers. Contain the labeled amount, within ±7%. Meet the requirements for Identification, Dissolution (75% in 45 minutes in phosphate buffer [pH 7.5] in Apparatus 1 at 100 rpm), and Uniformity of dosage units.

Sulfinpyrazone Tablets USP—Preserve in well-closed containers. Contain the labeled amount, within ±7%. Meet the requirements for Identification, Dissolution (75% in 45 minutes in phosphate buffer [pH 7.5] in Apparatus 1 at 100 rpm), and Uniformity of dosage units.

SULFISOXAZOLE

Chemical name:

Sulfisoxazole—Benzenesulfonamide, 4-amino-*N*-(3,4-dimethyl-5-isoxazolyl)-.

Sulfisoxazole acetyl—Acetamide, *N*-[(4-aminophenyl)-sulfonyl]-*N*-(3,4-dimethyl-5-isoxazolyl)-.

Sulfisoxazole diolamine—Benzenesulfonamide, 4-amino-*N*-(3,4-dimethyl-5-isoxazolyl)-, compd. with 2,2′-iminobis-[ethanol] (1:1).

Molecular formula:

Sulfisoxazole—$C_{11}H_{13}N_3O_3S$.

Sulfisoxazole acetyl—$C_{13}H_{15}N_3O_4S$.

Sulfisoxazole diolamine—$C_{11}H_{13}N_3O_3S \cdot C_4H_{11}NO_2$.

Molecular weight:

Sulfisoxazole—267.30.

Sulfisoxazole acetyl—309.34.

Sulfisoxazole diolamine—372.44.

Description:

Sulfisoxazole USP—White to slightly yellowish, odorless, crystalline powder.

Sulfisoxazole Acetyl USP—White or slightly yellow, crystalline powder.

Sulfisoxazole Diolamine USP—White to off-white, fine crystalline, odorless powder.

Solubility:

Sulfisoxazole USP—Very slightly soluble in water; soluble in boiling alcohol and in 3 *N* hydrochloric acid.

Sulfisoxazole Acetyl USP—Practically insoluble in water; sparingly soluble in chloroform; slightly soluble in alcohol.

Sulfisoxazole Diolamine USP—Freely soluble in water; soluble in alcohol.

Other characteristics: Sulfonamides have certain chemical similarities to some goitrogens, diuretics (acetazolamide and thiazides), and oral antidiabetic agents.

USP requirements:

Sulfisoxazole USP—Preserve in tight, light-resistant containers. Contains not less than 99.0% and not more than 101.0% of sulfisoxazole, calculated on the dried basis. Meets the requirements for Identification, Melting range (194–199 °C), Loss on drying (not more than 0.5%), Residue on ignition (not more than 0.1%), Selenium (not more than 0.003%), Heavy metals (not more than 0.002%), and Ordinary impurities.

Sulfisoxazole Tablets USP—Preserve in well-closed, light-resistant containers. Contain the labeled amount, within ±5%. Meet the requirements for Identification, Dissolution (70% in 30 minutes in dilute hydrochloric acid [1 in 12.5] in Apparatus 1 at 100 rpm), and Uniformity of dosage units.

Sulfisoxazole Acetyl USP—Preserve in tight, light-resistant containers. Contains not less than 98.0% and not more than 100.5% of sulfisoxazole acetyl, calculated on the dried basis. Meets the requirements for Identification, Melting range (192–195 °C), Loss on drying (not more than 0.5%), Ordinary impurities, and Organic volatile impurities, and for Residue on ignition, Selenium, and Heavy metals under Sulfisoxazole

Sulfisoxazole Acetyl Oral Suspension USP—Preserve in tight, light-resistant containers. Contains an amount of sulfisoxazole acetyl equivalent to the labeled amount of sulfisoxazole, within ±7%. Meets the requirements for Identification and pH (5.0–5.5).

Sulfisoxazole Acetyl Oral Syrup—Not in USP.

Sulfisoxazole Diolamine USP—Preserve in tight, light-resistant containers. Contains not less than 99.0% and not more than 101.0% of sulfisoxazole diolamine, calculated on the dried basis. Meets the requirements for Identification, Melting range (119–124 °C), Loss on drying (not more than 0.2%), Residue on ignition (not more than 0.1%), and Heavy metals (not more than 0.002%).

Sulfisoxazole Diolamine Injection USP—Preserve in single-dose or in multiple-dose containers, preferably of Type I glass, protected from light. A sterile solution of Sulfisoxazole Diolamine in Water for Injection. Contains an amount of sulfisoxazole diolamine equivalent to the labeled amount of sulfisoxazole, within ±10%. Meets the requirements for Identification, Pyrogen, pH (7.0–8.5), Particulate matter, and Injections.

Sulfisoxazole Diolamine Ophthalmic Ointment USP—Preserve in collapsible ophthalmic ointment tubes. A sterile ointment. Contains an amount of sulfisoxazole diolamine equivalent to the labeled amount of sulfisoxazole, within ±10%. Meets the requirements for Identification, Sterility, Minimum fill, Leakage, and Metal particles.

Sulfisoxazole Diolamine Ophthalmic Solution USP—Preserve in tight, light-resistant containers. A sterile solution. Contains an amount of sulfisoxazole diolamine equivalent to the labeled amount of sulfisoxazole, within −10% to +15%. Meets the requirements for Identification, Sterility, and pH (7.2–8.2).

SULFISOXAZOLE AND PHENAZOPYRIDINE

For *Sulfisoxazole* and *Phenazopyridine*—See individual listings for chemistry information.

USP requirements: Sulfisoxazole and Phenazopyridine Hydrochloride Tablets—Not in USP.

SULFUR

Chemical name: Precipitated sulfur—Sulfur.

Molecular formula: Precipitated sulfur—S.

Molecular weight: Precipitated sulfur—32.07.

Description: Precipitated Sulfur USP—Very fine, pale yellow, amorphous or microcrystalline powder. Is odorless.

Solubility: Precipitated Sulfur USP—Practically insoluble in water; very soluble in carbon disulfide; slightly soluble in olive oil; very slightly soluble in alcohol.

USP requirements:

Precipitated Sulfur USP—Preserve in well-closed containers. Contains not less than 99.5% and not more than 100.5% of sulfur, calculated on the anhydrous basis. Meets the requirements for Identification, Reaction, Water (not more than 0.5%), Residue on ignition (not more than 0.3%), and Other forms of sulfur.

Sulfur Cream—Not in USP.

Sulfur Lotion—Not in USP.

Sulfur Ointment USP—Preserve in well-closed containers, and avoid prolonged exposure to excessive heat. Contains not less than 9.5% and not more than 10.5% of Sulfur.

Prepare Sulfur Ointment as follows: 100 grams of Precipitated Sulfur, 100 grams of Mineral Oil, and 800 grams of White Ointment, to make 1000 grams. Levigate the sulfur with the Mineral Oil to a smooth paste, and then incorporate with the White Ointment.

Sulfur Bar Soap—Not in USP.

SUBLIMED SULFUR

Chemical name: Sulfur.

Molecular formula: S.

Molecular weight: 32.07.

Description: Sublimed Sulfur USP—Fine, yellow, crystalline powder, having a faint odor.

Solubility: Sublimed Sulfur USP—Practically insoluble in water and in alcohol; sparingly soluble in olive oil.

USP requirements: Sublimed Sulfur USP—Preserve in well-closed containers. Dried over phosphorus pentoxide for 4 hours, contains not less than 99.5% and not more than 100.5% of sulfur. Meets the requirements for Solubility in carbon disulfide, Identification, Residue on ignition (not more than 0.5%), and Arsenic (not more than 4 ppm).

SULFUR DIOXIDE

Chemical name: Sulfur dioxide.

Molecular formula: SO_2.

Molecular weight: 64.07.

Description: Sulfur Dioxide NF—Colorless, non-flammable gas, possessing a strong suffocating odor characteristic of burning sulfur. Under pressure, it condenses readily to a colorless liquid that boils at –10 °C and has a density of approximately 1.5.

NF category: Antioxidant.

Solubility: Sulfur Dioxide NF—At 20 °C and at standard pressure, approximately 36 volumes dissolve in 1 volume of water, and approximately 114 volumes dissolve in 1 volume of alcohol. Soluble also in ether and in chloroform.

NF requirements: Sulfur Dioxide NF—Preserve in cylinders. Note: Sulfur Dioxide is used most in the form of a gas in pharmaceutical applications, and the monograph deals with it for such purposes. However, it is usually packaged under pressure; hence, the NF specifications are designed for testing it in liquid form. Contains not less than 97.0%, by volume, of sulfur dioxide. Meets the requirements for Water (not more than 2.0%), Limit of nonvolatile residue (not more than 0.0025%), and Sulfuric acid (not more than 0.002%).

Caution: Sulfur Dioxide is poisonous.

SULFURIC ACID

Chemical name: Sulfuric acid.

Molecular formula: H_2SO_4.

Molecular weight: 98.08.

Description: Sulfuric Acid NF—Clear, colorless, oily liquid. Very caustic and corrosive. Specific gravity is about 1.84.

NF category: Acidifying agent.

Solubility: Sulfuric Acid NF—Miscible with water and with alcohol with the generation of much heat.

NF requirements: Sulfuric Acid NF—Preserve in tight containers. Contains not less than 95.0% and not more than 98.0%, by weight, of sulfuric acid. Meets the requirements for Identification, Residue on ignition (not more than 0.005%), Chloride (not more than 0.005%), Arsenic (not more than 1 ppm), Heavy metals (not more than 5 ppm), and Reducing substances.

Caution: When Sulfuric Acid is to be mixed with other liquids, always add it to the diluent, and exercise great caution.

SULINDAC

Chemical group: Indeneacetic acid derivative.

Chemical name: 1*H*-Indene-3-acetic acid, 5-fluoro-2-methyl-1-[[4-(methylsulfinyl)phenyl]methylene]-, (*Z*)-.

Molecular formula: $C_{20}H_{17}FO_3S$.

Molecular weight: 356.42.

Description: Sulindac USP—Yellow, crystalline powder, which is odorless or practically so.

Solubility: Sulindac USP—Slightly soluble in methanol, in alcohol, in acetone, and in chloroform; very slightly soluble in isopropanol and in ethyl acetate; practically insoluble in hexane and in water.

USP requirements:

Sulindac USP—Preserve in well-closed containers. Contains not less than 99.0% and not more than 101.0% of sulindac, calculated on the dried basis. Meets the requirements for Identification, Loss on drying (not more than 0.5%), Residue on ignition (not more than 0.1%), Heavy metals (not more than 0.001%), Chromatographic purity, and Organic volatile impurities.

Sulindac Tablets USP—Preserve in well-closed containers. Contain the labeled amount, within ±10%. Meet the requirements for Identification, Dissolution (80% in 45 minutes in 0.1 *M* phosphate buffer [pH 7.2] in Apparatus 2 at 50 rpm), Uniformity of dosage units, and Related compounds.

SUMATRIPTAN

Chemical name: Sumatriptan succinate—1*H*-Indole-5-methanesulfonamide, 3-[2-(dimethylamino)ethyl]-*N*-methyl-, butanedioate (1:1).

Molecular formula: Sumatriptan succinate—$C_{14}H_{21}N_3O_2S \cdot C_4H_6O_4$.

Molecular weight: Sumatriptan succinate—413.50.

Description: Sumatriptan succinate—White to off-white powder.

Solubility: Sumatriptan succinate—Readily soluble in water and in saline.

USP requirements:

Sumatriptan Succinate Injection—Not in USP.

Sumatriptan Succinate Tablets—Not in USP.

SUPROFEN

Chemical name: Benzeneacetic acid, alpha-methyl-4-(2-thienylcarbonyl)-.

Molecular formula: $C_{14}H_{12}O_3S$.

Molecular weight: 260.32.

Description: Suprofen USP—White to off-white powder, odorless to having a slight odor.

Solubility: Suprofen USP—Sparingly soluble in water.

USP requirements:

Suprofen USP—Preserve in well-closed containers. Contains not less than 98.0% and not more than 102.0% of suprofen, calculated on the dried basis. Meets the requirements for Clarity of solution, Identification, Melting range (118–125 °C, within a range of less than 4 °C), Loss on drying (not more than 0.5%), Residue on ignition (not more than 0.2%), Heavy metals (not more than 0.002%), and Ordinary impurities.

Suprofen Ophthalmic Solution USP—Preserve in tight containers. A sterile, buffered, aqueous solution of Suprofen adjusted to a suitable tonicity. Contains a suitable antimicrobial preservative. Contains the labeled amount, within −10% to +15%. Meets the requirements for Identification, Sterility, and pH (6.5–8.0).

SUTILAINS

Chemical name: Sutilains.

Description: Sutilains USP—Cream-colored powder.

USP requirements:

Sutilains USP—Preserve in tight containers, and store in a refrigerator. Allow to reach room temperature before opening container. A substance containing proteolytic enzymes, derived from the bacterium *Bacillus subtilis.* When assayed as in *USP/NF,* contains not less than 2,500,000 USP Casein Units of proteolytic activity per gram, calculated on the dried basis. Meets the requirements for Solubility test, pH (6.1–7.1, in a solution [1 in 100]), Loss on drying (not more than 5.0%), Nitrogen (11.0–13.5%), and Organic volatile impurities.

Note: One USP Casein Unit of proteolytic activity is contained in the amount of sutilains which, when incubated with 35 mg of denatured casein at 37 °C, produces in 1 minute a hydrolysate whose absorbance at 275 nanometers is equal to that of a tyrosine solution containing 1.5 mcg of USP Tyrosine Reference Standard per mL.

Sutilains Ointment USP—Preserve in collapsible tubes or in tight containers, and store in a refrigerator. Contains the labeled potency of sutilains, within −15% to +25%, in a suitable ointment base. Meets the requirement for Sterility.

Note: One USP Casein Unit of proteolytic activity is contained in the amount of sutilains which, when incubated with 35 mg of denatured casein at 37 °C, produces in 1 minute a hydrolysate whose absorbance at 275 nanometers is equal to that of a tyrosine solution containing 1.5 mcg of USP Tyrosine Reference Standard per mL.

ABSORBABLE SURGICAL SUTURE

USP requirements: Absorbable Surgical Suture USP—Preserve dry or in fluid, in containers (packets) so designed that sterility is maintained until the container is opened. A number of such containers may be placed in a box. A sterile, flexible strand prepared from collagen derived from healthy mammals, or from a synthetic polymer. Suture prepared from synthetic polymer may be in either monofilament or multifilament form. It is capable of being absorbed by living mammalian tissue, but may be treated to modify its resistance to absorption. Its diameter and tensile strength correspond to the size designation indicated on the label, within the limits prescribed in *USP/NF.* May be modified with respect to body or texture. May be impregnated or treated with a suitable coating, softening, or antimicrobial agent. May be colored by a color additive approved by the U.S. Food and Drug Administration. The collagen suture is designated as either *Plain Suture* or *Chromic Suture.* Both types consist of processed strands of collagen, but *Chromic Suture* is processed by physical or chemical means so as to provide greater resistance to absorption in living mammalian tissue. The label of each individual container (packet) of Suture indicates the size, length, type of Suture, kind of needle (if a needle is included), number of sutures (if multiple), lot number, and name of the manufacturer or distributor. If removable needles are used, the labeling so indicates. Suture size is designated by the metric size (gauge number) and the corresponding USP size. The label of the box indicates also the address of the manufacturer, packer, or distributor, and the composition of any packaging fluids used. Note: If the Suture is packaged with a fluid, make the required measurements for the following tests within 2 minutes after removing it from the fluid—Length, Diameter, Tensile strength, and Needle attachment. Meets the requirements for Length (not less than 95.0% of length stated on label), Diameter, Tensile strength, Needle attachment, Sterility, Extractable color (if Suture is dyed), and Soluble chromium compounds.

NONABSORBABLE SURGICAL SUTURE

USP requirements: Nonabsorbable Surgical Suture USP—Preserve non-sterilized Suture in well-closed containers. Preserve sterile Suture dry or in fluid, in containers (packets) so designed that sterility is maintained until the container is opened. A number of such containers may be placed in a box. A flexible strand of material that is suitably resistant to the action of living mammalian tissue. It may be in either monofilament or multifilament form. If it is a multifilament strand, the individual filaments may be combined by spinning, twisting, braiding, or any combination thereof. May be either sterile or nonsterile. Its diameter and tensile strength correspond to the size designation indicated on the label, within the limits prescribed in *USP/NF.* May be modified with respect to body or texture, or to reduce capillarity, and may be suitably bleached. May be impregnated or treated with a suitable coating, softening, or antimicrobial agent. May be colored by a color additive approved by the U.S. Food and Drug Administration. Nonabsorbable Surgical Suture is classed and typed as follows: *Class I* Suture is composed of silk or synthetic fibers of monofilament, twisted or braided construction where the coating, if any, does not significantly affect thickness (e.g., braided silk, polyester, or nylon; microfilament nylon, or polypropylene). *Class II* Suture is composed of cotton or linen fibers or coated natural or synthetic fibers where the coating significantly affects thickness but does not contribute significantly to strength (e.g., virgin silk sutures). *Class III* Suture is composed of monofilament or multifilament metal wire. The label of each individual container (packet) of Suture indicates the material from which the Suture is made, the size, construction, and length of the Suture, whether it is sterile or non-sterile, kind of needle (if a needle is included), number of sutures (if multiple), lot number, and name of the manufacturer or distributor. If removable needles are used, the labeling so indicates. Suture size is designated by the metric size (gauge number) and the corresponding USP size. The label of the box indicates also the address of the manufacturer, packer, or distributor, and the composition of any packaging fluids used. Note: If the Suture is packaged with a fluid, make the required measurements for the following tests within 2 minutes after removing it from the fluid—Length, Diameter,

Tensile strength, and Needle attachment. Meets the requirements for Length (not less than 95.0% of length stated on label), Diameter, Tensile strength, Needle attachment, Sterility, and Extractable color (if Suture is dyed).

SYRUP

Description: Syrup NF—NF category: Sweetening agent; tablet binder; flavored and/or sweetened vehicle.

NF requirements: Syrup NF—Preserve in tight containers, preferably in a cool place. A solution of Sucrose in Purified Water. Contains a preservative unless it is used when freshly prepared.

Prepare Syrup as follows: 850 grams of Sucrose and a sufficient quantity of Purified Water to make 1000 mL. May be prepared by the use of boiling water or, preferably, without heat, by the following process. Place the Sucrose in a suitable percolator, the neck of which is nearly filled with loosely packed cotton, moistened, after packing, with a few drops of water. Pour carefully about 450 mL of Purified Water upon the Sucrose, and regulate the outflow to a steady drip of percolate. Return the percolate, if necessary, until all of the Sucrose has been dissolved. Then wash the inside of the percolator and the cotton with sufficient Purified Water to bring the volume of the percolate to 1000 mL, and mix.

Meets the requirements for Specific gravity (not less than 1.30) and Organic volatile impurities.

TACRINE

Chemical name: Tacrine hydrochloride—9-Acridinamine, 1,2,3,4-tetrahydro-, monohydrochloride.

Molecular formula: Tacrine hydrochloride—$C_{13}H_{14}N_2 \cdot HCl$.

Molecular weight: Tacrine hydrochlordie—234.73.

Description: Tacrine hydrochloride—White solid.

Solubility: Tacrine hydrochloride—Freely soluble in distilled water, in 0.1 *N* hydrochloric acid, in acetate buffer (pH 4.0), in phosphate buffer (pH 7.0–7.4), in methanol, in dimethylsulfoxide, in ethanol, and in propylene glycol; sparingly soluble in linoleic acid and in PEG 400.

USP requirements: Tacrine Hydrochloride Capsules—Not in USP.

TACROLIMUS

Chemical name: 15,19-Epoxy-3*H*-pyrido[2,1-*c*][1,4]oxaazacyclotricosine-1,7,20,21(4*H*,23*H*)-tetrone, 5,6,8,11,12,13,14,15,16,17,18,19,24,25,26,26a-hexadecahydro-5,19-dihydroxy-3-[2-(4-hydroxy-3-methoxycyclohexyl)-1-methylethenyl]-14,16-dimethoxy-4,10,12,18-tetramethyl-8-(2-propenyl)-, monohydrate, [3*S*-[3*R**,[*E*(1*S**,3*S**,4*S**)],4*S**,5*R**,8*S**,9*E*,12*R**,14*R**,15*S**,16*R**,18*S**,19*S**,26a*R**]]-.

Molecular formula: $C_{44}H_{69}NO_{12} \cdot H_2O$.

Molecular weight: 822.05.

Description: White crystals or crystalline powder.

Solubility: Practically insoluble in water; freely soluble in ethanol; very soluble in methanol and in chloroform.

USP requirements:

Tacrolimus Capsules—Not in USP.
Tacrolimus Injection—Not in USP.

TALC

Description: Talc USP—Very fine, white or grayish-white, crystalline powder. It is unctuous, adheres readily to the skin, and is free from grittiness.

NF category: Glidant and/or anticaking agent; tablet and/or capsule lubricant.

USP requirements: Talc USP—Preserve in well-closed containers. A native, hydrous magnesium silicate, sometimes containing a small proportion of aluminum silicate. Meets the requirements for Identification, Microbial limit, Loss on ignition (not more than 6.5%), Acid-soluble substances (not more than 2.0%), Reaction and soluble substances (not more than 0.1%), Water-soluble iron, Arsenic, Heavy metals, and Lead (not more than 3 ppm for arsenic, not more than 0.004% for heavy metals, and not more than 0.001% for lead).

TAMOXIFEN

Chemical name: Tamoxifen citrate—Ethanamine, 2-[4-(1,2-diphenyl-1-butenyl)phenoxy]-*N*,*N*-dimethyl, (*Z*)-, 2-hydroxy-1,2,3-propanetricarboxylate (1:1).

Molecular formula: Tamoxifen citrate—$C_{26}H_{29}NO \cdot C_6H_8O_7$.

Molecular weight: Tamoxifen citrate—563.65.

Description: Tamoxifen Citrate USP—White, fine, crystalline powder. Melts at about 142 °C, with decomposition.

pKa: Tamoxifen citrate—8.85.

Solubility: Tamoxifen Citrate USP—Very slightly soluble in water, in acetone, in chloroform, and in alcohol; soluble in methanol.

USP requirements:

Tamoxifen Citrate USP—Preserve in well-closed, light-resistant containers. Contains not less than 99.0% and not more than 101.0% of tamoxifen citrate, calculated on the dried basis. Meets the requirements for Identification, Loss on drying (not more than 0.5%), Residue on ignition (not more than 0.2%), *E*-isomer (not more than 0.3% of tamoxifen citrate), Related impurities, Iron (not more than 0.005%), Arsenic (not more than 2 ppm), Heavy metals (not more than 0.001%), and Organic volatile impurities.

Tamoxifen Citrate Tablets USP—Preserve in well-closed, light-resistant containers. Contain an amount of tamoxifen citrate equivalent to the labeled amount of tamoxifen, within ±10%. Meet the requirements for Identification, Dissolution (75% in 30 minutes in 0.02 *N* hydrochloric acid in Apparatus 1 at 100 rpm), and Uniformity of dosage units.

Tamoxifen Citrate Enteric-coated Tablets—Not in USP.

TANNIC ACID

Chemical name: Tannin.

Description: Tannic Acid USP—Amorphous powder, glistening scales, or spongy masses, varying in color from yellowish white to light brown. Is odorless or has a faint, characteristic odor.

Solubility: Tannic Acid USP—Very soluble in water, in acetone, and in alcohol; freely soluble in diluted alcohol, and only slightly soluble in dehydrated alcohol; practically insoluble in chloroform, in ether, and in solvent hexane; 1 gram dissolves in about 1 mL of warm glycerin.

USP requirements: Tannic Acid USP—Preserve in tight, light-resistant containers. A tannin usually obtained from nutgalls, the excrescences produced on the young twigs of *Quercus infectoria* Oliver, and allied species of *Quercus* Linné (Fam. Fagaceae), from the seed pods of Tara (*Caesalpinia spinosa*), or from the nutgalls or leaves of sumac (any of a genus *Rhus*). Meets the requirements for Identification, Loss on drying (not more than 12.0%), Residue on ignition (not more than 1.0%), Arsenic (not more than 3 ppm), Heavy metals (not more than 0.004%), Gum or dextrin, Resinous substances, and Organic volatile impurities.

ADHESIVE TAPE

USP requirements: Adhesive Tape USP—Preserve in well-closed containers, and prevent exposure to excessive heat and to sunlight. Adhesive Tape that has been rendered sterile is so packaged that the sterility of the contents of the package is maintained until the package is opened for use. Consists of fabric and/or film evenly coated on one side with a pressure-sensitive, adhesive mixture. Its length is not less than 98.0% of that declared on the label, and its average width is not less than 95.0% of the declared width. If Adhesive Tape has been rendered sterile, it is protected from contamination by appropriate packaging. The package label of Adhesive Tape that has been rendered sterile indicates that the contents may not be sterile if the package bears evidence of damage or previously has been opened. The package label indicates the length and width of the Tape, and the name of the manufacturer, packer, or distributor. Meets the requirements for Dimensions (length, not less than 98.0% of labeled length; width, average of 5 measurements not less than 95% of the labeled width of Tape), Tensile strength, Adhesive strength, and Sterility.

TARTARIC ACID

Chemical name: Butanedioic acid, 2,3-dihydroxy-; Butanedioic acid, 2,3-dihydroxy-, [*R*-(*R**,*R**)]-.

Molecular formula: $C_4H_6O_6$.

Molecular weight: 150.09.

Description: Tartaric Acid NF—Colorless or translucent crystals, or white, fine to granular, crystalline powder. Odorless. Stable in air.

NF category: Acidifying agent.

Solubility: Tartaric Acid NF—Very soluble in water; freely soluble in alcohol.

NF requirements: Tartaric Acid NF—Preserve in well-closed containers. Dried over phosphorus pentoxide for 3 hours, contains not less than 99.7% and not more than 100.5% of tartaric acid. Meets the requirements for Identification, Specific rotation (+12.0° to +13.0°, calculated on the dried basis), Loss on drying (not more than 0.5%), Residue on ignition (not more than 0.1%), Oxalate, Sulfate, Heavy metals (not more than 0.001%), and Organic volatile impurities.

TECHNETIUM Tc 99m ALBUMIN

USP requirements: Technetium Tc 99m Albumin Injection USP—Preserve in single-dose or in multiple-dose containers, at a temperature between 2 and 8 °C. A sterile, aqueous solution, suitable for intravenous administration, of Albumin Human that is labeled with ^{99m}Tc. Label it to include the following, in addition to the information specified for Labeling under Injections: the time and date of calibration; the amount of ^{99m}Tc as albumin expressed as total megabecquerels (or microcuries or millicuries) and concentration as megabecquerels (or microcuries or millicuries) per mL at the time of calibration; the expiration date; and the statement, "Caution—Radioactive Material." The labeling indicates that in making dosage calculations, correction is to be made for radioactive decay, and also indicates that the radioactive half-life of ^{99m}Tc is 6.0 hours. Contains the labeled amount of ^{99m}Tc, within ±10%, as albumin expressed in megabecquerels (or microcuries or millicuries) per mL at the time indicated in the labeling. Other chemical forms of radioactivity do not exceed 10.0% of the total radioactivity. Its production and distribution are subject to U.S. regulations. Meets the requirements for Bacterial endotoxins, pH (2.5–5.0), Radiochemical purity, and Biological distribution, for Radionuclide identification and Radionuclidic purity under Sodium Pertechnetate Tc 99m Injection, and for Injections (except that it may be distributed or dispensed prior to completion of the test for Sterility, the latter test being started on the day of final manufacture, and except that it is not subject to the recommendation on Volume in Container).

TECHNETIUM Tc 99m ALBUMIN AGGREGATED

Description: Technetium Tc 99m Albumin Aggregated Injection USP—Milky suspension, from which particles settle upon standing.

USP requirements: Technetium Tc 99m Albumin Aggregated Injection USP—Preserve in single-dose or in multiple-dose containers, at a temperature between 2 and 8 °C. A sterile, aqueous suspension of Albumin Human that has been denatured to produce aggregates of controlled particle size that are labeled with ^{99m}Tc. Suitable for intravenous administration. Label it to include the following, in addition to the information specified for Labeling under Injections: the time and date of calibration; the amount of ^{99m}Tc as aggregated albumin expressed as total megabecquerels (or millicuries or microcuries) and concentration as megabecquerels (or microcuries or millicuries) per mL at the time of calibration; the expiration date; and the statement, "Caution—Radioactive Material." The labeling indicates that in making dosage calculations, correction is to be made for radioactive decay, and also indicates that the radioactive half-life of ^{99m}Tc is 6.0 hours. In addition, the labeling states that it is not to be used if clumping of the albumin is observed and directs that the container be agitated before the contents are withdrawn into a syringe. Its production and distribution are subject to U.S. regulations. Contains the labeled amount of ^{99m}Tc, within ±10%, as aggregated albumin expressed in megabecquerels (or microcuries or millicuries) per mL at the time indicated in the labeling. Other chemical forms of radioactivity do not exceed 10.0% of the total radioactivity. Meets the requirements for Particle size, Bacterial endotoxins, pH (3.8–8.0), Radiochemical purity, Protein concentration, and Biological distribution, for Radionuclide identification and Radionuclidic purity under Sodium Pertechnetate Tc 99m Injection, and for Injections (except that it may be distributed or dispensed prior to completion of the test for Sterility, the latter test being started on the day of final manufacture, and except that it is not subject to the recommendation on Volume in Container).

TECHNETIUM Tc 99m ALBUMIN COLLOID

USP requirements: Technetium Tc 99m Albumin Colloid Injection USP—Preserve in single-dose or in multiple-dose containers, at a temperature between 2 and 8 °C. A sterile, pyrogen-free, aqueous suspension of Albumin Human that has been denatured to produce colloids of controlled particle size and that are labeled with ^{99m}Tc. Label it to include the following, in addition to the information specified for Labeling under Injections: the time and date of calibration; the amount of ^{99m}Tc expressed as total megabecquerels (or millicuries) and concentration as megabecquerels (or millicuries) per mL at the time of calibration; the expiration date and time and a statement, "Caution—Radioactive Material." The labeling indicates that in making dosage calculations, correction is to be made for radioactive decay, and also indicates that the radioactive half-life of ^{99m}Tc is 6.0 hours. In addition, the labeling states that it is not to be used if clumping of the albumin is observed, and directs that the container be agitated before the contents are withdrawn into a syringe. Contains the labeled amount of ^{99m}Tc, within ±10%, as albumin colloid complex, expressed in megabecquerels (or millicuries) per mL at the time indicated on the label. The vials are sealed under a suitable inert atmosphere. Its production and distribution are subject to U.S. regulations. Other chemical forms of radioactivity do not exceed 10.0% of the total radioactivity. Meets the requirements for Bacterial endotoxins, pH (7.5–8.5), Radiochemical purity, Particle size distribution, Biological distribution, and Albumin content, for Radionuclide identification and Radionuclidic purity under Sodium Pertechnetate Tc 99m Injection, and for Injections (except that it may be distributed or dispensed prior to completion of the test for Sterility, the latter test being started on the date of manufacture, and except that it is not subject to the recommendation on Volume in Container).

TECHNETIUM Tc 99m DISOFENIN

Chemical group: Disofenin—derivative of iminodiacetic acid (IDA).

Chemical name: Disofenin—Glycine, *N*-[2-[[2,6-bis(1-methylethyl)phenyl]amino]-2-ox-oethyl]-*N*-(carboxymethyl)-.

Molecular formula: Disofenin—$C_{18}H_{26}N_2O_5$.

Molecular weight: Disofenin—350.41.

USP requirements: Technetium Tc 99m Disofenin Injection USP—Preserve in single-dose or in multiple-dose containers sealed under a suitable inert atmosphere. A sterile, aqueous solution, suitable for intravenous administration, of disofenin that is labeled with ^{99m}Tc. Label it to include the following, in addition to the information specified for Labeling under Injections: the time and date of preparation; the amount of ^{99m}Tc expressed as total megabecquerels (or microcuries or millicuries) and concentration as megabecquerels (or microcuries or millicuries) per mL at the time of preparation; the expiration date and time; and a statement, "Caution—Radioactive Material." The labeling indicates that in making dosage calculations, correction is to be made for radioactive decay, and also indicates that the radioactive half-life of ^{99m}Tc is 6.0 hours. Contains the labeled amount of ^{99m}Tc, within ±10%, as a disofenin complex, expressed in megabecquerels (or microcuries or millicuries) per mL at the time indicated on the labeling. Contains a suitable reducing agent. Meets the requirements for pH (4.0–5.0), Radiochemical purity, and Biological distribution, for Radionuclide identification, Radionuclidic purity, and Bacterial endotoxins under Sodium Pertechnetate Tc 99m Injection, and for Injections (except that it may be distributed or dispensed prior to completion of the test for Sterility, the latter test being started on the date of preparation, and except that it is not subject to the recommendation on Volume in Container).

TECHNETIUM Tc 99m ETIDRONATE

USP requirements: Technetium Tc 99m Etidronate Injection USP—Preserve in single-dose or in multiple-dose containers. A sterile, clear, colorless solution, suitable for intravenous administration, of radioactive technetium (^{99m}Tc) in the form of a chelate of etidronate sodium. Label it to include the following, in addition to the information specified for Labeling under Injections: the time and date of calibration; the amount of ^{99m}Tc as labeled etidronate expressed as total megabecquerels (or microcuries or millicuries) and concentration as megabecquerels (or microcuries or millicuries) per mL at the time of calibration; the expiration date and time; and the statement, "Caution—Radioactive Material." The labeling indicates that in making dosage calculations, correction is to be made for radioactive decay, and also indicates that the radioactive half-life of ^{99m}Tc is 6.0 hours. Contains the labeled amount of ^{99m}Tc, within ±10%, as chelate expressed in megabecquerels (or microcuries or millicuries) per mL at the time indicated in the labeling. Other chemical forms of radioactivity do not exceed 10.0% of the total radioactivity. Meets the requirements for pH (2.5–7.0), and for Bacterial endotoxins, Radiochemical purity, Biological distribution, and Other requirements under Technetium Tc 99m Pyrophosphate Injection.

TECHNETIUM Tc 99m EXAMETAZIME

Chemical name: Exametazime—2-Butanone, 3,3′-[(2,2-dimethyl-1,3-propanediyl)diimino]bis-, dioxime, [*R**,*R**-(*E*,*E*)]-(±)-.

Chemical formula: Exametazime—$C_{13}H_{28}N_4O_2$.

Molecular weight: Exametazime—272.39.

USP requirements: Technetium Tc 99m Exametazime Injection—Not in USP.

TECHNETIUM Tc 99m FERPENTETATE

Chemical name: Iron, ascorbic acid and *N*,*N*-bis[2-[bis-(carboxymethyl)amino]ethyl]glycine complex, metastable technetium-99 labeled.

Description: Technetium Tc 99m Ferpentetate Injection USP—Clear, light brown to yellow solution.

USP requirements: Technetium Tc 99m Ferpentetate Injection USP—Preserve in single-dose or in multiple-dose containers, at a temperature between 2 and 8 °C. Protect from light. A sterile, aqueous solution of iron ascorbate pentetic acid that is complexed with ^{99m}Tc. Suitable for intravenous administration. Label it to include the following, in addition to the information specified for Labeling under Injections: the time and date of calibration; the amount of ^{99m}Tc as labeled ferpentetate expressed as total megabecquerels (or microcuries or millicuries) and concentration as megabecquerels (or microcuries or millicuries) per mL at the time of calibration; the expiration date; and the statement, "Caution—Radioactive Material." The labeling indicates that in making dosage calculations, correction is to be made for radioactive decay, and also indicates that the radioactive half-life of ^{99m}Tc is 6.0 hours. Contains the labeled amount of ^{99m}Tc, within ±10%, as the ferpentetate expressed in megabecquerels (or microcuries or millicuries) per mL at the time indicated in the labeling. Other chemical forms of radioactivity do not exceed 10.0% of the total radioactivity. Meets the requirements for Bacterial endotoxins, pH (4.0–5.5), Radiochemical purity, and Biological distribution, for Radionuclide identification and Radionuclidic purity under Sodium Pertechnetate Tc 99m Injection, and for Injections (except that it may be distributed or dispensed prior to completion of test for Sterility, the latter test being started on the day of manufacture, and except that it is not subject to the recommendation on Volume in Container).

TECHNETIUM Tc 99m GLUCEPTATE

Chemical name: D-*glycero*-D-*gulo*-Heptonic acid, technetium-^{99m}*Tc* complex.

USP requirements: Technetium Tc 99m Gluceptate Injection USP—Preserve in single-dose or in multiple-dose containers, at a temperature between 2 and 8 °C. A sterile, aqueous solution, suitable for intravenous administration, of sodium gluceptate and stannous chloride that is labeled with ^{99m}Tc. Label it to include the following, in addition to the information specified for Labeling under Injections: the time and date of calibration; the amount of ^{99m}Tc as labeled stannous gluceptate expressed as total megabecquerels (or microcuries or millicuries) and concentration as megabecquerels (or microcuries or millicuries) per mL at the time of calibration; the expiration date and time; and the statement, "Caution—Radioactive Material." The labeling indicates that in making dosage calculations, correction is to be made for radioactive decay, and also indicates that the radioactive half-life of ^{99m}Tc is 6.0 hours. Contains the labeled amount of ^{99m}Tc, within ±10%, as stannous gluceptate complex expressed in megabecquerels (or microcuries or millicuries) per mL at the time indicated in the labeling. Other chemical forms of radioactivity do not exceed 10.0% of the total radioactivity. Meets the requirements for Bacterial endotoxins, pH (4.0–8.0), Radiochemical purity, and Biological distribution, for Radionuclide identification and Radionuclidic purity under Sodium Pertechnetate Tc 99m Injection, and for Injections (except that it may be distributed or dispensed prior to completion of the test for Sterility, the latter test being started on the date of manufacture, and except that it is not subject to the recommendation on Volume in Container).

TECHNETIUM Tc 99m LIDOFENIN

Chemical group: Lidofenin—Derivative of iminodiacetic acid (IDA).

Chemical name: Lidofenin—Glycine, *N*-(carboxymethyl)-*N*-[2-[(2,6-dimethylphenyl)amino]-2-oxoethyl]-.

Molecular formula: Lidofenin—$C_{14}H_{18}N_2O_5$.

Molecular weight: Lidofenin—294.31.

Description: Lidofenin—Possesses both a lipophilic component and a hydrophilic group; forms an anionic bis-complex with Tc 99m.

USP requirements: Technetium Tc 99m Lidofenin Injection USP—Preserve in single-dose or in multiple-dose containers at a temperature between 2 and 8 °C. A sterile, clear, colorless solution of lidofenin complexed to radioactive technetium (^{99m}Tc) in the form of a chelate. Label it to include the following, in addition to the information specified for Labeling under Injections: the time and date of calibration; the amount of ^{99m}Tc as labeled lidofenin expressed as total megabecquerels (or millicuries) per mL at the time of calibration; the expiration date and time; the storage temperature and the statement, "Caution—Radioactive Material." The labeling indicates that, in making dosage calculations, correction is to be made for radioactive decay, and also indicates that the radioactive half-life of ^{99m}Tc is 6.0 hours. Contains the labeled amount of ^{99m}Tc, within ±10%, as the lidofenin chelate, expressed in megabecquerels (or millicuries) per mL at the time indicated in the labeling. Other chemical forms of radioactivity do not exceed 10.0% of the total radioactivity. Meets the requirements for Bacterial endotoxins, pH (3.5–5.0), Radiochemical purity, and Biological distribution, for Radionuclide identification and Radionuclidic purity under Sodium Pertechnetate Tc 99m Injection, and for Injections (except that it may be distributed or dispensed prior to completion of the test for Sterility, the latter test being started on the day of manufacture, and except that it is not subject to the recommendation on Volume in Container).

TECHNETIUM Tc 99m MEBROFENIN

Chemical group: Mebrofenin—Derivative of iminodiacetic acid (IDA).

Chemical name: Mebrofenin—Glycine, *N*-[2-[(3-bromo-2,4,6-trimethylphenyl)amino]-2-oxoethyl]-*N*-(carboxymethyl)-.

Molecular formula: Mebrofenin—$C_{15}H_{19}BrN_2O_5$.

Molecular weight: Mebrofenin—387.23.

Description: Mebrofenin—Possesses both a lipophilic component and a hydrophilic group; forms an anionic bis-complex with Tc 99m.

USP requirements: Technetium Tc 99m Mebrofenin Injection—Not in USP.

TECHNETIUM Tc 99m MEDRONATE

Chemical group: Sodium medronate—A biphosphonate compound.

USP requirements: Technetium Tc 99m Medronate Injection USP—Preserve in single-dose or in multiple-dose containers at a temperature specified in the labeling. A sterile, aqueous solution, suitable for intravenous administration, of sodium medronate and stannous chloride or stannous fluoride that is labeled with radioactive Tc 99m. Contains the labeled amount of Tc 99m, within ±10%, as stannous medronate complex expressed in megabecquerels (or microcuries or millicuries) per mL at the date and time indicated in the labeling. Other chemical forms of radioactivity do not exceed 10.0% of the total radioactivity. Meets the requirements for Bacterial endotoxins, pH (4.0–7.8), and Radiochemical purity, for Radionuclide identification and Radionuclidic purity under Sodium Pertechnetate Tc 99m Injection, for Labeling and Biological distribution under Technetium Tc 99m Pyrophosphate Injection, and for Injections (except that it may be distributed or dispensed prior to completion of the test for Sterility, the latter test being started on the day of manufacture, and except that it is not subject to the recommendation on Volume in Container).

TECHNETIUM Tc 99m MERTIATIDE

Chemical name: Technetate(2–)-^{99m}*Tc*, [*N*-[*N*-[*N*-(mercaptoacetyl)glycyl]glycyl]glycinato(5–)-*N*,*N*′, *N*″,*S*]-oxo-, disodium, (*SP*-5-25)-.

Molecular formula: $C_8H_8N_3Na_2O_6S^{99m}Tc$.

USP requirements: Technetium Tc 99m Mertiatide Injection—Not in USP.

TECHNETIUM Tc 99m OXIDRONATE

Chemical group: Oxidronate sodium—A biphosphonate compound.

USP requirements: Technetium Tc 99m Oxidronate Injection USP—Preserve in single-dose or in multiple-dose containers. A sterile, clear, colorless solution, suitable for intravenous administration, of radioactive technetium (^{99m}Tc) in the form of a chelate of oxidronate sodium. Label it to include the following, in addition to the information specified for Labeling under Injections: the time and date of calibration; the amount of ^{99m}Tc as labeled oxidronate expressed as total megabecquerels (or microcuries or millicuries) and concentration as megabecquerels (or microcuries or millicuries) per mL at the time of calibration; the expiration date and time; and the statement, "Caution—Radioactive Material." The labeling indicates that in making dosage calculations, correction is to be made for radioactive decay, and also indicates that the radioactive half-life of ^{99m}Tc is 6.0 hours. Contains the labeled amount of ^{99m}Tc, within ±10%, as chelate expressed in megabecquerels (or microcuries or millicuries) per mL at the date and time indicated in the labeling. Other chemical forms of radioactivity do not exceed 10.0% of the total radioactivity. Meets the requirements for pH (2.5–7.0), and for Bacterial endotoxins, Radiochemical purity, Biological distribution, and Other requirements under Technetium Tc 99m Pyrophosphate Injection.

TECHNETIUM Tc 99m PENTETATE

Chemical name: Technetate(1-)^{99m}*Tc*, [*N,N*-bis[2-bis(carboxymethyl)amino]ethyl]glycinato(5-)]-, sodium.

Molecular formula: $C_{14}H_{18}N_3NaO_{10}{}^{99m}Tc$.

Description: Technetium Tc 99m Pentetate Injection USP—Clear, colorless solution.

USP requirements: Technetium Tc 99m Pentetate Injection USP—Preserve in single-dose or in multiple-dose containers, at a temperature between 2 and 8 °C. A sterile solution of pentetic acid that is complexed with ^{99m}Tc in Sodium Chloride Injection. Suitable for intravenous administration. Label it to include the following, in addition to the information specified for Labeling under Injections: the time and date of calibration; the amount of ^{99m}Tc as labeled pentetic acid complex expressed as total megabecquerels (or millicuries or microcuries) and concentration as megabecquerels (or microcuries or millicuries) per mL at the time of calibration; the expiration date; and the statement, "Caution—Radioactive Material." The labeling indicates that in making dosage calculations, correction is to be made for radioactive decay, and also indicates that the radioactive half-life of ^{99m}Tc is 6.0 hours. Contains the labeled amount of ^{99m}Tc, within ±10%, as the pentetic acid complex, expressed in megabecquerels (or microcuries or millicuries) per mL at the time indicated on the labeling. Other chemical forms of radioactivity do not exceed 10.0% of the total radioactivity. Meets the requirements for pH (3.8–7.5) and Radiochemical purity, for Radionuclide identification and Radionuclidic purity under Sodium Pertechnetate Tc 99m Injection, for Bacterial endotoxins and Biological distribution under Technetium Tc 99m Ferpentetate Injection, and for Injections (except that it may be distributed or dispensed prior to completion of the test for Sterility, the latter test being started on the day of manufacture, and except that it is not subject to the recommendation on Volume in Container).

SODIUM PERTECHNETATE Tc 99m

Chemical name: Pertechnetic acid ($H^{99m}TcO_4$), sodium salt.

Molecular formula: $Na^{99m}TcO_4$.

Description: Sodium Pertechnetate Tc 99m Injection USP—Clear, colorless solution.

USP requirements: Sodium Pertechnetate Tc 99m Injection USP—Preserve in single-dose or in multiple-dose containers. A sterile solution, suitable for intravenous or oral administration, containing radioactive technetium (^{99m}Tc) in the form of sodium pertechnetate and sufficient Sodium Chloride to make the solution isotonic. Technetium 99m is a radioactive nuclide formed by the radioactive decay of molybdenum 99. Molybdenum 99 is a radioactive isotope of molybdenum and may be formed by the neutron bombardment of molybdenum 98 or as a product of uranium fission. If intended for intravenous use, label it with the information specified for Labeling under Injections. Label it also to include the following: the time and date of calibration; the amount of ^{99m}Tc as sodium pertechnetate expressed as total megabecquerels (or millicuries) and as megabecquerels (or millicuries) per mL on the date and at the time of calibration; a statement of the intended use, whether oral or intravenous; the expiration date; and the statement, "Caution—Radioactive Material." If the Injection has been prepared from molybdenum 99 produced from uranium fission, the label so states. The labeling indicates that in making dosage calculations, correction is to be made for radioactive decay, and also indicates that the radioactive half-life of ^{99m}Tc is 6.0 hours. Contains the labeled amount of ^{99m}Tc, within ±10%, at the date and hour stated on the label. Other chemical forms of ^{99m}Tc do not exceed 5% of the total radioactivity. Meets the requirements for Radionuclide identification, Bacterial endotoxins, pH (4.5–7.5), Radiochemical purity, Radionuclidic purity, Chemical purity, and Injections (except that the Injection may be distributed or dispensed prior to the completion of the test for Sterility, the latter test being started on the day of manufacture, and except that it is not subject to the recommendation on Volume in Container).

TECHNETIUM Tc 99m PYROPHOSPHATE

Chemical name:
Sodium pyrophosphate—Diphosphoric acid, tetrasodium salt.
Stannous chloride—Tin chloride ($SnCl_2$) dihydrate.

Molecular formula:
Sodium pyrophosphate—$Na_4P_2O_7$.
Stannous chloride—$SnCl_2 \cdot 2H_2O$.

Molecular weight:
Sodium pyrophosphate—265.90.
Stannous chloride—225.65.

USP requirements: Technetium Tc 99m Pyrophosphate Injection USP—Preserve in single-dose or in multiple-dose containers, at a temperature between 2 and 8 °C. A sterile aqueous solution, suitable for intravenous administration, of pyrophosphate that is labeled with ^{99m}Tc. Label it to include the following, in addition to the information specified for Labeling under Injections: the time and date of calibration; the amount of ^{99m}Tc as labeled tetrasodium pyrophosphate expressed as total megabecquerels (or microcuries or millicuries) and concentration as megabecquerels (or microcuries or millicuries) per mL at the time of calibration; the expiration date and time; and the statement, "Caution—Radioactive Material." The labeling indicates that in making dosage calculations, correction is to be made for radioactive decay, and also indicates that the radioactive half-life of ^{99m}Tc is 6.0 hours. Contains the labeled amount of ^{99m}Tc, within ±10%, as pyrophosphate expressed in megabecquerels (or microcuries or millicuries) per mL at the time indicated in the labeling. Other chemical forms of radioactivity do not exceed 10.0% of the total radioactivity. Meets the requirements for Bacterial endotoxins, pH (4.0–7.5), Radiochemical purity, and Biological distribution, for Radionuclide identification and Radionuclidic purity under Sodium Pertechnetate Tc 99m Injection, and for Injections (except that it may be distributed or dispensed prior to completion of the test for Sterility, the latter test being started on the day of final manufacture, and except that it is not subject to the recommendation on Volume in Container).

TECHNETIUM Tc 99m (PYRO- AND TRIMETA-) PHOSPHATES

Chemical name:
Sodium pyrophosphate—Diphosphoric acid, tetrasodium salt.
Sodium trimetaphosphate—Metaphosphoric acid ($H_3P_3O_9$), trisodium salt.
Stannous chloride—Tin chloride ($SnCl_2$) dihydrate.

Molecular formula:
Sodium pyrophosphate—$Na_4P_2O_7$.
Sodium trimetaphosphate—$Na_3P_3O_9$.
Stannous chloride—$SnCl_2 \cdot 2H_2O$.

Molecular weight:
Sodium pyrophosphate—265.90.
Sodium trimetaphosphate—305.89.
Stannous chloride—225.65.

Description: Technetium Tc 99m (Pyro- and Trimeta-) Phosphates Injection USP—Clear solution.

USP requirements: Technetium Tc 99m (Pyro- and trimeta-) Phosphates Injection USP—A sterile, aqueous solution, suitable for intravenous administration, composed of sodium pyrophosphate, sodium trimetaphosphate, and stannous chloride labeled with radioactive Tc 99m. Contains the labeled amount of ^{99m}Tc, within ±10%, as phosphate expressed in megabecquerels (or microcuries or millicuries) per mL at the time indicated in the labeling. Other chemical forms of radioactivity do not exceed 10.0% of the total radioactivity. Meets the requirements for pH (4.0–7.0) and Radiochemical purity, for Radionuclide identification and Radionuclidic purity under Sodium Pertechnetate Tc 99m Injection, for Packaging and storage, Labeling, Bacterial endotoxins, and Biological distribution under Technetium Tc 99m Pyrophosphate Injection, and for Injections (except that it may be distributed or dispensed prior to completion of the test for Sterility, the latter test being started on the day of final manufacture, and except that it is not subject to the recommendation on Volume in Container).

TECHNETIUM Tc 99m SESTAMIBI

Chemical name: Technetium(1+)-*^{99m}Tc*, hexakis(1-isocyano-2-methoxy-2-methylpropane)-, (*OC*-6-11)-.

Molecular formula: $C_{36}H_{66}N_6O_6{}^{99m}Tc$.

USP requirements: Technetium Tc 99m Sestamibi Injection—Not in USP.

TECHNETIUM Tc 99m SUCCIMER

Chemical name: meso-2,3-Dimercaptosuccinic acid, *^{99m}Tc* complex.

USP requirements: Technetium Tc 99m Succimer Injection USP—Preserve in single-dose containers, at a temperature between 15 and 30 °C. Do not freeze or store above 30 °C. Protect from light. A sterile, clear, colorless, aqueous solution of succimer complexed with ^{99m}Tc. Suitable for intravenous administration. Label it to include the following, in addition to the information specified for Labeling under Injections: the time and date of calibration; the amount of ^{99m}Tc as labeled succimer expressed as total megabecquerels (or microcuries or millicuries) and concentration as megabecquerels (or microcuries or millicuries) per mL at the time of calibration; the expiration date and time; and the statement, "Caution—Radioactive Material." The labeling indicates that in making dosage calculations, correction is to be made for radioactive decay, and also indicates that the radioactive half-life of ^{99m}Tc is 6.0 hours. In addition, the labeling states that it is not to be used if discoloration or particulate matter is observed. (Note: A beyond-use time of 30 minutes shall be stated on the label upon constitution with Sodium Pertechnetate Tc 99m Injection.) Contains not less than 85% of the labeled amount of ^{99m}Tc as the succimer complex expressed in megabecquerels (or microcuries or millicuries) per mL at the time indicated in the labeling. Other chemical forms of radioactivity do not exceed 15.0% of the total radioactivity. Meets the requirements for Bacterial endotoxins, pH (2.0–3.0), Radiochemical purity, and Biological distribution, for Radionuclide identification and Radionuclidic purity under Sodium Pertechnetate Tc 99m Injection, and for Injections (except that it may be distributed or dispensed prior to completion of the test for Sterility, the latter test being started on the day of final manufacture, and except that it is not subject to the recommendation on Volume in Container).

TECHNETIUM Tc 99m SULFUR COLLOID

Description: Technetium Tc 99m Sulfur Colloid Injection USP—Colloidal dispersion. Slightly opalescent, colorless to light tan liquid.

USP requirements: Technetium Tc 99m Sulfur Colloid Injection USP—Store in single-dose or in multiple-dose containers. A sterile, colloidal dispersion of sulfur labeled with radioactive ^{99m}Tc, suitable for intravenous administration. Label it to include the following, in addition to the information specified for Labeling under Injections: the time and date of calibration; the amount of ^{99m}Tc as sulfur colloid expressed as total megabecquerels (or microcuries or millicuries) and concentration as megabecquerels (or microcuries or millicuries) per mL at the time of calibration; the expiration date; and the statement, "Caution—Radioactive Material." The labeling indicates that in making dosage calculations, correction is to be made for radioactive decay, and also indicates that the radioactive half-life of ^{99m}Tc is 6.0 hours; in addition, the labeling states that it is not to be used if flocculent material is visible and directs that the container be agitated before the Injection is withdrawn into a syringe. Contains the labeled amount of ^{99m}Tc, within ±10%, as sulfur colloid expressed in megabecquerels (or microcuries or millicuries) per mL at the time indicated in the labeling. Other chemical forms of radioactivity do not exceed 8% of the total radioactivity. Meets the requirements for Bacterial endotoxins, pH (4.5–7.5), Radionuclidic purity under Sodium Pertechnetate Tc 99m Injection, Radiochemical purity, Biological distribution, and Injections (except that the Injection may be distributed or dispensed prior to completion of the test for Sterility, the latter test being started on the day of final manufacture, and except that it is not subject to the recommendation on Volume in Container).

Note: Agitate the container before withdrawing the Injection into a syringe.

TECHNETIUM Tc 99m TEBOROXIME

Chemical name: Technetium-*^{99m}Tc*, [bis[(1,2-cyclohexanedione dioximato)(1-)-*O*][(1,2-cyclohexanedione dioximato)(2-)-*O*]methylborato(2-)-*N,N′,N″,N‴,N⁗,N‴″*]-chloro-, (*TPS*-7-1-232′4′54)-.

Molecular formula: $C_{19}H_{29}BClN_6O_6{}^{99m}Tc$.

USP requirements: Technetium Tc 99m Teboroxime Injection—Not in USP.

TEMAZEPAM

Chemical name: 2*H*-1,4-Benzodiazepin-2-one, 7-chloro-1,3-dihydro-3-hydroxy-1-methyl-5-phenyl-.

Molecular formula: $C_{16}H_{13}ClN_2O_2$.

Molecular weight: 300.74.

Description: Temazepam USP—White or nearly white crystalline powder. Melts between 157 and 163 °C, within a 3 °C range.

Solubility: Temazepam USP—Very slightly soluble in water; sparingly soluble in alcohol.

USP requirements:

Temazepam USP—Preserve in well-closed, light-resistant containers. Contains not less than 98.0% and not more than 102.0% of temazepam, calculated on the dried basis. Meets the requirements for Identification, Loss on drying (not more than 0.5%), Residue on ignition (not more than 0.1%), Heavy metals (not more than 20 ppm), and Chromatographic purity.

Caution: Temazepam is a potent sedative—its powder should not be inhaled.

Temazepam Capsules USP—Preserve in well-closed, light-resistant containers. Contain the labeled amount, within ±10%. Meet the requirements for Identification, Dissolution (80% in 30 minutes in sodium acetate buffer with 0.05% polysorbate 80 in Apparatus 2 at 75 rpm), and Uniformity of dosage units.

Caution: Temazepam is a potent sedative—its powder should not be inhaled.

Temazepam Tablets—Not in USP.

TENIPOSIDE

Chemical name: Furo[3′,4′:6,7]naphtho[2,3-*d*]-1,3-dioxol-6(5a*H*)-one, 5,8,8a,9-tetrahydro-5-(4-hydroxy-3,5-dimethoxyphenyl)-9-[[4,6-*O*-(2-thienylmethylene)-beta-D-glucopyranosyl]-oxy]-, [5*R*-[5 alpha,5a beta,8a alpha,9 beta(*R**)]]-.

Molecular formula: $C_{32}H_{32}O_{13}S$.

Molecular weight: 656.66.

Description: White to off-white crystalline powder.

Solubility: Insoluble in water and in ether; slightly soluble in methanol; very soluble in acetone and in dimethylformamide.

USP requirements: Teniposide Injection—Not in USP.

TENOXICAM

Chemical name: 2*H*-Thieno[2,3-*e*]-1,2-thiazine-3-carboxamide, 4-hydroxy-2-methyl-*N*-2-pyridinyl-, 1,1-dioxide.

Molecular formula: $C_{13}H_{11}N_3O_4S_2$.

Molecular weight: 337.37.

Description: Yellow, practically odorless, crystalline powder which melts with decomposition at approximately 205 °C.

pKa: Approximately 1.1 and 5.3.

Solubility: Quite insoluble in water and in common organic solvents.

USP requirements: Tenoxicam Tablets—Not in USP.

TERAZOSIN

Chemical group: Quinazoline derivative.

Chemical name: Terazosin hydrochloride—Piperazine, 1-(4-amino-6,7-dimethoxy-2-quinazolinyl)-4-[(tetrahydro-2-furanyl)carbonyl]-, monohydrochloride, dihydrate. Is a racemic mixture, both components of which are active.

Molecular formula: Terazosin hydrochloride—$C_{19}H_{25}N_5O_4 \cdot HCl \cdot 2H_2O$.

Molecular weight: Terazosin hydrochloride—459.93.

Description: Terazosin hydrochloride—White, crystalline substance.

pKa: 7.04.

Solubility: Terazosin hydrochloride—Freely soluble in water and in isotonic saline.

USP requirements: Terazosin Hydrochloride Tablets—Not in USP.

TERBINAFINE

Chemical name: Terbinafine hydrochloride—(E)-*N*-(6,6-dimethyl-2-hepten-4-ynyl)-*N*-methyl-1-naphthalenemethanamine hydrochloride.

Molecular formula: Terbinafine hydrochloride—$C_{21}H_{26}ClN$.

Molecular weight: Terbinafine hydrochloride—327.90.

Description: Terbinafine hydrochloride—White to off-white fine crystalline powder.

Solubility: Terbinafine hydrochloride—Freely soluble in methanol and in methylene chloride; soluble in ethanol; slightly soluble in water.

USP requirements: Terbinafine Hydrochloride Cream—Not in USP.

TERBUTALINE

Chemical name: Terbutaline sulfate—1,3-Benzenediol, 5-[2-[(1,1-dimethylethyl)amino]-1-hydroxyethyl]-, sulfate (2:1) (salt).

Molecular formula: Terbutaline sulfate—$(C_{12}H_{19}NO_3)_2 \cdot H_2SO_4$.

Molecular weight: Terbutaline sulfate—548.66.

Description: Terbutaline Sulfate USP—White to gray-white, crystalline powder. Is odorless or has a faint odor of acetic acid.

Solubility: Terbutaline Sulfate USP—Soluble in water and in 0.1 *N* hydrochloric acid; slightly soluble in methanol; insoluble in chloroform.

USP requirements:

Terbutaline Sulfate USP—Preserve in well-closed, light-resistant containers, at controlled room temperature. Contains not less than 98.0% and not more than 101.0% of terbutaline sulfate, calculated on the dried basis. Meets the requirements for Identification, Acidity, Loss on drying (not more than 0.5%), Residue on ignition (not more than 0.2%), Heavy metals (not more than 0.0025%), 3,5-Dihydroxy-*omega-tert*-butylaminoacetophenone sulfate, and Organic volatile impurities.

Terbutaline Sulfate Inhalation Aerosol USP—Preserve in small, nonreactive, light-resistant aerosol containers equipped with metered-dose valves and provided with oral inhalation actuators. Store at controlled room temperature. A suspension of microfine Terbutaline Sulfate in suitable propellants in a pressurized container. Contains the labeled amount, within ±10%. Meets the requirements for Identification, Uniformity of dosage units, Water (not more than 0.02%), Uniformity of unit spray content, and Particle size, and for Leakage testing and Minimum fill under Aerosols.

Terbutaline Sulfate Injection USP—Preserve in single-dose containers, preferably of Type I glass, protected from light, at controlled room temperature. A sterile solution of Terbutaline Sulfate in Water for Injection. Contains the labeled amount, within ±10%. Meets the requirements for Identification, Bacterial endotoxins, and pH (3.0–5.0), and for Injections.

Note: Do not use the Injection if it is discolored.

Terbutaline Sulfate Tablets USP—Preserve in tight containers, at controlled room temperature. Contain the labeled amount, within ±10%. Meet the requirements for Identification, Dissolution (75% in 45 minutes in water in Apparatus 1 at 100 rpm), and Uniformity of dosage units.

TERCONAZOLE

Chemical name: Piperazine, 1-[4-[[2-(2,4-dichlorophenyl)-2-(1*H*-1,2,4-triazol-1-ylmethyl)-1,3-dioxolan-4-yl]methoxy]phenyl]-4-(1-methylethyl)-, *cis*-.

Molecular formula: $C_{26}H_{31}Cl_2N_5O_3$.

Molecular weight: 532.47.

Description: White to almost white powder.

Solubility: Soluble in butanol; sparingly soluble in ethanol; insoluble in water.

USP requirements:

Terconazole Vaginal Cream—Not in USP.
Terconazole Vaginal Suppositories—Not in USP.

TERFENADINE

Chemical group: Butyrophenone derivative.

Chemical name: 1-Piperidinebutanol, alpha-[4-(1,1-dimethylethyl)phenyl]-4-(hydroxydiphenylmethyl)-.

Molecular formula: $C_{32}H_{41}NO_2$.

Molecular weight: 471.68.

Description: Terfenadine USP—White to off-white, crystalline powder.

Solubility: Terfenadine USP—Slightly soluble in water, in hexane, and in 0.1 *N* hydrochloric acid; freely soluble in chloroform; soluble in alcohol, in methanol, in octanol, and in toluene.

USP requirements:

Terfenadine USP—Preserve in tight, light-resistant containers. Contains not less than 98.0% and not more than 101.5% of terfenadine, calculated on the dried basis. Meets the requirements for Identification, Melting range (145–151 °C), Loss on drying (not more than 0.5%), Residue on ignition (not more than 0.1%), and Chromatographic purity.

Terfenadine Oral Suspension—Not in USP.

Terfenadine Tablets USP—Preserve in tight, light-resistant containers. Contain the labeled amount, within ±10%. Meet the requirements for Identification, Dissolution (75% in 45 minutes in 0.1 *N* hydrochloric acid in Apparatus 2 at 50 rpm), and Uniformity of dosage units.

TERFENADINE AND PSEUDOEPHEDRINE

For *Terfenadine* and *Pseudoephedrine*—See individual listings for chemistry information.

USP requirements: Terfenadine and Pseudoephedrine Hydrochloride Extended-release Tablets—Not in USP.

TERIPARATIDE

Source: Teriparatide acetate—A synthetic polypeptide hormone consisting of the 1–34 fragment of human parathyroid hormone, the biologically active N-terminal region of the 84-amino-acid native hormone.

Chemical name: Teriparatide acetate—L-Phenylalanine, L-seryl-L-valyl-L-seryl-L-alpha-glutamyl-L-isoleucyl-L-glutaminyl-L-leucyl-L-methionyl-L-histidyl-L-asparaginyl-L-leucylglycyl-L-lysyl-L-histidyl-L-leucyl-L-asparaginyl-L-seryl-L-methionyl-L-alpha-glutamyl-L-arginyl-L-valyl-L-alpha-glutamyl-L-tryptophyl-L-leucyl-L-arginyl-L-lysyl-L-lysyl-L-leucyl-L-glutaminyl-L-alpha-aspartyl-L-valyl-L-histidyl-L-asparaginyl-, acetate (salt) hydrate.

Molecular formula: Teriparatide acetate—$C_{181}H_{291}N_{55}O_{51}S_2 \cdot xH_2O \cdot yC_2H_4O_2$.

USP requirements: Teriparatide Acetate for Injection—Not in USP.

TERPIN HYDRATE

Chemical name: Cyclohexanemethanol, 4-hydroxy-alpha,alpha,-4-trimethyl-, monohydrate.

Molecular formula: $C_{10}H_{20}O_2 \cdot H_2O$.

Molecular weight: 190.28.

Description: Terpin Hydrate USP—Colorless, lustrous crystals or white powder. Has a slight odor, and effloresces in dry air. A hot solution (1 in 100) is neutral to litmus. When dried in vacuum at 60 °C for 2 hours, it melts at about 103 °C.

Solubility: Terpin Hydrate USP—Slightly soluble in water, in chloroform, and in ether; very soluble in boiling alcohol; soluble in alcohol; sparingly soluble in boiling water.

USP requirements:

Terpin Hydrate USP—Preserve in tight containers. Contains not less than 98.0% and not more than 100.5% of terpin hydrate, calculated on the anhydrous basis. Meets the requirements for Identification, Water (9.0–10.0%), Residue on ignition (not more than 0.1%), and Residual turpentine.

Terpin Hydrate Elixir USP—Preserve in tight containers. Contains, in each 100 mL, not less than 1.53 grams and not more than 1.87 grams of terpin hydrate. Meets the requirement for Alcohol content (within ±10% of labeled amount).

TERPIN HYDRATE AND CODEINE

For *Terpin Hydrate* and *Codeine*—See individual listings for chemistry information.

USP requirements: Terpin Hydrate and Codeine Elixir USP—Preserve in tight containers. Contains, in each 100 mL, not less than 1.53 grams and not more than 1.87 grams of terpin hydrate, and not less than 180 mg and not more than 220 mg of codeine. Meets the requirements for Identification and Alcohol content (within ±10% of labeled amount).

TERPIN HYDRATE AND DEXTROMETHORPHAN

For *Terpin Hydrate* and *Dextromethorphan*—See individual listings for chemistry information.

USP requirements: Terpin Hydrate and Dextromethorphan Hydrobromide Elixir USP—Preserve in tight containers. Contains, in each 100 mL, not less than 1.53 grams and not more than 1.87 grams of terpin hydrate, and not less than 180 mg and not more than 220 mg of dextromethorphan hydrobromide. Meets the requirements for Identification and Alcohol content (within ±10% of labeled amount).

TESTOLACTONE

Chemical name: D-Homo-17a-oxaandrosta-1,4-diene-3,17-dione.

Molecular formula: $C_{19}H_{24}O_3$.

Molecular weight: 300.40.

Description: Testolactone USP—White to off-white, practically odorless, crystalline powder. Melts at about 218 °C.

Solubility: Testolactone USP—Slightly soluble in water and in benzyl alcohol; soluble in alcohol and in chloroform; insoluble in ether and in solvent hexane.

USP requirements:

Testolactone USP—Preserve in tight containers. Contains not less than 95.0% and not more than 105.0% of testolactone, calculated on the dried basis. Meets the requirements for Identification, Specific rotation (−44° to −52°, calculated on the dried basis), Loss on drying (not more than 1.0%), Residue on ignition (not more than 0.1%), Heavy metals (not more than 0.003%), Chromatographic impurities, Ordinary impurities, and Organic volatile impurities.

Sterile Testolactone Suspension USP—Preserve in single-dose or in multiple-dose containers, preferably of Type I glass. A sterile suspension of Testolactone in a suitable aqueous medium. Contains the labeled amount, within −10% to +20%. Meets the requirements for Identification, Uniformity of dosage units, Bacterial endotoxins, pH (5.0–7.5), and Injections.

Testolactone Tablets USP—Preserve in tight containers. Contain the labeled amount, within ±10%. Meet the requirements for Identification, Dissolution (80% in 120 minutes in 0.1 *N* hydrochloric acid in Apparatus 2 at 75 rpm), and Uniformity of dosage units.

TESTOSTERONE

Chemical group:

Testosterone—Naturally occurring androgen.

Testosterone cypionate, testosterone enanthate, and testosterone propionate—Semi-synthetic androgens.

Chemical name:

Testosterone—Androst-4-en-3-one, 17-hydroxy-, (17 beta)-.

Testosterone cypionate—Androst-4-en-3-one, 17-(3-cyclopentyl-1-oxopropoxy)-, (17 beta)-.

Testosterone enanthate—Androst-4-en-3-one, 17-[(1-oxoheptyl)oxy]-, (17 beta)-.

Testosterone propionate—Androst-4-en-3-one, 17-(1-oxopropoxy)-, (17 beta)-.

Molecular formula:

Testosterone—$C_{19}H_{28}O_2$.

Testosterone cypionate—$C_{27}H_{40}O_3$.

Testosterone enanthate—$C_{26}H_{40}O_3$.

Testosterone propionate—$C_{22}H_{32}O_3$.

Molecular weight:

Testosterone—288.43.

Testosterone cypionate—412.61.

Testosterone enanthate—400.60.

Testosterone propionate—344.49.

Description:

Testosterone USP—White or slightly creamy white crystals or crystalline powder. Is odorless, and is stable in air.

Testosterone Cypionate USP—White or creamy white, crystalline powder. Is odorless or has a slight odor, and is stable in air.

Testosterone Enanthate USP—White or creamy white, crystalline powder. Is odorless or has a faint odor characteristic of heptanoic acid.

Testosterone Propionate USP—White or creamy white crystals or crystalline powder. Is odorless and is stable in air.

Solubility:

Testosterone USP—Practically insoluble in water; freely soluble in dehydrated alcohol and in chloroform; soluble in dioxane and in vegetable oils; slightly soluble in ether.

Testosterone Cypionate USP—Insoluble in water; freely soluble in alcohol, in chloroform, in dioxane, and in ether; soluble in vegetable oils.

Testosterone Enanthate USP—Insoluble in water; very soluble in ether; soluble in vegetable oils.

Testosterone Propionate USP—Insoluble in water; freely soluble in alcohol, in dioxane, in ether, and in other organic solvents; soluble in vegetable oils.

USP requirements:

Testosterone USP—Preserve in well-closed containers. Contains not less than 97.0% and not more than 103.0% of testosterone, calculated on the dried basis. Meets the requirements for Identification, Melting range (153–157 °C), Specific rotation (+101° to +105°, calculated on the dried basis), Loss on drying (not more than 1.0%), and Organic volatile impurities.

Testosterone Pellets USP—Preserve in tight containers holding one pellet each and suitable for maintaining sterile contents. They are sterile pellets composed of Testosterone in compressed form, without the presence of any binder, diluent, or excipient. Contain the labeled amount, within ±3%. Meet the requirements for Identification, Melting range, and Specific rotation under Testosterone, Solubility in chloroform, Sterility, and Weight variation (within ±5% of labeled weight of testosterone for average weight of 5 Pellets, and within ±10% of labeled weight of testosterone for each Pellet).

Sterile Testosterone Suspension USP—Preserve in single-dose or in multiple-dose containers, preferably of Type I glass. A sterile suspension of Testosterone in an aqueous medium. Contains the labeled amount, within ±10%. Meets the requirements for Identification, Uniformity of dosage units, Bacterial endotoxins, pH (4.0–7.5), and Injections.

Testosterone Cypionate USP—Preserve in well-closed, light-resistant containers. Contains not less than 97.0% and not more than 103.0% of testosterone cypionate, calculated on the dried basis. Meets the requirements for Identification, Melting range (98–104 °C), Specific rotation (+85° to +92°, calculated on the dried basis), Loss on drying (not more than 0.5%), Residue on ignition (not more than 0.2%), Free cyclopentanepropionic acid (not more than 0.20%), and Organic volatile impurities.

Testosterone Cypionate Injection USP—Preserve in single-dose or in multiple-dose containers, preferably of Type I glass, protected from light. A sterile solution of Testosterone Cypionate in a suitable vegetable oil. Contains the labeled amount, within ±10%. Meets the requirements for Identification and Injections.

Testosterone Enanthate USP—Preserve in well-closed containers, in a cool place. Contains not less than 97.0% and not more than 103.0% of testosterone enanthate. Meets the requirements for Identification, Melting range (34–39 °C), Specific rotation (+77° to +82°, calculated on the anhydrous basis), Water (not more than 0.05%), Free heptanoic acid (not more than 0.16%), Ordinary impurities, and Organic volatile impurities.

Testosterone Enanthate Injection USP—Preserve in single-dose or in multiple-dose containers, preferably of Type I glass. A sterile solution of Testosterone Enanthate in a suitable vegetable oil. Contains the labeled amount, within ±10%. Meets the requirements for Identification and Injections.

Testosterone Propionate USP—Preserve in well-closed, light-resistant containers. Contains not less than 97.0% and not more than 103.0% of testosterone propionate, calculated on the dried basis. Meets the requirements for Identification, Melting range (118–123 °C), Specific rotation (+83° to +90°, previously dried), and Loss on drying (not more than 0.5%).

Testosterone Propionate Injection USP—Preserve in single-dose or in multiple-dose containers, preferably of Type I glass. A sterile solution of Testosterone Propionate in a suitable vegetable oil. Contains the labeled amount, within ±12%. Meets the requirements for Identification and Injections.

Testosterone Propionate Ointment—Not in USP.

TESTOSTERONE AND ESTRADIOL

Chemical name:

Testosterone cypionate—Androst-4-en-3-one, 17-(3-cyclopentyl-1-oxopropoxy)-, (17 beta)-.

Testosterone enanthate—Androst-4-en-3-one, 17-[(1-oxoheptyl)oxy]-, (17 beta)-.

Estradiol cypionate—Estra-1,3,5(10)-triene-3,17-diol, (17 beta)-, 17-cyclopentanepropanoate.

Estradiol valerate—Estra-1,3,5(10)-triene-3,17-diol(17 beta)-, 17-pentanoate.

Estradiol benzoate—Estra-1,3,5(10)-triene-3,17-diol, (17 beta)-, 3-benzoate.

Molecular formula:

Testosterone cypionate—$C_{27}H_{40}O_3$.

Testosterone enanthate—$C_{26}H_{40}O_3$.

Estradiol cypionate—$C_{26}H_{36}O_3$.

Estradiol valerate—$C_{23}H_{32}O_3$.

Estradiol benzoate—$C_{25}H_{28}O_3$.

Molecular weight:

Testosterone cypionate—412.61.

Testosterone enanthate—400.60.

Estradiol cypionate—396.57.

Estradiol valerate—356.51.

Estradiol benzoate—376.50.

Description:

Testosterone Cypionate USP—White or creamy white, crystalline powder. Is odorless or has a slight odor, and is stable in air.

Testosterone Enanthate USP—White or creamy white, crystalline powder. Is odorless or has a faint odor characteristic of heptanoic acid.

Estradiol Cypionate USP—White to practically white, crystalline powder. Is odorless or has a slight odor.

Estradiol Valerate USP—White, crystalline powder. Is usually odorless but may have a faint, fatty odor.

Estradiol benzoate—Colorless crystals or a white or almost white crystalline powder.

Solubility:

Testosterone Cypionate USP—Insoluble in water; freely soluble in alcohol, in chloroform, in dioxane, and in ether; soluble in vegetable oils.

Testosterone Enanthate USP—Insoluble in water; very soluble in ether; soluble in vegetable oils.

Estradiol Cypionate USP—Insoluble in water; soluble in alcohol, in acetone, in chloroform, and in dioxane; sparingly soluble in vegetable oils.

Estradiol Valerate USP—Practically insoluble in water; soluble in castor oil, in methanol, in benzyl benzoate, and in dioxane; sparingly soluble in sesame oil and in peanut oil.

Estradiol benzoate—Practically insoluble in water; slightly soluble in alcohol and in fixed oils; soluble 1 in 50 of acetone.

USP requirements:

Testosterone Cypionate and Estradiol Cypionate Injection—Not in USP.

Testosterone Enanthate and Estradiol Valerate Injection—Not in USP.

Testosterone Enanthate Benzilic Acid Hydrazone, Estradiol Dienanthate, and Estradiol Benzoate Injection—Not in USP.

TETANUS ANTITOXIN

Description: Tetanus Antitoxin USP—Transparent or slightly opalescent liquid, faint brownish, yellowish, or greenish in color and practically odorless or having an odor because of the antimicrobial agent.

USP requirements: Tetanus Antitoxin USP—Preserve at a temperature between 2 and 8 °C. A sterile, non-pyrogenic solution of the refined and concentrated proteins, chiefly globulins, containing antitoxic antibodies obtained from the blood serum or plasma of healthy horses that have been immunized against tetanus toxin or toxoid. Label it to state that it was prepared from horse serum or plasma. Has a potency of not less than 400 antitoxin units per mL based on the U.S. Standard Tetanus Antitoxin and the U.S. Control Tetanus Test Toxin, tested in guinea pigs. Meets the requirement for Expiration date (for Antitoxin containing a 20% excess of potency, not later than 5 years after date of issue from manufacturer's cold storage [5 °C, 1 year; or 0 °C, 2 years]). Conforms to the regulations of the U.S. Food and Drug Administration concerning biologics.

TETANUS IMMUNE GLOBULIN

Description: Tetanus Immune Globulin USP—Transparent or slightly opalescent liquid, practically colorless and practically odorless. May develop a slight granular deposit during storage.

USP requirements: Tetanus Immune Globulin USP—Preserve at a temperature between 2 and 8 °C. A sterile, non-pyrogenic solution of globulins derived from the blood plasma of adult human donors who have been immunized with tetanus toxoid. Label it to state that it is not for intravenous injection. Has a potency of not less than 50 antitoxin units per mL based on the U.S. Standard Tetanus Antitoxin and the U.S. Control Tetanus Test Toxin, tested in guinea pigs. Contains not less than 10 grams and not more than 18 grams of protein per 100 mL, of which not less than 90% is gamma globulin. Contains 0.3 *M* glycine as a stabilizing agent, and contains a suitable preservative. Meets the requirement for Expiration date (for Tetanus Immune Globulin containing a 10% excess of potency, not later than 3 years after date of issue from manufacturer's cold storage [5 °C, 1 year]). Conforms to the regulations of the U.S. Food and Drug Administration concerning biologics.

TETANUS TOXOID

Source: Tetanus toxoid adsorbed and fluid are prepared by growing the tetanus bacilli *Clostridium tetani* on a protein-free, semi-synthetic medium. The tetanus toxin produced by these bacilli is detoxified using formaldehyde and forms the tetanus toxoid. Thimerosal is added as a preservative. In addition, for tetanus toxoid adsorbed, aluminum phosphate or aluminum potassium sulfate is used as a mineral adjuvant to adsorb the tetanus antigens. This prolongs and enhances the antigenic properties by retarding the rate of absorption of the injected toxoid into the body.

Description:
Tetanus Toxoid USP—Clear, colorless to brownish yellow, or slightly turbid liquid, free from evident clumps or particles, having a characteristic odor or an odor of formaldehyde.
Tetanus Toxoid Adsorbed USP—Turbid, white, slightly gray, or slightly pink suspension, free from evident clumps after shaking.

USP requirements:
Tetanus Toxoid USP—Preserve at a temperature between 2 and 8 °C. A sterile solution of the formaldehyde-treated products of growth of the tetanus bacillus (*Clostridium tetani*). Label it to state that it is not to be frozen. Meets the requirements of the specific guinea pig potency test of antitoxin production based on the U.S. Standard Tetanus Antitoxin and the U.S. Control Tetanus Test Toxin. Meets the requirements of the specific guinea pig detoxification test. Contains not more than 0.02% of residual free formaldehyde. Contains a preservative other than a phenoloid compound. Meets the requirement for Expiration date (not later than 2 years after date of issue from manufacturer's cold storage [5 °C, 1 year]). Conforms to the regulations of the U.S. Food and Drug Administration concerning biologics.
Tetanus Toxoid Adsorbed USP—Preserve at a temperature between 2 and 8 °C. A sterile preparation of plain tetanus toxoid that meets all of the requirements for that product with the exception of those for potency, and that has been precipitated or adsorbed by alum, aluminum hydroxide, or aluminum phosphate adjuvants. Label it to state that it is to be well shaken before use and that it is not to be frozen. Meets the requirements of the specific mouse or guinea pig potency test of antitoxin production based on the U.S. Standard Tetanus Antitoxin and the U.S. Control Test Tetanus Toxin. Meets the requirements of the specific guinea pig detoxification test. Meets the requirements for Expiration date (not later than 2 years after date of issue from manufacturer's cold storage [5 °C, 1 year]) and Aluminum content. Conforms to the regulations of the U.S. Food and Drug Administration concerning biologics.

TETANUS AND DIPHTHERIA TOXOIDS ADSORBED FOR ADULT USE

Description: Tetanus and Diphtheria Toxoids Adsorbed for Adult Use USP—Turbid, white, slightly gray, or cream-colored suspension, free from evident clumps after shaking.

USP requirements: Tetanus and Diphtheria Toxoids Adsorbed for Adult Use USP—Preserve at a temperature between 2 and 8 °C. A sterile suspension prepared by mixing suitable quantities of adsorbed diphtheria toxoid and adsorbed tetanus toxoid using the same precipitating or adsorbing agent for both toxoids. The antigenicity or potency and the proportions of the toxoids are such as to provide, in each dose prescribed in the labeling, an immunizing dose of Tetanus Toxoid Adsorbed as defined for that product, and one-tenth of the immunizing dose of Diphtheria Toxoid Adsorbed as defined for that product for children, such that in the specific guinea pig antigenicity test it meets the requirement of production of not less than 0.5 unit of diphtheria antitoxin per mL and each immunizing dose has an antigen content of not more than 2 Lf (flocculating units) value as measured with the U.S. Reference Diphtheria Antitoxin for Flocculation Test. Each component meets the other requirements for those products. Contains not more than 0.02% of residual free formaldehyde. Label it to state that it is to be well shaken before use and that it is not to be frozen. Meets the requirement for Expiration date (not later than 2 years after date of issue from manufacturer's cold storage [5 °C, 1 year]). Conforms to the regulations of the U.S. Food and Drug Administration concerning biologics.

TETRACAINE

Chemical group: Ester, aminobenzoic acid (PABA)–derivative.

Chemical name:
Tetracaine—Benzoic acid, 4-(butylamino)-, 2-(dimethylamino)ethyl ester.
Tetracaine hydrochloride—Benzoic acid, 4-(butylamino)-, 2-(dimethylamino)ethyl ester, monohydrochloride.

Molecular formula:
Tetracaine—$C_{15}H_{24}N_2O_2$.
Tetracaine hydrochloride—$C_{15}H_{24}N_2O_2 \cdot HCl$.

Molecular weight:
Tetracaine—264.37.
Tetracaine hydrochloride—300.83.

Description:
Tetracaine USP—White or light yellow, waxy solid.
Tetracaine Hydrochloride USP—Fine, white, crystalline, odorless powder. Its solutions are neutral to litmus. Melts at about 148 °C, or may occur in either of two other polymorphic modifications that melt at about 134 °C and 139 °C, respectively. Mixtures of the forms may melt within the range of 134 to 147 °C. Is hygroscopic.
Sterile Tetracaine Hydrochloride USP—Fine, white, crystalline, odorless powder. Its solutions are neutral to litmus. Melts at about 148 °C, or may occur in either of two other polymorphic modifications that melt at about 134 °C and 139 °C, respectively. Mixtures of the forms may melt within the range of 134 to 147 °C. Is hygroscopic.

pKa: Tetracaine hydrochloride—8.39.

Solubility:
Tetracaine USP—Very slightly soluble in water; soluble in alcohol, in ether, and in chloroform.
Tetracaine Hydrochloride USP—Very soluble in water; soluble in alcohol; insoluble in ether.
Sterile Tetracaine Hydrochloride USP—Very soluble in water; soluble in alcohol; insoluble in ether.

USP requirements:
Tetracaine USP—Preserve in tight, light-resistant containers. Contains not less than 98.0% and not more than 101.0% of tetracaine, calculated on the dried basis. Meets the requirements for Identification, Melting range (41–46 °C), Loss on drying (not more than 0.5%), Residue on ignition (not more than 0.1%), and Chromatographic purity.
Tetracaine Ointment USP—Preserve in collapsible ointment tubes. Contains the labeled amount, within ± 10%, in a suitable ointment base. Meets the requirements for Identification, Microbial limits, and Minimum fill.
Tetracaine Ophthalmic Ointment USP—Preserve in collapsible ophthalmic ointment tubes. A sterile ointment. Contains not less than 0.45% and not more than 0.55% of Tetracaine in White Petrolatum. Meets the requirements for Identification, Sterility, Minimum fill, and Metal particles.

Tetracaine Topical Aerosol Solution—Not in USP.

Tetracaine Hydrochloride USP—Preserve in tight, light-resistant containers. Contains not less than 98.5% and not more than 101.0% of tetracaine hydrochloride, calculated on the anhydrous basis. Meets the requirements for Identification, Water (not more than 2.0%), Residue on ignition (not more than 0.1%), and Chromatographic purity.

Tetracaine Hydrochloride Cream USP—Preserve in collapsible, lined metal tubes. Contains an amount of tetracaine hydrochloride equivalent to the labeled amount of tetracaine, within ±10%, in a suitable water-miscible base. Meets the requirements for Identification, Microbial limits, Minimum fill, and pH (3.2–3.8).

Tetracaine Hydrochloride Injection USP—Preserve in single-dose or in multiple-dose containers, preferably of Type I glass, under refrigeration and protected from light. It may be packaged in 100-mL multiple-dose containers. Injection supplied as a component of spinal anesthesia trays may be stored at room temperature for 12 months. A sterile solution of Tetracaine Hydrochloride in Water for Injection. Label it to indicate that the Injection is not to be used if it contains crystals, or if it is cloudy or discolored. Contains the labeled amount, within ±5%. Meets the requirements for Identification, Bacterial endotoxins, pH (3.2–6.0), Particulate matter, and Injections.

Tetracaine Hydrochloride Ophthalmic Solution USP—Preserve in tight, light-resistant containers. A sterile, aqueous solution of Tetracaine Hydrochloride. Label it to indicate that the Ophthalmic Solution is not to be used if it contains crystals, or if it is cloudy or discolored. Contains the labeled amount, within ±10%. Meets the requirements for Identification, Sterility, and pH (3.7–6.0).

Sterile Tetracaine Hydrochloride USP—Preserve in Containers for Sterile Solids, preferably of Type I glass. It is Tetracaine Hydrochloride suitable for parenteral use. Contains not less than 98.0% and not more than 101.0% of tetracaine hydrochloride, calculated on anhydrous basis. Meets the requirements for Completeness of solution, Constituted solution, Identification, Container content variation, Bacterial endotoxins, pH (5.0–6.0, in a solution [1 in 100]), Water (not more than 2.0%), Residue on ignition (not more than 0.1%), and Chromatographic purity, and for Sterility tests and Labeling under Injections.

Tetracaine Hydrochloride Topical Solution USP—Preserve in tight, light-resistant containers. An aqueous solution of Tetracaine Hydrochloride. Contains a suitable antimicrobial agent. Label it to indicate that the Topical Solution is not to be used if it contains crystals, or if it is cloudy or discolored. Contains the labeled amount, within ±5%. Meets the requirements for Identification and pH (4.5–6.0).

TETRACAINE AND DEXTROSE

For *Tetracaine* and *Dextrose*—See individual listings for chemistry information.

USP requirements: Tetracaine Hydrochloride in Dextrose Injection USP—Preserve in single-dose or in multiple-dose containers, preferably of Type I glass, under refrigeration and protected from light. It may be packaged in 100-mL multiple-dose containers. Injection supplied as a component of spinal anesthesia trays may be stored at room temperature for 12 months. A sterile solution of Tetracaine Hydrochloride and Dextrose in Water for Injection. Label it to indicate that the Injection is not to be used if it contains crystals, or if it is cloudy or discolored. Contains the labeled amounts, within ±5%. Meets the requirements for Identification, Bacterial endotoxins, pH (3.5–6.0), Particulate matter under Small-volume injections, and Injections.

TETRACAINE AND MENTHOL

For *Tetracaine* and *Menthol*—See individual listings for chemistry information.

USP requirements: Tetracaine and Menthol Ointment USP—Preserve in collapsible ointment tubes. Contains the labeled amounts, within ±10%, in a suitable ointment base. Meets the requirements for Identification and Minimum fill.

TETRACYCLINE

Chemical name:

Tetracycline—2-Naphthacenecarboxamide, 4-(dimethylamino)-1,4,4a,5,5a,6,11,12a-octahydro-3,6,10,12,12a-pentahydroxy-6-methyl-1,11-dioxo-, [4*S*-(4 alpha,4a alpha,5a alpha,6 beta,12a alpha)]-.

Tetracycline hydrochloride—2-Naphthacenecarboxamide, 4-(dimethylamino)-1,4,4a,5,5a,6,11,12a-octahydro-3,6,-10,12,12a-pentahydroxy-6-methyl-1,11-dioxo-, monohydrochloride, [4*S*-(4 alpha,4a alpha,5a alpha,6 beta,12a alpha)]-.

Tetracycline phosphate complex—2-Naphthacenecarboxamide, 4-(dimethylamino)-1,4,4a,5,5a,6,11,12a-octahydro-3,6,10,12,12a-pentahydroxy-6-methyl-1,11-dioxo, [4*S*-(4 alpha,4a alpha,5a alpha,6 beta,12a alpha)]-, phosphate complex.

Molecular formula:

Tetracycline—$C_{22}H_{24}N_2O_8$.

Tetracycline hydrochloride—$C_{22}H_{24}N_2O_8 \cdot HCl$.

Molecular weight:

Tetracycline—444.44.

Tetracycline hydrochloride—480.90.

Description:

Tetracycline USP—Yellow, odorless, crystalline powder. Is stable in air, but exposure to strong sunlight causes it to darken. It loses potency in solutions of pH below 2, and is rapidly destroyed by alkali hydroxide solutions.

Tetracycline Hydrochloride USP—Yellow, odorless, crystalline powder. Is moderately hygroscopic. Is stable in air, but exposure to strong sunlight in moist air causes it to darken. It loses potency in solution at a pH below 2, and is rapidly destroyed by alkali hydroxide solutions.

Tetracycline Phosphate Complex USP—Yellow, crystalline powder, having a faint, characteristic odor.

Solubility:

Tetracycline USP—Very slightly soluble in water; freely soluble in dilute acid and in alkali hydroxide solutions; sparingly soluble in alcohol; practically insoluble in chloroform and in ether.

Tetracycline Hydrochloride USP—Soluble in water and in solutions of alkali hydroxides and carbonates; slightly soluble in alcohol; practically insoluble in chloroform and in ether.

Tetracycline Phosphate Complex USP—Sparingly soluble in water; slightly soluble in methanol; very slightly soluble in acetone.

USP requirements:

Tetracycline USP—Preserve in tight, light-resistant containers. Label it to indicate that it is to be used in the manufacture of nonparenteral drugs only. Has a potency equivalent to not less than 975 mcg of tetracycline hydrochloride per mg, calculated on the anhydrous basis. Meets the requirements for Identification, Crystallinity, pH (3.0–7.0, in an aqueous suspension containing 10 mg per mL), Water (not more than 13.0%), and 4-Epianhydrotetracycline (not more than 2.0%).

Tetracycline Boluses USP—Preserve in tight containers. Label Boluses to indicate that they are intended for veterinary use only. Contain the equivalent of the labeled amount of tetracycline hydrochloride, within −10% to +20%. Meet the requirements for Identification, Uniformity of dosage units, and Loss on drying (not more than 3.0%; or for Boluses greater than 15 mm in diameter, not more than 6.0%).

Tetracycline Oral Suspension USP—Preserve in tight, light-resistant containers. It is Tetracycline with or without one or more suitable buffers, preservatives, stabilizers, and suspending agents. Contains the equivalent of the labeled amount of tetracycline hydrochloride, within −10% to +25%. Meets the requirements for Identification, pH (3.5–6.0), 4-Epianhydrotetracycline (not more than 5.0%), Uniformity of dosage units (single-unit containers), and Deliverable volume.

Tetracycline Hydrochloride USP—Preserve in tight, light-resistant containers. Has a potency of not less than 900 mcg of tetracycline hydrochloride per mg. Meets the requirements for Identification, Crystallinity, pH (1.8–2.8, in a solution containing 10 mg per mL), Loss on drying (not more than 2.0%), and 4-Epianhydrotetracycline (not more than 2.0%).

Tetracycline Hydrochloride Capsules USP—Preserve in tight, light-resistant containers. Contain the labeled amount, within −10% to +25%. Meet the requirements for Identification, Dissolution (70% in 60 minutes in water in Apparatus 2 at 75 rpm), Uniformity of dosage units, Loss on drying (not more than 4.0%), and 4-Epianhydrotetracycline (not more than 3.0%).

Tetracycline Hydrochloride for Injection USP—Preserve in Containers for Sterile Solids, protected from light. A sterile, dry mixture of Sterile Tetracycline Hydrochloride, one form of which contains Magnesium Chloride or magnesium ascorbate and one or more suitable buffers, and the other form of which contains one or more suitable stabilizing agents. Label Tetracycline Hydrochloride for Injection that contains an anesthetic agent to indicate that it is intended for intramuscular administration only. Contains the labeled amount, within −10% to +15%. Meets the requirements for Constituted solution, Identification, Bacterial endotoxins, Sterility, pH (2.0–3.0, in a solution containing 10 mg per mL), Loss on drying (not more than 5.0%), Particulate matter, and 4-Epianhydrotetracycline (not more than 3.0%), and for Uniformity of dosage units and Labeling under Injections. Where it is labeled for intravenous use it meets the requirements for Depressor substances under Sterile Tetracycline Hydrochloride.

Tetracycline Hydrochloride Ointment USP—Preserve in well-closed containers, preferably at controlled room temperature. Contains the labeled amount, within −10% to +25%. Meets the requirements for Identification, Minimum fill, and Water (not more than 1.0%).

Tetracycline Hydrochloride Ophthalmic Ointment USP—Preserve in collapsible ophthalmic ointment tubes. Contains the labeled amount, within −10% to +25%. Meets the requirements for Sterility, Minimum fill, Water (not more than 0.5%), and Metal particles.

Tetracycline Hydrochloride Soluble Powder USP—Preserve in tight containers. Label it to indicate that it is intended for veterinary use only. Contains the labeled amount, within −10% to +25%. Meets the requirements for Identification and Loss on drying (not more than 2.0%).

Tetracycline Hydrochloride for Topical Solution USP—Preserve in tight, light-resistant containers. A dry mixture of Tetracycline Hydrochloride and Epitetracycline Hydrochloride with Sodium Metabisulfite packaged in conjunction with a suitable aqueous vehicle. Contains the labeled amount of tetracycline hydrochloride, within −10% to +30%, when constituted as directed. Meets the requirements for Identification, pH (1.9–3.5, in the solution constituted as directed in the labeling), Loss on drying (not more than 5.0%), and Epitetracycline hydrochloride content.

Sterile Tetracycline Hydrochloride USP—Preserve in Containers for Sterile Solids, protected from light. It is Tetracycline Hydrochloride suitable for parenteral use. Has a potency of not less than 900 mcg of tetracycline hydrochloride per mg and, where packaged for dispensing, contains the equivalent of the labeled amount of tetracycline hydrochloride, within −10% to +15%. Meets the requirements for Constituted solution, Depressor substances, Bacterial endotoxins, Sterility, and Particulate matter, for Identification tests, Crystallinity, pH, Loss on drying, and 4-Epianhydrotetracycline under Tetracycline Hydrochloride, and, where packaged for dispensing, for Uniformity of dosage units and Labeling under Injections.

Tetracycline Hydrochloride Ophthalmic Suspension USP—Preserve in tight, light-resistant containers of glass or plastic, containing not more than 15 mL. The containers or individual cartons are sealed and tamper-proof so that sterility is assured at time of first use. A sterile suspension of Sterile Tetracycline Hydrochloride in a suitable oil. Contains the labeled amount, within −10% to +25%. Meets the requirements for Identification, Sterility, and Water (not more than 0.5%).

Tetracycline Hydrochloride Tablets USP—Preserve in tight, light-resistant containers. Contain the labeled amount, within −10% to +25%. Meet the requirements for Identification, Dissolution (70% in 60 minutes in water in Apparatus 2 at 75 rpm), Uniformity of dosage units, Loss on drying (not more than 3.0%), and 4-Epianhydrotetracycline (not more than 3.0%).

Tetracycline Phosphate Complex USP—Preserve in tight, light-resistant containers. Label it to indicate that it is to be used in the manufacture of nonparenteral drugs only. Has a potency equivalent to not less than 750 mcg of tetracycline hydrochloride per mg, calculated on the anhydrous basis. Meets the requirements for Identification, Crystallinity, pH (2.0–4.0, in an aqueous suspension containing 10 mg per mL), Water (not more than 9.0%), Chloride (not more than 0.2%), Tetracycline (not more than 1.0%), and 4-Epianhydrotetracycline (not more than 2.0%).

Tetracycline Phosphate Complex Capsules USP—Preserve in tight, light-resistant containers. Contain an amount of tetracycline phosphate complex equivalent to the labeled amount of tetracycline hydrochloride, within −10% to +25%. Meet the requirements for Identification, Dissolution (75% in 30 minutes in 0.1 *N* hydrochloric acid in Apparatus 1 at 100 rpm), Uniformity of dosage units, Loss on drying (not more than 9.0%), and 4-Epianhydrotetracycline (not more than 3.0%).

Tetracycline Phosphate Complex for Injection USP—Preserve in Containers for Sterile Solids, protected from light. A sterile, dry mixture of Sterile Tetracycline Phosphate Complex and Magnesium Chloride or magnesium ascorbate, and one or more suitable buffers. Contains an amount of tetracycline phosphate complex equivalent to the labeled amount of tetracycline hydrochloride, within −10% to +15%. Meets the requirements for Constituted solution, Identification, Bacterial endotoxins, Sterility, pH (2.0–3.0, in a solution containing 10 mg per mL), Loss on drying (not more than 5.0%), Particulate matter, and 4-Epianhydrotetracycline (not more than 3.0%), and for Uniformity of dosage units and Labeling under Injections.

Sterile Tetracycline Phosphate Complex USP—Preserve in Containers for Sterile Solids, protected from light. It is

Tetracycline Phosphate Complex suitable for parenteral use. Has a potency equivalent to not less than 750 mcg of tetracycline hydrochloride per mg, calculated on the anhydrous basis. Meets the requirements for Depressor substances and Sterility, and for Identification tests, pH, Water, Chloride, Crystallinity, Tetracycline, and 4-Epianhydrotetracycline under Tetracycline Phosphate Complex.

TETRACYCLINE AND NOVOBIOCIN

For *Tetracycline* and *Novobiocin*—See individual listings for chemistry information.

USP requirements:

Tetracycline Hydrochloride and Novobiocin Sodium Tablets USP—Preserve in tight containers. Label Tablets to indicate that they are intended for veterinary use only. Contain amounts of tetracycline hydrochloride and novobiocin sodium equivalent to the labeled amounts of tetracycline hydrochloride and novobiocin, within −10% to +25%. Meet the requirements for Identification, Disintegration (60 minutes, simulated gastric fluid TS being substituted for water in the test), Uniformity of dosage units, Loss on drying (not more than 6.0%), and 4-Epianhydrotetracycline (not more than 2.0%).

Tetracycline Phosphate Complex and Novobiocin Sodium Capsules USP—Preserve in tight containers. Label Capsules to indicate that they are intended for veterinary use only. Contain amounts of tetracycline phosphate complex and novobiocin sodium equivalent to the labeled amounts of tetracycline hydrochloride and novobiocin, within −10% to +20%. Meet the requirements for Identification, Uniformity of dosage units, Loss on drying (not more than 9.0%), and 4-Epianhydrotetracycline (not more than 3.0%).

TETRACYCLINE, NOVOBIOCIN, AND PREDNISOLONE

For *Tetracycline, Novobiocin,* and *Prednisolone*—See individual listings for chemistry information.

USP requirements: Tetracycline Hydrochloride, Novobiocin Sodium, and Prednisolone Tablets USP—Preserve in tight containers. Label Tablets to indicate that they are intended for veterinary use only. Contain amounts of tetracycline hydrochloride and novobiocin sodium equivalent to the labeled amounts of tetracycline hydrochloride and novobiocin, within −10% to +25%, and the labeled amount of prednisolone, within ±10%. Meet the requirements for Disintegration (60 minutes, simulated gastric fluid TS being substituted for water in the test), Uniformity of dosage units, and 4-Epianhydrotetracycline (not more than 2.0%), and for Identification test and Loss on drying under Tetracycline Hydrochloride and Novobiocin Sodium Tablets.

TETRACYCLINE AND NYSTATIN

For *Tetracycline* and *Nystatin*—See individual listings for chemistry information.

USP requirements: Tetracycline Hydrochloride and Nystatin Capsules USP—Preserve in tight, light-resistant containers. Contain the labeled amount of tetracycline hydrochloride, within −10% to +25%, and the labeled amount of USP Nystatin Units, within −10% to +35%. Meet the requirements for Identification, Dissolution (70% in 60 minutes in water in Apparatus 2 at 75 rpm), Loss on drying (not more than 4.0%), and 4-Epianhydrotetracycline (not more than 3.0%).

TETRAHYDROZOLINE

Chemical name: Tetrahydrozoline hydrochloride—1*H*-Imidazole, 4,5-dihydro-2-(1,2,3,4-tetrahydro-1-naphthalenyl)-, monohydrochloride.

Molecular formula: Tetrahydrozoline hydrochloride—$C_{13}H_{16}N_2 \cdot HCl$.

Molecular weight: Tetrahydrozoline hydrochloride—236.74.

Description: Tetrahydrozoline Hydrochloride USP—White, odorless solid. Melts at about 256 °C, with decomposition.

Solubility: Tetrahydrozoline Hydrochloride USP—Freely soluble in water and in alcohol; very slightly soluble in chloroform; practically insoluble in ether.

USP requirements:

Tetrahydrozoline Hydrochloride USP—Preserve in tight containers. Contains not less than 98.0% and not more than 100.5% of tetrahydrozoline hydrochloride, calculated on the dried basis. Meets the requirements for Identification, Loss on drying (not more than 1.0%), Residue on ignition (not more than 0.1%), Heavy metals (not more than 0.005%), and Ordinary impurities.

Tetrahydrozoline Hydrochloride Nasal Solution USP—Preserve in tight containers. A solution of Tetrahydrozoline Hydrochloride in water adjusted to a suitable tonicity. Contains the labeled amount, within ±10%. Meets the requirements for Identification, Microbial limits, and pH (5.3–6.5).

Tetrahydrozoline Hydrochloride Ophthalmic Solution USP—Preserve in tight containers. A sterile, isotonic solution of Tetrahydrozoline Hydrochloride in water. Contains the labeled amount, within ±10%. Meets the requirements for Identification, Sterility, and pH (5.8–6.5).

THALLOUS CHLORIDE Tl 201

Chemical name: Thallium chloride ($^{201}TlCl$).

Molecular formula: $^{201}TlCl$.

USP requirements: Thallous Chloride Tl 201 Injection USP—Preserve in single-dose or in multiple-dose containers. A sterile, isotonic, aqueous solution of radioactive thallium (^{201}Tl) in the form of thallous chloride suitable for intravenous administration. Label it to include the following, in addition to the information specified for Labeling under Injections: the time and date of calibration; the amount of ^{201}Tl as labeled thallous chloride expressed as total megabecquerels (or microcuries or millicuries) and concentration as megabecquerels (or microcuries or millicuries) per mL at the time of calibration; the expiration date and time; and the statement, "Caution—Radioactive Material." The labeling indicates that in making dosage calculations, correction is to be made for radioactive decay, and also indicates that the radioactive half-life of ^{201}Tl is 73.1 hours. Contains the labeled amount of ^{201}Tl, within ±10%, as chloride, expressed in megabecquerels (or microcuries or millicuries) per mL, at the time indicated in the labeling. Other chemical forms of radioactivity do not exceed 5.0% of the total radioactivity. Meets the requirements for Radionuclide identification, Bacterial endotoxins, pH (4.5–7.5), Radiochemical purity, Radionuclidic purity, Thallium, Iron, Copper, and Injections (except that the Injection may be distributed or dispensed prior to completion of the test for Sterility, the latter test being started on the day of final manufacture, and except that it is not subject to the recommendation on Volume in Container).

THEOPHYLLINE

Source: Theophylline sodium glycinate—An equimolar mixture of theophylline sodium and aminoacetic acid (glycine).

Chemical name:
Theophylline—1*H*-Purine-2,6-dione, 3,7-dihydro-1,3-dimethyl-, monohydrate.
Theophylline sodium glycinate—Glycine, mixt. with 3,7-dihydro-1,3-dimethyl-1*H*-purine-2,6-dione, monosodium salt.

Molecular formula: $C_7H_8N_4O_2 \cdot H_2O$ (hydrous); $C_7H_8N_4O_2$ (anhydrous).

Molecular weight: 198.18 (hydrous); 180.17 (anhydrous).

Description:
Theophylline USP—White, odorless, crystalline powder. Is stable in air.
Theophylline Sodium Glycinate USP—White, crystalline powder having a slight ammoniacal odor.

Solubility:
Theophylline USP—Slightly soluble in water, but more soluble in hot water; freely soluble in solutions of alkali hydroxides and in ammonia; sparingly soluble in alcohol, in chloroform, and in ether.
Theophylline Sodium Glycinate USP—Freely soluble in water; very slightly soluble in alcohol; practically insoluble in chloroform.

USP requirements:
Theophylline USP—Preserve in well-closed containers. Contains one molecule of water of hydration or is anhydrous. Label it to indicate whether it is hydrous or anhydrous. Contains not less than 97.0% and not more than 102.0% of theophylline, calculated on the dried basis. Meets the requirements for Identification, Melting range (270–274 °C, the range between beginning and end of melting not more than 3 °C), Acidity, Loss on drying (7.5–9.5% for the hydrous form and not more than 0.5% for the anhydrous form), Residue on ignition (not more than 0.15%), and Organic volatile impurities.
Theophylline Capsules USP—Preserve in well-closed containers. Contain the labeled amount of anhydrous theophylline, within ±10%. Meet the requirements for Identification, Dissolution (80% in 60 minutes in water in Apparatus 2 at 50 rpm), and Uniformity of dosage units.
Theophylline Extended-release Capsules USP—Preserve in well-closed containers. The labeling indicates whether the product is intended for dosing every 12 or 24 hours, and states with which in-vitro *Drug Release Test* the product complies. Contain the labeled amount of anhydrous theophylline, within ±10%. Meet the requirements for Identification, Drug release, and Uniformity of dosage units.
Theophylline Elixir—Not in USP.
Theophylline Oral Solution—Not in USP.
Theophylline Oral Suspension—Not in USP.
Theophylline Syrup—Not in USP.
Theophylline Tablets USP—Preserve in well-closed containers. Contain the labeled amount of anhydrous theophylline, within ±6%. Meet the requirements for Identification, Dissolution (80% in 45 minutes in water in Apparatus 2 at 50 rpm), and Uniformity of dosage units.
Theophylline Extended-release Tablets—Not in USP.
Theophylline Sodium Glycinate USP—Preserve in tight containers. An equilibrium mixture containing Theophylline Sodium and Glycine in approximately equimolecular proportions buffered with an additional mole of Glycine. Dried at 105 °C for 4 hours, contains theophylline sodium glycinate equivalent to not less than 44.5% and not more than 47.3% of anhydrous theophylline. Meets the requirements for Identification, pH (8.5–9.5, in a saturated solution), Loss on drying (not more than 2.0%), Glycine content (42.0–48.0%, on the dried basis), and Organic volatile impurities.
Theophylline Sodium Glycinate Elixir USP—Preserve in tight containers. Label Elixir to state both the content of theophylline sodium glycinate and the content of anhydrous theophylline. Contains an amount of theophylline sodium glycinate equivalent to the labeled amount of anhydrous theophylline, within ±7%. Meets the requirements for Identification, pH (8.3–9.1), and Alcohol content (17.0–23.0%).
Theophylline Sodium Glycinate Tablets USP—Preserve in well-closed containers. Label Tablets to state both the content of theophylline sodium glycinate and the content of anhydrous theophylline. Contain an amount of theophylline sodium glycinate equivalent to the labeled amount of anhydrous theophylline, within ±7%. Meet the requirements for Identification, Dissolution (75% in 45 minutes in water in Apparatus 1 at 100 rpm), and Uniformity of dosage units.

THEOPHYLLINE AND DEXTROSE

For *Theophylline* and *Dextrose*—See individual listings for chemistry information.

USP requirements: Theophylline in Dextrose Injection USP—Preserve in single-dose containers, preferably of Type I or Type II glass, or of a suitable plastic material. A sterile solution of Theophylline and Dextrose in Water for Injection. Contains the labeled amount of anhydrous theophylline, within ±7%, and the labeled amount of dextrose, within ±5%. Meets the requirements for Identification, Bacterial endotoxin, pH (3.5–6.5), 5-Hydroxymethylfurfural and related substances, and Injections.

THEOPHYLLINE, EPHEDRINE, GUAIFENESIN, AND BUTABARBITAL

For *Theophylline, Ephedrine, Guaifenesin,* and *Butabarbital*—See individual listings for chemistry information.

USP requirements:
Theophylline, Ephedrine Hydrochloride, Guaifenesin, and Butabarbital Capsules—Not in USP.
Theophylline, Ephedrine Hydrochloride, Guaifenesin, and Butabarbital Elixir—Not in USP.

THEOPHYLLINE, EPHEDRINE, GUAIFENESIN, AND PHENOBARBITAL

For *Theophylline, Ephedrine, Guaifenesin,* and *Phenobarbital*—See individual listings for chemistry information.

USP requirements:
Theophylline, Ephedrine Hydrochloride, Guaifenesin, and Phenobarbital Elixir—Not in USP.
Theophylline, Ephedrine Hydrochloride, Guaifenesin, and Phenobarbital Tablets—Not in USP.
Theophylline, Ephedrine Sulfate, Guaifenesin, and Phenobarbital Elixir—Not in USP.
Theophylline, Ephedrine Sulfate, Guaifenesin, and Phenobarbital Tablets—Not in USP.

THEOPHYLLINE, EPHEDRINE, AND HYDROXYZINE

For *Theophylline, Ephedrine,* and *Hydroxyzine*—See individual listings for chemistry information.

USP requirements:
Theophylline, Ephedrine Sulfate, and Hydroxyzine Hydrochloride Syrup—Not in USP.
Theophylline, Ephedrine Sulfate, and Hydroxyzine Hydrochloride Tablets—Not in USP.

THEOPHYLLINE, EPHEDRINE, AND PHENOBARBITAL

For *Theophylline, Ephedrine,* and *Phenobarbital*—See individual listings for chemistry information.

USP requirements:
Theophylline, Ephedrine Hydrochloride, and Phenobarbital Elixir—Not in USP.
Theophylline, Ephedrine Hydrochloride, and Phenobarbital Suspension—Not in USP.
Theophylline, Ephedrine Hydrochloride, and Phenobarbital Tablets USP—Preserve in tight containers. Contain the labeled amounts of anhydrous theophylline, ephedrine hydrochloride, and phenobarbital, within ±10%. Meet the requirements for Identification, Dissolution (75% of each active ingredient in 30 minutes in water in Apparatus 1 at 100 rpm), and Uniformity of dosage units.
Theophylline, Ephedrine Hydrochloride, and Phenobarbital Extended-release Tablets—Not in USP.

THEOPHYLLINE AND GUAIFENESIN

For *Theophylline* and *Guaifenesin*—See individual listings for chemistry information.

USP requirements:
Theophylline and Guaifenesin Capsules USP—Preserve in tight containers. Contain the labeled amounts of anhydrous theophylline and guaifenesin, within ±10%. Meet the requirements for Identification and Uniformity of dosage units.
Theophylline and Guaifenesin Elixir—Not in USP.
Theophylline and Guaifenesin Oral Solution USP—Preserve in tight containers. Contains the labeled amount of anhydrous theophylline, within ±10%, and the labeled amount of guaifenesin, within ±13.3%. Meets the requirements for Identification and Alcohol content (if present, within ±10% of labeled amount).
Theophylline and Guaifenesin Syrup—Not in USP.
Theophylline and Guaifenesin Tablets—Not in USP.
Theophylline Sodium Glycinate and Guaifenesin Elixir—Not in USP.
Theophylline Sodium Glycinate and Guaifenesin Syrup—Not in USP.
Theophylline Sodium Glycinate and Guaifenesin Tablets—Not in USP.

THIABENDAZOLE

Chemical group: Benzimidazole derivative; structurally related to mebendazole.

Chemical name: 1*H*-Benzimidazole, 2-(4-thiazolyl)-.

Molecular formula: $C_{10}H_7N_3S$.

Molecular weight: 201.25.

Description: Thiabendazole USP—White to practically white, odorless or practically odorless powder.

Solubility: Thiabendazole USP—Practically insoluble in water; slightly soluble in acetone and in alcohol; very slightly soluble in chloroform and in ether.

USP requirements:
Thiabendazole USP—Preserve in well-closed containers. Contains not less than 98.0% and not more than 101.0% of thiabendazole, calculated on the anhydrous basis. Meets the requirements for Identification, Melting range (296–303 °C), Water (not more than 0.5%), Residue on ignition (not more than 0.1%), Selenium (not more than 0.003%), Heavy metals (not more than 0.001%), and Chromatographic purity.

Note: Thiabendazole labeled solely for veterinary use is exempt from the requirements of the tests for Residue on igniton, Selenium, Heavy metals, and Chromatographic purity.

Thiabendazole Oral Suspension USP—Preserve in tight containers. Contains the labeled amount, within ±10%. Meets the requirements for Identification and pH (3.4–4.2).
Thiabendazole Topical Suspension—Not in USP.
Thiabendazole Tablets USP—Preserve in tight containers. Label the Tablets to indicate that they are to be chewed before swallowing. Contain the labeled amount, within ±10%. Meet the requirements for Identification and Uniformity of dosage units.

THIAMINE

Chemical name:
Thiamine hydrochloride—Thiazolium, 3-[(4-amino-2-methyl-5-pyrimidinyl)methyl]-5-(2-hydroxyethyl)-4-methyl-, chloride, monohydrochloride.
Thiamine mononitrate—Thiazolium, 3-[(4-amino-2-methyl-5-pyrimidinyl)methyl]-5-(2-hydroxyethyl)-4-methyl-, nitrate (salt).

Molecular formula:
Thiamine hydrochloride—$C_{12}H_{17}ClN_4OS \cdot HCl$.
Thiamine mononitrate—$C_{12}H_{17}N_5O_4S$.

Molecular weight:
Thiamine hydrochloride—337.27.
Thiamine mononitrate—327.36.

Description:
Thiamine Hydrochloride USP—White crystals or crystalline powder, usually having a slight, characteristic odor. When exposed to air, the anhydrous product rapidly absorbs about 4% of water. Melts at about 248 °C, with some decomposition.
Thiamine Mononitrate USP—White crystals or crystalline powder, usually having a slight, characteristic odor.

pKa: 4.8 and 9.0.

Solubility:
Thiamine Hydrochloride USP—Freely soluble in water; soluble in glycerin; slightly soluble in alcohol; insoluble in ether.
Thiamine Mononitrate USP—Sparingly soluble in water; slightly soluble in alcohol and in chloroform.

USP requirements:
Thiamine Hydrochloride USP—Preserve in tight, light-resistant containers. Contains not less than 98.0% and not more than 102.0% of thiamine hydrochloride, calculated on the anhydrous basis. Meets the requirements for Identification, pH (2.7–3.4, in a solution [1 in 100]), Water (not more than 5.0%), Residue on ignition (not more than 0.2%), Absorbance of solution (not more than 0.025), and Nitrate.
Thiamine Hydrochloride Elixir USP—Preserve in tight, light-resistant containers. Contains the labeled amount, within −5% to +35%. Meets the requirements for Identification and Alcohol content (within ±10% of labeled amount).
Thiamine Hydrochloride Injection USP—Preserve in single-dose or in multiple-dose containers, preferably of Type I glass, protected from light. A sterile solution of Thiamine Hydrochloride in Water for Injection. Contains the labeled amount, within ±10%. Meets the requirements for Identification, Bacterial endotoxins, pH (2.5–4.5), and Injections.

Thiamine Hydrochloride Tablets USP—Preserve in tight, light-resistant containers. Contain the labeled amount, within ±10%. Meet the requirements for Identification, Disintegration (30 minutes), and Uniformity of dosage units.

Thiamine Mononitrate USP—Preserve in tight, light-resistant containers. Contains not less than 98.0% and not more than 102.0% of thiamine mononitrate, calculated on the dried basis. Meets the requirements for Identification, pH (6.0–7.5, in a solution [1 in 50]), Loss on drying (not more than 1.0%), Residue on ignition (not more than 0.2%), and Chloride (not more than 0.06%).

Thiamine Mononitrate Elixir USP—Preserve in tight, light-resistant containers. Contains the labeled amount, within −5% to +15%. Meets the requirements for Identification and Alcohol content (within ±10% of labeled amount).

THIAMYLAL

Chemical group: Thiamyl sodium—A thiobarbiturate.

Chemical name:

Thiamylal—Dihydro-5-(1-methylbutyl)-5-(2-propenyl)-2-thioxo-4,6-(1*H*,5*H*)-pyrimidinedione.

Thiamylal sodium—4,6-(1*H*,5*H*)-Pyrimidinedione, dihydro-5-(1-methylbutyl)-5-(2-propenyl)-2-thioxo-, monosodium salt.

Molecular formula:

Thiamylal—$C_{12}H_{18}N_2O_2S$.

Thiamylal sodium—$C_{12}H_{17}N_2NaO_2S$.

Molecular weight:

Thiamylal—254.35.

Thiamylal sodium—276.33.

Description: Thiamylal Sodium for Injection USP—Pale yellow, hygroscopic powder, having a disagreeable odor.

USP requirements:

Thiamylal USP—Preserve in well-closed containers. Contains not less than 98.0% and not more than 102.0% of thiamylal, calculated on the dried basis. Meets the requirements for Identification, Melting range (135–139 °C), Loss on drying (not more than 1.0%), and Ordinary impurities.

Thiamylal Sodium for Injection USP—Preserve in Containers for Sterile Solids. A sterile mixture of thiamylal with anhydrous Sodium Carbonate as a buffer. Contains the labeled amount, within ±7%. Meets the requirements for Labeling under injections, Completeness of solution, Constituted solution, Identification, Sterility, Uniformity of dosage units, Bacterial endotoxins, pH (10.7–11.5, in the solution prepared as directed in the test for Completeness of solution), Loss on drying (not more than 2.0%), and Heavy metals (not more than 0.003%).

Thiamylal Sodium for Rectal Solution—Not in USP.

THIETHYLPERAZINE

Chemical name:

Thiethylperazine malate—10*H*-Phenothiazine, 2-(ethylthio)-10-[3-(4-methyl-1-piperazinyl)propyl]-, 2-hydroxy-1,4-butanedioate (1:2).

Thiethylperazine maleate—10*H*-Phenothiazine, 2-(ethylthio)-10-[3-(4-methyl-1-piperazinyl)propyl]-, (*Z*)-2-butenedioate (1:2).

Molecular formula:

Thiethylperazine malate—$C_{22}H_{29}N_3S_2 \cdot 2C_4H_6O_5$.

Thiethylperazine maleate—$C_{22}H_{29}N_3S_2 \cdot 2C_4H_4O_4$.

Molecular weight:

Thiethylperazine malate—667.79.

Thiethylperazine maleate—631.76.

Description:

Thiethylperazine malate—White to faintly yellow crystalline powder with not more than a slight odor.

Thiethylperazine Maleate USP—Yellowish, granular powder. Odorless or has not more than a slight odor. Melts at about 183 °C, with decomposition.

Solubility:

Thiethylperazine malate—Soluble 1 in 40 of water, 1 in 90 of alcohol, 1 in 525 of chloroform, and 1 in 3400 of ether.

Thiethylperazine Maleate USP—Practically insoluble in water; slightly soluble in methanol; practically insoluble in chloroform.

USP requirements:

Thiethylperazine Malate USP—Preserve in tight, light-resistant containers. Contains not less than 98.0% and not more than 101.5% of thiethylperazine malate, calculated on the dried basis. Meets the requirements for Identification, pH (2.8–3.8, in a freshly prepared solution [1 in 100]), Loss on drying (not more than 0.5%), Residue on ignition (not more than 0.1%), Selenium (not more than 0.003%), and Organic volatile impurities.

Thiethylperazine Malate Injection USP—Preserve in single-dose containers, preferably of Type I glass, protected from light. A sterile solution of Thiethylperazine Malate in Water for Injection. Contains the labeled amount, within ±10%. Meets the requirements for Identification, Bacterial endotoxins, pH (3.0–4.0), and Injections.

Thiethylperazine Maleate USP—Preserve in tight, light-resistant containers. Contains not less than 98.0% and not more than 101.5% of thiethylperazine maleate, calculated on the dried basis. Meets the requirements for Identification, pH (2.8–3.8), Loss on drying (not more than 0.5%), Residue on ignition (not more than 0.1%), Selenium (not more than 0.003%), Chromatographic purity, and Organic volatile impurities.

Thiethylperazine Maleate Suppositories USP—Preserve in tight containers at temperatures below 25 °C. Do not expose unwrapped Suppositories to sunlight. Contain the labeled amount, within ±10%. Meet the requirement for Identification.

Thiethylperazine Maleate Tablets USP—Preserve in tight, light-resistant containers. Contain the labeled amount, within ±10%. Meet the requirements for Identification, Dissolution (75% in 30 minutes in 0.1 *N* hydrochloric acid in Apparatus 1 at 120 rpm), and Uniformity of dosage units.

THIMEROSAL

Chemical name: Mercury, ethyl (2-mercaptobenzoato-*S*)-, sodium salt.

Molecular formula: $C_9H_9HgNaO_2S$.

Molecular weight: 404.81.

Description:

Thimerosal USP—Light cream-colored, crystalline powder, having a slight characteristic odor. Affected by light. The pH of a solution (1 in 100) is about 6.7.

NF category: Antimicrobial preservative.

Thimerosal Topical Solution USP—Clear liquid, having a slight characteristic odor. Affected by light.

Thimerosal Tincture USP—Transparent, mobile liquid, having the characteristic odor of alcohol and acetone. Affected by light.

Solubility: Thimerosal USP—Freely soluble in water; soluble in alcohol; practically insoluble in ether.

USP requirements:
Thimerosal USP—Preserve in tight, light-resistant containers. Contains not less than 97.0% and not more than 101.0% of thimerosal, calculated on the dried basis. Meets the requirements for Identification, Loss on drying (not more than 0.5%), Ether-soluble substances (not more than 0.8%), Mercury ions (not more than 0.70%), and Readily carbonizable substances.
Thimerosal Topical Aerosol USP—Preserve in tight, light-resistant, pressurized containers, and avoid exposure to excessive heat. An alcoholic solution of Thimerosal mixed with suitable propellants in a pressurized container. Contains the labeled amount, within ±15%. Meets the requirements for Identification and Alcohol content (18.7–25.3% [w/w]), and for Leak testing and Pressure testing under Aerosols.
Note: Thimerosal Topical Aerosol is sensitive to some metals.
Thimerosal Topical Solution USP—Preserve in tight, light-resistant containers, and avoid exposure to excessive heat. Contains, in each 100 mL, not less than 95 mg and not more than 105 mg of thimerosal. Meets the requirements for Identification and pH (9.6–10.2).
Note: Thimerosal Topical Solution is sensitive to some metals.
Thimerosal Tincture USP—Preserve in tight, light-resistant containers, and avoid exposure to excessive heat. Contains, in each 100 mL, not less than 90 mg and not more than 110 mg of thimerosal. Meets the requirements for Identification and Alcohol content (45.0–55.0%).
Note: Thimerosal Tincture is sensitive to some metals.

THIOGUANINE

Chemical name: 6*H*-Purine-6-thione, 2-amino-1,7-dihydro-.

Molecular formula: $C_5H_5N_5S \cdot xH_2O$.

Molecular weight: 167.19 (anhydrous).

Description: Thioguanine USP—Pale yellow, odorless or practically odorless, crystalline powder.

pKa: 8.1.

Solubility: Thioguanine USP—Insoluble in water, in alcohol, and in chloroform; freely soluble in dilute solutions of alkali hydroxides.

USP requirements:
Thioguanine USP—Preserve in tight containers. It is anhydrous or contains one-half molecule of water of hydration. Label it to indicate its state of hydration. Contains not less than 97.0% and not more than 100.5% of thioguanine, calculated on the dried basis. Meets the requirements for Identification, Loss on drying (not more than 6.0%), Selenium (not more than 0.003%), Phosphorus-containing substances, Free sulfur, Nitrogen content (40.6–43.1%, calculated on the dried basis), and Organic volatile impurities.
Thioguanine Tablets USP—Preserve in tight containers. Contain the labeled amount, within ±7%. Meet the requirements for Identification, Dissolution (75% in 45 minutes in water in Apparatus 2 at 50 rpm), and Uniformity of dosage units.

THIOPENTAL

Chemical group: A thiobarbiturate, the sulfur analog of pentobarbital sodium.

Chemical name: Thiopental sodium—4,6(1*H*,5*H*)-Pyrimidinedione, 5-ethyldihydro-5-(1-methylbutyl)-2-thioxo-, monosodium salt.

Molecular formula: Thiopental sodium—$C_{11}H_{17}N_2NaO_2S$.

Molecular weight: Thiopental sodium—264.32.

Description:
Thiopental Sodium USP—White to off-white, crystalline powder, or yellowish-white to pale greenish-yellow, hygroscopic powder. May have a disagreeable odor. Its solutions are alkaline to litmus. Its solutions decompose on standing, and on boiling precipitation occurs.
Thiopental Sodium for Injection USP—White to off-white, crystalline powder, or yellowish-white to pale greenish-yellow, hygroscopic powder. May have a disagreeable odor. Its solutions are alkaline to litmus. Its solutions decompose on standing, and on boiling precipitation occurs.

pKa: Thiopental sodium—7.4.

Solubility: Thiopental Sodium USP—Soluble in water and in alcohol; insoluble in absolute ether and in solvent hexane.

USP requirements:
Thiopental Sodium USP—Preserve in tight containers. Contains not less than 97.0% and not more than 102.0% of thiopental sodium, calculated on the dried basis. Meets the requirements for Identification, Loss on drying (not more than 2.0%), Heavy metals (not more than 0.002%), and Ordinary impurities.
Thiopental Sodium for Injection USP—Preserve in Containers for Sterile Solids, preferably of Type III glass. A sterile mixture of Thiopental Sodium and anhydrous Sodium Carbonate as a buffer. Contains the labeled amount, within ±7%. Meets the requirements for Completeness of solution, Constituted solution, Bacterial endotoxins, and pH (10.2–11.2), for Identification tests and Heavy metals under Thiopental Sodium, and for Sterility tests, Uniformity of dosage units, and Labeling under Injections.
Thiopental Sodium for Rectal Solution—Not in USP.
Thiopental Sodium Rectal Suspension—Not in USP.

THIOPROPAZATE

Chemical group: Piperazine phenothiazine derivative.

Chemical name: Thiopropazate hydrochloride—4-[3-(2-Chlorophenothiazin-10-yl)propyl]-1-piperazineethanol acetate dihydrochloride.

Molecular formula: Thiopropazate hydrochloride—$C_{23}H_{28}ClN_3O_2S \cdot 2HCl$.

Molecular weight: Thiopropazate hydrochloride—518.93.

Description: Thiopropazate hydrochloride—White or pale yellow crystalline powder with a faint odor.

Solubility: Thiopropazate hydrochloride—Soluble 1 in 4 of water, 1 in 130 of alcohol, and 1 in 65 of chloroform; practically insoluble in ether.

USP requirements: Thiopropazate Hydrochloride Tablets—Not in USP.

THIOPROPERAZINE

Chemical group: Phenothiazine.

Chemical name: Thioproperazine mesylate—*NN*-Dimethyl-10-[3-(4-methylpiperazin-1-yl)propyl]phenothiazine-2-sulphonamide dimethanesulphonate.

Molecular formula: Thioproperazine mesylate—$C_{22}H_{30}N_4O_2S_2 \cdot 2CH_4O_3S$.

Molecular weight: Thioproperazine mesylate—638.8.

Description: Thioproperazine mesylate—Slightly hygroscopic white powder with a yellowish tint.

Solubility: Thioproperazine mesylate—Readily soluble in water; slightly soluble in ethanol; practically insoluble in methanol and in dimethylformamide.

USP requirements: Thioproperazine Mesylate Tablets—Not in USP.

THIORIDAZINE

Chemical group: Phenothiazine.

Chemical name:
Thioridazine—10*H*-Phenothiazine, 10-[2-(1-methyl-2-piperidinyl)ethyl]-2-(methylthio)-.
Thioridazine hydrochloride—10*H*-Phenothiazine, 10-[2-(1-methyl-2-piperidinyl)ethyl]-2-(methylthio)-, monohydrochloride.

Molecular formula:
Thioridazine—$C_{21}H_{26}N_2S_2$.
Thioridazine hydrochloride—$C_{21}H_{26}N_2S_2 \cdot HCl$.

Molecular weight:
Thioridazine—370.57.
Thioridazine hydrochloride—407.03.

Description:
Thioridazine USP—White to slightly yellow, crystalline or micronized powder, odorless or having a faint odor.
Thioridazine Hydrochloride USP—White to slightly yellow, granular powder, having a faint odor.

Solubility:
Thioridazine USP—Practically insoluble in water; freely soluble in dehydrated alcohol and in ether; very soluble in chloroform.
Thioridazine Hydrochloride USP—Freely soluble in water, in methanol, and in chloroform; insoluble in ether.

USP requirements:
Thioridazine USP—Preserve in well-closed, light-resistant containers. Contains not less than 99.0% and not more than 101.0% of thioridazine, calculated on the dried basis. Meets the requirements for Identification, Loss on drying (not more than 0.5%), Residue on ignition (not more than 0.1%), Chromatographic purity, and Organic volatile impurities.
Thioridazine Oral Suspension USP—Preserve in tight, light-resistant containers, at a temperature not exceeding 30 °C. Contains the labeled amount, within ±10%. Meets the requirements for Identification, Specific gravity (1.180–1.310), and pH (8.0–10.0).
Thioridazine Hydrochloride USP—Preserve in tight, light-resistant containers. Contains not less than 99.0% and not more than 101.0% of thioridazine hydrochloride, calculated on the dried basis. Meets the requirements for Identification, Melting range (159–165 °C, the range between beginning and end of melting not more than 3 °C), pH (4.2–5.2, in a solution [1 in 100]), Loss on drying (not more than 0.4%), Residue on ignition (not more than 0.1%), Selenium (not more than 0.003%), Chromatographic purity, and Organic volatile impurities.
Thioridazine Hydrochloride Oral Solution USP—Preserve in tight, light-resistant containers, at controlled room temperature. Label it to indicate that it is to be diluted to appropriate strength with water or other suitable fluid prior to administration. Contains the labeled amount, within ±10%. Meets the requirements for Identification and Alcohol content (not more than 4.75%).
Thioridazine Hydrochloride Tablets USP—Preserve in tight, light-resistant containers. Contain the labeled amount, within ±10%. Meet the requirements for Identification, Dissolution (75% in 60 minutes in 0.1 *N* hydrochloric acid in Apparatus 2 at 75 rpm), and Uniformity of dosage units.

THIOSTREPTON

Molecular formula: $C_{72}H_{85}N_{19}O_{18}S_5$.

Molecular weight: 1664.88.

Description: Thiostrepton USP—White to off-white, crystalline solid.

Solubility: Thiostrepton USP—Practically insoluble in water, in the lower alcohols, in nonpolar organic solvents, and in dilute aqueous acids or alkali; soluble in glacial acetic acid, in chloroform, in dimethylformamide, in dimethyl sulfoxide, in dioxane, and in pyridine.

USP requirements: Thiostrepton USP—Preserve in tight containers. An antibacterial substance produced by the growth of strains of *Streptomyces azureus* (Fam. Streptomycetaceae). Has a potency of not less than 900 USP Thiostrepton Units per mg, calculated on the dried basis. Meets the requirements for Identification, Loss on drying (not more than 5.0%), and Residue on ignition (not more than 1.0%).

THIOTEPA

Chemical name: Aziridine,1,1′,1″-phosphinothioylidynetris-.

Molecular formula: $C_6H_{12}N_3PS$.

Molecular weight: 189.22.

Description:
Thiotepa USP—Fine, white, crystalline flakes, having a faint odor.
Thiotepa for Injection USP—White powder.

Solubility: Thiotepa USP—Freely soluble in water, in alcohol, in chloroform, and in ether.

USP requirements:
Thiotepa USP—Preserve in tight, light-resistant containers, and store in a refrigerator. Contains not less than 97.0% and not more than 102.0% of thiotepa, calculated on the anhydrous basis. Meets the requirements for Identification, Melting range (52–57 °C), and Water (not more than 2.0%).
Caution: Great care should be taken to prevent inhaling particles of Thiotepa or exposing the skin to it.
Thiotepa for Injection USP—Preserve in Containers for Sterile Solids, and store in a refrigerator, protected from light. It is Thiotepa, with or without added substances, that is suitable for parenteral use. Contains the labeled amount, within −5% to +10%. Meets the requirements for Completeness of solution, Identification, pH (7.0–8.6, in a solution, constituted as directed in the labeling, containing 10 mg of thiotepa per mL), Loss on drying (not more than 0.5%), and Bacterial endotoxins, and for Sterility tests, Uniformity of dosage units, and Labeling under Injections.

THIOTHIXENE

Chemical group: Thioxanthene derivative.

Chemical name:
Thiothixene—9*H*-Thioxanthene-2-sulfonamide, *N,N*-dimethyl-9-[3-(4-methyl-1-piperazinyl)propylidene]-, (*Z*)-.
Thiothixene hydrochloride—9*H*-Thioxanthene-2-sulfonamide, *N,N*-dimethyl-9-[3-(4-methyl-1-piperazinyl)propylidene]-, dihydrochloride, dihydrate (*Z*)-.

Molecular formula:
Thiothixene—$C_{23}H_{29}N_3O_2S_2$.
Thiothixene hydrochloride—$C_{23}H_{29}N_3O_2S_2 \cdot 2HCl \cdot 2H_2O$.

Molecular weight:
Thiothixene—443.62.
Thiothixene hydrochloride—552.57.

Description:
Thiothixene USP—White to tan, practically odorless crystals. Is affected by light.
Thiothixene Hydrochloride USP—White, or practically white, crystalline powder, having a slight odor. Is affected by light.

Solubility:
Thiothixene USP—Practically insoluble in water; very soluble in chloroform; slightly soluble in methanol and in acetone.
Thiothixene Hydrochloride USP—Soluble in water; slightly soluble in chloroform; practically insoluble in acetone and in ether.

Other characteristics: Structurally and pharmacologically similar to the piperazine phenothiazines.

USP requirements:
Thiothixene USP—Preserve in tight, light-resistant containers. Contains not less than 96.0% and not more than 101.5% of thiothixene, calculated on the dried basis. Meets the requirements for Identification, Melting range (147–153.5 °C), Loss on drying (not more than 2.0%), Residue on ignition (not more than 0.2%), Selenium (not more than 0.003%), Heavy metals (not more than 0.0025%), Limit of (*E*)-thiothixene (not more than 1.0%), and Organic volatile impurities.
Thiothixene Capsules USP—Preserve in well-closed, light-resistant containers. Contain the labeled amount, within ±10%. Meet the requirements for Identification, Dissolution (75% in 15 minutes in solution of 2.0 grams of sodium chloride and 7 mL of hydrochloric acid in water to make 1000 mL in Apparatus 1 at 150 rpm), and Uniformity of dosage units.
Thiothixene Hydrochloride USP—Preserve in tight, light-resistant containers. Contains two molecules of water of hydration or is anhydrous. Contains not less than 97.0% and not more than 102.5% of thiothixene hydrochloride, calculated on the anhydrous basis. Meets the requirements for Identification, Water (6.2–7.5% for the dihydrate and not more than 1.0% for the anhydrous form), Residue on ignition (not more than 0.2%), Heavy metals (not more than 0.0025%), Selenium (not more than 0.003%), Limit of (*E*)-thiothixene (not more than 1.0%), and Organic volatile impurities.
Thiothixene Hydrochloride Injection USP—Preserve in single-dose containers, preferably of Type I glass, protected from light. A sterile solution of Thiothixene Hydrochloride in Water for Injection. Contains an amount of thiothixene hydrochloride equivalent to the labeled amount of thiothixene, within ±10%. Meets the requirements for Identification, Bacterial endotoxins, pH (2.5–3.5), and Injections.
Thiothixene Hydrochloride for Injection USP—Preserve in light-resistant Containers for Sterile Solids. A sterile, dry mixture of Thiothixene Hydrochloride and Mannitol. Contains an amount of thiothixene hydrochloride equivalent to the labeled amount of thiothixene, within ±10%. Meets the requirements for Identification, Bacterial endotoxins, pH (2.3–3.7, in the solution constituted as directed in the labeling), Water (not more than 4.0%), and Injections.
Thiothixene Hydrochloride Oral Solution USP—Preserve in tight, light-resistant containers. Contains an amount of thiothixene hydrochloride equivalent to the labeled amount of thiothixene, within ±10%. Meets the requirements for Identification, pH (2.0–3.0), and Alcohol content (if present, within ±10% of the labeled amount, the labeled amount being not more than 7.0%).

THONZONIUM

Chemical name: Thonzonium bromide—1-Hexadecanaminium, *N*-[2-[[(4-methoxyphenyl)methyl]-2-pyrimidinylamino]-ethyl]-*N,N*-dimethyl-, bromide.

Molecular formula: Thonzonium bromide—$C_{32}H_{55}BrN_4O$.

Molecular weight: Thonzonium bromide—591.72.

USP requirements: Thonzonium Bromide USP—Preserve in tight containers. Contains not less than 97.0% and not more than 103.0% of thonzonium bromide, calculated on the anhydrous basis. Meets the requirements for Identification, Melting range (93–97 °C), Water (not more than 0.5%), Residue on ignition (not more than 0.2%), Ordinary impurities, and Organic volatile impurities.

THREONINE

Chemical name: L-Threonine.

Molecular formula: $C_4H_9NO_3$.

Molecular weight: 119.12.

Description: Threonine USP—White, odorless crystals.

Solubility: Threonine USP—Freely soluble in water; insoluble in absolute alcohol, in ether, and in chloroform.

USP requirements: Threonine USP—Preserve in well-closed containers. Contains not less than 98.5% and not more than 101.5% of threonine, as L-threonine, calculated on the dried basis. Meets the requirements for Identification, Specific rotation (−26.7° to −29.1°, calculated on the dried basis), pH (5.0–6.5, in a solution [1 in 20]), Loss on drying (not more than 0.2%), Residue on ignition (not more than 0.4%), Chloride (not more than 0.05%), Sulfate (not more than 0.03%), Arsenic (not more than 1.5 ppm), Iron (not more than 0.003%), Heavy metals (not more than 0.0015%), and Organic volatile impurities.

THROMBIN

Description: Thrombin USP—White to grayish, amorphous substance dried from the frozen state.

USP requirements: Thrombin USP—Preserve at a temperature between 2 and 8 °C. Dispense it in the unopened container in which it was placed by the manufacturer. A sterile, freeze-dried powder derived from bovine plasma containing the protein substance prepared from prothrombin through interaction with added thromboplastin in the presence of calcium. It is capable, without the addition of other substances, of causing the clotting of whole blood, plasma, or a solution of fibrinogen. Its potency is determined in U.S. Units in terms of the U.S. Standard Thrombin in a test comparing clotting times of fibrinogen solution. Label it to indicate that solutions of Thrombin are to be used within a few hours after preparation, and are not to be injected into or otherwise allowed to enter large blood vessels. Meets the requirement for Expiration date (not more than 3 years after date of manufacture). Conforms to the regulations of the U.S. Food and Drug Administration concerning biologics.

THYMOL

Chemical name: Phenol, 5-methyl-2-(1-methylethyl)-.

Molecular formula: $C_{10}H_{14}O$.

Molecular weight: 150.22.

Description: Thymol NF—Colorless, often large, crystals, or white, crystalline powder, having an aromatic, thyme-like odor. Affected by light. Its alcohol solution is neutral to litmus.

NF category: Antimicrobial preservative; flavors and perfumes.

Solubility: Thymol NF—Very slightly soluble in water; freely soluble in alcohol, in chloroform, in ether, and in olive oil; soluble in glacial acetic acid and in fixed and volatile oils.

NF requirements: Thymol NF—Preserve in tight, light-resistant containers. Contains not less than 99.0% and not more than 101.0% of thymol. Meets the requirements for Identification, Melting range (48–51 °C, but when melted, Thymol remains liquid at a considerably lower temperature), and Nonvolatile residue (not more than 0.05%).

THYROGLOBULIN

Chemical name: Thyroglobulin.

Description: Thyroglobulin USP—Cream to tan-colored, free-flowing powder, having a slight, characteristic odor.

Solubility: Thyroglobulin USP—Insoluble in water, in dimethylformamide, in alcohol, in hydrochloric acid, in chloroform, and in carbon tetrachloride.

USP requirements:

Thyroglobulin USP—Preserve in tight containers. An extract obtained by the fractionation of thyroid glands from the hog, *Sus scrofa* Linné var. *domesticus* Gray (Fam. Suidae). On hydrolysis yields the labeled amounts of levothyroxine and liothyronine, within ±10%. Free from iodine in inorganic or any form of combination other than that peculiar to thyroglobulin. Meets the requirements for Identification, Microbial limits, Loss on drying (not more than 5.0%), Residue on ignition (not more than 4.0%), and Inorganic iodides.

Thyroglobulin Tablets USP—Preserve in tight containers. Contain the labeled amount of levothyroxine, within ±15%, and the labeled amount of liothyronine, within ±10%, the labeled amounts being 36 mcg of levothyroxine and 12 mcg of liothyronine for each 65 mg of the labeled content of thyroglobulin. Meet the requirements for Identification, Microbial limits, Disintegration (15 minutes), and Uniformity of dosage units.

THYROID

Description: Thyroid USP—Yellowish to buff-colored, amorphous powder, having a slight, characteristic, meat-like odor.

USP requirements:

Thyroid USP—Preserve in tight containers. The cleaned, dried, and powdered thyroid gland previously deprived of connective tissue and fat. Obtained from domesticated animals that are used for food by man. On hydrolysis yields the labeled amounts of levothyroxine and liothyronine, within ±10%, calculated on the dried basis. It is free from iodine in inorganic or any form of combination other than that peculiar to the thyroid gland. Meets the requirements for Identification, Microbial limits, Loss on drying (not more than 6.0%), and Inorganic iodides (not more than 0.004%).

Thyroid Tablets USP—Preserve in tight containers. Contain the labeled amount of levothyroxine, within ±15%, and the labeled amount of liothyronine, within ±10%, the labeled amounts being 38 mcg of levothyroxine and 9 mcg of liothyronine for each 65 mg of the labeled content of thyroid. Meet the requirements for Microbial limit, Disintegration (15 minutes), Uniformity of dosage units, and Inorganic iodides (not more than 0.004%).

Thyroid Enteric-coated Tablets—Not in USP.

THYROTROPIN

Source: Thyroid stimulating hormone (TSH) isolated from bovine anterior pituitary.

Molecular weight: Range of 28,000–30,000.

Solubility: Dissolves readily in physiologic saline.

USP requirements: Thyrotropin for Injection—Not in USP.

TIAPROFENIC ACID

Chemical group: Propionic acid derivative.

Chemical name: 5-Benzoyl-alpha-methyl-2-thiopheneacetic acid.

Molecular formula: $C_{14}H_{12}O_3S$.

Molecular weight: 260.31.

Description: White, microcrystalline powder. Melts at about 95 °C.

pKa: 3.0.

Solubility: Readily soluble in alcohol, in chloroform, and in acetone; sparingly soluble in water.

USP requirements:

Tiaprofenic Acid Extended-release Capsules—Not in USP.

Tiaprofenic Acid Tablets—Not in USP.

TICARCILLIN

Chemical name:

Ticarcillin disodium—4-Thia-1-azabicyclo[3.2.0]heptane-2-carboxylic acid, 6-[(carboxy-3-thienylacetyl)amino]-3,3-dimethyl-7-oxo-, disodium salt, [2*S*-[2 alpha,5 alpha,6 beta(*S**)]]-.

Ticarcillin monosodium—4-Thia-1-azabicyclo[3.2.0]heptane-2-carboxylic acid, 6-[(carboxy-3-thienylacetyl)amino]-3,3-dimethyl-7-oxo, monosodium salt, [2*S*-[2 alpha,5 alpha,6 beta(*S**)]]-, monohydrate.

Molecular formula:

Ticarcillin disodium—$C_{15}H_{14}N_2Na_2O_6S_2$.

Ticarcillin monosodium monohydrate—$C_{15}H_{15}N_2NaO_6S_2 \cdot H_2O$.

Molecular weight:

Ticarcillin disodium—428.39.

Ticarcillin monosodium monohydrate—424.42.

Description: Sterile Ticarcillin Disodium USP—White to pale yellow powder, or white to pale yellow solid having the characteristic appearance of products prepared by freeze-drying.

Solubility: Sterile Ticarcillin Disodium USP—Freely soluble in water.

USP requirements:
Sterile Ticarcillin Disodium USP—Preserve in Containers for Sterile Solids. It is ticarcillin disodium suitable for parenteral use. Has a potency equivalent to not less than 800 mcg of ticarcillin per mg, calculated on the anhydrous basis, and, where packaged for dispensing, contains an amount of ticarcillin disodium equivalent to the labeled amount of ticarcillin, within −10% to +15%. Meets the requirements for Constituted solution, Identification, Specific rotation (+172° to +187°, calculated on the anhydrous basis), Bacterial endotoxins, Sterility, pH (6.0–8.0, in a solution containing 10 mg of ticarcillin per mL [or in the solution constituted as directed in the labeling]), Water (not more than 6.0%), Particulate matter, Dimethylaniline, and Ticarcillin content (80.0–94.0%, calculated on the anhydrous basis). Where packaged for dispensing, meets the requirements for Uniformity of dosage units and Labeling under Injections.
Ticarcillin Monosodium USP—Preserve in tight containers. Contains the equivalent of not less than 890 mcg of ticarcillin per mg, calculated on the anhydrous basis. Meets the requirements for Identification, Specific rotation (+181° to +197°, calculated on the anhydrous basis), Crystallinity, pH (2.5–4.0, in a solution containing the equivalent of 10 mg of ticarcillin per mL), Water (4.0–6.0%), and Dimethylaniline.

TICARCILLIN AND CLAVULANATE

For *Ticarcillin* and *Clavulanate*—See individual listings for chemistry information.

USP requirements:
Ticarcillin Disodium and Clavulanate Potassium Injection USP—Preserve in Containers for Injections. Maintain in the frozen state. A sterile isoosmotic solution of Ticarcillin Monosodium and Clavulanate Potassium in Water for Injection. Contains one or more suitable buffering agents and a tonicity-adjusting agent. The label states that it is to be thawed just prior to use, describes conditions for proper storage of the resultant solution, and directs that the solution is not to be refrozen. Contains an amount of ticarcillin disodium equivalent to the labeled amount of ticarcillin, within −10 to +15%, and an amount of clavulanate potassium equivalent to the labeled amount of clavulanic acid, within −15% to +20%. Meets the requirements for Identification, Pyrogen, Sterility, pH (5.5–7.5), and Particulate matter, for Uniformity of dosage units, and for Labeling under Injections.
Sterile Ticarcillin Disodium and Clavulanate Potassium USP—Preserve in Containers for Sterile Solids. A sterile, dry mixture of Sterile Ticarcillin Disodium and Sterile Clavulanate Potassium. Contains amounts of ticarcillin disodium and clavulanate potassium equivalent to the labeled amount of ticarcillin, within −10% to +15%, and clavulanic acid, within −15% to +20%, the labeled amounts representing proportions of ticarcillin to clavulanic acid of 15:1 or 30:1. Where the proportion is 15:1, contains not less than 733 mcg of ticarcillin per mg, calculated on the anhydrous basis. Where the proportion is 30:1, contains not less than 755 mcg of ticarcillin per mg, calculated on the anhydrous basis. Meets the requirements for Constituted solution, Identification, Bacterial endotoxins, Sterility, pH (5.5–7.5, in a solution [1 in 10]), Water (not more than 4.2%), and Particulate matter, for Uniformity of dosage units, and for Labeling under Injections.

TICLOPIDINE

Chemical name: Ticlopidine hydrochloride—Thieno[3,2-*c*]pyridine, 5-[(2-chlorophenyl)methyl]-4,5,6,7-tetrahydro-, hydrochloride.

Molecular formula: Ticlopidine hydrochloride—$C_{14}H_{14}ClNS \cdot HCl$.

Molecular weight: Ticlopidine hydrochloride—300.25.

Description: Ticlopidine hydrochloride—White crystalline solid.

Solubility: Ticlopidine hydrochloride—Freely soluble in water and in self buffers to a pH of 3.6, and in methanol; sparingly soluble in methylene chloride and in ethanol; slightly soluble in acetone; insoluble in a buffer solution of pH 6.3.

USP requirements: Ticlopidine Hydrochloride Tablets—Not in USP.

TIMOLOL

Chemical name: Timolol maleate—2-Propanol, 1-[(1,1-dimethylethyl)amino]-3-[[4-(4-morpholinyl)-1,2,5-thiadiazol-3-yl]oxy]-, (*S*)-, (*Z*)-2-butenedioate (1:1) (salt).

Molecular formula: Timolol maleate—$C_{13}H_{24}N_4O_3S \cdot C_4H_4O_4$.

Molecular weight: Timolol maleate—432.49.

Description: Timolol Maleate USP—White to practically white, odorless or practically odorless, powder.

pKa: Timolol maleate—Approximately 9 in water at 25 °C.

Solubility: Timolol Maleate USP—Freely soluble in water; soluble in alcohol and in methanol; sparingly soluble in chloroform and in propylene glycol; insoluble in ether and in cyclohexane.

Other characteristics: Lipid solubility—Moderate.

USP requirements:
Timolol Maleate USP—Preserve in well-closed containers. Contains not less than 98.0% and not more than 101.0% of timolol maleate, calculated on the dried basis. Meets the requirements for Identification, Specific rotation (−11.7° to −12.5°, calculated on the dried basis), pH (3.8–4.3, in a solution containing 20 mg per mL), Loss on drying (not more than 0.5%), Residue on ignition (not more than 0.1%), Heavy metals (not more than 0.002%), Chromatographic purity, and Organic volatile impurities.
Timolol Maleate Ophthalmic Solution USP—Preserve in tight, light-resistant containers. A sterile aqueous solution of Timolol Maleate. Contains an amount of timolol maleate equivalent to the labeled amount of timolol, within ±10%. Meets the requirements for Identification, Sterility, and pH (6.5–7.5).
Timolol Maleate Ophthalmic Gel-forming Solution—Not in USP.
Timolol Maleate Tablets USP—Preserve in well-closed containers. Contain the labeled amount, within ±10%. Meet the requirements for Identification, Dissolution (80% in 20 minutes in 0.1 *N* hydrochloric acid in Apparatus 1 at 100 rpm), and Uniformity of dosage units.

TIMOLOL AND HYDROCHLOROTHIAZIDE

For *Timolol* and *Hydrochlorothiazide*—See individual listings for chemistry information.

USP requirements: Timolol Maleate and Hydrochlorothiazide Tablets USP—Preserve in well-closed, light-resistant containers. Contain the labeled amounts, within ±10%. Meet the requirements for Identification, Dissolution (80% of each active ingredient in 20 minutes in 0.1 *N* hydrochloric acid in Apparatus 2 at 50 rpm), Limit of 4-amino-6-chloro-1,3-benzenedisulfonamide (not more than 1.0%), and Uniformity of dosage units.

TIOCONAZOLE

Chemical name: 1*H*-Imidazole, 1-[2-[(2-chloro-3-thienyl)methoxy]-2-(2,4-dichlorophenyl)ethyl]-.

Molecular formula: $C_{16}H_{13}Cl_3N_2OS$.

Molecular weight: 387.71.

Description: White to off-white crystalline solid.

Solubility: Moderately soluble in chloroform, in methanol, in ethanol, and in ethyl acetate; virtually insoluble in water.

USP requirements:

Tioconazole USP—Preserve in tight containers. Contains not less than 97.0% and not more than 103.0% of tioconazole. Meets the requirements for Identification, Water (not more than 0.5%), Residue on ignition (not more than 0.2%), Chloride (not more than 0.05%), Heavy metals (not more than 0.005%), and Related compounds (not more than 1.0% for each related compound).

Tioconazole Cream USP—Preserve in tight containers. Contains the labeled amount, within ±10%, in a suitable cream base. Meets the requirements for Identification, Microbial limits, Minimum fill, and pH (3.0–6.0, in a 1:1 aqueous suspension of the Cream).

Tioconazole Vaginal Ointment—Not in USP.

Tioconazole Vaginal Suppositories—Not in USP.

TIOPRONIN

Chemical name: *N*-(2-Mercaptopropionyl)glycine.

Molecular formula: $C_5H_9NO_3S$.

Molecular weight: 163.19.

Description: A white, crystalline powder with a characteristic sulphurous odor.

Solubility: Soluble in water.

Other characteristics: Chemically similar to penicillamine.

USP requirements: Tiopronin Tablets—Not in USP.

TITANIUM DIOXIDE

Chemical name: Titanium oxide (TiO_2).

Molecular formula: TiO_2.

Molecular weight: 79.88.

Description: Titanium Dioxide USP—White, odorless powder. Its 1 in 10 suspension in water is neutral to litmus.

NF category: Coating agent.

Solubility: Titanium Dioxide USP—Insoluble in water, in hydrochloric acid, in nitric acid, and in 2 *N* sulfuric acid. Dissolves in hydrofluoric acid and in hot sulfuric acid. It is rendered soluble by fusion with potassium bisulfate or with alkali carbonates or hydroxides.

USP requirements: Titanium Dioxide USP—Preserve in well-closed containers. Contains not less than 99.0% and not more than 100.5% of titanium dioxide, calculated on the dried basis. Meets the requirements for Identification, Loss on drying (not more than 0.5%), Loss on ignition (not more than 0.5%), Water-soluble substances (not more than 0.25%), Acid-soluble substances (not more than 0.5%), Arsenic (not more than 1 ppm), and Organic volatile impurities.

Note: The U.S. Food and Drug Administration requires the content of lead to be not more than 10 ppm, that of antimony to be not more than 2 ppm, and that of mercury to be not more than 1 ppm.

TOBRAMYCIN

Source: Derived from *Streptomyces tenebrarius*.

Chemical group: Aminoglycoside.

Chemical name:

Tobramycin—D-Streptamine, *O*-3-amino-3-deoxy-alpha-D-glucopyranosyl-(1→6)-*O*-[2,6-diamino-2,3,6-trideoxy-alpha-D-*ribo*-hexopyranosyl-(1→4)]-2-deoxy-.

Tobramycin sulfate—D-Streptamine, *O*-3-amino-3-deoxy-alpha-D-glucopyranosyl-(1→6)-*O*-[2,6-diamino-2,3,6-trideoxy-alpha-D-*ribo*-hexopyranosyl-(1→4)]-2-deoxy-, sulfate (2:5) (salt).

Molecular formula:

Tobramycin—$C_{18}H_{37}N_5O_9$.

Tobramycin sulfate—$(C_{18}H_{37}N_5O_9)_2 \cdot 5H_2SO_4$.

Molecular weight:

Tobramycin—467.52.

Tobramycin sulfate—1425.41.

Description:

Tobramycin USP—White to off-white, hygroscopic powder.

Tobramycin Sulfate Injection USP—Clear, colorless solution.

Solubility: Tobramycin USP—Freely soluble in water; very slightly soluble in alcohol; practically insoluble in chloroform and in ether.

USP requirements:

Tobramycin USP—Preserve in tight containers. Has a potency of not less than 900 mcg of tobramycin per mg, calculated on the anhydrous basis. Meets the requirements for Identification, pH (9–11, in a solution [1 in 10]), Water (not more than 8.0%), Residue on ignition (not more than 1.0%), Heavy metals (not more than 0.003%), and Related compounds.

Tobramycin Ophthalmic Ointment USP—Preserve in collapsible ophthalmic ointment tubes. Contains the labeled amount, within −10% to +20%. Meets the requirements for Identification, Sterility, Minimum fill, Water (not more than 1.0%), and Metal particles.

Tobramycin Ophthalmic Solution USP—Preserve in tight containers, and avoid exposure to excessive heat. Contains the labeled amount, within −10% to +20%. Meets the requirements for Identification, Sterility, and pH (7.0–8.0).

Tobramycin Sulfate USP—Preserve in tight containers. Has a potency of not less than 634 mcg and not more than 739 mcg of tobramycin per mg. Meets the requirements for Identification, Bacterial endotoxins, pH (6.0–8.0, in a solution containing 40 mg per mL), and Water (not more than 2.0%), and for Residue on ignition and Heavy metals under Tobramycin.

Tobramycin Sulfate Injection USP—Preserve in single-dose or in multiple-dose glass or plastic containers. Glass containers are preferably of Type I glass. A sterile solution of Tobramycin Sulfate or of Sterile Tobramycin Sulfate in Water for Injection, or of Tobramycin in Water for Injection prepared with the aid of Sulfuric Acid. Contains an amount of tobramycin sulfate equivalent to the labeled amount of tobramycin, within −10% to +20%. Meets the requirements for Identification, Bacterial endotoxins, Sterility, pH (3.0–6.5), Particulate matter, and Injections.

Sterile Tobramycin Sulfate USP—Preserve in Containers for Sterile Solids. It is tobramycin sulfate suitable for parenteral use. Has a potency of not less than 634 mcg and not more than 739 mcg of tobramycin per mg and, where packaged for dispensing, contains an amount of tobramycin sulfate equivalent to the labeled amount of tobramycin within −10% to +15%. Meets the requirements for Identification, Constituted solution, Bacterial endotoxins, Sterility, pH (6.0–8.0, in a solution containing 40 mg per mL [or, where packaged for dispensing, in the solution constituted as directed in the labeling]), Water (not more than 2.0%), and Particulate matter, for Residue on ignition and Heavy metals under Tobramycin, and for Uniformity of dosage units (where packaged for dispensing) and Labeling under Injections.

TOBRAMYCIN AND DEXAMETHASONE

For *Tobramycin* and *Dexamethasone*—See individual listings for chemistry information.

USP requirements:

Tobramycin and Dexamethasone Ophthalmic Ointment USP—Preserve in collapsible ophthalmic ointment tubes. Contains the labeled amount of tobramycin, within −10% to +20%, and the labeled amount of dexamethasone, within ±10%. Meets the requirements for Identification, Sterility, Minimum fill, Water (not more than 1.0%), and Metal particles.

Tobramycin and Dexamethasone Ophthalmic Suspension USP—Preserve in tight containers. A sterile aqueous suspension containing Tobramycin and Dexamethasone. Contains the labeled amount of tobramycin, within −10% to +20%, and the labeled amount of dexamethasone, within ±10%. Meets the requirements for Identification, Sterility, and pH (5.0–6.0).

TOBRAMYCIN AND FLUOROMETHOLONE

For *Tobramycin* and *Fluorometholone*—See individual listings for chemistry information.

USP requirements: Tobramycin and Fluorometholone Acetate Ophthalmic Suspension USP—Preserve in tight containers. A sterile aqueous suspension of Tobramycin and Fluorometholone Acetate. Contains the labeled amount of tobramycin, within −10% to +20%, and the labeled amount of fluorometholone acetate, within −10% to +15%. Meets the requirements for Identification, Sterility, and pH (6.0–7.0).

TOCAINIDE

Chemical name: Tocainide hydrochloride—Propanamide, 2-amino-*N*-(2,6-dimethylphenyl)-, hydrochloride.

Molecular formula: Tocainide hydrochloride—$C_{11}H_{16}N_2O \cdot HCl$.

Molecular weight: Tocainide hydrochloride—228.72.

Description: Tocainide Hydrochloride USP—Fine, white, odorless powder.

pKa: Tocainide hydrochloride—7.8.

Solubility: Tocainide Hydrochloride USP—Freely soluble in water and in alcohol; practically insoluble in chloroform and in ether.

USP requirements:

Tocainide Hydrochloride USP—Preserve in well-closed containers. Contains not less than 98.0% and not more than 101.0% of tocainide hydrochloride, calculated on the dried basis. Meets the requirements for Identification, Loss on drying (not more than 0.5%), Residue on ignition (not more than 0.1%), Heavy metals (not more than 0.002%), Chromatographic purity, and Organic volatile impurities.

Tocainide Hydrochloride Tablets USP—Preserve in well-closed containers. Contain the labeled amount, within ±5%. Meet the requirements for Identification, Dissolution (80% in 30 minutes in water in Apparatus 2 at 50 rpm), and Uniformity of dosage units.

TOCOPHEROLS EXCIPIENT

Description: Tocopherols Excipient NF—Brownish red to red, clear, viscous oil, having a mild, characteristic odor. May show a slight separation of waxlike constituents in microcrystalline form. Oxidizes and darkens slowly in air and on exposure to light, particularly in alkaline media.

NF category: Antioxidant.

Solubility: Tocopherols Excipient NF—Insoluble in water; soluble in alcohol; miscible with acetone, with chloroform, with ether, and with vegetable oils.

NF requirements: Tocopherols Excipient NF—Preserve in tight containers, protected from light. Protect with a blanket of an inert gas. A vegetable oil solution containing not less than 50.0% of total tocopherols, of which not less than 80.0% consists of varying amounts of beta, gamma, and delta tocopherols. Label it to indicate the content, in mg per gram, of total tocopherols, and of the sum of beta, gamma, and delta tocopherols. Meets the requirements for Identification and Acidity.

TOLAZAMIDE

Chemical group: Sulfonylurea.

Chemical name: Benzenesulfonamide, *N*-[[(hexahydro-1*H*-azepin-1-yl)amino]carbonyl]-4-methyl-.

Molecular formula: $C_{14}H_{21}N_3O_3S$.

Molecular weight: 311.40.

Description: Tolazamide USP—White to off-white, crystalline powder, odorless or having a slight odor. Melts with decomposition in the approximate range of 161 to 173 °C.

pKa: 3.6 at 25 °C and 5.68 at 37.5 °C.

Solubility: Tolazamide USP—Very slightly soluble in water; freely soluble in chloroform; soluble in acetone; slightly soluble in alcohol.

USP requirements:

Tolazamide USP—Preserve in well-closed containers. Contains not less than 97.5% and not more than 102.5% of tolazamide, calculated on the dried basis. Meets the requirements for Identification, Loss on drying (not more than 0.5%), Residue on ignition (not more than 0.2%), Selenium (not more than 0.003%, a 200-mg specimen being used), Heavy metals (not more than 0.002%), *N*-Aminohexamethyleneimine (not more than 0.005%), Chromatographic purity, and Organic volatile impurities.

Tolazamide Tablets USP—Preserve in tight containers. Contain the labeled amount, within ±5%. Meet the requirements for Identification, Dissolution (70% in 30 minutes in 0.05 *M* Tris(hydroxymethyl)aminomethane, adjusted, if necessary, with hydrochloric acid to a pH of 7.6, in Apparatus 2 at 75 rpm), and Uniformity of dosage units.

TOLAZOLINE

Chemical group: Imidazoline derivative, structurally related to phentolamine.

Chemical name: Tolazoline hydrochloride—1*H*-Imidazole, 4,5-dihydro-2-(phenylmethyl)-, monohydrochloride.

Molecular formula: Tolazoline hydrochloride—$C_{10}H_{12}N_2 \cdot HCl$.

Molecular weight: Tolazoline hydrochloride—196.68.

Description: Tolazoline Hydrochloride USP—White to off-white, crystalline powder. Its solutions are slightly acid to litmus.

pKa: 10.5.

Solubility: Tolazoline Hydrochloride USP—Freely soluble in water and in alcohol.

USP requirements:

Tolazoline Hydrochloride USP—Preserve in well-closed containers. Contains not less than 98.0% and not more than 101.0% of tolazoline hydrochloride, calculated on the dried basis. Meets the requirements for Identification, Melting range (172.0–176.0 °C), Loss on drying (not more than 0.2%), Residue on ignition (not more than 0.1%), Heavy metals (not more than 0.001%), and Chromatographic purity.

Tolazoline Hydrochloride Injection USP—Preserve in single-dose or in multiple-dose containers, preferably of Type I glass. A sterile solution of Tolazoline Hydrochloride in Water for Injection. Contains the labeled amount, within ±5%. Meets the requirements for Identification, Bacterial endotoxins, pH (3.0–4.0), and Injections.

Tolazoline Hydrochloride Tablets USP—Preserve in well-closed containers. Contain the labeled amount, within ±5%. Meet the requirements for Identification, Dissolution (75% in 45 minutes in water in Apparatus 2 at 50 rpm), and Uniformity of dosage units.

TOLBUTAMIDE

Chemical group: Sulfonylurea.

Chemical name:

Tolbutamide—Benzenesulfonamide, *N*-[(butylamino)carbonyl]-4-methyl-.

Tolbutamide sodium—Benzenesulfonamide, *N*-[(butylamino)carbonyl]-4-methyl-, monosodium salt.

Molecular formula:

Tolbutamide—$C_{12}H_{18}N_2O_3S$.

Tolbutamide sodium—$C_{12}H_{17}N_2NaO_3S$.

Molecular weight:

Tolbutamide—270.35.

Tolbutamide sodium—292.33.

Description:

Tolbutamide USP—White, or practically white, crystalline powder. Is practically odorless.

Sterile Tolbutamide Sodium USP—White to off-white, practically odorless, crystalline powder.

pKa: 5.3.

Solubility:

Tolbutamide USP—Practically insoluble in water; soluble in alcohol and in chloroform.

Sterile Tolbutamide Sodium USP—Freely soluble in water; soluble in alcohol and in chloroform; very slightly soluble in ether.

USP requirements:

Tolbutamide USP—Preserve in well-closed containers. Contains not less than 97.0% and not more than 103.0% of tolbutamide, calculated on the dried basis. Meets the requirements for Identification, Melting range (126–130 °C), Loss on drying (not more than 0.5%), Selenium (not more than 0.003%), Heavy metals (not more than 0.002%), and Non-sulfonyl urea.

Tolbutamide Tablets USP—Preserve in well-closed containers. Contain the labeled amount, within ±10%. Meet the requirements for Identification, Dissolution (70% in 30 minutes in phosphate buffer [pH 7.4] in Apparatus 2 at 75 rpm), and Uniformity of dosage units.

Sterile Tolbutamide Sodium USP—Preserve in Containers for Sterile Solids. It is prepared from Tolbutamide with the aid of Sodium Hydroxide. Suitable for parenteral use. Contains an amount of tolbutamide sodium equivalent to the labeled amount of tolbutamide, within ±5%. Meets the requirements for Constituted solution, Identification, Bacterial endotoxins, pH (8.0–9.8, in a solution containing 50 mg per mL), and Loss on drying (not more than 1.0%), and for Sterility, Uniformity of dosage units, and Labeling under Injections.

TOLMETIN

Chemical group: Pyrroleacetic acid derivative.

Chemical name: Tolmetin sodium—1*H*-Pyrrole-2-acetic acid, 1-methyl-5-(4-methylbenzoyl)-, sodium salt, dihydrate.

Molecular formula: Tolmetin sodium—$C_{15}H_{14}NNaO_3 \cdot 2H_2O$.

Molecular weight: Tolmetin sodium—315.30.

Description: Tolmetin Sodium USP—Light yellow to light orange, crystalline powder.

pKa: 3.5.

Solubility: Tolmetin Sodium USP—Freely soluble in water and in methanol; slightly soluble in alcohol; very slightly soluble in chloroform.

USP requirements:

Tolmetin Sodium USP—Preserve in well-closed containers. Contains not less than 98.0% and not more than 102.0% of tolmetin sodium, calculated on the dried basis. Meets the requirements for Identification, Loss on drying (10.4–12.4%), Heavy metals (not more than 0.002%), Chromatographic purity, and Organic volatile impurities.

Tolmetin Sodium Capsules USP—Preserve in tight containers. Contain an amount of tolmetin sodium equivalent to the labeled amount of tolmetin, within ±7%. Meet the requirements for Identification, Dissolution (85% in 30 minutes in phosphate buffer [pH 4.5] in Apparatus 2 at 50 rpm), and Uniformity of dosage units.

Tolmetin Sodium Tablets USP—Preserve in well-closed containers. Contain an amount of tolmetin sodium equivalent to the labeled amount of tolmetin, within ±10%. Meet the requirements for Identification, Dissolution (75% in 30 minutes in phosphate buffer [pH 4.5] in Apparatus 2 at 50 rpm), and Uniformity of dosage units.

TOLNAFTATE

Chemical name: Carbamothioic acid, methyl(3-methylphenyl)-, *O*-2-naphthalenyl ester.

Molecular formula: $C_{19}H_{17}NOS$.

Molecular weight: 307.41.

Description: Tolnaftate USP—White to creamy white, fine powder, having a slight odor.

Solubility: Tolnaftate USP—Practically insoluble in water; freely soluble in acetone and in chloroform; sparingly soluble in ether; slightly soluble in alcohol.

USP requirements:
Tolnaftate USP—Preserve in tight containers. Contains not less than 98.0% and not more than 102.0% of tolnaftate, calculated on the dried basis. Meets the requirements for Identification, Melting range (110–113 °C), Loss on drying (not more than 0.5%), Residue on ignition (not more than 0.1%), and Heavy metals (not more than 0.002%).
Tolnaftate Cream USP—Preserve in tight containers. Contains the labeled amount, within ±10%. Meets the requirements for Identification and Minimum fill.
Tolnaftate Gel USP—Preserve in tight containers. Contains the labeled amount, within ±10%. Meets the requirements for Identification and Minimum fill.
Tolnaftate Topical Powder USP—Preserve in tight containers. Contains the labeled amount, within ±10%. Meets the requirements for Identification and Minimum fill.
Tolnaftate Topical Aerosol Powder USP—Preserve in tight, pressurized containers, and avoid exposure to excessive heat. A suspension of powder in suitable propellants in a pressurized container. Contains the labeled amount, within ±10%. Meets the requirements for Identification and for Leak testing and Pressure testing under Aerosols.
Tolnaftate Topical Solution USP—Preserve in tight containers. Contains the labeled amount, within −10% to +15%. Meets the requirement for Identification.
Tolnaftate Topical Aerosol Solution—Not in USP.

TOLU BALSAM

Description:
Tolu Balsam USP—Brown or yellowish-brown, plastic solid, transparent in thin layers and brittle when old, dried, or exposed to cold temperatures. Has a pleasant, aromatic odor resembling that of vanilla.

NF category: Flavors and perfumes.

Tolu Balsam Syrup NF—NF category: Flavored and/or sweetened vehicle.
Tolu Balsam Tincture NF—NF category: Flavors and perfumes.

Solubility: Tolu Balsam USP—Practically insoluble in water and in solvent hexane; soluble in alcohol, in chloroform, and in ether, sometimes with a slight residue or turbidity.

USP requirements: Tolu Balsam USP—Preserve in tight containers, and avoid exposure to excessive heat. A balsam obtained from *Myroxylon balsamum* (Linné) Harms (Fam. Leguminosae). Meets the requirements for Rosin, rosin oil, and copaiba, Acid value (112–168), and Saponification value (154–220).

NF requirements:
Tolu Balsam Syrup NF—Preserve in tight containers, at a temperature not above 25 °C.

Prepare Tolu Balsam Syrup as follows: 50 mL of Tolu Balsam Tincture, 10 grams of Magnesium Carbonate, 820 grams of Sucrose and a sufficient quantity of Purified Water to make 1000 mL. Add the tincture all at once to the Magnesium Carbonate and 60 grams of the Sucrose in a mortar, and mix. Gradually add 430 mL of Purified Water with trituration, and filter. Dissolve the remainder of the Sucrose in the clear filtrate with gentle heating, strain the syrup while warm, and add sufficient Purified Water through the strainer to make the product measure 1000 mL. Mix.

Meets the requirements for Alcohol content (3.0–5.0%) and Organic volatile impurities.

Note: Tolu Balsam Syrup may be prepared also as follows: Place 760 grams of the Sucrose in a suitable percolator, the neck of which is nearly filled with loosely-packed cotton, moistened after packing with a few drops of water. Pour the filtrate, obtained as directed in the preceding instructions, upon the Sucrose, and regulate the outflow to a steady drip of percolate. When all of the liquid has run through, return portions of the percolate, if necessary, to dissolve all the Sucrose. Then pass enough Purified Water through the cotton to make the product measure 1000 mL. Mix.

Tolu Balsam Tincture NF—Preserve in tight, light-resistant containers, and avoid exposure to direct sunlight and to excessive heat.

Prepare Tolu Balsam Tincture as follows: 200 grams of Tolu Balsam to make 1000 mL. Prepare a tincture by Process M, using alcohol as the menstruum.

Meets the requirements for Alcohol content (77.0–83.0%) and Organic volatile impurities.

TORSEMIDE

Chemical name: 3-Pyridinesulfonamide, *N*-[[(1-methylethyl)-amino]carbonyl]-4-[(3-methylphenyl)amino]-.

Molecular formula: $C_{16}H_{20}N_4O_3S$.

Molecular weight: 348.43.

Description: White to off-white crystalline powder.

pKa: 7.1

USP requirements:
Torsemide Injection—Not in USP.
Torsemide Tablets—Not in USP.

TRAGACANTH

Description: Tragacanth NF—Odorless.
NF category: Suspending and/or viscosity-increasing agent.

NF requirements: Tragacanth NF—Preserve in well-closed containers. The dried gummy exudation from *Astragalus gummifer* Labillardière, or other Asiatic species of *Astragalus* (Fam. Leguminosae). Meets the requirements for Botanic characteristics, Identification, Microbial limits, Arsenic (not more than 3 ppm), Lead (not more than 0.001%), Heavy metals (not more than 0.004%), and Karaya gum.

TRANEXAMIC ACID

Chemical name: Cyclohexanecarboxylic acid, 4-(aminomethyl)-, *trans*-.

Molecular formula: $C_8H_{15}NO_2$.

Molecular weight: 157.21.

Description: White, odorless or almost odorless, crystalline powder.

Solubility: Freely soluble in water and in glacial acetic acid; practically insoluble in alcohol and in ether.

USP requirements:
Tranexamic Acid Injection—Not in USP.
Tranexamic Acid Tablets—Not in USP.

TRANYLCYPROMINE

Chemical group: Nonhydrazine derivative structurally similar to amphetamine, with the exception of a cyclopropyl rather than an isopropyl side chain.

Chemical name: Tranylcypromine sulfate—Cyclopropanamine, 2-phenyl-, *trans*-(±)-, sulfate (2:1).

Molecular formula: Tranylcypromine sulfate—$(C_9H_{11}N)_2 \cdot H_2SO_4$.

Molecular weight: Tranylcypromine sulfate—364.46.

Description: Tranylcypromine sulfate—White or almost white crystalline powder, odorless or having a faint odor of cinnamaldehyde.

Solubility: Tranylcypromine sulfate—Soluble 1 in 20 of water; very slightly soluble in alcohol and in ether; practically insoluble in chloroform.

USP requirements: Tranylcypromine Sulfate Tablets—Not in USP.

TRAZODONE

Chemical group: Triazolopyridine derivative.

Chemical name: Trazodone hydrochloride—1,2,4-Triazolo[4,3-*a*]pyridin-3(2*H*)-one, 2-[3-[4-(3-chlorophenyl)-1-piperazinyl]-propyl]-, monohydrochloride.

Molecular formula: Trazodone hydrochloride—$C_{19}H_{22}ClN_5O \cdot HCl$.

Molecular weight: Trazodone hydrochloride—408.33.

Description: Trazodone Hydrochloride USP—White to off-white crystalline powder. Melts between 231 and 234 °C when the melting point determination is carried out in an evacuated capillary tube; otherwise melts with decomposition over a broad range below 230 °C.

Solubility: Trazodone Hydrochloride USP—Sparingly soluble in chloroform and in water.

Other characteristics: Not chemically related to tricyclic, tetracyclic, or other known antidepressants.

USP requirements:
Trazodone Tablets USP—Preserve in tight, light-resistant containers. Contain the labeled amount of trazodone hydrochloride, within ±10%. Label the Tablets to state both the content of the active moiety and the content of the salt used in formulating the article. Meet the requirements for Identification, Dissolution (80% in 60 minutes in 0.01 *N* hydrochloric acid in Apparatus 2 at 50 rpm), and Uniformity of dosage units.
Trazodone Hydrochloride USP—Preserve in tight, light-resistant containers. Contains not less than 97.0% and not more than 102.0% of trazodone hydrochloride, calculated on the dried basis. Meets the requirements for Identification, Loss on drying (not more than 0.5%), Residue on ignition (not more than 0.2%), Chromatographic purity, and Ordinary impurities.

TRETINOIN

Chemical name: Retinoic acid.

Molecular formula: $C_{20}H_{28}O_2$.

Molecular weight: 300.44.

Description: Tretinoin USP—Yellow to light-orange, crystalline powder.

Solubility: Tretinoin USP—Insoluble in water; slightly soluble in alcohol and in chloroform.

USP requirements:
Tretinoin USP—Preserve in tight containers, preferably under an atmosphere of an inert gas, protected from light. Contains not less than 97.0% and not more than 103.0% of tretinoin, calculated on the dried basis. Meets the requirements for Identification, Loss on drying (not more than 0.5%), Residue on ignition (not more than 0.1%), Limit of isotretinoin (not more than 5.0%), and Heavy metals (not more than 0.002%).
Tretinoin Cream USP—Preserve in collapsible tubes or in tight, light-resistant containers. Contains the labeled amount, within −10% to +20%. Meets the requirements for Identification and Minimum fill.
Tretinoin Gel USP—Preserve in tight containers, protected from light. Contains the labeled amount, within −10% to +30%. Meets the requirements for Identification and Minimum fill.
Tretinoin Topical Solution USP—Preserve in tight, light-resistant containers. A solution of Tretinoin in a suitable nonaqueous, hydrophilic solvent. Contains the labeled amount (w/w), within −10% to +35%. Meets the requirements for Identification and Alcohol content (50.0–60.0%).

TRIACETIN

Chemical name: 1,2,3-Propanetriol triacetate.

Molecular formula: $C_9H_{14}O_6$.

Molecular weight: 218.21.

Description: Triacetin USP—Colorless, somewhat oily liquid having a slight fatty odor.
NF category: Plasticizer.

Solubility: Triacetin USP—Soluble in water; slightly soluble in carbon disulfide. Miscible with alcohol, with ether, and with chloroform.

USP requirements: Triacetin USP—Preserve in tight containers. Contains not less than 97.0% and not more than 100.5% of triacetin, calculated on the anhydrous basis. Meets the requirements for Identification, Specific gravity (1.152–1.158), Refractive index (1.429–1.430), Acidity, and Water (not more than 0.2%).

TRIAMCINOLONE

Chemical name:
Triamcinolone—Pregna-1,4-diene-3,20-dione, 9-fluoro-11,16,-17,21-tetrahydroxy-, (11 beta,16 alpha).
Triamcinolone acetonide—Pregna-1,4-diene-3,20-dione, 9-fluoro-11,21-dihydroxy-16,17-[(1-methylethylidene)bis-(oxy)]-, (11 beta,16 alpha)-.
Triamcinolone diacetate—Pregna-1,4-diene-3,20-dione, 16,-21-bis(acetyloxy)-9-fluoro-11,17-dihydroxy-, (11 beta,16 alpha)-.
Triamcinolone hexacetonide—Pregna-1,4-diene-3,20-dione, 21-(3,3-dimethyl-1-oxobutoxy)-9-fluoro-11-hydroxy-16,17-[(1-methylethylidene)bis(oxy)]-, (11 beta,16 alpha)-.

Molecular formula:
Triamcinolone—$C_{21}H_{27}FO_6$.
Triamcinolone acetonide—$C_{24}H_{31}FO_6$.
Triamcinolone diacetate—$C_{25}H_{31}FO_8$.
Triamcinolone hexacetonide—$C_{30}H_{41}FO_7$.

Molecular weight:
Triamcinolone—394.44.
Triamcinolone acetonide—434.50.
Triamcinolone diacetate—478.51.
Triamcinolone hexacetonide—532.65.

Description:
Triamcinolone USP—White or practically white, odorless, crystalline powder.
Triamcinolone Acetonide USP—White to cream-colored, crystalline powder, having not more than a slight odor.
Triamcinolone Diacetate USP—Fine, white to off-white, crystalline powder, having not more than a slight odor.
Triamcinolone Hexacetonide USP—White to cream-colored powder.

Solubility:
Triamcinolone USP—Very slightly soluble in water, in chloroform, and in ether; slightly soluble in alcohol and in methanol.
Triamcinolone Acetonide USP—Practically insoluble in water; sparingly soluble in dehydrated alcohol, in chloroform, and in methanol.
Triamcinolone Diacetate USP—Practically insoluble in water; soluble in chloroform; sparingly soluble in alcohol and in methanol; slightly soluble in ether.
Triamcinolone Hexacetonide USP—Practically insoluble in water; soluble in chloroform; slightly soluble in methanol.

USP requirements:
Triamcinolone USP—Preserve in well-closed containers. Contains not less than 97.0% and not more than 102.0% of triamcinolone, calculated on the dried basis. Meets the requirements for Identification, Specific rotation (+65° to +72°, calculated on the dried basis), Loss on drying (not more than 2.0%), Residue on ignition (not more than 0.5%), and Heavy metals (not more than 0.0025%).
Triamcinolone Tablets USP—Preserve in well-closed containers. Contain the labeled amount, within ±10%. Meet the requirements for Identification, Dissolution (75% in 45 minutes in 0.1 *N* hydrochloric acid in Apparatus 1 at 100 rpm), and Uniformity of dosage units.
Triamcinolone Acetonide USP—Preserve in well-closed containers. Contains not less than 97.0% and not more than 102.0% of triamcinolone acetonide, calculated on the dried basis. Meets the requirements for Identification, Specific rotation (+118° to +130°, calculated on the dried basis), Loss on drying (not more than 1.5%), and Heavy metals (not more than 0.0025%).
Triamcinolone Acetonide Inhalation Aerosol—Not in USP.
Triamcinolone Acetonide Nasal Aerosol—Not in USP.
Triamcinolone Acetonide Topical Aerosol USP—Preserve in pressurized containers, and avoid exposure to excessive heat. A solution of Triamcinolone Acetonide in a suitable propellant in a pressurized container. Contains the labeled amount, within −10% to +15%. Meets the requirements for Identification and Microbial limits, and for Leak testing and Pressure testing under Aerosols.
Triamcinolone Acetonide Cream USP—Preserve in tight containers. It is Triamcinolone Acetonide in a suitable cream base. Contains the labeled amount, within −10% to +15%. Meets the requirements for Identification, Microbial limits, and Minimum fill.
Triamcinolone Acetonide Lotion USP—Preserve in tight containers. It is Triamcinolone Acetonide in a suitable lotion base. Contains the labeled amount, within ±10%. Meets the requirements for Identification, Microbial limits, and Minimum fill.
Triamcinolone Acetonide Ointment USP—Preserve in well-closed containers. It is Triamcinolone Acetonide in a suitable ointment base. Contains the labeled amount, within −10% to +15%. Meets the requirements for Identification, Microbial limits, and Minimum fill.
Triamcinolone Acetonide Dental Paste USP—Preserve in tight containers. It is Triamcinolone Acetonide in a suitable emollient paste. Contains the labeled amount, within −10% to +15%. Meets the requirements for Identification, Microbial limits, and Minimum fill.
Sterile Triamcinolone Acetonide Suspension USP—Preserve in single-dose or in multiple-dose containers, preferably of Type I glass, protected from light. A sterile suspension of Triamcinolone Acetonide in a suitable aqueous medium. Contains the labeled amount, within −10% to +15%. Meets the requirements for Identification, Bacterial endotoxins, pH (5.0–7.5), and Injections.
Triamcinolone Diacetate USP—Preserve in well-closed containers. Contains not less than 97.0% and not more than 103.0% of triamcinolone diacetate, calculated on the dried basis. Meets the requirements for Identification, Specific rotation (+39° to +45°, calculated on the dried basis), Loss on drying (not more than 6.0%), Residue on ignition (not more than 0.5%), and Heavy metals (not more than 0.0025%).
Sterile Triamcinolone Diacetate Suspension USP—Preserve in single-dose or in multiple-dose containers, preferably of Type I glass. A sterile suspension of Triamcinolone Diacetate in a suitable aqueous medium. Contains the labeled amount, within −10% to +15%. Meets the requirements for Identification, Uniformity of dosage units, Bacterial endotoxins, pH (4.5–7.5), and Injections.
Triamcinolone Diacetate Syrup USP—Preserve in tight, light-resistant containers. Contains the labeled amount, within ±10%. Contains a suitable preservative. Meets the requirement for Identification.
Triamcinolone Hexacetonide USP—Preserve in well-closed containers. Contains not less than 97.0% and not more than 102.0% of triamcinolone hexacetonide, calculated on the dried basis. Meets the requirements for Identification, Specific rotation (+85° to +95°, calculated on the dried basis), Loss on drying (not more than 2.0%), and Heavy metals (not more than 0.002%).
Sterile Triamcinolone Hexacetonide Suspension USP—Preserve in single-dose or in multiple-dose containers, preferably of Type I glass. A sterile suspension of Triamcinolone Hexacetonide in a suitable aqueous medium. Contains the labeled amount, within −10% to +15%. Meets the requirements for Identification, Bacterial endotoxins, pH (4.0–8.0), and Injections.

TRIAMTERENE

Chemical name: 2,4,7-Pteridinetriamine, 6-phenyl-.

Molecular formula: $C_{12}H_{11}N_7$.

Molecular weight: 253.27.

Description: Triamterene USP—Yellow, odorless, crystalline powder.

pKa: 6.2.

Solubility: Triamterene USP—Practically insoluble in water, in chloroform, in ether, and in dilute alkali hydroxides; soluble in formic acid; sparingly soluble in methoxyethanol; very slightly soluble in acetic acid, in alcohol, and in dilute mineral acids.

USP requirements:
Triamterene USP—Preserve in tight, light-resistant containers. Contains not less than 98.0% and not more than 102.0% of triamterene, calculated on the dried basis. Meets the requirements for Identification, Loss on drying (not

more than 1.0%), Ordinary impurities, and Limit for 2,4,6-triamino-5-nitrosopyrimidine (not more than 0.1%).

Triamterene Capsules USP—Preserve in tight, light-resistant containers. Contain the labeled amount, within ±7%. Meet the requirements for Identification and Uniformity of dosage units.

Triamterene Tablets—Not in USP.

TRIAMTERENE AND HYDROCHLOROTHIAZIDE

For *Triamterene* and *Hydrochlorothiazide*—See individual listings for chemistry information.

USP requirements:

Triamterene and Hydrochlorothiazide Capsules USP—Preserve in tight, light-resistant containers. Label Capsules to indicate the Dissolution test with which the product complies. Contain the labeled amounts, within ±10%. Meet the requirements for Identification, Dissolution (80% of each active ingredient in 120 minutes in 0.1 *M* acetic acid containing 1% of polysorbate 20 in Apparatus 2 at 100 rpm for Test 1 and 70% of triamterene and 80% of hydrochlorothiazide in 8 hours in 4.0% tetrasodium ethylenediaminetetraacetate, 2.0% polysorbate 40, 0.05% pancreatin in Apparatus 1 [use 10-mesh baskets] at 100 rpm for Test 2), Related compounds (not more than 1.0%), and Uniformity of dosage units.

Note: The Capsules and Tablets dosage forms should not be considered bioequivalent. If patients are to be transferred from one dosage form to the other, retitration and appropriate changes in dosage may be necessary.

Triamterene and Hydrochlorothiazide Tablets USP—Preserve in tight, light-resistant containers. Contain the labeled amounts, within ±10%. Meet the requirements for Identification, Dissolution (80% of each active ingredient in 30 minutes in 0.1 *N* hydrochloric acid in Apparatus 2 at 75 rpm), Related compounds (not more than 1.0%), and Uniformity of dosage units.

Note: The Capsules and Tablets dosage forms should not be considered bioequivalent. If patients are to be transferred from one dosage form to the other, retitration and appropriate changes in dosage may be necessary.

TRIAZOLAM

Chemical name: 4*H*-[1,2,4]Triazolo[4,3-*a*][1,4]benzodiazepine, 8-chloro-6-(2-chlorophenyl)-1-methyl-.

Molecular formula: $C_{17}H_{12}Cl_2N_4$.

Molecular weight: 343.22.

Description: Triazolam USP—White to off-white, practically odorless, crystalline powder.

Solubility: Triazolam USP—Soluble in chloroform; slightly soluble in alcohol; practically insoluble in ether and in water.

USP requirements:

Triazolam USP—Preserve in well-closed containers. Contains not less than 97.0% and not more than 103.0% of triazolam, calculated on the dried basis. Meets the requirements for Identification, Loss on drying (not more than 0.5%), Residue on ignition (not more than 0.5%), Heavy metals (not more than 0.002%), and Chromatographic purity.

Caution: Exercise care to prevent inhaling particles of triazolam and to prevent its contacting any part of the body.

Triazolam Tablets USP—Preserve in tight, light-resistant containers. Contain the labeled amount, within ±10%. Meet the requirements for Identification, Dissolution (70% in 30 minutes in water in Apparatus 2 at 50 rpm), and Uniformity of dosage units.

TRICHLORFON

Chemical name: Dimethyl(2,2,2-trichloro-1-hydroxyethyl)phosphonate.

Molecular formula: $C_4H_8Cl_3O_4P$.

Molecular weight: 257.44.

Description: Trichlorfon USP—White crystalline powder. Decomposed by alkali. Melts at about 78 °C with decomposition.

Solubility: Trichlorfon USP—Freely soluble in acetone, in alcohol, in chloroform, in ether, and in water; very soluble in methylene chloride; very slightly soluble in hexane and in pentane.

USP requirements: Trichlorfon USP—Preserve in well-closed containers at a temperature not exceeding 25 °C. Label it to indicate that it is for veterinary use only. Contains not less than 98.0% and not more than 100.5% of trichlorfon, calculated on the anhydrous basis. Meets the requirements for Completeness of solution, Color of solution, Identification, Acidity, Limit of free chloride, Water (not more than 0.3%), Heavy metals (not more than 0.001%), and Chromatographic purity.

TRICHLORMETHIAZIDE

Chemical name: 2*H*-1,2,4-Benzothiadiazine-7-sulfonamide, 6-chloro-3-(dichloromethyl)-3,4-dihydro-, 1,1-dioxide.

Molecular formula: $C_8H_8Cl_3N_3O_4S_2$.

Molecular weight: 380.65.

Description: Trichlormethiazide USP—White or practically white, crystalline powder. Is odorless, or has a slight characteristic odor. Melts at about 274 °C, with decomposition.

pKa: 8.6.

Solubility: Trichlormethiazide USP—Very slightly soluble in water, in ether, and in chloroform; freely soluble in acetone; soluble in methanol; sparingly soluble in alcohol.

USP requirements:

Trichlormethiazide USP—Preserve in well-closed containers. Dried at 105 °C for 3 hours, contains not less than 98.0% and not more than 102.0% of trichlormethiazide. Meets the requirements for Identification, Loss on drying (not more than 0.5%), Residue on ignition (not more than 0.1%), Selenium (not more than 0.003%), Heavy metals (not more than 0.002%), and Diazotizable substances (not more than 2.5%).

Trichlormethiazide Tablets USP—Preserve in tight containers. Contain the labeled amount, within ±10%. Meet the requirements for Identification, Dissolution (65% in 60 minutes in water in Apparatus 2 at 50 rpm), and Uniformity of dosage units.

TRICHLOROMONOFLUOROMETHANE

Chemical name: Methane, trichlorofluoro-.

Molecular formula: CCl_3F.

Molecular weight: 137.37.

Description: Trichloromonofluoromethane NF—Clear, colorless gas, having a faint, ethereal odor. Its vapor pressure at 25 °C is about 796 mm of mercury (1 psig).

NF category: Aerosol propellant.

NF requirements: Trichloromonofluoromethane NF—Preserve in tight cylinders, and avoid exposure to excessive heat. Meets the requirements for Identification, Boiling temperature (approximately 24 °C), Water (not more than 0.001%), High-boiling residues (not more than 0.01%), and Inorganic chlorides.

TRICITRATES

For *Sodium Citrate, Potassium Citrate,* and *Citric Acid*—See individual listings for chemistry information.

USP requirements: Tricitrates Oral Solution USP—Preserve in tight containers. A solution of Sodium Citrate, Potassium Citrate, and Citric Acid in a suitable aqueous medium. Contains, in each 100 mL, not less than 2.23 grams and not more than 2.46 grams of sodium, equivalent to not less than 9.5 grams and not more than 10.5 grams of sodium citrate dihydrate; not less than 3.78 grams and not more than 4.18 grams of potassium, equivalent to not less than 10.45 grams and not more than 11.55 grams of potassium citrate monohydrate; not less than 12.20 grams and not more than 13.48 grams of citrate as sodium citrate and potassium citrate; and not less than 6.34 grams and not more than 7.02 grams of citric acid monohydrate. Meets the requirements for Identification and pH (4.9–5.4).

Note: The sodium and potassium ion contents of Tricitrates Oral Solution are each approximately 1 mEq per mL.

TRIDIHEXETHYL

Chemical group: Quaternary ammonium compound.

Chemical name: Tridihexethyl chloride—Benzenepropanaminium, gamma-cyclohexyl-*N,N,N*-triethyl-gamma-hydroxy-, chloride.

Molecular formula: Tridihexethyl chloride—$C_{21}H_{36}ClNO$.

Molecular weight: Tridihexethyl chloride—353.98.

Description: Tridihexethyl Chloride USP—White, odorless, crystalline powder.

Solubility: Tridihexethyl Chloride USP—Freely soluble in water, in methanol, and in chloroform; practically insoluble in ether and in acetone.

USP requirements:

Tridihexethyl Chloride USP—Preserve in tight containers. Dried at 105 °C for 2 hours, contains not less than 98.0% and not more than 100.5% of tridihexethyl chloride. Meets the requirements for Identification, Melting range (196–202 °C), Loss on drying (not more than 0.5%), Residue on ignition (not more than 0.1%), Sulfate (not more than 0.04%), Heavy metals (not more than 0.002%), Ordinary impurities, Chloride content (9.81–10.06%), and Organic volatile impurities.

Tridihexethyl Chloride Injection USP—Preserve in single-dose containers, preferably of Type I glass. A sterile solution of Tridihexethyl Chloride in Water for Injection. Contains the labeled amount, within ±10%. Meets the requirements for Identification, Bacterial endotoxins, pH (5.0–7.5), and Injections.

Tridihexethyl Chloride Tablets USP—Preserve in tight containers. Contain the labeled amount, within ±10%. Meet the requirements for Identification, Dissolution (75% in 45 minutes in water in Apparatus 1 at 100 rpm), and Uniformity of dosage units.

TRIENTINE

Chemical name: Trientine hydrochloride—1,2-Ethanediamine, *N,N'*-bis(2-aminoethyl)-, dihydrochloride.

Molecular formula: Trientine hydrochloride—$C_6H_{18}N_4 \cdot 2HCl$.

Molecular weight: Trientine hydrochloride—219.16.

Description: Trientine Hydrochloride USP—White to pale yellow, crystalline powder. Melts at about 117 °C.

Solubility: Trientine Hydrochloride USP—Insoluble in chloroform and in ether; slightly soluble in alcohol; soluble in methanol; freely soluble in water.

USP requirements:

Trientine Hydrochloride USP—Preserve under an inert gas in tight, light-resistant containers, and store in a refrigerator. Contains not less than 97.0% and not more than 103.0% of trientine hydrochloride, calculated on the dried basis. Meets the requirements for Identification, pH (7.0–8.5, in a solution [1 in 100]), Loss on drying (not more than 2.0%), Residue on ignition (not more than 0.15%), Heavy metals (not more than 0.001%), Chromatographic purity, and Organic volatile impurities.

Trientine Hydrochloride Capsules USP—Preserve in tight containers, and store in a refrigerator. Contain the labeled amount, within ±10%. Meet the requirements for Identification, Dissolution (80% in 30 minutes in water in Apparatus 2 at 50 rpm), and Uniformity of dosage units.

TRIETHYL CITRATE

Molecular formula: $C_{12}H_{20}O_7$.

Molecular weight: 276.29.

Description: Triethyl Citrate NF—Odorless, practically colorless, oily liquid.

NF category: Plasticizer.

Solubility: Triethyl Citrate NF—Slightly soluble in water; miscible with alcohol and with ether.

NF requirements: Triethyl Citrate NF—Preserve in tight containers. Contains not less than 99.0% and not more than 100.5% of triethyl citrate, calculated on the anhydrous basis. Meets the requirements for Specific gravity (1.135–1.139), Refractive index (1.439–1.441), Acidity, and Water (not more than 0.25%).

TRIETHANOLAMINE

USP requirements: Triethanolamine Salicylate Cream—Not in USP.

TRIFLUOPERAZINE

Chemical group: Phenothiazine derivative of piperazine.

Chemical name: Trifluoperazine hydrochloride—10*H*-Phenothiazine, 10-[3-(4-methyl-1-piperazinyl)propyl]-2-(trifluoromethyl)-, dihydrochloride.

Molecular formula: Trifluoperazine hydrochloride—$C_{21}H_{24}F_3N_3S \cdot 2HCl$.

Molecular weight: Trifluoperazine hydrochloride—480.42.

Description: Trifluoperazine Hydrochloride USP—White to pale yellow, crystalline powder. Is practically odorless. Melts at about 242 °C, with decomposition.

Solubility: Trifluoperazine Hydrochloride USP—Freely soluble in water; soluble in alcohol; sparingly soluble in chloroform; insoluble in ether.

USP requirements:

Trifluoperazine Hydrochloride USP—Preserve in tight, light-resistant containers. Dried in vacuum at 60 °C for 4 hours, contains not less than 98.0% and not more than 101.0% of trifluoperazine hydrochloride. Meets the requirements for Identification, pH (1.7–2.6, in a solution [1 in 20]), Loss on drying (not more than 1.5%), Residue on ignition (not more than 0.1%), and Organic volatile impurities.

Trifluoperazine Hydrochloride Injection USP—Preserve in multiple-dose containers, preferably of Type I glass, protected from light. A sterile solution of Trifluoperazine Hydrochloride in Water for Injection. Contains an amount of trifluoperazine hydrochloride equivalent to the labeled amount of trifluoperazine, within ±10%. Meets the requirements for Identification, Bacterial endotoxins, pH (4.0–5.0), and Injections.

Trifluoperazine Hydrochloride Oral Solution—Not in USP.

Trifluoperazine Hydrochloride Syrup USP—Preserve in tight, light-resistant containers. Contains an amount of trifluoperazine hydrochloride equivalent to the labeled amount of trifluoperazine, within ±7%. Meets the requirements for Identification and pH (2.0–3.2).

Trifluoperazine Hydrochloride Tablets USP—Preserve in well-closed, light-resistant containers. Contain an amount of trifluoperazine hydrochloride equivalent to the labeled amount of trifluoperazine, within ±7%. Meet the requirements for Identification, Dissolution (75% in 30 minutes in 0.1 *N* hydrochloric acid in Apparatus 1 at 50 rpm), and Uniformity of dosage units.

TRIFLUPROMAZINE

Chemical group: Phenothiazine.

Chemical name:

Triflupromazine—10*H*-Phenothiazine-10-propanamine, *N,N*-dimethyl-2-(trifluoromethyl)-.

Triflupromazine hydrochloride—10*H*-Phenothiazine-10-propanamine, *N,N*-dimethyl-2-(trifluoromethyl)-, monohydrochloride.

Molecular formula:

Triflupromazine—$C_{18}H_{19}F_3N_2S$.

Triflupromazine hydrochloride—$C_{18}H_{19}F_3N_2S \cdot HCl$.

Molecular weight:

Triflupromazine—352.42.

Triflupromazine hydrochloride—388.88.

Description:

Triflupromazine USP—Viscous, light amber-colored, oily liquid, which crystallizes on prolonged standing into large, irregular crystals.

Triflupromazine Hydrochloride USP—White to pale tan, crystalline powder, having a slight characteristic odor. Melts between 170 and 178 °C.

Solubility:

Triflupromazine USP—Practically insoluble in water.

Triflupromazine Hydrochloride USP—Soluble in water, in alcohol, and in acetone; insoluble in ether.

USP requirements:

Triflupromazine USP—Preserve in tight, light-resistant containers. Contains not less than 97.0% and not more than 103.0% of triflupromazine. Meets the requirements for Identification, Residue on ignition (not more than 0.2%), Ordinary impurities, and Organic volatile impurities.

Triflupromazine Oral Suspension USP—Preserve in tight, light-resistant, glass containers. Contains an amount of triflupromazine equivalent to the labeled amount of triflupromazine hydrochloride, within ±10%. Meets the requirement for Identification.

Triflupromazine Hydrochloride USP—Preserve in tight, light-resistant glass containers. Contains not less than 97.0% and not more than 103.0% of triflupromazine hydrochloride, calculated on the dried basis. Meets the requirements for Identification, Loss on drying (not more than 0.5%), Residue on ignition (not more than 0.1%), Ordinary impurities, and Organic volatile impurities.

Triflupromazine Hydrochloride Injection USP—Preserve in single-dose or in multiple-dose containers, preferably of Type I glass, protected from light. A sterile solution of Triflupromazine Hydrochloride in Water for Injection. Contains the labeled amount, within −10% to +12%. Meets the requirements for Identification, Bacterial endotoxins, pH (3.5–5.2), and Injections.

Triflupromazine Hydrochloride Tablets USP—Preserve in well-closed, light-resistant containers. Contain the labeled amount, within ±10%. Meet the requirements for Identification, Dissolution (75% in 45 minutes in 0.1 *N* hydrochloric acid in Apparatus 1 at 100 rpm), and Uniformity of dosage units.

TRIFLURIDINE

Chemical group: Fluorinated pyrimidine nucleoside.

Chemical name: Thymidine, alpha,alpha,alpha-trifluoro-.

Molecular formula: $C_{10}H_{11}F_3N_2O_5$.

Molecular weight: 296.20.

Description: White crystals melting at about 188 °C.

Solubility: Soluble in water and in alcohol.

USP requirements: Trifluridine Ophthalmic Solution—Not in USP.

TRIHEXYPHENIDYL

Chemical group: Tertiary amine.

Chemical name: Trihexyphenidyl hydrochloride—1-Piperidinepropanol, alpha-cyclohexyl-alpha-phenyl-, hydrochloride.

Molecular formula: Trihexyphenidyl hydrochloride—$C_{20}H_{31}NO \cdot HCl$.

Molecular weight: Trihexyphenidyl hydrochloride—337.93.

Description: Trihexyphenidyl Hydrochloride USP—White or slightly off-white, crystalline powder, having not more than a very faint odor. Melts at about 250 °C.

Solubility: Trihexyphenidyl Hydrochloride USP—Slightly soluble in water; soluble in alcohol and in chloroform.

USP requirements:

Trihexyphenidyl Hydrochloride USP—Preserve in tight containers. Contains not less than 98.0% and not more than 102.0% of trihexyphenidyl hydrochloride, calculated on the dried basis. Meets the requirements for Identification, Loss on drying (not more than 0.5%), Residue on ignition (not more than 0.1%), Heavy metals (not more than 0.002%), Chloride content (10.3–10.7%, calculated on the dried basis), and Chromatographic purity.

Trihexyphenidyl Hydrochloride Extended-release Capsules USP—Preserve in tight containers. Contain the labeled amount, within ±10%. Meet the requirements for Identification, Drug release (20–50% at 0.25*D* hours, 40–70% at 0.50*D* hours, and not less than 70% at 1.00*D* hours in water in Apparatus 1 at 100 rpm), and Uniformity of dosage units.

Trihexyphenidyl Hydrochloride Elixir USP—Preserve in tight containers. Contains the labeled amount, within ±10%. Meets the requirements for Identification, pH (2.0–3.0), and Alcohol content (within ±10% of labeled amount).

Trihexyphenidyl Hydrochloride Tablets USP—Preserve in tight containers. Contain the labeled amount, within ±10%. Meet the requirements for Identification, Dissolution (75% in 45 minutes in acetate buffer [pH 4.5] in Apparatus 1 at 100 rpm), and Uniformity of dosage units.

TRIKATES

For *Potassium Acetate, Potassium Bicarbonate,* and *Potassium Citrate*—See individual listings for chemistry information.

USP requirements: Trikates Oral Solution USP—Preserve in tight, light-resistant containers. A solution of Potassium Acetate, Potassium Bicarbonate, and Potassium Citrate in Purified Water. Contains the labeled amount of potassium, within ±10%. Meets the requirement for Identification.

TRILOSTANE

Chemical name: Androst-2-ene-2-carbonitrile, 4,5-epoxy-3,17-dihydroxy-, (4 alpha,5 alpha,17 beta)-.

Molecular formula: $C_{20}H_{27}NO_3$.

Molecular weight: 329.44.

Description: White to nearly white crystalline powder.

Solubility: Practically insoluble in water.

USP requirements: Trilostane Capsules—Not in USP.

TRIMEPRAZINE

Chemical group: Phenothiazine derivative.

Chemical name: Trimeprazine tartrate—10*H*-Phenothiazine-10-propanamine *N,N*,beta-trimethyl-, [*R*-(*R**,*R**)]-2,3-dihydroxybutanedioate (2:1).

Molecular formula: Trimeprazine tartrate—$(C_{18}H_{22}N_2S)_2 \cdot C_4H_6O_6$.

Molecular weight: Trimeprazine tartrate—746.98.

Description: Trimeprazine Tartrate USP—White to off-white, odorless, crystalline powder.

Solubility: Trimeprazine Tartrate USP—Freely soluble in water and in chloroform; soluble in alcohol; very slightly soluble in ether.

USP requirements:

Trimeprazine Tartrate USP—Preserve in tight, light-resistant containers. Contains not less than 98.0% and not more than 101.0% of trimeprazine tartrate, calculated on the dried basis. Meets the requirements for Identification, Loss on drying (not more than 0.5%), Residue on ignition (not more than 0.1%), Heavy metals (not more than 0.002%), and Ordinary impurities.

Trimeprazine Tartrate Extended-release Capsules—Not in USP.

Trimeprazine Tartrate Syrup USP—Preserve in tight, light-resistant containers. Contains an amount of trimeprazine tartrate equivalent to the labeled amount of trimeprazine, within ±10%. Meets the requirements for Identification and Alcohol content (4.5–6.5%).

Trimeprazine Tartrate Tablets USP—Preserve in well-closed, light-resistant containers. Contain an amount of trimeprazine tartrate equivalent to the labeled amount of trimeprazine, within ±7%. Meet the requirements for Identification, Dissolution (75% in 45 minutes in 0.1 *N* hydrochloric acid in Apparatus 1 at 100 rpm), and Uniformity of dosage units.

TRIMETHADIONE

Chemical group: Oxazolidinedione.

Chemical name: 2,4-Oxazolidinedione, 3,5,5-trimethyl-.

Molecular formula: $C_6H_9NO_3$.

Molecular weight: 143.14.

Description: Trimethadione USP—White, crystalline granules. Has a slight camphor-like odor.

Solubility: Trimethadione USP—Soluble in water; freely soluble in alcohol, in ether, and in chloroform.

USP requirements:

Trimethadione USP—Preserve in tight containers, preferably at controlled room temperature. Contains not less than 98.0% and not more than 102.0% of trimethadione, calculated on the dried basis. Meets the requirements for Identification, Melting range (45–47 °C), Loss on drying (not more than 0.5%), Residue on ignition (not more than 0.1%), Urethane (not more than 1 ppm), and Organic volatile impurities.

Trimethadione Capsules USP—Preserve in tight containers, preferably at controlled room temperature. Contain the labeled amount, within ±6%. Meet the requirements for Identification, Dissolution (80% in 30 minutes in water in Apparatus 1 at 100 rpm), and Uniformity of dosage units.

Trimethadione Oral Solution USP—Preserve in tight containers, preferably at controlled room temperature. An aqueous solution of trimethadione. Contains the labeled amount, within ±6%. Meets the requirements for Identification and pH (3.0–5.0).

Trimethadione Tablets USP—Preserve in tight containers, preferably at a temperature not exceeding 25 °C. Contain the labeled amount, within ±6%. Meet the requirements for Identification, Disintegration (30 minutes), and Uniformity of dosage units.

TRIMETHAPHAN

Chemical name: Trimethaphan camsylate—Thieno[1′,2′:1,2]-thieno[3,4-*d*]imidazol-5-ium, decahydro-2-oxo-1,3-bis(phenylmethyl)-, salt with (+)-7,7-dimethyl-2-oxobicyclo[2.2.1]-heptane-1-methanesulfonic acid (1:1).

Molecular formula: Trimethaphan camsylate—$C_{32}H_{40}N_2O_5S_2$.

Molecular weight: Trimethaphan camsylate—596.80.

Description: Trimethaphan Camsylate USP—White crystals or white, crystalline powder. Is odorless or has a slight odor. Its solution (1 in 10) is clear and practically colorless. Melts at about 232 °C, with decomposition.

Solubility: Trimethaphan Camsylate USP—Freely soluble in water, in alcohol, and in chloroform; insoluble in ether.

USP requirements:
Trimethaphan Camsylate USP—Preserve in tight containers, in a cold place. Contains not less than 99.0% and not more than 101.5% of trimethaphan camsylate, calculated on the dried basis. Meets the requirements for Identification, Specific rotation (+20° to +23°), Loss on drying (not more than 0.1%), Residue on ignition (not more than 0.1%), and Selenium (not more than 0.003%).
Trimethaphan Camsylate Injection USP—Preserve in single-dose or in multiple-dose containers, preferably of Type I glass. Store in a refrigerator, but avoid freezing. A sterile solution of Trimethaphan Camsylate in Water for Injection. Label it to indicate that it is to be appropriately diluted prior to administration. Contains the labeled amount, within ±7%. Meets the requirements for Identification, Bacterial endotoxins, pH (4.9–5.6), Particulate matter, and Injections.

TRIMETHOBENZAMIDE

Chemical group: Trimethobenzamide hydrochloride—Ethanolamine derivative.

Chemical name: Trimethobenzamide hydrochloride—Benzamide, *N*-[[4-[2-(dimethylamino)ethoxy]phenyl]methyl]-3,4,5-trimethoxy-, monohydrochloride.

Molecular formula: Trimethobenzamide hydrochloride—$C_{21}H_{28}N_2O_5 \cdot HCl$.

Molecular weight: Trimethobenzamide hydrochloride—424.92.

Description: Trimethobenzamide Hydrochloride USP—White, crystalline powder having a slight phenolic odor.

Solubility: Trimethobenzamide Hydrochloride USP—Soluble in water and in warm alcohol; insoluble in ether.

USP requirements:
Trimethobenzamide Hydrochloride USP—Preserve in well-closed containers. Dried at 105 °C for 4 hours, contains not less than 98.5% and not more than 100.5% of trimethobenzamide hydrochloride. Meets the requirements for Identification, Melting range (186–190 °C), Loss on drying (not more than 0.5%), Residue on ignition (not more than 0.1%), and Heavy metals (not more than 0.002%).
Trimethobenzamide Hydrochloride Capsules USP—Preserve in well-closed containers. Contain the labeled amount, within ±10%. Meet the requirements for Identification, Dissolution (75% in 45 minutes in water in Apparatus 1 at 100 rpm), and Uniformity of dosage units.
Trimethobenzamide Hydrochloride Injection USP—Preserve in single-dose or in multiple-dose containers, preferably of Type I glass. A sterile solution of Trimethobenzamide Hydrochloride in Water for Injection. Contains the labeled amount, within ±5%. Meets the requirements for Identification, Bacterial endotoxins, pH (4.5–5.5), and Injections.
Trimethobenzamide Hydrochloride Suppositories—Not in USP.

TRIMETHOPRIM

Chemical name: 2,4-Pyrimidinediamine, 5-[(3,4,5-trimethoxyphenyl)methyl]-.

Molecular formula: $C_{14}H_{18}N_4O_3$.

Molecular weight: 290.32.

Description: Trimethoprim USP—White to cream-colored, odorless crystals, or crystalline powder.

Solubility: Trimethoprim USP—Very slightly soluble in water; soluble in benzyl alcohol; sparingly soluble in chloroform and in methanol; slightly soluble in alcohol and in acetone; practically insoluble in ether and in carbon tetrachloride.

USP requirements:
Trimethoprim USP—Preserve in tight, light-resistant containers. Contains not less than 98.5% and not more than 101.0% of trimethoprim, calculated on the dried basis. Meets the requirements for Identification, Melting range (199–203 °C), Loss on drying (not more than 0.5%), Residue on ignition (not more than 0.1%), and Chromatographic impurities.
Trimethoprim Tablets USP—Preserve in tight, light-resistant containers. Contain the labeled amount, within ±10%. Meet the requirements for Identification, Dissolution (75% in 45 minutes in 0.01 *N* hydrochloric acid in Apparatus 2 at 50 rpm), and Uniformity of dosage units.

TRIMETREXATE

Chemical group: A dihydrofolate reductase inhibitor with general properties similar to those of methotrexate.

Chemical name: Trimetrexate glucuronate—2,4-Quinazolinediamine, 5-methyl-6-[[(3,4,5-trimethoxyphenyl)amino]-methyl]-, mono-D-glucuronate.

Molecular formula: Trimetrexate glucuronate—$C_{19}H_{23}N_5O_3 \cdot C_6H_{10}O_7$.

Molecular weight: Trimetrexate glucuronate—563.56.

Description:
Trimetrexate glucuronate—Tan-colored solid.
Trimetrexate glucuronate for injection—Pale greenish-yellow powder or cake.

pKa: 8.0 in 50% methanol/water.

Solubility: Trimetrexate glucuronate—Soluble in water.

USP requirements: Trimetrexate Glucuronate for Injection—Not in USP.

TRIMIPRAMINE

Chemical group: Dibenzazepine.

Chemical name: Trimipramine maleate—5*H*-Dibenz[*b,f*]-azepine-5-propanamine, 10,11-dihydro-*N,N*,beta-trimethyl-, (*Z*)-2-butenedioate (1:1).

Molecular formula: Trimipramine maleate—$C_{20}H_{26}N_2 \cdot C_4H_4O_4$.

Molecular weight: Trimipramine maleate—410.51.

Description: Trimipramine maleate—Almost odorless, white or slightly cream-colored, crystalline substance, melting at 140–144 °C.

pka: 8.0.

Solubility: Trimipramine maleate—Very slightly soluble in ether and in water; slightly soluble in ethyl alcohol and in acetone; freely soluble in chloroform and in methanol at 20 °C.

Other characteristics: Tertiary amine.

USP requirements:
Trimipramine Maleate Capsules—Not in USP.
Trimipramine Maleate Tablets—Not in USP.

TRIOXSALEN

Chemical name: 7*H*-Furo[3,2-*g*][1]benzopyran-7-one, 2,5,9-trimethyl-.

Molecular formula: $C_{14}H_{12}O_3$.

Molecular weight: 228.25.

Description: Trioxsalen USP—White to off-white or grayish, odorless, crystalline solid. Melts at about 230 °C.

Solubility: Trioxsalen USP—Practically insoluble in water; sparingly soluble in chloroform; slightly soluble in alcohol.

USP requirements:

Trioxsalen USP—Preserve in well-closed, light-resistant containers. Contains not less than 97.0% and not more than 103.0% of trioxsalen, calculated on the dried basis. Meets the requirements for Identification, Loss on drying (not more than 0.5%), Residue on ignition (not more than 0.5%), Related substances, and Organic volatile impurities.

Caution: Avoid exposing the skin to Trioxsalen.

Trioxsalen Tablets USP—Preserve in well-closed, light-resistant containers. Contain the labeled amount, within ±7%. Meet the requirements for Identification, Dissolution (75% in 60 minutes in dilute simulated intestinal fluid [1 in 12 solution of simulated intestinal fluid TS and water] in Apparatus 2 at 100 rpm), and Uniformity of dosage units.

TRIPELENNAMINE

Chemical group: Ethylenediamine derivative.

Chemical name:

Tripelennamine citrate—1,2-Ethanediamine, *N,N*-dimethyl-*N′*-(phenylmethyl)-*N′*-2-pyridinyl-, 2-hydroxy-1,2,3-propanetricarboxylate (1:1).

Tripelennamine hydrochloride—1,2-Ethanediamine, *N,N*-dimethyl-*N′*-(phenylmethyl)-*N′*-2-pyridinyl-, monohydrochloride.

Molecular formula:

Tripelennamine citrate—$C_{16}H_{21}N_3 \cdot C_6H_8O_7$.

Tripelennamine hydrochloride—$C_{16}H_{21}N_3 \cdot HCl$.

Molecular weight:

Tripelennamine citrate—447.49.

Tripelennamine hydrochloride—291.82.

Description:

Tripelennamine Citrate USP—White, crystalline powder. Its solutions are acid to litmus. Melts at about 107 °C.

Tripelennamine Hydrochloride USP—White, crystalline powder. Slowly darkens on exposure to light. Its solutions are practically neutral to litmus.

pKa: 3.9 and 9.0.

Solubility:

Tripelennamine Citrate USP—Freely soluble in water and in alcohol; very slightly soluble in ether; practically insoluble in chloroform.

Tripelennamine Hydrochloride USP—Freely soluble in water, in alcohol, and in chloroform; slightly soluble in acetone; insoluble in ether and in ethyl acetate.

USP requirements:

Tripelennamine Citrate USP—Preserve in well-closed, light-resistant containers. Contains not less than 98.0% and not more than 100.5% of tripelennamine citrate, calculated on the dried basis. Meets the requirements for Identification, Loss on drying (not more than 0.5%), Residue on ignition (not more than 0.1%), Ordinary impurities, and Organic volatile impurities.

Tripelennamine Citrate Elixir USP—Preserve in tight, light-resistant containers. Contains, in each 100 mL, not less than 705 mg and not more than 795 mg of tripelennamine citrate. Meets the requirements for Identification and Alcohol content (11.0–13.0%).

Tripelennamine Hydrochloride USP—Preserve in well-closed, light-resistant containers. Contains not less than 98.0% and not more than 100.5% of tripelennamine hydrochloride, calculated on the dried basis. Meets the requirements for Identification, Melting range (188–192 °C), Loss on drying (not more than 1.0%), Residue on ignition (not more than 0.1%), Ordinary impurities, and Organic volatile impurities.

Tripelennamine Hydrochloride Tablets USP—Preserve in well-closed containers. Contain the labeled amount, within ±5%. Meet the requirements for Identification, Dissolution (75% in 45 minutes in water in Apparatus 1 at 100 rpm), and Uniformity of dosage units.

Tripelennamine Hydrochloride Extended-release Tablets—Not in USP.

TRIPROLIDINE

Chemical group: Propylamine derivative (alkylamine).

Chemical name: Triprolidine hydrochloride—Pyridine, 2-[1-(4-methylphenyl)-3-(1-pyrrolidinyl)-1-propenyl]-, monohydrochloride, monohydrate, (*E*)-.

Molecular formula: Triprolidine hydrochloride—$C_{19}H_{22}N_2 \cdot HCl \cdot H_2O$.

Molecular weight: Triprolidine hydrochloride—332.87.

Description: Triprolidine Hydrochloride USP—White, crystalline powder, having no more than a slight, unpleasant odor. Its solutions are alkaline to litmus, and it melts at about 115 °C.

pKa: 3.6 and 9.3.

Solubility: Triprolidine Hydrochloride USP—Soluble in water, in alcohol, and in chloroform; insoluble in ether.

USP requirements:

Triprolidine Hydrochloride USP—Preserve in tight, light-resistant containers. Contains not less than 98.0% and not more than 101.0% of triprolidine hydrochloride, calculated on the anhydrous basis. Meets the requirements for Identification, Water (4.0–6.0%), Residue on ignition (not more than 0.1%), Arsenic (not more than 4 ppm), Heavy metals (not more than 0.002%), Chromatographic purity, and Organic volatile impurities.

Triprolidine Hydrochloride Syrup USP—Preserve in tight, light-resistant containers. Contain the labeled amount, within ±10%. Meets the requirements for Identification, pH (5.6–6.6), and Alcohol content (3.0–5.0%).

Triprolidine Hydrochloride Tablets USP—Preserve in tight, light-resistant containers. Contain the labeled amount, within ±10%. Meet the requirements for Identification, Dissolution (80% in 30 minutes in acetate buffer [pH 4.0 ±0.05] in Apparatus 1 at 50 rpm), and Uniformity of dosage units.

TRIPROLIDINE AND PSEUDOEPHEDRINE

For *Triprolidine* and *Pseudoephedrine*—See individual listings for chemistry information.

USP requirements:

Triprolidine Hydrochloride and Pseudoephedrine Hydrochloride Capsules—Not in USP.

Triprolidine Hydrochloride and Pseudoephedrine Hydrochloride Extended-release Capsules—Not in USP.

Triprolidine and Pseudoephedrine Hydrochlorides Syrup USP—Preserve in tight, light-resistant containers. Contains the labeled amounts of triprolidine hydrochloride and pseudoephedrine hydrochloride, within ±10%. Meets the requirement for Identification.

Triprolidine and Pseudoephedrine Hydrochlorides Tablets USP—Preserve in tight, light-resistant containers. Contain the labeled amounts of triprolidine hydrochloride and pseudoephedrine hydrochloride, within ±10%. Meet the requirements for Identification, Dissolution (75% of each active ingredient in 45 minutes in water in Apparatus 2 at 50 rpm), and Uniformity of dosage units.

TRIPROLIDINE, PSEUDOEPHEDRINE, AND ACETAMINOPHEN

For *Triprolidine, Pseudoephedrine,* and *Acetaminophen*—See individual listings for chemistry information.

USP requirements: Triprolidine Hydrochloride, Pseudoephedrine Hydrochloride, and Acetaminophen Tablets—Not in USP.

TRIPROLIDINE, PSEUDOEPHEDRINE, AND CODEINE

For *Triprolidine, Pseudoephedrine,* and *Codeine*—See individual listings for chemistry information.

USP requirements:

Triprolidine Hydrochloride, Pseudoephedrine Hydrochloride, and Codeine Phosphate Syrup—Not in USP.

Triprolidine Hydrochloride, Pseudoephedrine Hydrochloride, and Codeine Phosphate Tablets—Not in USP.

TRIPROLIDINE, PSEUDOEPHEDRINE, CODEINE, AND GUAIFENESIN

For *Triprolidine, Pseudoephedrine, Codeine,* and *Guaifenesin*—See individual listings for chemistry information.

USP requirements: Triprolidine Hydrochloride, Pseudoephedrine Hydrochloride, Codeine Phosphate, and Guaifenesin Oral Solution—Not in USP.

TRIPROLIDINE, PSEUDOEPHEDRINE, AND DEXTROMETHORPHAN

For *Triprolidine, Pseudoephedrine,* and *Dextromethorphan*—See individual listings for chemistry information.

USP requirements: Triprolidine Hydrochloride, Pseudoephedrine Hydrochloride, and Dextromethorphan Oral Solution—Not in USP.

TRISULFAPYRIMIDINES

For *Sulfadiazine, Sulfamerazine,* and *Sulfamethazine*—See individual listings for chemistry information.

USP requirements:

Trisulfapyrimidines Oral Suspension USP—Preserve in tight containers, at a temperature above freezing. Its label indicates the presence and proportion of any sodium citrate or sodium lactate and any antimicrobial agent. Contains, in each 100 mL, not less than 3.0 grams and not more than 3.7 grams of sulfadiazine, of sulfamerazine, and of sulfamethazine. May contain either Sodium Citrate or Sodium Lactate, and may contain a suitable antimicrobial agent. Meets the requirement for Identification.

Trisulfapyrimidines Tablets USP—Preserve in well-closed containers. Contain the labeled amount of each of the sulfapyrimidines, consisting of equal amounts of sulfadiazine, sulfamerazine, and sulfamethazine, within ±5%. Meet the requirements for Identification, Dissolution (70% of labeled amount of total sulfapyrimidines in 60 minutes in 0.1 *N* hydrochloric acid in Apparatus 2 at 50 rpm), and Uniformity of dosage units.

TROLAMINE

Chemical name: Ethanol, 2,2′,2″-nitrilotris-.

Molecular formula: $C_6H_{15}NO_3$.

Molecular weight: 149.19.

Description: Trolamine NF—Colorless to pale yellow, viscous, hygroscopic liquid, having a slight ammoniacal odor.

NF category: Alkalizing agent; emulsifying and/or solubilizing agent.

Solubility: Trolamine NF—Miscible with water and with alcohol. Soluble in chloroform.

NF requirements: Trolamine NF—Preserve in tight, light-resistant containers. A mixture of alkanolamines consisting largely of triethanolamine containing some diethanolamine and monoethanolamine. Contains not less than 99.0% and not more than 107.4% of alkanolamines, calculated on the anhydrous basis as triethanolamine. Meets the requirements for Identification, Specific gravity (1.120–1.128), Refractive index (1.481–1.486 at 20 °C), Water (not more than 0.5%), Residue on ignition (not more than 0.05%), and Organic volatile impurities.

TROLEANDOMYCIN

Chemical name: Oleandomycin, triacetate (ester).

Molecular formula: $C_{41}H_{67}NO_{15}$.

Molecular weight: 813.98.

Description: Troleandomycin USP—White, odorless, crystalline powder.

Solubility: Troleandomycin USP—Freely soluble in alcohol; soluble in chloroform; slightly soluble in ether and in water.

USP requirements:

Troleandomycin USP—Preserve in tight containers. Contains the equivalent of not less than 750 mcg of oleandomycin per mg. Meets the requirements for Identification, Crystallinity, pH (7.0–8.5, in a solution of alcohol and water [1:1] containing 100 mg per mL), Loss on drying (not more than 1.0%), Residue on ignition (not more than 0.1%), and Acetyl content (15.3–16.0%).

Troleandomycin Capsules USP—Preserve in tight containers. Contain an amount of troleandomycin equivalent to the labeled amount of oleandomycin, within −10% to +20%. Meet the requirements for Identification and Loss on drying (not more than 5.0%).

Troleandomycin Oral Suspension USP—Preserve in tight containers, in a cool place. Contains an amount of troleandomycin equivalent to the labeled amount of oleandomycin, within −10% to +25%. Contains one or more suitable buffers, colors, dispersants, and preservatives. Meets the requirements for Identification, Uniformity of dosage units (single-unit containers), Deliverable volume (multiple-unit containers), and pH (5.0–8.0).

TROMETHAMINE

Chemical name: 1,3-Propanediol, 2-amino-2-(hydroxymethyl)-.

Molecular formula: $C_4H_{11}NO_3$.

Molecular weight: 121.14.

Description: Tromethamine USP—White, crystalline powder, having a slight characteristic odor.

Solubility: Tromethamine USP—Freely soluble in water and in low molecular weight aliphatic alcohols; practically insoluble in chloroform and in carbon tetrachloride.

USP requirements:

Tromethamine USP—Preserve in tight containers. Contains not less than 99.0% and not more than 101.0% of tromethamine, calculated on the dried basis. Meets the requirements for Identification, Melting range (168–172 °C), pH (10.0–11.5, in a solution [1 in 20]), Loss on drying (not more than 1.0%), Residue on ignition (not more than 0.1%), Heavy metals (not more than 0.001%), and Organic volatile impurities.

Tromethamine for Injection USP—Preserve in Containers for Sterile Solids. A sterile, lyophilized mixture of tromethamine with Potassium Chloride and Sodium Chloride. Contains the labeled amount of tromethamine, within ±7%, and the labeled amounts of potassium chloride and sodium chloride, within ±10%. Meets the requirements for Constituted solution, Identification, Bacterial endotoxins, pH (10.0–11.5, in a solution constituted as directed in the labeling), Water (not more than 1.0%), Particulate matter, Potassium chloride content, and Sodium chloride content, and for Sterility tests, Uniformity of dosage units, and Labeling under Injections.

TROPICAMIDE

Chemical name: Benzeneacetamide, *N*-ethyl-alpha-(hydroxymethyl)-*N*-(4-pyridinylmethyl)-.

Molecular formula: $C_{17}H_{20}N_2O_2$.

Molecular weight: 284.36.

Description: Tropicamide USP—White or practically white, crystalline powder, odorless or having not more than a slight odor.

Solubility: Tropicamide USP—Slightly soluble in water; freely soluble in chloroform and in solutions of strong acids.

USP requirements:

Tropicamide USP—Preserve in tight, light-resistant containers. Contains not less than 99.0% and not more than 101.0% of tropicamide, calculated on the dried basis. Meets the requirements for Identification, Melting range (96–100 °C), Loss on drying (not more than 0.5%), and Heavy metals (not more than 0.002%).

Tropicamide Ophthalmic Solution USP—Preserve in tight containers, and avoid freezing. A sterile aqueous solution of Tropicamide. Contains the labeled amount, within ±5%. Contains a suitable antimicrobial agent, and may contain suitable substances to increase its viscosity. Meets the requirements for Identification, Sterility, and pH (4.0–5.8).

TRYPSIN

Description:

Crystallized Trypsin USP—White to yellowish white, odorless, crystalline or amorphous powder.

Crystallized Trypsin for Inhalation Aerosol—White to yellowish white, crystalline or amorphous powder.

USP requirements:

Crystallized Trypsin USP—Preserve in tight containers, and avoid exposure to excessive heat. A proteolytic enzyme crystallized from an extract of the pancreas gland of the ox, *Bos taurus* Linné (Fam. Bovidae). When assayed as directed in *USP/NF,* contains not less than 2500 USP Trypsin Units in each mg, calculated on the dried basis, and not less than 90.0% and not more than 110.0% of the labeled potency. Meets the requirements for Solubility test, Microbial limit, Loss on drying (not more than 5.0%), Residue on ignition (not more than 2.5%), and Chymotrypsin (not more than approximately 5%).

Note: Determine the suitability of the substrates and check the adjustment of the spectrophotometer by performing the Assay using USP Crystallized Trypsin Reference Standard.

Crystallized Trypsin for Inhalation Aerosol USP—Preserve in single-dose containers, preferably of Type I glass, and avoid exposure to excessive heat. Prepared by cryodesiccation. Contains the labeled potency, within ±10%. Meets the requirements for Identification and Solubility test.

TRYPTOPHAN

Chemical name: L-Tryptophan.

Molecular formula: $C_{11}H_{12}N_2O_2$.

Molecular weight: 204.23.

Description: Tryptophan USP—White to slightly yellowish white crystals or crystalline powder.

Solubility: Tryptophan USP—Soluble in hot alcohol and in dilute hydrochloric acid.

USP requirements: Tryptophan USP—Preserve in well-closed containers. Contains not less than 98.5% and not more than 101.5% of tryptophan, as L-tryptophan, calculated on the dried basis. Meets the requirements for Identification, Specific rotation (−29.4° to −32.8°, calculated on the dried basis), pH (5.5–7.0, in a solution [1 in 100]), Loss on drying (not more than 0.3%), Residue on ignition (not more than 0.1%), Chloride (not more than 0.05%), Sulfate (not more than 0.03%), Arsenic (not more than 1.5 ppm), Iron (not more than 0.003%), Heavy metals (not more than 0.0015%), and Organic volatile impurities.

TUAMINOHEPTANE

Chemical name: 2-Heptanamine.

Molecular formula: $C_7H_{17}N$.

Molecular weight: 115.22.

Description: Tuaminoheptane USP—Volatile, colorless to pale yellow liquid, having an amine-like odor. On exposure to air it may absorb carbon dioxide with the formation of a white precipitate of tuaminoheptane carbonate.

Solubility: Tuaminoheptane USP—Sparingly soluble in water; freely soluble in alcohol, in chloroform, and in ether.

USP requirements:

Tuaminoheptane USP—Preserve in tight containers, and store in a cool place. Contains not less than 99.0% and not more than 100.5% of tuaminoheptane. Meets the requirements for Identification, Specific gravity (0.760–0.763), Refractive index (1.415–1.417), and Nonvolatile residue (not more than 0.2%).

Tuaminoheptane Inhalant USP—Preserve in tight containers (inhalers), and avoid exposure to excessive heat. Consists of cylindrical rolls of suitable fibrous material impregnated with Tuaminoheptane (as the carbonate), usually aromatized, and contained in a suitable inhaler.

The inhaler contains the labeled amount of tuaminoheptane, within −10% to +25%. Meets the requirement for Identification.

TUBERCULIN

Description: Tuberculin USP—Old Tuberculin is a clear, brownish liquid and has a characteristic odor. Purified Protein Derivative (PPD) of Tuberculin is a very slightly opalescent, colorless solution. Old Tuberculin and PPD concentrates contain 50% of glycerin for use with various application devices. Old Tuberculin and PPD are also dried on the tines of multiple-puncture devices.

Solubility: Tuberculin USP—Old Tuberculin is readily miscible with water.

USP requirements: Tuberculin USP—Preserve at a temperature between 2 and 8 °C. Multiple-puncture devices may be stored at a temperature not exceeding 30 °C. A sterile solution derived from the concentrated, soluble products of growth of the tubercle bacillus (*Mycobacterium tuberculosis* or *Mycobacterium bovis*) prepared in a special medium. Provided either as Old Tuberculin, a culture filtrate adjusted to the standard potency based on the U.S. Standard Tuberculin, Old, by addition of glycerin and isotonic sodium chloride solution, or as Purified Protein Derivative (PPD), a further purified protein fraction standardized with the U.S. Standard Tuberculin, Purified Protein Derivative. Has a potency, tested by comparison with the corresponding U.S. Standard Tuberculin, on intradermal injection of sensitized guinea pigs, of between 80–120% of that stated on the label. Free from viable *Mycobacteria* as shown by injection into guinea pigs. Meets the requirement for Expiration date (for concentrated Old Tuberculin containing 50% of glycerin, not later than 5 years after date of issue from manufacturer's cold storage [5 °C, 1 year; or 0 °C, 2 years]; for diluted Old Tuberculin, not later than 1 year after date of issue from manufacturer's cold storage [5 °C, 1 year; or 0 °C, 2 years]; for concentrated PPD containing 50% of glycerin, not later than 2 years after date of issue from manufacturer's cold storage [5 °C, 1 year]; for diluted PPD, not later than 1 year after date of issue by the manufacturer; for Old Tuberculin and PPD dried on multiple-puncture devices, not later than 2 years after date of issue from manufacturer's cold storage [30 °C, 1 year], provided the recommended storage is at a temperature not exceeding 30 °C). Conforms to the regulations of the U.S. Food and Drug Administration concerning biologics.

TUBOCURARINE

Chemical name: Tubocurarine chloride—Tubocuraranium, 7′,12′-dihydroxy-6,6′-dimethoxy-2,2′,2′-trimethyl-, chloride, hydrochloride, pentahydrate.

Molecular formula: Tubocurarine chloride—$C_{37}H_{41}ClN_2O_6 \cdot HCl \cdot 5H_2O$ (pentahydrate); $C_{37}H_{41}ClN_2O_6 \cdot HCl$ (anhydrous).

Molecular weight: Tubocurarine chloride—771.73 (pentahydrate); 681.65 (anhydrous).

Description: Tubocurarine Chloride USP—White or yellowish white to grayish white, crystalline powder. Melts at about 270 °C, with decomposition.

Solubility: Tubocurarine Chloride USP—Soluble in water; sparingly soluble in alcohol.

USP requirements:

Tubocurarine Chloride USP—Preserve in tight containers. Contains not less than 95.0% and not more than 105.0% of tubocurarine chloride, calculated on the anhydrous basis. Meets the requirements for Identification, Specific rotation (+210° to +224°, calculated on the anhydrous basis), Water (not more than 12.0%), Residue on ignition (not more than 0.25%), Related substances, and Chloride content (9.9–10.7%, calculated on the anhydrous basis).

Tubocurarine Chloride Injection USP—Preserve in single-dose or in multiple-dose containers. A sterile solution of Tubocurarine Chloride in Water for Injection. Contains the labeled amount, within ±7%. Meets the requirements for Identification, Angular rotation (+0.32° to +0.48° for each mg of tubocurarine chloride per mL claimed on the label), Bacterial endotoxins, pH (2.5–5.0), and Injections.

TYLOXAPOL

Chemical name: Phenol, 4-(1,1,3,3-tetramethylbutyl)-, polymer with formaldehyde and oxirane.

Description: Tyloxapol USP—Viscous, amber liquid, having a slight, aromatic odor. May exhibit a slight turbidity.

NF category: Wetting and/or solubilizing agent.

Solubility: Tyloxapol USP—Slowly but freely miscible with water. Soluble in glacial acetic acid, in toluene, in carbon tetrachloride, in chloroform, and in carbon disulfide.

USP requirements: Tyloxapol USP—Preserve in tight containers. A nonionic liquid polymer of the alkyl aryl polyether alcohol type. Meets the requirements for Identification, Cloud point (92–97 °C), pH (4.0–7.0, in a solution [1 in 20]), Residue on ignition (not more than 1.0%), Free phenol, Limit of anionic detergents (not more than 0.075%), Absence of cationic detergents, Limit of formaldehyde (not more than 0.0075%), Limit of ethylene oxide (not more than 10 ppm), and Organic volatile impurities.

Note: Precautions should be exercised to prevent contact of Tyloxapol with metals.

TYPHOID VACCINE

Description: Typhoid Vaccine USP—More or less turbid, milky fluid, practically odorless or having a faint odor due to the antimicrobial agent, or white solid having the characteristic appearance of freeze-dried products.

USP requirements: Typhoid Vaccine USP—Preserve at a temperature between 2 and 8 °C. A sterile suspension or solid containing killed typhoid bacilli (*Salmonella typhosa*) of the Ty 2 strain. Label it to state that it is to be well shaken before use and that it is not to be frozen. Has a labeled potency of 8 units per mL. Geometric mean potency, determined by the specific mouse potency test based on the U.S. Standard Typhoid Vaccine using the Ty 2 strain for challenge, from at least 2 assays is not less than 3.9 units per mL. Aqueous vaccine and any constituting fluid supplied with dried vaccine contains a preservative. Dried vaccine contains no preservative. Meets the requirements for Expiration date (not later than 18 months after date of issue from manufacturer's cold storage [5 °C, 1 year]) and Nitrogen content (total not more than 35.0 mcg per mL for non-extracted bacteria preparations and not more than 23.0 mcg per mL for acetone-extracted bacteria preparations). Conforms to the regulations of the U.S. Food and Drug Administration concerning biologics.

TYPHOID VACCINE LIVE ORAL

Source: Typhoid vaccine Ty21a is a live attenuated vaccine for oral administration. The vaccine contains the attenuated strain *Salmonella typhi* Ty21a. The vaccine strain is grown under controlled conditions in a medium containing dextrose, galactose, a digest of bovine tissues, and an acid digest of casein. The bacteria are collected by centrifugation, mixed with a stabilizer containing lactose and amino acids, and then lyophilized. The lyophilized bacteria mixture is placed in gelatin capsules, which are coated with an organic solution to render them resistant to dissolution by stomach acids.

USP requirements: Typhoid Vaccine Live Oral Enteric-coated Capsules—Not in USP.

TYROPANOATE

Chemical group: Triiodinated benzoic acid derivative.

Chemical name: Tyropanoate sodium—Benzenepropanoic acid, alpha-ethyl-2,4,6-triiodo-3-[(1-oxobutyl)amino]-, monosodium salt.

Molecular formula: Tyropanoate sodium—$C_{15}H_{17}I_3NNaO_3$.

Molecular weight: Tyropanoate sodium—663.01.

Description: Tyropanoate Sodium USP—White, hygroscopic, odorless powder.

Solubility: Tyropanoate Sodium USP—Soluble in water, in alcohol, and in dimethylformamide; very slightly soluble in acetone and in ether.

USP requirements:

Tyropanoate Sodium USP—Preserve in tight, light-resistant containers. Contains not less than 98.0% and not more than 102.0% of tyropanoate sodium, calculated on the anhydrous basis. Meets the requirements for Identification, Water (not more than 3.0%), Iodine and iodide, and Heavy metals (not more than 0.003%).

Tyropanoate Sodium Capsules USP—Preserve in tight, light-resistant containers. Contain the labeled amount, within ±6%. Meet the requirements for Identification, Iodine and iodide, and Uniformity of dosage units.

TYROSINE

Chemical name: L-Tyrosine.

Molecular formula: $C_9H_{11}NO_3$.

Molecular weight: 181.19.

Description: Tyrosine USP—White, odorless crystals or crystalline powder.

Solubility: Tyrosine USP—Very slightly soluble in water; insoluble in alcohol and in ether.

USP requirements: Tyrosine USP—Preserve in well-closed containers. Contains not less than 98.5% and not more than 101.5% of tyrosine, as L-tyrosine, calculated on the dried basis. Meets the requirements for Identification, Specific rotation (−9.8° to −11.2°, calculated on the dried basis), Loss on drying (not more than 0.3%), Residue on ignition (not more than 0.4%), Chloride (not more than 0.04%), Sulfate (not more than 0.04%), Arsenic (not more than 1.5 ppm), Iron (not more than 0.003%), Heavy metals (not more than 0.0015%), and Organic volatile impurities.

TYROTHRICIN

USP requirements: Tyrothricin USP—Preserve in tight containers. An antibacterial substance produced by the growth of *Bacillus brevis* Dubos (Fam. *Bacteriaceae*). Consists principally of gramicidin and tyrocidine, the tyrocidine usually being present as the hydrochloride. Contains not less than 900 mcg and not more than 1400 mcg of tyrothricin per mg. Meets the requirements for Identification and Loss on drying (not more than 5.0%).

UNDECYLENIC ACID

Chemical name: 10-Undecenoic acid.

Molecular formula: $C_{11}H_{20}O_2$.

Molecular weight: 184.28.

Description: Undecylenic Acid USP—Clear, colorless to pale yellow liquid having a characteristic odor.

Solubility: Undecylenic Acid USP—Practically insoluble in water; miscible with alcohol, with chloroform, with ether, and with fixed and volatile oils.

USP requirements: Undecylenic Acid USP—Preserve in tight, light-resistant containers. Contains not less than 97.0% and not more than 100.5% of undecylenic acid. Meets the requirements for Identification, Specific gravity (0.910–0.913), Congealing range (not lower than 21 °C), Refractive index (1.447–1.448), Residue on ignition (not more than 0.15%), Water-soluble acids, Heavy metals (not more than 0.001%), and Iodine value (131–138).

COMPOUND UNDECYLENIC ACID

For *Calcium Undecylenate, Undecylenic Acid,* and *Zinc Undecylenate*—See individual listings for chemistry information.

USP requirements:

Compound Undecylenic Acid Topical Aerosol Foam—Not in USP.

Compound Undecylenic Acid Topical Aerosol Powder—Not in USP.

Compound Undecylenic Acid Cream—Not in USP.

Compound Undecylenic Acid Ointment USP—Preserve in tight containers, and avoid prolonged exposure to temperatures exceeding 30 °C. Contains not less than 18.0% and not more than 22.0% of zinc undecylenate and not less than 4.5% and not more than 5.5% of free undecylenic acid, in a suitable ointment base.

Compound Undecylenic Acid Topical Powder—Not in USP.

Compound Undecylenic Acid Topical Solution—Not in USP.

URACIL MUSTARD

Chemical name: 2,4(1*H*,3*H*)-Pyrimidinedione, 5-[bis(2-chloroethyl)amino]-.

Molecular formula: $C_8H_{11}Cl_2N_3O_2$.

Molecular weight: 252.10.

Description: Off-white, odorless, crystalline powder. Melts at about 200 °C, with decomposition.

Solubility: Very slightly soluble in water; slightly soluble in acetone and in alcohol; practically insoluble in chloroform.

USP requirements: Uracil Mustard Capsules—Not in USP.

UREA

Chemical name: Urea.

Molecular formula: CH_4N_2O.

Molecular weight: 60.06.

Description:

Urea USP—Colorless to white, prismatic crystals, or white, crystalline powder, or small white pellets. Is practically odorless, but may gradually develop a slight odor of ammonia upon long standing. Its solutions are neutral to litmus.

Sterile Urea USP—Colorless to white, prismatic crystals, or white, crystalline powder, or small white pellets. Is practically odorless, but may gradually develop a slight odor of ammonia upon long standing. Its solutions are neutral to litmus.

Solubility: Urea USP—Freely soluble in water and in boiling alcohol; practically insoluble in chloroform and in ether.

USP requirements:

Urea USP—Preserve in well-closed containers. Contains not less than 99.0% and not more than 100.5% of urea. Meets the requirements for Identification, Melting range (132–135 °C), Residue on ignition (not more than 0.1%), Alcohol-insoluble matter (not more than 0.04%), Chloride (not more than 0.007%), Sulfate (not more than 0.010%), and Heavy metals (not more than 0.002%).

Sterile Urea USP—Preserve in Containers for Sterile Solids. It is Urea suitable for parenteral use. Meets the requirements for Completeness of solution, Constituted solution, and Bacterial endotoxins, for Identification tests, Melting range, Residue on ignition, Alcohol-insoluble matter, Chloride, Sulfate, and Heavy metals under Urea, and for Sterility tests, Uniformity of dosage units, and Labeling under Injections.

UROFOLLITROPIN

Source: A preparation of purified extract of human postmenopausal urine containing follicle-stimulating hormone (FSH).

Chemical name: Urofollitropin.

Description: Urofollitropin for injection—White to off-white powder or pellets.

USP requirements: Urofollitropin for Injection—Not in USP.

UROKINASE

Source: An enzyme obtained from human kidney cells by tissue culture techniques.

Chemical name: Kinase (enzyme-activating), uro-.

Molecular weight: 34,000 daltons.

Solubility: Soluble in water.

USP requirements: Urokinase for Injection—Not in USP.

URSODIOL

Source: Ursodeoxycholic acid, a naturally occurring human bile acid found in small quantities in normal human bile and in larger quantities in the biles of certain species of bears.

Chemical name: Cholan-24-oic acid, 3,7-dihydroxy-, (3 alpha,5 beta,7 beta)-.

Molecular formula: $C_{24}H_{40}O_4$.

Molecular weight: 392.58.

Description: White powder.

Solubility: Practically insoluble in water; freely soluble in ethanol and in glacial acetic acid; slightly soluble in chloroform; sparingly soluble in ether.

USP requirements: Ursodiol Capsules—Not in USP.

VACCINIA IMMUNE GLOBULIN

Description: Vaccinia Immune Globulin USP—Transparent or slightly opalescent liquid. Practically colorless and practically odorless. May develop a slight granular deposit during storage.

USP requirements: Vaccinia Immune Globulin USP—Preserve at a temperature between 2 and 8 °C. A sterile, non-pyrogenic solution of globulins derived from the blood plasma of adult human donors who have been immunized with vaccinia virus (Smallpox Vaccine). It is standardized for viral neutralizing activity in eggs or tissue culture with the U.S. Reference Vaccinia Immune Globulin and a specified vaccinia virus. Label it to state that it is not intended for intravenous injection. Contains not less than 15 grams and not more than 18 grams of protein per 100 mL, not less than 90.0% of which is gamma globulin. Contains 0.3 *M* glycine as a stabilizing agent, and contains a suitable antimicrobial agent. Meets the requirement for Expiration date (not later than 3 years after date of issue). Conforms to the regulations of the U.S. Food and Drug Administration concerning biologics.

VALINE

Chemical name: L-Valine.

Molecular formula: $C_5H_{11}NO_2$.

Molecular weight: 117.15.

Description: Valine USP—White, odorless crystals.

Solubility: Valine USP—Soluble in water; practically insoluble in ether, in alcohol, and in acetone.

USP requirements: Valine USP—Preserve in well-closed containers. Contains not less than 98.5% and not more than 101.5% of valine, as L-valine, calculated on the dried basis. Meets the requirements for Identification, Specific rotation (+26.6° to +28.4°, calculated on the dried basis), pH (5.5–7.0, in a solution [1 in 20]), Loss on drying (not more than 0.3%), Residue on ignition (not more than 0.1%), Chloride (not more than 0.05%), Sulfate (not more than 0.03%), Arsenic (not more than 1.5 ppm), Iron (not more than 0.003%), Heavy metals (not more than 0.0015%), and Organic volatile impurities.

VALPROIC ACID

Chemical name: Pentanoic acid, 2-propyl-.

Molecular formula: $C_8H_{16}O_2$.

Molecular weight: 144.21.

Description: Valproic Acid USP—Colorless to pale yellow, slightly viscous, clear liquid, having a characteristic odor. Refractive index: about 1.423 at 20 °C.

pKa: 4.8.

Solubility: Valproic Acid USP—Slightly soluble in water; freely soluble in 1 *N* sodium hydroxide, in methanol, in alcohol, in acetone, in chloroform, in ether, and in *n*-heptane; slightly soluble in 0.1 *N* hydrochloric acid.

USP requirements:

Valproic Acid USP—Preserve in tight, glass, stainless steel or polyethylene (HDPE) containers. Contains not less than 98.0% and not more than 102.0% of valproic acid, calculated on the anhydrous basis. Meets the requirements for Identification, Water (not more than 1.0%), Residue on ignition (not more than 0.1%), Heavy metals (not more than 0.002%), Chromatographic purity, and Organic volatile impurities.

Valproic Acid Capsules USP—Preserve in tight containers, at controlled room temperature. Contain the labeled amount, within ±10%. Meet the requirements for Identification, Disintegration (15 minutes, determined as directed for Soft Gelatin Capsules), and Uniformity of dosage units.

Valproic Acid Syrup USP—Preserve in tight containers. Contains the labeled amount, within ±10%. It is prepared with the aid of Sodium Hydroxide. Meets the requirements for Identification and pH (7.0–8.0).

VANCOMYCIN

Source: Derived from *Amycolatopsis orientalis* (formerly *Nocardia orientalis*).

Chemical group: High-molecular-weight tricyclic glycopeptide.

Chemical name: Vancomycin hydrochoride—Vancomycin, monohydrochloride.

Molecular formula: Vancomycin hydrochloride—$C_{66}H_{75}Cl_2N_9O_{24} \cdot HCl$.

Molecular weight: Vancomycin hydrochloride—1485.74.

Description:

Vancomycin Hydrochloride USP—Tan to brown, free-flowing powder, odorless.

Sterile Vancomycin Hydrochloride USP—Tan to brown, free-flowing powder, odorless.

Solubility:

Vancomycin Hydrochloride USP—Freely soluble in water; insoluble in ether and in chloroform.

Sterile Vancomycin Hydrochloride USP—Freely soluble in water; insoluble in ether and in chloroform.

USP requirements:

Vancomycin Hydrochloride USP—Preserve in tight containers. The hydrochloride salt of a kind of vancomycin, a substance produced by the growth of *Streptomyces orientalis* (Fam. Streptomycetaceae), or a mixture of two or more such salts. Has a potency equivalent to not less than 900 mcg of vancomycin per mg, calculated on the anhydrous basis. Meets the requirements for Identification, pH (2.5–4.5, in a solution containing 50 mg per mL), Water (not more than 5.0%), and Chromatographic purity.

Vancomycin Hydrochloride Capsules USP—Preserve in tight containers. Contain a dispersion of Vancomycin Hydrochloride in Polyethylene Glycol. Contain an amount of vancomycin hydrochloride equivalent to the labeled amount of vancomycin, within −10% to +15%. Meet the requirements for Identification, Dissolution (85% in 45 minutes in water in Apparatus 1 at 100 rpm), Water (not more than 8.0%), and Uniformity of dosage units.

Vancomycin Hydrochloride for Injection USP—Preserve in Containers for Sterile Solids. A sterile dry mixture of Vancomycin Hydrochloride and a suitable stabilizing agent. Has a potency equivalent to not less than 925 mcg of vancomycin per mg, calculated on the anhydrous basis. In addition, contains an amount of vancomycin hydrochloride equivalent to the labeled amount of vancomycin, within −10% to +15%. Meets the requirements for Constituted solution, Pyrogen, Sterility, Particulate matter, Heavy metals (not more than 0.003%), and Chromatographic purity, for Identification test, pH, and Water under Vancomycin Hydrochloride, and for Uniformity of dosage units and Labeling under Injections.

Vancomycin Hydrochloride for Oral Solution USP—Preserve in tight containers. Contains an amount of vancomycin hydrochloride equivalent to the labeled amount of vancomycin, within −10% to +15%. Meets the requirements for pH (2.5–4.5, for the solution constituted as directed in the labeling) and Water (not more than 5.0%).

Sterile Vancomycin Hydrochloride USP—Preserve in Containers for Sterile Solids. Has a potency equivalent to not less than 900 mcg per mg, calculated on the anhydrous basis and, where packaged for dispensing, contains an amount of vancomycin hydrochloride equivalent to the labeled amount of vancomycin, within −10% to +15%. Meets the requirements for Constituted solution, Bacterial endotoxins, Sterility, Particulate matter, and Heavy metals (not more than 0.003%), for Identification test, pH, Water, and Chromatographic purity under Vancomycin Hydrochloride, and for Uniformity of dosage units and Labeling under Injections.

VANILLIN

Chemical name: Benzaldehyde, 4-hydroxy-3-methoxy-.

Molecular formula: $C_8H_8O_3$.

Molecular weight: 152.15.

Description: Vanillin NF—Fine, white to slightly yellow crystals, usually needle-like, having an odor suggestive of vanilla. It is affected by light. Its solutions are acid to litmus.

NF category: Flavors and perfumes.

Solubility: Vanillin NF—Slightly soluble in water; freely soluble in alcohol, in chloroform, in ether, and in solutions of the fixed alkali hydroxides; soluble in glycerin and in hot water.

NF requirements: Vanillin NF—Preserve in tight, light-resistant containers. Contains not less than 97.0% and not more than 103.0% of vanillin, calculated on the dried basis. Meets the requirements for Identification, Melting range (81–83 °C), Loss on drying (not more than 1.0%), and Residue on ignition (not more than 0.05%).

VARICELLA-ZOSTER IMMUNE GLOBULIN

USP requirements: Varicella-Zoster Immune Globulin USP—Preserve at a temperature between 2 and 8 °C. A sterile 15 to 18% solution of pH 7.0 containing the globulin fraction of human plasma consisting of not less than 99% of immunoglobulin G with traces of immunoglobulin A and immunoglobulin M, in 0.3 *M* glycine as a stabilizer and 1:10,000 thimerosal as a preservative. Derived from adult human plasma selected for high titers of varicella-zoster antibodies. Each unit of blood or plasma has been found non-reactive for hepatitis B surface antigen by a suitable method. The proteins of the plasma pools are fractionated by the cold ethanol precipitation method. The content of specific antibody is not less than 125 units, deliverable from a vial containing not more than 2.5 mL solution. The unit is defined as equivalent to 0.01 mL of a Varicella-Zoster Immune Globulin lot found effective in clinical trials and used as a reference for potency determinations, based on a fluorescent-antibody membrane antigen (FAMA) method for antibody titration. Label it to state that it is to be administered by intramuscular injection, in the recommended dose based on body weight. Meets the requirement for Expiration date (not later than 2 years after date of issue from manufacturer's cold storage). Conforms to the regulations of the U.S. Food and Drug Administration concerning biologics.

VASOPRESSIN

Chemical name: Vasopressin, 8-L-arginine- (arginine form); Vasopressin, 8-L-lysine- (lysine form).

Molecular formula: $C_{46}H_{65}N_{15}O_{12}S_2$ (arginine form); $C_{46}H_{65}N_{13}O_{12}S_2$ (lysine form).

Molecular weight: 1084.2 (arginine form); 1056.2 (lysine form).

Description: Vasopressin Injection USP—Clear, colorless or practically colorless liquid, having a faint, characteristic odor.

USP requirements: Vasopressin Injection USP—Preserve in single-dose or in multiple-dose containers, preferably of Type I glass. Do not freeze. A sterile solution, in a suitable diluent, of material containing the polypeptide hormone having the properties of causing the contraction of vascular and other smooth muscle, and of antidiuresis, which is prepared by synthesis or obtained from the posterior lobe of the pituitary of healthy, domestic animals used for food by man. Each mL of Vasopressin Injection possesses a pressor activity stated in the label in USP Posterior Pituitary Units, within −15% to +20%. Meets the requirements for pH (2.5–4.5), Limit of oxytocic activity, and Injections.

VECURONIUM

Chemical name: Vecuronium bromide—Piperidinium, 1-[(2 beta,3 alpha,5 alpha,16 beta,17 beta)-3,17-bis(acetyloxy)-2-(1-piperidinyl)androstan-16-yl]-1-methyl-, bromide.

Molecular formula: Vecuronium bromide—$C_{34}H_{57}BrN_2O_4$.

Molecular weight: Vecuronium bromide—637.75.

Description: Vecuronium bromide—White to off-white or slightly pink crystals or crystalline powder.

Solubility: Vecuronium bromide—Solubilities of 9 and 23 mg/mL in water and in alcohol, respectively.

USP requirements: Vecuronium Bromide for Injection—Not in USP.

HYDROGENATED VEGETABLE OIL

Description: Hydrogenated Vegetable Oil NF—Fine, white powder at room temperature, and a pale yellow, oily liquid above its melting temperature.

NF category:
Type I—Tablet and/or capsule lubricant.
Type II—Ointment base.

Solubility: Hydrogenated Vegetable Oil NF—Insoluble in water; soluble in hot isopropyl alcohol, in hexane, and in chloroform.

NF requirements: Hydrogenated Vegetable Oil NF—Preserve in tight containers, in a cool place. A mixture of triglycerides of fatty acids. The melting range, heavy metals limit, iodine value, and saponification value differ, depending on Type, as set forth in the accompanying table.

	Type I	Type II
Melting range	57–70 °C	20–50 °C
Heavy metals	10 ppm	0.001%
Iodine value	0–5	55–80
Saponification value	175–205	185–200

Label it to state whether it is Type I or Type II. Meets the requirements for Loss on drying (not more than 0.1%), Acid value (not more than 4.0), and Unsaponifiable matter (not more than 0.8%).

VENLAFAXINE

Chemical name: Venlafaxine hydrochloride—Cyclohexanol, 1-[2-(diemethylamino)-1-(4-methoxyphenyl)ethyl]-, hydrochloride.

Molecular formula: Venlafaxine hydrochloride—$C_{17}H_{27}NO_2 \cdot HCl$.

Molecular weight: Venlafaxine hydrochloride—313.87.

Description: Venlafaxine hydrochloride—White to off-white crystalline solid.

Solubility: Venlafaxine hydrochloride—Solubility of 572 mg/mL in water (adjusted to ionic strength of 0.2 *M* with sodium chloride).

Other characteristics: Venlafaxine hydrochloride—Octanol:water (0.2 *M* sodium chloride) partition coefficient: 0.43.

USP requirements: Venlafaxine Hydrochloride Tablets—Not in USP.

VERAPAMIL

Chemical name: Verapamil hydrochloride—Benzeneacetonitrile, alpha-[3-[[2-(3,4-dimethoxyphenyl)ethyl]methylamino]-propyl]-3,4-dimethoxy-alpha-(1-methylethyl)-, monohydrochloride.

Molecular formula: Verapamil hydrochloride—$C_{27}H_{38}N_2O_4 \cdot HCl$.

Molecular weight: Verapamil hydrochloride—491.07.

Description: Verapamil Hydrochloride USP—White or practically white, crystalline powder. It is practically odorless.

Solubility: Verapamil Hydrochloride USP—Soluble in water; freely soluble in chloroform; sparingly soluble in alcohol; practically insoluble in ether.

USP requirements:

Verapamil Hydrochloride USP—Preserve in tight, light-resistant containers. Contains not less than 99.0% and not more than 100.5% of verapamil hydrochloride, calculated on the dried basis. Meets the requirements for Identification, Melting range (140–144 °C), pH (4.5–6.5, in a solution, prepared with gentle heating, containing 50 mg per mL), Loss on drying (not more than 0.5%), Residue on ignition (not more than 0.1%), Chromatographic purity, and Organic volatile impurities.

Verapamil Hydrochloride Injection USP—Preserve in single-dose containers, preferably of Type I glass, protected from light. A sterile solution of Verapamil Hydrochloride in Water for Injection. Contains the labeled amount, within ±10%. Meets the requirements for Identification, Bacterial endotoxins, pH (4.0–6.5), Particulate matter, Related compounds, and Injections.

Verapamil Hydrochloride Tablets USP—Preserve in tight, light-resistant containers. Contain the labeled amount, within ±10%. Meet the requirements for Identification, Dissolution (75% in 30 minutes in 0.1 *N* hydrochloric acid in Apparatus 2 at 50 rpm), Uniformity of dosage units, and Related compounds.

Verapamil Hydrochloride Extended-release Capsules—Not in USP.

Verapamil Hydrochloride Extended-release Tablets—Not in USP.

VIDARABINE

Source: Obtained from fermentation cultures of *Streptomyces antibioticus*.

Chemical group: Purine nucleoside.

Chemical name: 9*H*-Purin-6-amine, 9-beta-D-arabinofuranosyl-, monohydrate.

Molecular formula: $C_{10}H_{13}N_5O_4 \cdot H_2O$.

Molecular weight: 285.26.

Description: Sterile Vidarabine USP—White to off-white powder.

Solubility: Sterile Vidarabine USP—Very slightly soluble in water; slightly soluble in dimethylformamide.

USP requirements:

Vidarabine Concentrate for Injection USP—Preserve in single-dose or in multiple-dose containers, preferably of Type I glass. Label it to indicate that it is to be solubilized in a suitable parenteral vehicle prior to intravenous infusion. Contains an amount of vidarabine equivalent to the labeled amount of anhydrous vidarabine, within −10% to +20%, in a sterile, aqueous suspension intended for solubilization with a suitable parenteral vehicle prior to intravenous infusion. Contains suitable buffers and preservatives. Meets the requirements for Depressor substances, Bacterial endotoxins, Sterility, and pH (5.0–6.2, in the undiluted suspension).

Sterile Vidarabine USP—Preserve in tight containers. Has a potency equivalent to not less than 845 mcg and not more than 985 mcg of vidarabine per mg. Meets the requirements for Identification, Specific rotation (−56.0° to −65.0°), Bacterial endotoxins, Sterility, and Loss on drying (5.0–7.0%).

Vidarabine Ophthalmic Ointment USP—Preserve in collapsible ophthalmic ointment tubes. Contains an amount of vidarabine equivalent to the labeled amount of anhydrous vidarabine, within −10% to +20%. Meets the requirements for Sterility, Minimum fill, and Metal particles.

VINBLASTINE

Source: Salt of an alkaloid extracted from *Vinca rosea* Linn, a common flowering herb known as the periwinkle.

Chemical name: Vinblastine sulfate—Vincaleukoblastine, sulfate (1:1) (salt).

Molecular formula: Vinblastine sulfate—$C_{46}H_{58}N_4O_9 \cdot H_2SO_4$.

Molecular weight: Vinblastine sulfate—909.07.

Description:

Vinblastine Sulfate USP—White or slightly yellow, odorless, amorphous or crystalline powder. Is hygroscopic.

Sterile Vinblastine Sulfate USP—Yellowish white solid, having the characteristic appearance of products prepared by freeze-drying.

pKa: 5.4 and 7.4 in water.

Solubility: Vinblastine Sulfate USP—Freely soluble in water.

USP requirements:

Vinblastine Sulfate USP—Preserve in tight, light-resistant containers, in a freezer. Contains not less than 96.0% and not more than 102.0% of vinblastine sulfate, corrections being applied for loss in weight. Meets the requirements for Identification, pH (3.5–5.0, in a solution prepared by dissolving 3 mg in 2 mL of water), Loss on drying (not more than 15.0%), and Related compounds.

Caution: Handle Vinblastine Sulfate with great care since it is a potent cytotoxic agent.

Vinblastine Sulfate Injection—Not in USP.

Sterile Vinblastine Sulfate USP—Preserve in Containers for Sterile Solids, in a refrigerator. It is Vinblastine Sulfate suitable for parenteral use. Contains the labeled amount, within ±10%. Meets the requirements for Completeness of solution, Constituted solution, Bacterial endotoxins, Uniformity of dosage units, and Related compounds, for Identification test under Vinblastine Sulfate, and for Sterility tests and Labeling under Injections.

Caution: Handle Sterile Vinblastine Sulfate with great care, since it is a potent cytotoxic agent.

VINCRISTINE

Source: Salt of an alkaloid extracted from *Vinca rosea* Linn, a common flowering herb known as the periwinkle.

Chemical name: Vincristine sulfate—Vincaleukoblastine, 22-oxo-, sulfate (1:1) (salt).

Molecular formula: Vincristine sulfate—$C_{46}H_{56}N_4O_{10} \cdot H_2SO_4$.

Molecular weight: Vincristine sulfate—923.06.

Description:

Vincristine Sulfate USP—White to slightly yellow, odorless, amorphous or crystalline powder. Is hygroscopic.

Vincristine Sulfate for Injection USP—Yellowish white solid, having the characteristic appearance of products prepared by freeze-drying.

pKa: 5.1 and 7.5 in water.

Solubility: Vincristine Sulfate USP—Freely soluble in water; soluble in methanol; slightly soluble in alcohol.

USP requirements:

Vincristine Sulfate USP—Preserve in tight, light-resistant containers, in a freezer. Contains not less than 95.0% and not more than 105.0% of vincristine sulfate, corrections being applied for loss in weight. Meets the requirements for Identification, pH (3.5–4.5, in a solution [1 in 1000]), Loss on drying (not more than 12.0%), and Related compounds.

Caution: Handle Vincristine Sulfate with great care since it is a potent cytotoxic agent.

Vincristine Sulfate Injection USP—Preserve in light-resistant, glass containers, in a refrigerator. A sterile solution of Vincristine Sulfate in Water for Injection. The label states: "FATAL IF GIVEN INTRATHECALLY. FOR INTRAVENOUS USE ONLY." Where labeled as containing more than 2 mg, it must also be labeled as a Pharmacy bulk package. The labeling directs that the drug be dispensed only in containers enclosed in an overwrap labeled as directed below. When packaged in a Pharmacy bulk package, it is exempt from the requirement under Injections, that the closure be penetrated only one time after constitution with a suitable sterile transfer device or dispensing set, when it contains a suitable substance or mixture of substances to prevent the growth of microorganisms. When dispensed, the container or syringe (holding the individual dose prepared for administration to the patient) must be enclosed in an overwrap bearing the statement "DO NOT REMOVE COVERING UNTIL MOMENT OF INJECTION. FATAL IF GIVEN INTRATHECALLY. FOR INTRAVENOUS USE ONLY." Contains the labeled amount, within ±10%. Meets the requirements for Identification, Bacterial endotoxins, pH (3.5–5.5), and Related compounds, for Sterility tests, and for Labeling under Injections.

Caution: Handle Vincristine Sulfate Injection with great care, since it is a potent cytotoxic agent.

Vincristine Sulfate for Injection USP—Preserve in Containers for Sterile Solids, in a refrigerator. A sterile mixture of Vincristine Sulfate with suitable diluents. The label states: "FATAL IF GIVEN INTRATHECALLY. FOR INTRAVENOUS USE ONLY." Where labeled as containing more than 2 mg, it must also be labeled as a Pharmacy bulk package. The labeling directs that the drug be dispensed only in containers enclosed in an overwrap labeled as directed below. When packaged in a Pharmacy bulk package, it is exempt from the requirement under Injections, that the closure be penetrated only one time after constitution with a suitable sterile transfer device or dispensing set, when it contains a suitable substance or mixture of substances to prevent the growth of microorganisms. When dispensed, the container or syringe (holding the individual dose prepared for administration to the patient) must be enclosed in an overwrap bearing the statement "DO NOT REMOVE COVERING UNTIL MOMENT OF INJECTION. FATAL IF GIVEN INTRATHECALLY. FOR INTRAVENOUS USE ONLY." Contains the labeled amount, within ±10%. Meets the requirements for Constituted solution, Identification, Bacterial endotoxins, Uniformity of dosage units, and Related compounds, for Sterility tests, and for Labeling under Injections.

Caution: Handle Vincristine Sulfate for Injection with great care since it is a potent cytotoxic agent.

VINDESINE

Chemical name: Vindesine sulfate—Vincaleukoblastine, 3-(aminocarbonyl)-*O*[4]-deacetyl-3-de(methoxycarbonyl)sulfate (1:1) (salt).

Molecular formula: Vindesine sulfate—$C_{43}H_{55}N_5O_7 \cdot H_2SO_4$.

Molecular weight: Vindesine sulfate—852.02.

Description: Vindesine sulfate—Amorphous solid melting at less than 250 °C.

USP requirements: Vindesine Sulfate for Injection—Not in USP.

VITAMIN A

Chemical name: Retinol—3,7-Dimethyl-9-(2,6,6-trimethyl-1-cyclohexen-1-yl)-2,4,6,8-nonate-traen-1-ol.

Molecular formula: Retinol—$C_{20}H_{30}O$.

Molecular weight: Retinol—286.46.

Description: Vitamin A USP—In liquid form, a light-yellow to red oil that may solidify upon refrigeration. In solid form, has the appearance of any diluent that has been added. May be practically odorless or may have a mild fishy odor, but has no rancid odor. Is unstable to air and light.

Solubility: Vitamin A USP—In liquid form, insoluble in water and in glycerin; very soluble in chloroform and in ether; soluble in absolute alcohol and in vegetable oils. In solid form, may be dispersible in water.

USP requirements:

Vitamin A USP—Preserve in tight containers, preferably under an atmosphere of an inert gas, protected from light. Label it to indicate the form in which the vitamin is present, and to indicate the presence of any antimicrobial agent, dispersant, antioxidant, or other added substance, and to indicate the vitamin A activity in terms of the equivalent amount of retinol, in mg per gram. The vitamin A activity may be stated also in USP Units, on the basis that 1 USP Vitamin A Unit equals the biological activity of 0.3 mcg of the all-*trans* isomer of retinol. Contains a suitable form of retinol (vitamin A alcohol) and possesses vitamin A activity equivalent to not less than 95.0% of that declared on the label. May consist of retinol or esters of retinol formed from edible fatty acids, principally acetic and palmitic acids. May be diluted with edible oils, or it may be incorporated in solid, edible carriers or excipients. Meets the requirements for Identification for vitamin A and Absorbance ratio.

Vitamin A Capsules USP—Preserve in tight, light-resistant containers. Label Capsules to indicate the form in which the vitamin is present, and to indicate the vitamin A activity in terms of the equivalent amount of retinol in mg. The vitamin A activity may be stated also in USP Units per Capsule, on the basis that 1 USP Vitamin A Unit equals the biological activity of 0.3 mcg of the all-*trans* isomer of retinol. Contain the labeled amount, within −5% to +20%. Meet the requirements for Uniformity of dosage units, for Identification tests for vitamin A, and for the Absorbance ratio test under Vitamin A.

Vitamin A Injection—Not in USP.

Vitamin A Oral Solution—Not in USP.

Vitamin A Tablets—Not in USP.

VITAMIN E

Molecular formula:

d- or *dl*-Alpha tocopherol—$C_{29}H_{50}O_2$.

d- or *dl*-Alpha tocopheryl acetate—$C_{31}H_{52}O_3$.

d- or *dl*-Alpha tocopheryl acid succinate—$C_{33}H_{54}O_5$.

Description:

Vitamin E USP—Practically odorless. The alpha tocopherols and alpha tocopheryl acetates occur as clear, yellow, or greenish-yellow, viscous oils. *d*-Alpha tocopheryl acetate may solidify in the cold. Alpha tocopheryl acid succinate occurs as a white powder; the *d*-isomer melts at about 75 °C, and the *dl*-form melts at about 70 °C. The alpha tocopherols are unstable to air and to light, particularly when in alkaline media. The esters are stable to air and to light, but are unstable to alkali; the acid succinate is also unstable when held molten.

Vitamin E Preparation USP—The liquid forms are clear, yellow to brownish-red, viscous oils. The solid forms are white to tan-white granular powders.

Solubility:

Vitamin E USP—Alpha tocopheryl acid succinate is insoluble in water; slightly soluble in alkaline solutions; soluble in alcohol, in ether, in acetone, and in vegetable oils; very soluble in chloroform. The other forms of Vitamin E are insoluble in water; soluble in alcohol; miscible with ether, with acetone, with vegetable oils, and with chloroform.

Vitamin E Preparation USP—The liquid forms are insoluble in water; soluble in alcohol; and miscible with ether, with acetone, with vegetable oils, and with chloroform. The solid forms disperse in water to give cloudy suspensions.

USP requirements:

Vitamin E USP—Preserve in tight containers, protected from light. Protect *d*- or *dl*-alpha tocopherol with a blanket of an inert gas. A form of alpha tocopherol. Includes the following: *d*- or *dl*-alpha tocopherol; *d*- or *dl*-alpha tocopheryl acetate; *d*- or *dl*-alpha tocopheryl acid succinate. Label Vitamin E to indicate the chemical form and to indicate whether it is the *d*- or the *dl*- form. The Vitamin E activity may be expressed in terms of the equivalent amount of *d*-alpha tocopherol, in mg per gram, based on the relationship between the former USP Units (equal to the former International Units) and mass. Contains not less than 96.0% and not more than 102.0% of *d*- or *dl*-alpha tocopherol, *d*- or *dl*-alpha tocopheryl acetate, or *d*- or *dl*-alpha tocopheryl acid succinate, respectively. Meets the requirements for Identification and Acidity.

Vitamin E Preparation USP—Preserve in tight containers, protected from light. Protect Preparation containing *d*- or *dl*-alpha tocopherol with a blanket of an inert gas. A combination of a single form of Vitamin E with one or more inert substances. May be in a liquid or solid form. Label it to indicate the chemical form of Vitamin E present, and to indicate whether the *d*- or the *dl*-form is present, excluding any different forms that may be introduced as a minor constituent of the vehicle. Designate the quantity of Vitamin E present. Contains the labeled amount of Vitamin E, within −5% to +20%. Vitamin E Preparation labeled to contain a *dl*-form of Vitamin E may contain also a small amount of a *d*-form occurring as a minor constituent of an added substance. Meets the requirements for Identification and Acidity.

Vitamin E Capsules USP—Preserve in tight containers, protected from light. Contain Vitamin E or Vitamin E Preparation. The Capsules meet the requirements for Labeling under Vitamin E Preparation. Contain the labeled amount, within −5% to +20%. Meet the requirements for Identification and Uniformity of dosage units.

Vitamin E Oral Solution—Not in USP.

Vitamin E Tablets—Not in USP.

Vitamin E Chewable Tablets—Not in USP.

VITAMINS A, D, AND C AND FLUORIDE

Chemical name:

Retinol—3,7-Dimethyl-9-(2,6,6-trimethyl-1-cyclohexen-1-yl)-2,4,6,8-nonate-traen-1-ol.

Calcifediol—9,10-Secocholesta-5,7,10(19)-triene-3,25-diol monohydrate, (3 beta,5*Z*,7*E*)-.

Calcitriol—9,10-Secocholesta-5,7,10(19)-triene-1,3,25-triol, (1 alpha,3 beta,5*Z*,7*E*)-.

Ergocalciferol—9,10-Secoergosta-5,7,10(19),22-tetraen-3-ol, (3 beta,5*Z*,7*E*,22*E*)-.

Ascorbic acid—L-Ascorbic acid.

Sodium fluoride—Sodium fluoride.

Pyridoxine hydrochloride—3,4-Pyridinedimethanol, 5-hydroxy-6-methyl-, hydrochloride.

Molecular formula:

Retinol—$C_{20}H_{30}O$.

Calcifediol—$C_{27}H_{44}O_2 \cdot H_2O$.

Calcitriol—$C_{27}H_{44}O_3$.

Ergocalciferol—$C_{28}H_{44}O$.

Ascorbic acid—$C_6H_8O_6$.

Sodium fluoride—NaF.

Potassium fluoride—FK.

Pyridoxine hydrochloride—$C_8H_{11}NO_3 \cdot HCl$.

d- or *dl*-Alpha tocopherol—$C_{29}H_{50}O_2$.

d- or *dl*-Alpha tocopheryl acetate—$C_{31}H_{52}O_3$.

d- or *dl*-Alpha tocopheryl acid succinate—$C_{33}H_{54}O_5$.

Molecular weight:

Retinol—286.46.

Calcifediol—418.66.

Calcitriol—416.65.

Ergocalciferol—396.66.

Ascorbic acid—176.13.

Sodium fluoride—41.99.

Potassium fluoride—58.10.

Pyridoxine hydrochloride—205.64.

Description:

Vitamin A USP—In liquid form, a light-yellow to red oil that may solidify upon refrigeration. In solid form, has the appearance of any diluent that has been added. May be practically odorless or may have a mild fishy odor, but has no rancid odor. Is unstable to air and light.

Calcifediol—A white powder. It has a melting point of about 105 °C.

Calcitriol—A practically white crystalline compound with a melting range of 111–115 °C.

Ergocalciferol USP—White, odorless crystals. Is affected by air and by light.

Ascorbic Acid USP—White or slightly yellow crystals or powder. On exposure to light it gradually darkens. In the dry state, is reasonably stable in air, but in solution rapidly oxidizes. Melts at about 190 °C.

NF category: Antioxidant.

Sodium Fluoride USP—White, odorless powder.

Potassium fluoride—White, deliquescent powder or solid. Melting point 859.9 °C.

Pyridoxine Hydrochloride USP—White to practically white crystals or crystalline powder. Is stable in air, and is slowly affected by sunlight. Its solutions have a pH of about 3.

Vitamin E USP—Practically odorless. The alpha tocopherols and alpha tocopheryl acetates occur as clear, yellow, or greenish-yellow, viscous oils. *d*-Alpha tocopheryl acetate may solidify in the cold. Alpha tocopheryl acid succinate occurs as a white powder; the *d*-isomer melts at about 75 °C, and the *dl*-form melts at about 70 °C. The alpha tocopherols are unstable to air and to light, particularly when in alkaline media. The esters are stable to air and to light, but are unstable to alkali; the acid succinate is also unstable when held molten.

Solubility:

Vitamin A USP—In liquid form, insoluble in water and in glycerin; very soluble in chloroform and in ether; soluble in absolute alcohol and in vegetable oils. In solid form, may be dispersible in water.

Calcifediol—Practically insoluble in water; soluble in organic solvents.

Calcitriol—Insoluble in water; soluble in organic solvents.

Ergocalciferol USP—Insoluble in water; soluble in alcohol, in chloroform, in ether, and in fatty oils.

Ascorbic Acid USP—Freely soluble in water; sparingly soluble in alcohol; insoluble in chloroform and in ether.

Sodium Fluoride USP—Soluble in water; insoluble in alcohol.

Potassium fluoride—Soluble in water (92.3 grams per 100 mL at 18 °C and 96.4 grams per 100 mL at 21 °C); very freely soluble in boiling water; insoluble in alcohol unless water is present.

Pyridoxine Hydrochloride USP—Freely soluble in water; slightly soluble in alcohol; insoluble in ether.

Vitamin E USP—Alpha tocopheryl acid succinate is insoluble in water; slightly soluble in alkaline solutions; soluble in alcohol, in ether, in acetone, and in vegetable oils; very soluble in chloroform. The other forms of Vitamin E are insoluble in water; soluble in alcohol; miscible with ether, with acetone, with vegetable oils, and with chloroform.

USP requirements:

Vitamins A, D, and C and Sodium or Potassium Fluoride Oral Solution—Not in USP.

Vitamins A, D, and C and Sodium or Potassium Fluoride Chewable Tablets—Not in USP.

MULTIPLE VITAMINS AND FLUORIDE

Chemical name:

Ascorbic acid—L-Ascorbic acid.

Cyanocobalamin—Vitamin B_{12}.

Folic acid—L-Glutamic acid, *N*-[4-[[(2-amino-1,4-dihydro-4-oxo-6-pteridinyl)methyl]amino]benzoyl]-.

Niacin—3-Pyridinecarboxylic acid.
Pyridoxine hydrochloride—3,4-Pyridinedimethanol, 5-hydroxy-6-methyl-, hydrochloride.
Riboflavin—Riboflavine.
Thiamine hydrochloride—Thiazolium, 3-[(4-amino-2-methyl-5-pyrimidinyl)methyl]-5-(2-hydroxyethyl)-4-methyl-, chloride, monohydrochloride.
Retinol—3,7-Dimethyl-9-(2,6,6-trimethyl-1-cyclohexen-1-yl)-2,4,6,8-nonate-traen-1-ol.
Calcifediol—9,10-Secocholesta-5,7,10(19)-triene-3,25-diol monohydrate, (3 beta,5*Z*,7*E*)-.
Calcitriol—9,10-Secocholesta-5,7,10(19)-triene-1,3,25-triol, (1 alpha,3 beta,5*Z*,7*E*)-.
Ergocalciferol—9,10-Secoergosta-5,7,10(19),22-tetraen-3-ol, (3 beta,5*Z*,7*E*,22*E*)-.
Sodium fluoride—Sodium fluoride.

Molecular formula:
Ascorbic acid—$C_6H_8O_6$.
Cyanocobalamin—$C_{63}H_{88}CoN_{14}O_{14}P$.
Folic acid—$C_{19}H_{19}N_7O_6$.
Niacin—$C_6H_5NO_2$.
Pyridoxine hydrochloride—$C_8H_{11}NO_3 \cdot HCl$.
Riboflavin—$C_{17}H_{20}N_4O_6$.
Thiamine hydrochloride—$C_{12}H_{17}ClN_4OS \cdot HCl$.
Retinol—$C_{20}H_{30}O$.
Calcifediol—$C_{27}H_{44}O_2 \cdot H_2O$.
Calcitriol—$C_{27}H_{44}O_3$.
Ergocalciferol—$C_{28}H_{44}O$.
d- or *dl*-Alpha tocopherol—$C_{29}H_{50}O_2$.
d- or *dl*-Alpha tocopheryl acetate—$C_{31}H_{52}O_3$.
d- or *dl*-Alpha tocopheryl acid succinate—$C_{33}H_{54}O_5$.
Sodium fluoride—NaF.
Potassium fluoride—FK.

Molecular weight:
Ascorbic acid—176.13.
Cyanocobalamin—1355.38.
Folic acid—441.40.
Niacin—123.11.
Pyridoxine hydrochloride—205.64.
Riboflavin—376.37.
Thiamine hydrochloride—337.27.
Retinol—286.46.
Calcifediol—418.66.
Calcitriol—416.65.
Ergocalciferol—396.66.
Sodium fluoride—41.99.
Potassium fluoride—58.10.

Description:
Ascorbic Acid USP—White or slightly yellow crystals or powder. On exposure to light it gradually darkens. In the dry state, is reasonably stable in air, but in solution rapidly oxidizes. Melts at about 190 °C.
NF category: Antioxidant.
Cyanocobalamin USP—Dark red crystals or amorphous or crystalline red powder. In the anhydrous form, it is very hygroscopic and when exposed to air it may absorb about 12% of water.
Folic Acid USP—Yellow, yellow-brownish, or yellowish orange, odorless, crystalline powder.
Niacin USP—White crystals or crystalline powder. Is odorless, or has a slight odor. Melts at about 235 °C.
Pyridoxine Hydrochloride USP—White to practically white crystals or crystalline powder. Is stable in air, and is slowly affected by sunlight. Its solutions have a pH of about 3.
Riboflavin USP—Yellow to orange-yellow, crystalline powder having a slight odor. Melts at about 280 °C. Its saturated solution is neutral to litmus. When dry, it is not appreciably affected by diffused light, but when in solution, light induces quite rapid deterioration, especially in the presence of alkalies.
Thiamine Hydrochloride USP—White crystals or crystalline powder, usually having a slight, characteristic odor. When exposed to air, the anhydrous product rapidly absorbs about 4% of water. Melts at about 248 °C, with some decomposition.
Vitamin A USP—In liquid form, a light-yellow to red oil that may solidify upon refrigeration. In solid form, has the appearance of any diluent that has been added. May be practically odorless or may have a mild fishy odor, but has no rancid odor. Is unstable to air and light.
Calcifediol—A white powder. It has a melting point of about 105 °C.
Calcitriol—A practically white crystalline compound with a melting range of 111–115 °C.
Ergocalciferol USP—White, odorless crystals. Is affected by air and by light.
Vitamin E USP—Practically odorless. The alpha tocopherols and alpha tocopheryl acetates occur as clear, yellow, or greenish-yellow, viscous oils. *d*-Alpha tocopheryl acetate may solidify in the cold. Alpha tocopheryl acid succinate occurs as a white powder; the *d*-isomer melts at about 75 °C, and the *dl*-form melts at about 70 °C. The alpha tocopherols are unstable to air and to light, particularly when in alkaline media. The esters are stable to air and to light, but are unstable to alkali; the acid succinate is also unstable when held molten.
Sodium Fluoride USP—White, odorless powder.
Potassium fluoride—White, deliquescent powder or solid. Melting point 859.9 °C.

Solubility:
Ascorbic Acid USP—Freely soluble in water; sparingly soluble in alcohol; insoluble in chloroform and in ether.
Cyanocobalamin USP—Sparingly soluble in water; soluble in alcohol; insoluble in acetone, in chloroform, and in ether.
Folic Acid USP—Very slightly soluble in water; insoluble in alcohol, in acetone, in chloroform, and in ether; readily dissolves in dilute solutions of alkali hydroxides and carbonates, and is soluble in hot, 3 *N* hydrochloric acid and in hot, 2 *N* sulfuric acid. Soluble in hydrochloric acid and in sulfuric acid, yielding very pale yellow solutions.
Niacin USP—Sparingly soluble in water; freely soluble in boiling water, in boiling alcohol, and in solutions of alkali hydroxides and carbonates; practically insoluble in ether.
Pyridoxine Hydrochloride USP—Freely soluble in water; slightly soluble in alcohol; insoluble in ether.
Riboflavin USP—Very slightly soluble in water, in alcohol, and in isotonic sodium chloride solution; very soluble in dilute solutions of alkalies; insoluble in ether and in chloroform.
Thiamine Hydrochloride USP—Freely soluble in water; soluble in glycerin; slightly soluble in alcohol; insoluble in ether.
Vitamin A USP—In liquid form, insoluble in water and in glycerin; very soluble in chloroform and in ether; soluble in absolute alcohol and in vegetable oils. In solid form, may be dispersible in water.
Calcifediol—Practically insoluble in water; soluble in organic solvents.
Calcitriol—Insoluble in water; soluble in organic solvents.
Ergocalciferol USP—Insoluble in water; soluble in alcohol, in chloroform, in ether, and in fatty oils.
Vitamin E USP—Alpha tocopheryl acid succinate is insoluble in water; slightly soluble in alkaline solutions; soluble in alcohol, in ether, in acetone, and in vegetable oils; very soluble in chloroform. The other forms of Vitamin E are insoluble in water; soluble in alcohol; miscible with ether, with acetone, with vegetable oils, and with chloroform.

Sodium Fluoride USP—Soluble in water; insoluble in alcohol.

Potassium fluoride—Soluble in water (92.3 grams per 100 mL at 18 °C and 96.4 grams per 100 mL at 21 °C); very freely soluble in boiling water; insoluble in alcohol unless water is present.

USP requirements:

Multiple Vitamins and Sodium or Potassium Fluoride Oral Solution—Not in USP.

Multiple Vitamins and Sodium or Potassium Fluoride Chewable Tablets—Not in USP.

OIL-SOLUBLE VITAMINS

For *Vitamin A, Vitamin D* (Cholecalciferol, Ergocalciferol), *Vitamin E, Phytonadione,* and *Beta Carotene*—See individual listings for chemistry information.

USP requirements:

Oil-soluble Vitamins Capsules USP—Preserve in tight, light-resistant containers. Label the Capsules to state that the product is Oil-soluble Vitamins Capsules. The label states also the quantity of each vitamin in terms of metric units per dosage unit and, where necessary, the chemical form in which it is present. Where the product contains vitamin A, the label indicates the Vitamin A activity in terms of the equivalent amount of retinol, in mg per Capsule. Where the product contains beta carotene, the label indicates the content of beta carotene, in mg per Capsule, and the vitamin A activity in terms of the equivalent amount of the all-*trans* isomer of retinol, in mg per Capsule. Where the product contains both vitamin A and beta carotene, the label indicates also the total vitamin A activity per Capsule in terms of the all-*trans*-retinol equivalents of vitamin A and beta carotene. The vitamin A activity may be stated also in USP Units per Capsule, on the basis that 1 USP Vitamin A Unit equals the biological activity of 0.3 mcg of the all-*trans* isomer of retinol. Where the product contains vitamin D, the vitamin D activity may be stated also in USP Units per Capsule, on the basis that 1 USP Vitamin D Unit equals 0.25 mcg of cholecalciferol or ergocalciferol. Where the product contains vitamin E, the label indicates also whether it is the *d*- or *dl*- form and indicates also the content, in mg per Capsule, of vitamin E expressed as the *d*-alpha tocopherol equivalent. Contain two or more of the following oil-soluble vitamins: Vitamin A, Vitamin D as Ergocalciferol (Vitamin D_2) or Cholecalciferol (Vitamin D_3), Vitamin E, Phytonadione (Vitamin K_1), and Beta Carotene. Capsules contain the labeled amounts of Vitamin A, as retinol or esters of retinol in the form of retinyl acetate or retinyl palmitate; Vitamin D, as ergocalciferol or cholecalciferol; Vitamin E as alpha tocopherol, alpha tocopheryl acetate, or alpha tocopheryl acid succinate; phytonadione; and beta carotene, within −10% to +65%. Oil-soluble Vitamins Capsules contain no other vitamins, or any minerals or any other ingredient for which nutritional value is claimed. Do not contain any other physiologically active substances. May contain other labeled added substances that are generally recognized as safe, in amounts that are unobjectionable. Meet the requirements for Microbial limits, Disintegration and dissolution, and Weight variation.

Oil-soluble Vitamins Tablets USP—Preserve in tight, light-resistant containers. Label the Tablets to state that the product is Oil-soluble Vitamins Tablets. The label states also the quantity of each vitamin in terms of metric units per dosage unit and where necessary the chemical form in which it is present. Where the product contains vitamin A, the label indicates the Vitamin A activity in terms of the equivalent amount of retinol, in mg per Tablet. Where the product contains beta carotene, the label indicates the content of beta carotene, in mg per Tablet, and the vitamin A activity in terms of the equivalent amount of the all-*trans* isomer of retinol, in mg per Tablet. Where the product contains both vitamin A and beta carotene, the label indicates also the total vitamin A activity per Tablet in terms of the all-*trans*-retinol equivalents of vitamin A and beta carotene. The vitamin A activity may be stated also in USP Units per Tablet, on the basis that 1 USP Vitamin A Unit equals the biological activity of 0.3 mcg of the all-*trans* isomer of retinol. Where the product contains vitamin D, the vitamin D activity may be stated also in USP Units per Tablet, on the basis that 1 USP Vitamin D Unit equals 0.25 mcg of cholecalciferol or ergocalciferol. Where the product contains Vitamin E, the label indicates whether it is the *d*- or *dl*- form and indicates also the content, in mg per Tablet, of vitamin E, expressed as the *d*-alpha tocopherol equivalent. Contain two or more of the following oil-soluble vitamins: Vitamin A, Vitamin D as Ergocalciferol (Vitamin D_2) or Cholecalciferol (Vitamin D_3), Vitamin E, Phytonadione (Vitamin K_1), and Beta Carotene. Tablets contain the labeled amounts of Vitamin A, as retinol or esters of retinol in the form of retinyl acetate or retinyl palmitate; Vitamin D, as ergocalciferol or cholecalciferol; Vitamin E as alpha tocopherol, alpha tocopheryl acetate, or alpha tocopheryl acid succinate; phytonadione; and beta carotene, within − 10% to +65%. Oil-soluble Vitamins Tablets contain no other vitamins or any minerals or any other ingredient for which nutritional value is claimed. Do not contain any other physiologically active substances. May contain other labeled added substances that are generally recognized as safe, in amounts that are unobjectionable. Meet the requirements for Microbial limits, Disintegration and dissolution, and Weight variation.

OIL- AND WATER-SOLUBLE VITAMINS

For *Vitamin A, Cholecalciferol* or *Ergocalciferol, Vitamin E, Phytonadione, Beta Carotene, Ascorbic Acid, Calcium Ascorbate, Sodium Ascorbate, Biotin, Cyanocobalamin, Folic Acid, Niacin* or *Niacinamide, Dexpanthenol* or *Panthenol, Calcium Pantothenate, Pyridoxine, Riboflavin,* and *Thiamine*—See individual listings for chemistry information.

USP requirements:

Oil- and Water-soluble Vitamins Capsules USP—Preserve in tight, light-resistant containers. Contain one or more of the following oil-soluble vitamins: Vitamin A, Vitamin D as Ergocalciferol (Vitamin D_2) or Cholecalciferol (Vitamin D_3), Vitamin E, Phytonadione (Vitamin K_1), and Beta Carotene, and one or more of the following water-soluble vitamins: Ascorbic Acid or its equivalent as Calcium Ascorbate or Sodium Ascorbate, Biotin, Cyanocobalamin, Folic Acid, Niacin or Niacinamide, Dexpanthenol or Panthenol, Pantothenic Acid (as Calcium Pantothenate or Racemic Calcium Pantothenate), Pyridoxine Hydrochloride, Riboflavin, and Thiamine Hydrochloride or Thiamine Mononitrate. The label states that the product is Oil- and Water-soluble Vitamins Capsules. The label states also the quantity of each vitamin in terms of metric units per dosage unit and where necessary the chemical form in which it is present. Where the product contains vitamin A, the label indicates the Vitamin A activity in terms of the equivalent amount of retinol, in mg per Capsule. Where the product contains both vitamin A and beta carotene, the label indicates the content of beta carotene, in mg per Capsule, as well as the Vitamin A activity of beta carotene in terms of the equivalent amount of the all-*trans* isomer of retinol, and the potential vitamin A content from conversion of beta carotene is expressed as the equivalent amount of retinol, in mg per Capsule, and included in the total vitamin A activity. The vitamin A activity may be stated also in USP Units per Capsule, on the basis that 1 USP Vitamin A Unit equals the biological activity of 0.3 mcg of the all-*trans* isomer of retinol. Where the product contains vitamin D, the vitamin D activity may be stated also in USP Units per Capsule, on the basis that 1 USP Vitamin D Unit equals 0.25 mcg of cholecalciferol or ergocalciferol. Where the product contains vitamin E, the label indicates whether it is the *d*- or *dl*- form and indicates also the content, in mg per Capsule, of vitamin E expressed as the *d*-alpha tocopherol equivalent. Where more than one *Assay* method is given for a particular vitamin, the labeling states with which *Assay* method the product complies only if *Method 1* is not used. Contain the labeled amounts of vitamin A as retinol or esters of retinol in the form of retinyl acetate or retinyl palmitate and of beta carotene, within −10% to +65%. Contain the labeled amounts of Vitamin D as ergocalciferol or cholecalciferol, Vitamin E as alpha tocopherol, alpha tocopheryl acetate, or alpha tocopheryl acid succinate, phytonadione, ascorbic acid or its salts as calcium ascorbate or sodium ascorbate, biotin, cyanocobalamin, folic acid, niacin or niacinamide, dexpanthenol or panthenol, calcium pantothenate, pyridoxine, riboflavin, and thiamine as thiamine hydrochoride or thiamine mononitrate, within −10% to +50%. Meet the requirements for Disintegration and dissolution, Weight variation, and Microbial limits.

Oil- and Water-soluble Vitamins Tablets USP—Preserve in tight, light-resistant containers. Contain one or more of the following oil-soluble vitamins: Vitamin A, Vitamin D as Ergocalciferol (Vitamin D_2) or Cholecalciferol (Vitamin D_3), Vitamin E, Phytonadione (Vitamin K_1), and Beta Carotene, and one or more of the following water-soluble vitamins: Ascorbic Acid or its equivalent as Calcium Ascorbate or Sodium Ascorbate, Biotin, Cyanocobalamin, Folic Acid, Niacin or Niacinamide, Pantothenic Acid (as Calcium Pantothenate or Racemic Calcium Pantothenate), Pyridoxine Hydrochloride, Riboflavin, and Thiamine Hydrochloride or Thiamine Mononitrate. The label states that the product is Oil- and Water-soluble Vitamins Tablets. The label states also the quantity of each vitamin in terms of metric units per dosage unit and where necessary the chemical form in which it is present. Where the product contains vitamin A, the label indicates the Vitamin A activity in terms of the equivalent amount of retinol, in mg per Tablet. Where the product contains both vitamin A and beta carotene, the label indicates the content of beta carotene, in mg per Tablet, as well as the vitamin A activity of beta carotene in terms of the equivalent amount of the all-*trans* isomer of retinol, and the potential vitamin A content from conversion of beta carotene is expressed as the equivalent amount of retinol, in mg per Tablet, and included in the total vitamin A activity. The vitamin A activity may be stated also in USP Units per Tablet, on the basis that 1 USP Vitamin A Unit equals the biological activity of 0.3 mcg of the all-*trans* isomer of retinol. Where the product contains vitamin D, the vitamin D activity may be stated also in USP Units per Tablet, on the basis that 1 USP Vitamin D Unit equals 0.25 mcg of cholecalciferol or ergocalciferol. Where the product contains vitamin E, the label indicates whether it is the *d*- or *dl*- form and indicates also the content, in mg per Tablet, of vitamin E expressed as the *d*-alpha tocopherol equivalent. Where more than one *Assay* method is given for a particular vitamin, the labeling states with which *Assay* method the product complies only if *Method 1* is not used. Contain the labeled amounts of vitamin A as retinol or esters of retinol in the form of retinyl acetate or retinyl palmitate and of beta carotene, within −10% to +65%. Contain the labeled amounts of Vitamin D as ergocalciferol or cholecalciferol, Vitamin E as alpha tocopherol, alpha tocopheryl acetate, or alpha tocopheryl acid succinate, phytonadione, ascorbic acid or its salts, as calcium ascorbate or sodium ascorbate, biotin, cyanocobalamin, folic acid, niacin or niacinamide, calcium pantothenate, pyridoxine, riboflavin, and thiamine as thiamine hydrochoride or thiamine mononitrate, within −10% to +50%. Meet the requirements for Disintegration and dissolution, Weight variation, and Microbial limits.

OIL- AND WATER-SOLUBLE VITAMINS WITH MINERALS

USP requirements:

Oil- and Water-soluble Vitamins with Minerals Capsules USP—Preserve in tight, light-resistant containers. Contain one or more of the following oil-soluble vitamins: Vitamin A, Vitamin D as Ergocalciferol (Vitamin D_2) or Cholecalciferol (Vitamin D_3), Vitamin E, Phytonadione (Vitamin K_1), and Beta Carotene; one or more of the following water-soluble vitamins: Ascorbic Acid or its equivalent as Calcium Ascorbate or Sodium Ascorbate, Biotin, Cyanocobalamin, Folic Acid, Niacin or Niacinamide, Dexpanthenol or Panthenol, Pantothenic Acid (as Calcium Pantothenate or Racemic Calcium Pantothenate), Pyridoxine Hydrochloride, Riboflavin, and Thiamine Hydrochloride or Thiamine Mononitrate; and one mineral or more, furnishing one or more of the following elements in ionic form: calcium, chromium, copper, fluorine, iodine, iron, magnesium, manganese, molybdenum, phosphorus, potassium, selenium, and zinc, derived from substances generally recognized as safe. The label states that the product is Oil- and Water-soluble Vitamins with Minerals Capsules. The label states also the quantity of each vitamin and mineral in terms of metric units per dosage unit and where necessary the chemical form in which a vitamin is present and states also the salt form of the mineral used as the source of each element. Where the product contains vitamin A, the label indicates the vitamin A activity in terms of the equivalent amount of retinol, in mg per Capsule. Where the product contains both vitamin A and beta carotene, the label indicates the content of beta carotene, in mg per Capsule, as well as the vitamin A activity of beta carotene in terms of the equivalent amount of the all-*trans* isomer of retinol, and the potential vitamin A content from conversion of beta carotene is expressed as the equivalent amount of retinol, in mg per Capsule, and included in the total vitamin A activity. The vitamin A activity may be stated also in USP Units per Capsule, on the basis that 1 USP Vitamin A Unit equals the biological activity of 0.3 mcg of the all-*trans* isomer of retinol. Where the product contains vitamin E, the label indicates whether it is the *d*- or *dl*- form and indicates also the content, in mg per Capsule, of vitamin E expressed as the *d*-alpha tocopherol equivalent. Where more than one *Assay* method is given for a particular vitamin or mineral, the labeling states with which *Assay* method the product complies only if *Method 1* is not used. Contain the labeled amounts of vitamin A as retinol or esters of retinol in the form of retinyl acetate or retinyl palmitate and of beta carotene, within −10% to +65%. Contain the labeled amounts of vitamin D as ergocalciferol or cholecalciferol, vitamin E as alpha tocopherol or alpha tocopheryl acetate or alpha tocopheryl acid succinate, phytonadione, ascorbic acid or its salts as calcium ascorbate or sodium ascorbate, biotin, cyanocobalamin, folic acid, niacin or niacinamide, dexpanthenol or panthenol, calcium pantothenate, pyridoxine hydrochloride, riboflavin, and thiamine as thiamine hydrochoride or thiamine mononitrate, within −10% to +50%. Contain the labeled amounts of calcium, copper, iron, magnesium, manganese, phosphorus, potassium, and zinc, within −10% to +25%, and the labeled amounts of chromium, fluorine, iodine, molybdenum, and selenium, within −10% to +100%. Do not contain any other ingredient for which nutritional value is claimed. Do not contain any other physiologically active substances. May contain other labeled added substances that are generally recognized as safe, in amounts that are unobjectionable. Meet the requirements for Disintegration and dissolution, Weight variation, and Microbial limits.

Oil- and Water-soluble Vitamins with Minerals Tablets USP—Preserve in tight, light-resistant containers. Contain one or more of the following oil-soluble vitamins: Vitamin A, Vitamin D as Ergocalciferol (Vitamin D_2) or Cholecalciferol (Vitamin D_3), Vitamin E, Phytonadione (Vitamin K_1), and Beta Carotene; one or more of the following water-soluble vitamins: Ascorbic Acid or its equivalent as Calcium Ascorbate or Sodium Ascorbate, Biotin, Cyanocobalamin, Folic Acid, Niacin or Niacinamide, Pantothenic Acid (as Calcium Pantothenate or Racemic Calcium Pantothenate), Pyridoxine Hydrochloride, Riboflavin, and Thiamine Hydrochloride or Thiamine Mononitrate; and one or more minerals derived from substances generally recognized as safe, furnishing one or more of the following elements in ionic form: calcium, chromium, copper, fluorine, iodine, iron, magnesium, manganese, molybdenum, phosphorus, potassium, selenium, and zinc. The label states that the product is Oil- and Water-soluble Vitamins with Minerals Tablets. The label states also the quantity of each vitamin and mineral in terms of metric units per dosage unit and where necessary the chemical form in which a vitamin is present and states also the salt form of the mineral used as the source of each element. Where the product contains vitamin A, the label indicates the Vitamin A activity in terms of the equivalent amount of retinol, in mg per Tablet. Where the product contains both vitamin A and beta carotene, the label indicates the content of beta carotene, in mg per Tablet, as well as the Vitamin A activity of beta carotene in terms of the equivalent amount of the all-*trans* isomer of retinol, and the potential Vitamin A content from conversion of beta carotene is expressed as the equivalent amount of retinol, in mg per Tablet, and included in the total vitamin A activity. The vitamin A activity may be stated also in USP Units per Tablet, on the basis that 1 USP Vitamin A Unit equals the biological activity of 0.3 mcg of the all-*trans* isomer of retinol. Where the product contains vitamin D, the vitamin D activity may be stated also in USP Units per Tablet, on the basis that 1 USP Vitamin D Unit equals 0.25 mcg of cholecalciferol or ergocalciferol. Where the product contains vitamin E, the label indicates whether it is the *d*- or *dl*-form and indicates also the content, in mg per Tablet, of Vitamin E expressed as the *d*-alpha tocopherol equivalent. Where more than one *Assay* method is given for a particular vitamin, the labeling states with which *Assay* method the product complies only if *Method 1* is not used. Contain the labeled amounts of Vitamin A as retinol or esters of retinol in the form of retinyl acetate or retinyl palmitate and of beta carotene, within −10% to +65%. Contain the labeled amounts of Vitamin D, as ergocalciferol or cholecalciferol, Vitamin E as alpha tocopherol or alpha tocopheryl acetate or alpha tocopheryl acid succinate, phytonadione, ascorbic acid or its salts as calcium ascorbate or sodium ascorbate, biotin, cyanocobalamin, folic acid, niacin or niacinamide, dexpanthenol or panthenol, calcium pantothenate, pyridoxine, riboflavin, and thiamine as thiamine hydrochoride or thiamine mononitrate, within −10% to +50%. Contain the labeled amounts of calcium, copper, iron, magnesium, manganese, phosphorus, potassium, and zinc, within −10% to +25%, and the labeled amounts of chromium, fluorine, iodine, molybdenum, and selenium, within −10% to +100%. Do not contain any other ingredient for which nutritional value is claimed. Do not contain any other physiologically active substances. May contain other labeled added substances that are generally recognized as safe, in amounts that are unobjectionable. Meet the requirements for Disintegration and dissolution, Weight variation, and Microbial limits.

WATER-SOLUBLE VITAMINS

For *Ascorbic Acid* (or *Sodium Ascorbate* or *Calcium Ascorbate*), *Biotin, Cyanocobalamin, Folic Acid, Niacin* or *Niacinamide, Dexpanthenol* or *Panthenol, Calcium Pantothenate* or *Racemic Calcium Pantothenate, Pyridoxine, Riboflavin,* and *Thiamine*—See individual listings for chemistry information.

USP requirements:

Water-soluble Vitamins Capsules USP—Preserve in tight, light-resistant containers. The label states that the product is Water-soluble Vitamins Capsules. The label states also the quantity of each vitamin in terms of metric units per dosage unit and where necessary the salt form in which it is present. Where more than one *Assay* method is given for a particular vitamin, the labeling states which *Assay* method is used only if *Method I* is not used. Where products are labeled to contain panthenol, the label states the equivalent content of dexpanthenol. Contain two or more of the following water-soluble vitamins: Ascorbic Acid or its equivalent as Sodium Ascorbate or Calcium Ascorbate, Biotin, Cyanocobalamin, Folic Acid, Niacin or Niacinamide, Dexpanthenol or Panthenol, Pantothenic Acid (as Calcium Pantothenate or Racemic Calcium Pantothenate), Pyridoxine Hydrochloride, Riboflavin, and Thiamine Hydrochloride or Thiamine Mononitrate. Contain the labeled amounts of ascorbic acid, biotin, cyanocobalamin, folic acid, niacin or niacinamide, dexpanthenol or panthenol, calcium pantothenate, pyridoxine hydrochloride, riboflavin, and thiamine as the hydrochloride or mononitrate, within −10% to +50%. Do not contain any form of Vitamins A, D, E, K, or Beta Carotene. Do not contain any minerals for which nutritional value is claimed. May contain other labeled added substances in amounts that are unobjectionable. Meet the requirements for Microbial limits, Disintegration and dissolution, and Weight variation.

Water-soluble Vitamins Tablets USP—Preserve in tight, light-resistant containers. The label states that the product is Water-soluble Vitamins Tablets. The label states also the quantity of each vitamin in terms of metric units per dosage unit and where necessary the salt form in which it is present. Where more than one *Assay* method is given for a particular vitamin, the labeling states which *Assay* method is used only if *Method I* is not used. Contain two or more of the following water-soluble vitamins: Ascorbic Acid or its equivalent as Sodium Ascorbate or Calcium Ascorbate, Biotin, Cyanocobalamin, Folic Acid, Niacin or Niacinamide, Pantothenic Acid (as Calcium Pantothenate or Racemic Calcium Pantothenate), Pyridoxine Hydrochloride, Riboflavin, and Thiamine Hydrochloride or Thiamine Mononitrate. Contain the labeled amounts of ascorbic acid or its equivalent as sodium ascorbate or calcium ascorbate, biotin, thiamine as the hydrochloride or mononitrate, cyanocobalamin, folic acid, niacin or niacinamide, calcium pantothenate, pyridoxine hydrochloride, and riboflavin, within −10% to +50%. Do not contain any form of Vitamins A, D, E, K, or Beta Carotene. Do not contain any minerals for which nutritional value is claimed. May contain other labeled added substances in amounts that are unobjectionable. Meet the requirements for Microbial limits, Disintegration and dissolution, and Weight variation.

WATER-SOLUBLE VITAMINS WITH MINERALS

USP requirements:

Water-soluble Vitamins with Minerals Capsules USP—Preserve in tight, light-resistant containers. Contain one or more of the following water-soluble vitamins: Ascorbic Acid or its equivalent as Calcium Ascorbate or Sodium Ascorbate, Biotin, Cyanocobalamin, Folic Acid, Niacin or Niacinamide, Dexpanthenol or Panthenol, Pantothenic Acid (as Calcium Pantothenate or Racemic Calcium Pantothenate), Pyridoxine Hydrochloride, Riboflavin, and Thiamine Hydrochloride or Thiamine Mononitrate; and one mineral or more, furnishing one or more of the following elements in ionic form: calcium, chromium, copper, fluorine, iodine, iron, magnesium, manganese, molybdenum, phosphorus, potassium, selenium, and zinc, derived from substances generally recognized as safe. The label states that the product is Water-soluble Vitamins with Minerals Capsules. The label states also the quantity of each vitamin and mineral in terms of metric units per dosage unit and where necessary the chemical form in which a vitamin is present and states also the salt form of the mineral used as the source of each element. Where more than one *Assay* method is given for a particular vitamin or mineral, the labeling states with which *Assay* method the product complies only if *Method 1* is not used. Contain the labeled amounts of ascorbic acid or its salts as calcium ascorbate or sodium ascorbate, biotin, cyanocobalamin, folic acid, niacin or niacinamide, dexpanthenol or panthenol, calcium pantothenate, pyridoxine, riboflavin, and thiamine as thiamine hydrochoride or thiamine mononitrate, within −10% to +50%. Contain the labeled amounts of calcium, copper, iron, magnesium, manganese, phosphorus, potassium, and zinc, within −10% to +25%, and the labeled amounts of chromium, fluorine, iodine, molybdenum, and selenium, within −10% to +100%. Do not contain any form of Vitamins A, D, E, or K, or Beta Carotene. Do not contain any other ingredient for which nutritional value is claimed. Do not contain any other physiologically active substances. May contain other labeled added substances that are generally recognized as safe, in amounts that are unobjectionable. Meet the requirements for Disintegration and dissolution, Weight variation, and Microbial limits.

Water-soluble Vitamins with Minerals Tablets USP—Preserve in tight, light-resistant containers. Contain one or more of the following water-soluble vitamins: Ascorbic Acid or its equivalent as Calcium Ascorbate or Sodium Ascorbate, Biotin, Cyanocobalamin, Folic Acid, Niacin or Niacinamide, Pantothenic Acid (as Calcium Pantothenate or Racemic Calcium Pantothenate), Pyridoxine Hydrochloride, Riboflavin, and Thiamine Hydrochloride or Thiamine Mononitrate; and one or more minerals derived from substances generally recognized as safe, furnishing one or more of the following elements in ionic form: calcium, chromium, copper, fluorine, iodine, iron, magnesium, manganese, molybdenum, phosphorus, potassium, selenium, and zinc. The label states that the product is Water-soluble Vitamins with Minerals Tablets. The label states also the quantity of each vitamin and mineral in terms of metric units per dosage unit and where necessary the chemical form in which a vitamin is present and states also the salt form of the mineral used as the source of each element. Where more than one *Assay* method is given for a particular vitamin, the labeling states with which *Assay* method the product complies only if *Method 1* is not used. Contain the labeled amounts of ascorbic acid or its salts as calcium ascorbate or sodium ascorbate, biotin, cyanocobalamin, folic acid, niacin or niacinamide, calcium pantothenate, pyridoxine, riboflavin, and thiamine as thiamine hydrochoride or thiamine mononitrate, within −10% to +50%. Contain the labeled amounts of calcium, copper, iron, manganese, magnesium, phosphorus, potassium, and zinc, within −10% to +25%, and the labeled amounts of chromium, fluorine, iodine, molybdenum, and selenium, within −10% to +100%. Do not contain any form of Vitamins A, D, E, K, or Beta Carotene. Do not contain any other ingredient for which nutritional value is claimed. Do not contain any other physiologically active substances. May contain other labeled added substances that are generally recognized as safe, in amounts that are unobjectionable. Meet the requirements for Disintegration and dissolution, Weight variation, and Microbial limits.

WARFARIN

Chemical group: Coumarin derivative.

Chemical name: Warfarin sodium—2*H*-1-Benzopyran-2-one, 4-hydroxy-3-(3-oxo-1-phenylbutyl)-, sodium salt.

Molecular formula: Warfarin sodium—$C_{19}H_{15}NaO_4$.

Molecular weight: Warfarin sodium—330.32.

Description: Warfarin Sodium USP—White, odorless, amorphous or crystalline powder. Is discolored by light.

Solubility: Warfarin Sodium USP—Very soluble in water; freely soluble in alcohol; very slightly soluble in chloroform and in ether.

USP requirements:

Warfarin Sodium USP—Preserve in well-closed, light-resistant containers. An amorphous solid or a crystalline clathrate. Label it to indicate whether it is the amorphous or the crystalline form. The clathrate form consists principally of warfarin sodium and isopropyl alcohol, in a 2:1 molecular ratio; contains not less than 8.0% and not more than 8.5% of isopropyl alcohol. Contains not less than 97.0% and not more than 102.0% of warfarin sodium, calculated on the anhydrous basis for the amorphous form or on the anhydrous and isopropyl alcohol-free basis for the crystalline form. Meets the requirements for Identification, pH (7.2–8.3, in a solution [1 in 100]), Water (not more than 4.5% for the amorphous form and not more than 0.3% for the crystalline clathrate form), Absorbance in alkaline solution, Heavy metals (not more than 0.001%), Isopropyl alcohol content, and Organic volatile impurities.

Warfarin Sodium for Injection USP—Preserve in light-resistant Containers for Sterile Solids. A sterile, freeze-dried mixture of Warfarin Sodium and suitable added substances. Contains the labeled amount, within ±5%. Meets the requirements for Completeness of solution, Constituted solution, Bacterial endotoxins, and Water (not more than 4.5%), for Identification tests A and B, pH, and Heavy metals under Warfarin Sodium, and for Sterility tests, Uniformity of dosage units, and Labeling under Injections.

Warfarin Sodium Tablets USP—Preserve in tight, light-resistant containers. Contain the labeled amount, within

±5%. Meet the requirements for Identification, Dissolution (80% in 30 minutes in water in Apparatus 2 at 50 rpm), and Uniformity of dosage units.

WATER

Chemical name: Purified water—Water.

Molecular formula: Purified water—H_2O.

Molecular weight: Purified water—18.02.

Description:

Water for Injection USP—Clear, colorless, odorless liquid.

NF category: Solvent.

Bacteriostatic Water for Injection USP—Clear, colorless liquid, odorless, or having the odor of the antimicrobial substance.

NF category: Vehicle (sterile).

Sterile Water for Inhalation USP—Clear, colorless solution.

Sterile Water for Injection USP—Clear, colorless, odorless liquid.

NF category: Solvent.

Sterile Water for Irrigation USP—Clear, colorless, odorless liquid.

NF category: Solvent.

Purified Water USP—Clear, colorless, odorless liquid.

NF category: Solvent.

USP requirements:

Water for Injection USP—Where packaged, preserve in tight containers. Where packaged, it may be stored at a temperature below or above the range in which microbial growth occurs. It is water purified by distillation or by reverse osmosis. Contains no added substance. Meets the requirement for Bacterial endotoxins.

Note: Water for Injection is intended for use as a solvent for the preparation of parenteral solutions. Where used for the preparation of parenteral solutions subject to final sterilization, use suitable means to minimize microbial growth, or first render the Water for Injection sterile and thereafter protect it from microbial contamination. For parenteral solutions that are prepared under aseptic conditions and are not sterilized by appropriate filtration or in the final container, first render the Water for Injection sterile and, thereafter, protect it from microbial contamination.

Bacteriostatic Water for Injection USP—Preserve in single-dose or in multiple-dose containers, preferably of Type I or Type II glass, of not larger than 30-mL size. It is Sterile Water for Injection containing one or more suitable antimicrobial agents. Label it to indicate the name(s) and proportion(s) of the added antimicrobial agent(s). Label it also to include the statement, "**NOT FOR USE IN NEWBORNS**," in boldface capital letters on the label immediately under the official name, printed in a contrasting color, preferably red. Alternatively, the statement may be placed prominently elsewhere on the label if the statement is enclosed within a box. Meets the requirements for Antimicrobial agent(s), Bacterial endotoxins, Sterility, pH (4.5–7.0), and Particulate matter, and for Sulfate, Calcium, Carbon dioxide, and Heavy metals under Sterile Water for Injection.

Note: Use Bacteriostatic Water for Injection with due regard for the compatibility of the antimicrobial agent or agents it contains with the particular medicinal substance that is to be dissolved or diluted.

Sterile Water for Inhalation USP—Preserve in single-dose containers. It is water purified by distillation or by reverse osmosis and rendered sterile. Label it to indicate that it is for inhalation therapy only and that it is not for parenteral administration. Contains no antimicrobial agents, except where used in humidifiers or other similar devices and where liable to contamination over a period of time, or other added substances. Meets the requirements for Bacterial endotoxins, Sterility, pH (4.5–7.5), and Chloride (not more than 0.5 ppm), for Sulfate, Calcium, Carbon dioxide, and Heavy metals under Purified Water, and for Ammonia, Oxidizable substances, and Total solids under Sterile Water for Injection.

Note: Do not use Sterile Water for Inhalation for parenteral administration or for other sterile compendial dosage forms.

Sterile Water for Injection USP—Preserve in single-dose glass or plastic containers, of not larger than 1-liter size. Glass containers are preferably of Type I or Type II glass. It is Water for Injection sterilized and suitably packaged. Contains no antimicrobial agent or other added substance. Label it to indicate that no antimicrobial or other substance has been added, and that it is not suitable for intravascular injection without its first having been made approximately isotonic by the addition of a suitable solute. Meets the requirements for Bacterial endotoxins, Sterility, Particulate matter, Ammonia, Chloride, Oxidizable substances, and Total solids, and for pH, Sulfate, Calcium, Carbon dioxide, and Heavy metals under Purified water.

Sterile Water for Irrigation USP—Preserve in single-dose glass or plastic containers. Glass containers are preferably of Type I or Type II glass. The container may contain a volume of more than 1 liter, and may be designed to empty rapidly. It is Water for Injection sterilized and suitably packaged. Contains no antimicrobial agent or other added substance. Label it to indicate that no antimicrobial or other substance has been added. The designations "For irrigation only" and "Not for injection" appear prominently on the label. Meets the requirements of all of the tests under Sterile Water for Injection except the test for Particulate matter.

Purified Water USP—Where packaged, preserve in tight containers. It is water obtained by distillation, ion-exchange treatment, reverse osmosis, or other suitable process. Prepared from water complying with the regulations of the U.S. Environmental Protection Agency with respect to drinking water. Contains no added substance. Where packaged, label it to indicate the method of preparation. Meets the requirements for pH (5.0–7.0), Chloride, Sulfate, Limit of ammonia (not more than 0.3 ppm), Calcium, Carbon dioxide, Heavy metals, Oxidizable substances, and Total solids (not more than 0.001%).

Note: Purified Water is intended for use as an ingredient in the preparation of compendial dosage forms. Where used for sterile dosage forms, other than for parenteral administration, process the article to meet the requirements under Sterility tests, or first render the Purified Water sterile and thereafter protect it from microbial contamination. Do not use Purified Water in preparations intended for parenteral administration. For such purposes use Water for Injection, Bacteriostatic Water for Injection, or Sterile Water for Injection.

CARNAUBA WAX

Description: Carnauba Wax NF—Light brown to pale yellow, moderately coarse powder or flakes, possessing a characteristic bland odor, and free from rancidity. Specific gravity is about 0.99.

NF category: Coating agent.

Solubility: Carnauba Wax NF—Insoluble in water; soluble in warm chloroform and in toluene; slightly soluble in boiling alcohol.

NF requirements: Carnauba Wax NF—Preserve in well-closed containers. Obtained from the leaves of *Copernicia cerifera* Mart. (Fam. Palmae). Meets the requirements for Melting range (81–86 °C), Residue on ignition (not more than 0.25%), Heavy metals (not more than 0.004%), Acid value (2–7), and Saponification value (78–95).

EMULSIFYING WAX

Description: Emulsifying Wax NF—Creamy white, wax-like solid, having a mild characteristic odor.

NF category: Emulsifying and/or solubilizing agent; stiffening agent.

Solubility: Emulsifying Wax NF—Insoluble in water; freely soluble in ether, in chloroform, in most hydrocarbon solvents, and in aerosol propellants; soluble in alcohol.

NF requirements: Emulsifying Wax NF—Preserve in well-closed containers. A waxy solid prepared from Cetostearyl Alcohol containing a polyoxyethylene derivative of a fatty acid ester of sorbitan. Meets the requirements for Melting range (50–54 °C), pH (5.5–7.0, in a dispersion [3 in 100]), Hydroxyl value (178–192), Iodine value (not more than 3.5), and Saponification value (not more than 14).

MICROCRYSTALLINE WAX

Description: Microcrystalline Wax NF—White or cream-colored, odorless, waxy solid.

NF category: Coating agent.

Solubility: Microcrystalline Wax NF—Insoluble in water; sparingly soluble in dehydrated alcohol; soluble in chloroform, in ether, in volatile oils, and in most warm fixed oils.

NF requirements: Microcrystalline Wax NF—Preserve in tight containers. A mixture of straight-chain, branched-chain, and cyclic hydrocarbons, obtained by solvent fractionation of the still bottom fraction of petroleum by suitable dewaxing or deoiling means. Label it to indicate the name and proportion of any added stabilizer. Meets the requirements for Color, Melting range (54–102 °C), Consistency (0.3–10.0 mm), Acidity, Alkalinity, Residue on ignition (not more than 0.1%), Organic acids, and Fixed oils, fats, and rosin.

WHITE WAX

Description: White Wax NF—Yellowish white solid, somewhat translucent in thin layers. Has a faint, characteristic odor, and is free from rancidity. Specific gravity is about 0.95.

NF category: Stiffening agent.

Solubility: White Wax NF—Insoluble in water; sparingly soluble in cold alcohol. Boiling alcohol dissolves the cerotic acid and a portion of the myricin, which are constituents of White Wax. Completely soluble in chloroform, in ether, and in fixed and volatile oils. Partly soluble in cold carbon disulfide, and completely soluble in this liquid at about 30 °C.

NF requirements: White Wax NF—Preserve in well-closed containers. The product of bleaching and purifying Yellow Wax that is obtained from the honeycomb of the bee (*Apis mellifera* Linné [Fam. Apidae]) and that meets the requirements for the Saponification cloud test. Meets the requirements for Melting range (62–65 °C), Saponification cloud test, Fats or fatty acids, Japan wax, rosin, and soap, Acid value (17–24), and Ester value (72–79).

YELLOW WAX

Description: Yellow Wax NF—Solid varying in color from yellow to grayish brown. Has an agreeable, honey-like odor. Somewhat brittle when cold, and presents a dull, granular, noncrystalline fracture when broken. It becomes pliable from the heat of the hand. Specific gravity is about 0.95.

NF category: Stiffening agent.

Solubility: Yellow Wax NF—Insoluble in water; sparingly soluble in cold alcohol. Boiling alcohol dissolves the cerotic acid and a portion of the myricin, which are constituents of Yellow Wax. Completely soluble in chloroform, in ether, in fixed oils, and in volatile oils. Partly soluble in cold carbon disulfide, and completely soluble in this liquid at about 30 °C.

NF requirements: Yellow Wax NF—Preserve in well-closed containers. The purified wax from the honeycomb of the bee (*Apis mellifera* Linné [Fam. Apidae]). Meets the requirements for Melting range, Saponification cloud test, Fats or fatty acids, Japan wax, rosin, and soap, Acid value, and Ester value under White Wax.

Note: To meet specifications of this monograph, the crude beeswax used to prepare Yellow Wax conforms to the Saponification cloud test.

WHITE LOTION

USP requirements: White Lotion USP—Dispense in tight containers.

Prepare White Lotion as follows: 40 grams of Zinc Sulfate, 40 grams of Sulfurated Potash, and a sufficient quantity of Purified Water to make 1000 mL. Dissolve the Zinc Sulfate and the Sulfurated Potash separately, each in 450 mL of Purified Water, and filter each solution. Add the sulfurated potash solution slowly to the zinc sulfate solution with constant stirring. Then add the required amount of purified water, and mix.

Note: Prepare the Lotion fresh, and shake it thoroughly before dispensing.

WITCH HAZEL

USP requirements: Witch Hazel USP—Preserve in tight containers, and avoid exposure to excessive heat. A clear, colorless distillate prepared from recently cut and partially dried dormant twigs of *Hamamelis virginiana* Linné.

Prepare Witch Hazel as follows. Macerate a weighed amount of the twigs for about 24 hours in about twice their weight of water, then distil until not less than 800 mL and not more than 850 mL of clear, colorless distillate is obtained from each 1000 grams of the twigs taken. Add 150 mL of Alcohol to each 850 mL of distillate, and mix thoroughly.

Meets the requirements for Specific gravity (0.979–0.983), pH (3.0–5.0), Nonvolatile residue (not more than 0.025%), Limit of tannins, and Alcohol content (14.0–15.0%).

XANTHAN GUM

Description: Xanthan Gum NF—Cream-colored powder. Its solutions in water are neutral to litmus.

NF category: Suspending and/or viscosity-increasing agent.

Solubility: Xanthan Gum NF—Soluble in hot or cold water.

NF requirements: Xanthan Gum NF—Preserve in well-closed containers. A high molecular weight polysaccharide gum produced by a pure-culture fermentation of a carbohydrate with *Xanthomonas campestris*, then purified by recovery with Isopropyl Alcohol, dried, and milled. Contains D-glucose and D-mannose as the dominant hexose units, along with D-glucuronic acid, and is prepared as the sodium, potassium, or calcium salt. Yields not less than 4.2% and not more than 5.0% of carbon dioxide, calculated on the dried basis, corresponding to not less than 91.0% and not more than 108.0% of Xanthan Gum. Meets the requirements for Identification, Viscosity (not less than 600 centipoises at 24 °C), Microbial limits, Loss on drying (not more than 15.0%), Ash (6.5–16.0%, calculated on the dried basis), Arsenic (not more than 3 ppm), Heavy metals (not more than 0.003%), Lead (not more than 5 ppm), Isopropyl alcohol (not more than 0.075%), and Pyruvic acid (not less than 1.5%).

XENON Xe 127

Description: Xenon Xe 127 USP—Clear, colorless gas.

USP requirements: Xenon Xe 127 USP—Preserve in single-dose vials having leak-proof stoppers, at room temperature. The vials are enclosed in appropriate lead radiation shields. The vial content may be diluted with air and is packaged at atmospheric pressure. A gas suitable for inhalation in diagnostic studies. Xenon 127 is a radioactive nuclide that may be prepared from the bombardment of a cesium 133 target with high-energy protons. Label it to include the following: the name of the preparation; the container volume, MBq (or mCi) of ^{127}Xe per container; the amount of ^{127}Xe expressed as megabecquerels (or millicuries) per mL; the intended route of administration; recommended storage conditions; the date of calibration; the expiration date; the name, address, and batch number of the manufacturer; the statement "Caution—Radioactive Material"; and a radioactive symbol. The labeling contains a statement of radionuclide purity, identifies probable radionuclidic impurities, and indicates permissible quantities of each impurity. The labeling indicates that in making dosage calculations, correction is to be made for radioactive decay, and also indicates that the radioactive half-life of ^{127}Xe is 36.41 days. Contains the labeled amount of ^{127}Xe, within $\pm 15\%$, at the calibration date indicated in the labeling. Meets the requirements for Radionuclide identification and Radionuclidic purity.

XENON Xe 133

Chemical name: Xenon, isotope of mass 133.

Description: Xenon Xe 133 Injection USP—Clear, colorless solution.

USP requirements:

Xenon Xe 133 USP—Preserve in single-dose or in multiple-dose vials having leak-proof stoppers, at room temperature. A gas suitable for inhalation in diagnostic studies. Xenon 133 is a radioactive nuclide that may be prepared from the fission of uranium 235. Contains the labeled amount of ^{133}Xe, within $\pm 15\%$, at the date and time indicated in the labeling. Meets the requirements for Labeling (except for the information specified for Labeling under Injections), for Radionuclide identification, and for Radionuclidic purity under Xenon 133 Injection (except to determine the radioactivity in MBq [or mCi] per container).

Xenon Xe 133 Injection USP—Preserve in single-dose containers that are totally filled, so that any air present occupies not more than 0.5% of the total volume of the container. Store at a temperature between 2 and 8 °C. If there is free space above the solution, a significant amount of the xenon 133 is present in the gaseous phase. Glass containers may darken under the effects of radiation. A sterile, isotonic solution of Xenon 133 in Sodium Chloride Injection suitable for intravenous administration. Xenon 133 is a radioactive nuclide prepared from the fission of uranium 235. Label it to include the following, in addition to the information specified for Labeling under Injections: the time and date of calibration; the amount of xenon 133 expressed as total megabecquerels (or microcuries or millicuries), and concentration as megabecquerels (or microcuries or millicuries), per mL at the time of calibration; the expiration date; the name and amount of any added bacteriostatic agent; and the statement, "Caution—Radioactive Material." The labeling indicates that in making dosage calculations, correction is to be made for radioactive decay, and also indicates that the radioactive half-life of ^{133}Xe is 5.24 days. Contains the labeled amount of Xenon 133, within $\pm 10\%$, at the date and time stated on the label. Meets the requirements for Radionuclide identification, Bacterial endotoxins, pH (4.5–8.0), Radionuclidic purity, and Injections (except that the Injection may be distributed or dispensed prior to the completion of the test for Sterility, the latter test being started on the day of manufacture, and except that it is not subject to the recommendation on Volume in Container).

XYLITOL

Chemical name: Xylitol.

Molecular formula: $C_5H_{12}O_5$.

Molecular weight: 152.15.

Description: Xylitol NF—White crystals or crystalline powder. Crystalline xylitol has a melting range between 92 and 96 °C.

Solubility: Xylitol NF—One gram dissolves in about 0.65 mL of water. Sparingly soluble in alcohol.

NF requirements: Xylitol NF—Preserve in well-closed containers. Contains not less than 98.5% and not more than 101.0% of xylitol, calculated on the anhydrous basis. Meets the requirements for Identification, Water (not more than 0.5%), Residue on ignition (not more than 0.5%), Arsenic (not more than 3 ppm), Heavy metals (not more than 0.001%), Reducing sugars, Organic volatile impurities, and Limit of other polyols (not more than 2.0%).

XYLOMETAZOLINE

Chemical name: Xylometazoline hydrochloride—1*H*-Imidazole, 2-[[4-(1,1-dimethylethyl)-2,6-dimethylphenyl]methyl]-4,5-dihydro-, monohydrochloride.

Molecular formula: Xylometazoline hydrochloride—$C_{16}H_{24}N_2 \cdot HCl$.

Molecular weight: Xylometazoline hydrochloride—280.84.

Description: Xylometazoline Hydrochloride USP—White to off-white, odorless, crystalline powder. Melts above 300 °C, with decomposition.

Solubility: Xylometazoline Hydrochloride USP—Soluble in water; freely soluble in alcohol; sparingly soluble in chloroform; practically insoluble in ether.

USP requirements:

Xylometazoline Hydrochloride USP—Preserve in tight, light-resistant containers. Contains not less than 99.0% and not more than 101.0% of xylometazoline hydrochloride, calculated on the dried basis. Meets the requirements for Identification, pH (5.0–6.6, in a solution [1 in 20]), Loss on drying (not more than 0.5%), Residue on ignition (not more than 0.1%), and Chromatographic purity.

Xylometazoline Hydrochloride Nasal Solution USP—Preserve in tight, light-resistant containers. An isotonic solution of Xylometazoline Hydrochloride in Water. Contains the labeled amount, within ±10%. Meets the requirements for Identification and pH (5.0–7.5).

XYLOSE

Chemical name: D-Xylose.

Molecular formula: $C_5H_{10}O_5$.

Molecular weight: 150.13.

Description: Xylose USP—Colorless needles or white, crystalline powder. Is odorless.

Solubility: Xylose USP—Very soluble in water; slightly soluble in alcohol.

USP requirements: Xylose USP—Preserve in tight containers at controlled room temperature. Contains not less than 98.0% and not more than 102.0% of xylose, calculated on the dried basis. Meets the requirements for Color of solution, Identification, Specific rotation (+18.2° to +19.4°), Loss on drying (not more than 0.1%), Residue on ignition (not more than 0.05%), Arsenic (not more than 1 ppm), Iron (not more than 5 ppm), Heavy metals (not more than 0.001%), Chromatographic purity, and Organic volatile impurities.

YELLOW FEVER VACCINE

Description: Yellow Fever Vaccine USP—Slightly dull, light-orange colored, flaky or crustlike, desiccated mass.

USP requirements: Yellow Fever Vaccine USP—Preserve in nitrogen-filled, flame-sealed ampuls or suitable stoppered vials at a temperature preferably below 0 °C but never above 5 °C, throughout the dating period. Preserve it during shipment in a suitable container adequately packed in solid carbon dioxide, or provided with other means of refrigeration, so as to insure a temperature constantly below 0 °C. The attenuated strain that has been tested in monkeys for viscerotropism, immunogenicity, and neurotropism, of living yellow fever virus selected for high antigenic activity and safety. Prepared by the culturing of the virus in the living embryos of chicken eggs, from which a suspension is prepared, processed with aseptic precautions, and finally dried from the frozen state. Meets the requirements of the specific mouse potency test in titer of mouse LD_{50} (quantity of virus estimated to produce fatal specific encephalitis in 50% of the mice) or the requirements for plaque-forming units in a suitable cell-culture system, such as a Vero cell system for which the relationship between mouse LD_{50} and plaque-forming units has been established, in which cell monolayers in 35 mm petri dishes are inoculated for a specified time with dilutions of Vaccine, after which the dilutions are replaced with 0.5% agarose-containing medium. Following adsorption and incubation for five days an overlay is added of the 0.5% agarose medium containing 1:50,000 neutral red and the plaques are counted on the sixth day following inoculation. Label it to state that it is to be well shaken before use and that the constituted vaccine is to be used entirely or discarded within 1 hour of opening the container. Label it also to state that it is the living yellow fever vaccine virus prepared from chicken embryos and that the dose is the same for persons of all ages, but that it is not recommended for infants under six months of age. It is sterile and contains no human serum and no antimicrobial agent. Yellow Fever Vaccine is constituted, with Sodium Chloride Injection containing no antimicrobial agent, just prior to use. Meets the requirement for Expiration date (not later than 1 year after the date of issue from manufacturer's cold storage [−20 °C, 1 year]). Conforms to the regulations of the U.S. Food and Drug Administration concerning biologics.

YOHIMBINE

Source: Yohimbine hydrochloride—Obtained from the principal alkaloid of the bark of the yohimbe tree.

Chemical name: Yohimbine hydrochloride—Methyl 17 alpha-hydroxy-yohimban-16 alpha-carboxylate hydrochloride.

Molecular formula: Yohimbine hydrochloride—$C_{21}H_{26}N_2O_3 \cdot HCl$.

Molecular weight: Yohimbine hydrochloride—390.9.

USP requirements: Yohimbine Hydrochloride Tablets—Not in USP.

ZALCITABINE

Chemical name: Cytidine, 2′,3′-dideoxy-.

Molecular formula: $C_9H_{13}N_3O_3$.

Molecular weight: 211.22.

Description: White to off-white crystalline powder.

Solubility: Aqueous solubility of 76.4 mg/mL at 25 °C.

USP requirements: Zalcitabine Tablets—Not in USP.

ZEIN

Description: Zein NF—White to yellow powder.
NF category: Coating agent.

Solubility: Zein NF—Soluble in aqueous alcohols, in glycols, in ethylene glycol ethyl ether, in furfuryl alcohol, in tetrahydrofurfuryl alcohol, and in aqueous alkaline solutions of pH 11.5 or greater. Insoluble in water and in acetone; readily soluble in acetone-water mixtures between the limits of 60% and 80% of acetone by volume; insoluble in all anhydrous alcohols except methanol.

NF requirements: Zein NF—Preserve in tight containers. A prolamine derived from corn (*Zea mays* Linné [Fam. Gramineae]). Meets the requirements for Identification, Microbial limits, Loss on drying (not more than 8.0%), Residue on ignition (not more than 2.0%), Arsenic (not more than 3 ppm), Heavy metals (not more than 0.002%), and Nitrogen content (13.1–17.0%, on the dried basis).

ZIDOVUDINE

Chemical group: Dideoxynucleoside analog; also a thymidine analog.

Chemical name: Thymidine, 3′-azido-3′-deoxy-.

Molecular formula: $C_{10}H_{13}N_5O_4$.

Molecular weight: 267.25.

Description: White to beige, odorless, crystalline solid.

USP requirements:
Zidovudine Capsules—Not in USP.

Zidovudine Injection—Not in USP.
Zidovudine Syrup—Not in USP.

ZINC ACETATE

Chemical name: Acetic acid, zinc salt, dihydrate.

Molecular formula: $C_4H_6O_4Zn \cdot 2H_2O$.

Molecular weight: 219.51.

Description: Zinc Acetate USP—White crystals or granules, having a slight acetous odor. Is slightly efflorescent.

Solubility: Zinc Acetate USP—Freely soluble in water and in boiling alcohol; slightly soluble in alcohol.

USP requirements: Zinc Acetate USP—Preserve in tight containers. Contains not less than 98.0% and not more than 102.0% of zinc acetate. Meets the requirements for Identification, pH (6.0–8.0, in a solution [1 in 20]), Insoluble matter (not more than 0.005%), Arsenic (not more than 3 ppm), Lead (not more than 0.002%), Chloride (not more than 0.005%), Sulfate (not more than 0.010%), Alkalies and alkaline earths (not more than 0.2%), and Organic volatile impurities.

ZINC CARBONATE

Chemical name: Bis[carbonato(2–)]hexahydroxypentazinc.

Molecular formula: $3Zn(OH)_2 \cdot 2ZnCO_3$.

Molecular weight: 549.02.

USP requirements: Zinc Carbonate USP—Preserve in tight containers. Contains the equivalent of not less than 70.0% of zinc oxide. Meets the requirements for Identification, Insoluble matter (not more than 0.02%), Chloride (not more than 0.002%), Sulfate (not more than 0.01%), Iron (not more than 0.002%), Lead (not more than 5 ppm), and Substances not precipitated by ammonium sulfide (not more than 0.4%).

ZINC CHLORIDE

Chemical name: Zinc chloride.

Molecular fomula: $ZnCl_2$.

Molecular weight: 136.30.

Description: Zinc Chloride USP—White or practically white, odorless, crystalline powder, or white or practically white crystalline granules. May also be in porcelain-like masses or molded into cylinders. Very deliquescent. A solution (1 in 10) is acid to litmus.

Solubility: Zinc Chloride USP—Very soluble in water; freely soluble in alcohol and in glycerin. Its solution in water or in alcohol is usually slightly turbid, but the turbidity disappears when a small quantity of hydrochloric acid is added.

USP requirements:

Zinc Chloride USP—Preserve in tight containers. Contains not less than 97.0% and not more than 100.5% of zinc chloride. Meets the requirements for Identification, Limit of oxychloride, Sulfate (not more than 0.03%), Limit of ammonium salts, Lead (not more than 0.005%), Alkalies and alkaline earths (not more than 1.0%), and Organic volatile impurities.

Zinc Chloride Injection USP—Preserve in single-dose or in multiple-dose containers, preferably of Type I or Type II glass. A sterile solution of Zinc Chloride in Water for Injection. Label the Injection to indicate that it is to be diluted with Water for Injection or other suitable fluid to appropriate strength prior to administration. Contains an amount of zinc chloride equivalent to the labeled amount of zinc, within ±5%. Meets the requirements for Identification, Bacterial endotoxins, pH (1.5–2.5), Particulate matter, and Injections.

ZINC GLUCONATE

Chemical name: Bis(D-gluconato-O^1,O^2) zinc.

Molecular formula: $C_{12}H_{22}O_{14}Zn$.

Molecular weight: 455.69.

Description: Zinc Gluconate USP—White or practically white powder or granules.

Solubility: Zinc Gluconate USP—Soluble in water; very slightly soluble in alcohol.

USP requirements:

Zinc Gluconate USP—Preserve in well-closed containers. Contains not less than 97.0% and not more than 102.0% of zinc gluconate, calculated on the anhydrous basis. Meets the requirements for Identification, pH (5.5–7.5, in a solution [1 in 100]), Water (not more than 11.6%), Chloride (not more than 0.05%), Sulfate (not more than 0.05%), Arsenic (not more than 3 ppm), Reducing substances (not more than 1.0%), Cadmium (not more than 5 ppm), Lead (not more than 0.001%), and Organic volatile impurities.

Zinc Gluconate Tablets—Not in USP.

ZINC OXIDE

Chemical name: Zinc oxide.

Molecular formula: ZnO.

Molecular weight: 81.39.

Description: Zinc Oxide USP—Very fine, odorless, amorphous, white or yellowish white powder, free from gritty particles. Gradually absorbs carbon dioxide from air.

Solubility: Zinc Oxide USP—Insoluble in water and in alcohol; soluble in dilute acids.

USP requirements:

Zinc Oxide USP—Preserve in well-closed containers. Freshly ignited, contains not less than 99.0% and not more than 100.5% of zinc oxide. Meets the requirements for Identification, Alkalinity, Loss on ignition (not more than 1.0%), Carbonate and color of solution, Arsenic (not more than 6 ppm), Iron and other heavy metals, and Lead.

Zinc Oxide Ointment USP—Preserve in well-closed containers, and avoid prolonged exposure to temperatures exceeding 30 °C. Contains not less than 18.5% and not more than 21.5% of zinc oxide.

Zinc Oxide Ointment may be prepared as follows: 200 grams of Zinc Oxide, 150 grams of Mineral Oil, and 650 grams of White Ointment, to make 1000 grams. Levigate the Zinc Oxide with the Mineral Oil to a smooth paste, and then incorporate the White Ointment.

Meets the requirements for Identification, Minimum fill, and Calcium, magnesium, and other foreign substances.

Zinc Oxide Paste USP—Preserve in well-closed containers, and avoid prolonged exposure to temperatures exceeding 30 °C. Contains not less than 24.0% and not more than 26.0% of zinc oxide.

Zinc Oxide Paste may be prepared as follows: 250 grams of Zinc Oxide, 250 grams of Starch, and 500 grams of

White Petrolatum, to make 1000 grams. Mix the ingredients.

Meets the requirements for Identification and Minimum fill.

ZINC OXIDE AND SALICYLIC ACID

For *Zinc Oxide* and *Salicylic Acid*—See individual listings for chemistry information.

USP requirements: Zinc Oxide and Salicylic Acid Paste USP—Preserve in well-closed containers. Contains not less than 23.5% and not more than 25.5% of zinc oxide, and not less than 1.9% and not more than 2.1% of salicylic acid.

Zinc Oxide and Salicylic Acid Paste may be prepared as follows: 20 grams of Salicylic Acid, in fine powder, and a sufficient quantity of Zinc Oxide Paste to make 1000 grams. Thoroughly triturate the Salicylic Acid with a portion of the paste, then add the remaining paste, and triturate until a smooth mixture is obtained.

Meets the requirements for Identification and Minimum fill.

ZINC STEARATE

Chemical name: Octadecanoic acid, zinc salt.

Description: Zinc Stearate USP—Fine, white, bulky powder, free from grittiness. Has a faint, characteristic odor. Is neutral to moistened litmus paper.

NF category: Tablet and/or capsule lubricant.

Solubility: Zinc Stearate USP—Insoluble in water, in alcohol, and in ether.

USP requirements: Zinc Stearate USP—Preserve in well-closed containers. A compound of zinc with a mixture of solid organic acids obtained from fats, consisting chiefly of variable proportions of zinc stearate and zinc palmitate. Contains the equivalent of not less than 12.5% and not more than 14.0% of zinc oxide. Meets the requirements for Identification, Arsenic (not more than 1.5 ppm), Lead (not more than 0.001%), and Alkalies and alkaline earths (not more than 1.0%).

ZINC SULFATE

Chemical name: Sulfuric acid, zinc salt (1:1), hydrate.

Molecular formula: $ZnSO_4 \cdot xH_2O$.

Molecular weight: 179.46 (monohydrate); 287.56 (heptahydrate); 161.46 (anhydrous).

Description: Zinc Sulfate USP—Colorless, transparent prisms, or small needles. May occur as a granular, crystalline powder. Odorless; efflorescent in dry air. Its solutions are acid to litmus.

Solubility: Zinc Sulfate USP—Very soluble in water (heptahydrate); freely soluble in water (monohydrate); freely soluble in glycerin (heptahydrate); practically insoluble in alcohol (monohydrate); insoluble in alcohol (heptahydrate).

USP requirements:

Zinc Sulfate USP—Preserve in tight containers. Contains one or seven molecules of water of hydration. The label indicates whether it is the monohydrate or the heptahydrate. Label any oral or parenteral preparations containing Zinc Sulfate to state the content of elemental zinc. The monohydrate contains not less than 89.0% and not more than 90.4% of anhydrous zinc sulfate, corresponding to not less than 99.0% and not more than 100.5% of zinc sulfate (monohydrate), and the heptahydrate contains not less than 55.6% and not more than 61.0% of anhydrous zinc sulfate, corresponding to not less than 99.0% and not more than 108.7% of zinc sulfate (heptahydrate). Meets the requirements for Identification, Acidity, Arsenic (not more than 14 ppm), Lead (not more than 0.002%), and Alkalies and alkaline earths (not more than 0.9%).

Zinc Sulfate Capsules—Not in USP.

Zinc Sulfate Injection USP—Preserve in single-dose or in multiple-dose containers. A sterile solution of Zinc Sulfate in Water for Injection. Label the Injection in terms of its content of anhydrous zinc sulfate and in terms of its content of elemental zinc. Label it to state that it is not intended for direct injection but is to be added to other intravenous solutions. Contains an amount of zinc sulfate equivalent to the labeled amount of zinc, within ±5%. Meets the requirements for Identification, Bacterial endotoxins, pH (2.0–4.0), Particulate matter, and Injections.

Zinc Sulfate Ophthalmic Solution USP—Preserve in tight containers. A sterile solution of Zinc Sulfate in Water rendered isotonic by the addition of suitable salts. Contains the labeled amount, within ±5%. Meets the requirements for Identification, Sterility, and pH (5.8–6.2; or, if it contains sodium citrate, 7.2–7.8).

Zinc Sulfate Tablets—Not in USP.

ZINC UNDECYLENATE

Chemical name: 10-Undecenoic acid, zinc(2+) salt.

Molecular formula: $C_{22}H_{38}O_4Zn$.

Molecular weight: 431.94.

Description: Zinc Undecylenate USP—Fine, white powder.

Solubility: Zinc Undecylenate USP—Practically insoluble in water and in alcohol.

USP requirements: Zinc Undecylenate USP—Preserve in well-closed containers. Contains not less than 98.0% and not more than 102.0% of zinc undecylenate, calculated on the dried basis. Meets the requirements for Identification, Loss on drying (not more than 1.25%), and Alkalies and alkaline earths (not more than 1.0%).

ZOLPIDEM

Chemical name: Zolpidem tartrate—Imidazo[1,2-*a*]pyridine-3-acetamide, *N,N*,6-trimethyl-2-(4-methylphenyl)-, [*R*-(*R**,*R**)]-2,3-dihydroxybutanedioate (2:1).

Molecular formula: Zolpidem tartrate—$(C_{19}H_{21}N_3O)_2 \cdot C_4H_6O_6$.

Molecular weight: Zolpidem tartrate—764.88.

Description: Zolpidem tartrate—White to off-white crystalline powder.

Solubility: Zolpidem tartrate—Sparingly soluble in water, in alcohol, and in propylene glycol.

USP requirements: Zolpidem Tartrate Tablets—Not in USP.

Section IV

THE USP PRACTITIONERS' REPORTING NETWORK℠ (USP PRN℠): AN FDA MEDWATCH PARTNER

Health care professionals are encouraged to report reactions or problems that they observe with the use of medications or medical devices. Without such input, manufacturers, government, the compendia, and colleagues may not be aware of problems that are experienced. This exchange of meaningful information is an integral part of improving the safety, efficacy, and quality of medical products. The individual practitioner is in the best position to recognize that a problem may exist and to report it.

The USP Practitioners' Reporting Network is the umbrella system that encompasses all four USP coordinated reporting programs. By participating in these programs you can play an active part in helping to protect your patients from unreliable drug and radiopharmaceutical products, defective medical devices and diagnostics, and possible future medication errors. Unlike any other quality reporting program, the USP PRN can directly impact the development and revision of *USP-NF* standards of quality, purity, strength, packaging and labeling, and information monographs in the *USP DI*. There is no charge for reporting through this service.

(1) **The USP Drug Product Problem Reporting (DPPR) Program:** This program alerts manufacturers, labelers, the FDA, and the USP Committee of Revision to your observations of poor product quality, unclear labeling, defective packaging, therapeutic ineffectiveness, suspected counterfeiting, and possible product tampering for over-the-counter and prescription drugs.

When you detect a drug product problem, submit your report using the convenient USP DPPR reporting form, or call 1-800-4-USP PRN (1-800-487-7776).

(2) **The USP Medication Errors Reporting (MER) Program:** Since 1991, the USP in cooperation with the Institute for Safe Medication Practices (ISMP), has enabled health professionals to confidentially report any actual or potential medication errors they observe. This nationwide program, founded by ISMP in 1975, encompasses a wide variety of problems, such as mis-administrations, unclear instruction-for-use information, and similar or confusing product names or packaging.

To report a medication error call 1-800-23-ERROR or submit your report on the MER form.

(3) **The USP Drug Product Problem Reporting Program for Radiopharmaceuticals:** This program has enabled health professionals to report adverse reactions, quality problems, and altered biodistribution to a responsive nationwide network. Jointly sponsored by USP and the Society of Nuclear Medicine (SNM), the program shares reports with the FDA, SNM, and product manufacturers on radionuclide and radiochemical impurities, packaging and labeling problems, quality concerns, and patient reactions. Information is also shared with the European Association of Nuclear Medicine.

To report radiopharmaceutical problems call 1-800-4-USP PRN or submit your report on the USP-SNM DPPR form.

(4) **The Veterinary Practitioners' Reporting (VPR) Program:** In June 1994, the USP, in cooperation with the American Veterinary Medical Association, established the Veterinary Practitioners' Reporting (VPR) Program. The VPR Program is designed to detect product quality problems, medication mishaps, and adverse reactions with drugs, biologics, chemicals, pesticides, medical devices, and other products used not only for companion animals, but also for food-producing, zoo, and exotic animals.

Reports are shared with the FDA Center for Veterinary Medicine, EPA, USDA, and othe regulatory agencies. To report product problems, receive information, or request reporting forms call 1-800-4-USP PRN or use the VPR form.

The USP Practitioners' Reporting Network is a partner in MedWatch, the Food and Drug Administration's medical products reporting program. This means that your report is shared with the FDA on a daily basis (immediately for perceived health hazards like product mix-ups).

MedWatch, the FDA Medical Products Reporting Program

For health care providers wishing to report serious adverse events or product problems directly to the FDA, a MedWatch form is provided.

Report experiences with:
- medications (drugs or biologics)
- medical devices (including *in vitro* diagnostics)
- special nutritional products (dietary supplements, medical foods, infant formulas)
- other products regulated by FDA

Report SERIOUS adverse events. An event is serious when the patient outcome is:
- death
- life-threatening (real risk of dying)
- hospitalization (initial or prolonged)
- disability (significant, persistent or permanent)
- congenital anomaly
- required intervention to prevent permanent impairment or damage

How to report:
- fill in the sections that apply to your report
- use section C for all products except medical devices
- attach additional blank pages if needed
- use a separate form for each patient
- report either to FDA or the manufacturer (or both)

Important numbers:
- 1-800-FDA-0178 to FAX report
- 1-800-FDA-7737 to report by modem
- 1-800-FDA-1088 for more information or to report quality problems
- 1-800-822-7967 for a VAERS form for vaccines

If your report involves a serious adverse event with a device and it occurred in a facility outside a doctor's office, that facility may be legally required to report to FDA and/or the manufacturer. Please notify the person in that facility who would handle such reporting.

To report a medical device problem, you may submit an FDA MedWatch form.

Confidentiality: The patient's identity is held in strict confidence by FDA and protected to the fullest extent of the law. The reporter's identity may be shared with the manufacturer unless requested otherwise. However, FDA will not disclose the reporter's identity in reponse to a request from the public pursuant to the Freedom of Information Act.

USP PRACTITIONERS' REPORTING NETWORK℠

An FDA MEDWATCH partner

DRUG PRODUCT PROBLEM REPORTING PROGRAM

1. PRODUCT NAME (include generic name)

2. DOSAGE FORM (tablet, capsule, injectable, etc.)	3. SIZE/TYPE OF CONTAINER	4. STRENGTH	5. NDC NUMBER

6. LOT NUMBER(S)	7. EXPIRATION DATE(S)

8. NAME AND ADDRESS OF THE MANUFACTURER	9. NAME AND ADDRESS OF LABELER (if different from manufacturer)

10. PROBLEMS NOTED OR SUSPECTED (if more space is needed, please attach separate page)

11. YOUR NAME AND TITLE (please type or print)

12. YOUR PRACTICE LOCATION (include establishment name, address and zip code)

Days and times available________________

13. PHONE NUMBER AT PRACTICE LOCATION (include area code)

14. A copy of your report is routinely sent to the manufacturer/labeler and to the FDA. USP may release my identity to: (check boxes that apply)

- ❑ The manufacturer and/or labeler as listed above.
- ❑ The Food and Drug Administration.
- ❑ Other persons requesting a copy of this report.
- ❑ None of the above.

15a. If requested, will the actual product involved be available for examination by the manufacturer or FDA? ❑ Yes ❑ No (Do not send samples to USP)

b. This event has been reported to: ❑ Manufacturer ❑ FDA

Other ________________

c. Date problem occurred or observed: ________________

16. SIGNATURE OF REPORTER (as listed in question 11)	17. DATE

Return to:

USP PRN℠

12601 Twinbrook Parkway
Rockville, Maryland 20852-1790

Call Toll Free:

1-800-4-USP PRN (1-800-487-7776)
or FAX 1-301-816-8532

File Access Number:

Date Received by USP:

Additional forms can be found in the *USP DI Vol. I* and *Vol. III* and in all monthly *Updates*.

USP DI

USP PRACTITIONERS' REPORTING NETWORK℠

MEDICATION ERRORS REPORTING PROGRAM

Coordinated by the United States Pharmacopeial Convention, Inc. for the Institute for Safe Medication Practices, Inc., Huntingdon Valley, PA

1. For errors relating to drug labeling, packaging or the naming of drug products, please complete the following:

DRUG #1	**DRUG #2**
Brand Name ____	Brand Name ____
Generic Name ____	Generic Name ____
Manufacturer ____	Manufacturer ____
Labeler *(if different from mfr.)* ____	Labeler *(if different from mfr.)* ____
Dosage Form ____	Dosage Form ____
Strength/Concentration ____	Strength/Concentration ____
Type and Size of Container ____	Type and Size of Container ____
Lot Number ____	Lot Number ____
NDC # ____	NDC # ____

2. Please describe the medication error or potential error ***(if more space is needed, please attach separate page)***
Please note the type of personnel involved *(R.Ph., R.N., M.D., student, etc.)*

3. Please include any pertinent patient information that may be relevant including patient age, sex, diagnosis, etc.
(patient identification not necessary)

4. Was error caught prior to patient administration? ☐ Yes ☐ No
If injury or mortality occured, please be specific.

5. Date and time incident occurred.

6. When and how was the error discovered?

7. Reports are most useful when materials such as product label, physician's order copy, graphics, etc., can be reviewed by the Institute. Do you have such materials available? ☐ Yes ☐ No
If yes, please specify ____
Please retain these materials/samples if possible for 60 days.

8. This incident has been reported to:
(check all boxes that apply)
- ☐ Institution *(via incident report)*
- ☐ Peers
- ☐ Supervisor
- ☐ Manufacturer
- ☐ State regulatory board/department of health
- ☐ Coroner
- ☐ Not reported to anyone else
- ☐ Other ____

This Section Is Optional

The Institute on occasion needs to conduct follow-up analysis on reports. Kindly provide the contact information below. You may use your home address and telephone number should you prefer. The USP and the Institute will not voluntarily disclose your identity in processing this report without your permission.

Name ____
Title ____
May we contact you by mail? ☐ Yes ☐ No
Address to be used: ____
May we contact you by telephone? ☐ Yes ☐ No
Phone number: (   ) ____

9. Do you have any recommendations to prevent recurrence of this error?

RETURN TO:
The Medication Errors Reporting Program
c/o The United States Pharmacopeial Convention, Inc.
12601 Twinbrook Parkway
Rockville, MD 20852

or call toll free anytime
1-800-23-ERROR
FAX 1-301-816-8532

File Access Number
Date Received by USP

USP DI

RADIO PHARMACEUTICALS DRUG PRODUCT PROBLEM REPORTING PROGRAM

USP PRACTITIONERS' REPORTING NETWORK[SM]

An FDA MEDWATCH *partner*

The DPPR for Radiopharmaceuticals is presented in cooperation with The Society of Nuclear Medicine

RADIOPHARMACEUTICAL IDENTIFICATION

1. Name of radiopharmaceutical prepared agent __________

Manufacturer's name and address __________

Central pharmacy name and address (if applicable) __________

Radioactivity concentration ______ Assay date and time ______ Preparation time ______

Calibration date ______ Expiration date ______

2a. Tc-99m generator ☐ Check here if not applicable

Brand name ______ Size ______ Ci Lot # ______

Calibration date and time ______ Date and time of current and last elution ______; ______ Exp. date ______

Amount and volume Tc-99m added to kit or given to patient ______

Manufacturer's name and address ______

Central pharmacy name and address (if applicable) ______

2b. Kit ☐ Check here if not applicable

Name of kit ______ Lot # ______ Volume diluted to ______ Expiration date ______

Kit heated ☐ No ☐ Yes duration ______

Manufacturer's name and address ______

Central pharmacy name and address (if applicable) ______

2c. Were manufacturer drug preparation methods strictly adhered to? ☐ Yes ☐ No ☐ Not applicable

2d. If non-radioactive drugs were used in association with radiopharmaceuticals, please list here ______

PRODUCT ADMINISTERED TO PATIENT

☐ Yes, go to #3 ☐ No, go to #8

3. Problem noted or suspected

☐ Adverse reaction ☐ Other ______

☐ Altered biodistribution

☐ Product quality ☐ Patient physiology ☐ Concomitant drugs

4. Describe the problem (Please give time sequence of events, attach additional pages if necessary.)

4a. Was interpretation of image possible? ☐ Yes ☐ No ☐ Not applicable

5. Patient information

a. Patient initials ____ **b.** Suspected disease ______

c. Concurrent drugs, doses and frequency ______

d. Other disease states ______

6. Administration information

Activity administered ______ mCi / μCi (Circle one) Volume administered ______ mL Route of administration ______

Date and time of administration (indicate AM or PM) ______ Site of administration ______

Other patients received dose from same lot ☐ Yes ☐ No

Did they experience any reaction or altered biodistribution? ☐ Yes ☐ No

If yes, please file a report for each reaction. Number of patients ____

FILE ACCESS NUMBER:	DATE RECEIVED BY USP:

USP DI

7. Adverse reaction information

Date and time of reaction onset ____________________

☐ Recovered, no treatment necessary
☐ Alive, with sequelae
☐ Recovered, required treatment

☐ Died (date ______)
☐ due to product
☐ due to other cause
☐ unknown

Your interpretation of reaction cause

☐ Allergic
☐ Pyrogenic ____________________
☐ Pharmacologic effect ____________________

How classified (briefly) ____________________

8. Problem noted or suspected (check all that apply)

☐ Product identification incorrect
☐ Radiochemical impurity
☐ pH high ☐ pH low
☐ Packaging compromised
☐ Radionuclide impurity
☐ Other ____________________
☐ Compounding error
☐ Color/clarity/foreign matter
☐ Particle size/number
☐ Heating period too long or short

9. Describe the problem

10. Test(s) if any (include ITLC data, particle size, etc.), performed to confirm problem

REPORTER IDENTIFICATION

11a. Your name and title

11b. Name and address of institution

11c. Phone number, please indicate times you are available at workplace.

12. Please indicate to whom USP may voluntarily disclose your identity (check boxes that apply).

☐ Involved manufacturer(s)
☐ Food and Drug Administration (FDA)
☐ Society of Nuclear Medicine
☐ Other persons requesting a copy of this report

13. If requested, is sample of involved product available for examination?

☐ Yes ☐ No ☐ Sent to manufacturer

14. Signature and date

Evaluation by SNM Committee

Reviewer:

Return To:

USP Practitioners' Reporting Network[SM]
12601 Twinbrook Parkway
Rockville, Maryland 20852

OR

Call Toll Free Anytime

1-800-4-USP PRN

(FAX 1-301-816-8532)

USP PRACTITIONERS' REPORTING NETWORK℠

An FDA MEDWATCH partner

The Veterinary Practitioners' Reporting Program is presented in cooperation with the American Veterinary Medical Association (AVMA)

VETERINARY PRACTITIONERS' REPORTING PROGRAM

1. Product Name (brand and generic)	2. Dosage Form/Strength	3. Lot Number/Exp. Date
4. Name and Address of Manufacturer/Labeler		

5. Diagnosis and/or Reason for Product Usage	6. Administered by ❑ Veterinarian ❑ Owner

7. Product Administration

Dose & interval:

Route:

Length of treatment:

No. of animals treated:

Concurrent clinical problems/products administered including pesticides, chemicals, feed additives, etc.:

8. Species	9. Breed	10. Age	11. Sex	12. Weight ______kg. ______lbs.

13. Reaction/Problem Information
   a. Number of animals affected ______________
   b. Time between initiation of therapy with suspected product and onset of reaction was ______________
   c. Time between last administration of suspected product and onset of reaction was ______________
   d. Outcome: ❑ Recovered from reaction ❑ Died from reaction ❑ Other (comment below)
   e. Was the reaction treated? ❑ No ❑ Yes (comment below)
   f. When the reaction appeared, treatment with suspected product:
      ❑ Had already been completed
      ❑ Was discontinued due to reaction
      ❑ Was discontinued and replaced with another product
      ❑ Was discontinued and reintroduced later
      ❑ Was continued at altered dose
   g. The reaction:
      ❑ Continued ❑ Stopped ❑ Recurred ❑ Other (comment below)
   h. Level of suspicion that drug caused the reaction:
      ❑ High ❑ Medium ❑ Low

14. Describe the reaction or product quality problem. Add details about case history including laboratory results, and outcome (attach separate sheet if necessary)

15. Veterinarian's Name and Address Telephone Number	16. Case ID

17. A copy of your report is routinely sent to the manufacturer/labeler and to the appropriate agency [FDA, USDA, or EPA]. Please indicate to whom USP may voluntarily disclose your identity (check box(es) that apply)

❑ The manufacturer and/or labeler as listed above ❑ The Food and Drug Administration or appropriate agency ❑ AVMA ❑ Other persons requesting a copy of this report ❑ None of these

Signature of Reporter	Date

Return to: **USP Practitioners' Reporting Network (USP PRN℠)**
12601 Twinbrook Parkway
Rockville, Maryland 20852
or FAX to: 1-301-816-8532

or Call Toll Free **1-800-4-USP PRN (1-800-487-7776)**

File Access Number:
Date Received by USP:

VT694

MEDWATCH

THE FDA MEDICAL PRODUCTS REPORTING PROGRAM

For VOLUNTARY reporting by health professionals of adverse events and product problems

Page ____ of ____

Form Approved: OMB No. 0910-0291 Expires: 12/31/94
See OMB statement on reverse

FDA Use Only (USP)

Triage unit sequence #

PLEASE TYPE OR USE BLACK INK

A. Patient information

1. Patient identifier — In confidence
2. Age at time of event: ______ or Date of birth:
3. Sex ☐ female ☐ male
4. Weight ____ lbs or ____ kgs

B. Adverse event or product problem

1. ☐ Adverse event and/or ☐ Product problem (e.g., defects/malfunctions)
2. Outcomes attributed to adverse event (check all that apply)
   - ☐ death ______ (mo/day/yr)
   - ☐ life-threatening
   - ☐ hospitalization – initial or prolonged
   - ☐ disability
   - ☐ congenital anomaly
   - ☐ required intervention to prevent permanent impairment/damage
   - ☐ other: ______
3. Date of event (mo/day/yr)
4. Date of this report (mo/day/yr)
5. Describe event or problem
6. Relevant tests/laboratory data, including dates
7. Other relevant history, including preexisting medical conditions (e.g., allergies, race, pregnancy, smoking and alcohol use, hepatic/renal dysfunction, etc.)

C. Suspect medication(s)

1. Name (give labeled strength & mfr/labeler, if known)
   #1
   #2
2. Dose, frequency & route used
   #1
   #2
3. Therapy dates (if unknown, give duration) from/to (or best estimate)
   #1
   #2
4. Diagnosis for use (indication)
   #1
   #2
5. Event abated after use stopped or dose reduced
   #1 ☐ yes ☐ no ☐ doesn't apply
   #2 ☐ yes ☐ no ☐ doesn't apply
6. Lot # (if known)
   #1
   #2
7. Exp. date (if known)
   #1
   #2
8. Event reappeared after reintroduction
   #1 ☐ yes ☐ no ☐ doesn't apply
   #2 ☐ yes ☐ no ☐ doesn't apply
9. NDC # (for product problems only)
   – –
10. Concomitant medical products and therapy dates (exclude treatment of event)

D. Suspect medical device

1. Brand name
2. Type of device
3. Manufacturer name & address
4. Operator of device
   - ☐ health professional
   - ☐ lay user/patient
   - ☐ other: ______
5. Expiration date (mo/day/yr)
6. model # ______
   catalog # ______
   serial # ______
   lot # ______
   other #
7. If implanted, give date (mo/day/yr)
8. If explanted, give date (mo/day/yr)
9. Device available for evaluation? (Do not send to FDA)
   ☐ yes ☐ no ☐ returned to manufacturer on ______ (mo/day/yr)
10. Concomitant medical products and therapy dates (exclude treatment of event)

E. Reporter (see confidentiality section on back)

1. Name & address — phone #
2. Health professional? ☐ yes ☐ no
3. Occupation
4. Also reported to
   - ☐ manufacturer
   - ☐ user facility
   - ☐ distributor
5. If you do NOT want your identity disclosed to the manufacturer, place an " X " in this box. ☐

FDA

Mail to: MEDWATCH
5600 Fishers Lane
Rockville, MD 20852-9787

or FAX to:
1-800-FDA-0178

FDA Form 3500 (6/93)

Submission of a report does not constitute an admission that medical personnel or the product caused or contributed to the event.

Section V

THE MEDICINE CHART

The Medicine Chart presents photographs of the most frequently prescribed medicines in the United States. In general, commonly used brand name products and a representative sampling of generic products have been included. The pictorial listing is not intended to be inclusive and does not represent all products on the market. Only selected solid oral dosage forms (capsules and tablets) have been included. The inclusion of a product does not mean the USPC has any particular knowledge that the product included has properties different from other products, nor should it be interpreted as an endorsement by USPC. Similarly, the fact that a particular product has not been included does not indicate that the product has been judged by the USPC to be unsatisfactory or unacceptable.

The drug products in *The Medicine Chart* are listed alphabetically by generic name of active ingredient(s). To quickly locate a particular medicine, check the product listing index that follows. This listing provides brand and generic names and directs the user to the appropriate page and chart location. In addition, any identifying code found on the surface of a capsule or tablet that might be useful in making a correct identification is included in the parentheses that follow the product's index entry. Please note that these codes may change as manufacturers reformulate or redesign their products. In addition, some companies may not manufacture all of their own products. In some of these cases, the imprinting on the tablet or capsule may be that of the actual manufacturer and not of the company marketing the product.

An inverted cross-index has also been included to help identify products by their identifying codes. These codes may not be unique to a given product; they are intended for use in initial identification only. In this cross-index, the codes are listed first in alpha-numeric order, accompanied by their generic or brand names and page and chart location.

Brand names are in *italics*. An asterisk next to the generic name of the active ingredient(s) indicates that the solid oral dosage forms containing the ingredient(s) are available only from a single source with no generic equivalents currently available in the U.S. Where multiple source products are shown, it must be kept in mind that other products may also be available.

The size and color of the products shown are intended to match the actual product as closely as possible; however, there may be some differences due to variations caused by the photographic process. Also, manufacturers may occasionally change the color, imprinting, or shape of their products, and for a period of time both the "old" and the newly changed dosage form may be on the market. Such changes may not occur uniformly thoughout the different dosages of the product. These types of changes will be incorporated in subsequent versions of the chart as they are brought to our attention.

> Use of this chart is limited to serving as an initial guide in identifying drug products. The identity of a product should be verified further before any action is taken.

Cephalexin *(continued)*
Biocraft Capsules—
500 mg (117) MC-4, C2
Cephradine MC-4, C5–7
Barr Capsules—
250 mg (550) MC-4, C6
500 mg (551) MC-4, C6
Biocraft Capsules—
250 mg (112) MC-4, C7
500 mg (113) MC-4, C7
Chlordiazepoxide MC-4, D1–2
Chlordiazepoxide and
Amitriptyline MC-4, D3–4
Mylan Tablets—
5/12.5 mg (211) MC-4, D3
10/25 mg (277) MC-4, D3
Chlordiazepoxide and
Clidinium MC-4, D5
Chlorpheniramine and
Phenylpropanolamine MC-4, D6
Chlorpheniramine, Phenylpropanolamine,
Phenylephrine, and Phenyl-
toloxamine MC-4, D7–MC-5, A1
Geneva Extended-release Tablets—
40/10/15/5 mg
(GG 118) MC-5, A1
Chlorpromazine MC-5, A2–4
Geneva Tablets—
100 mg (GG 437) MC-5, A2
200 mg (GG 457) MC-5, A2
Chlorpropamide MC-5, A5–7
Geneva Tablets—
100 mg (GG 61) MC-5, A5
250 mg (GG 144) MC-5, A5
Schein/Danbury Tablets—
100 mg (5579) MC-5, A7
250 mg (5455) MC-5, A7
Chlorthalidone MC-5, B1–3
Barr Tablets—
25 mg (267) MC-5, B1
50 mg (268) MC-5, B1
Chlorzoxazone MC-5, B4–6
Barr Tablets—
500 mg (555 585) MC-5, B4
Mutual Tablets—
500 mg (MP 74) MC-5, B6
Cimetidine MC-5, B7–C1
Ciprofloxacin MC-5, C2–3
Cipro Tablets—
250 mg (250) MC-5, C2
500 mg (500) MC-5, C3
750 mg (750) MC-5, C3
Cisapride MC-5, C4
Clarithromycin MC-5, C5
Claritin Tablets—
10 mg (458) MC-13, D7
Clemastine MC-5, C6
Cleocin Capsules—
75 mg (75 mg) MC-5, D2
150 mg (150 mg) MC-5, D2
300 mg (300 mg) MC-5, D2
Clindamycin MC-5, C7–D2
Biocraft Capsules—
150 mg (149) MC-5, C7
Schein/Danbury Capsules—
150 mg (DAN 5708) MC-5, D1
Clinoril Tablets—
150 mg (MSD 941) MC-21, D2
200 mg (MSD 942) MC-21, D2
Clomipramine MC-5, D3
Clonidine MC-5, D4–MC-6, A3
Geneva Tablets—
0.1 mg (GG 81) MC-5, D5
0.2 mg (GG 82) MC-5, D5
0.3 mg (GG 83) MC-5, D5
Lederle Tablets—
0.1 mg (C 42) MC-5, D6
0.2 mg (C 43) MC-5, D6
0.3 mg (C 44) MC-5, D6
Clonidine *(continued)*
Mylan Tablets—
0.1 mg (152) MC-5, D7
0.2 mg (186) MC-5, D7
0.3 mg (199) MC-5, D7
Purepac Tablets—
0.1 mg (127) MC-6, A1
0.2 mg (128) MC-6, A1
0.3 mg (129) MC-6, A1
Schein/Danbury Tablets—
0.1 mg (DAN 5609) MC-6, A2
0.2 mg (DAN 5612) MC-6, A2
0.3 mg (DAN 5613) MC-6, A2
Warner Chilcott Tablets—
0.1 mg (443) MC-6, A3
0.2 mg (444) MC-6, A3
0.3 mg (WC 445) MC-6, A3
Clonidine and Chlorthalidone . . MC-6, A4–5
Mylan Tablets—
0.1/15 mg (M 1) MC-6, A5
0.2/15 mg (M 27) MC-6, A5
0.3/15 mg (M 72) MC-6, A5
Clorazepate MC-6, A6–B2
Mylan Tablets—
3.75 mg (M 30) MC-6, B1
7.5 mg (M 40) MC-6, B1
15 mg (M 70) MC-6, B1
Purepac Tablets—
3.75 mg (078) MC-6, B2
7.5 mg (081) MC-6, B2
15 mg (083) MC-6, B2
Clotrimazole MC-6, B3
Clozapine MC-6, B4
Clozaril Tablets—
25 mg (25) MC-6, B4
100 mg (100) MC-6, B4
Cogentin Tablets—
0.5 mg (MSD 21) MC-3, A5
1 mg (MSD 635) MC-3, A5
2 mg (MSD 60) MC-3, A5
Cognex Capsules—
10 mg (10) MC-21, D6
20 mg (20) MC-21, D6
30 mg (30) MC-21, D6
40 mg (40) MC-21, D6
Combipres Tablets—
0.1/15 mg (BI 8) MC-6, A4
0.2/15 mg (BI 9) MC-6, A4
0.3/15 mg (BI 10) MC-6, A4
Compazine
Extended-release Capsules—
10 mg (SKF C44) MC-20, A1
15 mg (SKF C46) MC-20, A1
Tablets—
5 mg (SKF C66) MC-20, A2
10 mg (SKF C67) MC-20, A2
Cordarone Tablets—
200 mg (4188) MC-1, C6
Corgard Tablets—
20 mg (PPP 232) MC-16, A1
40 mg (PPP 207) MC-16, A1
80 mg (PPP 241) MC-16, A1
120 mg (PPP 208) MC-16, A1
160 mg (PPP 246) MC-16, A2
Cortef Tablets—
5 mg (5) MC-11, D2
10 mg (10) MC-11, D2
20 mg (20) MC-11, D2
Corzide Tablets—
40/5 mg (283) MC-16, A3
80/5 mg (284) MC-16, A3
Coumadin Tablets—
2 mg (2) MC-24, D4
2.5 mg (2½) MC-24, D4
5 mg (5) MC-24, D4
7.5 mg (7½) MC-24, D4
10 mg (10) MC-24, D5
Cromolyn MC-6, B5
Cyclobenzaprine MC-6, B6–C1
Mylan Tablets—
10 mg (710) MC-6, B7
Cyclobenzaprine *(continued)*
Schein/Danbury Tablets—
10 mg (5658) MC-6, C1
Cyclosporine MC-6, C2
Cytotec Tablets—
0.1 mg (1451) MC-15, D4
0.2 mg (1461) MC-15, D4
Dalmane Capsules—
15 mg (15) MC-10, C4
30 mg (30) MC-10, C4
Danazol MC-6, C3
Danocrine Capsules—
50 mg (D 03) MC-6, C3
100 mg (D 04) MC-6, C3
200 mg (D 05) MC-6, C3
Dantrium Capsules—
25 mg (0149 0030) MC-6, C4
50 mg (0149 0031) MC-6, C4
100 mg (0149 0033) MC-6, C4
Dantrolene MC-6, C4
Darvocet-N Tablets—
50/325 mg (50) MC-20, A7
100/650 mg (100) MC-20, A7
Daypro Tablets—
600 mg (1381) MC-17, C7
Decadron Tablets—
0.25 mg (MSD 20) MC-6, D1
0.5 mg (MSD 41) MC-6, D1
0.75 mg (MSD 63) MC-6, D1
1.5 mg (MSD 95) MC-6, D2
4 mg (MSD 97) MC-6, D2
6 mg (MSD 147) MC-6, D2
Deltasone Tablets—
2.5 mg (2.5) MC-19, C4
5 mg (5) MC-19, C4
10 mg (10) MC-19, C4
20 mg (20) MC-19, C4
50 mg (50) MC-19, C4
Demerol Tablets—
50 mg (D 35) MC-14, B7
100 mg (D 37) MC-14, B7
Demi-Regroton Tablets—
0.125/25 mg (32) MC-20, A3
Demulen 1/35-21 and -28 Tablets—
1/0.035 mg (151) MC-9, D3
Inert (P) MC-9, D3
Demulen 1/50-21 and -28 Tablets—
1/0.05 mg (71) MC-9, D4
Inert (P) MC-9, D4
Depakene Capsules—
250 mg MC-24, B4
Depakote Sprinkle Capsules—
125 mg (125 mg) MC-8, A7
Depakote Delayed-release Tablets—
125 mg (NT) MC-8, B1
250 mg (NR) MC-8, B1
500 mg (NS) MC-8, B1
Desipramine MC-6, C5–7
Geneva Tablets—
100 mg (GG 167) MC-6, C5
150 mg (GG 168) MC-6, C5
Desyrel Tablets—
50 mg (MJ 775) MC-23, D2
100 mg (MJ 776) MC-23, D2
150 mg Dividose (MJ 778) . . . MC-23, D2
Dexamethasone MC-6, D1–4
Roxane Tablets—
0.5 mg (54 299) MC-6, D3
0.75 mg (54 960) MC-6, D3
1 mg (54 489) MC-6, D3
1.5 mg (54 943) MC-6, D4
2 mg (54 662) MC-6, D4
4 mg (54 892) MC-6, D4
DiaBeta Tablets—
1.25 mg MC-11, A1
2.5 mg MC-11, A1
5 mg MC-11, A1
Diabinese Tablets—
100 mg (393) MC-5, A6
250 mg (394) MC-5, A6

Zocor Tablets—
5 mg (MSD 726) MC-21, B2
10 mg (MSD 735) MC-21, B2
Zofran Tablets—
4 mg (4) MC-17, C5
8 mg (8) MC-17, C5
Zoloft Tablets—
50 mg (50 MG) MC-21, B1
100 mg (100 MG) MC-21, B1
Zolpidem MC-24, D7
Zovirax
Capsules—
200 mg (200) MC-1, A5
Zovirax (continued)
Tablets—
400 mg MC-1, A6
800 mg (800) MC-1, A6
Zyloprim Tablets—
100 mg (100) MC-1, B4
300 mg (300) MC-1, B4

*In thousands of units of lipase/amylase/protease, respectively.

INVERTED CROSS-INDEX

AHR—*Donnatal* Extended-release Tablets 0.0582/0.3111/0.0195/48.6 mg MC-2, D1
AHR—*Quinidex* Extended-release Tablets 300 mg MC-20, D7
AHR—*Robaxin* Tablets 500 mg MC-14, C4
AHR—*Robaxisal* Tablets 400/325 mg MC-14, C5
AHR 10—*Reglan* Tablets 10 mg MC-15, A7
AHR 4207—*Donnatal* Capsules 0.0194/0.1037/0.0065/16.2 mg MC-2, C6
AHR 5720—*Micro-K* Extended-release Capsules 600 mg MC-19, B1
AHR 5730—*Micro-K* Extended-release Capsules 750 mg MC-19, B1
AHR 6242—*Phenaphen with Codeine* Capsules 325/15 mg MC-1, A3
AHR 6257—*Phenaphen with Codeine* Capsules 325/30 mg MC-1, A3
Ast 10—*Hismanal* Tablets 10 mg MC-2, B2
A2C—*Lanoxicaps* Capsules 0.05 mg MC-7, B6
A3 250—*Achromycin V* Capsules 250 mg MC-22, B4
A5 500—*Achromycin V* Capsules 500 mg MC-22, B4
A7—Lederle Atenolol Tablets 25 mg MC-2, B5
A 49—Lederle Atenolol Tablets 50 mg MC-2, B5
A 51—Lederle Alprazolam Tablets 0.25 mg MC-1, C1
A 52—Lederle Alprazolam Tablets 0.5 mg MC-1, C1
A 53—Lederle Alprazolam Tablets 1 mg MC-1, C1
A54—Lederle Alprazolam Tablets 2 mg MC-1, C1
A 71—Lederle Atenolol Tablets 100 mg MC-2, B5
BI 6—*Catapres* Tablets 0.1 mg MC-5, D4
BI 7—*Catapres* Tablets 0.2 mg MC-5, D4
BI 8—*Combipres* Tablets 0.1/15 mg MC-6, A4
BI 9—*Combipres* Tablets 0.2/15 mg MC-6, A4
BI 10—*Combipres* Tablets 0.3/15 mg MC-6, A4
BI 11—*Catapres* Tablets 0.3 mg MC-5, D4
BI 17—*Persantine* Tablets 25 mg MC-7, D7
BI 18—*Persantine* Tablets 50 mg MC-7, D7
BI 19—*Persantine* Tablets 75 mg MC-7, D7
BI 72—*Alupent* Tablets 20 mg MC-14, C2
BI 74—*Alupent* Tablets 10 mg MC-14, C2
BL N1—*Naldecon* Extended-release Tablets 40/10/15/5 mg MC-4, D7
BL 512—*Quibron-T Dividose* Tablets 300 mg MC-22, C2
BL 519—*Quibron-T/SR Dividose* Extended-release Tablets 300 mg MC-22, C3
BMP 140—*Totacillin* Capsules 250 mg MC-2, A5
BMP 141—*Totacillin* Capsules 500 mg MC-2, A5
BMP 189—*Augmentin* Chewable Tablets 125/31.25 mg MC-2, A3
BMP 190—*Augmentin* Chewable Tablets 250/62.5 mg MC-2, A3
B1—*Zebeta* Tablets 5 mg MC-3, B2
B2C—*Lanoxicaps* Capsules 0.1 mg MC-7, B6
B3—*Zebeta* Tablets 10 mg MC-3, B2
B 12—*Zinc* Tablets 2.5/6.25 mg MC-3, B3
B 13—*Ziac* Tablets 5/6.25 mg MC-3, B3
B 14—*Ziac* Tablets 10/6.25 mg MC-3, B3
CHEW EZ—*EryPed* Chewable Tablets 200 mg MC-9, C2
C2C—*Lanoxicaps* Capsules 0.2 mg MC-7, B6
C 42—Lederle Clonidine Tablets 0.1 mg MC-5, D6
C 43—Lederle Clonidine Tablets 0.2 mg MC-5, D6
C 44—Lederle Clonidine Tablets 0.3 mg MC-5, D6
DAN 10mg—Schein/Danbury Nortriptyline Capsules 10 mg MC-17, C1
DAN 25mg—Schein/Danbury Nortriptyline Capsules 25 mg MC-17, C1
DAN 50mg—Schein/Danbury Nortriptyline Capsules 50 mg MC-17, C2
DAN 75mg—Schein/Danbury Nortriptyline Capsules 75 mg MC-17, C2
DAN 5026—Schein/Danbury Procainamide Capsules 250 mg MC-19, D6
DAN 5162—Schein Tetracycline Capsules 250 mg Orange/Yellow MC-22, B6
DAN 5333—Schein/Danbury Procainamide Capsules 500 mg MC-19, D6
DAN 5350—Schein/Danbury Procainamide Capsules 375 mg MC-19, D6
DAN 5440—Schein/Danbury Doxycycline Capsules 100 mg MC-8, D3
DAN 5535—Schein/Danbury Doxycycline Capsules 50 mg MC-8, D3
DAN 5554—Schein/Danbury Propranolol Tablets 10 mg MC-20, B7
DAN 5555—Schein/Danbury Propranolol Tablets 20 mg MC-20, B7
DAN 5556—Schein/Danbury Propranolol Tablets 40 mg MC-20, B7
DAN 5557—Schein/Danbury Propranolol Tablets 80 mg MC-20, B7
DAN 5609—Schein/Danbury Clonidine Tablets 0.1 mg MC-6, A2
DAN 5612—Schein/Danbury Clonidine Tablets 0.2 mg MC-6, A2
DAN 5613—Schein/Danbury Clonidine Tablets 0.3 mg MC-16, A2
DAN 5614—Schein/Danbury Flurazepam Capsules 15 mg MC-10, C5
DAN 5615—Schein/Danbury Flurazepam Capsules 30 mg MC-10, C5
DAN 5616—Schein/Danbury Oxazepam Capsules 15 mg MC-17, D4
DAN 5617—Schein/Danbury Oxazepam Capsules 10 mg MC-17, D4
DAN 5618—Schein/Danbury Oxazepam Capsules 30 mg MC-17, D4
DAN 5619—Schein/Danbury Diazepam Tablets 5 mg MC-7, A1
DAN 5620—Schein/Danbury Diazepam Tablets 10 mg MC-7, A1
DAN 5621—Schein/Danbury Diazepam Tablets 2 mg MC-7, A1
DAN 5622—Schein/Danbury Lorazepam Tablets 2 mg MC-14, A3
DAN 5624—Schein/Danbury Lorazepam Tablets 1 mg MC-14, A3
DAN 5625—Schein/Danbury Lorazepam Tablets 0.5 mg MC-14, A3
DAN 5629—Schein/Danbury Doxepin Capsules 10 mg MC-8, C2
DAN 5630—Schein/Danbury Doxepin Capsules 25 mg MC-8, C2
DAN 5631—Schein/Danbury Doxepin Capsules 50 mg MC-8, C3
DAN 5632—Schein/Danbury Doxepin Capsules 75 mg MC-8, C3
DAN 5633—Schein/Danbury Doxepin Capsules 100 mg MC-8, C3
DAN 5642—Schein/Danbury Minoxidil Tablets 2.5 mg MC-15, D2
DAN 5643—Schein/Danbury Minoxidil Tablets 10 mg MC-15, D2
DAN 5682—Schein/Danbury Triamterene and Hydrochlorothiazide Tablets 75/50 mg MC-24, D2
DAN 5693—Schein/Danbury Prazosin Capsules 5 mg MC-19, B7

DAN 5696—Schein/Danbury Prazosin Capsules 2 mg ... MC-19, B7
DAN 5697—Schein/Danbury Prazosin Capsules 1 mg ... MC-19, B7
DAN 5708—Schein/Danbury Clindamycin Capsules 150 mg ... MC-5, D1
DAN 5730—Schein/Danbury Baclofen Tablets 10 mg ... MC-2, D7
DAN 5731—Schein/Danbury Baclofen Tablets 20 mg ... MC-2, D7
DAN 5782—Schein/Danbury Atenolol and Chlorthalidone Tablets 50/25 mg ... MC-2, C3
DAN 5783—Schein/Danbury Atenolol and Chlorthalidone Tablets 100/25 mg ... MC-2, C3
DF—*Hytrin* Tablets 1 mg ... MC-22, A5
DH—*Hytrin* Tablets 2 mg ... MC-22, A5
DI—*Hytrin* Tablets 10 mg ... MC-22, A5
DJ—*Hytrin* Tablets 5 mg ... MC-22, A5
dp 25—*Levoxine* Tablets 0.025 mg ... MC-13, B6
dp 50—*Levoxine* Tablets 0.05 mg ... MC-13, B6
dp 75—*Levoxine* Tablets 0.075 mg ... MC-13, B6
dp 88—*Levoxine* Tablets 0.088 mg ... MC-13, B6
dp 100—*Levoxine* Tablets 0.1 mg ... MC-13, B6
dp 112—*Levoxine* Tablets 0.112 mg ... MC-13, B7
dp 125—*Levoxine* Tablets 0.125 mg ... MC-13, B7
dp 150—*Levoxine* Tablets 0.15 mg ... MC-13, B7
dp 175—*Levoxine* Tablets 0.175 mg ... MC-13, B7
dp 200—*Levoxine* Tablets 0.2 mg ... MC-13, B7
dp 300—*Levoxine* Tablets 0.3 mg ... MC-13, B7
DS—*Anaprox* Tablets 500 mg ... MC-16, A7
DS 02C—*Septra* Tablets 800/160 mg ... MC-21, C4
D 03—*Danocrine* Capsules 50 mg ... MC-6, C3
D 04—*Danocrine* Capsules 100 mg ... MC-6, C3
D 05—*Danocrine* Capsules 200 mg ... MC-6, C3
D 35—*Demerol* Tablets 50 mg ... MC-14, B7
D 37—*Demerol* Tablets 100 mg ... MC-14, B7
EA—Abbott Erythromycin Tablets 500 mg ... MC-9, A7
EB—Abbott Erythromycin Tablets 250 mg ... MC-9, A7
EC—*Ery-Tab* Delayed-release Tablets 250 mg ... MC-9, B1
ED—*Ery-Tab* Delayed-release Tablets 500 mg ... MC-9, B1
EE—*E.E.S.* Tablets 400 mg ... MC-9, C1
EH—*Ery-Tab* Delayed-release Tablets 333 mg ... MC-9, B1
EK—*PCE* Delayed-release Tablets 500 mg ... MC-9, B2
ER—Abbott Erythromycin Delayed-release Capsules 250 mg ... MC-9, A6
ES—*Erythrocin* Tablets 250 mg ... MC-9, C4
ET—*Erythrocin* Tablets 500 mg ... MC-9, C4
GG 27—Geneva Hydrochlorothiazide Tablets 50 mg ... MC-11, C4
GG 28—Geneva Hydrochlorothiazide Tablets 25 mg ... MC-11, C4
GG 35—Geneva Thioridazine Tablets 150 mg ... MC-22, D6
GG 36—Geneva Thioridazine Tablets 200 mg ... MC-22, D6
GG 45—Geneva Dipyridamole Tablets 50 mg ... MC-8, A1
GG 49—Geneva Dipyridamole Tablets 25 mg ... MC-8, A1
GG 51—Geneva Trifluoperazine Tablets 1 mg ... MC-24, A5
GG 53—Geneva Trifluoperazine Tablets 2 mg ... MC-24, A5
GG 55—Geneva Trifluoperazine Tablets 5 mg ... MC-24, A5
GG 56—Geneva Disopyramide Capsules 100 mg ... MC-8, A4
GG 57—Geneva Disopyramide Capsules 150 mg ... MC-8, A4
GG 58—Geneva Trifluoperazine Tablets 10 mg ... MC-24, A5
GG 61—Geneva Chlorpropamide Tablets 100 mg ... MC-5, A5
GG 71—Geneva Propranolol Tablets 10 mg ... MC-20, B3
GG 72—Geneva Propranolol Tablets 20 mg ... MC-20, B3
GG 73—Geneva Propranolol Tablets 40 mg ... MC-20, B3
GG 74—Geneva Propranolol Tablets 60 mg ... MC-20, B3
GG 75—Geneva Propranolol Tablets 80 mg ... MC-20, B3
GG 81—Geneva Clonidine Tablets 0.1 mg ... MC-5, D5
GG 82—Geneva Clonidine Tablets 0.2 mg ... MC-5, D5
GG 83—Geneva Clonidine Tablets 0.3 mg ... MC-5, D5
GG 85—Geneva Spironolactone Tablets 25 mg ... MC-21, B4
GG 95—Geneva Spironolactone and Hydrochlorothiazide Tablets 25/25 mg ... MC-21, B7
GG 101—Geneva Methocarbamol Tablets 750 mg ... MC-14, C3
GG 103—Geneva Metronidazole Tablets 250 mg ... MC-15, C2
GG 104—Geneva Methyldopa Tablets 125 mg ... MC-14, D1
GG 111—Geneva Methyldopa Tablets 250 mg ... MC-14, D1
GG 118—Geneva Chlorpheniramine, Phenylpropanolamine, Phenylephrine, and Phenyltoloxamine Extended-release Tablets 40/10/15/5 mg ... MC-5, A1
GG 119—Geneva Butalbital, Aspirin, and Caffeine Tablets 50/325/40 mg ... MC-3, C3
GG 124—Geneva Haloperidol Tablets 2 mg ... MC-11, B1
GG 125—Geneva Haloperidol Tablets 5 mg ... MC-11, B1
GG 126—Geneva Haloperidol Tablets 10 mg ... MC-11, B1
GG 132—Geneva Verapamil Tablets 80 mg ... MC-24, C3
GG 133—Geneva Verapamil Tablets 120 mg ... MC-24, C3
GG 134—Geneva Haloperidol Tablets 20 mg ... MC-11, B1
GG 141—Geneva Meclizine Tablets 12.5 mg ... MC-14, A7
GG 144—Geneva Chlorpropamide Tablets 250 mg ... MC-5, A5
GG 167—Geneva Desipramine Tablets 100 mg ... MC-6, C5
GG 168—Geneva Desipramine Tablets 150 mg ... MC-6, C5
GG 172—Geneva Triamterene and Hydrochlorothiazide Tablets 75/50 mg ... MC-23, D7
GG 190—Geneva Methocarbamol Tablets 500 mg ... MC-14, C3
GG 195—Geneva Metronidazole Tablets 500 mg ... MC-15, C2
GG 219—Geneva Methyldopa and Hydrochlorothiazide Tablets 250/15 mg ... MC-14, D5
GG 242—Geneva Methyclothiazide Tablets 5 mg ... MC-14, C7
GG 243—Geneva Methyldopa and Hydrochlorothiazide Tablets 500/30 mg ... MC-14, D6
GG 244—Geneva Methyclothiazide Tablets 2.5 mg ... MC-14, C7
GG 254—Geneva Fenoprofen Tablets 600 mg ... MC-10, A5
GG 261—Geneva Meclizine Tablets 25 mg ... MC-14, A7
GG 263—Geneva Atenolol Tablets 50 mg ... MC-2, B3
GG 264—Geneva Atenolol Tablets 100 mg ... MC-2, B3
GG 265—Geneva Methyldopa and Hydrochlorothiazide Tablets 250/25 mg ... MC-14, D5
GG 270—Geneva Tolazamide Tablets 100 mg ... MC-23, B7
GG 271—Geneva Tolazamide Tablets 250 mg ... MC-23, B7
GG 272—Geneva Tolazamide Tablets 500 mg ... MC-23, B7
GG 289—Geneva Methyldopa and Hydrochlorothiazide Tablets 500/50 mg ... MC-14, D6
GG 437—Geneva Chlorpromazine Tablets 100 mg ... MC-5, A2
GG 457—Geneva Chlorpromazine Tablets 200 mg ... MC-5, A2
GG 464—Geneva Dipyridamole Tablets 75 mg ... MC-8, A1
GG 471—Geneva Methyldopa Tablets 500 mg ... MC-14, D1
GG 472—Geneva Procainamide Extended-release Tablets 250 mg ... MC-19, C7
GG 473—Geneva Procainamide Extended-release Tablets 500 mg ... MC-19, C7
GG 474—Geneva Procainamide Extended-release Tablets 750 mg ... MC-19, C7
GG 501—Geneva Nitroglycerin Extended-release Capsules 6.5 mg ... MC-16, D2
GG 511—Geneva Nitroglycerin Extended-release Capsules 2.5 mg ... MC-16, D2
GG 512—Geneva Nitroglycerin Extended-release Capsules 9 mg ... MC-16, D2
GG 517—Geneva Indomethacin Capsules 25 mg ... MC-12, C2
GG 518—Geneva Indomethacin Capsules 50 mg ... MC-12, C2
GG 533—Geneva Diphenhydramine Capsules 25 mg ... MC-7, D1
GG 541—Geneva Diphenhydramine Capsules 50 mg ... MC-7, D1
GG 551—Geneva Procainamide Capsules 250 mg ... MC-19, C6
GG 552—Geneva Procainamide Capsules 375 mg ... MC-19, C6
GG 553—Geneva Procainamide Capsules 500 mg ... MC-19, C6
GG 558—Geneva Fenoprofen Capsules 200 mg ... MC-10, A4
GG 559—Geneva Fenoprofen Capsules 300 mg ... MC-10, A4
GG 572—Geneva Doxepin Capsules 25 mg ... MC-8, B3
GG 573—Geneva Doxepin Capsules 50 mg ... MC-8, B4
GG 574—Geneva Doxepin Capsules 75 mg ... MC-8, B4
GG 576—Geneva Doxepin Capsules 10 mg ... MC-8, B3
GG 577—Geneva Doxepin Capsules 100 mg ... MC-8, B4
GG 589—Geneva Thiothixene Capsules 1 mg ... MC-23, A5
GG 596—Geneva Thiothixene Capsules 2 mg ... MC-23, A5
GG 597—Geneva Thiothixene Capsules 5 mg ... MC-23, A5
GG 598—Geneva Thiothixene Capsules 10 mg ... MC-23, A5
H09—*Ilosone* Capsules 250 mg ... MC-9, B6
H11—Lederle Hydralazine Tablets 25 mg ... MC-11, B6
H12—Lederle Hydralazine Tablets 50 mg ... MC-11, B6
H69—*Keflex* Capsules 250 mg ... MC-4, C3
H71—*Keflex* Capsules 500 mg ... MC-4, C3
H76—*Nalfon* Capsules 200 mg ... MC-10, A2
H77—*Nalfon* Capsules 300 mg ... MC-10, A2
H 203—Schein Tetracycline Capsules 500 mg ... MC-22, B6
H 214—Schein Tetracycline Capsules 250 mg Blue/Yellow ... MC-22, B6
IBU 400—Boots Laboratories Ibuprofen Tablets 400 mg ... MC-12, A4
IBU 600—Boots Laboratories Ibuprofen Tablets 600 mg ... MC-12, A4
IBU 800—Boots Laboratories Ibuprofen Tablets 800 mg ... MC-12, A4
J10—*Eskalith CR* Extended-release Tablets 450 mg ... MC-13, D2
KL—*Biaxin* Tablets 500 mg ... MC-5, C5
KT—*Biaxin* Tablets 250 mg ... MC-5, C5

K2—*Dilaudid* Tablets 2 mg ... MC-11, D3
K4—*Dilaudid* Tablets 4 mg ... MC-11, D3
LL 200—*Suprax* Tablets 200 mg ... MC-4, B4
L 9—*Ledercillin VK* Tablets 500 mg ... MC-18, B7
L 10—*Ledercillin VK* Tablets 250 mg ... MC-18, B7
MJ 5—*BuSpar* Tablets 5 mg ... MC-3, C1
MJ 10—*BuSpar* Tablets 10 mg ... MC-3, C1
MJ 10 mEq 770—*Klotrix* Extended-release Tablets 750 mg ... MC-19, A6
MJ 755—*Estrace* Tablets 1 mg ... MC-9, C6
MJ 756—*Estrace* Tablets 2 mg ... MC-9, C6
MJ 775—*Desyrel* Tablets 50 mg ... MC-23, D2
MJ 776—*Desyrel* Tablets 100 mg ... MC-23, D2
MJ 778—*Desyrel* Tablets 150 mg Dividose ... MC-23, D2
MJ 784—*Duricef* Capsules 500 mg ... MC-4, B2
MJ 785—*Duricef* Tablets 1 gram ... MC-4, B3
MO—*Toprol XL* Extended-release Tablets 50 mg ... MC-15, B5
MP 44—Mutual Benztropine Tablets 1 mg ... MC-3, A6
MP 50—Mutual Tolmetin Tablets 200 mg ... MC-23, C6
MP 71—Purepac Allopurinol Tablets 100 mg ... MC-1, B5
MP 74—Mutual Chlorzoxazone Tablets 500 mg ... MC-5, B6
MP 80—Mutual Allopurinol Tablets 300 mg ... MC-1, B5
MP 112—Mutual Sulindac Tablets 150 mg ... MC-21, D3
MP 114—Mutual Trazodone Tablets 100 mg ... MC-23, D3
MP 116—Mutual Sulindac Tablets 200 mg ... MC-21, D3
MP 118—Mutual Trazodone Tablets 50 mg ... MC-23, D3
MP 142—Mutual Benztropine Tablets 2 mg ... MC-3, A6
MP 146—Mutual Atenolol Tablets 50 mg ... MC-2, B6
MP 147—Mutual Atenolol Tablets 100 mg ... MC-2, B6
MP 152—Mutual Atenolol and Chlorthalidone Tablets 100/25 mg ... MC-2, C2
MP 153—Mutual Atenolol and Chlorthalidone Tablets 50/25 mg ... MC-2, C2
MP 178—Mutual Pindolol Tablets 5 mg ... MC-19, A1
MP 183—Mutual Pindolol Tablets 10 mg ... MC-19, A1
MP 184—Mutual Metoprolol Tartrate Tablets 50 mg ... MC-15, B7
MP 185—Mutual Metoprolol Tartrate Tablets 100 mg ... MC-15, B7
MS—*Toprol XL* Extended-release Tablets 100 mg ... MC-15, B5
MSD 14—*Vasotec* Tablets 2.5 mg ... MC-8, D6
MSD 19—*Prinivil* Tablets 5 mg ... MC-13, C2
MSD 20—*Decadron* Tablets 0.25 mg ... MC-6, D1
MSD 21—*Cogentin* Tablets 0.5 mg ... MC-3, A5
MSD 23—*Elavil* Tablets 10 mg ... MC-1, D2
MSD 25—*Indocin* Capsules 25 mg ... MC-12, C3
MSD 41—*Decadron* Tablets 0.5 mg ... MC-6, D1
MSD 42—*HydroDIURIL* Tablets 25 mg ... MC-11, C5
MSD 45—*Elavil* Tablets 25 mg ... MC-1, D2
MSD 50—*Indocin* Capsules 50 mg ... MC-12, C3
MSD 59—*Blocadren* Tablets 5 mg ... MC-23, B3
MSD 60—*Cogentin* Tablets 2 mg ... MC-3, A5
MSD 63—*Decadron* Tablets 0.75 mg ... MC-6, D1
MSD 72—*Proscar* Tablets 5 mg ... MC-10, B2
MSD 95—*Decadron* Tablets 1.5 mg ... MC-6, D2
MSD 97—*Decadron* Tablets 4 mg ... MC-6, D2
MSD 102—*Elavil* Tablets 50 mg ... MC-1, D2
MSD 105—*HydroDIURIL* Tablets 50 mg ... MC-11, C5
MSD 106—*Prinivil* Tablets 10 mg ... MC-13, C2
MSD 135—*Aldomet* Tablets 125 mg ... MC-14, D2
MSD 136—*Blocadren* Tablets 10 mg ... MC-23, B3
MSD 140—*Prinzide* Tablets 20/12.5 mg ... MC-13, C4
MSD 142—*Prinzide* Tablets 20/25 mg ... MC-13, C4
MSD 147—*Decadron* Tablets 6 mg ... MC-6, D2
MSD 207—*Prinivil* Tablets 20 mg ... MC-13, C2
MSD 237—*Prinivil* Tablets 40 mg ... MC-13, C2
MSD 401—*Aldomet* Tablets 250 mg ... MC-14, D2
MSD 410—*HydroDIURIL* Tablets 100 mg ... MC-11, C5
MSD 423—*Aldoril* Tablets 250/15 mg ... MC-14, D7
MSD 430—*Elavil* Tablets 75 mg ... MC-1, D2
MSD 435—*Elavil* Tablets 100 mg ... MC-1, D2
MSD 437—*Blocadren* Tablets 20 mg ... MC-23, B3
MSD 451—*Plendil* Tablets 5 mg ... MC-10, A1
MSD 452—*Plendil* Tablets 10 mg ... MC-10, A1
MSD 456—*Aldoril* Tablets 250/25 mg ... MC-14, D7
MSD 516—*Aldomet* Tablets 500 mg ... MC-14, D2
MSD 517—*Triavil* Tablets 4/50 mg ... MC-18, C7
MSD 635—*Cogentin* Tablets 1 mg ... MC-3, A5
MSD 673—*Elavil* Tablets 150 mg ... MC-1, D2
MSD 675—*Dolobid* Tablets 250 mg ... MC-7, B5
MSD 693—*Indocin SR* Extended-release Capsules 75 mg ... MC-12, C4
MSD 694—*Aldoril* Tablets 500/30 mg ... MC-15, A1
MSD 697—*Dolobid* Tablets 500 mg ... MC-7, B5
MSD 705—*Noroxin* Tablets 400 mg ... MC-17, B3
MSD 707—*Tonocard* Tablets 400 mg ... MC-23, B6
MSD 709—*Tonocard* Tablets 600 mg ... MC-23, B6
MSD 712—*Vasotec* Tablets 5 mg ... MC-8, D6
MSD 713—*Vasotec* Tablets 10 mg ... MC-8, D6
MSD 714—*Vasotec* Tablets 20 mg ... MC-8, D6
MSD 720—*Vaseretic* Tablets 10/25 mg ... MC-8, D7
MSD 726—*Zocor* Tablets 5 mg ... MC-21, B2
MSD 731—*Mevacor* Tablets 20 mg ... MC-14, A5
MSD 732—*Mevacor* Tablets 40 mg ... MC-14, A5
MSD 735—*Zocor* Tablets 10 mg ... MC-21, B2
MSD 742—*Prilosec* Delayed-release Capsules 20 mg ... MC-17, C4
MSD 914—*Triavil* Tablets 2/10 mg ... MC-18, C6
MSD 917—*Moduretic* Tablets 5/50 mg ... MC-1, C5
MSD 921—*Triavil* Tablets 2/25 mg ... MC-18, C6
MSD 931—*Flexeril* Tablets 10 mg ... MC-6, B6
MSD 934—*Triavil* Tablets 4/10 mg ... MC-18, C6
MSD 935—*Aldoril* Tablets 500/50 mg ... MC-15, A1
MSD 941—*Clinoril* Tablets 150 mg ... MC-21, D2
MSD 942—*Clinoril* Tablets 200 mg ... MC-21, D2
MSD 946—*Triavil* Tablets 4/25 mg ... MC-18, C7
MSD 963—*Pepcid* Tablets 20 mg ... MC-9, D6
MSD 964—*Pepcid* Tablets 40 mg ... MC-9, D6
MT 4—*Pancrease* Delayed-release Capsules 4/20/25 ... MC-18, B1
MT 10—*Pancrease* Delayed-release Capsules 10/30/30 ... MC-18, B1
MT 16—*Pancrease* Delayed-release Capsules 16/48/48 ... MC-18, B2
MT 25—*Pancrease* Delayed-release Capsules 25/75/75 ... MC-18, B2
MY—*Toprol XL* Extended-release Capsules 200 mg ... MC-15, B5
M 1—Mylan Clonidine and Chlorthalidone Tablets 0.1/15 mg ... MC-6, A5
M2—Schein/Danbury Furosemide Tablets 20 mg ... MC-10, D4
M 3—*Minocin* Tablets 50 mg ... MC-15, C7
M 5—*Minocin* Tablets 100 mg ... MC-15, C7
M8—*Maxzide* Tablets 75/50 mg ... MC-24, A1
M9—*Maxzide* Tablets 37.5/25 mg ... MC-24, A1
M 27—Mylan Clonidine and Chlorthalidone Tablets 0.2/15 mg ... MC-6, A5
M 30—Mylan Clorazepate Tablets 3.75 mg ... MC-6, B1
M 31—Mylan Allopurinol Tablets 100 mg ... MC-1, B6
M 40—Mylan Clorazepate Tablets 7.5 mg ... MC-6, B1
M 45—*Minocin* Capsules 50 mg ... MC-15, C6
M 46—*Minocin* Capsules 100 mg ... MC-15, C6
M 54—Mylan Thioridazine Tablets 10 mg ... MC-22, D7
M 55—Mylan Timolol Tablets 5 mg ... MC-23, B4
M 58—Mylan Thioridazine Tablets 25 mg ... MC-22, D7
M 59—Mylan Thioridazine Tablets 50 mg ... MC-22, D7
M 61—Mylan Thioridazine Tablets 100 mg ... MC-22, D7
M 70—Mylan Clorazepate Tablets 15 mg ... MC-6, B1
M 71—Mylan Allopurinol Tablets 300 mg ... MC-1, B6
M 72—Mylan Clonidine and Chlorthalidone Tablets 0.3/15 mg ... MC-6, A5
M 221—Mylan Timolol Tablets 10 mg ... MC-23, B4
NE—*Asacol* Delayed-release Tablets 400 mg ... MC-14, C1
NE—*Entex PSE* Tablets 120/600 mg ... MC-20, D2
NE—*Nicolar* Tablets 500 mg ... MC-16, B3
NR—*Depakote* Delayed-release Tablets 250 mg ... MC-8, B1
NS—*Depakote* Delayed-release Tablets 500 mg ... MC-8, B1
NT—*Depakote* Delayed-release Tablets 125 mg ... MC-8, B1
N 21—*NegGram* Tablets 250 mg ... MC-16, A4
N 22—*NegGram* Tablets 500 mg ... MC-16, A4
N 23—*NegGram* Tablets 1 gram ... MC-16, A5
P—*Demulen 1/35-28* Tablets Inert ... MC-9, D3
P—*Demulen 1/50-28* Tablets Inert ... MC-9, D4
PAA—*Trinalin* Extended-release Tablets 1/120 mg ... MC-2, D3
P-D 007—*Dilantin* Chewable Tablets 50 mg ... MC-18, D6
P-D 204—*Procan SR* Extended-release Tablets 500 mg ... MC-19, D1
P-D 205—*Procan SR* Extended-release Tablets 750 mg ... MC-19, D2
P-D 207—*Procan SR* Extended-release Tablets 1 gram ... MC-19, D2
P-D 362—*Dilantin* Capsules 100 mg ... MC-18, D7
P-D 365—*Dilantin* Capsules 30 mg ... MC-18, D7
P-D 471—*Benadryl* Capsules 25 mg ... MC-7, D2
P-D 473—*Benadryl* Capsules 50 mg ... MC-7, D2
P-D 622—*Loestrin Fe 1/20* Tablets 75 mg ... MC-17, A6
P-D 622—*Loestrin Fe 1.5/30* Tablets 75 mg ... MC-17, A7

P-D 696—*Eryc* Delayed-release Capsules 250 mg ... MC-9, B5
P-D 915—*Loestrin Fe 1/20* Tablets 1/0.02 mg ... MC-17, A6
P-D 915—*Loestrin 21 1/20* Tablets 1/0.02 mg ... MC-17, A4
P-D 916—*Loestrin Fe 1.5/30* Tablets 1.5/0.03 mg ... MC-17, A7
P-D 916—*Loestrin 21 1.5/30* Tablets 1.5/0.03 mg ... MC-17, A5
PPP 207—*Corgard* Tablets 40 mg ... MC-16, A1
PPP 208—*Corgard* Tablets 120 mg ... MC-16, A1
PPP 232—*Corgard* Tablets 20 mg ... MC-16, A1
PPP 241—*Corgard* Tablets 80 mg ... MC-16, A1
PPP 246—*Corgard* Tablets 160 mg ... MC-16, A2
PPP 606—*Naturetin* Tablets 5 mg ... MC-3, A3
PPP 618—*Naturetin* Tablets 10 mg ... MC-3, A3
PPP 775—*Pronestyl-SR* Extended-release Tablets 500 mg ... MC-19, D5
PPP 863—*Prolixin* Tablets 1 mg ... MC-10, B6
PPP 864—*Prolixin* Tablets 2.5 mg ... MC-10, B6
PPP 877—*Prolixin* Tablets 5 mg ... MC-10, B6
PPP 956—*Prolixin* Tablets 10 mg ... MC-10, B6
P7F—*Mepron* Tablets 250 mg ... MC-2, C5
P10—*Propulsid* Tablets 10 mg ... MC-5, C4
P20—*Propulsid* Tablets 20 mg ... MC-5, C4
P 44—Lederle Propranolol Tablets 10 mg ... MC-20, B4
P 45—Lederle Propranolol Tablets 20 mg ... MC-20, B4
P 46—Lederle Propranolol Tablets 40 mg ... MC-20, B4
P 47—Lederle Propranolol Tablets 80 mg ... MC-20, B4
P 65—Lederle Propranolol Tablets 60 mg ... MC-20, B4
rPr 351—*Slo-Phyllin* Tablets 100 mg ... MC-22, D1
rPr 352—*Slo-Phyllin* Tablets 200 mg ... MC-22, D1
R021—Purepac Flurazepam Capsules 15 mg ... MC-10, C3
R022—Purepac Flurazepam Capsules 30 mg ... MC-10, C3
R1—*Risperdal* Tablets 1 mg ... MC-21, A6
R2—*Risperdal* Tablets 2 mg ... MC-21, A6
R3—*Risperdal* Tablets 3 mg ... MC-21, A6
R4—*Risperdal* Tablets 4 mg ... MC-21, A6
R 497—Purepac Nifedipine Capsules 10 mg ... MC-16, C3
R 520—Purepac Tolmetin Capsules 400 mg ... MC-23, C7
R 530—Purepac Nifedipine Capsules 20 mg ... MC-16, C3
SKF—*Dyazide* Capsules 50/25 mg ... MC-24, A3
SKF—*Ornade* Extended-release Capsules 75/12 mg ... MC-4, D6
SKF C44—*Compazine* Extended-release Capsules 10 mg ... MC-20, A1
SKF C46—*Compazine* Extended-release Capsules 15 mg ... MC-20, A1
SKF C66—*Compazine* Tablets 5 mg ... MC-20, A2
SKF C67—*Compazine* Tablets 10 mg ... MC-20, A2
SR 80—*Calan SR* Extended-release Tablets 180 mg ... MC-24, D3
SR 120—*Calan SR* Extended-release Tablets 120 mg ... MC-24, D3
SR 240—*Calan SR* Extended-release Tablets 240 mg ... MC-24, D3
S04—*Stelazine* Tablets 2 mg ... MC-24, A6
S 5—*Eldepryl* Tablets 5 mg ... MC-21, A7
TL—*Tranxene T-Tab* Tablets 3.75 mg ... MC-6, A7
TM—*Tranxene T-Tab* Tablets 7.5 mg ... MC-6, A7
TN—*Tranxene T-Tab* Tablets 15 mg ... MC-6, A7
TX—*Tranxene SD* Tablets 11.25 mg ... MC-6, A6
TY—*Tranxene SD* Tablets 22.5 mg ... MC-6, A6
T9A—*Lanoxin* Tablets 0.5 mg ... MC-7, B7
T37—*Talacen* Tablets 25/650 mg ... MC-18, C3
T 51—*Talwin-Nx* Tablets 50/0.5 mg ... MC-18, C4
T64—*Thorazine* Extended-release Capsules 75 mg ... MC-5, A3
T74—*Thorazine* Tablets 25 mg ... MC-5, A4
UC—ProSom Tablets 1 mg ... MC-9, C5
UD—ProSom Tablets 2 mg ... MC-9, C5
U05—*Ilosone* Chewable Tablets 125 mg ... MC-9, B7
U25—*Ilosone* Chewable Tablets 250 mg ... MC-9, B7
U 121—*Loniten* Tablets 2.5 mg ... MC-15, D3
V7—*Verelan* Extended-release Capsules 180 mg ... MC-24, C4
V8—*Verelan* Extended-release Capsules 120 mg ... MC-24, C4
V9—*Verelan* Extended-resease Capsules 240 mg ... MC-24, C5
WC 242—Warner Chilcott Carbamazepine Chewable Tablets 100 mg ... MC-4, A1
WC 407—Warner Chilcott Tetracycline Capsules 250 mg ... MC-22, C1
WC 445—Warner Chilcott Clonidine Tablets 0.3 mg ... MC-6, A3
WC 607—Warner Chilcott Phenobarbital Tablets 60 mg ... MC-18, D1
WC 615—Warner Chilcott Minocycline Capsules 50 mg ... MC-15, D1
WC 616—Warner Chilcott Minocycline Capsules 100 mg ... MC-15, D1
WC 697—Warner Chilcott Tetracycline Capsules 500 mg ... MC-22, C1
WC 698—Warner Chilcott Phenobarbital Tablets 100 mg ... MC-18, D1
WC 699—Warner Chilcott Phenobarbital Tablets 15 mg ... MC-18, D1
WC 700—Warner Chilcott Phenobarbital Tablets 30 mg ... MC-18, D1
WC 773—Warner Chilcott Sulindac Tablets 150 mg ... MC-21, D5
WC 774—Warner Chilcott Sulindac Tablets 200 mg ... MC-21, D5
WHR 1354—*Slo-Phyllin* Extended-release Capsules 60 mg ... MC-22, C7
WHR 1356—*Slo-Phyllin* Extended-release Capsules 250 mg ... MC-22, C7
X3A—*Lanoxin* Tablets 0.25 mg ... MC-7, B7
Y2B—*Septra* Tablets 400/80 mg ... MC-21, C4
Y3B—*Lanoxin* Tablets 0.125 mg ... MC-7, B7
Y9C 100—*Retrovir* Capsules 100 mg ... MC-24, D6
Z 2931—Rugby Methyldopa Tablets 250 mg ... MC-14, D3
Z 2932—Rugby Methyldopa Tablets 500 mg ... MC-14, D3
0051—*Lopurin* Tablets 100 mg ... MC-1, B3
0052—*Lopurin* Tablets 300 mg ... MC-1, B3
0.125—*Halcion* Tablets 0.125 mg ... MC-24, A4
0.25—*Halcion* Tablets 0.25 mg ... MC-24, A4
0.25—*Xanax* Tablets 0.25 mg ... MC-1, C3
0.3—*Premarin* Tablets 0.3 mg ... MC-9, C7
0.5—*Bumex* Tablets 0.5 mg ... MC-3, B6
0.5—*Xanax* Tablets 0.5 mg ... MC-1, C3
0.5/35—*Genora 0.5/35-21* Tablets 0.5/0.035 mg ... MC-17, A2
0.625—*Premarin* Tablets 0.625 mg ... MC-9, C7
0.9—*Premarin* Tablets 0.9 mg ... MC-9, C7
039—Purepac Alprazolam Tablets 2 mg ... MC-1, C2
04 30—*Felbatol* Tablets 400 mg ... MC-9, D7
04 31—*Felbatol* Tablets 600 mg ... MC-9, D7
051—Purepac Diazepam Tablets 2 mg ... MC-6, D5
052—Purepac Diazepam Tablets 5 mg ... MC-6, D5
053—Purepac Diazepam Tablets 10 mg ... MC-6, D5
058—Barr Diphenhydramine Capsules 25 mg ... MC-7, C7
059—Barr Diphenhydramine Capsules 50 mg ... MC-7, C7
063—Purepac Lorazepam Tablets 2 mg ... MC-14, A2
067—Purepac Oxazepam Capsules 10 mg ... MC-17, D3
069—Purepac Oxazepam Capsules 15 mg ... MC-17, D3
073—Purepac Oxazepam Capsules 30 mg ... MC-17, D3
076—Purepac Temazepam Capsules 15 mg ... MC-22, A3
077—Purepac Temazepam Capsules 30 mg ... MC-22, A3
078—Purepac Clorazepate Tablets 3.75 mg ... MC-6, B2
081—Purepac Clorazepate Tablets 7.5 mg ... MC-6, B2
083—Purepac Clorazepate Tablets 15 mg ... MC-6, B2
085—Purepac Propoxyphene Napsylate and Acetaminophen Tablets 100/650 mg ... MC-20, B2
094—*Vibramycin* Capsules 50 mg ... MC-8, C6
095—*Mycelex Troche* Lozenges 10 mg ... MC-6, B3
095—*Vibramycin* Capsules 100 mg ... MC-8, C6
099—*Vibra-Tabs* Tablets 100 mg ... MC-8, C7
09A—*Proloprim* Tablets 100 mg ... MC-24, B1
0115 3875—Rugby Meclizine Chewable Tablets 25 mg ... MC-14, B2
0149 0007—*Macrodantin* Capsules 25 mg ... MC-16, C7
0149 0008—*Macrodantin* Capsules 50 mg ... MC-16, C7
0149 0009—*Macrodantin* Capsules 100 mg ... MC-16, C7
0149 0030—*Dantrium* Capsules 25 mg ... MC-6, C4
0149 0031—*Dantrium* Capsules 50 mg ... MC-6, C4
0149 0033—*Dantrium* Capsules 100 mg ... MC-6, C4
0149 0412—*Entex* Capsules 5/45/200 mg ... MC-18, D4
0149 0436—*Entex LA* Extended-release Tablets 75/400 mg ... MC-18, D5
0230—Rugby Doxycycline Capsules 100 mg ... MC-8, D2
0280—Rugby Doxycycline Capsules 50 mg ... MC-8, D2
0665 4160—Solvay Lithium Capsules ... MC-13, D3
0920—*Dilatrate-SR* Extended-release Capsules 40 mg ... MC-12, C5
½—*Haldol* Tablets 0.5 mg ... MC-11, B2
½—*Mykrox* Tablets 0.5 mg ... MC-15, B3
1—*Bumex* Tablets 1 mg ... MC-3, B6
1—*Haldol* Tablets 1 mg ... MC-11, B2
1—IPR Pharmaceuticals Atenolol Tablets 25 mg ... MC-2, B4
1—*Tenex* Tablets 1 mg ... MC-11, A5
1—*Tylenol with Codeine* Tablets 300/7.5 mg ... MC-1, A1
1.0—*Xanax* Tablets 1 mg ... MC-1, C3
1.25—*Micronase* Tablets 1.25 mg ... MC-11, A2
1.25—*Premarin* Tablets 1.25 mg ... MC-9, D1
1.25 mg—*Altace* Capsules 1.25 mg ... MC-21, A1
1/35—*Genora 1/35-28* Tablets 1/0.035 mg ... MC-17, A3

1/50—*Genora 1/50-28* Tablets 1/0.05 mg ... MC-17, B2
1A—*Cartrol* Tablets 2.5 mg ... MC-4, A7
1C—*Cartrol* Tablets 5 mg ... MC-4, A7
1 mg—*Cardura* Tablets 1 mg ... MC-8, B2
2—*Bumex* Tablets 2 mg ... MC-3, B6
2—*Coumadin* Tablets 2 mg ... MC-24, D4
2—*Haldol* Tablets 2 mg ... MC-11, B2
2—*Halotestin* Tablets 2 mg ... MC-10, B5
2—*Medrol* Tablets 2 mg ... MC-15, A4
2—*Tenex* Tablets 2 mg ... MC-11, A5
2—*Tylenol with Codeine* Tablets 300/15 mg ... MC-1, A1
2—*Valium* Tablets 2 mg ... MC-6, D7
2—*Ventolin* Tablets 2 mg ... MC-1, A7
2—*Xanax* Tablets 2 mg ... MC-1, C3
2 mg—*Cardura* Tablets 2 mg ... MC-8, B2
.25—*Rocaltrol* Capsules 0.25 mcg ... MC-3, C7
2½—*Coumadin* Tablets 2.5 mg ... MC-24, D4
2½—*Zaroxolyn* Tablets 2.5 mg ... MC-15, B4
2.5—*Deltasone* Tablets 2.5 mg ... MC-19, C4
2.5—*DynaCirc* Capsules 2.5 mg ... MC-13, A1
2.5—*Micronase* Tablets 2.5 mg ... MC-11, A2
2.5—*Norvasc* Tablets 2.5 mg ... MC-1, D4
2.5—*Premarin* Tablets 2.5 mg ... MC-9, D1
2.5—*Provera* Tablets 2.5 mg ... MC-14, B5
2.5 mg—*Altace* Capsules 2.5 mg ... MC-21, A1
3—*Empirin with Codeine* Tablets 325/30 mg ... MC-2, B1
3—*Ritalin* Tablets 10 mg ... MC-15, A2
3—*Tylenol with Codeine* Tablets 300/30 mg ... MC-1, A1
4—*Empirin with Codeine* Tablets 325/60 mg ... MC-2, B1
4—*Medrol* Tablets 4 mg ... MC-15, A4
4—Mylan Fluphenazine Tablets 1 mg ... MC-10, B7
4—*Tylenol with Codeine* Tablets 300/60 mg ... MC-1, A1
4—*Ventolin* Tablets 4 mg ... MC-1, A7
4—*Zofran* Tablets 4 mg ... MC-17, C5
4 mg—*Cardura* Tablets 4 mg ... MC-8, B2
.5—*Rocaltrol* Capsules 0.5 mcg ... MC-3, C7
5—*Accupril* Tablets 5 mg ... MC-20, D4
5—*Cortef* Tablets 5 mg ... MC-11, D2
5—*Coumadin* Tablets 5 mg ... MC-24, D4
5—*Deltasone* Tablets 5 mg ... MC-19, C4
5—*Dyna Circ* Capsules 5 mg ... MC-13, A1
5—*Glucotrol XL* Extended-release Tablets ... MC-10, D7
5—*Haldol* Tablets 5 mg ... MC-11, B2
5—*Halotestin* Tablets 5 mg ... MC-11, B5
5—*Isordil* Sublingual Tablets 5 mg ... MC-12, D1
5—*Libritabs* Tablets 5 mg ... MC-4, D2
5—*Librium* Capsules 5 mg ... MC-4, D1
5—*Lotensin* Tablets 5 mg ... MC-3, A1
5—*Micronase* Tablets 5 mg ... MC-11, A2
5—*Norvasc* Tablets 5 mg ... MC-1, D4
5—*Provera* Tablets 5 mg ... MC-14, B5
5—*Reglan* Tablets 5 mg ... MC-15, A7
5—*Valium* Tablets 5 mg ... MC-6, D7
5—*Zaroxolyn* Tablets 5 mg ... MC-15, B4
5 mg—*Altace* Capsules 5 mg ... MC-21, A1
6—*Rufen* Tablets 600 mg ... MC-12, A5
6—*Serax* Capsules 15 mg ... MC-17, D5
7—*Lozol* Tablets 1.25 mg ... MC-12, C1
7—*Ritalin* Tablets 5 mg ... MC-15, A2
7.5—*Doral* Tablets 7.5 mg ... MC-20, D3
7.5 mg—*Restoril* Capsules 7.5 mg ... MC-22, A4
7½—*Coumadin* Tablets 7.5 mg ... MC-24, D4
8—*Dilaudid* Tablets 8 mg ... MC-11, D3
8—*Klor-Con* Extended-release Tablets 600 mg ... MC-19, B3
8—*Lozol* Tablets 2.5 mg ... MC-12, C1
8—*Medrol* Tablets 8 mg ... MC-15, A4
8—*Rufen* Tablets 800 mg ... MC-12, A5
8—*Zofran* Tablets 8 mg ... MC-17, C5
8 mg—*Cardura* Tablets 8 mg ... MC-8, B2
9—Mylan Fluphenazine Tablets 2.5 mg ... MC-10, B7
10—*Accupril* Tablets 10 mg ... MC-20, D4
10—*Accutane* Capsules 10 mg ... MC-12, D7
10—*Atarax* Tablets 10 mg ... MC-11, D7
10—*Bentyl* Capsules 10 mg ... MC-7, A7
10—*Cognex* Capsules 10 mg ... MC-21, D6
10—*Cortef* Tablets 10 mg ... MC-11, D2
10—*Coumadin* Tablets 10 mg ... MC-24, D5
10—*Deltasone* Tablets 10 mg ... MC-19, C4
10—*Glucotrol XL* Extended-release Tablets ... MC-10, D7
10—*Haldol* Tablets 10 mg ... MC-11, B2
10—*Halotestin* Tablets 10 mg ... MC-10, B5
10—*Inderal* Tablets 10 mg ... MC-20, C3
10—*Isordil* Sublingual Tablets 10 mg ... MC-12, D1
10—*K-Dur* Extended-release Tablets 750 mg ... MC-19, A7
10—*Kerlone* Tablets 10 mg ... MC-3, B1
10—*Klor-Con* Extended-release Tablets 750 mg ... MC-19, B3
10—*Librium* Capsules 10 mg ... MC-4, D1
10—*Loniten* Tablets 10 mg ... MC-15, D3
10—*Lotensin* Tablets 10 mg ... MC-3, A1
10—*Norvasc* Tablets 10 mg ... MC-1, D4
10—*Pravachol* Tablets 10 mg ... MC-19, B4
10—*Provera* Tablets 10 mg ... MC-14, B5
10—*Valium* Tablets 10 mg ... MC-6, D7
10—*Zaroxolyn* Tablets 10 mg ... MC-15, B4
10-0364—Schein Nifedipine Capsules 10 mg ... MC-16, C4
10 mg—*Altace* Capsules 10 mg ... MC-21, A1
11—*Tri-Levlen 28* Tablets Inert ... MC-13, B1
15—Biocraft Penicillin V Tablets 250 mg Round ... MC-18, B6
15—*Dalmane* Capsules 15 mg ... MC-10, C4
15—*Doral* Tablets 15 mg ... MC-20, D3
15—*Ionamin* Capsules 15 mg ... MC-18, D2
15—*Valrelease* Extended-release Capsules 15 mg ... MC-6, D6
16—Biocraft Penicillin V Tablets 250 mg Oval ... MC-18, B6
16—*Medrol* Tablets 16 mg ... MC-15, A4
16—*Ritalin-SR* Extended-release Tablets 20 mg ... MC-15, A3
17—Biocraft Penicillin V Tablets 500 mg Round ... MC-18, B6
17 12—*Carafate* Tablets 1 gram ... MC-21, C3
18—*Didrex* Tablets 25 mg ... MC-3, A4
19—*Phenergan* Tablets 12.5 mg ... MC-20, A3
20—*Accupril* Tablets 20 mg ... MC-20, D4
20—*Accutane* Capsules 20 mg ... MC-12, D7
20—*Bentyl* Tablets 20 mg ... MC-7, B1
20—*Cognex* Capsules 20 mg ... MC-21, D6
20—*Cortef* Tablets 20 mg ... MC-11, D2
20—*Deltasone* Tablets 20 mg ... MC-19, C4
20—*Haldol* Tablets 20 mg ... MC-11, B2
20—*Inderal* Tablets 20 mg ... MC-20, C3
20—*ISMO* Tablets 20 mg ... MC-12, D6
20—*K-Dur* Tablets 1500 mg ... MC-19, A7
20—*Kerlone* Tablets 20 mg ... MC-3, B1
20—*Lescol* Capsules 20 mg ... MC-10, C7
20—*Lotensin* Tablets 20 mg ... MC-3, A1
20—*Paxil* Tablets 20 mg ... MC-18, B3
20—*Pravachol* Tablets 20 mg ... MC-19, B4
20—*Tofranil-PM* Capsules 75 mg ... MC-12, B5
20-0364—Schein Nifedipine Capsules 20 mg ... MC-16, C4
20 (R)—*Hygroton* Tablets 50 mg ... MC-5, B3
21—*Hygroton* Tablets 100 mg ... MC-5, B3
21—*Levlen 21 and 28* Tablets 0.15/0.03 mg ... MC-13, A7
22—*Esidrix* Tablets 25 mg ... MC-11, C3
22—*Levatol* Tablets 20 mg ... MC-18, B4
22—*Tofranil-PM* Capsules 150 mg ... MC-12, B6
22 (R)—*Hygroton* Tablets 25 mg ... MC-5, B3
23—*Lioresal* Tablets 10 mg ... MC-2, D6
25—*Atarax* Tablets 25 mg ... MC-11, D7
25—*Clozaril* Tablets 25 mg ... MC-6, B4
25—*Isordil* Sublingual Tablets 2.5 mg ... MC-12, D1
25—*Libritabs* Tablets 25 mg ... MC-4, D2
25—*Librium* Capsules 25 mg ... MC-4, D1
25—*Norpramin* Tablets 25 mg ... MC-6, C6
25—*Synthroid* Tablets 0.025 mg ... MC-13, B4
25—*Tenuate* Tablets 25 mg ... MC-7, B3
25—*Videx* Tablets 25 mg ... MC-7, B2
25—*Voltaren* Tablets 25 mg ... MC-7, A2
25 mg—*Anafranil* Capsules 25 mg ... MC-5, D3
25 mg DAN—Schein/Danbury Nitrofurantoin Capsules 25 mg ... MC-16, D1
26—*Ludiomil* Tablets 50 mg ... MC-14, A6
27—*Phenergan* Tablets 25 mg ... MC-20, A3
27—Purepac Propranolol Tablets 10 mg ... MC-20, B5
27 27—*Tegretol* Tablets 200 mg ... MC-3, D5
28—*Levlen 28* Tablets Inert ... MC-13, A7
29—Purepac Propranolol Tablets 20 mg ... MC-20, B5
30—*Cognex* Capsules 30 mg ... MC-21, D6
30—*Dalmane* Capsules 30 mg ... MC-10, C4
30—*Ionamin* Capsules 30 mg ... MC-18, D2
30—*Paxil* Tablets 30 mg ... MC-18, B3
30—*Procardia XL* Extended-release Tablets 30 mg ... MC-16, C2
31—*Regroton* Tablets 0.25/50 mg ... MC-21, A4
32—*Demi-Regroton* Tablets 0.125/25 mg ... MC-20, A3
32—*Medrol* Tablets 32 mg ... MC-15, A5
32—*Tofranil* Tablets 10 mg ... MC-12, B7

33—*Lioresal* Tablets 20 mg MC-2, D6
34—*Ritalin* Tablets 20 mg MC-15, A2
35 35—*Lopressor HCT* Tablets 50/25 mg MC-15, C1
37—*Apresoline* Tablets 10 mg MC-11, B5
37—Geneva Hydroxyzine Tablets 10 mg MC-11, D5
37-0713—*Rynatan* Tablets 25/8/25 mg MC-18, D3
37-2001—*Soma* Tablets 350 mg MC-4, A4
38—Geneva Hydroxyzine Tablets 25 mg MC-11, D5
39—*Apresoline* Tablets 25 mg MC-11, B5
39—Geneva Hydroxyzine Tablets 50 mg MC-11, D5
40—*Accupril* Tablets 40 mg MC-20, D4
40—*Accutane* Capsules 40 mg MC-12, D7
40—*Calan* Tablets 40 mg MC-24, D2
40—*Cognex* Capsules 40 mg MC-21, D6
40—*Inderal* Tablets 40 mg MC-20, C3
40—*Isoptin* Tablets 40 mg MC-24, B7
40—*Lasix* Tablets 40 mg MC-10, D3
40—*Lescol* Capsules 40 mg MC-10, C7
40—*Lotensin* Tablets 40 mg MC-3, A1
40—*Pravachol* Tablets 40 mg MC-19, B4
40—*Tofranil-PM* Capsules 100 mg MC-12, B5
40/25—*Inderide* Tablets 40/25 mg MC-20, D1
45—IPR Pharmaceuticals Atenolol Tablets 50 mg MC-2, B4
45—*Tofranil-PM* Capsules 125 mg MC-12, B6
46—*Esidrix* Tablets 50 mg MC-11, C3
49—Biocraft Penicillin V Tablets 500 mg Oval MC-18, B6
50—*Atarax* Tablets 50 mg MC-11, D7
50—*Darvocet-N* Tablets 50/325 mg MC-20, A7
50—*Deltasone* Tablets 50 mg MC-19, C4
50—*Didrex* Tablets 50 mg MC-3, A4
50—*Diflucan* Tablets 50 mg MC-10, B3
50—*Imuran* Tablets 50 mg MC-2, D4
50—*Norpramin* Tablets 50 mg MC-6, C6
50—*Slo-bid* Extended-release Capsules 50 mg MC-22, C5
50—*Synthroid* Tablets 0.05 mg MC-13, B4
50—*Voltaren* Tablets 50 mg MC-7, A2
50 mg—*Anafranil* Capsules 50 mg MC-5, D3
50 mg—*Ansaid* Tablets 50 mg MC-10, C6
50 MG—*Zoloft* Tablets 50 mg MC-21, B1
50 mg DAN—Schein/Danbury Nitrofurantoin Capsules 50 mg MC-16, D1
50 PD—*Meclomen* Capsules 50 mg MC-14, B4
51—*Serax* Capsules 10 mg MC-17, D5
51 51—*Lopressor* Tablets 50 mg MC-15, B6
52—*Serax* Capsules 30 mg MC-17, D5
52—*Tegretol* Chewable Tablets 100 mg MC-3, D6
53—*Omnipen* Capsules 250 mg MC-2, A6
53 53—*Lopressor HCT* Tablets 100/25 mg MC-15, C1
54 092—Roxane Prednisone Tablets 1 mg MC-19, C2
54 213—Roxane Lithium Capsules 150 mg MC-13, C6
54 299—Roxane Dexamethasone Tablets 0.5 mg MC-6, D3
54 339—Roxane Prednisone Tablets 2.5 mg MC-19, C2
54 343—Roxane Prednisone Tablets 50 mg MC-19, C2
54 452—Roxane Lithium Tablets 300 mg MC-13, C7
54 463—Roxane Lithium Capsules 300 mg MC-13, C6
54 489—Roxane Dexamethasone Tablets 1 mg MC-6, D3
54 582—*Roxicodone* Tablets 5 mg MC-18, A1
54 612—Roxane Prednisone Tablets 5 mg MC-19, C2
54 662—Roxane Dexamethasone Tablets 2 mg MC-6, D4
54 702—Roxane Lithium Capsules 600 mg MC-13, C6
54 730—*Roxicet* Tablets 5/500 mg MC-18, A4
54 760—Roxane Prednisone Tablets 20 mg MC-19, C2
54 892—Roxane Dexamethasone Tablets 4 mg MC-6, D4
54 899—Roxane Prednisone Tablets 10 mg MC-19, C2
54 902—*Roxiprin* Tablets 4.88/325 mg MC-18, A7
54 943—Roxane Dexamethasone Tablets 1.5 mg MC-6, D4
54 960—Roxane Dexamethasone Tablets 0.75 mg MC-6, D3
55 63—Schein/Danbury Procainamide Extended-release Tablets 500 mg MC-19, D7
55 64—Schein/Danbury Procainamide Extended-release Tablets 750 mg MC-19, D7
55 126—Barr Dicyclomine Tablets 20 mg MC-7, A6
56—*Ovral-21 and -28* Tablets 0.5/0.05 mg MC-17, B5
57—Purepac Lorazepam Tablets 0.5 mg MC-14, A2
59—*Pen-Vee K* Tablets 250 mg MC-18, C2
59—Purepac Lorazepam Tablets 1 mg MC-14, A2
60—*Inderal LA* Extended-release Capsules 60 mg MC-20, C1
60—*Inderal* Tablets 60 mg MC-20, C3
60—*Procardia XL* Extended-release Tablets 60 mg MC-16, C2
60 mg—*Cardizem SR* Capsules 60 mg MC-7, C3
61—*Lomotil* Tablets 2.5/0.025 mg MC-7, D5
64—*Ativan* Tablets 1 mg MC-14, A4
65—*Ativan* Tablets 2 mg MC-14, A4
68-7—*Norpramin* Tablets 10 mg MC-6, C6
71—*Demulen 1/50-21 and -28* Tablets 1/0.05 mg MC-9, D4
71—*Ser-Ap-Es* Tablets 0.1/25/15 mg MC-21, A5
71 71—*Lopressor* Tablets 100 mg MC-15, B6
72—*Brethine* Tablets 2.5 mg MC-22, A6
73—*Apresoline* Tablets 50 mg MC-11, B5
73—*Wytensin* Tablets 4 mg MC-11, A4
73 73—*Lopressor HCT* Tablets 100/50 mg MC-15, C1
74—Mylan Fluphenazine Tablets 5 mg MC-10, C1
74—*Wytensin* Tablets 8 mg MC-11, A4
75—*Nordette-21 and -28* Tablets 0.15/0.03 mg MC-13, B2
75—*Norpramin* Tablets 75 mg MC-6, C7
75—*Ortho-Novum 7/7/7-21 and -28* Tablets 0.75/0.035 mg MC-17, A1
75—*Synthroid* Tablets 0.075 mg MC-13, B4
75—*Tenuate* Extended-release Tablets 75 mg MC-7, B4
75—*Voltaren* Tablets 75 mg MC-7, A2
75—*Wellbutrin* Tablets 75 mg MC-3, B7
75 mg—*Anafranil* Capsules 75 mg MC-5, D3
75 mg—*Cleocin* Capsules 75 mg MC-5, D2
75 mg—*Slo-bid* Extended-release Capsules 75 mg MC-22, C5
76—*Thalitone* Tablets 25 mg MC-5, B2
78—*Lo-Ovral-21 and -28* Tablets 0.3/0.03 mg MC-17, B4
78-2—*Mellaril* Tablets 10 mg MC-23, A1
78-3—*Mellaril* Tablets 25 mg MC-23, A1
78-4—*Mellaril* Tablets 50 mg MC-23, A1
78-5—*Mellaril* Tablets 100 mg MC-23, A2
78-6—*Mellaril* Tablets 150 mg MC-23, A2
78-7—*Mellaril* Tablets 200 mg MC-23, A2
78-8—*Mellaril* Tablets 15 mg MC-23, A1
78-17—*Parlodel* Tablets 2.5 mg MC-3, B5
78-34—*Cafergot* Tablets 1/100 mg MC-9, A5
78-72—*Tavist* Tablets 2.68 mg MC-5, C6
78-73—*Visken* Tablets 10 mg MC-19, A2
78-75—*Tavist* Tablets 1.34 mg MC-5, C6
78-78—*Pamelor* Capsules 50 mg MC-17, B7
78-79—*Pamelor* Capsules 75 mg MC-17, B7
78-84—*Fioricet* Tablets 50/325/40 mg MC-3, C2
78-86—*Pamelor* Capsules 10 mg MC-17, B6
78-87—*Pamelor* Capsules 25 mg MC-17, B6
78-98—*Restoril* Capsules 15 mg MC-22, A4
78-99—*Restoril* Capsules 30 mg MC-22, A4
78-101—*Hydergine LC* Capsules 1 mg MC-9, A2
78-102—*Parlodel* Capsules 5 mg MC-3, B4
78-103—*Fiorinal* Capsules 50/325/40 mg MC-3, C4
78-104—*Fiorinal* Tablets 50/325/40 mg MC-3, C5
78-107—*Fiorinal with Codeine* Capsules 50/325/30/40 mg MC-3, C6
78-111—*Visken* Tablets 5 mg MC-19, A2
78 240—*Sandimmune SGC* Capsules 25 mg MC-6, C2
78 241—*Sandimmune SGC* Capsules 100 mg MC-6, C2
80—*Calan* Tablets 80 mg MC-24, D2
80—*Inderal LA* Extended-release Capsules 80 mg MC-20, C1
80—*Inderal* Tablets 80 mg MC-20, C3
80—*Isoptin* Tablets 80 mg MC-24, B7
80—*Lasix* Tablets 80 mg MC-10, D3
80 mg—*Betapace* Tablets 80 mg MC-21, B3
80/25—*Inderide* Tablets 80/25 mg MC-20, D1
80/50—*Inderide LA* Extended-release Capsules 80/50 mg MC-20, C6
81—*Ativan* Tablets 0.5 mg MC-14, A4
90—IPR Pharmaceuticals Atenolol Tablets 100 mg MC-2, B4
90—*Procardia XL* Extended-release Tablets 90 mg MC-16, C2
90 mg—*Cardizem SR* Capsules 90 mg MC-7, C3
90 mg—*Cardizem* Tablets 90 mg MC-7, C5
95—*Tri-Levlen 21 and 28* Tablets 0.05/0.03 mg MC-13, B1
96—*Tri-Levlen 21 and 28* Tablets 0.075/0.04 mg MC-13, B1
97—Mylan Fluphenazine Tablets 10 mg MC-10, C1
97—*Tri-Levlen 21 and 28* Tablets 0.125/0.03 mg MC-13, B1
100—*Atarax* Tablets 100 mg MC-11, D7
100—*Clozaril* Tablets 100 mg MC-6, B4
100—*Darvocet-N* Tablets 100/650 mg MC-20, A7
100—*Diflucan* Tablets 100 mg MC-10, B3
100—*Norpramin* Tablets 100 mg MC-6, C7
100—*Sporanox* Capsules 100 mg MC-13, A2
100—*Synthroid* Tablets 0.1 mg MC-13, B4
100—*Theo-Dur* Extended-release Tablets 100 mg MC-22, C4
100—*Tigan* Capsules 100 mg MC-24, A7

100—*Tolinase* Tablets 100 mg ... MC-23, C1
100—*Trandate* Tablets 100 mg ... MC-13, A5
100—*Wellbutrin* Tablets 100 mg ... MC-3, B7
100—*Zyloprim* Tablets 100 mg ... MC-1, B4
100 mg—*Ansaid* Tablets 100 mg ... MC-10, C6
100 mg—*Neurontin* Capsules 100 mg ... MC-10, D5
100 mg—*Slo-bid* Extended-release Capsules 100 mg ... MC-22, C5
100 MG—*Zoloft* Tablets 100 mg ... MC-21, B1
100 mg DAN—Schein/Danbury Nitrofurantoin Capsules 100 mg ... MC-16, D1
100 PD—*Meclomen* Capsules 100 mg ... MC-14, B4
101—*Apresoline* Tablets 100 mg ... MC-11, B5
101—*Azulfidine* Tablets 500 mg ... MC-21, C7
101—*Gastrocrom* Capsules 100 mg ... MC-6, B5
101—*Tenormin* Tablets 100 mg ... MC-2, C1
102—*Azulfidine EN-Tabs* Enteric-coated Tablets 500 mg ... MC-21, D1
105—*Brethine* Tablets 5 mg ... MC-22, A6
105—Geneva Haloperidol Tablets 0.5 mg ... MC-11, B1
105—*Tenormin* Tablets 50 mg ... MC-2, C1
107—*Tenormin* Tablets 25 mg ... MC-2, C1
110—*Ludiomil* Tablets 25 mg ... MC-14, A6
112—Biocraft Cephradine Capsules 250 mg ... MC-4, C7
112—*Synthroid* Tablets 0.112 mg ... MC-13, B4
113—Biocraft Cephradine Capsules 500 mg ... MC-4, C7
113—*Velosef* Capsules 250 mg ... MC-4, C5
114—*Velosef* Capsules 500 mg ... MC-4, C5
115—*Tenoretic* Tablets 50/25 mg ... MC-2, C4
117—Biocraft Cephalexin Capsules 500 mg ... MC-4, C2
117—*Tenoretic* Tablets 100/25 mg ... MC-2, C4
120—*Calan* Tablets 120 mg ... MC-24, D2
120—*Inderal LA* Extended-release Capsules 120 mg ... MC-20, C2
120—*Isoptin* Tablets 120 mg ... MC-24, B7
120 mg—*Cardizem SR* Capsules 120 mg ... MC-7, C3
120 mg—*Cardizem* Tablets 120 mg ... MC-7, C5
120 mg—*Dilacor XR* Extended-release Capsules 120 mg ... MC-7, C6
120 SR—*Isoptin SR* Extended-release Tablets 120 mg ... MC-24, C1
120/50—*Inderide LA* Extended-release Capsules 120/50 mg ... MC-20, C6
123—Geneva Haloperidol Tablets 1 mg ... MC-11, B1
125—*Amoxil* Chewable Tablets 125 mg ... MC-1, D7
125—*Depakote Sprinkle* Capsules 125 mg ... MC-8, A7
125—*Synthroid* Tablets 0.125 mg ... MC-13, B5
125—*V-Cillin K* Tablets 125 mg ... MC-18, C1
125 mg—*Nicobid* Extended-release Capsules 125 mg ... MC-16, B1
125 mg—*Slo-bid* Extended-release Capsules 125 mg ... MC-22, C6
125 mg—*Slo-Phyllin* Extended-release Capsules 125 mg ... MC-22, C7
127—Purepac Clonidine Tablets 0.1 mg ... MC-6, A1
127—Schein/Danbury Propranolol Tablets 60 mg ... MC-20, B7
128—Barr Dicyclomine Capsules 10 mg ... MC-7, A5
128—Purepac Alprazolam Tablets 0.25 mg ... MC-1, C2
128—Purepac Alprazolam Tablets 0.5 mg ... MC-1, C2
128—Purepac Clonidine Tablets 0.2 mg ... MC-6, A1
129—Purepac Clonidine Tablets 0.3 mg ... MC-6, A1
130—*Zestril* Tablets 5 mg ... MC-13, C3
131—*Zestril* Tablets 10 mg ... MC-13, C3
132—*Zestril* Tablets 20 mg ... MC-13, C3
134—*Zestril* Tablets 40 mg ... MC-13, C3
135—*Ludiomil* Tablets 75 mg ... MC-14, A6
135—*Ortho-Novum 1/35-21 and -28* Tablets 1/0.035 mg ... MC-16, D7
135—*Ortho-Novum 7/7/7-21 and -28* Tablets 1/0.035 mg ... MC-17, A1
136—*Tofranil* Tablets 50 mg ... MC-12, B7
139—*Apresazide* Capsules 25/25 mg ... MC-11, B7
140—*Tofranil* Tablets 25 mg ... MC-12, B7
142—*Zestoretic* Tablets 20/12.5 mg ... MC-13, C5
143—*Geocillin* Tablets 382 mg ... MC-4, A2
143—Purepac Carbamazepine Tablets 200 mg ... MC-3, D7
145—*Zestoretic* Tablets 20/25 mg ... MC-13, C5
149—*Apresazide* Capsules 50/50 mg ... MC-11, B7
149—Biocraft Clindamycin Capsules 150 mg ... MC-5, C7
150—*Norpramin* Tablets 150 mg ... MC-6, C7
150—*Ortho-Novum 1/50-21 and -28* Tablets 1/0.05 mg ... MC-17, B1
150—*Rythmol* Tablets 150 mg ... MC-20, A4
150—*Synthroid* Tablets 0.15 mg ... MC-13, B5
150—*Zantac* Tablets 150 mg ... MC-21, A2
150 mg—*Cleocin* Capsules 150 mg ... MC-5, D2
151—*Demulen 1/35-21 and -28* Tablets 1/0.035 mg ... MC-9, D3
152—Mylan Clonidine Tablets 0.1 mg ... MC-5, D7
155—*Medrol* Tablets 24 mg ... MC-15, A4
155—Mylan Propoxyphene Napsylate and Acetaminophen Tablets 100/65 mg Pink ... MC-20, B1
158—*Monopril* Tablets 10 mg ... MC-10, D1
159—*Apresazide* Capsules 100/50 mg ... MC-11, B7
160—*Inderal LA* Extended-release Capsules 160 mg ... MC-20, C2
160 mg—*Betapace* Tablets 60 mg ... MC-21, B3
160/50—*Inderide LA* Extended-release Capsules 160/50 mg ... MC-20, C7
165—Mutual Piroxicam Capsules 10 mg ... MC-19, A3
166—Mutual Piroxicam Capsules 20 mg ... MC-19, A3
170—Barr Furosemide Tablets 20 mg ... MC-10, D2
175—*Synthroid* Tablets 0.175 mg ... MC-13, B5
179—Mutual Tolmetin Capsules 400 mg ... MC-23, C5
180 mg—*Cardizem CD* Capsules 180 mg ... MC-7, C1
180 mg—*Dilacor XR* Extended-release Capsules 180 mg ... MC-7, C6
180 MG—*Isoptin SR* Extended-release Tablets 180 mg ... MC-24, C2
181—Apothecon Cephalexin Capsules 250 mg ... MC-4, C1
183—Purepac Dipyridamole Tablets 50 mg ... MC-8, A2
185—Purepac Dipyridamole Tablets 75 mg ... MC-8, A2
186—Mylan Clonidine Tablets 0.2 mg ... MC-5, D7
191—Purepac Diphenhydramine Capsules 25 mg ... MC-7, D3
192—*Esidrix* Tablets 100 mg ... MC-11, C3
192—Purepac Diphenhydramine Capsules 50 mg ... MC-7, D3
193—Purepac Dipyridamole Tablets 25 mg ... MC-8, A2
194—Purepac Doxycycline Capsules 50 mg ... MC-8, D1
195—Purepac Doxycycline Capsules 100 mg ... MC-8, D1
199—Mylan Clonidine Tablets 0.3 mg ... MC-5, D7
200—*Diflucan* Tablets 200 mg ... MC-10, B3
200—*Ethmozine* Tablets 200 mg ... MC-15, D5
200—*Proloprim* Tablets 200 mg ... MC-24, B1
200—*Synthroid* Tablets 0.2 mg ... MC-13, B5
200—*Theo-Dur* Extended-release Tablets 200 mg ... MC-22, C4
200—*Tolectin* Tablets 200 mg ... MC-23, C4
200—*Trandate* Tablets 200 mg ... MC-13, A5
200—*Vascor* Tablets 200 mg ... MC-3, A7
200—*Zovirax* Capsules 200 mg ... MC-1, A5
200 mg—*Floxin* Tablets 200 mg ... MC-17, C3
200 mg—*Lodine* Capsules 200 mg ... MC-9, D5
200 mg—*Slo-bid* Extended-release Capsules 200 mg ... MC-22, C6
200 SKF—*Tagamet* Tablets 200 mg ... MC-5, B7
210—*Antivert* Tablets 12.5 mg ... MC-14, B1
211—*Antivert* Tablets 25 mg ... MC-14, B1
211—*Grifulvin V* Tablets 250 mg ... MC-11, A3
211—Mylan Chlordiazepoxide and Amitriptyline Tablets 5/12.5 mg ... MC-4, D3
214—*Antivert* Tablets 50 mg ... MC-14, B1
214—*Grifulvin V* Tablets 500 mg ... MC-11, A3
214—Mylan Haloperidol Tablets 2 mg ... MC-11, B3
227—*Phenergan* Tablets 50 mg ... MC-20, A3
239—Apothecon Cephalexin Capsules 500 mg ... MC-4, C1
240 mg—*Betapace* Tablets 240 mg ... MC-21, B3
240 mg—*Cardizem CD* Capsules 240 mg ... MC-7, C1
240 mg—*Dilacor XR* Extended-release Capsules 240 mg ... MC-7, C6
244—*Normodyne* Tablets 100 mg ... MC-13, A6
250—*Amoxil* Capsules 250 mg ... MC-1, D6
250—*Amoxil* Chewable Tablets 250 mg ... MC-1, D7
250—*Cipro* Tablets 250 mg ... MC-5, C2
250—*Ethmozine* Tablets 250 mg ... MC-15, D5
250—*Keftab* Tablets 250 mg ... MC-4, C4
250—*Lorelco* Tablets 250 mg ... MC-19, C5
250—*Naprosyn* Tablets 250 mg ... MC-16, A6
250—*Orinase* Tablets 250 mg ... MC-23, C2
250—*Slo-Niacin* Extended-release Tablets 250 mg ... MC-16, B4
250—*Ticlid* Tablets 250 mg ... MC-23, B2
250—*Tigan* Capsules 250 mg ... MC-24, A7
250—*Tolinase* Tablets 250 mg ... MC-23, C1
250—*V-Cillin K* Tablets 250 mg ... MC-18, C1
250mg—*E-Mycin* Delayed-release Tablets 250 mg ... MC-9, B4
250 mg—*Nicobid* Extended-release Capsules 250 mg ... MC-16, B1
250 mg—*Panmycin* Capsules 250 mg ... MC-22, B7
250/125—*Augmentin* Tablets 250/125 mg ... MC-2, A2
252—Barr Dipyridamole Tablets 25 mg ... MC-7, D6
257—Mylan Haloperidol Tablets 1 mg ... MC-11, B3

259—Barr Erythromycin Ethylsuccinate Tablets 400 mg MC-9, C3
260—Barr Thioridazine Tablets 10 mg MC-22, D4
260—*Procardia* Capsules 10 mg MC-16, C1
261—Barr Thioridazine Tablets 25 mg MC-22, D4
261—*Procardia* Capsules 20 mg MC-16, C1
262—Barr Thioridazine Tablets 50 mg MC-22, D4
263—Barr Thioridazine Tablets 100 mg MC-22, D4
267—Barr Chlorthalidone Tablets 25 mg MC-5, B1
268—Barr Chlorthalidone Tablets 50 mg MC-5, B1
269—Purepac Metoclopramide Tablets 10 mg MC-15, A6
274—*Anaprox* Tablets 275 mg MC-16, A7
277—Mylan Chlordiazepoxide and Amitriptyline Tablets 10/25 mg MC-4, D3
280—Purepac Haloperidol Tablets 1 mg MC-11, B4
281—Purepac Haloperidol Tablets 2 mg MC-11, B4
282—Purepac Haloperidol Tablets 5 mg MC-11, B4
283—*Corzide* Tablets 40/5 mg MC-16, A3
284—*Corzide* Tablets 80/5 mg MC-16, A3
285—Barr Dipyridamole Tablets 50 mg MC-7, D6
286—Barr Dipyridamole Tablets 75 mg MC-7, D6
286—Purepac Haloperidol Tablets 10 mg MC-11, B4
287—Purepac Haloperidol Tablets 20 mg MC-11, B4
289—Purepac Alprazolam Tablets 1 mg MC-1, C2
289—Purepac Haloperidol Tablets 0.5 mg MC-11, B4
295—Barr Doxycycline Tablets 100 mg MC-8, C5
296—Barr Doxycycline Capsules 50 mg MC-8, C4
297—Barr Doxycycline Capsules 100 mg MC-8, C4
300—*Ethmozine* Tablets 300 mg MC-15, D6
300—*Rythmol* Tablets 300 mg MC-20, A4
300—*Synthroid* Tablets 0.3 mg MC-13, B5
300—*Theo-Dur* Extended-release Tablets 300 mg MC-22, C4
300—*Trandate* Tablets 300 mg MC-13, A5
300—*Vascor* Tablets 300 mg MC-13, A7
300—*Zantac* Tablets 300 mg MC-20, A2
300—*Zyloprim* Tablets 300 mg MC-1, B4
300mg—*Motrin* Tablets 300 mg MC-12, B3
300 MG—*Actigall* Capsules 300 mg MC-24, B3
300 mg—*Cardizem CD* Capsules 300 mg MC-7, C2
300 mg—*Cleocin* Capsules 300 mg MC-5, D2
300 mg—*Floxin* Tablets 300 mg MC-17, C3
300 mg—*Lodine* Tablets 300 mg MC-9, D5
300 mg—*Neurontin* Capsules 300 mg MC-10, D5
300 mg—*Slo-bid* Extended-release Capsules 300 mg MC-22, C6
300 SKF—*Tagamet* Tablets 300 mg MC-5, B7
302—Schein/Danbury Furosemide Tablets 80 mg MC-10, D4
305—*Zithromax* Capsules 250 mg MC-2, D5
309—*Omnipen* Capsules 500 mg MC-2, A6
317—Barr Propoxyphene Napsylate and Acetaminophen Tablets 50/325 mg MC-20, A6
317—Purepac Fenoprofen Tablets 600 mg MC-10, A6
317—*Serax* Tablets 15 mg MC-17, D6
318—Barr Propoxyphene Napsylate and Acetaminophen Tablets 100/650 mg White MC-20, A6
321—Purepac Propranolol Tablets 60 mg MC-20, B5
322—*Feldene* Capsules 10 mg MC-19, A4
323—*Feldene* Capsules 20 mg MC-19, A4
327—Barr Thioridazine Tablets 150 mg MC-22, D5
327—Mylan Haloperidol Tablets 5 mg MC-11, B3
328—Barr Thioridazine Tablets 200 mg MC-22, D5
331—Barr Disopyramide Capsules 100 mg MC-8, A3
331—Purepac Propranolol Tablets 40 mg MC-20, B5
332—Barr Disopyramide Capsules 150 mg MC-8, A3
333—Purepac Propranolol Tablets 80 mg MC-20, B5
333mg—*E-Mycin* Delayed-release Tablets 333 mg MC-9, B4
338—*Capozide* Tablets 25/15 mg MC-3, D3
349—*Capozide* Tablets 25/25 mg MC-3, D3
351—Mylan Haloperidol Tablets 0.5 mg MC-11, B3
358—Purepac Propranolol and Hydrochlorothiazide Tablets 40/25 mg MC-20, C4
360—Purepac Propranolol and Hydrochlorothiazide Tablets 80/25 mg MC-20, C4
370—Barr Lorazepam Tablets 0.5 mg MC-14, A1
371—Barr Lorazepam Tablets 1 mg MC-14, A1
372—Barr Lorazepam Tablets 2 mg MC-14, A1
373—Barr Oxazepam Tablets 15 mg MC-17, D2
374—Barr Oxazepam Capsules 10 mg MC-17, D1
375—Barr Oxazepam Capsules 15 mg MC-17, D1
375—*Naprosyn* Tablets 375 mg MC-16, A6
376—Barr Oxazepam Capsules 30 mg MC-17, D1
377—Barr Flurazepam Capsules 15 mg MC-10, C2
378—Barr Flurazepam Capsules 30 mg MC-10, C2
381—Barr Meperidine Tablets 50 mg MC-14, B6
382—Barr Meperidine Tablets 100 mg MC-14, B6
384—*Capozide* Tablets 50/15 mg MC-3, D4
387—*Ceftin* Tablets 250 mg MC-4, B6
388—Purepac Spironolactone Tablets 25 mg MC-21, B5
390—*Capozide* Tablets 50/25 mg MC-3, D4
390—*Pen-Vee K* Tablets 500 mg MC-18, C2
393—*Diabinese* Tablets 100 mg MC-5, A6
394—*Ceftin* Tablets 500 mg MC-4, B7
394—*Diabinese* Tablets 250 mg MC-5, A6
395—*Ceftin* Tablets 125 mg MC-4, B6
400—*Maxaquin* Tablets 400 mg MC-13, D4
400—*Rufen* Tablets 400 mg MC-12, A5
400—*Suprax* Tablets 400 mg MC-4, B4
400—*Vascor* Tablets 400 mg MC-3, A7
400 mg—*Floxin* Tablets 400 mg MC-17, C3
400 mg—*Neurontin* Capsules 400 mg MC-10, D5
400mg—*Motrin* Tablets 400 mg MC-12, B3
400 SKF—*Tagamet* Tablets 400 mg MC-5, C1
404—Purepac Tetracycline Capsules 250 mg MC-22, B5
406—Purepac Tetracycline Capsules 500 mg MC-22, B5
419—Barr Ibuprofen Tablets 400 mg MC-12, A3
420—Barr Ibuprofen Tablets 600 mg MC-12, A3
425—Barr Verapamil Tablets 80 mg MC-24, B6
430—*Minizide* Capsules 1/0.5 mg MC-19, C1
431—*Minipress* Capsules 1 mg MC-19, A5
431—*Pronestyl* Tablets 250 mg MC-19, D4
431—*Proventil* Extended-release Tablets 4 mg MC-1, B2
432—*Minizide* Capsules 2/0.5 mg MC-19, C1
434—*Pronestyl* Tablets 375 mg MC-19, D4
436—*Minizide* Capsules 5/0.5 mg MC-19, C1
437—*Minipress* Capsules 2 mg MC-19, A5
438—*Minipress* Capsules 5 mg MC-19, A5
438—*Normodyne* Tablets 300 mg MC-13, A6
438—*Pronestyl* Tablets 500 mg MC-19, D4
439—Purepac Trazodone Tablets 50 mg MC-23, D4
441—Purepac Trazodone Tablets 100 mg MC-23, D4
443—Warner Chilcott Clonidine Tablets 0.1 mg MC-6, A3
444—Warner Chilcott Clonidine Tablets 0.2 mg MC-6, A3
445—*Ovral-28* Tablets Inert MC-17, B5
450—*Capoten* Tablets 12.5 mg MC-3, D1
452—*Capoten* Tablets 25 mg MC-3, D1
455—Barr Verapamil Tablets 120 mg MC-24, B6
458—*Claritin* Tablets 10 mg MC-13, D7
470—Barr Propoxyphene Napsylate and Acetaminophen Tablets 100/650 mg Pink MC-20, A6
473—Purepac Verapamil Tablets 80 mg MC-24, C6
475—Purepac Verapamil Tablets 120 mg MC-24, C6
477—Barr Haloperidol Tablets 0.5 mg MC-11, A6
478—Barr Haloperidol Tablets 1 mg MC-11, A6
479—Barr Haloperidol Tablets 2 mg MC-11, A6
480—Barr Haloperidol Tablets 5 mg MC-11, A6
481—Barr Haloperidol Tablets 10 mg MC-11, A7
482—Barr Haloperidol Tablets 20 mg MC-11, A7
482—*Capoten* Tablets 50 mg MC-3, D2
485—*Capoten* Tablets 100 mg MC-3, D2
486—*Lo-Ovral-21 and -28* Tablets Inert MC-17, B4
486—*Nordette-28* Tablets Inert MC-13, B2
487—Barr Temazepam Capsules 15 mg MC-22, A1
488—Barr Temazepam Capsules 30 mg MC-22, A1
499—Barr Ibuprofen Tablets 800 mg MC-12, A3
500—*Amoxil* Capsules 500 mg MC-1, D6
500—*Cipro* Tablets 500 mg MC-5, C3
500—*Flagyl* Tablets 500 mg MC-15, C5
500—*Keftab* Tablets 500 mg MC-4, C4
500—*Lorelco* Tablets 500 mg MC-19, C5
500—*Naprosyn* Tablets 500 mg MC-16, A6
500—*Nicobid* Extended-release Capsules 500 mg MC-16, B2
500—*Orinase* Tablets 500 mg MC-23, C2
500—Purepac Prazosin Capsules 1 mg MC-19, B6
500—*Relafen* Tablets 500 mg MC-15, D7
500—*Slo-Niacin* Extended-release Tablets 500 mg MC-16, B4
500—*Tolinase* Tablets 500 mg MC-23, C1
500—*V-Cillin K* Tablets 500 mg MC-18, C1
500/125—*Augmentin* Tablets 500/125 mg MC-2, A2
501—Purepac Prazosin Capsules 2 mg MC-19, B6
502—Purepac Prazosin Capsules 5 mg MC-19, B6
515—*Quibron* Capsules 300/180 mg MC-22, D3
516—*Quibron* Capsules 150/90 mg MC-22, D3
521—*Lufyllin* Tablets 200 mg MC-8, D5

521—Mylan Propoxyphene Napsylate and Acetaminophen Tablets 100/65 mg White.......... MC-20, B1
534—*Sinequan* Capsules 10 mg.......................... MC-8, B5
535—*Ortho-Novum 7/7/7-21 and -28* Tablets 0.5/0.035 mg.................................. MC-17, A1
535—*Sinequan* Capsules 25 mg.......................... MC-8, B5
536—*Sinequan* Capsules 50 mg.......................... MC-8, B5
537—*Sinequan* Capsules 150 mg.......................... MC-8, B6
538—*Sinequan* Capsules 100 mg.......................... MC-8, B6
539—*Sinequan* Capsules 75 mg.......................... MC-8, B6
541—*Vistaril* Capsules 25 mg MC-11, D6
542—*Vistaril* Capsules 50 mg MC-11, D6
543—*Roxicet* Tablets 5/325 mg MC-18, A4
543—*Vistaril* Capsules 100 mg MC-11, D6
550—Barr Cephradine Capsules 250 mg MC-4, C6
551—Barr Cephradine Capsules 500 mg MC-4, C6
555 19—Barr Hydrochlorothiazide Tablets 25 mg MC-11, C2
555 20—Barr Hydrochlorothiazide Tablets 50 mg MC-11, C2
555 169—Barr Furosemide Tablets 40 mg............. MC-10, D2
555 192—Barr Hydrochlorothiazide Tablets 100 mg MC-11, C2
555 196—Barr Furosemide Tablets 80 mg.............. MC-10, D2
555 444—Barr Triamterene and Hydrochlorothiazide Tablets 75/50 mg.................................. MC-23, D6
555 585—Barr Chlorzoxazone Tablets 500 mg MC-5, B4
559—*Wymox* Capsules 250 mg MC-2, A1
560—*Wymox* Capsules 500 mg MC-2, A1
571—*Navane* Capsules 1 mg MC-22, A6
572—*Navane* Capsules 2 mg MC-22, A6
573—*Navane* Capsules 5 mg MC-22, A6
574—*Navane* Capsules 10 mg MC-22, A7
577—*Navane* Capsules 20 mg MC-22, A7
583—*Ovcon 35-21 and -28* Tablets 0.4/0.035 mg....... MC-16, D5
584—Barr Erythromycin Delayed-release Capsules 250 mg.. MC-9, B3
584—*Ovcon 50-21 and -28* Tablets 1/0.05 mg MC-16, D6
600—*Nolvadex* Tablets 10 mg.......................... MC-21, D7
600—*Tolectin* Tablets 600 mg.......................... MC-23, C4
600mg—*Motrin* Tablets 600 mg MC-12, B4
601—*Pro-Banthine* Tablets 15 mg.......................... MC-20, A5
603—*Sumycin* Tablets 500 mg MC-22, B3
609—*Monopril* Tablets 20 mg.......................... MC-10, D1
611—*Pro-Banthine* Tablets 7.5 mg MC-20, A5
641—*Triphasil-21 and -28* Tablets 0.05/0.03 mg.......... MC-13, B3
642—*Triphasil-21 and -28* Tablets 0.075/0.04 mg....... MC-13, B3
643—*Triphasil-21 and -28* Tablets 0.125/0.03 mg....... MC-13, B3
647—*Sinemet* Tablets 10/100 mg.......................... MC-4, A3
648—*Veetids* Tablets 500 mg.......................... MC-18, B5
650—*Sinemet* Tablets 25/100 mg.......................... MC-4, A3
650—*Triphasil-28* Tablets Inert MC-13, B3
654—*Sinemet* Tablets 25/250 mg.......................... MC-4, A3
655—*Sumycin* Capsules 250 mg MC-22, B2
663—*Sumycin* Tablets 250 mg MC-22, B3
684—*Veetids* Tablets 250 mg.......................... MC-18, B5
701—*Effexor* Tablets 25 mg MC-24, B5
703—*Effexor* Tablets 50 mg MC-24, B5
703—*Trinalin* Extended-release Tablets 1/120 mg........ MC-2, D3
704—*Effexor* Tablets 75 mg MC-24, B5
705—*Effexor* Tablets 100 mg MC-24, B5
710—Mylan Cyclobenzaprine Tablets 10 mg............ MC-6, B7
715—Mylan Timolol Tablets 20 mg MC-23, B4
731—*Lufyllin* Tablets 400 mg MC-8, D5
750—*Cipro* Tablets 750 mg MC-5, C3
750—*Relafen* Tablets 750 mg MC-15, D7
750—*Robaxin* Tablets 750 mg.......................... MC-14, C4
750—*Slo-Niacin* Extended-release Tablets 750 mg MC-16, B4
752—*Normodyne* Tablets 200 mg.......................... MC-13, A6
756—*Pronestyl* Capsules 375 mg MC-19, D3
757—*Pronestyl* Capsules 500 mg MC-19, D3
758—*Pronestyl* Capsules 250 mg MC-19, D3
760—*Sorbitrate* Sublingual Tablets 5 mg MC-12, D5
761—*Sorbitrate* Sublingual Tablets 10 mg MC-12, D5
763—*Sumycin* Capsules 500 mg MC-22, B2
770—*Sorbitrate* Tablets 5 mg MC-12, D2
773—*Sorbitrate* Tablets 30 mg MC-12, D3
774—*Sorbitrate* Tablets 40 mg MC-12, D3
780—*Sorbitrate* Tablets 10 mg MC-12, D2
781—*Effexor* Tablets 37.5 mg MC-24, B5
800—*Zovirax* Tablets 800 mg.......................... MC-1, A6
800mg—*Motrin* Tablets 800 mg MC-12, B4
800 SKF—*Tagamet* Tablets 800 mg.......................... MC-5, C1
810—*Sorbitrate* Chewable Tablets 5 mg MC-12, D4
811—*Adalat* Capsules 10 mg.......................... MC-16, B7
815—*Sorbitrate* Chewable Tablets 10 mg MC-12, D4
820—*Sorbitrate* Tablets 20 mg MC-12, D2
821—*Adalat* Capsules 20 mg.......................... MC-16, B7
850—*Ovcon 35-28* Tablets Inert MC-16, D5
850—*Ovcon 50-28* Tablets Inert MC-16, D6
853—*Sorbitrate* Sublingual Tablets 2.5 mg............. MC-12, D5
855—*Nimotop* Capsules 30 mg MC-16, C5
901—*Lortab* Tablets 2.5/500 mg MC-11, D1
902—*Lortab* Tablets 5/500 mg MC-11, D1
903—*Lortab* Tablets 7.5/500 mg MC-11, D1
1001—*Aldactone* Tablets 25 mg MC-21, B6
1011—*Aldactazide* Tablets 25/25 mg MC-21, C2
1021—*Aldactazide* Tablets 50/50 mg MC-21, C2
1031—*Aldactone* Tablets 100 mg MC-21, B6
1041—*Aldactone* Tablets 50 mg MC-21, B6
1375—*Ditropan* Tablets 5 mg MC-17, D7
1381—*Daypro* Tablets 600 mg MC-17, C7
1451—*Cytotec* Tablets 0.1 mg.......................... MC-15, D4
1461—*Cytotec* Tablets 0.2 mg.......................... MC-15, D4
1771—*Cardizem* Tablets 30 mg.......................... MC-7, C4
1772—*Cardizem* Tablets 60 mg.......................... MC-7, C4
1800—*Ortho-Est* Tablets 1.25 mg.......................... MC-9, D2
1801—*Ortho-Est* Tablets 0.625 mg.......................... MC-9, D2
1831—*Flagyl* Tablets 250 mg MC-15, C5
2103—*Soma Compound* Tablets 200/325 mg............ MC-4, A6
2150—Mylan Meclofenamate Capsules 50 mg MC-14, B3
2403—*Soma Compound with Codeine* Tablets 200/325/16 mg MC-4, A6
2440—*Cardene SR* Extended-release Capsules 30 mg ... MC-16, B5
2441—*Cardene SR* Extended-release Capsules 45 mg ... MC-16, B5
2442—*Cardene SR* Extended-release Capsules 60 mg ... MC-16, B5
2732—*Norpace CR* Extended-release Capsules 100 mg... MC-8, A6
2742—*Norpace CR* Extended-release Capsules 150 mg... MC-8, A6
2752—*Norpace* Capsules 100 mg MC-8, A5
2762—*Norpace* Capsules 150 mg MC-8, A5
2832—*Theo-24* Extended-release Capsules 100 mg MC-22, D2
2842—*Theo-24* Extended-release Capsules 200 mg MC-22, D2
2852—*Theo-24* Extended-release Capsules 300 mg MC-22, D2
3000—Mylan Meclofenamate Capsules 100 mg MC-14, B3
3061—*Ceclor* Capsules 250 mg MC-4, B1
3062—*Ceclor* Capsules 500 mg MC-4, B1
3071—Rugby Amitriptyline Tablets 10 mg MC-1, C7
3072—Rugby Amitriptyline Tablets 25 mg MC-1, C7
3073—Rugby Amitriptyline Tablets 50 mg MC-1, C7
3074—Rugby Amitriptyline Tablets 75 mg MC-1, C7
3075—Rugby Amitriptyline Tablets 100 mg MC-1, D1
3076—Rugby Amitriptyline Tablets 150 mg MC-1, D1
3105—*Prozac* Capsules 20 mg.......................... MC-20, D2
3144—*Axid* Capsules 150 mg MC-16, D4
3145—*Axid* Capsules 300 mg MC-16, D4
3170—*Lorabid* Capsules 200 mg.......................... MC-13, D6
3597—*Diphenhist* Tablets 25 mg.......................... MC-7, D4
3736—Rugby Doxepin Capsules 10 mg MC-8, B7
3737—Rugby Doxepin Capsules 75 mg MC-8, C1
3738—Rugby Doxepin Capsules 150 mg MC-8, C1
3874—Rugby Hydroxyzine Tablets 10 mg.................. MC-12, A1
3875—Rugby Hydroxyzine Tablets 25 mg.................. MC-12, A1
3876—Rugby Hydroxyzine Tablets 50 mg.................. MC-12, A1
3952—Rugby Levothyroxine Tablets 0.1 mg............... MC-13, C1
3953—Rugby Levothyroxine Tablets 0.15 mg............. MC-13, C1
3958—Rugby Levothyroxine Tablets 0.3 mg............... MC-13, C1
3977—Rugby Ibuprofen Tablets 400 mg MC-12, A6
3978—Rugby Ibuprofen Tablets 600 mg MC-12, A6
3979—Rugby Ibuprofen Tablets 800 mg MC-12, A7
4010—Mylan Temazepam Capsules 15 mg MC-22, A2
4018—Rugby Metronidazole Tablets 250 mg MC-15, C3
4019—Rugby Metronidazole Tablets 500 mg MC-15, C3
4042—Rugby Metoclopramide Tablets 10 mg.............. MC-15, B1
4125—*Isordil* Extended-release Tablets 40 mg MC-12, C7
4132—*Surmontil* Capsules 25 mg.......................... MC-24, B2
4133—*Surmontil* Capsules 50 mg.......................... MC-24, B2
4152—*Isordil* Tablets 5 mg MC-12, C6
4153—*Isordil* Tablets 10 mg MC-12, C6
4154—*Isordil* Tablets 20 mg MC-12, C6
4158—*Surmontil* Capsules 100 mg.......................... MC-24, B2
4159—*Isordil* Tablets 30 mg MC-12, C6
4188—*Cordarone* Tablets 200 mg.......................... MC-1, C6
4191—*Synalgos-DC* Capsules 356.4/30/16 mg MC-2, A7
4192—*Isordil* Tablets 40 mg MC-12, C6

4250—*Donnatal* Tablets 0.0194/0.1037/0.0065/16.2 mg MC-2, C7
4309—Rugby Propranolol Tablets 10 mg MC-20, B6
4313—Rugby Propranolol Tablets 20 mg MC-20, B6
4314—Rugby Propranolol Tablets 40 mg MC-20, B6
4315—Rugby Propranolol Tablets 60 mg MC-20, B6
4316—Rugby Propranolol Tablets 80 mg MC-20, B6
4325—Rugby Prednisone Tablets 10 mg MC-19, C3
4326—Rugby Prednisone Tablets 20 mg MC-19, C3
4381—Rugby Levothyroxine Tablets 0.2 mg MC-13, C1
4402—Rugby Propranolol and Hydrochlorothiazide Tablets 40/25 mg MC-20, C5
4403—Rugby Propranolol and Hydrochlorothiazide Tablets 80/25 mg MC-20, C5
4564—Rugby Doxepin Capsules 25 mg MC-8, B7
4565—Rugby Doxepin Capsules 50 mg MC-8, B7
4566—Rugby Doxepin Capsules 100 mg MC-8, C1
4812—Rugby Verapamil Tablets 80 mg MC-24, C7
4932—Rugby Verapamil Tablets 120 mg MC-24, C7
5050—Mylan Temazepam Capsules 30 mg MC-22, A2
5100—*Penetrex* Tablets 200 mg MC-9, A1
5140—*Penetrex* Tablets 400 mg MC-9, A1
5401—*Ambien* Tablets 5 mg MC-24, D7
5421—*Ambien* Tablets 10 mg MC-24, D7
5455—Schein/Danbury Chlorpropamide Tablets 250 mg MC-5, A7
5496—Schein/Danbury Spironolactone and Hydrochlorothiazide Tablets 25/25 mg MC-21, C1
5522—Schein/Danbury Hydroxyzine Tablets 10 mg MC-12, A2
5523—Schein/Danbury Hydroxyzine Tablets 25 mg MC-12, A2
5538—Schein/Danbury Quinidine Gluconate Extended-release Tablets 324 mg MC-20, D6
5540—Schein/Danbury Metronidazole Tablets 250 mg MC-15, C4
5542—Schein/Danbury Thioridazine Tablets 25 mg MC-23, A3
5543—Schein/Danbury Allopurinol Tablets 100 mg MC-1, B7
5544—Schein/Danbury Allopurinol Tablets 300 mg MC-1, B7
5546—Schein/Danbury Sulfamethoxazole and Trimethoprim Tablets 400/80 mg MC-21, C6
5547—Schein/Danbury Sulfamethoxazole and Trimethoprim Tablets 800/160 mg MC-21, C6
5552—Schein/Danbury Metronidazole Tablets 500 mg MC-15, C4
5553—Schein/Danbury Doxycycline Tablets 100 mg MC-8, D4
5562—Schein/Danbury Procainamide Extended-release Tablets 250 mg MC-19, D7
5565—Schein/Danbury Hydroxyzine Tablets 50 mg MC-12, A2
5566—Schein/Danbury Thioridazine Tablets 10 mg MC-23, A3
5568—Schein/Danbury Thioridazine Tablets 50 mg MC-23, A3
5569—Schein/Danbury Thioridazine Tablets 100 mg MC-23, A4
5575—Schein/Danbury Furosemide Tablets 40 mg MC-10, D4
5579—Schein/Danbury Chlorpropamide Tablets 100 mg MC-5, A7
5580—Schein/Danbury Thioridazine Tablets 150 mg MC-23, A4
5581—Schein/Danbury Thioridazine Tablets 200 mg MC-23, A4
5584—Schein/Danbury Ibuprofen Tablets 400 mg MC-12, B1
5585—Schein/Danbury Ibuprofen Tablets 200 mg MC-12, B1
5586—Schein/Danbury Ibuprofen Tablets 600 mg MC-12, B2
5587—Schein/Danbury Methyldopa Tablets 500 mg MC-14, D4
5588—Schein/Danbury Methyldopa Tablets 250 mg MC-14, D4
5589—Schein/Danbury Metoclopramide Tablets 10 mg MC-15, B2
5592—Schein/Danbury Thiothixene Capsules 2 mg MC-23, B1
5593—Schein/Danbury Thiothixene Capsules 1 mg MC-23, B1
5594—Schein/Danbury Thiothixene Capsules 10 mg MC-23, B1
5595—Schein/Danbury Thiothixene Capsules 5 mg MC-23, B1
5599—Schein/Danbury Trazodone Tablets 100 mg MC-23, D5
5600—Schein/Danbury Trazodone Tablets 50 mg MC-23, D5
5601—Schein/Danbury Verapamil Tablets 80 mg MC-24, D1
5602—Schein/Danbury Verapamil Tablets 120 mg MC-24, D1
5644—Schein/Danbury Ibuprofen Tablets 800 mg MC-12, B2
5658—Schein/Danbury Cyclobenzaprine Tablets 10 mg MC-6, C1
5660—Schein/Danbury Sulindac Tablets 200 mg MC-21, D4
5661—Schein/Danbury Sulindac Tablets 150 mg MC-21, D4
5704—Schein/Danbury Fenoprofen Tablets 600 mg MC-10, A7
5710—Schein/Danbury Albuterol Tablets 2 mg MC-1, B1
5711—Schein/Danbury Albuterol Tablets 4 mg MC-1, B1
5736—Schein/Danbury Timolol Tablets 5 mg MC-23, B5
5737—Schein/Danbury Timolol Tablets 10 mg MC-23, B5
5738—Schein/Danbury Timolol Tablets 20 mg MC-23, B5
5777—Schein/Danbury Atenolol Tablets 50 mg MC-2, B7
5778—Schein/Danbury Atenolol Tablets 100 mg MC-2, B7
7278—*Trimox* Capsules 250 mg MC-1, D5
7279—*Trimox* Capsules 500 mg MC-1, D5
7658—*Dynapen* Capsules 500 mg MC-6, A4
7720—*Cefzil* Tablets 250 mg MC-4, B5
7721—*Cefzil* Tablets 500 mg MC-4, B5
7892—*Dynapen* Capsules 125 mg MC-6, A3
7893—*Dynapen* Capsules 250 mg MC-6, A3
7977—*Prostaphlin* Capsules 250 mg MC-17, C6
7982—*Prostaphlin* Capsules 500 mg MC-17, C6
7992—*Principen* Capsules 250 mg MC-2, A4
7993—*Principen* Capsules 500 mg MC-2, A4

A B C D

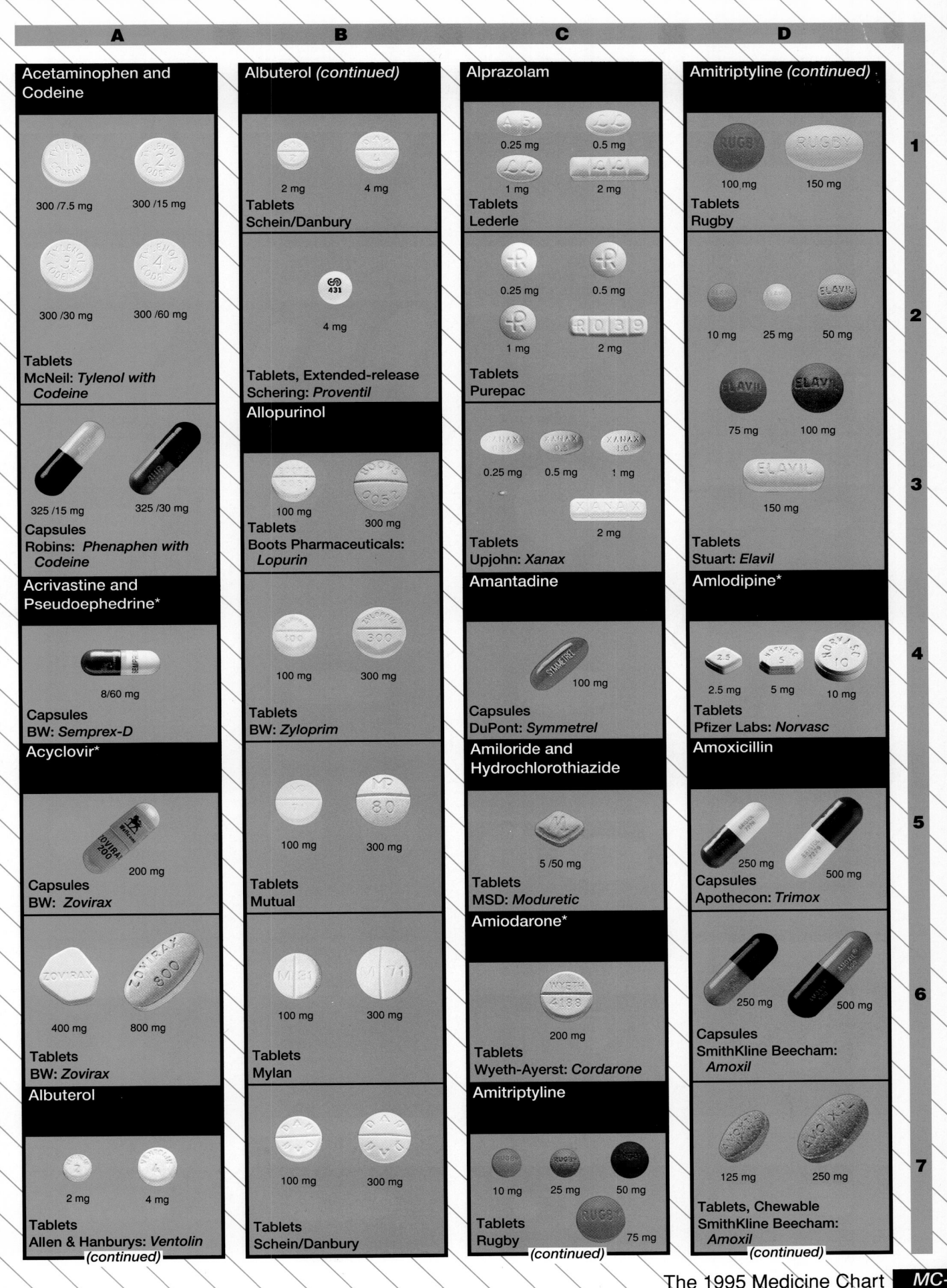

Acetaminophen and Codeine

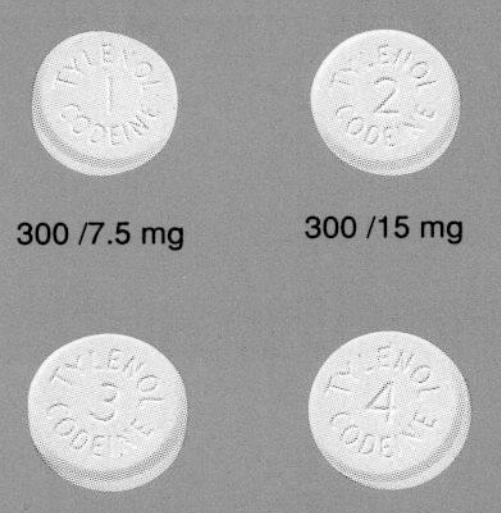

300 /7.5 mg · 300 /15 mg · 300 /30 mg · 300 /60 mg

Tablets
McNeil: *Tylenol with Codeine*

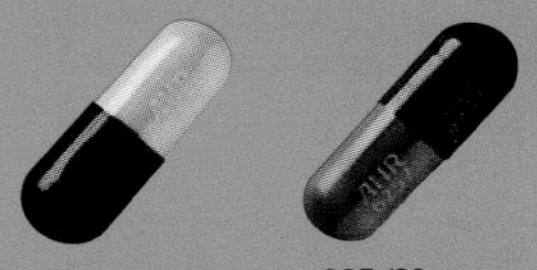

325 /15 mg · 325 /30 mg

Capsules
Robins: *Phenaphen with Codeine*

Acrivastine and Pseudoephedrine*

8/60 mg

Capsules
BW: *Semprex-D*

Acyclovir*

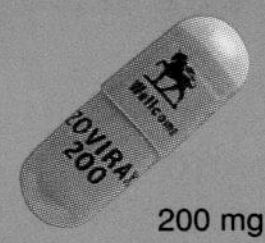

200 mg

Capsules
BW: *Zovirax*

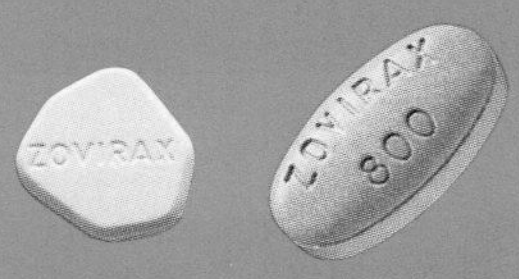

400 mg · 800 mg

Tablets
BW: *Zovirax*

Albuterol

2 mg · 4 mg

Tablets
Allen & Hanburys: *Ventolin*

(continued)

Albuterol *(continued)*

2 mg · 4 mg

Tablets
Schein/Danbury

4 mg

Tablets, Extended-release
Schering: *Proventil*

Allopurinol

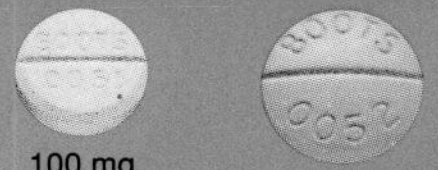

100 mg · 300 mg

Tablets
Boots Pharmaceuticals: *Lopurin*

100 mg · 300 mg

Tablets
BW: *Zyloprim*

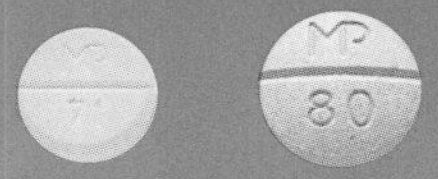

100 mg · 300 mg

Tablets
Mutual

100 mg · 300 mg

Tablets
Mylan

100 mg · 300 mg

Tablets
Schein/Danbury

Alprazolam

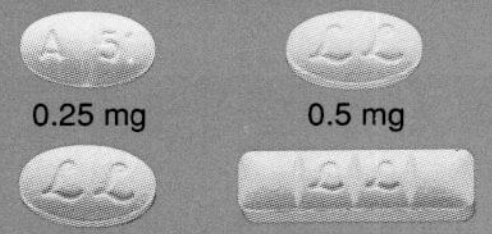

0.25 mg · 0.5 mg · 1 mg · 2 mg

Tablets
Lederle

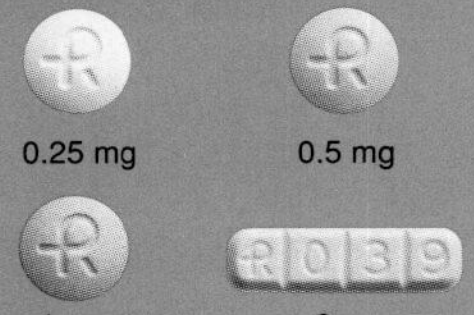

0.25 mg · 0.5 mg · 1 mg · 2 mg

Tablets
Purepac

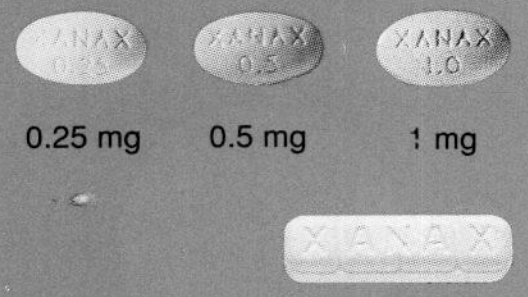

0.25 mg · 0.5 mg · 1 mg · 2 mg

Tablets
Upjohn: *Xanax*

Amantadine

100 mg

Capsules
DuPont: *Symmetrel*

Amiloride and Hydrochlorothiazide

5 /50 mg

Tablets
MSD: *Moduretic*

Amiodarone*

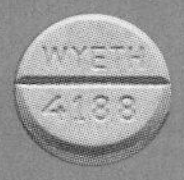

200 mg

Tablets
Wyeth-Ayerst: *Cordarone*

Amitriptyline

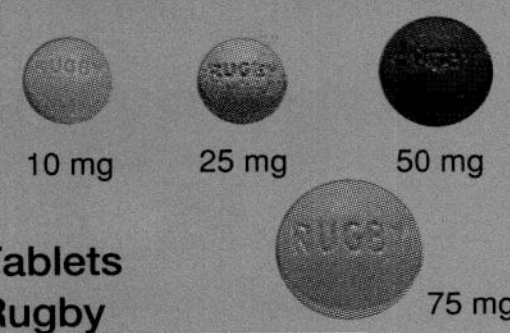

10 mg · 25 mg · 50 mg · 75 mg

Tablets
Rugby

(continued)

Amitriptyline *(continued)*

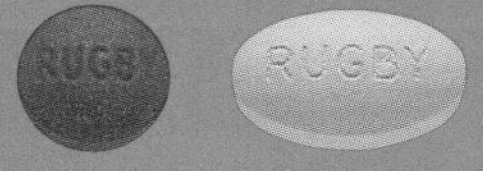

100 mg · 150 mg

Tablets
Rugby

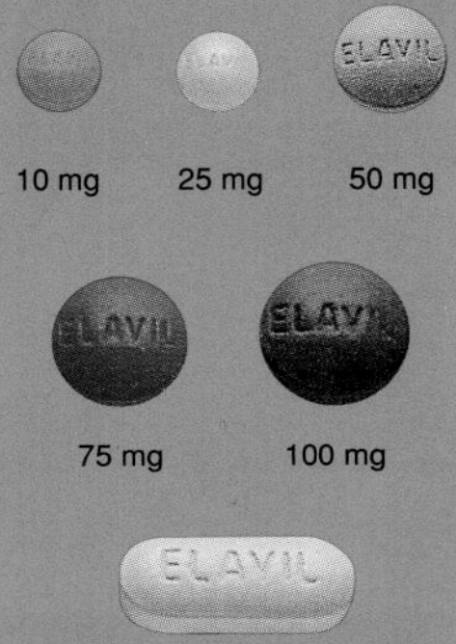

10 mg · 25 mg · 50 mg · 75 mg · 100 mg · 150 mg

Tablets
Stuart: *Elavil*

Amlodipine*

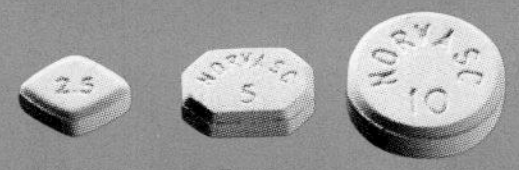

2.5 mg · 5 mg · 10 mg

Tablets
Pfizer Labs: *Norvasc*

Amoxicillin

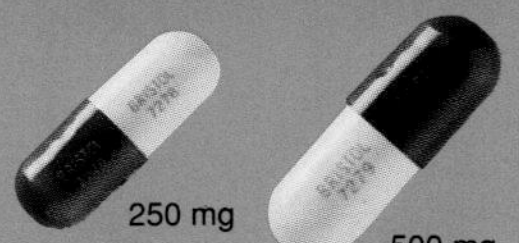

250 mg · 500 mg

Capsules
Apothecon: *Trimox*

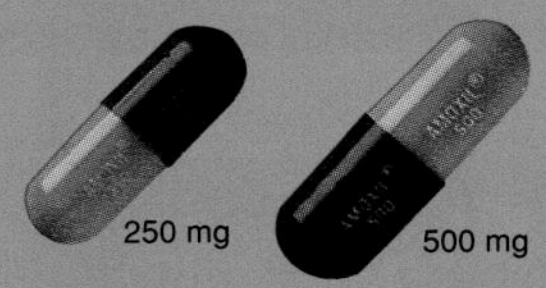

250 mg · 500 mg

Capsules
SmithKline Beecham: *Amoxil*

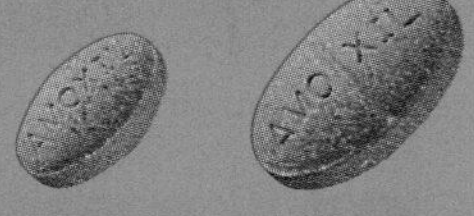

125 mg · 250 mg

Tablets, Chewable
SmithKline Beecham: *Amoxil*

(continued)

*Single source product for solid oral dosage forms in the U.S.

A

Amoxicillin *(continued)*

1

250 mg 500 mg
Capsules
Wyeth-Ayerst: *Wymox*

Amoxicillin and Clavulanate*

2
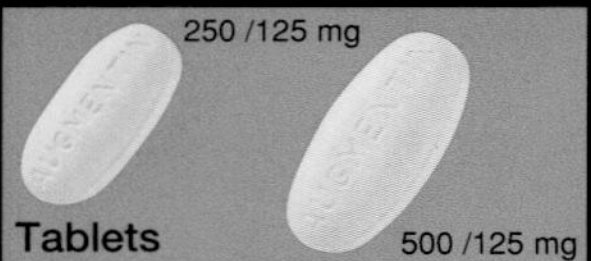
250 /125 mg 500 /125 mg
Tablets
SmithKline Beecham: *Augmentin*

3
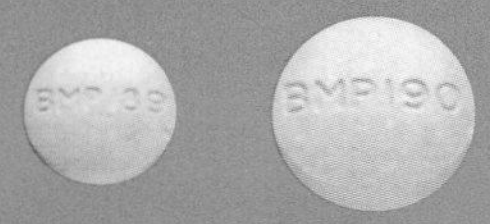

125 /31.25 mg 250 /62.5 mg
Tablets, Chewable
SmithKline Beecham: *Augmentin*

Ampicillin

4
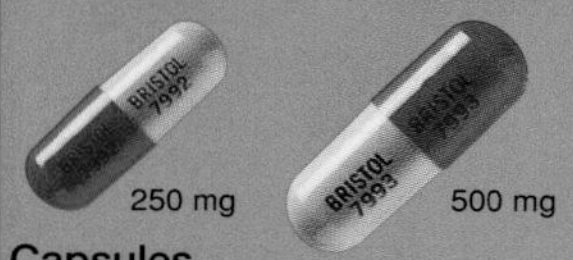
250 mg 500 mg
Capsules
Apothecon: *Principen*

5

250 mg 500 mg
Capsules
SmithKline Beecham: *Totacillin*

6
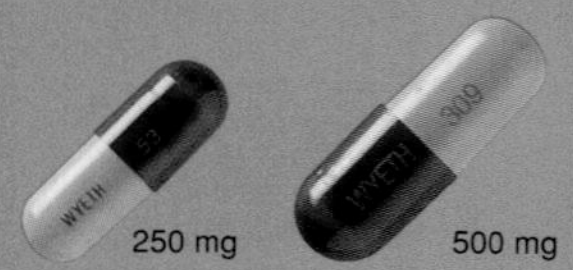
250 mg 500 mg
Capsules
Wyeth-Ayerst: *Omnipen*

Aspirin, Caffeine, and Dihydrocodeine

7
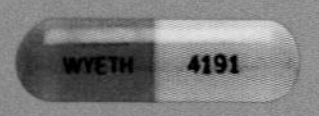

356.4/30/ 16 mg
Capsules
Wyeth-Ayerst: *Synalgos-DC*

B

Aspirin and Codeine

1

325 /30 mg 325 /60 mg
Tablets
BW: *Empirin with Codeine*

Astemizole*

2

10 mg
Tablets
Janssen: *Hismanal*

Atenolol

3

50 mg 100 mg
Tablets
Geneva

4
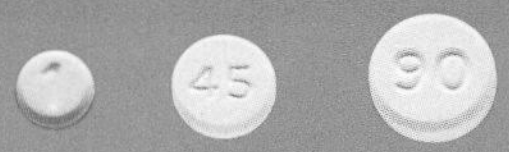

25 mg 50 mg 100 mg
Tablets
IPR Pharmaceuticals

5

25 mg 50 mg 100 mg
Tablets
Lederle

6
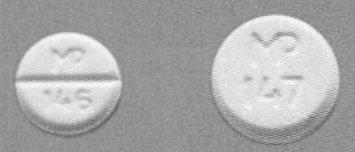
50 mg 100 mg
Tablets
Mutual

7
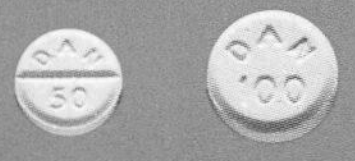
50 mg 100 mg
Tablets
Schein/Danbury

(continued)

C

Atenolol *(continued)*

1

25 mg 50 mg 100 mg
Tablets
ZENECA: *Tenormin*

Atenolol and Chlorthalidone

2

50/25 mg 100/25 mg
Tablets
Mutual

3

50/25 mg 100/25 mg
Tablets
Schein/Danbury

4
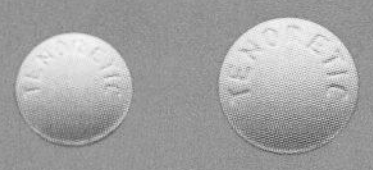
50 /25 mg 100 /25 mg
Tablets
ZENECA: *Tenoretic*

Atovaquone*

5
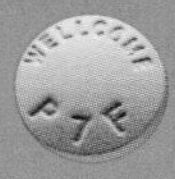
250 mg
Tablets
BW: *Mepron*

Atropine, Hyoscyamine, Scopolamine, and Phenobarbital

6
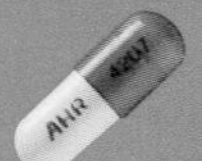
0.0194/0.1037/0.0065/16.2 mg
Capsules
Robins: *Donnatal*

7

0.0194/0.1037/0.0065/16.2 mg
Tablets
Robins: *Donnatal*

(continued)

D

Atropine, Hyoscyamine, Scopolamine, and Phenobarbital *(continued)*

1

0.0582/0.3111/0.0195/48.6 mg
Tablets, Extended-release
Robins: *Donnatal*

Auranofin*

2
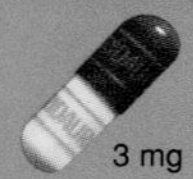
3 mg
Capsules
SmithKline Beecham: *Ridaura*

Azatadine and Pseudoephedrine*

3

1/120 mg
Tablets, Extended-release
Schering: *Trinalin*

Azathioprine

4
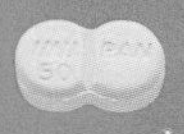
50 mg
Tablets
BW: *Imuran*

Azithromycin*

5

250 mg
Capsules
Pfizer: *Zithromax*

Baclofen

6

10 mg 20 mg
Tablets
Geigy: *Lioresal*

7
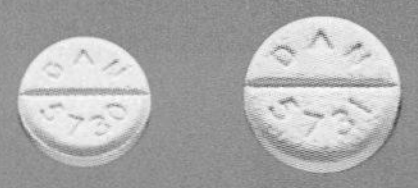
10 mg 20 mg
Tablets
Schein/Danbury

*Single source product for solid oral dosage forms in the U.S.

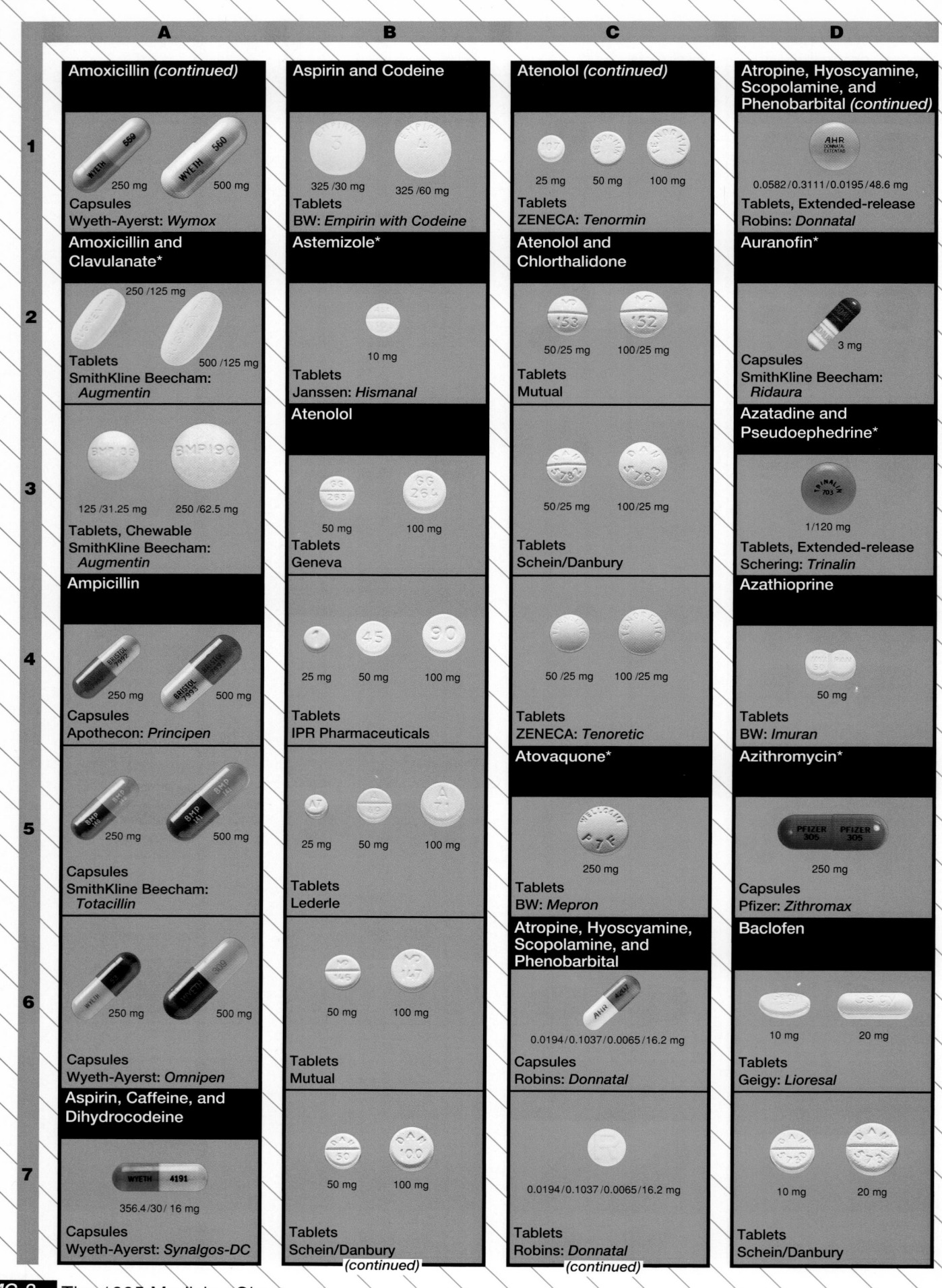

A

Benazepril*

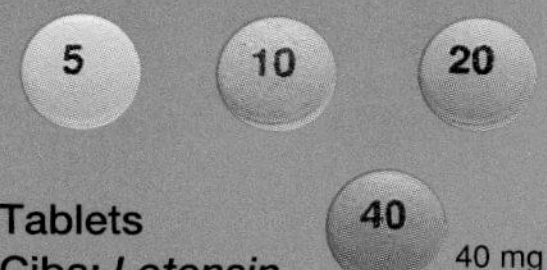
5 mg 10 mg 20 mg 40 mg

Tablets
Ciba: *Lotensin*

Benazepril and Hydrochlorothiazide*

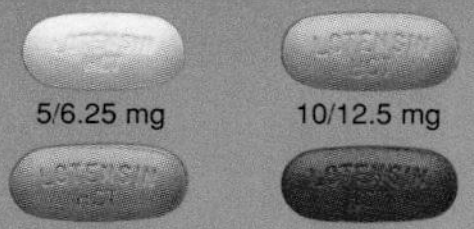
5/6.25 mg 10/12.5 mg 20/12.5 mg 20/25 mg

Tablets
Ciba: *Lotensin HCT*

Bendroflumethiazide

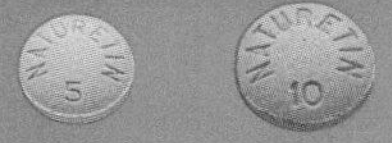
5 mg 10 mg

Tablets
Apothecon: *Naturetin*

Benzphetamine*

25 mg 50 mg

Tablets
Upjohn: *Didrex*

Benztropine

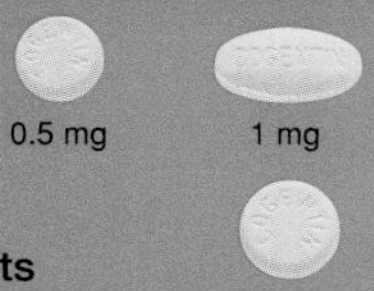
0.5 mg 1 mg 2 mg

Tablets
Merck: *Cogentin*

1 mg 2 mg

Tablets
Mutual

Bepridil*

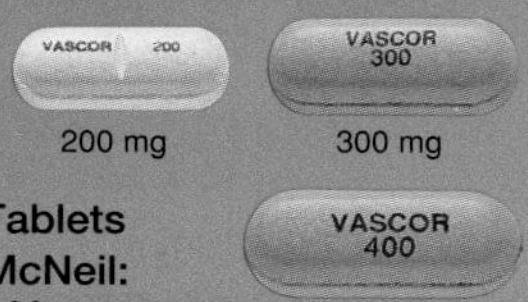
200 mg 300 mg 400 mg

Tablets
McNeil: *Vascor*

B

Betaxolol*

10 mg 20 mg

Tablets
Searle: *Kerlone*

Bisoprolol*

5 mg 10 mg

Tablets
Lederle: *Zebeta*

Bisoprolol and Hydrochlorothiazide*

2.5/6.25 mg 5/6.25 mg 10/6.25 mg

Tablets
Lederle: *Ziac*

Bromocriptine*

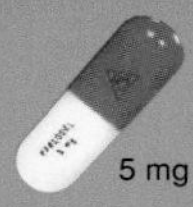
5 mg

Capsules
Sandoz: *Parlodel*

2.5 mg

Tablets
Sandoz: *Parlodel*

Bumetanide*

0.5 mg 1 mg 2 mg

Tablets
Roche: *Bumex*

Bupropion*

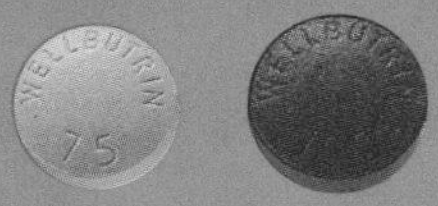
75 mg 100 mg

Tablets
BW: *Wellbutrin*

C

Buspirone*

5 mg 10 mg

Tablets
Mead Johnson: *BuSpar*

Butalbital, Acetaminophen, and Caffeine

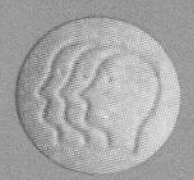
50/325/40 mg

Tablets
Sandoz: *Fioricet*

Butalbital, Aspirin, and Caffeine

50/325/40 mg

Tablets
Geneva

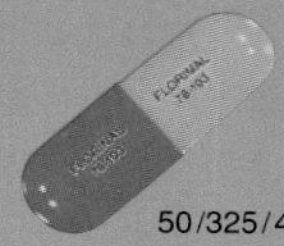
50/325/40 mg

Capsules
Sandoz: *Fiorinal*

50/325/40 mg

Tablets
Sandoz: *Fiorinal*

Butalbital, Aspirin, Codeine, and Caffeine

50/325/30/40 mg

Capsules
Sandoz: *Fiorinal with Codeine*

Calcitriol

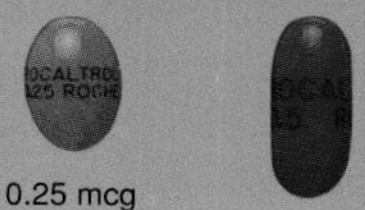
0.25 mcg 0.5 mcg

Capsules
Roche: *Rocaltrol*

D

Captopril*

1

12.5 mg 25 mg

2

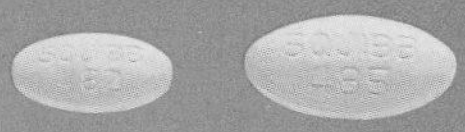
50 mg 100 mg

Tablets
Squibb: *Capoten*

Captopril and Hydrochlorothiazide*

3

25/15 mg 25/25 mg

4

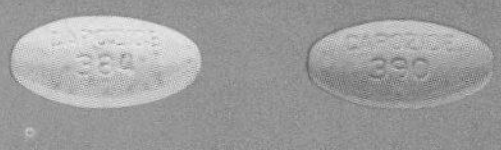
50/15 mg 50/25 mg

Tablets
Squibb: *Capozide*

Carbamazepine

5

200 mg

Tablets
Basel: *Tegretol*

6

100 mg

Tablets, Chewable
Basel: *Tegretol*

7

200 mg

Tablets
Purepac

(continued)

*Single source product for solid oral dosage forms in the U.S.

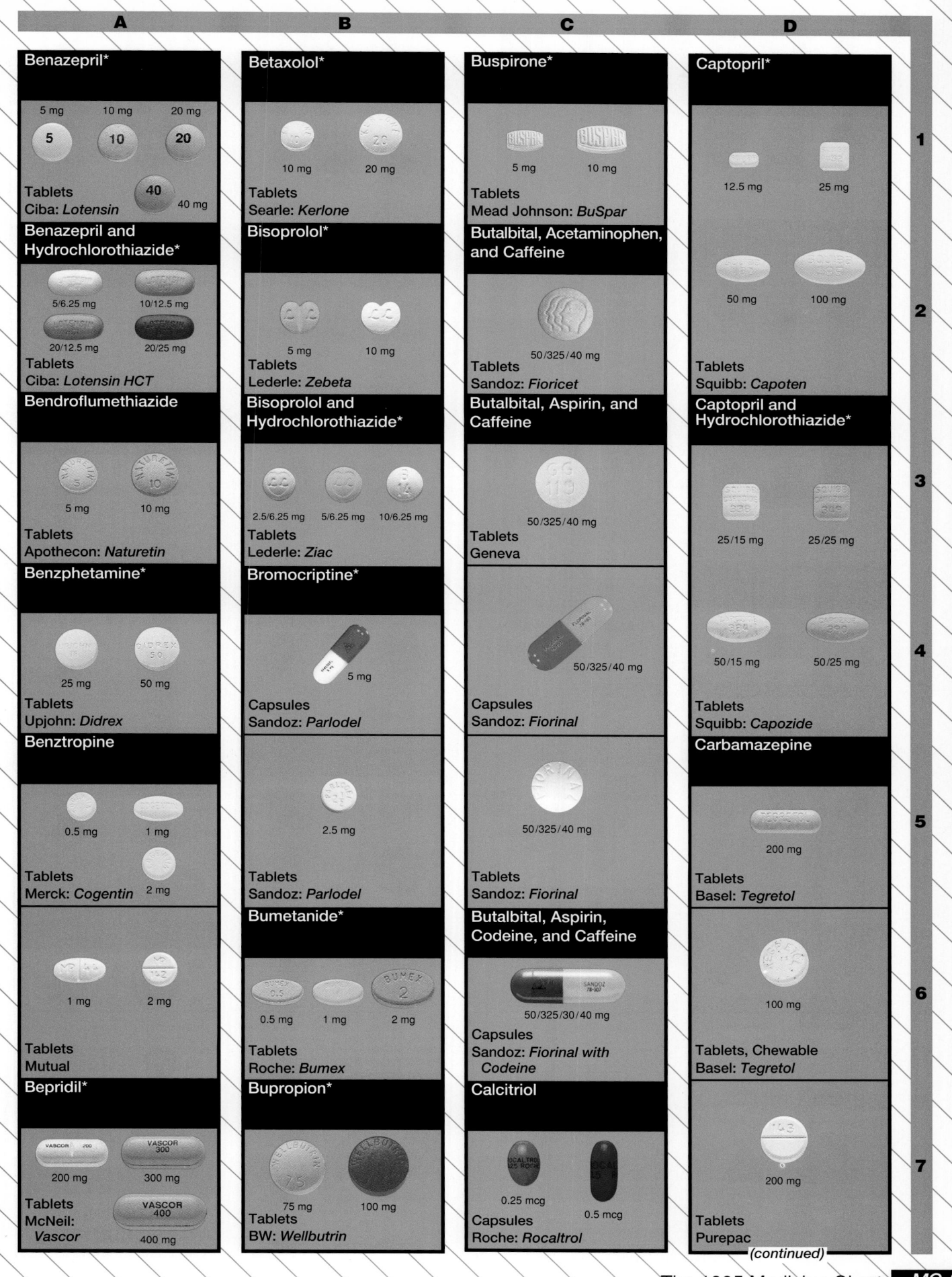

A

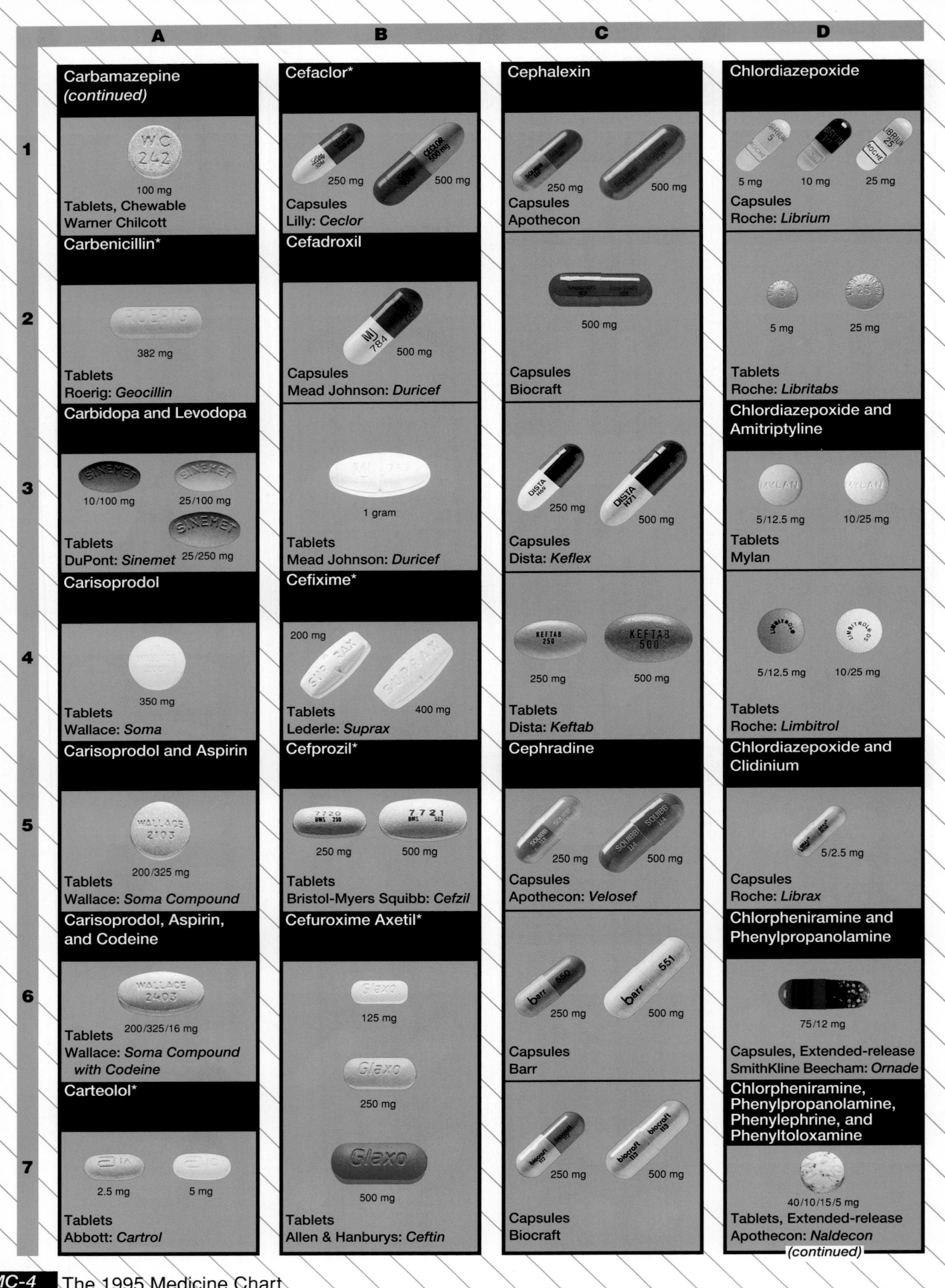

Carbamazepine *(continued)*

1

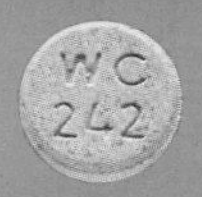

100 mg

Tablets, Chewable
Warner Chilcott

Carbenicillin*

2

382 mg

Tablets
Roerig: *Geocillin*

Carbidopa and Levodopa

3

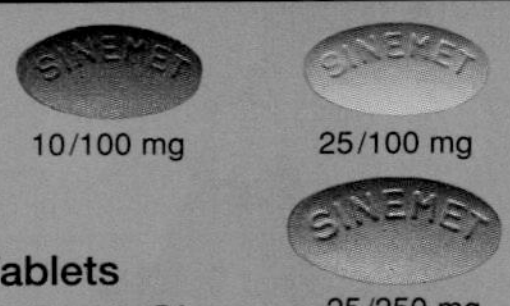

10/100 mg — 25/100 mg — 25/250 mg

Tablets
DuPont: *Sinemet*

Carisoprodol

4

350 mg

Tablets
Wallace: *Soma*

Carisoprodol and Aspirin

5

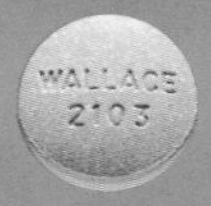

200/325 mg

Tablets
Wallace: *Soma Compound*

Carisoprodol, Aspirin, and Codeine

6

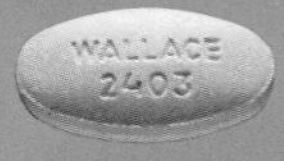

200/325/16 mg

Tablets
Wallace: *Soma Compound with Codeine*

Carteolol*

7

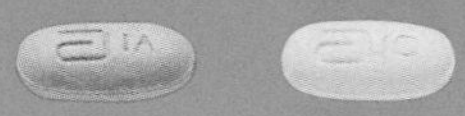

2.5 mg — 5 mg

Tablets
Abbott: *Cartrol*

B

Cefaclor*

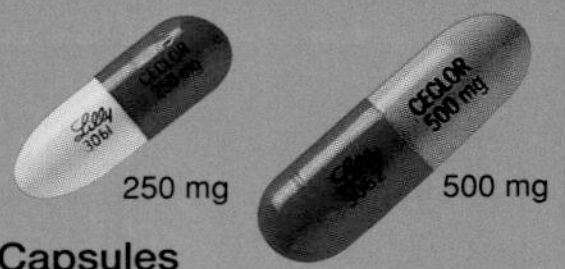

250 mg — 500 mg

Capsules
Lilly: *Ceclor*

Cefadroxil

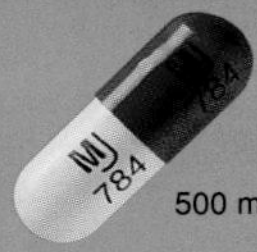

500 mg

Capsules
Mead Johnson: *Duricef*

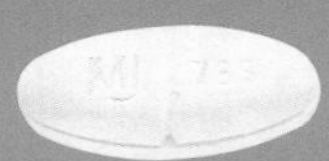

1 gram

Tablets
Mead Johnson: *Duricef*

Cefixime*

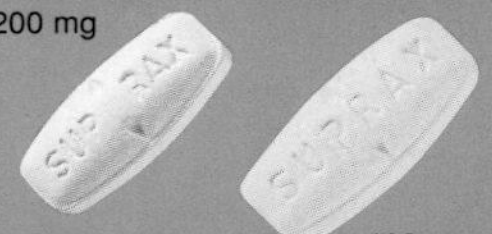

200 mg — 400 mg

Tablets
Lederle: *Suprax*

Cefprozil*

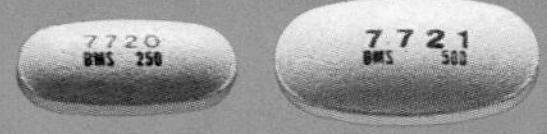

250 mg — 500 mg

Tablets
Bristol-Myers Squibb: *Cefzil*

Cefuroxime Axetil*

125 mg

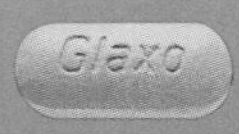

250 mg

500 mg

Tablets
Allen & Hanburys: *Ceftin*

C

Cephalexin

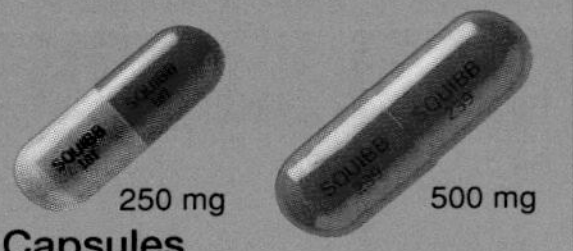

250 mg — 500 mg

Capsules
Apothecon

500 mg

Capsules
Biocraft

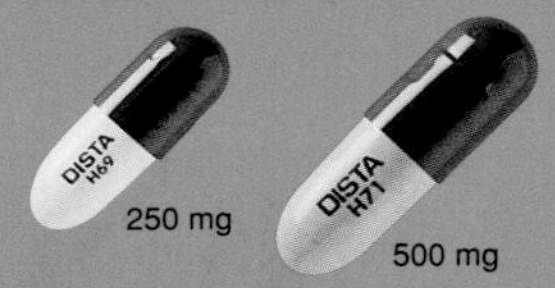

250 mg — 500 mg

Capsules
Dista: *Keflex*

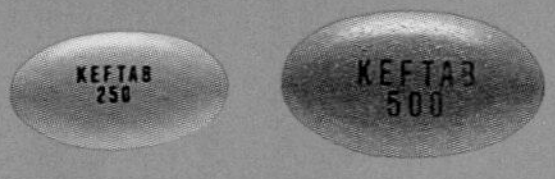

250 mg — 500 mg

Tablets
Dista: *Keftab*

Cephradine

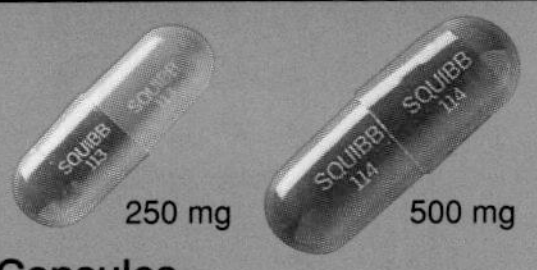

250 mg — 500 mg

Capsules
Apothecon: *Velosef*

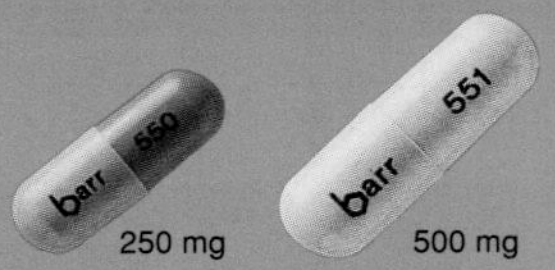

250 mg — 500 mg

Capsules
Barr

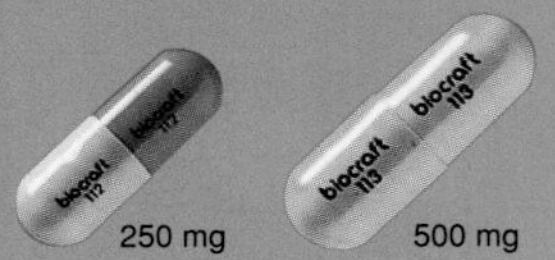

250 mg — 500 mg

Capsules
Biocraft

D

Chlordiazepoxide

5 mg — 10 mg — 25 mg

Capsules
Roche: *Librium*

5 mg — 25 mg

Tablets
Roche: *Libritabs*

Chlordiazepoxide and Amitriptyline

5/12.5 mg — 10/25 mg

Tablets
Mylan

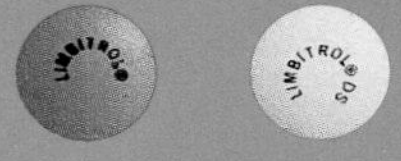

5/12.5 mg — 10/25 mg

Tablets
Roche: *Limbitrol*

Chlordiazepoxide and Clidinium

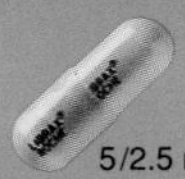

5/2.5 mg

Capsules
Roche: *Librax*

Chlorpheniramine and Phenylpropanolamine

75/12 mg

Capsules, Extended-release
SmithKline Beecham: *Ornade*

Chlorpheniramine, Phenylpropanolamine, Phenylephrine, and Phenyltoloxamine

40/10/15/5 mg

Tablets, Extended-release
Apothecon: *Naldecon*

(continued)

*Single source product for solid oral dosage forms in the U.S.

A B C D

Chlorpheniramine, Phenylpropanolamine, Phenylephrine, and Phenyltoloxamine *(cont.)*

40/10/15/5 mg

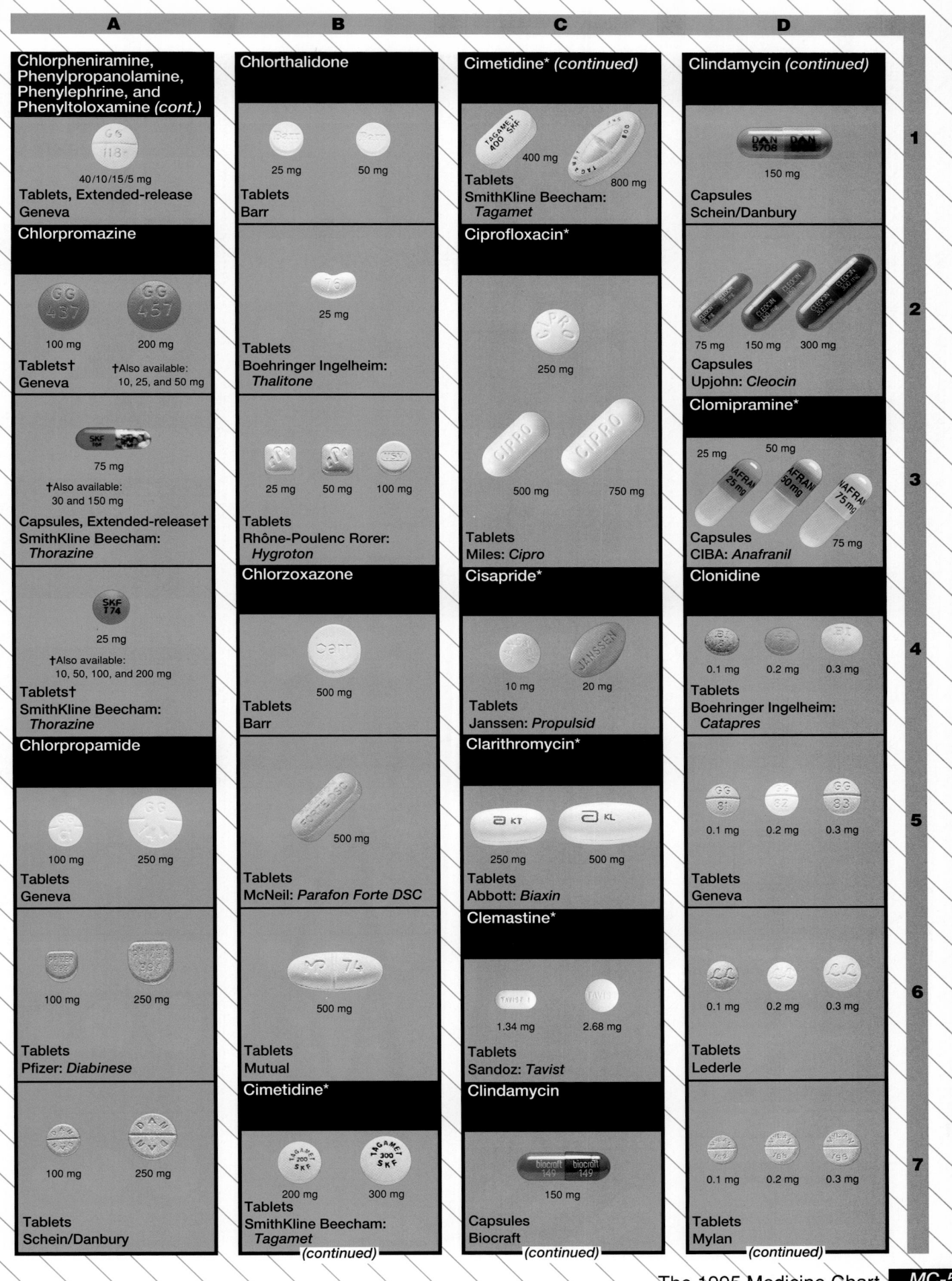

Tablets, Extended-release
Geneva

Chlorpromazine

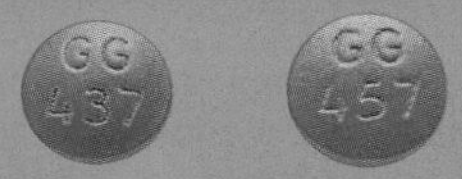

100 mg 200 mg

Tablets† †Also available: 10, 25, and 50 mg
Geneva

75 mg

†Also available: 30 and 150 mg

Capsules, Extended-release†
SmithKline Beecham: *Thorazine*

25 mg

†Also available: 10, 50, 100, and 200 mg

Tablets†
SmithKline Beecham: *Thorazine*

Chlorpropamide

100 mg 250 mg

Tablets
Geneva

100 mg 250 mg

Tablets
Pfizer: *Diabinese*

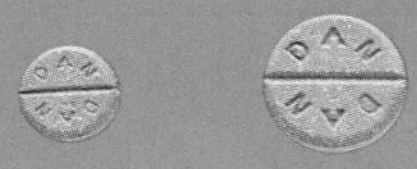

100 mg 250 mg

Tablets
Schein/Danbury

Chlorthalidone

25 mg 50 mg

Tablets
Barr

25 mg

Tablets
Boehringer Ingelheim: *Thalitone*

25 mg 50 mg 100 mg

Tablets
Rhône-Poulenc Rorer: *Hygroton*

Chlorzoxazone

500 mg

Tablets
Barr

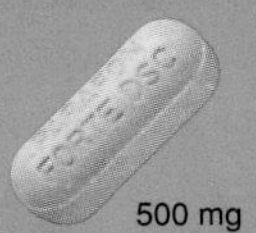

500 mg

Tablets
McNeil: *Parafon Forte DSC*

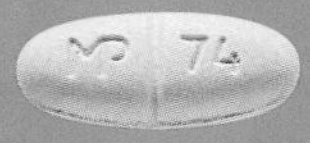

500 mg

Tablets
Mutual

Cimetidine*

200 mg 300 mg

Tablets
SmithKline Beecham: *Tagamet*

(continued)

Cimetidine* *(continued)*

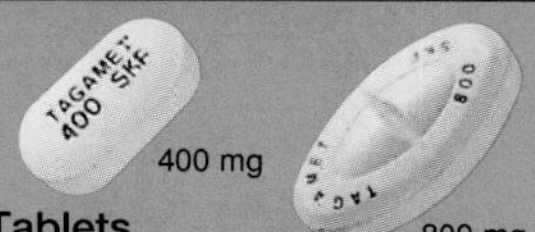

400 mg 800 mg

Tablets
SmithKline Beecham: *Tagamet*

Ciprofloxacin*

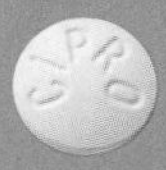

250 mg

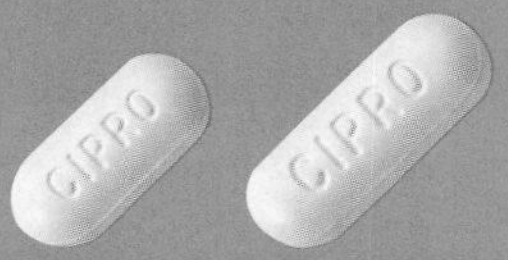

500 mg 750 mg

Tablets
Miles: *Cipro*

Cisapride*

10 mg 20 mg

Tablets
Janssen: *Propulsid*

Clarithromycin*

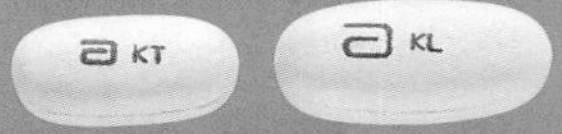

250 mg 500 mg

Tablets
Abbott: *Biaxin*

Clemastine*

1.34 mg 2.68 mg

Tablets
Sandoz: *Tavist*

Clindamycin

150 mg

Capsules
Biocraft

(continued)

Clindamycin *(continued)*

150 mg

Capsules
Schein/Danbury

75 mg 150 mg 300 mg

Capsules
Upjohn: *Cleocin*

Clomipramine*

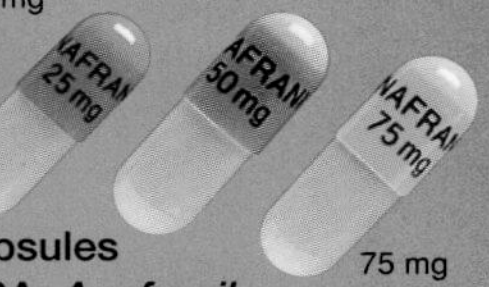

25 mg 50 mg 75 mg

Capsules
CIBA: *Anafranil*

Clonidine

0.1 mg 0.2 mg 0.3 mg

Tablets
Boehringer Ingelheim: *Catapres*

0.1 mg 0.2 mg 0.3 mg

Tablets
Geneva

0.1 mg 0.2 mg 0.3 mg

Tablets
Lederle

0.1 mg 0.2 mg 0.3 mg

Tablets
Mylan

(continued)

1 2 3 4 5 6 7

*Single source product for solid oral dosage forms in the U.S.

A	B	C	D

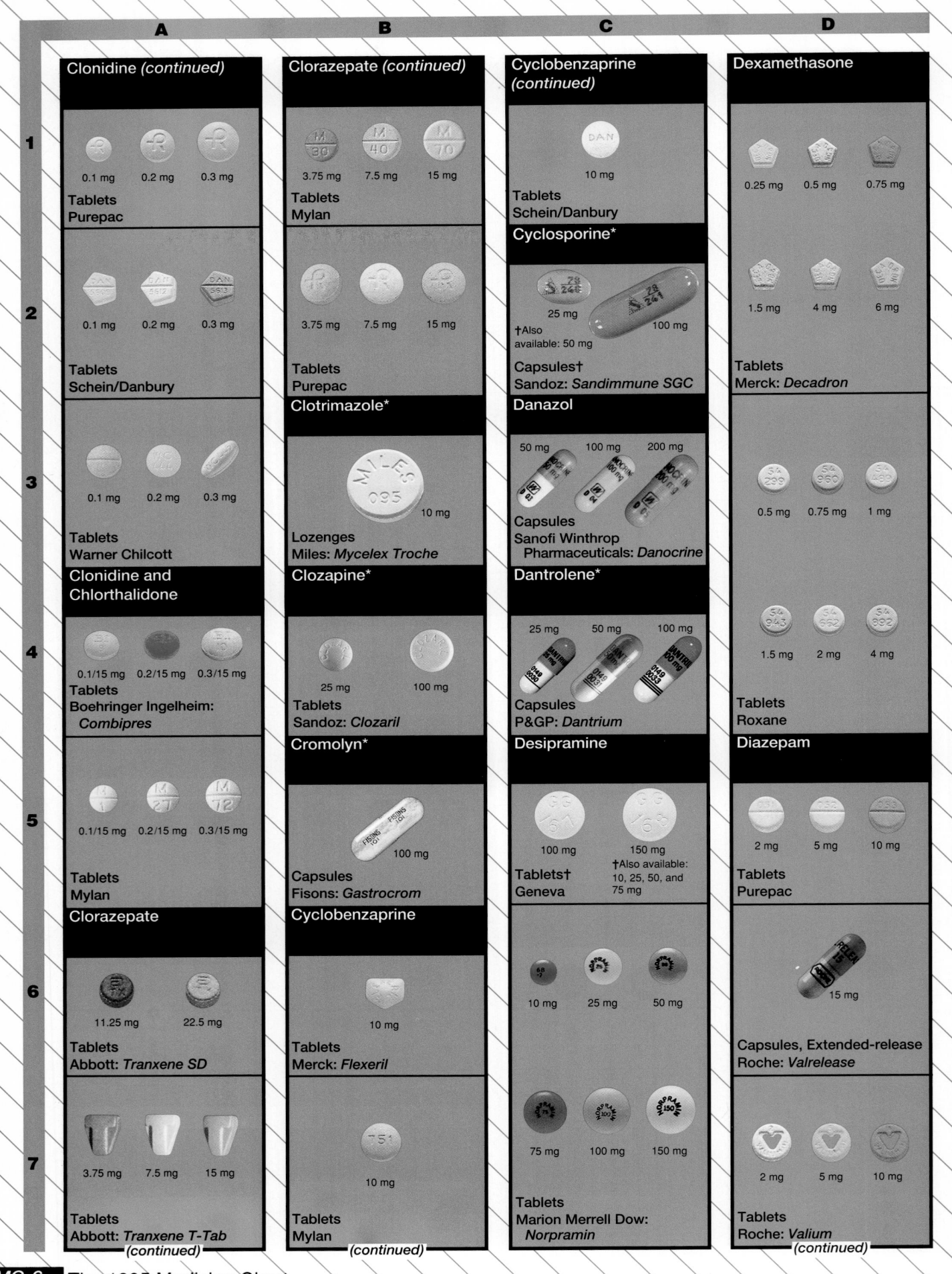

Clonidine *(continued)*

1

0.1 mg 0.2 mg 0.3 mg

Tablets
Purepac

2

0.1 mg 0.2 mg 0.3 mg

Tablets
Schein/Danbury

3

0.1 mg 0.2 mg 0.3 mg

Tablets
Warner Chilcott

Clonidine and Chlorthalidone

4

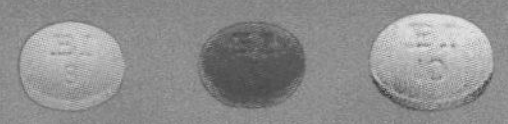

0.1/15 mg 0.2/15 mg 0.3/15 mg

Tablets
Boehringer Ingelheim: *Combipres*

5

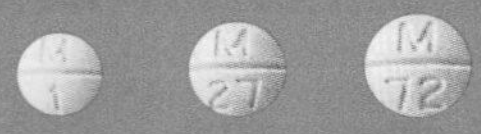

0.1/15 mg 0.2/15 mg 0.3/15 mg

Tablets
Mylan

Clorazepate

6

11.25 mg 22.5 mg

Tablets
Abbott: *Tranxene SD*

7

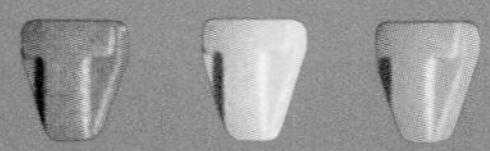

3.75 mg 7.5 mg 15 mg

Tablets
Abbott: *Tranxene T-Tab*

(continued)

Clorazepate *(continued)*

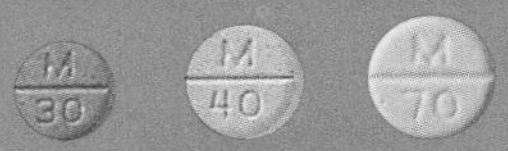

3.75 mg 7.5 mg 15 mg

Tablets
Mylan

3.75 mg 7.5 mg 15 mg

Tablets
Purepac

Clotrimazole*

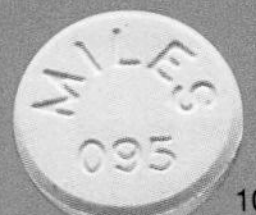

10 mg

Lozenges
Miles: *Mycelex Troche*

Clozapine*

25 mg 100 mg

Tablets
Sandoz: *Clozaril*

Cromolyn*

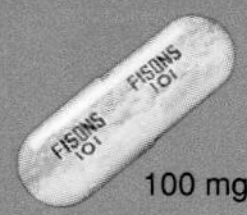

100 mg

Capsules
Fisons: *Gastrocrom*

Cyclobenzaprine

10 mg

Tablets
Merck: *Flexeril*

10 mg

Tablets
Mylan

(continued)

Cyclobenzaprine *(continued)*

10 mg

Tablets
Schein/Danbury

Cyclosporine*

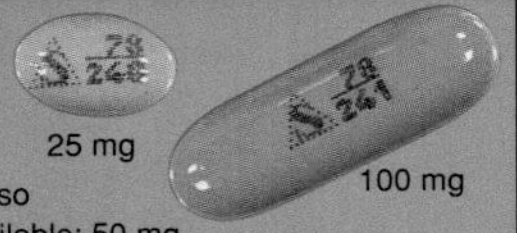

25 mg 100 mg

†Also available: 50 mg

Capsules†
Sandoz: *Sandimmune SGC*

Danazol

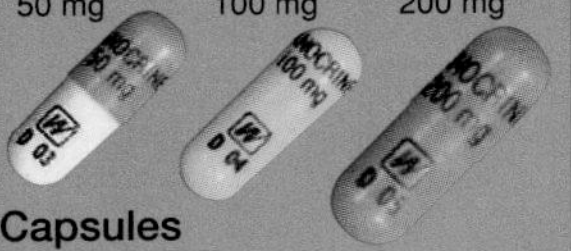

50 mg 100 mg 200 mg

Capsules
Sanofi Winthrop Pharmaceuticals: *Danocrine*

Dantrolene*

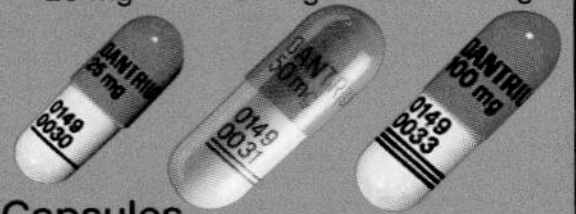

25 mg 50 mg 100 mg

Capsules
P&GP: *Dantrium*

Desipramine

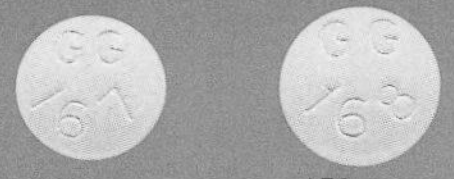

100 mg 150 mg

Tablets†
Geneva

†Also available: 10, 25, 50, and 75 mg

10 mg 25 mg 50 mg

75 mg 100 mg 150 mg

Tablets
Marion Merrell Dow: *Norpramin*

Dexamethasone

0.25 mg 0.5 mg 0.75 mg

1.5 mg 4 mg 6 mg

Tablets
Merck: *Decadron*

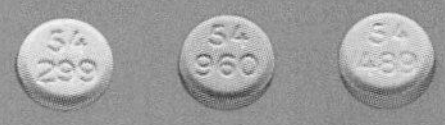

0.5 mg 0.75 mg 1 mg

1.5 mg 2 mg 4 mg

Tablets
Roxane

Diazepam

2 mg 5 mg 10 mg

Tablets
Purepac

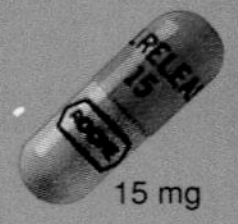

15 mg

Capsules, Extended-release
Roche: *Valrelease*

2 mg 5 mg 10 mg

Tablets
Roche: *Valium*

(continued)

*Single source product for solid oral dosage forms in the U.S.

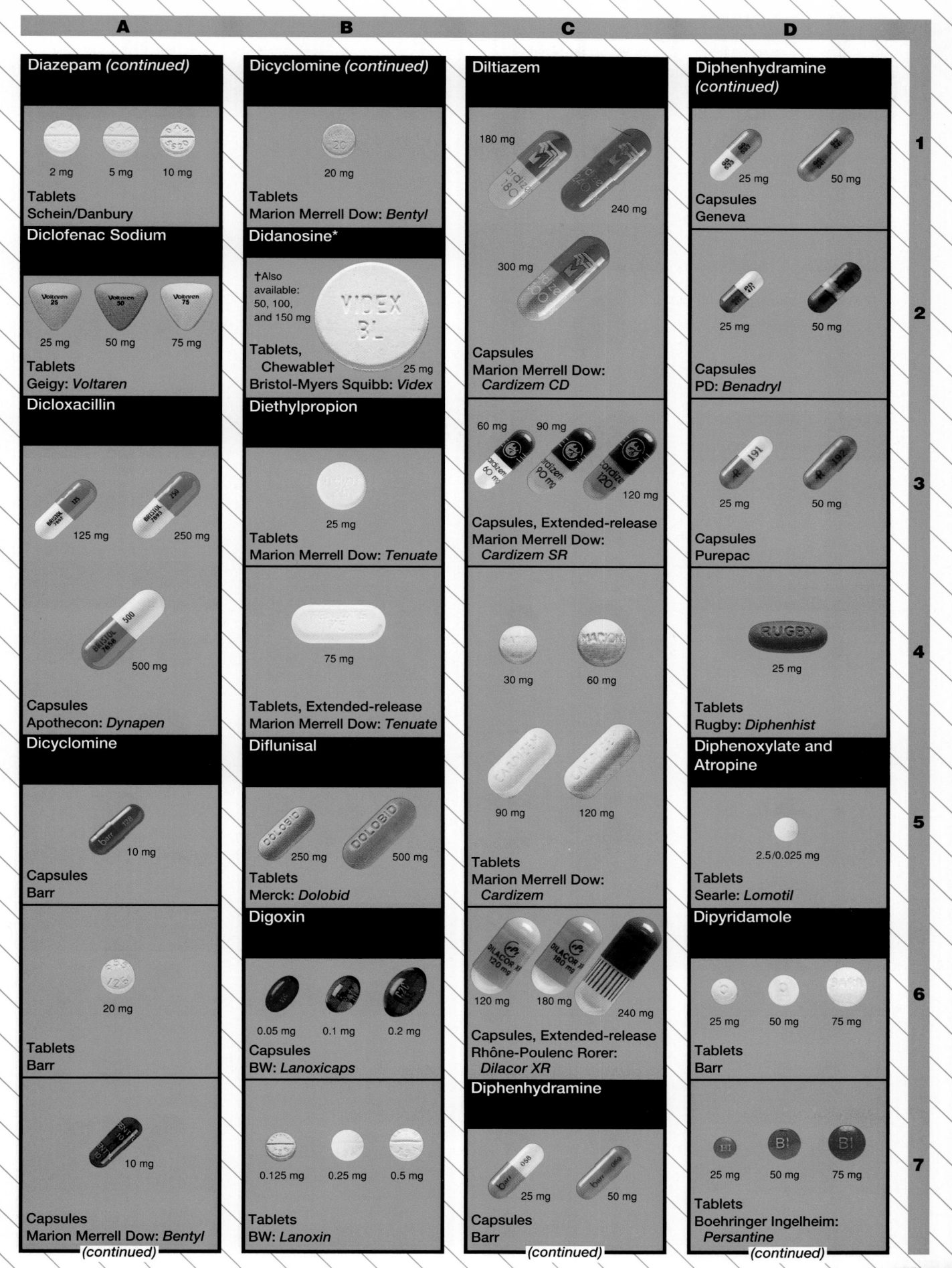

Diazepam *(continued)*

2 mg 5 mg 10 mg

Tablets
Schein/Danbury

Diclofenac Sodium

25 mg 50 mg 75 mg

Tablets
Geigy: *Voltaren*

Dicloxacillin

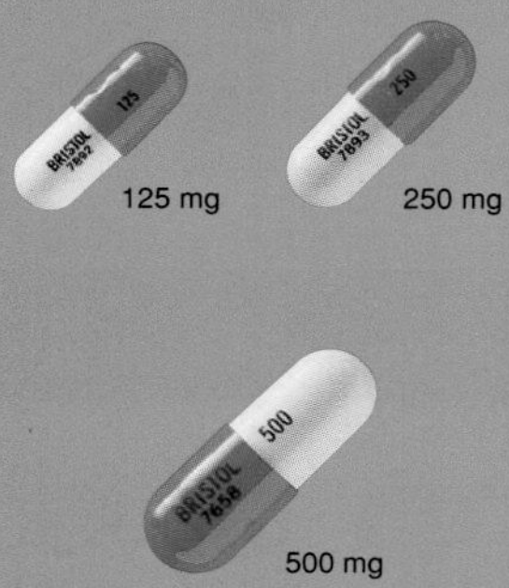

125 mg 250 mg 500 mg

Capsules
Apothecon: *Dynapen*

Dicyclomine

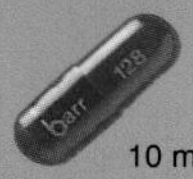

10 mg

Capsules
Barr

20 mg

Tablets
Barr

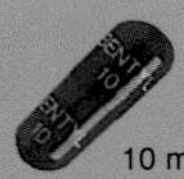

10 mg

Capsules
Marion Merrell Dow: *Bentyl*

(continued)

Dicyclomine *(continued)*

20 mg

Tablets
Marion Merrell Dow: *Bentyl*

Didanosine*

†Also available: 50, 100, and 150 mg

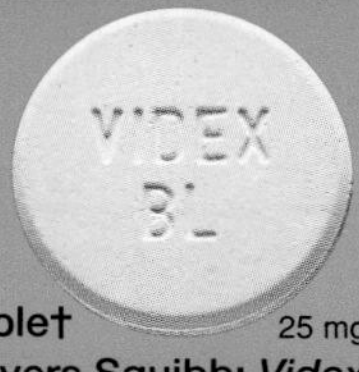

25 mg

Tablets, Chewable†
Bristol-Myers Squibb: *Videx*

Diethylpropion

25 mg

Tablets
Marion Merrell Dow: *Tenuate*

75 mg

Tablets, Extended-release
Marion Merrell Dow: *Tenuate*

Diflunisal

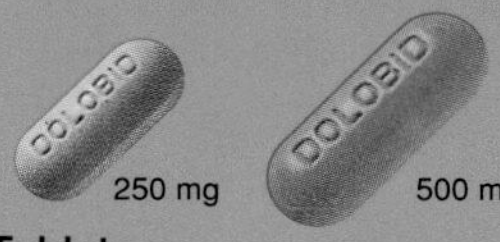

250 mg 500 mg

Tablets
Merck: *Dolobid*

Digoxin

0.05 mg 0.1 mg 0.2 mg

Capsules
BW: *Lanoxicaps*

0.125 mg 0.25 mg 0.5 mg

Tablets
BW: *Lanoxin*

Diltiazem

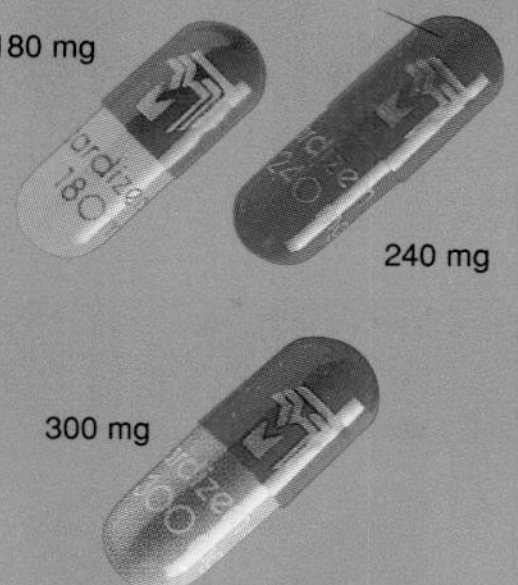

180 mg 240 mg 300 mg

Capsules
Marion Merrell Dow: *Cardizem CD*

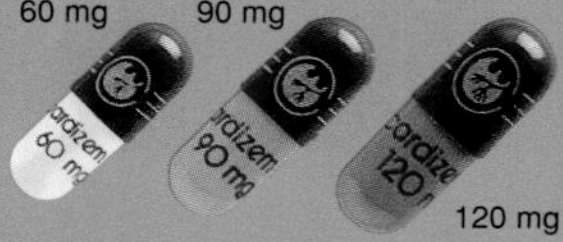

60 mg 90 mg 120 mg

Capsules, Extended-release
Marion Merrell Dow: *Cardizem SR*

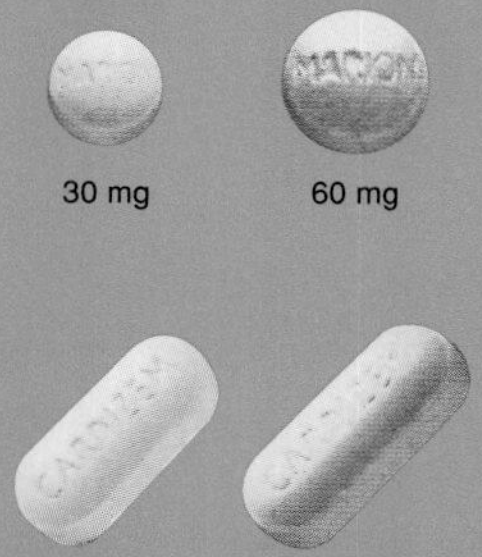

30 mg 60 mg 90 mg 120 mg

Tablets
Marion Merrell Dow: *Cardizem*

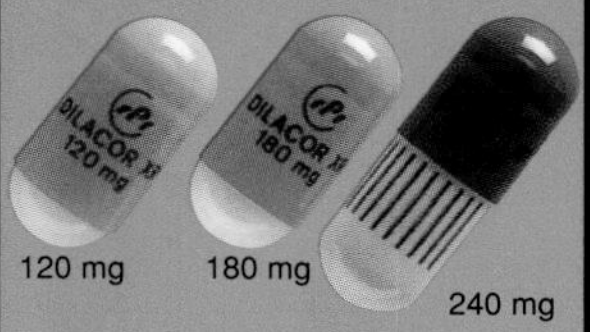

120 mg 180 mg 240 mg

Capsules, Extended-release
Rhône-Poulenc Rorer: *Dilacor XR*

Diphenhydramine

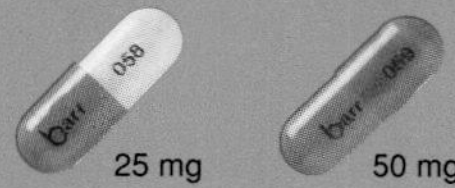

25 mg 50 mg

Capsules
Barr

(continued)

Diphenhydramine *(continued)*

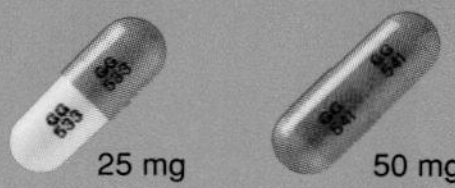

25 mg 50 mg

Capsules
Geneva

25 mg 50 mg

Capsules
PD: *Benadryl*

25 mg 50 mg

Capsules
Purepac

25 mg

Tablets
Rugby: *Diphenhist*

Diphenoxylate and Atropine

2.5/0.025 mg

Tablets
Searle: *Lomotil*

Dipyridamole

25 mg 50 mg 75 mg

Tablets
Barr

25 mg 50 mg 75 mg

Tablets
Boehringer Ingelheim: *Persantine*

(continued)

A B C D

A

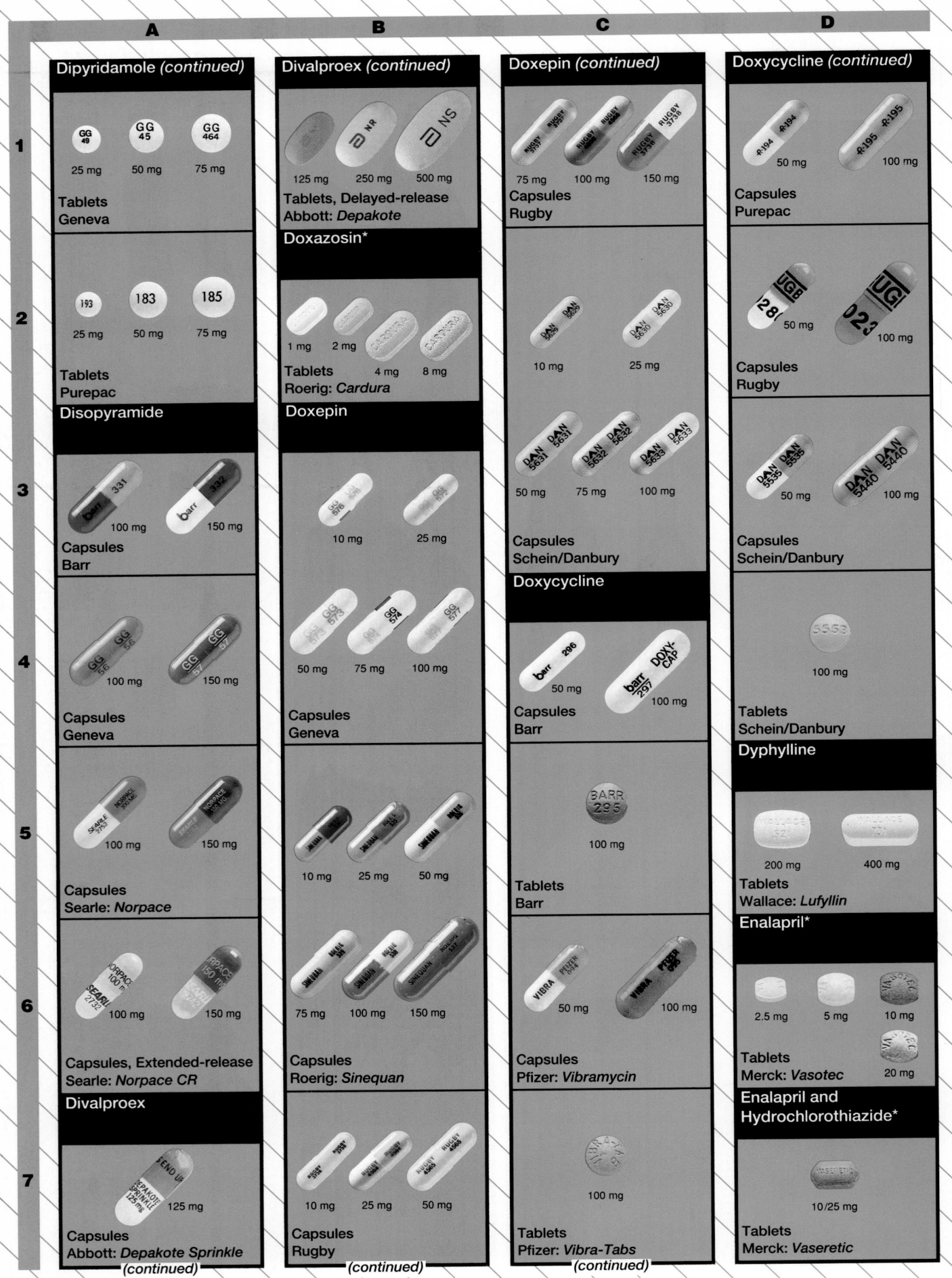

Dipyridamole (continued)

1

25 mg 50 mg 75 mg

Tablets
Geneva

2

25 mg 50 mg 75 mg

Tablets
Purepac

Disopyramide

3

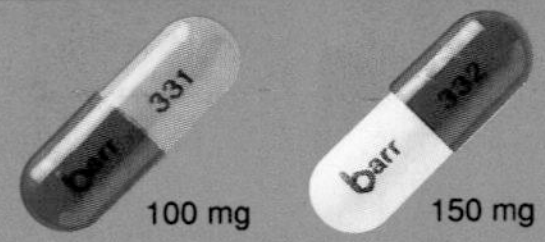

100 mg 150 mg

Capsules
Barr

4

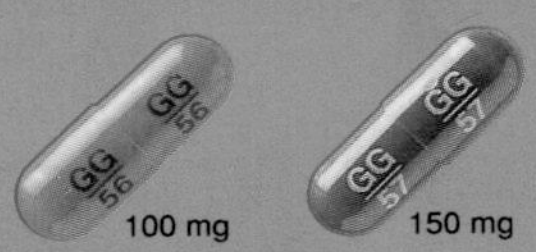

100 mg 150 mg

Capsules
Geneva

5

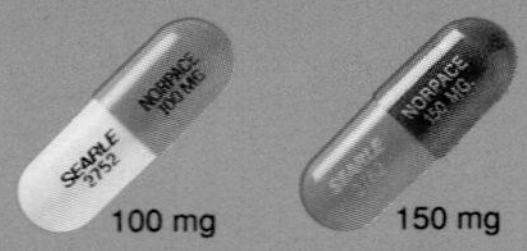

100 mg 150 mg

Capsules
Searle: *Norpace*

6

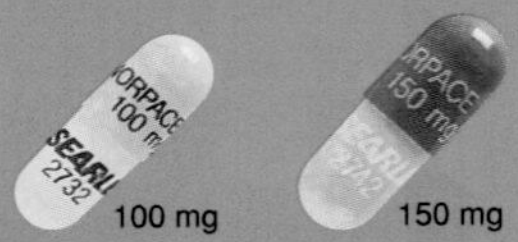

100 mg 150 mg

Capsules, Extended-release
Searle: *Norpace CR*

Divalproex

7

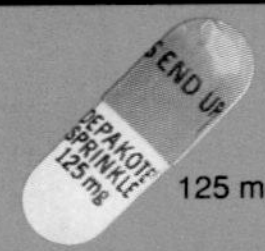

125 mg

Capsules
Abbott: *Depakote Sprinkle*

(continued)

B

Divalproex (continued)

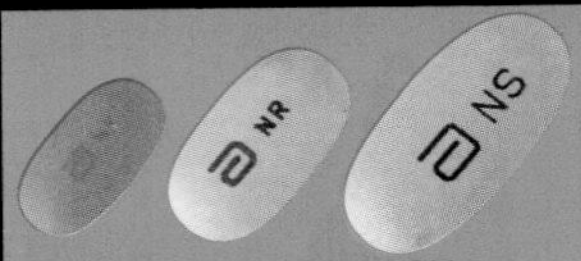

125 mg 250 mg 500 mg

Tablets, Delayed-release
Abbott: *Depakote*

Doxazosin*

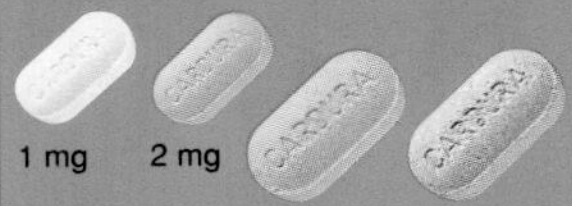

1 mg 2 mg 4 mg 8 mg

Tablets
Roerig: *Cardura*

Doxepin

10 mg 25 mg

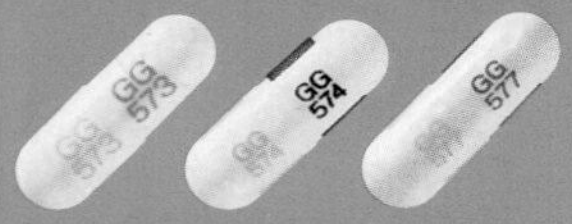

50 mg 75 mg 100 mg

Capsules
Geneva

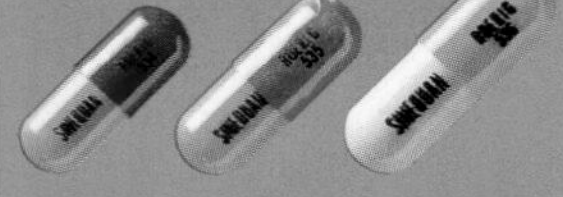

10 mg 25 mg 50 mg

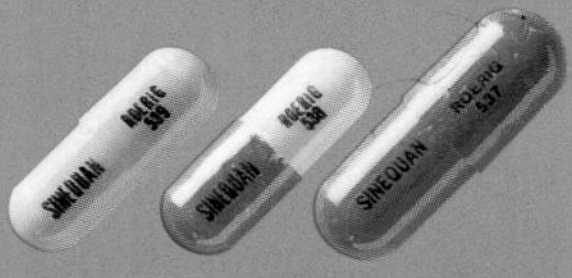

75 mg 100 mg 150 mg

Capsules
Roerig: *Sinequan*

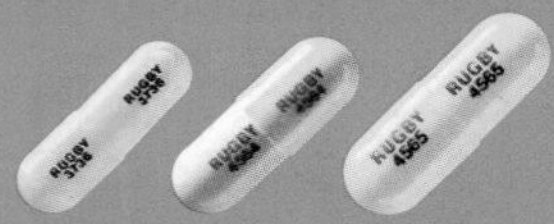

10 mg 25 mg 50 mg

Capsules
Rugby

(continued)

C

Doxepin (continued)

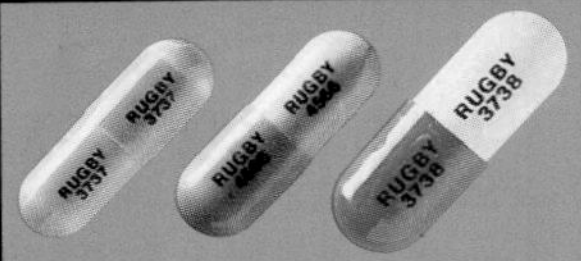

75 mg 100 mg 150 mg

Capsules
Rugby

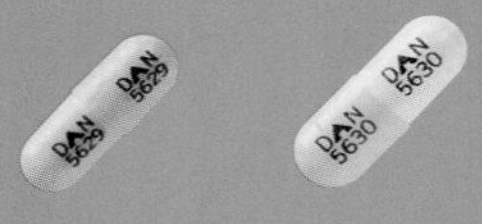

10 mg 25 mg

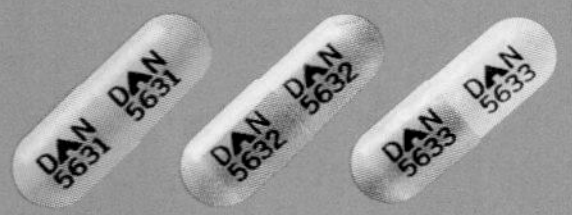

50 mg 75 mg 100 mg

Capsules
Schein/Danbury

Doxycycline

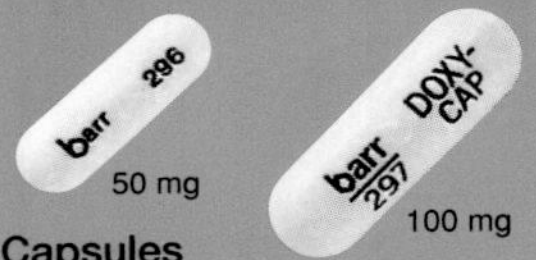

50 mg 100 mg

Capsules
Barr

100 mg

Tablets
Barr

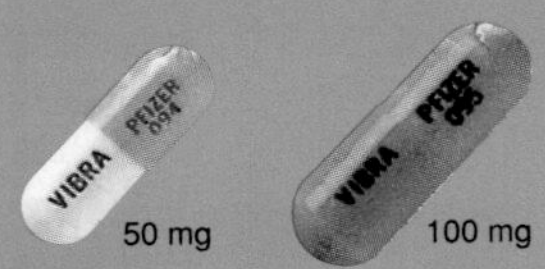

50 mg 100 mg

Capsules
Pfizer: *Vibramycin*

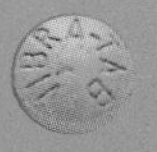

100 mg

Tablets
Pfizer: *Vibra-Tabs*

(continued)

D

Doxycycline (continued)

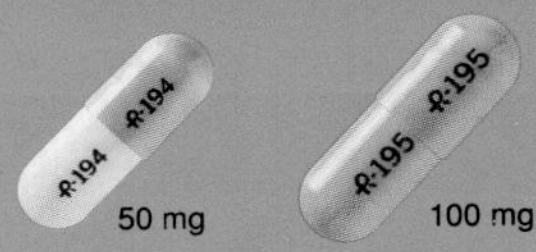

50 mg 100 mg

Capsules
Purepac

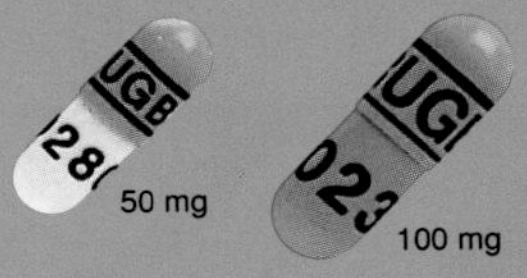

50 mg 100 mg

Capsules
Rugby

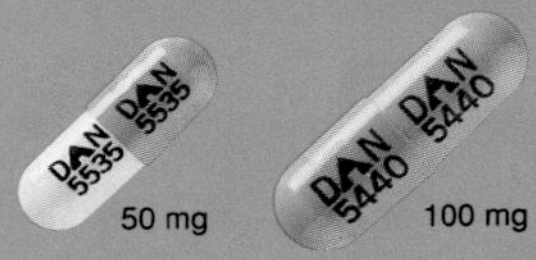

50 mg 100 mg

Capsules
Schein/Danbury

100 mg

Tablets
Schein/Danbury

Dyphylline

200 mg 400 mg

Tablets
Wallace: *Lufyllin*

Enalapril*

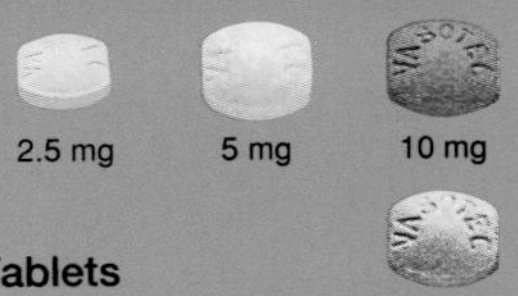

2.5 mg 5 mg 10 mg 20 mg

Tablets
Merck: *Vasotec*

Enalapril and Hydrochlorothiazide*

10/25 mg

Tablets
Merck: *Vaseretic*

*Single source product for solid oral dosage forms in the U.S.

A

Enoxacin*

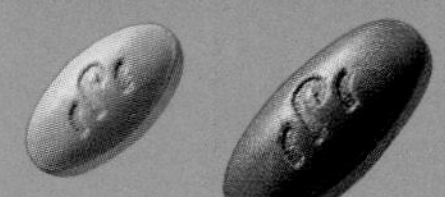

200 mg 400 mg
Tablets
Rhône-Poulenc Rorer: *Penetrex*

Ergoloid Mesylates

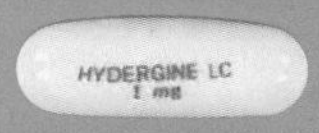

1 mg
Capsules
Sandoz: *Hydergine LC*

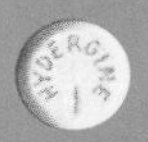

1 mg
Tablets
Sandoz: *Hydergine*

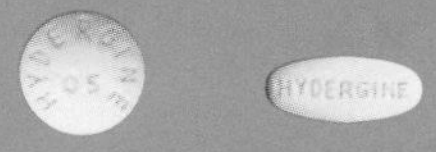

0.5 mg 1 mg
Tablets, Sublingual
Sandoz: *Hydergine*

Ergotamine and Caffeine

1/100 mg
Tablets
Sandoz: *Cafergot*

Erythromycin

250 mg
Capsules, Delayed-release
Abbott

250 mg 500 mg
Tablets
Abbott

(continued)

B

Erythromycin *(continued)*

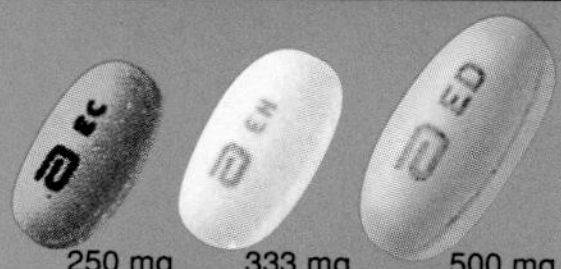

250 mg 333 mg 500 mg
Tablets, Delayed-release
Abbott: *Ery-Tab*

333 mg 500 mg
Tablets
Abbott: *PCE*

250 mg
Capsules, Delayed-release
Barr

250 mg 333 mg
Tablets, Delayed-release
Boots Pharmaceuticals: *E-Mycin*

250 mg
Capsules, Delayed-release
PD: *Eryc*

Erythromycin Estolate

250 mg
Capsules
Dista: *Ilosone*

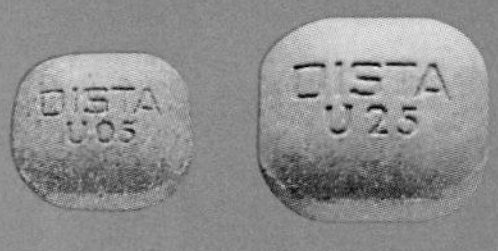

125 mg 250 mg
Tablets, Chewable
Dista: *Ilosone*

C

Erythromycin Ethylsuccinate

400 mg
Tablets
Abbott: *E.E.S.*

200 mg
Tablets, Chewable
Abbott: *EryPed*

400 mg
Tablets
Barr

Erythromycin Stearate

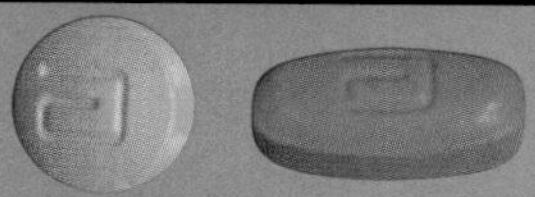

250 mg 500 mg
Tablets
Abbott: *Erythrocin*

Estazolam*

1 mg 2 mg
Tablets
Abbott: *ProSom*

Estradiol

1 mg 2 mg
Tablets
Mead Johnson: *Estrace*

Estrogens, Conjugated

0.3 mg 0.625 mg 0.9 mg
Tablets
Wyeth-Ayerst: *Premarin*

(continued)

D

Estrogens, Conjugated *(continued)*

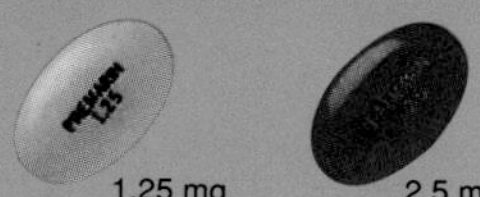

1.25 mg 2.5 mg
Tablets
Wyeth-Ayerst: *Premarin*

Estropipate

0.625 mg 1.25 mg
Tablets
Ortho: *Ortho-Est*

Ethynodiol Diacetate and Ethinyl Estradiol*

1/0.035 mg Inert ‡
‡ Included only in 28-day pack
Tablets
Searle: *Demulen 1/35-21 and -28*

1/0.05 mg Inert ‡
‡ Included only in 28-day pack
Tablets
Searle: *Demulen 1/50-21 and -28*

Etodolac*

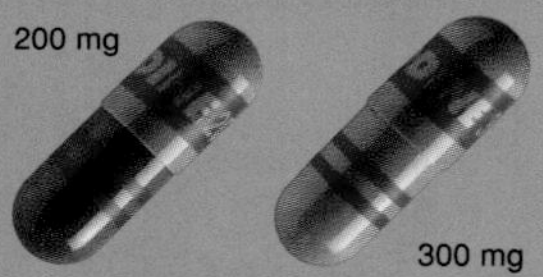

200 mg 300 mg
Capsules
Wyeth-Ayerst: *Lodine*

Famotidine*

20 mg 40 mg
Tablets
Merck: *Pepcid*

Felbamate*

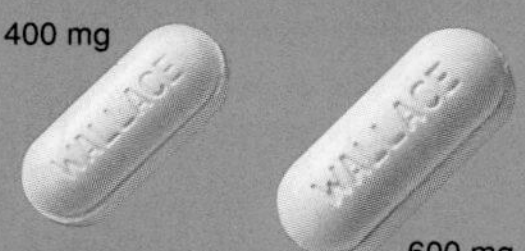

400 mg 600 mg
Tablets
Wallace: *Felbatol*

*Single source product for solid oral dosage forms in the U.S.

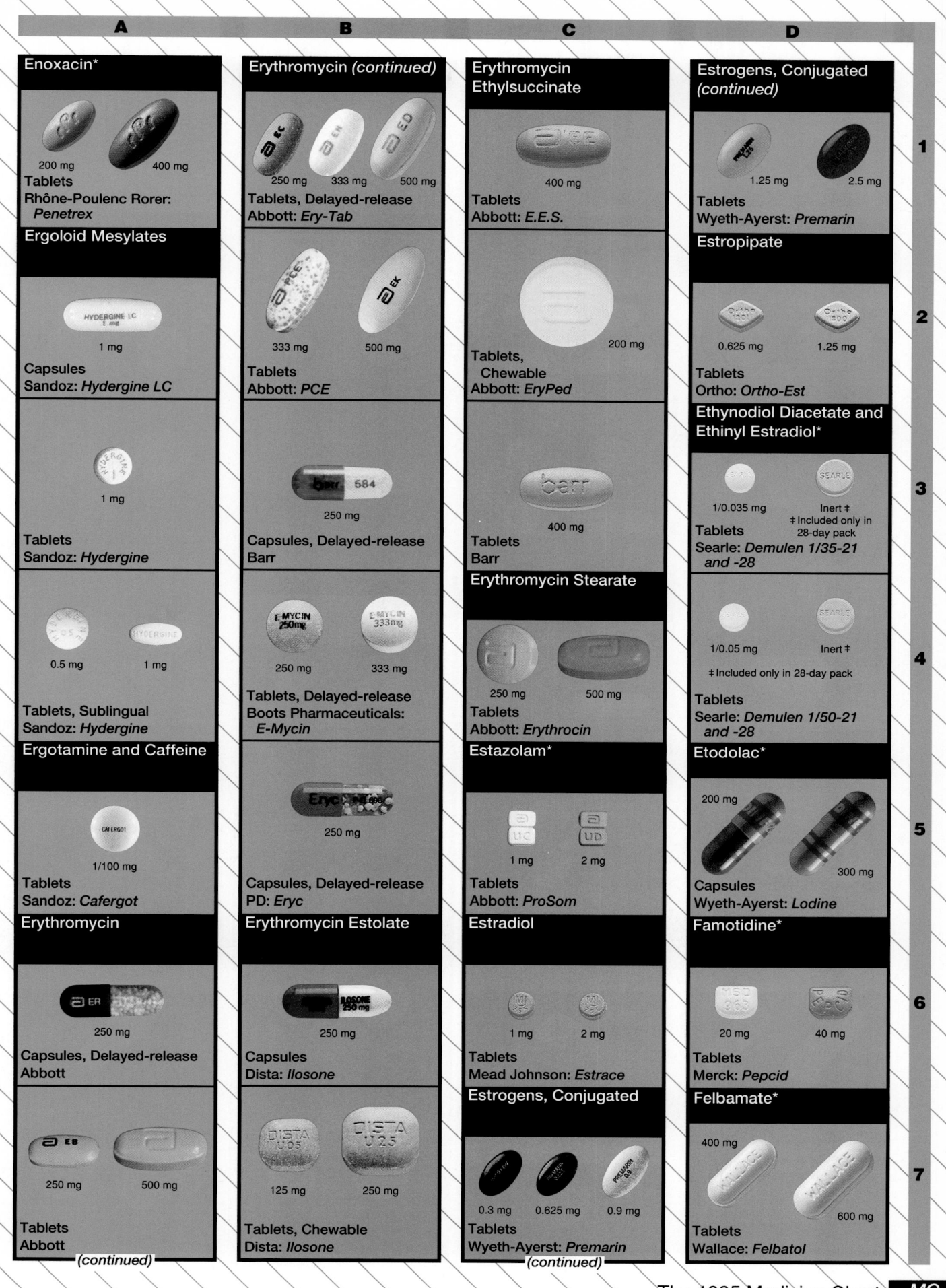

	A	B	C	D

1

A

Felodipine*

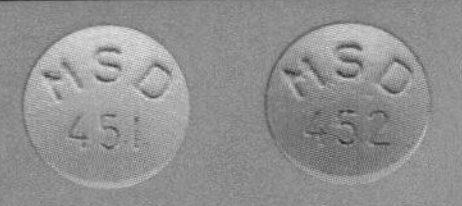

5 mg 10 mg

Tablets
Merck: *Plendil*

Fenoprofen

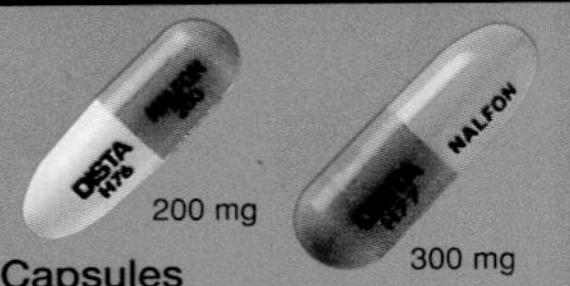

200 mg 300 mg

Capsules
Dista: *Nalfon*

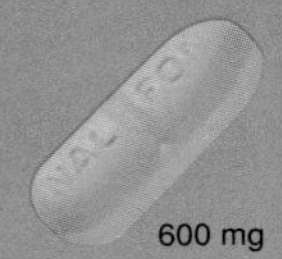

600 mg

Tablets
Dista: *Nalfon*

200 mg 300 mg

Capsules
Geneva

600 mg

Tablets
Geneva

600 mg

Tablets
Purepac

600 mg

Tablets
Schein/Danbury

B

Ferrous Sulfate

300 mg

Tablets
Upsher-Smith

Finasteride*

5 mg

Tablets
Merck: *Proscar*

Fluconazole*

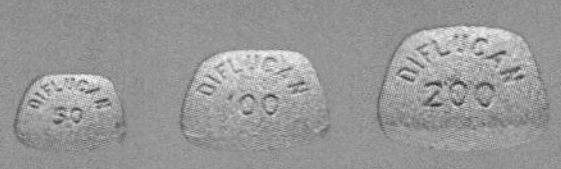

50 mg 100 mg 200 mg

Tablets
Roerig: *Diflucan*

Fluoxetine*

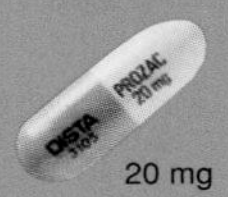

20 mg

Capsules
Dista: *Prozac*

Fluoxymesterone

2 mg 5 mg 10 mg

Tablets
Upjohn: *Halotestin*

Fluphenazine

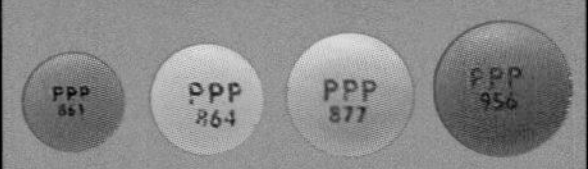

1 mg 2.5 mg 5 mg 10 mg

Tablets
Apothecon: *Prolixin*

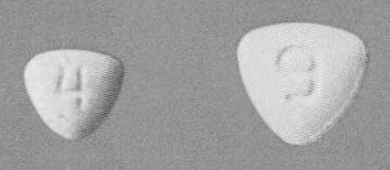

1 mg 2.5 mg

Tablets
Mylan

(continued)

C

Fluphenazine *(continued)*

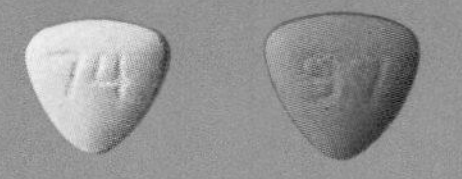

5 mg 10 mg

Tablets
Mylan

Flurazepam

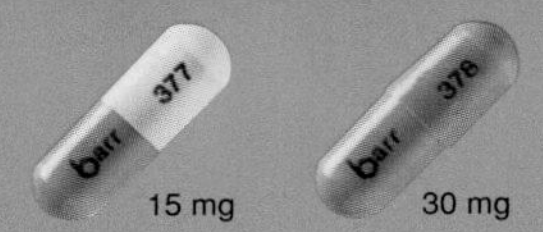

15 mg 30 mg

Capsules
Barr

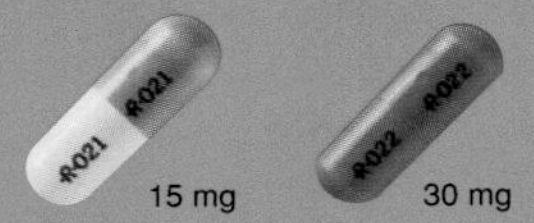

15 mg 30 mg

Capsules
Purepac

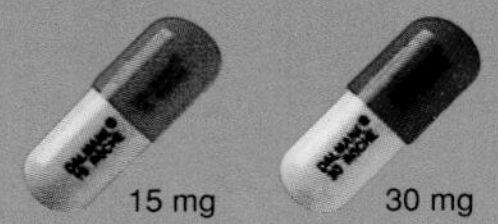

15 mg 30 mg

Capsules
Roche: *Dalmane*

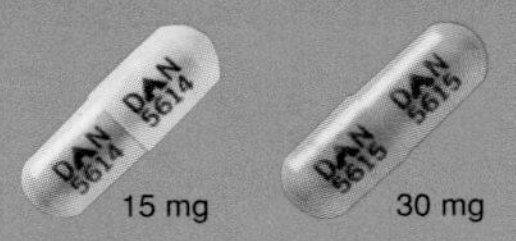

15 mg 30 mg

Capsules
Schein/Danbury

Flurbiprofen*

50 mg 100 mg

Tablets
Upjohn: *Ansaid*

Fluvastatin*

20 mg 40 mg

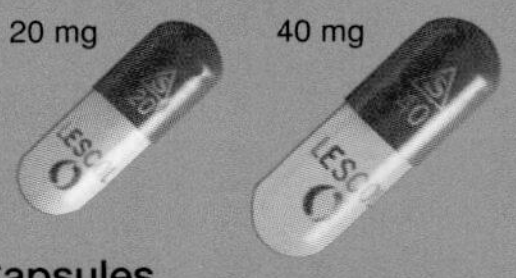

Capsules
Sandoz: *Lescol*

D

Fosinopril*

10 mg 20 mg

Tablets
Mead Johnson: *Monopril*

Furosemide

20 mg 40 mg 80 mg

Tablets
Barr

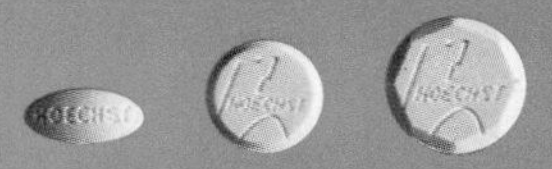

20 mg 40 mg 80 mg

Tablets
Hoechst-Roussel: *Lasix*

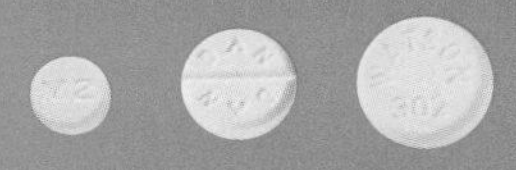

20 mg 40 mg 80 mg

Tablets
Schein/Danbury

Gabapentin*

100 mg 300 mg 400 mg

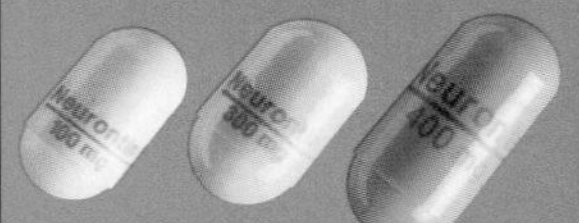

Capsules
PD: *Neurontin*

Gemfibrozil

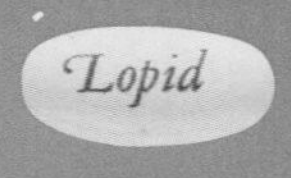

600 mg

Tablets
PD: *Lopid*

Glipizide*

5 mg 10 mg

Tablets, Extended-release
Pratt: *Glucotrol XL*

*Single source product for solid oral dosage forms in the U.S.

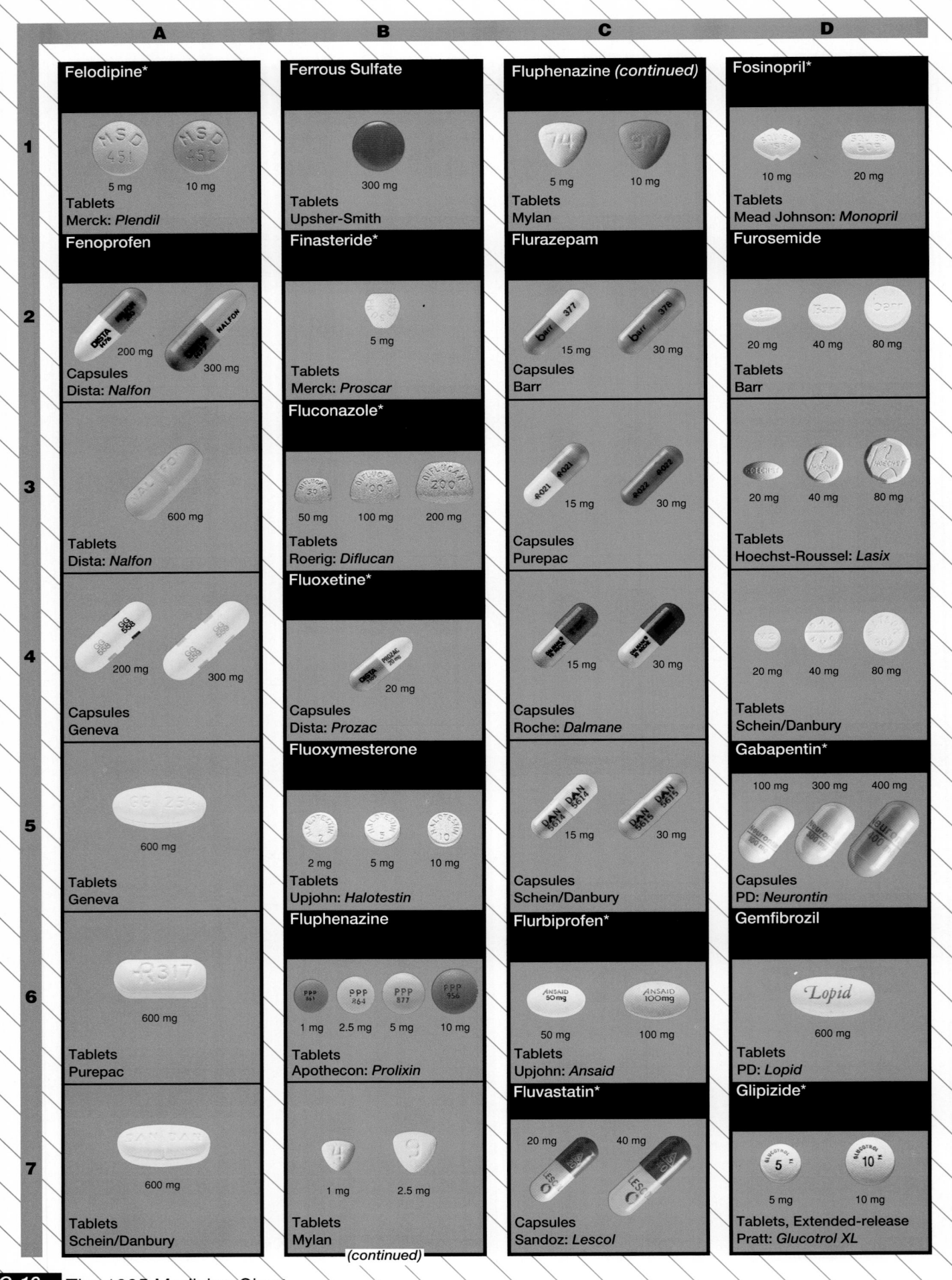

A | B | C | D

Glyburide

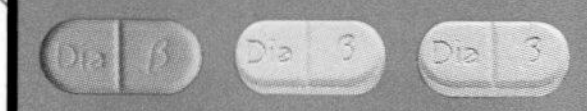

1.25 mg 2.5 mg 5 mg

Tablets
Hoechst-Roussel: *DiaBeta*

1.25 mg 2.5 mg 5 mg

Tablets
Upjohn: *Micronase*

Griseofulvin

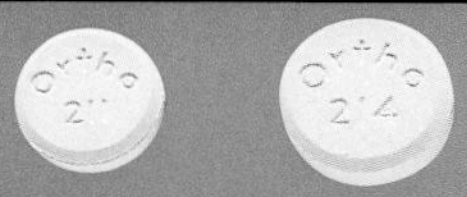

250 mg 500 mg

Tablets
Ortho: *Grifulvin V*

Guanabenz*

4 mg 8 mg

Tablets
Wyeth-Ayerst: *Wytensin*

Guanfacine*

1 mg 2 mg

Tablets
Robins: *Tenex*

Haloperidol

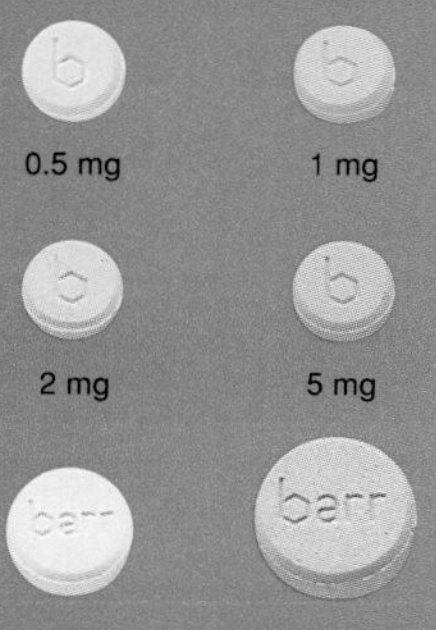

0.5 mg 1 mg 2 mg 5 mg 10 mg 20 mg

Tablets
Barr

(continued)

Haloperidol *(continued)*

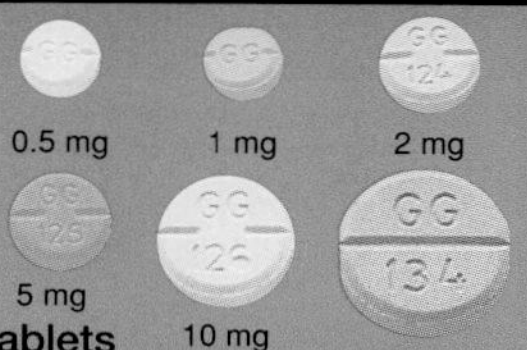

0.5 mg 1 mg 2 mg 5 mg 10 mg 20 mg

Tablets
Geneva

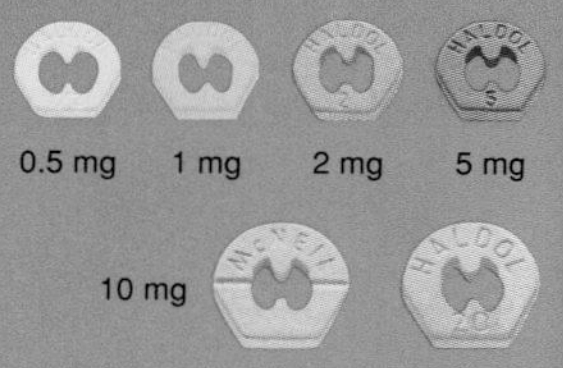

0.5 mg 1 mg 2 mg 5 mg 10 mg 20 mg

Tablets
McNeil: *Haldol*

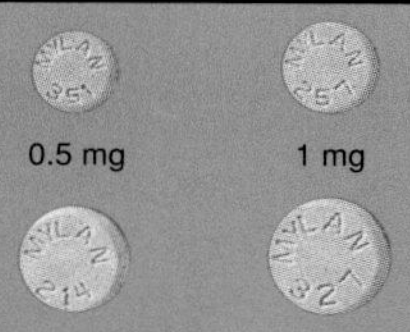

0.5 mg 1 mg 2 mg 5 mg

Tablets
Mylan

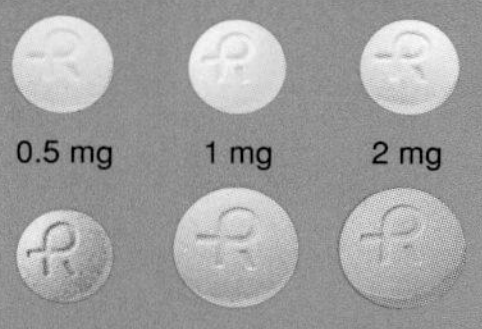

0.5 mg 1 mg 2 mg 5 mg 10 mg 20 mg

Tablets
Purepac

Hydralazine

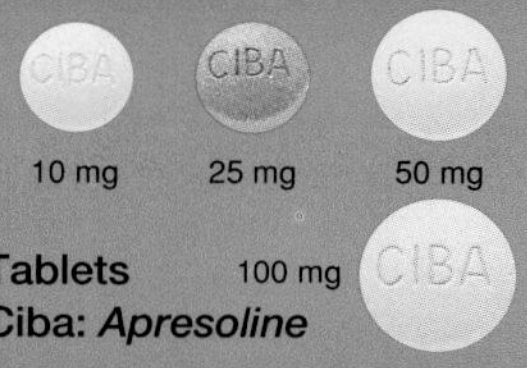

10 mg 25 mg 50 mg 100 mg

Tablets
Ciba: *Apresoline*

25 mg 50 mg

Tablets
Lederle

Hydralazine and Hydrochlorothiazide

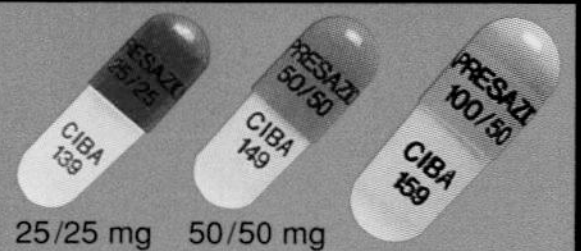

25/25 mg 50/50 mg 100/50 mg

Capsules
Ciba: *Apresazide*

Hydrochlorothiazide

25 mg 50 mg

Tablets
Abbott: *Oretic*

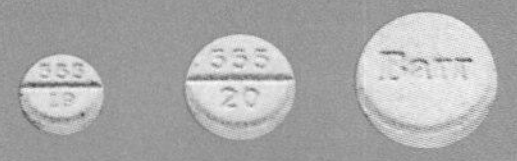

25 mg 50 mg 100 mg

Tablets
Barr

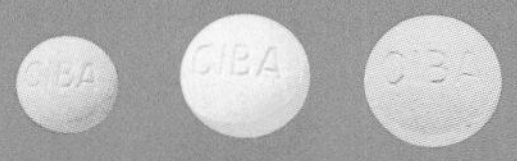

25 mg 50 mg 100 mg

Tablets
Ciba: *Esidrix*

25 mg 50 mg

Tablets
Geneva

25 mg 50 mg 100 mg

Tablets
Merck: *HydroDIURIL*

Hydrocodone and Acetaminophen

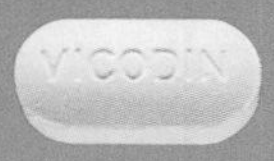

5/500 mg

Tablets
Knoll: *Vicodin*

7.5/750 mg

Tablets
Knoll: *Vicodin ES*

(continued)

Hydrocodone and Acetaminophen *(continued)*

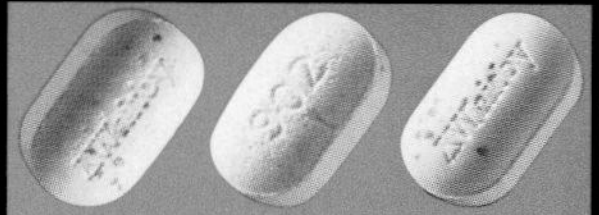

2.5/500 mg 5/500 mg 7.5/500 mg

Tablets
Whitby: *Lortab*

Hydrocortisone

5 mg 10 mg 20 mg

Tablets
Upjohn: *Cortef*

Hydromorphone

2 mg 4 mg 8 mg

Tablets
Knoll: *Dilaudid*

Hydroxychloroquine*

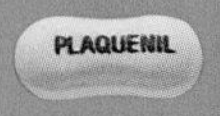

200 mg

Tablets
Sanofi Winthrop Pharmaceuticals: *Plaquenil*

Hydroxyzine

10 mg 25 mg 50 mg

Tablets
Geneva

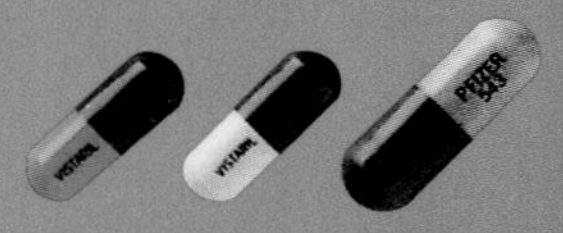

25 mg 50 mg 100 mg

Capsules
Pfizer: *Vistaril*

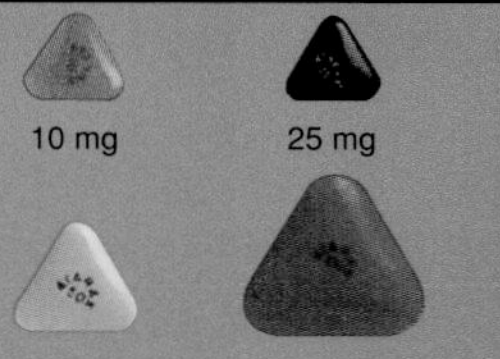

10 mg 25 mg 50 mg 100 mg

Tablets
Roerig: *Atarax*

(continued)

1 2 3 4 5 6 7

*Single source product for solid oral dosage forms in the U.S.

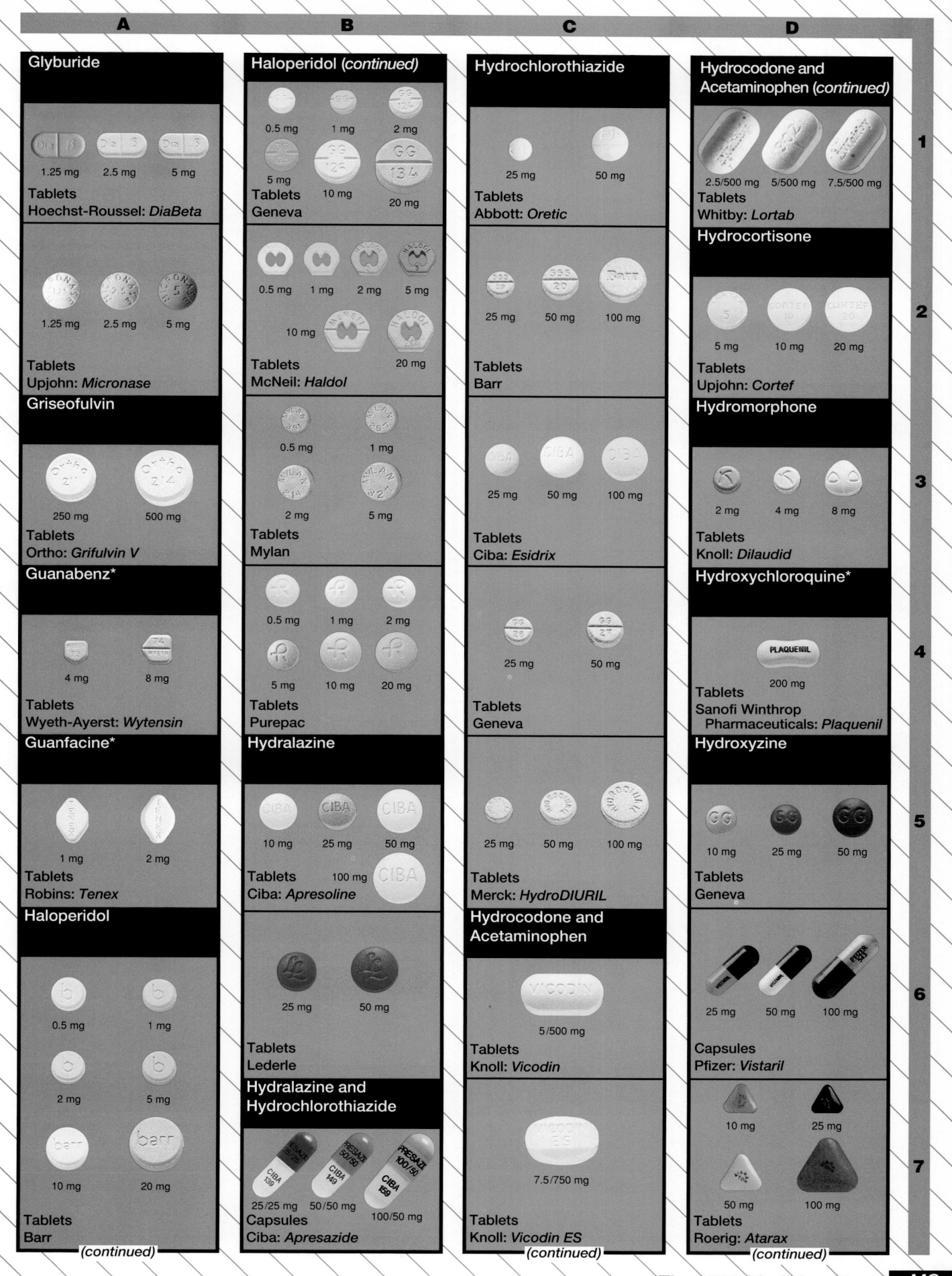

A

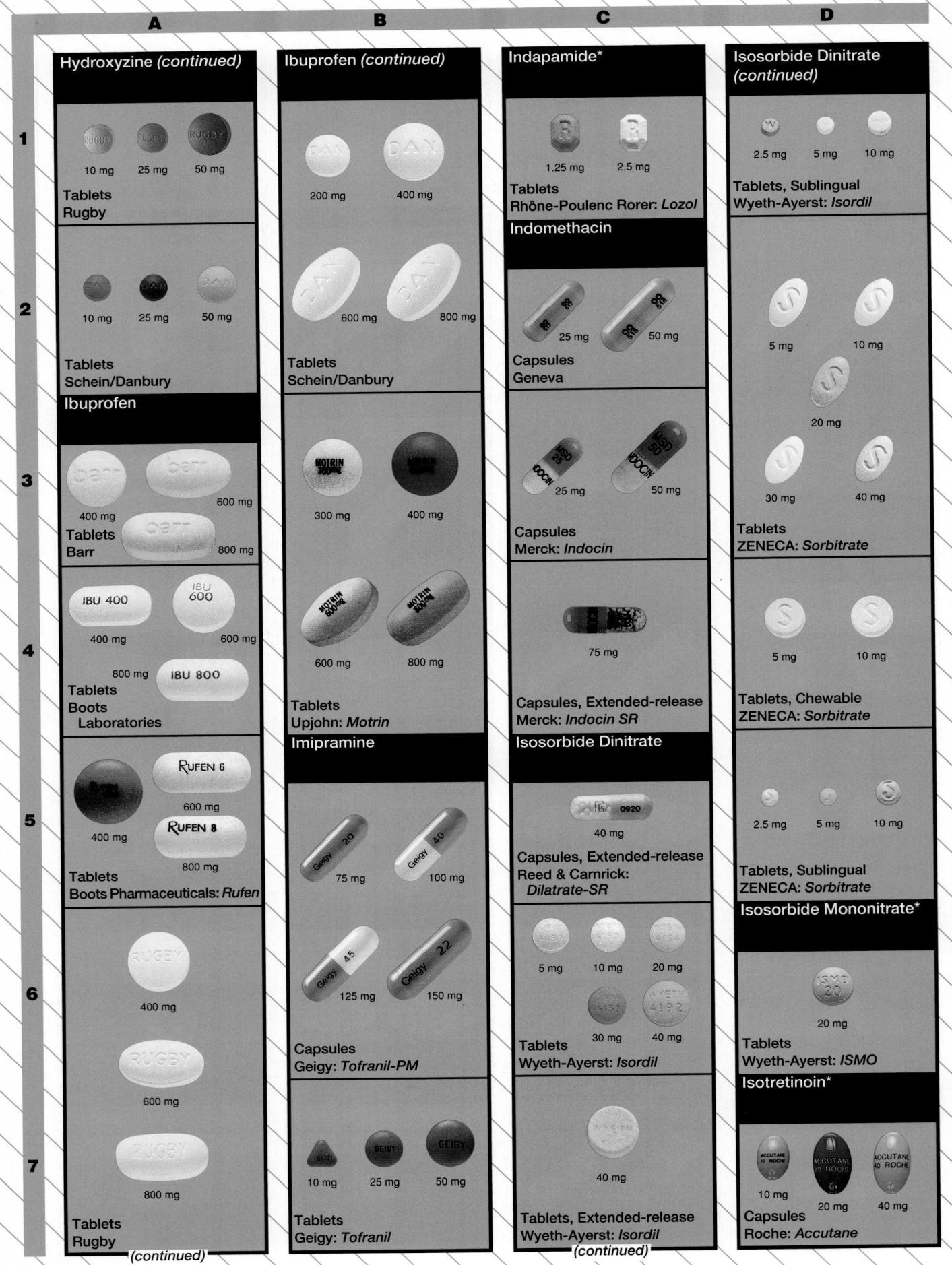

Hydroxyzine *(continued)*

10 mg 25 mg 50 mg

Tablets
Rugby

10 mg 25 mg 50 mg

Tablets
Schein/Danbury

Ibuprofen

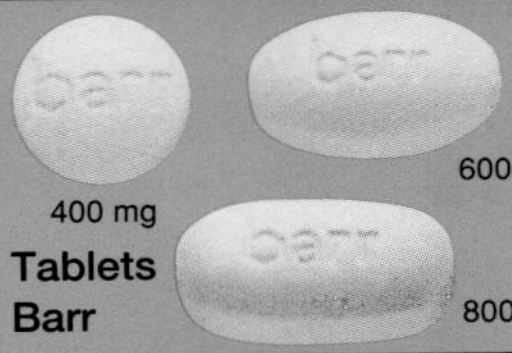

400 mg 600 mg 800 mg

Tablets
Barr

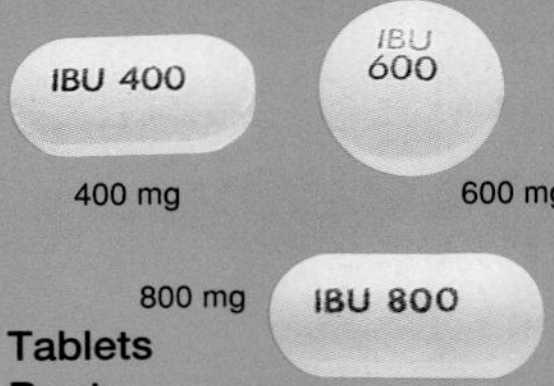

400 mg 600 mg 800 mg

Tablets
Boots Laboratories

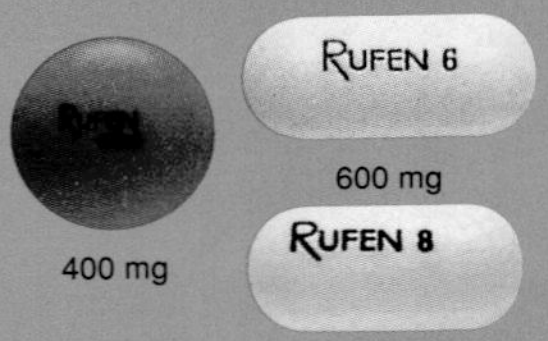

400 mg 600 mg 800 mg

Tablets
Boots Pharmaceuticals: *Rufen*

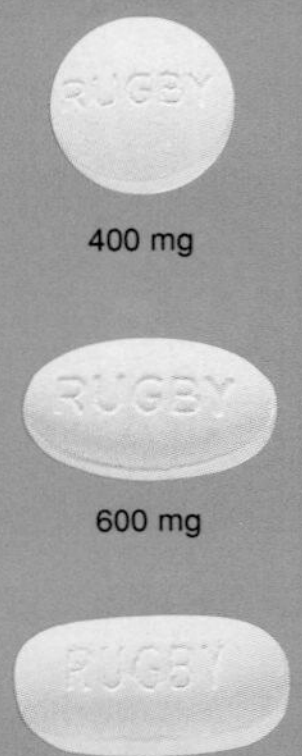

400 mg 600 mg 800 mg

Tablets
Rugby

(continued)

B

Ibuprofen *(continued)*

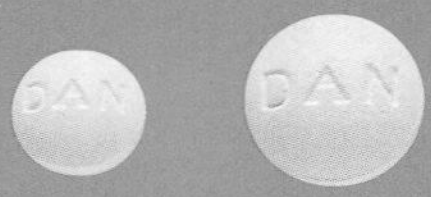

200 mg 400 mg

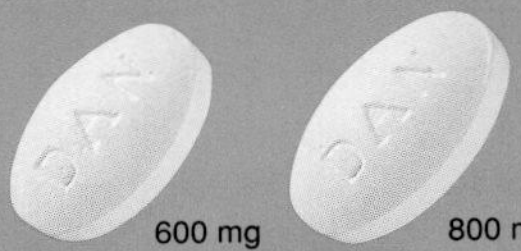

600 mg 800 mg

Tablets
Schein/Danbury

300 mg 400 mg

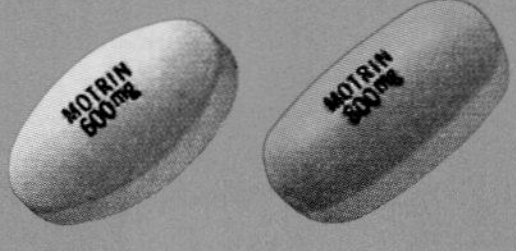

600 mg 800 mg

Tablets
Upjohn: *Motrin*

Imipramine

75 mg 100 mg

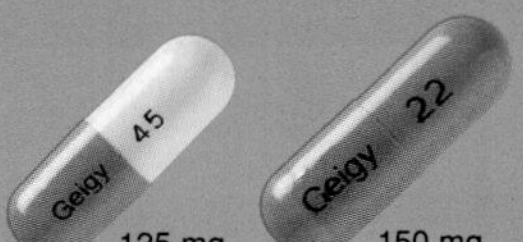

125 mg 150 mg

Capsules
Geigy: *Tofranil-PM*

10 mg 25 mg 50 mg

Tablets
Geigy: *Tofranil*

C

Indapamide*

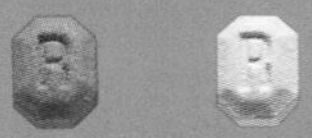

1.25 mg 2.5 mg

Tablets
Rhône-Poulenc Rorer: *Lozol*

Indomethacin

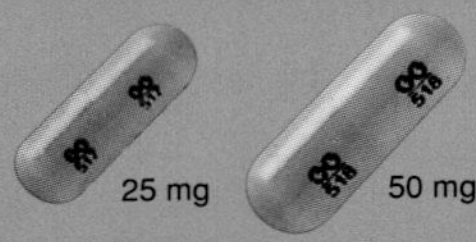

25 mg 50 mg

Capsules
Geneva

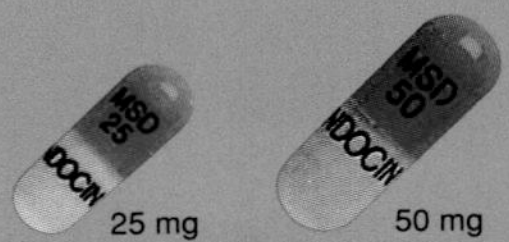

25 mg 50 mg

Capsules
Merck: *Indocin*

75 mg

Capsules, Extended-release
Merck: *Indocin SR*

Isosorbide Dinitrate

40 mg

Capsules, Extended-release
Reed & Carnrick: *Dilatrate-SR*

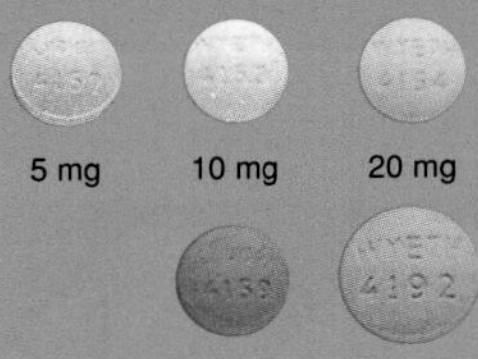

5 mg 10 mg 20 mg 30 mg 40 mg

Tablets
Wyeth-Ayerst: *Isordil*

40 mg

Tablets, Extended-release
Wyeth-Ayerst: *Isordil*

(continued)

D

Isosorbide Dinitrate *(continued)*

2.5 mg 5 mg 10 mg

Tablets, Sublingual
Wyeth-Ayerst: *Isordil*

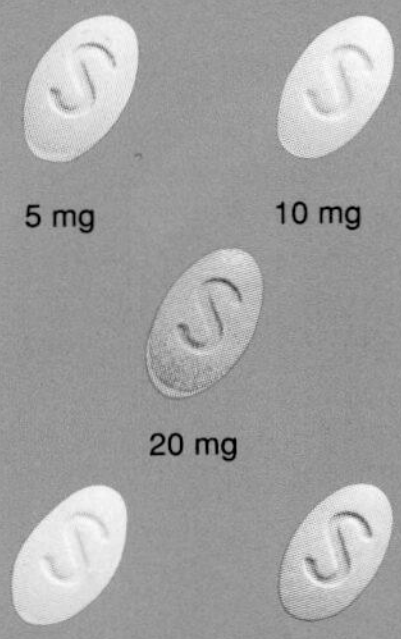

5 mg 10 mg 20 mg 30 mg 40 mg

Tablets
ZENECA: *Sorbitrate*

5 mg 10 mg

Tablets, Chewable
ZENECA: *Sorbitrate*

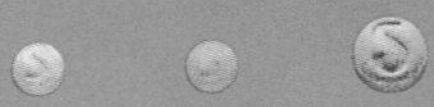

2.5 mg 5 mg 10 mg

Tablets, Sublingual
ZENECA: *Sorbitrate*

Isosorbide Mononitrate*

20 mg

Tablets
Wyeth-Ayerst: *ISMO*

Isotretinoin*

10 mg 20 mg 40 mg

Capsules
Roche: *Accutane*

*Single source product for solid oral dosage forms in the U.S.

A B C D

Isradipine*

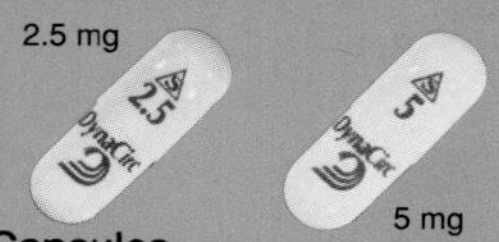

2.5 mg

5 mg

Capsules
Sandoz: *DynaCirc*

Itraconazole*

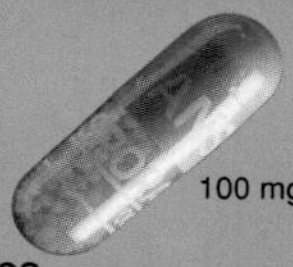

100 mg

Capsules
Janssen: *Sporanox*

Ketoconazole*

200 mg

Tablets
Janssen: *Nizoral*

Ketorolac*

10 mg

Tablets
Syntex: *Toradol*

Labetalol

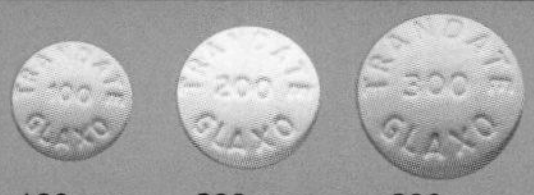

100 mg 200 mg 300 mg

Tablets
Allen & Hanburys: *Trandate*

100 mg 200 mg 300 mg

Tablets
Schering: *Normodyne*

Levonorgestrel and Ethinyl Estradiol

0.15/0.03 mg Inert ‡

‡ Included only in 28-day pack

Tablets
Berlex: *Levlen 21 and 28*

(continued)

Levonorgestrel and Ethinyl Estradiol *(cont.)*

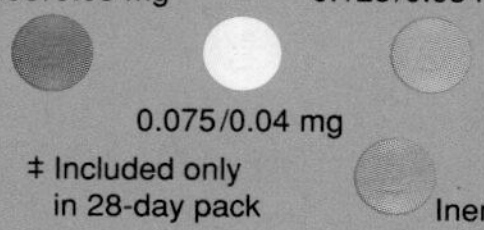

0.05/0.03 mg 0.125/0.03 mg

0.075/0.04 mg

‡ Included only in 28-day pack

Inert ‡

Tablets
Berlex: *Tri-Levlen 21 and 28*

0.15/0.03 mg Inert ‡

‡ Included only in 28-day pack

Tablets
Wyeth-Ayerst: *Nordette-21 and -28*

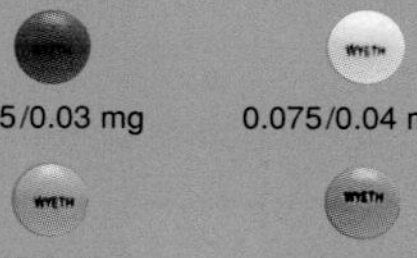

0.05/0.03 mg 0.075/0.04 mg

0.125/0.03 mg Inert ‡

‡ Included only in 28-day pack

Tablets
Wyeth-Ayerst: *Triphasil-21 and -28*

Levothyroxine

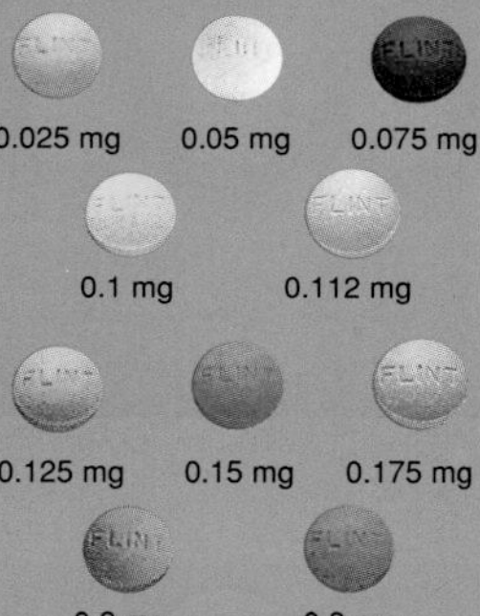

0.025 mg 0.05 mg 0.075 mg

0.1 mg 0.112 mg

0.125 mg 0.15 mg 0.175 mg

0.2 mg 0.3 mg

Tablets
Boots Pharmaceuticals: *Synthroid*

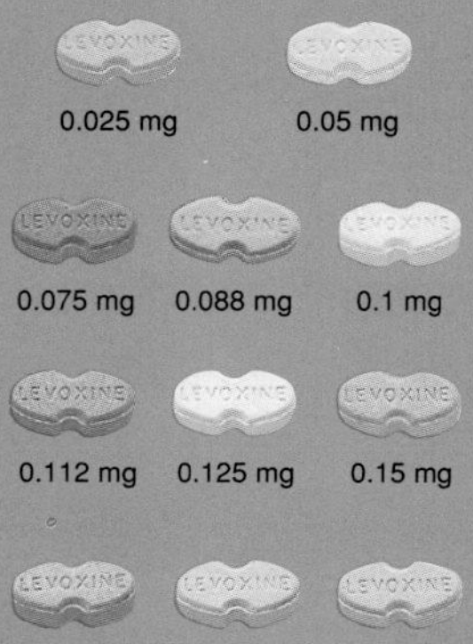

0.025 mg 0.05 mg

0.075 mg 0.088 mg 0.1 mg

0.112 mg 0.125 mg 0.15 mg

0.175 mg 0.2 mg 0.3 mg

Tablets
Daniels: *Levoxine*

(continued)

Levothyroxine *(continued)*

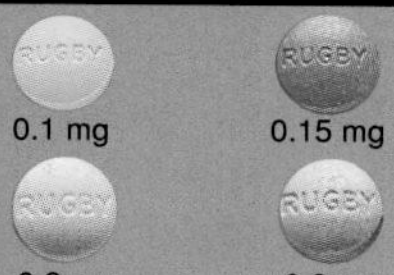

0.1 mg 0.15 mg

0.2 mg 0.3 mg

Tablets
Rugby

Lisinopril

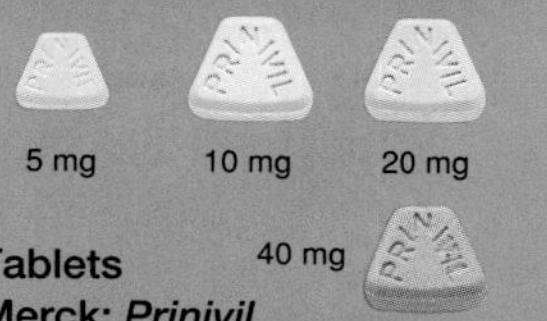

5 mg 10 mg 20 mg

40 mg

Tablets
Merck: *Prinivil*

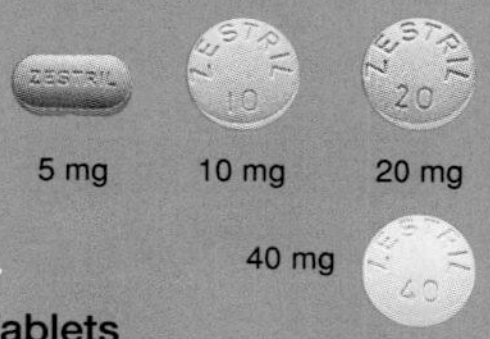

5 mg 10 mg 20 mg

40 mg

Tablets
Stuart: *Zestril*

Lisinopril and Hydrochlorothiazide

20/12.5 mg 20/25 mg

Tablets
Merck: *Prinzide*

20/12.5 mg 20/25 mg

Tablets
Stuart: *Zestoretic*

Lithium

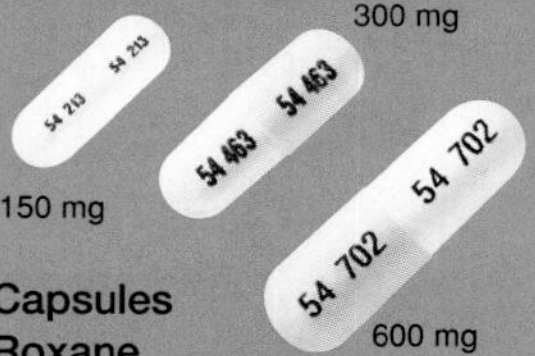

300 mg

150 mg

600 mg

Capsules
Roxane

300 mg

Tablets
Roxane

(continued)

Lithium *(continued)*

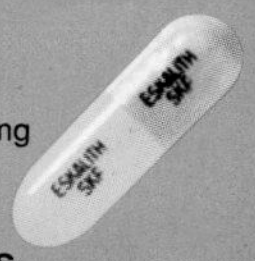

300 mg

Capsules
SmithKline Beecham: *Eskalith*

450 mg

Tablets, Extended-release
SmithKline Beecham: *Eskalith CR*

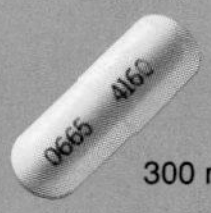

300 mg

Capsules
Solvay

Lomefloxacin*

400 mg

Tablets
Searle: *Maxaquin*

Loperamide

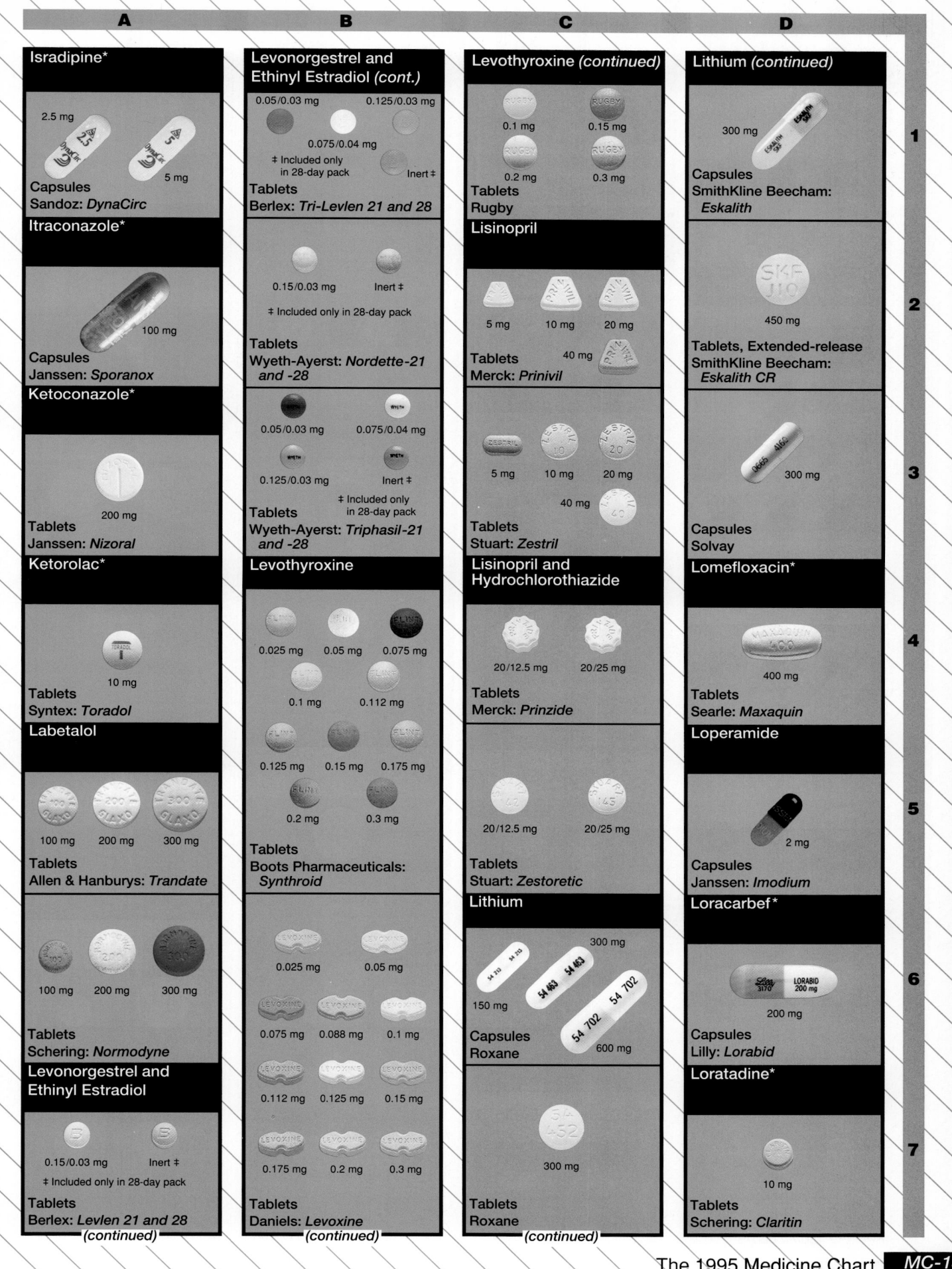

2 mg

Capsules
Janssen: *Imodium*

Loracarbef*

200 mg

Capsules
Lilly: *Lorabid*

Loratadine*

10 mg

Tablets
Schering: *Claritin*

1 2 3 4 5 6 7

*Single source product for solid oral dosage forms in the U.S.

A

Lorazepam

1

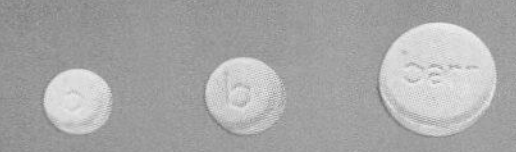

0.5 mg 1 mg 2 mg

Tablets
Barr

2

0.5 mg 1 mg 2 mg

Tablets
Purepac

3

0.5 mg 1 mg 2 mg

Tablets
Schein/Danbury

4

0.5 mg 1 mg 2 mg

Tablets
Wyeth-Ayerst: *Ativan*

Lovastatin*

5

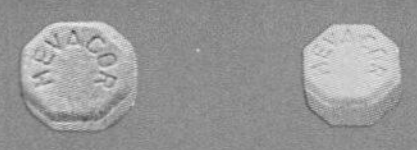

20 mg 40 mg

Tablets
Merck: *Mevacor*

Maprotiline

6

25 mg 50 mg 75 mg

Tablets
Ciba: *Ludiomil*

Meclizine

7

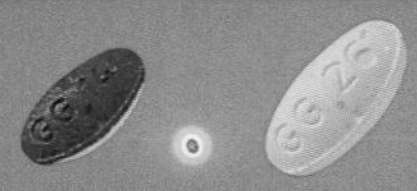

12.5 mg 25 mg

Tablets
Geneva

(continued)

B

Meclizine *(continued)*

1

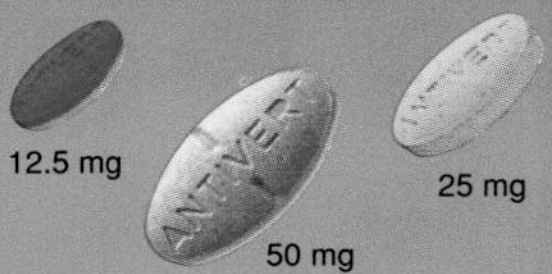

12.5 mg 50 mg 25 mg

Tablets
Roerig: *Antivert*

2

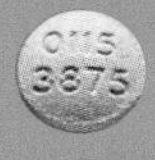

25 mg

Tablets, Chewable
Rugby

Meclofenamate

3

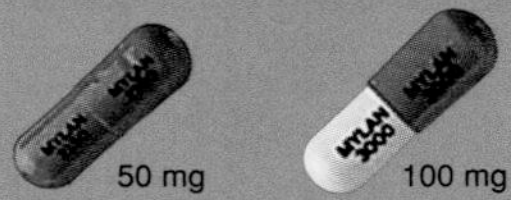

50 mg 100 mg

Capsules
Mylan

4

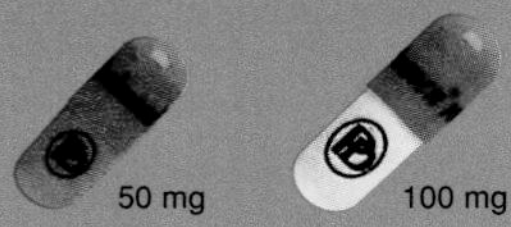

50 mg 100 mg

Capsules
PD: *Meclomen*

Medroxyprogesterone

5

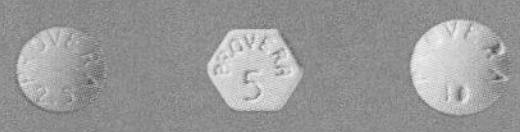

2.5 mg 5 mg 10 mg

Tablets
Upjohn: *Provera*

Meperidine

6

50 mg 100 mg

Tablets
Barr

7

50 mg 100 mg

Tablets
Sanofi Winthrop Pharmaceuticals: *Demerol*

C

Mesalamine

1

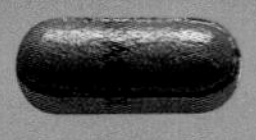

400 mg

Tablets, Delayed-release
P&GP: *Asacol*

Metaproterenol

2

10 mg 20 mg

Tablets
Boehringer Ingelheim: *Alupent*

Methocarbamol

3

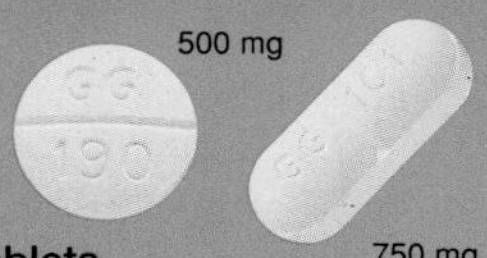

500 mg 750 mg

Tablets
Geneva

4

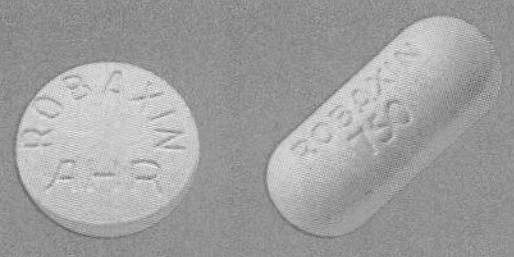

500 mg 750 mg

Tablets
Robins: *Robaxin*

Methocarbamol and Aspirin

5

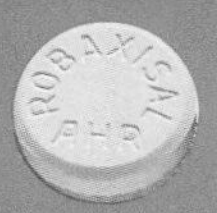

400/325 mg

Tablets
Robins: *Robaxisal*

Methyclothiazide

6

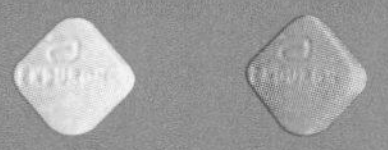

2.5 mg 5 mg

Tablets
Abbott: *Enduron*

7

2.5 mg 5 mg

Tablets
Geneva

D

Methyldopa

1

125 mg 250 mg 500 mg

Tablets
Geneva

2

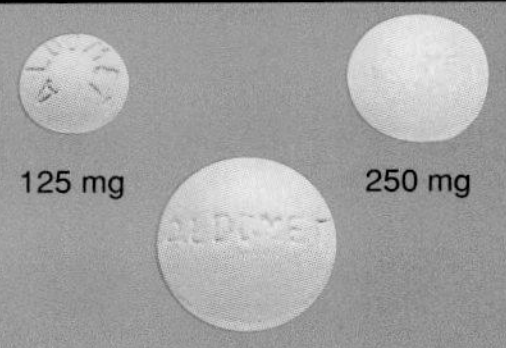

125 mg 250 mg 500 mg

Tablets
Merck: *Aldomet*

3

250 mg 500 mg

Tablets
Rugby

4

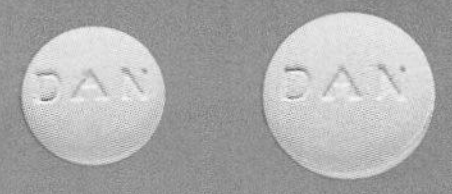

250 mg 500 mg

Tablets
Schein/Danbury

Methyldopa and Hydrochlorothiazide

5–6

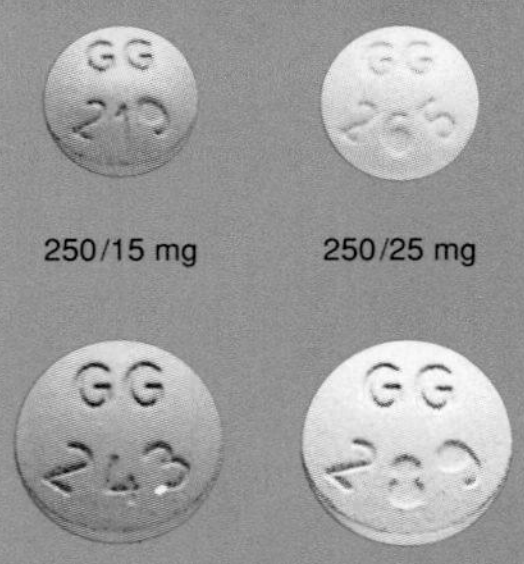

250/15 mg 250/25 mg
500/30 mg 500/50 mg

Tablets
Geneva

7

250/15 mg 250/25 mg

Tablets
Merck: *Aldoril*

(continued)

*Single source product for solid oral dosage forms in the U.S.

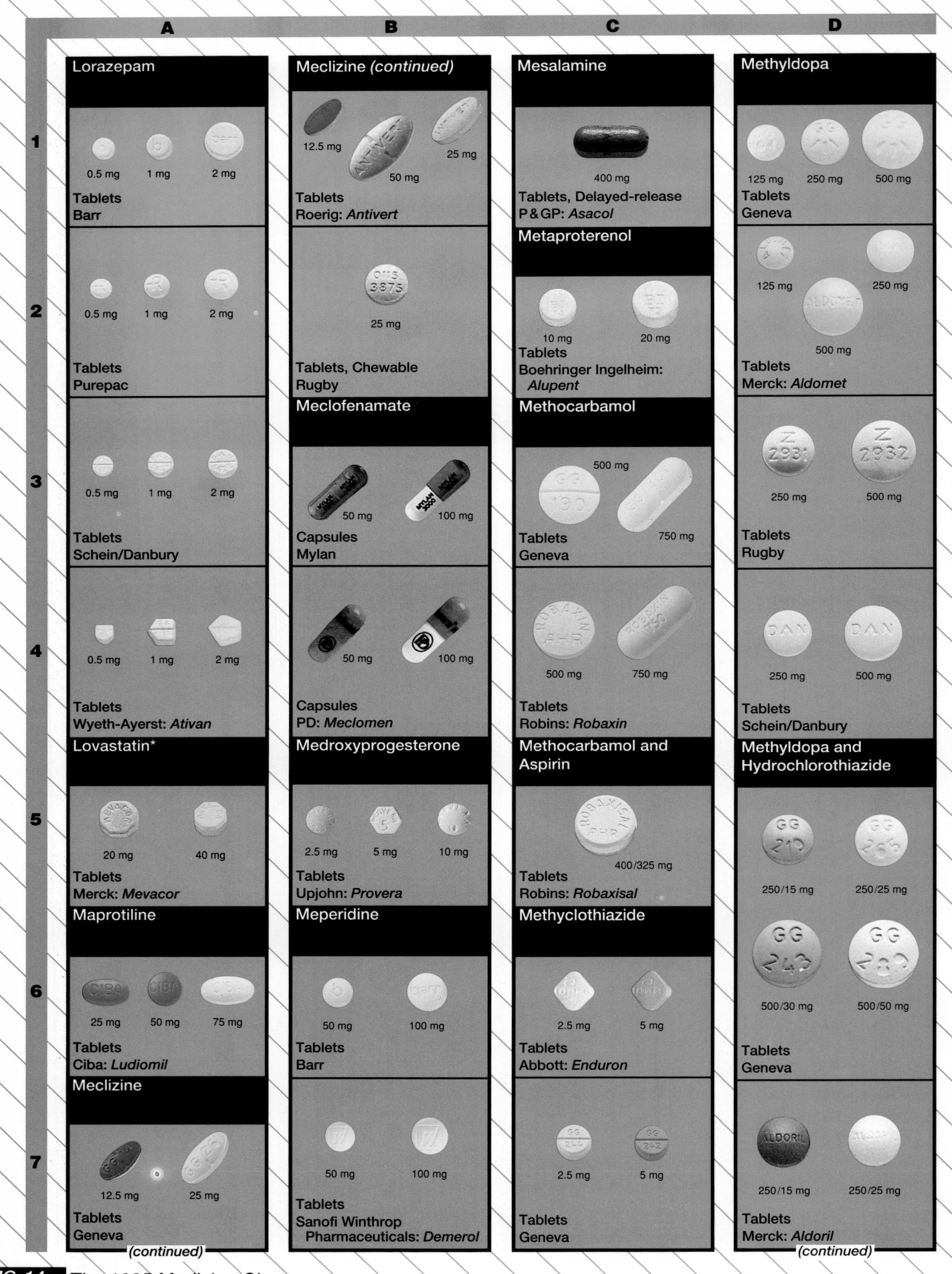

A | B | C | D

Methyldopa and Hydrochlorothiazide *(cont.)*

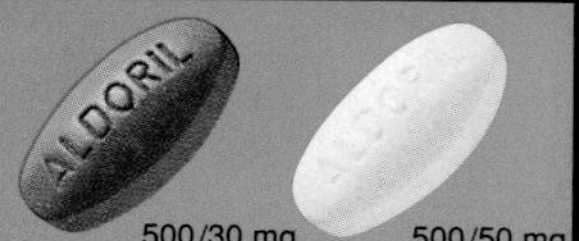

500/30 mg 500/50 mg

Tablets
Merck: *Aldoril*

Methylphenidate

5 mg 10 mg 20 mg

Tablets
Ciba: *Ritalin*

20 mg

Tablets, Extended-release
Ciba: *Ritalin-SR*

Methylprednisolone

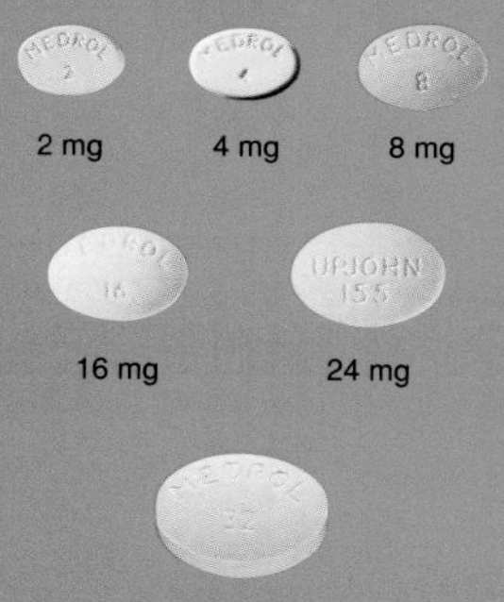

2 mg 4 mg 8 mg
16 mg 24 mg
32 mg

Tablets
Upjohn: *Medrol*

Metoclopramide

10 mg

Tablets
Purepac

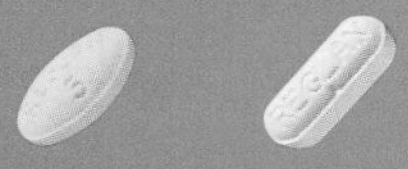

5 mg 10 mg

Tablets
Robins: *Reglan*

(continued)

Metoclopramide *(continued)*

10 mg

Tablets
Rugby

10 mg

Tablets
Schein/Danbury

Metolazone

0.5 mg

Tablets
Fisons: *Mykrox*

2.5 mg 5 mg 10 mg

Tablets
Fisons: *Zaroxolyn*

Metoprolol Succinate

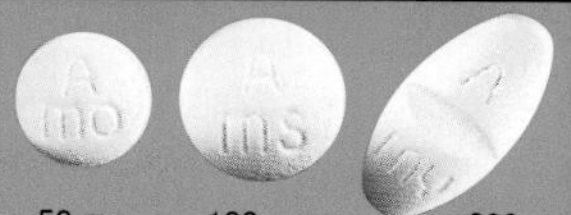

50 mg 100 mg 200 mg

Tablets, Extended-release
Astra: *Toprol XL*

Metoprolol Tartrate

50 mg 100 mg

Tablets
Geigy: *Lopressor*

50 mg 100 mg

Tablets
Mutual

Metoprolol and Hydrochlorothiazide*

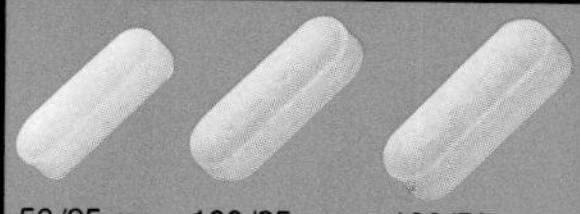

50/25 mg 100/25 mg 100/50 mg

Tablets
Geigy: *Lopressor HCT*

Metronidazole

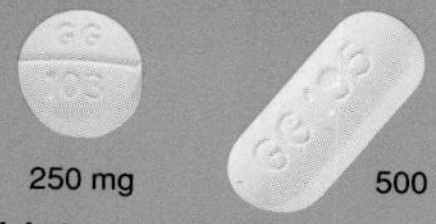

250 mg 500 mg

Tablets
Geneva

250 mg 500 mg

Tablets
Rugby

250 mg 500 mg

Tablets
Schein/Danbury

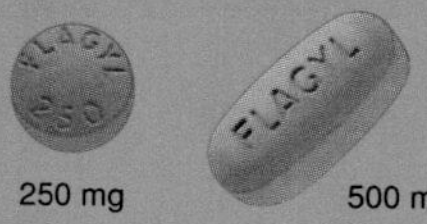

250 mg 500 mg

Tablets
Searle: *Flagyl*

Minocycline

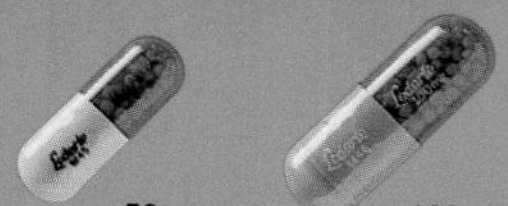

50 mg 100 mg

Capsules
Lederle: *Minocin*

50 mg 100 mg

Tablets
Lederle

(continued)

Minocycline *(continued)*

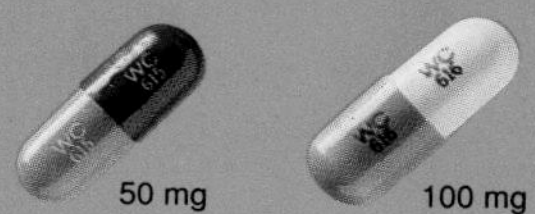

50 mg 100 mg

Capsules
Warner Chilcott

Minoxidil

2.5 mg 10 mg

Tablets
Schein/Danbury

2.5 mg 10 mg

Tablets
Upjohn: *Loniten*

Misoprostol*

0.1 mg 0.2 mg

Tablets
Searle: *Cytotec*

Moricizine*

200 mg

250 mg

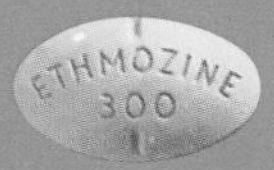

300 mg

Tablets
DuPont: *Ethmozine*

Nabumetone*

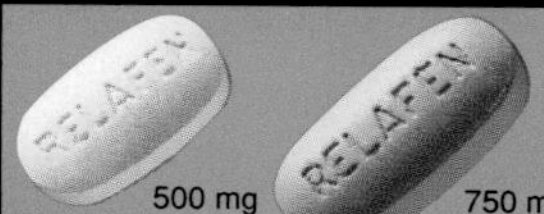

500 mg 750 mg

Tablets
SmithKline Beecham: *Relafen*

1 2 3 4 5 6 7

*Single source product for solid oral dosage forms in the U.S.

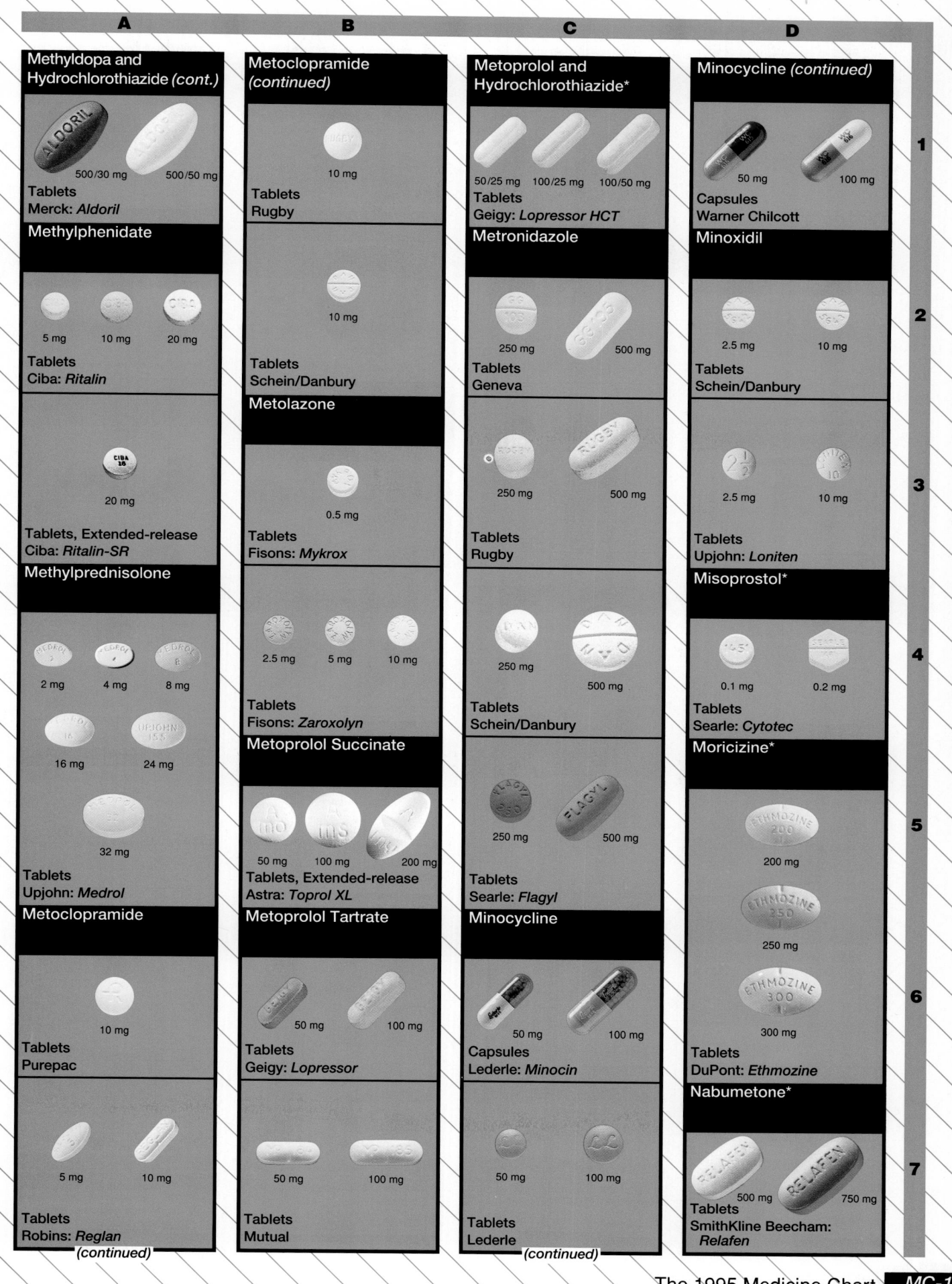

A

Nadolol*

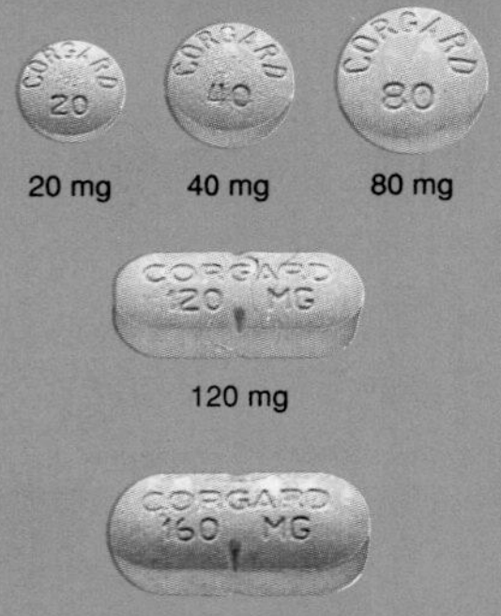

20 mg 40 mg 80 mg

120 mg

160 mg

Tablets
Bristol: *Corgard*

Nadolol and Bendroflumethiazide*

40/5 mg 80/5 mg

Tablets
Bristol: *Corzide*

Nalidixic Acid*

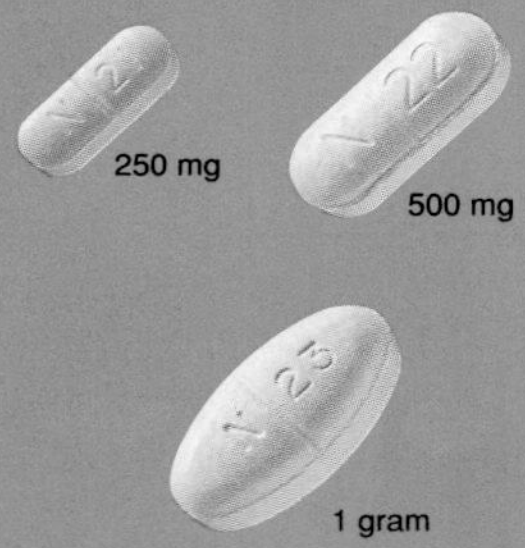

250 mg 500 mg

1 gram

Tablets
Sanofi Winthrop Pharmaceuticals: *NegGram*

Naproxen

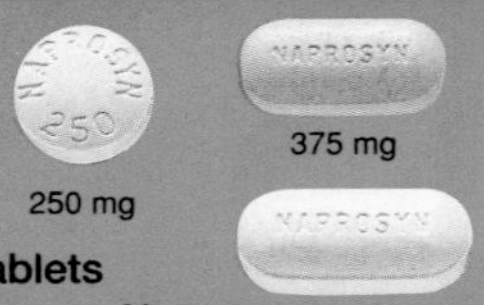

250 mg 375 mg 500 mg

Tablets
Syntex: *Naprosyn*

Naproxen Sodium

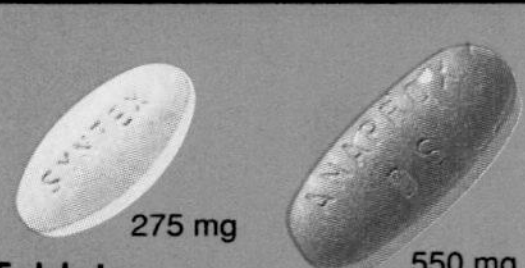

275 mg 550 mg

Tablets
Syntex: *Anaprox*

B

Niacin

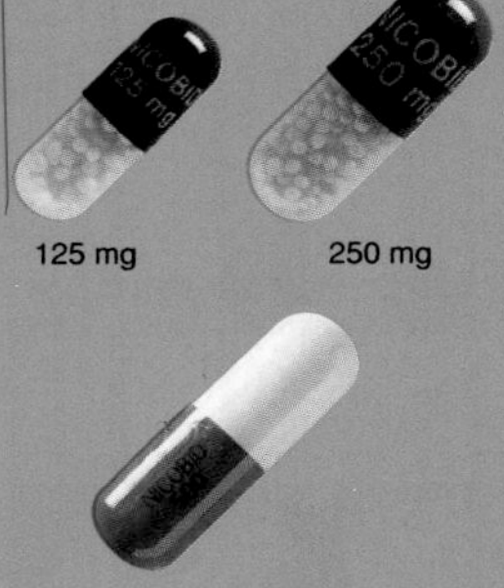

125 mg 250 mg

500 mg

Capsules, Extended-release
Rhône-Poulenc Rorer: *Nicobid*

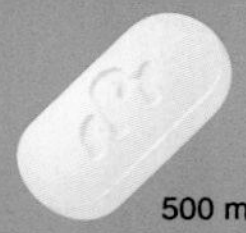

500 mg

Tablets
Rhône-Poulenc Rorer: *Nicolar*

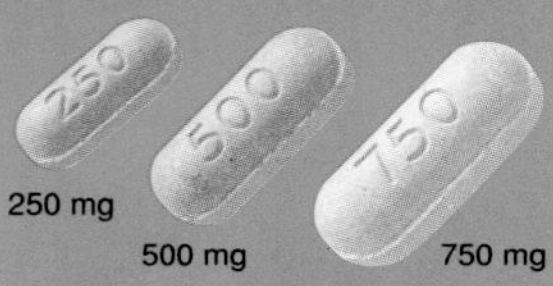

250 mg 500 mg 750 mg

Tablets, Extended-release
Upsher-Smith: *Slo-Niacin*

Nicardipine*

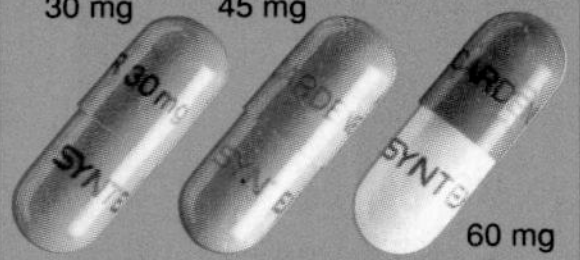

30 mg 45 mg 60 mg

Capsules, Extended-release
Syntex: *Cardene SR*

Nicotine*

2 mg

Tablets, Chewing Gum
SmithKline Beecham: *Nicorette*

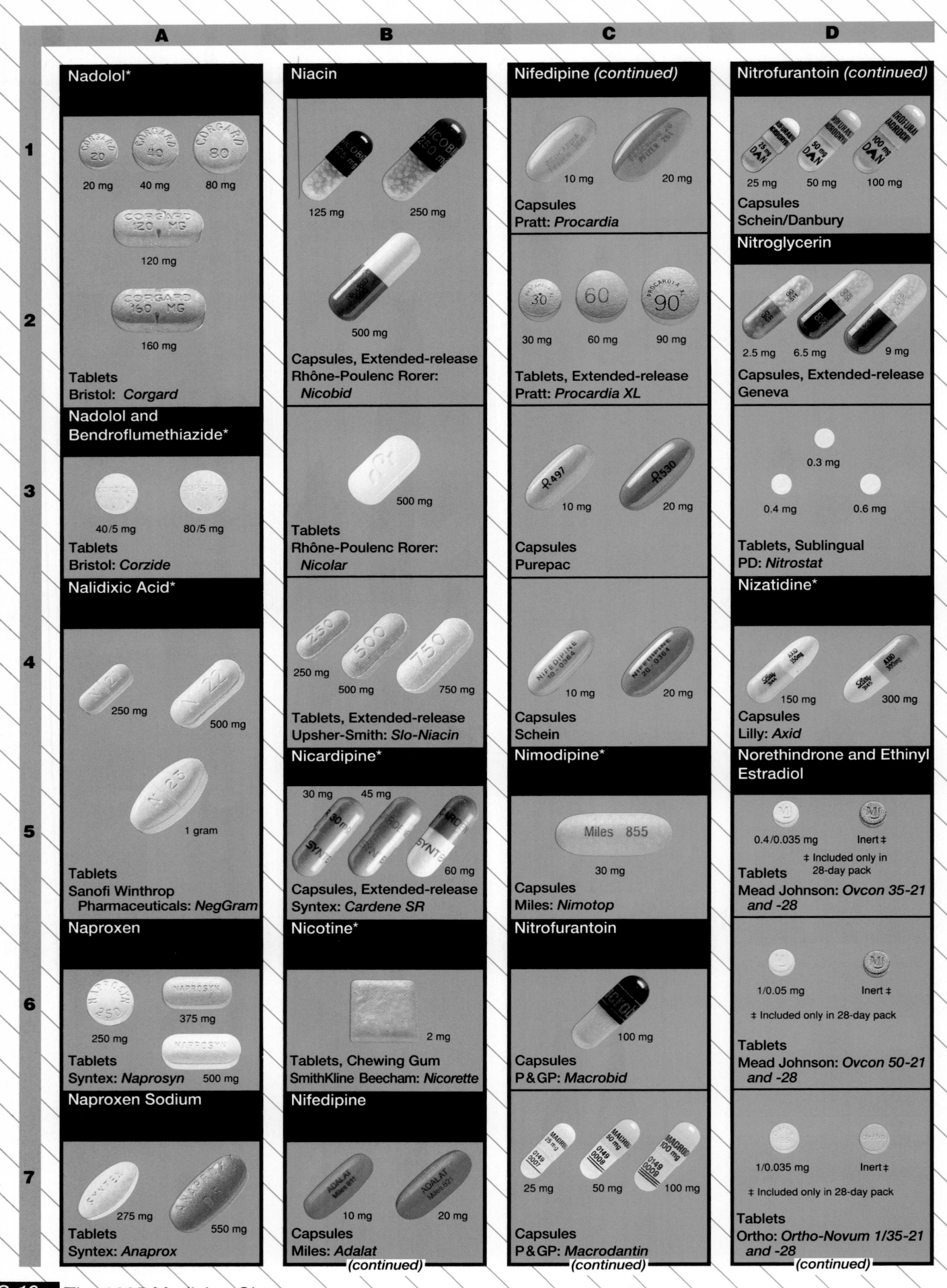

Nifedipine

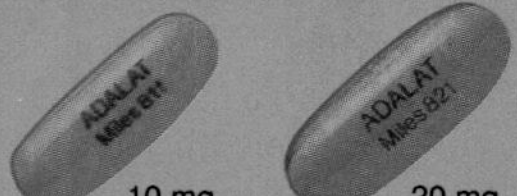

10 mg 20 mg

Capsules
Miles: *Adalat*

(continued)

C

Nifedipine *(continued)*

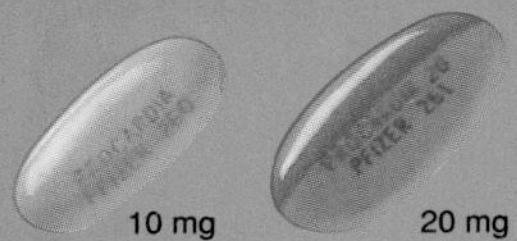

10 mg 20 mg

Capsules
Pratt: *Procardia*

30 mg 60 mg 90 mg

Tablets, Extended-release
Pratt: *Procardia XL*

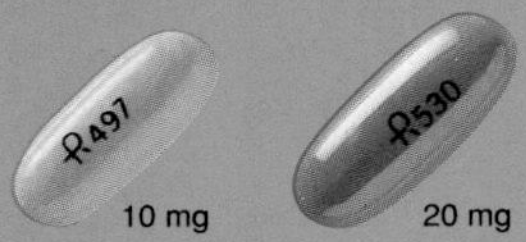

10 mg 20 mg

Capsules
Purepac

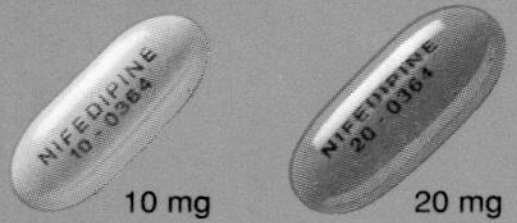

10 mg 20 mg

Capsules
Schein

Nimodipine*

30 mg

Capsules
Miles: *Nimotop*

Nitrofurantoin

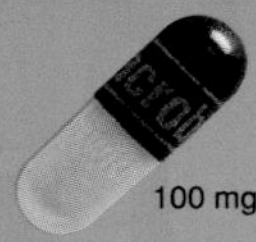

100 mg

Capsules
P&GP: *Macrobid*

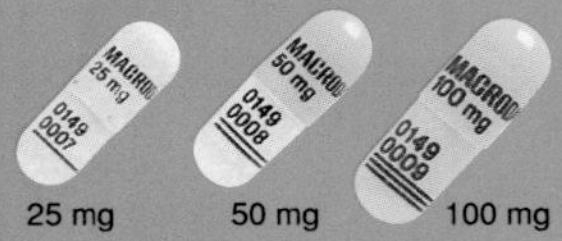

25 mg 50 mg 100 mg

Capsules
P&GP: *Macrodantin*

(continued)

D

Nitrofurantoin *(continued)*

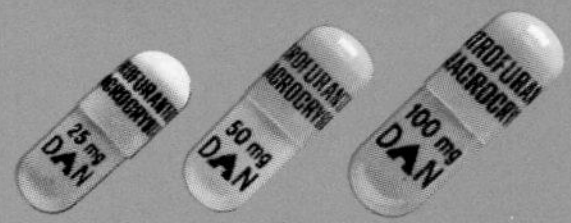

25 mg 50 mg 100 mg

Capsules
Schein/Danbury

Nitroglycerin

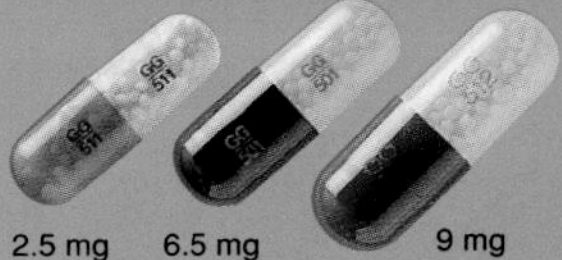

2.5 mg 6.5 mg 9 mg

Capsules, Extended-release
Geneva

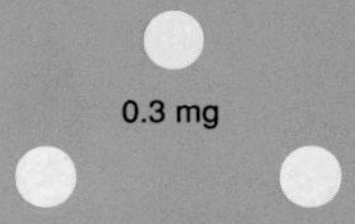

0.3 mg

0.4 mg 0.6 mg

Tablets, Sublingual
PD: *Nitrostat*

Nizatidine*

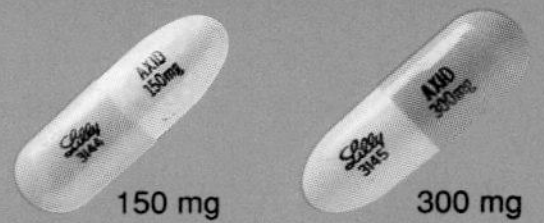

150 mg 300 mg

Capsules
Lilly: *Axid*

Norethindrone and Ethinyl Estradiol

0.4/0.035 mg Inert ‡

‡ Included only in 28-day pack

Tablets
Mead Johnson: *Ovcon 35-21 and -28*

1/0.05 mg Inert ‡

‡ Included only in 28-day pack

Tablets
Mead Johnson: *Ovcon 50-21 and -28*

1/0.035 mg Inert ‡

‡ Included only in 28-day pack

Tablets
Ortho: *Ortho-Novum 1/35-21 and -28*

(continued)

*Single source product for solid oral dosage forms in the U.S.

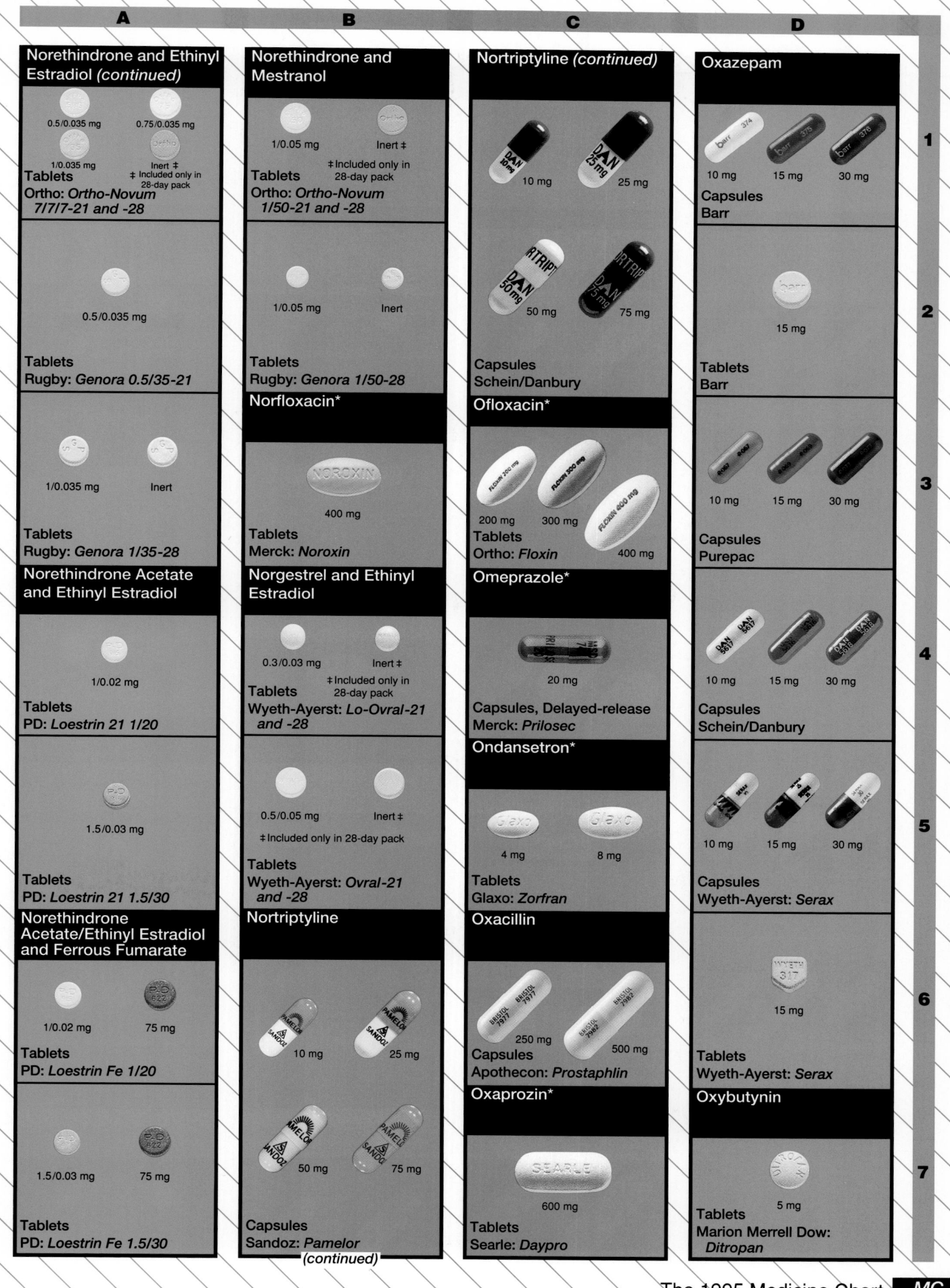

Norethindrone and Ethinyl Estradiol *(continued)*

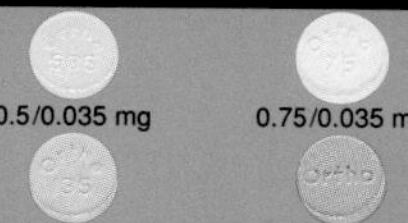

0.5/0.035 mg 0.75/0.035 mg

1/0.035 mg Inert ‡

‡ Included only in 28-day pack

Tablets
Ortho: *Ortho-Novum 7/7/7-21 and -28*

0.5/0.035 mg

Tablets
Rugby: *Genora 0.5/35-21*

1/0.035 mg Inert

Tablets
Rugby: *Genora 1/35-28*

Norethindrone Acetate and Ethinyl Estradiol

1/0.02 mg

Tablets
PD: *Loestrin 21 1/20*

1.5/0.03 mg

Tablets
PD: *Loestrin 21 1.5/30*

Norethindrone Acetate/Ethinyl Estradiol and Ferrous Fumarate

1/0.02 mg 75 mg

Tablets
PD: *Loestrin Fe 1/20*

1.5/0.03 mg 75 mg

Tablets
PD: *Loestrin Fe 1.5/30*

Norethindrone and Mestranol

1/0.05 mg Inert ‡

‡Included only in 28-day pack

Tablets
Ortho: *Ortho-Novum 1/50-21 and -28*

1/0.05 mg Inert

Tablets
Rugby: *Genora 1/50-28*

Norfloxacin*

400 mg

Tablets
Merck: *Noroxin*

Norgestrel and Ethinyl Estradiol

0.3/0.03 mg Inert ‡

‡Included only in 28-day pack

Tablets
Wyeth-Ayerst: *Lo-Ovral-21 and -28*

0.5/0.05 mg Inert ‡

‡Included only in 28-day pack

Tablets
Wyeth-Ayerst: *Ovral-21 and -28*

Nortriptyline

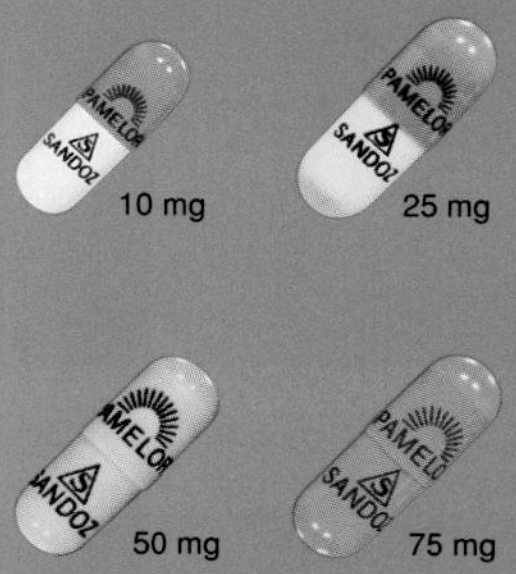

10 mg 25 mg

50 mg 75 mg

Capsules
Sandoz: *Pamelor*

(continued)

Nortriptyline *(continued)*

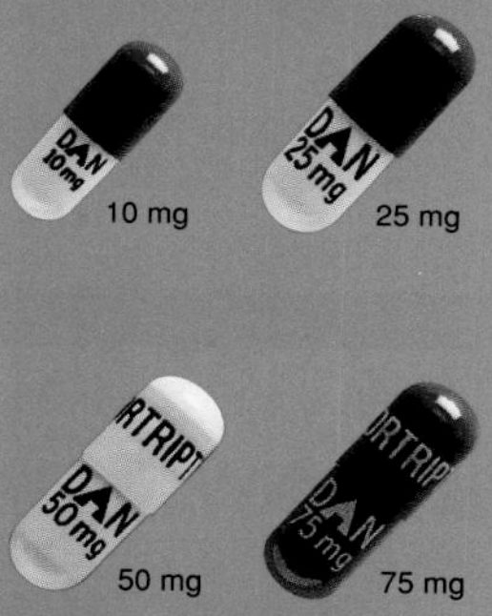

10 mg 25 mg

50 mg 75 mg

Capsules
Schein/Danbury

Ofloxacin*

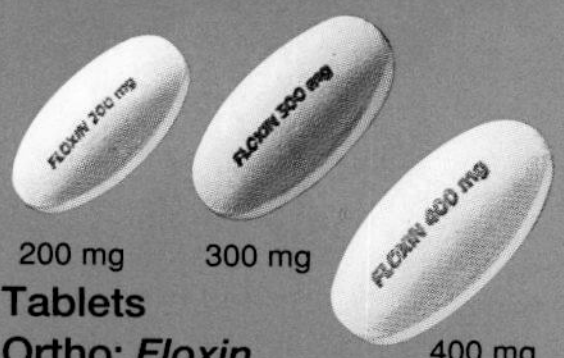

200 mg 300 mg 400 mg

Tablets
Ortho: *Floxin*

Omeprazole*

20 mg

Capsules, Delayed-release
Merck: *Prilosec*

Ondansetron*

4 mg 8 mg

Tablets
Glaxo: *Zorfran*

Oxacillin

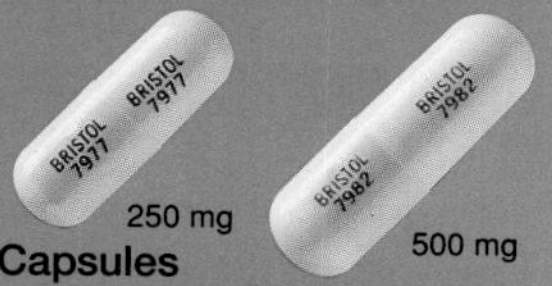

250 mg 500 mg

Capsules
Apothecon: *Prostaphlin*

Oxaprozin*

600 mg

Tablets
Searle: *Daypro*

Oxazepam

10 mg 15 mg 30 mg

Capsules
Barr

15 mg

Tablets
Barr

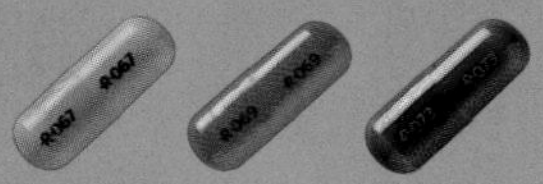

10 mg 15 mg 30 mg

Capsules
Purepac

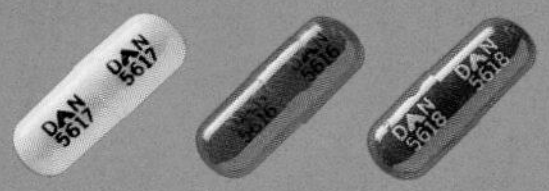

10 mg 15 mg 30 mg

Capsules
Schein/Danbury

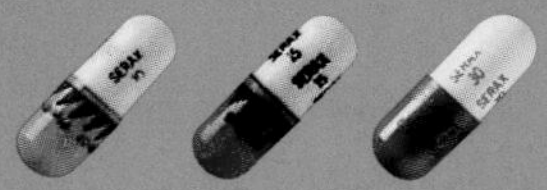

10 mg 15 mg 30 mg

Capsules
Wyeth-Ayerst: *Serax*

15 mg

Tablets
Wyeth-Ayerst: *Serax*

Oxybutynin

5 mg

Tablets
Marion Merrell Dow: *Ditropan*

*Single source product for solid oral dosage forms in the U.S.

A B C D

Oxycodone*

5 mg

Tablets
Roxane: *Roxicodone*

Oxycodone and Acetaminophen

5/325 mg

Tablets
DuPont: *Percocet*

5/500 mg

Capsules
McNeil: *Tylox*

5/325 mg   5/500 mg

Tablets
Roxane: *Roxicet*

Oxycodone and Aspirin

4.88/325 mg

Tablets
DuPont: *Percodan*

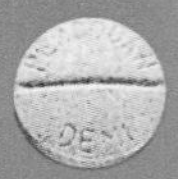
2.44/325 mg

Tablets
DuPont: *Percodan-Demi*

4.88/325 mg

Tablets
Roxane: *Roxiprin*

Pancrelipase

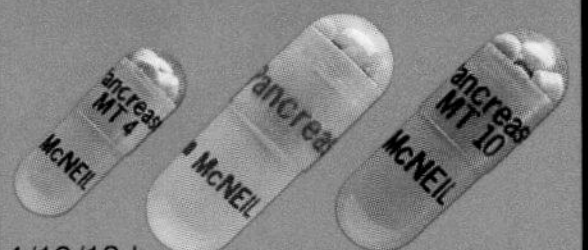
4/12/12 ‡   4/20/25 ‡   10/30/30 ‡

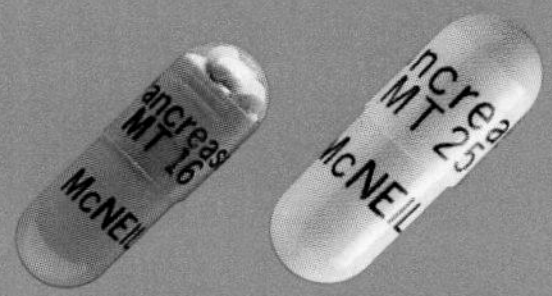
16/48/48 ‡   25/75/75 ‡

‡ In thousands of units of lipase/amylase/protease, respectively

Capsules, Delayed-release
McNeil: *Pancrease*

Paroxetine*

20 mg   30 mg

Tablets
SmithKline Beecham: *Paxil*

Penbutolol*

20 mg

Tablets
Reed & Carnrick: *Levatol*

Penicillin V

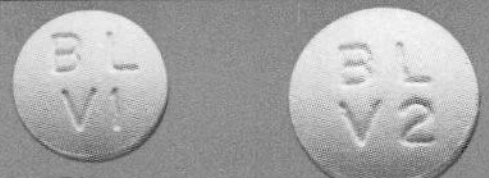
250 mg   500 mg

Tablets
Apothecon: *Veetids*

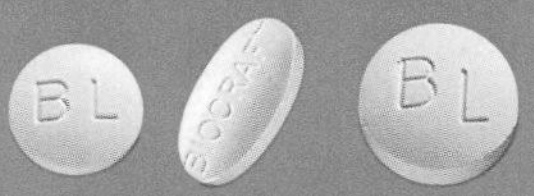
250 mg   250 mg   500 mg

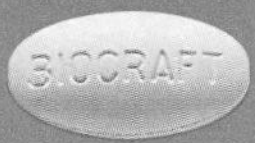
500 mg

Tablets
Biocraft

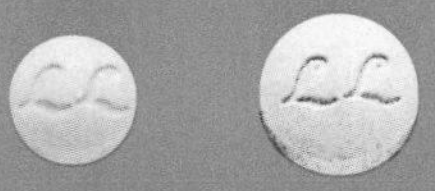
250 mg   500 mg

Tablets
Lederle: *Ledercillin VK*

(continued)

Penicillin V *(continued)*

125 mg   250 mg   500 mg

Tablets
Lilly: *V-Cillin K*

250 mg   500 mg

Tablets
Wyeth-Ayerst: *Pen-Vee K*

Pentazocine and Acetaminophen*

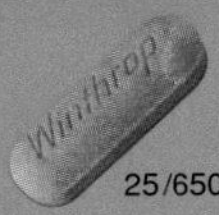
25/650 mg

Tablets
Sanofi Winthrop Pharmaceuticals: *Talacen*

Pentazocine and Naloxone*

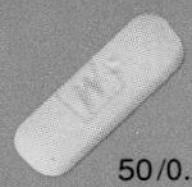
50/0.5 mg

Tablets
Sanofi Winthrop Pharmaceuticals: *Talwin-Nx*

Pentoxifylline*

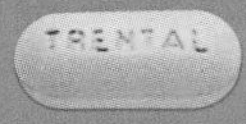
400 mg

Tablets, Extended-release
Hoechst-Roussel: *Trental*

Perphenazine and Amitriptyline

2/10 mg   2/25 mg   4/10 mg

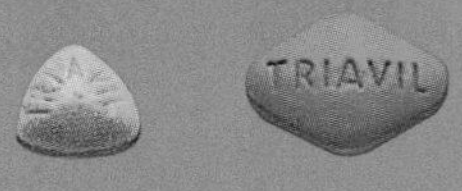
4/25 mg   4/50 mg

Tablets
Merck: *Triavil*

Phenobarbital

15 mg   30 mg   60 mg

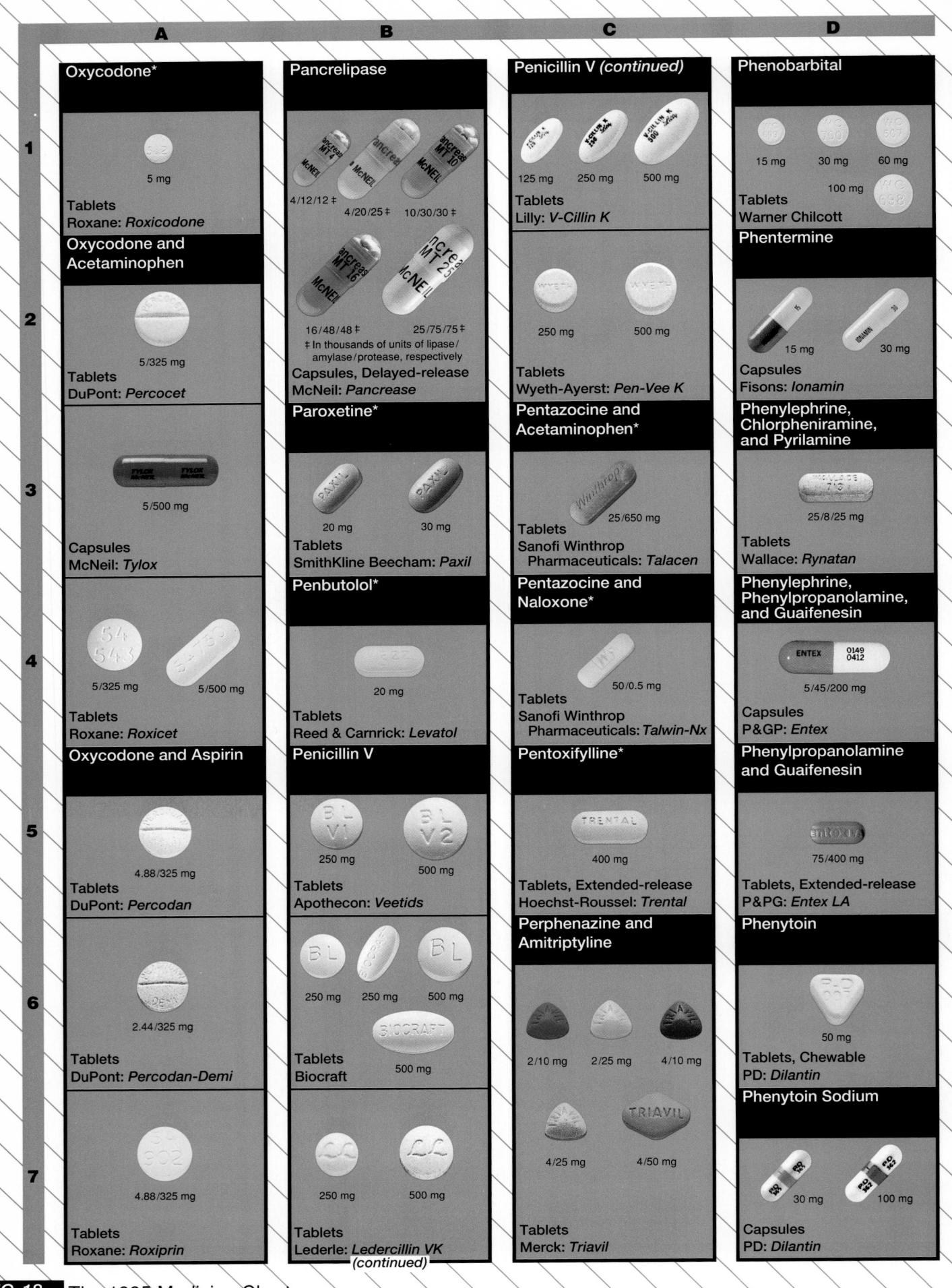
100 mg

Tablets
Warner Chilcott

Phentermine

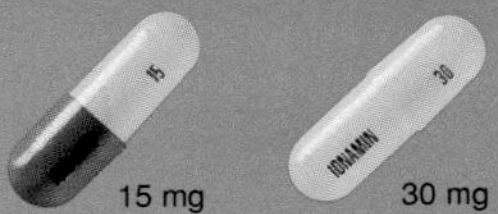
15 mg   30 mg

Capsules
Fisons: *Ionamin*

Phenylephrine, Chlorpheniramine, and Pyrilamine

25/8/25 mg

Tablets
Wallace: *Rynatan*

Phenylephrine, Phenylpropanolamine, and Guaifenesin

5/45/200 mg

Capsules
P&GP: *Entex*

Phenylpropanolamine and Guaifenesin

75/400 mg

Tablets, Extended-release
P&PG: *Entex LA*

Phenytoin

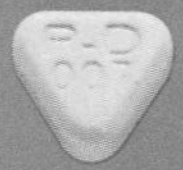
50 mg

Tablets, Chewable
PD: *Dilantin*

Phenytoin Sodium

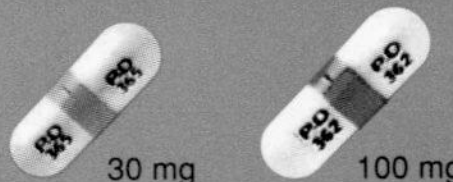
30 mg   100 mg

Capsules
PD: *Dilantin*

*Single source product for solid oral dosage forms in the U.S.

A | B | C | D

A

Pindolol

5 mg | 10 mg

Tablets
Mutual

5 mg | 10 mg

Tablets
Sandoz: *Visken*

Piroxicam

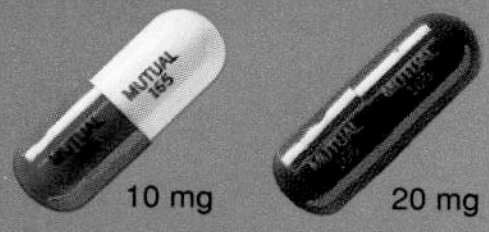
10 mg | 20 mg

Capsules
Mutual

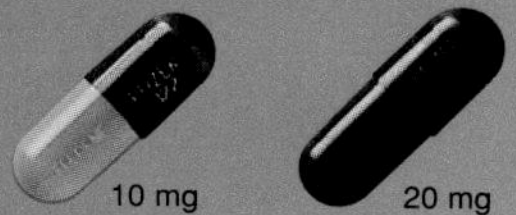
10 mg | 20 mg

Capsules
Pratt: *Feldene*

Potassium Chloride

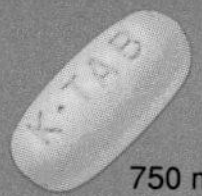
750 mg

Tablets, Extended-release
Abbott: *K-Tab*

750 mg

Tablets, Extended-release
Apothecon: *Klotrix*

750 mg | 1500 mg

Tablets, Extended-release
Key: *K-Dur*

(continued)

B

Potassium Chloride *(cont.)*

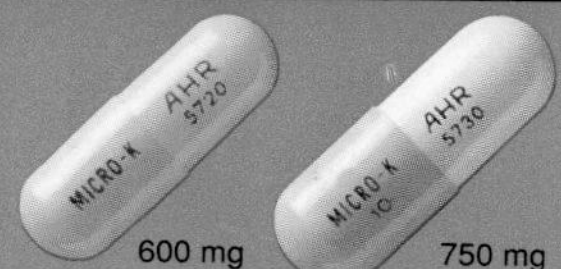
600 mg | 750 mg

Capsules, Extended-release
Robins: *Micro-K*

600 mg

Tablets, Extended-release
Summit: *Slow-K*

600 mg | 750 mg

Tablets, Extended-release
Upsher-Smith: *Klor-Con*

Pravastatin

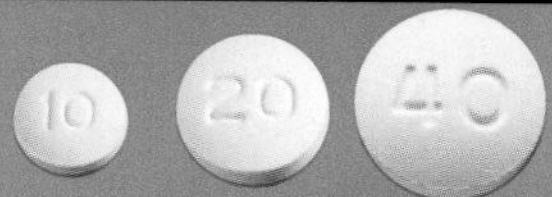
10 mg | 20 mg | 40 mg

Tablets
Squibb: *Pravachol*

Prazosin

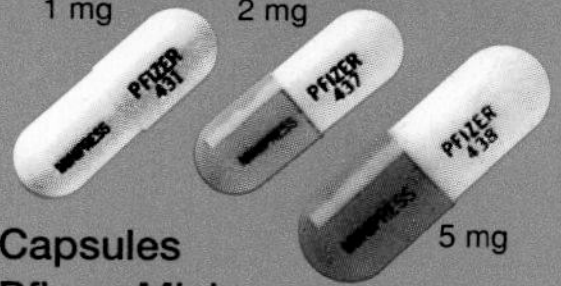
1 mg | 2 mg | 5 mg

Capsules
Pfizer: *Minipress*

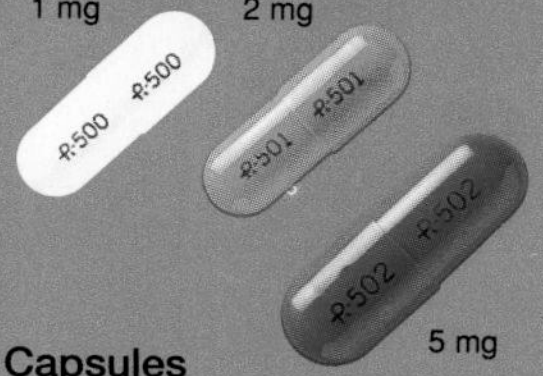
1 mg | 2 mg | 5 mg

Capsules
Purepac

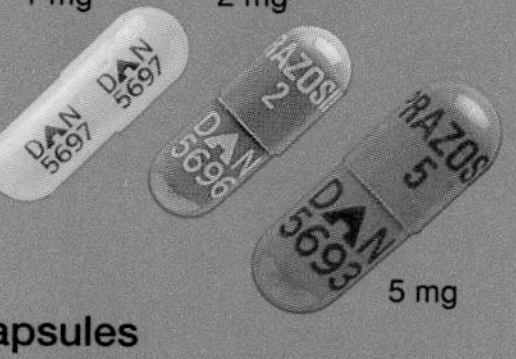
1 mg | 2 mg | 5 mg

Capsules
Schein/Danbury

C

Prazosin and Polythiazide*

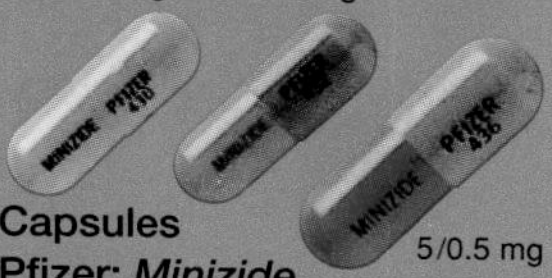
1/0.5 mg | 2/0.5 mg | 5/0.5 mg

Capsules
Pfizer: *Minizide*

Prednisone

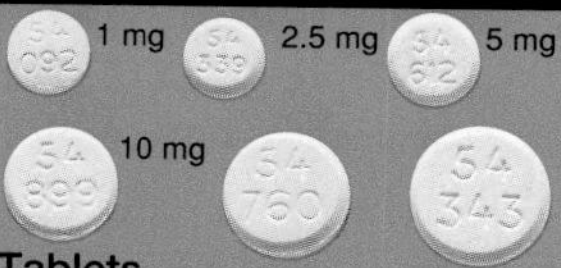
1 mg | 2.5 mg | 5 mg | 10 mg | 20 mg | 50 mg

Tablets
Roxane

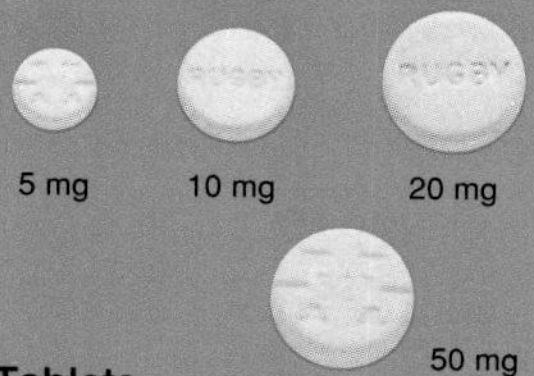
5 mg | 10 mg | 20 mg | 50 mg

Tablets
Rugby

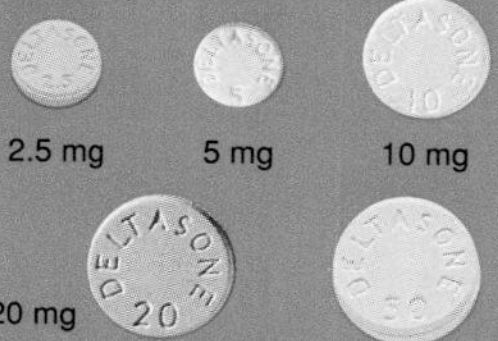
2.5 mg | 5 mg | 10 mg | 20 mg | 50 mg

Tablets
Upjohn: *Deltasone*

Probucol*

250 mg | 500 mg

Tablets
Marion Merrell Dow: *Lorelco*

Procainamide

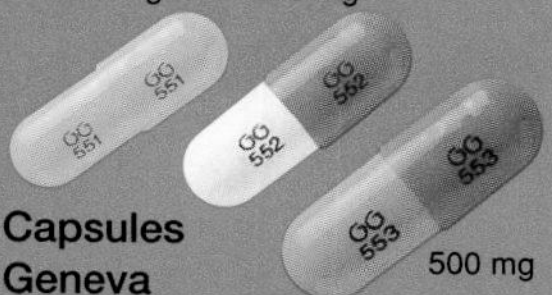
250 mg | 375 mg | 500 mg

Capsules
Geneva

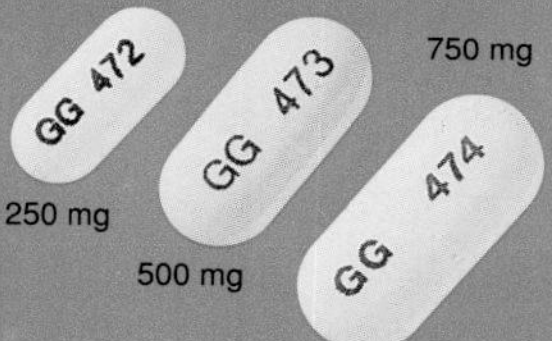

250 mg | 500 mg | 750 mg

Tablets, Extended-release
Geneva

(continued)

D

Procainamide *(continued)*

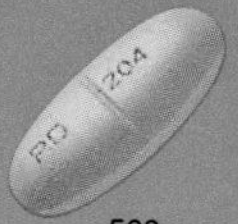
500 mg

Tablets, Extended-release
PD: *Procan SR*

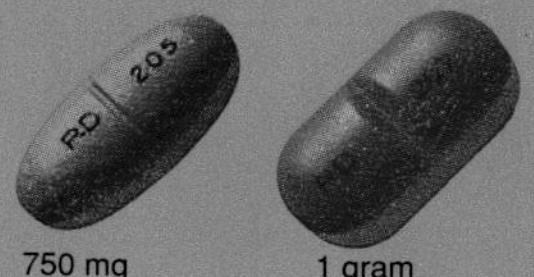
750 mg | 1 gram

Tablets, Extended-release
PD: *Procan SR*

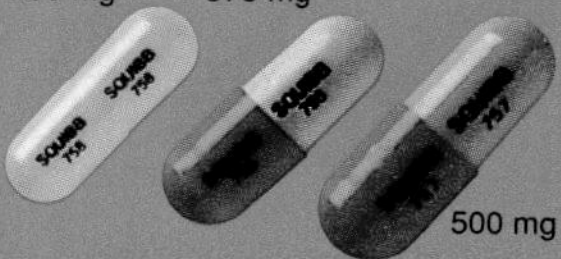
250 mg | 375 mg | 500 mg

Capsules
Apothecon: *Pronestyl*

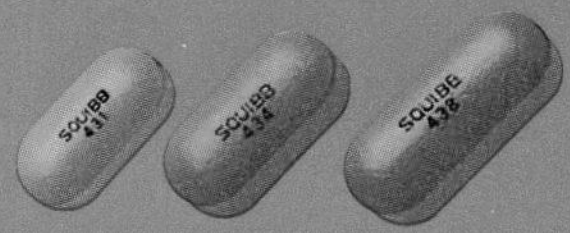
250 mg | 375 mg | 500 mg

Tablets
Apothecon: *Pronestyl*

500 mg

Tablets, Extended-release
Apothecon: *Pronestyl-SR*

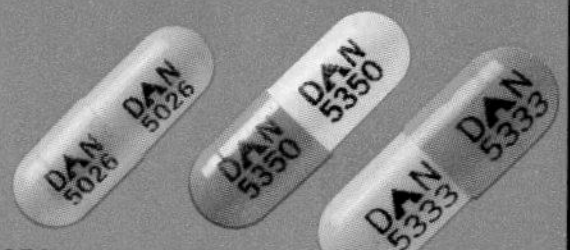
250 mg | 375 mg | 500 mg

Capsules
Schein/Danbury

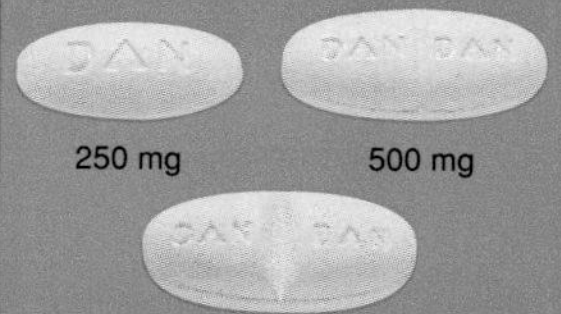
250 mg | 500 mg | 750 mg

Tablets, Extended-release
Schein/Danbury

1 2 3 4 5 6 7

*Single source product for solid oral dosage forms in the U.S.

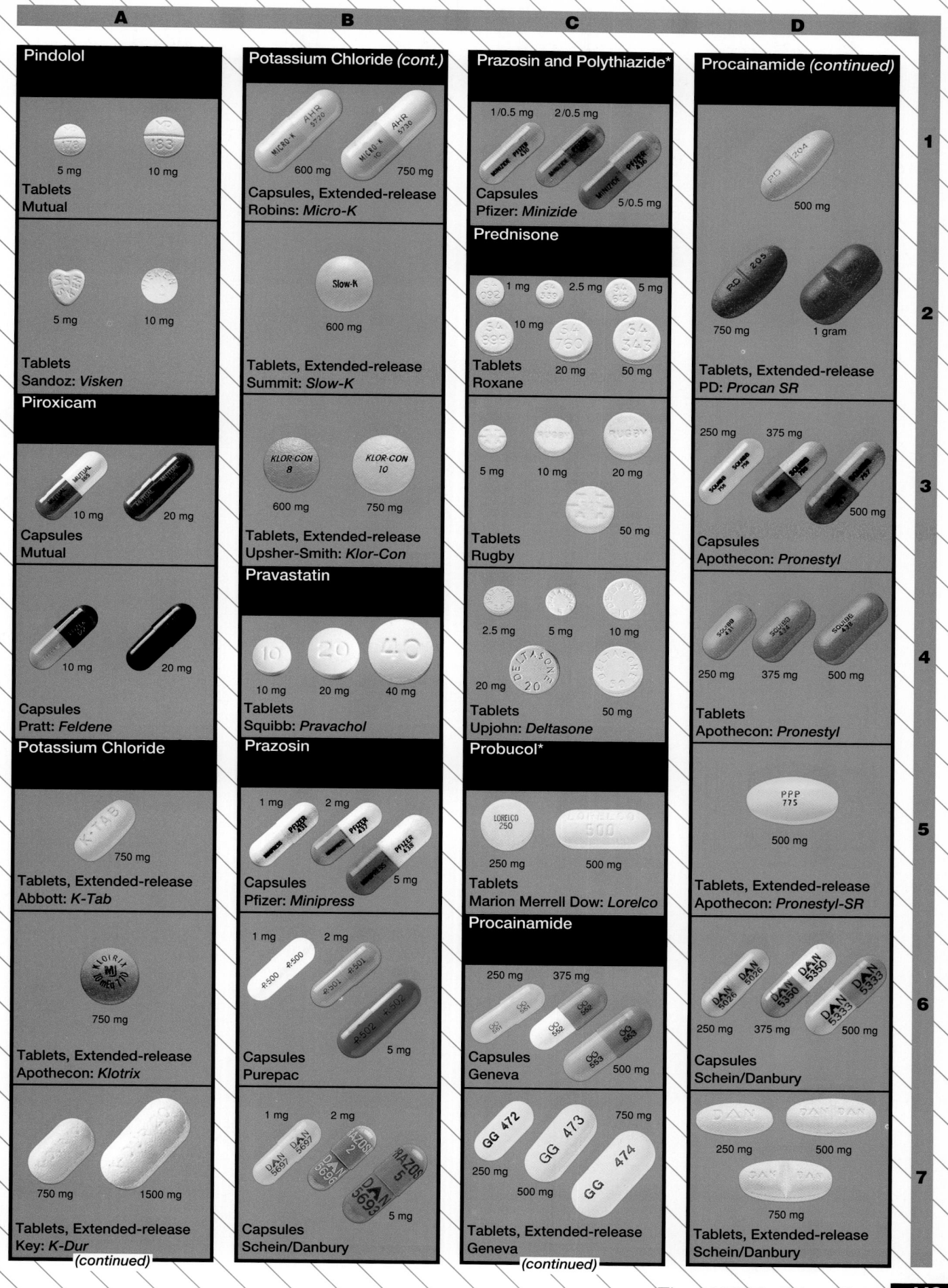

A

Prochlorperazine

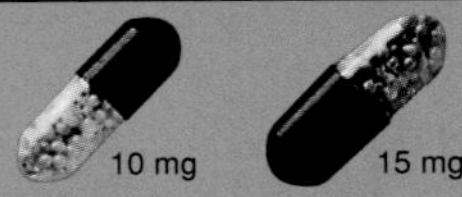
10 mg 15 mg

Capsules, Extended-release
SmithKline Beecham: *Compazine*

5 mg 10 mg

Tablets
SmithKline Beecham: *Compazine*

Promethazine

12.5 mg 25 mg 50 mg

Tablets
Wyeth-Ayerst: *Phenergan*

Propafenone*

150 mg 300 mg

Tablets
Knoll: *Rythmol*

Propantheline

7.5 mg 15 mg

Tablets
Roberts: *Pro-Banthine*

Propoxyphene Napsylate and Acetaminophen

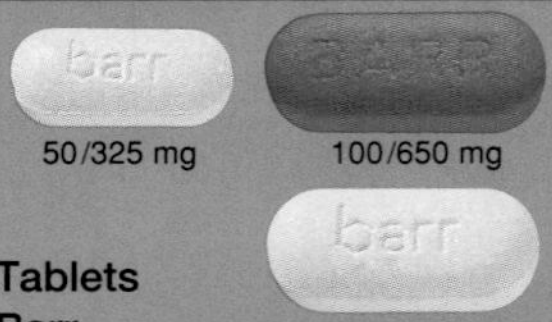
50/325 mg 100/650 mg 100/650 mg

Tablets
Barr

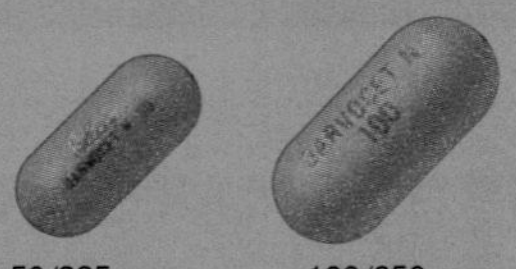
50/325 mg 100/650 mg

Tablets
Lilly: *Darvocet-N*

(continued)

B

Propoxyphene Napsylate and Acetaminophen *(cont.)*

100/650 mg

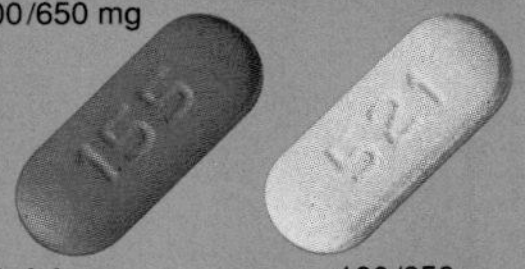
100/650 mg

Tablets
Mylan

100/650 mg

Tablets
Purepac

Propranolol

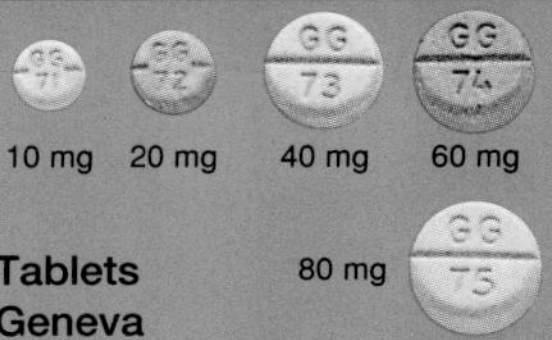
10 mg 20 mg 40 mg 60 mg 80 mg

Tablets
Geneva

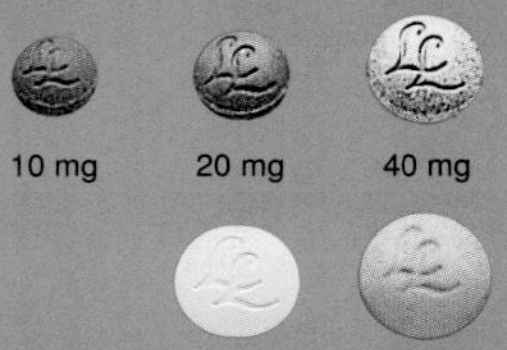
10 mg 20 mg 40 mg 60 mg 80 mg

Tablets
Lederle

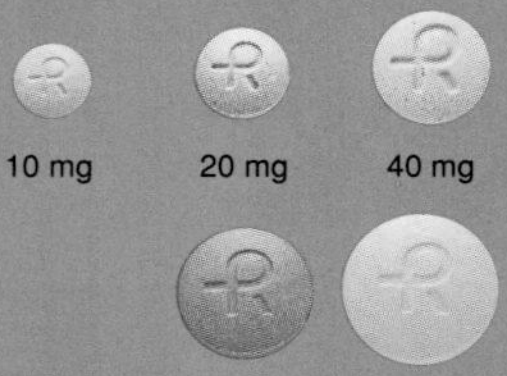
10 mg 20 mg 40 mg 60 mg 80 mg

Tablets
Purepac

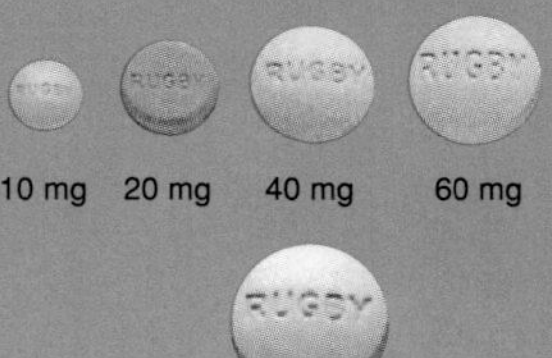
10 mg 20 mg 40 mg 60 mg 80 mg

Tablets
Rugby

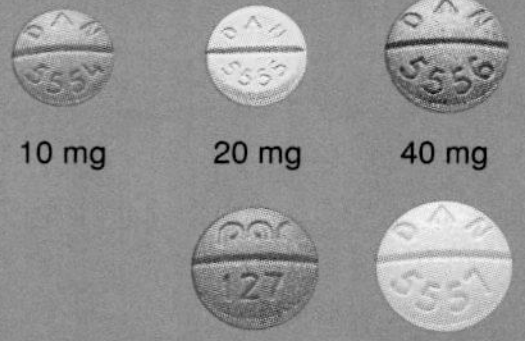
10 mg 20 mg 40 mg 60 mg 80 mg

Tablets
Schein/Danbury

(continued)

C

Propranolol *(continued)*

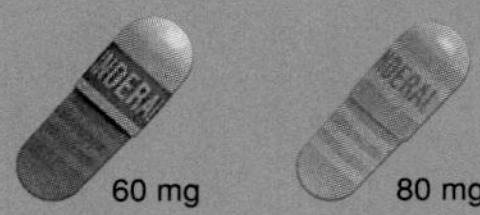
60 mg 80 mg

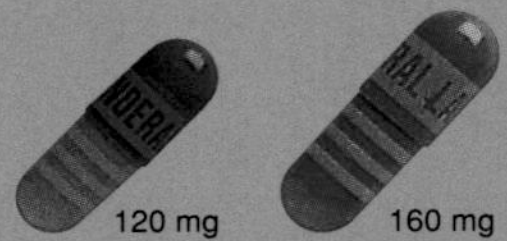
120 mg 160 mg

Capsules, Extended-release
Wyeth-Ayerst: *Inderal LA*

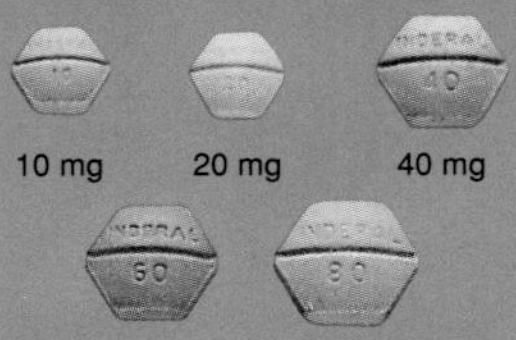
10 mg 20 mg 40 mg 60 mg 80 mg

Tablets
Wyeth-Ayerst: *Inderal*

Propranolol and Hydrochlorothiazide

40/25 mg 80/25 mg

Tablets
Purepac

40/25 mg 80/25 mg

Tablets
Rugby

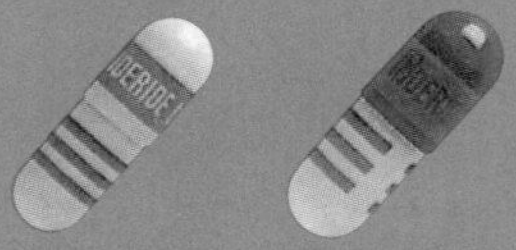
80/50 mg 120/50 mg

160/50 mg

Capsules, Extended-release
Wyeth-Ayerst: *Inderide LA*

(continued)

D

Propranolol and Hydrochlorothiazide *(continued)*

40/25 mg 80/25 mg

Tablets
Wyeth-Ayerst: *Inderide*

Pseudoephedrine and Guaifenesin

120/600 mg

Tablets
P&GP: *Entex PSE*

Quazepam*

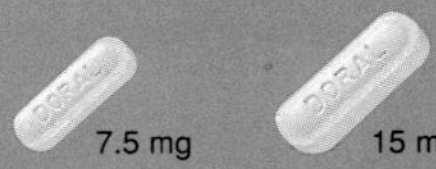
7.5 mg 15 mg

Tablets
Wallace: *Doral*

Quinapril*

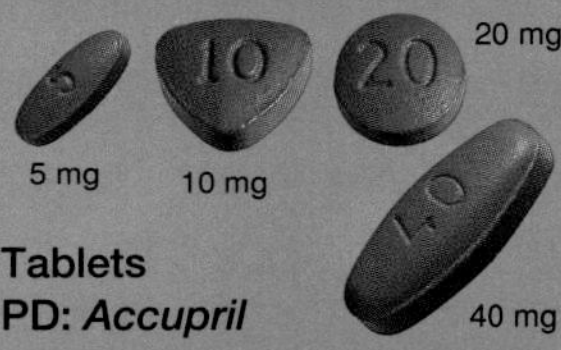
5 mg 10 mg 20 mg 40 mg

Tablets
PD: *Accupril*

Quinidine Gluconate

324 mg

Tablets, Extended-release
Berlex: *Quinaglute Dura-Tabs*

324 mg

Tablets, Extended-release
Schein/Danbury

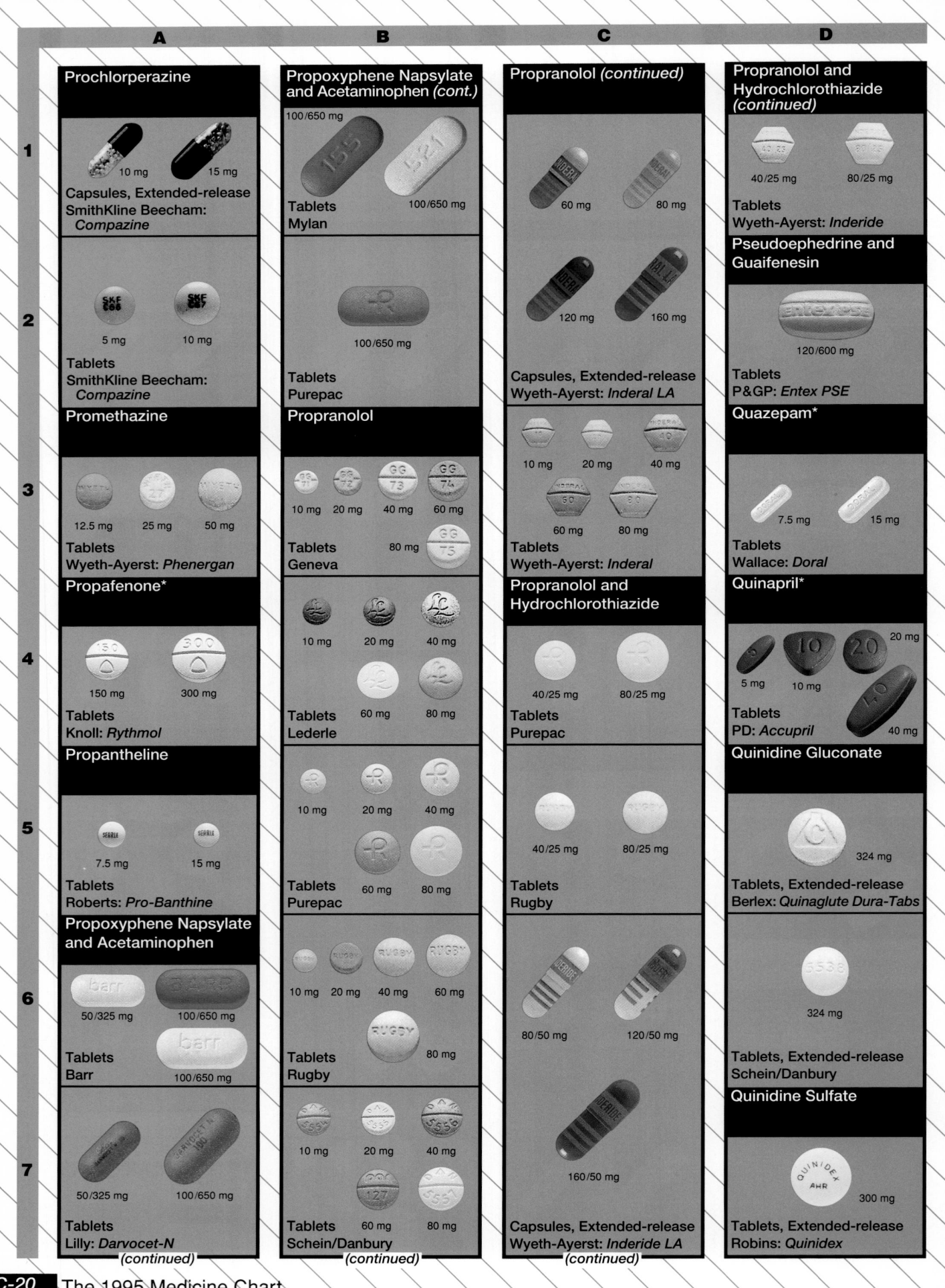

Quinidine Sulfate

300 mg

Tablets, Extended-release
Robins: *Quinidex*

*Single source product for solid oral dosage forms in the U.S.

A	B	C	D

Ramipril*

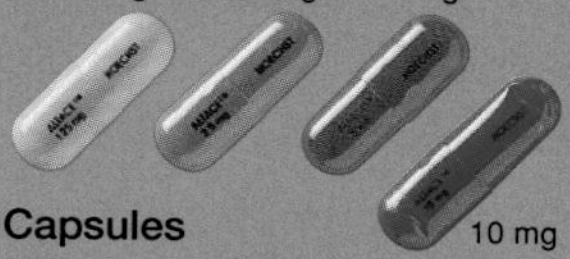

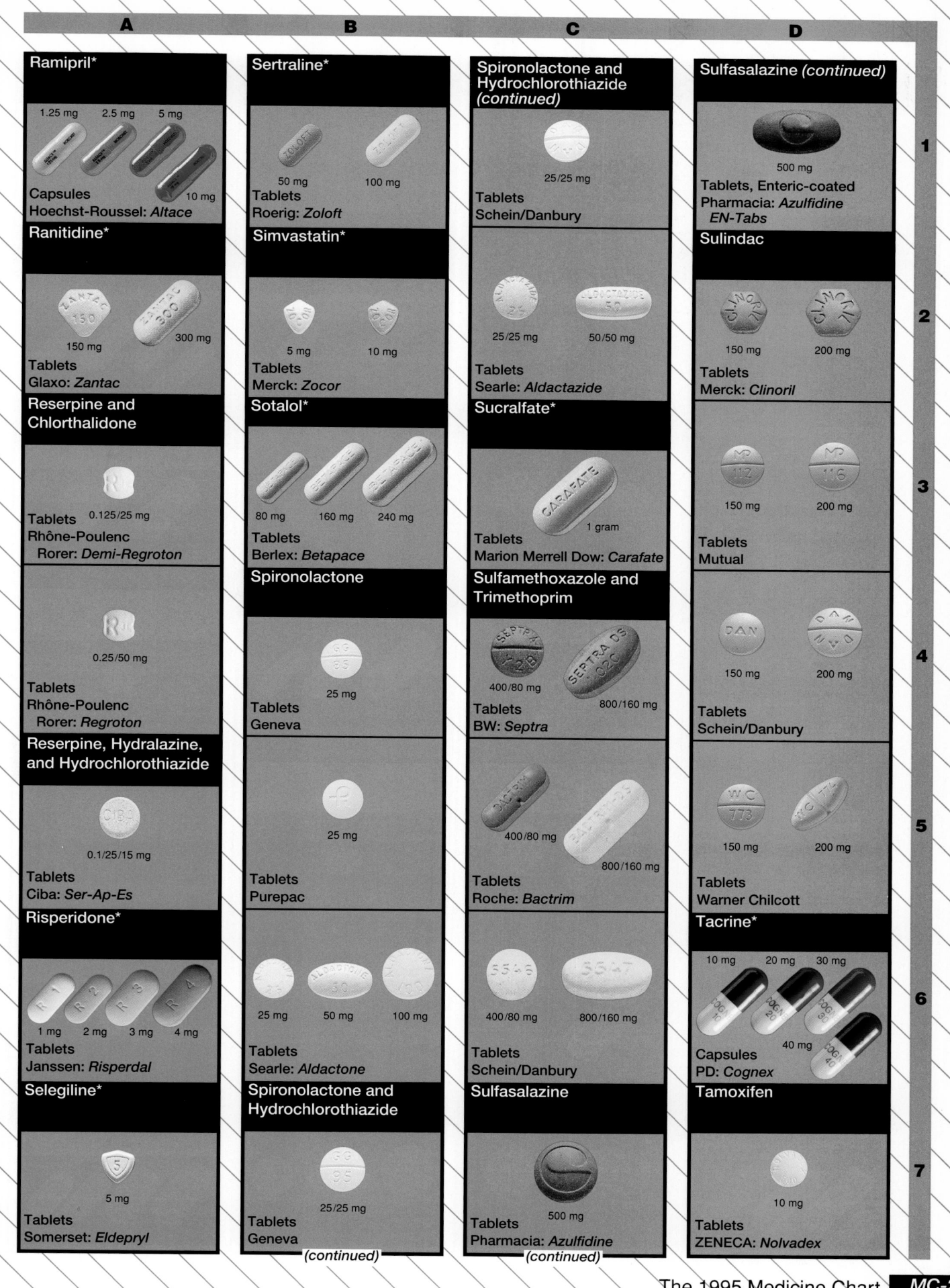

1.25 mg 2.5 mg 5 mg 10 mg

Capsules
Hoechst-Roussel: *Altace*

Ranitidine*

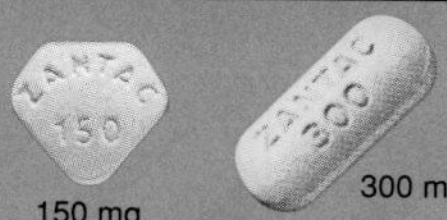

150 mg 300 mg

Tablets
Glaxo: *Zantac*

Reserpine and Chlorthalidone

0.125/25 mg

Tablets
Rhône-Poulenc Rorer: *Demi-Regroton*

0.25/50 mg

Tablets
Rhône-Poulenc Rorer: *Regroton*

Reserpine, Hydralazine, and Hydrochlorothiazide

0.1/25/15 mg

Tablets
Ciba: *Ser-Ap-Es*

Risperidone*

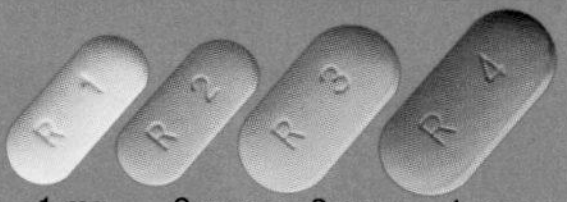

1 mg 2 mg 3 mg 4 mg

Tablets
Janssen: *Risperdal*

Selegiline*

5 mg

Tablets
Somerset: *Eldepryl*

Sertraline*

50 mg 100 mg

Tablets
Roerig: *Zoloft*

Simvastatin*

5 mg 10 mg

Tablets
Merck: *Zocor*

Sotalol*

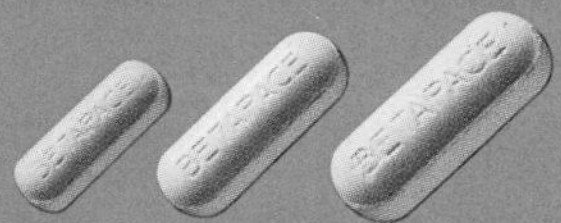

80 mg 160 mg 240 mg

Tablets
Berlex: *Betapace*

Spironolactone

25 mg

Tablets
Geneva

25 mg

Tablets
Purepac

25 mg 50 mg 100 mg

Tablets
Searle: *Aldactone*

Spironolactone and Hydrochlorothiazide

25/25 mg

Tablets
Geneva

(continued)

Spironolactone and Hydrochlorothiazide *(continued)*

25/25 mg

Tablets
Schein/Danbury

25/25 mg 50/50 mg

Tablets
Searle: *Aldactazide*

Sucralfate*

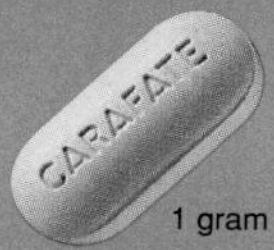

1 gram

Tablets
Marion Merrell Dow: *Carafate*

Sulfamethoxazole and Trimethoprim

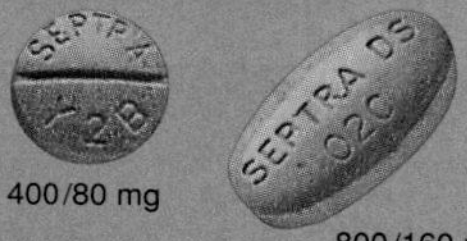

400/80 mg 800/160 mg

Tablets
BW: *Septra*

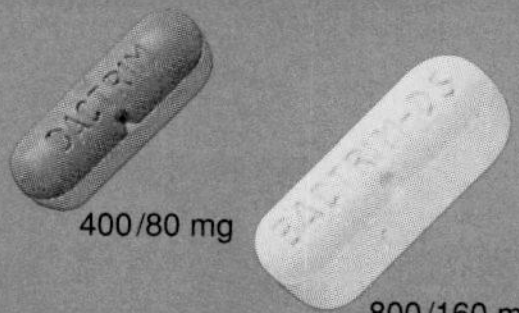

400/80 mg 800/160 mg

Tablets
Roche: *Bactrim*

400/80 mg 800/160 mg

Tablets
Schein/Danbury

Sulfasalazine

500 mg

Tablets
Pharmacia: *Azulfidine*

(continued)

Sulfasalazine *(continued)*

500 mg

Tablets, Enteric-coated
Pharmacia: *Azulfidine EN-Tabs*

Sulindac

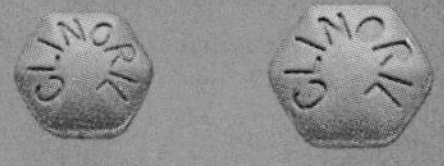

150 mg 200 mg

Tablets
Merck: *Clinoril*

150 mg 200 mg

Tablets
Mutual

150 mg 200 mg

Tablets
Schein/Danbury

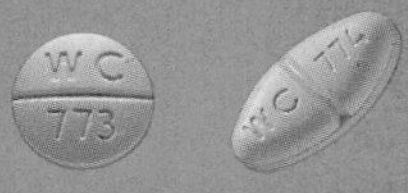

150 mg 200 mg

Tablets
Warner Chilcott

Tacrine*

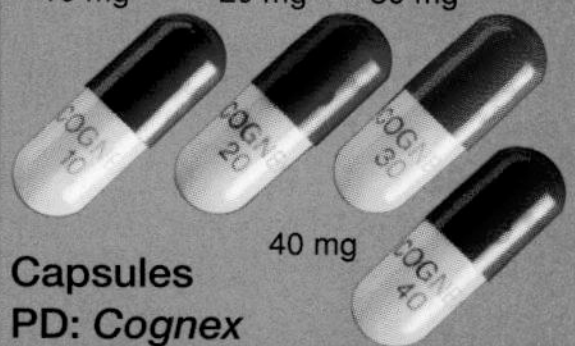

10 mg 20 mg 30 mg 40 mg

Capsules
PD: *Cognex*

Tamoxifen

10 mg

Tablets
ZENECA: *Nolvadex*

Row markers: 1 2 3 4 5 6 7

*Single source product for solid oral dosage forms in the U.S.

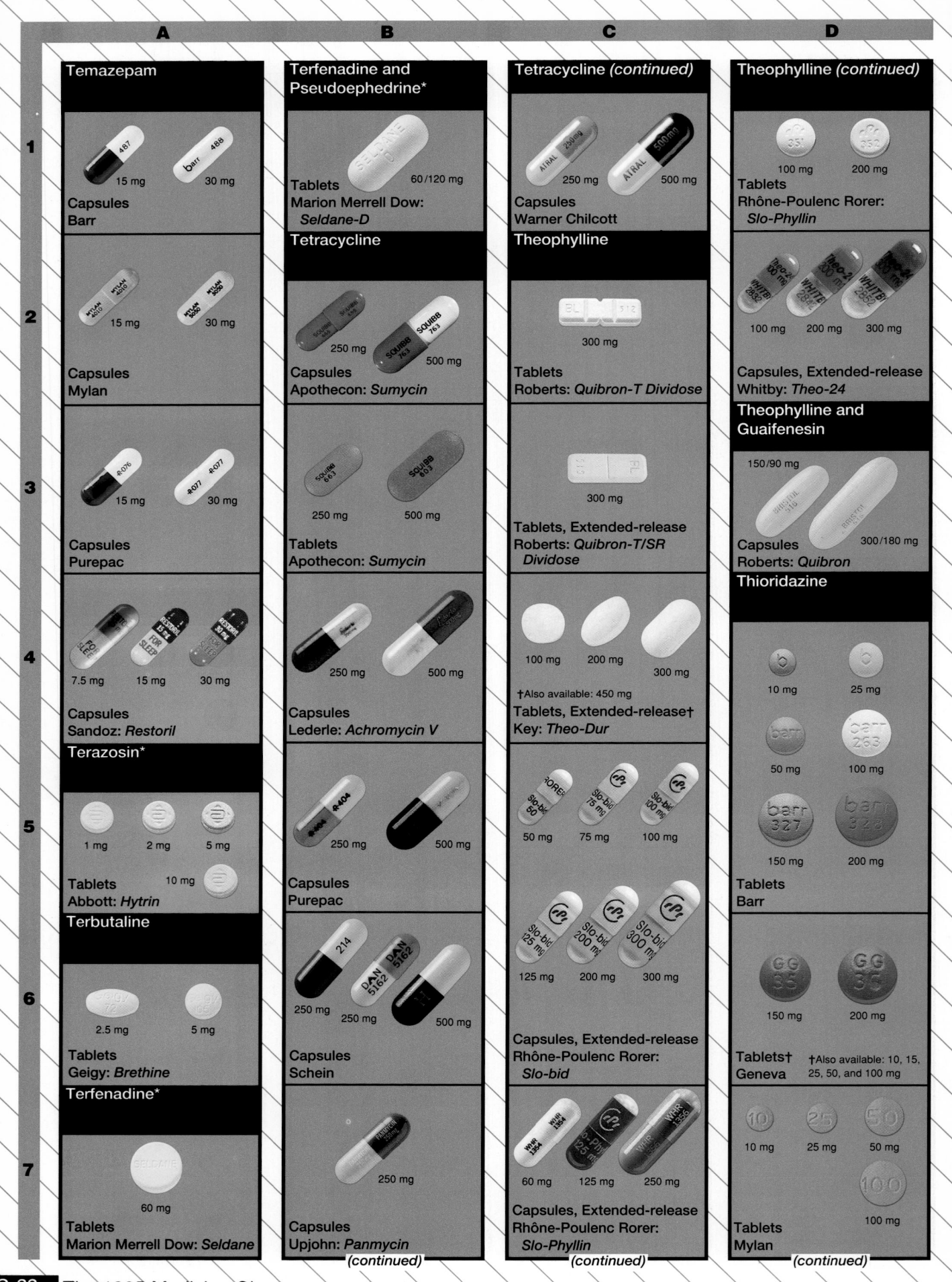

A B C D

Temazepam

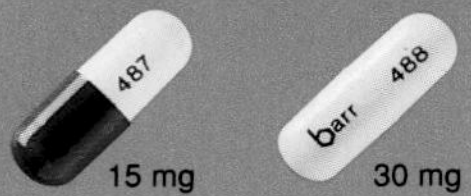
15 mg 30 mg
Capsules
Barr

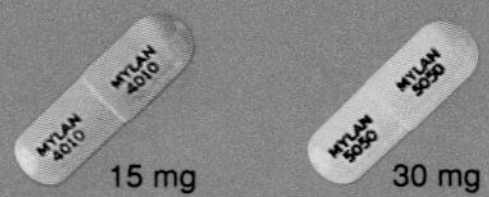
15 mg 30 mg
Capsules
Mylan

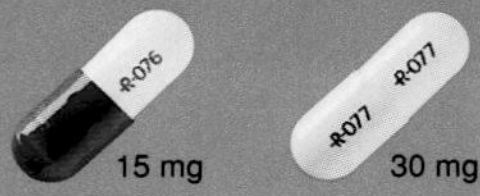
15 mg 30 mg
Capsules
Purepac

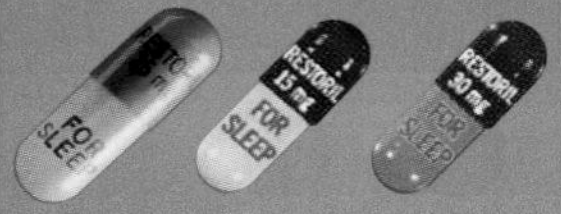
7.5 mg 15 mg 30 mg
Capsules
Sandoz: *Restoril*

Terazosin*

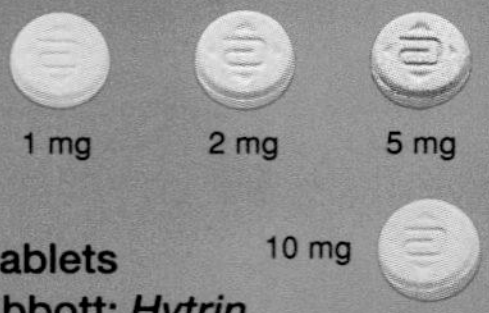
1 mg 2 mg 5 mg
10 mg
Tablets
Abbott: *Hytrin*

Terbutaline

2.5 mg 5 mg
Tablets
Geigy: *Brethine*

Terfenadine*

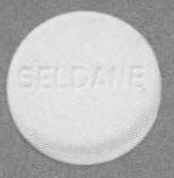
60 mg
Tablets
Marion Merrell Dow: *Seldane*

Terfenadine and Pseudoephedrine*

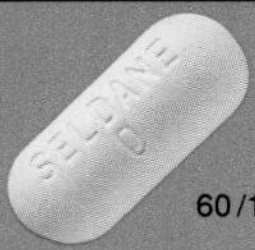
60/120 mg
Tablets
Marion Merrell Dow:
Seldane-D

Tetracycline

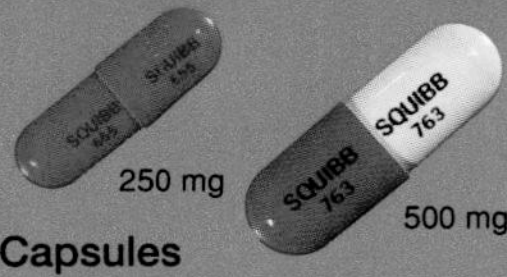
250 mg 500 mg
Capsules
Apothecon: *Sumycin*

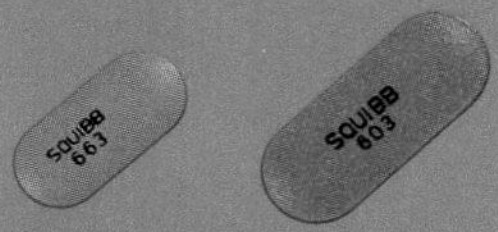
250 mg 500 mg
Tablets
Apothecon: *Sumycin*

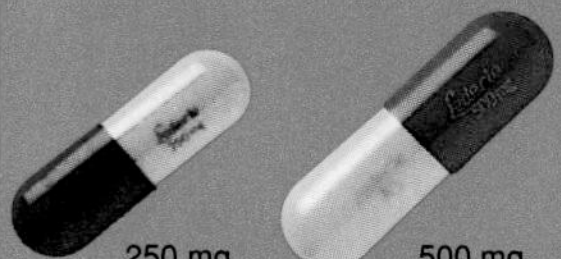
250 mg 500 mg
Capsules
Lederle: *Achromycin V*

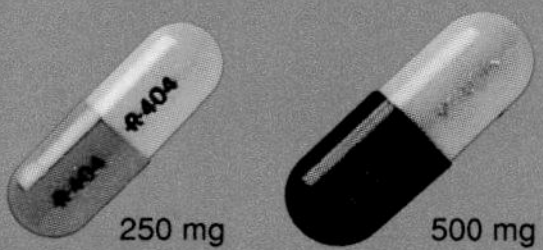
250 mg 500 mg
Capsules
Purepac

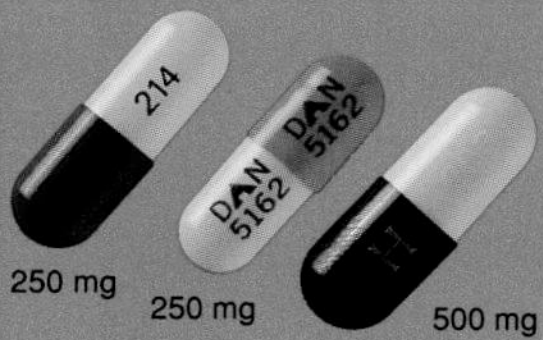
250 mg 250 mg 500 mg
Capsules
Schein

250 mg
Capsules
Upjohn: *Panmycin*

(continued)

Tetracycline *(continued)*

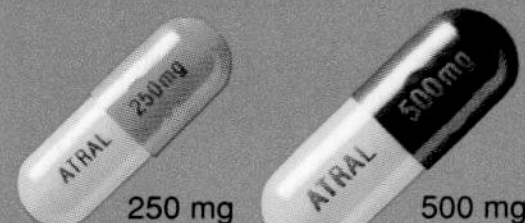
250 mg 500 mg
Capsules
Warner Chilcott

Theophylline

300 mg
Tablets
Roberts: *Quibron-T Dividose*

300 mg
Tablets, Extended-release
Roberts: *Quibron-T/SR Dividose*

100 mg 200 mg 300 mg
†Also available: 450 mg
Tablets, Extended-release†
Key: *Theo-Dur*

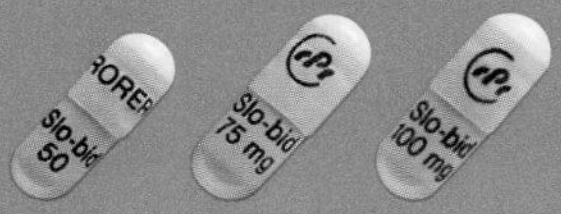
50 mg 75 mg 100 mg

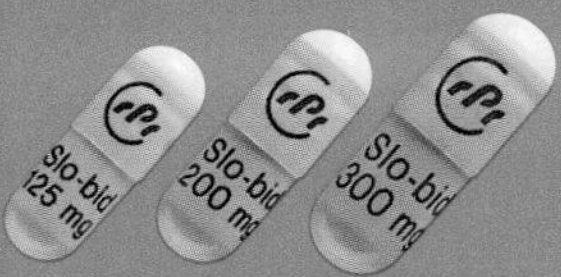
125 mg 200 mg 300 mg
Capsules, Extended-release
Rhône-Poulenc Rorer:
Slo-bid

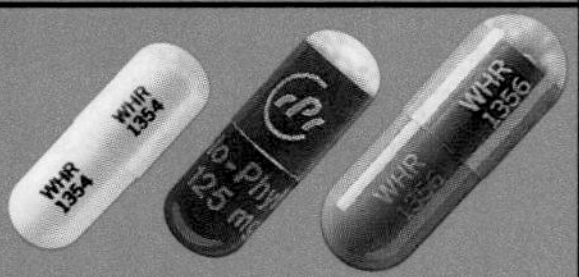
60 mg 125 mg 250 mg
Capsules, Extended-release
Rhône-Poulenc Rorer:
Slo-Phyllin

(continued)

Theophylline *(continued)*

100 mg 200 mg
Tablets
Rhône-Poulenc Rorer:
Slo-Phyllin

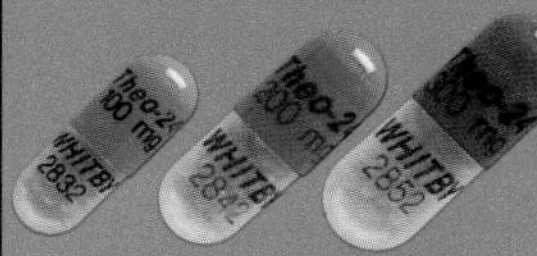
100 mg 200 mg 300 mg
Capsules, Extended-release
Whitby: *Theo-24*

Theophylline and Guaifenesin

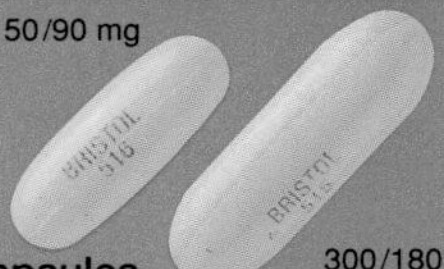
150/90 mg 300/180 mg
Capsules
Roberts: *Quibron*

Thioridazine

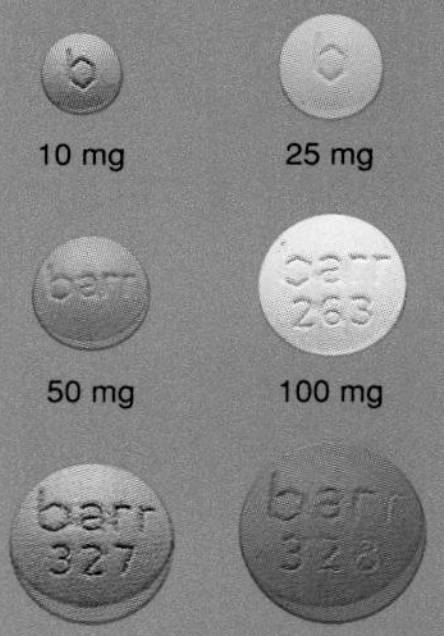
10 mg 25 mg
50 mg 100 mg
150 mg 200 mg
Tablets
Barr

150 mg 200 mg
Tablets†
Geneva
†Also available: 10, 15, 25, 50, and 100 mg

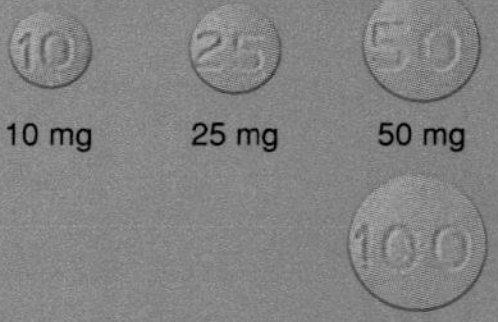
10 mg 25 mg 50 mg
100 mg
Tablets
Mylan

(continued)

*Single source product for solid oral dosage forms in the U.S.

Thioridazine *(continued)*

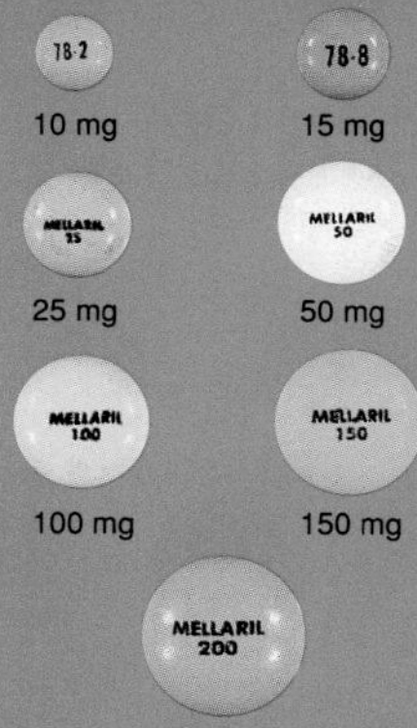

10 mg · 15 mg · 25 mg · 50 mg · 100 mg · 150 mg · 200 mg

Tablets
Sandoz: *Mellaril*

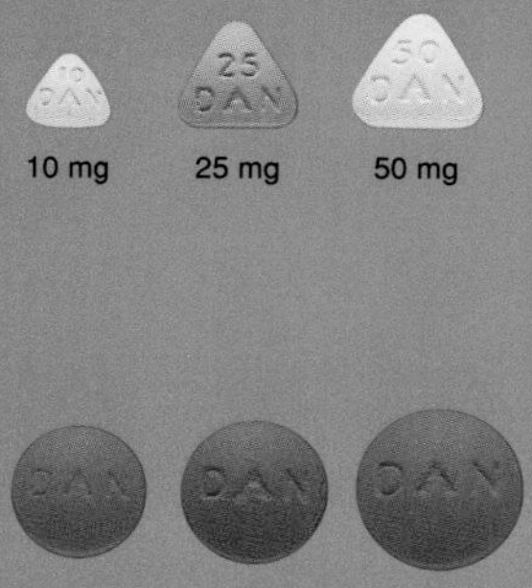

10 mg · 25 mg · 50 mg · 100 mg · 150 mg · 200 mg

Tablets
Schein/Danbury

Thiothixene

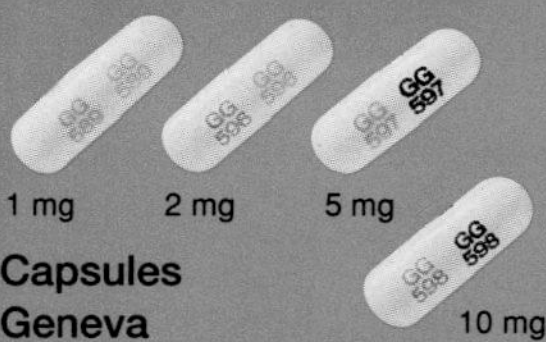

1 mg · 2 mg · 5 mg · 10 mg

Capsules
Geneva

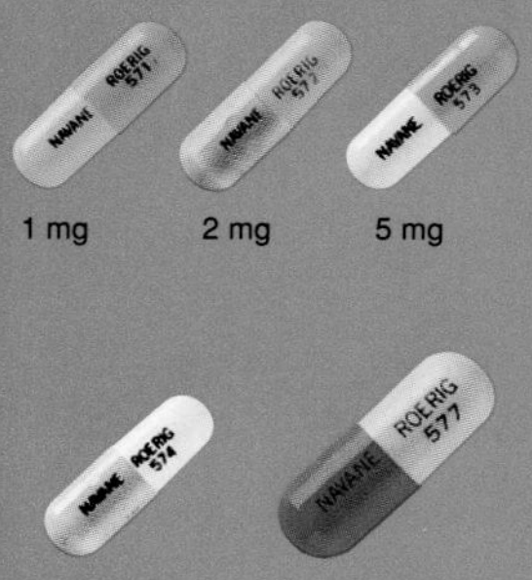

1 mg · 2 mg · 5 mg · 10 mg · 20 mg

Capsules
Roerig: *Navane*

(continued)

Thiothixene *(continued)*

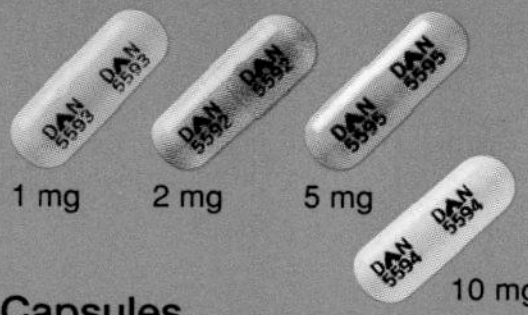

1 mg · 2 mg · 5 mg · 10 mg

Capsules
Schein/Danbury

Ticlopidine*

250 mg

Tablets
Syntex: *Ticlid*

Timolol

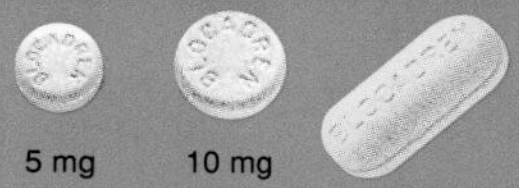

5 mg · 10 mg · 20 mg

Tablets
Merck: *Blocadren*

5 mg · 10 mg · 20 mg

Tablets
Mylan

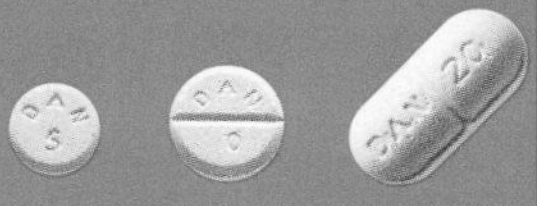

5 mg · 10 mg · 20 mg

Tablets
Schein/Danbury

Tocainide*

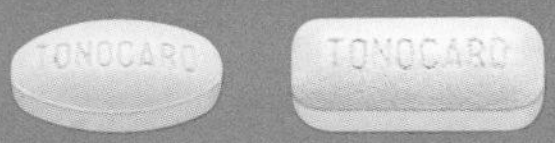

400 mg · 600 mg

Tablets
Merck: *Tonocard*

Tolazamide

100 mg · 250 mg · 500 mg

Tablets
Geneva

(continued)

Tolazamide *(continued)*

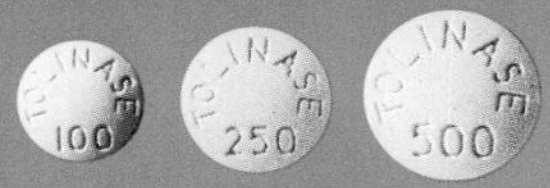

100 mg · 250 mg · 500 mg

Tablets
Upjohn: *Tolinase*

Tolbutamide

250 mg · 500 mg

Tablets
Upjohn: *Orinase*

Tolmetin*

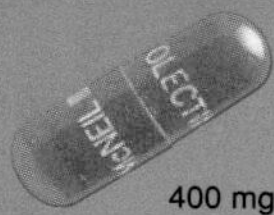

400 mg

Capsules
McNeil: *Tolectin DS*

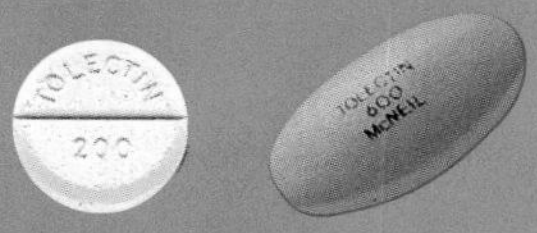

200 mg · 600 mg

Tablets
McNeil: *Tolectin*

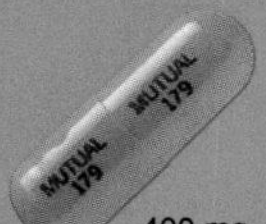

400 mg

Capsules
Mutual

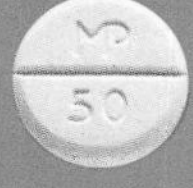

200 mg

Tablets
Mutual

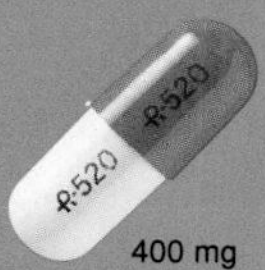

400 mg

Capsules
Purepac

Tranylcypromine*

10 mg

Tablets
SmithKline Beecham: *Parnate*

Trazodone

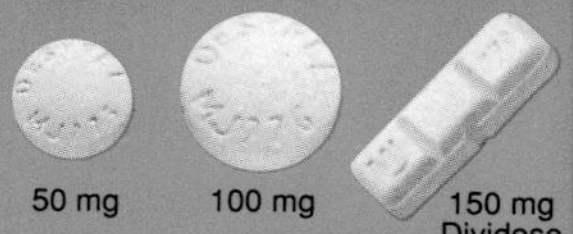

50 mg · 100 mg · 150 mg Dividose

†Also available in 300 mg Dividose

Tablets†
Apothecon: *Desyrel*

50 mg · 100 mg

Tablets
Mutual

50 mg · 100 mg

Tablets
Purepac

50 mg · 100 mg

Tablets
Schein/Danbury

Triamterene and Hydrochlorothiazide

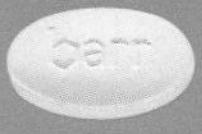

75/50 mg

Tablets
Barr

75/50 mg

Tablets
Geneva

(continued)

*Single source product for solid oral dosage forms in the U.S.

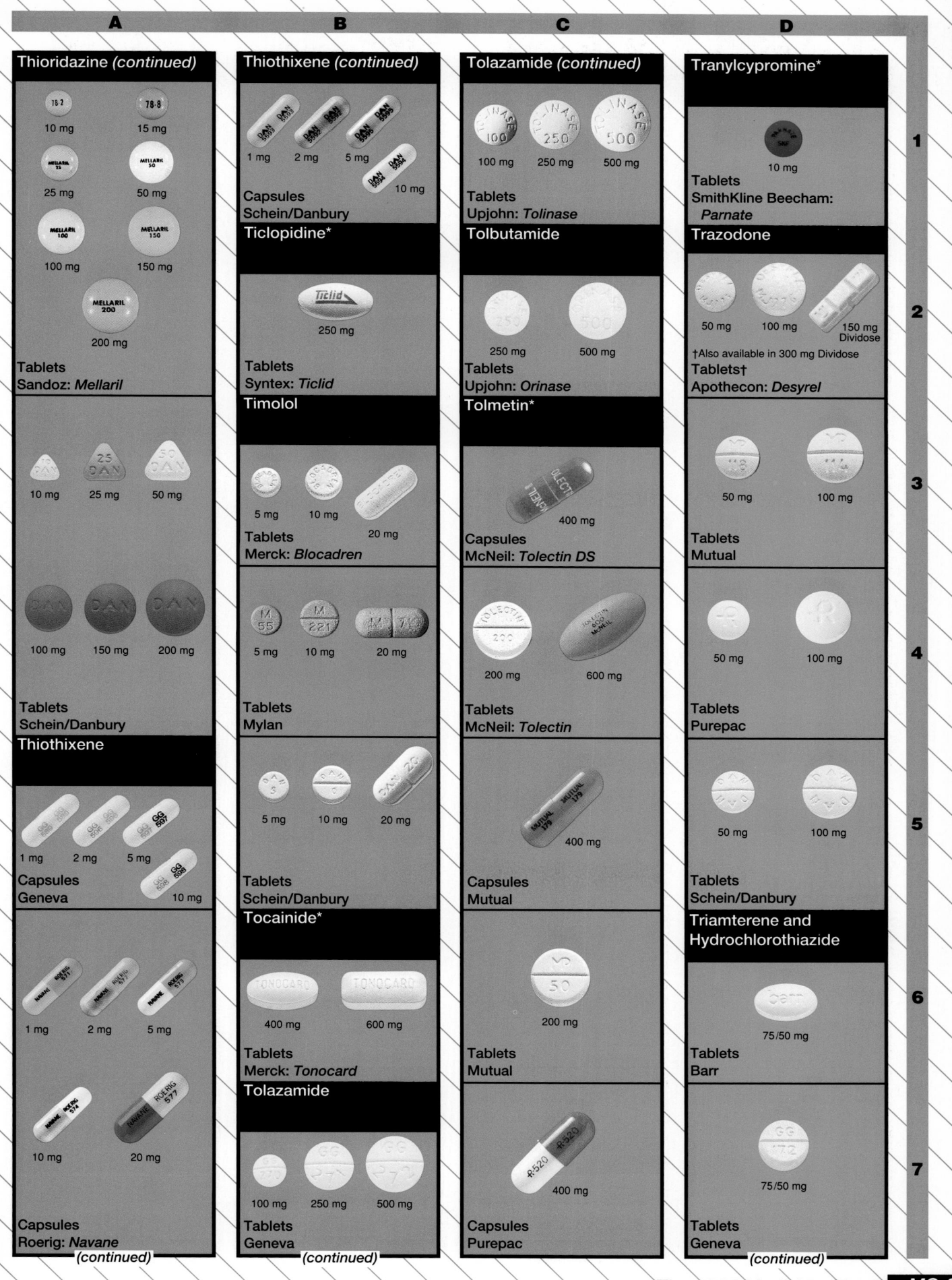

A

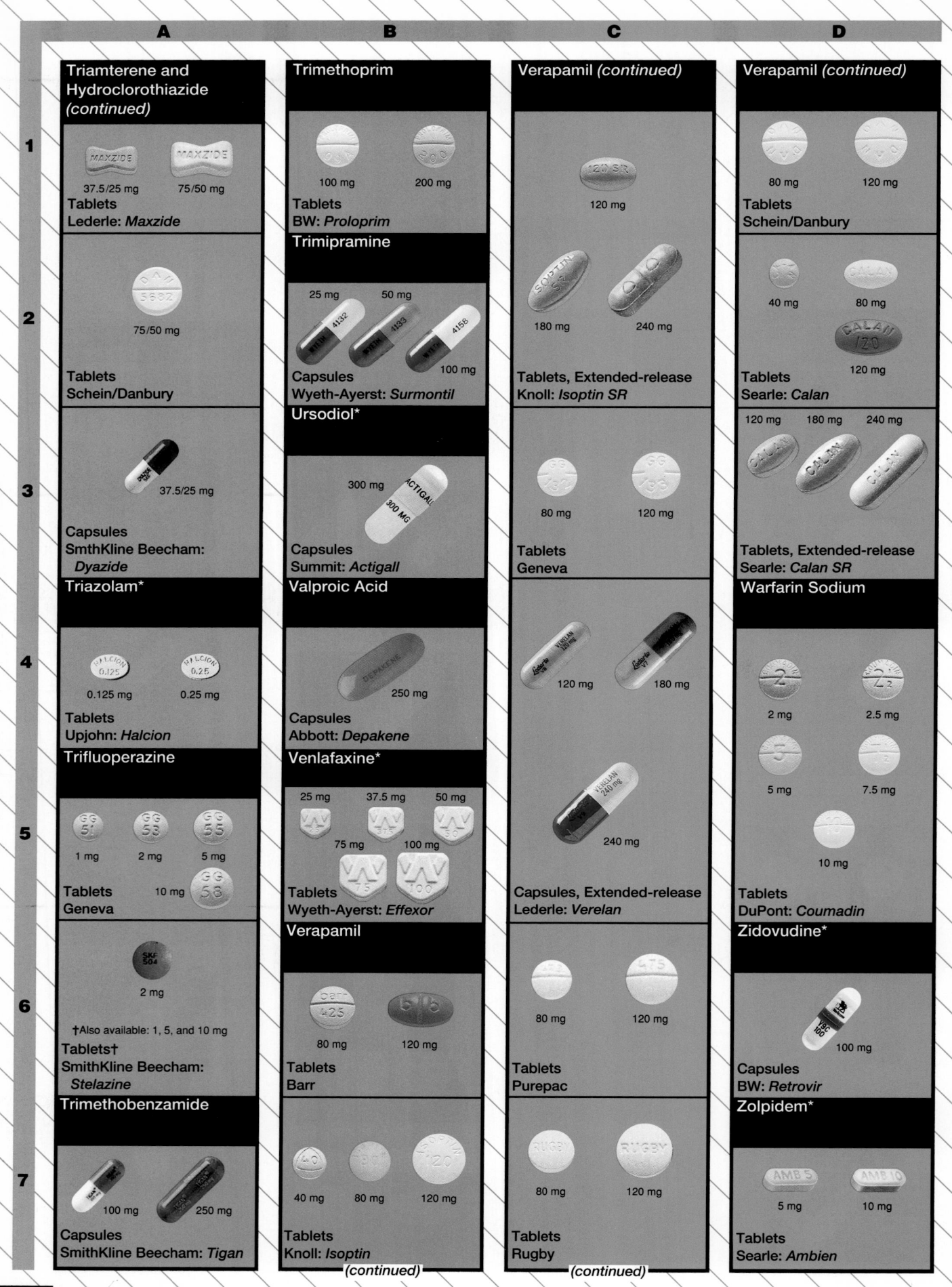

Triamterene and Hydroclorothiazide *(continued)*

1

37.5/25 mg — 75/50 mg

Tablets
Lederle: *Maxzide*

2

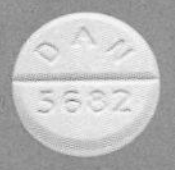

75/50 mg

Tablets
Schein/Danbury

3

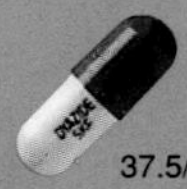

37.5/25 mg

Capsules
SmthKline Beecham: *Dyazide*

Triazolam*

4

0.125 mg — 0.25 mg

Tablets
Upjohn: *Halcion*

Trifluoperazine

5

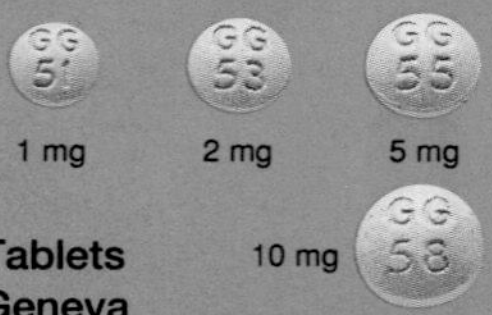

1 mg — 2 mg — 5 mg — 10 mg

Tablets
Geneva

6

2 mg

†Also available: 1, 5, and 10 mg

Tablets†
SmithKline Beecham: *Stelazine*

Trimethobenzamide

7

100 mg — 250 mg

Capsules
SmithKline Beecham: *Tigan*

B

Trimethoprim

100 mg — 200 mg

Tablets
BW: *Proloprim*

Trimipramine

25 mg — 50 mg — 100 mg

Capsules
Wyeth-Ayerst: *Surmontil*

Ursodiol*

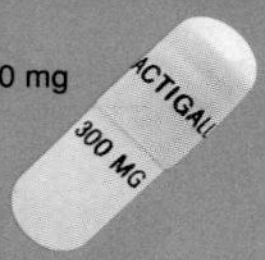

300 mg

Capsules
Summit: *Actigall*

Valproic Acid

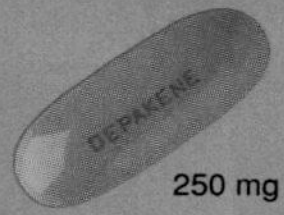

250 mg

Capsules
Abbott: *Depakene*

Venlafaxine*

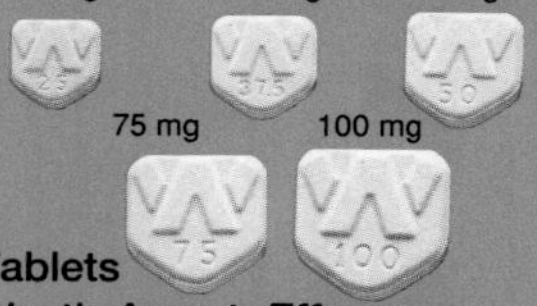

25 mg — 37.5 mg — 50 mg — 75 mg — 100 mg

Tablets
Wyeth-Ayerst: *Effexor*

Verapamil

80 mg — 120 mg

Tablets
Barr

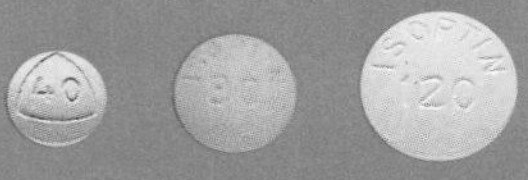

40 mg — 80 mg — 120 mg

Tablets
Knoll: *Isoptin*

(continued)

C

Verapamil *(continued)*

120 mg

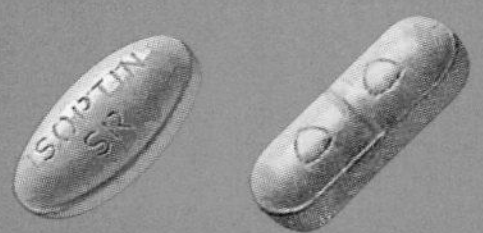

180 mg — 240 mg

Tablets, Extended-release
Knoll: *Isoptin SR*

80 mg — 120 mg

Tablets
Geneva

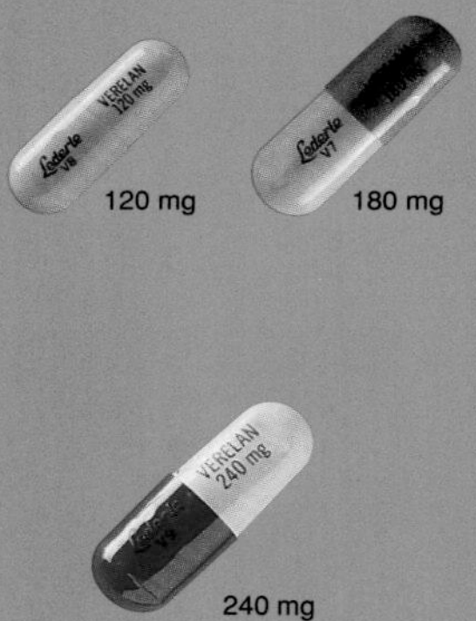

120 mg — 180 mg — 240 mg

Capsules, Extended-release
Lederle: *Verelan*

80 mg — 120 mg

Tablets
Purepac

80 mg — 120 mg

Tablets
Rugby

(continued)

D

Verapamil *(continued)*

80 mg — 120 mg

Tablets
Schein/Danbury

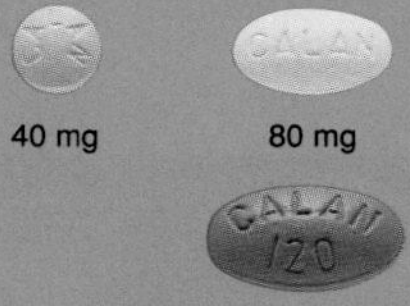

40 mg — 80 mg — 120 mg

Tablets
Searle: *Calan*

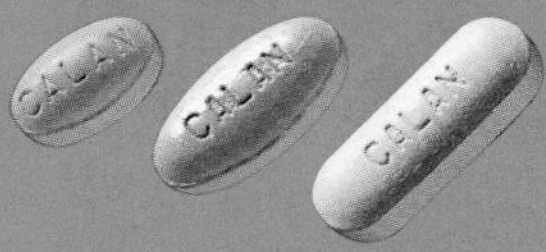

120 mg — 180 mg — 240 mg

Tablets, Extended-release
Searle: *Calan SR*

Warfarin Sodium

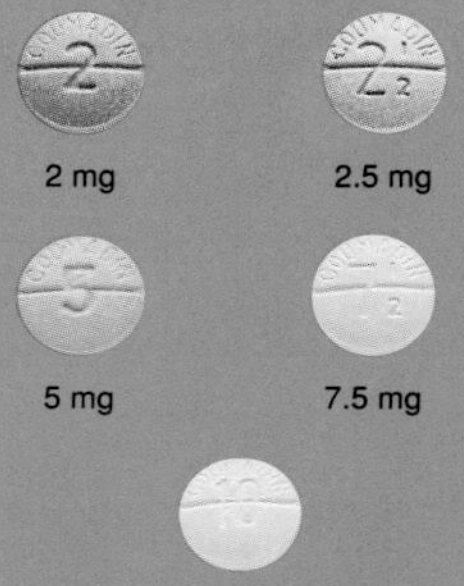

2 mg — 2.5 mg — 5 mg — 7.5 mg — 10 mg

Tablets
DuPont: *Coumadin*

Zidovudine*

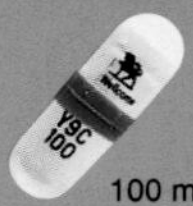

100 mg

Capsules
BW: *Retrovir*

Zolpidem*

5 mg — 10 mg

Tablets
Searle: *Ambien*

*Single source product for solid oral dosage forms in the U.S.

Section VI

SELECTED USP GENERAL NOTICES AND CHAPTERS

This Section is intended to provide convenient access to portions of the *USP-NF* that are most often used by Volume III subscribers. The information is arranged in the following manner:

Selected General Notices and Requirements

Applying to Standards, Tests, Assays, and Other Specifications of the United States Pharmacopeia

"OFFICIAL" AND "OFFICIAL ARTICLES"

The word "official," as used in this Pharmacopeia or with reference hereto, is synonymous with "Pharmacopeial," with "USP," and with "compendial."

The designation USP in conjunction with the official title on the label of an article means that the article purports to comply with USP standards; such specific designation on the label does not constitute a representation, endorsement, or incorporation by the manufacturer's labeling of the informational material contained in the USP monograph, nor does it constitute assurance by USP that the article is known to comply with USP standards. The standards apply equally to articles bearing the official titles or names derived by transposition of the definitive words of official titles or transposition in the order of the names of two or more active ingredients in official titles, whether or not the added designation "USP" is used. Names considered to be synonyms of the official titles may not be used for official titles.

Where an article differs from the standards of strength, quality, and purity, as determined by the application of the assays and tests set forth for it in the Pharmacopeia, its difference shall be plainly stated on its label. Where an article fails to comply in identity with the identity prescribed in the USP, or contains an added substance that interferes with the prescribed assays and tests, such article shall be designated by a name that is clearly distinguishing and differentiating from any name recognized in the Pharmacopeia.

Articles listed herein are official and the standards set forth in the monographs apply to them only when the articles are intended or labeled for use as drugs, as nutritional supplements, or as medical devices and when bought, sold, or dispensed for these purposes or when labeled as conforming to this Pharmacopeia.

An article is deemed to be recognized in this Pharmacopeia when a monograph for the article is published in it, including its supplements, addenda, or other interim revisions, and an official date is generally or specifically assigned to it.

The following terminology is used for distinguishing the articles for which monographs are provided: an *official substance* is an active drug entity, a recognized nutrient, or a pharmaceutic ingredient (see also *NF 18*) or a component of a finished device for which the monograph title includes no indication of the nature of the finished form; an *official preparation* is a *drug product*, a *nutritional supplement*, or a *finished device*. It is the finished or partially finished (e.g., as in the case of a sterile solid to be constituted into a solution for administration) preparation or product of one or more official substances formulated for use on or for the patient or consumer; an *article* is an item for which a monograph is provided, whether an official substance or an official preparation.

Nutritional Supplements—The designation of an official preparation containing recognized nutrients as "USP" or the use of the designation "USP" in conjunction with the title of such nutritional supplement preparation may be made only if the article contains two or more of the recognized nutrients and the preparation meets the applicable requirements contained in the individual Class Monograph and General Chapters. Any additional ingredient in such article that is not recognized in the pharmacopeia and for which nutritional value is claimed, shall not be represented nor imply that it is of USP quality or recognized by USP. If a preparation does not comply with applicable requirements but contains nutrients that are recognized in the USP, the article may not designate the individual nutrients as complying with USP standards or being of USP quality without designating on the label that the article itself does not comply with USP standards.

Tolerances—The limits specified in the monographs for Pharmacopeial articles are established with a view to the use of these articles as drugs, except where it is indicated otherwise. The use of the molecular formula for the active ingredient(s) named in defining the required strength of a Pharmacopeial article is intended to designate the chemical entity or entities, as given in the complete chemical name of the article, having absolute (100 percent) purity.

A dosage form shall be formulated with the intent to provide 100 percent of the quantity of each ingredient declared on the label. Where the content of an ingredient is known to decrease with time, an amount in excess of that declared on the label may be introduced into the dosage form at the time of manufacture to assure compliance with the content requirements of the monograph throughout the expiration period. The tolerances and limits stated in the definitions in the monographs for Pharmacopeial articles allow for such overages and for analytical error, for unavoidable variations in manufacturing and compounding, and for deterioration to an extent considered acceptable under practical conditions.

The specified tolerances are based upon such attributes of quality as might be expected to characterize an article produced from suitable raw materials under recognized principles of good manufacturing practice.

The existence of compendial limits or tolerances does not constitute a basis for a claim that an official substance that more nearly approaches 100 percent purity "exceeds" the Pharmacopeial quality. Similarly, the fact that an article has been prepared to closer tolerances than those specified in the monograph does not constitute a basis for a claim that the article "exceeds" the Pharmacopeial requirements.

Interpretation of Requirements—Analytical results observed in the laboratory (or calculated from experimental measurements) are compared with stated limits to determine whether there is conformance with compendial assay or test requirements. The observed or calculated values usually will contain more significant figures than there are in the stated limit, and an observed or calculated result is to be rounded off to the number of places that is in agreement with the limit expression by the following procedure. [NOTE—Limits, which are fixed numbers, are not rounded off.]

When rounding off is required, consider only one digit in the decimal place to the right of the last place in the limit expression. If this digit is smaller than 5, it is eliminated and the preceding digit is unchanged. If this digit is greater than 5, it is eliminated and the preceding digit is increased by one. If this digit equals 5, the 5 is eliminated and the preceding digit is increased by one.

Illustration of Rounding Numerical Values for Comparison with Requirements

Compendial Requirement	Unrounded Value	Rounded Result	Conforms
Assay limit ≥98.0%	97.96%	98.0%	Yes
	97.92%	97.9%	No
	97.95%	98.0%	Yes
Assay limit ≤101.5%	101.55%	101.6%	No
	101.46%	101.5%	Yes
	101.45%	101.5%	Yes
Limit test ≤0.02%	0.025%	0.03%	No
	0.015%	0.02%	Yes
	0.027%	0.03%	No
Limit test ≤3 ppm	0.00035%	0.0004%	No
	0.00025%	0.0003%	Yes
	0.00028%	0.0003%	Yes

GENERAL CHAPTERS

Each general chapter is assigned a number that appears in brackets adjacent to the chapter name (e.g., ⟨601⟩ *Aerosols*). General chapters that include general *requirements* for tests and assays are numbered from ⟨1⟩ to ⟨999⟩, chapters that are *informational* are numbered from ⟨1000⟩ to ⟨1999⟩, and chapters pertaining to *nutritional supplements* are numbered above ⟨2000⟩.

The use of the general chapter numbers is encouraged for the identification and rapid access to general tests and information. It is especially helpful where monograph section headings and chapter names are not the same (e.g., *Ultraviolet absorption* ⟨197U⟩ in a monograph refers to method ⟨197U⟩ under general tests chapter ⟨197⟩ *Spectrophotometric Identification Tests; Specific rotation* ⟨781S⟩ in a monograph refers to method ⟨781S⟩ under general tests chapter ⟨781⟩ *Optical Rotation;* and *Calcium* ⟨191⟩ in a monograph refers to the tests for *Calcium* under general tests chapter ⟨191⟩ *Identification Tests—General*).

UNITS OF POTENCY

For substances that cannot be completely characterized by chemical and physical means, it may be necessary to express quantities of activity in biological units of potency, each defined by an authoritative, designated reference standard.

Units of biological potency defined by the World Health Organization (WHO) for International Biological Standards and International Biological Reference Preparations are termed International Units (IU). Units defined by USP Reference Standards are USP Units, and the individual monographs refer to these. Unless otherwise indicated, USP Units are equivalent to the corresponding International Units, where such exist. Such equivalence is usually established on the basis solely of the compendial assay for the substance.

For antibiotics (see *Antibiotics—Microbial Assays* ⟨81⟩), USP Units are defined by the corresponding USP Reference Standards in terms of the units of activity established by the FDA. Each unit is established through the corresponding antibiotic master standard, which in many instances is the basis also for the definition of the WHO International Unit. For most antibiotics, however, biological units of potency are not necessary, and their activity is expressed in metric units (micrograms or milligrams) in terms of the chemically defined substances described in the individual monographs.

For biological products, whether or not International Units or USP Units do exist (see *Biologics* ⟨1041⟩), units of potency are defined by the corresponding US Standard established by the FDA.

INGREDIENTS AND PROCESSES

Official preparations are prepared from ingredients that meet the requirements of the compendial monographs for those individual ingredients for which monographs are provided (see also *NF 18*).

Official substances are prepared according to recognized principles of good manufacturing practice and from ingredients complying with specifications designed to assure that the resultant substances meet the requirements of the compendial monographs (see also *Foreign Substances and Impurities* under *Tests and Assays*).

Preparations for which a complete composition is given in this Pharmacopeia, unless specifically exempted herein or in the individual monograph, are to contain only the ingredients named in the formulas. However, there may be deviation from the specified processes or methods of compounding, though not from the ingredients or proportions thereof, provided the finished preparation conforms to the relevant standards laid down herein and to preparations produced by following the specified process.

Where a monograph on a preparation calls for an ingredient in an amount expressed on the dried basis, the ingredient need not be dried prior to use if due allowance is made for the water or other volatile substances present in the quantity taken.

Unless specifically exempted elsewhere in this Pharmacopeia, the identity, strength, quality, and purity of an official article are determined by the definition, physical properties, tests, assays, and other specifications relating to the article, whether incorporated in the monograph itself, in the *General Notices*, or in the section *General Chapters*.

Water—Water used as an ingredient of official preparations meets the requirements for *Purified Water*, for *Water for Injection*, or for one of the sterile forms of water covered by a monograph in this Pharmacopeia.

Potable water meeting the requirements for drinking water as set forth in the regulations of the federal Environmental Protection Agency may be used in the preparation of official substances.

Alcohol—All statements of percentages of alcohol, such as under the heading *Alcohol content* refer to percentage, by volume, of C_2H_5OH at 15.56°. Where reference is made to "C_2H_5OH," the chemical entity possessing absolute (100 percent) strength is intended.

Alcohol—Where "alcohol" is called for in formulas, tests, and assays, the monograph article *Alcohol* is to be used.

Denatured Alcohol—Specially denatured alcohol formulas are available for use in accordance with federal statutes and regulations of the Internal Revenue Service. A suitable formula of specially denatured alcohol may be substituted for Alcohol in the manufacture of Pharmacopeial preparations intended for internal or topical use, provided that the denaturant is volatile and does not remain in the finished product. A finished product that is intended for topical application to the skin may contain specially denatured alcohol, provided that the denaturant is either a normal ingredient or a permissible added substance; in either case the denaturant must be identified on the label of the topical preparation. Where a process is given in the individual monograph, the preparation so made must be identical with that prepared by the given process.

Added Substances—An official substance, as distinguished from an official preparation, contains no added substances except where specifically permitted in the individual monograph. Where such addition is permitted, the label indicates the name(s) and amount(s) of any added substance(s).

Unless otherwise specified in the individual monograph, or elsewhere in the *General Notices*, suitable substances such as antimicrobial agents, bases, carriers, coatings, colors, flavors, preservatives, stabilizers, and vehicles may be added to an official preparation to enhance its stability, usefulness, or elegance or to facilitate its preparation. Such substances are regarded as unsuitable and are prohibited unless (a) they are harmless in the amounts used, (b) they do not exceed the minimum quantity required to provide their intended effect, (c) their presence does not impair the bioavailability or the therapeutic efficacy or safety of the official preparation, and (d) they do not interfere with the assays and tests prescribed for determining compliance with the Pharmacopeial standards.

Nutritional Supplements—Unless otherwise specified in the individual monograph, or elsewhere in the *General Notices*, consistent with applicable regulatory requirements, suitable added substances such as bases, carriers, coatings, colors, flavors, preservatives, and stabilizers may be added to a nutritional supplement preparation to enhance its stability, usefulness, or elegance, or to facilitate its preparation. Such added substances shall be regarded suitable and shall be permitted unless they interfere with the assays and tests prescribed for determining compliance with Pharmacopeial standards.

Additional Ingredients—Additional ingredients, including excipients, may be added to nutritional supplement preparations containing *recognized nutrients*, consistent with applicable regulatory requirements, provided that (a) they do not interfere with the assays and tests prescribed for determining compliance with Pharmacopeial standards, and (b) that such additional ingredients are listed separately on the label from those ingredients recognized in the definition of the USP article.

Inert Headspace Gases—The air in a container of an article for parenteral use may be evacuated or be replaced by carbon dioxide, helium, or nitrogen, or by a mixture of these gases, which fact need not be declared in the labeling.

Colors—Added substances employed solely to impart color may be incorporated into official preparations, except those intended for parenteral or ophthalmic use, in accordance with the regulations pertaining to the use of colors issued by the FDA provided such added substances are otherwise appropriate in all respects. (See also *Added Substances* under *Injections* ⟨1⟩.)

Ointments and Suppositories—In the preparation of ointments and suppositories, the proportions of the substances constituting the base may be varied to maintain a suitable consistency under different climatic conditions, provided the concentrations of active ingredients are not varied.

TESTS AND ASSAYS

Foreign Substances and Impurities—Tests for the presence of foreign substances and impurities are provided to limit such substances to amounts that are unobjectionable under conditions in which the article is customarily employed (see also *Impurities in Official Articles* ⟨1086⟩).

While one of the primary objectives of the Pharmacopeia is to assure the user of official articles of their identity, strength, quality, and purity, it is manifestly impossible to include in each monograph a test for every impurity, contaminant, or adulterant that might be present, including microbial contamination. These may arise from a change in the source of material or from a change in the processing, or may be introduced from extraneous sources. Tests suitable for detecting such occurrences, the presence of which is inconsistent with applicable manufacturing practice or good pharmaceutical practice, should be employed in addition to the tests provided in the individual monograph.

Procedures—Assay and test procedures are provided for determining compliance with the Pharmacopeial standards of identity, strength, quality, and purity.

Every compendial article in commerce shall be so constituted that when examined in accordance with these assay and test procedures, it meets all of the requirements in the monograph defining it. However, it is not to be inferred that application of every analytical procedure in the monograph to samples from every production batch is necessarily a prerequisite for assuring compliance with Pharmacopeial standards before the batch is released for distribution. Data derived from manufacturing *process validation* studies and from *in-process controls* may provide greater assurance that a batch meets a particular monograph requirement than analytical data derived from an examination of finished units drawn from that batch. On the basis of such assurances, the analytical procedures in the monograph may be omitted by the manufacturer in judging compliance of the batch with the Pharmacopeial standards.

Automated procedures employing the same basic chemistry as those assay and test procedures given in the monograph are recognized as being equivalent in their suitability for determining compliance. Conversely, where an automated procedure is given in the monograph, manual procedures employing the same basic chemistry are recognized as being equivalent in their suitability for determining compliance. Compliance may be determined also by the use of alternative methods, chosen for advantages in accuracy, sensitivity, precision, selectivity, or adaptability to automation or computerized data reduction or in other special circumstances. Such alternative or automated procedures or methods shall be validated. However, Pharmacopeial standards and procedures are interrelated; therefore, where a difference appears or in the event of dispute, only the result obtained by the procedure given in this Pharmacopeia is conclusive.

Odor—Terms such as "odorless," "practically odorless," "a faint characteristic odor," or variations thereof, apply to examination, after exposure to the air for 15 minutes, of either a freshly opened package of the article (for packages containing not more than 25 g) or (for larger packages) of a portion of about 25 g of the article that has been removed from its package to an open evaporating dish of about 100-mL capacity. An odor designation is descriptive only and is not to be regarded as a standard of purity for a particular lot of an article.

Test Results, Statistics, and Standards—Interpretation of results from official tests and assays requires an understanding of the nature and style of compendial standards, in addition to an understanding of the scientific and mathematical aspects of laboratory analysis and quality assurance for analytical laboratories.

Confusion of compendial standards with release tests and with statistical sampling plans occasionally occurs. Compendial standards define what is an acceptable article and give test procedures that demonstrate that the article is in compliance. These standards apply at any time in the life of the article from production to consumption. The manufacturer's release specifications, and compliance with good manufacturing practices generally, are developed and followed to assure that the article will indeed comply with compendial standards until its expiration date, when stored as directed. Thus, when tested from the viewpoint of commercial or regulatory compliance, any specimen tested as directed in the monograph for that article shall comply (see *Test and Assays* under *General Notices*).

Tests and assays in this Pharmacopeia prescribe operation on a single specimen, that is, the singlet determination, which is the minimum sample on which the attributes of a compendial article should be measured. Some tests, such as those for *Dissolution* and *Uniformity of dosage units*, require multiple dosage units in conjunction with a decision scheme. These tests, albeit using a number of dosage units, are in fact the singlet determinations of those particular attributes of the specimen. These procedures should not be confused with statistical sampling plans. The compendial procedures demonstrate compliance of the attributes of an article with compendial standards for a specimen (of one or more dosage units) that is subjected to analysis. Repeats, replicates, statistical rejection of outliers, or extrapolations of results to larger populations are neither specified nor proscribed by the compendia; such decisions are dependent on the objectives of the testing. Commercial or regulatory compliance testing, or manufacturer's release testing, may or may not require examination of additional specimens, in accordance with predetermined guidelines or sampling strategies. Treatments of data handling are available from organizations such as ISO, IUPAC, and AOAC.

Description—Information on the "description" pertaining to an article, which is relatively general in nature, is provided in the reference table *Description and Relative Solubility of USP and NF Articles* in this Pharmacopeia for those who use, prepare, and dispense drugs and/or related articles, solely to indicate properties of an article complying with monograph standards. The properties are not in themselves standards or tests for purity even though they may indirectly assist in the preliminary evaluation of an article.

Solubility—The statements concerning solubilities given in the reference table *Description and Relative Solubility of USP and NF Articles* for Pharmacopeial articles are not standards or tests for purity but are provided primarily as information for those who use, prepare, and dispense drugs and/or related articles. Only where a quantitative solubility test is given, and is designated as such, is it a test for purity.

The approximate solubilities of Pharmacopeial substances are indicated by the descriptive terms in the accompanying table.

Descriptive Term	Parts of Solvent Required for 1 Part of Solute
Very soluble	Less than 1
Freely soluble	From 1 to 10
Soluble	From 10 to 30
Sparingly soluble	From 30 to 100
Slightly soluble	From 100 to 1000

Descriptive Term	Parts of Solvent Required for 1 Part of Solute
Very slightly soluble	From 1000 to 10,000
Practically insoluble, or Insoluble	10,000 and over

Soluble Pharmacopeial articles, when brought into solution, may show traces of physical impurities, such as minute fragments of filter paper, fibers, and other particulate matter, unless limited or excluded by definite tests or other specifications in the individual monographs.

PRESCRIBING AND DISPENSING

Prescriptions for compendial articles shall be written to state the quantity and/or strength desired in metric units unless otherwise indicated in the individual monograph (see also *Units of Potency* in these *General Notices*). If an amount is prescribed by any other system of measurement, only an amount that is the metric equivalent of the prescribed amount shall be dispensed.

PRESERVATION, PACKAGING, STORAGE, AND LABELING

Containers—The *container* is that which holds the article and is or may be in direct contact with the article. The *immediate container* is that which is in direct contact with the article at all times. The *closure* is a part of the container.

Prior to its being filled, the container should be clean. Special precautions and cleaning procedures may be necessary to ensure that each container is clean and that extraneous matter is not introduced into or onto the article.

The container does not interact physically or chemically with the article placed in it so as to alter the strength, quality, or purity of the article beyond the official requirements.

The Pharmacopeial requirements for the use of specified containers apply also to articles as packaged by the pharmacist or other dispenser, unless otherwise indicated in the individual monograph.

Tamper-resistant Packaging—The container or individual carton of a sterile article intended for ophthalmic or otic use, except where extemporaneously compounded for immediate dispensing on prescription, shall be so sealed that the contents cannot be used without obvious destruction of the seal.

Articles intended for sale without prescription are also required to comply with the tamper-resistant packaging and labeling requirements of the FDA where applicable.

Preferably, the immediate container and/or the outer container or protective packaging utilized by a manufacturer or distributor for all dosage forms that are not specifically exempt is designed so as to show evidence of any tampering with the contents.

Light-resistant Container (see *Light Transmission* under *Containers* ⟨661⟩)—A light-resistant container protects the contents from the effects of light by virtue of the specific properties of the material of which it is composed, including any coating applied to it. Alternatively, a clear and colorless or a translucent container may be made light-resistant by means of an opaque covering, in which case the label of the container bears a statement that the opaque covering is needed until the contents are to be used or administered. Where it is directed to "protect from light" in an individual monograph, preservation in a light-resistant container is intended.

Where an article is required to be packaged in a light-resistant container, and if the container is made light-resistant by means of an opaque covering, a single-use, unit-dose container or mnemonic pack for dispensing may not be removed from the outer opaque covering prior to dispensing.

Well-closed Container—A well-closed container protects the contents from extraneous solids and from loss of the article under the ordinary or customary conditions of handling, shipment, storage, and distribution.

Tight Container—A tight container protects the contents from contamination by extraneous liquids, solids, or vapors, from loss of the article, and from efflorescence, deliquescence, or evaporation under the ordinary or customary conditions of handling, shipment, storage, and distribution, and is capable of tight re-closure. Where a tight container is specified, it may be replaced by a hermetic container for a single dose of an article.

A gas cylinder is a metallic container designed to hold a gas under pressure. As a safety measure, for carbon dioxide, cyclopropane, helium, nitrous oxide, and oxygen, the Pin-index Safety System of matched fittings is recommended for cylinders of Size E or smaller.

NOTE—Where packaging and storage in a *tight container* or a *well-closed container* is specified in the individual monograph, the container utilized for an article when dispensed on prescription meets the requirements under *Containers—Permeation* ⟨671⟩.

Hermetic Container—A hermetic container is impervious to air or any other gas under the ordinary or customary conditions of handling, shipment, storage, and distribution.

Single-unit Container—A single-unit container is one that is designed to hold a quantity of drug product intended for administration as a single dose or a single finished device intended for use promptly after the container is opened. Preferably, the immediate container and/or the outer container or protective packaging shall be so designed as to show evidence of any tampering with the contents. Each single-unit container shall be labeled to indicate the identity, quantity and/or strength, name of the manufacturer, lot number, and expiration date of the article.

Single-dose Container (see also *Containers for Injections* under *Injections* ⟨1⟩)—A single-dose container is a single-unit container for articles intended for parenteral administration only. A single-dose container is labeled as such. Examples of single-dose containers include pre-filled syringes, cartridges, fusion-sealed containers, and closure-sealed containers when so labeled.

Unit-dose Container—A unit-dose container is a single-unit container for articles intended for administration by other than the parenteral route as a single dose, direct from the container.

Multiple-unit Container—A multiple-unit container is a container that permits withdrawal of successive portions of the contents without changing the strength, quality, or purity of the remaining portion.

Multiple-dose Container (see also *Containers for Injections* under *Injections* ⟨1⟩)—A multiple-dose container is a multiple-unit container for articles intended for parenteral administration only.

Storage Temperature—Specific directions are stated in some monographs with respect to the temperatures at which Pharmacopeial articles shall be stored, when stability data indicate that storage at a lower or a higher temperature produces undesirable results. Such directions apply except where the label on an article states a different storage temperature on the basis of stability studies of that particular formulation. The conditions are defined by the following terms.

Freezer—A place in which the temperature is maintained thermostatically between −20° and −10° (−4° and 14°F).

Cold—Any temperature not exceeding 8° (46°F). A *refrigerator* is a cold place in which the temperature is maintained thermostatically between 2° and 8° (36° and 46°F).

Cool—Any temperature between 8° and 15° (46° and 59°F). An article for which storage in a *cool place* is directed may, alternatively, be stored in a *refrigerator*, unless otherwise specified by the individual monograph.

Room Temperature—The temperature prevailing in a working area.

Controlled Room Temperature—A temperature maintained thermostatically that encompasses the usual and customary working environment of 20° to 25° (68° to 77°F); that results in a mean kinetic temperature calculated to be not more than 25°; and that allows for excursions between 15° and 30° (59° and 86°F) that are experienced in pharmacies, hospitals, and warehouses. Articles may be labeled for storage at "controlled room temperature" or at "up to 25°", or other wording based on the same mean kinetic temperature. The mean kinetic temperature is a calculated value that may be used as an isothermal storage temperature that simulates the nonisothermal effects of storage temperature variations. (See also *Stability* under *Pharmaceutical Dosage Forms* ⟨1151⟩.)

An article for which storage at *Controlled room temperature* is directed may, alternatively, be stored in a *cool place*, unless otherwise specified in the individual monograph or on the label.

Warm—Any temperature between 30° and 40° (86° and 104°F).

Excessive Heat—Any temperature above 40° (104°F).

Protection from Freezing—Where, in addition to the risk of breakage of the container, freezing subjects an article to loss of strength or potency, or to destructive alteration of its characteristics, the container label bears an appropriate instruction to protect the article from freezing.

Storage under Nonspecific Conditions—For articles, regardless of quantity, where no specific storage directions or limitations are provided in the individual monograph, it is to be understood that conditions of storage and distribution include protection from moisture, freezing, and excessive heat.

Labeling—The term "labeling" designates all labels and other written, printed, or graphic matter upon an immediate container of an article or upon, or in, any package or wrapper in which it is enclosed, except any outer shipping container. The term "label" designates that part of the labeling upon the immediate container.

A shipping container, unless such container is also essentially the immediate container or the outside of the consumer package, is exempt from the labeling requirements of this Pharmacopeia.

Articles in this Pharmacopeia are subject to compliance with such labeling requirements as may be promulgated by governmental bodies in addition to the Pharmacopeial requirements set forth for the articles.

Amount of Ingredient per Dosage Unit—The strength of a drug product is expressed on the container label in terms of micrograms or milligrams or grams or percentage of the therapeutically active moiety or drug substance, whichever form is used in the title. Both the active moiety and drug substance names and their equivalent amounts are then provided in the labeling.

Pharmacopeial articles in capsule, tablet, or other unit dosage form shall be labeled to express the quantity of each active ingredient or recognized nutrient contained in each such unit. Pharmacopeial drug products not in unit dosage form shall be labeled to express the quantity of each active ingredient in each milliliter or in each gram, or to express the percentage of each such ingredient (see *Percentage Measurements*), except that oral liquids or solids intended to be constituted to yield oral liquids may, alternatively, be labeled in terms of each 5-milliliter portion of the liquid or resulting liquid. Unless otherwise indicated in a monograph or chapter, such declarations of strength or quantity shall be stated only in metric units (see also *Units of Potency* in these *General Notices*.

In order to help minimize the possibility of errors in the dispensing and administration of drugs, the quantity of active ingredient when expressed in whole numbers shall be shown without a decimal point that is followed by a terminal zero (e.g., express as 4 mg [not 4.0 mg]). The quantity of active ingredient when expressed as a decimal number smaller than one shall be shown with a zero preceding the decimal point (e.g., express as 0.2 mg [not .2 mg]).

Labeling of Salts of Drugs—It is an established principle that Pharmacopeial articles shall have only one official name. For purposes of saving space on labels, and because chemical symbols for the most common inorganic salts of drugs are well known to practitioners as synonymous with the written forms, the following alternatives are permitted in labeling official articles that are salts: HCl for hydrochloride; HBr for hydrobromide; Na for sodium; and K for potassium. The symbols Na and K are intended for use in abbreviating names of the salts of organic acids; but these symbols are not used where the word Sodium or Potassium appears at the beginning of an official title (e.g., Phenobarbital Na is acceptable, but Na Salicylate is not to be written).

Labeling Vitamin-containing Products—The vitamin content of Pharmacopeial preparations shall be stated on the label in metric units per dosage unit. The amounts of vitamins A, D, and E may be stated also in USP Units. Quantities of vitamin A declared in metric units refer to the equivalent amounts of retinol (vitamin A alcohol). The label of a nutritional supplement shall bear an identifying lot number, control number, or batch number.

Labeling Parenteral and Topical Preparations—The label of a preparation intended for parenteral or topical use states the names of all added substances (see *Added Substances* in these General Notices, and see *Labeling* under *Injections* ⟨1⟩), and, in the case of parenteral preparations, also their amounts or proportions, except that for substances added for adjustment of pH or to achieve isotonicity, the label may indicate only their presence and the reason for their addition.

Labeling Electrolytes—The concentration and dosage of electrolytes for replacement therapy (e.g., sodium chloride or potassium chloride) shall be stated on the label in milliequivalents (mEq). The label of the product shall indicate also the quantity of ingredient(s) in terms of weight or percentage concentration.

Labeling Alcohol—The content of alcohol in a liquid preparation shall be stated on the label as a percentage (v/v) of C_2H_5OH.

Special Capsules and Tablets—The label of any form of Capsule or Tablet intended for administration other than by swallowing intact bears a prominent indication of the manner in which it is to be used.

Expiration Date—The label of an official drug product or nutritional supplement shall bear an expiration date. All articles shall display the expiration date so that it can be read by an ordinary individual under customary conditions of purchase and use. The expiration date shall be prominently displayed in high contrast to the background or sharply embossed, and easily understood (e.g., "EXP 6/89," "Exp. June 89," "Expires 6/89"). [NOTE—For additional information and guidance, refer to the Nonprescription Drug Manufacturers Association's *Voluntary Codes and Guidelines of the OTC Medicines Industry*.]

The monographs for some preparations state how the expiration date that shall appear on the label is to be determined. In the absence of a specific requirement in the individual monograph for a drug product or nutritional supplement, the label shall bear an expiration date assigned for the particular formulation and package of the article, with the following exception: the label need not show an expiration date in the case of a drug product or nutritional supplement packaged in a container that is intended for sale without prescription and the labeling of which states no dosage limitations, and which is stable for not less than 3 years when stored under the prescribed conditions.

Where an official article is required to bear an expiration date, such article shall be dispensed solely in, or from, a container labeled with an expiration date, and the date on which the article is dispensed shall be within the labeled expiry period. The expiration date identifies the time during which the article may be expected to meet the requirements of the Pharmacopeial monograph provided it is kept under the prescribed storage conditions. The expiration date limits the time during which the article may be dispensed or used. Where an expiration date is stated only in terms of the month and the year, it is a representation that the intended expiration date is the last day of the stated month.

For articles requiring constitution prior to use, a suitable beyond-use date for the constituted product shall be identified in the labeling.

In determining an appropriate period of time during which a prescription drug may be retained by a patient after its dispensing, the dispenser shall take into account, in addition to any other relevant factors, the nature of the drug; the container in which it was packaged by the manufacturer and the expiration date thereon; the characteristics of the patient's container, if the article is repackaged for dispensing; the expected storage conditions to which the article may be exposed; and the expected length of time of the course of therapy. Unless otherwise required, the dispenser may, on taking into account the foregoing, place on the label of a multiple-unit container a suitable beyond-use date to limit the patient's use of the article. Unless otherwise specified in the individual monograph, such beyond-use date shall be not later than (a) the expiration date on the manufacturer's container, or (b) one year from the date the drug is dispensed, whichever is earlier.

WEIGHTS AND MEASURES

The International System of Units (SI) is used in this Pharmacopeia. The SI metric and other units, and the symbols commonly employed, are as follows.

Ci	= curie	Eq	= gram-equivalent weight (equivalent)
mCi	= millicurie	mEq	= milliequivalent
μCi	= microcurie	mol	= gram-molecular weight (mole)
nCi	= nanocurie		
Mrad	= megarad	Da	= dalton (relative molecular mass)
m	= meter	mmol	= millimole
dm	= decimeter	Osmol	= osmole
cm	= centimeter	mOsmol	= milliosmole
mm	= millimeter	Hz	= hertz
μm	= micrometer (0.001 mm)	kHz	= kilohertz
		MHz	= megahertz
nm	= nanometer*	MeV	= million electron volts
kg	= kilogram		
g	= gram **	keV	= kilo-electron volt
mg	= milligram	mV	= millivolt
μg; mcg	= microgram†	psi	= pounds per square inch
ng	= nanogram		
pg	= picogram	Pa	= pascal

dL = deciliter	kPa = kilopascal
L = liter	*g* = gravity (in centrifugation)
mL = milliliter; ‡	
μL = microliter	

---

* Formerly the symbol mμ (for millimicron) was used.

** The gram is the unit of mass that is used to measure quantities of materials. Weight, which is a measure of the gravitational force acting on the mass of a material, is proportional to, and may differ slightly from, its mass due to the effects of factors such as gravity, temperature, latitude, and altitude. The difference between mass and weight is considered to be insignificant for compendial assays and tests, and the term "weight" is used throughout *USP* and *NF*.

† Formerly the abbreviation mcg was used in the Pharmacopeial monographs; however, the symbol μg now is more widely accepted and thus is used in this Pharmacopeia. The term "gamma," symbolized by γ, is frequently used for microgram in biochemical literature.

NOTE—The abbreviation mcg is still commonly employed to denote microgram(s) in labeling and in prescription writing. Therefore, for purposes of labeling, "mcg" may be used to denote microgram(s).

‡ One milliliter (mL) is used herein as the equivalent of 1 cubic centimeter (cc).

The International System of Units (SI) is also used in all radiopharmaceutical monographs. The symbols commonly employed are as follows.

Bq = becquerel	GBq = gigabecquerel
kBq = kilobecquerel	Gy = gray
MBq = megabecquerel	mGy = milligray

CONCENTRATIONS

Percentage Measurements—Percentage concentrations are expressed as follows:

Percent weight in weight—(w/w) expresses the number of g of a constituent in 100 g of solution or mixture.

Percent weight in volume—(w/v) expresses the number of g of a constituent in 100 mL of solution, and is used regardless of whether water or another liquid is the solvent.

Percent volume in volume—(v/v) expresses the number of mL of a constituent in 100 mL of solution.

The term *percent* used without qualification means, for mixtures of solids and semisolids, percent weight in weight; for solutions or suspensions of solids in liquids, percent weight in volume; for solutions of liquids in liquids, percent volume in volume; and for solutions of gases in liquids, percent weight in volume. For example, a 1 percent solution is prepared by dissolving 1 g of a solid or semisolid, or 1 mL of a liquid, in sufficient solvent to make 100 mL of the solution.

In the dispensing of prescription medications, slight changes in volume owing to variations in room temperatures may be disregarded.

Drug and Dosage Form Requirements

⟨1⟩ INJECTIONS

INTRODUCTION

Parenteral articles are preparations intended for injection through the skin or other external boundary tissue, rather than through the alimentary canal, so that the active substances they contain are administered, using gravity or force, directly into a blood vessel, organ, tissue, or lesion. Parenteral articles are prepared scrupulously by methods designed to ensure that they meet Pharmacopeial requirements for sterility, pyrogens, particulate matter, and other contaminants, and, where appropriate, contain inhibitors of the growth of microorganisms. An Injection is a preparation intended for parenteral administration and/or for constituting or diluting a parenteral article prior to administration.

NOMENCLATURE AND DEFINITIONS

Nomenclature

The following nomenclature pertains to five general types of preparations, all of which are suitable for, and intended for, parenteral administration. They may contain buffers, preservatives, or other added substances.

1. [*DRUG*] *Injection*—Liquid preparations that are drug substances or solutions thereof.
2. [*DRUG*] *for Injection*—Dry solids that, upon the addition of suitable vehicles, yield solutions conforming in all respects to the requirements for *Injections*.
3. [*DRUG*] *Injectable Emulsion*—Liquid preparations of drug substances dissolved or dispersed in a suitable emulsion medium.
4. [*DRUG*] *Injectable Suspension*—Liquid preparations of solids suspended in a suitable liquid medium.
5. [*DRUG*] *for Injectable Suspension*—Dry solids that, upon the addition of suitable vehicles, yield preparations conforming in all respects to the requirements for *Injectable Suspensions*.

Definitions

PHARMACY BULK PACKAGE

A *Pharmacy bulk package* is a container of a sterile preparation for parenteral use that contains many single doses. The contents are intended for use in a pharmacy admixture program and are restricted to the preparation of admixtures for infusion or, through a sterile transfer device, for the filling of empty sterile syringes.

The closure shall be penetrated only one time after constitution with a suitable sterile transfer device or dispensing set which allows measured dispensing of the contents. The *Pharmacy bulk package* is to be used only in a suitable work area such as a laminar flow hood (or an equivalent clean air compounding area).

Designation as a *Pharmacy bulk package* is limited to preparations from *Nomenclature* categories 1, 2, or 3 as defined above. *Pharmacy bulk packages*, although containing more than one single dose, are exempt from the multiple-dose container volume limit of 30 mL and the requirement that they contain a substance or suitable mixture of substances to prevent the growth of microorganisms.

Where a container is offered as a *Pharmacy bulk package*, the label shall (a) state prominently "Pharmacy Bulk Package—Not for direct infusion," (b) contain or refer to information on proper techniques to help assure safe use of the product, and (c) bear a statement limiting the time frame in which the container may be used once it has been entered, provided it is held under the labeled storage conditions.

LARGE- AND SMALL-VOLUME INJECTIONS

Where used in this Pharmacopeia, the designation *Large-volume intravenous solution* applies to a single-dose injection that is intended for intravenous use and is packaged in containers labeled as containing more than 100 mL. The designation *Small-volume Injection* applies to an Injection that is packaged in containers labeled as containing 100 mL or less.

BIOLOGICS

The Pharmacopeial definitions for sterile preparations for parenteral use generally do not apply in the case of the biologics because of their special nature and licensing requirements (see *Biologics* ⟨1041⟩).

INGREDIENTS
Vehicles and Added Substances

Aqueous Vehicles—The vehicles for aqueous Injections meet the requirements of the *Pyrogen Test* ⟨151⟩ or the *Bacterial Endotoxins Test* ⟨85⟩, whichever is specified. *Water for Injection* generally is used as the vehicle, unless otherwise specified in the individual monograph. Sodium chloride may be added in amounts sufficient to render the resulting solution isotonic; and *Sodium Chloride Injection*, or *Ringer's Injection*, may be used in whole or in part instead of *Water for Injection* unless otherwise specified in the individual monograph. For conditions applying to other adjuvants, see *Added Substances* in this chapter.

Other Vehicles—Fixed oils used as vehicles for nonaqueous injections are of vegetable origin, are odorless or nearly so, and have no odor suggesting rancidity. They meet the requirements of the test for *Solid paraffin* under *Mineral Oil*, the cooling bath being maintained at 10°, have a *Saponification value* of between 185 and 200 (see *Fats and Fixed Oils* ⟨401⟩), have an *Iodine value* of between 79 and 128 (see *Fats and Fixed Oils* ⟨401⟩), and meet the requirements of the following tests.

Unsaponifiable Matter—Reflux on a steam bath 10 mL of the oil with 15 mL of sodium hydroxide solution (1 in 6) and 30 mL of alcohol, with occasional shaking until the mixture becomes clear. Transfer the solution to a shallow dish, evaporate the alcohol on a steam bath, and mix the residue with 100 mL of water: a clear solution results.

Free Fatty Acids—The free fatty acids in 10 g of oil require for neutralization not more than 2.0 mL of 0.020 *N* sodium hydroxide (see *Fats and Fixed Oils* ⟨401⟩).

Synthetic mono- or diglycerides of fatty acids may be used as vehicles, provided they are liquid and remain clear when cooled to 10° and have an *Iodine value* of not more than 140 (see *Fats and Fixed Oils* ⟨401⟩).

These and other nonaqueous vehicles may be used, provided they are safe in the volume of injection administered, and also provided they do not interfere with the therapeutic efficacy of the preparation or with its response to prescribed assays and tests.

Added Substances—Suitable substances may be added to preparations intended for injection to increase stability or usefulness, unless proscribed in the individual monograph, provided they are harmless in the amounts administered and do not interfere with the therapeutic efficacy or with the responses to the specified assays and tests. No coloring agent may be added, solely for the purpose of coloring the finished preparation, to a solution intended for parenteral administration (see also *Added Substances* under *General Notices* and *Antimicrobial Preservatives—Effectiveness* ⟨51⟩).

Observe special care in the choice and use of added substances in preparations for injection that are administered in a volume exceeding 5 mL. The following maximum limits prevail unless otherwise directed: for agents containing mercury and the cationic, surface-active compounds, 0.01%; for those of the types of chlorobutanol, cresol, and phenol, 0.5%; and for sulfur dioxide, or an equivalent amount of the sulfite, bisulfite, or metabisulfite of potassium or sodium, 0.2%.

A suitable substance or mixture of substances to prevent the growth of microorganisms must be added to preparations intended for injection that are packaged in multiple-dose containers, regardless of the method of sterilization employed, unless otherwise directed in the individual monograph, or unless the active ingredients are themselves antimicrobial. Such substances are used in concentrations that will prevent the growth of or kill microorganisms in the preparations for injection. Such substances also meet the requirements of *Antimicrobial Preservatives—Effectiveness* ⟨51⟩ and *Antimicrobial Agents—Content* ⟨341⟩. Sterilization processes are employed even though such substances are used (see also *Parenteral and Topical Preparations* in the section *Added Substances* under *General Notices* and *Sterilization and Sterility Assurance of Compendial Articles* ⟨1211⟩). The air in the container may be evacuated or be displaced by a chemically inert gas. Where specified in a monograph, information regarding sensitivity of the article to oxygen is to be provided in the labeling.

LABELS AND LABELING

Labeling—[NOTE—See definitions of "label" and "labeling" under *Labeling* in the section *Preservation, Packaging, Storage, and Labeling* of the *General Notices*.]

The label states the name of the preparation; in the case of a liquid preparation, the percentage content of drug or amount of drug in a specified volume; in the case of a dry preparation, the amount of *active* ingredient; the route of administration; a statement of storage conditions and an expiration date; the name of the manufacturer and distributor; and an identifying lot number. The lot number is capable of yielding the complete manufacturing history of the specific package, including all manufacturing, filling, sterilizing, and labeling operations.

Where the individual monograph permits varying concentrations of active ingredients in the large-volume parenteral, the concentration of each ingredient named in the official title is stated as if part of the official title, e.g., Dextrose Injection 5%, or Dextrose (5%) and Sodium Chloride (0.2%) Injection.

The labeling includes the following information if the complete formula is not specified in the individual monograph: (1) In the case of a liquid preparation, the percentage content of each ingredient or the amount of each ingredient in a specified volume, except that ingredients added to adjust to a given pH or to make the solution isotonic may be declared by name and a statement of their effect; and (2) in the case of a dry preparation or other preparation to which a diluent is intended to be added before use, the amount of each ingredient, the composition of recommended diluent(s) [the name(s) alone, if the formula is specified in the individual monograph], the amount to be used to attain a specific concentration of active ingredient and the final volume of solution so obtained, a brief description of the physical appearance of the constituted solution, directions for proper storage of the constituted solution, and an expiration date limiting the period during which the constituted solution may be expected to have the required or labeled potency if it has been stored as directed.

Containers for Injections that are intended for use as dialysis, hemofiltration, or irrigation solutions and that contain a volume of more than 1 liter are labeled to indicate that the contents are not intended for use by intravenous infusion.

Injections intended for veterinary use are labeled to that effect.

The container is so labeled that a sufficient area of the container remains uncovered for its full length or circumference to permit inspection of the contents.

PACKAGING

Containers for Injections

Containers, including the closures, for preparations for injections do not interact physically or chemically with the preparations in any manner to alter the strength, quality, or purity beyond the official requirements under the ordinary or customary conditions of handling, shipment, storage, sale, and use. The container is made of material that permits inspection of the contents. The type of glass preferable for each parenteral preparation is usually stated in the individual monograph.

For definitions of single-dose and multiple-dose containers, see *Containers* under *General Notices*. Containers meet the requirements under *Containers* ⟨661⟩.

Containers are closed by fusion, or by application of suitable closures, in such manner as to prevent contamination or loss of contents. Closures for multiple-dose containers permit the withdrawal of the contents without removal or destruction of the closure. The closure permits penetration by a needle, and, upon withdrawal of the needle, at once recloses the container against contamination.

The use of a black closure system on a vial (e.g., a black flip-off button and a black ferrule to hold the elastomeric closure), or the use of a black band or series of bands above the constriction on an ampul, is prohibited except for *Potassium Chloride for Injection Concentrate*.

Containers for Sterile Solids

Containers, including the closures, for dry solids intended for parenteral use do not interact physically or chemically with the preparation in any manner to alter the strength, quality, or purity beyond the official requirements under the ordinary or customary conditions of handling, shipment, storage, sale, and use.

A container for a sterile solid permits the addition of a suitable solvent and withdrawal of portions of the resulting solution or suspension in such manner that the sterility of the product is maintained.

Where the *Assay* in a monograph provides a procedure for *Assay preparation* in which the total withdrawable contents are to be withdrawn from a single-dose container with a hypodermic needle and syringe, the contents are to be withdrawn as completely as possible into a dry hypodermic syringe of a rated capacity not exceeding three times the volume to be withdrawn and fitted with a 21-gauge needle not less than 2.5 cm (1 inch) in length, care being taken to expel any air bubbles, and discharged into a container for dilution and assay.

Volume in Container—Each container of an Injection is filled with a volume in slight excess of the labeled "size" or that volume which is to be withdrawn. The excess volumes recommended in the accompanying table are usually sufficient to permit withdrawal and administration of the labeled volumes.

DETERMINATION OF VOLUME OF INJECTION IN CONTAINERS

Select 1 or more containers if the volume is 10 mL or more, 3 or more if the volume is more than 3 mL and less than 10 mL, or 5 or more if the volume is 3 mL or less. Take up individually the contents of each container selected into a dry hypodermic syringe of a rated capacity not exceeding three times the volume to be measured, and fitted with a 21-gauge needle not less than 2.5 cm (1 inch) in length. Expel any air bubbles from the syringe and needle, and then discharge the contents of the syringe, without emptying the needle, into a standardized, dry cylinder (graduated to contain rather than to deliver the designated volumes) of such size that the volume to be measured occupies at least 40% of its rated volume. Alternatively, the contents of the syringe may be discharged into a dry, tared beaker, the volume, in mL, being calculated as the weight, in g, of Injection taken divided by its density. The contents of two or three 1-mL or 2-mL containers may be pooled for the measurement, provided that a separate, dry syringe assembly is used for each container. The content of containers holding 10 mL or more may be determined by means of opening them and emptying the contents directly into the graduated cylinder or tared beaker.

The volume is not less than the labeled volume in the case of containers examined individually or, in the case of 1-mL and 2-mL containers, is not less than the sum of the labeled volumes of the containers taken collectively.

For Injections in multiple-dose containers labeled to yield a specific number of doses of a stated volume, proceed as directed in the foregoing, using the same number of separate syringes as the number of doses specified. The volume is such that each syringe delivers not less than the stated dose.

For Injections containing oil, warm the containers, if necessary, and thoroughly shake them immediately before removing the contents. Cool to 25° before measuring the volume.

Packaging and Storage

The volume of Injection in single-dose containers provides the amount specified for parenteral administration at one time and in no case is more than sufficient to permit the withdrawal and administration of 1 liter.

Preparations intended for intraspinal, intracisternal, or peridural administration are packaged only in single-dose containers.

Unless otherwise specified in the individual monograph, no multiple-dose container contains a volume of Injection more than sufficient to permit the withdrawal of 30 mL.

Injections packaged for use as irrigation solutions or for hemofiltration or dialysis or for parenteral nutrition are exempt from the 1-liter restriction of the foregoing requirements relating to packaging. Containers for Injections packaged for use as hemofiltration or irrigation solutions may be designed to empty rapidly and may contain a volume of more than 1 liter.

Injections labeled for veterinary use are exempt from packaging and storage requirements concerning the limitation to single-dose containers and the limitation on the volume of multiple-dose containers.

FOREIGN MATTER AND PARTICLES

Foreign Matter

Every care should be exercised in the preparation of all products intended for injection, to prevent contamination with microorganisms and foreign material. Good pharmaceutical practice requires also that each final container of Injection be subjected individually to a physical inspection, whenever the nature of the container permits, and that every container whose contents show evidence of contamination with visible foreign material be rejected.

Particulate Matter

All large-volume Injections for single-dose infusion, and those small-volume Injections for which the monographs specify such requirements, are subject to the particulate matter limits set forth under *Particulate Matter in Injections* ⟨788⟩. An article packaged as both a large-volume and a small-volume Injection meets the requirements set forth for *Small-volume Injections* where the container is labeled as containing 100 mL or less if the individual monograph includes a test for *Particulate matter;* it meets the requirements set forth for *Large-volume Injections for Single-dose Infusion* where the container is labeled as containing more than 100 mL. Injections packaged and labeled for use as irrigating solutions are exempt from requirements for *Particulate matter.*

	Recommended Excess Volume	
Labeled Size	For Mobile Liquids	For Viscous Liquids
0.5 mL	0.10 mL	0.12 mL
1.0 mL	0.10 mL	0.15 mL
2.0 mL	0.15 mL	0.25 mL
5.0 mL	0.30 mL	0.50 mL
10.0 mL	0.50 mL	0.70 mL
20.0 mL	0.60 mL	0.90 mL
30.0 mL	0.80 mL	1.20 mL
50.0 mL or more	2%	3%

STERILITY

Sterility Tests—Preparations for injection meet the requirements under *Sterility Tests* ⟨71⟩.

CONSTITUTED SOLUTIONS

Dry solids from which constituted solutions are prepared for injection bear titles of the form [*DRUG*] *for Injection.* Since these dosage forms are constituted at the time of use by the health care practitioner, tests and standards pertaining to the solution as constituted for administration are not included in the individual monographs on sterile dry solids or liquid concentrates. However, in the interest of assuring the quality of injection preparations as they are actually administered, the following nondestructive tests are provided for demonstrating the suitability of constituted solutions when they are prepared just prior to use.

Completeness and Clarity of Solution—Constitute the solution as directed in the labeling supplied by the manufacturer for the sterile dry dosage form.

A: The solid dissolves completely, leaving no visible residue as undissolved matter.

B: The constituted solution is not significantly less clear than an equal volume of the diluent or of Purified Water contained in a similar vessel and examined similarly.

Particulate Matter—Constitute the solution as directed in the labeling supplied by the manufacturer for the sterile dry dosage form: the solution is essentially free from particles of foreign matter that can be observed on visual inspection.

⟨751⟩ METAL PARTICLES IN OPHTHALMIC OINTMENTS

The following test is designed to limit to a level considered to be unobjectionable the number and size of discrete metal particles that may occur in ophthalmic ointments.

Procedure—Extrude, as completely as practicable, the contents of 10 tubes individually into separate, clear, flat-bottom, 60-mm petri dishes that are free from scratches. Cover the dishes, and heat at 85° for 2 hours, increasing the temperature slightly if necessary to ensure that a fully fluid state is obtained. Taking precautions against disturbing the melted sample, allow each to cool to room temperature and to solidify.

Remove the covers, and invert each petri dish on the stage of a suitable microscope adjusted to furnish 30 times magnification and equipped with an eye-piece micrometer disk that has been calibrated at the magnification being used. In addition to the usual source of light, direct an illuminator from above the ointment at a 45° angle. Examine the entire bottom of the petri dish for metal particles. Varying the intensity of the illuminator from above allows such metal particles to be recognized by their characteristic reflection of light.

Count the number of metal particles that are 50 μm or larger in any dimension: the requirements are met if the total number of such particles in all 10 tubes does not exceed 50, and if not more than 1 tube is found to contain more than 8 such particles. If these results are not obtained, repeat the test on 20 additional tubes: the requirements are met if the total number of metal particles that are 50 μm or larger in any dimension does not exceed 150 in all 30 tubes tested, and if not more than 3 of the tubes are found to contain more than 8 such particles each.

⟨771⟩ OPHTHALMIC OINTMENTS

Added Substances—Suitable substances may be added to ophthalmic ointments to increase stability or usefulness, unless proscribed in the individual monograph, provided they are harmless in the amounts administered and do not interfere with the therapeutic efficacy or with the responses to the specified assays and tests. No coloring agent may be added, solely for the purpose of coloring the finished preparation, to an article intended for ophthalmic use (see also *Added Substances* under *General Notices* and under *Antimicrobial Preservatives—Effectiveness* ⟨51⟩).

A suitable substance or mixture of substances to prevent the growth of microorganisms must be added to ophthalmic ointments that are packaged in multiple-use containers, regardless of the method of sterilization employed, unless otherwise directed in the individual monograph, or unless the formula itself is bacteriostatic. Such substances are used in concentrations that will prevent the growth of or kill microorganisms in the ophthalmic ointments (see also *Antimicrobial Preservatives—Effectiveness* ⟨51⟩ and *Antimicrobial Agents—Content* ⟨341⟩). Sterilization processes are employed for the finished ointment or for all ingredients, if the ointment is manufactured under rigidly aseptic conditions, even though such substances are used (see also *Parenteral and Topical Preparations* in the section *Added Substances*, under *General Notices*, and *Sterilization and Sterility Assurance of Compendial Articles* ⟨1211⟩). Ophthalmic ointments that are packaged in single-use containers are not required to contain antibacterial agents; however, they meet the requirements for *Sterility Tests* ⟨71⟩.

Containers—Containers, including the closures, for ophthalmic ointments do not interact physically or chemically with the preparation in any manner to alter the strength, quality, or purity beyond the official requirements under the ordinary or customary conditions of handling, shipment, storage, sale, and use (see also *Containers for Articles Intended for Ophthalmic Use* under *General Notices*).

Metal Particles—Follow the *Procedure* set forth under *Metal Particles in Ophthalmic Ointments* ⟨751⟩.

Leakage—Select 10 tubes of the Ointment, with seals applied when specified. Thoroughly clean and dry the exterior surfaces of each tube with an absorbent cloth. Place the tubes in a horizontal position on a sheet of absorbent blotting paper in an oven maintained at a temperature of 60 ± 3° for 8 hours. No significant leakage occurs during or at the completion of the test (disregard traces of ointment presumed to originate externally from within the crimp of the tube or from the thread of the cap). If leakage is observed from one, but not more than one, of the tubes, repeat the test with 20 additional tubes of the Ointment. The requirement is met if no leakage is observed from the first 10 tubes tested, or if leakage is observed from not more than one of 30 tubes tested.

⟨785⟩ OSMOLARITY

Osmotic pressure is fundamentally related to all biological processes that involve diffusion of solutes or transfer of fluids through membranes. Thus, knowledge of the osmolar concentrations of parenteral fluids is essential. The labels of Pharmacopeial solutions that provide intravenous replenishment of fluid, nutrient(s), or electrolyte(s), as well as of the osmotic diuretic Mannitol Injection, are required to state the osmolar concentration.

The declaration of osmolar concentration on the label of a parenteral solution serves primarily to inform the practitioner whether the solution is hypo-osmotic, iso-osmotic, or hyper-osmotic. A quantitative statement facilitates calculation of the dilution required to render a hyperosmotic solution iso-osmotic. It also simplifies many calculations involved in peritoneal dialysis and hemodialysis procedures. The osmolar concentration of an extemporaneously compounded intravenous solution prepared in the pharmacy (e.g., a hyperalimentation solution) from osmolar-labeled solutions also can be obtained simply by summing the osmoles contributed by each constituent.

The units of osmolar concentration are usually expressed as milliosmoles (abbreviation: mOsmol) of solute per liter of solution. In general terms, the weight of an osmole is the gram molecular weight of a substance divided by the number of ions or chemical species (n) formed upon dissolution. In ideal solutions, for example, $n = 1$ for glucose, $n = 2$ for sodium chloride or magnesium sulfate, $n = 3$ for calcium chloride, and $n = 4$ for sodium citrate.

The ideal osmolar concentration may be determined according to the formula:

$$\text{osmolar concentration (mOsmol/liter)} = \text{mOsM}$$

$$= \frac{\text{wt. of substance (g/liter)}}{\text{mol. wt. (g)}} \times \text{number of species} \times 1000.$$

As the concentration of the solute increases, interaction among solute particles increases, and actual osmolar values decrease when compared to ideal values. Deviation from ideal conditions is usually slight in solutions within the physiologic range and for more dilute solutions, but for highly concentrated solutions the actual osmolarities may be appreciably lower than ideal values. For example, the ideal osmolarity of 0.9% Sodium Chloride Injection is $9/58.4 \times 2 \times 1000 = 308$ milliosmoles per liter. In fact, however, n is slightly less than 2 for solutions of sodium chloride at this concentration, and the actual measured osmolarity of 0.9% Sodium Chloride Injection is about 286 milliosmoles per liter.

The theoretical osmolarity of a complex mixture, such as Protein Hydrolysate Injection, cannot be readily calculated. In such instances, actual values of osmolar concentration are to be used to meet the labeling requirement set forth in the individual monograph. They are determined by calculating the osmolarity from measured values of osmolal concentration and water content. Each osmole of solute added to 1 kg of water lowers the freezing point approximately 1.86° and lowers the vapor pressure approximately 0.3 mm of mercury (at 25°). These physical changes are measurable, and they permit accurate estimations of osmolal concentrations.

Where osmometers that measure the freezing-point depression are employed, a measured volume of solution (usually 2 mL) is placed in a glass tube immersed in a temperature-controlled bath. A thermistor and a vibrator are lowered into the mixture, and the temperature of the bath is decreased until the mixture is super-cooled. The vibrator is activated to induce crystallization of the water in the test solution, and the released heat of fusion raises the temperature of the mixture to its freezing point. By means of a Wheatstone bridge, the recorded freezing point is converted to a measurement in terms of milliosmolality, or its near equivalent for dilute solutions, milliosmolarity. The instrument is calibrated by using two standard solutions of sodium chloride that span the expected range of osmolarities.

Osmometers that measure the vapor pressures of solutions are less frequently employed. They require a smaller volume of specimen (generally about 5 µL), but the accuracy and precision of the resulting osmolality determination are comparable to those obtained by the use of osmometers that depend upon the observed freezing points of solutions.

Labeling—Where an osmolarity declaration is required in the individual monograph, the label states the total osmolar concentration in milliosmoles per liter. Where the contents are less than 100 mL, or where the label states that the article is not for direct injection but is to be diluted before use, the label alternatively may state the total osmolar concentration in milliosmoles per milliliter.

Drug and Dosage Form Information

⟨1121⟩ NOMENCLATURE

The USP (or NF) titles are legally recognized as the designations for use in labeling the articles to which they apply.

The value of designating each drug by one and only one nonproprietary[1] name is obvious, in terms of achieving simplicity and uniformity in drug nomenclature. In support of the U. S. Adopted Names program (see *Preface*), of which the U. S. Pharmacopeial Convention is a co-sponsor, the USP Committee of Revision gives consideration to the adoption of the U. S. Adopted Name, if any, as the official title for any compound that attains compendial recognition.

A compilation of the U. S. Adopted Names (USAN) published from the start of the USAN program in 1961, as well as other names for drugs, both current and retrospective, is provided in *USAN and the USP Dictionary of Drug Names*. This publication is intended to serve as a book of names useful for identifying and distinguishing all kinds of names for drugs, whether public or proprietary or chemical or code-designated names.[2]

A nonproprietary name of a drug serves numerous and varied purposes, its principal function being to identify the substance to which it applies by means of a designation that may be used by the professional and lay public free from the restrictions associated with registered trademarks. Teaching in pharmacy and medicine requires a common designation, especially for a drug that is available from several sources or is incorporated into a combination drug product; nonproprietary names facilitate communication among physicians; nonproprietary names must be used as the titles of the articles recognized by official drug compendia; a nonproprietary name is essential to the pharmaceutical manufacturer as a means of protecting trademark rights in the brand name for the article concerned; and, finally, the manufacturer is obligated by federal law to include the established nonproprietary name in advertising and labeling.

[1] The term "generic" has been widely used in place of the more accurate and descriptive term "nonproprietary," with reference to drug nomenclature.

[2] *USAN and the USP Dictionary of Drug Names* is obtainable on order from the USAN Division, USP Convention, Inc., 12601 Twinbrook Parkway, Rockville, MD 20852.

Under the terms of the Drug Amendments of 1962 to the Federal Food, Drug, and Cosmetic Act, which became law October 10, 1962, the Secretary of Health and Human Services is authorized to designate an official name for any drug wherever deemed "necessary or desirable in the interest of usefulness and simplicity." [3]

The Commissioner of Food and Drugs and the Secretary of Health and Human Services published in the *Federal Register* regulations effective November 26, 1984, which state, in part:

Sec. 299.4 Established names of drugs.

(e) "The Food and Drug Administration will not routinely designate official names under section 508 of the act. As a result, the established name under section 502(e) of the act will ordinarily be either the compendial name of the drug or, if there is no compendial name, the common or usual name of the drug. Interested persons, in the absence of the designation by the Food and Drug Administration of an official name, may rely on as the established name for any drug the current compendial name or the USAN adopted name listed in *USAN and the USP Dictionary of Drug Names*. . . ." [4]

It will be noted that the monographs on the biologics, which are produced under licenses issued by the Secretary of the U. S. Department of Health and Human Services, represent a special case. Although efforts continue toward achieving uniformity, there may be a difference between the respective title required by federal law and the USP title. Such differences are fewer than in past revisions of the Pharmacopeia. The USP title, where different from the FDA Bureau of Biologics title, does not constitute a synonym for labeling purposes; the conditions of licensing the biologic concerned require that each such article be designated by the name appearing in the product license issued to the manufacturer. Where a USP title differs from the title in the federal regulations, the former has been adopted with a view to usefulness and simplicity and conformity with the principles governing the selection of monograph titles generally.

⟨1151⟩ PHARMACEUTICAL DOSAGE FORMS

Dosage forms are provided for most of the Pharmacopeial drug substances, but the processes for the preparation of many of them are, in general, beyond the scope of the Pharmacopeia. In addition to defining the dosage forms, this section presents the general principles involved in the manufacture of some of them, particularly on a small scale. Other information that is given bears on the use of the Pharmacopeial substances in extemporaneous compounding of dosage forms.

BIOAVAILABILITY

Bioavailability, or the extent to which the therapeutic constituent of a pharmaceutical dosage form intended for oral or topical use is available for absorption is influenced by a variety of factors. Among the inherent factors known to affect absorption are the method of manufacture or method of compounding; the particle size and crystal form or polymorph of the drug substance; and the diluents and excipients used in formulating the dosage form, including fillers, binders, disintegrating agents, lubricants, coatings, solvents, suspending agents, and dyes. Lubricants and coatings are foremost among these. The maintenance of a demonstrably high degree of bioavailability requires particular attention to all aspects of production and quality control that may affect the nature of the finished dosage form.

STABILITY

The term "stability," with respect to a drug dosage form, refers to the chemical and physical integrity of the dosage unit, and, when appropriate, the ability of the dosage unit to maintain protection against microbiological contamination. The shelf life of the dosage form is the time lapse from initial preparation to the specified expiration date. The monograph specifications of identity, strength, quality, and purity apply throughout the shelf life of the product.

The stability parameters of a drug dosage form can be influenced by environmental conditions of storage (temperature, light, air, and humidity), as well as the package components. Pharmacopeial articles should include required storage conditions on their labeling. These are the conditions under which the expiration date shall apply. The storage requirements specified in the labeling for the article must be observed throughout the distribution of the article (i.e., beyond the time it leaves the manufacturer up to and including its handling by the dispenser or seller of the article to the consumer). Although labeling for the consumer should indicate proper storage conditions, it is recognized that control beyond the dispenser or seller is difficult.

Stability Protocols—Stability of manufactured dosage forms must be demonstrated by the manufacturer by the use of methods adequate for the purpose. Monograph assays may be used for stability testing if they are stability-indicating (i.e., if they accurately differentiate between the intact drug molecules and their degradation products). Stability considerations should include not only the specific compendial requirements, but also changes in physical appearance of the product that would warn users that the product's continued integrity is questionable.

Stability studies on active substances and packaged dosage forms are conducted by means of "real-time," long-term tests at specific temperatures and relative humidities representing storage conditions experienced in the distribution chain of the climatic zone(s) of the country or region of the world concerned. Labeling of the packaged active substance or dosage form should reflect the effects of temperature, relative humidity, air, and light on its stability. Label temperature storage warnings will reflect both the results of the real-time storage tests and also allow for expected seasonal excursions of temperature.

Controlled room temperature (see the *Storage Temperature* section under *General Notices and Requirements—Preservation, Packaging, Storage, and Labeling*) delineates the allowable tolerance in storage circumstances at any location in the chain of distribution (e.g., pharmacies, hospitals, and warehouses). This terminology also allows patients or consumers to be counseled as to appropriate storage for the product. Products may be labeled either to store at "Controlled room temperature" or to store at temperatures "up to 25°" where labeling is supported by long-term stability studies at the designated storage condition of 25°. *Controlled room temperature* limits the permissible excursions to those consistent with the maintenance of a mean kinetic temperature calculated to be not more than 25°. See *Mean Kinetic Temperature*. The common international guideline for long-term stability studies specifies 25 ± 2° at 60 ± 5% relative humidity. Accelerated studies are specified at 40 ± 2° and at 75 ± 5% relative humidity. Accelerated studies also allow the interpretation of data and information on short-term spikes in storage conditions in addition to the excursions allowed for by controlled room temperature.

The term "room temperature" is used in different ways in different countries, and it is usually preferable for product labeling for products to be shipped outside the continental U.S. to refer to a maximum storage temperature or temperature range in degrees Celsius.

Mean Kinetic Temperature—Mean kinetic temperature is defined as a single calculated temperature at which the degradation of an article would be equivalent to the actual degradation that would result from temperature fluctuations during the storage period. It is not a simple arithmetic mean. The mean kinetic temperature is calculated from average storage temperatures recorded over a one-year period, with a minimum of twelve equally spaced average storage temperature observations being recorded. Average temperature may be determined using automated recording devices or as the arithmetic mean of the highest and lowest temperatures attained during the observation period as measured on a high-low thermometer. The mean kinetic temperature is calculated by the following equation (derived from the Arrhenius equation):

$$T_k = \frac{\Delta H/R}{-\ln\left(\dfrac{e^{-\Delta H/RT_1} + e^{-\Delta H/RT_2} + \ldots + e^{-\Delta H/RT_n}}{n}\right)},$$

in which T_k is the mean kinetic temperature; ΔH is the heat of activation, 83.144kJ · mole^{-1} (unless more accurate information is available from experimental studies); R is the universal gas constant, 8.3144 × 10^{-3} kJ · mole^{-1} · degree^{-1}; T_1 is the average storage temperature during the first time period (e.g., month); T_2 is the average storage temperature during the second time period; T_n is the average storage temperature during the nth time period, n being the total number of average storage temperatures recorded (minimum of twelve) during the observation period; and all temperatures (T) being absolute temperatures in degrees Kelvin (°K).

[3] F.D.&C. Act, Sec. 508 [358].

[4] 53 Fed. Reg. 5369 (1988) amending 21 CFR § 299.4.

Climatic Zones—For convenience in planning for packaging and storage, and for stability studies, international practice identifies four climatic zones, which are described in Table 1. The United States, Europe, and Japan are characterized by zones I and II. The values in Table 1 are based on observed temperatures and relative humidities, both outside and in rooms, from which mean kinetic temperatures and average humidity values are calculated.[1] Derived values are based on inspection of data from individual cities and on allowances for a margin of safety in assignment of these specified conditions.

A discussion of aspects of drug product stability that are of primary concern to the pharmacist in the dispensing of medications may be found under *Stability Considerations in Dispensing Practice* ⟨1191⟩.

Inasmuch as this chapter is for purposes of general information only, no statement herein is intended to modify or supplant any of the specific requirements pertinent to pharmaceutical preparations, which are given elsewhere in this Pharmacopeia.

TERMINOLOGY

Occasionally it is necessary to add solvent to the contents of a container just prior to use, usually because of instability of some drugs in the diluted form. Thus, a solid diluted to yield a suspension is called [*DRUG*] *for Suspension;* a solid dissolved and diluted to yield a solution is called [*DRUG*] *for Solution*; and a solution or suspension diluted to yield a more dilute form of the drug is called [*DRUG*] *Oral Concentrate.* After dilution, it is important that the drug be homogeneously dispersed before administration.

AEROSOLS

Pharmaceutical aerosols are products that are packaged under pressure and contain therapeutically active ingredients that are released upon activation of an appropriate valve system. They are intended for topical application to the skin as well as local application into the nose (nasal aerosols), mouth (lingual aerosols), or lungs (inhalation aerosols).

The term "aerosol" refers to the fine mist of spray that results from most pressurized systems. However, the term has been broadly misapplied to all self-contained pressurized products, some of which deliver foams or semisolid fluids. In the case of *Inhalation Aerosols*, the particle size of the delivered medication must be carefully controlled and the average size of the particles should be under 10 μm. These products are also known as metered-dose inhalers (MDIs). (See *Inhalations.*) Other aerosol sprays may contain particles up to several hundred micrometers in diameter.

[1] The source of the data and information in Table 1 is the International Conference on Harmonization sponsored by the International Federation of Pharmaceutical Manufacturers Associations.

The basic components of an aerosol system are the container, the propellant, the concentrate containing the active ingredient(s), the valve, and the actuator. The nature of these components determines such characteristics as particle size distribution, uniformity of valve delivery for metered valves, delivery rate, wetness and temperature of the spray, foam density, or fluid viscosity.

Types of Aerosols

Aerosols consist of two-phase (gas and liquid) or three-phase (gas, liquid, and solid or liquid) systems. The two-phase aerosol consists of a solution of active ingredients in liquefied propellant and the vaporized propellant. The solvent is composed of the propellant or a mixture of the propellant and co-solvents such as alcohol, propylene glycol, and polyethylene glycols, which are often used to enhance the solubility of the active ingredients.

Three-phase systems consist of a suspension or emulsion of the active ingredient(s) in addition to the vaporized propellants. A suspension consists of the active ingredient(s) that may be dispersed in the propellant system with the aid of suitable excipients such as wetting agents and/or solid carriers such as talc or colloidal silicas.

A foam aerosol is an emulsion containing one or more active ingredients, surfactants, aqueous or nonaqueous liquids, and the propellants. If the propellant is in the internal (discontinuous) phase (i.e., of the oil-in-water type), a stable foam is discharged; and if the propellant is in the external (continuous) phase (i.e., of the water-in-oil type), a spray or a quick-breaking foam is discharged.

Propellants

The propellant supplies the necessary pressure within an aerosol system to expel material from the container and, in combination with other components, to convert the material into the desired physical form. Propellants may be broadly classified as liquefied or compressed gases having vapor pressures generally exceeding atmospheric pressure. Propellants within this definition include various hydrocarbons, especially fluorochloro-derivatives of methane and ethane, low molecular weight hydrocarbons such as the butanes and pentanes, and compressed gases such as carbon dioxide, nitrogen, and nitrous oxide. Mixtures of propellants are frequently used to obtain desirable pressure, delivery, and spray characteristics. A good propellant system should have the proper vapor pressure characteristics consistent with the other aerosol components.

Table 1. International Climatic Zones.

Climatic Zone	Calculated Data °C*	°C MKT**	%	mbar***	Derived Data °C	%	mbar
I. *Temperate* United Kingdom Northern Europe Canada Russia	20.0	20.0	42	9.9	21	45	11.2
II *Mediterranean, Subtropical* United States Japan Southern Europe (Portugal-Greece)	21.6	22.0	52	13.5	25	60	19.0
III. *Hot, Dry* Iran Iraq Sudan	26.4	27.9	35	11.9	30	35	15.0
IV. *Hot, Humid* Brazil Ghana Indonesia Nicaragua Philippines	26.7	27.4	76	26.6	30	70	30.0

* Data recorded as <19° calculated as 19°.
** Calculated mean kinetic temperature.
***Partial pressure of water vapor.

Valves

The primary function of the valve is to regulate the flow of the therapeutic agent and propellant from the container. The spray characteristics of the aerosol are influenced by orifice dimension, number, and location. Most aerosol valves provide for continuous spray operation and are used on most topical products. However, pharmaceutical products for oral or nasal inhalation often utilize metered-dose valves that must deliver a uniform quantity of spray upon each valve activation. The accuracy and reproducibility of the doses delivered from metering valves are generally good, comparing favorably to the uniformity of solid dosage forms such as tablets and capsules. However, when aerosol packages are stored improperly, or when they have not been used for long periods of time, valves must be primed before use. Materials used for the manufacture of valves should be inert to the formulations used. Plastic, rubber, aluminum, and stainless steel valve components are commonly used. Metered-dose valves must deliver an accurate dose within specified tolerances.

Actuators

An actuator is the fitting attached to an aerosol valve stem which, when depressed or moved, opens the valve, and directs the spray containing the drug preparation to the desired area. The actuator usually indicates the direction in which the preparation is dispensed and protects the hand or finger from the refrigerant effects of the propellant. Actuators incorporate an orifice which may vary widely in size and shape. The size of this orifice, the expansion chamber design, and the nature of the propellant and formulation influence the physical characteristics of the spray, foam, or stream of solid particles dispensed. For inhalation or oral dose aerosols, an actuator capable of delivering the medication in the proper particle size range is utilized.

Containers

Aerosol containers usually are made of glass, plastic, or metal, or a combination of these materials. Glass containers must be precisely engineered to provide the maximum in pressure safety and impact resistance. Plastics may be employed to coat glass containers for improved safety characteristics, or to coat metal containers to improve corrosion resistance and enhance stability of the formulation. Suitable metals include stainless steel, aluminum, and tin-plated steel.

Manufacture

Aerosols are usually prepared by one of two general processes. In the "cold-fill" process, the concentrate (generally cooled to a temperature below 0°) and the refrigerated propellant are measured into open containers (usually chilled). The valve-actuator assembly is then crimped onto the container to form a pressure-tight seal. During the interval between propellant addition and crimping, sufficient volatilization of propellant occurs to displace air from the container. In the "pressure-fill" method, the concentrate is placed in the container, and either the propellant is forced under pressure through the valve orifice after the valve is sealed, or the propellant is allowed to flow under the valve cap and then the valve assembly is sealed ("under-the-cap" filling). In both cases of the "pressure-fill" method, provision must be made for evacuation of air by means of vacuum or displacement with a small amount of propellant. Manufacturing process controls usually include monitoring of proper formulation and propellant fill weight, and pressure testing and leak testing of the finished aerosol.

Labeling

Medicinal aerosols should contain at least the following warning information on the label as in accordance with appropriate regulations.

Warning—Avoid inhaling. Keep away from eyes or other mucous membranes.

NOTE—The statement "Avoid inhaling" is not necessary for preparations specifically designed for use by inhalation. The phrase "or other mucous membranes" is not necessary for preparations specifically designed for use on mucous membranes.

Warning—Contents under pressure. Do not puncture or incinerate container. Do not expose to heat or store at temperatures above 120° F (49° C). Keep out of reach of children.

In addition to the aforementioned warnings, the label of a drug packaged in an aerosol container in which the propellant consists in whole or in part of a halocarbon or hydrocarbon shall, where required under regulations of the FDA, bear either of the following warnings:

Warning—Do not inhale directly; deliberate inhalation of contents can cause death.

Warning—Use only as directed; intentional misuse by deliberately concentrating and inhaling the contents can be harmful or fatal.

CAPSULES

Capsules are solid dosage forms in which the drug is enclosed within either a hard or soft soluble container or "shell." The shells are usually formed from gelatin; however, they also may be made from starch or other suitable substances. Hard shell capsule sizes range from No. 5, the smallest, to No. 000, which is the largest, except for veterinary sizes. However, size No. 00 generally is the largest size acceptable to patients. Size 0 hard gelatin capsules having an elongated body (known as size OE) also are available, which provide greater fill capacity without an increase in diameter. Hard gelatin capsules consist of two, telescoping cap and body pieces. Generally, there are unique grooves or indentations molded into the cap and body portions to provide a positive closure when fully engaged, which helps prevent the accidental separation of the filled capsules during shipping and handling. Positive closure also may be affected by spot fusion ("welding") of the cap and body pieces together through direct thermal means or by application of ultrasonic energy. Factory-filled hard gelatin capsules may be completely sealed by banding, a process in which one or more layers of gelatin are applied over the seam of the cap and body, or by a liquid fusion process wherein the filled capsules are wetted with a hydroalcoholic solution that penetrates into the space where the cap overlaps the body, and then dried. Hard shell capsules made from starch consist of two, fitted cap and body pieces. Since the two pieces do not telescope or interlock positively, they are sealed together at the time of filling to prevent their separation. Starch capsules are sealed by the application of a hydroalcoholic solution to the recessed section of the cap immediately prior to its being placed onto the body.

The banding of hard shell gelatin capsules or the liquid sealing of hard shell starch capsules enhances consumer safety by making the capsules difficult to open without causing visible, obvious damage, and may improve the stability of contents by limiting O_2 penetration. Industrially filled hard shell capsules also are often of distinctive color and shape or are otherwise marked to identify them with the manufacturer. Additionally, such capsules may be printed axially or radially with strengths, product codes, etc. Pharmaceutical grade printing inks are usually based on shellac and employ FDA-approved pigments and lake dyes.

In extemporaneous prescription practice, hard shell capsules may be hand-filled; this permits the prescriber a latitude of choice in selecting either a single drug or a combination of drugs at the exact dosage level considered best for the individual patient. This flexibility gives hard shell capsules an advantage over compressed tablets and soft shell capsules as a dosage form. Hard shell capsules are usually formed from gelatins having relatively high gel strength. Either type may be used, but blends of pork skin and bone gelatin are often used to optimize shell clarity and toughness. Hard shell capsules also may be formed from starch or other suitable substances. Hard shell capsules may also contain colorants, such as D&C and FD&C dyes or the various iron oxides, opaquing agents such as titanium dioxide, dispersing agents, hardening agents such as sucrose, and preservatives. They normally contain between 10% and 15% water.

Hard gelatin capsules are made by a process that involves dipping shaped pins into gelatin solutions, after which the gelatin films are dried, trimmed, and removed from the pins, and the body and cap pieces are joined. Starch capsules are made by injection molding a mixture of starch and water, after which the capsules are dried. A separate mold is used for caps and bodies, and the two parts are supplied separately. The empty capsules should be stored in tight containers until they are filled. Since gelatin is of animal origin and starch is of vegetable origin, capsules made with these materials should be protected from potential sources or microbial contamination.

Hard shell capsules typically are filled with powder, beads, or granules. Inert sugar beads (nonpareils) may be coated with active ingredients and coating compositions that provide extended-release profiles or enteric properties. Alternatively, larger dose active ingredients themselves may be suitably formed into pellets and then coated. Semisolids or liquids also may be filled into hard shell capsules; however, when the latter are encapsulated, one of the sealing techniques must be employed to prevent leakage.

In hard gelatin capsule filling operations, the body and cap of the shell are separated prior to dosing. In hard starch shell filling operations, the bodies and caps are supplied separately and are fed into separate hoppers of the filling machine. Machines employing various dosing principles may be employed to fill powders into hard shell capsules; however, most fully automatic machines form powder plugs by compression and eject them into empty capsule bodies. Accessories to these machines generally are available for the other types of fills. Powder formulations often require adding fillers, lubricants, and glidants to the active ingredients to facilitate encapsulation. The formulation, as well as the method of filling, particularly the degree of compaction, may influence the rate of drug release. The addition of wetting agents to the powder mass is common where the active ingredient is hydrophobic. Disintegrants also may be included in powder formulations to facilitate deaggregation and dispersal of capsule plugs in the gut. Powder formulations often may be produced by dry blending; however, bulky formulations may require densification by roll compaction or other suitable granulation techniques.

Powder mixtures that tend to liquefy may be dispensed in hard shell capsules if an absorbent such as magnesium carbonate, colloidal silicon dioxide, or other suitable substance is used. Potent drugs are often mixed with an inert diluent before being filled into capsules. Where two mutually incompatible drugs are prescribed together, it is sometimes possible to place one in a small capsule and then enclose it with the second drug in a larger capsule. Incompatible drugs also can be separated by placing coated pellets or tablets, or soft shell capsules of one drug into the capsule shell before adding the second drug.

Thixotropic semisolids may be formed by gelling liquid drugs or vehicles with colloidal silicas or powdered high molecular weight polyethylene glycols. Various waxy or fatty compounds may be used to prepare semisolid matrices by fusion.

Soft shell capsules made from gelatin (sometimes called softgels) or other suitable material require large-scale production methods. The soft gelatin shell is somewhat thicker than that of hard shell capsules and may be plasticized by the addition of a polyol such as sorbitol or glycerin. The ratio of dry plasticizer to dry gelatin determines the "hardness" of the shell and may be varied to accommodate environmental conditions as well as the nature of the contents. Like hard shells, the shell composition may include approved dyes and pigments, opaquing agents such as titanium dioxide, and preservatives. Flavors may be added and up to 5% sucrose may be included for its sweetness and to produce a chewable shell. Soft gelatin shells normally contain 6% to 13% water. Soft shell capsules also may be printed with a product code, strength, etc. In most cases, soft shell capsules are filled with liquid contents. Typically, active ingredients are dissolved or suspended in a liquid vehicle. Classically, an oleaginous vehicle such as a vegetable oil was used; however, nonaqueous, water-miscible liquid vehicles such as the lower molecular weight polyethylene glycols are more common today due to fewer bioavailability problems.

Available in a wide variety of sizes and shapes, soft shell capsules are both formed, filled, and sealed in the same machine; typically, this is a rotary die process, although a plate process or reciprocating die process also may be employed. Soft shell capsules also may be manufactured in a bubble process that forms seamless spherical capsules. With suitable equipment, powders and other dry solids also may be filled into soft shell capsules.

Liquid-filled capsules of either type involve similar formulation technology and offer similar advantages and limitations. For instance, both may offer advantages over dry-filled capsules and tablets in content uniformity and drug dissolution. Greater homogeneity is possible in liquid systems, and liquids can be metered more accurately. Drug dissolution may benefit because the drug may already be in solution or at least suspended in a hydrophilic vehicle. However, the contact between the hard or soft shell and its liquid content is more intimate than exists with dry-filled capsules, and this may enhance the chances for undesired interactions. The liquid nature of capsule contents presents different technological problems than dry-filled capsules in regard to disintegration and dissolution testing. From formulation, technological, and biopharmaceutical points of view, liquid-filled capsules of either type have more in common than liquid-filled and dry-filled capsules having the same shell composition. Thus, for compendial purposes, standards and methods should be established based on capsule contents rather than on whether the contents are filled into hard or soft shell capsules.

ENTERIC-COATED CAPSULES

Capsules may be coated, or, more commonly, encapsulated granules may be coated to resist releasing the drug in the gastric fluid of the stomach where a delay is important to alleviate potential problems of drug inactivation or gastric mucosal irritation. The term "delayed-release" is used for Pharmacopeial monographs on enteric-coated capsules that are intended to delay the release of medicament until the capsule has passed through the stomach, and the individual monographs include tests and specifications for *Drug release* (see *Drug Release* ⟨724⟩).

EXTENDED-RELEASE CAPSULES

Extended-release capsules are formulated in such manner as to make the contained medicament available over an extended period of time following ingestion. Expressions such as "prolonged-action," "repeat-action," and "sustained-release" have also been used to describe such dosage forms. However, the term "extended-release" is used for Pharmacopeial purposes and requirements for *Drug release* (see *Drug Release* ⟨724⟩) typically are specified in the individual monographs.

CREAMS

Creams are semisolid dosage forms containing one or more drug substances dissolved or dispersed in a suitable base. This term has traditionally been applied to semisolids that possess a relatively fluid consistency formulated as either water-in-oil (e.g., *Cold Cream*) or oil-in-water (e.g., *Fluocinolone Acetonide Cream*) emulsions. However, more recently the term has been restricted to products consisting of oil-in-water emulsions or aqueous microcrystalline dispersions of long chain fatty acids or alcohols that are water washable and more cosmetically and aesthetically acceptable. Creams can be used for administering drugs via the vaginal route (e.g., *Triple Sulfa Vaginal Cream*).

ELIXIRS

See *Solutions*.

EMULSIONS

Emulsions are two-phase systems in which one liquid is dispersed throughout another liquid in the form of small droplets. Where oil is the dispersed phase and an aqueous solution is the continuous phase, the system is designated as an oil-in-water emulsion. Conversely, where water or an aqueous solution is the dispersed phase and oil or oleaginous material is the continuous phase, the system is designated as a water-in-oil emulsion. Emulsions are stabilized by emulsifying agents that prevent coalescence, the merging of small droplets into larger droplets and, ultimately, into a single separated phase. Emulsifying agents (surfactants) do this by concentrating in the interface between the droplet and external phase and by providing a physical barrier around the particle to coalescence. Surfactants also reduce the interfacial tension between the phases, thus increasing the ease of emulsification upon mixing.

Natural, semisynthetic, and synthetic hydrophilic polymers may be used in conjunction with surfactants in oil-in-water emulsions as they accumulate at interfaces and also increase the viscosity of the aqueous phase, thereby decreasing the rate of formation of aggregates of droplets. Aggregation is generally accompanied by a relatively rapid separation of an emulsion into a droplet-rich and droplet-poor phase. Normally the density of an oil is lower than that of water, in which case the oil droplets and droplet aggregates rise, a process referred to as creaming. The greater the rate of aggregation, the greater the droplet size and the greater the rate of creaming. The water droplets in a water-in-oil emulsion generally sediment because of their greater density.

The consistency of emulsions varies widely, ranging from easily pourable liquids to semisolid creams. Generally oil-in-water creams are prepared at high temperature, where they are fluid, and cooled to room temperature, whereupon they solidify as a result of solidification of the internal phase. When this is the case, a high internal-phase volume to external-phase volume ratio is not necessary for semisolid character, and, for example, stearic acid creams or vanishing creams are semisolid with as little as 15% internal phase. Any semisolid character with water-in-oil emulsions generally is attributable to a semisolid external phase.

All emulsions require an antimicrobial agent because the aqueous phase is favorable to the growth of microorganisms. The presence of a preservative is particularly critical in oil-in-water emulsions where contamination of the external phase occurs readily. Since fungi and yeasts are found with greater frequency than bacteria, fungistatic as well as bacteriostatic properties are desirable. Bacteria have been shown to degrade nonionic and anionic emulsifying agents, glycerin, and many natural stabilizers such as tragacanth and guar gum.

Complications arise in preserving emulsion systems, as a result of partitioning of the antimicrobial agent out of the aqueous phase where it is most needed, or of complexation with emulsion ingredients that reduce effectiveness. Therefore, the effectiveness of the preservative system should always be tested in the final product. Preservatives commonly used in emulsions include methyl-, ethyl-, propyl-, and butylparabens, benzoic acid, and quaternary ammonium compounds.

See also *Creams* and *Ointments*.

EXTRACTS AND FLUIDEXTRACTS

Extracts are concentrated preparations of vegetable or animal drugs obtained by removal of the active constituents of the respective drugs with suitable menstrua, by evaporation of all or nearly all of the solvent, and by adjustment of the residual masses or powders to the prescribed standards.

In the manufacture of most extracts, the drugs are extracted by percolation. The entire percolates are concentrated, generally by distillation under reduced pressure in order to subject the drug principles to as little heat as possible.

Fluidextracts are liquid preparations of vegetable drugs, containing alcohol as a solvent or as a preservative, or both, and so made that, unless otherwise specified in an individual monograph, each mL contains the therapeutic constituents of 1 g of the standard drug that it represents.

A fluidextract that tends to deposit sediment may be aged and filtered or the clear portion decanted, provided the resulting clear liquid conforms to the Pharmacopeial standards.

Fluidextracts may be prepared from suitable extracts.

GELS

Gels (sometimes called Jellies) are semisolid systems consisting of either suspensions made up of small inorganic particles or large organic molecules interpenetrated by a liquid. Where the gel mass consists of a network of small discrete particles, the gel is classified as a two-phase system (e.g., *Aluminum Hydroxide Gel*). In a two-phase system, if the particle size of the dispersed phase is relatively large, the gel mass is sometimes referred to as a magma (e.g., *Bentonite Magma*). Both gels and magmas may be thixotropic, forming semisolids on standing and becoming liquid on agitation. They should be shaken before use to ensure homogeneity and should be labeled to that effect. (See *Suspensions*.)

Single-phase gels consist of organic macromolecules uniformly distributed throughout a liquid in such a manner that no apparent boundaries exist between the dispersed macromolecules and the liquid. Single-phase gels may be made from synthetic macromolecules (e.g., *Carbomer*) or from natural gums (e.g., *Tragacanth*). The latter preparations are also called mucilages. Although these gels are commonly aqueous, alcohols and oils may be used as the continuous phase. For example, mineral oil can be combined with a polyethylene resin to form an oleaginous ointment base.

Gels can be used to administer drugs topically or into body cavities (e.g., *Phenylephrine Hydrochloride Nasal Jelly*).

IMPLANTS (PELLETS)

Implants or pellets are small sterile solid masses consisting of a highly purified drug (with or without excipients) made by compression or molding. They are intended for implantation in the body (usually subcutaneously) for the purpose of providing continuous release of the drug over long periods of time. Implants are administered by means of a suitable special injector or surgical incision. This dosage form has been used to administer hormones such as testosterone or estradiol. They are packaged individually in sterile vials or foil strips.

INFUSIONS, INTRAMAMMARY

Intramammary infusions are suspensions of drugs in suitable oil vehicles. These preparations are intended for veterinary use only, and are administered by instillation via the teat canals into the udders of milk-producing animals.

INHALATIONS

Inhalations are drugs or solutions or suspensions of one or more drug substances administered by the nasal or oral respiratory route for local or systemic effect.

Solutions of drug substances in sterile water for inhalation or in sodium chloride inhalation solution may be nebulized by use of inert gases. Nebulizers are suitable for the administration of inhalation solutions only if they give droplets sufficiently fine and uniform in size so that the mist reaches the bronchioles. Nebulized solutions may be breathed directly from the nebulizer or the nebulizer may be attached to a plastic face mask, tent, or intermittent positive pressure breathing (IPPB) machine.

Another group of products, also known as metered-dose inhalers (MDIs) are propellant driven drug suspensions or solutions in liquified gas propellant with or without a cosolvent and are intended for delivering metered doses of the drug to the respiratory tract. An MDI contains multiple doses, often exceeding several hundred. The most common single-dose volumes delivered are from 25 to 100 μL (also expressed as mg) per actuation.

Examples of MDIs containing drug solutions and suspensions in this pharmacopeia are *Epinephrine Inhalation Aerosol* and *Isoproterenol Hydrochloride and Phenylephrine Bitartrate Inhalation Aerosol*, respectively.

Powders may also be administered by mechanical devices that require manually produced pressure or a deep inhalation by the patient (e.g., *Cromolyn Sodium for Inhalation*).

A special class of inhalations termed inhalants consists of drugs or combination of drugs, that by virtue of their high vapor pressure, can be carried by an air current into the nasal passage where they exert their effect. The container from which the inhalant generally is administered is known as an inhaler.

INJECTIONS

See *Injections* ⟨1⟩.

IRRIGATIONS

Irrigations are sterile solutions intended to bathe or flush open wounds or body cavities. They are used topically, never parenterally. They are labeled to indicate that they are not intended for injection.

LOTIONS

See *Solutions* or *Suspensions*.

LOZENGES

Lozenges are solid preparations, which are intended to dissolve or disintegrate slowly in the mouth. They contain one or more medicaments, usually in a flavored, sweetened base. They can be prepared by molding (gelatin and/or fused sucrose or sorbitol base) or by compression of sugar based tablets. Molded lozenges are sometimes referred to as pastilles while compressed lozenges are often referred to as troches. They are usually intended for treatment of local irritation or infections of the mouth or throat but may contain active ingredients intended for systemic absorption after swallowing.

OINTMENTS

Ointments are semisolid preparations intended for external application to the skin or mucous membranes.

Ointment bases recognized for use as vehicles fall into four general classes: the hydrocarbon bases, the absorption bases, the water-removable bases, and the water-soluble bases. Each therapeutic ointment possesses as its base a representative of one of these four general classes.

Hydrocarbon Bases

These bases, which are known also as "oleaginous ointment bases," are represented by *White Petrolatum* and *White Ointment*. Only small amounts of an aqueous component can be incorporated into them. They serve to keep medicaments in prolonged contact with the skin and act as occlusive dressings. Hydrocarbon bases are used chiefly for their emollient effects, and are difficult to wash off. They do not "dry out" or change noticeably on aging.

Absorption Bases

This class of bases may be divided into two groups: the first group consisting of bases that permit the incorporation of aqueous solutions with the formation of a water-in-oil emulsion (*Hydrophilic Petrolatum* and *Lanolin*), and the second group consisting of water-in-oil emulsions that permit the incorporation of additional quantities of aqueous solutions (*Lanolin*). Absorption bases are useful also as emollients.

Water-removable Bases

Such bases are oil-in-water emulsions, e.g., *Hydrophilic Ointment*, and are more correctly called "creams." (See *Creams*.) They are also described as "water-washable," since they may be readily washed from the skin or clothing with water, an attribute that makes them more acceptable for cosmetic reasons. Some medicaments may be more effective in these bases than in hydrocarbon bases. Other advantages of the water-removable bases are that they may be diluted with water and that they favor the absorption of serous discharges in dermatological conditions.

Water-soluble Bases

This group of so-called "greaseless ointment bases" is comprised of water-soluble constituents. *Polyethylene Glycol Ointment* is the only Pharmacopeial preparation in this group. Bases of this type offer many of the advantages of the water-removable bases and, in addition, contain no water-insoluble substances such as petrolatum, anhydrous lanolin, or waxes. They are more correctly called "Gels." (See *Gels*.)

Choice of Base—The choice of an ointment base depends upon many factors, such as the action desired, the nature of the medicament to be incorporated and its bioavailability and stability, and the requisite shelf-life of the finished product. In some cases, it is necessary to use a base that is less than ideal in order to achieve the stability required. Drugs that hydrolyze rapidly, for example, are more stable in hydrocarbon bases than in bases containing water, even though they may be more effective in the latter.

OPHTHALMIC PREPARATIONS

Drugs are administered to the eyes in a wide variety of dosage forms, some of which require special consideration. They are discussed in the following paragraphs.

Ointments

Ophthalmic ointments are ointments for application to the eye. Special precautions must be taken in the preparation of ophthalmic ointments. They are manufactured from sterilized ingredients under rigidly aseptic conditions and meet the requirements under *Sterility Tests* ⟨71⟩.If the specific ingredients used in the formulation do not lend themselves to routine sterilization techniques, ingredients that meet the sterility requirements described under *Sterility Tests* ⟨71⟩, along with aseptic manufacture, may be employed. Ophthalmic ointments must contain a suitable substance or mixture of substances to prevent growth of, or to destroy, microorganisms accidentally introduced when the container is opened during use, unless otherwise directed in the individual monograph, or unless the formula itself is bacteriostatic (see *Added Substances* under *Ophthalmic Ointments* ⟨771⟩). The medicinal agent is added to the ointment base either as a solution or as a micronized powder. The finished ointment must be free from large particles and must meet the requirements for *Leakage* and for *Metal Particles* under *Ophthalmic Ointments* ⟨771⟩. The immediate containers for ophthalmic ointments shall be sterile at the time of filling and closing. It is mandatory that the immediate containers for ophthalmic ointments be sealed and tamper-proof so that sterility is assured at time of first use.

The ointment base that is selected must be nonirritating to the eye, permit diffusion of the drug throughout the secretions bathing the eye, and retain the activity of the medicament for a reasonable period under proper storage conditions.

Petrolatum is mainly used as a base for ophthalmic drugs. Some absorption bases, water-removable bases, and water-soluble bases may be desirable for water-soluble drugs. Such bases allow for better dispersion of water-soluble medicaments, but they must be nonirritating to the eye.

Solutions

Ophthalmic solutions are sterile solutions, essentially free from foreign particles, suitably compounded and packaged for instillation into the eye. Preparation of an ophthalmic solution requires careful consideration of such factors as the inherent toxicity of the drug itself, isotonicity value, the need for buffering agents, the need for a preservative (and, if needed, its selection), sterilization, and proper packaging. Similar considerations are also made for nasal and otic products.

ISOTONICITY VALUE

Lacrimal fluid is isotonic with blood, having an isotonicity value corresponding to that of a 0.9% sodium chloride solution. Ideally, an ophthalmic solution should have this isotonicity value; but the eye can tolerate isotonicity values as low as that of a 0.6% sodium chloride solution and as high as that of a 2.0% sodium chloride solution without marked discomfort.

Some ophthalmic solutions are necessarily hypertonic in order to enhance absorption and provide a concentration of the active ingredient(s) strong enough to exert a prompt and effective action. Where the amount of such solutions used is small, dilution with lacrimal fluid takes place rapidly so that discomfort from the hypertonicity is only temporary. However, any adjustment toward isotonicity by dilution with tears is negligible where large volumes of hypertonic solutions are used as collyria to wash the eyes; it is therefore important that solutions used for this purpose be approximately isotonic.

BUFFERING

Many drugs, notably alkaloidal salts, are most effective at pH levels that favor the undissociated free bases. At such pH levels, however, the drug may be unstable so that compromise levels must be found and held by means of buffers. One purpose of buffering some ophthalmic solutions is to prevent an increase in pH caused by the slow release of hydroxyl ions by glass. Such a rise in pH can affect both the solubility and the stability of the drug. The decision whether or not buffering agents should be added in preparing an ophthalmic solution must be based on several considerations. Normal tears have a pH of about 7.4 and possess some buffer capacity. The application of a solution to the eye stimulates the flow of tears and the rapid neutralization of any excess hydrogen or hydroxyl ions within the buffer capacity of the tears. Many ophthalmic drugs, such as alkaloidal salts, are weakly acidic and have only weak buffer capacity. Where only 1 or 2 drops of a solution containing them are added to the eye, the buffering action of the tears is usually adequate to raise the pH and prevent marked discomfort. In some cases pH may vary between 3.5 and 8.5. Some drugs, notably pilocarpine hydrochloride and epinephrine bitartrate, are more acid and overtax the buffer capacity of the lacrimal fluid. Ideally, an ophthalmic solution should have the same pH, as well as the same isotonicity value, as lacrimal fluid. This is not usually possible since, at pH 7.4, many drugs are not appreciably soluble in water. Most alkaloidal salts precipitate as the free alkaloid at this pH. Additionally, many drugs are chemically unstable at pH levels approaching 7.4. This instability is more marked at the high temperatures employed in heat sterilization. For this reason, the buffer system should be selected that is nearest to the physiological pH of 7.4 and does not cause precipitation of the drug or its rapid deterioration.

An ophthalmic preparation with a buffer system approaching the physiological pH can be obtained by mixing a sterile solution of the drug with a sterile buffer solution using aseptic technique. Even so, the possibility of a shorter shelf-life at the higher pH must be taken into consideration, and attention must be directed toward the attainment and maintenance of sterility throughout the manipulations.

Many drugs, when buffered to a therapeutically acceptable pH, would not be stable in solution for long periods of time. These products are lyophilized and are intended for reconstitution immediately before use (e.g., *Acetylcholine Chloride for Ophthalmic Solution*).

STERILIZATION

The sterility of solutions applied to an injured eye is of the greatest importance. Sterile preparations in special containers for individual use on one patient should be available in every hospital, office, or other installationwhereaccidentallyorsurgicallytraumatizedeyesaretreated.The method of attaining sterility is determined primarily by the character of the particular product (see *Sterilization and Sterility Assurance of Compendial Articles* ⟨1211⟩).

Whenever possible, sterile membrane filtration under aseptic conditions is the preferred method. If it can be shown that product stability is not adversely affected, sterilization by autoclaving in the final container is also a preferred method.

Buffering certain drugs near the physiological pH range makes them quite unstable at high temperature.

Avoiding the use of heat by employing a bacteria-retaining filter is a valuable technique, provided caution is exercised in the selection, assembly, and use of the equipment. Single-filtration, presterilized disposable units are available and should be utilized wherever possible.

PRESERVATION

Ophthalmic solutions may be packaged in multiple-dose containers when intended for the individual use of one patient and where the ocular surfaces are intact. It is mandatory that the immediate containers for ophthalmic solutions be sealed and tamper-proof so that sterility is assured at time of first use. Each solution must contain a suitable substance or mixture of substances to prevent the growth of, or to destroy, microorganisms accidentally introduced when the container is opened during use.

Where intended for use in surgical procedures, ophthalmic solutions, although they must be sterile, should not contain antibacterial agents, since they may be irritating to the ocular tissues.

THICKENING AGENT

A pharmaceutical grade of methylcellulose (e.g., 1% if the viscosity is 25 centipoises, or 0.25% if 4000 centipoises) or other suitable thickening agents such as hydroxypropyl methylcellulose or polyvinyl alcohol occasionally are added to ophthalmic solutions to increase the viscosity and prolong contact of the drug with the tissue. The thickened ophthalmic solution must be free from visible particles.

Suspensions

Ophthalmic suspensions are sterile liquid preparations containing solid particles dispersed in a liquid vehicle intended for application to the eye (see *Suspensions*). It is imperative that such suspensions contain the drug in a micronized form to prevent irritation and/or scratching of the cornea. Ophthalmic suspensions should never be dispensed if there is evidence of caking or aggregation.

Strips

Fluorescein sodium solution should be dispensed in a sterile, single-use container or in the form of a sterile, impregnated paper strip. The strip releases a sufficient amount of the drug for diagnostic purposes when touched to the eye being examined for a foreign body or a corneal abrasion. Contact of the paper with the eye may be avoided by leaching the drug from the strip onto the eye with the aid of sterile water or sterile sodium chloride solution.

PASTES

Pastes are semisolid dosage forms that contain one or more drug substances intended for topical application. One class is made from a single phase aqueous gel (e.g., *Carboxymethylcellulose Sodium Paste*). The other class, the fatty pastes (e.g., *Zinc Oxide Paste*), consists of thick, stiff ointments that do not ordinarily flow at body temperature, and therefore serve as protective coatings over the areas to which they are applied.

The fatty pastes appear less greasy and more absorptive than ointments by reason of a high proportion of drug substance(s) having an affinity for water. These pastes tend to absorb serous secretions, and are less penetrating and less macerating than ointments, so that they are preferred for acute lesions that have a tendency towards crusting, vesiculation, or oozing.

A dental paste is intended for adhesion to the mucous membrane for local effect (e.g., *Triamcinolone Acetonide Dental Paste*).

PELLETS

See *Implants*.

POWDERS

Powders are intimate mixtures of dry, finely divided drugs and/or chemicals that may be intended for internal (Oral Powders) or external (Topical Powders) use. Because of their greater specific surface area, powders disperse and dissolve more readily than compacted dosage forms. Children and those adults who experience difficulty in swallowing tablets or capsules may find powders more acceptable. Drugs that are too bulky to be formed into tablets or capsules of convenient size may be administered as powders. Immediately prior to use, oral powders are mixed in a beverage or apple sauce.

Often, stability problems encountered in liquid dosage forms are avoided in powdered dosage forms. Drugs that are unstable in aqueous suspensions or solutions may be prepared in the form of granules or powders. These are intended to be constituted by the pharmacist by the addition of a specified quantity of water just prior to dispensing. Because these constituted products have limited stability, they are required to have a specified expiration date after constitution and may require storage in a refrigerator.

Oral powders may be dispensed in doses premeasured by the pharmacist, i.e., divided powders, or in bulk. Traditionally, divided powders have been wrapped in materials such as bond paper and parchment. However, the pharmacist may provide greater protection from the environment by sealing individual doses in small cellophane or polyethylene envelopes.

Bulk oral powders are limited to relatively nonpotent drugs such as laxatives, antacids, dietary supplements, and certain analgesics that the patient may safely measure by the teaspoonful or capful. Other bulky powders include douche powders, tooth powders, and dusting powders. Bulk powders are best dispensed in tight, wide-mouth glass containers to afford maximum protection from the atmosphere and to prevent the loss of volatile constituents.

Dusting powders are impalpable powders intended for topical application. They may be dispensed in sifter-top containers to facilitate dusting onto the skin. In general, dusting powders should be passed through at least a 100-mesh sieve to assure freedom from grit that could irritate traumatized areas (see *Powder Fineness* ⟨811⟩).

SOLUTIONS

Solutions are liquid preparations that contain one or more chemical substances dissolved, i.e., molecularly dispersed, in a suitable solvent or mixture of mutually miscible solvents. Since molecules in solutions are uniformly dispersed, the use of solutions as dosage forms generally provides for the assurance of uniform dosage upon administration, and good accuracy when diluting or otherwise mixing solutions.

Substances in solutions, however, are more susceptible to chemical instability than the solid state and dose for dose, generally require more bulk and weight in packaging relative to solid dosage forms. For all solutions, but particularly those containing volatile solvents, tight containers, stored away from excessive heat, should be used. Consideration should also be given to the use of light-resistant containers when photolytic chemical degradation is a potential stability problem. Dosage forms categorized as "Solutions" are classified according to route of administration, such as "Oral Solutions" and "Topical Solutions," or by their solute and solvent systems, such as "Spirits," "Tinctures," and "Waters." Solutions intended for parenteral administration are officially entitled, "Injections" (see *Injections* ⟨1⟩).

Oral Solutions

Oral Solutions are liquid preparations, intended for oral administration, that contain one or more substances with or without flavoring, sweetening, or coloring agents dissolved in water or cosolvent-water mixtures. Oral Solutions may be formulated for direct oral administration to the patient or they may be dispensed in a more concentrated form that must be diluted prior to administration. It is important to recognize that dilution with water of Oral Solutions containing cosolvents, such as alcohol, could lead to precipitation of some ingredients. Hence, great care must be taken in diluting concentrated solutions when cosolvents are present. Preparations dispensed as soluble solids or soluble mixtures of solids, with the intent of dissolving them in a solvent and administering them orally, are designated "for Oral Solution" (e.g., *Potassium Chloride for Oral Solution*).

Oral Solutions containing high concentrations of sucrose or other sugars traditionally have been designated as Syrups. A near-saturated solution of sucrose in purified water, for example, is known as Syrup or "Simple Syrup." Through common usage the term, syrup, also has been used to include any other liquid dosage form prepared in a sweet and viscid vehicle, including oral suspensions.

In addition to sucrose and other sugars, certain polyols such as sorbitol or glycerin may be present in Oral Solutions to inhibit crystallization and to modify solubility, taste, mouth-feel, and other vehicle properties. Antimicrobial agents to prevent the growth of bacteria, yeasts, and molds are generally also present. Some sugarless Oral Solutions contain sweetening agents such as sorbitol or aspartame, as well as thickening agents such as the cellulose gums. Such viscid sweetened solutions, containing no sugars, are occasionally prepared as vehicles for administration of drugs to diabetic patients.

Many oral solutions, which contain alcohol as a cosolvent, have been traditionally designated as Elixirs. Many others, however, designated as Oral Solutions, also contain significant amounts of alcohol. Since high concentrations of alcohol can produce a pharmacologic effect when administered orally, other cosolvents, such as glycerin and propylene glycol, should be used to minimize the amount of alcohol required. To be designated as an Elixir, however, the solution must contain alcohol.

Topical Solutions

Topical Solutions are solutions, usually aqueous but often containing other solvents, such as alcohol and polyols, intended for topical application to the skin, or as in the case of Lidocaine Oral Topical Solution, to the oral mucosal surface. The term "lotion" is applied to solutions or suspensions applied topically.

Otic Solutions

Otic Solutions, intended for instillation in the outer ear, are aqueous, or they are solutions prepared with glycerin or other solvents and dispersing agents (e.g., *Antipyrine and Benzocaine Otic Solution* and *Neomycin and Polymyxin B Sulfates and Hydrocortisone Otic Solution*).

Ophthalmic Solutions

(See *Ophthalmic Preparations*.)

Spirits

Spirits are alcoholic or hydroalcoholic solutions of volatile substances prepared usually by simple solution or by admixture of the ingredients. Some spirits serve as flavoring agents while others have medicinal value. Reduction of the high alcoholic content of spirits by admixture with aqueous preparations often causes turbidity.

Spirits require storage in tight, light-resistant containers to prevent loss by evaporation and to limit oxidative changes.

Tinctures

Tinctures are alcoholic or hydroalcoholic solutions prepared from vegetable materials or from chemical substances.

The proportion of drug represented in the different chemical tinctures is not uniform but varies according to the established standards for each. Traditionally, tinctures of potent vegetable drugs essentially represent the activity of 10 g of the drug in each 100 mL of tincture, the potency being adjusted following assay. Most other vegetable tinctures represent 20 g of the respective vegetable material in each 100 mL of tincture.

PROCESS P

Carefully mix the ground drug or mixture of drugs with a sufficient quantity of the prescribed solvent or solvent mixture to render it evenly and distinctly damp, allow it to stand for 15 minutes, transfer it to a suitable percolator, and pack the drug firmly. Pour on enough of the prescribed solvent or solvent mixture to saturate the drug, cover the top of the percolator and, when the liquid is about to drip from the percolator, close the lower orifice, and allow the drug to macerate for 24 hours or for the time specified in the monograph. If no assay is directed, allow the percolation to proceed slowly, or at the specified rate, gradually adding sufficient solvent or solvent mixture to produce 1000 mL of tincture, and mix (for definitions of flow rates, see under *Fluidextracts*). If an assay is directed, collect only 950 mL of percolate, mix this, and assay a portion of it as directed. Dilute the remainder with such quantity of the prescribed solvent or solvent mixture as calculation from the assay indicates is necessary to produce a tincture that conforms to the prescribed standard, and mix.

PROCESS M

Macerate the drug with 750 mL of the prescribed solvent or solvent mixture in a container that can be closed, and put in a warm place. Agitate it frequently during 3 days or until the soluble matter is dissolved. Transfer the mixture to a filter, and when most of the liquid has drained away, wash the residue on the filter with a sufficient quantity of the prescribed solvent or solvent mixture, combining the filtrates, to produce 1000 mL of tincture, and mix.

Tinctures require storage in tight, light-resistant containers, away from direct sunlight and excessive heat.

Waters, Aromatic

Aromatic waters are clear, saturated aqueous solutions (unless otherwise specified) of volatile oils or other aromatic or volatile substances. Their odors and tastes are similar, respectively, to those of the drugs or volatile substances from which they are prepared, and they are free from empyreumatic and other foreign odors. Aromatic waters may be prepared by distillation or solution of the aromatic substance, with or without the use of a dispersing agent.

Aromatic waters require protection from intense light and excessive heat.

SUPPOSITORIES

Suppositories are solid bodies of various weights and shapes, adapted for introduction into the rectal, vaginal, or urethral orifice of the human body. They usually melt, soften, or dissolve at body temperature. A suppository may act as a protectant or palliative to the local tissues at the point of introduction or as a carrier of therapeutic agents for systemic or local action. Suppository bases usually employed are cocoa butter, glycerinated gelatin, hydrogenated vegetable oils, mixtures of polyethylene glycols of various molecular weights, and fatty acid esters of polyethylene glycol.

The suppository base employed has a marked influence on the release of the active ingredient incorporated in it. While cocoa butter melts quickly at body temperature, it is immiscible with body fluids and this inhibits the diffusion of fat-soluble drugs to the affected sites. Polyethylene glycol is a suitable base for some antiseptics. In cases where systemic action is expected, it is preferable to incorporate the ionized rather than the nonionized form of the drug, in order to maximize bioavailability. Although un-ionized drugs partition more readily out of water-miscible bases such as glycerinated gelatin and polyethylene glycol, the bases themselves tend to dissolve very slowly and thus retard release in this manner. Oleaginous vehicles such as cocoa butter are seldom used in vaginal preparations because of the nonabsorbable residue formed, while glycerinated gelatin is seldom used rectally because of its slow dissolution. Cocoa butter and its substitutes (Hard Fat) are superior for allaying irritation, as in preparations intended for treating internal hemorrhoids.

Cocoa Butter Suppositories

Suppositories having cocoa butter as the base may be made by means of incorporating the finely divided medicinal substance into the solid oil at room temperature and suitably shaping the resulting mass, or by working with the oil in the melted state and allowing the resulting suspension to cool in molds. A suitable quantity of hardening agents may be added to counteract the tendency of some medicaments such as chloral hydrate and phenol to soften the base. It is important that the finished suppository melt at body temperature.

The approximate weights of suppositories prepared with cocoa butter are given below. Suppositories prepared from other bases vary in weight and generally are heavier than the weights indicated here.

Rectal Suppositories for adults are tapered at one or both ends and usually weigh about 2 g each.

Vaginal Suppositories are usually globular or oviform and weigh about 5 g each. They are made from water soluble or water miscible vehicles such as polyethylene glycol or glycerinated gelatin.

Suppositories with cocoa butter base require storage in well-closed containers, preferably at a temperature below 30° (controlled room temperature).

Cocoa Butter Substitutes

Fat-type suppository bases can be produced from a variety of vegetable oils, such as coconut or palm kernel, which are modified by esterification, hydrogenation, and fractionation to obtain products of varying composition and melting temperatures (e.g., *Hydrogenated Vegetable Oil* and *Hard Fat*). These products can be so designed as to reduce rancidity. At the same time, desired characteristics such as narrow intervals between melting and solidification temperatures, and melting ranges to accommodate various formulation and climatic conditions, can be built in.

Glycerinated Gelatin Suppositories

Medicinal substances may be incorporated into glycerinated gelatin bases by addition of the prescribed quantities to a vehicle consisting of about 70 parts of glycerin, 20 parts of gelatin, and 10 parts of water.

Glycerinated gelatin suppositories require storage in tight containers, preferably at a temperature below 35°.

Polyethylene Glycol–Base Suppositories

Several combinations of polyethylene glycols having melting temperatures that are above body temperature have been used as suppository bases. Inasmuch as release from these bases depends on dissolution rather than on melting, there are significantly fewer problems in preparation and storage than exist with melting-type vehicles. However, high concentrations of higher molecular weight polyethylene glycols may lengthen dissolution time, resulting in problems with retention. Labels on polyethylene glycol suppositories should contain directions that they be moistened with water before inserting. Although they can be stored without refrigeration, they should be packaged in tightly closed containers.

Surfactant Suppository Bases

Several nonionic surface-active agents closely related chemically to the polyethylene glycols can be used as suppository vehicles. Examples of such surfactants are polyoxyethylene sorbitan fatty acid esters and the polyoxyethylene stearates. These surfactants are used alone or in combination with other suppository vehicles to yield a wide range of melting temperatures and consistencies. One of the major advantages of such vehicles is their water-dispersibility. However, care must be taken with the use of surfactants, because they may either increase the rate of drug absorption or interact with drug molecules, causing a decrease in therapeutic activity.

Tableted Suppositories or Inserts

Vaginal suppositories occasionally are prepared by the compression of powdered materials into a suitable shape. They are prepared also by encapsulation in soft gelatin.

SUSPENSIONS

Suspensions are liquid preparations that consist of solid particles dispersed throughout a liquid phase in which the particles are not soluble. Dosage forms officially categorized as Suspensions are designated as such if they are not included in other more specific categories of suspensions, such as Oral Suspensions, Topical Suspensions, etc. (see these other categories). Some suspensions are prepared and ready for use, while others are prepared as solid mixtures intended for constitution just before use with an appropriate vehicle. Such products are designated "for Oral Suspension," etc. The term, Milk, is sometimes used for suspensions in aqueous vehicles intended for oral administration (e.g., *Milk of Magnesia*). The term, Magma, is often used to describe suspensions of inorganic solids such as clays in water, where there is a tendency for strong hydration and aggregation of the solid, giving rise to gel-like consistency and thixotropic rheological behavior (e.g., *Bentonite Magma*). The term, Lotion, has been used to categorize many topical suspensions and emulsions intended for application to the skin (e.g., *Calamine Lotion*). Some suspensions are prepared in sterile form and are used as Injectables, as well as for ophthalmic and otic administration. These may be of two types, ready to use or intended for constitution with a prescribed amount of Water for Injection or other suitable diluent before use by the designated route. Suspensions should not be injected intravenously or intrathecally.

Suspensions intended for any route of administration should contain suitable antimicrobial agents to protect against bacteria, yeast, and mold contamination (see *Emulsions* for some consideration of antimicrobial preservative properties that apply also to Suspensions). By its very nature, the particular matter in a suspension may settle or sediment to the bottom of the container upon standing. Such sedimentation may also lead to caking and solidification of the sediment with a resulting difficulty in redispersing the suspension upon agitation. To prevent such problems, suitable ingredients that increase viscosity and the gel state of the suspension, such as clays, surfactants, polyols, polymers, or sugars, should be added. It is important that suspensions always be shaken well before use to ensure uniform distribution of the solid in the vehicle, thereby ensuring uniform and proper dosage. Suspensions require storage in tight containers.

Oral Suspensions

Oral Suspensions are liquid preparations containing solid particles dispersed in a liquid vehicle, with suitable flavoring agents, intended for oral administration. Some suspensions labeled as Milks or Magmas fall into this category.

Topical Suspensions

Topical Suspensions are liquid preparations containing solid particles dispersed in a liquid vehicle, intended for application to the skin. Some suspensions labeled as Lotions fall into this category.

Otic Suspensions

Otic Suspensions are liquid preparations containing micronized particles intended for instillation in the outer ear.

Ophthalmic Suspensions

(See *Ophthalmic Preparations*).

SYRUPS

See *Solutions*.

SYSTEMS

In recent years, a number of dosage forms have been developed using modern technology that allows for the uniform release or targeting of drugs to the body. These products are commonly called delivery systems. The most widely used of these are Transdermal Systems.

Transdermal Systems

Transdermal drug delivery systems are self-contained, discrete dosage forms that, when applied to intact skin, are designed to deliver the drug(s) through the skin to the systemic circulation. Systems typically comprise an outer covering (barrier), a drug reservoir, which may have a rate controlling membrane, a contact adhesive applied to some or all parts of the system and the system/skin interface, and a protective liner that is removed before applying the system. The activity of these systems is defined in terms of the release rate of the drug(s) from the system. The total duration of drug release from the system and the system surface area may also be stated.

Transdermal drug delivery systems work by diffusion: the drug diffuses from the drug reservoir, directly or through the rate controlling membrane and/or contact adhesive if present, and then through the skin into the general circulation. Typically, modified-release systems are designed to provide drug delivery at a constant rate, such that a true steady state blood concentration is achieved and maintained until the system is removed. At that time, blood concentration declines at a rate consistent with the pharmacokinetics of the drug.

Transdermal drug delivery systems are applied to body areas consistent with the labeling for the product(s). As long as drug concentration at the system/skin interface remains constant, the amount of drug in the dosage form does not influence plasma concentrations. The functional lifetime of the system is defined by the initial amount of drug in the reservoir and the release rate from the reservoir.

NOTE—Drugs for local rather than systemic effect are commonly applied to the skin embedded in glue on a cloth or plastic backing. These products are defined traditionally as plasters or tapes.

Ocular System

Another type of system is the ocular system, which is intended for placement in the lower conjunctival fornix from which the drug diffuses through a membrane at a constant rate over a seven-day period (e.g., *Pilocarpine Ocular System*).

Intrauterine System

An intrauterine system, based on a similar principle but intended for release of drug over a much longer period of time, i.e., one year, is also available (e.g., *Progesterone Intrauterine Contraceptive System*).

TABLETS

Tablets are solid dosage forms containing medicinal substances with or without suitable diluents. They may be classed, according to the method of manufacture, as compressed tablets or molded tablets .

The vast majority of all tablets manufactured are made by compression, and compressed tablets are the most widely used dosage form in this country. Compressed tablets are prepared by the application of high pressures, utilizing steel punches and dies, to powders or granulations. Tablets can be produced in a wide variety of sizes, shapes, and surface markings, depending upon the design of the punches and dies. Capsule-shaped tablets are commonly referred to as caplets. Boluses are large tablets intended for veterinary use, usually for large animals.

Molded tablets are prepared by forcing dampened powders under low pressure into die cavities. Solidification depends upon crystal bridges built up during the subsequent drying process, and not upon the compaction force.

Tablet triturates are small, usually cylindrical, molded or compressed tablets. Tablet triturates were traditionally used as dispensing tablets in order to provide a convenient, measured quantity of a potent drug for compounding purposes. Such tablets are rarely used today. Hypodermic tablets are molded tablets made from completely and readily water-soluble ingredients and formerly were intended for use in making preparations for hypodermic injection. They are employed orally, or where rapid drug availability is required such as in the case of *Nitroglycerin Tablets*, sublingually.

Buccal tablets are intended to be inserted in the buccal pouch, and sublingual tablets are intended to be inserted beneath the tongue, where the active ingredient is absorbed directly through the oral mucosa. Few drugs are readily absorbed in this way, but for those that are (such as nitroglycerin and certain steroid hormones), a number of advantages may result.

Soluble, effervescent tablets are prepared by compression and contain, in addition to active ingredients, mixtures of acids (citric acid, tartaric acid) and sodium bicarbonate, which release carbon dioxide when dissolved in water. They are intended to be dissolved or dispersed in water before administration. Effervescent tablets should be stored in tightly closed containers or moisture-proof packs and labeled to indicate that they are not to be swallowed directly.

Chewable Tablets

Chewable tablets are intended to be chewed, producing a pleasant tasting residue in the oral cavity that is easily swallowed and does not leave a bitter or unpleasant after-taste. These tablets have been used in tablet formulations for children, especially multivitamin formulations, and for the administration of antacids and selected antibiotics. Chewable tablets are prepared by compression, usually utilizing mannitol, sorbitol, or sucrose as binders and fillers, and containing colors and flavors to enhance their appearance and taste.

Preparation of Molded Tablets

Molded tablets are prepared from mixtures of medicinal substances and a diluent usually consisting of lactose and powdered sucrose in varying proportions. The powders are dampened with solutions containing high percentages of alcohol. The concentration of alcohol depends upon the solubility of the active ingredients and fillers in the solvent system and the desired degree of hardness of the finished tablets. The dampened powders are pressed into molds, removed, and allowed to dry. Molded tablets are quite friable and care must be taken in packaging and dispensing.

Formulation of Compressed Tablets

Most compressed tablets consist of the active ingredient and a diluent (filler), binder, disintegrating agent, and lubricant. Approved FD&C and D&C dyes or lakes (dyes adsorbed onto insoluble aluminum hydroxide), flavors, and sweetening agents may also be present. Diluents are added where the quantity of active ingredient is small or difficult to compress. Common tablet fillers include lactose, starch, dibasic calcium phosphate, and microcrystalline cellulose. Chewable tablets often contain sucrose, mannitol, or sorbitol as a filler. Where the amount of active ingredient is small, the overall tableting properties are in large measure determined by the filler. Because of problems encountered with bioavailability of hydrophobic drugs of low water-solubility, water-soluble diluents are used as fillers for these tablets.

Binders give adhesiveness to the powder during the preliminary granulation and to the compressed tablet. They add to the cohesive strength already available in the diluent. While binders may be added dry, they are more effective when added out of solution. Common binders include acacia, gelatin, sucrose, povidone, methylcellulose, carboxymethylcellulose, and hydrolyzed starch pastes. The most effective dry binder is microcrystalline cellulose, which is commonly used for this purpose in tablets prepared by direct compression.

A disintegrating agent serves to assist in the fragmentation of the tablet after administration. The most widely used tablet disintegrating agent is starch. Chemically modified starches and cellulose, alginic acid, microcrystalline cellulose, and cross-linked povidone, are also used for this purpose. Effervescent mixtures are used in soluble tablet systems as disintegrating agents. The concentration of the disintegrating agent, method of addition, and degree of compaction play a role in effectiveness.

Lubricants reduce friction during the compression and ejection cycle. In addition, they aid in preventing adherence of tablet material to the dies and punches. Metallic stearates, stearic acid, hydrogenated vegetable oils, and talc are used as lubricants. Because of the nature of this function, most lubricants are hydrophobic, and as such tend to reduce the rates of tablet disintegration and dissolution. Consequently, excessive concentrations of lubricant should be avoided. Polyethylene glycols and some lauryl sulfate salts have been used as soluble lubricants, but such agents generally do not possess optimal lubricating properties, and comparatively high concentrations are usually required.

Glidants are agents that improve powder fluidity, and they are commonly employed in direct compression where no granulation step is involved. The most effective glidants are the colloidal pyrogenic silicas.

Colorants are often added to tablet formulations for esthetic value or for product identification. Both D&C and FD&C dyes and lakes are used. Most dyes are photosensitive and they fade when exposed to light. The federal Food and Drug Administration regulates the colorants employed in drugs.

Manufacturing Methods

Tablets are prepared by three general methods: wet granulation, dry granulation (roll compaction or slugging), and direct compression. The purpose of both wet and dry granulation is to improve flow of the mixture and/or to enhance its compressibility.

Dry granulation (slugging) involves the compaction of powders at high pressures into large, often poorly formed tablet compacts. These compacts are then milled and screened to form a granulation of the desired particle size. The advantage of dry granulation is the elimination of both heat and moisture in the processing. Dry granulations can be produced also by extruding powders between hydraulically operated rollers to produce thin cakes which are subsequently screened or milled to give the desired granule size.

Excipients are available that allow production of tablets at high speeds without prior granulation steps. These directly compressible excipients consist of special physical forms of substances such as lactose, sucrose, dextrose, or cellulose, which possess the desirable properties of fluidity and compressibility. The most widely used direct-compaction fillers are microcrystalline cellulose, anhydrous lactose, spray-dried lactose, compressible sucrose, and some forms of modified starches. Direct compression avoids many of the problems associated with wet and dry granulations. However, the inherent physical properties of the individual filler materials are highly critical, and minor variations can alter flow and compression characteristics so as to make them unsuitable for direct compression.

Physical evidence of poor tablet quality is discussed under *Stability Considerations in Dispensing Practice* ⟨1191⟩.

WEIGHT VARIATION AND CONTENT UNIFORMITY

Tablets are required to meet a weight variation test (see *Uniformity of Dosage Units* ⟨905⟩) where the active ingredient comprises a major portion of the tablet and where control of weight may be presumed to be an adequate control of drug content uniformity. Weight variation is not an adequate indication of content uniformity where the drug substance comprises a relatively minor portion of the tablet, or where the tablet is sugar-coated. Thus, the Pharmacopeia generally requires that coated tablets and tablets containing 50 mg or less of active ingredient, comprising less than 50% by weight of the dosage-form unit, pass a content uniformity test (see *Uniformity of Dosage Units* ⟨905⟩), wherein individual tablets are assayed for actual drug content.

DISINTEGRATION AND DISSOLUTION

Disintegration is an essential attribute of tablets intended for administration by mouth, except those intended to be chewed before being swallowed and except some types of extended-release tablets. A disintegration test is provided (see *Disintegration* ⟨701⟩), and limits on the times in which disintegration is to take place, appropriate for the types of tablets concerned, are given in the individual monographs.

For drugs of limited water-solubility, dissolution may be a more meaningful quality attribute than disintegration. A dissolution test (see *Dissolution* ⟨711⟩) is required in a number of monographs on tablets. In many cases, it is possible to correlate dissolution rates with biological availability of the active ingredient. However, such tests are useful mainly as a means of screening preliminary formulations and as a routine quality-control procedure.

Coatings

Tablets may be coated for a variety of reasons, including protection of the ingredients from air, moisture, or light, masking of unpleasant tastes and odors, improvement of appearance, and control of the site of drug release in the gastrointestinal tract.

PLAIN COATED TABLETS

Classically, tablets have been coated with sugar applied from aqueous suspensions containing insoluble powders such as starch, calcium carbonate, talc, or titanium dioxide, suspended by means of acacia or gelatin. For purposes of identification and esthetic value, the outside coatings may be colored. The finished coated tablets are polished by application of dilute solutions of wax in solvents such as chloroform or powdered mix. Water-protective coatings consisting of substances such as shellac or cellulose acetate phthalate are often applied out of nonaqueous solvents prior to application of sugar coats. Excessive quantities should be avoided. Drawbacks of sugar coating include the lengthy time necessary for application, the need for waterproofing, which also adversely affects dissolution, and the increased bulk of the finished tablet. These factors have resulted in increased acceptance of film coatings. Film coatings consist of water-soluble or dispersible materials such as hydroxypropyl methylcellulose, methylcellulose, hydroxypropylcellulose, carboxymethylcellulose sodium, and mixtures of cellulose acetate phthalate and polyethylene glycols applied out of nonaqueous or aqueous solvents. Evaporation of the solvents leaves a thin film that adheres directly to the tablet and allows it to retain the original shape, including grooves or identification codes.

ENTERIC-COATED TABLETS

Where the drug may be destroyed or inactivated by the gastric juice or where it may irritate the gastric mucosa, the use of "enteric" coatings is indicated. Such coatings are intended to delay the release of the medication until the tablet has passed through the stomach. The term "delayed-release" is used for Pharmacopeial purposes, and the individual monographs include tests and specifications for *Drug release* (see *Drug Release* ⟨724⟩).

EXTENDED-RELEASE TABLETS

Extended-release tablets are formulated in such manner as to make the contained medicament available over an extended period of time following ingestion. Expressions such as "prolonged-action," "repeat-action," and "sustained-release" have also been used to describe such dosage forms. However, the term "extended-release" is used for Pharmacopeial purposes, and requirements for *Drug release* typically are specified in the individual monographs.

⟨1191⟩ STABILITY CONSIDERATIONS IN DISPENSING PRACTICE

NOTE—Inasmuch as this chapter is for purposes of general information only, no statement in the chapter is intended to modify or supplant any of the specific requirements pertinent to Pharmacopeial articles, which are given elsewhere in this Pharmacopeia.

Aspects of drug product stability that are of primary concern to the pharmacist in the dispensing of medications are discussed herein.

Stability is defined as the extent to which a product retains, within specified limits, and throughout its period of storage and use (i.e., its shelf-life), the same properties and characteristics that it possessed at the time of its manufacture. Five types of stability generally recognized are shown in the accompanying table.

Criteria for Acceptable Levels of Stability

Type of Stability	Conditions Maintained Throughout the Shelf-Life of the Drug Product
Chemical	Each active ingredient retains its chemical integrity and labeled potency, within the specified limits.
Physical	The original physical properties, including appearance, palatability, uniformity, dissolution, and suspendability are retained.
Microbiological	Sterility or resistance to microbial growth is retained according to the specified requirements. Antimicrobial agents that are present retain effectiveness within the specified limits.
Therapeutic	The therapeutic effect remains unchanged.
Toxicological	No significant increase in toxicity occurs.

Factors Affecting Product Stability

Each ingredient, whether therapeutically active or inactive, in a dosage form can affect stability. Environmental factors, such as temperature, radiation, light, air (specifically oxygen, carbon dioxide, and water vapor), and humidity also can affect stability. Similarly, such factors as particle size, pH, the properties of water and other solvents employed, the nature of the container, and the presence of other chemicals resulting from contamination or from the intentional mixing of different products can influence stability.

Stability Studies in Manufacturing

The scope and design of a stability study vary according to the product and the manufacturer concerned. Ordinarily the formulator of a product first determines the effects of temperature, light, air, pH, moisture, and trace metals, and commonly used excipients or solvents on the active ingredient(s). From this information, one or more formulations of each dosage form are prepared, packaged in suitable containers, and stored under a variety of environmental conditions, both exaggerated and normal. See *Stability* under *Pharmaceutical Dosage Forms* ⟨1151⟩. At appropriate time intervals, samples of the product are assayed for potency by use of a stability-indicating method, observed for physical changes, and, where applicable, tested for sterility and/or for resistance to microbial growth and for toxicity and bioavailability. Such a study in combination with clinical and toxicological results enables the manufacturer to select the optimum formulation and container, and to assign recommended storage conditions and an expiration date for each dosage form in its package.

Responsibility of the Pharmacist

The pharmacist helps to ensure that the products under his supervision meet acceptable criteria of stability by (1) dispensing oldest stock first and observance of expiration dates; (2) storing products under the environmental conditions stated in the individual monographs and/or in the labeling; (3) observing products for evidence of instability; (4) properly treating and labeling products that are repackaged, diluted, or mixed with other products; (5) dispensing in the proper container with the proper closure; and (6) informing and educating patients concerning the proper storage and use of the products, including the disposition of outdated or excessively aged prescriptions.

Rotating Stock and Observance of Expiration Dates—Proper rotation of stock is necessary to ensure the dispensing of suitable products. A product that is dispensed on an infrequent basis should be closely monitored so that old stocks are given special attention, particularly with regard to expiration dates. The manufacturer can guarantee the quality of a product up to the time designated as its expiration date only if the product has been stored in the original container under recommended storage conditions.

Storage under Recommended Environmental Conditions—In most instances, the recommended storage conditions are stated on the label, in which case it is imperative to adhere to those conditions. They may include a specified temperature range or a designated storage place or condition (e.g., "refrigerator," or "controlled room temperature") as defined in the *General Notices*. Supplemental instructions, such as a direction to protect the product from light, also should be followed carefully. Where a product is required to be protected from light and is in a clear or translucent container enclosed in an opaque outer covering, such outer covering is not to be removed and discarded until the contents have been used. In the absence of specific instructions, the product should be stored at controlled room temperature (see *Storage Temperature* in the *General Notices*). The product should be stored away from locations where excessive or variable heat, cold, or light prevails, such as near heating pipes or fluorescent lighting.

Observing Products for Evidence of Instability—Loss of potency usually results from a chemical change, the most common reactions being hydrolysis, oxidation-reduction, and photolysis. Chemical changes may occur also through interaction between ingredients within a product, or rarely between product and container. An apparent loss of potency in the active ingredient(s) may result from diffusion of the drug into or its combination with the surface of the container-closure system. An apparent gain in potency usually is caused by solvent evaporation or by leaching of materials from the container-closure system.

The chemical potency of the active ingredient(s) is required to remain within the limits specified in the monograph definition. Potency is determined by means of an assay procedure that differentiates between the intact molecule and its degradation products; and chemical stability data should be available from the manufacturer. Although chemical degradation ordinarily cannot be detected by the pharmacist, excessive chemical degradation sometimes is accompanied by observable physical changes. In addition, some physical changes not necessarily related to chemical potency, such as change in color and odor, or formation of a precipitate, or clouding of solution, may serve to alert the pharmacist to the possibility of a stability problem. It should be assumed that a product that has undergone a physical change not explained in the labeling may also have undergone a chemical change and such a product is never to be dispensed. Excessive microbial growth and/or contamination also may appear as a physical change. A gross change in a physical characteristic such as color or odor is a sign of instability in any product. Other common physical signs of deterioration of dosage forms include the following.

SOLID DOSAGE FORMS—Many solid dosage forms are designed for storage under low-moisture conditions. They require protection from environmental water, and therefore should be stored in tight containers (see *Containers* in the *General Notices*) or in the container supplied by the manufacturer. The appearance of fog or liquid droplets, or clumping of the product, inside the container signifies improper conditions. The presence of a desiccant inside the manufacturer's container indicates that special care should be taken in dispensing. Some degradation products, for example, salicylic acid from aspirin, may sublime and be deposited as crystals on the outside of the dosage form or on the walls of the container.

Hard and Soft Gelatin Capsules—Since the capsule formulation is encased in a gelatin shell, a change in gross physical appearance or consistency, including hardening or softening of the shell, is the primary evidence of instability. Evidence of release of gas, such as a distended paper seal, is another sign of instability.

Uncoated Tablets—Evidence of physical instability in uncoated tablets may be shown by excessive powder and/or pieces (i.e., crumbling as distinct from breakage) of tablet at the bottom of the container (from abraded, crushed, or broken tablets); cracks or chips in tablet surfaces; swelling; mottling; discoloration; fusion between tablets; or the appearance of crystals that obviously are not part of the tablet itself on the container walls or on the tablets.

Coated Tablets—Evidence of physical instability in coated tablets is shown by cracks, mottling, or tackiness in the coating and the clumping of tablets.

Dry Powders and Granules—Dry powders and granules that are not intended for constitution into a liquid form in the original container may cake into hard masses or change color, which may render them unacceptable.

Powders and Granules Intended for Constitution as Solutions or Suspensions—Dry powders and granules intended for constitution into solutions or suspensions require special attention. Usually such forms are those antibiotics or vitamins that are particularly sensitive to moisture. Since they are always dispensed in the original container, they generally are not subject to contamination by moisture. However, an unusual caked appearance necessitates careful evaluation, and the presence of a fog or liquid droplets inside the container generally renders the preparation unfit for use. Presence of an objectionable odor also may be evidence of instability.

Effervescent Tablets, Granules, and Powders—Effervescent products are particularly sensitive to moisture. Swelling of the mass or development of gas pressure is a specific sign of instability, indicating that some of the effervescent action has occurred prematurely.

LIQUID DOSAGE FORMS—Of primary concern with respect to liquid dosage forms are homogeneity and freedom from excessive microbial contamination and growth. Instability may be indicated by cloudiness or precipitation in a solution, breaking of an emulsion, nonresuspendable caking of a suspension, or organoleptic changes. Microbial growth may be accompanied by discoloration, turbidity, or gas formation.

Solutions, Elixirs, and Syrups—Precipitation and evidence of microbial or chemical gas formation are the two major signs of instability.

Emulsions—The breaking of an emulsion (i.e., separation of an oil phase that is not easily dispersed) is a characteristic sign of instability; this is not to be confused with creaming, an easily redispersible separation of the oil phase that is a common occurrence with stable emulsions.

Suspensions—A caked solid phase that cannot be resuspended by a reasonable amount of shaking is a primary indication of instability in a suspension. The presence of relatively large particles may mean that excessive crystal growth has occurred.

Tinctures and Fluidextracts—Tinctures, fluidextracts, and similar preparations usually are dark in color because they are concentrated, and thus they should be scrutinized carefully for evidence of precipitation.

Sterile Liquids—Maintenance of sterility is of course critical for sterile liquids. The presence of microbial contamination in sterile liquids usually cannot be detected visually, but any haze, color change, cloudiness, surface film, particulate or flocculent matter, or gas formation is sufficient reason to suspect possible contamination. Clarity of sterile solutions intended for ophthalmic or parenteral use is of utmost importance. Evidence that the integrity of the seal has been violated on such products should make them suspect.

SEMISOLIDS (CREAMS, OINTMENTS, AND SUPPOSITORIES)—For creams, ointments, and suppositories, the primary indication of instability is often either discoloration or a noticeable change in consistency or odor.

Creams—Unlike ointments, creams usually are emulsions containing water and oil. Indications of instability in creams are emulsion breakage, crystal growth, shrinking due to evaporation of water, and gross microbial contamination.

Ointments—Common signs of instability in ointments are a change in consistency and excessive "bleeding" (i.e., separation of excessive amounts of liquid) and formation of granules or grittiness.

Suppositories—Excessive softening is the major indication of instability in suppositories, although some suppositories may dry out and harden or shrivel. Evidence of oil stains on packaging material should warn the pharmacist to examine individual suppositories more closely by removing any foil covering if necessary. As a general rule (although there are exceptions), suppositories should be stored in a refrigerator (see *Storage Temperature* in the *General Notices*).

Proper Treatment of Products Subjected to Additional Manipulations—In repackaging, diluting, or mixing a product with another product, the pharmacist may become responsible for its stability.

REPACKAGING—In general, repackaging is inadvisable. However, if repackaging is necessary, the manufacturer should be consulted concerning potential problems. In the filling of prescriptions, it is essential that suitable containers be used. Appropriate storage conditions and, where appropriate, an expiration date, should be indicated on the label of the prescription container. Single-unit packaging calls for care and judgment, and for strict observance of the following guidelines: (1) use appropriate packaging materials; (2) where stability data on the new package are not available, repackage at any one time only sufficient stock for a limited time; (3) include on the unit-dose label a lot number and an appropriate expiration date; (4) where a sterile product is repackaged from a multiple-dose vial into unit-dose (disposable) syringes, discard the latter if not used within 24 hours, unless data are available to support longer storage; (5) where quantities are repackaged in advance of immediate needs, maintain suitable repackaging records showing name of manufacturer, lot number, date, and designation of persons responsible for repackaging and for checking; (6) where safety closures are required, use container closure systems that ensure compliance with compendial and regulatory standards for storage.

DILUTION OR MIXING—Where a product is diluted, or where two products are mixed, the pharmacist should observe good professional and scientific procedures to guard against incompatibility and instability. For example, tinctures such as those of belladonna and digitalis contain high concentrations of alcohol to dissolve the active ingredient(s), and they may develop a precipitate if they are diluted or mixed with aqueous systems. Pertinent technical literature and labeling should be consulted routinely; it should be current literature, because at times formulas are changed by the manufacturer. If a particular combination is commonly used, consultation with the manufacturer(s) is advisable. Since the chemical stability of extemporaneously prepared mixtures is unknown, the use of such combinations should be discouraged; if such a mixture involved an incompatibility, the pharmacist might be responsible. Oral antibiotic preparations constituted from powder into liquid form should never be mixed with other products.

Combining parenteral products necessitates special care, particularly in the case of intravenous solutions, primarily because of the route of administration. This area of practice demands the utmost in care, aseptic technique, judgment, and diligence. Because of potential unobservable problems with respect to sterility and chemical stability, all extemporaneous parenteral preparations should be used within 24 hours unless data are available to support longer storage.

Informing and Educating the Patient—As a final step in meeting responsibility for the stability of drugs dispensed, the pharmacist is obligated to inform the patient regarding the proper storage conditions (for example, in a cool, dry place—not in the bathroom), for both prescription and nonprescription products, and to suggest a reasonable estimate of the time after which the medication should be discarded. Where expiration dates are applied, the pharmacist should emphasize to the patient that the dates are applicable only when proper storage conditions are used. Patients should be encouraged to clean out their drug storage cabinets periodically.

⟨1206⟩ STERILE DRUG PRODUCTS FOR HOME USE

A home-use sterile drug product (HSD) is a drug product requiring sterility, such as injectables and ophthalmics, that is prepared in and dispensed from a licensed pharmacy for intended administration by the patient or by a family member or other caregiver in a setting other than an organized, professionally staffed health care facility. The residence or other location to which an HSD is delivered typically is not equipped to ensure injectable drug quality as described in this chapter and is not under the *direct supervision* of the dispensing pharmacist.

This chapter explains in detail various procedures necessary to prepare and dispense sterile drug products intended for home use: the validation of sterilization and aseptic processes, the quality and control of environmental conditions for aseptic operations, personnel training, aseptic techniques, finished product release testing, storage and expiration dating, the control of product quality beyond the pharmacy, patient or caregiver training, patient monitoring and complaints, and finally, a quality assurance program. This information is not prescriptive, nor does it exclude alternate practices. However, alternatives when used should be shown on the basis of valid evidence to be at least as suitable, effective, and reliable as the practices provided herein.

RESPONSIBILITY OF THE DISPENSING PHARMACIST

A pharmacist dispensing any HSD is responsible for ensuring that the product has been prepared, labeled, controlled, stored, dispensed, and distributed properly. This includes the responsibility for ensuring that the HSD is kept under appropriate controlled conditions at the location of use and that it is administered properly through adequate labeling and verbal or written instructions. The dispensing pharmacist is also responsible for ensuring that the HSD retains its quality attributes within acceptable limits through a written quality assurance program. This program should ensure that for the entire labeled life of the product, or until manipulated by the patient or caregiver, the potency, pH, sterility, freedom from pyrogens, particulate limits, container integrity, appearance, and other qualities or characteristics that the HSD is expected to have do exist. The quality assurance program should encompass every HSD under the pharmacy's control and includes all phases of its preparation, distribution, storage, administration, and use. The dispensing pharmacy should employ proper analytical testing, where appropriate, to ensure the microbiological, chemical, and physical quality of all HSDs. These responsibilities apply equally to commercially available injectable drug products that are dispensed to patients without compounding or other manipulation and to HSDs that have been repackaged, reconstituted, diluted, admixed, blended, or otherwise manipulated (collectively referred to as "Compounded") in any way prior to dispensing. Emphasis in this chapter is placed upon the quality and the control of the processes utilized, personnel performance, and the environmental conditions under which the processes are performed. Other factors, such as testing and stability, are addressed to the extent necessary for the limited quantities of products with relatively short expiration dating periods normally associated with home care pharmacy practice. This chapter is not intended to address issues concerning the manufacture of sterile drug products.

RISK LEVELS

With reference to the microbiological quality (i.e., sterility) of the finished drug product, an HSD, in general, is compounded under either relatively *low-risk* or *high-risk* conditions, as determined by the potential for the introduction of microbial contamination. This contamination may result from the use of nonsterile components; novel, complex, or prolonged aseptic processes; or open exposure of the drug product or product containment devices to the atmosphere. In addition, long storage time between compounding and initiation of administration may affect the microbiological quality of the finished drug product.

The characteristics itemized below to distinguish between the high-risk and low-risk levels are intended to provide conceptual guidance and are not intended to be prescriptive. The pharmacist is expected to exercise professional judgment on a case-by-case basis when determining the risk level that would be appropriate for a particular process.

Low-Risk

An HSD is considered to be aseptically processed under low-risk conditions when all of the following conditions prevail:

(1) The finished product is compounded with commercially available, sterile drug products.
(2) Compounding involves only basic, and relatively few, aseptic manipulations that are promptly executed.
(3) "Closed system" transfers are used: the container-closure system remains essentially intact throughout the aseptic process, compromised only by the penetration of a sterile, pyrogen-free needle or cannula through the designated stopper or port to affect transfer, withdrawal, or delivery in accordance with the labeled instructions for the pertinent, commercially available devices.

Examples of low-risk processes include the following:

(1) Transferring sterile drug products from vials or ampuls into sterile final containers using a sterile needle and syringe.
(2) Transferring sterile drug products into sterile elastomeric infusion containers with the aid of a mechanical pump and an appropriate sterile transfer tubing device, with or without the subsequent addition of sterile drug products to the infusion container with a sterile needle and syringe.
(3) Compounding sterile nutritional solutions by combining *Dextrose Injection* and *Amino Acids Injection* via gravity transfer into sterile empty containers, with or without the subsequent addition of sterile drug products to the final container with a sterile needle and syringe.

High-Risk

Category I—A high-risk HSD may fall into either of two subclassifications. High-risk HSDs in *Category I* are those prepared from commercially available, sterile components where one or more of the following conditions prevail:

(1) Compounding involves the intermediate closed system pooling of sterile drug products.
(2) Compounding includes complex and/or numerous aseptic manipulations executed over a prolonged period.
(3) An individual finished product is administered as a multi-day infusion via a portable pump or reservoir.

Examples of high-risk category I processes include the following:

(1) Compounding sterile nutritional solutions using an automated compounding device involving repeated attachment of fluid containers to proximal openings of the compounder tubing set and of empty final containers to the distal opening. The process concludes with the transfer of additives into the filled final container from individual drug product containers or from a pooled additive solution.

(2) Preparing ambulatory pump reservoirs by adding more than one drug product with the evacuation of air from the reservoir prior to dispensing.
(3) Preparing ambulatory pump reservoirs for multi-day (i.e., ambient temperature) administration.

Category II—High-risk HSDs in *Category II* are those involving either of the following:
(1) A nonsterile drug substance or an injectable drug product prepared in-house from a nonsterile substance is used to compound the HSD.
(2) "Open systems" are used, for example, when combining ingredients in a nonsealed reservoir before filling or when fluid passes through the atmosphere during a fill-seal operation.

Examples of high-risk category II processes include the following:
(1) Compounding injectable morphine solutions from nonsterile morphine substance and suitable vehicles.
(2) Compounding sterile nutritional solutions from nonsterile ingredients with initial mixing in a nonsealed or nonsterile reservoir.

Key factors for *building quality into products* include at least the following general principles:
(1) Personnel are capable and qualified to perform their assigned duties.
(2) Ingredients used in compounding have their expected identity, quality, and purity.
(3) Critical processes are validated to ensure that procedures, when used, will consistently result in the expected qualities in the finished product.
(4) The production environment is suitable for its intended purpose (addressing such matters as environmental cleanliness, control, monitoring, and the setting of action limits, as appropriate).
(5) Appropriate release checks or testing procedures are performed to ensure that finished products have their expected potency, purity, quality, and characteristics at the time of release.
(6) Appropriate stability evaluation is performed for establishing reliable expiration dating to ensure that finished products have their expected potency, purity, quality, and characteristics at least until the labeled expiration date.
(7) There is assurance that processes are always carried out as intended or specified and are under control.
(8) Preparation conditions and procedures are adequate for preventing mixups.
(9) There are adequate procedures and records for investigating and correcting failures or problems in preparation, testing, or in the product itself.
(10) There is adequate separation of quality control functions and decisions from those of production.

VALIDATION

The sterilization or aseptic processing of an HSD should be in accordance with properly designed and validated written procedures. The act of validation of a sterilization or aseptic process involves planned testing designed to demonstrate that microorganisms will be effectively destroyed, removed, or prevented from inadvertently being introduced by personnel or by process-related activities.

Sterilization Processes

A high-risk HSD prepared from nonsterile ingredients or components should be sterilized using an appropriate sterilization process, such as filtration or heat sterilization. In general, each sterilization process should be validated to demonstrate suitability for its intended purpose and specific manner of intended uses.

STERILIZATION BY FILTRATION

A sterilizing filtration process should be capable of removing microorganisms from the liquid HSD. Commercially available presterilized filtration devices should be certified to be appropriate for human use in sterile pharmaceutical applications, have a pore size of 0.2 μm or smaller (generally recognized as a sterilizing filter), and have been lot tested for retention of *Pseudomonas diminuta* at a minimum concentration of 10^7 organisms per cm^2 under specified operating parameters. The individual devices should be tested for membrane and housing integrity, nonpyrogenicity, and extractables by the manufacturer. Such devices should be capable of sterilizing an HSD (see *Sterilization and Sterility Assurance of Compendial Articles* ⟨1211⟩). Before using such devices, the pharmacist should thoroughly evaluate their suitability for the intended HSD and conditions of use.

The size and configuration of filtration devices should accommodate the volume being filtered to permit complete filtration within a reasonable period of time and without clogging to the point where mid-process filter changes would be required.

Filters and associated devices and apparatus (housing, gaskets, etc.) should be physically and chemically compatible with the product to be filtered and should be capable of withstanding the temperatures, pressures, and hydrostatic stresses imposed on the system. These capabilities are to be established through appropriate product-specific testing. To establish compatibility, the pharmacy may rely on vendor certification or on definitive evidence, specific to product and filter, obtained from a critical review of the literature or from reliable unpublished research.

Validation should be established experimentally for all filtration apparatus involving assembly in the pharmacy of the membrane (filtration medium) into its housing or holder. The pharmacy may rely on vendor certification of validation for commercially available presterilized ready-to-use filter devices or for pharmacy-assembled apparatus. (The sterilization process used for pharmacy-assembled apparatus must be properly validated.) When relying on vendor certification of filtration validation, the pharmacy should request data from the vendor sufficient to ensure that an adequate challenge was used (minimum concentration of 10^7 organisms *Pseudomonas diminuta* per cm^2 of filter surface); and to ensure that the filtration apparatus and configuration, duration of filtration, filtration operating conditions (filtration rate and temperature), and the critical product formulation parameters (pH, viscosity, ionic strength, and osmolarity) used to generate the supplied data are representative of the pharmacy's product, apparatus, specified operating parameters, etc., in regard to the factors that might physically or chemically alter filter integrity, affect microbial capture mechanisms, or shrink the microorganism during filtration.

Each filter device used for product sterilization should be checked for integrity at the time of use. Integrity testing of commercially available, sterile, self-contained filter devices requiring no preuse assembly may be performed at the conclusion of the filtration process. Filter integrity test kits suitable for pharmacy use (for example, those consisting of a small gauge and a three-way stopcock assembly) are commercially available for testing the bubble point of small disk-type filters. For pharmacy-assembled apparatus, as defined above, prefiltration integrity testing is recommended in addition to postfiltration testing. Quantitative integrity testing, such as the bubble-point or forward flow tests (see *Sterilization and Sterility Assurance of Compendial Articles* ⟨1211⟩) should be used, as appropriate for larger filtration devices or when *Category II* high-risk HSDs are sterilized.

Filtration should be performed in accordance with written procedures that list those filters determined to be acceptable for the various HSDs to be filtered in the pharmacy or in accordance with master batch formulas that include definitive filter specifications. Filtration procedures and master batch formulas should also describe acceptable techniques for using and for checking the integrity of all listed filters. Fluid-filter compatibility must be established prior to the filtration of any HSD not included in the procedure.

HEAT STERILIZATION

Terminal sterilization should be used when sterilizing *Category II* high-risk HSDs. Sterilization may be accomplished in the final sealed container as a validated, controlled moist heat process (see *Sterilization and Sterility Assurance of Compendial Articles* ⟨1211⟩). In the absence of heat sterilization capabilities, or where heat labile drug products or container-closure systems preclude heat sterilization, an HSD may be sterilized by filtration and aseptically processed and controlled in accordance with the standards set forth in this chapter.

Heat sterilization processes should be validated to ensure that the likelihood of survival of the most resistant microorganisms likely to constitute product bioburden is no greater than 10^{-6} under the specified operating conditions and parameters, such as sterilization time and temperature, size and nature of load, and chamber loading configuration. The validation and monitoring of heat sterilization processes should be in writing with all critical parameters specified, should be followed each time of use, and should be supervised by a pharmacist knowledgeable of the technology involved in the sterilization of drug products. Monitoring data should be recorded properly to ensure, retrospectively, that

[7] Dishes meeting these specifications are obtainable from laboratory supply houses as Rodac brand, or use the equivalent.

the processes were carried out as specified and that all critical parameters were within specified limits during processing.[1]

Aseptic Processing

All aseptic processing operations and configurations should be adequately established by media-fill validation.[2] Media fills should simulate as closely as possible actual aseptic operations. All manipulations, handling, environmental conditions, and other factors likely to influence the risk of process-associated contamination should be represented by the media-fill simulations. The intensity of such challenges should represent the greatest risk that would be expected during normal production. Media-fill validations should be repeated with sufficient frequency to ensure the ongoing capability of performing properly each aseptic processing operation used in the pharmacy. The frequency and results of media-fill runs should be documented.

The culture medium selected should be capable of supporting the growth of a broad spectrum of microorganisms likely to be production-associated contaminants in the pharmacy. Commercially available media can be obtained that, when reconstituted as directed by the manufacturer, are certified to have growth-promoting properties. Soybean-Casein Digest Medium is acceptable (see *Sterility* ⟨71⟩). Incubation of medium-filled units should take at least 14 days and may be at room temperature for 14 days or may be at room temperature for the first 7 days, with the final 1 to 7 days at 30° to 35°. Alternate suitable incubation schedules may be used as determined by the pharmacy to ensure enough growth of any potential contaminating microorganisms to be visually detectable. Microorganisms in all medium-filled units showing visible evidence of microbial growth should be promptly identified, and if this growth exceeds the action limits, an immediate investigation should be made with prompt correction of any identifiable causes of the failure. Review of environmental monitoring data obtained during the media fill should be included in the investigation, as well as a review of the cleaning, sanitizing, disinfection, production procedures, aseptic technique, personnel practices, and other factors as appropriate. Revalidation should occur after all media-fill failures (see Table 1).

Table 1. Validation of Aseptic Processing.

Validation Purpose	Validation Requirements: Low Risk	High Risk*
General	Personnel validation	Process validation
Initial	3 consecutive media-fill runs without contamination	3 consecutive media-fill runs without contamination
Revalidation	1 media-fill run quarterly without contamination	annual media-fill run without contamination
Failure revalidation	3 consecutive media-fill runs without contamination	3 consecutive media-fill runs without contamination

* NOTE—Personnel should have first passed low-risk validation.

Low-Risk Operations

The primary objective of the validation of aseptic processing involving low-risk operations is to ensure that personnel are capable of using effective aseptic technique to compound an HSD successfully under the most rigorous conditions encountered during normal work assignments. In carrying out validation of the process, personnel should perform media fills consisting of a planned repetitive sequence of compounded or repackaged units. The number of manipulations of each unit and the number of units in each media fill should reflect the most complex and prolonged aseptic manipulations likely to be encountered by an operator as a normal workload requirement. The number of units per media-fill run should be enough to ensure that the operator is capable of replicating acceptable aseptic procedures. Media transfers could be used to represent procedures such as syringe transfers, use of automated compounding devices, multiple additive procedures, and various aseptic assemblies and connections (see *Example of a Validation Procedure for Low-risk Operations*).

EXAMPLE OF A VALIDATION PROCEDURE FOR LOW-RISK OPERATIONS

Scenario—A pharmacy prepares antibiotics, hydration solutions, and parenteral nutrition solutions for home use. The most complex and prolonged aseptic manipulations are required for the parenteral nutrition solutions. The parenteral nutrition solution is made by combining the amino acid and dextrose by gravity transfer into 2-liter empty flexible bags, and then adding a maximum of 10 additives to a bag via syringe transfer. Typically, the pharmacy prepares no more than a 2- or 3-week supply of the solutions at one time.

Example of a validation procedure—One hundred mL of sterile Soybean Casein Digest Medium is transferred via gravity into plastic bags. Twenty units are completed in this manner, to approximate the number of units typically compounded at one time. After all twenty units have been filled, the media containers are lined up in pairs. One mL of media is drawn from one container and transferred aseptically by syringe transfer to another media unit and repeated for a total of ten transfers. Then media from the other units is syringe transferred to the first unit for a total of ten syringe transfers. This process is continued until all twenty units have undergone ten syringe transfers. The media fill units are incubated at room temperature for a total of fourteen days, with frequent checks for growth.

Media fills should be representative of peak periods of fatigue, stress, and pacing demands. For example, media fills could be scheduled immediately after normal production activity has ended. Media fills should not be performed during normal production.

Operators should pass an initial validation, performing three media fills with no contamination, before they are allowed to make HSDs for patients. Subsequently, each operator should perform at least one media fill involving low-risk operations quarterly. If one contaminated unit results from a media fill, the operator should be retrained and then perform three consecutive media fills with no contaminated unit before again being allowed to compound HSDs for patients. Operators should also be revalidated if the nature of their aseptic compounding assignments changes to the extent that their previous media fills are not representative of their revised assignments.

High-Risk Operations

In the case of high-risk operations, the focus of validation is on the process as well as personnel capability. Thus, the primary objective of the validation of aseptic processing for high-risk operations is to ensure that the aseptic process is capable of being carried out consistently under control by any qualified operator, before the process is utilized for production of units intended for administration to patients. Accordingly, each type of high-risk operation should be validated independently, rather than having operators perform representative sets of aseptic activities, as is the case with low-risk aseptic operations.

Personnel assigned to high-risk aseptic operations should be validated for low-risk operations as described above. In addition, these personnel should participate at least annually in the validation of each high-risk aseptic operation to which assigned.

For example, for high-risk operations involving nonsterile components, the media-fill run should simulate as closely as possible the most intensive conditions likely to be encountered during the normal production activities. The number of units in a media-fill run should be no less than the largest number of units encountered during production involving the process being validated. However, the fill volume of media-fill units need not equal the fill volume of finished product units.

A media-fill run should be performed at least annually for each unique high-risk batch processing procedure and configuration. A media-fill failure for most home care operations (less than 1000 units) is one or more contaminated units after incubation. For batches equal to or greater than 1000 units, a media-fill failure is greater than one contaminated unit. When a media-fill failure occurs, three consecutive successful media fills should occur before the process failing the media fill may be used for the compounding of an HSD for patients.

[1] PDA Technical Monograph No. 1, Validation of Steam Sterilization Cycles, 1978.

[2] FDA Guideline on Sterile Drug Products Produced by Aseptic Processing, June 1987, pp. 20–27; PDA Technical Monograph No. 2, Validation of Aseptic Filling for Solution Drug Products, 1980.

ENVIRONMENTAL QUALITY AND CONTROL

Achieving and maintaining sterility and overall freedom from contamination of a pharmaceutical product is dependent upon the quality status of the components incorporated, the process utilized, personnel performance, and the environmental conditions under which the process is performed. The standards required for the environmental conditions depend upon the amount of exposure of the HSD to the immediate environment anticipated during processing. The quality and control of environmental conditions for low-risk and high-risk operations is explained in this section. In addition, operations using nonsterile components require the use of a method of preparation designed to produce a sterile product.

Critical Site Exposure

The degree of exposure of the product during processing will be affected by the length of time of exposure, the size of the critical site exposed, and the nature of the critical site.

A critical site is any opening providing a direct pathway between a sterile product and the environment or any surface coming in direct contact with the product and the environment. The risk of such a site picking up contamination from the environment increases with time of exposure. Therefore, the processing plan and the intent of the operator should give due consideration to organization, efficiency, and speed in order to keep such exposure time to a minimum. For example, an ampul should not be opened unnecessarily in advance of use.

The size of the critical site affects the risk of contamination entering the product: the greater the exposed area, the greater the risk. An open vial or bottle exposes to contamination a critical site of much larger area than the tip of a 26-gauge needle. Therefore, the risk of contamination when entering an open vial or bottle is much greater than during the momentary exposure of a needle tip.

The nature of a critical site also affects the risk of contamination. The relatively rough, permeable surface of a rubber closure retains microorganisms and other contaminants, after wiping with an alcohol pad, more readily than does the smooth glass surface of the neck of an ampul. Therefore, the surface disinfection can be expected to be more effective for an ampul.

The prevention or elimination of airborne particles must be given high priority. Mobile or airborne contaminants are much more likely to reach critical sites than contaminants that are adhering to the floor or other surfaces below the work level. Further, particles that are relatively large or of high density settle from the airspace more quickly and thus can be removed from the vicinity of critical sites.

Environmentally Controlled Workspaces

LAFW AND BUFFER ROOM

An environmentally controlled workspace suitable for the aseptic processing of an HSD consists of a suitably constructed, properly functioning, and regularly certified device, which sweeps the workspace or an entire room with HEPA-filtered air at a velocity of 90 feet per minute ± 20%, such as a laminar airflow workbench (LAFW). Such a workspace is required for both low-risk and high-risk operations. The air blower for the workspace should be operated without interruption in order to sweep the workspace continually. Since the airflow velocity is relatively gentle, an LAFW must be located in an environmentally controlled room or a space otherwise separated from less controlled work areas, such as the main pharmacy, by partitions, plastic curtains, or preferably, a solid wall. Hereinafter, this area surrounding an LAFW shall be called the "Buffer Room." Clean and sanitized supplies may be accumulated and stored for a limited period of time in the Buffer Room in order to be conveniently available for use in preparing products in the LAFW.

Table 2. Class Limits in Particles per Cubic Foot.
(Size equal to or greater than particle sizes shown.)*

Class	Measured Particle Size (micrometers) 0.1	0.2	0.3	0.5	5.0
1	35	7.5	3	1	—
10	350	75	30	10	—
100	—	750	300	100	—
1,000	—	—	—	1,000	7
10,000	—	—	—	10,000	70
100,000	—	—	—	100,000	700

* The Class limit particle concentrations shown in Table 2 are defined for class purposes only and do not necessarily represent the size distribution to be found in any particular situation. Federal Standard No. 209E, General Services Administration, Washington, DC 20407, September 11, 1992.

Since an LAFW is normally a self-contained unit, the air circulated is drawn from the Buffer Room and does not contribute fresh air. Therefore, such a unit does not create positive air pressure in the Buffer Room. However, units can be installed to draw in fresh outside air through an HEPA filter and provide positive air pressure, but they cannot be movable.

The direction of flow may be horizontal or vertical. (A suitable biological safety cabinet with vertical airflow should be used for processing cytotoxic and other hazardous agents to protect the operator as well as the product.) The air quality within the LAFW adjacent to critical sites should meet a Class 100 (MCB-1) clean room specification during normal work activity. (See Table 2 for the definition of clean room classes. Also, see *Microbiological Evaluation and Classification of Clean Rooms and Clean Zones* ⟨1116⟩.)

The environmental quality within the Buffer Room should be demonstrably better than that of adjacent areas, such as the main pharmacy, to reduce the risk of contaminants being blown, dragged, or otherwise introduced into the LAFW. For example, strong air currents from briefly opened doors, personnel walking past the LAFW, or the airstream from the heating, ventilating, and air-conditioning (HVAC) system can easily exceed the velocity of clean air from the LAFW. Also, operators introducing supplies into the LAFW or reaching in with their arms can drag contaminants along with those movements.

The level of cleanliness of the air in the Buffer Room, in conjunction with the expertise of the operator, is critical to maintaining the Class 100 (MCB-1) conditions within the LAFW. The air entering the Buffer Room should be fresh, HEPA-filtered, conditioned air. The air in the Buffer Room should meet the requirements for at least a Class 100,000 (see Table 2) clean room for low-risk operations and a Class 10,000 (MCB-2) for high-risk operations. In addition to cleaning the inflowing air and providing at least 10 air changes per hour, cooling is essential because of the continual buildup of heat from the circulation of air through the blower and HEPA filter of the LAFW. It should be noted that the circulation of air from the Buffer Room through the HEPA filter of the LAFW enhances the cleanliness of the air, particularly during nonuse periods.

Tasks carried out within the Buffer Room should be limited to those for which a controlled environment is necessary. Only the furniture, equipment, supplies, and other goods required for the tasks to be performed may be brought into this room, and they should be nonpermeable, nonshedding, and resistant to disinfectants. Whenever such items are brought into the room, they should first be cleaned and sanitized. Whenever possible, equipment and other items used in the Buffer Room should not be taken from the room except for calibration, servicing, or other activity associated with the proper maintenance of the item.

The surfaces of ceilings, walls, floors, fixtures, shelving, counters, and cabinets in the Buffer Room should be smooth, impervious, free from cracks and crevices, and nonshedding, thereby promoting cleanability and minimizing spaces in which microorganisms and other contaminants may accumulate. The surfaces should be resistant to damage by sanitizing agents. Junctures of ceilings to walls should be coved or caulked to avoid cracks and crevices where dirt can accumulate. If ceilings consist of inlaid panels, the panels should be impregnated with a polymer to render them impervious and hydrophobic, and they should be caulked around each perimeter to seal them to the support frame. Walls may be of panels locked together and sealed or of epoxy-coated gypsum board. Preferably, floors are overlaid with wide sheet vinyl flooring with heat-welded seams and coving to the sidewall. Dust-collecting overhangs, such as ceiling utility pipes, or ledges, such as window sills, should be avoided. The exterior lens surface of ceiling lighting fixtures should be smooth, mounted flush, and sealed. Any other penetrations through the ceiling or walls should be sealed.

The Buffer Room should contain no sinks or floor drains. Work surfaces should be constructed of smooth, impervious materials, such as stainless steel or molded plastic, so that they are readily cleanable and sanitizable. Carts should be of stainless steel wire or sheet metal construction with good quality, cleanable casters to promote mobility. Storage shelving, counters, and cabinets should be smooth, impervious, free from cracks and crevices, nonshedding, cleanable, and sanitizable. Their number, design, and manner of installation should promote effective cleaning and sanitizing.

ACCESS CONTROL TO THE BUFFER ROOM (ANTEROOM)

Access to the Buffer Room should be planned and strictly controlled because of the need to protect the aseptic operations performed in an LAFW from contaminating substances, while permitting supplies and personnel to enter the area from relatively uncontrolled storerooms, from the main pharmacy, or from administrative areas. Access should be strictly limited to only designated, qualified personnel. The number of personnel in the Buffer Room at any one time should not exceed those essential to perform the required tasks.

An Anteroom or other separated area should be available for the decontamination of supplies, equipment, and personnel before they enter the Buffer Room. (This decontamination area is hereafter referred to as the Anteroom.) The size of the room should be sufficient to accommodate this activity with the heaviest work load anticipated. Minimally this would require space for two or more carts and space for personnel to clean, sanitize, and transfer supplies from the stockroom cart to the clean room cart. A floor demarcation should identify the maximum distance into the room that stockroom carts can penetrate.

The Anteroom should also be designed for uncartoning and disinfecting large-volume parenteral (LVP) bottles, pouches of hypodermic syringes, ampuls, vials, pouches of LVP bags, transfer set packages, and other required supplies. Here, also, carts for use in the Buffer Room should be cleaned and disinfected.

One or more sinks and a forced air hand dryer or disposable nonshedding towels should be available near the entrance door to the Buffer Room so that personnel can scrub their hands and arms before donning hair covers, shoe covers, clean gowns, and face masks. After donning hair and shoe covers, foamed alcohol may be used to resanitize the hands. Faucet handles should be designed so that they can be shut off with the elbows or feet. An alternate procedure being used increasingly is to disinfect the hands and arms with a foamed alcohol, or other effective sanitizer, instead of scrubbing with detergent and water. The hot air hand dryer is then not needed. A means of demarcation should be provided between the Buffer Room side and the general entry side of the Anteroom to enhance the gowning procedure. One option, a movable bench (preferably of stainless steel), provides a barrier and place for personnel to sit down to don shoe covers just before entering the Buffer Room. A storage area for clean gowning supplies should be conveniently located nearby. The door into the Buffer Room should remain automatically, positively closed and capable of being opened with elbow hooks or other means without using clean hands. The Anteroom should be designed to reduce to as low as possible the risk of recontamination of cleaned and sanitized supplies and personnel prior to entry into the Buffer Room.

An Anteroom as just described is necessary for high-risk operations. For low-risk operations, a carefully controlled area adjacent to the Buffer Room but without rigid walls may be acceptable. However, essentially the same attention for organization and cleanliness of the anteroom area is to be given in conjunction with both high- and low-risk operations.

Cleaning and Sanitizing the Workspaces

The cleaning, sanitizing, and organizing of the LAFW should be the responsibility of trained operators (pharmacists and technicians) following written procedures and should be performed at the beginning of each shift. All items should be removed from the LAFW and all surfaces wiped clean with a freshly prepared mild detergent followed by an approved sanitizing agent,[3] allowing sufficient time for the agent to exert its antimicrobial effect. The chosen sanitizing agent should be rotated with one of a different action at least quarterly. Recleaning should be performed if spillage or other events indicate the need.

Work surfaces near the LAFW in the Buffer Room should be cleaned in a similar manner, including counter tops and supply carts. Storage shelving should be emptied of all supplies and then cleaned and sanitized at least weekly, using approved agents.

Floors in the Buffer Room should be cleaned by mopping once daily when no aseptic operations are in progress. Mopping may be performed by trained and supervised custodial personnel using approved agents described in the written procedures. Only approved cleaning and sanitizing agents should be utilized, with careful consideration of compatibilities, effectiveness, and inappropriate or toxic residues. Their schedules of use and methods of application should be in accord with written procedures. All cleaning tools, such as wipers, sponges, and mops, should be nonshedding and dedicated to use in the Buffer Room. Floor mops may be used in both the Buffer Room and the Anteroom, but only in that order. Most wipers should be discarded after one use. If cleaning tools are reused, their cleanliness should be maintained by thorough rinsing and sanitization after use and by storing in a clean environment between uses. Trash should be collected in suitable plastic bags and removed with minimal agitation.

In the Anteroom supplies and equipment removed from shipping cartons should be wiped with a sanitizing agent, such as sterile 70% isopropyl alcohol (IPA[4]), which is checked periodically for contamination. Alternatively, if supplies are planned to be received in sealed pouches, the pouches can be removed as the supplies are introduced into the Buffer Room without the need to sanitize the individual supply items. No shipping or other external cartons may be taken into the Buffer Room. Cleaning and sanitizing of the Anteroom should be performed at least weekly by trained and supervised custodial personnel, in accordance with written procedures. However, floors are cleaned and sanitized daily, always proceeding from the Buffer Room to the Anteroom. Storage shelving should be emptied of all supplies and cleaned and sanitized at planned intervals, preferably monthly.

These cleaning and sanitizing procedures apply to both low-risk and high-risk operations.

Personnel and Gowning

Personnel are critical keys to the maintenance of asepsis when carrying out their assigned responsibilities. They must be thoroughly trained in aseptic techniques and be highly motivated to maintain these standards each time they prepare a sterile product.

Prior to entering the Buffer Room, operators should remove outer lab jackets or the like, makeup, and jewelry and should thoroughly scrub hands and arms to the elbow. After drying hands and arms they should properly don clean, nonshedding uniform components, including hair covers, shoe covers, knee-length coats or coveralls, and sterile latex gloves, in that order. The coats should fit snugly at the wrists and be zipped or snapped closed in the front. Shoe covers should be donned so that feet then touch the floor only on the clean side of the bench or other demarcation. Face masks should be donned just prior to beginning work at the horizontal LAFW, as talking, sneezing, or coughing normally generates an air velocity that exceeds the velocity of air from the LAFW. When working at a vertical LAFW, the wearing of a mask is optional where a solid transparent shield establishes a physical barrier between the face of the operator and the workspace. However, any facial hair should be completely covered in all instances.

Sterile latex gloves should be put on, aseptically—being sure to protect the outer surfaces from contamination—as the last uniform component. Latex gloves are effective in containing bacteria, skin scales, and other particles shed by the most scrupulously scrubbed hands. However, the outer sterile surfaces do not remain sterile since they will contact the room air, sanitized supply items, work counters, and other surfaces that, while clean, are not sterile. Therefore, operators must perform aseptic manipulations in a manner designed to prevent touching critical sites with the gloved fingers or hands. Further, operators should attempt to maintain gloved hand surfaces as free from contamination as possible by repeated rinsing with a sterile sanitizing agent, such as IPA, during use.

Sterile latex gloves must be worn when operator protection as well as product protection is essential, such as during operations involving cytotoxic or otherwise hazardous sterile products.

Proper scrubbing and gowning immediately prior to entry into the Buffer Room is required of all personnel, without exception. Should the operator find it necessary to leave the room, the coat may be carefully removed at the entrance and hung inside out for redonning upon re-entry, but only during the same shift. However, hair covers, masks, shoe covers, and gloves should be discarded and new ones donned prior to re-entry.

For high-risk operations, it is especially critical to minimize the risk of contamination on lab coats, coveralls, and other garb to be worn in the Buffer Room. Preferably, fresh clean garb should be donned upon each entry into the Buffer Room to avoid liberating contaminants from previously worn garb. Alternatively, garb that has been worn may be removed with the intention of regarbing for re-entry into the Buffer Room and stored during the interim under proper control and protection

[3] Approved by the pharmacist in charge.

[4] NOTE—70% isopropyl alcohol (IPA) may harbor resistant microbial spores. Therefore, IPA used in aseptic areas should always be filtered through a 0.2-μm hydrophobic filter to render it sterile.

in the Anteroom. Garb worn or taken outside the confines of the Anteroom should not be worn in the Buffer Room.

Dispersion of particles from body surfaces, such as from skin rashes, sunburn, or cosmetics, increases the risk of contamination of critical sites and should be appropriately controlled or minimized. If severe, the operator should be excluded from the Buffer Room until the condition is remedied, especially for high-risk operations.

Suggested Standard Operating Procedures (SOPs)

The pharmacy should have written, properly approved SOPs designed to ensure the quality of the environment in which an HSD is prepared. The following procedures are recommended:

(1) Access to the Buffer Room should be restricted to qualified personnel with specific responsibilities or assigned tasks in the area.
(2) All cartoned supplies should be decontaminated in the Anteroom by removing them from shipping cartons and wiping with a disinfecting agent, such as sterile IPA, while being transferred to a clean, sanitized cart or other conveyance for introduction into the Buffer Room. Individual pouched supplies need not be wiped because the pouches can be removed as these supplies are introduced into the Buffer Room.
(3) Supplies required frequently or otherwise needed close at hand but not necessarily needed for the scheduled operations of the shift should be decontaminated and stored on the shelving in the Anteroom.
(4) Carts used to bring supplies from the storeroom should not be rolled beyond the demarcation line in the Anteroom, and carts used in the Buffer Room should not be rolled outward beyond the demarcation line unless cleaned and sanitized before returning.
(5) Generally, supplies required for the scheduled operations of the shift should be prepared and brought into the Buffer Room, preferably on one or more movable carts. Supplies that are required for back-up or general support of operations may be stored on the designated shelving in the Buffer Room, but excessive accumulation of supplies should be avoided.
(6) Objects that shed particles should not be brought into the Buffer Room, including pencils, cardboard cartons, paper towels, and cotton items.
(7) Traffic flow into and out of the Buffer Room should be minimized.
(8) All personnel preparing to enter the Buffer Room should remove all jewelry from hands and arms.
(9) All personnel entering the Buffer Room should first scrub hands and arms with soap, including using a scrub brush on the fingers and nails. An air dryer or disposable nonshedding towels should be used to dry hands and arms after washing.
(10) All personnel entering the Buffer Room, after scrubbing, should don attire as described under *Personnel and Gowning*.
(11) No chewing gum, candy, or food items may be brought into the Buffer Room.
(12) At the beginning of each shift and when spillage occurs, the LAFW surface should be wiped with a clean, nonlinting wiper or sponge dampened with distilled water. The entire inside of the LAFW should then be wiped with another clean wiper wet with an approved disinfectant, such as IPA.
(13) The blower of the LAFW should be operated continuously. However, in the event of a long period of nonuse, the blower may be turned off and the opening covered with a plastic curtain or other shield. Before reuse, all internal surfaces should be sanitized and the blower operated for a minimum of 30 minutes.
(14) Traffic in the area of the LAFW should be minimized and controlled. The LAFW should be shielded from all less clean air currents that are of higher velocity than the clean laminar airflow.
(15) Supplies to be utilized in the LAFW for the planned procedures should be accumulated and then decontaminated by wiping the outer surface with IPA or removing the outer wrap at the edge of the LAFW as the item is introduced into the aseptic work area.
(16) After proper introduction into the LAFW of supply items required for and limited to the assigned operations, they should be so arranged that a clear, uninterrupted path of HEPA-filtered air will bathe all critical sites at all times during the planned procedures. That is, no objects may be placed behind an exposed critical site in a horizontal position or above in the vertical laminar flow workbench.
(17) All supply items should be arranged in the LAFW to reduce clutter and to provide maximum efficiency and order for the flow of work.
(18) All procedures should be performed in a manner designed to minimize the risk of touch contamination. Gloves should be sanitized with adequate frequency.
(19) All rubber stoppers of vials and bottles and the neck of ampuls should be sanitized with IPA prior to the introduction of a needle or spike for the removal of product.
(20) After the preparation of every admixture, the contents of the container should be thoroughly mixed and then inspected for the presence of particulate matter, evidence of incompatibility, or other defects.
(21) After procedures are completed, used syringes, bottles, vials, and other supplies should be removed, but with a minimum of exit and re-entry into the LAFW to minimize the risk of dragging contamination into the aseptic workspace.

Environmental Control and Monitoring Program

Because achieving or maintaining sterility is essential in the preparation of sterile products, the assessment of the level of control of the environment in which those products are prepared is recommended. The level of environmental control achieved may be evaluated by measuring the viable and the total (viable and nonviable) number of particles in the environment. Viable particle counting is recommended for environmental assessment in conjunction with the preparation of an HSD. Total particle counting is recommended for facility classification.

Viable particle counts are indicative of the portion of the total particle counts that represent microorganisms, normally reported as Colony Forming Units (cfu's), since typical viable particle counting results do not distinguish between single microorganisms and clusters. The difficulties in obtaining consistent and quantitative growth of microorganisms and the time lag between sampling and obtaining results because of growth time are important environmental monitoring limitations.

Total particle counts are usually performed by means of electronic instruments that give results instantly, based upon the measurement of particles in a prescribed volume of air. Clean room classifications (see Table 2) are based upon such measurements. A number of different types of instruments are available. Measurements can be made one at a time, or, with most instruments, automatically obtained on a planned, ongoing schedule. Instantaneous results permit assessment of environmental particulates at any given time and permit rapid changes in the control program should the results indicate a problem. However, these results do not distinguish between viable and nonviable particulates.

This section focuses on the measurement and monitoring of programs for viable particles.[5]

TESTING PROGRAM

A testing program is based upon the use of various methods for collecting an environmental sample on a nutrient, usually solid, culture medium, incubating at a temperature and for a time period conducive to the multiplication of any collected microorganisms, and then counting the discrete colonies that have developed on the surface of the medium. The count, reported as cfu's, is a measure of microbial contamination of the environment at the time and under the conditions of sampling. For more details, see *Microbiological Evaluation and Classification of Clean Rooms and Clean Zones* ⟨1116⟩.

In general, test methods for airborne environmental microbial contaminants either determine the number of cfu's collected in a measured volume of air ("quantitative" or "volumetric") or during a specified period of time. Any test method sensitive enough to show trends in environmental quality under specified conditions of the sampling used is acceptable. In general, quantitative methods are preferred over nonquantitative methods. When using either approach, the sample size should be sufficient to give a result of statistical significance. The testing program should also include surface sampling.

Dynamic monitoring, that is, testing under operating conditions during work activity, should be used routinely in order to give a cfu count during the processing of an HSD that demonstrates the critical effects

[5] The PDA Technical Report No. 13, 1990, may be consulted for details and monitoring methods not covered in this section.

of the presence and movement of operators. The latter is possible when comparing results from dynamic monitoring with results from static monitoring when no processing is being performed. Static monitoring generally evaluates the status of the facilities, operating equipment, and housekeeping.

The greatest value of ongoing microbial monitoring is achieved when microbial recoveries show trends. For a given environmental area, a baseline count is determined under the best environmental control believed to be possible for the area. Sampling should be done in selected locations and in a manner intended to reflect best the environmental conditions in the area. To establish the baseline count, a large number of samples should be taken in multiple locations over a period of time to reflect time of day and week, workload conditions, and, preferably, seasonal variations. Analysis of these results would give counts normally expected to be achievable and the identification of a reduced number of selected sites expected to reflect the environmental conditions in the area with subsequent monitoring. This analysis then becomes the basis for ongoing monitoring. The baseline count limits may be slightly higher for low-risk operations than for high-risk operations. Subsequently, any significant change in the counts obtained, either as a single spike or a gradual rise in the cfu count, would require investigation into the cause.

When counts exceed the established baseline count by a determined amount (the action level), a written plan of action should be initiated. The plan would usually call for a repeat of the monitoring tests the next day and an investigation into the cause, and may include such actions as review of decontamination procedures, resanitization of the LAFW and the Buffer Room, a change to a different sanitizing agent, or retraining of operators. It should be remembered that microbial monitoring results are not available until after incubation, usually 48 hours, thus causing a delay in taking any corrective action. Therefore, trends should be detected as early as possible. Action levels would be slightly higher for low-risk operations than for high-risk operations.

The workspace in an LAFW is the only environment required to meet Class 100 (MCB-1) conditions, with the exception of specialized rooms (e.g., laminar flow rooms) specifically designed to achieve Class 100 conditions. To ensure that Class 100 conditions are met continuously, the LAFW (or room) should be certified after installation and recertified at least annually and after the unit is moved. This certification process includes testing for HEPA filter leaks and the laminar airflow velocity. The microbial counts normally anticipated within the LAFW (or room) will average less than one per 10 cubic feet, even under dynamic testing conditions. However, culture media exposed to the airstream tends to dry and, therefore, should not be exposed for more than one hour. Table 3 provides examples of microbial environmental test limits, and is presented as a guide.[6]

Table 3. A Sample Dynamic Environmental Microbial Monitoring Program.

Site	Baseline cfu	Low-risk Action Level	High-risk Action Level
Settling Plates*			
A	0,1	3	2
D	2,3	6	4
E	4,5	10	6
J	5	10	7
L	8	15	10
Contact Plates			
D	2,3	6	4
E	4,6	10	7
J	6	12	8
L	8	15	10
STA or Impaction Sampler**			
A	0,1	3	2
E	5	10	7
H	8	15	10

* Based on 3-hour exposure, except 1-hour for "A." See Fig. 1 for site locations.

** Based on 10 cu. ft. samples.

TEST METHODS

A well-known test method is the exposure of settling plates, that is, petri dishes with solid nutrient agar medium congealed in the bottom section of the plate. These 100-mm diameter plates are simply opened and allowed to rest on a surface for a planned period of time. They do not sample a known volume of air; rather, viable particles collect on the agar surface as they fall from the environment or are impacted by the movement of air currents. Three-hour exposure of settling plates in a room is an appropriate, easy, and inexpensive way to obtain a representation of the contamination that could be expected to settle from the air at the sampling site.

Well-known volume-of-air samplers include the slit-to-agar (STA) sampler and the Reuter centrifugal air sampler (RCS). The STA sampler utilizes a revolving nutrient agar plate under a slit orifice to impinge the air sample particles on the surface of the nutrient agar in the plate. While the unit is portable, it requires a vacuum and an electrical source. The unit can be sanitized but not sterilized. The RCS draws air with an impeller into the head of the unit and centrifugally impacts any particles on a nutrient agar strip around the perimeter of the head. The unit samples in multiples of 40 liters per minute and is sanitizable and portable, with a self-contained battery power unit. Both of these units are relatively expensive but, unlike settling plates, have the advantage of quantitative sampling.

Surface sampling is most frequently done with contact plates[7] to detect accumulated microbial contamination on a flat surface. These plates are 60 mm in diameter and filled with nutrient agar medium to form a convex surface. The agar usually contains additives to help neutralize residues of disinfectants that may be on the test surface. The agar is pressed onto a flat surface lifting any microorganisms present onto the surface of the agar. This method can be considered to be relatively quantitative when contaminants are residing superficially on a flat, smooth surface. However, residual agar must be thoroughly removed from the test surface.

AN EXAMPLE OF AN ENVIRONMENTAL MONITORING PROGRAM

The following is a suggestion for one possible environmental monitoring program consisting of multiple tests to determine the baseline count and subsequent reduced testing for ongoing monitoring of the environmental control conditions.[8]

Settling plates should be uncovered and exposed for 3 hours both under static and dynamic conditions. This test should be repeated each day and each shift for at least one week, preferably two weeks. If STA or RCS air samplers are used, at least 10 cu. ft. (280 liters) air samples should be taken at certain sites. The nutrient agar plates or strips are then incubated at 30° to 35° for 48 hours and the colonies counted. These tests should be repeated about six months later. The average number of colonies at each site is computed to give baseline counts, being sure that housekeeping and other environmental control procedures are functioning at maximum efficiency.

Similarly, at the end of each shift and before any clean-up sanitization is done, perform surface sampling with contact plates at the same sites, being careful to remove any residual medium from the surfaces with an alcohol wipe. In addition, at least the index finger of each operator should be rolled on a contact plate.

The results of these evaluations are critically reviewed. Using the data given in Table 3 as an example, a reduced number of sites for monitoring, which give the best evidence of the level of microbial control maintained during facility operation, can be selected. Monitoring tests under dynamic conditions should then be performed at least weekly during the shift of highest activity at the selected sites (sites that give

[6] These test limits were compiled from suggested values in Technical Monograph No. 2, the Parenteral Society (Great Britain), 1989, and other sources. They were also correlated with the USP proposed data in *Microbiological Evaluation and Classification of Clean Rooms and Clean Zones* ⟨1116⟩.

[7] Dishes meeting these specifications are obtainable from laboratory supply houses as Rodac brand, or use the equivalent.

[8] See also *Am. J. Hosp. Pharm.* 1980; 37:668.

evidence of being representative of the true environmental control conditions). At least monthly another shift should be monitored in the same manner. Volume-of-air samples might be reduced to one site in each room weekly. However, the number of monitoring sites or the sampling frequency should be increased if there is any indication that the monitoring program is inadequate. Action levels are determined by making a reasoned judgment. A 50% increase above the baseline count is probably reasonable for high-risk operations. For low-risk operations an increase of 100% probably would be acceptable. However, whenever a rising trend appears to be in progress, the operations should be closely monitored with more frequent sampling being performed to confirm whether or not a trend is occurring.

PROCESSING

Personnel Training and Evaluation

The pharmacy should follow a written program of training and performance evaluation designed to ensure that each person working in the aseptic area has the appropriate knowledge and skills necessary to perform the assigned tasks properly. Each person assigned to the aseptic area must successfully complete specialized training in aseptic technique and aseptic area practices.

Training should include didactic material and practical skills activities. Evaluation should include written testing and a written protocol of frequent routine performance checks involving random direct observation of critical operations and adherence to all aseptic area procedures and codes. Prompt appropriate action should occur to correct performance deviations, whether detected during a performance check or informally. At six-month intervals each person's continuing training needs should be reassessed, then documented, to ensure that skill levels are maintained.

Aseptic Technique

All critical operations are carried out by appropriately trained and qualified personnel in an LAFW using proper aseptic technique described in a written procedure (see the section *Suggested Standard Operating Procedures*). Aseptic technique is equally applicable to the preparation of sterile sensitizing and chemotoxic agents. However, it should be recognized that additional precautions must be used to protect the compounder and the compounding environment from the adverse effects of the agents being processed. A vertical laminar flow workbench (VLFW) with biohazard control capabilities, the protective capabilities of garb and gloves, sprayback and spill control techniques, the use of specialized compounding devices, and proper disposal are some of the additional measures to be considered.

Components

The pharmacy should follow written procedures to ensure that all items used to compound sterile drug products retain their purported or expected qualities at the time of use.

STERILE COMPONENTS

Commercially available sterile drug products, sterile ready-to-use containers and devices are examples of sterile components. A written procedure for unit-by-unit physical inspection preparatory to use should be followed to ensure that these components are sterile, free from defects, and otherwise suitable for their intended use.

NONSTERILE COMPONENTS

Drug components should meet compendial standards. Certificates of analysis from reputable manufacturers of bulk drug substances may be used to establish that each lot of bulk drug substance received by the pharmacy meets its specifications. Bulk drug substances stored properly in the pharmacy can be expected to retain their quality until the manufacturer's labeled expiration date. Bulk drug substances that are not labeled with a manufacturer's expiration date should be dated upon receipt, stored properly, dated when opening the container, used within a reasonable period of time, and visually inspected by the pharmacist upon use. The conditions under which containers of bulk drug substances are opened and the technique of the contents' withdrawal should be strictly controlled. Additionally, the devices used to withdraw the contents should be clean to preclude contamination of the remaining contents. The pharmacy may repackage bulk drug substances into smaller, suitable, and properly sealed containers (e.g., using a shrink seal) to minimize the risk of contamination. Upon receipt of each lot of bulk drug substance used to compound an HSD, the pharmacy should perform an inspection of the lot for any visual evidence of deterioration, other types of unacceptable quality, and wrong identity. Visual inspection of bulk drug substances should be performed routinely.

Because finished compounded HSDs are not usually tested for pyrogens, nonsterile bulk drug substances could impart pyrogenic properties to the finished product. Therefore, the pharmacy should have a procedure to ensure that the final product does not exceed specified endotoxin limits. See *Bacterial Endotoxins Test* ⟨85⟩ for procedural details concerning endotoxin testing.

Equipment

The pharmacy should ensure that equipment, apparatus, and devices used to compound an HSD are capable of consistently operating properly and within acceptable tolerance limits. Written procedures should be established and followed that include equipment calibration, annual maintenance, monitoring, and control. Routine maintenance checks should be documented. Personnel should be qualified through an appropriate combination of specific training and experience to operate or manipulate any item of equipment, apparatus, or device to which they will be assigned to use when preparing drug products for patients. Training should include the ability to determine whether any item of equipment is operating properly or is malfunctioning.

FINISHED PRODUCT RELEASE CHECKS AND TESTS

All HSDs should be subjected to appropriate checks or tests to ensure that only those HSDs free from defects and meeting all quality specifications will be distributed. An HSD should not be released until all quality specifications have been reviewed and it is determined that all release requirements are met.

Physical Inspection

All finished HSDs should be individually inspected in accordance with written procedures after compounding and, if not distributed promptly, prior to leaving the pharmacy. Immediately after compounding and as a condition of release, each product unit, where possible, should be inspected against lighted white and black backgrounds for evidence of visible particulates or other foreign matter. Pre-release inspection should also include container-closure integrity and any other apparent visual defect. Products with observed defects should be immediately discarded or marked and segregated from acceptable products in a manner that prevents their administration to patients. When products are not distributed promptly after preparation, a predistribution inspection should be conducted to ensure that an HSD with defects, such as precipitation, cloudiness, and leakage, which may develop between the time of release and the time of distribution, is not released.

Compounding Accuracy Checks

Written procedures for double checking compounding accuracy should be followed for every HSD prior to release. The double check system should meet state regulations and include label accuracy and accuracy of the addition of all drug products or ingredients used to prepare the finished product and their volumes or quantities. The used additive containers and, for those additives for which the entire container was not expended, the syringes used to measure the additive, should be quarantined with the final products until the final product check is completed. Syringe plungers should be drawn back to the volume mark used for each additive, if the additive volume was not checked prior to the addition. Automated pump settings should be verified just prior to or just after pumping and mixing. In addition, the volumes of each ingredient actually pumped should be checked to establish that the accuracy of the automated pump is within the limits set by the manufacturer. Written procedures for accountability of all drug product units used in the preparation of HSDs should be followed.

Additional finished product tests should be performed on *high-risk HSDs*, as follows.

Sterility Testing

Sterility testing should be performed on *Category II* high-risk HSDs promptly upon the completion of preparation. The sterility test, including the sampling scheme, should be conducted according to one of the USP methods (see *Sterility* ⟨71⟩). Membrane filtration is the method of choice where feasible. A method not described in the USP may be used if validation results demonstrate that the alternative is at least as effective and reliable as the USP membrane filtration method or the direct transfer method where the membrane filtration method is not feasible.

Normally, the HSD should not be released for patient use until test results show no evidence of microbial contamination of the product. However, when the HSD must be released on the same day of compounding prior to the completion of the sterility testing, the HSD can be conditionally released. In such a case the pharmacy should have a procedure requiring daily observation of the media and requiring an immediate recall if there is any evidence of microbial growth. In addition, the physicians of those patients to whom a potentially contaminated HSD was administered should be notified as to the potential risk to the patient. Positive sterility test results should prompt an investigation of aseptic technique, environmental control, and other sterility assurance controls to identify and correct problems as much as possible.

Pyrogen Testing

Each HSD prepared from nonsterile drug components or from an intermediate compounded for a nonsterile component should be tested for pyrogen or endotoxin according to the recommended methods (see *Bacterial Endotoxins Test* ⟨85⟩). The product should not be released until it has been determined that the endotoxin limit specified for the product is not exceeded.

Potency Testing

The pharmacy should have a procedure for a pre-release check of the potency of the active ingredients in HSDs prepared from nonsterile bulk active ingredients. The procedure should include at least the following verifications by a pharmacist:

(1) The lot of the active ingredient used for compounding has the necessary identity, potency, purity, and other relevant qualities. For example, this can be established for official drug substances by comparing the information stated on the lot's certificate of analysis with the requirements specified in the USP monograph for the substance.

(2) All weighings, volumetric measurements, and additions of ingredients were carried out properly. This can be established by reviewing compounding records to ensure that these steps were confirmed and initialed by a second person during compounding.

(3) The compounding or control records include documentation that the fill volumes of all units available for release were checked and were correct.

(4) The final yield is confirmed to be consistent with the theoretical yield.

In addition, instrumental analysis of potency should be performed to support expiration dating periods greater than 30 days assigned to HSDs prepared from nonsterile drug substances.

STORAGE AND EXPIRATION DATING

Each finished drug product unit should bear labeling that specifies the product's storage requirements and expiration date, and where appropriate, the time of day beyond which the product is not to be used. Unless otherwise indicated, HSDs should be refrigerated until time of use, with allowance for adequate time to equilibrate to room temperature before administering to the patient. HSDs intended for administration promptly after compounding may be retained at room temperature from the time of compounding.

Even under the best of conditions, there is always the likelihood that unsuspected microorganisms might inadvertently gain entry into the HSD during aseptic processing. Thus, as an adjunct sterility assurance measure, HSDs not intended for prompt use should be stored at a temperature no greater than 4°, that is, at a temperature expected to inhibit microbial growth. The multi-day HSDs (injections prepared for administration by a portable infusion pump or reservoir) should be started promptly after preparation, and administration should be completed within 7 days. Those HSDs, such as 5-fluorouracil, that cannot be refrigerated after preparation should be used within 28 hours of preparation as further assurance of sterility.

Pharmacists should also consider the effect of "cumulative" room temperature storage on the physical-chemical stability and characteristics of the HSD. For example, an HSD may be removed from the refrigerator and allowed to equilibrate to room temperature, only to be replaced into the refrigerator. This could happen any number of times before the product is ultimately used by the patient. Thus, the original expiration date assigned by the pharmacist could easily be invalidated under these circumstances. A procedure should be in place that details what is to be done when this situation occurs. Should this situation arise, the pharmacist needs to determine what the actual stability of the product will be, keeping in mind the cumulative effects of room temperature storage upon the product. The drug product's manufacturer or other credible stability reference source should be consulted, particularly for expensive biotechnology or chemotherapeutic drugs.

Additionally, some HSDs may be subjected to elevated temperature conditions, (e.g., body temperature) for continuous or novel drug delivery devices such as ambulatory infusion pumps, implantable infusion devices, and elastomeric infusion devices. Pharmacists should have adequate stability reference data to ensure that the product's potency characteristics are maintained when stored at these elevated temperatures during the labeled period of time chosen. HSDs may be frozen if adequate stability evidence to support freezing is available.

All light-sensitive products should be suitably protected from light from the time of preparation until the time of use or, where indicated, until the conclusion of administration.

Determining Expiration Dates

Where possible, the expiration date should be in accordance with allowances specified in the approved labeling. However, reliable, published stability information is sometimes lacking for many types of drugs. In these instances, pharmacists should consult with the drug's manufacturer to establish an expiration date. Because of compelling patient-care needs, a pharmacist may be unable to stay within the approved labeling and product guidelines stated in the package insert. For example, a higher concentration of drug may be prescribed; different diluent, container, etc., may be necessary; or the patient may require the HSD for longer periods of time. The pharmacist should communicate the deviations from the package insert to the manufacturer when requesting stability information. Otherwise, the pharmacist should ensure that the manufacturer's stability information is product specific, that is, the exact strength, diluent, fill volume, and container type (PVC bag, plastic syringe, elastomeric infusion device, etc.) will be used by the pharmacist when preparing the HSD. Pharmacists should obtain a letter from the manufacturer certifying the expiration dating period provided. Information provided by the manufacturer is usually for the HSD's chemical and physical stability only and would therefore not be relevant to sterility assurance imparted by the pharmacist each time the product is made. Therefore, it is the pharmacist's responsibility to ensure that compounding methods are validated to ensure final product sterility. Expiration dating not specifically referenced in the product's approved labeling should be limited to 30 days.

To ensure consistent practices in determining and assigning expiration dates, the pharmacy should have written policies and procedures governing the determination of the expiration dates for all of its compounded products. The following information may be helpful in providing a basis for these policies and procedures.

Product-specific, experimentally determined stability data based on sound stability evaluation protocols are preferable to published stability information for the prediction of expiration dates. Pharmacists should consult the general information chapter *Pharmaceutical Dosage Forms* ⟨1151⟩ for the appropriate stability parameters to be considered when initiating or evaluating a product-specific stability study. However, the use of professional judgment based on accumulated information may also be acceptable for determining expiration dates.

It should be recognized that the only truly valid evidence of stability for predicting expiration dating is from product-specific (appropriate bracketing is acceptable) experimental studies. Predictions based on other evidence, such as publications, charts, tables, etc., would result in theoretical expiration dates. Theoretically predicted expiration dating introduces varying degrees of assumptions and hence a likelihood of error, or at least inaccuracy. The degree of error or inaccuracy would be dependent upon the extent of differences between the HSD's characteristics (e.g., composition, concentration of ingredients, fill volume, container type and material, etc.) and the characteristics of the products from which stability data or information are to be extrapolated. Thus, the greater the doubt of the accuracy of theoretically predicted expiration dating, the greater the need to determine dating periods experimentally. Theoretically predicted expiration dating periods should be seriously considered for HSDs prepared from nonsterile bulk active ingredients having therapeutic activity, especially where these HSDs are expected to be compounded routinely. Semi-quantitative procedures, such as thin-layer chromatography (TLC), may be acceptable for many HSDs. However, quantitative stability-indicating assays, such as high-performance liquid chromatography (HPLC), would be more appropriate for certain critical HSDs. Examples include HSDs with a narrow therapeutic dosage range or a narrow therapeutic index where close monitoring or titering is required to ensure therapeutic effectiveness or to avoid toxicity; where a theoretically established expiration dating period is supported by only marginal evidence; or where a significant margin of safety cannot be verified for the proposed theoretical expiration dating period.

Additionally, conditions to which the finished product may be subjected during in-home use (e.g., in homes without air-conditioning in a hot climate) should be considered on a patient-by-patient basis. Thus, the possible need to shorten a general expiration date should be considered at the time of dispensing based on the particular circumstances of the patient.

In all instances where alternate informational resources are used to establish an expiration date for a drug product, the pharmacist should ensure that those resources have undergone critical evaluation in conjunction with the specific product for which an expiration date is established. Expiration dates predicted from alternate informational resources should be conservative and not extend beyond the realistic and practical patient care needs of the pharmacy. Pharmacists should subsequently maintain a record of the specific basis used to establish the expiration date for each compounded drug product. Pharmacists should utilize an exception log for products with expiration dates that fall outside of the pharmacy's established SOPs on stability and expiration dating. Alternatively, the exceptional reasons for changing the product's expiration date may also be documented in the patient's chart.

Monitoring Controlled Storage Areas

To ensure that product potency is retained through the expiration date, pharmacists must monitor the drug storage areas within the pharmacy. Controlled temperature storage areas in the pharmacy (refrigerators, 2° to 8°, freezers, −20° to −10°, and incubators, 30° to 35°, etc.) should be monitored at least once daily and the results documented on a temperature log. Additionally, pharmacy personnel should note the storage temperature when placing the product into or removing the product from the storage unit in order to monitor for any temperature aberrations. Suitable temperature recording devices may include a calibrated continuous recording device or an NBS calibrated thermometer that has adequate accuracy and sensitivity for the intended purpose and should be properly calibrated at suitable intervals. If the pharmacy uses a continuous temperature recording device, pharmacy personnel should verify at least once daily that the recording device itself is functioning properly.

The temperature sensing mechanism should be suitably placed in the controlled temperature storage space to reflect accurately its true temperature. In addition, the pharmacy should adhere to appropriate procedures of all controlled storage spaces to ensure that such spaces are not subject to significantly prolonged temperature fluctuations as may occur, for example, by leaving a refrigerator door open too long.

MAINTAINING PRODUCT QUALITY AND CONTROL AFTER IT LEAVES THE PHARMACY

Packing

The pharmacy is responsible for ensuring that the HSDs are suitably packed for transport. Packing should provide adequate control of the conditions under which HSDs are transported to the patient. Packing specifications, including configuration and materials, should be appropriate, as determined on a product-by-product basis, to maintain the storage conditions necessary to protect the product against adverse physical conditions such as temperatures beyond the range allowable for the HSD and, where indicated, exposure to light. Packing should retain adequate effectiveness for the duration of, and under the environmental conditions expected during, transit.

In-transit temperatures of HSDs should be maintained near the midpoint of the HSDs' specified upper and lower limits, recognizing that some temperature excursion, not to exceed the product's specified limits, is permissible during transit. Under no circumstances may excursions exceed the limits specified in the *General Notices* under *Storage Temperatures* for the defined temperature conditions.

The pharmacy should have and follow written procedures that specify packing techniques, configurations, and materials for groups of products with common storage characteristics and for specific products where unique storage conditions are required to retain adequate stability and product quality. It must be recognized that additional precautions should be used to protect the shipper, patient, and caregiver from adverse effects from any leakage of sensitizing or chemotoxic agents. Although written procedures should also ensure that biohazard controls are adequate for transit conditions and for meeting all OSHA and local requirements, this topic is beyond the scope of this chapter, and other references should be consulted.

The pharmacy should ensure that transit specifications and procedures are effective. For example, post-transit determinations of internal pack temperatures following several trial shipments of goods packed with new or modified materials, configurations, or techniques provide an indicator of packing suitability under actual transit conditions. Following the initial determination of packing suitability, occasional shipments should be subsequently checked, especially whenever transit conditions vary, such as from seasonal temperature changes or transit times. Because different packing configurations, pack size, internal packing matrices (e.g., insulated coolers or containers, styrofoam, bubble wrap, freezer packs, etc.) and pack thickness differ in their resistance to heat penetration or loss, packing should not vary from established procedures and specifications without evaluation.

Transit

Unlike the selection of the adherence to packing specifications, the pharmacy may lack complete control over transit time and conditions. However, the pharmacy can establish reasonable expectations of transit time and conditions and can carry out procedures to ensure that expectations are usually met. The determination of packing suitability is based on these expectations. Where possible, delivery personnel should be trained by the pharmacist on how to transport HSDs.

When common carriers are utilized, the pharmacy is responsible for choosing a reliable carrier capable of consistently fulfilling the pharmacy's requirements for delivery schedules, transit time duration, handling, care, external temperature controls, and special handling that may be required. The pharmacy should provide the carrier with a written statement of shipping requirements and should obtain from the carrier an assurance of capability and commitment for fulfilling these requirements before the pharmacy engages the carrier's services.

Delivery personnel, whether employees of the pharmacy, the parent organization, or the common carrier, should know the shipping requirements of each package consigned. Printed labels, prominently displayed on the exterior of each package, are usually sufficient. Supplementary printed instructions may be necessary in some instances.

The pharmacy should have an effective system for the routine evaluation of shipping performance. For example, the pharmacy might periodically review delivery receipts or conduct periodic shipment follow-ups by telephoning patients or caregivers. Delivery time, internal temperature (temperature indicators such as strips or probes inside packages provide objective evidence for determining the adequacy of temperature control), condition of goods upon receipt, and courteousness of personnel are some key determinants of acceptable shipping performance.

In The Home

The pharmacy's basic responsibilities for ensuring that HSDs in the home maintain their quality until administered include the following:

(1) The immediate labeling of the HSD container displays prominently and understandably the requirements for proper storage and expiration dating.

(2) Adequate information is obtained to assure the pharmacist that the storage conditions existing in the home are suitable for the HSD's specified storage requirements. (It is acceptable for the pharmacist to obtain this information through documentation by nursing or delivery personnel.)

(3) The patient has an acceptable temperature measurement device in the refrigerator and understands the importance of its use for maintaining proper storage temperature.

(4) A separate information sheet is issued and includes instructions for proper storage, interpretation of the expiration dating, and how to look for signs of unsuitability for use.

The patient or caregiver should be informed of the need to notify the pharmacy promptly of any actual or suspected malfunction of the refrigerator, freezer, or temperature measurement device. The pharmacy should assist patients or caregivers as necessary to ensure that proper storage conditions for HSDs are maintained with little or no interruption.

The pharmacy is responsible for ensuring that the home is visited at regular intervals to confirm compliance with appropriate drug storage conditions, cleanliness, separation of food and drug items, avoidance of improper re-use of multiple dose containers or supplies such as tubing or syringes, avoidance of the use of single-dose products as multiple-dose containers, and product inventory as indicative of product usage compliance. Inappropriately stored, exteriorly soiled, expired, or visibly defective drug products should be removed from the patient's possession, using the opportunity to instruct the patient or caregiver or to reinforce storage and handling responsibilities. Similarly, the home visit should also assess compliance with waste containment and disposal. The pharmacy may entrust the home visit to another health professional or paraprofessional.

PATIENT OR CAREGIVER TRAINING

A formal training program should be provided as a means to ensure understanding and compliance with the many special and complex responsibilities placed upon the patient or caregiver for the storage, handling, and administration of HSDs. The instructional objectives for the training program should include all home care responsibilities expected of the patient or caregiver and should be specified in terms of patient or caregiver competencies.

Upon the conclusion of the training program, the patient or caregiver should, correctly and consistently, be able to do the following:

(1) Describe the therapy involved, including the disease or condition for which the HSD is prescribed, goals of therapy, expected therapeutic outcome, and potential side effects of the HSD.
(2) Inspect all drug products, devices, equipment, and supplies on receipt to ensure that proper temperatures were maintained during transport and that goods received show no evidence of deterioration or defects.
(3) Handle, store, and monitor all drug products and related supplies and equipment in the home, including all special requirements related to same.
(4) Visually inspect all drug products, devices, and other items the patient or caregiver is required to use immediately prior to administration in a manner to ensure that all items are acceptable for use. For example, HSDs should be free from leakage, container cracks, particulates, precipitate, haziness, discoloration, or other deviations from the normal expected appearance, and the immediate packages of sterile devices should be completely sealed with no evidence of loss of package integrity.
(5) Check labels immediately prior to administration to ensure the right drug, dose, patient, and time of administration.
(6) Clean the in-home preparation area, scrub hands, use proper aseptic technique, and manipulate all containers, equipment, apparatus, devices, and supplies used in conjunction with administration.
(7) Employ all techniques and precautions associated with HSD administration, for example, preparing supplies and equipment, handling of devices, priming the tubing, and discontinuing an infusion.
(8) Care for catheters, change dressings, and maintain site patency as indicated.
(9) Monitor for and detect occurrences of therapeutic complications such as infection, phlebitis, electrolyte imbalance, and catheter misplacement.
(10) Respond immediately to emergency or critical situations such as catheter breakage or displacement, tubing disconnection, clot formation, flow blockage, and equipment malfunction.
(11) Know when to seek and how to obtain professional emergency services or professional advice.
(12) Handle, contain, and dispose of wastes, such as needles, syringes, devices, biohazardous spills or residuals, and infectious substances.

Training programs should include hands-on demonstration and practice with actual items that the patient or caregiver is expected to use, such as HSD containers, devices, and equipment. The patient or caregiver should practice aseptic and injection technique under the direct observation of a health professional.

The pharmacy is responsible for ensuring initially and on an ongoing basis that the patient or caregiver understands, has mastered, and is capable of and willing to comply with all of these home care responsibilities. This should be achieved through a formal, written assessment program. All specified competencies in the patient or caregiver's training program should be formally assessed. The patient or caregiver should be expected to demonstrate to appropriate health care personnel their mastery of their assigned activities before being allowed to administer HSDs unsupervised by a health professional.

Printed material such as checklists or instructions provided during training may serve as continuing post-training reinforcement of learning or as reminders of specific patient or caregiver responsibilities. Post-training verbal counseling should also be used periodically, as appropriate, to reinforce training and to ensure continuing correct and complete fulfillment of responsibilities.

PATIENT MONITORING AND COMPLAINT SYSTEM

The pharmacy must have written policies and procedures describing the monitoring of patients using HSDs and the handling of reports of adverse events.

Outcome Monitoring

The pharmacy is responsible for developing a patient monitoring plan, which includes written outcome measures and systems for routine patient assessment. The outcome monitoring system should provide information suitable for the evaluation of the quality of patient care and of pharmaceutical services. Examples of assessment parameters include infection rates, rehospitalization rates, incidence of adverse drug reactions, catheter complications, and other variables that may serve as meaningful indicators of the effectiveness and suitability of the home use of HSDs. In selecting suitable outcome measures, the focus should be on high-risk, high-volume, or problem-prone factors.

Reports

The pharmacy should have policies and procedures for the receipt, documentation, handling, and disposition of reports of patient problems, complaints, adverse drug reactions, drug product or device defects, and other adverse events reported by patients, caregivers, family members, pharmacists, or other health professionals. The pharmacy should have a procedure to ensure that the patient receives prompt and appropriate medical attention as necessary in response to all adverse incidents from HSDs or devices. When a complaint or problem prompts a suspicion that an HSD or a device may be defective, the pharmacy should also be able to identify and recall the potentially defective item to the patient level whenever appropriate.

Procedures should also include a mechanism for periodic review of reports received to determine any need for correction of underlying systems problems. All reports received should be maintained in a log, file, or binder dedicated for this purpose and readily retrievable as needed for subsequent analysis, legal or regulatory inquiry, or quality assurance audit. Standardized forms or formats for the reporting and recording of incidents, complaints, etc., should be used. Reports should be completed and signed by the individual receiving it or by the individual involved in the situation. Procedures should depict the classification, documentation, investigation, and resolution of all reports and should provide a mechanism for participation in various federal and state reporting programs such as USP or FDA programs for reporting reaction problems, or defects with drug products or medical devices.

THE QUALITY ASSURANCE PROGRAM

A provider of HSDs should have in place a formal Quality Assurance (QA) Program[9] intended to provide a mechanism for monitoring, evaluating, correcting, and improving the activities and processes described in this chapter. Emphasis in the QA Program should be placed on maintaining and improving the quality of systems and the provision of patient care. In addition, the QA program should ensure that any plan

[9] Other accepted terms that describe activities aimed at assessing and improving the quality of care rendered include Continuous Quality Improvement, Quality Assessment and Improvement, and Total Quality Management.

aimed at correcting identified problems also includes appropriate follow-up to make certain that effective corrective actions were performed.[10]

Characteristics of a QA plan include the following:

(1) Formalization in writing;
(2) Consideration of all aspects of the preparation and dispensing of products as described in this chapter, including environmental testing, validation results, etc.;
(3) Description of specific monitoring and evaluation activities;
(4) Specification of how results are to be reported and evaluated;
(5) Identification of appropriate follow-up mechanisms when action limits or thresholds are exceeded; and
(6) Delineation of the individuals responsible for each aspect of the QA program.

In developing a specific plan, focus should be on establishing objective, measurable indicators for monitoring activities and processes that are deemed high-risk, high-volume, or problem-prone. Appropriate evaluation of environmental monitoring might include, for example, the trending of an indicator such as settling plate counts. In general, the selection of indicators and the effectiveness of the overall QA plan should be reassessed on an annual basis.

⟨1211⟩ STERILIZATION AND STERILITY ASSURANCE OF COMPENDIAL ARTICLES

This informational chapter provides a general description of the concepts and principles involved in the quality control of articles that must be sterile. Any modifications or variations in sterility test procedures from those described under *Sterility Tests* ⟨71⟩ should be validated in the context of the entire sterility assurance program and are not intended to be alternative methods to those described in that chapter.

Within the strictest definition of sterility, a specimen would be deemed sterile only when there is complete absence of viable microorganisms from it. However, this absolute definition cannot currently be applied to an entire lot of finished compendial articles because of limitations in testing. Absolute sterility cannot be practically demonstrated without complete destruction of every finished article. The sterility of a lot purported to be sterile is therefore defined in probabalistic terms, where the likelihood of a contaminated unit or article is acceptably remote. Such a state of sterility assurance can be established only through the use of adequate sterilization cycles and subsequent aseptic processing, if any, under appropriate current good manufacturing practice, and not by reliance solely on sterility testing. The basic principles for validation and certification of a sterilizing process are enumerated as follows.

(1) Establish that the process equipment has capability of operating within the required parameters.

(2) Demonstrate that the critical control equipment and instrumentation are capable of operating within the prescribed parameters for the process equipment.

(3) Perform replicate cycles representing the required operational range of the equipment and employing actual or simulated product. Demonstrate that the processes have been carried out within the prescribed protocol limits and finally that the probability of microbial survival in the replicate processes completed is not greater than the prescribed limits.

(4) Monitor the validated process during routine operation. Periodically as needed, requalify and recertify the equipment.

(5) Complete the protocols, and document steps (1) through (4) above.

The principles and implementation of a program to validate an aseptic processing procedure are similar to the validation of a sterilization process. In aseptic processing, the components of the final dosage form are sterilized separately and the finished article is assembled in an aseptic manner.

Proper validation of the sterilization process or the aseptic process requires a high level of knowledge of the field of sterilization and clean room technology. In order to comply with currently acceptable and achievable limits in sterilization parameters, it is necessary to employ appropriate instrumentation and equipment to control the critical parameters such as temperature and time, humidity, and sterilizing gas concentration, or absorbed radiation. An important aspect of the validation program in many sterilization procedures involves the employment of biological indicators (see *Biological Indicators* ⟨1035⟩). The validated and certified process should be revalidated periodically; however, the revalidation program need not necessarily be as extensive as the original program.

A typical validation program, as outlined below, is one designed for the steam autoclave, but the principles are applicable to the other sterilization procedures discussed in this informational chapter. The program comprises several stages.

The *installation qualification* stage is intended to establish that controls and other instrumentation are properly designed and calibrated. Documentation should be on file demonstrating the quality of the required utilities such as steam, water, and air. The *operational qualification* stage is intended to confirm that the empty chamber functions within the parameters of temperature at all of the key chamber locations prescribed in the protocol. It is usually appropriate to develop heat profile records, i.e., simultaneous temperatures in the chamber employing multiple temperature-sensing devices. A typical acceptable range of temperature in the empty chamber is $\pm 1°$ when the chamber temperature is not less than 121°. The *confirmatory* stage of the validation program is the actual sterilization of materials or articles. This determination requires the employment of temperature-sensing devices inserted into samples of the articles as well as *either*, samples of the articles to which appropriate concentrations of suitable test microorganisms have been added *or*, separate biological indicators in operationally fully loaded autoclave configurations. The effectiveness of heat delivery or penetration into the actual articles and the time of the exposure are the two main factors that determine the lethality of the sterilization process. The *final* stage of the validation program requires the documentation of the supporting data developed in executing the program.

It is generally accepted that terminally sterilized injectable articles or critical devices purporting to be sterile, when processed in the autoclave, attain a 10^{-6} microbial survivor probability, i.e., assurance of less than one chance in one million that viable microorganisms are present in the sterilized article or dosage form. With heat-stable articles, the approach often is to considerably exceed the critical time necessary to achieve the 10^{-6} microbial survivor probability (overkill). However, with an article where extensive heat exposure may have a damaging effect, it may not be feasible to employ this overkill approach. In this latter instance, the development of the sterilization cycle depends heavily on knowledge of the microbial burden of the product based on examination, over a suitable time period, of a substantial number of lots of the presterilized product.

The D value is the time (in minutes) required to reduce the microbial population by 90% or 1 log cycle (i.e., to a surviving fraction of 1/10), at a specific temperature. Therefore, where the D value of a biological indicator preparation of, for example, *Bacillus stearothermophilus* spores is 1.5 minutes under the total process parameters, e.g. at 121°, if it is treated for 12 minutes under the same conditions, it can be stated that the lethality input is 8D. The effect of applying this input to the product would depend on the initial microbial burden. Assuming that its resistance to sterilization is equivalent to that of the biological indicator, if the microbial burden of the product in question is 10^2 microorganisms, a lethality input of 2D yields a microbial burden of 1 (10^0 theoretical) and a further 6D yields a calculated microbial survivor probability of 10^{-6}. (Under the same conditions, a lethality input of 12D may be used in a typical "overkill" approach.) Generally the survivor probability achieved for the article under the validated sterilization cycle is not completely correlated with what may occur with the biological indicator. For valid use, therefore, it is essential that the resistance of the biological indicator be greater than that of the natural microbial burden of the article sterilized. It is then appropriate to make a worst-case assumption and treat the microbial burden as though its heat resistance were equivalent to that of the biological indicator, although it is not likely that the most resistant of a typical microbial burden isolates will demonstrate a heat resistance of the magnitude shown by this species, frequently employed as a biological indicator for steam sterilization. In the above example, a 12-minute cycle is considered adequate for sterilization if the product had a microbial burden of 10^2 microorganisms. However, if the indicator originally had 10^6 microorganisms content, actually a 10^{-2} probability of survival could be expected; i.e., 1 in 100 biological indicators may yield positive results. This type of situation may be avoided by selection of the appropriate biological indicator. Alternatively, high content indicators may be used on the basis of a predetermined acceptable count reduction.

The D value for the *Bacillus stearothermophilus* preparation determined or verified for these conditions should be re-established when a specific program of validation is changed. Determination of survival

[10] The use of additional resources, such as the Accreditation Manual for Home Care from the Joint Commission on Accreditation of Healthcare Organizations, may prove helpful in the development of a QA plan.

curves (see under *Biological Indicators* ⟨1035⟩) or what has been called the fractional cycle approach may be employed to determine the D value of the biological indicator preferred for the specific sterilization procedure. The fractional cycle approach may also be used to evaluate the resistance of the microbial burden. Fractional cycles are studied either for microbial count-reduction or for fraction negative achievement. These numbers may be used to determine the lethality of the process under production conditions. The data can be used in qualified production equipment to establish appropriate sterilization cycles. A suitable biological indicator such as the *Bacillus stearothermophilus* preparation may be employed also during routine sterilization. Any microbial burden method for sterility assurance requires adequate surveillance of the microbial resistance of the article to detect any changes, in addition to periodic surveillance of other attributes.

Methods of Sterilization

In this informational chapter five methods of terminal sterilization, including removal of microorganisms by filtration, and guidelines for aseptic processing are described. Modern technological developments, however, have led to the use of additional procedures. These include blow-molding (at high temperatures), forms of moist heat other than saturated steam and ultraviolet irradiation, as well as on-line continuous filling in aseptic processing. The choice of the appropriate process for a given dosage form or component requires a high level of knowledge of sterilization techniques and information concerning any effects of the process on the material being sterilized.[1]

STEAM STERILIZATION

The process of thermal sterilization employing saturated steam under pressure is carried out in a chamber called an autoclave. It is probably the most widely employed sterilization process.[2] The basic principle of operation is that the air in the sterilizing chamber is displaced by the saturated steam, achieved by employing vents or traps. In order to displace air more effectively from the chamber and from within articles, the sterilization cycle may include air and steam evacuation stages. The design or choice of a cycle for given products or components depends on a number of factors, including the heat lability of the material, knowledge of heat penetration into the articles, and other factors described under the validation program (see above). Apart from that description of sterilization cycle parameters, using a temperature of 121°, the F_0 concept may be appropriate. The F_0, at a particular temperature other than 121°, is the time (in minutes) required to provide the lethality equivalent to that provided at 121° for a stated time. Modern autoclaves generally operate with a control system that is significantly more responsive than the steam reduction valve of older units that have been in service for many years. In order for these older units to achieve the precision and level of control of the cycle discussed in this chapter, it may be necessary to upgrade or modify the control equipment and instrumentation on these units. This modification is warranted only if the chamber and steam jacket are intact for continued safe use and if deposits that interfere with heat distribution can be removed.

DRY-HEAT STERILIZATION

The process of thermal sterilization of Pharmacopeial articles by dry heat is usually carried out by a batch process in an oven designed expressly for that purpose. A modern oven is supplied with heated, filtered air, distributed uniformly throughout the chamber by convection or radiation and employing a blower system with devices for sensing, monitoring, and controlling the critical parameters. The validation of a dry-heat sterilization facility is carried out in a manner similar to that for a steam sterilizer described earlier. Where the unit is employed for sterilizing components such as containers intended for intravenous solutions, care should be taken to avoid accumulation of particulate matter in the chamber. A typical acceptable range in temperature in the empty chamber is ±15° when the unit is operating at not less than 250°.

In addition to the batch process described above, a continuous process is frequently employed to sterilize and depyrogenate glassware as part of an integrated continuous aseptic filling and sealing system. Heat distribution may be by convection or by direct transfer of heat from an open flame. The continuous system usually requires a much higher temperature than cited above for the batch process because of a much shorter dwell time. However, the total temperature input during the passage of the product should be equivalent to that achieved during the chamber process. The continuous process also usually necessitates a rapid cooling stage prior to the aseptic filling operation. In the qualification and validation program, in view of the short dwell time, parameters for uniformity of the temperature, and particularly the dwell time, should be established.

A microbial survival probability of 10^{-12} is considered achievable for heat-stable articles or components. An example of a biological indicator for validating and monitoring dry-heat sterilization is a preparation of *Bacillus subtilis* spores. Since dry heat is frequently employed to render glassware or containers free from pyrogens as well as viable microbes, a pyrogen challenge, where necessary, should be an integral part of the validation program, e.g., by inoculating one or more of the articles to be treated with 1000 or more USP Units of bacterial endotoxin. The test with *Limulus* lysate could be used to demonstrate that the endotoxic substance has been inactivated to not more than 1/1000 of the original amount (3 log cycle reduction). For the test to be valid, both the original amount and, after acceptable inactivation, the remaining amount of endotoxin should be measured. For additional information on the endotoxin assay, see *Bacterial Endotoxins Test* ⟨85⟩.

GAS STERILIZATION

The choice of gas sterilization as an alternative to heat is frequently made when the material to be sterilized cannot withstand the high temperatures obtained in the steam sterilization or dry-heat sterilization processes. The active agent generally employed in gaseous sterilization is ethylene oxide of acceptable sterilizing quality. Among the disadvantages of this sterilizing agent are its highly flammable nature unless mixed with suitable inert gases, its mutagenic properties, and the possibility of toxic residues in treated materials, particularly those containing chloride ions. The sterilization process is generally carried out in a pressurized chamber designed similarly to a steam autoclave but with the additional features (see below) unique to sterilizers employing this gas. Facilities employing this sterilizing agent should be designed to provide adequate post-sterilization degassing, to enable microbial survivor monitoring, and to minimize exposure of operators to the potentially harmful gas.[3]

Qualification of a sterilizing process employing ethylene oxide gas is accomplished along the lines discussed earlier. However, the program is more comprehensive than for the other sterilization procedures, since in addition to temperature, the humidity, vacuum/positive pressure,

---

[1] A number of guidelines dealing particularly with the development and validation of sterilization cycles and related topics have been published. These include, of the Parenteral Drug Association, Inc. (PDA) *Validation of Steam Sterilization Cycles* (Technical Monograph No. 1), *Validation of Aseptic Filling For Solution Drug Products* (Technical Monograph No. 2) and *Validation of Dry Heat Processes Used for Sterilization and Depyrogenation* (Technical Monograph No. 3), and of the Pharmaceutical Manufacturers Association (PMA) *Validation of Sterilization of Large-Volume Parenterals—Current Concepts* (Science and Technology Publication No. 25). Other series of technical publications on these subjects of the Health Industry Manufacturers Association (HIMA) include *Validation of Sterilization Systems* (Report No. 78-4.1), *Sterilization Cycle Development* (Report No. 78-4.2), *Industrial Sterility: Medical Device Standards and Guidelines* (Document #9, Vol. 1) and *Operator Training* . . . . for *Ethylene Oxide Sterilization*, for *Steam Sterilization Equipment*, for *Dry Heat Sterilization Equipment* and for *Radiation Sterilization Equipment* Report Nos. 78-4.5 through 4.8). Recommended practice guidelines published by the Association for the Advancement of Medical Instrumentation (AAMI) include *Guideline for Industrial Ethylene Oxide Sterilization of Medical Devices—Process Design, Validation, Routine Sterilization* (No. OPEO-12/81) and *Process Control Guidelines for the Radiation Sterilization of Medical Devices* (No. RS-P 10/82). These detailed publications should be consulted for more extensive treatment of the principles and procedures described in this chapter.

[2] An autoclave cycle, where specified in the compendia for media or reagents, is a period of 15 minutes at 121°, unless otherwise indicated.

[3] See *Ethylene Oxide*, Encyclopedia of Industrial Chemical Analysis, 1971, *12*, 317–340, John Wiley & Sons, Inc., and *Use of Ethylene Oxide as a Sterilant in Medical Facilities*, NIOSH Special Occupational Hazard Review with Control Recommendations, August 1977, U. S. Department of Health and Human Services, Public Health Service, Center for Disease Control, National Institute for Occupational Safety and Health, Division of Criteria Documentation and Standards Development, Priorities and Research Analysis Branch, Rockville, MD.

and ethylene oxide concentration also require rigid control. An important determination is to demonstrate that all critical process parameters in the chamber are adequate during the entire cycle. Since the sterilization parameters applied to the articles to be sterilized are critical variables, it is frequently advisable to precondition the load to achieve the required moisture content, to minimize the time of holding at the required temperature, prior to placement of the load in the ethylene oxide chamber. The validation process is generally made employing product inoculated with appropriate biological indicators such as spore preparations of *Bacillus subtilis*. For validation they may be used in full chamber loads of product, or simulated product. The monitoring of moisture and gas concentration requires the utilization of sophisticated instrumentation that only knowledgeable and experienced individuals can calibrate, operate, and maintain. The biological indicators may be employed also in monitoring routine runs.

As is indicated elsewhere in this chapter, the biological indicator may be employed in a fraction negative mode to establish the ultimate microbiological survivor probability in designing an ethylene oxide sterilization cycle using inoculated product or inoculated simulated product.

One of the principal limitations of the ethylene oxide sterilization process is the limited ability of the gas to diffuse to the innermost product areas that require sterilization. Package design and chamber loading patterns therefore must be determined so that there is minimal resistance to gas diffusion.

STERILIZATION BY IONIZING RADIATION

The rapid proliferation of medical devices unable to withstand heat sterilization and the concerns about the safety of ethylene oxide have resulted in increasing applications of radiation sterilization. It is, however, applicable also to drug substances and final dosage forms. The advantages of sterilization by irradiation include low chemical reactivity, low measurable residues, and the fact that there are fewer variables to control. In fact, radiation sterilization is unique in that the basis of control is essentially that of the absorbed radiation dose, which can be precisely measured. Because of this characteristic, new procedures have been developed to determine the sterilizing dose. These, however, are still under review and appraisal, particularly with regard to the need, or otherwise, for additional controls and safety measures. Irradiation causes only a minimal temperature rise, but can affect certain grades and types of plastics and glass.

The two types of ionizing radiation in use are radioisotope decay (gamma radiation) and electron-beam radiation. In either case the radiation dose to yield the required degree of sterility assurance should be established such that within the range of minimum and maximum doses set, the properties of the article being sterilized are acceptable.

For gamma irradiation, the validation of a procedure includes the establishment of article materials compatibility, establishment of product loading pattern and completion of dose mapping in the sterilization container (including identification of the minimum and maximum dose zones), establishment of timer setting, and demonstration of the delivery of the required sterilization dose. For electron-beam irradiation, in addition the on-line control of voltage, current, conveyor speed, and electron beam scan dimension must be validated.

For gamma radiation sterilization, an effective sterilizing dose which is tolerated without damaging effect should be selected. Although 2.5 megarads (Mrad) of absorbed radiation was historically selected, it is desirable and acceptable in some cases to employ lower doses for devices, drug substances, and finished dosage forms. In other cases, however, higher doses are essential. In order to validate the efficacy particularly of the lower exposure levels, it is necessary to determine the magnitude (number and/or degree) of the natural radiation resistance of the microbial population of the product. Specific product loading patterns must be established and absorbed minimum and maximum dosage distribution must be determined by use of chemical dosimeters. (These dosimeters are usually dyed plastic cylinders, slides, or squares that show color intensification based directly on the amount of absorbed radiation energy; they require careful calibration.)

The setting of the preferred absorbed dose has been carried out on the basis of pure cultures of resistant microorganisms and employing inoculated product, e.g., with spores of *Bacillus pumilus* as biological indicators. A fractional experimental cycle approach provides the data to be utilized to determine the D_{10} value of the biological indicator. This information is then applied in extrapolating the amount of absorbed radiation to establish an appropriate microbial survivor probability. The most recent procedures for gamma radiation sterilization, base the dose upon the radiation resistance of the natural heterogeneous microbial burden contained on the product to be sterilized. Such procedures are currently being refined but may provide a more representative assessment of radiation resistance, especially where significant numbers of radiation-resistant organisms are present.[4] These range from inoculation with standard resistant organisms such as *Bacillus pumilus* to subprocess (sublethal) dose exposure of finished product samples taken from production lines. Certain hypotheses are common to all of these methods. While the total microbial population present on an article generally consists of a mixture of microorganisms of differing sensitivity to radiation, the step of subjecting the article to a less than totally lethal sterilization dose eliminates the less resistant microbial fraction. This results in a residual relatively homogeneous population with respect to radiation resistance, and yields consistent and reproducible results of determinations with the residual population. The amount of laboratory manipulation required is dependent upon the particular procedure used.

One such procedure requires the enumeration of the microbial population on representative samples of independently manufactured lots of the article. The resistance of the microbial population is not determined and dose setting is based on a standard arbitrary radiation resistance assigned to the microbial population, derived from data obtained from manufacturers and from the literature. The assumption is made that the distribution of resistances chosen represents a more severe challenge than the natural microbial population on the product to be sterilized. This assumption, however, is verified by experiment. After verification the appropriate radiation sterilization dose is read from a table.

Another, more elaborate, method does not require the enumeration of the microbial population but uses a series of incremental dose exposures to allow a dose to be established such that approximately one out of 100 samples irradiated at that dose will be nonsterile. This is not the ultimate sterilization dose, but provides the basis to determine the sterilization dose by extrapolation from the dose yielding one out of 100 nonsterile samples, using an appropriate resistance factor which characterizes the remaining microorganism-resistant population. A periodic audit is conducted to check that the findings continue to be operative.

More elaborate procedures, requiring more experimentation and including the isolation of microbial cultures, include one where, after determining the substerilization dose (yielding one out of 100 nonsterile samples), the resistance of the surviving microorganisms is used to determine the sterilizing dose. Another is based on different determinations, starting with a substerilization incremental dose which results in not more than 50% of the samples being nonsterile. After irradiation of sufficient samples at this dose, a number of microbial isolates are obtained. The radiation resistance of each of these is determined. The sterilization dose is then calculated using the resistance determinations and the 50% sterilizing dose initially determined. Audit procedures are required for these methods as for the others described.

Where the required minimum radiation dose has been determined and delivery of that dose has been confirmed (by chemical or physical dosimeters), release of the article being sterilized could be effected within the overall validation of sterility assurance (which may include such confirmation of applied dosage, the use of biological indicators, and other means).

STERILIZATION BY FILTRATION

Filtration through microbial retentive materials is frequently employed for the sterilization of heat-labile solutions by physical removal of the contained microorganisms. A filter assembly generally consists of a porous matrix sealed or clamped into an impermeable housing. The effectiveness of a filter medium or substrate depends upon the pore size of the porous material and may depend upon adsorption of bacteria on or in the filter matrix or upon a sieving mechanism. There is some evidence to indicate that sieving is the more important component of the mechanism. Fiber-shedding filters, particularly those containing asbestos, are to be avoided unless no alternative filtration procedures are possible. Where a fiber-shedding filter is required, it is obligatory that the process include a nonfiber-shedding filter introduced downstream or subsequent to the initial filtration step.

Filter Rating—Rating the pore size of filter membranes is by a nominal rating that reflects the capability of the filter membrane to retain

[4] Detailed descriptions of these procedures have been published by the Association for the Advancement of Medical Instrumentation (AAMI) in the document entitled "*Process Control Guidelines for Radiation Sterilization of Medical Devices*" (No. AAMI RS-P 10/82).

microorganisms of size represented by specified strains, not by determination of an average pore size and statement of distribution of sizes. Sterilizing filter membranes (those which are used for removing a majority of contaminating microorganisms) are membranes capable of retaining 100% of a culture of 10^7 microorganisms of a strain of *Pseudomonas diminuta* (ATCC 19146) per square centimeter of membrane surface under a pressure of not less than 30 psi (2.0 bar). Such filter membranes are nominally rated 0.22 μm or 0.2 μm, depending on the manufacturer's practice.[5] This rating of filter membranes is also specified for reagents or media that have to be sterilized by filtration (see treatment of Isopropyl Myristate under *Ointments and Oils Soluble in Isopropyl Myristate* in the chapter *Sterility Tests* ⟨71⟩). Bacterial filter membranes (also known as analytical filter membranes), which are capable of retaining only larger microorganisms, are labeled with a nominal rating of 0.45 μm. No single authoritative method for rating 0.45-μm filters has been specified, and this rating depends on conventional practice among manufacturers; 0.45-μm filters are capable of retaining particular cultures of *Serratia marcescens* (ATCC 14756) or *Ps. diminuta*. Test pressures used vary from low (5 psi, 0.33 bar for *Serratia*, or 0.5 psi, 0.34 bar for *Ps. diminuta*) to high (50 psi, 3.4 bar). They are specified for sterility testing (see *Test Procedures Using Membrane Filtration* under the chapter *Sterility Tests* ⟨71⟩), where less exhaustive microbial retention is required. There is a small probability of testing specimens contaminated solely with small microorganisms). Filter membranes with a very low nominal rating may be tested with a culture of *Acholeplasma laidlawii* or other strain of *Mycoplasma*, at a pressure of 7 psi (0.7 bar) and be nominally rated 0.1 μm. The nominal ratings based on microbial retention properties differ when rating is done by other means, e.g., by retention of latex spheres of various diameters. It is the user's responsibility to select a filter of correct rating for the particular purpose, depending on the nature of the product to be filtered. It is generally not feasible to repeat the tests of filtration capacity in the user's establishment. Microbial challenge tests are preferably performed under a manufacturer's conditions on each lot of manufactured filter membranes.

The user must determine whether filtration parameters employed in manufacturing will significantly influence microbial retention efficiency. Some of the other important concerns in the validation of the filtration process include product compatibility, sorption of drug, preservative and/or other additives, and initial effluent endotoxin content.

Since the effectiveness of the filtration process is also influenced by the microbial burden of the solution to be filtered, the determination of the microbiological quality of solutions prior to filtration is an important aspect of the validation of the filtration process in addition to establishment of the other parameters of the filtration procedure, such as pressures, flow rates, and filter unit characteristics. Hence another method of describing filter-retaining capability is by the log reduction value (LRV). For instance, a 0.2-μm filter that can retain 10^7 microorganisms of a specified strain will have an LRV of not less than 7, under the stated conditions.

The process of sterilization of solutions by filtration has recently achieved new levels of proficiency, largely as a result of the development and proliferation of membrane filter technology. This class of filter media lends itself to more effective standardization and quality control and also gives the user greater opportunity to confirm the characteristics or properties of the filter assembly before and after use. The fact that membrane filters are thin polymeric films offers many advantages but also some disadvantages when compared to depth filters such as porcelain or sintered material. Since much of the membrane surface is a void or open space, the properly assembled and sterilized filter offers the advantage of a high flow rate. A disadvantage is that since the membrane is usually fragile, it is essential to determine that the assembly was properly made and that the membrane was not ruptured during assembly, sterilization, or use. The housings and filter assemblies that are chosen to be used should first be validated for compatibility and integrity by the user. While it may be possible to mix assemblies and filter membranes produced by different manufacturers, the compatibility of these hybrid assemblies should first be validated. Additionally, there are other tests to be made by the manufacturer of the membrane filter, which are not usually repeated by the user. These include microbiological challenge tests. Results of these tests on each lot of manufactured filter membranes should be obtained from the manufacturer by the user for his records.

[5] Consult "Microbiological Evaluation of Filters for Sterilizing Liquids," Health Industry Manufacturers Association, Document No. 3, Vol. 4, 1982.

Filtration for sterilization purposes is usually carried out with assemblies having membranes of nominal pore size rating of 0.2 μm or less, based on the validated challenge of not less than 10^7 *Pseudomonas diminuta* (ATCC No. 19146) suspension per square centimeter of filter surface area. Membrane filter media which are now available include cellulose acetate, cellulose nitrate, fluorocarbonate, acrylic polymers, polycarbonate, polyester, polyvinyl chloride, vinyl, nylon, polytef, and even metal membranes, and they may be reinforced or supported by an internal fabric. A membrane filter assembly should be tested for initial integrity prior to use, provided that such test does not impair the validity of the system, and should be tested after the filtration process is completed to demonstrate that the filter assembly maintained its integrity throughout the entire filtration procedure. Typical use tests are the bubble point test, the diffusive airflow test, the pressure hold test, and the forward flow test. These tests should be correlated with microorganism retention.

ASEPTIC PROCESSING

While there is general agreement that sterilization of the final filled container as a dosage form or final packaged device is the preferred process for assuring the minimal risk of microbial contamination in a lot, there is a substantial class of products that are not terminally sterilized but are prepared by a series of aseptic steps. These are designed to prevent the introduction of viable microorganisms into components, where sterile, or once an intermediate process has rendered the bulk product or its components free from viable microorganisms. This section provides a review of the principles involved in producing aseptically processed products with a minimal risk of microbial contamination in the finished lot of final dosage forms.

A product defined as aseptically processed is likely to consist of components that have been sterilized by one of the processes described earlier in this chapter. For example, the bulk product, if a filterable liquid, may have been sterilized by filtration. The final empty container components would probably be sterilized by heat, dry heat being employed for glass vials and an autoclave being employed for rubber closures. The areas of critical concern are the immediate microbial environment where these presterilized components are exposed during assembly to produce the finished dosage form and the aseptic filling operation.

The requirements for a properly designed, validated and maintained filling or other aseptic processing facility are mainly directed to (i) an air environment free from viable microorganisms, of a proper design to permit effective maintenance of air supply units and (ii) the provision of trained operating personnel who are adequately equipped and gowned. The desired environment may be achieved through the high level of air filtration technology now available, which contributes to the delivery of air of the requisite microbiological quality.[6] The facilities include both primary (in the vicinity of the exposed article) and secondary (where the aseptic processing is carried out) barrier systems.

For a properly designed aseptic processing facility or aseptic filling area, consideration should be given to such features as non-porous and smooth surfaces, including walls and ceilings that can be sanitized frequently; gowning rooms with adequate space for personnel and storage of sterile garments; adequate separation of preparatory rooms for personnel from final aseptic processing rooms, with the availability where necessary of such devices as airlocks and/or air showers; proper pressure differentials between rooms, the most positive pressure being in the aseptic processing rooms or areas; the employment of laminar (unidirectional) air-flow in the immediate vicinity of exposed product or components, and filtered air exposure thereto, with adequate air change frequency; appropriate humidity and temperature environmental controls; and a documented sanitization program. Proper training of personnel in hygienic and gowning techniques should be undertaken so that, for example, gowns, gloves, and other body coverings substantially cover exposed skin surfaces.

Certification and validation of the aseptic process and facility are achieved by establishing the efficiency of the filtration systems, by employing microbiological environmental monitoring procedures, and by processing of sterile culture medium as simulated product.

[6] Available published standards for such controlled work areas include the following: (1) Federal Standard No. 209B, Clean Room and Work Station Requirements for a Controlled Environment, Apr. 24, 1973. (2) NASA Standard for Clean Room and Work Stations for Microbially Controlled Environment, publication NHB5340.2, Aug. 1967. (3) Contamination Control of Aerospace Facilities, U. S. Air Force, T.O. 00-25-203 1 Dec. 1972, change 1–1 Oct. 1974.

Monitoring of the aseptic facility should include periodic environmental filter examination as well as routine particulate and microbiological environmental monitoring, and may include periodic sterile culture medium processing.

Sterility Testing of Lots

It should be recognized that the referee sterility test might not detect microbial contamination if present in only a small percentage of the finished articles in the lot because the specified number of units to be taken imposes a significant statistical limitation on the utility of the test results. This inherent limitation, however, has to be accepted since current knowledge offers no nondestructive alternatives for ascertaining the microbiological quality of every finished article in the lot, and it is not a feasible option to increase the number of specimens significantly.

The primary means of supporting the claim that a lot of finished articles purporting to be sterile meets the specifications consist of the documentation of the actual production and sterilization record of the lot and of the additional validation records that the sterilization process possesses the capability of totally inactivating the established product microbial burden or a more resistant challenge. Further, it should be demonstrated that any processing steps involving exposed product following the sterilization procedure are performed in an aseptic manner, to prevent contamination. If data derived from the manufacturing process sterility assurance validation studies and from in-process controls are judged to provide greater assurance that the lot meets the required low probability of containing a contaminated unit (compared to sterility testing results from finished units drawn from that lot), any sterility test procedures adopted may be minimal, or dispensed with on a routine basis. However, assuming that all of the above production criteria have been met, it may still be desirable to perform sterility testing on samples of the lot of finished articles. Such sterility testing is usually carried out directly after the lot is manufactured as a final product quality control test.[7] Sterility tests employed in this way in manufacturing control should not be confused with those described under *Sterility Tests* ⟨71⟩. The procedural details may be the same with regard to media, inocula and handling of specimens, but the number of units and/or incubation time(s) selected for testing may differ. The number should be chosen relative to the purpose to be served, i.e., according to whether greater or lesser reliance is placed on sterility testing in the context of all the measures for sterility assurance in manufacture. Also, longer times of incubation would make the test more sensitive to slow-growing microorganisms. In the growth promotion tests for media, such slow growers, particularly if isolated from the product microbial burden, should be included with the other test stains. Negative or satisfactory sterility test results serve only as further support of the existing evidence concerning the quality of the lot if all of the pertinent production records of the lot are in order and the sterilizing or aseptic process is known to be effective. Unsatisfactory test results, however, in manufacturing quality control indicate a need for further action (see under *Performance, Observation, and Interpretation*).

DEFINITION OF A LOT AND SELECTION OF SPECIMENS FOR STERILITY TEST PURPOSES

Articles may be terminally sterilized either in a chamber or by a continuous process. In the chamber process, a number of articles are sterilized simultaneously under controlled conditions, for example, in a steam autoclave, so that for the purpose of sterility testing, the lot is considered to be the contents of a single chamber. In the continuous process, the articles are sterilized individually and consecutively, for example, by exposure to electron-beam radiation, so that the lot is considered to be not larger than the total number of similar items subjected to uniform sterilization for a period of not more than 24 hours.

For aseptic fills, the term "filling operation" describes a group of final containers, identical in all respects, that have been aseptically filled with the same product from the same bulk within a period of time not longer than 24 consecutive hours without an interruption or change that would affect the integrity of the filling assembly. The items tested should be representative of each filling assembly and should be selected at appropriate intervals throughout the entire filling operation. If more than three filling machines, each with either single or multiple filling stations, are used for filling a single lot, a minimum of 20 filled containers (not less than 10 per medium) should be tested for each filling machine, but the total number generally need not exceed 100 containers.

For small lots, in the case of either aseptic filling or terminal sterilization, if the number of final containers in the lot is between 20 and 200, about 10% of the containers should usually be tested. If the number of final containers in the lot is 20 or less, not fewer than 2 final containers should be tested.

Performance, Observation, and Interpretation

The facility for sterility testing should be such as to offer no greater a microbial challenge to the articles being tested than that of an aseptic processing production facility. The sterility testing procedure should be performed by individuals having a high level of aseptic technique proficiency. The test performance records of these individuals should be documented.

The extensive aseptic manipulations required to perform sterility testing may result in a probability of nonproduct-related contamination of the order of 10^{-3}, a level similar to the overall efficiency of an aseptic operation and comparable to the microbial survivor probability of aseptically processed articles. This level of probability is significantly greater than that usually attributed to a terminal sterilization process, namely one in one million or 10^{-6} microbial survivor probability. Appropriate, known-to-be-sterile, finished articles should be employed periodically as negative controls as a check on the reliability of the test procedure. Preferably the technicians performing the test should be unaware that they are testing negative controls. Of these tests a false positive frequency not exceeding 2% is desirable.

For aseptically processed articles, these facts support the routine use of the test set forth under *Sterility Tests* ⟨71⟩ or a more elaborate one. The production and validation documentation should be acceptable and complete. For effectively terminally sterilized products, however, the lower microbial survivor probability may direct the use of a less extensive test than the compendial procedure specified under *Sterility Tests* ⟨71⟩, or even preclude the necessity altogether for performing one. This added reliability of sterility assurance of terminal sterilization depends upon a properly validated and documented sterilization process. Sterility testing alone is no substitute.

Interpretation of Quality Control Tests—The overall responsibility for the operation of the test unit and the interpretation of test results in relation to acceptance or rejection of a lot should be in the hands of those who have appropriate formal training in microbiology and have knowledge of industrial sterilization, aseptic processing, and the statistical concepts involved in sampling. These individuals should be knowledgeable also concerning the environmental control program in the test facility to assure that the microbiological quality of the air and critical work surfaces are consistently acceptable.

Quality control sterility tests (either according to the official referee test or modified tests) may be carried out in two separate stages in order to rule out false positive results. *First Stage.* Regardless of the sampling plan used, if no evidence of microbial growth is found, the results of the test may be taken as indicative of absence of intrinsic contamination of the lot.

If microbial growth is found, proceed to the *Second Stage* (unless the *First Stage* test can be invalidated). Evidence for invalidating a *First Stage* test in order to repeat it as a *First Stage* test may be obtained from a review of the testing environment and the relevant records thereto. Finding of microbial growth in negative controls need not be considered the sole grounds for invalidating a *First Stage* test. When proceeding to the *Second Stage*, particularly where depending on the results of the test for lot release, concurrently, initiate and document a complete review of all applicable production and control records. In this review consideration should be paid to the following: (1) a check on monitoring records of the validated sterilization cycle applicable to the product; (2) sterility test history relating to the particular product for both finished and in-process samples, as well as sterilization records of supporting equipment, containers/closures, and sterile components, if any; (3) environmental control data, including those obtained from media fills, exposure plates, filtering records, any sanitization records and microbial monitoring records of operators, gowns, gloves, and garbing practices.

Failing any lead from the above review, the current microbial profile of the product should be checked against the known historical profile for possible change. Records should be checked concomitantly for any

[7] *Radioactive Pharmaceutical Products*—Because of rapid radioactive decay, it is not feasible to delay the release of some radioactive pharmaceutical products in order to complete sterility tests on them. In such cases, results of sterility tests provide only retrospective confirmatory evidence for sterility assurance, which therefore depends on the primary means thereto established in the manufacturing and validation/certification procedures.

changes in source of product components and/or in-processing procedures that might be contributory. Depending on the findings, and in extreme cases, consideration may have to be given to re-validation of the total manufacturing process. For the *Second Stage* it is not possible to specify a particular number of specimens to be taken for testing. It is usual to select double the number specified for the *First Stage* under *Sterility Tests* ⟨71⟩, or other reasonable number. The minimum volumes tested from each specimen, the media, and the incubation periods are the same as those indicated for the *First Stage*.

If no microbial growth is found in the *Second Stage*, and the documented review of appropriate records and the indicated product investigation does not support the possibility of intrinsic contamination, the lot may meet the requirements of a test for sterility. If growth is found, the lot fails to meet the requirements of the test. As was indicated for the *First Stage* test, the *Second Stage* test may similarly be invalidated with appropriate evidence, and, if so done, repeated as a *Second Stage* test.

⟨1231⟩ WATER FOR PHARMACEUTICAL PURPOSES

Water is the most copiously and widely used substance in pharmaceutical manufacturing. Control of the chemical and microbiological quality of water for pharmaceutical purposes is difficult because its basic sources—municipal and nonmunicipal water systems—are influenced by many factors.

Monitoring of quality parameters in source water is necessary to ensure an acceptable water supply.

Water is required for a variety of purposes ranging from the needs of manufacturing processes to the final preparation of therapeutic agents just prior to their administration to patients.

Drinking water, which is subject to federal Environmental Protection Agency regulations and which is delivered by the municipal or other local public system or drawn from a private well or reservoir, is the starting material for most forms of water covered by Pharmacopeial monographs. Water prepared from other starting material may have to be processed to meet drinking water standards. Drinking water may be used in the preparation of USP drug substances but not in the preparation of dosage forms, or in the preparation of reagents or test solutions.

The Pharmacopeia provides several monographs for water. Of these, *Purified Water* and *Water for Injection* represent ingredient materials, while the other monographs for water provide standards for compendial pharmaceutical articles in themselves.

Purified Water (see USP monograph)—This article represents water rendered suitable for pharmaceutical purposes by processes such as distillation, ion-exchange treatment (deionization or demineralization), or reverse osmosis. It meets rigid specifications for chemical purity, the requirements of the federal Environmental Protection Agency with respect to drinking water, and it contains no added substances. However, the various methods of production each present different potential for contaminating products. Purified Water produced by distillation is sterile, provided the production equipment is suitable and is sterile. On the other hand, ion-exchange columns and reverse osmosis units require special attention in that they afford sites for microorganisms to foul the system and to contaminate the effluent water. Thus, frequent monitoring may be called for, particularly with the use of these units following periods of shutdown of more than a few hours.

Water for Injection (see USP monograph)—By definition, this article is water purified by distillation or by reverse osmosis, and it meets the purity requirements under *Purified Water*. Although not intended to be sterile, it meets a test for a limit of bacterial endotoxin. It must be produced, stored, and distributed under conditions designed to prevent production of endotoxin.

Sterile Water for Injection (see USP monograph)—As a form in which water is distributed in sterile packages, Sterile Water for Injection is intended mainly for use as a solvent for parenteral products such as sterile solids that must be distributed dry because of limited stability of their solutions. It must be packaged only in single-dose containers of not larger than 1-liter size.

Bacteriostatic Water for Injection (see USP monograph)—Inasmuch as it serves the same purposes as Sterile Water for Injection, it meets the same standards, with the exception that it may be packaged in either single-dose or multiple-dose containers of not larger than 30-mL size.

Sterile Water for Irrigation (see USP monograph)—This form of water meets most, but not all, of the requirements for Sterile Water for Injection. The exceptions are with respect to the following: (1) container size (i.e., the container may contain a volume of more than 1 liter of Sterile Water for Irrigation), (2) container design (i.e., the container may be designed so as to empty rapidly the contents as a single dose), (3) *Particulate matter* requirements (i.e., it need not meet the requirement for particulate matter for Large-volume Injections for single-dose infusions), and (4) *Labeling* requirements (e.g., the designations "For irrigation only" and "Not for injection" appear prominently on the label).

ACTION GUIDELINES FOR THE MICROBIAL CONTROL OF INGREDIENT WATER—Criteria for controlling the microbial quality of Purified Water and Water for Injection may vary according to the method of production, distribution and/or storage and use. The suitability of water systems to produce water of acceptable microbiological quality should be validated prior to production. Suitable microbiological, chemical, and operating controls should be in place. The compendial *Microbial Limit Tests* ⟨61⟩ have not been designed for testing of ingredient waters. Suitable standard methods are found elsewhere.*

A total microbial (aerobic) count that may be used for source drinking water is 500 colony-forming units (cfu) per mL. Since *Purified Water* is used to manufacture a variety of products, the action limit set should be based on the intended use of the water, the nature of the product to be made, and the effect of the manufacturing process on the fate of the microorganisms. A general guideline for *Purified Water* may be 100 cfu/mL. Since ingredient waters are not produced as a lot or batch, these numbers, when exceeded or approached, serve as an alert for corrective action. In practice, the supply of ingredient water and manufacture of pharmaceutical articles are usually carried out concurrently, and the results of the microbial tests made may be available only after some pharmaceutical articles have already been manufactured. The actions to be taken to bring the microbial quality of the ingredient water into desired conformance may include sanitization of the system, for example, flushing with hot water, steam, or suitable disinfectants. Further sampling and monitoring to ensure that the corrective action has been adequate should be conducted.

* Standard Methods for the Examination of Water and Wastewater—American Public Health Association, Current Edition, Washington, DC 20005.

Packaging Requirements

⟨661⟩ CONTAINERS

Many Pharmacopeial articles are of such nature as to require the greatest attention to the containers in which they are stored or maintained even for short periods of time. While the needs vary widely and some of them are not fully met by the containers available, objective standards are essential. It is the purpose of this chapter to provide such standards as have been developed for the materials of which pharmaceutical containers principally are made, i.e., glass and plastic.

A container intended to provide protection from light or offered as a "light-resistant" container meets the requirements for *Light Transmission*, where such protection or resistance is by virtue of the specific properties of the material of which the container is composed, including any coating applied thereto. A clear and colorless or a translucent container that is made light-resistant by means of an opaque enclosure (see *General Notices*) is exempt from the requirements for *Light Transmission*.

Containers composed of glass meet the requirements for *Chemical Resistance—Glass Containers*, and containers composed of plastic and intended for packaging products prepared for parenteral use meet the requirements under *Biological Tests—Plastics* and *Physicochemical Tests—Plastics*.

Where dry oral dosage forms, not meant for constitution into solution, are intended to be packaged in a container defined in the section *Polyethylene Containers*, the requirements given in that section are to be met.

Guidelines and requirements under *Single-unit Containers and Unit-dose Containers for Non-sterile Solid and Liquid Dosage Forms* apply to official dosage forms that are repackaged into single-unit or unit-dose containers or mnemonic packs for dispensing pursuant to prescription.

LIGHT TRANSMISSION

Table 1. Limits for Glass Types I, II, and III and Plastic Classes I–VI.

Nominal Size (in mL)	Maximum Percentage of Light Transmission at Any Wavelength Between 290 and 450 nm	
	Flame-sealed Containers	Closure-sealed Containers
1	50	25
2	45	20
5	40	15
10	35	13
20	30	12
50	15	10

NOTE—Any container of a size intermediate to those listed above exhibits a transmission not greater than that of the next larger size container listed in the table. For containers larger than 50 mL, the limits for 50 mL apply.

CHEMICAL RESISTANCE—GLASS CONTAINERS

Glass Types—Glass containers suitable for packaging Pharmacopeial preparations may be classified as in Table 2 on the basis of the tests set forth in this section. Containers of Type I borosilicate glass are generally used for preparations that are intended for parenteral administration. Containers of Type I glass, or of Type II glass (i.e., soda-lime glass that is suitably dealkalized) are usually used for packaging acidic and neutral parenteral preparations. Type I glass containers, or Type II glass containers (where stability data demonstrate their suitability), are used for alkaline parenteral preparations. Type III soda-lime glass containers usually are not used for parenteral preparations, except where suitable stability test data indicate that Type III glass is satisfactory for the parenteral preparations that are packaged therein. Containers of Type NP glass are intended for packaging nonparenteral articles i.e., those intended for oral or topical use.

Table 2. Glass Types and Test Limits.

Type	General Description[a]	Type of Test	Limits: Size,[b] mL	Limits: mL of 0.020 *N* Acid
I	Highly resistant, borosilicate glass	*Powdered Glass*	All	1.0
II	Treated soda-lime glass	*Water Attack*	100 or less	0.7
			Over 100	0.2
III	Soda-lime glass	*Powdered Glass*	All	8.5
NP	General-purpose soda-lime glass	*Powdered Glass*	All	15.0

[a] The description applies to containers of this type of glass usually available.

[b] Size indicates the overflow capacity of the container.

CONTAINERS FOR OPHTHALMICS—PLASTICS

Plastics for ophthalmics are composed of a mixture of homologous compounds, having a range of molecular weights. Such plastics frequently contain other substances such as residues from the polymerization process, plasticizers, stabilizers, antioxidants, pigments, and lubricants. Factors such as plastic composition, processing and cleaning procedures, contacting media, inks, adhesives, absorption, adsorption and permeability of preservatives, and conditions of storage may also affect the suitability of a plastic for a specific use.

Definition—For the purposes of this chapter, a *container* is that which holds the drug and is or may be in direct contact with the drug.

Biological Tests—Plastics and other polymers used for containers for ophthalmics meet the requirements set forth in the section *Biological Tests—Plastics and Other Polymers.*

POLYETHYLENE CONTAINERS

The standards and tests provided in this section characterize high-density and low-density polyethylene containers that are interchangeably suitable for packaging dry oral dosage forms not meant for constitution into solution.

Where stability studies have been performed to establish the expiration date of a particular dry oral dosage form not meant for constitution into solution in a container meeting the requirements set forth herein for either high- or low-density polyethylene containers, then any other polyethylene container meeting the same sections of these requirements may be similarly used to package such dosage form, provided that the appropriate stability programs are expanded to include the alternative container, in order to assure that the identity, strength, quality, and purity of the dosage form are maintained throughout the expiration period.

Both high- and low-density polyethylene are long-chain polymers synthesized under controlled conditions of heat and pressure, with the aid of catalysts from not less than 85.0% ethylene and not less than 95.0% total olefins. The other olefin ingredients most frequently used are butene, hexene, and propylene. The ingredients used to manufacture the polyethylene, and those used in the fabrication of the containers, conform to the requirements in the applicable sections of the Code of Federal Regulations, Title 21.

High-density polyethylene and low-density polyethylene both have an infrared absorption spectrum that is distinctive for polyethylene, and each possesses characteristic thermal properties. High-density polyethylene has a density between 0.941 and 0.965 g per cm^3. Low-density polyethylene has a density between 0.850 and 0.940 g per cm^3. The permeation properties of molded polyethylene containers may be altered when re-ground polymer is incorporated, depending upon the proportion of re-ground material in the final product. Other properties that may affect the suitability of polyethylene used in containers for packaging drugs are: oxygen and moisture permeability, modulus of elasticity, melt index, environmental stress crack resistance, and degree of crystallinity after molding. The requirements in this section are to be met when dry oral dosage forms, not meant for constitution into solution, are intended to be packaged in a container defined by this section.

POLYETHYLENE TEREPHTHALATE BOTTLES AND POLYETHYLENE TEREPHTHALATE G BOTTLES

The standards and tests provided in this section characterize polyethylene terephthalate (PET) and polyethylene terephthalate G (PETG) bottles that are interchangeably suitable for packaging liquid oral dosage forms.

Where stability studies have been performed to establish the expiration date of a particular liquid oral dosage form in a bottle meeting the requirements set forth herein for either PET or PETG bottles, any other PET or PETG bottle meeting these requirements may be similarly used to package such dosage form, provided that the appropriate stability programs are expanded to include the alternative bottle in order to assure that the identity, strength, quality, and purity of the dosage form are maintained throughout the expiration period.

The suitability of a specific PET or PETG bottle for use in the dispensing of a particular pharmaceutical liquid oral dosage form must be established by appropriate testing.

PET resins are long-chain crystalline polymers prepared by the condensation of ethylene glycol with dimethyl terephthalate or terephthalic acid. PET copolymer resins are prepared in a similar way, except that they may also contain a small amount of either isophthalic acid (not more than 3 mole percent) or 1,4-cyclohexanedimethanol (not more than 5 mole percent). Polymerization is conducted under controlled conditions of heat and vacuum, with the aid of catalysts and stabilizers.

PET copolymer resins have physical and spectral properties similar to PET and for practical purposes are treated as PET. The tests and specifications provided in this section to characterize PET resins and bottles apply also to PET copolymer resins and to bottles fabricated from them.

PET and PET copolymer resins generally exhibit a large degree of order in their molecular structure. As a result, they exhibit characteristic composition-dependent thermal behavior, including a glass transition temperature of about 76° and a melting temperature of about 250°. These resins have a distinctive infrared absorption spectrum that allows them to be distinguished from other plastic materials (e.g., polycarbonate, polystyrene, poly-ethylene, and PETG resins). PET and PET copolymer resins have a density between 1.3 and 1.4 g per cm^3 and a minimum intrinsic viscosity of 0.7 dL per g, which corresponds to a number average molecular weight of about 23,000 daltons.

PETG resins are high molecular weight polymers prepared by the condensation of ethylene glycol with dimethyl terephthalate or terephthalic acid and 15 to 34 mole percent of 1,4-cyclohexanedimethanol. PETG resins are clear, amorphous polymers, having a glass transition temperature of about 81° and no crystalline melting point, as determined by differential scanning calorimetry. PETG resins have a distinctive infrared absorption spectrum that allows them to be distinguished from other plastic materials, including PET. PETG resins have a density of approximately 1.27 g per cm^3 and a minimum instrinsic viscosity of 0.65 dL per g, which corresponds to a number average molecular weight of about 16,000 daltons.

PET and PETG resins, and other ingredients used in the fabrication of these bottles, conform to the requirements in the applicable sections of the Code of Federal Regulations, Title 21, regarding use in contact with food and alcoholic beverages. PET and PETG resins do not contain any plasticizers, processing aids, or antioxidants. Colorants, if used in the manufacture of PET and PETG bottles, do not migrate into the contained liquid.

SINGLE-UNIT CONTAINERS AND UNIT-DOSE CONTAINERS FOR NONSTERILE SOLID AND LIQUID DOSAGE FORMS

An official dosage form is required to bear on its label an expiration date assigned for the particular formulation and package of the article. This date limits the time during which the product may be dispensed or used. Because the expiration date stated on the manufacturer's or distributor's package has been determined for the drug in that particular package and may not be applicable to the product where it has been repackaged in a different container, repackaged drugs dispensed pursuant to a prescription are exempt from this label requirement. It is necessary, therefore, that other precautions be taken by the dispenser to preserve the strength, quality, and purity of drugs that are repackaged for ultimate distribution or sale to patients.

The following guidelines and requirements are applicable where official dosage forms are repackaged into single-unit or unit-dose containers or mnemonic packs for dispensing pursuant to prescription.

Labeling—It is the responsibility of the dispenser, taking into account the nature of the drug repackaged, the characteristics of the containers, and the storage conditions to which the article may be subjected, to determine a suitable beyond-use date to be placed on the label. In the absence of stability data to the contrary, such date should not exceed (1) 25% of the remaining time between the date of repackaging and the expiration date on the original manufacturer's bulk container, or (2) a six-month period from the date the drug is repackaged, whichever is earlier. Each single-unit or unit-dose container bears a separate label, unless the device holding the unit-dose form does not allow for the removal or separation of the intact single-unit or unit-dose container therefrom.

Storage—Store the repackaged article in a humidity-controlled environment and at the temperature specified in the individual monograph or in the product labeling. Where no temperature or humidity is specified in the monograph or in the labeling of the product, controlled room temperature and a relative humidity corresponding to 75% at 23° are not to be exceeded during repackaging or storage.

A refrigerator or freezer shall not be considered to be a humidity-controlled environment, and drugs that are to be stored at a cold temperature in a refrigerator or freezer shall be placed within an outer container that meets the monograph requirements for the drug contained therein.

CUSTOMIZED PATIENT MEDICATION PACKAGES

In lieu of dispensing two or more prescribed drug products in separate containers, a pharmacist may, with the consent of the patient, the patient's caregiver, or a prescriber, provide a customized patient medication package (patient med pak).[1]

A patient med pak is a package prepared by a pharmacist for a specific patient comprising a series of containers and containing two or more prescribed solid oral dosage forms. The patient med pak is so designed or each container is so labeled as to indicate the day and time, or period of time, that the contents within each container are to be taken.

It is the responsibility of the dispenser to instruct the patient or caregiver on the use of the patient med pak.

Label—

(A) The patient med pak shall bear a label stating:

(1) the name of the patient;

(2) a serial number for the patient med pak itself and a separate identifying serial number for each of the prescription orders for each of the drug products contained therein;

(3) the name, strength, physical description or identification, and total quantity of each drug product contained therein;

(4) the directions for use and cautionary statements, if any, contained in the prescription order for each drug product therein;

(5) any storage instructions or cautionary statements required by the official compendia;

(6) the name of the prescriber of each drug product;

(7) the date of preparation of the patient med pak and the beyond-use date or period of time assigned to the patient med pak (such beyond-use date or period of time shall be not longer then the shortest recommended beyond-use date for any dosage form included therein or not longer than 60 days from the date of preparation of the patient med pak and shall not exceed the shortest expiration date on the original manufacturer's bulk containers for the dosage forms included therein); alternatively, the package label shall state the date of the prescription(s) or the date of preparation of the patient med pak, provided the package is accompanied by a record indicating the start date and the beyond-use date;

(8) the name, address, and telephone number of the dispenser (and the dispenser's registration number where necessary); and

(9) any other information, statements, or warnings required for any of the drug products contained therein.

(B) If the patient med pak allows for the removal or separation of the intact containers therefrom, each individual container shall bear a label identifying each of the drug products contained therein.

Labeling—The patient med pak shall be accompanied by a patient package insert, in the event that any medication therein is required to be dispensed with such insert as accompanying labeling. Alternatively, such required information may be incorporated into a single, overall educational insert provided by the pharmacist for the total patient med pak.

Packaging—In the absence of more stringent packaging requirements for any of the drug products contained therein, each container of the patient med pak shall comply with the moisture permeation requirements for a Class B single-unit or unit-dose container (see *Containers—Permeation* ⟨671⟩). Each container shall be either not reclosable or so designed as to show evidence of having been opened.

Guidelines—It is the responsibility of the dispenser, when preparing a patient med pak, to take into account any applicable compendial requirements or guidelines and the physical and chemical compatibility of the dosage forms placed within each container, as well as any therapeutic incompatibilities that may attend the simultaneous administration of the medications. In this regard, pharmacists are encouraged to report to USP headquarters any observed or reported incompatibilities.

Recordkeeping—In addition to any individual prescription filing requirements, a record of each patient med pak shall be made and filed. Each record shall contain, as a minimum:

(1) the name and address of the patient;

---

[1] It should be noted that there is no special exemption for patient med paks from the requirements of the Poison Prevention Packaging Act. Thus the patient med pak, if it does not meet child-resistant standards, shall be placed in an outer package that does comply, or the necessary consent of the purchaser or physician, to dispense in a container not intended to be child-resistant, shall be obtained.

(2) the serial number of the prescription order for each drug product contained therein;
(3) the name of the manufacturer or labeler and lot number for each drug product contained therein;
(4) information identifying or describing the design, characteristics, or specifications of the patient med pak sufficient to allow subsequent preparation of an identical patient med pak for the patient;
(5) the date of preparation of the patient med pak and the beyond-use date that was assigned;
(6) any special labeling instructions; and
(7) the name or initials of the pharmacist who prepared the patient med pak.

⟨671⟩ CONTAINERS—PERMEATION

The tests that follow are provided to determine the moisture permeability of containers utilized for drugs being dispensed on prescription. The section *Multiple-unit Containers for Capsules and Tablets* applies to multiple-unit containers (see *Preservation, Packaging, Storage, and Labeling* under *General Notices*). The section *Single-unit Containers and Unit-dose Containers for Capsules and Tablets* applies to single-unit and unit-dose containers (see *Single-unit Containers and Unit-dose Containers for Nonsterile Solid and Liquid Dosage Forms* under *Containers* ⟨661⟩). As used herein, the term "container" refers to the entire system comprising, usually, the container itself, the liner (if used), the closure in the case of multiple-unit containers, and the lidding and blister in the case of single-unit and unit-dose containers.

Where the manufacturer's unopened multiple-unit, single-unit, or unit-dose packages are used for dispensing the drug, such containers are exempt from the requirements of this test.

Torque Applicable to Screw-Type Container

Closure Diameter[1] (mm)	Suggested Tightness Range with Manually Applied Torque[2] (inch-pounds)
8	5
10	6
13	8
15	5–9
18	7–10
20	8–12
22	9–14
24	10–18
28	12–21
30	13–23
33	15–25
38	17–26
43	17–27
48	19–30
53	21–36
58	23–40
63	25–43
66	26–45
70	28–50
83	32–65
86	40–65
89	40–70
100	45–70
110	45–70
120	55–95
132	60–95

[1] The torque designated for the next larger closure diameter is to be applied in testing containers having a closure diameter intermediate to the diameters listed.

[2] A suitable apparatus is available from Owens-Illinois, Toledo, OH 43666. (Model 25 torque tester is used for testing between 0 and 25; Model 50 for testing between 0 and 50; and Model 100 for testing between 0 and 100 inch-pounds of torque.) The torque values refer to application, not removal, of the closure. For further detail regarding instructions, reference may be made to "Standard Method of Measuring Application and Removal Torque of Threaded Closures," ASTM Designation D 3198-73, published by the American Society for Testing and Materials, 1916 Race St., Philadelphia, PA 19103.

MULTIPLE-UNIT CONTAINERS FOR CAPSULES AND TABLETS

Desiccant—Place a quantity of 4- to 8-mesh, anhydrous calcium chloride[1] in a shallow container, taking care to exclude any fine powder, then dry at 110° for 1 hour, and cool in a desiccator.

Procedure—Select 12 containers of a uniform size and type, clean the sealing surfaces with a lint-free cloth, and close and open each container 30 times. Apply the closure firmly and uniformly each time the container is closed. Close screw-capped containers with a torque that is within the range of tightness specified in the accompanying table. Add *Desiccant* to 10 of the containers, designated *test containers*, filling each to within 13 mm of the closure if the container volume is 20 mL or more, or filling each to two-thirds of capacity if the container volume is less than 20 mL. If the interior of the container is more than 63 mm in depth, an inert filler or spacer may be placed in the bottom to minimize the total weight of the container and *Desiccant;* the layer of *Desiccant* in such a container shall be not less than 5 cm in depth. Close each immediately after adding *Desiccant*, applying the torque designated in the accompanying table when closing screw-capped containers. To each of the remaining 2 containers, designated *controls*, add a sufficient number of glass beads to attain a weight approximately equal to that of each of the *test containers*, and close, applying the torque designated in the accompanying table when closing screw-capped containers. Record the weight of the individual containers so prepared to the nearest 0.1 mg if the container volume is less than 20 mL; to the nearest mg if the container volume is 20 mL or more but less than 200 mL; or to the nearest centigram (10 mg) if the container volume is 200 mL or more; and store at 75 ± 3% relative humidity and a temperature of 23 ± 2°. [NOTE—A saturated system of 35 g of sodium chloride with each 100 mL of water placed in the bottom of a desiccator maintains the specified humidity. Other methods may be employed to maintain these conditions.] After 336 ± 1 hours (14 days), record the weight of the individual containers in the same manner. Completely fill 5 empty containers of the same size and type as the containers under test with water or a noncompressible, free-flowing solid such as well-tamped fine glass beads, to the level indicated by the closure surface when in place. Transfer the contents of each to a graduated cylinder, and determine the average container volume, in mL. Calculate the rate of moisture permeability, in mg per day per liter, taken by the formula:

$$(1000/14V)[(T_f - T_i) - (C_f - C_i)],$$

in which V is the volume, in mL, of the container, $(T_f - T_i)$ is the difference, in mg, between the final and initial weights of each *test container*, and $(C_f - C_i)$ is the average of the differences, in mg, between the final and initial weights of the 2 *controls*. The containers so tested are *tight containers* if not more than one of the 10 *test containers* exceeds 100 mg per day per liter in moisture permeability, and none exceeds 200 mg per day per liter.

The containers are *well-closed containers* if not more than one of the 10 *test containers* exceeds 2000 mg per day per liter in moisture permeability, and none exceeds 3000 mg per day per liter.

SINGLE-UNIT CONTAINERS AND UNIT-DOSE CONTAINERS FOR CAPSULES AND TABLETS

To permit an informed judgment regarding the suitability of the packaging for a particular type of product, the following procedure and classification scheme are provided for evaluating the moisture-permeation characteristics of single-unit and unit-dose containers. Inasmuch as equipment and operator performance may affect the moisture permeation of a container formed or closed, the moisture-permeation characteristics of the packaging system being utilized shall be determined.

Desiccant—Dry suitable desiccant pellets[2] at 110° for 1 hour prior to use. Use pellets weighing approximately 400 mg each and having a

[1] Suitable 4- to 8-mesh, anhydrous calcium chloride is available commercially as Item JT1313-1 from VWR Scientific. Consult the VWR Scientific catalog for ordering information or call 1-800-234-9300.

[2] Suitable moisture-indicating desiccant pellets are available commercially from sources such as Medical Packaging, Inc., 470 Route 31, Ringoes, NJ 08551-1409 [Telephone 800-257-5282; in NJ, 609-466-8991; FAX 609-466-3775], as Indicating Desiccant Pellets, Item No. TK-1002.

diameter of approximately 8 mm. [NOTE—If necessary due to limited unit-dose container size, pellets weighing less than 400 mg each and having a diameter of less than 8 mm may be used.]

Procedure—

Method I—Seal not less than 10 unit-dose containers with 1 pellet in each, and seal 10 additional, empty unit-dose containers to provide the controls, using finger cots or padded forceps to handle the sealed containers. Number the containers, and record the individual weights[3] to the nearest mg. Weigh the controls as a unit, and divide the total weight by the number of controls to obtain the average. Store all of the containers at 75 ± 3% relative humidity and at a temperature of 23 ± 2°. [NOTE—A saturated system of 35 g of sodium chloride with each 100 mL of water placed in the bottom of a desiccator maintains the specified humidity. Other methods may be employed to maintain these conditions.] After a 24-hour interval, or a multiple thereof (see *Results*), remove the containers from the chamber, and allow them to equilibrate for 15 to 60 minutes in the weighing area. Again record the weight of the individual containers and the combined controls in the same manner. [NOTE—If any indicating pellets turn pink during this procedure, or if the pellet weight increase exceeds 10%, terminate the test, and regard only earlier determinations as valid.] Return the containers to the humidity chamber. Calculate the rate of moisture permeation, in mg per day, of each container taken by the formula:

$$(1/N)[(W_f - W_i) - (C_f - C_i)],$$

in which N is the number of days expired in the test period, $(W_f - W_i)$ is the difference, in mg, between the final and initial weights of each test container, and $(C_f - C_i)$ is the average of the difference, in mg, between the final and initial weights of the controls, the data being calculated to two significant figures. [NOTE—Where the permeations measured are less than 5 mg per day, and where the controls are observed to reach a steady state in 7 days, the individual permeations may be determined more accurately after an initial 7 days of equilibration by using that weight as W_i, zero time, in the calculation.]

Method II—Use this procedure for packs (e.g., punch-out cards) that incorporate a number of separately sealed unit-dose containers or blisters. Seal a sufficient number of packs, such that not less than 4 packs and a total of not less than 10 unit-dose containers or blisters filled with 1 pellet in each unit are tested. Seal a corresponding number of empty packs, each pack containing the same number of unit-dose containers or blisters as used in the test packs, to provide the controls. Store all of the containers at 75 ± 3% relative humidity and at a temperature of 23 ± 2°. [See *Note* under *Method I*.] After 24 hours, and at multiples thereof (see *Results*), remove the packs from the chamber, and allow them to equilibrate for approximately 45 minutes. Record the weights of the individual packs, and return them to the chamber. Weigh the control packs as a unit, and divide the total weight by the number of control packs to obtain the average empty pack weight. [NOTE—If any indicating pellets turn pink during the procedure, or if the average pellet weight increase in any pack exceeds 10%, terminate the test, and regard only earlier determinations as valid.] Calculate the average rate of moisture permeation, in mg per day, for each unit-dose container or blister in each pack taken by the formula:

$$(1/NX)[(W_f - W_i) - (C_f - C_i)],$$

in which N is the number of days expired in the test period (beginning after the initial 24 hour equilibration period), X is the number of separately sealed units per pack, $(W_f - W_i)$ is the difference, in mg, between the final and initial weights of each test pack, and $(C_f - C_i)$ is the average of the difference, in mg, between the final and initial weights of the control packs, the rates being calculated to two significant figures.

Results—The individual unit-dose containers as tested in *Method I* are designated *Class A* if not more than 1 of 10 containers tested exceeds 0.5 mg per day in moisture permeation rate and none exceeds 1 mg per day; they are designated *Class B* if not more than 1 of 10 containers tested exceeds 5 mg per day and none exceeds 10 mg per day; they are designated *Class C* if not more than 1 of 10 containers tested exceeds 20 mg per day and none exceeds 40 mg per day; and they are designated *Class D* if the containers tested meet none of the moisture permeation rate requirements.

The packs as tested in *Method II* are designated *Class A* if no pack tested exceeds 0.5 mg per day in average blister moisture permeation rate; they are designated *Class B* if no pack tested exceeds 5 mg per day in average blister moisture permeation rate; they are designated *Class C* if no pack tested exceeds 20 mg per day in average blister moisture permeation rate; and they are designated *Class D* if the packs tested meet none of the above average blister moisture permeation rate requirements.

With the use of the *Desiccant* described herein, suitable test intervals for the final weighings, W_f, are: 24 hours for *Class D;* 48 hours for *Class C;* 7 days for *Class B;* and not less than 28 days for *Class A*.

[3] Accurate comparisons of *Class A* containers may require test periods in excess of 28 days if weighings are performed on a *Class A* prescription balance (see *Prescription Balances and Volumetric Apparatus* ⟨1176⟩). The use of an analytical balance on which weights can be recorded to 4 or 5 decimal places may permit more precise characterization between containers and/or shorter test periods.

⟨1091⟩ LABELING OF INACTIVE INGREDIENTS

This informational chapter provides guidelines for labeling of inactive ingredients present in dosage forms.

Within the past few years a number of trade associations representing pharmaceutical manufacturers have adopted voluntary guidelines for the disclosure and labeling of inactive ingredients. This is helpful to individuals who are sensitive to particular substances and who wish to identify the presence or confirm the absence of such substances in drug products. Because of the actions of these associations, the labeling of therapeutically inactive ingredients currently is deemed to constitute good pharmaceutical practice.

Although the manufacturers represented by these associations produce most of the products sold in this country, not all manufacturers, repackagers, or labelers here or abroad are members of these associations. Further, there are some differences in association guidelines. The guidelines presented here are designed to help promote consistency in labeling.

In accordance with good pharmaceutical practice, all dosage forms [NOTE—for requirements on parenteral and topical preparations, see the General Notices] should be labeled to state the identity of all added substances (therapeutically inactive ingredients) present therein, including colors, except that flavors and fragrances may be listed by the general term "flavor" or "fragrance." Such listing should be in alphabetical order by name and be distinguished from the identification statement of the active ingredient(s).

The name of an inactive ingredient should be taken from the current edition of one of the following reference works (in the following order of precedence): (1) the *United States Pharmacopeia* or the *National Formulary;* (2) *USAN and the USP Dictionary of Drug Names;* (3) CTFA *Cosmetic Ingredient Dictionary;* (4) *Food Chemicals Codex*. An ingredient not listed in any of the aforementioned reference works should be identified by its common or usual name (the name generally recognized by consumers or health-care professionals) or, if no common or usual name is available, by its chemical or other technical name.

An ingredient that may be, but not always is, present in a product should be qualified by words such as "or" or "may also contain."

The name of an ingredient whose identity is a trade secret may be omitted from the list if the list states "and other ingredients." For the purposes of this guideline, an ingredient is considered to be a trade secret only if its presence confers a significant competitive advantage upon its manufacturer and if its identity cannot be ascertained by the use of modern analytical technology.

An incidental trace ingredient having no functional or technical effect on the product need not be listed unless it has been demonstrated to cause sensitivity reactions or allergic responses.

Inactive ingredients should be listed on the label of a container of a product intended for sale without prescription, except that in the case of a container too small, such information may be contained in other labeling on or within the package.

Weight and Measures

⟨1176⟩ PRESCRIPTION BALANCES AND VOLUMETRIC APPARATUS

Prescription Balances

NOTE—Balances other than the type described herein may be used provided these afford equivalent or better accuracy. This includes micro-, semimicro-, or electronic single-pan balances (see *Weights and*

Balances ⟨41⟩). Some balances offer digital or direct-reading features. All balances should be calibrated and tested frequently using appropriate test weights, both singly and in combination.

Description—A prescription balance is a scale or balance adapted to weighing medicinal and other substances required in prescriptions or in other pharmaceutical compounding. It is constructed so as to support its full capacity without developing undue stresses, and its adjustment is not altered by repeated weighings of the capacity load. The removable pans or weighing vessels should be of equal weight. The balance should have leveling feet or screws. The balance may feature dial-in weights and also a precision spring and dial instead of a weighbeam. A balance that has a graduated weighbeam must have a stop that halts the rider or poise at the "zero" reading. The reading edge of the rider is parallel to the graduations on the weighbeam. The distance from the face of the index plate to the indicator pointer or pointers should be not more than 1.0 mm, the points should be sharp, and when there are two, their ends should be separated by not more than 1.0 mm when the scale is in balance. The indicating elements and the lever system should be protected against drafts, and the balance lid should permit free movement of the loaded weighing pans when the lid is closed. The balance must have a mechanical arresting device.

Definitions—

Capacity—Maximum weight, including the weight of tares, to be placed on one pan. The *N.B.S. Handbook 44*, 4th ed., states: "*In the absence of information to the contrary*, the nominal capacity of a Class *A* balance shall be assumed to be 15.5 g (½ apothecaries' ounce)." Most of the commercially available Class *A* balances have a capacity of 120 g and bear a statement to that effect.

Weighbeam or Beam—A graduated bar equipped with a movable poise or rider. Metric graduations are in 0.01-g increments up to a maximum of 1.0 g.

Tare Bar—An auxiliary ungraduated weighbeam bar with a movable poise. This can be used to correct for variations in weighing-glasses or papers.

Balance Indicator—A combination of elements, one or both of which will oscillate with respect to the other, to indicate the equilibrium state of the balance during weighing.

Rest Point—The point on the index plate at which the indicator or pointer stops when the oscillations of the balance cease; or the index plate position of the indicator or pointer calculated from recorded consecutive oscillations in both directions past the "zero" of the index plate scale. If the balance has a two-pointer indicating mechanism, the position or the oscillations of only one of the pointers need be recorded or used to determine the rest point.

Sensitivity Requirements (*SR*)—The maximum change in load that will cause a specified change, one subdivision on the index plate, in the position of rest of the indicating element or elements of the balance.

Class A Prescription Balance—A balance that meets the tests for this type of balance has a sensitivity requirement of 6 mg or less with no load and with a load of 10 g on each pan. The Class *A* balance should be used for all of the weighing operations required in prescription compounding.

In order to avoid errors of 5 percent or more that might be due to the limit of sensitivity of the Class *A* prescription balance, do not weigh less than 120 mg of any material. If a smaller weight of dry material is required, mix a larger known weight of the ingredient with a known weight of dry diluent, and weigh an aliquot portion of the mixture for use.

Testing the Prescription Balance—A Class *A* prescription balance meets the following four basic tests. Use a set of test weights, and keep the rider on the weighbeam at zero unless directed to change its position.

1. *Sensitivity Requirement*—Level the balance, determine the rest point, and place a 6-mg weight on one of the empty pans. Repeat the operation with a 10-g weight in the center of each pan. The rest point is shifted not less than one division on the index plate each time the 6-mg weight is added.

2. *Arm Ratio Test*—This test is designed to check the equality of length of both arms of the balance. Determine the rest point of the balance with no weight on the pans. Place in the center of each pan a 30-g test weight, and determine the rest point. If the second rest point is not the same as the first, place a 20-mg weight on the lighter side; the rest point should move back to the original place on the index plate scale or farther.

3. *Shift Tests*—These tests are designed to check the arm and lever components of the balance.

A. Determine the rest point of the indicator without any weights on the pans.

B. Place one of the 10-g weights in the center of the left pan, and place the other 10-g weight successively toward the right, left, front, and back of the right pan, noting the rest point in each case. If in any case the rest point differs from the rest point determined in Step *A*, add a 10-mg weight to the lighter side; this should cause the rest point to shift back to the rest point determined in Step *A* or farther.

C. Place a 10-g weight in the center of the right pan, and place a 10-g weight successively toward the right, left, front, and back of the left pan, noting the rest point in each case. If in any case the rest point is different from that obtained with no weights on the pans, this difference should be overcome by addition of the 10-mg weight to the lighter side.

D. Make a series of observations in which both weights are simultaneously shifted to off-center positions on their pans, both toward the outside, both toward the inside, one toward the outside, and the other toward the inside, both toward the back, and so on until all combinations have been checked. If in any case the rest point differs from that obtained with no weights on the pan, the addition of the 10-mg weight to the lighter side should overcome this difference.

A balance that does not meet the requirements of these tests must be adjusted.

4. *Rider and Graduated Beam Tests*—Determine the rest point for the balance with no weight on the pans. Place on the left pan the 500-mg test weight, move the rider to the 500-mg point on the beam, and determine the rest point. If it is different from the zero rest point, add a 6-mg weight to the lighter side. This should bring the rest point back to its original position or farther. Repeat this test, using the 1-g test weight and moving the rider to the 1-g division on the beam. If the rest point is different, it should be brought back at least to the zero rest point position by addition of 6 mg to the lighter pan. If the balance does not meet this test, the weighbeam graduations or the rider must be corrected.

Metric or apothecaries' weights for use with a prescription balance should be kept in a special rigid and compartmentalized box and handled with plastic or plastic-tipped forceps to prevent scratching or soiling. For prescription use, analytical weights (Class P or better) are recommended. However, Class Q weights have tolerances well within the limits of accuracy of the prescription balance, and they retain their accuracy for a long time with proper care. Coin-type (or disk-shaped) weights should not be used.

Test weights consisting of two 20-g or two 30-g, two 10-g, one 1-g, one 500-mg, one 20-mg, one 10-mg, and one 6-mg (or suitable combination totaling 6 mg) weights, adjusted to N.B.S. tolerances for analytical weights (Class P or better) should be used for testing the prescription balances. These weights should be kept in a tightly closed box and should be handled only with plastic or plastic-tipped forceps. The set of test weights should be used only for testing the balance or constantly used weights. If properly cared for, the set lasts indefinitely.

Volumetric Apparatus

Pharmaceutical devices for measuring volumes of liquids, including burets, pipets, and cylinders graduated either in metric or apothecary units meet the standard specifications for glass volumetric apparatus described in NTIS COM-73-10504 of the National Technical Information Service.[1] Conical graduates meet the standard specifications described in N.B.S. *Handbook 44*, 4th Edition, of the National Institute of Standards and Technology.[2] Graduated medicine droppers meet the specifications (see *Medicine Dropper* ⟨1101⟩). An acceptable ungraduated medicine dropper has a delivery end 3 mm in external diameter and delivers 20 drops of water, weighing 1 g at a temperature of 15°. A tolerance of ±10% of the delivery specification is reasonable.

Selection and Use of Graduates—

Capacity—The capacity of a graduate is the designated volume, at the maximum graduation, that the graduate will contain, or deliver, as indicated, at the specified temperature.

Cylindrical and Conical Graduates—The error in a measured volume caused by a deviation of ±1 mm, in reading the lower meniscus in a graduated cylinder remains constant along the height of the uniform

[1] NTIS COM-73-10504 is for sale by the National Technical Information Service, Springfield, VA 22151.

[2] N.B.S. Handbook 44, 4th ed. (1971) is for sale by the Superintendent of Documents, U. S. Government Printing Office, Washington, DC 20402.

column. The same deviation of ±1 mm causes a progressively larger error in a conical graduate, the extent of the error being further dependent upon the angle of the flared sides to the perpendicular of the upright graduate. A deviation of ±1 mm in the meniscus reading causes an error of approximately 0.5 mL in the measured volume at any mark on the uniform 100-mL cylinder graduate. The same deviation of ±1 mm can cause an error of 1.8 mL at the 100-mL mark on an acceptable conical graduate marked for 125 mL.

A general rule for selection of a graduate for use is to use the graduate with a capacity equal to or *just exceeding* the volume to be measured. Measurement of small volumes in large graduates tends to increase errors, because the larger diameter increases the volume error in a deviation of ±1 mm from the mark. The relation of the volume error to the internal diameters of graduated cylinders is based upon the equation $V = \pi r^2 h$. An acceptable 10-mL cylinder having an internal diameter of 1.18 cm holds 109 µL in 1 mm of the column. Reading 4.5 mL in this graduate with a deviation of ±1 mm from the mark causes an error of about ±2.5%, while the same deviation in a volume of 2.2 mL in the same graduate causes an error of about ±5%. Minimum volumes that can be measured within certain limits of error in graduated cylinders of different capacities are incorporated in the design details of graduates in N.B.S. *Handbook 44*, 4th ed., of the National Institute of Standards and Technology. Conical graduates having a capacity of less than 25 mL should not be used in prescription compounding.

⟨1101⟩ MEDICINE DROPPER

The Pharmacopeial medicine dropper consists of a tube made of glass or other suitable transparent material that generally is fitted with a collapsible bulb and, while varying in capacity, is constricted at the delivery end to a round opening having an external diameter of about 3 mm. The dropper, when held vertically, delivers water in drops each of which weighs between 45 mg and 55 mg.

In using a medicine dropper, one should keep in mind that few medicinal liquids have the same surface and flow characteristics as water, and therefore the size of drops varies materially from one preparation to another.

Where accuracy of dosage is important, a dropper that has been calibrated especially for the preparation with which it is supplied should be employed. The volume error incurred in measuring any liquid by means of a calibrated dropper should not exceed 15%, under normal use conditions.

⟨1221⟩ TEASPOON

For household purposes, an American Standard Teaspoon has been established by the American National Standards Institute* as containing 4.93 ± 0.24 mL. In view of the almost universal practice of employing teaspoons ordinarily available in the household for the administration of medicine, the teaspoon may be regarded as representing 5 mL. Preparations intended for administration by teaspoon should be formulated on the basis of dosage in 5-mL units. Any dropper, syringe, medicine cup, special spoon, or other device used to administer liquids should deliver 5 mL wherever a teaspoon calibration is indicated. Under ideal conditions of use, the volume error incurred in measuring liquids for individual dose administration by means of such calibrated devices should be not greater than 10% of the indicated amount.

Household units are used often to inform the patient of the size of the dose. Fifteen milliliters should be considered 1 standard tablespoonful; 10 mL, 2 standard teaspoonfuls; and 5 mL, 1 standard teaspoonful. Doses of less than 5 mL are frequently stated as fractions of a teaspoonful or in drops.

Because of the difficulties involved in measuring liquids under normal conditions of use, patients should be cautioned that household spoons are not appropriate for measuring medicines. They should be directed to use the standard measures in the cooking-and-baking measuring spoon sets or, preferably, oral dosing devices that may be provided by the practitioner. It must be kept in mind that the actual volume of a spoonful of any given liquid is related to the latter's viscosity and surface tension, among other influencing factors. These factors can also cause variability in the true volumes contained in or delivered by medicine cups. Where accurate dosage is required, a calibrated syringe or dropper should be used.

---

* American National Standards Institute, 1430 Broadway, New York, NY 10018.

EQUIVALENTS OF WEIGHTS AND MEASURES

Metric, Avoirdupois, and Apothecaries

NOTE—These values are for water at the temperature of 4 °C (39.2 °F) in vacuum. For practical purposes the values may be used without correction.

This table of exact equivalents should not be confused with the table of *approximate* dose equivalents, which appears on the next page. The latter table is provided only as a convenience to physicians for prescribing.

For the conversion of specific quantities in pharmaceutical formulas, use the exact equivalents. For prescription compounding, use the exact equivalents rounded to three significant figures.

Weights					Metric Equivalents	Measures		
Apothecaries		Avoirdupois				Fluid		Decimal
oz	grains	lb	oz	grains	g or mL	ounces	minims	Equivalent
32	72.4	2	3	119.9	**1000**	33	391.1	33.815
30	204.1	2	1	166.6	946.333	**32**	....	32
29	80.0	**2**	..	....	907.185	30	324.6	30.676
16	36.2	1	1	278.7	**500**	16	435.6	16.907
15	102.1	1	..	302.1	473.167	**16**	....	16
14	280.0	**1**	..	....	453.592	15	162.3	15.338
12	....	..	13	72.5	373.242	12	298.1	12.621
8	....	..	8	340.0	248.828	8	198.7	8.414
7	291.0	..	8	151.0	236.583	8	....	8
7	140.0	..	8	....	226.796	7	321.1	7.669
6	206.5	..	7	24.0	**200**	6	366.2	6.763
4	....	..	4	170.0	124.414	4	99.4	4.207
3	385.5	..	4	75.5	118.292	**4**	....	4
3	310.0	..	**4**	....	113.398	3	400.6	3.835
3	103.2	..	3	230.7	**100**	3	183.1	3.381
2	....	..	2	85.0	62.207	2	49.7	2.104
1	432.8	..	2	37.8	59.146	**2**	....	2
1	395.0	..	**2**	....	56.699	1	440.3	1.917
1	291.6	..	1	334.1	**50**	1	331.5	1.691
1	....	..	1	42.5	31.1035	1	24.9	1.052
..	456.380	..	1	18.88	29.5729	**1**	....	1
..	437.5	..	**1**	....	28.350	..	460.15	0.959
..	385.8	..	..	....	**25**	..	405.78	0.845
..	308.6	..	..	....	**20**	..	324.62	0.676
..	154.3	..	..	....	**10**	..	162.31	0.338
..	19.02	..	..	....	1.232	..	**20**	....
..	15.4324	..	..	....	**1**	..	16.23	....
..	9.51	..	..	....	0.616	..	**10**	....
..	**5**	..	..	....	0.324	..	....	....
..	4.75	..	..	....	0.308	..	**5**	....
..	**1**	..	..	....	0.06480	..	1.0517	....

Laws and Regulations

⟨1071⟩ CONTROLLED SUBSTANCES ACT REGULATIONS

Selected portions of the regulations promulgated under the Controlled Substances Act that are believed to be of most concern to practitioners and students of pharmacy and medicine are presented here as a service to the professions and at the suggestion of the Drug Enforcement Administration in accordance with its registrant information and self-regulation program.

The publication of these regulations in the *United States Pharmacopeia* is for purposes of information and does not impart to them any legal effect.

The Drug Enforcement Administration was established July 1, 1973, through the merging of various Bureaus and offices of the federal government with the Bureau of Narcotics and Dangerous Drugs.

INDEX TO THE PORTIONS OF CONTROLLED SUBSTANCES ACT REGULATIONS PRESENTED HEREIN

General Provisions

§ 290.05 Drugs; statement of required warning.

The label of any drug listed as a "controlled substance" in Schedule II, III, or IV of the Federal Controlled Substances Act shall, when dispensed to or for a patient, contain the following warning: "Caution: Federal law prohibits the transfer of this drug to any person other than the patient for whom it was prescribed." This statement is not required to appear on the label of a controlled substance dispensed for use in clinical investigations which are "blind."

§ 290.06 Spanish-language version of required warning.

By direction of section 305(c) of the Federal Controlled Substances Act, § 290.05, promulgated under section 503(b) of the Federal Food, Drug, and Cosmetic Act, requires the following warning on the label of certain drugs when dispensed to or for a patient: "Caution: Federal law prohibits the transfer of this drug to any person other than the patient for whom it was prescribed." The Spanish version of this is: "Precaucion: La ley Federal prohibe el transferir de esta droga a otra persona que no sea el paciente para quien fue recetada." (Secs. 502, 503; 53 Stat. 854, 65 Stat. 648; 21 U.S.C. 352, 353)

§ 290.10 Definition of emergency situation.

For the purposes of authorizing an oral prescription of a controlled substance listed in Schedule II of the Federal Controlled Substances Act, the term "emergency situation" means those situations in which the prescribing practitioner determines:

(a) That immediate administration of the controlled substance is necessary, for proper treatment of the intended ultimate user; and

(b) That no appropriate alternative treatment is available, including administration of a drug which is not a controlled substance under Schedule II of the Act, and

(c) That it is not reasonably possible for the prescribing practitioner to provide a written prescription to be presented to the person dispensing the substance, prior to the dispensing.

General Information

§ 1301.01 Scope of Part 1301.

Procedures governing the registration of manufacturers, distributors, and dispensers of controlled substances pursuant to sections 1301 through 1304 of the Act (21 U.S.C. 821–824) are set forth generally by those sections and specifically by the sections of this part.

§ 1301.02 Definitions.

As used in this part, the following terms shall have the meanings specified:

(a) The term "Act" means the Controlled Substances Act (84 Stat. 1242; 21 U.S.C. 801) and/or the Controlled Substances Import and Export Act (84 Stat. 1285; 21 U.S.C. 951).

(b) The term "basic class" means, as to controlled substances listed in Schedules I and II:

(1) Each of the opiates, including its isomers, esters, ethers, salts, and salts of isomers, esters, and ethers whenever the existence of such isomers, esters, ethers, and salts is possible within the specific chemical designation, listed in § 1308.11(b) of this chapter;

(2) Each of the opium derivatives, including its salts, isomers, and salts of isomers whenever the existence of such salts, isomers, and salts of isomers is possible within the specific chemical designation, listed in § 1308.11(c) of this chapter;

(3) Each of the hallucinogenic substances, including its salts, isomers, and salts of isomers whenever the existence of such salts, isomers, and salts of isomers is possible within the specific chemical designation, listed in § 1308.11(d) of this chapter;

(4) Each of the following substances, whether produced directly or indirectly by extraction from substances of vegetable origin, or independently by means of chemical synthesis, or by a combination of extraction and chemical synthesis:

(i) Opium, including raw opium, opium extracts, opium fluid extracts, powdered opium, granulated opium, deodorized opium and tincture of opium;
(ii) Apomorphine;
(iii) Codeine;
(iv) Etorphine hydrochloride;
(v) Ethylmorphine;
(vi) Hydrocodone;
(vii) Hydromorphone;
(viii) Metopon;
(ix) Morphine;
(x) Oxycodone;
(xi) Oxymorphone;
(xii) Thebaine;
(xiii) Mixed alkaloids of opium listed in § 1308.12(b)(2) of this chapter;
(xiv) Cocaine; and
(xv) Ecgonine.

(5) Each of the opiates, including its isomers, esters, ethers, salts, and salts of isomers, esters, and ethers whenever the existence of such isomers, esters, ethers, and salts is possible within the specific chemical designation, listed in § 1308.12(c) of this chapter; and

(6) Methamphetamine, its salts, isomers, and salts of its isomers;

(7) Amphetamine, its salts, optical isomers, and salts of its optical isomers;

(8) Phenmetrazine and its salts;

(9) Methylphenidate;

(10) Each of the substances having a depressant effect on the central nervous system, including its salts, isomers, and salts of isomers whenever the existence of such salts, isomers, and salts of isomers is possible within the specific chemical designation, listed in § 1308.12(e) of this chapter.

(c) The term "Administration" means the Drug Enforcement Administration.

(d) The term "compounder" means any person engaging in maintenance or detoxification treatment who also mixes, prepares, packages or changes the dosage form of a narcotic drug listed in Schedules II, III, IV or V for use in maintenance or detoxification treatment by another narcotic treatment program.

(e) The term *detoxification treatment* means the dispensing, for a period of time as specified below, of a narcotic drug or narcotic drugs in decreasing doses to an individual to alleviate adverse physiological or psychological effects incident to withdrawal from the continuous or sustained use of a narcotic drug and as a method of bringing the individual to a narcotic drug-free state within such period of time. There are two types of detoxification treatments: Short-term detoxification treatment and long-term detoxification treatment.

(1) *Short-term detoxification treatment* is for a period not in excess of 30 days.

(2) *Long-term detoxification treatment* is for a period more than 30 days but not in excess of 180 days.

(f) The term "Administrator" means the Administrator of the Drug Enforcement Administration. The Administrator has been delegated authority under the Act by the Attorney General (28 CFR 0.100).

(g) The term "hearing" means any hearing held pursuant to this part for the granting, denial, revocation, or suspension of a registration pursuant to sections 303 and 304 of the Act (21 U.S.C. 823–824).

(h) The term "maintenance treatment" means the dispensing for a period in excess of twenty-one days, of a narcotic drug or narcotic drugs in the treatment of an individual for dependence upon heroin or other morphine-like drug.

(i) The term "narcotic treatment program" means a program engaged in maintenance and/or detoxification treatment with narcotic drugs.

(j) The term "person" includes any individual, corporation, government or governmental subdivision or agency, business trust, partnership, association, or other legal entity.

(k) The terms "register" and "registration" refer only to registration required and permitted by section 303 of the Act (21 U.S.C. 823).

(l) The term "registrant" means any person who is registered pursuant to either section 303 or section 1008 of the Act (21 U.S.C. 823 or 958).

(m) Any term not defined in this section shall have the definition set forth in section 102 of the Act (21 U.S.C. 802).

§ 1301.03 Information; special instructions.

Information regarding procedures under these rules and instructions supplementing these rules will be furnished upon request by writing to the Registration Unit, Drug Enforcement Administration, Department of Justice, Post Office Box 28083, Central Station, Washington, DC 20005.

Fees for Registration and Reregistration

§ 1301.11 Fee amounts.

(c) For each registration or reregistration to dispense, or to conduct instructional activities with, controlled substances listed in Schedules II through V, the registrant shall pay an application fee of $60 for a three-year registration.

(d) For each registration to conduct research or instructional activities with a controlled substance listed in Schedule I, or to conduct research with a controlled substance in Schedules II through V, the registrant shall pay an application fee of $20.

(f) For each registration or reregistration to engage in a narcotic treatment program, including a compounder, the registrant shall pay an application fee of $5.

§ 1301.12 Time and method of payment; refund.

Application fees shall be paid at the time when the application for registration or reregistration is submitted for filing. Payments should be made in the form of a personal, certified, or cashier's check or money order made payable to "Drug Enforcement Administration." Payments made in the form of stamps, foreign currency, or third party endorsed checks will not be accepted. These application fees are not refundable.

Requirements for Registration

§ 1301.21 Persons required to register.

Every person who manufactures, distributes, or dispenses any controlled substance or who proposes to engage in the manufacture, distribution, or dispensing of any controlled substance shall obtain annually a registration unless exempted by law or pursuant to §§ 1301.24–1301.29. Only persons actually engaged in such activities are required to obtain a registration; related or affiliated persons who are not engaged in such activities are not required to be registered. (For example, a stockholder or parent corporation of a corporation manufacturing controlled substances is not required to obtain a registration.)

§ 1301.22 Separate registration for independent activities.

(a) The following groups of activities are deemed to be independent of each other:

(1) Manufacturing controlled substances;

(2) Distributing controlled substances;

(3) Dispensing controlled substances listed in Schedules II through V;

(4) Conducting research with controlled substances listed in Schedules II through V;

(5) Conducting instructional activities with controlled substances listed in Schedules II through V;

(6) Conducting a narcotic treatment program using any narcotic drug listed in Schedules II, III, IV or V, however, pursuant to § 1301.24, employees, agents, or affiliated practitioners, in programs, need not register separately. Each program site located away from the principal location and at which place narcotic drugs are stored or dispensed must be separately registered and obtain narcotic drugs by use of order forms pursuant to § 1305.03;

(7) Conducting research and instructional activities with controlled substances listed in Schedule I;

(8) Conducting chemical analysis with controlled substances listed in any schedule;

(9) Importing controlled substances;

(10) Exporting controlled substances; and

(11) A compounder as defined by § 1301.02(d).

(b) Every person who engages in more than one group of independent activities shall obtain a separate registration for each group of activities, except as provided in this paragraph. Any person, when registered to engage in the group of activities described in each subparagraph in this paragraph, shall be authorized to engage in the coincident activities described in that subparagraph without obtaining a registration to engage in such coincident activities, provided that, unless specifically exempted, he complies with all requirements and duties prescribed by law for persons registered to engage in such coincident activities;

(6) A person registered to dispense controlled substances listed in Schedules II through V shall be authorized to conduct research and to conduct instructional activities with those substances, except that a mid-level practitioner, as defined in 1304.02 (f), may conduct research coincident to his/her practitioner registration only to the extent expressly authorized by state statute.

(c) A single registration to engage in any group of independent activities may include one or more controlled substances listed in the schedules authorized in that group of independent activities. A person registered to conduct research with controlled substances listed in Schedule I may conduct research with any substance listed in Schedule I for which he has filed and had approved a research protocol.

§ 1301.23 Separate registrations for separate locations.

(a) A separate registration is required for each principal place of business or professional practice at one general physical location where controlled substances are manufactured, distributed, or dispensed by a person.

(b) The following locations shall be deemed not to be places where controlled substances are manufactured, distributed, or dispensed:

(1) A warehouse where controlled substances are stored by or on behalf of a registered person, unless such substances are distributed directly from such warehouse to registered locations other than the registered location from which the substances were delivered or to persons not required to register by virtue of subsection 302(c)(2) of the Act (21 U.S.C. 822(c)(2));

(2) An office used by agents of a registrant where sales of controlled substances are solicited, made, or supervised but which neither contains such substances (other than substances for display purposes or lawful distribution as samples only) nor serves as a distribution point for filling sales orders; and

(3) An office used by a practitioner (who is registered at another location) where controlled substances are prescribed but neither administered nor otherwise dispensed as a regular part of the professional practice of the practitioner at such office, and where no supplies of controlled substances are maintained.

§ 1301.24 Exemption of agents and employees; affiliated practitioners.

(a) The requirement of registration is waived for any agent or employee of a person who is registered to engage in any group of independent activities, if such agent or employee is acting in the usual course of his business or employment.

(b) An individual practitioner, as defined in § 1304.02 of this chapter (other than an intern, resident, foreign-trained physician, or physician on the staff of a Veterans Administration facility or physician who is an agent or employee of the Health Bureau of the Canal Zone Government), who is an agent or employee of another practitioner (other than a mid-level practitioner) registered to dispense controlled substances may, when acting in the usual course of his/her employment, administer and dispense (other than by issuance of prescription) controlled substances if and to the extent that such individual practitioner is authorized or permitted to do so by the jurisdiction in which he/she practices under the registration of the employer or principal practitioner in lieu of being registered him/herself. (For example, a staff physician employed by a hospital need not be registered individually to administer and dispense, other than by prescribing, controlled substances within the hospital.)

(c) An individual practitioner, as defined in § 1304.02 of this chapter, who is an intern, resident, mid-level practitioner, foreign-trained physician or physician on the staff of a Veterans Administration facility or physician who is an agent or employee of the Health Bureau of the Canal Zone Government, may dispense, administer and prescribe controlled substances under the registration of the hospital or other institution which is registered and by whom he/she is employed in lieu of being registered him/herself, provided that:

(1) Such dispensing, administering, or prescribing is done in the usual course of his professional practice;

(2) Such individual practitioner is authorized or permitted to do so by the jurisdiction in which he is practicing;

(3) The hospital or other institution by whom he is employed has verified that the individual practitioner is so permitted to dispense, administer, or prescribe drugs within the jurisdiction;

(4) Such individual practitioner is acting only within the scope of his employment in the hospital or institution;

(5) The hospital or other institution authorizes the intern, resident, or foreign-trained physician to dispense or prescribe under the hospital registration and designates a specific internal code number for each intern, resident, or foreign-trained physician so authorized. The code number shall consist of numbers, letters, or a combination thereof and shall be a suffix to the institution's DEA registration number, preceded by a hyphen (e.g., APO 123456-10 or APO 123456-A12); and

(6) A current list of internal codes and the corresponding individual practitioners is kept by the hospital or other institution and is made available at all times to other registrants and law enforcement agencies upon request for the purpose of verifying the authority of the prescribing individual practitioner.

§ 1301.25 Exemption of certain military and other personnel.

(a) The requirement of registration is waived for any official of the U.S. Army, Navy, Marine Corps, Air Force, Coast Guard, Public Health Service, or Bureau of Prisons who is authorized to prescribe, dispense, or administer, but not to procure or purchase, controlled substances in the course of his official duties. Such officials shall follow procedures set forth in Part 1306 of this chapter regarding prescriptions, but shall state the branch of service or agency (e.g., "U.S. Army" or "Public Health Service") and the service identification number of the issuing official in lieu of the registration number required on prescription forms. The service identification number for a Public Health Service employee is his Social Security identification number.

(b) If any official exempted by this section also engages as a private individual in any activity or group of activities for which registration is required, such official shall obtain a registration for such private activities.

§ 1301.28 Registration regarding ocean vessels.

(a) If acquired by and dispensed under the general supervision of a medical officer described in paragraph (b) of this section, or the master or first officer of the vessel under the circumstances described in paragraph (d) of this section, controlled substances may be held for stocking, be maintained in, and dispensed from medicine chests, first aid packets, or dispensaries:

(1) On board any vessel engaged in international trade or in trade between ports of the United States and any merchant vessel belonging to the U.S. Government;

(2) On board any aircraft operated by an air carrier under a certificate of permit issued pursuant to the Federal Aviation Act of 1958 (49 U.S.C. 1301); and

(3) In any other entity of fixed or transient location approved by the Administrator as appropriate for application of this section (e.g., emergency kits at field sites of an industrial firm).

(b) A medical officer shall be:

(1) Licensed in a state as a physician;

(2) Employed by the owner or operator of the vessel, aircraft or other entity; and

(3) Registered under the Act at either of the following locations:

(i) The principal office of the owner or operator of the vessel, aircraft or other entity or

(ii) At any other location provided that the name, address, registration number, and expiration date as they appear on his Certificate of Registration (DEA Form 223) for this location are maintained for inspection at said principal office in a readily retrievable manner.

(c) A registered medical officer may serve as medical officer for more than one vessel, aircraft, or other entity under a single registration, unless he serves as medical officer for more than one owner or operator, in which case he shall either maintain a separate registration at the location of the principal office of each such owner or operator or utilize one or more registrations pursuant to paragraph (b)(3)(ii) of this section.

(d) If no medical officer is employed by the owner or operator of a vessel, or in the event such medical officer is not accessible and the acquisition of controlled substances is required, the master or first officer of the vessel, who shall not be registered under the Act, may purchase controlled substances from a registered manufacturer or distributor, or from an authorized pharmacy as described in paragraph (f) of this section, by following the procedure outlined below:

(1) The master or first officer of the vessel must personally appear at the vendor's place of business, present proper identification (e.g., Seaman's photographic identification card) and a written requisition for the controlled substances.

(2) The written requisition must be on the vessel's official stationery or purchase order form and must include the name and address of the vendor, the name of the controlled substance, description of the controlled substance (dosage form, strength and number or volume per container), number of containers ordered, the name of the vessel, the vessel's official number and country of registry, the owner or operator of the vessel, the port at which the vessel is located, signature of the vessel's officer who is ordering the controlled substances and the date of the requisition.

(3) The vendor may, after verifying the identification of the vessel's officer requisitioning the controlled substances, deliver the control substances to that officer. The transaction shall be documented, in triplicate, on a record of sale in a format similar to that outlined in paragraph (d)(4) of this section. The vessel's requisition shall be attached to copy 1 of the record of sale and filed with the controlled substances records of the vendor, copy 2 of the record of sale shall be furnished to the officer of the vessel and retained aboard the vessel, copy 3 of the record of sale shall be forwarded to the nearest DEA Division Office within 15 days after the end of the month in which the sale is made.

(4) The vendor's record of sale should be similar to, and must include all the information contained in, the below listed format.

Sale of Controlled Substances to Vessels

(Name of registrant) ____________

(Address of registrant) ____________

(DEA registration number) ____________

Line No.	Number of packages ordered	Size of packages	Name of product	Packages distributed	Date distributed
1					
2					
3					

Line numbers may be continued according to needs of the vendor.

Number of lines completed ____________

Name of vessel ____________

Vessel's official number ____________

Vessel's country of registry ____________

Owner or operator of the vessel ____________

Name and title of vessel's officer who presented the requisition ____________

Signature of vessel's officer who presented the requisition ____________

(e) Any medical officer described in paragraph (b) of this section shall, in addition to complying with all requirements and duties prescribed for registrants generally, prepare an annual report as of the date on which his registration expires, which shall give in detail an accounting for each vessel, aircraft, or other entity, and a summary accounting for all vessels, aircraft, or other entities under his supervision for all controlled substances purchased, dispensed or disposed of during the year. The medical officer shall maintain this report with other records required to be kept under the Act and, upon request, deliver a copy of the report to the Administration. The medical officer need not be present when controlled substances are dispensed, if the person who actually dispensed the controlled substances is responsible to the medical officer to justify his actions.

(f) Any registered pharmacy which wishes to distribute controlled substances pursuant to this section shall be authorized to do so, provided that:

(1) The registered pharmacy notifies the nearest Division Office of the Administration of its intention to so distribute controlled substances prior to the initiation of such activity. This notification shall be by registered mail and shall contain the name, address, and registration number of the pharmacy as well as the date upon which such activity will commence; and

(2) Such activity is authorized by State law; and

(3) The total number of dosage units of all controlled substances distributed by the pharmacy during any calendar year in which the pharmacy is registered to dispense does not exceed the limitations imposed upon such distribution by § 1307.11(a)(4) and (b) of this chapter.

(g) Owners or operators of vessels, aircraft, or other entities described in this section shall not be deemed to possess or dispense any controlled substance acquired, stored and dispensed in accordance with this section.

(h) The Master of a vessel shall prepare a report for each calendar year which shall give in detail an accounting for all controlled substances purchased, dispensed, or disposed of during the year. The Master shall file this report with the medical officer employed by the owner or operator of his vessel, if any, or, if not, he shall maintain this report with other records required to be kept under the Act and, upon request, deliver a copy of the report to the Administration.

(i) Controlled substances acquired and possessed in accordance with this section shall not be distributed to persons not under the general supervision of the medical officer employed by the owner or operator of the vessel, aircraft, or other entity, except in accordance with § 1307.21 of this chapter.

§ 1301.29 Provisional registration of narcotic treatment programs; compounders.

(a) All persons currently approved by the Food and Drug Administration under § 310.505 (formerly § 130.44) of this title to conduct a methadone treatment program and who are registered by the Drug Enforcement Administration under this section will be granted a Provisional Narcotic Treatment Program Registration.

(b) The provisions of §§ 1301.45–1301.57 relating to revocation and suspension of registration, shall apply to a provisional registration.

(c) Unless sooner revoked or suspended under paragraph (b) of this section, a provisional registration shall remain in effect until (1) the date on which such person has registered under this section or has had his registration denied, or (2) such date as may be prescribed by written notification to the person from the Drug Enforcement Administration for the person to become registered to conduct a narcotic treatment program, whichever occurs first.

Applications for Registration

§ 1301.31 Time for application for registration; expiration date.

(a) Any person who is required to be registered and who is not so registered may apply for registration at any time. No person required to be registered shall engage in any activity for which registration is required until the application for registration is granted and a Certificate of Registration is issued by the Administrator to such person.

(b) Any person who is registered may apply to be reregistered not more than 60 days before the expiration date of his registration.

(c) At the time a manufacturer, distributor, researcher, analytical lab, importer, exporter or narcotic treatment program is first registered, that business activity shall be assigned to one of twelve groups, which shall correspond to the months of the year. The expiration date of the registrations of all registrants within any group will be the last date of the month designated for that group. In assigning any of the above business activities to a group, the Administration may select a group the expiration date of which is less than one year from the date such business activity was registered. If the business activity is assigned to a group which has an expiration date less than three months from the date on which the business activity is registered, the registration shall not expire until one year from that expiration date; in all other cases, the registration shall expire on the expiration date following the date on which the business activity is registered.

(d) At the time a retail pharmacy, hospital/clinic, practitioner or teaching institution is first registered, that business activity shall be assigned to one of twelve groups, which shall correspond to the months of the year. The expiration date of the registrations of all registrants within any group will be the last day of the month designated for that group. In assigning any of the above business activities to a group, the Administration may select a group the expiration date of which is not less than 28 months nor more than 39 months from the date such business activity was registered. After the initial registration period, the registration shall expire 36 months from the initial expiration date.

§ 1301.32 Application forms; contents; signature.

(a) If any person is required to be registered, and is not so registered and is applying for registration:

(1) To manufacture or distribute controlled substances, he shall apply on DEA Form 225;

(2) To dispense controlled substances listed in Schedules II through V, he shall apply on DEA Form 224;

(9) To conduct a narcotic treatment program, including a compounder, he shall apply on DEA Form 363.

(b) If any person is registered and is applying for reregistration:

(1) To manufacture or distribute controlled substances, he shall apply on DEA Form 225a;

(2) To dispense controlled substances listed in Schedules II through V, he shall apply on DEA Form 224A;

(9) To conduct a narcotic treatment program, including a compounder, he shall apply on DEA Form 363a (Renewal Form).

(c) DEA (or BND) Forms 224 and 225 may be obtained at any regional office of the Administration or by writing to the Registration Unit, Drug Enforcement Administration, Department of Justice, Post Office Box 28083, Central Station, Washington, DC 20005. DEA Forms 224a, 225a and 363a will be mailed, as applicable, to each registered person approximately 60 days before the expiration date of his registration; if any registered person does not receive such forms within 45 days before the expiration date of his registration, he must promptly give notice of such fact and request such forms by writing to the Registration Unit of the Administration at the foregoing address.

(d) Each application for registration to handle any basic class of controlled substance listed in Schedule I (except to conduct chemical analysis with such classes) and each application for registration to manufacture a basic class of controlled substance listed in Schedule II shall include the Administration Controlled Substances Code Number, as set forth in Part 1308 of this chapter, for each basic class to be covered by such registration.

(e) Each application for registration to conduct research with any basic class of controlled substance listed in Schedule II shall include the Administration Controlled Substances Code Number, as set forth in Part 1308 of this chapter, for each such basic class to be manufactured or imported as a coincident activity of that registration. A statement listing the quantity of each such basic class or controlled substance to be imported or manufactured during the registration period for which application is being made shall be included with each such application. For purposes of this paragraph only, manufacturing is defined as the production of a controlled substance by synthesis, extraction or by agricultural/horticultural means.

(f) Each application shall include all information called for in the form, unless the item is not applicable, in which case this fact shall be indicated.

(g) Each application, attachment, or other document filed as part of an application, shall be signed by the applicant, if an individual; by a partner of the applicant, if a partnership; or by an officer of the applicant, if a corporation, corporate division, association, trust or other entity. An applicant may authorize one or more individuals, who would not otherwise be authorized to do so, to sign applications for the applicant by filing with the Registration Unit of the Administration a power of attorney for each such individual. The power of attorney shall be signed by a person who is authorized to sign applications under this paragraph and shall contain the signature of the individual being authorized to sign applications. The power of attorney shall be valid until revoked by the applicant.

§ 1301.34 Filing of application; joint filings.

(a) All applications for registration shall be submitted for filing to the Registration Unit, Drug Enforcement Administration, Department of Justice, Post Office Box 28083, Central Station, Washington, DC 20005. The appropriate registration fee and any required attachments must accompany the application.

(b) Any person required to obtain more than one registration may submit all applications in one package. Each application must be complete and should not refer to any accompanying application for required information.

§ 1301.35 Acceptance for filing; defective applications.

(a) Applications submitted for filing are dated upon receipt. If found to be complete, the application will be accepted for filing. Applications failing to comply with the requirements of this part will not generally be accepted for filing. In the case of minor defects as to completeness, the Administrator may accept the application for filing with a request to the applicant for additional information. A defective application will be returned to the applicant within 10 days following its receipt with a statement of the reason for not accepting the application for filing. A defective application may be corrected and resubmitted for filing at any time; the Administrator shall accept for filing any application upon resubmission by the applicant, whether complete or not.

(b) Accepting an application for filing does not preclude any subsequent request for additional information pursuant to § 1301.36 and has no bearing on whether the application will be granted.

§ 1301.36 Additional information.

The Administrator may require an applicant to submit such documents or written statements of fact relevant to the application as he deems necessary to determine whether the application should be granted. The failure of the applicant to provide such documents or statements within a reasonable time after being requested to do so shall be deemed to be a waiver by the applicant of an opportunity to present such documents or facts for consideration by the Administrator in granting or denying the application.

§ 1301.37 Amendments to and withdrawal of applications.

(a) An application may be amended or withdrawn without permission of the Administrator at any time before the date on which the applicant receives an order to show cause pursuant to § 1301.48, or before the date on which a notice of hearing on the application is published pursuant to § 1301.43, whichever is sooner. An application may be amended or withdrawn with permission of the Administrator at any time where good cause is shown by the applicant or where the amendment or withdrawal is in the public interest.

(b) After an application has been accepted for filing, the request by the applicant that it be returned or the failure of the applicant to respond to official correspondence regarding the application, when sent by registered or certified mail, return receipt requested, shall be deemed to be a withdrawal of the application.

§ 1301.38 Special procedures for certain applications.

(a) If, at the time of application for registration of a new pharmacy, the pharmacy has been issued a license from the appropriate State licensing agency, the applicant may include with his application an affidavit as to the existence of the State license in the following form:

AFFIDAVIT FOR NEW PHARMACY

I, ______________, the ______________________
(Title of officer, official, partner,

______________ of ______________________________
or other position) (Corporation, partnership, or sole

__________, doing business as ____________ at ____________
proprietor) (Store name) (Number

____,
and Street) (City) (State) (Zip code)

hereby certify that said store was issued a pharmacy permit No. ________ by the ______________________________
(Board of Pharmacy or Licensing Agency)

of the State of ______________ on ______________.
(Date)

This statement is submitted in order to obtain a Drug Enforcement Administration registration number. I understand that if any information is false, the Administration may immediately suspend the registration for this store and commence proceedings to revoke under 21 U.S.C. 824(a) because of the danger to public health and safety. I further understand that any false information contained in this affidavit may subject me personally and the above-named corporation/partnership/business to prosecution under 21 U.S.C. 843, the penalties for conviction of which include imprisonment for up to 4 years, a fine of not more than $30,000 or both.

____
Signature (Person who Signs Application for Registration)

State of ______________

County of ______________

Subscribed to and sworn before me this ______________ day of ______________, 19______.

____
Notary Public

(b) Whenever the ownership of a pharmacy is being transferred from one person to another, if the transferee owns at least one other pharmacy licensed in the same State as the one the ownership of which is being transferred, the transferee may apply for registration prior to the date of transfer. The Administrator may register the applicant and authorize him to obtain controlled substances at the time of transfer. Such registration shall not authorize the transferee to dispense controlled substances until the pharmacy has been issued a valid State license. The transferee shall include with his application the following affidavit:

AFFIDAVIT FOR TRANSFER OF PHARMACY

I, ______________, the ______________________
(Title of officer, official, partner

______________ of ______________________________
or other position) (Corporation, partnership, or sole

__________, doing business as ______________________,
proprietor) (Store name)

hereby certify:

(1) That said company was issued a pharmacy permit No. ________ by the ______________________________
(Board of Pharmacy or Licensing Agency)

of the State of ______________ and a DEA Registration Number ________ for a pharmacy located at ______________________
(Number and Street)

______________________________________; and
(City) (State) (Zip code)

(2) That said company is acquiring the pharmacy business of ______________ doing business as ______________
(Name of Seller)

with DEA Registration Number ______________ on or about ______________ and that said company has applied (or will
(Date of Transfer)

apply) on ______________ for a pharmacy permit from the
(Date)

board of pharmacy (or licensing agency) of the State of ______________ to do business as ______________________
(Store name)

at ____.
(Number and Street) (City) (State) (Zip code)

This statement is submitted in order to obtain a Drug Enforcement Administration registration number.

I understand that if a DEA registration number is issued, the pharmacy may acquire controlled substances but may not dispense them until a pharmacy permit or license is issued by the State board of pharmacy or licensing agency.

I understand that if any information is false, the Administration may immediately suspend the registration for this store and commence proceedings to revoke under 21 U.S.C. 824(a) because of the danger to public health and safety. I further understand that any false information contained in this affidavit may subject me personally to prosecution under 21 U.S.C. 843, the penalties for conviction of which include imprisonment for up to 4 years, a fine of not more than $30,000 or both.

____
Signature (Person who Signs Application for Registration)

State of __________
County of __________
Subscribed to and sworn before me this __________ day of __________, 19 ____.

____
Notary Public

(c) The Administrator shall follow the normal procedures for approving an application to verify the statements in the affidavit. If the statements prove to be false, the Administrator may revoke the registration on the basis of section 1304(a)(1) of the Act [21 U.S.C. 824(a)(1)] and suspend the registration immediately by pending revocation on the basis of section 1304(d) of the Act [21 U.S.C. 824(d)]. At the same time, the Administrator may seize and place under seal all controlled substances possessed by the applicant under section 1304(f) of the Act [21 U.S.C. 824(f)]. Intentional misuse of the affidavit procedure may subject the applicant to prosecution for fraud under section 403(a)(4) of the Act [21 U.S.C. 843(a)(4)], and obtaining controlled substances under a registration fraudulently gotten may subject the applicant to prosecution under section 403(a)(3) of the Act [21 U.S.C. 843(a)(3)]. The penalties for conviction of either offense include imprisonment for up to 4 years, a fine not exceeding $30,000 or both.

Action on Applications for Registration: Revocation or Suspension of Registration

§ 1301.41 Administrative review generally.

The Administrator may inspect, or cause to be inspected, the establishment of an applicant or registrant, pursuant to Subpart A of Part 1316 of this chapter. The Administrator shall review the application for registration and other information gathered by the Administrator regarding an applicant in order to determine whether the applicable standards of section 1303 of the Act (21 U.S.C. 823) have been met by the applicant.

§ 1301.44 Certificate of registration; denial of registration.

(a) The Administrator shall issue a Certificate of Registration (DEA Form 223) to an applicant if the issuance of registration or reregistration is required under the applicable provisions of section 303 of the Act (21 U.S.C. 823). In the event that the issuance of registration or reregistration is not required, the Administrator shall deny the application. Before denying any application, the Administrator shall issue an order to show cause pursuant to § 1301.48 and, if requested by the applicant, shall hold a hearing on the application pursuant to § 1301.51.

(b) The Certificate of Registration (DEA Form 223) shall contain the name, address, and registration number of the registrant, the activity authorized by the registration, the schedules and/or Administration Controlled Substances Code Number (as set forth in Part 1308 of this chapter) of the controlled substances which the registrant is authorized to handle, the amount of fee paid (or exemption), and the expiration date of the registration. The registrant shall maintain the certificate of registration at the registered location in a readily retrievable manner and shall permit inspection of the certificate by any official, agent or employee of the Administration or of any Federal, State, or local agency engaged in enforcement of laws relating to controlled substances.

§ 1301.47 Extension of registration pending final order.

In the event that an applicant for reregistration (who is doing business under a registration previously granted and not revoked or suspended) has applied for reregistration at least 45 days before the date on which the existing registration is due to expire, and the Administrator has issued no order on the application on the date on which the existing registration is due to expire, the existing registration of the applicant shall automatically be extended and continue in effect until the date on which the Administrator so issues his order. The Administrator may extend any other existing registration under the circumstances contemplated in this section even though the registrant failed to apply for reregistration at least 45 days before expiration of the existing registration, with or without request by the registrant, if the Administrator finds that such extension is not inconsistent with the public health and safety.

Modification, Transfer and Termination of Registration

§ 1301.61 Modification in registration.

Any registrant may apply to modify his registration to authorize the handling of additional controlled substances or to change his name or address, by submitting a letter of request to the Registration Unit, Drug Enforcement Administration, Department of Justice, Post Office Box 28083, Central Station, Washington, DC 20005. The letter shall contain the registrant's name, address, and registration number as printed on the certificate of registration, and the substances and/or schedules to be added to his registration or the new name or address and shall be signed in accordance with § 1301.32(f). If the registrant is seeking to handle additional controlled substances listed in Schedule I for the purpose of research or instructional activities, he shall attach three copies of a research protocol describing each research project involving the additional substances, or two copies of a statement describing the nature, extent, and duration of such instructional activities, as appropriate. No fee shall be required to be paid for the modification. The request for modification shall be handled in the same manner as an application for registration. If the modification in registration is approved, the Administrator shall issue a new certificate of registration (DEA Form 223) to the registrant, who shall maintain it with the old certificate of registration until expiration.

§ 1301.62 Termination of registration.

The registration of any person shall terminate if and when such person dies, ceases legal existence, or discontinues business or professional practice. Any registrant who ceases legal existence or discontinues business or professional practice shall notify the Administrator promptly of such fact.

§ 1301.63 Transfer of registration.

No registration or any authority conferred thereby shall be assigned or otherwise transferred except upon such conditions as the Administrator may specifically designate and then only pursuant to his written consent.

Security Requirements

§ 1301.71 Security requirements generally.

(a) All applicants and registrants shall provide effective controls and procedures to guard against theft and diversion of controlled substances. In order to determine whether a registrant has provided effective controls against diversion, the Administrator shall use the security requirements set forth in §§ 1301.72–1301.76 as standards for the physical security controls and operating procedures necessary to prevent diversion. Materials and construction which will provide a structural equivalent to the physical security controls set forth in §§ 1301.72, 1301.73, and 1301.75 may be used in lieu of the materials and construction described in those sections.

§ 1301.72 Physical security controls for nonpractitioners; narcotic treatment programs and compounders for narcotic treatment programs; storage areas.

(a) *Schedules I* and *II*. Raw materials, bulk materials awaiting further processing, and finished products which are controlled substances listed in Schedule I or II shall be stored in one of the following secure storage areas:

(1) Where small quantities permit, a safe or steel cabinet:

(i) Which safe or steel cabinet shall have the following specifications or the equivalent: 30 man-minutes against surreptitious entry, 10 man-minutes against forced entry, 20 man-hours against lock manipulation, and 20 man-hours against radiological techniques;

(ii) Which safe or steel cabinet, if it weighs less than 750 pounds, is bolted or cemented to the floor or wall in such a way that it cannot be readily removed; and

(iii) Which safe or steel cabinet, if necessary, depending upon the quantities and type of controlled substances stored, is equipped with an alarm system which, upon attempted unauthorized entry, shall transmit a signal directly to a central protection company or a local or State police agency which has a legal duty to respond, or a 24-hour control station operated by the registrant, or such other protection as the Administrator may approve.

(2) A vault constructed before, or under construction on, September 1, 1971, which is of substantial construction with a steel door, combination or key lock, and an alarm system; or

(3) A vault constructed after September 1, 1971:

(i) The walls, floors, and ceilings of which vault are constructed of at least 8 inches of reinforced concrete or other substantial masonry, reinforced vertically and horizontally with ½-inch steel rods tied 6 inches on center, or the structural equivalent to such reinforced walls, floors, and ceilings;

(ii) The door and frame unit of which vault shall conform to the following specifications or the equivalent: 30 man-minutes against surreptitious entry, 10 man-minutes against forced entry, 20 man-hours against lock manipulation, and 20 man-hours against radiological techniques;

(iii) Which vault, if operations require it to remain open for frequent access, is equipped with a "day-gate" which is self-closing and self-locking, or the equivalent, for use during the hours of operation in which the vault door is open;

(iv) The walls or perimeter of which vault are equipped with an alarm, which upon unauthorized entry shall transmit a signal directly to a central station protection company, or a local or State police agency which has a legal duty to respond, or a 24-hour control station operated by the registrant, or such other protection as the Administrator may approve, and, if necessary, holdup buttons at strategic points of entry to the perimeter area of the vault;

(v) The door of which vault is equipped with contact switches; and

(vi) Which vault has one of the following: complete electrical lacing of the walls, floor and ceilings; sensitive ultrasonic equipment within the vault; a sensitive sound accumulator system; or such other device designed to detect illegal entry as may be approved by the Administration.

(b) *Schedules III, IV, and V.* Raw materials, bulk materials awaiting further processing, and finished products which are controlled substances listed in Schedules III, IV, and V shall be stored in the following secure storage areas:

(1) A safe or steel cabinet as described in paragraph (a)(1) of this section;

(2) A vault as described in paragraph (a)(2) or (3) of this section equipped with an alarm system as described in paragraph (b)(4)(v) of this section;

(3) A building used for storage of Schedules III through V controlled substances with perimeter security which limits access during working hours and provides security after working hours and meets the following specifications:

(i) Has an electronic alarm system as described in paragraph (b)(4)(v) of this section,

(ii) Is equipped with self-closing, self-locking doors constructed of substantial material commensurate with the type of building construction, provided, however, a door which is kept closed and locked at all times when not in use and when in use is kept under direct observation of a responsible employee or agent of the registrant is permitted in lieu of a self-closing, self-locking door. Doors may be sliding or hinged. Regarding hinged doors, where hinges are mounted on the outside, such hinges shall be sealed, welded or otherwise constructed to inhibit removal. Locking devices for such doors shall be either of the multiple-position combination or key lock type and:

(a) In the case of key locks, shall require key control which limits access to a limited number of employees, or;

(b) In the case of combination locks, the combination shall be limited to a minimum number of employees and can be changed upon termination of employment of an employee having knowledge of the combination;

(4) A cage, located within a building on the premises, meeting the following specifications:

(i) Having walls constructed of not less than No. 10 gauge steel fabric mounted on steel posts, which posts are:

(a) At least one inch in diameter;

(b) Set in concrete or installed with lay bolts that are pinned or brazed; and

(c) Which are placed no more than ten feet apart with horizontal one and one-half inch reinforcements every sixty inches.

(ii) Having a mesh construction with openings of not more than two and one-half inches across the square,

(iii) Having a ceiling constructed of the same material, or in the alternative, a cage shall be erected which reaches and is securely attached to the structural ceiling of the building. A lighter gauge mesh may be used for the ceilings of large enclosed areas if walls are at least 14 feet in height,

(iv) Is equipped with a door constructed of No. 10 gauge steel fabric on a metal door frame in a metal door flange, and in all other respects conforms to all the requirements of 21 CFR 1301.72(b)(3)(ii), and

(v) Is equipped with an alarm system which upon unauthorized entry shall transmit a signal directly to a central station protection agency or a local or State police agency, each having a legal duty to respond, or to a 24-hour control station operated by the registrant, or to such other source of protection as the Administrator may approve;

(5) An enclosure of masonry or other material, approved in writing by the Administrator as providing security comparable to a cage;

(6) A building or enclosure within a building which has been inspected and approved by DEA or its predecessor agency, BNDD, and continues to provide adequate security against the diversion of Schedule III through V controlled substances, of which fact written acknowledgment has been made by the Special Agent in Charge of DEA for the area in which such building or enclosure is situated;

(7) Such other secure storage areas as may be approved by the Administrator after considering the factors listed in § 1301.71(b), (1) through (14);

(8)(i) Schedule III through V controlled substances may be stored with Schedules I and II controlled substances under security measures provided by 21 CFR 1301.72(a);

(ii) Noncontrolled drugs, substances and other materials may be stored with Schedule III through V controlled substances in any of the secure storage areas required by 21 CFR 1301.72(b), provided that permission for such storage of noncontrolled items is obtained in advance, in writing, from the Special Agent in Charge of DEA for the area in which such storage area is situated. Any such permission tendered must be upon the Special Agent in Charge's written determination that such nonsegregated storage does not diminish security effectiveness for Schedule III through V controlled substances.

(c) *Multiple storage areas.* Where several types or classes of controlled substances are handled separately by the registrant or applicant for different purposes (e.g., returned goods or goods in process), the controlled substances may be stored separately, provided that each storage area complies with the requirements set forth in this section.

(d) *Accessibility to storage areas.* The controlled substances storage areas shall be accessible only to an absolute minimum number of specifically authorized employees. When it is necessary for employee maintenance personnel, nonemployee maintenance personnel, business guests, or visitors to be present in or pass through controlled substances storage areas, the registrant shall provide for adequate observation of the area by an employee specifically authorized in writing.

§ 1301.73 Physical security controls for nonpractitioners; compounders for narcotic treatment programs; manufacturing and compounding areas.

All manufacturing activities (including processing, packaging and labeling) involving controlled substances listed in any schedule and all activities of compounders shall be conducted in accordance with the following:

(a) All in-process substances shall be returned to the controlled substances storage area at the termination of the process. If the process is not terminated at the end of a workday (except where a continuous process or other normal manufacturing operation should not be interrupted), the processing area or tanks, vessels, bins, or bulk containers containing such substances shall be securely locked, with adequate security for the area or building. If such security requires an alarm, such alarm, upon unauthorized entry, shall transmit a signal directly to a central station protection company, or local or State police agency which has a legal duty to respond, or a 24-hour control station operated by the registrant.

(b) Manufacturing activities with controlled substances shall be conducted in an area or areas of clearly defined limited access which is under surveillance by an employee or employees designated in writing as responsible for the area. "Limited access" may be provided, in the absence of physical dividers such as walls or partitions, by traffic control lines or restricted space designation. The employee designated as responsible for the area may be engaged in the particular manufacturing operation being conducted: *Provided,* That he is able to provide continuous surveillance of the area in order that unauthorized persons may not enter or leave the area without his knowledge.

(c) During the production of controlled substances, the manufacturing areas shall be accessible to only those employees required for efficient operation. When it is necessary for employee maintenance personnel, nonemployee maintenance personnel, business guests, or visitors to be present in or pass through manufacturing areas during production of controlled substances, the registrant shall provide for adequate observation of the area by an employee specifically authorized in writing.

§ 1301.74 Other security controls for nonpractitioners; narcotic treatment programs and compounders for narcotic treatment programs.

(c) The registrant shall notify the Field Division Office of the Administration in his area of any theft or significant loss of any controlled substances upon discovery of such theft or loss. The supplier shall be responsible for reporting in-transit losses of controlled substances by the common or contract carrier selected pursuant to § 1301.74(e), upon discovery of such theft or loss. The registrant shall also complete DEA Form 106 regarding such theft or loss. Thefts must be reported whether or not the controlled substances are subsequently recovered and/or the responsible parties are identified and action taken against them.

(h) The acceptance of delivery of narcotic substances by a narcotic treatment program shall be made only by a licensed practitioner employed at the facility or other authorized individuals designated in writing. At the time of delivery, the licensed practitioner or other authorized individual designated in writing (excluding persons currently or previously dependent on narcotic drugs), shall sign for the narcotics and place his specific title (if any) on any invoice. Copies of these signed invoices shall be kept by the distributor.

(i) Narcotics dispensed or administered at a narcotic treatment program will be dispensed or administered directly to the patient by either (1) the licensed practitioner, (2) a registered nurse under the direction of the licensed practitioner, (3) a licensed practical nurse under the direction of the licensed practitioner, or (4) a pharmacist under the direction of the licensed practitioner.

(j) Persons enrolled in a narcotic treatment program will be required to wait in an area physically separated from the narcotic storage and dispensing area. This requirement will be enforced by the program physician and employees.

(k) All narcotic treatment programs must comply with standards established by the Secretary of Health and Human Services (after consultation with the Administration) respecting the quantities of narcotic drugs which may be provided to persons enrolled in a narcotic treatment program for unsupervised use.

(l) DEA may exercise discretion regarding the degree of security required in narcotic treatment programs based on such factors as the location of a program, the number of patients enrolled in a program and the number of physicians, staff members and security guards. Similarly, such factors will be taken into consideration when evaluating existing security or requiring new security at a narcotic treatment program.

§ 1301.75 Physical security controls for practitioners.

(a) Controlled substances listed in Schedule I shall be stored in a securely locked, substantially constructed cabinet.

(b) Controlled substances listed in Schedules II, III, IV, and V shall be stored in a securely locked, substantially constructed cabinet. However, pharmacies and institutional practitioners [as defined in § 1304.02(e) of this chapter] may disperse such substances throughout the stock of noncontrolled substances in such a manner as to obstruct the theft or diversion of the controlled substances.

(d) Carfentanil, etorphine hydrochloride, and diprenorphine shall be stored in a safe or steel cabinet equivalent to a U.S. Government Class V security container.

§ 1301.76 Other security controls for practitioners.

(a) The registrant shall not employ, as an agent or employee who has access to controlled substances, any person who has been convicted of a felony offense relating to controlled substances or who, at any time, had an application for registration with the DEA denied, had a DEA registration revoked or has surrendered a DEA registration for cause. For purposes of this subsection, the term "for cause" means a surrender in lieu of, or as a consequence of, any federal or state administrative, civil or criminal action resulting from an investigation of the individual's handling of controlled substances.

(b) The registrant shall notify the Field Division Office of the Administration in his area of the theft or significant loss of any controlled substances upon discovery of such loss or theft. The registrant shall also complete DEA (or BND) Form 106 regarding such loss or theft.

(c) Whenever the registrant distributes a controlled substance [without being registered as a distributor, as permitted in § 1301.22(b) and/or §§ 1307.11–1307.14], he shall comply with the requirements imposed on nonpractitioners in § 1301.74(a), (b), and (e).

Labeling and Packaging Requirements for Controlled Substances

§ 1302.02 Definitions.

As used in this part, the following terms shall have the meanings specified:

(a) The term "commercial container" means any bottle, jar, tube, ampule, or other receptacle in which a substance is held for distribution or dispensing to an ultimate user, and in addition, any box or package in which the receptacle is held for distribution or dispensing to an ultimate user. The term "commercial container" does not include any package liner, package insert or other material kept with or within a commercial container, nor any carton, crate, drum, or other package in which commercial containers are stored or are used for shipment of controlled substances.

(b) The term "label" means any display of written, printed, or graphic matter placed upon the commercial container of any controlled substance by any manufacturer of such substance.

(c) The term "labeling" means all labels and other written, printed, or graphic matter (1) upon any controlled substance or any of its commercial containers or wrappers, or (2) accompanying such controlled substance.

(d) The term "manufacture" means the producing, preparation, propagation, compounding, or processing of a drug or other substance or the packaging or repackaging of such substance, or the labeling or relabeling of the commercial container of such substance, but does not include the activities of a practitioner who, as an incident to his administration or dispensing such substance in the course of his professional practice, prepares, compounds, packages or labels such substance. The term "manufacturer" means a person who manufactures a drug or other substance, whether under a registration as a manufacturer or under authority of registration as a researcher or chemical analyst.

§ 1302.03 Symbol required; exceptions.

(a) Each commercial container of a controlled substance (except for a controlled substance excepted by the Administrator pursuant to § 1308.31 of this chapter) shall have printed on the label the symbol designating the schedule in which such controlled substance is listed. Each such commercial container, if it otherwise has no label, must bear a label complying with the requirement of this part.

(b) Each manufacturer shall print upon the labeling of each controlled substance distributed by him the symbol designating the schedule in which such controlled substance is listed.

(c) The following symbols shall designate the schedule corresponding thereto:

Schedule	*Symbol*
Schedule I	CI or C-I.
Schedule II	CII or C-II.
Schedule III	CIII or C-III.
Schedule IV	CIV or C-IV.
Schedule V	CV or C-V.

The word "schedule" need not be used. No distinction need be made between narcotic and nonnarcotic substances.

(d) The symbol is not required on a carton or wrapper in which a commercial container is held if the symbol is easily legible through such carton or wrapper.

(e) The symbol is not required on a commercial container too small or otherwise unable to accommodate a label, if the symbol is printed on the box or package from which the commercial container is removed upon dispensing to an ultimate user.

(f) The symbol is not required on a commercial container containing, or on the labeling of, a controlled substance being utilized in clinical research involving blind and double blind studies.

§ 1302.04 Location and size of symbol on label.

(a) The symbol shall be prominently located on the right upper corner of the principal panel of the label of the commercial container and/or the panel of the commercial container normally displayed to dispensers of any controlled substance listed in Schedules I through V. The symbol must be at least two times as large as the largest type otherwise printed on the label.

(b) In lieu of locating the symbol in the corner of the label, as prescribed in paragraph (a) of this section, the symbol may be overprinted on the label, in which case the symbol must be printed at least one-half the height of the label and in a contrasting color providing clear visibility against the background color of the label.

(c) In all cases the symbol shall be clear and large enough to afford easy identification of the schedule of the controlled substance upon inspection without removal from the dispenser's shelf.

§ 1302.05 Location and size of symbol on labeling.

The symbol shall be prominently located on all labeling other than labels covered by § 1302.04. In all cases the symbol shall be clear and large enough to afford prompt identification of the controlled substance upon inspection of the labeling.

§ 1302.07 Sealing of controlled substances.

(a) On each bottle, multiple-dose vial, or other commercial container of any controlled substance listed in Schedule I or II or of any narcotic controlled substance listed in Schedule III or IV, there shall be securely affixed to the stopper, cap, lid, covering, or wrapper of such container a seal to disclose upon inspection any tampering or opening of the container.

Records and Reports of Registrants

§ 1304.02 Definitions.

As used in this part, the following terms shall have the meanings specified:

(a) The term "Act" means the Controlled Substances Act (84 Stat. 1242; 21 U.S.C. 801) and/or the Controlled Substances Import and Export Act (84 Stat. 1285; 21 U.S.C. 951).

(b) The term "commercial container" means any bottle, jar, tube, ampule, or other receptacle in which a substance is held for distribution or dispensing to an ultimate user, and in addition, any box or package in which the receptacle is held for distribution or dispensing to an ultimate user. The term "commercial container" does not include any package liner, package insert or other material kept with or within a commercial container, nor any carton, crate, drum, or other package in which commercial containers are stored or are used for shipment of controlled substances.

(c) The term "dispenser" means an individual practitioner, institutional practitioner, pharmacy or pharmacist who dispenses a controlled substance.

(d) The term "individual practitioner" means a physician, dentist, veterinarian, or other individual licensed, registered, or otherwise permitted, by the United States or the jurisdiction in which he practices, to dispense a controlled substance in the course of professional practice, but does not include a pharmacist, a pharmacy, or an institutional practitioner.

(e) The term "institutional practitioner" means a hospital or other person (other than an individual) licensed, registered, or otherwise permitted, by the United States or the jurisdiction in which it practices, to dispense a controlled substance in the course of professional practice, but does not include a pharmacy.

(f) The term "mid-level practitioner" means an individual practitioner (as defined in section "3" 1304.02(d)), other than a physician, dentist, veterinarian, or podiatrist, who is licensed, registered, or otherwise permitted by the United States or the jurisdiction in which he/she practices, to dispense a controlled substance in the course of professional practice. Examples of mid-level practitioners include, but are not limited to, health care providers such as nurse practitioners, nurse midwives, nurse anesthetists, clinical nurse specialists, and physician assistants who are authorized to dispense controlled substances by the state in which they practice.

(g) The term mid-level practitioner means an individual practitioner (as defined in § 1304.02(d)), other than a physician, dentist, veterinarian, or podiatrist, who is licensed, registered, or otherwise permitted by the United States of the jurisdiction in which he/she practices, to dispense a controlled substance in the course of professional practice. Examples of mid-level practitioners include, but are not limited to, health care providers such as nurse practitioners, nurse midwives, nurse anesthetists, clinical nurse specialists and physician assistants who are authorized to dispense controlled substances by the state in which they practice.

(h) The term "name" means the official name, common or usual name, chemical name, or brand name of a substance.

(i) The term "pharmacist" means any pharmacist licensed by a State to dispense controlled substances, and shall include any other person (e.g., pharmacist intern) authorized by a State to dispense controlled substances under the supervision of a pharmacist licensed by such State.

(j) The term "readily retrievable" means that certain records are kept by automatic data processing systems or other electronic or mechanized record keeping systems in such a manner that they can be separated out from all other records in a reasonable time and/or records are kept on which certain items are asterisked, redlined, or in some other manner visually identifiable apart from other items appearing on the records.

§ 1304.03 Persons required to keep records and file reports.

(a) Each registrant shall maintain the records and inventories and shall file the reports required by this part, except as exempted by this section. Any registrant who is authorized to conduct other activities without being registered to conduct those activities, either pursuant to § 1301.22(b) of this chapter or pursuant to §§ 1307.11–1307.15 of this chapter, shall maintain the records and inventories and shall file the reports required by this part for persons registered to conduct such activities. This latter requirement should not be construed as requiring stocks of controlled substances being used in various activities under one registration to be stored separately, nor that separate records are required for each activity. The intent of the Administration is to permit the registrant to keep one set of records which are adapted by the registrant to account for controlled substances used in any activity. Also, the Administration does not wish to require separate stocks of the same substance to be purchased and stored for separate activities. Otherwise, there is no advantage gained by permitting several activities under one registration. Thus, when a researcher manufactures a controlled item, he must keep a record of the quantity manufactured; when he distributes a quantity of the item, he must use and keep invoices or order forms to document the transfer; when he imports a substance, he keeps as part of his records the documentation required of an importer; and when substances are used in chemical analysis, he need not keep a record of this because such a record would not be required of him under a registration to do chemical analysis. All of these records may be maintained in one consolidated record system. Similarly, the researcher may store all of his controlled items in one place, and every two years take inventory of all items on hand, regardless of whether the substances were manufactured by him, imported by him, or purchased domestically by him, or whether the substances will be administered to subjects, distributed to other researchers, or destroyed during chemical analysis.

(b) A registered individual practitioner is required to keep records, as described in § 1304.04 of controlled substances in Schedules II, III, IV, and V which are dispensed, other than by prescribing or administering in the lawful course of professional practice.

(c) A registered individual practitioner is not required to keep records of controlled substances in Schedules II, III, IV, and V which are prescribed in the lawful course of professional practice, unless such substances are prescribed in the course of maintenance or detoxification treatment of an individual.

(d) A registered individual practitioner is not required to keep records of controlled substances listed in Schedules II, III, IV and V which are administered in the lawful course of professional practice unless the practitioner regularly engages in the dispensing or administering of controlled substances and charges patients, either separately or together with charges for other professional services, for substances so dispensed or administered. Records are required to be kept for controlled substances administered in the course of maintenance or detoxification treatment of an individual.

(e) Each registered mid-level practitioner shall maintain in a readily retrievable manner those documents required by the state in which he/she practices which describe the conditions and extent of his/her authorization to dispense controlled substances and shall make such documents available for inspection and copying by authorized employees of the Administration. Examples of such documentation include protocols, practice guidelines, or practice agreements.

(f) Each registered mid-level practitioner shall maintain in a readily retrievable manner those documents required by the statae in which he/she practices which describe the conditions and extent of this/her authorization to dispense controlled substances and shall make such documents available for inspection and copying by authorized employees of the Administration. Examples of such documentation include protocols, practice guidelines or practice agreements.

§ 1304.04 Maintenance of records and inventories.

(a) Every inventory and other records required to be kept under this Part shall be kept by the registrant and be available, for at least 2 years from the date of such inventory or records, for inspection and copying by authorized employees of the Administration, except that financial and shipping records (such as invoices and packing slips but not executed order forms subject to paragraph 1305.13 of this chapter) may be kept at a central location, rather than at the registered location, if the registrant has notified the Administration of his intention to keep central records. Written notification must be submitted by registered or certified mail, return receipt requested, in triplicate, to the Special Agent in Charge of the Administration in the area in which the registrant is located. Unless the registrant is informed by the Special Agent in Charge that permission to keep central records is denied, the registrant may maintain central records commencing 14 days after receipt of his notification by the Special Agent in Charge.

All notifications must include:

(1) The nature of the records to be kept centrally.

(2) The exact location where the records will be kept.

(3) The name, address, DEA registration number and type of DEA registration of the registrant whose records are being maintained centrally.

(4) Whether central records will be maintained in a manual, or computer readable form.

(b) All registrants that are authorized to maintain a central record keeping system shall be subject to the following conditions:

(1) The records to be maintained at the central record location shall not include executed order forms, prescriptions and/or inventories which shall be maintained at each registered location.

(2) If the records are kept on microfilm, computer media or in any form requiring special equipment to render the records easily readable, the registrant shall provide access to such equipment with the records. If any code system is used (other than pricing information), a key to the code shall be provided to make the records understandable.

(3) The registrant agrees to deliver all or any part of such records to the registered location within two business days upon receipt of a written request from the Administration for such records, and if the Administration chooses to do so in lieu of requiring delivery of such records to the registered location, to allow authorized employees of the Administration to inspect such records at the central location upon request by such employees without a warrant of any kind.

(4) In the event that a registrant fails to comply with these conditions, the Special Agent in Charge may cancel such central recordkeeping authorization, and all other central record keeping authorizations held by the registrant without a hearing or other procedures. In the event of a cancellation of central recordkeeping authorizations under this sub-paragraph the registrant shall, within the time specified by the Special Agent in Charge, comply with the requirements of this section that all records be kept at the registered location.

(c) Registrants need not notify the Special Agent in Charge or obtain central record keeping approval in order to maintain records on an in-house computer system.

(d) ARCOS participants who desire authorization to report from other than their registered locations must obtain a separate central reporting identifier. Request for central reporting identifiers will be submitted to: ARCOS Unit, P.O. Box 28293, Central Station, Washington, DC 20005.

(e) All central record keeping permits previously issued by the Administration will expire on September 30, 1980. Registrants who desire to continue maintaining central records will make notification to the local Special Agent in Charge as provided in (a) above.

(f) Each registered manufacturer, distributor, importer, exporter, narcotic treatment program and compounder for narcotic treatment program shall maintain inventories and records of controlled substances as follows:

(1) Inventories and records of controlled substances listed in Schedules I and II shall be maintained separately from all of the records of the registrant; and

(2) Inventories and records of controlled substances listed in Schedules III, IV, and V shall be maintained either separately from all other records of the registrant or in such form that the information required is readily retrievable from the ordinary business records of the registrant.

(g) Each registered individual practitioner required to keep records and institutional practitioner shall maintain inventories and records of controlled substances in the manner prescribed in paragraph (f) of this section.

(h) Each registered pharmacy shall maintain the inventories and records of controlled substances as follows:

(1) Inventories and records of all controlled substances listed in Schedules I and II shall be maintained separately from all other records of the pharmacy, and prescriptions for such substances shall be maintained in a separate prescription file; and

(2) Inventories and records of controlled substances listed in Schedules III, IV, and V shall be maintained either separately from all other records of the pharmacy or in such form that the information required is readily retrievable from ordinary business records of the pharmacy, and prescriptions for such substances shall be maintained either in a separate prescription file for controlled substances listed in Schedules III, IV, and V only or in such form that they are readily retrievable from the other prescription records of the pharmacy. Prescriptions will be deemed readily retrievable if, at the time they are initially filed, the face of the prescription is stamped in red ink in the lower right corner with the letter "C" no less than 1-inch high and filed either in the prescription file for controlled substances listed in Schedules I and II or in the usual consecutively numbered prescription file for noncontrolled substances.

Inventory Requirements

§ 1304.11 General requirements for inventories.

(a) Each inventory shall contain a complete and accurate record of all controlled substances on hand on the date the inventory is taken. Controlled substances shall be deemed to be "on hand" if they are in the possession of or under the control of the registrant, including substances returned by a customer, substances ordered by a customer but not yet invoiced, substances stored in a warehouse on behalf of the registrant, and substances in the possession of employees of the registrant and intended for distribution as complimentary samples.

(b) A separate inventory shall be made by a registrant for each registered location. In the event controlled substances are in the possession or under the control of the registrant at a location for which he is not registered, the substances shall be included in the inventory of the registered location to which they are subject to control or to which the person possessing the substance is responsible. Each inventory for a registered location shall be kept at the registered location.

(c) A separate inventory shall be made by a registrant for each independent activity for which he is registered, except as provided in § 1304.18.

(d) A registrant may take an inventory on a date that is within 4 days of his biennial inventory date pursuant to § 1304.13 if he notifies in advance the Special Agent in Charge of the Administration in his area of the date on which he will take the inventory. A registrant may take an inventory either as of the opening of business or as of the close of business on the inventory date. The registrant shall indicate on the inventory records whether the inventory is taken as of the opening or as of the close of business and the date the inventory is taken.

(e) An inventory must be maintained in a written, typewritten or printed form. An inventory taken by use of an oral recording device must be promptly transcribed.

§ 1304.12 Initial inventory date.

(b) Every person required to keep records who is registered after May 1, 1971, and who was not provisionally registered on that date, shall take an inventory of all stocks of controlled substances on hand on the date he first engages in the manufacture, distribution, or dispensing of controlled substances, in accordance with §§ 1304.15–1304.19, as applicable. In the event a person commences business with no controlled substances on hand, he shall record this fact as his initial inventory.

§ 1304.13 Biennial inventory date.

Every 2 years following the date on which the initial inventory is taken by a registrant pursuant to § 1304.12, the registrant shall take a new inventory of all stocks of controlled substances on hand. The biennial inventory may be taken (a) on the day of the year on which the initial inventory was taken or (b) on the registrant's regular general physical inventory date, if any, which is nearest to and does not vary by more than 6 months from the biennial date that would otherwise apply or (c) on any other fixed date which does not vary by more than 6 months from the biennial date that would otherwise apply. If the registrant elects to take the biennial inventory on his regular general physical inventory date or another fixed date, he shall notify the Administration of this election and of the date on which the biennial inventory will be taken.

§ 1304.14 Inventory date for newly controlled substances.

On the effective date of a rule by the Administrator pursuant to §§ 1308.48–1308.49, or 1308.50 of this chapter adding a substance to any schedule of controlled substances, which substance was, immediately prior to that date, not listed on any such schedule, every registrant required to keep records who possesses that substance shall take an inventory of all stocks of the substance on hand. Thereafter such substance shall be included in each inventory made by the registrant pursuant to § 1304.13.

§ 1304.15 Inventories of manufacturers.

Each person registered or authorized [by § 1301.22(b), § 1307.12, or § 1307.15 of this chapter] to manufacture controlled substances shall include the following information in his inventory:

(a) For each controlled substance in bulk form to be used in (or capable of use in) the manufacture of the same or other controlled or noncontrolled substances in finished form:

(1) The name of the substance; and

(2) The total quantity of the substance to the nearest metric unit weight consistent with unit size (except that for inventories made in 1971, avoirdupois weights may be utilized where metric weights are not readily available).

(b) For each controlled substance in the process of manufacture on the inventory date:

(1) The name of the substance;

(2) The quantity of the substance in each batch and/or stage of manufacture, identified by the batch number or other appropriate identifying number;

(3) The physical form which the substance is to take upon completion of the manufacturing process (e.g., granulations, tablets, capsules, or solutions), identified by the batch number or other appropriate identifying number, and if possible the finished form of the substance (e.g., 10-milligram tablet or 10-milligram concentration per fluid ounce or milliliter) and the number or volume thereof; and

(c) For each controlled substance in finished form:

(1) The name of the substance;

(2) Each finished form of the substance (e.g., 10-milligram tablet or 10-milligram concentration per fluid ounce or milliliter);

(3) The number of units or volume of each finished form in each commercial container (e.g., 100-tablet bottle or 3-milliliter vial); and

(4) The number of commercial containers of each such finished form (e.g., four 100-tablet bottles or six 3-milliliter vials).

(d) For each controlled substance not included in paragraphs (a), (b) or (c) of this section (e.g., damaged, defective, or impure substances awaiting disposal, substances held for quality control purposes, or substances maintained for extemporaneous compoundings):

(1) The name of the substance;

(2) The total quantity of the substance to the nearest metric unit weight or the total number of units of finished form; and

(3) The reason for the substance being maintained by the registrant and whether such substance is capable of use in the manufacture of any controlled substance in finished form.

§ 1304.17 Inventories of dispensers and researchers.

Each person registered or authorized [by § 1301.22(b) of this chapter] to dispense or conduct research with controlled substances and required to keep records pursuant to § 1304.03 shall include in his inventory the same information required of manufacturers pursuant to § 1304.15(c) and (d). In determining the number of units of each finished form of a controlled substance in a commercial container which has been opened, the dispenser shall do as follows:

(a) If the substance is listed in Schedule I or II, he shall make an exact count or measure of the contents; and

(b) If the substance is listed in Schedule III, IV, or V, he shall make an estimated count or measure of the contents, unless the container holds more than 1000 tablets or capsules in which case he must make an exact count of the contents.

Continuing Records

§ 1304.21 General requirements for continuing records.

(a) On and after May 1, 1971, every registrant required to keep records pursuant to § 1304.03 shall maintain on a current basis a complete and accurate record of each such substance manufactured, imported, received, sold, delivered, exported, or otherwise disposed of by him, except that no registrant shall be required to maintain a perpetual inventory.

(b) Separate records shall be maintained by a registrant for each registered location except as provided in § 1304.04(a). In the event controlled substances are in the possession or under the control of a registrant at a location for which he is not registered, the substances shall be included in the records of the registered location to which they are subject to control or to which the person possessing the substance is responsible.

(c) Separate records shall be maintained by a registrant for each independent activity for which he is registered, except as provided in §§ 1304.25 and 1304.26.

(d) In recording dates of receipt, importation, distribution, exportation, or other transfers, the date on which the controlled substances are actually received, imported, distributed, exported, or otherwise transferred shall be used as the date of receipt or distribution of any documents of transfer (e.g., invoices or packing slips).

§ 1304.23 Records for distributors.

Each person registered or authorized [by § 1301.22(b) or §§ 1307.11–1307.14 of this chapter] to distribute controlled substances shall maintain records with the following information for each controlled substance:

(a) The name of the substance;

(b) Each finished form (e.g., 10-milligram tablet or 10-milligram concentration per fluid ounce or milliliter) and the number of units or volume of finished form in each commercial container (e.g., 100-tablet bottle or 3-milliliter vial);

(c) The number of commercial containers of each such finished form received from other persons, including the date of and number of containers in each receipt and the name, address, and registration number of the person from whom the containers were received;

(d) The number of commercial containers or each such finished form imported directly by the person (under a registration or authorization to import), including the date of, the number of commercial containers in, and the import permit or declaration number for, each importation;

(e) The number of commercial containers of each such finished form distributed to other persons, including the date of and number of containers in each distribution and the name, address, and registration number of the person to whom the containers were distributed;

(f) The number of commercial containers of each such finished form exported directly by the person (under a registration or authorization to export), including the date of, the number of commercial containers in, and the export permit or declaration number for, each exportation; and

(g) The number of units or volume of finished forms and/or commercial containers distributed or disposed of in any other manner by the person (e.g., by distribution as complimentary samples or by destruction) including the date and manner of distribution or disposal, the name, address, and registration number of the person to whom distributed, and the quantity of the substance in finished form distributed or disposed.

§ 1304.24 Records for dispensers and researchers.

Each person registered or authorized [by § 1301.22(b) of this chapter] to dispense or conduct research with controlled substances and required to keep records pursuant to § 1304.03 shall maintain records with the following information for each controlled substance:

(a) The name of the substance;

(b) Each finished form (e.g., 10-milligram tablet or 10-milligram concentration per fluid ounce or milliliter) and the number of units or volume of finished form in each commercial container (e.g., 100-tablet bottle or 3-milliliter vial);

(c) The number of commercial containers of each such finished form received from other persons, including the date of and number of containers in each receipt and the name, address, and registration number of the person from whom the containers were received;

(d) The number of units or volume of such finished form dispensed, including the name and address of the person to whom it was dispensed, the date of dispensing, the number of units or volume dispensed, and the written or typewritten name or initials of the individual who dispensed or administered the substance on behalf of the dispenser; and

(e) The number of units or volume of such finished forms and/or commercial containers disposed of in any other manner by the registrant, including the date and manner of disposal and the quantity of the substance in finished form disposed.

§ 1304.28 Records for maintenance treatment programs and detoxification treatment programs.

(a) Each person registered or authorized (by § 1301.22 of this chapter) to maintain and/or detoxify controlled substance users in a narcotic treatment program shall maintain records with the following information for each narcotic controlled substance:

(1) Name of substance;
(2) Strength of substance;
(3) Dosage form;
(4) Date dispensed;
(5) Adequate identification of patient (consumer);
(6) Amount consumed;
(7) Amount and dosage form taken home by patient; and
(8) Dispenser's initials.

(b) The records required by paragraph (a) of this section will be maintained in a dispensing log at the narcotic treatment program site and will be maintained in compliance with § 1304.24 without reference to § 1304.03.

(c) All sites which compound a bulk narcotic solution from bulk narcotic powder to liquid for on-site use must keep a separate batch record of the compounding.

(d) Records of identity, diagnosis, prognosis, or treatment of any patients which are maintained in connection with the performance of a narcotic treatment program shall be confidential, except that such records may be disclosed for purposes and under the circumstances authorized by Part 310 and Part 1401 of this title.

§ 1304.29 Records for treatment programs which compound narcotics for treatment programs and other locations.

Each person registered or authorized by § 1301.22 of this chapter to compound narcotic drugs for off-site use in a narcotic treatment program shall maintain records which include the following information for each narcotic drug:

(a) For each narcotic controlled substance in bulk form to be used in, or capable of use in, or being used in, the compounding of the same or other noncontrolled substances in finished form:

(1) The name of the substance;

(2) The quantity compounded in bulk form by the registrant, including the date, quantity and batch or other identifying number of each batch compounded;

(3) The quantity received from other persons, including the date and quantity of each receipt and the name, address, and registration number of the other person from whom the substance was received;

(4) The quantity imported directly by the registrant (under a registration as an importer) for use in compounding by him, including the date, quantity and import permit or declaration number of each importation;

(5) The quantity used to compound the same substance in finished form, including:

(i) The date and batch or other identifying number of each compounding;
(ii) The quantity used in the compound;
(iii) The finished form (e.g., 10-milligram tablets or 10-milligram concentration per fluid ounce or milliliter);
(iv) The number of units of finished form compounded;
(v) The quantity used in quality control;
(vi) The quantity lost during compounding and the causes therefore, if known;
(vii) The total quantity of the substance contained in the finished form;
(viii) The theoretical and actual yields; and
(ix) Such other information as is necessary to account for all controlled substances used in the compounding process;

(6) The quantity used to manufacture other controlled and noncontrolled substances; including the name of each substance manufactured and the information required in paragraph (a)(5) of this section;

(7) The quantity distributed in bulk form to other programs, including the date and quantity of each distribution and the name, address and registration number of each program to whom a distribution was made;

(8) The quantity exported directly by the registrant (under a registration as an exporter), including the date, quantity, and export permit or declaration number of each exportation; and

(9) The quantity disposed of by destruction, including the reason, date and manner of destruction. All other destruction of narcotic controlled substances will comply with § 1307.22.

(b) For each narcotic controlled substance in finished form:

(1) The name of the substance;

(2) Each finished form (e.g., 10-milligram tablet or 10-milligram concentration per fluid ounce or milliliter) and the number of units or volume or finished form in each commercial container (e.g., 100-tablet bottle or 3-milliliter vial);

(3) The number of containers of each such commercial finished form compounded from bulk form by the registrant, including the information required pursuant to paragraph (a)(5) of this section;

(4) The number of units of finished forms and/or commercial containers received from other persons, including the date of and number of units and/or commercial containers in each receipt and the name, address and registration number of the person from whom the units were received;

(5) The number of units of finished forms and/or commercial containers imported directly by the person (under a registration or authorization to import), including the date of, the number of units and/or commercial containers in, and the import permit or declaration number for, each importation;

(6) The number of units and/or commercial containers compounded by the registrant from units in finished form received from others or imported, including:

(i) The date and batch or other identifying number of each compounding;
(ii) The operation performed (e.g., repackaging or relabeling);
(iii) The number of units of finished form used in the compound, the number compounded and the number lost during compounding, with the causes for such losses, if known; and
(iv) Such other information as is necessary to account for all controlled substances used in the compounding process;

(7) The number of containers distributed to other programs, including the date, the number of containers in each distribution, and the name, address and registration number of the program to whom the containers were distributed;

(8) The number of commercial containers exported directly by the registrant (under a registration as an exporter), including the date, number of containers and export permit or declaration number for each exportation; and

(9) The number of units of finished forms and/or commercial containers destroyed in any manner by the registrant, including the reason, the date and manner of destruction. All other destruction of narcotic controlled substances will comply with §1307.22.

NOTE—A complete set of the regulations appears in Volume 21, part 1300 to end, of the *Code of Federal Regulations*, revised annually, and covers regulations pertaining to manufacturers, distributors, researchers, exporters, and importers.

Information regarding procedures under these regulations and instructions implementing them are obtainable from the Drug Enforcement Administration, Department of Justice, 1405 I Street, N.W., Washington, DC 20537.

Order Forms

§ 1305.02 Definitions.

As used in this part, the following terms shall have the meanings specified:

(b) The term "purchaser" means any registered person entitled to obtain and execute order forms pursuant to § 1305.04 and § 1305.06.

(c) The term "supplier" means any registered person entitled to fill order forms pursuant to § 1305.08.

§ 1305.03 Distributions requiring order forms.

An order form (DEA Form 222) is required for each distribution of a controlled substance listed in Schedule I or II, except for the following:

(a) The exportation of such substances from the United States in conformity with the Act;

(b) The delivery of such substances to or by a common or contract carrier for carriage in the lawful and usual course of its business, or to or by a warehouseman for storage in the lawful and usual course of its business (but excluding such carriage or storage by the owner of the substance in connection with the distribution to a third person);

(c) The procurement of a sample of such substances by an exempt law enforcement official pursuant to § 1301.26(b) of this chapter, provided that the receipt required by that section is used and is preserved in the manner prescribed in this part for order forms;

(d) The procurement of such substances by a civil defense or disaster relief organization, pursuant to § 1301.27 of this chapter, provided that the Civil Defense Emergency Order Form required by that section is used and is preserved with other records of the registrant; and

(e) The purchase of such substances by the master or first officer of a vessel pursuant to § 1301.28 of this chapter: Provided, that copies of the record of sale are generated, distributed, and preserved by the vendor according to that section.

(f) The delivery of such substances to a registered analytical laboratory, or its agent approved by DEA, from an anonymous source for the analysis of the drug sample, provided the laboratory has obtained a written waiver of the order form requirement from the Regional Director[1] of the Region in which the laboratory is located, which waiver may be granted upon agreement of the laboratory to conduct its activities in accordance with Administration guidelines.

§ 1305.04 Persons entitled to obtain and execute order forms.

(a) Order forms may be obtained only by persons who are registered under section 303 of the Act (21 U.S.C. 823) to handle controlled substances listed in Schedules I and II, and by persons who are registered under section 1008 of the Act (21 U.S.C. 958) to export such substances. Persons not registered to handle controlled substances listed in Schedule I or II and persons registered only to import controlled substances listed in any schedule are not entitled to obtain order forms.

(b) An order form may be executed only on behalf of the registrant named thereon and only if his registration as to the substances being purchased has not expired or been revoked or suspended.

§ 1305.05 Procedure for obtaining order forms.

(a) Order Forms are issued in mailing envelopes containing either seven or fourteen forms, each form containing an original duplicate and triplicate copy (respectively, Copy 1, Copy 2, and Copy 3). A limit, which is based on the business activity of the registrant, will be imposed on the number of order forms which will be furnished on any requisition unless additional forms are specifically requested and a reasonable need for such additional forms is shown.

(b) Any person applying for a registration which would entitle him to obtain order forms may requisition such forms by so indicating on the application form; order forms will be supplied upon the registration of the applicant. Any person holding a registration entitling him to obtain order forms may requisition such forms for the first time by contacting any Division Office or the Registration Unit of the Administration. Any person already holding order forms may requisition additional forms on DEA Form 222a which is mailed to a registrant approximately 30 days after each shipment of order forms to that registrant or by contacting any Division Office or the Registration Unit of the Administration. All requisition forms (DEA Form 222a) shall be submitted to the Registration Unit, Drug Enforcement Administration, Department of Justice, Post Office Box 28083, Central Station, Washington, DC 20005.

(c) Each requisition shall show the name, address, and registration number of the registrant and the number of books of order forms desired. Each requisition shall be signed and dated by the same person who signed the most recent application for registration or for reregistration, o- by any person authorized to obtain and execute order forms by a power of attorney pursuant to § 1305.07.

(d) Order forms will be serially numbered and issued with the name, address and registration number of the registrant, the authorized activity and schedules of the registrant. This information cannot be altered or changed by the registrant; any errors must be corrected by the Registration Unit of the Administration by returning the forms with notification of the error.

§ 1305.06 Procedure for executing order forms.

(a) Order forms shall be prepared and executed by the purchaser simultaneously in triplicate by means of interleaved carbon sheets which are part of the DEA Form 222 . Order forms shall be prepared by use of a typewriter, pen, or indelible pencil.

(b) Only one item shall be entered on each numbered line. There are ten lines on each order form. If one order form is not sufficient to include all items in an order, additional forms shall be used. Order forms for carfentanil, etorphine hydrochloride, and diprenorphine shall contain only these substances. The total number of items ordered shall be noted on that form in the space provided.

(c) An item shall consist of one or more commercial or bulk containers of the same finished or bulk form and quantity of the same substance; a separate item shall be made for each commercial or bulk container of different finished or bulk form, quantity or substance. For each item the form shall show the name of the article ordered, the finished or bulk form of the article (e.g., 10-milligram tablet, 10-milligram concentration per fluid ounce or milliliter, or USP), the number of units or volume in each commercial or bulk container (e.g., 100-tablet bottle or 3-milliliter vial) or the quantity or volume of each bulk container (e.g., 10 kilograms), the number of commercial or bulk containers ordered, and the name and quantity per unit of the controlled substance or substances contained in the article if not in pure form. The catalogue number of the article may be included at the discretion of the purchaser.

(d) The name and address of the supplier from whom the controlled substances are being ordered shall be entered on the form. Only one supplier may be listed on any one form.

(e) Each order form shall be signed and dated by a person authorized to sign a requisition for order forms on behalf of the purchaser pursuant to § 1305.05(c). The name of the purchaser, if different from the individual signing the order form, shall also be inserted in the signature space. Unexecuted order forms may be kept and may be executed at a location other than the registered location printed on the form, provided that all unexecuted forms are delivered promptly to the registered location upon an inspection of such location by any officer authorized to make inspections, or to enforce, any Federal, State, or local law regarding controlled substances.

§ 1305.07 Power of attorney.

Any purchaser may authorize one or more individuals, whether or not located at the registered location of the purchaser, to obtain and execute order forms on his behalf by executing a power of attorney for each such individual. The power of attorney shall be signed by the same person who signed (or was authorized to sign, pursuant to § 1301.32(f) of this chapter or § 1311.32(f) of this chapter) the most recent application for registration or reregistration and by the individual being authorized to obtain and execute order forms. The power of attorney shall be filed with the executed order forms of the purchaser, and shall be retained for the same period as any order form bearing the signature of the attorney. The power of attorney shall be available for inspection together with other order form records. Any power of attorney may be revoked at any time by executing a notice of revocation, signed by the person who signed (or was authorized to sign) the power of attorney or by a successor, whoever signed the most recent application for registration or reregistration, and filing it with the power of attorney being revoked. The form for the power of attorney and notice of revocation shall be similar to the following:

POWER OF ATTORNEY FOR DEA ORDER FORMS

____
(Name of registrant)

____
(Address of registrant)

____
(DEA registration number)

I, ____________________, the undersigned,
(Name of person granting power)

who is authorized to sign the current application for registration of the above-named registrant under the Controlled Substances Act or Controlled Substances Import and Export Act, have made, constituted, and appointed, and by these presents, do make, constitute, and appoint ____________,
(Name of attorney-in-fact)

my true and lawful attorney for me in my name, place, and stead, to execute applications for books of official order forms and to sign such order forms in requisition for Schedule I and II controlled substances, in accordance with section 308 of the Controlled Substances Act (21 U.S.C. 828) and Part 305 of Title 21 of the Code of Federal Regulations. I hereby ratify and confirm all that said attorney shall lawfully do or cause to be done by virtue hereof.

____
(Signature of person granting power)

[1] Special Agent in Charge.

I, ______________, hereby affirm that
(Name of attorney-in-fact)
I am the person named herein as attorney-in-fact and that the signature affixed hereto is my signature.

______________ (Signature of attorney-in-fact)

Witnesses:

1. ______________.
2. ______________.

Signed and dated on the ______ day of ______, 19___, at ______________.

NOTICE OF REVOCATION

The foregoing power of attorney is hereby revoked by the undersigned, who is authorized to sign the current application for registration of the above-named registrant under the Controlled Substances Act or the Controlled Substances Import and Export Act. Written notice of this revocation has been given to the attorney-in-fact ______________ this same day.

______________ (Signature of person revoking power)

Witnesses:

1. ______________.
2. ______________.

Signed and dated on the ______ day of ______________, 19___, at ______________.

§ 1305.08 Persons entitled to fill order forms.

An order form may be filled only by a person registered as a manufacturer or distributor of controlled substances listed in Schedule I or II under section 303 of the Act (21 U.S.C. 823) or as an importer of such substances under section 1008 of the Act (21 U.S.C. 958), except for the following:

(a) A person registered to dispense such substances under section 303 of the Act, or to export such substances under section 1008 of the Act, if he is discontinuing business or if his registration is expiring without reregistration, may dispose of any controlled substances listed in Schedule I or II in his possession pursuant to order forms in accordance with § 1307.14 of this chapter;

(b) A person who has obtained any controlled substance in Schedule I or II by order form may return such substance, or portion thereof, to the person from whom he obtained the substance or the manufacturer of the substance pursuant to the order form of the latter person;

(c) A person registered to dispense such substances may distribute such substances to another dispenser pursuant to, and only in the circumstances described in, § 1307.11 of this chapter; and

(d) A person registered or authorized to conduct chemical analysis or research with controlled substances may distribute a controlled substance listed in Schedule I or II to another person registered or authorized to conduct chemical analysis, instructional activities, or research with such substances pursuant to the order form of the latter person, if such distribution is for the purpose of furthering such chemical analysis, instructional activities, or research.

(e) A person registered as a compounder of narcotic substances for use at off-site locations in conjunction with a narcotic treatment program at the compounding location, who is authorized to handle Schedule II narcotics, is authorized to fill order forms for distribution of narcotic drugs to off-site narcotic treatment programs only.

§ 1305.09 Procedure for filling order forms.

(a) The purchaser shall submit Copy 1 and Copy 2 of the order form to the supplier, and retain Copy 3 in his own files.

(b) The supplier shall fill the order, if possible and if he desires to do so, and record on Copies 1 and 2 the number of commercial or bulk containers furnished on each item and the date on which such containers are shipped to the purchaser. If an order cannot be filled in its entirety, it may be filled in part and the balance supplied by additional shipments within 60 days following the date of the order form. No order form shall be valid more than 60 days after its execution by the purchaser, except as specified in paragraph (f) of this section.

(c) The controlled substances shall only be shipped to the purchaser and at the location printed by the Administration on the order form, except as specified in paragraph (f) of this section.

(d) The supplier shall retain Copy 1 of the order form for his own files and forward Copy 2 to the Special Agent in Charge of the Drug Enforcement Administration in the area in which the supplier is located. Copy 2 shall be forwarded at the close of the month during which the order is filled; if an order is filled by partial shipments, Copy 2 shall be forwarded at the close of the month during which the final shipment is made or during which the 60-day validity period expires.

(e) The purchaser shall record on Copy 3 of the order form the number of commercial or bulk containers furnished on each item and the dates on which such containers are received by the purchaser.

(f) Order forms submitted by registered procurement officers of the Defense Personnel Support Center of Defense Supply Agency for delivery to armed services establishments within the United States may be shipped to locations other than the location printed on the order form, and in partial shipments at different times not to exceed six months from the date of the order, as designated by the procurement officer when submitting the order.

§ 1305.10 Procedure for endorsing order forms.

(a) An order form made out to any supplier who cannot fill all or a part of the order within the time limitation set forth in § 1305.09 may be endorsed to another supplier for filling. The endorsement shall be made only by the supplier to whom the order form was first made, shall state (in the spaces provided on the reverse sides of Copies 1 and 2 of the order form) the name and address of the second supplier, and shall be signed by a person authorized to obtain and execute order forms on behalf of the first supplier. The first supplier may not fill any part of an order on an endorsed form. The second supplier shall fill the order, if possible and if he desires to do so, in accordance with § 1305.09 (b), (c), and (d), including shipping all substances directly to the purchaser.

(b) Distributions made on endorsed order forms shall be reported by the second supplier in the same manner as all other distributions except that where the name of the supplier is requested on the reporting form, the second supplier shall record the name, address and registration number of the first supplier.

§ 1305.11 Unaccepted and defective order forms.

(a) No order form shall be filled if it:

(1) Is not complete, legible, or properly prepared, executed, or endorsed; or

(2) Shows any alteration, erasure, or change of any description.

(b) If an order form cannot be filled for any reason under this section, the supplier shall return Copies 1 and 2 to the purchaser with a statement as to the reason (e.g., illegible or altered). A supplier may for any reason refuse to accept any order and if a supplier refuses to accept the order, a statement that the order is not accepted shall be sufficient for purposes of this paragraph.

(c) When received by the purchaser, Copies 1 and 2 of the order form and the statement shall be attached to Copy 3 and retained in the files of the purchaser in accordance with § 1305.13. A defective order form may not be corrected; it must be replaced by a new order form in order for the order to be filled.

§ 1305.12 Lost and stolen order forms.

(a) If a purchaser ascertains that an unfilled order form has been lost, he shall execute another in triplicate and a statement containing the serial number and date of the lost form, and stating that the goods covered by the first order form were not received through loss of that order form. Copy 3 of the second form and a copy of the statement shall be retained with Copy 3 of the order form first executed. A copy of the statement shall be attached to Copies 1 and 2 of the second order form sent to the supplier. If the first order form is subsequently received by the supplier to whom it was directed, the supplier shall mark upon the face thereof "Not accepted" and return Copies 1 and 2 to the purchaser, who shall attach it to Copy 3 and the statement.

(b) Whenever any used or unused order forms are stolen from or lost (otherwise than in the course of transmission) by any purchaser or supplier, he shall immediately upon discovery of such theft or loss, report the same to the Registration Unit, Drug Enforcement Administration, Department of Justice, Post Office Box 28083, Central Station, Washington, DC 20005, stating the serial number of each form stolen or lost. If the theft or loss includes any original order forms received from purchasers and the supplier is unable to state the serial numbers of such order forms, he shall report the date or approximate date of receipt thereof and the names and addresses of the purchasers. If an entire book of order forms is lost or stolen, and the purchaser is unable to state the serial numbers of the order forms contained therein, he shall report, in lieu of the numbers of the forms contained in such book, the date or approximate date of issuance thereof. If any unused order form reported stolen or lost is subsequently recovered or found, the Registration Unit of the Administration shall immediately be notified.

§ 1305.13 Preservation of order forms.

(a) The purchaser shall retain Copy 3 of each order form which has been filled. He shall also retain in his files all copies of each unaccepted or defective order form and each statement attached thereto.

(b) The supplier shall retain Copy 1 of each order form which he has filled.

(c) Order forms must be maintained separately from all other records of the registrant. Order forms are required to be kept available for inspection for a period of 2 years. If a purchaser has several registered locations, he must retain Copy 3 of the executed order forms and any attached statements or other related documents [not including unexecuted order forms which may be kept elsewhere pursuant to § 1305.06(e)] at the registered location printed on the order form.

(d) The supplier of carfentanil, etorphine hydrochloride, and diprenorphine shall maintain order forms for these substances separately from all other order forms and records required to be maintained by the registrant.

§ 1305.14 Return of unused order forms.

If the registration of any purchaser terminates (because the purchaser dies, ceases legal existence, discontinues business or professional practice, or changes his name or address as shown on his registration) or is suspended or revoked pursuant to §§ 1301.45 or 1301.46 of this chapter as to all controlled substances listed in Schedules I and II for which he is registered, he shall return all unused order forms for such substance to the nearest office of the Administration.

§ 1305.15 Cancellation and voiding of order forms.

(a) A purchaser may cancel part or all of an order on an order form by notifying the supplier in writing of such cancellation. The supplier shall indicate the cancellation on Copies 1 and 2 of the order form by drawing a line through the canceled items and printing "canceled" in the space provided for number of items shipped.

(b) A supplier may void part or all of an order on an order form by notifying the purchaser in writing of such voiding. The supplier shall indicate the voiding in the manner prescribed for cancellation in paragraph (a) of this section.

(c) No cancellation or voiding permitted by this section shall affect in any way contract rights of either the purchaser or the supplier.

Prescriptions

§ 1306.02 Definitions.

As used in this part, the following terms shall have the meanings specified:

(b) The term "individual practitioner" means a physician, dentist, veterinarian, or other individual licensed, registered, or otherwise permitted, by the United States or the jurisdiction in which he practices, to dispense a controlled substance in the course of professional practice, but does not include a pharmacist, a pharmacy, or an institutional practitioner.

(c) The term "institutional practitioner" means a hospital or other person (other than an individual) licensed, registered, or otherwise permitted, by the United States or the jurisdiction in which it practices, to dispense a controlled substance in the course of professional practice, but does not include a pharmacy.

(d) The term "pharmacist" means any pharmacist licensed by a State to dispense controlled substances, and shall include any other person (e.g., a pharmacist intern) authorized by a State to dispense controlled substances under the supervision of a pharmacist licensed by such State.

(e) A "Long Term Care Facility" (LTCF) means a nursing home, retirement care, mental care or other facility or institution which provides extended health care to resident patients.

(f) The term "prescription" means an order for medication which is dispensed to or for an ultimate user but does not include an order for medication which is dispensed for immediate administration to the ultimate user. (e.g., an order to dispense a drug to a bed patient for immediate administration in a hospital is not a prescription.)

(g) The terms "register" and "registered" refer to registration required and permitted by section 303 of the Act (21 U.S.C. 823).

§ 1306.03 Persons entitled to issue prescriptions.

(a) A prescription for a controlled substance may be issued only by an individual practitioner who is:

(1) Authorized to prescribe controlled substances by the jurisdiction in which he is licensed to practice his profession and

(2) Either registered or exempted from registration pursuant to §§ 1301.24(c) and 1301.25 of this chapter.

(b) A prescription issued by an individual practitioner may be communicated to a pharmacist by an employee or agent of the individual practitioner.

§ 1306.04 Purpose of issue of prescription.

(a) A prescription for a controlled substance to be effective must be issued for a legitimate medical purpose by an individual practitioner acting in the usual course of his professional practice. The responsibility for the proper prescribing and dispensing of controlled substances is upon the prescribing practitioner, but a corresponding responsibility rests with the pharmacist who fills the prescription. An order purporting to be a prescription issued not in the usual course of professional treatment or in legitimate and authorized research is not a prescription within the meaning and intent of section 309 of the Act (21 U.S.C. 829) and the person knowingly filling such a purported prescription, as well as the person issuing it, shall be subject to the penalties provided for violations of the provisions of law relating to controlled substances.

(b) A prescription may not be issued in order for an individual practitioner to obtain controlled substances for supplying the individual practitioner for the purpose of general dispensing to patients.

(c) A prescription may not be issued for the dispensing of narcotic drugs listed in any schedule for "detoxification treatment" or "maintenance treatment" as defined in Section 102 of the Act (21 U.S.C. 802).

§ 1306.05 Manner of issuance of prescriptions.

(a) All prescriptions for controlled substances shall be dated as of, and signed on, the day when issued and shall bear the full name and address of the patient, the drug name, strength, dosage form, quantity prescribed, directions for use, and the name, address, and registration number of the practitioner. A practitioner may sign a prescription in the same manner as he would sign a check or legal document (e.g., J. H. Smith or John H. Smith). Where an oral order is not permitted, prescriptions shall be written with ink or indelible pencil or typewriter and shall be manually signed by the practitioner. The prescriptions may be prepared by a secretary or agent for the signature of a practitioner, but the prescribing practitioner is responsible in case the prescription does not conform in all essential respects to the law and regulations. A corresponding liability rests upon the pharmacist who fills a prescription not prepared in the form prescribed by these regulations.

(b) An intern, resident, or foreign-trained physician, or physician on the staff of a Veterans Administration facility, exempted from registration under § 1301.24(c) shall include on all prescriptions issued by him the registration number of the hospital or other institution and the special internal code number assigned to him by the hospital or other institution as provided in § 1301.24(c), in lieu of the registration number of the practitioner required by this section. Each written prescription shall have the name of the physician stamped, typed, or handprinted on it, as well as the signature of the physician.

(c) An official exempted from registration under § 1301.25 shall include on all prescriptions issued by him his branch of service or agency (e.g., "U.S. Army" or "Public Health Service") and his service identification number, in lieu of the registration number of the practitioner required by this section. The service identification number for a Public Health Service employee is his Social Security identification number. Each prescription shall have the name of the officer stamped, typed, or handprinted on it, as well as the signature of the officer.

§ 1306.06 Persons entitled to fill prescriptions.

A prescription for controlled substances may only be filled by a pharmacist acting in the usual course of his professional practice and either registered individually or employed in a registered pharmacy or registered institutional practitioner.

§ 1306.07 Administering or dispensing of narcotic drugs.

(a) The administering or dispensing directly (but not prescribing) of narcotic drugs listed in any schedule to a narcotic drug dependent person for "detoxification treatment" or "maintenance treatment" as defined in section 102 of the Act (21 U.S.C. 802) shall be deemed to be within the meaning of the term "in the course of his professional practice or research" in section 308(e) and section 102(20) of the Act [21 U.S.C. 828(e)]: *Provided*, That the practitioner is separately registered with the Attorney General as required by section 303(g) of the Act [21 U.S.C. 823(g)] and then thereafter complies with the regulatory standards imposed relative to treatment qualification, security, records and unsupervised use of drugs pursuant to such Act.

(b) Nothing in this section shall prohibit a physician who is not specifically registered to conduct a narcotic treatment program from administering (but not prescribing) narcotic drugs to a person for the purpose of relieving acute withdrawal symptoms when necessary while arrangements are being made for referral for treatment. Not more than one day's medication may be administered to the person or for the person's use at one time. Such emergency treatment may be carried out for not more than three days and may not be renewed or extended.

(c) This section is not intended to impose any limitations on a physician or authorized hospital staff to administer or dispense narcotic drugs in a hospital to maintain or detoxify a person as an incidental adjunct to medical or surgical treatment of conditions other than addiction, or to administer or dispense narcotic drugs to persons with intractable pain in which no relief or cure is possible or none has been found after reasonable efforts.

Controlled Substances Listed in Schedule II

§ 1306.11 Requirement of prescription.

(a) A pharmacist may dispense directly a controlled substance listed in Schedule II, which is a prescription drug as determined under the Federal Food, Drug, and Cosmetic Act, only pursuant to a written prescription signed by the prescribing individual practitioner, except as provided in paragraph (d) of this section.

(b) An individual practitioner may administer or dispense directly a controlled substance listed in Schedule II in the course of his professional practice without a prescription, subject to § 1306.07.

(c) An institutional practitioner may administer or dispense directly (but not prescribe) a controlled substance listed in Schedule II only pursuant to a written prescription signed by the prescribing individual practitioner or to an order for medication made by an individual practitioner which is dispensed for immediate administration to the ultimate user.

(d) In the case of an emergency situation, as defined by the Secretary in § 290.10 of this title, a pharmacist may dispense a controlled substance listed in Schedule II upon receiving oral authorization of a prescribing individual practitioner, provided that:

(1) The quantity prescribed and dispensed is limited to the amount adequate to treat the patient during the emergency period (dispensing beyond the emergency period must be pursuant to a written prescription signed by the prescribing individual practitioner);

(2) The prescription shall be immediately reduced to writing by the pharmacist and shall contain all information required in § 1306.05, except for the signature of the prescribing individual practitioner;

(3) If the prescribing individual practitioner is not known to the pharmacist, he must make a reasonable effort to determine that the oral authorization came from a registered individual practitioner, which may include a callback to the prescribing individual practitioner using his phone number as listed in the telephone directory and/or other good faith efforts to ensure his identity; and

(4) Within 72 hours after authorizing an emergency oral prescription, the prescribing individual practitioner shall cause a written prescription for the emergency quantity prescribed to be delivered to the dispensing pharmacist. In addition to conforming to the requirements of § 1306.05, the prescription shall have written on its face "Authorization for Emergency Dispensing," and the date of the oral order. The written prescription may be delivered to the pharmacist in person or by mail, but if delivered by mail it must be postmarked within the 72-hour period. Upon receipt, the dispensing pharmacist shall attach this prescription to the oral emergency prescription which had earlier been reduced to writing. The pharmacist shall notify the nearest office of the Administration if the prescribing individual practitioner fails to deliver a written prescription to him; failure of the pharmacist to do so shall void the authority conferred by this paragraph to dispense without a written prescription of a prescribing individual practitioner.

§ 1306.12 Refilling prescriptions.

The refilling of a prescription for a controlled substance listed in Schedule II is prohibited.

§ 1306.13 Partial filling of prescriptions.

(a) The partial filling of a prescription for a controlled substance listed in Schedule II is permissible, if the pharmacist is unable to supply the full quantity called for in a written or emergency oral prescription and he makes a notation of the quantity supplied on the face of the written prescription (or written record of the emergency oral prescription). The remaining portion of the prescription may be filled within 72 hours of the first partial filling; however, if the remaining portion is not or cannot be filled within the 72-hour period, the pharmacist shall so notify the prescribing individual practitioner. No further quantity may be supplied beyond 72 hours without a new prescription.

(b) A prescription for a Schedule II controlled substance written for a patient in a Long Term Care Facility (LTCF) or for a patient with a medical diagnosis documenting a terminal illness may be filled in partial quantities to include individual dosage units. If there is any question whether a patient may be classified as having a terminal illness, the pharmacist must contact the practitioner prior to partially filling the prescription. Both the pharmacist and prescribing practitioner have a corresponding responsibility to assure that the controlled substance is for a terminally ill patient. The pharmacist must record on the prescription whether the patient is "terminally ill" or an "LTCF patient." A prescription that is partially filled and does not contain the notation "terminally ill" or "LTCF patient" shall be deemed to have been filled in violation of the Act. For each partial filling, the dispensing pharmacist shall record on the back of the prescription (or on another appropriate record, uniformly maintained, and readily retrievable) the date of the partial filling, quantity dispensed, remaining quantity authorized to be dispensed, and the identification of the dispensing pharmacist. Prior to any subsequent partial filling the pharmacist is to determine that the additional partial filling is necessary. The total quantity of Schedule II controlled substances dispensed in all partial fillings must not exceed the total quantity prescribed. Schedule II prescriptions for patients in a LTCF or patients with a medical diagnosis documenting a terminal illness shall be valid for a period not to exceed 60 days from the issue date unless sooner terminated by the discontinuance of medication.

(c) Information pertaining to current Schedule II prescriptions for patients in a LTCF or for patients with a medical diagnosis documenting a terminal illness may be maintained in a computerized system if this system has the capability to permit:

(1) Output (display or printout) of the original prescription number, date of issue, identification of prescribing individual practitioner, identification of patient, address of the LTCF or address of the hospital or residence of the patient, identification of medication authorized (to include dosage, form, strength, and quantity), listing of the partial fillings that have been dispensed under each prescription and the information required in § 1306.13(b).

(2) Immediate (real time) updating of the prescription record each time a partial filling of the prescription is conducted.

(3) Retrieval of partially filled Schedule II prescription information is the same as required by § 1306.22(b)(4) and (5) for Schedule III and IV prescription refill information.

§ 1306.14 Labeling of substances.

(a) The pharmacist filling a written or emergency oral prescription for a controlled substance listed in Schedule II shall affix to the package a label showing date of filling, the pharmacy name and address, the serial number of the prescription, the name of the patient, the name of the prescribing practitioner, and directions for use and cautionary statements, if any, contained in such prescription or required by law.

(b) The requirements of paragraph (a) of this section do not apply when a controlled substance listed in Schedule II is prescribed for administration to an ultimate user who is institutionalized: *Provided*, That:

(1) Not more than a 7-day supply of the controlled substance listed in Schedule II is dispensed at one time;

(2) The controlled substance listed in Schedule II is not in the possession of the ultimate user prior to the administration;

(3) The institution maintains appropriate safeguards and records regarding the proper administration, control, dispensing, and storage of the controlled substance listed in Schedule II; and

(4) The system employed by the pharmacist in filling a prescription is adequate to identify the supplier, the product, and the patient, and to set forth the directions for use and cautionary statements, if any, contained in the prescription or required by law.

§ 1306.15 Filing of prescriptions.

All written prescriptions and written records of emergency oral prescriptions shall be kept in accordance with requirements of § 1304.04(h) of this chapter.

Controlled Substances Listed in Schedules III and IV

§ 1306.21 Requirement of prescription.

(a) A pharmacist may dispense directly a controlled substance listed in Schedule III or IV, which is a prescription drug as determined under the Federal Food, Drug, and Cosmetic Act, only pursuant to either a written prescription signed by a prescribing individual practitioner or an oral prescription made by a prescribing individual practitioner and promptly reduced to writing by the pharmacist containing all information required in § 1306.05, except for the signature of the prescribing individual practitioner.

(b) An individual practitioner may administer or dispense directly a controlled substance listed in Schedule III or IV in the course of his professional practice without a prescription, subject to § 1306.07.

(c) An institutional practitioner may administer or dispense directly (but not prescribe) a controlled substance listed in Schedule III or IV pursuant to a written prescription signed by a prescribing individual practitioner, or pursuant to an oral prescription made by a prescribing individual practitioner and promptly reduced to writing by the pharmacist (containing all information required in § 1306.05 except for the signature of the prescribing individual practitioner), or pursuant to an order for medication made by an individual practitioner which is dispensed for immediate administration to the ultimate user, subject to § 1306.07.

§ 1306.22 Refilling of prescriptions.

(a) No prescription for a controlled substance listed in Schedule III or IV shall be filled or refilled more than 6 months after the date on which such prescription was issued and no such prescription authorized to be refilled may be refilled more than five times. Each refilling of a prescription shall be entered on the back of the prescription or on another appropriate document. If entered on another document, such as a medication record, the document must be uniformly maintained and readily retrievable. The following information must be retrievable by the prescription number consisting of the name and dosage form of the controlled substance, the date filled or refilled, the quantity dispensed, initials of the dispensing pharmacist for each refill, and the total number of refills for that prescription. If the pharmacist merely initials and dates the back of the prescription it shall be deemed that the full face amount of the prescription has been dispensed. The prescribing practitioner may authorize additional refills of Schedule III or IV controlled substances on the original prescription through an oral refill authorization transmitted to the pharmacist provided the following conditions are met:

(1) The total quantity authorized, including the amount of the original prescription, does not exceed five refills nor extend beyond six months from the date of issue of the original prescription.

(2) The pharmacist obtaining the oral authorization records on the reverse of the original prescription the date, quantity of refill, number of additional refills authorized, and initials the prescription showing who received the authorization from the prescribing practitioner who issued the original prescription.

(3) The quantity of each additional refill authorized is equal to or less than the quantity authorized for the initial filling of the original prescription.

(4) The prescribing practitioner must execute a new and separate prescription for any additional quantities beyond the five refill, six-month limitation.

(b) As an alternative to the procedures provided by subsection (a), an automated data processing system may be used for the storage and retrieval of refill information for prescription orders for controlled substances in Schedules III and IV, subject to the following conditions:

(1) Any such proposed computerized system must provide on-line retrieval (via CRT display or hard-copy printout) of original prescription order information for those prescription orders which are currently authorized for refilling. This shall include, but is not limited to, data such as the original prescription number, date of issuance of the original prescription order by the practitioner, full name and address of the patient, name, address, and DEA registration number of the practitioner, and the name, strength, dosage form, quantity of the controlled substance prescribed (and quantity dispensed if different from the quantity prescribed), and the total number of refills authorized by the prescribing practitioner.

(2) Any such proposed computerized system must also provide on-line retrieval (via CRT display or hard-copy printout) of the current refill history for Schedule III or IV controlled substance prescription orders (those authorized for refill during the past six months). This refill history shall include, but is not limited to, the name of the controlled substance, the date of refill, the quantity dispensed, the identification code, or name or initials of the dispensing pharmacist for each refill and the total number of refills dispensed to date for that prescription order.

(3) Documentation of the fact that the refill information entered into the computer each time a pharmacist refills an original prescription order for a Schedule III or IV controlled substance is correct must be provided by the individual pharmacist who makes use of such a system. If such a system provides a hard-copy printout of each day's controlled substance prescription order refill data, that printout shall be verified, dated, and signed by the individual pharmacist who refilled such a prescription order. The individual pharmacist must verify that the data indicated is correct and then sign this document in the same manner as he would sign a check or legal document (e.g., J. H. Smith, or John H. Smith). This document shall be maintained in a separate file at that pharmacy for a period of two years from the dispensing date. This printout of the day's controlled substance prescription order refill data must be provided to each pharmacy using such a computerized system within 72 hours of the date on which the refill was dispensed. It must be verified and signed by each pharmacist who is involved with such dispensing. In lieu of such a printout, the pharmacy shall maintain a bound log book, or separate file, in which each individual pharmacist involved in such dispensing shall sign a statement (in the manner previously described) each day, attesting to the fact that the refill information entered into the computer that day has been reviewed by him and is correct as shown. Such a book or file must be maintained at the pharmacy employing such a system for a period of two years after the date of dispensing the appropriately authorized refill.

(4) Any such computerized system shall have the capability of producing a printout of any refill data which the user pharmacy is responsible for maintaining under the Act and its implementing regulations. For example, this would include a refill-by-refill audit trail for any specified strength and dosage form of any controlled substance (by either brand or generic name or both). Such a printout must indicate name of the prescribing practitioner, name and address of the patient, quantity dispensed on each refill, date of dispensing for each refill, name or identification code of the dispensing pharmacist, and the number of the original prescription order. In any computerized system employed by a user pharmacy the central recordkeeping location must be capable of sending the printout to the pharmacy within 48 hours, and if a DEA Special Agent or Compliance Investigator requests a copy of such printout from the user pharmacy, it must, if requested to do so by the Agent or Investigator, verify the printout transmittal capability of its system by documentation (e.g., postmark).

(5) In the event that a pharmacy which employs such a computerized system experiences system down-time, the pharmacy must have an auxiliary procedure which will be used for documentation of refills of Schedule III and IV controlled substance prescription orders. This auxiliary procedure must ensure that refills are authorized by the original prescription order, that the maximum number of refills has not been exceeded, and that all of the appropriate data are retained for on-line data entry as soon as the computer system is available for use again.

(c) When filing refill information for original prescription orders for Schedule III or IV controlled substances, a pharmacy may use only one of the two systems described in paragraph (a) or (b) of this section.

§ 1306.23 Partial filling of prescriptions.

The partial filling of a prescription for a controlled substance listed in Schedule III or IV is permissible, provided that:

(a) Each partial filling is recorded in the same manner as a refilling,

(b) The total quantity dispensed in all partial fillings does not exceed the total quantity prescribed, and

(c) No dispensing occurs after 6 months after the date on which the prescription was issued.

§ 1306.24 Labeling of substances.

(a) The pharmacist filling a prescription for a controlled substance listed in Schedule III or IV shall affix to the package a label showing the pharmacy name and address, the serial number and date of initial filling, the name of the patient, the name of the practitioner issuing the prescription, and directions for use and cautionary statements, if any, contained in such prescription as required by law.

(b) The requirements of paragraph (a) of this section do not apply when a controlled substance listed in Schedule III or IV is prescribed for administration to an ultimate user who is institutionalized: *Provided*, That:

(1) Not more than a 34-day supply or 100 dosage units, whichever is less, of the controlled substance listed in Schedule III or IV is dispensed at one time;

(2) The controlled substance listed in Schedule III or IV is not in the possession of the ultimate user prior to administration;

(3) The institution maintains appropriate safeguards and records the proper administration, control, dispensing, and storage of the controlled substance listed in Schedule III or IV; and

(4) The system employed by the pharmacist in filling a prescription is adequate to identify the supplier, the product and the patient, and to set forth the directions for use and cautionary statements, if any, contained in the prescription or required by law.

§ 1306.25 Filing prescriptions.

All prescriptions for controlled substances listed in Schedules III and IV shall be kept in accordance with § 1304.04(h) of this chapter.

§ 1306.26 Transfer between pharmacies of prescription information for Schedules III, IV, and V controlled substances for refill purposes.

(a) The transfer of original prescription information for a controlled substance listed in Schedules III, IV or V for the purpose of refill dispensing is permissible between pharmacies on a one time basis subject to the following requirements:

(1) The transfer is communicated directly between two licensed pharmacists and the transferring pharmacist records the following information:

(i) Write the word "VOID" on the face of the invalidated prescription.

(ii) Record on the reverse of the invalidated prescription the name, address and DEA registration number of the pharmacy to which it was transferred and the name of the pharmacist receiving the prescription information.

(iii) Record the date of the transfer and the name of the pharmacist transferring the information.

(b) The pharmacist receiving the transferred prescription information shall reduce to writing the following:

(1) Write the word "transfer" on the face of the transferred prescription.

(2) Provide all information required to be on a prescription pursuant to 21 CFR 1306.05 and include:

(i) Date of issuance of original prescription;

(ii) Original number of refills authorized on original prescription;

(iii) Date of original dispensing;

(iv) Number of valid refills remaining and date of last refill;

(v) Pharmacy's name, address, DEA registration number and original prescription number from which the prescription information was transferred;

(vi) Name of transferor pharmacist.

(3) Both the original and transferred prescription must be maintained for a period of two years from the date of last refill.

(c) Pharmacies electronically accessing the same prescription record must satisfy all information requirements of a manual mode for prescription transferral.

(d) The procedure allowing the transfer of prescription information for refill purposes is permissible only if allowable under existing state or other applicable law.

Controlled Substances Listed in Schedule V

§ 1306.31 Requirement of prescription.

(a) A pharmacist may dispense directly a controlled substance listed in Schedule V pursuant to a prescription as required for controlled substances listed in Schedules III and IV in § 1306.21. A prescription for a controlled substance listed in Schedule V may be refilled only as expressly authorized by the prescribing individual practitioner on the prescription; if no such authorization is given, the prescription may not be refilled. A pharmacist dispensing such substance pursuant to a prescription shall label the substance in accordance with § 1306.24 and file the prescription in accordance with § 1306.25.

(b) An individual practitioner may administer or dispense directly a controlled substance listed in Schedule V in the course of his professional practice without a prescription, subject to § 1306.07.

(c) An institutional practitioner may administer or dispense directly (but not prescribe) a controlled substance listed in Schedule V only pursuant to a written prescription signed by the prescribing individual practitioner, or pursuant to an oral prescription made by a prescribing individual practitioner and promptly reduced to writing by the pharmacist (containing all information required in § 1306.05 except for the signature of the prescribing individual practitioner), or pursuant to an order for medication made by an individual practitioner which is dispensed for immediate administration to the ultimate user, subject to § 1306.07.

§ 1306.32 Dispensing without prescription.

A controlled substance listed in Schedule V, and a controlled substance listed in Schedule II, III, or IV which is not a prescription drug as determined under the Federal Food, Drug, and Cosmetic Act, may be dispensed by a pharmacist without a prescription to a purchaser at retail, provided that:

(a) Such dispensing is made only by a pharmacist (as defined in § 1306.02(d)), and not by a nonpharmacist employee even if under the supervision of a pharmacist (although after the pharmacist has fulfilled his professional and legal responsibilities set forth in this section, the actual cash, credit transaction, or delivery, may be completed by a nonpharmacist);

(b) Not more than 240 cc. (8 ounces) of any such controlled substance containing opium, nor more than 120 cc. (4 ounces) of any other such controlled substance nor more than 48 dosage units of any such controlled substance containing opium, nor more than 24 dosage units of any other such controlled substance may be dispensed at retail to the same purchaser in any given 48-hour period;

(c) The purchaser is at least 18 years of age;

(d) The pharmacist requires every purchaser of a controlled substance under this section not known to him to furnish suitable identification (including proof of age where appropriate);

(e) A bound record book for dispensing of controlled substances under this section is maintained by the pharmacist, which book shall contain the name and address of the purchaser, the name and quantity of controlled substance purchased, the date of each purchase, and the name or initials of the pharmacist who dispensed the substance to the purchaser (the book shall be maintained in accordance with the recordkeeping requirement of § 1304.04 of this chapter); and

(f) A prescription is not required for distribution or dispensing of the substance pursuant to any other Federal, State, or local law.

Miscellaneous

§ 1307.02 Application of State law and other Federal law.

Nothing in Parts 1301–1308, 1311, 1312, or 1316 of this chapter shall be construed as authorizing or permitting any person to do any act which such person is not authorized or permitted to do under other Federal laws or obligations under international treaties, conventions or protocols, or under the law of the State in which he desires to do such act nor shall compliance with such Parts be construed as compliance with other Federal or State laws unless expressly provided in such other laws.

§ 1307.03 Exceptions to regulations.

Any person may apply for an exception to the application of any provision of Parts 1301–1308, 1311, 1312, or 1316 of this chapter by filing a written request stating the reasons for such exception. Requests shall be filed with the Administrator, Drug Enforcement Administration, Department of Justice, Washington, DC 20537. The Administrator may grant an exception in his discretion, but in no case shall he be required to grant an exception to any person which is not otherwise required by law or the regulations cited in this section.

Special Exceptions for Manufacture and Distribution of Controlled Substances

§ 1307.11 Distribution by dispenser to another practitioner.

(a) A practitioner who is registered to dispense a controlled substance may distribute (without being registered to distribute) a quantity of such substance to another practitioner for the purpose of general dispensing by the practitioner to his or its patients: *Provided*, That:

(1) The practitioner to whom the controlled substance is to be distributed is registered under the Act to dispense that controlled substance;

(2) The distribution is recorded by the distributing practitioner in accordance with § 1304.24(e) of this chapter and by the receiving practitioner in accordance with § 1304.24(c) of this chapter;

(3) If the substance is listed in Schedule I or II, an order form is used as required in Part 1305 of this chapter;

(4) The total number of dosage units of all controlled substances distributed by the practitioner pursuant to this section and § 1301.28 of this chapter during each calendar year in which the practitioner is registered to dispense does not exceed 5 percent of the total number of dosage units of all controlled substances distributed and dispensed by the practitioner during the same calendar year.

(b) If, during any calendar year in which the practitioner is registered to dispense, the practitioner has reason to believe that the total number of dosage units of all controlled substances which will be distributed by him pursuant to this section and § 1301.28 of this chapter will exceed 5 percent of the total number of dosage units of all controlled substances distributed and dispensed by him during that calendar year, the practitioner shall obtain a registration to distribute controlled substances.

§ 1307.12 Manufacture and distribution of narcotic solutions and compounds by a pharmacist.

As an incident to a distribution under § 1307.11, a pharmacist may manufacture (without being registered to manufacture) an aqueous or oleaginous solution or solid dosage form containing a narcotic controlled substance in a proportion not exceeding 20 percent of the complete solution, compound, or mixture.

§ 1307.13 Distribution to supplier.

Any person lawfully in possession of a controlled substance listed in any schedule may distribute (without being registered to distribute) that substance to the person from whom he obtained it or to the manufacturer of the substance, provided that a written record is maintained which indicates the date of the transaction, the name, form and quantity of the substance, the name, address, and registration number, if any, of the person making the distribution, and the name, address, and registration number, if known, of the supplier or manufacturer. In the case of returning a controlled substance listed in Schedule I or II, an order form shall be used in the manner prescribed in Part 1305 of this chapter and be maintained as the written record of the transaction. Any person not required to register pursuant to sections 302(c) or 1007(b)(1) of the Act [21 U.S.C. 823(c) or 957(b)(1)] shall be exempt from maintaining the records required by this section.

§ 1307.14 Distribution upon discontinuance or transfer of business.

(a) Any registrant desiring to discontinue business activities altogether or with respect to controlled substances (without transferring such business activities to another person) shall return for cancellation his certificate of registration, and any unexecuted order forms in his possession, to the Registration Unit, Drug Enforcement Administration, Department of Justice, Post Office Box 28083, Central Station, Washington, DC 20005. Any controlled substances in his possession may be disposed of in accordance with § 1307.21.

(b) Any registrant desiring to discontinue business activities altogether or with respect to controlled substances (by transferring such business activities to another person) shall submit in person or by registered or certified mail, return receipt requested, to the Special Agent in Charge in his area, at least 14 days in advance of the date of the proposed transfer (unless the Special Agent in Charge waives this time limitation in individual instances), the following information:

(1) The name, address, registration number, and authorized business activity of the registrant discontinuing the business (registrant-transferor);

(2) The name, address, registration number, and authorized business activity of the person acquiring the business (registrant-transferee);

(3) Whether the business activities will be continued at the location registered by the person discontinuing business, or moved to another location (if the latter, the address of the new location should be listed);

(4) Whether the registrant-transferor has a quota to manufacture or procure any controlled substance listed in Schedule I or II (if so, the basic class or class of the substance should be indicated); and

(5) The date on which the transfer of controlled substances will occur.

(c) Unless the registrant-transferor is informed by the Regional Administrator,[1] before the date on which the transfer was stated to occur, that the transfer may not occur, the registrant-transferor may distribute (without being registered to distribute) controlled substances in his possession to the registrant-transferee in accordance with the following:

(1) On the date of transfer of the controlled substances, a complete inventory of all controlled substances being transferred shall be taken in accordance with §§ 1304.11–1304.19 of this chapter. This inventory shall serve as the final inventory of the registrant-transferor and the initial inventory of the registrant-transferee, and a copy of the inventory shall be included in the records of each person. It shall not be necessary to file a copy of the inventory with the Administration unless requested by the Regional Administrator.[1] Transfers of any substances listed in Schedule I or II shall require the use of order forms in accordance with Part 1305 of this chapter.

(2) On the date of transfer of the controlled substances, all records required to be kept by the registrant-transferor with reference to the controlled substances being transferred, under Part 1304 of this chapter, shall be transferred to the registrant-transferee. Responsibility for the accuracy of records prior to the date of transfer remains with the transferor, but responsibility for custody and maintenance shall be upon the transferee.

(3) In the case of registrants required to make reports pursuant to Part 1304 of this chapter, a report marked "Final" will be prepared and submitted by the registrant-transferor showing the disposition of all the controlled substances for which a report is required; no additional report will be required from him, if no further transactions involving controlled substances are consummated by him. The initial report of the registrant-transferee shall account for transactions beginning with the day next succeeding the date of discontinuance or transfer of business by the transferor-registrant and the substances transferred to him shall be reported as receipts in his initial report.

Disposal of Controlled Substances

§ 1307.21 Procedure for disposing of controlled substances.

(a) Any person in possession of any controlled substance and desiring or required to disposed of such substance may request the Special Agent in Charge of the Administration in the area in which the person is located for authority and instructions to dispose of such substance. The request should be made as follows:

(1) If the person is a registrant required to make reports pursuant to Part 1304 of this chapter, he shall list the controlled substance or substances which he desires to dispose of on the "b" subpart of the report normally filed by him, and submit three copies of that subpart to the Special Agent in Charge of the Administration in his area;

(2) If the person is a registrant not required to make reports pursuant to Part 1304 of this chapter, he shall list the controlled substance or substances which he desires to dispose of on DEA Form 41, and submit three copies of that form to the Special Agent in Charge in his area; and

(3) If the person is not a registrant, he shall submit to the Special Agent in Charge a letter stating:

(i) The name and address of the person;

(ii) The name and quantity of each controlled substance to be disposed of;

(iii) How the applicant obtained the substance, if known; and

(iv) The name, address, and registration number, if known, of the person who possessed the controlled substances prior to the applicant, if known.

(b) The Special Agent in Charge shall authorize and instruct the applicant to dispose of the controlled substance in one of the following manners:

(1) By transfer to person registered under the Act and authorized to possess the substance;

(2) By delivery to an agent of the Administration or to the nearest office of the Administration;

(3) By destruction in the presence of an agent of the Administration or other authorized person; or

(4) By such other means as the Special Agent in Charge may determine to assure that the substance does not become available to unauthorized persons.

(c) In the event that a registrant is required regularly to dispose of controlled substances, the Special Agent in Charge may authorize the registrant to dispose of such substances, in accordance with paragraph (b) of this section, without prior approval of the Administration in each instance, on the condition that the registrant keep records of such disposals and file periodic reports with the Special Agent in Charge

[1] Special Agent in Charge.

summarizing the disposals made by the registrant. In granting such authority, the Special Agent in Charge may place such conditions as he deems proper on the disposal of controlled substances, including the method of disposal and the frequency and detail of reports.

(d) This section shall not be construed as affecting or altering in any way the disposal of controlled substances through procedures provided in laws and regulations adopted by any State.

Schedules of Controlled Substances

§ 1308.02 Definitions.

(b) The term *anabolic steroid* means any drug or hormonal substance, chemically and pharmacologically related to testosterone (other than estrogens, progestins, and corticosteroids) that promotes muscle growth, and includes:

(1) Boldenone;
(2) Chlorotestosterone (4-chlortestosterone);
(3) Clostebol;
(4) Dehydrochlormethyltestosterone;
(5) Dihydrotestosterone (4-dihydrotestosterone);
(6) Drostanolone;
(7) Ethylestrenol;
(8) Fluoxymesterone;
(9) Formebulone (formebolone);
(10) Mesterolone;
(11) Methandienone;
(12) Methandranone;
(13) Methandriol;
(14) Methandrostenolone;
(15) Methenolone;
(16) Methyltestosterone;
(17) Mibolerone;
(18) Nandrolone;
(19) Norethandrolone;
(20) Oxandrolone;
(21) Oxymesterone;
(22) Oxymetholone;
(23) Stanolone;
(24) Stanozolol;
(25) Testolactone;
(26) Testosterone;
(27) Trenbolone; and
(28) Any salt, ester, or isomer of a drug or substance described or listed in this paragraph, if that salt, ester, or isomer promotes muscle growth. Except such term does not include an anabolic steroid which is expressly intended for administration through implants to cattle or other nonhuman species and which has been approved by the Secretary of Health and Human Services for such administration. If any person prescribes, dispenses, or distributes such steroid for human use, such person shall be considered to have prescribed, dispensed, or distributed an anabolic steroid within the meaning of this paragraph.

(d) The term "isomer" means the optical isomer, except as used in § 1308.11(d) and § 1308.12(b)(4). As used in § 1308.11(d), the term "isomer" means the optical, positional, or geometric isomer. As used in § 1308.12(b)(4), the term "isomer" means the optical or geometric isomer.

(e) The term "interested person" means any person adversely affected or aggrieved by any rule or proposed rule issuable pursuant to section 201 of the Act.

(f) The term "narcotic drug" means any of the following whether produced directly or indirectly by extraction from substances of vegetable origin or independently by means of chemical synthesis or by a combination of extraction and chemical synthesis:

(1) Opium, opiates, derivatives of opium and opiates, including their isomers, esters, ethers, salts, and salts of isomers, esters, and ethers whenever the existence of such isomers, esters, ethers and salts is possible within the specific chemical designation. Such term does not include the isoquinoline alkaloids of opium.

(2) Poppy straw and concentrate of poppy straw.

(3) Coca leaves, except coco leaves and extracts of coca leaves from which cocaine, ecgonine and derivatives of ecgonine or their salts have been removed.

(4) Cocaine, its salts, optical and geometric isomers, and salts of isomers.

(5) Ecgonine, its derivatives, their salts, isomers and salts of isomers.

(6) Any compound, mixture, or preparation which contains any quantity of any of the substances referred to in subparagraphs (1) through (5).

§ 1308.11 Schedule I.

(a) Schedule I shall consist of the drugs and other substances, by whatever official name, common or usual name, chemical name, or brand name designated, listed in this section. Each drug or substance has been assigned the DEA Controlled Substances Code Number set forth opposite it.

(b) *Opiates.* Unless specifically excepted or unless listed in another schedule, any of the following opiates, including their isomers, esters, ethers, salts, and salts of isomers, esters and ethers, whenever the existence of such isomers, esters, ethers, and salts is possible within the specific chemical designation [for purposes of paragraph (b)(34) only, the term isomer includes the optical and geometric isomers]:

(1)	Acetyl-alpha-methylfentanyl (*N*-[1-(1-methyl-2-phenethyl)-4-piperidinyl]-*N*-phenylacetamide)	9815
(2)	Acetylmethadol	9601
(3)	Allylprodine	9602
(4)	Alphacetylmethadol	9603
(5)	Alphameprodine	9604
(6)	Alphamethadol	9605
(7)	Alpha-methylfentanyl (*N*-[1-(alpha-methyl-beta-phenyl)ethyl-4-piperidyl] propionanilide; 1-(1-methyl-2-phenylethyl)-4-(N-propanilido) piperidine)	9814
(8)	Alpha-methylthiofentanyl (*N*-[1-methyl-2-(2-thienyl)ethyl-4-piperidinyl]-*N*-phenylpropanamide)	9832
(9)	Benzethidine	9606
(10)	Betacetylmethadol	9607
(11)	Beta-hydroxyfentanyl (*N*-[1-(2-hydroxy-2-phenethyl)-4-piperidinyl]-*N*-phenylpropanamide)	9830
(12)	Beta-hydroxy-3-methylfentanyl (other name: *N*-[1-(2-hydroxy-2-phenethyl)-3-methyl-4-piperidinyl]-*N*-phenylpropanamide)	9831
(13)	Betameprodine	9608
(14)	Betamethadol	9609
(15)	Betaprodine	9611
(16)	Clonitazene	9612
(17)	Dextromoramide	9613
(18)	Diampromide	9615
(19)	Diethylthiambutene	9616
(20)	Difenoxin	9168
(21)	Dimenoxadol	9617
(22)	Dimepheptanol	9618
(23)	Dimethylthiambutene	9619
(24)	Dioxaphetyl butyrate	9621
(25)	Dipipanone	9622
(26)	Ethylmethylthiambutene	9623
(27)	Etonitazene	9624
(28)	Etoxeridine	9625
(29)	Furethidine	9626
(30)	Hydroxypethidine	9627
(31)	Ketobemidone	9628
(32)	Levomoramide	9629
(33)	Levophenacylmorphan	9631
(34)	3-Methylfentanyl(*N*-[3-methyl-1-(2-phenylethyl)-4-piperidyl]-*N*-phenylpropanamide)	9813
(35)	3-Methylthiofentanyl (*N*-[(3-methyl-1-(2-thienyl)ethyl-4-piperidinyl]-*N*-phenylpropanamide)	9833
(36)	Morpheridine	9632
(37)	MPPP (1-methyl-4-phenyl-4-propionoxypiperidine)	9661
(38)	Noracymethadol	9633
(39)	Norlevorphanol	9634
(40)	Normethadone	9635

(41) Norpipanone 9636
(42) Para-fluorofentanyl (*N*-(4-fluorophenyl)-*N*-[1-(2-phenethyl)-4-piperidinyl]-propanamide) 9812
(43) Phenadoxone 9637
(44) PEPAP (1-(-2-phenethyl)-4-phenyl-4-acetoxypiperidine) 9663
(45) Phenampromide 9638
(46) Phenomorphan 9647
(47) Phenoperidine 9641
(48) Piritramide 9642
(49) Proheptazine 9643
(50) Properidine 9644
(51) Propiram 9649
(52) Racemoramide 9645
(53) Thiofentanyl (*N*-phenyl-*N*-[1-(2-thienyl)-ethyl-4-piperidinyl]-propanamide) 9835
(54) Tilidine 9750
(55) Trimeperidine 9646

(c) *Opium derivatives.* Unless specifically excepted or unless listed in another schedule, any of the following opium derivatives, its salts, isomers, and salts of isomers whenever the existence of such salts, isomers, and salts of isomers is possible within the specific chemical designation:

(1) Acetorphine 9319
(2) Acetyldihydrocodeine 9051
(3) Benzylmorphine 9052
(4) Codeine methylbromide 9070
(5) Codeine-N-Oxide 9053
(6) Cyprenorphine 9054
(7) Desomorphine 9055
(8) Dihydromorphine 9145
(9) Drotebanol 9335
(10) Etorphine (except hydrochloride salt) 9056
(11) Heroin 9200
(12) Hydromorphinol 9301
(13) Methyldesorphine 9302
(14) Methyldihydromorphine 9304
(15) Morphine methylbromide 9305
(16) Morphine methylsulfonate 9306
(17) Morphine-N-Oxide 9307
(18) Myrophine 9308
(19) Nicocodeine 9309
(20) Nicomorphine 9312
(21) Normorphine 9313
(22) Pholcodine 9314
(23) Thebacon 9315

(d) *Hallucinogenic substances.* Unless specifically excepted or unless listed in another schedule, any material, compound, mixture, or preparation, which contains any quantity of the following hallucinogenic substances, or which contains any of its salts, isomers, and salts of isomers whenever the existence of such salts, isomers, and salts of isomers is possible within the specific chemical designation (for purposes of this paragraph only, the term "isomer" includes the optical, position, and geometric isomers):

(1) 4-bromo-2,5-dimethoxyamphetamine 7391
Some trade or other names: 4-bromo-2,5-dimethoxy-α-methylphenethyl amine; 4-bromo-2,5-DMA.
(2) 2,5-dimethoxyamphetamine 7396
Some trade or other names: 2,5-dimethoxy-α-methylphenethylamine; 2,5-DMA.
(3) 2,5-dimethoxy-4-ethylamphetamine 7399
Some trade or other names: DOET
(4) 4-methoxyamphetamine 7411
Some trade or other names: 4-methoxy-α-methylphenethylamine; paramethoxy-amphetamine; PMA.
(5) 5-methoxy-3,4-methylenedioxyamphetamine 7401
(6) 4-methyl-2,5-dimethoxyamphetamine 7395
Some trade and other names: 4-methyl-2,5-dimethoxy-α-methylphenethyl amine; "DOM"; and "STP."
(7) 3,4-methylenedioxy amphetamine 7400
(8) 3,4-methylenedioxymethamphetamine (MDMA) 7405
(9) 3,4-methylenedioxy-*N*-ethylamphetamine (also known as *N*-ethyl-alpha-methyl-3,4(methylenedioxy)phen ethylamine, *N*-ethyl MDA, MDE, MDEA 7404
(10) *N*-hydroxy-3,4-methylenedioxyamphetamine (also known as *N*-hydroxy-alpha-methyl-3,4(methylenedioxy)-phenethylamine, and *N*-hydroxy MDA 7402
(11) 3,4,5-trimethoxy amphetamine 7390
(12) Bufotenine 7433
Some trade and other names: 3-(β-Dimethylaminoethyl)-5-hydroxyindole; 3-(2-dimethylaminoethyl)-5-indolol; *N*,*N*-dimethylserotonin; 5-hydroxy-*N*,*N*-dimethyltryptamine; mappine.
(13) Diethyltryptamine 7434
Some trade and other names: *N*,*N*-Diethyltryptamine; DET.
(14) Dimethyltryptamine 7435
Some trade or other names: DMT.
(15) Ibogaine 7260
Some trade and other names: 7-Ethyl-6,6β,7,8,9,10,12,13-octahydro-2-methoxy-6,9-methano-5*H*-pyrido [1′,2′:1,2]azepino [5,4-b] indole; tabernanthe iboga.
(16) Lysergic acid diethylamide 7315
(17) Marijuana 7360
(18) Mescaline 7381
(19) Parahexyl 7374
Some trade or other names: 3-Hexyl-1-hydroxy-7,8,9,10-tetrahydro-6,6,9-trimethyl-6*H*-dibenzo[b,d]pyran; Synhexyl.
(20) Peyote 7415
Meaning all parts of the plant presently classified botanically as *Lophophora Williamsii Lemaire*, whether growing or not, the seeds thereof, any extract from any part of such plant, and every compound, manufacture, salt, derivative, mixture, or preparation of such plant, its seeds or extracts.
[Interprets 21 U.S.C. 812(c), Schedule I(c)(12)]
(21) *N*-ethyl-3-piperidyl benzilate 7482
(22) *N*-methyl-3-piperidyl benzilate 7484
(23) Psilocybin 7437
(24) Psilocyn 7438
(25) Tetrahydrocannabinols 7370
Synthetic equivalents of the substances contained in the plant, or in the resinous extractives of Cannabis, sp. and/or synthetic substances, derivatives, and their isomers with similar chemical structure and pharmacological activity such as the following:
Δ1 cis or trans tetrahydrocannabinol, and their optical isomers.
Δ6 cis or trans tetrahydrocannabinol, and their optical isomers.
Δ3,4 cis or trans tetrahydrocannabinol, and its optical isomers.
(Since nomenclature of these substances is not internationally standardized, compounds of these structures, regardless of numerical designation of atomic positions covered.)
(26) Ethylamine analog of phencyclidine 7455
Some trade or other names: *N*-ethyl-1-phenylcyclohexylamine, (1-phenylcyclohexyl)-ethylamine, *N*-(1-phenylcyclohexyl)-ethylamine, cyclohexamine, PCE.
(27) Pyrrolidine analog of phencyclidine 7458

Some trade or other names: 1-(1-phenylcyclohexyl)-pyrrolidine, PCPy, PHP.

(28) Thiophene analog of phencyclidine 7470
Some trade or other names: 1-[1-(2-thienyl)-cyclohexyl]-piperidine, 2-thienyl analog of phencyclidine, TPCP, TCP.

(29) 1-[1-(2-thienyl)cyclohexyl]pyrrolidine 7473
Some other names: TCPY

(e) *Depressants.* Unless specifically excepted or unless listed in another schedule, any material compound, mixture, or preparation which contains any quantity of the following substances having a depressant effect on the central nervous system, including its salts, isomers, and salts of isomers whenever the existence of such salts, isomers, and salts of isomers is possible within the specific chemical designation:

(1) Mecloqualone 2572
(2) Methaqualone 2565

(f) *Stimulants.* Unless specifically excepted or unless listed in another schedule, any material, compound, mixture, or preparation which contains any quantity of the following substances having a stimulant effect on the central nervous system, including its salts, isomers, and salts of isomers:

(1) Cathinone 1235
Some trade or other names: 2-amino-1-phenyl-1-propanone, alpha-aminopropiophenone, 2-aminopropiophenone, and norephedrone.

(2) Fenethylline 1503
(3) (±)*cis*-4-methylaminorex((±)*cis*-4,5-dihydro-4-methyl-5-phenyl-2-oxazolamine) 1590
(4) *N*-ethylamphetamine 1475
(5) *N,N*-dimethylamphetamine (also known as *N,N*,alpha-trimethylbenzeneethanamine: *N,N*,alpha-trimethylphenethylamine) 1480

(g) Temporary listing of substances subject to emergency scheduling. Any material, compound, mixture, or preparation which contains any quantity of the following substances:

(1) *N*-[1-benzyl-4-piperidyl]-*N*-phenylpropanamide (benzylfentanyl), its optical isomers, salts, and salts of isomers 9818
(2) *N*-[1-(2-thienyl)methyl-4-piperidyl]-*N*-phenylpropanamide (thenylfentanyl), its optical isomers, salts, and salts of isomers 9834
(3) Methcathinone (Some other names: 2-Methylamino-1-Phenylpropan-1-one; Ephedrone; Monomethylpropion; UR 1431, its salts, optical isomers, and salts of optical isomers—1237).
(4) Aminorex (Some other names: aminoxaphen, 2-amino-5-phenyl-2-oxazoline, or 4,5-dihydro-5-phenyl-2-oxazolamine, its salts, optical isomers, and salts of optical isomers—1585).
(5) Alpha-ethyltryptamine, its optical isomers, salts and salts of isomers 7249
Some other names: etryptamine; α-methyl-1H-indole-3-ethanamine; 3-(2-ami-nobutyl) indole.

§ 1308.12 Schedule II.

(a) Schedule II shall consist of the drugs and other substances, by whatever official name, common or usual name, chemical name, or brand name designated, listed in this section. Each drug or substance has been assigned the Controlled Substances Code Number set forth opposite it.

(b) *Substances, vegetable origin, or chemical synthesis.* Unless specifically excepted or unless listed in another schedule, any of the following substances whether produced directly or indirectly by extraction from substances of vegetable origin, or independently by means of chemical synthesis, or by a combination of extraction and chemical synthesis:

(1) Opium and opiate, and any salt, compound, derivative, or preparation of opium or opiate, excluding apomorphine, thebaine-derived butorphanol, dextrorphan, nalbuphine, nalmefene, naloxone, and naltrexone, and their respective salts, but including the following:

(1) Raw opium 9600
(2) Opium extracts 9610
(3) Opium fluid extracts 9620
(4) Powdered opium 9639
(5) Granulated opium 9640
(6) Tincture of opium 9630
(7) Codeine 9050
(8) Ethylmorphine 9190
(9) Etorphine hydrochloride 9059
(10) Hydrocodone 9193
(11) Hydromorphone 9150
(12) Metopon 9260
(13) Morphine 9300
(14) Oxycodone 9143
(15) Oxymorphone 9652
(16) Thebaine 9333

(2) Any salt, compound, derivative, or preparation thereof which is chemically equivalent or identical with any of the substances referred to in paragraph (b)(1) of this section, except that these substances shall not include the isoquinoline alkaloids of opium.

(3) Opium poppy and poppy straw.

(4) Coca leaves (9040) and any salt, compound, derivative or preparation of coca leaves [including cocaine (9041) and ecgonine (9180) and their salts, isomers, derivatives and salts of isomers and derivatives], and any salt, compound, derivative, or preparation thereof which is chemically equivalent or identical with any of these substances, except that the substances shall not include decocainized coca leaves or extraction of coca leaves, which extractions do not contain cocaine or ecgonine.

(5) Concentrate of poppy straw (the crude extract of poppy straw in either liquid, solid or powder form which contains the phenanthrine alkaloids of the opium poppy), 9670.

(c) *Opiates.* Unless specifically excepted or unless in another schedule any of the following opiates, including its isomers, esters, ethers, salts and salts of isomers, esters and ethers whenever the existence of such isomers, esters, ethers, and salts is possible within the specific chemical designation, dextrorphan and levopropoxyphene excepted:

(1) Alfentanil 9737
(2) Alphaprodine 9010
(3) Anileridine 9020
(4) Benzitramide 9800
(5) Bulk Dextropropoxyphene (nondosage forms) 9273
(6) Carfentanil 9743
(7) Dihydrocodeine 9120
(8) Diphenoxylate 9170
(9) Fentanyl 9801
(10) Isomethadone 9226
(11) Levomethorphan 9210
(12) Levorphanol 9220
(13) Metazocine 9240
(14) Methadone 9250
(15) Methadone-Intermediate, 4-cyano-2-dimethyl amino-4,4-diphenyl butane 9254
(16) Moramide-Intermediate, 2-methyl-3-morpholino-1,1-diphenylpropane-carboxylic acid ... 9802
(17) Pethidine (meperidine) 9230
(18) Pethidine-Intermediate-A, 4-cyano-1-methyl-4-phenylpiperidine 9232
(19) Pethidine-Intermediate-B, ethyl-4-phenyl-piperidine-4-carboxylate 9233
(20) Pethidine-Intermediate-C, 1-methyl-4-phenyl-piperidine-4-carboxylic acid 9234
(21) Phenazocine 9715
(22) Piminodine 9730
(23) Racemethorphan 9732
(24) Racemorphan 9733
(25) Sufentanil 9740

(d) *Stimulants.* Unless specifically excepted or unless listed in another schedule, any material, compound, mixture, or preparation which contains any quantity of the following substances having a stimulant effect on the central nervous system:

(1) Amphetamine, its salts, optical isomers, and salts of its optical isomers 1100
(2) Methamphetamine, its salts, isomers, and salts of its isomers 1105
(3) Phenmetrazine and its salts 1631
(4) Methylphenidate 1724

(e) *Depressants.* Unless specifically excepted or unless listed in another schedule, any material, compound, mixture, or preparation which contains any quantity of the following substances having a depressant effect on the central nervous system, including its salts, isomers, and salts of isomers whenever the existence of such salts, isomers, and salts of isomers is possible within the specific chemical designation:

(1) Amobarbital 2125
(2) Glutethimide 2250
(3) Pentobarbital 2270
(4) Phencyclidine 7471
(5) Secobarbital 2315

(f) *Hallucinogenic substances.*

(1) Dronabinol (synthetic) in sesame oil and encapsulated in a soft gelatin capsule in a U.S. Food and Drug Administration approved drug product[2] 7369
Some other names for dronabinol: (6a*R*-*trans*)-6a,7,8,10a-tetrahydro-6,6,9-trimethyl-3-pentyl-6*H*-dibenzo-[*b,d*]pyran-1-ol, or (−)-delta-9-(trans)-tetrahydrocannabinol
(2) Nabilone 7379
Another name for nabilone: (±)-*trans*-3-(1,1-dimethylheptyl)-6,6a,7,8,10,10a-hexahydro-1-hydroxy-6,6-dimethyl-9H-dibenzo[b,d]pyran-9-one.

(g) *Immediate precursors.* Unless specifically excepted or unless listed in another schedule, any material, compound, mixture, or preparation which contains any quantity of the following substances:

(1) Immediate precursor to amphetamine and methamphetamine:
(i) Phenylacetone 8501
Some trade or other names: phenyl-2-propanone; P2P; benzyl methyl ketone; methyl benzyl ketone;
(2) Immediate precursors to phencyclidine (PCP):
(i) 1-phenylcyclohexylamine 7460
(ii) 1-piperidinocyclohexanecarbonitrile (PCC) 8603

§ 1308.13 Schedule III.

(a) Schedule III shall consist of the drugs and other substances, by whatever official name, common or usual name, chemical name, or brand name designated, listed in this section. Each drug or substance has been assigned the DEA Controlled Substances Code Number set forth opposite it.

(b) *Stimulants.* Unless specifically excepted or unless listed in another schedule, any material, compound, mixture, or preparation which contains any quantity of the following substances having a stimulant effect on the central nervous system, including its salts, isomers (whether optical, position, or geometric), and salts of such isomers whenever the existence of such salts, isomers, and salts of isomers is possible within the specific chemical designation:

(1) Those compounds, mixtures, or preparations in dosage unit form containing any stimulant substances listed in Schedule II which compounds, mixtures, or preparations were listed on August 25, 1971, as excepted compounds under § 308.32, and any other drug of the quantitative composition shown in that list for those drugs or which is the same except that it contains a lesser quantity of controlled substances 1405
(2) Benzphetamine 1228
(3) Chlorphentermine 1645
(4) Clortermine 1647
(5) Phendimetrazine 1615

(c) *Depressants.* Unless specifically excepted or unless listed in another schedule, any material, compound, mixture, or preparation which contains any quantity of the following substances having a depressant effect on the central nervous system:

(1) Any compound, mixture, or preparation containing:
(i) Amobarbital 2128
(ii) Secobarbital 2316
(iii) Pentobarbital 2271
or any salt thereof and one or more other active medicinal ingredients which are not listed in any schedule.
(2) Any suppository dosage form containing:
(i) Amobarbital 2126
(ii) Secobarbital 2316
(iii) Pentobarbital 2271
or any salt of any of these drugs and approved by the Food and Drug Administration for marketing only as a suppository.
(3) Any substance which contains any quantity of a derivative of barbituric acid or any salt thereof 2100
(4) Chlorhexadol 2510
(5) Lysergic acid 7300
(6) Lysergic acid amide 7310
(7) Methyprylon 2575
(8) Sulfondiethylmethane 2600
(9) Sulfonethylmethane 2605
(10) Sulfonmethane 2610
(11) Tiletamine and zolazepam or any salt thereof 7295
Some trade or other names for a tiletamine-zolazepam combination product: Telazol.
Some trade or other names for tiletamine: 2-(ethylamino)-2-(2-thienyl)-cyclohexanone.
Some trade or other names for zolazepam: 4-(2-fluorophenyl)-6,8-dihydro-1,3,8-trimethylpyrazolo-[3,4-*e*][1,4]-diazepin-7(1*H*)-one, flupyrazapon.

(d) *Nalorphine* 9400

(e) *Narcotic drugs.* Unless specifically excepted or unless listed in another schedule, any material, compound, mixture, or preparation containing any of the following narcotic drugs, or their salts calculated as the free anhydrous base or alkaloid, in limited quantities as set forth below:

(1) Not more than 1.8 grams of codeine per 100 milliliters or not more than 90 milligrams per dosage unit, with an equal or greater quantity of an isoquinoline alkaloid of opium 9803
(2) Not more than 1.8 grams of codeine per 100 milliliters or not more than 90 milligrams per dosage unit, with one or more active, nonnarcotic ingredients in recognized therapeutic amounts 9804

[2] DEA Statement of Policy: *Any person registered by DEA to distribute, prescribe, administer, or dispense controlled substances in Schedule II who engages in the distribution or dispensing of dronabinol for medical indications outside the approved use associated with cancer treatment, except within the confines of a structured and recognized research program, may subject his or her controlled substances registration to review under the provisions of 21 U.S.C. 823(f) and 824(a)(4) as being inconsistent with the public interest. DEA will take action to revoke that such distribution or dispensing constitutes a threat to the public health and safety, and in addition will pursue any criminal sanctions which may be warranted under 21 U.S.C. 841(a)(1).* See *United States* v. *Moore*, 423 U.S. 122 (1975).

(3) Not more than 300 milligrams of dihydrocodeinone (hydrocodone) per 100 milliliters or not more than 15 milligrams per dosage unit, with a fourfold or greater quantity of an isoquinoline alkaloid of opium	9805
(4) Not more than 300 milligrams of dihydrocodeinone (hydrocodone) per 100 milliliters or not more than 15 milligrams per dosage unit, with one or more active nonnarcotic ingredients in recognized therapeutic amounts	9806
(5) Not more than 1.8 grams of dihydrocodeine per 100 milliliters or not more than 90 milligrams per dosage unit, with one or more active nonnarcotic ingredients in recognized therapeutic amounts	9807
(6) Not more than 300 milligrams of ethylmorphine per 100 milliliters or not more than 15 milligrams per dosage unit, with one or more active, nonnarcotic ingredients in recognized therapeutic amounts	9808
(7) Not more than 500 milligrams of opium per 100 milliliters or per 100 grams or not more than 25 milligrams per dosage unit, with one or more active, nonnarcotic ingredients in recognized therapeutic amounts	9809
(8) Not more than 50 milligrams of morphine per 100 milliliters or per 100 grams, with one or more active, nonnarcotic ingredients in recognized therapeutic amounts	9810

(f) *Anabolic steroids.* Unless specifically excepted or unless listed in another schedule, any material, compound, mixture, or preparation containing any quantity of the following substances, including its salts, isomers, and salts of isomers whenever the existence of such salts of isomers is possible within the specific chemical designation:

(1) Anabolic Steroids	4000

§ 1308.14 Schedule IV.

(a) Schedule IV shall consist of the drugs and other substances, by whatever official name, common or usual name, chemical name, or brand name designated, listed in this section. Each drug or substance has been assigned the DEA Controlled Substances Code Number set forth opposite it.

(b) *Narcotic drugs.* Unless specifically excepted or unless listed in another schedule, any material, compound, mixture, or preparation containing any of the following narcotic drugs, or their salts calculated as the free anhydrous base or alkaloid, in limited quantities as set forth below:

(1) Not more than 1 milligram of difenoxin (DEA Drug Code No. 9618) and not less than 25 micrograms of atropine sulfate per dosage unit.	
(2) Dextropropoxyphene (alpha-(+)-4-dimethylamino-1,2-diphenyl-3-methyl-2-propionoxybutane)	9273

(c) *Depressants.* Unless specifically excepted or unless listed in another schedule, any material, compound, mixture, or preparation which contains any quantity of the following substances, including its salts, isomers, and salts of isomers whenever the existence of such salts, isomers, and salts of isomers is possible within the specific chemical designation:

(1) Alprazolam	2882
(2) Barbital	2145
(3) Bromazepam	2748
(4) Camazepam	2749
(5) Chloral betaine	2460
(6) Chloral hydrate	2465
(7) Chlordiazepoxide	2744
(8) Clobazam	2751
(9) Clonazepam	2737
(10) Clorazepate	2768
(11) Clotiazepam	2752
(12) Cloxazolam	2753
(13) Delorazepam	2754
(14) Diazepam	2765
(15) Estazolam	2756
(16) Ethchlorvynol	2540
(17) Ethinamate	2545
(18) Ethyl loflazepate	2758
(19) Fludiazepam	2759
(20) Flunitrazepam	2763
(21) Flurazepam	2767
(22) Halazepam	2762
(23) Haloxazolam	2771
(24) Ketazolam	2772
(25) Loprazolam	2773
(26) Lorazepam	2885
(27) Lormetazepam	2774
(28) Mebutamate	2800
(29) Medazepam	2836
(30) Meprobamate	2820
(31) Methohexital	2264
(32) Methylphenobarbital (mephobarbital)	2250
(33) Midazolam	2884
(34) Nimetazepam	2837
(35) Nitrazepam	2834
(36) Nordiazepam	2838
(37) Oxazepam	2835
(38) Oxazolam	2839
(39) Paraldehyde	2585
(40) Petrichloral	2591
(41) Phenobarbital	2285
(42) Pinazepam	2883
(43) Prazepam	2764
(44) Quazepam	2881
(45) Temazepam	2925
(46) Tetrazepam	2886
(47) Triazolam	2887
(48) Zolpidem	2783

(d) *Fenfluramine.* Any material, compound, mixture, or preparation which contains any quantity of the following substances, including its salts, isomers (whether optical, position, or geometric), and salts of such isomers whenever the existence of such salts, isomers, and salts of isomers is possible:

(1) Fenfluramine	1670

(e) *Stimulants.* Unless specifically excepted or unless listed in another schedule, any material, compound, mixture, or preparation which contains any quantity of the following substances having a stimulant effect on the central nervous system, including its salts, isomers and salts of isomers:

(1) Cathine ((+)-norpseudoephedrine)	1230
(2) Diethylpropion	1610
(3) Fencamfamin	1760
(4) Fenproporex	1575
(5) Mazindol	1605
(6) Mefenorex	1580
(7) Pemoline (including organometallic complexes and chelates thereof)	1530
(8) Phentermine	1640
(9) Pipradrol	1750
(10) SPA ((−)-1-dimethylamino-1,2-diphenylethane)	1635

(f) *Other substances.* Unless specifically excepted or unless listed in another schedule, any material, compound, mixture, or preparation which contains any quantity of the following substances, including its salts:

(1) Pentazocine	9709

§ 1308.15 Schedule V.

(a) Schedule V shall consist of the drugs and other substances, by whatever official name, common or usual name, chemical name, or brand name designated, listed in this section.

(b) *Narcotic drugs.* Unless specifically excepted or unless listed in another schedule, any material, compound, mixture, or preparation containing any of the following narcotic drugs and their salts, as set forth below:

(1) Buprenorphine 9064

(c) Narcotic drugs containing nonnarcotic active medicinal ingredients. Any compound, mixture, or preparation containing any of the following narcotic drugs, or their salts calculated as the free anhydrous base or alkaloid, in limited quantities as set forth below, which shall include one or more nonnarcotic active medicinal ingredients in sufficient proportion to confer upon the compound, mixture, or preparation valuable medicinal qualities other than those possessed by narcotic drugs alone:

(1) Not more than 200 milligrams of codeine per 100 milliliters or per 100 grams.

(2) Not more than 100 milligrams of dihydrocodeine per 100 milliliters or per 100 grams.

(3) Not more than 100 milligrams of ethylmorphine per 100 milliliters or per 100 grams.

(4) Not more than 2.5 milligrams of diphenoxylate and not less than 25 micrograms of atropine sulfate per dosage unit.

(5) Not more than 100 milligrams of opium per 100 milliliters or per 100 grams.

(6) Not more than 0.5 milligram of difenoxin (DEA Drug Code No. 9618) and not less than 25 micrograms of atropine sulfate per dosage unit.

(d) *Stimulants.* Unless specifically exempted or excluded or unless listed in another schedule, any material, compound, mixture, or preparation which contains any quantity of the following substances having a stimulant effect on the central nervous system, including its salts, isomers and salts of isomers:

(1) Pyrovalerone 1485

Inspections

§ 1316.02 Definitions.

As used in this Subpart, the following terms shall have the meanings specified:

(c) The term "controlled premises" means—(1) Places where original or other records or documents required under the Act are kept or required to be kept, and

(2) Places, including factories, warehouses, or other establishments, and conveyances, where persons registered under the Act or exempted from registration under the Act may lawfully hold, manufacture, or distribute, dispense, administer, or otherwise dispose of controlled substances.

(e) The term "inspector" means an officer or employee of the Administration authorized by the Administrator to make inspections under the Act.

(f) The term "register" and "registration" refer to registration required and permitted by sections 303 and 1008 of the Act (21 U.S.C. 823 and 958).

§ 1316.03 Authority to make inspections.

In carrying out his functions under the Act, the Administrator, through his inspectors, is authorized in accordance with sections 510 and 1015 of the Act (21 U.S.C. 880 and 965) to enter controlled premises and conduct administrative inspections thereof, for the purpose of:

(a) Inspecting, copying, and verifying the correctness of records, reports, or other documents required to be kept or made under the Act and regulations promulgated under the Act, including, but not limited to, inventory and other records required to be kept pursuant to Part 1304 of this chapter, order form records required to be kept pursuant to Part 1305 of this chapter, prescription and distribution records required to be kept pursuant to Part 1306 of this chapter, tableting machines, and encapsulating machines required to be kept pursuant to part 1310 of this chapter, import/export records of listed chemicals required to be kept pursuant to part 1313 of this chapter, shipping records identifying the name of each carrier used and the date and quantity of each shipment, and storage records identifying the name of each warehouse used and the date and quantity of each storage;

(b) Inspecting within reasonable limits and in a reasonable manner all pertinent equipment, finished and unfinished controlled substances and other substances or materials, containers, and labeling found at the controlled premises relating to this Act;

(c) Making a physical inventory of all controlled substances on-hand at the premises;

(d) Collecting samples of controlled substances or precursors (in the event any samples are collected during an inspection, the inspector shall issue a receipt for such samples on DEA Form 84 to the owner, operator, or agent in charge of the premises);

(e) Checking of records and information on distribution of controlled substances by the registrant as they relate to total distribution of the registrant (i.e., has the distribution in controlled substances increased markedly within the past year, and if so why); and

(f) Except as provided in § 1316.04, all other things therein (including records, files, papers, processes, controls and facilities) appropriate for verification of the records, reports, documents referred to above or otherwise bearing on the provisions of the Act and the regulations thereunder.

§ 1316.04 Exclusion from inspection.

(a) Unless the owner, operator or agent in charge of the controlled premises so consents in writing, no inspection authorized by these regulations shall extend to:

(1) Financial data;

(2) Sales data other than shipping data; or

(3) Pricing data.

§ 1316.05 Entry.

An inspection shall be carried out by an inspector. Any such inspector, upon (a) stating his purpose and (b) presenting to the owner, operator or agent in charge of the premises to be inspected (1) appropriate credentials, and (2) written notice of his inspection authority under § 1314.06 of this chapter, and (c) receiving informed consent under § 1316.08 or through the use of administrative warrant issued under §§ 1316.09–1316.14, shall have the right to enter such premises and conduct inspections at reasonable times and in a reasonable manner.

§ 1316.06 Notice of inspection.

The notice of inspection [DEA (or DNB) Form 82] shall contain:

(a) The name and title of the owner, operator, or agent in charge of the controlled premises;

(b) The controlled premises name;

(c) The address of the controlled premises to be inspected;

(d) The date and time of the inspection;

(e) A statement that a notice of inspection is given pursuant to section 510 of the Act (21 U.S.C. 880);

(f) A reproduction of the pertinent parts of section 510 of the Act; and

(g) The signature of the inspector.

§ 1316.07 Requirement for administrative inspection warrant; exceptions.

In all cases where an inspection is contemplated, an administrative inspection warrant is required pursuant to section 510 of the Act (21 U.S.C. 880), except that such warrant shall not be required for establishments applying for initial registration under the Act, for the inspection of books and records pursuant to an administrative subpoena issued in accordance with section 506 of the Act (21 U.S.C. 876) nor for entries in administrative inspections (including seizures of property):

(a) With the consent of the owner, operator, or agent in charge of the controlled premises as set forth in § 1316.08;

(b) In situations presenting imminent danger to health or safety;

(c) In situations involving inspection of conveyances where there is reasonable cause to obtain a warrant;

(d) In any other exceptional or emergency circumstance or time or opportunity to apply for a warrant is lacking; or

(e) In any other situations where a warrant is not constitutionally required.

§ 1316.08 Consent to inspection.

(a) An administrative inspection warrant shall not be required if informed consent is obtained from the owner, operator, or agent in charge of the controlled premises to be inspected;

(b) Wherever possible, informed consent shall consist of a written statement signed by the owner, operator, or agent in charge of the premises to be inspected and witnessed by two persons. The written consent shall contain the following information:

(1) That he (the owner, operator, or agent in charge of the premises) has been informed of his constitutional right not to have an administrative inspection made without an administrative inspection warrant;

(2) That he has right to refuse to consent to such an inspection;

(3) That anything of an incriminating nature which may be found may be seized and used against him in a criminal prosecution;

(4) That he has been presented with a notice of inspection as set forth in § 1316.06;

(5) That the consent given by him is voluntary and without threats of any kind; and

(6) That he may withdraw his consent at any time during the course of inspection.

(c) The written consent shall be produced in duplicate and be distributed as follows:

(1) The original will be retained by the inspector; and

(2) The duplicate will be given to the person inspected.

§ 1316.11 Execution of warrants.

An administrative inspection warrant shall be executed and returned as required by, and any inventory or seizure made shall comply with the requirements of, section 510(d)(3) of the Act [21 U.S.C. 880(d)(3)]. The inspection shall begin as soon as is practicable after the issuance of the administrative inspection warrant and shall be completed with reasonable promptness. The inspection shall be conducted during regular business hours and shall be completed in a reasonable manner.

§ 1316.12 Refusal to allow inspection with an administrative warrant.

If a registrant or any person subject to the Act refuses to permit execution of an administrative warrant or impedes the inspector in the execution of that warrant, he shall be advised that such refusal or action constitutes a violation of section 402(a)(6) of the Act [21 U.S.C. (a)(6)]. If he persists and the circumstances warrant, he shall be arrested and the inspection shall commence or continue.

§ 1316.13 Frequency of administrative inspections.

Except where circumstances otherwise dictate, it is the intent of the Administration to inspect all manufacturers of controlled substances listed in Schedules I and II and distributors of controlled substances listed in Schedule I once each year; and to inspect all distributors of controlled substances listed in Schedules II through V and manufacturers of controlled substances listed in Schedules III through V once every 3 years.

⟨1076⟩ FEDERAL FOOD, DRUG, AND COSMETIC ACT REQUIREMENTS RELATING TO DRUGS FOR HUMAN AND ANIMAL USE

Selected portions of the Federal Food, Drug, and Cosmetic Act as it relates to the regulation of drugs for human use are presented here as a service to practitioners and students of pharmacy and medicine. The complete text of the Act can be found in Title 21 of the United States Code. The corresponding section number of the code appear in brackets after the section number of the Act.

In addition to federal requirements, statutes governing drugs and their quality have been enacted by various states. In many cases, state requirements parallel those of the federal law. However, this should not be assumed to be the case and individual state laws and requirements should be consulted also.

It should be noted that many provisions of the Act make no distinction between drugs for animal use or drugs for human use, but simply refer to drugs. For ease of reference, those sections of the Act which specifically relate to drugs for animal use are indexed separately and appear at the end of this chapter.

Publication of these sections in the United States Pharmacopeia is for purposes of information and does not impart to them any legal effect.

Inquiries regarding these requirements should be directed to the U.S. Food and Drug Administration, 5600 Fishers Lane, Rockville, MD 20857.

INDEX TO SELECTED PORTIONS OF THE FEDERAL FOOD, DRUG, AND COSMETIC ACT RELATED TO DRUGS FOR HUMAN USE PRESENTED HEREIN

(o) unregistered establishment or failure to bear identification symbol
(p) failure to comply with Poison Prevention Packaging Act

§ 503 Exemptions from Labeling and Packaging Requirements; Sales Restrictions of Drug Samples

(a) exemptions for repacking
(b) (1) prescription drug classification
(b) (2) dispensed prescription drug labeling requirements
(b) (4) federal caution statement required
(c) (1) drug sample marketing prohibited
(c) (2) coupon marketing prohibited
(c) (3) hospital or charity resale restrictions
(d) (1) restrictions on distribution of drug samples
(d) (2) requirements for sampling by mail
(d) (3) other distribution requirements
(e) (1) wholesale distributor restrictions
(e) (2) state licensure requirements
(e) (3) distributor and wholesale distribution definitions

§ 505 New Drugs

§ 506 Certification of Drugs Containing Insulin

§ 507 Certification of Antibiotics

§ 508 Authority to Designate Official Names

§ 510 Registration Requirements

(g) nonapplicability to pharmacies and practitioners

§ 525 Recommendations for Investigations of Drugs for Rare Diseases or Conditions

§ 526 Designation of Drugs for Rare Diseases or Conditions

§ 527 Protection of Unpatented Drugs for Rare Diseases or Conditions

§ 528 Open Protocols for Investigations of Drugs for Rare Diseases or Conditions

§ 703 Records of Interstate Shipment

§ 704 Inspections

Cooperation in Revision of USP and Development of Analytical Methods

INDEX TO SELECTED PORTIONS OF THE FEDERAL FOOD, DRUG, AND COSMETIC ACT RELATED TO DRUGS FOR ANIMAL USE

§ 201 Definitions

(s) food additive
(w) new animal drug
(x) animal feed
(bb) abbreviated drug application

§ 501 Adulterated Drugs

(a) (5) unsafe new animal drug
(a) (6) unsafe animal feed

§ 503 Exemptions From Labeling and Packaging Requirements

(f) (1) (a) prescription drug classification
(2) dispensed prescription drug labeling requirements
(4) Federal caution statement required

§ 512 New Animal Drugs

Short Title

§ 1 This Act may be cited as the Federal Food, Drug, and Cosmetic Act.

Definitions

§ 201 [321] For the purposes of this Act—

(e) The term "person" includes individual, partnership, corporation, and association.

(g) (1) The term "drug" means (A) articles recognized in the official United States Pharmacopeia, official Homeopathic Pharmacopeia of the United States, or official National Formulary, or any supplement to any of them; and (B) articles intended for use in the diagnosis, cure, mitigation, treatment, or prevention of disease in man or other animals; and (C) articles (other than food) intended to affect the structure or any function of the body of man or other animals; and (D) articles intended for use as a component of any articles specified in clause (A), (B), or (C); but does not include devices or their components, parts, or accessories.

(2) The term "counterfeit drug" means a drug which, or the container or labeling of which, without authorization, bears the trademark, trade name, or other identifying mark, imprint, or device, or any likeness thereof, of a drug manufacturer, processor, packer, or distributor other than the person or persons who in fact manufactured, processed, packed, or distributed such drug and which thereby falsely purports or is represented to be the product of, or to have been packed or distributed by, such other drug manufacturer, processor, packer, or distributor.

(j) The term "official compendium" means the official United States Pharmacopeia, official Homeopathic Pharmacopeia of the United States, official National Formulary, or any supplement to any of them.

(k) The term "label" means a display of written, printed, or graphic matter upon the immediate container of any article; and a requirement made by or under authority of this Act that any word, statement, or other information appear on the label shall not be considered to be complied with unless such word, statement, or other information also appears on the outside container or wrapper, if any there be, of the retail package of such article, or is easily legible through the outside container or wrapper.

(l) The term "immediate container" does not include package liners.

(m) The term "labeling" means all labels and other written, printed, or graphic matter (1) upon any article or any of its containers or wrappers, or (2) accompanying such article.

(n) If an article is alleged to be misbranded because the labeling or advertising is misleading, then in determining whether the labeling or advertising is misleading there shall be taken into account (among other things) not only representations made or suggested by statement, word, design, device, or any combination thereof, but also the extent to which the labeling or advertising fails to reveal facts material in the light of such representations or material with respect to consequences which may result from the use of the article to which the labeling or advertising relates under the conditions of use prescribed in the labeling or advertising thereof or under such conditions of use as are customary or usual.

(o) The representation of a drug, in its labeling, as an antiseptic shall be considered to be a representation that it is a germicide, except in the case of a drug purporting to be, or represented as, an antiseptic for inhibitory use as a wet dressing, ointment, dusting powder, or such other use as involves prolonged contact with the body.

(p) The term "new drug" means—

(1) Any drug (except a new animal drug or an animal feed bearing or containing a new animal drug) the composition of which is such that such drug is not generally recognized, among experts qualified by scientific training and experience to evaluate the safety and effectiveness of drugs, as safe and effective for use under the conditions prescribed, recommended, or suggested in the labeling thereof, except that such a drug not so recognized shall not be deemed to be a "new drug" if at any time prior to the enactment of this Act it was subject to the Food and Drugs Act of June 30, 1906, as amended, and if at such time its labeling contained the same representations concerning the conditions of its use; or

(2) Any drug (except a new animal drug or an animal feed bearing or containing a new animal drug) the composition of which is such that such drug, as a result of investigations to determine its safety and effectiveness for use under such conditions, has become so recognized, but which has not, otherwise than in such investigations, been used to a material extent or for a material time under such conditions.

(t) (1) The term "color additive" means a material which—

(A) is a dye, pigment, or other substance made by a process of synthesis or similar artifice, or extracted, isolated, or otherwise derived, with or without intermediate or final change of identity, from a vegetable, animal, mineral, or other source, and

(B) when added or applied to a food, drug, or cosmetic, or to the human body or any part thereof, is capable (alone or through reaction with another substance) of imparting color thereto:

except that such term does not include any material which the Secretary, by regulation, determines is used (or intended to be used) solely for a purpose or purposes other than coloring.

(2) The term "color" includes black, white, and intermediate grays.

(u) The term "safe," as used in paragraph(s) of this section and in sections 409, 512, and 706, has reference to the health of man or animal.

Prohibited Acts

§ **301** [331] The following acts and the causing thereof are hereby prohibited:

(a) The introduction or delivery for introduction into interstate commerce of any food, drug, device, or cosmetic that is adulterated or misbranded.

(b) The adulteration or misbranding of any food, drug, device, or cosmetic in interstate commerce.

(c) The receipt in interstate commerce of any food, drug, device, or cosmetic that is adulterated or misbranded, and the delivery or proffered delivery thereof for pay or otherwise.

(d) The introduction or delivery for introduction into interstate commerce of any article in violation of section 404 or 505.

(e) The refusal to permit access to or copying of any record as required by section 703; or the failure to establish or maintain any record, or make any report, required under section 505 (i) or (j), 507 (d) or (g), 512 (j), (l) or (m), 515 (f) or 519, or the refusal to permit access to or verification or copying of any such required record.

(f) The refusal to permit entry or inspection as authorized by section 704.

(g) The manufacture within any Territory of any food, drug, device, or cosmetic that is adulterated or misbranded.

(h) The giving of a guaranty or undertaking referred to in section 303 (c) (2), which guaranty or undertaking is false, except by a person who relied upon a guaranty or undertaking to the same effect signed by, and containing the name and address of, the person residing in the United States from whom he received in good faith the food, drug, device, or cosmetic; or the giving of a guaranty or undertaking referred to in section 303 (c) (3), which guaranty or undertaking is false.

(i) (1) Forging, counterfeiting, simulating, or falsely representing, or without proper authority using any mark, stamp, tag, label, or other identification device authorized or required by regulations promulgated under the provisions of section 404, 506, 507, or 706.

(2) Making, selling, disposing of, or keeping in possession, control, or custody, or concealing any punch, die, plate, stone, or other thing designed to print, imprint, or reproduce the trademark, trade name, or other identifying mark, imprint, or device of another or any likeness of any of the foregoing upon any drug or container or labeling thereof so as to render such drug a counterfeit drug.

(3) The doing of any act which causes a drug to be a counterfeit drug, or the sale or dispensing, or the holding for sale or dispensing, of a counterfeit drug.

(k) The alteration, mutilation, destruction, obliteration, or removal of the whole or any part of the labeling of, or the doing of any other act with respect to, a food, drug, device, or cosmetic, if such act is done while such article is held for sale (whether or not the first sale) after shipment in interstate commerce and results in such article being adulterated or misbranded.

(l) The using, on the labeling of any drug or device or in any advertising relating to such drug or device, of any representation or suggestion that approval of an application with respect to such drug or device is in effect under section 505, 515, or 520 (g), as the case may be, or that such drug or device complies with the provisions of such action.

(n) The using, in labeling, advertising or other sales promotion of any reference to any report or analysis furnished in compliance with section 704.

(p) The failure to register in accordance with section 510, the failure to provide any information required by section 510 (j) or 510 (k), or the failure to provide a notice required by section 510 (j) (2).

(t) The importation of a drug in violation of section 801 (d) (1), the sale, purchase, or trade of a drug or drug sample or the offer to sell, purchase, or trade a drug or drug sample in violation of section 503 (c), the sale, purchase, or trade of a coupon, the offer to sell, purchase, or trade such a coupon, or the counterfeiting of such a coupon in violation of section 503 (c) (2), the distribution of a drug sample in violation of section 503 (d) or the failure to otherwise comply with the requirements of section 503 (d), or the distribution of drugs in violation of section 503 (e) or the failure to otherwise comply with the requirements of section 503 (e).

Penalties

§ **303** [333] (a) (1) Any person who violates a provision of section 301 shall be imprisoned for not more than one year or fined not more than $1,000, or both.

(2) Notwithstanding the provisions of paragraph (1) of this section, if any person commits such a violation after a conviction of him under this section has become final, or commits such a violation with the intent to defraud or mislead, such person shall be imprisoned for not more than three years or fined not more than $10,000 or both.

(b) (1) Notwithstanding subsection (a), any person who violates section 301 (t) because of an importation of a drug in violation of section 801 (d) (1), because of a sale, purchase, or trade of a drug or drug sample or the offer to sell, purchase, or trade a drug or drug sample in violation of section 503 (c), because of the sale, purchase, or trade of a coupon, the offer to sell, purchase, or trade such a coupon, or the counterfeiting of such a coupon in violation of section 503 (c) (2), or the distribution of drugs in violation of section 503 (e) (2) (A) shall be imprisoned for not more than 10 years or fined not more than $250,000, or both.

(2) Any manufacturer or distributor who distributes drug samples by means other than the mail or common carrier whose representative, during the course of the representative's employment or association with the manufacturer or distributor, violated section 301 (t) because of a violation of section 503 (c) (1) or violated any State law prohibiting the sale, purchase, or trade of a drug sample subject to section 503 (b) or the offer to sell, purchase, or trade such a drug sample shall, upon conviction of the representative for such violation, be subject to the following civil penalties:

(A) A civil penalty of not more than $50,000 for each of the first two such violations resulting in a conviction of any representative of the manufacturer or distributor in any 10-year period.

(B) A civil penalty of not more than $1,000,000 for each violation resulting in a conviction of any representative after the second conviction in any 10-year period.

For the purposes of this paragraph, multiple convictions of one or more persons arising out of the same event or transaction, or a related series of events or transactions, shall be considered as one violation.

(3) Any manufacturer or distributor who violates section 301 (t) because of a failure to make a report required by section 503 (d) (3) (E) shall be subject to a civil penalty of not more than $100,000.

(4) (A) If a manufacturer or distributor or any representative of such manufacturer or distributor provides information leading to the arrest and conviction of any representative of that manufacturer or distributor for a violation of section 301 (t) because of a sale, purchase, or trade or offer to purchase, sell, or trade a drug sample in violation of section 503 (c) (1) or for a violation of State law prohibiting the sale, purchase, or trade or offer to sell, purchase, or trade a drug sample, the conviction of such representative shall not be considered as a violation for purposes of paragraph (2).

(B) If, in an action brought under paragraph (2) against a manufacturer or distributor relating to the conviction of a representative of such manufacturer or distributor for the sale, purchase, or trade of a drug or the offer to sell, purchase, or trade a drug, it is shown, by clear and convicting evidence—

(i) that the manufacturer or distributor conducted, before the arrest of such representative for the violation which resulted in such conviction, an investigation of events or transactions which would have led to the reporting of information leading to the arrest and conviction of such representative for such purchase, sale, or trade or offer to purchase, sell, or trade, or

(ii) that, except in the case of the conviction of a representative employed in a supervisory function, despite diligent implementation by the manufacturer or distributor of an independent audit and security system designed to detect such a violation, the manufacturer or distributor could not reasonably have been expected to have detected such violation, the conviction of such representative shall not be considered as a conviction for purpose of paragraph (2).

(5) If a person provides information leading to the arrest and conviction of a person for a violation of section 301 (t) because of the sale, purchase, or trade of a drug sample or the offer to sell, purchase, or trade a drug sample in violation of section 503 (c) (1), such person shall be entitled to one-half of the criminal fine imposed and collected for such violation but not more than $125,000.

(c) No person shall be subject to the penalties of subsection (a) of this section, (1) for having received in interstate commerce any article and delivered it or proffered delivery of it, if such delivery or proffer was made in good faith, unless he refuses to furnish on request of an officer or employee duly designated by the Secretary the name and address of the person from whom he purchased or received such article and copies of all documents, if any there be, pertaining to the delivery of the article to him; or (2) for having violated section 301 (a) or (d), if he establishes a guaranty or undertaking signed by, and containing the name and address of, the person residing in the United States from whom he received in good faith the article, to the effect, in case of an alleged violation of section 301 (a), that such article is not adulterated or misbranded, within the meaning of this Act, designating this Act, or to the effect, in case of an alleged violation of section 301 (d), that such article is not an article which may not, under the provisions of section 404 or 505, be introduced into interstate commerce; or (3) for having violated section 301 (a), where the violation exists because the article is adulterated by reason of containing a color additive not from a batch certified in accordance with regulations promulgated by the Secretary under this Act, if such person establishes a guaranty or undertaking signed by, and containing the name and address of, the manufacturer of the color additive, to the effect that such color additive was from a batch certified in accordance with the applicable regulations promulgated by the Secretary under this Act; or (4) for having violated section 301 (b), (c), or (k) by failure to comply with section 502 (f) in respect to an article received in interstate commerce to which neither section 503 (a) nor section 503 (b) (1) is applicable if the delivery or proffered delivery was made in good faith and the labeling at the time thereof contained the same directions for use and warning statements as were contained in the labeling at the time of such receipt of such article; or (5) for having violated section 301 (i) (2) if such person acted in good faith and had no reason to believe that use of the punch, die, plate, stone, or other thing involved would result in a drug being a counterfeit drug, or for having violated section 301 (i) (3) if the person doing the act or causing it to be done acted in good faith and had no reason to believe that the drug was a counterfeit drug.

Adulterated Drugs

§ **501** [351] A drug or device shall be deemed to be adulterated—

(a) (1) if it consists in whole or in part of any filthy, putrid, or decomposed substance; or (2) (A) if it has been prepared, packed, or held under insanitary conditions whereby it may have been contaminated with filth, or whereby it may have been rendered injurious to health; or (B) if it is a drug and the methods used in, or the facilities or controls used for, its manufacture, processing, packing, or holding do not conform to or are not operated or administered in conformity with current good manufacturing practice to assure that such drug meets the requirements of this Act as to safety and has the identity and strength, and meets the quality and purity characteristics, which it purports or is represented to possess; or (3) if its container is composed, in whole or in part, of any poisonous or deleterious substance which may render the contents injurious to health; or (4) if (A) it bears or contains, for purposes of coloring only, a color additive which is unsafe within the meaning of section 706 (a), or (B) it is a color additive the intended use of which in or on drugs or devices is for purposes of coloring only and is unsafe within the meaning of section 706 (a);

(b) If it purports to be or is represented as a drug the name of which is recognized in an official compendium, and its strength differs from, or its quality or purity falls below, the standards set forth in such compendium. Such determination as to strength, quality, or purity shall be made in accordance with the tests or methods of assay set forth in such compendium, except that whenever tests or methods of assays have not been prescribed in such compendium, or such tests or methods of assay as are prescribed are, in the judgment of the Secretary, insufficient for the making of such determination, the Secretary shall bring such fact to the attention of the appropriate body charged with the revision of such compendium, and if such body fails within a reasonable time to prescribe tests or methods of assay which, in the judgment of the Secretary, are sufficient for purposes of this paragraph, then the Secretary shall promulgate regulations prescribing appropriate tests or methods of assay in accordance with which such determination as to strength, quality, or purity shall be made. No drug defined in an official compendium shall be deemed to be adulterated under this paragraph because it differs from the standard of strength, quality, or purity therefor set forth in such compendium, if its difference in strength, quality, or purity from such standards is plainly stated on its label. Whenever a drug is recognized in both the United States Pharmacopeia and the Homeopathic Pharmacopeia of the United States it shall be subject to the requirements of the United States Pharmacopeia unless it is labeled and offered for sale as a homeopathic drug, in which case it shall be subject to the provisions of the Homeopathic Pharmacopeia of the United States and not to those of the United States Pharmacopeia.

(c) If it is not subject to the provisions of paragraph (b) of this section and its strength differs from, or its purity or quality falls below, that which it purports or is represented to possess.

(d) If it is a drug and any substance has been (1) mixed or packed therewith so as to reduce its quality or strength or (2) substituted wholly or in part therefor.

Misbranded Drugs

§ **502** [352] A drug or device shall be deemed to be misbranded—

(a) If its labeling is false or misleading in any particular.

(b) If in a package form unless it bears a label containing (1) the name and place of business of the manufacturer, packer, or distributor; and (2) an accurate statement of the quantity of the contents in terms of weight, measure, or numerical count: *Provided*, That under clause (2) of this paragraph reasonable variations shall be permitted, and exemptions as to small packages shall be established, by regulations prescribed by the Secretary.

(c) If any word, statement, or other information required by or under authority of this Act to appear on the label or labeling is not prominently placed thereon with such conspicuousness (as compared with other words, statements, designs, or devices, in the labeling) and in such terms as to render it likely to be read and understood by the ordinary individual under customary conditions of purchase and use.

(d) If it is for use by man and contains any quantity of the narcotic or hypnotic substance alpha-eucaine, barbituric acid, beta-eucaine, bromal, cannabis, carbromal, chloral, coca, cocaine, codeine, heroin, marijuana, morphine, opium, paraldehyde, peyote, or sulfonmethane; or any chemical derivative of such substance, which derivative has been by the Secretary, after investigation, found to be, and by regulations designated as, habit forming; unless its label bears the name, and quantity or proportion of such substance or derivative and in juxtaposition therewith the statement "Warning—May be habit forming."

(e) (1) If it is a drug, unless (A) its label bears, to the exclusion of any other nonproprietary name (except the applicable systematic chemical name or the chemical formula), (i) the established name (as defined in subparagraph (3)) of the drug, if such there be, and (ii) in case it is fabricated from two or more ingredients, the established name and quantity of each active ingredient, including the quantity, kind, and proportion of any alcohol, and also including whether active or not, the established name and quantity or proportion of any bromides, ether, chloroform, acetanilide, acetophenetidin, amidopyrine, antipyrine, atropine, hyoscine, hyoscyamine, arsenic, digitalis, digitalis glucosides, mercury, ouabain, strophanthin, strychnine, thyroid, or any derivative or preparation of any such substances, contained therein: *Provided*, That the requirement for stating the quantity of the active ingredients, other than the quantity of those specifically named in this paragraph, shall apply only to prescription drugs; and (B) for any prescription drug the established name of such drug or ingredient, as the case may be, on such label (and on any labeling on which a name for such drug or ingredient is used) is printed prominently and in type at least half as large as that used thereon for any proprietary name or designation for such drug or ingredient: and *Provided*, That to the extent that compliance with the requirements of clause (A) (ii) or clause (B) of this subparagraph is impracticable, exemptions shall be established by regulations promulgated by the Secretary.

(3) As used in paragraph (l) the term "established name," with respect to a drug or ingredient thereof, means (A) the applicable official name designated pursuant to section 508, or (B) if there is no such name and such drug, or such ingredient, is an article recognized in an official compendium, then the official title thereof in such compendium or (C) if neither clause (A) nor clause (B) of this subparagraph applies, then the common or usual name, if any, of such drug or of such ingredient: *Provided further*, That where clause (B) of this subparagraph applies to an article recognized in the United States Pharmacopeia and in the Homeopathic Pharmacopeia under different official titles, the official title used in the United States Pharmacopeia shall apply unless it is labeled and offered for sale as a homeopathic drug, in which case the official title used in the Homeopathic Pharmacopeia shall apply.

(f) Unless its labeling bears (1) adequate directions for use; and (2) such adequate warnings against use in those pathological conditions or by children where its use may be dangerous to health, or against unsafe dosage or methods or duration of administration or application, in such manner and form, as are necessary for the protection of users: *Provided*, That where any requirement of clause (1) of this paragraph, as applied to any drug or device, is not necessary for the protection of the public health, the Secretary shall promulgate regulations exempting such drug or device from such requirement.

(g) If it purports to be a drug the name of which is recognized in an official compendium, unless it is packaged and labeled as prescribed therein: *Provided*, That the method of packing may be modified with the consent of the Secretary. Whenever a drug is recognized in both the United States Pharmacopeia and the Homeopathic Pharmacopeia of the United States, it shall be subject to the requirements of the United States Pharmacopeia with respect to packaging, and labeling unless it is labeled and offered for sale as a homeopathic drug, in which case it shall be subject to the provisions of the Homeopathic Pharmacopeia of the United States, and not to those of the United States Pharmacopeia: *Provided further*, That, in the event of inconsistency between the requirements of this paragraph and those of paragraph (e) as to the name by which the drug or its ingredients shall be designated, the requirements of paragraph (e) shall prevail.

(h) If it has been found by the Secretary to be a drug liable to deterioration, unless it is packaged in such form and manner, and its label bears a statement of such precautions, as the Secretary shall by regulations require as necessary for the protection of the public health. No such regulation shall be established for any drug recognized in an official compendium until the Secretary shall have informed the appropriate body charged with the revision of such compendium of the need for such packaging or labeling requirements and such body shall have failed within a reasonable time to prescribe such requirements.

(i) (1) If it is a drug and its container is so made, formed, or filled as to be misleading; or (2) if it is an imitation of another drug; or (3) if it is offered for sale under the name of another drug.

(j) If it is dangerous to health when used in the dosage or manner, or with the frequency or duration prescribed, recommended, or suggested in the labeling thereof.

(k) If it is, or purports to be, or is represented as a drug composed wholly or partly of insulin, unless (1) it is from a batch with respect to which a certificate or release has been issued pursuant to section 506, and (2) such certificate or release is in effect with respect to such drug.

(l) If it is, or purports to be, or is represented as a drug (except a drug for use in animals other than man) composed wholly or partly of any kind of penicillin, streptomycin, chlortetracycline, chloramphenicol, bacitracin, or any other antibiotic drug, or any derivative thereof, unless (1) it is from a batch with respect to which a certificate or release has been issued pursuant to section 507, and (2) such certificate or release is in effect with respect to such drug; *Provided*, That this paragraph shall not apply to any drug or class of drugs exempted by regulations promulgated under section 507 (c) or (d).

(m) If it is a color additive the intended use of which is for the purpose of coloring only, unless its packaging and labeling are in conformity with such packaging and labeling requirements applicable to such color additive, as may be contained in regulations issued under section 706.

(n) In the case of any prescription drug distributed or offered for sale in any State, unless the manufacturer, packer, or distributor thereof includes in all advertisements and other descriptive printed matter issued or caused to be issued by the manufacturer, packer, or distributor with respect to that drug a true statement of (1) the established name as defined in section 502 (e), printed prominently and in type at least half as large as that used for any trade or brand name thereof, (2) the formula showing quantitatively each ingredient of such drug to the extent required for labels under section 502 (e), and (3) such other information in brief summary relating to side effects, contraindications, and effectiveness as shall be required in regulations which shall be issued by the Secretary in accordance with the procedure specified in section 701 (e) of this Act: *Provided*, That (A) except in extraordinary circumstances, no regulation issued under this paragraph shall require prior approval by the Secretary of the content of any advertisement, and (B) no advertisement of a prescription drug, published after the effective date of regulations issued under this paragraph applicable to advertisements of prescription drugs, shall, with respect to the matters specified in this paragraph or covered by such regulations, be subject to the provisions of sections 12 through 17 of the Federal Trade Commission Act, as amended (15 U.S.C. 52–57). This paragraph (n) shall not be applicable to any printed matter which the Secretary determines to be labeling as defined in section 201 (m) of this Act. Nothing in the Convention on Psychotropic Substances, signed at Vienna, Austria, on February 21, 1971, shall be construed to prevent drug price communications to consumers.

(o) If it was manufactured, prepared, propagated, compounded, or processed in an establishment in any State not duly registered under section 510, if it was not included in a list required by section 510 (j), if a notice or other information respecting it was not provided as required by such section or section 510 (k), or if it does not bear such symbols from the uniform system for identification of devices prescribed under section 510 (e) as the Secretary by regulation requires.

(p) If it is a drug and its packaging or labeling is in violation of an applicable regulation issued pursuant to section 3 or 4 of the Poison Prevention Packing Act of 1970.

Exemptions in Case of Drugs

§ **503** [353] (a) The Secretary is hereby directed to promulgate regulations exempting from any labeling or packaging requirement of this Act drugs and devices which are, in accordance with the practice of the trade, to be processed, labeled, or repacked in substantial quantities at establishments other than those where originally processed or packed, on condition that such drugs and devices are not adulterated or misbranded under the provisions of this Act upon removal from such processing, labeling, or repacking establishment.

(b) (1) A drug intended for use by man which—

(A) is a habit-forming drug to which section 502 (d) applies; or

(B) because of its toxicity or other potentiality for harmful effect, or the method of its use, or the collateral measures necessary to its use, is not safe for use except under the supervision of a practitioner licensed by law to administer such drug; or

(C) is limited by an approved application under section 505 to use under the professional supervision of a practitioner licensed by law to administer such drug; shall be dispensed only (i) upon a written prescription of a practitioner licensed by law to administer such drug, or (ii) upon an oral prescription of such practitioner which is reduced promptly to writing and filed by the pharmacist, or (iii) by refilling any such written or oral prescription if such refilling is authorized by the prescriber either in the original prescription or by oral order which is reduced promptly to writing and filed by the pharmacist. The act of dispensing a drug contrary to the provisions of this paragraph shall be deemed to be an act which results in the drug being misbranded while held for sale.

(2) Any drug dispensed by filling or refilling a written or oral prescription of a practitioner licensed by law to administer such drug shall be exempt from the requirements of section 502, except paragraphs (a), (i) (2) and (3), (k), and (l), and the packaging requirements of paragraphs (g), (h), and (p), if the drug bears a label containing the name and address of the dispenser, the serial number and date of the prescription or of its filling, the name of the prescriber, and, if stated in the prescription, the name of the patient, and the directions for use and cautionary statements, if any, contained in such prescription. This exemption shall not apply to any drug dispensed in the course of the conduct of a business of dispensing drugs pursuant to diagnosis by mail, or to a drug dispensed in violation of paragraph (1) of this subsection.

(3) The Secretary may by regulation remove drugs subject to section 502 (d) and section 505 from the requirements of paragraph (1) of this subsection when such requirements are not necessary for the protection of the public health.

(4) A drug which is subject to paragraph (1) of this subsection shall be deemed to be misbranded if at any time prior to dispensing its label fails to bear the statement "Caution: Federal law prohibits dispensing without prescription." A drug to which paragraph (1) of this subsection does not apply shall be deemed to be misbranded if at any time prior to dispensing its label bears the caution statement quoted in the preceding sentence.

(5) Nothing in this subsection shall be construed to relieve any person from any requirement prescribed by or under authority of law with respect to drugs now included or which may hereafter be included within the classifications stated in section 3220 of the Internal Revenue Code (26 U.S.C. 3220), or to marijuana as defined in section 3238 (b) of the Internal Revenue Code (26 U.S.C. 3238 (b)).

(c) (1) No person may sell, purchase, or trade or offer to sell, purchase, or trade any drug sample. For purpose of this paragraph and subsection (d), the term 'drug sample' means a unit of a drug, subject to subsection (b), which is not intended to be sold and is intended to promote the sale of the drug. Nothing in this paragraph shall subject an officer or executive of a drug manufacturer or distributor to criminal liability solely because of a sale, purchase, trade, or offer to sell, purchase, or trade in violation of this paragraph by other employees of the manufacturer or distributor.

(2) No person may sell, purchase, or trade, offer to sell, purchase, or trade, or counterfeit any coupon. For purposes of this paragraph, the term 'coupon' means a form which may be redeemed, at no cost or at a reduced cost, for a drug which is prescribed in accordance with section 503 (b).

(3) (A) No person may sell, purchase, or trade, or offer to sell, purchase, or trade, any drug—

(i) which is subject to subsection (b), and

(ii) (I) which was purchased by a public or private hospital or other health care entity, or

(II) which was donated or supplied at a reduced price to a charitable organization described in section 501 (c) (3) of the Internal Revenue Code of 1954.

(B) Subparagraph (A) does not apply to—

(i) the purchase or other acquisition by a hospital or other health care entity which is a member of a group purchasing organization of a drug for its own use from the group purchasing organization or from other hospitals or health care entities which are members of such organization,

(ii) the sale, purchase, or trade of a drug or an offer to sell, purchase, or trade a drug by an organization described in subparagraph (A) (ii) (II) to a nonprofit affiliate of the organization to the extent otherwise permitted by law,

(iii) a sale, purchase, or trade of a drug or an offer to sell, purchase, or trade a drug among hospitals or other health care entities which are under common control,

(iv) a sale, purchase, or trade of a drug or an offer to sell, purchase, or trade a drug for emergency medical reasons, or

(v) a sale, purchase, or trade of a drug, an offer to sell, purchase, or trade a drug, or the dispensing of a drug pursuant to a prescription executed in accordance with section 503 (b).

For purposes of this paragraph, the term 'entity' does not include a wholesale distributor of drugs or a retail pharmacy licensed under State law and the term 'emergency medical reasons' includes transfers of a drug between health care entities or from a health care entity to a retail pharmacy undertaken to alleviate temporary shortages of the drug arising from delays in or interruptions of regular distribution schedules.

(d) (1) Except as provided in paragraphs (2) and (3), no representative of drug manufacturer or distributor may distribute any drug sample.

(2) (A) The manufacturer or distributor of a drug subject to subsection (b) may, in accordance with this paragraph, distribute drug samples by mail or common carrier to practitioners licensed to prescribe such drugs, or, at the request of a licensed practitioner, to pharmacies of hospitals or other health care entities. Such a distribution of drug samples may only be made—

(i) in response to a written request for drug samples made on a form which meets the requirements of subparagraph (B), and

(ii) under a system which requires the recipient of the drug sample to execute a written receipt for the drug sample upon its delivery and the return of the receipt to the manufacturer or distributor.

(B) A written request for a drug sample required by subparagraph (A) (i) shall contain—

(i) the name, address, professional designation, and signature of the practitioner making the request,

(ii) the identity of the drug sample requested and the quantity requested,

(iii) the name of the manufacturer of the drug sample requested, and

(iv) the date of the request.

(C) Each drug manufacturer or distributor which makes distributions by mail or common carrier under this paragraph shall maintain, for a period of 3 years, the request forms submitted for such distributions and shall maintain a record of distributions of drug samples which identifies the drugs distributed and the recipients of the distributions. Forms, receipts, and records required to be maintained under this subparagraph shall be made available by the drug manufacturer or distributor to Federal and State officials engaged in the regulation of drugs and in the enforcement of laws applicable to drugs.

(3) The manufacturer or distributor of a drug subject to subsection (b) may, by means other than mail or common carrier, distribute drug samples only if the manufacturer or distributor makes the distributions in accordance with subparagraph (A) and carries out the activities described in subparagraphs (B) through (F) as follows:

(A) Drug samples may only be distributed—

(i) to practitioners licensed to prescribe such drugs if they make a written request for the drug samples, or

(ii) at the written request of such a licensed practitioner, to pharmacies of hospitals or other health care entities.

A written request for drug samples shall be made on a form which contains the practitioner's name, address, and professional designation, the identity of the drug sample requested, the quantity of drug samples requested, the name of the manufacturer or distributor of the drug sample, the date of the request and signature of the practitioner making the request.

(B) Drug manufacturers or distributors shall store drug samples under conditions that will maintain their stability, integrity, and effectiveness and will assure that the drug samples will be free of contamination, deterioration, and adulteration.

(C) Drug manufacturers or distributors shall conduct, at least annually, a complete and accurate inventory of all drug samples in the possession of representatives of the manufacturer or distributor. Drug manufacturers or distributors shall maintain lists of the names and addresses of each of their representatives who distribute drug samples and of the sites where drug samples are stored. Drug manufacturers or distributors shall maintain records for at least 3 years of all drug samples distributed, destroyed, or returned to the manufacturer or distributor, of all inventories maintained under this subparagraph, of all thefts or significant losses of drug samples, and of all requests made under subparagraph (A) for drug samples. Records and lists maintained under this subparagraph shall be made available by the drug manufacturer or distributor to the Secretary upon request.

(D) Drug manufacturers or distributors shall notify the Secretary of any significant loss of drug samples and any known theft of drug samples.

(E) Drug manufacturers or distributors shall report to the Secretary any conviction of their representatives for violations of section 503 (c) (1) or a State law because of the sale, purchase, or trade of a drug sample or the offer to sell, purchase, or trade a drug sample.

(F) Drug manufacturers or distributors shall provide to the Secretary the name and telephone number of the individual responsible for responding to a request for information respecting drug samples.

(e) (1) Each person who is engaged in the wholesale distribution of drugs subject to subsection (b) and who is not an authorized distributor of record of such drugs shall provide to each wholesale distributor of such drugs a statement identifying each sale of the drug (including the date of the sale) before the sale to such wholesale distributor. Each manufacturer shall maintain at its corporate offices a current list of such authorized distributors.

(2) (A) No person may engage in the wholesale distribution in interstate commerce of drugs subject to subsection (b) in a State unless such person is licensed by the State in accordance with the guidelines issued under subparagraph (B).

(B) The Secretary shall by regulation issue guidelines establishing minimum standards, terms, and conditions for the licensing of persons to make wholesale distributions in interstate commerce of drugs subject to subsection (b). Such guidelines shall prescribe requirements for the storage and handling of such drugs and for the establishment and maintenance of records of the distributions of such drugs.

(3) For the purposes of this subsection—

(A) the term 'authorized distributors of record' means those distributors with whom a manufacturer has established an ongoing relationship to distribute such manufacturer's products, and

(B) the term 'wholesale distribution' means distribution of drugs subject to subsection (b) to other than the consumer or patient but does not include intracompany sales and does not include distributions of drugs described in subsection (c) (3) (B).

New Drugs

§ **505** [355] (a) No person shall introduce or deliver for introduction into interstate commerce any new drug, unless an approval of an application filed pursuant to subsection (b) or (j) is effective with respect to such drug.

(b) (1) Any person may file with the Secretary an application with respect to any drug subject to the provisions of subsection (a). Such persons shall submit to the Secretary as a part of the application (A) full reports of investigations which have been made to show whether or not such drug is safe for use and whether such drug is effective in use; (B) a full list of the articles used as components of such drug; (C) a full statement of the composition of such drug; (D) a full description of the methods used in, and the facilities and controls used for, the manufacture, processing, and packing of such drug; (E) such samples of such drug and of the articles used as components thereof as the Secretary may require; and (F) specimens of the labeling proposed to be used for such drug. The applicant shall file with the application the patent number and the expiration date of any patent which claims the drug for which the applicant submitted the application or which claims a method of using such drug and with respect to which a claim of patent infringement could reasonably be asserted if a person not licensed by the owner engaged in the manufacture, use, or sale of the drug. If an application is filed under this subsection for a drug and a patent which claims such drug or a method of using such drug is issued after the filing date but before approval of the application, the applicant shall amend the application to include the information required by the preceding sentence. Upon approval of the application, the Secretary shall publish information submitted under the two preceding sentences.

(2) An application submitted under paragraph (1) for a drug for which the investigations described in clause (A) of such paragraph and relied upon by the applicant for approval of the application were not conducted by or for the applicant and for which the applicant has not obtained a right of reference or use from the person by or for whom the investigations were conducted shall also include—

(A) a certification, in the opinion of the applicant and to the best of his knowledge, with respect to each patent which claims the drug for which such investigations were conducted or which claims a use for such drug for which the applicant is seeking approval under this subsection and for which information is required to be filed under paragraph (1) or subsection (c)—

(i) that such patent information has not been filed,

(ii) that such patent has expired,

(iii) of the date on which such patent will expire, or

(iv) that such patent is invalid or will not be infringed by the manufacture, use, or sale of the new drug for which the application is submitted; and

(B) if with respect to the drug for which investigations described in paragraph (1) (A) were conducted information was filed under paragraph (1) or subsection (c) for a method of use patent which does not claim a use for which the applicant is seeking approval under this subsection, a statement that the method of use patent does not claim such a use.

(3) (A) An applicant who makes a certification described in paragraph (2) (A) (iv) shall include in the application a statement that the applicant will give the notice required by subparagraph (B) to—

(i) each owner of the patent which is the subject of the certification or the representative of such owner designated to receive such notice, and

(ii) the holder of the approved application under subsection (b) for the drug which is claimed by the patent or a use of which is claimed by the patent or the representative of such holder designated to receive such notice.

(B) The notice referred to in subparagraph (A) shall state that an application has been submitted under this subsection for the drug with respect to which the certification is made to obtain approval to engage in the commercial manufacture, use, or sale of the drug before the expiration of the patent referred to in the certification. Such notice shall include a detailed statement of the factual and legal basis of the applicant's opinion that the patent is not valid or will not be infringed.

(C) If an application is amended to include a certification described in paragraph (2) (A) (iv), the notice required by subparagraph (B) shall be given when the amended application is submitted.

(c) (1) Within one hundred and eighty days after the filing of an application under subsection (b), or such additional period as may be agreed upon by the Secretary and the applicant, the Secretary shall either—

(A) approve the application if he then finds that none of the grounds for denying approval specified in subsection (d) applies, or

(B) give the applicant notice of an opportunity for a hearing before the Secretary under subsection (d) on the question whether such application is approvable. If the applicant elects to accept the opportunity for hearing by written request within thirty days after such notice, such hearing shall commence not more than ninety days after the expiration of such thirty days unless the Secretary and the applicant otherwise agree. Any such hearing shall thereafter be conducted on an expedited basis and the Secretary's order thereon shall be issued within ninety days after the date fixed by the Secretary for filing final briefs.

(2) If the patent information described in subsection (b) could not be filed with the submission of an application under subsection (b) because the application was filed before the patent information was required under subsection (b) or a patent was issued after the application was approved under such subsection, the holder of an approved application shall file with the Secretary the patent number and the expiration date of any patent which claims the drug for which the application was submitted or which claims a method of using such drug and with respect to which a claim of patent infringement could reasonably be asserted if a person not licensed by the owner engaged in the manufacture, use, or sale of the drug. If the holder of an approved application could not file patent information under subsection (b) because it was not required at the time the application was approved, the holder shall file such information under this subsection not later than thirty days after the date of the enactment of this sentence, and if the holder of an approved application could not file patent information under subsection (b) because no patent had been issued when an application was filed or approved, the holder shall file such information under this subsection not later than thirty days after the date the patent involved is issued. Upon the submission of patent information under this subsection, the Secretary shall publish it.

(3) The approval of an application filed under subsection (b) which contains a certification required by paragraph (2) of such subsection shall be made effective on the last applicable date determined under the following:

(A) If the applicant only made a certification described in clause (i) or (ii) of subsection (b) (2) (A) or in both such clauses, the approval may be made effective immediately.

(B) If the applicant made a certification described in clause (iii) of subsection (b) (2) (A), the approval may be made effective on the date certified under clause (iii).

(C) If the applicant made a certification described in clause (iv) of subsection (b) (2) (A), the approval shall be made effective immediately unless an action is brought for infringement of a patent which is the subject of the certification before the expiration of forty-five days from the date the notice provided under paragraph (3) (B) is received. If such an action is brought before the expiration of such days, the approval may be made effective upon the expiration of the thirty-month period beginning on the date of the receipt of the notice provided under paragraph (3) (B) or such shorter or longer period as the court may order because either party to the action failed to reasonably cooperate in expediting the action, except that—

(i) if before the expiration of such period the court decides that such patent is invalid or not infringed, the approval may be made effective on the date of the court decision,

(ii) if before the expiration of such period the court decides that such patent has been infringed, the approval may be made effective on such date as the court orders under section 271 (e) (4) (A) of title 35, United States Code, or

(iii) if before the expiration of such period the court grants a preliminary injunction prohibiting the applicant from engaging in the commercial manufacture or sale of the drug until the court decides the issues of patent validity and infringement and if the court decides that such patent is invalid or not infringed, the approval shall be made effective on the date of such court decision.

In such an action, each of the parties shall reasonably cooperate in expediting the action. Until the expiration of forty-five days from the date the notice made under paragraph (3) (B) is received, no action may be brought under section 2201 of title 28, United States Code, for a declaratory judgment with respect to the patent. Any action brought under such section 2201 shall be brought in the judicial district where the defendent has its principal place of business or a regular and established place of business.

(D) (i) If an application (other than an abbreviated new drug application) submitted under subsection (b) for a drug, no active ingredient (including any ester or salt of the active ingredient) of which has been approved in any other application under subsection (b), was approved during the period beginning January 1, 1982, and ending on the date of the enactment of this subsection, the Secretary may not make the approval of another application for a drug for which the investigations described in clause (A) of subsection (b) (1) and relied upon by the applicant for approval of the application were not conducted by or for the applicant and for which the applicant has not obtained a right of reference or use from the person by or for whom the investigations were conducted effective before the expiration of ten years from the date of the approval of the application previously approved under subsection (b).

(ii) If an application submitted under subsection (b) for a drug, no active ingredient (including any ester or salt of the active ingredient) of which has been approved in any other application under subsection (b), is approved after the date of the enactment of this clause, no application which refers to the drug for which the subsection (b) application was submitted and for which the investigations described in clause (A) of subsection (b) (1) and relied upon by the applicant for approval of the application were not conducted by or for the applicant and for which the applicant has not obtained a right of reference or use from the person by or for whom the investigations were conducted may be submitted under subsection (b) before the expiration of five years from the date of the approval of the application under subsection (b), except that such an application may be submitted under subsection (b) after the expiration of four years from the date of the approval of the subsection (b) application if it contains a certification of patent invalidity or noninfringement described in clause (iv) of subsection (b) (2) (A). The approval of such an application shall be made effective in accordance with this paragraph except that, if an action for patent infringement is commenced during the one-year period beginning forty-eight months after the date of the approval of the subsection (b) application, the thirty-month period referred to in subparagraph (C) shall be extended by such amount of time (if any) which is required for seven and one-half years to have elapsed from the date of approval of the subsection (b) application.

(iii) If an application submitted under subsection (b) for a drug, which includes an active ingredient (including any ester or salt of the active ingredient) that has been approved in another application approved under subsection (b), is approved after the date of the enactment of this clause and if such application contains reports of new clinical investigations (other than bioavailability studies) essential to the approval of the application and conducted or sponsored by the applicant, the Secretary may not make the approval of an application submitted under subsection (b) for the conditions of approval of such drug in the approved subsection (b) application effective before the expiration of three years from the date of the approval of the application under subsection (b) if the investigations described in clause (A) of subsection (b) (1) and relied upon by the applicant for approval of the application were not conducted by or for the applicant and if the applicant has not obtained a right of reference or use from the person by or for whom the investigations were conducted.

(iv) If a supplement to an application approved under subsection (b) is approved after the date of enactment of this clause and the supplement contains reports of new clinical investigations (other than bioavailability studies) essential to the approval of the supplement and conducted or sponsored by the person submitting the supplement, the Secretary may not make the approval of an application submitted under subsection (b) for a change approved in the supplement effective before the expiration of three years from the date of the approval of the supplement under subsection (b) if the investigations described in clause (A) of subsection (b) (1) and relied upon by the applicant for approval of the application were not conducted by or for the applicant and if the applicant has not obtained a right of reference or use from the person by or for whom the investigations were conducted.

(v) If an application (or supplement to an application) submitted under subsection (b) for a drug, which includes an active ingredient (including any ester or salt of the active ingredient) that has been approved in another application under subsection (b), was approved during the period beginning January 1, 1982, and ending on the date of the enactment of this clause, the Secretary may not make the approval of an application submitted under this subsection and for which the investigations described in clause (A) of subsection (b) (1) and relied upon by the applicant for approval of the application were not conducted by or for the applicant and for which the applicant has not obtained a right of reference or use from the person by or for whom the investigations were conducted and which refers to the drug for which the subsection (b) application was submitted effective before the expiration of two years from the date of enactment of this clause.

(d) If the Secretary finds, after due notice to the applicant in accordance with subsection (c) and giving him an opportunity for a hearing, in accordance with said subsection, that (1) the investigations, reports of which are required to be submitted to the Secretary pursuant to subsection (b), do not include adequate tests by all methods reasonably applicable to show whether or not such drug is safe for use under the conditions prescribed, recommended, or suggested in the proposed labeling thereof; (2) the results of such tests show that such drug is unsafe for use under such conditions or do not show that such drug is safe for use under such conditions; (3) the methods used in, and the facilities and controls used for, the manufacture, processing, and packing of such drug are inadequate to preserve its identity, strength, quality, and purity; (4) upon the basis of the information submitted to him as part of the application, or upon the basis of any other information before him with respect to such drug, he has insufficient information to determine whether such drug is safe for use under such conditions; or (5) evaluated on the basis of the information submitted to him as part of the application and any other information before him with respect to such drug, there is a lack of substantial evidence that the drug will have the effect it purports or is represented to have under the conditions of use prescribed, recommended, or suggested in the proposed labeling thereof; or

(6) the application failed to contain the patent information prescribed by subsection (b); or

(7) based on a fair evaluation of all material facts, such labeling is false or misleading in any particular; he shall issue an order refusing to approve the application. If, after such notice and opportunity for hearing, the Secretary finds that clauses (1) through (6) do not apply, he shall issue an order approving the application. As used in this subsection and subsection (e), the term "substantial evidence" means evidence consisting of adequate and well-controlled investigations, including clinical investigations, by experts qualified by scientific training and experience to evaluate the effectiveness of the drug involved, on the basis of which it could fairly and responsibly be concluded by such experts that the drug will have the effect it purports or is represented to have under the conditions of use prescribed, recommended, or suggested in the labeling or proposed labeling thereof.

(e) The Secretary shall, after due notice and opportunity for hearing to the applicant, withdraw approval of an application with respect to any drug under this section if the Secretary finds (1) that clinical or other experience, tests, or other scientific data show that such drug is unsafe for use under the conditions of use upon the basis of which the application was approved; (2) that new evidence of clinical experience, not contained in such application or not available to the Secretary until after such application was approved, or tests by new methods, or tests by methods not deemed reasonably applicable when such application was approved, evaluated together with the evidence available to the Secretary when the application was approved, shows that such drug is not shown to be safe for use under the conditions of use upon the basis of which the application was approved; or (3) on the basis of new information before him with respect to such drug, evaluated together with the evidence available to him when the application was approved, that there is a lack of substantial evidence that the drug will have the effect it purports or is represented to have under the conditions of use prescribed, recommended, or suggested in the labeling thereof; or

(4) the patent information prescribed by subsection (c) was not filed within thirty days after the receipt of written notice from the Secretary specifying the failure to file such information; or

(5) that the application contains any untrue statement of a material fact: *Provided*, That if the Secretary (or in his absence the officer acting as Secretary) finds that there is an imminent hazard to the public health, he may suspend the approval of such application immediately, and give the applicant prompt notice of his action and afford the applicant the opportunity for an expedited hearing under this subsection; but the authority conferred by this proviso to suspend the approval of an application shall not be delegated. The Secretary may also, after due notice and opportunity for hearing to the applicant, withdraw the approval of an application submitted under subsection (b) or (j) with respect to any drug under this section if the Secretary finds (1) that the applicant has failed to establish a system for maintaining required records, or has repeatedly or deliberately failed to maintain such records or to make required reports, in accordance with a regulation or order under subsection (k) or to comply with the notice requirements of section 510 (k) (2), or the applicant has refused to permit access to, or copying or verification of, such records as required by paragraph (2) of such subsection; or (2) that on the basis of new information before him, evaluated together with the evidence before him when the application was approved, the methods used in, or the facilities and controls used for, the manufacture, processing, and packing of such drug are inadequate to assure and preserve its identity, strength, quality, and purity and were not made adequate within a reasonable time after receipt of written notice from the Secretary specifying the matter complained of; or (3) that on the basis of new information before him, evaluated together with the evidence before him when the application was approved, the labeling of such drug, based on a fair evaluation of all material facts, is false or misleading in any particular and was not corrected within a reasonable time after receipt of written notice from the Secretary specifying the matter complained of. Any order under this subsection shall state the findings upon which it is based.

(f) Whenever the Secretary finds that the facts so require, he shall revoke any previous order under subsection (d) or (e) refusing, withdrawing, or suspending approval of an application and shall approve such application or reinstate such approval, as may be appropriate.

(g) Orders of the Secretary issued under this section shall be served (1) in person by any officer or employee of the Department designated by the Secretary or (2) by mailing the order by registered mail or by certified mail addressed to the applicant or respondent at his last-known address in the records of the Secretary.

(h) An appeal may be taken by the applicant from an order of the Secretary refusing or withdrawing approval of an application under this section. Such appeal shall be taken by filing in the United States court of appeals for the circuit wherein such applicant resides or has his principal place of business, or in the United States Court of Appeals for the District of Columbia Circuit, within sixty days after the entry of such order, a written petition praying that the order of the Secretary be set aside. A copy of such petition shall be forthwith transmitted by the clerk of the court to the Secretary, or any officer designated by him for that purpose, and thereupon the Secretary shall certify and file in the court the record upon which the order complained of was entered, as provided in section 2112 of title 28, United States Code. Upon the filing of such petition such court shall have exclusive jurisdiction to affirm or set aside such order, except that until the filing of the record the Secretary may modify or set aside his order. No objection to the order of the Secretary shall be considered by the court unless such objection shall have been urged before the Secretary or unless there were reasonable grounds for failure so to do. The finding of the Secretary as to the facts, if supported by substantial evidence, shall be conclusive. If any person shall apply to the court for leave to adduce additional evidence, and shall show to the satisfaction of the court that such additional evidence is material and that there were reasonable grounds for failure to adduce such evidence in the proceeding before the Secretary, the court may order such additional evidence to be taken before the Secretary and to be adduced upon the hearing in such manner and upon such terms and conditions as to the court may seem proper. The Secretary may modify his findings as to the facts by reason of the additional evidence so taken, and he shall file with the court such modified findings which, if supported by substantial evidence, shall be conclusive, and his recommendation, if any, for the setting aside of the original order. The judgment of the court affirming or setting aside any such order of the Secretary shall be final, subject to review by the Supreme Court of the United States upon certiorari or certification as provided in section 1254 of title 28 of the United States Code. The commencement of proceedings under this subsection shall not, unless specifically ordered by the court to the contrary, operate as a stay of the Secretary's order.

(i) The Secretary shall promulgate regulations for exempting from the operation of the foregoing subsections of this section drugs intended solely for investigational use by experts qualified by scientific training and experience to investigate the safety and effectiveness of drugs. Such regulations may, within the discretion of the Secretary, among other conditions relating to the protection of the public health, provide for conditioning such exemption upon—

(1) the submission to the Secretary, before any clinical testing of a new drug is undertaken, of reports, by the manufacturer or the sponsor of the investigation of such drug, or preclinical tests (including tests on animals) of such drug adequate to justify the proposed clinical testing;

(2) the manufacturer or the sponsor of the investigation of a new drug proposed to be distributed to investigators for clinical testing obtaining a signed agreement from each of such investigators that patients to whom the drug is administered will be under his personal supervision, or under the supervision of investigators responsible to him, and that he will not supply such drug to any other investigator, or to clinics, for administration to human beings; and

(3) the establishment and maintenance of such records, and the making of such reports to the Secretary, by the manufacturer or the sponsor of the investigation of such drug, of data (including but not limited to analytical reports by investigators) obtained as the result of such investigational use of such drug, as the Secretary finds will enable him to evaluate the safety and effectiveness of such drug in the event of the filing of an application pursuant to subsection (b).

Such regulations shall provide that such exemption shall be conditioned upon the manufacturer, or the sponsor of the investigation, requiring that experts using such drugs for investigational purposes certify to such manufacturer or sponsor that they will inform any human beings to whom such drugs, or any controls used in connection therewith, are being administered, or their representatives, that such drugs are being used for investigational purposes and will obtain the consent of such human beings or their representatives, except where they deem it not feasible or, in their professional judgment, contrary to the best interests of such human beings. Nothing in this subsection shall be construed to require any clinical investigator to submit directly to the Secretary reports on the investigational use of drugs.

(j) (1) Any person may file with the Secretary an abbreviated application for the approval of a new drug.

(2) (A) An abbreviated application for a new drug shall contain—

(i) information to show that the conditions of use prescribed, recommended, or suggested in the labeling proposed for the new drug have been previously approved for a drug listed under paragraph (6) (hereinafter in this subsection referred to as a listed drug);

(ii) (I) if the listed drug referred to in clause (i) has only one active ingredient, information to show that the active ingredient of the new drug is the same as that of the listed drug;

(II) if the listed drug referred to in clause (i) has more than one active ingredient, information to show that the active ingredients of the new drug are the same as those of the listed drug, or

(III) if the listed drug referred to in clause (i) has more than one active ingredient and if one of the active ingredients of the new drug is different and the application is filed pursuant to the approval of a petition filed under subparagraph (C), information to show that the other active ingredients of the new drug are the same as the active ingredients of the listed drug, information to show that the different active ingredient is an active ingredient of a listed drug or of a drug which does not meet the requirements of section 201 (p), and such other information respecting the different active ingredient with respect to which the petition was filed as the Secretary may require;

(iii) information to show that the route of administration, the dosage form, and the strength of the new drug are the same as those of the listed drug referred to in clause (i) or, if the route of administration, the dosage form, or the strength of the new drug is different and the application is filed pursuant to the approval of a petition filed under subparagraph (C), such information respecting the route of administration, dosage form, or strength with respect to which the petition was filed as the Secretary may require;

(iv) information to show that the new drug is bioequivalent to the listed drug referred to in clause (i), except that if the application is filed pursuant to the approval of a petition filed under subparagraph (C), information to show that the active ingredients of the new drug are of the same pharmacological or therapeutic class as those of the listed drug referred to in clause (i) and the new drug can be expected to have the same therapeutic effect as the listed drug when administered to patients for a condition of use referred to in clause (i);

(v) information to show that the labeling proposed for the new drug is the same as the labeling approved for the listed drug referred to in clause (i) except for changes required because of differences approved under a petition filed under subparagraph (C) or because the new drug and the listed drug are produced or distributed by different manufacturers;

(vi) the items specified in clauses (B) through (F) of subsection (b) (1);

(vii) a certification, in the opinion of the applicant and to the best of his knowledge, with respect to each patent which claims the listed drug referred to in clause (i) or which claims a use for such listed drug for which the applicant is seeking approval under this subsection and for which information is required to be filed under subsection (b) or (c)—

(I) that such patent information has not been filed,

(II) that such patent has expired,

(III) of the date on which such patent will expire, or

(IV) that such patent is invalid or will not be infringed by the manufacture, use, or sale of the new drug for which the application is submitted; and

(viii) if with respect to the listed drug referred to in clause (i) information was filed under subsection (b) or (c) for a method of use patent which does not claim a use for which the applicant is seeking approval under this subsection, a statement that the method of use patent does not claim such a use.

The Secretary may not require that an abbreviated application contain information in addition to that required by clauses (i) through (viii).

(B) (i) An applicant who makes a certification described in subparagraph (A) (vii) (IV) shall include in the application a statement that the applicant will give the notice required by clause (ii) to—

(I) each owner of the patent which is the subject of the certification or the representative of such owner designated to receive such notice, and

(II) the holder of the approved application under subsection (b) for the drug which is claimed by the patent or a use of which is claimed by the patent or the representative of such holder designated to receive such notice.

(ii) The notice referred to in clause (i) shall state that an application, which contains data from bioavailability or bioequivalence studies, has been submitted under this subsection for the drug with respect to which the certification is made to obtain approval to engage in the commercial manufacture, use, or sale of such drug before the expiration of the patent referred to in the certification. Such notice shall include a detailed statement of the factual and legal basis of the applicant's opinion that the patent is not valid or will not be infringed.

(iii) If an application is amended to include a certification described in subparagraph (A) (vii) (IV), the notice required by clause (ii) shall be given when the amended application is submitted.

(C) If a person wants to submit an abbreviated application for a new drug which has a different active ingredient or whose route of administration, dosage form, or strength differ from that of a listed drug, such person shall submit a petition to the Secretary seeking permission to file such an application. The Secretary shall approve or disapprove a petition submitted under this subparagraph within ninety days of the date the petition is submitted. The Secretary shall approve such a petition unless the Secretary finds—

(i) that investigations must be conducted to show the safety and effectiveness of the drug or of any of its active ingredients, the route of administration, the dosage form, or the strength, which differs from the listed drug; or

(ii) that any drug with a different active ingredient may not be adequately evaluated for approval as safe and effective on the basis of the information required to be submitted in an abbreviated application.

(3) Subject to paragraph (4), the Secretary shall approve an application for a drug unless the Secretary finds that—

(A) the methods used in, or the facilities and controls used for, the manufacture, processing, and packing of the drug are inadequate to assure and preserve its identity, strength, quality, and purity;

(B) the information submitted with the application is insufficient to show that each of the proposed conditions of use have been previously approved for the listed drug referred to in the application;

(C) (i) if the listed drug has only one active ingredient, information submitted with the application is insufficient to show that the active ingredient is the same as that of the listed drug;

(ii) if the listed drug has more than one active ingredient, information submitted with the application is insufficient to show that the active ingredients are the same as the active ingredients of the listed drug, or

(iii) if the listed drug has more than one active ingredient and if the application is for a drug which has an active ingredient different from the listed drug, information submitted with the application is insufficient to show—

(I) that the other active ingredients are the same as the active ingredients of the listed drug, or

(II) that the different active ingredient is an active ingredient of a listed drug or a drug which does not meet the requirements of section 201 (p), or no petition to file an application for the drug with the different ingredient was approved under paragraph (2) (C);

(D) (i) if the application is for a drug whose route of administration, dosage form, or strength of the drug is the same as the route of administration, dosage form, or strength of the listed drug referred to in the application, information submitted in the application is insufficient to show that the route of administration, dosage form, or strength is the same as that of the listed drug, or

(ii) if the application is for a drug whose route of administration, dosage form, or strength of the drug is different from that of the listed drug referred to in the application, no petition to file an application for the drug with the different route of administration, dosage form, or strength was approved under paragraph (2) (C);

(E) if the application was filed pursuant to the approval of a petition under paragraph (2) (C), the application did not contain the information required by the Secretary respecting the active ingredient, route of administration, dosage form, or strength which is not the same;

(F) information submitted in the application is insufficient to show that the drug is bioequivalent to the listed drug referred to in the application or, if the application was filed pursuant to a petition approved under paragraph (2) (C), information submitted in the application is insufficient to show that the active ingredients of the new drug are of the same pharmacological or therapeutic class as those of the listed drug referred to in paragraph (2) (A) (i) and that the new drug can be expected to have the same therapeutic effect as the listed drug when administered to patients for a condition of use referred to in such paragraph;

(G) information submitted in the application is insufficient to show that the labeling proposed for the drug is the same as the labeling approved for the listed drug referred to in the application except for changes required because of differences approved under a petition filed under paragraph (2) (C) or because the drug and the listed drug are produced or distributed by different manufacturers;

(H) information submitted in the application or any other information available to the Secretary shows that (i) the inactive ingredients of the drug are unsafe for use under the conditions prescribed, recommended, or suggested in the labeling proposed for the drug, or (ii) the composition of the drug is unsafe under such conditions because of the type or quantity of inactive ingredients included or the manner in which the inactive ingredients are included;

(I) the approval under subsection (c) of the listed drug referred to in the application under this subsection has been withdrawn or suspended for grounds described in the first sentence of subsection (e), the Secretary has published a notice of opportunity for hearing to withdraw approval of the listed drug under subsection (c) for grounds described in the first sentence of subsection (e), the approval under this subsection of the listed drug referred to in the application under this subsection has been withdrawn or suspended under paragraph (5), or the Secretary has determined that the listed drug has been withdrawn from sale for safety or effectiveness reasons;

(J) the application does not meet any other requirement of paragraph (2) (A); or

(K) the application contains an untrue statement of material fact.

(4) (A) Within one hundred and eighty days of the initial receipt of an application under paragraph (2) or within such additional period as may be agreed upon by the Secretary and the applicant, the Secretary shall approve or disapprove the application.

(B) The approval of an application submitted under paragraph (2) shall be made effective on the last applicable date determined under the following:

(i) If the applicant made a certification described in subclause (I) or (II) of paragraph (2) (A) (vii) or in both such subclauses, the approval may be made effective immediately.

(ii) If the applicant made a certification described in subclause (III) of paragraph (2) (A) (vii), the approval may be made effective on the date certified under subclause (III).

(iii) If the applicant made a certification described in subclause (IV) of paragraph (2) (A) (vii), the approval shall be made effective immediately unless an action is brought for infringement of a patent which is the subject of the certification before the expiration of forty-five days from the date the notice provided under paragraph (2) (B) (i) is received. If such an action is brought before the expiration of such days, the approval shall be made effective upon the expiration of the thirty-month period beginning on the date of the receipt of the notice provided under paragraph (2) (B) (i) or such shorter or longer period as the court may order because either party to the action failed to reasonably cooperate in expediting the action, except that—

(I) if before the expiration of such period the court decides that such patent is invalid or not infringed, the approval shall be made effective on the date of the court decision,

(II) if before the expiration of such period the court decides that such patent has been infringed, the approval shall be made effective on such date as the court orders under section 271 (e) (4) (A) of title 35, United States Code, or

(III) if before the expiration of such period, the court grants a preliminary injunction prohibiting the applicant from engaging in the commercial manufacture or sale of the drug until the court decides the issues of patent validity and infringement, and if the court decides that such patent is invalid or not infringed, the approval shall be made effective on the date of such court decision.

In such an action, each of the parties shall reasonably cooperate in expediting the action. Until the expiration of forty-five days from the date the notice made under paragraph (2) (B) (i) is received, no action may be brought under section 2201 of title 28, United States Code, for a declaratory judgment with respect to the patent. Any action brought under section 2201 shall be brought in the judicial district where the defendant has its principal place of business or a regular and established place of business.

(iv) If the application contains a certification described in subclause (IV) of paragraph (2) (A) (vii) and is for a drug for which a previous application has been submitted under this subsection continuing such a certification, the application shall be made effective not earlier than one hundred and eighty days after—

(I) the date the Secretary receives notice from the applicant under the previous application of the first commercial marketing of the drug under the previous application, or

(II) the date of a decision of a court in an action described in clause (iii) holding the patent which is the subject of the certification to be invalid or not infringed, whichever is earlier.

(C) If the Secretary decides to disapprove an application, the Secretary shall give the applicant notice of an opportunity for a hearing before the Secretary on the question of whether such application is approvable. If the applicant elects to accept the opportunity for hearing by written request within thirty days after such notice, such hearing shall commence not more than ninety days after the expiration of such thirty days unless the Secretary and the applicant otherwise agree. Any such hearing shall thereafter be conducted on an expedited basis and the Secretary's order thereon shall be issued within ninety days after the date fixed by the Secretary for filing final briefs.

(D) (i) If an application (other than an abbreviated new drug application) submitted under subsection (b) for a drug, no active ingredient (including any ester or salt of the active ingredient) of which has been approved in any other application under subsection (b), was approved during the period beginning January 1, 1982, and ending on the date of the enactment of this subsection, the Secretary may not make the approval of an application submitted under this subsection which refers to the drug for which the subsection (b) application was submitted effective before the expiration of ten years from the date of the approval of the application under subsection (b).

(ii) If an application submitted under subsection (b) for a drug, no active ingredient (including any ester or salt of the active ingredient) of which has been approved in any other application under subsection (b), is approved after the date of the enactment of this subsection, no application may be submitted under this subsection which refers to the drug for which the subsection (b) application was submitted before the expiration of five years from the date of the approval of the application under subsection (b), except that such an application may be submitted under this subsection after the expiration of four years from the date of the approval of the subsection (b) application if it contains a certification of patent invalidity or noninfringement described in subclause (IV) of paragraph (2) (A) (vii). The approval of such an application shall be made effective in accordance with subparagraph (B) except that, if an action for patent infringement is commenced during the one-year period beginning forty-eight months after the date of the approval of the subsection (b) application, the thirty-month period referred to in subparagraph (B) (iii) shall be extended by such amount of time (if any) which is required for seven and one-half years to have elapsed from the date of approval of the subsection (b) application.

(iii) If an application submitted under subsection (b) for a drug, which includes an active ingredient (including any ester or salt of the active ingredient) that has been approved in another application approved under subsection (b), is approved after the date of enactment of this subsection and if such application contains reports of new clinical investigations (other than bioavailability studies) essential to the approval of the application and conducted or sponsored by the applicant, the Secretary may not make the approval of an application submitted under this subsection for the conditions of approval of such drug in the subsection (b) application effective before the expiration of three years from the date of the approval of the application under subsection (b) for such drug.

(iv) If a supplement to an application approved under subsection (b) is approved after the date of enactment of this subsection and the supplement contains reports of new clinical investigations (other than bioavailability studies) essential to the approval of the supplement and conducted or sponsored by the person submitting the supplement, the Secretary may not make the approval of an application submitted under this subsection for a change approved in the supplement effective before the expiration of three years from the date of the approval of the supplement under subsection (b).

(v) If an application (or supplement to an application) submitted under subsection (b) for a drug, which includes an active ingredient (including any ester or salt of the active ingredient) that has been approved in another application under subsection (b), was approved during the period beginning January 1, 1982, and ending on the date of the enactment of this subsection, the Secretary may not make the approval of an application submitted under this subsection which refers to the drug for which the subsection (b) application was submitted or which refers to a change approved in a supplement to the subsection (b) application effective before the expiration of two years from the date of enactment of this subsection.

(5) If a drug approved under this subsection refers in its approved application to a drug the approval of which was withdrawn or suspended for grounds described in the first sentence of subsection (e) or was withdrawn or suspended under this paragraph or which, as determined by the Secretary, has been withdrawn from sale for safety or effectiveness reasons, the approval of the drug under this subsection shall be withdrawn or suspended—

(A) for the same period as the withdrawal or suspension under subsection (e), or this paragraph, or

(B) if the listed drug has been withdrawn from sale, for the period of withdrawal from sale or, if earlier, the period ending on the date the Secretary determines that the withdrawal from sale is not for safety or effectiveness reasons.

(6) (A) (i) Within sixty days of the date of the enactment of this subsection, the Secretary shall publish and make available to the public—

(I) a list in alphabetical order of the official and proprietary name of each drug which has been approved for safety and effectiveness under subsection (c) before the date of the enactment of this subsection;

(II) the date of approval if the drug is approved after 1981 and the number of the application which was approved; and

(III) whether in vitro or in vivo bioequivalence studies, or both such studies, are required for applications filed under this subsection which will refer to the drug published.

(ii) Every thirty days after the publication of the first list under clause (i) the Secretary shall revise the list to include each drug which has been approved for safety and effectiveness under subsection (c) or approved under this subsection during the thirty-day period.

(iii) When patent information submitted under subsection (b) or (c) respecting a drug included on the list is to be published by the Secretary the Secretary shall, in revisions made under clause (ii), include such information for such drug.

(B) A drug approved for safety and effectiveness under subsection (c) or approved under this subsection shall, for purposes of this subsection, be considered to have been published under subparagraph (A) on the date of its approval or the date of enactment, whichever is later.

(C) If the approval of a drug was withdrawn or suspended for grounds described in the first sentence of subsection (e) or was withdrawn or suspended under paragraph (5) or if the Secretary determines that a drug has been withdrawn from sale for safety or effectiveness reasons, it may not be published in the list under subparagraph (A) or, if the withdrawal or suspension occurred after its publication in such list, it shall be immediately removed from such list—

(i) for the same period as the withdrawal or suspension under subsection (e) or paragraph (5), or

(ii) if the listed drug has been withdrawn from sale, for the period of withdrawal from sale or, if earlier, the period ending on the date the Secretary determines that the withdrawal from sale is not for safety or effectiveness reasons.

A notice of the removal shall be published in the Federal Register.

(7) For purposes of this subsection:

(A) The term 'bioavailability' means the rate and extent to which the active ingredient or therapeutic ingredient is absorbed from a drug and becomes available at the site of drug action.

(B) A drug shall be considered to be bioequivalent to a listed drug if—

(i) the rate and extent of absorption of the drug do not show a significant difference from the rate and extent of absorption of the listed drug when administered at the same molar dose of the therapeutic ingredient under similar experimental conditions in either a single dose or multiple doses; or

(ii) the extent of absorption of the drug does not show a significant difference from the extent of absorption of the listed drug when administered at the same molar dose of the therapeutic ingredient under similar experimental conditions in either a single dose or multiple doses and the difference from the listed drug in the rate of absorption of the drug is intentional, is reflected in its proposed labeling, is not essential to the attainment of effective body drug concentrations on chronic use, and is considered medically insignificant for the drug.

(k) (1) In the case of any drug for which an approval of an application filed under subsection (b) or (j) is in effect, the applicant shall establish and maintain such records, and make such reports to the Secretary, of data relating to clinical experience and other data or information, received or otherwise obtained by such applicant with respect to such drug, as the Secretary may by general regulation, or by order with respect to such application, prescribe on the basis of a finding that such records and reports are necessary in order to enable the Secretary to determine, or facilitate a determination, whether there is or may be ground for invoking subsection (e) of this section: *Provided, however,* That regulations and orders issued under subsection and under subsection (i) shall have due regard for the professional ethics of the medical profession and the interests of patients and shall provide, where the Secretary deems it to be appropriate, for the examination, upon request, by the persons to whom such regulations or orders are applicable, of similar information received or otherwise obtained by the Secretary.

(2) Every person required under this section to maintain records, and every person in charge or custody thereof, shall, upon request of an officer or employee designated by the Secretary, permit such officer or employee at all reasonable times to have access to and copy and verify such records.

(l) Safety and effectiveness data and information which has been submitted in an application under subsection (b) for a drug and which has not previously been disclosed to the public shall be made available to the public, upon request, unless extraordinary circumstances are shown—

(1) if no work is being or will be undertaken to have the application approved,

(2) if the Secretary has determined that the application is not approvable and all legal appeals have been exhausted,

(3) if approval of the application under subsection (c) is withdrawn and all legal appeals have been exhausted,

(4) if the Secretary has determined that such drug is not a new drug, or

(5) upon the effective date of the approval of the first application under subsection (j) which refers to such drug or upon the date upon which the approval of an application under subsection (j) which refers to such drug could be made effective if such an application had been submitted.

(m) For purposes of this section, the term 'patent' means a patent issued by the Patent and Trademark Office of the Department of Commerce.

Certification of Drugs Containing Insulin

§ **506** [356] (a) The Secretary, pursuant to regulations promulgated by him, shall provide for the certification of batches of drugs composed wholly or partly of insulin. A batch of any such drug shall be certified if such drug has such characteristics of identity and such batch has such characteristics of strength, quality, and purity, as the Secretary prescribes in such regulations as necessary to adequately insure safety and efficacy of use, but shall not otherwise be certified. Prior to the effective date of such regulations the Secretary, in lieu of certification, shall issue a release for any batch which, in his judgment, may be released without risk as to the safety and efficacy of its use. Such release shall prescribe the date of its expiration and other conditions under which it shall cease to be effective as to such batch and as to portions thereof.

(b) Regulations providing for such certification shall contain such provisions as are necessary to carry out the purposes of this section, including provisions prescribing (1) standards of identity and of strength, quality, and purity; (2) tests and methods of assay to determine compliance with such standards; (3) effective periods for certificates, and other conditions under which they shall cease to be effective as to certified batches and as to portions thereof; (4) administration and procedure; and (5) such fees, specified in such regulations, as are necessary to provide, equip, and maintain an adequate certification service. Such regulations shall prescribe no standard of identity or of strength, quality, or purity for any drug different from the standard of identity, strength, quality, or purity set forth for such drug in an official compendium.

(c) Such regulations, insofar as they prescribe tests or methods of assay to determine strength, quality, or purity of any drug, different from the tests or methods of assay set forth for such drug in an official compendium, shall be prescribed, after notice and opportunity for revision of such compendium, in the manner provided in the second sentence of section 501 (b). The provisions of subsections (e), (f), and (g) of section 701 shall be applicable to such portion of any regulation as prescribes any such different test or method, but shall not be applicable to any other portion of any such regulation.

Certification of Antibiotics

§ **507** [357] (a) The Secretary, pursuant to regulations promulgated by him, shall provide for the certification of batches of drugs (except drugs for use in animals other than man) composed wholly or partly of any kind of penicillin, streptomycin, chlortetracycline, chloramphenicol, bacitracin, or any other antibiotic drug, or any derivative thereof. A batch of any such drug shall be certified if such drug has such characteristics of identity and such batch has such characteristics of strength, quality, and purity, as the Secretary prescribes in such regulations as necessary to adequately insure safety and efficacy of use, but shall not otherwise be certified. Prior to the effective date of such regulations the Secretary, in lieu of certification, shall issue a release for any batch which, in his judgment, may be released without risk as to the safety and efficacy of its use. Such release shall prescribe the date of its expiration and other conditions under which it shall cease to be effective as to such batch and as to portions thereof. For purposes of this section and of section 502 (l), the term "antibiotic drug" means any drug intended for use by man containing any quantity of any chemical substance which is produced by a microorganism and which has the capacity to inhibit or destroy microorganisms in dilute solution (including the chemically synthesized equivalent of any such substance).

(b) Regulations providing for such certification shall contain such provisions as are necessary to carry out the purposes of this section, including provisions prescribing (1) standards of identity and of strength, quality, and purity; (2) tests and methods of assay to determine compliance with such standards; (3) effective periods for certificates, and other conditions under which they shall cease to be effective as to certified batches and as to portions thereof; (4) administration and procedure; and (5) such fees, specified in such regulations, as are necessary to provide, equip, and maintain an adequate certification service. Such regulations shall prescribe only such tests and methods of assay as will provide for certification or rejection within the shortest time consistent with the purposes of this section.

(c) Whenever in the judgment of the Secretary, the requirements of this section and of section 502 (l) with respect to any drug or class of drugs are not necessary to insure safety and efficacy of use, the Secretary shall promulgate regulations exempting such drug or class of drugs from such requirements. In deciding whether an antibiotic drug, or class of antibiotic drugs, is to be exempted from the requirement of certification the Secretary shall give consideration, among other relevant factors, to—

(1) whether such drug or class of drugs is manufactured by a person who has, or hereafter shall have, produced fifty consecutive batches of such drug or class of drugs in compliance with the regulations for the certification thereof within a period of not more than eighteen calendar months, upon the application by such person to the Secretary; or

(2) whether such drug or class of drugs is manufactured by any person who has otherwise demonstrated such consistency in the production of such drug or class of drugs, in compliance with the regulations for the certification thereof, as in the judgment of the Secretary is adequate to insure the safety and efficacy of use thereof. When an antibiotic drug or a drug manufacturer has been exempted from the requirement of certification, the manufacturer may still obtain certification of a batch or batches of that drug if he applies for and meets the requirements for certification. Nothing in this Act shall be deemed to prevent a manufacturer or distributor of an antibiotic drug from making a truthful statement in labeling or advertising of the product as to whether it has been certified or exempted from the requirement of certification.

(d) The Secretary shall promulgate regulations exempting from any requirement of this section and of section 502 (l), (1) drugs which are to be stored, processed, labeled, or repacked at establishments other than those where manufactured, on condition that such drugs comply with all such requirements upon removal from such establishments; (2) drugs which conform to applicable standards of identity, strength, quality, and purity prescribed by these regulations and are intended for use in manufacturing other drugs; and (3) drugs which are intended solely for investigational use by experts qualified by scientific training and experience to investigate the safety and efficacy of drugs. Such regulations may, within the discretion of the Secretary, among other conditions relating to the protection of the public health, provide for conditioning the exemption under clause (3) upon—

(1) the submission to the Secretary, before any clinical testing of a new drug is undertaken, of reports, by the manufacturer or the sponsor of the investigation of such drug, of preclinical tests (including tests on animals) of such drug adequate to justify the proposed clinical testing;

(2) the manufacturer or the sponsor of the investigation of a new drug proposed to be distributed to investigators for clinical testing obtaining a signed agreement from each of such investigators that patients to whom the drug is administered will be under his personal supervision, or under the supervision of investigators responsible to him, and that

he will not apply such drug to any other investigator, or to clinics, for administration to human beings; and

(3) the establishment and maintenance of such records, and the making of such reports to the Secretary, by the manufacturer or the sponsor of the investigation of such drug, of data (including but not limited to analytical reports by investigators) obtained as the result of such investigational use of such drug, as the Secretary finds will enable him to evaluate the safety and effectiveness of such drug in the event of the filing of an application for certification or release pursuant to subsection (a).

Such regulations shall provide that such exemption shall be conditioned upon the manufacturer, or the sponsor of the investigation, requiring that experts using such drugs for investigational purposes certify to such manufacturer or sponsor that they will inform any human beings to whom such drugs, or any controls used in connection therewith, are being administered, or their representatives, that such drugs are being used for investigational purposes and will obtain the consent of such human beings or their representatives, except where they deem it not feasible or, in their professional judgment, contrary to the best interests of such human beings. Nothing in this subsection shall be construed to require any clinical investigator to submit directly to the Secretary reports on the investigational use of drugs.

(e) No drug which is subject to section 507 shall be deemed to be subject to any provision of section 505 except a new drug exempted from the requirements of this section and of section 502 (l) pursuant to regulations promulgated by the Secretary: *Provided*, That, for purposes of section 505, the initial request for certification, as thereafter duly amended, pursuant to section 507, of a new drug so exempted shall be considered a part of the application filed pursuant to section 505 (b) with respect to the person filing such request and to such drug as of the date of the exemption. Compliance of any drug subject to section 502 (l) or 507 with section 501 (b) and 502 (g) shall be determined by the application of the standards of strength, quality, and purity, the tests and methods of assay, and the requirements of packaging, and labeling, respectively, prescribed by regulations promulgated under section 507.

(f) Any interested person may file with the Secretary a petition proposing the issuance, amendment, or repeal of any regulation contemplated by this section. The petition shall set forth the proposal in general terms and shall state reasonable grounds therefor. The Secretary shall give public notice of the proposal and an opportunity for all interested persons to present their views thereon, orally or in writing, and as soon as practicable thereafter shall make public his action upon such proposal. At any time prior to the thirtieth day after such action is made public any interested person may file objections to such action, specifying with particularity the changes desired, stating reasonable grounds therefor, and requesting a public hearing upon such objections. The Secretary shall thereupon, after due notice, hold such public hearing. As soon as practicable after completion of the hearing, the Secretary shall by order make public his action on such objections. The Secretary shall base his order only on substantial evidence of record at the hearing and shall set forth as part of the order detailed findings of fact on which the order is based. The order shall be subject to the provision of section 701 (f) and (g).

(g) (1) Every person engaged in manufacturing, compounding, or processing any drug within the purview of this section with respect to which a certificate or release has been issued pursuant to this section shall establish and maintain such records, and make such reports to the Secretary, of data relating to clinical experience and other data or information, received or otherwise obtained by such person with respect to such drug, as the Secretary may by general regulation, or by order with respect to such certification or release, prescribe on the basis of a finding that such records and reports are necessary in order to enable the Secretary to make, or to facilitate, a determination as to whether such certification or release should be rescinded or whether any regulation issued under this section should be amended or repealed: *Provided, however*, That regulations and orders issued under this subsection and under clause (3) of subsection (d) shall have due regard for the professional ethics of the medical profession and the interests of patients and shall provide, where the Secretary deems it to be appropriate, for the examination, upon request, by the persons to whom such regulations or orders are applicable, of similar information received or otherwise obtained by the Secretary.

(2) Every person required under this section to maintain records, and every person having charge or custody thereof, shall, upon request of an officer or employee designated by the Secretary, permit such officer or employee at all reasonable times to have access to and copy and verify such records.

(h) In the case of a drug for which, on the day immediately preceding the effective date of this subsection, a prior approval of an application under section 505 had not been withdrawn under section 505 (e), the initial issuance of regulations providing for certification or exemption of such drug under this section 507 shall, with respect to the conditions of use prescribed, recommended, or suggested in the labeling covered by such application, not be conditioned upon an affirmative finding of the efficacy of such drug. Any subsequent amendment or repeal of such regulations so as no longer to provide for such certification or exemption on the ground of a lack of efficacy of such drug for use under such conditions of use may be effected only on or after that effective date of clause (3) of the first sentence of section 505 (e) which would be applicable to such drug under such conditions of use if such drug were subject to section 505 (e), and then only if (1) such amendment or repeal is made in accordance with the procedure specified in subsection (f) of this section (except that such amendment or repeal may be initiated either by a proposal of the Secretary or by a petition of any interested person) and (2) the Secretary finds, on the basis of new information with respect to such drug evaluated together with the information before him when the application under section 505 became effective or was approved, that there is a lack of substantial evidence (as defined in section 505 (d)) that the drug has the effect it purports or is represented to have under such conditions of use.

Authority to Designate Official Names

§ **508** [358] (a) The Secretary may designate an official name for any drug or device if he determines that such action is necessary or desirable in the interest of usefulness and simplicity. Any official name designated under this section for any drug or device shall be the only official name of that drug or device used in any official compendium published after such name has been prescribed or for any other purpose of this Act. In no event, however, shall the Secretary establish an official name so as to infringe a valid trademark.

(b) Within a reasonable time after the effective date of this section, and at such other times as he may deem necessary, the Secretary shall cause a review to be made of the official names by which drugs are identified in the official United States Pharmacopeia, the official Homeopathic Pharmacopeia of the United States, and the official National Formulary, and all supplements thereto and at such times as he may deem necessary shall cause a review to be made of the official names by which devices are identified in any official compendium (and all supplements thereto), to determine whether revision of any of those names is necessary or desirable in the interest of usefulness and simplicity.

(c) Whenever he determines after any such review that (1) any such official name is unduly complex or is not useful for any other reason, (2) two or more official names have been applied to a single drug or device, or to two or more drugs which are identical in chemical structure and pharmacological action and which are substantially identical in strength, quality, and purity or to two or more devices which are substantially equivalent in design and purpose, or (3) no official name has been applied to a medically useful drug or device, he shall transmit in writing to the compiler of each official compendium in which that drug or drugs or device are identified and recognized his request for the recommendation of a single official name for such drug or drugs or device which will have usefulness and simplicity. Whenever such a single official name has not been recommended within one hundred and eighty days after such request, or the Secretary determines that any name so recommended is not useful for any reason, he shall designate a single official name for such drug or drugs or device. Whenever he determines that the name so recommended is useful, he shall designate that name as the official name of such drug or drugs or device. Such designation shall be made as a regulation upon public notice and in accordance with the procedure set forth in section 4 of the Administrative Procedure Act (5 U.S.C. 1003).

(d) After each such review, and at such other times as the Secretary may determine to be necessary or desirable, the Secretary shall cause to be compiled, published, and publicly distributed a list which shall list all revised official names of drugs or devices designated under this section and shall contain such descriptive and explanatory matter as the Secretary may determine to be required for the effective use of those names.

(e) Upon a request in writing by any compiler of an official compendium that the Secretary exercise the authority granted to him under section 508 (a), he shall upon public notice and in accordance with the procedure set forth in section 4 of the Administrative Procedure Act (5 U.S.C. 1003) designate the official name of the drug or device for which the request is made.

Registration Requirements

§ **510** [360] (a) As used in this section—

(1) the term "manufacture, preparation, propagation, compounding, or processing" shall include repackaging or otherwise changing the container, wrapper, or labeling of any drug package or device package in furtherance of the distribution of the drug or device from the original place of manufacture to the person who makes final delivery or sale to the ultimate consumer or user; and

(2) the term "name" shall include in the case of a partnership the name of each partner and, in the case of a corporation, the name of each corporate officer and director, and the State of incorporation.

(b) On or before December 31 of each year every person who owns or operates any establishment in any State engaged in the manufacture, preparation, propagation, compounding, or processing of a drug or drugs or a device or devices shall register with the Secretary his name, places of business, and all such establishments.

(c) Every person upon first engaging in the manufacture, preparation, propagation, compounding, or processing of a drug or drugs or a device or devices in any establishment which he owns or operates in any State shall immediately register with the Secretary his name, place of business, and such establishment.

(d) Every person duly registered in accordance with the foregoing subsections of this section shall immediately register with the Secretary any additional establishment which he owns or operates in any State and in which he begins the manufacture, preparation, propagation, compounding, or processing of a drug or drugs or a device or devices.

(e) The Secretary may assign a registration number to any person or any establishment registered in accordance with this section. The Secretary may also assign a listing number to each drug or class of drugs listed under subsection (j). Any number assigned pursuant to the preceding sentence shall be the same as that assigned pursuant to the National Drug Code. The Secretary may by regulation prescribe a uniform system for the identification of devices intended for human use and may require that persons who are required to list such devices pursuant to subsection (j) shall list such devices in accordance with such system.

(f) The Secretary shall make available for inspection, to any person so requesting, any registration filed pursuant to this section, except that any list submitted pursuant to paragraph (3) of subsection (j) and the information accompanying any list or notice filed under paragraph (1) or (2) of that subsection shall be exempt from such inspection unless the Secretary finds that such an exemption would be inconsistent with protection of the public health.

(g) The foregoing subsections of this section shall not apply to—

(1) pharmacies which maintain establishments in conformance with any applicable local laws regulating the practice of pharmacy and medicine and which are regularly engaged in dispensing prescription drugs or devices, upon prescriptions of practitioners licensed to administer such drugs or devices to patients under the care of such practitioners in the course of their professional practice, and which do not manufacture, prepare, propagate, compound, or process drugs or devices for sale other than in the regular course of their business of dispensing or selling drugs or devices at retail;

(2) practitioners licensed by law to prescribe or administer drugs or devices and who manufacture, prepare, propagate, compound, or process drugs or devices solely for use in the course of their professional practice;

(3) persons who manufacture, prepare, propagate, compound, or process drugs or devices solely for use in research, teaching, or chemical analysis and not for sale;

(4) such other classes of persons as the Secretary may by regulation exempt from the application of this section upon a finding that registration by such classes of persons in accordance with this section is not necessary for the protection of the public health.

(h) Every establishment in any State registered with the Secretary pursuant to this section shall be subject to inspection pursuant to section 704 and every such establishment engaged in the manufacture, propagation, compounding, or processing of a drug or drugs or of a device or devices classified in class II or III shall be so inspected by one or more officers or employees duly designated by the Secretary at least once in the two-year period beginning with the date of registration of such establishment pursuant to this section and at least once in every successive two-year period thereafter.

(i) Any establishment within any foreign country engaged in the manufacture, preparation, propagation, compounding, or processing of a drug or drugs or a device or devices shall be permitted to register under this section pursuant to regulations promulgated by the Secretary. Such regulations shall require such establishment to provide the information required by subsection (j) and shall require such establishment to provide the information required by subsection (j) in the case of a device or devices and shall include provisions for registration of any such establishment upon condition that adequate and effective means are available, by arrangement with the government of such foreign country or otherwise, to enable the Secretary to determine from time to time whether drugs or devices manufactured, prepared, propagated, compounded or processed in such establishment, if imported or offered for import into the United States, shall be refused admission on any of the grounds set forth in section 801 (a) of this Act.

(j) (1) Every person who registers with the Secretary under subsection (b), (c), or (d) shall, at the time of registration under any such subsection, file with the Secretary a list of all drugs and a list of all devices and a brief statement of the basis for believing that each device included in the list is a device rather than a drug (with each drug and device in each list listed by its established name as defined in section 502 (e) and by any proprietary name) which is being manufactured, prepared, propagated, compounded, or processed by him for commercial distribution and which he has not included in any list of drugs or devices filed by him with the Secretary under this paragraph or paragraph (2) before such time of registration. Such list shall be prepared in such form and manner as the Secretary may prescribe and shall be accompanied by—

(A) in the case of a drug contained in the applicable list and subject to section 505, 506, 507, or 523, or a device intended for human use contained in the applicable list with respect to which a performance standard has been established under section 514 or which is subject to section 515, a reference to the authority for the marketing of such drug or device and a copy of all labeling for such drug or device;

(B) in the case of any other drug or device contained in an applicable list—

(i) which drug is subject to section 503 (b) (1), or which device is a restricted device, a copy of all labeling for such drug or device, a representative sampling of advertisements for such drug or device, and, upon request made by the Secretary for good cause, a copy of all advertisements for a particular drug product or device, or

(ii) which drug is not subject to section 503 (b) (1) or which device is not a restricted device, the label and package insert for such drug or device and a representative sampling of any other labeling for such drug or device;

(C) in the case of any drug contained in an applicable list which is described in subparagraph (B), a quantitative listing of its active ingredient or ingredients, except that with respect to a particular drug product the Secretary may require the submission of a quantitative listing of all ingredients if he finds that such submission is necessary to carry out the purposes of this Act; and

(D) if the registrant filing a list has determined that a particular drug product or device contained in such list is not subject to section 505, 506, 507, or 512, or the particular device contained in such list is not subject to a performance standard established under section 514 or to section 515 or is not a restricted device, a brief statement of the basis on which the registrant made such determination if the Secretary requests such a statement with respect to that particular drug product or device.

(2) Each person who registers with the Secretary under this subsection shall report to the Secretary once during the month of June of each year and once during the month of December of each year the following information:

(A) A list of each drug or device introduced by the registrant for commercial distribution which has not been included in any list previously filed by him with the Secretary under this subparagraph or paragraph (1) of this subsection. A list under this subparagraph shall list a drug or device by its established name (as defined in section 502 (e)) and by any proprietary name it may have and shall be accompanied by the other information required by paragraph (1).

(B) If since the date the registrant last made a report under this paragraph (or if he has not made a report under this paragraph, since the effective date of this subsection) he has discontinued the manufacture, preparation, propagation, compounding, or processing for commercial distribution of a drug or device included in a list filed by him under subparagraph (A) or paragraph (1); notice of such discontinuance, the date of such discontinuance, and the identity (by established name as defined in section 502 (e) and by any proprietary name) of such drug or device.

(C) If since the date the registrant reported pursuant to subparagraph (B) a notice of discontinuance he has resumed the manufacture, preparation, propagation, compounding, or processing for commercial distribution of the drug or device with respect to which such notice of discontinuance was reported; notice of such resumption, the date of such resumption, the identity of such drug or device (each by established name (as defined in section 502 (e)) and by any proprietary name), and the other information required by paragraph (1), unless the registrant has previously reported such resumption to the Secretary pursuant to this subparagraph.

(D) Any material change in any information previously submitted pursuant to this paragraph or paragraph (1).

(3) The Secretary may also require each registrant under this section to submit a list of each drug product which (A) the registrant is manufacturing, preparing, propagating, compounding, or processing for commercial distribution, and (B) contains a particular ingredient. The Secretary may not require the submission of such a list unless he has made a finding that the submission of such a list is necessary to carry out the purposes of this Act.

Drugs for Rare Diseases or Conditions

RECOMMENDATIONS FOR INVESTIGATIONS OF DRUGS FOR RARE DISEASES OR CONDITIONS

§ **525** [360aa] (a) The sponsor of a drug for a disease or condition which is rare in the States may request the Secretary to provide written recommendations for the non-clinical and clinical investigations which must be conducted with the drug before—

(1) it may be approved for such disease or condition under section 505, or

(2) if the drug is a biological product, before it may be licensed for such disease or condition under section 351 of the Public Health Service Act.

If the Secretary has reason to believe that a drug for which a request is made under this section is a drug for a disease or condition which is rare in the States, the Secretary shall provide the person making the request written recommendations for the non-clinical and clinical investigations which the Secretary believes, on the basis of information available to the Secretary at the time of the request under this section, would be necessary for approval of such drug for such disease or condition under section 505 or licensing under section 351 of the Public Health Service Act for such disease or condition.

(b) The Secretary shall by regulation promulgate procedures for the implementation of subsection (a).

DESIGNATION OF DRUGS FOR RARE DISEASES OR CONDITIONS

§ **526** [360bb] (a) (1) The manufacturer or the sponsor of a drug may request the Secretary to designate the drug as a drug for a rare disease or condition. If the Secretary finds that a drug for which a request is submitted under this subsection is being or will be investigated for a rare disease or condition and—

(A) if an application for such drug is approved under section 505, or

(B) if the drug is a biological product, a license is issued under section 351 of the Public Health Service Act, the approval or license would be for use for such disease or condition, the Secretary shall designate the drug as a drug for such disease or condition. A request for a designation of a drug under this subsection shall contain the consent of the applicant to notice being given by the Secretary under subsection (b) respecting the designation of the drug.

(2) For purposes of paragraph (1), the term 'rare disease or condition' means any disease or condition *which (A) affects less than 200,000 persons in the U.S. or (B) affects more than 200,000 persons in the U.S. and for which* there is no reasonable expectation that the cost of developing and making available in the United States a drug for such disease or condition will be recovered from sales in the United States of such drug. Determinations under the preceding sentence with respect to any drug shall be made on the basis of the facts and circumstances as of the date the request for designation of the drug under this subsection is made.

(b) Notice respecting the designation of a drug under subsection (a) shall be made available to the public.

(c) The Secretary shall by regulation promulgate procedures for the implementation of subsection (a).

PROTECTION FOR UNPATENTED DRUGS FOR RARE DISEASES OR CONDITIONS

§ **527** [360cc] (a) Except as provided in subsection (b), if the Secretary—

(1) approves an application filed pursuant to section 505 (b), or

(2) issues a license under section 351 of the Public Health Service Act for a drug designated under section 526 for a rare disease or condition and for which a United States Letter of Patent may not be issued, the Secretary may not approve another application under section 505 (b) or issue another license under section 351 of the Public Health Service Act for such drug for such disease or condition for a person who is not the holder of such approved application or of such license until the expiration of seven years from the date of the approval of the approved application or the issuance of the license. Section 505 (c) (2) does not apply to the refusal to approve an application under the preceding sentence.

(b) If an application filed pursuant to section 505 (b) is approved for a drug designated under section 526 for a rare disease or condition or a license is issued under section 351 of the Public Health Service Act for such a drug and if a United States Letter of Patent may not be issued for the drug, the Secretary may, during the seven-year period beginning on the date of the application approval or of the issuance of the license, approve another application under section 505 (b), or, if the drug is a biological product, issue a license under section 351 of the Public Health Service Act, for such drug for such disease or condition for a person who is not the holder of such approved application or of such license if—

(1) The Secretary finds, after providing the holder notice and opportunity for the submission of views, that in such period the holder of the approved application or of the license cannot assure the availability of sufficient quantities of the drug to meet the needs of persons with the disease or condition for which the drug was designated; or

(2) such holder provides the Secretary in writing the consent of such holder for the approval of other applications or the issuance of other licenses before the expiration of such seven-year period.

OPEN PROTOCOLS FOR INVESTIGATIONS OF DRUGS FOR RARE DISEASES OR CONDITIONS

§ **528** [360dd] If a drug is designated under section 526 as a drug for a rare disease or condition and if notice of a claimed exemption under section 505 (i) or regulations issued thereunder is filed for such drug, the Secretary shall encourage the sponsor of such drug to design protocols for clinical investigations of the drug which may be conducted under the exemption to permit the addition to the investigations of persons with the disease or condition who need the drug to treat the disease or condition and who cannot be satisfactorily treated by available alternative drugs.

Records of Interstate Shipment

§ **703** [373] For the purpose of enforcing the provisions of this Act, carriers engaged in interstate commerce, and persons receiving foods, drugs, devices, or cosmetics in interstate commerce or holding such articles so received, shall, upon the request of an officer or employee duly designated by the Secretary, permit such officer or employee, at reasonable times, to have access to and to copy all records showing the movement in interstate commerce of any food, drug, device, or cosmetic, or the holding thereof during or after such movement, and the quantity, shipper, and consignee thereof; and it shall be unlawful for any such carrier or person to fail to permit such access to and copying of any such record so requested when such request is accompanied by a statement in writing specifying the nature or kind of food, drug, device, or cosmetic to which such request relates: *Provided*, That evidence obtained under this section, or any evidence which is directly or indirectly derived from such evidence, shall not be used in a criminal prosecution of the person from whom obtained: *Provided further*, That carriers shall not be subject to the other provisions of this Act by reason of their receipt, carriage, holding, or delivery of food, drugs, devices, or cosmetics in the usual course of business as carriers.

Inspections

§ **704** [374] (a) (1) For purposes of enforcement of this Chapter, officers or employees duly designated by the Secretary, upon presenting appropriate credentials and a written notice to the owner, operator, or agent in charge, are authorized (A) to enter, at reasonable times, any factory, warehouse, or establishment in which food, drugs, devices, or cosmetics are manufactured, processed, packed, or held, for introduction into interstate commerce or after such introduction, or to enter any vehicle being used to transport or hold such food, drugs, devices or cosmetics in interstate commerce; and (B) to inspect, at reasonable times and within reasonable limits and in a reasonable manner, such factory, warehouse, establishment, or vehicle and all pertinent equipment, finished and unfinished materials, containers, and labeling therein. In the case of any factory, warehouse, establishment, or consulting laboratory in which prescription drugs or restricted devices are manufactured, processed, packed, or held, the inspection shall extend to all things therein (including records, files, papers, processes, controls, and facilities) bearing on whether prescription drugs or restricted devices which are adulterated or misbranded within the meaning of this Chapter, or which may not be manufactured, introduced into interstate commerce, or sold, or offered for sale by reason of any provision of this Chapter, have been or are being manufactured, processed, packed, transported, or held in any such place, or otherwise bearing on violation of this Chapter. No inspection authorized by the preceding sentence or by paragraph (3) shall extend to financial data, sales data other than shipment data, pricing data, personnel data (other than data as to qualifications of technical and professional personnel performing functions subject to this Chapter, and research data (other than data relating to new drugs, antibiotic drugs, and devices and subject to reporting and inspection under regulations lawfully issued pursuant to section 505 (i) or (j), section 507 (d) or (g), section 519, or 520 (g), and data relating to other drugs or devices which in the case of a new drug would be subject to reporting or inspection under lawful regulations issued pursuant to section 505 (j) of the title). A separate notice shall be given for each such inspection, but a notice shall not be given for each such inspection, but a notice shall not be required for each entry made during the period covered by the inspection. Each such inspection shall be commenced and completed with reasonable promptness.

(2) The provisions of the second sentence of this subsection shall not apply to—

(A) pharmacies which maintain establishments in conformance with any applicable local laws regulating the practice of pharmacy and medicine and which are regularly engaged in dispensing prescription drugs, or devices upon prescriptions of practitioners licensed to administer such drugs or devices to patients under the care of such practitioners in the course of their professional practice, and which do not, either through a subsidiary or otherwise, manufacture, prepare, propagate, compound, or process drugs or devices for sale other than in the regular course of their business of dispensing or selling drugs or devices at retail;

(B) practitioners licensed by law to prescribe or administer drugs or prescribe or use devices, as the case may be, and who manufacture, prepare, propagate, compound, or process drugs or manufacture or process devices solely for use in the course of their professional practice;

(C) persons who manufacture, prepare, propagate, compound, or process drugs or manufacture or process devices solely for use in research, teaching, or chemical analysis and not for sale;

(D) such other classes of persons as the Secretary may by regulation exempt from the application of this section upon a finding that inspection as applied to such classes of persons in accordance with this section is not necessary for the protection of the public health.

(b) Upon completion of any such inspection of a factory, warehouse, consulting laboratory, or other establishment, and prior to leaving the premises, the officer or employee making the inspection shall give to the owner, operator, or agent in charge a report in writing setting forth any conditions or practices observed by him which, in his judgment, indicate that any food, drug, device, or cosmetic in such establishment (1) consists in whole or in part of any filthy, putrid, or decomposed substance, or (2) has been prepared, packed, or held under insanitary conditions whereby it may have become contaminated with filth, or whereby it may have been rendered injurious to health. A copy of such report shall be sent promptly to the Secretary.

(c) If the officer or employee making any such inspection of a factory, warehouse, or other establishment has obtained any sample in the course of the inspection, upon completion of the inspection and prior to leaving the premises he shall give to the owner, operator, or agent in charge a receipt describing the samples obtained.

Revision of United States Pharmacopeia; Development of Analysis and Mechanical and Physical Tests

The Secretary, in carrying into effect the provisions of this chapter, is authorized hereafter to cooperate with associations and scientific societies in the revision of the United States Pharmacopeia and in the development of methods of analysis and mechanical and physical tests necessary to carry out the work of the Food and Drug Administration.

Definitions

§ **201** [321] For purposes of this Act—

(s) The term "food additive" means any substance the intended use of which results or may reasonably be expected to result, directly or indirectly, in its becoming a component or otherwise affecting the characteristics of any food (including any substance intended for use in producing, manufacturing, packing, processing, preparing, treating, packaging, transporting, or holding food; and including any source of radiation intended for any such use), if such substance is not generally recognized, among experts qualified by scientific training and experience to evaluate its safety, as having been adequately shown through scientific procedures (or, in the case of a substance used in food prior to January 1, 1958, through either scientific procedures or experience based on common use in food) to be safe under the conditions of its intended use; except that such term does not include—

(1) a pesticide chemical in or on a raw agricultural commodity; or

(2) a pesticide chemical to the extent that it is intended for use or is used in the production, storage, or transportation of any raw agricultural commodity, or

(3) a color additive; or

(4) any substance used in accordance with a sanction or approval granted prior to the enactment of this paragraph [September 6, 1958] pursuant to this Act, the Poultry Products Inspection Act (21 U.S.C. 451 and the following) or the Meat Inspection Act of March 4, 1907 (34 Stat. 1260), as amended and extended (21 U.S.C. 71 and the following); or

(5) a new animal drug.

(w) The term "new animal drug" means any drug intended for use for animals other than man, including any drug intended for use in animal feed but not including such animal feed—

(1) the composition of which is such that such drug is not generally recognized, among experts qualified by scientific training and experience to evaluate the safety and effectiveness of animal drugs, as safe and effective for use under the conditions prescribed, recommended, or suggested in the labeling thereof; except that such a drug not so recognized shall not be deemed to be a "new animal drug" if at any time prior to June 25, 1938, it was subject to the Food and Drug Act of June 30, 1906, as amended, and if at such time its labeling contained the same representations concerning the conditions of its use; or

(2) the composition of which is such that such drug, as a result of investigations to determine its safety and effectiveness for use under such conditions, has become so recognized but which has not, otherwise than in such investigations, been used to a material extent or for a material time under such conditions.

(x) The term "animal feed", as used in paragraph (w) of this section, in section 512, and in provisions of this Act referring to such paragraph or section, means an article which is intended for use for food for animals other than man and which is intended for use as a substantial source of nutrients in the diet of the animal, and is not limited to a mixture intended to be the sole ration of the animal.

(bb) The term "abbreviated drug application" means an application submitted under section 505(j) or 507 for the approval of a drug that relies on the approved application of another drug with the same active ingredient to establish safety and efficacy, and

(1) in the case of section 306, includes a supplement to such an application for a different or additional use of the drug but does not include a supplement to such an application for other than a different or additional use of the drug, and

(2) in the case of sections 307 and 308, includes any supplement to such an application.

(ee) For purposes of sections 306 and 307, the term "drug product" means a drug subject to regulation under section 505, 507, 512, or 802 of this Act or under section 351 of the Public Health Service Act.

§ **501** [351] (a) A drug or device shall be deemed to be adulterated—

(5) if it is a new animal drug which is unsafe within the meaning of seciton 512; or (6) if it is an animal feed bearing or containing a new animal drug, and such animal feed is unsafe within the meaning of section 512.

§ **503** [353]

(f) (1) (A) A drug intended for use by animals other than man which—

(i) because of its toxicity or other potentiality for harmful effect, or the method of its use, or the collateral measures necessary for its use, is not safe for animal use except under the professional supervision of a licensed veterinarian, or

(ii) is limited by an approved application under subsection (b) of section 512 to use under the professional supervision of a licensed veterinarian, shall be dispensed only by or upon the lawful written or oral order of a licensed veterinarian in the course of the veterinarian's professional practice.

(B) For purposes of subparagraph (A), an order is lawful if the order—

(i) is a prescription or other order authorized by law,

(ii) is, if an oral order, promptly reduced to writing by the person lawfully filling the order, and filed by that person, and

(iii) is refilled only if authorized in the original order or in a subsequent oral order promptly reduced to writing by the person lawfully filling the order, and filed by that person.

(C) The act of dispensing a drug contrary to the provisions of this paragraph shall be deemed to be an act which results in the drug being misbranded while held for sale.

(2) Any drug when dispensed in accordance with paragraph (1) of this subsection—

(A) shall be exempt from the requirements of section 502, except subsections (a), (g), (h), (i)(2), (i)(3), and (p) of such section, and

(B) shall be exempt from the packaging requirements of subsections (g), (h), and (p) of such section if—

(i) when dispensed by a licensed veterinarian, the drug bears a label containing the name and address of the practitioner and any directions for use and cautionary statements specified by the practitioner, or

(ii) when dispensed by filling the lawful order of a licensed veterinarian, the drug bears a label containing the name and address of the dispenser, the serial number and date of the order or of its filling, the name of the licensed veterinarian, and the directions for use and cautionary statements, if any, contained in such order. The preceding sentence shall not apply to any drug dispensed in the course of the conduct of a business of dispensing drugs pursuant to diagnosis by mail. The Secretary may by regulation exempt drugs for animals other than man subject to section 512 from the requirements of paragraph (1) when such requirements are not necessary for the protection of the public health.

(4) A drug which is subject to paragraph (1) shall be deemed to be misbranded if at any time prior to dispensing its label fails to bear the statement "Caution: Federal law restricts this drug to use by or on the order of a licensed veterinarian." A drug to which paragraph (1) does not apply shall be deemed to be misbranded if at any time prior to dispensing its label bears the statement specified in the preceding sentence.

New Animal Drugs

§ **512** [360b] (a) (1) A new animal drug shall, with respect to any particular use or intended use of such drug, be deemed unsafe for the purposes of section 501(a)(5) and section 402(a)(2)(D) unless—

(A) there is in effect an approval of an application filed pursuant to subsection (b) of this section with respect to such use or intended use of such drug, and

(B) such drug, its labeling, and such use conform to such approved application.

(2) An animal feed bearing or containing a new animal drug shall, with respect to any particular use or intended use of such animal feed, be deemed unsafe for the purposes of section 501(a)(6) unless—

(A) there is in effect an approval of an application filed pursuant to subsection (b) of this section with respect to such drug, as used in such animal feed,

(B) there is in effect an approval of an application pursuant to subsection (m)(1) of this section with respect to such animal feed, and

(C) such animal feed, its labeling, and such use conform to the conditions and indications of use published pursuant to subsection (i) of this section and to the application with respect thereto approved under subsection (m) of this section.

(3) A new animal drug or an animal feed bearing or containing a new animal drug shall not be deemed unsafe for the purposes of section 501(a)(5) or (6) if such article is for investigational use and conforms to the terms of an exemption in effect with respect thereto under section 512(j).

(b) (1) Any person may file with the Secretary an application with respect to any intended use or uses of a new animal drug. Such person shall submit to the Secretary as a part of the application (A) full reports of investigations which have been made to show whether or not such drug is safe and effective for use; (B) a full list of the articles used as components of such drug; (C) a full statement of the composition of such drug; (D) a full description of the methods used in, and the facilities and controls used for, the manufacture, processing, and packing of such drug; (E) such samples of such drug and of the articles used as components thereof, of any animal feed for use in or on which such drug is intended, and of the edible portions or products (before or after slaughter) of animals to which such drug (directly or in or on animal feed) is intended to be administered, as the Secretary may require; (F) specimens of the labeling proposed to be used for such drug, or in case such drug is intended for use in animal feed, proposed labeling appropriate for such use, and specimens of the labeling for the drug to be manufactured, packed, or distributed by the applicant; (G) a description of practicable methods for determining the quantity, if any, of such drug in or on food, and any substance formed in or on food, because of its use; and (H) the proposed tolerance or withdrawal period or other use restrictions for such drug if any tolerance or withdrawal period or other use restrictions are required in order to assure that the proposed use of such drug will be safe. The applicant shall file with the application the patent number and the expiration date of any patent which claims the new animal drug for which the applicant filed the application or which claims a method of using such drug and with respect to which a claim of patent infringement could reasonably be asserted if a person not licensed by the owner engaged in the manufacture, use, or sale of the drug. If an application is filed under this subsection for a drug and a patent which claims such drug or a method of using such drug is issued after the filing date but before approval of the application, the applicant shall amend the application to include the information required by the preceding sentence. Upon approval of the application, the Secretary shall publish information submitted under the two preceding sentences.

(2) Any person may file with the Secretary an abbreviated application for the approval of a new animal drug. An abbreviated application shall contain the information required by subsection (n).

(2) (A) Subject to subparagraph (C), the Secretary shall approve an abbreviated application for a drug unless the Secretary finds—

(i) the methods used in, or the facilities and controls used for, the manufacture, processing, and packing of the drug are inadequate to assure and preserve its identity, strength, quality, and purity;

(ii) the conditions of use prescribed, recommended, or suggested in the proposed labeling are not reasonably certain to be followed in practice or, except as provided in subparagraph (B), information submitted with the application is insufficient to show that each of the proposed conditions of use or similar limitations [whether in the labeling or published pursuant to subsection (i)] have been previously approved for the approved new animal drug referred to in the application;

(iii) information submitted with the application is insufficient to show that the active ingredients are the same as those of the approved new animal drug referred to in the application;

(iv) (I) if the application is for a drug whose active ingredients, route of administration, dosage form, strength, or use with other animal drugs in animal feed is the same as the active ingredients, route of administration, dosage form, strength, or use with other animal drugs in animal feed of the approved new animal drug referred to in the application, information submitted in the application is insufficient to show that the active ingredients, route of administration, dosage form, strength, or use with other animal drugs in animal feed is the same as that of the approved new animal drug, or

(II) if the application is for a drug whose active ingredients, route of administration, dosage form, strength, or use with other animal drugs in animal feed is different from that of the approved new animal drug referred to in the application, no petition to file an application for the drug with the different active ingredients, route of administration, dosage form, strength, or use with other animal drugs in animal feed was approved under subsection (n)(3);

(v) if the application was filed pursuant to the approval of a petition under subsection (n)(3), the application did not contain the information required by the Secretary respecting the active ingredients, route of administration, dosage form, strength, or use with other animal drugs in animal feed which is not the same;

(vi) information submitted in the application is insufficient to show that the drug is bioequivalent to the approved new animal drug referred to in the application, or if the application is filed under a petition approved pursuant to subsection (n)(3), information submitted in the application is insufficient to show that the active ingredients of the new animal drug are of the same pharmacological or therapeutic class as the pharmacological or therapeutic class of the approved new animal drug and that the new animal drug can be expected to have the same therapeutic effect as the approved new animal drug when used in accordance with the labeling;

(vii) information submitted in the application is insufficient to show that the labeling proposed for the drug is the same as the labeling approved for the approved new animal drug referred to in the application except for changes required because of differences approved under a petition filed under subsection (n)(3), because of a different withdrawal period, or because the drug and the approved new animal drug are produced or distributed by different manufacturers;

(viii) information submitted in the application or any other information available to the Secretary shows that (I) the inactive ingredients of the drug are unsafe for use under the conditions prescribed, recommended, or suggested in the labeling proposed for the drug, (II) the composition of the drug is unsafe under such conditions because of the type or quantity of inactive ingredients included or the manner in which the inactive ingredients are included, or (III) in the case of a drug for food producing animals, the inactive ingredients of the drug or its composition may be unsafe with respect to human food safety;

(ix) the approval under subsection (b)(1) of the approved new animal drug referred to in the application filed under subsection (b)(2) has been withdrawn or suspended for grounds described in paragraph (1) of subsection (e), the Secretary has published a notice of a hearing to withdraw approval of the approved new animal drug for such grounds, the approval under this paragraph of the new animal drug for which the application under subsection (b)(2) was filed has been withdrawn or suspended under subparagraph (G) for such grounds, or the Secretary has determined that the approved new animal drug has been withdrawn from sale for safety or effectiveness reasons;

(x) the application does not meet any other requirement of subsection (n); or

(xi) the application contains an untrue statement of material fact.

(B) If the Secretary finds that a new animal drug for which an application is submitted under subsection (b)(2) is bioequivalent to the approved new animal drug referred to in such application and that residues of the new animal drug are consistent with the tolerances established for such approved new animal drug but at a withdrawal period which is different than the withdrawal period approved for such approved new animal drug, the Secretary may establish, on the basis of information submitted, such different withdrawal period as the withdrawal period for the new animal drug for purposes of the approval of such application for such drug.

(H) For purposes of this paragraph:

(i) The term "bioequivalence" means the rate and extent to which the active ingredient or therapeutic ingredient is absorbed from a new animal drug and becomes available at the site of drug action.

(ii) A new animal drug shall be considered to be bioequivalent to the approved new animal drug referred to in its application under subsection (n) if—

(I) the rate and extent of absorption of the drug do not show a significant difference from the rate and extent of absorption of the approved new animal drug referred to in the application when administered at the same dose of the active ingredient under similar experimental conditions in either a single dose or multiple doses;

(II) the extent of absorption of the drug does not show a significant difference from the extent of absorption of the approved new animal drug referred to in the application when administered at the same dose of the active ingredient under similar experimental conditions in either a single dose or multiple doses and the difference from the approved new animal drug in the rate of absorption of the drug is intentional, is reflected in its proposed labeling, is not essential to the attainment of effective drug concentrations in use, and is considered scientifically insignificant for the drug in attaining the intended purposes of its use and preserving human food safety or

(III) in any case in which the Secretary determines that the measurement of the rate and extent of absorption or excretion of the new animal drug in biological fluids is inappropriate or impractical, an appropriate acute pharmacological effects test or other test of the new animal drug and, when deemed scientifically necessary, of the approved new animal drug referred to in the application in the species to be tested or in an appropriate animal model does not show a significant difference between the new animal drug and such approved new animal drug when administered at the same dose under similar experimental conditions. If the approved new animal drug referred to in the application for a new animal drug under subsection (n) is approved for use in more than one animal species, the bioequivalency information described in subclause (I), (II), and (III) shall be obtained for one species, or if the Secretary deems appropriate based on scientific principles, shall be obtained for more than one species. The Secretary may prescribe the dose to be used in determining bioequivalency under subclause (I), (II), or (III). To assure that the residues of the new animal drug will be consistent with the established tolerances for the approved new animal drug referred to in the application under subsection (b)(2) upon the expiration of the withdrawal period contained in the application for the new animal drug, the Secretary shall require bioequivalency data or residue depletion studies of the new animal drug or such other data or studies as the Secretary considers appropriate based on scientific principles. If the Secretary requires one or more residue studies under the preceding sentence, the Secretary may not require that the assay methodology used to determine the withdrawal period of the new animal drug be more rigorous than the methodology used to determined the withdrawal period for the approved new animal drug referred to in the application. If such studies are required and if the approved new animal drug, referred to in the application for the new animal drug for which such studies are required, is approved for use in more than one animal species, such studies shall be conducted for one species, or if the Secretary deems appropriate based on scientific principles, shall be conducted for more than one species.

(d) (1) If the Secretary finds, after due notice to the applicant in accordance with subsection (c) and giving him an opportunity for a hearing, in accordance with said subsection, that —

(A) the investigations, reports of which are required to be submitted to the Secretary pursuant to subsection (b), do not include adequate tests by all methods reasonably applicable to show whether or not such drug is safe for use under the conditions prescribed, recommended or suggested in the proposed labeling thereof;

(B) the results of such tests show that such drug is unsafe for use under such conditions or do not show that such drug is safe for use under such conditions;

(C) the methods used in, and the facilities and controls used for, the manufacture, processing, and packing of such drug are inadequate to preserve its identity, strength, quality, and purity;

(D) upon the basis of the information submitted to him as part of the application, or upon the basis of any other information before him with respect to such drug, he has insufficient information to determine whether such drug is safe for use under such conditions;

(E) evaluated on the basis of the information submitted to him as part of the application and any other information before him with respect to such drug, there is a lack of substantial evidence that the drug will have the effect it purports or is represented to have under the conditions of use prescribed, recommended, or suggested in the proposed labeling thereof;

(F) upon the basis of the information submitted to him as part of the application or any other information before him with respect to such drug, the tolerance limitation proposed, if any, exceeds that reasonably required to accomplish the physical or other technical effect for which the drug is intended;

(G) the application failed to contain the patent information prescribed by subsection (b)(1);

(H) based on a fair evaluation of all material facts, such labeling is false or misleading in any particular; or

(I) such drug induces cancer when ingested by man or animal or, after tests which are appropriate for the evaluation for the safety of such drug, induces cancer in man or animal, except that the foregoing provisions of this subparagraph shall not apply with respect to such drug if the Secretary finds that, under the conditions of use specified in proposed labeling, and reasonably certain to be followed in practice (i) such drug will not adversely affect the animals, for which it is intended, and (ii) no residue of such drug will be found (by methods of examination prescribed or approved by the Secretary by regulations, which regulations shall not be subject to subsections (c), (d), and (h], in any edible portion of such animals after slaughter or in any food yielded by or derived from the living animals; he shall issue an order refusing to approve the application. If, after such notice and opportunity for hearing, the Secretary finds that subparagraphs (A) through (G) do not apply, he shall issue an order approving the application.

(2) In determining whether such drug is safe for use under the conditions prescribed, recommended, or suggested in the proposed labeling thereof, the Secretary shall consider, among other relevant factors, (A) the probable consumption of such drug and of any substance formed in or on food because of the use of such drug, (B) the cumulative effect on man or animal of such drug, taking into account any chemically or pharmacologically related substance, (C) safety factors which in the opinion of experts, qualified by scientific training and experience to evaluate the safety of such drugs, are appropriate for the use of animal experimentation data, and (D) whether the conditions of use prescribed, recommended, or suggested in the proposed labeling are reasonably certain to be followed in practice. Any order issued under this subsection refusing to approve an application shall state the findings upon which it is based.

(3) As used in this subsection and subsection (e), the term "substantial evidence" means evidence consisting of adequate and well-controlled investigations, including field investigation, by experts qualified by scientific training and experience to evaluate the effectiveness of the drug involved, on the basis of which it could fairly and reasonably be concluded by such experts that the drug will have the effect it purports or is represented to have under the conditions of use prescribed, recommended, or suggested in the labeling or proposed labeling thereof.

⟨1077⟩ GOOD MANUFACTURING PRACTICES

As is indicated in the *General Notices*, tolerances stated in the *United States Pharmacopeia* and in the *National Formulary* are based upon the consideration that the article is produced under recognized principles of good manufacturing practice. In the United States, a drug not produced in accordance with current good manufacturing practices may be considered to be adulterated. The U. S. Food and Drug Administration has published regulations setting forth minimum current good manufacturing practices for the preparation of drug products. While the regulations are directed primarily to drug manufacturers, the principles embodied therein may be helpful to those engaged in the practice of pharmacy and it is for this reason that these regulations are reproduced here.

Publication of these regulations in this *Pharmacopeia* is for purposes of information and does not impart to them any legal effect under the Federal Food, Drug, and Cosmetic Act.

Part 210—Current Good Manufacturing Practices in Manufacturing, Processing, Packing, or Holding of Drugs: General

§ 210.1 Status of current good manufacturing practice regulations.

(a) The regulations set forth in this part and in Parts 211 through 229 of this chapter contain the minimum current good manufacturing practice for methods to be used in, and the facilities or controls to be used for, the manufacture, processing, packing, or holding of a drug to assure that such drug meets the requirements of the act as to safety, and has the identity and strength and meets the quality and purity characteristics that it purports or is represented to possess.

(b) The failure to comply with any regulation set forth in this part and in Parts 211 through 229 of this chapter in the manufacture, processing, packing, or holding of a drug shall render such drug to be adulterated under section 501(a)(2)(B) of the act and such drug, as well as the person who is responsible for the failure to comply, shall be subject to regulatory action.

§ 210.2 Applicability of current good manufacturing practice regulations.

(a) The regulations in this part and in Parts 211 through 229 of this chapter as they may pertain to a drug and in Parts 600 through 680 of this chapter as they may pertain to a biological product for human use, shall be considered to supplement, not supersede, each other, unless the regulations explicitly provide otherwise. In the event that it is impossible to comply with all applicable regulations in these parts, the regulations specifically applicable to the drug in question shall supersede the more general.

(b) If a person engages in only some operations subject to the regulations in this part and in Parts 211 through 229 and Parts 600 through 680 of this chapter, and not in others, that person need only comply with those regulations applicable to the operations in which he or she is engaged.

§ 210.3 Definitions.

(a) The definitions and interpretations contained in section 201 of the act shall be applicable to such terms when used in this part and in Parts 211 through 229 of this chapter.

(b) The following definitions of terms apply to this part and to Parts 211 through 229 of this chapter.

(1) "Act" means the Federal Food, Drug, and Cosmetic Act, as amended (21 U.S.C. 301 et seq.).

(2) "Batch" means a specific quantity of a drug or other material that is intended to have uniform character and quality, within specified limits, and is produced according to a single manufacturing order during the same cycle of manufacture.

(3) "Component" means any ingredient intended for use in the manufacture of a drug product, including those that may not appear in such drug product.

(4) "Drug product" means a finished dosage form, for example, tablet, capsule, solution, etc., that contains an active drug ingredient generally, but not necessarily, in association with inactive ingredients. The term also includes a finished dosage form that does not contain an active ingredient but is intended to be used as a placebo.

(5) "Fiber" means any particulate contaminant with a length at least three times greater than its width.

(6) "Non-fiber-releasing filter" means any filter, which after any appropriate pretreatment such as washing or flushing, will not release fibers into the component or drug product that is being filtered. All filters composed of asbestos are deemed to be fiber-releasing filters.

(7) "Active ingredient" means any component that is intended to furnish pharmacological activity or other direct effect in the diagnosis, cure, mitigation, treatment, or prevention of disease, or to affect the structure of any function of the body of man or other animals. The term includes those components that may undergo chemical change in the manufacture of the drug product and be present in the drug product in a modified form intended to furnish the specified activity or effect.

(8) "Inactive ingredient" means any component other than an "active ingredient."

(9) "In-process material" means any material fabricated, compounded, blended, or derived by chemical reaction that is produced for, and used in the preparation of the drug product.

(10) "Lot" means a batch, or a specific identified portion of a batch, having uniform character and quality within specified limits; or, in the case of a drug product produced by continuous process, it is a specific identified amount produced in a unit of time or quantity in a manner that assures its having uniform character and quality within specified limits.

(11) "Lot number, control number, or batch number" means any distinctive combination of letters, numbers, or symbols, or any combination of them, from which the complete history of the manufacture, processing, packing, holding, and distribution of a batch or lot of drug product or other material can be determined.

(12) "Manufacture, processing, packing, or holding of a drug product" includes packaging and labeling operations, testing, and quality control of drug products.

(15) "Quality control unit" means any person or organizational element designated by the firm to be responsible for the duties relating to quality control.

(16) "Strength" means:

(i) The concentration of the drug substance (for example, weight/weight, weight/volume, or unit dose/volume basis), and/or

(ii) The potency, that is, the therapeutic activity of the drug product as indicated by appropriate laboratory tests or by adequately developed and controlled clinical data (expressed, for example, in terms of units by reference to a standard).

(17) "Theoretical yield" means the quantity that would be produced at any appropriate phase of manufacture, processing, or packing of a particular drug product, based upon the quantity of components to be used, in the absence of any loss or error in actual production.

(18) "Actual yield" means the quantity that is actually produced at any appropriate phase of manufacture, processing, or packing of a particular drug product.

(19) "Percentage of theoretical yield" means the ratio of the actual yield (at any appropriate phase of manufacture, processing, or

packing of a particular drug product) to the theoretical yield (at the same phase), stated as a percentage.

(20) "Acceptance criteria" means the product specifications and acceptance/rejection criteria, such as acceptable quality level and unacceptable quality level, with an associated sampling plan, that are necessary for making a decision to accept or reject a lot or batch (or any other convenient subgroups of manufactured units).

(21) "Representative sample" means a sample that consists of a number of units that are drawn based on rational criteria such as random sampling and intended to assure that the sample accurately portrays the material being sampled.

Part 211—Current Good Manufacturing Practice for Finished Pharmaceuticals

Subpart A—General Provisions

§ 211.1 Scope.

(a) The regulations in this part contain the minimum current good manufacturing practice for preparation of drug products for administration to humans or animals.

(b) The current good manufacturing practice regulations in this chapter, as they pertain to drug products, and in Parts 600 through 680 of this chapter, as they pertain to biological products for human use, shall be considered to supplement, not supersede, the regulations in this part unless the regulations explicitly provide otherwise. In the event it is impossible to comply with applicable regulations both in this part and in other parts of this chapter or in Parts 600 through 680 of this chapter, the regulation specifically applicable to the drug product in question shall supersede the regulation in this part.

§ 211.3 Definitions.

The definitions set forth in § 210.3 of this chapter apply in this part.

Subpart B—Organization and Personnel

§ 211.22 Responsibilities of quality control unit.

(a) There shall be a quality control unit that shall have the responsibility and authority to approve or reject all components, drug product containers, closures, in-process materials, packaging material, labeling, and drug products, and the authority to review production records to assure that no errors have occurred or, if errors have occurred, that they have been fully investigated. The quality control unit shall be responsible for approving or rejecting drug products manufactured, processed, packed, or held under contract by another company.

(b) Adequate laboratory facilities for the testing and approval (or rejection) of components, drug product containers, closures, packaging materials, in-process materials, and drug products shall be available to the quality control unit.

(c) The quality control unit shall have the responsibility for approving or rejecting all procedures or specifications impacting on the identity, strength, quality, and purity of the drug product.

(d) The responsibilities and procedures applicable to the quality control unit shall be in writing; such written procedures shall be followed.

§ 211.25 Personnel qualifications.

(a) Each person engaged in the manufacture, processing, packing, or holding of a drug product shall have education, training, and experience, or any combination thereof, to enable that person to perform the assigned functions. Training shall be in the particular operations that the employee performs and in current good manufacturing practice (including the current good manufacturing practice regulations in this chapter and written procedures required by these regulations) as they relate to the employee's functions. Training in current good manufacturing practice shall be conducted by qualified individuals on a continuing basis and with sufficient frequency to assure that employees remain familiar with CGMP requirements applicable to them.

(b) Each person responsible for supervising the manufacture, processing, packing, or holding of a drug product shall have the education, training, and experience, or any combination thereof, to perform assigned functions in such a manner as to provide assurance that the drug product has the safety, identity, strength, quality, and purity that it purports or is represented to possess.

(c) There shall be an adequate number of qualified personnel to perform and supervise the manufacture, processing, packing, or holding of each drug product.

§ 211.28 Personnel responsibilities.

(a) Personnel engaged in the manufacture, processing, packing, or holding of a drug product shall wear clean clothing appropriate for the duties they perform. Protective apparel, such as head, face, hand, and arm coverings, shall be worn as necessary to protect drug products from contamination.

(b) Personnel shall practice good sanitation and health habits.

(c) Only personnel authorized by supervisory personnel shall enter those areas of the buildings and facilities designated as limited-access areas.

(d) Any person shown at any time (either by medical examination or supervisory observation) to have an apparent illness or open lesions that may adversely affect the safety or quality of drug products shall be excluded from direct contact with components, drug product containers, closures, in-process materials, and drug products until the condition is corrected or determined by competent medical personnel not to jeopardize the safety or quality of drug products. All personnel shall be instructed to report to supervisory personnel any health conditions that may have an adverse effect on drug products.

§ 211.34 Consultants.

Consultants advising on the manufacture, processing, packing, or holding of drug products shall have sufficient education, training, and experience, or any combination thereof, to advise on the subject for which they are retained. Records shall be maintained stating the name, address, and qualifications of any consultants and the type of service they provide.

Subpart C—Buildings and Facilities

§ 211.42 Design and construction features.

(a) Any building or buildings used in the manufacture, processing, packing, or holding of a drug product shall be of suitable size, construction and location to facilitate cleaning, maintenance, and proper operations.

(b) Any such building shall have adequate space for the orderly placement of equipment and materials to prevent mixups between different components, drug product containers, closures, labeling, in-process materials, or drug products, and to prevent contamination. The flow of components, drug product containers, closures, labeling, in-process materials, and drug products through the building or buildings shall be designed to prevent contamination.

(c) Operations shall be performed within specifically defined areas of adequate size. There shall be separate or defined areas for the firm's operations to prevent contamination or mixups as follows:

(1) Receipt, identification, storage, and withholding from use of components, drug product containers, closures, and labeling, pending the appropriate sampling, testing, or examination by the quality control unit before release for manufacturing or packaging;

(2) Holding rejected components, drug product containers, closures, and labeling before disposition;

(3) Storage of released components, drug product containers, closures, and labeling;

(4) Storage of in-process materials;

(5) Manufacturing and processing operations;

(6) Packaging and labeling operations;

(7) Quarantine storage before release of drug products;

(8) Storage of drug products after release;

(9) Control and laboratory operations;

(10) Aseptic processing, which includes as appropriate:

(i) Floors, walls, and ceilings of smooth, hard surfaces that are easily cleanable;

(ii) Temperature and humidity controls;

(iii) An air supply filtered through high-efficiency particulate air filters under positive pressure, regardless of whether flow is laminar or nonlaminar;

(iv) A system for monitoring environmental conditions;

(v) A system for cleaning and disinfecting the room and equipment to produce aseptic conditions;

(vi) A system for maintaining any equipment used to control the aseptic conditions.

(d) Operations relating to the manufacture, processing, and packing of penicillin shall be performed in facilities separate from those used for other drug products for human use.

§ 211.44 Lighting.

Adequate lighting shall be provided in all areas.

§ 211.46 Ventilation, air filtration, air heating and cooling.

(a) Adequate ventilation shall be provided.

(b) Equipment for adequate control over air pressure, micro-organisms, dust, humidity, and temperature shall be provided when appropriate for the manufacture, processing, packing, or holding of a drug product.

(c) Air filtration systems, including prefilters and particulate matter air filters, shall be used when appropriate on air supplies to production areas. If air is recirculated to production areas, measures shall be taken to control recirculation of dust from production. In areas where air contamination occurs during production, there shall be adequate exhaust systems or other systems adequate to control contaminants.

(d) Air-handling systems for the manufacture, processing, and packing of penicillin shall be completely separate from those for other drug products for human use.

§ 211.48 Plumbing.

(a) Potable water shall be supplied under continuous positive pressure in a plumbing system free of defects that could contribute contamination to any drug product. Potable water shall meet the standards prescribed in the Environmental Protection Agency's Primary Drinking Water Regulations set forth in 40 CFR Part 141. Water not meeting such standards shall not be permitted in the potable water system.

(b) Drains shall be of adequate size and, where connected directly to a sewer, shall be provided with an air break or other mechanical device to prevent back-siphonage.

§ 211.50 Sewage and refuse.

Sewage, trash, and other refuse in and from the building and immediate premises shall be disposed of in a safe and sanitary manner.

§ 211.52 Washing and toilet facilities.

Adequate washing facilities shall be provided, including hot and cold water, soap or detergent, air driers or single-service towels, and clean toilet facilities easily accessible to working areas.

§ 211.56 Sanitation.

(a) Any building used in the manufacture, processing, packing, or holding of a drug product shall be maintained in a clean and sanitary condition. Any such building shall be free of infestation by rodents, birds, insects, and other vermin (other than laboratory animals). Trash and organic waste matter shall be held and disposed of in a timely and sanitary manner.

(b) There shall be written procedures assigning responsibility for sanitation and describing in sufficient detail the cleaning schedules, methods, equipment, and materials to be used in cleaning the buildings and facilities; such written procedures shall be followed.

(c) There shall be written procedures for use of suitable rodenticides, insecticides, fungicides, fumigating agents, and cleaning and sanitizing agents. Such written procedures shall be designed to prevent the contamination of equipment, components, drug product containers, closures, packaging, labeling materials, or drug products and shall be followed. Rodenticides, insecticides, and fungicides shall not be used unless registered and used in accordance with the Federal Insecticide, Fungicide, and Rodenticide Act (7 U.S.C. 135).

(d) Sanitation procedures shall apply to work performed by contractors or temporary employees as well as work performed by full-time employees during the ordinary course of operations.

§ 211.58 Maintenance.

Any building used in the manufacture, processing, packing, or holding of a drug product shall be maintained in a good state of repair.

Subpart D—Equipment

§ 211.63 Equipment design, size, and location.

Equipment used in the manufacture, processing, packing, or holding of a drug product shall be of appropriate design, adequate size, and suitably located to facilitate operations for its intended use and for its cleaning and maintenance.

§ 211.65 Equipment construction.

(a) Equipment shall be constructed so that surfaces that contact components, in-process materials, or drug products shall not be reactive, additive, or absorptive so as to alter the safety, identity, strength, quality, or purity of the drug product beyond the official or other established requirements.

(b) Any substances required for operation, such as lubricants or coolants, shall not come into contact with components, drug product containers, closures, in-process materials, or drug products so as to alter the safety, identity, strength, quality, or purity of the drug product beyond the official or other established requirements.

§ 211.67 Equipment cleaning and maintenance.

(a) Equipment and utensils shall be cleaned, maintained, and sanitized at appropriate intervals to prevent malfunctions or contamination that would alter the safety, identity, strength, quality, or purity of the drug product beyond the official or other established requirements.

(b) Written procedures shall be established and followed for cleaning and maintenance of equipment, including utensils, used in the manufacture, processing, packing, or holding of a drug product. These procedures shall include, but are not necessarily limited to, the following:

(1) Assignment of responsibility for cleaning and maintaining equipment;

(2) Maintenance and cleaning schedules, including, where appropriate, sanitizing schedules;

(3) A description in sufficient detail of the methods, equipment, and materials used in cleaning and maintenance operations, and the methods of disassembling and reassembling equipment as necessary to assure proper cleaning and maintenance;

(4) Removal or obliteration of previous batch identification;

(5) Protection of clean equipment from contamination prior to use;

(6) Inspection of equipment for cleanliness immediately before use.

(c) Records shall be kept of maintenance, cleaning, sanitizing, and inspection as specified in §§ 211.180 and 211.182.

§ 211.68 Automatic, mechanical, and electronic equipment.

(a) Automatic, mechanical, or electronic equipment or other types of equipment, including computers, or related systems that will perform a function satisfactorily, may be used in the manufacture, processing, packing, and holding of a drug product. If such equipment is so used, it shall be routinely calibrated, inspected, or checked according to a written program designed to assure proper performance. Written records of those calibration checks and inspections shall be maintained.

(b) Appropriate controls shall be exercised over computer or related systems to assure that changes in master production and control records or other records are instituted only by authorized personnel. Input to and output from the computer or related system of formulas or other records or data shall be checked for accuracy. A backup file of data entered into the computer or related system shall be maintained except where certain data, such as calculations performed in connection with laboratory analysis, are eliminated by computerization or other automated processes. In such instances a written record of the program shall be maintained along with appropriate validation data. Hard copy or alternative systems, such as duplicates, tapes, or microfilm, designed to assure that backup data are exact and complete and that it is secure from alteration, inadvertent erasures, or loss shall be maintained.

§ 211.72 Filters.

Filters for liquid filtration used in the manufacture, processing, or packing of injectable drug products intended for human use shall not release fibers into such products. Fiber-releasing filters may not be used in the manufacture, processing, or packing of these injectable drug products unless it is not possible to manufacture such drug products without the use of such filters. If use of a fiber-releasing filter is necessary, an additional non-fiber-releasing filter of 0.22 micron maximum mean porosity (0.45 micron if the manufacturing conditions so dictate) shall subsequently be used to reduce the content of particles in the injectable drug product. Use of an asbestos-containing filter, with or without subsequent use of a specific non-fiber-releasing filter, is permissible only upon submission of proof to the appropriate bureau of the Food and Drug Administration that use of a non-fiber-releasing filter will, or is likely to, compromise the safety or effectiveness of the injectable drug product.

Subpart E—Control of Components and Drug Product Containers and Closures

§ 211.80 General requirements.

(a) There shall be written procedures describing in sufficient detail the receipt, identification, storage, handling, sampling, testing, and approval or rejection of components and drug product containers and closures; such written procedures shall be followed.

(b) Components and drug product containers and closures shall at all times be handled and stored in a manner to prevent contamination.

(c) Bagged or boxed components of drug product containers, or closures shall be stored off the floor and suitably spaced to permit cleaning and inspection.

(d) Each container or grouping of containers for components or drug product containers, or closures shall be identified with a distinctive code for each lot in each shipment received. This code shall be used in recording the disposition of each lot. Each lot shall be appropriately identified as to its status (i.e., quarantined, approved, or rejected).

§ 211.82 Receipt and storage of untested components, drug product containers, and closures.

(a) Upon receipt and before acceptance, each container or grouping of containers of components, drug product containers, and closures shall be examined visually for appropriate labeling as to contents, container damage or broken seals, and contamination.

(b) Components, drug product containers, and closures shall be stored under quarantine until they have been tested or examined, as appropriate, and released. Storage within the area shall conform to the requirements of § 211.80.

§ 211.84 Testing and approval or rejection of components, drug product containers, and closures.

(a) Each lot of components, drug product containers, and closures shall be withheld from use until the lot has been sampled, tested, or examined, as appropriate, and released for use by the quality control unit.

(b) Representative samples of each shipment of each lot shall be collected for testing or examination. The number of containers to be sampled, and the amount of material to be taken from each container, shall be based upon appropriate criteria such as statistical criteria for component variability, confidence levels, and degree of precision desired, the past quality history of the supplier, and the quantity needed for analysis and reserve where required by § 211.170.

(c) Samples shall be collected in accordance with the following procedures:

(1) The containers of components selected shall be cleaned where necessary, by appropriate means.

(2) The containers shall be opened, sampled, and resealed in a manner designed to prevent contamination of their contents and contamination of other components, drug product containers, or closures.

(3) Sterile equipment and aseptic sampling techniques shall be used when necessary.

(4) If it is necessary to sample a component from the top, middle, and bottom of its container, such sample subdivisions shall not be composited for testing.

(5) Sample containers shall be identified so that the following information can be determined: name of the material sampled, the lot number, the container from which the sample was taken, the data on which the sample was taken, and the name of the person who collected the sample.

(6) Containers from which samples have been taken shall be marked to show that samples have been removed from them.

(d) Samples shall be examined and tested as follows:

(1) At least one test shall be conducted to verify the identity of each component of a drug product. Specific identity tests, if they exist, shall be used.

(2) Each component shall be tested for conformity with all appropriate written specifications for purity, strength, and quality. In lieu of such testing by the manufacturer, a report of analysis may be accepted from the supplier of a component, provided that at least one specific identity test is conducted on such component by the manufacturer, and provided that the manufacturer establishes the reliability of the supplier's analyses through appropriate validation of the supplier's test results at appropriate intervals.

(3) Containers and closures shall be tested for conformance with all appropriate written procedures. In lieu of such testing by the manufacturer, a certificate of testing may be accepted from the supplier, provided that at least a visual identification is conducted on such containers/closures by the manufacturer and provided that the manufacturer establishes the reliability of the supplier's test results through appropriate validation of the supplier's test results at appropriate intervals.

(4) When appropriate, components shall be microscopically examined.

(5) Each lot of a component, drug product container, or closure that is liable to contamination with filth, insect infestation, or other extraneous adulterant shall be examined against established specifications for such contamination.

(6) Each lot of a component, drug product container, or closure that is liable to microbiological contamination that is objectionable in view of its intended use shall be subjected to microbiological tests before use.

(e) Any lot of components, drug product containers, or closures that meets the appropriate written specifications of identity, strength, quality, and purity and related tests under paragraph (d) of this section may be approved and released for use. Any lot of such material that does not meet such specifications shall be rejected.

§ 211.86 Use of approved components, drug product containers, and closures.

Components, drug product containers, and closures approved for use shall be rotated so that the oldest approved stock is used first. Deviation from this requirement is permitted if such deviation is temporary and appropriate.

§ 211.87 Retesting of approved components, drug product containers, and closures.

Components, drug product containers, and closures shall be retested or reexamined, as appropriate, for identity, strength, quality, and purity and approved or rejected by the quality control unit in accordance with § 211.84 as necessary, e.g., after storage for long periods or after exposure to air, heat or other conditions that might adversely affect the component, drug product container, or closure.

§ 211.89 Rejected components, drug product containers, and closures.

Rejected components, drug product containers, and closures shall be identified and controlled under a quarantine system designed to prevent their use in manufacturing or processing operations for which they are unsuitable.

§ 211.94 Drug product containers and closures.

(a) Drug product containers and closures shall not be reactive, additive, or absorptive so as to alter the safety, identity, strength, quality, or purity of the drug beyond the official or established requirements.

(b) Container closure systems shall provide adequate protection against foreseeable external factors in storage and use that can cause deterioration or contamination of the drug product.

(c) Drug product containers and closures shall be clean and, where indicated by the nature of the drug, sterilized and processed to remove pyrogenic properties to assure that they are suitable for their intended use.

(d) Standards or specifications, methods of testing, and, where indicated, methods of cleaning, sterilizing, and processing to remove pyrogenic properties shall be written and followed for drug product containers and closures.

Subpart F—Production and Process Controls

§ 211.100 Written procedures; deviations.

(a) There shall be written procedures for production and process control designed to assure that the drug products have the identity, strength, quality, and purity they purport or are represented to possess. Such procedures shall include all requirements in this subpart. These written procedures, including any changes, shall be drafted, reviewed, and approved by the appropriate organizational units and reviewed and approved by the quality control unit.

(b) Written production and process control procedures shall be followed in the execution of the various production and process control functions and shall be documented at the time of performance. Any deviation from the written procedures shall be recorded and justified.

§ 211.101 Charge-in of components.

Written production and control procedures shall include the following, which are designed to assure that the drug products produced have the identity, strength, quality, and purity they purport or are represented to possess:

(a) The batch shall be formulated with the intent to provide not less than 100 percent of the labeled or established amount of active ingredient.

(b) Components for drug product manufacturing shall be weighed, measured, or subdivided as appropriate. If a component is removed from the original container to another, the new container shall be identified with the following information:

(1) Component name or item code;

(2) Receiving or control number;

(3) Weight or measure in new container;

(4) Batch for which component was dispensed, including its product name, strength, and lot number.

(c) Weighing, measuring, or subdividing operations for components shall be adequately supervised. Each container of component dispensed to manufacturing shall be examined by a second person to assure that:

(1) The component was released by the quality control unit;

(2) The weight or measure is correct as stated in the batch production records;

(3) The containers are properly identified.

(d) Each component shall be added to the batch by one person and verified by a second person.

§ 211.103 Calculation of yield.

Actual yields and percentages of theoretical yield shall be determined at the conclusion of each appropriate phase of manufacturing, processing, packaging, or holding of the drug product. Such calculations shall be performed by one person and independently verified by a second person.

§ 211.105 Equipment identification.

(a) All compounding and storage containers, processing lines, and major equipment used using the production of a batch of a drug product shall be properly identified at all times to indicate their contents and, when necessary, the phase of processing of the batch.

(b) Major equipment shall be identified by a distinctive identification number or code that shall be recorded in the batch production record to show the specific equipment used in the manufacture of each batch of a drug product. In cases where only one of a particular type of equipment exists in a manufacturing facility, the name of the equipment may be used in lieu of a distinctive identification number or code.

§ 211.110 Sampling and testing of in-process materials and drug products.

(a) To assure batch uniformity and integrity of drug products, written procedures shall be established and followed that describe the in-process controls, and tests, or examinations to be conducted on appropriate samples of in-process materials of each batch. Such control procedures shall be established to monitor the output and to validate the performance of those manufacturing processes that may be responsible for causing variability in the characteristics of in-process material and the drug product. Such control procedures shall include, but are not limited to, the following, where appropriate:

(1) Tablet or capsule weight variation;

(2) Disintegration time;

(3) Adequacy of mixing to assure uniformity and homogeneity;

(4) Dissolution time and rate;

(5) Clarity, completeness, or pH of solutions.

(b) Valid in-process specifications for such characteristics shall be consistent with drug product final specifications and shall be derived from previous acceptable process average and process variability estimates where possible and determined by the application of suitable statistical procedures where appropriate. Examination and testing of samples shall assure that the drug product and in-process material conform to specifications.

(c) In-process materials shall be tested for identity, strength, quality, and purity as appropriate, and approved or rejected by the quality control unit, during the production process, e.g., at commencement or completion of significant phases or after storage for long periods.

(d) Rejected in-process materials shall be identified and controlled under a quarantine system designed to prevent their use in manufacturing or processing operations for which they are unsuitable.

§ 211.111 Time limitations on production.

When appropriate, time limits for the completion of each phase of production shall be established to assure the quality of the drug product. Deviation from established time limits may be acceptable if such deviation does not compromise the quality of the drug product. Such deviation shall be justified and documented.

§ 211.113 Control of microbiological contamination.

(a) Appropriate written procedures, designed to prevent objectionable microorganisms in drug products not required to be sterile, shall be established and followed.

(b) Appropriate written procedures, designed to prevent microbiological contamination of drug products purporting to be sterile, shall be established and followed. Such procedures shall include validation of any sterilization process.

§ 211.115 Reprocessing.

(a) Written procedures shall be established and followed prescribing a system for reprocessing batches that do not conform to standards or specifications and the steps to be taken to insure that the reprocessed batches will conform with all established standards, specifications, and characteristics.

(b) Reprocessing shall not be performed without the review and approval of the quality control unit.

Subpart G—Packaging and Labeling Control

§ 211.122 Materials examination and usage criteria.

(a) There shall be written procedures describing in sufficient detail the receipt, identification, storage, handling, sampling, examination, and/or testing of labeling and packaging materials; such written procedures shall be followed. Labeling and packaging materials shall be representatively sampled, and examined or tested upon receipt and before use in packaging or labeling of a drug product.

(b) Any labeling or packaging materials meeting appropriate written specifications may be approved and released for use. Any labeling or packaging materials that do not meet such specifications shall be rejected to prevent their use in operations for which they are unsuitable.

(c) Records shall be maintained for each shipment received of each different labeling and packaging material indicating receipt, examination or testing, and whether accepted or rejected.

(d) Labels and other labeling materials for each different drug product, strength, dosage form, or quantity of contents shall be stored separately with suitable identification. Access to the storage area shall be limited to authorized personnel.

(e) Obsolete and outdated labels, labeling, and other packaging materials shall be destroyed.

(f) Gang printing of labeling to be used for different drug products or different strengths of the same drug product (or labeling of the same size and identical or similar format and/or color schemes) shall be minimized. If gang printing is employed, packaging and labeling operations shall provide for special control procedures, taking into consideration sheet layout, stacking, cutting, and handling during and after printing.

(g) Printing devices on, or associated with, manufacturing lines used to imprint labeling upon the drug product unit label or case shall be monitored to assure that all imprinting conforms to the print specified in the batch production record.

§ 211.125 Labeling issuance.

(a) Strict control shall be exercised over labeling issued for use in drug product labeling operations.

(b) Labeling materials issued for a batch shall be carefully examined for identity and conformity to the labeling specified in the master or batch production records.

(c) Procedures shall be utilized to reconcile the quantities of labeling issued, used, and returned, and shall require evaluation of discrepancies found between the quantity of drug product finished and the quantity of labeling issued when such discrepancies are outside narrow preset limits based on historical operating data. Such discrepancies shall be investigated in accordance with § 211.192.

(d) All excess labeling bearing lot or control numbers shall be destroyed.

(e) Returned labeling shall be maintained and stored in a manner to prevent mixups and provide proper identification.

(f) Procedures shall be written describing in sufficient detail the control procedures employed for the issuance of labeling; such written procedures shall be followed.

§ 211.130 Packaging and labeling operations.

There shall be written procedures designed to assure that correct labels, labeling, and packaging materials are used for drug products; such written procedures shall be followed. These procedures shall incorporate the following features:

(a) Prevention of mixups and cross-contamination by physical or spatial separation from operations on other drug products.

(b) Identification of the drug product with a lot or control number that permits determination of the history of the manufacture and control of the batch.

(c) Examination of packaging and labeling materials for suitability and correctness before packaging operations, and documentation of such examination in the batch production record.

(d) Inspection of the packaging and labeling facilities immediately before use to assure that all drug products have been removed from previous operations. Inspection shall also be made to assure that packaging and labeling materials not suitable for subsequent operations have been removed. Results of inspection shall be documented in the batch production records.

§ 211.132 Tamper-resistant packaging requirements for over-the-counter human drug products.

(a) *General.* The Food and Drug Administration has the authority under the Federal Food, Drug, and Cosmetic Act (the act) to establish a uniform national requirement for tamper-resistant packaging of OTC drug products that will improve the security of OTC drug packaging and help assure the safety and effectiveness of OTC drug products. An OTC drug product (except a dermatological, dentifrice, insulin, or throat lozenge product) for retail sale that is not packaged in a tamper-resistant package or that is not properly labeled under this section is adulterated under section 501 of the act or misbranded under section 502 of the act, or both.

(b) *Requirement for tamper-resistant package.* Each manufacturer and packer who packages an OTC drug product (except a dermatological, dentifrice, insulin, or throat lozenge product) for retail sale shall package the product in a tamper-resistant package, if this product is accessible to the public while held for sale. A tamper-resistant package is one having one or more indicators or barriers to entry which, if breached or missing, can reasonably be expected for provide visible evidence to consumers that tampering has occurred. To reduce the likelihood of successful tampering and to increase the likelihood that consumers will discover if a product has been tampered with, the package is required to be distinctive by design (e.g., an aerosol product container) or by the use of one or more indicators or barriers to entry that employ an identifying characteristic (e.g., a pattern, name, registered trademark, logo, or picture). For purposes of this section, the term "distinctive by design" means the packaging cannot be duplicated with commonly available materials or through commonly available processes. For purposes of this section, the term "aerosol product" means a product which depends upon the power of a liquefied or compressed gas to expel the contents from the container. A tamper-resistant package may involve an immediate-container and closure system or secondary-container or carton system or any combination of systems intended to provide a visual indication of package integrity. The tamper-resistant feature shall be designed to and shall remain intact when handled in a reasonable manner during manufacture, distribution, and retail display.

(1) For two-piece, hard gelatin capsule products subject to this requirement, a minimum of two tamper-resistant packaging features is required, unless the capsules are sealed by a tamper-resistant technology.

(2) For all other products subject to this requirement, including two-piece, hard gelatin capsules that are sealed by a tamper-resistant technology, a minimum of one tamper-resistant feature is required.

(c) *Labeling.* Each retail package of an OTC drug product covered by this section, except ammonia inhalant in crushable glass ampules, aerosol products as defined in paragraph (b) of this section, or containers of compressed medical oxygen, is required to bear a statement that is prominently placed so that consumers are alerted to the specific tamper-resistant feature of the package. The labeling statement is also required to be so placed that it will be unaffected if the tamper-resistant feature of the package is breached or missing. If the tamper-resistant feature chosen to meet the requirement in paragraph (b) of this section is one that uses an identifying characteristic, that characteristic is required to be referred to in the labeling statement. For example, the labeling statement on a bottle with a shrink band could say "For your protection, this bottle has an imprinted seal around the neck."

(d) *Request for exemptions from packaging and labeling requirements.* A manufacturer or packer may request an exemption from the packaging and labeling requirements of this section. A request for an exemption is required to be submitted in the form of a citizen petition under § 10.30 of this chapter and should be clearly identified on the envelope as a "Request for Exemption from Tamper-Resistant Rule." The petition is required to contain the following:

(1) The name of the drug product or, if the petition seeks an exemption for a drug class, the name of the drug class, and a list of products within that class.

(2) The reasons that the drug product's compliance with the tamper-resistant packaging or labeling requirements of this section is unnecessary or cannot be achieved.

(3) A description of alternative steps that are available, or that the petitioner has already taken, to reduce the likelihood that the product or drug class will be the subject of malicious adulteration.

(4) Other information justifying an exemption.

(e) *OTC drug products subject to approved new drug applications.* Holders of approved new drug applications for OTC drug products are required under § 314.70 of this chapter to provide the agency with notification of changes in packaging and labeling to comply with the requirements of this section. Changes in packaging and labeling required by this regulation may be made before FDA approval, as provided under § 314.70(c) of this chapter. Manufacturing changes by which capsules are to be sealed require prior FDA approval under § 314.70(b) of this chapter.

(f) *Poison Prevention Packaging Act of 1970.* This section does not affect any requirements for "special packaging" as defined under § 310.3(1) of this chapter and required under the Poison Prevention Packaging Act of 1970.

§ 211.134 Drug product inspection.

(a) Packaged and labeled products shall be examined during finishing operations to provide assurance that containers and packages in the lot have the correct label.

(b) A representative sample of units shall be collected at the completion of finishing operations and shall be visually examined for correct labeling.

(c) Results of these examinations shall be recorded in the batch production or control records.

§ 211.137 Expiration dating.

(a) To assure that a drug product meets applicable standards of identity, strength, quality, and purity at the time of use, it shall bear an expiration date determined by appropriate stability testing described in § 211.166.

(b) Expiration dates shall be related to any storage conditions stated on the labeling, as determined by stability studies described in § 211.166.

(c) If the drug product is to be reconstituted at the time of dispensing, its labeling shall bear expiration information for both the reconstituted and unreconstituted drug products.

(d) Expiration dates shall appear on labeling in accordance with the requirements of § 201.17 of this chapter.

(e) Homeopathic drug products shall be exempt from the requirements of this section.

(f) Allergenic extracts that are labeled "No U.S. Standard of Potency" are exempt from the requirements of this section.

(g) Pending consideration of a proposed exemption, published in the FEDERAL REGISTER of September 29, 1978, the requirements in this section shall not be enforced for human OTC drug products if their labeling does not bear dosage limitations and they are stable for at least 3 years as supported by appropriate stability data.

Subpart H—Holding and Distribution

§ 211.142 Warehousing procedures.

Written procedures describing the warehousing of drug products shall be established and followed. They shall include:

(a) Quarantine of drug products before release by the quality control unit.

(b) Storage of drug products under appropriate conditions of temperature, humidity, and light so that the identity, strength, quality, and purity of the drug products are not affected.

§ 211.150 Distribution procedures.

Written procedures shall be established, and followed, describing the distribution of drug products. They shall include:

(a) A procedure whereby the oldest approved stock of a drug product is distributed first. Deviation from this requirement is permitted if such deviation is temporary and appropriate.

(b) A system by which the distribution of each lot of drug product can be readily determined to facilitate its recall if necessary.

Subpart I—Laboratory Controls

§ 211.160 General requirements.

(a) The establishment of any specifications, standards, sampling plans, test procedures, or other laboratory control mechanisms required by this subpart, including any change in such specifications, standards, sampling plans, test procedures, or other laboratory control mechanisms, shall be drafted by the appropriate organizational unit and reviewed and approved by the quality control unit. The requirements in this subpart shall be followed and shall be documented at the time of performance. Any deviation from the written specifications, standards, sampling plans, test procedures, or other laboratory control mechanisms shall be recorded and justified.

(b) Laboratory controls shall include the establishment of scientifically sound and appropriate specifications, standards, sampling plans, and test procedures designed to assure that components, drug product containers, closures, in-process materials, labeling, and drug products conform to appropriate standards of identity, strength, quality, and purity. Laboratory controls shall include:

(1) Determination of conformance to appropriate written specifications for the acceptance of each lot within each shipment of components, drug product containers, closures, and labeling used in the manufacture, processing, packing, or holding of drug products. The specifications shall include a description of the sampling and testing procedures used. Samples shall be representative and adequately identified. Such procedures shall also require appropriate retesting of any component, drug product container, or closure that is subject to deterioration.

(2) Determination of conformance to written specifications and a description of sampling and testing procedures for in-process materials. Such samples shall be representative and properly identified.

(3) Determination of conformance to written descriptions of sampling procedures and appropriate specifications for drug products. Such samples shall be representative and properly identified.

(4) The calibration of instruments, apparatus, gauges, and recording devices at suitable intervals in accordance with an established written program containing specific directions, schedules, limits for accuracy and precision, and provisions for remedial action in the event accuracy and/or precision limits are not met. Instruments, apparatus, gauges, and recording devices not meeting established specifications shall not be used.

§ 211.165 Testing and release for distribution.

(a) For each batch of drug product, there shall be appropriate laboratory determination of satisfactory conformance to final specifications for the drug product, including the identity and strength of each active ingredient, prior to release. Where sterility and/or pyrogen testing are conducted on specific batches of short-lived radiopharmaceuticals, such batches may be released prior to completion of sterility and/or pyrogen testing, provided such testing is completed as soon as possible.

(b) There shall be appropriate laboratory testing, as necessary, of each batch of drug product required to be free of objectionable microorganisms.

(c) Any sampling and testing plans shall be described in written procedures that shall include the method of sampling and the number of units per batch to be tested; such written procedure shall be followed.

(d) Acceptance criteria for the sampling and testing conducted by the quality control unit shall be adequate to assure that batches of drug products meet each appropriate specification and appropriate statistical quality control criteria as a condition for their approval and release. The statistical quality control criteria shall include appropriate acceptance levels and/or appropriate rejection levels.

(e) The accuracy, sensitivity, specificity, and reproducibility of test methods employed by the firm shall be established and documented. Such validation and documentation may be accomplished in accordance with § 211.194 (a) (2).

(f) Drug products failing to meet established standards or specifications and any other relevant quality control criteria shall be rejected.

Reprocessing may be performed. Prior to acceptance and use, reprocessed material must meet appropriate standards, specifications, and any other relevant criteria.

§ 211.166 Stability testing.

(a) There shall be a written testing program designed to assess the stability characteristics of drug products. The results of such stability testing shall be used in determining appropriate storage conditions and expiration dates. The written program shall be followed and shall include:

(1) Sample size and test intervals based on statistical criteria for each attribute examined to assure valid estimates of stability;

(2) Storage conditions for samples retained for testing;

(3) Reliable, meaningful, and specific test methods;

(4) Testing of the drug product in the same container-closure system as that in which the drug product is marketed;

(5) Testing of drug products for reconstitution at the time of dispensing (as directed in the labeling) as well as after they are reconstituted.

(b) An adequate number of batches of each drug product shall be tested to determine an appropriate expiration date and a record of such data shall be maintained. Accelerated studies, combined with basic stability information on the components, drug products, and container-closure system, may be used to support tentative expiration dates provided full shelf life studies are not available and are being conducted. Where data from accelerated studies are used to project a tentative expiration date that is beyond a date supported by actual shelf life studies, there must be stability studies conducted, including drug product testing at appropriate intervals, until the tentative expiration date is verified or the appropriate expiration date determined.

(c) For homeopathic drug products, the requirements of this section are as follows:

(1) There shall be a written assessment of stability based at least on testing or examination of the drug product for compatibility of the ingredients, and based on marketing experience with the drug product to indicate that there is no degradation of the product for the normal or expected period of use.

(2) Evaluation of stability shall be based on the same container-closure system in which the drug product is being marketed.

(d) Allergenic extracts that are labeled "No U.S. Standard of Potency" are exempt from the requirements of this section.

§ 211.167 Special testing requirements.

(a) For each batch of drug product purporting to be sterile and/or pyrogen-free, there shall be appropriate laboratory testing to determine conformance to such requirements. The test procedures shall be in writing and shall be followed.

(b) For each batch of ophthalmic ointment, there shall be appropriate testing to determine conformance to specifications regarding the presence of foreign particles and harsh or abrasive substances. The test procedures shall be in writing and shall be followed.

(c) For each batch of controlled-release dosage form, there shall be appropriate laboratory testing to determine conformance to the specifications for the rate of release of each active ingredient. The test procedures shall be in writing and shall be followed.

§ 211.170 Reserve samples.

(a) An appropriately identified reserve sample that is representative of each lot in each shipment of each active ingredient shall be retained. The reserve sample consists of at least twice the quantity necessary for all tests required to determine whether the active ingredient meets its established specifications, except for sterility and pyrogen testing. The retention time is as follows:

(1) For an active ingredient in a drug product other than those described in paragraphs (a) (2) and (3) of this section, the reserve sample shall be retained for 1 year after the expiration date of the last lot of the drug product containing the active ingredient.

(2) For an active ingredient in a radioactive drug product, except for nonradioactive reagent kits, the reserve sample shall be retained for:

(i) Three months after the expiration date of the last lot of the drug product containing the active ingredient if the expiration dating period of the drug product is 30 days or less; or

(ii) Six months after the expiration date of the last lot of the drug product containing the active ingredient if the expiration dating period of the drug product is more than 30 days.

(3) For an active ingredient in an OTC drug product that is exempt from bearing an expiration date under § 211.137, the reserve sample shall be retained for 3 years after distribution of the last lot of the drug product containing the active ingredient.

(b) An appropriately identified reserve sample that is representative of each lot or batch of drug product shall be retained and stored under conditions consistent with product labeling. The reserve sample shall be stored in the same immediate container-closure system in which the drug product is marketed or in one that has essentially the same characteristics. The reserve sample consists of at least twice the quantity necessary to perform all the required tests, except those for sterility and pyrogens. Reserve samples, except those drug products described in paragraph (b) (2), shall be examined visually at least once a year for evidence of deterioration unless visual examination would affect the integrity of the reserve samples. Any evidence of reserve sample deterioration shall be investigated in accordance with § 211.192. The results of the examination shall be recorded and maintained with other stability data on the drug product. Reserve samples of compressed medical gases need not be retained. The retention time is as follows:

(1) For a drug product other than those described in paragraphs (b) (2) and (3) of this section, the reserve sample shall be retained for 1 year after the expiration date of the drug product.

(2) For a radioactive drug product, except for nonradioactive reagent kits, the reserve sample shall be retained for:

(i) Three months after the expiration date of the drug product if the expiration dating period of the drug product is 30 days or less; or

(ii) Six months after the expiration date of the drug product if the expiration dating period of the drug product is more than 30 days.

(3) For an OTC drug product that is exempt from bearing an expiration date under § 211.137, the reserve sample must be retained for 3 years after the lot or batch of drug product is distributed.

§ 211.173 Laboratory animals.

Animals used in testing components, in-process materials, or drug products for compliance with established specifications shall be maintained and controlled in a manner that assures their suitability for their intended use. They shall be identified, and adequate records shall be maintained showing the history of their use.

§ 211.176 Penicillin contamination.

If a reasonable possibility exists that a non-penicillin drug product has been exposed to cross-contamination with penicillin, the non-penicillin drug product shall be tested for the presence of penicillin. Such drug product shall not be marketed if detectable levels are found when tested according to procedures specified in 'Procedures for Detecting and Measuring Penicillin Contamination in Drugs,' which is incorporated by reference. Copies are available from the Bureau of Drugs (HFD-430), Food and Drug Administration, 200 C St., SW., Washington, DC 20204, or available for inspection at the Office of the Federal Register, 1100 L St. NW., Washington, DC 20408. [Ed. Note—The Bureau of Drugs (HFD-430) is now designated as National Center for Drugs and Biologics (HFN-416).]

Subpart J—Records and Reports

§ 211.180 General requirements.

(a) Any production, control, or distribution record that is required to be maintained in compliance with this part and is specifically associated with a batch of a drug product shall be retained for at least 1 year after the expiration date of the batch or, in the case of certain OTC drug products lacking expiration dating because they meet the criteria for exemption under § 211.137, 3 years after distribution of the batch.

(b) Records shall be maintained for all components, drug product containers, closures, and labeling for at least 1 year after the expiration date or, in the case of certain OTC drug products lacking expiration dating because they meet the criteria for exemption under § 211.137, 3 years after distribution of the last lot of drug product incorporating the component or using the container, closure, or labeling.

(c) All records required under this part, or copies of such records, shall be readily available for authorized inspection during the retention period at the establishment where the activities described in such records occurred. These records or copies thereof shall be subject to photocopying or other means of reproduction as part of such inspection. Records that can be immediately retrieved from another location by computer or other electronic means shall be considered as meeting the requirements of this paragraph.

(d) Records required under this part may be retained either as original records or as true copies such as photocopies, microfilm, microfiche, or other accurate reproductions of the original records. Where reduction techniques, such as microfilming, are used, suitable reader and photocopying equipment shall be readily available.

(e) Written records required by this part shall be maintained so that data therein can be used for evaluating, at least annually, the quality standards of each drug product to determine the need for changes in drug product specifications or manufacturing or control procedures. Written procedures shall be established and followed for such evaluations and shall include provisions for:

(1) A review of every batch, whether approved or rejected, and, where applicable, records associated with the batch.

(2) A review of complaints, recalls, returned or salvaged drug products, and investigations conducted under § 211.192 for each drug product.

(f) Procedures shall be established to assure that the responsible officials of the firm, if they are not personally involved in or immediately aware of such actions, are notified in writing of any investigations conducted under §§ 211.198, 211.204, or 211.208 of these regulations, any recalls, reports of inspectional observations issued by the Food and Drug Administration, or any regulatory actions relating to good manufacturing practices brought by the Food and Drug Administration.

§ 211.182 Equipment cleaning and use log.

A written record of major equipment cleaning, maintenance (except routine maintenance such as lubrication and adjustments), and use shall be included in individual equipment logs that show the date, time, product, and lot number of each batch processed. If equipment is dedicated to manufacture of one product, then individual equipment logs are not required, provided that lots or batches of such product follow in numerical order and are manufactured in numerical sequence. In cases where dedicated equipment is employed, the records of cleaning, maintenance, and use shall be part of the batch record. The persons performing and double-checking the cleaning and maintenance shall date and sign or initial the log indicating that the work was performed. Entries in the log shall be in chronological order.

§ 211.184 Component, drug product container, closure, and labeling records.

These records shall include the following:

(a) The identity and quantity of each shipment of each lot of components, drug product containers, closures, and labeling; the name of the supplier; the supplier's lot number(s) if known; the receiving code as specified in § 211.80; and the date of receipt. The name and location of the prime manufacturer, if different from the supplier, shall be listed if known.

(b) The results of any test or examination performed (including those performed as required by § 211.82 (a), § 211.84 (d), or § 211.122 (a)) and the conclusions derived therefrom.

(c) An individual inventory record of each component, drug product container, and closure and, for each component, a reconciliation of the use of each lot of such component. The inventory record shall contain sufficient information to allow determination of any batch or lot of drug product associated with the use of each component, drug product container, and closure.

(d) Documentation of the examination and review of labels and labeling for conformity with established specifications in accord with §§ 211.122 (c) and 211.130 (c).

(e) The disposition of rejected components, drug product containers, closure, and labeling.

§ 211.186 Master production and control records.

(a) To assure uniformity from batch to batch, master production and control records for each drug product, including each batch size thereof, shall be prepared, dated, and signed (full signature, handwritten) by one person and independently checked, dated, and signed by a second person. The preparation of master production and control records shall be described in a written procedure and such written procedure shall be followed.

(b) Master production and control records shall include:

(1) The name and strength of the product and a description of the dosage form;

(2) The name and weight or measure of each active ingredient per dosage unit or per unit of weight or measure of the drug product, and a statement of the total weight or measure of any dosage unit;

(3) A complete list of components designated by names or codes sufficiently specific to indicate any special quality characteristic;

(4) An accurate statement of the weight or measure of each component, using the same weight system (metric, avoirdupois, or apothecary) for each component. Reasonable variations may be permitted, however, in the amount of components necessary for the preparation in the dosage form, provided they are justified in the master production and control records;

(5) A statement concerning any calculated excess of component;

(6) A statement of theoretical weight or measure at appropriate phases of processing;

(7) A statement of theoretical yield, including the maximum and minimum percentages of theoretical yield beyond which investigation according to § z211.192 is required;

(8) A description of the drug product containers, closures, and packaging materials, including a specimen or copy of each label and all other labeling signed and dated by the person or persons responsible for approval of such labeling;

(9) Complete manufacturing and control instructions, sampling and testing procedures, specifications, special notations, and precautions to be followed.

§ 211.188 Batch production and control records.

Batch production and control records shall be prepared for each batch of drug product produced and shall include complete information relating to the production and control of each batch. These records shall include:

(a) An accurate reproduction of the appropriate master production or control record, checked for accuracy, dated, and signed;

(b) Documentation that each significant step in the manufacture, processing, packing, or holding of the batch was accomplished, including:

(1) Dates;

(2) Identity of individual major equipment and lines used;

(3) Specific identification of each batch of component or in-process material used;

(4) Weights and measures of components used in the course of processing;

(5) In-process and laboratory control results;

(6) Inspection of the packaging and labeling area before and after use;

(7) A statement of the actual yield and a statement of the percentage of theoretical yield at appropriate phases of processing;

(8) Complete labeling control records, including specimens or copies of all labeling used;

(9) Description of drug product containers and closures;

(10) Any sampling performed;

(11) Identification of the persons performing and directly supervising or checking each significant step in the operation;

(12) Any investigation made according to § 211.192;

(13) Results of examinations made in accordance with § 211.134.

§ 211.192 Production record review.

All drug product production and control records, including those for packaging and labeling, shall be reviewed and approved by the quality control unit to determine compliance with all established, approved written procedures before a batch is released or distributed. Any unexplained discrepancy (including a percentage of theoretical yield exceeding the maximum or minimum percentages established in master production and control records) or the failure of a batch or any of its components to meet any of its specifications shall be thoroughly investigated, whether or not the batch has already been distributed. The investigation shall extend to other batches of the same drug product and other drug products that may have been associated with the specific failure or discrepancy. A written record of the investigation shall be made and shall include the conclusions and followup.

§ 211.194 Laboratory records.

(a) Laboratory records shall include complete data derived from all tests necessary to assure compliance with established specifications and standards, including examinations and assays, as follows:

(1) A description of the sample received for testing with identification of source (that is, location from where sample was obtained), quantity, lot number or other distinctive code, date sample was taken, and date sample was received for testing.

(2) A statement of each method used in the testing of the sample. The statement shall indicate the location of data that establish that the methods used in the testing of the sample meet proper standards of accuracy and reliability as applied to the product tested. (If the method employed is in the current revision of the United States Pharmacopeia,

National Formulary, Association of Official Analytical Chemists, Book of Methods,* or in other recognized standard references, or is detailed in an approved new drug application and the referenced method is not modified, a statement indicating the method and reference will suffice.) The suitability of all testing methods used shall be verified under actual conditions of use.

(3) A statement of the weight or measure of sample used for each test, where appropriate.

(4) A complete record of all data secured in the course of each test, including all graphs, charts, and spectra from laboratory instrumentation, properly identified to show the specific component, drug product container, closure, in-process material, or drug product, and lot tested.

(5) A record of all calculations performed in connection with the test, including units of measure, conversion factors, and equivalency factors.

(6) A statement of the results of tests and how the results compare with established standards of identity, strength, quality, and purity for the component, drug product container, closure, in-process material, or drug product tested.

(7) The initials or signature of the person who performs each test and the date(s) the tests were performed.

(8) The initials or signature of a second person showing that the original records have been reviewed for accuracy, completeness, and compliance with established standards.

(b) Complete records shall be maintained of any modification of an established method employed in testing. Such records shall include the reason for the modification and data to verify that the modification produced results that are at least as accurate and reliable for the material being tested as the established method.

(c) Complete records shall be maintained of any testing and standardization of laboratory reference standards, reagents, and standard solutions.

(d) Complete records shall be maintained of the periodic calibration of laboratory instruments, apparatus, gauges, and recording devices required by § 211.160 (b) (4).

(e) Complete records shall be maintained of all stability testing performed in accordance with § 211.166.

§ 211.196 Distribution records.

Distribution records shall contain the name and strength of the product and a description of the dosage form, name and address of the consignee, date and quantity shipped, and lot or control number of the drug product.

§ 211.198 Complaint files.

(a) Written procedures describing the handling of all written and oral complaints regarding a drug product shall be established and followed. Such procedures shall include provisions for review by the quality control unit, of any complaint involving the possible failure of a drug product to meet any of its specifications and, for such drug products, a determination as to the need for an investigation in accordance with § 211.192.

(b) A written record of each complaint shall be maintained in a file designated for drug product complaints. The file regarding such drug product complaints shall be maintained at the establishment where the drug product involved was manufactured, processed, or packed, or such file may be maintained at another facility if the written records in such files are readily available for inspection at that other facility. Written records involving a drug product shall be maintained until at least 1 year after the expiration date of the drug product, or 1 year after the date that the complaint was received, whichever is longer. In the case of certain OTC drug products lacking expiration dating because they meet the criteria for exemption under § 211.137, such written records shall be maintained for 3 years after distribution of the drug product.

(1) The written record shall include the following information, where known: the name and strength of the drug product, lot number, name of complainant, nature of complaint, and reply to complainant.

(2) Where an investigation under § 211.192 is conducted, the written record shall include the findings of the investigation and followup. The record or copy of the record of the investigation shall be maintained at the establishment where the investigation occurred in accordance with § 211.180 (c).

(3) Where an investigation under § 211.192 is not conducted, the written record shall include the reason that an investigation was found not to be necessary and the name of the responsible person making such a determination.

Subpart K—Returned and Salvaged Drug Products

§ 211.204 Returned drug products.

Returned drug products shall be identified as such and held. If the conditions under which returned drug products have been held, stored, or shipped before or during their return, or if the condition of the drug product, its container, carton, or labeling, as a result of storage or shipping, casts doubt on the safety, identity, strength, quality or purity of the drug product, the returned drug product shall be destroyed unless examination, testing, or other investigations prove the drug product meets appropriate standards of safety, identity, strength, quality, or purity. A drug product may be reprocessed provided the subsequent drug product meets appropriate standards, specifications, and characteristics. Records of returned drug products shall be maintained and shall include the name and label potency of the drug product dosage form, lot number (or control number or batch number), reason for the return, quantity returned, date of disposition, and ultimate disposition of the returned drug product. If the reason for a drug product being returned implicates associated batches, an appropriate investigation shall be conducted in accordance with the requirements of § 211.192. Procedures for the holding, testing, and reprocessing of returned drug products shall be in writing and shall be followed.

§ 211.208 Drug product salvaging.

Drug products that have been subjected to improper storage conditions including extremes in temperature, humidity, smoke, fumes, pressure, age, or radiation due to natural disasters, fires, accidents, or equipment failures shall not be salvaged and returned to the marketplace. Whenever there is a question whether drug products have been subjected to such conditions, salvaging operations may be conducted only if there is (a) evidence from laboratory tests and assays (including animal feeding studies where applicable) that the drug products meet all applicable standards of identity, strength, quality, and purity and (b) evidence from inspection of the premises that the drug products and their associated packaging were not subjected to improper storage conditions as a result of the disaster or accident. Organoleptic examinations shall be acceptable only as supplemental evidence that the drug products meet appropriate standards of identity, strength, quality, and purity. Records including name, lot number, and disposition shall be maintained for drug products subject to this section.

Part 820—Good Manufacturing Practice for Medical Devices: General

Subpart A—General Provisions

Subpart B—Organization and Personnel

Subpart C—Buildings

Subpart D—Equipment

Subpart E—Control of Components

Subpart F—Production and Process Controls

---

* Copies may be obtained from: Association of Official Analytical Chemists, P. O. Box 540, Benjamin Franklin Station, Washington, DC 20204.

Subpart G—Packaging and Labeling Control

Subpart H—Holding, Distribution, and Installation

Subpart I—Device Evaluation

Subpart J—Records

Subpart A—General Provisions

§ 820.1 Scope.

The regulation set forth in this part describes current good manufacturing practices for methods used in, and the facilities and controls used for, the manufacture, packing, storage, and installation of all finished devices intended for human use. The regulation is intended to assure that such devices will be safe and effective and otherwise in compliance with the Federal Food, Drug, and Cosmetic Act. Part 820 establishes basic requirements applicable to finished devices, including additional requirements for critical devices. This regulation is not intended to apply to manufacturers of components or parts of finished devices, but such manufacturers are encouraged to use appropriate provisions of this regulation as guidelines. Manufacturers of human blood and blood components are not subject to this part, but are subject to Part 606 of this chapter.

(a) Authority. This Part 820 is established and promulgated under authority of sections 501, 502, 518, 519, 520(f), and 701(a) of the act [21 U.S.C. 351, 352, 360h, 360i, 360j(f), and 371(a)]. The failure to comply with any applicable provisions in Part 820 in the manufacture, packing, storage, or installation of a device renders the device adulterated under section 501(h) of the act. Such a device, as well as the person responsible for the failure to comply, is subject to regulatory action.

(b) Limitations. The current good manufacturing practice regulation in Part 820 supplements regulations in other parts of this chapter except where explicitly stated otherwise. In the event it is impossible to comply with applicable regulations both in this part and in other parts of this chapter, the regulations specifically applicable to the device in question shall supersede any other regulations.

(c) Applicability. The provisions of Part 820 shall be applicable to any finished device, as defined in this part, intended for human use, that is manufactured, imported, or offered for import in any State or territory of the United States, the District of Columbia, or the Commonwealth of Puerto Rico.

(d) Exemptions or variances. Any person who wishes to petition for an exemption or variance from any device good manufacturing practice requirement is subject to the requirements of section 520(f)(2) of the act. Petitions for an exemption or variance shall be submitted according to the procedures set forth in § 10.30 of this chapter, the Food and Drug Administration's administrative procedures. Guidance is available from the Center for Devices and Radiological Health, Division of Compliance Programs, Manufacturing Quality Assurance Branch (HFZ-332), 1390 Piccard Dr., Rockville, MD 20850; telephone 301-427-1128.

§ 820.3 Definitions.

(a) "Act" means the Federal Food, Drug, and Cosmetic Act, as amended [secs. 201–902, 52 Stat. 1040 et seq., as amended (21 U.S.C. 321–392)].

(b) "Audit" means a documented activity performed in accordance with written procedures on a periodic basis to verify, by examination and evaluation of objective evidence, compliance with those elements of the quality assurance program under review. "Audit" does not include surveillance or inspection activities performed for the purpose of conducting a quality assurance program or undertaking complaint investigations or failure analyses of a device.

(c) "Component" means any material, substance, piece, part, or assembly used during device manufacture which is intended to be included in the finished device.

(d) "Control number" means any distinctive combination of letters or numbers, or both, from which the complete history of the manufacture, control, packaging, and distribution of a production run, lot, or batch of finished devices can be determined.

(e) "Critical component" means any component of a critical device whose failure to perform can be reasonably expected to cause the failure of a critical device or to affect its safety or effectiveness.

(f) "Critical device" means a device that is intended for surgical implant process used into the body or to support or sustain life and whose failure to perform when properly used in accordance with instructions for use provided in the labeling can be reasonably expected to result in a significant injury to the user. Critical devices will be identified by the Commissioner after consultation with the Device Good Manufacturing Practice Advisory Committee authorized under section 520(f) of the act, and an illustrative list of critical devices will be available from the Center for Devices and Radiological Health, Food and Drug Administration.

(g) "Critical operation" means any operation in the manufacture of a critical device which, if improperly performed, can be reasonably expected to cause the failure of a critical device ,or to affect its safety or effectiveness.

(h) "Device history record" means a compilation of records containing the complete production history of a finished device.

(i) "Device master record" means a compilation of records containing the design, formulation, specifications, complete manufacturing procedures, quality assurance requirements, and labeling of a finished device.

(j) "Finished device" means a device, or any accessory to a device, which is suitable for use, whether or not packaged or labeled for commercial distribution.

(k) "Manufacturer" means any person, including any repacker and/or relabeler, who manufactures, fabricates, assembles, or processes a finished device. The term does not include any person who only distributes a finished device.

(l) "Manufacturing material" means any material such as a cleaning agent, mold-release agent, lubricating oil, or other substance used to facilitate a manufacturing process and which is not intended by the manufacturer to be included in the finished device.

(m) "Noncritical device" means any finished device other than a critical device.

(n) "Quality assurance" means all activities necessary to assure and verify confidence in the quality of the process used to manufacture a finished device.

§ 820.5 Quality assurance program.

Every finished device manufacturer shall prepare and implement a quality assurance program that is appropriate to the specific device manufactured and meets the requirements of this part.

Subpart B—Organization and Personnel

§ 820.20 Organization.

Each manufacturer shall have in place an adequate organizational structure and sufficient personnel to assure that the devices the manufacturer produces are manufactured in accordance with the requirements of this regulation. Each manufacturer shall prepare and implement quality assurance procedures adequate to assure that a formally established and documented quality assurance program is performed. Where possible, a designated individual(s) not having direct responsibility for the performance of a manufacturing operation shall be responsible for the quality assurance program.

(a) Quality assurance program requirements. The quality assurance program shall consist of procedures adequate to assure that the following functions are performed:

(1) Review of production records;

(2) Approval or rejection of all components, manufacturing materials, in-process materials, packaging materials, labeling, and finished devices; approval or rejection of devices manufactured, processed, packaged, or held under contract by another company;

(3) Identifying, recommending, or providing solutions for quality assurance problems and verifying the implementation of such solutions; and

(4) Assuring that all quality assurance checks are appropriate and adequate for their purpose and are performed correctly.

(b) Audit procedures. Planned and periodic audits of the quality assurance program shall be implemented to verify compliance with the quality assurance program. The audits shall be performed in accordance with written procedures by appropriately trained individuals not having direct responsibilities for the matters being audited. Audit results shall be documented in written audit reports, which shall be reviewed by management having responsibility for the matters audited. Follow-up corrective action, including reaudit of deficient matters, shall be taken when indicated. An employee of the Food and Drug Administration, designated by the Food and Drug Administration, shall have access to the written procedures established for the audit. Upon request of such an employee, a responsible official of the manufacturer shall certify in writing that the audits of the quality assurance program required under this paragraph have been performed and documented and that any required corrective action has been taken.

§ 820.25 Personnel.

Each manufacturer shall have sufficient personnel with the necessary education, background, training, and experience to assure that all operations are correctly performed.

(a) Personnel training. All personnel shall have the necessary training to perform their assigned responsibilities adequately. Where training programs are necessary to assure that personnel have a thorough understanding of their jobs, such programs shall be conducted and documented. All employees shall be made aware of device defects which may occur from the improper performance of their specific jobs. Quality assurance personnel shall be made aware of defects and errors likely to be encountered as part of their quality assurance functions.

(b) Personnel health and cleanliness. Personnel in contact with a device or its environment shall be clean, healthy, and suitably attired where lack of cleanliness, good health, or suitable attire could adversely affect the device. Any personnel who, by medical examination or supervisory observation, appear to have a condition which could adversely affect the device shall be excluded from affected operations until the condition is corrected. Personnel shall be instructed to report such conditions to their supervisors.

Subpart C—Buildings

§ 820.40 Buildings.

Buildings in which manufacturing, assembling, packaging, packing, holding, testing, or labeling operations are conducted shall be of suitable design and contain sufficient space to facilitate adequate cleaning, maintenance, and other necessary operations. The facilities shall provide adequate space designed to prevent mixups and to assure orderly handling of the following: Incoming components; rejected or obsolete components; in-process components; finished devices; labeling; devices that have been reprocessed, reworked, or repaired; equipment; molds, patterns, tools, records, drawings, blueprints; testing and laboratory operations; and quarantined products.

§ 820.46 Environmental control.

Where environmental conditions at the manufacturing site could have an adverse effect on a device's fitness for use, these environmental conditions shall be controlled to prevent contamination of the device and to provide proper conditions for each of the operations performed pursuant to § 820.40. Conditions to be considered for control are lighting, ventilation, temperature, humidity, air pressure, filtration, airborne contamination, and other contamination. Any environmental control system shall be periodically inspected to verify that the system is properly functioning. Such inspections shall be documented.

§ 820.56 Cleaning and sanitation.

There shall be adequate written cleaning procedures and schedules to meet manufacturing process specifications. Such procedures shall be provided to appropriate personnel.

(a) Personnel sanitation. Washing and toilet facilities shall be clean and adequate. Where special clothing requirements are necessary to assure that a device is fit for its intended use, clean dressing rooms shall be provided for personnel.

(b) Contamination control. There shall be procedures designed to prevent contamination of equipment, components, or finished devices by rodenticides, insecticides, fungicides, fumigants, hazardous substances, and other cleaning and sanitizing substances. Such procedures shall be documented.

(c) Personnel practices. Where eating, drinking, and smoking by personnel could have an adverse effect on a device's fitness for use, such practices shall be limited to designated areas selected so as to avoid such an adverse effect.

(d) Sewage and refuse disposal. Sewage, trash, by-products, chemical effluents, and other refuse shall be disposed of in a timely, safe, and sanitary manner.

Subpart D—Equipment

§ 820.60 Equipment.

Equipment used in the manufacturing process shall be appropriately designed, constructed, placed, and installed to facilitate maintenance, adjustment, and cleaning.

(a) Maintenance schedule. Where maintenance of equipment is necessary to assure that manufacturing specifications are met, a written schedule for the maintenance, adjustment, and cleaning of equipment shall be developed and adhered to. Such schedule shall be visibly posted on or near each piece of equipment, or be readily available to personnel performing maintenance activities. A written record shall be maintained documenting when scheduled maintenance activities are performed.

(b) Inspection. Periodic documented inspections shall be made to assure adherence to applicable equipment maintenance schedules.

(c) Adjustment. Any inherent limitations or allowable tolerances shall be visibly posted on or near equipment requiring periodic adjustments, or be readily available to personnel performing these adjustments.

(d) Manufacturing material. Manufacturing material, including a cleaning agent, mold-release agent, lubricating oil, or other substance used on or in the manufacturing equipment or the device, shall be subsequently removed from the device or limited to a specified amount that does not adversely affect the device's fitness for use. There shall be written procedures for the use and removal of such manufacturing material. The removal of such manufacturing material shall be documented.

§ 820.61 Measurement equipment.

All production and quality assurance measurement equipment, such as mechanical, automated, or electronic equipment, shall be suitable for its intended purposes and shall be capable of producing valid results. Such equipment shall be routinely calibrated, inspected, and checked according to written procedures. Records documenting these activities shall be maintained. When computers are used as part of an automated production or quality assurance system, the computer software programs shall be validated by adequate and documented testing. All program changes shall be made by a designated individual(s) through a formal approval procedure.

(a) Calibration. Calibration procedures shall include specific directions and limits for accuracy and precision. There shall be provisions for remedial action when accuracy and precision limits are not met. Calibration shall be performed by personnel having the necessary education, training, background, and experience.

(b) Calibration standards. Where practical, the calibration standards used for production and quality assurance measurement equipment shall be traceable to the national standards of the National Institute of Standards and Technology, Department of Commerce. If national standards are not practical for the parameter being measured, an independent reproducible standard shall be used. If no applicable standard exists, an in-house standard shall be developed and used.

(c) Calibration records. The calibration date, the calibrator, and the next calibration date shall be recorded and displayed, or records containing such information shall be readily available for each piece of equipment requiring calibration. A designated individual(s) shall maintain a record of calibration dates and of the individual performing each calibration.

Subpart E—Control of Components

§ 820.80 Components.

Components used in manufacturing shall be received, stored, and handled in a manner designed to prevent damage, mixup, contamination, and other adverse effects. Components shall be quarantined prior to acceptance or clearly identified as not yet accepted.

(a) Acceptance of components. There shall be a written procedure for acceptance of components. A designated individual(s) shall accept or reject components. A record shall be maintained of component acceptance and rejection. Upon receipt, each shipping container of components shall be visually examined for damage. Where deviations from component specifications could result in the device being unfit for its intended use, components shall be inspected, sampled, and tested for conformance to specifications.

(b) Storage and handling of components. If the quality or fitness for use of components deteriorates over time, the components shall be stored in a manner to facilitate proper stock rotation. Component control numbers or other identifications shall be easily viewable. All obsolete, rejected, or deteriorated components shall be clearly identified and segregated from accepted components. Records shall be maintained of the disposition of all obsolete, rejected, or deteriorated components.

§ 820.81 Critical devices, components.

In addition to the requirements of § 820.80, the following requirements apply to critical devices:

(a) Acceptance of critical components. There shall be written procedures for the accepting, sampling, testing, and inspecting of all lots of critical components to assure that critical components conform to specifications. The number of units sampled from each lot of critical components shall be based upon an acceptable statistical rationale, the past quality history of the supplier, and the quantity needed for analysis and reserve. Each lot of critical components shall be identified with a control number(s) upon receipt. The percentage of defective critical components for each lot and the percentage of lots rejected shall be recorded and identified by supplier name.

(b) Critical component supplier agreement. Where possible, the manufacturer shall secure from the critical component supplier a written agreement whereby the supplier agrees to notify the manufacturer of any proposed change in a critical component. Where such an agreement exists, the manufacturer shall not accept such a change until the manufacturer has determined the impact of the change on the finished device.

Subpart F—Production and Process Controls

§ 820.100 Manufacturing specifications and processes.

Written manufacturing specifications and processing procedures shall be established, implemented, and controlled to assure that the device conforms to its original design or any approved, specifications.

(a) Specification controls.

(1) Procedures for specification control measures shall be established to assure that the design basis for the device, components, and packaging is correctly translated into approved specifications.

(2) Specification changes shall be subject to controls as stringent as those applied to the original design specifications of the device. Such changes shall be approved and documented by a designated individual(s) and shall include the approval date and the date the change becomes effective.

(b) Processing controls.

(1) Where deviations from device specifications could occur as a result of the manufacturing process itself, there shall be written procedures describing any processing controls necessary to assure conformance to specifications.

(2) All processing control shall be conducted in a manner designed to assure that the device conforms to applicable specifications.

(3) There shall be a formal approval for any change in the manufacturing process of a device. Any approved change shall be communicated to appropriate personnel in a timely manner.

§ 820.101 Critical devices, manufacturing specifications, and processes.

In addition to the requirements of § 820.100, the following requirements apply to critical devices:

(a) Critical operation performance. Any critical operation shall be performed by a suitable designated individual(s) or suitable equipment and shall be verified.

(b) Record of critical operation. Any individual responsible for the performance of a critical operation shall record or reference that operation in the device history as required in § 820.185.

§ 820.115 Reprocessing of devices or components.

(a) Reprocessing procedures shall be established, implemented, and controlled to assure that the reprocessed device or component meets the original, or subsequently modified and approved, specifications.

(b) Any device rejected during finished device inspection and later reprocessed shall be subject to another complete final inspection for any characteristic of the device which may be adversely affected by such reprocessing.

§ 820.116 Critical devices, reprocessing of devices or components.

In addition to the requirements of § 820.115, the following requirements apply to critical devices:

(a) Reprocessing procedures. There shall be written procedures for any reprocessing associated with the production of a critical device or component. These procedures shall prescribe the equipment to be used in reprocessing and shall include any special quality assurance methods or tests. The procedures shall be designed so that the reprocessed device or component meets the original, or subsequently modified and approved, specifications. The procedures shall be designed to prevent adulteration, e.g., because of material, structural, or molecular change in the device or component due to reprocessing. Special care shall be taken to assure that the device or component to be reprocessed is clearly identified and separated from like devices or components not to be reprocessed. When there is constant reprocessing of a device or component, a determination of the effect of the reprocessing upon the device or component shall be made and documented. There shall be a formal approval procedure for instituting a new, or altering an approved, reprocessing procedure.

(b) Reprocessing control. Any critical device or component subject to reprocessing procedures shall conform to the original, or subsequently modified and approved, specifications. Written testing and sampling procedures to assure such conformity shall be contained or referenced in the device master record. Any prior quality assurance check shall be repeated on the reprocessed device or componenet if the reprocessing could adversely affect any performance characteristic previously inspected.

Subpart G—Packaging and Labeling Control

§ 820.120 Device labeling.

There shall be adequate controls to maintain labeling integrity and to prevent labeling mixups.

(a) Label integrity. Labels shall be designed, printed, and applied so as to remain legible during the customary conditions of processing, storage handling, distribution, and use. Labels and other labeling shall not be released to inventory until a designated individual has proofread samples of the labeling for accuracy.

(b) Separation of operations. Each labeling or packaging operation shall be separated physically or spatially in a manner designed to prevent mixups.

(c) Area inspection. Prior to the implementation of any labeling or packaging operation, there shall be an inspection of the area where the operation is to occur by a designated individual to assure that devices and labeling materials from prior operations do not remain in the labeling or packaging area. Any such items found shall be destroyed, disposed of, or returned to storage prior to the onset of a new or different labeling or packaging operation.

(d) Storage. Labels and labeling shall be stored and maintained in a manner that provides proper identification and is designed to prevent mixups.

(e) Labeling materials. Labeling materials issued for devices shall be examined for identity and, where applicable, the correct expiration date, control number, storage instructions, handling instructions, and additional processing instructions. A record of such examination, including the date and person performing the examination, shall be maintained in the device history record.

§ 820.121 Critical devices, device labeling.

In addition to the requirements of § 820.120, the following requirements apply to critical devices:

(a) Control number. Labels issued for critical devices shall contain a control number.

(b) Labeling check. The signature of the individual who proofreads the labels and other labeling, and the date of the proofreading, shall be recorded.

(c) Access restrictions. Access to the labels and other labeling shall be restricted to authorized personnel.

§ 820.130 Device packaging.

The device package and any shipping container for a device shall be designed and constructed to protect the device from alteration or damage during the customary conditions of processing, storage, handling, and distribution.

Subpart H—Holding, Distribution, and Installation

§ 820.150 Distribution.

There shall be written procedures for warehouse control and distribution of finished devices to assure that only those devices approved for release are distributed. Where a device's fitness for use or quality deteriorates over time, there shall be a system to assure that the oldest approved devices are distributed first.

§ 820.151 Critical devices, distribution records.

In addition to the requirements of § 820.150, adequate distribution records for critical devices shall include, or make reference to the location of: the name and address of the consignee, the name and quantity of devices, the date shipped, and the control number used. These records shall be retained as required by § 820.180(b).

§ 820.152 Installation.

Where a device is installed by the manufacturer or its authorized representative, the manufacturer or representative shall inspect the device after installation to assure that the device will perofrm as intended. Where a device is installed by a person other than the manufacturere or its authorized representative, the manufacturer shall provide adequate instructions and procedures for proper installation.

Subpart I—Device Evaluation

§ 820.160 Finished device inspection.

There shall be written procedures for finished device inspection to assure that device specifications are met. Prior to release for distribution, each production run, lot or batch shall be checked and, where necessary, tested for conformance with device specifications. Where practical, a device shall be selected from a production run, lot or batch and tested under simulated use conditions. Sampling plans for checking, testing, and release of a device shall be based on an acceptable statistical rationale. Finished devices shall be held in quarantine or otherwise adequately controlled until released.

§ 820.161 Critical devices, finished device inspection.

In addition to the requirements of § 820.160, the following requirement applies to critical devices. A critical device or component which does not meet its performance specifications shall be investigated. A written record of the investigation, including conclusions and followup, shall be made. A critical device shall not leave the control of the manufacturer for distribution until all acceptance records and test results have been checked by a designated individual(s). Such individual(s) shall assure that all records and documentation required for the device history record are present and complete, and show that release of the device was consistent with the release criteria. Such individual(s) shall authorize, by signature, the release of the device for distribution.

§ 820.162 Failure investigation.

After a device has been released for distribution, any failure of that device or any of its components to meet performance specifications shall be investigated. A written record of the investigation, including conclusions and followup, shall be made.

Subpart J—Records

§ 820.180 General requirements.

All records required by this part shall be maintained at the manufacturing establishment or other location that is reasonably accessible to responsible officials of the manufacturer and to employees of the Food and Drug Administration designated to perform inspections. Such records shall be available for review and copying by such employees. Except as specifically provided elsewhere, the following general provisions shall apply to all records required by this part.

(a) Confidentiality. Those records deemed confidential by the manufacturer may be marked to aid the Food and Drug Administration in determining whether information may be disclosed under the public information regulation in Part 20 of this chapter.

(b) Record retention period. All required records pertaining to a device shall be retained for a period of time equivalent to the design and expected life of the device, but in no case less than 2 years from the date of release for commercial distribution by the manufacturer. Photostatic or other reproductions of records required by this part may be used.

§ 820.181 Device master record.

The device master record shall be prepared, dated, and signed by a designated individual(s). Any changes in the device master record shall be authorized in writing by the signature of a designated individual(s). Any approval forms shall be part of the device master record. The device master record for each type of device shall include, or refer to the location of, the following information:

(a) Device specifications including appropriate drawings, composition, formulation, and component specifications.

(b) Production process specifications including the appropriate equipment specifications, production method production procedures, and production environment specifications.

(c) Quality assurance procedures and specifications including quality assurance checks used and the quality assurance apparatus used.

(d) Packaging and labeling specifications including methods and processes used.

§ 820.182 Critical devices, device master record.

In addition to the requirements of § 820.181, the device master record for a critical device shall include or refer to the location of the following information:

(a) Critical components and critical component suppliers. Full information concerning critical components and critical component suppliers, including the complete specifications of all critical components, the sources where they maybe obtained, and written copies of any-agreements made with suppliers under § 820.81(b).

(b) Labels and labeling. Complete labeling procedures for the individual device and copies of all approved labels and other labeling.

§ 820.184 Device history record.

A device history record shall be maintained to demonstrate that the device is manufactured in accordance with the device master record. The device history record shall include, or refer to the location of, the following information: The dates of manufacture, the quantity manufactured, the quantity released for distribution, and any control number used.

§ 820.185 Critical devices, device history record.

In addition to the requirements of § 820.184, the following requirements apply to critical devices. There shall be a critical device history record for each control number, which shall include complete information relating to the production unit. This record shall identify the specific label, labeling, and control number used for each production unit and shall be readily accessible and maintained by a designated individual(s). The device history record shall include, or refer to the location of, the following:

(a) Component documentation. The documentation of each critical component used in the manufacture of a device shall include:

(1) Control number. The control number designating each critical component or lot of critical components used in the manufacture of a device.

(2) Acceptance record. The acceptance record of the critical component, including acceptance date and signature of the recipient.

(b) Record of critical operation. The record of, or reference to, each critical operation, identifying the date performed, the designated individual(s) performing the operation and, when appropriate, the major equipment used.

(c) Inspection checks. The inspection checks performed, the methods and equipment used, results, the date, and signature of the inspecting individual.

§ 820.195 Critical devices, automated data processing.

When automated data processing is used for manufacturing or quality assurance purposes, adequate checks shall be designed and implemented prevent inaccurate data output, input, and programming errors.

§ 820.198 Complaint files.

(a) Written and oral complaints relative to the identity, quality, durability, reliability, safety, effectiveness, or performance of a device shall be reviewed, evaluated, and maintained by a formally designated unit. This unit shall determine whether or not an investigation is necessary. When no investigation is made, the unit shall maintain a record that includes the reason and the name of the individual responsible for the decision not to investigate.

(b) Any complaint involving the possible failure of a device to meet any of its performance specifications shall be reviewed, evaluated, and investigated. Any complaint pertaining to injury, death, or any hazard to safety shall be immediately reviewed, evaluated, and investigated by a designated individual(s) and shall be maintained in a separate portion of the complaint file.

(c) When an investigation is made, a written record of each investigation shall be maintained by the formally designated unit identified in paragraph (a) of this section. The record of investigation shall include the name of the device, any control number used, name of complainant, nature of complaint, and reply to complainant.

(d) Where the formally designated unit is located at a site separate from the actual manufacturing establishment, a duplicate copy of the record of investigation of any complaint shall be transmitted to and maintained at the actual manufacturing establishment in a file designated for device complaints.

⟨1141⟩ PACKAGING—CHILD-SAFETY

The Poison Prevention Packaging Act is administered and enforced by the Consumer Product Safety Commission of the federal government. The purpose of the law is to decrease the chance that children may obtain access to poisons. The act applies not only to drugs, but also to other household substances. The Commission is authorized to promulgate regulations providing standards for special packaging of any household substance where that special packaging will help to protect children from serious injury or illness resulting from the handling, using, or ingesting of such substance. Special packaging of this type is not necessarily packaging that all children under 5 years of age cannot open, but is packaging that makes it difficult for most children under the age of 5 to open or to obtain a harmful amount of the contents. On the other hand, the packaging should not be difficult for normal adults to open.

Not all hazardous household substances are subject to special packaging requirements. However, once a special packaging requirement is published, special packaging becomes the rule, and conventional packaging the exception. There are basically four ways by which exceptions are allowed for drugs:

(1) The substance is specifically exempted by regulation;

(2) If the drug is dispensed on prescription, the prescriber directs in the prescription order that it be dispensed in a noncomplying package;

(3) The purchaser of a prescription drug so requests;

(4) The manufacturer (or packer) of a drug for sale without prescription may provide a single-size, noncomplying package provided it bears conspicuous labeling stating, "This package for households without young children," or, if the package is small, stating, "Package not child-resistant," and provided the manufacturer also supplies the substance in complying packages.

The Commission has taken the view that in the case of prescription drugs, the manufacturer has the primary responsibility to provide special packaging where the manufacturer places the drug in a container clearly intended to be utilized in dispensing the drug for use in the home. If the pharmacist transfers a drug from the manufacturer's container to a dispensing container, the responsibility shifts to him. The fact that a manufacturer fails to provide suitable dispensing packaging does not relieve the pharmacist of this responsibility. It should be noted also that there is no special exemption for single-unit or unit-dose packages in the Act. Therefore, in order to comply, such unit packages, if they do not meet child-resistant standards, are to be placed in an outer package that does comply. Drugs placed in containers having dual-purpose closures must be dispensed in the child-resistant mode unless the physician has specified, or the patient has requested, the conventional mode.

Although special packaging should not be difficult for normal adults to open, it is recognized that some individuals having physical limitations, e.g., some elderly persons or arthritics, may have difficulties. Where pharmacists are aware of such infirmities, the proper procedure is to make the patient aware that non-complying packages are available for his or her prescription medication and that the choice is his or hers, with regard to the need for taking into account the likelihood of young children's gaining access to the medication.

Failure to dispense a drug in a child-resistant container where such is required may be a violation of the Federal Food, Drug, and Cosmetic Act (misbranding). Where a question may arise with regard to whether or not a particular container meets the requirements of the Poison Prevention Packaging Act, the manufacturer or the supplier should be consulted.

A child-resistant container that meets the requirements of the Poison Prevention Packaging Act is required to meet also the requirements of the Federal Food, Drug, and Cosmetic Act, and, if it is used to contain an official drug, the requirements of the official compendia. Because safety closures may lose their effectiveness through repeated opening and closing, replacement of the container and/or the cap should be made if the prescription is refilled.

There is no prohibition against utilizing safety packaging in those instances where the Consumer Product Safety Commission does not require it.

Where a non-complying container is dispensed upon the request of a patient, written documentation is advisable. Although there is no statutory requirement that this be done, such documentation might be important in the event that a subsequent question arises, such as in a negligence suit. A blanket waiver is permissible, but this option is limited to the purchaser.

Problems or defects with child-safety containers may be reported through the Drug Product Problem Reporting Program. Reports received through this program are forwarded to the Consumer Product Safety Commission by the Food and Drug Administration. Questions concerning compliance with the law should be directed to the Consumer Product Safety Commission, Washington, DC 20207.

Following are the standards and protocol for testing special packaging. (See also the first paragraph under *The Poison Prevention Packaging Act and Regulations.*)

§ 1700.15 Poison prevention packaging standards.

To protect children from serious personal injury or serious illness resulting from handling, using, or ingesting household substances, the Commission has determined that packaging designed and constructed to meet the following standards shall be regarded as "special packaging" within the meaning of section 2(4) of the act. Specific application of these standards to substances requiring special packaging is in accordance with § 1700.14.

(a) *General requirements.* The special packaging must continue to function with the effectiveness specifications set forth in paragraph (b) of this section when in actual contact with the substance contained therein. This requirement may be satisfied by appropriate scientific evaluation of the compatibility of the substance with the special packaging to determine that the chemical and physical characteristics of the substance will not compromise or interfere with the proper functioning of the special packaging. The special packaging must also continue to function with the effectiveness specifications set forth in paragraph (b) of this section for the number of openings and closings customary for its size and contents. This requirement may be satisfied by appropriate technical evaluation based on physical wear and stress factors, force required for activation, and other such relevant factors which establish that, for the duration of normal use, the effectiveness specifications of the packaging would not be expected to lessen.

(b) *Effectiveness specifications.* Special packaging, tested by the method described in § 1700.20, shall meet the following specifications:

(1) Child-resistant effectiveness of not less than 85 percent without a demonstration and not less than 80 percent after a demonstration of the proper means of opening such special packaging. In the case of unit packaging, child-resistant effectiveness of not less than 80 percent.

(2) Adult-use effectiveness of not less than 90 percent.

(c) *Reuse of special packaging.* Special packaging for substances subject to the provisions of this paragraph shall not be reused.

(d) *Restricted flow.* Special packaging subject to the provisions of this paragraph shall be special packaging from which the flow of liquid is so restricted that not more than 2 milliliters of the contents can be obtained when the inverted, opened container is shaken or squeezed once or when the container is otherwise activated once.

§ 1700.20 Testing procedure for special packaging.

(a) The protocol for testing "special packaging" as defined in section 2(4) of the act shall be as follows:

(1) Use 200 children between the ages of 42 and 51 months inclusive, evenly distributed by age and sex, to test the ability of the special packaging to resist opening by children. The even age distribution shall be determined by having 20 children (plus or minus 10 percent) whose nearest age is 42 months, 20 whose nearest age is 43 months, 20 at 44 months, etc., up to and including 20 at 51 months of age. There should be no more than a 10 percent preponderance of either sex in each age group. The children selected should be healthy and normal and should have no obvious or overt physical or mental handicap.

(2) The children shall be divided into groups of two each. The testing shall be done in a location that is familiar to the children; for example, their customary nursery school or regular kindergarten. No child shall test more than two special packages, and each package shall be of a different type. For each test, the paired children shall receive the same special packaging simultaneously. When more than one special packaging is being tested, they shall be presented to the paired children in random order, and this order shall be recorded. The special

packaging, each test unit of which, if appropriate, has previously been opened and properly resecured by the tester, shall be given to each of the two children with a request for them to open it. (In the case of unit packaging, it shall be presented exposed so that the individual units are immediately available to the child.) Each child shall be allowed up to 5 minutes to open the special packaging. For those children unable to open the special packaging after the first 5 minutes, a single visual demonstration, without verbal explanation, shall be given by the demonstrator. A second 5 minutes shall then be allowed for opening the special packaging. (In the case of unit packaging, a single visual demonstration, without verbal explanation, will be provided at the end of the first 5 minutes only for those test subjects who have not opened at least one unit package, and a second 5 minutes allowed for all subjects.) If a child fails to use his teeth to open the special packaging during the first 5 minutes, the demonstrator shall instruct him, before the start of the second 5-minute period, that he is permitted to use his teeth if he wishes.

(3) Records shall be kept on the number of children who were and were not able to open the special packaging, with and without demonstration. (In the case of unit packaging, records shall be kept on the number of individual units opened or gained access to by each child.) The percent of child-resistant effectiveness shall be the number of children tested, less the test failures, divided by two. A test failure shall be any child who opens the special packaging or gains access to its contents. In the case of unit packaging, however, a test failure shall be any child who opens or gains access to the number of individual units which constitute the amount that may produce serious personal injury or serious illness, or a child who opens or gains access to more than 8 individual units, whichever number is lower, during the full 10 minutes of testing. The determination of the amount of a substance that may produce serious personal injury or serious illness shall be based on a 25-pound child. Manufacturers or packagers intending to use unit packaging for a substance requiring special packaging are requested to submit such toxicological data to the Commission.

(4) One hundred adults, age 18 to 45 years inclusive, with no overt physical or mental handicaps, and 70 percent of whom are female, shall comprise the test panel for normal adults. The adults shall be tested individually, rather than in groups of two or more. The adults shall receive only such printed instructions on how to open and properly resecure the special packaging as will appear on the package as it is delivered to the consumer. Five minutes shall be allowed to complete the opening and, if appropriate, the resecuring process.

(5) Records shall be kept on the number of adults unable to open and the number of the other adults tested who fail to properly resecure the special packaging. The number of adults who successfully open the special packaging and then properly resecure the special packaging (if resecuring is appropriate) is the percent of adult-use effectiveness of the special packaging. In the case of unit packaging, the percent of adult-use effectiveness shall be the number of adults who successfully open a single package.

(b) The standards published as regulations issued for the purpose of designating particular substances as being subject to the requirements for special packaging under the act will stipulate the percent of child-resistant effectiveness and adult-use effectiveness required for each and, where appropriate, will include any other conditions deemed necessary and provided for in the act.

(c) It is recommended that manufacturers of special packaging, or producers of substances subject to regulations issued pursuant to the act, submit to the Commission summaries of data resulting from tests conducted in accordance with this protocol.

THE POISON PREVENTION PACKAGING ACT AND REGULATIONS

Selective portions of the Poison Prevention Packaging Act and Regulations promulgated thereunder that are believed to be of most interest to practitioners and students of pharmacy and medicine are presented here as a service to the professions and with the cooperation of the Consumer Product Safety Commission. The publication of these sections in The United States Pharmacopeia is for purposes of information and does not impart to them any legal effect.

SEC. 2. For the purpose of this Act—

(2) The term "household substance" means any substance which is customarily produced or distributed for sale for consumption or use, or customarily stored, by individuals in or about the household and which is—

(A) a hazardous substance as that term is defined in section 2(f) of the Federal Hazardous Substances Act (15 U.S.C. 1261(f));

(B) an economic poison as that term is defined in section 2a of the Federal Insecticide, Fungicide, and Rodenticide Act (7 U.S.C. 135(a));

(C) a food, drug, or cosmetic as those terms are defined in section 201 of the Federal Food, Drug, and Cosmetic Act (21 U.S.C. 321); or

(D) a substance intended for use as fuel when stored in a portable container and used in the heating, cooking, or refrigeration system of a house.

(3) The term "package" means the immediate container or wrapping in which any household substance is contained for consumption, use, or storage by individuals in or about the household, and, for purposes of section 4(a)(2) of this Act, also means any outer container or wrapping used in the retail display of any such substances to consumers. Such term does not include—

(A) any shipping container or wrapping used solely for the transportation of any household substance in bulk or in quantity to manufacturers, packers, or processors, or to wholesale or retail distributors thereof, or

(B) any shipping container or outer wrapping used by retailers to ship or deliver any household substance to consumers unless it is the only such container or wrapping.

(4) The term "special packaging" means packaging that is designed or constructed to be significantly difficult for children under five years of age to open or obtain a toxic or harmful amount of the substance contained therein within a reasonable time and not difficult for normal adults to use properly, but does not mean packaging which all such children cannot open or obtain a toxic or harmful amount within a reasonable time.

(5) The term "labeling" means all labels and other written, printed, or graphic matter (A) upon any household substance or its package, or (B) accompanying such substance.

SEC. 3. (a) The Secretary, after consultation with the technical advisory committee provided for in section 6 of this Act, may establish in accordance with the provisions of this Act, by regulation, standards for the special packaging of any household substance if he finds that—

(1) the degree or nature of the hazard to children in the availability of such substance, by reason of its packaging, is such that special packaging is required to protect children from serious personal injury or serious illness resulting from handling, using, or ingesting such substance; and

(2) the special packaging to be required by such standard is technically feasible, practicable, and appropriate for such substance.

(b) In establishing a standard under this section, the Secretary shall consider—

(1) the reasonableness of such standard;

(2) available scientific, medical, and engineering data concerning special packaging and concerning childhood accidental ingestions, illness, and injury caused by household substances;

(3) the manufacturing practices of industries affected by this Act; and

(4) the nature and use of the household substance.

(c) In carrying out this Act, the Secretary shall publish his findings, his reasons therefor, and citation of the sections of statutes which authorize his action.

(d) Nothing in this Act shall authorize the Secretary to prescribe specific packaging designs, product content, package quantity, or, with the exception of authority granted in section 4(a) (2) of this Act, labeling. In the case of a household substance for which special packaging is required pursuant to a regulation under this section, the Secretary may in such regulation prohibit the packaging of such substance in packages which he determines are unnecessarily attractive to children.

SEC. 4. (a) For the purpose of making any household substance which is subject to a standard established under section 3 readily available to elderly or handicapped persons unable to use such substance when packaged in compliance with such standard, the manufacturer or packer, as the case may be, may package any household substance, subject to such a standard, in packaging of a single size which does not comply with such standard if—

(1) the manufacturer (or packer) also supplies such substance in packages which comply with such standard; and

(2) the packages of such substances which do not meet such standard bear conspicuous labeling stating: "This package for households without young children"; except that the Secretary may by regulation prescribe a substitute statement to the same effect for packaging too small to accommodate such labeling.

(b) In the case of a household substance which is subject to such a standard and which is dispensed pursuant to an order of a physician, dentist, or other licensed medical practitioner authorized to prescribe, such substance may be dispensed in noncomplying packages only when directed in such order or when requested by the purchaser.

(c) In the case of a household substance subject to such a standard which is packaged under subsection (a) in a noncomplying package, if the Secretary determines that such substance is not also being supplied by a manufacturer (or packer) in popular size packages which comply with such standard, he may, after giving the manufacturer (or packer) an opportunity to comply with the purposes of this Act, by order require such substance to be packaged by such manufacturer (or packer) exclusively in special packaging complying with such standard if he finds, after opportunity for hearing, that such exclusive use of special packaging is necessary to accomplish the purposes of this Act.

SEC. 502 [352]. A drug or device shall be deemed to be misbranded—

"(p) If it is a drug and its packaging or labeling is in violation of an applicable regulation issued pursuant to section 3 or 4 of the Poison Prevention Packaging Act of 1970."

Poison Prevention Packaging Act of 1970 Regulations

§ 1700.14 Substances requiring special packaging.

(a) *Substances.* The Commission has determined that the degree or nature of the hazard to children in the availability of the following substances, by reason of their packaging, is such that special packaging is required to protect children from serious personal injury or serious illness resulting from handling, using, or ingesting such substances, and that the special packaging herein required is technically feasible, practicable, and appropriate for these substances:

(1) *Aspirin.* Any aspirin-containing preparation for human use in a dosage form intended for oral administration shall be packaged in accordance with the provisions of § 1700.15(a), (b), and (c), except the following:

(i) Effervescent tablets containing aspirin, other than those intended for pediatric use, provided the dry tablet contains not more than 15 percent aspirin and has an oral LD-50 in rats of 5 grams or more per kilogram of body weight.

(ii) Unflavored aspirin-containing preparations in powder form (other than those intended for pediatric use) that are packaged in unit doses providing not more than 15.4 grains of aspirin per unit dose and that contain no other substance subject to the provisions of this section.

(3) *Methyl salicylate.* Liquid preparations containing more than 5% by weight of methyl salicylate, other than those packaged in pressurized spray containers, shall be packaged in accordance with the provisions of § 1700.15(a), (b), and (c).

(4) *Controlled drugs.* Any preparation for human use that consists in whole or in part of any substance subject to control under the Comprehensive Drug Abuse Prevention and Control Act of 1970 (21 U.S.C. 801 et seq.) and that is in a dosage form intended for oral administration shall be packaged in accordance with the provisions of § 1700.15(a), (b), and (c).

(6) *Turpentine.* Household substances in liquid form containing 10% or more by weight of turpentine shall be packaged in accordance with the provisions of § 1700.15(a) and (b).

(10) *Prescription drugs.* Any drug for human use that is in a dosage form intended for oral administration and that is required by Federal law to be dispensed only by or upon an oral or written prescription of a practitioner licensed by law to administer such drug shall be packaged in accordance with the provisions of § 1700.15(a), (b), and (c), except for the following:

(i) Sublingual dosage forms of nitroglycerin.

(ii) Sublingual and chewable forms of isosorbide dinitrate in dosage strengths of 10 milligrams or less.

(iii) Erythromycin ethylsuccinate granules for oral suspension and oral suspensions in packages containing not more than 8 grams of the equivalent of erythromycin.

(iv) Cyclically administered oral contraceptives in manufacturers' mnemonic (memory-aid) dispenser packages that rely solely upon the activity of one or more progestogen or estrogen substances.

(v) Anhydrous cholestyramine in powder form.

(vi) All unit-dose forms of potassium supplements, including individually wrapped effervescent tablets, unit-dose vials of liquid potassium, and powdered potassium in unit-dose packets, containing not more than 50 milliequivalents of potassium per unit dose.

(vii) Sodium fluoride drug preparations, including liquid and tablet forms, containing no more than 264 milligrams of sodium fluoride per package and containing no other substances subject to this § 1700.14(a)(10).

(viii) Betamethasone tablets packaged in manufacturers' dispenser packages, containing no more than 12.6 milligrams betamethasone.

(ix) Pancrelipase preparations in tablet, capsule, or powder form and containing no other substances subject to this § 1700.14(a)(10).

(x) Prednisone in tablet form, when dispensed in packages containing no more than 105 mg of the drug, and containing no other substances subject to this § 1700.14(a)(10).

(xiii) Mebendazole in tablet form in packages containing not more than 600 mg of the drug, and containing no other substance subject to the provisions of this section.

(xiv) Methylprednisolone in tablet form in packages containing not more than 84 mg of the drug and containing no other substance subject to the provisions of this section.

(xv) Colestipol in powder form in packages containing not more than 5 grams of the drug and containing no other substance subject to the provisions of this section.

(xvi) Erythromycin ethylsuccinate tablets in packages containing no more than the equivalent of 16 grams erythromycin.

(xvii) Conjugated Estrogen Tablets, USP, when dispensed in mnemonic packages containing not more than 32 mg of the drug and containing no other substances subject to this § 1700.14(a)(10).

(xviii) Norethindrone Acetate Tablets, USP, when dispensed in mnemonic packages containing not more than 50 mg of the drug and containing no other substances subject to this § 1700.14(a)(10).

(xix) Medroxyprogesterone acetate tablets.

(12) *Iron-containing drugs.* With the exception of: (i) Animal feeds used as vehicles for the administration of drugs, and (ii) those preparations in which iron is present solely as a colorant, noninjectable animal and human drugs providing iron for therapeutic or prophylactic purposes, and containing a total amount of elemental iron, from any source, in a single package, equivalent to 250 mg or more elemental iron in a concentration of 0.025% or more on a weight to volume basis for liquids and 0.05% or more on a weight-to-weight basis for nonliquids (e.g., powders, granules, tablets, capsules, wafers, gels, viscous products, such as pastes and ointments, etc.) shall be packaged in accordance with the provisions of § 1700.15(a), (b), and (c).

(13) *Dietary supplements containing iron.* With the exception of those preparations in which iron is present solely as a colorant, dietary supplements, as defined in § 1700.1(a)(3), that contain an equivalent of 250 mg or more of elemental iron, from any source, in a single package in concentrations of 0.025% or more on a weight to volume basis for liquids and 0.05% or more on a weight-to-weight basis for nonliquids (e.g., powders, granules, tablets, capsules, wafers, gels, viscous products, such as pastes and ointments, etc.) shall be packaged in accordance with the provisions of § 1700.15(a), (b), and (c).

(16) *Acetaminophen.* Preparations for human use in a dosage form intended for oral administration and containing in a single package a total of more than one gram acetaminophen shall be packaged in accordance with the provisions of § 1700.15(a), (b), and (c), except the following:

(i) Effervescent tablets or granules containing acetaminophen, provided the dry tablet or granules contain less than 15% acetaminophen, the tablet or granules have an oral LD-50 of 5 grams or greater per kilogram of body weight, and the tablet or granules contain no other substance subject to the provisions of this section.

(ii) Unflavored acetaminophen-containing preparations in powder form (other than those intended for pediatric use) that are packaged in unit doses providing not more than 13 grains of acetaminophen per unit dose and that contain no other substance subject to this § 1700.14(a).

(17) *Diphenhydramine.* Preparations for human use in a dosage form intended for oral administration and containing more than the equivalent of 66 mg diphenhydramine base in a single package shall be packaged in accordance with the provisions of § 1700.15(a), (b), and (c), if packaged on or after February 11, 1985.

(20) *Ibuprofen.* Ibuprofen preparations for human use in a dosage form intended for oral administration and containing one gram (1,000 mg) or more of ibuprofen in a single package shall be packaged in accordance with the provisions § 1700.15(a), (b), and (c).

Guide to General Chapters

General Tests and Assays

General Requirements for Tests and Assays

⟨ 1⟩ Injections
⟨ 11⟩ USP Reference Standards

Apparatus for Tests and Assays

⟨ 16⟩ Automated Methods of Analysis
⟨ 21⟩ Thermometers
⟨ 31⟩ Volumetric Apparatus
⟨ 41⟩ Weights and Balances

Microbiological Tests

⟨ 51⟩ Antimicrobial Preservatives—Effectiveness
⟨ 61⟩ Microbial Limit Tests
⟨ 71⟩ Sterility Tests

Biological Tests and Assays

⟨ 81⟩ Antibiotics—Microbial Assays
⟨ 85⟩ Bacterial Endotoxins Test
⟨ 87⟩ Biological Reactivity Tests, In-vitro
⟨ 88⟩ Biological Reactivity Tests, In-vivo
⟨ 91⟩ Calcium Pantothenate Assay
⟨101⟩ Depressor Substances Test
⟨111⟩ Design and Analysis of Biological Assays
⟨115⟩ Dexpanthenol Assay
⟨121⟩ Insulin Assay
⟨141⟩ Protein—Biological Adequacy Test
⟨151⟩ Pyrogen Test
⟨161⟩ Transfusion and Infusion Assemblies
⟨171⟩ Vitamin B_{12} Activity Assay

Chemical Tests and Assays

IDENTIFICATION TESTS

⟨181⟩ Identification—Organic Nitrogenous Bases
⟨191⟩ Identification Tests—General
⟨193⟩ Identification—Tetracyclines
⟨197⟩ Spectrophotometric Identification Tests
⟨201⟩ Thin-layer Chromatographic Identification Test

LIMIT TESTS

⟨211⟩ Arsenic
⟨216⟩ Calcium, Potassium, and Sodium
⟨221⟩ Chloride and Sulfate
⟨223⟩ Dimethylaniline
⟨224⟩ Dioxane
⟨226⟩ 4-Epianhydrotetracycline
⟨231⟩ Heavy Metals
⟨241⟩ Iron
⟨251⟩ Lead
⟨261⟩ Mercury
⟨271⟩ Readily Carbonizable Substances Test
⟨281⟩ Residue on Ignition
⟨291⟩ Selenium

OTHER TESTS AND ASSAYS

⟨301⟩ Acid-neutralizing Capacity
⟨311⟩ Alginates Assay
⟨331⟩ Amphetamine Assay
⟨341⟩ Antimicrobial Agents—Content
⟨351⟩ Assay for Steroids
⟨361⟩ Barbiturate Assay
⟨371⟩ Cobalamin Radiotracer Assay
⟨381⟩ Elastomeric Closures for Injections
⟨391⟩ Epinephrine Assay
⟨401⟩ Fats and Fixed Oils
⟨411⟩ Folic Acid Assay
⟨421⟩ Hydroxypropoxy Determination
⟨425⟩ Iodometric Assay—Antibiotics
⟨431⟩ Methoxy Determination
⟨441⟩ Niacin or Niacinamide Assay
⟨451⟩ Nitrite Titration
⟨461⟩ Nitrogen Determination
⟨466⟩ Ordinary Impurities
⟨467⟩ Organic Volatile Impurities
⟨468⟩ Oxygen Determination
⟨471⟩ Oxygen Flask Combustion
⟨475⟩ Penicillin G Determination
⟨481⟩ Riboflavin Assay
⟨501⟩ Salts of Organic Nitrogenous Bases
⟨521⟩ Sulfonamides
⟨531⟩ Thiamine Assay
⟨541⟩ Titrimetry
⟨551⟩ Alpha Tocopherol Assay
⟨561⟩ Vegetable Drugs—Sampling and Methods of Analysis
⟨571⟩ Vitamin A Assay
⟨581⟩ Vitamin D Assay
⟨591⟩ Zinc Determination

Physical Tests and Determinations

⟨601⟩ Aerosols
⟨611⟩ Alcohol Determination
⟨621⟩ Chromatography
⟨631⟩ Color and Achromicity
⟨641⟩ Completeness of Solution
⟨651⟩ Congealing Temperature
⟨661⟩ Containers
⟨671⟩ Containers—Permeation
⟨691⟩ Cotton
⟨695⟩ Crystallinity
⟨698⟩ Deliverable Volume
⟨701⟩ Disintegration
⟨711⟩ Dissolution
⟨721⟩ Distilling Range
⟨724⟩ Drug Release
⟨726⟩ Electrophoresis
⟨731⟩ Loss on Drying
⟨733⟩ Loss on Ignition
⟨736⟩ Mass Spectrometry
⟨741⟩ Melting Range or Temperature
⟨751⟩ Metal Particles in Ophthalmic Ointments
⟨755⟩ Minimum Fill
⟨761⟩ Nuclear Magnetic Resonance
⟨771⟩ Ophthalmic Ointments
⟨781⟩ Optical Rotation
⟨785⟩ Osmolarity
⟨788⟩ Particulate Matter in Injections
⟨791⟩ pH
⟨801⟩ Polarography
⟨811⟩ Powder Fineness
⟨821⟩ Radioactivity
⟨831⟩ Refractive Index
⟨841⟩ Specific Gravity
⟨851⟩ Spectrophotometry and Light-scattering
⟨861⟩ Sutures—Diameter
⟨871⟩ Sutures—Needle Attachment
⟨881⟩ Tensile Strength
⟨891⟩ Thermal Analysis
⟨905⟩ Uniformity of Dosage Units
⟨911⟩ Viscosity

⟨921⟩ Water Determination
⟨941⟩ X-ray Diffraction

General Information

⟨1001⟩ Antacid Effectiveness
⟨1015⟩ Automated Radiochemical Synthesis Apparatus
⟨1035⟩ Biological Indicators
⟨1041⟩ Biologics
⟨1045⟩ Biotechnology-derived Articles
⟨1051⟩ Cleaning Glass Apparatus
⟨1061⟩ Color—Instrumental Measurement
⟨1071⟩ Controlled Substances Act Regulations
⟨1076⟩ Federal Food, Drug and Cosmetic Act Requirements Relating to Drugs for Human Use
⟨1077⟩ Good Manufacturing Practice for Finished Pharmaceuticals
⟨1081⟩ Gel Strength of Gelatin
⟨1086⟩ Impurities in Official Articles
⟨1088⟩ In vitro and In vivo Evaluation of Dosage Forms
⟨1090⟩ In vivo Bioequivalence Guidances
⟨1091⟩ Labeling of Inactive Ingredients
⟨1101⟩ Medicine Dropper
⟨1111⟩ Microbiological Attributes of Nonsterile Pharmaceutical Products
⟨1121⟩ Nomenclature
⟨1141⟩ Packaging—Child-safety
⟨1151⟩ Pharmaceutical Dosage Forms
⟨1171⟩ Phase-solubility Analysis
⟨1176⟩ Prescription Balances and Volumetric Apparatus
⟨1181⟩ Scanning Electron Microscopy
⟨1191⟩ Stability Considerations in Dispensing Practice
⟨1196⟩ Stability Testing of New Drug Substances and Products—The Tripartite Guideline
⟨1211⟩ Sterilization and Sterility Assurance of Compendial Articles
⟨1216⟩ Tablet Friability
⟨1221⟩ Teaspoon
⟨1225⟩ Validation of Compendial Methods
⟨1231⟩ Water for Pharmaceutical Purposes
⟨1241⟩ Water-solid Interactions in Pharmaceutical Systems

Guide to General Chapters—Nutritional Supplements

General Tests and Assays

⟨2021⟩ Microbial Limit Tests—Nutritional Supplements
⟨2040⟩ Disintegration and Dissolution of Nutritional Supplements
⟨2091⟩ Weight Variation of Nutritional Supplements
⟨2750⟩ Manufacturing Practices for Nutritional Supplements

Section VII

Index

A selected number of brand names *(italicized)* have been included. The inclusion of a brand name does not mean the USPC has any particular knowledge that the brand listed has properties different from other brands of the same drug, nor should it be interpreted as an endorsement by the USPC. Similarly, the fact that a particular brand has not been included does not indicate that the product has been judged to be unsatisfactory or unacceptable. Page numbers for MC-1 through MC-24 refer to the product identification photographs in *The Medicine Chart* (Section V).

See Appendix A (p. **I/489**) and Appendix B (p. **I/523**) of the "Approved Drug Products with Therapeutic Equivalence Evaluations" section of this volume for listings of the products included in the Orange Book.

A–B

C–D

E–G

H–L

L–O

P–Q

R–Z

"Fast-finder" Subject Guide

TO ORDER OTHER USP PUBLICATIONS, USE THIS FORM

See inside of back cover for full listing.

Send orders to:
United States Pharmacopeia
Customer Service Department
12601 Twinbrook Parkway, Rockville, MD 20852
SINCE 1820 Tel. (301) 881-0666 800-227-8772 (Toll-free ordering) FAX: 301-816-8148

NO RISK: Full Money Back Guarantee! If for any reason you are not satisfied after receipt of your order, you may return your purchase within 30 days for full refund.

TITLE	QTY	PRICE	SHIPPING (per subscription)	TOTAL
USP DI, Volume 1, Drug Information for the Health Care Professional 920155	_____	$109	$14*	________
USP DI, Volume II, Advice for the Patient 920257	_____	$54	$14*	________
USP DI, Volume III, Approved Drug Products and Legal Requirements 920359	_____	$98	$14*	________
Please call for foreign shipping rates.			Order total	________

Maryland residents add 5% sales tax.

Please allow 2-4 weeks for delivery. The 1995 USP DI is published in January 1995. Prices subject to change without notice.
*If DI Vol. 1 & 2 are shipped to the same address and individual in the U.S., shipping is $18 in total. If DI Vol. 1, 2, & 3 are shipped to the same address and individual in the U.S., shipping is $30 in total.

Please fill out the reverse side of this form.

Moving?

PLEASE SEND your new address, and your latest label, or an exact copy of it, to: USP, Customer Service Dept., 12601 Twinbrook Parkway, Rockville, MD 20852. Please allow 30 days notice for a change of address correction.

The POSTCARD BELOW is for your convenience if you wish to clip it along the dotted lines, affix postage, and mail it. Or, if you prefer not to clip, please send your new address and your latest label, or an exact copy of it, in a stamped envelope to the above address.

CHANGE OF ADDRESS

New Address

Company

Your Name

Address

City State Zip Code

Former Address

(attach latest label here)

ALL ORDERS MUST BE PAID IN ADVANCE IN U.S. DOLLARS DRAWN ON A U.S. BANK.
Inquire for foreign order shipping charges.

To place orders using your MasterCard or VISA, call Toll-free 1-800-227-8772. Payment is required in advance in U.S. dollars drawn on a U.S. bank. Any bank fees, custom duties, tariffs, and taxes are the responsibility of the customer.

Enclosed is my check or money order made payable to USP for $ ______________

Charge my order to: ❑ MasterCard ❑ VISA ($20 minimum)

Account Number ________________________ Expiration Date ________________

Signature ____

Company Name ____

Your Name ____

Street Address ____

City ____

State ________________ ZIP ____________ Phone Number (____) ________________

Fax Number (____) ________________

ATTACH
STAMP
HERE

The United States Pharmacopeia
Customer Service Dept.
12601 Twinbrook Parkway
Rockville, MD 20852